S0-BCI-334

تقدم الى حسان مع اصدق التمنيات

بالنجاح والتوفيق

نبيه

مونستر ١٩٦٦

Blakiston's

NEW GOULD MEDICAL DICTIONARY

Editorial Board

Normand L. Hoerr

A.B., Johns Hopkins University; Ph.D., M.D., University of Chicago; Henry Willson Payne Professor of Anatomy, School of Medicine, Western Reserve University. Cleveland, Ohio

Arthur Osol

Ph.G., B.Sc. [Chem.], Philadelphia College of Pharmacy and Science; M.Sc. [Chem.], Ph.D., University of Pennsylvania; Professor of Chemistry and Director of the Chemistry Department, Philadelphia College of Pharmacy and Science. Philadelphia, Pennsylvania

Samuel W. Chase

A.B., Bowdoin College; A.M., Ph.D., Harvard University; Professor of Histology and Embryology, School of Dentistry, and Associate Professor of Histology and Embryology, School of Medicine, Western Reserve University. Cleveland, Ohio

Carl C. Francis

A.B., Bethany College; M.D., School of Medicine, Western Reserve University; Associate Professor of Anatomy, School of Medicine, Western Reserve University. Cleveland, Ohio

Blakiston's

NEW GOULD MEDICAL DICTIONARY

A modern comprehensive dictionary of the terms used in all branches of medicine and allied sciences, including medical physics and chemistry, dentistry, pharmacy, nursing, veterinary medicine, zoology and botany, as well as medicolegal terms; with illustrations and tables

EDITORS

Normand L. Hoerr, M.D.
Arthur Osol, Ph.D.

WITH THE COOPERATION OF AN EDITORIAL BOARD AND 88 CONTRIBUTORS

252 ILLUSTRATIONS ON 45 PLATES, 129 IN COLOR

SECOND EDITION

The Blakiston Division
McGraw-Hill Book Company, Inc.
New York Toronto London

Library of Congress Catalog Card Number: 55-7269

GOULD'S MEDICAL DICTIONARY

Fifth Edition, 1941
Fourth Edition, 1935
Third Edition, 1931
Second Edition, 1928
First Edition, 1926

A DICTIONARY OF MEDICAL TERMS—GOULD

First Edition, 1904

AN ILLUSTRATED DICTIONARY OF
MEDICINE, BIOLOGY, AND ALLIED SCIENCES—GOULD

First Edition, 1894

A NEW MEDICAL DICTIONARY—GOULD

First Edition, 1890

"The use of portions of the text of the United States Pharmacopeia, Fifteenth Revision, official December 15, 1955, is by permission received from the Board of Trustees of the United States Pharmacopeial Convention. The said Board is not responsible for any inaccuracies of the text thus used."

"Permission to use for comment parts of the text of The National Formulary, Tenth Edition, in this volume has been granted by the Council of the American Pharmaceutical Association. The American Pharmaceutical Association is not responsible for any inaccuracy of quotation nor for any errors in the statement of quantities or percentage strengths."

VII

PRINTED IN THE UNITED STATES OF AMERICA

Contents

Contributors

Abbott, William E.

B.S., Washington and Jefferson College; M.D., School of Medicine, Western Reserve University; Associate Professor of Surgery, School of Medicine, Western Reserve University. Cleveland, Ohio. Special Field: *Gastrointestinal Surgery and Metabolism.*

Austen, George, Jr.

A.B., Princeton University; M.D., Harvard Medical School; Assistant Professor of Urology, School of Medicine, Western Reserve University; Associate Urologist, University Hospitals. Cleveland, Ohio. Special Field: *Urology.*

Bacon, Franklin J.

Ph.G., Ph.D. (Bot.), University of Wisconsin; Professor of Botany and Pharmacognosy and Head of the Biology Department, Western Reserve University. Cleveland, Ohio. Special Field: *Medicinal Plants.*

Badal, Daniel W.

A.B., Adelbert College, and M.D., School of Medicine, Western Reserve University; Assistant Professor of Psychiatry, School of Medicine, Western Reserve University. Cleveland, Ohio. Special Field: *Psychiatry and Psychoanalysis.*

Barnes, Allen C.

A.B., Princeton University; M.D., University of Pennsylvania School of Medicine; Professor and Chairman of the Department of Obstetrics and Gynecology, School of Medicine, Western Reserve University; Director, MacDonald House, University Hospitals. Cleveland, Ohio. Special Field: *Obstetrics and Gynecology.*

Beams, A. J.

A.B., Wittenberg College; M.D., School of Medicine, Western Reserve University; Clinical Professor of Medicine, School of Medicine, Western Reserve University. Cleveland, Ohio. Special Field: *Gastroenterology.*

Berne, Robert M.

A.B., University of North Carolina; M.D., Harvard Medical School; Associate Professor of Physiology and Instructor in Medicine, School of Medicine, Western Reserve University. Cleveland, Ohio. Special Field: *Cardiovascular and Renal Physiology.*

Binkley, George W.

A.B., Hiram College; M.D., School of Medicine, Western Reserve University; Assistant Clinical Professor of Dermatology and Syphilology, School of Medicine, Western Reserve University. Cleveland, Ohio. Special Field: *Dermatology and Pathology of the Skin.*

Bird, Brian

M.D., University of Manitoba; Associate Professor of Psychiatry, School of Medicine, Western Reserve University. Cleveland, Ohio. Special Field: *Psychiatry and Psychoanalysis.*

Bloch, Edward H.

A.B., University of Chicago; M.D., University of Tennessee College of Medicine; Ph.D., University of Chicago; Established Investigator of the American Heart Association; Assistant Professor of Anatomy, School of Medicine, Western Reserve University. Cleveland, Ohio. Special Field: *Microcirculatory Physiology and Pathology.*

Bochner, Alfred K.

M.D., University of Toronto; Assistant Professor of Psychiatry, School of Medicine, Western Reserve University. Cleveland, Ohio. Special Field: *Psychological Medicine.*

Bond, Douglas D.

A.B., Harvard University; M.D., University of Pennsylvania School of Medicine; Professor of Psychiatry, School of Medicine, Western Reserve University; Physician in Charge, Division of Psychiatry, University Hospitals. Cleveland, Ohio. Special Field: *Psychiatry.*

Bonte, Frederick J.

B.S., Western Reserve University; M.D., School of Medicine, Western Reserve University; Assistant Professor of Radiology, School of Medicine, Western Reserve University. Cleveland, Ohio. Special Field: *Radiation and Radioactive Isotope Therapy.*

Breed, Robert S.

B.S., Amherst College; M.S., University of Colorado; Ph.D., Harvard University; Emeritus Professor of Bacteriology, Cornell University. Geneva, New York. Special Field: *Bacteriology.*

Broadbent, B. Holly

D.D.S., Western Reserve University; Director of the Bolton Fund and Fellow of Dentofacial Anatomy, School of Medicine, and Professor of Dentofacial Morphology, School of Dentistry, Western Reserve University. Cleveland, Ohio. Special Field: *Orthodontics.*

Bruckner, Robert J.

D.D.S., University of Maryland; M.S., Western Reserve University; Associate Professor of Pathology, School of Dentistry, and Assistant Professor of Histology and Embryology, School of Medicine, Western Reserve University. Cleveland, Ohio. Special Field: *Oral Pathology.*

Bunts, Alexander Taylor

A.B., Yale University; M.D., Harvard Medical School; Associate Neurosurgeon, Cleveland Clinic. Cleveland, Ohio. Special Field: *Neurologic Surgery.*

Chase, Samuel W.

A.B., Bowdoin College; A.M., Ph.D., Harvard University; Professor of Histology and Embryology, School of Dentistry, and Associate Professor of Histology and Embryology, School of Medicine, Western Reserve University. Cleveland, Ohio. Special Fields: *Histology and Teratology.*

Clark, William S.

B.S., University of Dayton (Ohio); M.D., St. Louis University School of Medicine; Assistant Professor of Medicine, School of Medicine, Western Reserve University. Cleveland, Ohio. Special Field: *Rheumatic Diseases.*

Collins, William F., Jr.

B.S., Yale University; M.D., Yale University School of Medicine; Instructor Neurological Surgery, School of Medicine, Western Reserve University; Attending Neurosurgeon, University Hospitals. Cleveland, Ohio. Special Field: *Neurosurgery.*

Cover, Morris S.

V.M.D., University of Pennsylvania School of Veterinary Medicine; M.S., Kansas State College; Ph.D., University of Illinois; Associate Research Professor and Poultry Pathologist, University of Delaware. Newark, Delaware. Special Field: *Veterinary Pathology.*

Dupertuis, C. Wesley

B.S., M.A., Ph.D., Harvard University; Associate Professor of Clinical Anthropology, Western Reserve University. Cleveland, Ohio. Special Field: *Anthropology.*

Ecker, Enrique E.

Ph.D., University of Chicago; Professor of Immunology, School of Medicine, Western Reserve University. Cleveland, Ohio. Special Field: *Immunology and Bacteriology.*

Emmons, Chester W.

B.S., Penn College (Iowa); M.S., State University of Iowa; Ph.D., Columbia University; Principal Mycologist, U.S. Public Health Service. Bethesda, Maryland. Special Field: *Mycology.*

Faulkner, Robert L.

B.S., Allegheny College; M.D., Johns Hopkins University School of Medicine; Assistant Professor of Gynecology, School of Medicine, Western Reserve University. Cleveland, Ohio. Special Field: *Gynecology.*

Feil, Harold

A.B., University of Denver; M.D., Ohio Wesleyan University Medical Department; Clinical Professor of Medicine, School of Medicine, Western Reserve University. Cleveland, Ohio. Special Field: *Cardiovascular Diseases and Electrocardiography.*

Fortune, George F.

A.B., Western Reserve University; M.A., The Ohio State University; Director, The Cleveland Hearing and Speech Center affiliated with Western Reserve University; Lecturer, Speech and Hearing, Graduate School, Western Reserve University. Cleveland, Ohio. Special Field: *Speech and Hearing.*

Francis, Carl C.

A.B., Bethany College; M.D., School of Medicine, Western Reserve University; Associate Professor of Anatomy, School of Medicine, Western Reserve University. Cleveland, Ohio. Special Field: *Gross Anatomy.*

Friedell, Hymer L.

B.S., University of Minnesota; M.B., M.D., University of Minnesota Medical School; Professor of Radiology, School of Medicine, Western Reserve University. Cleveland, Ohio. Special Field: *Radiology and Clinical Applications of Radioisotopes.*

Garver, William P.

A.B., Cornell University; M.D., Cornell University Medical College; Visitant in Charge of Allergy, Cleveland City and St. Vincent's Charity Hospitals; Instructor of Medicine, School of Medicine, Western Reserve University. Cleveland, Ohio. Special Field: *Allergy.*

Ginsberg, Harold S.

A.B., Duke University; M.D., Tulane University School of Medicine; Associate Professor of Preventive Medicine and Assistant Professor of Medicine, School of Medicine, Western Reserve University. Cleveland, Ohio. Special Field: *Virology and Infectious Diseases.*

Glasser, Otto

Ph.D., University of Freiburg; Professor of Biophysics, Research Division, Cleveland Clinic Foundation. Cleveland, Ohio. Special Field, *Medical Physics.*

Goldblatt, Harry

B.A., McGill University; M.D., C.M., McGill University Faculty of Medicine; Professor of Experimental Pathology, School of Medicine, Western Reserve University; Director of Laboratories, Mt. Sinai Hospital. Cleveland, Ohio. Special Field: *Pathology.*

Ham, Thomas Hale

B.S., Dartmouth College; M.D., Cornell University Medical College; Professor of Medicine and Chairman of Committee on Medical Education, School of Medicine, Western Reserve University. Cleveland, Ohio. Special Field: *Internal Medicine.*

Hauser, Harry

A.B., University of Texas; M.D., University of Texas School of Medicine; Chief Radiologist, Cleveland City Hospital; Associate Professor of Radiology, School of Medicine, Western Reserve University. Cleveland, Ohio. Special Field: *Radiology.*

Hellerstein, Herman K.

A.B., Western Reserve University; M.D., School of Medicine, Western Reserve University; Assistant Professor of Medicine, School of Medicine, Western Reserve University; Assistant Physician, University Hospitals; Director, The Work Classification Clinic of the Cleveland Area Heart Society. Cleveland, Ohio. Special Field: *Cardiovascular Diseases, Electrocardiography, Vectorcardiography, and Cardiac Rehabilitation.*

HERNDON, CHARLES H.

B.A., University of Texas; M.D., Harvard Medical School; Associate Professor of Orthopedic Surgery, School of Medicine, Western Reserve University; Director, Department of Orthopedic Surgery, University Hospitals and Rainbow Hospital. Cleveland, Ohio. Special Field: *Orthopedics.*

HERSH, A. H.

A.B., Sc.D. (Hon.), Franklin and Marshall College; Ph.D., University of Illinois; Professor of Biology, Western Reserve University. Cleveland, Ohio. Special Field: *Biology and Genetics.* Deceased, 1955.

HINGSON, ROBERT A.

A.B., University of Alabama; M.D., Emory University School of Medicine; Professor of Anesthesia, School of Medicine, Western Reserve University. Cleveland, Ohio. Special Field: *Anesthesiology.*

HIRSCHMANN, HANS

M.D., University of Basel; Ph.D., Columbia University; Associate Professor of Biochemistry in the Department of Medicine, School of Medicine, Western Reserve University. Cleveland, Ohio. Special Field: *Steroid Chemistry.*

HOERR, NORMAND L.

A.B., Johns Hopkins University; Ph.D., University of Chicago; M.D., University of Chicago School of Medicine; Henry Willson Payne Professor of Anatomy, School of Medicine, Western Reserve University; Secretary-Treasurer, American Association of Anatomists; Editor, *Blakiston's New Gould Medical Dictionary.* Cleveland, Ohio. Special Field: *Anatomy.*

HORRIGAN, DANIEL L.

A.B., DePauw University; M.D., College of Medicine of the University of Cincinnati; Assistant Professor of Medicine, School of Medicine, Western Reserve University. Cleveland, Ohio. Special Field: *Hematology.*

HOVORKA, FRANK

B.A., Iowa State Teacher's College; M.S., Ph.D., University of Illinois; Hurlbut Professor of Chemistry and Chairman, Department of Chemistry, Western Reserve University. Cleveland, Ohio. Special Field: *Electrochemistry and Ultrasonics.*

JEFFRIES, WILLIAM McK.

B.A., Hampden-Sydney College; M.D., University of Virginia School of Medicine; Assistant Professor of Medicine, School of Medicine, Western Reserve University. Cleveland, Ohio. Special Field: *Endocrinology.*

JOHNSON, HERBERT H., JR.

A.B., Stanford University; M.D., Stanford University School of Medicine; Associate Clinical Professor of Dermatology and Syphilology, School of Medicine, Western Reserve University. Cleveland, Ohio. Special Field: *Dermatology and Syphilology.*

JOHNSON, LORAND V.

M.A., Boston University; M.D., Boston University School of Medicine; Clinical Professor of Ophthalmology, School of Medicine, Western Reserve University; Ophthalmologist in Charge, University Hospitals. Cleveland, Ohio. Special Field: *Ophthalmology.*

JONES, OLIVER P.

A.B., Temple University; Ph.D., University of Minnesota; Professor and Head of Anatomy, University of Buffalo School of Medicine. Buffalo, New York. Special Field: *Experimental and Morphologic Hematology.*

KARNOSH, LOUIS J.

B.S., Berea College; M.D., School of Medicine, Western Reserve University; Sc.D., Berea College; Director of Neuropsychiatry, Cleveland Clinic Foundation; Clinical Professor of Neurology, School of Medicine, Western Reserve University. Cleveland, Ohio. Special Field: *Neurology and Psychiatry.*

KEYS, THOMAS E.

A.B., Beloit College; M.A., Graduate Library School, University of Chicago; Librarian, The Mayo Clinic. Rochester, Minnesota. Special Field: *Medical Librarianship.*

KINNEY, THOMAS D.

A.B., University of Pennsylvania; M.D., Duke University School of Medicine; Professor of Pathology, School of Medicine, Western Reserve University. Cleveland, Ohio. Special Field: *Pathology.*

KOLETSKY, SIMON

B.A., Yale University; M.D., Yale University School of Medicine; Pathologist, University Hospitals; Professor of Pathology, School of Medicine, Western Reserve University. Cleveland, Ohio. Special Field: *Pathology.*

LAZAROW, ARNOLD

B.S., University of Chicago; M.D., University of Chicago School of Medicine; Ph.D., University of Chicago; Professor and Head of the Department of Anatomy, University of Minnesota Medical School. Minneapolis, Minnesota. Special Field: *Cytochemistry and Experimental Diabetes.*

LEUALLEN, E. E.

B.Sc. (Pharm.), M.Sc. (Chem.), D.Sc., Philadelphia College of Pharmacy and Science; Dean, Columbia University College of Pharmacy. New York, New York. Special Field: *Chemistry and Pharmacy.*

LITTELL, ARTHUR S.

A.B., Harvard University; A.M., Sc.D., Johns Hopkins University; Senior Instructor in Biostatistics, School of Medicine, Western Reserve University. Cleveland, Ohio. Special Field: *Biostatistics.*

LUDLOW, ALFRED I.

A.B., Adelbert College, and M.D., School of Medicine, Western Reserve University; M.A.

(Hon.), Western Reserve University; D.Sc. (Hon.), College of Wooster; Professor Emeritus of Surgery, Severance Union Medical College, Seoul, Korea. Cleveland, Ohio. Special Field: *Medical Editing.*

McCullagh, E. Perry

M.D., University of Manitoba; Head, Section of Endocrinology and Metabolism, Cleveland Clinic. Cleveland, Ohio. Special Field: *Endocrinology and Metabolism.*

McKay, Raymond C.

A.B., Brown University; M.D., School of Medicine, Western Reserve University; Medical Director, Division of Tuberculosis, Cleveland City Hospital; Associate Clinical Professor of Medicine, School of Medicine, Western Reserve University. Cleveland, Ohio. Special Field: *Chest Diseases.*

Mackrell, John S.

B.S., University of Pittsburgh; M.D., University of Pittsburgh School of Medicine; Senior Instructor in Pathology, School of Medicine, Western Reserve University; Pathologist, St. Vincent Charity Hospital. Cleveland, Ohio. Special Field: *Pathology and Clinical Pathology.*

Mendelsohn, Harvey J.

A.B., Western Reserve University; M.D., School of Medicine, Western Reserve University; Assistant Professor of Surgery, School of Medicine, Western Reserve University. Cleveland, Ohio. Special Field: *Thoracic Surgery.*

Miller, Genevieve

A.B., Goucher College; M.A., Johns Hopkins University; Ph.D., Cornell University; Assistant Professor of Medical History, School of Medicine, Western Reserve University. Cleveland, Ohio. Special Field: *Medical History.*

Miller, Max

B.S., Yale University; M.D., Yale University School of Medicine; Assistant Professor in Medicine, School of Medicine, Western Reserve University; Associate Physician, Lakeside Hospital. Cleveland, Ohio. Special Field: *Renal Diseases.*

Mommaerts, Wilfried F. H. M.

B.A., M.A., University of Leyden, Netherlands; Ph.D., University of Kolozsvar, Hungary; Associate Professor of Biochemistry, School of Medicine, Western Reserve University; Established Investigator for the American Heart Association. Cleveland, Ohio. Special Field: *Biochemistry.*

Moritz, Alan R.

S.B., M.A., University of Nebraska; M.D., University of Nebraska College of Medicine; Professor of Pathology and Director of the Institute of Pathology, Western Reserve University. Cleveland, Ohio. Special Field: *Pathology.*

Orbison, J. Lowell

A.B., Ottawa University (Kansas); M.S., Michigan State University; M.D., Northwestern University Medical School; Professor of Pathology, Rochester University School of Medicine and Dentistry. Rochester, New York. Special Field: *Pathology.*

Osol, Arthur

Ph.G., B.Sc. (Chem.), Philadelphia College of Pharmacy and Science; M.Sc. (Chem.), Ph.D., University of Pennsylvania; Professor of Chemistry and Director of the Chemistry Department, Philadelphia College of Pharmacy and Science; Editor-in-chief, *The Dispensatory of the United States of America;* Editor, *Blakiston's New Gould Medical Dictionary.* Philadelphia, Pennsylvania. Special Field: *Chemistry and Pharmacy.*

Parker, Robert F.

B.S., Washington University; M.D., Washington University School of Medicine; Professor of Microbiology and Associate Professor of Medicine, School of Medicine, Western Reserve University. Cleveland, Ohio. Special Field: *Cell Culture and Tissue Culture of Viruses.*

Perlich, Myron M.

A.B., Western Reserve University; M.D., College of Medicine, The Ohio State University; Senior Instructor in Medicine, School of Medicine, Western Reserve University. Cleveland, Ohio. Special Field: *Medicine.*

Persky, Lester

B.S., University of Michigan; M.D., Johns Hopkins University School of Medicine; Instructor in Urology, School of Medicine, Western Reserve University. Cleveland, Ohio. Special Field: *Genitourinary Diseases.*

Pillemer, Louis

B.S., Duke University; Ph.D., Western Reserve University; Professor of Biochemistry in Department of Pathology, Institute of Pathology, Western Reserve University. Cleveland, Ohio. Special Field: *Immunochemistry.*

Potts, Albert M.

A.B., Johns Hopkins University; Ph.D., University of Chicago; M.D., School of Medicine, Western Reserve University; Associate Professor of Ophthalmic Research, School of Medicine, Western Reserve University. Cleveland, Ohio. Special Field: *Ophthalmology, Clinical and Basic Science Aspects.*

Price, J. Waide

B.S., Butler University; M.A., Ph.D., University of Cincinnati; Assistant Professor of Pathological Chemistry, School of Medicine, Western Reserve University, Cleveland, Ohio. Special Field: *Biochemistry.*

Pritchard, Jack A.

B.S., Ohio Northern University; M.D., School of Medicine, Western Reserve University; Professor of Obstetrics and Gynecology, Southwestern Medical School of the University of Texas. Dallas, Texas. Special Field: *Obstetrics and Gynecology.*

Ratnoff, Oscar D.

A.B., Columbia University; M.D., College of Physicians and Surgeons, Columbia University; Assistant Professor of Medicine, School of Medicine, Western Reserve University. Cleveland, Ohio. Special Field: *Blood Coagulation and Hemorrhagic Disorders.*

Reagan, James W.

B.S., University of Pittsburgh; M.D., University of Pittsburgh School of Medicine; Associate Professor of Pathology, School of Medicine, Western Reserve University. Cleveland, Ohio. Special Field: *Pathology.*

Sassaman, William H.

A.B., Franklin and Marshall College; M.A., D.B., University of Chicago; Curator of Hamann Museum of Anatomy and Comparative Anthropology and Assistant Professor of Anatomy, School of Medicine, Western Reserve University. Cleveland, Ohio. Special Field: *Anatomy and Physical Anthropology.*

Sayers, George

B.S., Wayne University; M.S., University of Michigan; Ph.D., Yale University; Professor of Physiology, School of Medicine, Western Reserve University. Cleveland, Ohio. Special Field: *Pituitary-adrenal Physiology.*

Scott, Roger B.

A.B., B.S., West Virginia University; M.D., Johns Hopkins University School of Medicine; Associate Professor of Obstetrics and Gynecology, School of Medicine, Western Reserve University. Cleveland, Ohio. Special Field: *Gynecology.*

Sollmann, Torald

M.D., LL.D., School of Medicine, Western Reserve University; D.Sc. (Hon.), The Ohio State University; Professor Emeritus of Pharmacology, School of Medicine, Western Reserve University. Cleveland, Ohio. Special Field: *Pharmacology.*

Spector, Samuel

B.S., Columbia University; M.D., Long Island College of Medicine; Associate Professor of Pediatrics, School of Medicine, Western Reserve University. Cleveland, Ohio. Special Field: *Pediatrics.*

Stavitsky, Abram B.

A.B., University of Michigan; M.S., University of Michigan; Ph.D., University of Minnesota; V.M.D., University of Pennsylvania School of Veterinary Medicine; Associate Professor of Microbiology, School of Medicine, Western Reserve University. Cleveland, Ohio. Special Field: *Immunochemistry and Immunology.*

Stecher, Robert Morgan

B.S., Dartmouth College; M.D., Harvard Medical School; Associate Clinical Professor of Medicine, School of Medicine, Western Reserve University. Cleveland, Ohio. Special Field: *Rheumatic Diseases.*

Storaasli, John P.

B.S., M.B., University of Minnesota; M.D., University of Minnesota Medical School; Assistant Professor of Radiology, School of Medicine, Western Reserve University. Cleveland, Ohio. Special Field: *Therapeutic Radiology and Clinical Uses of Radioactive Isotopes and Radiobiology.*

Tager, Morris

Ph.B., Yale University; M.D., Yale University School of Medicine; Professor and Chairman of the Department of Bacteriology and Immunology, Emory University. Emory University, Georgia. Special Field: *Infectious Diseases and Microbiology.*

Thomas, Charles I.

A.B., Wesleyan University; M.D., School of Medicine, Western Reserve University; Associate Clinical Professor of Ophthalmology, Department of Surgery, School of Medicine, Western Reserve University. Cleveland, Ohio. Special Field: *Ophthalmology.*

Vosburgh, Gilbert J.

A.B., Princeton University; M.D., Johns Hopkins University School of Medicine; Professor of Obstetrics and Gynecology, College of Physicians and Surgeons, Columbia University. New York, New York. Special Field: *Obstetrics and Gynecology.*

Wallace, William M.

A.B., University of Pennsylvania; M.D., University of Pennsylvania School of Medicine; Gertrude Lee Chandler Tucker Professor of Pediatrics, School of Medicine, Western Reserve University; Director of Pediatrics, University Hospitals. Cleveland, Ohio. Special Field: *Electrolyte Metabolism.*

Weckesser, Elden C.

A.B., Western Reserve University; M.D., School of Medicine, Western Reserve University; Assistant Clinical Professor of Surgery, School of Medicine, Western Reserve University. Cleveland, Ohio. Special Field: *Surgery.*

Wedgwood, Ralph J.

M.D., Harvard Medical School; Senior Instructor in Pediatrics and in Biochemistry, Department of Pathology, School of Medicine, Western Reserve University. Cleveland, Ohio. Special Field: *Pediatrics and Immunochemistry.*

Weil, William B., Jr.

A.B., B.S., University of Minnesota; M.D., University of Minnesota Medical School; Senior Instructor in Pediatrics, School of Medicine, Western Reserve University. Cleveland, Ohio. Special Field: *Fluid and Electrolyte Metabolism.*

Weisberger, Austin S.

A.B., Adelbert College, and M.D., School of Medicine, Western Reserve University; Associate Professor of Medicine, School of Medicine, Western Reserve University. Cleveland, Ohio. Special Field: *Hematology.*

Weisman, Russell, Jr.

A.B., Western Reserve University; M.D., School of Medicine, Western Reserve University; Senior Instructor in Medicine and Instructor in Clinical Pathology, School of Medicine, Western Reserve University. Cleveland, Ohio. Special Field: *Hematology.*

Wiggers, Carl J.

M.D., University of Michigan Medical School; Sc.D., University of Michigan; Formerly Professor of Physiology and Director of the Department of Physiology, School of Medicine, Western Reserve University; Consultant in Physiology, Cleveland Clinic. Cleveland, Ohio. Special Field: *Physiology and Cardiology.*

Preface

The first edition of *Blakiston's New Gould Medical Dictionary* in 1949 was a major step in an evolutionary process that began with the publication of *A New Medical Dictionary* in 1890; its immediate predecessor was the fifth edition of *Gould's Medical Dictionary*. The present work carries on the scholarly tradition of its forerunners.

Careful selection of vocabulary entries has continued in this second edition. Professional literature has been studied for new words to be defined, and each entry in the first edition has been reconsidered and, if necessary, redefined or expanded to conform with today's usage. In particular the rapidly growing fields of chest surgery and psychiatry have been surveyed thoroughly in order that dictionary users may find definitions of new words. Oncology terms have been increased by several hundred; in microbiology the names of genera have been modernized to agree with latest terminology; new entries in infectious diseases, hematology, and cardiology can be mentioned as examples of the completeness of revision.

In the fields allied to medicine, extended coverage has been given to terms in dentistry and veterinary medicine, in addition to the inclusion of many new words in biochemistry, organic medicinal chemistry, and nuclear science that will increasingly become a part of the vocabulary of medical scientists. A useful new table, Radioactive and Other Isotopes Commonly Used in Medicine, has been added to the Appendix.

In pharmacology, drugs described in *The Pharmacopeia of the United States of America* (*United States Pharmacopeia*), *Fifteenth Revision* (1955), in *The National Formulary*, *Tenth Edition* (1955), and in *New and Nonofficial Remedies* (1955) have been defined; other drugs in *The Dispensatory of the United States of America* (*United States Dispensatory*), *Twenty-fifth Edition* (1955), and in various listings of medicinals bearing trade-marked, proprietary, or other trade names have been included. In so far as possible, drugs in various stages of animal and clinical investigation have also been defined, but no attempt has been made to establish their individual merit. Drug names known to be trade-marks have been thus indicated, while certain others have been designated as *trade names* or *proprietary names*. In applying such designations, it is understood that the use of a more general designation does not exclude the possibility that a more specific designation may properly apply.

In anatomy it has been possible to include not only the BNA (Basle Nomina Anatomica) terms with modifications and those BR (British Revision) terms that differ significantly from them, but also to retain that part of the old terminology (OT) still in current clinical usage and to include recent modifications suggested by the International Nomenclature Commission.

An explanation of the system of pronunciation used will be found on page xxiii, while Explanatory Notes on page xxi gives details of the arrangement of material.

The illustrative material has been treated as a functional part of the dictionary and, by a system of keyed cross-references, integrated with it; the terminology used in labeling conforms to the primary definitions in the text. The systematic arrangement of the illustrations and the advantages of presenting units large enough to indicate interrelationships will be readily evident.

The wide range of coverage in *Blakiston's New Gould Medical Dictionary* was far beyond the capabilities of the Editorial Board alone. As a consequence, ever-increasing demands were made upon the time and knowledge of their associates in many divergent fields. In this second edition will be found the work of a distinguished staff of 88 contributing editors in addition to the Editorial Board.

It is to be regretted that time and circumstance prevented the participation of Colonel Harold W. Jones, Dr. Robert M. Stecher, Dr. Max H. Fisch, and Mr. Thomas E. Keys as members of the Editorial Board. Their contribution to the first edition was outstanding and is gratefully acknowledged. Acknowledgment is also made to the Consulting Editor, Dr. Morris Fishbein, and to those contributing editors who worked on the first edition. It is because of space limitation only that the list of contributing editors appearing elsewhere in this book is confined to those who worked on this second edition. The Editors want to express here their deep appreciation for the constant and invaluable assistance they have received from many others in the medical and scientific world who are not specifically mentioned elsewhere.

THE EDITORS

Index of Tables and Lists

Names and folios set in **boldface** type refer to tables in the Appendix

Index of Illustrative Plates

Abbreviations Used in Definitions

Abbreviations with medical significance appear in their proper alphabetical sequence in the dictionary

adj.	adjective
adv.	adverb
AF.	Anglo-French
Amer.	American
Ar.	Arabic
AS.	Anglo-Saxon
at. wt.	atomic weight
b.	born
BNA	Basle Nomina Anatomica
BR	*In anatomy,* British Revision of BNA
ca.	[L. *circa*]. About
Chin.	Chinese
D.	Dutch
d.	died
dial.	dialect
E.	English
e.g.	[L. *exempli gratia*]. For example
F.	French
fl.	flourished
G.	Greek
Gael.	Gaelic
Ger.	German
Heb.	Hebrew
Hind.	Hindustani
Hung.	Hungarian
Icel.	Icelandic
i.e.	[L. *id est*]. That is
It.	Italian
Jap.	Japanese
L.	Latin
LG.	Low German
LL.	Late Latin
MD.	Middle Dutch
ME.	Middle English
mEq./l.	milliequivalents per liter
ML.	Middle Latin
MLG.	Middle Low German
n.	noun
N.F.	*The National Formulary*
NL.	New Latin
NNR	*New and Nonofficial Remedies*
obs.	obsolete
OF.	Old French
ON.	Old Norse
ONF.	Old North French
OT	*In anatomy,* Old Terminology
Per.	Persian
Pg.	Portuguese
pl.	plural
S. Afr. D.	South African Dutch
Scand.	Scandinavian
Skr.	Sanskrit
Sp.	Spanish
Swed.	Swedish
syn.	synonym
Teut.	Teutonic
U.S.D.	*United States Dispensatory*
U.S.P.	*United States Pharmacopeia*
v.	verb
v.i.	intransitive verb
VL.	Vulgar Latin
v.t.	transitive verb

Transliterations from the Greek

Greek Letter	Name	Transliteration	Greek Letter	Name	Transliteration
Α α	alpha	a	Ν ν	nu	n
Β β	beta	b	Ξ ξ	xi	x
Γ γ	gamma	g	Ο ο	omicron	o
Δ δ	delta	d	Π π	pi	p
Ε ε	epsilon	e	Ρ ρ	rho	r, rh
Ζ ζ	zeta	z	Σ σ	sigma	s
Η η	eta	ē	Τ τ	tau	t
Θ θ	theta	th	Υ υ	upsilon	y
Ι ι	iota	i	Φ φ	phi	ph
Κ κ	kappa	k	Χ χ	chi	ch
Λ λ	lambda	l	Ψ ψ	psi	ps
Μ μ	mu	m	Ω ω	omega	ō

Explanatory Notes

Vocabulary Entries

The word or term to be defined is set in **boldface** type and extends slightly to the left of the definition.

In polysyllabic words, the separation of the syllables is indicated either by a raised dot (·) or by a primary (′) or secondary (″) accent. Syllabification and pronunciation are not indicated for trade-marks, trade names, proprietaries, or eponymic entries.

Words spelled identically but derived from different roots appear as separate entries.

Definitions

The definitions of a term are numbered when there is more than one distinct meaning or use. The most inclusive definition is presented first, followed by the more restricted meanings.

Definitions restricted to specialized fields are preceded by field labels or glosses, such as *In psychiatry*, *In bacteriology*, *In dentistry*, etc. All definitions following a field label are in use in that field.

Etymology

The etymology appears in square brackets immediately following the vocabulary entry or the phonetic respelling. The root term, its language, and its meaning are given. The languages are indicated by abbreviations, a key to which appears on page xix.

Greek terms are transliterated into the Roman alphabet. A table of transliterations appears on page xix.

When the same root is carried down through an uninterrupted series of entries, its meaning and the abbreviation indicating its language are given only on its first occurrence. If, however, such a series is interrupted at any time by words of a different origin or an eponymic entry, the information about the root is repeated in full when the series is resumed. Derivations have been omitted in entries of a chemical nature as well as in trade names and compound or hyphenated words.

Abbreviations

Abbreviations with medical significance appear in their proper alphabetical sequence in the dictionary.

Abbreviations *used* in the dictionary—lexicographic and etymologic terms, etc.—are listed and defined on page xix.

Pronunciation

For a detailed explanation of pronunciation, see Notes on Pronunciation beginning on page xxiii. A Key to Pronunciation is printed facing page 1 of the vocabulary.

Chemical and Pharmaceutical Terms

Formulas: Definitions for chemical substances include the chemical formula of the substance when this is known. In an organic compound, this formula is of the type which shows the conventional structural arrangement.

Synonyms: The definition of a medicinal substance includes the synonyms applied to that substance.

Latin Names: Entries for older *official drugs*—those recognized in *The Pharmacopeia of the United States of America, Fifteenth Revision*, or *The National Formulary, Tenth Edition*—are followed by the Latin name in *italics* enclosed in parentheses.

Medicinal Plants: The definition for a drug representing a structural part of a plant includes its botanical origin, this being distinguished by the use of italicized type. The definition also includes a statement of the active constituents, if any, of the plant, and their approximate proportions. In the case of official drugs representing parts of plants, the quantitative limits of active constituents, such as alkaloids, are those established by *The Pharmacopeia of the United States of America, Fifteenth Revision*, or *The National Formulary, Tenth Edition.*

Dosage: The limits of dosage of medicinals are indicated in those cases where such limits have been established. The dose statement is given first in the metric system, this being followed by the approximate apothecary system equivalents. Unless otherwise stated, the limits are for a single adult dose. Where the dosage of a drug has not been definitely established, or in cases where there is marked variation in dosage according to different authorities, no statement of limits of dosage has been provided in the definition.

Run-ons

Derivative forms of a vocabulary entry are entered as run-ons following the definition or, when there is more than one definition for the main entry, the definition to which they are most closely related.

In general, the pronunciation of a run-on entry can be inferred from that of the main entry. Syllabification is, therefore, not indicated, but a primary accent is used when necessary to show that the position of the main stress in the run-on differs from that of the heading.

Tables and Lists

Lists, statistics, and other material most conveniently handled in tabular form are presented in the Appendix at the back of the book. An index of these and other tables and lists appears on page xv.

Groups or classes of definitions related by a common root term appear under that term: disease, method, operation, stain, etc. The series is slightly indented and each subentry to be defined is set in **boldface.**

Biographic Entries

Proper names, biographic entries, and eponymic terms appear in their proper alphabetical sequence. In those cases in which the eponymic term is fully defined elsewhere under another entry—as a disease described more fully in the *disease* list, for example—the user is directed to the proper entry by a cross-reference.

Names with prefixes have been alphabetized according to the customs of their languages. In general, in American and English names of foreign origin, prefix and name are treated as a unit, while in other languages the article or preposition is often ignored in alphabetizing. Names with two or more parts have been treated as single units. Biographic entries have been made under pen names when those names are more commonly used in medical literature than the true names. In all cases where confusion seemed possible, cross-references have been inserted.

Cross-references

Whenever it is desirable, the user is directed to additional or fuller information by such cross-reference terms as *see*, *see under*, *syn*. The entry to which the user is directed is italicized; in the case of compound terms, only the word or part of the term under which the information is entered is italicized.

THE EDITORS

Notes on Pronunciation

§1 The principle followed for pronunciation in this dictionary has been to record pronunciation in actual, current use, and not to presume to dictate standards of alleged correctness. The objective has been to show what usage is, not what somebody supposes it ought to be. Where more than one pronunciation is given for a word, the intention has been to give the most widely used variant first. Sometimes it has been possible to do this with a high degree of confidence. More often, the division of usage is not clear-cut, or the facts not readily ascertainable; so that the order in which variant pronunciations are given is more likely to be arbitrary than to be of any real significance. In any case, there is no implication of editorial preference intended.

§2 The manner of indicating pronunciation is such that the users of the dictionary can fit medical terminology into their own natural, everyday speech habits. The basis is the syllable. In whatever way a person may pronounce the syllable **car**, for instance, whether as the word **car** itself or as a syllable in a longer word like **reincarnation**, that is the way for him to pronounce it when it appears as one of the syllables in a medical word, such as **cardiogram** or **metacarpal.** The syllables in the phonetic respellings (see §§14–36, below) are to be treated the same way. For example, in the system used here, **merry** would be respelled (merr′ee) and **Mary** (mair′ee), similarly **ferry** (ferr′ee) and **fairy** (fair′ee). But if you pronounce **merry** and **Mary** the same, and likewise **ferry** and **fairy,** then you can consider pairs of syllables in the respellings like (merr) and (mair) or (ferr) and (fair) as meaning the same thing and as representing your own sounds in those words.

§3 The respellings for pronunciation are put in parentheses immediately following the entry term whose pronunciation is to be shown; but in the majority of instances no respellings have been needed. The pronunciation is clearly indicated by syllabification of the heading itself and by marking the accents. In all such cases each syllable is simply pronounced according to the most common values of the letters and letter sequences that make it up, with due regard to the preceding and following syllables and to the positions of the accents.

§4 The accent marks used are a single accent (′), denoting main stress, that is, the emphasis put on the most heavily pronounced syllable in a word, and a double accent (″) for secondary stress, that is, some degree of emphasis as found on syllables more strongly accented than neighboring "unstressed" syllables, but less prominently than the syllable that carries the main stress: **car″di·ol′o·gy, car′di·o·gram″, met″a·car′pal, su″per·al″i·men·ta′tion.**

§5 In the following paragraphs, lists of illustrative examples are given, showing how the various letters are to be interpreted in different groupings and with varying accentual conditions. Pronunciations according to these examples apply only to headings that have no respelling for pronunciation. It will also be noted that the pronunciation of a given letter often depends on what other letters immediately precede or follow.

§6 The vowels, if immediately followed by an accent, either the primary accent (′) or the secondary accent(″), have the following values: **a** as in **fla′vor, ca″pa·bil′i·ty, fa′cial, Ma′bel; e** as in **ce′dar, he′ro, se′ri·ous; i** and **y** as in **ti′ger, ny′lon, Hi′ram, ty′rant; o** as in **no′tice, no″to·ri′e·ty, sto′ry, mo″bi·li·za′tion, mo′lar; u** as in **mu′sic, du′ty, stu′di·o, Lu′cy, il·lu′sion, su′per·vise, ru′mor, fu′ry, tu′lip.**

§7 The same pronunciations are found in monosyllable words and accented syllables with final silent **e,** as in: **game, a·bate′ment, base′ment, gene, se·rene′ly, sin·cere′ly, nice, po·lite′ness, rhyme′ster, tire′less, lyre′bird, spoke, re·mote′ly, fore′man, cute, huge′ly, in·duce′·ment, par′a·chute″, pro·cure′ment, al·lure′·ment, ma·ture′ness.**

§8 Otherwise, if a vowel is followed immediately by a consonant in the same syllable, and that syllable is accented, then the vowel is pronounced as follows; **a** as in **bag, mag′ni·tude, car′ol, com·par′i·son; e** as in **led, let′ter, mer′it, her′ald; i** and **y** as in **glim′mer, sys′tem, spir′it, lyr′ic; o** as in **cop′per,** or before a single **r** as in **bor′ing,** before **rr** as in **bor′row; u** as in **num′·ber, cur′rent.**

§9 If a vowel in an accented syllable is followed by **r** and the next letter is another consonant, but not **r,** then the vowel is pronounced as follows: **a** as in **bar′ber; e, i, y,** and **u** as in **cer′tain, skir′mish, myr′tle, cur′tain; o** can be as in **for′tune, bor′der,** or **por′trait.**

§10 Unaccented syllables will give little difficulty. Their pronunciation ordinarily will be evident. It should be noted, however, that in the case of medical and other scientific words, much more than in the case of ordinary, everyday words, something like full vowel value is frequently heard in unaccented syllables. Thus the **o** in **biochemical** is more likely to have a clear **o** sound than is the **o** in **biographic.**

§11 Final syllables, accented or unaccented, follow the customary pronunciation of such syllables, for example: **re·late′, cor′re·late″, bro′·mate, syn′di·cate, pre·sage′, dam′age, py′·rene, re·plete′, con·fine′, de·cide′, con·spire′, an′o·dyne, re·mote′, re·morse′, al·lude′, al·lure′, fail′ure, na′ture, par·tic′u·lar, sa′ber, la′bor, le′mur, de·mur′, Ai′ken, ba′con, ca·reen′, ca·reer′, re·la′tion, con·fu′sion, fab′·u·lous, far″i·na′ceous, con·ta′gious, re·lent′, ma·lev′o·lent.** Some final groups can be pronounced as one syllable or as two, for example: **-gia** in **neu·ral′gi·a, -tia** in **or″tho·don′ti·a,** etc.

§12 A combination of two vowels, or of a vowel with **y** or **w,** will be understood as having its most common English pronunciation, thus: **ai** and **ay** as in **paid** or **pair, pray** or **prayer; au** and **aw** as in **faun, lawn; ea** as in **clean** or **clear; eu** as in **neuter** or **neural; ew** as in **few, new, dew, flew,**

chew; oa as in **boat** or **boar; oi** and **oy** as in **anoint, annoy; ou** as in **flout** or **flour.**

§13 The consonants are to be pronounced with their usual English values, whether singly, or in combinations like **sh** or **th,** or in syllable groups like **tion,** as the case may be; **c** before **e, i,** or **y** is like **s: Cecil, Cyril, cent, acid, cypress,** otherwise like **k: cab, cub, clay; g** before **e, i,** or **y** as in **ginger, gyrate, gem, agile,** otherwise as in **gargoyle, gun, glue, lignite; ch** ordinarily represents the sound in **chin, rich,** but before **l** or **r** it is pronounced like **k,** for example in **chloroform, chronic, achromatic.**

§14 When the pronunciation of a word is not apparent from its spelling, syllabification, and accentuation, in accordance with the examples given above, then a respelling for pronunciation is put in parentheses immediately after the vocabulary entry. These phonetic transcriptions are also based on the syllable as a unit and on ordinary values of letters. The syllables are designed for easy recognition. Often, in fact, a syllable is respelled, not arbitrarily, but in the form of some well-known English monosyllable, such as *buy, coal, cue, juice, view.* And syllables with a final silent *e* are used a great deal, whether they represent actual English words or not: *sole, tole, daze, dace, mate, nate, dyne, byne, styne, style.*

§15 There are some convenient combinations of letters that are used in the respellings more extensively than they actually occur in the writing of English syllables. Thus *igh,* representing "long *i*" in such words as *high, thigh, sigh, sight, flight,* is used for the same sound in other syllables, for example: *kigh, thrigh, smigh;* similarly *ye,* as found in *dye, lye, rye,* is also used for this sound elsewhere, for example: *pye, tye, chye, kwye.* On the same principle, *ew,* as in *few, pew, dew, new, flew, chew,* is extended to other syllables, such as *bew, thew, tew, lew.*

§16 The following points are to be particularly noted:

§17 In the phonetic respellings, as in the entry headings themselves, a single accent (**′**) marks the most strongly stressed syllable and double accent marks (**″**) are used for the secondary accents.

§18 An *s* always represents the sound in **dose** and **loose,** never the sound in **rose, choose,** and **lose.** Similarly, *f* always stands for the sound in **loaf,** never as in **of.** At the end of a syllable, again on the principle of clarity and ready recognition, *ss* is sometimes used for *s,* and *ff* for *f.*

§19 A *g* in the respellings always stands for the "hard *g*" sound, as in **gun** and **get,** never for the sound in **gem, gym·na′si·um** (jim·nay′-zi·um), and **reg″i·men·ta′tion** (redj″i·men·tay′-shun). To avoid possible ambiguity in certain syllables, *gh* is sometimes used instead of *g* for the "hard *g*" sound, for example, **gel′ding** (gheld′ing). An *ng* stands for the simple *ng* sound in **sing′er.** When used in combination with *g* or *k,* it is so transcribed: **fin′ger** (fing′gur), **link′age** (ling′kidj).

§20 A *ch* is as in **church;** *th* always as in **thin** and **both.** For the sound in **then** and **writhe** the symbol t̶h̶ is used; so the syllable respelled *thee* as in **ap′a·thy** (ap′uh·thee) or **the·ol′o·gy** (thee·ol′o·jee) is not the same as the English word **thee,** which would have to be respelled (t̶h̶ee).

§21 For the sound of *s* in **pleasure** and **usual,** *z* in **azure,** the symbol *zh* is used: **meas′ure** (mezh′ur), **vi′sion** (vizh′un), **clo′sure** (klo′zhur).

§22 Unless followed by a consonant in the same syllable, *ar* is to be pronounced as in **parish, charity, marathon, farinaceous,** and **tariff,** but, with a following consonant, as in **hard** and **garter;** and *ah* is used for the *a* in **fa′ther** (fah′-t̶h̶ur), **psalm,** and **balmy,** also **tar** (tahr) and **quar′an·tine** (kwahr′un·teen).

§23 The combinations *err* and *irr* are used as in **error, terror, merrily,** and **irrigate, cirrus, mirror,** respectively, and *orr* as in **borrow, horrible, tomorrow.**

§24 The *oo* in **boot** is represented by o͞o: **ru″mi·na′tion** (ro͞o″mi·nay′shun), but for the sound in **foot** o͝o is used: **sug′ar** (sho͝og′ur); while *oo* without any mark is used before *r,* as in **poor, Eu′rope** (yoor′up), and is also used in unaccented syllables unless the sound is clearly o͞o: **ma·nip′u·late** (ma·nip′yoo·late), but **a′gue** (ayg′yo͞o), **e·val′u·ate″** (i·val′yo͞o·ate″).

§25 In many unaccented syllables the somewhat obscure sound of *a* in **about, sofa, Manila, logarithm, organize, pentagon,** is represented in the respellings by *uh* or, before consonants, just by *u*: **pri″va·teer′** (pry″vuh·teer′), **Tex′as** (teck′sus).

§26 This sound is, of course, also commonly heard for the *e* of **enough, system, category,** the *i* of **directory, dilapidated, manifest,** and the *o* of **molasses, hypocrite, hammock.** A great many speakers of English do, however, use a vowel like the *i* of **bit** in many or most unaccented syllables spelled with **e, i,** or **y;** and a fairly clear, even though unstressed, *o* is not uncommon in syllables spelled with **o,** especially in scientific and other technical words. Therefore, the respellings for pronunciation in this dictionary regularly show *i* and *o,* and sometimes *e,* where sounds ordinarily represented by these letters can occur as well as the more obscure vowel here represented by *uh* or *u.* This does not mean that the Editors recommend such pronunciations, but merely that they recognize their occurrence, as no better and no worse than pronunciations of the *uh* variety.

§27 Similarly, in the first syllable of a word, again especially a scientific word, an **a** is often not pronounced *uh,* as in **about,** but may have some other *a* sound such as the **a** in **cat** or the **a** in **sardonic.** This is reflected in the respellings by the use of *a* instead of *uh* in initial syllables. Thus **fa·ri′na** would be transcribed (fa·ree′nuh) rather than (fuh·ree′nuh), it being understood that the latter is implied as one of the commonly heard variants.

§28 When **a** appears as the first letter in certain classes of words, it may often have the sound of *ay* in **pay,** and this is generally shown in the dictionary: **A·cho′ri·on** (a·kor′ee·on, ay·kor′-ee·on), **a·dip′sa** (ay·dip′suh, a·dip′suh).

§29 In general, where there are variant pronunciations the variations are shown by additional respellings of those portions of a word affected by the variations in question. Thus **chel″e·ryth′rine** (kel″i·rith′reen, ·rin, kel·err′ith·) indicates four different pronunciations in current use for this word: *kel″i·rith′reen, kel″i·rith′rin, kel·err′ith·reen, kel·err′ith·rin,* as well as variants with *kel″uh·* instead of *kel″i·,* and *·err′uth·* instead of *·err′ith·* (see §26, above).

§30 An indication like *·shuh, ·see·uh,* or *·zhuh, ·zee·uh,* for an ending is meant to cover a whole gradation of possibilities between the two extremes; for example: **am·ne′si·a** (am·nee′zhuh, ·zee·uh) is intended to include such intermediate forms as *am·nee′zhee·zuh, am·neez′yuh,* etc.

§31 Inasmuch as the termination **·ide,** common in chemical words, can be pronounced *·id* as well as *·ide,* this general rule is taken for granted and no respellings are inserted merely to show this variation. The variants are shown, however, when a word that has the **·ide** ending is respelled for some other reason. Similarly, the chemical ending **·ol** can be pronounced *·ole*, *·ol*, or *·awl;* also, **·yl** is *·il* or *·eel;* and names of enzymes in **·ase** are pronounced *·ace* or *·aze*.

§32 Names of diseases ending in **·i′tis** are always shown only with the *·eye′tis* pronunciation, which is used much more widely than *·ee′tis*. In every case, the latter is to be understood as also occurring and in no way less correct than the other.

§33 Very often the pronunciation of the beginning of a word is apparent from that of neighboring entries in the dictionary and, if the rest of the word is clear, no respelling is needed. Thus, the first syllable of **cy·tot′ro·phy** is seen to be *sigh·*, and not *si·*, from the respelling of **cy·tot′ro·pism** (sigh·tot′ro·piz·um), the pronunciation of **mi·ot′ic** is clear from that of **mi·o′sis** (migh·o′sis), etc.

§34 Many long compounds are not respelled, especially when there are variant pronunciations for each of several elements in the compound. And often, when a compound is respelled, a relatively uncommon variant pronunciation may be omitted. Such variants can be found under the individual elements themselves.

§35 Foreign words and phrases, and words recently taken into English from foreign languages, are pronounced in a great variety of ways, ranging from the original, native pronunciation to complete Anglicization. In this dictionary, a compromise Anglicization is frequently indicated in the respelling of such expressions.

§36. The pronunciation of Latin is usually given in the traditional Anglicization, but exceptions are made in cases where a given term is most commonly pronounced in some other way. And it is to be understood that other pronunciations of Latin—in particular the Roman pronunciation as taught in schools—are also used for Latin medical terms.

JOHN KEPKE

Key to Pronunciation

(Also see Notes on Pronunciation, page xxiii)

A single accent (′) marks the strongest accent, the most heavily stressed syllable in a word. A double accent (″) marks syllables with secondary stress, lighter accent than the primary.

When there is no respelling for pronunciation, the spelling of the entry itself gives the pronunciation. A vowel has its long sound if it is followed immediately by an accent mark. Consonants are pronounced according to the usual rules. For example, **c** followed by **e, i,** or **y** is pronounced as in **cent, de·cide′, cy′press;** otherwise as in **cab, cob, cub, clay, screw; ch** followed by **l** or **r** as in **chlo′ro·form, chron′ic;** otherwise as in **chin, rich, church; g** followed by **e, i,** or **y** as in **gin′ger, gy′rate, ag′ile, a·gil′i·ty;** otherwise as in **gag, gar′goyle, gun, glue, gray, lig′nite.**

When the ordinary rules do not apply, respellings are given in parentheses immediately after the boldface entries, using the common values of letters, like **aw** in **paw, ay** in **pay,** etc., and observing the conventions shown in the following table.

In the Respellings

ah	**calm, fa′ther** (fah′~~th~~ur), **Ja′va** (jah′vuh), **Na′ga** (nah′guh)
ahr	**hard, farm, smart, Dart′mouth** (dahrt′muth), **Scars′dale** (skahrz′dale)
ar	**par′ish, tar′iff, mar′a·thon, phar″yn·gec′to·my** (far″in·jeck′to·mee)
err	**mer′ry, ter′ror, dic′tion·ar″y** (dick′shuh·nerr″ee), **pal″a·to·pter′y·goid** (pal″uh·to·terr′i·goyd)
ew	**few, pew, Bu·chan′an** (bew·kan′un), **mu″co·hem″or·rhag′ic** (mew″ko·hem″o·radj′ick), **dew, new, du·plic′i·ty** (dew·plis′i·tee), **tu″me·fa′cient** (tew″mi·fay′shunt)
i	**bit, fas′ci·nate, ag″i·ta′tion** (adj″i·tay′shun), **my″ce·tog′e·nous** (migh″si·todj′i·nus)
igh	**high, sigh, flight, chi″ro·prac′tor** (kigh″ro·prack′tur), **chei″ma·pho′bi·a** (kigh″muh·fo′bee·uh)
ye	**dye, rye, lye, ty·phoi′dal** (tye·foy′dul), **pi·lo′sis** (pye·lo′sis)
irr	**ir′ri·gate, mir′ror, con·spir′a·cy** (kon·spirr′uh·see), **myr″in·gec′to·my** (mirr″in·jeck′to·mee)
orr	**bor′row, hor′rid, Hor′ace** (horr′is), **cor′o·nar″y** (korr′o·nerr″ee)
o͞o	**boot** (bo͞ot), **Hoo′ver** (ho͞o′vur), **u″ku·le′le** (yo͞o″kuh·lay′lee), **u′ni·tar″y** (yo͞o′ni·terr″ee)
o͝o	**foot** (fo͝ot), **Hook′er** (ho͝ok′ur), **pul′ley** (po͝ol′ee), **kous′so** (ko͝os′o)
oo	**poor, doc″u·men·ta′tion** (dock″yoo·men·tay′shun), **pleu′rae** (ploor′ee), **kie′sel·guhr″** (kee′zul-goor″), **fas·cic′u·lus** (fa·sick′yoo·lus)
uh	**so′fa** (so′fuh), **con″tra·vene′** (kon″truh·veen′), **plas′ma·cyte** (plaz′muh·sight), **hap″a·lo·nych′i·a** (hap″uh·lo·nick′ee·uh)
g	**gag, gig, ugly, gre·ga′ri·ous, ex·haus′tion** (eg·zaws′chun)
ng	**sing′er, link′age** (ling′kidj), **con′cha** (kong′kuh)
s	**sense, crease, con·tri′vance** (kon·try′vuns), **oc·cip′i·tal** (ock·sip′i·tul)
th	**thick, thin, path**
~~th~~	**then** (~~th~~en), **thee** (~~th~~ee), **weath′er** (we~~th~~′ur)
zh	**meas′ure** (mezh′ur), **con·fu′sion** (kon·few′zhun), **in·ci′sion** (in·sizh′un)

Syllables respelled as common words (e.g., *buy, coal, view*) are pronounced like those words: **vu″e·rom′e·ter** (view″i·rom′i·tur)

A

A 1. *In chemistry,* symbol for argon. 2. *In radiology,* symbol for area of heart shadow. 3. *In physics,* abbreviation for angstrom unit.

A. Abbreviation for absolute, accommodation, anode.

Å Abbreviation for angstrom unit.

A Symbol for absorbance.

a. Accommodation, ampere, anode, anterior, aqua, arteria.

a Symbol for absorptivity.

a-, an- [Greek alpha privative]. A prefix equivalent to *un-* or *in-* and signifying *absence, lack, -less, not.*

A.A. Abbreviation for achievement age.

ā, āā [G. *ana,* of each]. Symbol denoting the same quantity of each ingredient in a prescription.

āāā. Amalgam.

aaa dis·ease′. An endemic anemia of ancient Egypt, or hookworm disease, described in the Ebers Papyrus. *Obs.*

A. A. A. S. American Association for the Advancement of Science.

Ab Chemical symbol for alabamine.

ab-, a- [L., from]. A prefix meaning *from* or *away,* or signifying *separation* or *departure.*

Abadie, Jean Marie Charles [*French ophthalmologist,* 1842–1932]. Described a spasm of the levator palpebrae muscle, a sign significant of exophthalmic goiter; called *Abadie's sign.*

ab·a″li·en·a′tion [L. *abalienare,* to separate, transfer]. *In psychiatry,* mental deterioration or derangement; insanity. *Obs.*

a·ban′don·ment. *In medical jurisprudence,* the withdrawal of a physician from the care of a patient, without reasonable notice of such withdrawal or without discharge from the case by the patient.

ab·ap′i·cal [L. *ab,* from; *apex,* apex]. Away from or opposite the apex.

ab″ap·tis′ton [G. *abaptistos,* from *a-,* not; *baptistos,* immersed]. A conical trephine which cannot slip through the opening and injure the brain.

a·bar″og·no′sis [*a-*; G. *baros,* weight; *gnōsis,* knowledge]. Loss or lack of the ability to estimate weight; baragnosis.

ab″ar·tic′u·lar [L. *ab,* from; *articulus,* joint]. Not connected with or situated near a joint.

a·ba′si·a (a·bay′zhuh, ·zee·uh) [G. *a-,* not; *basis,* step]. Motor incoordination in walking. See *astasia.* —**aba′sic, abat′ic,** *adj.*

a.-astasia. See *astasia*-abasia.

ataxic a. Awkwardness and uncertainty displayed in locomotion.

choreic a. Inability to walk due to choreic spasm of muscles in the lower extremities.

paralytic a. Total inability of the legs to support the body in walking or standing, due to organic paralysis.

paroxysmal trepidant a. A form of astasia-abasia in which the legs become spastic when the patient attempts to walk.

trembling a. Incapacity to walk because of exaggerated trembling of the legs.

abasin. A brand of acetylcarbromal.

a·bate′ment [OF. *abattre,* from *a,* to; *battre,* to beat]. Lessening or moderation of the pain or untoward symptoms of a disease. —**abated,** *adj.;* **abate,** *v.t., v.i.*

a·bat·tage′, a·ba·tage′ (ah·buh·tahzh′) [F.]. 1. The slaughter of animals; specifically, the slaughter of diseased animals to prevent the infection of others. 2. Art of casting an animal preparatory to an operation.

ab″at·toir′ (ab″uh·twahr′) [F.]. Slaughterhouse or establishment for the killing and dressing of animals.

ab·ax′i·al [L. *ab,* from; *axis,* axle]. Not situated in the line of the axis.

Abbas, Haly. See *Haly Abbas.*

Abbe, Ernst [*German mathematician and physicist,* 1840–1905]. Celebrated for his introduction of the oil immersion lens (1878), and for his invention of a system of lenses, or condenser, attached to the microscope for concentrating light upon an object (1886); called *Abbe's condenser.*

Abbe, Robert [*American surgeon,* 1851–1928]. Pioneer abdominal surgeon, remembered for his work in intestinal anastomosis and for the development of the catgut ring. The technic of the so-called string operation for the relief of esophageal stricture is credited to his genius.

ab″bo·cil′lin. A trade-mark for certain preparations containing penicillin G.

Abbott, Edville Gerhardt [*American orthopedist,* 1871–1938]. In *Abbott's method* for the treatment of scoliosis, a series of plaster jackets and bandages is applied to achieve gradual overcorrection.

Abbott, William Osler [*American physician,* 1902–43]. Known for his development of two tubes: one, evolved in cooperation with Rawson, is a double-barreled gastroenterostomy tube; the other, on which he worked with T. Grier Miller, is an intestinal drainage tube called the *Miller-Abbott tube.*

Abbott's staining method. See under *stain.*

Abbotts, William [*English physician,* 1831–ca. 1900]. Originator of a paste made of arsenic trioxide, morphine, and creosote, used to devitalize the nerve of a tooth.

abbo-vac. A trade-mark for a blood-collecting unit, the container of which is evacuated.

abbr., abbrev. Abbreviation.

Abderhalden, Emil [*Swiss pathologist and physiological chemist in Germany,* 1877–1946]. Investigator of amino acids and proteins. Contributed to our knowledge of intracellular metabolism. See also Abderhalden's *test.*

ab·do′men, ab′do·men [L., belly]. The large, inferior cavity of the trunk, extending from the brim of the pelvis to the diaphragm. It is bounded in front and at the sides by the lower ribs and abdominal muscles, and behind by the vertebral column, the psoas, and the quadratus lumborum muscles. It is artificially divided into nine regions by two lines, the upper parallel with the cartilages of the ninth ribs, the lower with the iliac crests, and by two lines drawn vertically upward from the center of the inguinal ligament. These lines are situated differently by different writers. The regions thus formed are: above, the right hypochondriac, the epigastric, and the left hypochondriac; in the middle, the right lumbar, the umbilical, and the left lumbar; and below, the right inguinal, the hypogastric, and the left inguinal. See Plates 8, 14. —**abdom′inal,** *adj.*

a. obstipum. An abdominal deformity resulting from congenitally short recti muscles.

accordion a. A swelling of the abdomen attended with flattening of the arch of the diaphragm and increased respiration. It is not due to the presence of gas or to tumor, and disappears under anesthesia; nervous pseudotympany.

acute a. An acute pathologic condition within the belly, requiring prompt surgical intervention.

carinate a. A keel-shaped belly, prominent in the middle and receding at the sides, with a sharply convex contour.

navicular a. Boat-shaped abdomen. See scaphoid *a.*

pendulous a. A relaxed condition of the abdominal wall in which the anterior abdominal wall hangs down over the pubis.

scaphoid a. A belly characterized by sunken walls, presenting a concavity; seen in starvation and acute meningitis. Also called *navicular a.*

ab·dom′i·no- [*abdomen*]. A combining form signifying *relating to the abdomen.*

ab·dom″i·no·an·te′ri·or [*abdomen;* L. *anterior*, foremost]. *In obstetrics,* designating a fetal position in which the belly is forward.

ab·dom″i·no·cen·te′sis [*abdomen;* G. *kentēsis*, a pricking]. Paracentesis of the abdominal cavity.

ab·dom″i·no·hys″ter·ec′to·my. See *hysterectomy.*

ab·dom″i·no·hys″ter·ot′o·my [*abdomen;* G. *hystera*, womb; *tomē*, a cutting]. Hysterotomy through an abdominal incision.

ab·dom″i·no·per″i·ne′al [*abdomen;* G. *perineos*, space between the anus and the scrotum]. Relating to the abdominal and perineal regions.

ab·dom″i·no·pos·te′ri·or [*abdomen;* L. *posterior*, posterior]. *In obstetrics,* designating a fetal position in which the belly is toward the mother's back.

ab·dom″i·nos′co·py [*abdomen;* G. *skopein*, to examine]. Diagnostic examination of the abdomen externally by the generally practiced physical methods, and internally by endoscopic methods.

ab·dom′i·nous [*abdomen*]. Having a large abdomen.

ab·dom″i·no·u″ter·ot′o·my. See *abdominohysterotomy.*

ab·dom″i·no·ves′i·cal [*abdomen;* L. *vesica*, bladder]. Relating to the abdomen and the urinary bladder.

ab·du′cens (ab·dew′senz) [L. *abducere*, to lead away]. The sixth cranial nerve, whose fibers arise from the nucleus in the dorsal portion of the pons near the internal genu of the facial nerve and run a long course to supply the external rectus muscle which rotates the eyeball outward.

ab·du′cent [*abducere*]. Abducting.

ab·duct′ [L. *abductum*, from *abducere*]. To draw away from the median line.

ab·duc′tion [L. *abductio*, from *abducere*]. Withdrawal of a part from the axis of the body or of an extremity. *In ophthalmology,* turning of the eyes outward from the central position by the external rectus muscles. In refraction, the turning of the eyes outward beyond parallelism under the artificial stimulus of base in prisms and expressed in terms of prism diopters, the measurement being the strongest prism power with which the eyes can maintain single vision at infinity.

total a. The expression in prism diopters of the capacity for turning the eyes outward from the extreme point of inward or positive convergence to the extreme point of outward or negative convergence beyond parallelism. It is measured from convergence near point. A test of, and an exercise stimulus for, relaxation of the internal recti and convergence.

ab·duc′tor [*abducere*]. A muscle which, on contraction, draws a part away from the axis of the body or of an extremity. See Table of Muscles in the Appendix.

a. accessorius digiti quinti. A rare variant of the opponens digiti quinti (pedis) inserted into the base of the proximal phalanx of the little toe.

a. caudae. A muscle found in tailed animals, corresponding to the coccygeus muscle in man.

a. digiti minimi. The BR term for *abductor digiti quinti.*

a. digiti quinti. That of the little finger or toe.

a. hallucis. That of the great toe.

a. hallucis longus. A rare muscle of the anterior region of the leg inserted into the base of the first metatarsal.

a. indicis. The first dorsal interosseous muscle of the hand: variant term.

a. ossis metatarsi quinti. A variant slip of the *abductor digiti quinti* (pedis) muscle inserted into the tuberosity of the fifth metatarsal.

a. pollicis. One of the two abductor muscles of the thumb known as *abductor pollicis brevis* and *abductor pollicis longus.*

Abel, John Jacob [*American pharmacologist,* 1857–1938]. Studied and named epinephrine. With Rowntree, discovered that phenolsulfonphthalein is excreted by the kidney (1909).

ab″em″bry·on′ic [L. *ab*, from; G. *embryon*, embryo]. Away from or opposite the embryo.

ab″en·ter′ic [*ab;* G. *enteron*, intestine]. Affecting or involving organs and structures outside the intestine, said of pathologic conditions which are usually intestinal, as abenteric typhoid.

Abercrombie, John [*Scottish physician,* 1780–1844]. His name is associated with amyloid degeneration, called *Abercrombie's degeneration.*

Abernethy, John [*English surgeon,* 1764–1831]. The first to ligate the external iliac artery for aneurysm (1796); the operation bore his name for many years.

ab·er′rant [L. *aberrare*, to wander from]. Varying or deviating from the normal in form, structure, or course; especially anatomic organs, as aberrant ducts of the testis.

ab″er·ra′tion [L. *aberratio*, from *aberrare*]. 1. A wandering from the correct, the normal, the standard. 2. Slight mental disorder. 3. *In biology,* an abnormal part or individual; a sport. 4. *In optics,* any imperfection in the refraction or the focalization of a lens. —**aber′rant,** *adj.*

chromatic a. Unequal refraction of different parts of the spectrum producing indistinct images surrounded by a halo of colors.

chromosomal aberrations. Changes in the structure of chromosomes following their breakage and rearrangement.

dioptric a. See spherical *a.*

distantial a. Indistinct vision due to distance.

lateral a. Deviation of a ray in any direction from the axis, measured in the focal plane perpendicularly to the axis.

longitudinal a. Deviation of a ray from the focus, measured along the axis above or below the focal plane.

mental a. A deviation from normal mental function.

Newtonian a. See chromatic *a.*

spherical a. Unequal refraction of monochromatic light in different parts of a spherical lens, producing faulty images which show lack of sharpness or of flatness, or distortion. Also called *monochromatic a.*

ab″er·rom′e·ter [*aberrare;* G. *metron*, a measure]. An instrument for measuring aberration.

a·bey′ance (a·bay′uns) [OF. *abeance*, expectation, from *a*, to; *baer*, to gape]. 1. A cessation of activity or function. 2. A state of suspended animation.

ab′i·ent [L. *abire*, to go away]. Tending away from the source of a stimulus, as opposed to *adient.*

A′bi·es (ay′bee·eez, ab′ee·eez) [L., the silver fir]. A genus of evergreen trees belonging to the family Pinaceae; fir.

A. alba (A. pectinata). European silver fir. Yields Strasbourg turpentine.

A. balsamea. Balsam fir. Yields the oleoresin, fir balsam or Canada balsam, consisting chiefly of *l*-pinene, resin, and a bitter principle. It is used as a microscopical mounting medium.

ab″i·et′ic [*abies*]. Pertaining to the genus *Abies*, as abietic acid, which is present in the resin of *Abies* and other coniferous plants.

ab″i·et′ic ac′id, ab″i·e·tin′ic ac′id. $C_{19}H_{29}COOH$. An acid from the resin of various species of pine. The anhydride of the acid, or an isomeric form or modification of the anhydride, appears to be the chief constituent of rosin.

a·bi′o- [G. *abios*, from *a*-, not; *bios*, life]. A combining form meaning *without life*.

a·bi″o·gen′e·sis (a·buy″o·jen′i·sis), **a″bi·og′e·ny** (a·buy·odj′i·nee) [*abios;* G. *genesis*, production]. Theory of the production of living from nonliving matter; spontaneous generation. —**abiogenet′ic, abiog′enous,** *adj.;* **abiog′enist,** *n.*

a·bi″o·log′ic (a·buy″o·lodj′ick), **a·bi″o·log′i·cal** [*abios;* G. *logos*, word] Not pertaining to biology. —**abiol′ogy,** *n.*

a″bi·on′er·gy. See *abiotrophy.*

a″bi·o′sis [*abios;* G. *-ōsis*, condition]. 1. Absence of life. 2. Nonviability. —**abiot′ic,** *adj.*

a″bi·ot′ro·phy [*abios;* G. *trophē*, nourishment]. A genetically determined defect of the germinal layers, which may remain latent or which may become apparent and give rise to disordered functioning, as in Huntington's chorea: a controversial term. Also called *abionergy.* —**abiotroph′ic,** *adj.*

ab·ir′ri·tant [L. *ab*, from; *irritare*, to irritate]. 1. Tending to diminish irritation; soothing. 2. Relating to diminished sensitiveness. —**abirritative,** *adj.;* **abirritate,** *v.t.*

ab·ir′ri·tant. A remedy or agent that allays irritation.

ab·ir″ri·ta′tion [*ab; irritare*]. Diminished tissue irritability; atony or asthenia.

ab″lac·ta′tion [L. *ablactare*, from *ab; lactare*, to give suck]. 1. The weaning of an infant. 2. The end of the period of mammary secretion.

a·blast′in [G. *a*-, not; *blastos*, shoot, offspring]. An antibodylike substance, appearing in the blood of rats infected with trypanosomes, which inhibits reproduction of this organism.

ab·la′ti·o (ab·lay′shee·o) [L., a taking away]. Detachment; removal; ablation.

a. placentae. Premature separation of the placenta. Also called *abruptio placentae.*

a. retinae. Detachment of a nonpathologic retina.

ab·la′tion [*ablatio*]. Removal of a part, as a tumor, by amputation, excision, etc. —**ablate′,** *v.t.*

ab″le·pha′ri·a. See *ablephary.*

a·bleph′a·ron. See *ablephary.*

a·bleph′a·ry [G. *ablepharos*, from *a*-, not; *blepharon*, eyelid]. A congenital defect marked by partial or total absence of the eyelids or palpebral fissure. —**ablepharous,** *adj.;* **ablepharus,** *n.*

a·blep′si·a, a·blep′sy [G., blindness, from *a-; blepein*, to see]. Loss or absence of vision.

ab′lu·ent [L. *abluere*, to wash away]. Detergent; cleansing.

ab′lu·ent. A cleansing or washing agent, as a soap.

ab·lu′tion [*abluere*]. The act of washing or cleansing the body. Syn., *lavation.*

ab·mor′tal [L. *ab*, from; *mortalis*, subject to death]. Flowing away from the dead or dying toward the living tissue; applied to electric currents generated in an injured organ, as a muscle.

ab·nerv′al [*ab;* L. *nervus*, nerve]. Away from a nerve; denoting the direction of an electric current passing through muscle fibers away from the point of entrance of the nerve, as opposed to *adnerval.*

ab·neu′ral [*ab;* G. *neuron*, nerve]. 1. Remote from the spinal or dorsal aspect; ventral. 2. Abnerval.

ab·nor′mal [*ab;* L. *normalis*, from *norma*, a rule]. 1. Not normal. 2. Deviating in form, structure, or position; not conforming with the natural or general rule —**abnormity, abnormal′ity, abnormalism,** *n.*

ab″o·ma·si′tis [*ab;* L. *omasum*, paunch; G. *-itis*, inflammation]. Inflammation of the abomasum.

ab″o·ma′sum, ab″o·ma′sus [*ab; omasum*]. The true digestive stomach of ruminants. Also called *fourth stomach, read.*

ab·o′rad [*ab;* L. *os*, mouth]. Tending aborally; situated or directed away from the mouth.

ab·o′ral [*ab; os*]. Opposite to, or remote from, the mouth.

a·bort′ [L. *abortus*, from *ab; ortus*, from *oriri*, to be born]. 1. Miscarry; bring forth a nonviable fetus. 2. Prevent complete flare-up of a disease; nip a disease in the bud. 3. Check or fall short of maximal growth and development. —**a·bort′,** *n.*

a·bor′ti·cide [*abortus;* L. *caedere*, to kill]. 1. Killing of an unborn fetus. 2. The agent which destroys the fetus and produces abortion.

a·bor′tient. Causing abortion; abortifacient.

a·bor″ti·fa′cient (a·bor″ti·fay′shunt), **a·bor′tient** (a·bor′shunt) [*abortus;* L. *facere*, to make]. Drug or agent inducing expulsion of the fetus. —**a·bor″ti·fa′cient,** *adj.*

a·bor′tin [*abortus*]. A glycerin preparation of *Brucella abortus*, made like tuberculin; has been used for the diagnosis of brucellosis, but is of questionable usefulness in this respect.

a·bor′tion [L. *abortio*, from *abortus*]. 1. Expulsion of the product of conception before the child is viable. When this occurs during the first three months, it is termed *abortion;* from this time to viability, *immature delivery* or *miscarriage;* and from the period of viability to full term, *premature delivery.* 2. A prematurely expelled fetus. —**abortionist,** *n.*

accidental a. An unexpected premature termination of pregnancy.

artificial a. Intentional premature termination of pregnancy by medicinal or mechanical means.

complete a. One in which all the products of conception are shed or expelled.

criminal a. Interference with the progress of pregnancy which is not justified by the state of the mother's health; an illegal abortion.

habitual a. Accidental abortion recurring in successive pregnancies.

incomplete a. Partial expulsion of the product of conception, with some of the secundines remaining within the uterus.

induced a. See artificial *a.*

inevitable a. One which has advanced to a stage where termination of the pregnancy no longer can be prevented.

infectious a. An infectious disease in animals which causes premature termination of gestation. The specific organisms are *Brucella abortus* for cattle, *Salmonella abortus equi* for horses, and *Salmonella abortus ovis* for sheep.

justifiable a. See therapeutic *a.*

missed a. A condition in which the fetus has died but the products of conception are not expelled within two weeks.

partial a. Premature expulsion of one fetus in the presence of multiple gestation.

psychiatric a. A therapeutic abortion dictated by

the aggravation or inception of mental disease during pregnancy.

septic a. An abortion resulting in infection of the endometrium.

spontaneous a. Unexpected premature expulsion of the product of conception when no ecbolic agent has been employed.

therapeutic a. Termination of a pregnancy which is a hazard to the life of the mother.

threatened a. Occurrence of signs and symptoms of impending loss of the embryo. It may be prevented by treatment or may go on to inevitable abortion.

tubal a. Escape of the product of conception through the abdominal opening of the oviduct into the peritoneal cavity.

a·bor′tive [L. *abortivus*, from *abortus*]. 1. Prematurely born; undeveloped; immature; rudimentary. 2. Coming to an untimely end. 3. Checking the full development of a disease or cutting short its duration. Syn., *abortifacient, abortient.*

a·bor′tus [L.]. Aborted fetus; abortion.

a·bou′li·a (a·bōō′lee·uh). See *abulia.*

a·bou″lo·ma′ni·a (a·bōō″lo·may′nee·uh). See *abulomania.*

a·bra′chi·a (a·bray′kee·uh). Armlessness.

a·bra″chi·o·ceph′a·lus (a·bray″kee·o·sef′uh·lus) [G. *a-*, not; L. *brachium*, arm; G. *kephalē*, head]. Headless and armless monster. —**abrachiocepha′lia,** *n.*

a·bra′chi·us (a·bray′kee·us) [*a-; brachium*]. An armless monster.

ab·ra′dant. See *abrasive.*

Abrami, Pierre [*French physician,* 1879–1945]. Known for his description, with Widal, of acquired hemolytic jaundice (1907).

ab·ra′sion [L. *abrasum*, from *abradere*, to rub off]. 1. A spot denuded of skin, mucous membrane, or superficial epithelium by rubbing or scraping, as a corneal abrasion; an excoriation or attrition. 2. *In dentistry,* the mechanical wearing down of the teeth, as from chewing or by instruments (dental abrasion). —**abrade′,** *v.*

ab·ra′sive [*abradere*]. Agent which scrapes or rubs off the external layers of a part. —**ab·ra′sive,** *adj.*

ab·ra′sor (a·bray′zor) [L. *abrasum*, from *abradere*]. A surgeon's rasp or xyster; any file or instrument used in the surgical or dental abrasion of a surface; a rasp used in pharmacy.

a·bras′tol. See *asaprol.*

ab″re·ac′tion [L. *ab*, away; *re-*, again; *actus*, from *agere*, to do]. *In psychoanalysis,* the mental process by which repressed emotionally charged material is freed, and forgotten memories are brought to consciousness and relived with appropriate emotional release after insight is obtained; catharsis. It also occurs in hypnosis and narcoanalysis.

motor a. Motor or muscular expression of an unconscious impulse.

Abrikosov, Aleksei Ivanovich [*Russian pathologist,* 1875–]. Described granular-cell myoblastoma, called *Abrikosov's tumor.* Also spelled *Abrikossoff.*

a′brin [G. *habros*, graceful]. A phytotoxin obtained from *Abrus praecatorius.* It has been employed in treating corneal opacities and trachomatous pannus.

L-a′brine. $C_{12}H_{14}N_2O_2$; N-methyltryptophan, an amino acid derivative extracted from *Abrus praecatorius:* not to be confused with *abrin.*

a·bro′si·a (a·bro′zhuh, ·zee·uh) [G. *abrōsia*, fasting, from *a-*, not; *brōsis*, eating]. Abstinence from food; fasting.

ab·rup′ti·o (ab·rup′tee·o) [L., from *ab*, from; *ruptio*, breaking]. Abruption; a tearing away.

a. placentae. Premature separation of the placenta. Also called *ablatio placentae.*

A′brus [G. *habros*, graceful]. A genus of tropical vines; rosary-pea. The seeds of **A. praecatorius,** jequirity, are the source of the phytotoxin abrin.

ab′scess, ab·sces′sus [L. *abscessus*, a going away, departure]. Localized collection of pus in any part of the body. According to location, abscesses are named *dorsal, mammary, rectal,* etc. See also *microabscess.*

acute a. One resulting from an acute inflammation of the part in which it is formed.

alveolar a. One associated with the alveolar process and usually originating at the apex of a tooth as a *periapical abscess,* or along a lateral surface of the root of a tooth as a *lateral alveolar abscess.* The former is usually the result of pulpal disease, the latter of periodontal disease.

amebic a. A variety found in the liver and lung, containing amebas. It is a complication or sequel of amebic dysentery.

anorectal a. An abscess of the perirectal adipose tissue near the anus: also called *ischiorectal a., perirectal a.*

apical a. One occurring at the end of the root of a tooth.

appendiceal a. Pus formation about the vermiform process, secondary to acute suppurative inflammation of the appendix.

arthrifluent a. A wandering abscess having its origin in a diseased joint.

atheromatous a. A focus of softening, the result of degeneration and necrosis, in the wall of a vessel, the seat of simple intimal arteriosclerosis. Not a true abscess. Also called *atherocheumata.*

Bezold's a. See Friedrich *Bezold.*

blind a. One which does not point on a surface, as a dental granuloma.

Brodie's a. A localized infection of the bone occurring in chronic osteomyelitis. Most often seen in the tibia of young adults.

canalicular a. A mammary abscess that communicates with a milk duct.

caseous a. One in which the pus has a cheesy appearance, usually tuberculous.

cheesy a. See caseous *a.*

chronic a. One of slow development, generally about a bone or joint, or in a lymph node; usually tuberculous and containing cheesy material.

circumtonsillar a. Quinsy. Syn., *peritonsillar a.*

cold a. A slow-growing abscess attended by little or no inflammation. A tuberculous abscess. See chronic *a.*

Darier's a. See Pautrier's *microabscess.*

embolic a. One formed at the seat of a septic embolus.

epidural a. A localized suppuration and granulation outside the dura mater but within the cranium or spinal canal: also called *extradural a., pachymeningitis externa.*

fecal a. One containing feces and communicating with the lumen of the large intestine.

fixation a. One produced by the subcutaneous injection of a chemical irritant.

follicular a. One arising in a lymph nodule.

gravitation a. One in which pus formed in one part of the body tends to migrate, usually to portions deeper or lower down, in the direction gravity would take it.

helminthic a. One initiated by a worm, such as filaria.

hematic a. One due to an extravasated blood clot.

hemorrhagic a. One containing blood.

hypostatic a. See wandering *a.*
idiopathic a. One not attributable to any disease.
iliac a. A wandering abscess of the iliac region.
ischiorectal a. See anorectal *a.*
lacunar a. One involving a lacuna, usually of the urethra.
lumbar a. A wandering abscess of the lumbar region.
lymphatic a. The suppuration of a lymph node.
mammary a. One involving the essential breast tissue.
marginal a. One situated near the margin of an orifice, specifically, near the anal orifice.
metastatic a. One secondary to pyemia and acute or subacute bacterial endocarditis, but not occurring through septicemia. It is usually of embolic origin and generally located in the lungs or liver.
miliary a. A minute embolic abscess.
milk a. A mammary abscess occurring during lactation.
myocardial a. An abscess in the muscle of the heart.
ossifluent a. One arising from diseased bone.
otic cerebral a. An abscess of the brain following purulent disease of the inner ear.
palmar a. One in the palm of the hand, usually beneath the palmar fascia.
parametritic a. One occurring frequently between the folds of the broad ligaments of the uterus or in the neighboring cellular tissue.
paranephric a. See perinephric *a.*
pelvic a. One involving structures within the pelvis.
perianal a. One adjacent to the walls of the anal canal.
periapical a. An abscess originating at the apex of a tooth; a type of alveolar *abscess.*
pericemental a. One on the lateral surface of a tooth, unrelated to apical or gingival abscess.
perimetritic a. Pus within the peritoneum originating from inflammation of the peritoneal covering of the uterus.
perinephric a. One originating in the region immediately surrounding the kidney.
periodontal a. A lateral alveolar *abscess.*
periproctitic a. One involving the loose areolar tissue surrounding the lower rectum.
perirectal a. See anorectal *a.*
peritonsillar a. One forming in acute tonsillitis around one or both tonsils; quinsy: also called *retrotonsillar a.*
perityphlitic a. One involving the tissues surrounding the cecum and appendix.
phlegmonous a. An acute abscess in connective tissue, especially the subcutaneous.
pilonidal a. One in the sacrococcygeal area within, or resulting from, a pilonidal cyst or sinus.
postfascial a. See subfascial *a.*
postmammary a. See submammary *a.*
prelacrimal a. One from caries of a lacrimal or ethmoid bone, producing a swelling at the inner canthus just below the upper margin of the orbit.
primary a. One originating at the seat of a pyogenic infection.
psoas a. A cold abscess arising from diseased lumbar or lower thoracic vertebrae, the pus gravitating through the sheath of the psoas and pointing finally in the femoral triangle.
pyemic a. One occurring as a complication of pyemia.
residual a. One forming in or about the residue of a former infection.
retromammary a. See submammary *a.*
retrotonsillar a. See peritonsillar *a.*
retrovesical a. One situated behind the urinary bladder in the male or between the urinary bladder and the uterus in the female.
scrofulous a. A chronic abscess from infected bone or lymph nodes. *Obs.*
secondary a. An embolic abscess.
septicemic a. One resulting from septic infection or accompanying septicemia.
shirtstud a. One near the surface, communicating by means of a sinus with a deeper abscess.
spermatic a. One involving the seminiferous tubules.
spirillar a. One containing spirilla from the saliva.
stitch a. One formed about a stitch or suture.
subareolar a. One beneath the pigmented epithelium of the nipple, sometimes draining through the nipple.
subdiaphragmatic a. One situated below the diaphragm and above the dome of the liver.
subfascial a. One beneath a fascia; a postfascial abscess.
submammary a. One lying between the mammary gland and the chest wall. Syn., *postmammary a., retromammary a.*
subpectoral a. One beneath the chest muscles.
subperitoneal a. One arising between the parietal peritoneum and the abdominal wall. Also called *preperitoneal a.*
subphrenic a. One located beneath the diaphragm.
suburethral a. One located beneath the urethra; in the female it may protrude from the introitus as a bulge in the anterior vaginal wall.
sudoriparous a. One due to inflammation of obstructed sweat glands.
supralevator a. One located between the levator muscles and the reflection of the peritoneum.
sympathetic a. A secondary or metastatic abscess at a distance from the part in which the exciting cause has acted, as a bubo.
thecal a. One in the sheath of a tendon.
Tornwaldt's a. One located in the pharyngeal tonsil or surrounding structures and caused by an infection of the pharyngeal bursa. See also Gustav Ludwig *Tornwaldt.*
tropical a. Amebic abscess (usually of the liver) found in conjunction with amebic dysentery.
tuberculous a. See chronic *a.*
tympanitic a. One containing gas. Also called *abscessus flatuosus, gas a.*
urinary a. One resulting from extravasation of urine.
urinous a. One containing urine mingled with the pus.
verminous a. One containing worms from the intestine.
wandering a. One in which the pus has traveled along the connective-tissue planes and points at some locality distant from its origin. Syn., *hypostatic a.* Also called *abscessus per decubitum.*
worm a. See verminous *a.*

ab·scis′sa (ab·siss′uh) [L. *abscissum*, from *abscindere*, to cut off]. 1. The horizontal of the two coordinates used in plotting the interrelationship of two sets of data. The vertical line is called the ordinate. 2. *In optics*, the point where a ray of light crosses the principal axis.

ab·scis′sion (ab·sish′un, ab·sizh′un) [L. *abscissio*, from *abscindere*]. Removal of a part by cutting.

ab·scon′si·o (ab·skon′see·o, ·shee·o) [L. *abscondere*, to hide]. A cavity, depression, or recess—either normal or pathologic; especially one in bone which conceals the head of a contiguous bone. *Obs.*

ab′sence [L. *absentia*, absence]. 1. *In psychiatry*, indifference to one's environment. 2. Temporary loss of consciousness, as in epilepsy, melancholia, and individuals with central lesions. 3. Fleeting loss of consciousness occurring in hysterical attacks or at the climax of a completed or very intense sexual gratification (Freud).

ab″sen·tee′ism [L. *absens*, from *abesse*, to be absent]. The practice of industrial workers of absenting themselves from their jobs for minor illness or injury, or for personal reasons; the time lost from such practices.

abs. feb. *Absente febre;* in the absence of fever.

Ab·sid′i·a. See *Mucor.*

ab′sinthe, ab′sinth [L. *absinthium*, from G. *apsinthion*, wormwood]. A green, French liqueur; an alcoholic solution of absinthium, anise, and marjoram oils, and other aromatics. Its manufacture and use have been prohibited in France since 1915.

ab·sin′thic ac′id. An acid from wormwood oil; it may be identical with succinic acid.

ab·sin′thin. A bitter crystalline glycoside, $C_{20}H_{28}O_4$, obtained from wormwood. See *absinthium.*

ab′sinth·ism [*absinthium*]. A morbid state resulting from the habitual and excessive use of absinthe; characterized by neuritis, hyperesthesia, and hallucinations. Acute or chronic excess may cause convulsions, acute mania, or a general paralysis.

ab·sin′thi·um [L.]. Common wormwood; the leaves and tops of *Artemisia absinthium.* Absinthium contains a volatile oil and an intensely bitter principle, absinthin; it has been used as an aromatic bitter, diaphoretic, anthelmintic, and flavoring agent.

ab·sin′thol. $C_{10}H_{16}O$. Principal constituent of wormwood oil; it is isomeric with ordinary camphor.

ab′so·lute [L. *absolutus*, from *absolvere*, to set free]. 1. Simple; pure; free from admixture. 2. Unlimited and unqualified. 3. Complete; entire; real. 4. *In physics*, derived from basic data, not arbitrary.

ab′so·lute al′co·hol. See under *alcohol.*

ab′so·lute cell in′crease. A rise in the number of leukocytes of a particular type. The absolute number of the cells of a given variety equals the total white-cell count multiplied by the percentage of cells of that variety.

ab·sorb′ [L. *absorbere*, to suck up]. 1. *In physiology*, suck up; take in; imbibe, as fluids or gases, through osmosis and capillarity. 2. Infiltrate into the skin, as ultraviolet rays. 3. Incorporate into the body via the blood and lymph. 4. Stop radiant heat rays.

ab·sor′bance. In applied spectroscopy, the negative logarithm, to the base 10, of transmittance. The term *optical density*, sometimes used to express the absorbance of solutions, is recommended to be abandoned. Symbol, *A.* Sometimes written *absorbence.*

ab·sor″be·fa′cient (ab·sor″bi·fay′shunt) [*absorbere;* L. *facere*, to make]. Any agent which promotes absorption. —**ab·sor″be·fa′cient,** *adj.*

ab·sorb′ent [*absorbere*]. Anything capable of absorbing or sucking up fluids, gases, or light waves. 2. A drug, application, or dressing which promotes absorption of diseased tissues. —**ab·sorb′ent, absorp′tive,** *adj.*

ab·sorp″ti·om′e·ter (ab·sorp″shee·om′i·tur) [*absorbere;* G. *metron*, a measure]. 1. An instrument which determines the solubility of a gas, or the amount absorbed. 2. An apparatus which measures the thickness of a layer of fluid between tow parallel sheets of plate glass in apparent apposition. When used with a spectrophotometer it is a hematoscope.

ab·sorp′tion [L. *absorptio*, from *absorbere*]. 1. *In physiology*, sucking up, taking in, and assimilation of certain gases, fluids, and suitable matter by the skin, mucous membranes, lacteals, lymphatics, and blood vessels. 2. *In physics*, taking up of a specific gas by a given solid. 3. Extinction of white light or any of its component rays by black or colored objects. 4. *In physiological chemistry*, neutralization of an acid. 5. *In psychology*, inattention to all but a single thought or activity. 6. *In radiology*, reduction in intensity of a beam of radiation as it passes through matter: (a) particulate radiation loses energy through collisions with electrons or atomic nuclei, and (b) photons lose energy by transferring it to electrons by scattering or photoelectric processes.

a. band. A region of the absorption spectrum in which the absorptivity passes through a maximum or inflection.

bone a. See *osteoclasis*, 2.

cutaneous a. Absorption through the skin.

disjunctive a. Separation of a slough or necrotic part by the absorption of a thin layer of the healthy tissue immediately adjacent to and surrounding it.

external a. Taking up of foods, medicaments, and other matter by the skin and mucous membranes.

internal a. Normal digestive assimilation of foods, water, etc. Also called *molecular, nutritive,* and *organic a.*

interstitial a. Taking up of metabolites by the absorbent system.

pathologic a. Absorption by the blood of any morbid product or excretion, as pus or bile. Also called *excrementitial a., absorptio morbosa.*

self-a. *In radiobiology*, the absorption of radiation by the material from which the radiation is originating.

ab″sorp·tiv′i·ty. *In applied spectroscopy*, the ratio of the absorbance to the product of concentration and length of optical path; it is the absorbance per unit concentration and thickness. Symbol, *a.*

ab′sti·nence [L. *abstinentia*, from *abstinere*, to keep away]. Voluntary self-denial of or forbearance from indulgence of appetites, especially from food, alcoholic drink, or sex relations.

ab·strac′tion [L. *abstractio*, from *abstrahere*, to draw away]. 1. Removal or separation of one or more ingredients from a compound, as an abstract from a crude drug. 2. Bloodletting. 3. Absorption of the mind; absent-mindedness; inattention to ideas. 4. *In psychology*, isolation of a meaning or characteristic from a totality which is unique and inaccessible to comparison; may be performed by thinking, feeling, sensation, or intuition.

Abt's method. See Farmer and Abt's *method.*

ab·ter′mi·nal [L. *ab*, from; *terminalis*, from *terminus*, end]. From the tendinous end toward the center of the muscle, noting the direction of an electric current in muscle.

a·bu′li·a (ab·yoo′lee·uh, a·boo′·), **a·bou′li·a** (a·boo′lee·uh), **ab″u·le′ia** (ab″yoo·lee′yuh) [G. *a-*, not; *boulē*, will]. Loss or defect of the ability to make decisions, seen in an extreme form in the simple type of schizophrenic reaction. —**abu′lic,** *adj.*

a·bu″lo·ma′ni·a (ab·yoo″lo·may′nee·uh, a·boo″-lo·), **a·bou″lo·ma′ni·a** (a·boo″lo·may′nee·uh) [*a-; boulē;* G. *mania*, madness]. Abulia. *Obs.*

Abū-L-Qāsim. See *Albucasis.*

Abumeron. See *Avenzoar.*

a·buse′ [L. *abusus*, a using up]. 1. Wrong use, misuse, or, particularly, excessive use. 2. Rape.

a·but′ment, a·but′tal [OF. *abouter*, to fix the

limits of]. A tooth used to support or stabilize a prosthetic appliance. —**abut,** *v.i.*

AC Anodal closure.

A. C. Abbreviation for air conduction, anodal closure.

A.C., ac, a.c., a-c Abbreviations for alternating current.

Ac Chemical symbol for actinium; acetyl.

a. c. *Ante cibum;* before meals.

A·ca′cia (a·kay′shuh) [G. *akakia,* acacia tree]. A large genus of woody plants of the Mimosaceae, found in warm regions, many being native to Africa and Australia.

A. senegal. The most important of several African species yielding gum arabic.

a·ca′cia [*akakia*]. The dried gummy exudation from the stems and branches of *Acacia senegal* (Linné) Willdenow, or of some other African species of *Acacia,* occurring in translucent or somewhat opaque, white to yellowish-white spheroidal tears; it is almost completely soluble in water. It consists of calcium, magnesium, and potassium salts of the polysaccharide arabic acid (also known as *arabin*). In the form of acacia mucilage and acacia syrup, it is used as a demulcent; it has also been used, by intravenous injection, in treating shock and edema. The mucilage and syrup are valuable vehicles. Syn., *gum arabic.*

a·cal″ci·co′sis [G. *a-,* not; L. *calx,* lime; G. *-ōsis,* condition]. The condition resulting from a diet continuously low in calcium.

a″cal·cu′li·a, ac″al·cu′li·a [*a-;* L. *calculare,* to compute]. An aphasia marked by the inability to work even the simplest mathematical problems: also called *arithmetic disability.*

a·camp′si·a [*a-;* G. *kamptein,* to bend]. Inflexibility or rigidity of a joint or limb; an ankylosis.

acanth-. See *acantho-.*

a·can″thes·the′si·a, a·can″thaes·the′si·a (a·can″thess·thee′zhuh, ·zee·uh) [G. *akantha,* thorn; *aisthēsis,* sensation]. A sensation as of pricking with needles.

a·can′thi·on [G. *akanthion,* a little thorn]. A craniometric point named and located by von Török at the tip of the anterior nasal spine: also spelled *akanthion.* —**a·can′thi·al,** *adj.*

a·can′tho-, acanth- [G. *akantha,* thorn]. A combining form meaning *thorn, thorny, spine, spiny.*

a·can″tho·a·mel″o·blas·to′ma. An ameloblastoma in which the cells are of the squamous or prickle-cell type. The basal-cell layer resembles the ameloblasts.

A·can″tho·ceph′a·la [*akantha;* G. *kephalē,* head]. The proboscidal roundworms; common parasites of birds and fishes, found less frequently in other vertebrates.

a·can″tho·ceph″a·li′a·sis [*akantha; kephalē;* NL. *-iasis,* condition]. Infestation by *Acanthocephala.*

A·can″tho·chei″lo·ne′ma (·kigh″lo·nee′muh) [*akantha;* G. *cheilos,* lip; *nēma,* thread]. A genus of filarial worms.

A. perstans. A species found extensively in tropical regions, with man the definitive host.

a·can″tho·chei″lo·ne·mi′a·sis (·kigh″lo·ni·migh′-uh·sis) [*akantha; cheilos; nēma;* NL. *-iasis,* condition]. Infestation by the *Acanthocheilonema perstans;* characterized by fever, malaise, edema, and headache.

a·can′thoid [*akantha;* G. *eidos,* form]. Resembling a spine, spinous.

a·can″tho·ker″a·to·der′mi·a [*akantha;* G. *keras,* horn; *derma,* skin]. Thickening of the horny layer of the skin of the hands or feet.

ac″an·thol′y·sis [*akantha;* G. *lysis,* a loosing]. Any skin disease in which there is an atrophy of the prickle-cell layer.

a. bullosa. A congenital or neonatal skin disease with bullae and vesicles. See *epidermolysis bullosa.*

ac″an·tho′ma [*akantha;* G. *-ōma,* tumor]. A highly differentiated form of epidermoid carcinoma, rich in keratinized epithelium and epithelial pearls.

a. adenoides cysticum. See *trichoepithelioma.*

a·can″tho·pel′vis [*akantha;* L. *pelvis,* basin]. A rachitic pelvis having a sharp, prominent pubic crest. Also called *acanthopelyx, pelvis spinosa.*

A·can′tho·phis [*akantha;* G. *ophis,* serpent]. A genus of snakes of the Elapidae.

A. antarcticus. The death adder of Australia and New Guinea which possesses a neurotoxic venom.

ac″an·tho′sis [*akantha;* G. *-ōsis,* condition]. A thickening of the germinative layer of the epidermis seen in many skin diseases and caused by hyperplasia of the cells. —**acanthot′ic,** *adj.*

a. nigricans. A generalized pigmentation of the skin accompanied by papillary and verrucous growths, in about half of the cases with adenocarcinoma of internal organs; in the benign type, onset occurs at birth, early childhood, or puberty.

juvenile a. One characterized by obesity, hypogenitalism, and metabolic disorders. The neck, throat, axillae, epigastrium, pubis, back, interscapular and sacral regions are affected, and the gray-brown lesions are hyperkeratotic, rugose, and are not shed. Also called *papular papillomatosis.*

a·can′thro·cyte [*akantha;* ery*throcyte*]. A genetically malformed erythrocyte characterized in wet preparations by several irregularly spaced, large, coarse, spiculated cytoplasmic projections, giving the cells a thorny or star-shaped appearance, and exhibiting marked increase in mechanical fragility.

a·can″thro·cy·to′sis. An association of the predominating presence in blood of acanthrocytes, the celiac syndrome in early childhood, and diffuse ataxic neuropathy, with or without retinitis pigmentosa: considered to be hereditary on the basis of consanguinity of the parents.

a·can′thu·lus [*akantha*]. An instrument for removing thorns from wounds.

a·cap′ni·a [G. *a-,* not, without; *kapnos,* smoke]. The complete absence of CO_2: commonly used incorrectly for *hypocapnia.* —**a·cap′ni·al,** *adj.*

a·cap′su·lar [*a-;* L. *capsula,* a small box]. *In biology,* without a capsule.

a·car′di·a [G. *akardios,* from *a-, kardia,* heart]. Congenital absence of the heart. —**acardiac,** *adj., n.*

a″car·di′a·cus (ay″car·dye′uh·kus, a″car·) [*a-;* G.; *kardiakos,* belonging to the heart]. Omphalosite completely lacking a heart.

a. acephalus. An omphalosite without a head.

a. amorphus. A shapeless omphalosite with only rudiments of organs. Also called *a. anceps.*

a·car″di·o·he′mi·a, a·car″di·o·hae′mi·a [G. *akardios,* from *a-, kardia,* heart; *haima,* blood]. Lack of blood in the heart.

a·car″di·o·ner′vi·a [*akardios;* L. *nervus,* nerve]. A deficiency or absence of nervous stimulation to the heart.

a·car″di·o·tro′phi·a [*akardios;* G. *trophē,* nourishment]. Atrophy of the heart.

a·car′di·us [*akardios*]. Monster lacking a heart, occurring as a parasitic twin. —**acardiac,** *adj.*

ac″a·ri′a·sis [G. *akari,* mite, from *a-,* not; *keirein,* to cut; NL. *-iasis,* condition]. Infestation with acarids or mites and the resulting diseased condition. Also called *acarinosis.*

a·car′i·cide [*akari;* L. *caedere,* to kill]. Agent that destroys acarids.

ac′a·rid [*akari*]. A tick or mite. —**aca′rian, acar′idan, acarid′ian,** *adj., n.*

Ac″a·ri′na [*akari*]. An order of Arachnida comprising the ticks and mites. Many species are important vectors of bacterial, protozoan, rickettsial, and spirochetal diseases. In addition, severe reactions may result from their bites.

a·car″i·no′sis. See *acariasis.*

a·car″i·o′sis. See *acariasis.*

ac′a·ro- [*akari*]. A combining form denoting *mites* or *itch.*

ac″a·ro·der″ma·ti′tis [*akari;* G. *derma,* skin; *-itis,* inflammation]. Dermatitis caused by acarids.

a. urticarioides. An urticarial and pruritic dermatitis due to infestation by the acarine mite *Pediculoides ventricosus,* whose normal hosts are insect larvae. It is seen in man exposed to grain or straw. Also called *grain itch.*

ac′a·roid [*akari;* G. *eidos,* form]. Mitelike.

ac″a·ro·pho′bi·a [*akari;* G. *phobos,* fear]. Morbid fear of mites or of certain small animate or inanimate things, as worms or pins.

ac″a·ro·tox′ic [*akari;* G. *toxikon,* poison]. Poisonous, or destructive, to acarids.

a·car′pi·a [G. *akarpia,* unfruitfulness]. Sterility, barrenness, unfruitfulness.

a·car′pous [G. *akarpos,* without fruit]. 1. Having no elevations; not nodular. 2. Producing no fruit; sterile, barren.

Ac′a·rus [G. *akari,* mite]. A genus of mites.

A. folliculorum. Synonym for *Demodex folliculorum.*

A. scabiei. Synonym for *Sarcoptes scabiei.*

a·car′y·ote [G. *a-,* not; *karyon,* nucleus]. Nonnucleated. See *akaryote.*

a·cat″a·lep′si·a, a·cat′a·lep″sy [*a-;* G. *katalambanein,* to comprehend]. 1. Mental impairment; dementia. *Obs.* 2. Uncertainty in diagnosis. *Obs.* **—acatalep′tic,** *adj., n.*

a·cat″a·ma·the′si·a (a·cat″uh·muth·ee′zhuh, ·zee·uh) [*a-;* G. *katamathēsis,* thorough knowledge]. 1. An inability to understand conversation. 2. A morbid blunting or deterioration of the senses, as in mental deafness and blindness.

a·cat″a·pha′si·a (·fay′zhuh, ·zee·uh) [*a-;* G. *kataphasis,* affirmation]. Syntactic aphasia; characterized by an inability to construct a sentence properly.

ac″a·tap′o·sis [*a-;* G. *kataposis,* swallowing down]. A difficulty in swallowing; dysphagia.

ac″a·tas·ta′si·a (ack″uh·tas·tay′zhuh, ·zee·uh, ·shuh, ·see·uh) [G., instability, from *a-; katastasis,* a standing firm]. Irregularity; nonconformation to type; variation from the normal. **—acatastat′ic,** *adj.*

ac″a·thex′i·a [*a-;* G. *kathexis,* a holding back]. Failure or inability to retain bodily secretions and excretions. **—acathec′tic,** *adj.*

ac·a·thex′is [*a-; kathexis*]. *In psychiatry,* lack of affect toward some thing or idea which unconsciously is very important to the individual.

ac·a·thi′si·a. See *akathisia.*

a·cau′dal (ay·kaw′dul, a·kaw′dul), **a·cau′date** [*a-;* L. *cauda,* tail]. Tailless.

ACC Anodal closure contraction.

Acc. Accommodation.

ac·cel′er·ans (ack·sel′ur·anz) [L. *accelerare,* to hasten]. Old term for accelerator nerve. See under *nerve.*

ac·cel′er·ant. See *accelerator.*

ac·cel″er·a′tion (ack·sel″uh·ray′shun) [L. *acceleratio,* from *accelerare*]. 1. Quickening, as of the pulse or the respiration. 2. Change of velocity (**linear acceleration**) or of direction of movement (**centrifugal acceleration**); important in aviation medicine. See *blackout; G,* 2.

ac·cel′er·a″tor, ac·cel′er·ant [*accelerare*]. 1. That which hastens. 2. Any agent or part which quickens the speed of a function. 3. A catalyst. **—accel′erate,** *v.*

electrostatic a. Any device making use of electrostatic forces to establish a large potential difference that can be used to accelerate positive or negative charges; condenser-rectifier circuits or a Van de Graaff generator can accomplish this.

particle a. Any device for accelerating atomic or nuclear particles, such as the cyclotron, etc.

ac·cel′er·a″tor u·ri′nae (yoor·eye′nee). Old term for the bulbocavernosus muscle. See Table of Muscles in the Appendix.

ac·cel′er·in. A factor in plasma or serum which accelerates the conversion of prothrombin to thrombin by thromboplastin; it is present as a precursor, *proaccelerin.* Syn., *factor VI, serum accelerator globulin, labile factor.*

ac·cel″er·om′e·ter [*accelerare;* G. *metron,* a measure]. An instrument for measuring acceleration in gravity units.

ac·cen′tu·a″tor (ack·sen′chōō·ay″tur, ack·sent′-yōō·) [L. *accentus,* accentuation]. A chemical substance which intensifies the action of a tissue stain.

ac·cep′tor (ack·sep′tur, ·tor) [L. *accipere,* to accept]. A substance which accepts or combines with a product of a chemical reaction; applied especially to those substances which increase the rate of a reaction by acting as intermediaries in transferring another substance, such as hydrogen, from a reactant to the final product. See *hydrogen* acceptor.

ac″ces·so′ri·us [L. *accessum,* from *accedere,* to be added]. Accessory; supernumerary; assisting.

ac″ces·so′ri·us. Any muscle which contributes to or reinforces the function of another.

a. ad flexorem digitorum profundum. An occasional additional slip of the flexor digitorum profundus muscle, originating from the coronoid process of the ulna and usually associated with the tendons for middle and index fingers.

a. of gluteus minimus. An occasional slip of muscle lying under the gluteus minimus and inserted into the capsule of the hip joint.

a. muscle. (a) Old name for quadratus plantae muscle. (b) Old name for iliocostalis dorsi muscle.

a. pterygoid. An occasional slip of muscle extending from the body of the sphenoid to the lateral pterygoid plate.

accessorone. Trade-mark for a preparation containing vitamins A and D, red bone marrow extract, iron and ammonium citrates, malt and yeast extracts.

ac·ces′so·ry (ack·sess′o·ree) [*accessum*]. Auxiliary, assisting; applied to a lesser organ or part which supplements a similar organ or part.

ac′ci·dent [L. *accidere,* to occur]. 1. *In legal medicine,* an event occurring to an individual without his expectation, and without the possibility of his preventing it at the moment of its occurrence. 2. An intercurrent or complicating symptom or event, not to be looked for in the regular progression of an attack of disease.

cerebral a. A sudden, unexpected event of an injurious nature that occurs within the cerebrum, as cerebral hemorrhage or apoplexy.

cerebrovascular, cerebral vascular a. See *apoplexy,* 1.

serum a. A serious allergic reaction which immediately follows the introduction of a foreign serum into a hypersensitive individual. Dyspnea and flushing occur, soon followed by shock and occasionally by fatal termination.

ac″ci·den′tal·ism [*accidere*]. A system of medicine based on symptoms only, disregarding etiology or pathology.

ac′ci·dent-prone. *In psychosomatic medicine,* of, pertaining to, or describing a person or group of persons who may have a low incidence of somatic illnesses but an unusually high incidence rate of accidents. The accidents are considered to be subconsciously caused by emotional or personality conflicts, and may represent unconscious hostility or desire for punishment.

ac·cip′i·ter (ack·sip′i·tur) [L., hawk]. A facial bandage with tails radiating like the claws of a hawk.

ac·cli″ma·ti·za′tion, ac″cli·ma′tion [F. *acclimater*, from *à*, to; *climat*, climate]. Process of adjusting to a strange or foreign climate, soil, water, etc., applied to plants, animals, and people. —**accli′mate, ac′climate, accli′matize,** *v.t., v.i.*

ac″co·lé′ (ack″o·lay′). A form of the malaria parasite, *Plasmodium falciparum*, in which it appears as a thin strip of cytoplasm adhering to the surface of the erythrocyte.

ac·com″mo·da′tion [L. *accommodare*, to adapt]. Adaptation or adjustment of an organ, part, or organism, especially that of the eye. It includes the changes in the ciliary muscle and the lens in bringing light rays from various distances to focus upon the retina. Abbreviated, a., Acc. —**accom′modative,** *adj.*

absolute a. Accommodation of each eye considered individually.

a. phosphene. Peripheral light-streak seen in the dark after accommodation.

a. reflex. Changes which occur when the vision is focused from a distant to a near object; namely, contraction of the pupil, convergence of the eyes, and increased refraction by the lens.

binocular a. Simultaneous accommodation of the two eyes.

Helmholtz's theory of a. The increased convexity of the lens is produced by a relaxation of the suspensory ligament, thus removing the influence which tends to flatten the lens and permitting the latter, by its elasticity, to become more convex.

histologic a. Microscopic changes in the form, structure, and function of cells and tissues after adapting to new conditions.

negative a. Lessening of the accommodation for distant vision.

obstetric a. Fetal conformation to the cavity of the uterus, particularly during the last third of pregnancy.

positive a. Adjustment required for near vision.

region of a. Span of clear vision through which the eye can focus (that is, from its far point to its near point).

relative a. Extent of accommodation possible for any particular degree of convergence.

spasm of a. Excessive or persistent contraction of the ciliary muscle, following the attempt to overcome error of refraction. It stimulates myopia.

Tscherning's theory of a. By the contraction of the anterior part of both the radiating and circular fibers of the ciliary muscle, the ciliary processes are drawn backward and the suspensory ligament pulled backward and outward; pressure of the anterior portion of the muscle causes increased convexity of the lens.

ac·com′plish·ment quo′tient. See *achievement q.* under *quotient*.

ac·couche′ment (a·kōōsh′mahng, uh·kōōsh′munt. *See* Notes § 35) [F.]. Childbirth; parturition.

a. forcé. Rapid delivery by manual dilation of the cervix followed by version or application of forceps and immediate extraction.

ac″cou·cheur′ (ack″ōō·shur′) [F.]. Obstetrician; a professionally trained person attending women in childbirth.

ac″cou·cheuse′ (ack″ōō·shuz′) [F.]. A female obstetrician; a midwife.

ac″cre·men·ti′tion (ack″ri·men·tish′un) [L. *accrescere*, to grow; *incrementum*, growth]. Increase and growth characterized by the addition of like tissue by: simple fission, cellular division, and budding or gemmation. —**accrementitial,** *adj.*

accretin. Trade-mark for an anterior pituitary growth hormone preparation; administered intramuscularly.

ac·cre′ti·o cor′dis (a·kree′shee·o kor′dis). A serious form of adherent pericarditis with fibrous bands extending from the mediastinal surface of the parietal pericardium to the pleura, diaphragm, and chest wall.

ac·cre′tion [L. *accrescere*, to grow]. 1. Growth characterized by addition to the periphery, as in crystalline and certain organic compounds. 2. Adherence of parts normally separate. 3. A growing together; adhesion. 4. An accumulation of foreign matter, as about a tooth (tartar) or within any cavity. —**accrete′,** *adj., v.i.;* **accretive,** *adj.*

a. lines. Linear markings showing the addition of successive layers of enamel, seen in microscopic sections of a tooth; incremental lines.

ac·cu′mu·la″tor [L., from *ad*, to; *cumulare*, to heap]. 1. A device which stores electricity, as a storage battery or cell. 2. Condenser.

A.C.D. solution. Abbreviation for anticoagulant acid citrate dextrose solution: used to prevent coagulation of blood in preparation of plasma or whole blood for indirect transfusions.

-a′ce·ae (-ay′see·ee) [L., suffix meaning *of the nature of*]. *In botany*, a suffix used in combination with the name of one of the principal genera to form the names of families of plants.

a·ce′li·a. See *acoelia*.

A. C. E. mix′ture. Inhalation anesthetic composed of a mixture of *a*lcohol, *c*hloroform, and *e*ther: now rarely used.

a″ce·naes·the′si·a. See *acenesthesia*.

ac″e·naph′thene (ass″i·naf′theen). 1,8-Ethylenenaphthalene; $C_{12}H_{10}$; a tricyclic solid hydrocarbon occurring in coal tar: used as an insecticide and fungicide, a dye intermediate, and in the manufacture of plastics.

a″ce·nes·the′si·a, a″ce·naes·the′si·a (ay″seh-ness·thee′zhuh, ·zee·uh, a·sen″ess·) [G. *a-*, Not; *koinos*, common; *aisthēsis*, feeling]. Loss of body sense or well-being; absence of visceral sense, said to occur in melancholia and hypochondriasis. See *cenesthesia*.

a·cen′tric (a·sen′trick) [*a-;* G. *kentron*, center]. 1. Not central; peripheral; eccentric. 2. Not arising centrally, as from a nerve center.

ac″e·pha′li·a (ass″i·fay′lee·uh). See *acephaly*.

a·ceph′a·lism. See *acephaly*.

a·ceph″a·lo·bra′chi·a (a·sef″uh·lo·bray′kee·uh) [*a-;* G. *kephalē*, head; L. *brachium*, arm]. Congenital absence of the head and arms.

a·ceph″a·lo·bra′chi·us [*a-; kephalē; brachium*]. A monster exhibiting acephalobrachia.

a·ceph″a·lo·car′di·a [*a-; kephalē;* G. *kardia*, heart]. Congenital absence of the head and heart.

a·ceph″a·lo·car′di·us [*a-; kephalē; kardia*]. A monster with neither head nor heart.

a·ceph″a·lo·chei′rus. See *acephalochirus*.

a·ceph″a·lo·chi′ri·a [*a-; kephalē;* G. *cheir*, hand]. Congenital absence of the head and hands.

a·ceph″a·lo·chi′rus, a·ceph″a·lo·chei′rus (a·sef″uh·lo·kigh′rus) [*a-; kephalē; cheir*]. A monster with neither head nor hands.

a·ceph′a·lo·cyst″ (a·sef′uh·lo·sist″) [*a-; kephalē;* G. *kystis*, bladder]. A sterile hydatid, without scolices or brood capsules, found in the human liver and other organs, representing aberrant development of the larval stage of *Echinococcus granulosus*.

a·ceph″a·lo·cys′tis pla′na. Various concretions found in the tendon sheaths and muscles.

a·ceph″a·lo·gas′ter [*a-; kephalē;* G. *gastēr*, belly]. A parasitic monster with neither head, thorax, nor belly. It consists of a pelvis and legs.

a·ceph″a·lo·gas·te′ri·a [*a-; kephalē; gastēr*]. Congenital absence of the head and the upper part of the abdomen.

a·ceph″a·lo·po′di·a [*a-; kephalē;* G. *pous*, foot]. Congenital absence of head and feet.

a·ceph″a·lo·po′di·us [*a-; kephalē; pous*]. A monster with neither head nor feet.

a·ceph″a·lo·ra′chus. See *acephalorrhachus.*

a·ceph″a·lor·rha′chi·a (a·sef″uh·lo·ray′kee·uh) [*a-; kephalē;* G. *rhachis*, spine]. Congenital absence of head and vertebral column.

a·ceph″a·lor′rha·chus, a·ceph″a·lo·ra′chus (·ray′kus) [*a-; kephalē; rhachis*]. Monster with neither head nor vertebral column. —**acephalorrhachia,** *n.*

a·ceph″a·lo·sto′mi·a [*a-; kephalē;* G. *stoma*, mouth]. A condition marked by congenital absence of a head, with a mouthlike aperture present at the upper part of the neck or chest.

a·ceph″a·los′to·mus [*a-; kephalē; stoma*]. A monster exhibiting acephalostomia.

a·ceph″a·lo·tho·ra′ci·a [*a-; kephalē;* G. *thōrax*, thorax]. Congenital absence of the head and thorax.

a·ceph″a·lo·tho′rax, a·ceph″a·lo·tho′rus [*a-; kephalē; thōrax*]. A monster with neither head nor thorax.

a·ceph′a·lus [G. *akephalos*, from *a-; kephalē*]. Any one of a group of omphalositic monsters characterized by absence of the head. —**acephalous,** *adj.*

a·ceph′a·ly [*a-; kephalē*]. Absence of the head.

ac′er·ate (ass′ur·ayt) [L. *acer*, sharp]. Sharp-pointed, acicular.

Acerbi, Francesco Enrico [*Italian pathologist,* 1785–1827]. Precursor of the modern bacteriologist. He held the belief that the cause of contagious disease is a specific, organized substance capable of reproduction.

a·cer′bi·ty [L. *acerbitas*, sharpness, sourness]. Acidity combined with astringency.

a·cer″bo·pho′bi·a (a·sur″bo·), **a·cer″o·pho′bi·a** (a·serr″o·) [L. *acerbus*, sour; G. *phobos*, fear]. Morbid fear of sourness.

ac′er·dol (ass′ur·dole, ·dol, ·dawl). $Ca(MnO_4)_2.4H_2O$. Calcium permanganate; used to disinfect water.

a·cer′ic [L. *acer*, maple tree]. Pertaining to, or derived from, the maple, as aceric acid.

a·cer″o·pho′bi·a. See *acerbophobia.*

a·cer′vu·line (a·sur′view·line, ·leen) [L. *acervulus*, a little heap]. Agminated or aggregated, as certain mucous glands.

a·cer′vu·lus [L.]. Old term for brain sand.

a·ces′cent (a·sess′int) [L. *acescere*, to turn sour]. Acid or tart; acidulous. —**acescence,** *n.*

a·ces′o·dyne [G. *akesōdynos*, from *akeisthai*, to cure; *odynē*, pain]. A pain-relieving agent; an anodyne. —**acesod′ynous,** *adj.*

a″ces·to′ma [*akeisthai;* G. *-ōma*, tumor]. Granulation tissue which later becomes organized into scar tissue.

acet-. See *aceto-.*

ac″e·tab″u·lec′to·my (ass″i·tab″yoo·leck′to·mee) [L. *acetabulum*, cup-shaped vessel, orig. vessel for vinegar, *acetum;* G. *ektomē*, excision]. Excision of the acetabulum.

ac″e·tab′u·lo·plas″ty [*acetabulum;* G. *plassein*, to form]. Any plastic operation on the acetabulum, especially an operation aimed at restoring or enlarging the acetabular cavity.

ac″e·tab′u·lum [L.]. 1. Cup-shaped depression on the outer aspect of the hipbone for the reception of the head of the femur. 2. The sucking cup of flukes. —**acetabular,** *adj.*

ac′e·tal (ass″i·tal). 1. $C_6H_{14}O_2$; ethidene diethylate; a colorless liquid with an ethereal odor, produced by the reaction of alcohol with acetaldehyde. It is moderately soluble in water, and has been used as a soporific in human and veterinary medicine. 2. Generic name for products of the interaction of aldehydes and alcohol.

ac″et·al′de·hyde (ass″it·al′di·hyde, a·seet″al′di·hyde). $CH_3.CHO$. A clear, colorless liquid with a characteristic pungent odor. It results from the oxidation of ethyl alcohol or reduction of acetic acid; when taken internally, it causes narcosis and other noxious effects. Also called *acetic aldehyde, ethanal.*

ac″et·am′ide (ass″i·tam′ide, ·id, a·seet′uh·mide, ·mid). CH_3CONH_2. A white, crystalline solid produced by distilling ammonium acetate or by heating ethyl acetate with strong aqueous ammonia. It combines with both acids and bases to form unstable compounds.

ac″et·a·mi″no·flu′o·rene (ass″it·uh·mee″no·flōō′o·reen, ass″it·am″i·no·). $C_6H_4CH_2C_6H_3NH.CO.CH_3$. A compound said to produce cancer when administered orally.

p-a·cet″a·mi″no·phe′nol. $OH.C_6H_4.NHCH_3CO$, occurring in crystals and practically insoluble in water: used in medicine as an analgesic and antipyretic. Also called *p-acetylaminophenol, N-acetyl-p-aminophenol, p-hydroxyacetanilid.*

ac″et·an′i·lid (ass″i·tan′i·lid) (*acetanilidum*). $C_6H_5NH.OC.CH_3$. Monoacetylaniline, occurring as colorless, shiny crystals, but more often as white scales or a white, crystalline powder. It is odorless, stable in air, and soluble in boiling water and alcohol; used in neuralgia and rheumatism; an analgesic and antipyretic. Dose, 0.13–0.65 Gm. (2–10 gr.). Prolonged use may lead to toxic symptoms. Syn., *antifebrin.*

ac″e·tan′nin. See *acetyl* tannin, *acetyltannic acid.*

ac″et·ar′sol. The British Pharmacopoeia name for acetarsone.

ac″et·ar′sone (ass″i·tahr′sohn) (*acetarsonum*). $CH_3CO.NH.C_6H_3(OH)AsO(OH)_2$. 3-Acetylamino-4-hydroxyphenylarsonic acid; a white or yellowish powder, slightly soluble in water; used in treatment of amebiasis, also in prophylaxis and treatment in certain cases of syphilis. Dose, 0.25 Gm. (4 gr.) two or three times daily for seven days. Syn., *acetarsol.* See *spirocid, stovarsol.*

ac′e·tate. Any salt of acetic acid.

active a. Acetyl coenzyme A.

a·cet″a·zole·am′ide. Generic name for 2-acetylamino-1,3,4-thiadiazole-5-sulfonamide, a renal carbonic anhydrase inhibitor, supplied under the trade-mark *diamox.*

a·cet′-di·a-mer-sul·fon′a·mides. Generic name for a sulfonamide mixture containing equal weights of sulfacetamide, sulfadiazine, and sulfamerazine, to which there may or may not be added a suitable compatible agent to increase the pH of the urine.

a·ce′tic ac′id (a·see′tick) (*acidum aceticum*). An aqueous solution containing 36–37% CH_3COOH. It is occasionally used, when diluted, as an astringent and styptic.

diluted a. a. (*acidum aceticum dilutum*). An aqueous solution containing 5.7–6.3% (w/v) CH_3COOH. Dose, 2–4 cc. (30–60 minims).

glacial a. a. (*acidum aceticum glaciale*). A colorless liquid containing not less than 99.4% CH_3COOH; formerly used as a caustic for removing warts and corns.

a·ce′tic ac′id am′ide. Acetamide.

a·ce′tic al′de·hyde. Acetaldehyde.

a·ce′tic an·hy′dride. $(CH_3CO)_2O$. The anhydride

of acetic acid; a colorless, mobile liquid having the odor of acetic acid.

a·ce'tic e'ther. Ethyl acetate.

a·ce'tic fer"men·ta'tion. Any process of fermentation resulting in the formation of acetic acid.

acetidine. Trade-mark for a combination of acetylsalicylic acid, acetophenetidin, and caffeine.

a·cet"i·fi·ca'tion [L. *acetum*, vinegar, from *acere*, to be sour; *facere*, to make]. The production of vinegar by acetic fermentation. —**acet'ify,** *v.*

ac"e·tim'e·ter (ass"i·tim'i·tur), **ac"e·tom'e·ter** [*acetum;* G. *metron*, measure]. A device for determining the amount of acetic acid present in vinegar or other solutions. —**acetimet'ric, acetomet'ric,** *adj.;* **acetimetry, acetometry,** *n.*

ac'e·tin (ass'i·tin). An ester formed by glycerin with one, two, or three molecules of acetic acid.

ac'e·to- (ass'i·to-, a·see'to-), **acet-** [*acetum*]. A combining form denoting *connection with*, or *derivation from, acetic acid* or *acetyl.*

ac"e·to·a·ce'tic ac'id (ass"i·to·a·see'tick, a·see"to-a·see'tick). $CH_3CO.CH_2COOH$. A monobasic ketone acid eliminated in the urine. It is believed to be a normal product of fat metabolism and is found especially when fatty acids are incompletely oxidized, as in diabetes. Syn., *diacetic acid; beta-ketohydroxybutyric acid.*

ac"e·to·a·ce'tic es'ter. $CH_3CO.CH_2.COOC_2H_5$. Ethyl acetoacetate; a colorless liquid of characteristic odor; used in the synthesis of many important medicinals. Also called *ethyl diacetate.*

A·ce"to·bac'ter [L., *acetum*, vinegar; *G. baktērion*, little staff]. A genus of aerobic bacteria with high oxidative powers, oxidizing various organic compounds to organic acids and other oxidation products, such as ethyl alcohol to acetic acid. The cells may be ellipsoidal to long and rod-shaped, and may occur singly, in pairs, or in long or short chains. They are widely distributed in nature, especially where alcoholic fermentation is taking place, and are important to man in the production of wine, beer, and vinegar. *Acetobacter aceti* is the principal and typical species.

A. aceti. Aerobic rods with marked oxidative powers causing the rapid oxidation of such substrates as glucose and ethyl alcohol. They oxidize acetic acid to carbon dioxide and water, and are found in vinegar, souring fruits, vegetables, and beverages.

a·cet'o·in. Acetylmethylcarbinol.

ac'e·tol (ass'i·tole, ·tol, ·tawl). See *acetyl* carbinol.

ac"e·tol'y·sis [*acetum;* G. *lysis*, a loosing]. The breakdown of an organic compound by acetic anhydride or acetic acid. An acetyl radical may be attached to one of the breakdown products as part of the reaction.

a·cet'o·mel. See *oxymel.*

ac"e·to·me·naph'thone. Menadiol diacetate or 2-methyl-1,4-naphthohydroquinone diacetate; a white, crystalline powder, almost insoluble in water: used orally for its vitamin-K effect.

ac"e·to·mer·oc'tol (ass"e·to·mer·ock'tawl, a·see"-to·). Generic name assigned to 2-acetoxymercuri-4-(1,1,3,3-tetramethylbutyl)phenol, an organomercurial topical antiseptic supplied in tincture form under the trade-marked name *merbak.*

ac"e·tom'e·ter. See *acetimeter.*

ac"e·to·mor'phine (ass"i·to·). Heroin.

ac"e·to·nae'mi·a. See *acetonemia.*

ac"e·ton·asth'ma (ass"i·ton·az'muh, ·ass'muh) [*acetum;* G. *asthma*, panting]. Dyspnea associated with acetonuria, sometimes called uremic asthma. It is marked by restlessness, headache, nausea, vomiting, and transient blindness.

ac'e·tone (ass'i·tone) (*acetonum*). $CH_3.CO.CH_3$. Dimethylketone, propanone. A colorless, inflammable liquid, miscible with water, alcohol, and ether, and having a sweetish, ethereal odor and a burning taste. Normally it occurs in the blood and urine in minute quantities which may become greatly increased in diabetics.

a. bodies. See *ketone bodies* under *body.*

a. bromoform. Brometone.

a. chloroform. Chlorobutanol.

ac"e·to·ne'mi·a, ac"e·to·nae'mi·a (ass"i·to·nee'-mee·uh) [*acetum;* G. *haima*, blood]. The presence of large amounts of acetone bodies in the blood. —**acetone'mic,** *adj.*

ac"e·to·ni'trile (ass"i·to·nigh'trile, ·tril, a·see"to·). CH_3CN. Methyl cyanide. A colorless liquid, having an agreeable odor, miscible with water and alcohol. Also called *carbamine.*

ac"e·to'num. See *acetone.*

ac"e·to·nu'ri·a (ass"i·to·new'ree·uh) [*acetum;* G. *ouron*, urine]. Abnormal increase in the amount of acetone bodies in the urine, found during fevers, diabetic acidosis, malignancy, and intestinal disorders.

a·cet'o·nyl. $CH_3.CO.CH_2$—. A univalent radical representing acetone less one atom of hydrogen.

acetophen. Trade name of a preparation containing acetylsalicylic acid, acetophenetidin, caffeine, phenobarbital, and hyoscyamus extract; used as an analgesic and sedative.

ac"et·o·phe·net'i·din (ass"i·to·fi·net'i·din, a·see"-to·) (*acetophenetidinum*). $C_2H_5O.C_6H_4.NH.COCH_3$. Paraethoxyacetanilid. Occurs as white crystals or as a fine, white, crystalline powder; 1 Gm. dissolves in 1300 cc. of water and in 15 cc. of alcohol. Used as antipyretic and analgesic. Dose, 0.26–1.0 Gm. (4–15 gr.). Syn., *phenacetin.*

ac"e·to·phe·none' (ass"i·to·fi·nohn', ·fee'nohn, a·see"to·). $CH_3.CO.C_6H_5$. Phenylmethylketone. A liquid coal-tar derivative with the odor of bitter almond, which has been used as an antiseptic and hypnotic: also called *hypnone.*

a·cet'o·sal. See *acetylsalicylic acid.*

ac'e·tous (ass'i·tus, a·see'tus) [*acetum*]. Pertaining to, resembling, forming, or containing, vinegar or acetic acid.

ac"et·ox'ime (ass"et·ock'seem, ·sim). $(CH_3)_2C:NOH$; the crystalline oxime resulting from the interaction of acetone and hydroxylamine.

ac"et·par"a·phe·net'i·dine (ass"it·par"uh·fi·net'-i·deen, ·din). See *acetophenetidin.*

a"cet·ri·zo'ic ac'id. The official generic name for 3-acetylamino-2,4,6-triiodobenzoic acid; $C_9H_6I_3NO_3$, the sodium salt of which, sodium acetrizoate, marketed under the trade-marked name *urokon sodium*, is employed as a contrast medium. Acetrizoic acid occurs as a white powder, slightly soluble in water.

a·ce'tum [L.]. 1. Vinegar; an impure, dilute acetic acid produced by acetous fermentation of fruit juices, as in wine or cider. 2. *In pharmacy*, a solution of the active principles of certain drugs in dilute acetic acid. See *vinegar.* —**acetic,** *adj.*

a. acerrimum. Concentrated acetic acid.

a. Saturni. Lead subacetate solution.

ac'e·tyl (ass'i·til, ·teel, a·see'til). C_2H_3O. The univalent radical CH_3CO—. The aldehyde may be regarded as the hydride, and acetic acid as the hydroxide of acetyl.

a. benzene. See *acetophenone.*

a. carbinol. $CH_3CO.CH_2OH$. Hydroxyacetone. A colorless oil possessing a weak, peculiar odor; boils at 145°–150° C. Also called *pyroracemic alcohol, oxyacetone, methyl ketol, acetol.*

a. coenzyme A. A compound of acetic acid and coenzyme A combined by a thioester linkage. Syn. *active acetate.* Abbreviated *a. Co A.*

a. number. The number of milligrams of potassium hydroxide required to combine with the acetic acid liberated by the saponification of 1 Gm. of acetylated fat.

a. peroxide. $(C_2H_3O)_2O_2$. A heavy, unstable liquid, insoluble in water but soluble in alcohol and ether. It is a powerful oxidizing agent, decomposes in sunlight, and explodes when heated.

a. tannin. A grayish yellow powder, slightly hygroscopic, odorless, and tasteless. It is soluble in alcohol, slightly soluble in hot water and ether, and insoluble in cold water and acts as an astringent. Used internally for treating chronic diarrhea, and externally for chronic pharyngitis. Syn., *acetannin, acetyltannic acid, tannigen.*

ac″e·tyl·a·ce′tic ac′id (ass″e·til·a·see′tik). Acetoacetic acid.

ac″e·tyl·a·mi″no·hy·drox″y·phen″yl·ar·son′ic acid. Acetarsone.

acetylarsan. A proprietary arsenical for treating syphilis, said to contain diethylamine oxyacetylaminophenylarsonate.

a·cet″y·la′tion. See *acetylization.*

ac″e·tyl-be″ta-meth·yl·cho′line. A choline compound characterized by sufficient stability in the body and effectiveness, even when administered orally, to produce increased gastrointestinal tone and motion, and vascular dilation. It is used, in the form of water-soluble salts, for treating tachycardia, peripheral vascular diseases, abdominal distention, etc.

a. bromide. $(CH_3)_3N(Br)CH_2.CH(CH_3).O.COCH_3$. Less hygroscopic than the chloride, this form is preferred for use in tablets. Dose, 0.2–0.6 Gm. (3–10 gr.). See *mecholyl bromide.*

a. chloride. $(CH_3)_3N(Cl)CH_2.CH(CH_3).O.COCH_3$. The preferred form for administration subcutaneously or by iontophoresis. Dose (subcutaneously), 0.01–0.04 Gm. (1/6–2/3 gr.). Syn., *methacholine chloride.* See *mecholyl chloride.*

ac″e·tyl·car′bro·mal. The acetyl derivative of carbromal; a white, crystalline powder slightly soluble in water. Used as a sedative. Dose, 0.25–0.5 Gm. (4–8 gr.). See *abasin.*

ac″e·tyl·cho′line (ass″i·til·ko′leen, ·lin, ·kol′een, ·in, a·see″til·). Acetylethanol-trimethylammonium hydroxide. $(CH_3)_3N(OH)CH_2.CH_2.O.CO.CH_3$. First synthesized by Baeyer in 1867, this base has been identified in certain ergot extracts; it lowers blood pressure, increases peristalsis, and commonly is regarded as the substance released from nerves to activate the muscles (Dale). The compound is liberated from parasympathetic postganglionic and all preganglionic nerve terminals, and at synapses in the central nervous system.

a. bromide. The salt formed by addition of HBr to acetylcholine.

a. chloride. The salt formed by addition of HCl to acetylcholine and the form in which the latter substance is most frequently employed. Occurs as a white, odorless, hygroscopic crystalline powder; very soluble in water and in alcohol. Dose, 0.06–0.2 Gm. (1–3 gr.) subcutaneously or intramuscularly.

a. esterase. See under *esterase.*

a·cet′y·lene. C_2H_2. A colorless gas with a characteristic, unpleasant odor; burns with a luminous, smoky flame. It is produced by the action of water on calcium carbide. Syn., *ethine, ethyne.*

a. dichloride. CHCl:CHCl; an ethereal liquid employed as a solvent for fats and other organic substances. Syn., *sym.-dichloroethylene.*

a. tetrachloride. $CHCl_2.CHCl_2$; an ethereal liquid, nonflammable, employed as a solvent for fats and other organic substances, and in the manufacture of paint and varnish removers, insecticides, etc. Syn., *sym.-tetrachloroethane.*

a·cet′y·lide (a·set′i·lyde, ·lid). A derivative of acetylene formed by replacing its hydrogen atoms by a metal, as cuprous acetylide, C_2Cu_2.

a·cet″y·li·za′tion, a·cet″y·la′tion. Chemical introduction of an acetyl radical ($CH_3.CO$—) into the molecular structure of an organic compound, usually by reaction with acetic acid.

ac″e·tyl·meth″yl·car′bi·nol. $CH_3.CHOH.CO.CH_3$; 3-hydroxy-2-butanone: a product of bacterial fermentation in foodstuffs.

ac″e·tyl·mor′phine (ass″i·til·mor′feen, ·mor′fin, ·mor·feen′, a·see″til·). Monoacetyl morphine. An analgesic said to be four times as effective as morphine sulfate in the control of cutaneous and ischemic pain.

ac″e·tyl·phe″nyl·hy′dra·zine (ass″i·til·fee″nil-high′druh·zeen, ·zin). $C_6H_5(NH)_2.C_2H_3O$. A powerful but dangerous antipyretic, causing destruction of red blood cells. Has been suggested for use in polycythemia.

ac″e·tyl·sal″i·cyl′ic ac′id. $C_6H_4.O(CH_3CO).COOH$. A white, crystalline powder, hydrolyzing in moist air to acetic and salicylic acids; 1 Gm. dissolves in 300 cc. of water and in 5 cc. of alcohol. Used internally as antirheumatic, analgesic, and antipyretic; locally in acute pharyngitis and tonsillitis. Dose, 0.3–1.0 Gm. (5–15 gr.). A common allergen. Syn., *aspirin.*

ac″e·tyl·sal′ol. Phenyl acetylsalicylate.

ac″e·tyl·sul·fon′a·mide (ass″i·til·sul·fon′uh·mide, ·mid, ·fo′nuh·, ·sul″fo·nam′ide, ·id). A sulfonamide in which the hydrogen atom of the NH_2 group, attached directly to the benzene ring, is replaced by an acetyl group; a conjugation which occurs in the liver of man and other species, except the canine. The resulting acetyl compounds are therapeutically ineffective and are sometimes less soluble than the parent sulfonamides. Harmful effects may be produced in the renal tubules and urinary tract by the precipitation of these compounds. This can be prevented if urine is kept alkaline, excepting with acetylsulfapyridine and acetylsulfathiazole.

ac″e·tyl·tan′nic ac′id (ass″i·til·tan′ick, a·see″til·). An acetylated tannic acid; a yellowish or grayish powder, only slightly soluble in water. In the lower intestine it is gradually hydrolyzed with liberation of tannic acid which acts as an astringent. Used in the treatment of diarrheas. Dose, 0.3–1.0 Gm. (5–15 gr.). Syn., *diacetyltannin.* See *tannigen.*

ach″a·la′si·a (ack″uh·lay′zhuh, ·zee·uh) [G. *a*-, not; *chalasis*, relaxation]. Inability to relax, said of a hollow muscular organ.

a. of the cardia. Dilatation of the esophagus, due to spasmodic constriction of the lower portion; cardiospasm.

a. of the esophagus. See *megaesophagus.*

sphincteral a. Failure to relax on the part of one or more sphincter muscles.

Achard, Emile Charles [*French physician*, 1860–1944]. Known with Bensaude for their description of paratyphoid fever and isolation of the *Bacillus paratyphosus B* (1896), now classified as *Salmonella paratyphi B.* Described, with Thiers, a syndrome of diabetes associated with female hirsutism, called *Achard-Thiers syndrome.* Developed, with Castaigne, a methylene blue test known as the *Achard-Castaigne method* for renal permeability. See methylene blue *test.*

ache [AS. *acan*, to ache]. A constant or fixed pain, dull to severe in character. **—ache,** *v.i.*

a·chei′li·a (a·kigh′lee·uh) [G. *a*-, not; *cheilos*, lip]. A condition marked by congenital absence of the lips.

a·chei′lus, a·chi′lus (a·kigh′lus) [*a-; cheilos*]. A monster exhibiting acheilia. —**acheilous,** *adj.*

a·chei′ri·a, a·chi′ri·a (a·kigh′ree·uh) [G. *acheir*, from *a-; cheir*, hand]. 1. Congenital absence of the hands. 2. Loss of sensation in, together with the loss of the sense of possession of, one or both hands—a hysterical symptom. 3. Inability to determine from which side a stimulus is applied. See *dyschiria.* —**acheirous,** *adj.*

a·chei′rus (a·kigh′rus) [*acheir*]. An individual without hands.

a·chieve′ment age. See under *age.*

a·chieve′ment quo′tient. See under *quotient.*

Ach″il·le′a (ack″i·lee′uh) [L., from G. *Achilles*, who is said to have used the plant]. A genus of herbs of the Carduaceae; the milfoil or yarrow. A composite-flowered herb, **A. millefolium,** containing a bitter, aromatic, astringent principle, achillein, and a volatile oil, has been used as stimulant and tonic.

ach″il·le′in (ack″i·lee′in). $C_{20}H_{38}N_2O_{15}$. A glycoside obtained from *Achillea millefolium.* Occurs as a brownish red, amorphous mass with a strongly bitter taste; soluble in water, less soluble in alcohol, insoluble in ether.

A·chil′les [*Greek legendary hero*]. According to Homer's *Iliad*, Achilles was vulnerable only in one heel. His name designates the tendon of the gastrocnemius and soleus muscles (also called *tendo calcaneus* [BNA]) and is applied to certain ailments of the heel. The Achilles jerk or reflex is the ankle clonus reflex. See Achilles tendon *reflex.*

Achillini, Alessandro [*Italian anatomist*, 1463–1512]. Said to have been the first to recognize the function of the first pair of cranial nerves, and to have discovered the fourth cranial nerve and the malleus and incus of the middle ear.

a·chil″lo·bur·si′tis (a·kill″o·bur·sigh′tis) [*Achilles;* LL. *bursa*, bag; G. *-itis*, inflammation]. Inflammation of the Achilles bursa.

a·chil″lo·dyn′i·a (a·kill″o·din′ee·uh) [*Achilles;* G. *odynē*, pain]. Pain in the Achilles tendon or bursa; achillobursitis.

ach″il·lor′rha·phy (ack″il·or′uh·fee) [*Achilles;* G. *rhaphē*, a seam]. Any suturing operation on the Achilles tendon.

ach″il·lot′o·my (ack″i·lot′o·mee), **a·chil″lo·te·not′o·my** (a·kill″o·ti·not′o·mee) [*Achilles;* G. *tomē*, a cutting]. Surgical section of the Achilles tendon.

a·chi′lus. See *acheilus.*

ACH in′dex. An index of nutrition based on measurements of arm girth, chest depth, and hip width.

a·chi′ri·a. See *acheiria.*

a″chlor·hy′dri·a (ay″klor·high′dree·uh, ack″lor·) [G. *a-*, not; *chlōros*, green; *hydrios*, from *hydōr*, water]. The absence of free hydrochloric acid in the stomach, even after the administration of histamine.

a·chlo′rides. Salts which are not chlorides; specifically, salts other than chlorides occurring in the urine.

a″chlor·op′si·a (ay″klor·op′see·uh, ack″lor·), **a·chlo″ro·blep′si·a** [*a-; chlōros;* G. *opsis, blepsis*, vision]. Green blindness.

ach″lu·o·pho′bi·a (ack″lo͞o·o·fo′bee·uh) [G. *achlus*, darkness; *phobos*, fear]. Morbid fear of darkness.

a·cho′li·a (ay·ko′lee·uh, a·ko′·) [G. *a-*, not; *cholē*, bile]. 1. Absence or suppression of biliary secretion. 2. Any condition obstructing the escape of the bile into the small intestine. 3. A mild temperament. —**achol′ic, ach′olous,** *adj.*

pigmentary a. A deficiency of bile marked by clay-colored feces but no jaundice.

ach″o·lu′ri·a (ack″o·lew′ree·uh) [*a-; cholē;* G. *ouron*, urine]. The absence of bile pigments in the urine. —**acholuric,** *adj.*

a·chon″dro·pla′si·a (ay·kon″dro·play′zhuh, ·zee·uh, a·kon″dro·), **a·chon′dro·plas″ty** [*a-;* G. *chondros*, cartilage; *plassein*, to form]. A condition of abnormal osteogenesis resulting in the typical congenital dwarf. The pathologic process begins early in intrauterine life as disordered chondrification and ossification of the ends of the long bones; the membrane bones develop normally. Syn., *chondrodystrophia foetalis.* —**achondroplas′tic,** *adj.*

a′chor (ay′kor, ack′or) [G. *achōr*, dandruff]. 1. A papular or pustular eruption of the hairy parts. 2. An eczematoid eruption affecting the face and scalp of infants with many scales and scabs, as a milk crust. 3. An acuminate pustule. 4. Barber's itch; tinea barbae.

A″chor·da′ta (ay″kor·day′tuh, ack″or·day′tuh) [G. *a-*, not; *chordē*, chord]. Animals without a notochord; invertebrates. —**achor′dal,** *adj.;* **achor′date,** *n., adj.*

ach″o·re′sis (ack″or·ee′sis, ay″kor·) [*a-;* G. *chōrēsis*, from *chōrein*, to make room]. Permanent diminution in the volume of any hollow organ, as the stomach or urinary bladder.

A·cho′ri·on (a·kor′ee·on, ay·kor′ee·on) [G., dim. of *achōr*, dandruff]. A former name for a genus of dermatophytes.

A. gallinae. Old synonym for *Trichophyton megnini.*

A. gypseum. Synonym for *Microsporum gypseum.*

A. quinckeanum. Old synonym for *Trichophyton mentogrophytes.*

A. schoenleini. Old synonym for *Trichophyton schoenleini.*

a·chre″o·cy·the′mi·a (a·kree″o·sigh·thee′mee·uh) [G. *achroia*, absence of color; *kytos*, cell; *haima*, blood]. Paleness of the red blood cells due to a deficiency of hemoglobin; anemia.

a·chro′a·cyte (ay·kro′uh·sight, a·kro′·) [*achroia; kytos*]. A colorless cell, or lymphocyte.

a·chro″a·cy·to′sis (ay·kro″uh·sigh·to′sis, a·kro″·), **a·chro″o·cy·to′sis** [*achroia; kytos;* G. *-ōsis*, increase]. An increase in the number of colorless or lymphocytic cells in the blood; lymphocythemia.

a·chroi″o·cy·the′mi·a (a·kroy″o·sigh·thee′mee·uh) [*achroia; kytos;* G. *haima*, blood]. 1. Achreocythemia. 2. The general condition associated with this anemia.

a·chro′ma·cyte (ay·kro′muh·sight, a·kro′·), **a·chro·mat′o·cyte″** [G. *a-*, not; *chrōma*, color; *kytos*, cell]. A decolorized erythrocyte; a ghost or shadow corpuscle due to loss of hemoglobin. Also called *Ponfick's shadow, Bizzozero's blood platelet, Hayem's corpuscle.*

a″chro·ma′si·a (ay·kro·may′zhuh, ·zee·uh, ·shuh, ·see·uh) [*a-; chrōma*]. 1. Loss or absence of normal skin pigmentation, as in albinism, leukoderma, vitiligo. 2. Pallor of cachexia. 3. Failure of cells or tissues to stain normally.

achromat-. See *achromato-.*

a′chro·mate (ay′kro·mate) [*a-; chrōma*]. A totally colorblind person.

a″chro·mat′ic (ay″kro·mat′ick) [*a-; chrōma*]. 1. Without color. 2. Containing achromatin. 3. Not decomposing light into its constituent colors. 4. Staining with difficulty, said of cells or tissues.

a·chro′ma·tin (ay·kro′muh·tin, a·kro′·) [*a-; chrōma*]. The faintly staining substance of the cell nucleus exclusive of the hyaloplasm; essentially, the linin network which supports the chromatin granules. —**achromatin′ic,** *adj.*

a·chro′ma·tism [*a-; chrōma*]. 1. Absence of chromatic aberration. 2. Absence of color.

a·chro′ma·to- (ay·kro′muh·to-, a·kro′muh·to-),

achromat- [*a-; chrōma*]. A combining form denoting *achromatic, colorless.*

a·chro″ma·tol′y·sis [*a-; chrōma;* G. *lysis*, solution]. Dissolution of the achromatin of a cell; plasmolysis.

a·chro′ma·to·phil″ [*a-; chrōma;* G. *philein*, to love]. A microorganism or histologic element which does not stain readily. —**achromatophil, achromatophil′ic,** *adj.;* **achromatophil′ia,** *n.*

a·chro″ma·top′si·a [*a-; chrōma;* G. *opsis*, vision]. Total colorblindness.

a·chro″ma·to′sis [*a-; chrōma;* G. *-ōsis*, condition]. Any condition characterized by a deficiency of natural pigment, as albinism, leukoderma, vitiligo.

a·chro′ma·tous (ay·kro′muh·tus, a·kro′·), **a·chro′mic** [*a-; chrōma*]. Deficient in color; nonpigmented.

a·chro″ma·tu′ri·a [*a-; chrōma;* G. *ouron*, urine]. A very pale or waterlike urine.

a·chro′mi·a (ay·kro′mee·uh, a·kro′·), **a·chro′ma** [*a-; chrōma*]. Absence of color; pallor; achromatosis. —**achromic, achromous,** *adj.*

a. cutis. Leukoderma; vitiligo.

a. parasitica. A type of dermatophytosis (pityriasis versicolor) in which fungi disturb the process of skin pigmentation.

congenital a. Albinism.

a·chro′mic. See *achromatous.*

A·chro″mo·bac·te″ri·a′ce·ae [*a-; chrōma;* G. *baktērion*, dim. of *baktron*, staff]. A family of bacteria of the order Eubacteriales.

a·chro″mo·der′mi·a, a·chro″mo·der′ma [*a-; chrōma;* G. *derma*, skin]. A deficiency or lack of pigment in the skin; leukoderma.

a·chro″mo·trich′i·a (ay·kro″mo·trick′ee·uh, a·kro″·) [*a-; chrōma;* G. *thrix*, hair]. Absence of pigment from the hair.

achromycin. Trade-mark for the crystalline antibiotic substance *tetracycline* prepared by catalytic hydrogenation of chlortetracycline but also obtainable by fermentation. The antibiotic is commonly available as the hydrochloride salt.

a·chron′y·chous. See *acronychous.*

ach″ro·o·am′y·loid (ack″ro·o·am′i·loyd) [G. *achroos*, colorless; *amylon*, starch; *eidos*, form]. Recently deposited amyloid which does not form a blue color with iodine.

a·chro″o·cy·to′sis. See *achroacytosis.*

a″chro·o·dex′trin. A reducing dextrin formed by the action of the diastatic ferment of saliva or of acid upon starch. It is a modification of dextrin and may be precipitated by alcohol; it is not converted into sugar by ptyalin, nor colored by iodine.

Achucárro, Nicolás [*Spanish histologist*, 1881–1918]. Remembered for his method of preparing histologic sections of connective tissue by impregnation with silver tannin. See under *stain.*

a·chyl″a·ne′mi·a, a·chyl″a·nae′mi·a (a·kigh″-luh·nee′mee·uh). See achlorhydric *anemia.*

a·chy′li·a (a·kigh′lee·uh) [*a-; chylos*]. Absence of chyle. —**achylous,** *adj.*

a. gastrica. Absence of gastric secretion of enzymes (rennin, pepsin) and of hydrochloric acid, even after stimulation with histamine: frequently associated with atrophic gastritis.

a. pancreatica. An absence of pancreatic juice resulting in fatty stools, intestinal indigestion, and malnutrition.

ach″y·lo′sis (ack″i·lo′sis). See *achylia.*

a·chy′mi·a (a·kigh′mee·uh) [*a-;* G. *chymos*, juice]. Deficient formation of chyme. Also called *achymosis.* —**achymous,** *adj.*

a·cic′u·lar (a·sick′yoo·lur) [L. *acus*, needle]. Needlelike; shaped like a needle.

ac′id [L. *acidus*, from *acere*, to be sour]. 1. A substance having a sour taste. 2. A substance containing hydrogen replaceable by metals to form salts, and capable of dissociating in aqueous solution to form hydrogen ions (Arrhenius). 3. A substance, ionic or molecular, capable of yielding a proton to another substance (Brönsted and Lowry). This definition has the advantage over Arrhenius' in that it is applicable also to nonaqueous mediums. 4. A substance, ionic or molecular, capable of accepting a share in an electron pair, made available by a base, to form a coordinate covalent bond between the two substances (G. N. Lewis). This definition has the advantage over those of Arrhenius and of Brönsted and Lowry in being applicable also to substances which do not contain a proton (hydrogen ion).

a. stain. See under *stain.*

alcohol a. Any substance containing both an alcohol (—CH_2OH, =CHOH, or ≡COH) group and a carboxyl (—COOH) group.

aldehyde a. Any substance containing both an aldehyde (—CHO) group and a carboxyl (—COOH) group.

aldonic a. Any of a group of monobasic sugar acids, having the general formula CH_2OH-$(CHOH)_nCOOH$, obtained when the aldehyde group of an aldose is oxidized to carboxyl, without oxidizing the primary alcohol group.

aliphatic a. An acid derived from open chain organic compounds.

amino a. See *amino acid.*

aromatic a. Any acid derived from benzene or other carbon ring compound. Many such acids are found in balsams and resins and other odoriferous substances.

carboxylic a. A substance containing the —COOH group.

fatty a. An acid derived from the saturated series of open chain hydrocarbons. See Table of Normal Values of Blood Constituents in the Appendix.

inorganic a. Any acid, except H_2CO_3, which does not contain carbon.

ketone a. Any substance containing both a ketone (=CO) group and a carboxyl (—COOH) group. Also called *keto acid.*

mineral a. An inorganic acid.

organic a. Any acid containing the carboxyl group —COOH.

ac′id al·bu′min. A protein which has been acted upon or dissolved by the stronger acids, and which gives an acid reaction.

ac′id al′co·hol. Alcohol containing various percentages of alcohol. In histological techniques, a common mixture is one-tenth per cent of hydrochloric acid in 95% alcohol.

ac″id·am″in·u′ri·a (ass″id·am″i·new′ree·uh) [*acidus; ammonia; -ine;* G. *ouron*, urine]. Presence of an excess of amino acids in the urine.

ac″i·de′mi·a, ac″i·dae′mi·a (ass″i·dee′mee·uh) [*acidus;* G. *haima*, blood]. A condition of decreased alkalinity of the blood, demonstrated by a lowered pH. See *acidosis.*

ac′id-fast″. Denoting certain bacteria which are not decolorized by mineral acids after staining with aniline dyes, as the bacilli of tuberculosis, leprosy, and smegma.

ac′id-form″ing. 1. Designating nonmetallic elements or oxides which are acidic in water. 2. *In nutrition*, designating those foods which yield an acid ash or residue when metabolized. Syn., *acidogenic.*

ac′id fuch′sin (fo͝ok′sin, fo͝ok′sin) (C.C.). See under *stain.*

a·cid″i·fi·ca′tion [*acidus;* L. *facere*, to make]. Conversion into an acid; process of becoming acid; addition of acid. —**acid′ifiable,** *adj.;* **acid′ify,** *v.*

ac″i·dim′e·ter (ass″i·dim′i·tur), **ac″i·dom′e·ter** [*acidus;* G. *metron,* a measure]. An instrument for determining the degree of acidity of a liquid or the strength of an acid. —**acidimet′ric, acidomet′ric,** *adj.;* **acidimetry, acidometry,** *n.*

ac′id in·tox″i·ca′tion. A toxic condition of the body resulting from an excess of acids accumulated from within or introduced from without.

ac′id·ism [*acidus*]. Acid intoxication.

a·cid′i·ty [*acidus*]. 1. Quality of being acid; sourness; excess of acid. 2. Acid content of any substance.

a. of the stomach. Sourness of the stomach due to oversecretion of acid or to fermentation of food. Associated with heartburn, acid eructations, and epigastric pain and distress.

ac′id num′ber. The number of milligrams of potassium hydroxide required to neutralize the free fatty acids in 1 Gm. of fat, or to neutralize naturally occurring acids in 1 Gm. of other substances, e.g., a resin.

a·cid′o·cyte [*acidus;* G. *kytos,* cell]. An acidophilic leukocyte; an eosinophil.

ac″i·do·cy″to·pe′ni·a (ass″i·do·sigh″to·pee′nee·uh) [*acidus; kytos;* G. *penia,* poverty]. Morbid decrease in the number of circulating eosinophils. Also called *acidopenia.*

ac″i·do·cy·to′sis (ass″i·do·sigh·to′sis) [*acidus; kytos;* G. *-ōsis,* increase]. Morbid increase in the number of circulating eosinophils.

acidogen. COOH.CH_2.CH_2.CH(NH_2).COOH.HCl. Trade-mark for glutamic acid hydrochloride; the preparation liberates hydrochloric acid in the stomach.

ac″i·do·gen′ic (ass″i·do·jen′ick) [*acidus;* G. *genesthai,* from *gignesthai,* to be produced]. Forming acids, especially an acid urine.

acidol. Trade-mark for betaine hydrochloride, ClN(CH_3)$_3$.CH_2.COOH. Administered as a source of hydrochloric acid.

acidolate. A proprietary skin detergent prepared from sulfated vegetable oils, liquid petrolatum, and water.

ac″i·dom′e·ter (ass″i·dom′i·tur). See *acidimeter.*

ac″i·do·pe′ni·a. Acidocytopenia.

a·cid′o·phil″ (a·sid′o·fil″, ass′i·do·fil″) [*acidus;* G. *philein,* to love]. 1. A cell, element, or substance having an affinity for acid stains. 2. One of a group of acid-staining cells found in the anterior pituitary body. 3. The alpha cells found in the adenohypophysis. Syn., *eosinophil, oxyphil.* —**acidophil′ic, acidoph′ilous,** *adj.*

a·cid″o·phil′i·a. See *eosinophilia.*

ac″i·doph′i·lism (ass″i·dof′i·liz·um) [*acidus; philein*]. A condition of overabundance or overactivity of the acidophilic cells of the adenohypophysis.

ac″i·do·re·sist′ant (ass″i·do·ri·ziss′tunt), **ac″id-re·sist′ant** [*acidus;* L. *resistere,* to resist]. Not readily decolorized by acids, applied to certain microorganisms. See *acid-fast.* —**acidoresistance, acid-resistance,** *n.*

acidoride. A trade-mark for *glutamic acid hydrochloride.*

ac″i·do′sis (ass″i·do′sis) [*acidus;* G. *-ōsis,* condition]. Reduction of the alkali reserve; acidemia; due to an excess of acid metabolites which are incompletely oxidized or poorly eliminated. When toxic symptoms develop, the condition is called acid intoxication. —**acidot′ic,** *adj.*

carbon-dioxide a. The result of CO_2 retention, as in drowning. Also called *gaseous a.*

compensated a. A condition of reduced blood bicarbonate with the H_2CO_3 to $NaHCO_3$ ratio unchanged because of the blood buffers. In compensated CO_2 acidosis, the blood bicarbonate may be increased, but pH is normal.

diabetic a. That occurring in diabetes mellitus, due to loss of base in the urine in combination with ketone acids and as a result of polyuria. It may become extremely severe, characterized by air hunger and eventually coma.

gaseous a. Carbon-dioxide acidosis.

idiopathic hyperchloremic a. Acidosis resulting from defective renal tubular mechanisms for acidifying the urine. Glomerular function is either normal or relatively less impaired than tubular function, so that azotemia generally does not appear. Filtered phosphorus is normal, but tubular resorption fails and hypophosphotemia follows. Skeletal demineralization and nephrocalcinosis may appear.

metabolic a. A condition characterized by a decreased pH and bicarbonate content of the body fluids, caused either by the accumulation of excess acids stronger than carbonic or by abnormal losses of fixed base from the body, as in diarrhea or renal disease.

renal tubular a. A condition resulting from a defect of the distal tubules of the kidney, characterized by inability to acidify urine. This may result in renal rickets and dwarfism in children, and in osteomalacia (Milkman's syndrome) in adults: also described as *hyperchloremic acidosis with nephrocalcinosis.*

respiratory a. Acidosis resulting from an increase of the carbonic acid of blood relative to the bicarbonate fraction with resultant decrease of pH; this occurs whenever elimination of carbon dioxide is impaired, as in respiratory obstruction or paralysis.

uncompensated a. A condition of reduced blood bicarbonate in which there is a change in the blood pH. In uncompensated CO_2 acidosis, the blood bicarbonate may be normal.

ac″i·dos′te·o·phyte″ [G. *akis,* point; *osteon,* bone; *phyton,* plant]. A sharp-pointed bony projection or outgrowth; an osseous spicule.

ac′id·proof″. See *acid-fast.*

ac″id-re·sist′ant. See *acidoresistant.*

ac′id tide. The temporary increase in the acidity of urine and body fluids which follows the alkaline tide.

a·cid′u·late [L. *acidulus,* dim. of *acidus,* from *acere,* to be sour]. Render sour or acid in reaction; pour acid into; acidify. —**acid′ulant,** *adj., n.;* **acidulated, acidulous,** *adj.*

acidulin. Trade-mark for glutamic acid hydrochloride.

ac″i·du′ric (ass″i·dew′rick) [*acidus;* L. *durare,* to endure]. Referring to bacteria which can grow in an acid medium but which grow better in an alkaline medium.

ac′id·yl. The radical of an organic acid, particularly from hydrocarbons of the formula C_nH_{2n+2}.

a·cid′y·la″ted. Combined with the residue of an organic acid (acidyl).

ac″i·e′sis. See *acyesis.*

aciform. A proprietary arthritis remedy reported to contain formic acid, iodine, sulfur, and terpene in a hydroalcoholic medium.

aci-jel. Trade name of a vaginal jelly containing acetic acid, ricinoleic acid, oxyquinoline sulfate, and glycerin in a vegetable gum base for use in vaginal infections causing leukorrhea.

ac″i·ne′si·a (ass″i·nee′zhuh, ·zee·uh, ·shuh, ·see·uh). See *akinesia.*

ac′i·ni (ass′i·nigh). Plural of acinus.

ac″i·no·tu′bu·lar [L. *acinus,* grape; *tubulus,* dim. of *tubus,* pipe]. Consisting of tubular acini.

ac′i·nus (ass′i·nus) (pl. *acini*) [L.]. A saccular terminal division of a compound gland having a narrow lumen, as contrasted with an alveolus. Several acini combine to form a lobule. —**acinal, acinar, acinic, acinous,** *adj.*

acitrin. Trade-mark of the ethyl ester of cinchophen; $C_6H_5.C_9H_5N.CO.O.C_2H_5$: used in gout.

ack′ee. Fruit of the tree *Blighia sapida,* native to Jamaica.

a. poisoning. An acute, sometimes fatal, poisoning, caused by eating the unripe fruit of the ackee tree. Characterized by vomiting and collapse.

a·cla″di·o′sis (a·clay″dee·o′sis, a·clad″ee·) [*Acladium;* G. *-ōsis,* condition]. An ulcerative dermatomycosis occurring on the palms of the hands and soles of the feet; due to the fungus *Acladium castellanii;* characterized by sharply defined round or oval ulcers with granulating centers. —**acladiot′ic,** *adj.*

A·cla′di·um. A genus of conidiospore fungi found in Ceylon, the Malay States, and Macedonia.

A. castellanii. The species which causes acladiosis.

ac′la·sis, a·cla′si·a (a·clay′zhuh, ·zee·uh, ·shuh, ·see·uh) [G. *a-,* not; *klasis,* a breaking]. Morbid continuity of structure, as in chondrodystrophia; especially diaphysial aclasis, marked by imperfect bone formation in cartilage and abnormal cartilaginous growths near the epiphyses, causing multiple exostoses.

a·clas′tic [G. *aklastos,* from *a-; klan,* to break]. Not refracting.

a·cleis″to·car′di·a (ay·kly″sto·car′dee·uh, a·kly″sto·, a·klis″to·) [*a-;* G. *kleiein,* to close; *kardia,* heart]. A condition in which the foramen ovale of the heart fails to close.

aclor. Trade-mark for glutamic acid hydrochloride.

ac·mas′tic [G. *akmastikos,* from *akmē,* point]. Designating a disease with a period of progressive symptoms (*epacmastic*), followed by a period of abatement (*paracmastic*).

ac′me (ack′mee) [*akmē*]. 1. Highest point. 2. Crisis or critical stage of a disease.

ac′ne (ack′nee) [NL., perhaps from G. *achnē,* chaff]. A chronic inflammatory condition of the pilosebaceous structures commonly involving the face, back, and chest. The lesions are papular, pustular, or nodular; they affect persons between the age of puberty and 30 years of age, generally are worse in winter, and often are associated with menstrual and gastrointestinal disorders. The primary lesion is the comedo, or blackhead, later developing into a pink, acuminate papule, a pustule, or nodule. Syn., *a. vulgaris.* Also called *adolescent a., a. varis.*

a. agminata. A facial eruption of small, dusky, reddish papules which develop into pustules and leave scars when healed. Also called *acnitis.*

a. albida. See *milium.*

a. artificialis. A type of acneform eruption which disappears when its cause is removed.

a. atrophica. See *a.* varioliformis.

a. cachecticorum. An acneform eruption seen in debilitated persons after long wasting diseases, such as tuberculosis. The lesions occur on the trunk and legs, appearing as flat, dull-red papules and pustules varying in size from that of a pinhead to that of a lentil.

a. coagminata. A pustular acneform eruption often seen after administering any of the halogens or their salts and among industrial workers exposed to hydrochloric acid, tar, tar vapor, oil, wax, or paraffin. The skin is pigmented with many comedos. The pustules form thick clusters and are covered with crusts and scabs involving, in addition to the usual sites, the extensor surfaces of the arms and legs, the scalp, the inner thighs, and the genitalia. Syn., *bromine a., chlorine a., iodine a., tar a., a. medicamentosa, a. picealis.*

a. conglobata. A severe chronic inflammation of the pilosebaceous structures of the face, chest, and back with many lesions on the lower back, buttocks, and thighs, occurring in men long after puberty. There are common acne lesions, double comedones, cysts, fluctuant plaques and sinuses; resulting scars are often keloidal.

a. contagiosa. An infectious pustular eruption of horses, said to differ from horsepox.

a. decalvans. A purulent inflammation of the hair follicles of the scalp causing destruction of the hair with irregular patches of baldness and scarring or atrophy of the skin. Syn., *folliculitis decalvans.*

a. erythematosa. See *a.* rosacea.

a. frontalis. See *a.* varioliformis.

a. hordeolans, a. hordeolaris. A nodular eruption in which the lesions are hard, tough, and arranged in rows.

a. hypertrophica. A stage in the development of acne rosacea in which there is a permanent, intensely red, noninflammatory, nodular thickening of the sides of the nose and the lips. Syn., *rhinophyma.*

a. indurata. Acne vulgaris in which the lesions are hard and livid due to perifollicular infiltration, and are very resistant to treatment.

a. keloid. Acneform eruption with minute red papules that suppurate and heal by hypertrophic granulations. See *folliculitis keloidalis.*

a. keratosa. A rare acne with horny plugs taking the place of the comedos causing inflammation. Also called *lichen spinulosus.*

a. medicamentosa. That which results from medication with certain drugs, as the iodides and bromides. See *a.* coagminata.

a. miliaris. See *milium.*

a. necrotica. See *a.* varioliformis.

a. neonatorum. Acne vulgaris in newborn infants, considered to be due to placental transfer of hormones.

a. of the cornea. See *a.* keratosa.

a. pancreatica. Small cysts in the pancreas due to obstruction of the smaller ducts.

a. papulosa. A papular form commonly seen on the foreheads of young adults.

a. picealis. See tar *a.*

a. punctata. A superficial papular eruption with pointed lesions marked by slight inflammation about the comedos.

a. pustulosa. A variety of acne vulgaris with a predominance of small abscesses.

a. rodens. See *a.* varioliformis.

a. rosacea. A chronic hyperemic skin affection of the nose, forehead, and cheeks, marked by hypertrophy, erythema and flushing, and telangiectasis. Also called *rosacea, telangiectasis faciei, whisky nose.*

a. scrofulosorum. A variety of acne cachecticorum affecting tuberculous children.

a. sebacea. Syn., *seborrhea.*

a. simplex. Acne vulgaris.

a. sycosiformis. See *sycosis.*

a. tarsi. An inflammatory affection of the large sebaceous glands of the eyelids (tarsal glands).

a. tropica. A severe form having all the symptoms of acne conglobata, but induced by tropical climate and improving in a cooler climate.

a. urticata. An eruption of the face and scalp characterized by small wheals and vesicles associated with itching and burning.

a. varioliformis. An uncommon skin affection, usually found on the forehead, that sometimes extends beyond the hairline onto the scalp. The lesions are pustular, covered with hard crusts and scabs. These fall off, leaving small craterlike ulcers that heal as scarred pits.

a. vermoulante. See *folliculitis ulerythematosa reticulata.*

a. vulgaris. The common type of acne occurring in sexually maturing and mature individuals, and related to disturbances in hormonal balance.

adolescent a. Acneform eruptions which occur in young adolescents.

bromine a. The acneform eruption which frequently exists in bromine poisoning. See *a.* coagminata. Also called *bromine eruptions.*

chlorine a. A pustular acne following the administration of chlorine compounds. See *a.* coagminata.

congestive a. See *a.* rosacea.

cystic a. That distinguished by cyst formation, each enclosing hard, inspissated sebum.

halogen a. See *a.* coagminata.

iodine a. A skin eruption often following administration of iodine and related compounds. See *a.* coagminata.

tar a. An acneform pustular eruption usually involving the extensor surfaces of the legs of industrial workers exposed to tar, tar vapor, and related compounds. See chlorine *a.*, *a.* coagminata.

varicose a. That associated with dilated superficial capillaries.

ac′ne·form, ac·ne′i·form [*acne;* L. *forma,* form]. Resembling acne.

ac·ne′mi·a [G. *a-,* not; *knēmē,* leg]. 1. Atrophy of the calves of the legs. 2. Congenital absence of the legs. **—acnemous,** *adj.*

ac·ni′tis. Acne agminata.

acnomel. Trade-mark for a preparation for the treatment of acne, containing resorcinol and sulfur in a base including bentonite, propylene glycol, alcohol, and titanium dioxide.

ac″o·as′ma (ack″o·ass′muh, ·az′muh), **ac′o·asm.** See *acousma.*

a·coe′li·a, a·ce′li·a (a·see′lee·uh) [*a-;* G. *koilia,* cavity of the body]. Absence of a body cavity or coelom. **—acoelious, acelomate, acoelomate, acoelous,** *adj.*

ac′o·ine (ack′o·een, ·in), **ac′o·in.** Hydrochloride of diparaanisylmonoparaphenetylguanidine, a white powder, used in infiltration anesthesia by Schleich's method in a 1:1000 solution with 0.8% sodium chloride; also in 1% aqueous solution in ophthalmology.

Ac″o·kan′ther·a [G. *akōkē,* a point; *anthēros,* blooming]. A genus of apocynaceous herbs native to Africa. Juices from the leaves and stems of several species furnish the natives with arrow poison, since they contain a principle, acokantherin, similar to or identical with ouabain.

ac″o·kan′ther·in. $C_{32}H_{50}O_{12}$. The poisonous glycoside of *Acokanthera,* similar to digitalis and ouabain in its action.

acolake. Trade name for vitamin A capsules.

ac″o·la′si·a (ack″o·lay′zhuh, ·zee·uh) [G. *akolasia,* intemperance]. Unrestrained self-indulgence; lust; intemperance. *Obs.* **—acolas′tic,** *adj.*

acolite. A proprietary casting material used in dentistry.

a·co′lous (ay·ko′lus, a·ko′lus) [G. *a-,* not; *kōlon,* limb]. Having no limbs.

a·co′mi·a [*a-;* G. *komē,* hair]. Baldness. A deficiency of hair from any cause. Syn., *alopecia.* **—acomous,** *adj.*

acon. Trade-mark for a water-dispersible preparation of vitamin A.

a·con′a·tive [*a-;* L. *conatus,* from *conari,* to try]. Having no wish or desire to act. See *conation.*

ac′o·nine (ack′o·neen, ·nin). $C_{25}H_{41}O_9N$. An alkaloid obtained from aconitine; much less toxic.

a·con′i·tase. The enzyme that catalyzes the breakdown of citric acid to *cis*-aconitic and *l*-isocitric acids.

ac′o·nite [G. *akoniton,* leopard's bane] (*aconitum*). A very poisonous drug obtained from the roots of *Aconitum napellus.* It has a bitter, pungent taste and leaves a sensation of numbness and tingling on the lips and tongue. Physiologically, it is a cardiac, respiratory, and circulatory depressant and produces sensory paralysis. The principal alkaloid is aconitine. It acts as a diaphoretic, antipyretic, and diuretic.

ac″o·nit′ic ac′id. COOH.CH.C(COOH):CH.COOH; 1,2,3-propenetricarboxylic acid, representing citric acid minus a molecule of water; it occurs in two modifications, *cis-* and *trans-*. *Cis*-aconitic acid is believed to be an intermediate product in Krebs cycle explaining aerobic oxidation of carbohydrates. Aconitic acid, presumably of *trans*-configuration, occurs in a number of plants, including species of *Aconitum,* beets, and sugar cane.

a·con′i·tin. See *aconitine.*

a·con′i·tine (a·kon′i·teen, ·tin), **a·con′i·tin** (*aconitina*). $C_{34}H_{47}O_{11}N$. An extremely poisonous alkaloid derived from *Aconitum napellus* and other species; it occurs as white, flat crystals of slightly bitter taste. Dose, 0.0002 Gm. (1/300 gr.).

a. hydrobromide. $C_{34}H_{47}O_{11}N.HBr$. From crystalline aconitine, occurring as small white crystals; soluble in water and alcohol. Dose, the same as the crystalline alkaloid.

a. hydrochloride. $C_{34}H_{47}O_{11}N.HCl$. A white, crystalline powder from crystalline aconitine; soluble in water and alcohol. Dose, about the same as the alkaloid.

a. nitrate. $C_{34}H_{47}O_{11}N.HNO_3$. Fine, white prisms or rhombic crystals; highly poisonous; used in neuralgia and rheumatism. Dose, about the same as the alkaloid. Syn., *Duquesnel's a.*

amorphous a. A mixture of several bases found in the bulbs of *Aconitum napellus.* Its principal constituents are aconitine and picroaconitine. It is 15 or 20 times less poisonous than pure, crystallized aconitine.

British a. A yellowish white, crystalline alkaloid prepared by Morson from *Aconitum ferox.* Also called *English aconitine, acraconitine, Morson's napelline* or *pure aconitine, Hubschmann's pseudaconitine, Flückiger's nepaline.*

Duquesnel's a. See *a.* nitrate.

Ac″o·ni′tum [*akoniton*]. A genus of poisonous ranunculaceous plants, whose species are the source of aconite.

a·con″u·re′sis [G. *akōn,* involuntary; *ourēsis,* urination]. Involuntary passage of urine.

a″co·pro′sis (ay″ko·pro′sis, ack″o·) [G. *a-,* not; *koprōsis,* from *kopros,* excrement]. Marked deficiency or absence of feces in the intestine. **—acop′rous,** *adj.*

ac″o·re′a [*a-;* G. *korē,* pupil]. Absence of the pupil.

a·co′ri·a [*a-;* G. *koros,* satiety]. 1. A form of hunger due to the absence of the feeling of satiety following a meal, to be differentiated from bulimia. 2. Greedy or insatiable appetite because the patient never feels full; a constant desire for food although the appetite may not be large.

ac′o·rin. A bitter, nonnitrogenous substance, possibly $C_{36}H_{60}O_6$; found in the root of *Acorus calamus,* or sweet flag.

a·cor′mus [*a-;* G. *kormos,* trunk]. An acardiac monster lacking a trunk.

Ac′o·rus [G. *akoron,* yellow flag]. A genus of araceous plants.

A. calamus. A species from which calamus is obtained.

Acosta, José de [*Spanish missionary and author,* ca.1539–1600]. A Jesuit father who first described the syndrome of mountain sickness (1590), called *Acosta's disease.*

a·cos′tate [G. *a-*, not; L. *costatus,* from *costa,* rib]. Without ribs.

acou- (a·kōō-), **acouo-** [G. *akouein,* to hear]. A combining form denoting *relation to hearing.*

a·cou″aes·the′si·a. See *acouesthesia.*

a·cou″es·the′si·a (a·kōō″ess·thee′zhuh, ·zee·uh) [*akouein;* G. *aisthēsis,* sensation]. The hearing sense; usually a very acute sense of hearing.

ac″ou·la′li·on (ack″ōō·lay′lee·on) [*akouein;* G. *lalia,* speech]. An instrument used in teaching speech to deaf-mutes.

a·cou′me·ter (a·kōō′mi·tur), **ac″ou·om′e·ter, ac″ou·tom′e·ter** [*akouein;* G. *metron,* a measure]. Instrument for measuring the acuteness of hearing. —**acoumet′ric, acoumomet′ric,** *adj.;* **acou′metry,** *n.*

ac″ou·oph′o·ny (ack″ōō·off′o·nee), **a·cou″o·pho′ni·a** (a·kōō″o·fo′nee·uh) [*akouein;* G. *phōnē,* sound]. Auscultatory percussion.

-a·cou′si·a (-a·kōō′zhuh, ·zee·uh, ·shuh, ·see·uh), **-a·cou′sis** [G. *akousis,* hearing]. A combining form denoting *hearing.*

a·cous′ma (a·kōōs′muh, a·kōōz′muh, a·kouz′muh) [G. *akousma,* thing heard]. *In psychopathology,* a simple auditory hallucination, as of buzzing or ringing. A borderline condition between illusion and true hallucinosis.

a·cous″mat·ag·no′sis (a·kōōs″mat·ag·no′sis, a·kōōz″·) [*akousma;* G. *a-*, not; *gnōsis,* recognition]. Inability to recognize sounds or understand spoken words; mind deafness.

a·cous″mat·am·ne′si·a (a·kōōs″mat·am·nee′-zhuh, ·zee·uh) [*akousma;* G. *amnēsia,* from *a-; mnēsios,* pertaining to memory]. Inability to remember sounds.

a·cous′tic [*akoustikos*]. Pertaining to sound or hearing.

acoustic (eighth cranial) nerve. A composite sensory nerve having two roots and two branches: *cochlear* (for hearing) and *vestibular* (for movement and position of head in space).

a·cous″ti·co·pho′bi·a (a·kōōs″ti·ko·) [G. *akoustikos,* from *akouein,* to hear; *phobos,* fear]. Morbid fear of sounds.

a·cous′tics (a·kōōs′ticks) [*akoustikos*]. 1. *In physics,* the science of sound. 2. *In psychology,* that branch dealing with hearing.

ac″ou·tom′e·ter. See *acoumeter.*

ac·quired′ [L. *acquirere,* to acquire]. 1. *In psychology,* gained from experience or learning, as an acquired idea; in contradistinction to innate. 2. *In biology,* developed as a result of environment, or of use or disuse, as an acquired characteristic; in contradistinction to an inherited characteristic.

ac·quired′ a·tel·ec′ta·sis. See under *atelectasis.*

ac′ral [G. *akron,* extremity]. Relating to, or affecting, the limbs or extremities.

a·cra′ni·a (ay·kray′nee·uh, a·kray′·) [G. *a-*, not; *kranion,* skull]. Partial or complete absence of the cranium at birth. —**acranial,** *adj.;* **acranius,** *n.*

a·cra′si·a (a·kray′zhuh, ·zee·uh) [G., from *a-; kratos,* power]. Intemperance; lack of self-control.

a·cra′ti·a (a·kray′shee·uh) [*a-; kratos*]. Impotence, loss of power.

a·crat″u·re′sis [*a-; kratos;* G. *ourēsis,* urination]. Inability to micturate due to atony of the bladder.

ac″re·mo″ni·o′sis [*Acremonium;* G. *-ōsis,* condition]. A fungus infection caused by *Acremonium potroni;* characterized by fever and gummalike swellings.

ac″ren·ceph′a·lon. The portion of the central nervous system of vertebrates whose development is induced by the roof of the stomodeum; the prosencephalon; no sulcus limitans occurs. Also see *chordencephalon.*

ac″ri·bom′e·ter [G. *akribēs,* exact; *metron,* a measure]. A device for measuring minute objects.

ac′rid [L. *acer,* sharp]. Pungent; irritating.

ac′ri·dine (ack′ri·deen, ·din). $CH:(C_6H_4)_2:N$. A solid hydrocarbon obtained from coal tar. It is employed in the synthesis of various dyes, certain of which (acriflavine, diflavine, proflavine) are used as antiseptics.

ac″ri·fla′vine (ack″ri·flay′veen, ·vin, ·flav′een, ·in) (*acriflavina*). A mixture of 3,6-diamino-10-methylacridinium chloride and 3,6-diaminoacridine; a deep orange, granular powder, freely soluble in water. It is used chiefly as a local antiseptic, but has been administered intravenously in treating various infections. Also called *a. base, neutral a.* See *trypaflavin.*

a. hydrochloride A mixture of the hydrochlorides of 3,6-diamino-10-methylacridinium chloride and 3,6-diaminoacridine; a strong reddish-brown powder, freely soluble in water. It is used for the same purposes as acriflavine, but is more irritant because of its acid reaction. Also called *acid a.*

ac′ri·nyl sul″fo·cy′a·nate. An acrid and vesicating substance found in white mustard.

a·crit′i·cal (ay·krit′i·kul, a·krit′·) [G. *a-*, not; *krisis,* crisis]. 1. Without a crisis; not relating to a crisis; applied to diseases which resolve by lysis. 2. Indeterminate, as regards prognosis.

a·crit″o·chro′ma·cy [G. *akritos,* from *a-; kritos,* distinguished; *chrōma,* color]. Colorblindness; achromatopsia.

ac′ro-, acr- [G. *akron,* extremity]. A combining form meaning *pertaining to extremes* or *to the extremities.*

ac″ro·aes·the′si·a. See *acroesthesia.*

ac″ro·ag·no′sis [*akron;* G. *a-*, not; *gnōsis,* knowledge]. Absence of sense perception in a limb.

ac″ro·an″es·the′si·a, ac″ro·an″aes·the′si·a (ack″ro·an″ess·thee′zhuh, ·zee·uh) [*akron;* G. *anaisthēsia,* lack of sensation]. Anesthesia of the extremities.

ac″ro·ar·thri′tis [*akron;* G. *arthron,* joint; *-itis,* inflammation]. Arthritis of the extremities.

ac″ro·as·phyx′i·a [*akron;* G. *asphyxia,* from *a-*, *sphyxis,* pulse]. Early symptom of Raynaud's syndrome characterized by coldness and pallor alternating with heat and redness of the hands and feet.

ac″ro·a·tax′i·a [*akron;* G. *ataxia,* disorder]. Incoordination of the muscles of the fingers and toes, as opposed to *proximoataxia,* incoordination of the proximal portions of the extremities.

ac′ro·blast [*akron;* G. *blastos,* germ]. Golgi remnant; part of the Golgi material in the spermatid forms the acrosome of the spermatozoon, part becomes the acroblast.

ac″ro·ce·pha′li·a. See *acrocephaly.*

ac″ro·ceph·a·lop′a·gus. Synonym for *craniopagus parietalis.*

ac″ro·ceph″a·lo·syn″dac·tyl′i·a, ac″ro·ceph″a-lo·syn·dac′ty·ly [*akron;* G. *kephalē,* head; *syn,* together; *daktylos,* digit]. Congenital malformation consisting of a pointed top of the head and syndactyly of the hands and feet. Also called *acrosphenosyndactylia, Apert's syndrome, acrocephalosyndactylism.*

ac″ro·ceph′a·ly, ac″ro·ce·pha′li·a [*akron; kephalē*]. Deformity of the head, in which the top is more or less pointed. See *oxycephaly.* —**acrocephal′ic, acrocephalous,** *adj.*

ac″ro·chor·do′ma. See *chordoma.*

ac″ro·chor′don (ack″ro·kor′don) [G. *akrochordōn,* wart with a thin neck, from *akron; chordē,* cord]. Pedunculated wart. Syn., *molluscum fibrosum.*

ac″ro·ci·ne′sis (ack″ro·sin·ee′sis) [*akron;* G. *kinēsis,* movement]. Markedly excessive motion, as in certain cases of hysteria. —**acrocinet′ic,** *adj.*

ac″ro·con·trac′ture [*akron;* L. *contractura,* contracting]. Contracture of the joints of the hands or feet.

ac″ro·cy″a·no′sis [*akron;* G. *kyanos,* blue; *-ōsis,* condition]. Blueness of the extremities due to vasomotor disturbance. In chronic progressive acrocyanosis there is hypertrophy of the soft tissues of the hands and feet, associated with cyanosis or intense redness.

ac″ro·der″ma·ti′tis [*akron;* G. *derma,* skin; *-itis,* inflammation]. Inflammation of the skin of an extremity.

a. atrophicans chronica. An atrophic dermatitis which begins as an inflammation and is followed by atrophy; it is progressive, but usually limited to the extremities; its cause is unknown.

a. continua (*of Hallopeau*). A chronic relapsing vesicopustular dermatosis, of uncertain cause, primarily of the extremities, chiefly the hands, with secondary eruptions of erythematous and desquamating types: also called *a. perstans.*

a. enteropathica. A rare, chronic, relapsing vesiculobullous dermatitis asociated with mucous-membrane lesions, diarrhea, and alopecia, appearing in infants during the first year of life.

a. hiemalis. A skin affection seen in cold weather, consisting of indolent and indurated papulopustules over the fingers and about the knuckles; probably a tuberculid.

a. pustulosa. See *pustulosis palmaris et plantaris.*

a. vesiculosa tropica. A rare dermatitis of the fingers, marked by atrophy of the skin and an eruption of small vesicles; the fingers may show a tapering shape.

ac″ro·dig′i·ta·lin (ack″ro·didj′i·tuh·lin, ·didj″i-tay′lin). A digitalis substance which does not possess the general characteristics of a glycoside.

ac″ro·dol″i·cho·me′li·a (ack″ro·dol″i·ko·mee′-lee·uh) [*akron;* G. *dolichos,* long; *melos,* limb]. Condition in which the hands and feet grow disproportionately long or large.

ac′ro·dont [*akron;* G. *odous,* tooth]. 1. Denoting a tooth which is ankylosed by its root to a bony eminence, and not inserted in a socket or alveolus. 2. Having teeth of this kind.

ac″ro·dyn′i·a, ac″ro·dy′ni·a. See *erythredema polyneuropathy.*

ac″ro·e·de′ma [*akron;* G. *oidēma,* swelling]. 1. Swelling of the extremities, sometimes accompanied by erythredema polyneuropathy: seen particularly in neuropathic individuals. 2. Permanent posttraumatic swelling of a hand or foot.

ac″ro·es·the′si·a, ac″ro·aes·the′si·a (ack″ro·ess-thee′zhuh, ·zee·uh) [*akron;* G. *aisthēsis,* sensation]. 1. Exaggerated sensitiveness or sensibility. 2. Pain in one or more of the extremities.

ac″ro·ger′i·a (ack″ro·jerr′ee·uh, ·jeer′ee·uh) [*akron;* G. *gerōn,* old man]. Premature aging of the skin of the hands and feet, marked by looseness and wrinkling.

ac″rog·no′sis [*akron;* G. *gnōsis,* knowledge]. Cenesthesia of the extremities and of their parts.

ac″ro·hy″per·hi·dro′sis (ack″ro·high″pur·hi·dro′-sis, ·high″pur·high·dro′sis) [*akron;* G. *hyper,* over; *hidrōsis,* sweating]. Increased perspiration of the hands and feet.

ac″ro·hy′po·ther″my [*akron;* G. *hypo,* under; *thermē,* heat]. Abnormal coldness of the extremities.

ac″ro·ker″a·to′sis ver·ru″ci·for′mis. Form of epithelial nevus; discrete verrucous lesions occurring chiefly on the dorsum of the hands and feet; the palms, wrists, and knees also may be involved.

a·cro′le·in. CH_2:CH.CHO. Acrylic aldehyde. A colorless, mobile liquid with a pungent odor, resulting from the decomposition of glycerin. Syn., *allyl aldehyde.*

ac″ro·mac′ri·a [*akron;* G. *makros,* long]. Spider fingers. See *arachnodactyly.*

ac″ro·ma′ni·a [*akron;* G. *mania,* madness]. A violent form of mania. *Obs.*

ac″ro·mas·ti′tis [*akron;* G. *mastos,* breast; *-itis,* inflammation]. Inflammation of the nipple.

ac″ro·meg′a·loid·ism [*akron;* G. *megas,* great; *eidos,* form]. State or condition of the body in which the form resembles that of an acromegalic, but is not caused by hyperpituitarism.

ac″ro·meg′a·ly, ac″ro·me·ga′li·a [*akros; megas*]. Chronic condition resulting from hyperfunction and hyperplasia of the eosinophilic cells of the adenohypophysis. The characteristic features are: increase in size of the viscera (splanchnomegaly), the soft parts, and the bones, especially the short and flat bones (acromegaly), without increase in height, the hands, feet, and face showing most change; metabolic disturbances, chief of which is a change in sugar tolerance; secondary changes in the function of other endocrine organs; and so-called neighborhood symptoms such as bitemporal hemianopsia. *Acromegaloid, forme fruste, transient acromegaly,* and *fugitive acromegaly* are terms which have been used to designate incomplete, arrested, or rapidly changing types of the disease. See *gigantism.* Also called *Marie's syndrome.* —**acromegal′ic,** *adj., n.*

ac″ro·mel·al′gi·a [*akron;* G. *melos,* limb; *algos,* pain]. A peripheral vascular disease. See *erythromelalgia.*

ac″ro·met″a·gen′e·sis [*akron;* G. *meta,* beyond; *genesis,* origin]. Undue growth of the extremities.

ac″ro·mic′ri·a [*akron;* G. *mikros,* small]. Underdevelopment of the extremities and of the skull as contrasted with visceral development.

a. congenita. A term introduced by Benda for mongolism.

a·cro″mi·o·cla·vic′u·lar [*akron;* G. *ōmos,* shoulder; L. *clavicula,* dim. of *clavis,* key]. Pertaining to the acromion and the clavicle; applied to the articulation between these two bones and the ligaments joining them. See Table of Joints and Ligaments in the Appendix.

a·cro″mi·o·cor′a·coid [*akron; ōmos;* G. *korakoeidēs,* like a raven]. Pertaining to the acromion and the coracoid process. Also *coracoacromial.*

a·cro″mi·o·hu′mer·al [*akron; ōmos;* L. *humerus,* upper bone of the arm]. Relating to the acromion and the humerus.

a·cro′mi·on [*akron; ōmos*]. The flat, somewhat triangular bony process formed by the lateral extension of the scapular spine, and situated just above the glenoid cavity. It articulates with the clavicle, and serves as a point of attachment for some of the fibers of the deltoid and trapezius muscles. See Plate 1. —**acromial,** *adj.*

a·cro″mi·o·tho·rac′ic (a·kro″mee·o·thor·ass′ick) [*akron; ōmos;* G. *thōrax,* chest]. Relating to the shoulder and thorax; designating a branch of the axillary artery.

a·crom′pha·lus [*akron;* G. *omphalos,* navel]. 1. The center of the umbilicus, where the cord attaches. 2. Unusual prominence of the navel, often the first sign of an umbilical hernia. 3. Remains of the umbilical cord attached to the child.

ac″ro·my″o·to′ni·a (ack″ro·my″o·to′nee·uh, ack″-ro·mee″o·), **ac″ro·my·ot′o·nus** (ack″ro·mee·ot′o·

nus, ·my·ot′o·nus) [*akron;* G. *mys,* muscle; *tonos,* tension]. Tonic muscular spasm of the extremities, usually causing deformity of the hands or feet.

ac″ro·nar·cot′ic [L. *acer,* sharp; G. *narkē,* numbness]. An agent which combines a local irritant effect, by acting directly on the peripheral nerves, with a general obtunding effect, by affecting the brain and vital centers in the cord. —**ac″ro-nar·cot′ic,** *adj.*

ac″ro·neu·rop′a·thy [G. *akron,* extremity; *neuron,* nerve; *pathos,* disease]. The simultaneous degeneration of the peripheral nerves in their most distal parts, usually symmetrical. Most common causes: alcohol, arsenic, lead or mercury poisoning, or a deficiency disease such as beriberi. Syn., *polyneuropathy, polyneuritis.*

ac″ro·neu·ro′sis [*akron; neuron;* G. *-ōsis,* condition]. Any neurosis manifesting itself in the extremities, usually vasomotor in nature or due to deficiency disease.

a·cron′y·chous, a·chron′y·chous (a·kron′i·kus) [G. *acrōnychos,* with nails, from *akron; onyx,* nail]. Having claws, nails, or hoofs.

ac′ro·nyx [*akron; onyx*]. Ingrowing of a nail.

ac′ro·os″te·ol′y·sis. Myelodysplasia with osseous lesions.

ac′ro·pach″y (ack′ro·pack″ee) [*akron;* G. *pachys,* thick]. Old term for secondary hypertrophic osteoarthropathy.

ac″ro·pach″y·der′ma (ack″ro·pack″i·dur′muh) [*akron; pachys;* G. *derma,* skin]. Old term for pachyacria.

ac″ro·pa·ral′y·sis [*akron;* G. *paralysis,* from *para,* beside; *luein,* to loosen]. Paralysis of the extremities.

ac″ro·par″es·the′si·a, ac″ro·par″aes·the′si·a (·par″ess·thee′zhuh, ·zee·uh) [*akron;* G. *paraisthēsis,* misperception]. A vasomotor neurosis, seen chiefly in middle-aged women; characterized by tingling or crawling sensations in the hands, hyperesthesia and hyperalgesia of the fingers, coldness, and pallor or cyanosis of the hands.

ac″ro·pa·thol′o·gy [*akron;* G. *pathos,* disease; *logos,* word]. The pathology of the extremities, especially the morbid changes occurring in orthopedic diseases.

a·crop′a·thy [*akron; pathos*]. Any disease of the extremities.

a·crop′e·tal [*akron;* L. *petere,* to seek]. Tending upward to a summit, applied to an inflorescence and certain infections.

ac″ro·pho′bi·a [*akron;* G. *phobos,* fear]. Morbid dread of being at a great height.

ac″ro·pig·men·ta′tion. Increased melanin pigmentation of the distal parts of the extremities. See *acropigmentatio reticularis.*

ac″ro·pig·men·ta′ti·o re·tic″u·lar′is. A genodermatosis characterized by small evenly brown-pigmented, rough-surfaced, slightly depressed macules located on the extensors of the distal parts of the extremities.

ac″ro·pos·thi′tis [*akron;* G. *posthē,* foreskin; *-itis,* inflammation]. Inflammation of the prepuce. See *posthitis.*

ac″ro·scle″ro·der′ma (ack″ro·skleer″o·dur′muh, ·sklerr″o·dur′muh). See *sclerodactylia.*

ac″ro·scle·ro′sis [*akron;* G. *sklērōsis,* hardening]. Scleroderma affecting the hands and extending to the upper extremities and the face; seen usually as a sequel of Raynaud's syndrome.

ac′rose. A saccharine substance resulting from the polymerization or other reaction of such substances as glycerin, glycollic aldehyde, etc.; the chief constituent is DL-fructose: frequently designated *α-acrose.*

ac′ro·some [*akron;* G. *sōma,* body]. A crescent-shaped body molded to the nucleus, forming the anterior part of the sperm head; the apical body.

ac″ro·sphe″no·syn″dac·tyl′i·a. See *acrocephalosyndactylia.*

ac″ros·te·al′gi·a [*akron;* G. *osteon,* bone; *algos,* pain]. Pain in one or more of the bones of an extremity.

ac″ro·ter′ic [G. *akrōterion,* extremity]. Relating to the periphery or most distal parts, as the tips of the toes, fingers, nose, etc. —**acrote′ria,** *n.*

Ac″ro·the′ci·um floc·co′sum. Synonym for *Epidermophyton floccosum.*

a·crot′ic [G. *a-,* not; *krotos,* a striking]. Exhibiting any defective beating of the pulse; distinguished by absent or barely perceptible pulse.

a·crot′ic [G. *akron,* extremity]. Relating to the glands of the skin; affecting the surface or periphery.

ac′ro·tism [G. *a-,* not; *krotos,* a striking]. Absence or imperceptibility of the pulse.

ac″ro·tro″pho·neu·ro′sis [G. *akron,* extremity; *trophē,* nourishment; *neuron,* nerve; *-ōsis,* condition]. A trophic disturbance of the extremities caused by a nerve lesion.

a·cryl′ic ac′id. CH_2:CH.COOH. A liquid acid resulting from oxidation of acrolein.

a·cryl′ic al′de·hyde. See *acrolein.*

a·cryl′ics. A group of thermoplastic substances prepared by reaction and polymerization of sodium cyanide, acetone, methyl alcohol, and acid; methyl methacrylates. They resemble clear glass, but are lighter in weight and permit the passage of ultraviolet rays; used in making dental prostheses and temporary artificial eyes. Lucite and plexiglas are commercial forms.

ac′ry·lo-, acryl- [L. *acer,* sharp; G. *hylē,* wood, material]. A combining form denoting *relationship to acrylic acid* or *acrylics.*

ac″ry·lo·ni·trile′ (ack″ri·lo·nigh·trill′, ·nigh·treel′, ·nigh′tryle, ·nigh′trill, ·nigh′treel). A colorless liquid, H_2C:CH.CN, used in the manufacture of synthetic rubber. Its toxic action has been said to be due to the formation of hydrocyanic acid. An increase in serum thiocyanates is observed in workers exposed to it. Syn., *vinyl cyanide.*

ACS Antireticular cytotoxic serum; a specific cytotoxic antiserum produced by the intravenous injection of an antigen prepared from human or heterologous animal spleen and bone marrow. Minute doses are said to have a stimulating effect, and large doses a depressing effect, on the reticuloendothelial system. This is the basis for its use in the treatment of such unrelated conditions as wounds, fractures, arthritis, ozena, and even cancer.

act [L. *actus,* from *agere,* to do]. 1. Any deed, action, or performance. 2. Fulfillment of a purpose or function.

compulsive a. Any conscious deed or act of an individual performed on irresistible impulse: usually the result of an obsession.

reflex a. Any action innervated through a reflex arc.

sexual a. Coitus; cohabitation; sexual intercourse.

actamer. Trade-mark for the bacteriostatic agent bithionol.

ACTH The adrenocorticotropic hormone from the anterior pituitary; it stimulates the adrenal cortex to secrete its entire spectrum of hormones. Syn., *corticotropin.* See *acthar.*

acthar. Trade-mark for a preparation of corticotropin.

ac″ti·di′one. Antibiotic substance produced by *Streptomyces griseus,* highly active against yeasts but relatively innocuous to other microorganisms.

ac′tin. Protein constituent of the muscle fibril,

occurring side by side with myosin as actomyosin. It can undergo a reversible transformation between a globular or monomeric (**G-actin**) and a fibrous or polymeric (**F-actin**) state.

actin-. See *actino-*.

ac·tin′ic [G. *aktis*, ray]. Pertaining to, or designating, the rays of the spectrum which produce chemical change.

ac′tin·ide. Any of the group of related chemical elements starting with actinium and including thorium, palladium, uranium, neptunium, plutonium, americium, curium, berkelium, and californium.

ac·tin′i·form [*aktis;* L. *forma*, form]. Exhibiting radiate form or structure, such as the ray fungus or sea anemone.

ac·tin″i·o·he′ma·tin (ack·tin″ee·o·hee′muh·tin, ·hem′uh·tin) [*aktis;* G. *haima*, blood]. A red, respiratory pigment found in various sea anemones.

ac′tin·ism [*aktis*]. 1. Property of producing chemical changes possessed by spectral rays, especially those from beyond the violet end of the visible spectrum. 2. The science which treats of the chemical changes produced by radiation.

ac·tin′i·um [*aktis*]. Ac = 227. A radioactive element found in uranium ores, as pitchblende. Half-life 20 years.

a. X. The disintegration product of radioactinium.

ac′ti·no-, actin- [*aktis*]. A combining form meaning *ray, rays*, or *radiated structure*.

ac″ti·no·bac″il·lo′sis (ack″ti·no·bas″i·lo′sis) [*aktis;* L. *bacillus*, little stick; G. *-ōsis*, disease]. An actinomycosislike disease of bovine and other domestic animals caused by the *Actinobacillus lignieresi;* characterized by the formation of morbid, radiate bodies in the affected tissues.

Ac″ti·no·ba·cil′lus [*aktis; bacillus*]. A genus of the family Parvobacteriaceae; small, Gram-negative bacteria which attack the soft tissues of cattle and swine, causing a disease resembling actinomycosis. Important species of the group are **A. actinoides, A. actinomycetum-comitans, A. lignieresi.**

ac″ti·no·chem′is·try [*aktis;* G. *chēmeia*, alchemy]. Branch of chemistry concerned with the reactions produced by light.

ac″ti·no·der″ma·ti′tis. See *dermatitis* actinica.

ac·tin′o·gen [*aktis;* G. *genesthai*, from *gignesthai*, to be produced]. Any substance producing radiation. —**actinogen′ic,** *adj.;* **actinogen′esis, actinogen′ics,** *n.*

ac·tin′o·graph [*aktis;* G. *graphein*, to write]. 1. An instrument which records variations in the actinic strength of the sun's rays, hence permits the determination of proper time of exposure of a photographic plate; an exposure meter. 2. A roentgenogram. *Obs.*

ac·tin′o·lite. See *actinolyte*.

ac″ti·nol′o·gy [*aktis;* G. *logos*, word]. 1. The homology existing between the successive segments, regions, or parts of a radially symmetrical organ or organism. 2. Study of the chemical action of light.

ac·tin′o·lyte, ac·tin′o·lite [*aktis;* G. *lytos*, from *lyein*, to loose]. 1. An apparatus designed for use in actinotherapy. 2. A device which generates ultraviolet rays. 3. Any substance which undergoes a rather marked change when exposed to light.

ac″ti·nom′e·ter [*aktis;* G. *metron*, a measure]. 1. An apparatus for determining the intensity of chemical rays. 2. A device which determines the degree of penetration of such rays. —**actinometry,** *n.*

ac″ti·no·my·ce′li·al (ack″ti·no·migh·see′lee·ul) [*aktis;* G. *mykēs*, fungus]. 1. Relating to the mycelium of *Actinomyces*. 2. Actinomycetic.

Ac″ti·no·my′ces (ack″ti·no·migh′seez) [*aktis; mykēs*]. A genus of anaerobic vegetable parasites belonging to the family Actinomycetaceae. In tissue they resemble rosettes of fine filaments, each clubbed at the distal end, surrounding a central group of coccuslike spores. Also called *ray fungus, asteroid bodies*. See also *Discomyces*. —**actinomyce′tic, actinomyce′tous,** *adj.*

A. antibioticus. A species of fungi living in the soil and possessing antibacterial properties.

A. asteroides. Synonym for *Nocardia asteroides*.

A. bovis. The organism which produces actinomycosis in man and lumpy jaw in cattle, the majority of cases being reported in the United States. See Table of the Most Common Microorganisms Pathogenic to Man in the Appendix.

A. hominis. The organism thought by some to be the cause of actinomycosis in man, believed by others to be a contaminant.

A. keratolyticus. The organism which causes cracked heels in India.

A. madurae. Synonym for *Nocardia madurae*.

A. minutissimus. Synonym for *Nocardia minutissima*.

A. mycetoma. See *mycetoma*.

A. necrophorus. A species found in lung and liver abscesses and in chronic ulcerative colitis in man; produces necrobacillosis in domestic animals.

A. somaliensis. Synonym for *Nocardia somaliensis*.

A. venezuelae. The organism which elaborates biosynthetic chloramphenicol.

Ac″ti·no·my″ce·ta′ce·ae (·migh″see·tay′see·ee) [*aktis; mykēs*]. A family of the order Actinomycetales.

Ac″ti·no·my″ce·ta′les (·migh″see·tay′leez) [*aktis; mykēs*]. Any of an order of fungi belonging to the class Schizomycetes, consisting of moldlike, rod-shaped, filamentous, or clubbed forms, many showing considerable branching. The order contains three families: Actinomycetaceae, Mycobacteriaceae, and Streptomycetaceae.

ac″ti·no·my·ce′tin (ack″ti·no·migh·see′tin, ·migh′si·tin) [*aktis; mykēs*]. An antibacterial substance synthesized by several strains of *Actinomyces*, and effective against certain Gram-negative and Gram-positive organisms.

actinomycin. An antibiotic substance elaborated by *Streptomyces antibioticus* and other *Streptomyces* species, originally described as consisting of actinomycin A and actinomycin B. But the latter has been found to be an inactive oil contaminated with the antibiotic. It contains nitrogen, occurs as red platelets, and is active against a number of bacteria and fungi.

ac″ti·no·my·co′ma (ack″ti·no·migh·ko′muh) [*aktis; mykēs;* G. *-ōma*, tumor]. A tumor produced by the *Actinomyces*.

ac″ti·no·my·co′sis (·migh·ko′sis) [*aktis; mykēs;* G. *-ōsis*, condition]. A parasitic, infectious, inoculable disease affecting cattle, hogs, and sometimes communicated to man; caused by *Actinomyces bovis*, an anaerobe, and species of *Nocardia*, which are aerobic. The jaw is commonly involved (cervicofacial form) although other organs and systems may be infected (abdominal and thoracic or mediastinal forms). The disease is characterized by the formation of slow-growing granulomatous tumors which usually suppurate, discharging through multiple draining sinuses a thick oily pus containing yellowish granules, and by constitutional symptoms of sepsis. Also called *lumpy jaw, clyers, wooden tongue*. —**actinomycot′ic,** *adj.*

ac″ti·no·my′co·tin [*aktis; mykēs*]. An extract of cultures of *Actinomyces*, prepared like tuberculin and used in cases of actinomycosis.

ac'ti·non [*aktis*]. An = 219. Actinium emanation, an isotope of radon. Half-life 3.9 seconds.

ac"ti·no·neu·ri'tis [*aktis;* G. *neuron*, nerve; *-itis*, inflammation]. Neuritis from exposure to x-rays or radium.

ac"ti·no·phy·to'sis (ack"ti·no·figh·to'sis) [*aktis;* G. *phyton*, plant; *-ōsis*, condition]. A disease, usually caused by *Staphylococcus aureus*, characterized by granulomatous abscesses with granules simulating those of actinomycosis or streptothricosis. Syn., *botryomycosis.*

ac"tin·o·rho'dine. An antibiotic substance, possibly $C_{23}H_{20}O_{10}$, produced by a species of *Actinomyces;* it inhibits *Staphylococcus aureus.*

ac"tin·o·ru'bin. An antibiotic substance produced by a species of *Actinomyces* and named from its characteristic red mycelium; the substance is active against various organisms but is relatively toxic.

ac"ti·nos'co·py [*aktis;* G. *skopein*, to examine]. Examination of the body by x-rays. Syn., *skiascopy, radioscopy, fluoroscopy, roentgenoscopy.*

ac"ti·no·ther'a·py [*aktis;* G. *therapeia*, therapy]. Therapeutic use of chemical rays or radiant energy, including sunlight, ultraviolet light, x-rays, and emanations of radium or other radioactive matter. Syn., *radiotherapy.* —**actinotherapeu'tic,** *adj.*

ac'tion [L. *actio*, from *agere*, to do or to perform]. 1. Performance of a function or a movement. 2. Application or wielding of a force—physical, chemical, or mental. 3. *In pathology*, production of a morbid process. Syn., *activity.*

a. of arrest. Inhibition.

a. time. The duration of stimulation of the retina required to produce a visual sensation of maximum strength.

afteraction. The temporary negative variation of the electric current in a tetanized muscle after stimulation ceases.

antagonistic a. (a) Counteraction; opposition. (b) The effect of an opposing agent or principle. See *antagonism.*

ball-valve a. The alternate blocking and opening of a narrow passage by a floating object acting as a valve, as a gallstone in the common bile duct.

buffer a. That exhibited by certain chemical substances which, when added to a fluid, tend to maintain its reaction (pH) within narrow limits.

calorigenic a. (a) Specific dynamic action. (b) The total heat liberated by a food or food constituent when metabolized by the body.

capillary a. Capillary attraction; capillarity.

chemical a. The molecular change produced in any substance through the action of heat, light, electricity, or another chemical.

contact a. Catalysis.

cumulative a. Sudden and marked action of a drug after administration of a number of ineffectual or slightly effective doses.

electrocapillary a. The electric phenomena resulting from the chemical reaction between dissimilar fluids connected by a capillary medium.

hydrotropic a. Action which confers water-solubility on substances ordinarily not soluble in water, such as that of bile salts on fatty acids.

oligodynamic a. Toxicity of heavy metals in very dilute solution for Algae and other microorganisms.

opsonic a. The effect produced upon susceptible microorganisms and other cells by opsonins, which renders them vulnerable to phagocytes.

radiobiological a. The action of radiation on living things.

reflex a. A response of some peripheral organ to stimulation of the sensory branch of a reflex arc, the action occurring immediately, without the aid of the will or without even entering consciousness. Also called *automatic a.*

specific a. The action of certain remedial agents which possess exclusive curative powers for a particular disease symptom, or microorganism, as arsphenamine for syphilis, quinine for malaria, or biologicals like antimeningococcic and antipneumococcic serums.

specific dynamic a. The stimulating effect upon the metabolism produced by the ingestion of food, especially proteins, causing the metabolic rate to rise above basal levels.

synergistic a. See *synergy.*

thermogenic a. The action of various drugs and foods in raising the body temperature.

trigger a. A sudden stimulus which initiates a physiologic or pathologic process having nothing in common with the action that started it.

vital a. Physiologic activity or functions which are necessary for maintaining life, as the action of the heart, lungs, and vital centers of the brain and cord.

ac'tion po·ten'tial. See under *potential.*

ac"ti·thi·az'ic ac'id. $C_9H_{10}NO_3S$; an antibiotic substance, (−)-2-(5-carboxypentyl)-4-thiazolidone, isolated from a species of *Streptomyces* and also synthesized; it is effective *in vitro* against *Mycobacterium tuberculosis.*

ac"ti·va'tion [L. *activus*, active]. 1. The process of activating or rendering active. 2. Stimulation of general cellular activity by the use of nonspecific therapy; plasma activation. 3. Stimulation of the ovum by the sperm or other agents causing cell division. 4. *In chemistry*, the transformation of any substance into a more reactive form, including the renewal of activity of a catalyst. —**ac'tivate,** *v.*

a. analysis. See under *analysis.*

ac'ti·va"tor [*activus*]. 1. An agent which is necessary to activate another substance, as a coenzyme to an enzyme; applied to biochemical reactions. An enzyme activator is called *coenzyme* or *kinase.* 2. Internal secretion of the pancreas. 3. Substance which stimulates the development of an embryonic structure. Also called *inductor* or *organizer.* 4. Apparatus which charges water with radium emanations. 5. A catalyst.

ac'tive [*activus*]. 1. Energetic, decisive, as active treatment. 2. Due to an intrinsic as distinguished from a passive force, as active hyperemia. 3. *In optics*, possessing the ability to rotate the plane of a polarized light beam. 4. *In psychoanalysis*, pertaining to masculine qualities. 5. *In biochemistry*, referring or pertaining to a presumed derivative of a substance regarded as the participating form in biological reactions in which the parent compound itself does not exhibit full activity.

ac'tive cen'ter, ac'tive site. 1. That part of the enzyme to which the substrate or necessary cofactor is linked in normal enzymatic function. 2. That part of an antibody to which the antigen or hapten is linked in a normal antigen-antibody reaction.

activin. Trade-mark for an injectable solution containing casein in combination with sodium iodohydroxyquinoline sulfonate: used in nonspecific protein therapy.

ac·tiv'i·ty [*activus*]. Capacity for acting; sensibility; vitality; potency; energy.

optical a. The ability of a substance to rotate the plane of vibration of polarized light. It is characteristic of compounds having an asymmetric atom, usually of carbon.

specific a. *In radiobiology*, the number of disintegrations per unit time per unit mass of radioactive subsatnce.

actol. Trade name for silver lactate.

ac″to·my′o·sin. A protein complex consisting of myosin and actin, forming the major constituent of the muscle fibril and, presumably, of the contractile mechanism. Actomyosin is soluble in concentrated salt solutions (e.g. 0.5 M KCl) in which state, as evidenced by high viscosity, turbidity, and flow birefringence, it consists of large molecular swarms. Adenosinetriphosphate (ATP) affects these physical properties and is able to cause contraction of actomyosin fibers in a suitable electrolyte medium.

actophen. Trade-mark for a preparation containing purified activated ergosterol (vitamin D_2) and bile salts; used when high dosage of the vitamin is required.

ac′tu·al [L. *actualis*, active, from *agere*, to do]. Real, existent; effective; not potential, as actual cautery.

ac′u- [L. *acus*, needle]. A combining form meaning *needle*.

a·cu″es·the′si·a. Acoustic sensibility; hearing.

a·cu′i·ty [L. *acuere*, to sharpen]. 1. Sharpness; clearness; keenness; distinctness, as of vision. 2. *In optics*, sharpness and clarity, as of a visual image when a lens is in focus.

auditory a. The degree of acuteness or clearness of hearing.

darkness a. Acuity of vision in comparative darkness.

displacement threshold a. Minimal displacement of a line necessary to produce doubling.

minimal separable a. Minimal angle of separation between two points to produce doubling. At the fovea, the measurements are from 50 to 64 seconds of arc.

minimal visual a. Smallest image to which the brain responds, threshold illumination being present.

vernier a. The ability of the eye to perceive a break in contour; the aligning discrimination of the eye, accurate on an average to a few seconds of arc (3.0–3.5), or less than the diameter of a single foveal cone.

visual a. Extent of visual perception, dependent upon the clarity of the retinal focus, integrity of the nervous elements, and cerebral interpretation of the stimulus. It is tested usually with Snellen's letters at 20 feet.

a·cu′le·ate [L. *aculeus*, a sting, prickle]. 1. *In botany*, armed with prickles, as the rose or other brier. 2. *In zoology*, having a sting.

a·cu′me·ter (a·cue′mi·tur, a·kōō′·). See *acoumeter*.

a·cu′mi·nate [L. *acuminatus*, from *acuminare*, to make pointed]. Sharp-pointed; conical; tapering to a point.

ac′u·pres″sure [L. *acus*, needle; *pressura*, pressure]. An operation to stop hemorrhage by compressing the artery with a needle inserted into the tissues upon either side.

ac′u·punc″ture [*acus*; L. *punctura*, a pricking]. Puncture of the tissues with long fine needles; used for centuries for relief of neuralgic pain or the release of fluid.

a′cus [L.]. A surgical needle.

ac″u·sec′tor [*acus*; L. *sector*, a cutter]. An electric needle, operating on a high-frequency current, which cuts tissues like a scalpel. —**acusec′tion,** *n.*

-a·cu′si·a (-a·cue′zhuh, ·zee·uh, ·shuh, ·see·uh, -a·kōō′·). See *-acousia*.

a·cus′ti·cus (a·kōōs′ti·kus) [G. *akoustikos*, from *akouein*, to hear]. The auditory or eighth cranial nerve.

a·cute′ [L. *acutus*, sharp]. 1. Sharp; severe. 2. Having a rapid onset, a short course, and pronounced symptoms; not chronic.

a·cute′ness [*acutus*]. 1. The quality of being acute, rapid, or sharp. 2. *In ophthalmology*, acuity; keenness of vision.

a·cu″ti·cos′tal [*acutus*; L. *costa*, a rib]. Having projecting ribs.

a·cu′to- [*acutus*]. A combining form meaning *acute*.

a·cy″a·no·blep′si·a (ay·sigh″uh·no·blep′see·uh, a·sigh″·). See *acyanopsia*.

a·cy″a·nop′si·a [G. *a-*, not; *kyanos*, blue; *opsis*, sight]. Inability to see blue colors. Also called *acyanoblepsia, acyoblepsia*.

a·cy″a·not′ic [*a-*; *kyanos*; G. *-ōsis*, condition]. Without cyanosis, as an acyanotic congenital cardiovascular defect.

a·cy′cli·a (ay·sigh′klee·uh, a·sigh′·, ay·sick′lee·uh, a·sick′·) [*a-*; G. *kyklios*, from *kyklein*, to revolve]. State of arrested circulation of body fluids.

a·cy′clic (ay·sigh′click, a·sigh′click, ay·sick′lick, a·sick′lick) [*a-*; G. *kyklikos*, from *kyklein*]. 1. Not occurring in cycles; not characterized by a self-limited course; nonintermittent. See *cyclic*. 2. *In chemistry*, denoting organic compounds with an open-chain structure; aliphatic. 3. *In botany*, not whorled.

ac″y·e′sis, ac″i·e′sis (ass″ee·ee′sis, ass″eye·ee′sis) [*a-*; G. *kyēsis*, pregnancy]. 1. Sterility of the female. 2. Nonpregnancy. 3. Incapacity for natural delivery. —**acyet′ic,** *adj.*

ac′yl (ass′il, ass′eel). An organic radical derived by removal of a hydroxyl group (OH) from an organic acid: thus, R.CO is derived from R.CO.OH.

ac″yl·a′tion (ass″i·lay′shun). Introduction of an acyl radical into a compound.

a·cys′ti·a (ay·sis′tee·uh, a·sis′·) [*a-*; G. *kystis*, bladder]. Absence of the urinary bladder.

A d Abbreviation for anistropic disk.

a.d. *Auris dextra;* right ear.

ad- [L.]. A prefix signifying *to, toward, near, addition to*, and *more intense*.

-ad [G. *-as, -ados*, a fem. suffix]. 1. A suffix used to form *collective numerals*. 2. *In chemistry*, a suffix used to form the names of *elements, atoms*, or *radicals*. 3. *In botany*, a suffix used to form the names of *individual members of groups*.

-ad [L. *ad*, to, toward]. *In anatomy* and *zoology*, an adverbial suffix indicating *direction toward*.

A. D. A. American Dental Association, American Dietetic Association.

a·dac′ry·a (ay·dack′ree·uh, a·dack′·) [G. *a-*, not; *dakryon*, tear]. Absence or deficiency of tears.

a·dac·tyl′i·a (ay·dack·til′ee·uh, a·dack·) [*a-*; G. *daktylos*, finger]. Congenital absence of fingers or toes, or both. —**adac′tylous,** *adj.;* **adac′tylism, adac′tylus,** *n.;* **adac′tyl,** *adj., n.*

adagol. Trade-mark for a vitamin A and D concentrate of fish-liver oils.

Adair-Dighton syndrome. See under *syndrome*.

adalin. Trade-mark for a brand of carbromal.

ad″a·man′tine (ad″uh·man′teen, ·tyne) [G. *adamas*, adamant]. Pertaining to dental enamel; very hard.

ad″a·man″ti·no·car″ci·no′ma [*adamas*; G. *karkinos*, crab; *-ōma*, tumor]. A malignant ameloblastoma.

ad″a·man″ti·no′ma, ad″a·man·to′ma. See *ameloblastoma*.

ad″a·man′to·blast. See *ameloblast*.

ad″a·man″to·blas·to′ma. See *ameloblastoma*.

Adami, John George [*English pathologist in Canada*, 1862–1926]. Remembered for his studies concerning cardiac overstrain and heredity, and for his advancement of a theory of immunity similar to Ehrlich's side-chain theory.

Adamkiewicz, Albert [*Austrian pathologist*, 1850–1921]. Known for his description of the crescent-shaped cells found beneath the neurilemma of medullated nerve fibers, and for his protein reaction using sulfuric and glacial acetic acids.

Adams, James Alexander [*Scottish surgeon*, 1857–1930]. Devised an operation similar to the Alexander operation for retroversion of the uterus (1882).

Adams, Robert [*Irish physician*, 1791–1875]. Gave a classic description of heart block (1826). The characteristic syndrome of syncope and heart block, with or without convulsive seizures, is known as *Stokes-Adams syndrome, Spens syndrome.*

Adams, William [*English surgeon*, 1820–1900]. Remembered for his subtrochanteric osteotomy for correction of deformity due to bony ankylosis of the hip (1871). This operation, as performed by Adams, followed the principle set forth by Barton (1826), and later became standardized under Gant's technique.

Adam's apple. Common term for the laryngeal prominence. Also called *pomum Adami.*

ad'ams·ite (ad'um·zite, ·sight). A poison gas used in chemical warfare; diphenylaminechloroarsine.

adanon hydrochloride. A trade-marked name for methadon hydrochloride.

Ad"an·so'ni·a [after Michel *Adanson*, French naturalist, 1727–1806]. A genus of trees of the Bombacaceae.

A. digitata. The baobab of Africa and India, whose dried leaves are used by the natives as an antipyretic.

ad"ap·ta'tion [L. *adaptare*, to adjust]. 1. *In biology,* any change in structure, form, or habits of an organism to suit a new environment. 2. *In ophthalmology,* normal ability of the eye to adjust to varying intensities of light. See *biophotometer*. 3. Immunization. 4. In reflex action, decline in the frequency of impulses when the sensory nerve is stimulated repeatedly. 5. *In dentistry,* proper fitting of a denture or accurate adjustment of bands to teeth; close approximation of filling material to the walls of a tooth cavity. 6. *In psychiatry,* those changes experienced by an individual which lead to adjustment.

catalyzed a. *In psychoanalysis,* the best response to stress which the therapist can elicit from the patient.

dark a. Adjustment of the iris and retina for night vision. In a clinical test for the determination of vitamin-A sufficiency, the eye is exposed to a standard light and its adjustment to darkness is measured.

a·dap·ta'tion di·sease'. According to Selye, a biochemical or metabolic disorder due to physical or emotional stress, with a reversability which may be effected spontaneously, therapeutically, or accidentally.

a·dapt'er, a·dap'tor [*adaptare*]. 1. A device which permits the fitting of one part of an instrument or apparatus to another, as a glass or rubber tube or metal collar. 2. An apparatus which converts the electric current to the form required in the various types of electrotherapy, or for a particular electric appliance.

ad"ap·tom'e·ter [*adaptare;* G. *metron*, a measure]. An instrument for measuring the time taken for retinal adaptation or for regeneration of the rhodopsin (visual purple); used to determine the minimum light threshold and to diagnose night blindness.

Aero Medical Laboratory radium-plaque a. One consisting of a radium plaque of constant brightness in the scotopic range; the test object is a Landolt ring, the effective size of which is varied by changing the testing distance.

ad'at"om [L. *ad*, to; G. *atomos*, indivisible]. An atom held on a surface by adsorption.

ad·ax'i·al [*ad;* L. *axis*, axis]. On the side of, or directed toward, the axis.

ADC Anodal duration contraction.

add. Abbreviation for *adde* or *additur* in prescription writing, meaning *add*, or *let there be added.*

ad'de [imperative sing. of L. *addere*, to add]. Add; a direction used in prescription writing.

ad de·liq'. *Ad deliquium (animi);* to the point of fainting.

ad"de·pha'gi·a. See *adephagia.*

ad'der [AS. *nǣdre*]. The common name of several genera of snakes, especially the *Vipera berus* of Britain and Europe, or of species of other genera of terrestrial snakes.

death a. See *Acanthophis antarcticus.*

puff a. See *Bitis lachesis.*

ad'dict [L. *addictum*, from *addicere*, to devote]. One who is habituated to some practice, especially the alcohol or drug habit. A **drug addict** is one who uses habitually a narcotic drug for the comfort such indulgence affords, and who has no illness or other legitimate reasons for such practice. —**addict'**, *v.t., v.i.;* **addic'tion,** *n.*

ad'di·ment [L. *addere*, to add]. Complement. —**addimen'tary,** *adj.*

Addis' method. See under *method.*

Addis and Shevky's test. See under *test.*

ad'dis·in. A substance in the gastric juice which stimulates the hematopoietic functions of the bone marrow. An extract of the gastric mucosa of swine is used in treating pernicious anemia. Also called *biermerin.*

Addison, Christopher [*English anatomist*, 1869–]. Described a series of planes, known as *Addison's planes*, which are used as landmarks in the topographic anatomy of the abdomen and thorax.

Addison, Thomas [*English physician, diagnostician, and teacher*, 1793–1860]. Described pernicious anemia (called *Addison's anemia*) and studied diseases of the ductless glands, particularly the adrenals. Adrenal cortical hypofunction is also known as *Addison's disease, adrenal insufficiency.*

Ad'di·son·ism [after Thomas *Addison*]. A syndrome sometimes present in pulmonary tuberculosis, consisting of dark pigmentation of the skin, loss of weight and strength; somewhat resembles true Addison's disease.

ad·di'tion [L. *additio*, from *addere*, to add]. *In chemistry,* a reaction in which two elements or compounds unite without the loss or substitution of any atoms, or any loss of valence, as $H_2O + CO_2 = H_2CO_3$, $HCl + NH_3 = NH_4Cl$. Also called *a. reaction.*

ad·du'cent [L. *adducere*, to lead to]. Adducting.

ad·duct' [L. *adductum*, from *adducere*]. 1. Draw toward the median line of a body. 2. *In optics,* turn the eyes inward from the central position.

ad·duc'tion [*adductum*]. 1. Any movement whereby one part is brought toward another or toward the median line of the body. 2. *In ophthalmology,* turning of the eyes inward from the central position, through contraction of the medial rectus muscles. This action may be voluntary, but usually is subconscious, following the stimulus of accommodation. The power of adduction, provoked by fixation of the gaze upon an object placed at the near point, is called **convergence-stimulus adduction.**

ad·duc'tor [*adductum*]. Any muscle which draws a part toward the median line of the body. See Table of Muscles in the Appendix.

a. brevis. The short adductor of the femur.

a. digiti secundi. A rare variant slip of muscle associated with the adductor hallucis and inserted into the lateral side of base of proximal phalanx of second toe.

a. hallucis. The adductor of the great toe.

a. hallucis transversus. Old name for the transverse head of the adductor of the great toe.

a. longus. The long adductor of the femur.

a. magnus. The largest adductor of the femur.

a. minimus. A variable portion of the adductor magnus muscle of the thigh.

a. pollicis. That of the thumb.

a. pollicis obliquus. The oblique or carpal head of the adductor pollicis muscle.

a. pollicis transversus. Old name for transverse or metacarpal head of the adductor pollicis muscle.

A″de·cid″u·a′ta [G. *a-*, not; L. *deciduus*, falling off]. A division of mammals including those not having a deciduate placenta.

a·de″lo·mor′phous, a·de″lo·mor′phic (a·dee″lo·, ad″i·lo·) [*a-;* G. *dēlos*, visible; *morphē*, form]. Not clearly defined; applied to certain cells in the gastric glands.

a·del′pho·site [G. *adelphos*, brother; *sitos*, food]. An acardiac monster. Syn., *acardius, acardiacus, omphalosite.*

a·del′pho·tax″is, a·del′pho·tax″y [*adelphos;* G. *taxis*, arrangement]. The tendency of motile cells to arrange themselves into definite positions.

-a·del′phus [*adelphos*]. Suffix used by I. Geoffroy St. Hilaire to signify inferior duplicity in conjoined twins.

ad′en-. See *adeno-*.

ad″en·al′gi·a [G. *adēn*, gland; *algos*, pain]. Pain due to an inflamed gland.

ad′e·nase. A deaminizing enzyme which converts adenine to hypoxanthine. It is secreted by the liver, pancreas, and spleen.

ad″en·as·the′ni·a [*adēn;* G. *astheneia*, want of strength]. Functional deficiency of a gland.

ad″en·drit′ic, a·den′dric [G. *a-*, not; *dendron*, tree]. Lacking dendrites, applied to certain spinal ganglion cells.

ad″en·ec′to·my [G. *adēn*, gland; *ektomē*, excision]. The excision of a gland.

ad″en·ec·to′pi·a [*adēn;* G. *ektopos*, away from a place]. Occurrence of a gland in an abnormal place.

A′den fe′ver. Dengue.

a·de′ni·a [*adēn*]. A chronic affection of the lymph nodes characterized by marked hypertrophy but no leukocytosis.

angibromic a. Any affection of the lymphatic tissue of the digestive tract.

leukemic a. Enlargement of lymph nodes associated with a leukemia.

simple a. Lymphomatosis without leukocytosis; Hodgkin's disease.

a·den′i·form [*adēn; -form*]. Glandlike; shaped like a gland.

ad′e·nine (ad′i·neen, ·nin). $C_5H_5N_5$. 6-Aminopurine; the simplest member of the uric acid group of leucomaines. It occurs with other purine bases as a nonpoisonous decomposition product of nuclein, and is found in animal and vegetable tissues rich in nucleated cells, as the liver, pancreas, kidneys, and spleen, and in the urine of leukemic patients.

a. hypoxanthine. $C_5H_5N_5 + C_5H_4N_4O$. A compound of adenine and hypoxanthine, belonging to the leucomaines.

a. sulfate. $(C_5H_5N_5)_2H_2SO_4$. A compound used in the nucleotide treatment of acute agranulocytosis, and in pneumonia.

ad″e·ni′tis [*adēn;* G. *-itis*, inflammation]. Inflammation of a gland or lymph node.

acute salivary a. An infectious disease epidemic about Naples, Italy, affecting the parotid and other salivary glands and causing splenomegaly and pain in the axillary lymph nodes.

cervical a. One of a number of various inflammatory conditions, acute and chronic, which affect the lymph nodes of the neck, especially in children. It is often secondary to acute infections of the mouth, throat, and ears; to lice infestation of the scalp; and is associated with contagious diseases, such as rubella, measles, scarlet fever, etc. In chronic tuberculosis, leukemias, and syphilis, it occurs as part of a generalized lymph-node involvement.

infectious a. See infectious *mononucleosis.*

lacrimal a. Dacryoadenitis.

paratracheal a. Inflammation of the paratracheal lymph nodes: a common complication of tuberculosis.

phlegmonous a. Inflammation of a gland and the adjacent connective tissue.

primitive syphilitic a. Enlarged lymph nodes associated with a primary lesion, which follow a slow indolent course of six months or more.

tropical a. Climatic bubo; venereal lymphogranuloma.

universal a. Widespread induration of the lymph nodes, associated with primary syphilis.

venereal a. Venereal lymphogranuloma.

A·de′ni·um. A genus of the Apocynaceae, the various species of which have provided arrow poisons for the African natives. Glycosides have been obtained which have a digitalislike action on the heart but cause tetanic convulsions.

ad′e·no-, ad′en- [*adēn*]. A combining form denoting *gland, glandular*, or *relation to glands.*

ad″e·no·ac″an·tho′ma [*adēn;* G. *akantha*, prickle; *-ōma*, tumor]. An adenocarcinoma, usually of low malignancy, in which much of the cylindrical epithelium of the acinic spaces is replaced by squamous epithelium: frequent in the uterus.

ad″e·no·a·me″lo·blas·to′ma. An ameloblastoma in which the epithelium exhibits a glandular structure and arrangement.

ad″e·no·an″gi·o·sar·co′ma. A malignant *mesenchymoma.*

ad″e·no·can′croid. Adenoacanthoma.

ad″e·no·car″ci·no′ma. One originating in glandular or ductal epithelium and tending to produce acinic structures. Differentiation of the adenocarcinomas depends on the degree of resemblance which the acinic structures bear to the gland; the completely undifferentiated form is the *carcinoma simplex*, and the most highly differentiated tumor is sometimes named *malignant adenoma.*

a. of lung. A form of bronchogenic *carcinoma.*

a. of testis. See embryonal *carcinoma* of testis.

alveolar a. of thyroid. See follicular *a.* of thyroid.

comedo a. See *comedo-carcinoma.*

cystic mucoid a. See pseudomucinous *cystadenocarcinoma.*

feminizing a. A malignant feminizing tumor.

follicular a. of thyroid. A glandular carcinoma showing follicles and invasion grossly as well as microscopically: also called *alveolar a. of thyroid.*

mucoid a. See pseudomucinous *cystadenocarcinoma.*

papillary a. See papilliferous *carcinoma.*

papillary a. of thyroid. A glandular carcinoma of the thyroid, often cystic, which produces papillae and shows gross and microscopic evidence of invasion: also called *papillary cystadenocarcinoma of thyroid.*

virilizing a. A malignant masculinizing tumor of an ovary.

ad′e·no·cele [*adēn;* G. *kēlē*, tumor]. A cystic tumor containing adenomatous tissue. See *adenoma.*

ad″e·no·cel″lu·li′tis [*adēn;* L. *cellula,* dim. of *cella,* cavity; G. *-itis,* inflammation]. Inflammation of a gland and the surrounding cellular tissue.

ad″e·no·chon·dro′ma (ad″i·no·kon·dro′muh) [*adēn;* G. *chondros,* cartilage; *-ōma,* tumor]. A tumor consisting of both glandular and cartilaginous tissue. Also see mixed *tumor* of salivary gland type.

ad″e·no·cys·to′ma (ad″i·no·sis·to′muh). See *cystadenoma.*

papillary a. of thyroid. See papillary *adenoma* of thyroid.

teratoid a. See *mesonephroma.*

ad″e·no·cys″to·sar·co′ma. See *cystadenosarcoma.* Also see *cystosarcoma phylloides.*

ad″e·no·fi·bro′ma (·figh·bro′muh) [*adēn;* L. *fibra,* fiber; G. *-ōma,* tumor]. Combination of adenoma and fibroma frequently occurring in the uterus. See also *fibroadenoma.*

pseudomucinous a. See pseudomucinous *cystadenoma.*

ad″e·no·fi·bro′sis (·figh·bro′sis) [*adēn; fibra;* G. *-ōsis,* condition]. Fibroid degeneration of a gland, particularly the replacement fibrosis following inflammation. See *fibrosis.*

endometrioid a. See *adenomyosis.* Obs.

ad″e·no·gen′e·sis [*adēn;* G. *genesis,* production]. Development of a gland.

ad″e·nog′e·nous (ad″i·nodj′i·nus), **ad″e·no·gen′ic** [*adēn;* G. *genesthai,* from *gignesthai,* to be produced]. Originating from a gland.

ad″e·no·hy″per·sthe′ni·a [*adēn;* G. *hyper,* over; *sthenos,* strength]. Excessive activity of the glands.

a. gastrica. A condition in which the secretion of gastric juice is greatly increased or excessively acid.

ad″e·no·hy·poph′y·sis (ad″i·no·high·pof′i·sis) [*adēn;* G. *hypophysis,* from *hypo,* under, *physis,* growth]. The glandular part of the pituitary gland, developing from somatic ectoderm of the posterior nasopharynx (Rathke's pouch). It has three subdivisions: anteriorly the *pars distalis* (*pars anterior, anterior lobe of the hypophysis,* 1), medially the *pars intermedia* (*intermediate lobe of the hypophysis*), and superiorly the *pars tuberalis.* Formerly called *pars buccalis, pars glandularis.* See also *neurohypophysis.*

ad′e·noid [*adēn;* G. *eidos,* form]. 1. A structure consisting of reticular connective tissue supporting masses of small lymphocytes, as found in lymph nodes, spleen, red bone marrow, and other lymphoid organs. *Rare.* 2. Hypertrophied lymphoid tissue often present in the nasopharynx; occurs especially in children. Also called *pharyngeal tonsil.* See Plate 12. —**ad′e·noid,** *adj.*

ad″e·noi·dec′to·my [*adēn; eidos;* G. *ektomē,* excision]. The surgical removal of adenoids.

ad″e·noid′es per″i·to·ni′tis. See *adenomyosis.*

ad′e·noid·ism [*adēn; eidos*]. Series of changes in respiration, facial contour, and tooth arrangement resulting from the presence of adenoids.

ad″e·noi·di′tis [*adēn; eidos;* G. *-itis,* inflammation]. Inflammation of adenoids.

ad′e·noids. See *adenoid,* 2.

ad″e·no·lei″o·my″o·fi·bro′ma, ad″e·no·li″o·my″o·fi·bro′ma (ad″i·no·lye″o·my″o·figh·bro′muh) [*adēn;* G. *leios,* smooth; *mys,* muscle; L. *fibra,* fiber; G. *-ōma,* tumor]. A leiomyofibroma containing glandular tissue.

ad″e·no·li·po′ma [*adēn;* G. *lipos,* fat; *-ōma*]. A combination of adenoma and lipoma.

ad″e·no·li·po″ma·to′sis [*adēn; lipos; -ōma;* G. *-ōsis,* condition]. Diffuse symmetrical lipomatosis; the fatty masses are large, disfiguring, and not encapsulated. More common in men than in women.

ad″e·no·log″a·di′tis (·log″uh·dye′tis, ·lo″guh·dye′tis) [*adēn;* G. *logades,* whites of the eyes; *-itis,* inflammation]. 1. Ophthalmia neonatorum. 2. Inflammation of the glands and conjunctiva of the eyes.

ad″e·no·lym·phi′tis [*adēn;* L. *lympha,* water; *-itis*]. Lymphadenitis.

ad″e·no·lym′pho·cele (ad″i·no·lim′fo·seel) [*adēn; lympha;* G. *kēlē,* tumor]. Widening of the lymphatics and cystic dilatation of the lymph nodes, from obstruction.

ad″e·no·lym·pho′ma [*adēn; lympha;* G. *-ōma,* tumor]. Adenoma of a lymph node. See *lymphadenoma.*

ad″e·no′ma [*adēn; -ōma*]. A benign tumor of glandular origin which in its growth more or less reduplicates acini, tubules, or both.

acidophilic a. 1. An eosinophilic adenoma of the pituitary gland. 2. A sweat-gland tumor.

a. of bronchus. A slowly growing, at first circumscribed but later sometimes invasive or slowly metastasizing, polypoid or sessile, epithelial neoplasm involving the subepithelial tissues, usually of proximal bronchi. Two forms occur: (a) the **carcinoid** form, made up of uniformly small cells with finely granular acidophilic cytoplasm and nuclei finely stippled with chromatin. The cells are situated about delicate sinusoidal vessels. Argentaffin granules are rare. An infrequent variant of this form, seen in older individuals, is a tumor consisting partially or wholly of oncocytes. (b) the **cylindroid** form, made up of basophilic staining epithelial cells arranged in branching cylinders or tubules. Also called *adenocystic* or *adenoid basal-cell carcinoma, adenomatoid tumor, bronchial adenoma, mixed tumor, mucoepidermoid tumor, reserve-cell tumor, vascular adenoma* (all of *bronchus*)*: benign glandular* (*bronchiogenic*) *tumor.*

a. destruens. A destructive, invasive form, really adenocarcinoma.

a. malignum. See malignant *a.*

a. pseudosarcomatodes. See *cystosarcoma phylloides.*

a. rete ovarii. See adrenocorticoid *a.* of the ovary.

a. sebaceum. Localized hyperplasia of sebaceous glands forming distinct papules, usually seen on the skin of the nose and cheeks, and frequently associated with tuberous sclerosis: also called *Pringle's tumor.*

a. substantiae corticalis suprarenalis. Cortical *a.*

a. sudoriparum. One derived from and reproducing tissue of sweat glands. Syn., *hidradenoma.*

a. testiculi ovotestes. See adrenocorticoid *a.* of the ovary.

a. tubulare ovarii, a. tubulare ovarii testiculare. See adrenocorticoid *a.* of the ovary.

adrenal a. See cortical *a., pheochromocytoma.*

adrenocorticoid a. of the ovary. One of a rare group of closely related masculinizing tumors of the ovary, clinically characterized by production of defemination or virilism, and composed of cells resembling those of the adrenal cortex. Special stains, in many instances, disclose fat and glycogen droplets and sometimes fuchsinophilic granules, but histologic appearance varies from tumor to tumor and even within the same neoplasm. Malignant transformation is rare. This classification includes lesions formerly designated as *a. rete ovarii, a. testiculi ovotestes, a. tubulare ovarii, a. tubulare ovarii testiculare, testicular* (*tubular*) *a. of ovary, tubular a., tubular a. of ovary, Wolffian a., tubular hamartoma of ovary, masculinoma, masculinovoblastoma, struma androblastoma of ovary, suprarenalis aberrata of ovary, adrenal clear-cell tumor of ovary, adrenocortical tumor of ovary,* *androgenic hilar-cell tumor or hilus-cell tumor, Grawitz tumor of ovary, hypernephroid tumor, sympathotropic-cell tumor, virilizing lipoid-cell tumor.*

basophilic a. Adenoma of the pituitary gland made up of basophilic cells.

chromophobe a. Adenoma of the pituitary gland made up of chromophobe cells, neither basophilic nor acidophilic.

colloid a. of thyroid. An encapsulated adenoma containing excessive colloid within greatly distended follicles, which may vary markedly in size: also called *macrofollicular a.*

cortical a. A benign encapsulated neoplasm composed principally of cells resembling those of the adrenal cortex, but with little or no tendency to form acini: also called *adenoma subtantiae corticalis suprarenalis, adrenal hypernephroma, functioning cortical tumor, granular cell tumor of adrenal cortex.*

cystic a. One in which the acini are enlarged or distended to form cysts.

embryonal a. of thyroid. A poorly differentiated follicular adenoma characterized by columnlike arrangement of small, closely packed thyroid cells. Follicles are either absent or small, and rarely contain colloid. Also called *trabecular a.*

eosinophilic a. 1. Adenoma of the pituitary gland, characterized by multiplication of eosinophilic or acidophilic cells. In early life, often accompanied by gigantism: in later life, by acromegaly. 2. A sweat-gland tumor.

feminizing a. See feminizing *tumor.*

fetal a. of thyroid. A follicular adenoma of the thyroid made up of numerous small follicles of a primitive or fetal type, containing little or no colloid: also called *microfollicular a.*

follicular a. of thyroid. A benign epithelial neoplasm with cells and gross patterns similar to those seen in normal or embryonic thyroid glands. Follicles are usually present.

Hürthle cell a. See Hürthle cell *tumor.*

islet a. See islet-cell *tumor.*

Langerhansian a. See islet-cell *tumor.*

macrofollicular a. See colloid *a.* of thyroid.

malignant a. A well-differentiated adenocarcinoma: also called *a. malignam.*

malignant a. of thyroid. See follicular *carcinoma* of thyroid.

medullary a. of the adrenal. See *pheochromocytoma.*

microfollicular a. See fetal *a.* of thyroid.

papillary a. One which grows from a surface in papillary form. Also see serous *cystadenoma.*

papillary a. of thyroid. A tumor of the thyroid which produces papillae and has a tendency to form cysts: also called *adenocystoma* or *cystadenoma of thyroid.*

papilliferous a. One in which papillary projections grow into the acini.

pleomorphic (salivary) a. See mixed *tumor* of salivary gland type.

pseudomucinous (solid) a. See pseudomucinous *cystadenoma.*

pseudomucinous tubular a. See pseudomucinous *cystadenoma.*

pseudosolid a. of the ovary. See pseudomucinous *cystadenoma.*

simple a. of thyroid. Encapsulated adenoma made up of well-differentiated thyroid tissue with follicles and colloid content comparable to that of a normal gland.

testicular a. See *androblastoma.*

testicular (tubular) a. of the ovary. See adrenocorticoid *a.* of the ovary.

thyroid a. A benign tumor arising from glandular epithelium which can be differentiated into follicular and papillary types.

trabecular a. See embryonal *a.* of thyroid.

tubular a. One in which the spaces are elongated in the form of tubules.

tubular a. of the ovary. See adrenocorticoid *a.* of the ovary.

Wolffian a. See adrenocorticoid *a.* of the ovary.

ad″e·no·ma·la′ci·a [*adēn;* G. *malakia,* softness]. Abnormal softening of a gland.

ad″e·no′ma·tome [*adēn;* G. *-ōma,* tumor; *tomos,* cutting]. Cutting forceps or scissors for use in the removal of adenomatous growths; surgical instrument for excising adenoids.

ad″e·no·ma·to′sis [*adēn; -ōma;* G. *-ōsis,* condition]. Condition characterized by multiple overgrowths of glandular tissue.

cancerous pulmonary a. A more malignant form of bronchiolar carcinoma.

fibrosing a. Adenosis of the breast.

polypoid a. See acquired multiple *polyposis.*

pulmonary a. A relatively benign, slowly progressive form of bronchiolar carcinoma.

ad″e·nom′a·tous, ad″e·nmo′a·toip [*adēn; -ōma*]. Pertaining to an adenoma; characteristic of glandular hyperplasia.

ad′e·no·mere [*adēn;* G. *meros,* part]. That portion of a developing gland which will be responsible for its functioning.

ad″e·no·my″o·hy·per·pla′si·a. See isthmic nodular *salpingitis.*

ad″e·no·my·o′ma (ad″i·no·migh·o′muh) [*adēn;* G. *mys,* muscle; *-ōma,* tumor]. Tumor which occurs in the uterus, adnexa, parametrial structures, and rectum; composed of leiomyoma in which adenomatous acini are incorporated.

ad″e·no·my″o·me·tri′tis [*adēn; mys;* G. *mētra,* womb; *-itis,* inflammation]. Inflammatory thickening of the uterine wall, resembling an adenomyoma.

ad″e·no·my″o·sar·co′ma [*adēn; mys;* G. *sarkōma,* fleshy excrescence; *-ōma,* tumor]. Malignant tumor composed of muscular and glandular elements.

embryonal a. A malignant mesenchymoma.

ad″e·no·my·o′sis (ad″i·no·migh·o′sis) [*adēn; mys;* G. *-ōsis,* condition]. The invasion of the uterine musculature by endometrial tissue through direct extension from the mucosa of the uterus: formerly called *endometrioid adenofibrosis.* Syn., *internal endometriosis.* See also *endometriosis.*

a. of fallopian tube. See isthmic nodular *salpingitis.*

ad″e·no·myx″o·chon″dro·sar·co′ma. See mixed *tumor* of salivary gland type.

ad″e·no·myx·o′ma [*adēn;* G. *myxa,* mucus; *-ōma,* tumor]. A growth having the characters of glandular and mucoid tissues.

ad″e·no·myx″o·sar·co′ma [*adēn; myxa;* G. *sarkōma,* fleshy excrescence]. A rare type of rapidly growing, malignant, mixed tumor arising from glandular and mucoid tissue, the latter undergoing sarcomatous change.

ad″e·non′cus [*adēn;* G. *ogkos,* mass]. An enlargement or tumor of a gland. *Obs.*

ad″e·nop′a·thy [*adēn;* G. *pathos,* disease]. Any glandular disease, especially the swelling and enlargement of lymph nodes.

ad″e·no·phar″yn·gi′tis [*adēn;* G. *pharygx,* pharynx; *-itis,* inflammation]. Inflammation of the tonsils and pharynx.

ad″e·no·phleg′mon [*adēn;* G. *phlegmonē,* inflammation]. Suppurative inflammation of a gland.

ad″e·no·sal″pin·gi′tis. See isthmic nodular *salpingitis.*

ad″e·no·sar·co′ma [*adēn;* G. *sarkōma,* fleshy excrescence]. A tumor with the characters of adenoma and sarcoma combined.

a. of kidney. See Wilms's *tumor*.

ad″e·no·sar″co·rhab″do·my·o′ma (·sahr″ko-rab″do·migh·o′muh) [*adēn;* G. *sarx*, flesh; *rhabdos*, rod; *mys*, muscle; *-ōma*, tumor]. A tumor composed of the elements of sarcoma, adenoma, and rhabdomyoma.

ad″e·no·scle·ro′sis [*adēn;* G. *sklērōsis*, a hardening]. A hardening of a gland, with or without swelling.

ad′e·nose (ad′i·noce, ·noze) [*adēn;* L. *-osus*, suffix meaning *fullness*]. Glandular; abounding in glands; glandlike.

a·den′o·sine (a·den′o·seen, ·sin, ad′i·no·seen″, ·sin″). $C_5H_4N_5.C_5H_9O_4$. A mononucleoside composed of adenine and D-ribose produced by the hydrolysis of adinosinemonophosphate.

a·den″o·sine·di·phos′phate (·dye·fos′fate). A compound of one molecule each of adenine and D-ribose and two molecules of phosphoric acid. It is an intermediate compound in the production of energy for muscular and perhaps other types of cellular work. Abbreviated ADP. Syn., *adenosinediphosphoric acid.* See *adenosinetriphosphate.*

adenosinediphosphoric acid. Adenosinediphosphate.

a·den″o·sine·mon″o·phos′phate. A compound of one molecule each of adenine, D-ribose, and phosphoric acid. It occurs in muscle and other tissues, as well as in yeast; that from the former source is adenosine-5-phosphate, while that from the latter is adenosine-3-phosphate. The acid is an intermediate product in the release of energy for muscular and perhaps other types of cellular work. Abbreviated AMP. Syn., *adenosinemonophosphoric acid, adenylic acid.*

a·den″o·sine·mon″o·phos·phor′ic ac′id. Adenosinemonophosphate.

a·den″o·sine·tri·phos′pha·tase (·try·fos′fuh-tace, ·taze). An enzyme catalyzing the hydrolysis of adenosinetriphosphate. Several different enzymes exist, one of them related to myosin. The decomposition of adenosinetriphosphate is believed to provide the energy for cellular activities such as muscular contraction. Abbreviated ATPase. Syn. *adenylpyrophosphatase.*

a·den″o·sine·tri·phos′phate. A compound of one molecule each of adenine and D-ribose with three molecules of phosphoric acid. Hydrolysis of it to similar compounds containing one or two molecules of phosphoric acid is accompanied by release of energy for muscular and perhaps other types of cellular work. Abbreviated ATP. Syn., *adenosinetriphosphoric acid, adenylpyrophosphoric acid.* Also called *adenylpyrophosphate.* See *adenosinetriphosphatase.*

a·den″o·sine·tri″phos·phor′ic ac′id. Adenosinetriphosphate.

ad″e·no′sis [*adēn;* G. *-ōsis*, condition]. 1. Any glandular disease, especially one involving the lymph nodes. 2. Nonneoplastic proliferation of glandular elements.

a. of the breast. A condition affecting women, commonly between the ages of 35 and 45, who usually are nulliparous and give a history of menstrual irregularity, characterized by the presence in one or both breasts of multiple small hard nodules distributed mostly about the periphery of the upper or outer hemisphere, which on histologic examination show an increase in fibrous tissue, little or no fat, dilatation of ducts, and foci of epithelial proliferation. Incidence of carcinoma following this condition is greatly increased. Also called *adenocystic disease, microcystic disease.* Syn., *fibrosing adenomatosis, fibrosing a., sclerosing a., a. scleroticans mammae, Schimmelbusch's disease.*

ad′e·no·tome [*adēn;* G. *tomos*, cutting]. 1. An instrument for incising a gland. 2. An instrument for removing adenoids.

ad″e·not′o·my [*adēn;* G. *tomē*, a cutting]. Dissection, incision, or surgical removal of a gland.

A′den ul′cer. See tropical *ulcer*.

ad′e·nyl. $C_5H_4N_5$—. The radical present in adenine.

ad″e·nyl′ic ac′id. Adenosinemonophosphate.

ad″e·nyl·py″ro·phos′pha·tase (ad″i·nil·py″ro-fos′fuh·tace, ·taze). Adenosinetriphosphatase.

ad″e·nyl·py″ro·phos′phate. Adenosinetriphosphate.

ad″e·nyl·py″ro·phos·phor′ic ac′id. Adenosinetriphosphate.

ad″e·pha′gi·a, ad″de·pha′gi·a [G. *hadēn*, to one's fill; *phagein*, to eat]. Old term for *bulimia.*

ad′eps [L., lard]. 1. Lard; the purified omental fat of the hog. It contains 38% stearin and margarin, and 62% olein; used in ointments. 2. Animal fat.

a. anserinus. Goose grease.

a. benzoinatus. Benzoinated lard containing 1% benzoin.

a. ex fele. Cat's grease.

a. lanae. Wool fat; the purified, anhydrous, fatty substance from sheep's wool; anhydrous lanolin.

a. lanae hydrosus. Hydrous wool fat containing 25–30% water; lanolin.

a. ovillus. Mutton suet or tallow.

a. praeparatus. Purified hog fat.

a. suillus. Hog lard.

a·der′mi·a [G. *a-*, not; *derma*, skin]. Absence or defect of the skin.

a·der′min. Old term for pyridoxine.

a·der″mo·gen′e·sis [*a-; derma;* G. *genesis*, production]. 1. Deficient cutaneous development. 2. Imperfect healing of a skin defect.

a·der″mo·tro′phi·a [*a-; derma;* G. *trophē*, nourishment]. Atrophy of the skin.

Ad·hat′o·da [Tamil]. A genus of plants of the family Acanthaceae. The fruit, leaves, and root of the East Indian plant, **A. vasica,** or Malabar nut tree, are used in India as an expectorant and antispasmodic.

ad·he′sion [L. *adhaesio*, from *adhaerere*, to stick to]. 1. *In physics*, molecular force exerted between two surfaces in contact. 2. Abnormal union of an organ or part to another. 3. *In dentistry*, force which holds an upper denture in place without the aid of vacuum cups. —**adher′ent,** *adj.;* **adher′ence,** *n.;* **adhere′,** *v.*

amniotic a. Attachment of the amnion to various portions of the germinal disk or embryo by means of fibrous bands.

fibrinous a. Loose attachment of adjacent serous membranes due to the presence of fibrinous exudate.

fibrous a. Firm attachment of adjacent serous membranes by bands or masses of fibrous connective tissue; due to organization and cicatrization of exudates, resulting from infection or partial destruction of the surfaces.

ad·he″si·ot′o·my (ad·hee″zee·ot′o·mee) [*adhaesio;* G. *tomē*, a cutting]. Surgical cutting or division of adhesions.

ad·he′sive [L. *adhaesum*, from *adhaerere*]. 1. Sticky; tenacious; tending to cling or stick. 2. Resulting in or attended with adhesion.

ad·he′sive. A plaster or emplastrum.

a″di·ac·tin′ic [G. *a-*, not; *dia*, through; *aktis*, ray]. Impervious to, or not penetrated by, actinic rays.

a″di·ad″o·cho·ki·ne′sis (a″dee·ad″o·ko·ki·nee′sis), **a″di·ad″o·ko·ci·ne′sis** (a″dee·ad″o·ko·si·nee′sis), **a″di·ad″o·ko·ki·ne′sis** [*a-;* G. *diadochos*, succeeding; *kinēsis,* motion]. 1. Inability to perform rapidly alternating movements, such as pronation and supination—seen in cerebellar disease. 2. Incessant movement. Also spelled *adiadokocinesia, adiadokokinesia.*

Ad″i·an′tum [*a-;* G. *diantos,* from *diainein,* to wet]. A genus of ferns, commonly called maidenhair. The North American species, **A. capillus-veneris** and **A. pedatum,** formerly were used as remedies for coughs.

a·di″a·pho·ret′ic. [*a-;* G. *diaphorētikos,* promoting perspiration, from *dia,* through, *pherein,* to carry]. Reducing, checking, or preventing perspiration; anhidrotic. —**adiaphore′sis,** *n.*

a·di″a·pho·ret′ic. Any agent or drug which reduces, checks, or prevents perspiration.

a″di·as′to·le (ay″dye·ass′to·lee, ad″eye·) [*a-;* G. *diastolē,* a drawing apart]. Absence or imperceptibility of diastole.

a″di·a·ther′mic (ad″ee·uh·thur′mick, ay″dye·uh·, ad″eye·uh·) [*a-;* G. *dia,* through; *thermē,* heat]. Impervious to radiant heat. —**adiathermance, adiathermancy,** *n.*

a″di·a·thet′ic, a″di·a·the′sic [*a-;* G. *diathetikos,* from *diatithenai,* to arrange]. Without relation to any diathesis or constitutional tendency; applied to a symptom or disease.

a·dic′i·ty. *In chemistry,* valence.

Adie, William John (1886–1935). Australian physician who described in detail a syndrome of tonic pupils and absent tendon reflexes, called *Adie's syndrome.*

ad′i·ent [L. *adire,* to approach]. Tending toward or approaching the source of a stimulus, as opposed to *abient.*

adiphenine. See *trasentine.*

a·dip′ic [L. *adeps,* lard]. Of, or belonging to, fat.

a·dip′ic ac′id. $COOH(CH_2)_4COOH$; a dibasic acid, occurring as colorless or yellowish needles, obtained by oxidation of various fats, as with nitric acid. Syn., *hexanedioic acid.*

ad′i·po-, adip- [*adeps*]. A combining form denoting *fat, fats, fatty tissue.*

ad′i·po·cele″ (ad′i·po·seel″) [*adeps;* G. *kēlē,* tumor]. A true hernia with hernial sac, containing only fatty tissue. Also called *lipocele.*

ad″i·po·cel′lu·lar [*adeps;* L. *cellula,* dim. of *cella,* cavity]. Made up of fat and connective tissue.

ad′i·po·cere″ (ad′i·po·seer″) [*adeps;* L. *cera,* wax]. A waxlike substance which occurs during the decomposition of dead animal tissues (corpses) at suitable temperatures, in the presence of moisture, and in the absence of air, as under earth or water. It consists chiefly of fatty acids and their salts. —**adipocer′atous,** *adj.*

ad″i·po·fi·bro′ma (ad″i·po·figh·bro′muh) [*adeps;* L. *fibra,* fiber; G. *-ōma,* tumor]. Lipofibroma.

ad″i·pol′y·sis [*adeps;* G. *lysis,* a loosing]. Cleavage or hydrolysis of fats during digestion, by fat-splitting enzymes. —**adipolyt′ic,** *adj.*

ad″i·po′ma [*adeps;* G. *-ōma,* tumor]. Lipoma.

ad″i·po·ne·cro′sis ne″o·na·to′rum. Necrosis of fatty tissue. A self-limiting, localized process, occurring usually in large, well-nourished infants born after difficult labor, characterized by bluish red lesions, becoming manifest 2 to 20 days after birth as deep subcutaneous indurations, and disappearing completely within four months.

ad″i·po·pex′is, ad″i·po·pex′i·a [*adeps;* G. *pēxis,* fixation]. Fixation of fats; storage of fats. —**adipopec′tic, adipopexic,** *adj.*

ad″i·po′sa dys·tro′phi·a gen″i·ta′lis. See adiposogenital *dystrophy.*

ad′i·pose [*adeps*]. Fatty, fatlike, fat.

ad″i·po′sis [*adeps;* G. *-ōsis,* condition]. 1. Corpulence; obesity. 2. Excessive accumulation of fat in the body, local or general; fatty infiltration. Syn., *adiposity.*

a. dolorosa. A disease marked by deposition of symmetrical masses of fat in various parts accompanied by more or less pain. It affects women oftener than men and may cause death from pulmonary complications. Also called *Dercum's disease.*

a. hepatica. Old term for fatty degeneration or infiltration of the liver.

a. orchalis. See adiposogenital *dystrophy.*

a. tuberosa simplex. Disease resembling adiposis dolorosa but marked by small nodular fatty tumors, painful or tender to the touch, and found mostly on the abdomen and extremities. Also called *Anders' disease.*

ad″i·pos′i·tas cer″e·bral′is. Disturbances of fat deposition due to intracranial lesions or associated with deficient function of the hypophysis.

ad″i·po·si′tis [*adeps;* G. *-itis,* inflammation]. Inflammation of the subcutaneous fatty tissue.

ad″i·pos′i·ty. See *adiposis.*

ad″i·po″so·gen′i·tal [*adeps;* L. *genitalis,* genital]. Pertaining to superficial fat of the body and the external genitalia, as adiposogenital dystrophy.

ad″i·po·su′ri·a [*adeps;* G. *ouron,* urine]. Presence of fat in the urine; lipuria.

a·dip′sa (ay·dip′suh, a·dip′suh) [G. *adipson,* from *a-,* not; *dipsa,* thirst]. 1. Remedies to allay thirst. 2. Foods which do not produce thirst.

a·dip′si·a (ay·dip′see·uh, a·dip′·), **a·dip′sy** [*a-; dipsa*]. Absence of thirst; avoidance of drinking.

ad′i·tus [L., entrance]. *In anatomy,* an entrance.

a. ad antrum. Outer side of the attic, opening upward, backward, and outward into the mastoid antrum. It gives lodgment to the head of the malleus and the greater part of the incus.

ad·just′ed death rate. Standardized death rate.

ad·just′ment [F. *ajuster,* from *à,* to, *juste,* from L. *justus,* right]. 1. Mechanism of a microscope which brings the objective into focus. 2. Chiropractic treatment aimed at reduction of subluxated vertebrae. 3. *In biology,* changes undergone by a plant or animal better to adapt it to the environment. 4. *In psychology,* the establishment of a relationship between the individual and his environment.

absolute a. Accommodation of each eye, considered alone. Also called *absolute accommodation.*

mental a. *In psychology,* an adjustment involving an individual's attitudes, traits, or feelings. Also called *intrapsychic a.*

social a. *In psychiatry,* adaptation of an individual to society and to his social environment.

ad·jus′tor [*ajuster*]. The central neuron, or neurons, of a reflex arc in the nervous system.

ad′ju·vant [L. *adjuvare,* to assist]. A material administered with and enhancing the action of a drug or antigenic substance.

a. elixir. See *glycyrrhiza* elixir.

Adler, Alfred (1870–1937). Austrian psychiatrist; founder of the school of individual psychology. See under *psychology.*

ad lib. *Ad libitum;* at pleasure; the amount desired.

ad·me′di·al, ad·me′di·an [L. *ad,* near; *medius,* middle]. Located near or approaching the median plane or central axis.

ad″mi·nic′u·lum [L., support, from *ad,* to, *manus,* hand]. 1. A supporting structure; adjuvant; auxiliary. 2. A triangular fibrous expansion which extends from the superior pubic ligament to the posterior surface of the linea alba. Also called *a. lineae albae.*

ad·mis′sion rate. Number of admissions to a hospital per thousand of population; often refers to a military population.

ad·na′sal (ad·nay′zul, ad·nay′sul) [*ad;* L. *nasus*, nose]. Pertaining to the nose; situated near the nose; toward the nose.

ad′nate [L. *adnatus*, connected by birth]. Congenitally attached or united.

ad nau′se·am (ad naw′shee·um, ·see·um) [L.]. To the point of producing nausea.

adnephrin. Trade-mark for an encapsulated bronchial antispasmodic and sedative containing phenobarbital, aminophylline, and neo-synephrine hydrochloride.

ad·ner′val, ad·neu′ral [L. *ad*, near; *nervus*, nerve]. 1. Near or toward a nerve. 2. Denoting an electric current which passes through the muscle fibers toward the entrance point of the nerve.

ad·nex′a [L. *adnexum*, from *adnectere*, to tie to]. Accessory parts or appendages of an organ. Also called *annexa.* —**adnexal,** *adj.*

a. oculi. Appendages of the eye, as the lids and the lacrimal apparatus.

a. uteri. The uterine tubes and the ovaries.

fetal a. The extraembryonic membranes.

ad″nex·i′tis [*adnexum;* G. *-itis*, inflammation]. Inflammation of the adnexa uteri. Also called *annexitis.*

ad·nex″o·gen′e·sis [*adnexum;* G. *genesis*, production]. The forming of the extraembryonic membranes of the embryo.

ad″o·don′ti·a [L. *ad*, prefix meaning *addition;* G. *odous*, tooth]. An excessive number of teeth.

ad″o·les′cence [L. *adolescere*, to grow]. The youth period, extending from puberty to maturity. —**adolescent,** *adj., n.*

ad″o·les′cent mam″mo·pla′si·a. Enlargement of the male breasts during adolescence, caused by the action of androgen without the presence of inhibin. Later, inhibin is produced, and the breasts return to normal size.

adoleum. Trade name for a mixture of refined fish-liver oils of high vitamin-A and -D potency.

a·don′i·din. A mixture of glycosides and adonic acid derived from *Adonis vernalis*, a plant indigenous in Europe and Asia. It has been recommended in cardiac dropsy.

a·do′nin. A glycoside from *Adonis autumnalis.* It is a powerful heart stimulant.

A·do′nis, A·don′is [a handsome youth in Greek mythology]. A genus of European herbs belonging to the order Ranunculaceae.

A. aestivalis. A plant much used in Italy as a cardiac tonic.

A. vernalis. A species used as a cardiac stimulant and diuretic. Dose, 0.06–0.3 Gm. (1–5 gr.).

ad·o′ral [L. *ad*, near; *os*, mouth]. Situated near the mouth; toward the mouth.

ad·or′bit·al [*ad;* L. *orbita*, track]. Situated near the orbit; toward the orbit.

ADP Adenosinediphosphate.

ad·re′nal [*ad;* L. *renalis*, of the kidneys]. The adrenal gland. —**ad·re′nal,** *adj.*

ad·re′nal cor′tex. Cortical substance of the adrenal gland.

ad·re′nal cor′tex in·jec′tion. The U.S.P. designation of a sterile solution in water for injection containing a mixture of the endocrine principles derived from the cortex of adrenal glands of healthy domestic animals used for food by man; each milliliter is required to have biological activity equivalent to that of 100 micrograms of U.S.P. hydrocortisone acetate reference standard, and a suitable antibacterial agent is required.

ad·re′nal cor′ti·cal ex′tract. An extract of the cortex of adrenal glands obtained from slaughtered domesticated animals, containing the cortical steroids (corticosterone, dehydrocorticosterone, desoxycorticosterone, etc.) essential for the maintenance of life in adrenalectomized animals. Only traces of epinephrine are present.

ad·re′nal cor′ti·cal hy″po·func′tion. A progressively fatal disease due to a deficiency of the adrenal cortex, usually from tuberculous infection, characterized by anemia, marked weakness and prostration, low blood pressure, feeble heart action, frequent dizziness, and fainting. There are also gastrointestinal disorders, nervous irritability, psychic changes, and often bronzing of the skin and pigmentation of the mucous membranes. Death occurs in two to three years. Also called *Addison's disease, asthenia pigmentosa, melanoma suprarenale, bronzed skin.*

ad·re″nal·ec′to·my. Surgical removal of an adrenal gland.

bilateral a. The surgical removal of both adrenal glands.

adrenalin. Trade-mark for epinephrine.

adrenalin chloride. Trade-mark for epinephrine hydrochloride.

ad·ren′al·ine. The official British Pharmacopoeia name for epinephrine. See also *adrenalin.*

ad·ren″al·in·e′mi·a, ad·ren″al·in·ae′mi·a [*ad; renalis;* G. *haima*, blood]. Presence of epinephrine in the blood.

ad·ren″al·in·u′ri·a [*ad; renalis;* G. *ouron*, urine]. Presence of epinephrine in the urine.

ad·re′nal·ism [*ad; renalis*]. A condition due to dysfunction of the adrenal gland. See *hyperadrenalism.* Also called *suprarenalism.*

ad·re″na·li′tis, ad″re·ni′tis [*ad; renalis;* G. *-itis*, inflammation]. Inflammation of the adrenal glands.

ad·ren″al·og′ra·phy. See *adrenogram.*

ad′ren·arch′e. The time in the development of a child at which an increased output of adrenocortical hormones occurs, manifested by the appearance of pubic and axillary hair and increase in urinary steroid excretion. It usually occurs about the eighth or ninth year of life.

ad″ren·er′gic [*ad;* L. *renes*, kidneys; G. *ergon*, work]. Of, pertaining to, or designating the type of chemical activity characteristic of epinephrine and epinephrinelike substances: term introduced by H. H. Dale (1934). See adrenergic *nerves.*

ad″re·ner′gic block′ing a′gent. See under *agent.*

adrenine, adrenin. Trade name for epinephrine.

ad·re·ni′tis. See *adrenalitis.*

ad·ren′o·chrom, ad·ren′o·chrome. $C_9H_9O_3N$. A quinone-type oxidation product of epinephrine. It occurs as a brick-red substance which has the power of converting hemoglobin into methemoglobin.

ad·ren″o·cor″ti·co·mi·met′ic. Pertaining to an activity or effect similar to that of an adrenal cortical steroid.

ad·ren″o·cor″ti·co·tro′phic. See *adrenocorticotropic.*

ad·ren″o·cor″ti·co·tro′pic [*ad; renes;* L. *cortex*, bark; G. *tropikos*, from *trepein*, to turn]. Exhibiting a hormonal influence on the adrenal cortex: formerly spelled *adrenocorticotrophic.*

ad·ren″o·cor″ti·co·tro′pin [*ad; renes; cortex; tropikos*]. The adenohypophyseal hormone which stimulates the adrenal cortex: also called *adrenotropin, corticotropin.* See *ACTH.*

adreno-cortin. Trade-mark for an injectable extract of adrenal glands containing cortical steroids but substantially free of epinephrine.

ad·re″no·gen′i·tal [*ad; renes;* L. *genitalis*, genital]. Pertaining to the adrenal glands and the gonads.

ad·re′no·gram [*ad; renes;* G. *gramma*, writing]. A roentgenogram of the adrenal glands made after perirenal insufflation; used for adrenal examination.

ad·re″no·lyt′ic. Term formerly used to describe any adrenergic blocking agent.

ad·ren′o·pause [*ad; renes;* G. *pausis,* a stopping]. The hypothetical age of reduction of production of certain adrenocortical hormones, occurring in old age.

ad″ren·os′te·rone (ad″ren·os′ti·rohn, ad″ri·nos′·). $C_{19}H_{24}O_3$; 4-androstene-3,11,17-trione; a steroid hormone with androgenic properties; obtained from the adrenal cortex. See Table of Hormones in the Appendix. —**ad″ren·os′teroid,** *adj.*

ad·re″no·tox′in (ad·ree″no·tock′sin, ad·ren″o·) [*ad; renes;* G. *toxikon,* poison]. 1. An antibody produced when adrenal tissue is introduced into an animal. 2. Anything that is toxic to the adrenals.

ad·ren′o·trope [*ad; renes;* G. *tropos,* a turn]. A person with the adrenal type of endocrine diathesis.

ad·ren″o·tro′phic. See *adrenotropic.*

ad·ren″o·tro′pic [*ad; renes;* G. *tropikos,* from *trepein,* to turn]. Of, pertaining to, or denoting adrenocorticotropin: formerly spelled *adrenotrophic.* See Table of Hormones in the Appendix.

ad·ren″o·tro′pin, ad·ren″o·troph′in. See *adrenocorticotropin.*

ad″re·not′ro·pism (ad″ree·not′ro·piz·um, ad″ren·o·tro′piz·um) [*ad; renes;* G. *tropos,* a turn]. Dominance of the adrenal in the endocrine functions.

adrephine. Trade-mark for adrenalin-ephedrine compounds.

Adrian, Edgar Douglas (1889–). English neurophysiologist, known for his investigations of the sense organs by electrical methods, and his writings on the nervous basis for sensation and perception; Nobel prize winner in physiology and medicine, with Charles Sherrington, for discoveries regarding the function of the neuron (1932).

adrin. Trade-mark for an injectable preparation of epinephrine hydrochloride.

adrocaine. Trade-mark for adrenalin-procaine compounds, used to produce local anesthesia and to inhibit hemorrhage.

a·dro′mi·a [G. *a-,* not; *dromos,* a running]. Complete failure of impulse conduction in muscle or nerve.

ad·ru′e (ad·roo′uh). See *flatsedge.*

Adson, Alfred Washington [*American surgeon,* 1887–1951]. Associated with many procedures in surgery of the brain and spinal cord, especially with operations for the removal of the cervicothoracic ganglions and for the relief of trigeminal neuralgia; credited with the development of scalenotomy to relieve symptoms due to cervical ribs, and with being a pioneer in the surgical treatment of protruded intervertebral disks.

ad·sor′bate [L. *ad,* to; *sorbere,* to suck]. Any substance which is adsorbed.

ad·sorb′ent [*ad; sorbere*]. Any substance which produces adsorption, as activated charcoal, silica gel. See *adsorption.*

adsorl. Trade-mark for a water-dispersible solution of vitamins A and D.

ad·sorp′tion [*ad; sorbere*]. 1. The power possessed by certain substances (*adsorbents*) of taking up fluids, apart from capillary attraction. 2. The process whereby a solid (*adsorbent*) attracts and concentrates upon its surface, in a thin layer, molecules of a gas, liquid, or dissolved substance (*adsorbate*) by adhesion. —**adsorptive,** *adj.;* **adsorb′,** *v.t., v.i.*

ad·ster′nal [*ad;* G. *sternon,* breast]. Situated near the sternum; toward the sternum.

ad·ter′mi·nal [*ad;* L. *terminus,* end]. Moving toward the insertion of a muscle; said of electric currents in muscular fiber.

ad·tor′sion [*ad;* L. *torsio,* from *torquere,* to twist]. Convergent squint. Also called *conclination.*

a·dult′ [L. *adultus,* from *adolescere,* to grow]. Mature; having attained full size and strength; of full legal age.

ad′ult. A person of mature age.

a·dul′ter·ant [L. *adulterare,* to pollute]. Any substance that adulterates.

a·dul″ter·a′tion [*adulterare*]. Admixture or substitution of inferior, impure, inert, or cheaper ingredients for gain, deception, or concealment. —**adul′terate,** *v.t.*

ad·vance′, ad·vance′ment [OF. *avancer,* from L. *ab,* away; *ante,* before]. 1. A tenotomy followed by reattachment of the tendon at a more advanced point. 2. *In ophthalmology,* operative correction of strabismus. The muscle tendon opposite to the direction of the squint is removed at its insertion and sutured to the sclera anterior to the original attachment. A modification in which the shortened muscle, rather than its tendon, is attached anterior to the stump, is called **Lancaster's advancement.**

ad″ven·ti′ti·a (ad″ven·tish′ee·uh) [L. *adventicius,* foreign]. The external covering of an organ derived from adjacent connective tissue, as the external coat of a blood vessel or other organ. See Plate 6.

ad″ven·ti′tious (ad″ven·tish′us) [*adventicius*]. 1. Accidental, foreign, acquired, as opposed to natural or hereditary. 2. Occurring in unusual or abnormal places. 3. Pertaining to the adventitia.

ad″y·na′mi·a (ad″i·nay′mee·uh, ·nam′ee·uh, ay″·di·), **a·dyn′a·my** [G. *a-,* not; *dynamis,* power]. Loss of vital strength or muscular power; weakness; debility; asthenia. —**adynam′ic,** *adj.*

ae-. For words beginning with *ae-* not found here, see words beginning *e-.*

Aeby, Christoph Theodor [*Swiss anatomist,* 1835–85]. *Aeby's plane* is a craniometric plane passing through the nasion and basion perpendicular to the median plane.

A·ë′des (ay·ee′deez) [G. *aēdēs,* from *a-,* not; *ēdos,* pleasure]. A genus of mosquitoes, belonging to the family Culicidae, having north temperate distribution. Many species are noxious and troublesome biters. In North America, the species **A. vexans** is found near fresh water; **A. aldrichi, A. dorsalis, A. sollicitans, A. squamiger,** and **A. taeniorhynchus** are found near salt marshes. **A. aegypti** is the principal vector of yellow fever and dengue. It has urban breeding habits.

ae″doe·o·ceph′a·lus (ee″dee·o·sef′uh·lus, ed″ee·o·) [G. *aidoia,* genitals; *kephalē,* head]. See *edocephalus.*

ae″lu·rop′sis (ee″lew·rop′sis, el″yoo·) [G. *ailouros,* cat; *opsis,* vision]. Obliquity of the eye or of the palpebral fissure.

ae′quum (ee′kwum) [L., equal]. Amount of food necessary to maintain weight with normal physical activity. It varies with the individual's size and the nature of his activity.

a′er·ate [G. *aēr,* air]. Charge with air or gas; oxygenate, carbonate, etc.; arterialize. —**aerated,** *adj.;* **aerator,** *n.*

a″er·a′tion [*aēr*]. 1. Exposure to air. 2. Saturation of a fluid with air or a gas, as carbon dioxide. 3 Conversion of venous to arterial blood.

a·er·e′mi·a. See caisson *disease.*

a″er·en″do·car′di·a [*aēr;* G. *endon,* within; *kardia,* heart]. Presence of air within the heart.

a″er·en″ter·ec·ta′si·a (ay″ur·en″tur·eck·tay′zhuh, ·zee·uh, ·shuh, ·see·uh) [*aēr;* G. *enteron,* intestine; *ektasis,* extension]. Excessive amount of air or gas in the intestines; tympanites; meteorism.

a·e′ri·al (ay·eer′ee·ul, air′ee·ul) [G. *aerios*, from *aēr*]. Pertaining to the air, as aerial conduction, hearing through air vibrations.

a″er·if′er·ous [*aēr*; L. *ferre*, to bear]. Conveying air, as the trachea and its branches.

a′er·i·form″ (ay′ur·i·form″, ay·eer′·, ay·air′·) [*aēr*; L. *forma*, form]. Airlike; gaseous.

a′er·o- (ay′ur·o-, air′o-), **aer-** [*aēr*]. A combining form denoting *air*, *aerial*, or *gas, gases*.

a″er·o·an·a″er·o′bic (ay″ur·o·an·ay″ur·o′bick, ·ob′ick) [*aēr*; G. *a-*, not; *aēr*; *bios*, life]. Of or pertaining to organisms which are both aerobic and anaerobic.

A″er·o·bac′ter [*aēr*; G. *bakterion*, little staff]. A genus of nonpathogenic, Gram-negative, saprophytic bacteria of the Enterobacteriaceae.

A. aerogenes. A species of coliform bacteria widely distributed in nature, which closely resembles the *Escherichia coli*; a lactose-fermenter. Also called *Bacterium aerogenes*, *Bacterium lactis aerogenes*.

a′er·obe [*aēr*; G. *bios*, life]. A microorganism which requires air as free oxygen for the maintenance of life. Also called *aerobion*.

facultative aerobes. Organisms normally or usually anaerobic but which, under certain circumstances, acquire aerobic power.

obligate aerobes. Organisms dependent upon free oxygen at all times; never anaerobic.

a″er·o′bic (ay″ur·o′bick, ·ob′ick), **a″er·o′bi·an** [*aēr*; *bios*]. 1. Requiring air or free oxygen in order to live. 2. Relating to or produced by aerobes.

a″er·o·bi·ol′o·gy. The study of air-borne substances such as pollens, molds, dust, and bacteria.

a″er·o·bi′o·scope [*aēr*; *bios*; G. *skopein*, to examine]. Apparatus for collecting and filtering bacteria from the air to determine the bacterial content.

a″er·o·bi·o′sis (ay″ur·o·buy·o′sis) [*aēr*; *bios*; G. *-ōsis*, condition]. Life that requires the presence of air, or free oxygen. —**aerobiot′ic,** *adj*.

a′er·o·cele″ (ay′ur·o·seel″) [*aēr*; G. *kēlē*, tumor]. A tumor caused by the escape of air into an adventitious pouch usually connected with the trachea or larynx, hence its size may vary with respiration. Also called *tracheocele*, *laryngocele*, *pneumatocele*.

epidural a. An intracranial extradural accumulation of air or gas, usually resulting from a fracture of the skull.

a″er·o·col′pos [*aēr*; G. *kolpos*, vagina]. Distention of the vagina with air or gas.

a″er·o·cys·tos′co·py [*aēr*; G. *kystis*, bladder; *skopein*, to examine]. Examination of the interior of the urinary bladder with a cystoscope, the bladder being distended with air. —**aerocys′toscope,** *n*.

a″er·o″don·tal′gi·a. See *barodontalgia*.

a″er·o·don′ti·a [*aēr*; *odous*]. Aviation dentistry.

a″er·o·duc′tor [*aēr*; L. *ducere*, to lead]. Apparatus to prevent asphyxia of the fetus when the aftercoming head is retained.

a″er·o·dy·nam′ics (ay″ur·o·dye·nam′icks, ·dinam′icks, air″o·) [*aēr*; G. *dynamis*, power]. The branch of physics that deals with gases in motion.

a″er·o·em′bo·lism [*aēr*; L. *embolismus*, from G. *en*, in; *ballein*, to throw]. A condition caused by an abrupt drop from normal to low atmospheric pressure; occurs in aviators in rapid ascents to high altitudes; marked by the formation of nitrogen bubbles in the blood and body tissues. Symptoms include severe pain in the joints and chest, itching of the skin, pulmonary edema, urticaria, paralysis, convulsions, and sometimes coma. Symptoms may be relieved by descent to lower altitude. Syn., *aeroemphysema*, *chokes*, *decompression sickness*, *dysbarism*. Also see caisson *disease*.

a″er·o·em″phy·se′ma (·em″fi·see′muh, ·zee′muh, ·em″figh·). Aeroembolism.

a′er·o·gen″ [*aēr*; G. *genesthai*, from *gignesthai*, to be produced]. Any gas-producing microorganism.

a″er·o·gen′e·sis [*aēr*; G. *genesis*, production]. Gas formation. —**aerogenic, aerog′enous,** *adj*.

a′er·o·gram″ [*aēr*; G. *gramma*, letter]. An x-ray film of an organ inflated with air.

a″er·og′ra·phy [*aēr*; G. *graphein*, to write]. Description of air and its qualities.

a″er·o·hy·drop′a·thy (·high·drop′uth·ee) [*aēr*; G. *hydōr*, water; *pathos*, disease]. Use of air and water in the treatment of disease. Also called *aerohydrotherapy*.

a″er·o·i″on·i·za′tion [*aēr*; G. *ion*, from *ienai*, to go]. The process of electrically charging particles, such as oil drops, suspended in the air. Inhalation of air with such charges is recommended for treatment of respiratory diseases.

a″er·o·i″on·o·ther′a·py [*aēr*; *ion*; G. *therapeia*, treatment]. Inhalation of electric charges in the treatment of disease.

aerolin. Trade-mark for a preparation containing clopane hydrochloride, aludrine hydrochloride, atropine sulfate, and procaine hydrochloride: used for inhalation therapy in bronchial asthma.

a″er·o·mam·mog′ra·phy [*aēr*; G. *mammē*, breast; *graphein*, to write]. X-ray examination of the breast after injecting the retromammary space with carbon dioxide or air.

A′er·o Med′i·cal Lab′o·ra·to″ry. A laboratory in the Air Force where flight surgeons, physiologists, and aeronautical engineers work upon problems associated with aviation, as anoxia, aeroembolism, etc.

a″er·o·med′i·cine. Aviation medicine.

a″er·om′e·ter [*aēr*; G. *metron*, a measure]. Instrument for determining the density of gases.

a″er·o·neu·ro′sis [*aēr*; G. *neuron*, nerve; *-ōsis*, condition]. A form of psychoneurosis found in aviators, characterized by anxiety, restlessness, and various physical manifestations.

a″er·op′a·thy [*aēr*; G. *pathos*, disease]. Any pathologic condition brought about by changes in atmospheric pressure, as caisson disease or aeroembolism.

a′er·o·pause″. That region of the atmosphere where its various functions (e.g., supplying breathing air and climate, filtrating cosmic factors, offering mechanical support) for man and aircraft begin to cease and conditions equivalent to outer space are gradually approached.

a″er·o·per″i·to·ne′um, a″er·o·per·i·to′ni·a [*aēr*; G. *peritonaion*, from *peri*, around; *tenein*, to stretch]. Air or gas in the peritoneal cavity.

a″er·o·pha′gi·a, a″er·oph′a·gy [*aēr*; G. *phagein*, to eat]. Imbibing and swallowing of air followed by noisy eructations, especially in hysterical patients. Aspiration of air by the rectum is called **rectal aerophagia.**

a′er·o·phil″ [*aēr*; G. *philein*, to love]. 1. Loving the open air. 2. Aerobic.

a″er·o·pho′bi·a [*aēr*; G. *phobos*, fear]. Morbid fear of drafts or of fresh air.

a′er·o·phore″ [*aēr*; G. *phoros*, bearing, from *pherein*, to bear]. 1. Device for inflating the lungs with air in the case of a stillborn child or in any case of asphyxia. 2. Apparatus which purifies air for rebreathing, used by firemen and others.

a′er·o·phyte″ [*aēr*; G. *phyton*, plant]. A plant living on other plants but deriving its moisture from the air, as an orchid; an epiphyte.

a″er·o·pi·e″so·ther′a·py (·pye·ee″so·therr′uh·pee) [*aēr*; G. *piezein*, to press; *therapeia*, therapy]. Use of compressed or rarefied air in the treatment of disease.

a″er·o·ple·thys′mo·graph [*aēr;* G. *plēthysmos*, enlargement; *graphein*, to write]. Apparatus for registering graphically the amount of air respired.

a″er·o·pleu′ra (ay″ur·o·ploor′uh) [*aēr;* G. *pleura*, side]. Air or gas in the pleural cavity; pneumothorax.

a′er·o·scope″ [*aēr;* G. *skopein*, to examine]. Instrument for the examination of air dust and for estimating the purity of the air.

a″er·os′co·py [*aēr; skopein*]. Investigation of atmospheric conditions.

a″er·o·si·al·oph′a·gy [*aēr;* G. *sialon*, saliva; *phagein*, to eat]. The habit of constantly swallowing, and so taking air and saliva into the stomach.

a″er·o·si″nus·i′tis (ay″ur·o·sigh″nuh·sigh′tis, ·sin″yoo·sigh′tis, ·sigh″new·sigh′tis) [*aēr;* L. *sinus*, a hollow; G. *-itis*, inflammation]. An acute or chronic inflammation of one or more of the nasal accessory sinuses; caused by a difference in barometric pressure between the gas inside the sinus and that of the surrounding atmosphere: also called *barosinusitis*.

a·er·o′sis [*aēr;* G. *-ōsis*, condition]. Formation of gas in any of the body tissues.

a′er·o·sol″ [*aēr;* hydro*sol*, confused with Ger. *sole*, salt water]. 1. Atomized particles suspended in the air. 2. Any solution or compressed gas containing an agent for the treatment of the air to remove or destroy insects or microorganisms. 3. *In chemistry*, a colloid in which gas is the dispersion medium.

aerosol OT dry. Trade-mark for dioctyl sodium sulfosuccinate.

a′er·o·spo″rin [*aēr;* G. *spora, seed*]. Trade-mark for a brand of polymyxin B sulfate administered internally and topically in the treatment of various systemic, meningeal, urinary, and topical infections.

a″er·o·stat′ics [*aēr;* G. *statikos*, bringing to a standstill]. The branch of physics that treats of the properties of gases at rest, or in equilibrium.

a″er·o·tax′is [*aēr;* G. *taxis*, order]. Tendency of living organisms, especially aerobes and anaerobes, to be attracted or repelled by oxygen or air.

a″er·o·ther″a·peu′tics, a″er·o·ther′a·py [*aēr;* G. *therapeuein*, to treat medically]. A mode of treating disease by varying the pressure or the composition of the air breathed.

a″er·o·ther″mo·ther′a·py [*aēr;* G. *thermē*, heat; *therapeia*, therapy]. Treatment with hot air.

a″er·o·ti′tis me′di·a. Extrusion of blood serum and cells into the middle ear due to an uncompensated low pressure in this cavity during descent from an air flight. Syn., *aviator's ear, otic barotrauma, barotitis media.*

a″er·o·to·nom′e·ter [*aēr;* G. *tonos*, tension; *metron*, a measure]. Instrument for determining the tension of gases in the blood. —**aerotonometry,** *n.*

a·er·ot′ro·pism [*aēr;* G. *tropos*, from *trepein*, to turn]. The inherent tendency of an organism to be attracted to a supply of air, as various bacteria and protozoa collect about an air bubble. —**aerotrop′ic,** *adj.*

a″er·o·tym′pa·nal [*aēr;* G. *tympanon*, drum]. Pertaining to the air in the tympanum, especially in regard to forcing air through the auditory tube, as in politzerization.

a″er·o·u·re′thro·scope [*aēr;* G. *ourēthra*, urethra; *skopein*, to examine]. A modified endoscope which permits viewing the urethra after it is inflated with air. —**aerourethros′copy,** *n.*

ae·ru′go (ee·rōō′go) [L., rust]. 1. Rust of a metal. 2. Copper rust; verdigris.

aes (eez) [L.]. Copper or brass. See *copper.*

Aesculapius. Latin name of the Greek physician *Asklepios.*

aes·the′si·o-. See *esthesio-.*

aes′ti·val. See *estival.*

aes′tus (es′tus) [L.]. Heat; especially a flushing, or sudden glow of heat.

a. volaticus. Wildfire rash; strophulus; especially a temporary rash in infants.

aet. *Aetatis, aetate;* of age, at the age of.

ae′ther. See *ether.*

Ae·thu′sa (eeth·yōō′suh, ·zuh) [G. *aithousa*, fem. pres. part. of *aithein*, to burn]. A genus of the Umbelliferae. The fruit of **A. cynapium,** or fool's-parsley, yields a volatile alkaloid, cynapine, related to coniine.

ae″ti·o·por′phy·rin. Etioporphyrin.

Aetius of Amida [*Byzantine medical writer and compiler*, 502–75]. Author of a compendium containing writings of many authors, including his own description of an original treatment of aneurysm of the brachial artery by ligation. His treatise on diseases of the eye was all-inclusive for the time.

afaxin. A trade-mark for oleovitamin A.

a·fe′brile (ay·fee′bril, a·fee′·, ay·feb′ril, a·feb′·) [G. *a-*, not; L. *febris*, fever]. Without fever.

afenil. Trade name for calcium chloride-urea, $CaCl_2.4(NH_2)_2CO$, white crystals used intravenously in calcium therapy.

a·fe′tal (ay·fee′tul, a·fee′tul) [*a-;* L. *fetus*, an offspring]. Without a fetus.

af′fect [L. *affectus*, from *afficere*, to affect]. *In psychology*, feeling; emotion as it influences a mental state or idea (Freud); the feeling element in emotion; mood. —**affec′tive,** *adj.*

af·fect″a·bil′i·ty [*affectus*]. Capacity for responding to stimulation.

af″fec·ta′tion [L. *affectare*, to strive after]. Artificiality of manner or behavior.

af·fec′tion [L. *affectus*, from *afficere*, to affect]. 1. Any pathologic state or condition. 2. *In psychology*, the emotional factor in consciousness. —**affective,** *adj.*

af″fec·tiv′i·ty [*affectus*]. 1. Susceptibility to emotional stimuli. 2. *In psychology*, that part of consciousness comprising affection and affect.

af·fec″to·mo′tor [*affectus;* L. *motor*, from *movere*, to move]. Exhibiting emotional tension and muscular activity.

af·fekt′ep·i·lep″sie [Ger.]. A psychogenic convulsion which occurs in functional neuroses and obsessive states.

af′fer·ent [L. *afferre*, to carry to]. Carrying toward; centripetal.

af·fil″i·a′tion [L. *ad*, to; *filius*, son]. *In legal medicine*, imputing or fixing the paternity of a child in order to provide for its maintenance.

af·fi′nal, af′fi·nal [L. *affinis*, adjoining]. 1. Connected through marriage. 2. Having the same origin.

af′fi·nin. An insecticidal amide isolated from the roots of *Erigeron affinis.*

af·fin′i·ty [*affinis*]. 1. Inherent attraction and relationship. 2. *In biology*, the relationship between members of species or more specialized groups, which depends upon their mutual resemblance in structure and form, indicating a similarity of origin.

chemical a. The force of attraction between atoms which causes them to enter into and maintain certain combinations.

genetic a. Relationship by direct descent.

morbid a. The tendency for certain affections to exist simultaneously with, or as sequels of, a particular disease.

vital a. The selective action or chemotaxis exhibited by the several tissues of an organism for their particular pabulum.

af″fir·ma′tion [L. *affirmare*, to affirm]. During autosuggestion, the stage in which the subject acquires a positive reactive tendency; facilitation of positive reaction tendency.

af′flux, af·flux′ion [L. *affluxum*, from *affluere*, to flow toward]. Flow of blood or other fluid to a part. Syn., *congestion.* —**af′fluent,** *adj.;* **af′fluence,** *n.*

af·fu′sion [L. *affusum*, from *affundere*, to pour upon]. Pouring of water upon a part or upon the body, as in fever, to reduce temperature and calm nervous symptoms. The method of treating fevers by pouring cold water over the patient is called **cold affusion.**

a·fi″brin·o·gen·e′mi·a, a·fi″brin·o·gen·ae′mia [a-; L. *fibra*, fiber; G. *gignesthai*, to produce; *haima*, blood]. Complete absence of fibrinogen in the blood. See *fibrinogenopenia.*

a·foe′tal (ay·fee′tul, a·fee′tul). See *afetal.*

af′ri·dol. Sodium hydroxymercuric toluate; an antiseptic used in soap.

af′tan·nin. An infusion of herbs with formaldehyde and glycerin; used in veterinary medicine.

aft′er·birth″ [AS. *aefter;* ME. *burth*]. The placenta and membranes; normally expelled from the uterus following birth of the child.

aft′er·brain″. See *hindbrain, metencephalon.*

aft′er·care″ [*aefter;* AS. *caru*]. Care or nursing of convalescents, especially the postoperative treatment of surgical patients. Syn., *aftertreatment.*

aft′er·cat″a·ract [*aefter;* G. *kataraktēs*, a waterfall]. 1. A portion of lens substance or of lens capsule retained after the extraction of an extracapsular cataract. 2. Any membrane in the area of the pupil following removal or absorption of the lens. Syn., *secondary cataract.*

aft′er·cur″rent [*aefter;* L. *currere*, to run]. An electric current induced in a muscle or nerve following the cessation of a stimulating current through these organs.

aft′er·damp″ [*aefter;* MLG. *damp*, vapor]. A poisonous mixture of gases, containing principally carbon dioxide and nitrogen, found in coal mines after an explosion of inflammable gases.

aft″er·dis·charge′ [*aefter;* OF. *deschargier*]. A discharge of impulses by nerve elements which continues for a short period after reflex stimulation ceases because of the discharge of the central excitatory state,.

aft′er·ef·fect″ [*aefter;* L. *effectus*, from *efficere*, to bring about]. A delayed response to a stimulus or agent, appearing only after the subsidence of the primary response.

aft′er·gild″ing [*aefter;* AS. *gyldan*]. Application of gold salts to histologic preparations of nerve tissue after fixation and hardening.

aft′er·hear″ing [*aefter;* AS. *hīeran*]. A sensation of hearing a sound after the stimulus which produces it has ceased; may be a symptom of some neuroses.

aft′er·im″age [*aefter;* L. *imago*, image]. A retinal impression continued after the stimulus of the light or image has ceased to act. A **positive afterimage** is a simple prolongation of the sensation; a **negative afterimage** is the appearance of the image in complementary colors. Syn., *accidental image.*

aft′er·im·pres″sion [*aefter;* L. *impressio*, from *imprimere*, to press into]. An aftersensation.

aft′er·pains″ [*aefter;* G. *poinē*, penalty]. Pains from uterine contractions following delivery.

aft′er·per·cep″tion [*aefter;* L. *perceptio*, from *percipere*, to perceive]. Perception of a sensation after the stimulus has passed away.

aft″er·po·ten′tial. See under action *potential.*

aft′er·sen·sa″tion [*aefter;* ML. *sensatio*, from L. *sensus*, sense]. A sensation lasting longer than the stimulus producing it.

aft′er·sound″. See *afterhearing.*

aft′er·stain″ [*aefter;* OF. *desteindre*, to take away color]. A counterstain.

aft′er·taste″ [*aefter;* OF. *taster*, to feel]. A gustatory sensation continuing for some time after the stimulus has been removed.

aft′er·treat″ment. See *aftercare.*

aft′er·vi″sion [*aefter;* L. *visio*, from *videre*, to see]. Perception of an afterimage.

a·func′tion (ay·funk′shun, a·funk′shun) [G. *a-*, not; L. *functio*, a performing]. Loss or lack of function. —**afunctional,** *adj.*

Ag Chemical symbol for *argentum*, silver.

AGA *In embryology*, abbreviation for accelerated growth area.

a″ga·lac′ti·a, a″ga·lax′i·a, a″ga·lax′y [*a-;* G. *gala*, milk]. Nonsecretion or imperfect secretion of milk after childbirth. Also called *agalasia.* —**agalactous,** *adj.*

a. contagiosa. An epidemic, contagious disease of sheep and goats, marked by drying-up of the milk due to inflammation of the udders. The eyes and joints are also affected.

ag″a·lor·rhe′a, ag″a·lor·rhoe′a [*a-; gala;* G. *rhein*, to flow]. A cessation of the flow of milk.

a·gam′ete [*a-;* G. *gametēs*, husband]. Any protozoan which reproduces asexually.

a·gam′ic, ag′a·mous [*a-;* G. *gamos*, marriage]. *In biology*, asexual; reproducing without union of sexual cells.

a·gam″ma-glob″u·lin·e′mi·a. Near or complete absence of gamma-globulin in human serum with relatively normal serum total proteins. Thought to be congenital and sex-linked, affecting males only, the condition is characterized by a failure to produce antibodies and may be treated by specific replacement therapy.

a·gam″o·cy·tog′o·ny (a·gam″o·sigh·tog′o·nee, ag″uh·mo·) [*a-; gamos;* G. *kytos*, cell; *gonē*, offspring]. Agamogenesis.

Ag″a·mo·fi·la′ri·a [*a-; gamos;* L. *filum*, thread]. A genus of little-known filarial worms of man.

a·gam″o·gen′e·sis [*a-; gamos;* G. *genesis*, production]. 1. Asexual reproduction. 2. Parthenogenesis. Syn., *agamogony, agamocytogony.* —**agamogenet′ic,** *adj.*

ag″a·mog′o·ny [*a-; gamos;* G. *gonē*, offspring]. Agamogenesis.

a·gam′o·spore [*a-; gamos;* G. *spora*, offspring]. *In biology*, an asexually produced spore.

ag′a·mous. See *agamic.*

a′gar (ay′gahr, ag′ahr, ah′gahr) [Malay]. 1. A seaweed of the genus *Gelideum*, especially *G. cartilagineum.* 2. Any of various culture mediums containing agar-agar. Special agar mediums, as blood agar, may be made for fastidious organisms.

a. hanging block. *In bacteriology*, a small block of nutrient agar cut from a poured plate and placed on a cover glass, the surface next to the glass first having been touched with a loop from a young fluid culture or with a dilution from the same. It is examined upside down, the same as a hanging-drop culture.

a. plaque. A plug of agar, previously inoculated with an antibiotic producer, removed under sterile conditions, after incubation, and placed on an agar plate seeded with the test organisms, in order to measure the zone of inhibition which develops around the agar plug after further incubation.

a. spot. A drop of seeded nutrient agar in a sterile petri dish, used for the quantitative determination of antibiotic activity by subculturing to which successive increments of antibiotics have been added.

a.-streak plate. A petri dish containing agar, for a technique of antibiotic assay in which a series of solutions containing various concentrations of an antibiotic are incorporated in the nutrient agar, and the test organisms are subsequently streaked on the surface of the agar.

a.-streak slant. A hardened, slanted agar in a test tube, for a technique of antibiotic assay in which a series of antibiotic concentrations are incorporated in the test medium, followed by the streaking of the test organisms on the agar surface.

a. wells. The holes made in seeded agar into which antibiotics may be introduced to determine the extent of the inhibition (of microorganisms) which results from the diffusion of the antibiotic from the well into the surrounding agar in the course of subsequent incubation.

cornmeal a. A medium for the culture of yeasts, which encourages the production of *mycelium* and *chlamydospores.*

desoxycholate-citrate a. A medium for the culture of organisms of the enteric, *Salmonella,* and dysentery groups.

malt a. A medium for the culture of fungi.

penicillin-streptomycin blood a. A bacteria-inhibiting medium for the culture of fungi.

Simmon's citrate a. A medium for the culture and identification of *Salmonella.*

a′gar-a′gar [Malay]. 1. A dried mucilaginous extract obtained from certain species of seaweeds, especially agar; used in bacteriology to solidify culture mediums. Used as laxative because of its marked increase in bulk when moist. 2. See *agar.*

a·gar′ic (a·gar′ick, ag′ur·ick) [G. *agarikon,* tree-fungus]. Touchwood; spunk; tinder; the product of different basidia fungi, mostly *Polyporus.*

fly a. Poisonous mushroom which contains the alkaloid muscarine. Also called *Amanita muscaria.*

larch a. *Polyporus officinalis;* has been used as an anhidrotic. Syn., *white a.*

surgeons' a. *Agaricus chirurgorum, Boletus chirurgorum;* a parasitic fungus formerly used for moxa. It forms spunk when soaked in a solution of potassium nitrate.

white a. See larch *a.*

a·gar′ic ac′id (a·gar′ick). See *agaricin,* 1.

a·gar′i·cin. 1. $C_{19}H_{36}OH(COOH)_3.1\frac{1}{2}H_2O$. A white, crystalline substance; the active principle of larch agaric. It has proved useful in the night sweats of pulmonary tuberculosis and in arresting perspiration in phthisis. Syn., *agaric acid.* 2. An impure alcoholic extract of larch agaric, *Polyporus officinalis;* used as an anhidrotic.

A·gar′i·cus [G. *agarikon,* tree-fungus]. A large genus of fungi.

A. campestris. The common, nonpoisonous or edible mushroom.

A. muscarius. Fly agaric.

a·gar′y·thrine (a·gar′i·threen, ·thrin, ag″ur·ith′-rin). A yellow alkaloid extracted by ether from *Agaricus rubra.*

a·gas′tric (ay·gas′trick, a·gas′·) [G. *a-,* not; *gastēr,* stomach]. Without an alimentary canal, as the tapeworms. —**agastria,** *n.*

a·gas″tro·neu′ri·a [*a-; gastēr;* G. *neuron,* nerve]. Lowered or deficient nervous tone of the stomach.

A·ga′ve (a·gay′vee) [G. *agauos,* noble]. A large genus of the Amaryllidaceae, native North American plants.

A. americana. American aloe; the leaves of this plant; has been used as diuretic, antisyphilitic, and antiscorbutic.

Ag″chy·los′to·ma (ag″ki·los′to·muh). See *Ancylostoma.*

age [OF. *aage,* from L. *aetas*]. 1. The time elapsed from birth to the present in a living individual. 2. A particular period of life distinguished by development, equilibrium, or involution; especially old age. 3. *In psychology,* a measure of development expressed in terms of the age of an average individual of an equivalent development.

achievement a. Educational accomplishment expressed as equivalent to the age in years of the average child showing similar attainments; determined by tests. Also see accomplishment *quotient.*

a. critique. The menopause.

a. de retour. Old age, simple senile deterioration.

a. of consent. *In legal medicine,* the age at which a minor is considered capable of legally assenting to marriage or to sexual intercourse, varying from 13 years upward according to statute.

anatomic a. Age as judged by body development.

Binet a. Mental age as estimated by Binet tests.

bone a. Age as judged roentgenologically from bone development, when compared with the normal ossification for that chronologic age.

climacteric a. (a) Puberty. (b) The time of the cessation of the catamenia.

mental a. The score obtained on an intelligence test. An adult whose score is the equivalent of that of a normal child of 12 has a mental age of 12.

physiologic a. Age as judged by the functional development.

age. To grow old. 2. To age artificially, as wine.

a·gen′e·sis, ag″e·ne′si·a [G. *a-,* not; *genesis,* production]. 1. Incomplete and imperfect development; aplasia. 2. Impotence; barrenness. —**agenet′ic,** *adj.*

ovarian a. Failure of development of the ovaries. See also Turner's *syndrome.*

a·gen″i·o·ce·pha′li·a, a·gen″i·o·ceph′a·ly [*a-;* G. *geneion,* chin; *kephalē,* head]. A minor degree of otocephalus, described by Blanc, with the brain, cranial vault, and sense organs intact. —**ageniocephʹalus,** *n.*

a·gen′i·tal·ism [*a-;* L. *genitalis,* genital]. Symptom complex found in persons who lack testes or ovaries.

a·gen″o·so′mi·a [*a-;* G. *genesthai,* from *gignesthai,* to be produced; *sōma,* body]. Defective development of the genitals.

a·gen″o·so′mus [*a-; genesthai; sōma*]. Fetal monster with extrusion of the lower abdominal viscera because of a deficiency of the abdominal wall (celosoma); the genitalia are lacking or rudimentary.

a′gent [L. *agens,* from *agere,* to do, to act]. A substance or force which, by its action, effects changes.

adrenergic blocking a. Any agent which blocks the action of epinephrine or epinephrinelike substances, i.e. which blocks the impulse of postganglionic sympathetic nerves: also called *adrenolytic* or *sympatholytic agent.*

biological a. A virus; any of certain classifications of microorganisms and toxic substances derived from living organisms used to produce death or disease in man, animals, and growing plants.

chemical a. *In military medicine,* a solid, liquid, or gas which through its chemical properties produces lethal, injurious, or irritant effects; a screening or colored smoke, or an incendiary agent. War gases, smokes, and incendiaries are the three main groups.

chemical warfare a. Any agent used in chemical warfare, especially toxic gas. See war *gas.*

clearing a. *In microscopy,* a substance used to render tissues transparent for mounting.

dealcoholization a. A liquid used for getting

rid of the alcohol in preserved specimens; also one that facilitates the penetration of paraffin in microtomy.

radiomimetic a. Any agent, such as nitrogen mustards, urethane, benzol and hydrogen peroxide, capable of duplicating many of the radiation-induced effects in tissue.

wetting a. A substance which causes a liquid to spread more readily upon a solid surface, chiefly through a reduction of surface tension. Wetting agents are either ionic or non-ionic, the former being further classified as cationic or anionic, depending on whether the characteristic activity is inherent in the cation or anion.

a″ge·ra′si·a (ay″juh·ray′see·uh, ·zee·uh, adj″uh·) [G., eternal youth, from *a-*, not; *gēras*, old age]. Vigorous, healthy old age.

a·geu′si·a (ag·yōō′see·uh, a·jew′see·uh, ·shuh), **a·geus′ti·a** (ag·yōōs′tee·uh, a·juice′tee·uh) [*a-;* G. *geusis*, sense of taste]. Loss or impairment of the sense of taste. When due to a cortical lesion, it is called **central ageusia;** when due to a disorder of the nerve endings, **peripheral ageusia;** when due to a lesion in the nerve between its origin and distribution, **conduction ageusia.**

ag′ger (ag′ur, ad′jur) [L., mound]. *In anatomy*, a projection, eminence, or mound.

a. nasi. An oblique ridge on the inner surface of the nasal process of the maxilla; the anterior part of the ethmoidal crest.

ag·glom′er·ate [L. *agglomerare*, to wind on a ball]. Grouped or clustered. Syn., *agminate, aggregate.* —**agglomera′tion,** *n.*

ag·glu″ti·na′tion [L. *agglutinare*, to glue]. A joining together; an aggregation of suspended particles. —**agglu′tinable, agglu′tinative,** *adj.*

cold a. Phenomenon caused by presence of cold *agglutinin.*

specific a. Reaction between the suspension of an antigen (bacteria or cells) and its specific antiserum, leading to the clumping of the suspended elements. Used in the diagnosis of certain diseases, as the Widal test for typhoid.

ag·glu′ti·nin [*agglutinare*]. An antibody occurring in a normal or immune serum which, when added to a suspension of its homologous, particulate antigen, causes the antigen elements to adhere to one another, forming clumps.

anti-Rh a. An antibody not found normally in man, but only as the result of sensitization. See *Rh sensitization, blood groups.*

chief a. An agglutinating antibody in the blood of an individual immunized against a specific disease or microorganism. It is active at higher dilutions than are the group or partial agglutinins. Syn., *major a.* See also *antibody.*

cold a. A nonspecific panagglutinin found in normal human sera which produces maximum clumping of erythrocytes at 4° C. and none at 37° C. These hemagglutinins increase in titer in one-third to one-half of patients with primary atypical pneumonia, and are found in high titer in some patients with acquired hemolytic anemia. Syn., *cold hemagglutinin.*

flagellar a. See H *a.*

group a. One which acts as a specific toward one species and which will agglutinate other related species. Syn., *minor a., partial a.*

H a. One which is specific for the flagella of an organism only. Also called *flagellar a.*

major a. See chief *a.*

minor a. An agglutinin acting on other related organisms to the one utilized for immunization, but in lower dilution. Also called *group a.*

O a. One specific for the body of a microorganism. Also called *somatic a.*

partial a. See group *a.*

somatic a. See O *a.*

ag″glu·tin′o·gen (ag″lew·tin′o·jen, a·glew′in·ot·jen) [*agglutinare;* G. *genesthai*, from *gignesthai*, to be produced]. An antigen which, when injected into the animal body, stimulates the formation of a specific agglutinin. This, in turn, has the capacity to agglutinate the antigen.

ag·glu′ti·noid [*agglutinare;* G. *eidos*, form]. 1. An agglutinin which has lost its zymophore group through the action of heat, age, acids, etc., but still possesses its haptophore group. 2. An agglutinin which, as the result of certain chemical or physical treatment, has lost the ability to clump its homologous antigen but retains the capacity to combine with it. 3. *In hematology*, incomplete antibodies.

ag·glu′ti·no·phore″ [*agglutinare;* G. *phorein*, to bear]. Factor present in an agglutinin, which causes clumping; the zymophore of an agglutinin.

ag″glu·tin′o·scope (ag″lew·tin′o·scope, a·glew′tin·o·scope″) [*agglutinare;* G. *skopein*, to examine]. Instrument used to observe the process of agglutination in a test tube and to facilitate the reading of the result.

ag′gre·gate [L. *aggregare*, to add to]. The mass formed by certain antibodies and their homologous antigens; a clump. —**aggregate,** *adj., v.*

ag″gre·ga′tion [*aggregare*]. Agmination; a massing together of materials; a congeries or collection of particles, parts, or bodies, usually of a similar nature.

ag·gres′sin [L. *aggressus*, from *aggredi*, to attack]. A soluble substance of bacterial origin which promotes infection by combining with specific antibodies which uncombined would enhance phagocytosis and destruction of the bacteria.

ag·gres′sion [L. *aggressio*, from *aggredi*]. *In psychiatry*, an act or attitude of hostility, commonly arising out of frustration or feelings of inferiority.

ag′i·tat″ed de·pres′sion. A type of manic-depressive or involutional psychosis; characterized by marked restlessness, continual activity, despondency, and anxiety.

ag″i·ta′tion [L. *agitatio*, the state of being in motion, from *agitare*]. 1. Fatiguing restlessness with violent motion. 2. Mental disturbance. 3. Stirring or shaking a mixture, as in pharmacy.

a″gi·ta′tor caud′ae. An occasional additional slip of the gluteus maximus muscle arising from the coccyx.

ag″i·to·graph′i·a (adj″i·to·graf′ee·uh) [*agitare;* G. *graphein*, to write]. A condition characterized by excessive speed in writing, with unconscious omissions of words, syllables, or letters.

ag″i·to·la′li·a (adj″i·to·lay′lee·uh). See *agitophasia.*

ag″i·to·pha′si·a (adj″i·to·fay′zhuh, ·zee·uh) [*agitare;* G. *phasis*, speech]. A condition marked by excessive rapidity of speech, with sounds or syllables unconsciously slurred, omitted, or distorted. Syn., *agitolalia.*

Ag·kis′tro·don (ang·kis′tro·don) [NL; G. *agkistron*, fishhook; *odōn*, tooth]. A genus of Crotalidae, the pit vipers.

A. acutus. A well-known species found in China.

A. bilineatus. A well-known species found in Mexico.

A. halys. A common eastern European species.

A. mokasen. The copperhead; found in the eastern half of the United States. Attains a length of about three feet; its bite is common, but seldom fatal except in children.

A. piscivorus. The water moccasin or cottonmouth; found in swamps in the southeastern United States.

A. rhodastoma. A species commonly found in Siam.

a·glan′du·lar [G. *a-*, not; L. *glandulae*, glands]. Having no glands; without glands, as the brain.

a·glau·cop′si·a, a·glau·kop′si·a (ay·glaw·cop′-see·uh, a·glaw·) [*a-;* G. *glaukos*, bluish green; *opsis*, vision]. Green blindness. See *colorblindness*.

ag′li·a [G. *agliē*, incorrect form for *aigis*, speck in the eye]. A speck or spot upon the cornea or the sclera.

a″glo·mer′u·lar (ay″glo·merr′yoo·lur, ag″lo·, ah″-glo·) [G. *a-*, not; L. *glomerulus*, dim. of *glomus*, ball]. Without glomeruli, as aglomerular kidney.

a·glos′si·a (ay·glos′ee·uh, a·glos′·) [*a-;* G. *glōssa*, tongue]. 1. Congenital absence of the tongue. 2. Loss of the ability to speak; mutism.

a·glos″so·sto′mi·a [*a-; glōssa;* G. *stoma*, mouth]. A condition in a monster in which the tongue is lacking and the mouth is imperforate.

a·glos′sus (ay·glos′us, a·glos′us) [*a-; glōssa*]. A person without a tongue.

a·glu′cone (ay·glue′cone, a·glue′cone). 1. An older term for the nonsugar portion of a glycoside, now called aglycone. 2. The nonsugar portion of a glucoside.

ag″lu·ti′tion (ag″loo·tish′un) [*a-;* L. *glutire*, to swallow]. Difficulty in swallowing; inability to swallow; dysphagia.

a·gly·cae′mic. See *aglycemic.*

a·gly·ce′mic (ay·glye·see′mick, a·glye·) [*a-;* G. *glykys*, sweet; *haima*, blood]. Having no sugar in the blood. —**aglycemia,** *n.*

a·gly′cone (ay·gly′cone, a·gly′cone) [*a-; glykys*]. The nonsugar portion of a glycoside. Also called *genin.*

a·gly″co·su′ric (ay·gly″ko·sue′rick, a·gly″ko·) [*a-; glykys;* G. *ouron*, urine]. Free from glycosuria; exhibiting no urinary sugar. —**aglycosuria,** *n.*

Ag′ly·pha [G. *aglyphos*, unhewn]. A subdivision of the Colubridae family of snakes, distinguished from venomous varieties by the absence of enlarged, front fangs.

ag′ma·tine (ag′muh·teen, ·tin). $C_5H_{14}N_4$. Aminobutyl guanidine, an amine isolated from ergot and from herring spawn.

ag′mi·nate, ag′mi·nat″ed [L. *agmen*, a crowd, a band]. Gathered into clumps or clusters; aggregate, as agminated lymph nodules of the intestine.

ag·na′thi·a [G. *a-*, not; *gnathos*, jaw]. Absence or deficient development of the jaws. —**ag′nathous,** *adj.;* **ag′nathus, ag′nathy,** *n.*

ag·na″tho·ceph′a·lus [*a-; gnathos;* G. *kephalē*, head]. Type of otocephalus in which the eyes are situated low on the face with approximation or fusion of the zygomas. —**agnathocepha′lia, agnathocephaly,** *n.*

ag′na·thus (ag′nuth·us, ag·nay′thus) [*a-; gnathos*]. An individual exhibiting agnathia.

ag·ne′a, ag·noe′a [G. *agnoia*, want of perception]. A condition in which the patient does not recognize things or persons.

Agnew, Cornelius Rea [*American ophthalmologist,* 1830–88]. Invented surgical instruments and devised operative procedures, such as canthoplasty, for the correction of strabismus and for chalazion.

Agnew, David Hayes [*American surgeon,* 1818–92]. Devised an amputation, a method of operating for inguinal hernia, operations for the relief of salivary fistula and for webbed fingers, and a special splint for fracture of the patella.

ag·noe′a. See *agnea.*

ag″no·gen′ic [G. *agnostos*, unknowing, unknown; *-genic* from *genesthai*, to become, be born]. Of unknown etiology. Syn. *cryptogenic, idiopathic.*

ag·no′si·a [G. *a-*, not; *gnōsis*, a recognizing]. Total or partial loss of the perceptive faculty by which persons and things are recognized. It is commonly classified as **auditory agnosia, optic agnosia, tactile agnosia,** etc., according to the sense or senses affected.

ag·nos′ter·ol [L. *agnus*, lamb; G. *stereos*, hard; *-ol*, from L. *oleum*, oil]. $C_{30}H_{47}OH$. A complex terpene alcohol found in wool fat. Formerly considered to be a sterol but now shown not to possess the structure characteristic of this group of compounds. See also *isocholesterol.*

ag″om·phi′a·sis, ag″om·pho′sis [G. *a-*, not; *gomphios*, tooth; NL. *-iasis*, condition]. 1. Looseness of the teeth. 2. Absence of teeth. —**agom′-phious,** *adj.*

a·gon′ad·ism. Absence of the ovaries or testes, or their functions, and the resulting physiologic changes; it may be congenital or acquired. See *eunuchoidism.*

ag′o·nal [G. *agōn*, a struggle]. Struggling; relating to the death struggle or to agony.

a·go′ni·a [G. *agōnia*, a struggle]. Distress of mind; extreme anguish.

a·go′ni·a [G. *agonos*, barren]. Sterility; barrenness; impotence.

ag″o·ni′a·din [NL., Sp., and Pg., from *agonio*, wavy algae, from L. *agere*, to set in motion]. Plumierin. The active principle in the bark of *Plumeria succuba* or pagoda tree. Formerly used as antiperiodic.

ag′o·nist [G. *agōnistēs*, combatant, from *agōn*, a struggle]. A contracting muscle engaged in the movement of a part and opposed by an antagonistic muscle. Thus, when flexing the elbow, the biceps is the *agonist* and the triceps is the *antagonist.* Also called *protagonist.*

ag′o·ny [*agōn*]. 1. Violent pain; extreme anguish. 2. The death struggle.

agoral. Trade-mark for certain emulsions containing mineral oil and agar gel: formerly spelled *agarol.*

ag″o·ra·pho′bi·a [G. *agora*, market place, assembly; *phobos*, fear]. Morbid fear of open places or spaces, as opposed to claustrophobia.

-ag′ra [G. *agra*, a catching]. A combining form denoting *gout, a gouty affection,* or *a seizure of pain.*

a·gram″ma·pha′si·a Agrammatism.

a·gram′ma·tism [*a-; gramma*, letter]. A type of aphasia in which the patient is unable to frame a grammatical or intelligible sentence, although able to utter words. Also called *jargon aphasia.* Syn., *agrammaphasia, paraphasia.*

Agramonte y Simoni, Aristide [*Cuban parasitologist,* 1869–1931]. Member with Reed, Carroll, and Lazear of the U. S. Army Yellow Fever Commission which proved that yellow fever is transmitted to man by mosquitoes (1900–01).

a·gran′u·lo·cyte″ (ay·gran′yoo·lo·sight″, a·gran′·) [*a-;* L. *granulum*, a small grain; G. *kytos*, cell]. A nongranular leukocyte. —**agranulocyt′ic,** *adj.*

a·gran″u·lo·cy·the′mi·a. Agranulocytosis.

a·gran″u·lo·cy·to′sis (a·gran″yoo·lo·sigh·to′sis, ay·gran″yoo·lo·) [*a-; granulum;* G. *kytos*, cell; *-ōsis*, condition]. An acute febrile disease, affecting females oftener than males, frequently caused by coal-tar drugs and some of the sulfonamides. It is characterized by prostration, high fever, ulcerative lesions of the mucous membranes in the mouth, throat, and other areas, and a marked reduction in the number of the granular leukocytes. Before the introduction of pentnucleotide treatment, the mortality rate was very high. Also called *agranulocythemia, agranulocytic angina, agranulosis, granulocytic hypoplasia, granulocytopenia, granulopenia, hypogranulocytis,* and *idiopathic, malignant,* or *pernicious leukopenia.*

a·gran″u·lo·plas′tic [*a-; granulum;* G. *plassein,* to form]. 1. Not forming granular cells. 2. Forming nongranular cells only.

a·gran″u·lo′sis. Agranulocytosis.

a·graph′i·a (ay·graf′ee·uh, a·graf′·) [*a-;* G. *graphein,* to write]. Loss of ability to write; a form of aphasia.

absolute a. Inability to write even unconnected letters. Also called *atactic a., literal a.*

acoustic a. Inability to write from dictation.

amnemonic a. Inability to write connected sentences, although letters and words can be written.

cerebral a. Incapacity to express a thought in writing. Also called *mental a.*

congenital a. Developmental *a.*

developmental a. Marked deficiency in learning to write, not based on any obvious skeletal or neuromuscular defect, and out of line with the individual's mental age, accomplishment quotient in other subjects, and general manual dexterity. Syn. *congenital a.*

motor a. Loss of ability to write because of ataxia.

musical a. Loss of ability to write musical notes.

optic a. Inability to copy.

verbal a. Inability to write words, although single letters can be written.

ag′ri·mo″ny [L. *agrimonia,* for *argemonia,* from G. *argemōnē,* a kind of poppy]. Specifically, the root of *Agrimonia eupatoria,* a mild astringent.

ag′ri·us, a′gri·us [G. *agrios,* wild]. Having a red or angry look, as in certain dermatoses.

Ag″ro·bac·te′ri·um [L. *ager,* soil; G. *baktērion,* little staff]. Name proposed by Conn for a genus of bacteria of the Rhizobiaceae, including *Alcaligenes fecalis, Bacterium radicicola,* and the bacterium of hairy root disease.

ag″ro·ma′ni·a [*ager;* G. *mania,* madness]. A morbid desire to live in the open country or in isolation.

a·gryp′ni·a (ay·grip′nee·uh, a·grip′·) [G., sleeplessness]. Sleeplessness; insomnia. *Obs.*

a. excitata. That associated with mental excitement and disinterest in surroundings.

a. pertaesa. That due to physical disorder.

a. senilis. That appearing with old age.

ag″ryp·not′ic [*agrypnia*]. Inducing, relating to, or characterized by insomnia.

a″gua·miel′ (ah″gwahm·yell′, ag″wuh·mee·el′) [Sp. *agua,* water; *miel,* honey]. The sap of *Agave atrovirens* and *A. mexicana,* from which pulque, the fermented drink, is made. It is said to have diuretic, laxative, galactagogue, and nutrient properties.

a′gue (ayg′yōō) [F. *aigu,* sharp, from L. *acutus*]. 1. Old term for an attack of malaria. 2. A recurrent chill. 3. Neuralgia, as **face ague,** tic douloureux.

a. cake. The enlarged spleen of chronic malaria.

brass founder's a. Severe chills which follow the inhalation of fumes of finely divided metal, especially fumes of cadmium, lead, manganese, mercury, magnesium, and zinc (brass). Syn., *metal fume fever, galvo.*

catenating a. Chills associated with other diseases.

dumb a. Subacute malaria without definite chills, and only slight periodicity.

agurin. A brand of theobromine and sodium acetate.

a″gyi·o·pho′bi·a (adj″ee·o·fo′bee·uh) [G. *agyia,* street; *phobos,* fear]. Morbid fear of streets, as fear of crossing the street.

a·gy′ri·a (ay·jy′ree·uh, a·jy′·) [G. *a-,* not; *gyros,* ring, circle]. Congenital absence of cerebral convolutions.

ah Abbreviation for hypermetropic astigmatism.

a·hyp′ni·a (ay·hip′nee·uh, a·hip′·), **a·hyp·no′sis** (ay·hip·no′sis, a·hip·) [*a-;* G. *hypnos,* sleep]. Pathologic insomnia; extreme wakefulness. Also called *agrypnia.*

aich″mo·pho′bi·a (ayk″mo·fo′bee·uh, ike″mo·) [G. *aichmē,* point of a spear; *phobos,* fear]. Morbid dread of sharp or pointed objects, or of being touched by them or by a finger.

aid man. An enlisted man of the U. S. Army Medical Service, attached to a company, battery, troop, and other units, who gives emergency medical treatment to casualties.

ai·doi′o- (ay·doy′o-, eye·doy′o-). For words beginning *aidoio-* not found here, see words beginning *edeo-.*

Ai·lan′thus (ay·lanth′us) [*aylanto,* tree of heaven, name of the tree in the Moluccas]. A genus of trees of the order Simarubaceae.

ail′ing [AS. *eglan,* to trouble, pain]. Indisposed; in ill health; not well.

ail′ment [*eglan*]. A disease; sickness; complaint.

ai·lu″ro·pho′bi·a (ay·lew″ro·fo′bee·uh, eye″lew-ro·) [G. *ailouros,* cat; *phobos,* fear]. A morbid fear of cats.

ain′hum (ayn′hum, in′yoom. *See* NOTES § 35) [Yoruba *ayun*]. A tropical disease peculiar to male Negroes, in which a toe is slowly and spontaneously amputated by a fibrous ring. Etiology unknown. Syn., *dactylolysis spontanea.*

air [G. *aēr,* air]. Atmospheric air is a simple nonchemical mixture of gases 78.03 parts by volume or 75.51 parts by weight of nitrogen, 20.98 parts by volume or 23.15 parts by weight of oxygen, and 0.03 part by volume of carbon dioxide. Air also contains small amounts of ammonia, nitrates, organic matter, and the rare gases argon, neon, krypton, and xenon. By virtue of its oxygen content it is able to sustain respiration. The density of air at 32° F. and 14.7 pounds pressure is 0.081 pound per cubic foot. The pressure of air at sea level is 14.7 pounds per square inch. Syn., *atmosphere.*

alkaline a. Free or volatile ammonia.

alveolar a. That contained in the air sacs and pulmonary alveoli.

complemental, complementary a. The amount that can still be inhaled after a normal inspiration. See also inspiratory reserve *volume.*

expired a. That which is exhaled from the lungs by expiration.

functional residual a. See functional residual *capacity.*

inspired a. That which is taken in by inspiration.

liquid a. That which has been liquefied by subjecting it to great pressure; extreme cold is produced by its evaporation.

minimal a. The small amount left in an excised or collapsed lung.

reserve a. Expiratory reserve volume.

residual a. Residual volume.

stationary a. That remaining in the lungs during normal respiration.

supplemental a. Expiratory reserve volume.

tidal a. Tidal volume.

air con·di′tion·ing. The modification of the air—by the control of its temperature and humidity, the removal of particulate water, and the sterilization of pathogenic organisms—for better health, bodily comfort, and industrial needs.

air my·e·log′ra·phy. Radiographic examination of the spinal cord after injecting air into the subarachnoid space.

airol. A trade-mark for a brand of suppositories containing bismuth oxyiodide-subgallate, formula approximately $C_6H_2(OH)_3CO.O.Bi(OH)I$.

air pi′lots′ dis·ease′. Acute emotional shock; aeroneurosis.

air′sick″ness [G. *aēr*, air; AS. *sēoc*]. A form of motion sickness occurring in airplane flights, principally as a result of acceleration; characterized by vertigo, nausea, headache, mental depression and anxiety, pallor, cold sweats, tremor, and vomiting; a feeling of nervous and muscular tenseness is followed by muscular weakness, faintness, and prostration. Airsickness is the same as seasickness and car sickness in etiology and symptoms, but should not be confused with altitude sickness.

air′way″ [*aer;* AS. *weg*]. 1. *In anesthesia*, any of several devices used to maintain a clear and unobstructed respiratory passage during general anesthesia. 2. A respiratory passage.

endobronchial a. One extending down to one of the bronchi.

endotracheal a. One extending into the trachea.

nasal a. One through the nose.

oral a. One through the mouth.

pharyngeal a. One extending down into the pharynx.

Aitken, John A. [*Scottish surgeon*, d. 1790]. Described a bilateral pelviotomy for dystocia.

Aitken, William [*Scottish physician*, 1825–92]. Introduced a pill of iron, quinine, strychnine, and arsenic, called *Aitken's pill.*

a·ja′cine (a·jay′seen, ·sin, adj′uh·seen, ·sin). $C_{15}H_{24}NO_4$. An alkaloid from larkspur, *Delphinium ajacis.*

a·jac′o·nine (a·jack′o·neen, ·nin). $C_{17}H_{29}NO_2$. An alkaloid from larkspur, *Delphinium ajacis.*

aj·mal′i·cine. An alkaloid from *Rauwolfia serpentina.*

aj′ma·line. An alkaloid, sometimes called *rauwolfine*, isolated from *Rauwolfia serpentina.*

aj·mal′i·nine. An alkaloid from *Rauwolfia serpentina.*

ak-. For words beginning with *ak-* not found here, see words beginning *ac-*.

a″ka·mu′shi (ah″kah·mōō′shee, ·mew′shee, ack″-uh·) [Jap. *aka*, red; *mushi*, bug or insect]. Tsutsugamushi disease.

a·kan″thes·the′si·a, a·kan″thaes·the′si·a. See *acanthesthesia.*

a·kar′y·o·cyte [G. *a-*, not; *karyon*, kernel; *kytos*, cell]. An erythrocyte; erythroplastid.

a·kar′y·ote [*a-; karyon*]. A nonnucleated cell. Also *akaryota.* —**a·kar′y·ote,** *adj.*

ak″a·thi′si·a, ac″a′thi′si·a [*a-;* G. *kathisis*, a sitting down]. 1. A condition seen in parkinsonism; because of the severe muscular rigidity, the patient is compelled to change position at frequent intervals or to rise and pace the floor. 2. *In psychiatry*, inability to sit down; intense anxiety about sitting.

a·ker″a·to′sis (a·ker″uh·to′sis) [G. *a-*, not; *keras*, horn; *-osis*, condition]. A deficiency or absence of horny tissue, as of the nails.

Åkerlund, Åke Olof [*Swedish roentgenologist*, 1887–]. His name is associated with a deformity or irregularity of the duodenal cap, observed in roentgenograms of ulcers; called *Åkerlund's deformity.*

a·kin″aes·the′si·a. See *akinesthesia.*

ak″i·ne′si·a (ack″i·nee′shuh, ·see·uh), **ak″i·ne′sis, ac″i·ne′si·a** [G., from *a-; kinēsis*, motion]. Loss of or impaired motor function; immobility from any cause.

a. algera. A form of hysteria characterized by painfulness associated with any kind of movements.

a. amnestica. Immobility from disuse of the muscles.

a. iridis. Rigidity or immobility of the iris.

cerebral a. Loss of motion associated with a cerebral lesion.

crossed a. A motor paralysis on the side opposite that in which the lesion exists.

reflex a. Impairment or loss of reflex action.

spinal a. Motor impairment due to a lesion of the cord.

a·kin″es·the′si·a, a·kin″aes·the′si·a (ay·kin″-ess·thee′zhuh, ·zee·uh, a·kin″·), **a·ki·naes′thi·a** (ay·ki·ness′thee·uh, a·ki·) [*a-; kinēsis;* G. *aisthēsis*, sensation]. Loss of muscular sense or sense of movement.

ak″i·net′ic, ak″i·ne′sic [*a-;* G. *kinētikos*, relating to motion]. 1. Relating to or affected with akinesia. 2. Amitotic.

A′kis spi·no′sa. A beetle belonging to the family Tenebrionidae. Serves as an intermediate host for the cysticercoid of *Hymenolepis diminuta.*

ak′o·asm (ack′o·az·um). See *acousma.*

Al Chemical symbol for aluminum.

al-. A combining form from *all.*

al- [Ar.]. A combining form from the Arabic definite article *the.*

al- [L.]. A form of *ad-* assimilated in Latin before *l.*

-al [*al*dehyde]. *In chemistry*, a suffix indicating *the presence of the aldehyde group.*

-al [L. *-alis*, a suffix forming adjectives from nouns]. An adjective suffix denoting *belonging to, of* or *pertaining to, having the character of, appropriate to.*

a′la (pl. *alae*) [L., wing]. 1. A wing. 2. Any winglike process. —**alar, al′iform, alate,** *adj.*

a. auris. Pinna of the ear.

a. cinerea. A triangular eminence on the floor of the fourth ventricle of the brain, overlying the dorsal nucleus of the vagus nerve.

alae laterales. (a) Great wings of the sphenoid bone. (b) Winglike processes on each side of the frontal bone.

a. ethmoidalis. Alar process of the ethmoid.

a. lobuli centralis [BNA]. Lateral part of the median cerebellar lobe.

a. magna. Great wing of the sphenoid.

a. nasi. Lower portion of the side of the nose; a wing of the nose.

a. of the sacrum. Flat, triangular surface of bone extending outward from the base of the sacrum.

a. of the vomer. Either of the two lateral expansions of the superior border of the vomer.

a. parva. Small wing of the sphenoid.

al″a·bam′ine (al″uh·bam′een, ·in) [after *Alabama*]. A rare element found in monazite sand; now called astatine.

al′a·bas″ter [G. *alabastros*, from *alabastos*, a box for holding perfumes, often made of alabaster]. 1. Hydrous calcium sulfate. 2. Calcium carbonate. —**al″a·bas′trine,** *adj.*

al″a·bas′trine (al″uh·bas′trin) [*alabastros*]. Naphthalene.

a′lae (ay′lee). Plural of ala.

a·la′li·a [G. *a-*, not; *lalia*, talk]. 1. Impairment or loss of speech due to any organic defect or paralysis. 2. Aphasia due to psychic disorder. —**alal′ic,** *adj.*

mental a. Speech impairment caused by stammering, especially in children. Also called *relative a.*

al-amphylline. Trade-mark for a tablet preparation containing aminophylline, aluminum hydroxide, and magnesium trisilicate, characterized by reduced tendency of the aminophylline to produce nausea, and thus allowing increased oral dosage of the same.

a·lan′gine (a·lan′jeen, ·jin, al′un·jeen, ·jin). An alkaloid obtained from *Alangium salviifolium;* it is a parasympathetic stimulant and has been employed as a febrifuge and emetic.

al′a·nine (al′uh·neen, ·nin). $CH_3CH(NH_2).COOH$; alpha-aminopropionic acid or 2-aminopropanoic acid. The L-form is a constituent of many proteins; it is classified as a nonessential amino acid. It is also called *alpha*-alanine (not to be confused with *beta*-alanine, $CH_2NH_2.CH_2.COOH$, or 3-aminopropanoic acid), *lactamic acid, lactamine.*

Alanson, Edward [*English surgeon,* 1747–1823]. Remembered for his development of a method of amputation in which a division of the skin and muscles is made in the form of a hollow cone.

a·lan′tic [Ger. *alant*, elecampane]. Pertaining to or derived from elecampane.

a·lan′tol (a·lan′tole, ·tol, ·tawl, al′un·tole, ·tol, ·tawl). $C_{10}H_{16}O$. An aromatic liquid obtained from elecampane; formerly used like creosote in pulmonary tuberculosis.

a·lan″to·lac′tone. $C_{15}H_{20}O_2$. One of the crystalline principles found in alant camphor, obtained by steam distillation of inula; said to have anthelmintic action.

al′a·nyl. The univalent radical, $CH_3CH(NH_2)CO$—, of the amino acid alanine.

al″a·nyl·gly·cine′ (al″uh·nil·glye·seen′, ·glye′seen, ·sin). A dipeptide formed by the combination of two amino acids, alanine and glycine.

a·larm′ re·ac′tion. See under *reaction.*

a·las′trim [Pg., from *alastrar*, to spread, cover]. Mild smallpox.

a·la′tus [L.]. An individual in whom there is a marked backward projection of the scapulas.

al′ba [L. *albus*, white]. The white fibrous tissue of the brain; the white matter as opposed to the gray.

reticular a. The reticulated layer of alba on the anterior half of the uncinate gyrus. *O.T.*

Albarran y Dominguez, Joaquin [*Cuban surgeon and urologist in France,* 1860–1912]. Associated with inventions of special cystoscopes, with operations for the removal of the median lobe of the prostate, and with a test of renal function (1905) known as the *polyuria test.* See subcervical *gland.*

al·bas′pi·din [*albus;* G. *aspidion*, little shield]. An anthelmintic substance extracted from aspidium (male fern).

Albee, Fred Houdlett [*American surgeon,* 1876–1945]. Noted for his application of mechanical methods to bone operations; for his method of stabilizing tuberculous or fractured spines by the insertion of a tibial graft into the split spinous processes of the vertebrae (spinal fusion); for his bundle-of-reeds technic in which parallel strips of bone are taken from the tibia and used as a bone graft; and for his fracture table, which has had wide use in orthopedic surgery. See also Albee's *saw.*

Albers-Schönberg, Heinrich Ernst [*German surgeon,* 1865–1921]. His name is associated with osteopetrosis, called *Albers-Schönberg disease* (1903). Also remembered for his invention of the compression diaphragm, which intensifies the action of roentgen rays (1903).

Albert, Eduard [*Austrian surgeon,* 1841–1900]. Remembered for his description of painful heel (achillodynia), once known as *Albert's disease, Swediaur's disease.* His original work (1882) on arthrodesis of the joints for the partial relief of disability in flaccid paralysis paved the way for the modern operations of joint fusion.

Albert's stain. See under *stain.*

al·bes′cent [L. *albescere*, to become white]. Whitish.

al′bi·cans (al′bi·kanz) (pl. *albicantia*) [L. *albicare*, to make white]. White; whitish.

al′bi·cans. One of the corpora albicantia of the ovary.

albicol. Trade name of a preparation of colloidal aluminum silicate, betanaphthyl benzoate, bismuth subsalicylate, and aromatics: used as a gastric antacid, astringent, and protective.

al″bi·du′ri·a, al″bi·nu′ri·a [L. *albidus*, white; G. *ouron*, urine]. 1. Passage of very pale, almost colorless urine, of low specific gravity. 2. Chyluria.

al″bi·fac′tion [L. *albus*, white; *facere*, to make]. Act or process of blanching or rendering white.

Albini, Giuseppe [*Italian physiologist,* 1827–1911]. His name is associated with small nodules found on the free edge of the atrioventricular valves in infants.

al′bi·nism, al″bi·nis′mus (al′bin·izm, al″bi·niz′mus), **al·bi′no·ism** [*albus*]. Congenital absence of pigment from the skin, hair, choroid coat, and iris. It may be localized, in **partial albinism,** or generalized, in **total albinism.** The latter form is associated with astigmatism, nystagmus, and photophobia. Also called *leukoderma, achromodermia, congenital achroma, achromatosis.*

al·bi′no (al·buy′no, al·bee′no) [Pg., from *albus*]. A person affected with albinism. —**albinot′ic,** *adj.*

al·bi′no·ism. See *albinism.*

al″bi·nu′ri·a. See *albiduria.*

al′bo-, alb- [*albus*]. A combining form meaning *white, whitish.*

al″bo·ci·ne′re·ous [*albus;* L. *cinereus*, ash-colored]. Having both white and gray matter.

albolene. Trade-mark for a brand of liquid petrolatum and certain products containing the same.

Albright, Fuller [*American physician,* 1900–]. His name is associated with the syndrome of polyostotic fibrous dysplasia (usually asymmetrical and segmental), pigmentation (often segmental), and precocious puberty in females: also called *osteitis fibrosa disseminata, Albright-McCune-Sternberg syndrome.* See *fibrous dysplasia.*

Albucasis (Abū-L-Qāsim, Alsaharavius) [*Arabian surgical writer in Cordoba,* 936–ca. 1013]. The greatest exponent of the Arabian school. Author of *al-Tasrīf*, a treatise on medicine and surgery, the medical portion of which contains the earliest description of hemophilia. For a time in the Middle Ages, the surgical portion was the leading textbook on surgery.

albucid. $NH_2.C_6H_4.SO_2.NH.CH_3CO$. Trade name for sulfacetimide. Para-aminobenzenesulfonacetamide, a sulfonamide employed in the treatment of meningitis, gonorrhea, and other urinary infections.

al″bu·gin′e·a [L. *albugo*, from *albus*]. A layer of white fibrous tissue investing an organ or part.

a. oculi. Sclerotic coat of the eye.

a. ovarii. Tunica albuginea of the ovary.

a. testis. Tunica albuginea of the testis.

al″bu·gin′e·ous [*albugo*]. 1. Whitish. 2. Belonging to a tunica albuginea.

al″bu·gi·ni′tis [*albugo;* G. *-itis*, inflammation]. Inflammation of a tunica albuginea.

al·bu′go [L.]. A white spot upon the cornea; a corneal opacity.

al·bu′men [L.]. 1. Egg white, consisting chiefly of albumin. 2. The stored food matter in a vegetable seed. 3. Albumin.

al·bu′min [L. *albus*, white]. One of a group of protein substances, the chief constituents of animal tissues. They are soluble in water, coagulable by heat, and composed of carbon, hydrogen, nitrogen, oxygen, and sulfur. Some varieties are named after their sources or characteristic reactions: *acid a., alkali a., muscle a., ovum a., serum a., vegetable a.* See American Classification of Proteins in the Appendix. —**albuminous,** *adj.*

acid a. That changed by the action of acid.

a. tannate. An astringent used in diarrheas.
blood a. See serum *a.*
circulating a. That found in the fluids of the body.
derived a. A modified albumin resulting from the action of certain reagents upon native albumin.
egg a. The form found in egg white.
imperfect a. One which fails to give all the ordinary reactions.
lactalbumin. The albumin found in milk.
muscle a. A variety found in muscle.
native a. Any albumin occurring normally in the tissues.
organic a. That forming an integral part of the tissue.
serum a. The chief protein of blood plasma and other serous fluids. See Table of Normal Values of Blood Constituents in the Appendix.
urinary a. Serum albumin, globulin, and other proteins occurring in the urine to produce albuminuria.
vegetable a. That found in plant or vegetable matter.

al·bu′mi·nate. Any compound of albumin with an acid or base; a product of the hydrolysis of albumin or globulin. These compounds are soluble in dilute acids or bases, and are insoluble in dilute salt solutions, water, and alcohol.

al·bu″mi·nif′er·ous. Containing or yielding albumin.

al·bu″mi·nim′e·ter, al·bu″mi·nom′e·ter. An instrument for the quantitative estimation of albumin in a fluid, as in urine. —**albuminimetry, albuminometry,** *n.*

al·bu″mi·nog′e·nous (alb·yōō″mi·nodj′i·nus). Producing albumin.

al·bu′mi·noid, al′bu·moid, al·bu′moid. Resembling albumin; applied to certain compounds having many of the characteristics of albumin.

al·bu′mi·noid. Any scleroprotein, a simple protein characterized by being insoluble in neutral solvents, such as collagen, elastin, keratin, etc. See American Classification of Proteins in the Appendix. Also spelled *albumoid.*

al·bu″mi·nol′y·sin. A lysin which decomposes proteins. Also called *proteolysin.* —**albuminolysis,** *n.*

al·bu″mi·nom′e·ter. See *albuminimeter.*

al·bu′mi·nose (alb·yōō′mi·noce, ·noze). A product of the digestion of fibrin or of any albuminoid in very dilute hydrochloric acid; acid albumin.

al·bu″min·u·ret′ic, al·bu″mi·nu′ric [L. *albus,* white; G. *ouron,* urine]. A drug which causes albuminuria. —**albuminuret′ic,** *adj.*

al·bu″mi·nu′ri·a [*albus; ouron*]. The presence in the urine of serum albumin, globulin, and other proteins which may result from disease of the kidneys or from the admixture of blood or pus with the urine; proteinuria. —**al·bu″mi·nu′ric,** *adj.*
accidental a. See false *a.*
adventitious a. See pseudoalbuminuria under *albuminuria.*
a. acetonica. That due to asphyxia. Also called *anoxemic a.*
a. of adolescence. See cyclic *a.*
alimentary a. That following the ingestion of a heavy protein meal.
cardiac a. That due to chronic valvular disease.
colliquative a. A form seen in convalescence from severe fevers.
consumptive a. See colliquative *a.*
cyclic a. The albuminuria of adolescence, in which a small quantity of albumin appears in the urine at stated times of the day. Also called *physiologic a., simple a., functional a.*
dietetic a. That due to the ingestion of certain forms of food.
emulsion a. That in which the urine has a milky turbidity which does not clear on heating, filtration, or acidification.
exudative a. An albuminuria partially due to the filtration of albumin through the membranes of the kidney and also to the presence in the urine of products of inflammation, as in cases of nephritis.
false a. A mixture of albumin with the urine during its transit through the urinary passages, where it may be derived from blood, pus, or special secretions that contain albumin.
febrile a. That due to fever, or associated with acute infectious diseases, slight changes occurring in the glomeruli without organic lesion.
functional a. See cyclic *a.*
globular a. That due to destruction of blood cells or dependent upon the presence of blood in the urine.
hematogenous a. That occurring in diseases which cause some change in the quality and quantity of the normal protein of the blood.
hypostatic a. That which is present when the patient lies flat on his back, but which disappears when he is erect.
intermittent a. Cyclic albuminuria.
intrinsic a. See true *a.*
march a. That following prolonged walking or running, as in soldiers or marathon runners.
nephrogenous a. That due to renal disease.
neurotic a. That which is present in epilepsy, exophthalmic goiter, apoplexy, neurasthenia, injuries to the brain, and various psychoses.
orthostatic a. A form dependent upon an upright posture.
paroxysmal a. Cyclic albuminuria.
partial a. A form in which it is assumed that only certain tubules are affected. Also called *a. parcellaire.*
pathologic a. That which results from a diseased condition, such as that due to degenerative change in the kidneys or to an acute febrile disease.
physiologic a. Albumin in normal urine, without appreciable coexisting renal lesion or diseased condition.
pseudoalbuminuria. That dependent upon the presence of such fluids as blood, pus, lymph, spermatic fluid, or the contents of an abscess cavity, in the urine. Syn., *adventitious a.*
residual a. A form in which a small amount of albumin may persist after nephritis.
true a. That due to the excretion of some albuminous constituents of the blood with the water and salts of the urine. Syn., *intrinsic a.*

al·bu″mi·nu′ric. See *albuminuretic.*

al′bu·moid, al·bu′moid. See *albuminoid.*

al·bu′mo·scope′. See *horismascope.*

al′bu·mose (alb′yōō·moce, alb·yōō′moze). An albuminous substance, among the first of the decomposition products of proteolysis, not coagulated by heat.

al″bu·mo·su′ri·a [*albumin;* G. *ouron,* urine]. The presence of Bence-Jones protein in the urine. Formerly called *Bence-Jones albumose.*

al″bu·tan′nin. Albumin tannate, a yellowish white powder, almost insoluble in water; used in treating diarrhea. See *tannalbin.*

Al″ca·lig′e·nes fe·cal′is (al″kuh·lidj′i·neez fi·kal′-iss). A species of bacteria found in feces and water, which resembles the typhoid bacillus. Conn has proposed a new genus, *Agrobacterium,* to include this organism.

al·cap″to·nu′ri·a. See *alkaptonuria.*

al′che·my [ML. *alchimia*, from Ar. *al-kīmiyā′*, perhaps from G. *chymos*, juice]. The chemical science of the Middle Ages, which attempted to transmute base metals into gold and to find a remedy for all diseases.

Alcock's canal. See under *canal.*

al′co·gel. An alcoholic, colloidal suspension with the dispersion medium a gel.

al′co·hol [ML., from Ar. *al-kuhl*, a fine powder for painting the eyelids]. 1. A derivative of an aliphatic hydrocarbon which contains a hydroxyl (OH) group. Alcohols are classified on the basis of the number of hydroxyl groups present in the molecule, i.e., monohydric (monatomic), dihydric (diatomic), trihydric (triatomic); or on the basis of the presence of a —CH_2OH (primary alcohol), a =CHOH (secondary alcohol), or a ≡COH (tertiary alcohol) group. 2. Ethyl alcohol, C_2H_5OH (*alcohol*). A liquid containing not less than 92.3% by weight, corresponding to 94.9% by volume, at 15.56° C., of C_2H_5OH. It may be obtained by distillation of fermented grain, starchy substances, or saccharine liquids; it is also prepared by synthesis. It is inflammable, colorless, and possesses a pungent odor and a burning taste. The effects of its ingestion are well known, but are generally misinterpreted, since the initial euphoria, increased pulse rate, and sense of warmth give rise to the belief in its value as a stimulant. Larger doses cause increasing exaltation and excitement with muscular incoordination, and, depending on the individual, eventually lead to sleep, stupor, or active delirium. All these manifestations are due to its action as a central nervous system depressant. *In medicine*, it is used internally for its fuel value in the debilitated, and for its cutaneous vasodilative and euphoric effect. On the skin it is antiseptic and astringent. In 70% solution it is used as an antiseptic for instruments. It exists in wine, whisky, brandy, gin, rum, beer, etc. See *alcoholism.*

absolute a. (*alcohol dehydratum*). Ethyl alcohol deprived of most of its water.

aliphatic a. One derived from a hydrocarbon of the aliphatic or open-chain type.

amino a. See *amino* alcohol.

aromatic a. One obtained from a hydrocarbon of the aromatic series.

batyl a. $CH_2OH.CHOH.CH_2O(CH_2)_{17}CH_3$; 3-(octadecyloxy)-1,2-propanediol; a mono-octadecyl ether of glycerin, a solid substance occurring in shark-liver oil.

fatty a. One obtained from a hydrocarbon of the fatty series.

grain a. Alcohol prepared by distillation of fermented grain. See *alcohol*, def. 2.

rubbing a. Any of a variety of preparations used as a rubefacient and containing a specially denatured ethyl alcohol, or isopropyl alcohol. It is poisonous.

wood a. See *methyl alcohol.*

al′co·hol·ase (al′ko·haul·ace, ·aze, al′ko·hol·). See alcohol *dehydrogenase.*

al′co·hol·ate. 1. A derivative of an alcohol in which the hydroxyl hydrogen is replaced by a base. 2. A preparation made with alcohol.

al″co·hol′a·ture. An alcoholic tincture.

al′co·hol de″hy·dra′tum (dee″high·dray′tum). Dehydrated alcohol; absolute alcohol.

al′co·hol de·o″dor·a′tum. Ethyl alcohol from which odorous and coloring matters have been removed by filtration through charcoal.

al″co·hol′ic [*al-kuhl*]. Pertaining to, containing, or producing alcohol.

Al″co·hol′ics A·non′y·mous. A fellowship of persons formerly addicted to alcohol who have banded together to cure others of alcoholism.

al′co·hol·ism [*al-kuhl*]. 1. Alcohol poisoning. 2. Morbid results of excessive or prolonged use of alcoholic liquors. —**al″co·hol′ic,** *n.*

acute a. Inebriety; drunkenness. Also called *ebrietas.*

chronic a. A state produced by repeated and long-continued excesses of alcoholic indulgence, and associated with severe disturbances of the digestive and nervous systems. Syn., *dipsorrhexia, dipsomania, temulence.*

al″co·hol·om′e·ter [*al-kuhl;* G. *metron*, a measure]. A hydrometer or other instrument for determining the amount of alcohol in a liquid. —**alcoholometry,** *n.*

al″co·hol″o·phil′i·a [*al-kuhl;* G. *philein*, to love]. An appetite for strong alcoholic drink; a craving for intoxicants. *Rare.*

al″co·hol·u′ri·a [*al-kuhl;* G. *ouron*, urine]. Presence of alcohol in voided urine.

al″co·hol′y·sis. Any interaction of alcohol with another substance in which the alcohol also undergoes chemical change.

alcometer. Trade name for the apparatus devised by Greenberg and Keator for use in their breath alcohol method of determining the concentration of alcohol in the blood. See breath alcohol *method.*

al′co·sol (al′ko·sol, ·sawl, ·sole). A colloidal solution in which alcohol is the dispersion medium.

aldarsone. A proprietary arsenical consisting chiefly of sodium 3-amino-4-hydroxyphenylarsonate-N-methanal sulfoxylate, used by insufflation or in the form of a suppository in the treatment of *Trichomonas vaginalis* vaginitis, and by intravenous injection for central nervous system syphilis. It contains 17.0–18.5% of pentavalent arsenic. Dose, 0.25 Gm. (4 gr.) increased to 1 Gm. (15 gr.) intravenously once a week. See *phenarsone sulfoxylate.*

al′de·hyde [abbr. from *al*cohol *dehyd*rogenatum, alcohol deprived of hydrogen]. A class of organic compounds intermediate between alcohols and acids, derived from their corresponding primary alcohols by oxidation and removal of two atoms of hydrogen, and converted into acids by the addition of an atom of oxygen. They contain the group —CHO.

aliphatic a. One derived from a hydrocarbon of the aliphatic or open-chain type.

thioaldehyde. An aldehyde in which the oxygen of the —CHO radical is replaced by sulfur.

Alder, Kurt (1907–). German chemist who shared the Nobel prize in chemistry in 1950 with Otto Diels for the development of the Diels-Alder reaction. See Otto *Diels.*

Alderotti, Taddeo (Thaddeus of Florence, Florentinus) [*Italian physician and teacher*, 1223–1303]. Introduced a new form of medical literature, the so-called consilia, or collections of clinical records.

aldinamide. Trade-mark for a brand of pyrazinamide, an antituberculosis drug having the composition of pyrazine-carboxylic acid amide.

al″do·bi·on′ic ac′id (al″do·buy·on′ick). $C_{12}H_{20}O_{12}$. An acid produced by the hydrolysis of gum arabic and other gums, as well as of the specific carbohydrate of Type 3 pneumococcus. Its components are D-glucuronic acid and D-galactose.

al″do·hex′ose. A hexose that contains an aldehyde group; examples are glucose, galactose, and mannose.

al′dol (al′dole, ·dol, ·dawl). 1. $CH_3.CH(OH).CH_2$.-CHO. Beta-hydroxybutyric aldehyde, a condensation product of acetaldehyde. 2. One of a class of condensation products formed from an aldehyde.

al′dol·ase. An enzyme occurring in muscle and capable of splitting fructose-1,6-diphosphate into dihydroxyacetone phosphate and phosphoglyceraldehyde. Syn., *zymohexase.*

al·don′ic ac′id. See under *acid.*

al″do·pen′tose. A pentose containing an aldehyde group; examples are arabinose, ribose, and xylose.

Aldor's test. See von Aldor's *test.*

al′dose (al′dose, al′doze). Any carbohydrate containing the aldehyde group —CHO.

al′do·side. A glycoside resulting from the condensation of an aldose and a compound containing a hydroxyl group.

al·dos′ter·one. 11β-21-Dihydroxy-3,20-diketo-4-pregnene-18-al; a potent adrenocortical hormone which, in very small amounts, maintains the life of adrenalectomized animals. It is isolated from adrenal venous blood and also from the amorphous residue of adrenal extracts after separation of other crystalline hormones. It is a very potent regulator of the metabolism of sodium and potassium, many times more active than desoxycorticosterone in its effect on electrolyte metabolism, less effective in regulating carbohydrate metabolism. Formerly known as *electrocortin.*

al″do·tet′rose. A tetrose, such as threose, containing an aldehyde group.

al·dox′ime (al·docks′im, ·docks′eem). 1. The product derived from an aldehyde when the oxygen of the —CHO group is replaced by —NOH, forming the —CHNOH group. 2. Acetaldoxime, CH_3.-CHNOH.

Aldrich's test. See Hench and Aldrich's *test.*

al′drin. Common name for an insecticide containing not less than 95% of 1,2,3,4,10,10-hexachloro-1,4,4a,5,8,8a-hexahydro-1,4,5,8-dimethanonaphthalene; the crystals are soluble in most organic solvents but insoluble in water. It is readily absorbed through the skin and is toxic.

a·lec′i·thal (a·less′i·thul) [G. *a-*, not; *lekithos*, yolk]. Having little or no yolk, as the eggs of placental mammals.

a·lem′bic [Ar. *al-inbīq*, the still, from G. *ambix*, cap of still]. A vessel that was formerly used for distillation.

A·lep′po boil. See *oriental sore.*

A·lep′po but′ton. See *oriental sore.*

alerdex. Trade-mark for a protein-free carbohydrate mixture used in modifying milk formulas for infant feeding.

al′e·trin. A concentrate of *Aletris farinosa.*

al′e·tris [G., a female slave who grinds corn]. 1. Star grass; unicorn root; starwort; colic root. 2. The dried rhizome and roots of *Aletris farinosa.* It is tonic, diuretic, and anthelmintic. Formerly a popular remedy in colic, dropsy, and chronic rheumatism.

al′eu·drin (al′yoo·drin, al·yōō′drin). Dichloroisopropyl carbamate, $C_4H_7O_2NCl_2$, a white crystalline substance, used as a hypnotic and sedative. It is sparingly soluble in water, but dissolves readily in alcohol, chloroform, ether, and fatty oils.

al″eu·ke′mi·a. See aleukemic *leukemia.*

al·eu′ki·a he″mor·rhag′i·ca. See primary refractory *anemia.*

a·leu′ro·nat. A vegetable protein used as a substitute for flour in diabetes.

a·leu′rone (a·lew′rohn) [G. *aleuron*, wheat-meal]. Small protein particles found in the endosperm of ripe seeds and in a special layer in a grain of wheat.

Alexander, William [*English surgeon*, 1844–1919]. Noted for his operation for displacement of the uterus by extraperitoneal shortening of the uterine round ligaments.

Alexander of Tralles [*Byzantine physician and writer*, 525–605]. Author of a highly original treatise on intestinal worms and their eradication. Has been referred to as the first parasitologist.

Alexander's test. See *Hemophilus influenzae* antibody *test.*

a·lex′i·a [G. *a-*, not; *lexis*, word]. Word blindness; a form of aphasia in which the patient is unable to recognize or comprehend written or printed words. Also called *optic a.*, *sensory a.*, *visual aphasia.*

congenital a. Developmental *a.*

cortical a. A variety of sensory aphasia produced by lesions of the left angular gyrus.

developmental a. Marked deficiency in learning to read, not based on obvious visual disturbance and out of line with the individual's mental age and accomplishment quotients in other subjects. Syn. *congenital a.*

motor a. That in which written or printed words are understood, but cannot be read aloud.

musical a. Loss of ability to read music.

a·lex′in [G. *alexein*, to ward off]. Complement.

a·lex″i·phar′mac [*alexein;* G. *pharmakon*, drug]. A defensive remedy against poison, venom, or infection.

a·ley′dig·ism (a·lye′dig·ism). Absence of interstitial-cell function: usually synonymous with *hypoleydigism.*

Al′gae (al′jee) [L.]. Group name for one of the major divisions of primitive plants, the Thallophyta, including numerous marine plants, such as the seaweeds, rockweeds, etc., fresh-water pond scums, the stoneworts, and others. Because the algae can synthesize food they are separated from the fungi which are saprophytic or parasitic.

al″ga·ro′ba, al″gar·ro′ba. See *mesquite.*

al″ge·don′ic [G. *algos*, pain; *hēdonē*, pleasure]. Pertaining to pain associated with pleasure. —**algedonics,** *n.*

al·ge′si·a (al·jee′zee·uh, ·see·uh) [G. *algēsis*, sense of pain]. 1. Sensitivity to pain. 2. Hyperesthesia. Syn., *algesthesia.* —**algesic,** *adj.*

al″ge·sim′e·ter [*algēsis;* G. *metron*, a measure]. Instrument for determining the acuteness of the sense of pain. —**algesimetry,** *n.*

al″ges·the′si·a. Algesia.

al·get′ic [G. *algos*, pain]. Pertaining to or producing pain.

-al′gi·a [*algos*]. A suffix denoting *pain.*

al′gid [L. *algidus*, cold]. 1. Cold or chilly. 2. Denoting a pernicious type of malaria in which the patient is in shock. —**algid′ity,** *n.*

al′gin. See *alginic acid.*

al′gin·ate. A salt of alginic acid extracted from marine kelp, believed to be a polymer of D-manuronic acid. Certain such salts form viscous sols in water and may then react with calcium compounds to form a rigid insoluble gel. It is an essential component of hydrocolloid impression material.

al·gin′ic ac′id. A gelatinous polysaccharide derived from marine algae of the *Fucus* type; it appears to consist entirely of D-mannuronic acid residues. The sodium salt produces with water a transparent mucilage, for which reason it is used as a suspending agent in pharmacy.

al″gi·o·mo′tor [G. *algos*, pain; L. *motor*, from *movere*, to move]. Causing movements attended with pain.

al″gi·o·mus′cu·lar [*algos;* L. *musculus*, muscle]. Causing pain in the muscles.

alglyn. A trade-mark for the gastric antacid substance, dihydroxyaluminum aminoacetate.

al′go-, al′gi·o-, alg- [*algos*]. A combining form signifying *pain*, or *of* or *pertaining to pain.*

algodin. Trade name of an injectable solution of iodine, sodium iodide, and sodium chloride; used in hay fever, catarrhal acute otitis media, sinusitis, and rhinitis.

al″go·gen′e·sis, al″go·ge·ne′si·a [*algos;* G. *genesis*, production]. The source or origin of pain.

al″go·gen′ic [*algos;* G. *genesthai*, from *gignesthai*, to be produced]. Causing pain.

al″go·gen′ic [L. *algidus*, cold; G. *genesthai*]. Lowering the body temperature.

al″go·lag′ni·a [G. *algos*, pain; *lagneia*, coition]. A sexual perversion in which the experiencing or infliction of pain heightens sexual gratification, or gives sexual pleasure without intercourse. —**al′golagnist,** *n.*

active a. Sadism.

passive a. Masochism.

al·gom′e·ter [*algos;* G. *metron*, a measure]. An instrument for recording the amount of pain suffered by a patient.

al″go·pho′bi·a [*algos;* G. *phobos*, fear]. Unreasonable or morbid dread of pain.

al′gor [L.]. A sense of chilliness or coldness.

a. mortis. Chill of death.

al′go·spasm [G. *algos*, pain; *spasmos*, spasm]. Painful spasm or cramp. —**algospas′tic,** *adj.*

Alhazen (ibn al-Haitham) [*Arabian physicist and optician*, ca. 965–1039]. Important figure in the history of optics. He maintained that the visual rays pass from the object to the eye, and not vice versa.

Alibert, Jean Louis Marc [*French dermatologist*, 1766–1837]. Classified skin diseases. His name has been given to mycosis fungoides (1806), keloid (1810), sycosis vulgaris (1825), and oriental sore (1829).

al′i·ble [L. *alibilis*, nutritive]. Nutritive; absorbable and assimilable, as a food.

al′i·bour wa′ter (al′i·boor). A lotion containing copper sulfate 10, zinc sulfate 35, camphor 1, alcohol 9, saffron tincture 1, and distilled water to 1000. Used (well diluted) as a wet dressing in eczema.

al″i·cy′clic (al″i·sigh′click, ·sick′lick) [G. *aleiphar*, fat; *kyklos*, circle]. Having the properties of both aliphatic (open-chain) and cyclic (closed-chain) compounds.

alidase. Trade-mark for *hyaluronidase.*

a″lien·a′tion (ay″lyen·ay′shun, ay″lee·en·, al″yen·) [L. *alienatio*, alienation]. *In psychiatry*, mental derangement; insanity.

a′lien·ist (ayl′yuh·nist, ay′lee·uh·nist) [L. *alienus*, of another, foreign, strange]. 1. A psychiatrist; a physician who is expert in the diagnosis and treatment of mental disorders. 2. *In legal medicine*, a medical expert testifying in an insanity hearing. —**alienism,** *n.*

ʻAli ibn al ʻAbbas. See *Haly Abbas.*

ʻAli ibn ʻĪsa. See *Jesu Haly.*

al′i·ment [L. *alimentum*, from *alere*, to nourish]. Any food or nutritive substance.

al″i·men′ta·ry [L. *alimentarius*, from *alere*]. 1. Nourishing, nutritious. 2. Of or relating to food and nutrition. 3. Pertaining to or caused by diet.

al″i·men·ta′tion [*alere*]. Act of nourishing with food; feeding.

artificial a. See artificial *feeding.*

forced a. See forced *feeding.*

parenteral a. Feeding other than via the alimentary tract, such as subcutaneously or intravenously.

rectal a. The nourishing of a patient by the administration of small quantities of food through the rectum.

voluntary a. Nourishment of those who are willing to be fed, but are incapacitated.

al″i·men″to·ther′a·py [*alere;* G. *therapeia*, treatment]. The treatment of disease by systematic feeding; dietary treatment.

al″i·na′sal (al″i·nay′zul, ·nay′sul) [L. *ala*, wing; *nasus*, nose]. Pertaining to the wing of the nose.

al″i·phat′ic [G. *aleiphar*, fat]. 1. Pertaining to a fat. 2. Belonging to the open-chain series of organic compounds.

al′i·quot. 1. A number which will divide a larger number without a remainder. 2. *In quantitative chemistry*, a definite known fraction of a larger sample, used to facilitate volumetric analysis.

al″i·sphe′noid [L. *ala*, wing; G. *sphēnoeidēs*, wedge-shaped]. 1. Pertaining to the greater wing of the sphenoid bone. 2. The bone that in adult life forms the main portion of the greater wing of the sphenoid.

a·liz′a·rin. $C_6H_4(CO)_2C_6H_2(OH)_2$. 1,2-Dihydroxyanthraquinone. The reddish coloring matter of *Rubia tinctorum*, dyers' madder. Prepared synthetically from anthracene, it is a brownish yellow powder or orange-red crystals, insoluble in cold water, soluble in alcohol or ether. Used in dyeing and in the manufacture of dyestuffs; also as pH indicator.

a. blue. $C_6H_4{:}(CO)_2{:}C_9H_3N{:}(OH)_2$. Dihydroxyanthraquinone-quinoline. Dark blue, lustrous crystals used as dye and pH indicator. Syn., *anthracene blue.*

a. carmine. See *a.* red S.

a. red S. (C.C.). An acid aniline dye, sodium alizarin sulfonate; an ingredient in some mitochondrial staining methods and used as a stain for bone. Also called *alizarin red, water soluble; alizarin carmine.*

a. yellow. Sodium *p*-nitraniline salicylate, used as pH indicator.

a. yellow C. See *gallacetophenone.*

a. yellow GG. $O_2N.C_6H_4.N{:}N.C_6H_3(OH)$-COONa, sodium *m*-nitrobenzene-azosalicylate. A yellow powder used as pH indicator. Also called *salicyl yellow.*

a. yellow R. The *p*-derivative corresponding to *a. yellow GG*, used as pH indicator.

alkagel. Trade-mark for aluminum hydroxide supplied in tablet form.

al″ka·lae′mi·a (al″kuh·lee′mee·uh). See *alkalemia.*

al″ka·le′mi·a [Ar. *al-qili*, ashes of saltwort; G. *haima*, blood]. Increase of the hydrogen-ion concentration in the blood; increased alkalinity of the blood.

al″ka·les′cent (al″kuh·less′unt). Somewhat alkaline. —**alkalescence,** *n.*

al′ka·li (al′kuh·lye) (pl. *alkalies, alkalis*) [Ar. *al-qili*]. 1. Essentially a hydroxide of an alkali metal. 2. A class of compounds which react with acids to form salts, turn red litmus blue, saponify fats, and form soluble carbonates. 3. The term is sometimes applied also to carbonates of alkali metals.

a. albuminate. A compound of albumin and an alkali metal. A soluble powder used as a culture medium.

a. reserve. See under *reserve.*

caustic a. Commonly the hydroxide of potassium or sodium.

fixed a. Any metallic hydroxide.

volatile a. Ammonium hydroxide; also ammonium carbonate.

al′ka·li blue. Sodium triphenylrosaniline sulfonate; a dye.

al″ka·lim′e·ter [*al-qili;* G. *metron*, a measure]. An instrument for estimating the alkali in a substance. —**alkalimet′ric,** *adj.;* **alkalimetry,** *n.*

al′ka·line (al′kuh·lyne, ·lin) [*al-qili*]. 1. Containing more hydroxyl than hydrogen ions. 2. Having the qualities of, or pertaining to, an alkali.

al′ka·line-earth met′als. The divalent elements, calcium, strontium, and barium. Some include magnesium in the group.

al′ka·line earths. The oxides of calcium, strontium, and barium. Some also include magnesium oxide.

al′ka·line tide. The temporary decrease in acidity of urine and body fluids after eating, attributed by some to the withdrawal of acid from the blood for gastric digestion.

al″ka·lin′i·ty [*al-qili*]. Quality of being alkaline.

al′ka·lin·ize, al′ka·lize [*al-qili*]. Render alkaline. —**alkaliniza′tion, alkaliza′tion,** *n.*

al″ka·li·nu′ri·a [*al-qili;* G. *ouron*, urine]. Alkalinity of the urine.

al″ka·li·pe′ni·a (al″kuh·lye·pee′nee·uh) [*al-qili;* G. *penia*, poverty]. A condition in which the body alkali is under normal levels.

al″ka·li·ther′a·py (al″kuh·lye·), **al″ka·lo·ther′a·py** [*al-qili;* G. *therapeia*, treatment]. 1. Use of alkalis in treating disease. 2. Administration of large doses of alkaline medicaments, as in peptic ulcer.

al′ka·lize. See *alkalinize.*

al′ka·loid. A term applied to naturally occurring, basic, organic, nitrogenous compounds, usually of plant origin. Most plant alkaloids are found in phanerogams, rarely in cryptogams. They occur generally as salts of organic acids, sometimes as free bases, esters, amides, or in glycosidic combination. Alkaloids are usually colorless, crystalline compounds containing carbon, hydrogen, oxygen, and nitrogen. A few are liquids and, as a rule, contain no oxygen; some are colored. Most are insoluble in water, soluble in organic solvents, and react with acids to form salts which are soluble in water and insoluble in organic solvents. Many alkaloids are medicinally valuable. —**alkaloi′dal,** *adj.*

animal a. See *ptomaine* and *leucomaine.*

cadaveric a. See *ptomaine.*

putrefactive a. See *ptomaine.*

al″ka·lo′sis [*al-qili;* G. *-ōsis*, condition]. A condition in which the bicarbonate content of the blood is relatively high and there is a tendency toward alkalemia. It may be the result of the ingestion of large amounts of sodium bicarbonate, persistent vomiting with the loss of hydrochloric acid, or forced breathing with the reduction of carbon dioxide from blood. (The last is also called *respiratory, acapnial,* or *gaseous alkalosis.*) It is marked by slow pulse, vertigo, and jerky muscular action.

altitude a. A type of respiratory alkalosis resulting from hyperventilation during accommodation to increased altitude.

compensated a. Increased blood bicarbonate without a change of the H_2CO_3:$NaHCO_3$ ratio, and hence no change in pH.

metabolic a. A condition characterized by an increased pH and bicarbonate concentration in the body fluids, caused either by the accumulation of alkaline salts or by the loss of fixed acid from the body, as in the excessive ingestion of alkali or loss of chloride by vomiting. Hyperfunction of the adrenals is often accompanied by metabolic alkalosis.

respiratory a. Alkalosis resulting from a decrease of the carbonic acid fraction of blood relative to the bicarbonate fraction with resultant increase in pH; this occurs in excessive elimination of carbon dioxide, as in hyperventilation.

uncompensated a. Increased blood bicarbonate with a change in the ratio H_2CO_3:$NaHCO_3$, and hence an upward shift of the pH.

al″ka·lo·ther′a·py. Alkalitherapy.

alkamid. Trade name for tablets containing sulfanilamide and sodium bicarbonate.

alk′a·mine. An amino alcohol.

al′kane. Any member of the paraffin series of hydrocarbons. See *paraffin.*

al′ka·net [Sp., dim. of *alcana*, henna, from Ar. *al-hinnā*]. The root of the herb, *Alkanna tinctoria*, yielding a red dye used in staining wood and to give a red color to various pharmaceutical preparations.

al·kan′nin, al·kan′in [*alcana*]. Alkanna-red, a valuable coloring matter obtained from alkanet.

al′ka·nol (al′ka·nol, al·ka′nol). An alcohol derived from any alkane.

al″ka·nol′a·mine. An amino alcohol.

al·kap′ton, al·kap′tone [*alkali;* G. *haptein*, to possess]. A yellowish, resinous, nitrogenous substance occasionally found in urine. It is identified as homogentisic acid.

al·kap″to·nu′ri·a [*al-qili; haptein;* G. *ouron*, urine]. The presence of alkapton (homogentisic acid) in the urine. A hereditary defect of metabolism characterized by the incomplete oxidation of phenylalanine and tyrosine, resulting in the excretion of homogentisic acid in the urine, which may turn dark. In time, ochronosis may develop.

al″ka·ver′vir. Generic name for a fraction of the alkaloids of veratrum viride obtained by a process involving selective extraction of the crude drug and selective precipitation of the extract: supplied under the trade-mark *veriloid.*

al″ke·ken′gi (al″kee·ken′jee) [Ar. *al-kakanj;* Per. *kāknaj*, a resin]. The *Physalis alkekengi*, the winter cherry or strawberry tomato, whose leaves have been used as diuretic.

al′kene. Any member of the series of unsaturated aliphatic hydrocarbons (ethylene series) having one double bond and represented by the general formula, C_nH_{2n}.

al·ke′nol (al·ke′nol). An alcohol derived from any alkene.

al·ker′mes (al·kur′meez, al′kur·meez). See *kermes.*

alk·ox′ide. Any of a class of salts produced when the hydrogen atom of the hydroxyl group of an aliphatic alcohol is replaced by a metal; specific salts are named for the particular alcohol involved, as sodium methoxide for CH_3ONa. Syn., *alcoholate* (definition 1).

alk·ox′y. Of or pertaining to alkoxyl.

alk·ox′y-. *In chemistry,* a combining form for *alkoxyl.*

alk·ox′yl. Any of a class of univalent radicals representing an aliphatic alcohol from which the hydrogen atom of the hydroxyl group is omitted; specific radicals are named for the particular alcohol involved, as methoxyl for CH_3O—. Syn., *alkoxy.*

al′kyl. Any one of the univalent saturated hydrocarbon radicals of the general formula C_nH_{2n+1}; as methyl (CH_3), ethyl (C_2H_5), propyl (C_3H_7).

al″kyl·a·mine′ (al″kil·uh·meen′, al″kil·am′in). A substance having the constitution of ammonia in which an alkyl replaces hydrogen; one, two, or three hydrogen atoms of the ammonia molecule may be replaced, yielding *primary* or *monalkylamines, secondary* or *dialkylamines,* and *tertiary* or *trialkylamines,* respectively.

al′kyl·ate. A compound derived from a monohydric alcohol by replacement of the hydroxyl hydrogen by a metal.

al″kyl·a′tion. The replacement of a hydrogen atom in a cyclic compound by an alkyl radical, as by the introduction of a side chain into an aromatic compound.

al″kyl·ol′a·mine (al″kill·ol′a·meen). An aliphatic

compound which contains both a hydroxyl and an amino group.

al·kyl′o·gen. Any one of the alkyl halides.

al′kyne (al′kyne). Any member of the series of unsaturated aliphatic hydrocarbons having a triple bond and represented by the general formula, C_nH_{2n-2}. Acetylene is the first hydrocarbon of the series, hence sometimes called acetylene series.

al·ky′nol. An alcohol derived from any alkyne.

al″la·ches·the′si·a, al″la·chaes·the′si·a (al″uh-kess·thee′zhuh), **al″lo·ches·the′si·a, al″lo·chaes·the′si·a** [G. *allachē*, elsewhere; *aisthēsis*, feeling]. A tactile sensation experienced remote from the point of stimulation. Syn., *allesthesia*.

al″laes·the′si·a (al″ess·thee′zhuh, ·zee·uh). See *allachesthesia*.

allansol. Trade name for a saturated solution of allantoin.

al·lan′to-, allant- [G. *allas*, sausage]. A combining form usually meaning *allantoic* or *allantoid* (see under *allantois*).

al·lan″to·cho′ri·on (a·lan″to·kor′ee·on) [*allas;* G. *chorion*, membrane]. The allantois and chorion fused together and thus forming a single structure; a chorion supplied by allantoic blood vessels. Syn., *chorion allantoideum*.

al·lan″to·en·ter′ic [*allas;* G. *enteron*, intestine]. Pertaining to the allantois and to the enteron.

al·lan″to·gen′e·sis [*allas;* G. *genesis*, production]. The development of the allantois.

Al″lan·toi′de·a [*allas;* G. *eidos*, form]. Amniota. **—allantoidean, allantoidian,** *adj.*

al·lan·toi″do·an·gi·op′a·gous [*allas; eidos;* G. *aggeion*, vessel; *pagos*, that which is fixed]. Denoting the parasitic individual in cases of unequal, monochorionic twins, the lesser of which is a placental parasite (omphalosite) dependent for its existence on the circulation of the larger (autosite). See *acardiacus*. Syn., *omphaloangiopagous*.

al·lan′to·in. $NH_2CO.NH.\overline{CHCO.NH.CO.NH}$. A crystallizable substance found in allantoic fluid, fetal urine, amniotic fluid, and some plants. It is produced by the oxidation of uric acid; used as local application to wounds, ulcers, osteomyelitis, etc., to accelerate cell proliferation.

al·lan′tois (a·lan′toyss, a·lan′to·iss) [*allas; eidos*]. An extraembryonic membrane arising as an outgrowth of the cloaca in amniotes. It functions as an organ of respiration and excretion in birds and reptiles and plays an important part in the development of the placenta in most mammals, its blood vessels forming the important pathways for the circulation of the blood between fetus and placenta. **—allanto′ic, allantoid,** *adj.*

allantomide. A proprietary combination of allantoin and sulfanilamide used as cell proliferant and bacteriostatic agent.

allanturea. Trade-mark for an ointment of allantoin, urea, chlorobutanol, and benzocaine.

al·las″so·ther′a·py [G. *allassein*, to change; *therapeia*, treatment]. Treatment which requires changing the general biologic conditions of the individual.

allatuss. Trade-mark for an expectorant preparation containing chloroform, potassium citrate, potassium guaiacolsulfonate, ipecac fluidextract, and dilute phosphoric acid.

al·lax′is [G., from *allassein*]. Metamorphosis; transformation.

al″le·gor″i·za′tion [G. *allēgorein*, to speak allegorically]. *In psychiatry*, the formation of apparently meaningless new words or sentences, frequently demonstrated in the schizophrenic reactions, especially the hebephrenic type; neologisms.

al·lele′, al·lel′ [G. *allēlōn*, of one another]. One of a pair, or any one of a series, of genes having the same locus on homologous chromosomes. **—allelic,** *adj.*

al·le′lo- (a·lee′lo-, a·lel′o-) [*allēlōn*]. A combining form denoting *of one another, reciprocally*.

al·lel″o·cat″a·lyt′ic [*allēlōn;* G. *katalytikos*, from *katalyein*, to dissolve]. 1. Denoting two substances, each decomposing in the presence of the other; mutually catalytic or destructive. 2. Promoting reproduction; when two or more unicellular organisms are placed in a drop of culture medium, reproduction proceeds more rapidly than when one organism is present. **—allelocatal′ysis,** *n.*

al·le′lo·morph (a·lee′lo·morf, a·lel′o·) [*allēlōn;* G. *morphē*, form]. 1. One of a pair of sharply contrasted Mendelian characteristics. Also, the genes in identical loci of homologous chromosomes, upon which the characteristics depend. 2. *In chemistry*, one of two or more isomorphic substances which contain the same atoms and of the same valences but differing in the manner of their linkage. 3. *In chemistry*, the first of a mixture of isomers in a solution to separate or crystallize. **—allelomor′phic,** *adj.*; **allelomor′phism,** *n.*

al·lel″o·tax′is (a·lel″o·tack′sis, a·llee′lo·), **al·lel′o·tax″y** [*allēlōn;* G. *taxis*, arrangement]. The development of an organ or part from several different embryonic structures.

Allen, Edgar [*American anatomist*, 1892–1943]. Known for his work with Doisy in isolating the active principle from ovarian hormones (1923).

Allen, Frederick Madison (1879–), American physician who discovered the nature of hydropic degeneration of the pancreatic islands (1912). He introduced caloric restriction in diabetic treatment (1914), salt-free diet for hypertension (1920), surgical refrigeration (1937), saline infusions and reduced temperature for shock (1939).

Allen, Willard Myron [*American physician*, 1904–]. With Corner, discovered progesterone, the hormone of the corpus luteum (1929).

al′lene. The gaseous hydrocarbon $CH_2{:}C{:}CH_2$. Syn., *propadiene*.

Allen's test. See under *test*.

al·len′the·sis [G. *allos*, other; *enthesis*, a putting in]. Introduction of foreign substances into the body.

al′ler·gen [*allos;* G. *ergon*, work; *genesthai*, from *gignesthai*, to be produced]. Any agent capable of producing a state or manifestation of allergy. The commonest allergens are drugs, pollens, fungi, animal hair, and foods. The drugs most frequently causing allergy are: aspirin, aminopyrine, quinine, morphine, barbiturates, sedormid, sulfanilamide, dinitrophenol, arsphenamine, phenolphthalein. The pollens most frequently causing allergy are: ragweed, sagebrush, goosefoot, pigweed, amaranth, grass, and some trees and shrubs. The most frequent fungi allergens are: *Alternaria, Hormodendrum, Helminthosporium, Aspergillus, Penicillium, Chaetomium, Phoma*, ergot, yeasts, torulae, *Cephalosporium, Trichoderma, Candida, Botrytis, Fusarium*, smuts, rusts, *Mucor, Rhizopus, Trichophyton, Candida albicans*, and mushrooms. Horse dander, the hair of cats, dogs, cows, rabbits, sheep, goats, and guinea pigs, and feathers are common allergens. The foods most frequently causing allergy are: egg, wheat, milk, peas, beans, nuts, fish, onion, white potato, chocolate, and fruits, as berries and cantaloupe. **—allergen′ic,** *adj.*; **allergenic′ity,** *n.*

epidermal a. The dander of animal hairs or feathers which causes allergic reactions.

al′ler·gid. A cutaneous eruption caused by an allergen. Also see *bacterid*.

nodular dermal a. The allergid, possibly a bacterid, characterized by nodules, purpuric macules, and erythematopapules. Syn., *Gougerot's trisymptomatic disease.*

al′ler·gin [*allos; ergon*]. The antibody which is produced by a certain allergen, and which is specific to it. *Rare.*

al′ler·gist [*allos; ergon*]. One skilled in the diagnosis and treatment of allergic diseases.

al″ler·gi·za′tion [*allos; ergon*]. Sensitization; the introduction of foreign substances into an organism.

al″ler·go·der′mi·a [*allos; ergon;* G. *derma*, skin]. An allergic skin affection.

al″ler·go′sis [*allos; ergon;* G. *-osis*, condition]. Any allergic disease.

al′ler·gy [*allos; ergon*]. Altered reaction capacity to a specific substance (which causes no symptoms of hypersensitivity in the nonsensitive. In the strict sense, this is an antigen-antibody mechanism, although the antibody is not always demonstrable. The allergens (antigens) may be proteins, carbohydrates, lipids, and haptens. There are four types of allergic diseases: (a) Anaphylaxis, a response induced by previous sensitization, usually refers to the state of hypersensitivity which occurs in experimental animals. (b) Atopic diseases, which depend upon an inherited constitutional capacity, include hay fever, vasomotor rhinitis, asthma, urticaria, infantile-type eczema, drug sensitivities, and other rare expressions. (c) Serum sickness. (d) Contact dermatitis. 3. Acquired sensitivities to drugs and biologicals (may be true anaphylaxis). **—aller′gic,** *adj.*

bacterial a. A hypersensitivity to bacteria or parts or products thereof; allergic exposure is characterized by either immediate (anaphylaxis) or delayed (tuberculin-type reaction) allergy.

cardiovascular a. Allergic reactions in which the cardiovascular system, or parts thereof, act as the shock organ.

cerebral a. Symptoms of bizarre and unusual cerebral disturbances occurring in allergic persons.

delayed a. See delayed *hypersensitivity.*

entomogenous a. Allergic reaction to insects and their products.

extrinsic a. An allergic reaction caused by an allergen that originates outside the body.

familial nonreaginic a. A hypersensitivity to foods occurring upon a hereditary basis; no antibody is demonstrable either by skin testing or the Prausnitz-Küstner reaction. Symptoms of allergic exposure are asthma, urticaria, anginal pain, fatigue, petit mal.

immediate a. See immediate *hypersensitivity.*

infectious a. Delayed hypersensitivity in which the antigen is part or product of an infecting microorganism, including bacteria, spirochetes, fungi, protozoa, rickettsias, or viruses.

intrinsic a. An allergic reaction in which the allergen may possibly originate within the body.

physical a. The response of some individuals to various physical factors, as cold, heat, sunlight, or mechanical irritation, manifested by urticaria, edema, and varying systemic reactions.

Al″les·che′ri·a (al″ess·keer′ee·uh). A genus of fungi of the class Ascomycetes.

A. boydii. The species regarded as one of the causes of mycetoma; it produces white or yellowish white granules.

al″les·the′si·a, al″laes·the′si·a. See *allachesthesia.*

al″le·thrin′. A coined generic name for the liquid insecticidal chemical representing *dl*-2-allyl-4-hydroxy-3-methyl-2-cyclopenten-1-one esterified with a mixture of cis- and trans-*dl*-chrysanthemum monocarboxylic acid; the chemical is an allyl homolog of cinerin I, which is an active insecticidal constituent of pyrethrum flowers.

al′li·cin [L. *allium*, garlic]. The antibacterial principle obtained from common garlic (*Allium sativum*). It contains about 40% sulfur.

al″li·ga′tion [L. *alligatio*, a binding to]. *In pharmacy,* the formula for solving problems concerning the mixing of solutions of different percentages; the rule of mixtures. If two substances when mixed retain the specific values of a property, the value for the mixture can be calculated from the equation, $\frac{aA + bB}{a + b}$, where a and b are the proportions and A and B equal the respective values for the property.

al′li·ga″tor for′ceps. *In surgery,* a toothed instrument, one jaw of which operates with a double lever.

allimin. A proprietary tablet of garlic and parsley used as vasodilator.

Allingham, Herbert William [*English surgeon,* 1862–1904]. Introduced his operation for inguinal colostomy just above the inguinal ligament; called *Allingham's operation.*

Allingham, William [*English surgeon,* 1830–1908]. Introduced a radical operation, called *Allingham's operation,* which illustrates a type of rectal extirpation for cancer; making an oval incision around the bowel into both ischiorectal fossae, he isolated the bowel above the tumor and removed it in toto with scissors or cautery. Described anal fissure, called *Allingham's painful ulcer.*

Allis, Oscar Huntington [*American surgeon,* 1836–1921]. Invented an inhalation device for administration of anesthetics by the drop method, and a surgical forceps with fine, blunt, interlocking teeth which are adapted especially to securing and holding intestine, stomach wall, and hollow viscera at the incised edges during surgical operations. Described a sign indicative of fracture of the femur. See Allis' *sign.*

allisatin. Trade name for a tablet containing the active principles of fresh garlic (*Allium sativum);* used as sedative-antispasmodic in intestinal disorders.

al·lit″er·a′tion [L. *ad*, to; *litera*, letter]. A form of dysphrasia in which the patient chooses words with the same consonant sounds.

Al′li·um [L. garlic]. A genus of bulbous plants of the Liliaceae family, species of which include garlic, onion, leek, and chives.

al′li·um. Any plant, bulb, or flower of the genus *Allium;* specifically, the bulb of garlic (*Allium sativum*): used medicinally as a hypotensive, pectoral, antiseptic, anthelmintic, and rubefacient.

al′lo-, all- [G. *allos*, other]. 1. A combining form denoting *differentiation from the normal, extraneousness,* or *reversal.* 2. *In chemistry,* a combining form denoting *an isomer, close relative,* or *variety of a compound;* or denoting *the more stable of two isomers.*

al″lo·chaes·the′si·a. See *allachesthesia.*

al″lo·chei′ri·a (al″o·kigh′ree·uh) [*allos;* G. *cheir*, hand]. A form of allachesthesia occurring rarely in tabes dorsalis; if one extremity is pricked, the sensation is felt in the opposite.

al″lo·ches·the′si·a. See *allachesthesia.*

al″lo·che′zi·a (al″o·kee′zee·uh), **al″lo·che′ti·a** (al″o·kee′shee·uh, ·kee′tee·uh) [*allos;* G. *chezein*, to ease oneself]. 1. The passage of feces from the body through an abnormal opening. 2. The passing of nonfecal matter from the bowels.

al″lo·cho·les′ter·ol (al″o·ko·les′tur·ole, ·ol, ·awl) [*allos;* G. *cholē*, bile; *stereos*, stiff]. A sterol found in wool fat.

allochrysine. Trade-mark for a solution of gold

sodium thiopropanolsulfonate used by intramuscular injection in phthisis.

al″lo·cor′tex [*allos;* L. *cortex,* bark]. Those areas or portions of the cerebral cortex where lamination is absent or incomplete, as the olfactory cortex, representing less developed or more primitive areas. Syn., *heterogenetic cortex, heterotypical cortex.*

al″loe·o′sis (al″ee·o′sis) [G. *alloiōsis,* alteration]. Change; alterative effect; recovery from illness. —**alloeot′ic,** *adj., n.*

al″lo·er′o·tism, al″lo·e·rot′i·cism [G. *allos,* other; *erōs,* love]. Sexual excitement that is induced by and directed to another, not oneself; opposed to autoerotism.

al·lom′e·try [*allos;* G. *metron,* a measure]. 1. The quantitative relation between a part and the whole or another part, as the organism increases in size. Syn., *heterauxesis.* 2. The quantitative relation between the size of a part and the whole or another part, in a series of related organisms that differ in size. Syn., *allomorphosis.*

al″lo·mor′phism [*allos;* G. *morphē,* form]. The property possessed by certain substances of assuming a different form while remaining unchanged in constitution. —**allomorphic, allomorphous,** *adj.*

al″lo·mor′pho·sis (al″o·mor′fo·sis, ·mor·fo′sis) [*allos;* G. *morphōsis,* a shaping]. A type of allometry which deals with the relation of a part to the whole, or to another part, in a series of organisms that differ in size and in genetic constitution; as the relation of jaw length to skull length of the adult in a series of breeds of dogs. Also see *heterauxesis.*

allonal. Trade-mark for a tablet containing allyl isopropyl barbituric acid and acetophenetidin.

al′lo·path, al·lop′a·thist [*allos;* G. *pathos,* disease]. An incorrect designation for a regular medical practitioner.

al·lop′a·thy [*allos; pathos*]. System of medical treatment using remedies that produce effects upon the body differing from those produced by disease; the opposite of the homeopathic system. It has been applied erroneously to the so-called regular medical profession. —**allopath′ic,** *adj.*

al·loph′a·sis [*allos;* G. *phasis,* speech]. Incoherency of speech; delirium. *Obs.*

al′lo·plasm [*allos;* G. *plasma,* from *plassein,* to form]. *In biology,* a supposedly less fundamental form of protoplasm from which nonindependent flagella and various cytoplasmic fibrils are formed. —**alloplasmat′ic,** *adj.*

al′lo·plast [*allos;* G. *plastos,* from *plassein*]. *In biology,* a plastic compound of two or more tissues, as opposed to homoplast.

al′lo·plas″ty [*allos; plastos*]. 1. A plastic operation in which material from outside the human body is utilized, such as ivory, animal bone, gold, silver, plastics, etc. Distinguished from autoplasty and heteroplasty. 2. *In psychoanalysis,* the process whereby the libido of the growing individual directs its energies away from self and toward other individuals and objects. —**al·lo·plas′tic,** *adj.*

al″lo·pol′y·ploid [*allos;* G. *polys,* many; *-ploos,* -fold; *eidos,* form]. A hybrid with more than two complete sets of chromosomes derived from different species.

al″lo·preg′nane. $C_{21}H_{36}$; 17-ethylandrostane; a saturated, solid, steroid hydrocarbon, the parent substance of adrenal cortical and certain other hormones. Syn., *5-α-pregnane.*

al″lo·psy′che (al″o·sigh′kee) [*allos;* G. *psychē,* soul]. The mind or psyche of another.

al″lo·psy′chic (al″o·sigh′kick) [*allos; psychē*]. Pertaining to mental processes in their relation to the outside world, as opposed to autopsychic.

β-D-al″lo·py′ran·ose. Allose.

al″lo·rhyth′mi·a (al″o·rith′mee·uh, ·rith′mee·uh) [*allos;* G. *rhythmos,* rhythm]. An irregularity of the pulse which is repeated continuously. —**allorhythmic,** *adj.*

all′-or-noth′ing. Occurring either completely or not at all, as the response of a single nerve or muscle unit to a stimulus.

al′lose. $C_6H_{12}O_6$; an aldohexose sugar, stereoisomeric with D-glucose, prepared by synthesis; it is more exactly denoted as D-*allose,* or *β-D-allopyranose.*

al′lo·some [*allos;* G. *sōma,* body]. 1. Originally any chromosome distinguished from ordinary chromosomes (autosomes) by certain peculiarities of form, size, and behavior, but now the term is usually used as synonymous with sex chromosome; an accessory chromosome. Syn., *heterochromosome.* 2. A cytoplasmic inclusion introduced from without.

paired a. One of a pair of similar allosomes; a diplosome.

unpaired a. A monosome; an accessory chromosome.

al″lo·ste″a·to′des (al″o·stee″uh·to′deez) [*allos;* G. *steatōdēs,* like tallow]. A perversion or disturbance of the sebaceous secretion.

al″lo·syn·ap′sis [*allos;* G. *synapsis,* contact]. A form of synapsis in hybrids, characterized by pairing between the chromosomes of both species.

al′lo·therm [*allos;* G. *thermē,* heat]. An organism whose temperature is directly dependent upon that of its environment.

al·lot″ri·o·don′ti·a [G. *allotrios,* belonging to another; *odōn,* tooth]. 1. Transplanting of teeth. 2. Occurrence of teeth in abnormal places, as in teratomas.

al·lot″ri·o·geu′si·a (a·lot″ree·o·gew′see·uh, ·jew′see·uh) [*allotrios;* G. *geuein,* to taste]. 1. Perversion of taste sense. 2. Abnormal appetite.

al″lo·tri′o·lith (al″o·try′o·lith, a·lot′ree·o·lith) [*allotrios;* G. *lithos,* stone]. A stone or calculus found in an unusual location.

al·lot″ri·oph′a·gy, al·lot″ri·o·pha′gi·a [*allotrios;* G. *phagein,* to eat]. 1. Depraved or unnatural appetite. 2. Eating of unusual or injurious substances. See *pica.*

al·lot″ri·u′ri·a [*allotrios;* G. *ouron,* urine]. Abnormality of the urine.

al′lo·trope [G. *allos,* other; *tropos,* turn]. One of the forms in which an element capable of assuming different forms may appear.

al″lo·troph′ic [*allos;* G. *trophē,* nourishment]. Altered or modified by digestion so as to become innutritious.

al″lo·trop′ic [*allos;* G. *tropos,* turn]. 1. Pertaining to, or exhibiting, allotropy. 2. *In psychiatry,* denoting a personality which is concerned about others; not egocentric.

al·lot′ro·py (a·lot′ro·pee, al′o·tro″pee), **al·lot′ro·pism** [*allos; tropos*]. 1. Occurrence of an element in two or more distinct forms with differences in physical properties, as carbon, phosphorus, and sulfur. 2. Appearance in an unusual or abnormal form. 3. An attraction or tropism between different cells or structures, as between sperms and ova. 4. Adolf Meyer's term for allopsyche.

al″lo·tryl′ic [G. *allotrios,* strange; *hylē,* matter]. Caused by a strange or foreign principle or material; enthetic.

allox- [G. *allas,* sausage; *oxys,* sharp]. A combining form for *alloxan.*

al″lox·an′ (al″ock·san′, a·lock′sun). $C_4H_2N_2O_4$.

Mesoxalyl urea. A crystalline substance produced by the oxidation of uric acid. It has been found in the intestinal mucus during diarrhea and is used for the production of experimental diabetes through selective necrosis of the islets of Langerhans.

al″lox·an′ di″a·be′tes. Severe hyperglycemia, following the experimental administration of alloxan. In animals, the symptoms and the degeneration of pancreatic islets are similar to those seen in human diabetes mellitus.

al″lox·an′ic ac′id. $NH_2CO.NH.CO.COOH$. A crystalline acid obtained by treating alloxan with alkali.

al″lox·an′tin. $C_8H_6O_8N_4.2H_2O$. A substance obtained by the reduction of alloxan. Syn., *uroxin.*

al·lox′a·zine (a·lock′suh·zeen). 1. $C_{10}H_6N_4O_2$. The three-ring heterocylic compound pyrimido[4,5-b]-quinoxaline-2,4(1H,3H)-dione. 2. A term loosely applied to derivatives of (1) and, sometimes, to isoalloxazine and its derivatives.

al″lox·u′ri·a [*allas; oxys;* G. *ouron,* urine]. Old term used to designate the presence of purines in the urine. —**allox′ur, alloxuric,** *adj.*

al·lox″y·pro·te′ic ac′id (a·lock′see·pro·tee′ick). An acid, containing nitrogen and sulfur, said to be sometimes found in urine.

al′loy [F. *aloyer,* to mix metals, from L. *alligare,* to bind]. The product of the fusion of two or more metals. —**al·loy′,** *v.*

all′spice″ [AS. *all;* L. *species,* sort]. 1. The fruit of *Pimenta officinalis.* 2. Any of several other aromatic shrubs, such as the **Carolina allspice,** the leaves of which have the properties of an aromatic stimulant. It contains two toxic alkaloids.

al′lyl [L. *allium,* garlic; G. *hylē,* matter]. The univalent radical $—CH_2.CH{:}CH_2$ or $C_3H_5—$.

a. alcohol. C_3H_5OH. A colorless, inflammable liquid, with pungent odor, boiling at 97° C.

a. aldehyde. See *acrolein.*

a. isothiocyanate. C_3H_5NCS. Volatile oil of mustard, a colorless or pale yellow liquid, soluble in alcohol. Also called *a. mustard oil, a. isosulfocyanate.*

a. sulfide. $(C_3H_5)_2S$. A liquid of garliclike odor, possibly present in garlic; formerly used in cholera and tuberculosis.

a. thiourea. See *thiosinamine.*

a. tribromide. $C_3H_5Br_3$. 1,2,3-Tribromopropane, a colorless liquid, has been used as an antispasmodic. Dose, 0.3–0.6 cc. (5–10 min.).

al″lyl·a·mine′ (al″il·uh·meen′, al″il·am′in, a·lil′-uh·meen, ·min). $CH_2{:}CH.CH_2.NH_2$. 2-Propenylamine. A yellowish, caustic liquid.

al″lyl·bar″bi·tur′ic ac′id. The official generic name of 5-allyl-5-isobutylbarbituric acid, marketed under the trade-marked name *sandoptal.*

al′lyl·ene. $HC{\equiv}CCH_3$; a gaseous hydrocarbon of the alkyne series. Syn., *methylacetylene, propyne.*

al″lyl·i″so·pro″pyl·bar″bi·tur′ic ac′id. $(CH_3)_2$-$CH.(CH_2{:}CHCH_2).C.CO.NH.CO.NH.CO;$ a white, crystalline powder, very slightly soluble in water; it is a sedative and hypnotic, characterized by intermediate duration of action. Syn., *aprobarbital.* See *alurate.*

N-al″lyl·nor·mor′phine. A derivative of morphine in which the methyl group attached to the nitrogen atom in the latter has been replaced by an allyl group; occurs as a crystalline compound, sparingly soluble in water. It antagonizes most of the actions of morphine, and is used as an analeptic in the treatment of acute narcotic poisoning.

almag. Trade-mark for a preparation containing aluminum hydroxide powder and magnesium trisilicate.

al″ma·gu′cin. Generic name applied to antacid mixtures of gastric mucin, dried aluminum hydroxide gel, and magnesium trisilicate. See *mucotin.*

alminate. A trade-mark for dihydroxyaluminum aminoacetate.

al′mond (ah′mund, am′und, al′mund) [OF., from G. *amygdalē,* almond]. The seed of *Prunus amygdalus,* a small tree widely cultivated in warm temperate regions of the world.

bitter a. oil (*oleum amygdalae amarae*). The volatile oil obtained from dried ripe kernels of *Prunus amygdalus* or from other kernels containing amygdalin by maceration with water and subsequent distillation with steam. It contains not less than 80% of benzaldehyde and from 2–4% of hydrogen cyanide. It acts physiologically like hydrocyanic acid; externally, it is used, mixed with water, in pruritus senilis and other forms of itching.

expressed a. oil (*oleum amygdalae expressum*). The fixed oil expressed from the kernels of several varieties of *Prunus amygdalus:* employed as an emollient, a demulcent, and a nutrient. Syn., *sweet a. oil.*

al′mond-eyed″. Having eyes of elliptical form and slanting eyelids, as various Mongolian peoples.

a·lo′chi·a (a·lo′kee·uh) [G. *a-,* not; *lochia,* discharge after childbirth]. Absence of the lochia.

Al′o·e (al′o·ee, al′o) [G. *aloē,* the aloe]. A genus of liliaceous plants.

A. americana. See *Agave.*

A. barbadensis. See *A. vera.*

A. vera. A tropical plant, the milk or sap of which is used as a dressing for x-ray or radium dermatitis, especially where ulceration occurs. Has been used in ointments or by direct application of inner surface of the leaf. Syn., *A. barbadensis.*

al′oe (al′o, al′o·ee) [*aloē*]. The dried juice of the leaves of *Aloe Perryi, A. barbadensis, A. ferox,* and hybrids of this species with *A. africana* and *A. spicata.* Its purgative properties are due to three pentosides (barbaloin, iso-barbaloin, and beta-barbaloin) and to a resin. It is cathartic and tonic, particularly useful in chronic constipation, and has been used in amenorrhea. Local application of the leaves is of benefit in the treatment of x-ray burns. Dose, 0.13–0.65 Gm. (2–10 gr.). Syn., *aloes.* —**al″o·et′ic,** *adj.*

a. and mastic pills (*pilulae aloes et mastiches*). 0.13 Gm. (2 gr.) aloe and 0.04 Gm. (⅔ gr.) mastic per pill. Syn., *Lady Webster dinner pills.*

a. and myrrh tincture (*tinctura aloes et myrrhae*), 10% each of aloe, myrrh, and glycyrrhiza.

caballine a. An inferior aloe. Syn., *fetid a., horse a.*

Cape a. From *A. ferox* and hybrids of this species with *A. africana* and *A. spicata.*

Curaçao a. From *A. barbadensis.*

fetid a. An inferior aloe.

hepatic a. An inferior, liver-colored aloe

horse a. An inferior aloe.

Socotrine a. From *A. Perryi.*

West Indian a. From *A. barbadensis.* Syn., *Curaçao a.*

Zanzibar a. A hepatic variety of Socotrine aloe made by slow evaporation of the juice.

al″oe-em′o·din. $C_{15}H_{10}O_5$; 1,8-dihydroxy-3-hydroxymethylanthraquinone, occurring in the free state and as glycoside in various species of aloe, also in rhubarb and in senna. It is an irritant cathartic.

al′oes (al′oze). See *aloe.*

al″o·et′ic [*aloē*]. A medication containing aloe.

al″o·e′tin [*aloē*]. 1. Aloe resin. 2. A yellow, crystalline principle obtainable from aloes.

a·lo′gi·a [G. *a-,* not; *logos,* word]. 1. Motor or expressive aphasia. 2. Stupid or senseless behavior.

al′o·in [G. *aloē*, the aloe] (*aloinum*). A mixture of active principles, chiefly barbaloin and iso-barbaloin, obtained from aloe. It is a yellow, microcrystalline powder with an intensely bitter taste. Used as laxative and purgative. Dose, 10–60 mg. (1/6–1 gr.). Syn., *barbaloin.*

alomin. Trade-mark for a gastric antacid and adsorbent containing kaolin, aluminum hydroxide, calcium carbonate, bismuth subnitrate, sodium chloride, acacia, aromatics, and dextrose.

al″o·pe′ci·a (al″o·pee′shee·uh, ·see·uh) [G. *alōpekia*, a disease like mange in foxes, from *alōpēx*, fox]. Loss of hair; baldness. The loss may be partial or total; congenital, premature, or senile. Alopecia may complicate various systemic affections. Syn., *calvities, baldness.* Also called *defluvium capillorum.* —**alopecic,** *adj.*

a. areata. Loss of hair in circumscribed patches with little or no inflammation. The scalp and beard areas are usually involved. Syn., *a. circumscripta.* Also called *area Celsi.*

a. cachectica. Baldness due to general malnutrition.

a. cicatrisata. Circular and irregular patches of alopecia due to atrophy of the skin, causing permanent baldness. Syn., *pseudopelade.*

a. circumscripta. See *a.* areata.

a. congenitalis. An unusual form appearing congenitally due to partial or complete absence of hair follicles.

a. furfuracea. See *a.* seborrheica.

a. neuritica. Baldness of trophoneurotic origin.

a. pityrodes. See *a.* seborrheica.

a. prematura. Baldness which occurs any time after puberty and resembles the senile type. The hair gradually thins and falls out, often beginning at the temples. Also called *presenile a.*

a. prematura symptomatica. Loss of hair in the course of some diseases, or following prolonged, debilitating fevers, or with changes in endocrine secretion. When baldness follows acute illnesses, it is usually temporary.

a. seborrheica. Baldness associated with seborrheic dermatitis. Scaliness and varying degrees of inflammation are present. Itching is often associated, and the hair is dry and lusterless. This condition is quite common. Syn., *a. pityrodes, pityriasis simplex.* Also called *seborrhea capillitii.*

a. senilis. That which occurs in old age and is preceded by gradual thinning of the hair.

a. syphilitica. In this form, the hair presents a moth-eaten appearance prior to falling out.

a. unguialis, a. unguis. Shedding of the nails. Syn., *onychoptosis, defluvium unguium.*

a. universalis. Loss of hair from all parts of the body. Also called *a. totalis.*

traumatic marginal a. Partial alopecia involving the marginal area of the scalp above and anterior to the ears, caused by continued traction on the hair from braiding or hair straightening procedures. Prognosis is good if the cause is eliminated early.

alopectose. A proprietary adsorbent and antacid tablet containing kaolin, aluminum hydroxide, pectin, and betalactose.

alophen. Trade-mark for a laxative preparation containing aloin, belladonna extract, ipecac, and phenolphthalein.

al′pha [G.]. 1. The first letter of the Greek alphabet (A, α). 2. *In chemistry*, it is often combined with the name of a compound to indicate the first of a series, as of isomers or otherwise related substances. 3. In other sciences, it is often employed to differentiate between the members of various groups or series. For many terms so designated, see under the specific noun.

al″pha-hy·poph′a·mine (-high·pof′uh·meen, ·min). The oxytocin obtained from the posterior portion of the pituitary gland.

al″pha-i′o·dine. Thyroxin.

alphalin. A trade-mark for preparations containing vitamin A.

al″pha-lo′be·line (-lo′bi·leen, ·lin, -lo·bee′leen, ·lin). An alkaloid from lobelia used in asphyxia.

al″pha·naph′thol. An isomer of betanaphthol; used as a local antiseptic, occasionally as an intestinal antiseptic.

a. salicylate. A white, crystalline powder used as an antiseptic and antirheumatic. Also called *alphol, alphanaphthyl salicylate.*

al″pha-naph·thyl·thi″o·u·re′a. ANTU.

al″pha·pro′dine hy″dro·chlo′ride. Generic name for *dl*-alpha-1,3-dimethyl-4-phenyl-4-propionoxypiperidine hydrochloride, a synthetic narcotic used to relieve pain. Syn., *prisilidene hydrochloride.* See *nisentil hydrochloride.*

al″pha·to·coph′er·ol. See under *tocopherol.*

al″pho·der′mi·a [G. *alphos*, dull-white leprosy; *derma*, skin]. Achromatosis; any disease marked by lack of pigmentation.

al′phos, al′phus [*alphos*]. 1. Psoriasis. 2. Leprosy. *Obs.*

al·pho′sis [*alphos;* G. *-ōsis*, condition]. Albinism; leukoderma.

al′pho·zone. Succinyl peroxide, $(HOOC.CH_2.-CH_2.CO)_2O_2$. A white crystalline powder derived from hydrogen peroxide by action of succinic acid. It is used as a germicide in dilute aqueous solutions.

al′phus. See *alphos.*

alphyllin. Trade-mark for a preparation containing allylphenylbarbituric acid and aminophylline.

Alpino, Prospero (Alpinus) [*Italian physician, botanist, and writer*, 1553–1617]. Supported the theory of contagion in typhus and left an important work on Egyptian medicine (1591). Also wrote a classic pamphlet on prognosis of disease (1601).

alrac. Trade-mark for a preparation containing dihydroxyaluminum aminoacetate and magnesium trisilicate.

Alsaharavius. See *Albucasis.*

alsol. A brand of aluminum acetotartrate.

Al·sto′ni·a [NL., after Charles *Alston*, Scottish physician, 1683–1760]. A genus of apocynaceous trees and shrubs.

A. constricta. The quinine alstonia of Australia; yields the alkaloid *alstonine.* The bark is tonic, antiperiodic, and antipyretic, and has been used in intermittent fevers.

A. scholaris. The devil's-tree of eastern Asia and the Philippines; it furnishes dita bark; it is tonic, astringent, antiperiodic, and anthelmintic.

al′sto·nine. $C_{21}H_{20}N_2O_3$; an alkaloid from *Alstonia constricta.*

al′ter·ant (awl′tur·unt). Alterative.

al″ter·a′tion cav·i·taire′. Intercellular edema of epidermal cells, resulting in the formation of multilocular bullae.

al′ter·a·tive (awl′tur·uh·tiv) [ML. *alterativus*, from L. *alter*, other (of two)]. Any medicine that alters the processes of nutrition, restoring, in some unknown way, the normal functions of an organ or of the system. Arsenic, iodine, the iodides, mercury, and gold formerly were classed as alteratives, but the term has little if any application now. *Obs.*

al′ter·a·tive. Changing; alterant; reestablishing healthy nutritive processes. *Obs.*

al″ter·e′go·ism (al″tur·ee′go·iz·um, ·eg′o·iz·um) [*alter;* L. *ego*, I]. An altruistic feeling for only those who are in the same situation as oneself.

Al″ter·na′ri·a [L. *alternare*, to alternate]. A genus

of atmospheric fungi of the Dematiaceae family, clinically significant as the cause of atopy.

al″ter·nar′ic ac′id. An antibiotic substance derived from the fungus *Alternaria solani;* it has negligible antibacterial activity but is inhibitory to some fungi.

al′ter·nate case meth′od. See under *method.*

al′ter·nate paired case meth′od. See *method.*

al′ter·nat″ing [*alternare*]. Occurring turn and turn about, or alternately.

al″ter·na′tion [*alternare*]. 1. The act of alternating or of performing alternately. 2. *In neurology,* the phenomenon whereby only every other impulse is carried over the eighth cranial (auditory) nerve when the exciting impulse is from 900 to 1800 cycles. Because of the refractory period of nerve impulses, the maximum frequency that can be carried by a nerve is about 900 per second. —**al′ternate,** *adj., n.,* —**al′ter·nate″,** *v.*

al″ter·na′tion of gen″er·a′tions. *In biology,* the succession of asexual and sexual individuals in a life history, such as the alternation of polyp and medusa in the life cycle of many coelenterates; metagenesis.

al′ter·na″tor [*alternare*]. An apparatus for converting direct current into alternating current.

Althausen test. See galactose tolerance *test.*

Althausen-Mancke's test. See under *test.*

al·the′a [L. *althaea*] (*althaea*). Marshmallow root. The peeled root of *Althaea officinalis,* a plant of the mallow family. It consists chiefly of starch and gum with some pectin and sugar and contains up to 2% of asparagin. Used in the form of a decoction as a demulcent; also as a pill excipient.

a. syrup (*syrupus althaeae*). Represents 5% althea; used as a vehicle.

alt. hor. Abbreviation for L. *alternis horis,* every other hour.

al′ti·tude sick′ness. A symptom complex resulting from anoxia during airplane flights at high altitudes, due to lowered partial pressure of oxygen in the inspired air. **Acute altitude sickness** may occur as the result of a single flight; it is marked by symptoms of acute anoxia, as headache, increased lung ventilation, general bodily distress, mental anxiety, lassitude, sleepiness, fatigue, depression, or euphoria. **Chronic altitude sickness** results from repeated flights at high altitudes; it is characterized by headache, mental and physical fatigue, increased appetite, irritability, nervousness, insomnia, poor mental concentration, lack of volition, disregard for danger in the air, and is accompanied by some nausea, anorexia, indigestion, and vertigo.

Altmann, Richard [*German histologist,* 1852–1900]. *Altmann's theory* states that the fundamental units of protoplasm are granular particles. See Altmann's *stain* for mitochondria, formerly called *Altmann's granules.* His method for tissue fixation was later modified by Gersh. See Altmann-Gersh *method.*

al″tri·gen′der·ism [L. *alter,* the other (of two); *genus,* race]. The nonsexual, nonamorous activities between members of opposite sexes.

altrisil. Trade-mark for a gastric antacid and adsorbent containing magnesium trisilicate, aluminum hydroxide, and pectin.

al′trose. $C_6H_{12}O_6$; an aldohexose sugar, stereoisomeric with D-glucose, prepared by synthesis: more exactly denoted as **D-altrose,** or **D-altropyranose.**

al-u-creme. A trade-mark for a flavored suspension of aluminum hydroxide.

aludrine hydrochloride. A trade name for isopropylarterenol hydrochloride, a sympathomimetic amine salt employed in the treatment of asthma.

aludrox. A trade-mark for preparations containing aluminum hydroxide gel and magnesium hydroxide.

alugel. Trade-mark for tablets containing dried aluminum hydroxide gel.

alulotion. Trade-mark for an adsorbent and protective lotion containing ammoniated mercury, kaolin, and aluminum hydroxide gel.

al′um. 1. Any one of a class of double salts of general formula $M_2'SO_4.M_2'''(SO_4)_3.24H_2O$ or $M'M'''(SO_4)_2.12H_2O$, in which M′ is a univalent metal or group, and M‴ is a trivalent metal. 2. The official alum (*alumen*), which may be ammonium alum, $AlNH_4(SO_4)_2.12H_2O$, or potassium alum, $AlK(SO_4)_2.12H_2O$. Both forms occur as colorless, odorless crystals or as powder; soluble in water, insoluble in alcohol. It is astringent and emetic. Dose as astringent, 0.3–1.0 Gm. (5–15 gr.); as emetic, 4 Gm. (60 gr.).

a. hematoxylin. A purple stain for tissues; obtained from an alcoholic solution of hematoxylin by adding an aqueous solution of potassium alum.

a. whey. A preparation obtained by boiling 2 dr. of alum in a pint of milk and straining; formerly used as an astringent and internal hemostatic in wineglassful doses.

ammonioferric a. $FeNH_4(SO_4)_2.12H_2O$. It is astringent and styptic. Dose, 0.3–0.6 Gm. (5–10 gr.). Also called *ferric ammonium sulfate, ferric a., iron a.*

ammonium a. See *alum,* 2.

burnt a. See exsiccated *a.*

dried a. See exsiccated *a.*

exsiccated a. Official alum (see *alum,* 2) which has been deprived of most of its water of crystallization. It is more powerful and irritant than the hydrated salt. Occasionally applied to exuberant granulations. Syn., *burnt a., dried a.*

potassium a. One containing potassium, particularly ordinary alum or aluminum and potassium sulfate. Also called *potash a.*

sodium a. One containing the double sulfate of sodium and aluminum.

a·lu′min·a. Aluminum oxide; Al_2O_3, occurring naturally in many minerals, or prepared artificially.

al″u·min′i·um. See *aluminum.*

a·lu′mi·num, al″u·min′i·um [L. *alumen,* alum]. Al = 26.98. Valence, 3. A silver-white, light, ductile metal occurring abundantly in nature, chiefly in combination with silica and metallic oxides. It is soluble in acids and alkalis and, on exposure to air, takes on a coating of oxide. Because of its lightness (sp. gr. 2.7) and relative stability, it is used extensively for manufacturing and construction purposes. It readily forms alloys, some of which are of great importance, as *duralumin* and *magnalium.* Powdered aluminum is variously used as a protective in treating ulcers, fissures, etc., and has been used in treating silicosis. See *thermite.*

a. acetate solution (*liquor alumini acetatis*). A solution prepared by the reaction of lead acetate with aluminum sulfate; an astringent and antiseptic used after dilution with from 10 to 40 parts of water as a gargle or a local application for ulcerative conditions. Also called *Burow's solution.* Also see *a.* subacetate solution.

a. acetoglycerate. A glycerite of aluminum acetate used as an antiseptic astringent in the nose and throat.

a. acetotartrate. Colorless crystals or white powder used as an antiseptic astringent in 1–3% solution.

a. ammonium sulfate. See *alum.*

a. betanaphthol disulfonate. See *alumnol*.

a. chloride (*alumini chloridum*). A white or yellow-white, deliquescent, crystalline powder with a sweetish, astringent taste; easily soluble in water. An astringent and antiseptic, especially in hyperhidrosis, applied as a 25% solution.

a. chloride solution (*liquor alumini chloridi*). A 25% solution.

a. citrate. A white, crystalline powder, sparingly soluble in cold water. A 6% solution has been recommended as the approximate equivalent of the aluminum acetate solution.

a. formate. Used in 1–3% solution as an antiseptic wash for suppurating cavities or as a vaginal douche. See *ormicet*.

a. hydroxide. $Al(OH)_3$; a white, bulky, amorphous powder, insoluble in water; a protective and astringent dusting powder or ointment ingredient.

a. hydroxide gel (*gelatum alumini hydroxidi*). A white, viscous suspension of aluminum hydroxide equivalent to 4% of Al_2O_3, used as gastric antacid, especially in the treatment of peptic ulcers. It is advantageous in that it does not produce a reactive secretion of acid in the stomach. Dose, 4–12 cc. (1–3 fluidrachms). See *amphojel, creamalin, fluagel, hydrogel, lactalumina*.

a. oleate. A yellowish, viscid mass, used in ointments for skin diseases.

a. oxide. Al_2O_3; a white, amorphous powder, insoluble in water and, if it has been ignited, in acids. It is used for absorbing gases, water vapor, and in chromatographic analysis. Hydrated aluminum oxide, known as *aluminum hydroxide*, is employed as a gastric antacid.

a. paste. A paste containing 10% of powdered aluminum, 5% liquid petrolatum, and 85% zinc oxide ointment; used locally as a protective, especially around intestinal fistulae to protect surrounding skin against digestive action of intestinal fluids.

a. phenolsulfonate. $Al(C_6H_4.OH.SO_3)_3$. White or reddish white powder; used as an antiseptic astringent. Syn., *a. sulfocarbolate*.

a. phosphate. $AlPO_4$. A white powder, insoluble in water; used in the manufacture of dental and other cements and in ceramics.

a. phosphate gel (*gelatum alumini phosphatis*). A white, viscous suspension containing 4.2% of $AlPO_4$, used like aluminum hydroxide gel, but does not interfere with phosphate absorption. See *phosphaljel*.

a. potassium sulfate. See *alum*.

a. salicylate. A white or pink powder used as an antiseptic insufflation in nasal catarrh and ozena.

a. silicate. Approximately $Al_2O_3.3SiO_2$. White powder or lumps; used for preparing dental cements, in ceramics, etc.

a. silicofluoride. A white, insoluble powder used occasionally as an insecticide and in the glass industry. Also called *a. fluorosilicate*.

a. subacetate. See basic *a.* acetate.

a. subacetate solution (*liquor alumini subacetatis*). A clear, colorless, or faintly yellow liquid, with an acetous odor; used, after dilution with 20 to 40 parts of water, as an astringent and antiseptic wash, especially as a gargle.

a. sulfate (*alumini sulfas*). $Al_2(SO_4)_3.18H_2O$. A white, crystalline, odorless powder freely soluble in water, used in 5% solution as an astringent and antiseptic.

a. sulfocarbolate. See *a.* phenolsulfonate.

a. tannate. A brownish yellow powder, insoluble in water; used as an astringent dusting powder or in insufflation.

a. tannotartrate. A yellow-white powder, soluble in water; used as an astringent in rhinology and laryngology.

a. zinc sulfate. $Al_2Zn(SO_4)_4.24H_2O$. White crystals, soluble in water; used as caustic.

basic a. acetate. Approximately $Al_2O(CH_3COO)_4.4H_2O$. White powder, incompletely soluble in water, soluble in mineral acids and the alkalis. Used as desiccant and deodorant dusting powder; a mordant in dyeing; in fireproofing and waterproofing fabrics. Syn., *a. subacetate, printer's acetate*. Also called *lenicet*.

dried a. hydroxide gel (*gelatum alumini hydroxidi siccum*). A white, odorless, tasteless, amorphous powder yielding on ignition not less than 50% of Al_2O_3. Used as antacid. Dose, 0.3–1.0 Gm. (5–15 gr.).

soluble a. silicate. A mixture of aluminum and sodium silicates used in hyperchlorhydria. See *ludozan*.

alumnol. Brand of aluminum betanaphthol disulfonate. $Al_2[C_{10}H_5OH(SO_3)_2]_3$; used as an astringent and antiseptic in 0.5–5.0% solution.

alupec. Trade-mark for gastric antacid preparations containing aluminum hydroxide gel, pectin, and magnesium carbonate.

alurate. Trade-mark for 5-allyl-5-isopropylbarbituric acid, officially designated *aprobarbital*. The substance is a white, crystalline powder, very slightly soluble in water; it is used as a long-acting sedative and hypnotic. Dose, 65–130 mg. (1–2 gr.).

sodium a. Trade-marked name for the sodium derivative of 5-allyl-5-isopropylbarbituric acid, which substance is soluble in water.

a·lu′si·a [G. *alyein*, to be at a loss, to wander]. Hallucination; morbid state of mind.

alutabs. Trade-mark for an effervescent tablet which hydrates in water to form an aluminum hydroxide gel; used as a gastric antacid.

Alvarez, Walter Clement [*American physician*, 1884–]. Author of numerous significant contributions to the study of diseases of the gastrointestinal system and to the physiology of the digestive tract; a pioneer in calling attention to the importance of the nervous system in producing these diseases, and in psychosomatic medicine.

al′ve·at·ed [L. *alveatus*, hollowed out like a trough]. Honeycombed; channeled; vaulted.

al′ve·in. An antibiotic substance derived from *Bacillus alvei;* it is active against many bacteria but also produces hemolysis of red blood cells.

alveol-. See *alveolo-*.

al″ve·o·la′bi·al. See *alveololabial*.

al·ve′o·lar [L. *alveolus*, dim. of *alveus*, trough]. Pertaining to an alveolus.

al·ve′o·late [*alveolus*]. Pitted like a honeycomb.

al″ve·o·lec′to·my [*alveolus;* G. *ektomē*, excision]. Surgical removal of part of the alveolar process of the upper or lower jaw.

al·ve′o·li″. Plural of alveolus.

al″ve·o·lin′gual, al·ve″o·lo·lin′gual [L. *alveus*, trough; *lingua*, tongue]. Pertaining to the lingual aspects of the alveolar processes.

al″ve·o·li′tis [L. *alveolus*, dim. of *alveus;* G. *-itis*, inflammation]. Inflammation of a dental alveolus; especially the inflamed condition following the removal of a tooth. A frequent complication of tooth extraction. See dry *socket*.

al·ve′o·lo-, alveol- [*alveolus*]. A combining form denoting *alveolus, alveolar*.

al·ve″o·lo·cla′si·a (al·vee″o·lo·clay′zhuh, ·zee·uh, al″vee·o·lo·) [*alveolus;* G. *klasis*, a breaking]. *In dentistry*, a nonspecific breaking-down of the alveolar process, causing loosening of the teeth. Also see *periodontosis, pyorrhea*.

al·ve″o·lo·con·dyl′e·an [*alveolus;* G. *kondylos*, knuckle of a joint]. *In craniometry*, pertaining to the anterior portion of the maxillary alveolus and the occipital condyles.

al·ve″o·lo·den′tal [*alveolus;* L. *dens*, tooth]. Pertaining to the teeth and their sockets.

al·ve″o·lo·la′bi·al, al″ve·o·la′bi·al [*alveolus;* L. *labia*, lip]. Pertaining to the alveolar processes and the lips, or to the labial aspect of the alveolar process.

al·ve″o·lo·lin′gual. See *alveolingual.*

al·ve′o·lon [*alveolus*]. That point at which a straight line tangent to the posterior surfaces of the maxillary alveolar processes intersects the midline of the hard palate, or the median palatine suture. There will be found many specimens in which the line just defined will fall posterior to the tip of the posterior nasal spine. In these cases, the midline of the hard palate is to be prolonged till it intersects the line tangent to the posterior surfaces of the maxillary alveolar processes.

al·ve·ol′o·plas″ty. *In dentistry*, surgical alteration of the shape or size of the alveolar ridge to aid in the construction of prosthetic appliances.

al·ve″o·lo·sub·na′sal (·sub·nay′zul) [*alveolus;* L. *sub*, under; *nasus*, nose]. Pertaining to the alveolar portion of the maxilla that lies below the anterior bony aperture of the nose.

al″ve·o·lot′o·my [*alveolus;* G. *tomē*, a cutting]. Incision into a dental alveolus.

al·ve′o·lus (pl. *alveoli*) [L.]. 1. Bony socket of a tooth; also called *phatne.* 2. An air cell of the lung. 3. A cavity, depression, pit, cell, or recess. 4. A terminal acinus of a racemose gland.

pulmonary a. See *alveolus*, 2.

al″ve·ol′y·sis [L. *alveus*, trough; G. *lysis*, a loosing]. Periodontosis.

alvesen. Trade-mark for an effervescent alkalizing agent containing sodium bicarbonate, calcium lactophosphate, potassium bicarbonate, anhydrous magnesium sulfate, and sodium chloride.

al′ve·us [L.]. 1. A trough, tube, or canal; applied to ducts and vessels of the body. 2. A cavity or excavation. See *alvus.*

a. hippocampi. A bundle of nerve fibers in the cerebral hemisphere investing the convexity of the hippocampus.

al′vi. Plural of alvus.

al·vi′no·lith, al′vi·no·lith [L. *alvus*, the bowels; G. *lithos*, stone]. An intestinal concretion, usually formed from calcareous salts and debris.

al′vus (pl. and gen. *alvi*) [L.]. The abdomen or its contained viscera. —**alvine,** *adj.*

a·lym′phi·a (ay·lim′fee·uh, a·lim′·) [G. *a-*, not; L. *lympha*, water]. Absence or deficiency of lymph.

a·lym″pho·cy·to′sis (ay·lim″fo·sigh·to′sis, a·lim″·) [*a-; lympha;* G. *kytos*, cell; *-ōsis*, condition]. A very marked decrease or absence of lymphocytes in the blood.

alypin hydrochloride. Trade-mark for a brand of the hydrochloride of benzoyl 1,3-tetramethyl-diamino-2-ethyl-isopropyl alcohol; $C_6H_5COOC(C_2H_5)(CH_2N(CH_3)_2)_2.HCl$; a white, crystalline, soluble powder used as a local anesthetic in strengths of 2–5%. See *amydricaine hydrochloride.*

alysine. Trade-mark of an antipyretic and analgesic powder containing natural sodium salicylate, natural magnesium salicylate, natural calcium salicylate, sodium bicarbonate, calcium carbonate, and magnesium carbonate.

a·lys′mus [G. *alysmos*, disquiet]. The natural anxiety and restlessness which accompanies any physical disease. Also called *alysm.*

al″ys·o′·sis [G. *alys*, boredom; *-ōsis*, condition]. Boredom.

a·lys′sous, a·lys′sus [G. *alysson*, Galen's madwort]. Curing or preventing rabies.

Alzheimer, Alois [*German physician*, 1864–1915]. Described presenile dementia associated with cortical cerebral sclerosis (1907), called *Alzheimer's disease.* See presenile *sclerosis.*

alzinox. A trade-mark for preparations containing the gastric antacid substance, dihydroxyaluminum aminoacetate.

Am Chemical symbol for americium.

A. M. A. American Medical Association.

am′a·dou (am′uh·doo͞) [F. *amadouer*, to coax]. German tinder or touchwood; spunk; used as a hemostatic. See *agaric.*

a·mai·o′sis (a·migh·o′sis, ay″migh·). See *ameiosis.*

a·mal′gam [G. *malagma*, emollient, from *malassein*, to soften]. 1. An alloy of mercury with any other metal. 2. Any soft alloy. Symbol, āāā.

a. carrier. An instrument designed for carrying and introducing amalgam into the cavity of a tooth.

a. plugger. See *a.* carrier.

dental a. Compounds of a basal alloy of silver and tin with mercury, used for filling teeth. Gold, platinum, copper, zinc, or bismuth is frequently added as a third metal to the basal alloy.

a·mal′gam·ate [*malagma*]. 1. Unite a metal in an alloy with mercury. 2. Unite two dissimilar substances. 3. Cover the zinc elements of a galvanic battery with mercury.

a·mal″gam·a′tion [*malagma*]. 1. Formation of an amalgam. 2. Formation of an alloy of mercury with another metal.

a. process. A method of extracting certain metals, especially gold and silver, from ores by alloying them with mercury.

a·man′din, am′an·din. A globulin contained in certain fruit kernels, such as sweet almonds and peach seeds.

Am″a·ni′ta [G. *amanitai*, a kind of fungus]. A genus of mushrooms belonging to the Agaricaceae.

A. muscaria. Fly agaric.

A. phalloides. A very poisonous species; the source of amanita toxin and amanita hemolysin.

a·man′i·tin, a·man′i·tine [*amanitai*]. 1. A principle identical with choline, obtained from fly agaric. 2. A poisonous glycoside obtainable from various species of poisonous mushrooms.

a·ma′ra [L. *amarus*, bitter]. Drug used for its bitter taste, chiefly to increase appetite; bitters.

am′a·ranth [G. *amarantos*, from *a-*, not; *marainein*, to wither]. 1. Any plant of the genus *Amaranthus.* An important cause of hay fever in the states west of Missouri and Iowa. 2. (*amaranthum*). $C_{10}H_6(SO_2.ONa).N{:}N.C_{10}H_4(SO_2.ONa)_2.OH$. A dark, red-brown powder used as a color for foods, drugs, and cosmetics, and in dyeing. Also called *F.D.* and *C. Red No.* 2.

a. solution (*liquor amaranthi*). A 1% aqueous solution of amaranth, 2.

am′a·rine (am′uh·reen, ·rin), **am′a·rin.** Triphenyl dihydroglyoxaline:

$$C_6H_5\overline{CH.N{:}C(C_6H_5)NH.CH}.C_6H_5$$

A white, lustrous, crystalline powder, which occurs in bitter almond oil and can be prepared synthetically.

am′a·roid [L. *amarus*, bitter; G. *eidos*, form]. Any distinctly bitter vegetable extractive of definite chemical composition other than an alkaloid or a glycoside. The names of specific amaroids end in *-in* or *-inum.* Also called *bitter principle.*

am″a·se′sis [G. *a-*, not; *masēsis*, a chewing]. Inability to chew.

a·mas′ti·a, a·ma′zi·a [*a-;* G. *mastos*, breast]. Congenital absence of the mammae.

am″a·tho·pho′bia [G. *amathos*, dust; *phobos*, fear]. A morbid fear of dust.

am′a·tive·ness [L. *amare*, to love]. The sexual passion; disposition to love. Syn., *erotism*. —**amative, amatory,** *adj.*

am′a·tol (am′uh·tole, ·tol, ·tawl). An explosive mixture of trinitrotoluene and ammonium nitrate.

am″au·ro′sis [G., a darkening]. Partial or total blindness from any cause. —**am″au·rot′ic,** *adj.*

a. fugax. Temporary blindness resulting from sudden acceleration, as in aerial flight. Syn., *blackout*.

a. partialis fugax. Partial blindness associated with headache, vertigo, and scotomas. It is usually sudden and transitory.

congenital a. Condition of total blindness existing at birth when no change can be seen in the eye to account for it.

toxic a. Blindness which follows the introduction of various poisons and toxic products into the body, as ethyl and methyl alcohol, tobacco, lead, arsenic, quinine, etc., and the metabolites of uremia and diabetes.

uremic a. A toxic *a.*

am″au·rot′ic [*amaurōsis*]. One suffering from amaurosis.

a. cat's-eye. A light reflex through the pupil in suppurative choroiditis or intraocular neoplasm.

a. familial idiocy. (a) A familial disease occurring almost exclusively in Jewish children, and manifesting symptoms in the fourth month of life; characterized by flaccid muscles, convulsions, decerebrate rigidity, and blindness marked by the appearance of a cherry-red spot at the macula lutea; associated with optic atrophy. Also called *cerebromacular degeneration, Tay-Sachs disease.* (b) A late infantile type in which the symptoms first appear at the age of three or four years. The patient may live about four years. (c) A juvenile type beginning between seven and twelve years, running a longer course; not associated with macular changes; occurring in Gentiles: also called *Batten-Mayou's disease.*

am″a·xo·pho′bi·a (am″uk·so·fo′bee·uh, a·mack″-so·) [G. *amaxa*, wagon; *phobos*, fear]. Morbid dread of being in, or riding upon, any vehicle.

Ambard, Léon [*French pharmacologist*, 1876–]. Associated with a coefficient for estimating renal activity, the formula showing the relations between the amount of urea in the blood and that excreted by the kidneys. $K = \frac{Ur}{\sqrt{D \times \frac{70}{P} \times \frac{\sqrt{C}}{25}}}$

Ur = grams of urea in a liter of blood; D = grams of urea excreted in 24 hours; C = grams of urea in the urine; P = weight of the patient in kilograms. An increase above normal (0.06–0.08) equals renal insufficiency. The formula is seldom used today. He is also known for his laws: (a) the output of urea varies directly with the square of the concentration of the blood urea when the urinary urea concentration is constant; (b) when the blood urea concentration is constant, the output of urea varies inversely as the square root of its urinary concentration.

am′ber [OF. *ambre*, from Ar. *'anbar*]. A fossil resin found in alluvial soils and lignite beds in various parts of the world, and especially along the southern shores of the Baltic Sea. It is an amorphous solid, insoluble in water and incompletely soluble in any solvent, and assumes a negative charge through friction.

a. oil (*oleum succini*). A product of the dry distillation of amber, formerly used as rubefacient and, internally, in amenorrhea, hysteria, and whooping cough.

am′ber·gris (am′bur·greece, ·griss) [*ambre;* F. *gris*, gray]. An intestinal concretion of the sperm whale, *Physeter macrocephalus*, found floating on the sea, particularly in the southern hemisphere. It is usually gray in color with brown, white, or yellow streaks. It is used in perfumes, particularly as a fixative for floral odors, and has been used as a cordial and antispasmodic in adynamic fevers and various nervous diseases. See *ambrein.*

amberlite. Trade-mark applied to a group of ion-exchange resins of the cation-exchange type and anion-exchange type; certain of the purified resins are used medicinally. See *carbacrylic resin* and *polyamine-methylene resin.*

am′bi- [L. *ambo*, both]. A combining form meaning *both.*

am′bi-, amb- [L. *ambi-*, around]. A prefix meaning *about, around.*

am″bi·dex′trous [L. *ambo*, both; *dexter*, right]. Able to use both hands equally well. —**ambidexter, ambidexter′ity, ambidextrism, ambidextral′ity,** *n.*

am″bi·lat′er·al [*ambo;* L. *latus*, side]. Relating to or affecting both sides.

am″bi·le′vous [*ambo;* L. *laevus*, left]. Clumsy in the use of both hands. Syn., *ambisinister.*

ambinon. A proprietary extract of the anterior pituitary gland.

am″bi·oc·u·lar′i·ty [*ambo;* L. *oculus*, eye]. Ability to use both eyes equally well.

am″bi·o′pi·a [*ambo;* G. *ōps*, eye]. Diplopia.

am″bi·sex′u·al, am″bo·sex′u·al [*ambo;* L. *sexus*, sex]. 1. Denoting feelings and behavior which are neither strictly masculine nor feminine, but common to both sexes. 2. Designating organs, extracts, and substances which evoke activity common to both sexes, as opposed to *bisexual* or *hermaphroditic.* 3. Denoting an individual in whom exist undifferentiated primordia of both sexes. Should both sets develop, hermaphroditism would result. —**ambisexual′ity, ambosexual′ity,** *n.*

am″bi·sin′is·ter [*ambo;* L. *sinister*, left]. Ambilevous.

am″bi·tend′en·cy [*ambo;* L. *tendere*, to direct one's course]. A trend in instinctual human behavior which arouses a countertrend.

am·biv′a·lence, am″bi·va′lence, am·biv′a·len·cy [*ambo;* L. *valere*, to be powerful]. *In psychiatry*, the coexistence, conscious or unconscious, of the feelings or attitudes of love and hate toward the same person or object. —**ambivalent,** *adj.*

am′bi·vert [*ambo;* L. *vertere*, to turn]. Both introvert and extrovert; or, intermediate between the two. —**ambiver′sion,** *n.*

am′bi·vert. A personality type intermediate between extrovert and introvert.

am′bly- [G. *amblys*, dulled]. A combining form meaning *obtuse* or *dulled, faint.*

am″bly·a·cou′si·a (am″bli·a·kōō′zhuh, ·zee·uh, ·shuh, ·see·uh) [*amblys;* G. *akouein*, to hear]. Dullness of hearing.

am″bly·chro·ma′si·a (am″bli·kro·may′zhuh, ·zee·uh) [*amblys;* G. *chrōma*, color]. *In bacteriology* a deficiency in nuclear chromatin which causes the cell to stain faintly. —**amblychromat′ic,** *adj.*

Am″bly·om′ma [*amblys;* G. *omma*, eye]. A genus of hard-bodies ticks of the Ixodidae. Several species act as vectors of rickettsial diseases of man and of heartwater fever of ruminants.

am′bly·ope [*amblys;* G. *ōps*, eye]. A person with amblyopia.

am″bly·o′pi·a [*amblys;* *ōps*]. Dimness of vision, especially that not due to refractive errors or organic disease of the eye. It may be congenital or acquired. —**amblyop'ic,** *adj.*

a. albinismus. That associated with albinism.

a. ex anopsia. That from disuse or from nonuse.

color a. Partial colorblindness.

crossed a., a. cruciata. That occurring through lesion of the brain. See *hemianopsia.*

hysterical a. A unilateral or bilateral disturbance of vision involving great variations in the extent of the visual fields, and, occasionally, inversion of the color fields; seen in hysteria.

toxic a. A chronic optic neuritis due to poisons, usually alcohol and tobacco.

uremic a. Loss of vision without disease of the retina, sometimes accompanying an attack of uremia, and presumably due to central suppression by edema of the occipital cortex.

am"bly·o"pi·at'rics [*amblys; ōps;* G. *iatrikos,* pertaining to medicine]. The therapeutics of amblyopia. See *orthoptics.*

am'bly·o·scope" [*amblys; ōps;* G. *skopein,* to examine]. A device which presents a separate image of an artificial target to each eye: used in diagnosis and in some aspects of the treatment of disturbances of binocular vision.

am"bo·cep'toid [L. *ambo,* both; *capere,* to take; G. *eidos,* form]. A degenerated amboceptor which has lost its binding group (haptophore) for the cell, or for the complement. *Obs.*

am'bo·cep"tor [*ambo; capere*]. According to the Ehrlich theory, an antibody present in the blood of immunized animals which contains two specialized elements: a cytophile group that unites with a cellular antigen, and a complementophile group that joins with the complement. Syn., *sensitizer.*

a. unit. The smallest quantity of amboceptor in the presence of which a given quantity of red blood cells will be dissolved by an excess of complement.

ambodryl hydrochloride. Trade-marked name for the antihistaminic substance bromodiphenhydramine hydrochloride or bromazine hydrochloride.

am'bon. Old term for labrum glenoidale.

am"bo·sex'u·al. See *ambisexual.*

am"bo·tox'oid [*ambo;* G. *toxikon,* poison; *eidos,* form]. An immunization agent prepared by reinoculating bacterial toxin with pooled cultures of the bacteria and their bacteriophage, then detoxicating the mixture with formalin and merthiolate. Used especially as a staphylococcus preparation.

Am·boy'na but'ton. See *yaws.*

am'bre·in, am'bra·in. A crystalline, fatty substance, probably a polymer of cholesterol, obtained from ambergris.

Am·bro'si·a (am·bro'zhuh, ·zee·uh) [G., food of the gods]. A genus of composite-flowered herbs. The common ragweed of North America, or **A. artemisiaefolia,** is used by the eclectics as a stimulant, tonic, antiperiodic, and astringent; properties of **A. trifida** are similar. The pollen of these two species is generally regarded as a frequent cause of hay fever.

am'bu·lance [L. *ambulare,* to go about, walk]. 1. In foreign countries, the staff and equipment of an army medical unit in the field. 2. In the United States, a vehicle for the transportation of the sick or wounded.

air a. See *a.* plane.

a. basic relay post. *In U. S. Army medicine,* the relay post farthest to the rear in an ambulance shuttle where the bulk of unemployed ambulances are dispersed awaiting use.

a. company. Field unit in the U. S. Army Medical Department made up of staff and equipment for the evacuation of the sick and wounded.

a. control post. *In U. S. Army medicine,* the point at a road junction at which a soldier is stationed to direct ambulances along the proper route.

a. insert. *In U. S. Army medicine,* a special frame installed in a motor vehicle to support loaded stretchers; it converts a regular truck into a field ambulance.

a. loading post. *In U. S. Army medicine,* a point on the ambulance shuttle, normally the point farthest forward, where one or more ambulances are stationed to receive patients for transportation. It is usually located at the collecting station. An advanced ambulance loading post is a point forward of the collecting station at which casualties are loaded for evacuation to the rear.

a. plane. An airplane designed for the evacuation of troop casualties. Syn., *air a.*

a. relay post. *In U. S. Army medicine,* a point on the ambulance shuttle where one or more ambulances are stationed ready to advance to replace one which has left the post forward.

hi-lift a. An ambulance body on a truck chassis with a controlled hydraulic, built-in lift mechanism. It can be loaded at the hospital, driven to the plane, and the body of the ambulance elevated to the door of the plane.

veterinary a. One designed to transport sick or injured animals, especially horses.

am'bu·lance chas'er. An unethical lawyer who endeavors to exploit injury cases.

am'bu·la·to"ry, am'bu·lant [*ambulare*]. Walking or able to walk; designating a patient not confined to bed, but requiring medical care.

am·bus'tion [L. *ambustio,* a burn]. A burn or scald.

amdelate. Trade-mark for preparations of ammonium mandelate.

a·me'ba, a·moe'ba (pl. *amebas, amoebae*) [G. *amoibē,* change]. A colorless, jellylike, unicellular organism found in sea and fresh waters. It constantly undergoes change in form, progressing by means of pseudopodia, reproducing by simple fission, obtaining nourishment by engulfing tiny neighboring particles. —**amebic, amoebic,** *adj.*

am"e·bi'a·sis [*amoibē;* NL. *-iasis,* condition]. Infection with *Endamoeba histolytica.*

a. cutis. Ulceration of the skin due to amebas, especially in association with visceral amebiasis.

intestinal a. See amebic *colitis.*

a·me'bi·cide, a·moe'bi·cide [*amoibē;* L. *caedere,* to kill]. An agent fatal to amebas, usually applied to one fatal to *Endamoeba histolytica.* —**amebicid'al,** *adj.*

a·me'bid [*amoibē*]. An allergic, cutaneous reaction due to infection with *Endamoeba histolytica.*

a·me'bo·cyte, a·moe'bo·cyte [*amoibē;* G. *kytos,* cell]. 1. Old terminology for leukocyte. 2. A cell found in the coelomic fluid of echinoderms or among the tissues of various invertebrates. 3. Any ameboid cell.

a·me'boid [*amoibē;* G. *eidos,* form]. Resembling an ameba in form or in movement, as the leukocytes.

a·me'boid·ism [*amoibē*]. Movements in certain body cells, notably of the central nervous system, which resemble the movements of an ameba. —**ameboid,** *adj.*

am·e·bo'ma. See amebic *granuloma.*

a·me'bu·la, a·moe'bu·la [*amoibē;* L. *-ulus,* diminutive suffix]. A merozoite having the power of ameboid movement.

am"e·bu'ri·a, am"oe·bu'ri·a [*amoibē;* G. *ouron,* urine]. Presence of amebas in the urine.

a·mei·o'sis, a·mi·o'sis, a·mai·o'sis (a·migh·o'·sis, ay"migh·) [G. *a-,* not; *meiōsis,* diminution]. Aberrant miosis, forming diploid spores or gametes.

am·el′e·ia [G. *ameleia*, indifference]. Morbid apathy; indifference.

a·mel″i·fi·ca′tion [OF. *amel*, enamel]. The formation of dental enamel.

a·mel′o·blast (a·mel′o·blast, a·mee′lo·, am′i·lo·) [*amel;* G. *blastos*, germ]. An enamel cell; one of the columnar cells of the enamel organ which helps in forming dental enamel. Syn., *adamantoblast, ganoblast.*

a·mel″o·blas·to′ma. A tumor derived from epithelium associated with the enamel organ and composed of islands of cells whose basal layers resemble the ameloblast. It may be solid, monocystic, or polycystic. No enamel is formed. The tumor is usually found in the mandible, and rarely in the tibia and pituitary gland. Also called *adamantinoma, adamantoma.*

am″el·o·blas″to·sar·co′ma. A malignant tumor derived from epithelial and mesenchymal odontogenic tissues.

am″e·lo·gen′e·sis [*amel;* G. *genesis*, production]. Histogenesis of the dental enamel.

a·me′lus [G. *a-*, not; *melos*, limb]. An individual with congenital absence of all extremities. —**amel′ia,** *n.*

a·me′ni·a. Amenorrhea.

a·men″o·ma′ni·a, a·moen″o·ma′ni·a [L. *amoenus*, pleasant; G. *mania*, madness]. A mild form of mania in which the symptoms are manifested in gaiety, fondness of dress, exaggeration of social condition and the like; a cheerful or joyous delirium; a morbid elevation of the spirits; manic phase of manic-depressive psychosis.

a·men″or·rhe′a, a·men″or·rhoe′a [G. *a-*, not; *mēn*, month; *rhoia*, flow]. Absence of menstruation. Syn., *amenia.* —**amenorrheal, amenorrhoeal,** *adj.*

emotional a. That which results from sympathetic vasomotor disturbances caused by fright, emotional causes, or hysteria.

endocrinopathic a. An abnormal amenorrhea due to unphysiologic function or dysfunction of one or more of the endocrine glands. It does not include such cessation of function as normal menopause or lactation amenorrhea.

functional a. A type lacking definite or known organic, endocrine, or nutritional causes, which often results from a psychologic disturbance.

hypothalamic a. Emotional *a.*

lactation a. Postpartum amenorrhea due to lactation and nursing. It is probably a result of pituitary inhibition of the ovaries and indirectly or directly related to the lactogenic hormone.

pathologic a. That due to pathologic conditions, such as hysterectomy, oophorectomy, absence of or damage to endometrium, ovarian failure, debility, or sympathetic vasomotor disturbances.

premenopausal a. A prolongation of the intermenstrual intervals for weeks or months which may occur for a considerable time prior to the menopausal cessation of menstrual flow.

primary a. Term applied to those cases in which menstruation has not appeared at the proper time. Also called *radical a., primitive a.*

secondary a. That which occurs after menstruation has been established.

a′ment, am′ent [L. *amens*, out of one's senses, from *a*, from; *mens*, mind]. A person suffering from amentia; an idiot.

diplegic a. An individual with congenital spastic diplegia and amentia or failure of brain to develop.

a·men′ti·a (a·men′shee·uh, ·shuh) [L., madness]. Subnormal mental development; especially, congenital intellectual incapacity. Contrasted with dementia: term proposed by the Viennese school for temporary mental disorder, acute hallucinatory confusion; not generally accepted in U.S.A.

nevoid a. That associated with a face or scalp nevus, calcification of parts of the brain, glaucoma, epilepsy, and defects of the pyramidal tracts. Also called *encephalotrigeminal audiomatosis, Sturge-Weber-Dimitri disease* or *syndrome, Kalischer disease.*

phenylpyruvic a. See phenylpyruvic *oligophrenia.*

American National Red Cross. A quasi-governmental agency and member of the Red Cross Society, whose principal services are to the armed forces in peace and war, to the civilian population in disaster, and community services such as the teaching of first aid, life saving, maintenance of blood banks, and many volunteer services.

American Type Culture Collection. A quasi-official organization suggested by the Society of American Bacteriologists, by groups from industry, and the United States Public Health Service, as a repository for standard bacterial cultures. Abbreviated ATCC.

am″er·i′ci·um (am″ur·ish′ee·um) [named after the *Americas*]. Chemical element No. 95, symbol Am, produced artificially.

am″er·is′tic [G. *a-*, not; *meros*, portion]. Not segmented. —**am′erism,** *n.*

amesec. Trade-mark for a bronchial antispasmodic and sedative preparation containing aminophylline, ephedrine hydrochloride, and amytal.

a·me″si·al′i·ty (a·mee″zee·al′i·tee) [*a-;* G. *mesos*, middle]. Shifting of a part, as the pelvis, to one side of the long axis of the body.

a″me·tab′o·lous [*a-;* G. *metabolē*, change]. Referring to a mode of insect development in which the insect resembles the adult when it hatches from the egg, as in the silverfish and the springtail.

amethocaine hydrochloride. British Pharmacopoeia name for tetracaine hydrochloride.

amethone. Trade-mark for 3-(beta-diethylaminoethyl)-3-phenyl-2-benzofuranone hydrochloride. The drug has antispasmodic action on smooth muscle, especially of the kidney vessels, ureter, and urinary bladder.

amethopterin. Trade-mark for 4-aminomethylpteroylglutamic acid or 4-aminomethylfolic acid, a folic acid antagonist useful in treating certain types of leukemia.

a·me′tri·a, a·met′ri·a [*a-;* G. *mētra*, womb]. Congenital absence of the uterus. —**ametrous,** *adj.*

a·me″tro·he′mi·a, a·me″tro·hae′mi·a (a·mee″tro·, a·met″ro·) [*a-; mētra;* G. *haima*, blood]. Deficiency in uterine blood supply.

am″e·tro′pi·a [*a-;* G. *metron*, a measure; *ōps*, eye]. Imperfect refractive ability due to defects of the media or the structures of the eye, which causes images to fail to focus directly upon the retina. See *myopia, hypermetropia, astigmatism, presbyopia, aphakia.*—**ametrop′ic,** *adj.;* **am′etrope,** *n.*

amfetin. Trade-mark for a solution of a purified fraction of bovine amniotic fluid; the product is a tissue stimulant: administered by peritoneal cavity instillation during abdominal operations.

am″i·an″thi·nop′sy [*a-;* G. *ianthinos*, violet-colored; *opsis*, sight]. Violet blindness; inability to distinguish violet rays.

am″i·an′thoid [G. *amiantos*, asbestos]. Resembling asbestos; asbestoslike: said of certain fibers seen in degeneration of hyalin cartilage and called *amiantine degeneration.*

am″i·an·tho′sis [*amiantos;* G. *-ōsis*, condition]. Asbestosis.

a″mi·cet′in. An antibiotic substance isolated from cultures of a species of *Streptomyces* found in soil. It is markedly inhibitory to *Mycobacterium tuber-*

culosis var. *hominis*, *Proteus vulgaris*, *Escherichia coli*, and *Micrococcus pyogenes* var. *aureus*.

Amici, Giovanni Battista [*Italian astronomer and physicist*, 1784–1863]. Said to have been the first to construct a microscope with an achromatic lens (1817–18). Credited with the invention of an immersion objective (1850). Also remembered for his contribution to our knowledge of muscle.

a″mi·cro′bic (ay″migh·kro′bick, ·krob′ick, a″migh·, am″i·) [G. *a*-, not; *mikros*, small; *bios*, life]. Pertaining to the absence of microorganisms.

a·mi′cron, a·mi′crone (ay·migh′kron, ·krone, ay-mick′ron, ·rone, a·migh′, a·mick′·) [*a*-; *mikros*]. A colloid particle, measuring about 10^{-7} cm. or less than 5 $m\mu$ in diameter, so small as to be just barely visible through the ultramicroscope.

a·mi″cro·scop′ic [*a*-; *mikros*; G. *skopein*, to examine]. Too small to be observed by the ultramicroscope.

a·mic′u·lum [L., a mantle or cloak thrown around the body]. A dense plexus of fibers around the dentate nucleus of the cerebellum formed by fibers from the Purkinje cells of the cerebellar cortex.

am′i·dase. Any enzyme catalyzing the hydrolysis of nonpeptide C═N linkages, generally with elimination of ammonia. Syn., *desamidase*. See Table of Enzymes in the Appendix.

am′ide. 1. Any organic compound containing the univalent radical, —CO.NH_2. Amides are derived from acids by replacing the —OH group of the —COOH group by —NH_2, or by the replacement of a hydrogen of ammonia by an acyl group, R.CO—, where R indicates any organic radical, forming R.CO.NH_2. 2. A compound formed by the replacement of a hydrogen of ammonia by a metal, such as sodamide, $NaNH_2$. Syn., *ammono base*.

am′i·din. The part of starch that is soluble in water; soluble starch.

am′i·dine (am′i·deen, ·din). Any compound containing the univalent radical —C(NH_2):NH; any amide in which the oxygen is replaced by the divalent imide group, ═NH.

a·mi′do′ (a·mee′do-, am′i·do-), **amid-** [*amide*]. A prefix denoting *a compound containing the —CO.NH_2 radical*. Also see *amino-*.

a·mi″do·az″o·tol′u·ene (a·mee″do·, am″i·do·). See *aminoazotoluene*.

a·mi″do·ben′zene, a·mi″do·ben′zol (a·mee″do·, am″i·do·). See *aniline*.

am′i·dol. Diaminophenol hydrochloride, C_6H_3-(OH):(NH_2.HCl)$_2$. Colorless or grayish white crystals, freely soluble in water. Used as photographic developer and in dyeing fur and hair. May be irritating.

am′i·done hy″dro·chlo′ride. Methadone hydrochloride.

amidophen. Trade-mark for an antipyretic and analgesic preparation containing aminopyrine, acetophenetidin, caffeine, and hyoscyamus extract.

a·mi″do·py′rine (a·mee″do·pye′reen, ·rin, am″-i·do·). Aminopyrine.

am″i·dox′ime, am″i·dox′im (am″i·dock′seem, ·sim). A compound containing the group —C(NH_2):N.OH; it is an amidine in which the hydrogen of the imide group has been replaced by an —OH; as ethenyl- or acetamidoxime, CH_3-C(NH_2):N.OH. Syn., *oxamidine*.

amigen. Trade-mark for certain preparations of protein hydrolysate.

a·mim′i·a [G. *a*-, not; *mimos*, mimic]. 1. Loss of the ability to communicate by gestures or signs. It may be an **amnesic amimia** when the meanings of the signs are not remembered, or an **ataxic amimia** when gestures cannot be made because of muscular defects. 2. *In neurology*, a paralysis of the facial muscles, affecting chiefly the angles of the mouth, apparent when the patient attempts an emotional grimace, as in paralysis agitans.

am′in. Amine.

a·mi′na·crine. Aminoacridine.

am″i·na′tion. The process of introducing an amino group into a molecule; also, the formation of an amine.

a·mine′ (a·meen′, am′een, am′in), **am′in.** Any member of the group of compounds formed by replacing one or more of the hydrogens of ammonia by one or more organic radicals, such as R.NH_2, R.NH.R′, and R.N.(R′)R″, where R, R′, and R″ may or may not represent the same radical. The amines are classified as *primary*, *secondary*, and *tertiary* depending on whether one, two, or three hydrogens are replaced.

quaternary a. A compound derived from ammonium hydroxide by replacement of the four hydrogens of the —NH_4 group by radicals; tetra-alkyl ammonium bases.

tertiary a. An amine of the type R_3N or R′(R″)-NR‴.

aminet. Trade-mark for a suppository containing aminophylline and pentobarbital sodium.

a·mi′no- (a·mee′no-, am′i·no-) [from *amine*]. *In chemistry*, a prefix meaning *pertaining to* or *containing the group NH_2 united to a radical other than an acid radical*.

a·mi″no·a·ce′tic ac′id (*acidum aminoaceticum*). $H_2N.CH_2.COOH$. White, odorless, crystalline powder with a sweetish taste; 1 Gm. dissolves in about 2 cc. of water; it is slightly soluble in alcohol. It is a constituent of many proteins from which it may be obtained by hydrolysis. It is also prepared synthetically. Used in muscular dystrophy and myasthenia gravis. Dose, 4–8 Gm. (60–120 gr.) t.i.d. Syn., *glycocoll*, *glycine*.

a·mi″no·ac″e·to·phe·none′ (a·mee′no·ass″i·to·fi-nohn′, ·fee′nohn, am′i·no·) (para-). $NH_2.C_6H_4$.-$COCH_3$. A yellow, crystalline compound used in a colorimetric assay of thiamine hydrochloride.

a·mi′no ac′id (a·mee′no, am′i·no). Any one of a large group of organic compounds with the basic formula NH_2—R—COOH, R representing any aliphatic radical. These compounds are amphoteric in reaction and represent the end products of protein hydrolysis. From amino acids, the body resynthesizes its proteins. Ten of them are considered essential to life: arginine, histidine, isoleucine, leucine, lysine, methionine, phenylalanine, threonine, tryptophan, and valine. See Table of Normal Values of Blood Constituents in the Appendix.

D-a·mi′no ac′id ox′i·dase. A flavoprotein enzyme present in animal tissues, responsible for oxidative deamination of the D- or unnatural form of amino acids but not acting upon the L- or natural form.

L-a·mi′no ac′id ox′i·dase. A flavoprotein enzyme present in animal tissues, responsible for oxidative deamination of the L- or natural form of amino acids but not acting upon the D- or unnatural form.

a·mi′no·a″cid·u′ri·a. The presence of amino acids in the urine, especially in excess amounts.

a·mi″no·ac′ri·dine (a·mee″no·ack′ri·deen, ·din, am″i·no·). An amino derivative of acridine; of the several possible isomers the 9-aminoacridine (or 5-aminoacridine in the British numbering system) possesses useful bacteriostatic and bactericidal powers. The hydrochloride, $C_{13}H_{10}N_2$.-$HCl.H_2O$, a yellow, crystalline powder, soluble in 300 parts of water, is the form in which the compound is used. Syn., *aminacrine*.

α-a·mi″no·a·dip′ic ac′id. COOH.CH(NH_2).-(CH_2)$_3$.COOH; a dibasic amino acid produced in the metabolism of lysine by liver homogenates, and also isolated from *Cholera vibrio.*

a·mi′no al′co·hol. Any of a group of compounds containing both an alcoholic hydroxyl group and an amino group. Syn., *alkamine, alkanolamine.*

amino-an-fol. Trade-mark for 4-aminopteroyl-aspartic acid, a folic acid antagonist useful in treating certain types of leukemia.

a·mi″no·az″o·tol′u·ene (a·mee″no·, am″i·no·) (ortho-). $CH_3.C_6H_4.N{:}N.C_6H_3(NH_2).CH_3$. Golden leaflets or plates once used in ointment or as dusting powder to stimulate granulation in wounds. It may cause systemic poisoning.

a·mi″no·az″o·tol′u·ol. Aminoazotoluene.

a·mi″no·ben′zene (a·mee″no·ben′zeen, ·ben·zeen′, am″i·no·). See *aniline.*

p-a·mi″no·ben″zene·ar·son′ic ac′id. Arsanilic acid.

a·mi″no·ben′zene·sul·fon′a·mide. See *sulfanilamide.*

4-a·mi″no·ben·zo′ic ac′id. Para-aminobenzoic acid.

4-a·mi″no·ben″zo·yl gly′cine. *p*-Aminohippuric acid.

α-a·mi″no·bu·tyr′ic ac′id. $CH_3CH_2CH(NH_2)$-COOH; the L-stereoisomer, a dextrorotatory crystalline substance, isolated from certain proteins. Syn., *2-aminobutanoic acid.*

2-a·mi″no·bu·tyr′ic acid. α-Aminobutyric acid.

aminocaine. Trade-mark for *p*-amino-benzoyl-diethylamino-ethanolphenyl carboxylate, used as a local anesthetic in 1–2% solution.

α-a·mi″no·ca·pro′ic ac′id. Norleucine.

2-a·mi″no-D-glu′cose. Glucosamine.

2-a mi″no·eth″ane·sul·fon′ic ac′id. Taurine.

2-a·mi″no·eth′a·nol. Cholamine.

a·mi″no·flu′o·rene (a·mee″no·, am″i·no·). Fluoreneamine.

4-a·mi″no·fo′lic ac′id. See *aminopterin.*

a·mi″no·glu′cose. 2-Amino-D-glucose. See *glucosamine.*

α-a·mi″no·glu·tar′ic ac′id. Glutamic acid.

2-a·mi″no·hep′tane. A chemical name for the sympathomimetic agent known by the generic name *tuaminoheptane,* and supplied under the trade-marked name *tuamine.* Syn., *1-methylhexylamine.*

2-a·mi″no·hex″a·no′ic ac′id. Norleucine.

p-a·mi″no·hip·pu′ric ac′id. $NH_2.C_6H_4.CONH-CH_2COOH$; a white, crystalline substance, sparingly soluble in water: employed in kidney function tests. Syn., *4-aminobenzoylglycine.*

α-a·mi″no·hy″dro·cin·nam′ic ac′id. Phenylalanine.

2-a·mi″no-3-hy·drox″y·bu″ta·no′ic ac′id. Threonine.

α-a·mi″no-β-hy·drox″y·bu·tyr′ic ac′id (al″fuh-a·mee″no-bay″tuh-high·drock″si·bew·tirr′ick, -am″i·no-). Threonine.

2-a·mi″no-3-hy·drox″y·pro″pa·no′ic ac′id. Serine.

α-a·mi″no-β-hy·drox″y·pro″pi·on′ic ac′id. Serine.

aminoids. A proprietary nutrient containing amino acids, dipeptides, carbohydrates, inorganic salts.

α-a·mi″no-3-in″dole·pro″pi·on′ic ac′id. L-Tryptophan.

α-a·mi″no·i″so·ca·pro′ic ac′id. Leucine.

α-a·mi″no·i″so·va·ler′ic ac′id. Valine.

a·mi″no·lip′id (a·mee″no·lip′id, am″i·no·). A fatty acid ester of an alcohol containing nitrogen in the amino form.

2-a·mi″no-3-mer·cap″to·pro·pa·no′ic ac′id. Cysteine.

a·mi″no·meth″an·am′i·dine (·am′i·deen, ·din). Guanidine.

2-a·mi″no-3-meth·yl·bu″ta·no′ic ac′id. Valine.

4-a·mi″no·meth″yl·pter″o·yl·glu·tam′ic ac′id. See *amethopterin.*

aminonat. Trade-mark for a protein hydrolyzate prepared from lactalbumin.

a·mi″no·pent′a·mide. Generic name for the anticholinergic substance α,α-diphenyl-γ-dimethylaminovaleramide. See *centrine.*

a·mi″no·pep′ti·dase. An enzyme occurring in intestinal mucosa, yeast, and certain bacteria. Catalyzes polypeptides at the end having a free amino group, producing an amino acid and a smaller peptide which may undergo further hydrolysis under the influence of the enzyme.

a·mi″no·pep′to·drate. Generic name for an enzymatic digest of extracted liver and beef muscle, wheat gluten, soya, yeast, casein, and lactalbumin with dextrose, maltose, and sucrose, containing amino acids and polypeptides equivalent to 45% proteins and 40% carbohydrates. See *caminoids.*

α-a·mi″no-β-phen″yl·pro″pi·on′ic ac′id. Phenylalanine.

a·mi″no·pher′ase. Transaminase: occasional usage.

a·mi″no·phyl′line (·fil′een, ·fil′in). $(C_7H_8N_4O_2)_2$-$C_2H_4(NH_2)_2.2H_2O$; a salt of theophylline and ethylenediamine, occuring as white or slightly yellowish granules or powder, soluble in water. It has the action and uses of theophylline, modifying blood flow, relaxing bronchial and other smooth musculature, and producing diuresis. Dose, orally, 100–200 mg. (1½–3 gr.); rectally, 500 mg. (7½ gr.); intravenously, 500 mg. (7½ gr.). Syn., *theophylline ethylenediamine.*

a·mi″no·pol″y·pep′ti·dase. A proteolytic enzyme occurring in yeast, intestinal mucosa, kidney, spleen, and liver. Its action is the cleavage of polypeptides which contain either a free amino group or a basic nitrogen atom carrying at least one hydrogen atom.

2-a·mi″no·pro″pa·no′ic ac′id. Alanine.

α-a·mi″no·pro″pi·on′ic ac′id. Alanine.

a·mi″no·pro′te·ase. An enzyme which will hydrolyze a protein and unite with the free amino group of its substrate.

aminopterin. Trade-mark for 4-aminopteroyl-glutamic acid or 4-aminofolic acid; a folic acid antagonist useful in treating certain types of leukemia.

4-a·mi″no·pter″o·yl·as·par′tic ac′id. See *amino-an-fol.*

4-a·mi″no·pter″o·yl·glu·tam′ic ac′id. See *aminopterin.*

a·mi″no·pu′rine (a·mee″no·pew′reen, ·rin, am″-i·no·). A purine in which one or more hydrogens are replaced by amino groups, as *adenine, guanine.*

a·mi″no·py′rine (a·mee″no·pye′reen, ·rin, am″i-no·) (*aminopyrina*). Dimethylaminophenyl-dimethyl pyrazolone; $C_{13}H_{17}N_3O$. An antipyretic and analgesic used in neuralgia, neuritis, migraine, and colds. Its continued use may lead to agranulocytosis. A common allergen. Dose, 0.12–0.3 Gm. (2–5 gr.). Syn., *amidopyrine.* See *pyramidon.*

a·mi′no·quin naph′tho·ate. Pamaquine naphthoate.

aminosal. Trade-mark for a partial acid hydrolyzate of blood fibrin, consisting of a mixture of approximately two-thirds free amino acids and one-third small peptides: used to maintain positive nitrogen balance in patients unable to ingest or digest food.

a·mi″no·sal″i·cyl′ic ac′id. The U.S.P. official name for para-aminosalicylic acid.

aminosol. Trade-mark for certain preparations of protein hydrolyzate prepared from modified fibrin.

a·mi″no·suc″cin·am′ic ac′id (a·mee″no·suck″-sin·am′ick, am″i·no·). Asparagin.

a·mi′no su′gar. Any of a class of sugars in which one or more hydroxyl groups have been replaced by amino groups, as, for example, glucosamine and galactosamine.

a·mi″no·su′ri·a (a·mee″no·sue′ree·uh, am″i·no·), **am″i·nu′ri·a** [*ammoniac; -ine;* G. *ouron,* urine]. The presence of amines in the urine.

a·mi″no·tol′u·ene. See *toluidine.*

α-a·mi″no·va·ler′ic ac′id. Norvaline: also written *α-amino-n-valeric acid.*

am″i·nu′ri·a. See *aminosuria.*

amiodoxyl benzoate. A brand of ammonium orthoiodoxybenzoate, $C_6H_4(IO_2)COONH_4$, used as antiarthritic.

a·mi·o′sis (a·migh·o′sis, ay″migh·). See *ameiosis.*

am″i·thi′o·zone. Generic name for the tuberculostatic agent *p*-formylacetanilid thiosemicarbazone or *p*-acetylaminobenzaldehyde thiosemicarbazone; $CH_3CO.NH.C_6H_4.CH{:}N.NH.CS(NH_2)$; a pale yellow crystalline substance, insoluble in water: supplied under various trade-marked names, including *conteben, myvizone, panrone, tibione.* Syn., *thiacetazone.*

a″mi·to′sis [G. *a-,* not; *mitos,* thread; *-ōsis,* condition]. Reproduction by direct nuclear cleavage or simple fission. —**amitot′ic,** *adj.*

Amman, Jan Coenraad [*Dutch educator and scientist,* 1669–1730]. Remembered for his work in the education of deaf-mutes (1692–1700).

am′me″ter [André Marie *Am*père, French physicist, 1755–1836; G. *metron,* a measure]. A type of galvanometer in which the electric current is measured directly in amperes.

am′mi·din. $C_{16}H_{14}O_4$; a hydroxy-furocoumarin ether from *Ammi majus* which, like ammoidin but to a lesser degree, induces normal pigmentation in patients with leukodermic areas. The substance is identical with *imperatorin.*

am′mine. A complex compound characterized by containing ammonia molecules linked to a metal (not to be confused with *amine,* which is a substituted ammonia).

am′mism [G. *ammos,* sand]. Ammotherapy; psammism; treatment of disease with sand baths.

ammivin. A trade-mark for pure crystalline khellin.

am′mo-, amm- [*ammos*]. A combining form meaning *sand.*

am·moi′din. $C_{12}H_8O_4$; the methyl ether of 8-hydroxy-4,′5′,6,7-furocoumarin, obtained from the fruits of the herb *Ammi majus;* when given internally or applied externally, followed by exposure to sunlight, it induces normal pigmentation in patients with leukodermic areas. The substance is identical with *xanthotoxin.*

Ammon, Friedrich August von [*German ophthalmologist and surgeon,* 1799–1861]. Known for his many ophthalmic operations and for his anatomic observations. Described the posterior scleral protuberance, the pyriform scleral fissure of early fetal life, etc. His atlas of diseases of the eye is considered the most complete summary written before the introduction of the ophthalmoscope.

am′mo·nate. A compound containing ammonia of crystallization, analogous to one containing water of crystallization.

am″mo·na′tion. A process of combining a compound with ammonia. —**am′monate,** *v.*

Am′mon's horn. Old term for hippocampus.

am·mo′ni·a [sal *ammoniac,* named from Temple of Jupiter Ammon]. A colorless, pungent gas, NH_3, very soluble in water, a portion combining with it to form ammonium hydroxide. The ammonia of commerce is produced synthetically from nitrogen and hydrogen or obtained by the destructive distillation of nitrogenous organic matter. It is used as a detergent, a saponifying agent, in refrigeration, and for other industrial applications. See also *ammonium.* —**ammoniated, ammoni′acal,** *adj.*

a. liniment (*linimentum ammoniae*). A rubefacient prepared from diluted solution of ammonia, oleic acid, and sesame oil. Syn., *hartshorn liniment.* Also called *volatile liniment.*

a. water (*aqua ammoniae*). See diluted *a.* solution.

aromatic a. spirit (*spiritus ammoniae aromaticus*). A flavored, hydroalcoholic solution of ammonia and ammonium carbonate having an aromatic, pungent odor. Dose, 2–4 cc. (30–60 min.), well diluted.

diluted a. solution (*liquor ammoniae dilutus*). A 10% solution of ammonia in water; used as local irritant, stimulant, and antacid. Dose, 0.6–2.0 cc. (10–30 min.), greatly diluted.

strong a. solution (*liquor ammoniae fortis*). A 28% solution of ammonia in water.

stronger a. water (*aqua ammoniae fortior*). See strong *a.* solution.

am·mo′ni·ac. A gum resin from a Persian umbelliferous plant, *Dorema ammoniacum,* which has been employed in chronic bronchitis as a stimulating expectorant and counterirritant.

African a. A gum resin derived from *Ferula communis* var. *brevifolia,* used chiefly as incense.

a. emulsion (*emulsum ammoniaci*). A 4% emulsion in water. Dose, 15–30 cc. (½–1 fluidounce).

a. mixture (*mistura ammoniaci*). A 3% emulsion in water flavored with tolu balsam syrup.

am·mo″ni·e′mi·a, am·mo″ni·ae′mi·a [sal *ammoniac;* G. *haima,* blood]. The presence in the blood of ammonia compounds believed to be the result of urea decomposition. The condition is attended by subnormal temperature, digestive disorders, weakened pulse, and coma.

am·mon″i·fi·ca′tion (a·mon″i·fi·kay′shun, a·mo″-ni·). Production of ammonia by bacterial action.

am·mo′ni·um. The univalent radical, NH_4. It exists only in combination.

acid a. carbonate. Ammonium bicarbonate.

a. acetate solution (*liquor ammonii acetatis*). Mindererus spirit, dilute acetic acid neutralized with ammonium carbonate. Dose, 4–30 cc. (1 dr.–1 oz.). Used as diaphoretic.

a. alum. See *alum* (definition 2).

a. arsenate. $(NH_4)_2HAsO_4$. It has been used as an alterative in skin diseases.

a. benzoate. $C_6H_5COONH_4$. Stimulant and diuretic. Dose, 0.3–1.0 Gm. (5–15 gr.).

a. bicarbonate. NH_4HCO_3, occurring in white crystals as a fine white crystalline powder, or in colorless crystalline lumps, freely soluble in water: used like ammonium carbonate, and in the same dosage. Syn., *acid ammonium carbonate.*

a. bifluoride. $NH_4F.HF$, occurring as crystals, freely soluble in water; it etches glass in the solid state. Solutions are germicidal and have been used for this effect in pyorrhea alveolaris.

a. bitartrate. $NH_4HC_4H_4O_6$. A white, crystalline, acid powder. An ingredient of baking powder.

a. bromide (*ammonii bromidum*). NH_4Br. Used as sedative and somnifacient. Dose, 0.6–2.0 Gm. (10–30 gr.).

a. carbamate. $NH_2.COO.NH_4$. A white, crystalline, volatile powder.

a. carbonate (*ammonii carbonas*). A compound of ammonium acid carbonate (NH_4HCO_3) and ammonium carbamate ($NH_2.COO.NH_4$) in varying proportions. It is a stimulant expectorant and reflex stimulant. Dose, 0.2–0.6 Gm. (3–10 gr.).

a. chloride (*ammonii chloridum*). NH_4Cl. When used as a saline expectorant, the dose is 0.3–0.6 Gm. (5–10 gr.); and for the acidification of urine, the dose is 1–4 Gm. (15–60 gr.) per day.

a. hydroxide. NH_4OH; a weakly-ionizing base formed to some extent when ammonia (NH_3) is dissolved in water. The term is frequently applied, not entirely correctly, to aqueous solutions of ammonia.

a. hypophosphite (*ammonii hypophosphis*). $NH_4PH_2O_2$; it has been used in treating bronchitis and laryngitis. Dose, 0.13–0.3 Gm. (2–5 gr.), 3 times daily.

a. ichthosulfonate. Ichthammol.

a. iodide (*ammonii iodidum*). NH_4I; it has been used in treating asthma and in chronic bronchitis when exudate is fibrinous. Dose, 0.13–0.6 Gm. (2–10 gr.).

a. mandelate. $C_6H_5CH(OH)COONH_4$. A white deliquescent powder, soluble in water. Used as a urinary antiseptic. Dose, 3–4 Gm. (45–60 gr.). Syn., *mandamon.*

a. muriate. Ammonium chloride.

a. nitrate. NH_4NO_3. Used in preparing nitrous oxide.

a. oxalate. $(NH_4)_2C_2O_4.H_2O$, occurring in colorless crystals or white granules, soluble in water; it is of importance as an analytical reagent.

a. persulfate. $(NH_4)_2S_2O_8$. Colorless crystals, soluble in water. It is a disinfectant and deodorizer. Application, 0.5–2.0% solution.

a. phosphate, dibasic. $(NH_4)_2HPO_4$, occurring in crystals, freely soluble in water; it gradually loses ammonia on exposure to air; has been used medicinally. Also called *secondary ammonium phosphate, diammonium hydrogen phosphate.*

a. phosphate, monobasic. $(NH_4)H_2PO_4$, occurring in crystals, freely soluble in water, permanent in air: has been used medicinally. Also called *primary ammonium phosphate, ammonium biphosphate, ammonium dihydrogen phosphate.*

a. picrate. A yellow salt which, like other picrates, is explosive and should be handled with care.

a. salicylate (*ammonii salicylas*). $C_6H_4.OH.COONH_4$. An antirheumatic and antipyretic. Dose, 0.13–1.3 Gm. (2–20 gr.).

a. sulfate. $(NH_4)_2SO_4$. Used as a protein precipitant.

a. urate. $NH_4C_5H_3N_4O_3$, occurring as a crystalline powder, almost insoluble in water; an occasional constituent of urine. It has been used in the local treatment of eczema.

a. valerate. Has been used as a sedative in hysteria. Dose, 0.06–0.3 Gm. (1–5 gr.).

am·mo″ni·u′ri·a [sal *ammoniac;* G. *ouron,* urine]. Presence of an excess of ammonia in the urine.

am·mo′no base. An inorganic amide obtained by replacing a hydrogen of ammonia with a metal, as $NANH_2$, sodium amide.

am″mo·nol′y·sis. Any interaction of ammonia with another substance in which the ammonia also undergoes chemical change.

am″mon·o·tel′ic [*ammono-*, combining form from ammonia; Gr. *telikos,* from *telos,* end, or purpose]. Having ammonia as the principal compound of its nitrogenous waste: said of aquatic invertebrates and tadpoles.

am″mo·ther′a·py [G. *ammos,* sand; *therapeia,* treatment]. The use of sand baths in the treatment of disease.

am″ne·mon′ic (am″nee·mon′ick) [G. *a-*, not; *mnēmonikos,* relating to memory]. Relating to impairment of the memory.

am·ne′si·a (am·nee′zhuh, ·zee·uh) [G., forgetfulness]. Loss of memory, especially of the ideas represented by words. —**amnesic, amnes′tic,** *adj.*

anterograde a. Loss of memory for the period immediately following trauma, shock, or a confused state.

auditory a. Word deafness. Inability to recognize the spoken word.

lacunar a. Loss of memory for only certain isolated events, not a complete memory loss.

retroanterograde a. A perversion of memory in which recent events are referred to the past, and conversely.

retrograde a. Loss of memory for events occurring before the onset of the current disease.

tactile a. Inability to recognize objects by the sense of touch; astereognosis.

visual a. Word blindness. Inability to recognize the written or printed word, or objects previously seen.

amnestrogen. Trade-mark for a preparation of conjugated (water-soluble) estrogenic substances derived from gravid mares' urine.

am′ni·a. Plural of amnion.

am′ni·o- [G. *amnion,* membrane around the fetus, dim. of *amnos,* lamb]. A combining form denoting *amnion, amnionic.*

am″ni·o·cho′ri·al (am″nee·o·kor′ee·ul) [*amnion;* G. *chorion,* chorion]. Pertaining to both amnion and chorion.

am″ni·o·em″bry·on′ic [*amnion;* G. *embryon,* embryo]. Pertaining to the embryo and the amnion.

am″ni·o·gen′e·sis [*amnion;* G. *genesis,* production]. The development or formation of the amnion.

am″ni·og′ra·phy [*amnion;* G. *graphein,* to write]. Radiography of the fetus by injection of a solution of strontium iodide through the abdominal wall and into the amniotic sac; usually used as a diagnostic aid in suspected placenta previa.

am′ni·on (pl. *amnia*) [G.]. The innermost of the fetal membranes forming a fluid-filled sac for the protection of the embryo. Its thin, translucent wall is composed of an inner layer of ectoderm and an outer layer of mesoderm continuous with the embryonic somatopleure at the umbilicus. After the second month of development, it obliterates the extraembryonic coelom, forms a sheath about the umbilical cord, and fuses loosely with the chorionic mesoderm. —**amnion′ic, amniot′ic,** *adj.*

false a. A temporary cavity in the trophoblastic knob, resembling the early true amnion. Syn., *false amniotic cavity, ectoplacental cavity.*

true a. The inner amniotic folds of avian, reptilian, and certain mammalian embryos; the amnion proper.

am″ni·or·rhe′a, am″ni·or·rhoe′a [*amnion;* G. *rhoia,* flow]. The premature escape or discharge of the liquor amnii.

Am″ni·o′ta [*amnion*]. Group of animals with an amnion and allantois, comprising mammals, birds, and reptiles. Syn., *Allantoidea.* —**am′niote,** *adj., n.*

amniotin. Trade-mark for an estrogenic preparation derived from gravid mares' urine, containing estrone as the principal active constituent.

am″ni·o·ti′tis [*amnion;* G. *-itis,* inflammation]. Inflammation of the amnion.

am′ni·o·tome [*amnion;* G. *tomos,* cutting]. An instrument for puncturing the fetal membranes.

am″ni·ot′o·my. Rupture of the fetal membranes by a surgical procedure.

am″o·bar′bi·tal. The official generic name of 5-ethyl-5-isoamylbarbituric acid, introduced under the trade-marked name *amytal.* **Amobarbital so-**

dium is the official generic name of the water-soluble sodium derivative of amobarbital.

am″o·di′a·quin. Generic name for the antimalarial drug 4-(7-chloro-4-quinolylamino)-α-diethylamino-*o*-cresol, the dihydrochloride of which is supplied under the trade-marked name *camoquin hydrochloride*.

amodrine. Trade-mark for a bronchial antispasmodic and sedative containing aminophylline, racephedrine hydrochloride, and phenobarbital.

A·moe′ba. See *Endamoeba.*

a·moe′ba. See *ameba.*

a·mok′, a·muck′ [Malay *amoq*, furious]. In a state of murderous frenzy. Certain Orientals, mostly Malays, attack with knives and kill while in this state of wild fury.

A·mo′mum [G. *amōmon*, Indian spice plant]. A genus of plants of the Zingiberaceae.

A. cardamomum. Source of the cardamom.

A. granum paradisi. Source of the grains of paradise; possessing diuretic properties.

a′mor [L.]. Love, especially physical attraction and union.

a. insanus. Erotomania.

a. lesbicus. Lesbianism; sapphism.

a. sui. Love of self; vanity.

a·mo·ral′i·a [G. *a-*, not; L. *moralis*, moral]. Moral imbecility. *Obs.*

a·mor′phic. See *amorphous.*

a·mor′phin·ism [*a-;* G. *Morpheus*, god of dreams]. State resulting when morphine is withdrawn from an addict.

a·mor′phous, a·mor′phic [*a-;* G. *morphē*, form]. 1. Formless, shapeless. 2. *In biology*, without visible differentiation in structure. 3. *In chemistry*, not crystalline. —**amorphism, amorphia,** *n.*

a·mor′phus [*a-; morphē*]. An acardiac monster without head or extremities; a similar parasitic monster which is but a shapeless mass, sometimes called *amorphus globulus*. See *anideus.*

amoryn. Trade-mark for a preparation of conjugated or free estrogens derived from gravid mares' urine.

a·mo′ti·o ret′i·nae (a·mo′tee·o ret′i·nee) [L.]. Detachment of the retina.

AMP Adenosinemonophosphate.

amp. Ampere; amperage.

am·per′age (am·peer′idj, am′pi·ridj, am·pair′idj) [after André Marie *Ampère*, French physicist, 1775–1836]. The number of amperes passing in a given electric circuit. Abbreviated, amp.

am′pere (am′peer, am·peer′) [*Ampère*]. A unit of current electricity; one-tenth of the unit of current of the centimeter-gram-second system of electromagnetic units; the current produced by one volt through a resistance of one ohm. The international ampere is the value of a steady current depositing 0.001118 Gm. of silver per second from a solution of silver nitrate. Abbreviated, a., amp.

am′pere·me″ter. See *ammeter.*

amphedroxyn hydrochloride. A trade-marked name for *methamphetamine hydrochloride.*

am″pher·ot′o·ky, am·phit′o·ky [irreg., from G. *amphoteros*, both of two; *tokos*, offspring]. Production of both sexes in a single parthenogenetic brood. —**ampherot′okous, amphit′okal,** *adj.*

am·phet′a·mine (am·fet′uh·meen, ·min). Racemic 1-phenyl-2-aminopropane, $C_6H_5.CH_2.CHNH_2.CH_3$, a colorless, volatile, mobile liquid. Inhalation of its vapors causes shrinking of the nasal mucosa in head colds, sinusitis, and hay fever. Also see *benzedrine.*

a. phosphate. $C_9H_{13}N.H_3PO_4$; a white, crystalline powder, freely soluble in water: used as a central stimulant. Syn., *racemic amphetamine phosphate, dl-monobasic amphetamine phosphate.*

a. sulfate. $(C_9H_{13}N)_2.H_2SO_4$; a white, crystalline powder, freely soluble in water: used as a central stimulant. Syn., *racemic amphetamine sulfate.*

dextro-a. The dextrorotatory form of amphetamine phosphate and sulfate, salts of which are used; a more powerful cerebral stimulant than the levo form. See *dexedrine.*

dibasic a. phosphate. $(C_9H_{13}N)_2.H_3PO_4$; a white, crystalline powder, soluble in water: used as a central stimulant. Syn., *racemic dibasic amphetamine phosphate, dl-dibasic amphetamine phosphate.*

am′phi-, amph- [G., on both sides]. A prefix signifying *both, of both kinds, on both sides, about, around.*

am″phi·ar·thro′sis [*amphi;* G. *arthron*, joint]. An articulation of contiguous bony surfaces which are connected by either fibrocartilage, as the vertebrae, or an interosseous ligament, as the tibiofibular junction. They permit only slight motion. —**am″phi·ar·throt′ic,** *adj.*

am′phi·as″ter [*amphi; astēr*, star]. The achromatic figure in mitosis, consisting of two asters connected by a spindle: formerly called *diaster.*

Am·phib′i·a [G. *amphibios*, from *amphi; bios*, life]. A class of vertebrates which includes the salamanders and newts, frogs and toads, the tropical Apoda, and certain extinct orders: distinguished by scaleless skin, paired limbs with toes, gills in at least larval stages, lungs in most orders, and a three-chambered heart.

am·phib′i·ous [*amphi; bios*]. Capable of living both on land and in water.

am″phi·blas′tic [*amphi;* G. *blastos*, germ]. *In biology*, designating the complete but unequal segmentation of telolecithal eggs.

am″phi·blas′tu·la [*amphi;* dim. from *blastos*]. 1. A ciliated larval stage of many sponges. 2. A blastula produced by amphiblastic or unequal cleavage, as in amphibia.

am″phi·bles·tro′des (am″fi·bles·tro′deez) [G. *amphiblestron*, fishnet; *eidos*, form]. The retina. *Obs.*

am″phi·chro′ic [G. *amphi*, on both sides; *chroia*, color]. Having the power to turn blue litmus paper red and red litmus paper blue. *Obs.*

am″phi·coe′lous (am″fi·see′lus) [*amphi;* G. *koilos*, hollow]. Biconcave; applied to the centrum of the vertebra of certain fishes.

am″phi·cra′ni·a [*amphi;* G. *kranion*, skull]. Headache affecting both sides of the head, as opposed to *hemicrania.*

am″phi·cre′a·tine (am″fi·kree′uh·teen, ·tin) [*amphi;* G. *kreas*, flesh]. One of the tissue leucomaines of the creatine type.

am″phi·cre·at′i·nine (·kree·at′i·neen, ·nin) [*amphi; kreas*]. One of the tissue leucomaines of the creatinine type.

am′phi·cyte [*amphi;* G. *kytos*, cell]. A satellite cell.

am″phi·des′mic, am″phi·des′mous [*amphi;* G. *desmos*, bond]. Furnished with a double ligament.

am″phi·di″ar·thro′sis [*amphi;* G. *diarthrōsis*, articulation]. A mixed articulation such as that of the lower jaw, which partakes of the nature of both amphiarthrosis and diarthrosis.

am″phi·er′o·tism [*amphi;* G. *erōs*, love]. A condition in which an individual can conceive of himself as being either male or female or both at the same time.

am″phi·gas′tru·la [*amphi;* dim. from G. *gastēr*, stomach]. A gastrula having blastomeres of different size in the two hemispheres as a result of total unequal cleavage.

am″phi·gen′e·sis [*amphi;* G. *genesis*, production]. The capacity of a predominantly homosexual person to carry on normal sexual relations with the opposite sex. —**amphigenet′ic,** *adj.*

am·phig′o·ny [*amphi;* G. *gonē*, offspring]. Sexual reproduction.

am″phi·kar′y·on [*amphi;* G. *karyon*, kernel]. A diploid nucleus.

am″phi·mix′is [*amphi;* G. *mixis*, a mingling]. 1. *In genetics*, interbreeding. 2. *In psychoanalysis*, urethral and anal erotism combined.

am″phi·mor′u·la [*amphi;* dim. from G. *moron*, mulberry]. A morula resulting from unequal segmentation, the cells of the hemispheres being unlike in size. Syn., *unequal stereoblastula.*

am″phi·ox′us [G. *amphi*, both; *oxus*, sharp]. A lancelet (genus *Amphioxus*), a primitive marine chordate belonging to the subphylum Cephalochorda, regarded by many as a connecting link between the invertebrates and vertebrates.

Am″phi·sto′ma·ta [*amphi;* G. *stoma*, mouth]. A suborder of trematode worms, distinguished by a prominent posterior ventral sucking disk.

am′phi·tene [*amphi;* G. *tainia*, filament]. The stage of mitosis in which the homologous chromosomes are in the process of conjugation. Syn., *synaptene, zygotene.*

am′phi·the″a·ter, am′phi·the″a·tre [G. *amphitheatron*, amphitheater]. A room with seats arranged in tiers; used for students or others to attend surgical operations, lectures, demonstrations, etc.

am·phit′o·ky. See *ampherotoky.*

am·phit′ri·chous (am·fit′ri·kus), **am·phit′ri·chate** (am·fit′ri·kit, ·kate, am″fi·try′kate) [*amphi;* G. *thrix*, hair]. Having flagella at both ends.

am′pho- [G., both]. A combining form meaning *both.*

amphocillin. Trade-mark for a package containing a vial of penicillin and a bottle of amphojel: used, after mixing, as oral penicillin therapy.

am″pho·di·plo′pi·a, am·phot″er·o·di·plo′pi·a [*amphō;* G. *diploos*, double; *ōps*, eye]. Double vision affecting each of the eyes.

amphojel. Trade-mark for a suspension of aluminum hydroxide used in gastric hyperacidity.

am′pho·lyte [G. *amphoteros*, both; *lytos*, soluble]. An amphoteric electrolyte.

amphomate. Trade-mark for ampuls of methenamine, partly combined with camphoric acid, administered intravenously as a urinary antiseptic.

am·phor′ic [G. *amphoreus*, jar with narrow neck]. Resembling the sound produced by blowing across the mouth of a large, narrow-mouthed jar or bottle.

am·phor′ic breath′ing. See amphoric *respiration.*

am″pho·ril′o·quy [*amphoreus;* L. *loqui*, to speak]. The production of hollow, blowing sounds in speaking.

am″pho·roph′o·ny [*amphoreus;* G. *phōnē*, voice]. An amphoric resonance of the voice.

am″pho·ter′ic. Having both acid and basic properties; capable of behaving either as a weak acid or as a weak base; as aluminum hydroxide, $Al(OH)_3 \rightleftharpoons H_3AlO_3$. Having the power of altering the color of both red and blue litmus paper. —**amphot′erism,** *n.*

am·phot″er·o·di·plo′pi·a. See *amphodiplopia.*

amphotropin. Trade-mark for methenamine camphorate; a white, crystalline powder, soluble in water: used as a urinary antiseptic.

am″pli·fi·ca′tion [L. *amplificare*, to enlarge]. 1. *In microscopy*, the enlargement of the visual area, as *amplification 200×*, or *200 diameters.* 2. *In sound* or *radio*, the magnification of sound. 3. *In electricity*, the increase of electric current in either voltage or amperage, as of a transformer.

am′pli·fi″er [*amplificare*]. 1. Any device which enlarges, magnifies, or increases the size, strength, or power of an object or force. 2. The concavo-convex lens between the objective and ocular of a microscope. 3. An electron tube in radio or radiotherapy. 4. A transformer.

am′pli·tude [L. *amplitudo*, breadth]. One-half the range of a periodic variation for symmetric vibrations; the maximum displacement from the normal for asymmetric vibrations; largeness; extent; range.

am″pro·tro′pine phos′phate. Generic name for the phosphate of the *dl*-tropic acid ester of 3-diethylamino-2,2-dimethyl-1-propanol. See *syntropan.*

am′pul (am′pul, am′pōōl), **am′pule** (am′pewl, am′pōōl), **am·poule′** (am·pōōl′, am′pōōl) [L. *ampulla*, bottle]. 1. A container, commonly made of glass and capable of being hermetically sealed, intended to hold sterile preparations usually intended for parenteral use. 2. Any of a class of preparations consisting of a sealed container holding a medicament. Such preparations are now more commonly known as injections (*injectiones*).

am·pul′la (pl. *ampullae*) [L.]. The dilated extremity of a canal or duct, as of the mammary ducts and semicircular canals. —**ampullar, am′pullary, ampullate,** *adj.*

a. lactifera. A dilatation of a milk duct near its opening on the nipple.

a. of the ductus deferens. That of the ductus deferens just before its junction with the duct of the seminal vesicle. See Plate 44.

a. of the lacrimal duct. A slight dilatation of the lacrimal duct beyond the punctum.

a. of the uterine tube. The dilated end of a uterine tube.

a. of the vagina. The dilated upper end of the vagina, where it joins the cervix of the uterus.

a. of Vater. The dilatation of the common bile duct and pancreatic duct where they join the duodenum.

membranous ampullae. Those occurring at one end of the membranous semicircular canals near their junction with the utricle, and containing the end organs of the sense of equilibrium.

osseous ampullae. Those parts of the bony labyrinth of the internal ear which house the membranous ampullae.

rectal a. The dilated part of the rectum situated just above the anal canal.

am·pul′lu·la [L., dim. of *ampulla*]. A minute ampulla, as in the lymphatic or lacteal vessels.

am″pu·ta′tion [L. *amputare*, to cut away]. The removal, generally by surgical means, of a limb, wholly or in part, a projecting part or process, or an organ of the body. Amputation may occur in the course of pathologic processes, such as gangrene or constriction, or as the result of accident.

amniotic a. Amputation of a fetal limb by a portion of the amnion.

a. appliance. A prosthesis for an amputated limb.

a. by transfixion. That performed by thrusting an amputating knife through a limb and cutting the flaps from within out.

a. center. *In military medicine*, a general hospital in home territory where, prior to discharge, amputees are sent for prosthetic appliances, training in the use of artificial limbs, and rehabilitation.

a. in contiguity. That performed through a joint (disarticulation, dismemberment).

a. in continuity. That performed elsewhere than at a joint.

a. neuroma. A painful bulbous enlargement of the end of a nerve divided at amputation, occurring after the formation of the stump.

a. stump. The rounded and shaped lower portion of an amputated limb or organ.

aperiosteal a. One in which all periosteum is removed in the vicinity of the divided bone ends.
bloodless a. One in which, owing to control, but little blood is lost, or, because of crushing or other circumstance, the circulation has ceased within the field of operation. Also called *dry a.*
central a. One in which the flaps are joined so that the suture line runs across the end of the stump.
chop a. One by a circular cut through the soft parts and bone without provision for flaps.
Chopart's a. An amputation of the foot consisting of a dislocation of the tarsal bones, leaving only the talus and calcaneus.
cinematic a. One in which a muscular stump is left so as to allow for movement of an artificial limb.
cineplastic a. One in which tendons are arranged in the stump to permit their use in moving parts of the prosthetic appliance. Types of cineplastic amputations include the *club*, the *loop*, the *tendon tunnel*, and the *muscle tunnel*.
circular a. An operation performed with the use of a flap by circular sweeps or incisions around the limb vertical to the long axis of the bone, Syn., *guillotine a.*
coat-sleeve a. One in which one long skin flap, like a coat sleeve, is left to enclose the stump.
congenital a. One which takes place in the uterus as the result of some pathologic or accidental process. Syn., *intrauterine a.*
double-flap a. One in which there are two opposing skin and muscle flaps.
elliptic a. One similar in performance to the circular, but in which the incision is elliptic.
Gritti-Stokes a. A supracondylar osteoplastic operation in which the patella, after removal of its articular surface, is retained in the flap and attached to the divided end of the femur, the skin and muscle flap being closed posteriorly.
guillotine a. See circular *a.*
Hey's a. The same as Lisfranc's amputation except that the medial cuneiform bone is sawed through in a line with the articulation of the second metatarsal bone, instead of being disarticulated.
interpelvioabdominal a. Amputation of the thigh with a portion of the adjoining half of the pelvis.
interthoracicoscapular a. Amputation of the upper extremity at the shoulder girdle with disarticulation of the humerus. It includes removal of the scapula and outer portion of the clavicle.
intrauterine a. See congenital *a.*
Lisfranc's a. A disarticulation of the tarsometatarsal joints.
Mackenzie a. A modified Syme amputation in which the flap of skin is taken from the medial aspect of the ankle.
major a. Any amputation through the long bones of the upper or lower extremities; disarticulation at the hip joint or shoulder girdle.
mammary a. Removal of the breast, either simple or radical.
mediotarsal a. See Chopart's *a.* Also called *midtarsal a.*
osteoplastic a. One in which there is a portion of bone fitted to the amputated bone end. See Gritti-Stokes *a.*
partial a. One in which only a portion of a member, part, or organ has been removed.
pathologic a. One occurring as a result of some pathologic process.
Pirogoff's a. A partial osteoplastic operation in which the calcaneus is sawed through obliquely from above downward and forward, and the posterior portion is brought up and secured against the surface made by sawing off the lower ends of the tibia and fibula.
primary a. One performed immediately after injury, during the period of reaction from shock and before the onset of suppuration.
racket a. A variety of elliptic or oval amputation with a long cut, like a racket handle, below the elliptic incision.
renal auto-a. The condition in which a kidney is cut off functionally by a diseased or obstructed ureter.
secondary a. One performed after suppuration has occurred or for the purpose of improving a temporary circular amputation with flaps left open.
spontaneous a. (a) Congenital amputation. (b) Amputation not caused by external trauma or injury, as in ainhum.
subperiosteal a. One in which the divided bone ends are covered by neighboring periosteum.
supracondylar a. An operation in which the femur is sawed through above the condyles. See Gritti-Stokes *a.*
Syme's a. Amputation above the ankle joint, the malleoli being sawed through, and a flap made with the skin of the heel.
thigh a. One through the femur below the hip joint.
traumatic a. One resulting from direct trauma.
two-stage a. See secondary *a.*

am″pu·tee′ [L. *amputare*, to cut away]. One who has had a major amputation of one or more limbs.

a·muck′. See *amok.*

a·mu′si·a (a·mew′zee·uh, ·see·uh) [G. *a-*, not; *mousa*, muse]. Loss of the ability to produce or comprehend music or musical sounds; an abnormality in regard to music, analogous to aphasia in regard to the faculty of speech.
motor a. That in which music is understood, but the power of singing or otherwise reproducing music is lost.
sensory a. Musical deafness, or the loss of the power of comprehension of musical sounds.

Amussat, Jean Zuléma [*French surgeon*, 1796–1856]. Remembered for his operation of lumbar colostomy (1839), said to have been the first performed for the relief of intestinal obstruction.

am″y·cho·pho′bi·a (am″i·ko·fo′bee·uh) [G. *amychē*, a tearing; *phobos*, fear]. Morbid fear of laceration, as of being scratched or clawed.

am″y·dri′a·sis [G. *a-*, not; *mydriasis*, dilatation of the pupil]. Pupillary contraction. See *mydriasis.*

a·myd′ri·caine hy″dro·chlo′ride (a·mid′ri·kane, ·ka·een, ·ka·in). See *alypin hydrochloride.*

a·my″e·len·ceph′a·lus [*a-*; G. *myelos*, marrow; *egkephalos*, brain]. A monster having neither brain nor spinal cord. —**amyelencephal′ic,** *adj.*; **amyelencepha′lia,** *n.*

am″y·e′li·a (am″eye·ee′lee·uh, ·el′ee·uh, am″ee·) [*a-; myelos*]. Congenital absence of the spinal cord. —**amyel′ic, amy′elous,** *adj.*

am″y·el″in·at′ed. Having no myelin sheath, as sympathetic nerve fibers; nonmedullated.

a·my′e·lus [*a-; myelos*]. A monster with partial or complete absence of the spinal cord.

a·myg′da·la. See *almond.*

a·myg′da·lase. Emulsin.

a·myg·dal′ic ac′id. Mandelic acid.

a·myg′da·lin. $C_{20}H_{27}O_{11}N.3H_2O$. A glycoside of mandelonitrile, $C_6H_5.CHOH.CN$, and the disaccharide gentiobiose, occurring in the bitter almond and other sources. In the presence of water, the enzyme emulsin causes its hydrolysis into glucose, benzaldehyde, and hydrocyanic acid.

a·myg′da·loid. See amygdaloid *nucleus.*

a·myg″da·loid·ec′to·my. Surgical excision of the amygdaloid nucleus, sometimes used to control olfactory hallucinations.

a·myg′da·lo·lith, am″yg·dal′o·lith. Tonsillar calculus.

A·myg′da·lus [G. *amygdalē*, almond]. See *almond.*

am′yl, a′myl [G. *amylon*, starch]. The univalent radical, —C_5H_{11}, derived from pentane. Three structural arrangements are possible, as follows: *normal amyl*, written *n-amyl*, the radical CH_3.-CH_2.CH_2.CH_2.CH_2—; *isoamyl*, the radical $(CH_3)_2$:CH.CH_2.CH_2—; *tertiary amyl*, the radical CH_3.CH_2.$(CH_3)_2$C—. Syn., *pentyl.* —**amyl′ic,** *adj.*

a. acetate. Isoamyl acetate. CH_3.COO.C_5H_{11}. A colorless liquid, miscible with alcohol, having a characteristic pearlike odor and taste; used as flavor, perfume, and solvent. Syn., *banana oil.* Also called *pear oil.*

a. alcohol. Any of eight isomeric alcohols of the composition $C_5H_{11}OH$, variously denominated. Commercial amyl alcohol, also known as *fusel oil*, consists predominantly of isoamyl alcohol (3-methyl-1-butanol).

a. bromide. Isoamyl bromide. $C_5H_{11}Br$. A colorless liquid, miscible with alcohol. Antiseptic and slightly anesthetic.

a. butyrate. Isoamyl *n*-butyrate. C_3H_7COO.-C_5H_{11}. A colorless liquid, soluble in alcohol; used in fruit essences. *n-Amyl n-butyrate* is similar.

a. nitrite (*amylis nitris*). Isoamyl nitrite. C_5H_{11}.ONO. A yellowish liquid, having an ethereal, fruity odor and a pungent, aromatic taste; used by inhalation to relax arterial spasms and of especial value in angina pectoris. Its action is immediate but fleeting. Dose, by inhalation, 0.2–0.3 cc. (3–5 min.).

a. valerate, a. valerianate. Isoamyl isovalerate. C_4H_9.COO.C_5H_{11}. A colorless liquid, miscible with alcohol, having an applelike odor and an artificial apple flavor.

tertiary a. alcohol. See *amylene* hydrate.

amyl-. See *amylo-.*

am″y·la′ceous [*amylon*]. Containing starch; starchlike.

am″yl·a·mine′ hy″dro·chlo′ride (am″il·uh-meen′, am″il·am′in, ·am′een, a·mil′uh·meen, ·min). C_5H_{11}.NH_2.HCl. Colorless crystals, soluble in water; has been used as an antipyretic. See *isoamylamine.*

am′yl·ase (am′i·lace, ·laze). Any amylolytic enzyme which hydrolyzes starch to sugar. See Table of Normal Values of Blood Constituents in the Appendix.

pancreatic a. Amylopsin.

salivary a. Ptyalin.

vegetable a. Diastase.

amylcaine hydrochloride. See *amylsine hydrochloride.*

am′yl·ene. C_5H_{10}. A liquid hydrocarbon having anesthetic properties but too dangerous to use.

a. chloral. Chloral amylene hydrate.

a. hydrate (*amyleni hydras*). Tertiary amyl alcohol, C_2H_5.$(CH_3)_2$C.OH. A narcotic substance; rarely used by itself, but employed as a solvent for and synergist with tribromoethanol.

am′y·lo-, amyl- [*amylon*]. A combining form denoting *pertaining to starch.*

am′y·lo-, a·my′lo-, amyl- [*amylon*; G. *hylē*, wood, material]. A combining form denoting *amyl*, the radical.

am″y·lo·bar′bi·tone, a·myl″o·bar′bi·tone. British generic name for *amobarbital.*

am″y·lo·caine′ hy″dro·chlo′ride. C_6H_5.CO_2.C-$(CH_3)(C_2H_5)$.$CH_2N(CH_3)_2$.HCl. The hydrochloride of the benzoyl ester of methylethyldimethylaminomethylcarbinol, a colorless, crystalline powder, soluble in water. Used as a local and spinal anesthetic in concentrations of 1 to 10 per cent. See *stovaine.*

am″y·lo·dex′trin [*amylon;* L. *dexter*, right]. Soluble starch.

am″y·lo·dys·pep′si·a [*amylon;* G. *dyspeptein*, to digest with difficulty]. Inability to digest starchy foods.

a·myl′o·gen [*amylon;* G. *genesthai*, from *gignesthai*, to be produced]. Soluble starch.

am′y·loid [*amylon;* G. *eidos*, form]. A complex protein deposited in tissues, characterized physically by its hyaline structureless nature, and chemically by special staining reactions. Its exact composition is unknown, and probably variable. It is starchlike only in that it stains brown with iodine. Amyloid results from degeneration of tissue and infiltration of unknown substances. It stains brown with iodine in watery solutions and turns a mahogany brown, almost black, when treated subsequently with dilute sulfuric acid. It takes a red tinge when heated in the metachromatic aniline dyes, such as gentian violet, methylrosaniline chloride, and methyl green.

am′y·loid de″gen·er·a tion. See secondary *amyloidosis.*

am″y·loi·do′sis [*amylon; eidos;* G. *-ōsis*, condition]. Widespread deposit of amyloid in various organs of the body or, less commonly, deposit in a particular organ, as amyloidosis of the kidney.

a. cutis. The presence of amyloid in the skin in the form of papules or plaques; it is not necessarily associated with systemic amyloidosis.

lichenoid a. A primary amyloidosis involving only the skin, usually of the legs. The papules resemble those of lichen planus, are conical or flat, discrete, brownish-red, and may coalesce to form plaques. The amyloid deposits are small and are found only in the subepidermal region of the skin.

primary a. A rare disease without known cause, characterized by more or less widespread deposit of amyloid in mesodermal structures, including skeletal muscle, tongue, bone, tendons, cartilage, cardiac muscle, lips, and other sites. This amyloid has less uniform staining reactions than the common secondary forms.

secondary a. Deposit of amyloid in various organs of the body—especially liver, spleen, and kidney—secondary to chronic diseases, such as chronic ulcerative tuberculosis of the lungs, chronic tuberculosis of the bones, chronic suppurative osteomyelitis, leprosy, tertiary syphilis, and malignant tumors. The material is first found immediately around capillaries and vascular sinuses, then around small arteries and veins, and then later more widely distributed in the organ. Staining reactions are regular and characteristic. Syn., *amyloid degeneration.*

am″y·lol′y·sis [*amylon;* G. *lysis*, a loosing]. The digestion of starch, or its conversion into maltose. —**amylolyt′ic,** *adj.*

am′y·lon [G.]. 1. Starch. 2. Glycogen.

am″y·lo·pec′tin. The outer, almost insoluble, phosphorus-containing portion of starch granules. It stains violet with iodine and forms a paste with water. See *amylose.* Also called *α-amylose, α-starch.*

am″y·lop′sin. An enzyme which changes starch into maltose; found in the pancreatic juice.

am′yl·ose (am′i·loce, ·loze). 1. The inner, relatively soluble portion of starch granules. It is stained blue by iodine. See *amylopectin.* 2. A polysaccharide. Also called *β-amylose, β-starch, granulose.*

amylsine hydrochloride. Trade-mark for the local anesthetic substance *naepine hydrochloride*, used to produce corneal anesthesia.

am′y·lum. See *starch.*

am″y·lu′ri·a [*amylon;* G. *ouron,* urine]. Presence of starch in the urine.

a·my″o·es·the′si·a, a·my″o·aes·the′si·a (·ess-thee′zhuh, ·zee·uh), **a·my″o·es·the′sis, a·my″-o·aes·the′sis** [G. *a-,* not; *mys,* muscle; *aisthēsis,* sense]. State of being without muscle sense; lack of the sense of motion, weight, and position.

a·my″o·pla′si·a (a·my″o·play′zhuh, ·zee·uh, ·shuh, ·see·uh) [*a-; mys;* G. *plassein,* to form]. Lack of muscle formation and development. —**amyo-plas′tic,** *adj.*

a. congenita. A congenital muscle deficiency attended by joint fixation, malpresentation, and difficult delivery.

a·my″o·sta′si·a (a·my″o·stay′zhuh, ·zee·uh, ·shuh, ·see·uh) [*a-; mys;* G. *stasis,* a standing]. A tremor of the muscles causing difficulty in standing, often seen in locomotor ataxia. —**amyostat′ic,** *adj.*

a·my″o·tax′i·a, a·my″o·tax′y [*a-; mys;* G. *taxis,* arrangement]. Muscular ataxia or incoordination of spinal or cerebellar origin. —**amyotax′ic,** *adj.*

a·my″o·to′ni·a [*a-; mys;* G. *tonos,* tone]. Lack of muscular tone; myatonia.

a. congenita. A rare congenital disease of the brain stem and spinal cord of infants; marked by absence of postural tone in the voluntary muscles, absence of reflexes, and with no reaction of degeneration in electrical tests. Mental development is rarely retarded, but the ability to sit up, stand, or walk is badly impaired. Also called *Oppenheim's disease.*

a·my″o·tro′phi·a, a·my″ot′ro·phy [*a-; mys;* G. *trophē,* nourishment]. Muscular atrophy. —**amyo-troph′ic,** *adj.*

a. spinalis progressiva. See myelopathic muscular *atrophy.*

syphilitic a. Progressive muscular atrophy due to syphilitic motor neuron degeneration or associated with a recognized syndrome of neurosyphilis: also called *amyotrophic syphilitic myelitis, syphilitic poliomyelitis.*

am′y·rin. $C_{24}H_{39}O$. A crystalline, resinous principle, derived from Mexican elemi and other gums.

Am′y·ris [*a-;* G. *myron,* balsam]. A genus of tropical trees and shrubs producing fragrant resins and gums, such as elemi.

amytal. Trade-mark for 5-ethyl-5-isoamylbarbituric acid, officially designated *amobarbital.* The substance is a white, crystalline powder, very slightly soluble in water; it is used as a sedative and hypnotic, having an intermediate duration of action. Dose, 20–300 mg. (⅓–5 gr.).

sodium a. Trade-marked name for the sodium derivative of 5-ethyl-5-isoamylbarbituric acid or amobarbital, the substance being soluble in water.

a·myx′i·a [*a-;* G. *myxa,* mucus]. Absence or deficiency of mucous secretion.

a·myx″or·rhe′a, a·myx″or·rhoe′a [*a-; myxa;* G. *rhoia,* flow]. Absence of the normal flow of mucous secretion.

An Chemical symbol for actinon.

an. Abbreviation for anode.

an-. See *a-.*

-an. *In chemistry,* a suffix which indicates *a sugar-like substance, a glycoside,* or *a gum.*

A. N. A. American Nurses' Association.

an′a [G., a preposition used distributively with numerals]. So much of each. Contracted in prescriptions to *āā.*

an′a- [G., on, up]. A prefix meaning *back, up, again, through, excessively.*

-a′na (-ay′nuh, -ah′nuh, -an′uh) [L., neuter plural of adjectives in *-anus*]. A suffix meaning *belonging to, connected with, derived from.* In the naming of subsections or groups of species it is added to the name of a species around which other species naturally cluster.

a·nab′a·sine (a·nab′uh·seen, ·sin). An alkaloid from the Russian herb *Anabasis aphylla.* It has effects similar to those of nicotine.

a. sulfate. The commercial mixture of the alkaloids of anabasis, used as an insecticide.

an″a·bi·ot′ic (an″uh·buy·ot′ick) [G. *anabioein,* to come to life again]. Apparently lifeless, but capable of being revived. —**anabio′sis,** *n.*

an″a·bi·ot′ic. Any agent used to effect restoration or revival.

an″a·bol′er·gy [G. *anabolē,* from *anaballein,* to throw up; *ergon,* work]. The work performed in anabolism.

a·nab′o·lin [*anabolē*]. Any substance formed during the anabolic process.

an·ab′o·lism [*anabolē*]. Synthetic or constructive metabolism; the conversion of nutritive material into more complex living matter. —**anabol′ic,** *adj.*

an″a·camp′tics [G. *anakamptein,* to bend back]. The study of reflection of light or of sound. *Obs.* —**anacamptic,** *adj.*

An″a·car″di·a′ce·ae (an″uh·car″dee·ay′see·ee) [G. *ana,* similar to; *kardia,* heart]. A family of plants, found mostly in the tropics, reported to cause dermatitis on contact, including poison ivy, poison oak.

an″a·car′dic ac′id. An acid from cashew nut; has been employed as an anthelmintic.

anacardone. Trade-mark for *nikethamide.*

an″a·cat″a·did′y·mus. See *anakatadidymus.*

an″a·ce″li·a·del′phous [G. *ana,* up; *koilia,* cavity; *adelphos,* brother]. Designating a paired monstrosity united by the thorax or upper part of the abdomen. *Obs.* —**anaceliadelphus,** *n.*

an″a·cid′i·ty [G. *a-,* not; L. *acidus,* from *acere,* to be sour]. The complete absence of hydrochloric acid in the stomach, demonstrated by lack of response to all secretory stimulants, particularly to histamine; achlorhydria. See *hypoacidity.*

a·nac′la·sis [G. *anaklasis,* a bending back]. Reflection or refraction of light or sound. —**anaclas′-tic,** *adj.*

a·nac′li·sis [G. *anaklisis,* a lying back]. 1. The act of reclining; decubitus. 2. *In psychiatry,* state of being emotionally dependent upon others. 3. *In psychoanalysis,* state in which the satisfaction of the sex libido is conditioned by some other instinct, such as hunger. —**anaclit′ic,** *adj.*

an·ac′me·sis [G. *a-,* not; *akmē,* culminating point]. The arrest of development in certain bone-marrow cells.

an″a·cou′si·a. See *anacusia.*

a·nac″ro·a′si·a (a·nack″ro·ay′zhuh, ·zee·uh, ·shuh, ·see·uh, an″uh·kro·) [*a-;* G. *akroasis,* a hearing]. Inability to understand spoken language.

an″a·crot′ic in″ci·su′ra (in″sigh·sue′ruh). In kymographic tracings, a sharp notch in the upstroke of the central arterial pulse seen in cases of aortic stenosis.

a·nac′ro·tism [G. *ana,* up; *krotos,* rattling noise]. The condition in which one or more notches occur on the ascending limb of the pulse curve. —**ana-crot′ic,** *adj.*

an″a·cu′si·a (an″uh·cue′zhuh, ·zee·uh, ·shuh, ·see·uh, an″uh·kōō′·), **an″a·cu′sis** (an″uh·cue′sis, ·kōō′sis), **an″a·cou′si·a** (an″uh·kōō′zhuh, ·zee·uh, ·shuh, ·see·uh), **an″a·ku′sis** [G. *a-,* not; *akouein,* to hear]. Complete deafness.

an″a·de′ni·a [*a-;* G. *adēn,* gland]. 1. Deficient glandular activity. 2. Absence of glands.

an″a·did′y·mus [G. *ana,* up; *didymos,* twin]. A monster showing inferior duplicity but union above. Syn., *dipygus*. Also called *inferior duplicity*. —**anadidymous,** *adj*.

an″a·dip′si·a [G. *ana*, intensive; *dipsa*, thirst]. Intense thirst. See *polydipsia*.

a·nae′mi·a. See *anemia*.

an′aer·obe (an′air·ohb, an·air′ohb, an·ay′ur·ohb) [G. *a-*, not; *aēr*, air; *bios*, life]. A microorganism that will grow in the absence of molecular oxygen. Also called *anaerobion*. —**anaero′bic,** *adj*.

facultative a. An organism which will grow in the presence or absence of molecular oxygen.

obligatory a. One which grows only when oxygen is rigorously excluded.

an″aer·o·bi′ase (an″air·o·buy′ace, ·aze, an·air″o·, an·ay″ur·o·). A proteolytic enzyme which acts under anaerobic conditions and is present in a number of anaerobes.

an″aer·o·bi·o′sis (an″air·o·buy·o′sis, an·air″o·, an-ay″ur·o·) [*a-; aēr; bios*; G. *ōsis*, condition]. Life sustained in the absence of molecular oxygen. See *anaerobe*. —**anaerobiot′ic,** *adj*.

an″aer·o·gen′ic [*a-; aēr*; G. *genesthai*, from *gignesthai*, to be produced]. Not gas-producing.

an′aer·o·phyte″ (an′air·o·fight″, an·air′o·, an·ay′-ur·o·) [*a-; aēr*; G. *phyton*, plant]. *In botany*, a plant capable of living without a direct supply of oxygen.

an″aes·the′si·a. See *anesthesia*.

an″a·gen′e·sis [G. *anagennēsis*, regeneration]. Reparation or reproduction of tissues, regeneration.

Anagnostakis, Andreas [*Cretan surgeon*, 1826–97]. Remembered for his description of a plastic operation for entropion by resection of a strip of orbicularis muscle through an incision the length of the tarsal plate.

an″a·go′ge (an″uh·go′jee), **an″a·go′gy** [G. *anagōgē*, a bringing up, lifting up]. Spiritual, moral, or idealistic phases of thought.

an″a·gog′ic (an″uh·godj′ick) [*anagōgē*]. 1. Relating to the mystical or anagoge. 2. *In psychoanalysis*, pertaining to the efforts of the subconscious to achieve the moral, ideal, or uplifting; also, pertaining to dream material which expresses idealistic and spiritual ideas, as contrasted with that representing the sexual forces of the unconscious.

an″a·gy′rine (an″uh·jy′reen, ·rin, an·adj′i·reen, ·rin). $C_{15}H_{18}N_2O$. An alkaloid from the seeds of the shrub, *Anagyris foetida*. It decreases the heart rate and the force of the systole in the frog but is said to have little effect on mammalian blood pressure. Large doses cause respiratory paralysis.

anahemin, anahaemin. A proprietary preparation containing the hematopoietic factors of liver.

an″a·kat″a·did′y·mus [G. *ana*, up; *kata*, down; *didymos*, twin]. A conjoined twin monster exhibiting both inferior and superior duplicity. —**anakatadidymous,** *adj*.

an″a·ku′sis. See *anacusia*.

a′nal char′ac·ter. A type of personality in which anal erotic traits dominate beyond the period of childhood.

an″a·lep′sis. Restoration, especially of respiration and wakefulness.

an″a·lep′tic [G. *analēptikos*, restorative]. 1. Restoring consciousness in fainting or coma. 2. Hastening convalescence.

an″a·lep′tic. A restorative drug, used especially for restoration of respiration and wakefulness.

an·al′gen. Ortho-ethoxy-monobenzoyl aminoquinoline; a white, crystalline, insoluble powder used as an anodyne for headaches, neuralgia, and rheumatism.

an″al·ge′si·a (an″al·jee′zee·uh, ·see·uh), **an·al′gi·a** [G. *a-*, not; *algos*, pain]. Insensibility to pain without loss of consciousness.

a. algera. Severe pain in a part with loss of general sensibility.

a. dolorosa. See *a*. algera.

continuous caudal a. See continuous caudal *anesthesia*.

fractional caudal a. See continuous caudal *anesthesia*.

infiltration a. Paralyzing the nerve endings at the site of operation by subcutaneous injection of an anesthetic.

intermittent caudal a. See continuous caudal *anesthesia*.

obstetrical a. That induced to relieve the pain of childbirth; perception of pain is diminished or obliterated without necessarily affecting cerebration or motor nerve activity.

permeation a. See surface *a*.

serial caudal a. See continuous caudal *anesthesia*.

surface a. Topical application on mucous membranes for local analgesia.

an″al·ge′sic (an″al·jee′zick, ·jess′ick, ·jee′sick), **an″al·get′ic, an·al′gic** [*a-; algos*]. 1. Anodyne; relieving pain. 2. Not affected by pain. —**analge′sist,** *n.*; **an′algize,** *v.t.*

analgesin, analgesine. A brand of antipyrine.

an·al′gi·a. See *analgesia*.

an″al·ler′gic [*a-*; G. *allos*, other; *ergon*, work]. Not producing allergy, anaphylaxis, or hypersensitivity; applied to especially refined serums which cause no reactions.

an′a·log, an′a·logue [G. *analogos*, conformable]. 1. Organ or part having the same function as another but differing in structure and origin, as the wing of an insect and the wing of a bird. 2. One of a group of compounds with similar electronic structure, but with different atoms, as an isolog.

a·nal′o·gy [*analogos*]. 1. Resemblance in two or more attributes between two things which differ in other respects. 2. *In biology*, a similarity in function without correspondence in structure and origin. —**analogous,** *adj*.

a·nal′y·sand [G. *analyein*, to unloose]. One who is being psychoanalyzed.

a·nal′y·ses. Plural of *analysis*.

a·nal′y·sis [G., a loosing]. 1. The determination of the nature, properties, or composition of a substance. 2. The resolution of a compound body into its constituent parts. 3. *In psychiatry*, psychoanalysis.

activation a. A method of analysis by which a small amount of an element, otherwise difficult to identify and quantitatively determine, is made radioactive by bombardment with neutrons or other activating particles, and then qualitatively identified by observing the half-life of one or more of its radioisotopes and the characteristics of its radiations. Quantitative analysis is achieved through similar treatment of reference material containing a known amount of the element found to be present.

chromatographic a. Separation of chemical constituents by differential adsorption. The adsorbent is usually packed in a column and the solution percolated through the column.

clinical a. (a) Thorough examination of symptoms, lesions, and history to determine the nature of a disease and its cause. (b) Examination of body fluids and tissues for the diagnosis of diseases.

colorimetric a. Determination of substances by means of the intensity of color of their reaction products.

densimetric a. Analysis for a substance by determining the density of its solution, thus estimating the amount of dissolved matter.

distributive a. Analysis of a subject's symptoms

and complaints according to the concepts of psychobiology, as distinguished from psychoanalysis.

gasometric a. Analysis of a solid or liquid substance by conversion to a gas, or the determination of the constituents of gaseous compounds. Also called *eudiometric a.*

gravimetric a. Quantitative determination, by weight, of the elements of a body.

inorganic a. Determination of the chemical composition of inorganic matter.

microchemical a. (a) Chemical analysis with the aid of a microscope. (b) Chemical analysis using small quantities of materials, but employing the conventional reactions.

nephelometric a. Quantitative determination of a substance by observation of the degree of turbidity produced by it in a suitable dispersion medium.

organic a. Analysis of organic chemical substances.

polariscopic a. Analysis by polariscope.

proximate a. Determination of gross constituents, as alkaloids, glycosides, fat, protein, carbohydrate, etc., in drugs.

qualitative a. Determination of the elements that compose a substance.

quantitative a. Determination of the amount of an element or compound in a substance.

radiometric a. Determination of an element that is not itself radioactive by means of an interaction (e.g. precipitation) with a radioactive element.

spectrophotometric a. Identification and determination of substances through study of the adsorption of energy in the ultraviolet, visible, or infrared spectrum.

spectrum a. The determination of the composition of certain substances from a study of their spectrums.

thermometric a. Analysis by means of observation of the varying temperatures produced by the interaction of substances combined together.

ultimate a. Resolution of a compound into its ultimate elements.

volumetric a. Quantitative determination of a constituent by titration with standardized volumetric solutions.

an′a·lyst [G. *analyein*, to unloose]. 1. One experienced in performing analyses. 2. *In psychiatry,* one who analyzes the psyche, usually one who adheres to the formulations of the psychoanalytic school of Freud. See *psychoanalyst.*

an″a·lyt′ic psy·chol′o·gy. Psychology which analyzes the psyche according to the concepts of Carl Jung; it differs from the psychoanalysis of Freud in that the emphasis in diagnosing and treating a neurosis is not on early complexes but on current maladjustments.

an′a·ly″zer [G. *analysis*, a loosing]. 1. An analyst. 2. In a polariscope, the Nicol prism which exhibits the properties of light after polarization. 3. An apparatus for recording the excursions of tremor movements.

An″a·mir′ta (an″uh·mur′tuh) [Skr. *an*, not; *amṛta*, immortal]. A genus of the Menispermaceae.

A. cocculus. The source of cocculus, yielding picrotoxin.

an″am·ne′sis [G., a calling to mind]. 1. Faculty of memory. 2. Information gained from the patient and others regarding the past history of a case. **—anamnes′tic,** *adj.*

An·am″ni·o′ta [G. *a-*, not; *amnion*, inner membrane around the fetus]. A group of vertebrates having no amnion; it includes the fishes and the amphibia.

an·am″ni·ot′ic [*a-; amnion*]. Without an amnion.

an″a·mor′pho·sis (an″uh·mor′fo·sis, ·mor·fo′sis) [G. *amamorphōsis*, a forming anew]. 1. The tendency toward increasing complication and differentiation of animate systems: contrasted with catamorphosis in inanimate systems. 2. *In optics,* that process by which a distorted image is corrected by means of a curved mirror.

catoptric a. The correction of a distorted optical image by means of a conic or cylindric mirror.

dioptric a. The correction of a distorted optical image by means of a pyramidal glass.

an·an″a·ba′si·a (an·an″uh·bay′zhuh, ·zee·uh, ·shuh, ·see·uh) [G. *a-*, not; *anabasis*, an ascending]. Inability to ascend to heights.

an·an″a·phy·lax′is [*a-;* G. *ana*, backward; *phylaxis*, protection]. A condition neutralizing anaphylaxis; antianaphylaxis.

an·an″as·ta′si·a (·ass·tay′zhuh, ·zee·uh, ·shuh, ·see·uh) [*a-;* G. *anastasis*, a rising up]. Abulic inability to rise from a sitting posture.

a·nan·cas′ti·a [G. *anagkastos*, forced]. The constrained feeling in the obsessive neurosis of psychasthenia.

an·an′dri·a [G. *a-*, not; *anēr*, man]. Lack of virility; impotence.

an·an″gi·o·pla′si·a (an·an″jee·o·play′zhuh, ·zee·uh, ·shuh, ·see·uh) [*a-;* G. *aggeion*, vessel; *plassein*, to form]. Congenital narrowing of the caliber of the blood vessels. *Obs.*

an·an″gi·o·plas′tic [*a-; aggeion; plassein*]. Characterized by defective development of the cardiovascular system.

an″a·pau′sis [G., rest]. Hypnotic inducement of calm sleep by allaying excitement.

an″a·pei·rat′ic (an″uh·pye·rat′ick) [G. *anapeiraesthai*, to try again]. Denoting a condition which results from overuse, as writer's cramp.

an″a·phal″an·ti′a·sis [G., forehead-baldness]. The loss or absence of the eyebrows. *Obs.*

an′a·phase (an′uh·fayz) [G. *ana*, up; *phasis*, phase]. The stage of mitosis between the metaphase and telophase, in which the daughter chromosomes move apart toward the poles of the spindle, to form the diaster. See *mitosis.*

an·a′phi·a, an·aph′i·a [G. *a-*, not; *haphē*, touch]. 1. Defective or absent sense of touch. 2. A state of abnormal sensitiveness to touch. 3. A state in which nothing is learned by palpation. **—anap′tic,** *adj.*

an″a·pho·re′sis [*a-;* G. *diaphorēsis*, perspiration]. 1. Diminished activity of the sweat glands. 2. The migration of electropositive particles, or ions, into tissues under the influence of an electric field. **—anaphoret′ic,** *adj.*

an″a·pho′ri·a [G. *ana*, up; *pherein*, to bear]. A tendency toward upward turning of the eyes and of the visual axes. Syn., *anatropia.*

an·aph″ro·dis′i·a (an·af″ro·diz′ee·uh) [G. *a-*, not; *Aphroditē*, Venus]. Impairment of sexual appetite. **—an·aph″ro·dis′i·ac,** *adj.;* **anaph′rodite,** *n.*

an·aph″ro·dis′i·ac [*a-;* G. *aphrodisiakos*, sexual]. An agent that allays the sexual desire.

an″a·phy·lac′tic [G. *ana*, backward; *phylaktos*, from *phylassein*, to watch, defend]. 1. Relating to the production or state of anaphylaxis. 2. Increasing sensitivity.

an″a·phy·lac′tin [*ana; phylaktos*]. The antibody concerned in anaphylaxis; an allergin. Has been confused with allergen.

an″a·phy·lac′to·gen [*ana; phylaktos;* G. *genesthai*, from *gignesthai*, to be produced]. A substance which is capable of producing a state of anaphylaxis in a subject previously sensitized to it. **—anaphylactogen′ic,** *adj.*

an″a·phy·lac′toid [*ana; phylaktos;* G. *eidos,* form]. Anaphylactoid reaction.

an″a·phyl″a·tox′in, an″a·phyl″o·tox′in [*ana;* G. *phylaxis,* protection; *toxikon,* poison]. A poisonous substance liberated in the tissues of a sensitized animal when antigen and antibody react; claimed by some to be histaminelike.

an″a·phy·lax′is [*ana; phylaxis*]. A state of increased susceptibility, or hypersensitivity, following the parenteral injection of an antigen in an animal. Upon the reintroduction of the antigen after a lapse of time (10 to 12 days) there is manifested a series of characteristic symptoms, including spasm of smooth muscle, capillary dilatation, glandular secretion, altered permeability of the vessels, and varying degrees of shock. The reaction is believed to be due to fixation of a specific antibody in certain tissues, rendering them sensitive to subsequently injected antigen. Also called *active a.*

active a. Hypersensitization produced by the direct introduction of an antigen.

local a. A reaction at the site of injections, dependent upon the union in the tissues of the circulating precipitin and its specific antigen, as edema, induration, and necrosis caused by repeated subcutaneous injections of horse serum into rabbits. Also called *Arthus' phenomenon.*

passive a. Hypersensitivity produced in an animal by parenteral injection of serum from another previously sensitized animal.

reverse passive a. A type in which the antigen is injected first, then followed by the specific antibody, causing shock.

an″a·phyl″o·tox′in. See *anaphylatoxin.*

an″a·pla′si·a (an″uh·play′zhuh, ·zee·uh, ·shuh, ·see·uh) [G. *anaplasis,* from *ana, plassein,* to form]. Reversion of form of a cell or cells toward the embryonal, together with increased capacity for multiplication: term often used by morphologists to indicate reversion of form only, without reference to capacity for multiplication.

an″a·plas·mo′sis (an″uh·plaz·mo′sis) [*ana;* G. *plasma,* anything formed; *-ōsis,* condition]. A term sometimes used to indicate infection with *Anaplasma;* a disease of cattle.

an″a·plas′tic [G. *anaplastikos,* from *anaplasis*]. 1. Relating to or affected with anaplasia. 2. Pertaining to the replacement of a lost or absent part by surgery.

an′a·plas″ty [G. *ana,* again; *plassein,* to form]. An operation for the restoration of lost parts; plastic surgery.

an″a·ple·ro′sis [G., a filling up]. The restoration or repair of a wound or lesion in which there has been a loss of substance. *Obs.*

an″a·poph′y·sis [G. *ana,* back; *apophysis,* offshoot]. An accessory process of a lumbar or thoracic vertebra, corresponding to the inferior tubercle of the transverse process of a typical thoracic vertebra.

an″a·rith′mi·a [G. *a-,* not; *arithmein,* to count]. An inability to count.

an·ar′thri·a [*a-;* G. *arthron,* joint]. Defective articulation in speaking. —**anarthric,** *adj.*

a. centralis. Partial aphasia due to a central lesion.

a. literalis. Stammering.

an″a·sar′ca [G. *ana,* throughout; *sarx,* flesh]. An accumulation of serum in the subcutaneous connective tissue and the serous cavities of the body; generalized edema. —**anasarcous,** *adj.*

a. hystericum. A transient swelling in a hysterical individual.

an″a·schist′ic (an″uh·skis′tick, ·shis′tick) [G. *ana,* up; *schizein,* to cleave]. *In biology,* applied to bivalents or tetrads that split longitudinally in miosis. See *diaschistic.*

an″a·stal′sis [G., from *ana; stalsis,* constriction]. 1. Antiperistalsis. 2. Styptic action.

a·nas′ta·sis [G., a rising up]. Recovery; convalescence. —**anastat′ic,** *adj.*

an″as·tig·mat′ic, an·as″tig·mat′ic [G. *a-,* not; *a-; stigma,* point]. Free from astigmatism; corrected for astigmatism, said especially of photographic objectives which are also corrected for spherical and chromatic aberration.

a·nas″to·mo′sis (pl. *anastomoses*) [G., an opening]. 1. The intercommunication of blood vessels by the natural anatomic arrangement which, as a result of an interruption of the chief arterial blood supply, provides alternate pathways for blood supply to a peripheral part. Occasionally, anastomosis of blood vessels is secured by a direct surgical operation upon the vessels themselves. 2. The establishment by surgical means of a communication between two hollow organs or two parts of the same organ, as between the jejunum and stomach, the hepatic duct and small intestine, the ureter and colon. 3. The joining of a nerve to another nerve or to a portion of the same nerve. —**anastomot′ic,** *adj.;* **anas′tomose,** *v.i., v.t.*

arteriovenous a. A modified vessel which connects an artery with a vein without the intervention of capillaries. Such structures are particularly numerous in the palm, the sole, and the skin of terminal phalanges.

cruciate a. An arterial anastomosis in the upper thigh, formed by the inferior gluteal, medial circumflex femoral, lateral circumflex femoral, and first perforating arteries. It is important in the formation of collateral circulation after ligation of the femoral artery.

en Y a. See *Roux, César.*

intersubcardinal a. A transverse anastomosis between the paired subcardinal veins of the early embryo, ventral to the aorta.

portacaval a. One joining the portal vein to the inferior vena cava; also known as *Eck's fistula.*

postcostal a. A longitudinal anastomosis between successive intersegmental arteries, the first through the seventh cervical, which forms the vertebral artery.

posttransverse a. A longitudinal anastomosis between intersegmental arteries, dorsal to the transverse process forming the deep cervical artery.

precostal a. A longitudinal anastomosis between cervical and thoracic intersegmental arteries, which forms the thyrocervical trunk and the superior intercostal artery.

a·nas″to·mot′i·ca [*anastomōsis*]. A communicating artery or vein.

an·as′tral [G. *a-,* not; *astēr,* star]. Without an aster; pertaining to an achromatic figure without asters.

anat. Anatomic, anatomical, anatomy.

a·nat′a·bine (a·nat′uh·bean, ·bin). An alkaloid found in tobacco.

a·nat′o·mist [G. *anatomē,* dissection]. One who specializes or is skilled in anatomy.

a·nat′o·mist's snuff′box″. A hollow, triangular space on the dorsum of the hand at the base of the metacarpal of the thumb, when it is extended. It is formed on the sides by the tendons of the long and short extensor pollicis muscles. Syn., *tabatière anatomique.*

a·nat′o·my [*anatomē*]. 1. Science or branch of morphology which treats of the structure of animals and the relation of their parts. 2. Dissection of the various parts of a plant or animal. —**anatom′ic, anatom′ical,** *adj.*

applied a. Anatomy as a factor in diagnosis and treatment.

artistic a. That branch of anatomy which treats of the external form of man and animals, their osseous and muscular systems, and their relation to painting and sculpture.

clastic a. Study of anatomy by means of models in which the different layers can be removed to show the position and relations of the structures underneath.

comparative a. Investigation and comparison of the anatomy of different orders of animals or of plants, one with another.

descriptive a. Study of the separate and individual portions of the body.

general a. That which treats of the structure and physiologic properties of the tissues and their arrangement into systems without regard to the disposition of the organs of which they form a part.

gross a. That which deals with the naked-eye appearance of tissues.

homologic a. Study of the correlations of the several parts of the body.

microscopic a. Histology. Also called *minute a.*

pathologic a. Study of the changes in structure caused by disease. Also called *morbid a.*

physiologic a. Anatomic study of tissues in respect to their functions.

regional a. Study of limited parts or regions of the body.

surface a. Study of superficial landmarks for the location of internal structures.

surgical a. Application of anatomy to surgery.

topographic a. Anatomy of a part in its relation to other parts.

an″a·tox′in [G. *ana*, backward; *toxikon*, poison]. A toxoid.

an″a·tro′pi·a [G. *ana*, up; *tropē*, a turning]. A tendency of the eyes to turn upward when at rest; anaphoria.

an·au′di·a. Aphonia.

an″a·vac′cine [*ana; L. vaccinus*, of cows]. A detoxified vaccine.

an″a·ven′in [G. *ana*, throughout; L. *venenum*, poison]. Venoms which have been altered by physical or chemical agents that eliminate their toxic property but make little or no change in their antigenic qualities.

anayodin. Trade-mark for a brand of chiniofon.

an·az″o·tu′ri·a [G. *a-*, not; *a-; zōē*, life; *ouron*, urine]. An absence or deficiency of nitrogenous elements in the urine, affecting chiefly urea.

AnCC Anodal closure contraction; also ACC.

an′chor·age [L. *ancora*, anchor, from G. *agkyra*]. 1. The fixation of a floating or displaced viscus, whether by a natural process or by surgical means. 2. *In dentistry*, the means of retaining a dental filling, particularly its initial portion; also, the means by which a bridge or artificial crown is secured. 3. *In orthodontics*, a tooth or teeth used for resistance in applying a regulating force.

an′chy·lo- (ang′ki·lo-), **an′cy·lo-** (an′ki·lo-). For words beginning *anchylo-* or *ancylo-* not found here, see words beginning *ankylo-*.

an′chy·lops (ang′ki·lops) [G. *agkylos*, curved; *ōps*, eye]. Abscess at the inner angle of the eye.

An·cis′tro·don. See *Agkistrodon.*

an″co·ne′us, an·co′ne·us [G. *agkōn*, elbow]. A small triangular muscle at the back of the elbow joint. See Table of Muscles in the Appendix.

a. internus. The epitrochleo-olecranonis muscle.

an′co·noid [*agkōn;* G. *eidos*, form]. Resembling the elbow. *Obs.*

An″cy·los′to·ma [G. *agkylos*, curved; *stoma*, mouth]. A genus of nematodes; the hookworms.

A. braziliense. A species which infests cats and dogs; instances of human infestation, producing larva migrans or creeping eruption, have been reported in South America, Africa, and the Orient.

A. caninum. A common species of parasite of dogs and cats found particularly in the Northern Hemisphere; human infestation is very rare.

A. duodenale. A species of hookworm which infests man, the principal and optimum host. Occasionally hogs, dogs, felines, and gorillas are infested.

An″cy·los″to·mat′i·dae (an″ki·los″to·mat′i·dee) [*agkylos; stoma*]. A family of hookworms of the superfamily Strongyloidea, characterized by oral cutting organs. The hookworms of man of the genera *Ancylostoma* and *Necator* belong to this family.

an″cy·los″to·mi′a·sis [*agkylos; stoma;* NL. *-iasis*, condition]. Infestation of the human intestine with *Ancylostoma duodenale* and the resulting morbid state.

Andernach. See *Guenther von Andernach.*

Anders' disease. See *adiposis* tuberosa simplex.

Anderson, John F. [*American physician*, 1871–]. Reported the existence of spotted fever in the Rocky Mountains (1903). Made valuable contributions, with Rosenau, concerning sudden death following injection of horse serum (1906). Made notable experimental researches, with Goldberger, on production of measles in monkeys (1911).

Anderson, Roger [*American orthopedic surgeon*, 1891–]. His name is associated with the treatment of fracture of the femur at various levels by means of a well-leg countertraction apparatus, both legs being encased in plaster. It permits ambulatory treatment. Called *Anderson splint* or *method.*

Anderson-Nightingale dilution test. See under *test.*

Andral, Gabriel [*French physician*, 1797–1876]. Editor of Laennec's works and a vigorous opponent of bloodletting. Said to have originated the terms anemia and hyperemia.

an″dra·nat′o·my [G. *anēr*, man; *anatomē*, dissection]. Human anatomy; the anatomy or dissection of a male. *Obs.*

André, Nicolas (Andry) [*French physician*, 1658–1742]. Author of what is said to be the first book devoted to orthopedics, a term he coined. Made many important observations and gave sound advice on the value of correct posture for prevention of scoliosis (1741).

André Thomas' sign. See under *sign.*

an″drei·o·blas·to′ma. See *androblastoma.*

an″drei·o′ma (an″drye·o′muh) [G. *andreios*, from *anēr; -ōma*, tumor]. Androblastoma.

Andrews, Edward Wyllys [*American surgeon*, 1856–1927]. Distinguished for his contributions to the surgery of inguinal hernia. His modification of Bassini's method is known as the *Wyllys Andrews method.*

an″dri·at′rics, an·dri′a·try [G. *andreios*, from *anēr; iatrikos*, skilled in the medical art]. A branch of medicine dealing with those disorders peculiar to men, especially those of the male genitalia.

an′dro-, andr- [G. *anēr*, *andros*, man]. A combining form signifying *man* or *male, masculine, relating to the male sex.*

an″dro·blas·to′ma. A rare tumor, resembling fetal testis, which is the testicular homolog of ovarian arrhenoblastoma. It may be associated with feminizing characteristics in the male. Also called *testicular adenoma, andreioblastoma, andreioma.*

an″dro·ga·lac″to·ze′mi·a [*anēr;* G. *gala,* milk; *zēmia,* loss]. The oozing of milk from the male mamma.

an″dro·gam′one. A gamone present in a spermatozoon.

an′dro·gen [*anēr;* G. *genesthai,* from *gignesthai,* to be produced]. A hormone which controls the physiologic status of the secondary sex characteristics of males. —**androgen′ic, androg′enous,** *adj.*

an″dro·gen′e·sis [*anēr;* G. *genesis,* production]. Activation of the egg by the sperm followed by development without the participation of the egg nucleus (Wilson).

an·drog′e·nous [*anēr;* G. *genesthai,* from *gignesthai,* to be produced]. Giving birth to males.

an′dro·gyne (an′dro·jyne, ·jin), **an·drog′y·nus** (an·drodj′i·nus), **an·drog′y·na** (an·drodj′i·nuh) [*anēr;* G. *gynē,* woman]. A pseudohermaphrodite. —**androg′ynous,** *adj.*

an·drog′y·nism (an·drodj′i·niz·um) [*anēr; gynē*]. Hermaphroditism.

an·drog′y·ny (an·drodj′i·nee), **an″dro·gy·ne′i·ty** [*anēr; gynē*]. Hermaphroditism. —**androg′ynoid,** *adj., n.*

an′droid [*anēr;* G. *eidos,* form]. Resembling the male.

an″dro·ma′ni·a. Nymphomania.

an·drom″e·do·tox′in [G. *Andromeda; toxikon,* poison]. A toxic principle found in *Andromeda* (*Pieris*) *japonica* and other ericaceous plants. It has potent hypotensive action, and causes convulsions, labored respiration, and cardiac paralysis.

an″dro·mor′phous [G. *anēr,* man; *morphē,* form]. Having the form of a man.

an″droph′i·lous [*anēr, andros,* man; G. *philein,* to love]. Anthropophilic.

an″dro·pho′bi·a [*anēr;* G. *phobos,* fear]. Morbid fear or dislike of men or of the male sex.

an′dros·tane. $C_{19}H_{32}$. A saturated, solid, steroid hydrocarbon, the parent substance of androgenic hormones. Also called *etioallocholane.*

an″dro·stene′di·ol (an″dro·steen′dye·ole, ·dee·ole, ·dye·ol, ·dee·ol, ·dye·awl, ·dee·awl). $C_{19}H_{28}(OH)_2$. Any one of three isomeric derivatives of androstane characterized by the presence of two alcohol groups and an unsaturated linkage (C=C).

an″dro·stene′di·one (an″dro·steen′dye·ohn, ·dee·ohn). $C_{19}H_{26}O_2$. Any one of three isomeric derivatives of androstane characterized by the presence of two ketone groups and an unsaturated linkage (C=C).

an·dros′ter·one. $C_{19}H_{30}O_2$; 3(α)-hydroxy-17-ketoandrostane, an androgenic steroid found in the urine of men and women. See also *isoandrosterone.*

androstine. A proprietary testicular extract available in tablets and ampuls.

andrusol. A trade-mark for *testosterone propionate.*

Andry. See *André.*

a·ne′de·ous [G. *a-,* not; *aidoia,* genitals]. Lacking external genital organs.

Anel, Dominique [*French surgeon,* ca. 1679–ca. 1730]. Remembered for his ligation of traumatic aneurysm (1710) and for his original treatment of stenosis of the lacrimal duct by dilatation with a probe of his own invention (1712).

an″e·lec·trot′o·nus [G. *ana,* up; *ēlektron,* amber; *tonos,* tone]. Decreased irritability present in a nerve in the neighborhood of the anode during the passage of an electric current. —**anelectroton′ic,** *adj.*

a·ne′mi·a [G. *a-,* not; *haima,* blood]. A significant reduction below normal in the number of erythrocytes per cubic millimeter, the hemoglobin concentration, and the volume of packed red cells per 100 cc. of blood, resulting in a decrease in the oxygen-carrying capacity of a given volume of blood. Anemia may be due to an imbalance between the productive and the destructive blood processes, or to chronic or acute blood loss. Symptoms, when present, vary greatly; they may be general, such as weakness, pallor, and poor appetite, or relate to the underlying disease process. Microscopically, anemias may be classified according to cell size (macrocytic, microcytic, normocytic), shape (e.g., sickle cell, anisocytosis, poikilocytosis), and color (normochromic, "hyperchromic," and hypochromic). Anemia is to be distinguished from *oligemia* (reduction in total amount of blood), *oligocythemia* (deficiency in total quantity of erythrocytes), and *oligochromemia* (reduction in total quantity of hemoglobin). —**anemic,** *adj.*

achlorhydric a. A chronic hypochromic microcytic anemia, probably due to poor iron absorption, in which hydrochloric acid is frequently not secreted even after injection of histamine. The intrinsic factor is present. Also called *achylanemia, anemia achylica, Faber's syndrome.*

achrestic a. A rare macrocytic anemia due to an inability of the body to utilize the antianemia factor.

acquired hemolytic a. Any hemolytic normocytic anemia due to the action of an external agent or disease process upon normally constructed erythrocytes.

Addison's a. Pernicious *a.*

American nutritional megaloblastic a. A macrocytic anemia due to defective diet.

a. pseudoleukemia infantum. See infantile pseudoleukemic *a.*

aplastic a. That resulting from defects of the bone marrow, as hypoplasia, aplasia, and degenerative changes. It is marked by a deficiency of red cells, hemoglobin and granular cells, and a predominance of lymphocytes. Also called *aleukia hemorrhagica, atrophic a.*

aregenerative a., aregeneratory a. See primary refractory *a.*

asiderotic a. See hypochromic microcytic *a.*

Baghdad spring a. A form of acute hemolytic anemia thought to be caused by acquired sensitivity to inhaled pollens of certain plants native to the Middle East.

Belgian Congo a. Kasai.

Biermer's a. See Anton *Biermer,* pernicious *a.*

Bothriocephalus a. Tapeworm *a.*

chlorotic a. See *chlorosis.*

cryptogenic a. See primary refractory *a.*

deficiency a. See hypochromic microcytic *a.*

drepanocytic a. See sickle-cell *a.*

essential a. See pernicious *a.,* idiopathic *a.*

familial erythroblastic a. Thalassemia.

familial hemolytic a. See hereditary *spherocytosis.*

familial microcytic a. Thalassemia.

globe-cell a. See *spherocytosis.*

goat's-milk a. A macrocytic nutritional anemia observed in infants fed goat's milk exclusively, and probably due to folic acid deficiency.

hemolytic a. Any anemia characterized by a short life span of the erythrocytes. It may be due to extracorpuscular causes, as infectious agents, chemical agents and drugs, thermal burns, vegetable or animal poisons, immune body reactions, acquired hemolytic anemias without presence of antibodies or secondary to some malignancy or lupus erythematosus; or it may be due to intracorpuscular defects, as in sickle-cell anemia, hereditary spherocytosis, thalassemia, and paroxysmal hemoglobinuria.

hemolytic a. of pregnancy. See hyperchromic *a.* of pregnancy.
hemorrhagic a. That following gross hemorrhage.
Herrick's a. See sickle-cell *a.*
hyperchromic a. That in which the hemoglobin deficiency is comparatively less than that of the red cells (where the color index is high).
hyperchromic a. of pregnancy. A condition characterized by pallor, asthenia, edema, and later by stomatitis, dyspepsia, diarrhea, and vomiting; erythrocyte count and hemoglobin are low; the spleen may be enlarged. It is progressive while the pregnancy lasts, and is often associated with premature labor, after which recovery is often spontaneous. Syn., *hemolytic a. of pregnancy, megalocytic a. of pregnancy, pernicious a. of pregnancy.*
hypochromic microcytic a. An anemia in which the hemoglobin and to a lesser degree the volume of packed red cells are comparatively more reduced than the erythrocyte count, due to the erythrocytes being smaller than normal and greatly deficient in hemoglobin (MCH, MCV, and especially MCHC are reduced.) It is readily remedied by iron therapy and may be due to chronic blood loss, disorders of the alimentary tract, and extremely faulty diet, particularly in infants and females, or to thalassemia. Also called *asideratic a., nutritional hypochromic a., chronic* or *idiopathic hypochromic a., hypochromic a. of prematurity, infancy, childhood, or pregnancy.* Syn. *iron-deficiency a.*
hypoplastic a. See primary refractory *a.*
idiopathic a. That in which the lesion is in the blood or blood-forming organs. Syn., *primary a., essential a.*
infantile pseudoleukemic a. A symptom complex characterized by anemia, abnormal erythrocytes, leukocytosis, lymphocytosis, and enlargement of spleen, liver, and lymph nodes, seen in infants and young children. It was described by Rudolf von Jaksch (1889) and is now known to be associated with many different conditions, such as malnutrition, gastrointestinal disturbances, syphilis, tuberculosis, and other infections.
infectious a. A refractory anemia secondary to an infection.
infectious a. of horses. A virus disease of horses which may be acute or chronic, characterized by fever, progressive anemia, edema, and emaciation. The acute phase lasts from four days to three weeks, the chronic for years. The disease is rarely transmitted to man, but if this occurs it causes fever, anemia, diarrhea, and nephritic pain. Transmission may be by parenteral injection, by the bite of the fly, *Stomoxys calcitrans,* or by contact of the virus with abraded skin or mucous membranes. Syn., *equine malaria, swamp fever of horses.*
iron-deficiency a. Hypochromic microcytic *a.*
lead a. Anemia resulting from lead poisoning. The basic cause is thought to be due to inhibition of hemoglobin synthesis through failure of iron to enter the porphyrin ring. There is also increased rate of erythrocyte destruction.
Lederer's acute a. An autoacquired acute hemolytic anemia of unknown causation, sometimes with hemoglobinuria and variable osmotic fragility. Most cases seem to occur in childhood. Therapy is blood transfusion.
leukoerythroblastic a. See myelophthisic *a.*
local a. Deficient blood supply to a particular organ or part. See *ischemia.*
lymphatic a. Hodgkin's disease.
macrocytic a. Any anemia characterized by the presence in the blood of abnormally large erythrocytes (MCV greater than 96 $\mu\mu^3$). This may occur in megaloblastic anemia, in anemias in which production of erythrocytes is increased without deficiency of iron, and in hypothyroidism. See also *megaloblastic a.*
Mediterranean a. Thalassemia.
megaloblastic a. Any anemia characterized by the presence of megaloblasts in the bone marrow and due to a dietary deficiency or abnormal utilization of one or more hematopoietic factors (vitamin B_{12} or folic acid and related substances). This includes pernicious anemia, sprue syndrome, nutritional macrocytic anemias, the macrocytic anemias of pregnancy and the puerperium, of infancy, of primary gastrointestinal disorders, and the anemia associated with the fish-tapeworm infestation.
megalocytic a. of pregnancy. A megaloblastic anemia of pregnancy of unknown cause.
metastatic a. See myelophthisic *a.*
microcytic a. That in which the erythrocytes are smaller than normal. See hypochromic microcytic *a.*
myelopathic a. See myelophthisic *a.*
myelophthisic a. An anemia associated with space-occupying disorders of the bone marrow, as in metastatic carcinoma, leukemia, multiple myeloma, myelo- or osteosclerosis, Hodgkin's disease, and primary xanthomatoses. Immature precursor cells of both the erythrocytic and the granulocytic series may appear in the blood, Syn., *leukoerythroblastosis.* Also called *leukoerythroblastic a., metastatic a., myelopathic a., myelosclerotic a., osteosclerotic a.*
myelosclerotic a. See myelophthisic *a.*
normochromic a. (a) A type in which the hemoglobin content of the red blood cell is normal. (b) One with a normal color index and a normal mean corpuscular hemoglobin.
normocytic a. That in which the erythrocytes are of normal size.
nutritional a. See hypochromic microcytic *a.*
osteosclerotic a. See myelophthisic *a.*
oval-cell a. See *elliptocytosis.*
pernicious a. A macrocytic anemia characterized by increased blood destruction, achylia gastrica, nervous and digestive disorders, and frequently glossitis. It is thought to be caused by a permanent gastric defect associated with atrophy and failure of secretion of an intrinsic factor, and resultant failure of absorption of vitamin B_{12} Also called *Addison's a., Biermer's disease, primary a.*
pernicious a. of pregnancy. A megaloblastic anemia of pregnancy of unknown cause.
physiologic a. That affecting most infants at about the second month and disappearing usually before the end of the first year.
postoperative cerebral a. Cerebral dysfunction after the ligation of the common carotid artery, often resulting in hemiplegia.
primary a. Pernicious *a.*
primary refractory a. Any persistent and often severe anemia, refractory to any treatment other than transfusion of blood. The bone marrow may be hypoplastic, normally cellular, or even hyperplastic. It is not associated with any infection, chronic systemic disease, malignancy, or malnutrition. Also called *aregeneratory a., cryptogenic a., hypoplastic a., aleukia hemorrhagica, progressive hypocythemia.*
radiation a. A plastic or hypoplastic anemia following excessive exposure to ionizing radiation: also called *roentgen-ray a.*
refractory megaloblastic a. A macrocytic anemia of unknown cause and unresponsive

to any therapy (e.g. iron, liver, vitamin B_{12}, folic acid, ascorbic acid, citrovorum factor) other than blood transfusion.

roentgen-ray a. See radiation *a.*

secondary a. That following or resulting from a pathologic condition, as malignancy, poisoning, trauma, or hemorrhagic disease.

secondary refractory a. Anemia alleviated only by transfusion and associated with known infections, chronic kidney disease or malignancy.

sickle-cell a. Hereditary, familial, chronic hemolytic anemia, peculiar to Negroes and sometimes seen in other dark-skinned peoples, but rarely in whites, characterized by the sickling of erythrocytes when hemoglobin is deoxygenated. It is due to a specific gene for sickle-cell hemoglobin (S), and is found in persons homozygous for the gene; sickling without anemia (trait) occurs in those who are heterozygous. Also called *Herrick's a.*, *drepanocytosis*, *meniscocytosis*, *sicklanemia.* Syn. *sicklemia.*

spherocytic a. See *spherocytosis.*

splenic a. See chronic congestive *splenomegaly.*

tapeworm a. A clinical syndrome which resembles, or may be coincidental with, pernicious anemia, observed in persons harboring the fish tapeworm. *Diphyllobothrium latum.* The role of the parasite with respect to the anemia is unknown; free hydrochloric acid may be present. Also called *Bothriocephalus a.*

target-cell a. Thalassemia.

toxic a. Any hemolytic anemia due to toxins and poisons.

tropical macrocytic a. Macrocytic anemia, observed primarily among natives of tropical and subtropical regions, due to dietary deficiency, and relieved by yeast, autolyzed yeast, liver, or folic acid. Clinically it resembles pernicious anemia, but achlorhydria and nervous disorders are not characteristic features.

tunnel a. Ancylostomiasis.

von Jaksch's a. Infantile pseudoleukemic *a.*

an″e·mom′e·ter [G. *anemos*, wind; *metron*, a measure]. An instrument for measuring the velocity of the wind.

A·nem′o·ne (a·nem′o·nee) [G., mountain windflower]. A genus of the Ranunculaceae, most of the species of which have active medicinal and poisonous qualities.

a·nem′o·nin. $C_{10}H_8O_4$. Yellowish white crystals, insoluble in water, soluble in hot alcohol, from *Anemone pulsatilla* and some other members of the Ranunculaceae; has been used as antispasmodic, sedative, and anodyne in asthma and pulmonary affections. Syn., *pulsatilla camphor.*

a·ne″mo·pho′bi·a (a·nee″mo·fo′bee·uh, an″i·mo·) [G. *anemos*, wind; *phobos*, fear]. Morbid dread of drafts or of winds.

an·en″ce·pha′li·a, an″en·ceph′a·ly [G. *a-*, not; *egkephalos*, brain]. Absence of cerebrum and cerebellum with absence of the flat bones of the skull. **—anenceph′alous, anencephal′ic,** *adj.*

an″en·ceph′a·lus [*a-; egkephalos*]. A monster showing partial or complete anencephalia.

an·en′ter·ous [*a-;* G. *enteron*, intestine]. *In biology*, having no intestine, as a tapeworm.

an·ep′i·a, an·e′pi·a [G. *anepēs*, speechless]. Inability to speak.

an·ep″i·plo′ic [G. *a-*, not; *epiploon*, omentum]. Having no epiploon or omentum.

an″er·ga′si·a (an″ur·gay′zhuh, ·zee·uh, ·shuh, ·see·uh) [G., unemployment, idleness]. *In psychiatry*, the term coined by Adolf Meyer for a psychosis caused by organic lesions of the nervous system. See organic brain *syndrome.*

an′er·gy [*a-;* G. *ergon*, work]. 1. Lack of energy or activity. 2. Absence of reaction to a specific antigen or allergen. The capacity to resist the effects of potentially harmful agents. **—aner′gic,** *adj.*

an′er·oid [*a-;* G. *nēros*, water; *eidos*, form]. Working without a fluid, as an aneroid barometer.

anertan. Trade-mark for testosterone propionate.

an″e·ryth″ro·blep′si·a. See *anerythropsia.*

an″e·ryth′ro·cyte [*a-;* G. *erythros*, red; *kytos*, cell]. An erythrocyte without hemoglobin.

an″e·ryth″ro·pla′si·a (an″i·rith″ro·play′zhuh, ·zee·uh, ·shuh, ·see·uh, an·err″ith·ro·) [*a-; erythros;* G. *plassein*, to form]. Inadequate formation of erythrocytes.

an″e·ryth·rop′si·a [*a-; erythros;* G. *opsis*, sight]. Impaired color perception of red; red blindness.

an·es″the·ki·ne′sis (an·ess″thi·ki·nee′sis, ·kigh-nee′·), **an·es″the·ki·ne′si·a** (·ki·nee′shuh, ·see·uh, ·zhuh, ·zee·uh, ·kigh·nee′·) [*a-;* G. *aisthēsis*, feeling; *kinēsis*, movement]. Sensory and motor paralysis, combined.

an″es·the′si·a, an″aes·the′si·a (an″ess·thee′-zhuh, ·zee·uh) [G. *anaisthēsia*, lack of sensation]. Loss of sensation.

a. dolorosa. Severe pain experienced after complete motor and sensory paralysis; observed in certain diseases of the spinal cord.

angiospastic a. Loss of sensibility due to spasm of the blood vessels.

balanced a. That produced by safe doses of two or more agents or methods of anesthesia.

basal a. An incomplete anesthesia; supplementary anesthetics are usually required. Thus, preliminary narcosis may be induced with an injected drug, requiring but a small amount of inhalation anesthetic to produce surgical anesthesia. Among basal anesthetics are the barbiturates, amytal, sodium amytal, avertin.

block a. Anesthesia produced by injecting an anesthetic solution into the nerve trunks supplying the operative field (regional block), or infiltrating close to the nerves (infiltration block), or by a wall of anesthetic solution injected about the field (field block). In all these methods the nerve conduction is *blocked*, and painful impulses fail to reach the brain.

bulbar a. That due to a lesion in the medulla.

carbon-dioxide absorption a. See closed *a.*

caudal a. That induced by injection of the anesthetic into the sacral canal: also called *extradural sacral a.*

central a. That due to disease of the central nervous system.

closed a. Inhalation anesthesia with complete rebreathing of the anesthetic gases. Soda-lime generally is used to absorb the excess CO_2.

closed circuit a. That produced by an anesthetizing apparatus in which explosive agents used in anesthesia are prevented from coming in contact with sparks or flame.

combined a. (a) Anesthesia produced by a combination of anesthetics—as chloroform, ether, and nitrous oxide—or of methods. (b) That produced by anesthetics plus somnifacient drugs.

conduction a. See block *a.*

continuous caudal a. The caudal needle or plastic catheter is inserted through the caudal hiatus into the sacrum for serial intermittent injections of the anesthetic agent, for producing a continuous anesthesia, also called *fractional spinal a.*

continuous sacral a. A continuous caudal needle is inserted into the second posterior sacral foramen and attached to apparatus for periodical injections.

continuous spinal a. The spinal needle is left

in place so that the anesthetic drug can be administered periodically as needed.

crossed a. Anesthesia on one side of the body due to a central lesion on the other side.

cryanesthesia. See refrigeration *a.*

dental a. Anesthesia of the teeth for dental operations.

dissociated a. Loss of pain and temperature sensations, the tactile sense being still present.

electric a. Transient anesthesia caused by the passage of an electric current through a part.

endotracheal a. General anesthesia in which the anesthetic is administered by means of a tube which conducts the vapor directly into the trachea.

epidural a. See peridural *a.*

extradural a. See peridural *a.*

fractional caudal a. See continuous caudal *a.*

fractional spinal a. See continuous spinal *a.*

gauntlet a. Glove *a.*

general a. Loss of sensation with loss of consciousness. See stages of general *a.*

girdle a. A zone of anesthesia encircling the body.

glove a. A loss of sensation in an area corresponding to that covered by a glove; usually a hysterical phenomenon.

hypospray a. That produced by hypospray or jet-injector.

hysterical a. A loss of pain sense in areas of the skin; dictated by suggestion and usually taking on geometric configuration or conforming to zones covered by various articles of apparel. See glove *a.*

ice a. Refrigeration anesthesia.

infiltration a. That induced by the injection of the anesthetic solution directly into the tissues that are to be anesthetized.

inhalation a. That produced by the inhalation of anesthetic gases or vapors.

insufflation a. That produced by the delivery of anesthetic gases under pressure into the respiratory system.

intermittent caudal a. See continuous caudal *a.*

intravenous a. The injection of an anesthetic into a vein, as pentothal sodium.

local a. Anesthesia limited to a local area. See regional *a.*

mixed a. That produced by two or more anesthetics.

morphine-scopolamine a. See *twilight sleep.*

muscular a. Loss of the muscular sense.

nerve a. Block anesthesia.

olfactory a. Anosmia.

open a. Inhalation anesthesia with a minimum amount of rebreathing.

optic a. Temporary amaurosis.

parasacral a. Anesthetization of the sacral nerves near the anterior sacral foramen by injection through the pelvic tissue inferiorly. Syn., *presacral block.*

partial a. Anesthesia in which some degree of sensibility is still present.

peridural a. A form of regional anesthesia resulting from the deposition of a local anesthetic solution, such as procaine, beneath the ligamentum flavum and into the peridural space. Syn., *epidural a., extradural a.*

peripheral a. Loss of sensation due to changes in the peripheral nerves.

pharyngeal a. Anesthesia of the pharynx occasionally complicating nervous disorders; most common in hysterical patients.

planes of a. Subdivisions of the stages of surgical anesthesia, based on Guedel's classification (1937) of the clinical signs of the stages of general anesthesia. The *first plane* is marked by loss of the eyelid reflex; the *second plane* by cessation of eyeball movement; the *third plane* by beginning of intercostal paralysis; and the *fourth plane* by complete intercostal paralysis and purely diaphragmatic respiration.

pressure a. The topical application of an anesthetic using pressure to force it into the tissue.

primary a. The transient anesthesia resulting from a small amount of anesthetic.

pudendal a. Local anesthesia for obstetrical delivery induced by blocking the pudendal nerves near the spinous process of the ischium.

rectal a. That induced by placing the anesthetic agent, such as avertin, paraldehyde, or barbiturate, in the rectum with a catheter.

refrigeration a. A method of rendering a lower limb insensitive by the use of cracked ice applied to the member so as to surround it completely. After two and a half hours of this application, amputation may be performed without medication or anesthesia.

regional a. That limited to a part of the body by blocking nerve conduction from the area. See block *a.*

segmental a. Loss of sensation of an area supplied by one or a limited group of spinal nerves.

semiopen a. Inhalation anesthesia with partial rebreathing.

serial caudal a. See continuous caudal *a.*

sexual a. Anaphrodisia.

spinal a. (a) That due to a lesion of the spinal cord. (b) That produced by the injection of an anesthetic into the spinal subarachnoid space.

stages of general a. Divisions of the sequence of physiologic responses of the patient to a circulating general anesthetic, based on Guedel's classification (1937) of clinical signs which are the expression of progressive depression of the central nervous system. The stages of anesthesia are: I. *Analgesia* or *altered consciousness* (higher cortical centers): from the beginning of the administration of the anesthetic to the loss of consciousness, in which there is progressive loss of sensation. II. *Delirium* or *excitement* (basal ganglia and cerebellum): from the loss of consciousness to the onset of muscular relaxation, in which the patient tends to exhibit hyperactivity. III. *Surgical anesthesia* (spinal cord, motor and sensory); in this stage, which is divided into four *planes*, there is sufficient muscular paralysis to permit surgical manipulation. IV. *Medullary paralysis* (brain stem): usually paralysis of the respiratory center followed by paralysis of the cardiac center.

subarachnoid a. That state of conduction nerve block produced by the deposition of a local anesthetic agent in suitable mixture into the cerebrospinal fluid of the vertebral canal. The anesthetic acts upon contact with and depolarization of the sensory motor and vasomotor axones. Syn., *spinal and intrathecal anesthesia.*

surface a. See topical *a.*

surgical a. Stage III of general anesthesia where muscles are sufficiently relaxed. See stages of general *a.*

synergistic a. That combining several anesthetics used simultaneously.

tactile a. Loss of sense of touch.

terminal a. That state of insensitivity produced by the deposition of the local anesthetic agent about the terminal arborizations of the afferent axone. These are designated as anociceptors. This anesthetic works best through very thin mucous membrane surfaces, such as conjunctiva, urethra, urinary bladder, larynx, peritoneum, pleura. Syn., *topical anesthesia.*

thalamic hyperesthetic a. See thalamic *syndrome.*

thermic a. Loss of temperature sense.

topical a. Application of an anesthetic to one of the body surfaces, as with a swab.

traumatic a. Loss of sensation due to injury of a nerve.

unilateral a. Hemianesthesia.

an·es″the·sim′e·ter, an″es·the″si·om′e·ter (an″ess·thee″zee·om′i·tur) [*anaisthēsia;* G. *metron,* a measure]. 1. An instrument that measures the amount of an anesthetic administered in a given time. 2. An instrument that determines the degree of insensibility of a part. Also called *anesthetometer, esthesiometer.*

anesthesin. Brand of ethyl aminobenzoate; used as local anesthetic. See *benzocaine.*

an″es·the″si·ol′o·gy (an″ess·thee″zee·ol′o·jee) [*anaisthēsia;* G. *logos,* word]. The art and science of administering local and general anesthetics to produce the various types of anesthesia. —**anesthesiologist,** *n.*

an″es·the″si·om′e·ter. See *anesthesimeter.*

an″es·thet′ic, an″aes·thet′ic [*anaisthēsia*]. 1. Causing anesthesia. 2. Insensible to touch, pain, or other stimulation.

an″es·thet′ic, an″aes·thet′ic. A drug which produces local or general loss of sensibility.

general a. An agent which produces general anesthesia either by injection or by inhalation.

local a. A drug which, topically applied or injected into the tissues, causes local insensibility to pain.

an·es′the·tize [*anaisthēsia*]. Subject or place under the influence of an anesthetic; induce anesthesia; render anesthetic. —**anesthetist, anesthetiza′tion, anesthetizer,** *n.*

an·es′trum, an·oes′trum, an·es′trus, an·oes′trus [G. *a-,* not; *oistros,* gadfly]. The interval between the periods of sexual heat of female mammals; diestrum. —**anestrous,** *adj.*

an′e·thole. $CH_3O.C_6H_4.C_3H_5$. The chief constituent of anise and fennel oils; used as flavor and carminative.

a·ne′thum [G. *anēthon,* dill]. Dill; the dried fruit of *Anethum graveolens,* indigenous to southern Europe; used as a carminative and flavoring.

an″e·to·der′ma. Degeneration and disappearance of the elastic fibers of the derma, resulting in wrinkling and flabbiness of the skin; macular atrophy.

an·eu′ploid (a·new′ployd) [G. *a-,* not; *eu,* well; *-ploos,* fold; *eidos,* form]. Having an uneven multiple of the basic number of chromosomes; opposed to euploid. —**aneu′ploid,** *n.*

a·neu′ri·a [*a-;* G. *neuron,* nerve]. Lack of nervous energy. —**aneuric,** *adj.*

an′eu·rin (an′yoor·in), **a·neu′rin** [*a-; neuron*]. Name given to vitamin B_1 by Jansen and Donath who first isolated it in crystalline form. See *thiamine hydrochloride.*

a·neu′rine hy″dro·chlo′ride. The British Pharmacopoeia title for thiamine hydrochloride.

an′eu·rysm, an′eu·rism [G. *aneurysma,* dilatation]. A circumscribed axial or laterally communicating dilatation of the wall of an artery forming a blood-containing tumor which pulsates with each systole, produces a bruit, and often is associated with pain, pressure symptoms, and absorption of contiguous parts. Most common in the aorta as a result of syphilis. —**aneurys′mal, aneurysmat′ic,** *adj.*

ampullary a. A small saccular aneurysm; it is most common in the arteries of the brain. See berry *a.*

anastomotic a. See cirsoid *a.*

aortic a. An aneurysm of the aorta. It occurs most frequently in the ascending aorta where it may cause severe pressure symptoms and eventually may rupture. The usual cause is syphilitic aortitis.

arteriovenous a. Any abnormal communication between arteries and veins, congenital or acquired. Gunshot wounds of the larger vessels of the extremities are the most common cause. A *varicose aneurysm* is produced by the rupture of an aneurysm into a vein. An *aneurysmal varix* results from the establishment of a communication between an artery and a vein, the latter becoming dilated and pulsating. Also called arteriovenous *fistula.*

atherosclerotic a. Dilatation especially of the basilar and internal carotid arteries and the circle of Willis in cases of severe atherosclerosis.

berry a. A saccular aneurysm formed from a congenital defect of the media of a cerebral artery, rupture of which is the most common source of subarachnoid hemorrhage: also called *intracranial aneurysm.*

cardiac a. An aneurysm of the heart wall.

carotid a. Aneurysm of the internal carotid, which may cause, by pressure on nerves, defects in the sense of smell, ptosis, convergent strabismus, dilated pupil, and amaurosis. By pressure on the cavernous sinus, it may cause ocular congestion and swelling of the facial veins. Enlargement of the sac may lead to deafness, facial paralysis, and crossed hemiplegia.

carotid-cavernous fistulous a. An aneurysm in the carotid artery at the point where it transverses the cavernous sinus. It is most often the result of a head injury, but a few arise spontaneously. Cephalic bruit and exophthalmos are two common symptoms.

cirsoid a. (a) A tortuous lengthening and dilatation of a part of an artery. (b) A dilatation of a group of vessels (arteries, veins, and capillaries), the whole forming a pulsating subcutaneous tumor, occurring most often in the scalp.

circumscribed a. An aneurysm, either true or false, in which the contents are still within the arterial wall though there may be rupture of one or more of its coats.

compound a. One in which one or several of the coats of the artery are ruptured and the others merely dilated.

congenital a. One due to a developmental defect.

consecutive a. One following rupture of all the arterial coats, with infiltration of surrounding tissues with blood.

Crisp's a. Aneurysm of the splenic artery.

cylindric, cylindrical a. An aneurysm of the same transverse diameter throughout the dilatation returning fairly abruptly to the normal diameter of the artery: similar to a *fusiform a.*

developmental a. See congenital *a.*

diffused a. See consecutive *a.*

dissecting a. One in which the blood forces its way between the coats of an artery. Syn., *intramural a., dissecting hematoma.*

ectatic a. An expansion of a portion of an artery due to yielding of all the coats.

embolic a. One caused by embolism.

endogenous a. One formed by disease of the vessel walls.

erosive a. An aneurysm due to extension of inflammation from an infected valve (aortic or pulmonic) breaking down the vessel wall.

exogenous a. One due to traumatism.

external a. (a) One remote from the great body cavities. (b) One in which the cavity of the tumor is entirely or chiefly outside the inner coat of the artery, similar to cylindric *a.*

false a. One due to a rupture of all the coats of

an artery, the effused blood being retained by the surrounding tissues.

fusiform a. Spindle-shaped dilatation of an artery, similar to cylindric *a.*

hernial a. One in which the internal coat of the artery, with or without the middle coat, forms the aneurysmal sac which has forced its way through an opening in the outer coat.

intracavernous a. A nonfistulous aneurysm of the internal carotid artery within the cavernous sinus, which, upon enlargement, suddenly produces a unilateral pain of the head or face which may continue for a period of weeks. Following the pain, a sensation of numbness is often felt over the forehead and infraorbital region. This aneurysm may rupture when quite small and produce a fistulous carotid-cavernous aneurysm. Syn., *subclinoid a.*

intracranial a. An aneurysm located on any of the cerebral arteries. Treatment is intracranial ligation of the affected artery. The most frequent is berry aneurysm.

intramural a. See dissecting *a.*

lateral a. One projecting on one side of a vessel, the rest of the circumference being intact.

malignant bone a. See osteogenic *sarcoma.*

medical a. One which cannot be treated surgically.

miliary a. A minute saclike dilatation of an arteriole.

mural a. See cardiac *a.*

mycotic a. One caused by bacterial infection and inflammation of the wall of a blood vessel.

osteoid a. Pulsating tumor of a bone.

partial a. (a) See lateral *a.* (b) Aneurysmal dilatation of a portion of the heart.

peripheral a. One involving the circumference of an artery.

primary a. An aneurysm in which the disease of the arterial wall which predisposes to the dilatation is unknown: also called *spontaneous a.*

racemose a. See cirsoid *a.*

saccular a. A saclike dilatation of an artery communicating with the main arterial trunk by an opening that is relatively small.

spontaneous a. See primary *a.*

spurious a. See false *a.*

subclinoid a. Intracavernous a.

supraclinoid a. One occurring just above the sphenoid bone.

surgical a. One which can be treated surgically.

syphilitic a. One occurring in a vessel as a result of syphilitic lesions in its wall. It is most common in the ascending aorta.

traction a. One due to traction on the aorta by an incompletely atrophied ductus arteriosus.

traumatic a. One produced by injury, as crushing, or following a gunshot wound, as distinguished from one resulting from disease.

true a. One in which the sac is formed of one, two, or all of the arterial coats.

varicose a. An arteriovenous aneurysm in which the sac of a hematoma intervenes between the arteries and veins.

an″eu·rys·mec′to·my (an″yoor·iz·meck′to·mee) [*aneurysma;* G. *ektomē,* excision]. Excision of an aneurysmal sac.

an″eu·rys′mo·graph [*aneurysma;* G. *graphein,* to write]. An x-ray film of an aneurysm.

an″eu·rys′mo·plas″ty [*aneurysma;* G. *plassein,* to form]. Restoration of an artery in aneurysm; reconstructive endoaneurysmorrhaphy.

an″eu·rys·mor′rha·phy (an″yoor·iz·mor′uh·fee) [*aneurysma;* G. *rhaphē,* suture]. Repair of aneurysm of an artery by means of an obliterative operation of the sac.

an″eu·rys·mot′o·my [*aneurysma;* G. *tomē,* a cutting]. Incision of an aneurysm for the purpose of suturing or to promote granulation.

an″eu·tha·na′si·a (an″yo͞o·thuh·nay′zhuh, ·zee·uh) [G. *a-,* not; *euthanasia,* easy death]. A painful or difficult death.

an·frac″tu·os′i·ty [L. *anfractus,* a bending round]. 1. Any one of the furrows or sulci between the cerebral convolutions. *Obs.* 2. Any spiral turn or winding.

ethmoidal a. An ethmoidal cell. *Obs.*

an·frac′tu·ous [*anfractus*]. Winding, turning, sinuous.

an·gei′al [G. *aggeion,* vessel]. Vascular.

an′gei·o- (an′jye·o-). For words beginning *angeio-,* see words beginning *angio-.*

an·gel′i·ca, an″ge·lique′ (an″ji·leek′) [G. *aggelikos,* pertaining to messengers, angelic]. An aromatic plant of the genus *Angelica,* especially *Angelica archangelica.* The fruit, roots, and rhizomes were formerly used, chiefly in household medicine, as a carminative, diuretic, and emmenagogue. The seeds were supposed to have antimalarial properties.

an·gel′ic ac′id. An unsaturated acid from the roots of *Angelica archangelica;* has been used in the treatment of rheumatism.

an′gel's wing. Winged scapula; a condition in which the scapula projects posteriorly because of weakness or paralysis of the serratus anterior muscle. Syn. *alar scapula.*

an′gi-. See *angio-.*

an″gi·ec′ta·sis, an″gi·ec·ta′si·a [G. *aggeion,* vessel; *ektasis,* extension]. Abnormal dilatation of a vessel; enlargement of capillaries. —**angiectat′ic,** *adj.*

an″gi·ec′tid. An abnormal intradermal venous dilataion, consisting of a circumscribed conglomerate mass of venules, which causes a frequently tense and tender elevation of the skin. Angiectids usually occur in the skin of the lower extremities of pregnant women, and are to be distinguished from varicose veins, which are subcutaneous.

an″gi·ec′to·my. See *arteriectomy; venectomy.*

an″gi·ec·to′pi·a [*aggeion;* G. *ektopos,* away from a place]. Displacement or abnormal position of a vessel. —**angiectop′ic,** *adj.*

an″gi·i′tis [*aggeion;* G. *-itis,* inflammation]. Inflammation of a blood or lymph vessel.

consecutive a. Inflammation of vessels by extension from adjacent tissues.

an·gi′na, an′gi·na [L., from *angere,* to strangle]. 1. Any disease marked by attacks of choking or suffocation, particularly an affection of the fauces or throat. 2. Sore throat. 3. Spasmodic, cramplike pain or attack. —**angi′nal, an′ginoid, an′ginose, an′ginous,** *adj.*

agranulocytic a. Agranulocytosis.

a. abdominis. Acute attacks of severe, colicky, intraabdominal pain associated with increased pulse and tension; attributed to sclerosis of the abdominal blood vessels or abdominal aneurysm.

a. cordis. See *a.* pectoris.

a. cruris. Intermittent lameness with pain and cyanosis caused by arterial obstruction. See intermittent *claudication.*

a. diphtheritica. Diphtheria of the pharynx or larynx. Also called *a. membranacea, suffocative a.*

a. epiglottidea. Inflammation of the epiglottis.

a. hypercyanotica. Severe precordial or substernal pain with cyanosis, occurring in patients with mitral stenosis, due probably to myocardial anoxia.

a. maligna. (a) Gangrenous or necrotic pharyngitis. See gangrenous *a.* (b) Septic sore throat.

a. necrotica. See gangrenous *a.*

a. parotidea. That form due to mumps. Also called *a. externa, a. maxillaris.*

a. pectoris. Paroxysmal pain of psychosomatic origin, characterized by a sense of oppression and severe constriction about the chest. The pain radiates from the precordium to the left shoulder and down the arm along the ulnar nerve. Associated is a sense of apprehension of impending death. The pain is caused by myocardial ischemia and occurs suddenly because of emotional stress or physical exertion. The condition chiefly affects men over 40, and is rare in women. Syn., *a. cordis, cardiac a.*

a. pectoris vasomotoria. Angina pectoris in which the breast pain is comparatively mild but is attended by pallor and cyanosis, with marked coldness and numbness of the extremities. Also called *mock a., a. notha, spurious a., false a.*

a. simplex. Simple sore throat. Also called *a. acuta.*

a. tonsillaris. Quinsy. Syn., *a. vera.*

a. vera. Quinsy.

aphthous a. Throat inflammation associated with the formation of small ulcers.

cardiac a. See *a.* pectoris.

exudative a. Croup. Also called *a. canina.*

fibrinous a. A noninfectious, diphtherialike disease of the throat, characterized by a fibrinous exudate especially over the tonsillar area. Also called *croupous a., pseudomembranous a.*

follicular a. Follicular tonsillitis.

gangrenous a. That form characterized by necrotic patches of the fauces, occasionally following scarlet fever or diphtheria. Syn., *a. maligna, a. necrotica.*

herpetic a. That type marked by the formation of vesicles in the throat, associated with patches of exudation.

hypoleukocytic a. Agranulocytic angina; acute agranulocytosis.

Ludwig's a. An acute streptococcic infection of the floor of the mouth. It begins suddenly with marked constitutional symptoms and swelling under the jaw, rapidly extending into the neck. The floor of the mouth becomes swollen and indurated and the tongue pushed upward. Speech and swallowing are impeded, and the disease may be fatal.

lymphocytic a. See infectious *mononucleosis.*

monocytic a. Infectious mononucleosis.

nerve a. Neuralgic angina due to spasm of the nutrient arteries of the nerves.

phlegmonous a. (a) Inflammation of the mucous and submucous tissues of the throat with edema. (b) Acute inflammation of the deep structures of the throat with a tendency to suppuration.

pseudoangina. A neurosis affecting anemic women, simulating angina pectoris but less severe and never terminating fatally.

pultaceous a. An affection of the throat with whitish or grayish patches which detach easily and are not true exudates.

serous a. (a) Edema of the glottis. (b) Catarrhal pharyngitis.

thymic a. (a) Laryngismus stridulus. (b) Allergic asthma.

Vincent's a. An extension of necrotizing ulcerative gingivitis to the faucial and tonsillar region. See also Vincent's *stomatitis.*

an·gi″no·pho′bi·a (an·jye″no·fo′bee·uh, an″ji·no·) [*angina;* G. *phobos,* fear]. Morbid fear of angina pectoris.

an′gi·o- (an′jee·o-), **an′gi-** [G. *aggeion,* vessel]. A combining form meaning *a vessel* or denoting *a seed, blood vessel,* or *pertaining to* or *covered by* (such) *a vessel.*

an′gi·o·blast″ [*aggeion;* G. *blastos,* germ]. 1. Special primordium derived from extraembryonic endoderm, which gives rise to the blood cells and blood vessels in the early embryo. 2. That part of the mesenchyme, especially extraembryonic, from which the first blood cells and blood vessels arise. 3. A vasoformative cell of the mesenchyme. —**angioblas′tic,** *adj.*

an″gi·o·blas·to′ma [*aggeion; blastos;* G. *-ōma,* tumor]. See *hemangioendothelioma.*

an″gi·o·car′di·o·gram″ [*aggeion;* G. *kardia,* heart; *gramma,* letter]. A radiograph of the heart and large vessels.

an″gi·o·car″di·og′ra·phy [*aggeion; kardia;* G. *graphein,* to write]. Roentgenographic visualization of the thoracic vessels and the heart chambers after intravenous injection of radiopaque material (diodrast). —**angiocardiograph′ic,** *adj.*

an″gi·o·car″di·op′a·thy. Abnormalities of the heart and great vessels.

an″gi·o·cav″er·no′ma. A cavernous angioma.

an″gi·o·cav′ern·ous [*aggeion;* L. *cavernosus,* full of hollows]. Relating to cavernous angioma.

an″gi·o·chei′lo·scope (an″jee·o·kigh′lo·scope) [*aggeion;* G. *cheilos,* lip; *skopein,* to examine]. An instrument which magnifies the capillary circulation of the lips, permitting observation.

an″gi·o·cho·li′tis (an″jee·o·ko·lye′tis) [*aggeion;* G. *cholē,* bile; *-itis,* inflammation]. Cholangitis.

an″gi·o·chon·dro′ma. A mesenchymoma.

malignant a. A malignant mesenchymoma.

an″gi·o·der′ma pig″men·to′sum. Xeroderma pigmentosum.

an″gi·o·der″ma·ti′tis [*aggeion;* G. *derma,* skin; *-itis*]. Inflammation of the vessels of the skin.

an″gi·o·di′a·ther″my. Obliteration of blood vessels by diathermy.

an″gi·o·dys·tro′phi·a, an″gi·o·dys′tro·phy [*aggeion;* G. *dys,* bad; *trophē,* nourishment]. Defective nutrition of the blood vessels.

an″gi·o·e·de′ma. See angioneurotic *edema.*

an″gi·o·el″e·phan·ti′a·sis [*aggeion;* G. *elephantiasis,* elephantiasis]. Nodular or lobulated masses of vascular tumors (angiomas), especially of the subcutaneous tissues, which commonly bleed on pressure, may pulsate, and sometimes are erectile.

an″gi·o·en″do·the″li·o′ma [*aggeion;* G. *endon,* within; *thēlē,* nipple; *-ōma,* tumor]. A tumor composed of endothelial cells and blood or lymph vessels: also called *Ewing's tumor.*

a. of bone. See Ewing's *sarcoma.*

an″gi·o·fi″bro·blas·to′ma [*aggeion;* L. *fibra,* fiber; G. *blastos,* germ; *-ōma*]. An angioma with fibroblastic tissue between the vascular structures.

an″gi·o·fi·bro′ma (an″jee·o·figh·bro′muh) [*aggeion; fibra; -ōma*]. A fibroma rich in blood vessels or lymphatics.

an″gi·o·gen′e·sis [*aggeion;* G. *genesis,* generation]. The development of the blood vessels. —**angiogenic,** *adj.*

an″gi·o·gli·o′ma (an″jee·o·glye·o′muh) [*aggeion;* G. *glia,* glue; *-ōma,* tumor]. A glioma which is rich in blood vessels.

an″gi·o·gli·o″ma·to′sis (·glye·o″muh·to′sis) [*aggeion; glia; -ōma;* G. *-ōsis,* condition]. The presence of numerous foci of proliferating capillaries and neuroglia.

an″gi·og′ra·phy [*aggeion;* G. *graphein,* to write]. 1. Determination of the arrangement of blood or lymph vessels without dissection, as by capillaroscopy, fluoroscopy, or radiography. 2. In radiology, the visualization of blood vessels by injection of a nontoxic radiopaque substance.

intracranial a. Roentgenography of the blood vessels within the cranial cavity following the injection of a radiopaque material.

an″gi·o·hy″per·to′ni·a [*aggeion;* G. *hyper*, over; *tonos*, tension]. A condition in which the walls of the blood vessels are constricted; vasoconstriction.

an″gi·o·hy″po·to′ni·a [*aggeion;* G. *hypo*, under; *tonos*]. A condition in which the walls of the blood vessels are relaxed; vasodilatation.

an′gi·oid [*aggeion;* G. *eidos*, form]. Linear; in appearance resembling a blood vessel.

an″gi·o·ker″a·toi·di′tis [*aggeion;* G. *keras*, horn; *-itis*, inflammation]. Vascular keratitis.

an″gi·o·ker″a·to′ma [*aggeion; keras;* G. *-ōma*, tumor]. A rare disease of the skin, usually of the extremities; characterized by telangiectatic warty growths; often preceded by chilblains.

a. corporis diffusum. A metabolic genodermatosis marked by the presence on the trunk of small telangiectatic verrucous growths, and usually associated with internal lesions, as degeneration of the muscle fibers of blood vessels and the heart.

a. Mibelli. A progressive condition beginning in childhood in which small, vascular, verrucous growths are seen on the backs of the fingers and toes and over the knees.

an″gi·o·li·po′ma [*aggeion;* G. *lipos*, fat; *-ōma*]. A mixed tumor of vascular and fatty tissue.

an′gi·o·lith″ [*aggeion;* G. *lithos*, stone]. A calculus of a blood vessel. —**angiolith′ic,** *adj.*

an″gi·ol′o·gy [*aggeion;* G. *logos*, word]. The science dealing with blood vessels and lymphatics.

an″gi·o·lu′poid [*aggeion;* L. *lupus*, wolf; G. *eidos*, form]. A cutaneous sarcoid of the type seen in generalized sarcoidosis; usually found on the face; marked by small bluish-red nodules with capillary dilatation: also called *a. of Brocq and Pautrier.*

an″gi·ol′y·sis [*aggeion;* G. *lysis*, a loosing]. Obliteration of a blood vessel during embryonal, fetal, or postnatal life; by progressive fibrosis, or by thrombosis followed by organization and cicatrization, as obliteration of the ductus arteriosus.

an″gi·o′ma [*aggeion;* G. *-ōma*, tumor]. A tumor composed of blood or lymphatic vessels; a hemangioma or lymphangioma. Probably derived from embryonal isolation of mesenchymal structures; it is essentially a hamartoma, but many consider it a neoplasm. —**angiom′atous,** *adj.*

a. arteriale racemosum. A complex meshwork of small blood vessels, near or attached to an artery.

capillary a. See capillary *hemangioma.*

cavernous a. One in which the vascular spaces are large or cystic, like the erectile tissue of the penis. Also called *angiocavernoma.*

fissural a. A vascular nevus occurring at the site of embryonal fissures, as on the face or neck.

plexiform a. One consisting of tortuous capillaries, and sometimes of arteries and veins; usually subcutaneous; produces sessile or wartlike superficial masses.

senile a. See papillary *varix.*

serpiginous a. A skin disease in which tiny red vascular dots appear in groups on the skin; called *Hutchinson's disease.*

spider a. See spider *nevus.*

telangiectatic a. One in which the component vessels are large, as in angioma of the bone.

an″gi·o·ma·la′ci·a (an″jee·o·ma·lay′shee·uh, ·see·uh) [*aggeion;* G. *malakia*, softness]. Softening of the blood vessels.

an″gi·o·ma·to′sis [*aggeion;* G. *-ōma*, tumor; *-ōsis*, condition]. A pathologic state of the blood vessels marked by the formation of multiple angiomas.

a. retinae. An uncommon disease of the retina marked by areas of proliferating capillaries and neuroglia, indicating a neoplasm. Also called *von Hippel's disease, angiogliomatosis.*

encephalotrigeminal a. Nevoid amentia.

an″gi·o·meg′a·ly [*aggeion;* G. *megas*, large]. Enlargement of blood vessels, occurring chiefly in the eyelid.

an″gi·om′e·ter [*aggeion;* G. *metron*, a measure]. An instrument for measuring the diameter or tension in a vessel. See *sphygmograph.*

an″gi·o·my″o·lip·o′ma. A mesenchymoma.

an″gi·o·my·o′ma (an″jee·o·migh·o′muh) [*aggeion;* G. *mys*, muscle; *-ōma*, tumor]. A myoma rich in blood vessels or lymphatics.

an″gi·o·my·op′a·thy (·migh·op′uth·ee) [*aggeion; mys;* G. *pathos*, disease]. Any affection of the vessels involving the musculature.

an″gi·o·my″o·sar·co′ma [*aggeion; mys;* G. *sarkōma*, fleshy excrescence]. A myosarcoma rich in blood vessels or lymphatics.

an″gi·o·neu·rec′to·my [*aggeion;* G. *neuron*, nerve; *ektomē*, excision]. Excision of blood vessels and nerves.

an″gi·o·neu·ro′ma [*aggeion; neuron;* G. *-ōma*, tumor]. A benign tumor composed of vascular tissue and nerve fibers.

an″gi·o·neu″ro·my·o′ma (·new″ro·migh·o′muh) [*aggeion; neuron;* G. *mys*, muscle; *-ōma*]. Glomus tumor.

an″gi·o·neu·ro′sis [*aggeion; neuron;* G. *-ōsis*, condition]. A psychoneurosis which partially expresses itself by a disturbance of the vasomotor system, either of the nature of a spasm of the peripheral blood vessels (*angiospasm*), of a paralysis (*angioparalysis*), or of a paresis (*angioparesis*): formerly called *vasomototrophoneurosis.* —**angioneurotic,** *n.* and *adj.*

an″gi·o·no′ma [*aggeion;* G. *-ōma*, tumor]. Ulceration of a vessel.

an″gi·o·pa·ral′y·sis [*aggeion;* G. *paralysis*, paralysis]. Paralysis of blood vessels caused by vasomotor defect. —**angioparalyt′ic,** *adj., n.*

an″gi·o·pa·re′sis (an″jee·o·pa·ree′sis, ·par′i·sis) [*aggeion;* G. *paresis*, slackening]. Partial paralysis of the vasomotor apparatus.

an″gi·op′a·thy [*aggeion;* G. *pathos*, disease]. Any disease of the vascular system.

an″gi·o·pla′ni·a, an′gi·o·pla″ny [*aggeion;* G. *planē*, a wandering]. Irregularity or abnormality in the course of a vessel; angiectopia.

an′gi·o·plas″ty [*aggeion;* G. *plassein*, to form]. Plastic surgery upon blood vessels.

an″gi·o·pneu·mog′ra·phy [*aggeion;* G. *pneumon*, lung; *graphein*, to write]. Radiographic visualization of the pulmonary artery by means of a nontoxic radiopaque substance.

an″gi·o·poi·e′sis [*aggeion;* G. *poiēsis*, production]. The process by which certain cells cause the formation of blood vessels in new tissue.

an″gi·o·poi·et′ic [*aggeion;* G. *poiein*, to make]. Forming blood vessels, as in new tissue.

an′gi·o·pres″sure [*aggeion;* L. *pressura*, pressure]. The production of hemostasia without ligation, by angiotribe, hemostat, or other pressure.

an″gi·or′rha·phy [*aggeion;* G. *rhaphē*, suture]. Plastic suture of a blood vessel or vessels.

an″gi·or·rhex′is [*aggeion;* G. *rhēxis*, a breaking]. Rupture of a blood vessel.

an″gi·o·sar·co′ma [*aggeion;* G. *sarkōma*, fleshy excrescence]. Sarcoma derived from an angioma or a sarcoma rich in blood vessels or lymphatics.

multiplex a. See multiple idiopathic hemorrhagic *sarcoma.*

an″gi·o·scle·ro′sis (an″jee·o·skli·ro′sis) [*aggeion;* G. *sklērōsis*, hardening]. Induration and thickening of the walls of the blood vessels.

an′gi·o·scope″ [*aggeion;* G. *skopein*, to examine]. An instrument for examining the capillary vessels.

an″gi·o·sco·to′ma [*aggeion;* G. *skotōma*, dizziness]. Defects in the visual field due to the presence of retinal vessels.

an″gi·o′sis [*aggeion;* G. *-ōsis,* condition]. Angiopathy. See *angiitis.*

an′gi·o·spasm″ [*aggeion;* G. *spasmos,* spasm]. A segmental contracture of a blood vessel. —**angiospas′tic,** *adj.*

an′gi·o·sperm″ [*aggeion;* G. *sperma,* seed]. A plant the seeds of which are protected by a pericarp.

an″gi·o·stax′is [*aggeion;* G. *staxis,* a dropping]. The oozing of blood. See *hemophilia.*

an″gi·o·ste·no′sis [*aggeion;* G. *stenōsis,* a being straitened]. Narrowing of the lumen of a blood vessel.

an″gi·os″te·o′sis [*aggeion;* G. *osteon,* bone; *-ōsis,* condition]. Ossification of blood vessels.

an″gi·o·tel″ec·ta′si·a (·tel″eck·tay′zhuh, ·zee·uh, ·shuh, ·see·uh) [*aggeion;* G. *telos,* end; *ektasis,* a stretching out]. A condition in which there is dilatation of groups of capillaries; telangiectasis.

an″gi·o·ten′ic [*aggeion;* G. *teinein,* to stretch]. Due to or marked by distention of the blood vessels.

an″gi·o·ti′tis [*aggeion;* G. *ous,* ear; *-itis,* inflammation]. Inflammation of blood vessels of the ear.

an″gi·ot′o·my [*aggeion;* G. *tomē,* a cutting]. Incision into a blood vessel.

an″gi·ot′o·nase. One of a group of enzymes capable of destroying angiotonin. Syn., *hypertensinase.*

an″gi·o·ton′ic [*aggeion;* G. *tonos,* tension]. Tending to increase arterial tension.

an″gi·ot′o·nin. A polypeptide, the product of the action of the enzyme renin on renin substrate, a pseudoglobulin in the blood plasma. The injection of angiotonin into the blood stream causes an abrupt, fleeting rise of blood pressure. Syn., *hypertensin.*

an″gi·o·to′nin·ase. See *angiotonase.*

an′gi·o·tribe″ [*aggeion;* G. *tribein,* to grind, to bruise]. A clamp with powerful jaws used to crush arteries embedded in tissue.

an″gi·o·troph′ic [*aggeion;* G. *trophē,* nourishment]. Relating to nutrition of blood vessels.

an·gi·ox′yl. An acidified alcoholic pancreatic extract used as a treatment for hypertension.

an·gi′tis. Angiitis.

Angle, Edward Hartley [*American orthodontist,* 1855–1930]. Celebrated for his classification of the various forms of malocclusion; for his wire splint, designed to hold the lower teeth to the upper in fracture of the mandible; and for his clamp band, used with his regulating appliances.

an′gle [L. *angulus,* an angle]. 1. Degree of divergence of two lines or planes that meet each other; the space between two such lines. 2. A corner. —**angular,** *adj.*

acromial a. That formed between the head of the humerus and the clavicle.

alveolar a. That formed between a line passing through a point beneath the nasal spine and the most prominent point of the lower edge of the alveolar process of the maxilla and the cephalic horizontal line.

a. alpha. The angle formed by intersection of the optic and visual axes at the nodal point of the eye. In myopia, the alpha angle is smaller than normal and the eye appears to converge; in hypermetropia, the angle is larger than normal and the eye appears to diverge.

a. of aberration. See *a.* of deviation.

a. of anomaly. Angular degree of the shift from the normal to the abnormal retinal correspondence observed in squint.

a. of aperture. *In optics,* that included between two lines joining the opposite points of the periphery of a lens and the focus.

a. of circulatory efficiency. The angle of elevation of a limb at which color returns after ischemia or blanching.

a. of convergence. The angle between the two visual axes, when the eyes are turned inward. See *meter-a.*

a. of deviation. (a) *In magnetism,* the angle traversed by the needle when disturbed by some magnetic force. (b) *In optics,* that formed by a refracted ray and the prolongation of the incident ray.

a. of elevation. *In optics,* that made by the visual plane with its primary position when moved upward or downward.

a. of eye. See *canthus.*

a. of incidence. *In optics,* the acute angle between a ray, incident upon a surface, and the perpendicular to the surface at the point of incidence.

a. of inclination of pelvic canal. *In obstetrics,* that formed by the anterior wall of the pelvis with the anteroposterior diameter of the pelvic inlet.

a. of inclination of pelvis. *In obstetrics,* that formed by the pelvis with the general line of the trunk, or that formed by the plane of the inferior strait with the horizon.

a. of iris. The iridial angle; the angulus iridis [BNA]. That formed by the iris and cornea. Also called filtration *a.*

a. of jaw. The junction of the base of the body of the mandible with the posterior border of its ramus.

a. of lips. That formed by the union of the lips at each extremity of the oral opening.

a. of Ludwig. See *a. of sternum.*

a. of polarization. *In optics,* the angle of reflection at which light is most completely polarized.

a. of pubes. That formed by the junction of the pubic bones at the symphysis.

a. of reflection. *In optics,* that which a reflected ray of light makes with a line drawn perpendicular to the point of incidence.

a. of refraction. *In optics,* that which exists between a refracted ray of light and a line drawn perpendicular to the point of incidence.

a. of rib. An angle of the body of a rib at the attachment of the iliocostalis muscle and the point at which the rib bends ventrally.

a. of sternum. That between the manubrium and body of the sternum. Also called *a. of Louis, a. of Ludwig.*

a. of supination of the hand, a. of supination of the radius. The extent to which the hand is capable of being supinated; about 180°.

angles of the scapula. The three angles of the triangular scapula. The **inferior angle of the scapula** is that formed by the junction of its axillary and vertebral borders. The **lateral angle of the scapula** is that formed by the junction of its axillary and superior borders; it includes the head of the scapula, bearing the glenoid cavity. The **medial** (or *superior*) **angle of the scapula** is that formed by the junction of its superior and vertebral borders.

a. of Sylvius. See Sylvian *a.*

beta a. That formed between the radius fixus and a line joining the bregma and hormion.

biorbital a. *In optics,* that formed by the intersection of the axes of the orbits.

cardiohepatic a. The angle formed by the junction of the upper limit of hepatic dullness with the right lateral line of cardiac dullness.

carrying a. Angle between the longitudinal axis of the forearm and that of the arm when the forearm is extended.

cavosurface a. That formed by the meeting of a cavity wall with the surface of the tooth.

cerebellopontine a. A region bounded laterally by the petrous portion of the temporal bone, medially by the cerebellum and brain stem, below by the floor of the posterior fossa of the skull, and above by the tentorium cerebelli. An area in which tumors frequently occur.

colic a. The angle formed by the junction of abdominal and umbilical colon in the fetus.

costal a. The angle formed by the right and left costal cartilages at the xiphoid process: also called *infrasternal a., subcostal a.*

costophrenic a. That formed by the ribs and diaphragm.

critical a. *In optics*, the least angle of incidence at which there is total reflection. It exists when light, traveling in one medium, is incident upon another medium which is less refracting.

distal a. *In dentistry*, that formed by the junction of the distal surface with any one of the other surfaces of the crown of a tooth.

distoincisal a. Angle formed by the distal surface and the incisive edge of an incisor.

distoocclusal a. The angle of a premolar or molar formed by the junction of its distal and occlusal surfaces. It forms the distal marginal ridge of the occlusal surfaces of these teeth.

epigastric a. See costal *a.*

facial a. That formed by the union of a line connecting nasion and gnathion with the Frankfort horizontal plane of the head. This may be measured on the dead skull with a craniostat, or on the living head with the aid of a lateral roentgenogram.

filtration a. The iridial angle, at which point filtration of the aqueous humor supposedly occurs.

frontal a. That determined by connecting the point that lies highest in the sagittal curvature of the frontal bone by straight lines with nasion and bregma respectively. This angle is greater in a skull with a low, receding forehead.

gamma a. *In ophthalmology*, the angle formed by the line of fixation and the optic axis.

gastric a. See angular *notch.*

genial a. The angle formed by the ramus and the body of the mandible.

great a. of eye. The inner canthus of the eye.

incisal a. *In dentistry*, the junction of the incisal edge of an anterior tooth with a proximal surface.

infrasternal a. The costal angle.

iridial a. See *a.* of iris.

kappa a. The angle formed by the visual and pupillary axes; when the pupillary axis is temporal to the visual axis, the angle is positive.

labial a. See *a.* of lips.

limiting a. See critical *a.*

line a. One formed by the meeting of two tooth surfaces.

mesial a. The junction of the mesial surface of a crown of a tooth with one of the other surfaces.

mesioocclusal a. That formed by the junction of the mesial and occlusal surfaces of a premolar or molar tooth.

metafacial a. That between the base of the skull and the pterygoid process. Also called *Serres' a.*

meter-a. *In optics*, the degree of convergence of the eyes when centered on an object one meter distant from each.

nasal a. The inner canthus of the eye.

occipital a. That determined by connecting the point in the sagittal curvature of the occipital bone by straight lines with lambda and the point of the external occipital protuberance respectively. The more convex the occipital bone, the smaller is this angle.

optic a. That included between lines joining the extremities of an object and the nodal point. The smallest is about 30 seconds.

parietal a. That determined by connecting the highest point in the sagittal curvature that lies highest above the plane passing from right to left through bregma and lambda, by straight lines with bregma and lambda, respectively. The greater the angle, the less convex the vault of the skull.

pelvivertebral a. See *a.* of inclination of pelvis.

point a. *In dentistry*, that formed by the meeting of three surfaces. Syn., *solid a.*

principal a. The angle formed by that side of a prism receiving the incident ray with the side from which the refracted ray escapes.

prism a. The angle made by the two refracting sides of a prism at its apex.

Rolandic a. The acute angle formed by the central sulcus (fissure of Rolando) with the superior border of the cerebral hemisphere.

sacrolumbar a. Old term for sacrovertebral angle.

sacrovertebral a. That which the sacrum forms with the last lumbar vertebra.

sigma a. One between the radius fixus and a line from the hormion to the staphylion.

solid a. One formed by the junction of three surfaces.

sternoclavicular a. That existing between the clavicle and the sternum.

subcostal a. See costal *a.*

subpubic a. That formed at the pubic arch.

Sylvian a. The angle formed by the posterior limb of the Sylvian fissure (lateral cerebral fissure) with a line perpendicular to the superior border of the hemisphere.

temporal a. The outer canthus of the eye.

uranal a. That determined by connecting the point that lies highest in the sagittal curvature of the hard palate by straight lines with the premaxillary point and the posterior nasal spine, respectively. The less arched the palate, the greater is this angle.

visual a. See optic *a.*

xiphoid a. That formed by the sides of the xiphoid notch.

An′gli·cus su′dor [L.]. English sweating fever.

an″go·phra′si·a (ang″go·fray′zhuh, ·zee·uh) [G. *agchein*, to choke; *phrasis*, utterance]. A halting, choking, and drawling type of speech occurring in paralytic dementia.

an′gor [L. *angor*, a strangling]. Angina, 3; extreme distress.

a. animi. A sense of imminent dissolution.

a. nocturnus. Night terrors. Syn., *pavor nocturnus.*

a. pectoris. Angina pectoris.

an″gos·tu′ra [Sp., former name of town in Venezuela, from L. *angustus*, narrow]. The bark of *Galipea cusparia.* It is a stimulant bitter tonic.

ang′strom, ång′ström (ang′strum, awng′strem. *See* Notes § 35) [after A. J. *Ångström*, Swedish physicist, 1814–74]. An angstrom unit; a unit of length equal to 10^{-8} cm. (1⁄100 millionth of a centimeter); used for measuring wavelengths, as of visible light, x-rays, and radium radiation. Designated by the symbol A, Å, A.U., Å.U., A.u., Å.u., or a.u.

An·guil′lu·la (ang·gwil′yoo·luh, ang·gwil′oo·luh) [L., dim. of *anguilla*, eel]. Synonym for *Strongyloides.*

an″guil·lu·li′a·sis, an″guil·lu·lo′sis [*Anguillula;* NL. *-iasis*, condition]. Old term for strongyloidiasis.

an″gu·la′tion [L. *angulatus*, from *angulus*, angle]. 1. The formation of an unnatural angle in a hollow organ (as of the intestine or ureter). These angles often become sites of obstruction. 2. Deviation from the normal long axis, as in a fractured bone healed out of line.

an′gu·lus. See *angle.*

a. iridis. See *angle* of iris.

an″ha·la·mine′ (an″huh·luh·meen′, an·hal′uh·meen, ·min). $C_{11}H_{15}O_3N$. An alkaloid from mescal buttons.

an′ha·line (an′huh·leen, ·lin). An alkaloid from mescal buttons. It is identical with hordenine found in barley.

an″ha·lon′i·dine (an″huh·lon′i·deen, ·din). $C_{12}H_{17}O_3N$. An alkaloid from mescal buttons.

an″ha·lo′nine (an″huh·lo′neen, ·nin, an·hal′o·) (*anhalonium*). An alkaloid, $C_{12}H_{15}O_3N$, from mescal buttons.

An″ha·lo′ni·um. The former name of a genus of cactus.

A. lewinii. Old term for *Lophophora williamsii.*

an″he·do′ni·a [G. *a-*, not; *hēdonē*, pleasure]. *In psychology,* a diminution or disappearance of pleasure in life; apathy in the performance of acts which normally give pleasure.

an·hem″a·to·poi·e′sis, an·haem″a·to·poi·e′sis (an·hem″uh·to·poy·ee′sis, an·hee″muh·to·) [*a-;* G. *haima*, blood; *poiēsis*, production]. Defective formation of blood, the result of hypofunction of the bone marrow.

an·he″ma·to′sis [*a-; haima;* G. *-ōsis*, condition]. Anhematopoiesis.

an·he″mo·lyt′ic (an·hee″mo·lit′ick, an·hem″o·) [*a-; haima;* G. *lysis*, a loosing]. Not hemolytic; not destructive of blood corpuscles.

an″hi·dro′sis (an″hi·dro′sis, an″high·) [*a-;* G. *hidrōs*, sweat; *-ōsis*, condition]. Deficiency or absence of sweat secretion; also, loosely, deficiency or absence of salivation. —**anhidrot′ic,** *adj.*

hereditary a. See hereditary anhidrotic ectodermal *dysplasia.*

thermogenic a. See sweat-retention *syndrome.*

anhydr-. See *anhydro-.*

an″hy·drae′mi·a (an″high·dree′mee·uh). See *anhydremia.*

an·hy′drase. Any enzyme catalyzing a reaction involving removal of water.

carbonic a. The enzyme, found in red blood cells and in parietal cells of gastric mucosa, which catalyzes the reaction: $H_2CO_3 \rightleftharpoons H_2O + CO_2$.

an″hy·dra′tion. See *dehydration.*

an″hy·dre′mi·a (an″high·dree′mee·uh) [*a-;* G. *hydōr*, water; *haima*, blood]. A deficiency of the fluid portion of the blood.

an·hy′dride. A compound resulting from the abstraction of water from a substance.

acid a. An oxide of a nonmetal; it forms an acid with water.

basic a. An oxide of a metal; it forms a base with water.

inner a. A compound resulting from withdrawal of the elements of water from a molecule, with simultaneous formation of a ring structure within the molecule.

an·hy′drite. Anhydrous calcium sulfate.

an·hy′dro-, anhydr- [G. *anydros*, from *a-*, *hydōr*]. A combining form meaning *waterless;* used to denote *deficiency of water* or *an anhydride of a compound.*

an·hy″dro·git′a·lin (·jit′uh·lin, ·ji·tay′lin, ·ji·tal′in). Gitoxin.

an·hy″dro·hy·drox″y·pro·ges′ter·one (*anhydrohydroxyprogesteronum*). $C_{21}H_{28}O_2$. 17-Ethinyltestosterone or pregneninolone, the synthetic steroid resulting from elimination of a molecule of water and introduction of a hydroxyl group into the molecule of progesterone. It is used like progesterone but is active when given orally. Dose, 5–75 mg. (1⁄12–1¼ gr.) daily. Syn., *ethisterone.* See *lutocylol, pranone, progestoral.*

anhydrone. A trade-mark for anhydrous magnesium perchlorate; the substance is used in various chemical procedures for absorption of water.

an·hy′drous. *In chemistry,* denoting the absence of water, especially of water of crystallization.

an″hyp·no′sis [G. *a-*, not; *hypnos*, sleep; *ōsis*, condition]. Sleeplessness; insomnia.

a·ni″a·ci·no′sis [*a-;* Jean *Nicot*, who introduced tobacco into France, 1560; L. *acidus*, sour; *-in*, chemical suffix; *-ōsis*]. The syndrome produced by a deficiency of niacin (nicotinic acid) in the diet. Also called *niacinamidosis.*

an″i·an′thi·nop·sy [*a-;* G. *ianthinos*, violet-colored; *opsis*, sight]. Inability to recognize violet tints.

an·ic·ter′ic. Without jaundice, as in anicteric hepatitis.

an·id′e·us [*a-;* G. *eidos*, form]. The lowest form of omphalosite, in which the parasitic fetus is a shapeless mass of flesh covered with skin. Syn., *acardiacus amorphus, holoacardius amorphus.* —**anidian, anidean, ani′dous,** *adj.*

an′i·lide, an′i·lid. 1. Any member of the group of compounds containing the radical $C_6H_5.NH—$. They may be formed by the action of an acid chloride or acid anhydride on aniline. 2. A term sometimes applied to compounds having the group $NH_2.C_6H_4—$.

an′i·line (an′i·leen, ·lin, ·lyne), **an′i·lin** [Ar. *al-nīl*, the indigo plant]. $C_6H_5NH_2$. A colorless liquid with a faint, characteristic odor, obtained from coal tar and other nitrogenous substances or prepared by the reduction of nitrobenzene. It is slightly soluble in water, miscible with alcohol and ether, and forms soluble, crystallizable salts with acids. Various derivatives constitute the aniline dyes or coal tar colors. See *anilide.* Formerly it was used in chorea and epilepsy. Syn., *aminobenzene, phenylamine, cyanol.*

a. oil. A solvent consisting of a mixture of aniline, toluidine, xylidine, and other products resulting from the distillation of coal; used in histologic technic.

a. sulfate. $(C_6H_5NH_2)_2.H_2SO_4$. White crystals, soluble in water or alcohol; formerly used in chorea and epilepsy.

an′i·line black. See *nigraniline.*

an′i·line blue, W. S. (C.C.). An acid, aniline dye of the triphenylmethane series, a mixture of trisulfonates of diphenyl rosaniline and triphenyl pararosaniline: used to stain collagenous fibers and as a general stain, usually a 0.2 to 1.0% solution of aniline blue in water or in 90% alcohol. Also called *China blue, soluble blue 3M* or *2R, marine blue V, cotton blue, water blue, Berlin blue.*

a·ni·lin′gus [L. *anus*, anus; *lingua*, tongue]. *In psychiatry,* one who applies mouth to anus.

an′il·ism. Aniline poisoning, usually incurred industrially by inhaling fumes or fine dust for long periods of time.

a·nil′i·ty [L. *anilis*, from *anus*, an old woman]. Imbecility or childishness. —**an′ile,** *adj.*

an′i·ma [L., breath, spirit, soul]. 1. The soul; the vital principle. 2. The active principle of a drug or medicine. 3. In Jung's analytical psychology, the inner personality; the soul: differentiated into *anima* (feminine soul) and *animus* (masculine soul).

an′i·mal [L.]. 1. Any member of the higher of the two major classes of living things (plants and animals). There is no special test for a strict separation of all plants from all animals. In general, however, animals are distinguished by their mode of nutrition, by a neuromuscular system which permits locomotion, and by a more complex form of development from the egg and a more determinate type of growth. 2. The physical and organic as contrasted with the mental and spiritual. —**an'imal,** *adj.*

control a. (a) One serving as a check or standard of comparison in experimental studies. (b) A nonimmune animal. See *control.*

decerebrate a. One in which the brain and higher centers have been removed or disconnected.

experimental a. One which is the subject of experimentation.

Houssay a. One in which the pancreas and hypophysis both have been excised.

laboratory a. See experimental *a.*

spinal a. One with the cord severed, cutting off connections to the brain.

thalamic a. One with the brain stem severed just above the thalamus.

an"i·mal'cule [dim. from *animal*]. A minute or microscopic animal; a protozoan.

an'i·mal heat. The heat generated in a living organism by metabolism. Animals fall into two great classes regarding temperature: poikilothermic—those whose temperature varies but seldom exceeds that of the environment, and homothermic—those whose temperature is maintained at a level which varies within narrow limits. In man, the normal temperature is 98.6° F. (37° C.) with a normal fluctuation of 1°–3° in 24 hrs.

an'i·mal mag'net·ism. 1. A form of magnetic healing, characterized by a belief that certain men, like certain metals, have remedial powers by virtue of a spiritlike effluvium emanating from their bodies. 2. Mesmer's universal fluid which, he believed, emanates from heavenly bodies and influences the health of man. *Obs.*

an"i·mas'tic [L. *anima*, soul]. Pertaining to the psyche or soul.

an"i·ma'tion [L. *animatum*, from *animare*, to fill with breath]. 1. State of being alive, animate. 2. Liveliness; high spirits.

suspended a. A state of interrupted respiration and loss of consciousness; temporary period of apparent death.

an'i·ma·tism [L. *anima*, soul]. The attribution of personality (not soul) to the animate and inanimate phenomena of nature.

an'i·mism [*anima*]. 1. The belief that all animals, inanimate objects, and natural phenomena possess conscious souls: a characteristic of many primitive religions. 2. The theory of the *anima mundi*, soul of the world (G. E. Stahl, 1720): that all the phenomena of nature are the product of an immaterial, activating soul or spirit.

an'i·mus [L., mind]. 1. A spirit or feeling of hatred or hostility. 2. For the psychoanalytical meaning, see *anima* 3.

an'i"on. An ion carrying one or more negative charges, and migrating to the anode on electrolysis. Examples: acetate ($C_2H_3O_2^-$), chloride (Cl^-), hydroxide (OH^-), phosphate (PO_4^{---}), sulfate (SO_4^{--}).

an"i·rid'i·a (an"eye·rid'ee·uh, an"i·rid'ee·uh) [G. *a-*, not; *iris*, rainbow, iris]. Absence or defect of the iris.

an"is·al'de·hyde. $CH_3.O.C_6H_4.CHO$. A volatile oil obtained on oxidizing various essential oils, as anise, fennel, etc. Also called *anisic aldehyde.*

an'ise (an'iss) [G. *anison*, anise] (*anisum*). The dried ripe fruit of *Pimpinella anisum;* a mild aromatic carminative by virtue of its content of volatile oil. Also called *anise seed, aniseed.*

a. oil (*oleum anisi*). The volatile oil from anise or star anise; used as carminative in flatulent colic, as flavor, and for its expectorant action. Dose, 0.2–0.3 cc. (3–5 min.).

a. spirit (*spiritus anisi*). A 10% alcoholic solution used as stomachic and carminative. Dose, 1–4 cc. (15–60 min.) well diluted.

a. water (*aqua anisi*). A vehicle. Dose, 4–16 cc. (1–4 dr.).

star a. The fruit of *Illicium verum.* It yields a volatile oil. See *a.* oil.

an'i·seed. See *anise.*

an"is·ei·kom'e·ter (an"iss·eye·kom'i·tur) [G. *anisos*, unequal; *eikōn*, image; *metron*, a measure]. A device for measuring the inequality of size, when the two retinal images differ. Also called *eikonometer.*

an"i·sei·ko'ni·a [*anisos; eikōn*]. A condition in which the image seen by one eye is different from that seen by the other. See iseikonic *lens.* Also spelled *anisokonia.* —**aniseikon'ic,** *adj.*

meridional a. That form in which one image is larger than the other in one meridian.

overall a. That type in which one image is larger than the other in all meridians.

a·nis'ic ac'id (a·niss'ick, a·nigh'sick). $CH_3O.C_6H_4.COOH$. *p*-Methoxybenzoic acid. A crystalline acid obtainable from anise and fennel; has been used as an antiseptic, antipyretic, and antirheumatic.

an·i'so-, an'i·so-, anis- [*anisos*]. A combining form denoting *unequal, unsymmetrical, dissimilar.*

an·i"so·chro·ma'si·a (an·eye"so·kro·may'zhuh, ·zee·uh, an"i·so·) [*anisos;* G. *chrōma*, color]. A variation in the color of erythrocytes in which only the peripheral zone of the cell is colored. Occurs as a result of iron deficiency in certain types of anemia.

an·i"so·chro'mi·a [*anisos; chrōma*]. 1. Variation in the intensity of staining of erythrocytes; due to differences in hemoglobin content. 2. See *heterochromia.* —**anisochromic, anisochromat'ic,** *adj.*

an·i"so·co'ri·a [*anisos;* G. *korē*, pupil]. Inequality in the diameter of the pupils.

an·i"so·cy·to'sis (a·nigh"so·sigh·to'sis, an"i·so·) [*anisos;* G. *kytos*, cell; *-ōsis*, condition]. Inequality in the size of the erythrocytes.

an·i"so·dac'ty·lous [*anisos;* G. *daktylos*, finger]. With unequal digits. —**anisodactylus,** *n.*

an·i'so·dont [*anisos;* G. *odous*, tooth]. Possessing irregular teeth of unequal length.

an·i"so·ga·mete' (a·nigh"so·ga·meet', ·gam'eet, an"i·so·) [*anisos;* G. *gametē*, wife, *gametēs*, husband, from *gamein*, to marry]. A macrogamete or a microgamete.

an"i·sog'a·my [*anisos;* G. *gamos*, marriage]. The conjugation of gametes having unequal size but the same general morphology. See *isogamous.* —**anisogamous,** *adj.*

an"i·sog'na·thous [*anisos;* G. *gnathos*, jaw]. Having jaws which do not match, one being considerably wider than the other, especially in the molar region.

an"i·so·gyn"e·co·mas'ti·a. See under *gynecomastia.*

an'i·sole. $C_6H_5.O.CH_3$. Methyl phenyl ether, a colorless, ethereal-smelling liquid used in perfume, in the manufacture of chemicals, and for destruction of vermin.

an·i"so·me'li·a [*anisos;* G. *melos*, limb]. An inequality between corresponding limbs.—**anisom'elous,** *adj.*

an·i"so·me'ri·a [*anisos;* G. *meros*, part]. Irregularity between the successive segments of organs or parts. —**anisomer'ic,** *adj.*

an·i"so·me·tro'pi·a [*anisos;* G. *metron*, a measure; *ōps*, eye]. A difference in the refraction of the two eyes. —**anisometrop'ic,** *adj.;* **anisomet'rope,** *n.*

a·nis"o·my'cin. An antibiotic substance isolated from cultures of two different species of *Streptomyces*, active, in vitro, against *Trichomonas vaginalis* and *Endamoeba histolytica.* See *flagecidin.*

an″i·so′pi·a [*anisos; ōps*]. See *anisometropia.*

an″i·so·sphyg′mi·a [*anisos;* G. *sphygmos,* pulse]. Inequality of the pulses in symmetrical vessels, as the two radial or dorsalis pedis arteries.

an″i·sos·then′ic [*anisos;* G. *sthenos,* strength]. Not of equal power, said of pairs of muscles.

an·i″so·ton′ic [*anisos;* G. *tonos,* tension]. Denoting unequal osmotic pressure.

an″i·sot′ro·py [*anisos;* G. *tropē,* a turning]. 1. The quality of being doubly refractive or unequally refractive in different directions; or of being unequally responsive to external influences. 2. *In biology,* variation in irritability in different parts or organs. 3. In an ovum, possession of a predetermined axis or axes. —**anisotrop′ic,** *adj.*

a·ni′sum. See *anise.*

an″i·su′ri·a [*anisos;* G. *ouron,* urine]. A condition characterized by alternate polyuria and oliguria.

a″ni·trog′e·nous (ay″nigh·trodj′i·nus, a·nigh·, an″-eye·) [G. *a-,* not; *nitron,* sodium bicarbonate; *genesthai,* from *gignesthai,* to be produced]. Nonnitrogenous.

An·kis′tro·don. See *Agkistrodon.*

an′kle [AS. *anclēo*]. The joint between the leg and the foot. It is a ginglymus joint, with four ligaments: anterior, posterior, medial, and lateral. See Table of Joints and Ligaments in the Appendix.

a. mortise. The space in the ankle joint, between the lateral and medial malleoli, occupied by the talus.

tailor's a. A ganglion or abnormal bursa over the lateral malleolus in tailors, due to pressure from sitting on the floor with crossed legs.

an′ky·lo- (ang′ki·lo-), **an′kyl-** [G. *agkylos,* crooked]. A combining form denoting *crooked* or *crookedness, bent; adhesion* or *growing together of parts.*

an″ky·lo·bleph′a·ron [*agkylos;* G. *blepharon,* eyelid]. The adhesion of the ciliary edges of the eyelids to each other.

an″ky·lo·chei′li·a, an″ky·lo·chi′li·a (ang″ki·lo-kigh′lee·uh) [*agkylos;* G. *cheilos,* lip]. Adhesion of the lips to each other.

an″ky·lo·col′pos, an″ky·lo·kol′pos [*agkylos;* G. *kolpos,* vagina]. Atresia of the vagina or the vulva.

an″ky·lo·dac·tyl′i·a [*agkylos;* G. *daktylos,* finger]. A deformity resulting from the adhesion of fingers or toes to one another.

an″ky·lo·don′ti·a [*agkylos;* G. *odous,* tooth]. Fusion of the dental roots. See *concrescence.*

an″ky·lo·glos′si·a [*agkylos;* G. *glōssa,* tongue]. Tongue-tie.

an″ky·lo·kol′pos. See *ankylocolpos.*

an′ky·losed [ang′kil·ohzd, ·ohst) [G. *agkylōsis,* stiffening of joints]. Stiff; firmly united; bound down with adhesions; designating a joint immobilized by some pathologic or operative process within or outside the capsule. —**ankylose,** *v.t., v.i.*

an″ky·lo′sis [*agkylōsis*]. Stiffness or fixation of a joint. —**an′kylose,** *v.t., v.i.;* **an′kylosed,** *adj.*

bony a. Complete fixation of a joint due to fusion of the bones. Also called *true a.*

capsular a. That due to cicatricial thickening or shortening of the joint capsule.

congenital fibrous a. Fibrosis affecting many of the joints; due to a variety of causes manifested as clubfoot, extension of knees and ankles.

extracapsular a. That due to rigidity of the parts external to the joint; such as interference resulting from bony block, adhesions of tendons and tendon sheaths, contractures due to muscles, scars, or thickening of skin from scleroderma. Also called *false a., spurious a.*

fibrous a. That due to fibrosis in the joint capsule or fibrous adhesions between the joint surfaces.

intracapsular a. That due to rigidity of structures within the joints.

ligamentous a. See fibrous *a.*

operative a. Arthrodesis.

partial a. That producing limitation of joint motion but not complete fixation.

tooth a. Fixation of the joint formed by a tooth and the alveolus. See *synostosis, concrescence.*

an″ky·los″to·mi′a·sis. See *ancylostomiasis.*

An″ky·los′to·mum [G. *agkylos,* crooked; *stoma,* mouth]. Old term for a genus of nematode worms.

A. americanum. See *Necator americanus.*

A. duodenale. See *Ancylostoma duodenale.*

an′ky·lo·tome (ang′kil·o·tome, ang·kil′o·) [*agkylos; tomos,* cutting]. 1. A knife for operating on tongue tie. 2. Any curved knife.

an″ky·lot′o·my [*agkylos;* G. *tomē,* a cutting]. An operation for the relief of tongue-tie.

an′la·ge (ahn′lah·guh) [Ger., arrangement]. 1. A rudiment; the indifferent embryonic cells or tissue from which an organ or part develops. Syn., *primordium, blastema.* 2. *In genetics,* the hereditary predisposition for a given trait (such as a talent or disorder) or even for the entire genotype of an individual.

embryonic a. The germ or embryonic disk.

vesicourethral a. That part of the urogenital tube, cephalad to the opening of the mesonephric ducts, which forms the urinary bladder and primary urethra. Syn., *vesicourethral canal.*

An·nam′ ul′cer. See tropical *ulcer.*

an·nat′to (ah·nah′to, a·nat′o), **an·not′to** [Galibi *annoto,* name of the tree]. A coloring matter obtained from the pulp surrounding the seeds of the *Bixa orellana;* used to color plasters and butter.

an·neal′ [AS. *anǣlan,* from *an,* on; *ǣlan,* to kindle]. Temper; apply a regulated process of heating and subsequent cooling to glass or metal to render it less brittle.

an·nec′tent, an·nec′tant [L. *adnectere,* to bind to]. Linking, joining, or binding together, as annectent convolutions.

An·nel′i·da [L. *anellus,* a little ring]. A phylum of segmented worms including the earthworms and many other worms. —**an′nelid,** *n., adj.*

an′ne·lism [*anellus*]. The state of being ringed; ringed structure.

an·not′to. See *annatto.*

An″nu·la′ta [*L. annulatus,* ringed]. Old name for the phylum Annelida.

an′nu·late [L. *anulus,* ring]. 1. Characterized by, made up of, or surrounded by, rings. 2. Pertaining to the Annelida.

an′nu·late. One of the Annelida.

an′nu·lose [*anulus*]. Possessing rings.

an″nu·lo·spi′ral [*anulus;* L. *spira,* coil, twist]. Afferent nerve endings, with bandlike branches winding around the muscle fiber, found in muscle spindles.

an′nu·lus (pl. *annuli*) [*anulus*]. A ring of tissue about an opening. —**an′nular, annulate,** *adj.*

a. cruralis. See femoral *ring.*

a. femoris. See femoral *ring.*

a. fibrocartilagineus membranae tympani [BNA]. Margin of the tympanic membrane fixed in the tympanic sulcus.

a. fibrosus. (a) External part of an intervertebral disk. Also called *a. fibrosus fibrocartilaginis intervertebralis* [BNA]. (b) Firm connective tissue containing elastic fibers surrounding the atrioventricular (*a. fibrosus atrioventricularis*), aortic, and pulmonary openings of the heart. (c) Circular fibrous attachment of the tympanic membrane to the tympanic sulcus. Syn., *a. fibrocartilagineus membranae tympani* [BNA]. (d) Fibrous loop holding a tendon in place.

a. inguinalis abdominalis. See abdominal inguinal *ring.*

a. inguinalis subcutaneous (externus). BNA term for subcutaneous inguinal *ring*.

a. iridis major. BNA term for the *greater ring of the iris*. See under *ring*.

a. iridis minor. BNA term for the *lesser ring of the iris*. See under *ring*.

a. migrans. Disease of the tongue marked by red patches with yellow borders which spread over its dorsal surface and sometimes over its margins and under surface.

a. ovalis. Rounded or oval margin of the foramen ovale of the heart. Syn., *limbus fossae ovalis* [BNA].

a. tendineus communis [BNA]. Fibrous ring from which arise the four rectus muscles of the eye. It is attached to the dural sheath of the optic nerve and to the upper and medial margins of the optic foramen; it bridges the superior orbital fissure. Also called *ligament of Zinn, tendon of Zinn*.

a. tympanicus. BNA term for tympanic *ring*.

a. urethralis. BNA term for the urethral *ring*.

an′o- [G. *anō*, up, upper, upward]. A combining form meaning *up, upper, upward*.

a′no- [L. *anus*, anus]. A combining form signifying *anus* or *anal*.

AnOC Anodal opening contraction.

an″o·chro·ma′si·a (an″o·kro·may′zhuh, ·zee·uh) [G. *anō*, up; *chrōma*, color]. 1. Concentration of hemoglobin about the periphery of the red cells with the centers pale; a condition noted in certain types of anemia. 2. Absence of the usual staining reaction in a cell or tissue; achromasia.

a·no″ci·as·so″ci·a′tion, a·no″ci·a′tion [G. *a-*, not; L. *nocere*, to injure; *associare*, to join to]. An anesthetic procedure whereby surgical shock, fear, and postoperative neuroses are minimized greatly by excluding most of the painful and harmful stimuli. Syn., *anocithesia*.

a·no″ci·cep′tor. See *nociperceptor*.

a·no″ci·the′si·a (a·no″sith·ee′zhuh, ·zee·uh) [*a-; nocere;* G. *aisthēsis*, feeling]. Anociassociation.

a″no·coc·cyg′e·al (ay″no·cock·sidj′ee·ul, an″o·) [L. *anus*, anus; G. *kokkyx*, coccyx]. Pertaining to the anus and the coccyx.

an·o′dal clos′ure. The closure of an electric circuit with the anode placed in relation to the muscle or nerve which is to be affected. Abbreviated AC.

an·o′dal con·trac′tion. See under *contraction*.

an·o′dal o′pen·ing. The opening of an electric circuit at the anode, as in stimulating a nerve or muscle. Abbreviated AO.

an′ode [G. *anō*, up; *hodos*, way]. The positive pole of a galvanic battery or other electric device. Abbreviated, a., An. —**ano′dal,** *adj*.

an′ode block. An increase of the positive charge on the outside of a nerve membrane, which diminishes depolarization of the nerve membrane and blocks nerve impulse conduction.

an′ode ex·ci·ta′tion. Excitation of the nerve at the anode when the anode block is removed.

an″o·der′mous [G. *a-*, not; *derma*, skin]. Without the appearance of an epidermis.

a·nod′ic ox″i·da′tion. See under *oxidation*.

an·od′mi·a [*a-;* G. *odmē*, smell]. Anosmia.

an″o·don′ti·a [*a-;* G. *odous*, tooth]. Absence of the teeth.

a. vera. That due to failure of development of the tooth buds.

senile a. Absence of the teeth because of their removal, in older persons.

an″o·don′tous, an′o·dous [*a-; odous*]. Toothless.

an′o·dyne [*a-; odynē*, pain]. A medicine that eases pain. —**an′o·dyne,** *adj*.

an″o·dyn′i·a (an″o·din′ee·uh, ·dye′nee·uh) [*a-; odynē*]. Absence of pain. —**anod′ynous,** *adj*.

an″o·e′si·a (an″o·ee′zhuh, ·zee·uh) [G., want of sense]. Want of understanding; idiocy.

an·oes′trum. See *anestrum*.

an″o·et′ic [G. *anoēsia*, want of sense]. 1. Not entirely conscious; pertaining to the fringe of consciousness. 2. Affected with, or of the nature of, anoesia.

a·noi′a [G., want of understanding]. Idiocy; anoesia.

a·nom′a·lo·scope″ [G. *anōmalos*, irregular; *skopein*, to examine]. Instrument used for the detection of color blindness.

a·nom′a·ly [G. *anōmalia*, irregularity]. Any deviation from the usual; any organ or part existing in an abnormal form, structure, or location. For representative anomalies, see Table in the Appendix. See Plate 25. —**anomalous,** *adj*.

Pelger's a. See Karel *Pelger*.

a·no′mi·a [G. *a-*, not; *onoma*, name]. Loss of ability to name objects or to recognize names, usually associated with a hemianopsia. Also called *optic aphasia*.

an·o′mous [*a-;* G. *ōmos*, the shoulder]. Without shoulders.

an″o·nych′i·a (an″o·nick′ee·uh) [*a-;* G. *onyx*, nail]. Absence of the nails.

a·non′y·ma [*a-;* G. *onyma*, name]. The innominate artery.

an″o·op′si·a [G. *anō*, upward; *opsis*, vision]. Strabismus in which the eye is turned upward.

a″no·per″i·ne′al [L. *anus*, anus; G. *perineos*, space between the anus and scrotum]. Relating to the anus and the perineum.

A·noph′e·les (a·nof′i·leez) [G. *anōphelēs*, harmful]. A genus of mosquitoes belonging to the family Culicidae. They alone transmit malaria and are important vectors of dengue and filariasis and may transmit yellow fever.

A. albimanus. A species of mosquito native to tropical America, characterized by white hind feet; a common malarial vector.

A. argyritarsis. A South American vector of malaria.

A. crucians. A species carrying the malaria parasite; infrequently molests man.

A. culicifacies. A species common to Arabia, India, and Siam. The most important vector of malaria in India.

A. darlingi. A species from Brazil and British Guiana. A domestic species; it is highly androphilous.

A. gambiae. A South African and Brazilian species which transmits a very virulent type of malaria.

A. hyrcanus. A species found from South Europe to China and Japan. Important transmitter of malaria and filariasis.

A. maculipennis. The type species of this genus, found throughout Europe and many other parts of the world; it is an active vector of malaria.

A. quadrimaculatus. A species which serves as the chief vector of human malaria in the United States.

an″o·phel′i·cide [*anōphelēs;* L. *caedere*, to kill]. An agent which is destructive to anopheles mosquitoes.

an″o·phel′i·fuge [*anōphelēs;* L. *fugare*, to put to flight]. An agent which prevents the bite or attack of anopheles mosquitoes.

A·noph″e·li′ni (a·nof″i·lye′nigh) [*anōphelēs*]. A tribe of the subfamily Culicinae of mosquitoes, including three genera, of which *Anopheles* is important as a vector of malaria.

an″o·pho′ri·a [G. *anò*, upward; *pherein*, to bear]. Anotropia.

an″oph·thal′mi·a [G. *a-*, not; *ophthalmos*, eye]. Anophthalmos.

an″oph·thal′mos [*a-; ophthalmos*]. 1. Congenital absence of the eyes. 2. A person born without eyes.

an·o′pi·a [*a-;* G. *ōps*, eye]. 1. Absence of sight, especially that due to defect of the eyes. 2. Anoopsia.

a′no·plas·ty [L. *anus*, anus; G. *plassein*, to form]. Plastic surgery or repair of the anus or anal canal.

An″o·plu′ra [NL., from G. *anoplos*, unarmed]. An order of the Insecta; parasitic, sucking insects without wings; lice.

an·op′si·a [G. *a-*, not; *opsis*, sight]. 1. Failure to use visual capacity. 2. Upward strabismus; anoopsia.

an·or′chism (an·or′kiz·um, an′or·), **an·or′chi·a** (an·or′kee·uh), **an·or′chid·ism** (an·or′ki·diz·um) [*a-;* G. *orchis*, testis]. Absence of the testes. —**anorchous,** *adj.*

an·or′chus (an·or′kus) [*a-; orchis*]. A person showing congenital absence of the testes.

a″no·rec′tal [L. *anus*, anus; *rectus*, straight]. Pertaining to the anus and the rectum. —**anorec′tum,** *n.*

a″no·rec″to·plas′ty. Surgical repair or reconstruction of the anus and rectum.

an″o·rex′i·a [G. *a-*, not; *orexis*, appetite]. Absence of appetite. —**anorec′tic, anorec′tous,** *adj.*

a. nervosa. A hysterical aversion to food, which may lead to serious malnutrition.

false a. A condition found in hysteria, in which the patient apparently eats nothing, but consumes large quantities of food in secret.

an·or·gas′my (an·or·gaz′mee) [*a-;* G. *orgasmos*, swelling]. A condition, usually psychic, in which there is a failure to reach a climax during coitus.

an″or·thog′ra·phy [*a-;* G. *orthos*, straight; *graphein*, to write]. Incapacity to write correctly; motor agraphia.

an″or·tho′pi·a [*a-; orthos;* G. *ōps*, eye]. 1. A defect in vision in which straight lines do not seem straight, and parallelism or symmetry is not properly perceived. 2. Squinting; obliquity of vision. See *strabismus.*

an″or·tho′sis [*a-;* G. *orthōsis*, a making straight]. Absence or defect of erectility. *Obs.*

a′no·scope [L. *anus*, anus; G. *skopein*, to examine]. Instrument for examining the rectum and anal canal. —**anos′copy,** *n.*

an·os′mi·a (an·oz′mee·uh, an·oss′mee·uh) [G. *a-*, not; *osmē*, smell]. Absence of the sense of smell. In type, it is *afferent* when due to the loss of conductivity of the olfactory nerves; *central*, if due to cerebral disease; *organic*, if due to disease of the nasal olfactory membrane; *peripheral*, if due to disease of the peripheral ends of the olfactory nerves. —**anosmic, anosmat′ic,** *adj.*

an·o″sog·no′si·a (an·o″sog·no′zhuh, ·zee·uh, ·shuh, ·see·uh) [*a-;* G. *nosos*, disease; *gnōsis*, knowledge]. Inability on the part of the patient to recognize that he is hemiplegic.

a″no·spi′nal [L. *anus*, anus; *spina*, spine]. Relating to the anus and the spinal cord.

an″os·to′sis [G. *a-*, not; *osteon*, bone; *-ōsis*, condition]. Defective development of bone.

an·o′ti·a (an·o′shuh, ·shee·uh) [*a-;* G. *ous*, ear]. Congenital absence of the pinnae or external ears. See *anotus.*

an″o·tro′pi·a [G. *anō*, upward; *trepein*, to turn]. The tendency of one eye to latent upward deviation. Syn., *anophoria.*

an·o′tus [G. *a-*, not; *ous*, ear]. A person showing congenital absence of the ears. —**anotous,** *adj.*

a″no·ves′i·cal [L. *anus*, anus; *vesica*, the bladder]. Pertaining conjointly to the anus and urinary bladder.

an·ov′u·lar (an·ov′yoo·lur), **an·o′vu·la·to″ry** (an.-ov′yoo·) [G. *a-*, not; L. *ovum*, egg]. Not associated with ovulation, applied to menstruation. See anovular *menstruation.*

an″ox·e′mi·a [*a-;* G. *oxys*, sharp; *haima*, blood]. A lack of oxygen in the blood from insufficient aeration due to high elevation, low partial pressure of oxygen in anesthesia, cardiac failure, or strangling.

an·ox′i·a [*a-; oxys*]. 1. Absence of oxygen: a condition incompatible with many forms of life. 2. Failure of tissue either to receive or to utilize an adequate amount of oxygen: former term now more properly *hypoxia*, and classified into **anemic, anoxic, stagnant,** and **histotoxic anoxia.** 3. The disturbance of bodily and mental functions resulting from hypoxia. —**anox′ic,** *adj.*

an′sa (pl. *ansae*) [L., a handle]. A loop.

a. hypoglossi. A loop formed at the side of the neck by the junction of the descendens hypoglossi and descendens cervicis nerves.

a. lenticularis. A bundle of efferent fibers from the globus pallidus, passing around the medial border of the internal capsule to join the fasciculus lenticularis. Syn., *a. lentiformis, lenticular loop.*

a. lentiformis. See *a.* lenticularis.

a. peduncularis. Fibers from the medial and basal surface of the thalamus passing below the lenticular nucleus and radiating to the cortex of the temporal lobe and insula.

a. sacralis. One joining the coccygeal ganglion with the sympathetic trunks of the two sides.

a. subclavia. A loop, between the inferior and middle cervical ganglions of the sympathetic chain, passing around the subclavian artery. Also called *a. of Vieussens.*

a. vitellina. See vitelline *a.*

cervical a. One of the intercommunicating branches between the anterior rami of the first four cervical nerves.

supramaxillary a. One of the communications between the anterior and posterior superior alveolar nerves.

vitelline a. Yolk-sac vein uniting with the umbilical vein in young embryos. Syn., *a. vitellina.*

ansadol. A trade-mark for salicylanilide, the substance being supplied in ointment form for use as a fungicide.

an′sae (an′see). Plural of ansa.

an′sate [L. *ansatus*, from *ansa*, handle]. Having a handle; handle-shaped; loop-shaped, ansiform.

an′ser·ine [L. *anser*, a goose]. (an′sur·yne, ·in) Pertaining to or like a goose.

an′ser·ine. (an′sur·een, ·in) $C_{10}H_{16}N_4O_3$; N-methylcarnosine; a dipeptide found in muscles of birds, reptiles, and fishes.

an′si·form [L. *ansa*, a handle; *forma*, shape]. Loop-shaped; ansate.

ansolysen. Trade-mark for pentamethylene-1:5-bis-(1′-methylpyrrolidinium bitartrate), known also by the generic name *pentolinium bitartrate,* a ganglionic blocking agent used in the management of hypertension.

ant-. See *anti-.*

antabuse. Trade-mark for tetraethylthiuram disulfide, used in the treatment of alcoholism.

ant·ac′id [G. *anti*, against; L. *acidus*, sour]. A substance which neutralizes acids or relieves acidity.

an·tag′o·nism [G. *antagōnizesthai*, to struggle against]. Opposition; the mutually opposing or resisting action seen between organisms (antibiosis), muscles, functions, diseases, and drugs; or between drugs and functions; or drugs and diseases. —**antagonis′tic,** *adj.*

bacterial a. The adverse effect produced by one species of microorganism upon the growth and development of another, as the action of actinomycosis on many Gram-positive organisms.

an·tag′o·nist [G. *antagōnistēs*, from *anti*, against, *agōn*, struggle]. 1. A drug that neutralizes the effects of another. 2. *In anatomy*, a muscle that acts in opposition to another. 3. *In dentistry*, a tooth that meets one in the opposing dental arch during occlusion or mastication.

associated a. One of two muscles or groups of muscles which pull in almost opposite directions. When they contract simultaneously, the affected part moves in a path between their divergent lines of action.

ant·al′ka·line [*anti;* Ar. *al-qili*, ashes of saltwort]. An agent which neutralizes alkalies. —**ant·al′ka·line,** *adj.*

ant″aph·ro·dis′i·ac (ant″af·ro·diz′ee·ack) [*anti;* G. *aphrodisiakos*, sexual]. An agent that lessens sexual desire; an anaphrodisiac. —**antaphrodis′iac,** *adj.*

an·taz′o·line hy″dro·chlo′ride. Generic name for the hydrochloride salt of the antihistaminic substance 2-(N-benzylanilinomethyl)-2-imidazoline hydrochloride, preparations of which are supplied under the trade-marked name *antistine hydrochloride.*

an′te- [L., before]. A prefix denoting *before, preceding, in front of, prior to, anterior to.*

an″te·au′ral [*ante;* L. *auris*, ear]. In front of the ear.

an″te·bra′chi·um. See *antibrachium.*

an′te ci′bum [L.]. Before meals. Abbreviated, a. c.; used in prescriptions.

an″te·cu′bi·tal [*ante;* L. *cubitum*, elbow]. Situated in front of the elbow.

an″te·cur′va·ture [*ante;* L. *curvare*, to bend]. A forward curvature.

an″te·flex′ion [*ante;* L. *flectere*, to bend]. A bending forward.

a. of the uterus. A condition in which the fundus of the uterus is bent excessively forward on the cervix.

an″te·hy·poph′y·sis (an″tee·high·pof′i·sis, ·hi-pof′i·sis) [*ante;* G. *hypophysis*, attachment underneath]. The anterior lobe of the pituitary, as differentiated from its posterior portion.

an″te mor′tem [L.]. Before death. —**ante-mortem,** *adj.*

an″te·na′ri·al [*ante;* L. *nares*, the nostrils]. Situated in front of the nostrils.

an″te·na′tal [*ante;* L. *natus*, born]. Occurring or existing before birth; prenatal.

an″te par′tum [L.]. Before delivery. —**ante-partum,** *adj.*

antergan. Trade-mark for the antihistaminic substance N-benzyl-N′, N′-dimethyl-N-phenylethylenediamine, commonly employed in the form of the hydrochloride salt.

an·te′ri·or [L., foremost, former]. Situated before or in front of; toward the ventral aspect of the body; noting the forward part of an organ. Abbreviated, a. —**anteriad, anteriorly,** *adv.*

an′ter·o-, anter- [*anterior*]. A combining form meaning *anterior, front, from front to.*

an″ter·o·dor′sal [*anterior;* L. *dorsum*, back]. *In embryology*, pertaining to the dorsal aspect of the head region.

an″ter·o·ex·ter′nal [*anterior;* L. *externus*, outward]. Situated in front to the outer side.

an′ter·o·grade″ [*anterior;* L. *gradi*, to go]. Proceeding forward.

an″ter·o·in·fe′ri·or [*anterior;* L. *inferior*, lower]. Situated in front and below.

an″ter·o·in·te′ri·or [*anterior;* L. *interior*, inner]. Located ventrally and internally.

an″ter·o·in·ter′nal [*anterior;* L. *internus*, inward]. Situated in front to the inner side.

an″ter·o·lat′er·al [*anterior;* L. *latus*, side]. In front and to one side; from the front to one side.

an″ter·o·me′di·an [*anterior;* L. *medius*, middle]. In front and toward the middle.

anteron. A proprietary gonadotropic extract from pregnant mares' serum.

an″ter·o·pa·ri′e·tal [*anterior;* L. *paries*, wall]. Forward and parietal, as the anteroparietal area of the cranium.

an″ter·o·pi·tu′i·tar·y [*anterior;* L. *pituita*, phlegm]. Referring to the anterior lobe of the pituitary gland.

an″ter·o·pos·te′ri·or [*anterior;* L. *posterior*, backward]. Extending from before backward; relating to both front and back.

an″ter·o·su·pe′ri·or [*anterior;* L. *superior*, upper]. Situated in front and above.

an″te·ver′sion [L. *ante*, before; *vertere*, to turn]. A tipping, tilting, or displacement forward of an organ or part, especially of the uterus. —**antevert′ed,** *adj.;* **antevert′,** *v.t., v.i.*

anthallan. Trade-mark for the antihistaminic substance 3-dibutylaminomethyl-4,5,6-trihydroxy-1-isobenzofuranone.

ant·he′lix, an″ti·he′lix [*anti; helix*, coil]. The curved ridge of the pinna just anterior to the helix and following through most of the course of the helix.

ant″hel·min′tic, an″thel·min′tic [G. *anti*, against; *helmins*, worm]. A remedy for the destruction or elimination of intestinal worms. —**ant″hel·min′tic, an″thel·min′tic,** *adj.*

an′thel·one. The principle or principles extractable from the mucosa of the small intestine (*enteroanthelone*) and from urine (*uroanthelone*) which exerts an anti-ulcer effect in Mann-Williamson dogs and has been used in the treatment of human peptic ulcer patients.

an·the′ma, an′the·ma (pl. *anthemata*) [G., from *anthein*, to bloom]. 1. An exanthema. 2. An elementary lesion of the skin.

an′the·mis [G., camomile]. English or Roman camomile. The flower heads of *Anthemis nobilis*, the properties of which are due to a volatile oil, anthemic acid, and a bitter principle. It has been used in coughs and spasmodic infantile complaints, and as a stomachic tonic. Dose, 2–4 Gm. (30–60 gr.).

ant″hem·or·rhag′ic (ant″hem·o·radj′ick) [G. *anti*, against; *haima*, blood; *rhēgnynai*, to burst]. Checking or preventing hemorrhage.

an′ther [G. *antheros*, flowery, blooming]. *In biology*, that part of the stamen which contains pollen.

anthiomaline. Trade-mark for antimony lithium thiomalate, approximately $Li_6C_{12}H_9O_{12}SbS_3$.-$9H_2O$, used for the treatment of filariasis, trypanosomiasis, lymphogranuloma, and schistosomiasis.

anthisan. A trade-mark for the antihistaminic substance pyrilamine maleate.

an′tho-, anth- [G. *anthos*, flower]. A combining form meaning *flower, floral, flowerlike.*

an″tho·cy·an′i·din. See *anthocyanin.*

an″tho·cy′a·nin. Any of a class of glycosides comprising the soluble coloring matter of blue, red, and violet flowers, and the reds and purples of autumn leaves. See *xanthophyll.*

An″tho·my′ia [*anthos;* G. *myia*, fly]. A genus of flies which, depositing their ova on food, especially on vegetable material, cause intestinal myiasis.

Anthony's method. See under *stain.*

an″tho·pho′bi·a [*anthos;* G. *phobos*, fear]. A morbid fear of flowers.

an′thra-, anthr- [G. *anthrax*, coal]. A combining form denoting *the presence of the anthracene nucleus.*

an″thra·ce′mi·a, an″thra·cae′mi·a [*anthrax;* G. *haima,* blood]. A disease due to the presence in the blood of *Bacillus anthracis;* woolsorter's disease; anthrax; splenic fever of animals.

an′thra·cene. $C_{14}H_{10}$. A colorless, solid hydrocarbon obtained by distillation from coal tar and other carbon compounds.

a. blue. See *alizarin* blue.

an′thra·co-, anthrac- [*anthrax*]. A combining form meaning *coal* or *carbuncle.*

an′thra·coid [*anthrax;* G. *eidos,* form]. Resembling carbon, anthrax, or the carbuncle (gem).

an″thra·co·ne·cro′sis [*anthrax;* G. *nekrōsis,* death]. Necrosis occurring in a focus of anthracosis. *Obs.*

an″thra·co·sil″i·co′sis [*anthrax;* L. *silex,* flint; G. *-ōsis,* condition]. Diffuse fibrosis of the lungs accompanied by black pigmentation, caused by the prolonged inhalation of dusts containing silicon dioxide and carbon; a form of pneumonoconiosis. Syn., *coal miner's disease, miner's phthisis, miner's asthma.*

an″thra·co′sis [*anthrax; -ōsis*]. Black pigmentation of the lungs associated with a mild degree of chronic inflammation; due to the inhalation of carbon dust. A form of pneumonoconiosis. —**anthracot′ic,** *adj.*

an″thra·gal′lol (an″thruh·gal′ole, ·ol, ·awl). $C_{14}H_8O_5$. A reaction product of benzoic, gallic, and sulfuric acids. It occurs as a dark-brown paste or orange-red acicular crystals, soluble in alcohol; used in dyeing. Syn., *trihydroxyanthraquinone.*

an″thra·glu·co′rhe·in. A glycoside found in rhubarb; used as a cathartic.

an′thra·lin. $C_{14}H_{10}O_3$; 1,8-dihydroxyanthranol, a crystalline, yellowish-brown powder, insoluble in water. It is used externally for treatment of various skin diseases. Syn., *dithranol.* See *cignolin.*

an″thra·nil′ic ac′id. $NH_2.C_6H_4.COOH$; *o*-aminobenzoic acid, first obtained from indigo, but synthesized in other ways; it is an important intermediate in many syntheses.

an′thra·nol. $C_{14}H_{10}O$; 9-hydroxyanthracene, derivatives of which are used medicinally. See *anthralin, anthrarobin.*

an″thra·pur′pu·rin. 1,2,8-Trihydroxyanthraquinone. Orange-colored needles used in the manufacture of dyes. See *purpurin.*

a. acetate. A fine, yellow, tasteless powder, sparingly soluble in alcohol; insoluble in water; used as aperient and laxative (it colors the urine red). Dose, 0.5 Gm. (7½ gr.). Also called *a. diacetate, purgatin, purgatol.*

an″thra·qui·none′ (an″thruh·kwi·nohn′, ·kwin′-ohn). $C_{14}H_8O_2$. A substance produced by oxidizing anthracene with HNO_3. Derivatives of it occur in aloe, cascara sagrada, rhubarb and senna and are responsible for the cathartic action.

an″thra·ro′bin. 3,4-Dihydroxyanthranol. Yellowish brown crystals used externally in alcoholic solution or as an ointment in skin diseases.

anthrasol. A proprietary, colorless, coal-tar preparation; used in the form of an ointment for pruritus and other skin affections.

an′thrax [G.]. 1. A carbuncle. 2. An acute infectious disease of cattle and sheep, transmissible to man and caused by *Bacillus anthracis.* Syn., *charbon, woolsorter's disease, malignant pustule, malignant a., milzbrand, ragpicker's disease, tanner's disease.* Also called *splenic fever.* See Plate 31.

a. polypeptide. A basic polypeptide of cellular origin isolated from fluids and tissues of species insusceptible to *Bacillus anthracis* and capable of killing this organism.

cerebral a. A complication of intestinal or pulmonary anthrax in which the organisms invade the brain. This form is marked by raging and violent delirium.

contagious a. See malignant *a.*

hemorrhoidal a. A contagious type of anthrax affecting the rectum of animals and marked by dark bloody evacuations.

malignant a. Infectious and fatal disease of sheep and cattle marked by ulceration or hard edema at the point of inoculation, followed by symptoms of general sepsis, prostration, and collapse. Transmissible to man. See *anthrax,* 2.

pulmonary a. The form usually called woolsorter's disease, acquired by inhalation of contaminated dust, resulting in pulmonary gangrene with grave symptoms of systemic infection, coughing, dyspnea, and prostration.

symptomatic a. An infection of cattle and sheep characterized by subcutaneous, emphysematous swellings and nodules, due to infection by *Clostridium feseri.* Also called *emphysematous a.*

an′throne. $C_{14}H_{10}O$; 9,10-dihydro-9-oxoanthracene, occurring in needlelike crystals: used in the determination of sugar in body fluids.

an″thro·pho′bi·a. See *anthropophobia.*

an′thro·po-, anthrop- [G. *anthrōpos,* a human being]. A combining form meaning *human being, man.*

an″thro·po·bi·ol′o·gy (an″thro·po·buy·ol′o·jee) [*anthrōpos;* G. *bios,* life; *logos,* word]. The biologic study of man and the anthropoid apes.

an″thro·po·gen′e·sis, an″thro·pog′e·ny (an″-thro·podj′i·nee) [*anthrōpos;* G. *genesis,* production]. The evolution and development of man, as a race (phylogenesis), and as an individual (ontogenesis). —**anthropogen′ic, anthropogenet′ic,** *adj.*

an′thro·poid [*anthrōpos;* G. *eidos,* form]. Pertaining to or resembling the primates, i.e., man, the apes, and the monkeys.

An″thro·poi′de·a [*anthrōpos; eidos*]. A suborder of Primates, including man, apes, and monkeys.

an″thro·pol′o·gy [*anthrōpos;* G. *logos,* word]. The science of man, in all of its ramifications, both physical and cultural.

criminal a. The study of man in relation to the habitual criminal, utilizing all of the measurements and identification data of anthropology; bertillonage. See A. *Bertillon.*

cultural a. The study of prehistoric and contemporary man in relation to his customs, technologies, his social, political and economic life, his religions, languages, folklores, and arts, and his adaptation to his own specific setting.

physical a. The study of prehistoric and contemporary man on a purely biological basis, including his organic growth, development, and degeneration, inheritance of body traits, the influences of environment, and his physical types and racial differences.

an″thro·pom′e·ter [*anthrōpos;* G. *metron,* a measure]. A somatometric caliper used in taking the larger measurements of the human body. —**anthropom′etrist,** *n.*

an″thro·pom′e·try [*anthrōpos; metron*]. The scientific measurement of the human body, its various parts, and the skeleton. The metric data thus obtained are used extensively in serial and comparative studies and in systems of identification.

an″thro·po·mor′phic [*anthrōpos;* G. *morphē,* form]. Manlike; having a human form.

an″thro·poph′a·gy [*anthrōpos;* G. *phagein,* to eat]. 1. Cannibalism. 2. Sexual perversion leading to rape, mutilation, and cannibalism.

an″thro·po·phil′ic [*anthrōpos;* G. *philein,* to love]. Showing a preference for human beings over animals; androphilous; man-loving.

an″thro·po·pho′bi·a [*anthrōpos;* G. *phobos*, fear]. Morbid fear of people or society.

an″thro·po·so″ma·tol′o·gy [*anthrōpos;* G. *sōma*, body; *logos*, word]. The science of the development, structure, and functions of the human body.

ant″hyp·not′ic [G. *anti*, against; *hypnos*, sleep]. An agent that tends to induce wakefulness or prevent sleep. —**ant″hyp·not′ic,** *adj.*

an′ti-, ant- [G.]. A prefix meaning *against, in return, opposed to, instead, counter.*

an″ti·ac′id. Antacid.

an″ti·ag·glu′ti·nin [*anti;* L. *agglutinare*, to glue]. A substance having the power of neutralizing the corresponding agglutinin.

an″ti·ag·gres′sin [*anti;* L. *aggressus*, from *aggredi*, to attack]. An antibody which neutralizes an aggressin or spreading agent produced by microorganisms.

an″ti·al′bu·mate, an″ti·al·bu′mi·nate. A product resulting from the incomplete digestion of albumin formed during gastric digestion. Syn., *parapeptone.*

an″ti·al·bu′min (an″tee·al·bew′min, ·al′bew·min) [*anti;* L. *albus*, white]. A poorly defined product of partial digestion of albumin.

an″ti·a·lex′in. See *anticomplement.*

an″ti·am″bo·cep′tor. See *antiantibody.*

an″ti·am′yl·ase (an″tee·am′i·lace, ·laze). A substance which neutralizes the action of amylase.

an″ti·an″a·phy·lax′is [*anti;* G. *ana*, backward; *phylaxis*, a watching, guarding]. A condition in which a sensitized animal (guinea pig) is refractory to anaphylaxis because of a saturation or exhaustion of fixed antibodies, or because of an excess of free antibodies which prevents the antigen from making contact with the fixed antibodies.

an″ti·a·ne′mi·a prin′ci·ple. A substance counteracting or preventing anemia; usually the specific principle in liver used in treating pernicious anemia.

an″ti·a·ne′mic [*anti;* G. *a-*, not; *haima*, blood]. A substance which relieves anemia. See antianemia *factor.* —**an″ti·a·ne′mic,** *adj.*

an″ti·an′thrax pol″y·pep′tide. See *anthrax polypeptide.*

an″ti·an′ti·bod″y [*anti; anti;* AS. *bodig*]. An antibody to an antibody.

an″ti·ar″ach·nol′y·sin (an″tee·ar″ack·nol′i·sin) [*anti;* G. *arachnē*, spider; *lysis*, a loosing]. An antivenin counteracting spider venom.

an′ti·a·rin (an′tee·uh·rin, an·tee′uh·rin, an″tee-air′in). $C_{14}H_{20}O_5.2H_2O$. An alkaloid from the gum-resinous exudate known as upas antiar, obtained from the East Indian tree *Antiaris toxicaria* or deadly upas tree. It is a violent poison, causing vomiting, evacuation, irregular heart action, prostration, and death.

an″ti·a′ris. An arrow poison produced from the resinous exudate of the upas tree of the East Indies. Its action is similar to that of curare.

an″ti·ar·thrit′ic [*anti;* G. *arthron*, joint; *-itis*, inflammation]. Tending to relieve or cure arthritis. —**an″ti·ar·thrit′ic,** *n.*

an″ti·bac·te′ri·al [*anti;* G. *baktērion*, little staff]. Preventing the growth of bacteria or destroying bacteria by physical and chemical agents. —**an″ti·bac·te′ri·al,** *n.*

an″ti·bi·o′sis (an″ti·buy·o′sis) [*anti;* G. *bios*, life; *-ōsis*, condition]. An association between two or more organisms which is harmful to one of them; the opposite of symbiosis.

an″ti·bi·ot′ic (an″ti·buy·ot′ick) [*anti; bios*]. 1. Pertaining to antibiosis. 2. Tending to destroy life; designating the extracts of certain organisms, or their synthetic equivalents, employed against infections caused by other organisms—that most commonly used is penicillin.

an″ti·bi·ot′ic. An antibiotic substance.

broad-spectrum a. One effective against a variety of microorganisms.

an″ti·bi′o·tin. See *avidin.*

an″ti·black′out″ suit. A flying suit in which the limbs may be compressed by inflating airtight chambers. This prevents the blackout ensuing from an undue amount of blood leaving the brain and entering the extremities during rapid deceleration in aerial flight.

an″ti·blas′tic [*anti;* G. *blastos*, germ]. Antagonistic to bacterial growth.

an′ti·bod″y [*anti;* AS. *bodig*]. One of a class of substances, natural or induced by exposure to an antigen, which have the capacity to react as agglutinins, lysins, precipitins, etc., with the specific or related antigens. In the serum, they are intimately associated with certain globulin fractions. Also see *antigen.* For specific antibodies (agglutinins) in blood, see under *blood group.*

anaphylactic a. The antibody concerned in anaphylaxis. Also called *anaphylactin.*

complete antibodies. *In hematology*, bivalent antibodies which usually occur early in the course of immunization. They are relatively thermolabile, are active in saline as well as plasma, and readily clump erythrocytes carrying the corresponding specific antigen. Also called *first-order antibodies* or *agglutinins.*

heterophile a. Antibody to the heterophile antigen. This antibody (agglutinin), found in the serum of patients with infectious mononucleosis, agglutinates sheep red cells often in high titers.

incomplete antibodies. *In hematology*, the forms in which antibodies of any specificity may occur. They tend to appear late in the course of immunization, are relatively thermolabile and combine specifically (in saline) with the erythrocytes carrying the specific antigens but without clumping of these cells. In media containing plasma or albumin clumping occurs. Syn. *blocking, hyperimmune, albumin-acting, second-order*, or *univalent antibodies; glutinins, agglutinoids.*

inhibiting a. A thermostable antibody sometimes produced in both allergic (atopic) and nonallergic individuals as a response to specific immunization which is believed to prevent the union of antigen (atopen, allergen) and reagin. Clinical tolerance in allergy following various desensitizing procedures may depend upon the titer of this antibody.

natural a. *In hematology*, an isoagglutinin.

sensitizing a. An anaphylactic antibody.

third-order a. Cryptagglutinoid.

an″ti·bra′chi·um (an″ti·bray′kee·um, ·brack′-ee·um) [BNA] [L. *anti*, opposed; *brachium*, arm]. The forearm. —**antibrachial,** *adj.*

an″ti·car·cin′o·gen [G. *anti*, against; *karkinos*, cancer; *genesthai*, from *gignesthai*, to be produced]. A substance or agent which opposes the action of carcinogens.

an″ti·car′i·ous (an″ti·kair′ee·us) [*anti;* L. *caries*, decay]. Inhibiting or preventing dental caries.

an″ti·cat′a·lyst, an″ti·cat′a·lyz·er [*anti;* G. *katalyein*, to dissolve]. Any substance which retards the action of a catalyst by acting directly upon it.

an″ti·ca·thex′is [*anti;* G. *kathexis*, from *katechein*, to hold]. A condition in which an emotional charge is released from one impulse and shifted to an impulse of an opposite nature. Also called *counterinvestment.*

an″ti·cath′ode, an″ti·kath′ode [*anti;* G. *kathodos*, descent]. The metal plate or target of a Crookes or x-ray tube. It is situated opposite the cathode and is struck by the cathode rays, giving rise to the x-rays.

an″ti·ceph′a·lin [*anti;* G. *kephalē*, head]. An inhibitor in plasma of thromboplastin, obtained from the hemophiliac in a form several times more active than normal.

an″ti·chei·rot′o·nus, an″ti·chi·rot′o·nous (an″-ti·kigh·rot′o·nus) [G. *anticheir*, thumb; *tonos*, tension]. Forcible and steady inflexion of the thumb, seen at times in or before attacks of epilepsy.

an′ti·chlor. Sodium thiosulfate.

an″ti·chol·in·er′gic. Pertaining to, designating, or caused by a cholinergic blocking agent.

an″ti·cho″lin·es′ter·ase (an″ti·ko″lin·es′tur·ace, ·aze). A substance which inhibits the enzyme activity of cholinesterase. Eserine (physostigmine) is a powerful anticholinesterase.

an″ti·chro·mat′ic re·spons′es. See under *response.*

an″ti·co·ag′u·lant [*anti;* L. *coagulare*, to cause a fluid to curdle]. Opposed to or preventive of coagulation. —**anticoag′ulant,** *n.;* **anticoag′ulative,** *adj.*

an″ti·col·la·gen·ase′. An antibody capable of neutralizing collagenase found in the commercial preparations of *Clostridium perfringens* antitoxin.

an″ti·com′ple·ment [*anti;* L. *complementum*, complement]. A substance having the capacity to neutralize, inhibit, or destroy a complement; antialexin. —**anticomplemen′tary,** *adj.*

an″ti·con·cep′tive [*anti;* L. *concipere*, to conceive]. Contraceptive.

an″ti·con·cus′sion plug. A device fitted into the external auditory meatus and worn in battle during artillery fire to protect the ears from injury.

an″ti·con·vul′sive [*anti;* L. *convulsus*, from *convellere*, to shake]. An agent which arrests or prevents convulsions. —**anticonvul′sive,** *adj.*

an′ti·cus [L., in front]. Anterior; in front of. *O.T.*

an″ti·cu′tin. Any substance capable of specifically inhibiting or reducing the capacity of an excitant to produce reaction in the sensitive skin, or of specifically inhibiting or reducing the capacity of the skin to react to an excitant.

an″ti·di″a·bet′ic [G. *anti*, against; *diabētēs*, siphon]. Efficient against diabetes, as the antidiabetic hormone, insulin. —**antidiabet′ic,** *n.*

an″ti·di″ar·rhe′al [*anti;* G. *diarrhein*, to flow through]. Preventing or overcoming diarrhea.

an″ti·di″u·ret′ic [*anti;* G. *diourētikos*, from *diourein*, to pass urine]. Opposing or preventing excretion of urine. —**antidiure′sis,** *n.;* **antidiuret′ic,** *n.*

an′ti·dote [G. *antidotos*, from *anti; didonai*, to give]. Any agent administered to prevent or counteract the action of a poison. —**an′tidotal,** *adj.*

chemical a. One that changes the chemical nature of the poison so that it becomes an insoluble or harmless compound.

mechanical a. An agent which prevents absorption of the poison.

physiologic a. One that counteracts the physiologic effects of a poison.

an″ti·drom′ic [*anti;* G. *dromos*, a running]. Conducting nerve impulses in a direction opposite to the normal, as when vasodilatation follows peripheral stimulation of an afferent nerve, or dispatching impulses to the spinal cord via the anterior roots by experimental stimulation.

an″ti·dys″en·ter′ic [*anti;* G. *dysenteria*, from *dys-*, difficult; *enteron*, intestine]. A remedy for or preventive of dysentery. —**antidysenter′ic.** *adj.*

an″ti·e·met′ic [*anti;* G. *emetikos*, provoking sickness]. Relieving or preventing nausea and vomiting. —**antiemet′ic,** *n.*

an″ti·en′zyme. 1. A substance of enzymatic nature which exerts a specific inhibiting action upon another enzyme. 2. An immune body formed by the injection of an enzyme into an animal; it acts as a defense against the injected enzyme.

an″ti·fe′brile (an″ti·fee′bril, ·feb′ril) [*anti;* L. *febris*, fever]. Relieving or reducing fever.

antifebrin. A proprietary name for acetanilid.

an″ti·fer′ment [*anti;* L. *fermentum*, leaven]. 1. An agent that prevents fermentation. 2. Any substance which counteracts an enzyme. Syn., *antienzyme.* —**antiferment′ative,** *adj.*

an″ti·fi″bri·nol′y·sin. The inhibitors of plasmin in serum or plasma; formerly, antistreptokinase.

an″ti·fi·bro″ma·to·gen′ic (·figh·bro″muh·to·jen′-ick) [*anti;* L. *fibra*, fiber; G. *-ōma*, tumor; *genesthai*, from *gignesthai*, to be produced]. Acting to prevent the formation of fibromas.

an″ti-flash′ gear. Equipment worn by naval gun crews for protection against flash burns.

antiformin. Trade name for a strongly alkaline solution of sodium hypochlorite used as a disinfectant and as an aid in the recognition of tubercle bacilli in sputum. It liquefies the sputum and dissolves other bacteria.

antifungin. A brand of magnesium borate. A white powder, slightly soluble in water; used as a preservative and gargle.

an″ti·ga·lac′tic [*anti;* G. *gala*, milk]. A drug or agent that lessens the flow of milk. —**antigalac′tic,** *adj.*

an′ti·gen [*anti;* G. *genesthai*, from *gignesthai*, to be produced]. 1. Any substance which stimulates the production of antibodies or reacts with them. A **complete antigen** performs both functions. An **incomplete antigen** (**hapten,** or **partial antigen**) is that part of an antigenic complex responsible for its specificity. Separate from the complex, it reacts with antibodies in vitro, but cannot stimulate their production. 2. A lipoid substance, incapable of eliciting antibodies, employed in syphilis tests; as **beef heart antigen,** that obtained from beef heart by alcoholic extraction. **Acetone-insoluble antigen** is that part of beef heart antigen insoluble in acetone; redissolved in alcohol and reinforced by the addition of cholesterol, it is known as **cholesterinized antigen.** Also see *antibody.* —**an·ti·gen′ic,** *adj.*

a. A A group of red blood cell antigens (A_1, A_2, etc.) occurring in types A and AB blood.

a. B The red blood cell antigen occurring in types B and AB blood.

artificial a. (a) A conjugated antigen prepared by compounding an incomplete antigen with a protein, as an azoprotein. (b) An antigen, the specificity of which has been altered through physical or chemical treatment, as through denaturation, nitration, or oxidation.

Boivin a. A nondialyzable, toxic complex consisting of a specific polysaccharide, fatty acids, phosphoric and acetic acid.

cat-scratch a. Material from an infected lymph node or a bubo of a known case of cat-scratch disease, used in an intradermal skin test.

conjugated a. An antigen in which an acyl group or a simple compound is attached to the protein.

diphasic antigens. Antigens such as those found in *Salmonella*, which exist in two phases—a specific phase and a group phase.

flagellar a. The antigenic component or components of flagella.

Forssman a. A heterophil antigen, found in the tissues of the guinea pig, cat, and horse, the red cells of the sheep and man, the tissues and red cells of certain birds, and many species of bacteria, including *Diplococcus pneumoniae* and *Salmonella typhosa*, also in certain plant tissues. It is not found in other animals, such as the rabbit. Injection of emulsions of tissues containing this antigen into an animal not containing the antigen results in the formation of antibodies which are hemolytic for sheep red cells.

H a. A thermolabile, flagellar antigen which confers type specificity like the capsular polysaccharides.

heterogenetic a. See heterophil *a.*

heterophil a. One occurring in entirely unrelated species of animals and having similar or identical serologic properties. Also called *heterogenetic a.* Also see Forssman *a.*

Kveim a. Emulsified material from a lymph node proved to be sarcoid, which, on injection into an individual with sarcoidosis, usually results in the formation of sarcoid tubercles: used in the Nickerson-Kveim *test.*

O a. The thermostable, somatic antigen of flagellated organisms.

pollen a. The antigenic protein or polypeptide extracted from pollen and used for diagnosis and specific pollen desensitization in hay fever.

Vi-antigen. A thermolabile antigen demonstrated in freshly isolated, virulent cultures of *Salmonella typhosa.*

an″ti·ge·nic′i·ty (an″ti·ji·nis′i·tee) [*anti; genesthai*]. The property of certain substances to produce antibodies.

an″ti-g′ suit. A suit worn by an aviator to avoid the deleterious effects of rapid changes in velocity and direction of flight, consisting of rubber bladders which, when rapidly inflated, exert pressure over the abdomen and lower extremities, thus preventing venous pooling in those areas and a lowering of arterial pressure in the head: also called *g suit.*

an″ti·he′lix. See *anthelix.*

an″ti·he″mo·lyt′ic (an″ti·hee″mo·lit′ick, ·hem″-o·lit′ick) [*anti;* G. *haima,* blood; *lysis,* a loosing]. 1. Relating to an antihemolysin. 2. Not capable of dissolving blood cells preventing hemolysis.

an″ti·he″mo·phil′ic fac′tor. See under *factor.*

an″ti·hem″or·rhag′ic (·hem″o·radj′ick) [*anti; haima;* G. *rhēgnynai,* to burst forth]. 1. Checking hemorrhage. 2. Pertaining to vitamin K.

an″ti·hem″or·rhoi′dal [*anti;* G. *haimorrois,* piles]. A drug or agent that prevents or relieves hemorrhoids. —**antihemorrhoi′dal,** *adj.*

an″ti·hi·drot′ic (·hi·drot′ick, ·high·drot′ick) [*anti;* G. *hidrōs,* sweat]. Diminishing the secretion of sweat. —**antihidrot′ic,** *n.*

an″ti·his′ta·mine. A substance capable of preventing or diminishing several of the pharmacologic effects of histamine, by a mechanism other than the production of pharmacologic responses diametrically opposed to those produced by histamine. —**antihistamin′ic,** *adj.*

an″ti·hor′mone [*anti;* G. *hormainein,* to set in motion]. A substance in the blood of animals which antagonizes the action of certain pituitary hormones.

an″ti·hy″a·lu·ron′i·dase. An antienzyme which destroys hyaluronidase. Syn., *antinvasin I.*

an″ti·hy·drop′ic, ant″hy·drop′ic (·high·drop′ick) [*anti;* G. *hydrōpikos,* suffering from dropsy]. Relieving dropsical states or conditions. —**antihydrop′ic, anthydrop′ic,** *n.*

antihypo. $K_2C_2O_6.H_2O$. A trade name for *potassium percarbonate.*

an″ti·in·fec′tive [*anti;* L. *infectus,* from *inficere,* to infect]. A substance that counteracts infection. —**antiinfec′tive,** *adj.*

antikamnia. A proprietary preparation containing acetanilid, caffeine, and sodium bicarbonate; used as analgesic.

an″ti·kath′ode. See *anticathode.*

an″ti·ke″to·gen′e·sis [*anti;* Ger. *keton,* from F. *acétone,* L. *acetum,* vinegar; G. *genesis,* production]. The diminution of acidosis by the oxidation of sugar and allied substances in the body. —**antiketogenic,** *adj.;* **antike′togen,** *n.*

an″ti·li′pase (an″ti·lye′pace, ·lip′ace). A substance inhibiting or counteracting a lipase.

an″ti·lip·fa·no′gen. An agent in blood serum which opposes the formation of fat granules from lipfanogens.

an″ti·lu·et′ic [*anti;* L. *lues,* plague]. Efficacious against the *Treponemia pallidum.* Syn. *antisyphilitic.*

an″ti·lu·et′ic. An agent used to treat syphilis. See *antisyphilitic.*

an″ti·lyt′ic [*anti;* G. *lysis,* a loosing]. A term applied to the secretion arising in a control gland as a result of experimental denervation of the gland of the opposite side; used in contradistinction to "paralytic," a term applied to secretion arising in the denervated gland. Syn., *antiparalytic.*

an″ti·ma·lar′i·al [*anti;* It. *mala aria,* bad air]. Preventing or suppressing malaria. —**antimalar′ial,** *n.*

an″ti·mel′lin. A glycoside from the bark of *Eugenia jambolana* or jambul.

an″ti·men·or·rhag′ic. A medication or method which will control profuse prolonged menstrual flow. —**antimenorrhag′ic,** *adj.*

an′ti·mer. Enantiomorph; enantiomer.

an′ti·mere [*anti;* G. *meros,* part]. 1. Any one of the segments of the body that are bounded by planes typically at right angles to the long axis of the body. 2. A segment exhibiting bilateral symmetry with respect to the longitudinal axis.

an″ti·me·tab′o·lite [*anti;* G. *metabolē,* change]. A substance having a molecular structure similar to but a pharmacologic effect antagonistic to an essential metabolite. The mechanism of antagonism is considered to be a competition between antimetabolite and metabolite for a specific protein in an organism.

an″ti·me·tro′pi·a [*anti;* G. *metron,* a measure; *ōps,* eye]. A condition characterized by opposing states of refraction in the two eyes, as the existence of myopia in one eye and of hypermetropia in the other.

antimonial powder. See *antimony* powder.

an″ti·mo′nic (an″ti·mo′nick, ·mon′ick) [ML. *antimonium*]. Relating to compounds of pentavalent antimony. See *antimony* pentoxide.

an′ti·mo·nous, an″ti·mo′ni·ous [*antimonium*]. Denoting compounds of trivalent antimony.

an′ti·mo·nous acid. See *antimony* trioxide.

an′ti·mo″ny [*antimonium*] (*stibium*). Sb = 121.76. A metallic, crystalline element possessing a bluish white luster. Found native, as the sulfide, Sb_2S_3, and the oxide; it is a constituent of many minerals. Used commercially chiefly for making alloys where its property of expanding on solidification is of considerable value. Type metal, Britannia metal, and Babbitt antifriction metal are alloys of antimony. The actions of antimony compounds resemble those of arsenic, but they are less toxic. They produce nausea, emesis, enteritis, and nephritis. The nauseant action is used in expectorant and diaphoretic mixtures; they were formerly employed to produce circulatory depression in fever, and for catharsis and emesis. Certain complex antimony compounds are valuable antiprotozoan agents.

a. aniline tartrate. Colorless crystals, soluble in water and alcohol, containing 22% of antimony. Used in sleeping sickness. Dose, 15 mg. (1/4 gr.) intravenously.

a. butter. Antimony chloride, $SbCl_3$.

a. chloride. $SbCl_3$, the so-called antimony butter; a strong caustic.

a. lithium thiomalate. See *anthiomaline.*

a. pentoxide. Sb_2O_5. Antimonic acid; combines with bases to form salts called antimoniates.

a. potassium tartrate. $2KSbOC_4H_4O_6.H_2O$, so-called tartar emetic. Occurs in colorless, transparent crystals or as a white powder; soluble in water and in glycerin. Dose, as a diaphoretic or expectorant, 1.5–8.0 mg. (1/40–1/8 gr.); as an emetic, 30–60 mg. (1/2–1 gr.); as a protozoacide, 30–120 mg. (1/2–2 gr.) intravenously in 1 or 2% solution.

a. powder (*pulvis antimonialis*). Antimonial powder, James's powder; consists of antimony trioxide and calcium phosphate and is diaphoretic, emetic in large doses, and cathartic. Has been used in a dose of 0.2–0.3 Gm. (3–5 gr.).

a. sodium tartrate. Used the same as the potassium compound but more soluble in water and better suited for intravenous use.

a. sodium thioglycollate. $NaOOC.CH_2.S.Sb.S.CH_2.COO$. White or faintly pink powder, soluble in water, insoluble in alcohol, used in the treatment of granuloma inguinale, kala-azar, and filariasis. Dose, 0.05–0.1 Gm. in 10–20 cc. of sterile water intramuscularly or intravenously.

a. sulfide. Sb_2S_3. Black sulfide of antimony. Dose, 0.015–0.06 Gm. (1/4–1 gr.).

a. tartrate. $(SbO)_2C_4H_4O_6 + H_2O$. A white, crystalline powder: has been used internally as a substitute for arsenic in affections of the skin.

a. thioglycollamide. $Sb(S.CH_2CONH_2)_3$. White crystals, soluble in about 200 parts of water, used in the treatment of granuloma inguinale, kala-azar, and filariasis. Dose, 0.08 Gm. in 20 cc. of sterile water intramuscularly or intravenously.

a. trioxide. Antimonous acid, Sb_2O_3; soluble in hydrochloric and tartaric acids. Dose, 0.06–0.12 Gm. (1–2 gr.). It is an ingredient of antimony powder.

a. wine (*vinum antimonii*). Boiling water, 60; tartar emetic, 4; stronger white wine, 1000 parts. It contains about 2 gr. of tartar emetic to the ounce. Dose, 0.3–1.0 cc. (5–15 min.).

black a. Purified antimony sulfide, Sb_2S_3.

compound a. pills. Plummer's pills; contain calomel and sulfurated antimony, of each, 0.03 Gm. (1/2 gr.).

golden a. sulfide. Sb_2S_5. A fine, odorless, orange-yellow powder, soluble in alkaline solutions: has been used as an alterative, diaphoretic, emetic, and expectorant.

sulfurated a. The sulfide with a small but indefinite amount of the oxide.

vegetable a. Boneset.

an'ti·mo·nyl. SbO. The univalent radical of antimonous compounds.

an"ti·my'cin A An antibiotic substance, isolated from a *Streptomyces* species possessing also insecticidal and miticidal activity.

an"ti·my·cot'ic (an"ti·migh·cot'ick) [G. *anti*, against; *mykēs*, a fungus]. Preventing the growth of fungi or the destruction of fungi by physical and chemical agents.

an"ti·nar·cot'ic [*anti;* G. *narkōsis*, a benumbing]. Preventing narcosis.

an"ti·neu·ral'gic [*anti;* G. *neuron*, nerve; *algos*, pain]. Alleviating neuralgia.

an"ti·neu·rit'ic [*anti; neuron;* G. *-itis*, inflammation]. Efficient in neuritis. —**antineurit'ic,** *n.*

an·tin'i·on [*anti;* G. *inion*, occipital bone]. The glabella; the point in the sagittal plane farthest removed from the inion. —**antinial,** *adj.*; **antiniad,** *adv.*

an"tin·va'sin I. An enzyme found in normal blood plasma of all animals, including man. It acts by destroying the hyaluronidase of bacteria and other sources and, by this action, counteracts invasion and spreading of those organisms and toxins which elaborate hyaluronidase.

an"tin·va'sin II. A protective enzyme observed in normal blood plasma which causes rapid destruction of proinvasin I in pathogenic organisms and venoms. With proinvasin I inactivated, antinvasin I is left intact to destroy hyaluronidase, the enzyme which aids invasion and spreading.

an"ti·o·be'sic [*anti;* L. *obesus*, from *obedere*, to devour]. Efficient against corpulence or obesity. —**antiobe'sic,** *n.*

an"ti·o·don·tal'gic [*anti;* G. *odous*, tooth; *algos*, pain]. Relieving or preventing toothache.

an"ti·op'so·nin. A substance retarding or destroying the action of an opsonin.

an"ti·ox'i·dant. Any substance which delays the process of oxidation.

an"ti·par"a·lyt'ic. Antilytic.

an"ti·par"a·sit'ic [*anti;* G. *parasitos*, parasite]. Destroying parasites. —**antiparasit'ic,** *n.*

an"ti·pep'sin. A hypothetical antiferment or a substance which inhibits the action of pepsin.

an"ti·pep'tone [*anti;* G. *peptos*, cooked]. A variety of peptone not acted upon by trypsin.

an"ti·per"i·od'ic. A medicinal preparation for the treatment of a periodic disease, especially malaria.

an"ti·per"i·od'ic. Of, pertaining to, or preventing attacks of a periodic disease, as of malaria.

an"ti·per"i·stal'sis [*anti;* G. *peri*, around; *stalsis*, constriction]. Reversed peristalsis.

an"ti·phag"o·cyt'ic [*anti;* G. *phagein*, to eat; *kytos*, cell]. Preventing phagocytosis.

an"ti·phlo·gis'tic [*anti;* G. *phlogōsis*, burning heat]. An agent subduing or reducing inflammation or fever. —**antiphlogis'tic,** *adj.*

antiphlogistine. Trade-mark for certain proprietary medicinals, including an analgesic poultice containing clay, glycerin, and antiseptic and aromatic substances.

an'ti·phone [*anti;* G. *phōnē*, sound]. An appliance worn in the auditory meatus and intended to protect the wearer from noises.

an"ti·phthi'ri·ac, an"ti·phthei'ri·ac (an"ti-tigh'ree·ack, an"tif·thigh'·, an"ti·thigh'·) [*anti;* G. *phtheir*, louse]. Efficient against lice or the condition caused by them. *Obs.*

an"ti·plas'min. A substance or substances found in plasma which inhibit plasmin (a plasma proteolytic enzyme). Syn. *plasmin inhibitor.*

an"ti·plas'tic [*anti;* G. *plassein*, to form]. 1. Unfavorable to granulation or to the healing process. 2. Preventing or checking plastic exudation. Not to be confused with *aplastic.*

an"ti·pneu"mo·coc'cic (·new"mo·cock'sick) [*anti;* G. *pneumōn*, lungs; *kokkos*, berry]. Destructive to *Diplococcus pneumoniae.*

an·tip'o·dal [*anti;* G. *pous*, foot]. Situated directly opposite.

an"ti·pro·throm'bin [*anti;* G. *pro*, before; *thrombos*, clot]. An agent present in the blood which prevents coagulation by neutralizing prothrombin. Substances having similar action are heparin, hirudin, and dicoumarin.

an"ti·pro'ton. A postulated elementary particle which differs from a proton only in having a negative charge.

an″ti·pru·rit′ic [*anti;* L. *pruritus,* itching]. Relieving or preventing itching. —**antiprurit′ic,** *n.*

an″ti·py″o·gen′ic [*anti;* G. *pyon,* pus; *genesthai,* from *gignesthai,* to be produced]. Preventing or inhibiting suppuration.

an″ti·py·ret′ic (an″ti·pye·ret′ick) [*anti;* G. *pyretos,* burning heat]. An agent reducing fever. The most important antipyretic agents are cold, diaphoretics, quinine, and many coal-tar products, such as salicylates, antipyrine, acetanilid, acetophenetidin. —**antipyre′sis,** *n.;* **antipyret′ic,** *adj.*

an″ti·py′rine (an″ti·pye′rin, ·reen, an″ti·pye·reen′) (*antipyrina*). $C_{11}H_{12}N_2O$. 1-Phenyl-2,3-dimethyl-5-pyrazolone. A white, crystalline powder with a slightly bitter taste; soluble in water or alcohol; used as antipyretic and analgesic. Locally its anesthetic and vasoconstrictive actions are useful in various mucous-membrane inflammations. May cause giddiness, sweating, skin eruption, or other toxic symptoms. Dose, 0.3–1.0 Gm. (5–15 gr.). Syn., *phenazone.*

a. amygdalate. See *a.* mandelate.

a. chloralhydrate. See *hypnal.*

a. mandelate. A white, crystalline powder used in whooping cough. See *tussol.*

a. salicylate. A white, odorless, crystalline powder, used as analgesic, antipyretic, and antirheumatic. Syn., *salipyrazolone.* See *salipyrin.*

an″ti·py″rin·o·ma′ni·a [*anti;* G. *pyrinos,* fiery; *mania,* madness]. A condition similar to morphinism, due to excessive use of antipyrine. It is marked by nervous excitement.

an″ti·ra′bic, an″ti·rab′ic [*anti;* L. *rabies,* madness]. Preventing rabies, as the Pasteur treatment.

an″ti·ra·chit′ic (an″ti·ra·kit′ick) [*anti;* G. *rhachis,* spine]. An agent for the prevention or cure of rickets. —**antirachit′ic,** *adj.*

an″ti·ren′net. Antirennin.

an″ti·ren′nin [*anti;* ME., from *rennen,* to run]. An antibody which is capable of neutralizing the milk-curdling action of rennin.

an″ti·re·tic′u·lar [*anti;* L. *reticulum,* net]. Pertaining to a factor operating against the reticuloendothelial system.

an″ti·rhe′o·scope [G. *antirroia,* back current; *skopein,* to examine]. A device for observing the manifestations of visual vertigo.

an″ti·rheu·mat′ic [G. *anti,* against; *rheumatikos,* subject to a flux]. Preventing or useful in treating rheumatism. —**antirheumat′ic,** *n.*

an′ti-Rh se′rum. See *Rh factor.*

an″ti·ri″bo·fla′vin (·rye″bo·flay′vin, ·flav′in, ·rib″o·). Any compound which interferes with the action of riboflavin in the organism.

an″ti·ri′cin (an″ti·rye′sin, ·riss′in) [*anti;* L. *ricinus,* castor-oil plant]. The antibody to ricin.

an″ti·sca·bet′ic [*anti;* L. *scabies,* itch]. Effective against the *Sarcoptes scabiei,* which causes scabies.

an″ti·scor·bu′tic [*anti;* L. *scorbutus.* scurvy]. An agent which prevents or cures scurvy; see *vitamin* C. —**antiscorbu′tic,** *adj.*

an″ti·scor·bu′tic vi′ta·min. See *ascorbic acid.*

an″ti·sep′sis [*anti;* G. *sēpsis,* decay]. Prevention of sepsis or poisoning by the destruction of microorganisms or their exclusion from the body tissues and fluids, or by preventing or checking their growth and multiplication.

an″ti·sep′tic [*anti; sēpsis*]. Any one of a large group of organic and inorganic compounds which stops or inhibits the growth of bacteria without necessarily killing them, thus checking putrefaction; as alcohol, mercuric chloride, phenol, sodium chloride, phenylmercuric salts, etc. —**antisep′tic,** *adj.*

an″ti·sep′tol. Cinchonine iodosulfate; a reddish brown, insoluble powder used like iodoform.

an″ti·se′rum [*anti;* L. *serum,* whey, watery part]. 1. The serum of man or animal immunized against bacteria or their products, or other antigenic agents, and therefore containing antibodies specific for these agents. 2. Serum containing natural antibodies such as hemagglutinins. 3. An immune therapeutic agent, such as diphtheria or tetanus antitoxin.

Rh antiserums. Antiserums reacting with one or more of the Rh factors.

an″ti·si·al′a·gogue, an″ti·si·al′a·gog (·sigh·al′-uh·gog) [*anti;* G. *sialon,* saliva; *agōgos,* leading]. Preventing or checking salivation.

an″ti·si·al′ic (·sigh·al′ick) [*anti; sialon*]. An agent that checks the secretion of saliva. —**antisial′ic,** *adj.*

an″ti·so′cial [*anti;* L. *socius,* comrade]. Denoting a psychopathic state marked by the refusal to accept the obligations and restraints imposed by society. —**antisocialism,** *n.*

an″ti·spas·mod′ic [*anti;* G. *spasmōdēs,* spasmodic]. An agent relieving convulsions or spasmodic pains, as the narcotics, diphenylhydantoin sodium, the nitrites, atropine. Syn., *spasmolytic.* —**antispasmod′ic,** *adj.*

an″ti·spas′tic [*anti;* G. *spastikos,* drawing in, absorbing]. Antispasmodic.

an″ti·spi″ro·che′tic (·spy″ro·kee′tick, ·ket′ick) [*anti;* G. *speira,* coil; *chaitē,* hair]. Arresting the growth and development of spirochetes. —**antispiroche′tic,** *n.*

an″ti·ster′num [*anti;* G. *sternon,* breast]. The part of the back opposite the breast. *Obs.*

antistine hydrochloride. Trade-marked name for the antihistaminic substance known by the generic name *antazoline hydrochloride.*

an″ti·strep″to·coc′cic (·strep″to·cock′sick) [*anti;* G. *streptos,* twisted; *kokkos,* berry]. Antagonistic to or preventing the growth of streptococci.

an″ti·strep″to·dor′nase. An antibody capable of neutralizing streptodornase.

an″ti·strep″to·he″mo·ly′sin (·hee″mo·lye′sin, ·hem″o·, ·hem·ol′i·sin) [*anti; streptos;* G. *haima,* blood; *lysis,* a loosing]. An antibody formed in response to the antigen streptohemolysin.

an″ti·strep″to·ki′nase. An antibody present in the serum which prevents the activation of plasminogen by streptokinase. It may be introduced into the serum by infection with hemolytic streptococci containing sufficient streptokinase or by injections of streptokinase for therapeutic reasons.

an″ti·strep″to·ly′sin [*anti; streptos; lysis*]. An antibody which operates against the hemotoxin of hemolytic streptococci.

an″ti·su″dor·if′ic [*anti;* L. *sudor,* sweat; *facere,* to make]. An agent that checks excretion of sweat: also called *antisudoral.* —**antisudorif′ic,** *adj.*

an″ti·syph″i·lit′ic [*anti-;* NL. *syphilis,* syphilis]. A remedy used in the treatment of syphilis. —**antisyphilit′ic,** *adj.*

an″ti·the′nar [*anti;* G. *thenar,* palm of the hand, flat of the foot]. Old term for hypothenar.

an″ti·ther′mic [*anti;* G. *thermē,* heat]. Cooling; antipyretic.

an″ti·ther′min. Phenylhydrazine-levulinic acid. $C_6H_5.NH.N{:}C(CH_3).CH_2.CH_2.COOH$. A white, crystalline powder formerly used as antipyretic, analgesic, and antiseptic. It is a vasomotor depressant causing pallor, sweating, and other toxic effects.

an″ti·throm′bin [*anti;* G. *thrombos,* clot]. A substance present in blood plasma, neutralizing thrombin.

an″ti·throm″bo·plas′tin [*anti; thrombos;* G. *plas-*

sein, to form]. A substance which inactivates thromboplastin.

an″ti·tox′i·gen, an″ti·tox·in′o·gen [*anti;* G. *toxikon*, poison; *genesthai*, from *gignesthai*, to be produced]. Any antigen, or toxin, which promotes antitoxin elaboration.

an″ti·tox′in [*anti; toxikon*]. 1. A substance elaborated in the body capable of neutralizing a given toxin (bacterial, plant, or animal toxin). 2. One of the class of specific antibodies. —**antitoxic,** *adj.*

an″ti·trag′i·cus. A vestigial slip of muscle associated with the antitragus.

an″ti·tra′gus [*anti;* G. *tragos*, goat]. The projection of the pinna just opposite and posterior to the tragus. —**antitrag′ic,** *adj.*

an″ti·tris′mus [*anti;* G. *trismos*, a grinding]. A condition of tonic spasm in which the mouth cannot be closed.

an′ti·trope [*anti;* G. *trepein*, to turn]. 1. Either one of a pair of symmetrical organs. 2. An antibody.

an″ti·tryp′sin [*anti;* G. *tryein*, to rub down; pe*psin*]. An antibody inhibiting the action of trypsin.

an″ti·tryp′tase. See *antitrypsin.*

antitussin. A proprietary ointment containing 5% of difluorodiphenyl; applied by inunction in whooping cough.

an″ti·tus′sive. Decreasing or relieving the amount and severity of coughing; or of pertaining to any agent which reduces or relieves coughing.

an″ti tus′sive. Any medication designed to reduce the amount and severity of coughing.

an″ti·ty′phoid [*anti;* G. *typhos*, fever; *eidos*, form]. Counteracting or preventing typhoid fever.

an″ti·ty′phoid. An antityphoid serum.

an″ti·u′re·ase (an″ti·yoor′ee·ace, ·aze). An antibody to urease.

an″ti·ven′ene. See *antivenin.*

an″ti·ve·ne′re·al [*anti;* L. *venereus*, venereal]. Preventive or curative of venereal disease.

an″ti·ven′in, an″ti·ven′ene (·ven′een, ·vi·neen′) [*anti;* L. *venenum*, poison]. 1. An antitoxin to a venin. 2. An antitoxic serum prepared by immunizing animals against the venom of snakes, insects, or other animals.

bothropic a. Polyvalent serum for the venom of pit vipers of the genus *Bothrops.*

Crotalus a. Polyvalent serum for the venom of rattlesnakes.

an″ti·vi′ral [*anti;* L. *virus*, poison]. Antagonistic to a virus, weakening or destroying its pathogenicity.

an″ti·vi·rot′ic. A substance which is detrimental to viruses and can be used to treat virus diseases.

an″ti·vir′u·lin. 1. A substance counteracting virulin. 2. The antibodylike substance elaborated in animals injected with rabies virus, inactivating the pathogenicity of the virus.

an″ti·vi′rus [*anti; virus*]. A broth culture, filtered of its bacteria and heated to attenuate its toxicity, used in producing local immunity.

an″ti·vi′ta·min. Any substance that prevents the normal metabolic functioning of vitamins; a vitamin-destroying enzyme, or a chemical substance that renders the vitamin unabsorbable or ineffective.

an″ti·viv″i·sec′tion [*anti;* L. *vivus*, living; *secare*, to cut]. Opposition to vivisection or animal experimentation. —**antivivisectionist,** *n.*

an″ti·xen′ic (an″ti·zen′ick) [*anti;* G. *xenos*, foreign]. Relating to the reaction which occurs when a foreign substance is introduced into living tissue.

an″ti·xe″roph·thal′mic [*anti;* G. *xēros*, dry; *ophthalmos*, eye]. Preventive of xerophthalmia. See *vitamin* A.

an″ti·xe·rot′ic [*anti; xēros*]. Preventing dryness of the skin.

an″ti·zy·mot′ic (·zye·mot′ic) [*anti;* G. *zymōtikos*, causing to ferment]. Preventing or checking fermentation. —**antizymot′ic,** *n.*

ant″lo·pho′bi·a [G. *antlos*, flood; *phobos*, fear]. A morbid fear of floods.

antodyne. Trade-mark for phenyl glyceryl ether, $C_6H_5O.CH_2.CHOH.CH_2OH$; an analgesic in neuralgia, migraine, etc.

an·trec′to·my [G. *antron*, cave; *ektomē*, excision]. Surgical removal of the walls of an antrum, especially the mastoid antrum.

antrenyl bromide. Trade-marked name for the anticholinergic agent *oxyphenonium bromide.*

an·tri′tis [*antron;* G. *-itis*, inflammation]. See maxillary *sinusitis.*

an′tro-, antr- [*antron*]. A combining form meaning *cavern, cavity.*

an″tro·at″ti·cot′o·my [*antron;* F. *attique*, G. *Attikos;* G. *tomē*, a cutting]. *In surgery*, the opening of the mastoid antrum and the attic of the tympanum.

an′tro·cele, an′tra·cele [*antron;* G. *kēlē*, tumor]. An accumulation of fluid in the maxillary sinus.

an″tro·na′sal [*antron;* L. *nasus*, nose]. Pertaining to the maxillary sinus and the nasal cavity.

ant′ro·phose (an′tro·foze) [*antron;* G. *phōs*, light]. A phose having its origin in the central ocular mechanism.

an′tro·scope″ [*antron;* G. *skopein*, to examine]. An instrument for examining the maxillary sinus. —**antros′copy,** *n.*

an·tros′to·my, an·trot′o·my [*antron;* G. *stoma*, mouth]. Opening of an antrum for drainage.

an″tro·tym·pan′ic [*antron;* G. *tympanon*, drum]. Relating to the mastoid antrum and the cavity of the middle ear.

an′trum [L.]. 1. A cavity or hollow space, especially in a bone. 2. The maxillary sinus. Formerly called *a. of Highmore.* —**antral,** *adj.*

a. of the ear. The mastoid antrum.

a. of the testis. See *mediastinum* testis.

a. of the tube. A saclike dilatation of the uterine tube about an inch from the fimbriated extremity; regarded by some as occurring only in pregnancy.

cardiac a. A dilatation sometimes found in the esophagus immediately above its passage through the diaphragm.

dental a. The pulp chamber of a tooth. *Obs.*

duodenal a. The normal dilatation presented by the duodenum near its origin. See duodenal *cap.*

ethmoidal a. An ethmoid sinus.

mastoid a. See tympanic *a.*

maxillary a. The maxillary sinus.

pyloric a. The cavity of the pylorus (3); the first part of the pyloric region of the stomach, proximal to the pyloric canal.

tympanic a. The pneumatic space between the epitympanic recess and the mastoid cells. Syn., *mastoid a.*

antrycide. Trade-mark for various 4-amino-6-(2-amino-6-methyl-4-pyrimidylamino)quinaldine-1, 1′-dimetho salts having trypanocidal action in animals.

antrypol. See *suramin.*

ANTU Alpha-naphthylthiourea, a gray powder, insoluble in water, with little odor or taste. It is harmless to human beings, unless ingested in large quantities, but is a highly specific poison for the common brown, or Norway, rat by causing accumulation of fluid in the lungs with strangulation. It is less effective against other rats and against mice. Poisonous to domestic pets.

antuitrin-growth. Trade-mark for a preparation of growth hormone extracted from the anterior pituitary.

antuitrin-S. Trade-mark for a preparation of chorionic gonadotropin extracted from the urine of pregnancy.

Antyllus (**Antyllos**) [*Greek physician and surgeon, second or third century*]. One of the great surgeons of antiquity, best known today for having recognized two forms of aneurysm: the congenital and the traumatic.

a·nu′cle·ar (ay·new′klee·ur, a·new′·) [G. *a*-, not; L. *nucleus*, kernel]. Without a nucleus: applied to an erythrocyte.

an·u′ri·a, an′u·ry, an″u·re′sis [*a*-; G. *ouron*, urine]. Arrest of urinary output, resulting from lack of renal function (*secretory type*) or from obstruction in the urinary tract (*excretory type*). —**anuret′ic, anu′ric,** *adj.*

compression a. See compression *syndrome.*

postrenal a. Anuria on the basis of urinary tract obstruction.

prerenal a. That characterized by disturbances in blood flow to the kidney, as in shock and renal vascular thrombosis.

renal a. Failure of urine formation due to bilateral intrinsic renal dysfunction.

traumatic a. That in lower nephron nephrosis following injury.

an·u′rous [*a*-; G. *oura*, tail]. Without a tail; applied to frogs and toads.

a′nus [L.]. The termination of the rectum; the outlet of the alimentary canal. See Plates 14, 41, 44. —**anal,** *adj.*

a. vesicalis. An anomaly in which the anus is imperforate, the rectum opening into the urinary bladder.

a. vulvovaginalis. An anal opening communicating with the vulva.

artificial a. A permanent artificial opening made surgically from the exterior into the intestine.

fissure of a. A slight tear in the mucous membrane at the anus, usually due to passage of hardened feces.

fistula of a. Fistula in ano, a sinus opening from the rectum into the connective tissue about the rectum or discharging externally.

imperforate a. Absence of the anus, the natural opening being closed by a membranous septum.

infundibuliform a. A relaxed condition of the anus with destruction of the natural folds.

preternatural a. An abnormal aperture serving as an anus, whether congenital, made by operation, or due to disease or injury.

preternatural ileovaginal a., preternatural vaginal a., a. praeternaturalis vestibularis. The rare abnormality of the rectum opening through the vulva.

vulvar a. An anomalous condition in which the anus is imperforate, the rectum opening into the vulva.

umbilical a. A preternatural anus located in the umbilical region.

anusol. Trade-mark for suppositories containing bismuth subgallate, bismuth-resorcin compound, and other ingredients; used for relief of hemorrhoids.

an′vil [AS. *anfilt*]. An ossicle of the middle ear. See *incus.*

anx·i′e·ty [L. *anxietas*, anxiety]. The awareness of the physiologic reactions to the perception of a dangerous situation calling for fight-or-flight responses. It may be produced by a fear of impulses within the personality as well as by external situations. Causes include social dangers such as loss of love or prestige. The person in the anxiety reaction manifests not only the signs and symptoms of anxiety but also his individual defense mechanisms against anxiety. Also see under *complex, neurosis, reaction.*

castration a. A fear of the young male child based on the phantasy that he will lose his penis.

negative a. Anxiety which leads to the breakdown of the defensive mechanisms of the individual.

positive a. The anxiety for growth.

anx·i′e·ty at·tack′. *In psychoanalysis*, a feeling of impending death or physical collapse, acute panic or crisis; occurs in an anxiety reaction.

AO 1. Anodal opening. 2. Opening of the atrioventricular valves.

AOC, AnOC Anodal opening contraction.

aolan. A proprietary injection prepared from milk; used in nonspecific protein therapy.

A. O. M. *Artium Obstetricarum Magister*, Master of Obstetric Art.

aort-. See *aorto-.*

a·or′ta (ay·or′tuh) [G. *aortē*, aorta, from *aeirein*, to raise]. The large vessel arising from the left ventricle and distributing, by its branches, arterial blood to every part of the body. It ends by bifurcating into the common iliacs at the fourth lumbar vertebra. The arch extending from the heart to the third thoracic vertebra is divided into an *ascending*, a *transverse*, and a *descending* part. The *thoracic* portion extends to the diaphragm; the *abdominal*, to the bifurcation. See Plates 5, 8. See Table of Arteries in the Appendix. —**aortal, aortic,** *adj.*

ascending a. The first part of the aorta. See Plate 5.

cardiac a. That part of the embryonic vascular system giving rise to the aortic arches. Sometimes refers to the bulbus arteriosus. Syn., *ventral a., aortic sac.*

descending a. The thoracic and abdominal portions of the aorta. See Plates 5, 7, 8, 14.

dorsal a. (a) See primitive *a.* (b) Thoracic aorta.

double a. Persistence of both right and left fourth aortic arches and dorsal aortas.

left a. The left primitive or dorsal aorta, especially in the aortic arch region where fusion of the aortas does not occur.

main a. See primitive *a.*

pericardial a. The part of the aorta within the pericardial cavity; the bulbus arteriosus.

primitive a. (a) That part of the aorta extending from its origin to the point where it first branches. (b) Two embryonic branches of the cardiac aorta extending through the first visceral arch and uniting to form the dorsal aorta.

right a. The embryonic division of the aortic bulb which finally forms the pulmonary artery.

root of a. The origin of the aorta at the heart. Also called *radix aortae.*

systemic a. See left *a.*

throbbing a. Exaggerated pulsation of the abdominal aorta, perceptible to the patient.

ventral a. The arterial trunk or trunks between the heart and first aortic arch in embryos or lower vertebrates.

a″or·tal′gi·a [*aortē*; G. *algos*, pain]. Severe, constant ache in the upper thorax, neck, and shoulders; due to pressure of an aneurysm against the surrounding tissues, or to periaortitis of syphilitic origin.

a·or″ti·co·re′nal (ay·or″ti·ko·ree′nul) [*aortē*; L. *renes*, kidneys]. Near the aorta and kidney, as the aorticorenal ganglion.

a″or·ti′tis (ay″or·tye′tis) [*aortē*; G. *-itis*, inflammation]. Inflammation of the aorta.

acute a. Inflammation usually observed in the intima, as an infiltration of lymphocytes, plasma cells, large mononuclear cells, and a few polymorphonuclear leukocytes.

acute bacterial a. See *mycotic aortitis.*

mycotic a. A form of infectious aortitis usually due to lodgment of infected emboli; a complication of bacterial endocarditis, tuberculosis, rheumatic fever, typhoid fever. Syn., *bacterial aortitis.*

rheumatic a. A form of intimal arteriosclerosis with large sausagelike plaques, due presumably to rheumatic fever.

suppurative a. Suppuration of the wall of the aorta as a result of extension of a neighboring pyogenic infection.

syphilitic a. Inflammation of the aorta due to syphilis. It affects the proximal part of the aorta but may be more extensive. The principal lesion is destruction of parts of the media as a result of syphilitic inflammation around the medial arterioles. The intima shows stellate lines of depression and often hyaline plaques. It begins probably as deforming or obliterative endarteritis of the vasa vasorum. Also called *syphilitic mesaortitis.*

verrucous (verrucose) a. Inflammation of the intima with the formation of verrucae.

a·or′to- (ay·or′to-), **aort-** [*aortē*]. A combining form meaning *aorta.*

a″or·tog′ra·phy. Roentgenography of the aorta.

a″or·tot′o·my. Cutting or opening the aorta.

A. O. T. A. American Occupational Therapy Association.

ap-. See *apo-.*

A. P. A. American Physiotherapy Association.

a·pal″laes·the′si·a. See *apallesthesia.*

a·pal″les·the′si·a (a·pal″ess·thee′zhuh, ·zee·uh) [G. *a-*, not; *pallein,* to sway; *aisthēsis,* feeling]. Loss of vibration sense. Syn., *pallanesthesia.*

a·pan′cre·a (ay·pang′kree·uh, a·pang′·) [*a-;* G. *pas,* all *kreas,* flesh]. Absence of the pancreas. —**apancreat′ic,** *adj.*

a·pan′dri·a [G. *apo,* from; *anēr,* man]. Morbid dislike of the male sex.

ap″an·thro′pi·a, a·pan′thro·py [*apo;* G. *anthrōpos,* man]. 1. Morbid desire for solitude. 2. Morbid aversion to human associations.

a·par″a·lyt′ic (ay·par″uh·lit′ick, a·par″·) [G. *a-*, not; *paralysis,* paralysis]. Without paralysis.

ap″ar·thro′sis [G., articulation]. Diarthrosis. *Obs.*

a·pas′ti·a [G., abstaining from food]. Abstinence from food; seen in mental disorder. —**apastic,** *adj.*

ap′a·thism [G. *apatheia,* apathy, from *a-; pathos,* feeling]. Slowness in reacting, as opposed to *erethism.*

ap′a·thy [*apatheia*]. 1. Want of passion or feeling. 2. Indifference. —**apathet′ic,** *adj.*

ap′a·tite [G. *apatē,* deceit, since it has been mistaken for other minerals]. A type of mineral having the formula $[Ca_3(PO_4)_2]_3.CaX_2$, where X_2 may be CO_3, $(OH)_2$, Cl_2, F_2, O, or SO_4. The inorganic component of bones and teeth contains a form of apatite.

ap·at′ro·pine (a·pat′ro·peen, ·pin). See *apoatropine.*

APC Common abbreviation for therapeutic formulations of acetylsalicylic acid, acetophenetidin (phenacetin), and caffeine.

ape [AS. *apa*]. A manlike, tailless primate.

a·pei″ro·pho′bi·a (a·pye″ro·fo′bee·uh) [G. *apeiros,* boundless; *phobos,* fear]. A morbid fear of infinity.

a·pel′lous [G. *a-*, not; L. *pellis,* skin]. 1. Skinless; not cicatrized, applied to wounds. 2. Without a prepuce; circumcised.

Apelt's test. See Nonne-Apelt's *test.*

ap″en·ter′ic. Abenteric.

a·pe′ri·ent [L. *aperire,* to open]. Laxative; mildly purgative. —**ape′rient,** *n.*

a·pe″ri·od′ic (ay·peer″ee·od′ick, a·peer″·) [G. *a-*, not; *periodos,* a going round]. Devoid of periodicity or rhythm. —**aperiodic′ity,** *n.*

a·per″i·stal′sis (ay·perr″i·stal′sis, a·perr″·) [*a-;* G. *peri,* around; *stalsis,* constriction]. Absence of the peristaltic movements of the intestine.

a·per′i·tive (a·perr′i·tiv) [L. *aperire,* to open]. 1. Aperient. 2. Deobstruent. 3. Stimulating the appetite.

Apert's syndrome. See *acrocephalosyndactylia.*

ap″er·tom′e·ter [*aperire;* G. *metron,* a measure]. An optic device for determining the angle of aperture of microscopic objectives.

ap″er·tu′ra (pl. *aperturae*) [L., from *aperire*]. An opening.

a. aquaeductus cochleae. Opening of the aqueduct of the cochlea on the petrous bone.

a. canalis inguinalis. Inguinal ring.

a. externa aquaeductus vestibuli. External opening of the aqueduct of the vestibule.

a. lateralis ventriculi quarti. Aperture at the tip of the lateral recesses of the fourth ventricle. Also called *foramen of Luschka.*

a. medialis ventriculi quarti. Medial aperture in the roof of the fourth ventricle: also called *foramen of Magendie.*

a. pelvis inferior [BNA]. Lower opening of the true pelvis (*O.T.*, pelvic outlet).

a. pelvis superior [BNA]. Upper opening of the true pelvis (*O.T.*, pelvic inlet).

a. piriformis [BNA]. Anterior nasal openings of the skull.

a. sinus sphenoidalis. Opening of the sphenoid sinus.

ap′er·ture [*apertura*]. 1. An opening; orifice. 2. *In optics,* the diameter of the exposed portion of a lens, designated as the ratio of the focal length to this diameter, as F/4, in which the aperture is one inch and the focal length is 4 in.

angular a. Diameter of a microscope objective measured by the angle made by lines from the most divergent rays capable of entering the objective from the focal point.

a. of the lens. See angular *a.*

lateral apertures of the fourth ventricle. Two openings at the lateral recesses of the fourth ventricle through which cerebrospinal fluid passes into the subarachnoid space. Also called *foramens of Luschka.*

medial a. of the fourth ventricle. One in the posterior central portion of the roof of the fourth ventricle through which cerebrospinal fluid passes into the subarachnoid space. Also called *foramen of Magendie.*

numerical a. Capacity of the objective to receive and transmit light rays to the image, expressed by the formula N.A. = sin $\frac{1}{2}\angle a \times n$ in which $\angle a$ = angular aperture and n = index of refraction of the medium in front of the lens.

urogenital a. External opening of the embryonic urogenital sinus after rupture of the urethral plate.

apestrin. Trade-mark for a brand of chorionic gonadotrophin obtained from human pregnancy urine. See *antuitrin-S.*

a′pex [L., the extreme end]. 1. Summit or top of anything; point or extremity of a cone. 2. *In optics,* junction of the two refractive sides of a prism. 3. *In craniometry,* the highest point in the transverse vertical section of the vault of a skull oriented on the Frankfort horizontal plane, the plane of section passing through the poria. —**ap′ical, apic′iform,** *adj.*

a. auriculae Darwini. Old term for auricular tubercle of Darwin, thought to correspond to the apex of the ear in lower mammals.

a. of the head of the fibula. Apex capituli fibulae [BNA]; the pointed proximal extremity of the fibula; the styloid process of the fibula.

a. of the lung. Upper extremity of the lung behind the border of the first rib.

a. radicis dentis. Radicular end of a tooth.

apexol. A trade-mark for vitamin A.

APF *A*nimal *p*rotein *f*actor. A substance, present in animal protein, necessary for normal growth of many animal species. The factor may be vitamin B_{12}.

aph-. See *apo-*.

A. P. H. A. American Public Health Association.

A. Ph. A. American Pharmaceutical Association.

a·pha′ci·a (a·fay′shee·uh, ·see·uh). See *aphakia.*

a·pha′gi·a [G. *a-*, not; *phagein*, to eat]. Loss of the ability to swallow.

a. algera. Inability or refusal to swallow because of pain.

a·pha′ki·a [*a-;* G. *phakos*, lentil]. Condition in which the lens is absent from the dioptric system. —**aphakic, aphakial,** *adj.*

aph″a·lan′gi·a, a·pha″lan·gi′a·sis [*a-;* G. *phalagx*, bone between two joints of the fingers and toes]. Loss or absence of fingers or toes. See *ainhum.*

aph″al·ge′si·a (af″al·jee′zee·uh, ·see·uh) [G. *apo*, from; *algos*, pain]. A hysterical state wherein pain is induced by contact with a harmless object having symbolic significance.

a·phan′i·sis [G., from *aphanizein*, to do away with]. Absence of all phases of sexuality in the individual.

a·pha′si·a (a·fay′zhuh, ·zee·uh) [G., from *a-*, not; *phasis*, speech]. Loss or impairment of the capacity to use words as symbols of ideas. Aphasia is organic and is caused by a lesion or lesions in the cortex and association paths of the dominant hemisphere. It does not refer to a defect in the mechanics of hearing or speaking but to an impairment of the highest function of the use of language as translating thought. Hysterical speech defects may imitate the symptoms of aphasia. There are many subdivisions according to the degree of loss and specific language function affected. Aphasia may be partial or total (global). The predominant defect may affect the ability to speak, called **motor, verbal,** or **expressive aphasia.** The lesion responsible is located in the parolfactory area at the posterior end of the third frontal convolution. The failure may be a lack of comprehension of the spoken word, or **auditory aphasia.** This is a form of **sensory** or **receptive aphasia.** Words are evoked with difficulty, used incorrectly, and do not translate ideas accurately. Sometimes words are uttered fluently but inappropriately, as in **jargon** or **paraphasia;** this is allied to **amnesic aphasia,** which is a loss of memory for specific words, with hesitant and fragmentary speech. The lesions which cause these types of aphasia lie in the parietal lobe at or near the angular gyrus. Expressive and receptive aphasia are the two most common types, and may occur together in mixed forms. Other varieties are **acalculia** (loss of ability to do mathematical reckoning); **agraphia** (inability to write); **alexia** or **visual aphasia** (loss of ability to understand the written word); **nominal aphasia** (anomia, dysnomia, loss of ability to name objects); **semantic aphasia** (loss of meaning of words); **syntactic aphasia** (loss of correct grammatical construction). —**aphasiac,** *adj., n.*

Broca's a. Motor aphasia.

congenital a. Developmental *a.*

developmental a. A deficiency in learning to speak which is not commensurate with the individual's (child's) mental age or development and accomplishment quotients along other lines. Syn. *congenital a.*

dysarthric a. Faulty articulation or a speech disturbance due to paresis of the peripheral nerves to the tongue, lips, and throat.

global a. Total loss of all sensory and motor functions of communication by speech or writing.

Wernicke's a. Cortical sensory aphasia in which both auditory aphasia and visual aphasia are present.

a·phelx′i·a [G. *aphelkein*, to draw away]. Absentmindedness; inattention or indifference to external impressions. —**aphelot′ic,** *adj.*

a·phe′mi·a [G. *a-*, not; *phēmē*, voice].Motor aphasia; inability to articulate words or sentences, due to a central lesion. See *aphasia.* —**aphem′ic,** *adj.*

aph″e·pho′bi·a [G. *haphē*, touch; *phobos*, fear]. Morbid fear of physical contact with other persons.

aph′e·ter [G., starting-point]. A hypothetic substance, believed to be a catabolite, which initiates the decomposition of inogen, thus beginning muscular contraction. In a general sense, any trigger substance which initiates a function may be an apheter. See trigger *action.*

a″phil·an′thro·py [G. *a-*, not; *philein*, to love; *anthrōpos*, man]. Loss or absence of social feeling; a frequent sign of approaching psychosis.

Aph″i·o·chae′ta (af″ee·o·kee′tuh). A genus of flies of the family Phoridae. The species **A. ferruginea** and **A. scalaris** produce intestinal myiasis.

a·pho′ni·a (ay·fo′nee·uh, a·fo′nee·uh) [*a-;* G. *phōnē*, voice]. 1. Loss of speech due to some peripheral lesion. 2. Hysterical loss of the power of speech. 3. Voicelessness. —**aph′onous, aphon′ic,** *adj.*

a. clericorum. Clergyman's sore throat.

a. paranoica. The stubborn silence sometimes encountered in the insane.

paralytic a. Paralysis of the speech muscles. Syn., *phonetic paralysis.*

spastic a. Spasm of the vocal muscles initiated by efforts to speak. Syn., *dysphonia spastica.*

a′phose (ay′fohz, a·fohz′, af′ohz) [*a-;* G. *phōs*, light]. A subjective dark spot or shadow in the field of vision. See *phose.*

a·phra′si·a (a·fray′zhuh, ·zee·uh) [*a-;* G. *phrazein*, to declare]. Loss of the power to utter connected phrases.

aph″ro·dis′i·a (af″ro·diz′ee·uh) [G., from *Aphroditē*, goddess of love]. 1. Sexual desire, especially when morbid or immoderate. 2. Sexual union.

aph″ro·dis′i·ac (af″ro·diz′ee·ack) [*aphrodisia*]. Stimulating the sexual appetite; erotic.

aph·ro·dis′i·ac. Any preparation or agent stimulating the sexual passion.

aph″ro·dis″i·o·ma′ni·a [*aphrodisia;* G. *mania*, madness]. Exaggerated sexual interest and excitement. Syn., *erotomania.*

aph″ro·ne′si·a (af″ro·nee′zhuh, ·zee·uh, ·shuh, ·see·uh) [G. *a-*, not; *phronēsis*, good sense]. Foolishness, silliness, madness.

aph′tha (pl. *aphthae*) [G., thrush]. 1. A round, pearly speck found in the mouth and gastrointestinal tract, and on the lips, caused by fungi; characteristic of certain diseases, as sprue, aphthous stomatitis. 2. Aphthous stomatitis.

a. anginosa. A form of sore throat attended by slight fever, redness, enlargement of the fauces, and the formation of small white specks on the tongue and mucosa of the throat.

a. epizootica. See foot-and-mouth *disease.*

aphthae tropicae. A disease of the tropics marked by epigastric fullness, pain, vomiting, diarrhea, and redness of the tongue, with the formation of small, white, painful spots. Also called *anguilluliasis, gastroenteritis aphthosa indica, phlegmasia membranae mucosae gastropulmonalis, psilosis, tropical sprue.*

a. febrilis. Ulceration of the mouth, extending to

the esophagus and stomach, and accompanied by fever.

aphthae Riga. See cachetic *a.*

a. serpens. See gangrenous *stomatitis.*

Bednar's aphthae. Two symmetrically placed ulcers, seen at times on the hard palate of cachectic infants, one on each side of the median line.

cachectic aphthae. Those appearing beneath the tongue, and associated with grave constitutional symptoms. Also called *Cardarelli's aphthae, Valleix's aphthae, apthae Riga.* See Bednar's *aphthae.* Syn., *Riga's disease.*

aph·thenx'i·a [G. *a-*, not; *phthegxis*, utterance]. An aphasia in which articulate sounds are poorly enunciated or expressed.

aph'thoid. See *aphthous.*

aph·thon'gi·a [*a-;* G. *phthoggos*, a sound]. A rare aphasia due to spasm of the muscles of speech controlled by the hypoglossal nerves.

aph·tho'sis. A degenerative disease of a mucous membrane with the development of ulcers. See *aphtha.*

Touraine's a. A condition in which small round or oval ulcers with yellow sloughs develop in the mouth, vulva, or glans penis. It is associated with keratitis, conjunctivitis, or scleritis.

aph'thous, aph'thoid [G. *aphtha*, thrush]. Relating to, affected with, or resembling, aphthae.

a'pi- [L. *apis*, bee]. A combining form meaning *bee.*

a″pi·cec'to·my (ay″pi·seck'to·mee, ap″i·) [L. *apex*, top; G. *ektomē*, excision]. 1. Resection of a tooth. 2. Exenteration of the air cells of the apex of the petrous pyramid.

ap″i·ci'tis [*apex;* G. *-itis*, inflammation]. Inflammation of any apex, as of a tooth root or of a lung.

ap″i·co·ec'to·my [*apex;* G. *ektomē*, excision]. Removal of the root of a tooth. See *apicectomy.*

ap″i·co·lo'ca·tor, ap″i·lo'ca·tor [*apex;* L. *locus*, place]. Instrument for locating the apex of a tooth.

ap″i·col'y·sis [*apex;* G. *lysis*, a loosing]. Artificial collapse of the upper portion of a lung by separation of the parietal pleura from the chest wall; used in the treatment of pulmonary tuberculosis with apical cavities.

apicosan. A proprietary preparation of bee venom; used in rheumatism.

a″pi·cot'o·my. See *apicectomy.*

a'pi·in [L. *apium*, parsley]. A substance, perhaps a glycoside, which is obtained from curly garden parsley, *Petroselinum crispum.*

ap″i·lo'ca·tor. See *apicolocator.*

A. P. I. M. Association Professionnelle Internationale des Médecins.

ap'i·nol. A product, chiefly levo-menthone, $C_{10}H_{18}O$, obtained by the destructive distillation of the wood of the pine, *Pinus palustris.* A clear, amber-colored oil with a pine odor. Has been used locally as antiseptic and anesthetic; internally as expectorant in chronic respiratory catarrh.

a'pi·ol, ap'i·ol. $C_{12}H_{14}O_4$. White, crystalline powder with faint odor of parsley; obtained from oleoresin of parsley and from celery. It has been used in dysmenorrhea and other uterine disorders. Syn., *parsley camphor.*

liquid a. A green or yellow, oily liquid with parsley odor, used as apiol; it consists of oleoresin of parsley fruit, made by percolating the fruit with ether. It is sometimes called *apiol.* Syn., *parsley oleoresin, parsley-seed oil.*

a″pi·o·ther'a·py [L. *apis*, bee; G. *therapeia*, therapy]. Treatment of disease, especially rheumatism, with bee venom.

a″pi·pho'bi·a (ay″pi·fo'bee·uh, ap″i·) [*apis;* G. *phobos*, fear]. Morbid terror of bees and their sting.

A'pis [L.]. A genus of hymenopterous insects.

A. mellifera. The honeybee.

apis pura. A proprietary preparation of bee venom; used by intracutaneous injection in rheumatism.

A'pi·um [L., parsley]. A genus of herbs of the carrot family.

A. graveolens. Wild celery; source of apiol.

A.P.L. 1. Abbreviation for anterior pituitarylike (see anterior pituitarylike *substance*). 2. Designation of a proprietary preparation of chorionic gonadotropic hormone used intramuscularly.

a″pla·cen'tal, ap″la·cen'tal [G. *a-*, not; L. *placenta*, a cake]. Without a placenta.

ap″la·nat'ic [*a-;* G. *planasthai*, to wander]. Corrected for spherical aberration, as an aplanatic focus, or an aplanatic lens (rectilinear lens). —**aplana'sia, aplan'atism,** *n.*

a·pla'si·a (a·play'zhuh, ·zee·uh, ·shuh, ·see·uh) [*a-;* G. *plassein*, to form]. 1. Defective development or congenital absence of a part. Syn., *agenesia.* 2. In the somatotype, a physique in which the whole body or a region of the body, is poorly developed.

a. axialis extracorticalis congenita. A heredofamilial disorder appearing in early infancy, manifested by rotary movements of the eyes and head, by spasticity of all limbs, cerebellar ataxia, intention tremor, slurring speech, and dementia; a noninflammatory degeneration of the white matter of the brain and brain stem. Also called *Merzbacher-Pelizaeus disease.*

nuclear a. A congenital defect in which certain cranial nerve nuclei are absent or imperfectly developed: also called *cranial nerve a.*

a·plas'tic (ay·plas'tick, a·plas'tick) [*a-; plassein*]. 1. Structureless; formless. 2. Incapable of forming new tissue. 3. Relating to aplasia. 4. Defective in fibrin. 5. Designating an inflammation with little or no production of granulation tissue.

a·pleu'ri·a (a·ploor'ee·uh, ay·ploor'·) [*a-;* G. *pleura*, rib]. Congenital absence of the ribs; ecostatism.

ap·ne'a, ap·noe'a [*a-;* G. *pnein*, to breathe]. A transient suspension of respiration because of a decrease of carbon dioxide tension of the blood with the resultant absence of stimulation of the respiratory center. Also called *a. vera.*

a. vagi. Temporary cessation of breathing due to vagal stimulation.

cardiac a. The temporary period of suspended breathing in Cheyne-Stokes respiration.

ap·neu″ma·to'sis. See *atelectasis.*

ap·neu'mi·a [*a-;* G. *pneumōn*, the lungs]. Congenital absence of the lungs.

ap·neu'sis [*a-;* G. *pneuma*, breath; *-osis*, state or condition]. A state of maintained contraction of the inspiratory muscles observed when rhythmic inhibitory influences are prevented from reaching the inspiratory center in the brain.

ap'o-, ap-, aph- [G., from]. A prefix meaning *away from, from.* It implies deprivation or separation.

ap″o·at'ro·pine, ap·at'ro·pine (·at'ro·peen, ·pin). A chemical substance, $C_{17}H_{21}O_2N$, derived from atropine by the action of nitric acid.

ap″o·cam·no'sis [G. *apokamnein*, to grow quite weary; *-ōsis*, condition]. Intense and readily induced fatigue.

ap″o·car″te·re'sis [G. *apokarterēsis*, suicide by hunger]. Suicide by self-starvation.

ap″o·chro·mat'ic [G. *apo*, from; *chrōma*, color]. *In optics*, corrected for spherical and chromatic aberration, as an apochromatic lens.

ap″o·clei'sis (ap″o·kly'sis) [G. *apokleisis*, a shutting up]. Aversion to eating.

ap″o·co'de·ine (·ko'dee·een, ·in, ·ko'deen). An alkaloid, $C_{18}H_{19}NO_2$, derived from codeine, and having expectorant and emetic qualities.

ap'o·crine (ap'o·kryne, ·krin) [G. *apo*, from; *krinein*, to separate]. Designating a type of secretion in which the secretion-filled free end of a gland cell is pinched off, leaving the nucleus and most of the cytoplasm to recover and repeat the process.

ap″o·cy·nam′a·rin. A bitter principle obtained from *Apocynum androsaemifolium;* probably identical with the aglycone of cymarin. It is emetic and diuretic.

new a. See *cymarin.*

ap·o·cyn′e·in (ap·o·sin′ee·in, ·sigh′nee·in). A glycoside from apocynum; it acts like digitalin.

a·poc′y·nin (a·poss′i·nin). A principle, chemically acetovanillone, 4-hydroxy-3-methoxy acetophenone, from apocynum; colorless prisms, slightly soluble in water.

a·poc′y·num (a·poss′i·num) [G. *apokynon,* dog's-bane]. The dried rhizome and roots of *Apocynum cannabinum* or of *Apocynum androsaemifolium.* Its most important constituent is cymarin, a glycoside closely related to many glycosides of the digitalis group. The physiologic actions of apocynum are similar to those of digitalis. It is more irritant to mucous membranes than either digitalis or strophanthus, and therefore may cause nausea and catharsis. Dose, 0.06–0.3 Gm. (1–5 gr.). Syn., *black Indian hemp, Canada hemp.*

ap″o·de″mi·al′gi·a [G. *apodēmein,* to be away from home; *algos,* pain]. A morbid dislike of home life, with a desire for wandering; wanderlust.

a·po′di·a, a·pod′i·a [G. *a-,* not; *pous,* foot]. Congenital absence of feet. —**ap′odal, ap′odous, ap′ous,** *adj.*

ap″o·en′zyme (ap″o·en′zime, ·zim). The purely protein part of an enzyme which, with the coenzyme, forms the complete or *holoenzyme.*

a″po·er′y·thein. A protein fraction which is apparently the same as the "intrinsic factor" of pernicious anemia. It is present in normal gastric juice, but absent in the gastric juice of patients with pernicious anemia. Although it is present in the saliva it is destroyed in the stomach of such patients.

ap″o-β-e·ryth·roi′dine. $C_{15}H_{15}NO_2$; a degradation product of β-erythroidine.

ap″o·fer′ment [G. *apo,* from; L. *fermentum,* leaven]. Apozymase.

ap″o·fer′ri·tin [*apo;* L. *ferrum,* iron]. The protein resulting when iron is removed from ferritin.

a·pog′a·my, ap″o·gam′i·a [*apo;* G. *gamos,* marriage]. The production of a sporophyte from the gametophyte without the formation or union of gametes. Syn., *apomixis, parthenogenesis.* —**apogam′ic, apog′amous,** *adj.*

ap″o·mix′is, ap″o·mix′i·a [*apo;* G. *mixis,* a mingling]. Apogamy. Syn., *parthenogenesis.*

ap″o·mor′phine (ap″o·mor′feen, ·fin, ·mor·feen′). $C_{17}H_{17}NO_2$. An artificial alkaloid, derived from morphine by the abstraction of a molecule of water.

a. bromomethylate. See *a.* methylbromide.

a. hydrochloride (*apomorphinae hydrochloridum*). The salt is a grayish, crystalline powder. It is an emetic of prompt action. Dose, 3–6 mg. (1/20–1/10 gr.) hypodermically. It is expectorant in doses of 1–2 mg. (1/60–1/30 gr.). The salt should not be used if it at once imparts a green color to 100 parts of distilled water when shaken with it.

a. methylbromide. $C_{17}H_{17}NO_2.CH_3Br.H_2O$. It is used like the hydrochloride. Its solution is said to be more stable. Dose, 3–5 mg. (1/20–1/12 gr.). Syn., *apomorphine bromomethylate, euporphin.*

ap″o·myt·to′sis [G. *apomyttesthai,* to blow one's nose; *-ōsis,* condition]. Any disease marked by stertor or sneezing.

ap′o·nal. Tertiary amyl carbamate, $C_2H_5(CH_3)_2$-$C.CO_2NH_2$: has been used as a sedative and hypnotic.

a·pon″eu·ror′rha·phy [G. *apo,* from; *neuron,* tendon; *rhaphē,* a suture]. Suturing of an aponeurosis, as of the abdominal wall.

a·pon″eu·ro′ses (a·pon″yoor·o′seez). Plural of aponeurosis.

a·pon″eu·ro′sis, ap″o·neu·ro′sis [*apo; neuron;* G. *-ōsis,* condition]. An expanded tendon consisting of a fibrous or membranous sheet, serving as a means of attachment for flat muscles at their origin or insertion, or as a fascia to enclose or bind a group of muscles. —**aponeurot′ic,** *adj.*

abdominal a. The wide, tendinous expanse by which the external oblique, internal oblique, and transversus muscles are inserted.

a. of insertion. A wide tendon serving as an insertion for a wide muscle.

a. of investment. A wide tendon serving as a fascia to bind or enclose groups of muscles.

a. of occipitofrontalis muscle. The galea aponeurotica.

a. of origin. One serving as an attachment of origin.

a. of soft palate. A thin, firm, fibrous layer attached above to the hard palate and becoming gradually thinner toward the free margin of the velum.

bicipital a. The lacertus fibrosus.

epicranial a. The galea aponeurotica [BNA]. Syn., *a. of the occipitofrontalis muscle.*

palatal a. See *a. of soft palate.*

pharyngeal a. The submucous layer of the pharynx.

subscapular a. The thin membrane attached to the entire circumference of the subscapular fossa, affording attachment by its inner surface to some of the fibers of the subscapularis muscle.

supraspinous a. A thick and dense membranous layer that completes the osseofibrous case in which the supraspinatus muscle is contained, affording attachment by its inner surface to some of the fibers of the muscle.

vertebral a. A thin aponeurotic lamina extending along the whole length of the back part of the thoracic region, serving to bind down the sacrospinalis muscle and separating it from those muscles that unite the spine to the upper extremity.

a·pon″eu·ro·si′tis (a·pon″yoor·o·sigh′tis, ap″o-new·ro·) [*apo; neuron; -ōsis;* G. *-itis,* inflammation]. Inflammation of an aponeurosis.

a·pon″eu·rot′o·my (a·pon″yoor·ot′o·mee, ap″o-new·rot′o·mee) [*apo; neuron;* G. *tomē,* a cutting]. Incision of an aponeurosis.

a·pon′i·a [G. *a-,* not; *ponos,* toil]. 1. Abstention from work; nonexertion. 2. Absence of pain.

a·poph′y·sate [G. *apo,* from; *physis,* growth]. Provided with an apophysis.

a·poph′y·sis [G.]. A process, outgrowth, or projection of some part or organ, as of a bone. —**apophys′eal, apophys′ial,** *adj.*

basilar a. Basilar process of the occipital bone.

calcaneal a. Epiphysis of the posterior part of calcaneus.

cerebral a. Pineal gland.

false a. See *epiphysis.*

lenticular a. The lenticular process.

mammillary a. Olfactory bulb.

true a. One which has never been an epiphysis.

a·poph″y·si′tis [*apophysis;* G. *-itis,* inflammation]. Inflammation of an apophysis.

ap″o·plas′mi·a (ap″o·plaz′mee·uh) [G. *apo,* from; *plasma,* from *plassein,* to form]. Deficiency of the blood plasma.

ap″o·plec′ti·form [G. *apoplēssein,* to cripple by a stroke; L. *forma,* form]. Resembling apoplexy.

ap′o·plex″y [G. *apoplēxia,* from *apoplēssein*]. 1. The symptom complex resulting from hemorrhage into or upon the brain, or from embolism or thrombosis of the cerebral vessels, consisting of sudden onset of coma, and focal neurological signs. 2. Gross hemorrhage into any organ, as the lungs, spleen, ovary, eye, etc.; designated as apoplexy of the affected organ. *Rare.* —**apoplec'tic, apoplec'tiform,** *adj.*

asthenic a. That due to vital depression or debility.

bulbar a. That due to hemorrhage into the substance of the medulla oblongata or pons, causing paralysis of one or both sides of the body, inability to swallow, difficulty in protruding the tongue, dyspnea, gastric disorders, and disturbed heart action.

capillary a. That resulting from the rupture of capillaries.

cerebellar a. That affecting the cerebellum.

cerebral a. That affecting the cerebrum.

embolic a. Apoplexy resulting from the plugging of a cerebral vessel by an embolus.

fulminant a. A sudden and fatal form of cerebral hemorrhage.

ingravescent a. A form in which there is a slowly progressing loss of consciousness, owing to a gradual leakage of blood from a ruptured vessel, or to a thrombosis. Also called *progressive a.*

nervous a. (a) Acute anemia of the brain. (b) A condition simulating apoplexy caused by some functional nervous condition, as hysteria. Also called *functional a.*

placental a. Escape of blood into the placental substance.

pulmonary a. Escape of blood into the pulmonary parenchyma.

renal a. A misuse of the word "apoplexy," commonly used for ischuria, or suppression of urine from hemorrhage into the substance of the kidney or other renal lesion.

retinal a. Hemorrhage into the retina.

sanguineous a. Hemorrhage into or upon the brain; true apoplexy.

serous a. (a) That due to an effusion of serous matter into or upon the brain; usually by effusion into the ventricles causing distention. (b) Serous meningitis. Also called *pituitous a.*

simple a. Fatal coma in which no cerebral accident can be found.

spinal a. Rupture of a blood vessel into the substance of the spinal cord.

splenic a. Hemorrhage into the splenic substance.

suppurative a. That due to purulent processes.

uterine a. Escape of blood into the muscular tissue of the uterus.

uteroplacental a. See Couvelaire *uterus.*

a·pop·nix'is [G. *apopnigein,* to choke]. A choking sensation. Syn., *globus hystericus.*

ap·o·qui'nine (ap·o·kwye'nine, ·kwi·neen'). $C_{19}H_{22}N_2O_2$; an alkaloid obtained by demethylation of quinine.

ap"or·rhip'sis [G., from *aporrhiptein,* to throw away]. The throwing off of the clothes or the bedclothes; a symptom seen in some cases of mental disorder.

a·po'si·a (a·po'zhuh, ·zee·uh) [G. *a-,* not; *posis,* a drinking]. Absence of thirst or of the feeling of thirst; adipsia.

ap"o·sid'er·in. A brown, granular, iron-negative pigment apparently formed from hemosiderin by action of acid fixatives.

ap"o·si'ti·a (ap"o·sish'ee·uh, ·sit'ee·uh) [G. *apo,* from; *sitos,* food]. Aversion to or loathing of food. —**aposit'ic,** *adj.*

ap'o·some [*apo;* G. *sōma,* body]. A cytoplasmic cellular inclusion produced by the cell itself.

a·pos'po·ry [*apo;* G. *sporos,* spore]. Apogamy involving the replacement of spores by unspecialized cells not undergoing miosis.

a·pos'ta·sis [G., defection]. End or crisis of an attack of disease; termination by crisis.

a·pos'thi·a [G. *a-,* not; *posthē,* foreskin]. Congenital absence of the prepuce.

a·poth'e·car"ies' weight. A system of weights and measures used in compounding medicines. The troy pound of 5760 grains is the standard. It is subdivided into 12 ounces. The ounce is subdivided into 8 drachms, the drachm into 3 scruples, and the scruple into 20 grains. For fluid measure the quart of 32 fluidounces is subdivided into 2 pints, the pint into 16 fluidounces, the fluidounce into 8 fluidrachms, and the fluidrachm into 60 minims. The following symbols and abbreviations are used:

♏, *minim.*
℈, *scrupulus,* a scruple (20 gr.).
ʒ, *drachma,* a drachm (60 gr.).
℥, *uncia,* an ounce (480 gr.).
℔., *libra,* a pound.
C., *congius,* a gallon.
O., *octarius,* a pint.
gr., *granum,* a grain.
ss., *semissis,* one-half.

See Tables of Weights and Measures, Appendix.

a·poth'e·car"y [G. *apothēkē,* storehouse]. 1. A druggist or pharmacist; one who prepares and sells drugs, fills prescriptions, etc. 2. In Great Britain, a physician filling his own prescriptions; especially one licensed by the Society of Apothecaries of London, or by the Apothecaries' Hall of Ireland. *Obs.*

apothesine hydrochloride. Trade-mark for a local anesthetic, gamma-diethylaminopropyl cinnamate hydrochloride. It is effective for injection anesthesia but relatively inefficient when applied to mucous membranes.

ap"ox·e'me·na [G. *apoxein,* to scrape off]. The group of substances removed from a pocket in the treatment of pericementoclasia.

ap"ox·e'sis [G., smoothing, from *apoxein*]. The act of removing apoxemena from the periodontoclasial pocket, and rendering the denuded cementum smooth.

ap"o·zy'mase. The residue from yeast after drying and extracting the cozymase with water.

ap"pa·ra'tus [L., preparation]. 1. A collection of instruments or devices used for a special purpose. 2. *In anatomy,* used to designate collectively the organs or parts of organs performing a certain function; a mechanism.

canalicular a. See internal reticular *a.*

Golgi a. See internal reticular *a.*

Guthrie-Smith a. One used to facilitate exercises in cases of poliomyelitis. The limb or trunk is suspended in slings, and exercises are controlled by adjusting the point of suspension.

Hertel a. An apparatus for measuring the degree of exophthalmos.

internal reticular a. An organoid, probably present in all cells, demonstrated by special staining methods. It may be important in cellular activities, especially in the secretion of gland cells. Syn., *Golgi a., canalicular a., vacuome.* Formerly called *trophospongium, segregation a.*

juxtaglomerular a. A cuff of epithelioid cells in the kidney around the afferent arteriole near its entrance into the glomerulus.

lacrimal a. The mechanism for secreting tears and draining them into the nose, consisting of the lacrimal gland, lake, puncta, canaliculi, sac, and the nasolacrimal duct. See Plate 19.

stereotaxic a. An apparatus which allows accurate insertion of long electrodes deep into the brain. This may be used in physiologic experimentation or in neurosurgery.

Tiselius a. An electrophoresis apparatus which permits the measurement of electric mobilities of proteins by use of the moving-boundary method. The cell is divided into compartments which permit easy isolation of the components separated by the electric current.

vestibular a. The anatomical parts concerned with the vestibular portion of the eighth cranial nerve, including the saccule, utricle, semicircular canals, vestibular nerve, and vestibular nuclei.

appella. A proprietary, dehydrated, concentrated apple powder for use in the treatment of diarrhea.

ap·pend′age [L. *appendere*, to weigh, hang]. Anything appended, usually of minor importance. —**appendic′ular, appendic′ulate,** *adj.*

appendages of the eye. The eyelashes, eyebrows, lacrimal gland, lacrimal sac and ducts, and conjunctiva.

auricular a. (a) The projecting part of either cardiac atrium. See *auricle*, 2. (b) See *auricle*, 1. (c) Any ear-shaped structure or appendage.

cecal a. Old term for the vermiform appendix.

cutaneous appendages. Nails, hair, sebaceous glands, mammary glands, and sweat glands.

epiploic appendages. See under *appendix.*

fetal appendages. Placenta, amnion, chorion, and umbilical cord.

ovarian a. Parovarium.

pineal a. Epiphysis.

pituitary a. The pituitary.

uterine appendages. Ovaries and oviducts.

ap″pen·dec′to·my, ap·pen″di·cec′to·my [L. *appendix*, appendage; G. *ektomē*, excision]. Excision of the vermiform appendix.

atrial a. Excision of an auricular appendage of a cardiac atrium, especially that of the left atrium as part of an operation for the relief of mitral stenosis.

ap·pen″di·ci′tis [*appendix;* G. *-itis*, inflammation]. Inflammation of the vermiform appendix.

actinomycotic a. That form due to infection with actinomyces.

acute a. That form characterized by sudden onset of abdominal pain, generalized at first, then becoming localized to the right lower quadrant, with nausea, vomiting, and constipation, fever, leukocytosis, localized tenderness, and rigidity. In the absence of operation the attack subsides or goes on to gangrene, perforation, and abscess formation or peritonitis.

acute catarrhal a. The early stage of the disease characterized by inflammation of the mucosa with a nonpurulent exudate. It may heal spontaneously or go on to the diffuse type. Also called *simple a.*

acute diffuse a. A later stage of the disease than the catarrhal form, characterized by more extensive inflammation, a purulent exudate, ulceration of the mucosa, and sometimes gangrene and rupture.

chronic a. That form characterized by recurring attacks of right-sided pain without the signs and symptoms of acute attacks. The appendicular origin of this ailment is doubted by many.

gangrenous a. Acute appendicitis with formation of pus and necrosis of the appendix.

obliterative a. That form in which the lumen is narrowed or closed; often found in so-called chronic appendicitis.

perforating a. This form follows acute gangrenous appendicitis with perforation of the appendix and peritonitis or abscess formation.

phlegmonous a. Abscess formation following perforating appendicitis.

purulent a. Suppurative appendicitis.

recurrent a. Repeated attacks of acute appendicitis.

subacute a. Mild acute appendicitis.

suppurative a. Acute appendicitis with formation of pus.

syncongestive a. Inflammation of the appendix due to disease of adjacent structures.

tuberculous a. Chronic ulcerative appendicitis of tuberculous origin.

ap·pen″di·clau′sis. Chronic appendicitis, especially of the obliterative type. See chronic *appendicitis*, obliterative *appendicitis.*

ap·pen″di·co·en″ter·os′to·my. See *appendicostomy.*

ap·pen′di·co·lith″ [*appendico-;* Gr. *lithos*, stone]. A concretion of dried mucus, bacteria, and cellular debris, or of fecal matter coated with mucus: often found in inflamed appendices.

ap·pen″di·cos′to·my [*appendix;* G. *stoma*, mouth]. Withdrawal of the appendix and mesoappendix through a McBurney incision, anchoring the former to the abdominal wall. The tip is then cut off and a catheter passed through the appendiceal lumen into the cecum for subsequent irrigation.

ap·pen′dix (pl. *appendixes, appendices*) [L.]. An appendage. —**appen′dical, appendicial, appendiceal,** *adj.*

appendices epiploicae. Fatty projections of the serous coat of the large intestine.

appendices epoophori. Vestigial remnants of the mesonephric tubules or ducts found in or on the broad ligament of the uterus or near the fimbriae of the uterine tube.

a. auricularis. See auricular *appendage.*

a. epididymidis. Vestigial mesonephric tubules or ducts attached to the head of the epididymis.

a. of the laryngeal ventricle. A blindly ending diverticulum of mucous membrane extending from the laryngeal ventricle upward, between the ventricular fold and the inner surface of the thyroid cartilage; saccule of the larynx.

a. testis. A remnant of the cranial part of Müller's duct, attached to the testis. Formerly called *hydatid of Morgagni.*

auricular a. See *auricle*, 2.

vermiform a. The small, blind gut projecting from the cecum. See Plate 13.

vesicular appendixes. Vestigial remnants of cranial mesonephric tubules, located in the distal end of the mesosalpinx or adjacent broad ligament.

xiphoid a. The third piece of the sternum: it becomes osseous in mature age. Also called *xiphoid cartilage, xiphoid process, ensiform process.*

ap″per·cep′tion [L. *ad*, to; *percipere*, to perceive]. Consciousness of the relation of new events, situations, or sensations to past experience. —**apperceptive,** *adj.*

ap″per·son″i·fi·ca′tion [*ad;* L. *persona*, person; *facere*, to make]. Unconscious transfer to one's own ego of certain qualities in other persons or objects. Syn., *identification.*

ap′pe·tite [L. *appetitus*, from *appetere*, to strive after]. Desire for food, not necessarily prompted by hunger; any natural desire or craving.

a. juice. Gastric juice, the flow of which is initiated by the sight, odor, or thought of food (psychic causes) and by tasting or chewing food, without swallowing it.

excessive a. Bulimia.

perverted a. A desire for unnatural or indigestible foods, seen occasionally during pregnancy; pica.

ap′pe·ti″zer [*appetere*]. A medicine or aperitif taken before a meal to stimulate the appetite.

ap′pla·nate [L. *ad*, to; *planus*, flat]. Horizontally flattened. —**applana′tion,** *n.*

ap′pli·ca″tor [L. *applicare*, to apply]. An instrument used in making local applications.

ap"po·si'tion [L. *appositus*, from *apponere*, to apply to]. The act of fitting together; the state of being fitted together; juxtaposition.

ap·proach' [OF. *approchier*, from L. *ad*, *propiare*, to draw near]. *In surgery*, the manner of securing access to a joint, cavity, part, or organ by a suitable incision through the overlying or neighboring structures, as the anterior axillary approach for exposing the shoulder joint.

a·pprox'i·mal, ap·prox'i·mate [L. *approximare*, to draw near to]. Situated close or near; contiguous; next to each other; as approximal fillings.

ap·prox"i·ma'tion [*approximare*]. The act or process of bringing together. —**approx'imate,** *v.*

a·prac"tog·no'si·a. A type of agnosia in which there is disorientation for right and left.

a·prax'i·a (ay·prack'see·uh, a·prack'·) [G., from *a-*, not; *prassein*, to do]. A disorder of the nervous system, caused by lesions in the cortical area; characterized by inability to perform purposeful movements, although no muscular paralysis or sensory disturbance is present. Also called *constructional apraxia.*

amnestic a. That due to inability to remember a command.

ideational a. That in which there is a lack of ideas for planning an act, or a distorted sequence of ideas or conception of how to use them; due to diffuse brain disease.

ideokinetic a. See ideomotor *a.*

ideomotor a. That in which simple single acts are correctly performed, but the sequence of associated acts is incorrect and a final, complex act cannot be carried out; due to interruption of the association pathways between ideational and motor kinesthetic areas. Syn., *ideokinetic a.*

kinetic a. See motor *a.*

motor a. Apraxia in which simple movements are clumsy and individual finger movements are often lost, caused by lesion of the precentral gyrus involving kinesthetic memory. Syn., *kinetic a.*

ocular motor a. A syndrome characterized by the absence of willed movements of the eyes laterally, retention of random movements, and fixation gaze accomplished by a jerky overshooting of the head.

apresoline hydrochloride. Trade-marked name for hydralazine hydrochloride or 1-hydrazinophthalazine hydrochloride, an antihypertensive agent.

a"pro·bar'bi·tal. Generic name for *allylisopropylbarbituric acid.* See *alurate.*

a·proc'ti·a (ay·prock'shee·uh, a·prock'·) [*a-*; G. *proktos*, anus]. Imperforate anus. —**aproctous,** *adj.*

a"pro·sex'i·a [G., want of attention]. A mental disturbance consisting in inability to fix attention upon a subject.

a. nasalis. Inattention and mental dullness often seen in chronic nasal catarrh, especially when associated with adenoids, in children.

a"pro·so'pi·a [G. *a-*, not; *prosōpon*, face]. Congenital absence of part or all of the face. —**apros'opous,** *adj.*; **apros'opus,** *n.*

ap·sel"a·phe'si·a (ap·sel"uh·fee'zhuh, ·zee·uh, ·shuh, ·see·uh) [*a-*; G. *psēlaphēsis*, a touching]. Loss of the tactile sense.

ap"si·thy'ri·a, ap"si·thu're·a [*a-*; G. *psithyrizein*, to whisper]. Hysterical aphonia, in which the patient loses the voice, being unable even to whisper.

ap·sych'i·a (ap·sick'ee·uh, ap·sigh'kee·uh, ay·sick'·, a·sigh'·) [*a-*; G. *psychē*, the conscious self]. Unconsciousness; a faint or swoon. *Obs.*

ap·ty'a·lism (ap·tye'u·liz·um, ay·tye'·), **ap"ty·a'li·a** (ap"tye·ay'lee·uh, ap"ti·) [*a-*; G. *ptyalizein*, to salivate]. Deficiency or absence of saliva.

a'pus [*a-*; G. *pous*, foot]. Lacking feet, or without the entire lower extremities.

a·py'e·tous [*a-*; G. *pyon*, pus]. Nonsuppurative; nonpurulent; without pus. *Obs.*

a·py'rene (ay·pye'reen) [*a-*; G. *pyrēn*, fruit-stone]. Descriptive of abnormal sperm cells in which all the chromosomes degenerate, so that they lack a nucleus. See *eupyrene, oligopyrene.*

a"py·rex'i·a (ay"pye·reck'see·uh, a·pye·) [*a-*; G. *pyressein*, to be feverish]. Absence of fever. —**apyrexial, apyret'ic,** *adj.*

AQ, A.Q. Achievement quotient.

aq. *Aqua;* water; water of crystallization.

A qrs *In electrocardiography*, symbol for the mean manifest magnitude of QRS determined algebraically and measured in microvolt seconds.

aq'ua (ack'wuh, ay'kwuh) (pl. *aquae*) [L., water]. Water; medicated water, as aromatic waters, saturated solutions of volatile oils or other volatile substances in water. Abbreviated, a., aq. —**a'que·ous,** *adj.*

aquacillin. A trade-mark for certain preparations of crystalline procaine penicillin G for administration by aqueous injection.

aq"uae·duc'tus. See *aqueduct.*

aquakay. Trade-mark for a water-soluble derivative of menadione.

aquaphor. A proprietary ointment base with the ability to absorb three times its own weight of water or aqueous solutions of medicaments.

aquasol A. Trade-mark for a water-dispersible preparation of vitamin A.

aq'ue·duct [*aqua;* L. *ductus*, a leading]. A canal for the passage of fluid; any canal.

a. of Fallopius. Old term for facial *canal.*

a. of Sylvius. See cerebral *a.*

a. of the cochlea. A canal which establishes a communication between the perilymphatic space of the osseous labyrinth and the subarachnoid space, and transmits a vein for the cochlea.

a. of the vestibule. A canal of the vestibule of the ear running from the vestibule and opening on the back of the petrous portion of the temporal bone and containing the endolymphatic duct and a small vein.

cerebral a. The elongated, slender cavity of the midbrain which connects the third and fourth ventricles. Also called *a. of Sylvius.* See Plate 18.

communicating a. A small canal sometimes found at the junction of the mastoid and petrous portions of the temporal bone; it gives passage to an emissary vein from the transverse sinus.

a'que·ous (ay'kwee·us, ack'wee·us) [*aqua*]. The aqueous humor; the transparent fluid of the anterior chamber of the eye.

aquinone. Trade-mark for menadione.

aq"uo-i'on. A complex ion containing one or more molecules of water.

ar-. 1. *In chemistry*, a combining form denoting *aromatic.* 2. A form of Latin *ad-* assimilated in English before *r.*

Ara's test. See Takata-Ara *test.*

ar'a·bic ac'id (ar'uh·bick, a·rab'ick). The chief constituent of acacia, in which it occurs in the form of calcium, magnesium, and potassium salts. It is a polysaccharide yielding on hydrolysis with dilute acid, L-arabinose, L-rhamnose, D-galactose, and an aldobionic acid containing D-glucuronic acid and D-galactose in glycosidal combination. Syn., *arabin.*

ar'a·bin [G. *Arabikos*, Arabic]. Arabic acid.

a·rab'i·nose, ar'a·bi·nose". $CHO(CHOH)_3CH_2OH$; an aldopentose which exists in two structural configurations having a mirror-image relationship to one another and differentiated as L-arabinose and D-arabinose. The former is dextrorotatory.

and hence is sometimes referred to as L(+)-arabinose; the latter is levorotatory, and is therefore designated D(−)-arabinose. The L-sugar, also called *pectinose, pectin sugar,* and *gum sugar,* is widely distributed in plants, usually as a component of a complex polysaccharide; thus, it may be obtained by hydrolysis of arabic acid from acacia. D-Arabinose may be obtained by degradation of dextrose (D-glucose).

a·rab′i·tol. $CH_2OH(CHOH)_3CH_2OH$; an alcohol derived from arabinose.

a·rach′ic, ar″a·chid′ic ac′id. $CH_3(CH_2)_{18}COOH$; a solid fatty acid obtained from peanut oil.

ar″a·chid′ic (ar″uh·kid′ick) [G. *arakos,* a leguminous plant]. Pertaining to the peanut, *Arachis hypogaea.*

a·rach″i·don′ic ac′id (a·rack″i·don′ick, a·rake″i·, ar″uh·ki·). $C_{20}H_{32}O_2$. An unsaturated, fatty acid occurring in lecithin and cephalin. It is one of the fatty acids which will cure the syndrome in the rat caused by dietary deficiency of essential fatty acids.

ar′a·chin (ar′uh·kin). A globulin from peanuts.

arachn-. See *arachno-.*

a·rach″ne·pho′bi·a (a·rack″ni·) [G. *arachnēs,* spider; *phobos,* fear]. Morbid fear of spiders.

A·rach′ni·da (a·rack′ni·duh) [*arachnēs*]. A large class of the Arthropoda which includes scorpions, spiders, mites, and ticks. They are wingless, usually lack antennae, and, as adults, have four pairs of legs.

a·rach′nid·ism, a·rach′noid·ism [*arachnēs;* G. *eidos,* form]. A condition produced by the bite of a poisonous spider; venom poisoning.

ar″ach·ni′tis (ar″ack·nigh′tis). See *arachnoiditis.*

a·rach′no- (a·rack′no-), **arachn-** [*arachnēs*]. A combining form meaning *spider.*

a·rach″no·dac′ty·ly [*arachnēs;* G. *daktylos,* finger]. Spider fingers; a condition in which the fingers, and sometimes the toes, are abnormally long; Marfan's syndrome. Syn., *dolichostenomelia.*

a·rach′noid (a·rack′noyd) [*arachnēs;* G. *eidos,* form]. The *arachnoidea encephali* [BNA], and *arachnoidea spinalis* [BNA]. The arachnoid membrane; the central of the three meninges covering the brain and spinal cord. It is very fine and delicate in structure, following the pia mater into each sulcus and around each convolution, but separated from it by the subarachnoid space. The two membranes are often considered as one organ, the piarachnoid. —**arachnoi′dal,** *adj.*

a·rach·noi′de·a [BNA]. The arachnoid membrane. See *arachnoid.*

a·rach′noid·ism. See *arachnidism.*

a·rach″noi·di′tis [*arachnēs; eidos;* G. *-itis,* inflammation]. Inflammation of the piarachnoid of the spinal cord and brain.

adhesive a. Adhesion of the arachnoid layers due to inflammation subsequent to infection, noxious agents, or trauma. The cicatrix may occur in any region of the central nervous system which is enveloped by arachnoid membrane.

a. of cerebral hemispheres. A collection of fluid in a thickened and opaque arachnoid in the surface of the brain. It is characterized by headache, monoplegia, speech disturbance, and changes in the visual fields, and later by focal epileptic attacks.

chiasmal a. Localized inflammation of the meninges around the optic chiasm and optic nerves and of the contained structures, formerly considered the pathogenetic factor in syphilitic optic atrophy. Syn., *optochiasmic a.*

chronic serous a. A form which may be local or generalized, similar to cerebellar tumor, with thickening of the arachnoid over the cerebellum and enlargement of the basilar cisterns causing internal hydrocephalus. Treatment is the surgical opening of the basal cisterns. Also called *cisternal arachnoiditis.*

cisternal a. Chronic serous arachnoiditis.

optochiasmic a. See chiasmal *a.*

posterior cranial fossa a. Inflammation of the arachnoid in the posterior cranial fossa, a common complication of mastoiditis, petrositis, lateral sinus thrombosis, chronic middle-ear disease, and leptomeningitis. It may increase intracranial pressure by impeding the escape of the cerebrospinal fluid from the fourth ventricle, thus causing obstructive internal hydrocephalus.

segmental a. A type in which arachnoidal adhesions connect the neighboring nerve roots with each other and with the dura mater.

a·rach′noid-u·re″ter·os′to·my. A one-stage operation for the relief of progressive hydrocephaly in infants, in which cerebrospinal fluid is shunted into the urinary tract. One kidney is removed and a polyethylene tube is inserted into the ureter. The other end of the tube is introduced into the subarachnoid space at the level of the second lumbar vertebra.

ar″ach·nol′y·sin (ar″ack·nol′i·sin) [*arachnēs;* G. *lysis,* a loosing]. A substance contained in the spider *Epeira diadema,* which reacts strongly with the blood of the rabbit and man but not with the blood of the horse or guinea pig.

aralen diphosphate. Trade-mark for chloroquine phosphate.

A·ra′li·a [perhaps Iroquoian in origin]. A genus of aromatic plants of the Araliaceae.

A. nudicaulis. Wild sarsaparilla; used similarly to *A. racemosa.*

A. racemosa. American spikenard, whose dried rhizome and roots yield a volatile oil and a saponin; formerly used as a stimulant, diaphoretic, and alterative.

Aran, François Amilcar [*French physician,* 1817–61]. Described progressive spinal muscular atrophy (1850) shortly after Duchenne (1849). This is called *Duchenne-Aran muscular atrophy, Cruveilhier's disease.*

Aranzi, Giulio Cesare (Arantius, Aranzio) [*Italian anatomist,* 1530–89]. Remembered for his description of the ductus venosus (called *duct of Arantius*), ligamentum venosum, semilunar valves, and Arantius' ventricle. The *nodules of Arantius* are those of the semilunar valves.

a·ra′phi·a. Dysraphism.

a″ra·ro′ba (ahr″uh·ro′buh, ar″uh·ro′buh) [Pg.]. Goa powder. An oxidation product of the resin found deposited in the wood of the trunk of *Andira Araroba,* of Brazil. From it is obtained chrysarobin, a complex mixture of reduction products of chrysophanol. It is used in skin affections.

ar″bor·i·za′tion [L. *arbor,* tree]. A conformation or arrangement resembling the branching of a tree. —**ar′borize,** *v.t., v.i.;* **arbo′real, arbo′reous, arbores′cent,** *adj.*

terminal a. (a) Branched end of a sensory nerve fiber. (b) A motor end plate. (c) Terminal ramifications of the Purkinje system of the heart.

vascular a. A treelike branching of blood vessels.

ar′bor vi′tae (ahr′bor vy′tee) [L., tree of life]. 1. Arborescent appearance of the white substance in a median section of the cerebellum. 2. Series of ridges and folds of the mucosa within the uterine cervix: also called *plicae palmatae cervicis.*

ar′bu·tin [L. *arbutus,* strawberry tree]. A bitter glycoside from the *Arctostaphylos Uva-ursi,* or bearberry. See *uva ursi.*

arc [L. *arcus,* a bow, an arch]. A part of the circumference of a circle; a more or less curved passageway.

a. de cercle. A pathologic posture in which there is extreme bending of the body forward or backward; sometimes seen in hysteria.

arterial a. of Riolan. An occasional artery situated in the posterior abdominal wall which forms a connection between the superior mesenteric artery and a branch of the inferior mesenteric artery.

bigonial a. (of lower jaw). A measurement around the anterior margin of the jaw.

binauricular a. A measurement from the center of one auditory meatus to the other, directly upward across the top of the head.

bregmatolambdoid a. A measurement along the sagittal suture from the bregma to the lambda.

frontal a. The measurement from the nasion to the bregma.

maximum transverse a. The measurement across the face from a point on each side just anterior to the external auditory meatus.

nasobregmatic a. A line measured from the root of the nose to the bregma.

nasomalar a. Measurement between the outer margins of the orbits over the nasion.

naso-occipital a. Measurement from the root of the nose to the lowest point of the occipital protuberance.

neural a. A nerve circuit consisting of two or more neurons, the receptor and the effector, with intercalated neurons between them.

nuclear a. Lens star.

occipital a. Measurement from the lambda to the opisthion.

parietal a. Measurement from the bregma to the lambda.

reflex a. The nervous pathway traversed by an impulse during reflex action, extending from a receptor to an effector.

ar·cade′ [*arcus*]. A series of arches; term used in reference to blood vessels.

crural a. The inguinal ligament.

inferior temporal a. The zygomatic arch.

superior temporal a. The upper margin of the orbit.

arcanol. A proprietary preparation in tablet form, containing atophan and acetylsalicylic acid.

ar·ca′num [L., a secret]. A secret medicine.

ar″ca·tu′ra [L. *arcus*, a bow, an arch]. A condition of horses marked by the undue outward curvature of the forelegs.

arch [*arcus*]. A structure having a curved outline resembling that of an arc or a bow.

abdominothoracic a. The lower boundary of the front of the thorax.

alveolar a. That formed by the alveolar process of each jaw.

anastomotic a. One uniting two veins or arteries.

aortic arches. Six pairs of embryonic vascular arches encircling the pharynx in the visceral arches. In mammals, the left fourth arch becomes a part of the systemic circulatory system and the sixth pair becomes incorporated in the pulmonary circulation.

arches of the foot. (a) The *metatarsal arch*, a transverse hollow on the inner part of the sole in the line of the tarsometatarsal articulations. (b) The *inner longitudinal arch*, consisting of the calcaneus, the talus, the navicular, three cuneiform bones, and the first three toes. (c) The *outer longitudinal arch*, made up of the calcaneus, the cuboid, and the fourth and fifth toes.

a. of the aorta. The transverse portion of the aorta between its ascending and descending portions. See Plates 5, 7.

axillary a. An occasional muscle slip in the axilla connecting the latissimus dorsi or teres major with the pectoralis major.

branchial a. (a) One of the posthyoid gill arches in lower vertebrates. (b) Any of the visceral arches in embryos of higher vertebrates.

carpal arches. See dorsal carpal *rete*.

cervical a. One of the second to sixth visceral arches forming part of the cervical region.

cortical a. The renal substance which stretches from one column to another and surrounds the base of a pyramid.

costal a. The arch of the ribs.

deep femoral a. A band of fibers originating apparently in the transversalis fascia, arching across the femoral sheath and attached to the middle of the inguinal ligament and the pectineal line.

deep palmar a. See deep volar *a*.

deep volar a. That formed by the anastomosis of the terminal part of the radial artery with the deep volar branch of the ulnar artery. Syn., *deep palmar a.*

dental a. The parabolic curve formed by the cutting edges and masticating surfaces of the teeth; the alveolar arch.

double aortic a. Failure of the right fourth branchial arch to disappear during normal embryological development, resulting in two aortic arches or an aortic ring.

facial a. The hyoid arch supplied by the facial nerve.

frontal a. *In comparative anatomy*, the ring formed by the presphenoid, orbitosphenoid, and frontal bones.

glossopalatine a. That formed by the projection of the glossopalatinus muscle covered with mucous membrane. Also called *palatoglossal a.* Formerly called *anterior pillar of the fauces.*

gluteal a. An opening in the gluteal fascia allowing passage for the gluteal vessels and nerves.

gothic a. A dental arch which is depressed laterally and pointed anteriorly.

hemal a. *In comparative anatomy*, the inferior loop of the typical vertebra, surrounding the essential portion of the vascular system. In man, the arch formed by the body of a vertebra together with the ribs and sternum.

hyoid a. The second visceral arch.

hypochordal a. A condensation of mesenchyme forming transverse bands connecting the ventral ends of the embryonic neural processes of the cervical vertebrae. Transitory except in the first cervical segment where it develops into the ventral arch of the atlas.

jugular a. A communicating vein between the anterior jugular veins situated in the suprasternal space.

lumbocostal a. A ligamentous arch from the twelfth rib to the first lumbar vertebra serving as part of the attachment of the diaphragm. The **lateral lumbocostal arch** is that lying anterior to the quadratus lumborum; the **medial lumbocostal arch** is that lying anterior to the psoas major.

mandibular a. The first visceral arch, including the maxillary process: also called *Meckel's bar.*

maxillary a. See palatomaxillary *a.*

nasal a. One uniting the two frontal veins.

neural a. (a) Vertebral arch. (b) *In comparative anatomy*, the superior loop of the typical vertebra including the neural canal.

occipital a. *In comparative anatomy*, the ring formed by the basioccipital, exoccipital, and supraoccipital bones.

palatal a. The concavity of the hard palate when seen in transverse section.

palatine arches. The glossopalatine and pharyngopalatine arches.
palatomaxillary a. One formed by the palatine, maxillary, and premaxillary bones.
palmar arches. See deep volar *a.* and superficial volar *a.*
parietal a. *In comparative anatomy,* the ring formed by the basisphenoid, alisphenoid, and parietal bones.
pharyngeal a. See visceral *a.*
pharyngopalatine a. That formed by the projection of the pharyngopalatinus muscle covered by mucous membrane. Also called *palatopharyngeal a.* Formerly called *posterior pillar of the fauces.*
plantar a. The arch, in the sole of the foot, made by the lateral plantar artery and the deep plantar branch of the dorsalis pedis artery.
postoral a. Any one of the second to sixth visceral arches.
pubic a. That formed by the conjoined inferior rami of the pubis and ischium.
sitting a. That representing the line of transfer of weight through the pelvis in the sitting position; from the sacrum through the ilia and ischia to the ischial tuberosities.
standing a. That representing the line of transfer of weight through the pelvis in the standing position; from the sacrum through the ilia to the acetabulums and heads of the femurs.
superciliary a. See supraorbital *a.*
superficial palmar a. See superficial volar *a.*
superficial volar a. That formed by the ulnar artery in the palm of the hand and completed by a branch of the radial artery. Syn., *superficial palmar a.* See Plate 7.
supraorbital a. The curved and prominent margin of the frontal bone that forms the upper boundary of the orbit.
tarsal arches. The arches of the palpebral arteries.
tendinous a. A thickened portion of the parietal pelvic fascia extending from the medial aspect of the body of the pubic bone to the spine of the ischium; the fibers of the iliococcygeal portion of the levator ani muscle attach to it. Syn., *arcus tendineus, white line of the pelvis.*
tonsillar a. The isthmus of the fauces.
vertebral a. That formed by the paired pedicles and laminas of a vertebra; the posterior part of a vertebra which together with the anterior part, the body, encloses the vertebral foramen in which the spinal cord is lodged.
visceral a. (a) One of the series of mesodermal ridges covered by epithelium bounding the lateral wall of the oral and pharyngeal region of vertebrates; embryonic in higher forms, they contribute to the formation of the face and neck. (b) The skeleton of a visceral arch. (c) In gill-bearing vertebrates, one of the first two arches as opposed to the remaining or branchial arches.
volar arches. See deep volar *a.* and superficial volar *a.*
zygomatic a. That formed by the zygomatic process of the temporal bone and the temporal process of the zygomatic bone.

arch- See *archi-.*

ar·cha′ic [G. *archaikos,* old-fashioned]. *In psychiatry,* designating elements in the unconscious which are remnants of man's prehistoric past, and which reappear in dreams and other symbolic manifestations.

ar″che·go′ni·um (ahr″ki·go′nee·um) [G. *archē,* beginning; *gonos,* race]. *In botany,* the structure which produces the egg in bryophytes and pteridophytes.

ar·chen′ter·on (ahr·ken′tur·on) [*archē;* G. *enteron, intestine*]. The embryonic alimentary cavity of the gastrula, lined by endoderm. Syn., *archigaster, coelenteron, gastrocoel, primitive* or *primary gut, progaster, primitive stomach.* —**archenter′ic,** *adj.*

ar″che·o·ki·net′ic (ahr″kee·o·ki·net′ick, ·kigh-net′ick) [G. *archaios,* ancient; *kinēsis,* motion]. Referring to an ancient or primitive type of motor function.

ar·che·py′on (ahr·ki·pye′on, ahr·kep′ee·on) [G. *archē,* beginning; *pyon,* pus]. Pus that has become caseated, or so thick that it does not flow.

ar′che·type (ahr′ki·type) [G. *archetypon,* pattern]. 1. A basic model; prototype. 2. *In comparative anatomy,* an ideal, generalized structural pattern of one of the main kinds of organisms, assumed to be the form of the original ancestor of the group.

ar′chi-, arch- [L.; G. prefix *archi-* from *archein,* to be first, and *archos,* chief]. 1. A prefix denoting *chief, first.* 2. *In anatomy* and *biology,* a prefix denoting *primitive, original, ancestral.*

ar″chi·a′ter [G. *archiatros,* court physician]. 1. The head physician at a court. 2. Chief physician of an institution. *Obs.*

ar′chi·coele (ahr′ki·seel) [G. *archē,* beginning; *koilia,* cavity]. The most primitive cavity of the embryo. Syn., *blastocoele.* Also called *segmentation cavity. Obs.*

ar′chi·gas″ter (ahr′ki·gas″tur). Archenteron.

ar″chi·gas′tru·la [*archē;* G. *gastēr,* belly]. A primitive ciliated type of gastrula formed largely by simple invagination.

ar″chi·neph′ron [*archē;* G. *nephros,* kidneys]. The primitive kidney; pronephros. —**archinephric,** *adj.*

ar″chi·pal′li·um [*archē;* L. *pallium,* cloak]. The olfactory pallium or the olfactory cerebral cortex; the rhinencephalon; the oldest part of the cerebral cortex. —**archipallial,** *adj.*

ar′chi·plasm. See *archoplasm.*

ar″chi·tec·ton′ic [G. *architektōn,* master-builder]. Pertaining to the structural arrangement or architectural construction of an organ or part. —**architectonics,** *n.*

ar′cho- (ahr′ko-) [G. *archos,* rectum]. A combining form formerly used to mean *rectal. Obs.*

ar′cho·plasm (ahr′ko·plaz·um), **ar″cho·plas′ma** (ahr″ko·plaz′muh), **ar′chi·plasm** (ahr′ki-plaz·um) [G. *archōn,* from *archein,* to be first; *plasma,* thing formed]. The protoplasmic matter from which the centrosomes, asters, and spindle fibers are derived and of which they are composed. Syn., *ergoplasm, kinoplasm.* —**archoplas′mic,** *adj.*

ar′chos [G.]. The anus. *Obs.*

ar·chu′si·a. An extractable substance which aids the migration, growth, and reproduction of cells: soluble in blood, serum, plasma, and isotonic salt solutions. The cells do not retain it, so its concentration depends upon the surrounding medium.

ar′ci·form [L. *arcus,* bow, arch; *forma,* form]. Arcuate, bow-shaped; especially used to designate certain sets of fibers in the medulla oblongata, and certain veins and arteries of the kidney. See Table of Arteries in the Appendix.

arc·ta′tion [L., from *arctare,* to draw close together]. Contraction of an opening or canal; stenosis.

ar′cu·ate, ar′cu·al [L. *arcuare,* to curve like a bow]. Arched; curved; bow-shaped, as the arcuate fibers of the cerebellum and the cerebrum which serve as association fibers.

ar″cu·a′tion [L. *arcuatio,* a bowing]. Curvature, especially of a bone. —**ar′cual,** *adj.*

ar′cus [L.]. An arch.
a. anterior atlantis [BNA]. The anterior arch of the atlas.
a. juvenilis. A white ring around the cornea

occurring in young individuals and resembling the arcus senilis.

a. posterior atlantis [BNA]. The posterior arch of the atlas.

a. senilis. An opaque ring at the edge of the cornea, seen in the aged.

a. senilis lentis. An opaque ring in the equator of the crystalline lens; it sometimes occurs in the aged.

a. superciliaris [BNA]. The supraorbital ridge.

a. tarseus inferior. An arterial arch along the edge of the lower eyelid.

a. tarseus superior. An arterial arch along the edge of the upper eyelid.

a. tendineus. See tendinous *arch.*

arc′-weld″er's dis·ease′. See *siderosis.*

ARD Abbreviation for acute respiratory disease.

Arderne. See *John of Arderne.*

a′re·a [L., an open space]. A limited extent of surface; a region; a structural or functional part of the cerebral cortex.

aortic a. The second right interspace near the sternum, where aortic sounds and murmurs are best heard.

a. acustica. An area in the lateral angle of the floor of the fourth ventricle overlying the nuclei of the vestibular nerve.

a. centralis. A thickened area of the retina in the center of which is the fovea centralis.

a. chorioidea. A thin-walled part of the embryonic brain, the site of the future choroid plexus of the third ventricle.

a. cribrosa. (a) A small perforated space in the internal auditory meatus through which pass filaments of the acoustic nerve. (b) The surface onto which the papillary ducts of a renal pyramid open into a minor calyx.

a. opaca. The opaque peripheral area of the blastoderm of birds and reptiles, continuous with the yolk.

a. paraterminalis. A space on the medial aspect of the embryonic cerebral hemisphere.

a. pellucida. The central transparent area of the blastoderm of birds and reptiles overlying the subgerminal cavity.

a. postrema. A narrow zone on the lateral wall of the fourth ventricle, separated from the ala cinerea by the funiculus separans.

a. vasculosa. The inner vascular zone of the area opaca; it consists of three layers.

a. vitellina. The outer nonvascular zone of the area opaca; it consists of ectoderm and endoderm.

association a. A term formerly used to designate cortical areas which supposedly had connections only with other parts of the cortex. Now used to designate many areas between the primary projection areas.

auditopsychic a. The auditory association area of the temporal cortex. Also called *Brodmann's a. 42.*

auditory projection a. The cortical receptive center for auditory impulses, located in the transverse temporal gyri. Also called *Brodmann's a. 41, auditosensory a., auditory cortex.*

auditosensory a. The primary auditory projection area of the temporal cortex. Also called *Brodmann's a. 41.*

bare a. of the liver. Triangular area on the superior surface of the liver devoid of peritoneum, enclosed by the coronary ligament.

Broca's a. See Pierre Paul *Broca.*

Brodmann's areas. Numbered regions of the cerebral cortex originally differentiated by histologic criteria, now used in discussions of cortical functions; as **areas 1, 2, 3,** the postcentral gyrus, the somesthetic area; **area 4,** the posterior part of the precentral gyrus, the motor area; **area 4S,** between areas 4 and 6, lesion of which causes spasticity of the muscles innervated by it: syn., *strip a., suppressor a.;* **area 6,** the anterior part of the precentral gyrus and the adjacent posterior superior part of the frontal cortex, the premotor area; **area 17,** the walls and margins of the calcarine fissure, the visual projection area; **area 41,** the two transverse temporal gyri, the auditory projection area.

buccopharyngeal a. That part of the embryonic disk anterior to the head process and devoid of mesoderm; the anlage of the buccopharyngeal membrane.

calcarine a. The visual projection area of the occipital cortex in the walls and margins of the calcarine fissure; Brodmann's area 17.

cardiogenic a. The region in the splanchnic mesoderm of the anterior part of the embryonic disk where the heart first appears in development.

dentofacial a. That portion of the face which includes the teeth and their supporting structures.

dermatomic a. The ringlike bands of the integument innervated by the segmental spinal nerves.

diffraction a. A clear area seen in the microscopic image around all bodies of greater or less refractive power.

embryonic a. That part of the blastoderm forming the embryo proper. Also called *embryonic disk, germinal disk.*

extrapyramidal motor areas. Those portions of the cortex other than the pyramidal cortex, from which motor responses can be obtained upon stimulation, or motor losses observed after ablation; Brodmann's areas 6, 5, 19, 22.

germ a. The germinal disk.

germinal a. The germinal disk.

hypothenar a. (a) The region of the hypothenar eminence. (b) The medial or ulnar palmar space.

infracochlear a. The posterior-inferior portion of the cochlear part of the otic capsule.

infranasal a. The ventral part of the median nasal process between the globular processes: forms the mobile septum of the nose.

Kiesselbach's a. See Wilhelm *Kiesselbach.*

limitrophic a. Limitrophic zone.

Little's a. See Wilhelm *Kiesselbach.*

mesobranchial a. The ventral pharyngeal region between the visceral arches and grooves.

motor a. The precentral gyrus containing centers for voluntary movement; characterized histologically by the presence of Betz cells. Also called *Brodmann's a. 4, pyramidal a., motor cortex.*

motor speech a. That located in the triangular and opercular portions of the inferior frontal gyrus; its destruction causes motor aphasia. Also called *Brodmann's a. 44, Broca's a., Broca's center.*

nasal a. The ventrolateral thickened ectoderm of the frontonasal process from which the olfactory placode arises. Syn., *nasal field, olfactory field.*

nonnucleated a. Hypothetic spaces found at times between the endothelial cells of blood vessels; they have no nuclei, are smaller than endothelial cells, and are considered to be due to the removal of parts of the surrounding endothelium.

Obersteiner-Redlich a. The zone of entrance of dorsal roots into the spinal cord, where they are constricted and devoid of myelin. Syn., *root entrance zone.*

olfactory a. See anterior perforated *substance.*

oval a. of Flechsig. See septomarginal *tract.*

parastriate a. The visual association area of the occipital cortex immediately surrounding the visual area. Also called *Brodmann's a. 18.*

parolfactory a. An area of the cerebral cortex separated by the posterior parolfactory sulcus from the subcallosal gyrus and, incompletely, by the anterior parolfactory sulcus from the superior frontal gyrus and gyrus cinguli.

peristriate a. The visual association area of the occipital cortex surrounding the parastriate area and extending to the borders of the occipital lobe; the second concentric area around the visual cortex. Also called *Brodmann's a. 19*.

piriform, pyriform a. The lateral olfactory gyrus, anterior part of hippocampal gyrus, and the uncus collectively.

portal a. See portal *space*.

precommisural a. See paraterminal *body*.

premotor a. The main cortical extrapyramidal motor area lying immediately in front of the motor area from which it differs histologically by the absence of Betz cells. Also called *Brodmann's a. 6*.

preoptic a. See preoptic *region*.

pretectal a. The area, rostral to the superior colliculus and lateral to the posterior commissure, which receives fibers from the optic tract.

projection a. An area of the cortex connected with lower centers by projection fibers. See under *fiber*.

psychoauditory a. The cortical area concerned in perception of sound.

pyramidal a. The motor area of the cerebral cortex characterized histologically by the presence of giant pyramidal, or Betz, cells; Brodmann's area 4.

seborrheic areas. The scalp, sides of the nose, chin, center of the chest, back, axillas, and groins.

sensory a. The general area of the cerebral cortex in which sensation is perceived.

septal a. See pararteminal *body*.

somesthetic a. The receptive center for proprioceptive or tactile sensation in the postcentral gyrus. Also called *Brodmann's areas 1, 2, 3*.

somesthetopsychic a. The somesthetic association area of the parietal cortex; Brodmann's areas 5 and 7.

striate a. The visual projection area of the occipital cortex characterized by the line of Gennari; Brodmann's area 17.

strip a. Area 4S of Brodmann's *areas*.

suppressor a. See suppressor *band*.

thenar a. (a) The region of the thenar eminence. (b) The lateral palmar space.

triangular a. That portion of the median nasal process between the nasofrontal sulcus and the future tip of the nose; forms the dorsum, or bridge, of the nose.

ulcer-bearing a. The posterior wall of the pyloric portion of the stomach, in which the great majority of all gastric ulcers occur.

vestibular a. A triangular area, lateral to the sulcus limitans, beneath which lie the terminal nuclei of the vestibular nerve.

viscerocutaneous areas. Areas of skin and viscera corresponding to different spinal segments.

visual a. See visual projection *a.*

visual projection a. The cortical receptive center for visual impulses, located in the walls and margins of the calcarine fissure of the occipital lobe, characterized by the line of Gennari. Also called *Brodmann's a. 17, visuosensory a., calcarine a., striate a., visual cortex, visual a.*

visuopsychic a. The visual association areas of the occipital cortex surrounding the visual projection area; Brodmann's area 18, the parastriate area, and Brodmann's area 19, the peristriate area, collectively.

visuosensory a. See visual projection *a.*

vocal a. The portion of the glottis lying between the vocal bands.

ar″e·a′tus [*area*]. Occurring in patches.

Ar′e·ca, A·re′ca [NL. *areca*, from Malayalam *adekka*]. A small genus of Palmae of tropical Asia and the Malay Archipelago; areca palm.

A. catechu. A species extensively cultivated in India, the Malay Archipelago, and the East Indies; betelnut palm. The dried ripe seeds contain several alkaloids, the most important being arecoline. The ground seeds are employed by veterinarians as a vermifuge. Dose, dogs, 2–4 Gm. (30–60 gr.); sheep, 4–8 Gm. (1–2 dr.). The seeds mixed with leaves of *Piper Betle* and lime are used as a masticatory.

ar′e·cin. Areca red; the red coloring matter from areca palm.

a·rec′o·line (a·reck′o·leen, ·lin, a·ree′ko·). $C_8H_{13}NO_2$. A liquid alkaloid isolated from the seeds of *Areca catechu*. It is a powerful poison, affecting the heart similarly to muscarine. It has anthelmintic properties. Dose, 4–6 mg. ($\frac{1}{15}$–$\frac{1}{10}$ gr.). *In veterinary medicine*, it is used also as a cathartic.

a″re·flex′i·a (ay″ri·fleck′see·uh, a·ri·) [G. *a-*, not; L. *reflectere*, to bend back]. Absence of reflexes.

a″re·gen″er·a′tion [*a*; LL. *regeneratio*, new growth, repair]. Failure of tissue to regenerate after disease or injury. —**aregen′erative,** *adj.*

ar″e·na′ceous [L. *arenaceus*, from *arena*, sand]. Sandy.

ar″e·na′tion [*arena*]. A sand bath. Therapeutic use of sand baths. Syn., *ammotherapy*.

ar′ene. Any aromatic hydrocarbon; any hydrocarbon in which at least one benzene ring is present.

a·re′o·la [L., dim. of *area*, area]. 1. Any minute interstice or space in a tissue. 2. A colored or pigmented ring surrounding some central point or space, as a nipple, pustule. 3. The part of the iris enclosing the pupil. —**areolar,** *adj.*

a. mammae. The pigmented area surrounding the nipple of the breast. This enlarges during pregnancy, producing the *second areola*. Also called *a. papillaris, mammary a.* See Plate 43.

umbilical a. A pigmented ring which surrounds the umbilicus in some individuals.

vaccinal a. A red ring surrounding a pustule.

Aretaeus the Cappadocian (Aretaeos) [*Greek physician and clinician in Rome*, fl. second or third century]. Second only to Hippocrates in descriptive power. Wrote on pneumonia, diabetes, tetanus, and diphtheria.

ar·gam″bly·o′pi·a, ar″gi·am″bly·o′pi·a [G. *argos*, idle; *amblys*, dull; *ōps*, eye]. Amblyopia due to disuse of the eye.

Ar′gas [NL., probably from G. *argos*, living without labor]. A genus of ticks.

A. persicus. A species primarily ectoparasitic on birds and occasionally man; believed to be the vector of tick fever.

Ar·gas′i·dae (ahr·gas′i·dee) [NL., probably from *argos*]. A family of soft-bodied ticks.

ar′ge·ma (pl. *argemata*) [G., an ulcer]. A white ulcer of the cornea, following phlyctenula.

argenitis. $AgCl.5CH_4N_2S$. Proprietary antiseptic consisting of a complex salt of silver chloride with thiourea; used topically as a 1:400 solution.

ar′gent-. See *argento-*.

ar·gen′taf·fin, ar·gen′taf·fine. Referring to the capacity of certain tissue elements to reduce silver in staining solution.

ar″gen·taf·fi·no′ma. See *carcinoid*.

ar·gen′tic [*argentum*]. Containing silver in higher valence state.

argentide. A proprietary solution of silver iodide; used locally as astringent and antiseptic.

ar·gen′to-, ar′gent- [*argentum*]. A combining form denoting *silver, containing silver.*

ar·gen′to·phile, ar·gen′to·phil. See *argentaffin.*

ar·gen′tous [*argentum*]. Containing silver in lower valence state.

ar·gen′tum [L.]. See *silver.*

ar″gi·am″bly·o′pi·a. See *argamblyopia.*

ar″gil·la′ceous (ahr″ji·lay′shus) [G. *argillos*, white clay]. Claylike; composed of clay.

ar′gi·nase (ar′ji·nace, ·naze). Enzyme found in the liver, kidney, and spleen of mammals and in the seeds of certain plants. Its action is to split arginine into ornithine and urea.

ar′gi·nine (ahr′ji·neen, ·nin). α-Amino-δ-guanidinovaleric acid. $NH_2C(:NH)NHCH_2CH_2CH_2CH(NH_2)COOH$. An essential amino acid obtained from both animal and vegetable proteins. It occurs as colorless crystals soluble in water.

ar′gi·nyl. The univalent radical, $H_2NC(:NH)NHCH_2CH_2CH_2CH(NH_2)CO—$, of the amino acid arginine.

ar′gol. The impure potassium bitartrate deposited during the fermentation of grape juice. See *tartar.*

ar′gon [G. *argos*, idle]. A = 39.944. An inert gaseous element present in the atmosphere. It may be obtained by fractionation of liquid air.

Argyll Robertson, Douglas Moray Cooper Lamb [*Scottish physician*, 1837–1909]. Remembered for his description of the pupil which reacts to accommodation but not to light, characteristic of certain diseases (1869); called *Argyll Robertson pupil.*

argyn. Colloidal compound of silver oxide and serum albumin; a brand of mild silver protein.

ar·gyr′i·a (ahr·jirr′ee·uh, ahr·jy′ree·uh) [G. *argyros*, silver]. A dusky-gray or bluish discoloration of the skin and mucous membranes produced by the prolonged administration or application of silver preparations, the granules of silver being deposited in much the same sites as those of the natural pigment of the skin. Syn. *argyrosis.* —**argyric,** *adj.*

ar′gy·ro-, argyr- [*argyros*]. A combining form meaning *silver.*

argyrol. Proprietary preparation somewhat similar to mild silver protein; used as a nonirritating antiseptic in infections of the mucous membranes.

ar·gy′ro·len·tis. A condition of the lens of the eye seen rarely in prolonged silver intoxication, characterized by a golden sheen to the anterior lens capsule.

ar·gy′ro·phile, ar·gy′ro·phil (ahr·jy′ro·, ahr′ji·ro·) [*argyros*; G. *philein*, to love]. Easily stained with silver. Syn. *argentaffin, argentophile, argentophil.*

ar″gy·ro′sis. Argyria.

a·rhin″en·ce·pha′li·a. See *arrhinencephalia.*

a·rhin′i·a. See *arrhinia.*

a·ri″bo·fla″vi·no′sis (a·rye″bo·flay″vi·no′sis, ·flav″i·no′sis, a·rib″o·) [*a-; ribose*, from Ger. transposition of *arabinose*, a pentose sugar; L. *flavus*, yellow; G. *-ōsis*, condition]. Deficiency of riboflavin, a condition formerly confused with pellagra. It is characterized by cheilosis, corneal and other eye changes, and dermatitis seborrheica.

ar′i·cine (ar′i·seen, ·sin). $C_{23}H_{26}N_2O_4$. An alkaloid obtained from several varieties of cinchona bark. Syn., *quinovatine.*

ariphon. Trade name for an analgesic and antipyretic preparation containing acetylsalicylic acid, sodium citrate, and citrated caffeine.

a·ris″to·gen′ic [G. *aristos*, best; *genos*, race]. Well endowed eugenically. —**aristogenics,** *n.*

aristol. Trade-mark for a brand of thymol iodide.

A·ris″to·lo′chi·a (a·ris″to·lo′kee·uh) [*aristos*; G. *locheia*, childbirth]. A genus of Aristolochiaceae, many species of which are reported to have active medicinal qualities.

A. cymbifera. Partial source of the drug guacin.

A. reticulata. Texas snakeroot. See *serpentaria.*

A. serpentaria. Virginia snakeroot. See *serpentaria.*

a·ris″to·lo′chine (a·ris″to·lo′keen, ·kin, ar·is·tol′o·) [*aristos; locheia*]. A poisonous alkaloid found in *Aristolochia serpentaria.*

Aristotle [*Greek philosopher and scientist*, 384–322 B.C.]. Tutor of Alexander the Great and founder of comparative anatomy. His influence on medical and scientific thought is felt to this day.

ar″ith·met′ic mean. The arithmetic average.

a·rith″mo·ma′ni·a [G. *arithmos*, number; *mania*, madness]. A morbid impulse to count objects; a preoccupation with numbers.

ar′ky·o·chrome″ [G. *arkys*, net; *chrōma*, color]. A nerve cell in which the stainable portion of the cytoplasm is in the form of network (Nissl).

Arlt, Carl Ferdinand von [*Bohemian ophthalmologist*, 1812–87]. Known for his operation for distichia, in which the ciliary bulbs are dissected from the tarsus by excision of a crescent-shaped piece of skin and transplanted away from the edge of the lid; this is known as *Arlt's operation, Arlt-Jaesche technic.* Arlt's name has been given to many operative procedures upon the eye and eyelid for the relief of entropion, ectropion, stricture of the lacrimal duct, and symblepharon (1854–56). He also introduced an operation for enucleation of the eye. The granular form of trachoma is called *Arlt's trachoma.*

arm [AS.]. 1. *In anatomy*, the upper extremity from the shoulder to the elbow. 2. Popularly, the arm and the forearm. 3. That portion of the stand connecting the body or tube of a microscope with the pillar.

ar″ma·men·tar′i·um (·tair′ee·um) [L., an arsenal]. All of the books, journals, medicines, instruments, and laboratory and therapeutic equipment possessed by a physician, surgeon, or medical institution to assist in the practice of his or its profession.

Ar·mil′li·fer [L. *armilla*, bracelet; *ferre*, to bear]. A genus of pentastomes (tongue worms) whose larvae have been found in the liver, lungs, and spleen of man. The medically important species are **A. armillatus** and **A. moniliformis.**

Ar′mor Med′i·cal Re·search′ Lab′o·ra·to″ry. An experimental station of the Army Medical Department, for research in the physiologic effects of armor equipment operation on personnel, and having for its object the reduction of operational hazards by the development of armor equipment.

arm′pit″ [AS. *arm*, arm; *pytt*, from L. *puteus*, well]. The axilla. See Plate 11.

Ar′my Med′i·cal Cen′ter. A centrally situated installation of the Army Medical Department where are located a general hospital, research facilities, training schools for service personnel, laboratories, etc.

Arnaldus. See *Arnold of Villanova.*

Arnatt, Neils [*Scottish physician*, 1788–1874]. Introduced local anesthesia maintained by the use of ice and salt, called *Arnatt's anesthesia.*

Arnaud de Villeneuve. See *Arnold of Villanova.*

Arndt, Rudolph [*German psychiatrist*, 1835–1900]. Remembered for his law in physiology that weak stimuli excite physiologic action, moderate ones favor it, and strong stimuli retard the action or abolish it altogether.

Arneth, Joseph (1873–) German physician who introduced a classification of the leukocytes of the myeloid series (1904) according to shape and lobulation of their nuclei by setting up five classes and a number of subdivisions. Arneth's formula gives the approximate class percentages found in healthy persons: I. Single-lobed neutrophils, 5%; II. Two-lobed, 35%; III. Three-lobed, 41%; IV. Four-lobed, 17%; V. Five- (or more) lobed, 2%. He correlated his classification of the neutrophils with their development, and shifts in class percentages with pathologic states. By tabulating the series from left (Class I) to right (Class V), he introduced the terms, *shift to left* to indicate a percentage increase of immature forms, and *shift to right* for an increase in older forms. He extended this system to the other formed cellular elements of the blood (leukocytes and erythrocytes) and to the platelets (1942). He also devised a phagocytic index based on the assumption that those neutrophils with three or more lobes possess the greatest phagocytic power (1904).

ar′ni·ca [perhaps corruption from G. *ptarmikē*, sneezewort]. The dried flower heads of the *Arnica montana*. Arnicin, arnidiol (or arnisterin), and a volatile oil have been isolated from it. Arnica is an irritant, and was popularly used as a tincture for sprains, bruises, and surface wounds. It is rarely used internally.

ar′ni·cin. A brownish, bitter neutral principle which is extracted from the flowers of *Arnica montana*.

Arnold, Friedrich [*German anatomist and physiologist*, 1803–90]. Known for his descriptions of the frontopontine bundle or tract of the brain which bears his name, and of the small canal in the petrous portion of the temporal bone which gives passage to the auricular branch of the vagus nerve. Also described the ligament connecting the body of the incus with the roof of the tympanic cavity.

Arnold, Julius [*German pathologist*, 1835–1915]. See *Arnold-Chiari syndrome* under *Chiari*.

Arnold of Villanova (**Arnaldus Catalonus, Arnaldus Villanovanus, Arnaud de Villeneuve**) [*Spanish or Catalan physician and alchemist*, ca. 1235–ca. 1312]. Credited with the introduction of tinctures into pharmacology.

Arnold and Gunning's method. See under *method*.

Arnold method. See Volhard-Arnold *method*.

Arnold sterilizer. See under *sterilizer*.

ar·not′to. See *annatto*.

Arnoux, Emile [*French gynecologist*, 1871–]. Published an important contribution to the study of kraurosis vulvae (1899). Distinguished the double and quadruple rhythmic sounds of the two fetal hearts beating in and out of unison in twin pregnancy; known as *Arnoux's sign*.

ar″o·mat′ic [G. *arōma*, spice]. 1. Having a spicy odor. 2. Characterized by a fragrant, spicy taste and odor, as cinnamon, ginger, or the essential oils. 3. A qualification applied to any carbon compound originating from benzene, C_6H_6.

ar·rec′tor (pl. *arrectores*) [L. *arrectus*, from *arrigere*, to erect]. *In anatomy*, an erector muscle.

arrectores pilorum. Minute, fanlike, involuntary muscles attached to the hair follicles which, by contraction, erect the hair and cause so-called goose flesh. See Table of Muscles in the Appendix.

ar·rest′ [L. *ad*, at; *restare*, to stop]. A stopping, checking, or restraining.

cardiac a. Standstill of the entire heart.

pelvic a. *In obstetrics*, a condition accompanying labor in which the presenting part of the fetus becomes fixed in its position in the maternal pelvis.

sinus a. See sinoatrial *heart block*.

transverse a. *In obstetrics*, a faulty condition in the mechanism of labor when a flat type of maternal pelvis causes a fixation of the fetal head in the transverse position.

Arrhenius, Svante August [*Swedish physicist and chemist*, 1859–1927]. Widely known for his work in the fields of chemistry and astronomy. Introduced the electrolytic dissociation theory. Nobel laureate (1903).

ar″rhe·no·blas·to′ma (ar″i·no·blas·to′muh, a·ree″no·) [G. *arrēn*, male; *blastos*, germ; *-ōma*, tumor]. An infrequent tumor of the ovary, moderate in size, encapsulated, nodular, firm, and nearly always unilateral, occurring most often in young adults: may be malignant. Three microscopic forms are observed: *testicular tubular adenoma*, a *sarcomatoid* form, and a *mixed tubular and sarcomatoid* form. The latter two forms, especially the sarcomatoid, are usually, if not always, accompanied by defemination and virilization, somewhat resembling that in Cushing's syndrome. Also called *arrhenoma, arrhenonoma*.

ar″rhe·no′ma, ar·rhen″o·no′ma. See *arrhenoblastoma*.

ar″rhe·not′o·ky, ar·rhe″no·to′ci·a [*arrēn*; G. *tokos*, childbirth]. *In zoology*, the parthenogenetic production of male individuals exclusively. —**arrhenot′okous,** *adj*.

ar·rhin″en·ce·pha′li·a [*a-*; G. *rhis*, nose; *egkephalos*, brain]. A form of partial anencephalia in which there is partial or total absence of the rhinencephalon and malformation of the nose. Also spelled *arhinencephalia*.

ar·rhin′i·a, a·rhin′i·a [G. *a-*, not; *rhis*, nose]. Congenital absence of the nose. —**arrhinic,** *adj*.

ar·rhyth′mi·a [*a-*; G. *rhythmos*, rhythm]. Absence of rhythm. —**arrhythmic,** *adj*.

neurogenic a. Phasic sinus *a*.

paroxysmal a. One caused by a stressful life situation which arouses anxiety, hostility, or depression.

phasic sinus a. Gradual waxing and waning of pulse rate, usually synchronous with the acts of breathing. May also be independent of respiration. Also called *neurogenic a., reflex a., vagal a.*

reflex a. Phasic sinus *a*.

respiratory a. Disturbed breathing.

vagal a. Phasic sinus *a*.

ar′row poi′son. See *curare*.

ar′row·root″ [ME. *arewe; roote*]. A variety of starch derived from *Maranta arundinacea* of the West Indies and southern United States.

ars a·man′di [L., art of loving]. Sexual prowess.

ar″sa·nil′ic ac′id. $NH_2.C_6H_4.AsO(OH)_2$. *p*-Aminobenzenearsonic acid. The starting compound for the synthesis of many useful medicinal arsenicals.

arsen-. See *arseno-*.

ar′se·nate, ar·se′ni·ate [G. *arsenikon*, yellow orpiment]. Any salt of arsenic acid.

ar′se·nic, ar·sen′i·cum, ar·se′num [*arsenikon*]. As = 74.91. 1. A brittle, usually steel-gray element of both metallic and nonmetallic properties. It exists in four allotropic modifications, the most important of which is the gray, or so-called metallic, arsenic. It sublimes readily, the vapor having a garlicky odor. Its salts are used in medicine for their tonic effect in wasting diseases; for their ability to increase the hematinic effect of iron; in skin diseases; in certain pulmonary diseases; for destruction of protozoan parasites; and as caustics. 2. Arsenic trioxide. —**arsen′ic,** *adj*.

a. bromide. $AsBr_3$. Arsenic tribromide, arsenous bromide. Dose, 1–4 mg. ($\frac{1}{60}$–$\frac{1}{15}$ gr.).

a. butter. See *a.* chloride.

a. chloride. $AsCl_3$. Arsenous chloride, arsenic trichloride; a colorless, oily liquid decomposed by water. Syn., *a. butter*.

a. disulfide. As_2S_2. Occurs native as *realgar*. Also called *red a., red a. sulfide*. An artificial product is known as *red a. glass* or *red orpiment*.

a. iodide. See *a.* triiodide.

a. test. The United States Pharmacopeia arsenic test involves a comparison of the stains produced on mercuric bromide test papers by a standard arsenic solution and by the sample being tested when the arsenic present is reduced to arsine (AsH_3) and the latter reacts with the test paper.

a. tribromide. See *a.* bromide.

a. trichloride. See *a.* chloride.

a. triiodide (*arseni triiodidum*). AsI_3. Arsenous iodide. Dose, 3–12 mg. (1/20–1/5 gr.). An ingredient in *arsenic and mercuric iodides solution* (*liquor arseni et hydrargyri iodidorum*), also known as *Donovan's solution*, which contains 1% each of arsenic triiodide and mercuric iodide: has been used in chronic skin diseases.

a. trioxide (*arseni trioxidum*). Arsenous oxide, As_2O_3. Dose, 1–3 mg. (1/60–1/20 gr.). Syn., *arsenous acid, white a.*

a. trisulfide. As_2S_3. Translucent, lemon-colored masses occurring in nature; formerly used as a depilatory. Syn., *orpiment, a. yellow sulfide, king's yellow.*

a. yellow sulfide. See *a.* trisulfide.

arsenious acid solution (*liquor acidi arseniosi*). A 1% arsenic trioxide solution in hydrochloric acid and distilled water. Dose, 0.12–0.5 cc. (2–8 min.). Also called *hydrochloric solution of a., a. chloride solution.*

white a. See *a.* trioxide.

ar·sen'ic ac'id. H_3AsO_4. Orthoarsenic acid; a white, hygroscopic powder used in the manufacture of medicinal and insecticidal arsenates.

ar·sen'i·cal. A drug, fungicide, or insecticide the effect of which depends on its arsenic content. —**arsen'ical,** *adj.*

ar·sen"i·co·der'ma. Dermatitis medicamentosa due to arsenic.

ar·sen'i·cum. See *arsenic.*

ar'se·nide. A compound of arsenic with another element in which the arsenic is negatively charged.

ar·se'ni·ous. Arsenous.

ar'se·nite. A salt of an arsenous acid.

ar·se'niu·ret"ted. Combined with arsenic so as to form an arsenide.

ar'se·no- (ahr'si·no-, ahr·sen'o-), **arsen-** [*arsenikon*]. A combining form designating *a drug combined with arsenic.*

arseno-bismulak. A trade name for the antisyphilitic substance bismuth sodium *p*-aminophenylarsonate.

arsenoferratose. Proprietary elixir containing iron and arsenic in organic combination; used as hematinic.

***p*-ar"sen·o"so·phen"yl·bu·tyr'ic ac'id.** C_6H_4-$AsO(CH_2CH_2CH_2COOH)$; a trivalent arsenical having trypanocidal activity. Syn., *butarsen.*

ar"se·no·ther'a·py [*arsenikon;* G. *therapeia*, treatment]. Treatment of disease by means of arsenical drugs.

ar'se·nous, ar·se'ni·ous [*arsenikon*]. Containing arsenic in the positive trivalent form.

ar'se·nous ac'id. See *arsenic* trioxide.

ar'se·nous bro'mide. See *arsenic* bromide.

ar'se·nous chlo'ride. See *arsenic* chloride.

ar'se·nous i'o·dide". See *arsenic* triiodide.

ar'se·nous ox'ide. See *arsenic* trioxide.

ar"se·nox'ide. 3-Amino-4-hydroxyphenyl-arsine oxide. $C_6H_6AsNO_2$. A breakdown product of arsphenamine which accounts for its activity. See *oxophenarsine hydrochloride.*

ar·se'num. See *arsenic.*

ar·sine' (ahr·seen', ahr'seen, ahr'sin). AsH_3. Hydrogen arsenide, or arsenous hydride. A poisonous gas with a garlicky odor.

ar·sin'ic ac'id. Any acid of the type of RHAs(:O)OH or of RR'As(:O)OH, where R is any hydrocarbon radical and R' is the same or a different hydrocarbon radical.

ar·son'ic ac'id. Any acid of the type of RAs(:O)(OH)$_2$, where R is any hydrocarbon radical.

Arsonval, Jacques Arsène d' [*French physiologist*, 1851–1940]. Introduced high-frequency currents in electrotherapy (1892). The high potential discharge of a current condenser through a large solenoid of wire is known as *d'Arsonval current.*

ar"son·val"i·za'tion [after Jacques Arsène d'*Arsonval*]. The therapeutic application of high-frequency currents. Three types are used: desiccating, coagulating, and cutting. Also called *darsonvalization.*

ars·phen'a·mine (ahrs·fen'uh·meen, ·min, ahrs"finam'een, ·in, ahrs"fen·uh·meen') (*arsphenamina*). Diaminodihydroxyarsenobenzene dihydrochloride, $C_{12}H_{12}As_2N_2O_2.2HCl.2H_2O$. A yellow hygroscopic crystalline powder, unstable in air, soluble in water with acid reaction. A specific in syphilis and other protozoan infections. This drug has been largely superseded by neoarsphenamine and other arsenicals (more conveniently and safely administered) and by antibiotics. Also called *606.* See *salvarsan.*

ars·phen'a·mized. Having been treated with arsphenamine.

ars'thin·ol. Generic name for the cyclic 3-hydroxypropylene ester of 3-acetamido-4-hydroxydithiobenzenearsonous acid, a trivalent arsenical supplied under the trade-mark *balarsen.* The substance is effective against intestinal amebiasis and yaws.

artane. Trade-mark for 3-(1-piperidyl)-1-phenyl-1-cyclohexyl-1-propanol hydrochloride, an antispasmodic drug. See *trihexyphenidyl.*

ar'tar root. A drug from West Africa, probably the root of *Xanthoxylum senegalense*, of the Rutaceae.

ar'te·fact, ar'ti·fact [L. *ars*, art; *facere*, to make]. 1. *In microscopy* and *histology*, a structure that has been produced by mechanical, chemical, or other artificial means; a structure or tissue that has been changed from its natural state. 2. *In electroencephalography*, a wave not originating in the brain.

Ar"te·mis'i·a (ahr"ti·miz'ee·uh, ·mish'ee·uh, ·miss'ee·uh) [G., plant of Artemis]. A genus of widely distributed plants of the Compositae. Various members have been used in folk medicine, the drugs of most recent importance being absinthium and santonica. Because the pollens of these plants are wind-borne, they are among the more important causes of hay fever, especially in the Mountain and Pacific States.

ar"ter·ec'to·my. See *arteriectomy.*

ar·ter'en·ol. Norepinephrine.

arteri-. See *arterio-.*

ar·te'ri·a (pl. *arteriae*). See *artery.*

ar·te"ri·al·i·za'tion [G. *artēria*, artery]. 1. The process of making or becoming arterial; the change from venous blood into arterial. 2. Vascularization. —**arte'rialize,** *v.*

ar·te"ri·arc'ti·a (ar·teer"i·ark'shee·uh, ·tee·uh) [*artēria;* NL. from L. *arctare*, to press together]. Vasoconstriction or stenosis of an artery.

ar"te·ri'a·sis [*artēria;* NL. *-iasis*, condition]. Degeneration of an artery.

ar·te"ri·ec'ta·sis, ar·te"ri·ec·ta'si·a (·eck·tay'zhuh, ·zee·uh, ·shuh, ·see·uh) [*artēria;* G. *ektasis*, a stretching out]. Arterial dilatation.

ar·te"ri·ec'to·my [*artēria;* G. *ektomē*, excision]. Excision of an artery or portion of an artery: used to treat intractable pain persisting after recovery from an acute arterial occlusion. Also spelled *arterectomy.*

ar·te"ri·ec·to'pi·a [*artēria;* G. *ektopos*, away from

a place]. Displacement or abnormality of the course of an artery.

ar·te′ri·o-, arteri- [*artēria*]. A combining form signifying *artery, arterial.*

ar·te″ri·o·cap′il·lar″y [*artēria;* L. *capillaris,* of the hair]. Blood vessel between an arteriole and a capillary, usually called arterial capillary. Syn., *precapillary, precapillary arteriole.*

ar·te″ri·o·fi·bro′sis (ahr·teer″ee·o·figh·bro′sis). See arteriocapillary *fibrosis.*

ar·te′ri·o·gram″ [*artēria;* G. *gramma,* letter]. 1. A roentgenogram of an artery after injection with a contrast material such as diodrast. 2. Arteriograph; a tracing of the arterial pulse.

ar·te′ri·o·graph [*artēria;* G. *graphein,* to write]. 1. Instrument which graphically presents the pulse. 2. Tracing of the arterial pulse. 3. Arteriogram.

ar·te″ri·og′ra·phy [*artēria; graphein*]. 1. Graphic presentation of the pulse; sphygmography. 2. Roentgenography of the arteries. —**arteriograph′ic,** *adj.*

carotid a. Roentgenography of the carotid artery.

vertebral a. Roentgenography of the vertebral artery.

ar·te″ri·o′la (pl. *arteriolae*) [L., dim. of *artēria*]. An arteriole.

a. recta. One of the straight arterioles going from the glomeruli to the pyramids of the kidney.

ar·te′ri·ole [*arteriola*]. A very small artery.

precapillary arterioles. See *precapillary.*

straight a. See *arteriola* recta.

ar·te′ri·o·lith″ [G. *artēria,* artery; *lithos,* stone]. A calculus in an artery.

ar·ter′i·o·li′tis. Inflammation of arterioles.

ar·te″ri·o″lo·ne·cro′sis [L. *arteriola,* dim. of *artēria;* G. *nekrōsis,* mortification]. Degeneration of the arterioles resulting in necrosis, as in nephrosclerosis. —**arteriolonecrot′ic,** *adj.*

ar·te″ri·o″lo·scle·ro′sis [*arteriola;* G. *sklērōsis,* a hardening]. Arteriolar sclerosis. —**arteriolosclerot′ic,** *adj.*

ar·te″ri·o·ma·la′ci·a (ahr·teer″ee·o·ma·lay′shee·uh, ·see·uh) [G. *artēria,* artery; *malakia,* softness]. Softening of an artery wall.

ar·te″ri·o·ne·cro′sis [*artēria;* G. *nekrōsis,* mortification]. Necrosis of an artery or arteries.

ar·te″ri·op′a·thy [*artēria;* G. *pathos,* disease]. Any disease of an artery or of arteries. *Obs.*

ar·te″ri·o·pla′ni·a [*artēria;* G. *planē,* a wandering]. A condition in which an anomaly is present in the course of an artery.

ar·te′ri·o·plas″ty [*artēria;* G. *plassein,* to form]. An operation for aneurysm in which the vessel is reconstructed by using the aneurysmal walls to restore its continuity. Syn., *aneurysmorrhaphy.* —**arterioplas′tic,** *adj.*

ar·te″ri·o·pres′sor [*artēria;* L. *pressor,* from *premere,* to press]. Causing increased blood pressure in the arteries.

ar·te′ri·o·punc″ture [*artēria;* L. *punctura,* puncture]. The surgical division or opening of an artery, chiefly for the abstraction of blood.

ar·te″ri·o·re′nal [*artēria;* L. *renes,* kidneys]. Pertaining to the renal arterial blood vessels.

ar·te″ri·or′rha·phy [*artēria;* G. *rhaphē,* suture]. Suture of an artery.

ar·te″ri·or·rhex′is [*artēria;* G. *rhēxis,* a breaking]. Rupture of an artery.

ar·te″ri·o·scle·ro′sis (ahr·teer″ee·o·skli·ro′sis) [*artēria;* G. *sklērōsis,* a hardening]. Any of various proliferative and degenerative changes in arteries, not necessarily related to each other, resulting in thickening of the walls, loss of elasticity, and in some instances, calcium deposition. —**arteriosclerot′ic,** *adj.*

a. obliterans. Arteriosclerosis associated with proliferation of the intima to the extent of obstructing the lumen.

cerebral a. That which affects the vessels of the brain.

decrescent a. Senile *a.*

diffuse a. See generalized *a.*

disuse a. Intimal fibrosis of an artery proximal to an occlusion, or in an organ or part that is atrophic, as in an atrophic ovary or leg. Syn. *involutional a.*

generalized a. A generalized thickening of the intimal portion of the smaller vessels. It is seen in chronic nephritis and essential hypertension.

intimal a. See *atherosclerosis.*

involutional a. See disuse *a.*

medial a. That which affects the middle coat of the small and medium-sized arteries, showing extensive destruction and atrophy of the muscular elements and deposition of calcium. Also called *Mönckeberg's a.*

Mönckeberg's a. Medial *a.*

senile a. That which often occurs in old age and affects the medium-sized arteries, especially those of the extremities.

syphilitic a. The arterial sclerosis due to syphilis. It affects chiefly the media, but also the adventitia.

ar·te′ri·o·spasm″ [*artēria;* G. *spasmos*]. Spasm of an artery.

ar·te″ri·o·ste·no′sis [*artēria;* G. *stenōsis,* a being straitened]. Narrowing of the caliber of an artery in any part.

ar·te″ri·os·to′sis [*artēria;* G. *osteon,* bone; *-ōsis,* condition]. Calcification of an artery.

ar·te″ri·o·strep′sis [*artēria;* G. *strepsis,* a twisting]. The twisting of an artery for the purpose of staying a hemorrhage.

ar·te′ri·o·tome″ [*artēria;* G. *tomos,* cutting]. Knife for use in arteriotomy. *Obs.*

ar·te″ri·ot′o·my [*artēria;* G. *tomē,* a cutting]. Cutting or opening of an artery for the purpose of bloodletting.

ar·te″ri·o·ve′nous [*artēria;* L. *vena,* vein]. Both arterial and venous; involving an artery and a vein, as an arteriovenous aneurysm.

ar·te″ri·o·ver′sion [*artēria;* L. *vertere,* to turn]. A method of arresting hemorrhage by turning vessels inside out. —**arteriovert′er,** *n.*

ar″te·ri′tis [*artēria;* G. *-itis,* inflammation]. Inflammation of an artery. See *endarteritis, periarteritis.*

a. deformans. A chronic endarteritis with calcareous infiltration. See *endarteritis.*

a. obliterans. Inflammation of arteries which leads to obstruction of the lumen. See *endarteritis.*

a. umbilicalis. Septic inflammation of the umbilical arteries.

gummatous a. See syphilitic *a.*

necrotizing a. See *polyarteritis nodosa.*

rheumatic a. A pathologic alteration of arteries caused by rheumatic fever, and occurring particularly in coronary arteries.

syphilitic a. A syphilitic infection of arteries characterized by destruction and fibrosis of the media and adventitia, and secondarily of the intima. In some instances the result is narrowing of the lumen by the intimal proliferation and in others by aneurysm formation. Also called *gummatous a.*

temporal a. A self-limiting disease of unconfirmed etiology, occurring in the fifth to eighth decade. It involves inflammation of arteries, particularly the temporal arteries. Symptoms include malaise, lassitude and weakness, anorexia, mental depression, aching and tenderness of muscles and joints, sciatic and brachial neuropathy, night sweats,

headache, and scalp tenderness. The disease usually lasts for several months, and the prognosis is generally good.
tuberculous a. Involvement of arteries by tuberculous inflammation, frequently resulting in thrombosis and occasionally in hemorrhage.

ar′ter·y [*artēria*]. A vessel conveying blood from the heart. It is composed of three coats: an outer *adventitia*, consisting of connective tissue and elastic fibers; an inner *intima* lined with endothelium and containing collagenous and elastic fibers; and a middle coat, the *media*, composed of elastic and muscular fibers. For arteries listed by name, see Table of Arteries in the Appendix. See Plates 7, 8. Abbreviated, a. —**arte′rial,** *adj.*
arciform a. An arterial arch at the base of a renal pyramid; a branch of a renal interlobar artery.
arcuate a. See arciform *a.*
axial a. The first main artery to a developing limb bud.
conducting a. One of large caliber and elastic walls, as the aorta, subclavian, common carotid.
copper wire a. One of the type of bright retinal vessels noted in arteriosclerosis.
corkscrew a. One of the smaller, tortuous, retinal vessels in the macular region, noted in hypertension.
dental a. 1. See *alveolar* artery in Table of Arteries. 2. A twig of an alveolar artery supplying a root of a tooth.
distributing a. Any of the arteries intermediate between the conducting arteries and arterioles. The muscular coat of the arterial wall is well developed. Also called *muscular a.*
end a. One without branches or anastomoses.
helicine a. A spiral vessel which empties into the cavernous sinuses of erectile tissue.
hyaloid a. In the embryo, a forward continuation of the central artery of the retina traversing the vitreous body to ramify on the posterior surface of the lens capsule.
interlobar a. One lying between the lobes of an organ. A branch of the renal artery, running in a renal column.
interlobular a. One lying between the lobules of an organ. One of the radial branches of an arciform artery, running in the renal radial cortex.
intralobular a. One lying within the lobule of an organ.
muscular a. A distributing artery.
nutrient a. One which supplies blood to a bone.
pipestem a. One with advanced calcification and stiffening, noted in senile arteriosclerosis.
radicular a. One which supplies the spinal cord, entering with the anterior and posterior nerve roots.
sheathed a. The thick-walled, second portion of one of the arterioles of a penicillus in the spleen.
stapedial a. An artery present in the middle ear of the embryo; the stapes develops around it.
terminal a. See end *a.*
venous a. One carrying venous blood, as the pulmonary artery.
vitelline a. One passing from the yolk sac to the primitive aorta of the embryo. Also called *omphalomesenteric a.*

arthr-. See *arthro-.*

arthralgen. Trade-mark for an antiarthritic preparation containing methacholine chloride, thymol, menthol, and methyl salicylate in an absorbable, washable ointment base.

ar·thral′gi·a [G. *arthron*, joint; *algos*, pain]. Pain in a joint. Syn., *articular neuralgia.* —**arthralgic,** *adj.*
a. hysterica. Pain in the joints of hysterical origin.
a. saturnina. Painful joints with rigidity and cramps in approximate muscles; symptomatic of lead poisoning.
gonorrheal a. Transient pain in joints occurring in gonorrhea without objective signs of disease.
menopausal a. See menopausal *arthritis* (b).

ar·threc′to·my [*arthron;* G. *ektomē*, excision]. Excision of a joint.

ar″thre·de′ma, ar″throe·de′ma [*arthron;* G. *oidēma*, swelling]. Edema affecting a joint.

ar″thres·the′si·a. Sensation in the joints.

ar·thrit′ic [*arthron;* G. *-itis*, inflammation]. An individual affected with arthritis.

ar·thrit′i·des (ahr·thrit′i·deez) [G., from *arthron; -itis*]. General term to include the various types of arthritis.

ar·thri′tis (pl. *arthrites*) [*arthron; -itis*]. Inflammation of a joint. —**arthrit′ic,** *adj.*
acromegalic a. A degenerative disease of the joints due to acromegaly.
acute a. Acute joint inflammation.
allergic a. (a) Intermittent hydrarthrosis, usually following ingestion of food allergens. (b) Serum sickness; usually occurring 7 to 10 days after injection of horse serum; characterized by fever and urticaria. There may be pain, redness, swelling, and stiffness of the joints resembling rheumatic fever.
a. deformans. Any chronic arthritis, usually a degenerative joint disease.
a. deformans juvenilis. See *osteochondritis deformans juvenilis.*
a. of rheumatic fever. Acute, reversible, migratory synovitis of short duration occurring during exacerbations of rheumatic fever.
atrophic a. See rheumatoid *a.*
blennorrhagic a. See gonorrheal *a.*
chronic a. A general term for any chronic joint disease, but usually rheumatoid arthritis or degenerative joint disease.
chronic infectious a. See rheumatoid *a.*
climacteric a. See menopausal *a.*
degenerative a. See degenerative joint *disease.*
foxhole a. See epidemic tropical acute *polyarthritis.*
fungous a. Tuberculous disease of the joints; white swelling.
gonorrheal a. A specific, blood-borne, gonococcal infection in joint tissue. May be very mild and transient, or may be severe, becoming purulent and leading to bony ankylosis.
gouty a. Arthritis due to gout; characterized by sudden, severe, painful attacks, often coming on in the night; affects one joint, and lasts weeks or months; followed by complete recovery. After repeated attacks in the same joint, degenerative joint disease results.
Heberden's a. Degenerative joint disease of the terminal joints of the fingers, producing enlargement and flexion deformities. Most common in women, occurring idiopathically and as a result of heredity. May result from trauma.
hematogenous a. An arthritis presumably caused most frequently by blood-borne pneumococcus or gonococcus infection.
hemophilic a. Inflammation due to blood in the joint of a hemophiliac. Repeated episodes lead to thickening of the synovial tissues and finally to degenerative joint disease.
hypertrophic a. See degenerative joint *disease.*
infectious a. An acute or chronic inflammatory disease of a joint caused by invasion of the articular tissue by microorganisms. Infection is usually hematogenous in origin, beginning in the

synovia or on subchondral marrow and spreading to other structures. Its course depends on the invading organism.

menopausal a. (a) Degenerative joint disease. (b) An arthralgia without objective or roentgenographic evidence of disease; it occurs in women at the menopause.

mixed a. A combination of features typical both of rheumatoid arthritis and of degenerative joint disease seen in the same patient or the same joint.

neurotrophic a. A trophic disease of joints; seen in tabes dorsalis, leprosy, syringomyelia, and other diseases of the nervous system. There is marked enlargement and disorganization of joint structures and hypermotility. It is usually painless. Also called *neuropathic a., Charcot's a.*

nonsuppurative a. Any inflammatory joint disease not associated with purulent synovial fluid and not progressing to suppuration; one of the varieties of inflammatory joint disease, e.g., rheumatoid arthritis, which are not known to be infectious in origin.

ochronotic a. A rare form of arthritis associated with ochronosis. See under *osteoarthritis.*

proliferative a. See rheumatoid *a.*

psoriatic a. (a) A type of rheumatoid arthritis associated with psoriasis. The cause and mechanisms of the association are not clear. (b) Rarely, a degenerative arthropathy, unrelated to rheumatoid arthritis, involving principally the phalangeal joints.

purulent a. An arthritis caused either by the spreading of a generalized infection through the blood, by the spread of osteomyelitic lesions of the bone, or by direct introduction through penetrating wounds.

rheumatic a. See *a.* of rheumatic fever.

rheumatoid a. A chronic arthritis of unknown etiology; affects multiple joints, producing constitutional effects such as debility, weakness, and loss of weight. The specific lesion is a proliferation of granulation or connective tissue in synovial and periarticular tissues over the joint surfaces and in subchondral spaces. There is pain, limitation of motion, deformity, and sometimes bony ankylosis. Syn., *atrophic a., chronic infectious a., proliferative a.*

rheumatoid a. of the spine. Ankylosing spondylitis.

scarlatinal a. A form common in scarlet fever epidemics, usually appearing at the end of 10 days, with redness, pain, and swelling of the wrists, hands, elbows, and knees due to synovial distention. Also called *scarlatinal synovitis.*

senescent a. See degenerative joint *disease.*

syphilitic a. (a) Painful and swollen joints due to syphilis, especially during the secondary stage or gumma of the joint. (b) Symmetrical synovitis associated with prenatal syphilis. See Henry Hugh *Clutton.*

traumatic a. Synovitis secondary to acute trauma.

tuberculous a. Invasion of synovial tissues or bone with *Mycobacterium tuberculosis;* it gives rise to tubercle formations, fibrosis, caseation, and causes marked destruction of articular structures; healing may occur through ankylosis.

ar′thro-, arthr- [*arthron*]. A combining form denoting *relation to the joints.*

ar·throc′a·ce (ahr·throck′uh·see) [*arthron;* G. *kakos,* bad]. Caries of a joint, as in tuberculous arthritis.

ar′thro·cele [*arthron;* G. *kēlē,* tumor]. 1. Any swollen joint. 2. Hernia of the synovial membrane through a joint capsule.

ar″thro·cen·te′sis [*arthron;* G. *kentēsis,* pricking]. Incision into or puncture through a joint capsule to relieve an effusion.

ar″thro·chon·dri′tis (ahr″thro·kon·dry′tis) [*arthron;* G. *chondros,* cartilage; *-itis,* inflammation]. Inflammation of the cartilaginous parts of a joint.

ar″thro·cla′si·a (ahr″thro·clay′zhuh, ·zee·uh, ·shuh, ·see·uh), **ar″thro·cla′sis** (ahr″thro·clay′-sis, ahr·throck′luh·sis) [*arthron;* G. *klaein,* to break]. The breaking down of ankylosis in order to produce free movement of a joint.

ar·thro·de′sis, ar″thro·de′si·a [*arthron;* G. *desis,* a binding together]. Fusion of a joint by removing the articular surfaces and securing bony union; operative ankylosis.

ar·thro′di·a [G., a kind of articulation]. A form of joint permitting a gliding movement. —**arthrodial,** *adj.*

ar″thro·dyn′i·a [G. *arthron,* joint; *odynē,* pain]. Pain in a joint; arthralgia. —**arthrodynic,** *adj.*

ar″thro·dys·pla′si·a (·dis·play′zhuh, ·zee·uh, ·shuh, ·see·uh) [*arthron;* G. *dys-,* bad; *plassein,* to form]. A familial disease in which the patellas are rudimentary, the heads of the radii dislocated, and the nails generally absent.

ar″throe·de′ma. See *arthredema.*

ar″thro·em·py·e′sis (·em·pye·ee′sis, ·em·pee·ee′-sis) [*arthron;* G. *empyēsis,* suppuration]. Suppuration in a joint.

ar″thro·en·dos′co·py [*arthron;* G. *endon,* within; *skopein,* to examine]. Examination of the interior of a joint by means of an endoscope.

ar″thro·er·ei′sis (ar″thro·er·eye′sis). Surgical reduction of the mobility of a joint.

ar·throg′ra·phy [*arthron;* G. *graphein,* to write]. 1. Roentgenography of a joint. 2. A treatise or monograph relating to the joints.

ar″thro·gry·po′sis (ahr″thro·grye·po′sis, ·gri·po′-sis) [*arthron;* G. *grypōsis,* a crooking]. 1. Permanent flexure of a joint; ankylosis. 2. Persistent idiopathic contracture of a joint.

ar″thro·ka·tad′y·sis [*arthron;* G. *katadysis,* a going down]. Intrapelvic protrusion of the acetabulum from thinning and eburnation of the pelvic wall; of undetermined etiology; Otto pelvis.

ar′thro·lith″ [*arthron;* G. *lithos,* stone]. A calcareous or gouty deposit or free body within a joint; a chalkstone. —**arthrolithi′asis,** *n.*

ar·throl′o·gy [*arthron;* G. *logos,* word]. The science which treats of joints.

ar·throl′y·sis [*arthron;* G. *lysis,* a loosing]. Surgical freeing of an ankylosed joint. *Obs.*

ar·throm′e·ter [*arthron;* G. *metron,* a measure]. An instrument for measuring and recording the extent of movement in a joint. Syn., *goniometer.* —**arthrometry,** *n.*

ar·thron′cus [*arthron;* G. *ogkos,* a mass]. A joint tumor; swelling of a joint. *Obs.*

ar·throp′a·thy [*arthron;* G. *pathos,* disease]. Any joint disease, especially a neurotrophic disorder associated with tabes dorsalis and syringomyelia, and rarely with general paralysis and disseminated sclerosis. —**arthropath′ic,** *adj.*

deforming a. Arthritis deformans.

inflammatory a. Any inflammatory condition affecting joints; arthritis.

neurogenic a. An osteoarthritis associated with swelling, hypermobility, bone destruction, and trophic disturbances. Also called *Charcot's joint, neuropathic a., tabetic a.*

osteopulmonary a. See hypertrophic pulmonary *osteoarthropathy.*

psoriatic a. A type of arthritis occurring in association with psoriasis. Also called *arthropathic psoriasis.*

tabetic a. See neurogenic *a.*

vertebral a. That associated with depressions and rugosities of the vertebrae.

ar′thro·phyte [*arthron;* G. *phyton*, a plant]. An abnormal growth occurring within a joint.

ar′thro plas″ty [*arthron;* G. *plassein*, to form]. 1. The making of an artificial joint. 2. Reconstruction of a new and functioning joint from an ankylosed one; a plastic operation upon a joint. —**arthroplas′tic,** *adj.*

Ar·throp′o·da [*arthron;* G. *pous*, foot]. The largest phylum of the animal kingdom; includes the crustacea, insects, myriopods, arachnids, and related forms. The members are bilaterally symmetrical, having a limited number of segments, a chitinous exoskeleton, and jointed appendages. —**ar′thropod,** *adj., n.;* **arthrop′odous,** *adj.*

ar″thror·rha′gi·a [*arthron;* G. *rhēgnynai*, to burst]. Hemorrhage into a joint.

ar′thro·scope [*arthron;* G. *skopein*, to examine]. An instrument used for the visualization of the interior of a joint.

ar·thros′co·py [*arthron; skopein*]. The act of examining the interior of a joint with an arthroscope.

ar·thro′sis [*arthron;* G. *-ōsis*, condition]. 1. Articulation or joint; a suture. 2. A degenerative process in a joint.

a. deformans. Degenerative joint disease.

ar′thro·spore [*arthron;* G. *sporos*, seed]. A cell functioning as a spore that forms by the breaking off of a hyphal cell from the parental hypha.

ar·thros′to·my [*arthron;* G. *stoma*, mouth]. Incision into a joint, as for drainage.

ar′thro·tome [*arthron;* G. *tomos*, cutting]. A stout knife used in joint surgery; a cartilage knife.

ar·throt′o·my [*arthron;* G. *tomē*, a cutting]. Incision into a joint.

ar″thro·tro′pi·a [*arthron;* G. *tropē*, a turning]. Torsion of a limb.

ar′throus [*arthron*]. Pertaining to a joint or joints; jointed.

Arthus, Nicolas Maurice [*French physiologist,* 1862–1945]. Known for his description of a generalized or local anaphylactic reaction, the result of the union of antigen and antibody within the tissues, manifested by local edema and inflammation (1903–06); called *Arthus' phenomenon.* Credited also with the first mention of the essential role of calcium in the mechanics of blood coagulation (1890).

ar·tic′u·lar, ar·tic″u·la′re [L. *articulare*, to divide in joints]. Os articulare; a bone of the lower jaw of fishes, amphibians, and reptiles which articulates with the quadrate bone to form the mandibular joint. Its homolog in man is the malleus. Syn., *articular bone.*

ar″tic·u·lar′is ge′nus. A small muscle arising from the distal fourth of the anterior surface of the femur and inserted into the capsule of the knee joint.

ar·tic′u·late [L. *articulare*, to divide in joints]. 1. Divided into joints. 2. Distinct, clear.

ar·tic′u·late. *In dentistry,* to position or adjust artificial teeth.

ar·tic′u·lat″ing pa′per. *In dentistry,* a carbon paper on which the patient bites, in order to show the relationship of the teeth in mastication.

ar·tic″u·la′ti·o (ahr·tick″yoo·lay′shee·o) (pl. *articulationes*) [L., the putting forth of new joints (belonging to the language of the vineyard)]. A joint. See *articulation.* See Table of Joints and Ligaments in the Appendix.

a. coxae [BNA]. Hip joint.

a. cubiti [BNA]. Elbow joint.

a. genus [BNA]. Knee joint.

a. manus [BNA]. Joint of the hand.

articulationes capitulorum [BNA]. Articulations between the heads of the ribs and the vertebrae.

articulationes digitorum manus [BNA]. Joints of the fingers.

articulationes digitorum pedis [BNA]. Joints of the toes.

a. pedis [BNA]. Joint of the foot.

a. sellaris [BNA] Saddle joint.

a. simplex [BNA]. Simple joint.

ar·tic″u·la′tion [*articulatio*]. 1. The enunciation of speech. 2. A joint; the junction of two or more bones. The articulations are divided into: *synarthroses,* or immovable joints, which are subdivided into (a) *schindyleses,* or grooved joints, (b) *gomphoses,* or sockets, as for the teeth, and (c) *suturae,* as the bones of the skull; *diarthroses,* or movable joints, which are subdivided into (a) *arthrodia,* or gliding joints, (b) *ginglymi,* or hinge-like joints, (c) *enarthroses,* or ball-and-socket joints; and *amphiarthroses,* or those of the mixed type. For articulations listed by name, see Table of Joints and Ligaments in the Appendix. 3. The positioning of artificial teeth. 4. Occlusion, 4: loose and improper usage. —**artic′ular,** *adj.*

compound a. A diarthrosis in which more than two bones are involved.

condyloid a. A type of diarthrosis in which an ovoid articular surface, or condyle, is received into an elliptical cavity. Syn., *ellipsoid a.*

congruent a. One in which the surfaces correspond in form and curvature.

ellipsoid a. See condyloid *a.*

false a. One formed between the end of a dislocated bone and the contiguous parts, or between fragments of a broken bone. Syn., *pseudarthrosis.*

hinge a. Ginglymus; an articulation in which a convex cylindrical surface is grooved at right angles to the axis of the cylinder, or trochlea, and meets a concave cylindrical surface which is ridged to fit the trochlea in such a manner as to permit motion in only one plane.

incongruent a. One in which two or more opposing surfaces may differ in form or present curves of unequal radii resulting in imperfect fitting.

irregular a. A type of diarthrosis in which the surfaces are small, irregular, flat, or slightly curved.

reciprocal a. A mode of articulation in which the articular surface is convex on one side and concave on the other. See condyloid *articulation.*

screw a. A hinge articulation in which the groove of the trochlea is in a plane not at right angles with the axis, and the hinge movement is accompanied by progression at right angles to the hinge plane. Also called *cochlear articulation* or *spiral joint.*

simple a. A diarthrosis in which only two bones are involved.

spheroid a. A type of diarthrosis in which a rounded head is lodged in a concave surface.

supplementary a. A false articulation in which the ends of the fragments become rounded and covered with a fibrous capsule.

trochoid a. A type of diarthrosis in which a pivotlike process rotates within a ring, or a ring rotates around a pivot, the ring being formed partly of bone, partly of ligament.

ar·tic″u·la″ti·o′nes (ahr·tick″yoo·lay″shee·o′neez). Plural of articulatio.

ar·tic′u·la″tor [L. *articulus*, joint]. An instrument used in dentistry for holding casts of the jaws or teeth in proper relation during the stages of the construction of artificial dentures. It may be adjusted so as to duplicate the mandibular movements of the patient.

ar·tic'u·lus (pl. and gen. *articuli*) [L.]. 1. A joint; a knuckle. 2. A segment; a part; a limb.

ar'ti·fact. See *artefact.*

ar"ti·fi'cial [L. *artificialis,* of or belonging to art, artificial]. Made or constructed by art; not natural.

ar"ti·fi'cial res"pi·ra'tion. The artificial promotion of normal breathing in one apparently dead, by the forcing of air into and out of the lungs to aerate the blood. Used in drowning, asphyxia neonatorum, asphyxia from smoke or toxic gases, electric shock, etc. Pulmotors or respirators are used for prolonged application, but numerous hand methods are employed. Chief methods are: *Buist's method* for asphyxia neonatorum, in which the child is alternately transferred from one hand of the obstetrician to the other, being supine in one and prone in the other; *Drinker's method,* which is the same as the Schafer method, with the addition of a second operator who kneels at the patient's head and raises the arms to assist in inspiration; *Eve's method,* in which the patient is tipped alternately head up and head down on a stretcher, inspiration and expiration occurring as the diaphragm moves up and down from shifting of the abdominal viscera; *Fell-O'Dwyer method,* in which air is forced into the lungs by a bellows through an intubation tube, expiration occurring spontaneously due to elasticity of the chest or being aided by external pressure; *hip-roll prone pressure method* or *hip-lift prone pressure method,* in which the Schafer method is combined with lifting the hips in expiration; the hips also may be rolled to one side, an action which is less effective but less exhausting for the operator; *Holger Nielsen's method,* in which the patient lies prone and the operator extends the patient's arms in inspiration and presses on the scapulae in expiration; *Howard's method,* in which the patient is placed on his back with his head lower than his abdomen and his hands over his head; rhythmic pressure is applied upward and inward against the lower lateral parts of the chest; *Laborde's method,* in which the respiratory center is stimulated by rhythmic traction of the tongue with the fingers or a specially designed forceps; *Marshall Hall's* method, in which the patient is alternately rolled from his side or back to his abdomen to expand or compress the lungs, expiration being augmented by pressure on the chest; *Prochownick's method,* for asphyxia neonatorum, in which the infant is suspended with the head extended, and intermittent pressure is applied to the chest; the *rocking method,* which is synonymous with Eve's method; the *rowing method,* in which the patient is supine with the operator at his head; the patient's arms are extended firmly above his head and then rapidly dropped back toward his chest at a rate of 10 to 12 times a minute; *Satterthwaite's method,* in which the patient is placed on his back, and there is alternate pressure and relaxation of the abdomen; *Schafer (prone pressure) method,* in which the patient is placed on his abdomen and his head turned to one side and rested on his arm; intermittent pressure over the lower part of the thorax 15 times per minute causes inspiration and expiration simulating natural breathing; *Schroeder's method* for asphyxia neonatorum, in which the infant is placed in a bath with its back supported by the operator, who then effects a forceful expiration by bending its body over the belly, thus compressing the thorax; *Schultze's method,* in which the newborn child is held by the shoulders from behind so that the operator has his thumbs on the front of the child's shoulders, the index fingers in the axillas, and the other fingers over the back. The child is gradually tipped up until the legs fall forward and the body is sharply flexed, so that the abdomen and chest are tightly compressed, thus producing a forcible expiration and allowing fluids to drain out of the nose and mouth; *Silvester's method,* in which the patient is placed on his back and his arms raised to the sides of his head and then turned down and pressed against the chest.

ar"y·ep"i·glot'tic, ar"y·ep"i·glot·tid'e·an, ar"-y·te"no-ep"i·glot'tic (ar"i·tee"no-, a·rit"i·no-) [G. *ary aina,* ladle; *epi,* upon; *glōttis,* glottis]. 1. Relating to the arytenoid cartilage and the epiglottis. 2. Designating two folds of mucous membrane extending between these structures (aryepiglottic folds), each containing an aryepiglottic muscle. See Table of Muscles in the Appendix.

ar'yl [G. *arōma,* aromatic herb; *hylē,* material]. An organic radical derived from an aromatic hydrocarbon by the removal of one hydrogen atom, as phenyl (C_6H_5—) from benzene.

ar"yl·ar'so·nate. Any aromatic organic salt of arsenic, as arsphenamine.

ar'yl·ene. Any bivalent radical derived from an aromatic hydrocarbon by removal of a hydrogen atom from each of two carbon atoms of the nucleus, as phenylene (C_6H_4=) from benzene.

ar"y·te"no·ep"i·glot'tic. See *aryepiglottic.*

ar"y·te"no·ep"i·glot'ti·cus. The continuation of the oblique arytenoid muscle: old term.

a·ryt'e·noid, ar"y·te'noid [G. *arytaina,* ladle; *eidos,* form]. 1. Resembling the mouth of a pitcher. 2. Pertaining to the arytenoid cartilages, glands, and muscles. See Table of Muscles in the Appendix.

ar"y·te"noi·dec'to·my (ar"i·tee"noy·deck'to·mee, a·rit"i·noy·) [*arytaina; eidos;* G. *ektomē,* excision]. Removal of an arytenoid cartilage.

ar"y·te"noi·di'tis (ar"i·tee"noy·dye'tis, a·rit"i-noy·) [*arytaina; eidos;* G. *-itis,* inflammation]. Inflammation of the arytenoid cartilages or muscles.

ar"y·te·noi'do·pex"y [*arytaina; eidos;* G. *pēxis,* a fixing]. Surgical fixation of the arytenoid cartilages.

ar"y·vo·cal'is. A portion of the vocalis muscle inserted into the vocal fold.

As Chemical symbol for arsenic.

As. Abbreviation for astigmatism; astigmatic.

As. h. Hyperopic astigmatism.

As. m. Myopic astigmatism.

a.s. *Auris sinistra;* left ear.

as"a·fet'i·da, as"a·foet'i·da [NL. *asa,* from Per. *azā,* mastic; L. *fetidus,* stinking]. An oleo-gum-resin obtained from the rhizomes and roots of *Ferula Assa-foetida, F. foetida,* and other species of *Ferula.* It consists of soft masses of yellow-brown color, bitter taste, and persistent, offensive odor. The odor is due to a volatile oil consisting largely of a mercaptan of the formula $C_7H_{14}S_2$. It is a carminative and psychic sedative. Dose, 0.32–0.65 Gm. (5–10 gr.), preferably in pill form. An emulsion prepared by shaking the drug in water has been used in infantile colic.

as"a·phi'a (ass"uh·figh'uh, a·saff'ee·uh, a·say'-fee·uh) [G. *asapheia,* want of clearness]. Indistinct speech; especially that due to cleft palate. *Obs.*

as'a·prol. $CaC_{20}H_{14}S_2O_8 + 3H_2O$. Calcium beta-naphthol-alpha-monosulfonate, a substance readily soluble in water and alcohol; employed as antipyretic and antirheumatic.

a·sar'ci·a [G. *a-,* not; *sarx,* flesh]. Emaciation; leanness.

as'a·ron. A stearopten from the oil of *Asarum europaeum.* It forms monoclinic prisms, has an aromatic taste, and smells like camphor.

as'a·rum [G. *asaron,* hazelwort]. The dried rhizome and roots of *Asarum canadense.* It contains an acrid, bitter resin and an aromatic volatile oil. It is carminative, but is used chiefly as a bitter aromatic flavor. Also called *Canada snakeroot, wild ginger.*

as·bes'tos [G., unquenchable]. A soft fibrous silicate mineral of flexible or elastic fibers; the best nonconductor of heat. Mixed with plaster, it is used in dentistry as a substitute for sand to form the investment preparatory to soldering. It is used by the military for making protective clothing against flash and gasoline burns. Workers in asbestos frequently acquire hyperkeratotic papules on their hands (asbestos corns, or warts), a foreign-body type of reaction caused by spicules of the substance.

as"bes·to'sis [*asbestos;* G. *-ōsis,* condition]. Pneumonoconiosis marked by fibrosis of the lungs from prolonged inhalation of dust laden with asbestos. See *silicatosis.*

as·bes'tos trans"for·ma'tion. A change in cartilage, especially of the hyaline type, often associated with advanced age, which leads to a softening of the tissue and to the formation of spaces in it.

as"ca·ri'a·sis [G. *askaris,* worm in the intestines; NL. *-iasis,* condition]. An infestation disease caused by the presence of the *Ascaris lumbricoides;* the intestine is most commonly affected but the infestation may spread to the stomach, liver, and lungs.

as·car'i·cide [*askaris;* L. *caedere,* to kill]. A medicine that kills ascarides.

As·car'i·dae (ass·kar'i·dee) [*askaris*]. A family of nematode worms, to which belong the roundworm (*Ascaris lumbricoides*) and the threadworm (*Enterobius vermicularis*).

as·car'i·dol, as·car'i·dole. $C_{10}H_{16}O_2$. An unsaturated terpene peroxide which constitutes from 45 to 70% of chenopodium oil. It is the active principle of the oil.

As'ca·ris [G.]. A genus of intestinal nematodes. **—ascarid,** *n.*

A. equorum. A species infesting horses; the maw worm.

A. lumbricoides. A species of roundworm causing ascariasis.

A. megalocephala. See *A. equorum.*

A. mystax. Synonym for *Toxocara cati,* the common ascarid of the domestic cat. Also see *Toxocara canis.*

A. suum. A species of roundworm causing ascariasis in the pig.

as·cend'ing [L. *ascendere,* to rise]. Taking an upward course; rising.

Asch, Morris Joseph [*American otolaryngologist,* 1833–1902]. Remembered for his operation for the correction of deviation of the nasal septum through a cruciate incision over the deflection. Also devised a perforated hard rubber nasal splint to fit the nasal passages; this had wide use in the treatment of fractures of the nasal bones.

Ascherson, Ferdinand Moritz [*German physician,* 1798–1879]. Long associated with the discovery of the casein coat surrounding milk globules and with the vesicles he described as being formed when oil and an albuminous fluid are agitated together.

Aschheim, Selmar [*German physician and biochemist,* 1878–]. Known as one of the discoverers of the gonadotropic hormone of the adenohypophysis. Introduced, with Zondek, test for pregnancy (1928); see Aschheim-Zondek *test, reaction.*

Aschner, Bernard [*Austrian gynecologist in America,* 1883–]. The oculocardiac reflex is called *Aschner's phenomenon.* See under *reflex.*

Aschoff, Karl Albert Ludwig [*German pathologist,* 1866–1942]. Studied the reticuloendothelial system. His writings on rheumatic myocarditis are regarded as classics. See Aschoff *nodule, cell.*

as·ci'tes (a·sigh'teez) [G. *askitēs,* a kind of dropsy, from *askos,* bag]. An abnormal accumulation of serous fluid in the peritoneal cavity caused by increased venous pressure or a decrease of plasma albumin. The clear, yellowish fluid coagulates on standing but may be turbid, sanguineous, or contain shreds. Physical examination reveals painless abdominal enlargement, dullness over fluid, shifting with position, and fluid wave. The condition is associated most frequently with cardiac failure, cirrhosis of the liver, and renal deficiency. Syn., *abdominal dropsy, hydroperitoneum.* **—ascit'ic,** *adj.*

acute a. A very sudden and large accumulation of fluid in the abdomen.

a. adiposus. An accumulation of milky fluid due to contained cells which have undergone fatty degeneration. Seen in chronic peritoneal inflammations as in tuberculosis, carcinoma, etc.

a. chylosus. Chyle in the peritoneal cavity due to rupture of the lacteals. Also called *chylous a.*

a. intercus. An effusion occurring between the skin and the peritoneum.

a. saccatus. (a) A form in which the effusion is prevented by adhesions or inflammatory exudate from entering the general peritoneal cavity. Syn., *encysted dropsy of the peritoneum.* (b) An ovarian cystoma.

a. vaginalis. A collection of liquid within the sheath of the rectus abdominis muscle.

a. vulgatior. A form apparently due to diseased kidneys, and preceded by scanty, highly colored urine.

gelatinous a. See *pseudomyxoma peritonaei.*

mechanical a. That due to portal obstruction. Also called *passive a.*

pseudochylous a. Presence in the peritoneal cavity of milky fluid which contains protein but no fat.

sanguineous a. A bloody form affecting sheep and lambs. Syn., *diarhemia.*

as'cle·pain (ass'kli·pane) [G. *asklēpias,* swallowwort, named from Asclepius]. A proteolytic enzyme derived from the latex of a species of *Asclepias.*

Asclepiades of Bithynia [*Greek physician,* b. ca. 124 B.C.]. Established Greek medicine in Rome. An opponent of Hippocrates, he held stubbornly to his own theories. Said to have been the first to mention tracheotomy.

as"cle·pi'ad·in (ass"kli·pye'uh·din). A bitter glycoside obtained from various species of *Asclepias.* It is poisonous, and has emetic, purgative, and sudorific properties.

as·cle'pi·as [G. *asklēpias,* swallow-wort, named from Asclepius]. Pleurisy root; the root of *Asclepias tuberosa,* a plant of the order Asclepiadaceae. A popular remedy in the southern states for pleurisy. It is diaphoretic, emetic, and cathartic.

as'co·carp [G. *askos,* bladder; *karpos,* fruit]. The developed fruit of Ascomycetes.

as"co·car'pic [*askos; karpos*]. Of, or relating to, an ascocarp.

as"co·go·nid'i·um [*askos;* root of G. *gignesthai,* to be produced]. A portion of the female sex organ in ascomycetous fungi which, after fertilization, develops into asci.

Ascoli test. See under *test.*

As"co·my·ce'tes (ass"ko·migh·see'teez) [*askos;* G. *mykēs,* fungus]. One of the four large classes of fungi. **—as"co·my·ce'tous,** *adj.*

a·scor′bate. A salt of ascorbic acid.

a·scor′bic ac′id (*acidum ascorbicum*). $C_6H_8O_6$; a substance, present in fresh green foods, citrus fruits, and various other uncooked materials, the lack of which in the body eventually leads to scurvy. It is a white or slightly yellowish, odorless, crystalline powder, optically active and fairly stable when dry, but rapidly destroyed by the oxygen of the air when in aqueous solution. Ascorbic acid functions in various oxidation-reduction reactions of the tissues and is essential for normal metabolism. It appears to be necessary for fibroblastic formation of collagenic connective tissue, and thus for wound-healing and tissue-repair. Dose, 25 mg. to 1 Gm. daily, depending on prophylactic or curative use. Also called L-*ascorbic acid.* Syn., *vitamin C, cevitamic acid, antiscorbutic vitamin.* See Tables of Vitamins and of Normal Values of Blood Constituents in the Appendix.

a. a. oxidase. (a) A general term for any enzyme capable of promoting the oxidation of ascorbic acid either directly or indirectly through the formation of a compound which acts as the oxidant. (b) More properly limited to an enzyme present in many vegetables, particularly squash and cucumber. In the presence of oxygen and water it causes ascorbic acid to take up two —OH radicals to form dehydroascorbic acid.

as′co·spore [*askos;* G. *sporos,* seed]. A spore produced in an ascus.

as′cus (pl. *asci*) [*askos*]. The characteristic spore case of the ascomycetes; usually consisting of a single terminal cell containing eight spores.

-ase (-ace, -aze) [diast*ase*, from G. *diastasis,* separation]. Suffix denoting *an enzyme.*

Aselli, Gasparo [*Italian physician and anatomist,* 1581–1626]. Discovered the lacteal vessels (lymphatics). *Aselli's glands* are the lymph nodes near the pancreas.

as″e·ma′si·a. See *asemia.*

a·se′mi·a [G. *a-,* not; *sēma,* sign]. An aphasia in which the patient is unable to understand or use speech, writing, or gestures as a means of communication. Syn., *asemasia, asymbolia.* —**asem′ic,** *adj.*

asepsin. A brand of bromoacetanilid. Also called *antisepsin.*

a·sep′sis [G. *a-,* not; *sēpsis,* putrefaction]. Exclusion of microorganisms producing decay. —**aseptic,** *adj.*

a·sex′u·al (ay·seck′shoo·ul, a·seck′shoo·ul) [*a-;* L. *sexus,* sex]. 1. Not involving the distinction between male and female. 2. Denoting reproduction without sexual union. —**asex′ually,** *adv.*

ash [AS. *asce*]. The incombustible mineral residue that remains when a substance is incinerated.

bone a. The white mineral constituents that remain after calcination or incineration of bone.

Ashford, Bailey Kelly [*American Army medical officer,* 1873–1934]. Discovered the great prevalence of ancylostomiasis in Puerto Rico (1900), and devoted his life to the eradication of the hookworm.

Ashhurst, John [*American surgeon,* 1839–1900]. Known for his introduction of a splint for use in leg fractures, called *Ashhurst's splint.*

a″si·a′li·a [G. *a-,* not; *sialon,* saliva]. Deficiency or failure of the secretion of saliva.

a″si·at′i·co·side″. An antibiotic substance derived from Madagascar varieties of the perennial umbelliferous herb *Centella asiatica* (*Hydrocotyle asiatica*); it is active against *Mycobacterium tuberculosis* in animals but is toxic.

Askenstedt's method. See under *method.*

Asklepios. Greek god of healing, son of Apollo; his cult was widespread in ancient Greece; his temples were houses of healing, precursors of the modern hospital; as Roman god of medicine, *Aesculapius.*

A. S. O. American Society of Orthodontists.

a·so′cial (ay·so′shul, a·so′shul) [*a-;* L. *socius,* companion]. Withdrawn from, not interested in others and their activities nor in realities.

a·so′ma [*a-;* G. *sōma,* body]. A placental parasite with an ill-formed head and only a rudimentary body. —**asomous,** *adj.;* **asomus,** *n.*

a·so′ni·a [*a-;* L. *sonus,* sound]. Tone deafness.

A. S. P. American Society of Pedodontists.

asp [G. *aspis,* asp]. A small venomous snake found in Africa and the Near East. *Vipera aspis.*

as″pal·a·so′ma [G. *aspalax,* blind rat; *sōma,* body]. A monster with median or lateral eventration of the lower abdomen, having three distinct openings for the urinary bladder, the rectum, and the sexual organs.

as·par′a·gin, as·par′a·gine. $COOH.CH(NH_2).CH_2.CONH_2$; the β-amide of asparaginic acid, found in the sprouts of dicotyledons and in many seeds; it occurs in white rhombic crystals, and is soluble in hot water, insoluble in alcohol or ether: a constituent of many proteins. Syn., *asparamide,* α*-aminosuccinamic acid.*

as·par′a·gin·ase. An enzyme, present in liver and other animal tissues as well as in plants, yeast, and bacteria, which catalyzes hydrolysis of asparagin to asparaginic acid and ammonia.

as·par″a·gin′ic ac′id. $COOH.CH(NH_2).CH_2.COOH$. Aminosuccinic acid, a hydrolysis product of asparagin and of many proteins. Syn., *aspartic acid.*

as·par′a·gi·nyl. The univalent radical, $H_2NCOCH_2CH(NH_2)CO$—, of asparagin, the monamide of asparaginic acid.

as·par·am′ide, as·par′am·ide. Asparagin

as·par′tase. An enzyme, present in several bacteria, which catalyzes the conversion of aspartic acid to fumaric acid and ammonia.

as·par′tic ac′id. Asparaginic acid.

as·par′to·yl. The divalent radical, $—COCH_2CH(NH_2)CO—$, of aspartic acid, an amino acid having two carboxyl groups.

as·par′tyl. The univalent radical, $HOOCCH_2CH(NH_2)CO$—, of aspartic acid, an amino acid having two carboxyl groups.

a·spas′tic [G. *a-,* not; *spasmos,* convulsion]. Not spastic.

a″spe·cif′ic [*a-;* ML. *specificus,* from *species,* sort, kind]. Nonspecific; not a specific.

as″per·gil′lic ac′id (ass″pur·jil′ick). An antibiotic substance produced by *Aspergillus flavus.*

as″per·gil′lin. 1. An antibiotic substance obtained from certain fungi; it is probably identical with flavacidin, flavatin, flavicin, gigantic acid, and parasiticin. 2. A pigment obtained from the spores of *Aspergillus niger.*

as·per″gil·lo′sis (ass·pur″ji·lo′sis, ass″pur·) [L. *aspergere,* to sprinkle; G. *-ōsis,* condition]. An infectious disease caused by any species of *Aspergillus.* Infections of lungs, bronchi, external ear, paranasal sinuses, orbit, bones, brain, and meninges have been described.

As″per·gil′lus (ass″pur·jil′us) [*aspergere*]. A genus of fungi important as a contaminant of lesions and as an agent of infection. The species **A. fumigatus** is the most common invader, but **A. flavus, A. nidulans,** and **A. niger** are also found in man.

a·sper′ma·tism (ay·spur′muh·tiz·um, a·spur′·), **a·sper′mi·a** (ay·spur′mee·uh, a·spur′·) [G. *a-,* not; *sperma,* seed]. 1. Nonemission of semen, whether owing to nonsecretion or to nonejaculation. 2. Defective secretion of semen or lack of formation of spermatozoa. —**aspermat'ic, aspermous,** *adj.*

a·sper"ma·to·gen'e·sis [*a-; sperma;* G. *genesis*, production]. Failure of maturation of spermatozoa.

as'per·ous [L. *asper*, rough]. Uneven; having a surface with distinct, minute elevations.

as·phyx'i·a [G., from *a-*, not; *sphyzein*, to throb]. Suffocation; coma the result of deprivation of oxygen causing anoxia in the body and an accumulation of carbon dioxide and fixed acids. Asphyxia should be differentiated from *anoxia* and *apnea.* —**asphyxial,** *adj.*

a. cyanotica. Traumatic asphyxia.

a. livida. Asphyxia neonatorum associated with cyanotic skin, strong pulse, and active reflexes. Syn., *blue a.*

a. neonatorum. Asphyxia of the newborn.

a. pallida. Asphyxia neonatorum attended by a slow, weak pulse, abolished reflexes, and a very pale skin.

blue a. See *a.* livida.

fetal a. Asphyxia of the fetus while in the uterus caused by interference with its blood supply, as by cord compression or premature placental separation. Syn., *intrauterine a.*

intrauterine a. Fetal *a.*

local a. Stagnation of the circulation in a part, as the fingers, hands, toes, or feet.

traumatic a. Cyanosis of the head and neck from sudden compression of the thorax, upper abdomen, or both. Also called *ecchymotic mask, traumatic apnea, pressure stasis.*

as·phyx'i·ant [*a-; sphyzein*]. An agent capable of producing asphyxia. —**asphyx'iant,** *adj.*; **asphyxiate,** *v.t., v.i.*

as'pi·din. $C_{23}H_{27}O_7$. An active principle obtained from aspidium, the rhizome and stipes of *Dryopteris Filix-mas.*

as·pid'i·um [G. *aspidion*, little shield]. The rhizome and stipes of European aspidium or male fern (*Dryopteris Filix-mas*) or of American aspidium or marginal fern (*D. marginalis*); both are sources of **aspidium oleoresin,** used for expelling tapeworm.

as"pi·do·sper'ma [G. *aspis*, shield; *sperma*, seed]. Quebracho. The dried bark of *Aspidosperma quebracho-blanco* containing the alkaloids aspidospermine, quebrachine, and others; it has been used as respiratory stimulant in asthmatic and cardiac dyspnea.

as"pi·do·sper'mine (ass"pi·do·spur'meen, ·min). $C_{23}H_{30}N_2O_2$. An alkaloid extracted from quebracho (aspidosperma). It stimulates respiration and depresses circulation.

as"pi·ra'tion [L. *aspirare*, to breathe upon]. 1. Act of sucking up or sucking in; inspiration; imbibition. 2. Act of using the aspirator. 3. The withdrawing of fluids and gases from a cavity. —**as'pirate,** *v.*

as'pi·ra"tor [*aspirare*]. A negative pressure apparatus for withdrawing liquids from cavities.

as'pi·rin. See *acetylsalicylic acid.*

As'pis [G. *aspis*, asp]. A genus of snakes of the Viperidae.

A. cornutus. The horned viper of the African deserts. The venom of this species is predominantly hemotoxic.

aspogen. A trade-mark for the gastric antacid substance *dihydroxyaluminum aminoacetate.*

a·spo"ro·gen'ic (ay·spor"o·jen'ick, a·spor"o·, ass"-po·ro·), **as"po·rog'e·nous** (ass"por·odj'i·nus) [G. *a-*, not; *sporos*, seed; *genesthai*, from *gignesthai*, to be produced]. 1. Producing no spores. 2. Reproduced without spores.

a·spo'rous (ay·spor'us, a·spor'us) [*a-; sporos*]. Without spores; especially without the resistant phase, as in the case of many bacteria.

a·spor'u·late (ay·spor'yoo·late, a·spor'·) [*a-; sporos*]. Producing no spores.

as·sault' [OF. *assaut*, from L. *ad*, to, *saltus*, a leaping]. An unlawful attempt to do bodily injury to another.

felonious a. A malicious attack showing criminal intent upon the person of another.

as·say', as'say [OF. *asai*, trial]. 1. Testing or analysis of a metal or drug to determine the relative proportion of its constituents. 2. Process of assaying. 3. Substance to be analyzed; also the report of the analysis. 4. Any substance to be analyzed.

Assézat, Jules [*French anthropologist*, 1832–76]. Remembered for his triangle formed by lines uniting the nasion and the basion and alveolar point; called *Assézat's triangle.*

as·sim"i·la'tion [L. *assimilatio*, similarity]. 1. Process of transforming food into a state suitable for absorption by the circulation and conversion into body tissue; synthetic or constructive metabolism; anabolism. 2. *In psychology,* mental reception of impressions, and their assignment by the consciousness to their proper place; mental assimilation. 3. The abnormal fusion of bones, as the fusion of the transverse processes of the last lumbar vertebra with the lateral masses of the first sacral vertebra, or the atlas with the occipital bone. —**assim'ilable,** *adj.*; **assim'ilate,** *v.t.*

a. limit. Amount of starchy or saccharine food which a person can ingest without the appearance of glycosuria.

primary a. Conversion of food into chyle.

secondary a. Conversion of food elements into body tissue.

as·so"ci·a'tion [L. *associare*, to join to]. 1. A connection, union, joining, or combination. 2. A society or united group of persons. 3. *In chemistry,* the correlation or aggregation of substances or functions. 4. *In psychology,* a mental linking, as that of objects, persons, or events with ideas, thoughts, or sensations.

a. of ideas. That established between two similar ideas or two ideas of simultaneous occurrence.

clang a. Association of words because of their similarity in sound; seen in manic patients.

controlled a. Directed association of relevant ideas, due to a specific stimulus.

free a. Spontaneous consciously unrestricted association of ideas or mental images. *In psychoanalysis,* the free-association method is used to gain an understanding of the organization of the content of the mind.

induced a. A form of controlled association in which the person to be tested calls out the first word coming to mind in response to a specific stimulus word.

as'so·nance [L. *assonare*, to respond to]. A morbid tendency to employ alliteration.

as'sue·tude (ass'wi·tewd, a·sue'i·tewd) [L. *assuetudo*, custom, habit]. 1. Habituation to disturbing influences. 2. Condition of an organism in which it has acquired such tolerance for a drug or poison that the effect is lost.

As'ta·cus [G. *astakos*, lobster, from *ostakos*]. A genus of crustaceans containing the crayfish. The species **A. japonicus** and **A. similis** are important second intermediate hosts of the *Paragonimus westermani.*

a·sta'si·a (a·stay'zhuh, ·zee·uh, ·shuh, ·see·uh) [G., from *a-*, not; *stasis*, standing]. Motor incoordination for standing.

a.-abasia. Apparent inability to walk or stand, due to some mental conflict; not accompanied with organic paralysis. It is a symptom of neurosis. Also called *hysterical ataxia*.

as′ta·tine (ass′tuh·teen, ·tin) [G. *astatos*, unstable]. At = 210. Element number 85, prepared in 1940 by bombarding bismuth with alpha particles; formerly called alabamine. It is radioactive and forms no stable isotopes.

as″ta·xan′thin. $C_{40}H_{52}O_4$; a carotenoid pigment found mostly in animal organisms, but also occurring in plants.

a·ste″a·to′sis, as″te·a·to′sis [*a-;* G. *stear*, suet; *-ōsis*, condition]. 1. A deficiency or absence of the sebaceous secretion. 2. Any skin disease (as xeroderma) characterized by scantiness or lack of sebaceous secretion, the skin becoming dry, scaly, and often fissured. Syn., *xerosis*. Also called *a. cutis*.

as′ter [G., a star]. The radiating structure surrounding the centrosome of the cell, seen at the beginning of mitosis. —**astral,** *adj*.

fibrin a. Radiation of fibrin lines from centers of platelets or leukocytes. Syn., *fibrin stars*.

a·ster″e·og·no′sis [G. *a-*, not; *stereos*, solid; *gnōsis*, knowledge]. Inability to recognize objects by the sense of touch. Also called *astereocognosy*.

as·te′ri·on [G. *asterios*, starry]. *In craniology*, the meeting point of the lambdoid, parietomastoid, and occipitomastoid sutures.

a·ster′nal (ay·stur′nul, a·stur′nul) [G. *a-*, not; *sternon*, breast]. 1. Not joined to the sternum, as the asternal ribs. 2. Without a sternum.

a·ster′ni·a [*a-; sternon*]. Absence of the sternum.

as′ter·o-, aster- [G. *astēr*, star]. A combining form meaning *star*.

as′ter·oid [*astēr;* G. *eidos*, form]. Star-shaped.

asterol dihydrochloride. Trade-marked name for the antifungal agent *diamthazole dihydrochloride*.

as·the′ni·a [G. *astheneia*, want of strength]. Absence or loss of strength; adynamia. —**asthen′ic,** *adj*.

a. pigmentosa. See *adrenal cortical hypofunction*.

a. universalis. Visceroptosis associated with neurasthenic tendency, vasomotor weakness, and intestinal atony.

grave hypophyseal a. A serious cachexia of pituitary origin marked by anorexia, emaciation, constipation, amenorrhea, subnormal temperature, hypotonia, and hypoglycemia. See *hypotonia*.

myalgic a. A state of generalized fatigue associated with muscular pains.

neurocirculatory a. A psychosomatic disorder characterized by dyspnea, palpitation, vertigo, faintness, fatigue, tremor, precordial pain, and tachycardia, occurring most frequently in soldiers during the stress and danger of training and combat. It may occur physiologically in untrained persons who exercise violently. Also called *effort syndrome, soldier's heart, irritable heart, disordered action of the heart, Da Costa's syndrome*. Abbreviated, N. C. A.

tropical anhidrotic a. Heat exhaustion due to inability to sweat. See sweat-retention *syndrome*.

as·then′ic type. A physical type (Kretschmer) marked by a tall, slender, flat-chested, angular form, and poor muscular development.

as′the·no-, asthen- [G. *asthenēs*, weak]. A combining form meaning *weak*.

as″the·no·bi·o′sis (ass″thi·no·buy·o′sis) [*asthenēs;* G. *bios*, life; *-ōsis*, condition]. A biologic state closely allied to hibernation or estivation, yet not induced by climate, temperature, or humidity.

as″the·no·co′ri·a [*asthenēs;* G. *korē*, pupil]. A sluggish pupillary light reflex, as in hypoadrenia.

as″the·no·ge′ni·a, as″the·no·gen′e·sis [*asthenēs;* G. *genesis*, production]. Production of asthenia. —**asthenogen′ic, asthenogenet′ic,** *adj*.

as″the·nol′o·gy [*asthenēs;* G. *logos*, word]. The theory that anatomic and functional anomalies are associated with constitutional weakness or debility.

as″the·nom′e·ter [*asthenēs;* G. *metron*, a measure]. An instrument for detecting and measuring asthenia; especially, a device for measuring muscular asthenopia.

as″the·no·pho′bi·a [*asthenēs;* G. *phobos*, fear]. Morbid fear of weakness.

as″the·no′pi·a [*asthenēs;* G. *ōps*, eye]. Weakness of the ocular muscles or of visual power, due to errors of refraction, heterophoria, overuse, etc. —**asthenop′ic,** *adj.;* **as′thenope,** *n*.

accommodative a. Subnormal power of the function of accommodation, or the pain or discomfort resulting from accommodative effort.

muscular a. That due to weakness, incoordination (heterophoria), or strain of the external ocular muscles.

as″the·no·sper′mi·a [*asthenēs;* G. *sperma*, seed]. Weakness or loss of vitality of the spermatozoa.

as″the·nox′i·a [*asthenēs;* G. *oxys*, sharp]. Insufficient oxidation of waste products, as ketosis from insufficient oxidation of fatty acids.

asth′ma (az′muh, ass′muh) [G., a panting]. Paroxysmal dyspnea. Commonly, however, it refers to **allergic asthma,** characterized by dyspnea, cough, wheezing, mucous sputum, and a sense of constriction of the chest. Pathologic changes consist of bronchiolar spasm, edema of mucosa, hypertrophy of glandular elements, and secretion of mucinlike substance. Is usually due to hypersensitiveness to inhaled or ingested substances, or bacteria. In allergic asthma, the name may include the etiologic factor; as **bacterial asthma, food asthma, horse asthma, pollen asthma.** —**asthmat′ic,** *adj*.

bronchial a. See allergic *a*.

cardiac a. Paroxysmal dyspnea due to cardiac failure occurring, usually at night, in patients with passive congestion of the lungs, secondary to failure of the left side of the heart; accompanied by characteristic rales.

fuller's a. A pulmonary affection due to the inhalation of lint and dust in the manufacture of wool cloth.

grinder's a. An interstitial pneumonia due to the inhalation of fine particles set free in grinding steel, etc. See fibroid *phthisis*.

intrinsic bronchitic a. A form due probably to infection resulting in structural changes.

miner's a. Dyspnea due to anthracosis.

potter's a. Pneumonoconiosis.

psychogenic a. An intrinsic asthma due to psychic causes, occurring usually in persons over thirty years of age.

renal a. Paroxysmal dyspnea occurring as a result of renal failure or uremia.

steam fitter's a. Asbestosis.

stone a. Pressure and pain in the chest due to the presence of a calculus in the bronchus.

symptomatic a. Asthma which is secondary to some other condition.

thymic a. A rare type due to an enlarged thymus.

asth′ma weed. Lobelia.

a·stig′ma·graph [G. *a-*, not; *stigma*, a point; *graphein*, to write]. An instrument for detecting astigmatism of the eye.

a·stig′ma·tism [*a-; stigma*]. The faulty vision which results from irregularity in the curvature of one or more refractive surfaces (cornea, anterior and posterior surfaces of the lens) of the eye. When such a condition occurs, rays emanating from a point are not brought into focus at a point on the retina, but appear to spread as a line in various directions depending upon the curvature. Abbreviated As. The condition may be **congenital** or **acquired.** When the irregularity is in the cornea, it is **corneal astigmatism;** when in the lens, **lenticular astigmatism.** When the greatest refractive power is along the horizontal meridian, it is called **astigmatism against the rule;** when along the vertical meridian, **astigmatism with the rule.** Astigmatism may complicate myopia or hypermetropia, causing **simple hypermetropic astigmatism,** where one principal meridian is hypermetropic, the other normal, or **compound hypermetropic astigmatism** with both meridians hypermetropic, one more so than the other. Abbreviated Ah. In the same manner, complicating myopia, there may be **simple myopic astigmatism** and **compound myopic astigmatism** (symbol, M + As). When one meridian is myopic and the other hypermetropic, **mixed astigmatism** is the result. Also, when the principal meridians are at right angles, the condition is known as **regular astigmatism,** and when different parts of the meridian have different refractive powers, **irregular astigmatism.** —**astigmat'ic, astig'mic,** *adj.*

retinal a. Changes in the localization of the fixation point, thought to be due to changes in light intensity.

a·stig"ma·tom'e·ter. See *astigmometer.*

as"tig·mat'o·scope. See *astigmoscope.*

as"tig·mom'e·ter, a·stig"ma·tom'e·ter [*a-; stigma;* G. *metron,* a measure]. An instrument which measures the degree of astigmatism. —**astigmom'etry,** *n.*

a·stig'mo·scope, as"tig·mat'o·scope [*a-; stigma;* G. *skopein,* to examine]. An instrument for measuring astigmatism. —**astigmos'copy,** *n.*

a·stom'a·tous (a·stom'uh·tus, a·sto'muh·tus), **as'-to·mous, a·sto'mous** [*a-;* G. *stoma,* mouth]. 1. Without a mouth or stoma. 2. *In botany,* without stomas.

a·sto'mi·a [*a-; stoma*]. Congenital absence of the mouth.

as·trag"a·lec'to·my [G. *astragalos,* ball of the ankle joint; *ektomē,* excision]. Excision of the astragalus, or talus.

As·trag'a·lus [G. *astragalos,* milk vetch]. A genus of leguminous plants some varieties of which yield gum tragacanth.

A. mollissimus is the locoweed. Several species of this genus produce peculiar intoxicating effects in horses and other animals.

as·trag'a·lus [G. *astragalos,* ball of the ankle joint]. The ankle bone, upon which the tibia rests. *O.T.* Syn., *talus* [BNA]. See Table of Bones in the Appendix. —**astragalar,** *adj.*

as"tra·pho'bi·a, as"tra·po·pho'bi·a [G. *astrapē,* lightning; *phobos,* fear]. Morbid fear of lightning and thunderstorms.

as·trin'gent [L. *astringere,* to bind together]. An agent that produces contraction of organic tissues, or arrests hemorrhages, diarrhea, etc. —**astringency,** *n.;* **astrin'gent,** *adj.*

as'tro-, astr- [G. *astron,* a star]. Combining form signifying *pertaining to the stars.*

as'tro·blast [*astron;* G. *blastos,* germ]. A primitive cell which develops into an astrocyte.

as"tro·blas"to-as"tro·cy·to'ma. See *astroblastoma.*

as"tro·blas·to'ma [*astron; blastos;* G. *-ōma,* tumor]. A glial tumor occurring in all parts of the central nervous system but with less frequency than the astrocytoma, and differing from it by being less fibrillar and having more numerous cells. The cells are larger, have thicker processes often extending to vessels, and have hyperchromatic nuclei. Also called *astroblasto-astrocytoma, ganglion-cell glioma, ganglion-celled neuroma, glioblastoma-astroblastoma, spongioblastoma, spongioblastoma polare* or *unipolare.* Syn., *astrocytoma, Grade 2.*

a. of the nose. See heterotopic *glioma.*

as'tro·cytes (ass'tro·sights) [*astron;* G. *kytos,* cell]. The many-processed stellate cells of the neuroglia, attached to the blood vessels of the brain and spinal cord by perivascular feet. Also called *astroglia, Cajal's cells, macroglia, spider cells.*

fibrous a. Those in the white matter, characterized by long, unbranched processes.

protoplasmic a. Those in the gray matter, characterized by numerous, freely branching protoplasmic processes.

as"tro·cy·to'ma (·sigh·to'muh) [*astron; kytos;* G. *-ōma,* tumor]. One of the commonest glial tumors of the central nervous system; formed of protoplasmic or fibrillary astrocytes. In a grading of this series of tumors, it is synonymous with *astrocytoma, Grade 1; astroblastoma,* with *astrocytoma, Grade 2;* and *glioblastoma multiforme,* with *astrocytoma, Grades 3* and *4.* Also called *gemistocytic a., pilocytic a., piloid a., astrocytic glioma, astroglioma, astroma, spongiocytoma.*

a. gigantocellulare. See *glioblastoma multiforme.*

a. of the nose. See heterotopic *glioma.*

fibrillary a. One in which the glial cells show abundant interlacing fibrils.

protoplasmic a. One in which the glial cells are rich in cytoplasm and the fibrils scanty or absent.

as·trog'li·a [*astron;* G. *glia,* glue]. Neuroglia composed of astrocytes.

as·trog"li·o'ma. A glial tumor of the central nervous system. See *astrocytoma.*

a. of the nose. See heterotopic *glioma.*

as'troid [*astron;* G. *eidos,* form]. Star-shaped.

as·tro'ma. See *astrocytoma.*

as"tro·pho'bi·a [*astron;* G. *phobos,* fear]. Morbid fear of the stars and celestial space.

as'tro·sphere [*astron;* G. *sphaira,* sphere]. 1. The central mass of the aster, exclusive of the filaments or rays. 2. The entire aster, exclusive of the centriole. Syn., *centrosphere, centrosome, attraction sphere.*

a·styph'i·a [G. *a-,* not; *styein,* to make stiff]. Sexual impotence; inability to erect the penis.

a·stys'i·a (ay·stizh'uh, ay·stiz'ee·uh, a·stizh'uh, a·stiz'ee·uh) [*a-; styein*]. Incomplete power to erect the penis; sexual impotence.

a"syl·la'bi·a [*a-;* G. *syllabē,* syllable]. A form of aphasia in which individual letters are recognized, but the formation of syllables and words is difficult or impossible.

a·sy'lum [L., a place of refuge]. An institution for the support, safekeeping, cure, or education of those incapable of caring for themselves, such as the insane, the blind, etc.

a"sym·bo'li·a [G. *a-,* not; *symbolon,* token]. See *asemia.*

a"sym·met'ric (ay"si·met'rick, ass"i·met'rick) [*a-;* G. *symmetria,* symmetry]. Pertaining to or exhibiting asymmetry.

a"sym·met'ric at'om. One which has each of its valence bonds satisfied by a different atom or radical; of special significance in respect to carbon and nitrogen atoms.

a·sym'me·try (ay·sim'i·tree, a·sim'·) [*a-; symmetria*]. 1. *In anatomy* and *biology,* lack of similarity or correspondence of the organs and parts on each side of an organism. 2. *In chemistry,* absence of symmetry in the arrangement of the atoms and radicals within a molecule. —**asymmet'ric, asymmet'rical,** *adj.*

a·sym'phy·tous [G. *asymphytos,* not growing together]. Distinct; not grown together.

a″symp·to·mat′ic (ay″simp·to·mat′ick, a·simp″-to·) [G. *a-*, not; *symptōmatikos*, from *symptōma*, symptom]. Symptomless; exhibiting no symptoms.

as″ymp·tot′ic [*a-;* G. *symptōsis*, a collapsing]. Of or pertaining to a straight line which an indefinitely extended curve continually approaches as a limit. Also see asymptotic *wish fulfilment.*

a·syn′chro·nism (ay·sing′kro·niz·um, a·sing′·) [*a-;* G. *sygchronismos*, agreement of time]. Absence of synchronism; disturbed coordination.

a·syn′cli·tism (ay·sing′kli·tiz·um, a·sing′·) [*a-;* G. *syn*, with; *klisis*, inclination]. An oblique presentation of the fetal head at superior strait of pelvis.
anterior a. Biparietal obliquity; the lateral inclination of the fetal head at the superior pelvic strait, which brings the sagittal suture nearer to the sacral promontory. Also called *Naegele's obliquity.*
posterior a. The lateral inclination of the fetal head at the superior pelvic strait which brings the sagittal suture toward the symphysis pubis while the posterior parietal bone occupies most of the superior strait: also called *Litzmann's obliquity.*

a·syn′de·sis [*a-;* G. *syndein*, to bind together]. Incoherency in syntax or sentence construction. —**asyndet′ic,** *adj.*

a″syn·ech′i·a (ay″si·neck′ee·uh, ·nee′kee·uh, a·si·, a·sin″i·kigh′uh) [*a-;* G. *synecheia*, from *synechein*, to hold together]. Absence of continuity in structure.

a·syn′er·gy, as″y·ner′gi·a [*a-;* G. *synergia*, cooperation]. Faulty coordination of groups of organs or muscles normally acting in unison; particularly, the abnormal state of muscle antagonism in cerebellar disease. Syn., *dyssynergy.* —**asyner′gic,** *adj.*
appendicular a. Asynergy of the limbs.
axial a. Asynergy of the axial musculature and muscles of the trunk. Syn., *trunkal a.*, *trunk ataxia.*
progressive cerebellar a. See cerebellofugal *degeneration.*
progressive locomotor a. See *tabes* dorsalis.
trunkal a. See axial *a.*
verbal a. Defective coordination of speech, as in aphasia, and in the scanning speech of multiple sclerosis.
vocal a. Faulty coordination of the muscles of the larynx, due to chorea.

a″syn·e′si·a [G., want of understanding]. Stupidity; loss or disorder of mental power. —**asynet′ic,** *adj.*

as″y·no′di·a [G. *a-*, not; *synodia*, a journey in company]. Sexual impotence.

a″syn·tax′i·a dor·sa′lis (ay″sin·tack′shuh, ·tack′-see·uh, a·sin·). Failure of the neural tube to close.

a·sys″tem·at′ic (ay·sis″ti·mat′ick, a·sis″·) [*a-;* G. *systēmatikos*, from *systēma*, system]. Diffuse; not restricted to any one of several systems of nerve fibers; applied to nervous diseases that are general.

a″sys·to′li·a (ay″sis·to′lee·uh, a·sis·), **a·sys′to·le** (ay·sis′to·lee, a·sis′·) [*a-;* G. *systolē*, contraction]. Faulty or imperfect contraction of the cardiac ventricles, especially of the right ventricle, as seen in the last stages of mitral disease. —**asystol′ic,** *adj.*
cardiataxic a. Temporary asystolia due to rapid heart rate.
cardioplegic a. That resulting from weakness or injury of the heart muscle.

A.T. 10 (*anti-tetany*). A preparation of dihydrotachysterol used in the treatment of parathyroid tetany.

A t *In electrocardiography*, symbol for the mean manifest magnitude of repolarization of the myocardium determined algebraically and measured in microvolt seconds.

At Chemical symbol for astatine.

atabrine dihydrochloride. Trade-mark for a brand of quinacrine hydrochloride. Also called *atabrine.*

at″a·bri·no·der′ma. Atabrine dermatitis.

a·tac′tic [G. *ataktos*, irregular]. Irregular; incoordinate. Pertaining to muscular incoordination, especially in aphasia; ataxic.

a·tac′ti·form [*ataktos;* L. *forma*, form]. Ataxialike; mildly ataxic.

a″tac·til′i·a (ay″tack·til′ee·uh, a·tack·) [G. *a-*, not; L. *tactilis*, from *tangere*, to touch]. Loss of tactile sense.

a·tav′i·cus [L. *atavus*, ancestor]. Not resembling either parent, but similar to a grandparent.

at′a·vism [*atavus*]. The reappearance of remote ancestral characteristics in an individual. Syn., *reversion.* —**atav′ic, atavis′tic,** *adj.*

a·tax″a·pha′si·a (a·tack″suh·fay′zhuh, ·zee·uh) [G. *ataxia*, disorder; *aphasia*, speechlessness]. Inability to arrange words into sentences.

a·tax′i·a [G.]. Incoordination of muscular action. —**ataxic,** *adj.*
acute a. That developing after a severe acute infection, presumably due to selective toxic effect on the spinocerebellar tracts: also called *Leyden's a.*, *Leyden-Westphal a.*
a. cordis. See *fibrillation.*
bulbar a. That due to a lesion in the pons or medulla oblongata.
cerebellar a. That due to disease of the cerebellum of the brain.
cerebellofugal degeneration a. Ataxia as the main manifestation of cerebellofugal degeneration.
diphtheritic a. A sequel of diphtheria preceding diphtheritic paralysis, in which the chief phenomena of tabes dorsalis are present.
Friedreich's a. A progressive, familial disease occurring in childhood and characterized by ataxia, absent deep reflexes, positive Babinski sign, speech disturbance, nystagmus, and clubfoot. The specific lesions are degenerations of lateral and posterior columns of the spinal cord and to some extent in the cerebellum and medulla.
hereditary cerebellar a. Inherited ataxia similar to Friedreich's ataxia but characterized by later onset (20–45 years), optic atrophy, incoordination of arms, legs, and trunk, speech disorders, and often mental deterioration. In contrast to Friedreich's ataxia, there may be hyperreflexia but no sensory disturbances and clubfoot. Also called *Marie's a.*, *Nonne-Marie's syndrome.*
hereditary spinal a. See Friedreich's *a.*
hysterical a. See *astasia-abasia.*
locomotor a. Tabes dorsalis.
Marie's a. See hereditary cerebellar *a.*
moral a. The inconstancy of ideas and will, attended with convulsions and pain, observed in hysterical subjects.
motor a. Inability to coordinate the muscles in walking.
spinal a. That due to disease of the spinal cord.
static a. Lack of muscular coordination in standing still, or in fixed positions of the limbs.
tabetic a. See *tabes dorsalis.*
thermal a. Large and irregular fluctuations of the body temperature.
trunk a. See axial *asynergy.*
vasomotor a. Instability of the circulatory mechanism, due to lack of coordination between the sympathetic and the parasympathetic nervous systems in relation to the vasomotor phenomena.

a·tax′i·a·graph″ [*ataxia;* G. *graphein*, to write]. A device for recording the degree of ataxia.

a·tax″i·o·pho′bi·a [*ataxia;* G. *phobos*, fear]. A morbid fear of disorder.

a·tax″o·phe′mi·a [*ataxia;* G. *phēmē,* speech]. Incoherence; faulty coordination of words.

ATCC American Type Culture Collection.

at′e·brin. See *atabrine dihydrochloride.*

at″e·lec′ta·sis [G. *atelēs,* imperfect; *ektasis,* extension]. Collapsed or airless state of all or part of a lung: also called *apneumatosis.* —**atelectat′ic,** *adj.*

acquired a. Obstructive or compression *a.*

a. of newborn. Imperfect expansion of the lungs at birth and for the first few days of life. Syn., *congenital a.*

compression a. Collapse of part or all of a lung due to pressure by extrinsic factors, as pleural effusion or the elevation of the diaphragm.

congenital a. *A.* of newborn.

lobular a. Airlessness in a group of lung lobules; patchy *a.*

massive a. See massive *collapse.*

obstructive a. Atelectasis caused by occlusion of a bronchus during inspiration by intrinsic factors, such as a tumor or mucous plug, with subsequent absorption of the trapped air and collapse of the alveoli.

patchy a. See lobular *a.*

a·tel″en·ce·pha′li·a, a·tel″en·ceph′a·ly, at″e·lo·en″ce·pha′li·a [*atelēs;* G. *egkephalos,* brain]. Imperfect development of the brain.

a·te″li·o′sis (a·tee″lee·o′sis, a·tel″ee·, a·tee″lye·o′·sis), **a·te″lei·o′sis** (a·tee″lye·o′sis) [G. *ateleia,* incompleteness; *-ōsis,* condition]. Infantilism or dwarfism; a generalized type of underdevelopment characterized by a childish face, thin voice, slender limbs, and normal intelligence. All parts are proportionately smaller, giving the impression of an adult in miniature, as differentiated from cretinism or achondroplastic dwarfs, where disproportion is the rule. —**ateliot′ic, ateleiot′ic, ate′lic,** *adj.*

at′el·o-, atel- [G. *atelēs,* imperfect]. Combining form signifying *imperfect* or *incomplete development.*

at″e·lo·car′di·a [*atelēs;* G. *kardia,* heart]. An imperfect or undeveloped state of the heart.

at″e·lo·ceph′a·lous [*atelēs;* G. *kephalē,* head]. Having the skull or head more or less imperfectly developed.

at″e·lo·chei′li·a (at″i·lo·kigh′lee·uh) [*atelēs;* G. *cheilos,* lip]. Defective development of the lip.

at″e·lo·chei′ri·a (·kigh′ree·uh) [*atelēs;* G. *cheir,* hand]. Defective development of the hand.

at″e·lo·en″ce·pha′li·a. See *atelencephalia.*

at″e·lo·glos′si·a [*atelēs;* G. *glōssa,* tongue]. Congenital defect in the tongue.

at″e·log·nath′i·a (at″i·log·nath′ee·uh, ·nayth′·ee·uh) [*atelēs;* G. *gnathos,* jaw]. Imperfect development of a jaw, especially of the lower jaw.

at″e·lo·mit′ic [*atelēs;* G. *mitos,* thread]. Nonterminal; applied to the spindle-fiber attachment of chromosomes.

at″e·lo·my·e′li·a (at″i·lo·migh·ee′lee·uh) [*atelēs;* G. *myelos,* marrow]. Congenital defect of spinal cord.

at″e·lo·po′di·a [*atelēs;* G. *pous,* foot]. Defective development of the foot.

at″e·lo·pro·so′pi·a [*atelēs;* G. *prosōpon,* face]. Incomplete facial development.

at″e·lo·ra·chid′i·a, at″e·lor·rha·chid′i·a (·ra·kid′ee·uh) [*atelēs;* G. *rhachis,* spine]. Imperfect development of the spinal column, as in spina bifida.

at″e·lo·sto′mi·a [*atelēs;* G. *stoma,* mouth]. Incomplete development of the mouth.

atepe. An antimalarial consisting of quinacrine hydrochloride and pamaquine naphthate in the ratio of 1:20.

at″e·pho′bi·a [G. *atē,* ruin; *phobos,* fear]. Morbid fear of ruin.

a·the′li·a [G. *a-,* not; *thēlē,* nipple]. Absence of the nipples.

ath″er·o·gen′e·sis. Production of fatty degeneration in arteries. —**atherogen′ic,** *adj.*

ath″er·o′ma [G. *athērē,* porridge; *-ōma,* tumor]. 1. A sebaceous cyst; steatoma. 2. The fatty degeneration and infiltration by lipids of the walls of the arteries in arteriosclerosis. —**atherom′atous,** *adj.*

capillary a. The formation of fatty granules in the walls of the capillaries.

ath″er·o″ma·to′sis [*athērē; -ōma;* G. *-ōsis,* condition]. Generalized atheromatous condition of the arteries.

ath″er·o″scle·ro′sis [*athērē;* G. *sklērōsis,* a hardening]. A form of simple intimal arteriosclerosis with atheromatous deposits within and beneath the intima. —**atherosclerogen′ic,** *adj.*

ath″e·to′sis [G. *athetos,* without position; *-ōsis,* condition]. A condition chiefly affecting children, characterized by recurrent, slow, and continual change of position of the fingers, toes, hands, feet, and other parts of the body, usually the result of a central brain lesion. Also called *Hammond's disease, posthemiplegic chorea.* —**ath′etoid, athetosic, athetot′ic,** *adj.*

double a. Bilateral congenital athetosis, usually nonprogressive, in which the face and neck muscles and those of all four extremities are involved; speech is distorted: also called *infantile spasmodic paraplegia, Vogt syndrome.*

pupillary a. Hippus.

a·thi″a·min·o′sis. See *beriberi.*

ath′lete's foot. See *dermatophytosis.*

a·threp′si·a. See *marasmus.*

a·thy′mic (ay·thy′mick, ath·im′ick) [G. *a-,* not; *thymos,* mind]. Without feeling, as an athymic psychopath.

a·thy·re·o′sis, a·thy·ro′sis. The condition associated with absence of secretion of thyroid hormone. If it occurs in infants, cretinism results; in older children or adults, myxedema. Syn., *athyrea, athyroidism.*

at·lan′to- [G. *atlas,* first of the neck vertebrae, from the Greek giant, *Atlas,* who supported the world on his shoulders]. A combining form signifying *relation to the atlas.*

at·lan″to·ax′i·al [*atlas;* L. *axis,* axis]. Pertaining to the atlas and the axis or epistropheus; applied to the joints between these two vertebrae and the ligaments which join them. Syn., *atlantoepistrophic.*

at·lan″to·bas·i·lar′is in·ter′nus. A rare variant of the longus capitis muscle arising from the anterior tubercle of the atlas and inserted into the basilar part of the occipital bone.

at·lan″to·ep″i·stroph′ic [*atlas;* G. *epistropheus,* turning on a pivot]. Pertaining to the atlas and the epistropheus or axis; applied to the joints between these two vertebrae and the ligaments joining them. Syn., *atlantoaxial.* See Table of Joints and Ligaments in the Appendix.

at·lan″to-oc·cip′i·tal (·ock·sip′i·tul) [*atlas;* L. *occiput,* back part of the head]. Pertaining to the atlas and the occipital bone; applied to the joints between these two bones and the ligaments joining them. See Table of Joints and Ligaments in the Appendix.

at′las [G.]. The first cervical vertebra. It articulates with the occipital bone of the skull and with the axis. See Table of Bones in the Appendix.

at′las as·sim″i·la′tion. See *platybasia.*

Atlee, Washington Lemuel [*American physician,* 1808–78]. One of the first to study surgical removal of uterine fibroids. With his brother, **John Light Atlee** (1799–1885), established the operation of ovariotomy.

at″lo·ax′oid. Atlantoaxial.

at·lod′y·mus, at″lo·did′y·mus [*atlas;* G. *didymos,*

twin]. A monster with two heads on one neck and a single body. Syn., *dicephalus monauchenos*.

atmo-, atm- [G. *atmos*, steam]. A combining form denoting *steam* or *vapor*.

at·mol'y·sis [*atmos;* G. *lysis*, a loosing]. A method of separating mixed gases or vapors by means of diffusion through a porous substance.

at·mom'e·ter [*atmos;* G. *metron*, a measure]. An instrument which measures the amount of water evaporated from a given surface in a given time, to determine the humidity of the atmosphere.

at'mos·phere [*atmos;* G. *sphaira*, sphere]. 1. Layer of air surrounding the earth to a height of approximately 200 miles. 2. A unit of pressure: the amount of pressure exerted by the air on one square inch of surface at sea level—about 15 lb. *In physics*, one atmosphere is equivalent to the pressure of a column of mercury 760 mm. high, at sea level and 0° C. 3. Climatic conditions of a locality. 4. *In chemistry*, gaseous medium surrounding a body. —**atmospher'ic,** *adj.*

at"mos·pher'ic blast. Blast injury.

a·to'ci·a (a·to'shee·uh, ·see·uh) [G. *atokia*, barrenness]. Sterility of the female.

at'om [G. *atomos*, uncut, indivisible]. The smallest particle of an element capable of existing individually or in combination with one or more atoms of the same or another element. It consists of a relatively heavy inner core, or nucleus, with a positive electric charge, and a number of lighter planetary particles, with negative charges, revolving or vibrating continuously around the nucleus in a vast empty space. The positive heavy particles in the nucleus are called *protons*, and the orbital particles are called *electrons*. The number of protons or of electrons in an electrically neutral atom is given by its *atomic number*. In addition to protons, the nucleus also contains *neutrons*, which are neutral particles resulting from the combination of a proton and an electron. The sum of protons and neutrons in the nucleus is called the mass number of the atom, or its mass or atomic weight. All atoms are constructed of these three fundamental building stones. —**atom'ic,** *adj.*

recoil a. The remainder of an atom still in motion after emission of an alpha particle, a beta particle, or a neutron.

a·tom'ic dis·in"te·gra'tion. The disintegration of atoms, either naturally, as in natural radioactivity, or artificially, as by the bombardment of atomic nuclei with protons, deuterons, alpha particles, neutrons, or photons, whereby new atoms are formed and more or less energy is liberated. Practically all elements have been disintegrated by artificial means. Generally the product differs only slightly from the original, but some atoms, as uranium of atomic weight 235, undergo fission into two atoms of approximately equal weight with release of much energy. See *isotope*.

at"o·mic'i·ty (at"o·miss'i·tee) [*atomos*]. Chemical valence.

a·tom'ic pile re·ac'tor. See *nuclear reactor*.

at"om·i·za'tion [*atomos*]. Mechanical process of breaking up a liquid into a fine spray. —**at'·omizer,** *n.*

a·to'ni·a, at'o·ny [G. *a-*, not; *tonos*, tone]. Abnormally low degree of tonus; absence of tonus. —**aton'ic,** *adj.;* **atonic'ity,** *n.*

a. of bladder. Inability to expel the urine, due to deficient muscular power.

at'o·pen [G. *atopos*, from *a-*, *topos*, place]. An antigen or allergen, usually inhaled or ingested, which produces an atopic disease.

atophan. Trade-mark identifying the original cinchophen.

a·top'ic (ay·top'ick, a·top'ick) [*atopos*]. 1. Pertaining to atopy or to an atopen. 2. Old term for ectopic.

a·top"og·no'si·a, a·top"og·no'sis [*atopos;* G. *gnōsis*, knowledge]. Lack of ability to locate a sensation accurately.

at'o·py. A peculiar form of allergy marked by a familial tendency to certain hypersensitivities, as hay fever, asthma, atopic dermatitis; an immediate vascularization and exudation of the sensitive tissue when exposed to the stimulant; and the presence of certain antibodies, called atopic reagins. Syn., *atopic hypersensitivity.*

a·tox'ic (ay·tock'sick, a·tock'sick) [G. *a-*, not; *toxikon*, poison]. Not venomous; not poisonous.

a·tox'yl (a·tock'sil, ay·tock'·). $C_6H_4NH_2.AsO.OH.$-$ONa.3H_2O$. Sodium arsanilate. A white, odorless, crystalline powder; formerly used in the treatment of syphilis, psoriasis, and trypanosomiasis. It may cause blindness.

ATP Adenosine triphosphate.

ATPase Adenosine triphosphatase.

a"tra·che'li·a (ay"tra·kee'lee·uh, a·tra·) [G. *atrachēlos*, from *a-; trachelos*, neck]. The condition of having little or no neck. —**atrach'elous,** *adj.*

a·trach"e·lo·ceph'a·lus (a·track"i·lo·sef'uh·lus) [*atrachēlos;* G. *kephalē*, head]. A monster with head and neck absent or poorly developed.

A'trax. A genus of Australian poisonous spiders related to the American tarantulas. They are similar to the black widow in effect; and treatment for their sting is similar.

a·tre'mi·a [G. *a-*, not; *tremein*, to tremble]. Hysterical inability to walk, stand, or sit without general discomfort and paresthesia of the head and back, all movements being readily executed without tremor in the recumbent posture. Also called *Neftel's disease*.

a·tre'si·a (a·tree'zhuh, ·zee·uh, ·shuh, ·see·uh) [*a-;* G. *trēsis*, perforation]. Imperforation or closure of a normal opening or canal, as of the anus, vagina, auditory meatus, or pupil. —**atresic, atret'ic,** *adj.*

aortic a. Defective development of the aortic orifice with coexisting patent ductus arteriosus: an extremely rare malformation in which the left ventricle may be absent or very poorly developed.

a. ani vaginalis. An anomaly in which there is imperforate anus, the rectum opening into the vagina. Also called *anus vaginalis*.

a. folliculi. The blighting of an ovarian follicle with degeneration of the ovum before maturation. The atresic follicle is characterized by a small cystic space, lined with thinned follicle cells, which subsequently progresses to complete obliteration.

a. of iter. See aqueduct *stenosis*.

tricuspid a. Failure in development of tricuspid valve, with diminutive right ventricle, and interatrial septal defect or patent foramen ovale.

a·tre'to- [G. *atrētos*, not perforated, from *a-*, *tetrainein*, to perforate]. A combining form meaning *imperforation; absence* or *closure of a passage*.

a·tre"to·ceph'a·lus [*atrētos;* G. *kephalē*, head]. A monster with imperforate nostrils or mouth.

a·tre"to·cor'mus [*atrētos;* G. *kormos*, trunk]. A monster having one or more of the body openings imperforate.

a·tre"to·cys'ti·a [*atrētos;* G. *kystis*, bladder]. Atresia of the urinary bladder.

a·tre"to·gas'tri·a [*atrētos;* G. *gastēr*, stomach]. Imperforation of the cardiac or pyloric orifice of the stomach.

a·tre"to·le'mi·a [*atrētos;* G. *laimos*, gullet]. Imperforation of the esophagus or pharynx.

a·tre"to·me'tri·a [*atrētos;* G. *mētra*, womb]. Atresia of the uterus.

at″re·top′si·a [*atrētos;* G. *opsis,* vision]. Imperforation of the pupil. Also called *membrana pupillaris persistens.*

a·tret″or·rhin′i·a [*atrētos;* G. *rhis,* nose]. Nasal atresia.

a·tre″to·sto′mi·a [*atrētos;* G. *stoma,* mouth]. Imperforation of the mouth.

a·tret″u·re′thri·a [*atrētos;* G. *ourēthra,* urethra]. Imperforate urethra.

a′tri·a. Plural of atrium.

at″ri·cho′sis (at″ri·ko′sis), **a·trich′i·a** (a·trick′-ee·uh) [G. *a-*, not; *thrix,* hair]. A condition characterized by absence of hair.

a. congenitalis. The congenital absence of hair.

at′ri·chous (at′ri·kus) [*a-; thrix*]. Denoting bacteria having no flagella.

at′ri·nal. $C_{17}H_{23}O_6NS$, atropinesulfuric acid; the sulfuric acid ester of atropine; occurs as white crystals; sparingly soluble in water; insoluble in alcohol. Its action is similar to that of atropine.

a′tri·o- [L. *atrium,* atrium]. A combining form denoting *atrium* or *atrial.*

a″tri·o·sep″to·pex′y [*atrium;* L. *saeptum,* partition; G. *pexis,* fixation]. Operation on the atrial septum of the heart for closure of defect.

a″tri·o·ven·tric′u·lar [*atrium;* L. *ventriculus,* ventricle]. Relating to the atria and the ventricles of the heart. Abbreviated **AV, A. V.**

a″tri·o·ven·tric″u·lar′is com′mu·nis. A malformation of the heart in which the atrial and ventricular septa have failed to fuse, leaving a free communication between all four chambers. The mitral and tricuspid leaflets are fused to form a single atrioventricular valve.

a′tri·um (pl. *atria*) [L.]. 1. The first chamber of the heart, which receives the blood from the veins. 2. The part of the tympanic cavity of the ear below the head of the malleus. *O.T.* 3. The end of an alveolar duct. See Plate 5. —**atrial,** *adj.*

a. cordis. An atrium of the heart.

a. cordis dextrum. Right atrium of the heart.

a. cordis sinistrum. Left atrium of the heart.

a. vaginae. The vestibule of the vulva.

infection a. The point of entrance of the bacteria in an infectious disease.

primitive a. The embryonic unpaired chamber of the heart between the sinus venosus and the primitive ventricle which becomes the adult atria. See *sinus venosus.*

At′ro·pa [G. *Atropos,* one of the Fates]. A genus of the Solanaceae; source of belladonna and atropine.

a·tro′phi·a ma·cu·lo′sa et stri·a′ta. See *atrophoderma* maculatum.

at″ro·pho·der′ma [G. *atrophia,* want of food, atrophy; *derma,* skin]. Atrophy of the skin.

a. albidum. A stockinglike type of atrophy affecting the extremities; usually starts in childhood and involves the lower limbs.

a. maculatum. 1. Primary macular atrophy of the skin, characterized by the formation of a macule which gradually disappears leaving a shiny white depressed spot. 2. Macular atrophy of the skin due to syphilis: also called *atrophia maculosa et striata.*

a. neuriticum. Glossy skin.

a. pigmentosum. Xeroderma pigmentosum.

a. reticulatum. See *folliculitis ulerythematosa reticulata.*

a. vermicularis. See *folliculitis ulerythematosa reticulata.*

at″ro·pho·der″ma·to′sis [*atrophia; derma;* G. *-ōsis,* condition]. A class of skin diseases characterized by atrophy of the cutis.

at′ro·phy [*atrophia*]. A reduction in size of an organ or cell which had previously reached mature size; hypoplastic organs may exhibit atrophy. It may be physiologic or pathologic, the latter type being accompanied by some degree of degeneration. —**atrophied, atroph′ic,** *adj.*

acute yellow a. See postnecrotic *cirrhosis.*

brown a. A form in which the atrophic organ is of a deeper brown than normal because of an increase of pigment (hemosiderin and hemofuscin); observed in the heart, skeletal muscles, and liver.

cardiac a. Atrophy of the heart observed especially in chronic, wasting diseases.

chronic spinal muscular a. See progressive muscular *dystrophy.*

circumscribed cerebral a. Atrophy and gliosis of cerebral tissue in parts of the frontal, temporal, or parietal lobe, or in combination, resulting in aphasia and progressive dementia: also called *convolutional cerebral a., Pick's disease* (for Arnold Pick). See also lobar *sclerosis.*

compression a. See pressure *a.*

concentric a. That which proceeds from without inward, as atrophy of bone beginning in the periosteal portion.

convolutional cerebral a. See circumscribed cerebral *a.*

correlated a. Atrophy secondary to the removal or destruction of other parts of the body, as atrophy of bone and muscle following amputation of an extremity.

cyanotic a. Atrophy of the liver accompanying prolonged passive hyperemia, largely degenerative.

degenerative a. A form in which cellular degeneration is conspicuous.

disuse a. That form resulting from inactivity, usually affecting glandular or muscular structures. Also called *inactivity a.*

eccentric a. That which proceeds from within outward, as atrophy of bone beginning next to the marrow cavity.

exhaustion a. That of an endocrine gland, presumably due to prolonged excessive stimulation.

facioscapulohumeral a. A hereditary progressive muscular dystrophy that usually begins early in life and affects the muscles of the face, shoulder girdle, and arm, but not of the forearm. The sacrospinalis may also be involved. Also called *facioscapulohumeral dystrophy, Landouzy-Dejerine a.*

gray a. Degeneration in the optic disk with assumption of a gray color.

gyrate a. of choroid and retina. A patchy destruction of the choroid and retina in which irregular patches of white sclera are visible on fundiscopic examination.

halisteretic a. Old term for atrophy of bone, or osteoporosis, thought to be due to a withdrawal of mineral salts from the bone.

hydronephrotic a. Loss of kidney substance secondary to formation of hydronephrosis.

inanition a. That due to inadequate nutrition.

infantile spinal muscular a. A disease of very young children characterized by extensive muscular atrophy as a result of degenerative changes in the anterior horn cells of the spinal cord. Death occurs within a year.

Kienböck's a. See Robert *Kienböck.*

Landouzy-Dejerine a. See facioscapulohumeral *a.*

Leber's optic a. A rare hereditary form of axial neuritis of the optic nerve.

linear a. Atrophy of the papillary layer of skin, resulting in striae atrophicae.

lobar a. See lobar *sclerosis.* See also circumscribed cerebral *a.*

macular a. See *anetoderma.*

muscular a. That in which muscle becomes atrophic, especially skeletal muscle; may be hereditary or acquired, idiopathic, myelopathic, myopathic, neuropathic, primary, secondary, simple, or progressive; often a part of a disease, such as progressive muscular atrophy, myasthenia gravis, and various forms of myotonia.
myelopathic muscular a. See progressive spinal muscular *a.*
myotonic a. A hereditary, progressive weakening and atrophy of muscles; usually begins in early life. Syn., *dystrophia myotonica.*
necrobiotic a. Atrophy resulting from slow disintegration and loss of cells by necrobiosis.
neuritic muscular a. See progressive neuropathic (peroneal) muscular *a.*
neurotrophic a. A form particularly observed in muscle as the result of interruption of motor nerve supply; due partly to inactivity and partly to absence of nutritional influences.
numerical a. Reduction in the number of cells of an organ; necrobiotic atrophy.
olivopontocerebellar a. A heredodegenerative disease occurring in the later decades of life; causes ataxia, hypotonia, and dysarthria.
olivorubrocerebellar a. A heredodegenerative disease involving the postural centers of the brain stem, particularly the superior cerebellar peduncle; causes ataxia, coarse tremor, and hypotonia.
optic a. Atrophy of the optic nerve.
overwork a. A type which follows hypertrophy and is due to excessive use of the part. It is often occupational, being seen, for example, in musicians, typists, and blacksmiths.
pathologic a. That due to disease or other abnormality.
periodontal a. Progressive resorption of alveolar bone with gingival recession and loss of the corresponding part of the periodontal membrane.
peroneal muscular a. See progressive neuropathic (peroneal) muscular *a.*
physiologic a. That which affects certain organs at different times of life, as atrophy of the thymus at puberty, atrophy of the mammary glands and ovaries after the menopause.
pressure a. That following prolonged pressure on a part, chiefly the result of local inanition.
progressive nervous a. Atrophy of spinal nerve roots due to pressure from fibrosis of the spinal arachnoid.
progressive neuropathic (peroneal) muscular a. A form of muscular atrophy due to degeneration of the cells of the posterior columns of the spinal cord and of the peripheral motor nerves. It begins in the muscles supplied by the peroneal nerves, progressing slowly to involve the muscles of the hands and arms. Also called *peroneal muscular a., Charcot-Marie-Tooth disease, progressive neural muscular a.*
progressive spinal muscular a. A chronic disease characterized by progressive wasting of individual muscles, or physiologic groups of muscles, and by an associated and proportional amount of paralysis; due to a degeneration and atrophy of the multipolar cells in the anterior gray horns of the spinal cord, with consecutive degeneration of the anterior nerve roots and muscles. Syn., *chronic anterior poliomyelitis, Cruveilhier's disease, Duchenne-Aran muscular a., myelopathic muscular a., wasting palsy.*
progressive unilateral facial a. Slowly progressive atrophy of skin, subcutaneous tissue, bone, and, less often, of the muscles of one side of the face.
red a. See cyanotic *a.*
senile a. That which occurs in old age.
serous a. Atrophy of fat associated with accumulation of serous fluid.
subacute yellow a. See postnecrotic *cirrhosis.*
Sudeck's a. Aseptic necrosis of bone following injury, described by Paul Herman Martin *Sudeck.*
sympathetic a. Rarely observed in one member of paired organs secondary to atrophy of its fellow.
syphilitic primary optic a. A condition involving pupillary abnormalities, which accompanies neurosyphilis. It occurs a number of years after infection, and is found predominantly in males.
syphilitic spinal muscular a. Progressive spinal muscular atrophy due to destruction of the anterior horn cells of the spinal cord by syphilis.
toxic a. Atrophy which appears in the course of prolonged wasting and infectious diseases, due probably to malnutrition rather than toxins.
trophoneurotic a. See neurotrophic *a.*
Wucher a. Fat replacement atrophy resulting from inflammatory infiltration into the subcutaneous tissue. This leads to degenerative or destructive changes of the fat cells.

at'ro·pic ac'id. See under *acid.*

at'ro·pine (at'ro·peen, ·pin) [G. *Atropos*, one of the Fates]. $C_{17}H_{23}O_3N$. A white, crystalline alkaloid obtained from *Atropa belladonna* and other solanaceous plants. It is soluble in alcohol and but sparingly soluble in water. It causes paralysis of all responses to parasympathetic stimulation, resulting in mydriasis, cycloplegia, suppression of sweat, tears, and mucus; quickening of the heart, and relaxation of the smooth muscles of the intestines, and bronchi, etc. Toxic doses cause motor restlessness, excitement, delirium, and coma. It is an antidote for morphine, pilocarpine, and hydrocyanic acid. Internally, it is used in treating acute attacks of bronchial asthma, intestinal and biliary colic, and pylorospasm; in cathartic pills; and in hypersecretion, especially of sweat. Topically, it is used extensively in ophthalmology for dilating the pupil and treating various eye conditions.
a. hydrobromide. $C_{17}H_{23}O_3N.HBr$. A white, crystalline powder, soluble in water or alcohol.
a. hydrochloride. $C_{17}H_{23}O_3N.HCl$. A white, crystalline powder, soluble in water or alcohol.
a. methylbromide. Methylatropine bromide. $C_{16}H_{20}O_3N(CH_3)_2Br$. Occurs as white crystals soluble in water or alcohol; used as is atropine. Dose, 1–3 mg. ($\frac{1}{60}$–$\frac{1}{20}$ gr.).
a. methylnitrate. Methylatropine nitrate. $C_{16}H_{20}O_3N(CH_3)_2NO_3$. Occurs as a white, crystalline powder, soluble in water or alcohol. Its action is essentially like that of atropine. Dose, 1–3 mg. ($\frac{1}{60}$–$\frac{1}{20}$ gr.). See *eumydrin.*
a. sulfate (*atropinae sulfas*). $(C_{17}H_{23}O_3N)_2.H_2SO_4.H_2O$. The most frequently used salt of atropine. A white, crystalline powder, soluble in 0.5 part of water, 5 parts of alcohol, or 2.5 parts of glycerin. Dose, 0.3–1.2 mg. ($\frac{1}{200}$–$\frac{1}{50}$ gr.).

at"ro·pine·sul·fu'ric ac'id. See *atrinal.*

at'ro·pin·ize [*Atropos*]. 1. Bring under the influence of, or treat with, atropine. 2. Administer belladonna or atropine until physiologic effects become manifest. —**atropiniza'tion,** *n.*

at'ro·scine (at'ro·seen, ·sin). $C_{17}H_{21}O_4N.H_2O$. *dl*-Scopolamine. An optically inert alkaloid prepared from several species of the Solanaceae. Used as mydriatic in 0.2–0.5% solution in oil.
a. hydrobromide. An atroscine salt, soluble in water and used in 1% solution as mydriatic.

A. T. S. Antitetanic serum; anxiety tension state; American Temperance Society.

at'tar [Per. *'aṭar*, from Ar. *'iṭr*, perfume]. A general name for any of the fragrant volatile oils.

at·ten′tion [L. *attentio*, from *attendere*, to direct the attention]. An act of consciousness directed toward external or internal stimuli; the application of intellectual energy in awareness and alertness.

at·ten″u·a′tion [L. *attenuare*, to weaken]. A thinning, weakening, or diluting; especially a reduction of the virulence of a virus or pathogenic microorganism, as by successive culture, repeated inoculation, or exposure to light, heat, air, or a weakening agent. —**atten′uant,** *adj., n.;* **atten′uate,** *v.t., v.i.;* **atten′uated,** *adj.*

at′tic [F. *attique*, G. *Attikos*]. Part of the tympanic cavity situated above the atrium. It contains the incus and the head of the malleus. Syn., *epitympanic recess.*

at′tic dis·ease′. Chronic suppurative inflammation of the attic of the tympanic cavity.

at″ti·co·an·trot′o·my [*Attikos;* G. *antron*, cave; *tomē*, a cutting]. Opening of the attic and mastoid air cells.

at″ti·co·mas′toid [*Attikos;* G. *mastoeidēs*, like a breast]. Relating to the attic and the mastoid.

at″ti·cot′o·my [*Attikos;* G. *tomē*, a cutting]. Surgical incision of the attic.

at′ti·tude [F., from L. *aptus*, suited]. Posture; the position of the body and limbs.

a. of fetus. Relation of the fetal members to one another *in utero.*

crucifixion a. In hysteroepilepsy, a rigid state of the body, the arms stretched out at right angles.

discobolus a. A position of the body assumed as a result of stimulation of one labyrinth. The trunk, head, and arms are turned toward the side stimulated in order to counteract the false sensation of falling in the opposite direction.

frozen a. A peculiar stiffness of the gait characteristic of disease of the spinal cord, especially of amyotrophic lateral sclerosis.

passionate a. Assumption of a dramatic or theatrical expression, a position assumed by some hysterical patients.

at′to·lens au′rem. Old name for the auricularis superior muscle.

at·ton′i·ty [L. *attonitus*, stunned]. A state of stupor with complete or partial immobility; occurs most frequently in the catatonic form of schizophrenia but also in some forms of melancholia.

at·trac′tion [L. *attractus*, from *attrahere*, to draw to]. The force exerted by one mass upon another, drawing them together. Syn., *gravitation, affinity, cohesion.*

capillary a. The force which draws fluids into and along the lumen of a capillary tube.

chemical a. The force which unites the atoms of one element to those of others, forming compounds. See *affinity.*

electric a. The tendency of bodies to draw together when carrying opposite charges of electricity. Also called *magnetic a.*

at′tra·hens au′rem. Old name for the auricularis anterior muscle.

at·tri′tion (a·trish′un) [L. *attritus*, from *atterere*, to rub against]. An abrasion, rubbing, or chafing of the skin or any surface; thus the wearing away of tooth enamel by mastication, brushing, or clasp friction is called attrition of enamel.

at. wt. Atomic weight.

a·typ′i·cal. Not typical; irregular. For **primary a. pneumonia,** see under *pneumonia.*

A.U., Å.U. Angstrom unit.

A.u., Å.u. Abbreviation for angstrom unit.

a.u., å.u. Abbreviation for angstrom unit.

Au Chemical symbol for gold.

Aubert, Hermann [*German physiologist*, 1826–92]. His name is associated with the optical illusion in which a vertical line inclines to one side as the head is inclined to the opposite side.

Auch″me·ro·my′ia (awk″mi·ro·my′uh) [G. *auchmēros*, dirty; *myia*, fly]. A genus of Diptera found in Africa.

A. luteola. A species whose larvae (Congo floor maggots) feed on blood and cause myiasis.

au″di·mu′tism [L. *audire*, to hear; *mutus*, mute]. Muteness not associated with deafness.

au′di·o-, au′di·to- [*audire*]. A combining form denoting *pertaining to hearing.*

au″di·o·ep″i·lep′tic sei′zure. See reflex *epilepsy.*

au″di·o·gen′ic [*audire;* G. *genesthai*, from *gignesthai*, to be produced]. Caused or induced by sound.

au′di·o·gram″ [*audire;* G. *gramma*, a letter]. A graphic record showing the variations of auditory acuity of an individual, as indicated by the audiometer. Syn., *audiometric curve.*

au″di·ol′o·gy [*audire;* G. *logos*, word]. The science of hearing.

au″di·om′e·ter [*audire;* G. *metron*, a measure]. An instrument for measuring the acuity and range of hearing. There are two main types: the pure tone audiometer and the speech or phonograph audiometer. Either may be used for an individual test or in screening large groups of people. —**audiomet′ric,** *adj.*

Békésy a. A self-recording and completely objective pure tone audiometer.

au″di·om′e·try. The quantitative and qualitative evaluation of a person's hearing by the use of an audiometer. —**audiom′etrist,** *n.*

air conduction a. Quantitative evaluation of hearing by introducing the stimulus through the air column in the external ear canal.

bone conduction a. Qualitative evaluation of hearing by introducing the stimulus directly to the skin over the mastoid process of the temporal bone.

au″di·o·vis′u·al [*audire;* L. *visus*, from *videre*, to see]. Pertaining to, or using, both sound and visual impressions, as the sound movies.

au·di′tion [L. *auditio*, hearing]. Hearing; ability to hear.

chromatic a. A condition in which certain sounds are said to produce subjective sensations of color.

gustatory a. A condition in which certain sounds are believed to cause a sensation of taste.

au′di·tive [L. *audire*, to hear]. Auditory.

au″di·tog·no′sis. Recognition of sounds.

au″di·to·psy′chic [*audire;* G. *psychē*, soul]. Pertaining to the auditory association area of the temporal cortex, Brodmann's area 42.

au′di·to″ry [L. *auditorius*, from *auditor*, a hearer]. Pertaining to the act or the organs of hearing.

au′di·to″ry mem′o·ry span. The number of individual speech sounds that a person is able to recall and to repeat in order after having heard them given once at the rate of one per second.

au″di·to·sen′so·ry [L. *audire*, to hear; *sentire*, to feel]. Pertaining to the auditory projection area of the temporal cortex, Brodmann's area 41.

Auenbrugger von Auenbrugg, Leopold Joseph [*Austrian physician*, 1722–1809]. Introduced percussion of the chest as a means of diagnosis. Also remembered for his description of the bulging of the epigastric region in cases of extensive pericardial effusion; called *Auenbrugger's sign.*

Auer, John [*American physician*, 1875–1948]. With Samuel J. Meltzer, demonstrated the anesthetic effects of magnesium salts (1906), and developed a method of anesthesia by intratracheal insufflation (1909). With Paul A. Lewis, described the physiologic reactions resulting in fatal anaphylactic shock (1910).

Auerbach, Leopold [*German anatomist*, 1828–97]. Noted for his description of the myenteric plexus and of the ganglion cells found therein (1863); called *Auerbach's plexus, ganglion.* Described the red-staining nuclear substance of cells, naming this *erythrophil.*

aug′ment, aug″men·ta′tion [L. *augmentare*, to increase]. 1. Exacerbation; aggravation of symptoms or signs. 2. Production by growths greater than normal. —**augment′,** *v.*

aug·men′tor [*augmentare*]. An agent which increases or accelerates the action of auxetics, though it is unable to initiate cell division when used alone.

a. nerves. Those which increase the force as well as the rate of cardiac contractions. See *accelerator.*

aug·na′thus [G. *au*, again; *gnathos*, jaw]. A rare anomaly in which a second lower jaw is parasitic on that of the host.

Aujeszky, Aladár [*Hungarian physician*, 1869–1933]. Known for his description of pseudorabies (bulbar paralysis or mad itch), caused by a filtrable virus and widely distributed in the animal world. It affects principally the central nervous system and is characterized by an intense pruritus; called *Aujeszky's disease.*

au″lo·pho′bi·a [G. *aulos*, tube; *phobos*, fear]. A morbid fear of flutes.

au′lo·phyte [*aulos;* G. *phyton*, plant]. A symbiotic plant; one that lives within another, but not as a parasite.

au′ra [G., breeze]. 1. A premonitory sensation preceding a convulsion, usually experienced by epileptics. 2. *In electricity*, the current of air which attends the receipt of a static electric discharge.

auditory a. An acoustic sensation which sometimes ushers in an epileptic seizure.

a. asthmatica. Oppression of the chest, flatulence, or other subjective phenomena which usher in an asthmatic attack.

a. hysterica. Sensation similar to those experienced in epilepsy, which introduce a hysterical attack.

cephalic a. A diffuse head sensation often described as heaviness, fullness, or pressure.

epigastric a. A midline sensation over the gastric area which may ascend to the throat.

olfactory a. A sudden disagreeable sensation of smell.

somatosensory a. A sensation of tingling, numbness, or of invisible movement in a part of the body.

vertiginous a. Dizziness announcing an epileptic seizure.

visual a. Flashing of bright light, whirling or colored light, or sudden darkness in the visual fields.

aurae. Plural of *aura:* also often **auras.**

au′ral [*aura*]. Relating to the air or to an aura.

au′ral [L. *auris*, ear]. Relating to the ear or to the hearing.

au′ra·mine″O (aw′ruh·meen″) (C.C.). A basic aniline dye of the diphenyl methane series used in fluorescence microscopy. Also called *canary yellow, pyoktanin yellow, pyoktaninum aureum.*

au·ran′ti·a. $C_6H_2(NO_2)_3.N:C_6H_2(NO_2)_2.N.O.-O.NH_4$. An orange coal-tar dye; an ammonium salt of hexanitrodiphenylamine.

au·ran″ti·am′a·rin [L. *aurantium*, orange; *amarus*, bitter]. A bitter glycoside obtained from orange peel.

aur″an·ti′a·sis cu′tis. Carotenosis.

au·ran′ti·um (aw·ran′shee·um) [L.]. Orange.

au′rate. A salt of auric acid.

aureomycin hydrochloride. Trade-marked name for the antibiotic substance *chlortetracycline hydrochloride.*

au′ri- [L. *auris*, ear]. A combining form denoting *the ear.*

au′ri- [L. *aurum*, gold]. A combining form denoting *gold*, and more precisely, *in chemistry, the presence of gold in the trivalent* or *auric state.*

au′ric [*aurum*]. 1. Pertaining to or containing gold. 2. *In chemistry*, referring to compounds of trivalent gold. See *aurous.*

au′ric ac′id. H_3AuO_3. Gold trihydroxide; insoluble in water but soluble in alkalis to form aurates.

au′ri·cle [L. *auricula*, the external ear]. 1. The pinna of the ear; the ear flap or external ear; auricula. 2. An appendage to an atrium of the heart; auricular appendage. 3. Any ear-shaped structure or appendage. 4. Commonly used mistakenly for atrium. —**auric′ular,** *adj.*

cervical a. Accessory auricle; a projection of the skin, sometimes containing cartilage, found over the sternocleidomastoid muscle; a developmental anomaly of the region around the second visceral groove: also called auricular *appendage* (c).

au·ric′u·la [L.]. Auricle.

au·ric″u·la′re (aw·rick″yoo·lair′ee, ·lahr′ay) [*auricula*]. A point on the root of the zygomatic process of the temporal bone lying perpendicularly above the center of the external auditory meatus.

au″ric·u·lar′is. Any of a number of vestigial muscles associated with the external ear. See Table of Muscles in the Appendix.

au·ric″u·lo·fron·tal′is. A portion of the auricularis anterior muscle.

au·ric″u·lo·tem′po·ral [*auricula;* L. *tempus*, temple]. Relating to the auricle and to the temporal region.

au·ric″u·lo·ven·tric′u·lar. See *atrioventricular.* Abbreviated **AV, A. V.**

au′rin. Rosalic acid.

au′ris [L.]. The ear. —**auriform,** *adj.*

a. dextra. Right ear. Abbreviated, a.d.

a. externa. The external ear, auricle, pinna.

a. interna. The internal ear, labyrinth.

a. media. The middle ear, tympanic cavity.

a. sinistra. Left ear. Abbreviated, a.s.

au′rist [*auris*]. A specialist in diseases of the ear.

au′ro- [L. *aurum*, gold]. A combining form denoting *gold*, and more precisely *in chemistry, the presence of gold in the univalent* or *aurous state.*

au·ro″ra·pho′bi·a [L. *aurora*, dawn; G. *phobos*, fear]. A morbid fear of northern lights.

au″ro·ther′a·py [L. *aurum*, gold; G. *therapeia*, treatment]. The administration of gold salts. Has been employed for the treatment of arthritis and various skin diseases.

au″ro·thi″o·glu′cose. $C_6H_{11}AuO_5S$; a compound of gold with thioglucose, linked through the sulfur atom of the latter, containing about 50% of gold; a yellow powder, freely soluble in water. It is used in the treatment of rheumatoid arthritis and nondisseminated lupus erythematosus, being administered in oil suspension. Syn., *gold thioglucose.* See *solganal.*

au″ro·thi″o·glyc′an·ide. Generic name for α-auromercaptoacetanilid; $C_6H_5.NHCO.CH_2SAu$; a water-insoluble gold compound administered in oil suspension for the treatment of rheumatoid arthritis. See *lauron.*

au′rous [*aurum*]. 1. Pertaining to gold and its compounds. 2. *In chemistry*, referring to compounds of univalent gold.

au′rum [L.]. See *gold.*

aus″cul·ta′tion [L. *auscultare*, to listen to]. The detection and study of sounds arising from various organs, chiefly the heart and lungs, to aid in the determination of their physical condition. —**auscul'tatory,** *adj.;* **auscult', aus'cultate,** *v.*

a. tube. *In otology,* an instrument for listening to the forced passage of air into the middle ear of a patient.

immediate a. The direct application of the examiner's ear to the patient's skin.

mediate a. Listening with the aid of a stethoscope.

Austin and Van Slyke's method. See under *method.*

Aus·tral'ian X dis·ease'. An epidemic virus encephalitis, prevalent in children; first appeared in Australia in 1917. It resembles poliomyelitis, and can be transmitted to some animals.

Aus"tra·lor'bis [L. *australis,* south; *orbis,* circle]. A genus of snails.

aut-. See *auto-.*

au'ta·coid [G. *autos,* self; *akos,* remedy; *eidos,* form]. A chemical messenger released into the blood by the cells of one organ to stimulate or inhibit activity in a remote organ (Schäfer). Thus hormones, for the most part, stimulate and chalones inhibit.

au·te'cious, au·toe'cious (aw·tee'shus), **au·te'cic, au·toe'cic** (aw·tee'sick) [*autos;* G. *oikos,* house]. Applied to parasitic fungi that pass through all the stages of their existence in the same host.

au·te·me'si·a (aw·ti·mee'shuh, ·see·uh, ·zhuh, ·zee·uh) [*autos;* G. *emesia,* disposition to vomit]. Idiopathic vomiting; vomiting at will by certain psychiatric patients.

au'tism [*autos*]. A tendency to morbid concentration on oneself; an interest in daydreaming and phantasy. —**autis'tic,** *adj.*

infantile a. That observed in young children. It often appears as excessive shyness and fearfulness and later as withdrawal and introspection. It may be an early manifestation or part of the childhood type of schizophrenic reaction.

au·tis'tic ges'ture. A muscular automatism. See *tic.*

au·tis'tic think'ing. A type of phantasy usually seen in schizophrenics.

au'to-, aut- [*autos*]. A combining form meaning *pertaining to, by,* or *for oneself or the same individual.*

au"to·ac"ti·va'tion [*autos;* L. *actus,* from *agere,* to do]. Activation of a gland by a kinase or hormone present in its own secretion.

au"to·ag·glu"ti·na'tion [*autos;* L. *agglutinare,* to glue]. 1. Agglutination which occurs without the addition of a specific antiserum. 2. Agglutination of the blood cells of an individual by his own serum.

au"to·ag·glu'ti·nin [*autos; agglutinare*]. An agglutinin contained in the serum of an individual which causes an agglutination of his red cells.

au"to·al"go·lag'ni·a [*autos;* G. *algos,* pain; *lagneia,* coition]. Self-inflicted pain serving as a source of sexual excitement.

au"to·a·nal'y·sis [*autos;* G. *analysis,* a loosing]. Analysis by a patient of his own mental disorder; employed as a psychotherapeutic method.

au"to·an"am·ne'sis [*autos;* G. *anamnēsis,* a recalling]. A history related by the patient alone.

au"to·an"ti·bi·o'sis (aw"to·an"ti·buy·o'sis) [*autos;* G. *anti,* against; *bios,* life; *-ōsis,* condition]. The self-inhibition of a culture medium as a result of the previous growth of the organism in the medium.

au"to·an'ti·bod"y. 1. An antibody produced by a host to his own tissues that ordinarily are not accessible to the blood stream, such as the lens of the eye. 2. *In hematology,* an antibody contained in the serum of a patient which causes agglutination or lysis of his erythrocytes: seen in paroxysmal hemoglobinuria, and other forms of hemolytic anemias.

au"to·au'di·ble [*autos;* L. *audire,* to hear]. Audible to the patient, applied to heart sounds.

au'to·blast [*autos;* G. *blastos,* germ]. An independent bioblast, as a bacterium.

au"to·ca·tal'y·sis. Process by which a chemical reaction is accelerated by one or more products of the reaction acting as catalysts. —**autocatalyt'ic,** *adj.;* **autocat'alyst,** *n.*

au"to·ca·thar'sis [*autos;* G. *katharsis,* a cleansing]. Psychotherapy by having the patient describe his difficulties, thus gaining insight into his mental complexes and conflicts.

au"to·cho"le·cys"to·du"o·de·nos'to·my [*autos;* G. *cholē,* bile; *kystis,* bladder; L. *duodeni,* twelve each; *stoma,* mouth]. The spontaneous formation of an opening between the gallbladder and duodenum, secondary to adhesions between the two organs; the opening permits the passage of gallstones into the duodenum.

au"to·cho"le·cys"to·trans·verse"co·los'to·my [*autos; cholē; kystis;* L. *transversus,* turned across; G. *kolon,* colon; *stoma,* mouth]. The spontaneous formation of an opening between the gallbladder and the transverse colon, secondary to adhesions between the two organs; the opening permits the passage of gallstones into the transverse colon.

au·toch'tho·nous (aw·tock'thon·us) [G. *autochthonos,* from *autos, chthōn,* land]. 1. Formed in the place where found, as a clot. 2. Native; aboriginal.

au·toc'la·sis [*autos;* G. *klasis,* a breaking]. A breaking up of a part due to causes developed within itself.

au'to·clave [*autos;* L. *clavis,* key]. An apparatus for sterilizing objects by steam heat at high pressure. —**au'toclave,** *v.*

au"to·con"den·sa'tion [*autos;* L. *condensare,* to condense]. An electrotherapeutic method of applying high-frequency currents in which the patient or affected part constitutes one plate of a capacitor.

au"to·con·duc'tion [*autos;* L. *conducere,* to bring together]. An electrotherapeutic method of applying high-frequency currents by induction. The patient or part is placed within a large solenoid which acts as the secondary of a transformer.

au"to·cy"to·tox'in [*autos;* G. *kytos,* cell; *toxikon,* poison]. A cell toxin produced against the cells of one's own body, due to retained degenerated and dead cells acting as an antigen.

au"to·di·ges'tion [*autos;* L. *digerere,* to digest]. Digestion of the stomach walls by gastric juice, in disease of the stomach, or after death; autolysis.

au"to·ech"o·la'li·a (aw"to·eck"o·lay'lee·uh) [*autos;* G. *ēchō,* echo; *lalia,* talk]. Stereotypy in which the patient continually repeats some word or phrase of his own.

au"to·ech"o·prax'i·a (·eck"o·prack'see·uh) [*autos; ēchō;* G. *praxis,* a doing]. Stereotypy in which the patient continually repeats some action he has previously experienced.

au·toe'cic. See *autecious.*

au"to·ec"ze·ma·ti·za'tion. The condition or process of suddenly becoming generally eczematized, presumably due to breakdown products of autogenous epidermis: clinically observed in individuals with chronic eczematous dermatoses, but not yet immunologically verified.

au"to·e·mas"cu·la'tion [*autos;* L. *emasculare,* to castrate]. Self-inflicted amputation of the external genitalia, a rare phenomenon confined to psychotic patients.

au"to·er'o·tism, au"to·e·rot'i·cism [*autos;* G. *erōs,* love]. 1. A combination of sexual emotion and self-admiration. 2. Self-gratification of sexual instinct. See *masturbation.* —**autoerot′ic,** *adj.*

au′to·fel·la′ti·o (·feh·lay′shee·o) [*autos;* L. *fellare,* to suck]. Fellatio practiced upon oneself.

au·tog′a·my [*autos;* G. *gamos,* marriage]. 1. *In botany,* self-fertilization. 2. A form of inbreeding marked by conjugation of closely related cells or nuclei. —**autogamous,** *adj.*

au·tog′e·nous (aw·todj′i·nus), **au″to·ge·net′ic, au″to·gen′ic** [*autos;* G. *genesthai,* from *gignesthai,* to be produced]. 1. Self-generated; endogenous. 2. Arising within the organism, applied to toxins, pathologic states, vaccines, and the like.

au′to·graft″. Any tissue removed from one part of a person's body and applied to another part: commonly used contraction for autogenous graft. Also called autoplastic *graft.*

au′to·graph″ [*autos, graphein*]. See *radioautograph.*

au″to·he·mol′y·sis, au″to·hae·mol′y·sis (aw″-to·hee·mol′i·sis, ·hem·ol′i·sis) [*autos;* G. *haima,* blood; *lysis,* a loosing]. Hemolysis of an individual's red blood cells by his own serum.

au″to·he″mo·ther′a·py, au″to·hae″mo·ther′-a·py (aw″to·hee″mo·therr′uh·pee, aw″to·hem″o·) [*autos; haima;* G. *therapeia,* therapy]. Treatment of disease with the patient's own blood, withdrawn through a venipuncture and injected directly into his body, usually intramuscularly.

au″to·hy·drol′y·sis (aw″to·high·drol′i·sis) [*autos;* G. *hydōr,* water; *lysis,* a loosing]. Spontaneous hydrolysis.

au″to·hyp′no·tism, au″to·hyp·no′sis [*autos;* G. *hypnos,* sleep]. Self-induced hypnosis. —**autohypnot′ic,** *adj., n.*

au″to·im·mun″i·za′tion [*autos;* L. *immunis,* free from]. Immunization obtained by natural processes within the body.

au″to·in·fec′tion [*autos;* L. *inficere,* to infect]. Infection by an organism existing within the body or transferred from one part of the body to another.

au″to·in·fu′sion [*autos;* L. *infundere,* to pour in]. Forcing of the blood toward the heart by applying firm bandages to the extremities distoproximally, compression of the abdominal aorta, etc., to raise blood pressure and get blood to the vital centers.

au″to·in·oc″u·la′tion [*autos;* L. *inoculare,* to ingraft an eye or bud of one tree into another]. Inoculation in one part of the body by an organism present in another part; self-inoculation.

au″to·in·tox′i·cant [*autos;* L. *in-,* in; G. *toxikon,* poison]. A poison originating within the system.

au″to·in·tox″i·ca′tion [*autos; in-; toxikon*]. Poisoning by faulty metabolic products elaborated within the body; generally synonymous with toxemia of morbid states. Formerly considered to occur in constipation.

au″to·i″so·ly′sin (aw″to·eye″so·lye′sin, ·eye·sol′i-sin, ·i·sol′i·sin) [*autos;* G. *isos,* equal; *lysis,* a loosing]. An antibody which dissolves the corpuscles of the individual from which it was obtained; also the red cells of others of the same species.

au″to·kin·e′sis. *In physiology,* movement as a result of internal stimuli; voluntary motion.

au·tol′o·gous [*autos;* G. *logos,* word]. Derived from, or a part of, an organism: contrasted with *homologous* (same species) and *heterologous* (different species).

au·tol′y·sate [*autos;* G. *lysis,* a loosing]. That which results from or is produced by autolysis.

au″to·ly′sin, au·tol′y·sin [*autos; lysis*]. A substance which produces autolysis, *q.v.*

au·tol′y·sis [*autos; lysis*]. 1. Self-digestion of tissues within the living body. 2. The chemical splitting-up of the tissue of an organ by the action of an enzyme peculiar to it. 3. The hemolytic action of the blood serum or plasma of an animal upon its own cells. —**autolyt′ic,** *adj.;* **au′tolyze,** *v.*

automat-. See *automato-.*

au″to·mat′ic [G. *automatos,* self-acting]. Performed without the influence of the will; spontaneous.

au·tom′a·tin [*automatos*]. 1. A theoretical substance present in the heart which normally initiates the contraction. 2. An extract of bovine heart muscle used therapeutically in various circulatory disorders.

au·tom″a·tin′o·gen, au″to·mat′o·gen [*automatos;* G. *genesthai,* from *gignesthai,* to be produced]. A substance said to occur in the heart and muscles which, through the action of potassium, is converted to automatin.

au·tom′a·tism [*automatos*]. 1. Performance of acts without apparent volition, as in somnambulism and in hysterical and epileptic states. 2. *In biology,* spontaneous activity of cells and tissues, as the spontaneous beating of a heart freed from its nervous connections.

ambulatory a. A condition in which the epileptic patient wanders around and functions effectively, but is unaware of his normal personality.

epileptic a. See paroxysmal *a.*

ictal a. That occurring during an epileptic seizure.

paroxysmal a. Automatic performance of certain simple acts, despite unconsciousness, seen in certain types of epileptic seizures, associated with typical cerebral electrical discharge in the slow range, 6 to 8 cycles per second. It is likely to occur in persons whose resting electroencephalogram (EEG) shows spike foci in the prefrontal region. Syn., epileptic *a.*

postictal a. That during the postepileptic state.

au·tom″a·ti·za′tion [G. *automatizein,* to act of oneself]. Automatic obedience to infantile impulses.

au·tom′a·to-, automat- [G. *automatos,* self-acting]. A combining form meaning *self-moving* or *self-acting;* used to denote *automatic.*

au″to·mat′o·gen. See *automatinogen.*

au·tom′a·ton [*automatos*]. One who acts in an involuntary or mechanical manner.

au″to·my″so·pho′bi·a [G. *autos,* self; *mysos,* uncleanness; *phobos,* fear]. Morbid fear of personal uncleanliness.

au″to·ne·phrec′to·my. The loss of kidney substance secondary to ureteral obstruction, usually on the basis of chronic infection, as tuberculosis.

au″to·no·ma′si·a (aw″to·no·may′zhuh, ·zee·uh) [*autos;* G. *onoma,* name]. Amnesic aphasia characterized by inability to recall substantives.

au″to·nom′ic [G. *autonomos,* from *autos, nomos,* law]. Autonomous: used specifically to designate the involuntary or sympathetic nervous system. See autonomic nervous *system.*

au·ton′o·mous. Independent in origin, action, or function; self-governing.

au″to-oph·thal′mo·scope, au″toph·thal′mo·scope [*autos;* G. *ophthalmos,* eye; *skopein,* to examine]. An ophthalmoscope for examining one's own eyes. —**auto-ophthalmos′copy, autophthalmos′copy,** *n.*

au′to-ox″i·da′tion. An oxidation reaction utilizing atmospheric oxygen without the aid of other oxidizing agents.

au·top′a·thy [*autos;* G. *pathos,* suffering]. Disease without apparent cause; idiopathy. —**autopath′ic,** *adj.*

au″to·pha′gi·a, au·toph′a·gy [*autos;* G. *phagein,* to eat]. 1. Self-consumption; emaciation. 2. Biting of one's own flesh, as in dementia.

au″to·phil′i·a [*autos;* G. *philia,* affection]. Morbid self-esteem.

au″to·pho′bi·a [*autos;* G. *phobos,* fear]. A morbid dread of one's self or of solitude.

au″to·pho″no·ma′ni·a [*autos;* G. *phonos,* murder; *mania,* madness]. Suicidal mania.

au·toph′o·ny, au″to·pho′ni·a [*autos;* G. *phōnē,* voice]. A condition in some middle-ear and auditory-tube diseases in which an individual's voice seems more resonant to himself.

au′to·plas″ty [*autos;* G. *plassein,* to form]. Repair of a defect by grafting tissue taken from another area of the patient's body. —**autoplas′tic,** *adj.;* **autoplast,** *n.*

au″to·pneu″mo·nec′to·my. The condition characterized by one lung being sequestrated by a pathological process such that the bronchus is completely occluded, so that the lung becomes functionless with little or no blood circulating through it. This can be the result of inflammation or injury.

au″to·pro·tol′y·sis. The process by which a molecule transfers a proton (hydrogen ion) to another identical molecule, as in the ionization of water: $2H_2O \rightleftarrows H_3O^+ + OH^-$.

au′top·sy [G. *autopsia,* seeing with one's own eyes]. A post-mortem examination of the body.

au″to·psy′che (aw″to·sigh′kee) [*autos;* G. *psychē,* soul]. The mind of one's self.

au″to·psy′chic [*autos; psychē*]. Pertaining to self-consciousness or to ideas relating to the individual's own personality.

au″to·psy·cho′sis [*autos;* G. *psychōsis,* from *psychē, -ōsis,* condition]. A mental derangement in which the patient's ideas about himself are distorted. —**autopsy′chic,** *adj.*

au″to·ra′di·o·gram. See *radioautograph.*

au″to·ra″di·og′ra·phy. The technique of locating and measuring the distribution of radioactive elements in a test material, such as tissue, by means of photographic registration of the emanations from the elements. —**autora′diograph,** *n.*

au″to·re·in·fu′sion [*autos;* L. *re-,* again, back; *infundere,* to pour into]. Intravenous infusion in a patient of his own blood.

au″to·sen″si·ti·za′tion [*autos;* L. *sentire,* to feel]. Process of rendering an organism sensitive to its own tissues; has been demonstrated in humans, as for lens tissue. Also called *autoallergization.*

au′to·site [*autos;* G. *sitos,* food]. 1. A monster with organs sufficiently developed to carry on a separate postnatal existence. 2. That member of an unequal twin monster which is capable of independent existence, and which nourishes the other twin (the parasite). The latter may be a complete fetus or accessory body parts attached to the autosite or to the placenta. —**autosit′ic,** *adj.*

au′to·some [*autos;* G. *sōma,* body]. Any ordinary chromosome as distinguished from an allosome. —**autosomal,** *adj.*

au″to·sug·ges′tion [*autos;* L. *suggestio,* from *suggerere,* to suggest]. 1. The acceptance of a thought or idea, predominantly from within one's own mind, which induces some mental or physical action or change. 2. Self-suggestion. The persistence in consciousness of impressions gained while in a hypnotic state. 3. The highly suggestible state of mind existing after accidents, where a very slight injury may be the cause of hysterical pain, paralysis, and other disorders. Also called *traumatic suggestion.* —**autosuggestibil′ity,** *n.*

au″to·syn′de·sis [G. *autos,* same; *syndesis,* binding together]. In polyploids, the pairing of chromosomes derived from the same parent.

au″to·syn·noi′a [G. *autos,* self; *synnoia,* meditation, from *syn,* with, *nous,* mind]. A state of introversion in which the subject is so concentrated in his thoughts or hallucinations that he loses all interest in the outside world.

Autotechnicon. An electrically timed machine for the automatic fixation, dehydration, and impregnation of tissue specimens, invented by Harry Goldblatt and Louis Gross (1929). It is also used for staining sections.

au·tot′o·my [*autos;* G. *tomē,* a cutting]. 1. Mechanism by means of which many organisms are able to cast off parts of their body. 2. Self-division; fission. 3. A surgical operation performed on one's own body. 4. *In psychiatry,* the act of scratching away some part of the body; occurs in catatonics and in patients with tics.

au″to·top·ag·no′si·a [*autos;* G. *topos,* place; *a-,* not; *gnōsis,* knowledge]. Loss of ability to orient parts of one's own body.

au″to·trans·form′er [*autos;* L. *transformare,* to transform]. A step-down transformer used extensively in varying the voltage to the primary windings of a high-voltage x-ray transformer.

au″to·trans·fu′sion [*autos;* L. *transfusio,* from *transfundere,* to pour off, transfer]. 1. Forcing of blood into vital regions after severe hemorrhage or to prevent shock, by elevation of, and application of Esmarch bandages to, three of the extremities. See *autoinfusion.* 2. Intravenous injection of blood or serum lost during an operation or hemorrhage, especially when it occurs in the abdominal cavity. See *autoreinfusion.*

au″to·trans″plan·ta′tion [*autos;* L. *transplantare,* to transplant]. The operation of transplanting to a part of the body tissue taken from another area in the same body.

au″to·troph′, au″to·trophe′, au′to·tro″phant. A bacterium able to grow in an inorganic environment by using carbon dioxide as its sole source of carbon for anabolic metabolism. There are *chemosynthetic* and *photosynthetic autotrophs.* See *chemotroph, phototroph.* —**autotro′phic,** *adj.*

au″to·vac″ci·na′tion [*autos;* L. *vaccinus,* from *vacca,* cow]. Revaccination of an individual using vaccine obtained from his own body.

au″to·vac′cine [*autos; vaccinus*]. Autogenous vaccine.

auxano- [G. *auxanein,* to increase]. A combining form denoting *growth.*

aux·an″o·dif″fer·en″ti·a′tion. See under *differentiation.*

aux·an′o·gram [*auxanein;* G. *gramma,* a letter]. A pure plate culture of microorganisms prepared by auxanography.

aux″a·nog′ra·phy [*auxanein;* G. *graphein,* to write]. A method for ascertaining the nutrient mediums most suited to the growth requirements of a particular strain of microorganisms. —**auxanograph′ic,** *adj.*

aux·e′sis [G. *auxēsis,* increase]. 1. Increase in size or bulk; growth. 2. Growth in size by cell expansion without cell division; hypertrophy. *Obs.*

aux·et′ic [*auxēsis*]. A hypothetical substance which excites cell reproduction; an agent which causes proliferation of human cells, especially leukocytes. —**aux·et′ic,** *adj.*

aux′in [G. *auxein,* to increase]. A plant hormone which governs cell extension or growth.

aux·i·om′e·ter. See *auxometer.*

aux′o- [*auxein*]. 1. A combining form signifying *increase.* 2. *In biochemistry,* a combining form denoting *accelerating* or *stimulating.* 3. *In biology,* a combining form denoting *concerned with,* or *due to, growth.*

aux″o·bar′ic [*auxein;* G. *baros,* weight]. Increasing pressure; denoting the developing pressure in the cardiac ventricles during the isometric and early ejection phases.

aux″o·car′di·a [*auxein;* G. *kardia,* heart]. 1. Normal increase of the volume of the heart during diastole, as differentiated from miocardia, the diminution during systole. 2. Cardiac enlargement from hypertrophy or dilatation.

aux′o·chrome [*auxein;* G. *chrōma,* color]. 1. That which increases color. 2. A chemical group which, added to a chromophore group, will produce a dye. 3. Increase or development of color. —**aux-och′romous,** *adj.*

aux′o·cyte [*auxein;* G. *kytos,* cell]. A spermatocyte, oocyte, or sporocyte during its early growth period.

aux′o·drome. A standard schedule of development.

aux·om′e·ter, aux·i·om′e·ter [*auxein;* G. *metron,* a measure]. A device for measuring the magnifying power of lenses.

A.V., AV Atrioventricular; auriculoventricular; arteriovenous.

AV block. See *atrioventricular block* under *heart block.*

Av. Avoirdupois weight.

av′a·lanche. The phenomenon or process, encountered when ionizing emanations are being measured whereby an ion produces another ion by collision, and these ions in turn produce other ions by further collisions, until an avalanche of ions and accompanying electrons results.

a·val′vu·lar (ay·valv′yoo·lur, a·valv′·) [G. *a-,* not; L. dim. of *valva,* folding-leaf of a door]. Lacking any structure for temporarily closing a passage or opening.

a·vas″cu·lar·i·za′tion (ay·vas″cue·lur·i·zay′shun, a·vas″·) [*a-;* L. *vasculum,* a small vessel]. Act of rendering a part bloodless, as by compression or bandaging. —**avas′cular,** *adj.;* **avas′cularize,** *v.t., v.i.*

Avellis, Georg [*German laryngologist,* 1864–1916]. Remembered for his description of ambiguospinothalamic paralysis affecting the same side of the larynx, pharynx, and uvula, with contralateral loss of pain and temperature sense; called *Avellis paralysis, Avellis' symptom complex* or *syndrome.*

A·ve′na [L., oats]. A genus of plants; the grain of **A. sativa,** one of the most important species, is the oat from which avenin is obtained.

a·ven″a·ce′in. An antibiotic substance produced by *Fusarium avenaceum;* it is a colorless compound, having the composition $C_{25}H_{44}N_2O_7$, and is active against a number of organisms.

a·ve′nin, av′e·nin. A nitrogenous principle obtained from oats; the glutelin of oats.

Avenzoar (Abumeron, ibn Zuhr) [*Arabian physician in Cordoba,* ca. 1091–ca. 1162]. Famous clinician. Noted the causal relationship of *Sarcoptes scabiei* (the itch mite) to scabies. Described gastric carcinoma, mediastinal abscess, and otitis media.

av′er·age [F. *avarie,* damage to ship or cargo, from Ar.]. The medial sum; the figure arrived at by adding together several quantities and dividing by the number of quantities; arithmetic mean.

av′er·age. Usual; typical of a group; ordinary.

Averroës (ibn Rushd) [*Arabian physician and philosopher in Cordoba,* 1126–98]. Last of the great Arabian physicians. Noted especially for his medical encyclopedia.

avertin. Trade-mark for tribromoethanol.

a. with amylene hydrate. Trade-marked name for tribromoethanol solution: used for basal anesthesia by rectal administration and for the control of certain convulsive conditions. See *bromethol.*

a′vi·an [L. *avis,* bird]. Pertaining to birds.

a′vi·an pneu″mo·en·ceph″a·li′tis Newcastle *disease.*

a′vi·an pseu′do·plague. Newcastle *disease.*

a″vi·a′tion med′i·cine. That branch of medicine concerned with the pathologic conditions and physiologic and emotional disturbances resulting from airplane flights.

a′vi·a″tor's ear. See *aerootitis media.*

Avicenna (ibn Sīnā) [*Persian physician, philosopher, and writer,* 980–1037]. The most illustrious physician in Arabian medicine of his time. Author of the *Canon,* a huge storehouse of learning, in which he attempted to codify the whole medical knowledge of the time and to square the facts with the systems of Aristotle and Galen. His ranking of surgery as an inferior branch of medical science halted its progress for many centuries.

av′i·din. A biotin-inactivating protein in raw egg white. It causes the syndrome known as egg white injury in rats fed a diet containing raw egg white as the source of protein. Heat renders it inert. It inhibits the growth of species of bacteria which require biotin but has no effect on the growth of those which do not require it. It has been suggested that the avidin-biotin complex plays a part in the physiology of avian reproduction.

a·vid′i·ty [L. *avidus,* eager, greedy]. 1. Obsolete term for chemical affinity. 2. *In immunology,* that characteristic of antitoxic serum which determines the rate of neutralization; it is distinct from the antitoxin content.

a·vir′u·lent (ay·virr′yoo·lunt, ·oo·lunt, a·virr′·) [G. *a-,* not; L. *virus,* poison]. Without virulence.

a·vi·tam′ic ac′id (ay·vye·tam′ic, ay·vi·, a·vye·, a·vi·). Ascorbic acid.

a·vi″ta·min·o′sis (ay·vy″tuh·mi·no′sis, a·vy″·, ay″vi·tam″i·no′sis) [*a-;* L. *vita,* life; G. *-ōsis,* condition]. Any disease resulting from a deficiency of one or more vitamins.

a·vo·ca′li·a (a·vo·kay′lee·uh, ay·vo·) [*a-;* L. *vocalis,* from *vox,* voice]. The inability to produce musical sounds, or sing in tune; motor amusia.

Avogadro, Amadeo [*Italian physicist,* 1776–1856]. Stated the physical law that equal volumes of all gases at the same temperature and pressure contain equal numbers of molecules (1811). **Avogadro's number** is the number of molecules of a substance in one gram-molecular weight; it is 6.06×10^{23}.

av″oir·du·pois′ (av″ur·duh·poyz′) [ME. *avoir de pois,* from OF. *avoir,* goods, *pois,* weight]. The English system of weights and measures. See Tables of Weights and Measures in the Appendix. Abbreviated, Av.

avosyl. A trade-mark for *mephenesin.*

a·vul′sion [L. *avellere,* to tear away]. A forcible tearing or wrenching away of a part, as a polyp or a limb.

a. of the bulb. Forcible separation of the eyeball by tearing the muscles, the tendons, and the optic nerve.

nerve a. Surgical tearing away of a nerve from its origin by traction, as a phrenic avulsion, for paralyzing one side of the diaphragm to obtain rest for a tuberculous lung.

ax. Axis.

ax-. See *axo-.*

ax″an·thop′si·a [G. *a-,* not; *xanthos,* yellow; *opsis,* vision]. Yellow blindness.

Axenfeld, Karl Theodor Paul Polykarpos [*German ophthalmologist,* 1867–1930]. Almost simultaneously with Morax, isolated *Hemophilus duplex,* also called *Moraxella lacunata, Morax-Axenfeld bacillus* (1896). This causes chronic conjunctivitis, known as *Morax-Axenfeld conjunctivitis.* He also described an anomalous loop of the ciliary nerve in the sclera, known as *Axenfeld's intrascleral nerve loop.*

axerophthol. A trade name for vitamin A.

ax″i·a′tion [L. *axis*, axis]. The formation or development of axial structures, such as notochord and neural tube.

ax·if′u·gal [*axis;* L. *fugere*, to flee]. Centrifugal.

ax″i·lem′ma. See *axolemma.*

ax·il′la [L.] The fossa between the arm and the thoracic wall, bounded anteriorly by the pectoralis major muscle, and posteriorly by the latissimus dorsi muscle; the armpit. See Plate 11. —**ax′illary,** *adj.*

ax′is (pl. *axes*) [L.]. 1. An imaginary line passing through the center of a body; also the line about which a rotating body turns. 2. The second cervical vertebra; the epistropheus [BNA]. See Table of Bones in the Appendix. 3. The spinal column. 4. The cerebrospinal nervous system. 5. The odontoid process of the epistropheus. 6. A very short artery which breaks up into several branches. Abbreviated, ax. —**axial,** *adj.*

a. uteri. (a) The long diameter of the uterus. (b) A line imagined to pass transversely through the uterus near its junction with the cervix, on which it is said to turn in retroversion.

basibregmatic a. The line connecting the basion and bregma.

basicranial a. A line connecting the basion to the midpoint of the sphenoethmoidal suture.

basifacial a. A line joining the subnasal point and the midpoint of the sphenoethmoidal suture.

binauricular a. *In craniometry,* the imaginary line joining the two auricular points.

bipolar a. *In electrocardiography,* that determined from standard limb leads.

brain a. The brain stem.

cardiac a. A line passing through the center of the base and apex of the heart.

celiac a. Celiac artery. See Plate 8.

cell a. An imaginary line passing through the nucleus and the central apparatus of a cell.

cerebrospinal a. The central nervous system.

conjugate a. The conjugate diameter of the pelvis.

cord a. See primitive *streak.*

craniofacial a. Axis through the bones forming the base of the skull.

electric a. The average direction of the activation or regression wave through the heart muscle at any instant; or the mean of the instantaneous values over a specified period (**mean electric axis**).

embryonic a. An imaginary line passing through the future anteroposterior regions of an egg or embryo.

encephalomyelonic a. Cerebrospinal axis. Also called *encephalospinal a.*

facial a. See basifacial *a.*

frontal a. 1. An imaginary transverse line passing through the center of both eyeballs. 2. *In electrocardiography,* an electric axis perpendicular to the ground when the patient is supine which is directed from the front of the thorax to the back.

hemal a. The aorta.

horizontal a. *In electrocardiography,* an electric axis parallel to the ground when the patient is supine which is directed from one side of the thorax to the other.

neural a. Cerebrospinal axis.

optic a. (a) An imaginary line on which the refracting surfaces of the eye are more or less centered; it passes from the midpoint (approximately) of the cornea (anterior pole) to the midpoint of the optic fundus (posterior pole); the principal axis of the eye.

pelvic a. An imaginary line passing through all the median anteroposterior diameters of the pelvic canal at their centers.

precordial a. *In electrocardiography,* an electric axis determined from precordial or chest leads.

principal a. *In optics,* a line which extends, through the center of a lens at a 90° angle to the surface of its lens. In *ophthalmology,* same as optic *axis.* Also called *optical center nodal point.*

pupillary a. An imaginary line through the center of the pupil of the eye and perpendicular to the cornea.

sagittal a. *In electrocardiography,* an electric axis parallel to the ground and directed from head to feet when the patient is supine.

sagittal a. of the eye. See visual *a.*

thoracic a. The thoracoacromial artery or vein.

unipolar a. *In electrocardiography,* that determined from the unipolar extremity leads.

vertical a. (a) The long axis of the body. (b) A vertical line passing through the center of the eyeball.

visual a. Line of vision; a line connecting the fixation point and fovea and passing through the nodal point of the eye.

Y a. The line joining the sella turcica and the gnathion.

ax′is cyl′in·der. The conducting or essential part of a nerve fiber.

ax′o-, ax- [*axis*]. A combining form meaning *axis* or denoting *the axis cylinder.*

ax″o·den·drit′ic. See under *synapse.*

ax″o·fu′gal, ax·of′u·gal [*axis;* L. *fugere,* to flee]. Pertaining to nerve impulses transmitted from the cell body to the periphery. Also *axifugal, centrifugal.*

ax′oid, ax·oi′de·an [*axis;* G. *eidos,* form]. 1. Pivot-shaped. 2. Relating to the second cervical joint.

ax″o·lem′ma [axis; G. *lemma,* sheath]. The plasma membrane surrounding the axon of a neuron, and reaching deep to the myelin sheath: first described by *Ludwig Mauthner.* Also spelled *axilemma.*

ax″o·mat′ic. See under *synapse.*

ax·om′e·ter [*axis;* G. *metron,* a measure]. An instrument for adjusting spectacles to the axes of the eyes.

ax′on, ax′one [G. *axōn,* axis]. The efferent process of a nerve cell. Also called *neuraxon, neurit, axis cylinder process.* —**axonal,** *adj.*

ax′o·neme″, ax″o·ne′ma. The axial filament of the flagellum of a protozoan.

ax″o·nom′e·ter [*axōn;* G. *metron,* a measure]. An instrument used for locating the axis of astigmatism, or for determining the axis of a cylindrical lens.

ax″on·ot·me′sis [*axōn;* G. *tmēsis,* a cutting]. The orderly and spontaneous regeneration of an axon, after a crushing injury which destroys the continuity of the axon, but not that of the supporting connective tissue.

ax·op′e·tal [*axōn;* L. *petere,* to seek]. Pertaining to nerve impulses transmitted along an axon toward the cell body. Also *axipetal, centripetal.*

ax′o·plasm″ [*axōn;* G. *plasma,* from *plassein,* to form]. Undifferentiated cytoplasm, neuroplasm, of the axon in which neurofibrils are embedded.

a″ya·huas′ca (ah″yah·woss′kah). A native name for *Banisteria caapi,* a Brazilian plant containing banisterine.

Ayala, A. G. [*Italian neurologist,* contemporary]. Described a congenital deformity due to the absence of the pectoral muscle, called *Ayala's disease.* Also devised a test for determining cerebrospinal pressure, called *Ayala quotient, Ayala test.* See under *test.*

a″ya·pa′na (ah″yah·pah′nah), **a″ya·pa′no** [Sp. and Pg., from Tupi *ayapana*]. The leaves of the herb *Eupatorium triplinerve,* native to tropical America. It is rich in tannin and has been used as a diaphoretic and a diuretic.

a″ya·pan′in. 7-Methoxycoumarin. One of the active principles of *Eupatorium ayapana,* an aromatic herb whose leaves have been used as a hemostatic agent.

a′ya·pin. 6,7-Methylenedioxycoumarin. One of the active principles of *Eupatorium ayapana,* an aromatic herb whose leaves have been used as a hemostatic agent.

Ayerza, Abel [*Argentinian physician,* 1861–1918]. Remembered for his description of the syndrome of chronic cyanosis, dyspnea, and sclerosis of the pulmonary artery (1901), called *Ayerza's disease, Ayerza's syndrome.* This is now classified as syphilis of the pulmonary artery, dilatation of the pulmonary artery due to mitral stenosis, hypertension of lesser circulation due to disease of the lungs, or arteriosclerosis of the pulmonary vessels.

ay·fi′vin. An impure polypeptide mixture, having antibiotic activity, obtained from cultures of *Bacillus licheniformis;* it yields the same amino acids as bacitracin.

a·yp′ni·a [G. *a-,* not; *hypnos,* sleep]. Insomnia.

az″a·gua′nine. 8-Azaguanine; guanine in which the —CH= group in position 8 is replaced by —N=. It interferes with the growth of certain mouse tumors, possibly because a nucleic acid containing 8-azaguanine functions as an antimetabolite for a corresponding nucleic acid containing guanine.

a·za′le·ine (a·zay′lee·een, ·in). See *fuchsin.*

a″za·ser′ine. $N_2CH.CO.O.CH_2.CHNH_2.COOH$; O-diazoacetyl-L-serine; a crystalline antibiotic substance isolated from broth cultures of a *Streptomyces* species and also synthesized. It powerfully inhibits growth of certain transplantable neoplasms in animals, possibly through competition with serine.

a·zed′a·rach (a·zed′uh·rack) [Per. *āzād dirakht,* free, or noble, tree]. Pride of China. The dried bark of the root of *Melia azedarach,* an Asiatic tree naturalized in the southern United States. It occurs in curved pieces or quills, having a sweetish taste. Preparations of it have been used as an anthelmintic against nematodes.

az″e·la′ic ac′id. $COOH(CH_2)_7COOH$; a solid acid produced by disruptive oxidation of oleic acid and certain other acids occurring in oils and fats. Syn., *nonanedioic acid.*

a·ze′o·trope (ay·zee′o·trope, a·zee′o·trope). The particular composition of a mixture of two or more substances exhibiting a minimum or a maximum boiling point for all possible mixtures of the particular substances, and thereby having a constant boiling point. Also called *az″e·o·trop′ic mix′ture.*

az′i- [G. *a-,* not; *zōē,* life]. A prefix denoting *the presence of the group* N_2.

az′ide (az′ide, ·id, ay′zide). A compound containing the univalent —N_3 group.

az′ine (az′een, ay′zeen). Any of a class of heterocyclic compounds containing six atoms in the ring, at least one of which is nitrogen. The number of nitrogen atoms is distinguished by prefixes, as *mono*azine, *di*azine, *tri*azine.

az′o- (az′o-, ay′zo-), **az-** [*a-; zōē*]. A combining form indicating *the presence of nitrogen* or *of the group —N:N— within a compound.*

az″o·ben′zene. $C_6H_5N:NC_6H_5$. A compound prepared by the reduction of nitrobenzene. It forms orange-red leaflets readily soluble in alcohol and ether, but sparingly soluble in water; used in organic synthesis.

az″o·car′mine G (az″o·kahr′min, ·myne, ay″zo·) (C.C.). A basic azine dye used in some methods for staining connective tissue.

azochloramid. Trade-mark for N,N′-dichloroazodicarbonamidine, $H_2N(ClN:)CN:NC(:NCl)NH_2$, or chloroazodin (*chloroazodinum*). The compound is a germicide available in solutions of various strengths and in a 1:1000 ointment.

az′o com′pound. *In chemistry,* a compound containing the group —N:N— united to two hydrocarbon groups.

az″o·der′min. An acetylated derivative of aminoazotoluene: used similarly.

az′o dyes (az′o, ay′zo). A group of synthetic organic dyes derivable from azobenzene, containing the chromophore —N:N—.

az″o·lit′min. A dark-red coloring matter obtained from litmus and used as an indicator, especially in routine bacteriologic work with milk.

a·zo″o·sper′mi·a, a·zo″o·sper′ma·tism [*a-; zōē;* G. *sperma,* seed]. Absence of spermatozoa in the semen.

az″o·pro′te·in. One of a group of synthetic antigens formed by coupling proteins with diazonium compounds.

az·o·ru′bin S. A dark-red dye injected intravenously; the time required for the dye to appear in the duodenal drainage after excretion by the liver can be used as a measure of liver function.

az″o·sul′fa·mide. See *neoprontosil.*

az″o·te′mi·a [*a-; zōē;* G. *haima,* blood]. The presence of excessive amounts of nitrogenous compounds in the blood; uremia.

alimentary a. Elevation of the blood urea nitrogen (BUN) secondary to the presence of a great amount of protein in the gastrointestinal tract, usually the result of hemorrhage.

a·zot′ic ac′id. Nitric acid.

a·zo″ti·fi·ca′tion [*a-; zōē;* L. *facere,* to make]. Fixation of atmospheric nitrogen.

az′o·tized. 1. Converted to an azo compound. 2. Nitrogenous; charged with nitrogen. —**azotize,** *v.t., v.i.*

Az″o·to·bac′ter. Soil and water bacteria capable of fixing atmospheric nitrogen. See also *nitrogen fixers.*

az″o·tom′e·ter [*a-; zōē;* G. *metron,* a measure]. A device for gasometrically measuring the nitrogen content of compounds in solution. —**azotom′etry,** *n.*

az″o·tor·rhe′a, az″o·tor·rhoe′a [*a-; zōē;* G. *rhoia,* flow]. Excess of nitrogenous matter in the urine or feces.

az″o·tu′ri·a [*a-; zōē;* G. *ouron,* urine]. An increase of the nitrogenous substances in the urine. —**azoturic,** *adj.*

az′u·lene. $C_{10}H_8$; cyclopentacycloheptene, forming intensely blue leaflets or plates, insoluble in water; it occurs in certain volatile oils.

azulfidine. Trade-mark for *salicylazosulfapyridine,* a sulfonamide derivative used in chronic ulcerative colitis.

az′ure (azh′ur, ay′zhur). A basic thiazine dye; used in blood and connective-tissue stains.

a. A (C.C.). Asymmetrical dimethyl thionine; used in 0.1–1.5% aqueous solution as a nuclear stain for sections of fixed tissue, or in combination with other dyes.

a. B (C.C.). The trimethyl derivative of thionine.

a. C A basic dye, monomethyl thionine.

a. I Trade name for a mixture of azure A and azure B. Syn., *methylene a.*

a. II A mixture of equal parts of azure I and methylene blue.

methylene a. See *a.* I.

az′u·rin. Theobromine sodium acetate; used as a diuretic. See *theobromine.*

a·zu′ro·phile″ (a·zhoor′o·file″, ·fil″, az·yoor′·), **a·zu′ro·phil″** [OF. *azure*, blue; G. *philein*, to love]. Staining promptly with an azure dye. **—azurophil′ic,** *adj.*

az″y·go·ag′na·thus, as″y·go·ag′na·thus. A form of otocephaly in which there is no mandible and the zygomas are absent or vestigial.

az′y·gos, a·zy′gos [G. *a*-, not; *zygon*, yoke]. An unpaired anatomic structure. **—az′ygos, az′ygous, azy′gous,** *adj.*

a. uvulae. Old name for the muscle of the uvula.

a·zy′mi·a, a·zym′i·a [*a*-; G. *zymē*, a leaven]. The absence of an enzyme or ferment.

a·zym′ic, a·zy′mic [*a*-; *zymē*]. 1. Not rising from a fermentation; unfermented. 2. Not containing enzymes.

B

B Chemical symbol for boron.

B. Abbreviation for *Bacillus;* formerly abbreviation for *Bacterium.*

Ba The chemical symbol for barium.

Bab′bitt met′al [after Isaac *Babbitt*, American inventor, 1799–1862]. *In dentistry*, an alloy of tin, antimony, and copper used in making dies and counterdies for swaging metallic artificial dentures.

Babcock, Stephen Moulton [*American agricultural chemist*, 1843–1931]. Remembered for his invention of a test for determining the percentage content of butterfat in milk by means of centrifuging a mixture of equal quantities of the specimen and sulfuric acid (1890).

Babcock, William Wayne [*American surgeon*, 1872–]. Known for his originality in devising a number of surgical procedures, as proctosigmoidectomy by the combined method; a plastic operation for relief of exstrophy of the urinary bladder; an operation for prognathism; a method for submucous perineorraphy; operations for aneurysm; a method of extirpating varicose veins. See also *Jackson-Babcock operation* under Chevalier *Jackson.*

Babcock-Levy test. See under *test.*

Babes, Victor [*Rumanian microbiologist*, 1854–1926]. With Ernst, described the metachromatic granules found in bacteria. These granules, called *Babes-Ernst bodies*, are more refractive than the surrounding cytoplasm, and take up dyes more avidly; developed the mallein test for glanders (1891). See under *test.*

Ba·be′si·a (ba·bee′zhuh, ·zee·uh, ba·bay′·, baybee′·) [L., after Victor *Babes*]. A genus of intracellular, nonpigmented sporozoa which invade the red blood cells of cattle, sheep, horses, rodents, dogs, and monkeys but not of man. Members of this genus are oval or pear-shaped.

B. bigemina. The species which causes Texas fever or bovine piroplasmosis in the United States; commonly transmitted to cattle by the tick *Boophilus annulatus.*

B. bovis. A species found in European countries which is slightly smaller than the *B. bigemina* and transmitted by the *Ixodes ricinus* and *Haemaphysalis punctata;* the disease is similar to Texas fever.

B. canis. The species which causes an icterus gravis known as canine piroplasmosis.

B. equi. The species which produces equine biliary fever in horses, mules, and donkeys.

B. ovis. The species which is the etiologic agent of a piroplasmosis of sheep.

bab″e·si′a·sis (bab″i·sigh′uh·sis, ·zigh′uh·sis, bay″bi·) [*Babesia;* NL. *-iasis*, condition]. Infestation of mammals other than man with a species of *Babesia.* Also see *piroplasmosis.*

Babinski, Joseph François Félix [*French neurologist*, 1857–1932]. Noted for his description of a reflex (extension of the great toe with fanning of the other toes on exciting the sole) connected with a lesion in the pyramidal tract and found in organic, but not in hysterical, hemiplegia: called *Babinski's sign.* He also described a sign in true sciatica, a diminution of the Achilles reflex, and a syndrome in which lightning pains, absent patellar reflex, Argyll Robertson pupil, and arterial disease indicate tabes. In association with Nageotte, he described a syndrome marked by contralateral hemiplegia and hemianesthesia with hemiasynergia and hemiataxia, due to multiple lesions of the pyramidal tracts and cerebral peduncle: known as the *Babinski-Nageotte syndrome.* He was the first to outline the syndrome of adiposogenital dystrophy (1900), called *Babinski-Froehlich's disease.*

ba′by [ME.]. An infant; a newborn child; a child up to the time he talks.

blue b. A newborn child suffering from cyanosis, transitory or permanent. The former is due to a passing obstruction, irregular respiration, or may follow crying or exercise; the latter occurs when venous blood is shunted to the arterial side because of a cardiac anomaly, as an open foramen ovale. See *cyanosis.*

Baccelli, Guido [*Italian physician and politician*, 1832–1916]. Regarded as a leading figure in Italian medicine of his time; remembered for his method of treating aneurysm by the insertion of a watch spring into the vessel to favor coagulation, and for his treatment of echinococcus cysts of the liver by aspiration and irrigation. See also Baccelli's *sign.*

Bac′cha·ris (back′uh·riss) [G. *bakkaris*, a plant with a fragrant root]. A genus of small trees or shrubs of the Carduceae: old classification, Compositae.

B. halimifolia. The groundsel tree, a shrub of North America. A decoction of the leaves and bark is a popular demulcent and pectoral medicine.

B. pilularis. Kidneywort or kidney root, a shrub of California: formerly used in cystitis and as a diuretic.

bac′ci·form (back′si·form) [L. *bacca*, berry; *forma*, form]. Berry-shaped.

Bachman test. See under *test.*

ba·cill′ (ba·sill′). A short rodlike lozenge.

bac′il·lar″y (bas′i·lerr″ee), **ba·cil′lar** [L. *bacillus*, dim. of *baculus*, stick]. 1. Relating to bacilli or to a bacillus. 2. Consisting of or containing rods.

bac″il·le′mi·a, bac″il·lae′mi·a (bas″i·lee′mee·uh) [*bacillus;* G. *haima*, blood]. Presence of bacilli in the blood.

ba·cil′li·form [*bacillus;* L. *forma*, form]. Having the shape or appearance of a bacillus; rod-shaped.

ba·cil′lo- (ba·sil′o-, bas′i·lo-), **ba·cil′li-** (ba·sil′ee-, bas′i·lee-) [*bacillus*]. A combining form meaning *bacillus*.

ba·cil″lo·my′cin [*bacillus;* G. *mykēs*, fungus]. An antibiotic substance isolated from cultures of *Bacillus subtilis;* it is active against a variety of fungi but has little effect against bacteria.

ba·cil″lo·pho′bi·a [*bacillus;* G. *phobos*, fear]. Morbid fear of bacilli.

bac″il·lu′ri·a (bas″i·lew′ree·uh) [*bacillus;* G. *ouron*, urine]. The presence of bacilli in the urine.

Ba·cil′lus (pl. *Bacilli*) [L.]. A genus of rod-shaped, nonflexuous forms of the family Bacillaceae, described by O. F. Müller before 1800; term first used by Cohn in 1872 with *Bacillus subtilis* as the type. They may occur as slender, short, straight, or slightly bent rods. Abbreviated B.

B. acidophilus. Lactobacillus acidophilus.

B. aerogenes capsulatus. Synonym for *Clostridium welchii.*

B. aertrycke. See *Salmonella typhimurium.*

B. agni. The lamb dysentery bacillus, which has also been designated as *Clostridium welchii B.*

B. anthracis. A species pathogenic to man, although in nature it is primarily a pathogen of cattle and horses. The *B. anthracis* is one of the largest of the pathogenic bacteria and is nonmotile. See Table of the Most Common Microorganisms Pathogenic to Man in the Appendix.

B. bifidus. See *Lactobacillus bifidus.*

B. botulinus. Synonym for *Clostridium botulinum.*

B. bovisepticus. Synonym for *Pasteurella boviseptica.*

B. brevis. A group of bacilli, widely distributed in soil, from which gramicidin, gramicidin S, and tyrocidine, powerful broad-spectrum antibiotic agents, have been extracted.

B. coli. Old term for *Escherichia coli.*

B. diphtheriae. *Corynebacterium diphtheriae.*

B. dysenteriae. See *Shigella dysenteriae.*

B. enteritidis. See *Salmonella enteritidis.*

B. erysipelatos-suis. Synonym for *Erysipelothrix rhusiopathiae.*

B. faecalis alcaligenes. See *Alcaligenes faecalis.*

B. fusiformis. Synonym for *Fusobacterium plauti-vincenti.*

B. gastrophilus. See *Lactobacillus acidophilus.*

B. hofmannii. Misnomer for *Corynebacterium pseudodiphtheriticum.*

B. influenzae. See *Hemophilus influenzae.*

B. lactis aerogenes. See *Aerobacter aerogenes.*

B. lacunatus. Synonym for *Moraxella lacunata.*

B. leprae. See *Mycobacterium leprae.*

B. mallei. See *Malleomyces mallei.*

B. mucosus capsulatum. Old term for *Klebsiella pneumoniae.*

B. oedematiens. Synonym for *Clostridium novyi.*

B. oedematis maligni. Synonym for *Clostridium novyi.*

B. ovitoxicus. Synonym for *Clostridium perfringens.*

B. paludis. Synonym for *Clostridium perfringens Type C.*

B. parabotulinus. Synonym for *Clostridium botulinum C.*

B. paratyphosus A. Synonym for *Salmonella paratyphi A.*

B. paratyphosus B. Synonym for *Salmonella paratyphi B.*

B. perfringens. Synonym for *Clostridium perfringens.*

B. pertussis. Synonym for *Hemophilus pertussis.*

B. pestis. See *Pasteurella pestis.*

B. phlegmonis emphysematosae. Synonym for *Clostridium perfringens.*

B. polymyxa. An aerobic, spore-forming, Gram-negative, sugar-fermenting rod, widely distributed in water, soil, milk, decaying vegetables, and the like: the source of polymyxin.

B. proteus. See *Proteus vulgaris.*

B. pyocyaneus. Synonym for *Pseudomonas aeruginosa.*

B. subtilis. The type species of the genus *Bacillus*, which infects human beings only rarely. Its medical importance lies in the fact that the antibiotic substance, subtilin, is prepared from this species.

B. suisepticus. Synonym for *Pasteurella suiseptica.*

B. tetani. *Clostridium tetani.*

B. tuberculosis. See *Mycobacterium tuberculosis.*

B. vaginalis. A common organism found in the vagina, contributing to the acidity of the vaginal secretions. It is thought to be identical with the *Lactobacillus acidophilus.*

B. whitmori. *Malleomyces pseudomallei.*

B. xerosis. See *Corynebacterium xerose.*

ba·cil′lus (pl. *bacilli*) [L.]. Loosely, any member of the class Schizomycetes.

abortus b. *Brucella abortus.*

anthrax b. *Bacillus anthracis.*

Barnsdale b. *Mycobacterium ulcerans.*

Bordet-Gengou b. *Hemophilus pertussis.*

colon b. *Escherichia coli.*

comma b. *Vibrio comma.*

diphtheria b. *Corynebacterium diphtheriae.*

diphtheroid bacilli. Bacilli similar to the diphtheria bacillus but which do not produce toxin.

Döderlein's b. *Bacillus vaginalis.*

Ducrey's b. *Hemophilus ducreyi.*

Duval's b. *Shigella sonnei.*

Flexner's b. *Shigella paradysenteriae.*

Friedländer's b. *Klebsiella pneumoniae.*

Frisch's b. See *Klebsiella rhinoscleromatis.*

fusiform b. A common designation for bacteria of spindle-shaped or cigar-shaped morphology, belonging to the genus *Fusobacterium.*

gas gangrene b. *Clostridium perfringens Type A.*

glanders b. *Malleomyces mallei.*

Hansen's b. *Mycobacterium leprae.*

hay b. *Bacillus subtilis.*

Hiss and Russell's Y b. *Shigella paradysenteriae.*

Hofmann's b. *Corynebacterium pseudodiphtheriticum.*

hog cholera b. See *Salmonella choleraesuis.*

Johne's b. See *Mycobacterium paratuberculosis* and *Johne's disease.*

Klebs-Loeffler b. *Corynebacterium diphtheriae.*

Koch-Weeks b. *Hemophilus aegyptius.*

Morax-Axenfeld b. *Moraxella lacunata.*

Morgan's b. *Proteus morganii.*

Much's b. See Hans Christian R. *Much.*

Perez' b. *Salmonella foetida.*

Pfeiffer's b. *Hemophilus influenzae.*

pneumobacillus. *Klebsiella pneumoniae.*

pseudodysentery b. *Shigella paradysenteriae.*

Schmitz's b. *Shigella ambigua.*

Shiga b. *Shigella dysenteriae.*

streptobacilli. Those bacilli which remain attached end to end producing a chainlike group.

tubercle b. *Mycobacterium tuberculosis.* Abbreviated, t. b.

typhoid b. Synonym for *Eberthella typhosa.*

vole b. A bacillus closely allied to *Mycobacterium tuberculosis* and causing a disease in voles resembling tuberculosis and rat leprosy. It is highly pathogenic for rats. Syn., *Mycobacterium tuberculosis var. muris.*

zur Nedden's b. See Max Wilhelm zur *Nedden.*

ba″ci·tra′cin [*bacillus; Tracy*]. An antibiotic obtained from *Bacillus subtilis* isolated from a wound (in the patient Margaret Tracy, after whom it was named). It is active against many Gram-positive organisms, such as streptococci, staphylococci, and pneumococci, and certain Gram-negative cocci, such as gonococci and meningococci; it is ineffective against most Gram-negative organisms.

back [AS. *baec*]. 1. Dorsum; posterior aspect. 2. The posterior part of the trunk from the neck to the pelvis.

b. rest. Any device used to support the back in an upright or semireclining position.

hollow b. One with excessive lumbar lordosis.

humpback. One with an abnormal prominence in the dorsal region due to kyphosis or scoliosis. Also called *hunchback*.

poker b. A back stiffened by ankylosing spondylitis.

saddleback. Lordosis.

sway-b. In humans, increased lumbar lordosis with compensatory increased thoracic kyphosis; in horses, sinking of the back or lordosis.

trench b. Dorsolumbar pain and rigidity experienced by troops engaged in trench warfare.

back′ache″ [*baec;* AS. *acan*, to ache]. Pain in the lower lumbar or lumbosacral regions of the back. Also called *lumbago, lumbosacral pain.*

back′bone″ [*baec;* AS. *bān*, bone]. The vertebral column.

primitive b. The notochord.

back′ward·ness. 1. Retarded growth or mental development due to any cause, as general illness or sense-deprivation, except mental deficiency. 2. Educational retardation due to extrinsic causes. —**backward,** *adj.*

Bact. Abbreviation for *Bacterium.*

bac″te·re′mi·a [G. *baktērion*, dim. of *baktron*, staff; *haima*, blood]. The presence of bacteria in the blood.

bac·te′ri·a (sing. *bacterium*) [*baktērion*]. 1. Formerly, the schizomycetes. 2. Large groups of unicellular, vegetable microorganisms existing morphologically as oval or spherical cells (cocci), rods (bacilli), spirals (spirilla), and a smaller group of comma-shaped organisms (vibrios). The first two forms occur singly or are grouped in pairs (diplococci), or chains (streptococci). Some cocci also appear in clusters. Bacteria are aerobic, requiring free oxygen, or anaerobic, living without oxygen. Some can flourish under both conditions, being facultative aerobes or anaerobes. The cells are either motile or nonmotile and exist as parasites on living hosts, or as saprophytes on dead hosts, some being facultative parasites while others are true parasites. A relatively small group is pathogenic, causing disease, while most are nonpathogenic. The organisms react differently to Gram's stain, being Gram-positive when they retain the stain, and Gram-negative when they decolorize. A few are acid-fast, retaining stain even when subjected to acid-alcohol. Some bacteria cause fermentation (zymogenic), others produce pigment (chromogenic), while another group produces gas (aerogenic). See bacterial *variation, colony.* See Table of the Most Common Microorganisms Pathogenic to Man in the Appendix. See Plate 30. —**bacterial,** *adj.*

cold-growing b. Psychrophilic bacteria; they develop optimally at 15°–20° C.

Bac·te″ri·a′ce·ae (back·teer″ee·ay′see·ee, back″-teer·ee·) [*baktērion*]. A family of Eubacteriales containing one genus: *Bacterium.*

bac·te′ri·cide (back·teer′i·side, ·terr′i·side, ·terr′i-sid) [*baktērion;* L. *caedere*, to kill]. An agent that destroys bacteria. —**bactericid′al,** *adj.*

bac″te·ri·ci′din, bac″te·ri·o·ci′din. An antibody that in the presence of complement kills bacteria.

bac′te·rid [*baktērion*]. A cutaneous hypersensitivity reaction, often limited to the hands and feet, due to absorption from a focus of bacterial infection. The mechanism is believed to be of infectious-allergic nature.

pustular b. See *pustulosis palmaris et plantaris.*

bac·te′ri·form. See *bacterioid.*

bac·te′ri·o-, bac·te′ri-, bac′te·ri- [*baktērion*]. A combining form denoting *relation to bacteria, bacterial.*

bac·ter″i·o·chlor′o·phyll. A pigment, similar in structure and function to green plant chlorophyll, found in the photosynthetic nonsulfur purple bacteria *Athiorhodaceae* and sulfur purple bacteria *Thiorhodaceae.*

bac·te″ri·o·ci′din [*baktērion;* L. *caedere*, to kill]. See *bactericidin.*

bac·te″ri·oc′la·sis [*baktērion;* G. *klasis*, a breaking]. The destruction or fragmentation of bacteria, a phenomenon similar to bacteriolysis by bacteriophage.

bac·te″ri·o·er′y·thrin [*baktērion;* G. *erythros*, red]. A red pigment present in certain bacteria.

bac·te″ri·o·flu″o·res′cin [*baktērion;* L. *fluere*, to flow]. A fluorescent coloring matter produced by the action of certain bacteria.

bac·te″ri·o·gen′ic, bac·te″ri·og′e·nous (back-teer″ee·odj′i·nus) [*baktērion;* G. *genesthai*, from *gignesthai*, to be produced]. Caused by bacteria; of bacterial origin.

bac·te″ri·o·he″mo·ly′sin, bac·te″ri·o·hae″mo-ly′sin (·hee″mo·lye′sin, ·hem″o·, ·hem·ol′i·sin) [*baktērion;* G. *haima*, blood; *lysis*, a loosing]. A very unstable substance which liberates hemoglobin from the red blood cells, and is formed in the body by bacterial action, as *streptolysins, staphylolysins, tetanolysins*, etc. A single bacterial strain may produce multiple hemolysins.

bac·te′ri·oid [*baktērion;* G. *eidos*, form]. A structure or organism resembling a bacterium. —**bacter′-ioid,** *adj.*

bac·te″ri·ol′o·gist [*baktērion;* G. *logos*, word; *-istes*, agent]. One versed in bacteriology. One whose profession is the study and practice of bacteriology.

bac·te″ri·ol′o·gy [*baktērion; logos*]. The science and study of bacteria. —**bacteriolog′ic,** *adj.*

bac·te″ri·o·ly′sin (back·teer″ee·o·lye′sin, ·ol′i·sin, back″teer·ee·ol′i·sin) [*baktērion;* G. *lysis*, a loosing]. A specific antibody which, in cooperation with other substances (complements), is capable of causing the dissolution of the homologous bacterium.

bac·te″ri·ol′y·sis [*baktērion; lysis*]. The intracellular or extracellular dissolution of bacteria. When mediated by a specific antibody and complement, it is called *immune bacteriolysis.* —**bacteriolyt′ic,** *adj.*

bac·te′ri·o·phage (back·teer′ee·o·faydj, ·o·fahzh″) [*baktērion;* G. *phagein*, to eat]. One of a group of viruses infecting bacteria. In some cases the infection results in lysis of the bacterial cell. —**bacteriophag′ic,** *adj.;* **bacterioph′agy,** *n.*

bac·te″ri·o·pha·gol′o·gy [*baktērion; phagein;* G. *logos*, word]. The study of bacteriophage in all its relations. Syn., *protobiology.*

bac·te″ri·o·pho′bi·a [*baktērion;* G. *phobos*, fear]. A morbid dread of bacteria or other microorganisms.

bac·te″ri·o·pro′te·in [*baktērion;* G. *prōtos*, first]. Any one of a number of protein substances contained in bacteria, often the cause of fever, inflammation, and suppuration.

bac·te″ri·op′so·nin [*baktērion;* G. *opsōnein*, to buy victuals]. An opsonin which acts upon bacteria, as distinguished from one affecting erythrocytes. —**bacteriopson'ic,** *adj.*

bac·te"ri·os'co·py [*baktērion;* G. *skopein,* to examine]. The microscopic study of bacteria. —**bacterioscop'ic,** *adj.*

bac·te"ri·os'ta·sis (back·teer"ee·os'tuh·sis, ·o·stay'sis) [*baktērion;* G. *stasis,* a standing still]. Arrest or hindrance of the growth of bacteria. —**bacteriostat'ic,** *adj.*

bac·te'ri·o·stat" [*baktērion; stasis*]. Any agent which arrests or hinders the growth of bacteria.

bac·te"ri·o·ther'a·py [*baktērion;* G. *therapeia,* treatment]. The treatment of disease by the introduction of bacteria or their products into the system. —**bacteriotherapeu'tic,** *adj.*

bac·te"ri·o·tox'in [*baktērion;* G. *toxikon,* poison]. 1. A toxin destructive to bacteria. 2. A toxin produced by bacteria. —**bacteriotoxic,** *adj.*

bac·te"ri·o·trop'ic [*baktērion;* G. *tropē,* a turning]. Denoting substances which render bacteria susceptible to phagocytosis.

bac·te"ri·ot'ro·pin [*baktērion; tropē*]. An immune opsonin; an antibody aiding the phagocytic action of certain cells, as leukocytes.

Bac·te'ri·um [*baktērion*]. A genus of the Bacteriaceae. Abbreviated, Bact.

Bact. aceti. Acetobacter aceti.

Bact. aerogenes. Synonym for *Aerobacter aerogenes.*

Bact. alkalescens. Synonym for *Shigella alkalescens.*

Bact. ambiguum. Synonym for *Shigella ambigua.*

Bact. avisepticum. Synonym for *Pasteurella avicida.*

Bact. bovisepticum. Synonym for *Pasteurella boviseptica.*

Bact. cholerae-suis. Synonym for *Salmonella choleraesuis.*

Bact. coli. Synonym for *Escherichia coli.*

Bact. dispar. Synonym for *Shigella madampensis.*

Bact. dysenteriae. Synonym for *Shigella dysenteriae.*

Bact. enteritidis. *Salmonella enteritidis.*

Bact. flexneri. Synonym for *Shigella paradysenteriae.*

Bact. friedländeri. Synonym for *Klebsiella pneumoniae.*

Bact. fusiformis. Synonym for *Fusobacterium plauti-vincenti.*

Bact. lactis aerogenes. Synonym for *Aerobacter aerogenes.*

Bact. monocytogenes. Synonym for *Listeria monocytogenes.*

Bact. paradysenteriae. Synonym for *Shigella paradysenteriae.*

Bact. paratyphosum A. Old term for *Salmonella paratyphi.*

Bact. paratyphosum B. Old term for *Salmonella schottmulleri.*

Bact. paratyphosum C. Old term for *Salmonella hirschfeldii.*

Bact. pneumoniae. Synonym for *Klebsiella pneumoniae.*

Bact. shigae. Synonym for *Shigella dysenteriae.*

Bact. sonnei. Synonym for *Shigella sonnei.*

Bact. suipestifer. Synonym for *Salmonella cholerae-suis.*

Bact. suisepticum. Synonym for *Pasteurella suiseptica.*

Bact. tularense. Synonym for *Pasteurella tularensis.*

Bact. typhimurium. Synonym for *Salmonella typhimurium.*

Bact. typhosum. Synonym for *Eberthella typhosa.*

bac·te'ri·um (pl. *bacteria*). See *bacteria.*

bac·te"ri·u'ri·a [*baktērion;* G. *ouron,* urine]. The presence of bacteria in the urine.

bac'ter·oid [*baktērion;* G. *eidos,* form]. A bacterium modified in form or structure. —**bac'teroid,** *adj.*

Bac"ter·o'i·des. A genus of obligate anaerobic, nonsporogenous Gram-negative bacilli, with rounded ends, which may be normal inhabitants of the genital, intestinal, and respiratory tracts, but may also cause severe infections, as, for example, *B. fundiliformis.*

B. fragilis. A species of *Bacteroides* found in some cases of appendicitis, lung gangrene, pelvic abscess, hepatic abscess, septicemia, and urinary-tract infection.

B. fundiliformis. An exceedingly pleomorphic, filamentous, often spindle-shaped rod, found in association with septicemias, puerperal infection, liver abscess, etc.

B. melaninogenicus. A species of *Bacteroides* found in the mouth, urine, feces, abdominal wounds, puerperal sepsis, focal kidney infections. In culture melanin pigment is produced.

B. pneumosintes. A minute, anaerobic, Gram-negative rod, which passes through Berkefeld V and N candles and has been recovered from nasopharyngeal washings of man. Officially it is classed in the genus *Dialister,* closely related to *Bacteroides.*

bactratycin. Trade-mark for an antibiotic ointment containing tyrothricin.

bael (bell, bay'el) [Hind.]. Bengal quince tree. See *bel.*

Baelz, Erwin von [*German physician,* 1849–1913]. Described the outbreak of beriberi (kakke) in Tokyo (1881) in one of the most important contributions to our early knowledge of the disease. His name is also associated with myxadenitis labialis, a disease marked by painless papules on the mucous membranes of the lips, also called *Baelz's disease.*

Baer, Karl Ernst von [*Estonian embryologist and anthropologist,* 1792–1876]. Celebrated as having promulgated, with Pander, the germ-layer theory (1817), and for his discovery of the mammalian ovum (1827). He is regarded as the father of modern embryology and, with Cuvier, is credited as the founder of modern morphology.

Baer's treatment. See under *treatment;* see also maggot *therapy.*

Baeyer, Johann Friedrich Wilhelm Adolf von [*German organic chemist,* 1835–1917]. Known for his discovery of a reaction for glucose, in which indigo is formed on boiling a glucose solution with orthonitrophenylpropionic acid and sodium bicarbonate; if the glucose is in excess, the blue is converted into indigo white. He also discovered a reaction for indole, in which a red liquid is yielded when fuming nitric acid, followed by a potassium nitrite solution, is added to a watery solution of indole (1883). Nobel laureate (1905).

baf·fle. A posterior bulge of the intervertebral disk which may simulate a defect radiographically, but which in reality is only a structural variation.

bag [ME. *bagge*]. 1. Sac or pouch. 2. The scrotum. 3. A cow's udder.

b. of waters. The amniotic sac and fluid which serve during pregnancy to protect the fetus and during labor to dilate the cervix. See *amnion.*

caked b. In cows, an inflammation of the udder.

colostomy b. One of rubber worn as a belt, especially constructed to receive the intestinal excreta from a colostomy opening.

Douglas b. The collecting bag used in open-circuit technique of determining basal metabolic rate. See also Claude Gordon *Douglas.*

ice b. One of rubber to hold cracked ice; used to reduce localized inflammation.

Lyster b. See water-sterilizing *b.*

Politzer b. A waterproof bag used to inflate the middle ear. One end is tightly fixed into one external naris while the other naris is held closed during the act of swallowing water or saying the letter *k.*

water-sterilizing b. *In military medicine,* a heavy canvas or rubberized-cloth bag for distributing disinfected water for use of troops; water bag: formerly called *Lyster b.*

ba″gas·so′sis, ba″gas·sco′sis [F. *bagasse;* G. *-ōsis,* condition]. A disease of the lungs occurring in workmen who handle bagasse, the dry residue of sugar cane after the juice has been expressed. It is characterized by abrupt onset, dyspnea, cough, fever; there is fine mottling in the roentgenogram, and the presence of small fibrils of sugar cane in the lungs. Also called *bagasse disease.*

Bag′dad boil. See *oriental sore.*

Ba·hi′a ul′cer (buh·high′uh, bah·ee′ah). See *leishmaniasis* americana.

Baillarger, Jules Gabriel François [*French neurologist,* 1809–90]. His name is associated with the white bands in the layer of large pyramidal cells of the cortex cerebri; he is also known for his sign, a difference in the size of the pupils noted in dementia paralytica. He pointed out that patients with aphasia who had lost the power of voluntary speech retained certain automatic expressions not always employed correctly; this is known as *Baillarger's principle.*

Baillou, Guillaume de (Ballonius) [*French physician,* 1538–1616]. Considered the first epidemiologist. In one posthumous publication (1640) he gave the first clear account of whooping cough, and in another (1642) apparently introduced the term rheumatism into the language. Advocated tracheotomy in diphtheria.

Bainbridge reflex. See under *reflex.*

Baker, William Morrant [*English surgeon,* 1839–96]. Described erythema serpens or erysipeloid (1873). His name is also associated with inflammation of the popliteal bursa, called *popliteal bursitis, Baker's cyst.*

bak′er [AS. *bacan*]. *In medicine,* a heating chamber for applying dry heat to a part: used especially in joint diseases. —**bake,** *v.*

bak′ing so′da. Sodium bicarbonate.

BAL $CH_2SH.CHSH.CH_2OH$. British anti-lewisite. 2,3-Dimercaptopropanol. Developed during World War II as an effective therapeutic agent against both the local and systemic actions of certain arsenic war gases; it is also effective as an antidote to arsenic poisoning following antisyphilitic therapy. It is useful as an antidote also to mercury and certain other metals. It is also used in the treatment of polyarteritis nodosa when it develops as a result of antisyphilitic treatment with organic arsenic drugs; it is administered intramuscularly as a 5–10% solution in peanut oil and benzyl benzoate. Syn., *dimercaprol, dithiopropanol-1.*

bal′ance [L. *bilanx,* having two scales]. 1. A device for weighing. 2. The normal, harmonious interaction between related parts and organs of the body; equilibrium.

acid-base b. The state of equilibrium of acids and bases maintained by physiologic processes, e.g., respiration, elimination and manufacture of buffers which keep the pH of the body constant: distinguished from the state of an excess of acid (acidosis) or an excess of alkali (alkalosis).

allergic b. A state of equilibrium between the patient and his environment, in which the amount of a specific noxious allergen does not exceed the patient's threshold of allergic tolerance.

calcium b. A state of equilibrium in the body between the outgo and intake of calcium, maintained by physiologic processes.

electromagnetic b. Apparatus for measuring electromagnetic forces by balancing them against gravity.

energy b. The relation of the amount of utilizable energy taken into the body to that which is employed for internal work, external work, and the growth and repair of tissues.

fluid b. A state of equilibrium in the body between the outgo and intake of water. Optimum water content is maintained by a special physiologic water-regulating mechanism.

heat b. The relation of the amount of heat produced in the body to that which is lost.

hemogenic-hemolytic b. The balance in the body between the production of normal erythrocytes and their destruction, which maintains the count and the hemoglobin at the optimum level by physiologic processes.

mineral b. The state of equilibrium of the body, maintained by physiologic processes, between the outgo and intake of any mineral or of any particular mineral constituent such as iron, calcium, or sodium.

nitrogen b. In a normal adult, the nitrogen excreted equals the nitrogen intake in the form of food. Syn., *nitrogen equilibrium.*

thermic b. See *bolometer.*

torsion b. Instrument which measures small torques by their torsional effect upon elastic fibers or wires.

vitamin b. The state of the body maintained by physiologic processes whereby there is an optimum content of the various vitamins in the body.

water b. See fluid *b.*

bal′a·nism [G. *balanos,* acorn, glans penis, suppository]. The application of a pessary or suppository. *Obs.*

bal″a·ni′tis [*balanos;* G. *-itis,* inflammation]. Inflammation of the glans penis, or glans clitoridis.

b. xerotica obliterans. A chronic, progressive, atrophic, sclerosing process of the penis which may eventuate in urethral stenosis or in epithelioma. The condition corresponds to kraurosis of the vulva in the female.

phagedenic b. A destructive balanitis leading to necrosis of the glans penis.

bal′a·no-, balan- [*balanos*]. A combining form meaning *relating to the glans penis* or *glans clitoridis.*

bal″a·no·chlam″y·di′tis [*balanos;* G. *chlamys,* cloak; *-itis,* inflammation]. Inflammation of the glans and prepuce of the clitoris: frequently called *balanitis.*

bal′a·no·plas″ty [*balanos;* G. *plassein,* to form]. Plastic surgery of the glans penis.

bal″a·no·pos·thi′tis [*balanos;* G. *posthē,* membrum virile; *-itis*]. Inflammation of the glans penis and of the prepuce.

bal″a·no·pre·pu′tial [*balanos;* L. *praeputium,* prepuce]. Relating to the glans penis and the prepuce.

bal″a·nor·rha′gi·a (bal″uh·no·ray′juh, ·jee·uh, ·radj′uh, ·radj′ee·uh) [*balanos;* G. *rhegnynai,* to burst forth]. Hemorrhage from the glans penis.

bal″an·or·rhe′a, bal″an·or·rhoe′a [*balanos;* G. *rhoia,* a flow]. Purulent balanitis.

bal″an·ti·di′a·sis. See balantidial *colitis.*

Bal″an·tid′i·um [G. *balantidion,* little bag]. A genus of ciliated, parasitic protozoans.

B. coli. A common parasite of the hog; occasionally infests man, causing severe dysentery

bal′a·nus [G. *balanos*, acorn]. The glans of the penis or of the clitoris.

Balard, Antoine Jérôme [*French chemist*, 1802–76]. Discoverer of amyl nitrite (1844) and also of bromine.

balarsen. Trade-mark for the arsenical compound *arsthinol*.

bal′ash. See *bejel*.

bald′ness [ME. *balled*]. Loss or absence of hair. Syn., *acomia, alopecia, calvities*. —**bald,** *adj*.

Baldwin, James Fairchild [*American gynecologist*, 1850–1936]. Remembered for his procedure for the formation of an artificial vagina by the transplantation of a loop of intestine between the urinary bladder and rectum.

Baldy, John Montgomery [*American gynecologist*, 1860–1934]. Known for his description of a uterine suspension operation in which the round ligaments are brought backward through an incision in the broad ligaments and plicated on the posterior aspect of the uterus: often referred to as *Baldy-Webster operation*. Said to have performed the first gastrectomy in America (1897).

Balfour, Andrew [*Scottish physician in Egypt*, 1873–1931]. Discoverer of a small, highly refractive, granular body observed in the red corpuscles of diseased fowls; this has received his name. It is thought to be a protozoan.

Balfour, Donald Church [*American surgeon*, 1882–]. Known for his association with the Mayo brothers and for his many contributions to the knowledge of surgery of the stomach and duodenum, including his technic of enteroenterostomy for the avoidance of the so-called vicious circle. Active in the development of educational features of the Mayo Foundation.

Balfour, Francis Maitland [*English embryologist*, 1851–82]. One of the greatest of comparative embryologists. His treatise on embryology (1880–81) contains the results of a vast amount of investigation and is regarded as a classic.

Bal′kan frame. An overhead quadrilateral supported by uprights fastened to the bedposts; used to suspend immobilized fractured limbs and to apply continuous traction by weights and pulleys.

Ball, Charles Bent [*Irish surgeon*, 1851–1916]. Described many procedures, including technics for iliac colostomy, for inguinal hernia, and for the relief of pruritus ani by division of the nerve filaments which supply the affected skin.

ball [ME. *bal*]. 1. An object having a globular or spherical shape. 2. *In anatomy*, any globular part. 3. *In veterinary medicine*, a pill or bolus.

chondrin balls. Isogenous cell groups in cartilage and their surrounding basophil matrix.

Ballance, Charles Alfred [*English surgeon*, 1856–1936]. One of the leaders of surgery in Great Britain. Remembered for his treatise on the ligation of the great arteries (1891); for his operation for anastomosis of the hypoglossal with the facial nerve; and for his description of a sign in rupture of the spleen. See Ballance's *sign*.

Ballet, Gilbert [*French ophthalmologist*, 1853–1916]. Remembered for his description of ophthalmoplegia externa. He also described a sign observed in hysteria and exophthalmic goiter: the loss of voluntary movements of the eyeball with preservation of the automatic movements and pupillary reflexes.

Ballingall, George [*English surgeon*, 1780–1855]. Remembered for his description of madura foot, called *Ballingall's disease*.

bal′lism (bal′iz·um), **bal·lis′mus** (ba·liz′mus) [G. *ballismos*, a jumping about]. 1. Chorea characterized by jerky, swinging movements of arms and legs. 2. Paralysis agitans. *Obs*.

bal·lis″to·car′di·o·graph [L. *ballista*, military machine for projectiles; G. *kardia*, heart; *graphein*, to write]. An instrument which records the movements of the body caused by the impact and recoil of the blood after ejection from the ventricles: used in estimating the cardiac output. The record made by this instrument is called a **ballistocardiogram.**

bal·lis″to·pho′bi·a [*ballista;* G. *phobos*, fear]. Morbid fear of projectiles or missiles.

ball mill. A grinding instrument used for breaking up cells, such as yeast cells.

Ballonius. See *Baillou*.

bal·lonne·ment′ (bal·awn·mahn′. *See* Notes § 35) [F.]. Ballooning.

bal·loon′ing [F. *ballon*, from It. *balla, palla*, ball]. Surgical distention of any body cavity by air or other means for examination or therapeutic purposes.

bal·lotte·ment′ (bal·awt·mahn′, ba·lot′munt. *See* Notes § 35) [F., a shaking about]. A diagnostic sign of pregnancy. The sensation perceived by the finger inserted into the vagina when sudden pressure applied through the uterine wall to the fetus is followed by its rise and rebound through the amniotic fluid. —**ballot′table,** *adj*.

b. of patella. A tapping sensation elicited when the patella is depressed against the femur in the presence of a knee-joint cavity distended with fluid.

cephalic b. The rebound of the fetal head against the hand when depressed through the abdominal wall: also called *abdominal b., external b.*

indirect b. See cephalic *b.*

internal b. See vaginal *b.*

ocular b. The falling of opaque particles in a vitreous body after the eye has moved.

renal b. The palpating of the kidney by pushing it suddenly forward with one hand against the other hand pressed into the abdominal wall.

vaginal b. The rebound of the fetus against a finger inserted into the vagina: also called *internal b.*

balm (bahm) [G. *balsamon*, balsam tree]. A popular synonym of balsam.

Gilead b. An oleoresin from the *Commiphora opobalsamum*.

Balme, Paul Jean (Balne) [*French physician*, 1857–]. His name is preserved in connection with a peculiar cough occurring in nasopharyngeal obstruction only when the patient is in the recumbent position.

bal″ne·ol′o·gy. The science of baths and their therapeutic uses. Also see *balneotherapy, bath.*

bal″ne·o·ther′a·py [L. *balneum*, bath; G. *therapeia*, treatment]. Therapeutic use of baths.

Baló, József [*Hungarian physician*, contemporary]. Described periaxial concentric encephalitis (1927), called *Baló's disease.*

balopticon. Trade-mark for a projector designed to throw on a screen magnified pictures of opaque objects.

bal′sam (bawl′sum) [G. *balsamon*, balsam tree]. 1. The resinous, aromatic, liquid, or semisolid substance obtained from certain trees by natural exudation or by artificial extraction and consisting chiefly of resins and volatile oils containing esters of cinnamic and benzoic acids. 2. The term is also applied to certain substances which are not true balsams in that they contain no cinnamic or benzoic acid, as copaiba balsam. —**bal·sam′ic,** *adj*.

b. apple. *Momordica balsamina*, and its warty, gourdlike fruit. It is purgative owing to the presence of momordicin, probably identical with elaterin.

b. tree. The *Abies balsamea* which yields Canada balsam.

b. vine. See *b.* apple.

Brazilian b. An oleoresin from *Myroxylon peruiferum;* resembles Peruvian balsam.

Canada b. A turpentine gathered from the natural blisters of the bark of *Abies balsamea;* used as a mounting medium by microscopists. Syn., *Canada turpentine.*

Cebur b. See Tagulaway *b.*

copaiba b. See *copaiba.*

friar's b. Compound benzoin tincture. Also called *Turlington's b.*

Gilead b. The resinous juice of *Commiphora opobalsum*, which grows on the shores of the Red Sea. Syn., *Gilead balm, Mecca b., opobalsam.*

gurjun b. An oleoresin from the East Indian tree, *Dipterocarpus turbinatus,* and other species: formerly used in gonorrhea and coughs. Syn., *gurjun oil, wood oil.*

Mecca b. See Gilead *b.*

Peruvian b. (*balsamum peruvianum*). That obtained from *Myroxylon Pereirae.* It contains not less than 53% of balsamic esters. A stimulating and antiseptic dressing for indolent ulcers, local tuberculosis, wounds, etc. It has been used as a stimulating expectorant in asthma and chronic bronchitis administered in emulsion. Also called *b. of Peru, Indian b.*

sulfur b. A mixture of eight parts of olive oil and one part of sublimed sulfur heated together. Linseed oil may be substituted for olive oil.

Tagulaway b., Tagulavay b. A yellow oil prepared in the Philippines by boiling the bark and twigs of *Parameria vulneraria* in coconut oil; used as a vulnerary and in skin diseases. Syn., *Cebur b.*

tolu b. (*balsamum tolutanum*). One obtained from *Myroxylon balsamum.* It is a feeble stimulant and expectorant. The syrup (*syrupus balsami tolutani*) is popular in cough mixtures because of its agreeable flavor.

white b. A semifluid substance obtained from the fruit of *Myroxylon Pereirae,* which also yields Peruvian balsam.

bal'sam·weed". The *Impatiens balsamina,* or touch-me-not.

Balser, W. [*German physician,* nineteenth century]. Described fat necrosis in acute pancreatitis (1882), called *Balser's fat necrosis.*

Bamberger, Eugen [*Austrian physician,* 1858–1921]. Described hypertrophic pulmonary osteoarthropathy (1889), called *Marie-Bamberger disease.*

Bamberger, Heinrich von [*Austrian physician,* 1822–88]. Associated with pericardial pseudocirrhosis of the liver, called *Bamberger's disease, Pick's disease.*

Banckes, Rycharde [*English physician,* sixteenth century]. Author of the earliest herbal printed in English (1525), called *Banckes' Herbal.*

Bancroft's filariasis. See *wuchereriasis.*

band [ME. *band*]. 1. That which binds. 2. *In zoology,* a stripe. 3. *In anatomy,* a ligament or long slender muscle. Also a disk of a striated muscle fiber as seen in longitudinal section. 4. *In dentistry,* a strip of thin metal, formed into a hoop, for encircling a natural tooth or its root.

absorption bands. See under *absorption.*

adjustable b. *In dentistry,* one provided with an adjusting screw or similar mechanism to permit alteration in size.

amniotic b. A fibrous band connecting amnion and fetus.

anchor b. That applied to one tooth as an anchor to aid in moving a second tooth.

anogenital b. The perineal raphe.

astigmatic b. In refraction, an apparent band of light seen under retinoscopy when one of the chief meridians is neutralized.

atrioventricular b. The atrioventricular bundle.

b. of Giacomini. See *frenulum* of Giacomini.

clamp b. A device made from a flat piece of metal for encircling a tooth; the ends are held in place by a nut and screw.

diagonal b. of Broca. See diagonal *gyrus.*

fetoamniotic b. See amniotic *b.*

furrowed b. A small band of gray matter uniting the uvula cerebelli with the cerebellar tonsils.

iliotibial b. A thickened portion of the fascia lata extending from the lateral condyle of the tibia to the iliac crest. See Plate 4.

lilac b. A dark violaceous strip forming a well-defined crescent behind the free border of the nail and parallel with it: said to be due to syphilis.

lip furrow b. See vestibular *lamina.*

mesocolic b. A longitudinal muscle band corresponding to the insertion of the mesocolon. Syn., *mesocolic taenia.*

moderator b. A muscle band in the right ventricle of the heart, between the interventricular septum and the base of the right anterior papillary muscle, transporting a fascicle of the atrioventricular bundle (of His). It was once thought to prevent overdistention of the right ventricle.

retention b. A thickening of the mesentery which fixes the cranial and the caudal end of the midgut to the dorsal abdominal wall, thus preventing herniation of the foregut and hindgut of the embryo.

seamless b. A nonadjustable ferrule stamped from a piece of metal, to be used as a plain or anchor band.

sternal b. One of the paired mesenchymal anlages of the sternal bones.

suppressor b. Any area on the cerebral cortex which suppresses the motor or projection response to stimulation of any other part of the cortex and its after-discharge. Narrow areas of cortex have been discovered by local stimulation with strychnine near Brodmann's areas 4, 8, 24, 2, and 19, and have been named areas 4s, 8s, 24s, 2s, and 19s. Also called *suppressor area.*

supraorbital bands. The embryonal thickenings above the eyes and to the outer side of them.

Z b. See Z *disk.*

band'age [F., from *bande*, a strip]. A strip of gauze, muslin, flannel, or other material, usually in the form of a roll, of various widths and lengths, but sometimes triangular or tailed. The chief functions of a bandage are: to hold dressings in place, to apply pressure, to immobilize a part, to support a dependent or injured part, to obliterate tissue cavities, and to check hemorrhage. See Plates 33, 34.

adhesive b. One composed of adhesive plaster or moleskin for immobilization or support of a part.

capeline b. One resembling a cap or hood, suitable for the head, shoulder, or amputation stump.

circular b. One in which the bandage is wound about the limb or part.

cohesive b. One of a number of bandages, sold under various trade names, which has the property of sticking to itself, but not to other substances.

compression b. One in which a high degree of compression is exerted on the tissues in order to shrink a part, as an amputation stump.

cravat b. A triangular bandage folded to form a band and wound about a part.

demigauntlet b. A bandage covering the wrist and hand but not the fingers.

double-headed roller b. A strip of material rolled from both ends to meet in the middle.

elastic b. One of rubber or woven elastic material. Used to exert continuous pressure on swollen extremities or joints, fractured ribs, the chest, or varicose veins.

Esmarch's b. A live rubber compression bandage with tourniquet, used to render a limb bloodless.

figure-of-eight b. One in which the successive turns cross like the figure eight. See Plates 33, 34.

four-tailed b. A strip of cloth with the ends split, used to cover prominent parts, as the elbow, chin, nose, or knee. See Plate 34.

gauntlet b. One which covers the hands and fingers, like a glove.

hammock b. One which retains scalp dressings. The dressings are covered by a broad strip of gauze brought down over the ears and anchored by a circular bandage around the head. The ends of the broad strip are then turned up over the circular bandage and secured by a few more turns.

immovable b. A bandage for immobilizing any part.

impregnated b. A wide-meshed bandage impregnated with such substances as plaster of Paris, sodium silicate, starch, or dextrin, put up in rolls and used for stiffening, immobilizing, and making molds of various parts of the body.

jelly b. A bandage used in treating varicose veins and ulcers. See *Unna's paste boot.*

many-tailed b. An irregular bandage having four or more cut or torn ends which are tied together to hold a dressing.

oblique b. A bandage which covers the part by oblique turns.

plaster b. An impregnated bandage.

pressure b. One used to stop hemorrhage or support varicose veins.

quadrangular b. A towel or large handkerchief, folded variously and used as a bandage.

recurrent b. One in which each turn comes back to the point of starting; used in bandaging the head or an amputation stump. See Plate 34.

reversed b. An oblique bandage applied to a limb; for each turn, the roll is given a half twist to make a snug fit over the expanded part of the limb.

roller b. A long strip of material from one-half to six inches in width, rolled on its short axis.

rubber b. An elastic bandage.

scultetus b. One used in compound fractures, usually of the lower extremity, composed of short pieces which overlap each other, thereby permitting their removal without movement of the limb. Also called *Scultet's b.*

silica b. A bandage impregnated with sodium silicate.

spica b. One with successive turns and crosses, as in a modified figure-of-eight bandage; so called because it resembles the folded edges of the husk of an ear of corn. See Plate 34.

spiral b. An oblique bandage. See Plate 33.

spiral reverse b. One in which the oblique turns are reversed and folded back at each turn, to adapt the bandage to the part. See Plate 33.

suspensory b. One for supporting the scrotum.

T b. A bandage with three arms which form a letter T: especially used about the waist and the perineum to hold a dressing.

triangular b. One made from a square of muslin cut diagonally to make two triangles, and used as a sling, and for inclusive dressing of a part, as a whole hand.

Velpeau's b. One which completely fixes the arm against the side, with the forearm flexed at an angle of 45°, the palm resting upon the midclavicular region opposite. By successive turns about the body, the bandage envelops the shoulder, arm, forearm, and hand. See Plate 34.

Bandl, Ludwig (1842–1892). German obstetrician who described a contraction ring resulting from obstructed labor. See retraction *ring,* 2.

bang, bangue. See *cannabis.*

Bang's disease. See under *disease.*

ban″i·ster′ine (ban″i·sterr′een, ·in, ba·nis′tuh·reen, ·rin). An alkaloid from ayahuasca, or *Banisteria caapi,* which has been employed in lethargic encephalitis.

bank [It. *banca,* bench]. A reserve stock of body fluids and parts usually maintained at a hospital or Red Cross Center under suitable storage facilities. The stocks kept now are: whole blood, plasma, blood vessels, arteries, nerves, bones, cartilage, and corneas (for corneal grafts).

Bannister, Henry Martyn [*American physician,* 1844–1920]. His name was once associated with angioneurotic edema.

banthine bromide. Trade-marked name for β-diethylaminoethylxanthene-9-carboxylate methobromide, an anticholinergic drug. See *methantheline bromide.*

Banti, Guido [*Italian physician,* 1852–1925]. Universally remembered for his description of splenomegaly of undetermined origin, which still bears his name (1882). It is often referred to as a syndrome, and is characterized by splenomegaly, anemia, leukopenia, hemorrhage, and cirrhosis of the liver: called *Banti's disease.* See chronic congestive *splenomegaly.*

Banting, Frederick Grant [*Canadian physician,* 1891–1941]. With C. H. Best, working in association with J. J. R. Macleod, discovered insulin (1922), and with Best, W. R. Campbell, J. B. Collip, and A. A. Fletcher, first used it in the treatment of diabetes (1922). Nobel laureate with Macleod (1923).

Banting, William [*English undertaker and coffin maker,* 1797–1878]. Celebrated for his advocacy of the withdrawal of sweets and carbohydrates in cases of obesity. Wrote his famous letter on reducing corpulence in 1863. His name has remained in the language (*Bantingism*) as synonymous with dieting for obesity.

bap·tis′i·a (bap·tizh′uh, ·tiz′ee·uh) [G. *baptizein,* to dip]. Wild indigo. The dried root of *Baptisia tinctoria,* containing baptisin, cytisine, and a blue dye. It was formerly used in the treatment of ulcers, as a gargle, and in some tooth powders.

bap′ti·sin (bap′ti·zin, ·sin). 1. A concentrate prepared from *Baptisia tinctoria;* antiseptic, purgative, ecbolic, resolvent. 2. A bitter glycoside obtainable from the plant *Baptisia tinctoria;* it has little medicinal activity.

bap″ti·tox′ine (bap″ti·tock′sin, ·seen). See *cytisine.*

bar [OF. *barre,* from LL. *barra*]. 1. A band or stripe. 2. A fetal or visceral arch. 3. That part of the horse's upper jaw which has no teeth. 4. That portion of the wall of a horse's hoof reflected sharply anteriorly onto the sole from each buttress. The two bars are separated by the frog. 5. A unit of atmospheric pressure representing one megadyne per square centimeter. 6. *In prosthetic dentistry,* a piece of metal connecting two parts of a bridge or partial denture. 7. *In orthodontics,* a wire or rod affixed to one or more teeth in the dental arch. The term has been applied to parts of various obsolete appliances; present use is limited to space maintainers.

arch b. *In orthodontics,* term used for a wire extending from one side of the dental arch to the other, to which intervening teeth can be attached.

b. of bladder. The transverse ridge joining the openings of the ureters on the inner surface of the urinary bladder; it forms the posterior boundary of the trigone: also called *Mercier's b.*

episternal b. See episternal *cartilage.*

hyoid bars. The pair of cartilaginous plates forming the second visceral arch; the hyoid arch.

hypochordal b. Hyoid arch.

interureteric b. Bar of the bladder.

lingual b. A metal bar on the lingual side of the mandibular arch, connecting the two saddles of a mandibular partial denture.

Meckel's b. Old term for mandibular *arch.*

median b. Contracture of the vesical neck, or constriction of the prostatic urethra, caused by prostatic hyperplasia (*glandular bar*) or by overgrowth of connective tissue across the posterior lip of the vesical orifice or of the vesical trigone (*fibrous bar*). A "muscular" bar due to congenital hypertrophy of muscle at the vesical neck, and a "prefibrotic" bar due to inflammatory changes associated with urethritis and prostatitis, have also been described.

Mercier's b. See *b.* of the bladder.

palatal b. A piece of metal extended across a portion of the hard palate for the purpose of joining and strengthening the two sections of a maxillary partial denture.

sternal b. One of the paired cartilaginous bars in the embryo that fuse to form the sternum.

terminal b. A thickening of the intercellular cement between the ends of epithelial cells.

bar″aes·the′si·a. See *baresthesia.*

bar″ag·no′sis (bar″ag·no′sis) [G. *baros*, weight; *a-*, not; *gnōsis*, knowledge]. Loss of the perception of weight; loss of barognosis.

baralyme. Trade name for a mixture of barium and calcium hydroxide: used to absorb CO_2 in closed inhalation anesthesia.

Bárány, Robert [*Austrian physician*, 1876–1936]. Noted for his studies of the pathology and physiology of the vestibular apparatus. Nobel laureate (1914). He introduced a number of ingenious tests, such as the caloric differential test for labyrinthine function and the pointing test for circumscribed cerebellar lesions. See caloric *test*, Bárány's pointing *test.* His name is associated with a syndrome characterized by unilateral deafness, vertigo, and pain in the occipital region. A special chair for testing air pilots has received his name.

barb [L. *barba*, beard]. *In dentistry*, one of the backward-projecting points on the side of a broach which opposes the withdrawal of the instrument, but does not interfere with its forward motion.

bar′ba [L.]. 1. The beard. 2. A hair of the beard. 3. The heavy beard which appears after puberty as a secondary male sex character [BNA].

bar·bal′o·in. The pentoside chiefly responsible for the purgative action of aloe. See *aloin.*

Barber's method. See under *method.*

Barberio's test. See under *test.*

bar′ber″ry. See *berberis.*

bar′bi·tal (bahr′bi·tol). Diethylmalonylurea. $(C_2H_5)_2$:C.CO.NH.CO.NH.CO. A white, crystalline powder, soluble in 15 parts of alcohol or 130 parts of water; used as hypnotic with prolonged action. Dose, 0.3–0.6 Gm. (5–10 gr.). Psychic habituation may result from its use, and toxic effects are produced by overdosage. Also called *barbitone, diethylbarbituric acid.* Also see *veronal.*

b. sodium (*barbitalum sodicum*). The sodium salt of barbital. It is a white powder soluble in 5 parts of water; aqueous solutions undergo hydrolysis and must, therefore, be frequently prepared. Also called *soluble b., sodium diethylbarbiturate.*

bar′bi·tone. British name for barbital.

bar·bit′u·rate, bar″bi·tu′rate. A general term denoting a derivative of barbituric acid, $C_4H_4O_3N_2$, formed by the substitution of an aliphatic or aromatic group on a carbon or nitrogen atom in the acid. Barbiturates are used in medicine as hypnotic and sedative drugs, but are not analgesics unless administered in relatively large doses. Modifications in their structure influence the power and rapidity of their effects. The therapeutic effects of these drugs are exerted upon the higher centers of the brain, and they do not usually cause injury to the heart, circulation, or kidneys. They are common allergens.

bar″bi·tu′ric ac′id. $C_4H_4O_3N_2$. Malonylurea, the parent compound of the barbiturates.

bar′bi·tu·rism [from L. *Usnea barbata*, the beard lichen; G. *ouron*, urine]. An acute intoxication following an overdose of drugs of the barbiturate group; often the result of attempted suicide. It is characterized by delirium, followed by coma and sometimes death. There are pathologic changes in the tissues; tremor, ataxia, and mental confusion are present, and cutaneous eruptions are sometimes observed.

bar·bo·tage′ (bahr·bo·tahzh′, ·tazh′) [F., from *barboter*, to dabble]. Method of spinal anesthesia; part of the anesthetic solution is injected into the subarachnoid space; spinal fluid is then aspirated into the syringe and reinjected. This may be repeated several times before the entire contents of the syringe is finally injected.

Barcroft, Joseph (1872–1947). English physiologist, known for his fundamental researches on the function of hemoglobin and the transport of respiratory gases in the blood, and for his important contributions to the knowledge of fetal circulation and human adaptation to high altitudes.

Bard, John [*American physician*, 1716–99]. Eminent practitioner remembered for his skill in directing the care of yellow fever. He performed the first successful operation for ectopic pregnancy in America (1759).

Bard, Louis [*Swiss physician*, 1857–1930]. Known for his sign, said to differentiate between organic and congenital nystagmus, the former displaying increased oscillations of the eyeball when the examiner's finger is moved before the eye from right to left and vice versa. In the congenital variety, the oscillations cease under the same conditions. His name is associated also with progressive icterus and cachexia due to primary carcinoma of the head of the pancreas: called *Bard-Pic syndrome.*

Bard, Samuel [*American physician*, 1742–1821]. Son of John Bard. Remembered for his part in founding King's College (later Columbia University) Medical School and for his book on diphtheria, a medical classic (1771).

Bardeleben, Adolf von [*German physician and surgeon*, 1861–1914]. Remembered for his operation for bilateral harelip, with protruding maxilla, in which he divided the vomer subperiosteally before making forcible reduction of the deformity.

Bardeleben, Karl von [*German anatomist*, 1849–1918]. Celebrated for the monumental handbook of anatomy which he edited (1896–1915). Originator of the bandage dressing which incorporates starch and which is used for burns, called *Bardeleben's bandage.*

Bardenheuer, Bernhard [*German surgeon*, 1839–1913]. Known for his numerous operative procedures, especially that for anchoring a floating spleen by making a pocket in the parietal peritoneum (splenopexy).

Bärensprung, Friedrich Wilhelm Felix von [*German dermatologist*, 1822–64]. Described eczema marginatum (1855), called *Bärensprung's disease.*

bar″es·the′si·a (bar″ess·thee′zhuh, ·zee·uh) [G. *baros*, weight; *aisthēsis*, perception]. Perception of weight or pressure; pressure sense.

bar″es·the″si·om′e·ter (bar″ess·thee″zee·om′i-tur) [*baros; aisthēsis;* G. *metron*, a measure]. An instrument for estimating the sensitivity of the weight or pressure sense.

Barfoed's test. See Barfoed's *reagent, test.*

Bargen, Jacob Arnold [*American physician*, 1894–]. Known for his work in diseases of the rectum and colon. Described a diplostreptococcus as a cause of ulcerative colitis (1924).

bar″i·to′sis [G. *baros*, weight; *-ōsis*, condition]. Chronic inflammation of the lungs due to the inhalation of barium: a form of pneumonoconiosis.

ba′ri·um, bar′i·um [G. *barys*, heavy]. Ba = 137.36. A metal belonging to the alkaline earths and occurring in nature only in the form of divalent compounds. All of its soluble salts are poisonous.

b. chloride. $BaCl_2.2H_2O$; a soluble salt, used as a test for sulfates, which it precipitates as barium sulfate. A violent stimulant of all smooth muscles; occasionally used to increase the force of cardiac contraction in atrioventricular dissociation (Adams-Stokes disease). Dose, usually 0.03 Gm. (½ gr.) three or four times daily.

b. hydroxide. $Ba(OH)_2 \cdot 8H_2O$; transparent crystals or masses, soluble in water: used as a chemical reagent.

b. sulfate (*barii sulfas*). $BaSO_4$; a white, odorless, tasteless powder, insoluble in water, employed as an opaque roentgenographic contrast medium.

b. sulfide. BaS; soluble in water, used in depilatories and in luminous paint.

bark [of Scand. origin]. 1. The covering of the wood of exogenous trees; all tissues outside the cambium. 2. Cinchona.

Barker, Arthur Edward James [*English surgeon*, 1850–1916]. Two operations have been described by him. In one, for excision of the talus, the incision runs from just above the tip of the lateral malleolus forward and a little inward, curving toward the dorsum of the foot. The other, for excision of the hip joint, is performed through an anterior incision commencing on the front of the thigh, one-half inch below the anterior superior iliac spine, and running downward and inward for three inches. Both are called *Barker's operation.*

Barker's method. See under *method.*

bar′ley [AS. *baerlic*]. Any cereal grass of the genus *Hordeum*, order Graminales: used as a food, and also in the preparation of malt.

b. water (*decoctum hordei*). A decoction prepared from 2 ounces of pearl barley boiled in 1½ pints of water: used as demulcent and food in children's diarrheas. Dose, 30–120 cc. (1–4 oz.).

pearl b. Husked barley grains, rounded and polished.

Barlow, Thomas [*English physician*, 1845–1945]. Known for his description of infantile scurvy, called *Barlow's disease, Moeller-Barlow disease.*

barn. A unit expressing the probability of a specific nuclear reaction occurring, stated in terms of cross-sectional area. It is equivalent to 10^{-24} sq. cm.

Barnard, Harold Leslie [*English physiologist*, 1868–1908]. With L. E. Hill, introduced a modification of the sphygmomanometer with a pressure gauge (1897).

Barnes, Robert [*English obstetrician*, 1817–1907]. Remembered for his definition of the cervical zone as the lowest fourth of the internal surface of the uterus, and for his description of a curve having for its center the sacral promontory. Known especially for his device, a series of graduated rubber bags for dilating the uterine cervix when labor is to be induced; called *Barnes's bags.*

bar′o- [G. *baros*, weight]. A combining form implying *heaviness.*

bar″o·cep′tor, bar″o·re·cep′tor. See *pressoreceptor.*

bar″o·don·tal′gi·a. Dental pain occurring in individuals exposed to decreased barometric pressures such as occur in high-altitude flying: also called *aerodontalgia.*

bar″og·no′sis [*baros;* G. *gnōsis*, knowledge]. The ability to estimate weight; the perception of weight.

bar′o·graph [*baros;* G. *graphein*, to write]. A self-registering barometer.

bar″o·ma·crom′e·ter [*baros;* G. *makros*, long; *metron*, a measure]. An apparatus to measure the weight and length of infants.

ba·rom′e·ter [*baros; metron*]. An instrument which measures atmospheric pressure; it consists of a capillary tube sealed at one end, filled with mercury, and inverted in a mercury reservoir. At sea level the height of the mercury column normally stands at 760 mm. or 30 inches, rising or falling directly as the atmospheric pressure. —**baro-met′ric,** *adj.;* **barom′etry,** *n.*

aneroid b. A barometer in which changes of pressure are indicated by the collapsing or bulging of a thin, corrugated cover of a partially evacuated metallic box.

bar″o·pho′bi·a [*baros;* G. *phobos*, fear]. A morbid fear of gravity.

bar′o·scope [*baros;* G. *skopein*, to examine]. 1. A sensitive barometer which indicates variations in atmospheric pressure, without accurately weighing them. 2. An instrument for the quantitative determination of urea.

bar″o·si″nus·i′tis. Aerosinusitis.

Ba·ros′ma (ba·roz′muh, ·ros′muh) [G. *barys*, heavy; *osmē*, smell]. A genus of plants of the Rutaceae, native to the Cape of Good Hope and vicinity, several species of which yield the buchu of commerce.

ba·ros′min (ba·roz′min, ·ros′min). 1. A glycoside obtained from buchu and other sources. Syn., *diosmin.* 2. A concentrate prepared from buchu.

bar″o·tal′gi·a. Pain arising in the middle ear caused by an inequality of air pressure between the middle ear and the surrounding atmosphere.

bar″o·ti′tis. Inflammation of the ear, or a part thereof, caused by changes in atmospheric pressure.

b. externa. An acute or chronic, traumatic ear condition resulting in inflammation of the external auditory canal and tympanic membrane, caused by a pressure differential between the external auditory canal and the middle ear; it is usually associated with imperforate plugging of the external ear.

b. media. Aerootitis media.

bar″o·trau′ma [G. *baros*, weight; *trauma*, wound]. Injury of certain organs due to a change in atmospheric pressure or water pressure.

otic b. Term used in England for aerootitis media.

Barraquer, Ignacio [*Spanish ophthalmologist*, 1884–]. Introduced a cataract extraction operation (phacoerisis), in which the lens is removed by suction by means of a special instrument: called *Barraquer's operation.*

Barraquer Roviralta, José Antonio [*Spanish*

physician, b. 1852]. Noted for his description of progressive lipodystrophy, marked by the deposit of fat in the trunk and extremities: called *Barraquer's disease, Barraquer-Simons disease.*

Barré, Jean Alexandre [*French neurologist,* 1880–]. Described a syndrome of diffuse, infectious disease of the nervous system; see Guillain-Barré *syndrome.* Also described a sign of disease of the corticospinal tract; see Barré's *sign.*

barrenness. Sterility in the female. Syn., *agenesia.*

bar'ri·er [F. *barrière,* from *barre,* bar]. An obstacle, barricade, or impediment.

blood-aqueous b. A functional barrier between the blood and aqueous humor: a concept formed to account for the fact that many small molecular electrolytes and all proteins have concentrations in the aqueous humor which vary markedly from those in the blood.

blood-brain b. The functional barrier between the blood supplying the central nervous system and the interstitial spaces of the neural tissue. Its existence depends upon the general property of all capillary walls for selective permeability, and results in physiologic obstruction to the free movement of various types of compounds. Syn. *hematoencephalic b., blood-cortical b.*

blood-cerebrospinal-fluid barriers. The functional barriers between the blood supplying the central nervous system and the cerebrospinal fluid. Varying from region to region, the barriers consist of the endothelial lining of the capillaries related in the several instances to the piaarachnoid membrane, the choroid plexuses invested by columnar epithelium, or the ependymal lining of the ventricular walls. Arachnoidal granulations also project into the dural sinuses. The selective permeability of the cells which make up the contiguous membranous surface of the barrier as well as the probable secretory activity of the choroidal and ependymal cells together comprise the physiologic obstruction to unimpeded entry of substances from the blood into the cerebrospinal fluid.

hematoencephalic b. Blood-brain *b.*

placental b. The tissues intervening between the maternal and the fetal blood of the placenta, which prevent or hinder certain substances or bacteria from passing from mother to fetus.

Barron, Moses [*American physician and pathologist,* 1883–]. Contributed important researches concerning the relation of the islets of the pancreas to diabetes (1920), leading to the discovery of insulin.

Barth, Jean Baptiste [*Alsatian physician,* 1383–84]. Remembered for his description of incarcerated loops of small intestine between the persistent vitelline duct and the abdominal wall: called *Barth's hernia.*

Barthez, Antoine Charles Ernest [*French physician,* 1811–91]. Noted as one of the earliest teachers of pediatrics in France. His treatise on diseases of children (1843) is important for its description of poliomyelitis.

Bartholin, Caspar [*Danish anatomist,* 1655–1738]. The son of the anatomist Thomas Bartholin (Bartholinus). His name is associated with the discovery of the major vestibular glands, *Bartholin's glands,* and with the major sublingual ducts.

Bartholin, Thomas (Bartholinus) [*Danish anatomist,* 1616–80]. Considered the greatest anatomist of his time. He discovered the thoracic duct (ca. 1651), and while his claim to have discovered the intestinal lymphatics was disputed by Rudbeck, he seems to have been the first to appreciate their significance. He published a well-known work on diseases mentioned in the Bible.

bar"tho·lin·i'tis (bahr"to·li·nigh'tis) [after Caspar *Bartholin;* G. *-itis,* inflammation]. Inflammation of the major vestibular glands.

Bartholow, Roberts (1831–1904). American physician, first to apply electrodes to the human cortex and to demonstrate that weak faradization of the cortex produced muscular contractions of the contralateral limbs and turning of the head to the same side (1874).

Bartisch, Georg [*German ophthalmologist,* 1535–1606]. Remembered for his famed Renaissance book on diseases of the eye, containing numerous anatomic plates illustrating operations and procedures. Includes meticulous details for enucleation of the eye and extraction of cataract. He is said to have been the first to describe excision of the eye in the living.

Barton, Clara [*American philanthropist and nurse,* 1821–1912]. Famed for her organization of nursing and medical aid during the American Civil War. First president of the American Red Cross Society (1881–1904).

Barton, John Rhea [*American surgeon,* 1794–1871]. Remembered for his skill and inventiveness in surgery. He devised a figure-of-eight bandage for fracture of the mandible, described a separation fracture of the lower articular surface of the radius, and is said to have been the originator of the operation of intertrochanteric osteotomy of the femur (1826). Inventor of a type of obstetric forceps called *Barton's forceps.*

Bar"to·nel'la [after Alberto L. *Barton,* Peruvian physician, contemporary]. A genus of microorganisms which multiply in fixed tissue cells and parasitize erythrocytes, consisting of minute, pleomorphic rods and cocci which invade erythrocytes and endothelium in man. They occur without an intermediate host in man and in arthropod vectors are found only as **B. bacilliformis,** the causative agent of bartonellosis. (Carrión's disease), manifesting itself either as Oroya fever or verruca peruviana.

bar"to·nel·lo'sis. An infection caused by *Bartonella bacilliformis,* endemic in the Andes of South America, and unique in having two distinct clinical and pathologic but immunologically cross-reacting forms: Oroya fever, and the more benign skin lesion, verruca peruviana. The two forms most probably represent successive immunologic states of the affected individual. Syn., *bartonelliasis, Carrión's disease.*

Baruch, Simon [*American physician,* 1840–1921]. Remembered for his interest in public bathing facilities and for his description of a sign observed in typhoid fever: that the fever as registered by a rectal thermometer persists after the patient has been subjected to a bath at 75° F. for 15 minutes.

bar'y- [G. *barys,* heavy]. A combining form signifying *heavy.*

bar"y·la'li·a [*barys;* G. *lalia,* talk]. An indistinct, thick speech; occurs in patients with organic brain disease: common in advanced general paresis.

bar"y·pho'ni·a [*barys;* G. *phōnē,* voice]. A heavy or deep quality of voice.

ba·ry'ta (ba·rye'tuh, bar'i·tuh), **ba·ry'tes** (ba·rye'teez, bar'i·teez). BaO; barium oxide.

b. water. An aqueous solution of barium hydroxide.

B. A. S. British Anatomical Society.

basaljel. A trade-mark for basic aluminum carbonate gel.

ba'sal met"a·bol'ic rate. The amount of energy expended per unit of time under basal conditions; usually expressed as large calories per square meter of body surface (or Kg. of body weight) per hour.

ba·sal″zell·füss′chen (bah·zahl″tsel·fiss′chen. *See* NOTES §35) [Ger. basal cell footlet]. See *root feet.*

Basch, Samuel Siegfried von [*German physician,* 1837–1905]. Pioneer in the science of recording blood pressure and first to make use of a reliable clinical sphygmomanometer.

bas″cu·la′tion [F. *basculer,* to seesaw]. Replacing a retroverted uterus by pressing upward on the fundus and downward on the cervix. *Obs.*

bas′cule move′ment. The recoil of the heart in its systolic motion.

base [G. *basis,* base]. 1. The lowest part of a body or the foundation upon which anything rests. 2. The principal ingredient of a substance or compound. 3. *In chemistry,* a compound which yields hydroxyl ions (OH^-) in aqueous solution and which reacts with an acid to produce a salt and water. A proton acceptor; a substance capable of taking up protons. A substance having an electron pair which may be shared by another substance which lacks such a pair, and is therefore called an acid, to form a coordinate covalent bond between the two substances. 4. *In dentistry,* the support for the teeth in an artificial denture; a baseplate.—**ba′sal, ba′sic, bas′ilar,** *adj.*

Of these three adjectives **basal** is usually used to indicate the lowest or least, as *basal* metabolic rate; **basic** is used to mean fundamental, as *basic* food requirements; **basilar** is used to denote relationship to the base of the skull, as the *basilar* portion of the occipital bone.

Bolton cranial b. A triangular base formed by the Bolton nasion plane and lines joining the center of sella turcica with the Bolton point and nasion.

cheoplastic b. *In dentistry,* the base of a denture; produced by filling a mold with metal in the molten state.

purine bases. The alkaloids derived from purine, as theobromine and caffeine.

bas′e·doid, bas′e·dow·oid [after Karl Adolph von *Basedow;* G. *eidos,* form]. Noting an atypical thyroid disease.

Basedow, Karl Adolph von [*German physician,* 1799–1854]. Famed for his early description of exophthalmic goiter (1840), called *Basedow's disease, Flajani's disease, Graves's disease, Parry's disease.* Described his syndrome of the disease: tachycardia, heat flashes, and sweating crises: called *Basedow's syndrome.*

bas′e·dow·oid. See *basedoid.*

Ba·sel′la [NL., prob. from a native name in Malabar]. A genus of plants of the Basellaceae. **B. rubra,** Malabar nightshade is an esculent herb cultivated throughout India, where the juice of the leaves is used for respiratory diseases of infants.

base′ment [G. *basis,* base; L. suffix *-mentum*]. Any base or fundamental part, as a basement membrane. See basement *membrane.*

basergin. Trade-mark for ergonovine, $C_{19}H_{23}O_2N_3$, an alkaloid from ergot.

bas-fond. A fundus; specifically, the depressed area in the posterior wall of the urinary bladder just behind and above the trigone. It enlarges and deepens when there is obstruction to urination. In the male, it is also called *postprostatic pouch.*

Basham's mixture. See *iron* and ammonium acetate solution.

ba′si- (bay′see-, bas′ee-) [G. *basis,* base]. A combining form meaning *basis, base, forming a base, relating to the basion,* or *walking.*

ba″si·al·ve′o·lar [*basis;* L. *alveolus,* small hollow]. Relating to the basion and the alveolar point.

ba″si·bran′chi·al (bay″si·brang′kee·ul) [*basis;* G. *bragchion,* gill]. A copula or unpaired skeletal element uniting the bases of each branchial arch skeleton.

ba″si·chro′ma·tin [*basis;* G. *chrōma,* color]. That portion of the nuclear reticulum stained by basic aniline dyes.

ba·sic′i·ty (bay·sis′i·tee) [*basis*]. 1. The quality of being basic. 2. The number of replaceable hydrogens of an acid.

ba″si·cra′ni·al [*basis;* G. *kranion,* skull]. Relating to the base of the skull.

ba·sid″i·o·ge·net′ic [NL. *basidium;* G. *genesthai,* from *gignesthai,* to be produced]. *In biology,* produced on a basidium.

Ba·sid″i·o·my·ce′tes (ba·sid″ee·o·migh·see′teez) [*basidium;* G. *mykēs,* fungus]. A large class of fungi comprising genera which produce spores upon basidia. It includes the smuts, rusts, mushrooms, puffballs, and their allies.

ba·sid′i·o·phore″ [*basidium;* G. *phoros,* bearing]. A branch or a portion of a thallus bearing a basidium.

ba·sid′i·o·spore″ [*basidium;* G. *spora,* seed]. A spore of the basidiomycetes, formed by a basidium.

ba·sid′i·um (pl. *basidia*) [NL., from G. *basidion,* dim. of *basis,* base]. *In botany,* the cell which produces basidiospores.

ba″si·fa′cial [*basis;* L. *facies,* face]. Pertaining to the lower portion of the face.

ba″si·hy′al [*basis;* G. *hyoeidēs,* shaped like the letter upsilon]. The ventral, unpaired bone of the hyoid arch, forming the copula or the body of the hyoid bone. Formerly called *copula.*

ba″si·lat′er·al [*basis;* L. *latus,* side]. Both basilar and lateral.

ba·sil′ic [G. *basilikos,* royal]. Important; prominent: said of a drug or of a structure, as the basilic vein. See Table of Veins in the Appendix.

ba·sil′i·con oint′ment. Rosin cerate.

ba·sil′ic vein. Large vein of the arm on the medial side of the biceps muscle.

ba·sil″o·breg·mat′ic [G. *basis,* base; *bregma,* front part of the head]. Pertaining to the base of the skull and the bregma.

ba·sil″o·men′tal [*basis;* L. *mens,* mind]. Pertaining to the base of the skull and to the chin.

ba·sil″o·pha·ryn′ge·al [*basis;* G. *pharygx,* throat]. Relating to the basilar process of the occipital bone and to the pharynx.

ba″si·na′sal, bas″i·lo·sub·na′sal (·nay′zul) [*basis;* L. *nasus,* nose]. Relating to the basion and the nasion.

ba″si·o·al·ve′o·lar [*basis;* L. *alveolus,* small hollow]. Relating to the basion and to the alveolar point.

ba″si·oc·cip′i·tal (bay″see·ock·sip′i·tul, bas″ee·) [*basis;* L. *occiput,* back part of the head]. Referring to the basilar process of the occipital bone.

ba″si·oc·cip′i·tal bone. In many of the lower vertebrate animals, the separate bone forming the central axis of the skull. In the human adult, the basilar process of the occipital bone.

ba′si·on [*basis*]. The craniometric point on the anterior margin of the foramen magnum where the midsagittal plane of the skull intersects the plane of the foramen magnum. —**basial,** *adj.*

ba′si·o·tribe″ (bay′see·o·, bas′ee·o·) [*basis;* G. *tribein,* to crush]. Instrument used for basiotripsy.

ba′si·o·trip″sy [*basis; tribein*]. The operation of crushing or perforating the fetal head to facilitate delivery. *Obs.*

ba″si·pho′bi·a [*basis;* G. *phobos,* fear]. A morbid fear of walking.

ba″si·pre·sphen′oid (bay″see·pree·sfee′noyd, bas″-ee·) [*basis;* L. *prae,* before; G. *sphēn,* wedge; *eidos,* form]. Relating to the basisphenoid and presphenoid bones.

ba″si·pre·sphen′oid. The basipresphenoid bone.

ba″si·rhi′nal, ba″sir·rhi′nal [*basis;* G. *rhis,* nose]. Designating a cerebral fissure located at the base of the rhinencephalon.

ba′sis [G.]. A base, foundation, or fundamental part; the part opposite the apex. —**bas′ilar,** *adj.*

b. cranii externa [BNA]. External aspect of the base of the skull.

b. cranii interna [BNA]. Internal aspect of the base of the skull.

b. linguae. See *root of the tongue* under *root.*

b. pedunculi [BNA]. The crus of the cerebrum which contains fiber tracts descending from the cerebral cortex to the pons: also called *crus cerebri, cerebral peduncle.*

ba″si·sphe′noid (bay″see·sfee′noyd, bas″ee·) [*basis;* G. *sphēn,* wedge; *eidos,* form]. The lower part of the sphenoid bone, which embryonically developed as a separate bone.

ba″si·syl′vi·an [*basis;* Franciscus *Sylvius*]. The transverse basilar portion or stem of the lateral (Sylvian) fissure of the cerebral hemisphere.

ba″si·tem′po·ral [*basis;* L. *temporalis,* from *tempus,* temple]. Relating to the lower part of the temporal bone.

ba″si·ver′te·bral [*basis;* L. *vertebra,* a joint]. Relating to the centrum of a vertebra.

bas′ket [ME.]. 1. The fibrillar network in which the Purkinje cell body rests, formed by large arborizations from the axis cylinder process of certain neurons. See basket *cells.* 2. A condensation of intracellular neurofibrils seen in senile dementia.

fiber baskets. The delicate fibrils extending from the outer limiting membrane of the retina to surround neighboring rods and cones.

Basle an″a·tom′i·cal no′men·cla″ture. A list of anatomic terms (in Latin) adopted by the German Anatomical Society in Basle, Switzerland, in 1895. Abbreviated, BNA (Basle Nomina Anatomica).

ba′so·phil, ba′so·phile [G. *basis,* base; *philein,* to love]. 1. A substance, cell, or tissue element showing an affinity for basic dyes. See *basophilia,* basophil *leukocyte.* See Plate 26. 2. One of the beta cells found in the adenohypophysis. —**basophil,** *adj.*

ba″so·phil′i·a [*basis; philein*]. 1. Increased number of basophils in the circulating blood. 2. Stippling of the red cells with basic staining granules, representing a degenerative condition as seen in severe anemia, leukemia, malaria, lead poisoning, and other toxic states. Syn., *granular degeneration, basophilic degeneration, stippling.* Also called *punctate b.*

ba″so·phil′ic, ba·soph′i·lous. Susceptible to staining by basic rather than by acid dyes.

ba·soph′i·lism. Basophilia.

pituitary b. A condition described and ascribed by H. Cushing to an excess of basophil cells (adenoma) of the anterior pituitary: now called Cushing's *disease* or *syndrome.*

ba·soph′i·lous. See *basophilic.*

ba″so·pho′bi·a (bay″so·fo′bee·uh, bas″o·) [*basis;* G. *phobos,* fear]. A morbid fear of walking or standing erect, without muscular impairment. —**basophobic,** *adj.;* **basophobiac,** *n.*

ba′so·plasm [*basis;* G. *plasma,* from *plassein,* to form]. The portion of the cytoplasm which readily takes a basic stain. *Obs.*

Bass, Charles Cassedy [*American bacteriologist and parasitologist,* 1875–]. Known for his investigations of ancylostomiasis, malaria, and pellagra. Devised a macroscopic typhoid agglutination test performed at the bedside of the patient: called *Bass-Watkins agglutination test.*

Basset, Antoine [*French surgeon,* 1882–]. Known for his advocacy of an operation he devised for the radical extirpation of carcinoma of the vulva. This includes the extirpation of the superficial and deep inguinal lymph nodes.

Bassi, Agostino [*Italian physician,* 1773–1856]. Noted as a microbiologist; he demonstrated the parasitic nature of a certain disease in silkworms, thus opening the way to acceptance of the doctrine of pathogenic microorganisms (1835).

bas″si·net′ [F., dim. of *bassin,* basin]. An infant's crib or bed; a wicker basket with a hood at one end, used as a cradle.

Bassini, Edoardo [*Italian surgeon,* 1844–1924]. Famed for having devised in 1889 a modern operation for the cure of inguinal hernia (hernioplasty). The technic includes ligation and excision of the sac and suturing of the conjoined tendon to the inguinal ligament under the spermatic cord. Called *Bassini operation.*

bas′so·ra gum. An inferior gum of uncertain origin; formerly used in adulterating tragacanth.

bas′so·rin. A tasteless, odorless, vegetable gum, insoluble in cold water, but rendered soluble by alkalies; found in gum tragacanth (of Bassora) and in cherry and plum gums.

Bastian, Henry Charlton [*English neurologist,* 1837–1915]. One of the founders of English neurology, he contributed valuable studies on diseases of the brain, the paralyses, word blindness, and word deafness. Remembered especially for his law that a transverse lesion of the spinal cord above the lumbar enlargement causes complete loss of tendon reflexes of the lower extremities; called *Bastian-Bruns law.*

Bateman, Thomas [*English physician,* 1778–1821]. Regarded as one of the founders of modern dermatology; continued the work of Willan in classifying skin diseases. Described urticaria papulosa (1816), and was the first to give a clear picture of molluscum contagiosum.

bath [AS. *baeth*]. 1. A bathing place or room. 2. Any yielding medium such as air, vapor, sand, or water, in which the body is wholly or partially immersed for therapeutic purposes. It may be designed to cleanse, to soothe, to stimulate, to irritate, to heat, or to cool.

air b. The therapeutic exposure of the naked body to air.

alcohol b. The sponging of the body with dilute alcohol for its soothing and cooling effect.

astringent b. One in which the body or a part is immersed in a solution of alum, tannic acid, or other astringent.

bed b. One given to a patient in bed.

bland b. Immersion in a bath containing bran or starch for relief of irritation, itching, or urticaria.

bran b. See bland *b.*

brine b. Immersion of the body in a strong solution of salt water.

cabinet b. An air bath given by placing the patient in a cabinet which is heated by means of numerous electric light bulbs.

cold b. One given in water of 50°–60° F.

continuous b. One in which a patient is restrained in a tub and immersed in water from 90°–98° F. for hours at a time. It is used for its sedative effect on agitated or maniacal patients. Also called *continuous tub.*

contrast b. The alternate immersion of the hands or feet in hot and cold water.

cool b. One in water 60°–75° F.

effervescent b. Immersion of the patient in water in which carbon dioxide is released. This may be natural or introduced.

electric cabinet b. See cabinet *b.*

foot b. One restricted to the feet.

full b. One in which the entire body except the head is immersed.

graduated b. One in which the temperature is gradually lowered.

hafussi b. A form of Nauheim bath in which only the hands and feet of the patient are immersed.

half b. One restricted to the lower half of the body. Also called *hip b.*

hot air b. Exposure of the whole body to hot air circulating in a bath cabinet.

hot b. One in which the water has a temperature of 98°–108° F.

hydroelectric b. The application of faradic, galvanic, or sinusoidal currents to a patient through water.

medicated b. One to which a medicinal substance has been added.

mustard b. One in which powdered mustard has been included.

Nauheim b. An effervescent bath popularized at Nauheim, using naturally hot, carbonated water.

needle b. Shower bath which throws very fine jets of water under forceful pressure.

oxygen b. An effervescent bath employing oxygen instead of carbon dioxide.

paraffin b. Apparatus for the infiltration of pieces of tissues or organs with molten paraffin before imbedding them for cutting sections.

radioactive b. One which is given in water having radioactive properties.

Russian b. Hot vapor bath followed by a rubdown and a cold plunge.

sand b. Covering the body with warm, dry sand.

Scotch b. Usually called *Scotch douche.* One given to a patient in the erect position by playing a forceful stream of alternately hot and cold water on the patient's body.

sea b. A bath in sea water, usually heated. Also called *salt water b.*

sedative b. A prolonged, warm, full bath.

sheet b. A cooling bath given by sprinkling tepid water on a sheet which is spread over the patient.

shower b. One given by spraying the patient with water from an overhead fixture.

sitz b. One given in a specially built tub so that only the patient's lower back, hips, and upper thighs are immersed.

sponge b. One in which the body is sponged one part at a time without being immersed.

starch b. A bland bath using starch.

stimulating b. One containing tonic, astringent, or aromatic substances which increase the cutaneous effect and stimulate the body circulation.

sun b. The exposure of part or all the body to the sun for the actinic effect.

sweat b. One given by any of several methods of applying heat to the body to produce sweating.

tannic acid b. The immersion of all or part of the body in a solution of tannic acid for its astringent effect; formerly used in the treatment of extensive burns.

tepid b. One employing water at about 80°–92° F.

tub b. Any bath in which the body is immersed in a tub.

Turkish b. One in which the bather is placed in steam rooms of successively higher temperature, then is rubbed and massaged and finally stimulated by a cold shower.

vapor b. One in which the bather is exposed to vapors.

water b. *In chemistry,* an apparatus utilizing the heat of boiling water for drying solids containing moisture or for evaporating fluids without subjecting them to a heat that will cause disintegration or dissipation of the contained substance.

whirlpool b. One in which an arm, or leg, or the greater part of the body is immersed in hot water which is agitated by a whirling or churning current of equally hot water mixed with air.

bath″es·the′si·a. Deep sensation; muscle, tendon, and joint sensation and deep touch sensibility.

bath″o·pho′bi·a [G. *bathos,* depth; *phobos,* fear]. Morbid fear of depths.

bath″y·car′di·a [G. *bathys,* deep; *kardia,* heart]. A condition in which the heart is in a lower position than usual; the condition is an anatomic one, and is not the result of disease.

bath·y·chro′mic effect. The shift of an absorption band to a lower frequency, caused by some external effect on the chromophore. See also *hypsochromic effect.*

bat″o·pho′bi·a [G. *batos,* passable; *phobos,* fear]. 1. Dread of passing high objects, as fear of passing near a high building or of going through a deep valley. 2. Morbid fear of being on something of great height.

bat′ta·rism, bat″ta·ris′mus (bat″uh·riz′mus). See *stammering.*

bat′ter·y [F. *batterie,* from *battre,* to beat]. 1. A device which converts chemical to electrical energy. 2. A series of two or more pieces of apparatus connected so as to augment their effects, as a battery of boilers, prisms, or galvanic cells.

faradic b. A device which produces induced electricity.

galvanic b. A device which produces electricity from chemical energy.

storage b. A galvanic cell which can be charged and discharged. On charge electrical energy is converted into chemical energy and on discharge the process is reversed.

Battey, Robert [*American surgeon,* 1828–95]. Advocated ovariotomy as a therapy in various conditions, including dysmenorrhea and bleeding due to fibromyoma. Called *Battey's operation.*

Battle, William Henry [*English surgeon,* 1855–1936]. See *Kammerer-Battle incision,* under *Kammerer.* See also Battle's *sign.*

bat′yl al′co·hol. $CH_2OH.CHOH.CH_2O(CH_2)_{17}CH_3$; 3-(octadecyloxy)-1,2-propanediol; a mono-octadecyl ether of glycerin, a solid substance occurring in shark-liver oil.

Baudelocque, Jean Louis [*French obstetrician,* 1745–1810]. An illustrious figure in French medicine and obstetrics, he invented the pelvimeter and advanced the science of pelvimetry. Known for his description of the external conjugate diameter of the pelvis.

Bauer's test. See galactose tolerance *test.*

Bauhin, Gaspard (Caspar Bauhinus) [*Swiss anatomist,* 1560–1624]. Author of works on human anatomy (1597). Described the ileocecal valve, formerly called *Bauhin's valve.*

Baumann, Eugen [*German physician and biochemist,* 1846–96]. Demonstrated the presence of iodine (organic combination) in the thyroid gland (1895), thus leading to the experimental work resulting in the isolation of thyroxin.

Baumann and Goldmann's test. See under *test.*

Baumès, Jean Baptiste Timothée [*French physician,* 1756–1828]. Described retrosternal pain in angina pectoris; called *Baumès' sign.*

Baumès, Pierre Prosper François [*French physician*, 1791–1871]. Stated, shortly after Colles, the law that a child with congenital syphilis, whose mother has no clinical evidence of the disease, will not infect the mother (1840); called *Baumès' law, Colles' law, Colles-Baumès law.*

Baumgarten, Walter [*American physician*, 1873–1945]. Known for his description of a syndrome of enlarged spleen, portal hypertension, and prominent umbilical circulation in the absence of hepatic enlargement (1908). Called *splenomegaly without enlargement of the liver, Baumgarten's syndrome.* Also described congenital cirrhosis of the liver, called *Cruveilhier-Baumgarten cirrhosis.*

Bau'ru ul'cer. See *leishmaniasis* americana.

bay'ber"ry. The wax myrtle *Myrica cerifera* or *M. pennsylvanica.* The dried bark of the root contains tannin, myricinic acid, and a volatile oil: formerly used as an astringent.

b. wax. That obtained from the fruit; used for making bayberry candles and in the manufacture of soap.

bay·cu'ru (buy·kōō'rōō) [Tupi]. The root of a Brazilian plant, *Limonium brasiliensis,* used by the natives as a discutient in glandular swellings and as an astringent gargle. It contains tannic acid.

Bayer 205. Trade name under which suramin was originally introduced.

Bayle, Antoine Laurent Jessé [*French physician and pathologist*, 1799–1858]. Gave the first classic description of dementia paralytica, long called *Bayle's disease.*

Bayle, Gaspard Laurent [*French physician*, 1774–1816]. Remembered for his description of tubercle (1810). The first to use the term miliary, he correlated tuberculosis of the lungs with that of other organs.

Bayliss, William Maddock [*English physician*, 1860–1924]. A general physiologist, he published a work important from the physical chemical viewpoint. Remembered for his discovery, with Starling, of secretin in the duodenal secretions (1902).

Bazett's index. See under *index.*

Bazin, Antoine Pierre Ernest [*French dermatologist*, 1807–78]. Remembered for his description of psoriasis buccalis and erythema induratum (1861). The latter is also called *Bazin's disease, tuberculosis indurativa.*

BCG Bacillus Calmette-Guérin, or the vaccine prepared from this organism. The vaccine is prepared from an avirulent strain of the *Mycobacterium tuberculosis* bacillus attenuated by extended cultivation on a medium containing bile, and is recommended for immunization against tuberculosis.

b.d. *Bis die;* twice a day; used in prescriptions.

B. D. A. British Dental Association.

bdel'li·um (del'ee·um) [L.; G. *bdellion;* from the Hebrew *bĕdhōlah*]. A resinous gum exuding from various species of *Commiphora.* It resembles myrrh.

bdel·yg'mi·a (del·ig'mee·uh) [G., nausea]. A morbid loathing of food.

B. D. J. British Dental Journal.

B.D.S. Bachelor of Dental Surgery.

B.D.Sc. Bachelor of Dental Science.

Be Chemical symbol for beryllium.

bead'ed [ME. *bede*, prayer, prayer bead]. 1. Having, or formed into, beads. 2. *In bacteriology*, the term is applied to the nonuniform appearance of certain organisms such as *Corynebacterium diphtheriae* when stained.

bead'ing of ribs. See *rachitic rosary.* Also called *rachitic beads.*

beam. *In radiobiology*, a directed stream of particles or photons.

bear'ber·ry [AS. *bera; berie*]. Uva ursi.

Beard, George Miller [*American physician*, 1839–83]. First to describe neurasthenia (1869), called *Beard's disease.*

bear'ing down. The feeling of weight or pressure in the pelvis in certain diseases.

b.-d. pains. Expulsive pains in labor.

beat [AS. *bēatan*]. An impulse or throb, as of the heart and blood vessels.

anomalous b. An abnormally distributed excitation wave in the ventricles.

apex b. See *point of maximal impulse.*

coupled b. See *bigeminy*, 2.

dropped b. Condition noted in extrasystoles, when an occasional ventricular beat is lost.

ectopic b. A beat or rhythmic series of beats initiated by ectopic impulses.

forced b. An extrasystole initiated by artificial stimulation.

idioventricular b. One following a long diastole, originating in the atrioventricular node or below it.

interpolated b. An isolated ectopic beat occurring between two normal beats, without disturbing the basic rhythm.

premature b. An extrasystole.

retrograde b. Excitation of the atrium by the ventricle; the P wave following the R of the electrocardiogram.

beat'ing. *In massage*, percussion movements in which the half-closed fists are brought down alternately in a rapid succession of blows. Movement is largely from the wrist.

Beau, Joseph Honoré Simon [*French physician*, 1806–65]. Described transverse rings seen on the fingernails after convalescence from exhausting diseases, called *Beau's lines.*

Beaumont, William [*American Army surgeon*, 1785–1853]. Internationally famous for his observations and experiments on human digestion (1822–33). By means of his access to the gastric fistula suffered by Alexis St. Martin, he was the first to study the process of digestion in life, and his work on this subject was the most important in existence, up to the time of Pavlov.

be·bee'rine (bi·bee'reen, ·rin, beb'i·reen, ·rin) [Sp. *bibiru*, tropical South American evergreen tree]. An alkaloid, $C_{18}H_{19}O_3N$, from the root of *Cissampelos pareira* or from *Ocotea rodioei* (*Nectandra*). Also called *chondodendrine.*

b. hydrochloride. A mixture of the hydrochlorides of the total alkaloids from the roots of the above; reddish brown scales, soluble in water or alcohol, and formerly used as antipyretic and bitter tonic.

b. sulfate. A mixture similar to the hydrochloride with like action.

be·bee'ru. See *Ocotea.*

Becher, Wolf [*German physician*, 1862–1906]. First to demonstrate experimentally, by roentgen rays, the outline of an animal stomach. Utilized a lead solution, thus assisting later studies leading to roentgenologic diagnosis of gastric lesions.

Bechterew, V. M. See V. M. *Bekhterev.*

Beck, Claude Schaeffer (1894–). American surgeon who, with Tichy, performed grafting operations upon the heart for improving circulation to the heart muscle. See *cardiomyopexy, cardiopericardiopexy. Beck I Operation* (for coronary artery occlusion) consists of abrasion of surface of the heart and lining of parietal pericardium, application of an inflammatory agent to these surfaces, and partial occlusion of the coronary sinus. *Beck II Operation* (for coronary artery occlusion) consists in revascularization of the heart by diverting arterial blood into the coronary sinus and its tributaries. He also described a triad of low arterial pressure, high venous pressure, and a quiet heart in acute cardiac compression, and another of ascites, high venous pressure, and a quiet heart in chronic cardiac compression. These are called *Beck's triads.* He also developed an operation whereby a free graft is placed between the aorta and coronary sinus. The latter is partially ligated. Arterial blood is directed into the myocardium for the relief of coronary artery disease. He developed and reported the first successful human defibrillation.

Beck, Emil G. [*American surgeon,* 1866–1932]. Remembered for his method of treating tuberculous sinuses and cavities by injecting bismuth paste, called *Beck's paste.*

Becker, Heinrich Otto [*German ophthalmologist,* 1828–90]. Described a sign in exophthalmic goiter of spontaneous pulsation of the retinal arteries. Invented a test for astigmatism, consisting of parallel lines in triplets to be placed in various meridians.

Béclard, Pierre Augustin [*French anatomist,* 1785–1825]. Remembered for his description of femoral hernia, which for a time bore his name. Credited with the first excision of the parotid gland (1823).

beclysyl. Trade-mark for a solution containing thiamine hydrochloride, riboflavin, niacinamide, dextrose, and sodium chloride.

becotin. Trade-mark for a preparation of B vitamins with liver and stomach concentrate.

Becquerel, Antoine Henri [*French physicist,* 1852–1908]. Discovered radioactivity in uranium (1896). Invented a disk or apparatus for estimating the difference in temperature between a sound limb and a paralyzed one. The rays bearing his name are invisible radiations of electrically charged particles or electromagnetic waves of very short wavelength, projected from radioactive bodies such as uranium, radium, polonium, or other salts. Nobel laureate with Marie and Pierre Curie (1903).

bed [AS *bed, bedd*]. The couch or support on which the body may rest in sleep or in sickness.

air b. One with an inflatable rubber mattress.

b. rest. See under *rest.*

fracture b. One especially devised for patients with broken bones.

hydrostatic b. One with a rubber mattress partially filled with water to prevent bedsores.

inactive beds. *In U. S. Army medicine,* those medical treatment facility bed spaces with beds, not necessarily set up, for which equipment and fixtures are on hand and installed, but for which operating staff is not provided.

metabolic b. One especially arranged to save fluid and solid waste of the patient.

mobilization b. capacity. *In U. S. Army medicine,* space for patients' beds measured in terms of the number of beds that can be set up in wards or rooms designed for patients' beds, spacing beds 6 feet between centers (approximately 72 sq. ft. per bed).

rocking b. A type of bed with attached motor which rocks the bed with a set rhythm as a means of artificial respiration: used instead of a respirator in some cases of respiratory paralysis. Also called *rapid-rocking b.*

surgical b. One equipped with a double windlass which raises and lowers, independently, the foot and the head of the bed.

vasoscillator b. One which may be tipped to provide postural vascular exercise. Also called *Sanders b.*

water b. Hydrostatic bed.

bed'bug" [*bedd;* ME. *bugge*]. A blood-sucking wingless bug of the genus *Cimex* which lives and lays its eggs in the crevices of bedsteads, upholstered furniture, and walls. It is apparently not a vector of pathogenic organisms, although it has been suspected. *Cimex lectularius* is the most common species in the temperate zone; *C. hemipterus* is the most common in the tropics.

bed cred'it. *In U. S. Army medicine,* the number of beds which a hospital is directed to make available for the receipt, care, and treatment of patients from the hospital, organization, or agency for which the credit is established.

bed'fast". Bedridden.

Bednar's aphthae. See under *aphtha.*

bed net. A mosquito bar or netting suspended over the bed, its edges being tucked in about the mattress to prevent the entrance of insects.

bed'pan" [*bedd;* AS. *panne*]. A shallow, suitably shaped receptacle for receiving solid and fluid waste from patients confined to bed.

bed'rid"den [AS. *bedreda,* from *bedd; rida,* a rider]. Confined to bed. Syn., *bedfast.*

bed'sore" [*bedd;* AS. *sār*]. An ulceration caused by pressure against the bed, generally occurring in those confined to bed for long periods; decubitus ulcer.

Beer, Edwin [*American surgeon,* 1876–1938]. Noted for having performed transurethral fulguration of urinary bladder tumors (1910). This was the forerunner of transurethral prostatic surgery.

Beer, Georg Joseph (1763–1821). Austrian ophthalmologist, known for his textbook on ophthalmology and his description of glaucoma. He established the first eye hospital in Europe (1786). The triangular-bladed knife for corneal and cataract operations bears his name.

bees'wax. Yellow wax.

bleached b. White wax.

Beevor's sign. See under *sign.*

Beggiatoa, Francesco Secondo [*Italian botanist,* 1806–83]. Remembered for his studies of a genus of bacteria bearing his name.

be·hen'ic acid. $CH_3(CH_2)_{20}COOH$; docosanoic acid, a waxy solid occurring as a glyceryl ester in many fats and oils.

beheparon. Trade-mark for capsules containing liver concentrate, exsiccated ferrous sulfate, pyridoxine, and thiamine hydrochloride.

Behre's test. See under *test.*

Behring, Emil Adolf von [*German bacteriologist,* 1854–1917]. With Kitasato, produced antitoxins for tetanus and diphtheria (1890). His discovery of passive immunization was the starting point of modern serotherapy. Nobel laureate (1901).

Beigel's disease. See under *piedra.*

bej'el [Colloq. Ar. *bajlah*]. An endemic nonvenereal spirochetal infection occurring in Arabs of the Near East. Thought to be identical with yaws.

Bekhterev, Vladimir Mikhailovich [*Russian neurologist,* 1857–1927]. Widely known for his many contributions in the fields of neurology, especially in cerebral localization and experimental psychology. Described ankylosing spondylitis (1892), called *Bekhterev's disease, Strümpell-Marie disease, atrophic spinal arthritis, rheumatoid spinal arthritis.* It is now identified as a chronic arthritis of unknown etiology, but with progressive deformity, stiffness, and bony fusion of vertebrae. Described a layer of fibers parallel to the tangential fibers in the cerebral cortex; called *Bekhterev's fibers.* He described a nucleus of the vestibular portion of the auditory nerve, called *Bekhterev's nucleus.* Described a reaction in tetany: repetition of the minimum strength of electric current necessary to initiate muscular contraction will cause tetanic contraction unless the strength is diminished at every interruption of current or change in density; called *Bekhterev's reaction.* See also Bekhterev's *reflex.*

bel [A. G. *Bell,* American inventor, 1847–1922]. A unit frequently used to measure the intensity of sound, commonly the intensity above the normal threshold of hearing. See *decibel.*

bel, bael (bell, bay'el) [Hind.]. The dried, half-ripe fruit of *Ægle marmelos,* or baelfruit, of India. It has been used as a remedy for chronic diarrhea and dysentery. The ripe fruit is slightly laxative: also called *belae fructus, Bengal quince.*

Bell, Charles [*Scottish physician,* 1774–1842]. Internationally known for his studies in anatomy, physiology, and neurology. His *System of Dissections* (1798–1803) was published while he was studying medicine. His experimental work on the motor functions of ventral spinal nerve roots is the earliest of its kind (1811). He demonstrated the sensory and motor functions of the fifth cranial nerve and the cause of facial palsy (1821); neuropathy of the facial nerve is also called *Bell's palsy.* His *System of Operative Surgery* (1807–09) revealed his qualities as a surgeon and anatomist and brought him fame as an artist. The posterior or the long thoracic nerve (external respiratory nerve) formerly was called *nerve of Bell.*

Bell, John [*Scottish surgeon and anatomist,* 1763–1820]. The brother of Charles Bell, he exercised great influence on the progress of surgery in England. Like his brother, he showed great talent as an illustrator. His name is associated with the short muscular ridge on the inner surface of the urinary bladder which passes forward from each ureteral opening.

Bell, William Blair [*English gynecologist,* 1871–1936]. Remembered for his treatment of epithelioma with colloidal lead. A founder of the Royal College of Obstetricians and Gynecologists. Described a method for determining the amount of calcium in blood; see Bell's *method, muscle* of Bell.

Bell's mania. Acute manic excitement.

bellabulgara. A proprietary tablet containing 0.4 mg. of total alkaloids from Bulgarian belladonna root.

belladenal. A proprietary combination of bellafoline and phenobarbital available as tablets and suppositories.

bel"la·don'na [It., fine lady]. Deadly nightshade. A perennial plant, *Atropa belladonna,* of the order Solanaceae, indigenous to southern Europe and Asia and cultivated in the United States. Its properties are due chiefly to its content of *hyoscyamine.* This substance under certain conditions is racemized to atropine. Both leaves and root are employed. It is used as an antispasmodic, as a cardiac and respiratory stimulant, to check secretions (as sweat and milk), and as an anodyne. See *atropine.*

b. extract (*extractum belladonnae*). One containing 1.15 to 1.35% of alkaloids, available in pilular or powdered form. Dose, 10–20 mg. (1/6–1/3 gr.). Also called *b.-leaf extract.*

b. leaf (*belladonnae folium*). The dried leaf and top, yielding not less than 0.35% of alkaloids. Dose, 0.03–0.12 Gm. (1/2–2 gr.).

b.-leaf fluidextract (*fluidextractum belladonnae folii*). One containing from 0.27 to 0.33% of alkaloids. Dose, 0.06 cc. (1 min.).

b. liniment (*linimentum belladonnae*). 5 Gm. of camphor in belladonna-root fluidextract to make 100 cc.

b. ointment (*unguentum belladonnae*). One composed of pilular belladonna extract 10 Gm., diluted alcohol 5 cc., yellow ointment 85 Gm. Applied externally, especially for hemorrhoids.

b. plaster (*emplastrum belladonnae*). One prepared from an extract of belladonna root and adhesive plaster mass: used as a local anodyne.

b. root (*belladonnae radix*). The root of *Atropa belladonna* containing not less than 0.45% of the alkaloids. Dose, 0.03–0.12 Gm. (1/2–2 gr.).

b.-root fluidextract (*fluidextractum belladonnae radicis*). The fluidextract contains from 0.405 to 0.495% of alkaloids. Dose, 0.06–0.12 cc. (1–2 min.).

b. tincture (*tinctura belladonnae*). It contains from 0.027 to 0.033% of alkaloids. Dose, 0.3–1.0 cc. (5–15 min.). Also called *b.-leaf tincture.*

bel"la·don'nine (bel"uh·don'een, ·in) [*bella donna*]. $C_{17}H_{21}O_2N$. An alkaloid found in solanaceous plants as belladonna, hyoscyamus. It is isomeric with apoatropine from the same sources.

bellafoline. Trade-mark for a combination of the malic acid salts of the total levorotatory alkaloids of belladonna leaves.

bell'-crowned. Having a long, wide crown tapering sharply toward the neck: said of a tooth.

bellergal. Trade-mark for a proprietary sedative in tablet form containing bellafoline, gynergen, and phenobarbital.

Belle'vue bridge. An adhesive dressing for the elevation of the scrotum in inflammatory lesions.

Belling's stain. See *acetocarmine* under *stain.*

Bellini, Lorenzo [*Italian anatomist,* 1643–1704]. Known for his classic description of the gross anatomy of the kidney and his discovery of the renal excretory ducts (1662). Advocated the chemical examination of the urine as an aid in diagnosis. Noteworthy, also, is his description of the organs of taste.

bel·lones' (bi·lohnz'). *In veterinary medicine,* partial nasal obstruction in horses; due to polyps in the posterior nares. Sometimes associated with roaring.

bel'ly [AS. *belg*]. The abdominal cavity or abdomen. See words beginning *celi-.*

b. button. Navel or umbilicus.

b. of a muscle. The most prominent, fleshy, central portion of a muscle.

frog-b. The flaccid abdomen of children suffering from rickets.

bel'ly·ache" [*belg;* AS. *acan,* to ache]. Pain in the abdomen; colic.

bel"o·ne·pho'bi·a [G. *belonē,* needle; *phobos,* fear]. A morbid dread of pins and needles, and of sharp-pointed objects in general.

bemax. A proprietary product prepared from whole wheat germ and intended as a food adjunct.

Ben'a·cus [NL.]. A genus of water bugs.

B. griscus. A species known as giant water bug which inflicts painful, but not poisonous, bites.

benadryl hydrochloride. Trade-marked name for the antihistaminic substance diphenhydramine hydrochloride.

Bence Jones's cylinders. See under *cylinder.*

Bence Jones protein. See under *protein.*

Bence Jones protein test. See under *test.*

Benda, Raymond [*French physician,* 1896–]. Pioneer in blood transfusion and in the study of blood types. Known for his contributions to the knowledge of pneumonia and pulmonary tuberculosis. Introduced a test for aplastic anemia; see Benda's *test.* Devised many stains and staining methods. See under *stain.*

bends. See caisson *disease.*

Beneden, Edouard van [*Belgian embryologist,* 1846–1910]. Discovered the centrosome independently of Flemming (1876). Gave first complete account of segmentation of mammalian ova.

Benedict's methods. See under *method.*
Benedict's quantitative test. See Benedict's *method* for glucose.
Benedict's reagents. See under *reagent.*
Benedict's solution. See under *solution.*
Benedict's test. See under *test.*
Benedict and Franke's method. See under *method.*
Benedict and Hitchcock's uric acid reagent. See under *reagent.*
Benedict and Newton's method. See under *method.*
Benedict and Theis's method. See under *method.*
Benedikt, Moritz [*Austrian physician,* 1835–1920]. Described tegmental mesencephalic paralysis, called *Benedikt syndrome.*
benemid. Trade-mark for *probenecid.*
be·nign′, be·nig′nant [L. *benignus,* kind]. Not endangering health or life; not malignant, innocent; applied to certain tumors.
Bennett, Edward Hallaran [*Irish surgeon,* 1837–1907]. Described a fracture of the thumb at the base of the first metacarpal (actually a fracture dislocation into the carpometacarpal joint), which still bears his name.
Bennett, James Henry [*English obstetrician,* 1816–91]. The first to differentiate between benign and malignant tumors of the uterus (1845). His name was once associated with the large, fatty, epithelial cells found in ovarian cysts which he described.
Bennhold's test. See Congo red *test.*
benodaine hydrochloride. Trade-marked name for *piperoxan hydrochloride.*
Bensaude, Raoul [*French physician,* 1866–1938]. With Achard, isolated the paratyphoid bacillus and first used the term paratyphoid fever. Remembered as having used quinine urea anesthesia in the treatment of anal fissure.
Bensley's formalin. See Zenker's *fixing fluid.*
Benson, A. H. [*English ophthalmologist,* contemporary]. Known for his description of astral hyalitis, an inflammation of the ocular vitreous body, marked by the presence of star-shaped bodies.
ben′ton·ite [from Fort *Benton,* Montana, after Thomas Hart *Benton,* American statesman] (*bentonitum*). A native, colloidal, hydrated aluminum silicate. It swells in water and is useful in the preparation of pastes and lotions and as a suspending agent for insoluble medicaments in mixtures and emulsions.

b. magma (*magma bentoniti*). A 5% suspension of bentonite in distilled water: used as a suspending agent.

bentyl hydrochloride. Trade-marked name for dicyclomine hydrochloride, an antispasmodic for smooth muscle.
ben·zac′o·nine (ben·zack′o·neen, ·nin). $C_{32}H_{45}O_{10}N$. An alkaloid from aconite. Also called *isaconitine, picroaconitine.*
benz·al′de·hyde [F. *benjoin,* ult. from Ar. *lubān jāwi,* frankincense of Jawa; *al*cohol *dehyd*rogenatum] (*benzaldehydum*). $C_6H_5.CHO$. A colorless liquid, used as a flavoring agent.
ben″zal·dox′ime (ben″zol·dock′seem, ·sim). C_6H_5-$CH:NOH$; the oxime resulting from the interaction of benzaldehyde and hydroxylamine; it exists in two isomeric forms, both of which are solids.
ben″zal·ko′ni·um chlo′ride (*benzalkonii chloridum*). A mixture of alkyl dimethyl-benzylammonium chlorides of the general formula, $C_6H_5CH_2N$-$(CH_3)_2RCl$, in which R represents a mixture of alkyl radicals from C_8H_{17} to $C_{18}H_{37}$. A white or yellowish white powder or in gelatinous pieces; soluble in water. In solution of proper concentration it is an effective surface disinfectant which is germicidal for many pathogenic, nonsporulating bacteria and fungi after several minutes' exposure. See *zephiran chloride.*
ben·zan′i·lide. $C_6H_5.CO.NH.C_6H_5$. Benzoyl anilide, phenylbenzamide. White to pink crystals, insoluble in water; formerly used as antipyretic.
ben·zan′thra·cenes. A group of hydrocarbons in which a benzene and anthracene ring have a double bond in common. Some of the benzanthracene compounds are estrogenic and many are carcinogenic.
benz′a·thine pen″i·cil′lin G. Generic name for N,N′-dibenzylethylenediamine dipenicillin G, an oral dosage form which yields higher blood levels of penicillin than are obtainable with equivalent amounts of other dosage forms of the antibiotic. See *benzethacil, bicillin, neolin, permapen.*
benz·az′o·line hy″dro·chlor′ide. Generic name for 2-benzylimidazoline hydrochloride, a vasodilator useful in treating peripheral vascular disorders: supplied under the trade-marked name *priscoline.*
benzedrex. Trade-mark for 1-cyclohexyl-2-methylaminopropane, employed by inhalation to shrink the nasal mucosa.
benzedrine. A trade-mark for amphetamine.
ben′zene, ben·zene′. A hydrocarbon, C_6H_6, obtained chiefly as a by-product in the manufacture of coke: formerly called *benzol.* An especially pure form is obtained by the dry distillation of benzoic acid with lime. It is a clear, colorless, highly inflammable liquid of characteristic odor, miscible with alcohol, chloroform, ether, acetone, and other organic solvents. It is extensively used as a solvent. Inhalation of its fumes may be toxic. It has been tried in the treatment of leukemia because of its action in depressing the hematopoietic system, but with inconstant success and with the grave danger of producing aplastic anemia. It is of chief importance in industrial toxicology. Acute **benzene poisoning** produces restlessness, excitement, inebriation, hyperpyrexia, coma, and, by arresting respiration, death. Continued exposure, as in industries, results in leukopenia, anemia, and purpura.

b. carboxylic acid. See *benzoic acid.*

b. hexachloride. The designation commonly, though incorrectly, applied to commercial mixtures of stereoisomers of 1,2,3,4,5,6-hexachlorocyclohexane ($C_6H_6Cl_6$), employed as insecticides. The gamma isomer, a purified grade of which is called *lindane,* is of greatest entomological and medical interest. Abbreviated, BHC. See *gammexane.*

ben·zes′trol. A synthetic estrogenic substance, 2,4-di(*p*-hydroxyphenyl)-3-ethyl-hexane, originally marketed under the trade-mark *octofollin.*
benzethacil. A trade-mark, formerly also used as a generic name, for N,N′-dibenzylethylenediamine dipenicillin G. See *benzathine penicillin G.*
ben″ze·tho′ni·um chlo′ride. Generic name for the detergent and antiseptic substance available under the trade-marked name *phemerol chloride.*
benz·hex′ol. British generic name for the basic form of the synthetic antispasmodic supplied as the hydrochloride salt under the trade-marked name *artane:* also known by the generic name (U. S.) *trihexyphenidyl.*
ben′zi·dine (ben′zi·deen, ·din). Diaminodiphenyl, $NH_2.C_6H_4.C_6H_4.NH_2$. A colorless crystalline compound; used in identification of occult blood. See under *test.*
benz″im·id′a·zole. $C_7H_6N_2$; a dicyclic compound representing the fusion of a benzene ring with an imidazole ring; also, any derivative of $C_7H_6N_2$,

ben′zin, ben′zine (ben′zin, ben′zeen, ben·zeen′). A mixture of hydrocarbons obtained in the fractional distillation of petroleum.

purified b. (*benzinum purificatum*). A purified distillate consisting chiefly of hydrocarbons of the methane series, predominantly pentanes and hexanes. A clear, colorless, volatile, and highly inflammable liquid; practically insoluble in water; miscible with ether, chloroform, benzene, volatile and fixed oils, except castor oil. It is a valuable solvent. Also called *petroleum b.*

ben′zo-, benz-. A combining form denoting *relation to benzene, presence of the benzene ring,* or *azo colors used for direct dyeing of cotton.*

ben′zo·ate. Any salt of benzoic acid, as sodium benzoate.

ben′zo·caine (ben′zo·cane, ·kay·in, ·kah·een). Ethyl aminobenzoate. See *anesthesin.*

ben·zo′ic ac′id (*acidum benzoicum*). C_6H_5COOH. White scales or needles, soluble in 275 parts of water, in three parts of ether or alcohol, or in five parts of chloroform; soluble in fixed and volatile oils. A mild antiseptic used as ointment or hydro-alcoholic solution; also as mouthwash. Occasionally used as a urinary antiseptic although its salts, being less irritant, are generally preferred. Dose, 0.6–2.0 Gm. (10–30 gr.).

ben·zo′ic al′de·hyde. See *benzaldehyde.*

ben″zo·di·ox′ane, ben″zo·di·ox′an. 1. Either of two isomeric substances: 1,3-benzodioxane,

```
        O——CH2
       /      |
  C6H4        |
       \      |
        CH2—O
```

or 1,4-benzodioxane,

```
          O—CH2
         /    |
  C6H4        |
         \    |
          O—CH2
```

2. Generic term for any derivative of the preceding.

ben′zo·in (ben′zo·in, ·zoyn, ben·zo′in) (*benzoinum*). A balsamic resin obtained from *Styrax benzoin, S. tonkinensis,* and other species of *Styrax.* It contains resins, free and combined cinnamic and benzoic acids, vanillin, and traces of other constituents; used as a stimulating expectorant, as an inhalant in respiratory-tract inflammations, and as an external antiseptic and protective. Syn., *gum benjamin.* Also called *gum b.* —**benzo′inated,** *adj.*

b. flowers. Benzoic acid, especially that obtained by sublimation from benzoin.

b. tincture (*tinctura benzoini*). 20% of benzoin in alcohol. Dose, 1–2 cc. (15–30 min.).

compound b. tincture (*tinctura benzoini composita*). A tincture prepared from benzoin 10, aloe 2, storax 8, tolu balsam 4, alcohol to make 100; used as an inhalant in bronchitis, etc., by steam vaporization; as an antiseptic and protective application to chapped hands, minor wounds, etc.; and occasionally as a stimulating expectorant in chronic bronchitis. Dose, 1–4 cc. (15–60 min.). Also called *friar's* or *Turlington's balsam.*

benzoinol. A proprietary petroleum product containing benzoin and intended as a soothing application to mucous membranes or as a vehicle for other ingredients.

ben′zol, ben′zole. See *benzene.*

ben′zo·lism. Benzene poisoning.

ben″zo·naph′tha·lene (ben″zo·naf′thuh·leen). A mixture of naphthalene and benzoic acid.

ben″zo·naph′thol. Betanaphthyl benzoate.

ben″zo·ni·trile′ (ben″zo·nigh·treel′, ·tril′, ·nigh′-tryle, ·tril). C_6H_5CN, phenyl cyanide. A colorless, inflammable liquid having an odor suggestive of bitter almond oil; used in synthesis of certain drugs and dyes.

ben″zo·phe·none′. $(C_6H_5)_2CO$; diphenyl ketone, the stable form of which occurs in crystals, insoluble in water, having a geraniumlike odor: used as a fixative for perfumes and in the manufacture of many medicinal agents.

1,2-ben″zo·py′ran. C H O; the parent substance of many plant pigments. Syn., *1,2-chromene.*

ben″zo·py′rene. $C_{20}H_{12}$. A carcinogenic substance obtained from tar.

ben″zo·qui·none″ a·ce′tic ac′id. $O.C_6H_3.O.$-CH_2COOH; an oxidation product of homogentisic acid; it occurs in urine in cases of scurvy and rheumatic fever.

ben″zo·qui·non′i·um chlo′ride. Generic name for 2,5-*bis*(3-diethylaminopropylamino)benzoquinone-*bis*-benzyl chloride, a skeletal-muscle relaxant supplied under the trade-marked name *mytolon chloride.*

benzosalin. A trade-mark for methyl benzoylsalicylate, which has been used as an intestinal antiseptic and as an antirheumatic.

benzosol. Trade-mark for guaiacol benzoate.

ben″zo·sul′fi·mide. Saccharin.

ben′zo·yl (ben′zo·il, ·eel). The univalent radical C_6H_5CO—, derived from benzoic acid.

b.-acetyl peroxide. Acetylbenzoyl peroxide, $C_6H_5CO.O.O.CO.CH_3$. A germicide. Also called *acetozone.*

b.-aconine. See *benzaconine.*

b. anilide. See *benzanilide.*

b. chloride. C_6H_5COCl. A colorless liquid of penetrating odor; has been used subcutaneously in leprosy and as a local application to ulcerating surfaces. Its chief use is in organic syntheses.

b. eugenol. A white, crystalline substance; insoluble in water but soluble in alcohol: formerly used in neuralgic headaches.

b.-glycocoll. Hippuric acid.

b.-glycolic acid. Mandelic acid.

b. green. Malachite green.

b.-guaiacol. Guaiacol benzoate.

b. peroxide. $(C_6H_5CO)_2O_2$. White crystals sparingly soluble in water or alcohol; used as dusting powder or in ointment or oily solution for application to skin diseases and burns.

b. salicin. Populin.

ben″zo·yl·ec′go·nine. $C_{16}H_{19}NO_4$; an alkaloidal constituent of certain varieties of coca leaves; also produced by boiling an aqueous solution of cocaine (benzoylmethylecgonine).

ben″zo·yl·meth″yl·ec′go·nine. Cocaine.

3,4-benz·py′rene. $C_{20}H_{12}$; a pentacyclic hydrocarbon constituent of coal tar.

benz″py·rin′i·um bro′mide. Generic name for 1-benzyl-3-(dimethylcarbamyloxy)pyridinium bromide, a cholinergic agent available under the trade-marked name *stigmonene bromide.*

ben′zyl (ben′zil, ·zeel). The univalent radical, $C_6H_5CH_2$—.

b. alcohol. $C_6H_5CH_2OH$. Phenyl methyl alcohol, occurring as an ester in tolu and other balsams, but produced synthetically. It is a colorless liquid, soluble in 25 volumes of water; employed as a local anesthetic by injection or by application to mucous membranes and as a bacteriostatic agent. Syn., *phenylcarbinol.*

b. benzoate (*benzylis benzoas*). $C_6H_5CO_2.CH_2$.-C_6H_5. Colorless crystals or oily liquid of faintly aromatic odor and pungent taste; insoluble in water or glycerin, soluble in alcohol. It occurs in certain balsamic resins or is prepared synthetically: formerly used as an antispasmodic. Dose,

0.2–0.4 cc. (3–6 min.). **Benzyl benzoate lotion** is used as a remedy for scabies.

b. bromide. $C_6H_5CH_2Br$. A colorless liquid used as a lacrimator in chemical warfare.

b. cinnamate. A constituent of cinnamein from Peruvian balsam.

b. fumarate. White, crystalline, odorless, and tasteless powder, which has been used as an antispasmodic.

b. succinate. The dibenzyl ester of succinic acid, which has been used as an antispasmodic.

benzylets. Trade-mark for a soluble gelatin globule containing benzyl benzoate.

ben·zyl′i·dene. The divalent radical, $C_6H_5CH=$.

2-ben″zyl·i·m·id·az′o·line hy″dro·chlor′ide. $NH.CCC_6H_5CH_2):N.CH_2.CH_2.HCl$. Benzazoline hydrochloride, a vasodilator available under the trade-marked name *priscoline.*

bepron. Trade-mark for a capsule containing the water-soluble constituents of beef liver with ferrous iron.

ber′ber·ine (bur′bur·een, ·in). $C_{20}H_{19}NO_5$. An alkaloid found in *Berberis* and many other plants.

ber′ber·is [L.]. Barberry; the dried rhizome and roots of various shrubs of the genus *Mahonia:* formerly used as a bitter tonic. The chief constituents are berberine and resin.

Bercovitz, Zacharias Taylor [*American physiologist,* 1895–]. Devised a test for pregnancy in which a few drops of the patient's citrated blood are instilled into one eye. If there is dilatation or contraction of the pupil, the test is regarded as positive; called *Bercovitz test.*

Berengario da Carpi, Jacopo (Berengarius, Berenger) [*Italian anatomist,* d. 1530]. Said to have been the first to describe the sphenoid sinuses, the vermiform process, and the arytenoid cartilages (1521). Also described the thymus (1522) and gave the first authentic account of excision of the uterus for prolapse (1522).

ber′ga·mot oil (*oleum bergamottae*). A volatile oil obtained by expression from the rind of the fresh fruit of *Citrus bergamia,* and yielding not less than 36% of esters calculated as linalyl acetate; used chiefly as a perfume. It is said to be a useful insecticide.

Bergenhem, Bengt Ludwig [*Swedish surgeon,* 1898–]. Known for his operation of implantation of the ureters into the rectum for the relief of exstrophy of the urinary bladder.

Berger, Emil [*Austrian ophthalmologist,* 1855–1926]. Described an irregularity of the pupil in which it exhibits an elliptical shape, a sign of early tabes dorsalis, called *Berger's sign.*

Berger, Hans [*German neurologist,* 1873–1941]. Remembered for his descriptions of the alpha rhythm and the waves recorded in encephalography, and for his early studies of bodily manifestations of psychic states.

Berger, Oskar [*German neurologist,* 1844–85]. Described a paresthesia involving the lower extremities, without objective symptoms, and accompanied by weakness; seen usually in juveniles; called *Berger's paresthesia.*

Berger, Paul [*French surgeon,* 1845–1908]. Remembered for his interthoracico-scapular amputation at the shoulder girdle, which is called *Berger's operation.*

Bergeron, Etienne Jules [*French physician,* 1817–1900]. Described the myoclonic form of epidemic encephalitis: called *Bergeron's disease.* Author of a classic description of ulcerative stomatitis (1855).

Bergey, David Hendricks [*American bacteriologist,* 1860–1937]. Celebrated for his systematic arrangement or key for the identification of the class Schizomycetes in his *Manual of Determinative Bacteriology* (1923).

Bergh's test. See van den Bergh's *test.*

Bergmann, Ernst von [*German surgeon,* 1836–1907]. Made important contributions to the development of brain surgery and of aseptic technic. *Von Bergmann's incision* to expose the kidney begins at the outer border of the sacrospinalis at the level of the twelfth rib and extends obliquely toward the junction of the outer and middle thirds of the inguinal ligament.

Bergmann, Gottlieb Heinrich [*German physician,* 1781–1861]. Described the processes of certain superficial neuroglia cells of the cerebellum; called *Bergmann's fibers.* Striae acusticae in the floor of the fourth ventricle are known as *Bergmann's cords, conductors.* (Description of these structures sometimes is ascribed erroneously to Ernst von Bergmann.)

ber′i·ber′i [Singhalese *beri,* weakness]. A disease due to deficiency of thiamine; seen endemically in those living mainly on a polished rice diet, and sporadically in other countries when the diet is similarly limited. Various manifestations occur, depending upon the severity and duration of the vitamin lack. Multiple neuritis, general weakness, paralysis, progressive edema, mental deterioration, and finally heart failure make up the classic picture. Also called *athiaminosis, kakke disease.*

Berkefeld, Wilhelm (1836–1897). German manufacturer who put on the market the Berkefeld filter candles, made of diatomaceous earth, designed for the separation of bacteria from viruses. The three grades were: V, which is coarse, from German *viel,* coarse; N, which is medium, from German *normal;* and W, which is fine, from German *wenig,* fine.

Berkefeld filter. See under *filter.*

berke′li·um [*named after Berkeley, California*]. Chemical element No. 97, symbol Bk, produced artificially in minute amounts.

Berlin, David Daniel [*American physician,* 1901–]. Associated with H. L. Blumgart and S. A. Levine in the treatment of angina pectoris by total thyroidectomy (1933).

Berlin, Rudolf [*German ophthalmologist,* 1833–97]. Known for his descriptions of word blindness, for which he chose the name dyslexia, and for his description of commotio retinae or traumatic edema of the retina.

Ber·lin′ blue. See *aniline blue.*

Berman, Samuel [*American electrical engineer,* 1895–]. Invented an apparatus for locating metallic foreign particles, as in the eye.

Bernard, Claude [*French physiologist,* 1813–78]. One of the greatest figures in the history of physiology, he introduced experimental methods (1855). Demonstrated nerve paralysis by the use of curare, showing the independent excitability of muscle. Discovered the vasoconstrictor and dilator nerves. Demonstrated the glycogenic function of the liver and the digestive action of pancreatic juice (1848). Showed that a slight wound in the floor of the fourth ventricle rendered an animal temporarily diabetic. He is said to have coined the term internal secretions (1855). The syndrome following section or paralysis of the cervical sympathetic trunk is known as the *Bernard-Horner syndrome, Horner's syndrome.* See *milieu intérieur.*

Bernhardt, Martin [*German neurologist,* 1844–1915]. Known for his description of meralgia paresthetica due to disease of the lateral cutaneous nerve of the thigh (1878); called *Bernhardt's disease, Roth-Bernhardt disease.*

Bernheim, Hippolyte [*French physician*, 1840–1919]. Widely known for his practical application of hypnotism to the treatment of neuroses. Author of a work on the subject of hypnotic suggestion (1891).

Bernreuter personality inventory. See under *test*.

Bernstein, Felix [*American biochemist of German birth*, 1878–]. Known for his theory regarding blood groups and heredity. This assumes three allelomorphic genes, A, B, and O (or R), one of which is present in each member of a certain pair of chromosomes. Each somatic cell possesses two of these genes, one derived from either parent. A and B factors are dominant over O. Called *Bernstein's theory*.

Berthelot, Pierre Eugene Marcelin [*French chemist*, 1827–1907]. Known for his investigation of the action of bacteria in soils, especially in reference to fixation of nitrogen. Remembered also for his test for phenol by treating an ammoniacal solution with sodium hypochlorite, which produces a blue coloration.

Ber″ti·el′la [L., after Paul *Bert*, French physiologist, 1833–86]. A genus of tapeworm parasites.

B. mucronata. A species parasitic to man, found in the intestine.

B. studeri. A species found in primates.

Bertillon, Alphonse [*French criminologist*, 1853–1914]. Inventor of the system of identification which bears his name (1886). It consists of selected measurements of various parts of the body. The *Bertillon system* has been largely superseded by the use of fingerprints.

ber·til·lon·age′ (bare·til·lon·azh′). The Bertillon system.

Bertin, column of. See renal *column*.

be·ryl″li·o′sis [G. *bēryllos*, beryl; *-ōsis*, condition]. Pneumonoconiosis due to inhalation of beryllium oxide dust.

acute b. Acute pneumonitis in beryllium workers.

chronic b. Chronic pulmonary granulomatosis in beryllium workers.

be·ryl′li·um [*bēryllos*]. Be = 9.013. A divalent metallic element occurring chiefly as beryllium aluminum silicate or beryl. Formerly called *glucinum*.

Berzelius, Jöns Jakob [*Swedish chemist*, 1779–1848]. Famous for his many scientific achievements, he discovered the elements selenium, thorium, and cerium, and introduced the modern system of writing chemical symbols and formulas.

bes″i·clom′e·ter [F. *besicles*, spectacles; G. *metron*, a measure]. An instrument used by opticians for measuring the forehead to obtain the proper width for spectacle frames.

Besnier, Ernest [*French dermatologist*, 1831–1909]. Described lupus pernio (1889), later classified by C. P. M. Boeck as benign sarcoid; called *lupus pernio of Besnier, Besnier-Boeck disease*. See *sarcoidosis*.

Besredka, Alexandre [*French physician*, 1870–1940]. Remembered for his work on anaphylaxis and antianaphylaxis (1907). Said to have introduced the term antivirus.

Best, Charles Herbert [*Canadian physician*, 1899–]. Famed for his part in the isolation of insulin (1922) with F. G. Banting, working in the laboratory of J. J. R. Macleod.

Best's carmine. See under *stain*.

Best's dis·ease′. Congenital macular degeneration.

bes″ti·al′i·ty [L. *bestialis*, from *bestia*, beast]. 1. Behavior resembling that of an animal. 2. *In psychiatry*, sexual relations between human beings and animals.

be′ta (bee′tuh, bay′tuh). The second letter of the Greek alphabet, β; used in chemical nomenclature to indicate the second of two isomeric compounds. For many words beginning *beta-*, see under the specific noun.

betabion. Trade-mark for synthetic thiamine hydrochloride.

be′ta·cism [*bēta*]. Overuse of the b-sound in speech, or conversion of other sounds into it.

be″ta·eu′caine hy″dro·chlo′ride. Eucaine hydrochloride.

be″ta-hy·poph′a·mine (-high·pof′a·meen, ·min). The pressor principle of posterior pituitary.

be′ta·ine (bee′tay·een, ·in, bee′tuh·een, ·in). $(CH_3)_3N.CH_2.COO$; a substance obtained from sugar-beet molasses or prepared synthetically. Colorless, deliquescent crystals of sweet taste, soluble in water or alcohol. It is an active methyl donor in the synthesis of choline and creatine, and is useful in preventing hepatic cirrhosis. Syn., *lycine, oxyneurine, trimethylglycine*.

b. hydrochloride. Colorless crystals, freely soluble in water into which it slowly liberates its hydrochloric acid. Used in gastric hypoacidity. Dose, 0.5 Gm. (8 gr.). See *acidol*.

be′ta·ines. A group of cyclic organic bases characterized by the group $(CH_3)_3N <$. They may be considered internal salts of quaternary ammonium bases, as trimethyl glycine betaine,

$$(CH_3)_3N.CH_2.COO;$$

croton betaine, $(CH_3)_3N.CH_2.CH{:}CH.COO$. See *betaine*.

be″ta·ke′to·hy·drox″y·bu·tyr′ic ac′id. Acetoacetic acid.

betalin S. Trade-mark for thiamine hydrochloride.

be″ta·naph′thol. $C_{10}H_7OH$. White to pale buff-colored, shining, crystalline leaflets or powder with faint phenol-like odor. Darkens on exposure to sunlight. It is an effective intestinal antiseptic and is useful in the form of an ointment or alcoholic solution as a parasiticide. It has been used as a vermifuge but the doses required are dangerous to the patient. Dose as an intestinal antiseptic, 0.13–0.32 Gm. (2–5 gr.). Also called *naphthol*.

b. sodium. Grayish white powder, soluble in three parts of water; used as antiseptic in 0.5–1.0% aqueous solution. See *microcidin*.

be″ta·naph′thyl. The radical $C_{10}H_7$—.

b. benzoate. $C_6H_5COO.C_{10}H_7$. White, crystalline powder; has been used as intestinal antiseptic and as parasiticide: also called *benzonaphthol, beta-naphthol benzoate*.

b. salicylate. $C_6H_4(OH).COO.C_{10}H_7$. White, odorless, tasteless, crystalline powder; has been used as an intestinal antiseptic. Syn., *betol*.

be″ta-ox″y·bu·tyr′ic ac′id. Beta-hydroxybutyric acid.

be′ta par′ticle. See under *particle*.

betaplexin. Trade-mark for an elixir containing the vitamin-B complex.

be″ta·to′pic. Of or pertaining to two atoms which differ by one in atomic number, so that by expulsion of a beta particle from the nucleus of the atom of an element of lower atomic number it is converted to an atom of the element having an atomic number greater by one unit.

be′ta·tron (bay′tuh·tron, bee′tuh·tron) [*bēta;* G. ēlek*tron*, amber]. An instrument with which electrons are accelerated to millions of electron volts by magnetic induction.

betaxin. Trade-mark for thiamine hydrochloride.

be′tel [Pg. *betle*, from Tamil *vettilai*]. A masticatory used in the East. A few grains of the nut of the catechu palm, *Areca Catechu*, are rolled up with a small amount of quicklime in a leaf of *Piper Betle*, and chewed.

be·thane′chol chlo′ride. The generic name for β-methylcholine carbamate chloride; $C_7H_{17}Cl-N_2O_2$; a parasympathomimetic agent not destroyed by cholinesterase. See *urecholine chloride.*

be′tol. Betanaphthyl salicylate.

Bets, Vladimir Aleksandrovich (Betz) [*Russian anatomist*, 1834–94]. Discovered the giant pyramidal cells of the cerebral cortex (1874), called *cells of Betz.*

Bettendorff's test. See under *test.*

Bettman, Adalbert G. [*American physician*, 1883–]. Known for his introduction of oxyquinoline sulfate Scarlet R Gauze for healing wounds (1931) and his tannic acid–silver nitrate treatment of burns (1935).

bet′u·lin. $C_{36}H_{60}O_3$, a diatomic alcohol contained in the bark of the white birch, *Betula alba.* Also called *betula camphor.*

be·tween′brain. See *diencephalon.*

Betz. See *Bets.*

Beurmann, Charles Lucien de [*French dermatologist*, 1851–1923]. With Gougerot, described sporotrichosis (1906), which also is called *de Beurmann-Gougerot disease, Schenck's disease. Sporotrichum beurmanni* is a species of the fungus which causes the disease.

bev Abbreviation for billion electron volts.

Bevan, Arthur Dean [*American surgeon*, 1861–1943]. Known for his inventiveness in the field of abdominal surgery. His operation for cholecystectomy through a vertical incision along the upper outer border of the rectus muscle still bears his name. Also devised a now superseded anchoring operation for undescended testis, and described a special operation for sliding hernia of the cecum.

be′va·tron. A contemplated apparatus for accelerating protons in the billion electron volt range.

bev′el [prob. from OF. *baer*, to gape]. A sloping edge.

cavosurface b. *In dentistry*, that portion of the enamel wall of a cavity which is cut back at an obtuse angle to the tooth surface in order to remove short and friable enamel rods at the cavity margin.

bewon. Trade-mark for a thiamine hydrochloride elixir.

Beyea, Henry Dorrance [*American surgeon*, 1867–1924]. Remembered for his suspension operation for gastroptosis, in which the gastrohepatic and gastrophrenic ligaments are plicated.

be′zoar (bee′zor, bee′zo·ar, bee·zo′ur) [F. *bézoard*, through Ar., from Per. *pād-zahr*, protecting against poison]. A concretion found in the stomach or intestine of some animals (especially ruminants), most commonly composed of ingested hair; may form a cast of the stomach large enough to cause obstruction. Also found in some psychopathic patients. Formerly believed to have magic medicinal properties.

Bezold, Albert von [*German physiologist*, 1836–68]. Discovered the accelerator nerve fibers of the heart and their origin in the spinal cord (1863). See also under *reflex.*

Bezold, Friedrich [*German otologist*, 1842–1908]. Celebrated for his contributions in the field of otology. Gave the first clear description of mastoiditis (1877), introduced an important test for audition in his monumental textbook, and described an abscess deep in the muscle planes of the neck, arising from the extension of a suppurative otitis media, sometimes with thrombosis of the transverse sinus. See Bezold's *sign.*

bhang. See *cannabis.*

BHC Abbreviation for the insecticide benzene hexachloride (hexachlorocyclohexane).

B-h fruc″to·si′dase. See *saccharase.*

Bi Chemical symbol for bismuth.

bi- (buy-) [L. *bis*, twice]. 1. A prefix meaning *two, twice, double.* 2. *In anatomy*, a prefix denoting *connection with* or *relation to each of two symmetrically paired parts.* 3. *In chemistry*, a prefix denoting *the presence of two atoms* or *equivalents* of the constituent to the name of which it is attached or *the presence* of this constituent *in double the usual proportion* or *in double the proportion of the other component.*

Bial's reagent. See under *reagent.*

Bial's test. See under *test.*

Bianchi, Giovanni Battista [*Italian anatomist*, 1681–1761]. Described the valve at the lower end of the nasolacrimal duct; called *Bianchi's valve.* The nodules of Arantius are sometimes known as *Bianchi's nodules.*

Bianchi, Leonardo (1848–1927). Italian psychiatrist and neurologist known for his experimental work on the neural mechanisms of the brain and his demonstration in monkeys that bilateral destruction of the frontal cortex resulted in significant alterations of character.

bi′ased er′rors. Those which tend in one direction.

bi′ased sam′ple. A sample which is not representative of its field.

bi″a·stig′ma·tism [L. *bis*, twice; G. *a-*, not; *stigma*, point]. Condition of the eye in which both corneal and lenticular astigmatism exist.

bi·ax′i·al [*bis;* L. *axis*, axis]. Furnished with two axes.

bib′li·o·clast″ [G. *biblion*, book; *klān*, to break]. One who mutilates books.

bib″li·o·klep″to·ma′ni·a [*biblion;* G. *kleptein*, to steal; *mania*, madness]. Morbid desire to steal books.

bib″li·o·ma′ni·a [*biblion; mania*]. An abnormal or intense desire to collect rare or curious books.

bib″li·o·pho′bi·a [*biblion;* G. *phobos*, fear]. A morbid fear or hatred of books.

bib″li·o·ther′a·py. Treatment of patients by advising reading of books.

bi·bo′rate. See *borate.*

bi·cap′i·tate [L. *bis*, twice; *caput*, head]. Having two heads; dicephalous.

bi·car′bon·ate. A salt of carbonic acid characterized by the radical —HCO_3, representing carbonic acid wherein one hydrogen has been replaced.

blood b. The amount of bicarbonate present in the blood indicating the alkali reserve. Also called *plasma b.*

bi·car′di·o·gram [*bis;* G. *kardia*, heart; *gramma*, letter]. The summated electrocardiogram yielded by the two ventricles beating normally.

bi·ceph′a·lous. See *dicephalous.*

bi′ceps [*bis; caput*]. A muscle having two heads, as the biceps brachii, the biceps femoris. See Table of Muscles in the Appendix. —**bicip′ital,** *adj.*

Bichat, Marie François Xavier [*French anatomist and physiologist*, 1771–1802]. Renowned for his treatise on anatomy in many volumes which he left unfinished at his death, and for his *Anatomie Générale*, which revolutionized descriptive anatomy and marked him as the founder of modern histology and histopathology.

bi·chlo′ride. 1. Any compound containing two atoms of chlorine, especially a salt having two chloride atoms. 2. A careless designation of mercury bichloride.

bi·chro′mate. A dichromate.

bicillin. A trade-mark for N,N′-dibenzylethylenediamine dipenicillin G. See *benzathine penicillin G.*

bi·cor′nate, bi·cor′nu·ate, bi″cor·nute′ (buy·kor′nate, buy·kor′nu·ate, -ker·newt′), **bi·cor′nous** [L. *bis*, twice; *cornutus*, horned]. Having two horns, as a bicornate uterus.

bi·cus′pid [*bis;* L. *cuspis*, point]. Having two cusps, as bicuspid teeth, or as the mitral (left atrioventricular) valve of the heart.

bi·cus′pid. A human premolar tooth.

b. i. d. *Bis in die;* twice daily.

bi·dac′ty·ly [*bis;* G. *daktylos*, finger]. Congenital absence of all fingers or toes except the first and fifth; lobster-claw deformity.

Bidder, Friedrich Heinrich [*German anatomist*, 1810–94]. Remembered for his description of an accumulation of ganglion cells in the frog's heart; called *Bidder's ganglion.* Contributed to our knowledge of the nature of free hydrochloric acid in the stomach.

bi·der·mo′ma. See *teratoma.*

Bie′brich scar′let (bee′brick). An acid disazo dye used in aqueous solution as a plasma stain. Also called *croceine scarlet, double scarlet BSF, Ponceau B, scarlet B* or *EC.*

Biedl, Artur [*Czechoslovakian physiologist*, 1869–1933]. Known for his work on the adrenal cortex (1910) and his contributions to the knowledge of endocrinology. Described the disease or syndrome of adiposogenital dystrophy, called *Laurence-Moon-Biedl syndrome.*

bi″e·lec·trol′y·sis [L. *bis*, twice; G. *ēlektron*, amber; *lysis*, a loosing]. The electrolysis of two substances, one at each pole.

Bielschowsky, Max [*German neuropathologist*, 1869–1940]. Known for his discoveries relating to tumors of the nervous and reticuloendothelial systems. Devised silver staining methods for the nervous system, called *Bielschowsky's silver methods;* see under *stain.* Described late infantile amaurotic familial idiocy, also called *Bielschowsky-Janský disease.*

Bier, August Karl Gustav [*German surgeon*, 1861–1949]. Remembered for his description of active and passive hyperemia as an aid in the treatment of inflammation in a part. Described the spots or blanched areas in the skin arising from diminution of the blood supply of an area; called *Bier's spots.* Introduced a method for producing anesthesia in a limb; see Bier's *method.*

Biermer, Anton [*German physician*, 1827–92]. Noted for his description of pernicious anemia (1872) and for being the first to observe retinal hemorrhage in the disease; called *Biermer's disease, anemia.*

Biernacki, Edmund Adolfovich [*Polish physician in Austria*, 1866–1911]. Described a sign diagnostic of tabes: severe pressure on the ulnar nerve is not productive of pronounced pain as in the case of a normal individual. Called *Biernacki's sign.*

Biesiadecki, Alfred von [*Polish physician*, 1839–88]. Described a fossa beneath the iliac fascia; called *Biesiadecki's fossa.*

Biett, Laurent Théodore [*Swiss physician in France*, 1781–1840]. Gave the first complete description of lupus erythematosus (1838); called *Biett's disease.*

bi′fid [L. *bis*, twice; L. *findere*, to cleave]. Divided into two parts; cleft, as bifid uvula.

bi·fo′cal [*bis;* L. *focus*, hearth]. Having two foci; applied to a system of lenses or spectacles.

bi·fo′cals. Lenses or spectacles used in the correction of presbyopia, where there is a refractive error for distant vision. The distance lens is above. Three types of bifocals are commonly used, the greater refractive power being obtained by: (a) cementing a wafer onto the front or back of the lens (**cement bifocals**); (b) fusing an insert of denser glass, as flint glass, into a crown-glass lens (**fused bifocals**); or (c) grinding the two different curvatures on one glass (**one-piece bifocals**).

bi·for′min. An antibiotic substance isolated from cultures of *Polyporus biformis*, a mushroom; it is active against a number of bacteria and possesses also antifungal activity.

bi″fur·ca′tion [L. *bifurcus*, having two prongs]. Division into two branches. —**bi′furcate,** *adj., v.t., v.i.*

Bigelow, Henry Jacob [*American surgeon*, 1818–90]. Developed a method of reducing dislocation of the hip, using the iliofemoral or Y ligament as a fulcrum; called *Bigelow's method.* Devised a special lithotrite, called *Bigelow's lithotrite*, for crushing large stones in the urinary bladder.

Bigelow, Jacob [*American physician and botanist*, 1787–1879]. One of the great botanists of America and celebrated as the author of a discourse on self-limited disease (1835). Said to have rescued medicine from the slavery of the drugging system.

bi·gem′i·nal [L. *bigeminus*, doubled]. Occurring in pairs; double; twin.

bi·gem′i·ny [L. *bigeminus*, doubled]. 1. The condition of occurring in pairs. 2. *In cardiology*, a premature beat coupled with each normal beat.

big jaw. Actinomycosis of cattle.

bi′labe [L. *bis*, twice; *labium*, lip]. A surgical instrument for removing foreign bodies from the urinary bladder through the urethra.

bi·lat′er·al [*bis;* L. *lateralis*, of the side]. Relating to two sides; pertaining to or affecting both sides of the body. —**bilateralism,** *n.*

bile [L. *bilis*]. A very bitter, alkaline, greenish yellow to golden-brown fluid, secreted by the liver and poured into the duodenum. It contains bile salts, cholesterol, lecithin, fat, various pigments, and mucin. Functionally, it aids in the emulsification, digestion, and absorption of fats, in the alkalinization of the intestines, and in the prevention of putrefaction.

A b. Bile collected from the common bile duct.

B b. Bile from the gallbladder.

b. pigments. Substances responsible for the color of bile, principally bilirubin and biliverdin, both derived from hemoglobin.

b. salts. Sodium salts of the bile acids, normally present in bile.

b. solubility. See under *test.*

C b. Bile from the hepatic duct.

cystic b. Bile stored in the gallbladder for some time; may be up to 10 times more concentrated than C bile.

ox b. See *ox bile.*

bile ac′id. Any one of the naturally occurring acids of bile formed by the conjugation of glycine or taurine with a cholic acid, forming glycocholic and taurocholic acids, respectively: also called *conjugated bile acid.*

unconjugated b. a. The residual cholic acid remaining when glycine or taurine is removed from a bile acid.

bilein. Trade-mark for a product containing sodium glycocholate and sodium taurocholate. Also spelled *bilene.*

Bil·har′zi·a [NL., after Theodor Maximilian *Bilharz*, German parasitologist, 1825–62]. Old term for *Schistosoma.*

bil″har·zi′a·sis. See *schistosomiasis*, 1.

bil′i- (bil′i-, buy′li-) [L. *bilis*, bile]. A combining form signifying *a relationship to bile* or *the biliary system.*

bil′i·ar″y [*bilis*]. Pertaining to or conveying bile, as a biliary duct.

bil″i·cy′a·nin [*bilis;* G. *kyanos*, dark blue]. A blue pigment obtained by the interaction of an ammoniacal solution of bilirubin and zinc chloride.

bil″i·fla′vin [*bilis;* L. *flavus,* yellow]. A yellow coloring matter derivable from biliverdin.

bil″i·ful′vin [*bilis;* L. *fulvus,* reddish yellow]. Bilirubin.

bil″i·fus′cin (bil″i·fuss′in, buy″li·) [*bilis;* L. *fuscus,* dark]. A normal fecal pigment (or possibly two isomeric substances) analogous to mesobilifuscin but having two vinyl groups in place of the two ethyl groups of mesobilifuscin.

bi·lig′u·late, bi·lig″u·la′tus [L. *bis,* twice; *ligula,* little tongue]. Formed like two tongues or having two tonguelike processes.

bil″i·hu′min [L. *bilis,* bile; L. *humus,* earth]. An insoluble residue left after treating gallstones with various solvents.

bil″i·leu′kan. A colorless precursor of bilifuscin.

bil″i·neu′rine (bil″i·new′reen, ·rin, buy″li·). Choline.

bil′ious [L. *biliosus,* full of bile]. 1. Pertaining to bile. 2. Popular term designating disorders arising from an excess of bile.

bil′ious·ness [*biliosus*]. Popular term for a condition marked by general malaise, headache, anorexia, indigestion, coated tongue, constipation, and lassitude; attributed to disorders of biliary secretions, but probably due to a digestive disorder.

bil″i·pha′in [L. *bilis,* bile; G. *phaios,* gray]. Bilirubin.

biliposol. A proprietary organic bismuth compound supplied in oil solution for use as antisyphilitic.

bil″i·pra′sin [*bilis;* G. *prasinos,* leek-green]. An intermediate bile pigment formed in the oxidation of bilirubin to biliverdin. Syn., *choleprasin.*

bil″i·pur′pu·rin. Cholehematin.

bil″i·ru′bic ac′id. $C_{17}H_{24}N_2O_3$; a cleavage product obtained, along with the isomeric isobilirubic acid, when bilirubin is reduced with hydriodic acid.

bil″i·ru′bin (bil″i·rōō′bin, buy″li·) [*bilis;* L. *ruber,* red]. $C_{33}H_{36}N_4O_6$. Orange-red crystals or powder. The principal pigment of bile, formed by reduction of biliverdin, normally present in feces and found in the urine in obstructive jaundice. It is insoluble in water, and is used intravenously as a test of liver function. See Table of Normal Values of Blood Constituents in the Appendix.

bil″i·ru″bi·ne′mi·a, bil″i·ru″bi·nae′mi·a (bil″i·rōō″bi·nee′mee·uh, buy″li·) [*bilis; ruber;* G. *haima,* blood]. The presence of bilirubin in the blood; jaundice, icterus.

bil′i·ru″bin-glo′bin. A transitional stage in the production of bilirubin from hemoglobin. It is the substance which remains after the removal of iron from the hemoglobin.

bil″i·ru″bi·nu′ri·a [*bilis; ruber;* G. *ouron,* urine]. Presence of bilirubin in the urine. Normally it occurs in small amounts and is increased in obstructive jaundice.

bil″i·u′ri·a [*bilis; ouron*]. The presence of bile salts in the urine.

bil″i·ver′din. $C_{33}H_{34}N_4O_6$; a dark green bile pigment, formed in the body from hemoglobin, but largely reduced in the liver to bilirubin, which is the principal pigment of bile. Biliverdin may also be obtained by oxidizing bilirubin.

bil″i·xan′thine (bil″i·zan′theen, ·thin, buy″li·), **bil″i·xan′thin.** See *choletelin.*

Billings, John Shaw [*American Army medical officer and librarian,* 1838–1913]. Well-known medical bibliographer and authority on public health and vital statistics. Compilation of the *Index-Catalogue of the Library of the Surgeon General* was begun under his direction (1880). With Robert Fletcher, founded the monthly *Index Medicus* (1879). Author of *History of Surgery* (1895). Responsible for the plans of the Johns Hopkins Hospital.

bill of health. An authenticated document issued by quarantine or other public health officials to a ship's master after inspection, to indicate the state of health of the ship's company and of the port.

Billroth, Christian Albert Theodor [*Austrian surgeon,* 1829–94]. Internationally recognized as an outstanding leader and founder of modern abdominal surgery. He was the first to excise the larynx (1874), the first to excise the esophagus (1872), and the first to excise a urinary bladder tumor by the abdominal route (1875). He resected the pylorus for cancer (1881) using his technic of excising the pyloric portion of the stomach, followed by anastomosis of the duodenal stump to the greater curvature (Billroth I operation). Later, he devised the operation of resection of the affected segment of the stomach with closure of the ends of the duodenum and stomach, followed by gastroenterostomy (Billroth II operation). His name is associated with the red cords of the spleen which he described, with an anesthetic mixture (alcohol, chloroform, and ether), and also with malignant lymphoma.

bi·lo′bate (buy·lo′bait) [L. *bis,* twice; G. *lobos,* lobe]. Having, or divided into, two lobes.

bi·loc′u·lar, bi·loc′u·late [*bis;* L. *loculus,* dim. of *locus,* place]. Having two cells, compartments, or chambers.

bilron. Trade-mark for a cholagogue composed of iron in combination with bile salts.

bi·man′u·al [*bis;* L. *manus,* hand]. Pertaining to both hands; done by both hands.

bi′na·ry [L. *binarius,* from *bini,* two by two]. 1. *In chemistry,* compounded of two elements. 2. *In anatomy,* separating into two branches or parts.

bi·na′sal (buy·nay′zul) [L. *bis,* twice; *nasus,* nose]. Referring to both nasal visual fields, as binasal hemianopsia.

bin·au′ral [L. *bini,* two by two; *auris,* ear]. Pertaining to or having two ears. Also *binauricular, binotic.*

bind [AS. *bindan*]. 1. To bandage; join together with a band. 2. *In chemistry,* unite with, as in the combination of two substances having affinity.

bind′er [*bindan*]. A wide bandage or girdle worn to support the abdomen or breasts after childbirth or operations, as an obstetric or abdominal binder.

Binet, Alfred [*French psychologist,* 1857–1911]. Devised an intelligence test, with Théodore Simon, in which the intellectual capacity of the subject is estimated by comparison with that of normal children and adolescents of various ages; the mental age divided by the chronologic age gives the intelligence quotient (I.Q.). Called *Binet's test, Binet-Simon test. Binet's formula* states that children under nine whose mental development is retarded by two years probably are mentally deficient, and that children of nine or more who are retarded by three years are definitely deficient.

bin·oc′u·lar [L. *bini,* two by two; *oculus,* eye]. *In optics,* an instrument with two eyepieces for use with both eyes at once. See *horopter.* —**binoc′ular,** *adj.*

bin·ox′ide. See *dioxide.*

Binswanger, Otto [*German neurologist,* 1859–1929]. Described chronic, progressive, subcortical encephalopathy with presenile dementia and loss of memory; called *Binswanger's dementia.*

Binz, Karl [*German chemist,* 1832–1912]. A pupil of Virchow, he founded the Pharmacological Institute at Bonn (1869). Remembered for his test for arsenic, now superseded.

bi′o-, bi- [G. *bios*, life]. A combining form denoting *relation to*, or *connection with, life, vital phenomena,* or *living organisms.*

bi′o-as·say″. Biological assay.

bi″o·aut·og′ra·phy. A technique, similar to autoradiography, in which the growth response (instead of the radioactivity) of specific micro-organisms is used for detection of a compound or compounds on a paper chromatogram. —**bio-autograph′ic,** *adj.*

bi′o·blast [*bios;* G. *blastos*, germ]. 1. Old term for mitochondria, thought by Altmann to be the vital unit of the cell. 2. Old term for any cell capable of living independently.

bi″o·cat′a·lyst [*bios;* G. *katalysis*, dissolution]. An enzyme; a biochemical catalyst.

bi″o·chem′is·try [*bios;* G. *chymeia*, perhaps a mingling, from *chymos*, juice]. The chemistry of the living tissues or of life; physiological chemistry. —**biochemical,** *adj.*

bi″o·chem·or′phic [*bios; chymos;* G. *morphē*, form]. Noting the relationship between chemical structure and biologic activity; relating to biochemorphology.

bi″o·chem″or·phol′o·gy [*bios; chymos; morphē;* G. *logos*, word]. The science dealing with the chemical structure of foods and drugs and their reactions on living organisms.

bi′o·chrome [*bios;* G. *chroma*, color]. Pigment synthesized in the metabolic processes of living organisms.

bi″o·cli″ma·tol′o·gy [*bios;* G. *klima*, slope; *logos*]. The study of the effect of climate on life. Also called *bioclimatics.*

bi″o·cy′tin. A complex of biotin occurring in yeast and possibly in other natural products.

bi″o·di·al′y·sate (buy″o·dye·al′i·sayt) [*bios;* G. *dialysis*, a separating]. The fluid bath after biodialysis, found to be inhibitory to gastric secretion upon intravenous or subcutaneous administration in dogs.

bi″o·di·al′y·sis (buy″o·dye·al′i·sis) [*bios; dialysis*]. In experimental physiology, the process of bathing the intestine for approximately one hour in Locke-Ringer's solution at 37° C.; the fluid bath is then known as the biodialysate.

bi″o-e·lec″tric′i·ty. Electric phenomena occurring in living tissues; effects of electric currents upon living tissues.

bi″o·en″er·get′ics [*bios;* G. *energētikos*, acting upon]. The science of the transformation of energy in biologic functions.

bi″o·flav′o·noids. Flavone compounds or derivatives having biological or pharmacological activity, such as vitamin P.

bi″o·gen′e·sis [*bios;* G. *genesis*, production]. 1. The doctrine that living things are produced only from living things—the reverse of abiogenesis. 2. Loosely, both ontogeny and phylogeny. —**bio-genet′ic, biog′enous,** *adj.*

bi·og′e·ny (buy·odj′i·nee) [*bios; genesis*]. Biogenesis.

bi″o·ki·net′ics (buy″o·ki·net′icks, ·kigh·net′icks) [*bios;* G. *kinētikos*, from *kinēsis*, motion]. The kinetics of life; the science of the movements of developing organisms. See *karyokinesis.*

bi″o·ki·net′ic tem′per·a·ture lim′its. The lowest and highest temperatures beyond which no form of life can be sustained: −273° C. to approximately 160° C.

Biol. Biology.

biolac. A proprietary, homogenized, modified milk; used as infant food.

bi″o·log′i·cal as·say′. A method of determining the potency of a substance by comparing its effects on living material quantitatively with those of a standard substance. Syn., *bio-assay.*

bi″o·log′i·cals [*bios;* G. *logos*, word]. Medicinal preparations of a complex biologic nature, their action depending on numerous phases of immunity. They include serums, vaccines, antitoxins, and antigens.

lyophilized b. Any biologic substance, such as blood plasma, antitoxins, toxins, serums, etc., which has been prepared in dry form by rapid freezing and dehydration, while in the frozen state, under high vacuum. Such a preparation is more stable than the product from which it is derived, does not require refrigeration, and is made ready for use by the addition of sterile, distilled water.

bi″o·log′i·cal war′fare. *In military medicine*, tactics and techniques of conducting warfare by use of biological agents.

bi·ol′o·gist [*bios; logos*]. One learned in biology.

bi·ol′o·gy [*bios; logos*]. The science of life. It includes botany, zoology, and all their branches. —**bio-log′ic, biolog′ical,** *adj.*

bi″o·lu″mi·nes′cence [*bios;* L. *lumen*, light]. Luminescence caused by living organisms; phosphorescence.

bi″o·math″e·mat′ics [*bios;* G. *mathēmatikos*, from *mathēma*, that which is learned, lesson]. Mathematics applied to biologic phenomena.

bi″o·me·chan′ics [*bios;* G. *mēchanē*, machine]. The science dealing with the mechanics of the living organism, especially of the levers and arches of the skeleton, and the forces applied to them by the muscles and by gravity.

bi·om′e·ter [*bios;* G. *metron*, a measure]. An instrument for measuring the amount of carbon dioxide given off by a small organism, tissue, etc.

bi·om′e·try [*bios; metron*]. 1. The statistical study of biologic problems; biometrics. 2. Calculation of the expectancy of life, for life insurance purposes.

bi″o·mi·cros′co·py [*bios;* G. *mikros*, small; *skopein*, to examine]. Microscopic study of living cell structures. —**biomi′croscope,** *n.*

Biondi's stain. See under *stain.*

bi′o·phore [*bios;* G. *phoros*, bearing]. A hypothetical vital unit in Weismann's theory of the architecture of the germ plasm, varying in complexity from that of a molecule to that of a cell, and with manifold properties and functions depending upon biologists' conceptions. Syn., *micelle.* —**biophor′ic,** *adj.*

bi″o·pho·tom′e·ter [*bios;* G. *phōs*, light; *metron*, a measure]. An instrument designed to measure the rate and degree of dark adaptation.

bi″o·phys′ics [*bios;* G. *physis*, nature]. The study of life processes by physical apparatus and methods; the physics of life processes.

bi·op′la·sis [*bios;* G. *plassein*, to form]. Anabolism. —**bioplas′tic,** *adj.*

bi′op·sy [*bios;* G. *opsis*, vision]. 1. Observation of the living subject, as opposed to necropsy. 2. The excision, during life, of tissue to establish a diagnosis by means of a microscopic examination of the excised piece.

aspiration b. A method for the aspiration of small amounts of tissue for biopsy, by the use of a trocar inserted into the desired tissue.

muscle b. The securing of biopsy material from a muscle.

needle b. The securing of biopsy material by means of a hollow needle.

ring b. Surgical excision of the entire circumference of the squamocolumnar junction of the cervix: used in the diagnosis of cancer.

surface b. Scraping of cells from the surface of tissues, especially from the squamocolumnar junction of the uterine cervix for microscopic examination in cancer diagnosis: also called *surface-cell biopsy.*

bi″o·psy·chol′o·gy. Psychobiology. —**biopsy′-chic,** *adj.*

bi′os I. Inositol.

bi′os IIb. Biotin.

bi′ose [L. *bis*, twice; *-ose*, chemical suffix]. 1. A disaccharide. 2. A sugar containing two carbon atoms.

bi″o·sta·tis′tics [G. *bios*, life; ML. *statisticus*]. The branch of biometry which deals with the laws and data of demography, natality, morbidity, and mortality; vital statistics.

bi·os′ter·ol. Old term for vitamin A.

bi″o·syn′the·sis. 1. The synthesis of a substance in living matter. 2. The formative reactions which take place during metabolism, such as the synthesis of enzymes, amino acids, or vitamins.

Biot, Camille [*French physician*, nineteenth century]. Remembered for his description of a type of shallow breathing interrupted by long pauses, seen in meningitis and sometimes in healthy persons.

bi·o′ta. The flora and fauna, collectively, of a region.

bi·ot′ic. 1. Pertaining to life or living matter. 2. Pertaining to biota.

bi·ot′ics. The science of vital activities.

bi′o·tin (buy′o·tin, buy·ot′in). $C_{10}H_{16}O_3N_2S$. A member of the vitamin-B complex, widely distributed in plant and animal tissues from which it is isolated by autolysis, digestion, or hydrolysis; essential for growth of certain bacteria and yeasts and a growth hormone for higher plants; of uncertain significance in animals and man. Syn., *vitamin H, coenzyme R, bios IIb.* See Table of Vitamins in Appendix.

bi′o·type [*bios;* G. *typos*, model]. 1. A group of individuals all of which have the same genotype. 2. Constitutional (body) type. —**biotyp′ic,** *adj.*

bi″o·ty·pol′o·gy (buy″o·tigh·pol′o·jee) [*bios; typos;* G. *logos*, word]. The systematic study of body types correlated with physiologic and psychologic aspects, as constitutional variations and inadequacies.

B.I.P. Bismuth iodoform paste.

bip′a·ra [L. *bis*, twice; *parere*, to bring forth]. A woman who has borne two children at different labors.

bi·par″a·sit′ic [*bis;* G. *parasitikos*, from *parasitein*, to board and lodge with]. Parasitic upon a parasite.

bi″pa·ri′e·tal [*bis;* L. *paries*, wall]. Relating to both parietal bones.

bi″pa·ri′e·tal di·am′e·ter. The distance from one parietal eminence to the other.

bip′a·rous [*bis;* L. *parere*, to bring forth]. Producing two at a birth.

bi′ped [*bis;* L. *pes*, foot]. An animal with two feet. —**bi′ped, bipedal,** *adj.*

bi·pen′ni·form (buy·pen′i·form), **bi·pen′nate** (buy·pen′ate) [*bis;* L. *penna*, feather]. Having the appearance of a feather with barbs on both sides, as certain muscles.

bi″po·lar′i·ty [*bis;* L. *polus*, pole]. 1. Condition of having two processes from opposite poles, as a nerve cell. 2. The use of the two electrodes in stimulation of muscle or nerve. —**bipo′lar,** *adj.*

bi″po·ten″ti·al′i·ty [*bis;* L. *potentia*, power]. The capacity of developing into two different types of tissues.

b. of gonad. Bisexual organization of the indifferent gonad; the medullary part is capable of forming the testis, the cortex, of forming the ovary. This bipotentiality forms the basis of sex reversal.

bipp. Dressing for wounds, composed of bismuth subnitrate 1 part, iodoform 2 parts, petrolatum 1 part. Also called *B.I.P., bismuth iodoform paste.*

birch [AS. *beorc, birce*]. Any tree of the genus *Betula*. Birch tar, or the tarry oil of *B. pendula*, has been used in certain skin diseases. The bark of *B. lenta*, the sweet birch, yields a fragrant volatile oil, which consists, like that of *Gaultheria procumbens*, almost entirely of methyl salicylate.

Birch-Hirschfeld, Felix Victor [*German pathologist*, 1842–99]. Known for his method of demonstrating amyloid degeneration by means of Bismarck brown and gentian violet stain, the amyloid material retaining the color while the normal tissue decolorizes with acetic acid.

Bird, Golding [*English physician*, 1814–54]. Said to have been the first to perform the operation for relief of obstruction of the small intestine. Oxaluria is still known as *Bird's disease.*

bi″re·frac′tive [L. *bis*, twice; *refractus*, from *refringere*, to break up]. Doubly refractive; anisotropic.

bi″re·frin′gence [*bis; refringere*]. Double refraction, in biologic objects three types occur: crystalline, form, and strain birefringences.

stream b. That occurring when solutions containing asymmetric particles are set into motion and the particles tend to orient as a result of the flow. When the flow stops, the solution becomes isotropic. The tobacco mosaic virus is such a particle.

bi·rhin′i·a, bir·rhin′i·a (buy·rin′ee·uh). See *dirrhinus.*

bi·ri′mose (buy·rye′moce, buy′rye·moce) [*bis;* L. *rima*, cleft]. Having two clefts or slits.

birth [ME. *burth, birth*]. 1. The delivery of offspring; parturition. 2. That which is born. See *labor.*

cross b. Transverse presentation.

multiple b. The occurrence of two or more offspring at a birth.

partial b. In labor, the incomplete expulsion of offspring, as the retention of a portion of a macerated fetus.

plural b. See multiple *b.*

premature b. See premature *labor.*

stillbirth. The birth of dead offspring.

birth cer·tif′i·cate. A legal form on which the date and place of birth, name and sex of child, names of parents, and other pertinent information are recorded.

birth con·trol′. The prevention or regulation of conception by whatever means; contraception.

birth in′ju·ry. Any injury suffered by a child during parturition, such as fracture of a bone, subluxation of a joint, injury to peripheral nerves, or intracranial hemorrhage.

birth′mark″. A nevus, either vascular, nonvascular, or pigmented.

birth rate. The proportion of births in a given year to the total population, known as the **crude birth rate. Specific birth rates** are figured for the female population, for the females of certain age or race groups, or for other variables.

birth reg″is·tra′tion a′re·a. That territory from which the United States Bureau of the Census collects birth records. Since 1933, this has been the entire United States.

bis- [L. *bis*, twice]. 1. A prefix meaning *twice, both.* 2. *In chemistry*, a prefix denoting *the doubling of a complex expression.*

Bischoff's test. See under *test.*

bi·sex′u·al (buy·seck′shoo·ul) [*bis;* L. *sexus*, sex]. 1. Biparental. 2. Hermaphroditic. 3. Referring or pertaining to an individual of mixed homosexual and heterosexual behavior. See also *gynandromorphy.*

bis·fe′ri·ous (biss·fear′i·us, ·ferr′i·us) [*bis;* L. *ferire*, to strike]. Having two peaks, as a bisferious pulse, in which the second peak is equal to, or often higher than, the first. See dicrotic *pulse.*

bis″hy·drox″y·cou′mar·in. The official generic

name for 3,3′-methylenebis(4-hydroxycoumarin); $C_{19}H_{12}O_6$, originally isolated from spoiled sweet clover, eating of which caused hemorrhagic disease in cattle. It occurs as a white crystalline powder, practically insoluble in water; it is therapeutically useful as a coagulant. Dose, 100–300 mg. (1½–5 gr.). Syn., *dicoumarin, dicoumarol, melitoxin.* See *dicumarol.*

Bis′kra but′ton. See *oriental sore.*

Bis′marck brown Y (C.C.). An aniline dye of the azo series; used in aqueous or saturated alcoholic solution as a contrast stain, as a mucin stain, for vital staining, and for staining in bulk. Also called *Vesuvin; phenylene brown; Manchester brown; Excelsior brown; leather brown; basic brown G, GX,* or *GXP; aniline brown.*

bismarsen. Trade-mark for bismuth arsphenamine sulfonate; used as antisyphilitic by intramuscular injection. Dose, 0.1 Gm. initially, followed by 0.2 Gm. weekly, later biweekly, for a total of 20 or more doses. Syn., *sulfarsphenamine bismuth.*

bismo-cymol. Trade-mark for a basic bismuth camphocarboxylate: has been used as an antisyphilitic.

bismoid. Trade-mark for a suspension of finely divided bismuth intended for intramuscular use as an antisyphilitic.

bismosol. Trade-mark for a solution of potassium sodium bismuthotartrate, piperazine, and glucose intended for intramuscular use as an antisyphilitic.

bis′muth (biz′muth) [Ger. *Wismut*]. Bi = 209.00. A white, crystalline metal with a reddish tint. Its insoluble salts are employed chiefly because of their protective action on mucous membranes; the salts are also feebly antiseptic. Various compounds of bismuth, soluble and insoluble, have been employed for the treatment of syphilis.

b. albuminate. A powder, incompletely soluble in water, containing about 22% bismuth; used in gastric or intestinal cramp. Dose, 0.3–1.0 Gm. (5–15 gr.).

b. and ammonium citrate. A water-soluble double salt. It is actively astringent and irritant, and is sometimes used in acute diarrheas. Dose, 0.06–0.2 Gm. (1–3 gr.).

b. and emetine iodide. A reddish orange salt, practically insoluble in water; used in the treatment of amebic colitis. Dose, 0.06–0.2 Gm. (1–3 gr.).

b. arsphenamine sulfonate. The sodium salt of a compound of bismuth and arsphenamine methylene sulfonic acid, containing about 13% arsenic and 24% bismuth. It is a brownish–yellow, water-soluble powder, and is employed in treating syphilis. Dose, by intramuscular injection, 0.1–0.2 Gm. (1½–3 gr.). See *bismarsen.*

b. betanaphthol. A compound of somewhat variable composition, employed in the treatment of enteritis because it is believed to yield betanaphthol in the intestinal tract. Dose, 0.3–1.3 Gm. (5–20 gr.). Syn., *orphol.*

b. bitannate. A light yellow powder, insoluble in water; believed to exercise astringent effect in the stomach. Dose, 0.3–2.0 Gm. (5–30 gr.). See *tannismut.*

b. bromide. $BiBr_3$. A yellow, crystalline powder, soluble in aqueous solutions of the potassium halides; used in veterinary medicine.

b. camphocarboxylate. A basic compound representing 37–40% bismuth. It is a white powder, insoluble in water but soluble in fixed oils. An oil solution has been employed intramuscularly as an antisyphilitic. See *bismo-cymol.*

b. carbolate. $Bi(OH)_2(C_6H_5O)$. A gray powder, insoluble in water; has been used as gastrointestinal antiseptic. Syn., *b. phenylate, phenol b.*

b. carbonate. The official British Pharmacopoeia name for bismuth subcarbonate.

b. citrate. Approximately $C_6H_5BiO_7$; a white powder insoluble in water: employed in the manufacture of bismuth and ammonium citrate but not used as such in medicine.

b. diasporal. A trade-mark for a 2% colloidal solution of bismuthyl-cordofanic acid employed as an antisyphilitic.

b. ethylcamphorate. $(C_{12}H_{19}O_4)_3Bi$. A white amorphous compound, insoluble in water but soluble in vegetable oils; an oil suspension of it is employed for the systemic effects of bismuth in the treatment of syphilis.

b. glycolylarsanilate. $HOCH_2.CO.HN.C_6H_4.$-$AsO(OH)(OBiO)$; a yellowish white to flesh-colored powder, very slightly soluble in water; it contains 15% arsenic (pentavalent) and 39% bismuth: used in the treatment of intestinal amebiasis. Syn., *glycobiarsol.* See *milibis.*

b. iodosubgallate. A basic compound of bismuth, iodine, and gallic acid; occurs as a grayish green powder, decomposed by water. It is a local antiseptic, liberating iodine in contact with body fluids. Syn., *b. oxyiodogallate.* See *airol.*

b. lactate. Approximately $C_3H_5O_3BiC_3H_4O_3$-$7H_2O$; a white salt of varying composition, formerly used in treating diarrhea.

b. oleate. A yellowish, soft mass, insoluble in water; used as a dusting powder with zinc oxide and starch, or in ointment, for application to skin infections. A suspension in olive oil is injected intramuscularly in the treatment of syphilis.

b. oxide. Bi_2O_3. A yellowish powder, insoluble in water; formerly used like other insoluble bismuth salts, especially in the treatment of enteritis.

b. oxybromide. Approximately BiOBr. A yellowish, water-insoluble powder; used in treating nervous dyspepsia.

b. oxychloride (*bismuthi oxychloridum*). A white, water-insoluble salt approximating the composition BiOCl; may be used internally for the same purposes as bismuth subcarbonate; has been used as an antisyphilitic by intramuscular injection. Dose, oral, 0.6–2.0 Gm. (10–30 gr.); intramuscular, 0.1–0.2 Gm. (1½–3 gr.).

b. oxyiodide. Approximately BiOI. A yellowish red powder, insoluble in water; formerly used as a local antiseptic and substitute for iodoform.

b. oxyiodogallate. See *b.* iodosubgallate.

b. permanganate. Approximately $Bi(MnO_4)_3$. A black powder, slightly soluble in water: has been employed as an antiseptic dusting powder for wounds and ulcers.

b. phenylate. See *b.* carbolate.

b. potassium tartrate. A water-soluble salt containing 60–64% bismuth. It is used principally as an antisyphilitic, an aqueous solution or oil suspension being injected intramuscularly.

b. quinine iodide. See *quinine* bismuth iodide.

b. salicylate. The name occasionally applied to bismuth subsalicylate, but used properly only for a mixture of salicylic acid and bismuth subsalicylate. The latter mixture is a white powder, insoluble in water, and acid in reaction; used as an intestinal astringent and antiseptic. Dose, 0.3–0.6 Gm. (5–10 gr.).

b. sodium iodide. See *sodium* iodobismuthite.

b. sodium tartrate. A water-soluble salt containing 35–42% bismuth (British Pharmacopoeia); a salt containing twice as much bismuth is also supplied under the same name in the United States. It is used principally as an antisyphilitic. Syn., *sodium bismuthyltartrate.*

b. sodium thioglycollate. See *thio-bismol.*

b. sodium triglycollamate. $C_{24}H_{28}BiN_4Na_7O_{25}$;

a white crystalline powder, very soluble in water; effective orally in the management of certain forms of syphilis and also in some cases of lupus erythematosus, lichen planus, and scleroderma. See *bistrimate.*

b. subbenzoate. A white powder, insoluble in water; used chiefly as a wound antiseptic.

b. subcarbonate (*bismuthi subcarbonas*). Approximately $(BiO)_2CO_3.\frac{1}{2}H_2O$; a white salt, insoluble in water: used as a protective in gastrointestinal diseases as well as for local application. Dose, 0.6–2.0 Gm. (10–30 gr.).

b. subgallate (*bismuthi subgallas*). Approximately $C_6H_2(OH)_3.COOBi(OH)_2$; a bright yellow powder, practically insoluble in water. It is used externally as a dusting powder, sometimes internally in treating enteritis. Dose, 0.45–2.0 Gm. (7–30 gr.). Syn., *dermatol.*

b. subnitrate (*bismuthi subnitras*). Approximately $4BiNO_3(OH)_2.BiO(OH)$; a white powder, practically insoluble in water. It is used like bismuth subcarbonate but yields some nitrite ions in the intestines. Dose, 0.3–2.0 Gm. (5–30 gr.).

b. subsalicylate (*bismuthi subsalicylas*). Approximately $C_6H_4(OH).COOBiO$; a white powder, practically insoluble in water. Its antiseptic action is superior to that of other basic bismuth salts. It is used in the treatment of enteritis, and has been used as an antisyphilitic. Dose, as a gastrointestinal protective, 0.6–2.0 Gm. (10–30 gr.); as an antisyphilitic, 0.06–0.12 Gm. (1–2 gr.), by intramuscular injection.

b. tribromphenate. Approximately $BiOH.(C_6H_2Br_3O)_2.Bi_2O_3$; a yellow powder, practically insoluble in water. It is used as an antiseptic, both internally and externally. Dose, 1–3 Gm. (15–45 gr.) per day to adults. Also called *b. tribromphenol.* See *xeroform.*

b. valerate, b. valerianate. Approximately $C_4H_9COOBiO.H_2O$; a white powder, practically insoluble in water; used as a sedative and antispasmodic. Dose, 0.03–0.2 Gm. (½–3 gr.).

b. violet. A proprietary dye used externally as a bactericide.

phenol b. See *b.* carbolate.

precipitated b. (*bismuthum praecipitatum*). A finely subdivided form of metallic bismuth, used as an injection (in 5% dextrose solution) in the treatment of syphilis.

bis·mu′thi·a. A blue discoloration of skin and mucous membranes resulting from administration of bismuth compounds.

bis″muth·o′sis (biz″muth·o′sis) [Ger. *Wismut;* G. *-ōsis,* condition]. Chronic bismuth poisoning.

bis″muth·o·tar′trate. A salt of tartaric acid in which a bismuthyl (—BiO) radical replaces the hydroxyl hydrogen of one or both of the secondary alcohol groups in the tartaric acid component of the salt.

bis′muth·yl (biz′muth·il, ·eel). The univalent radical —BiO.

bismutose. Trade-mark for a bismuth-albumin combination in powder form; it is antacid and astringent.

bisodol. A proprietary antacid and digestant.

bis′sa [prob. of African origin]. Affection of man and sheep, common in Egypt; characterized by the production of edema.

bis′sa·bol. A kind of myrrh from a species of trees of East Africa, genus *Commiphora,* used largely in finer grades of myrrh. Said to stimulate powerfully the flow of milk in cows.

bis″sy·no′sis. A benign pneumonia believed to be caused by inhalation of *Aerobacter cloacae,* an organism often found in stained, old cotton. The disease was formerly believed to be caused by inhalation of cotton fibers. Also called *gin fever, Monday morning fever.*

bis′tort [L. *bis,* twice; *tortus,* from *torquere,* to twist]. Snakeweed, adderwort; the rhizome of *Polygonum bistorta.* It contains about 20% tannin, and is used as astringent.

bis′tou·ry (biss′too·ree) [F. *bistouri*]. A long, narrow knife, either straight, curved, sharp-pointed, or probe-pointed, used for cutting from within outward. Its use in surgery is confined to the incision of abscesses, the opening of sinuses or fistulas, or, occasionally, the cutting of the constriction in strangulated hernia.

bistrimate. Trade-mark for a brand of *bismuth sodium triglycollamate,* a substance effective orally in treatment of syphilis and certain diseases of the skin.

bistrium bromide. A trade-marked name for a brand of hexamethonium bromide.

bi·sul′fide (buy·sul′fide, ·fid). A binary compound containing two atoms of sulfur. Syn., *disulfide.*

bi·sul′fite. Any compound containing the radical $—HSO_3$. An acid sulfite.

bit [AS. *bītan*]. *In dentistry,* a rotary drill.

bi·tar′trate. A salt of tartaric acid characterized by the radical $—HC_4H_4O_6$, representing tartaric acid wherein one hydrogen has been replaced.

bite [AS. *bītan*]. 1. The forcible closure of the lower against the upper teeth; the measure of force exerted by such closure as recorded in pounds by gnathodynamometer. 2. A skin puncture produced by the teeth or mouth parts of an insect, snake, or other animal. 3. *In dental prosthetics,* a plastic impression of the relationship of the upper and lower teeth in occlusion.

check b. A plastic impression of the teeth, serving as a guide for alignment in an articulator; used in orthodontics and dental prosthetics. It consists of bites taken in hard wax or soft modeling compound, which record centric, eccentric, and protrusive occlusion.

closed b. One in which the lower incisors and canines are posterior to the upper, almost touching the gum line when the jaws are closed; extreme overbite.

edge-to-edge b. The meeting of the cutting edges of the upper and lower anterior teeth. Also called *end-to-end b.*

jumping the b. A forcible shifting forward of a retruded lower jaw to obtain a normal occlusion.

locked b. Interdigitation of the teeth in such a manner that normal excursions of the mandible are restricted or prevented while the teeth are in occlusion.

mush b. An unfinished bite usually taken in beeswax, showing the correct relationship of the cusps in general, but with little or no reproduction of the outline of the teeth.

open b. A condition in which the upper and lower incisors do not occlude.

opening the b. Elevation of the occlusal plane of some or all of the posterior teeth by orthodontic manipulation or prosthetic restorations.

bite. To seize or grasp with the teeth. 2. To corrode or eat into by chemical action.

bite gauge. An instrument which helps to establish a correct bite.

bite′wing [*bītan;* ME. *winge*]. A type of dental x-ray film having a central fin or wing upon which the teeth can close to hold the film in place.

bi·thi′o·nol. $C_{12}H_6Cl_4O_2S$; 2,2′-thiobis(4,6-dichlorophenol); a white or grayish-white crystalline powder, insoluble in water; a bacteriostatic agent for use in soap formulations. See *actamer.*

Bi·thyn′i·a. A genus of snails whose species serve as intermediate hosts of the trematodes of man.

The species **B. tentaculata** of eastern Europe is the host of the cat liver fluke, *Opisthorchis felineus*. **B. fuchsiana** and **B. longicornis** of China are hosts of *Clonorchis sinensis*.

Bi'tis [NL.]. A genus of Viperidae, venomous snakes.

B. gabonica. The Gaboon viper of equatorial Africa; possesses powerful neurotoxic venom.

B. lachesis. The large-headed puff adder; a species found from South Africa to southern Arabia; possesses a hemotoxic venom.

B. nasicornis. The rhinoceros viper, one of the true vipers found in equatorial Africa. This viper also has a hemotoxic venom.

Bitot's spots. See under *spot*.

bit'ters [AS. *bīter*]. 1. Medicines characterized by a bitter taste. 2. An alcoholic drink, an appetizer.

angostura b. See *angostura*.

aromatic b. Medicines that unite the properties of aromatics with those of simple bitters.

astringent b. Medicines that add styptic and astringent properties to that of bitterness.

simple b. Medicines that stimulate the gastrointestinal tract without influencing the general system.

bit'ter·sweet". See *dulcamara*.

Bitt'ner milk fac'tor. See milk *factor*.

bi·tu'men (bi·tew'mun, buy·, bit'yoo·mun, bit'chew·mun). Any one of a group of native, solid, or semisolid hydrocarbons.

sulfonated b. An unofficial synonym for ichthammol.

bi·u'rate. An acid salt of uric acid.

bi"u·ret' (buy"yoo·ret', buy'yoo·ret). $NH(CO—NH_2)_2$. A compound obtained by heating urea. It is soluble in water and in alcohol, and crystallizes from water as monohydrate. The anhydrous form melts at 190° C. with decomposition.

bi"u·ret' re·ac'tion. A blue or blue-violet color given by biuret on the addition of copper sulfate and strong alkali. The test is given by protein solutions without heating, and by urea after prolonged heating.

bi·va'lent (buy·vay'lunt, biv'uh·lunt). 1. Denoting the ability to combine with or displace two atoms of hydrogen or their equivalent; having a valence of two. Syn., *divalent*. 2. *In biology:* see bivalent *chromosome*. 3. *In psychiatry:* see *ambivalence*. —**bivalence,** *n.*

bi'valve" [L. *bis*, twice; *valva*, leaf of a door]. A mollusk with double shells, as a clam or oyster. —**bi'valve", bi·val'vular,** *adj.*

bi·ven'ter (buy·ven'tur) [*bis;* L. *venter*, belly]. Having two bellies, as a muscle.

bi·ven'ter. A digastric muscle. See Table of Muscles in the Appendix. —**bi·ven'tral,** *adj.*

Bizzozero nodule. See under *nodule*.

Bizzozero's blood platelet. See *achromacyte*.

Bjerrum, Jannik [*Danish ophthalmologist*, 1827–92]. Invented a black screen one meter square, to be used at a distance of one meter to plot accurately the central field of vision; called *Bjerrum's screen*.

Bjerrum, Jannik Peterson [*Danish ophthalmologist*, 1851–1920]. Remembered for his description of a sign in scotoma, an arcuate area extending from the blind spot around the representation of the macula, considered pathognomonic of simple glaucoma. Called *Bjerrum's sign*.

Bk Chemical symbol for berkelium.

Black, Greene Vardiman (1836–1915). American dentist, known for his system of classification of cavities, development of the principles of cavity preparation, and investigations in the field of dental histology and pathology.

Black, J. A. [*English surgeon*, contemporary]. Adapted a formula or factor devised by Pignet, in which the figures are expressed in inches and pounds instead of centimeters and kilograms. F is the empirical factor and equals the weight in pounds (W) plus the chest measurement in inches at deep inspiration (C) minus the height in inches (H). $F = (W + C) - H$. If the result is over 120, the individual is rated very strong; between 100 and 110, good or average; between 90 and 100, only fair; under 80, very weak. The factor was designed originally (ca. 1908) for use in examining recruits for the French Army and is little used today. Called *Black's formula*.

Black, Joseph [*Scottish chemist*, 1728–99]. Remembered as the discoverer of carbon dioxide (1757).

Black's test. See under *test*.

Blackall, John [*English physician*, 1771–1860]. Remembered as having preceded Bright in observing albuminuria in cases of renal dropsy (1813).

black'damp". Carbon dioxide gas which collects in mines and deep shafts; chokedamp.

Black Death. The plague which ravaged Europe and Asia in the fourteenth century. See *plague*.

black haw. *Viburnum prunifolium*.

black'head". An enlarged, chronically disordered, sebaceous gland; comedo.

black'leg". A febrile, generally fatal, infectious disease; affects cattle and sheep and is characterized by diffuse, crepitating swelling in the muscles of the back and legs. *Clostridium feseri* is the principal causative organism, but *Clostridium septicum* or, more rarely, *Clostridium novyi* is sometimes found to be responsible.

black'out". *In aviation*, temporary loss of vision with preservation of consciousness, due to cessation of blood flow to the cranial cavity, caused by linear or centrifugal accelerations of considerable magnitudes. Syn., *amaurosis fugax, stagnant anoxia*.

black'tongue. A disease of dogs, due to a deficiency of niacin; similar to pellagra. Also see black, hairy *tongue*.

black'wa"ter fe'ver. A severe, usually fatal, form of malaria associated with bloody urine. See *hemoglobinuria*.

Blackwell, Elizabeth [*American physician*, 1821–1910]. The first woman to receive a medical degree in America (1849).

blad'der [AS. *blǣdre*]. 1. A membranous sac serving for the reception of fluids or gases. 2. The hollow organ which serves as a reservoir for the urine. The only adjective to mean: of, pertaining to, or affecting the bladder is **vesical.** See Plates 41, 44.

air b. See air *vesicle*.

allantoic b. A urinary bladder which develops as an evagination of the cloaca, homologous to the allantoic evagination.

atonic b. A urinary bladder in which the tonus of the detrusor muscle is markedly diminished or absent, usually as a result of partial or complete interruption of the sensory limb of the reflex arc (**sensory paralytic bladder**), as in tabes dorsalis, but occasionally as a result of prolonged overdistension secondary to injury of the motor neurones or nerves of the reflex arc (**motor paralytic bladder**) as seen in poliomyelitis.

autonomous b. A urinary bladder, functioning abnormally when both limbs of the reflex arc which controls it are destroyed by lesions of the sacral cord, conus medullaris or cauda equina. Rarely seen in its pure form, the autonomous bladder is found in patients with extensive destruction of the lumbosacral spinal cord or when there is destruction of both sensory and motor roots in the sacral plexus. The condition is marked by loss of voluntary and reflex micturition and by painless overflow incontinence.

bilocular b. A sacculated urinary bladder having two pouches.

b. bar. See *bar* of the bladder.

cord b. Dysfunction of the urinary bladder, due to a lesion in the spinal cord.

dwarf b. Hypoplasia of the urinary bladder.

encysted b. A urinary bladder with communicating cysts.

gallbladder. See *gallbladder*.

hourglass b. A urinary bladder in which there is a horizontal midvesical constriction.

hypertonic b. A condition of increased muscular activity of the urinary bladder which appears after recovery from the shock following section of its voluntary innervation.

hypotonic b. A urinary bladder in which the tonus of the detrusor muscle is diminished or absent as a result of either prolonged overdistension secondary to obstruction or of interruption, partial or complete, of the sensory limb of the reflex arc controlling normal vesical emptying.

irritable b. See nervous *b.*

motor paralytic b. See atonic *b.*

multilocular b. A sacculated urinary bladder having many pouches.

nervous b. A condition in which there is a frequent desire to urinate, with inability to perform the act perfectly. Syn., *irritable b.*

neurogenic b. A urinary bladder in a state of dysfunction due to lesions of the central or peripheral nervous system.

reflex b. A urinary bladder whose activity or function is dependent solely upon the primary (simple) reflex arc through the sacral cord, as the result of removal of suprasegmental control secondary to complete transection of the spinal cord, or gross lesions which result in profound disturbance of suprasegmental pathways, comparable to complete transection of the cord. Such a reflex bladder may have relatively normal capacity and may empty itself automatically at relatively normal intervals (**normal reflex b.**); or it may be contracted and spastic, with a limited capacity, and empty itself automatically at frequent and irregular intervals (**spastic reflex b.**). Syn., *spinal reflex b.*, *reflex neurogenic b.*

sacculated b. Condition due to overextension of the urinary bladder; pouches in which urine may be held are formed by the forcing out of the mucous coat between the muscular bundles.

sensory paralytic b. See atonic *b.*

spastic reflex b. See reflex *b.*

stammering b. Condition in which there is interruption of the urinary stream; may be nervous or pathologic in origin.

tabetic b. See atonic *b.*

uninhibited b. An abnormal urinary bladder which shows only a variable loss of cerebral inhibition over reflex bladder contractions, representing, of all neurogenic bladders, the least variance from normal. The vesical reflex is intact, and micturition can be initiated and interrupted voluntarily. It is seen normally in infants and abnormally in the adult enuretic, and in patients with subtotal destruction of the cerebral cortex or cortical regulatory system.

blad'der train'ing. Establishing the control of urination as a habit during infancy or early childhood.

blade [AS. *blaed*]. 1. The cutting portion of a surgical knife or of surgical scissors. 2. One of the two arms or limbs of forceps.

shoulder b. The scapula.

Blaes, Gérard (Blasius) [*Dutch anatomist*, 1625–92]. Celebrated comparative anatomist and author of the first comprehensive treatise on the subject (1681). His name was once associated with the parotid duct, discovered by his pupil Stensen.

Blainville, Henri Marie Ducrotay de [*French anthropologist and zoologist*, 1777–1850]. Described congenital asymmetry of the ears. Once called *Blainville's ears.*

Blair, Vilray Papin [*American plastic surgeon*, 1871–]. Introduced special operations for the correction of single harelip and for removal of the tongue and the floor of the mouth, this being preceded by tracheotomy. Devised procedures for skin grafting. Intermediate split graft is known as the *Blair-Brown graft*, for Blair and James Barrett Brown. The *Blair-Brown knife* is a special skin-grafting knife with a long, razorlike blade, detachable from the handle. It has gauges to regulate accurately the thickness of the graft.

Blakemore's operation. See arterial *bridge.*

Blalock, Alfred [*American surgeon*, 1899–]. Known for his work on traumatic shock and an operation for the relief of congenital obstruction at the origin of the pulmonary artery by the creation of an artificial ductus arteriosus. A surgical anastomosis is made of an artery arising from the aortic arch to the side of one of the pulmonary arteries, thus permitting a larger quantity of blood to reach the lungs. Called *Blalock-Taussig operation.*

Blancard. See *Blankaart.*

Blandin, Philippe Frédéric [*French surgeon*, 1798–1849]. His name is associated with the anterior lingual glands. Described an operation for double harelip in which he excised a triangular wedge of the vomer with reduction of the projecting maxillary process; also described an operation for deviated nasal septum, and one for excision of the maxilla.

Blane, Gilbert [*Scottish surgeon*, 1749–1834]. Physician to the British fleet. Improved living conditions among sailors, especially by adding fresh fruit to their diet and thus lessening the incidence of scurvy (1795). Assisted in bringing about the British Quarantine Act. Among the greatest names in the annals of naval medicine.

Blan·for'di·a. Synonym for *Oncomelania.*

Blankaart, Stephan (Blancard) [*Dutch physician*, 1650–1702]. Remembered for his preparation of pills of ferrous iodide. Author of a medical dictionary which, translated into English, was the first to be printed in the British Isles (1684).

Blasius, Ernst [*German surgeon*, 1802–75]. Remembered for his operation of blepharoplasty, in which a skin flap was taken from the nose and forehead to form a lower eyelid.

Blasius, Gerardus. See *Blaes.*

blast [AS. *blǣst*]. The compression or suction wave which is set up by the detonation of high explosives.

-blast [G. *blastos*, germ]. Combining form denoting *a sprout, shoot,* or *germ;* specifically, *in biology,* denoting *a formative cell, a germ layer,* or *a formative constituent of living matter.*

blas·te'ma (pl. *blastemata*) [G., offspring, excrescence]. 1. The formative cellular matrix from which an organ or part is derived. 2. A small bud of competent cells from which begins the regeneration of an organ or appendage. 3. Budding or sprouting part of a plant. 4. The formative lymph or fluid from which cells or organs are formed. *Obs.* —**blastemal, blastemat'ic, blastem'ic,** *adj.*

metanephric b. The caudal end of the nephrogenic cord.

blas′tin [G. *blastos*, germ]. A substance which stimulates cell growth and activity. A nutriment for cells.

blast in′ju·ry. Trauma resulting from short-range exposure to the detonation of high explosives.

atmospheric b. i. Trauma caused by pressure on the body, resulting in capillary hemorrhages of the lungs with hemoptysis; dyspnea and cyanosis are constant, lobar pneumonia may develop, and shock is often pronounced. The eardrums may be ruptured.

immersion b. i. Trauma caused by underwater explosion of a depth charge in close proximity. The abdominal viscera are most often injured, the injuries being serious due to the greater force exerted on the body in water. Symptoms and prognosis vary.

blas′to-, blast- [*blastos*]. A combining form denoting *connection with*, or *relation to*, *a bud*, *budding*, *a germ*, and especially *the early stages of the embryo*.

blas′to·cele. See *blastocoele*.

blas′to·chyle (blas′to·kile) [*blastos;* G. *chylos*, *juice*]. The fluid in the blastocoele.

blas′to·coele, blas′to·coel (blas′to·seel), **blas′to·cele** [*blastos;* G. *koilia*, cavity]. The central cavity of the blastula or blastocyst.

blas′to·cyst [*blastos;* G. *kystis*, bladder]. 1. A blastula. 2. The modified mammalian blastula consisting of trophoblast, inner cell mass, and blastocoele. See *blastula*.

Blas″to·cys′tis ho′mi·nis. A nonpathogenic fungous organism inhabiting the intestine of man and other animals.

blas′to·derm [*blastos;* G. *derma*, skin]. *In embryology:* 1. The cellular disk of blastomeres derived from the blastodisk of meroblastic ova. 2. The primitive germ layer or epithelium of a blastula or blastocyst from which the primary germ layers are derived. 3. By extension, the germinal membrane after the formation of the several germ layers. —**blastoder′mal, blastoder′mic,** *adj.*

bilaminar b. See bilaminar *blastodisk*.

embryonic b. That part of a blastoderm forming the embryo proper. Syn., *embryonic disk*, *embryonic shield*.

extraembryonic b. That part of a blastoderm forming the extraembryonic membranes.

trilaminar b. See trilaminar *blastodisk*.

blas′to·disk, blas′to·disc [*blastos;* G. *diskos*, disk]. 1. The uncleaved cytoplasmic disk capping the embryonic pole of meroblastic ova. 2. The embryonic or germinal disk of mammals.

bilaminar b. A two-layered embryonic disk before mesoderm formation. See *gastrula*.

trilaminar b. The early embryo at the time of the formation of the mesoderm and the head process.

blas″to·gen′e·sis [*blastos;* G. *genesis*, production]. 1. The early development of the embryo during cleavage and the formation of the germ layers. See *organogenesis*. 2. Weismann's theory of the origin and development of the germ plasm, in contradistinction to Darwin's theory of pangenesis. 3. Reproduction by budding. Syn., *blastogeny*. —**blastogenic, blastogenet′ic,** *adj.*

blas·tog′e·ny (blas·todj′i·nee) [*blastos;* G. *genesthai*, from *gignesthai*, to be produced]. 1. Blastogenesis. 2. The germ history of an organism (Haeckel); a division of ontogeny.

blas″to·ki·ne′sis (blas″to·ki·nee′sis, ·kigh·nee′sis) [*blastos;* G. *kinēsis*, motion]. A process of cephalocaudal reversal in the egg of insects and certain cephalopods.

blas·tok′o·lin. A substance isolated from the expressed juice of many fruits, including the apple, pear, quince, and fig, which retards the germination of various seeds. It has been shown to be a mixture of malic and citric acids.

blas·tol′y·sis [*blastos;* G. *lysis*, a loosing]. Destruction of a blastoderm or germ cell.

blas·to′ma [*blastos;* G. *-ōma*, tumor]. 1. A tumor which originates from embryonal cells, as fibroblastoma, chondroma. 2. A true tumor. —**blastom′atous,** *adj.*

b. ependymale. See *ependymoma*.

lymphoepitheliomatous b. See *lymphoepithelioma*.

-blas·to′ma. Suffix used to indicate a tumor that originates from embryonal cells.

blas·tom″a·to·gen′ic [*blastos;* *-ōma;* G. *genesthai*, from *gignesthai*, to be produced]. Pertaining to factors or agents which excite cellular multiplication resulting in neoplastic growth.

blas′to·mere [*blastos;* G. *meros*, part]. A cleavage or segmentation cell; any one of the cells into which the fertilized ovum divides.

formative b. One destined to form a part of the embryo, not its membranes.

Blas″to·my′ces (blas″to·my′seez) (pl. *Blastomycetes*) [*blastos;* G. *mykēs*, fungus]. A genus of fungi pathogenic to man. Syn., *Paracoccidioides*, *Zymonema*.

B. brasiliensis. A species which is the etiologic agent of South American blastomycosis. It reproduces in tissue and in culture at 37° C. by multiple-budding cells and thereby differs from the singly budding cells of the *B. dermatitidis*. Syn., *Paracoccidioides brasiliensis*.

B. dermatitidis. A fungus; the causative agent of North American blastomycosis, a cutaneous or systemic, suppurative, granulomatous disease. The organism is spheroid and budding in tissues; it produces aerial hyphae in culture. See Table of the Most Common Microorganisms Pathogenic to Man in the Appendix.

Blas″to·my·ce′tes (blas″to·migh·see′teez). Plural of *Blastomyces*.

blas″to·my·ce′tic [*blastos;* *mykēs*]. Pertaining to, or caused by, the budding fungi Blastomycetes.

Blas″to·my·coi′des (blas″to·migh·koy′deez) [*blastos;* *mykēs;* G. *eidos*, form]. Name proposed by Castellani for a genus of fungi.

B. dermatitidis. Synonym for *Blastomyces dermatitidis*.

B. immitis. Synonym for *Coccidioides immitis*.

blas″to·my·co′sis [*blastos;* *mykēs;* G. *-ōsis*, condition]. Originally this term represented a more or less definite clinical syndrome, but it has come to mean all diseases produced by budding, yeastlike organisms. Diseases vary in different countries and have different causative agents, but are similar in that they are granulomatous and may involve not only the skin but the viscera and bony structures as well.

European b. See *cryptococcosis*.

Jorge Lobo's b. A very rare chronic dermatomycosis, reported only in Brazil, characterized clinically by pseudo-keloid conglomerate cutaneous nodules, variable in number and size, which may become fistulous and suppurative.

North American b. A generalized mycosis, usually with skin lesions, caused by the *Blastomyces dermatitidis*. Also called *Gilchrist's disease*.

South American b. See *paracoccidioidal granuloma* under *granuloma*.

blas″to·neu′ro·pore [*blastos;* G. *neuron*, nerve; *poros*, passage]. The temporary aperture in certain embryos formed by the coalescence of the blastopore and neuropore.

blas′to·pore [*blastos;* *poros*]. External opening of

the archenteron in a gastrula. The avian and mammalian primitive streaks have been regarded by some as closed blastopores; hence the primitive pit, or the opening into the notochordal canal, may be considered a remnant of a blastopore. Also called *archistome, gastropore, primitive mouth.*

blas′to·sphere. See *blastula, blastocyst.*

blas′to·spore [*blastos;* G. *spora,* seed]. A spore formed by budding in the asexual reproduction of fungi; a type of thallospore. —**blastospor′ic,** *adj.*

blas·tot′o·my [*blastos;* G. *tomē,* a cutting]. The separation of blastomeres or groups of blastomeres, either naturally or artificially.

blas′tu·la [L., dim. from G. *blastos*]. A spherical mass consisting of a central cavity surrounded by a single layer of cells produced by the cleavage of the ovum; frequently modified by the presence of yolk. Syn., *blastodermic vesicle, germ* or *germinal vesicle, blastosphere, blastocyst.* Also called *vesicular morula.* —**blastular,** *adj.;* **blastula′tion,** *n.*

Bla·tel′la [L. *blatta,* an insect that shuns the light]. A genus of cockroaches whose species are important as transmitters of human pathogens.

B. germanica. A species which can serve as the intermediate host of *Hymenolepis diminuta.* Syn., *Croton bug.*

Blat′ta [L., an insect that shuns the light]. A genus of cockroaches of the Blattidae. The species **B. orientalis,** the oriental cockroach, has been incriminated as an intermediate host of *Hymenolepis diminuta.*

Blaud's pill. One containing ferrous carbonate, usually 60 mg.

bleach′ing pow′der. Chlorinated lime.

bleb [dialect E. from *blub,* suggesting a bubbling sound]. A skin blister or vesicle filled with serum or blood; bulla.

bleed′er [AS. *blēdan,* to bleed]. One who is subject to frequent hemorrhages, as a hemophiliac.

bleed′ing [*blēdan*]. The escape of blood from the vessels; venesection.

bleed′ing time. The time required for bleeding to cease from a puncture wound, usually of the ear lobe or ball of the finger. In the Ivy modification, the test is performed distal to an area compressed by a blood-pressure cuff inflated to 40 mm. Hg pressure. The normal value varies with the method. Also see *clotting time, clot retraction time, prothrombin time, recalcified clotting time.*

Blégny, Nicolaus de [*French physician,* 1652–1722]. Published the first medical journal in Paris (1679). Remembered for his invention of the truss for inguinal hernia (1676). Was one of the first in France to contribute to the study of legal medicine (1684).

blem′ma·trope [G. *blemma,* a glance; *trepein,* to turn]. Apparatus for showing the various positions of the eye in its orbit.

blend′ing. The mutual solubilization of two normally immiscible solvents by the addition of a colloidal electrolyte.

blen′no-, blenn- [G. *blenna,* mucus]. A combining form denoting *presence of,* or *relation to, mucus.*

blen″noph·thal′mi·a [*blenna;* G. *ophthalmia,* ophthalmia]. Catarrhal conjunctivitis.

blen″nor·rha′gi·a [*blenna;* G. *rhēgnynai,* to burst]. 1. An excessive mucous discharge. 2. Gonorrhea.

blen″nor·rhe′a [*blenna;* G. *rhoia,* flow]. Blennorrhagia.

inclusion b. See inclusion *conjunctivitis.*

neonatal b. See inclusion *conjunctivitis.*

bleph′a·ra. Plural of blepharon.

bleph″ar·ad″e·ni′tis, bleph″a·ro·ad″e·ni′tis [G. *blepharon,* eyelid; *adēn,* gland; *-itis,* inflammation]. Inflammation of the tarsal glands.

bleph′a·ral [*blepharon*]. Relating to the eyelids.

bleph″a·rec′to·my [*blepharon;* G. *ektomē,* excision]. Excision of a part or the whole of an eyelid.

bleph″ar·e·de′ma, bleph″a·ro·e·de′ma [*blepharon;* G. *oidēma,* swelling]. Swelling or edema of the eyelids.

bleph″ar·e·lo′sis. Entropion.

bleph′a·rism [G. *blepharizein,* to wink]. Rapid involuntary winking; spasmodic nictitation.

bleph″a·ri′tis [G. *blepharon,* eyelid; *-itis,* inflammation]. Inflammation of the eyelids.

b. angularis. That involving the medial commissure with blocking of puncta lacrimalia.

b. ciliaris. Inflammation of the hair follicles and sebaceous glands along the margins of the lids.

b. gangraenosa. Carbuncle of the lids.

b. marginalis. See *b.* ciliaris.

b. parasitica. Marginal blepharitis caused by lice and/or mites.

b. simplex. Mild inflammation of the borders of the eyelids with the formation of moist yellow crusts on the ciliary margins which glue the eyelids together.

b. squamosa. Marginal blepharitis with the formation of branny scales.

b. ulcerosa. Marginal blepharitis with ulcer formation.

bleph′a·ro-, blephar- [*blepharon*]. A combining form denoting *relating to the eyelid.*

bleph″a·ro·ad″e·ni′tis. See *blepharadenitis.*

bleph″a·ro·ad″e·no′ma [*blepharon;* G. *adēn,* gland; *-ōma,* tumor]. Adenoma of the eyelid.

bleph″a·ro·ath″er·o′ma [*blepharon;* G. *athērē,* porridge; *-ōma*]. Sebaceous cyst of the eyelid.

bleph″a·ro·blen″nor·rhe′a [*blepharon;* G. *blenna,* mucus; *rhoia,* a flow]. Conjunctivitis with a purulent discharge.

bleph″a·ro·chal′a·sis (blef″uh·ro·kal′uh·sis) [*blepharon;* G. *chalasis,* a slackening]. A redundance of the skin of the eyelids which causes the skin to fold over and hang down. In some persons it hides the tarsal margin when the lids are open.

bleph″a·ro·chrom″hi·dro′sis [*blepharon;* G. *chrōma,* color; *hidrōsis,* sweating]. Colored sweat of the eyelids, usually of a bluish tint.

bleph″a·ro·clei′sis (blef″uh·ro·kly′sis) [*blepharon;* G. *kleisis,* a closing]. Ankyloblepharon; abnormal closure of the eyelids.

bleph″a·roc′lo·nus [*blepharon;* G. *klonos,* agitation]. Spasm of the orbicularis oculi muscle.

bleph″a·ro·col″o·bo′ma. See *coloboma* palpebrae.

bleph″a·ro·con·junc″ti·vi′tis [*blepharon;* L. *conjunctiva;* G. *-itis,* inflammation]. Inflammation of both the eyelids and the conjunctiva.

bleph″a·ro·di·as′ta·sis (blef″uh·ro·dye·ass′tuh·sis) [*blepharon;* G. *diastasis,* separation]. Excessive separation of the eyelids; inability to close the eyelids completely.

bleph″a·ro·dys·chroi′a [*blepharon;* G. *dys-,* prefix meaning hard, bad, unlucky; *chroia,* skin]. Discoloration of the eyelid from nevus or from any other cause.

bleph″a·ro·e·de′ma. See *blepharedema.*

bleph″a·ro·me·las′ma [*blepharon;* NL., from G. *melasma,* black spot]. Seborrhea nigricans occurring on the eyelid.

bleph′a·ron (pl. *blephara*) [G.]. The eyelid; palpebra.

bleph″a·ron′cus (blef″uh·rong′kus) [*blepharon;* G. *ogkos,* a mass]. A tumor or swelling of the eyelid. —**blepharonco′sis,** *n.*

bleph″a·ro·pa·chyn′sis (blef″uh·ro·pa·kin′sis) [*blepharon;* G. *pachynsis,* thickening]. Morbid thickening of the eyelid.

bleph″a·ro·phi·mo′sis (blef″uh·ro·figh·mo′sis, ·fi-mo′sis) [*blepharon; G. phimōsis,* a muzzling]. Abnormal smallness of the palpebral aperture.

bleph″a·roph′ry·plas″ty [*blepharon;* G. *ophrys,* eyebrow; *plassein,* to form]. Plastic surgery of the eyebrow and eyelid. —**blepharophryplas′tic,** *adj.*

bleph″a·ro·phy′ma [*blepharon;* G. *phyma,* tumor]. A tumor of, or outgrowth from, the eyelid.

bleph′a·ro·plast″ [*blepharon; plassein*]. 1. A basal body from which a cilium or flagellum grows. 2. A centriole which forms such basal bodies.

bleph′a·ro·plas″ty [*blepharon; plassein*]. An operation for the restoration of any part of the eyelid. —**blepharoplas′tic,** *adj.*

bleph″a·ro·ple′gi·a [*blepharon;* G. *plēgē,* a stroke]. Paralysis of an eyelid.

bleph″a·rop·to′sis [*blepharon;* G. *ptōsis,* a falling]. Drooping of the upper eyelid.

bleph″a·ro·py″or·rhe′a [*blepharon;* G. *pyorroia,* discharge of matter]. A flow of pus from the eyelid.

bleph″a·ror′rha·phy [*blepharon;* G. *rhaphē,* a suture]. Repair by suturing of a cut or lacerated eyelid.

bleph′a·ro·spasm″ [*blepharon;* G. *spasmos,* spasm]. Spasm of the orbicularis oculi muscle; excessive winking.

bleph″a·ro·sphinc″ter·ec′to·my [*blepharon;* G. *sphigktēr,* binder; *ektomē,* excision]. An operation to lessen the pressure of the upper lid upon the cornea.

bleph′a·ro·stat″ [*blepharon;* G. *statos,* standing]. An instrument for holding the eyelids apart during operations upon the eyes or lids.

bleph″a·ro·ste·no′sis [*blepharon;* G. *stenos,* narrow; *-ōsis,* condition]. Pathologic narrowing of the space between the eyelids, or palpebral aperture.

bleph″a·ro·sym′phy·sis [*blepharon;* G. *symphysis,* a growing together]. The adhesion or growing together of the eyelids; blepharosynechia.

bleph″a·ro·syn·ech′i·a (blef″uh·ro·si·neck′ee·uh, ·sin″i·kigh′uh, ·si·nee′kee·uh) [*blepharon;* G. *synecheia,* a holding together]. Adhesion or growing together of the eyelids.

bleph″a·rot′o·my [*blepharon;* G. *tomē,* a cutting]. Incision into the eyelid.

blep″so·path′i·a, blep·sop′a·thy [G. *blepsis,* sight; *pathos,* suffering]. Eyestrain.

Blessig, Robert [*Russian physician,* 1830–78]. Remembered for his studies of the retina. Described a groove seen in the fundus of the optic cup and the tiny cystic spaces seen at the margin of the retina, which are called *Blessig-Ivanov cystoid degeneration of retina.*

blight. A fungus disease of plants.

blind [AS.]. Without sight; deprived of sight.

blind gut. The cecum.

blind′ness [AS. *blind*]. Loss or absence of vision; inability to see. Also called *caecitas, typhlosis.* See also *amaurosis.*

amnesic color b. See under *colorblindness.*

central b. Blindness in the central area of the visual field, or involving the normal point of fixation caused by a lesion and dysfunction of the macular region of the eye.

cerebral b. See psychic *b.*

color b. See *colorblindness.*

cortical b. That resulting from a lesion of the cortical visual center.

day b. A type of eye defect in which there is no sense of color and which is accompanied by photophobia. See *hemeralopia.*

eclipse b. Blindness after looking directly at an eclipse of the sun, caused by a hermal lesion in the retina.

electric-light b. A condition similar to snowblindness, due to exposure of the eyes to intense and prolonged electric illumination.

green b. A variety of colorblindness in which green is not distinguished; aglaucopsia.

night b. See *night blindness.*

psychic b. Loss of conscious visual sensation from destruction of the cerebral visual center while pupillary reactions remain intact.

red b. Defective vision for red. Also called *greensightedness.* See *protanopia.*

snow b. See *snowblindness.*

sun b. Blindness, either temporary or permanent, caused by retinal injury resulting from gazing at the sun without adequate protection: also called *photoretinitis.*

toxic b. See toxic *amaurosis.*

uremic b. See toxic *amaurosis.*

violet b. Amianthinopsy.

word b. See *aphasia.*

blind spot. That spot on the retina not affected by light; the place where the optic nerve leaves.

blink′ing [ME. *blenken*]. Involuntary winking.

blis′ter [ON. *blāstr,* a swelling]. 1. A vesicle resulting from the exudation of serous fluid between the epidermis and true skin. 2. The agent by which the blister is produced.

ambulant b. One that is shifted to different places.

blood b. One that contains blood.

fever b. Herpes simplex of the lips.

fly b. A blister of cantharides.

flying b. One that remains long enough to produce redness of the skin but not vesication.

pus b. One containing purulent matter, usually from infection of the serum in a blister.

water b. One with watery contents.

blis′ter·ing [*blāstr*]. Forming a vesicle upon the skin. Syn., *epispastic.*

Blix, Magnus Gustav [*German physiologist,* 1849–1904]. Author of an important work on the physiology of the cutaneous nerves and muscular contractions (1884). Devised a method of centrifuging blood specimens, separating white from red cells.

bloat [perhaps from AS. *blātian*]. 1. Puffiness; distention; edema; turgidity from any cause. 2. *In veterinary medicine,* an abnormal accumulation of gas in the stomach or intestines, resulting in distention of the abdomen. Also called *wind colic, hoven.*

Bloch, Felix (1905–). American physicist who discovered a technique which simplified the analysis of the atomic nucleus. With Edward M. Purcell he received the Nobel prize for physics in 1952.

Bloch, Oscar Thorvald [*Swedish surgeon,* 1847–1926]. Widely known in his time for his bold work on colonic surgery. Devised a two-stage removal of the rectum for carcinoma (1892).

block [OF. *bloc*]. To obstruct the path of sensory impressions by the injection of an anesthetic agent into the region of the nerve trunks in the area of surgical operation.

block. 1. Any obstruction of a passage or opening. 2. Any form of interference with the propagation of an impulse, as in heart or nerve block, or regional anesthesia. 3. *In dentistry,* a set of two or more artificial teeth (block teeth) carved as one piece on a porcelain base to which the corresponding section of the gum (gum block) has been added. 4. *In dentistry,* a mass of gold foil for filling teeth, made by folding a tape of foil upon itself several times to secure a block of the thickness desired. 5. *In histology,* a paraffin or celloidin block in which a slice of tissue is embedded to facilitate the cutting of thin sections by a microtome. 6. *In psychiatry*, see *blocking*. —**block,** *v.*

air b. An air leak from the lung alveoli into the pulmonary connective tissue and mediastinum, which obstructs the normal inflow and outflow of air and pulmonary blood.

arborization b. See *heart block.*

bite b. (a) *In dentistry*, a device for registering the proper interrelation of upper and lower jaws, with or without the presence of teeth. (b) Hard rubber device used in bronchoscopy.

bundle branch b. See *heart block.*

ear b. Trauma, inflammation and pain of the middle ear due to blocked auditory tube, observed in individuals subjected to sudden and extreme variations in barometric pressure.

field b. Regional anesthesia by surrounding an operative field with an anesthetic wall.

ganglionic b. That form of block anesthesia in which the anesthetic solution is infiltrated into the vicinity of a sympathetic or dorsal root ganglion. The two ganglions most frequently blocked are the semilunar and stellate.

heart b. See *heart block.*

manometric b. An obstruction to the free flow of cerebrospinal fluid as measured by a lumbar or cisternal puncture or both. The block may be partial or complete.

nerve b. See *nerve block.*

presacral b. See parasacral *anesthesia.*

sacral b. Anesthesia induced by injection of the anesthetic agent usually through the caudal hiatus.

saddle b. The appearance of a saddle-shaped area of anesthesia or bilateral sensation loss, which occurs in caudal anesthesia.

segmental b. Anesthesia producing blockage of both sensory supply of a visceral organ and somatic nerves of the region of approach.

sinoatrial b. See *heart block.*

spinal b. Obstruction to the flow of spinal fluid when the spinal canal is blocked.

subarachnoid b. A condition in which some obstructing mass prevents the normal flow of cerebrospinal fluid. Evidenced by failure of a rise of pressure in the lumbar manometer during jugular compression, the Queckenstedt-Stookey *test.*

transsacral b. Anesthesia of the sacral nerves approached through the posterior sacral foramens.

tubal b. Obstruction of the lumen of a tube. See ear *b.*

ventricular b. Block of the interventricular foramens, the cerebral aqueduct, or the lateral and medial apertures of the fourth ventricle; interfering with the flow of cerebrospinal fluid from the brain ventricles and causing internal hydrocephalus.

block′ing [*bloc*]. 1. Interference with the propagation of nerve currents in a certain direction. 2. *In psychoanalysis*, a sudden inhibition in both the progression and expression (speech, writing) of a flow of thought, occurring at times normally as the result of some strong affect, as anger or surprise. In free association it is due to revival of a painful complex. 3. *In psychiatry*, the process of sudden interruption of thought in schizophrenia, resulting in an abrupt change of subject, stopping or slowing down of speech or writing. 4. Fastening a histologic specimen on a microtome sproul, in preparation for cutting.

Blocq, Paul Oscar [*French physician*, 1860–96]. His name is often associated with the ataxic condition astasia-abasia.

blood [AS. *blōd*]. The fluid tissue which circulates through the heart, arteries, capillaries, and veins, supplies oxygen and food to the other tissues of the body, and removes from them carbon dioxide and waste products of metabolism. It is made up of plasma and cellular elements. The latter consists of erythrocytes, leukocytes, and blood platelets. One cu. mm. of normal blood contains about 6,000 white and 5,000,000 red cells. The bright red color of arterial blood is due to the oxyhemoglobin of the red cells, the darker red of venous blood to reduced hemoglobin or methemoglobin. The total amount of blood is equal to about $1/13$ of the body weight. On removal from the body and under abnormal conditions in the body, blood coagulates, forming a red clot from which a yellowish fluid, the serum, can be expressed. Healthy blood contains about 78% water and 22% solids. For normal values of blood constituents, see Table in the Appendix. Also see blood *island*, hematogenous *pigment, blood groups, serum, typing*. See Plate 5.

arterial b. The blood in the vascular system from the point of origin of the small venules in the lungs to the capillary beds in tissues where oxygen is released and carbon dioxide taken up. Normally the partial pressure of oxygen (pO_2) is higher and that of carbon dioxide (pCO_2) lower than in venous blood.

b. cell. See *erythrocyte; leukocyte.* See also Plate 26.

b. clot. A semisolid coagulum of blood.

b. corpuscle. See *erythrocyte; leukocyte.* See also Plate 26.

b. count. See *blood count.*

b. culture. Culture of blood on artificial media to determine the presence or absence of microorganisms.

b. groups. See *blood groups.*

b. platelets. Spheroidal or ovoid, light-gray bodies found in blood, about 1.0 to 2.5μ in diameter, and numbering about 300,000 per cubic millimeter; an important factor in blood coagulation. Syn., *thrombocytes, thromboplastids.* See Plate 26.

b. vessel. An artery, vein, or capillary.

cord b. Blood obtained from the umbilical cord.

defibrinated b. That from which the fibrin is removed.

laked b. That in which the red blood cells are hemolyzed.

occult b. Small amounts of blood, as in gastric contents, which are not visible. Their presence is determined by chemical tests.

sludged b. A change in vivo in the fluidity of blood from normal. This change may be produced by one or more of the following: aggregates of erythrocytes, leukocytes, platelets, or a change in the viscosity of the plasma.

venous b. The blood in the vascular system from the point of origin of the small venules in tissues to the capillary bed in the lungs where carbon dioxide is released and oxygen taken up. Normally the partial pressure of oxygen (pO_2) is lower, and that of carbon dioxide (pCO_2) higher than in arterial blood.

blood bank. A reserve stock of whole blood or plasma, obtained from suitable donors, stored under refrigeration for use in emergencies when erythrocytes, serum proteins, or antibodies are needed. See *bank.*

blood-brain bar′ri·er. See under *barrier.*

blood-cer″e·bro·spi′nal-fluid bar′ri·er. See under *barrier.*

blood-cor′ti·cal bar′ri·er. See blood-brain *barrier.*

blood count. The determination of the number of red and white cells per cubic millimeter of blood. This is done with a hemocytometer. The **differential blood count** is that made to estimate the percentage of each different type of leukocyte per cubic millimeter of blood. The **absolute blood count** determines the total number of each different type of leukocyte; this is obtained by multiplying the total leukocyte count per cubic millimeter by the percentage of each type, as shown by the differential count.

Arneth's blood c. See Joseph *Arneth.*

Schilling b. c. See Victor *Schilling.*

blood do′nor cen′ter. A central establishment where facilities are provided for the collection, processing, storage, and distribution of blood and plasma. During World War II, such a center was operated by the Red Cross in most large cities.

Bloodgood, Joseph Colt [*American surgeon,* 1867–1935]. Known for his operation for the radical cure of inguinal hernia by transplanting the rectus muscle and obliterating the conjoined tendon (1919). Remembered for his interest in chronic mastitis in connection with senile hypertrophy of the female breast and for his contributions to the knowledge of mammary cancer.

blood group′ing. Determination of an individual's blood group by laboratory tests; blood typing. Also see *cross-matching, antiglobulin* (*Coombs*) *test.*

blood groups. Immunologically distinct, genetically determined groups of human erythrocytes, depending on specific antigens (agglutinogens) in the erythrocytes for which the groups are named, and antibodies (agglutinins) in the serum. When incompatible bloods are mixed, agglutination results, which may be followed by hemolysis. Blood groups are of great importance in blood transfusions, hemolytic disease of the newborn (*erythroblastosis fetalis*), and in medicolegal problems.

In the **Standard** or **Universal grouping** (**Landsteiner's**), the agglutinogens, A and B, can be lacking, or one or both be present in a given individual; the serum contains those isoagglutinins (anti-A or α, anti-B or β antibodies) which react upon the agglutinogens not present in the individual's erythrocytes. Thus:

Antigens on cells	O	A	B	AB
Antibodies in serum	anti-A anti-B	anti-B	anti-A	

Group A has been split into various subgroups (A_1, A_2, etc.). Moss's grouping IV, II, III, I, and Janský's I, II, III, IV are equivalent to the Standard grouping. Commonly involved in erythroblastosis fetalis and in transfusion reactions are the

Rh——————**Hr** groups

Fischer-Race's nomenclature (preferred)		Wiener's (original) nomenclature
C		rh′
D		Rh_0
E		rh″
c		hr′
d	postulated	Hr_0
e		hr″

Other groups are: **Fy^a-Fy^b (Duffy), JKa-JKb (Kidd), K (Kell)-k (Celano), Le^a-Le^b (Lewis), Lu^a-Lu^b (Lutheran), M-N-S-s, P, U, Tj^a** (a tumor factor) and other rare groups. New groups are still being determined. Comparable, antigenically distinct blood groups are also found in certain species of animals.

b.g. in platelets. The presence of the A and B antigens in human blood platelets; from four to eight such antigens have been postulated.

Do b. group. A blood group in dogs, analogous to Rh in man; it may cause jaundice in the young because of incompatibility with the mother.

blood′less [AS. *blōdlēas*]. Without blood; blanched; exsanguinate.

blood′let″ting. Venesection.

blood poi′son·ing. Septicemia.

blood pres′sure. The pressure exerted by the blood within the arteries, depending upon the force of the heart beat, elasticity of the vessel walls, resistance of the capillary bed, and volume and viscosity of the blood. The systolic pressure depends upon the ventricular systole, and the diastolic upon the diastole. The difference between the systolic and the diastolic is the pulse pressure. Abbreviated B.P.

negative b. p. Pressure which is less than that of the atmosphere. It exists in the large veins near the heart, owing to the aspirating action of the thorax.

blood′root″. Sanguinaria.

blood sub′sti·tute. Some substance, or combination of substances, used in place of blood, such as dextran, polyvinylpyrrolidone, plasma, albumin, acacia, gelatin, or mineral salts.

blood typ′ing. Determination of an individual's blood group by laboratory tests. Also see *cross-matching, blood groups,* antiglobulin (Coombs) *test.*

blood ur·e′a ni′tro·gen. See under *nitrogen.*

Blot, Claude Philibert Hippolyte [*French obstetrician,* 1822–88]. Remembered for his invention of scissors designed for performing craniotomy in difficult labor; called *Blot's scissors.*

blow′fly″. See *Calliphoridae.*

blue baby. See blue *baby.*

blue drum. A distinct blue appearance of the tympanic membrane. It may be due to congenital prominence of the jugular bulb or to disease of the middle ear, which permits the jugular vein to be seen through the drum membrane.

blue mass. Massa hydrargyri, mercury mass. *Obs.*

Blumberg's sign. See under *sign.*

Blumenau, Leonid Vasilevich [*Russian neurologist,* 1862–1931]. Known for his description of the lateral part of the cuneate nucleus.

Blumenbach, Johann Friedrich [*German anthropologist,* 1752–1840]. Celebrated in the fields of medicine, physiology, and comparative anatomy. The founder of modern anthropology, his system of classification with a few changes is still good after the lapse of a century. His studies of human craniums are especially noteworthy.

Blu′mer's shelf. A pathological finding observed on rectal examination, due to a thickening of the peritoneum of the rectouterine pouch which produces a shelflike projection into the rectum. The thickening may be due to an inflammatory or neoplastic process. Also called *rectal shelf.*

Blumgart, Herrman Ludwig [*American physician,* 1895–]. Known for his original work with D. D. Berlin and S. A. Levine in the treatment of angina pectoris by total thyroidectomy (1933), for his studies of circulation time, and of coronary artery disease.

blunt′-hook″. An obstetric instrument, used mainly in embryotomy.

blutene chloride. Trade-marked name for the antiheparin-active dye tolonium chloride or toludine blue O; it is useful in treatment of idiopathic functional uterine bleeding.

blu″ter·krank′heit [Ger., bleeder's disease]. See *hemophilia.*

Blyth's test. See under *test.*

B. M. A. British Medical Association.

B. M. R. Basal metabolic rate.

BNA Basle Nomina Anatomica. See *Basle anatomical nomenclature.*

board of health. An official board in a municipality, state, or province, responsible for maintaining public health through sanitation and preventive medicine.

Boari, Achille [*Italian surgeon*, nineteenth century]. Described transplantation of the ductus deferens into the urethra for the relief of male sterility (1898). Called *Boari's operation.*

Boas, Ismar Isidor [*German physician*, 1858–1938]. Internationally famed gastroenterologist. Performed aspiration of the duodenum (1889) and introduced, with Ewald, the test meal (1885). He invented an algesimeter or apparatus to determine the relative sensitiveness over the epigastrium compared to the normal tolerance; said to be of value in the diagnosis of gastric ulcer. Described a tender point at the left of the twelfth thoracic vertebra, found in patients with gastric ulcer; known as *Boas' point.* Introduced tests for intestinal atony and for hydrochloric acid in the gastric contents. See Boas' *test*, Boas' *reagent.* Described a sign of cholecystitis. See Boas' *sign.* With Bruno Oppler, he described a Lactobacillus. See *Lactobacillus of Boas-Oppler.*

Boate. See *Bootius.*

Bobbs, John Stough [*American surgeon*, 1809–70]. The first to perform cholecystotomy for the removal of stones in the gallbladder (1868).

Bobroff, F. V. [*Russian surgeon*, 1858–]. Described osteoplastic closure of spina bifida, called *Bobroff's operation.*

Bochdalek, Victor [*Bohemian anatomist*, 1835–68]. Described the lumbocostal triangle, called *Bochdalek's triangle.*

Bochdalek, Vincent Alexander [*Bohemian anatomist*, 1801–83]. Described many anatomic structures which, for a time, bore his name, as the submaxillary ganglion, a muscle of the tongue, a cavity of the thyroglossal duct, and a fold of the lacrimal duct.

Bock'hart's im"pe·ti'go. See *impetigo follicularis.*

Bodansky's method. See under *method.*

Bodian, David [*American neurologist*, 1910–]. Known for his silver impregnation method for the demonstration of nerve fibers, in which protargol activated by metallic copper is used.

Bo'do [L.]. A genus of flagellate protozoa. Found in feces, urine, and ulcerations, but thought to be of little or no pathologic importance.

bod'y [AS. *bodig*]. 1. The animal frame with its organs. 2. A cadaver or corpse. 3. The largest and primarily central part of an organ, as the body of the uterus. 4. A mass of matter. 5. A small organ, as the carotid body. Also see *corpus, corpuscle.*

amyloid bodies. Microscopic, concentrically laminated, hyaline bodies occurring in the acini of the prostate, in the meninges, in diseased lungs, occasionally in other sites, and staining like amyloid with metachromatic aniline dyes. Syn., *corpora amylacea.*

anococcygeal b. 1. The anococcygeal muscle. 2. The coccygeal body.

aortic bodies. Irregular epithelioid masses associated with the aortic arch and innervated by the cardiac branches of the vagus; chemoreceptive in function; stimulated most importantly by arterial hypoxemia, but also responsive to other chemical changes: also called *glomera aortica.*

apical b. Acrosome.

asbestos bodies. Long, slender cylinders with a transparent capsule composed of protein and a core of altered asbestos fiber. They are found in the lungs, air passages, sputum, and feces in asbestosis.

Aschoff's bodies. See Aschoff's *nodule.*

asteroid bodies. 1. Star-shaped inclusion bodies found in the cytoplasm of giant cells in granulomas, as in sarcoidosis and berylliosis. 2. Ray fungus in tissues. Also see *Actinomyces* and *Nocardia.*

Auer bodies. Large granules, globules, or slender rods of azurophilic substance, which are peroxidase-positive and give positive reactions for protein, found in the cytoplasm of myeloblasts, myelocytes, monoblasts, monocytes, and histiocytes in acute leukemia.

basal bodies. Minute granules at the bases of cilia or flagella, derived from the centriole and producing the cilia or flagella. Also called *blepharoplast.*

b. of Retzius. A condensed protoplasmic mass with pigment granules found at the lower end of the hair cells.

Bracht-Wächter b. A small perivascular lesion found most frequently in the myocardium. Similar to the Aschoff nodule, it is characterized by the many lymphocytes surrounding an area of necrosis, the presence of many fibroblasts, and the small number of polymorphonuclear leukocytes.

Call-Exner bodies. Small central cavities surrounded by granulosa cells, seen in certain feminizing tumors of the ovary.

carotid bodies. Epithelioid masses similar in structure and function to the aortic bodies; situated at or near the carotid bifurcation, and innervated by the intercarotid or sinus branch of the glossopharyngeal nerve: formerly called *glomera carotica.*

cavernous bodies. The corpora cavernosa. See under *corpus.*

central b. Centrosome: sometimes incorrectly applied to centriole.

chromaffin bodies. Small bodies on either side of the abdominal aorta, which give a brown coloration with chromic acid or its salts. Also called *paraganglions.* Formerly called *Zuckerkandl's bodies.*

chromatin bodies. Chromosomes.

chromatoid bodies. Variously shaped dark bodies seen in the cystic stage of amebas when stained with hematoxylin.

ciliary b. The ciliary muscle and processes.

coccygeal b. A small, vascular nodule at the tip of the coccyx. Formerly called *glomus coccygeum.*

cytoid bodies. Knoblike swellings of nerve fibers visible on the retina, which may be degenerated masses isolated or continuous with neuroglial cells: also called *ganglioform swellings.*

Döhle bodies. Basophilic cytoplasmic bodies found in neutrophils, most often in scarlet fever, and sometimes in other infections.

Donovan bodies. Short rod- or oval-shaped capsulated organisms occurring in the cytoplasm of large mononuclear cells from ulcers of granuloma inguinale; better demonstrated by Wright's than Giemsa's stain.

epithelial b. A parathyroid gland. *Obs.*

foreign b. A substance occurring in any organ or tissue where it is not normally found.

fuchsin bodies. Inclusion bodies of keratohyalin, sometimes seen in the cytoplasm of epithelial tumor cells.

gamma-Favre bodies. Small cytoplasmic inclusions characteristic of venereal lymphogranuloma.

geniculate bodies. Four oval, flattened bodies on the posterior inferior aspect of the thalamus. The **medial geniculate bodies** receive auditory impulses by way of the brachia of the inferior colliculi and relay them to the temporal cortex via the auditory radiations. The **lateral geniculate bodies** receive optic impulses by way of the optic tracts and relay them to the occipital cortex via the geniculocalcarine tracts.

Guarnieri bodies. See Giuseppe *Guarnieri.*

Hassall's b. See thymic *corpuscle.*
Heinz-Ehrlich bodies. Highly refractile inclusion bodies in erythrocytes, found in association with hemolytic anemias due to oxidative toxic compounds. The inclusions do not stain with Wright's stain or the Romanovsky dyes, but are readily seen in wet preparations where they may exhibit Brownian motion.
Herring bodies. Granular bodies found in the neurohypophysis, thought to be terminal bulbs of fibers of the hypothalamo-hypophyseal tract, in which neurosecretory material has accumulated.
Howell-Jolly bodies. See William Henry *Howell.*
immune b. Old term for immune hemolysin. See *antibody.*
inclusion bodies. Those found in cells under special conditions.
inferior quadrigeminal b. Inferior colliculus.
intermediate b. of Flemming. In mitosis, a small, darkly staining, acidophilic body to which the two daughter cells are briefly attached during the telophase.
juxtarestiform b. The medial part of the inferior cerebellar peduncle which contains vestibulocerebellar and fastigiobulbar fibers; it is medial to the restiform body proper.
ketone b. A group name for any of the compounds, β-hydroxybutyric acid, acetoacetic acid, or acetone, which simultaneously increase in blood and urine in diabetic acidosis, starvation, pregnancy, after ether anesthesia, and in other conditions. See Table of Normal Values of Blood Constituents in the Appendix.
Kurlov b. See Mikhail Georgievich *Kurlov.*
L.C.L. bodies. Clusters of minute spherical or coccoid elementary inclusion bodies found within reticuloendothelial cells and in body fluids of birds and humans infected with psittacosis (ornithosis): so-called because described independently by Leventhal, Cole, and Lillie (1930).
Leishman-Donovan bodies. Small, parasitelike bodies on the liver and spleen of those suffering from kala-azar.
Lipschütz bodies. Eosinophilic intranuclear inclusions with margination of the nuclear chromatin commonly found in the vesicles of herpes: also called *Zoster bodies of Lipschütz.* Syn., *Type A inclusion bodies* (Cowdry).
lupus erythematosus (L.E.) b. See under *cell.*
Mallory bodies. Oval acidophilic hyalin inclusion bodies of cytoplasm of hepatic cells, observed in Laennec's cirrhosis.
Malpighian b. (a) A renal corpuscle. (b) A lymph nodule of the spleen. Also called *Malpighian corpuscle.*
mammillary bodies. Two small, spherical masses of gray matter in the interpeduncular space at the base of the brain. They receive olfactory impulses from the hippocampus by means of the fornix and relay them to the anterior nucleus of the thalamus via the mammillothalamic tract and to the tegmentum of the pons and medulla oblongata via the mammillotegmental bundle. Also called *corpora mammillaria.* See Plate 18.
Masson b. Granuloma in the alveolar ducts of the lung: usually associated with rheumatic pneumonia and considered equivalent to Aschoff nodules of the myocardium. It is considered nonspecific by other investigators and is observable in many pulmonary disorders. Nodules are budlike proliferations of pleomorphic cells in a loose stroma.
melonseed bodies. Bits of fibrin, cartilage, or of tuberculous or syphilitic granulation tissue found in enlarged bursae and ganglions.
metachromatic bodies. Granules in bacterial cells staining differently from the surrounding cytoplasm. Syn., *metachromatic granules.*
Michaelis-Gutmann bodies. Basophilic and often concentrically laminated bodies, which may contain iron and calcium, seen in malacoplakia.
molluscum bodies. The ovoid or spheroidal keratin bodies formed in the epithelium by the development of the inclusion bodies of molluscum contagiosum. They are much larger than the epithelial cells originally invaded by the virus of molluscum contagiosum.
Negri bodies. Inclusion bodies in the Purkinje cells and cells of the hippocampus of animals with rabies.
neutral red bodies. Bodies demonstrated in lymphocytes from peripheral blood supravitally stained with neutral red, closely associated with, if not identical to, the Golgi apparatus.
Nissl bodies. Chromophil substance of nerve cells.
olivary b. The inferior olive of the medulla oblongata.
Pacchionian bodies. See *arachnoidal granulations* under *granulation.*
Pappenheimer bodies. Iron-containing granules sometimes found in the cytoplasm of some normoblasts and red blood cells, particularly after splenectomy.
parabasal b. A kinetonucleus closely associated with the blepharoplast of hemoflagellates.
paraterminal b. The paraolfactory area and subcallosal gyrus collectively: also called *precommissural area, septal area.*
Paschen bodies. See Enrique *Paschen.*
perineal b. The dense connective tissue between the vulva and the anus or between the scrotum and the anus.
pineal b. A small cone-shaped body attached to the roof of the third ventricle between the superior colliculi; it appears to be a rudimentary gland of unknown function: formerly called *conarium, pineal gland.* See Plate 18. Syn., *epiphysis cerebri.*
pituitary b. Pituitary gland. See Plates 17, 18, 45.
polar bodies. The minute, abortive cells extruded by the oocyte in the process of maturation. Also called *polocytes.*
postbranchial bodies. Ultimobranchial *bodies.*
primitive perineal b. The primitive perineum; the projecting wedge formed by the urorectal septum, which separates the anus and the orifice of the primitive urogenital sinus after the rupture of the cloacal membrane.
Prowazek-Halberstaedter bodies. Homogeneous irregular inclusion bodies near the nuclei of epithelial cells of the conjunctival sac; found in trachomatous patients. Also called *trachoma bodies.*
psammoma bodies. Sandlike, laminated, calcareous deposits seen typically in the psammoma, a type of meningeal fibroma. Similar deposits are found in chronic inflammation, in benign and malignant tumors, and, as brain sand, in the pineal body. Also called *corpora arenacea.*
purine bodies. Compounds that contain the purine ring; compounds derived from purine by the substitution of their hydrogen atoms.
restiform b. The interior cerebellar peduncle.
rice bodies. Small free white bodies occurring in the synovial cavity of an arthritic joint (most commonly in tuberculous arthritis), composed of either compact masses of fibrin or necrotic villi.
ring bodies. Peculiar ring-shaped bodies found in the erythrocytes in pernicious anemia, leukemia, and lead poisoning: also called *Cabot's rings, Cabot's ring bodies.*

Russell bodies. See William *Russell.*
sand bodies. Corpora arenacea.
Schaumann bodies. Round or oval, doubly contoured and laminated, frequently calcified inclusion bodies seen in the giant cells of sarcoidosis, and occasionally, in the granuloma of berylliosis: so-called because they were described by J. Schaumann (1941).
segmenting b. The sporulating malarial parasite, when the schizont breaks up into the merozoites.
spongy b. The corpus cavernosum urethrae.
superior quadrigeminal b. Superior colliculus.
threshold b. Any substance in the blood plasma which, above a certain concentration, is excreted by the kidneys. The critical concentration is called the excretion threshold.
tigroid bodies. Chromophil substance.
trachoma bodies. See *Prowazek-Halberstaedter bodies* under *body.*
trapezoid b. Transverse decussating fibers in the ventral tegmental part of the pons, which connect the ventral cochlear nucleus of one side with the lateral lemniscus of the other side.
type A inclusion bodies. See Lipschütz *bodies.*
ultimobranchial bodies. Those considered by some to be rudimentary fifth pharyngeal pouches, by others, to be lateral thyroid primordia and fourth pouch derivatives. Syn., *postbranchial bodies.* Also called *lateral thyroids.*
Unna bodies. See *Russell bodies* under William *Russell.*
Verocay bodies. Small whorls of fibrils, surrounded by radially arranged elongated cells, seen in neurofibromas.
vertebral b. A short column of bone forming the anterior, weight-bearing segment of a vertebra.
vitreous b. The vitreous; the transparent, colorless, gelatinous body filling the space between the retina and the lens of the eye. See Plate 19.
Wolffian b. The mesonephros.
yellow b. The corpus luteum.
Zoster bodies. See Lipschütz *bodies.*

bod′y ar′mor. Clothing reinforced with armor; used by aviators as a protection against antiaircraft fire.

bod′y form. See *somatotype.*

bod′y snatch′ing. Unauthorized removal of a corpse from the grave.

Boë, de le. See Franciscus *Sylvius.*

Boeck, Caesar Peter Moeller [*Norwegian pathologist,* 1845–1917]. Described acne varioliformis (1889) and benign sarcoid (1899). The latter, previously called lupus pernio by Besnier, is now known as *sarcoidosis.*

Boeck, Carl Wilhelm [*Norwegian dermatologist,* 1808–75]. Described leprosy (1847), called *Danielssen-Boeck disease.* Described Norwegian scabies (1842), called *Boeck's scabies, scabies crustosa.* See under *scabies.*

Boerhaave, Hermann [*Dutch physician,* 1668–1738]. Celebrated as one of the greatest clinicians and the creator of modern clinical teaching. Published his greatest work, *Elementa Chemiae,* in 1732. Contributed greatly to knowledge of physiology and digestion (1708). Wrote his *Aphorisms* (1709). Described the sudoriparous or sweat glands, called *Boerhaave's glands.* Advocated discussion and consultations in the interest of the patient. Many of the greatest medical men of his time were his pupils.

Boerner, Jones, and Lukens test. A flocculation test for syphilis.

Boerner-Lukens test. A modification of the Wassermann test for syphilis.

Bogomolets, Aleksandr Aleksandrovich [*Russian physician and biochemist,* 1881–1946]. Introduced antireticular cytotoxic serum; see *ACS.*

Böhler, Lorenz [*Austrian surgeon,* 1885–]. Well known as a skilful and ingenious orthopedic surgeon. Devised special types of finger splints used with a plaster arm splint to permit traction of the phalanges in fracture. Introduced many new methods of treating fractures with special devices, including a walking iron for the ambulatory treatment of leg fractures.

Böhmer's hematoxylin. See under *stain.*

Bohr effect. The influence or effect exerted by carbon dioxide upon the dissociation of oxygen from hemoglobin and some related compounds.

boil [ME. *boilen,* to boil, or D. *buil*]. A furuncle; a localized inflammation of the skin and subcutaneous connective tissue, attended by suppuration; usually at the site of a hair follicle. It has but one opening for drainage in contrast to a carbuncle, which is larger and has several openings. See *furuncle.* Also see *sore.*
blind b. One not attended by the formation of a core; nonsuppurating.
Delhi b. See *oriental* sore.

Boivin antigen. See under *antigen.*

bol′do [Sp. *boldu*]. The dried leaves of the boldutree, *Peumus boldus,* formerly used as an aromatic stimulant and diuretic. Boldo contains a bitter alkaloid, boldine; a glycoside, boldoglucin; and a volatile oil.

Bol′du. Synonym for *Peumus.*

bole [G. *bōlos,* clod of earth]. A translucent, soft variety of clay formerly much used in medicine—internally as an astringent, externally as an absorbent. There are several varieties: the Armenian, the Lemnian, and the French bole.

Bo′ley gauge. *In dentistry,* a measuring instrument with a vernier scale.

Boll, Franz Christian [*German physiologist,* 1849–79]. Noted for his discovery of the coloring matter in the rods of the retina and for his description of visual purple.

Bollinger, Otto [*German pathologist,* 1843–1909]. Remembered as being the first to describe effectively actinomycosis (1877). Also described the yellowish-white granules in the granulation tissue of the abscess found in bovine mycosis; called *Bollinger's granules.*

Bollman, Jesse Louis [*American pathologist,* 1896–]. With Frank Charles Mann, introduced the Mann-Bollman *fistula,* used in animal experimentation.

bo·lom′e·ter [G. *bolē,* ray; *metron,* a measure]. A device for measuring minute differences in radiant heat. Syn., *thermic balance.*

Bolton point. See under *point.*

Bolt′worth skate. A non-weight-bearing device, mobile in all directions, with a wide base, usable when the leg is in plaster, after such surgical procedures as arthroplasty of the hip joint, consisting of a wide-grooved board lined with Sorbo rubber and diffusely perforated to facilitate fixation with bandages.

bo′lus [L. *bolus,* choice bit, nice morsel, possibly from G. *bōlos*]. 1. A large pill. 2. The rounded mass of food prepared by the mouth for swallowing, called an **alimentary bolus.** 3. Bole.

bonamine. Trade-mark for the dihydrochloride of *p*-chlorobenzylhydryl-4-*m*-methylbenzylpiperazine, a compound effective in preventing motion sickness. See *meclizine hydrochloride, postafene.*

bond [ME., var. of *band,* a fastening]. The linkage between atoms. holding these together, as in a compound, usually effected by the transfer of one or more electrons from one atom to another, or by the sharing, equally or unequally, of one or more pairs of electrons by two atoms.
coordinate covalent b. A bond consisting of a

pair of electrons shared by two atoms and thus joining them, both electrons being contributed by one of the atoms. Syn., *dative bond.*

dative b. A coordinate covalent bond.

energy-rich phosphate b. A phosphate bond, as in adenosinetriphosphate and phosphocreatine, which on cleavage by hydrolysis releases 11,000 calories per gram-molecule, as compared with the release of about 3000 calories from ordinary phosphate ester bonds. The symbol for such a bond is $\sim$. The bond provides a means of storing energy for subsequent use in muscular activity or biosynthesis.

hydrogen b. That formed between two molecules when the nucleus of a hydrogen atom, originally attached to a fluorine, nitrogen, or oxygen atom of a molecule, is attracted to the fluorine, nitrogen, or oxygen atom of a second molecule of the same or a different substance. Water molecules are joined to each other through hydrogen bond formation. Syn., *hydrogen bridge.*

ionic b. That formed between two atoms when one or more electrons are transferred from one atom to another, thereby completing a stable electron configuration for each.

normal covalent b. A bond consisting of a pair of electrons shared by two atoms and thus joining them, one electron being contributed by each atom.

peptide b. One joining two amino acids, in which the amino group of one acid is condensed with the carboxyl group of another with elimination of water and formation of a —CO.NH— linkage. The amino acids of proteins are joined in this manner.

Bondt, de. See *Bontius.*

bon′duc [Ar. *bunduq*, hazelnut]. The seeds of *Caesalpinia crista*, a tropical plant. They have been used as a bitter tonic and antiperiodic.

bone [AS. *bān*]. 1. Osseous tissue; a supportive, rigid connective tissue consisting of an abundant calcified matrix enclosing many much-branched cells, the osteocytes. The body of each osteocyte occupies an ovoid space, the lacuna; its branches lie in minute, branching tubules, the canaliculi. Many varieties of osseous tissue are differentiated according to method of formation, relation to other tissues, and architecture. See also *endosteum, ossein, ossification, osteogenesis, osteoid, periosteum.* 2. An element or individual member of the skeleton, as the femur, the parietal bone. For bones listed by name, see Table of Bones in the Appendix. See Plate 1. —**bony,** *adj.*

alveolar b. The alveolar processes of the maxilla and the mandible. Within the alveolar bone, a distinction should be made between the alveolar bone proper and the alveolar supporting bone because of their biologic and functional differences. The alveolar bone proper may be defined as that thin bony plate surrounding the root to which fibers of the periodontal membrane are attached. *In radiography,* this bony plate is called *lamina dura* as it appears more radiopaque than the surrounding spongy bone. The alveolar supporting bone consists of the compact alveolar plates and of the spongy bone of the alveolar processes, other than the alveolar bone proper.

ankle b. The talus.

articular b. See *articular.*

b. absorption. See *osteoclasis* 2.

b. of Bertin. The sphenoidal concha.

b. resorption. See *osteoclasis* 2.

brittle bones. See *osteogenesis imperfecta.*

bundle-b. Bone traversed by coarse collagenous fibers (Sharpey's perforating fibers), as where tendons or ligaments are affixed.

cancellous b. A form in which the matrix is arranged in a network of rods, plates, or tubes (the trabeculae), between which are spaces filled with marrow. Syn., *spongy b., substantia spongiosa.*

cartilage b. (a) Bone (1) preceded during development by a mass of hyaline cartilage which it largely replaces. (b) A bone (2) which has been preceded by a cartilaginous primordium.

coffin b. The distal phalanx of a horse's foot.

compact b. Bone (1) in which marrow spaces are replaced by cylindrical, concentrically laminated Haversian systems, each with an axial vascular channel, the Haversian canal. Syn., *substantia compacta.*

coronary b. The small pastern or second phalanx of a horse's foot.

cortical b. The compact bone next to the surface of a bone.

cotyloid b. See *os* acetabuli.

endochondral b. formation. See cartilage *bone.*

flat b. A bone (2) more or less in the form of a plate, as the parietal bone.

incisive b. The premaxilla or intermaxillary bone which bears the upper incisor teeth. Fused with the maxilla in man; a separate bone in most mammals.

interparietal b. A supernumerary bone occurring in the interparietal suture.

intracartilaginous b. formation. See endochondral *b.* formation.

intramembranous b. formation. The formation of bone by or within a connective tissue without involvement of a cartilage stage.

ivory bones. See *osteopetrosis.*

lamellar b. Bone (1) which exhibits microscopic laminations (lamellas) of its matrix.

long b. One in which the length markedly exceeds the width.

membrane b. Bone (1) formed by or within a connective tissue, as by a periosteum.

nonlamellar b. Bone in which the matrix is not layered.

omovertebral b. An aberrant bone extending from the upper medial angle of the scapula to the spines of the lower cervical vertebrae; it is sometimes present in congenital elevation of the scapula: also called *suprascapula.*

pastern b. The first phalanx (**great pastern bone**) or second phalanx (**small pastern bone**) of a horse's foot.

periosteal b. Membrane bone formed by the periosteum. Syn., *subperiosteal b.*

pneumatic bones. Those containing air cells, as the temporal bones, or air sacs, as in flying birds.

primary b. The first bone formed in a given location.

rider's b. Ossification occurring at or near the insertion of the adductor longus or magnus.

secondary b. Bone which replaces primary bone.

sesamoid b. A small bone developed in a tendon subjected to much pressure.

short b. One having the three dimensions nearly equal.

spongy b. See cancellous *b.*

spotted bones. Osteopoikilosis.

subperiosteal b. See periosteal *b.*

suprasternal b. An ossified, suprasternal cartilage not attached to the manubrium; anomalous in man, normal in some mammals.

sutural b. Any supernumerary bone occurring in a suture of the skull. Syn., *Wormian bone.*

tabular b. A flat bone; composed of an outer and an inner table of compact bone with cancellous bone or diploë between them.

Wormian b. See sutural *b.*

bone on′lay. A strip of transplanted bone laid

across a fracture and held in position by wires, pins, screws, or other device.

bone′set″. An herb used in making a therapeutic tea. See *Eupatorium.*

bone′set″ter. One who specializes in setting bones, especially an uneducated empiric, and often a pretender to hereditary skill in the business.

Bonet, Juan Pablo [*Spanish physician,* seventeenth century]. Remembered for his work in teaching the deaf to speak and the mute to write (1620).

bone wax. A material used for packing bone, especially during skull operations, for the arrest of bone bleeding.

Bonfils, Emile Adolphe [*French physician,* nineteenth century]. Known for his description of Hodgkin's disease.

Bonifacio, Giovanni [*Italian physician,* seventeenth century]. Originated a sign language for deaf-mutes (1616).

Bonjean's ergotin. See under *ergotin.*

Bonnet, Amédée [*French surgeon,* 1809–58]. Remembered for his operation for enucleation of the eye, in which injury to the soft parts of the orbit is avoided by the preservation of Tenon's capsule; called *Bonnet's operation.* Described a phenomenon in sciatica in which it was noted that passive flexion of the affected leg at both knee and hip produces no pain, but adduction of the flexed knee and hip immediately elicits pain if sciatica is present; called *Bonnet's phenomenon.*

Bonnier, Pierre [*French otolaryngologist,* 1861–1918]. Known for his study of a group of symptoms due to a lesion of the lateral ventricular nucleus in the medulla, consisting of paroxysmal vertigo, glossopharyngeal paralysis, tachycardia, somnolence, and contralateral hemiplegia; called *Bonnier's syndrome.*

Bontius, Jacobus (Jakob de Bondt) [*Dutch physician and naturalist,* 1592–1631]. Probably the first to regard tropical medicine as an important branch of medical science. In *De Medicini Indorum,* published posthumously (1642), he described beriberi and cholera.

Boogers. See *Boër.*

boom′slang″ [D. *boom,* tree; *slang,* snake]. *Dispholidus typus,* a rear-fanged, venomous snake of Africa.

Bo·öph′i·lus [G. *bous,* ox; *philein,* to love]. A genus of ticks.

B. annulatus. The cattle tick which carries the piroplasma responsible for Texas fever.

boos′ter dose. See under *dose.*

Bootius, Arnoldus (Boate, Arnaud de Boot) [*English physician,* 1606–50]. Early investigator of rickets (1649).

bo·rac′ic ac′id. Boric acid.

bor′age (bur′idj, borr′idj, boar′idj) [OF., from LL. *borrago,* from *burra,* rough hair]. The plant *Borago officinalis,* formerly used as a demulcent, mild refrigerant, and diaphoretic.

bo′rate. Any salt of boric acid.

bo′rat·ed. Containing or combined with sodium borate or boric acid.

bo′rax. Sodium borate.

bor″bo·ryg′mus [G. *borborygmos,* intestinal rumbling]. The rumbling noise caused by flatus in the intestines.

Bor″deaux′ mix′ture (boar″do′). A fungicide containing copper sulfate 1.5, calcium oxide 1.0, water to make 100.

Bor″deaux′ red. An acid monoazo dye, used as a plasma stain. Also called *acid Bordeaux; archelline 2B; azo-Bordeaux; cerasin R; fast red B, BN,* or *P.*

bor′der [OF. *bordure,* of Teut. origin]. *In anatomy,* the boundary of an area or surface.

brush b. The brushlike modification of the surface of cells lining the proximal convoluted tubules of the kidney.

striated b. The layer of modified cytoplasm, showing fine, perpendicular striations, found on the surface of the simple columnar intestinal epithelium.

vermilion b. Mucocutaneous junction of the lips.

Bordet, Jules Jean Baptiste Vincent [*Belgian bacteriologist and pathologist,* 1870–]. Known for his classic work on the properties of the serums of immunized animals (1895); also discovered hemolytic sera. He discovered the complement-fixation reaction (1900) and applied this reaction, with Gengou, to the diagnosis of several diseases. Also with Gengou he discovered the causative agent of whooping cough, *Hemophilus pertussis:* called *Bordet-Gengou bacillus.* The *Bordet-Gengou medium* is a bacterial culture of blood, potato extract, glycerin, and agar, used for the cultivation of the pertussis bacillus. He described a serum test, called *Bordet's test.* Nobel laureate (1919).

Bordeu, Théophile de [*French physician,* 1722–76]. Proponent of the idea that every organ, tissue, and cell discharges into the blood products which influence other parts of the body. Published his researches upon chronic disease and the medical analysis of blood (1775).

Borelli, Giovanni Alfonso [*Italian physiologist, physicist, and astronomer,* 1608–79]. A pupil of Galileo and teacher of Malpighi. Originated the neurogenic theory of the action of the heart. As a physiologist he was handicapped by the fact that he regarded physiology as a branch of physics; he considered the circulation a matter of hydraulics.

bo′ric ac′id (*acidum boricum*). H_3BO_3. Colorless scales, crystals, or a white crystalline powder, soluble in 18 parts of water, 18 of alcohol, or 4 of glycerin. Used as a mild antiseptic in saturated solution on mucous membranes, and as ointment on skin. Serious or fatal poisoning resulting from transcutaneous absorption may occur. Syn., *boracic acid, orthoboric acid.*

b. a. ointment (*unguentum acidi borici*). A preparation containing 10% of boric acid in liquid petrolatum and white ointment.

b. a. solution (*liquor acidi borici*). An aqueous solution containing not less than 4.25% of boric acid.

Born, Gustav Jacob [*German embryologist,* 1851–1900]. Remembered for his invention of the wax-plate reconstruction method used in embryology.

bor′ne·ol. $C_{10}H_{17}OH$. A substance which occurs as concrete masses in fissures in trees of the genus *Dryobalanops,* growing in Borneo and Sumatra, and occurring also as a constituent of certain volatile oils: used in the preparation of perfumes and incense. Syn., *Borneo camphor, Sumatra camphor.*

bor′nyl [*Borneo;* G. *hylē,* material]. The univalent $—C_{10}H_{17}$ radical derived from borneol by removing the hydroxyl-group.

bo′ro-, bor- [Ar. *bawraq,* from Per. *būrah,* borax]. A combining form for *boron.*

bo″ro·cal′cite. Native calcium borate.

bo″ro·cit′ric ac′id. A combination of boric and citric acids which has been used as a solvent for urates and phosphates in urinary calculi.

borofax. Trade-mark for an ointment of boric acid.

bo″ro·glyc′er·ide (boar″o·gliss′ur·ide, ·id). See *boroglycerin.*

bo″ro·glyc′er·in (boar″o·gliss′ur·in). A product formed by heating together boric acid and glycerin.

b. glycerite (*glyceritum boroglycerini*). A solution

of boroglycerin in glycerin. It is miscible with water. Also called *boric acid glycerin.*

bo′ron [Ar. *bawraq*]. B = 10.82. A nonmetallic element of the aluminum group; it is the characteristic element of boric acid, the borates, metaborates, and perborates.

bo″ro·sal″i·cyl′ic ac′id. A mixture of boric and salicylic acids which has been used externally like salicylic acid.

Bor·re′li·a, Bor·rel′i·a [NL., after Amádée *Borrel*, French bacteriologist, 1867–1936]. A genus of spirochetes, of many species, parasitic in man and other warm-blooded animals, and including the causative agents of relapsing fever.

B. buccale. A species of *Borrelia* found in the normal mouth, of no proved pathogenicity.

B. duttonii. The causative agent of tick-borne relapsing fever.

B. novyi. A species of *Borrelia:* causative agent of the American form of relapsing fever.

B. recurrentis. The causative agent of louse-borne relapsing fever: old designation, *Spirochaeta sogdianum.*

B. refringens. Nonpathogenic species of *Borrelia,* occurring on the external genitalia of both sexes.

B. vincentii. An anaerobic *Borrelia* found in the normal oral cavity and in conjunction with a fusiform bacillus associated with Vincent's angina.

bor·rel′i·din. An antibiotic substance produced by *Streptomyces rochei;* it is active against species of *Borrelia* in experimental animals.

Borsook, Henry (1897–). American biochemist, known for his work on the synthesis of creatine, the dynamic state of proteins, the applications of thermodynamics in biochemistry and physiology, and for his writings on vitamins.

boss [F. *bosse*]. A rounded or knoblike protuberance, as on the side of a bone or tumor; may result from disease of the spine (kyphosis). **—bos′selated,** *adj.;* **bossela′tion,** *n.*

parietal b. See parietal *eminence.*

Bossi, Luigi Maria [*Italian obstetrician,* 1859–1919]. Known for his method of induction of labor by means of forced dilatation of the cervical canal (1895). Invented a steel instrument for the rapid dilatation of the cervix, called *Bossi's dilator.*

Boston's sign. See under *sign.*

bos″try·coi′din. $C_{18}H_{14}O_7$; a brown or red, crystalline antibiotic substance, elaborated by *Fusarium bostrycoides,* active, in vitro, against the tubercle bacillus.

bot [perhaps from Irish *boiteag,* maggot]. The larva of the botfly, especially the species infesting the horse and related animals.

Botallo, Leonardo (Botallus) [*Italian anatomist in France,* b. ca. 1530]. Described the foramen ovale of the heart. He is sometimes erroneously credited with the discovery of the ductus arteriosus, called *Botallo's duct.*

bot′a·ny [G. *botanē,* herb]. That branch of biology dealing with plants. **—botan′ic,** *adj.*

bot′fly″. See *Oestridae, Gastrophilidae, Cuterebridae.*

Both respirator. See under *respirator.*

both·rid′i·um. See *bothrium.*

both′ri·o-, both′ri- [G. *bothrion,* dim. of *bothros,* trench]. A combining form signifying *bothrium.*

Both″ri·o·ceph′a·lus. Synonym for *Diphyllobothrium.*

both′ri·oid [*bothrion;* G. *eidos,* form]. Pitted; foveolated; covered with pitlike marks.

both′ri·um [*bothrion*]. A grooved sucker, such as is seen on the head of the tapeworm *Diphyllobothrium latum.* Syn., *bothrion.* Also called *bothridium.*

Bo′throps, Both′rops [G. *bothros,* trench]. A genus of pit vipers, Crotalidae, found chiefly in Central and South America.

B. alternata. Vibora de la cruz.

B. atrox. Fer-de-lance, having a powerful hemotoxic venom. This viper, the commonest cause of snakebite in Panama, may attain a length of eight feet. Also called *barba ammarilla.*

B. jararaca. Jararaca.

B. neuwiedii. White-tailed jararaca.

B. nummifer. Jumping pit viper.

bot″o·gen′in, bo″to·gen′in. A steroidal sapogenin obtained from the Mexican yam *Dioscorea mexicana:* a possible source for the synthesis of cortisone.

bot′ry·oid [G. *botrys,* bunch of grapes; *eidos,* form]. Resembling in shape a bunch of grapes, due to many rounded prominences.

bot″ry·o·my·co′sis (bot″ree·o·migh·ko′sis) [*botrys;* G. *mykēs,* fungus; *-ōsis,* condition]. A chronic infectious disease of horses and, rarely, of cattle; characterized by localized fibromatous tumors with occasional metastasis caused by the *Micrococcus ascoformans* (*Staphylococcus aureus, Staphylococcus albus*). **—botryomycot′ic,** *adj.*

Bo·try′tis [*botrys*]. A genus of fungi, members of whose species may act as allergens.

bots [perhaps from Irish *boiteay,* maggot]. *In veterinary medicine,* infestation with botflies, which pass through one period of development in the bodies of animals, as larvae. They infest the cavities of the facial bones, the stomach and intestine, and the subcutaneous connective tissue, causing severe damage to the affected animals. Also called *bot-larvae infestation.*

Böttcher, Arthur [*German anatomist,* 1831–89]. Remembered for his investigation of the endolymphatic circulation of the internal ear. Described dark polyhedral cells between the basilar membrane and the cells of Claudius, called *Böttcher's cells.* Described spermin crystals, called *Böttcher's crystals.*

Bottini, Enrico [*Italian surgeon,* 1837–1903]. Known for his use of galvanocautery for prostatic obstruction (1874). The operation consisted of intraurethral division of the enlarged portion of the gland. It is now superseded.

bot′tle [OF. *bouteille,* from LL. *buticula*]. A vessel, usually of glass, with a narrow neck.

b. nose. Popular name for acne rosacea.

b. stoop. *In pharmacy,* a grooved block which holds a wide-mouthed bottle obliquely while its powder content is being dispensed.

b. wax. A hard wax used to seal stoppers in bottles.

leather b. See under *stomach.*

Mariotte b. A device that delivers liquid under constant hydrostatic pressure.

nursing b. A feeding bottle; a narrow- or wide-mouthed flask with a rubber nipple attached; used for feeding infants.

bot′u·lism [L. *botulus,* sausage]. Food poisoning due to the production of toxins by *Clostridium botulinum* in improperly canned foods; characterized by the abrupt onset of violent symptoms; often fatal. **—botuli′nus, botuliform,** *adj.*

bou″gie′ (bo͞o″zhee′, bo͞o′zhee) [F., a candle]. 1. A slender cylindrical instrument of rubber, waxed silk, or other material, for introduction into body passages, as the urethra, anus, or other canal. It may be plain or tipped, angled or straight, being intended for use in exploration, in dilatation of strictures, as a guide for the passage of other instruments, or for the induction of labor. 2. A suppository, particularly for insertion into the urethra.

armed b. One having a caustic attached to the tip.

b. à boule. A bulbous or bulb-tipped instrument.

caustic b. See armed *b.*

cylindrical b. One which is circular in cross section.

dilatable b. One which can be increased in diameter for dilating a stricture. Also called *dilating b.*

elastic b. One made of some elastic material.

filiform b. One of very slender caliber and variously tipped.

fusiform b. One with a spindle-shaped shaft.

medicated b. One containing a medicinal agent. See *bougie,* 2.

olive-tipped b. A bulbous bougie with an olive- or acorn-shaped tip.

soluble b. One containing substances which dissolve at body temperature. See *bougie,* 2.

wax b. One made of linen or gauze impregnated with melted wax.

whip b. A variety of filiform bougie.

Bouillaud, Jean Baptiste [*French physician,* 1796–1881]. Known for his identification of the anterior cerebral lobes as the speech center and his demonstration that the brain controls equilibration and progression (1827). Rheumatic fever is known as *Bouillaud's syndrome.*

bouil″lon′ [F.]. Broth.

Bouin's fixing fluid. See under *fixing fluid.*

Bou·len″ge·ri′na. A genus of aquatic cobras inhabiting the rain forests of tropical Africa, possessing predominantly neurotoxic venom.

bou·lim′i·a (bōō·lim′ee·uh). See *bulimia.*

Boulton's solution. See phenolated *iodine* solution.

bour·donne·ment′ (boor·dun·mong′. *See* Notes § 35) [F., a buzzing]. A buzzing or humming sound heard during auscultation, or heard subjectively from any cause. The former is thought to be due to the contraction of muscle fibrils.

Bourgery, Marc Jean [*French anatomist and surgeon,* 1797–1869]. The posterior ligament of the knee joint is known as *Bourgery's ligament.*

Bourneville, Désiré Magloire [*French neurologist,* 1840–1909]. His name is associated with tuberous sclerosis, called *Bourneville's disease.*

Bourquin-Sherman unit. See under *unit.*

Boussingault, Jean Baptiste Joseph Dieudonné [*French physiological chemist,* 1802–87]. Made the first analyses of foodstuffs and fertilizers (1839). Discovered the excretion of urea and the existence of hippuric acid.

bou′ton ter′mi·nal (bōō′ton tur′mi·nul. *See* Notes § 35) (pl. *boutons terminaux*) [F.]. See *end-feet.*

Bouveret, Leon [*French physician,* 1850–1929]. Described auricular paroxysmal tachycardia, called *Bouveret's syndrome.*

Boveri, Piero [*Italian neurologist,* 1879–1932]. Discovered a test for excess of globulin in cerebrospinal fluid, called *Boveri's test.*

Boveri, Theodor [*German zoologist,* 1862–1915]. Remembered for his early research work on chromosomes. First to apply the term centrosomes (1888) to the bodies discovered by Flemming and van Beneden (1876).

bo′vine [L. *bovinus,* of an ox]. 1. Cattlelike. 2. Relating to, or derived from, a cow or ox.

bow′el [OF. *boel,* from L. *botellus,* a sausage]. The intestine.

bow′el com·plaint′. Diarrhea.

bow′el train′ing. The establishing of regular habits of defecation during early childhood.

Bowen, John Templeton [*American dermatologist,* 1857–1941]. First to describe precancerous dermatosis, now considered within the realm of epidermoid carcinoma; called *Bowen's disease, Bowen's epithelioma.*

Bowie's ethyl violet-Biebrich scarlet stain. See under *stain.*

bow′leg″ [AS. *boga;* ON. *leggr*]. An arching outward of the lower limbs, usually rachitic. Syn., *genu varum.*

Bowman, Donald E. (1908–). American biochemist, known for his extensive research on vitamins, endocrine factors, and enzymes. With Frank Evert Visscher he developed the Visscher-Bowman test for pregnancy.

Bowman, William [*English anatomist and ophthalmologist,* 1816–92]. Celebrated internationally for his classic description of striated muscle (1841) and for his description of the structure of the renal corpuscle (1857–60). Devised an operation for the formation of an artificial pupil and one for cataract, by dilaceration, separating the points of two needles inserted into the cataracts through the cornea. His operation for obstruction of the lacrimal sac by slitting of the canaliculus is well known. His name is associated with the double-walled vesicle surrounding the renal glomerulus, known as *Bowman's capsule.* Described the membrane separating the corneal epithelium from the substantia propria of the eye; called *Bowman's membrane.* Said to have been responsible, more than any other person, for the advancement of ophthalmic surgery in England.

box′er's ear. Lay term for an aural hematoma. Also see *cauliflower ear.*

Boyd's types of Shigella. See under *Shigella.*

Boyer, Alexis [*French surgeon,* 1757–1833]. Remembered for his operation for anal fissure by division of the external sphincter, called *Boyer's operation.*

Boyle, Henry Edmund Gaskin [*English surgeon,* 1875–1941]. Invented an anesthesia apparatus, standard in the British Isles, by which nitrous oxide gas, oxygen, chloroform, and ether may be administered. This has been adapted for use with cyclopropane also.

Boyle, Robert [*English physicist,* 1627–91]. Discovered the phenomenon, known as *Boyle's law:* at any given temperature the volume of a given mass of gas varies in inverse proportion to the pressure exerted upon it. Studied the elasticity and compressibility of air. His demonstration that air is necessary for life (1669) was an important contribution to the knowledge of respiration.

Boylston, Zabdiel [*American physician,* 1679–1766]. Distinguished leader of New England medicine and founder of the lectureship and prizes bearing his name. Said to have been the first to inoculate for smallpox in America (1721).

Bozeman, Nathan [*American surgeon,* 1825–1905]. Remembered for his invention of a double-current catheter and for his operation for relief of vesicouterovaginal fistula (1887); called *Bozeman's operation, hysterocystocleisis.* His invention is still known as *Bozeman's catheter.* Devised a position in which the patient rests on knees and elbows and is secured to the table by supports, called *Bozeman's position.*

Bozzini, Philipp [*Austrian surgeon,* 1773–1809]. Introduced an aural speculum with illumination and mirror reflection (1807). Is credited also with attempts at endoscopy of the urinary tract (1807).

Bozzolo, Camillo [*Italian physician,* 1845–1920]. Described lethargic encephalitis (1895–1900), called *Bozzolo's disease.* Was among the first to recognize the role of *Diplococcus pneumoniae* in meningitis and arthritis. Credited with the introduction of thymol as a vermifuge (1879).

B.P. Blood pressure.

B.P., B. Ph. British Pharmacopoeia.

B. P. C. British Pharmaceutical Codex.

BR Abbreviation for British Revision of the BNA terminology.

Br Chemical symbol for bromine.

brace [OF. *bracier*, to embrace]. Apparatus which gives support to any movable part of the body, intended for permanent use, in contradistinction to a splint; may assist in locomotion, and is frequently attached to clothing, as to shoes; sometimes jointed to permit flexion.

Brachet, Jean Louis [*Belgian physiologist*, 1789–1858]. Remembered for his description of the right leaf of the primitive ventral mesentery, which passes to the dorsal aspect of the right hepatic lobe, the free edge bounding the epiploic foramen: called *mesolateral fold of Brachet.*

bra′chi·a (bray′kee·uh, brack′ee·uh). Plural of brachium.

bra′chi·al ar′ter·y [*brachium;* G. *artēria*, artery]. An artery which originates at the axillary and has profunda brachii, nutrient, muscular, superior ulnar collateral, inferior ulnar collateral, radial, and ulnar branches. It distributes blood to the deltoid, triceps, brachioradialis, biceps brachii, brachialis, coracobrachialis, and anconeus muscles, the shaft of the humerus, the elbow joint, the forearm, and the hand.

bra″chi·al′gi·a (bray″kee·al′juh, ·jee·uh, brack″ee·) [L. *brachium*, arm; G. *algos*, pain]. Severe pain in the arm or in the brachial plexus.

bra″chi·a′lis (bray″kee·ah′liss, ·ay′liss, brack″ee·) [*brachium*]. A muscle lying under the biceps brachii and covering the front of the elbow joint. See Table of Muscles in the Appendix.

bra′chi·form [*brachium;* L. *forma*, form]. Arm-shaped.

bra′chi·o- (bray′kee·o-, brack′ee·o-), **bra′chi-** [*brachium*]. A combining form denoting *the arm* or *connection with the arm.*

bra″chi·o·cyl·lo′sis [*brachium;* NL. from G. *kyllōsis*, a crooking]. Crookedness of the humerus.

brach″i·o·ra″di·al′is. Pertaining to the arm and radius, as the brachioradialis muscle. See Table of Muscles in the Appendix.

bra″chi·ot′o·my [*brachium;* G. *tomē*, a cutting]. Surgical or obstetric cutting or removal of an arm.

bra′chi·um (bray′kee·um, brack′ee·um) (pl. *brachia*) [L., arm]. 1. The arm, especially the upper arm. 2. Any armlike structure. —**brachial,** *adj.*

brachia cerebelli. The cerebellar peduncles.

b. conjunctivum. The superior cerebellar *peduncle.*

b. of the inferior colliculus. A strand of fibers from the inferior colliculus together with fibers of the lateral lemniscus ending in the medial geniculate body. Syn., *inferior quadrigeminal b.*

b. of the superior colliculus. A strand of optic fibers which continue beyond the lateral geniculate body to end in the optic stratum of the superior colliculus and in the pretectal areas. Syn., *superior quadrigeminal b.*

b. pontis. The middle cerebellar peduncle.

inferior quadrigeminal b. See *b.* of the inferior colliculus.

superior quadrigeminal b. See *b.* of the superior colliculus.

Bracht, Erich Franz Eugen (1882–). German pathologist, known for his work on the pathology of rheumatic heart disease. See Bracht-Wächter *body.*

brach′y- (brack′i-) [G. *brachys*, short]. A combining form meaning *short.*

brach″y·car′di·a [*brachys;* G. *kardia*, heart]. Bradycardia.

brach″y·ce·pha′li·a, brach″y·ceph′a·lism, brach″y·ceph′a·ly [*brachys;* G. *kephalē*, head]. Shortness of the head, the cephalic index being 81.0 to 85.4. —**brachycephal′ic, brachyceph′alous,** *adj.*

brach″y·chei′li·a (brack″i·kigh′lee·uh), **brach″y·chi′li·a** (brack″i·kigh′lee·uh, ·kill′ee·uh), **bra·chych′il·y** (bra·kick′i·lee) [*brachys;* G. *cheilos*, lip]. Abnormal shortness of the lip. Syn., *microcheilia.*

brach″y·chei′rous, brach″y·chi′rous (brack″i·kigh′rus) [*brachys;* G. *cheir*, hand]. Having short hands. —**brachychiria, brachychirism,** *n.*

brach″y·dac·tyl′i·a, brach″y·dac′ty·ly [*brachys;* G. *daktylos*, finger]. Abnormal shortness of the fingers or toes. —**brachydac′tylous, brachydactyl′ic,** *adj.*

brach″y·glos′sal [*brachys;* G. *glōssa*, tongue]. Having a short tongue. —**brachyglossia,** *n.*

brach″yg·nath′ous (brack″ig·nath′us) [*brachys;* G. *gnathos*, jaw]. Having an abnormally short lower jaw. Syn., *micrognathus.* —**brachygna′thia, brachygnath′us,** *n.*

brach″y·ker′kic [*brachys;* G. *kerkis*, shuttle]. Denoting a forearm disproportionately shorter than the upper arm.

brach″y·me·tap′o·dy [*brachys;* G. *meta*, behind; *pous*, foot]. A condition in which the metatarsals are shorter than the average.

brach″y·mei·o′sis. The third division, i.e., the second reduction division, in the ascus of Ascomycetes.

brach″y·mor′phy [*brachys;* G. *morphē*, form]. Short stature. —**brachymorphic,** *adj.*

brach″y·pel′lic. Denoting an oval type of pelvis in which the transverse diameter exceeds the anteroposterior diameter by not more than three centimeters.

brach″y·pel′vic [*brachys;* L. *pelvis*, basin]. See *brachypellic.*

brach″y·pha·lan′gi·a, brach″y·pha·lan′gy [*brachys;* G. *phalanx*, bone between two joints of the fingers and toes]. A condition in which the phalanges are abnormally short. —**brachyphalangous,** *adj.*

brach″y·po′dous [*brachys;* G. *pous*, foot]. *In biology*, possessing a short foot or stalk.

brach″y·pro·sop′ic (brack″i·pro·sop′ick, ·so′pick) [*brachys;* G. *prosōpon*, face]. Having a short face.

brach″y·rhin′i·a [*brachys;* G. *rhis*, nose]. Abnormal shortness of the nose.

brach″y·rhyn′chus (brack″i·ring′kus) [*brachys;* G. *rhygchos*, snout]. Abnormal shortness of maxilla and nose; usually associated with cyclopia or cebocephaly, but occasionally occurring alone.

brach″y·skel′ic [*brachys;* G. *skelos*, leg]. Characterized by extreme shortness of the legs.

brach″y·staph′y·line [*brachys;* G. *staphylē*, uvula]. Having a short alveolar arch.

brach″y·sta′sis [*brachys;* G. *stasis*, a standing]. A process in which a muscle does not relax to its former length following a contraction and maintains its original degree of tension in its new state. Also called *brachystatic contraction.*

brach″y·u·ran′ic [*brachys;* G. *ouranos*, roof of the mouth]. Having a palatomaxillary index above 115.

Brackett, Elliott Gray [*American orthopedic surgeon*, 1860–1944]. Known for his operations in orthopedic surgery, especially for his method of fixing the fragments in fracture of the femoral neck. The head is retained and hollowed out to form a cap for the rounded-off end of the fractured femur; the greater trochanter is transplanted upward to the site of fracture. Called *Brackett's operation.*

Brade. See *Braid.*

Bradford, Edward Hickling [*American orthopedic surgeon*, 1848–1926]. Known for his invention of orthopedic appliances and especially for his canvas-covered, gas-pipe frame made in various sizes. It was devised originally for handling children with tuberculous disease of the spine, but was later extended to the care of joint disease and for immobilization after operations. Where young children are involved, restraint is imposed by webbing straps and a pelvic band.

brad'y- [G. *bradys*, slow]. A combining form meaning *slow*.

brad"y·ar'thri·a [*bradys;* G. *arthron*, joint]. Slow speech; due to organic disturbance of the speech apparatus.

brad"y·aux·e'sis [*bradys;* G. *auxēsis*, increase]. A type of relative growth in which a part grows at a slower rate than the whole organism or another part.

brad"y·car'di·a [*bradys;* G. *kardia*, heart]. Slowness of the heart; manifested in a pulse rate usually less than 60 per minute. Syn., *brachycardia.* —**bradycar'dic,** *adj.*

sinus b. Sinus rhythm with slow heart rate.

brad"y·crot'ic [*bradys;* G. *krotos*, rattling noise]. Characterized by a slow pulse.

brad"y·di·as'to·le (brad"i·dye·ass'to·lee), **brad"y·di"as·to'li·a** (brad"i·dye"ass·to'lee·uh) [*bradys;* G. *diastolē*, a drawing asunder]. Prolongation of the diastolic interval; associated with myocardial lesions.

brad"y·glos'si·a [*bradys;* G. *glōssa*, tongue]. Slow speech; due to difficulty in tongue movement.

brad"y·ki·ne'si·a (brad"i·ki·nee'shuh, ·see·uh, ·zhuh, ·zee·uh, brad"i·kigh·nee'·), **brad"y·ki·ne'sis** (·ki·nee'sis, ·kigh·nee'sis) [*bradys;* G. *kinēsis*, motion]. Slow or retarded movement, as in melancholia or catatonia. —**bradykinet'ic,** *adj.*

brad"y·la'li·a [*bradys;* G. *lalia*, talk]. Slowness of utterance.

brad"y·lex'i·a [*bradys;* G. *lexis*, word]. Abnormal slowness in reading.

brad"y·pha'si·a (brad"i·fay'zhuh, ·zee·uh) [*bradys;* G. *phasis*, utterance]. Slow speech.

brad"y·phre'ni·a [*bradys;* G. *phrēn*, mind]. Sluggish mental activity, such as that following lethargic encephalitis.

brad·y·pne'a (brad·i·nee'ah) [*bradys;* G. *pnoia*, breath]. A decreased breathing rate. It often follows the use of narcotics and sedatives or an increase in intracranial pressure.

brad"y·pra'gi·a [*bradys;* G. *prassein*, to do]. Abnormally slow action; usually applied to physical activity.

brad"y·prax'i·a [*bradys;* G. *praxis*, a doing, action]. Slow or retarded physical movement.

brad"y·rhyth'mi·a (brad"i·rith'mee·uh, ·rith'-mee·uh) [*bradys;* G. *rhythmos*, measured motion]. 1. Slowing of the heart or pulse rate; bradycardia. 2. *In electroencephalography*, slowing of the brain wave rate to one to six per second, the rate being normally about ten per second. See alpha *rhythm.*

brad"y·tel"e·o·ki·ne'sis (·tell"ee·o·ki·nee'sis, ·kigh·nee'sis, ·tee"lee·o·) [*bradys;* G. *teleos*, complete; *kinēsis*, movement]. The type of incoordination in which a movement is halted before completion, then completed slowly and irregularly.

Braid, James (**Brade**) [*Scottish physician in England*, 1795–1860]. Known as the inaugurator of hypnotism, a word he coined. Many of his theories concerning diseases of the mind were adopted by leaders in that field. The term *Braidist* was at one time used to indicate a person who used hypnotism.

Braille, Louis [*French teacher of the blind*, 1809–52]. Blinded by accident at the age of three, he invented (1837) the compact alphabet of raised dots in use for the blind today. This system had been suggested earlier by Charles Barbier but had not been perfected.

brain [AS. *bragen*]. The encephalon. That part of the central nervous system contained in the cranial cavity, consisting of the cerebrum, cerebellum, pons, and medulla oblongata. See Plates 17, 18.

afterbrain. Myelencephalon.

betweenbrain. Diencephalon; thalamus.

endbrain. Telencephalon.

forebrain. Prosencephalon.

hindbrain. Rhombencephalon.

midbrain. Mesencephalon.

smell b. Rhinencephalon.

walnut b. An atrophic *lobar sclerosis.*

wet b. Cerebral edema.

Brain's reflex. See under *reflex.*

brain sand. Psammoma bodies in the pineal body; corpora arenacea.

brain stem. See under *stem.* See Plates 17, 18.

Bramwell, Byron (1847–1931). English physician, known for his studies of intracranial tumors, and his early recognition of the functional significance of the hypothalamus (1888).

bran'chi·a (pl. *branchiae*) [*bragchia*]. See *gill.*

bran'chi·al (brang'kee·ul) [G. *bragchia*, gills]. 1. Pertaining to the branchiae or gills. 2. By extension, pertaining to the embryonic visceral arches. See under *arch, cyst, cleft.* See also lateral *fistula* of the neck.

branch'ing. *In radioactivity*, the occurrence of two or more processes by which atoms of a radioactive nuclide can undergo decay.

bran'chi·o- (brang'kee·o-), **bran'chi-** (brang'ki-) [*bragchia*]. A combining form denoting *connection with* or *relation to branchiae* or *gills.*

bran"chi·og'e·nous (brang"kee·odj'i·nus), **bran"-chi·o·gen'ic** [*bragchia;* G. *genesthai*, from *gignesthai*, to be produced]. Produced or developed from a branchial cleft or arch.

bran"chi·o'ma. See branchiogenic *carcinoma.*

bran'chi·o·mere" [*bragchia;* G. *meros*, part]. A segment of the visceral mesoderm which develops into a branchial or visceral arch.

bran"chi·om'er·ism [*bragchia; meros*]. Serial arrangement of the visceral arches or branchiomeres.

bran'dy [Dutch *brandewijn*, from *branden*, to burn, *wijn*, wine] (*spiritus vini vitis*). 1. The product of the distillation of fermented grape juice; it contains from 48 to 54%, by volume, of C_2H_5OH, ethyl alcohol. 2. The product of the distillation of a fermented fruit juice; as cherry, peach, and apricot brandies.

Branham, Henry H. [*American surgeon*, nineteenth century]. Remembered for his sign of bradycardia observed in certain cases of aneurysm.

Brasdor, Pierre [*French surgeon*, 1721–97]. Introduced his operation for aneurysm in which he ligated the vessel just distal to the dilatation.

bras'i·lin. Brazilin.

brass [AS. *braes*]. An alloy of copper with zinc.

brass chills. See metal fume *fever.*

brass found'er's a'gue (ayg'yoo). See metal fume *fever;* brass founder's *ague.*

brass poi'son·ing. Synonym for brass founder's ague. See metal fume *fever;* brass founder's *ague.*

Bratton, Andrew Calvin [*American biochemist and pharmacologist*, 1912–]. With E. K. Marshall, Jr., H. J. White, and J. T. Litchfield, introduced sulfaguanadine in the treatment of intestinal infections. With Marshall, L. B. Edwards, and E. Walker, introduced this treatment for acute bacillary dysentery in children (1941). See also Bratton and Marshall's *method* for determining concentrations of sulfonamides in blood and urine.

Brauer, Ludolph [*German surgeon,* 1865–]. Devised an operation for adherent pericardium in which he advocated removal of ribs, cartilages, and part of the sternum over the heart to relieve the condition described as angulation of the heart. Called *cardiolysis, Brauer operation.* His name is associated with the thoracoplasty described by Friedrich.

Braun, Christopher Heinrich [*German physician,* 1847–1911]. His name is associated with a test for glucose by the use of sodium hydroxide and picric acid, which produce a deep red color; called *Braun's test.*

Braun, Gustav August von [*Austrian obstetrician,* 1829–1911]. The inventor of a decapitation hook used in difficult labor, called *Braun's hook.*

Braun, Maximilian Gustav Christian Carl [*German anatomist and parasitologist,* 1850–1930]. Known primarily for his work in parasitology. The neurenteric canal is sometimes known as *Braun's canal.*

Braun's graft. Implant pinch graft.

Braune, Christian Wilhelm [*German anatomist,* 1831–92]. Known for his skill in preparing frozen sections for teaching purposes (1872), for his atlas of human anatomy (1884–89), and for his studies, with Otto Fischer, of the mechanics of body motion (1891) and human locomotion (1895). See retraction *ring,* 1.

brawn'y [OF. *braon,* fleshy part, muscle]. Fleshy; muscular.

Braxton Hicks's contractions. See under *contraction.*

Braxton Hicks's sign. See Hicks's *sign.*

Braxton Hicks's version. See under *version.*

brax'y. See *water-braxy.*

bra·ye'ra (bra·yair'uh, bray·yair'uh). The dried panicles of the pistillate flowers of *Hagenia abyssinica,* the kussotree. It contains tannic acid, a volatile oil, and kosotoxin, an active principle; has been used as an anthelmintic against tapeworms. In large doses it produces nausea and emesis. Also called *cusso, kousso, kusso.*

braz'i·lin. $C_{16}H_{14}O_5$; an amber-yellow crystalline substance from *Caesalpinia echinata* (Brazilwood) or certain other redwood trees: used as a dye.

break'bone" fe'ver. Dengue.

breast [AS. *braēst*]. 1. The front of the chest. 2. One of the mammary glands.

caked b. Colloquial term for puerperal mastitis.

carinate b. See pigeon *b.*

chicken b. See pigeon *b.*

funnel b. A thoracic wall anomaly characterized by a depression or groove involving the sternum and neighboring cartilages.

pigeon b. A chest with a prominent sternum due to rickets or obstructed infantile respiration: also called *chicken b.*

breast'bone" [*braēst;* AS. *bān*]. Sternum.

breath [AS. *brǣth*]. The air inhaled and exhaled during respiration.

pulse b. See *pulse breath.*

saturnine b. The peculiar sweet breath characteristic of lead poisoning.

breath al'co·hol meth'od. See under *method.*

breath'ing. See *respiration.*

breath'ing ma·chine'. Respirator.

Breda, Achille [*Italian dermatologist,* 1850–1933]. Discovered Brazilian yaws (1895), called *Breda's disease.*

breech [ME. *brech*]. The buttocks or nates.

b. presentation. See under *presentation.*

breg'ma (pl. *bregmata*) [G., front part of the head]. The junction of the coronal and sagittal sutures; in infants, the anterior fontanel. —**bregmat'ic,** *adj.*

breg·mat"o·dym'i·a [*bregma;* G. *didymos,* twin]. See *craniopagus parietalis.*

Breh and Gaebler's method. See under *method.*

brei (bry) [Ger. *brei,* mush]. Mush; soupy mixture; tissue ground to a pulp.

Breisky, August [*German gynecologist,* 1832–89]. Described kraurosis of the vulva (1885). In *Breisky's method* of determining the dimensions of the pelvis at its outlet, the distance between the ischial tuberosities, and that between the sacrococcygeal junction and the lower border of the pubis, are measured externally.

Bremer, Ludwig [*American physician,* 1844–1914]. Known for his test for diabetic blood, in which blood is prepared as in ordinary staining methods and, after drying in a hot-air sterilizer, is stained with methylene blue and eosin; the red cells appear greenish yellow whereas in normal blood they appear brownish. Called *Bremer's test.*

brems'strahl·en. *In radiobiology,* the secondary photon radiation produced by the interaction of energized electrons and the atomic nuclei of the material through which they pass: also called *bremsstrahlung.*

Brenner, Fritz (1887–). German physician who described a follicular ovarian tumor, called *Brenner tumor* (1907).

bren"ner·o'ma. See Brenner *tumor.*

Breschet, Gilbert [*French anatomist,* 1784–1845]. Described the veins and canals of the diploë, called *Breschet's veins, canals.*

Bretonneau, Pierre Fidèle [*French pathologist,* 1778–1862]. Identifying membranous croup, malignant angina, and certain affections of the gums as the same disease, he recognized diphtheria as a distinct disease entity (1826), and later coined the term. Said to have performed the first successful tracheotomy for diphtheria (1825).

Breuer, Josef [*Austrian psychiatrist,* 1842–1925]. With Sigmund Freud, he is credited with the theory of the unconscious mind. See also Hering-Breuer *reflex.*

Breus, Carl [*Austrian obstetrician,* 1852–1914]. Described a tuberous mole (1892), called *Breus's mole.*

brev"i·col'lis [L. *brevis,* short; *collum,* neck]. Congenital short neck; a deformity characterized by shortness or absence of the neck, limitation of head movements and sometimes of the facial muscles.

brev"i·lin'e·al [*brevis;* L. *linealis,* lineal]. Pertaining to a body type which is shorter and broader than normal. Syn., *brachymorphic.*

brev"i·ra'di·ate. See breviradiate *cell.*

bribe [OF., a lump of bread]. *In psychoanalysis,* a compromise in which the ego accepts the symptoms of a neurosis and, in turn, placates the superego by suffering.

bridge [AS. *brycg*]. 1. *In anatomy,* any ridge or spanlike structure. 2. *In dentistry,* a partial denture supported by one or more teeth. See *bridgework.* 3. *In electricity,* an apparatus for measuring the resistance of a conductor.

arterial b. A segment of vein, fresh or preserved by the rapid freeze technique, used to bridge a gap in an injured artery. The anastomosis between artery and vein is carried out by a nonsuture technique over two funnel-shaped vitallium tubes or one long vitallium tube through which the vein is threaded. Also called *Blakemore's operation.*

b. of the nose. That formed by the union of the two nasal bones.

cantilever b. One fixed at one end and with either no support or with a lug resting on the adjoining tooth at the other end.

intercellular bridges. Protoplasmic bridges which connect adjacent cells; plasmodesms.

Wheatstone b. An electric circuit containing four resistances in branches or arms. When the bridge is suitably adjusted or balanced, any one resistance can be calculated in terms of the other three.

bridge'work". *In dentistry:* 1. An appliance made of artificial crowns of teeth to replace missing natural teeth. Such crowns are connected to natural teeth or roots for anchorage by means of a bridge. A *fixed bridge* is one which is permanently fastened to its abutments; a *removable bridge* one which, though held firmly in place, may be removed by the wearer; a *removable fixed bridge* one which may be removed, without mutilation of any of its parts, by the dentist, but not by the patient. 2. The technique of making bridges.

Bridgman, Percy Williams (1882–). American physicist, noted investigator in the study of high-pressure physics and inventor of apparatus producing extremely high pressures. He made other studies on electrical conduction in metals, the properties of crystals, and the logic of modern physics. Nobel laureate in physics (1946).

bri'dle [AS. *bridel*]. 1. A band or filament stretching across the lumen of a passage, or from side to side of an ulcer, scar, abscess, etc. 2. A frenum.

Briggs, James Emmons [*American surgeon*, 1869–1942]. Inventor of the distensible rubber bag for controlling bleeding after suprapubic prostatectomy (1905); called *Briggs's bag*.

Bright, Richard [*English physician and clinician*, 1789–1858]. Known universally for his description of chronic nephritis, which received the name *Bright's disease* (1827). In his reports, he differentiated renal from cardiac dropsy. Described also status lymphaticus (1838) and pancreatic jaundice. Is said to have made the original description of acute yellow atrophy of the liver. The partial or complete loss of sight occasioned in uremia was once known as *Bright's blindness*.

bright'ness. The attribute of sensation by which an observer is aware of different luminances.

Brill, Nathan Edwin (1860–1925). American physician; first to describe (1910) a recrudescence of epidemic typhus occurring in a mild form years after initial infection among immigrants from eastern Europe: called *Brill's disease, recrudescent* or *sporadic typhus*. He also described follicular lymphoma, called *Brill-Symmers disease*.

bril'liance. *In color optics*, an old term for *brightness*.

bril'liant cres'yl blue (kress'il, kree'sil) (C.C.). A basic dye, having highly metachromatic properties; chiefly used for staining blood to demonstrate the platelets and reticulated corpuscles. Also called *brilliant blue C, cresyl blue 2RN* or *BBS*.

bril'liant green (C.C.). Tetraethyldiamino-triphenylcarbohydride sulfate; $C_{27}H_{34}N_2O_4S$; a surgical antiseptic used in 1:1000 aqueous solution: also called *ethyl green, malachite green G*.

bril'liant vi'tal red. See *vital red*.

brim'stone". See *sulfur*.

Brinton, William [*English physician*, 1823–67]. Gave early account of peptic ulcer with a review of many thousands of cases seen post mortem (1857). Described linitis plastica (1859), called *Brinton's disease*.

Briquet, Paul [*French physician*, 1796–1881]. Described hysterical ataxia (1859), called *Briquet's ataxia*. Described a syndrome of hysterical paralysis of the diaphragm with dyspnea and aphonia, called *Briquet's syndrome*.

Brissaud, Edouard [*French physician*, 1852–1909]. Remembered for having given the first clear description of dysthyroidal infantilism and for his description of a syndrome of hysterical glossolabial hemispasm, called *Brissaud-Marie syndrome*. See also Brissaud's *reflex*.

Brit'ish an"ti-lew'is·ite. BAL

broach [OF. *broche*]. *In dentistry*, a delicate, tapered, flexible steel instrument having a spring temper; used for removing the dental pulp and for opening, enlarging, and treating the root canals. Various forms are: the **barbed broach, hooked broach, smooth broach,** and **spiral broach,** all of which are operated by a removable handle. The **root canal broach** is used for root-canal surgery, and the **watchmaker's broach,** a four- or five-sided, very gradually tapering, sharp-angled instrument, is used as a reamer to enlarge the root canals.

Broadbent, William Henry [*English physician*, 1835–1907]. Author of *Heart Disease* with Sir J. F. H. Broadbent (1897). Celebrated for his contributions to clinical knowledge of the heart and pulse (1890–97). Described progressive cerebral hemorrhage, at first outside a brain ventricle and gradually advancing until it breaks into the ventricle: called *Broadbent's apoplexy*. Advanced his law that the upper motor neuron lesions produce a milder form of paralysis in those muscles generally concerned with bilateral contractions than in those muscles which act unilaterally: called *Broadbent's law*.

Broadbent's sign. See under *sign*.

broad-spec'trum an"ti·bi·ot'ic. An antibiotic effective in the treatment of various infections caused by different types of microorganisms.

Broca, Pierre Paul [*French surgeon and anthropologist*, 1824–80]. Known for his work in anatomy, physiology, and anthropology, and in brain surgery. He claimed discovery of the speech center in the third left frontal convolution. The dividing point of the Sylvian fissure, the parietal angle in craniotomy, and the visual plane drawn through the axes of the two orbits have all been known by his name. He also described cortical motor aphasia, called *Broca's aphasia*.

Brocq, Louis Anne Jean [*French dermatologist*, 1856–1928]. He proposed the term parapsoriasis to describe an exfoliative dermatitis not resulting from any known disease; called *Brocq's disease*. Also described an uncommon form of hyperpigmentation occurring about the mouth, especially in women, called *Brocq's syndrome*.

Broders, Albert Compton [*American pathologist*, 1885–]. Known for his classification of tumors, especially the epitheliomas, in which a division is made into four groups. The more nearly the cells approach the embryonic type, the more malignant the growth. The epitheliomas are graded from one to four, the latter being the most malignant.

Brodie, Benjamin Collins [*English surgeon*, 1783–1862]. Known for his descriptions of various pathologic conditions. *Brodie's abscess* is a chronic osteomyelitic focus, of tuberculous or other etiology. He described a chronic synovitis resulting in a pulpy degeneration of the joint tissue in the knee; a pseudo-fracture of the spine; a tumor of the breast, *cystosarcoma phylloides*, sometimes called *Brodie's serocystic disease of the breast, Brodie's tumor;* and a type of hemorrhoid. He also studied and made tests of the varicose veins, and is said to have been the first to describe intermittent claudication in man.

Brodmann, Korbinian (1868–1918). German neurologist; one of the founders of the modern science of comparative cytoarchitectonics of the mammalian cortex, and author of a map of the human cortex (1908). See *Brodmann's areas* under *area*.

Brodmann's map. The map of areas of the human cerebral cortex, differentiated by their cellular patterns, as drawn by Korbinian Brodmann. The numbers which he gave to these areas are still used for convenient reference.

brom-. See *bromo-*.

bro'mal. $CBr_3.CHO$. Tribromoacetaldehyde. The bromine analog of chloral; but unsuccessful therapeutically.

b. hydrate. $CBr_3.CH(OH)_2$. Colorless, deliquescent crystals; has been used as a sedative and antispasmodic.

brom·am'ide (bro·mam'id, ·ide, bro'muh·mide, ·mid). $C_6H_2Br_3.NH_2HBr$. Tribromoaniline hydrobromide. Has been used as an analgesic.

bro'mate [G. *brōmos*, stench]. A salt of bromic acid containing the univalent radical $—BrO_3$.

bro'mat·ed (bro'may·tid). Combined with or containing bromine; brominated.

bro"ma·tom'e·try [G. *brōma*, food; *metron*, a measure]. The estimation of the amount of food required for an individual.

bro"ma·to·ther'a·py [*brōma;* G. *therapeia*, treatment]. Dietotherapy.

bro"ma·to·tox'in [*brōma;* G. *toxikon*, poison]. A poison generated in food by the growth of microorganisms.

bro"ma·to·tox'ism [*brōma; toxikon*]. Poisoning with infected food.

bro'ma·zine hy"dro·chlo'ride. British generic name for the antihistaminic substance, bromodiphenhydramine hydrochloride. See *ambodryl hydrochloride.*

brom"di·eth"yl·ac"e·tyl·u·re'a (brohm"dye-eth"il·ass"i·til·yoo·ree'uh). Carbromal.

bro'me·lin, bro·mel'in. A protein-digesting enzyme from the pineapple.

bro'me·thol. British Pharmacopoeia title for solution of tribromoethanol. See *avertin.*

bro'me·tone. Tribromotertiarybutyl alcohol. Br_3-$C.C(OH)(CH_3)_2$. A fine, white, crystalline powder with sedative action similar to that of the bromides. Also *acetone bromoform.*

brom"hi·dro"si·pho'bi·a (brohm"hi·dro"si·fo'-bee·uh, ·dros"i·fo'bee·uh, brom"hi·) [G. *brōmos*, stench; *hidrōs*, sweat; *phobos*, fear]. Morbid dread of offensive personal smells, with hallucinations as to the perception of them.

brom"hi·dro'sis (brohm"hi·dro'sis, brom"hi·), **bro"mi·dro'sis** (bro"mi·dro'sis, brom"i·) [*brōmos; hidrōs*]. Excretion of sweat with an unpleasant odor. Various odors may occur, usually disagreeable. Syn., *osmidrosis, fetid perspiration.*

brom·hy'dric ac'id. Hydrobromic acid.

bro'mide, bro'mid. Any binary salt in which univalent bromine is the anion, as sodium bromide, NaBr. The bromides are used medicinally for several purposes, to check the convulsions of epilepsy and tetanus; as analgesics, particularly in combination with other drugs; and as sedatives in nervous excitation.

bro'mide poi'son·ing. See *bromine poisoning.*

bro"mi·dro'sis. See *bromhidrosis.*

bro'mine (bro'meen, ·min) [*brōmos*]. Br = 79.916. A reddish-brown liquid which, at ordinary temperatures, gives off a heavy, suffocating vapor. It is a very active escharotic and disinfectant and, internally, acts as a violent poison. —**bromated, brominated,** *adj.*

bro'mine poi'son·ing. A diseased state caused by the prolonged administration of bromides; characterized by headache, sleepiness, apathy, cold extremities, fetid breath, and a typical acneform eruption. There may be loss of strength and sexual drive, associated with atrophy of the testes or mammae.

bro'min·ism. See *bromine poisoning.*

bro'mi·pin. A liquid composed of bromine and sesame oil, containing 10% of bromine, formerly used as a sedative in epilepsy. A similar compound containing 33% of bromine was used as an x-ray contrast medium, especially in bronchography.

bro'mism, bro'min·ism. Bromine poisoning.

brom"i·so·val'um. Generic name for (α-bromoisovaleryl) urea, a sedative and hypnotic. See *bromural.*

bro'mite. 1. Native silver bromide. 2. A salt of bromous acid containing the radical $—BrO_2$.

bro'mo-, brom- [*brōmos*]. 1. A combining form denoting *a bad smell.* 2. *In chemistry,* a combining form denoting *the presence of bromine.*

bro"mo·ac"et·an'i·lid (bro"mo·ass"i·tan'i·lid). $C_6H_4Br.NH.CO.CH_3$. White crystals, almost insoluble in water, soluble in alcohol. Analgesic and antipyretic.

bro"mo·ben"zyl·cy'a·nide. $C_6H_5CHBrCN$. A lacrimator used in chemical warfare. Sometimes written *brombenzylcyanide.* See war *gas.*

bro"mo·cam'phor. See monobromated *camphor.*

bro"mo·cre'sol green. Tetrabromo-metacresolsulfonphthalein, an indicator used for determination of hydrogen-ion concentration. Its useful pH range is 3.8 to 5.4; the color varies from yellow at 3.8 to blue at 5.4. Sometimes written *bromcresol green.*

bro"mo·cre'sol pur'ple. Dibromo-orthocresolsulfonphthalein, an indicator used for determination of hydrogen-ion concentration. Its useful pH range is 5.2 to 6.8; the color varies from yellow at 5.2 to purple at 6.8. Sometimes written *bromcresol purple.*

bro"mo·der'ma [*brōmos;* G. *derma*, skin]. A skin eruption due to ingestion of bromides.

bro"mo·di"phen·hy'dra·mine hy"dro·chlo'ride. Generic name for a derivative of diphenhydramine hydrochloride in which a hydrogen atom of a phenyl group, in *para*-position, is replaced by an atom of bromine. The substance possesses higher antihistaminic potency and lower toxicity, as compared with diphenhydramine hydrochloride. Syn., *bromazine hydrochloride.* See *ambodryl hydrochloride.*

bro'mo·form. $CHBr_3$. Tribromomethane. A heavy, colorless, mobile liquid of sweetish taste; slightly soluble in water, miscible with alcohol. It has been used as a sedative in whooping cough and in seasickness but has produced dangerous effects.

bro"mo·hy"per·hi·dro'sis (·hi·dro'sis, ·high·dro'-sis), **bro"mo·hy"per·i·dro'sis** [*brōmos;* G. *hyper*, over; *hidrōsis*, sweating]. The excessive secretion of malodorous sweat.

bro"mo·ma'ni·a [*brōmos;* G. *mania*, madness]. Psychosis from the excessive use of bromides.

bro"mo·men"or·rhe'a, bro"mo·men"or·rhoe'a [*brōmos;* G. *mēn*, month; *rhoia*, flow]. Disordered menstruation marked by offensiveness of the flow.

bro"mo·phe'nol blue. Tetrabromophenolsulfonphthalein, an indicator used for determination of hydrogen-ion concentration. Its useful pH range is 3.0 to 4.6; the color varies from yellow at 3.0 to bluish violet at 4.6. Sometimes written *bromphenol blue.*

bro"mop·ne'a, bro"mop·noe'a [*brōmos;* G. *pnoia*, breath]. Fetid breath.

bro"mo·pro'pane. 1-Bromopropane, $BrCH_2.CH_2$-CH_3, and 2-bromopropane, $CH_3.CHBr.CH_3$; have been suggested as general inhalation anesthetics.

bro"mo·pro'pene. 1-Bromo-1-propene, $BrC{:}CH$.-CH_3, and 2-bromo-1-propene, $CH_2{:}CBr.CH_2$; have been suggested as general inhalation anesthetics.

bromoseltzer. A proprietary headache remedy in the form of a granulated, effervescent salt.

bro″mo·thy′mol blue. Dibromothymolsulfonphthalein, an indicator used for determination of hydrogen-ion concentration. Its useful pH range is from 6.0 to 7.6; the color varies from yellow at 6.0 to blue at 7.6. Sometimes written *bromthymol blue.*

bromsalizol. Trade-mark for the antispasmodic and local anesthetic substance monobromosalicyl alcohol.

bromsulphalein. Trade-mark for a brand of sulfobromophthalein sodium: the substance used for quantitative evaluation of liver function.

brom″te·trag′nost (brohm″ti·trag′nohst, ·nost). Sulfobromophthalein sodium: a diagnostic agent.

bromural. A trade-mark for bromisovalum: a sedative and hypnotic.

bro′mu·ra·ted [*brōmos*]. Containing bromine or a bromine salt.

bronch·ad″e·ni′tis (brong·kad″i·nigh′tis, brong″-kuh·di·) [G. *brogchos*, trachea; *adēn*, gland; *-itis*, inflammation]. Inflammation of the bronchial lymph nodes.

bron′chi (brong′kigh). Plural of bronchus.

bron″chi·ec′ta·sis (brong″kee·eck′tuh·sis) [G. *brogchia*, bronchial tubes; *ektasis*, extension]. Dilatation of bronchi due to an inflammatory or degenerative process, usually associated with chronic suppuration. —**bronchiectat′ic,** *adj.*

cylindrical b. A uniform dilatation of a tube.

sacculated b. Irregular dilatation in sacs or pockets.

bron′chi·o- (brong′kee·o-), **bron′chi-** (brong′ki-) [*brogchia*]. A combining form signifying *bronchial.*

bron″chi·o·gen′ic. Bronchogenic.

bron′chi·ole (brong′kee·ole) [dim. from *brogchia*]. One of the small (1 mm. or less in diameter) subdivisions of the bronchi. —**bron·chi′o·lar,** *adj.*

respiratory b. The last bronchiolar subdivision; one which has pulmonary alveoli in its wall.

terminal b. The next to the last bronchiolar subdivision; the last bronchiole without pulmonary alveoli in its wall.

bron″chi·o·lec′ta·sis [*brogchia;* G. *ektasis*, extension]. Dilatation of bronchioles. See *bronchiectasis.*

bron″chi·o·li′tis [*brogchia;* G. *-itis*, inflammation]. Inflammation of the bronchioles; capillary bronchitis.

acute obliterating b. Pulmonary cirrhosis affecting the smaller bronchioles, causing occlusion of the lumens by induration of the walls.

b. fibrosa obliterans. Bronchiolitis resulting in occlusion of the bronchioles by the growth of connective tissue from the terminal bronchi.

vesicular b. Bronchopneumonia.

bron·chi′tis (bron·kigh′tis, brong·kigh′tis) [*brogchia; -itis*]. Inflammation of the mucous membrane of the bronchial tubes. —**bronchit′ic,** *adj.*

acute b. That due to extension of an acute nasopharyngitis, to the inhalation of irritant vapors, or to certain infectious agents. It is characterized by fever, cough, substernal pain, and by dry rales in the early, and moist rales in the later, stages.

asthmatic b. (a) Asthmatic type of breathing, usually without acute dyspnea, associated with respiratory infections: believed to occur in individuals with an allergic constitution. (b) The syndrome of chronic bronchitis, emphysema, and secondary bronchiolar spasm, usually occurring in persons of middle age or older: an occasional use.

b. convulsiva. Whooping cough.

capillary b. An acute bronchitis of the bronchioles; bronchiolitis. Bronchopneumonia is a common complication.

catarrhal b. A form attended with profuse, mucopurulent discharges.

chronic b. A form of bronchitis usually occurring in middle or advanced life; characterized by cough and by dry and moist rales. It may be due to repeated attacks of acute bronchitis, to gout, rheumatism, or tuberculosis, or it may be secondary to cardiac and renal disease.

croupous b. A rare variety attended with the expectoration of casts of the bronchial tubes, containing Charcot-Leyden crystals and eosinophil cells, after a paroxysm of dyspnea and violent coughing.

dry b. That unattended by expectoration.

fibrinous b. See croupous *b.*

fusospirochetal b. A type of chronic bronchitis caused by a spirochete; it is amenable to treatment by neoarsphenamine.

mechanical b. A form caused by the inhalation of dust, etc.

phthisoid b. A tuberculous form with purulent sputum.

plastic b. See croupous *b.*

putrid b. A variety of chronic bronchitis characterized by the discharge of a copious, half-liquid, extremely offensive sputum.

secondary b. One which develops as a complication of some preceding disease.

bron′cho- (brong′ko-), **bronch-** [G. *brogchos*, trachea]. A combining form signifying *relating to a bronchus* or *to the bronchi.*

bron′cho·cele″ [*brogchos;* G. *kēlē*, tumor]. A dilatation of a bronchus.

bron″cho·con·stric′tor [*brogchos;* L. *constrictus*, from *constringere*, to draw together]. Any substance having the property of decreasing the caliber of the pulmonary air passages.

bron″cho·dil″a·ta′tion (brong″ko·dil″uh·tay′-shun, ·dye″luh·tay′shun) [*brogchos;* L. *dilatatio*, from *dilatare*, to dilate]. The widening of the caliber of the pulmonary air passages by the use of drugs or surgical instruments.

bron″cho·di·la′tor (·dye·lay′tor, ·di·lay′tor) [*brogchos; dilatare*]. 1. Any drug which has the property of increasing the caliber of the pulmonary air passages. 2. An instrument used for this purpose.

bron″cho·e·de′ma [*brogchos;* G. *oidēma*, swelling]. Swelling of the bronchial tubes which diminishes their lumens, hindering the passage of air through them, and causing dyspnea.

bron″cho·e·soph″a·ge′al. Pertaining to a bronchus and the esophagus, as the bronchoesophageal muscle, which is a small bundle of smooth muscle connecting the esophagus and the left main bronchus.

bron″cho·e·soph″a·gol′o·gy [*brogchos; oisō; phagein;* G. *logos*, word]. That field of medicine specializing in disorders of the esophagus and pulmonary respiratory tract, involving direct examination (bronchoesophagoescopy).

bron″cho·e·soph″a·gos′co·py [*brogchos;* perhaps G. *oisō*, I shall carry; *phagein*, to eat; *skopein*, to examine]. Visual examination of the interior of the larger tracheobronchial tubes and the esophagus with the aid of an instrument.

bron″cho·gen′ic, bron″chi·o·gen′ic [*brogchos;* G. *genesthai*, from *gignesthai*, to be produced]. 1. Arising in a bronchus or in the bronchi. 2. *In embryology*, capable of forming the bronchi.

bron′cho·gram [*brogchos;* G. *gramma*, letter]. Radiograph of the bronchial tree made after the injection of a radiopaque substance.

bron·chog′ra·phy (brong·cog′ruh·fee) [*brogchos;* G. *graphein*, to write]. Roentgenographic visualization of the bronchial tree after the introduction of an opaque contrast material, usually iodized oil.

ascending b. That of the pulmonary cavities.

bron′cho·lith (brong′ko·lith) [*brogchos;* G. *lithos,* stone]. A calculus or concretion in a pulmonary air passage. **—broncholithi′asis,** *n.*

bron·chol′o·gy. That special branch of medicine dealing with the study and treatment of the bronchial tree by means of bronchoscopy.

bron″cho·mo·ni·li′a·sis. See *bronchomycosis.*

bron″cho·mo′tor [*brogchos;* L. *motum,* from *movere,* to move]. Pertaining to the neuromuscular mechanism which controls the caliber of the pulmonary air passages.

bron″cho·my·co′sis (brong″ko·migh·ko′sis) [*brogchos;* G. *mykēs,* fungus; *-ōsis,* condition]. Bronchitis caused by any species of *Candida,* usually *Candida albicans.* Syn., *bronchomoniliasis.*

bron·chop′a·thy [*brogchos;* G. *pathos,* disease]. Any abnormality in a bronchus.

bron·choph′o·ny (brong·kof′o·nee) [*brogchos;* G. *phōnē,* voice]. An abnormal increase in the intensity of the voice sounds; heard by auscultation over the chest wall when the density of the lung tissue has been increased by disease. Also see *pectoriloquy.*

bron′cho·plas″ty [*brogchos;* G. *plassein,* to form]. *In surgery,* repair of a bronchial defect.

bron″cho·pleu′ral (brong″ko·ploor′ul) [*brogchos;* G. *pleura,* rib]. Pertaining to a bronchus and the pleural cavity, as bronchopleural fistula.

bron″cho·pneu·mo′ni·a [*brogchos;* G. *pneumonia,* disease of the lungs]. Inflammation of the lungs which has spread from infected bronchi; includes all forms of pneumonitis which are not suppurative or with lobar distribution. Common in the very young or very old, and may be due to a variety of causative organisms.

bron″cho·pneu″mo·ni′tis [*brogchos; pneumonia;* G. *-itis,* inflammation]. Bronchopneumonia.

bron″cho·pul′mo·na·ry [*brogchos;* L. *pulmonarius,* from *pulmo,* lung]. Relating to both the bronchi and the lungs.

bron·chor′rha·phy (brong·kor′uh·fee) [*brogchos;* G. *rhaphē,* a suture]. The suturing of a bronchus.

bron″chor·rhe′a, bron″chor·rhoe′a (brong″ko·ree′uh) [*brogchos;* G. *rhein,* to flow]. Excessive discharge from the bronchial mucous membranes. **—bronchorrheal,** *adj.*

bron′cho·scope [*brogchos;* G. *skopein,* to examine]. Instrument for the visual examination of the interior of the bronchi; also used for treatment and/or operation. **—bronchoscop′ic,** *adj.;* **bronchos′copy,** *n.*

bron′cho·spasm [*brogchos;* G. *spasma,* spasm]. Temporary narrowing of the bronchi due to violent, involuntary contraction of the bronchial muscles.

bron″cho·spi″ro·che·to′sis (brong″ko·spy″ro·kee·to′sis) [*brogchos;* G. *speira,* coil; *chaitē,* hair; *-ōsis,* condition]. Chronic bronchitis, usually complicated by bronchiectasis; caused by infection with a group of symbiotic anaerobic spirochetes and fusiform bacilli. Also called Castellani's *disease.*

bron″cho·spi·rog′ra·phy (·spy·rog′ruh·fee) [*brogchos;* L. *spirare,* to breathe; G. *graphein,* to write]. The graphic recording of the functional capacity of the lungs.

bron″cho·spi·rom′e·ter (·spy·rom′i·tur) [*brogchos; spirare;* G. *metron,* a measure]. A spirometer connected with a special type of catheter designed for intrabronchial use.

bron″cho·spi·rom′e·try [*brogchos; spirare; metron*]. The determination of various aspects of the functional capacity of a single lung.

differential b. Such determinations made of both lungs simultaneously, for comparison.

bron″cho·ste·no′sis [*brogchos;* G. *stenōsis,* a being straitened]. Narrowing of the lumen of one or more bronchi.

bron·chos′to·my [*brogchos;* G. *stoma,* mouth]. Fistulization of a bronchus through the chest wall.

bron·chot′o·my (brong·cot′o·mee) [*brogchos;* G. *tomē,* a cutting]. Incision into a bronchus.

bron″cho·ve·sic′u·lar [*brogchos;* L. *vesicula,* vesicle]. Pertaining to an intermediate stage in the transition from normal vesicular to completely bronchial breath sounds; characterized by elevation of pitch and prolongation of the expiratory phase.

bron′chus (brong′kus) (pl. *bronchi*) [*brogchos*]. One of the primary branches of the trachea or such of its branches within the lung as contain cartilage in their walls. See Plate 15. **—bronchial,** *adj.*

eparterial b. The first branch of the right primary bronchus, situated above the right pulmonary artery.

extrapulmonary b. One which is not surrounded by lung substance. Also called *primary b.*

hyparterial b. Any one of the first collateral branches of the stem bronchi except the eparterial bronchus.

stem b. The continuation of the main, or primary, bronchus which extends lengthwise in each lung, giving off anterior and posterior branches to the lobes.

Brönsted and Lowry substance. See *acid,* 3.

Brönsted theory. See under *theory.*

bron″to·pho′bi·a [G. *brontē,* thunder; *phobos,* fear]. Morbid fear of thunder.

bronze di″a·be′tes. Hemochromatosis.

brood cyst. A small papilla arising from the inner germinal layer of an *Echinococcus* cyst which in turn buds off 5 to 20 small oval buds or scolices from their inner layer. These latter represent the mature larval parasite. Also called *brood capsule.*

Brooke, Henry Ambrose Grundy [*English dermatologist,* 1854–1919]. Described an adenoid cystic epithelioma of skin usually involving the scalp, called *Brooke's tumor, cancer.*

Brooks, Clyde (1881–). American pharmacologist and physiologist, known for his discovery of the Brooks method for measuring blood sedimentation. A ½ mm.-bore glass tube 100 mm. long, with needle attached to end is flushed with anticoagulant; blood is drawn directly into the tube, which is set up in a holder in the erect position, and sedimentation observed and curve plotted.

Brophy, Truman William [*American oral surgeon,* 1848–1928]. Remembered for his inventiveness in plastic oral surgery and, especially, for his work in the repair of cleft palate which he closed by means of wire tension sutures reinforced by lead plates. Invented a special periosteal elevator for palate surgery.

broth [AS.]. A liquid nutritive medium for the culture of microorganisms, prepared from finely chopped lean meat or dehydrated meat extract. Syn., *bouillon.*

Sabouraud's b. See *Sabouraud's agar* under Raymond Jacques Adrien *Sabouraud.*

Bro′ti·a (bro′shee·uh). Synonym for *Melania.*

brow [AS. *brū*]. 1. The forehead; the upper anterior portion of the head. 2. The supraorbital ridge; the eyebrow.

brow a′gue (ayg′yoo). Old term for neuralgia of the first division of the trigeminal nerve.

Brown, James Barrett (1899–). American plastic surgeon, known for his contributions to the study of skin grafting. He was associated with V. P. Blair in devising an intermediate split graft known as the *Blair-Brown graft.*

Brown, Robert [*Scottish botanist,* 1773–1858]. Discovered the cell nucleus (1831). Credited also with the discovery of generation in plants by means of pollen. The so-called *Brownian movement,* an oscillatory movement of microscopic particles suspended in liquids, of unknown cause, was first described by him; also known as *pedesis, orthokinetic movement.*

Brown, Sanger [*American psychiatrist,* 1852–1928]. Described a hereditary spinocerebellar ataxia; called *Sanger Brown's ataxia.*

Brown personality inventory. See under *test.*

Brown's test. See cold pressor *test.*

Brown's test (*for arteriovenous fistula*). See under *test.*

Brown-Séquard, Charles Edouard [*British physiologist in France,* ca. 1817–94]. Widely known for his experimental work on internal secretions (1856), on the adrenal glands and testicular extracts (1889–90), on the functions of the sympathetic nerves (1852–54), and for his excellent exposition of the pathways of conduction in the spinal cord (1863). Described a lesion of one lateral half of the spinal cord, causing paralysis of motion on one side and of sensation on the opposite (1851); called *Brown-Séquard paralysis, syndrome.* He has been regarded as a successor of Claude Bernard and as one of the founders of modern endocrinology.

Browne, Donovan Clarence [*American physician,* 1898–]. Invented, with Gordon McHardy, an esophageal dilator (1939), called *Browne-McHardy's dilator.*

brown mix′ture. Compound opium and glycyrrhiza mixture. See *opium.*

Bruce, David [*British pathologist and bacteriologist,* 1855–1931]. Known internationally for his investigations of the causes of tropical diseases. Discovered the cause of nagana to be a trypanosome carried by the tsetse fly. Investigated, with Nabarro, the cause of sleeping sickness in Africa and showed the tsetse fly to be the vector.

Bru·cel′la [L., after David *Bruce*]. A genus of small, Gram-negative, nonmotile, short bacilli or coccobacilli which are not acid-fast and do not form endospores; the cause of brucellosis (undulant fever in man and infectious abortion in cattle). There are three species recognized: **Br. abortus,** the bovine strain; **Br. melitensis,** the goat strain; **Br. suis,** the porcine strain. These three species are the causative agents of infectious abortion and undulant fever. —**brucellar,** *adj.*

Br. tularensis. See *Pasteurella tularensis.*

brucellergen. Trade-mark for a suspension of *Brucella* nucleoproteins used in the intradermal test for the diagnosis of brucellosis; the preparation often causes general reactions.

bru″cel·li′a·sis. See *brucellosis.*

bru·cel′lin. A preparation from the combined cultures of the three species of *Brucella;* used in the diagnosis, prophylaxis, and treatment of brucellosis.

bru″cel·lo′sis [*Brucella;* G. *-ōsis,* condition]. A remittent febrile disease caused by infection with bacteria of the genus *Brucella.* In humans, brucellosis may occur in acute or chronic form and leads to weakness, loss of weight, and anemia. The disease is rarely transmitted from person to person, but spreads readily from animal to animal and from animal to man. Cattle, goats and hogs are the chief sources of infection. Syn., *brucelliasis, Malta fever, Mediterranean fever, undulant fever.*

Bruch's membrane. See basal *membrane* of Bruch.

bruc′ine (brew′seen, ·sin) [David *Bruce*]. $C_{23}H_{26}O_4N_2.4H_2O$. A poisonous alkaloid found in various species of *Strychnos,* including *S. nux-vomica, S. ignatia,* and others. It occurs as a white, crystalline powder with a bitter taste. It is used chiefly as a simple bitter, some difference of opinion existing as to its physiologic action. It is less poisonous than strychnine and appears to be depressant to the peripheral motor and sensory nerves. It is used as an alcohol denaturant.

b. sulfate (*brucinae sulfas*). $(C_{23}H_{26}O_4N_2)_2.H_2SO_4.7H_2O$. A white, crystalline powder of bitter taste, soluble in 70 parts of water. Dose, 2 mg. ($\frac{1}{30}$ gr.).

Bruck, Alfred [*German physician,* 1865–]. Described a rare disease of the bones characterized by multiple fractures, ankyloses, and muscle atrophy (1897), called *Bruck's disease.*

Brudzinski's reflex, signs. See *Brudzinski's signs* under *sign.*

bruise [AS. *brȳsan,* to break]. Contusion.

bruisse·ment′ (brwees·mong′. *See* NOTES § 35) [F., rustling noise]. A purring sound heard on auscultation.

bruit (broo·ee′) [F.]. Old term for an adventitious sound heard on auscultation. See *heart sound; heart murmur.*

b. de diable. See hemic *murmur.*

cephalic b. A loud, continuous heart sound with systolic accentuation heard on auscultation of the skull and face: a sign of a fistulous carotid-cavernous aneurysm which is markedly diminished or abolished by digital compression of the appropriate carotid artery in the neck.

placental b. Old term for placental *murmur.*

Brunfels, Otto [*German botanist,* 1488–1534]. Greatest botanist of the sixteenth century. Set a high standard of illustration in his work on plants (1530–34).

Brunn, Albert von [*German anatomist,* 1849–95]. Described the groups or nests of flat epithelial cells in the normal vesical mucosa, once called *Brunn's nests.*

Brunn, Fritz [*Austrian surgeon,* contemporary]. Introduced, with Mandl, the method of treating angina pectoris by paravertebral injection of alcohol (1924).

Brunner, Johann Conrad [*Swiss anatomist,* 1653–1727]. Remembered for his description of the duodenal glands, called *Brunner's glands.* He did pioneer work on internal secretions in the dog and observed thirst and polyuria following excision of the pancreas (1683).

Bruns, Ludwig von [*German neurologist,* 1858–1916]. Described a syndrome of vertigo, vomiting, and falling upon the ground as indicative of tumor of the fourth ventricle, when elicited by a sudden change in the position of the head; called *Bruns's syndrome.* See also *Bastian-Bruns law,* under *Bastian.*

Brunschwig, Alexander (1901–). American surgeon who introduced the operation of duodenopancreatectomy, sometimes known by his name (1937). He also introduced the operations of complete pelvic exenteration for advanced pelvic cancer (1946), and radical hysterectomy and pelvic lymph-node excision for cancer of the cervix (1947), and discovered gastric secretory depressant in the gastric juices of patients with pernicious anemia and gastric cancer.

Brunton, Thomas Lauder [*Scottish physician and pharmacologist,* 1844–1916]. Eminent for his work on the action of drugs on the cardiovascular system. Introduced amyl nitrite in the treatment of angina pectoris (1867).

brux′ism [G. *brychein,* to gnash the teeth]. Grinding of the teeth: an unconscious habit often limited to the sleeping period but sometimes occurring during mental or physical concentration or strain.

brux″o·ma′ni·a [*brychein;* G. *mania,* madness]. Grinding or pounding of the teeth as a manifestation of neurosis, usually occurring during sleep.

Bryant, Thomas [*English surgeon,* 1828–1914]. Widely known as an operating surgeon, he is remembered for his lumbar colostomy made between the last rib and the iliac crest, with permanent fixation of the bowel. He described the iliofemoral triangle and the third or vertical line forming the triangle, both sometimes indicated by his name.

Bryant's sign. See under *sign.*

bryg′mus [G. *brygmos,* biting]. Grinding of the teeth; odontoprisis.

bry·o′ni·a (brigh·o′nee·uh) [G., bryony]. The root of *Bryonia alba* or *B. dioica.* Its properties are due to the glycosides bryonin and bryonidin. It is an irritant emetic, drastic cathartic, and vesicant. Has been used in pleurisy, pleuropneumonia, rheumatic fever, and colds.

bry·on′i·din (brigh·on′i·din). A glycoside from *Bryonia alba* which causes paralysis of the central nervous system.

bry′o·nin. A glycoside from *Bryonia alba.*

bry′o·phyte [G. *bryon,* moss; *phytos,* grown]. A division of the plant kingdom, which includes liverworts and mosses.

BTPS *In respiratory physiology,* abbreviation for *b*ody *t*emperature, ambient *p*ressure, *s*aturated with water.

BTU, B.T.U., Btu, B.Th.U. British thermal unit.

bu′bas (bōō′bahss). Brazilian name for yaws.

b. braziliensis. See *leishmaniasis* americana.

bu′bo (bew′bo, bŏŏb′o, bōō′bo) [G. *boubōn,* groin]. Inflammation, swelling, and hypertrophy of one or more lymph nodes, often going on to suppuration, and usually located in the groin or axilla. It occurs commonly with chancroid, syphilis, and venereal lymphogranuloma. Syn., *sympathetic abscess.* Also called *inguinal adenitis.* —**bubon′ic,** *adj.*

climatic b. Venereal lymphogranuloma.

indolent b. One with enlargement and hyperplasia without the formation of pus or any tendency to break down.

parotid b. See *parotitis.*

pestilential b. One associated with the plague.

rheumatic b. A hard lump, occurring most frequently on the back of the neck, as a sequel of acute articular rheumatism.

serpiginous b. An ulcerated bubo which changes its seat or in which the ulceration extends in one direction while healing in another.

strumous b. Hypertrophied lymph node forming a large indolent swelling in a tuberculous subject.

syphilitic b. That which appears in syphilis a few days after the primary lesion.

venereal b. That due to venereal disease.

bu″bon·ad″e·ni′tis [*boubōn;* G. *adēn,* gland; *-itis,* inflammation]. Inflammation of an inguinal lymph node.

bu″bon·al′gi·a [*boubōn;* G. *algos,* pain]. Pain in the inguinal region.

bu·bon′ic plague. See under *plague.*

bu·bon′o·cele [*boubōn;* G. *kēlē,* hernia]. Inguinal hernia which is incomplete in that it does not extend beyond the inguinal canal.

bu·bon′u·lus [L., dim. from *boubōn*]. Focal suppurative lymphangitis, especially on the dorsum of the penis; a complication of chancroid. *Rare.*

bu·car′di·a (bew·kahr′dee·uh, boo·kahr′·) [G. *bous,* ox; *kardia,* heart]. Bovine heart; extreme hypertrophy of the heart.

buc′ca (pl. *buccae*) [L., cheek]. The cheek; the hollow of the cheek, or its inner surface. —**buccal,** *adj.*

buc′ci·na″tor (buck′si·nay″tor) [L., trumpeter]. The muscular foundation of the cheek. See Table of Muscles and Nerves in the Appendix.

buc′co- [L. *bucca,* cheek]. A combining form denoting *of* or *pertaining to the cheeks.*

buc″co·ax′i·al [*bucca;* L. *axis,* axis]. Pertaining to the buccal and axial walls of a dental cavity.

buc″coc·clu′sal [*bucca;* L. *occludere,* to close]. Pertaining to the buccal and occlusal walls of a dental cavity.

buc″co·cer′vi·cal [*bucca;* L. *cervix,* neck]. Pertaining to the cheek and the neck; also, pertaining to the buccal surface and neck of a tooth.

buc″co·dis′tal [*bucca;* L. *distare,* to be distant]. Pertaining to the buccal and distal walls of a dental cavity.

buc″co·fa′cial ob′tu·ra″tor. Any mechanical device for closing an opening through the cheek into the mouth.

buc″co·gin′gi·val (buck″o·jin′ji·vul, ·jin·jy′vul) [*bucca;* L. *gingiva,* gum]. Pertaining to the cheek and the gums.

buc″co·la′bi·al [*bucca;* L. *labium,* lip]. Pertaining to the cheek and the lip.

buc″co·lin′gual [*bucca;* L. *lingua,* tongue]. Relating to the cheek and the tongue. —**buccolingually,** *adv.*

buc″co·me′si·al (buck″o·mee′zee·ul, ·mess′ee·ul, ·mee′see·ul) [*bucca;* G. *mesos,* middle]. Pertaining to the buccal and mesial walls of a dental cavity.

buc″co·na′sal (buck″o·nay′zul) [*bucca;* L. *nasus,* nose]. Pertaining to the cheek and nose.

buc″co·na″so·pha·ryn′ge·al (·nay″zo·fa·rin′jul, ·jee·ul, ·far″in·jee′ul) [*bucca; nasus;* G. *pharygx,* throat]. Pertaining to the cheek and upper part of the pharynx.

buc″co·pha·ryn′ge·al [*bucca; pharygx*]. Relating to the cheek and to the pharynx.

buc″co·phar·yn′ge·us. A portion of the superior constrictor muscle of the pharynx.

buc″co·pulp′al [*bucca;* L. *pulpa,* fleshy part]. Pertaining to the buccal and pulpal walls of a dental cavity.

buc″co·ver′sion [*bucca;* L. *versum,* from *vertere,* to turn]. Condition of a tooth being out of the line of normal occlusion in the buccal direction.

buc′cu·la [L., little cheek]. The fleshy fold beneath the chin which forms what is called a double chin. *Obs.*

Buchner, Eduard [*German chemist,* 1860–1917]. Known for his work in enzyme action. Introduced a funnel with a perforated porcelain plate on which the filter paper is placed; called *Buchner filter, funnel.* Was awarded the Nobel prize for chemistry (1907).

Buchner, Hans [*German bacteriologist,* 1850–1902]. Demonstrated that bactericidal power of blood serums is lost when they are heated. Described the zymase expressed from dried yeast, called *yeast cell plasma, Buchner's zymase.*

bu′chu (bew′cue, bōō′kōō) [Zulu *bucu,* a mixture of aromatic leaves]. The leaves of several species of *Barosma,* yielding not less than 1.25% of a volatile oil, to which its properties are probably due. Formerly used as a diuretic in cystitis and other affections of the genitourinary mucous membrane.

bucillin. Trade-mark for a flavored penicillin troche.

Buck, Gurdon [*American surgeon,* 1807–77]. Eminent for his skill and invention in the treatment of fractures. Ligated the iliac and femoral arteries for aneurysm (1858). Invented an extension apparatus (1860–62) consisting of a weight and pulleys for the treatment of fractured femur, which was long in use; known as *Buck's extension.*

Devised an operation for the correction of bony ankylosis of the knee by removal of a wedge of bone including the patella and portions of the condyles (1845).

Bucky's diaphragm. See under *diaphragm.*

buc·ne'mi·a [G. *bous*, ox; *knēmē*, leg]. Phlegmasia alba dolens. *Obs.*

bud [ME. *budde*]. 1. *In embryology*, a protuberance or outgrowth which is the primordium of an appendage or an organ. 2. *In anatomy*, an organ or structure shaped like the bud of a plant. 3. *In mycology*, a gemma.

bronchial b. One of the outgrowths of the embryonic bronchi responsible for the continued growth and branching of the respiratory tree.

end b. A mass of indifferent cells produced by the remnant of Hensen's node; it develops into the caudal part of the trunk without forming distinctive germ layers.

gustatory b. A taste bud.

limb b. A lateral swelling of the embryonic trunk; the anlage of an appendage.

lung b. One of the primary outgrowths of the embryonic trachea whose growth and subsequent division produce a primary bronchus and all its branches.

periosteal b. Vascular osteogenic tissue from the cellular layer of the periosteum penetrating cartilage of a growing bone to help form a center of ossification.

tail b. (a) Anlage of the caudal appendage. (b) See end *b.*

taste b. End organ of the sense of taste; one of the oval, flask-shaped bodies embedded, most commonly, in the epithelium of the tongue. Also called *calyculus gustatorii.*

ureteric b. Dorsomedial outgrowth of a mesonephric duct; the anlage of a ureter, a renal pelvis and its calyxes, and the collecting tubules of a kidney.

Budd, George [*English physician*, 1808–82]. Described a variety of hepatic cirrhosis (1845), called *Budd's disease.*

Budd, William [*English physician*, 1811–80]. Known for his book on typhoid fever (1873) in which he insisted that the disease was spread by contagion. Established the fact that the disease is carried by contamination from the ejecta of individuals ill with typhoid and is probably waterborne. His work has been reprinted by the American Public Health Association (1931).

bud'ding [ME. *budde*]. *In biology*, a form of asexual reproduction occurring in the lower animals and plants, in which the parent organism develops projections which develop into new individuals.

Büdinger, Konrad [*Swiss physician in Austria*, 1867–]. Described a pathologic fracture of the cartilage of the patella, called *Büdinger-Ludloff-Läwen disease.*

Buerger, Leo [*American physician*, 1879–1943]. Known for his observations on thromboangiitis obliterans, a term he originated. His observations furnished the first clear report of the clinical course and the pathology of the disease, which is known as *Buerger's disease* (1908). Devised passive exercises as routine treatment of the condition.

Buergner, Otto von [*German neurologist*, 1858–1905]. Described cordlike tissues between the nerve fibers and associated structures, of the nature of connective tissue; called *Buergner's cords.* These have been identified as new cells of Schwann accompanying regeneration of an axon after an injury, arranged in bands, thus forming a tissue which acts as a pathway for the outgrowing nerve.

bu'fa·gins (bōō'fa·gins). The cardioactive genins present in the skin secretions of toads as, for example, bufalin and bufotalin.

bu'fa·lin (bōō'fa·lin). A cardioactive steroid aglycone, closely related to bufotalin, present in the skin secretions of toads.

buff'er [ME. *buffet*]. 1. A substance which, when added to a solution, causes resistance to any change of hydrogen-ion concentration when either acid or alkali is added. 2. Treat with a buffer.

buff'y coat. The white blood cells which separate and form a layer on top of the erythrocytes when whole blood is centrifuged.

bu"fo·tal'in. $C_{26}H_{36}O_6$; a cardioactive steroid aglycone present in the skin secretions of toads.

bu"fo·ten'i·dine. The betaine form of bufotenin; a component of the secretion of the skin glands of the toad, *Bufo vulgaris.*

bu·fot'e·nin, bu·fo'te·nin. 5-Hydroxy-N,N-dimethyltryptamine, a component of the secretion of the skin glands of the toad, *Bufo vulgaris.* It causes hypertension and strong and lasting vasoconstriction.

bu"fo·tox'in [L. *bufo*, toad; G. *toxikon*, poison]. $C_{40}H_{60}N_4O_{10}$; a suberylarginine ester of bufotalin; it is the principal toxin present in the skin secretions of toads and lizards.

bug [ME. *bugge*]. An insect of the order Hemiptera or suborder Heteroptera. See also *bedbug.*

assassin b. Any one of the Triatomidae. Syn., *conenose.* Also called *flying bedbug, kissing b., Mexican* or *Texas bedbug.*

Croton b. The cockroach. See *Blatella germanica.*

Miana b. Any tick of the genus *Argas.*

red b. Harvest mite; a mite of the *Trombicula.*

wheat b. A mite of the *Pediculoides.*

bug'gery [F. *bougre*, from ML. *Bulgarus*, a heretic]. *In legal medicine*, sodomy.

Buie, Louis Arthur [*American surgeon*, 1890–]. Known for devising an operation for the removal of hemorrhoids under caudal anesthesia with the patient in the prone position.

Buist's method. See under *artificial respiration.*

Bülau, Gotthard [*German physician*, 1835–1900]. Said to have originated the use of siphon drainage in treating empyema; called *Bülau drainage.*

bulb [L. *bulbus*, bulb]. 1. An oval or circular expansion of a cylinder or tube. 2. Old term for the medulla oblongata. —**bulb'ar,** *adj.*

aortic b. See *b.* of the heart.

arterial b. See *b.* of the heart.

brachial b. The expansion of the spinal cord at the place of distribution of the nerves forming the brachial plexus.

b. of the corpus cavernosum urethrae. See *b.* of the urethra.

b. of the eye. The eyeball.

b. of the heart (*bulbus cordis*). The anterior division of the embryonic heart within the pericardial cavity. Its proximal part is incorporated into the right ventricle; its distal part forms the aortic and pulmonary valve region of the heart. Syn., *aortic b., arterial b., bulbus arteriosus, bulbus cordis.*

b. of the penis. See *b.* of the urethra.

b. of the urethra. The expanded proximal portion of the corpus cavernosum urethrae. Syn., *b. of the penis.*

cerebral b. See *medulla* oblongata.

duodenal b. *In radiology*, the first part of the duodenum, immediately beyond the pylorus. Also called *duodenal cap.*

gustatory b. Old term for taste bud.

hair b. The swelling of the root of a hair at its deep end.

inferior b. of the internal jugular vein. An

enlargement of the jugular vein immediately above its union with the subclavian vein.

jugular b. See inferior *b.* of the internal jugular vein, superior *b.* of the internal jugular vein.

Krause's end-b. See Krause's *corpuscle*.

nerve b. An eminence of protoplasm within the sarcolemma of a muscular fiber, representing the termination of a motor nerve fiber.

olfactory b. The enlarged distal end of either olfactory tract situated on each side of the longitudinal fissure upon the undersurface of each anterior lobe of the cerebrum. See Plate 17.

sinovaginal b. One of the bilateral dorsal evaginations of the urogenital sinus forming the lower fifth of the vagina.

superior b. of the internal jugular vein. An enlargement of the internal jugular vein at the point of exit from the jugular foramen.

vaginal b. (a) One of the solid epithelial bulbs forming the lower part of the fetal vagina, regarded as of paramesonephric duct origin. (b) See vestibular *b.*

vestibular b. One of the paired masses of erectile tissue located on either side of the vestibule of the vagina, homologous to the bulb of the urethra and adjacent corpus cavernosum urethrae in the male.

bul'bo- [*bulbus*]. A combining form denoting *a bulb* or *bulbar*.

bul"bo·cap'nine (bul"bo·cap'neen, ·nin). $C_{19}H_{19}NO_4$. An alkaloid in the tubers of *Bulbocapnus cavus*. The phosphate and the hydrochloride have been used in certain diseases of the nervous system, such as paralysis agitans, chorea, and ataxic conditions.

bul"bo·cav"er·no'sus [*bulbus;* L. *caverna*, cavern]. A muscle encircling the bulb and adjacent, proximal parts of the penis in the male and encircling the orifice of the vagina and covering the lateral parts of the vestibular bulbs in the female. See Table of Muscles in the Appendix.

bul"bo·nu'cle·ar [*bulbus;* L. *nucleus*, kernel]. Relating to the medulla oblongata and its nerve nuclei.

bul"bo·spon"gi·o'sus. The BR name for the *bulbocavernosus muscle*.

bul"bo·u·re'thral [*bulbus;* G. *ourēthra*, urethra]. Relating to the bulb of the urethra, as the bulbourethral glands.

bulb'ous [*bulbus*]. Having or containing bulbs; bulb-shaped; swollen; terminating in a bulb.

bul"bo·ven·tric'u·lar [*bulbus;* L. *ventriculus*, belly]. Pertaining to the bulb and the ventricle of the heart.

bul'bus. See *bulb*.

bul'bus ar·te"ri·o'sus. See *bulb* of the heart.

bul'bus cor'dis. See *bulb* of the heart.

bu·le'sis [G. *boulēsis*, will]. The will, or an act of the will.

bu·lim'i·a (bew·lim'ee·uh, bo͞o·), **bou·lim'i·a** (bo͞o·lim'ee·uh) [G. *bous*, ox; *limos*, hunger]. Excessive, insatiable appetite, seen in psychotic states; a symptom of diabetes mellitus and of certain cerebral lesions. Syn., *adephagia, cynorexia, hyperphagia.* —**bulim'ic,** *adj.*

Bu·li'nus [L. *bulla*, bubble]. A genus of fresh-water snails, whose species serve as the intermediate hosts for *Schistosoma haematobium*.

bul'la (bo͝ol'uh, bul'uh) (pl. *bullae*) [L.]. A large bleb or blister forming either within or beneath the epidermis and filled with lymph.

auditory b. In certain mammals other than man, the bulbous accessory tympanic bone housing an expansion of the cavity of the middle ear. Syn., *tympanic b., b. tympani, otic b.*

b. ethmoidalis. A rounded projection into the middle meatus of the nose, due to an enlarged ethmoid cell.

b. tympani. Auditory *b.*

otic b. Auditory *b.*

tympanic b. Auditory bulla.

bul'late (bo͝ol'ate, bul'ate) [*bulla*]. 1. Blistered; marked by bullae. 2. Inflated, bladderlike, vesiculate. —**bulla'tion,** *n.*

Buller, Frank [*Canadian oculist,* 1844–1905]. Remembered for his invention of the eyeshield bearing his name and consisting of a watch crystal in a frame of adhesive plaster, so worn as to protect the sound eye from discharges from the infected one.

BuMed. The Bureau of Medicine and Surgery, U. S. Navy.

Bumke, Oswald Conrad Edward [*German neurologist,* 1877–1950]. Author of works on neurology. Described a peculiar dilatation of the pupil said to be caused by psychic stimuli; called *Bumke's pupil*.

BUN Blood urea nitrogen.

bun'dle [MD. *bondel*]. *In biology*, a fascicular grouping of elementary tissues, as nerve fibers or muscle fibers. Old term for *nerve fiber tract*.

atrioventricular b. That part of the conduction system of the heart arising from the atrioventricular node and dividing into two branches which run down either side of the interventricular septum and ramify among the muscle bundles of the ventricle. Syn., *b. of His*.

b. of His. See atrioventricular *b.*

b. of Kent. A bridge of muscular tissue joining the atria and ventricles at the right margin of the septum. It is considered an anomalous or aberrant atrioventricular bundle which, in some cases, may conduct impulses.

ground b. See *fasciculus* proprius.

Helweg's b. Olivospinal tract.

hook b. See uncinate *fasciculus*.

Bun'ga·rus (bung'guh·rus) [Telegu *bangaru*, golden]. A genus of venomous snakes found in southern Asia, commonly known as the kraits.

B. candidus. The common krait; especially dangerous because of its extremely virulent venom.

B. fasciatus. The Indian krait; one of the most venomous snakes in the world.

bun'ion [OF. *bugne*, a swelling]. A swelling of a bursa of the foot, especially of the metatarsophalangeal joint of the great toe; associated with a thickening of the adjacent skin and a forcing of the great toe into adduction.

bun"ion·ec'to·my [*bugne;* G. *ektomē*, excision]. Excision of a bunion; plastic repair of the first metatarsophalangeal joint.

Bunnell, Sterling [*American surgeon,* 1882–]. Known for his specialization in surgery of the hand for which he has devised many procedures.

Bunnell's test. See Paul-Bunnell *test*.

bu'no·dont [G. *bounos*, a mound; *odous*, tooth]. Provided with rounded or conical cusps, applied to molar teeth, as opposed to *lophodont*.

Bunsen, Robert Wilhelm [*German chemist and physicist,* 1811–99]. Celebrated for his invention of the gas burner which is provided with holes near the base, permitting admixture of air so that the gas is completely oxidized, giving a hot blue flame. His name is associated with one of the types of a galvanic cell, consisting of carbon in dilute nitric acid and zinc in dilute sulfuric acid, the solutions being separated by a porous partition; and also with a coefficient of absorption, *Bunsen's coefficient*. With Kirchhoff, discovered the elements cesium and rubidium (1860).

Bunyan, John (1907–). English naval surgeon; with William Stannard (1940) he evolved a method of irrigation with sodium hypochlorite through transparent envelopes in treatment of burns, wounds, and gross sepsis.

buph·thal′mi·a (bewf·thal′mee·uh, bōōf·thal′·), **buph·thal′mos** [G. *bous*, ox; *ophthalmos*, eye]. A globular enlargement of the eye with protrusion of the cornea, a condition noted in infantile glaucoma. Syn., *keratoglobus, hydrophthalmos.*

bur, burr [ME. *burre*]. 1. *In botany*, a rough, prickly shell or case. 2. The lobe of the ear. 3. *In dentistry*, a cutting instrument with a rounded, pointed, cylindrical, or ovoid head having numerous blades; used in the dental engine for excavating carious dentin and for other purposes. 4. *In surgery*, an instrument similar in form to a dental bur, but larger, designed for surgical operations upon the bones.

bur′bot. Fresh-water fish of the genus *Lota*, allied to the cod, which serves as the intermediate host of the tapeworm, *Diphyllobothrium latum.* The American species, called *ling* or *eelpout*, is found in New England and the Great Lakes.

bur′bot-liv′er oil. The oil extracted from the liver of the burbot, *Lota maculosa.*

Burchard's test. See Liebermann-Burchard *test.*

Burdach, Karl Friedrich [*German anatomist and physiologist*, 1776–1847]. Described the cuneate fasciculus in the spinal cord, called *column of Burdach.* He also published an important textbook of physiology (1826–40).

Burdenko, Nicolaj Nilovic [*Russian surgeon*, 1878–1946]. Introduced a treatment for purulent meningoencephalitis by injection of sulfonamides into the common carotid artery, called *Burdenko's method.*

Burdon-Sanderson, John Scott [*English physiologist*, 1828–1905]. With F. J. M. Page, studied the action currents of the heart (1879), and observed electric phenomena in the heart beat (1883). Measured the speed of nervous impulses (1891). His work contributed to the development of modern methods of electrocardiography.

Bu′reau of Med′i·cal Serv′ices. A division of the U. S. Public Health Service charged with the administration of Public Health Service hospitals (formerly known as marine hospitals), the national narcotics hospitals and leprosariums, medical services in federal prisons, and other related functions.

Bu′reau of State Serv′ices. A division of the U. S. Public Health Service charged with the administration of grants-in-aid to the states and with cooperation with state and local health authorities upon official request through the state health officer.

bu·ret′, bu·rette′. A graduated glass tube, commonly having a glass stopcock, used in volumetric analysis for measuring volumes of liquids.

Bur′gun·dy pitch. See under *pitch.*

Bur′ma boil. See *oriental sore.*

burn [AS. *baernan*]. The tissue reaction or injury resulting from application of heat, caustics, friction, or electricity and classified as simple hyperemic (*first degree*); vesicant (*second degree*); destructive of skin and underlying tissues (*third degree*).

atomic b. See radiation *b.*

brush b. Mechanical injury produced by friction.

chemical b. That produced by caustics (acid or alkaline), irritant gases, etc.

electric b. One caused by high-frequency currents.

flash b. One produced by ignition of high explosives such as cordite, especially in naval warfare. Also called *powder b.*

friction b. See brush *b.*

heat b. Thermal *b.*

inhalation b. A chemical or thermal burn of the respiratory tract due to inhalation.

radiation b. One resulting from exposure to radiant energy, as x-ray, radium, sunlight, or other form. These may be severe, and x-ray and radium burns heal very slowly.

sunburn. Injury to the skin of varying degrees of intensity, produced by actinic rays of the sun or sun lamps. See *sunburn.*

thermal b. An injury resulting from an excessive rise in tissue temperature.

x-ray b. See radiation *b.*

burn. 1. To feel the sensation of heat. 2. To char or destroy by fire. 3. *In chemistry*, to oxygenize.

Burnett, William [*Scottish surgeon*, 1779–1861]. Remembered for his disinfectant, consisting of zinc chloride in strong solution with ferrous chloride added.

bur′nish·er [OF. *burnir*, to polish]. *In dentistry*, an instrument for condensing and smoothing and for polishing the surface of a filling or inlay.

Burns, Allan [*Scottish physician and anatomist*, 1781–1813]. Known for his early description of endocarditis (1809); for his recognition of mitral stenosis; his description of the mechanism of cardiac murmurs; his suggestion that angina pectoris is connected with coronary occlusion (1809). Described the falciform process of the fascia lata. The triangular space above the manubrium within the superficial layer of deep cervical fascia, transmitting the anterior jugular vein, bears his name (1811). Is said to have recorded the first case of chloroma (1811).

Burow, Karl August [*German surgeon*, 1809–74]. Remembered for his operation for closure of triangular defects of the lip by lateral incisions at the corners of the mouth, with flaps raised at each side and sutured in the midline. Also devised a blepharoplastic operation for eyelid defect by a sliding flap, in which a triangular segment of skin is excised to secure mobility. Introduced a solution of alum and lead acetate for the treatment of ulcers.

burr. See *bur.*

Burri, Robert [*Swiss bacteriologist*, 1867–]. Remembered for his method or procedure in the microscopical examination of microorganisms in which India ink is mixed with the material to be observed: called *Burri's method.* This method replaces dark-field illumination.

bur′row. *In dermatology*, a cuniculus or tunnel in the skin, seen especially in scabies.

bur′sa (pl. *bursae*) [LL., from G. *byrsa*, wineskin]. A small sac filled with fluid interposed between parts that move upon one another. See Plate 2.

accidental b. An inconstant one due to friction or pressure: also called *adventitious b.*

Achilles b. The bursa lying between the Achilles tendon and the calcaneus. Also called *b. tendinis calcanei.*

anserine b. One under the insertion of the gracilis and semitendinosus muscles.

b. of the omentum. The omental bursa.

cystic b. A bursa which has become cystic.

gastrocnemius b. A bursa lying beneath the origin of either head of the gastrocnemius muscle. The lateral one is situated between the lateral head and the lateral condyle of the femur; the medial one lies between the medial head and medial condyle. Each communicates with the cavity of the knee joint.

gluteal b. One or more lying under the gluteus maximus.

gluteofascial b. One lying between the greater trochanter and the gluteus maximus. Also called *gluteotrochanteric b.*

iliac subtendinous b. One lying between the tendon of the iliopsoas muscle and the lesser trochanter.

iliopectineal b. One separating the tendon of the iliopsoas muscle from the iliopectineal eminence and the capsule of the hip joint.

infracardiac b. The cephalic end of the embryonic mesenteric recess lying in the mesentery between esophagus and right lung bud, or a small cyst in the right ligamentum pulmonis derived from it.

ischial b. One situated over the ischial tuberosity.

mucous b. A membranous sac filled with synovial fluid.

obturator b. One under the tendon of the obturator internus.

olecranon b. One lying between the olecranon process of the ulna and the skin.

omental b. The lesser peritoneal sac; formed in the embryo by a lateral outgrowth into the mesogastrium, dorsal to the stomach, and after rotation of the gut forming a cavity back of the stomach and opening into the great omentum at the epiploic foramen.

ovarian b. A small pocket containing the ovary; formed by a fold of the broad ligament.

patellar b. One of several bursae behind the patella which may communicate with the knee joint. See prepatellar *b.*

pharyngeal b. A small pit caudal to the pharyngeal tonsil, resulting from the ingrowth of epithelium along the course of the degenerating tip of the notochord. Also called *Luschka's b.*

popliteal b. A bursa situated between the tendon of origin of the popliteus muscle and the lateral condyle of the tibia. It is a tubular extension of the synovial membrane of the knee joint.

prepatellar b. A bursa situated over the patella and the upper part of the patellar ligament. See Plate 2.

radial b. The synovial bursa of the tendon of the flexor pollicis longus muscle.

rider's b. One resulting from inflammation; due to pressure on the adductor muscles of the thigh.

sacral b. One found in the aged, over the sacrococcygeal articulation or over the spine of the fourth or fifth sacral vertebra.

semimembranosus b. A bursa situated between the tendon of the semimembranosus muscle and the medial head of the gastrocnemius muscle and medial meniscus of the knee joint. It communicates with the medial gastrocnemius bursa.

subacromial b. See subdeltoid *b.*

subcutaneous acromial b. One lying over the acromion, between it and the skin.

subdeltoid b. One lying beneath the deltoid muscle and extending beneath the acromion and coracoacromial ligament; it separates these structures from the capsule of the shoulder joint. It is frequently inflamed. Syn., *subacromial b.* [BNA].

subhyoid b. One lying between the thyrohyoid membrane and hyoid bone and the conjoint insertion of the omohyoid and sternohyoid muscles.

subscapular b. One between the tendon of the subscapularis muscle and the capsule of the shoulder joint; it communicates with the shoulder joint cavity.

synovial b. One found between tendons and bony surfaces.

ulnar b. The synovial bursa of the tendons of the flexor digitorum sublimis and profundus muscles.

bur·sat'tee (bur·sat'ee, bur·sah'tee) [Hind. *barsātī*, relating to rain]. A fungus disease of horses, occurring in India and the southern United States, characterized by the formation of nodules underneath and in the skin, which eventually coalesce and form a raw surface, simulating cancer.

bur·sec'to·my [G. *byrsa*, wineskin; *ektomē*, excision]. The surgical removal of a bursa.

bur·si'tis [*byrsa*; G. *-itis*, inflammation]. Inflammation of a bursa.

Achilles b. Inflammation of the Achilles bursa.

olecranon b. That of the olecranon bursa.

omental b. Inflammation of the omental bursa.

popliteal b. Inflammation of the popliteal bursa. Syn., *Baker's cyst.*

prepatellar b. Inflammation of the bursa in front of the patella. Syn., *housemaid's knee.*

radiohumeral b. Inflammation of the olecranon bursa. See *epicondylitis, tennis arm.*

subdeltoid b. Inflammation of the subdeltoid bursa.

bur'so·lith [*byrsa*; G. *lithos*, stone]. A calculus formed within a bursa.

Burton, Henry [*English physician*, 1799–1849]. The first to note the blue line in the gums as a sign of chronic lead poisoning (1840); this sign once bore his name.

Bury, Judson Sykes [*English physician*, 1852–1944]. Described erythema elevatum (1889), called *Bury's disease.*

Buschke, Abraham [*German physician*, 1868–1943]. Known for his description of a disease of the skin, European blastomycosis or cryptococcosis (1895). This was described in the same year by Busse; called *Busse-Buschke's disease.* Also described scleredema adultorum, called *Buschke's scleredema.*

bush'mas"ter. See *Lachesis mutus.*

Busse, Otto [*German physician*, 1847–1922]. Known for his description of a disease of the skin, cryptococcosis (1895), called *Busse-Buschke's disease.*

but- [L. *butyrum*, butter, from G. *boutyron*]. *In chemistry*, a combining form denoting *the presence of a grouping containing four carbon atoms.*

bu"ta·bar'bi·tal. Generic name for 5-ethyl-5-*sec.*-butylbarbituric acid. See *butisol.*

bu-tabs. Trade-mark for vaginal tablets containing a viable culture of *Lactobacillus bulgaricus* with nutrient media, for use as a trichomonacide.

bu'ta·caine" sul'fate (bew'tuh·cane", bew"tuh·kay'een, ·in). γ-Di-*n*-butylaminopropyl-*p*-aminobenzoate sulfate, a water-soluble local anesthetic. See *butyn.*

bu"ta·di'ene. 1,3-Butadiene. $CH_2{:}CH.CH{:}CH_2$. A gaseous hydrocarbon derived from petroleum and used in the manufacture of synthetic rubber. In very high concentration, it has a narcotic effect when inhaled.

but"al·lyl'o·nal. Generic name for 5-*sec.*-butyl-5-β-bromallylbarbituric acid. See *pernoston.*

bu·tam'ben. Generic name for butyl aminobenzoate. See *butesin.*

butamin. See *tutocaine* hydrochloride.

bu'tane. The gaseous hydrocarbon $CH_3CH_2CH_2CH_3$, a colorless flammable gas occurring in natural gas and in solution in crude petroleum.

butanefrine. Trade-mark for the sympathomimetic amine *ethylnorepinephrine hydrochloride.*

butanefrine hydrochloride. Trade-marked name for ethylnorepinephrine hydrochloride or 1-(3,4-dihydroxyphenyl)-2-amino-1-butanol hydrochloride, a sympathomimetic agent used as a bronchial antispasmodic.

bu"ta·no'ic ac'id. Butyric acid.

bu'ta·nol. Butyl alcohol.

bu·tar'sen. *p*-Arsenosophenylbutyric acid; a trivalent arsenical having trypanocidal activity.

butazolidin. Trade-mark for *phenylbutazone*, a substance employed in the treatment of arthritis and allied disorders.

Butcher's saw. See under *saw.*

Butenandt, Adolf (1903–). German chemist noted for his work on sex hormones, their structure, and properties. Nobel laureate in chemistry (1939).

bu'tene. A four-carbon aliphatic hydrocarbon containing one double bond; two isomers are known: 1-butene or α-butylene, $CH_3CH_2CH{:}CH_2$; and 2-butene, or β-butylene, $CH_3CH{:}CHCH_3$. Both are gases occurring in oil or coal gas.

bu'ten·yl. The unsaturated radical C_4H_7, of which there are three isomeric forms: 1-butenyl is $CH_3CH_2CH{:}CH$—; 2-butenyl is $CH_3CH{:}CHCH_2$—; 3-butenyl is $CH_2{:}CHCH_2CH_2$—.

butesin. Trade-mark for a brand of butyl aminobenzoate. See *butamben.*

b. picrate. A trade-mark name for a compound of one molecule of trinitrophenol and two molecules of butyl aminobenzoate: used as 1% ointment in the treatment of burns and painful skin lesions, and in aqueous solution for anesthesia of the eye.

bu'te·thal. Generic name for 5-*n*-butyl-5-ethylbarbituric acid. See *neonal.*

bu·teth'a·mine. Generic name for 2-isobutylaminoethyl-*p*-aminobenzoate. See *monocaine.*

Bu'thus. A genus of scorpions.

B. cocitanus. A poisonous species found in North Africa; its bite is occasionally fatal.

B. martensi. A poisonous species of Manchuria.

butisol. A trade-mark for 5-ethyl-5-*sec.*-butylbarbituric acid, a sedative and hypnotic. See *butabarbital.*

b. sodium. Trade-mark name for the sodium derivative of 5-ethyl-5-*sec.*-butyl barbituric acid.

Butler and Tuthill's method. See under *method.*

butoben. A trade-mark for butyl parahydroxybenzoate.

bu"to·pyr"o·nox'yl. Butyl mesityl oxide, a yellowish liquid, insoluble in water: used as an insect repellent and toxicant. Syn., *indalone.*

Bütschli, Otto [*German zoologist,* 1848–1920]. Described the spindle-shaped figure observed in mitosis, called *Bütschli's nuclear spindle.*

but'ter [L. *butyrum,* butter, from G. *boutyron*]. 1. The fatty part of milk, obtained by rupturing the fat globules by churning or mechanical agitation. 2. Various vegetable fats having the consistency of butter. 3. Certain anhydrous chlorides having the appearance or consistency of butter: old usage.

antimony b. Antimony chloride.

cacao b. See *theobroma* oil.

tin b. Stannic chloride.

zinc b. Zinc chloride.

but'ter yel'low. $C_6H_5N{:}N.C_6H_4N(CH_3)_2$. *p*-Dimethylamino-azobenzene. A yellow, crystalline powder, insoluble in water and sparingly soluble in alcohol; used to color fats and in the preparation of Töpfer's reagent for the determination of free HCl in gastric juice.

but'tock [ME. *but,* end]. One of the two fleshy parts of the body posterior to the hip joints.

but'ton·hole" [OF. *boton,* button; AS. *hol,* hole]. *In surgery,* a small, straight opening into an organ or part.

mitral b. An advanced case of mitral stenosis, usually of rheumatic origin.

but'tress [OF. *bouterez,* from *bouter,* to thrust]. 1. A support or prop. 2. A thickening of the sole of the equine hoof between the frog and the posterior end of the bar.

bu'tyl. The univalent hydrocarbon radical, C_4H_9—. It occurs as **normal-b.,** $CH_3.CH_2.CH_2.CH_2$—, abbreviated *n*-butyl; **iso-b.,** $(CH_3)_2CH.CH_2$—, abbreviated *i*-butyl; **secondary-b.,** $CH_3.CH_2.(CH_3)CH$—, abbreviated *sec.*-butyl; and **tertiary-b.,** $(CH_3)_3C$—, abbreviated *tert.*-butyl.

b. acetate. Normal butyl acetate, a colorless liquid with fruity odor; used in manufacture of perfumes and as a solvent.

b. alcohol. $CH_3CH_2CH_2CH_2OH$. Normal butyl alcohol; used as a solvent, as a denaturant for ethyl alcohol, and in synthesis. Syn., *butanol.*

b. aminobenzoate (*butylis aminobenzoas*). Normal butyl aminobenzoate, $NH_2.C_6H_4.COO.C_4H_9$. An odorless and tasteless, white, crystalline powder, almost insoluble in water; used as anesthetic dusting powder or in the form of troches, ointment, suppositories, or oil solution. See *butesin.*

b.-chloral hydrate. $CH_3CHCl.CCl_2.CH(OH)_2$. Trichlorobutylidene glycol. White, lustrous scales with pungent odor, soluble in 50 parts of water or 1 of alcohol. It is an analgesic and hypnotic similar to chloral hydrate, used in facial neuralgia, migraine, spasms, etc. Dose, 0.3–1.3 Gm. (5–20 gr.). Syn., *croton chloral hydrate.*

b. parahydroxybenzoate. $HO.C_6H_4.COOC_4H_9$. White, crystalline powder with slight odor, soluble in 6500 parts of water; used as preservative of medicinals, foods, etc. See *butoben.*

bu'tyl·ene. Butene.

bu·tyl'i·dene. The radical $CH_3(CH_2)_2CH$=.

butyn sulfate. Trade-marked name for butacaine sulfate.

bu·ty'phus. See *rinderpest.*

bu"tyr·a'ceous (bew"ti·ray'shus) [L. *butyrum,* butter]. Resembling butter; containing or yielding butterlike substances.

bu'tyr·ate. A salt of butyric acid.

bu·tyr'ic. Pertaining to, or derived from, butter.

bu·tyr'ic ac'id. $CH_3.CH_2.CH_2.COOH$. Butanoic acid; a viscid liquid having a rancid smell. It occurs in butter as a glyceride and is found also in various plant and animal tissues.

bu'tyr·in. $(C_3H_7COO)_3C_3H_5$. Glyceryl tributyrate, a constituent of butterfat. Also called *tributyrin.*

bu'tyr·in·ase". An enzyme found in blood serum which hydrolyzes butyrin.

bu'tyr·o-, bu'tyr-. *In chemistry,* a combining form for *butyric.*

bu'tyr·oid [*butyrum;* G. *eidos,* form]. Buttery; having the consistency of butter.

bu'tyr·yl. The radical $CH_3.CH_2.CH_2.CO$— of butyric acid.

bux'ine (buck'seen, ·sin) [L. *buxus,* box-tree]. An alkaloid from the leaves of *Buxus sempervirens.*

Buzaglo's stain. See under *stain.*

by'nin [G. *bynē,* malt]. A protein which is derived from malt.

Byrd, Harvey Leonidas [*American physician,* 1820–84]. With Harvie Dew, described a method of artificial respiration in asphyxia of the newborn; called *Byrd-Dew method.*

bys"si·no'sis [G. *byssos,* flax; *-ōsis,* condition]. Irritation of the pulmonary air passages caused by the inhalation of cotton dust, formerly thought to be a form of pneumonoconiosis. Also called *Monday morning fever, gin fever.*

bys'soid [*byssos;* G. *eidos,* form]. Consisting of a filamentous fringe of which the strands are of unequal length.

bys"so·phthi'sis (biss"o·thigh'sis, ·tiss'is). See *byssinosis.*

bys'sus [*byssos*]. Charpie, lint, or cotton.

Bywaters, Eric George Lapthorne [*English physician,* 1910–]. With Desmond Beall, described crush syndrome with impairment of renal function (1941). See lower nephron *nephrosis.*

C

C 1. Chemical symbol for carbon. 2. Centimeter.
C. Abbreviation for canine of second dentition, Celsius, centigrade, closure, congius (L., gallon), contraction, cylinder, cylindrical lens.
C., c. Carbon, cathode, centigrade, centimeter, congius, (L. gallon), hundredweight.
c Centimeter.
c. 1. *Cum;* with. 2. *Centum;* one hundred. 3. Deciduous canine.
C′. Symbol for complement.
C5 A designation for pentamethonium, commonly the bromide or iodide salt.
C6 A designation for hexamethonium, commonly the bromide or iodide salt. See *bistrium bromide.*
C10 A designation for decamethonium, commonly the bromide salt. See *syncurine.*
Ca Chemical symbol for calcium.
ca. Abbreviation for cathode.
ca′ble [L. *capulum,* halter]. The flexible arm of the dental engine.
Cabot, Arthur Tracy [*American surgeon,* 1852–1912]. Remembered especially for his posterior wire splint with a footpiece at a right angle, designed for the treatment of fractures of the leg where traction is not required.
Cabot, Hugh [*American urologic surgeon,* 1872–1945]. Known for his many contributions to the knowledge of urology. Devised a method of nephropexy in which the renal capsule is split along the external border to form a capsular suspension, and the intercostal muscle of the last rib and the quadratus lumborum are used for anchorage.
Cabot, Richard Clarke [*American physician and clinician,* 1868–1939]. Widely known for his teachings of differential diagnosis by means of the case-history system and for his interest in the problems of social service. Remembered for his useful contributions to the knowledge of blood examination. The ringlike bodies, seen in red cells in some cases of severe anemia, are called *Cabot's ring bodies.*
ca·ca′o (ka·kay′o, ka·kah′o) [Sp., from Nahuatl *cacahuatl,* the seed]. Seeds from *Theobroma cacao* from which cacao butter, chocolate, and cocoa are prepared. See *Theobroma.*
c. butter. Theobroma oil, obtained from the roasted seeds of *T. cacao;* used in the preparation of suppositories, in ointments, and as an emollient.
CaCC, CCC Cathodal closure contraction.
cac″es·the′si·a, cac″aes·the′si·a (kack″ess·thee′-zhuh, ·zee·uh) [G. *kakos,* bad; *aisthēsis,* sensation]. Any morbid sensation. —**cacesthesic,** *adj.*
ca·chet′ (ka·shay′, cash′ay) [F., from *cacher,* to hide]. Two rounded or oblong, concave pieces of wafer (rice paper) enclosing an ill-tasting medication within the concavity formed when the opposing edges are pressed together.
ca·chex′i·a (ka·keck′see·uh) [G. *kakos,* bad; *hexis,* state]. Weakness and emaciation caused by some serious disease such as syphilis, tuberculosis, or carcinoma. —**cachec′tic,** *adj.*
African c. Wasting disease following earth eating. Also called *Negro c.*
aphthous c. Sprue.
c. exophthalmica. That associated with exophthalmic goiter.
c. hypophysiopriva. The symptoms of hypopituitary cachexia observed when the pituitary has been removed.
c. strumipriva. That following ablation of the thyroid. Also called *c. thyropriva.*
c. thyropriva. See *c. strumipriva.*
cancerous c. That associated with malignant disease.
hypophyseal c. See hypopituitary *c.*
hypopituitary c. A condition due to destruction of the adenohypophysis by infection, trauma, or tumors; characterized by emaciation, asthenia, psychic changes, and lowered temperature, blood pressure, and metabolism. Weight loss is extreme, body hair disappears, and there is general atrophy of organs, especially marked in adrenal and thyroid. The disease runs a progressive course and usually is fatal. Also called *hypophyseal c., Simmonds' disease.*
lymphatic c. See Hodgkin's *disease.*
malarial c. Anemia, weakness, mental depression, and emaciation associated with chronic malaria. Also called *paludal c.*
mercurial c. That which accompanies chronic mercury poisoning.
Negro c. See African *c.*
pachydermic c. Myxedematous cachexia.
paludal c. See malarial *c.*
Simmonds' c. See hypopituitary *c.*
strumous c. Tuberculous cachexia.
thyroid c. That associated with exophthalmic goiter.
urinary c. That associated with chronic suppurative infections of the urinary tract.
cach″in·na′tion (kack″i·nay′shun) [L. *cachinnare,* to laugh loudly]. Immoderate laughter, as in hysteria.
ca″chou′ (kah″shoo′, ka·shoo′) [F., catechu]. An aromatic pill or tablet for deodorizing the breath.
cac′o-, cac- [G. *kakos,* bad]. A combining form signifying *bad, diseased, deformed,* or *vitiated.*
cac″o·de·mo′ni·a, cac″o·de·mon″o·ma′ni·a [*kakos;* G. *daimōn,* spirit; *mania,* madness]. A psychosis in which the patient believes he is possessed by or of an evil spirit.
cac′o·dyl. $(CH_3)_2As\text{-}As(CH_3)_2$. Tetramethyldiarsenic. A colorless, heavy liquid with an extremely offensive odor; inflammable when exposed to air.
cac′o·dyl·ate. A salt of cacodylic acid. The sodium, calcium, and iron salts are used in medicine.
cac″o·dyl′ic ac′id. Dimethylarsinic acid, $AsO(CH_3)_2OH$.
cac″o·geu′si·a (kack″og·yoo′see·uh, kack″o·jew′-see·uh) [*kakos;* G. *geusis,* taste]. The sensation of bad taste; frequently a symptom in idiopathic epilepsy.
ca·coph′o·ny, cac″o·pho′ni·a [*kakos;* G. *phōnē,* voice]. An abnormally harsh or discordant voice. —**cacophon′ic,** *adj*
ca·cos′mi·a [*kakos;* G. *osme,* smell]. Imaginary odors, particularly putrefactive odors. See also *parosmia.*
cac′tus gran″di·flo′rus. The fresh, succulent stem of the wild-growing *Selenicereus grandiflorus,* night-blooming cereus, a plant indigenous to the West Indies and cultivated in North America and Europe. It has been used as a substitute for digitalis.

ca·dav′er [L., corpse, from *cadere*, to fall dead]. A dead body, especially that of a human being; a corpse. —**cadaveric,** *adj.*

ca·dav′er·ine (ka·dav′ur·een, ·in) [*cadaver*]. Pentamethylenediamine, a ptomaine formed by the action of the *Vibrio comma* on protein.

ca·dav′er·ous [*cadaver*]. Resembling a cadaver; of a deathly pallor.

cad′mi·um [G. *kadmeia*, calamine]. Cd = 112.41. A bluish white metal used as a constituent of easily fusible alloys. Its salts have physiologic actions similar to those of zinc, being astringent and, in concentrated solution, irritant. Internally, they are emetic.

c. iodide. CdI_2. Formerly used in ointment form for skin diseases.

c. salicylate. $(C_6H_4.OH.COO)_2Cd$: formerly used in 0.5–1.0% solution as antiseptic in ophthalmia.

c. sulfate. $CdSO_4.2\frac{2}{3}H_2O$: formerly used as astringent and stimulant wash in 0.5–1.0% solution.

c. sulfide. CdS; a yellow pigment. Syn., *cadmium yellow.*

c. yellow. See *c.* sulfide.

ca·du′ca [L. *caducus*, from *cadere*, to fall dead]. Decidua.

ca·du′ce·us (ka·dew′see·us) [L., herald's staff]. The symbol or insigne of medicine consisting of the staff of Asclepius about which a single serpent is coiled. The Medical Corps of the United States Army has modified the symbol to consist of a staff with two formal wings at the top, and two serpents entwined about the remainder. The latter is not regarded as a medical, but as an administrative emblem, implying neutral, noncombatant status.

ca·du′cous [L. *caducus*, from *cadere*, to fall dead]. *In botany*, dropping off very early, as compared with other parts.

Cadwalader, Thomas [*American physician*, 1708–79]. Contributed an early description of lead colic and lead palsy in his monograph on the dry gripes (1745), probably the first medical monograph published in the American Colonies. He is said to have given the first anatomic lecture in the Colonies (1730).

cae-. For words beginning with *cae-* not found here, see words beginning with *ce-*.

cae′ci·tas. See *blindness.*

cae′cum. See *cecum.*

Caelius Aurelianus [*Roman physician*, fifth century]. Remembered as the last of the medical writers of the Western Roman Empire.

cae″ru·lo·plas′min (see″roo·lo·plas′min). A plasma protein (alpha₂-globulin) which contains eight atoms of copper, probably in covalent linkage. It represents at least 90% of copper normally in plasma, and is estimated by its oxidase ability; blood values range from about 70–120 micromilligrams per 100 ml.

Caes″al·pin′i·a (sez″al·pin′ee·uh, ses″al·) [after Andrea *Cesalpino*, Italian botanist and physician, 1519–1603]. A genus of tropical trees of the Leguminosae.

C. coriaria. Divi divi, a South American shrub cultivated in India, where the dried powdered pods are used as antiperiodic.

C. crista. A prickly, trailing shrub of most tropical coasts. Its seeds (fever nuts, bonduc seeds) have been used as febrifuge, tonic, and antiperiodic. It contains bonducin.

C. echinata. A tree of Brazil whose wood is much used as a source of dye.

C. sappan. A tree of India whose wood is used for its coloring principle, related to that of hematoxylin.

Cae·sar′i·an sec′tion. See *Cesarian section.*

ca″fard′ (kah″fahr′, kaf′ahr, kaf′ard) [F., hypocrite]. A subacute melancholia, characterized by attacks of depression and irritability.

cafergone. Trade-mark for certain preparations containing ergotamine tartrate and caffeine.

caf′fe·a. Coffee.

caf·fe′ic ac′id. $(OH)_2.C_6H_3.CH{:}CH.COOH$. Dihydroxycinnamic acid, obtained from coffee.

caf′fe·ine (kaf′ee·in, kaf′een, kaf′ee·een) [Ar. *qahwah*, coffee, a decoction of berries] (*caffeina*). $C_8H_{10}N_4O_2 + H_2O$. An alkaloid, chemically 1,3,7-trimethylxanthine, found in the leaves and beans of the coffee tree, in tea, in Paraguay tea, and in guarana, the roasted pulp of the fruit of *Paullinia sorbilis*. It occurs, or is prepared synthetically, in long, silky needles, slightly soluble in cold water and alcohol, with a feebly bitter taste. It is a cerebrospinal, circulatory, and renal stimulant. Dose, 0.06–0.2 Gm. (1–3 gr.). See *coffee*. Syn., *guaranine, methyltheobromine, theine, trimethylxanthine.* Also called *psoraline.*

c. and sodium benzoate (*caffeina et sodii benzoas*). A white powder containing 47–50% of caffeine, soluble in two parts of water. It is a form of caffeine especially suited for subcutaneous injection. Dose, about double that of caffeine.

c. bromide. See *c.* hydrobromide.

c. hydrobromide. $C_8H_{10}N_4O_2.HBr.2H_2O$. Caffeine bromide. It occurs as transparent crystals, soluble in water; the solution is unstable. Has been used as a diuretic by subcutaneous injection.

c. salicylate. $C_8H_{10}N_4O_2.C_7H_6O_3$, occurring as white, crystalline masses, soluble in water and alcohol with decomposition. It is used for the same purposes and in the same dose as caffeine.

c. triiodide. $(C_8H_{10}N_4O_2I_2.HI)_2 + 3H_2O$. Dark-green prisms, of a metallic luster, soluble in alcohol. It was formerly used as a diuretic and alterative instead of potassium iodide.

c. with sodium salicylate (*caffeina cum sodii salicylate*). A white powder, soluble in two parts of water, and containing 48–52% of caffeine. It is used in the same manner and dosage as caffeine and sodium benzoate.

citrated c. (*caffeina citrata*). A mixture of equal parts of caffeine and citric acid, the latter increasing the solubility of caffeine in water. It is used like caffeine, but in double the dosage.

caf′fe·in·ism [*qahwah*]. Chronic poisoning due to the excessive use of coffee or other caffeine-containing preparations.

caf′fe·ol (kaf′ee·ole, ·ol, ·awl). A volatile oil, said to consist chiefly of furfuryl alcohol, in roasted coffee.

ca·hin′ca (ka·hing′kuh), **ca·in′ca** (ka·ing′ka) [Tupi]. The dried roots of *Chiococca alba*, and other species of *Chiococca*, a genus of shrubs of tropical America. It has been used as a diuretic, purgative, tonic, and emetic.

ca·in′cin (ka·in′sin) [Tupi]. Cainca bitter, cainca acid, $C_{40}H_{64}O_{18}$. A glycoside from *Chiococca alba* and *C. brachiata*. In small doses, it is reputedly diuretic and cathartic; in large doses, emetic.

cai″no·pho′bi·a (kigh″no·fo′bee·uh, kay″no·) [G. *kainos*, new; *phobos*, fear]. Neophobia; morbid fear of newness.

Cajal. See *Ramón y Cajal.*

cajandol. Trade-mark for a solution of cajeput oil with propyl-*p*-hydroxybenzoate in peanut oil: used as an analgesic in genitourinary-tract infections.

caj′e·put, caj′u·put (kadj′uh·putt) [Malay *kāyu-pūtih*, white tree]. An East Indian tree, *Melaleuca leucadendron*, which yields an aromatic, volatile oil containing cajeputol and cajeputene and resembling turpentine oil. Cajeput oil has been used in flatulent colic, hysteria, cutaneous disorders, and toothache.

caj'e·put·ol", caj'u·put·ol". Cineol; eucalyptol.

caked [ON. *kaka*]. Compressed, tense, or hardened, due to engorgement or induration.

Cal. Large or great calorie; kilocalorie. See *kcal.*

cal. Small calorie.

Cal'a·bar bean. The poisonous seed of a leguminous vine (*Physostigma venenosum*) of Africa. See *Physostigma.*

Cal'a·bar swel'lings. Edematous, egg-shaped, distended areas occurring in different parts of the body of natives of Calabar and other parts of West Africa. It is thought to be produced by the action of *Filaria loa* in the subcutaneous tissues.

cal'a·mine (kal'uh·myne, ·min) [G. *kadmeia*, calamine]. Native zinc carbonate. Official calamine, also called prepared calamine, is zinc oxide with a small amount of ferric oxide; occurs as a pink powder; insoluble in water. Used as a local application in the treatment of skin diseases. It is also used to impart a flesh color to ointments, washes, and powders.

c. liniment (*linimentum calaminae*). Contains calamine, 8 Gm.; zinc oxide, 8 Gm.; olive oil, 50 cc.; solution of calcium hydroxide, a sufficient quantity to make 100 cc. Used as a protective in various forms of dermatitis.

c. lotion (*lotio calaminae*). Contains calamine, 8 Gm.; zinc oxide, 8 Gm.; sodium carboxymethylcellulose, 2 Gm.; dioctyl sodium sulfosuccinate, 65 mg.; glycerin, 3 cc.; water, a sufficient quantity to make 100 cc.

c. ointment (*unguentum calaminae*). Contains calamine, 17 Gm.; yellow wax, 4 Gm.; wool fat, 4 Gm.; petrolatum, 75 Gm. Also called *Turner's cerate.*

phenolated c. lotion (*lotio calaminae phenolata*). Calamine lotion containing 1% of liquefied phenol. Also called *compound c. lotion.*

calamoin. Trade-mark for an antipruritic ointment containing calamine, zinc oxide, camphor, and phenol.

cal'a·mus [L., a reed]. Sweetflag. The rhizome of *Acorus calamus.* It contains a volatile oil and acorin, a bitter principle. The root is aromatic, stomachic, and tonic, and has been used as an ingredient of many popular bitters.

ca'la·mus scrip·to'ri·us. The inferior part of the rhomboid fossa; so named because it is shaped like a pen point.

calc-, calci-, calco-. Combining forms from Latin *calx, calcis*, lime: used to mean lime, calcium, or calcium salts.

cal·cae'mi·a. See *calcemia.*

cal·ca'ne·o- [L. *calcaneum*, heel]. A combining form signifying *pertaining to the calcaneus.*

cal·ca"ne·o·as·trag'a·lar [*calcaneum;* G. *astragalos*, ball of the ankle joint]. Old term for talocalcaneal.

cal·ca"ne·o·ca'vus [*calcaneum;* L. *cavus*, hollow]. A type of talipes.

cal·ca"ne·o·cu'boid [*calcaneum;* G. *kyboeidēs*, like a cube]. Pertaining to the calcaneus and the cuboid; applied to the joint between these two bones and the ligaments joining them. See Table of Joints and Ligaments in the Appendix.

cal·ca"ne·o·dyn'i·a, cal"ca·no·dyn'i·a [*calcaneum;* G. *odynē*, pain]. Pain in the heel, or calcaneus, when walking or standing. Syn., *achillodynia.*

cal·ca"ne·o·na·vic'u·lar [*calcaneum;* L. *navicula*, small boat]. Pertaining to the calcaneus and the navicular, as calcaneonavicular joint and ligaments.

cal·ca"ne·o·val"gus [*calcaneum;* L. *valgus*, bowlegged]. A type of talipes.

cal·ca'ne·um [L., heel]. BR term and OT for calcaneus.

cal·ca'ne·us [L.]. 1. The heel bone. See Table of Bones in the Appendix. 2. Clubfoot in which the heel alone touches the ground; talipes calcaneus. —**calca'neal, calca'nean,** *adj.*

cal"ca·no·dyn'i·a. See *calcaneodynia.*

cal'car (kal'kahr) (pl. *calcaria*) [L., a spur]. Any spur or spurlike point. —**calcarate, calcarine,** *adj.*

c. avis. A ridge in the wall of the posterior horn of the lateral ventricle, caused by the inward bulging of the floor of the calcarine fissure.

c. femorale. A plate of compact bone projecting almost vertically from the femoral shaft upward into the neck toward the greater trochanter; it is best seen in x-rays.

cal·car'e·ous (kal·kair'ee·us) [L. *calcarius*, from *calx*, lime]. 1. Pertaining to or of the nature of limestone. 2. Having a chalky appearance or consistence. 3. Containing calcium.

cal·car"i·u'ri·a [*calcarius;* G. *ouron*, urine]. The presence of calcium salts in the urine.

cal·ce'mi·a, cal·cae'mi·a (kal·see'mee·uh) [L. *calx*, lime; G. *haima*, blood]. The occurrence of an excessive amount of calcium in the blood. Syn., *hypercalcemia.*

calci-. See *calc-, calci-, calco-.*

cal'cic [*calx*]. Of or pertaining to lime or calcium.

cal"ci·co'sis [*calx;* G. *-ōsis*, condition]. A form of pneumonoconiosis due to the inhalation of marble dust.

calcidin. Trade-mark for a compound containing 15% iodine in combination with lime and starch: used chiefly in the treatment of respiratory infections.

cal·cif'er·ol. Vitamin D_2, obtained by irradiation of ergosterol. One mg. represents 40,000 units of vitamin-D activity.

cal·cif'ic [*calx;* L. *facere*, to make]. Forming lime.

cal"ci·fi·ca'tion [*calx; facere*]. The deposit of calcareous matter within the tissues of the body.

disseminated c. A streaming of calcified strands from the sides of the femoral and tibial epiphyses early in their development. This phenomenon is found upon radiologic examination in all children.

metastatic c. See pathologic *c.*

nodular c. See *denticle*, 2.

pathologic c. Abnormal deposition of calcium salts, of three forms: (a) *dystrophic*, deposition in degenerated or necrotic tissues; (b) *metastatic*, deposition of calcium salts mobilized from a natural site into tissues not demonstrably injured; commonly associated with destructive lesions of bone or in the late stages of chronic renal insufficiency; (c) *reversible metastatic*, calcinosis associated with long-standing peptic ulcer, mild hypercalcemia, and renal insufficiency, apparently related to protracted and excessive ingestion of milk and alkali. Dietary restriction of calcium intake results in marked improvement, particularly in regression of ocular and subcutaneous lesions but not of the renal symptoms. Syn., *milk-drinker's syndrome.*

cal·cig'er·ous (kal·sidj'ur·us) [*calx;* L. *gerere*, to bear]. Containing lime or a lime salt.

cal'ci·grade [L. *calx*, heel; *gradi*, to walk]. Walking on the heels. *Obs.*

cal·cim'e·ter [L. *calx*, lime; G. *metron*, a measure]. An apparatus for determining the amount of calcium in the blood.

cal"ci·na'tion [*calx*]. The process of driving off animal matter and volatile chemical constituents from inorganic compounds by heat. —**calcine',** *v.t.*

cal″ci·no′sis [*calx;* G. *-ōsis,* condition]. The deposition of calcium salts in the skin and subcutaneous tissues; presumed to be a disorder of hyperparathyroidism.

c. universalis. See diffuse *c.*

circumscribed c. Calcified nodules limited to the skin and subcutaneous tissues of the upper extremities, particularly the hands; frequently seen in scleroderma.

diffuse c. Widespread calcified nodules which tend to ulcerate and heal slowly, and involve subcutaneous tissues, muscles, tendons, and nerve sheaths; seen especially in children. Also called *universal c.*

cal″ci·pe′ni·a [*calx;* G. *penia,* need]. Calcium deficiency.

cal′cis. Old term for *calcaneus.*

cal′ci·um [*calx*]. Ca = 40.08. A brilliant, silver-white metal, characterized by strong affinity for oxygen and isolated with great difficulty. It is a very abundant element in nature.

c. acetate. $Ca(C_2H_3O_2)_2$. A white, amorphous powder, soluble in water; formerly used in tuberculosis and psoriasis.

c. acetylsalicylate. $(CH_3CO.OC_6H_4COO)_2Ca.2H_2O$. A white powder, readily soluble in water; used as an antirheumatic and analgesic. Dose, 0.5–1.0 Gm. (8–15 gr.).

c. aminosalicylate. United States Pharmacopeia name for *calcium para-aminosalicylate.*

c. arsenate. $Ca(AsO_4)_2$. A white powder slightly soluble in water; used as an insecticide.

c. benzoate. $Ca(C_7H_5O_2)_2$; $(C_6H_5COO)_2Ca.3H_2O$; white powder or crystals that have been used in nephritis and albuminuria of pregnancy.

c. borate. $CaB_4O_7.6H_2O$; a white powder that is antiseptic and has been used internally in children's diarrhea and externally in bromhidrosis and weeping eczema.

c. bromide (*calcii bromidum*). $CaBr_2$; a white, granular salt, very deliquescent and very soluble in water; a nerve sedative. Dose, 0.6–2.0 Gm. (10–30 gr.) twice daily.

c. cacodylate. $[(CH_3)_2AsO_2]_2Ca.H_2O$. A white, granular powder very soluble in water; used for the same purposes as sodium cacodylate. Dose, 0.03–0.06 Gm. (½–1 gr.).

c. carbide. CaC_2. A gray, crystalline solid, decomposed by water to yield acetylene.

c. carbonate. Any of the forms of $CaCO_3$, including chalk, marble, whiting, etc. See *precipitated calcium carbonate.*

c. caseinate. A pale-yellowish powder, containing 1.4–2.1% of calcium; used as an accessory food in diarrheas of infancy. See *casec.*

c. chloride (*calcii chloridum*). $CaCl_2.2H_2O$; it occurs as white, deliquescent fragments or granules, soluble in water; used therapeutically for the effects of calcium ion. Dose, 0.6–1.3 Gm. (10–20 gr.).

c. creosotate (*calcii creosotas*). A mixture of the calcium compounds of creosote, representing about 50% of creosote; used as an expectorant and intestinal antiseptic. Dose, 0.5–1.2 Gm. (8–20 gr.). See *calcreose.*

c. cresylate. A syrupy fluid obtained by treating calcium hydroxide with cresol; used as a disinfectant.

c. cyanamide. Ca:N.C:N. Gray lumps or powder. Reacts with water to produce ammonia. Used in fertilizers. Syn., *cyanamide.*

c. dibromobehenate. $(C_{22}H_{41}O_2Br_2)_2Ca$. A yellowish powder, insoluble in water. It liberates bromide slowly in the system, for which effect it is used. Dose, 0.3–1.2 Gm. (5–20 gr.).

c. fluoride. CaF_2. A white powder, insoluble in water; previously recommended for improving development of teeth, and in prevention of caries.

c. gluconate (*calcii gluconas*). $[CH_2OH(CHOH)_4.COO]_2Ca.H_2O$. A white, crystalline or granular powder, soluble in about 30 parts of water. It is less irritating than other calcium salts and can be given in large doses orally or intravenously. Dose (oral), 1–5 Gm. (15–75 gr.); (intravenous), 0.6–1.0 Gm. (10–15 gr.).

c. glycerophosphate (*calcii glycerophosphas*). $CaC_3H_5(OH)_2PO_4$. A white, crystalline powder, soluble in cold water; has been recommended as a nerve tonic. Dose, 0.3–1.2 Gm. (5–20 gr.).

c. hippurate. $Ca(C_9H_8NO_3)_2$. A white, crystalline powder slightly soluble in hot water. It has been employed in cystitis, phosphaturia, polyuria, etc.

c. hydrate. See *c.* hydroxide.

c. hydroxide (*calcii hydroxidum*). $Ca(OH)_2$. Slaked lime. It is the active ingredient of lime water. Syn., *c. hydrate.*

c. hypochlorite. $Ca(ClO)_2$. White cubes decomposing readily. It is antiseptic and is used as a disinfectant and strong bleaching agent.

c. hypophosphite (*calcii hypophosphis*). $Ca(PH_2O_2)_2$. A white, crystalline powder, lustrous scales, or transparent crystals, soluble in seven parts of water; has been used in tuberculosis, chlorosis, etc. Dose, 0.65–2.0 Gm. (10–30 gr.).

c. hyposulfite. See *c.* thiosulfate.

c. iodate. $Ca(IO_3)_2.6H_2O$. A white, crystalline powder, soluble in 400 parts of water, insoluble in alcohol. It has been used internally to check fermentation and also as a substitute for iodoform.

c. iodide. $CaI_2.6H_2O$. A white powder or yellowish white hygroscopic mass, soluble in water and alcohol; used like potassium iodide Dose, 0.13–0.3 Gm. (2–5 gr.).

c. iodobehenate (*calcii iodobehenas*). Contains principally $(C_{22}H_{42}O_2I)_2Ca$. It is a white or yellowish powder, insoluble in water. In the body, it slowly liberates iodide ions, for which effect it is used. Dose, 0.3–1.0 Gm. (5–15 gr.). See *calioben, sajodin.*

c. iodoricinoleate. A compound containing approximately 30% iodine. It has been used in prophylaxis and treatment of goiter, and in other conditions requiring iodine. See *iodicin.*

c. iodostearate. A cream-colored solid, insoluble in water, containing approximately 27% iodine; used as a prophylactic against goiter. Dose, 0.01 Gm. (⅙ gr.) weekly, or biannual series of six weeks' treatment in daily doses of 0.01 Gm. See *stearodine.*

c. lactate. $Ca(C_3H_5O_3)_2.5H_2O$. A white powder, soluble in water; used in diseases requiring calcium therapy. Dose, 1–2 Gm. (15–30 gr.).

c. lactophosphate. A mixture of calcium lactate, calcium acid lactate, and calcium acid phosphate; soluble in water. Formerly used therapeutically as a source of calcium. Dose, 0.3–0.6 Gm. (5–10 gr.).

c. levulinate. $Ca(CH_3.CO.CH_2.COO)_2.2H_2O$. A very soluble white powder mainly employed for intravenous administration of calcium. Dose, 0.5–1.0 Gm. (8–15 gr.).

c. mandelate (*calcii mandelas*). $(C_6H_5.CHOH.COO)_2Ca$. A white powder, slightly soluble in cold water. It is used for the effect of mandelic acid as urinary antiseptic and has the advantages of being comparatively tasteless and of not requiring an acidifier for the urine. Dose, 2–4 Gm. (30–60 gr.).

c. oxalate. $CaC_2O_4.H_2O$; a crystalline powder, practically insoluble in water. It is a constituent of normal urine but occurs in increased amounts in certain pathological conditions.

c. oxide. CaO. Lime; quicklime; burnt lime. It is not used medicinally.

c. pantothenate. [$CH_2OH.C(CH_3)_2.CH(OH)$.-$CO.NH.CH_2.CH_2.COO]_2Ca$; a white powder, slightly hygroscopic, soluble in water: employed for the effect of dextrorotatory pantothenic acid, one of the B-complex vitamins. It is supplied in dextrorotatory and racemic forms, the latter having half the activity of the former. See also *vitamin* B.

c. para-aminosalicylate. ($NH_3.C_6H_3.OH$.-$COO)_2Ca$; white to cream-colored crystals or powder, freely soluble in water: used as a tuberculostatic agent.

c. penicillin. See under *penicillin*.

c. perborate. Approximately $Ca(BO_3)_2.7H_2O$. A water-soluble powder; used in dentifrices.

c. permanganate. $Ca(MnO_4)_2.4H_2O$. It occurs as violet crystals, readily soluble in water; formerly used in gastroenteritis and diarrhea, and for purifying water.

c. peroxide. CaO_2. A cream-colored powder, practically insoluble in water; has been used as antacid and antiseptic in gastric and intestinal disorders.

c. phenolsulfonate. $(C_6H_4.OH.SO_3)_2Ca.H_2O$. A water-soluble powder; used as an intestinal antiseptic and astringent. Dose, 0.3–1.0 Gm. (5–15 gr.).

c. phosphate. See *monobasic c. phosphate, dibasic c. phosphate, tribasic c. phosphate* under *calcium*.

c. propionate. $Ca(C_3H_5O_2)_2$. A white powder, soluble in water; used to prevent molding of bread.

c. saccharate. A water-soluble powder; has been used as an antacid and increases the solubility of calcium gluconate, when the latter is to be used by injection.

c. salicylate. $(C_6H_4.OH.COO)_2Ca.2H_2O$. A white, crystalline powder, soluble with difficulty in water; it has been used in intestinal diseases. Dose, 0.5–1.3 Gm. (8–20 gr.).

c. santonate. $Ca(C_{15}H_{19}O_4)_2$. A white, odorless, insipid powder, insoluble in water or chloroform. It is anthelmintic. Dose, 0.03–0.1 Gm. (½–1½ gr.). Also called *c. santoninate*.

c. sulfate. This substance occurs in several forms: (a) $CaSO_4.2H_2O$. Found naturally as the minerals alabaster, gypsum, mineral white, satin spar, and selenite. (b) $CaSO_4.½H_2O$. Plaster of Paris, made by heating gypsum to 120° to 130° C. Plaster of Paris is used in making bandages and casts to provide mechanical support or to immobilize various parts of the body. (c) $CaSO_4$, completely dehydrated calcium sulfate prepared by heating gypsum or plaster of Paris above 200° C. It also occurs naturally as the mineral anhydrite. It has been recommended as an absorbent application for wounds and ulcers.

c. sulfhydrate. A hydrate of $Ca(SH)_2$; used as a depilatory.

c. sulfide. When pure, it has the composition CaS, occurring as colorless crystals. Crude calcium sulfide was formerly official. It was prepared by igniting calcium sulfate with carbonaceous matter. Medicinally, it was used both externally and internally for the treatment of various skin diseases. At present, it is used as depilatory. Sulfurated lime and liver of lime are terms occasionally applied to crude calcium sulfide. A calcium sulfide made by igniting a mixture of calcium carbonate, sulfur, and small quantities of various metallic salts, phosphoresces; used in making certain luminous paints. A solution of calcium sulfides (di-, penta-) is officially recognized by the name sulfurated lime solution (Vleminckx's solution) and is used in treating various skin diseases.

c. sulfite. $CaSO_3$. A white powder slightly soluble in water; antiseptic and has been used in flatulent diarrhea. It is sometimes used as a preservative.

c. sulfocarbolate. See *c.* phenolsulfonate.

c. thiosulfate. $CaS_2O_3.6H_2O$. White crystals, soluble in water; has been used as an internal antiseptic. Syn., *c. hyposulfite*.

c. tungstate. $CaWO_4$. It occurs naturally as the mineral scheelite, but is usually prepared by precipitation; used in preparing screens of fluoroscopes and in manufacturing fluorescent paints.

dibasic c. phosphate (*calcii phosphas dibasicus*). $CaHPO_4.2H_2O$. A white powder, almost insoluble in water; used in rickets and other bone diseases: sometimes called *dicalcium phosphate*. Dose, 0.5–5.0 Gm. (8–75 gr.).

liquid c. bisulfite. A solution of calcium sulfite ($CaSO_3$) in an aqueous solution of sulfurous acid; has been used, when diluted with water, as an antiseptic gargle or wash.

monobasic c. phosphate. $CaH_4(PO_4)_2.H_2O$. It occurs in granules or as a powder, partially soluble in water, used as an ingredient of certain baking powders and is the calcium superphosphate used as a fertilizer.

precipitated c. carbonate (*calcii carbonas praecipitatus*). $CaCO_3$. A white powder, without odor or taste, practically insoluble in water. It is antacid and is used for acidity of the stomach, and in treating diarrhea accompanied by acidity. Externally, it is used as a desiccant, dusting powder, and as an application to burns and ulcers. Dose, 0.65–2.0 Gm. (10–30 gr.).

tribasic c. phosphate (*calcii phosphas tribasicus*). $Ca_3(PO_4)_2$. A white powder, almost insoluble in water; used as an antacid in gastric hyperacidity. Dose, 1–4 Gm. (15–60 gr.). Also called *precipitated c. phosphate*.

cal"ci·u'ri·a. Calcium in the urine: often used to mean *hypercalciuria*.

calco-. See *calc-, calci-, calco-*.

cal"co·glob'u·lin [L. *calx*, lime; *globulus*, globule]. A combination of calcium with protein such as is found in calcospherites, probably representing an early stage in the process of laying down calcium salts in teeth and bone.

cal"co·sphe'rite, cal"co·sphae'rite [*calx;* L. *sphaera*, sphere]. One of the granules or globules formed in tissues like bone and shell by a loose combination of protein and blood-borne calcium salts.

calcreose. Trade-mark for calcium creosotate.

cal-c-tose. A proprietary chocolate-flavored vitamin nutritive in powder form.

cal"cu·lo·gen'e·sis. The origin or development of calculi.

cal"cu·lo'sis [L. *calculus*, small stone, dim. of *calx;* G. *-ōsis*, condition]. The presence of a calculus, or abnormal concretion.

cal'cu·lus (pl. *calculi*) [L., small stone, dim. of *calx*]. A solid concretion composed chiefly of mineral substances and salts found principally in ducts, passages, hollow organs, and cysts. Organic materials such as cells, mucus, etc., may form a centrum or nidus and may be dispersed as a matrix for the mineral deposits, as salts of calcium, of uric acid, of bile acids, etc. —**calculous,** *adj*.

alternating c. One composed of alternating layers of its constituents.

arthritic c. A deposit near a joint of salts of uric acid, as in gout.

articular c. See arthritic *c*.

aural c. Inspissated and sometimes calcified cerumen in the external auditory canal.

biliary c. One containing mineral material and originating in the biliary passages. If composed of cholesterol or pigment, or both, without mineral constituents, it is a concretion rather than a calculus.

blood c. One situated in a blood vessel, derived from a thrombus and infiltrated with salts of calcium; a phlebolith, an arteriolith.

bronchial c. A concretion of mucus or exudate, infiltrated with mineral salts, situated in the bronchial tree.

c. felleus. A gallstone.

chalky c. One made up principally of salts of calcium.

coral c. One that is branched, as in the formation of staghorn coral.

cutaneous c. See *milium.*

cystic c. One found in either the urinary bladder or the gallbladder.

cystine c. A urinary calculus composed largely of cystine, an infrequent form of calculus.

dendritic c. A coral or staghorn calculus.

dental c. Calcareous deposits on the teeth, consisting of organic and mineral matter: formerly divided into *salivary c.* and *serumal* (sanguinary) *c.* Syn., *tartar.*

encysted c. One confined in a localized dilatation or diverticulum of the urinary bladder or gallbladder.

extragingival c. See supragingival *c.*

fibrinous c. A mass of fibrin infiltrated with mineral salts; if not so infiltrated, it is a concretion.

fusible c. A urinary calculus composed of phosphates of ammonium, calcium, and magnesium; high degrees of heat transform it into a black mass.

hepatic c. A biliary calculus situated in the intrahepatic biliary passages.

incarcerated c. See encysted *c.*

intestinal c. See *enterolith.*

kidney c. Renal *c.*

lacteal c. See mammary *c.*

laminated c. One made up of layers of different materials.

mammary c. A calcified mass of secretion or exudate in the ducts of the mammary gland.

mulberry c. A urinary calculus with a finely nodular outer surface resembling a mulberry and usually composed largely of calcium oxalate.

nasal c. One found in the nasal cavity.

pancreatic c. One situated in the pancreatic duct and composed largely of calcium phosphate.

pineal c. A small calcified nodule in the pineal body.

podagric c. See arthritic *c.*

prostatic c. Calcified nodules in prostatic acini, probably derived from corpora amylacea.

renal c. A concretion in the kidney. Syn., *kidney stone.*

salivary c. One situated in the duct of a salivary gland, or a deposit upon the surfaces of the teeth.

sanguinary c. See serumal *c.*

serumal c. A dental calculus formerly believed to be a calcareous deposit formed about the teeth by exudation from diseased gums: also called *sanguinary c., serumnal c.*

spermatic c. One situated in the seminal vesicle, ductus deferens, or epididymis.

staghorn c. A large, irregularly branched calculus in the renal pelvis.

subgingival c. One deposited on the surface of a tooth below the level of the gum margin.

supragingival c. One deposited on the surface of a tooth above the level of the gum margin: also called *extragingival c.*

tonsillar c. A calcified mass of detritus in a tonsillar crypt.

urinary c. One situated in any part of the urinary system.

vesical c. A stone in the urinary bladder.

xanthine calculi. Brown to red, hard and laminated calculi; rare and found in the urinary bladder.

Caldani, Leopoldo Marco Antonio [*Italian physician and anatomist,* 1725–1813]. Known for his work in comparative anatomy and his early experiments with animals. Succeeded Morgagni at Padua.

Caldwell, George Walter [*American surgeon,* 1866–1946]. Devised an operation for the relief of severe disease of the maxillary sinus (1893). In addition to the usual nasomaxillary opening, an opening is made in the anterior wall through the canine fossa. Called *Caldwell-Luc operation.*

Caldwell, William Edgar [*American obstetrician,* 1880–1943]. Known for his modern classification of the varieties in the measurements and form of the female pelvis (1933), called *Caldwell-Moloy classification.*

cal″e·fa′cient (kal″i·fay′shunt) [L. *calefacere,* from *calidus,* warm; *facere,* to make]. A medicine, externally applied, that causes a sensation of warmth. —**calefa′cient,** *adj.*

ca·len′du·la [NL., from L. *calendae,* first day of the month, when the plant was supposed to blossom]. 1. A plant of the genus *Calendula,* of the Compositae. 2. The dried ligulate floret of plants of this genus, especially *C. officinalis.*

ca″len·tu′ra [Sp., from L. *calere,* to be warm]. Term used in the Philippine Islands for an epidemic disease of horses, possibly of trypanosome origin.

calevate. Trade-mark for a sterile aqueous solution of calcium levulinate, suitable for parenteral administration.

calf [ON. *kālfi*]. The thick, fleshy part of the back of the leg, formed by the gastrocnemius and soleus muscles and overlying tissues.

calf′-bone. The fibula.

calglucon. Trade-mark for a brand of calcium gluconate.

cal″i·bra′tion [F. *calibre,* from Ar. *qalib,* a form, mold]. 1. The specification and measurements of the properties or performance of a device, so that it may be used for subsequent measuring procedures. 2. The measurement of the caliber of a tube, or the determination or rectification of the graduations on a tube, pipet, or balance weights. —**cal′ibrator,** *n.,* **cal′ibrate,** *v.t.*

ca″li·ec′ta·sis. (kay″lee·ec′tah·sis). Dilatation of a calyx of the renal pelvis.

cal″i·for′ni·um. The chemical element of atomic number 98, symbol Cf, an isotope of which was produced by bombarding curium of atomic weight 244 with helium ions. This isotope, probably of atomic weight 246, is radioactive, with a half-life of 45 minutes.

calioben. Trade-mark for calcium iodobehenate.

cal′i·pers (kal′i·purz) [corruption of *caliber*]. Curved and hinged V-shaped instrument for measuring the thickness and the outside or inside diameters of objects. There are also other types, e.g., micrometer calipers.

cal″i·sa′ya [Sp.]. Cinchona bark, especially that of *Cinchona calisaya.* See *cinchona.*

cal″is·then′ics [G. *kallos,* beauty; *sthenos,* strength]. The practice of light gymnastics by various rhythmical movements of the body; intended to develop the muscles and graceful carriage.

ca′lix. See *calyx.*

Calkins, Leroy Adelbert [*American obstetrician,* 1894–]. Introduced a method of placental expression in which expression is delayed until the uterus assumes a globular shape; known as *Calkins' method.*

Call′-Ex′ner bod′ies. See under *body.*

cal″li·pe′di·a [G. *kallos,* beauty; *pais,* child]. The desire to give birth to a beautiful child.

Cal·liph′o·ra [*kallos;* G. *phoros,* bearing]. A genus of flies which feed chiefly on animal refuse. The maggots of these flies cause myiasis.

C. vomitoria. The common blowfly or bluebottle; may deposit ova in neglected wounds of man and other mammals.

Cal″li·phor′i·dae (kal″i·for′i·dee) [*kallos; phoros*]. A family of the Diptera which includes many large blue, green, or copper-colored species, commonly called bluebottle, greenbottle, and blowflies. They normally deposit their eggs or larvae in the decaying flesh of dead animals but may be secondary invaders of neglected wounds and sores.

cal″lo·ma′ni·a [*kallos;* G. *mania,* madness]. A mania characterized by delusions of beauty.

cal·lo′sal [L. *callosus,* hard-skinned]. Pertaining to the corpus callosum.

cal·los′i·tas [L.]. A hard, thickened patch of skin with hypertrophy of the horny layer caused by irritation, friction, or pressure. Syn., *callus,* 1, *keratoma, tyloma, tylosis.*

cal·los′i·ty [*callositas*]. A circumscribed area of thickened skin due to friction or pressure.

cal·lo″so·mar′gin·al [L. *callosus,* hard-skinned; *margo,* margin]. Relating to the callosal and marginal gyri of the brain.

cal·lo′sum. See *corpus* callosum.

cal′lus [L.]. 1. A callosity; an area of hardened and thickened skin, seen usually in the palm or the sole; a hypertrophic reaction of the epidermis to pressure and friction. 2. New growth of incompletely organized bony tissue surrounding the bone ends in fracture; a part of the reparative process. Where repair is complete, the bony thickening is known as **permanent callus.** —**callous,** *adj.*

fibrous c. The connective tissue which precedes formation of cartilage or bone in a *callus,* 2.

Calmette, Léon Charles Albert [*French bacteriologist,* 1863–1933]. Developed curative serum for the treatment of snakebite (1897); *Calmette's serum* is prepared from the blood of horses immunized against venom. With Camille Guérin, prepared a preventive vaccine for tuberculosis (1927); see *BCG.* See also Calmette *test.*

calmitol. Proprietary topical anesthetic and antipruritic, available as a liquid or an ointment.

cal′o·mel [G. *kalos,* beautiful; *melas,* black]. HgCl, mercurous chloride. A white, tasteless powder; formerly used popularly as a purgative, also as an alterative and antisyphilitic.

colloidal c. A finely divided form of calomel, usually stabilized by the addition of gelatin.

cal′or (kal′or, kay′lor) [L., heat]. 1. Heat; one of the four classic signs of inflammation: calor, rubor, tumor, dolor. 2. Body heat or moderate fever heat. 3. Localized heat associated with inflammation.

cal″o·ra′di·ance [*calor;* L. *radius,* ray]. Emission of heat rays ranging from 250 to 55,000 mμ.

cal″o·res′cence [*calor*]. The conversion of invisible heat rays into luminous heat rays.

calori- [*calor*]. A combining form signifying *heat.*

ca·lor′ic [*calor*]. Pertaining to a calorie, calories, or to heat.

cal′o·rie, cal′o·ry [F. *calorie,* from L. *calor*]. A heat unit; the amount of heat required to raise the temperature of 1 kg. of water from 0° to 1° C. This is also known as a **large calorie** or **kilocalorie,** and is the unit used in the study of metabolism. Abbreviated, Cal. The **small calorie** is the amount of heat required to raise the temperature of 1 Gm. of water 1° C., and is one one-thousandth of the large calorie. Abbreviated, cal.

cal″o·rif′ic [*calor;* L. *facere,* to make]. Heat-producing.

ca·lor″i·ge·net′ic. See *calorigenic.*

ca·lor″i·gen′ic, ca·lor″i·ge·net′ic [*calor;* G. *genesthai,* from *gignesthai,* to be produced]. Heat-producing; applied to certain foods.

cal″o·rim′e·ter [*calor;* G. *metron,* a measure]. Instrument for measuring the heat production of an individual or system.

bomb c. Apparatus for measuring the heat of combustion, as of foods and fuel.

respiration c. Apparatus which determines the heat production of an individual by measuring the gaseous exchange of the lungs.

cal″o·ri·met′ric e·quiv′a·lent. The amount of heat necessary to raise the temperature of the calorimeter 1° C.

cal″o·rim′e·try [*calor; metron*]. The determination of the heat change in any individual or system by use of the calorimeter. —**calorimet′ric,** *adj.*

direct c. Actual measurement of the heat produced by an animal enclosed in a box or suitable enclosure. Generally used experimentally.

indirect c. Measurement of heat produced by use of the respiration calorimeter.

calpurate. Trade-mark for a compound of the calcium salt of theobromine and calcium gluconate; the compound is a myocardial stimulant and diuretic.

calscorbate. Trade-mark for ampuls of calcium ascorbate with benzyl alcohol and dextrose.

ca·lum′ba [Mozambican *Kalumb*]. Colombo, the dried root of *Jateorrhiza palmata,* native to East Africa and Madagascar It is a simple bitter, its chief constituents being several alkaloids and the bitter glycoside columbin.

cal·va′ri·a (pl. *calvariae*) [L., skull, from *calva,* the scalp]. The upper part of the skull; the skullcap: also *calvarium.* —**calvarial,** *adj.*

Calvé, Jacques [*French surgeon,* 1875–]. Described osteochondritis deformans juvenilis and osteochondrosis involving primary growth centers of vertebral bodies.

cal·vi′ti·es (kal·vish′ee·eez) [L.]. Baldness. Loss of hair, especially of the upper part of the head. Syn., *alopecia.*

c. frontalis adolescentium. The loss of hair in males during puberty in the frontal region in two triangular areas on both sides of the midline, giving rise to the **M**-shaped hairline seen in most adult males. This development requires presence of male sex hormones.

cal′vous [L. *calvus,* bald]. Bald.

calx [L., heel]. Old term for the heel.

calx [L., lime]. Calx sodica, soda lime.

cal″y·can′thine. An alkaloid, $C_{22}H_{26}N_4$, found in several species of *Calycanthus* and elsewhere, having strychninelike action.

ca′lyx, ca′lix (kay′licks, kal′icks) (pl. *calyxes, calyces, calices*) [G. *kalyx,* cup]. 1. A cup. 2. *In anatomy,* one of the cuplike divisions of the pelvis of the kidney into which the pyramids project. —**cal′ycine, calyc′inal, calyc′iform, cal′icine,** *adj.*

c. of ovum. Wall of the Graafian follicle from which the ovum has escaped.

major c. A primary subdivision of the renal pelvis; derived from the embryonic pole tubules, usually two or three in number.

minor c. One of the 4 to 13 cuplike divisions of the major calyces; derived from tubules of the second, third, and fourth orders, each receiving one or more of the renal papillae.

cam′bi·um [LL.]. A layer of tissue formed between the wood and the bark of exogenous plants.

c. layer. The cellular layer of the periosteum.

cam·bo′gi·a. See *gamboge.*

camdelate. Trade-mark for calcium mandelate.

cam′er·a [L., from G. *kamara,* anything with an arched covering]. 1. Chamber or compartment. 2. Apparatus used for photography.

c. lucida. An optical device used to project onto paper the image of an object so that an accurate drawing can be made. There are two main types: (a) that equipped with a Wollaston prism which projects an image in reduced, enlarged, or natural size; (b) that equipped with an Abbe prism, mirror, and microscope, used where a magnified image is desired.

c. oculi. Chamber of the eye.

c. septi lucidi. The so-called fifth ventricle of the brain. *Obs.*

caminoids. Trade-marked name for a product conforming to the requirements established for aminopeptodrate.

cam′i·sole [F.]. A kind of straitjacket; a canvas shirt with very long sleeves; used to restrain violent psychotics.

Cammidge, Percy John [*English physician,* 1872–]. Known for his study of pancreatic disease, for which he described a test called the *Cammidge test.*

cam′o·mile. See *anthemis, matricaria.*

camoquin hydrochloride. Trade-marked name for the hydrochloride of the antimalarial drug known by the generic name *amodiaquin.*

Campbell, Alfred Walter (1868–1937). Australian neurologist and psychiatrist, known for his classic work, *Histological Studies on the Localization of Cerebral Function* (1905), and his map of the human brain, which have made him one of the founders of modern neurology.

Campbell, Willis Cohoon [*American orthopedic surgeon,* 1880–1941]. Introduced a method of bone grafting in which he used a massive onlay graft for nonunion in fractures. A section of endosteum bridges the bone defect, the cortical graft being placed on a prepared surface and held in place by bone pegs. Cancellous bone is placed about the site of the fracture. He perfected a method for the relief of recurrent dislocation of the patella by passing a flap of joint capsule through a tunnel in the quadriceps femoris above the patella.

Camper, Pieter [*Dutch anatomist,* 1722–89]. Noted for his work and research in anthropology and craniology. Contributed to the knowledge of the anatomy of the eye and the peritoneum. Famed as a great anatomic artist, he is remembered for his description of the facial angle, a term he originated (1791) and for Camper's fascia. The facial line is also called *Camper's line.*

cam·pes′ter·ol. $C_{28}H_{48}O$; a sterol occurring in small amounts in the fixed oil from rape seed, soybean, and wheat germ.

cam′phene [Malay *kāpūr,* camphor]. $C_{10}H_{16}$. Terpene hydrocarbon occurring in several volatile oils and obtained as an intermediate product in the synthesis of camphor from pinene.

chlorinated c. Toxaphene.

cam′pho-, camph- [*kāpūr*]. A combining form denoting *camphor.*

cam′phol. See *borneol.*

cam′phor (*camphora*). $C_{10}H_{16}O$. A ketone obtained from the volatile oil of *Cinnamomum camphora,* a tree indigenous to eastern Asia, or produced synthetically. It is a mild irritant and antiseptic and is used as a carminative and stimulant. Dose, 0.2 Gm. (3 gr.). —**camphorated, camphor′ic,** *adj.*

artificial c. Pinene hydrochloride or bornyl chloride. $C_{10}H_{16}.HCl$. A terpene hydrochloride obtained from turpentine oil by action of hydrochloric acid; it is a solid similar to camphor.

betula c. Betulin.

birch c. Birch resin. See *betulin.*

Borneo c. A camphor, chiefly dextroborneol, deposited in the wood of *Dryobalanops aromatica.*

c. and soap liniment. Contains 6% hard soap, 4.5% (w/v) camphor, rosemary oil, alcohol, and water; a rubefacient embrocation. Syn., *soap liniment.*

c. flowers. Camphor obtained by sublimation.

c. ice. A cosmetic preparation of camphor, spermaceti, white beeswax, and a vegetable oil.

c. liniment (*linimentum camphorae*). Contains 20% (w/v) camphor in cottonseed oil; a counterirritant embrocation. Syn., *camphorated oil.*

c. ointment (*unguentum camphorae*). Contains 22% camphor in white wax and lard.

c. spirit (*spiritus camphorae*). Contains 10% (w/v) camphor in alcohol. Dose, 1 cc. (15 min.).

c. water (*aqua camphorae*). A saturated solution of camphor in distilled water; used as a vehicle, an ingredient of eye washes, and sometimes for a supposed euphoric effect.

carbolated c. A mixture of two parts of camphor with one of phenol in liquid petrolatum; has germicidal and local anesthetic properties. Syn., *camphorated phenol.*

cedrene c. $C_{15}H_{26}O$. A camphor that separates from red cedar oil.

chloral c. A fluid prepared by mixing equal parts of camphor and chloral. It has been used externally as a local anodyne.

Japan c. The commercial variety brought from Japan. Also called *tub c., Dutch c.*

liquid c. Camphor oil.

monobromated c. $C_{10}H_{15}BrO$. Camphor in which one atom of hydrogen has been replaced by an atom of bromine. Formerly thought to be sedative. Dose, 0.13 Gm. (2 gr.).

pulsatilla c. See *anemonin.*

Sumatra c. See Borneo *c.*

cam″pho·ra′ceous [*kāpūr*]. Resembling or containing camphor.

cam′phor·ate. A salt of camphoric acid.

cam·phor′ic ac′id. $C_{10}H_{16}O_4$. A dibasic acid obtained by the oxidation of camphor; has been used in the night sweats of pulmonary tuberculosis.

cam′phor·ism [*kāpūr*]. Camphor poisoning; marked by gastritis, coma, and convulsions.

cam″phor·o·ma′ni·a [*kāpūr;* G. *mania,* madness]. The camphor habit; a morbid craving for camphor.

cam·pim′e·ter [L. *campus,* field; G. *metron,* measure]. Instrument for measuring the field of vision. See *perimeter.* —**campimetry,** *n.*

stereoscopic c. See *stereocampimeter.*

camp″to·cor′mi·a [G. *kamptein,* to bend; *kormos,* trunk]. A special form of hysteria, seen most often in soldiers; characterized by extreme forward flexion of the spine, the eyes usually being focused on the ground. The person affected apparently walks with great difficulty and frequently has associated tremors. Also called *bent back.*

camp″to·dac′ty·ly [*kamptein;* G. *daktylos,* finger]. A condition in which one or more fingers are constantly flexed at one or both phalangeal joints.

Can′a·da bal′sam. See under *balsam.*

can′a·dine (kan′uh·deen, ·din). *l*-Tetrahydroberberine. A colorless alkaloid from *Hydrastis canadensis.*

ca·nal′ [L. *canalis,* channel]. Any tubular channel; duct.

adductor c. A triangular, aponeurotic tunnel bounded by the sartorius, vastus medialis, and adductor muscles; it extends from the femoral triangle to the hiatus adductorius and gives passage to the femoral artery and vein, the saphenous nerve, and the nerve to the vastus medialis. Also called *Hunter's c., subsartorial c.*

Alcock's c. The pudendal *c.*

alimentary c. The whole digestive tube from the mouth to the anus; the gastrointestinal tract.

alveolar canals [BNA]. Those in the maxilla or mandible giving passage to vessels and nerves to the teeth. A **superior alveolar canal** is one located in the maxilla. The **inferior alveolar canal** is one located in the mandible. Syn., *dental canals.*

alveolodental c. Old term for any of the dental canals.

anal c. The terminal portion of the large intestine extending from the rectum to the anus.

atrioventricular c. The canal, originally unpaired, between atrium and ventricle in the embryo.

auditory c. Auditory meatus. The **external auditory canal** is that from the auricle to the tympanic membrane; the **internal auditory canal** is that beginning on the posterior surface of the petrous bone. It gives passage to the acoustic and facial nerves and the internal auditory artery.

auricular c. Old term for the external auditory canal.

basipharyngeal c. A small passage occasionally present on either side between the ala of the vomer and vaginal process of the sphenoid.

biliary intralobular c. A small intercellular bile canaliculus in a hepatic cord.

birth c. See parturient *c.*

blastoporic c. See neurenteric *c.*

c. of Corti. See *tunnel* of Corti.

c. of Nuck. A shallow, peritoneal invagination in the female corresponding to the vaginal process of the peritoneum in the male: also called *Nuck's diverticulum.*

c. of Petit. See *zonular spaces* under *space.*

c. of the cervix of the uterus. That portion of the uterine canal that extends between the internal and external os. See Plate 41.

c. of the chorda tympani. A small canal in each temporal bone, between its squamous and petrous portions, terminating in the petrotympanic fissure. It gives passage to a chorda tympani nerve.

c. of the greater superficial petrosal nerve. One opening into the hiatus of the facial canal for the passage of the nerve of that name.

c. of the lesser superficial petrosal nerve. One in the petrous portion of the temporal bone for the passage of the nerve of that name.

canals of cartilage. The canals in ossifying cartilage during its vascularization; intended to receive prolongations of the osteogenetic layer of the periosteum. They radiate in all directions from the center of ossification.

caroticotympanic canals. Two or three short canals extending from the carotid canal to the tympanic cavity; they give passage to branches of the carotid plexus.

carotid c. One in the petrous portion of the temporal bone; it gives passage to the internal carotid artery.

carpal c. The space beneath the flexor retinaculum of the wrist and above the volar aspect of the carpal bones; it transmits the tendons of the long flexor muscles and median nerve.

central c. of the spinal cord. The small canal that extends through the center of the spinal cord from the conus medullaris to the lower part of the fourth ventricle. It represents the embryonic neural tube.

cervical c. See *c.* of the cervix of the uterus.

cervico-axillary c. The region bounded anteriorly by the clavicle, posteriorly by the scapula, and medially by the thoracic brim, together with their attached muscles.

cervicouterine c. See uterine *c.*

chorda c. The canal in the head process or notochord of presomite embryos. Syn., *notochordal c., neurenteric c.*

ciliary c. See *Fontana's spaces* under *space.*

cochlear c. (a) The osseous cochlear canal. (b) Cochlear duct.

condylar c. A small canal occasionally present in the floor of the condylar fossa for the passage of a vein from the transverse sinus. This canal is sometimes called the *posterior condylar canal,* and the hypoglossal canal the *anterior condylar canal.* Also called *condylar* or *condyloid foramen.*

craniopharyngeal c. A fetal canal in the sphenoid bone formed by the growth of the bone about the stalk of the craniobuccal (Rathke's) pouch.

craniovertebral c. See vertebral *c.*

crural c. See femoral *c.*

cystic c. The cystic duct.

deferent c. The ductus deferens.

dental canals [BR]. The alveolar canals.

dentinal canals. The dentinal tubules.

digestive c. The gastrointestinal tract.

Dorello's c. A small canal between the apex of the petrosal process, the posterior clinoid, and the petrosphenoid ligament of the dura. The abducens nerve passes through it.

ethmoid canals. Canals between the ethmoid bone and the orbital plate of the frontal bone. The **anterior ethmoid canal** is one giving passage to the nasociliary nerve and the anterior ethmoid vessels. The **posterior ethmoid canal** is one giving passage to the posterior ethmoid nerve and vessels.

Eustachian c. Old term for the bony, or petrous, portion of the Eustachian (auditory) tube.

facial c. A canal in the temporal bone for the passage of the facial nerve: formerly called *aqueduct of Fallopius.*

femoral c. The medial compartment of the femoral sheath behind the inguinal ligament. Also called *crural c.*

Fontana's c. See *Fontana's spaces* under *space.*

galactophorous canals. The lactiferous tubules of the mammary gland. *Obs.*

gastric c. A groove of the mucous membrane of the lesser curvature of the stomach extending from esophagus to pylorus.

genital c. *In comparative anatomy,* any canal designated for copulation or for the discharge of ova or offspring.

gynecophoric c. A canal located on the ventral surface of the male of certain species of *Schistosoma* in which the female lies during copulation.

hair c. A canal in the epidermis through which a new hair shaft erupts.

Haversian canals. The canals penetrating the compact substance of bone in a longitudinal direction and anastomosing with one another by transverse or oblique branches. They contain blood vessels and connective tissue.

hemal c. The ventral of two canals of which the vertebrate animal is composed. It contains the heart and the other viscera, while the neural canal encloses the central nervous system.

hernial c. A canal giving passage to a hernia.

Huguier's c. See *iter chordae anterius.* See also Pierre Charles *Huguier.*

hyaloid c. A canal running posteroanteriorly through the vitreous through which, in the fetus, the hyaloid artery passes to ramify on the posterior surface of the crystalline lens. Formerly called *Cloquet's c.*

hypoglossal c. The anterior condyloid canal. See condylar *c.*

incisive c. The bifurcated bony passage from the floor of the nasal cavity to the incisive fossa. On each side, the branches open by a median and a lateral incisive foramen transmitting respectively the nasopalatine nerve and a branch of the greater palatine artery.

infraorbital c. A canal running obliquely through the bony floor of the orbit; it gives passage to the infraorbital artery and nerve.

inguinal c. A canal about one and one-half inches long, running obliquely downward and medially from the abdominal to the subcutaneous inguinal ring; the channel through which an inguinal hernia descends; it gives passage to the ilioinguinal nerve and to the spermatic cord in the male and to the round ligament of the uterus in the female.

intestinal c. The portion of the gastrointestinal tract extending from the pylorus to the anus.

lacrimal c. The nasolacrimal canal.

mandibular c. See alveolar *c.*

maxillary c. See alveolar *c.*

medullary c. The cavity of a long bone, containing the marrow.

membranous cochlear c. The cochlear duct.

membranous semicircular canals. That portion of the membranous labyrinth of the ear consisting of three loop-shaped tubes lying at right angles to one another and communicating with the utricle. The **superior** (*frontal*) **semicircular canal** and the **posterior** (*sagittal*) **semicircular canal** lie in the vertical plane, making a right angle which opens laterally. The **lateral** or **horizontal canal** lies in the horizontal plane. Syn., *semicircular ducts.*

musculotubal canals. The semicanals in the temporal bone which transmit the auditory tube and tensor tympani muscle considered together.

nasal c. (a) See nasolacrimal *c.* (b) An occasional canal found in the posterior portion of the nasal bone; it gives passage to the nasal nerves.

nasolacrimal c. The bony canal that lodges the nasolacrimal duct.

nasopalatine c. One of a pair of passages from the floor of the nasal cavities to the roof of the mouth, patent in most mammals but vestigial and normally occluded in man.

neural c. *In embryology,* syn. for vertebral *c.*

neurenteric c. See notochordal *c.*

notochordal c. A canal formed by a continuation of the primitive pit into the head process of mammals. It perforates the entoderm and opens into the yolk sac, thus forming a temporary connection between yolk sac and amnion. Syn., *blastoporic c., neurenteric c.*

nutritive canals. See *Haversian canals* under *canal.*

obstetric c. See parturient *c.*

obturator c. A gap in the obturator membrane which closes the obturator foramen in the hipbone; it gives passage to the obturator nerve and vessels.

olfactory canals. In the embryo, the nasal cavities at an early period of development.

omphalomesenteric c. In the embryo, a canal that connects the cavity of the intestine with the yolk sac.

optic c. In the embryo, the canal in the optic stalk.

orbital c. See ethmoid *c.*

osseous cochlear c. The bony canal in which the cochlear duct is housed.

osseous semicircular canals. That part of the bony labyrinth of the ear which houses the membranous semicircular canals: three loop-shaped canals in the petrous portion of the temporal bone, the **superior semicircular canal,** the **posterior semicircular canal,** and the **lateral** or **horizontal semicircular canal.** They lie at right angles to one another and communicate with the osseous vestibule. See Plate 20.

palatine canals. Canals in the palate bone, giving passage to branches of the descending palatine nerve and artery. The **greater palatine canal** is a continuation of the pterygopalatine canal. The **smaller palatine canals** branch from the greater palatine canal and open separately.

parturient c. The channel through which the fetus passes in parturition; the cavities of the uterus and vagina, considered as a single canal. Also called *birth c.*

pelvic c. The cavity of the true pelvis from inlet to outlet.

peritoneal c. The vaginal process.

pharyngeal c. A passage between the vaginal process of the sphenoid bone and the sphenoidal process of the palatine bone for the transmission of pharyngeal branches from the sphenopalatine ganglion and artery.

pharyngotracheal c. A narrow opening in the solid dorsal epithelium of the embryonic larynx which enlarges to form the cavity of the larynx.

pharyngotympanic c. The auditory tube.

pleural c. A narrow coelomic passage on either side of the mesentery dorsal to the transverse septum that connects pericardial and general coelom; it later develops into the pleural cavity.

pleuroperitoneal c. A dorsomedian opening between embryonic pleural and peritoneal cavities before closure by the pleuroperitoneal membrane.

portal c. An interlobular artery, vein, bile duct, nerve and lymph vessel, and the interlobular connective tissue in which they lie, between the corners of the anatomic lobules of the liver.

primitive c. The vertebral canal of the embryo.

pterygoid c. One in the sphenoid bone at the base of the medial pterygoid plate; it opens anteriorly into the pterygopalatine fossa. Also called *Vidian canal.*

pterygopalatine c. The connection between the pterygopalatine fossa and the mouth; it gives passage to the palatine nerves and vessels. Its inferior opening is the greater palatine foramen.

pudendal c. A passage within the inferior fascia of the obturator internus muscle for the transmission of the pudendal nerve and internal pudendal vessels: also called *Alcock's c.*

pyloric c. See *pylorus,* 3.

root c. of teeth. The cavity within the root of a tooth, occupied by pulp, nerves, and vessels.

sacculocochlear c. The ductus reuniens.

sacral c. The continuation of the vertebral canal in the sacrum.

Schlemm's c. An irregular space or plexiform series of spaces at the sclerocorneal junction in the eye. It drains the aqueous humor from the anterior chamber.

semicircular canals. (a) The osseous semicircular canals. See Plate 20. (b) The membranous semicircular canals.

sheathing c. The upper end of the vaginal process; it normally closes, leaving the lower end a closed sac, the tunica vaginalis.

spinal c. The vertebral canal.

spiral c. of the cochlea. (a) The osseous cochlear canal. (b) The cochlear duct. Also called *Rosenthal's canal.*

spiral c. of the modiolus. An irregular cavity of the bone extending along the line of attachment of the osseous spiral lamina to the modiolus; it lodges the spiral ganglion. Also called *canalis ganglionaris*.
suborbital c. The infraorbital canal.
subsartorial c. The adductor canal.
Sucquet-Hoyer c. The afferent arteriole of a glomus. It has a thick wall and a narrow lumen.
supraorbital c. One at the upper margin of the orbit, giving passage to the supraorbital nerve and vessels.
urogenital c. *In embryology*, one formed by the union of the embryonic urogenital sinus and the penile portion of the urethra. Also called *phallic urethra*.
uterine c. Cavity of the uterus, both of the body and cervix.
uterocervical c. Cavity of the cervix of the uterus.
uterovaginal c. (a) The common canal formed by the uterus and vagina. (b) *In embryology*, the single cavity formed by fusion of the paramesonephric ducts.
vaginal c. Canal of the vagina.
vertebral c. One formed by the foramens of the vertebrae; it contains the spinal cord and its meninges. Also called *spinal c.*, *neural c.* (in embryology).
vesicourethral c. That part of the primitive urogenital sinus, cranial to the openings of the mesonephric ducts, which develops into the bladder and primary urethra. Also called *vesicourethral anlage*.
Vidian c. The pterygoid canal.
Volkmann's canals. In compact bone, those vascular channels which lack the concentric lamellae of Haversian systems. The term is commonly erroneously applied to nutrient canals in compact bone, whether Haversian or Volkmann's.
zygomatico-orbital c. A canal or canals in the orbital process of the zygomatic bone for the passage of the zygomaticofacial and zygomaticotemporal branches of the zygomatic nerve.

can″a·lic′u·li (kan″uh·lick′yoo·lye). Plural of canaliculus.

can·al·ic″u·lo·plas′ty [L. *canaliculus*, small channel; G. *plassein*, to form]. Plastic repair of a canaliculus, especially that leading from the punctum to the lacrimal sac.

can″a·lic′u·lus (pl. *canaliculi*) [L., small channel]. 1. A small canal; especially that leading from the punctum lacrimale to the lacrimal sac of the eye. 2. Any one of the minute canals opening into the lacunas of bone. —**canalicular,** *adj.*; **canaliculiza′tion,** *n.*
accessory canaliculi. Inconstant canals at the outer edge of the anterior condyloid foramen giving passage to veins.
bile canaliculi. The intercellular channels in hepatic cords that convey bile toward the interlobular bile ducts.
canaliculi vasculosi. Old term for the Haversian canals.
c. chordae tympani. One in the petrous portion of the temporal bone for the passage of the chorda tympani.
innominate c. A small inconstant canal in the great wing of the sphenoid, which, when present, transmits the lesser superficial petrosal nerve: also called *foramen innominate*.
intracellular canaliculi. A system of fine canaliculi within certain gland cells which apparently drain their secretion, as those of the parietal cells of the gastric glands.
lacrimal canaliculi. A superior and inferior one; each extends from its lacrimal punctum to the sac to which it conveys tears: also called *lacrimal duct*.
mastoid c. One opening just above the stylomastoid foramen, giving passage to the auricular branch of the vagus nerve.
secretory canaliculi. Fine, intercellular canaliculi formed by grooves in adjoining gland cells, draining the secretion of the cells, and opening into the lumen of the gland. Also called *secretory capillaries*.
tympanic c. One that opens on the lower surface of the petrous portion of the temporal bone between the carotid canal and the jugular fossa. It gives passage to the tympanic branch of the glossopharyngeal nerve.

ca·na′lis (ka·nay′lis, ka·nal′is). See *canal*.

ca·nal″i·za′tion (ka·nal″i·zay′shun, kan″ul·i·zay′shun, kan″ul·eye·zay′shun) [L. *canalis*, channel]. 1. The formation of new channels in tissues, as the formation of new blood vessels in a thrombus. 2. A system of wound drainage without tubes.

can″al·og′ra·phy. Radiographic visualization of the spinal canal by epidural injection. A solution of contrast material containing water-soluble iodine is injected in the sacral hiatus and radiographs are made. The opaque material is absorbed by the epidural venous plexus and is excreted by the kidneys.

Canano, Giovanni Battista [*Italian anatomist*, 1515–79]. A great figure in the history of anatomy. Described the valves of the veins.

canary yellow. Auramine O.

Can″a·va′li·a [NL.]. A genus of tropical herbs having long pods with seeds or beans, which are used as a source of urease. The plant or the seed thereof is known as jack bean.

can″a·va′lin. A globulin found in jack beans, the seeds of *Canavalia*.

can·av′a·nine. $NH_2.C(:NH).NH.O.CH_2.CH_2.CH(NH_2)COOH$; an amino acid from jack beans; it is a potent inhibitor of L-arginine, as tested on various bacteria.

can′cel·late, can′cel·lat″ed. See *cancellous*.

can′cel·lous [L. *cancelli*, lattice]. Characterized by reticulated or latticed structure, as the spongy tissue of bones or, in botany, certain leaves consisting largely of veins. Syn., *cancellate, cancellated*. —**cancella′tion,** *n.*

can′cer [L., crab]. Any malignant tumor, including carcinoma and sarcoma; formerly a synonym of carcinoma.
alveolar (cell) c. See bronchiolar *carcinoma*.
black c. See *melanoma*.
Bowen's c. See Bowen's *disease*.
c. en cuirasse. Widely infiltrating carcinoma of the skin of the thorax, usually arising in mammary carcinoma; also applied to widespread carcinoma of the pleura.
c. of the lung. Bronchogenic carcinoma.
c. milk. A milky fluid which can be expressed or scraped from a cross section of certain carcinomas, especially those of the mammary gland.
c. nest. A small group of cells of carcinoma.
c. occultus. Carcinoma identified first by the appearance of metastasis.
claypipe c. Carcinoma of the lip and tongue, presumably due to the stem of the clay pipe. See smoker's *c.*
conjugal c. Cancer in both husband and wife, occurring simultaneously or successively. Almost certainly not due to conjugal transmission.
contact c. One occurring on a surface, as the lip, which has been in contact with a cancer of the

opposing surface. Rare and not proved to be due to direct implantation.

disseminated c. See under *carcinoma.*

dye workers' c. A carcinoma of the urinary bladder found among aniline-dye workers.

erysipeloid c. See inflammatory *carcinoma.*

"kangri basket" c. A nonmetastasizing squamous-cell carcinoma of the abdominal skin occurring in Kashmir and Tibet where people warm the belly by means of a basket of hot coals.

lobular c. See lobular *carcinoma.*

mule spinners' c. An epidermoid carcinoma of scrotum or vulva, occurring in textile workers and presumably due to exposure to machine oils.

osteolytic c. Metastasis of cancer in bone with destruction of bone.

osteoplastic c. Metastasis of cancer in bone which stimulates new production of bone in the immediate neighborhood.

Paget's c. See Paget's *disease,* (b).

primary c. An original malignant tumor as contrasted with a metastatic, or secondary, cancer.

radiation, radiologist c. See under *carcinoma.*

smoker's c. Squamous-cell carcinoma of the lip, usually the lower lip, observed in habitual smokers.

tar c. An epidermoid carcinoma associated with prolonged exposure to tar.

can″cer·o′gen. Any substance (or ray) which, applied in adequate quantity to a disposed individual, is apt either to produce cancer or to speed up its appearance, or which, acting upon a group, changes the group's total cancer-frequency, or at least the distribution of primary tumors by site and age. —**cancerogen′ic, cancerigen′ic,** *adj.*

can″cer·ol′o·gist [*cancer;* G. *logos,* word]. A cancer specialist.

can″cer·ol′o·gy [*cancer; logos*]. Study and science of cancer.

can″cer·o·pho′bi·a, can″cer·pho′bi·a [*cancer;* G. *phobos,* fear]. Morbid fear of acquiring a cancer.

can′croid [*cancer;* G. *eidos,* form]. An epidermoid carcinoma. —**can′croid,** *adj.*

can′crum o′ris. Canker of the mouth. Old term for gangrenous stomatitis.

can″di·ci′din. An antibiotic with antifungal properties in vitro.

Can′di·da [L. *candidus,* white]. A genus of yeastlike, pathogenic microorganisms.

C. albicans. A species of considerable importance which produces thrush and other types of moniliasis. Also called *Monilia albicans.*

can″di·did′. A secondary eruption characterized by sterile, grouped, vesicular lesions; a result of hypersensitivity and hematogenous spread from the primary focus which is caused by *Candida:* called *monilid.*

can·did′u·lin. An antibiotic substance, possibly $C_{11}H_{15}NO_3$, derived from *Aspergillus candidus;* it possesses some activity against many organisms but is inactivated by whole blood.

can′di·ru [Pg., from Tupi *candérú*]. Minute catfish of South America, which enters the urethra of unprotected bathers.

can′dle [L. *candela,* a light]. The unit of intensity of light, one-sixtieth of the intensity of 1 square centimeter of a perfect radiator.

ca·nel′la [ML., dim. of *canna,* a reed]. The bark of *Canella winterana,* native to the West Indies, dried and without the cork layer. It is called white cinnamon and is an aromatic tonic and bitter stomachic.

ca′nine [L. *canis,* dog]. 1. Relating to, resembling dogs. 2. Pertaining to the sharp tearing teeth of mammals, located between the incisors and the premolars.

ca′nine. A canine tooth.

ca·ni′nus. A muscle of facial expression arising above the canine tooth. See Table of Muscles in the Appendix.

ca·ni′ti·es (ka·nish′ee·eez) [L.]. Poliosis; hoariness; grayness or whiteness of the hair.

c. unguium. White spots, streaks, or bands of the nails.

can′ker [L. *cancer,* a crab]. 1. An ulceration, especially one of the mouth and lips; also a festering or gangrenous ulcer, as noma, gangrenous stomatitis. 2. Aphthous stomatitis; thrush. 3. *In veterinary medicine,* a disease of the horn-forming membrane of horse's hoofs, leading to destruction of the cells and loss of the horn-secreting function.

can′ker·root″. Coptis.

can″na·bid′i·ol [G. *kannabis,* hemp]. A constituent of cannabis which, on isomerization to a tetrahydrocannabinol, exhibits to a great degree the activity of cannabis.

can′na·bin, can′na·bine (kan′uh·bean, ·bin) [*kannabis*]. A resinous substance from Indian hemp; it is hypnotic but is no longer used medicinally.

can·nab′in·ol [*kannabis*]. A substance resulting from the spontaneous dehydrogenation of tetrahydrocannabinol in cannabis. Though commonly considered physiologically inactive, cannabinol recently has been demonstrated to possess some of the characteristic activity of cannabis.

can·nab′i·non, can·nab′i·none [*kannabis*]. An amorphous bitter resinoid from cannabis, formerly used as hypnotic.

can′na·bis [*kannabis*]. Hemp. The flowering tops of the pistillate plants of *Cannabis sativa,* of which there are two varieties, Indian and American, the former being the more potent. The active constituents appear to be tetrahydrocannabinols. Cannabis is antispasmodic and narcotic. In large doses it produces mental exaltation, intoxication, and a sensation of double consciousness. It is important as an intoxicant, but has no rational therapeutic use. *Bang, bhang, gunjah, charas, churrus, hashish,* and *marihuana* are among the various names by which the drug is known.

can′na·bism [*kannabis*]. Poisoning resulting from excessive or habitual use of cannabis.

can′na·bol [*kannabis*]. A constituent of cannabis; it is believed to be an isomer of cannabidiol.

can″ni·bal·is′tic [Carib *calina*]. Pertaining to the eating of human flesh, an impulse sometimes observed in psychotics.

Cannon, Walter Bradford (1871–1945). American physiologist, renowned as one of the great physiologists of his time. He demonstrated that hunger pains are due to cramplike contractions of the stomach (1912). With Binger and Fitz he showed that exophthalmic goiter could be produced artificially (1915). He was one of the first to produce evidence for the connection between bodily changes and emotional states as pain, hunger, fear, and rage (1915), and demonstrated that under certain conditions of physiological stress the sympathetic nervous system and the adrenal medulla produced visceral adjustments adapted to the preservation of the organism (fight-flight mechanism). This led to his concept of homeostasis, an extension of Claude Bernard's theory of the constancy of the *milieu interieur.* He pioneered in the field of chemical mediation of nerve impulses, and is credited with the discovery of sympathin (1931) and the establishment of the law of denervation. His book, *The Wisdom of the Body,* describing bodily mechanisms for homeostasis, is a classic in modern physiology.

can′non bone. One of the functional and complete

metacarpal or metatarsal bones of a hoofed quadruped, supporting the weight of the body upon the feet.

can′nu·la [L., dim. of *canna*, a reed]. An artificial tube often fitted with a trocar for insertion into a tube or cavity of the body, as an artery or the trachea. Clinically, numerous cannulas of various sizes and shapes have been devised for specific uses. —**cannular, cannulate,** *adj.*

perfusion c. A double cannula, one tube of which is used for the inflow of a fluid, the other for its escape; used in irrigating a cavity.

Cantani, Arnoldo [*Italian physician,* 1837–93]. Introduced an exclusive meat diet for diabetes, called *Cantani's diet.* Proposed a treatment for cholera consisting of injection into the rectum of large quantities of water containing tannic acid and opium; called *Cantani's treatment.*

cantaxin. Trade-mark for a brand of ascorbic acid.

can″tha·ri′a·sis [G. *kantharis,* a kind of beetle—probably blister beetle; NL. *-iasis,* condition]. The presence in the body of coleopterous insects or their larvae.

can·thar′i·date [*kantharis*]. Any salt of cantharidic acid.

can·thar′i·des (kan·thar′i·deez) [*kantharis*]. The dried insects, *Cantharis vesicatoria,* yielding not less than 0.6% cantharidin. Locally applied, cantharides is rubefacient and vesicant; internally, it is irritant, causing pain and vomiting. In toxic doses it produces severe gastroenteritis, strangury, and priapism. —**cantharidal, cantharidic,** *adj.*

c. cerate (*ceratum cantharidis*). An unction, containing 35% cantharides, used as vesicant.

c. plaster (*emplastrum cantharidis*). Cantharides cerate spread on plaster backing.

can·thar′i·dic ac′id (kan·thar′i·dick, kan″thuh-rid′ick). $C_{10}H_{14}O_5$. A cyclohexanedicarboxylic acid derivative; the hydrated form of cantharidin.

can·thar′i·din. $C_{10}H_{12}O_4$. The crystallizable, active principle contained in cantharides and other insects. Chemically, it is the anhydride of cantharidic acid.

can·thar′i·dism [*kantharis*]. Cantharidal poisoning. When caused by absorption from a cantharidal blister, it is called *external cantharidism.*

can′tha·ris. Singular of cantharides.

can·thec′to·my [G. *kanthos,* corner of the eye; *ektomē,* excision]. Excision of a canthus.

can·thi′tis [*kanthos;* G. *-itis,* inflammation]. Inflammation of a canthus.

can′tho-, canth- [*kanthos*]. A combining form denoting *canthal.*

can·thol′y·sis [*kanthos;* G. *lysis,* a loosing]. Canthotomy with section of the lateral palpebra ligament.

can′tho·plas″ty [*kanthos;* G. *plassein,* to form]. Increasing the length of the palpebral fissure by slitting the outer canthus. Also, any plastic restoration of a canthal defect.

can·thor′rha·phy [*kanthos;* G. *rhaphē,* a suture]. *In plastic surgery,* shortening of the palpebral fissure by suture of the canthus.

can·thot′o·my [*kanthos;* G. *tomē,* a cutting]. Surgical division of a canthus.

can′thus [*kanthos*]. Either of the two angles formed by the junction of the eyelids, designated outer or lateral, and inner or medial; palpebral angle. —**canthal,** *adj.*

CaOC Cathodal opening contraction.

caou′tchouc (kōō′chook) [F. from Tupi Indian *caú-uchú*]. Rubber. The terpene hydrocarbon substance dispersed in the milky juice that exudes upon incision of a number of tropical trees belonging to the families Euphorbiaceae, Artocarpaceae, and Apocynaceae. When pure, caoutchouc is nearly white, soft, elastic, and glutinous; it is soluble in organic solvents.

cap [AS. *caeppe,* from LL. *cappa*]. 1. A covering or coverlike organ; a tegmen. 2. *In dentistry,* a substance or structure designed to cover an exposed pulp.

abduction c. An orthopedic appliance of canvas or leather to maintain abduction in cases of subdeltoid bursitis.

c. of Zinn. X-ray shadow caused by patent ductus arteriosus (dilatation of the pulmonary artery proximal to ductus and dilatation of the conus arteriosus of the right ventricle).

cradle c. Seborrhea capitis seen in infants, perhaps a limited form of atopic dermatitis.

duodenal c. The first part of the duodenum, immediately beyond the pylorus. From radiographic appearance, it is called bishop's cap. Syn., *duodenal bulb.*

Dutch c. A contraceptive device to cover the cervix.

enamel c. The enamel covering the top of a growing dental papilla.

head c. The cap enclosing the sperm nucleus. It results from the fusion of the **anterior head cap** (the acrosome, especially the peripheral zone of the acrosome) and the **postnuclear head cap.**

knee c. Patella.

nuclear c. A small mass of chromophilic matter on one side of a cell nucleus.

phrygean c. The x-ray appearance of the gallbladder where kinking exists between the fundus and the body.

skull c. (a) Cranium. (b) Calvaria.

cap. 1. *Capiat;* let him take. 2. *Capsula;* a capsule.

ca·pac′i·tance (ka·pas′i·tunss) [L. *capax,* capacious]. The quantity of electricity which a condenser or other structure can hold per volt of electric pressure applied.

ca·pac′i·tor (ka·pas′i·tur) [*capax*]. An instrument for holding or storing charges of electricity; condenser.

ca·pac′i·ty [L. *capacitas,* capacity]. 1. The power of receiving, containing, holding, or absorbing. 2. Cubic volume. 3. Mental ability to acquire and hold knowledge, accomplish, or understand. 4. Physical ability to perform muscular work; maximum output. —**capacitate,** *v.t.*

cranial c. Volume of the cranial cavity.

electric c. (a) The amount of electricity a condenser can hold. (b) The amount of electricity that can be delivered under specific conditions, as by a battery or generator. (c) Maximum output of a generator. (d) Capacitance.

functional residual c. The amount of air remaining in the lungs after an involuntary expiration at any level of activity. It includes both the expiratory reserve volume and residual volume, and is important physiologically because it is the amount of air with which each tidal volume must be mixed.

heat c. See thermal *c.*

inspiratory c. That amount of air which can be inhaled after a normal expiration.

maximum breathing c. The greatest amount of air which can be voluntarily breathed during a 10–30-second period, and expressed as liters of air per minute. It is a test of many factors, including patient cooperation, his physical state, and muscular function. Adequately performed it is a reliable test of the ventilatory capacity of the thoracic bellows. Abbreviated, MBC.

"neutralization" c. The capacity of the skin surface to neutralize acids or alkali with which it comes in contact, thought by some to be related to sensitivity in contracting contact dermatitides.

pulmonary diffusing c. The number of milliliters of a gas transferred across the alveolar-capillary membrane per minute per millimeter difference in partial pressure of the gas in the alveolar air and capillary blood.

respiratory c. (a) Vital capacity. (b) The ability of the blood to combine with oxygen from the lungs, and with the carbon dioxide from the tissues.

testamentary c. *In medical jurisprudence,* the mental ability requisite to make a valid will.

thermal c. The amount of heat necessary to raise the temperature of a body from 15° to 16° C.

vital c. The volume of air that can be expelled from the lungs by the most forcible expiration after the deepest inspiration. It is the maximum stroke volume of the thoracic pump and is affected by any factor restricting either the amount of filling or emptying of the lungs. A **timed vital capacity** is a measure of rate of emptying of the lungs and aids greatly in determining the maximum ventilatory capacity. A normal individual can exhale three-fourths or more of his vital capacity in one second.

Capgras, Jean Marie Joseph (1873–1950) French psychiatrist, who with Paul Sérieux described a psychotic manifestation in which the subject fails to identify an individual but recognizes his appearance and behavior as familiar: called *Capgras' syndrome.*

cap″il·lar″ec·ta′si·a (kap″i·lar″eck·tay′zhuh, ·zee·uh, ·shuh, ·see·uh) [L. *capillaris,* from *capillus,* hair; G. *ektasis,* stretching out]. Dilatation of the capillaries.

cap″il·la·rim′e·ter [*capillaris;* G. *metron,* a measure]. A device for estimating the diameter of capillary tubes.

cap″il·lar′i·ty [*capillaris*]. Capillary attraction; elevation or depression of liquids in capillary tubes.

cap″il·la·ros′co·py, cap″il·lar″i·os′co·py [*capillaris;* G. *skopein,* to examine]. Microscopic examination of the cutaneous capillaries for diagnosis.

cap′il·lar″y (kap′i·lerr″ee) [*capillaris*]. Hairlike; relating to a hair, to a hairlike filament, or to a tube with a minute bore.

cap′il·lar″y. A minute blood vessel connecting the smallest ramifications of the arteries with those of the veins or one of the smallest lymph vessels.

arterial c. See *precapillary.*

c. fragility. Weakness of the capillaries, as in purpura.

c. respirometry. Measurement or determination of changes in the volume of gases in a capillary tube which leads from a chamber filled with a respiring sample to a chamber containing only media and reagents. The capillary tube contains an index droplet, the displacement of which serves to determine the changes in gas volume.

venous c. The terminal part of a capillary network, opening into a venule; a postcapillary.

cap″il·li′ti·um (kap″i·lish′ee·um) [L., the hair]. Protoplasmic threads forming a network in the spore capsule of *Myxomycetes.*

cap″il·lo·ve′nous [L. *capillus,* hair; *vena,* vein]. 1. Pertaining to a junctional vessel between a capillary and a venule. 2. Pertaining to the capillaries and first subpapillary venous plexus of the skin.

ca·pil′lus [L.]. A hair; specifically, a hair of the head.

cap′i·tate [L. *capitatus,* from *caput,* head]. 1. *In biology,* having a head or a headlike termination; head-shaped. 2. See Table of Bones, Appendix.

cap″i·ta′tum [*capitatus*]. The large bone of the wrist; the os magnum.

cap″i·tel′lum [L., dim. of *caput*]. A small head or rounded process of bone.

ca·pit′u·lum [L., dim. of *caput*]. A small head or small, bony eminence. —**capitular,** *adj.*

c. costae [BNA]. Head of a rib.

c. fibulae [BNA]. Proximal end of the fibula, articulating with the tibial lateral condyle.

c. humeri [BNA]. Radial head of the humerus.

c. mandibulae [BNA]. Posterior or articulating process of the lower jaw.

c. ossis metacarpalis. [BNA] The head of any of the metacarpal bones.

c. ossis metatarsalis. [BNA] The head of any of the metatarsal bones.

c. radii [BNA]. Disklike proximal head of the radius.

c. Santorinii. A small elevation at the apex of the arytenoid cartilage.

c. stapedis [BNA]. Articular head of the stapes.

c. ulnae [BNA]. Distal end or head of the ulna.

Capivaccio, Girolamo (Hieronymus Capivaccius) [*Italian surgeon,* d. 1589]. One of the first to describe gastric ulcer with malignant changes; called *Capivaccius' ulcer.*

capped hock. *In veterinary medicine,* the formation of a hygroma at the point of the hock in the horse, the result of continued irritation.

Capps's pleural reflex. See under *reflex.*

cap′rate. Any salt or ester of capric acid.

cap′re·o·late [L. *capreolus,* a tendril]. Resembling tendrils, furnished with tendrils. *Obs.*

ca′pri- [L. *caper,* goat]. A combining form meaning *goat.*

cap′ric ac′id. $CH_3(CH_2)_8COOH$. A solid fatty acid occurring as a glyceride in butter and other animal fats.

ca·pril′o·quism, ca·pri·lo′qui·um [*caper;* L. *loqui,* to speak]. Egophony.

ca·pro′ic ac′id. $CH_3(CH_2)_4COOH$. A liquid fatty acid occurring as a glyceride in butter and other animal fats.

caprokol. Trade-mark for a brand of hexylresorcinol.

cap′ro·ate. Any salt or ester of caproic acid.

cap′ro·in. Any of the caproic acid esters of glycerin.

cap′ryl·ate. Any salt or ester of caprylic acid.

ca·pryl′ic ac′id. $CH_3(CH_2)_6COOH$. A solid fatty acid occurring in butter, coconut oil, and other fats and oils. The sodium salt promises to be an effective agent for treating dermatomycosis of the feet.

cap·sa′i·cin. The vanillylamide of isodecenoic acid, the most important constituent of capsicum. See *capsicum.*

cap·san′thin [L. *capsa,* box]. A carotenoid pigment, $C_{40}H_{58}O$, in capsicum.

cap′si·cin [NL. *capsicum,* from *capsa*]. A resinous, fatty mixture, believed to be the active principle of capsicum.

cap′si·cum [*capsa*]. The dried fruit of *Capsicum frutescens* (bush red pepper) or of several other varieties (tabasco or Louisiana long or short peppers). Its characteristic pungent constituent is capsaicin, an extremely acrid substance; used internally as tonic and carminative, externally to produce counterirritation. Also called *Cayenne pepper, red pepper.*

c. ointment (*unguentum capsici*). It contains 5% of capsicum oleoresin; used as a counterirritant.

c. oleoresin (*oleoresina capsici*). An acetone or ether extract of the active principles of capsicum from which the solvent has been evaporated.

cap′su·la. See *capsule.*

cap′sule [L. *capsula,* small box]. 1. A membranous investment of a part. 2. An envelope surrounding certain organisms. 3. A soluble shell for administering medicines. 4. *In physiology*, an instrument used for the optical recording of pressure changes or vibrations, as pressure pulses or heart sounds. It consists of a cylindrical chamber closed on one end by a thin membrane to which is glued a small mirror. Pressure changes cause movement of the membrane and deflections of a beam of light which is reflected to a photokymograph. —**capsular,** *adj.*

acoustic c. See otic *c.*

adipose c. See *c.* of the kidney.

articular c. See joint *c.*

auditory c. See otic *c.*

Bowman's c. See glomerular *c.*

brood capsules. Stalked vesicles which develop from the germinative epithelium of a hydatid cyst. These brood capsules may detach from the mother cyst, become enlarged and produce brood capsules and scolices within themselves to form daughter cysts.

c. of a nerve cell. That portion of the neurilemma which covers a ganglion cell.

c. of the eyeball. The fascial envelope of the eyeball.

c. of the kidney. The fat-containing connective tissue encircling the kidney. It consists of an inner fibrous capsule and an outer adipose capsule (the perirenal fat).

c. of the lens. A transparent, structureless membrane enclosing the lens of the eye.

cartilage c. The matrix next to or near a lacuna.

cell c. A thick or unusually strong cell wall.

crystalline c. See *c.* of the lens.

external c. A layer of white nerve fibers forming part of the external boundary of the lenticular nucleus.

extreme c. A layer of white matter separating the claustrum from the insula.

Glisson's c. The coarse stroma of the liver that accompanies the vessels and bile ducts.

glomerular c. The sac surrounding the glomerulus of the kidney; the first part of the uriniferous tubule. Also called *Bowman's c.*

glutoid capsules. Gelatin capsules treated with formaldehyde.

hyaloid c. Limiting membrane of the vitreous body.

internal c. A layer of nerve fibers on the outer side of the thalamus and caudate nucleus, which it separates from the lenticular nucleus; it is continuous with the cerebral peduncles and the corona radiata and consists of fibers to and from the cerebral cortex.

joint c. The fibrous sheet enclosing a diarthrodial joint. See capsular *ligament.* See Plate 2.

Malpighian c. The commencement of the uriniferous tubule. *Obs.* See glomerular *c.*

nasal c. The cartilage around the embryonic nasal cavity.

olfactory c. See nasal *c.*

optic c. The embryonic structure forming the sclera.

otic c. The cartilage capsule that surrounds the developing auditory vesicle and later fuses with the sphenoidal and occipital cartilages.

periotic c. The structure surrounding the internal ear.

renal c. The capsule of the kidney.

segment c. A capsule used for the optical recording of pressure changes or vibrations, the cylindrical chamber being flattened on one side with a mirror pivoting on the chord of the circular membrane-covered surface. Also called *Frank's segment c.*

seminal c. Old term for the ampulla of the ductus deferens.

sense c. One of the cartilage capsules developing about the sense organs that form a part of the embryonic chondrocranium.

synovial c. See synovial *membrane.*

Tenon's c. The fascia of the eyeball.

cap″su·lec′to·my [*capsula;* G. *ektomē*, excision]. Surgical excision of a capsule.

cap″su·li′tis [*capsula;* G. *-itis*, inflammation]. Inflammation of a capsule, as that of the lens, liver (perihepatitis), or the labyrinth (otosclerosis).

adhesive c. See frozen *shoulder.*

cap′su·lo-, capsul- [*capsula*]. A combining form meaning *capsule*

cap′su·lo·plas″ty [*capsula;* G. *plassein*, to form]. Operation for plastic repair of a joint capsule.

cap″su·lor′rha·phy [*capsula;* G. *rhaphē*, a suture]. Suture of a capsule; especially suture of a joint capsule to repair a rent or to prevent dislocation.

cap′su·lo·tome″ [*capsula;* G. *tomos*, cutting]. 1. See *cystotome.* 2. Instrument used in capsulotomy of the crystalline lens.

cap″su·lot′o·my [*capsula;* G. *tomē*, a cutting]. The operation of incising the capsule of the crystalline lens in cataract operations, or a joint capsule.

renal c. Incision of the renal capsule.

cap·ta′tion [L. *captatio*, from *captare*, to seize]. The first or opening stage of hypnotism.

cap′ture. *In nuclear physics*, any process in which the nucleus of an atom acquires an additional elementary particle.

ca′put (kay′putt, kap′ut) [L.]. The head; also the chief part or beginning of an organ.

c. deformatum. See *osteochondritis deformans juvenilis.*

c. epididymidis. Head of the epididymis; the globus major.

c. galeatum. A child's head which emerges at birth covered with the caul, 1.

c. Medusae. The peculiar plexus of veins surrounding the umbilicus in portal obstruction of the liver. It represents collateral paths for the return of the venous blood from the abdominal viscera.

c. obstipum. Wryneck; torticollis.

c. quadratum. The rectangular head of rickets, flattened upon the top and at the sides, with projecting occiput and prominent frontal bosses.

c. succedaneum. A tumor composed of a serosanguineous infiltration of the connective tissue situated upon the presenting part of the fetus.

Carabelli, Georg [*Hungarian dentist*, 1787–1842]. Described a highly developed fifth cusp on the mesiolingual surface of upper molar teeth, always bilateral and usually hereditary, called *Carabelli cusp, tubercle.*

ca·ram′i·phen hy″dro·chlo′ride. Generic name for the hydrochloride of β-diethylaminoethyl-1-phenylcyclopentane-1-carboxylate, a drug possessing atropinelike action. See *panparnit.*

car′a·pace [F.]. A chitinous or bony shield covering the entire back or a portion of the back of certain lower animals.

ca·ra′te. See *pinta.*

car′a·way. See *carum.*

car′ba·chol (kahr′buh·coal, ·kol, ·kawl) (*carbacholum*). $NH_2.CO.O.CH_2.CH_2.N(CH_3)_3.Cl$. Carbamylcholine chloride, or carbaminoylcholine chloride. A synthetic choline derivative which is a potent parasympathomimetic and is effective orally. Used in peripheral vascular diseases, in threatened gangrene, in acute urinary retention following anesthesia or surgery or due to spinal-cord lesions. Dose, orally, 2 mg. (1/30 gr.) b.d. or t.i.d.; subcutaneously, 0.25–0.5 mg. (1/250–1/120 gr.). See *carcholin, doryl.*

car″ba·cryl′a·mine res′ins. The generic name for a combination of carbacrylic resin, potassium carbacrylate, and polyamine-methylene resin, the mixture being useful clinically for removal of sodium ion from intestinal fluid by processes of ion exchange with minimum or no disturbance of potassium-ion and hydrogen-ion equilibria. See *carbo-resin.*

car″ba·cryl′ic res′in. The generic name for the hydrogen form of cross-linked polyacrylic polycarboxylic cation exchange resins. Such a resin is useful clinically for its ability to remove sodium from intestinal fluid by a process of exchange with hydrogen in the resin; absorption of potassium by the resin is compensated for by inclusion of some potassium carbacrylate while the acidity resulting from liberation of hydrogen ion is neutralized with polyamine-methylene resin. See *carbacrylamine resins.*

car′ba·mate, car·bam′ate. A salt of carbamic acid; it contains the univalent radical, NH_2-COO—. See *ethyl* carbamate.

car·bam′ic ac′id. NH_2COOH. The mono-amide of carbonic acid existing only in the form of salts and esters, the latter known as urethanes.

car·bam′ide, car′ba·mide. Urea.

car·bam′i·dine (kahr·bam′i·deen, ·din). Guanidine.

car″ba·mi·no·he″mo·glo′bin. Hemoglobin united with carbon dioxide.

car·bam″i·no·yl·cho′line chlo′ride. Carbachol.

car″ba·myl·cho′line chlo′ride. Carbachol.

car′bar·sone (*carbarsonum*). $NH_2CO.NH.C_6H_4AsO(OH)_2$. A white powder containing from 28.1 to 28.8% of pentavalent arsenic, only slightly soluble in water or alcohol; used in the treatment of intestinal amebiasis either orally or, in resistant cases, by means of retention enemas. Adult dose, 0.25 Gm. (4 gr.). As a retention enema, 2 Gm. (30 gr.) dissolved in 200 cc. of warm 2% sodium bicarbonate solution. Also used in treatment of *Trichomonas vaginalis vaginitis.*

car′ba·sus [L., from G. *karpasos*, flax]. Gauze; thin muslin used in surgery. *O.T.*

c. absorbens. Absorbent gauze.

c. absorbens adhaesivus. Adhesive absorbent gauze.

c. absorbens sterilis. Sterile absorbent gauze.

c. carbolata. Carbolized gauze.

c. iodoformata. Iodoform gauze.

car″ba·zin·am′ide. See *semicarbazide.*

car″ba·zot′ic ac′id. Trinitrophenol.

carb·he″mo·glo′bin, car″bo·he″mo·glo′bin (·hee″mo·glo′bin, ·hem″o·glo′bin). Carbaminohemoglobin.

car′bi·nol. 1. Methyl alcohol. 2. The univalent radical, —CH_2OH, characteristic of primary alcohols. 3. A generic term for the primary alcohols; i.e., alcohols having the general formula $R.CH_2OH$, where R represents an organic radical.

dimethyl c. Isopropyl alcohol.

carbitol. 1. Trade-mark for diethylene glycol monoethyl ether, $C_2H_5OCH_2CH_2OCH_2CH_2OH$: used principally as a solvent. It injures the liver and kidneys. 2. Trade-mark for various ethers of diethylene glycol, the specific ether being indicated by a qualifying adjective, such as methyl or butyl.

car′bo [L.]. See *charcoal; carbon.*

car′bo-, carb- [L. *carbo*, coal]. A combining form signifying *carbon.*

car″bo·cy′clic (kahr″bo·sigh′click, ·sick′lick). *In chemistry*, pertaining to compounds of the closed-chain type in which all the ring atoms are carbon. See *heterocyclic, homocyclic.*

car″bo·he″mo·glo′bin. See *carbhemoglobin.*

car″bo·hy′drase. An enzyme capable of converting the higher carbohydrates into simple sugars. See Table of Enzymes in the Appendix.

car″bo·hy′drate [*carbo;* G. *hydōr*, water]. An organic substance belonging to the class of compounds represented by the sugars, dextrins, starches, and celluloses; it contains carbon, hydrogen, and oxygen. Formerly it was believed that the hydrogen and oxygen were always present in the proportion found in water; but this is not always the case. The carbohydrates form a large class of organic compounds; they may be further classified into monosaccharides, disaccharides, trisaccharides, tetrasaccharides, and polysaccharides.

car″bo·hy″dra·tu′ri·a [*carbo; hydōr;* G. *ouron*, urine]. Presence of an abnormally large proportion of carbohydrates in the urine; glycosuria.

car′bo·late. Phenate.

car′bo·late. To impregnate with phenol.

car·bol′ic ac′id. Phenol.

camphorated c. a. A mixture of 3 parts of phenol, 6 parts of camphor, and liquid petrolatum to 10 parts. Used as antiseptic and local anesthetic.

iodized c. a. A solution of 20 parts of iodine in 76 parts of phenol and 4 parts of glycerin. Used as an antiseptic and escharotic.

car″bo·li′gase. An enzyme found in animal and plant tissue which converts pyruvic acid to acetylmethylcarbinol.

car′bo·lism. Phenol poisoning.

car′bo·lized oil. Phenolated oil.

car″bo·lu′ri·a [*carbo;* L. *oleum*, oil; G. *ouron*, urine]. Presence of carbolic acid (phenol) in the urine, producing a dark discoloration.

car″bol·xy′lene (kahr″bol·zy′leen). A mixture of phenol, one part, and xylene, three parts; used for clearing sections for microscopy.

car″bo·my′cin. Generic name for the antibiotic substance, available under the trade-mark *magnamycin*, produced by selected strains of *Streptomyces halstedii.* The antibiotic possesses inhibitory activity especially against Gram-positive bacteria, and is also active against certain rickettsiae and large viruses. It may be used to treat infections caused by sensitive bacteria in patients who have become resistant to penicillin and other antibiotics; it is readily absorbed from the gastrointestinal tract.

car′bon [*carbo*]. C = 12.011. A nonmetallic element widely distributed in nature. Its three allotropic forms are exemplified by the diamond, graphite, and charcoal. It occurs in all organic compounds; the ability of its atoms to link to each other affords an innumerable variety of combinations.

c. bisulfide. See *c.* disulfide.

c. black. Finely divided carbon obtained by the incomplete combustion of natural gas, animal tissues, oils, wood, or other organic substances.

c. dioxide (*carbonei dioxidum*). CO_2. An odorless, colorless gas which neither burns nor supports combustion. It is useful as a respiratory stimulant when there is an insufficiency of carbon dioxide in the system. *Carbon dioxide snow*, or dry ice, is solid carbon dioxide used medicinally as an escharotic and commercially as a refrigerant. Also called *carbonic acid gas.* See *carbonic acid.* Also see Table of Normal Values of Blood Constituents, Appendix.

c. disulfide. CS_2. A colorless or slightly yellow, highly inflammable liquid; has been used externally as a counterirritant. A solvent of wide application.

c. monoxide. CO. A colorless, odorless, poisonous gas resulting from the combustion of carbonaceous compounds in an insufficient supply of oxygen. It combines firmly with hemoglobin, preventing subsequent union with oxygen. See *carboxyhemoglobin.*

c. tetrachloride. CCl_4. Tetrachloromethane. A colorless, noninflammable liquid, useful as an anthelmintic, especially against the hookworm. Dose, 2–3 cc. (30–45 min.), followed by a saline cathartic. It is also used as a fire extinguisher, a solvent, and an insecticide. See also carbon tetrachloride *poisoning*.

car′bon·ate. The divalent radical $=CO_3$; any salt containing this radical, as salts of carbonic acid.

acid c. See *bicarbonate*.

car′bon·a″ted. Containing or charged with carbon dioxide.

car·bon′ic ac′id. H_2CO_3. When carbon dioxide dissolves in water, a portion of it forms this feebly ionizing acid. Its salts are carbonates. See *carbon* dioxide.

car·bon′ic an·hy′drase. An enzyme, found in the erythrocytes and in tissues, which catalyzes the reaction $H_2O + CO_2 \rightleftharpoons H_2CO_3$. In the transport of CO_2 in the body, the reaction proceeds to the right in the tissues and to the left in the lungs, and in each instance is catalyzed by carbonic anhydrase.

car·bo′ni·um. A positively charged carbon radical: also called *carbonium ion*.

car″bon·i·za′tion [*carbo*]. 1. Decomposition of organic compounds by heat in the absence of air, driving off the volatile matter and leaving the carbon. 2. Charring. —**car′bonize,** *v.t.*

car″bon·om′e·ter [*carbo;* G. *metron*, a measure]. Apparatus for measuring the amount of carbon dioxide in a room or in exhaled breath. —**carbonom′etry,** *n.*

car″bon·u′ri·a [*carbo;* G. *ouron*, urine]. Presence of carbon compounds in the urine, particularly carbon dioxide.

car′bon·yl. The divalent radical $=CO$.

c. chloride. $COCl_2$. Phosgene.

carbo-resin. A trade-mark for a combination of ion exchange resins referred to by the generic designation *carbacrylamine resins*.

carborundum. A registered trade-mark for silicon carbide, SiC, a substance of extreme hardness.

carbowax. The trade-mark for certain polyethylene glycols, of the general formula $HOCH_2$-$(CH_2OCH_2)_xCH_2OH$, having a molecular weight above 1000. They are waxlike solids, are soluble in water and in many organic solvents; they are employed occasionally in preparing ointment bases.

carboxide. Trade-mark for a mixture of ethylene oxide and carbon dioxide, used as a fumigant.

car·box″y·hae″mo·glo′bin. See *carboxyhemoglobin*.

car·box″y·he″mo·glo′bin (kahr·bock″see·hee″mo-glo′bin, ·hem″o·glo′bin) [*carbo;* G. *oxys*, sharp; *haima*, blood; L. *globus*, globe]. The compound of carbon monoxide and hemoglobin formed when CO is present in the blood. The carbon monoxide displaces the oxygen and checks the respiratory function of erythrocytes.

car·box′yl. The group —COOH characteristic of organic acids. The hydrogen of this can be replaced by metals, forming salts.

car·box′yl·ase. 1. An enzyme, occurring in many plants and higher animals, also in bacteria, fungi, and yeast, capable of catalyzing decarboxylation of various α-keto acids, such as pyruvic and α-ketoglutaric. It is a complex of thiamine pyrophosphate (the coenzyme factor known as *cocarboxylase*), magnesium, and protein. Sometimes called *α-keto acid carboxylase* or *α-keto acid decarboxylase*. 2. Any of several enzymes, largely bacterial in origin, capable of catalyzing decarboxylation of various L-amino acids. Pyridoxal phosphate, known also as *codecarboxylase*, is the coenzyme or prosthetic component of these enzymes. Sometimes called *amino acid carboxylase* or *amino acid decarboxylase*.

carboxymethocel. Trade-mark for the sodium salt of carboxymethylcellulose.

car·box″y·meth″yl·cel′lu·lose. A substance obtained by the action of monochloroacetic acid on alkali cellulose; it is available as the sodium salt, a white, granular, odorless, and tasteless powder. It is dispersible in water to form viscous solutions useful for their thickening, suspending, and stabilizing properties. See *carboxymethocel*.

car·box″y·my″o·glo′bin. A compound of carbon monoxide and myoglobin.

car·box″y·pep′ti·dase. An enzyme, widely distributed but found especially in pancreatic juice, capable of catalyzing hydrolysis of polypeptides at the terminus having a free carboxyl group, producing an amino acid and a smaller peptide which may undergo further hydrolysis under the influence of the enzyme. Syn., *carboxypolypeptidase*.

car·box″y·pol″y·pep′ti·dase. Carboxypeptidase.

car·bro′mal (*carbromalum*). $(C_2H_5)_2$.CBr.CO.NH.-$CONH_2$. Bromodiethylacetylurea. A white, crystalline powder soluble in 18 parts of alcohol. A nerve sedative with marked analgesic power. Dose, 0.3–1.0 Gm. (5–15 gr.). See *adalin*.

car′bun·cle [L. *carbunculus*, dim. of *carbo*]. A hard, circumscribed, deep-seated, painful, suppurative inflammation of the subcutaneous tissue. It is larger than a boil, having a flat surface discharging pus from multiple points. There is usually fever with generalized constitutional reaction. Eventually, the entire mass sloughs away, healing as a scarred excavation. —**carbun′cular,** *adj.*

car·bun″cu·lo′sis [*carbunculus;* G. *-ōsis*, condition]. Condition characterized by the formation of carbuncles in rapid succession or simultaneously.

car″byl·a·mine′. An isocyanide.

carcholin. Trade-mark for carbachol supplied in powder form for preparing solutions and ointments for use in the treatment of simple glaucoma. The chemical reduces ocular tension, is a powerful miotic, and produces loss of accommodation through muscle spasm.

car′ci·no-, carcin- [G. *karkinos*, crab]. 1. *In zoology*, a combining form denoting *a crab*. 2. *In medicine*, a combining form denoting *cancer*.

car′ci·no·gen [*karkinos;* G. *genesthai*, from *gignesthai*, to be produced]. 1. A substance or agent causing development of a carcinoma or epithelioma. 2. Loosely, a substance or agent causing development of a malignancy of any sort: more properly called *cancerogen*. —**carcinogen′ic,** *adj.;* **carcinogenic′ity,** *n.*

car″ci·no·gen′e·sis [*karkinos;* G. *genesis*, production]. Origin or production of cancer. —**carcinogenet′ic,** *adj.*

car′ci·noid [*karkinos;* G. *eidos*, form]. A tumor derived from argentaffin (enterochromaffin) cells; it is usually benign, and commonly occurs in the appendix and ileum. Also called *argentaffin*, *argentaffinoma*, *argentaffin tumor*, *Kultschitzky's* or *spheroidal-cell carcinoma*.

c. of bronchus. See *adenoma* of bronchus.

car″ci·no′ma [G. *karkinōma*, from *karkinos;* *-ōma*, tumor]. An epithelial tumor which is malignant. The two principal varieties are **epidermoid carcinoma** and **cylindrical-cell carcinoma,** both of which may show various degrees of differentiation and may be graded accordingly. The chief forms of epidermoid carcinoma are **squamous-cell carcinoma, basal-cell carcinoma,** and **intermediate-cell carcinoma,** all derived from surface or lining epithelium. The principal form of cylindrical-cell carcinoma is the **adenocarcinoma,** derived from glandular epithelium. Completely undifferentiated carcinoma, or **carcinoma simplex,** is usually a cylindrical-cell carcinoma but may also be a form of epidermoid carcinoma. Metastasis is chiefly through lymphatics, either by embolism of cells or by permeation growth of the tumor through the vessels. Metastasis sometimes occurs through blood vessels; spread may also occur by direct extension or by surface implantation. —**carcinom'atoid, carcinom'atous,** *adj.*

actinic c. A basal-cell carcinoma of the face and other exposed surfaces of the body, seen in persons who spend prolonged periods of time in direct sunlight.

acute c. See inflammatory *c.*

adrenal cortical a. See cortical *c.*

alveolar (cell) c. See bronchiolar *c.*

aniline c. Carcinoma of the urinary bladder frequent among workers in anilines.

apocrine c. Extramammary Paget's disease.

appendage-cell c. Carcinoma originating in cutaneous appendages. See also *adenocarcinoma,* epidermoid *c.*

argentaffin c. See *carcinoid.*

arsenical c. A carcinoma of the skin following prolonged ingestion or exposure to arsenical compounds.

basal-cell c. See basal-cell *epithelioma.*

basosquamous c. A malignant growth of skin, composed of both squamous and basal cells: also called *basal squamous c., mixed c.*

betel-nut c. A squamous-cell carcinoma on the inside of the cheek: observed in peoples who chew betel. Syn., *sirih-chewer's c.*

branchiogenic c., branchial c. An epidermoid carcinoma arising from the epithelium of a branchial cyst or cysts. Numerous lymph nodules are characteristically present. Also called *branchioma, gill cleft c.*

bronchiolar c. A diffuse or focally distributed acinar tumor situated within alveoli and located mainly at the lung periphery. It is probably of multicentric origin, involving both lungs massively, yet slow to metastasize. Microscopically it shows peribronchiolar distribution, and often atypical, mucus-producing epithelium, and in the more benign forms, the characteristic cell is a tall columnar variety with finely granular cytoplasm. Also called *c. bronchiolorum; alveolar (cell) c.; alveolar (cell) cancer; diffuse lung c.; diffuse, multiple, solitary, terminal bronchiolar c.; cancerous pulmonary adenomatosis; carcinomatoides alveogenica multicentrica.*

bronchogenic c. A malignant tumor derived from the surface epithelium of bronchi, usually centrally or segmentally located, and more commonly seen in men after middle age. Implicated as causative factors are excessive amounts of inhaled tobacco smoke, arsenic, asbestos, chrome ores, nickel, radioactive gases and dusts, and less certainly tar, petroleum, and oil-shale distillates. Histologically, bronchogenic carcinomas may be classified as (a) **epidermoid,** in which the predominant cell type resembles stratified squamous epithelium in varying degrees of differentiation; (b) **anaplastic,** including the so-called reserve cell (oat-cell, round-cell, small-cell, and spindle-cell) carcinomas; (c) **adenocarcinoma,** in which there are mucus-producing cells; and (d) mixed forms; also included may be bronchiolar carcinoma. Syn., *bronchial c., bronchiogenic c., cancer of the lung.*

c. in situ. A neoplasm of the surface epithelium and/or the underlying gland spaces, whose component cells are morphologically identical with those in frank carcinoma: also called *intraepidermal c., intraepithelial c., preinvasive c.*

c. mucocellulare ovarii. See Krukenberg *tumor.*

c. occulta. Carcinoma which is unsuspected, or not subject to diagnosis.

c. of the corpus luteum. A malignant luteoma.

c. of the nipple. See Paget's *disease,* (b).

c. of sebaceous glands. A rare malignant epithelial tumor of the sebaceous and meibomian glands, most frequently found on the eyelids but may occur wherever there are sebaceous glands.

c. of the uterine cervix. A common carcinoma, either a squamous-cell one or, less frequently, adenocarcinoma, usually appearing in middle-aged women. On a clinical basis it has been internationally classified into: *Stage 0* carcinoma in situ, a microscopical diagnosis; *Stage I* carcinoma confined to cervix; *Stage II* carcinoma spread beyond cervix but not to pelvic wall (carcinoma involves vagina but not the lower third); *Stage III* carcinoma has reached pelvic wall (on rectal examination no cancer-free space is found between tumor and pelvic wall; carcinoma involves lower third of vagina); *Stage IV* carcinoma has involved urinary bladder, rectum, or both, or has extended beyond limits previously described.

c. simplex. Carcinoma in which differentiation is absent or poor. Usually a cylindrical-cell carcinoma but may be derived from epidermis or other lining epithelium. As a rule, highly malignant.

c. substantiae corticalis suprarenalis. Cortical *c.*

chimney-sweeps' c. An epidermoid carcinoma of the scrotum, known also as *chimney-sweeps' cancer* because of frequent association of this tumor with exposure to soot.

chorionic c. See *choriocarcinoma.*

clear-cell c. A carcinoma composed of large polyhedral, epithelial cells with clear cytoplasm. It is most commonly seen in the renal parenchyma, which tumor is also called *nephroma, solid-cell c., Grawitz tumor, hypernephroma.* Other sites are the ovary, adrenal, and thyroid.

colloid c. A misnomer for carcinomas of glandular or undifferentiated forms in which the cells produce mucin either in acinic spaces or within the cells. See also gelatinous *c.*

columnar-cell c. See *adenocarcinoma.*

comedo c. See *comedo-carcinoma.*

cortical c. A carcinoma composed mainly of cells resembling those of the adrenal cortex: also called *carcinoma substantiae corticalis suprarenalis, adrenal hypernephroma malignum.*

diffuse lung c. See bronchiolar *c.*

disseminated c. A carcinoma which has metastasized.

ductal c. Generally, a malignant tumor of the mammary gland, arising from the cells lining the ducts: also called *milk-duct c., ductal tumor.*

ductal papillary c. A papillary carcinoma of the mammary ducts.

embryonal c. of testis. A tumor of testis composed of highly malignant, multipotential, anaplastic cells, which may be entirely undifferentiated or show slight differentiation toward somatic or trophoblastic cell forms: also called *adenocarcinoma of testis, embryoma of testis, embryonic c., teratocarcinoma of testis, teratoid c. of testis.*

embryonic c. See malignant *teratoma.*

endometrial c. One of the endometrium, apparently related to genetic hormonal factors. Histologically the tumor is usually an adenocarcinoma and occasionally an adenoacanthoma.

epidermoid c. A type derived from surfaces covered by stratified squamous epithelium or by metaplasia from other types of epithelium. Tends to reproduce basal, intermediate, and squamous cells, but may be undifferentiated. The squamous cells may be concentrated in balls with concentric laminas, the so-called epithelial pearls. The most highly differentiated form is often called *acanthoma.* Another variety is the *basal-cell carcinoma.* Formerly called *epithelioma.*
erysipeloid c. See inflammatory *c.*
follicular c. of thyroid. A malignant tumor grossly resembling a benign follicular adenoma of the thyroid, but which microscopically shows evidence of invasion of blood or lymph vessels or of tumor capsule: also called *benign metastasizing goiter, metastasizing struma, struma maligna.*
fungating c. Rapidly growing carcinoma in which there is extensive necrosis.
gelatinous c. One which, arising within mammary ducts, is grossly characterized by the presence of colloid material. Syn., *colloid c., goblet-cell c., mucoid c., signet-ring-cell c.*
giant-cell c. of thyroid. A rapidly growing, undifferentiated carcinoma of the thyroid with numerous tumor giant cells: also called *spindle-cell carcinoma of thyroid, carcinosarcoma of thyroid.*
gill cleft c. See branchiogenic *c.*
glandular c. Adenocarcinoma.
goblet-cell c. See gelatinous *c.*
granular-cell c. A carcinoma of kidney parenchyma resembling the clear-cell carcinoma of the kidney, except that the cytoplasm is granular.
granulosa-cell c. A malignant granulosa-cell tumor.
hidradenoid c. See sweat-gland *tumor.*
Hürthle cell c. See Hürthle cell *tumor.*
infiltrating lobular c. A malignant tumor of the breast that grossly resembles scirrhous carcinoma but is characterized microscopically by thread-like strands of tumor cells, which tend to be small and compressed by the surrounding dense fibrous tissue.
inflammatory c. Clinically, a fast-spreading carcinoma associated with inflammation: also called *acute c., acute carcinosis, carcinomatous mastitis, erysipeloid cancer, erysipeloid c., telangiectatic c.*
intermediate-cell c. One derived from surface epithelium, but composed almost entirely of intermediate cells with intercellular bridges, the prickle cells: also called *intermediary c.*
intracystic papillary c. of the breast. A malignant tumor of the breast, characterized by a cyst or cysts containing serous or sanguineous fluid and a papillary component.
intraepidermal c. See *c.* in situ.
intraepithelial c. of the nipple. See Paget's *disease,* (b).
islet-cell c. A malignant islet-cell tumor.
Kultschitzky's c. See *carcinoid.*
liver-cell c. Hepatoma.
lobular c. One of the mammary lobules, divided into the lobular mammary carcinoma in situ and the noninfiltrating and the infiltrating lobular carcinoma.
lobular mammary c. in situ. A form of noninfiltrating carcinoma of the mammary lobules.
medullary c. A form of cylindrical-cell carcinoma which is soft in consistency because it is made up principally of carcinoma cells with little supporting connective tissue. Usually grows rapidly and metastasizes early and widely.
milk-duct c. See ductal *c.*
mixed basosquamous c. See basosquamous *c.*
mixed c. See basosquamous *c.*
mucinous c. See pseudomucinous *cystadenocarcinoma.*
mucoid c. See gelatinous *c.*
noninfiltrating lobular c. Carcinoma of the breast. It is confined to the lobules.
oat-cell c. See reserve-cell *c.*
papillary c. A carcinoma with trabeculae resembling the stalks of a papilloma, and usually grossly papillary in structure: commonly seen in transitional-cell carcinoma of the urinary tract.
papillary c. of thyroid. A tumor grossly appearing to be a benign papillary adenoma of the thyroid, but microscopically malignant.
papillary serous c. See serous *cystoadenocarcinoma.*
papilliferous c. An adenomatous or cystic carcinoma in which the epithelium is arranged in the form of papillae.
pleomorphic c. Any highly anaplastic carcinoma in which the cell type is highly undifferentiated and cannot be identified.
polypoid c. A carcinoma having a polypoid appearance on gross examination, seen commonly on mucous membranes of urinary and gastrointestinal tracts.
prickle-cell c. See intermediate-cell *c.*
pseudomucinous c. (*of ovary*). See pseudomucinous *cystadenocarcinoma.*
radiation c. An epidermoid carcinoma which is associated with overexposure to radiation.
reserve-cell c. A form of anaplastic bronchogenic carcinoma composed of undifferentiated small cells of round, oval, or spindle form: also called *oat-cell c., round-cell c., small-cell c., spindle-cell c.*
round-cell c. See reserve-cell *c.*
scirrhous c. Cylindrical-cell carcinoma which is hard, because the connective-tissue component is large in amount and collagenous, while the epithelial component is small in amount. Usually grows slowly and metastasizes late; the metastases usually have the same proportionate amount of the components. Syn., *scirrhus.*
self-healing squamous-cell carcinomata. An often familial genodermatosis, characterized by onset of benign tumors of the skin after puberty or in adult life. New lesions keep appearing and enlarge, ulcerate centrally, and heal spontaneously with a depressed scar. Histologically the findings resemble well-differentiated keratinizing squamous-cell carcinoma. Syn., *self-healing prickle-cell epithelioma of the skin.*
seminal c. See *seminoma.*
signet-ring-cell c. See gelatinous *c.*
sirih-chewer's c. See betel-nut *c.*
small-cell c. of thyroid. Anaplastic carcinoma of thyroid composed of small epithelial cells, which may grow either diffusely or compactly, and show little follicle or colloid formation: also called *solid c. of thyroid.*
solid c. of thyroid. See small-cell *c.* of thyroid.
solid-cell c. Clear-cell carcinoma of renal parenchyma.
spheroidal-cell c. of appendix. See *carcinoid.*
spindle-cell c. See reserve-cell *c.*
spindle-cell c. of thyroid. See giant-cell *c.* of thyroid.
spinous-cell c. Well-differentiated epidermoid *c.*
Spiroptera c. Carcinoma in the stomach of rats, associated with infestation by the nematode, *Spiroptera.* It was first demonstrated by J. Fibiger.
squamous-cell c. A form of epidermoid carcinoma.
syncytial c. See *choriocarcinoma.*
tar c. Carcinoma, usually epidermoid, produced experimentally by application of tar, its distilla-

tion products, or other agents of the same order.

telangiectatic c. See inflammatory *c.*

teratoid c. See malignant *teratoma.*

teratoid c. of testis. See embryonal *c.* of testis.

thymic c. A thymoma made up of cells resembling epithelium which may be so arranged as to resemble squamous-cell carcinoma but with little keratinization.

transitional-cell c. Derived from and made up of transitional epithelial cells. Prevalent in the urinary tract, especially the urinary bladder.

verrucal c. An epidermoid *c.*

villous c. See papillary *c.*

car″ci·nom′a·toid (kahr″si·nom′uh·toyd, ·no′-muh-toyd) [*karkinōma;* G. *eidos,* form]. *In experimental oncology,* epithelial proliferation in induced papillomas without invasion of adjacent tissue.

car″ci·nom″a·to′i·des al″ve·o·gen′i·ca mul″-ti·cen′tri·ca. See bronchiolar *carcinoma.*

car″ci·no″ma·to′sis [*karkinōma;* G. *-ōsis,* condition]. A condition of widespread dissemination of cancer throughout the body.

car″ci·no·sar·co′ma [G. *karkinos,* crab; *sarkōma,* fleshy excrescence]. A mixed tumor having the characteristics of carcinoma and sarcoma. Not to be confused with collision tumor, in which a sarcoma invades a carcinoma or vice versa.

c. of thyroid. See giant-cell *c.* of thyroid.

car″ci·no′sis. *Carcinomatosis.*

acute c. See inflammatory *carcinoma.*

car′da·mom (kahr′duh·mum, ·mom). The dried, ripe fruit or seed of *Elettaria cardamomum,* a plant of the ginger family of China and the East Indies. The flavor and therapeutic effect are due to the presence of 2–8% of volatile oil. It is an aromatic, carminative stomachic.

c. oil (*oleum cardamomi*). One used solely as a flavoring agent.

compound c. elixir (*elixir cardamomi compositum*). A vehicle containing compound cardamom spirit.

compound c. spirit (*spiritus cardamomi compositus*). An alcoholic solution of the oils of cardamom, orange, cinnamon, caraway, and clove, with anethole.

compound c. tincture (*tinctura cardamomi composita*). A tincture prepared from cardamom, cinnamon, caraway, and cochineal; a vehicle, occasionally used as a carminative.

Cardanus, Hieronymus (Jerome Cardan, Girolamo Cardano) [*Italian physician and mathematician,* 1501–76]. Remembered as a great clinician. Author of a remarkable work, with 800 illustrations, on the human face (1550).

Cardarelli, Antonio [*Italian physician,* 1831–1926]. Known for his important contributions to the knowledge of cardiology and remembered for his description of a sign significant of aortic aneurysm: tracheal tugging.

Carden, Henry Douglas [*English surgeon,* d. 1872]. Remembered for his single-flap operation through the condyles of the femur just above the articular surface (1864); called *Carden's amputation.* Advocated single flaps for amputations at other sites.

car′di·a [G. *kardia,* heart]. 1. The esophageal orifice of the stomach. 2. The fundus ventriculi [BNA].

car′di·ac [*kardia*]. 1. Relating to the heart. 2. Pertaining to the cardia.

car′di·ac. 1. A person with a heart lesion. 2. A tonic acting especially on the heart.

black c. A person with Ayerza's syndrome: also called *cardiaco negro.* See under Abel *Ayerza.*

car′di·ac fail′ure. The syndrome resulting from failure of the heart as a pump. The mechanism is varied, the symptoms depending on whether the left or right ventricle preponderantly fails. Dyspnea is most marked in left ventricular failure; and engorgement of organs with venous blood, edema, and ascites, most marked in right ventricular failure. **Forward cardiac failure** and **backward** or **congestive cardiac failure** refer to the mechanism which produces symptoms. Forward failure is due to the inability of the heart to furnish sufficient blood flow to the body; backward or congestive failure is due to the inability of the heart to pump out the blood being returned to it by the veins. Cardiac failure as seen clinically may be entirely of the backward type but more commonly represents a combination of these two. Also called *heart failure.* See *circulatory failure.*

car′di·ac in″suf·fi′cien·cy. See *cardiac failure.*

car″di·a′co ne′gro. Black cardiac. See under Abel *Ayerza.*

car′di·ac out′put″. Blood volume in liters ejected per minute by the left ventricle.

car″di·al′gi·a [*kardia;* G. *algos,* pain]. Pain in the region of the heart; heartburn.

car″di·am′e·ter [*kardia;* G. *metron,* a measure]. An apparatus for determining the position of the cardiac orifice of the stomach.

car″di·a·neu′ri·a [*kardia;* G. *a-,* not; *neuron,* nerve]. Lack of tone in the heart.

car″di·asth′ma (kahr″dee·az′muh, ·ass′muh) [*kardia;* G. *asthma,* asthma]. Asthmalike dyspnea from left ventricular failure. See cardiac *asthma.*

cardiazol. Trade-mark for pentamethylenetetrazol. See *metrazol.*

car″di·cen·te′sis. See *cardiocentesis.*

car′di·cin. An antibiotic substance produced mainly in the mycelium of species of the genus *Nocardia.* It has antimicrobial and antiviral properties.

car″di·ec′ta·sis [*kardia;* G. *ektasis,* a stretching out]. Dilatation of the heart.

car″di·ec′to·my [*kardia;* G. *ektomē,* excision]. Excision of the cardiac end of the stomach.

cardigin. Trade-mark for digitoxin.

car′di·nal flow′er. A common name for several species of *Lobelia,* chiefly *Lobelia cardinalis.*

car′di·o-, cardi- [*kardia*]. A combining form denoting *of,* or *pertaining to, the heart; cardiac.*

car″di·o·ac·cel′er·a″tor [*kardia;* L. *accelerare,* to accelerate]. An agent which quickens the action of the heart. —**car″dioaccel′erator,** *adj.*

car″di·o·ac′tive [*kardia;* L. *activus,* from *agere,* to act]. Affecting the heart.

car″di·o·an″gi·ol′o·gy (kahr″dee·o·an″jee·ol′o-jee) [*kardia;* G. *aggeion,* vessel; *logos,* word]. Branch of medicine dealing with the heart and blood vessels.

car″di·o-a·or′tic (-ay·or′tick) [*kardia;* G. *aortē,* aorta]. Relating to the heart and the aorta.

car″di·o·ar·te′ri·al [*kardia;* G. *artēria,* artery]. Pertaining to the heart and the arteries. See *interval.*

car′di·o·cele [*kardia;* G. *kēlē,* hernia]. Hernia of the heart.

car″di·o·cen·te′sis, car″di·cen·te′sis [*kardia;* G. *kentēsis,* a pricking]. Puncture of one of the chambers of the heart to relieve engorgement.

car″di·o·ci·net′ic (kahr″dee·o·si·net′ick). See *cardiokinetic.*

car″di·o·cir·rho′sis [*kardia;* G. *kirros,* orange-tawny; *-ōsis,* condition]. Cirrhosis of the liver due to chronic congestive heart failure.

car″di·oc′la·sis, car″di·o·cla′si·a (kahr″dee·o-clay′zhuh, ·zee·uh) [*kardia;* G. *klasis,* a breaking]. Rupture of the heart.

car″di·o·di·la′tor (kahr″dee·o·dye·lay′tur, ·di·lay′-tur) [*kardia;* L. *dilatare,* to extend]. Instrument for dilating the esophageal opening of the stomach.

car″di·o·di·o′sis (kahr″dee·o·dee·o′sis, ·dye·o′sis) [*kardia;* G. *diōsis*, a forcing open]. Dilatation of the cardiac end of the stomach by means of an instrument passed through the esophagus.

car″di·o·dy·nam′ics (kahr″dee·o·dye·nam′icks, ·di·nam′icks) [*kardia;* G. *dynamis*, power]. Kinetic mechanisms by means of which the heartbeat insures the circulation of the blood from the heart to the periphery and back to the heart. —**cardiodynamic,** *adj.*

car″di·o·dy″na·mom′et·ry. Plethysmographic measurement of cardiac flow in the upper extremities.

car″di·o·dyn′i·a [*kardia;* G. *odynē*, pain]. Pain in or about the heart.

car″di·o·e·soph″a·ge′al. Pertaining to the cardia of the stomach and the esophagus, usually to their junction.

car″di·o·gen′e·sis [*kardia;* G. *genesis*, production]. Development of the heart.

car″di·o·gen′ic [*kardia;* G. *genesthai*, from *gignesthai*, to be produced]. 1. Pertaining to the development of the heart. 2. Having an origin in the heart.

car′di·o·gram″ [*kardia;* G. *gramma*, a drawing]. A record of the heart's pulsation taken through the chest wall; the tracing made by the cardiograph.

car′di·o·graph″ [*kardia;* G. *graphein*, to write]. An instrument for registering graphically the cardiac cycle. —**cardiograph′ic,** *adj.*

car″di·og′ra·phy [*kardia; graphein*]. 1. Analysis of cardiac action by instrumental means, especially by tracings which record its movements. 2. A description of the heart.

car″di·o·he·pat′ic [*kardia;* G. *hēpar*, liver]. Pertaining to the heart and the liver, as the cardiohepatic angle.

car′di·oid [*kardia;* G. *eidos*, form]. Like a heart.

car″di·o·in·hib′i·to″ry [*kardia;* L. *inhibere*, to restrain]. Diminishing, restraining, or suppressing the heart's action, as the cardioinhibitory fibers which pass to the heart through the vagus nerves.

car″di·o·ki·net′ic (kahr″dee·o·ki·net′ick, ·kigh·net′ick) [*kardia;* G. *kinein*, to move]. Exciting the heart action.

car″di·o·ky·mog′ra·phy (·kigh·mog′ruh·fee) [*kardia;* G. *kyma*, wave; *graphein*, to write]. A method for recording changes in the size of the heart by kymographic means. See *kymography, radiokymography.*

car″di·o·lip′in [*kardia;* G. *lipos*, fat]. A class of phospholipids isolated from beef heart and consisting of a phosphorylated polysaccharide esterified with fatty acids. Essential for the reactivity of beef heart antigens in the serologic test for syphilis, and may be the pure antigen.

car′di·o·lith [*kardia;* G. *lithos*, a stone]. A cardiac concretion.

car″di·ol′o·gist [*kardia;* G. *logos*, word]. A specialist in the diagnosis and treatment of disorders of the heart.

car″di·ol′o·gy [*kardia; logos*]. The study of the heart.

car″di·ol′y·sis [*kardia;* G. *lysis*, a loosing]. 1. Resection of the precordial ribs and sternum to free the heart and its adherent pericardium from the anterior chest wall, to which they are bound by adhesions, as in adhesive mediastinopericarditis. 2. Cardiac degeneration or destruction.

car″di·o·ma·la′ci·a (kahr″dee·o·ma·lay′shee·uh, ·see·uh) [*kardia;* G. *malakia*, softness]. Pathologic softening of the heart musculature. *Obs.*

car″di·o·me·ga′li·a gly″co·gen′i·ca. See *glycogenosis.*

car″di·o·meg′a·ly. Enlargement of the heart.

car″di·o·mel″a·no′sis [*kardia;* G. *melas*, black; *-ōsis*, condition]. Deposition of pigment in the heart muscle.

car″di·o·men′su·ra·tor [*kardia;* L. *mensurator*, from *mensurare*, to measure]. An instrument for the detection of cardiac enlargement by direct correlation of the transverse diameter of the heart with body weight and height.

car″di·o·men′to·pex″y [*kardia;* L. *omentum*, omentum; G. *pēxis*, a fixing]. The operation of bringing vascular omentum through the diaphragm and attaching it to the heart for improving cardiac vascularization. Also called *O'Shaughnessy's operation.*

car″di·om′e·ter [*kardia;* G. *metron*, a measure]. An experimental apparatus which envelops the ventricles of a heart, recording their changes in volume during a cardiac cycle.

car″di·om′e·try [*kardia; metron*]. The measurement of the size of the heart, or of the force exerted with each contraction.

car″di·o·my′o·pex″y [*kardia;* G. *mys*, muscle; *pēxis*, a fixing]. The operation of suturing living muscular tissue, generally from the pectoral region, to the abraded surface of the heart, to provide improved vascularization of the heart. Also called *Beck's operation.*

car″di·o·my·ot′o·my (kahr″dee·o·migh·ot′o·mee) [*kardia; mys;* G. *tomē*, a cutting]. An operation for stenosis of the cardiac sphincter; consists of freeing the esophagus from the diaphragm and pulling it into the abdominal cavity, where the constricting muscle is divided anteriorly and posteriorly without dividing the mucous coat.

car″di·o·nec′tor [*kardia;* L. *nectere*, to fasten together]. All of those structures within the heart which regulate the heart beat, consisting of the sinoatrial node, the atrioventricular node, and the atrioventricular bundle.

car″di·o·neph′ric [*kardia;* G. *nephros*, kidneys]. Pertaining to the heart and the kidneys.

car″di·o·neu′ral [*kardia;* G. *neuron*, nerve]. Pertaining to the nervous control of the heart's mechanism.

car″di·o·pal′u·dism [*kardia;* L. *palus*, swamp]. Disturbance of the heart due to malaria, characterized by gallop rhythm, dilatation of the right heart, and reduplication of the diastolic sound.

car′di·o·path [*kardia;* G. *pathos*, disease]. A sufferer from heart disease; a cardiac. —**cardiopath′ic,** *adj.*

car″di·o·pa·thol′o·gy [*kardia; pathos;* G. *logos*, word]. Study of the diseases of the heart.

car″di·op′a·thy, car″di·o·path′i·a [*kardia; pathos*]. Any disease of the heart. The various types are: arteriosclerotic, hypertensive, inflammatory, nephropathic, thyrotoxic, toxic, and valvular.

car″di·o·per″i·car′di·o·pex″y. An operation to unite parietal pericardium to the surface of the heart for the purpose of improving the blood supply to the heart. See also Claude Schaeffer *Beck.*

car″di·o·per″i·car·di′tis [*kardia; perikardios;* G. *-itis*, inflammation]. Associated carditis and pericarditis; inflammation of the heart and pericardium.

car″di·o·pho′bi·a [*kardia;* G. *phobos*, fear]. Morbid fear of heart disease.

car′di·o·phone [*kardia;* G. *phōnē*, voice]. An instrument which makes the heart sounds audible; useful when presenting cases to a large group.

car′di·o·plas″ty [*kardia;* G. *plassein*, to form]. Plastic surgery of the cardiac sphincter of the stomach, as for cardiospasm.

car″di·o·ple′gi·a [*kardia;* G. *plēgē*, a stroke]. Paralysis of the heart. *Obs.*

car″di·o·pneu·mat′ic (kahr″dee·o·new·mat′ick) [*kardia;* G. *pneuma*, breath]. Pertaining to the heart and respiration, as the cardiopneumatic movements of the air in the lungs, caused by the pulsations of the heart and great vessels.

car″di·o·pneu′mo·graph [*kardia; pneuma;* G. *graphein,* to write]. An instrument designed for graphically recording cardiopneumatic movements. —**cardiopneumog′raphy,** *n.*

car″di·op·to′sis (kahr″dee·op·to′sis, kahr″dee·o-to′sis), **car″di·op·to′si·a** (kahr″dee·op·to′shuh, ·see·uh, kahr″dee·o·) [*kardia;* G. *ptōsis,* a falling]. Downward displacement of the heart from excessive mobility; prolapse of the heart.

car″di·o·pul′mo·nar·y [*kardia;* L. *pulmonarius,* from *pulmo,* lung]. Relating to the heart and lungs. Also *cardiopulmonic.*

car″di·o·punc′ture [*kardia;* L. *punctura,* a puncture]. 1. Cardiocentesis. 2. Any surgical or experimental puncture of the heart.

car″di·o·py·lor′ic (kahr″dee·o·pye·lor′ick, ·pi·lor′-ick) [*kardia;* G. *pylōros,* gatekeeper]. Referring to both the cardiac and the pyloric portions of the stomach.

car″di·o·re′nal [*kardia;* L. *renes,* kidneys]. Relating to the heart and kidneys.

car″di·o·re·spir′a·to″ry (kahr″dee·o·ri·spy′ruh-tor″ee, ·res′pi·ruh·tor″ee) [*kardia;* L. *respirare,* to breathe out]. Of or pertaining to the heart and respiration.

car″di·o·roent′gen·o·gram″ (·rent′ghin·o·gram″) [*kardia; Röntgen;* G. *gramma,* letter]. Roentgenogram of the heart.

car″di·o·roent″gen·og′ra·phy [*kardia; Röntgen;* G. *graphein,* to write]. Roentgenographic examination of the heart.

car″di·or′rha·phy [*kardia;* G. *rhaphē,* a suture]. Suturing of the heart.

car″di·or·rhex′is [*kardia;* G. *rhēxis,* a breaking]. Rupture of the heart. *Rare.*

car″di·os′chi·sis (kahr″dee·os′ki·sis) [*kardia;* G. *schisis,* cleavage]. Tearing apart of adhesions between the heart and chest wall in adhesive pericarditis.

car′di·o·scope″ [*kardia;* G. *skopein,* to examine]. A lag-screen belt electrocardiograph; the electrocardiogram can be visualized immediately for a few seconds' time on a rotating fluorescent belt.

car′di·o·spasm″ [*kardia;* G. *spasmos,* spasm]. Contraction of the cardiac sphincter, usually associated with spasm of the cardiac end of the stomach and dilatation and hypertrophy of the esophagus above the sphincter.

car″di·o·spec′tro·gram [*kardia; spectrum; graphein*]. The graphic record made by a cardiospectrograph of the heart sounds.

car″di·o·spec′tro·graph [*kardia;* L. *spectrum,* appearance; G. *graphein,* to write]. An instrument which picks up heart sounds by a microphone and then converts them into visual patterns and tracings.

car″di·o·ste·no′sis [*kardia;* G. *stenōsis,* a being straitened]. Constriction of the heart, especially of the conus arteriosus; the development of such a constriction.

car″di·o·sym′phy·sis. See *mediastinopericarditis.*

car″di·o·ta·chom′e·ter (kahr″dee·o·ta·kom′i·tur) [*kardia;* G. *tachos,* speed; *metron,* a measure]. Instrument that counts the total number of heartbeats over long periods of time.

car″di·o·ther′a·py [*kardia;* G. *therapeia,* treatment]. Treatment of heart disease.

car″di·ot′o·my [*kardia;* G. *tomē,* a cutting]. Dissection or incision of the heart or the cardiac end of the stomach.

car″di·o·ton′ic [*kardia;* G. *tonos,* a stretching]. Increasing the tonus of the cardiac muscle; generally applied to the effect of digitalis and related drugs. —**cardioton′ic,** *n.*

car″di·o·tox′ic [*kardia;* G. *toxikon,* poison]. Poisonous to the heart.

car″di·o·vas′cu·lar [*kardia;* L. *vasculum,* a small vessel]. Pertaining to the heart and the blood vessels.

car″di·o·vas′cu·lar-re′nal. Pertaining to the heart, blood vessels, and kidneys.

car″di·o·vec·tog′ra·phy [*kardia;* L. *vector,* from *vehere,* to carry; G. *graphein,* to write]. Technic of registering vectorcardiograms.

car″di·per″i·car·di′tis. See *cardiopericarditis.*

car·di′tis [*kardia;* G. *-itis,* inflammation]. Inflammation of the heart. —**cardit′ic,** *adj.*

internal c. Endocarditis.

car″di·val″vu·li′tis [*kardia;* NL. *valvula,* a little valve; *-itis*]. Endocarditis confined to the valves.

car″e·bar′i·a [G. *karē,* head; *barys,* heavy]. Unpleasant head sensations, such as pressure or heaviness. *Rare.*

car′ene. A dicyclic liquid hydrocarbon, $C_{10}H_{16}$, classed as a terpene, found in turpentine obtained from several *Pinus* species. Several isomers, differing in the position of a double bond, exist.

Carey's method. See under *stain.*

Cargile, Charles H. [*American surgeon,* 1853–1930]. Remembered for his introduction into surgery of animal membrane from the peritoneum to prevent adhesions and encourage the formation of artificial peritoneum; called *Cargile membrane.* The procedure is now obsolete.

Car′i·ca [L., a dry fig]. A genus of the Caricaceae.

C. papaya. The papaw tree of tropical America; contains in its leaves and fruit, besides the proteolytic enzyme papain (papayotin) and other enzymes, the alkaloid carpaine; the leaves also contain the glycoside carposide. The dried latex and leaves are used as a digestant.

ca′ri·es (kair′ee·eez, kair′eez) [L., decay]. A molecular death of bone or teeth, corresponding to ulceration in the soft tissues. —**car′ious,** *adj.*

c. of the spine. Tuberculous osteitis of the bodies of the vertebrae and intervertebral fibrocartilages, producing curvature of the spine. Also called *Pott's disease, tuberculosis of vertebra.*

c. of the teeth. See dental *c.*

c. sicca. A form of tuberculous caries characterized by absence of suppuration, obliteration of the cavity of a joint, and sclerosis and concentric atrophy of the articular extremities of the bones.

dental c. A localized, progressive, and molecular disintegration of the teeth, beginning with the solution of the enamel by lactic and pyruvic acids. The acids are the product of enzymic action of oral bacteria upon carbohydrates. [$C_6H_{12}O_6$ + bacterial enzymes = $2C_3H_6O_3$ (lactic acid).] The initial process is followed by bacterial invasion of the dentinal tubuli. The acids formed break down and remove the inorganic constituents of the enamel and dentin, and the unsupported organic matrix is gradually removed by proteolysis, leaving the so-called cavity of decay. Syn., *odontonecrosis.*

ca·ri′na [L., keel]. Any keel-like structure.

c. nasi. A narrow, cleftlike space between the agger nasi and the inner surface of the dorsum nasi.

c. tracheae. A ridge across the bottom of the trachea between the origins of the two bronchi.

urethral c. A continuation of the anterior column of the vagina in the vestibule as far as the external orifice of the urethra. Also called *c. vaginae.*

car·in′a·mide. 4′-Carboxyphenylmethanesulfonanilide, a white crystalline powder, sparingly soluble in water; it inhibits tubular excretion of penicillin, presumably by action on an enzyme system involved in transport of the antibiotic, and has been used in conjunction with penicillin to maintain therapeutic blood levels of the latter: formerly spelled *caronamide*. See *staticin*.

car″i·o·gen′ic. Conducive to the development of dental caries.

Carle, Antonio [*Italian surgeon*, 1854–1927]. Noted for his studies of the surgery of the brain and of the gastrointestinal and biliary tracts. With Rattone, demonstrated the transmissibility of tetanus (1884).

Carleton, Bukk G. [*American physician*, 1856–1914]. Described areas of sclerotic tissue in long bones, which are due to gonococcal bone lesions.

Carls′bad salt (karlz′bad, karls′baht, karlz′bahd). A mineral salt mixture from the Carlsbad springs, whose waters have been used for their supposed curative properties, or a similar synthetic salt.

Carlson, Anton Julius [*American physiologist*, 1875–   ]. Known for his contributions to the knowledge of the physiology of the stomach. Recorded stomach movements by means of a balloon inserted through a gastric fistula in experimental animals (1912). Studied control of hunger (1916).

carmacin. Trade name for a gastric antacid and carminative containing calcium carbonate, magnesium carbonate, sucrose, and peppermint oil.

car·min′a·tive (kahr·min′uh·tiv, kahr′min·, kahr′-mi·nay″tiv) [L. *carminare*, to card; hence, to cleanse]. Having the power to relieve flatulence and colic. Carminatives are generally aromatics.

car′mine (kahr′min, ·myne) (C.C.) [ML. *carminium*, carmine]. A bright red coloring matter prepared from cochineal, the active staining principle being carminic acid; of use in staining in toto, for staining tissues in bulk which are later sectioned; used as a specific stain for glycogen and for mucus and as a counterstain for blue vital dyes.

car″na·u′ba (kahr″nuh·ōō′buh) [Pg., of Tupian origin]. The root of *Copernicia cerifera*, a wax-producing palm tree of tropical America; used in Brazil as an alterative.

c. wax. The wax obtained from the leaf buds of *Copernicia cerifera*.

car″ni·fi·ca′tion [L. *caro*, flesh; *facere*, to make]. Alteration of tissue so that it resembles skeletal muscle in color and consistency. It sometimes affects the lungs.

car′ni·tine. $(CH_3)_3.N^+CH_2.CHOH.CH_2.COO^-$; the betaine of β-hydroxy-γ-aminobutyric acid, a water-soluble constituent of extracts of muscle. It appears to be identical with vitamin B_T.

Carnochan, John Murray [*American surgeon*, 1817–87]. Remembered as the first to excise the maxillary nerve for the relief of facial neuralgia; he removed the second division of the fifth cranial nerve together with the sphenopalatine ganglion as far back as the foramen rotundum. His operation for elephantiasis consisted in ligating main artery of limb involved.

car′no·sine (kahr′no·seen, ·sin). $C_9H_{14}N_4O_3$. Alanyl histidine, a dipeptide said to occur in muscle tissue; crystals of it have been isolated from meat extracts.

Carnoy's fixing fluid. See under *fixing fluid*.

car′ob [Ar. *karrūbah*]. A tree of the Near East, *Ceratonia siliqua*, whose pods yield **carob gum,** used in cosmetic preparation and as a pill excipient.

car·on′a·mide. Former spelling of *carinamide*.

car″o·te·nae′mi·a. See *carotenemia*.

car′o·tene [L. *carota*, carrot]. Any of three isomeric hydrocarbons, of the formula $C_{40}H_{56}$, distinguished by the prefixes α-, β-, and γ-. All are synthesized by plants, the α- and β-isomers being the more abundant. When pure they are red or purple crystalline solids, the color being due to the presence of a series of conjugated ethylenic linkages. The carotenes are precursors of vitamin A, β-carotene yielding two molecules of vitamin A, the others one molecule. Also spelled *carotin*.

car″o·te·ne′mi·a [*carota;* G. *haima*, blood]. Presence of carotene in the circulating blood. When excessive (*hypercarotenemia*), it may cause a yellowish pigmentation of the skin called pseudojaundice.

ca·rot′e·noid, ca·rot′i·noid (ka·rot′i·noyd, kar′o-ti·noyd) [*carota;* G. *eidos*, form]. One of a group of plant pigments occurring in carrots, tomatoes, and other vegetables, and in fruits and flowers. Chemically, carotenoids are unsaturated hydrocarbons of high molecular weight containing a series of conjugated ethylenic linkages or derivatives of such hydrocarbons. —**carot′enoid, carot′inoid,** *adj.*

car″o·te·no′sis [*carota;* G. *-ōsis*, condition]. Pigmentation of the skin due to carotene and carotenoids in the tissues. Syn., *aurantiasis cutis*.

ca·rot′ic [G. *karōtikos*, stupefying]. Pertaining to stupor.

ca·rot″i·co·cli′noid [*karōtikos;* G. *klinē*, bed; *eidos*, form]. Relating to an internal carotid artery and a clinoid process of the sphenoid bone.

ca·rot″i·co·tym·pan′ic [*karōtikos;* G. *tympanon*, drum]. Relating to the carotid canal and the tympanum. See Tables of Nerves and of Arteries in the Appendix.

ca·rot′id [G. *karōtides*, carotid arteries]. 1. The carotid artery, the principal large artery on each side of the neck. 2. A carotid nerve. —**carotid,** *adj.*

c. nerves. Sympathetic nerves, from the superior cervical ganglion, which innervate the smooth muscles and glands of the head. The **external carotid nerve** forms plexuses on the external carotid artery and its branches; the **internal carotid nerve** forms plexuses on the internal carotid artery and its branches.

common c. An artery which originates on the right from the innominate and on the left from the arch of the aorta, and has external and internal carotid, rarely superior thyroid, ascending pharyngeal, and even vertebral branches. It distributes blood to the region of the neck and head.

external c. An artery which originates at the common carotid and has superior thyroid, ascending pharyngeal, lingual, external maxillary (facial), sternocleidomastoid (occasionally), occipital, posterior auricular, superficial temporal, and internal maxillary branches. It distributes blood to the anterior portion of the neck, face, scalp, side of the head, ear, and dura mater.

internal c. An artery which originates at the common carotid and has three sets of branches: the *petrous portion* has a corticotympanic branch and the artery of the pterygoid canal (Vidian) (inconstant); the *cavernous portion* has cavernous, hypophyseal, semilunar, anterior meningeal, and ophthalmic branches; and the *cerebral portion* has anterior cerebral, middle cerebral, posterior communicating, and choroid branches. The artery distributes blood to the cerebrum, the eye and its appendages, the forehead, nose, internal ear, trigeminal nerve, dura mater, and hypophysis.

car″ot·i·dyn′i·a. See *carotodynia*.

car′o·tin. See *carotene*.

car″o·ti·ne′mi·a. Carotenemia.

ca·rot′i·noid. See *carotenoid*.

ca·rot′is [*karōtides*]. The carotid artery.

car″ot·o·dyn′i·a, car″ot·i·dyn′i·a (kar″rot·o-din′i·a; kar″rot·i·din′i·a). Pain in the malar region, around the eye and back of neck, due to pressure on the common carotid artery.

car′pa·ine (kahr′pay·een, ·in, kahr′puh·). $C_{14}H_{25}NO_2$. An alkaloid from the leaves of *Carica papaya.* It is said to slow the heart and depress the nervous system.

car′pal [G. *karpos*, wrist]. Pertaining to the wrist or carpus.

car·pec′to·my [*karpos;* G. *ektomē*, excision]. Excision of a carpal bone or bones.

car·phol′o·gy, car″pho·lo′gi·a [G. *karphos*, chips; *legein*, to collect]. Aimless picking and plucking at bedclothes, seen in delirious states, fevers, and exhaustion. Syn., *floccillation.*

Carpi, Berengario da. See *Berengario da Carpi.*

car′po-, carp- [G. *karpos*, wrist]. A combining form meaning *carpus* or *wrist.*

car″po·met″a·car′pal [*karpos;* G. *metakarpion*, from *meta*, beyond, *karpos*]. Pertaining to the carpal and the metacarpal bones; applied to the joints between them and to the ligaments joining them. See Table of Joints and Ligaments in the Appendix.

car″po·pe′dal (kahr″po·pee′dul, ·ped′ul) [*karpos;* L. *pes*, foot]. Affecting the wrists and feet, or the fingers and toes.

car″po·pha·lan′ge·al [*karpos;* G. *phalagx*, bone between the two joints of the fingers]. Pertaining to the wrist and the phalanges.

car′po·side. A crystalline glycoside from *Carica papaya.*

Carpue, Joseph Constantine [*English surgeon*, 1764–1846]. Pioneer in electrotherapy (1803). Known for his operations for stone in the urinary bladder. Popularized the so-called high operation which he described (1819). Revived the Hindu method of rhinoplasty in which he restored a nose by taking a heart-shaped flap from the forehead (1816).

carpule. Trade-mark for a glass cartridge containing a sterile solution of a drug which is loaded into a specially contrived syringe and is ready for hypodermic injection.

car′pus [G. *karpos*, wrist]. The wrist, consisting of eight wrist bones. See Table of Bones in the Appendix. —**carpal,** *adj.*

Carr, Francis Howard (1874–). English chemist, known for his published work on the alkaloids, and for his introduction with E. A. Price of the antimony trichloride test for vitamin A, formerly used as a standard and called *Carr-Price unit.*

car′ra·geen. Irish moss. See *Chondrus.*

Carrel, Alexis [*French surgeon*, 1873–1944]. Introduced the extravital cultivation of tissues. Demonstrated that arteries can be transplanted after being stored for some time. Successfully transplanted a kidney from one animal to another. Developed a method of suturing blood vessels end to end; correct apposition is maintained by three traction sutures, the site of suture assuming a triangular shape, called *Carrel method* or *suture.* With Dakin, developed a method of treating wounds by irrigation with a solution of chlorinated soda and sodium bicarbonate; called *Carrel-Dakin treatment.* He also devised various culture flasks (*Carrel flasks*) with slanting or horizontal necks for maintaining stable tissue cultures over long periods of time, and with Lindbergh, devised a perfusion apparatus with which organs can be kept alive outside the body, called *Carrel-Lindbergh pump.* Nobel laureate (1912).

car′ri·er [ONF. *carier*]. 1. A normal person or one convalescing from an infectious disease who shows no signs or symptoms of the disease but who harbors and eliminates the microorganism, and so spreads the disease. 2. A quantity of a naturally occurring element added to a minute amount of pure isotope to facilitate the chemical handling of the isotope.

bacteria c. A vector.

chronic c. One who eliminates the infectious element for an indefinite period.

temporary c. A convalescent who eliminates the infectious element for only a short time after recovery. Also called *transitory c.*

car′ri·er-free″. *In radiochemistry*, of, pertaining to, or describing a radioactive isotope to which none of the stable form of the isotope has been added as a carrier.

Carrión, Daniel Alcides (1859–1885). Peruvian medical student who inoculated himself with material from verruca peruviana and died 39 days later of Oroya fever, an experiment which offered suggestive evidence of the etiologic unity of the two conditions (1885), later shown to be caused by *Bartonella bacilliformis. Carrión's disease* or *bartonellosis* includes both forms.

Carroll, James [*American Army medical officer*, 1854–1907]. Served with Reed, Agramonte y Simoni, and Lazear on the United States Army Yellow Fever Commission which investigated the etiology of the disease and proved that it is transmitted to man by mosquitoes (1900–01).

car sick′ness. A form of motion sickness occurring as a result of movement of a train or automobile. See *airsickness, motion sickness.*

Carswell, Robert [*English physician*, 1793–1857]. Noted as a leading pathologist of his time and author of *Pathological Anatomy*, an atlas with 2000 hand-colored illustrations by himself, said to be unequaled in its excellence (1838). Gave one of the first comprehensive descriptions of disseminated sclerosis. Described pulmonary tubercles, called *Carswell's grapes.*

Carter, Henry Rose [*American public health officer*, 1852–1925]. Remembered for his investigations of yellow fever epidemics (1898); contributed valuable facts concerning its incubation period, influencing the work of Walter Reed at a later date.

Carter, Henry Vandyke [*English physician in India*, 1831–97]. Gave the first adequate descriptions of mycetoma of the foot, called *madura foot* (1861–74). Described spirillum fever (relapsing fever), which he reproduced in monkeys (1882). Described a minute organism, *Spirillum minus*, the cause of rat-bite fever (1887).

Carter, William Wesley [*American rhinologist, otolaryngologist, and plastic surgeon*, 1869–1950]. Known for his operation of rhinoplasty in which he used a portion of rib and rib cartilage to form a new bridge for the nose, and for devising the submucous operation for the correction of deflections of the nasal septum.

Cartesius. See *Descartes.*

Car′tha·mus [Ar. *qirṭim*]. A genus of Eurasian herbs of the Carduaceae.

C. tinctorius. Safflower; American or bastard saffron. The dried flowers are used in making an infusion used popularly as a diaphoretic.

car′ti·lage (kahr′ti·lidj) [L. *cartilago*, cartilage]. Gristle; a white, semiopaque, nonvascular connective tissue composed of a matrix containing nucleated cells which lie in cavities or lacunas of the matrix. When boiled, cartilage yields a substance called chondrin. —**cartilag′inous,** *adj.*

alar cartilages. The **major alar c.** is the lower lateral cartilage of the nose, and the **minor alar c.,** one of the lesser alar cartilages of the nose.

annular c. (a) Any ring-shaped cartilage. (b) The cricoid cartilage.

aortic c. The second costal cartilage on the right side.
arthrodial c. See articular *c.*
articular c. That covering the articular surfaces of bones. See Plate 2.
arytenoid c. One of two cartilages of the larynx regulating, by means of the attached muscles, the tension of the vocal folds.
auricular c. The cartilage of the pinna of the ear.
basilar c. The cartilage in the foramen lacerum.
bronchial c. Plates of cartilage, in some instances very minute, found in the bronchial tubes.
calcified c. That in which a calcareous deposit is contained in the matrix.
c. of Santorini. See corniculate *c.*
c. of Wrisberg. See cuneiform *c.*
circumferential c. The fibrocartilaginous rim about certain articulations.
corniculate cartilages. Cartilaginous nodules on the tips of the arytenoid cartilages. Also called *Santorini's cartilages.*
costal c. That occupying the interval between the true ribs and the sternum or adjacent cartilages.
cricoid c. The ring-shaped cartilage of the larynx.
cuneiform cartilages. Two small, rod-shaped cartilages of the larynx, located in the aryepiglottic folds anterior to the corniculate cartilages. Formerly called *Wrisberg's cartilages.*
diarthrodial c. See articular *c.*
ectethmoid c. See paranasal *c.*
elastic c. A type in which a feltwork of elastic fibers pervades the matrix.
embryonal c. Developing cartilage, usually cellular; young cartilage.
ensiform c. Old term for xiphoid process.
epactal cartilages. Small cartilaginous nodules on the upper edge of the alar cartilages of the nose.
epiglottal c. The cartilage of the epiglottis.
epiphyseal c. The cartilage of an epiphysis: also called *growth cartilage.*
episternal c. One of a pair of small embryonic cartilages articulating with the clavicle and forming part of the manubrium: also called (especially in some reptiles) *episternal bar.*
Eustachian c. That of the auditory tube. See tubal *c.*
fetal c. See temporary *c.*
floating c. A detached segment of cartilage in a joint cavity.
Huschke's c. See vomeronasal *c.*
hyaline c. That in which the matrix is clear and homogeneous.
innominate c. The cricoid cartilage.
interarticular cartilages. Flat fibrocartilages situated between the articulating surfaces of some of the joints. Also called *interarticular fibrocartilages, articular disks.*
interarytenoid c. An inconstant cartilage found between the arytenoid cartilages.
interhemal cartilages. Nodules of cartilage which aid in the formation of the hemal arch of a vertebra.
intermediary c. (a) Cartilage bone in process of transformation into true bone. (b) That interposed between the epiphysis and diaphysis of a bone; epiphyseal *c.*
interneural cartilages. Nodules of cartilage which aid in the formation of the neural arch of a vertebra.
intersphenoidal c. The cartilage between the basisphenoid and orbitosphenoid ossification centers in the fetus, which may persist until the thirteenth year.
intervertebral cartilages. See intervertebral *disks.*
investing c. See articular *c.*
Jacobson's c. See vomeronasal *c.*
laryngeal cartilages. The cartilages supporting the larynx.
lateral nasal cartilages. The upper lateral cartilage of the nose.
Luschka's c. An inconstant, small, cartilaginous nodule, enclosed in the front of the true vocal folds.
Luschka's subpharyngeal c. A small, inconstant body of hyaline cartilage, situated in the capsule or a septum of the palatine tonsil.
mandibular c. See Meckel's *c.*
meatal c. The U-shaped cartilaginous part of the external canal which is deficient superiorly and is continuous with the auricular cartilage.
Meckel's c. The cartilage bar of the mandibular arch.
palpebral c. Incorrect term for the connective tissue forming the framework of the eyelids; the tarsal plate. It is not composed of cartilage.
parachordal c. See *parachordal.*
paranasal c. The embryonic cartilage which gives rise to the inferior nasal conchae and all the ethmoid bone except the perpendicular plate.
paraseptal cartilages. Embryonic cartilages on either side of the inferior border of the septal cartilage of the nose. The vomeronasal cartilages are the persistent remains. Also called subvomerine *c.*
precricoid c. The interarytenoid cartilage.
quadrate cartilages. Several small cartilages passing out from the alar cartilages in the external part of the nostril.
Reichert's c. The cartilage of the hyoid arch.
Santorini's c. The corniculate cartilages.
semilunar cartilages. Two interarticular cartilages of the knee.
septal c. of the nose. Cartilage of the nasal septum.
sesamoid cartilages. A pair of small cartilages lying along the lateral margins of the arytenoid cartilages; they are constant in some animals and are occasionally found in man.
sphenobasilar c. See spheno-occipital *c.*
spheno-occipital c. The cartilage between the sphenoid and basilar part of the occipital, permitting growth of basis cranii until the twentieth year. Syn., *sphenobasilar c.*
subvomerine c. See vomeronasal *c.*
synarthrodial c. That of any fixed or slightly movable articulation.
tarsal c. See palpebral *c.*
temporary c. That which is ultimately replaced by bone.
thyroid c. The largest of the laryngeal cartilages, consisting of two laminas united at an angle in front called the laryngeal prominence. See Plates 13, 45.
trabecular cartilages. The prechordal primordia of the sphenoid, usually single in man.
triradiate c. The Y-shaped cartilage in the acetabulum between the ilium, pubis, and ischium; it disappears when the three bones fuse to form the adult hipbone.
triticeous c. A small, oblong cartilaginous nodule often found in the lateral thyrohyoid membrane.
tubal c. A rolled triangular cartilage running from the osseous part of the auditory tube to the pharynx: also called *Eustachian c.*
vomeronasal c. A strip of hyaline cartilage extending from the anterior nasal spine upward and backward on either side of the septal cartilage of the nose and attached to the anterior margin of the vomer: also called *Jacobson's cartilage.*
Wrisberg's cartilages. The cuneiform cartilages.

xiphoid c. The lower cartilaginous tip of the sternum.

yellow c. Elastic cartilage.

car″ti·la·gin″i·fi·ca′tion [*cartilago;* L. *facere,* to make]. A change into cartilage; chondrification.

ca′rum [G. *karon,* caraway]. Caraway; the dried ripe fruit of *Carum carvi.* Its odor and taste are due to a volatile oil containing carvone and *d*-limonene; used chiefly as a flavor.

car′un·cle, ca·run′cle [L. *caruncula,* a little piece of flesh]. A small, fleshy, red mass or nodule. **—carun′cular, carun′culate, carun′culated,** *adj.*

hymenal c. Any of the small irregular nodules which are the remains of the hymen.

lacrimal c. A small, reddish mass at the inner canthus. See Plate 19.

sublingual c. Any of the small papillae found along the sublingual fold where the ducts of the sublingual and the submaxillary glands empty.

urethral c. A small, benign, spherical or elliptical, strawberry-colored mass, sessile or pedunculated, situated on the posterior wall of the external urinary meatus of women; observed most frequently at the menopause, and a cause of pain and bleeding. Microscopically it is composed mainly of granulationlike tissue.

ca·run′cu·la [L.]. Caruncle.

Carus, Carl Gustav [*German obstetrician,* 1789–1869]. Remembered for his description of the longitudinal axis of the pelvic, or birth, canal which forms a curved line having as its center the symphysis pubis; called *curve of Carus.*

carvacrol. $C_{10}H_{14}O$. 2-Hydroxy-*p*-cymene, isomeric with thymol. It occurs in oils of marjoram and savory and is actively germicidal; has been proposed as an anthelmintic.

car′vone. $C_{10}H_{14}O$. A terpene ketone found in the volatile oils of caraway, dill, fennel, and spearmint.

car″y·en′chy·ma. See *karyenchyma.*

ca′ry·in [G. *karya,* nut-bearing tree]. A crystallizable principle from hickory bark.

car′y·o-, car′y- [G. *karyon,* nut]. A combining form signifying *nut* or *kernel.* Also see *kary-, karyo-.*

car″y·o·chrome′. See *karyochrome.*

car″y·o·clas′tic. Cell-nucleus splitting.

car″y·o·phyl′lin (kar″ee·o·fill′in, kar″ee·off′i·lin). A principle from cloves, identical with oleanolic acid.

car″y·o·phyl′lus (kar″ee·o·fill′us, ·off′i·lus). See *clove.*

Casal, Gaspar [*Spanish physician,* ca. 1681–1759]. In his book on the natural and medical history of Spain, written in 1735 but published posthumously (1762), he gave the first clear description of pellagra, which he called *mal de la rosa.* The skin lesions which occur in pellagra on the back of the neck are called *Casal's collar, necklace.* At first they are hyperemic and edematous; later they scale and leave a rough, red area.

Casares Gil's stain. See under *stain.*

cas′ca bark. Sassy bark; the bark of *Erythrophleum guineense,* an African tree. See *erythrophleine.*

cas·car′a (kas·kair′uh, kas·kar′uh) [Sp., bark]. Cascara sagrada.

aromatic c. sagrada fluidextract. One prepared from cascara sagrada debitterized with magnesium oxide, flavored and sweetened with saccharin: used as a cathartic. Dose, 2 cc, (30 min.).

c. amarga. Honduras bark. The bark of *Sweetia panamensis,* native to Mexico, which has been used as a bitter tonic.

c. sagrada. The bark of *Rhamnus Purshiana,* the chief constituents of which are anthraquinone derivatives. It is useful in chronic constipation. Also called *chittem bark, sacred bark.*

c. sagrada extract. A powdered extract representing 3 times its weight of cascara sagrada. Dose, 0.3 Gm. (5 gr.).

c. sagrada fluidextract. One prepared by extracting cascara sagrada with water; each cc. represents 1 Gm. of drug: used as a cathartic. Dose, 1 cc. (15 min.).

cas″ca·ril′la [Sp., dim. of *cáscara*]. The bark of *Croton eluteria,* native to the Bahama Islands; an aromatic bitter. Syn., *eleuthera bark.*

cas″ca·ril′lin. $C_{12}H_{18}O_4$. The bitter principle of cascarilla; white crystals, slightly soluble in water.

cas′ca·rin [*cáscara*]. A glycosidal cathartic fraction isolated from the bark of *Rhamnus Purshiana* (cascara sagrada); it occurs in granular masses or prisms.

case [L. *casus,* from *cadere,* to fall, happen]. 1. A single instance or example of a disease. 2. A covering; a boxlike structure.

brain c. Portion of the skull containing the brain.

c. history. Anamnesis.

c. taking. The collection of memoranda and notes of an individual case for service in diagnosis or prognosis, or for use in a medicolegal inquiry.

missed c. A mild or atypical case of a disease, which misses clinical recognition.

trial c. *In ophthalmology,* a case containing various lenses for refracting the eye.

ca′se·ase [L. *caseus,* cheese]. An enzyme from bacterial cultures which digests albumin and casein.

ca′se·ate [*caseus*]. 1. A lactate. 2. Caseinate, a casein compound.

ca′se·ate. To undergo caseous degeneration.

ca″se·a′tion [*caseus*]. 1. The precipitation of casein during the coagulation of milk. 2. A form of necrosis which changes tissue into a soft, cheeselike substance, characteristic of tuberculous infection.

casec. Trade-mark of a brand of calcium caseinate.

ca′se·ic ac′id (kay′see·ick, ka·see′ick). Lactic acid.

ca′se·i·form [*caseus;* L. *forma,* form]. Like cheese or casein.

ca′se·in [*caseus*]. A protein obtained from milk by the action of rennin or acids. Soluble in acids and alkalies.

c. iodine. A compound of milk casein with about 18% iodine in organic combination. Has been used in tertiary syphilis and for prophylaxis of goiter.

c. saccharide. A mixture of casein and sucrose used as an emulsifying agent.

c. sodium. A compound of casein and sodium hydroxide, used as nutrient.

gluten c. Vegetable casein.

saliva c. Ptyalin.

vegetable c. A protein of plant origin resembling the casein of milk, as legumin conglutin. Also called *gluten c.*

ca″se·in′o·gen [*caseus;* G. *genesthai,* from *gignesthai,* to be produced]. A compound protein of milk, yielding casein when acted upon by digestive enzymes; the precursor of casein, analogous to fibrinogen, myosinogen, etc.

ca′se·o-, ca′se- [*caseus*]. A combining form denoting *casein.*

ca′se·ose [*caseus*]. A product of the hydrolysis or gastric digestion of casein.

ca′se·ous [*caseus*]. Resembling, or having the nature or consistency of, cheese. See *caseation,* 2.

cas-evac. Trade-mark for a liquid laxative prepared from cascara sagrada.

case′worm″. See *Echinococcus.*

Cas″i·mi·ro′a (kas″i·mi·ro′uh, kas″i·mirr′o·uh) [after *Casimiro* Gómez de Ortega, Spanish botanist, 1740–1818]. A genus of plants belonging to the Rutaceae.

C. edulis. A species found in Mexico. The leaves have been used as an anthelmintic. Also called *white sapota.*

Casoni's test. See under *test.*

cas·sa′va (ka·sah′vuh) [Taino *casavi*]. 1. Any of several plants of the genus *Manihot.* 2. The starch obtained from rhizomes of *Manihot esculenta* and *Manihot aipi;* nutrient. Tapioca is prepared from it by heating while moist.

Casselberry, William Evans [*American laryngologist,* 1858–1916]. Devised a posture which the patient assumes after intubation. This prevents fluids from entering the tubes during the taking of liquids; known as *Casselberry's position.*

Casserius Placentinus, Julius (Giulio Casserio) [*Italian anatomist,* 1561–1616]. Outstanding leader in the field of comparative anatomy; teacher of Harvey. Described the structure and character of the auditory and vocal organs (1600–01). Noted the maxillary sinus, later described by Highmore. Described the posterior fontanel.

cas″sette′ (kah″set′, ka·zet′) [F., little box]. A holder for a roentgenographic film or plate.

Cas′si·a (cash′ee·uh, kas′ee·uh) [G. *kasia,* cassia]. A genus of the Leguminosae, several species of which provide senna.

C. alata. The ringworm shrub; a widely diffused tropical shrub. The juice of the leaves mixed with lime juice has been used in the treatment of ringworm.

C. beareana. A species indigenous to East Africa. The root and powdered bark have been used in native medicine.

C. fistula. See purging *cassia.*

C. marilandica. A species found in North America. Its leaves, American senna, are less active as a cathartic than the true senna.

cas′sia (cash′uh, cash′ee·uh) [*kasia*]. An old name, still used commercially, for the coarser varieties of cinnamon.

c. bark. Chinese cinnamon.

c. buds. The dried flowers of Chinese cinnamon; used chiefly as spice.

c. oil. The volatile cinnamon oil used in pharmacy and in perfumery; its chief constituent is cinnamic aldehyde.

purging c. *Cassia fistula.* The dried fruit of a tree growing in tropical regions. The pulp is a mild laxative, probably because of its high sugar content, although it contains a small amount of anthraquinone derivatives. Dose, 0.5 Gm. (8 gr.).

cas′sic ac′id. An antibiotic substance derived from the leaves of *Cassia reticulata:* active against a number of bacteria.

cast [ON. *kasta*]. 1. A mass of fibrous material or exudate that has taken the form of some cavity in which it has been molded. From their source, casts may be classified as bronchial, intestinal, nasal, esophageal, renal, tracheal, urethral, vaginal, etc. Of these, the renal casts, by reason of their significance in diseases of the kidney, are the most important. Classed according to their constitution, casts are blood, epithelial, fatty, fibrinous, granular, hyaline, mucous, waxy, etc. 2. An accurate reproduction in form of an object, structure, or part in some plastic substance which has taken form in an impression or mold. 3. A lay term for strabismus.

plaster c. See plaster of Paris *c.*

plaster of Paris c. A mixture of gypsum and water which becomes hard upon drying; when incorporated into gauze as a binder it may be used to immobilize fractured bones, arthritic joints, the spine, etc. Syn., *plaster c.*

waxy c. A tubal renal cast composed of translucent, usually amyloid, material.

Castaigne method. The Achard-Castaigne method for renal permeability. See methylene blue *test.*

Castañeda's rat lung method. See under *method.*

Castañeda vaccine. See under *vaccine.*

Castellani, Aldo (1878–). Italian pathologist; eminent authority in tropical medicine and microbiology; author of several books on tropical medicine. He discovered *Trypanosoma gambiense* in the spinal fluid of patients with Gambian trypanosomiasis or African sleeping sickness (1903), and was the first to establish a spirochete, *Treponema pertenue,* as the etiological agent of yaws (1905). He reported bronchospirochetosis (1920), called *Castellani's disease,* and contributed extensively to medical mycology. He also developed techniques of agglutination absorption and the symbiotic fermentation phenomenon.

cast′ing [ON. *kasta*]. 1. *In dentistry,* the act of forcing molten metal into a suitable mold. 2. *In veterinary medicine,* the act of throwing an animal on its side before administering an anesthetic.

Castle, William Bosworth (1897–). American physician, known for his experimental work and observations on human digestion, with special reference to the cause of pernicious anemia (1929). He also demonstrated the effectiveness of injectable liver extract in control of tropical sprue, and of iron in the treatment of anemia of hookworm disease without removal of parasites (1931).

cas′tor. Castoreum.

c. bean. The seed of *Ricinus communis.*

c. oil (*oleum ricini*). The fixed oil obtained from the seed of *Ricinus communis;* the oil contains glycerides of ricinoleic acid which impart its cathartic property. Dose, 15–60 cc. (½–2 fluidounces).

c. xylene. A mixture composed of castor oil, one part, and xylene, three parts; used for clearing or clarifying collodion or celloidin of objects embedded in them.

cas·to′re·um [G. *kastoreion,* from *kastōr,* beaver]. Dried preputial glands and their secretion, obtained from the beaver, *Castor fiber.* It is a reddish brown substance with a strong odor; formerly used in hysteria, its action resembling that of musk.

cas·tra′tion [L. *castrare,* to castrate]. Orchiectomy; the excision of one or both testes or ovaries. —**cas′trated,** *adj.;* **cas′trate,** *n., v.t.*

emotional c. See castration *anxiety* and castration *complex.*

female c. Removal of the ovaries; oophorectomy; spaying.

cas″tro·phre′ni·a [*castrare;* G. *phrēn,* mind]. A morbid fear or delusion, occasional in schizophrenic patients, that their thoughts are being sucked out of their brains by enemies. Syn., *nooklopia.*

Castroviejo, Ramón [*American ophthalmologist,* 1904–]. Known for his keratoplastic operation of transplantation of the cornea, in which a special double knife is used to outline a square on the cornea. A square plug is removed, after which the graft is similarly taken from the eye of the donor, being held in place with a cross stitch and conjunctival flap.

cas′u·al·ty [L. *casus,* from *cadere,* to fall, happen]. 1. An accident causing injury or death. 2. *In military medicine,* a member of the armed forces who is lost to a command, temporarily or permanently, by death, wounds, injury, sickness, internment, capture, missing in action.

cas″u·is′tics (kazh″o͞o·iss′ticks, kaz″yo͞o·) [*casus*].

Study of individual cases as a means of arriving at the general history of a disease.

cat′a-, cat-, cath- [G. *kata*, down]. A prefix denoting *downward, in accordance with, against, back, completely*. See also *kata-*.

cat″a·ba′si·al [*kata;* G. *basis*, base]. Noting skulls in which the basion is lower than the opisthion.

ca·tab′a·sis [G. *katabasis*, descent]. The decline of a disease. —**catabat′ic,** *adj.*

cat″a·bi·o′sis (cat″uh·buy·o′sis). See *catabolism.*

ca·tab′o·lin. Catabolite.

ca·tab′o·lism [*kata; ballein*]. Destructive phase of metabolism concerned with the breaking down by the body of complex compounds, often with the liberation of energy; the opposite of anabolism. —**catabol′ic,** *adj.*

ca·tab′o·lite. Any product of catabolism. Syn., *catabolin, catastate.*

cat″a·clei′sis (cat″uh·kly′sis) [G. *katakleisis*, a closing]. Closure of the eyelids by adhesion or by spasm.

cat″a·clo′nus [G. *kata*, down; *klonos*, confused motion]. Rhythmic convulsive movements which are of functional or hysterical nature rather than expressions of true epilepsy. —**cataclon′ic,** *adj.*

cat″a·cous′tics (cat″uh·kōōs′ticks) [*kata;* G. *akouein*, to hear]. The science of reflected sound; echolocation.

cat″a·crot′ic [G. *katakrotos*, from *kata; krotos*, a beat]. Designating the descending limb of the arterial pulse wave or any irregularities in it.

cat·ac′ro·tism [*kata; krotos*]. A condition of the arterial pulse characterized by significant oscillations in its descending, or catacrotic, limb.

cat″a·did′y·mus. See *katadidymus.*

cat″a·di·op′tric (cat″uh·dye·op′trick) [*kata;* G. *dioptrikos*, from *dia*, through, root of *opsomai*, I shall see]. Pertaining to both reflection and refraction of light rays.

cat″a·gel″o·pho′bi·a [G. *katagelōs*, derision; *phobos*, fear]. Morbid fear of ridicule.

cat′a·lase (cat′uh·lace, ·laze) [cf. G. *katallassein*, to change]. 1. An enzyme found in tissues, capable of decomposing peroxides. 2. Any one of a group of oxidizing enzymes.

cat′a·lep″sy [G. *katalēpsis*, a seizing]. A state of unconsciousness, usually trancelike, in which there is a loss of voluntary motion and a peculiar plastic rigidity of the muscles, by reason of which they retain for an indefinite time any position in which they are placed. The condition is associated with hysteria and the schizophrenic reactions, and is a stage of hypnotic sleep. In **local catalepsy,** a single organ or group of muscles is affected. Also called *catalepsis.* —**catalep′tiform, catalep′toid,** *adj.;* **catalep′tic,** *adj., n.;* **catalep′tize,** *v.*

cat″a·lep″to·le·thar′gic [*katalēpsis;* G. *lēthargos*, drowsiness]. Having the nature of catalepsy and lethargy.

Ca·tal′pa [Creek *kutuhlpa*]. A genus of American and Asiatic trees of the Bignoniaceae. The seeds of **C. bignonioides** and **C. speciosa,** of North America, have been used in asthma.

ca·tal′y·sis [G. *kata*, down; *lysis*, a loosing]. The process of change in the velocity of a chemical reaction through the presence of a substance which apparently remains chemically unaltered throughout the reaction. The velocity may be increased, in which case the process is described as *positive catalysis*, or it may be decreased, in which case the process is described as *negative catalysis.* —**catalyza′tion,** *n.*

cat′a·lyst [*kata; lysis*]. 1. A substance having the power to produce catalysis. 2. A substance which increases the velocity of a chemical reaction. Its concentration at the beginning of the reaction is equal to its concentration at the end. Syn., *catalyzer.* See *biocatalyst, enzyme.* —**catalyt′ic,** *adj.*

cat′a·ly″zer. Catalyst.

cat″a·me′ni·a [G. *kata*, according to; *mēn*, month]. Menstruation. —**catamenial,** *adj.*

cat″am·ne′sis [G. *kata*, down from; *mnēsis*, a remembering]. The medical history of a patient following an illness or a behavior disorder. —**catamnes′tic,** *adj.*

cat″a·mor′pho·sis [Gr. *kata*, down; Gr. *morphosis*, shaping, development]. The irreversible degradation of mechanical, chemical, and light energy to heat and the continual disappearance of heat gradients: a characteristic of closed physical systems and a necessary consequence of the second law of thermodynamics.

cat′a·pasm [G. *katapasma*, powder]. A dry powder to be sprinkled upon the skin or upon a sore.

cat″a·pha′si·a (cat″uh·fay′zhuh, ·zee·uh) [G. *kataphasis*, affirmation]. A speech disorder in which the patient keeps repeating the same word or series of words.

ca·taph′o·ra [G. *kataphora*, lethargic attack, from *katapheresthai*, to be brought down]. Lethargy associated with periods of imperfect remission; coma with intervals of imperfect consciousness.

cat″a·pho·re′sis (cat″uh·fo·ree′sis, ·for′i·sis) [G. *kata*, down; *phorēsis*, from *pherein*, to carry]. The migration of charged colloidal particles through the medium in which they are dispersed, when placed under the influence of an applied electric potential. Preferably called *electrophoresis.* The process of iontophoresis is sometimes erroneously called cataphoresis. —**cataphoret′ic,** *adj.*

cat″a·pho′ri·a [*kata;* G. *phoros*, tending]. A tendency of the visual axes of both eyes to incline below the horizontal plane.

cat″a·phor′ic [*kata; phoros*]. 1. Pertaining to cataphoresis. 2. Relating to cataphora.

cat″a·phy·lax′is [*kata;* G. *phylaxis*, a guarding]. Movement and transportation of phylactic agents (leukocytes, antibodies) to the site of an infection.

cat″a·pla′si·a (cat″uh·play′zhuh, ·zee·uh, ·shuh, ·see·uh), **ca·tap′la·sis** [*kata;* G. *plassein*, to form]. 1. Stage of decline in life. 2. Degenerative changes affecting cells and tissues, especially reversion to an earlier or embryonic type of cell or tissue. 3. Application of a plaster or coating. *Obs.*

cat′a·plasm [G. *kataplasma*, a poultice]. A poultice, of various substances and usually applied when hot.

kaolin c. A mixture of kaolin, glycerin, and boric acid, with small amounts of thymol, methyl salicylate, and peppermint oil.

cat′a·plex″y [G. *kataplēxis*, amazement, from *kataplēssein*, to strike down]. 1. A sudden and overwhelming emotion, fright, or shock causing muscular rigidity in some animals. 2. In man, the sudden loss of muscle tone provoked by exaggerated emotion, often associated with a tendency to narcolepsy. 3. Prostration by the sudden onset of disease. 4. Hypnotic sleep. —**cataplec′tic,** *adj.*

cat′a·ract [G. *katarraktēs*, cataract]. Partial or complete opacity of the crystalline lens or its capsule. —**catarac′tous,** *adj.*

allergic c. A cataract appearing in young persons who have had chronic and usually severe atopic dermatitis. Syn., *atopic c.*

aridosiliculose c. An overmature cataract with a dry, wrinkled capsule. Also called *aridosiliquate c.*

atomic c. See irradiation *c.*

black c. A nuclear cataract with a dark opacity.

blood c. A blood clot anterior to the lens and obstructing the pupil.

blue dot c. See cerulean *c.*
capsular c. Cataract due to opacity of the capsule.
capsulolenticular c. One involving both the capsule and the lens.
cerulean c. A cataract consisting of small, punctate opacities in the lens, which have a blue tint best seen with a slit lamp; it is usually congenital and not progressive. Also called *blue dot c.*
chalky c. See aridosiliculose *c.*
cholesterin c. One containing what are apparently crystals of cholesterin.
complicated c. Cataract secondary to intraocular disease.
concussion c. A soft cataract due to an explosion or some other concussion.
cortical c. One due to the loss of transparency of the outer layers of the lens.
cyclotron c. See irradiation *c.*
cystic c. See Morgagnian *c.*
diabetic c. A form associated with diabetes.
fibrinous c. A false cataract consisting of an effusion on the capsule during severe iridocyclitis.
fluid c. The breaking-up of an overmature cataract into a milky fluid.
glassblower's c. See irradiation *c.*
hard c. See senile *c.*
immature c. One in which only a part of the lens substance is cataractous.
incipient c. Forked linear opacities in the equatorial region of the lens seen in middle-aged persons and sometimes remaining unchanged for years.
intumescent c. An overmature cataract presenting a white, swollen appearance from having undergone degeneration.
irradiation c. One caused by the use of radium and roentgen rays in large doses or by exposure to intense radiation: also called *atomic c., cyclotron, c., radiation c.;* formerly called *glassblower's c., puddler's c.*
lacteal c. A cataract in which the lens is filled with fluid.
lamellar c. One due to opacity of certain layers between the cortex and nucleus, the remaining layers being transparent.
lenticular c. One occurring in the lens proper.
mature c. One in which the whole lens substance is cataractous.
membranous c. A fibrinous deposit from the iris upon the capsule, which becomes opaque.
Morgagnian c. One in which an overmature cataract shrinks and leaves a nucleus floating in the dissolved outer layers.
nuclear c. One of moderate extent beginning in the nucleus.
pigmented c. A spurious cataract due to an injury by which the pigment from the posterior surface of the iris has been detached. Also called *Vossius ring.*
polar c. Either anterior or posterior; a form in which the opacity is confined to one pole of the lens.
pupillary c. Congenital closure of the pupil.
pyramidal c. One in which the opacity is at the anterior pole and is conoid, the apex extending forward.
radiation c. See irradiation *c.*
ripe c. See mature *c.*
secondary c. Capsular cataract appearing after the extraction of the lens.
senile c. The cataract of old persons, the most frequent form, and that understood when not specified as congenital, juvenile, traumatic, soft, etc.
soft c. A form occurring especially in the young; the lens matter is of soft consistency and milky in appearance.
spindle c. One characterized by a spindle-shaped opacity extending from the posterior to the anterior portion of the lens capsule.
tetanic c. A cataract due to defect in calcium metabolism.
tremulous c. One associated with laceration of the ciliary zonule, causing trembling of the iris and of the cataract on movement of the eyeball.
true c. Lenticular cataract.
unripe c. See immature *c.*
zonular c. See lamellar *c.*

ca·tarrh' [G. *katarrhoos,* from *katarrhein,* to flow down]. Old term once widely used for inflammation of mucous membranes, particularly those of the air passages of the nose and throat, with an exudation containing mucin and epithelial cells. **—catarrhal,** *adj.*
spring c. Vernal conjunctivitis.

cat"a·stal'sis [G. *katastaltikos,* from *katastellein,* to check]. The downward moving wave of contraction occurring in the stomach during digestion. There is no preceding wave of inhibition.

cat'a·state [*cata;* G. *histanai,* to stand]. Catabolite.

cat"a·thy'mi·a [G. *katathymios,* from *kata,* down; *thymos,* mind]. The existence of a complex in the unconscious mind which is heavily charged with affect or feeling so as to produce a pronounced effect in consciousness.

cat"a·to'ni·a [*kata;* G. *tonos,* tension]. A phase or type of schizophrenic reaction in which the patient seems to lack the will to talk or move and stands or sits in one position, assumes fixed postures, and resists attempts to activate motion or speech. A benign stupor which frequently may be punctuated by violent outbursts, hallucinosis, and panic. **—cataton'ic,** *adj., n.*

cat"a·tro'pi·a [*kata;* G. *tropos,* turn]. Turning of both eyes downward; cataphoria.

cat'e·chin (cat'i·chin, ·kin). $C_{15}H_{14}O_6$. An acid substance from gambir (pale catechu) and other sources. An amorphous yellow powder, soluble in water, alcohol, or alkalis; used for tanning and in calico printing. Syn., *catechuic acid.*

cat'e·chol (cat'i·chole, ·coal, ·kol, ·kawl). See *pyrocatechol.*

cat'e·chu (cat'i·choo͞, ·koo͞) [Malay *kāchū*]. Extract prepared from the wood of *Acacia catechu,* a native tree of the East Indies. It contains about 25% catechutannic acid and hence is a powerful astringent. It was formerly used as a remedy for diarrhea of children and as a gargle and mouthwash. See *gambir.*

cat"e·chu'ic ac'id (cat"i·choo͞'ick, ·cue'ick). Catechin.

cat"e·lec"trot'o·nus [G. *kata,* down; *ēlektron,* amber; *tonos,* tension]. Increased irritability of a nerve or muscle near the cathode.

cat'er·pil"lar [L. *catta pilosa,* hairy cat]. The larval form of a moth or butterfly. Caterpillars of at least one family of butterflies and several families of moths have irritant hairs which produce caterpillar dermatitis.

cat'gut" [ME. *cat;* AS. pl. *guttas*]. A suture and ligature material made from the submucosa of sheep's intestine, cleansed, treated, and twisted. Put up aseptically in glass tubes, in sizes from 00000 to 8. Varieties are: *plain* (untreated), *chromicized* (treated with chromic trioxide), and *iodized* (immersed in a solution of iodine and potassium iodide).

ca·thaer'e·sis. See *catheresis.*

ca·thar'sis [G. *katharsis,* a cleansing]. 1. Purgation. 2. *In psychoanalysis,* mental and emotional purge by abreaction.

ca·thar'tic [G. *kathartikos*, from *katharsis*]. A medicine used to produce evacuations of the bowels; a purgative. —**cathar'tic,** *adj.*

ca·thar'tic ac'id. An active principle from several species of *Cassia.*

ca·thect', ca·thec'ti·cize [G. *kathektikos*, capable of holding or retaining]. *In psychiatry,* to charge ideas with affect or feeling.

ca·thep'sin [G. *kathepsein*, to boil down]. Any one of several proteolytic enzymes present in tissue, catalyzing the hydrolysis of high molecular weight proteins to proteoses and peptones, and having an optimum pH between 4 and 5. It is believed that after death the tissues become acid, and cathepsin produces autolysis (proteolysis).

ca·ther'e·sis, ca·thaer'e·sis (ka·therr'i·sis, ka·theer'i·sis, kath"i·ree'sis) [G. *kathairesis*, a pulling down, reducing]. 1. Prostration or weakness induced by medication. 2. A feebly caustic action.

cath"e·ret'ic [G. *kathairetikos*, reducing]. 1. Reducing; weakening; prostrating. 2. Caustic. —**catheret'ic,** *n.*

cath'e·ter [G. *kathetēr*, anything let down into]. A hollow tube of metal, glass, hard or soft rubber, rubberized silk, etc., for introduction into a cavity through a narrow canal, for the purpose of discharging the fluid contents of a cavity or for establishing the patency of a canal. Specifically, one intended to be passed into the bladder through the urethra for the relief of urinary retention.

angulated c. A catheter, the leading end or beak of which is bent or angulated so as to facilitate its passage.

bicoudé c. An angulated catheter with the tip or leading end bent at two points to form a double elbow or bicoudé tip.

c. fever. The rise in temperature ascribed to the passage of a catheter, associated especially with cystitis.

c. gauge. A metal sheet having circular holes punched in it which fit exactly certain sized catheters or sounds. See following illustration:

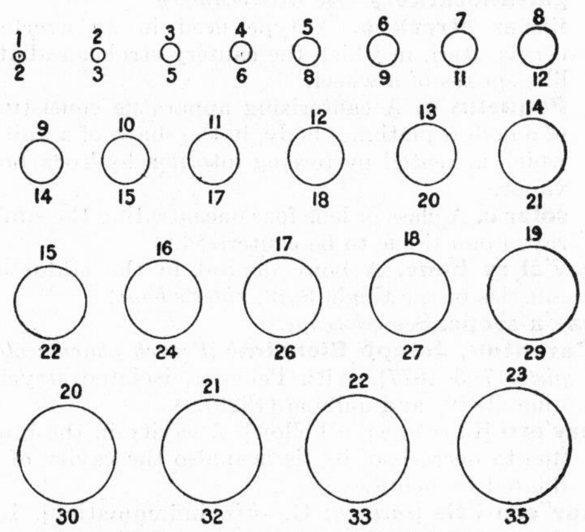

The upper number indicates the size of American catheters: the lower, the French.

c. life. A term employed to indicate constant employment of catheterization on the part of persons who are unable to void urine naturally or who can evacuate only a portion of the bladder contents because of high residual urine.

c. specimen. Urine obtained under aseptic technic, to insure its being uncontaminated when examined for diagnostic purposes.

coudé c. An angulated catheter with the tip or leading end bent at one point only to form an elbow or coudé tip.

elbow c. One of metal or stiff, rubberized material with one or two 45° bends at or near the proximal end.

eustachian c. A small catheter having a bend at the leading end: used for introduction into the auditory tube to relieve obstruction.

female c. A short catheter, usually of glass, for catheterizing women.

filiform c. A catheter the leading end of which is molded into an extremely slender or thread-shaped form in order to facilitate passage of the larger, following portion through a constricted or irregular passage: also called *whip c.*

Foley balloon c. An indwelling or self-retaining catheter which has near its beak a thin, distensible rubber balloon. After entering the urinary bladder, the balloon is inflated through a small side tube incorporated in the wall of the catheter, thereby retaining the catheter in the bladder without use of other fixing devices.

heart c. One which is inserted in the right side of the heart to obtain blood for gas analysis from the vena cava, right atrium, right ventricle, and pulmonary artery.

indwelling c. A catheter which, following its introduction, is held in position either by mechanisms incorporated in its own structure or by other fixing devices. It is used to establish constant drainage.

rat-tail c. A sharp, narrow-ended catheter shaped somewhat like a rat's tail and used in urethral strictures.

self-retaining c. A catheter so constructed that, following its introduction, it will be held in position by mechanisms incorporated in its particular structure.

sigmoid c. One shaped like an S, for passage into the female bladder.

two-way c. A double-current uterine catheter. Also called *Bozeman's catheter.*

wax-bulb c. One having a waxed tip, which, on being passed into the ureter, indicates the presence of nonopaque calculi by scratches on the wax.

whip c. See filiform *c.*

cath'e·ter·ism [*kathetēr*]. The habitual use of a catheter.

cath'e·ter·ize [*kathetēr*]. 1. Insert a catheter. 2. Withdraw urine by means of a ureteral catheter. —**catheteriza'tion,** *n.*

cath'e·ter·o·stat" (kath'i·tur·o·stat", kath·ee'tur·o·stat) [*kathetēr*; G. *statos*, placed]. Stand for holding and sterilizing catheters.

ca·thex'is [G. *kathexis*, retention]. *In psychoanalysis,* the investment of an object or idea with psychic energy, that is, with feelings and meanings. It may be qualitatively defined by terms, such as *ego, object, libidinal, instinctual,* or *erotic.*

cath'ode [G. *kathodos*, from *kata*, down; *hodos*, way]. The negative electrode or pole of an electric circuit. Abbreviated, C., c., ca. —**cathodal,** *adj.*

ca·thod'ic [*kathodos*]. 1. Relating to a cathode. 2. Proceeding downward; efferent or centrifugal (applied to a nerve current or nerve impulse).

cat'i"on [G. *katiōn*, descending, from *katienai*]. A positive ion moving toward, or being evolved at, the cathode in electrolytic cells or discharge tubes. —**cation'ic,** *adj.*

ca·ti'vi (ka·tee'vee). See *pinta.*

cat'lin, cat'ling [AS. *cat*; *-ling*, diminutive suffix]. A long, double-edged amputation knife especially adapted to the dividing of tissues between close-lying bones.

cat'o·dont [G. *kata*, down; *odous*, tooth]. Possessing teeth only in the lower jaw.

ca·top'trics [G. *katoptron*, mirror]. The branch of

physics dealing with the principles of reflected light.

ca·top′tro·scope [*katoptron;* G. *skopein,* to examine]. An instrument for examining objects by reflected light.

cat's′-ear″. A deformity of the human ear causing it to resemble somewhat a cat's ear; abnormal enlargement and folding forward of the superior part of the helix.

cat's purr. A peculiar purring sound heard on auscultation; due to stenosis of the mitral valve.

Cattell infant intelligence scale. See under *test.*

cau′da [L.]. A tail. —**caudal, caudate,** *adj.;* **cauda′tion,** *n.*

c. cerebelli. Old term for vermis.

c. epididymidis. The inferior part of the epididymis.

c. equina. A term applied collectively to the roots of the sacral and coccygeal nerves, from their resemblance to a horse's tail.

c. helicis. An appendage of the cartilage of the ear at the union of the helix and antihelix.

c. pancreatis. The tail of the pancreas, which has the largest amount of islet tissue and is most frequently the site of islet-cell tumors.

c. striati. The narrow, posterior portion of the caudate nucleus.

cau′dad [*cauda;* L. *ad,* toward]. Toward the tail or cauda; in man, downward; opposed to *cephalad.*

cau·da′tum [NL., from L. *cauda,* tail]. The caudate nucleus.

cau′do-, caud- [*cauda*]. A combining form denoting *caudal, connected with* or *related to the caudal vertebrae.*

cau″do·ceph′al·ad [*cauda;* G. *kephalē,* head; L. *ad,* toward]. In the direction from the tail toward the head.

caul [F. *cale*]. 1. A portion or all of the fetal membranes covering the head and carried out in advance of it in labor. 2. The great omentum.

cau′li·flow″er ear. Thickening and irregularity of the external ear following repeated blows; seen in pugilists.

cau′line (caw′lin, ·lyne) [G. *kaulos,* stem]. *In biology,* pertaining to the stem.

cau′lo-, caul- [*kaulos*]. A combining form meaning *stem.*

cau″lo·phyl′line (caw″lo·fill′een, ·in) [*kaulos;* G. *phyllon,* leaf]. The alkaloid of caulophyllum.

cau″lo·phyl′lum [*kaulos; phyllon*]. The dried rhizome and roots of *Caulophyllum thalictroides,* growing in Canada and the northern United States. It contains the alkaloid caulophylline, several glycosides, and two crystallizable saponins. It produces intermittent contractions of the gravid uterus and is also said to possess diuretic and anthelmintic properties. Syn., *blue cohosh, papoose root.* Also called *squaw root.*

cau″lo·ple′gi·a [*kaulos;* G. *plēgē,* a stroke]. Paralysis affecting the penis.

cau″mes·the′si·a (caw″mess·thee′zhuh, ·zee·uh) [G. *kauma,* burning heat; *aisthēsis,* sensation]. The experience of a sense of heat, when the temperature is not high.

cau·sal′gi·a [G. *kausos,* heat; *algos,* pain]. The burning pain that is sometimes present in injuries of the nerves, particularly those sensory nerves supplying the palms and soles. The disturbance may be associated with many vasomotor, trophic, and dermal changes in the affected parts.

cause [L. *causa,* reason]. The sources, conditions, and origins of a result. The preceding factors that unite to produce a given condition.

antecedent c. See predisposing *c.*

determining c. One that precipitates the action of another or other causes.

essential c. One that secures the effect independently of the action of other causes.

exciting c. The immediately preceding and conditioning factor.

immediate c. See proximate *c.*

predisposing c. That which favors the development of a condition.

proximate c. That one of several causes which is direct and effective.

secondary c. An ultimate cause.

ultimate c. One that eventually comes into play aided by a proximate cause.

caus′tic [G. *kaustikos,* from *kaiein,* to burn]. Very irritant; burning; capable of destroying tissue.

caus′tic. 1. A substance that destroys tissue. 2. *In optics,* a curve to which the rays of light reflected or refracted by another curve are tangent; it is called a *catacaustic* or a *catacaustic curve* when caused by reflection; and a *diacaustic* or a *diacaustic curve* when caused by refraction.

c. alcohol. Sodium ethylate.

c. alkali. The hydroxide of an alkali element.

c. potash. Potassium hydroxide.

c. soda. Sodium hydroxide.

lunar c. Toughened silver nitrate (*argenti nitras induratus*). See *silver* nitrate.

cau′ter·ant [G. *kautēr,* a burner]. A caustic or escharotic substance.

cau″ter·i·za′tion [G. *kautērion,* a branding iron, from *kaiein*]. The application of a cautery or a caustic; the effect of such an application. See *cautery.* —**cau′terize,** *v.*

cau′ter·y [*kautērion*]. 1. Destruction of tissue by the application of a cauterizing agent. 2. A device to produce tissue coagulation by chemical or mechanical means. See also *electrocautery.*

actual c. A white-hot or red-hot iron used for cauterization.

chemical c. A caustic substance used to destroy tissue.

cold c. Cauterization by extreme cold, as by carbon dioxide snow.

galvanocautery. See *electrocautery.*

linear streak c. A type used in an everted cervix uteri, in which the cautery strokes radiate like spokes of a wheel.

Paquelin c. A cauterizing apparatus consisting of a hollow platinum body, in the shape of a knife, which is heated by forcing into it a hydrocarbon vapor.

solar c. A glass or lens for concentrating the sun's rays upon tissue to be cauterized.

cav′al·ry bone. A bony deposit in the adductor muscles of the thigh. Syn., *rider's bone.*

cav′a·scope. See *celoscope.*

Caventou, Joseph Bienaimé [*French pharmacologist,* 1795–1877]. With Pelletier, isolated strychnine (1819) and quinine (1820).

cav′ern [L. *caverna,* a hollow]. A cavity in the lung due to necrosis of its tissues; also the cavity of a dilated bronchus.

cav″ern·i′tis [*caverna;* G. *-itis,* inflammation]. Inflammation of the corpora cavernosa penis. See Peyronie's *disease.*

cav″er·no′ma [*caverna;* G. *-ōma,* tumor]. A cavernous tumor; a cavernous hemangioma.

cav″er·no·si′tis. See *cavernitis.*

cav·er·nos′to·my [*caverna;* G. *stoma,* mouth]. The drainage of a pulmonary abscess or cavity through the chest wall by surgical or other means: also called *speleostomy.*

cav″er·no′sum (pl. *cavernosa*) [L. *cavernosus,* full of hollows]. See *corpora cavernosa* under *corpus.*

cav′ern·ous [*cavernosus*]. Having hollow spaces.

Ca′vi·a [F. *cabia;* of Cariban origin]. The genus of cavies, including the guinea pig.

cav′i·tas [L.]. A hollow, a cavity.
c. pulpae. The pulp cavity of a tooth.
cav″i·ta′tion [L. *cavus*, hollow]. 1. The formation of a cavity or cavities, as in tuberculosis of the lung. 2. The process of amnion formation in man and certain mammals. 3. Reduction of the hydrodynamic pressure within a liquid, as by subjecting it to ultrasonic vibration, to a value below the vapor pressure.
Ca·vi′te fe′ver (ka·vee′tay). See *dengue*.
cav′i·ty [*cavus*]. 1. A hole or hollow space. 2. *In dentistry*, the lesion produced by dental caries.
abdominal c. The space within the body between the diaphragm and the pelvic floor, containing the abdominal viscera.
amniotic c. The fluid-filled cavity of the amnion.
body c. The coelom; the peritoneal, pleural, and pericardial cavities, and that of the tunica vaginalis testis; any serous cavity.
brain c. The cavity of one of the embryonic brain vesicles.
c. of the septum pellucidum. A cavity in the septum pellucidum found occasionally between its two glial layers, extending from the genu of the corpus callosum anteriorly to the anterior limb and the pillars of the fornix posteriorly: misnamed *fifth ventricle.*
c. preparation. *In dentistry:* (a) the removal of carious tooth substance and the proper shaping of a cavity to receive and retain a filling material. (b) The cavity so prepared.
cerebral cavities. The ventricles of the brain.
cleavage c. The blastocoele. Syn., *segmentation c.*
cotyloid c. The acetabulum.
cranial c. The hollow of the skull.
cutigeral c. The gutterlike cavity situated at the upper and inner portion of the hoof wall in the horse.
ectoplacental c. See false amniotic *c.*
epidural c. The space between the dura mater of the spinal cord and the wall of the vertebral canal: also called *extradural cavity.*
extradural c. See epidural *c.*
false amniotic c. A cavity present in the trophoblastic knob. Also called *ectoplacental c., false amnion.*
glenoid c. The depression in the scapula for the reception of the head of the humerus.
head c. One of three specialized somites in the head region of lower vertebrate embryos that give rise to the somatic eye muscles; in man, represented only by a mesenchymal blastema.
lesser peritoneal c. The peritoneal space posterior to the stomach, communicating with the greater peritoneal cavity through the epiploic foramen.
magna c. A cavity in the extraembryonic mesoderm of the blastocyst.
Meckel's c. That occupied by the semilunar ganglion in the dura mater covering the trigeminal impression near the apex of the petrous part of the temporal bone: also called *cave of Meckel.*
nasal c. One of the pair of cavities between the anterior nares and nasopharynx. In the embryo, the two **primary nasal cavities** are derived from the nasal pits; and the **secondary nasal cavities,** in turn from them and from a part of the primary oral cavity, by the formation of the maxillary part of the palate. OT, nasal fossa. See Plate 12.
oral c. That of the mouth. The **primary oral cavity** is that derived from the stomodeum before it contributes to the nasal cavity; and the **secondary oral cavity,** the definitive oral cavity after the formation of the palate.
pelvic c. (a) The cavity within the bony pelvis, including both false and true pelves. (b) *In obstetrics*, the cavity of the true pelvis from inlet to outlet, containing the pelvic viscera.
pericardial c. A potential space within the pericardium between the serous layer of the pericardium and the epicardium of the heart and roots of the great vessels.
peritoneal c. A potential space between the visceral and parietal layers of the peritoneum.
pharyngotympanic c. The tubotympanic recess derived from the first and part of the second visceral pouches. The anlage of the middle ear and auditory tube.
pleural c. The potential space, included between the parietal and visceral layers of the pleura. Like the peritoneal and pericardial cavities, it is not an actual space unless opened.
pleuroperitoneal c. The coelom or body cavity.
pulp c. The space within the dentin of a tooth; it consists of a coronal portion, the pulp chamber, and a root canal for each root and contains the dental pulp.
respiratory c. The thoracic cavity; used as a general term to describe the air passages.
segmentation c. The blastocoele.
serous c. A potential space between two layers of serous membrane, as the pericardial, peritoneal, or pleural cavity or that of the tunica vaginalis testis.
somite c. The temporary lumen in the somite. Also called *myocoele.*
subgerminal c. The enlarged blastocoele of meroblastic ova lying between yolk and blastoderm.
thoracic c. The space within the walls of the thorax, between the base of the neck and the diaphragm, containing the thoracic viscera.
tympanic c. The cavity of the middle ear; an irregular, air-containing, mucous-membrane-lined space in the temporal bone. The chain of auditory ossicles extends from its lateral wall, the tympanic membrane, to its medial wall, the bony labyrinth. It communicates anteriorly with the nasopharynx through the auditory tube and posterosuperiorly with the mastoid cells through the tympanic antrum. See Plate 20.
vitreal c. The large posterior portion of the cavity of the eye between the posterior surface of the lens, the ciliary body, and the posterior wall of the eyeball. It is filled with the vitreous body.
ca′vo·sur″face [*cavus;* F. *surface*, from L. *superficies*]. *In dentistry,* the junction of the wall of a cavity preparation with the surface of a tooth.
ca″vo·val′gus [*cavus;* L. *valgus*, bow-legged]. Cavus combined with valgus. See *talipes.*
ca′vum [L.]. Cavity.
c. articulare. Joint cavity.
c. conchae. The inferior part of the concha of the ear.
c. dentis. The pulp cavity of a tooth.
c. hyaloideum. The vitreous chamber of the eye.
c. medullare. The medullary canal of bones.
c. Monroii. The most rostral part of the third ventricle.
c. pleuropericardiacoperitoneale. The embryonic coelom.
c. pleuropericardiale. The pleural and pericardial part of the coelom.
c. septi pellucidi. See *cavity* of septum pellucidum.
c. Vergae. A caudal extension of the cavity of the septum pellucidum from the fornix to the splenium of the corpus callosum: misnamed *sixth ventricle.*
ca′vus [L.]. 1. A hollow; a cavity. 2 Talipes cavus or pes cavus. See *talipes.*
ca′vy [*Cavia*, the generic name, of Cariban origin].

Any of several short-tailed, rough-haired rodents from the family Caviidae; usually, a guinea pig.

Cazenave, Pierre Louis Alphée [*French dermatologist*, 1795–1877]. Remembered for his description of pemphigus foliaceus (1844), called *Cazenave's disease.*

Cb Symbol for columbium.

C.C. Commission Certified; indicating that a sample of the stain so marked has been submitted to the Biological Stain Commission and has been found by them to be true to type, up to specification in respect to dye content, and satisfactory in the procedures listed on the label. Only one batch of dye may be sold under each certification number.

cc,cc. Cubic centimeter.

CCC Cathodal closure contraction.

Cd Symbol for cadmium.

Ce Symbol for cerium.

ceanothyn. Trade-mark for a hydroalcoholic extract of the alkaloids from the bark of the root of *Ceanothus americanus:* used as a hemostatic.

cebione. A trade-mark for ascorbic acid.

ce″bo·ce·pha′li·a (see″bo·si·fay′lee·uh) [G. *kēbos*, monkey; *kephalē*, head]. A condition, related to incipient cyclopia, in which there is absence or marked defect of the nose, with, however, two orbital cavities and two eyes, the region between the eyes being narrow and flat. Syn., *cebocephaly.*

ce″bo·ceph′a·lus [*kēbos; kephalē*]. An individual showing cebocephalia. **—cebocephal′ic, cebocephalous,** *adj.*

ce″bo·ceph′a·ly [*kēbos; kephalē*]. Cebocephalia.

ce·cec′to·my (see·seck′to·mee) [L. *caecus*, blind; G. *ektomē*, excision]. Excision of the cecum.

ce·ci′tis [*caecus;* G. *-itis*, inflammation]. Inflammation of the cecum. Syn., *typhlitis.*

ce′ci·ty [L. *caecitas*]. Blindness. *Rare.*

ce′co·cele (see′ko·seel) [L. *caecus*, blind; G. *kēlē*, hernia]. Herniation of the cecum.

ce″co·co·los′to·my [*caecus;* G. *kolon*, colon; *stoma*, mouth]. The formation of an anastomosis between the cecum and some part of the colon.

ce″co·il″e·os′to·my [*caecus;* G. *eilein*, to roll; *stoma*, mouth]. The formation of an anastomosis between the cecum and the ileum.

cecon. Trade-mark for a solution of ascorbic acid in propylene glycol.

ce′co·pex″y [*caecus;* G. *pēxis*, a fixing, putting together]. Fixation of the cecum by a surgical operation.

ce″co·pli·ca′tion [*caecus;* L. *plicare*, to fold]. Operation for the relief of dilated cecum, consisting in taking tucks or folds in the wall.

ce″cop·to′sis [*caecus;* G. *ptōsis*, a falling]. Downward displacement of the cecum.

ce·cor′rha·phy [*caecus;* G. *rhaphē*, a suture]. Suture of the cecum.

ce″co·sig″moid·os′to·my [*caecus;* G. *sigmoeidēs*, of the shape of sigma; *stoma*, mouth]. Establishment of anastomosis between the cecum and sigmoid colon.

ce·cos′to·my [*caecus; stoma*]. *In surgery*, the establishment of a permanent artificial opening into the cecum.

ce·cot′o·my [*caecus;* G. *tomē*, a cutting]. Incision into the cecum.

ce′cum, cae′cum (see′kum) [*caecus*]. 1. The large blind pouch or cul-de-sac in which the large intestine begins. See Plate 13. 2. The blind end of a tube. **—cecal,** *adj.*

c. cupulare. The blind end of the cochlear duct.

mobile c. Abnormal mobility of the cecum, so that it can be pushed up out of its normal situation.

vestibular c. A cecum formed at the beginning of the cochlear duct in the cochlear recess of the vestibule at the anterior end of the scala vestibuli.

ce′dar [G. *kedros*, cedar-tree]. A tree of the genus *Cedrus.*

c. oil. A transparent oil obtained from *Juniperus virginiana;* used as clearing agent in histology and for oil-immersion lenses.

cedilanid. Trade-mark for crystalline lanatoside C from *Digitalis lanata.* See *digoxin.*

ce′drene. $C_{15}H_{24}$. A volatile liquid hydrocarbon found in red cedar oil (*Juniperus virginiana*), clove oil, and cubeb oil.

ce′drin. A toxic, bitter, crystalline substance obtained from cedron.

ce′dron [*kedros*]. The seeds of *Simba cedron*, formerly considered antimalarial.

ceepryn chloride. Trade-marked name for certain antiseptic and detergent preparations containing cetylpyridinium chloride, $C_5H_5N\text{-}(C_{16}H_{33})Cl$.

cel′an·dine (sel′an·dyne). See *chelidonium.*

Ce·las′trus [G. *kēlastros*, holly]. A genus of trees and shrubs of the Celastraceae.

C. paniculata. A climbing shrub of India; the oil from the seeds (oleum nigrum) is reported to be a powerful stimulant and diaphoretic in gout and fever.

C. scandens. American bittersweet of North America; has been used as a cathartic, diuretic, and alterative.

-cele (-seel) [G. *kēlē*, tumor, hernia]. A suffix denoting *a tumor, hernia, pathologic swelling*, or *cavity.*

-cele. See *-coele.*

cel′er·y fruit. The dried, ripe fruit of *Apium graveolens*, containing a volatile oil; used as a stimulant and a condiment.

celi-. See *coelio-.*

ce′li·ac (see′lee·ack) [G. *koilia*, belly]. Abdominal; pertaining to the abdomen.

ce′li·ac ar′ter·y. See Table of Arteries in the Appendix.

ce″li·a·del′phus [*koilia;* G. *adelphos*, brother]. Conjoined twins united at the abdomen. Syn., *omphalopagus, gastrodidymus.*

ce″li·ec·ta′si·a, coe″li·ec·ta′si·a (see″lee·eck-tay′zhuh, ·zee·uh, ·shuh, ·see·uh) [*koilia;* G. *ektasis*, a stretching out]. Abnormal distention of the abdominal cavity.

ce′li·o-. See *coelio-.*

ce″li·o·col·pot′o·my, coe″li·o·col·pot′o·my [*koilia;* G. *kolpos*, vagina; *tomē*, a cutting]. The opening of the abdomen through the vagina, for the removal of a tumor or other body. *Rare.*

ce″li·o·en″ter·ot′o·my [*koilia;* G. *enteron*, intestine; *tomē*]. The opening of the intestine through an incision in the abdominal wall. *Obs.*

ce″li·o·gas·trot′o·my, coe″li·o·gas·trot′o·my [*koilia;* G. *gastēr*, belly; *tomē*]. The opening of the stomach through an abdominal incision. *Obs.*

ce″li·o·hys″ter·ec′to·my, coe″li·o·hys″ter·ec′-to·my [*koilia;* G. *hystera*, womb; *ektomē*, excision]. Removal of the uterus through an abdominal incision; abdominal hysterectomy. *Obs.*

ce″li·o·hys″ter·ot′o·my, coe″li·o·hys″ter·ot′-o·my [*koilia; hystera; tomē*]. Incision of the uterus through an abdominal section. *Obs.*

ce″li·o′ma. OT for *mesothelioma.*

ce″li·o·my″o·mec′to·my, coe″li·o·my″o·mec′-to·my [*koilia;* G. *mys*, muscle; *-ōma*, tumor; *ektomē*, excision]. *In surgery*, the removal of a myoma (of the uterus) through an abdominal incision. *Rare.*

ce″li·o·par″a·cen·te′sis, coe″li·o·par″a·cen·te′-sis [*koilia;* G. *parakentēsis*, tapping]. Tapping, or paracentesis of the abdomen.

ce″li·o·ple′gi·a, coe″li·o·ple′gi·a [*koilia;* G. *plēgē*, a stroke]. See *cholera.*

ce″li·or′rha·phy, coe″li·or′rha·phy [*koilia;* G. *rhaphē*, suture]. Suture of the abdominal wall. *Rare.*

ce′li·o·scope, coe′li·o·scope. See *celoscope.*

ce″li·os′co·py, coe″li·os′co·py [*koilia;* G. *skopein*, to examine]. Method of examining the peritoneal cavity by filling it with sterile filtered air through a hollow needle, plunging a trocar through the distended abdominal wall, and passing through the trocar a cystoscope by means of which the adjacent peritoneal surface may be inspected.

ce″li·ot′o·my [*koilia;* G. *tomē*, a cutting]. *In surgery*, the opening of the abdominal cavity.

ce·li′tis, coe·li′tis (see·lye′tis) [*koilia;* G. *-itis*, inflammation]. Inflammation of the abdominal organs. *Obs.*

cell [L. *cella*, stall, chamber]. 1. A mass of protoplasm containing a nucleus. The protoplasm of the nucleus is the nucleoplasm; that of the remainder of the cell (cytosome) is the cytoplasm. The cell body, or perikaryon, is the mass of cytoplasm exclusive of processes immediately surrounding the nucleus. 2. One of the units consisting of electrodes and an electrolyte in a voltaic battery. 3. A compartment; particularly, a hollow space in a bone. —**cell′ular,** *adj.*

acidophil c. One which stains with acid dyes.

acinar c. One of the cells lining a compound acinous gland. Also called *acinous c.*

adipose c. Lipoblast; fat cell.

adventitial c. A branched cell found in the perilymphatic and perivascular tissues; generally regarded as belonging to the reticuloendothelial system.

air c. A compartment of one of the air sinuses of the skull.

alpha cells. (a) Certain granular cells in the islets of the pancreas. (b) Cells containing acidophil granules in the adenohypophysis.

amacrine c. A retinal cell which apparently lacks an axon; its body is in one of the lower rows of the inner nuclear layer, and its dendritelike processes spread in the inner plexiform layer. Also called *inner horizontal c., association c.*

ameboid c. One capable of changing its form and moving about like an ameba.

ancestral c. An indefinite term applied to any formative cell, as a myeloblast, lymphoblast, blastomere.

Anitschkow c. Cardiac histiocyte having a characteristic bar of chromatin with fibrils radiating toward the nuclear membrane, normally present in connective tissue of the heart and coronary vessels; it proliferates in rheumatic inflammation and is seen in Aschoff nodules: also called *Anitschkow myocyte.*

anterior column cells. In general, all cells located in the anterior horn of the spinal cord; specifically, those in the anterior horn of the spinal cord whose axons extend to other parts and levels of the cord. See also anterior horn *c.*

anterior horn c. A large multipolar nerve cell in the anterior horn of the spinal cord whose axon constitutes an efferent fiber innervating a muscle. These cells are the most likely to be affected by the virus causing anterior poliomyelitis. Also called *motor c., motoneuron, root c.*

antipodal cells. A group of four cells formed in the lower end of the embryo sac of angiosperms, opposite to the cells constituting the ovum apparatus.

argentaffin c. A type of cell found in the intestinal and gastric glands which reduces silver salts in staining; enterochromaffin cell.

argyrophil c. Any cell which stains with a reduced silver method.

Aschoff c. The characteristic cell of the Aschoff nodule in rheumatic fever; a large, elongated cell with one or more vesicular nuclei having a central mass of chromatin from which fibrils radiate toward the nuclear membrane.

band c. A developmental stage of a granular leukocyte intermediate between the metamyelocyte and the adult segmented form. The nucleus is bandlike and nonfilamented; the cytoplasm and granules are those of the corresponding adult cell. Also called *staff c., stab c., rod (nuclear) c., stabkernige c., nonsegmented polymorphonuclear c., rhabdocyte.*

basal c. One of the cells of the deepest layer of a stratified epithelium.

basket cells. (a) Deep, stellate cells of the molecular layer of the cerebellar cortex. The terminal arborizations of their axons envelop Purkinje cells to form the baskets. (b) The myoepithelial cells of salivary, lacrimal, and sweat glands. (c) See *smudge c.*

basophil c. One in which basic dyes stain granules in the cytoplasm or all of the cytoplasm.

beta cells. (a) Cells in the pancreatic islets in which the cytoplasm contains alcohol-soluble granules. (b) Cells containing basophil granules in the adenohypophysis.

binucleated c. A cell, most commonly found in liver, whose nucleus has undergone mitosis without a division of the cytoplasm.

bipolar cells of the retina. Bipolar cells of the inner nuclear layer of the retina, connected with the rods and cones of the retina externally and ramifying internally in the middle of the molecular layer.

bipolar nerve c. One having two prolongations of the cytoplasm, as in the vestibular ganglion of the eighth nerve.

blast c. The most undifferentiated cell of any of the blood cell series: it refers to the stage of development as a whole without identifying the specific series to which it belongs.

blood c. See under *blood.*

bone c. A cell in a lacuna of bone; osteocyte.

burr c. A poikilocyte, having one or more spiny projections along its periphery, found in the blood of patients with uremia, carcinoma of the stomach, and bleeding peptic ulcer.

capsule c. See satellite *c.*

carmine c. A modified alpha cell of the adenohypophysis which stains deep red with azocarmine; ordinary acidophils are stained orange.

castration cells. Enlarged beta cells of the pars distalis of the pituitary, showing vacuolization and eccentric displacement of the nucleus following castration: sometimes called *signet-ring cells.*

c. of Cajal. See *astrocytes.*

c. of Meynert. See *solitary cells of Meynert* under *cell.*

c. of origin. A nerve cell body of the ganglion or nucleus from which a nerve fiber originates.

c. of termination. A nerve cell whose dendrites receive impulses from the axon of another cell or cells.

cells of Betz. Giant pyramidal cells of the fifth layer of the motor cortex.

cells of Böttcher. Dark polyhedral cells between the basilar membrane and the cells of Claudius.

cells of Claudius. Clear polygonal cells of varying heights, above the basilar membrane of the cochlear duct and beyond the cells of Hensen.

cells of Deiters. (a) The outer phalangeal cells of

the organ of Corti. (b) Large nerve cells in the lateral vestibular nucleus of the medulla.
cells of Hensen. Tall cells with a small base and an enlarged upper part outside the outer phalangeal cells of the organ of Corti.
cells of Kultschitzky. The argentaffin cells of the intestinal glands.
cells of Paneth. Coarsely granular cells found in the crypts of Lieberkühn in the small intestine.
cells of van Gehuchten. See Golgi *cells*, type II.
central c. See chief *c*.
centroacinar cells. Those of the intercalated ducts of the pancreas which, in certain planes of section, appear surrounded by the zymogenic cells of the pancreatic acini.
chief c. (a) One of the columnar, granular cells of the fundic glands of the stomach; the source of pepsin. Also called *zymogenic c., central c., adelomorphous c., peptic c.* (b) A chromophobe cell of the adenohypophysis. (c) The principal cell of the parathyroid, often divided into *dark chief cells* and *light chief cells.*
chromaffin cells. See *chromaffin*. Formerly called *pheochrome cells.*
chromophil cells. The alpha and beta cells of the adenohypophysis.
chromophobe cells. The faintly staining cells of the adenohypophysis, thought to give rise to alpha cells (a) and beta cells (b): also called *chief, principal, reserve,* or *mother cells.*
ciliated c. One provided with cilia.
clear c. (a) A nonstaining light chief cell of the parathyroid: also called *water-clear c.* (b) A cell considered to be of neural origin which has a small, darkly stained nucleus and clear, slightly basophilic cytoplasm in sections stained with hematoxylin and eosin. Syn., *celle claire, cellule claire.* See nevus *c., melanocyte.*
cleavage c. A blastomere.
columnar c. An epithelial cell in which the height is markedly greater than the width.
commissural c. A nerve cell of the gray matter of the spinal cord, the axon of which passes through one of the commissures and enters the white matter of the other side of the cord. Also called *heteromeric c.*
compound granule c. A rounded phagocytic microglia cell with cytoplasm distended with globules of lipid and other debris. Also called *gitter c., scavenger c.*
cone c. See *cone*, 3.
constant c. The galvanic element of a constant battery.
Conway c. A standard microdiffusion vessel consisting of two concentric petri-dish-like containers having the same floor. The outer wall is higher than the inner, and it is sealed with a square glass plate. A standard absorbing fluid, placed in the inner chamber, absorbs by simple gaseous diffusion the volatile substance placed in the outer chamber. It is used clinically in the determination of gases in body fluids, as alcohol in blood.
Councilman c. A liver parenchymal cell characteristic of yellow fever, globular in shape, which has undergone necrosis, nuclear chromatolysis, and has "punched-out" hyaline acidophil bodies in the cytoplasm.
counting c. A glass slide for counting, under the microscope, the cells in a blood dilution.
Crooke's c. Beta cells of the adenohypophysis exhibiting Crooke's change.
cuboidal c. An epithelial cell in which height and width are nearly equal.
cylindrical c. A columnar cell.
cytochrome c. See *cytochrome*, 1.
daughter c. A cell resulting from the division of a mother cell.
decidual c. One of the large, rounded, modified, connective-tissue cells characteristic of the deciduae in pregnancy and responsible for their hypertrophy.
Deiters' c. The outer phalangeal cells. See also *Deiters.*
delomorphous c. See parietal *c*.
delta c. 1. A possible third type of cell in the islets of the pancreas. 2. A second type of the beta cells (b) of the adenohypophysis.
demilune cells. Serous cells forming a cap at the end of a mucous tubule in mixed glands. Also called *cells of Giannuzzi, serous crescent.*
dendritic c. *In dermatology,* a melanocyte with many branched offshoots (as shown after impregnation with silver stains, provided a sufficient amount of melanin granules have migrated to the dendrites). Dendritic cells may be related to Langerhans cells.
dentinal c. See *odontoblast.*
disintegrated c. Any cell of any series in which the cytoplasmic outline has been disrupted or the nuclear chromatin is no longer surrounded by a membrane, excluding nuclear changes occurring during mitosis.
Dogiel's cells. Types of nerve cells found in the ganglions of the intramural plexuses of the gastrointestinal tract and in ganglions of the sympathetic chains. **Type I cells** are multipolar, have short branching dendrites synapsing with preganglionic parasympathetic fibers, and an axon terminating in a muscle or gland of the gastrointestinal tract. **Type II cells** are larger than type I, may be unipolar, bipolar, or multipolar, have long dendrites extending to the tunica submucosa, and an axon extending through several ganglions and terminating around a type I cell.
Dorothy Reed c. One of the extremely large cells observed in stained tissue specimens in Hodgkin's disease. See Reed-Sternberg *c*.
Downey cells. See atypical *lymphocytes.*
dust cells. Macrophages in the pulmonary alveoli.
elementary c. An embryonic cell.
embryonic c. An undifferentiated developmental cell. Also called *elementary c., formative c., primary c., primitive c., primordial c.* Also see *blastema.*
endothelial c. One of the thin, flat cells forming the lining (endothelium) of the heart and blood and lymph vessels.
endothelioid c. One resembling an endothelial cell: sometimes used improperly for epithelioid *c*.
enterochromaffin c. One of the chromaffin cells scattered throughout the epithelium of the glands of the small intestine and stomach; argentaffin cell.
ependymal c. (a) A cell of the ependymal zone in the developing neural tube. (b) A type of neuroglia cell lining the central canal of the spinal cord and brain.
epithelioid c. A large oval cell with a fairly large vesicular nucleus, resembling an epithelial cell, characteristic of the tubercles in tuberculosis and certain other granulomatous lesions, such as leprosy, tularemia, sarcoidosis: thought to be derived from the reticuloendothelial system (i.e., from the histiocyte), or from the lymphocyte or the plasma cell. Also called *alveolated cell.* Often also called *endothelioid c.*, a term more properly referring to *endothelial c.*
ethmoid cells. The paranasal air sinuses which lie in the ethmoid bone; also called *ethmoid sinuses.* See Plate 12.

fat c. A connective-tissue cell in which fat is stored.
fixed c. A reticular cell attached to the reticular fibers in reticuloendothelium.
floor cells. Those found in the floor of the organ of Corti.
foam c. A macrophage (histiocyte) containing lipids in small vacuoles, as seen in leprosy, xanthoma: also called *xanthoma c.*
follicular cells. The epithelial cells of the ovarian follicle exclusive of the ovum.
foreign-body giant c. A multinucleated giant cell with centrally placed nuclei; found in foreign-body reactions and in certain granulomatous lesions.
formative c. (a) An embryonic cell. (b) Any cell of the inner cell mass of the blastocyst concerned in the formation of the embryo proper.
free c. A reticular cell detached from the reticular mesh and indistinguishable from a free macrophage.
free rounded c. Myeloblast.
fusiform c. A spindle-shaped cell; a spindle cell.
ganglion c. A nerve cell in a ganglion. Formerly any neuron of the central nervous system.
Gaucher c. A large cell characteristic of Gaucher's disease and occurring in the bone marrow, spleen, or lymph nodes. The cytoplasm is abundant, fibrillar in appearance, and contains cerebroside. The nucleus is small, dense, frequently eccentric, and occasionally multiple.
genitaloid cells. Primary germ cells of the embryo.
germ c. A spermatozoon or an ovum, or a formative stage of either. Formerly called *gonoblast.*
germinal c. A cell from which other cells are derived, used specifically for dividing cells in the embryonic neural tube.
giant c. A large, multinucleate cell, as the megakaryocytes of bone marrow, the osteoclasts, and Langhans' giant cells of tubercles.
giant stellate cells of Meynert. See *solitary cells of Meynert* under *cell.*
gitter c. See compound granule *c.*
glia cells. See *neuroglia.*
goblet c. One of the unicellular mucous glands found in the epithelium of certain mucous membranes, notably those of the respiratory passages and the intestine.
Golgi cells. Nerve cells of two types: **type I,** those with long axons; **type II,** those with short axons that branch repeatedly and terminate near the cell body.
granule c. 1. One of the small nerve cells of the cerebellar and cerebral cortex. 2. See *reticulocyte.*
gryochrome c. See *gryochrome.*
gustatory c. A taste cell.
hair c. An epithelial cell with delicate, hairlike processes, as that of the organ of Corti, which responds to the stimuli of sound waves.
heart-failure cells. Macrophages containing hemosiderin granules found in the pulmonary alveoli and stroma of the lung in certain cardiac diseases. Also found in the sputum of patients with pulmonary congestion.
hecatomeric c. See *hecateromeric.*
heteromeric c. See *heteromeric.*
hilus cells. Cells in the hilus of the ovary, which may be functional, hormone-producing cells, related to, or identical with, the interstitial (Leydig) cells of the testis.
Hofbauer c. A large, sometimes binucleate, apparently phagocytic cell found in the connective tissue of the chorionic villi.
horizontal cells. Neurons of the inner nuclear layer of the retina, the axons of which run parallel to the retina.
Hortega c. See microglia *c.*
hyphal c. A cell of the hypha of a mold.
inflammatory c. Any cell appearing as an integral part of an inflammatory exudate; the term includes the neutrophil, eosinophil, lymphocyte, plasmacyte, and histiocyte.
interfollicular cells. (a) Tangential sections of acini of the thyroid gland simulating solid masses of cells between the acini. (b) See *parafollicular cells* under *cell.*
internuncial c. See *interneuron.*
interstitial c. (a) A cell which lies between the germ cells of a gonad. (b) A cell with short, branched processes in an enteric plexus, possibly of microglial nature.
juvenile c. A young *metamyelocyte.*
karyochrome c. See *karyochrome.*
Kupffer cells. Fixed macrophages lining the hepatic sinusoids.
Langerhans cells. Cells, demonstrable by gold impregnation, seen in the epidermis; they may be related to dendritic cells and celles claires, or they may be worn out melanocytes.
Langhans' c. One of the discrete cuboidal cells forming the cytotrophoblast layer of the chorionic villi during the first half of pregnancy.
Langhans' giant c. A multinucleated giant cell with peripheral, radially arranged nuclei found in certain granulomatous lesions, as tuberculosis, leprosy, tularemia.
LE c. See *lupus* erythematosus cell.
lepra c. Large mononuclear cell associated with lepromatous lesions, which contains the acid-fast organisms of leprosy.
Leydig c. One of the interstitial cells of the testis, thought to be the source of male sex hormone.
littoral cells. The macrophages which line lymph sinuses in lymphatic tissue, or the sinusoids of bone marrow. Also called *lining cells.*
lupus erythematosis c. See under *lupus.*
lutein cells. Cells of the corpus luteum. **Follicular (granulosa) lutein cells** are derived from the follicular cells of the ovarian follicle; **paralutein (theca lutein) cells** are modified connective-tissue cells from the theca folliculi.
lymphoblastic plasma c. See *plasmablast, proplasmacyte.*
lymphoid c. A mononuclear cell resembling a lymphocyte.
lymphoid stem cells. Lymphoblasts; hemocytoblasts.
lymphoid wandering cells. Lymphocytes or monocytes in connective tissue.
malakoplakia c. See *van Hansemann's cells* under *cell.*
Martinotti's c. See G. *Martinotti.*
mast c. One found in connective tissue; characterized by large, basophil, metachromatic granules.
mastoid c. One of the compartments in the mastoid part of the temporal bone, connected with the mastoid antrum and lined by a thin mucous membrane. Also called *mastoid air c.*
mesameboid c. A primitive cell. See stem *c.*
mesenchymal c. One found in mesenchyme and capable of differentiating into any of the special types of connective tissue: also called *fixed undifferentiated mesenchymal c.*
microglia c. A small glia cell which becomes phagocytic under pathologic conditions and acts to remove debris: also called *Hortega c.*
Mikulicz c. A large round or oval phagocytic cell with vacuolated cytoplasm and a small pycnotic nucleus, characteristic of rhinoscleroma.
mitral c. A large nerve cell in the olfactory bulb.
mother c. (a) The cell from which daughter cells

are formed by cell division. (b) The chromophobe cells of the adenohypophysis.
motor c. An efferent neuron; specifically, an anterior horn *c.*
mucin c. See mucous *c.*
mucoserous c. A cell intermediate in characteristics between mucous and serous cells. Also called *mucoalbuminous c.*
mucous c. One which secretes mucus.
mucous neck cells. Mucous cells in the necks of gastric glands.
multipolar c. One, usually a neuron, which has more than two processes.
myeloid c. See *osteoclast.*
myeloma c. See *plasmacyte; plasmablast.*
myoepithelial c. One of the smooth muscle cells of ectodermal origin in sweat, mammary, lacrimal, and salivary glands.
naked c. One which has no demonstrable cell membrane.
neuroglia cells. See *neuroglia.*
neutrophil c. See *neutrophil.*
nevus c. A cell, considered to be of neural origin, whose histologic appearance varies with location and stage of maturation. Transition appears to be from the clear cell (celle claire), found in greater number in the junction nevus of childhood, to a fusiform cell, found principally in the adult, which in many instances resembles a tactile corpuscle and is associated with structures resembling neurofibrils.
nonsegmented polymorphonuclear c. See band *c.*
olfactory c. One of the sensory nerve cells in the olfactory epithelium.
"owl eye" cells. Cells appearing in pairs, with large nuclei and prominent nucleoli, which are diagnostic of developing lesions in rheumatic fever.
oxyntic c. See parietal *c.*
oxyphil c. 1. See parietal *c.* 2. Acidophil cell found in the parathyroid, especially in the periphery.
parafollicular cells. Argyrophil cells in the thyroid epithelium.
paralutein cells. See *lutein cells* under *cell.*
parent c. See mother *cell* (b).
parietal c. One of those found in the periphery of the fundic glands of the stomach, immediately beneath the basement membrane. Their function is supposedly the secretion of hydrochloric acid. Also called *acid c., delomorphous c., oxyntic c.*
perithelial c. See adventitial *c.*
pessary c. An erythrocyte appearing in a stained smear as a pinkish halo with empty or pale centers: obsolete term.
phalangeal cells. Supporting cells in the organ of Corti. The **inner phalangeal cells** are arranged on the inner surface of the pillar cells; the **outer phalangeal cells,** called *Deiters' cells,* on the outer surface.
pheochrome c. See *chromaffin.*
photoelectric c. A cell or vacuum tube whose electrical properties can be modified by the intensity of light; light can vary the resistance (photoconductive cell), cause the emission of electrons (photoemissive cell), or generate an internal emf (photovoltaic cell), depending on the structure of the cell.
physaliphora cells. Spheroidal nucleated cells, containing glycogen or mucin, characteristic of chordoma.
Pick c. See foam *c.*
pigmented c. One containing granules of pigment.
pillar c. One of those bounding the tunnel in the organ of Corti.
plasma cells. See *plasmacyte.*
polar cells. See *polar bodies* under *body.*
porous c. A porous jar containing an electrolyte in a galvanic battery.
pregnancy cells. Alpha cells of the adenohypophysis distinguished by their smaller size and finer granules: seen during pregnancy.
prickle c. A cell possessing delicate rod-shaped processes by which it is connected with neighboring cells.
primary c. Embryonic or undifferentiated cell.
primary wandering c. A primitive cell. See stem *c.*
primordial germ c. One of the large spherical cells found in the germinal epithelium of the gonad, which are frequently considered to be primordia of the ova and spermatozoa.
principal cells. Chromophobe cells.
pro c. Any cell of the second stage of development of a blood cell, without identifying the specific series to which it belongs.
pseudoplasma cells. Old term for monocytes in the spleen.
pulp cells. Cells found in the pulp tissue of any organ.
Purkinje cells. (a) Cells of the cerebellar cortex with large, flask-shaped bodies forming a single cell layer between the molecular and granular layers. Their dendrites branch in the molecular layer in a plane at right angles to the long axis of the folia, and their axons run through the granular layer into the white substance to end in the central cerebellar nuclei. (b) See *Purkinje fibers* under *fiber.*
pus c. A degenerate or necrotic leukocyte; the characteristic cell of suppurative inflammation.
pyramidal c. A nerve cell of the cerebral cortex, usually somewhat triangular on longitudinal section, with one large apical dendrite and several smaller dendrites at the base. The axon is given off from the base of the cell or from one of the basal dendrites.
pyrrhol c. A mononuclear cell found in exudates, which stains supravitally with pyrrhol blue.
Rauber's c. One of the trophoblast cells overlying the inner cell mass in many mammals; they disappear, leaving the blastoderm superficial and continuous with the trophoblast.
red blood c. Erythrocyte. See Plate 26.
Reed-Sternberg c. The characteristic cell of Hodgkin's disease; a giant cell with homogeneous cytoplasm and one or more large oval vesicular nuclei; the nuclei in the multinuclear forms are overriding.
reserve cells. (a) Small undifferentiated epithelial cells at the base of the stratified columnar lining of the bronchial tree. (b) Chromophobe cells.
resting c. One in the interphase or vegetative stage of mitosis.
resting wandering c. Old term for *histiocyte.* See also fixed *macrophage.*
reticular c. (a) An undifferentiated cell of reticular tissue. (b) A reticulocyte or reticulated red blood cell of the bone marrow or peripheral blood.
reticuloendothelial c. See reticuloendothelial *system.* Also see *macrophage.*
Rieder's cells. Atypical, supposedly senile, lymphocytes. See Hermann *Rieder.*
rod c. (a) An elongated microglia cell found in the cerebral cortex in various pathologic conditions, especially general paralysis of the insane. (b) Band *c.* (c) See *rods of the retina* under *rod.*
root c. See anterior horn *c.*
Rouget cells. Branched cells on the external wall of capillaries which are contractile in the frog, but probably not in the mammal.

round c. A mononuclear phagocytic cell in an inflammatory lesion: also called *polyblast.*
sarcogenic c. Myoblast.
satellite cells. The neurilemmal cells around nerve cells in ganglions: also called *capsule cells.* Syn., *amphicytes.*
scavenger c. See compound granule *c.*
Schwann cells. See *neurilemma.*
segmentation c. Blastomere.
segmented c. Any mature granulocyte (basophil, eosinophil, neutrophil) in which the lobes of the nucleus are connected by a filament: also called *lobocyte.*
sensory c. One of those adapted for the reception and transmission of sensory impressions.
sensory epithelial c. One of the modified epithelial cells in an organ of sense connected with the nerves of that organ.
sensory nerve c. A nerve cell which receives sensory impulses from a sense organ.
septal cells. Macrophages in the interalveolar septa of the lung. See *heart-failure cells.*
serous fat c. An atrophic fat cell found in serous atrophy of adipose tissue.
serozymogenic c. That type of serous cell resembling pancreatic acinous cells and gastric chief cells, found in the parotid gland of most mammals and the submaxillary gland of man.
Sertoli cells. The sustentacular cells of seminiferous tubules.
shadow c. A cell characteristic of calcifying epithelioma, whose well-outlined cytoplasm stains pink with hematoxylin and eosin, but which shows a central unstained "shadow" in place of the nucleus.
sickle c. A crescent-shaped erythrocyte found in a form of anemia occurring almost exclusively in Negroes.
signet-ring c. A fat cell with an eccentrically placed nucleus in a thin rim of cytoplasm surrounding a large fat globule. The term is sometimes used also to describe castration cells.
sister c. One formed simultaneously with another in the division of a mother cell.
skein c. Ehrlich's term for *reticulocyte,* 1.
smudge c. Degenerate leukocytes in blood smears.
solitary cells of Meynert. Giant pyramidal cells arranged in a single row in the visual area of the cerebral cortex: also called *cells of Meynert, giant stellate cells of Meynert.*
somatic cells. All the cells of the body except the germ cells.
somatochrome c. See *somatochrome.*
Sorby's c. A narrow-lumen glass receptacle used for the spectroscopic examination of blood, made of barometer tubing, both ends of which are accurately ground to parallel surfaces, one end being cemented to a small polished glass plate.
sperm c. Spermatozoon.
spider c. Astrocyte.
spindle c. (a) A fibroblast or smooth muscle cell which is spindle-shaped. (b) A fusiform or spindle-shaped cell, typical of a variety of sarcoma.
squamous c. A thin, flat epithelial cell.
stab c., stab-kernige c. See band *c.*
staff c. See band *c.*
standard c. An electrolytic cell having a definite voltage, as the Weston cell.
star cells. The phagocytic, fixed macrophages lining the hepatic sinusoids. Syn., *Kupffer cells.*
stellate c. Any cell with numerous processes making it appear star-shaped, as a Kupffer cell or astrocyte. Also called *star c.*
stem c. (a) A formative cell. (b) A totipotential cell derived from the primitive mesenchyme, considered by proponents of the unitarian theory of hematopoiesis to be the primitive blood cell, giving rise to all other blood cells. Syn., *hemoblast, hamatogone, hemocytoblast, hemohistioblast, lymphoidocyte, mesameboid cell,* and *primary wandering cell.*
Sternberg c. See Reed-Sternberg *c.*
Sternheinner-Malbin cells. Leukocytes with cytoplasm containing granules agitated by brownian movement, seen in urinary sediments of patients with urological disorders, as in pyelonephritis.
stichochrome c. See *stichochrome.*
supporting c. See sustentacular *c.*
sustentacular c. One of the supporting cells of an epithelium as contrasted with other cells with special function, as the non-nervous cells of the olfactory epithelium or the Sertoli cells of the seminiferous tubules.
swarm cells. The motile reproductive cells of certain algae; swarm-spores; zoospores.
sympathetic c. A nerve cell of the sympathetic nervous system as contrasted with one of the central system.
sympathicotropic cells. Large, epithelioid, probably chromaffin cells associated with unmyelinated nerves in the hilus of the ovary.
sympathochromaffin c. One of the precursors of sympathetic and medullary cells in the adrenal medulla.
syncytial c. Any cell forming part of a syncytium, as cardiac and skeletal muscle cells, reticular connective-tissue cells, syncytiotrophoblast cells.
tactile c. An epithelial cell modified for reception of a tactile stimulus.
target c. An abnormal erythrocyte which, when stained, shows a central and peripheral zone of hemoglobin separated by an intermediate unstained area and thus resembles a bull's eye target. Found after splenectomy and in several types of anemia, etc. Also called *Mexican hat c.*
tart c. A polymorphonuclear leukocyte which has two nuclei, usually found in the bone marrow of patients with lymphoblastoma, pulmonary infections, or metastatic carcinoma.
taste c. An epithelial cell which receives a gustatory stimulus, as in the taste buds.
tautomeric c. See *tautomeral.*
trophochrome c. See mucoserous *c.*
Türk's irritation c. A lymphoid cell with eccentric, deeply staining nucleus related to the plasmacyte, but retaining the nuclear pattern of the myeloblast.
tympanic c. A mastoid air cell.
unipolar c. A nerve cell with one process only, as a cell of the dorsal root ganglions.
Unna cells. See *Russell bodies* under *Russell, William.*
van Hansemann's cells. Large multinuclear epithelioid cells with basophilic inclusion, seen in malakoplakia.
vasoformative c. A cell concerned in the development of blood vessels.
Virchow c. See lepra *c.*
visual c. One of the rods or cones of the retina.
wandering c. A leukocyte in connective tissue.
Warthin-Finkeldey giant cells. Multinucleated giant cells found in lymphoid tissue, particularly the tonsils and the appendix, in patients with measles. They contain many small, moderately vesicular nuclei closely clumped together and a relatively scanty cytoplasm. The nuclei may number 100 in a cell and give the so-called mulberry outline.
wasserhelle c. [Ger., clear-as-water]. A clear cell.
whip c. A flagellated cell.

white blood c. Leukocyte.

xanthoma c. See foam *c.*

zinc-carbon c. A galvanic cell in which the electrodes are zinc and carbon.

zinc-copper c. A galvanic cell in which the electrodes are zinc and copper.

zymogenic c. A cell which forms an enzyme, as that in a pancreatic acinus.

cel'la [L.]. The central part of the lateral ventricle of the brain, extending from the interventricular foramen to the splenium of the corpus callosum.

celle claire, cellule claire. See clear *cell,* (b).

cell mass. *In embryology,* a group of cells forming the primordium of an organ or of an organism.

inner c. m. That at the animal pole of the blastocyst, from which the embryo and certain adnexa are derived.

intermediate c. m. Nephrotome.

cel'lo- [*cella*]. *In chemistry,* a combining form denoting *cellulose.*

cel"lo·bi'ose. A disaccharide, $C_{12}H_{22}O_{11}$, formed by the partial hydrolysis of cellulose. On hydrolysis it yields two molecules of glucose.

cel"lo·dex'trin. Any of a mixture of dextrinlike substances resulting from partial hydrolysis of cellulose by acids.

cel·loi'din. One of many cellulose nitrates or cellulose acetates; used for embedding tissues in histologic technic. Also called *soluble guncotton, pyroxylin.*

cellophane. Trade-mark for a nonpermeable, transparent cellulose derivative used to maintain moisture in, or to protect, a surgical dressing.

cellosilk. See *cellophane.*

cel'lu·lase. Any of several enzymes, found in bacteria and other lower organisms, capable of catalyzing the hydrolysis of cellulose to cellobiose.

cel'lule [L. *cellula,* dim. of *cella*]. A small cell. *Rare.*

c. claire. See clear *cell,* (b).

cel"lu·lif'u·gal [*cellula;* L. *fugere,* to flee]. Pertaining to the transmission of impulses from a nerve cell. *Rare.*

cel'lu·lin. Cellulose.

cel"lu·li'tis [*cellula;* G. *-itis,* inflammation]. A diffuse inflammation of connective tissue.

ischiorectal c. Inflammation of the connective tissue in the ischiorectal fossa.

orbital c. A condition, occurring with acute sinusitis, in which the eyelids are red and edematous. The conjunctiva is very edematous, and proptosis, motion limitation, and diplopia eventually occur.

pelvic c. Inflammation of the connective tissue of the true pelvic cavity.

pneumococcus c. That due to the invasion of *Diplococcus pneumoniae.*

cel"lu·lo'sa [*cellula*]. A cellular coat.

c. chorioideae. The external layer of the choroid coat of the eye.

cel'lu·lose [*cellula*]. $(C_6H_{10}O_5)_n$. The principal carbohydrate constituent of the cell membranes of all plants. Absorbent cotton is one of the purest forms of cellulose; commercially, wood is the principal source of it. Pure cellulose is a white, amorphous mass, insoluble in most of the common solvents.

absorbable c. Oxidized cellulose.

c. acetate phthalate. A substance prepared by heating together phthalic anhydride and cellulose acetate: used for enteric coating of tablets and capsules. It is said to permit disintegration in the intestines within eight hours after ingestion.

c. ether. A product resulting from the reaction of a caustic alkali derivative of cellulose and an alkyl ester of an organic acid. An important compound of this type is methyl cellulose.

oxidized c. Cellulose, in the form of cotton or gauze, which has been oxidized by nitrogen dioxide so as to introduce carboxyl groups into the molecule, thereby imparting to the product a hemostatic effect and also the property of being absorbed when buried in tissues. It is useful for surgical hemostasis. Syn., *absorbable cellulose, cellulosic acid.* See *oxycel.*

cel"lu·lo'sic ac'id. The form of cellulose, characterized by the presence of carboxyl groups, present in oxidized cellulose.

ce'lom. See *coelom.*

ce'lo·scope, coe'lo·scope [G. *koilos,* hollow; *skopein,* to examine]. An instrument for illuminating and examining a cavity of the body.

ce"lo·so'ma [G. *kēlē,* hernia; *sōma,* body]. Congenital body cleft, with eventration; associated with various anomalies of the extremities, of the genitourinary apparatus, of the intestinal tract, and even of the whole trunk. Syn., *gastroschisis, abdominal fissure.*

ce"lo·so'mus [*kēlē; sōma*]. A monster with celosoma.

ce"lo·the"li·o'ma [G. *koilos,* hollow; *thēlē,* nipple; *-ōma,* tumor]. Old term for *mesothelioma.*

Cels. Celsius.

Cel'si·us [after Anders *Celsius,* Swedish astronomer, 1701–44]. A centigrade thermometer or scale. Abbreviated, C., Cels.

Celsus, Aulus Cornelius [*Roman physician and writer,* first century]. The first medical historian of note. Author of *De Medicina,* the oldest of medical documents after those of Hippocrates. His manuscript was not discovered until 1443. This provided the greater part of our information of the medicine of the Hellenic period, and contained the first translation of Greek medical terms into Latin. His method of performing amputation was to divide the skin in a circular incision and retract it, the muscles and bone being cut on a level with the retracted skin—an operation not unlike the modern circular amputation.

celtium. A supposed rare earth element which is probably identical with hafnium.

ce·ment' [L. *caementum,* a rough stone]. 1. Any plastic material capable of becoming hard and of binding together the objects that are contiguous to it. 2. Filling material for the teeth. 3. The cementum of the teeth. See *cementum.*

c. substance. The substance holding together the endothelial cells of the intima of blood vessels.

intercellular c. The substance holding epithelial cells together.

interprismatic c. The substance holding the enamel prisms together.

ce·men'ti·cle [dim. of *caementum*]. A calcified body found free in the connective tissue of the periodontal membrane, or fused with the cementum of a tooth.

ce·men"ti·fi·ca'tion [*caementum;* L. *facere,* to make]. Formation of cementum about the dental root.

ce·men'to·blast [*caementum;* G. *blastos,* germ]. An osteoblast that takes part in the development of the dental cementum.

ce·men"to·blas·to'ma. A benign odontogenic tumor made up principally of cementum-forming cells and varying amounts of cementum.

ce·men"to·den'ti·nal [*caementum;* L. *dens,* tooth]. Relating to the cementum and dentin of a tooth.

ce·men"to·gen'e·sis [*caementum;* G. *genesis,* production]. Formation of the cementum.

ce"men·to'ma (see"men·to'muh, sem"en·) [*caementum;* G. *-ōma,* tumor]. A benign odontogenic tumor made up of cementum.

ce·men"to·pa'thi·a [*caementum;* G. *pathos,* disease]. See *periodontosis.*

ce·men"to·per"i·os·ti'tis [*caementum;* G. *periosteos,* around the bones; *-itis,* inflammation]. Pyorrhea alveolaris.

ce"men·to'sis (see"men·to'sis, sem"en·) [*caementum;* G. *-ōsis,* increase]. A thickening of the cementum on the root of a tooth; sometimes associated with excess stresses, or may result from bacterial or other irritations. See *hypercementosis.*

ce·men'tum [*caementum*]. The bony tissue that covers chiefly the root of a tooth, in man, and may cover parts of the crown of a tooth in certain animals, such as the ungulates.

C. E. mix'ture. An inhalation anesthetic composed of a mixture of chloroform and ether; now rarely used.

cen"a·del'phus. See *diplopagus.*

ce"nes·the'si·a, ce"naes·the'si·a, coe"nes·the'si·a, coe"naes·the'si·a (see"ness·thee'zhuh, ·zee·uh, sen"ess·) [G. *koinos,* common; *aisthēsis,* sensation]. The general sense of bodily existence, the irreducible level of consciousness. —**cenesthet'ic,** *adj.*

ce"nes·thop'a·thy, coe"nes·thop'a·thy, ce"naes·thop'a·thy, coe"naes·thop'a·thy (see"ness·thop'uth·ee, sen"ess·) [*koinos; aisthēsis;* G. *pathos,* disease]. The general feeling of discomfort or fatigue in illness; it may be accompanied by a mild form of depersonalization.

ce"no·gen'e·sis, cae"no·gen'e·sis (see"no·jen'i·sis, sen"o·) [G. *kainos,* new; *genesis,* production]. The development of structures during ontogeny in adaptive response to the embryonic, larval, or fetal mode of life; opposed to *palingenesis.* See recapitulation *theory.* —**cenogenet'ic,** *adj.*

cenolate. Trade-mark for the methylglucamine salt of ascorbic acid, administered intramuscularly or subcutaneously.

cenolate-G. Trade-mark for ampuls of a methyl glucamine ascorbate used, by intramuscular or subcutaneous injection, in vitamin-C deficiencies.

cen"o·pho'bi·a (sen"o·fo'bee·uh, see"no·). See *kenophobia.*

ce'no·site (see'no·sight, sen'o·). See *coinosite.*

cen'sor·ship [L. *censor,* from *censere,* to value]. *In psychoanalysis,* the restrictions imposed upon a pure instinctual impulse by counterforces in the unconscious and conscious levels of the mind before it discharges itself upon the environment.

cen'tau·ry [G. *kentaurion,* from the centaur Chiron]. 1. A popular name for various plants of the genus *Centaurium.* 2. The dried flowering plant of *Centaurium umbellatum,* a small annual, native to Europe and cultivated in the United States. Centaury possesses the bitter properties of the gentians and has been used as a stomachic.

cen'ter [G. *kentron,* sharp point, center of a circle]. 1. The middle point of any surface or of a body. 2. A nucleus or collection of nuclei in the brain or spinal cord regulating a particular function. See also *area, nucleus.*

autonomic c. Any center of the brain or spinal cord regulating visceral functions by way of the parasympathetic and thoracolumbar outflows.

cardioaccelerator c. (a) See spinal cardioaccelerator *c.* (b) Any one of the three postulated higher centers. The precise locations of these centers are not known; they are thought to be in the floor of the fourth ventricle, in the posterior hypothalamic region, and in the motor and premotor areas of the cerebral cortex.

cardioinhibitory c. The dorsal motor nucleus of the vagus from which arise inhibitory fibers to the heart.

c. of curvature. *In ophthalmology,* the center of the sphere of which a lens curvature is the segment.

c. of ossification. A region at which bone first appears in cartilage or membrane.

c. of rotation. *In ophthalmology,* the point around which the eyeball rotates under the action of the extrinsic muscles.

chondrification c. A region at which cartilage is first formed.

ciliospinal c. The sympathetic nervous center in the eighth cervical and first three thoracic segments of the spinal cord; the origin of cervical sympathetic nerves which innervate the dilator muscle of the pupil of the eye.

convergence c. The medial group of cells of the oculomotor nucleus.

defecation centers. Those controlling the defecation reflex. The **medullary defecation center** is located in the floor of the fourth ventricle; the subsidiary **spinal defecation center,** in the second, third, and fourth sacral segments of the spinal cord.

division c. Centrosome. Also called *cell c.*

germinal c. The actively proliferating region of a lymphatic nodule in which lymphocytes are being formed. Also called *germ c.*

glycogenic c. One supposedly in the tegmental region of the pons; lesions in this area cause hyperglycemia.

gustatory c. The center for taste located in the anterior end of the nucleus of the tractus solitarius.

heat-regulating centers. Centers in the hypothalamus for the control of heat production and heat elimination and for regulating the relation of these.

higher c. A center usually located in the cerebrum; associated on the sensory side with consciousness, on the motor side with regulation of primary efferent nuclei.

hypothalamic centers. Superior centers for the autonomic nervous system. Those for the sympathetic system are located in the posterior group of hypothalamic nuclei; those for the parasympathetic system, in the anterior and middle nuclei.

lower c. A center of the brain stem or spinal cord, one concerned with a reflex pathway or one receiving impulses from a higher center.

median c. The centromedian nucleus of the thalamus. Also called *centrum medianum.*

medullary c. Centrum ovale.

micturition centers. Those governing the micturition reflex. Higher centers are located in the mesencephalon and in the medulla oblongata; the **spinal micturition center** is located in the second, third, and fourth sacral segments of the spinal cord.

optical c. The point where the secondary axes of a refractive system meet and cross the principal axis. See *Gaussian points* under *point.*

organization c. See *organizer.*

pneumotaxic c. A functional center which acts like the nucleus of the vagus in limiting inspiration and allowing expiration to begin.

projection c. Old term for projection area.

pupilloconstrictor c. Edinger-Westphal nucleus. See under *nucleus.*

pupillodilator c. See ciliospinal *c.*

reaction c. The actively proliferating region of a lymphatic nodule in which cells other than lymphocytes, e.g. macrophages, are being formed.

receptive centers. *In physiology* and *in psychophysics,* nerve centers which receive influences that may excite sensations or some kind of activity not associated with consciousness.

reflex c. Any nerve cell or group of nerve cells in

the central nervous system which transforms an afferent impulse into an efferent one.

respiratory c. A region at the calamus scriptorius, probably including the nucleus of the tractus solitarius and the dorsal sensory nucleus of the vagus, which regulates respiratory movements.

spinal cardioaccelerator c. That in the lateral column of the upper five thoracic segments of the spinal cord from which arise the preganglionic fibers of the accelerator nerves to the heart.

taste c. The gustatory nervous center, located in the anterior end of the nucleus of the solitary fasciculus.

trophic centers. Centers regulating the nutrition of nerves, or, through them, of organs.

vasoconstrictor c. That located in the floor of the fourth ventricle at the apex of the ala cinerea, regulating constriction of the blood vessels.

vasodilator c. That located in the floor of the fourth ventricle just lateral to the obex, regulating dilation of the blood vessels.

vasomotor centers. The vasoconstrictor and vasodilator centers.

vomiting c. A region located dorsolaterally in the reticular formation of the medulla oblongata; it includes the tractus solitarius and its nucleus of termination; this region is also concerned in associated activities such as salivation and respiratory movements.

cen′ter·ing, cen′tring [*kentron*]. 1. *In microscopy*, arrangement of an object or an accessory so that its center coincides with the optical axis of the microscope. 2. *In optics*, placing of the lens before the eye or in a spectacle frame so that the visual axis passes through the optical center of the lens. The decentering of the lens produces a prism effect.

cen·te′sis [G. *kentēsis*, a pricking]. Puncture; perforation.

cen′ti·bar [L. *centum*, hundred; G. *baros*, weight]. A unit of atmospheric pressure; it is one one-hundredth of a bar, 5.

cen′ti·grade [*centum;* L. *gradus*, a step]. Having 100 divisions or degrees. Abbreviated, C.

cen′ti·gram, cen′ti·gramme [F. *centigramme*]. The hundredth part of a gram, equal to 0.1543 grain. Abbreviated, cg, cg.

cen′ti·li″ter, cen′ti·li″tre (sen′ti·lee″tur) [F. *centilitre*]. The hundredth part of a liter, equal to 0.6102 cubic inch. Abbreviated, cl, cl.

cen′ti·me″ter, cen′ti·me″tre [L. *centum*, hundred; G. *metron*, a measure]. The hundredth part of a meter, equal to 0.3937 (or about ⅖) inch. Abbreviated, C, C., c, c., cm, cm.

cubic c. A unit of volume represented by a cube one centimeter on edge; for all practical purposes it is equivalent to a milliliter. Abbreviated, cc, cc.

cen″ti·nor′mal [*centum;* L. *normalis*, made according to the square]. Having one one-hundredth of the normal strength, said of a solution containing one one-hundredth of a gram equivalent of the solute in 1 liter of solution.

cen′ti·pede [L. *centipeda*, from *centum; pes*, foot]. Any myriapod of the class Chilopoda, with a pair of legs on each segment of the body except the last two. The claws of the first body segment have openings at the tips for expulsion of neurotoxic venom. Centipedes of temperate climates seldom produce more than mild, local symptoms in man. Tropical species cause necrotic local lesions as well as general symptoms of lymphangitis, vomiting, fever, and headache.

cen′ti poise. A unit of viscosity, one one-hundredth of a poise. It is the viscosity of water, at 20° C.

centr-. See *centro-*.

cen′trad [G. *kentron*, center of a circle; L. *ad*, to]. Toward the center, or toward the median line.

cen′trad. An angular measure, one one-hundredth of a radian; about 0.57°.

cen′trage (sen′traydj) [G. *kentron*, center of a circle]. Condition in which the centers of all the refracting surfaces of the eye are in one straight line.

cen′tra·phose (sen′truh·foze) [G. *kentron*, center of a circle; *a-*, not; *phōs*, light]. A subjective sensation of darkness originating in the optic centers.

cen″trax·o′ni·al [*kentron;* G. *axōn*, axis]. *In biology*, having a central axial line.

cen″tren·ce·phal′ic. A term introduced by W. G. Penfield (1950) to describe the neuron systems which are symmetrically connected with both cerebral hemispheres and which serve to coordinate their functions. These circuits are located in the higher brain stem and include the thalamus with the diencephalon, the mesencephalon, and rhombencephalon.

cen·tric′i·put (sen·triss′i·putt) [*kentron;* L. *caput*, head]. The midhead; the second cranial segment situated between the sinciput and the occiput. *O.T.* —**centricip′ital,** *adj.*

cen·trif′u·gal [*kentron;* L. *fugere*, to flee]. Proceeding from the center to the periphery.

cen·trif′u·gal ma·chine′. A centrifuge.

cen′tri·fuge [*kentron; fugere*]. An apparatus for separating substances of different densities by centrifugal force.

cen′tri·fuge. To submit (a substance) to the action of a centrifuge. See *ultracentrifuge.* —**centrifuga′tion, centrifugaliza′tion,** *n.*

centrine. Trade-mark for α,α-diphenyl-γ-dimethylaminovaleramide, an anticholinergic substance. See *aminopentamide.*

cen′tri·ole [*kentron;* L. *-olus*, dim. suffix]. A minute body, rod, or granule, usually found in the centrosome and frequently considered to be the active self-perpetuating, division center of the cell. See *blepharoplast, diplosome.*

anterior c. That giving rise to the axial filament of the spermatozoon.

posterior c. That forming the annulus of the center piece of the spermatozoon.

cen·trip′e·tal [*kentron;* L. *petere*, to seek]. Traveling toward the center from the periphery.

cen′tro-, centr- [*kentron*]. A combining form denoting *center* or *centrosome.*

cen′tro·cyte [*kentron;* G. *kytos*, cell]. A cell containing single and double granules of various sizes. Also called *Lipschütz cell.*

cen″tro·des′mose (sen″tro·des′moce, ·dez′moze), **cen″tro·des′mus** (·des′mus, ·dez′mus) [*kentron;* G. *desmos*, band]. The primary band which connects the centrosomes and gives rise to the central spindle in cell division.

cen″tro·don′tous [*kentron;* G. *odous*, tooth]. Furnished with sharp-pointed teeth.

cen″tro·lec′i·thal (sen″tro·less′i·thul) [*kentron;* G. *lekithos*, yolk]. Having the yolk in the center, as insect eggs.

cen′tro·mere [*kentron;* G. *meros*, part]. A small body at the constriction in a chromosome where it is attached to a spindle fiber.

cen′tro·phose (sen′tro·foze) [*kentron;* G. *phōs*, light]. A subjective sensation of light originating in the optic centers.

cen′tro·some [*kentron;* G. *sōma*, body]. The centrosphere together with the centriole or centrioles. Also called *central body.*

cen′tro·sphere″ [*kentron;* G. *sphaira*, sphere]. A hyaline body of differentiated cytoplasm found at the center of the astral rays in mitosis and miosis. Also called *astrosphere.*

cen″tro·the′ca. See *idiosome.*

cen'trum [*kentron*]. The center or middle part; the body of a vertebra, exclusive of the bases of the neural arches.

c. medianum. The *centromedian nucleus* of the thalamus; it lies between the medial and lateral nuclei.

c. ovale. Medullary center; the central white matter seen on making a section of the brain at the level of the upper surface of the corpus callosum.

c. semiovale. See *c.* ovale.

c. tendineum. Central tendon of the diaphragm.

Cen"tru·roi'des (sen"troo·roy'deez). A genus of Scorpionida, the true scorpions. Some species with seriously poisonous bites are the **C. suffusus** (the durango) and the **C. noxius,** found from the southern United States to Panama, and the **C. sculturatus,** found in Arizona.

ce·pha'ë·line. $C_{28}H_{38}N_2O_4$; an alkaloid of ipecac which, with emetine, is chiefly responsible for its emetic activity.

ceph'al-. See *cephalo-.*

ceph'al·ad [G. *kephalē*, head; L. *ad*, toward]. Toward the head.

ceph"a·lal'gi·a, ceph"a·lal'gy, ceph"al'gi·a [*kephalē;* G. *algos*, pain]. Headache.—**cephalalgic,** *adj.*

histaminic c. Intense headache with pain confined to the area of the external carotid artery (eye, temple, neck, and face), caused by histamine.

Ceph"a·lan'thus [*kephalē;* G. *anthos*, flower]. A genus of the Rubiaceae. **C. occidentalis** is the common buttonbush of North America; its bitter bark has been used as laxative and tonic and in periodic fevers and paralysis. The bark contains *cephalin*, a crystalline acid principle, *cephaletin*, a bitter principle, and a toxic glycoside, *cephalanthin.*

ceph"a·le'a [G. *kephalaia*, inveterate headache]. Headache; especially severe or chronic headache, with intolerance of light and sound.

ceph"al'gi·a. Cephalalgia.

ceph"al·he"ma·to'ma (·hee"muh·to'muh, ·hem"-uh·) [G. *kephalē*, head; *haima*, blood; *-ōma*, tumor]. 1. A collection of blood beneath the pericranium, forming a tumorlike swelling. 2. Caput succedaneum.

ceph"al·hy'dro·cele [*kephalē;* G. *hydōr*, water; *kēlē*, tumor]. Effusion of cerebrospinal fluid beneath the scalp in fractures of the skull.

ce·phal'ic [*kephalē*]. Pertaining to the head.

ce·phal'ic vein. A vein located on the lateral side of the arm which drains blood from the radial side of the hand and forearm into the axillary vein.

ceph'a·lin. [*kephalē*]. 1. Any of the phospholipids, found in brain and spinal tissues of mammals, which upon hydrolysis yield either β-aminoethyl alcohol (cholamine) or serine, with glycerin, phosphoric acid, and a mixture of saturated and unsaturated fatty acids. 2. A crystalline acid principle from the bark of *Cephalanthus.*

ceph"a·li'tis. See *encephalitis.*

ceph"a·li·za'tion [*kephalē*]. *In biology*, concentration of important organs at the head region of the body.

ceph'a·lo-, ceph'al- [*kephalē*]. A combining form denoting *the head.*

ceph"a·lo·cau'dal [*kephalē;* L. *cauda*, tail]. *In anatomy*, relating to the long axis of the body, head to tail.

ceph'a·lo·cele" (sef'uh·lo·seel", si·fal'o·) [*kephalē;* G. *kēlē*, tumor]. Hernia of the brain; protrusion of a mass of the cranial contents. See *encephalocele.*

ceph"a·lo·cen·te'sis [*kephalē;* G. *kentēsis*, a pricking]. Surgical puncture of the cranium.

ceph'a·lo·chord" [*kephalē;* G. *chordē*, string]. The cephalic portion of the notochord.

ceph"a·lo·di·pro'so·pus (·dye·pro'so·pus, ·dye"-pro·so'pus) [*kephalē;* G. *dis*, twice; *prosōpon*, face]. A monster having attached to its head a more or less incomplete parasitic head; a form of dicephalus parasiticus or diprosopus parasiticus.

ceph"a·lo·dym'i·a [*kephalē;* G. *-dymos*, -fold]. See *craniopagus.*

ceph"a·lo·gen'e·sis [*kephalē;* G. *genesis*, production]. The origin and development of the primordia of the head.

ceph'a·lo·graph" [*kephalē;* G. *graphein*, to write]. An instrument for diagrammatically recording the size and form of the head.

ceph"a·log'ra·phy [*kephalē; graphein*]. A method of diagrammatically recording the size and form of the head. Also see roentgenographic *cephalometer.*

ceph"a·lo·gy'ric [*kephalē;* G. *gyros*, circle]. Pertaining to or causing rotation of the head.

ceph"a·lo·hem'a·to·cele", ceph"a·lo·haem'a·to·cele" [*kephalē;* G. *haima*, blood; *kēlē*, tumor]. A hematocele beneath the scalp, communicating with a dural sinus.

ceph"a·lo·he·mom'e·ter, ceph"a·lo·hae·mom'e·ter [*kephalē; haima;* G. *metron*, a measure]. An instrument for noting changes in the intracranial blood pressure.

ceph'a·loid [*kephalē;* G. *eidos*, form]. Resembling the head; head-shaped.

ceph"a·lom'e·lus [*kephalē;* G. *melos*, limb]. A monster having a supernumerary limb attached to the head.

ceph"a·lo·me'ni·a [*kephalē;* G. *mēn*, month]. Vicarious menstruation through the nose.

ceph"a·lo·men"in·gi'tis [*kephalē;* G. *mēnigx*, membrane; *-itis*, inflammation]. Inflammation of the meninges of the brain.

ceph"a·lom'e·ter [*kephalē;* G. *metron*, a measure]. *In craniometry*, an instrument for measuring the head.

roentgenographic c. One combined with roentgenographic equipment for the production of complementary lateral and frontal roentgenograms for measuring head growth: also called *Broadbent-Bolton.*

ceph"a·lom'e·try [*kephalē; metron*]. *In plastic surgery and orthodontics*, use of the cephalometer for comparison with casts in facial reconstruction. —**cephalomet'ric,** *adj.*

roentgenographic c. Cephalometry utilizing a cephalometer which allows standardized x-rays to be made.

ceph"a·lo'ni·a [*kephalē*]. Macrocephaly with hypertrophy of the brain.

ceph"a·lo-or'bi·tal [*kephalē;* L. *orbita*, track]. Relating to the cranium and orbits.

ceph"a·lop'a·gus [*kephalē;* G. *pagos*, that which is fixed]. Craniopagus. —**cephalop'agous,** *adj.*

c. parietalis. Craniopagus parietalis.

ceph"a·lop'a·gy [*kephalē; pagos*]. See *craniopagus.*

ceph"a·lop'a·thy [*kephalē;* G. *pathos*, disease]. Any disease of the head.

ceph"a·lo·pel'vic [*kephalē;* L. *pelvis*, basin]. Relating to both the head of the fetus and the pelvis of the mother.

ceph"a·lo·pha·ryn'ge·us. Of or pretaining to cranium and pharynx, as the cephalopharyngeus muscle, which is a portion of the superior constrictor muscle of the pharynx.

ceph"a·lo·ple'gi·a [*kephalē;* G. *plēgē*, a stroke]. Paralysis of the muscles about the head and face.

ceph"a·los'co·py [*kephalē;* G. *skopein*, to examine]. Auscultation of the head.

ceph"a·lo·spo"ri·o'sis [*kephalē;* G. *sporos*, seed; *-ōsis*, condition]. An infection caused by a species of *Cephalosporium;* characterized by gummatous lesions.

Ceph″a·lo·spo′ri·um [*kephalē; sporos*]. A genus of fungi which are similar to *Aspergillus* or *Penicillium* in spore formation and to *Sporotrichum* in appearance; they are common allergens and contaminants.

ceph″a·lo·tho·rac′ic (sef″uh·lo·thor·ass′ick) [*kephalē;* G. *thōrax*, thorax]. Pertaining to the head and thorax; used to designate those arthropods having the head joined to the thorax.

ceph″a·lo·tho″ra·cop′a·gus [*kephalē; thōrax;* G. *pagos*, that which is fixed]. Conjoined twins (diplopagi) united by their heads, necks, and thoraxes. Syn., *janus, janiceps, syncephalus.*

c. disymmetros. A form in which the single head exhibits opposite, laterally directed, equal faces.

c. monosymmetros. A form in which the single head has one more or less complete, laterally directed face, opposite which is either no face or merely vestiges of a face.

ceph′a·lo·tome [*kephalē;* G. *tomos*, cutting]. An instrument for performing cephalotomy on the fetus.

ceph″a·lot′o·my [*kephalē;* G. *tomē*, a cutting]. The opening or division of the head of the fetus to facilitate delivery.

ceph″a·lo·trac′tor [*kephalē;* L. *tractum*, from *trahere*, to draw]. Obstetric forceps.

ceph′a·lo·tribe [*kephalē;* G. *tribein*, to rub]. An instrument for crushing the fetal head.

ceph″a·lo·trid′y·mus [*kephalē;* G. *tridymos*, threefold]. A three-headed monster. Syn., *tricephalus.*

ceph′a·lo·trip″sy [*kephalē;* G. *tripsis*, a rubbing]. The operation of crushing the fetal head when delivery is otherwise impossible. *Obs.*

ceph″a·lo·trip′tor. See *cephalotribe.*

ceph″a·lo·try·pe′sis (sef″uh·lo·trye·pee′sis, ·tri-pee′sis) [*kephalē;* G. *trypēsis*, a boring]. Trephining of the skull.

ceph″a·lox′i·a. Torticollis.

ce′ra [L.]. Wax; obtained from plants or made by insects; consists of esters of monohydric, high molecular-weight alcohols and/or alcohols, fatty acids, hydrocarbons, and possibly other substances, depending on the source. —**cera′ceous,** *adj.*

c. alba. White wax; prepared by bleaching yellow wax.

c. flava. Yellow wax; the purified wax from the honeycomb of the bee. Its chief constituent is myricyl palmitate.

cer′a·sin [G. *kerasos*, bird-cherry]. 1. A resin from the bark of cherry, peach, and plum trees. 2. A carbohydrate derived from cherry gum by hydrolysis. Cerasinose. 3. Kerasin; a cerebroside associated with phrenosin and nervon in brain tissue.

cer′a·si·nose (serr′uh·si·nohss, si·rass′i·nohss). A carbohydrate found in the gum of the cherry tree.

ce′rate [L. *cera*, wax]. *In pharmacy*, an unctuous preparation consisting of wax mixed with oils, fatty substances, or resins, and of such a consistence that at ordinary temperatures it can be spread readily upon linen or muslin, and yet so firm that it will not melt or run when applied to the skin. —**cerated,** *adj.*

cantharides c. See under *cantharides.*

lead subacetate c. See under *lead* subacetate solution.

rosin c. See under *rosin.*

cer′a·to-, cerat-. See *kerato-.*

cer″a·to·cri′coid. A variable slip of the posterior cricoarytenoid muscle, extending from the cricoid cartilage to the inferior cornu of the thyroid cartilage.

cer″a·to·hy′al. [G. *keras*, horn; *hyoeidēs*, shaped like the letter upsilon]. Old term for the lesser cornu of the hyoid bone.

Cer″a·to′ni·a [G. *keratōnia*, carob tree]. A genus of trees of the Leguminosae. The single species, **C. siliqua,** the carob, is a native of the regions about the Mediterranean. The falcate, fleshy beans, carob pods, of this tree are rich in sugar and have been used as a demulcent.

cer″a·to·phar·yn′geus. A portion of the superior constrictor muscle of the pharynx attached to the lesser cornu of the hyoid bone.

Cer″a·toph′yl·lus [G. *keras*, horn; *phyllon*, leaf]. A genus of fleas.

C. fasciatus. The common rat flea of the United States and Europe; a vector of typhus fever and a host of *Hymenolepis diminuta.*

ce·ra′tum. Cerate.

cer·ca′ri·a [G. *kerkos*, tail]. Any trematode worm in its second stage of larval life. —**cerca′rial,** *adj.;* **cerca′rian,** *adj., n.*

cer·clage′ (sair·klahzh′) [Fr. encirclement]. *In orthopedics*, application of wire encircling a bone; method of osteosynthesis in oblique and certain comminuted fractures.

cer″co·mo′nad (sur″ko·mo′nad, sur·kom′o·nad, sur″ko·mon′ad) [*kerkos;* G. *monas*, unit]. A member of the genus *Cercomonas.*

Cer″co·mo′nas (sur″ko·mo′nas, sur·kom′o·nas) [*kerkos; monas*]. A genus of coprozoic flagellates.

C. intestinalis. (a) Synonym for *Chilomastix mesnili.* (b) Synonym for *Giardia lamblia.*

ce′re·a flex″i·bil′i·tas [L.]. Muscular tension in the insane in which the limbs may be placed into any position. Typical of the catatonic type of schizophrenic reaction.

cer″e·bel·lif′u·gal [L. *cerebellum*, a small brain; *fugere*, to flee]. Tending from the cerebellum.

cer″e·bel·lip′e·tal [*cerebellum;* L. *petere*, to seek]. Tending toward the cerebellum.

cer″e·bel·li′tis [*cerebellum;* G. *-itis*, inflammation]. Inflammation of the cerebellum.

cer″e·bel″lo·ru′bral [*cerebellum;* L. *ruber*, red]. Pertaining to the tract of the brachium conjunctivum running from the dentate nucleus to the red nucleus.

cer″e·bel″lo·ru″bro·spi′nal [*cerebellum; ruber;* L. *spina*, spine]. Pertaining to the cerebellum, the red nucleus, and the spinal cord.

cer″e·bel″lo·spi′nal [*cerebellum; spina*]. Relating to the cerebellum and the spinal cord, a descending fiber tract.

cer″e·bel′lum [L.]. The inferior part of the brain lying below the cerebrum and above the pons and medulla, consisting of two lateral lobes and a middle lobe. See Plates 17, 18. —**cerebellar,** *adj.*

cer′e·bral (often pronounced cer·e′bral). Pertaining to the cerebrum.

cer″e·bra′tion [L. *cerebrum*, brain]. Mental activity.

cer′e·bric ac′id (serr′i·brick, si·reb′rick), **cer″e·brin′ic ac′id.** A fatty acid from brain tissue.

cer″e·brif′u·gal [*cerebrum;* L. *fugere*, to flee]. Efferent; transmitting or transmitted from the brain to the periphery; denoting nerve fibers or impulses.

cer′e·brin. $C_{17}H_{33}O_3N$. A nitrogenous glycoside obtained from brain and similar tissue. It is a light, colorless, exceedingly hygroscopic powder. As cerebrinin—a trade name for cerebrin obtained from brain tissue of calves and sheep—it has been used in chorea and neurasthenia.

cer″e·brin′ic ac′id. See *cerebric acid.*

cer″e·brip′e·tal [*cerebrum;* L. *petere*, to seek]. Afferent; transmitting or transmitted from the periphery to the brain; denoting nerve fibers or impulses.

cer″e·bri′tis [*cerebrum;* G. *-itis,* inflammation]. Old term for encephalitis.

cer′e·bro-, cerebr- [*cerebrum*]. A combining form denoting *the cerebrum* or *the brain.*

cer″e·bro·ma·la′ci·a (serr″i·bro·ma·lay′shuh, ·lay′see·uh). See *encephalomalacia.*

cer′e·brome. See *neuroastrocytoma.*

cer″e·bro·med′ul·lar″y (·med′yoo·lerr″ee) [*cerebrum;* L. *medulla,* marrow]. Relating to the brain and spinal cord.

cer′e·bron. See *phrenosin.*

cer″e·bron′ic ac′id. An acid obtained by hydrolysis of white brain substance.

cer″e·bro·phys″i·ol′o·gy [*cerebrum;* G. *physiologia,* from *physis,* growth, *logos,* word]. The physiology of the brain.

cer″e·bro·pon′tine (serr″i·bro·pon′tyne) [*cerebrum;* L. *pons,* bridge]. Relating to the cerebrum and the pons: formerly spelled *cerebropontile.*

cer″e·bro·scle·ro′sis [*cerebrum;* G. *sklērōsis,* a hardening]. Sclerosis of cerebral tissue.

cer′e·brose. $C_6H_{12}O_6$. Galactose.

cer′e·bro·side [*cerebrum*]. Any galactolipid found in the brain and, under certain conditions, possibly in other tissues.

cer″e·bro·spi′nal [*cerebrum;* L. *spina,* spine]. Pertaining to the brain and spinal cord.

cer″e·bro·to′ni·a [*cerebrum;* G. *tonos,* tension]. The behavioral counterpart of component III (ectomorphy) of the *somatotype,* manifested predominantly by extreme awareness of the external environment as well as of the internal self, with tendencies towards inhibition of bodily enjoyment and activity (the viscerotonic and somatotonic expressions).

cer″e·bro·to′nin. A pressor substance of cerebral origin, released by stimulation of afferent nerves.

cer′e·brum [L.]. The largest portion of the brain, occupying the whole upper part of the cranium, and consisting of the right and left hemispheres; the endbrain; telencephalon. See Plates 16, 17, 18. —**cerebral,** *adj.*

ce′re·ous [L. *cera,* wax]. Made of wax.

cer′e·sin, cer′e·sine (seer′i·sin, ·seen). A naturally occurring solid mixture of hydrocarbons somewhat resembling white beeswax. It occurs most abundantly in the Carpathian Mountains; a native source is southern Utah. Its uses are widespread: in the manufacture of candles, waxed paper, bottles for hydrogen fluoride, and other articles; waterproofing; as a modeling material, etc. Syn., *ozokerite, earth wax, mineral wax.*

cer′e·sine. See *ceresin.*

ce′rin. 1. $C_{30}H_{50}O_2$. A crystalline precipitate from an aqueous extract of cork by action of hot alcohol. 2. An ether of cerotic acid; one of the substances found in wax.

ce′ri·um [named from the asteroid *Ceres* in 1803 by Berzelius]. Ce = 140.13. One of the rarer metals. It forms two series of salts, cerous and ceric.

c. nitrate. $Ce(NO_3)_3.6H_2O$. White crystals, soluble in water; has been used as a nerve tonic in irritable dyspepsia and chronic vomiting. Also called *cerous nitrate.*

c. oxalate (*cerii oxalas*). A mixture of the oxalates of cerium, neodymium, praseodymium, lanthanum, and other associated elements; occurs as a fine, white, or slightly pink powder and is insoluble in water; useful in treating vomiting of pregnancy. Dose, 0.06–0.65 Gm. (1–10 gr.).

ce′ro- (seer′o-, serr′o-), **cer-** [L. *cera,* wax]. A combining form denoting *presence of,* or *resemblance to, wax.*

cer-o-cillin. Trade-mark for penicillin O, a biosynthetic penicillin useful for patients sensitive to penicillin G.

ce′roid [*cera;* G. *eidos,* form]. A substance found in the fat in experimental liver cirrhosis brought about by diet low in methionine. It gives the tinctorial reactions of lipid but is not soluble in any of the lipid solvents and is probably a combination of lipid and protein. It has a characteristic brown fluorescence when subjected to ultraviolet irradiation.

ce·ro′le·in. A substance found in beeswax, soluble in alcohol; it is probably a mixture of fatty acids.

ce′ro·sin. Cerosinyl cerosate. A waxlike substance forming a white or grayish green coating on some species of sugar cane.

ce·ro′sis [*cera;* G. *-ōsis,* condition]. Morbid condition of a membrane in which it seems to consist of waxlike scales.

cer′ti·fi″a·ble [L. *certus,* certain; *facere,* to make]. A term applied to certain infectious diseases which should be reported to the health authorities. See *notifiable.*

cer·tif′i·cate of lu′na·cy. A legal document which may originate from medical or judiciary authority asserting that a person is not legally sane.

ce·ru′men [L. *cera,* wax]. Wax of the ear; a combination of the secretion of the sweat glands and sebaceous gland of the external auditory (acustic) meatus. —**ceru′minous,** *adj.*

ce·ru″mi·no′sis [*cera;* G. *-ōsis,* increase]. An excessive secretion of cerumen.

cer″vi·cal′is as·cen′dens. Old term for *iliocostalis cervicis muscle.*

cer″vi·cec′to·my [L. *cervix,* neck; G. *ektomē,* excision]. Excision of the cervix of the uterus.

cer″vi·ci′tis [*cervix;* G. *-itis,* inflammation]. Inflammation of the cervix of the uterus.

cer′vi·co-, cervic- [*cervix*]. A combining form denoting *relation to the neck* or *cervix of an organ.*

cer″vi·co·ax′i·al [*cervix;* G. *axis,* axis]. *In dentistry,* pertaining to the cervical and axial walls of a cavity.

cer″vi·co·brach′i·al″gi·a. A condition in which pain extends from the cervical region to the arms or fingers.

cer″vi·co·buc′cal [*cervix;* L. *bucca,* cheek]. Pertaining to the buccal surface of the neck of a molar or premolar tooth.

cer″vi·co·buc″co·ax′i·al [*cervix; bucca;* G. *axis,* axis]. Pertaining to the cervical, buccal, and axial walls of a cavity in a tooth.

cer″vi·co·dyn′i·a [*cervix;* G. *odynē,* pain]. Cramp or neuralgia of the neck.

cer″vi·co·fa′cial [*cervix;* L. *facies,* face]. Pertaining to both the neck and the face.

cer″vi·co·la′bi·al [*cervix;* L. *labium,* lip]. Pertaining to the cervical portion of the labial surface of an incisor or canine tooth.

cer″vi·co·lin′gual [*cervix;* L. *lingua,* tongue]. Pertaining to the lingual surface of a tooth at or near the cervix.

cer″vi·co·pu′bic. Pertaining to the cervix of the uterus and the pubic bone, as cervicopubic muscle, a few strands of smooth muscle found in the pelvic fascia extending between the two structures.

cer″vi·co·rec′tal. Pertaining to the cervix of the uterus and the rectum, as cervicorectal muscle, a few strands of smooth muscle found in the pelvic fascia between these two structures.

cer″vi·co·u′ter·ine. Of or pertaining to the uterus and its cervix.

cer″vi·co·vag′i·nal (sur″vi·ko·vadj′i·nul, ·va·jy′·nul) [*cervix;* L. *vagina,* vagina]. Relating to the cervix of the uterus and to the vagina.

cer″vi·co·vag″i·ni′tis (·vadj″i·nigh′tis) [*cervix; vagina;* G. *-itis,* inflammation]. Inflammation involving the cervix of the uterus and the vagina.

cer″vi·co·ves′i·cal [*cervix;* L. *vesica,* bladder]. Pertaining to the cervix of the uterus and urinary bladder, as the cervicovesical muscle, a few strands of smooth muscle found in the pelvic fascia between these structures.

cer′vix [L.]. A constricted portion or neck. See Plate 41. —**cervical,** *adj.*

c. columnae posterioris griseae [BNA]. The constricted portion of the posterior column of gray matter in the spinal cord.

c. cornu. See *c.* columnae posterioris griseae.

c. obstipa. Torticollis.

c. of the uterus. The cylindrical lower portion of the uterus between the isthmus and internal os and the external os.

c. vesicae. The neck of the urinary bladder.

conoid c. Malformation of the cervix of the uterus marked by a conical shape and elongation, with constriction of the external os.

coring of c. Rotary coring of the cervix with electrocautery.

double c. A congenital malformation; usually associated with two uterine cavities.

erosion of the c. uteri. A reddened areola about the external cervical os; an extension of the columnar endocervical epithelium onto the vaginal portion of the cervix; it may be congenital or acquired.

eversion of c. A turning outward of the cervix of the uterus so that an excessive amount of endocervical tissue, which normally lies inside the external os, is visible; it usually follows unrepaired lacerations of the cervix at childbirth.

tapiroid c. A cervix of the uterus with a very elongated anterior lip.

ce′ryl. The univalent radical $C_{26}H_{53}$ of the alcohol component of certain waxes.

c.e.s. Central excitatory state.

Ce·sar′e·an sec′tion (si·zair′ee·un). Delivery of the fetus through an abdominal incision. Also spelled *Caesarian s.*

low cervical C. s. Delivery by the supravesical extraperitoneal route in contradistinction to the median abdominal route.

post-mortem C. s. Delivery of the fetus by section after the mother's death.

radical C. s. Section followed by hysterectomy.

Cesaris-Demel, Antonio [*Italian pathologist,* 1866–1938]. Described certain bodies observed in the leukocytes in anemia, called *Cesaris-Demel bodies.*

ce′si·um (see′zee·um) [L. *caesius,* bluish gray]. Cs = 132.91. A member of the alkali group of elements, which includes also sodium, potassium, lithium, and rubidium. Cesium forms a number of salts in which its valence is one. The physiologic actions of cesium are similar to those of potassium. Several of its salts have been used medicinally, largely experimentally.

Cestan, Raymond [*French neurologist,* 1872–1934]. With Chenais, described a syndrome produced by a tumor of the medulla oblongata (1903). The symptoms vary with the extent of the tumor and the involvement of the brain, and may or may not include miosis. Typically the symptoms are ipsilateral hemipalatolaryngoplegia with asynergy of the extremities and paralysis of the ocular sympathetic, plus crossed spastic paralysis of the extremities with hemianesthesia. Called *Cestan syndrome, Cestan-Chenais syndrome* or *paralysis.*

Ces·to′da [G. *kestos,* girdle]. The tapeworms.

ces′tode, ces′toid [*kestos*]. A parasitic worm; one of the Cestoda. —**ces′tode,** *adj.*

ces″to·di′a·sis [*kestos;* NL. *-iasis,* condition]. Infestation with tapeworms.

ces′toid. Resembling a tapeworm; caused by or consisting of tapeworms.

ce·ta′ce·um (see·tay′shee·um, ·see·um) [G. *kētos,* whale]. Spermaceti; a waxy substance obtained from the head of the sperm whale, *Physeter macrocephalus.* Its chief constituent is cetyl palmitate (cetin). It is soluble in ether, in chloroform, and in boiling alcohol, and is employed as a base for ointments and cerates.

cetavlon. Trade-mark for cetyltrimethylammonium bromide or cetrimide.

ce′tin. $C_{32}H_{64}O_2$. Cetyl palmitate, cetyl cetylate. The chief constituent of commercial, purified spermaceti. It is a fatty, crystalline substance, soluble in alcohol and ether, insoluble in water, melting at 49° C., and volatilizing at 360° C. Also called *cetinum.* —**cetic, cetin′ic,** *adj.*

Ce·tra′ri·a [L. *caetra,* short Spanish shield]. 1. A genus of lichens. 2. Iceland moss—a lichen, **C. islandica,** found in Iceland and other northern countries. It contains a starchlike substance, lichenin, that gelatinizes when boiled with water. It has been used as a demulcent and nutrient in the form of a jelly or decoction.

ce·trar′in (see·trair′in, set′ruh·rin). $C_{30}H_{30}O_{12}$. The bitter principle of Iceland moss, crystallizing in fine needles and nearly insoluble in water. Also called *cetraric acid.*

cet′ri·mide. $C_{16}H_{33}N(CH_3)_3Br$. Cetyltrimethylammonium bromide, a synthetic detergent having antiseptic power; useful for skin cleansing and washing of wounds. See *cetavlon; CTAB.*

cet′yl (set′il, see′til, set′eel) [G. *kētos,* whale; *hylē,* material]. The univalent radical $C_{16}H_{33}$, compounds containing which are found in beeswax and spermaceti.

c. cetylate. Cetin.

c. palmitate. $CH_3(CH_2)_{14}COOCH_2(CH_2)_{14}CH_3$; a white, fatty crystalline substance: the chief constituent of spermaceti.

cet′yl·al′co·hol. $C_{16}H_{33}OH$. A waxy solid, insoluble in water, soluble in alcohol; used as ingredient of many washable ointment bases. Also called *palmityl alcohol.*

cet″yl·pyr″i·din′i·um chlo′ride. $C_5H_5N(C_{16}H_{33})Cl$. A quaternary ammonium compound, soluble in water; used as a germicide and fungicide. See *ceepryn.*

cet″yl·tri·meth″yl·am·mo′ni·um bro′mide. See *cetrimide.*

cev″a·dil′la [Sp.]. Sabadilla.

cev′a·dine (sev′uh·deen), **cev′a·din** (·din). $C_{32}H_{49}NO_9$; an alkaloid isolated from both sabadilla seed and veratrum viride; formerly considered to be a tiglic acid ester of cevine, but now believed to be the same ester of veracevine. Syn., *veratrine.*

cev″a·gen′ine. A ketonic base, isomeric with cevine, produced when the latter is treated with alkali. See also *veracevine.*

cevalin. Trade-mark for ascorbic acid.

ce′vine (see′veen, ·vin, sev′een, ·in). An alkaloid, $C_{27}H_{43}NO_8$, found in sabadilla seed and veratrum. It is convulsant to mammals and causes reversible systolic stoppage in the isolated frog heart. Syn., *sabadinine.* See also *veracevine.*

ce″vi·tam′ic ac′id (see″vigh·tam′ick, see″vi·). Ascorbic acid.

Cf Chemical symbol for californium.

cg, cg. Centigram.

C. G. S. Centimeter-gram-second—denoting that system of scientific measurements which takes the centimeter, the gram, and the second as the units, respectively, of distance, mass (or weight), and time.

Chaddock's reflex. See under *reflex.*

Chadwick, Edwin (1800–1890). English sanitary reformer; pioneer in preventive medicine and public health legislation.

Chadwick, James Read [*American gynecologist,* 1844–1905]. Described a sign of pregnancy observed from about the sixth to the twelfth week, in which a blue coloration of the vaginal mucous membrane occurs; called *Chadwick's sign, Jacquemier's sign, Kluge's sign.*

chae·to′min (kee·to′min). A potent antibiotic active in vitro against a variety of microorganisms. It may be isolated from cultures of several species of the genus *Chaetomium:* sometimes written *chetomin.*

Chae·to′mi·um (kee·to′mee·um). A genus of fungi of which several species may act as allergens and are a source of a potent antibiotic called *chaetomin.*

cha′fing [OF. *chaufer,* from L. *calefacere,* to make warm]. Irritation of the skin, usually due to rubbing.

Chagas, Carlos [*Brazilian physician,* 1879–1934]. Known for his discovery of the cause of American trypanosomiasis: *Trypanosoma cruzi* (1909). This disease has since been shown to occur from a number of reduviids which constitute host and vector. Called *Chagas' disease, Cruz's disease.*

Cha′gres fe′ver (chah′gres, chag′rus, shag′rus). A malignant form of malaria, endemic on the Isthmus of Panama.

Chain, Ernst Boris (1906–). English biochemist, known for his study of enzymes and his systematic investigations of antibiotics, leading to the reinvestigation of penicillin (1938); Nobel prize winner in physiology and medicine with Sir Alexander Fleming and Howard W. Florey for their discovery of penicillin and its therapeutic effects (1945).

chain of e·vac″u·a′tion. A term used in the U. S. Army to denote the various medical installations through which a sick or wounded soldier passes in evacuation from the front line to the rear, such as the aid station, the surgical hospital, the evacuation hospital, the general hospital, etc.

chain saw. A surgeon's saw, the teeth of which are linked together like a chain.

cha·la′za (ka·lay′zuh) [G., hail, small knot like a hailstone]. 1. One of the two spiral opalescent cords formed as a prolongation of the dense albumen about the yolk toward the blunt and the narrow ends of the avian egg. 2. The place where the seed coats unite with the nucellus in the seed or ovule.

cha·la′zi·a (ka·lay′zee·uh) [G. *chalazion,* dim. of *chalaza*]. 1. Hailstone sputa. 2. A chalazion.

cha·la′zi·on (ka·lay′zee·on, kay·lay′·) [G.]. A tumor of the eyelid from retained secretion of the tarsal glands: also called *Meibomian cyst.*

cha·la″zo·der′mi·a (ka·lay″zo·dur′mee·uh, ka·laz″o·). See *dermatolysis.*

chal·ci′tis (kal·sigh′tis), **chal·ki′tis** (kal·kigh′tis). See *chalcosis.*

chal′co- (kal′co-) [G. *chalkos,* copper]. A combining form denoting *copper, brass.*

chal·co′sis (kal·ko′sis) [*chalkos;* G. *-ōsis,* condition]. A deposit of copper particles in the tissues, especially in the cornea and the lens of the eye.

ocular c. A characteristic inflammation, due to the effects of copper in the eye; seen in brass and copper workers.

chal″i·co′sis (kal″i·ko′sis) [G. *chalix,* gravel; *-ōsis*]. A type of pneumonoconiosis caused by inhalation of lime dust. Syn., *flint disease.*

chalk [AS. *cealc,* from L. *calx,* lime]. $CaCO_3$. An impure, native form of calcium carbonate.

aromatic c. powder (*pulvis cretae aromaticus*). Contains cinnamon, 8 Gm.; nutmeg, 6 Gm.; clove, 3 Gm.; cardamom seed, in fine powder, 2 Gm.; prepared chalk, 25 Gm.; sucrose, 56 Gm. Used as a warm stimulant and astringent, as well as an antacid and for diarrhea with acidity and without inflammation. Dose, 1–4 Gm. (15–60 gr.).

c. gout. Circumscribed calcinosis.

c. mixture (*mistura cretae*). Contains prepared chalk, 6 Gm.; saccharin sodium, 0.03 Gm.; bentonite magma, 50 cc.; cinnamon water, 40 cc.; purified water, a sufficient quantity to make 100 cc. Used for administering chalk in a palatable form. Dose, 15 cc. (4 fluidrachms).

compound c. powder (*pulvis cretae compositus*). Contains prepared chalk, 30 Gm.; acacia, 20 Gm.; sucrose, 50 Gm.; to make 100 Gm. Used as an antacid for gastric and intestinal conditions and in diarrhea associated with intestinal acidity. Dose, 2–8 Gm. (½–2 dr.).

mercury with c. (*hydrargyrum cum creta*). Contains mercury, 38 Gm.; honey, 10 Gm.; prepared chalk, 57 Gm.; occurs as light gray powder. Formerly used as a laxative and antisyphilitic. Syn., *gray powder.*

prepared c. (*creta praeparata*). A native form of calcium carbonate freed from most of its impurities by elutriation; occurs as a white to grayish white powder, often prepared in cones; insoluble in water. Used as an antacid and in diarrhea. Dose, 0.65–3.0 Gm. (10–45 gr.).

chalk′stone″ [*cealc;* ME. *ston*]. A gouty deposit in the fingers; a tophus.

chal′one (kal′on) [G. *kalaō,* to loosen]. An inhibitory autacoid; an internal secretion that depresses activity.

cha·lyb′e·ate (ka·lib′ee·ate) [G. *chalyps,* steel]. Containing iron; having the color or taste of iron.

cham′aer·rhine (kam′uh·ryne). See *platyrrhine.*

cham′ber [OF. *chambre,* G. *kamara,* anything with an arched cover]. 1. A cavity or space. 2. An apparatus in which material to be investigated may be enclosed.

air c. A vessel or tank in which air pressure can be increased or decreased at will.

air-equivalent ionization c. See air-wall ionization *c.*

air-wall ionization c. One in which the materials of the wall and electrodes are so selected as to produce ionization essentially equivalent to that found in a free-air ionization *c.:* also called *air-equivalent ionization c.*

anterior c. The space between cornea and iris.

aqueous c. of the eye. That between the posterior surface of the cornea and the anterior surface of the lens, containing aqueous humor. It is divided by the iris into the anterior and posterior chambers. See Plate 19.

Barach c. A pressure chamber which induces a type of artificial respiration. Oxygen is absorbed and carbon dioxide is eliminated without the use of any of the respiratory muscles.

c. of the heart. An atrium or a ventricle of the heart.

cloud c. Apparatus for studying ionizing rays. When nuclear particles, such as alpha particles, are shot into a chamber containing supersaturated water vapor, the particle produces gas ions, each of which condenses a droplet of water, thus marking the path of the particle.

counting c. An apparatus with a ruled chamber of fixed depth used for counting cells in a fluid; especially, that in which diluted blood is placed for counting the erythrocytes, leukocytes, and platelets.

decompression c. See *decompression chamber.*

extrapolation c. An ionization chamber for the measurement of roentgen-ray intensities arranged so that the enclosed volume of air may be altered and reduced almost to zero.

free-air ionization c. An ionization chamber in

which the beam of radiation passes between the electrodes without hitting them or other internal parts; the basic standard instrument for roentgen dosimetry in the range, 5-400 kv.

ionization c. An instrument for collecting and measuring ions produced in a definite volume of air by a beam of roentgen rays or rays emitted from radioactive substances.

moist c. A type of large culture plate made of heavy glass and having a loosely fitting cover; used in bacteriologic work.

monitor ionization c. 1. An ionization chamber, usually with large volume of air, employed for checking the constancy of performance of a roentgen-ray tube. 2. One which detects undesirable radiation: used in health protection.

posterior c. The space between iris and lens.

pulp c. The coronal portion of the central cavity in a tooth.

resonance c. One attached to a tuning fork for acoustic investigation.

respiratory c. A respiratory cavity.

thimble c. A small, thimble-sized, enclosed ionization chamber. An **air-wall thimble chamber** is one with walls of material having approximately the same effective atomic number as atmospheric air.

tissue equivalent ionization c. An ionization chamber in which the materials of the walls and electrodes are so selected as to produce ionization essentially equivalent to that characteristic of the tissue under consideration.

transparent c. See under *method.*

vitreous c. The portion of the globe of the eye posterior to the crystalline lens.

Chamberlaine, R. [*Jamaican surgeon,* nineteenth century]. Remembered for his method of ligation of the first portion of the axillary artery through a curved incision, its convexity downward across the supraclavicular fossa and extending just below the clavicle. Described ligation of the brachial artery through an incision along the lower margin of the clavicle joined near its middle by a second incision over the deltoid and pectoral muscles. Called *Chamberlaine's operation.*

Chamberland, Charles Édouard [*French bacteriologist,* 1851–1908]. Known for his filter of unglazed porcelain, which allowed only ultramicroscopic organisms to pass through. In association with Pasteur and Roux, he used attenuated bacterial cultures for therapeutic purposes (1880). Demonstrated, with Pasteur and Roux, the presence of rabies virus in the blood (1884). See also Pasteur-Chamberland *filter.*

Chamberlen, Peter [*English physician,* 1560–1631]. Famed in his time for his invention of a practical obstetric forceps constructed in a fenestrated form.

cham″e·ceph′a·lus (kam″i·sef′uh·lus) [G. *chamai,* on the ground; *kephalē,* head]. An individual with a flat head.

cham″e·ceph′a·ly, cham″ae·ceph′a·ly (kam″i-sef′uh·lee) [*chamai; kephalē*]. *In somatometry,* that condition of the head in which the length-height index, or the ratio of the height of the head to its greatest length, is 57.6 or less. A condition in which the vault of the head is low and receding. **—chamecephal′ic, chamecephalous,** *adj.*

cham′e·conch″, cham′ae·conch″ (kam′i-kongk″), **cham″e·con′cha, cham″ae·con′cha** (kam″i·kong′kuh) [*chamai;* G. *kogchē,* mussel, shell-like cavity]. *In craniometry,* designating orbits the index of which (the ratio of orbital height to orbital breadth) is 75.9 or less. Syn., *chameconchous.*

cham″e·cra′ni·al, cham″ae·cra′ni·al (kam″i-kray′nee·ul) [*chamai;* G. *kranion,* skull]. *In craniometry,* designating skulls with a length-height index of 69.9 or less.

cham″e·pro·sop′ic, cham″ae·pro·sop′ic (kam″i-pro·sop′ick, ·pro·so′pick) [*chamai;* G. *prosōpon,* face]. *In craniometry,* designating a facial skeleton that is relatively low and broad, with a total facial index of 74.9 or less. The index is the ratio of morphologic facial height, or distance from nasion to gnathion, to bizygomatic width.

cham′o·mile (kam′o·mile). See *anthemis, matricaria.*

cham′pa·col (cham′puh·kol). A sesquiterpene alcohol from champaca wood, *Michelia champaca.* Also called *champaca camphor, guaiol.*

Champetier de Ribes, Camille Louis Antoine [*French obstetrician,* 1848–1915]. Devised an obstetric dilating bag (1888); called the *de Ribes bag.*

Championnière. See *Lucas-Championnière.*

Champy's fixing fluid. See under *fixing fluid.*

Champy-Kull's method. See under *stain.*

chan′cre (shang′kur) [F., from L. *cancer,* crab]. The lesion formed at the site of primary inoculation; usually an ulcer. Generally refers to the initial lesion of syphilis, although the term may be used for the primary focus of such diseases as sporotrichosis and tularemia.

c. redux. A syphilitic lesion which is a recurrent ulcer at the site of a previous syphilitic chancre.

hard c. The primary lesion of syphilis. Also called *Hunterian c., true c.*

mixed c. See *mixed chancre.*

soft c. Chancroid.

chan′croid (shan′kroyd) [*cancer;* G. *eidos,* form]. A lesion produced by an infection with *Hemophilus ducreyi,* involving the genitalia, usually of venereal origin. The lesions are, as a rule, multiple and painful, and cause local lymph-node involvement with the formation of buboes. See *chancre.* Syn., *soft chancre, ulcus molle.* **—chancroi′dal,** *adj.*

ch′ang shan. A medicinal herb, probably originating from *Dichroa febrifuga* Lour., long used in China as an antimalarial. The isomeric alkaloids α-dichroine, β-dichroine, and γ-dichroine, as well as the isomer alkaloids febrifugine and isofebrifugine have been reported as constituents; β-dichroine and γ-dichroine may be crystalline modifications of febrifugine; α-dichroine may be identical with isofebrifugine.

chan′nel [L. *canalis,* water pipe]. Canal.

intercellular channels. Old term for irregular, communicating, intercellular spaces of the prickle-cell layer of the skin.

Channing, Walter [*American obstetrician,* 1786–1876]. Vigorous advocate of the use of anesthesia in obstetrics (1848).

cha·ot′ic heart ac′tion. See under *heart.*

Chaoul tube. See under *tube.*

Chapin, Charles Willard (1877–). American bacteriologist, who isolated the etiologic agent of tularemia, *Pasteurella tularensis,* with George W. McCoy.

Chapman, John [*English physician and publisher,* 1821–94]. Remembered for his invention of an elongated ice bag for application to the spine, called *Chapman bag.*

chapped [ME. *chappen*]. Cracked or roughened by cold, as chapped hands. **—chap,** *n., v.*

Chaput, Henri [*French surgeon,* 1857–1919]. Devised a method for treating osteomyelitis by curetting the cavity and filling it with fatty tissue obtained from the abdomen or thigh; called *Chaput's method.*

char′ac·ter [G., from *charassein,* to cut into furrows, to engrave]. *In biology,* any structural or functional property of an organism.

acquired c. A modification of the organism, caused by an environmental factor.

dominant c. The member of a pair of contrasted traits which manifests itself in the heterozygote.

primary sex characters. Those directly concerned with reproduction, as the gonads and genital apparatus.

recessive c. The member of a pair of contrasted traits which fails to manifest itself in the heterozygote.

secondary sex characters. Differences between males and females not directly concerned with reproduction, as those of voice, distribution of hair, of adipose tissue, and of muscularity.

char′as. Cannabis resin, especially as used for smoking.

char′bon (shahr′bon, shahr·bon′). See *anthrax.*

char′coal″ [possibly ME. *char*, a turning; AS. *col*]. The residue, largely amorphous carbon, obtained by incomplete combustion (destructive distillation) of animal or vegetable matter.

activated c. Charcoal which has been treated, as with steam and carbon dioxide or with other substances, to increase its adsorptive power. The medicinal grade is used to reduce hyperacidity, to adsorb toxins, and as an antidote to various poisons.

animal c. Charcoal derived from roasting animal bones and other tissue; largely used as a decolorizing agent. Also called *bone black.*

wood c. Charcoal prepared by incomplete combustion of wood.

Charcot, Jean Martin [*French neurologist and clinician*, 1825–93]. One of the greatest of neurologists, he created at La Salpêtrière the most famous neurologic clinic of modern times. Gave one of the earliest descriptions of intermittent claudication (1859), and the first description, with Abel Bouchard, of lightning pains in tabes dorsalis (1866). Contributed to geriatrics (1866), and to the knowledge of amyotrophic lateral sclerosis, of the cortical motor centers, and of diseases of the liver, bile ducts, and kidneys. Described neurogenic arthropathy (1868), also called *tabetic arthropathy, Charcot's joint.* With Joffroy, was first to demonstrate atrophy of the anterior horns of the spinal cord in poliomyelitis, and described the lesions of the spinal cord in muscular atrophy (1869). With Marie, described the peroneal type of progressive neuropathic muscular atrophy, called *Charcot-Marie-Tooth disease.* Angiospasm of the arteries of the leg and foot is known as *Charcot's syndrome.* Syphilitic spastic spinal paralysis is also called *Erb-Charcot disease.* He is renowned also for his pioneering work in modern psychopathology, particularly for his studies of hysteria and his scientific approach to hypnotism. See also *Charcot-Leyden crystals* under *crystal.*

charge [OF. *chargier*, from L. *carrus*, wagon]. A quantity of electricity.

electrostatic unit of c. Quantity of electricity which repels an equal and similar quantity at a distance of 1 cm. with a force of one dyne.

char′la·tan (shahr′luh·tun) [It. *ciarratano*, seller of papal indulgences]. One who claims to have more knowledge or skill than he really has; a quack.

char′la·tan·ism, char′la·tan·ry [*ciarratano*]. Unwarranted pretension to skill or knowledge; quackery.

char′ley horse. A rupture or strain of muscle or tendon fibers generally resulting from athletic efforts.

Charlton blanching test. See Schultz-Charlton blanching *test.*

Charrière, Joseph François Benôit [*French instrument maker*, 1803–76]. Remembered for his guillotine for excising the tonsil, and for his French scale for measuring the size of urethral sounds and catheters, the consecutive numbers differing by ⅓ mm. in diameter. See *catheter* gauge.

Charrin, Albert [*French pathologist*, 1857–1907]. Described infections caused by *Pseudomonas pyocyanea* (*Ps. aeruginosa*); called *Charrin's disease.*

char′ta (kahr′tuh) [L., from G. *chartēs*, papyrus]. *In pharmacy*, a strip of paper impregnated with a medicinal substance.

c. cantharidis. Blistering paper, impregnated with a preparation of cantharides: also called *c. epispastica.*

c. sinapis. Mustard paper.

char·treus′in. An antibiotic substance, $C_{18}H_{18}O_8 \cdot 2H_2O$, forming greenish-yellow crystals, isolated from cultures of *Streptomyces chartreusis;* it is active against certain Gram-positive organisms and mycobacteria.

char′tu·la (kahr′tew·luh) [L., dim. of *charta*]. A small paper, especially one containing a single dose of a medicinal powder.

Chassaignac, Edouard Pierre Marie [*French surgeon*, 1804–79]. Remembered for his introduction of rubber tube drains, said to have revolutionized surgical drainage (1859). Described the carotid tubercle on the transverse process of the sixth cervical vertebra, called *Chassaignac's tubercle.*

Chauffard, Anatole Marie Émile [*French physician*, 1855–1932]. Known for his contributions to the knowledge of pigmentary cirrhosis of bronze diabetes. Described increased fragility of erythrocytes in the disease now called *hereditary spherocytosis*, sometimes also called *Chauffard-Minkowski syndrome.*

Chauliac, Guy de. See *Guy de Chauliac.*

chaulmestrol. A brand of ethyl chaulmoograte used in the treatment of leprosy.

chaul·moo′gra oil [Bengali *cālmugrā*, from *cāl*, rice, *mugrā*, fibrous plant]. A yellow oil expressed from the seeds of *Taraktogenos Kurzii, Hydnocarpus Wightiana* or *Hydnocarpus anthelmintica*, trees of Burma and India. It contains chaulmoogric, gynocardic, and hydnocarpic acids; used in the treatment of leprosy. Dose, 1 cc. (15 min.) intramuscularly. See *hydnocarpus oil.*

chaul·moo′grate. An ester of chaulmoogric acid.

chaul·moo′gric ac′id. $CH_2.CH_2.CH{:}CH.CH(CH_2)_{12}COOH$. 13-(2-Cyclopenten-1-yl)tridecanoic acid. An unsaturated crystalline acid obtained from chaulmoogra and hydnocarpus oils.

Chaussier, François [*French physician*, 1746–1828]. Remembered for his description of the inflammatory areola about the anthrax pustule. He described also the raphe of the corpus callosum.

chav′i·cine. $C_{17}H_{19}NO_3$; a yellowish, oily mass, one of the active constituents of black pepper; it appears to be a stereoisomer of piperine.

chav′i·col. $CH_2{:}CHCH_2.C_6H_4.OH$; *p*-allylphenol, a constituent of the volatile oil from leaves of *Chavica betel.*

chay (chay, chye), **chay′a** (chay′uh, chye′uh), **choy, choy′a** [Malayalam *cāyavēr*, chayroot]. 1. The East Indian plant *Oldenlandia umbellata.* 2. The root of the *Oldenlandia umbellata*, which yields a madderlike dye.

Cheadle, Walter Butler [*English physician*, 1836–1910]. Remembered for his interest in the diagnosis of rickets and scurvy. He made a clear differentiation (1878) between these diseases. Scurvy is sometimes known as *Cheadle's disease.*

cheek [AS. *cēace*]. The side of the face: composed of skin, mucous membrane, and the fat, connective tissue, and muscles intervening. Syn., *bucca, gena.*

cheek′bone″ [*cēace;* AS. *bān*]. The zygoma.

chees′y [AS. *cēse*]. Of the nature of cheese; caseous.

chei·lal′gi·a (kigh·lal′juh, ·jee·uh) [G. *cheilos*, lip; *algos*, pain]. Neuralgia of the lips.

chei·lec′to·my (kigh·leck′to·mee) [*cheilos;* G. *ektomē*, excision]. Excision of a portion of the lip.

chei″lec·tro′pi·on (kigh″leck·tro′pee·on) [*cheilos;* G. *ektropion*, from *ektropos*, turning out of the way]. Eversion of the lips.

chei·li′tis (kigh·ligh′tis) [*cheilos;* G. *-itis*, inflammation]. Inflammation of the lips: also called *myxadenitis labialis*.

c. actinica. A form in which the lips are irritated by sunlight; usually seen in persons whose skin is sensitive to light.

c. exfoliativa. Persistent peeling of the lips.

c. glandularis. A chronic disorder of the lips; characterized by swelling due to hypertrophy of the labial glands and their ducts, with secondary inflammatory symptoms. Also called *c. glandularis apostematosa, myxadenitis labialis*.

c. venenata. A contact dermatitis of the lips, often caused by lipstick or cosmetics.

chei′lo- (kigh′lo-), **cheil-** (kyle-), **chi′lo-** (kigh′lo-), **chil-** (kyle-) [*cheilos*]. A combining form denoting *relation to the lips*.

chei″lo·an′gi·o·scope″ (kigh″lo·an′jee·o·scope″) [*cheilos;* G. *aggeion*, vessel; *skopein*, to examine]. Apparatus for observing the capillaries of the human lip.

chei·log″na·tho·pal″a·tos′chi·sis (kigh·log″na·tho·pal″uh·tos′ki·sis, kigh″lo·nay″tho·) [*cheilos;* G. *gnathos*, jaw; L. *palatum*, palate; G. *schisis*, a cleaving]. Unilateral or bilateral cleft of the upper lip, alveolar process, and palate.

chei·log″na·tho·pros″o·pos′chi·sis (kigh·log″nuth·o·pros″o·pos′ki·sis, kigh″lo·nayth″o·, kigh″lo·nath″o·) [*cheilos; gnathos;* G. *prosōpon*, face; *schisis*]. Oblique facial cleft involving also the upper lip and upper jaw.

chei·log″na·tho·u″ra·nos′chi·sis (kigh·log″nuth·o·yoor″uh·nos′ki·sis, kigh″lo·nayth″o·, kigh″lo·nath″o·) [*cheilos; gnathos;* G. *ouranos*, vault, palate; *schisis*]. A cleft which involves the upper lip, alveolar process, and palate.

chei′lo·plas″ty (kigh′lo·plas″tee) [*cheilos;* G. *plassein*, to form]. Any plastic operation upon the lip.

chei·lor′rha·phy (kigh·lor′uh·fee) [*cheilos;* G. *rhaphē*, a suture]. Suture of a cut or lacerated lip.

chei·los′chi·sis (kigh·los′ki·sis) [*cheilos;* G. *schisis*, a cleaving]. Harelip.

chei·lo′sis (kigh·lo′sis) [*cheilos;* G. *-ōsis*, condition]. A disorder of the lips; due to avitaminosis. There is pallor of the mucosa at the angles of the lips in the early stages, followed by maceration and piling up of tissue. Later, fissures appear which may become deep and extend into the cheek. Also called *riboflavin deficiency*.

chei·los″to·mat′o·plas″ty (kigh·los″to·mat′o·plas″tee, kigh″los·to·, kigh″lo·sto′mat·o·plas″tee) [*cheilos;* G. *stoma*, mouth; *plassein*, to form]. Plastic repair of the lips and mouth.

chei·lot′o·my (kigh·lot′o·mee) [*cheilos;* G. *tomē*, a cutting]. Excision of a part of the lip.

chei″ma·pho′bi·a (kigh″muh·fo′bee·uh) [G. *cheima*, winter weather; *phobos*, fear]. Morbid fear of cold.

chei·rag′ra (kigh·rag′ruh, ·ray′gruh, kigh′rag·ruh). See *chiragra*.

chei·ran′thin (kigh·ran′thin). A glycoside from the leaves and seeds of *Cheiranthus cheiri*, with action similar to that of digitalis.

chei′ro- (kigh′ro-), **cheir-**. See *chiro-*.

chek′an, chek′en [Araucan *chequeñ*]. The leaves of *Eugenia cheken*, a South American shrub. It was formerly used in bronchitis.

che′late (kee′late). Pertaining to the ring-type structure or the compound formed in chelation.

che′lat·ing (kee′lay·ting) **a′gent.** Any compound, usually organic, having two or more points of attachment at which an atom of a metal may be joined or coordinated in such a manner as to form a ring type of structure.

che·la′tion (kee·lay′shun). 1. A type of interaction between an organic compound (having two or more points at which it may coordinate with a metal) and the metal so as to form a ring-type structure. 2. A type of interaction, shown by organic compounds having both a carbonyl (CO) group and a hydroxyl (OH) group, in which by hydrogen bond formation involving generally two such molecules, but sometimes only one, a ring-type structure is produced.

chel″e·ryth′rine (kel″i·rith′reen, ·rin, kel·err′ith·). See *sanguinaria*.

chel′i·do·nine (kel′i·do·neen, ·nin, kel·id′o·, kel″·i·do′·). A crystalline alkaloid of celandine (*Chelidonium majus*), related to papaverine. It relaxes smooth muscle and depresses the central nervous system.

chel″i·do′ni·um (kel″i·do′nee·um) [G. *chelidonion*, celandine]. The leaves and stems of *C. majus*, with properties due to a number of alkaloids and acids. It is a drastic cathartic and, externally, irritant. Syn., *celandine*.

chel″i·do·xan′thin (kel″i·do·zan′thin, kee″li·do·). One of the bitter, crystalline constituents of celandine.

che′loid (kee′loid). See *keloid*.

chel′o·nin (kel′o·nin, ki·lo′nin). A bitter, amorphous powder, the concentrated balmony extract, from *Chelone glabra;* formerly used as a tonic.

Chel′sea pen′sion·er. Compound confection of guaiac; contains guaiac resin, rhubarb, acid potassium tartrate, nutmeg, sublimed sulfur, and clarified honey. It is a popular remedy in England for rheumatism and gout.

chem′i·cal [perhaps G. *chymeia*, a mingling, from *chymos*, juice]. Of or pertaining to chemistry. **—chem′i·cal,** *n.*

chem′i·cal a′gent de·tec′tor kit. *In military medicine*, a kit that reveals dangerous concentrations of certain war gases by color changes in tubes through which contaminated air is drawn and to which liquid reagents are added.

Chem′i·cal Corps. A department of the U. S. Army; responsible for the use and manufacture of toxic gases, incendiary materials, and chemicals used in warfare, and for defense apparatus used against such materials.

chem′i·cal war′fare″. The use in war of toxic gases, incendiary mixtures, and other chemicals, for defensive or offensive purposes. See war *gas*.

chem′i·co- [*chymos*]. A combining form signifying *relation to*, or *connection with, chemistry*.

chem″i·co·cau′ter·y [*chymos;* G. *kautērion*, branding iron]. Cauterization by means of chemical agents.

chem″i·lu″mi·nes′cence [*chymos;* L. *luminare*, to illuminate]. Light produced by means of a chemical reaction and entirely independent of any heat involved. The so-called cold light.

chem″i·o·tax′is. See *chemotaxis*.

chem′ist [*chymos*]. One skilled in chemistry.

chem′is·try [*chymos*]. The science of the structure of matter and the composition of substances, their transformation, analysis, synthesis, and manufacture.

analytical c. That concerned with the detection (qualitative analysis) and determination (quantitative analysis) of substances.

applied c. Chemistry applied to some useful end, as in industry.

biological c. The chemistry of life, or that which deals with the composition of animal and vegetable matter, the changes occurring in living organisms, the transformation of food into living tissues, and the elimination of waste products. Syn., *physiological c.*

colloid c. Study of the properties developed by substances in the colloidal state of subdivision.

fermentation c. Study of the reactions produced by enzymes and ferments.

food c. That dealing with the composition and examination of foods.

forensic c. The application of chemical knowledge in the solution of legal problems, especially in the detection of crime.

histological c. Chemistry of the tissues of plants and animals. See *histochemistry.*

iatrochemistry. See *medical c.*

immunochemistry. Chemistry of the changes associated with the phenomena of immunity.

industrial c. Chemistry applied to industry.

inorganic c. That branch which treats of substances other than carbon compounds.

medical c. Chemistry applied to medicine.

nuclear c. That dealing with changes occurring in the nucleus of an atom.

organic c. Chemistry of carbon compounds.

pathological c. Chemistry of abnormal tissues and the changes caused by disease.

pharmaceutical c. Chemistry applied to the preparation, the testing, and the composition of drugs.

physical c. That dealing with the generalizations or laws and the theories of chemistry.

physiological c. Study of the composition and chemical changes in plants and animals.

phytochemistry. Chemistry of plants and plant functions.

sanitary c. Application of chemistry to various problems of sanitation.

synthetic c. That dealing with synthesis of substances, especially organic compounds.

toxicological c. A branch of forensic chemistry dealing with the detection and estimation of poisons.

chem′o-, chem- [*chymos*]. A combining form denoting *relation to chemical action* or *to chemicals.*

chem′o·cep″tor, chem′o·re·cep″tor [*chymos;* L. *captum,* from *capere,* to take]. 1. One of the side chains or receptors in a living cell, having the power of fixing chemical substances in the same way that bacterial toxins are fixed. 2. A sensory end organ capable of reacting to a chemical stimulus.

chem″o·co·ag″u·la′tion [*chymos;* L. *coagulatio,* from *coagulare,* to cause a fluid to curdle]. The precipitation of proteins or colloids in a jellylike, soft mass caused by chemical agents.

chem″o·dec·to′ma. See carotid body *tumor.*

chem″o·pro″phy·lax′is [*chymos;* G. *prophylassein,* to guard against]. Prevention of disease by the administration of chemical drugs, as sulfanilamide.

chem′o·re·cep″tor. Chemoceptor.

chem″o·re′flex [*chymos;* L. *reflexus,* from *reflectere,* to turn back]. Denoting a reflex act initiated by a chemical stimulus.

che·mo′sis (ki·mo′sis) [G. *chēmōsis,* affection of the eyes, where the cornea swells like a cockleshell, *chēmē*]. Swelling of the conjunctiva. —**chemot′ic,** *adj.*

chem′o·stat (kem′·o·stat) [*chymos;* G. *statos,* standing]. A device used for keeping a bacterial population growing at a reduced rate over an indefinite period by controlling the inflow of nutrients and the outflow of the bacterial suspension: used in experimental bacteriology.

chem″o·sur′ger·y [G. *chymos,* juice; *cheirourgia,* a working by hand]. Removal of diseased or unwanted tissue by the application of chemicals.

chem″o·tax′is, chem′o·tax″y [G. *chymos,* juice; *taxis,* arrangement]. Response of organisms to chemical stimuli; attraction toward a substance is positive while repulsion is negative chemotaxis; chemotropism. —**chemotac′tic,** *adj.*

chem″o·ther′a·py [*chymos;* G. *therapeia,* treatment]. Prevention or treatment of infective diseases by chemicals which act as antiseptics within the body, without producing serious toxic effects on the patient.

che″mo·troph′. An autotrophic bacterium able to oxidize an inorganic substrate (as iron, sulfur, nitrate) specific to a particular species to secure energy for anabolic metabolism: also called *chemosynthetic autotroph.* —**chemotroph′ic,** *adj.*

che·mot′ro·pism [*chymos;* G. *trepein,* to turn]. 1. Attraction of cells by chemical substances. 2. *In immunology,* the positive attraction of phagocytes to microorganisms, cellular debris, and areas of inflammation. Syn., *chemotaxis.*

chem′ur·gy. Chemistry as applied specifically to the development of derivatives from raw materials, especially from agricultural products, for industry, e.g. the manufacture of paints from soybean oil, fire extinguishers from licorice root, etc.

Chenais, Louis Jean [*French physician,* 1872–1950]. See *Cestan-Chenais syndrome* under *Cestan.*

Che″no·po′di·um (kee″no·po′dee·um, ken″o·, chen″o·) [G. *chēn,* goose; *podion,* little foot]. A genus of herbs of the family Chenopodiaceae.

C. ambrosioides anthelminticum. The American wormseed; yields a volatile oil, chenopodium oil, which is an efficient anthelmintic against the roundworm. Dose, 0.32–1.0 cc. (5–15 min.).

che′o·plas·ty (kee′o·plas·tee) [G. *chein,* to pour; *plassein,* to mold]. *In dentistry,* the process of molding with low fusing metals or alloys. —**cheoplas′tic,** *adj.*

cheracol. Trade-mark for a liquid preparation used as an expectorant.

cher″o·ma′ni·a, chaer″o·ma′ni·a (kerr″o·may′-nee·uh, kee″ro·) [G. *chairein,* to rejoice; *mania,* madness]. Old term for amenomania.

cher″o·pho′bi·a (kerr″o·fo′bee·uh, keer″o·) [*chairein;* G. *phobos,* fear]. A morbid fear of gaiety or happiness.

cher′ry [G. *kerasos,* bird-cherry]. Any of a number of species of the genus *Prunus,* trees having typical globose drupes; family, Rosaceae.

c. laurel. European evergreen cherry, *P. laurocerasus.* Water distilled from its leaves has been used in the same way as dilute hydrocyanic acid.

wild c. (*prunus virginiana*). The stem bark of *Prunus serotina.* It contains an enzyme emulsin, which acts upon a cyanogenetic glycoside forming hydrocyanic acid. It also contains tannin and a bitter principle. Wild cherry has been employed in the treatment of bronchitis of various types, but is of no remedial value. It is frequently used as a flavoring agent, especially for cough syrups. Also called *wild black c. bark.*

Cherry and Crandall's test. See under *test.*

cher′u·bism. The characteristic facies of familial fibrous dysplasia of the jaws; chubby features with upturned eyes.

Cheselden, William [*English surgeon,* 1688–1752]. Famous surgeon of the eighteenth century and the chief representative of his period. Known also as an accomplished anatomist and author of two books on anatomy. His operation of lithotomy received much attention. By his iridotomy for the relief of a certain type of blindness, he made the most important contribution to ophthalmic surgery outside of the cataract operation.

chest [AS. *cest*, from G. *kistē*, basket]. The thorax.

emphysematous c. The altered contour caused by advanced pulmonary emphysema; characterized by fixation of the chest in the position of deep inspiration; the so-called *barrel chest.*

fissured c. A rare deformity of congenital origin; exists in two forms, vertical fissure of the thoracic wall along the sternum, and lateral fissure. It may be associated with hernia of the lungs or with ectopia cordis.

flail c. A condition in which there are multiple rib fractures, with or without fracture of the sternum, allowing the occurrence of paradoxical motion of the chest wall and the attendant physiological disturbances; "stove-in chest."

funnel c. The appearance produced by a deep funnel-like depression of the lower sternum, most commonly congenital, but sometimes the result of rickets in childhood.

phthisical c. A long, narrow, flat chest with winged scapulas, formerly thought to be characteristic of pulmonary tuberculosis.

pigeon c. See pigeon *breast.*

che·to′min. Chaetomin.

Chevreul, Michel Eugène [*French chemist*, 1786–1889]. Proved the sugar in diabetic urine to be glucose (1815). Discovered that fats consist of fatty acids and glyceryl (1823). Isolated creatine from muscle (1832).

Cheyne, John [*Scottish physician in Ireland*, 1777–1836]. Described a type of irregular breathing (1818) called *Cheyne-Stokes respiration.* See under *respiration.* Gave first description of acute hydrocephalus (1808). Contributed to the knowledge of croup (1809).

Chiari, Hans [*German pathologist*, 1851–1916] Widely known for his publication of one of the best works on the history of pathology (1903) and for his important study on gastric syphilis (1891); described obliterating endarteritis of the liver, called *Chiari's disease.* Described a downward elongation of the cerebellum and brain stem into the cervical portion of the spinal canal, associated with spina bifida. Called *Chiari's malformation* or *Arnold-Chiari syndrome.* Described fine fibers stretching across the right atrium of the heart, from the openings of the inferior vena cava and coronary sinus to the crista terminalis; these are thought to be inconstant remnants of embryonic valves. Called *Chiari's network.*

Chiarugi, Vincenzo [*Italian physician*, 1759–1820]. Known for his encouragement of fundamental reforms in the treatment of the insane. Said to have been the first in Europe to abandon the use of fetters in a mental hospital (1793).

chi·as′ma (kigh·az′muh) (pl. *chiasmata*) [G., from *chiazein*, to mark with two lines crossing like an X]. 1. The optic commissure. Also called *chiasm.* See Plates 17, 18. 2. A crossing. Also called *chiasm.* 3. *In genetics*, the crossing of two chromatids at the prophase of the first maturation division of the germ cells, as a result of crossing over.

chi·as′ma·ta. Plural of chiasma.

Chi·ca′go blue. An azo dye having a strong anticoagulant action when injected into the blood stream.

chick′en·pox″ [AS. *cīcen*, chicken; ME. *pokkes*]. An acute, contagious disease of childhood, characterized by a superficial eruption of macular transparent vesicles which appear in successive crops on different parts of the body. Varicella.

chig′ger [F. *chique*, of Cariban origin]. A larval mite of the genus *Trombicula;* the bite of the common chigger causes severe inflammatory lesions in warm-blooded animals, including man.

chig′oe, chig′o. See *Tunga* penetrans.

chil′blain″ [AS. *cele; blēgen*]. Congestion and swelling of the skin, due to cold, and followed by severe itching or burning; vesicles and bullae may form, and these may lead to ulceration. Syn., *erythema pernio, pernio.*

child [AS. *cild*]. One who has not reached the age of puberty.

child′bed″ [*cild;* AS. *bed*]. Condition of a woman being in labor; parturition.

c. fever. Puerperal fever.

child′birth″ [*cild;* ME. *burth*]. Parturition. See Plate 42.

natural c. A form of childbirth in which psychological and emotional aspects are emphasized in order to educate the patient for labor and, when possible, to reduce or eliminate the use of drugs: popular term. The expectant mother is prepared for natural childbirth by gaining an understanding of the labor process and sometimes by a regimen of exercises.

child′crow″ing [*cild;* AS. *crāwan*]. The sound characteristic of the respiratory effort in laryngismus stridulus.

Chil′dren's Bu′reau. A division of the Social Security Administration of the United States concerned with the health and welfare of the whole child. It provides grants to the states for maternal and child health, and makes available to national, state, and local organizations its publications and information service.

chi·li′tis (kigh·ligh′tis). See *cheilitis.*

chill [AS. *cele*]. A sensation of cold accompanied by shivering; frequently the initial symptom of acute infections, as pneumonia; a prominent symptom of various forms of malarial fever. The subjective sensation of chilliness results from constriction of the blood vessels of the skin and is accompanied by a rise of body temperature.

chi′lo- (kigh′lo-), **chil-** (kighl-). See *cheilo-.*

Chi″lo·mas′tix (kigh″lo·mas′ticks) [G. *cheilos*, lip; *mastix*, scourge]. A genus of flagellates parasitic in man and other animals.

C. mesnili. The species found in the intestine of man.

chi·lop′a. See *onyalai.*

Chi·lop′o·da [G. *cheilos*, lip; *poda*, feet]. The centipedes: a division of the arthropod group Myriapoda.

chi·maph′i·la (kigh·maf′i·luh, ki·maf′i·luh) [G. *cheima*, winter; *philein*, to love]. A preparation of dried leaves of *Chimaphila umbellata;* has been used as a diuretic, astringent, and urinary disinfectant.

chi·maph′i·line (kigh·maf′i·leen, ·lin, ki·maf′·). $C_{24}H_{21}O_4$. A crystalline neutral principle isolated from the leaves of *Chimaphila umbellata.*

chi·me′ra, chi·mae′ra (kigh·meer′uh, ki·meer′uh) [G. *chimaira*, she-goat]. 1. A plant composed of two genetically distinct types of tissue resulting from somatic mutation, segregation, or from artificial fusion, as in graft hybrids; mosaic. 2. A compound embryo produced by grafting approximately equal halves of two embryos, usually of different species.

chin [AS. *cin*]. The mentum; the lower part of the face, at or near the symphysis of the lower jaw.

c. reflex. See jaw-jerk *reflex.*

chinacrin hydrochloride. Trade name for quinacrine hydrochloride.

chin cough. See *whooping cough.*

chin′i·o·fon (kin′ee·o·fon, chin′ee·) (*chiniofonum*). A mixture of 7-iodo-8-hydroxyquinoline-5-sulfonic acid, its sodium salt, and sodium bicarbonate, containing 26.5–29.0% iodine. It is a canary yellow powder, soluble in 25 parts of water. It is employed as an amebicide in the treatment of dysentery; locally, it finds some use as a surgical dusting powder.

chin′o- (kin′o-, kee′no-), **chin-** (kin-) [Sp. *quina*, from Quechua *quinquina*, cinchona bark]. A combining form denoting *presence of* or *relation to quinine*.

chi·noi′dine (ki·noy′deen, ·din, chi·noy′·). Quinoidine. A mixture of amorphous alkaloids obtained in the manufacture of quinine. Occasionally employed as an inexpensive febrifuge, but has only slight antimalarial action.

chinosol. Trade name for 8-hydroxyquinoline sulfate (oxyquinoline sulfate), an active bactericide.

chin′o·vin (kin′o·vin, ki·no′vin). $C_{30}H_{48}O_8$. Quinovin; a glycoside obtained from cinchona.

chi″o·na·blep′si·a, chi″o·na·blep′sy (kigh″o-nuh·) [G. *chiōn*, snow; *ablepsia*, blindness]. Loss of sensibility of the retina resulting from the exposure of the eyes to reflection of the sunlight upon snow; snowblindness.

chi″o·na·blep′sy. See *chionablepsia*.

chi″o·nan′thin (kigh″o·nan′thin). $C_{22}H_{28}O_{10}$. A glycoside from the rootbark of *Chionanthus virginicus*, of the Oleaceae. See *Chionanthus*.

Chi″o·nan′thus (kigh″o·nan′thus) [*chiōn;* G. *anthos*, flower]. 1. Fringe-tree bark. The dried bark of the root of *Chionanthus virginicus*. It has been used as a bitter tonic, diuretic, and aperient. 2. A genus of the Oleaceae.

chi″o·no·pho′bi·a (kigh″o·no·fo′bee·uh) [*chiōn;* G. *phobos*, fear]. Morbid fear of snow.

chi·rag′ra (kigh·rag′ruh, ·ray′gruh, kigh′rag·ruh) [G. *cheir*, hand; *agra*, a seizure]. Pain in the hand.

chi·ral′gi·a (kigh·ral′juh, ·jee·uh) [*cheir;* G. *algos*, pain]. Neuralgic pain in the hand.

c. paresthetica. Numbness and spontaneous pain in that part of the hand supplied by the superficial branch of the radial nerve.

chi·rap′si·a (kigh·rap′see·uh) [*cheir;* G. *hapsis*, a touching]. Friction with the hand; massage.

chi′rap·sy, chei′rap·sy [*cheir;* G. *hapsis*, a touching]. The marking of a child in utero with the image of an object longed for and touched by the mother: an old belief.

chi″rar·thri′tis (kigh″rahr·thrigh′tis) [*cheir;* G. *arthritis*, from *arthron*, joint; *-itis*, inflammation]. Rheumatism or arthritis of the hand. *Rare.*

chi·ra′ta (kigh·ray′tuh, chi·rah′tuh, ki·ray′tuh) [Hindu *cirāytā*]. The dried plant of *Swertia chirayita;* has been used as a bitter tonic.

chi·ra′tin (kigh·ray′tin, ki·rat′in, kirr′uh·tin), **chi·ret′tin** (kigh·ret′in). $C_{26}H_{48}O_{15}$. A light yellow, crystalline, bitter glycoside, obtained from chirata.

chi·ris′mus (kigh·riz′mus) [G. *cheir*, hand]. Spasm of the hand.

chi′ro- (kigh′ro-), **chir-, chei′ro-** (kigh′ro-), **cheir-** [*cheir*]. A combining form denoting *pertaining to the hand.*

chi″ro·kin″es·thet′ic (kigh″ro·kin″ess·thet′ick) [*cheir;* G. *kinēsis*, motion; *aisthēsis*, sensation]. Relating to the subjective perception of the motions of the hand, particularly in writing.

chi·rol′o·gy (kigh·rol′o·jee) [*cheir;* G. *logos*, word]. 1. Method of communicating with deaf-mutes by means of the hands. *Obs.* 2. Study of the hand.

chi″ro·meg′a·ly (kigh″ro·meg′uh·lee) [*cheir;* G. *megas*, large]. Enlargement of one or both hands, but not of acromegalic nature. Also called *pseudoacromegaly*.

chi′ro·plas″ty (kigh′ro·plas″tee) [*cheir;* G. *plassein*, to form]. Plastic operation on the hand.

chi·rop′o·dist (kigh·rop′o·dist, ki·rop′·) [*cheir;* G. *pous*, foot]. One who treats minor ailments of the feet. Syn., *podiatrist*.

chi·rop′o·dy (kigh·rop′o·dee, ki·rop′·) [*cheir; pous*]. The medical specialty dealing with diseases of the feet.

chi″ro·pom′pho·lyx (kigh″ro·pom′fo·licks, ·pom-fo′licks) [*cheir;* G. *pompholyx*, bubble]. Dyshidrosis; pompholyx; an ill-defined, inflammatory, pruritic skin disease confined to the hands and feet, characterized by vesicles or blebs, arranged in groups. Often a dermatophytid associated with epidermophytosis of hands or feet.

chi″ro·prac′tic (kigh″ro·prack′tick) [*cheir;* G. *praktikos*, from *prassein*, to do]. A system of therapeutics based upon the theory that disease is caused by abnormal function of the nervous system; attempts to restore normal function are made through manipulation and treatment of the structures of the body, especially those of the spinal column.

chi′ro·scope (kigh′ro·scope) [*cheir;* G. *skopein*, to examine]. Device for correcting strabismus.

chi′ro·spasm (kigh′ro·spaz·um) [*cheir;* G. *spasmos*, spasm]. Writer's cramp. *Obs.*

chi·rur′geon (kigh·rur′jun) [G. *cheirourgos*, working by hand]. A surgeon. *Obs.*

chi·rur′ger·y (kigh·rur′juh·ree). Surgery. *Obs.* —**chirurgic, chirurgical,** *adj.*

chi′tin (kigh′tin). The structural material of skeletons of arthropoda, with few exceptions occurring only in invertebrates. It is a condensation product of acetylglucosamine molecules, as cellulose is a condensation product of glucose molecules. —**chitinous,** *adj.*

chi″to·bi′ose. A partial hydrolysis product of chitin; it contains two acetylglucosamine molecules linked in the same manner as the two glucose molecules of cellobiose.

Chittenden, Russell Henry [*American physiological chemist,* 1856–1943]. Remembered for his experimental work which advanced the knowledge of nutrition (1883). Founded the first laboratory of physiologic chemistry in the United States. Advocated a low protein diet as an aid to health (1904).

chlam″y·do·blas″to·my·co′sis (clam″i·do·blas″-to·migh·ko′sis) [G. *chlamys*, mantle; *blastos*, germ; *mykēs*, fungus; *-ōsis*, condition]. A form of chromoblastomycosis due to *Phialophora verrucosa*.

Chla·myd′o·phrys. A genus of coprozoic flagellates.

C. stercorea. A species found in the feces of man and other animals.

chlam′y·do·spore″ [*chlamys;* G. *spora*, seed]. A thick-walled spore of certain fungi; it is not produced on a basidium but represents a transformed vegetative cell.

Chlam″y·do·zo″a′ce·ae. Proposed name for the family of large viruses, which includes the genera *Chlamydozoon* and *Miyagawanella*, noncultivatable and cultivatable in chick embryos, respectively. Susceptibility of some species to treatment by sulfonamides and antibiotics separates this group from other viruses.

Chlam″y·do·zo′on. A genus of viruses, family *Chlamydozoaceae*, with limited host range and attacking primarily ocular and genital tissues, which form characteristic inclusion bodies. It includes the causative agent of trachoma (**C. trachomatosis**) and of inclusion conjunctivitis (**C. oculogenitale**), which may also cause inflammation of the lower genitourinary tract.

chlo·as′ma (klo·az′muh) [G., from *chloazein*, to be green]. Deposit of pigment in the skin, occurring in patches of various sizes and shapes, and of a yellow, brown, or black color; often associated with some endocrine derangement. Syn., *discolorations, melanoderma, melasma.*

c. gravidarum. See *c. uterinum.*

c. hepaticum. Liver spots, a term used by the laity for any pigmentation of the face or chest.

c. phthisicorum. Brown patches upon the skin of the forehead or upper portions of the cheeks in tuberculous patients.

c. uterinum. Located chiefly on the forehead, temples, cheeks, nipples, and median line of abdomen. They may be marked during pregnancy, menstruation, functional derangements of the uterus, or in ovarian disorders and tumors. Also called *c. gravidarum.*

chlor-. See *chloro-.*

chlor·ac′ne [G. *chlōros*, pale green; perhaps from G. *achnē*, chaff]. An acneform eruption caused by chlorine or paraffin.

chlo′ral. 1. Trichloroacetaldehyde, $CCl_3.CHO$. A colorless, caustic liquid of pungent odor. 2. Chloral hydrate.

camphorated c. (*chloral camphoratum*). A liquid prepared from equal parts of chloral hydrate and camphor; used as a counterirritant and anodyne. Syn., *chloral camphor.*

c. amylene hydrate. $CCl_3.CHOH.O.C(CH_3)_2$-C_2H_5. A hypnotic used in 50% solution. Dose, 0.5–2.0 cc. (8–30 min.). Syn., *amylene chloral.*

c. hydrate (*chloralis hydras*). $CCl_3.CH(OH)_2$. White crystals of penetrating odor and slightly bitter taste. 1 Gm. dissolves in 0.25 cc. of water or in 1.3 cc. of alcohol; used as rapid somnifacient, anticonvulsant, and as ingredient of anodyne liniments. Dose, 0.6–2.0 Gm. (10–30 gr.).

c. menthol. A liquid prepared from equal parts of chloral hydrate and menthol; has been used as counterirritant and local anesthetic.

chlo″ral·am′ide. See *chloralformamide.*

chlo″ral·form·am′ide (klor″ul·form·am′ide, ·id, ·form′uh·mide, ·mid). A crystalline solid, CCl_3.-$CHOH.NH.OC.H$; used as a hypnotic, somewhat slower-acting than chloral hydrate. Dose, 1–2 Gm. (15–30 gr.).

chlo·ral′i·mide. $CCl_3.CH{:}NH$. Colorless crystals soluble in alcohol; has been used as a hypnotic.

chlo′ral·ize. Put under the influence of chloral.

chlo′ral·ose (klor′ul·ohss, ·ohz). $C_8H_{11}Cl_3O_6$; an interaction product of chloral (anhydrous) and glucose (dextrose); white, bitter crystals. An uncertain and sometimes dangerous hypnotic. Dose, 0.2–0.6 Gm. (3–10 gr.). Syn., *glucochloral.*

chlor·am′ide, chlor′a·mide. See *chloralformamide.*

chlo″ra·mine′. Chloramine-T.

chlo″ra·mine′-B (klor″uh·meen′, ·min′, klor·am′in). Sodium benzenesulfonchloramide. A white, crystalline powder used like chloramine-T.

chlo″ra·mine′-T (*chloramina-T*). Sodium paratoluenesulfonchloramide. $CH_3.C_6H_4.SO_2.N(Na)$-$Cl.3H_2O$. A white or faintly yellow crystalline powder, unstable in air. A surgical disinfectant in 0.5–4.0% solution. Syn., *chlorazene, tosylchloramide sodium.*

chlor″am·phen′i·col. D(-)Threo-1-*p*-nitrophenyl-2-dichloroacetamido-1,3-propanediol; $NO_2.C_6H_4$.-$CH(OH).CH(CH_2OH).NH.C(O).CHCl_2$; an antibiotic substance produced by *Streptomyces venezuelae* Burkholder, and also synthetically. It is orally effective against Rickettsia and against certain Gram-negative organisms; it may produce serious blood dyscrasias. See *chloromycetin.*

chlo″ra·ne′mi·a, chlo″ro·a·ne′mi·a, chlo″ra·nae′mi·a. Chlorosis.

chlor·ar′se·nol. See *solarson.*

chlo′rate. A salt of chloric acid; the radical ClO_3^-.

chlo′ra·zene. Chloramine-T.

chlo′ra·zol. A highly toxic, oily liquid, obtained from proteins by action of strong acids.

chlo′ra·zol black E (C.C.). An acid poly-azo dye; used as a vital dye and as a nuclear stain. Also called *Erie black G X 00, Pontamine black E.*

chlor·bu′ta·nol. Chlorobutanol.

chlor·bu′tol. Chlorobutanol.

chlorcosane. Trade name of chlorinated paraffin.

chlor·cre′sol. See *chlorocresol.*

chlor·cy′cli·zine hy″dro·chlo′ride. Official name for 1-(*p*-chlorobenzhydryl)-4-methylpiperazine hydrochloride, $C_{18}H_{21}ClN_2.HCl$: an antihistaminic drug. See *di-paralene hydrochloride, perazil hydrochloride.*

chlordan, chlordane. Trade name for 1,2,4,5,6,7,-8,8-octachloro-2,3,3a,4,7,7a-hexahydro-4,7-methanoindene, an insecticide.

Chlor·el′la vul·gar′is. An alga, the source of the antibiotic chlorellin.

chlo·rel′lin. A substance produced by certain algae, notably species of *Chlorella*, which inhibits the growth of various Gram-positive and Gram-negative bacteria.

chlor″eph·i·dro′sis [G. *chlōros*, pale green; *ephidrōsis*, superficial perspiration]. A condition characterized by greenish perspiration.

chloresium. Trade-mark for certain medicinal products containing chlorophyll.

chlor-ethamin. Trade-mark for a urine acidifier, chemically ethylenediamine dihydrochloride.

chlor·eth′yl. See *ethyl* chloride.

chloretone. A trade-mark for chlorobutanol.

chlor·gua′nide hy″dro·chlo′ride. See *chloroguanide hydrochloride.*

chlor·hem′a·tin, chlor·haem′a·tin (klor·hem′-uh·tin, ·hee′muh·tin). See *hemin.*

chlor·hy′dri·a [*chlōros;* G. *hydōr*, water]. Excess of hydrochloric acid in the stomach.

chlo′ric ac′id. $HClO_3$. An acid known only in solution and in the form of its salts (chlorates).

chlo′ride. A salt of hydrochloric acid; a binary compound containing Cl^-.

lime c. Chlorinated lime.

chlo′ride shift. The exchange of chloride ion for bicarbonate ion between intracellular and extracellular fluid without a corresponding movement of cations.

chlo″ri·du′ri·a [*chlōros;* G. *ouron*, urine]. Excess of chlorides in the urine.

chlo″rin·a′tion [*chlōros*]. Act or process of treating or combining with chlorine, as for disinfecting sewage or drinking water.

chlo′rine (klo′reen, ·rin) [*chlōros*]. Cl = 35.457. A greenish yellow gas of suffocating odor; very irritant; prepared by the electrolysis of sodium chloride solutions. A powerful germicide only in the presence of moisture with which it forms hypochlorous and hydrochloric acids, the former decomposing with the liberation of nascent oxygen. This fact accounts for its germicidal as well as its bleaching and deodorant value. It has been used by inhalation in the treatment of acute coryza. **—chlorinated,** *adj.*

c. water. Saturated aqueous solution of chlorine.

chlo′rite. A salt containing the radical ClO_2^-, derived from chlorous acid.

chlor·mer′o·drin. Generic name for [3-(chloromercuri-2-methoxypropylurea; $NH_2.CO.NH$.-$CH_2.CH(OCH_3).CH_2.HgCl$; an orally effective mercurial diuretic. See *neohydrin.*

chlo′ro-, chlor- [*chlōros*]. 1. A combining form meaning *pale green.* 2. *In chemistry*, a combining form meaning *having chlorine as a substitute for hydrogen.*

chlo″ro·ac″e·to·phe′none (klor″o·ass″i·to·fee′-nohn). C_8H_7OCl. A white solid used as a lacrimator in chemical warfare. It has an odor resembling that of apple blossoms. See war *gas.*

chlo″ro·a·ne′mi·a. See *chloranemia.*

chlo″ro·az′o·din. Azochloramid.

c. solution (*liquor chloroazodini*). A solution of 2.6 Gm. of chloroazodin in sufficient glyceryl triacetate to make 1000 cc. Used as surgical antiseptic.

chlo″ro·bu′ta·nol. $Cl_3C.C.(CH_3)_2.OH$. White crystals with characteristic odor and taste. 1 Gm. dissolves in 125 cc. of water, in 1 cc. of alcohol, or in 10 cc. of glycerin. Hypnotic, sedative, and anticonvulsant. Externally, it is a local anesthetic and antiseptic. A preservative for injections and other pharmaceutical preparations. Syn., *chlorbutol, acetone-chloroform.*

chlo″ro·cre′sol. Parachlorometacresol, $CH_3.C_6H_3$-(Cl).OH. Colorless, slightly soluble crystals used for the sterilization and preservation of injections and, to some extent, as a surgical antiseptic.

chlo″ro·cru·or′in. Any of several iron-porphyrin proteins of extremely high molecular weight and containing a corresponding large number of iron atoms: found in some invertebrates. Dilute solutions of chlorocruorins are green; concentrated solutions are red.

chlo′ro·form. Trichloromethane, $CHCl_3$. A heavy, colorless liquid having a characteristic ethereal odor. The commercial article contains up to 2% by volume of alcohol. Chloroform boils at about 61° C.; at 25° C. has a specific gravity of 1.476; dissolves in 210 volumes of water. It should be kept in tight, light-resistant containers at a temperature below 30° C. It is used as an organic solvent and, medicinally, as an anesthetic, anodyne, and antispasmodic. It is administered chiefly by inhalation as a general anesthetic and is more potent and more rapid than ether, although generally not used because of its hepatotoxic and cardiotoxic properties. Locally, it is a penetrating and powerful irritant and, as such, is used in liniments. Administered orally, small doses are carminative and anodyne. Excessive oral doses produce unconsciousness and coma, results similar to those of inhalation. —**chloroform′ic,** *adj.*

acetone-c. Chlorobutanol.

alcoholized c. A mixture of chloroform and alcohol.

c. liniment (*linimentum chloroformi*). Chloroform, 300 cc.; camphor and soap liniment, 700 cc.

c. spirit (*spiritus chloroformi*). Chloroform 6 cc., alcohol 94 cc. Dose, 0.6–4.0 cc. (10–60 min.).

c. water (*aqua chloroformi*). A saturated solution of chloroform in water. Dose, 15–60 cc. (½–2 oz.).

gelatinized c. Equal parts of chloroform and white of egg shaken together.

chlo′ro·form·ism [*chlōros;* L. *formica,* ant]. 1. Habitual use of chloroform for its narcotic effect. 2. Symptoms produced by this use of the drug.

chlo″ro·form″i·za′tion [*chlōros; formica*]. 1. The act of administering chloroform as an anesthetic. 2. Anesthetic results from the inhalation of chloroform.

chlor″o·gua′nide hy″dro·chlo′ride. Generic name for N^1-(*p*-chlorophenyl)-N^5-isopropylbiguanide hydrochloride; $ClC_6H_4NHC(NH)NHC(NH)NHCH(CH_3)_2HCl$; an odorless, colorless, crystalline powder, soluble in alcohol, slightly soluble in water: useful for the prophylaxis, suppression, and treatment of malignant tertian (*Plasmodium falciparum*) malaria and for the suppression and treatment of tertian (*Plasmodium vivax*) malaria with strains so far studied. Dose, average, 0.3 Gm. (5 gr.) weekly to suppress falciparum and vivax malaria; 0.3 Gm. daily for 10 days to cure falciparum malaria. See *guanatol hydrochloride, paludrine hydrochloride.*

chlo″ro·lym·pho′ma. See *chloroma.*

chlo·ro′ma [*chlōros;* G. *-ōma,* tumor]. Multiple tumors of marrow of bones, and of soft tissues near bones, lymph nodes, and viscera. Grossly, the nodules are green; microscopically, they resemble focal lesions of leukemia. Chloroma is usually accompanied by the blood picture of leukemia.

chloromycetin. Trade-mark for the antibiotic substance *chloramphenicol.*

chlo″ro·naph′tha·lene (klor″o·naf′thuh·leen, ·nap′thuh·leen). $C_{10}H_7Cl$. The α-variety is a colorless liquid; the β-variety occurs as white scales. Various chlorinated naphthalenes are used industrially and have been the cause of severe liver necrosis among exposed workers.

chlo″ro·per′cha [*chlōros;* Malay *pĕrca,* tree producing gutta-percha]. Solution of gutta-percha in chloroform; used in dentistry as nonconducting cavity linings, pulp cappings, and for filling the roots of pulpless teeth.

chlo′ro·phane. A yellowish-green chromophane.

chlo″ro·phe′nol. Monochlorophenol. $C_6H_4Cl.OH$. The *ortho* variety is a colorless liquid; the *meta* and *para* isomers are crystalline. Antiseptic and caustic. *Trichlorophenol* occurs as white crystals; it is used as a 5–10% antiseptic ointment.

chlo″ro·phen′o·thane. United States Pharmacopeia name for the medicinal grade of DDT, chemically 1,1,1-trichloro-2,2-bis(*p*-chlorophenyl)-ethane, $Cl_3C.CH(C_6H_4Cl)_2$. The substance occurs as colorless to white crystals or as a white to slightly off-white powder, insoluble in water. It is used medicinally as a pediculicide, commonly in 5 to 10% concentration in an inert base. Syn., *dicophane.*

chlo″ro·phy′lase. An enzyme which splits or hydrolyzes chlorophyll.

chlo′ro·phyll [*chlōros;* G. *phyllon,* leaf]. The green coloring matter responsible for photosynthesis in plants. It consists of chlorophyll-α, $C_{55}H_{72}O_5N_4Mg$, which is bluish black in powder form, and chlorophyll-β, $C_{55}H_{70}O_6N_4Mg$, which is dark green. It is soluble in alcohol, chloroform, ether, and fixed and volatile oils; used as a coloring agent and, medicinally, in the treatment of various lesions, and as a deodorant. Also spelled *chlorophyl.*

crystalline c. Consists chiefly of ethyl chlorophyllide, a product of the extraction of green leaves with ethyl alcohol.

water-soluble c. A product of the hydrolysis of chlorophyll with sodium hydroxide; e.g., sodium magnesium chlorophyllin, $C_{34}H_{31}O_6N_4MgNa_3$. This substance has shown valuable anti-infective properties. Other water-soluble chlorophyllins containing iron or copper in place of magnesium have also been used medicinally. See *pheophytin.*

chlo·ro′pi·a. Chloropsia.

chlo″ro·pic′rin. Trichloronitromethane, CCl_3NO_2. A colorless, odorous liquid used as an insecticide and as a lacrimatory and emetic chemical warfare agent: also called *nitrochloroform, chlorpicrin.*

Chlo·rop′i·dae. Oscinidae.

chlo′ro·plast, chlo″ro·plas′tid [*chlōros;* G. *plassein,* to form]. An organelle bearing the chlorophyll of plant cells.

chlo″ro·plas′tin [*chlōros; plassein*]. The cytoplasm in chloroplasts.

chlo″ro·pro′pane. Both 1-chloropropane, $ClCH_2$-

$CH_2.CH_3$, and 2-chloropropane, $CH_3.CHCl.CH_3$, have been suggested as general inhalation anesthetics.

chlo″ro·pro′pene. 1-Chloro-1-propene, $ClC{:}CH.CH_3$, and 2-chloro-1-propene, $CH_2{:}CCl.CH_3$; have been suggested as general inhalation anesthetics.

chlo·rop′si·a, chlo·ro′pi·a [*chlōros;* G. *opsis*, vision, *ōps*, eye]. Defect of vision in which all objects appear green. It occurs occasionally in digitalis poisoning.

chlo″ro·pu′rine. $C_5H_3ClN_4$; 6-chloropurine; the chlorine analog of 6-aminopurine or adenine. It inhibits a strain of mouse sarcoma, possibly through ability to block a metabolic step in conversion of adenine to guanine, and is under investigation as a possible chemotherapeutic agent in human neoplastic diseases.

chlo′ro·quine phos′phate. Official title for 7-chloro-4-(4-diethylamino-1-methylbutylamino)-quinoline diphosphate, $C_{18}H_{26}ClN_3.2H_3PO_4$, a white, crystalline powder, freely soluble in water; produced by synthesis. It is effective in suppressive treatment of all types of malaria, also in hepatic amebiasis. Dose, as an antimalarial, 0.3–0.6 Gm. (5–10 gr.); as antiamebic, 0.5–1 Gm. (8–15 gr.). Chloroquine base was introduced as *SN 7618*. See *aralen diphosphate*.

chlo·ror′a·phin. $C_{13}H_{10}N_3O$; an antibiotic substance produced by *Pseudomonas chlororaphis*.

chlo″ro·sar·co′ma. See *chloroma*.

chlo·ro′sis [*chlōros;* G. *-ōsis*, condition]. Greensickness; a form of hypochromic microcytic anemia, most common in young women, characterized by a marked reduction of hemoglobin in the blood, with but a slight diminution in number of red cells: also called *chloranemia, achylic chloranemia*. —**chlorot′ic,** *adj*.

c. rubra. Anemia without pallor, due to dilatation of peripheral vessels.

Egyptian c. Incorrect term for ancylostomiasis.

chlo″ro·stig′ma [*chlōros;* G. *stigma*, spot]. The *Chlorostigma stuckertianum* (Asclepiadaceae), a South American plant, which contains an alkaloid, chlorostigmine, which has been used to stimulate the secretion of milk.

N-chlo″ro·suc″cin·im′ide. Succinchlorimide.

chlor′o·then cit′rate. $C_{14}H_{18}ClN_3S.C_6H_8O_7$; N,N-dimethyl-N′-(2-pyridyl)-N′-(5-chloro-2-thenyl)-ethylenediamine citrate; an antihistaminic substance. See *tagathin citrate*.

chlo″ro·thy′mol. Monochlorothymol, $CH_3.C_6H_3(Cl)(OH).CH(CH_3)_2$. A white, crystalline powder with characteristic odor and pungent taste, almost insoluble in water, very soluble in alcohol: used as a germicide. Also spelled *chlorthymol*.

chlo″ro·tri·an′i·sene. Generic name for tri-*p*-anisylchloroethylene, a synthetic estrogen, introduced under the trade-mark *tace:* employed in the treatment of prostatic carcinoma.

chlor′ous ac′id. $HClO_2$; an acid which has not been isolated, but salts of which, called *chlorites*, are known.

chlo″ro·vi″nyl·di″chlo·ro·ar′sine. $CHCl{:}CH.AsCl_2$. Lewisite; a potent lacrimator, lung irritant, and vesicant, developed for use as a chemical warfare agent. It is systemically toxic because of its arsenic content. See war *gas*.

chloroxyl. Trade-mark for cinchophen hydrochloride.

chlo″ro·xy′le·nol (klor″o·zy′li·nole, ·nol, ·nawl). 2-Chloro-5-hydroxy-1,3-dimethylbenzene, $HOC_6H_2(CH_3)_2Cl$. Creamy-white, crystalline powder used as an antiseptic in ointment form or in oil solution. It has been used as a urinary antiseptic, being administered by inunction.

chlor·phen·ir′amine ma·le′ate. Official name for 2-[*p*-chloro-α-(2-dimethylaminoethyl)benzyl]-pyridine maleate; $C_{16}H_{19}ClN_2.C_4H_4O_4$; an antihistaminic drug. Syn., *chlorprophenpyridamine maleate*. See *chlor-trimeton maleate*.

chlor·phe′nol. See *chlorophenol*.

chlor·pic′rin. See *chloropicrin*.

chlor·pro′ma·zine hy″dro·chlo′ride. Generic name for 10-(dimethylaminopropyl)-2-chlorophenothiazine hydrochloride; $C_{17}H_{19}ClN_2S.HCl$; a drug effective in suppressing nausea and vomiting associated with various pathologic states. See *largactil, thorazine hydrochloride*.

chlor″pro·phen·pyr·id′a·mine ma·le′ate. Chlorpheniramine maleate.

chlor″tet·ra·cy′cline hy″dro·chlo′ride. Generic name for the antibiotic substance, supplied under the trade-marked name *aureomycin hydrochloride*, biosynthesized by the actinomycete *Streptomyces aureofaciens;* a yellow, crystalline powder. Its composition is represented by $C_{22}H_{23}N_2O_8Cl.HCl$. It is a derivative of tetracycline in which a chlorine atom replaces a hydrogen atom in ring one of tetracycline. 1 Gm. dissolves in about 75 ml. of water. It is a broad-spectrum antibiotic, acting against many Gram-positive and Gram-negative bacteria and also against rickettsiae and certain viruses. It is effective when given orally, but may also be given intravenously.

chlor·thy′mol. See *chlorothymol*.

chlor-trimeton maleate. Trade-marked name for chlorpheniramine maleate, an antihistaminic compound.

chlorylen. Trade-mark for trichloroethylene.

cho′a·na (ko·ay′nuh, ko·ah′nuh) [G. *choanē*, funnel]. 1. A funnel-like opening. 2. Either of the posterior nasal orifices. Also called *internal naris*. —**cho′anal,** *adj*.

primary c. The embryonic opening between one of the olfactory sacs and the stomodeum; primitive choana.

primitive c. See primary *c*.

choke [ME. *choken*]. Suffocate; prevent access of air to the lungs by compression or obstruction of the trachea or larynx.

choke′damp″. A name given by miners to carbon dioxide gas; blackdamp.

choked disk. See *papilledema*.

chokes. A clinical manifestation of decompression sickness, characterized by a nonproductive cough, a deep, usually burning, substernal pain, and inability to take a deep breath.

chok′ing [*choken*]. Partial or complete suffocation from mechanical obstruction by a foreign body or external pressure, or from laryngeal spasm caused by an irritating gas or liquid.

chol-. See *cholo-*.

chol′a·gogue, chol′a·gog (kol′uh·gawg, ·gog, ko′luh·) [G. *cholē*, bile; *agōgos*, drawing forth]. Any agent that promotes the flow of bile. —**chol′agogue, chol′agog,** *adj*.

cho·lal′ic ac′id (ko·lal′ick, ko·lay′lick). See *cholic acid*, 1.

chol′a·mine. $CH_2OH.CH_2NH_2$; β-aminoethyl alcohol, a colorless oily liquid, miscible with water. In animals it may be formed by reduction of glycine or decarboxylation of serine; when methylated by methionine it forms choline. It is the basic component of certain cephalins. Syn., *2-aminoethanol, ethanolamine*.

cholan-DH. Trade-mark for dehydrocholic acid used as a choleretic.

cho′lane (ko′lane, kol′ane). $C_{24}H_{42}$. A hydrocarbon which may be considered as the parent substance of sterols, hormones, bile acids, and digitalis aglycones.

chol·an″e·re′sis (ko·lan″i·ree′sis) [*cholē;* G. *erēsis*, removal]. An increase in the output or elimination of cholic acid, its conjugates and their salts, such as sodium taurocholate and sodium glycocholate.

chol″an·gi·ec′ta·sis [*cholē;* G. *aggeion,* vessel; *ektasis,* a stretching out]. A dilatation of extrahepatic or intrahepatic biliary passages.

chol·an″gi·o·gas·tros′to·my (ko·lan″jee·o·gas-tros′to·mee) [*cholē; aggeion;* G. *gastēr,* belly; *stoma,* mouth]. The formation of an anastomosis between a bile duct and the stomach.

chol″an·gi·og′ra·phy (kol″an·jee·og′ruh·fee, ko″-lan·) [*cholē; aggeion;* G. *graphein,* to write]. Roentgenography of the bile ducts.

chol·an″gi·o·li′tis (ko·lan″jee·o·lye′tis) [*cholē; aggeion;* G. *-itis,* inflammation]. Inflammation of the bile ducts within the liver.

cho·lan″gi·o′ma. Adenocarcinoma of the bile ducts which characteristically has an abundant dense connective-tissue stroma.

chol″an·gi·os′to·my (kol″an·jee·os′to·mee, ko″-lan·) [*cholē; aggeion;* G. *stoma,* mouth]. *In surgery,* the drainage of any of the bile ducts by means of abdominal incision and penetration into the hepatic, cystic, or common duct.

chol″an·gi·ot′o·my (kol″an·jee·ot′o·mee, ko″lan·) [*cholē; aggeion;* G. *tomē,* a cutting]. Incision into any of the bile ducts, usually for removal of a calculus.

chol″an·gi′tis (kol″an·jy′tis, ko″lan·) [*cholē; aggeion;* G. *-itis,* inflammation]. Inflammation of the biliary ducts, especially the intrahepatic ducts in the portal canals. Syn., *angiocholitis.*

cho·lan′ic ac′id (ko·lan′ick). $C_{24}H_{40}O_2$. The hydroxyl-free, steroid parent substance of the unconjugated bile acids, the most important of which are *cholic acid,* 1, and *desoxycholic acid.*

chol·an″o·poi·e′sis (ko·lan″o·poy·ee′sis) [*cholē;* G. *poiēsis,* production]. The synthesis of cholic acid, or of its conjugates, or of natural bile salts.

chol·an″o·poi·et′ic (ko·lan″o·poy·et′ick) [*cholē;* G. *poiētikos,* productive]. Possessing the property of increasing the synthesis of cholic acid.

cho′late (ko′late). Any salt of cholic acid.

chol″e·bil″i·ru′bin (kol″i·bil″i·roo′bin, ·bye″li-roo′bin, ko″li·) [*cholē;* L. *bilis,* bile; *ruber,* red]. 1. Bilirubin after passage through the hepatic cells. 2. The form of bilirubin present in bile and blood in hepatic or obstructive jaundice, giving a positive direct van den Bergh test; determined quantitatively by the indirect reaction and not extracted by chloroform. It is not defined chemically. Also see *hemobilirubin.*

chol″e·cal·cif′er·ol. Recently adopted designation for vitamin D_3, prepared from cholesterol.

chol″e·chrom·e·re′sis (kol″i·kro·meh·ree′sis, ko″-li·) [*cholē;* G. *chrōma,* color; *erēsis,* removal]. Increased output or elimination of bile pigment.

chol″e·chro″mo·poi·e′sis (kol″i·kro″mo·poy·ee′-sis, ko″li·) [*cholē; chrōma;* G. *poiēsis,* production]. The synthesis of bile pigments.

chol″e·chry″o·cy·to′sis. A dissociation of the hepatic cords, accompanied by altered polarity and degenerative change of the hepatic cells.

chol″e·cy′a·nin (kol″i·sigh′uh·nin, ko″li·). Bilicyanin.

chol′e·cyst (kol′i·sist, ko′li·), **chol″e·cys′tis** [*cholē;* G. *kystis,* bladder]. The gallbladder. —**cholecys′tic,** *adj.*

chol″e·cyst′a·gogue (kol″i·sist′uh·gawg, ·gog, ko″-li·) [*cholē; kystis;* G. *agōgos,* leading]. An agent or agency which causes or promotes the evacuation of the gallbladder, by inducing contraction of its musculature, or by relaxation of the sphincter of Oddi.

chol″e·cyst·al′gi·a (kol″i·sist·al′juh, ·jee·uh, ko″-li·) [*cholē; kystis;* G. *algos,* pain]. Biliary colic.

chol″e·cyst·ec·ta′si·a (·eck·tay′zhuh, ·zee·uh, ·shuh, ·see·uh) [*cholē; kystis;* G. *ektasis,* a stretching out]. Distention or dilatation of the gallbladder. *Obs.*

chol″e·cyst·ec′to·my [*cholē; kystis;* G. *ektomē,* excision]. Excision of the gallbladder and cystic duct.

chol″e·cyst·en″ter·or′rha·phy [*cholē; kystis;* G. *enteron,* intestine; *rhaphē,* a suture]. *In surgery,* suturing the gallbladder to the small intestine.

chol″e·cyst·en″ter·os′to·my [*cholē; kystis; enteron;* G. *stoma,* mouth]. *In surgery,* the establishment of a communication between the gallbladder and the small intestine.

chol″e·cys·ti′tis [*cholē; kystis;* G. *-itis,* inflammation]. Inflammation of the gallbladder.

chol″e·cys″to·co·los′to·my [*cholē; kystis;* G. *kolon,* colon; *stoma,* mouth]. Formation, by operation, of an anastomosis between the gallbladder and some portion of the upper colon.

chol″e·cys″to·du″o·de′nal (kol″i·sis″to·dew″o-dee′nul, ·dew·odd′i·nul, ko″li·) [*cholē; kystis;* L. *duodeni,* twelve each]. Pertaining to the gallbladder and duodenum.

chol″e·cys″to·du″o·de·nos′to·my [*cholē; kystis; duodeni;* G. *stoma,* mouth]. *In surgery,* the establishment of a communication between the gallbladder and the duodenum.

chol″e·cys″to·e·lec″tro·co·ag″u·lec′to·my [*cholē; kystis;* G. *ēlektron,* amber; L. *coagulare,* to coagulate; G. *ektomē,* excision]. Electrosurgical obliteration of the gallbladder.

chol″e·cys″to·gas·tros′to·my [*cholē; kystis;* G. *gastēr,* belly; *stoma,* mouth]. *In surgery,* formation of anastomosis between the gallbladder and the stomach.

chol″e·cys′to·gram [*cholē; kystis;* G. *gramma,* letter]. A roentgen-ray picture of the gallbladder.

chol″e·cys·tog′ra·phy [*cholē; kystis;* G. *graphein,* to write]. Roentgenography of the gallbladder after it has been visualized by ingestion or intravenous injection of radiopaque substances, which are excreted into it.

chol″e·cys″to·il·e·os′to·my [*cholē; kystis;* L. *ileum,* entrails; G. *stoma,* mouth]. *In surgery,* establishment of a communication between the gallbladder and the ileum.

chol″e·cys″to·jej″u·nos′to·my [*cholē; kystis;* L. *jejunus,* empty; *stoma*]. *In surgery,* the establishment of a communication between the gallbladder and the jejunum.

chol″e·cys″to·ki·net′ic (kol″i·sis″to·ki·net′ick, ·kigh·net′ick, ko″li·) [*cholē; kystis;* G. *kinein,* to move]. Possessing the property of causing or promoting gallbladder contraction.

chol″e·cys″to·ki′nin (kol″i·sis″to·kigh′nin, ·kin′in, ·tok′i·nin, ko″li·) [*cholē; kystis; kinein*]. A hormone produced by the upper intestinal mucosa. It causes the gallbladder to contract. See Table of Hormones in the Appendix.

chol″e·cys″to·li·thi′a·sis [*cholē; kystis;* G. *lithos,* stone; NL. *-iasis,* condition]. Presence of one or more gallstones in the gallbladder.

chol·e·cys″to·lith·ot′o·my. The surgical removal of stones from the gallbladder.

chol″e·cys′to·pex″y [*cholē; kystis;* G. *pēxis,* a putting together]. Suture of the gallbladder to the abdominal wall. *Obs.*

chol″e·cys·tor′rha·phy [*cholē; kystis;* G. *rhaphē,* a suture]. Suture of the gallbladder, especially to the abdominal wall.

chol″e·cys·tos′to·my [*cholē; kystis;* G. *stoma,* mouth]. *In surgery,* establishment of an opening into the gallbladder, usually for drainage of its contents.

chol″e·cys·tot′o·my [*cholē; kystis;* G. *tomē,* a cutting]. Incision into the gallbladder to remove gallstones, etc.

cho·led′o·chal, cho·le·doch′al [*cholē;* G. *dochos,* from *dechesthai,* to receive]. Pertaining to the common bile duct.

cho·led″o·chec·ta′si·a (ko·led″o·keck·tay′zhuh, ·zee·uh, ·shuh, ·see·uh) [*cholē; dochos;* G. *ektasis,* a stretching out]. Dilatation of the common bile duct. *Rare.*

cho·led″o·chec′to·my (ko·led″o·keck′to·mee) [*cholē; dochos;* G. *ektomē,* excision]. Excision of a part of the common bile duct.

cho·led″o·chi′tis (ko·led″o·kigh′tis) [*cholē; dochos;* G. *-itis,* inflammation]. Inflammation of the common bile duct.

cho·led″o·cho·do·chor′rha·phy (ko·led″o·ko·do·kor′uh·fee) [*cholē; dochos; dochos;* G. *rhaphē,* a suture]. The operation of uniting the ends of a divided bile duct over an indwelling catheter.

cho·led″o·cho·du″o·de·nos′to·my [*cholē; dochos;* L. *duodeni,* twelve each; G. *stoma,* mouth]. *In surgery,* the establishment of a passage between the common bile duct and the duodenum.

cho·led″o·cho·en″ter·os′to·my [*cholē; dochos;* G. *enteron,* intestine; *stoma*]. *In surgery,* establishment of a passage between the common bile duct and the small intestine.

cho·led″o·cho·gas·tros′to·my [*cholē; dochos;* G. *gastēr,* belly; *stoma*]. The formation of an anastomosis between the common bile duct and the stomach.

cho·led″o·cho·lith·i′a·sis [*cholē; dochos;* G. *lithos,* stone; NL. *-iasis,* condition]. Formation of a calculus in the common bile duct.

cho·led″o·cho·li·thot′o·my [*cholē; dochos; lithos;* G. *tomē,* a cutting]. Surgical removal of a calculus by incision of the common bile duct.

transduodenal c. Removal of a biliary calculus in the common bile duct through an opening made into the duodenum.

cho·led″o·cho·lith′o·trip″sy (ko·led″o·ko·lith′o·trip″see, ·li·thot′rip·see) [*cholē; dochos; lithos;* G. *tripsis,* a rubbing]. Crushing of a gallstone in the common bile duct without opening the duct. *Obs.*

cho·led′o·cho·plas″ty [*cholē; dochos;* G. *plassein,* to form]. A plastic operation upon the common bile duct.

cho·led″o·chor′rha·phy (ko·led″o·kor′uh·fee) [*cholē; dochos;* G. *rhaphē,* a suture]. Repair of the divided common bile duct.

cho·led″o·chos′to·my (ko·led″o·kos′to·mee) [*cholē; dochos;* G. *stoma,* mouth]. *In surgery,* draining of the common bile duct through the abdominal wall.

cho·led″o·chot′o·my (ko·led″o·kot′o·mee) [*cholē; dochos;* G. *tomē,* a cutting]. An incision into the common bile duct.

transduodenal c. Incision for the removal of gallstones from the ampulla of Vater.

cho·led′o·chus (ko·led′o·kus) [*cholē; dochos*]. The ductus choledochus or common bile duct.

chol″e·glo′bin. Bile pigment-hemoglobin, i.e., combined native protein (globin) and open-ring iron-porphyrin; a precursor of biliverdin. Syn., *verdoglobin.*

chol″e·he′ma·tin (kol″i·hee′muh·tin, ·hem′uh·tin) [*cholē;* G. *haima,* blood]. Bilipurpurin; pigment found in the bile and biliary concretions of ruminants. It is identical with the pigment phylloerythrin, a porphyrin pigment obtained from the degradation of chlorophyll.

cho·le′ic (ko·lee′ick, kol′ee·ick), **cho′lic** (ko′lick, kol′ick) [*cholē*]. Pertaining to the bile.

cho·le′ic ac′id. Any one of the several stable molecular compounds formed by desoxycholic acid with other substances, especially fatty acids.

chol′e·lith (kol′i·lith, ko′li·lith) [*cholē;* G. *lithos,* stone]. A biliary calculus or gallstone.

chol″e·li·thi′a·sis [*cholē; lithos;* NL. *-iasis,* condition]. The presence of, or a condition associated with, calculi in the gallbladder or in a bile duct.

chol″e·li·thot′o·my [*cholē; lithos;* G. *tomē,* a cutting]. Incision for the removal of gallstones.

chol″e·lith′o·trip″sy [*cholē; lithos;* G. *tripsis,* a rubbing]. The crushing of a gallstone without opening the gallbladder. *Obs.* Also called *cholelithotrity.*

cho·lem′e·sis [*cholē;* G. *emesis,* vomiting]. Vomiting of bile.

cho·le′mi·a (ko·lee′mee·uh) [*cholē;* G. *haima,* blood]. 1. An ill-defined, usually fatal syndrome characterized by confusion, excitement, delirium, stupor and coma, and by protean neurologic abnormalities. No pathognomonic anatomic alterations have been described in the nervous system, and the symptom complex is usually ascribed to metabolic alterations resulting from the hepatic disease. 2. Presence of bile in the blood. *Obs.* —**cholemic,** *adj.*

chol″e·poi·e′sis (kol″i·poy·ee′sis, ko″li·) [*cholē;* G. *poiēsis,* production]. The process of formation of bile by the liver.

chol″e·poi·et′ic [*cholē;* G. *poiētikos,* productive]. Possessing the property of stimulating the processes or a process concerned in the formation of bile. —**chol″e·poi·et′ic,** *n.*

chol″e·pra′sin (kol″i·pray′zin, ·pray′sin, ko″li·) [*cholē;* G. *prasinos,* leek-green]. Biliprasin; a bile pigment.

chol″e·pyr′rhin [*cholē;* G. *pyrros,* yellowish red]. Bilirubin.

chol′er·a [G., cholera]. An acute, specific, infectious disease caused by *Vibrio comma;* characterized by profuse, effortless diarrhea, rice-water stools, vomiting, collapse, muscular cramps, and suppression of urine. Case fatality varies from 10 to over 50 per cent. The source is exclusively human. Food or water may be the vehicle. Epidemics are common in the tropical Orient, especially in India. A vaccine prepared from the causative organism killed by heat probably gives protection for several months. Also called *Asiatic c., c. indica.* —**cholera′ic,** *adj.*

chicken c. A highly fatal epidemic disease of fowls, caused by *Pasteurella avicida.*

c. indica. Old term for cholera.

c. infantum. Old term applied indiscriminately to diarrheal conditions in infants and young children.

c. morbus. Old term applied to any inflammatory enteritis with pain and purging.

c. nostras. Old term for *salmonellosis.*

c. sicca. Fatal cholera without diarrhea. At autopsy, the bowel is often found filled with rice-water material.

hog c. An infectious disease caused by a filtrable virus. *Salmonella choleraesuis* is a common secondary invader. The disease is characterized by a patchy redness of the skin with inflammation and ulceration of the intestines, abdominal lymphadenitis, and pulmonary congestion. Also called *swine fever.*

chol·er·e′sis (kol·ur·ee′sis, ko·lur·ee′sis) [G. *cholē,* bile; *erēsis,* removal]. Increased secretion of bile by the liver. —**choleret′ic,** *adj., n.*

chol′er·ic [*cholē*]. Easily angered; irritable.

chol′er·i·form″ (kol′ur·i·form″, ko·lerr′i·form) [G. *cholera,* cholera; L. *forma,* form]. Resembling or appearing like cholera.

chol″er·i·za′tion (kol″ur·eye·zay′shun, kol″ur·i·) [*cholera*]. Inoculation with cholera vaccine as a measure of protection against the disease. *Rare.*

chol′er·oid [*cholera;* G. *eidos,* form]. Resembling cholera; choleriform.

chol″er·o·ma′ni·a. See *cholerophobia.*

chol″er·o·pho′bi·a [*cholera;* G. *phobos,* fear]. Morbid fear of cholera.

chol″er·rha′gi·a (kol″uh·ray′juh, ·jee·uh, ·radj′-ee·uh) [G. *cholē,* bile; *rhēgnynai,* to break]. A flow of bile.

cho″les·cin′ti·gram. A scintigram of the gallbladder.

chol′es·tane (kol′es·tane, ko′les·tane). $C_{27}H_{48}$; a fully saturated hydrocarbon derivative of cyclopentenophenanthrene containing in addition two methyl groups (at carbon atoms 10 and 13) and a C_8H_{17} aliphatic group (at carbon atom 17). It may be considered a parent hydrocarbon from which many sterols, including cholesterol, are derived.

cho·les′ta·nol (ko·les′tuh·nole, ·nol, ·nawl). 1. $C_{27}H_{47}OH$; 3β-cholestanol, cholestan-3β-ol, or 3β-hydroxycholestane, occurring in various tissues; it represents cholesterol in which the double bond is saturated and may be prepared by reducing cholesterol. Syn., *dihydrocholesterol.* 2. Any hydroxyl derivative of cholestane of the general formula $C_{27}H_{47}OH$.

cho·les″te·a·to′ma (ko·les″tee·uh·to′muh, ko″les·, kol″es·) [*cholē;* G. *stear,* fat; *-ōma,* tumor]. Pearly tumor; a tumor derived from embryonal inclusions of ectoderm, lined by stratified squamous epithelium, and containing squames and a mixture of lipids including cholesterol and, occasionally, other structures, such as sebaceous glands; it occurs in the middle ear, and rarely, in the brain, about the base, and in the spinal cord. —**cholesteatom′atous,** *adj.*

c. of ovary. A teratoma.

cho·les″te·a·to′sis [*cholē; stear;* G. *-ōsis,* condition]. The presence of an abundance of cholesterol or its esters in a focus of degeneration or necrosis, usually the intima of the aorta.

chol′es·tene (kol′es·teen, ko′les·teen). Any of several hydrocarbons of the formula $C_{27}H_{46}$, resulting from introduction of a double bond in cholestane; the position of the double bond characterizes specific cholestenes. 5,6-Cholestene is the immediate parent hydrocarbon of cholesterol.

cho·les′te·nol. Any hydroxyl derivative of a cholestene, having the general formula $C_{27}H_{45}OH$. An important cholestenol is cholesterol, which is 5,6-cholesten-3-ol.

chol·es′ter·ase. An enzyme, present in blood and other tissues, which hydrolyzes cholesterol esters to form cholesterol and fatty acids.

cho·les″ter·e′mi·a. See *cholesterolemia.*

cho·les′ter·in (ko·les′tur·in). Old term for cholesterol.

cho·les″ter·i·nu′ri·a [*cholē; stear;* G. *ouron,* urine]. The presence of cholesterol in the urine.

cho·les′ter·ol. $C_{27}H_{45}OH$; 5,6-cholesten-3-ol, an unsaturated monohydric alcohol of the class of sterols; a constituent of all animal fats and oils, of bile, gallstones, nervous tissue, egg yolk, and blood, and sometimes found in foci of fatty degeneration. It is a glistening, white, crystalline substance, soapy to the touch, crystallizing in fine needles and rhombic plates. It is insoluble in water; soluble in hot alcohol, ether, acetone, and chloroform. It is important in metabolism and can be activated to form a vitamin D. See Table of Normal Values of Blood Constituents in the Appendix.

cho·les′ter·ol·ase″. An enzyme found in the liver which catalyzes the hydrolysis of cholesterol esters. The same enzyme is found in serum, in which it catalyzes the esterification of cholesterol.

cho·les″ter·ol·e′mi·a. The presence of cholesterol in the blood. The term is sometimes incorrectly used for *hypercholesterolemia.*

cho·les″ter·ol·er′e·sis [*cholē;* G. *stereos,* stiff; *erēsis,* removal]. An increased elimination of cholesterol in the bile.

cho·les″ter·ol·o·poi·e′sis [*cholē; stereos;* G. *poiēsis,* production]. The synthesis of cholesterol.

cho·les″ter·ol·o′sis. See *cholesterosis.*

cho·les″ter·o′sis [*cholē, stear;* G. *-ōsis,* condition]. A condition marked by an abnormal deposition of cholesterol in some region, as in the gallbladder.

extracellular c. A disturbance of lipoid metabolism, in which reddish blue nodules appear on the hands and other areas of the body. Lipoid deposits are seen about the vessels, and the tissue is vascular.

cho·les′ter·yl. $C_{27}H_{45}$. The radical of cholesterol.

cho·let′e·lin (ko·let′i·lin). $C_{16}H_{18}N_2O_6$. An amorphous, soluble, yellow pigment and oxidation product derived from biliverdin. It is readily soluble in alkalis, alcohol, and chloroform.

chol″e·ver′din (kol″i·vur′din, ko″li·). See *biliverdin.*

cho′lic (ko′lick, kol′ick). Choleic.

cho′lic ac′id. 1. $C_{24}H_{40}O_5$. The 3,7,12-trihydroxycholanic acid, one of the unconjugated bile acids. In bile it occurs as the sodium salt of the conjugated taurocholic or glycocholic acid. Syn., *cholalic acid.* 2. Any one of the several unconjugated bile acids which are hydroxy derivatives of cholanic acid.

cho′line (ko′leen, ·lin, kol′een, ·in). $(CH_3)_3N(OH)$.-$CH_2.CH_2OH$; (β-hydroxyethyl)trimethylammonium hydroxide, a liquid base widely distributed in nature as a component of lecithin and other phospholipids. Choline may be a member of the vitamin-B complex, as an insufficient supply of this or other lipotropic factors in the diet results in accumulation of fat in the liver and other body dysfunctions. See Table of Vitamins in the Appendix. A derivative of choline, acetylcholine, plays an important role in the chemical transmission of nervous impulses. Used as a drug, choline has an effect similar to that of parasympathetic stimulation.

c. bitartrate. $[(CH_3)_3N^+CH_2CH_2OH]HC_4H_4O_6^-$; white, crystalline powder, freely soluble in water: used clinically as a lipotropic agent.

c. chloride. $[(CH_3)_3N^+CH_2CH_2OH]Cl^-$; white, deliquescent crystals, very soluble in water: used clinically as a lipotropic agent.

c. dihydrogen citrate. $[(CH_3)_3N^+CH_2CH_2OH]$-$H_2C_6H_5O_7^-$; white, hygroscopic crystals, freely soluble in water: used clinically as a lipotropic agent.

cho″line·a·cet′y·lase (·a·set′i·lace, ·laze). An enzyme obtained from brain which catalyzes the synthesis of acetylcholine in the presence of adenosinetriphosphate as an energy source.

cho″lin·er′gic (ko″lin·ur′jick, kol″in·) [*cholē;* G. *ergon,* work]. Of, pertaining to, or designating the type of chemical activity characteristic of acetylcholine or agents which mimic the actions of acetylcholine: term introduced by H. H. Dale (1934). **Cholinergic nerves** are those nerves which, upon stimulation, release a cholinergic substance (acetylcholine) at their terminations; this includes all autonomic preganglionic nerves (sympathetic and parasympathetic), postganglionic parasympathetic nerves, somatic motor nerves to skeletal muscles, and fibers to sweat glands, and certain blood vessels. Also see *parasympathomimetic.*

cho″lin·er′gic block′ing a′gent. Any agent which blocks the action of acetylcholine or acetylcholinelike substances, i.e. which blocks the action of cholinergic nerves. Also see *parasympatholytic.*

cho″lin·es′ter·ase (ko″li·nes′tur·ace, ·aze). An enzyme found in blood and in various other tissues, which catalyzes the hydrolysis of acetylcholine to acetic acid and choline. Cholinesterase prevents the accumulation of acetylcholine at nerve endings and thus plays an important role in the chemical transmission of nervous impulses. Most of the pharmacologic properties of eserine (physostigmine) are believed to be due to inhibition of cholinesterase by extremely small concentrations of the drug.

chol′o- (kol′o-, ko′lo-), **chol-** [*cholē*]. A combining form denoting *bile* or *gall.*

chol′o·chrome [*cholē;* G. *chrōma,* color]. Any bile pigment.

chol′o·gogue [*cholē;* G. *agōgos,* leading]. A substance which stimulates the flow of bile.

chol″oi·din′ic ac′id. $C_{24}H_{38}O_4$. A decomposition product of cholic acid.

chol′o·lith [*cholē;* G. *lithos,* stone]. A gallstone. —**chololith′ic,** *adj.*

chol″o·li·thi′a·sis. See *cholelithiasis.*

chol·or·rhe′a [*cholē;* G. *rhoia,* flow]. Profuse secretion of bile.

cho·lu′ri·a (ko·lew′ree·uh) [*cholē;* G. *ouron,* urine]. The presence of bile in the urine.

Chon″do·den′dron. A genus of South American climbing plants of the Menispermaceae. **C. tomentosum** is the source of pareira.

chon′dral (kon′drul) [G. *chondros,* cartilage]. Cartilaginous; relating to cartilage.

chon·drec′to·my (kon·dreck′to·mee) [*chondros;* G. *ektomē,* excision]. *In surgery,* the excision of cartilage.

chon′dri·fy (kon′dri·figh) [*chondros;* L. *facere,* to make]. To convert into cartilage; to become cartilage or cartilaginous. —**chondrifica′tion,** *n.*

chon′dri·gen (kon′dri·jen) [*chondros;* G. *genesthai,* from *gignesthai,* to be produced]. The protein of cartilage which is converted by boiling into chondrin; similar to collagen.

chon′drin (kon′drin) [*chondros*]. A protein material obtained by boiling cartilage; primarily gelatin obtained from the collagen component of the cartilage.

chon′dri·o- (kon′dree·o-) [G. *chondrion,* dim. of *chondros*]. *In biology,* a combining form denoting *grit, grain, cartilage, chondriosome,* or *chondriosomal.*

chon′dri·o·cont″ [*chondrion;* G. *kontos,* pole]. Mitochondria in the form of rods or fibrils.

chon′dri·o·gene″. A hereditary factor thought to be present in mitochondria.

chon″dri·o·kin·e′sis. The division of the chondriome.

chon′dri·ome [*chondrion*]. The total chondriosomal content of a cell.

chon′dri·o·mite″. Old term for threadlike mitochondria.

chon′dri·o·some″ (kon′dree·o·sohm″) [*chondrion;* G. *sōma,* body]. Old term for mitochondria. —**chondrioso′mal,** *adj.*

chon·dri′tis (kon·dry′tis) [G. *chondros,* cartilage; *-itis,* inflammation]. Inflammation of a cartilage.

chon′dro- (kon′dro-), **chondr-** [*chondros*]. A combining form denoting *grain, cartilage, composed of cartilage,* or *connection with cartilage.*

chon″dro·al·bu′mi·noid. An insoluble protein component of cartilage matrix similar to elastin.

chon″dro·an″gi·o·path′i·a cal·car′e·a sen punc·ta′ta. See *dysplasia epiphysialis punctata.*

chon′dro·blast [*chondros;* G. *blastos,* germ]. A cartilage-forming cell.

chon″dro·blas·to′ma [*chondros; blastos;* G. *-ōma,* tumor]. A rare, benign tumor derived from cartilage cells or cartilage-forming connective tissue, occurring in the first two decades in life, and more frequently in males. It is usually seen in the lower end of the femur and upper end of the tibia, microscopically composed of compact, round, or polyhedral cells of moderate size with relatively large nucleus; it may contain multinucleated cells. Also called *calcifying giant-cell tumor, epiphyseal chondromatous giant-cell tumor, Codman's tumor.*

chon″dro·car″ci·no′ma (salivary-gland type). See mixed *tumor* of salivary-gland type.

chon·dro·cla′sis (kon″dro·clay′sis) [*chondros;* G. *klasis,* fracture]. 1. Crushing of a cartilage. 2. Resorption of cartilage.

chon′dro·clast (kon′dro·klast) [*chondros;* G. *klastēs,* from *klan,* to break]. A cell concerned in the resorption of cartilage.

chon″dro·cos′tal [*chondros;* L. *costa,* rib]. Relating to the ribs and their cartilages.

chon″dro·cra′ni·um [*chondros;* G. *kranion,* skull]. The embryonic cartilaginous cranium.

chon′dro·cyte [*chondros;* G. *kytos,* cell]. A cartilage cell.

chon″dro·der″ma·ti′tis [*chondros;* G. *derma,* skin; *-itis,* inflammation]. Inflammation of a cartilage and overlying skin.

c. nodularis helicis. Painful nodules of the ear; usually seen in men on the rim of the ear. Frostbite has often preceded their occurrence.

chon″dro·dys·pla′si·a (kon″dro·dis·play′zhuh, ·zee·uh, ·shuh, ·see·uh). See *dyschondroplasia.*

chon″dro·dys·tro′phi·a [*chrondos;* G. *dys-,* bad; *trophē,* nutrition]. A defect in the formation of bone from cartilage, congenital in origin.

c. calcificans congenita. See *dysplasia epiphysialis punctata.*

c. fetalis calcarea or **hypoplastica.** See *dysplasia epiphysialis punctata.*

c. foetalis. Achondroplasia.

c. hyperplastica. Enlarged cartilage with possible formation of massive, nodular, irregularly ossified projections at the ends of poorly developed bones. Also called *multiple osteocartilaginous exostoses.*

c. hypoplastica. Undeveloped cartilage, showing little or no proliferation.

c. malacia. Cartilage like chondrodystrophia hypoplastica, except that the cartilage is soft.

chon″dro·dys′tro·phy. 1. Chondrodystrophia. 2. See *gargoylism.*

calcareous c. See *dysplasia epiphysialis punctata.*

chon″dro·ec″to·der′mal [*chondros;* G. *ektos,* outside; *derma,* skin]. Pertaining to cartilage developed from ectoderm, as certain branchial arch cartilages from the neural crest.

chon″dro·ep″i·tro·chle′a·ris. Pertaining to rib cartilages and the region above the trochlea of the humerus.

chon″dro·ep″i·tro·chle′a·ris mus′cle. An occasional slip of muscle found in the axillary fascia.

chon″dro·fi·bro′ma. A fibroma containing cartilaginous tissue.

chon″dro·fi″bro·sar·co′ma. A variant term for *chondrosarcoma.*

chon′dro·gen. See *chondrigen.*

chon″dro·gen′e·sis [*chondros;* G. *genesis,* production]. Formation of cartilage. —**chondrogenic,** *adj.*

chon·drog′e·nous (kon·drodj′i·nus) [*chondros;* G. *genesthai,* from *gignesthai,* to be produced]. Of the nature of chondrogen; producing cartilage.

chon″dro·glos′sus. Pertaining to the cartilaginous tip of the hyoid and the tongue.

chon″dro·glos′sus mus′cle. A variable portion of the hyoglossus muscle.

chon″dro·hu·mer·al′is. Pertaining to the cartilages of the ribs and the humerus.

chon″dro·hu·mer·al′is mus′cle. An occasional slip of muscle found in the axillary fascia.

chon′droid (kon′droyd) [*chondros;* G. *eidos*, form]. Resembling cartilage.

chon″dro·it′ic ac′id (kon″dro·it′ick). Chondroitinsulfuric acid.

chon·dro′i·tin (kon·dro′i·tin). A complex nitrogenous substance which, in the form of chondroitinsulfuric acid, occurs combined with protein as chondromucoid, a constituent of cartilage.

chon·dro″i·tin·sul·fu′ric ac′id. A compound which on hydrolysis yields sulfuric acid, acetic acid, chondrosamine and glucuronic acid. It is the prosthetic group of the glycoprotein, chondromucoid. Heparin, the anticoagulant, has a chemical structure similar to chondroitinsulfuric acid. Syn., *chondroitic acid.*

chon″dro·lip″o·sar·co′ma. A variant term for *chondrosarcoma.*

chon·dro′ma (kon·dro′muh) [*chondros;* G. *-ōma*, tumor]. A benign tumor which in its growth simulates the structure of cartilage (either hyaline cartilage or fibrocartilage); may grow from bone, cartilage, or other tissue. Also see *ecchondroma, enchondroma.*

medullary c. See *enchondroma.*

chon″dro·ma·la′ci·a (kon″dro·muh·lay′shuh, ·see·uh) [*chondros;* G. *malakia*, softness]. Softening of a cartilage.

chon″dro·ma·to′sis. The presence of multiple chondromas.

synovial c. A chronic villous synovitis in which some of the synovial villi are converted into cartilage. They may break off and form loose bodies in the articular cavity.

chon·dro′mat·ous [*chondros; -ōma*, tumor]. Relating to or of the nature of cartilage.

chon′dro·mere [*chondros;* G. *meros*, part]. A cartilaginous segment of the embryonic vertebral column; a cartilage vertebra.

chon″dro·mu′coid [*chondros;* L. *mucus*, mucus; G. *eidos*, form]. A mucoid found in cartilage; a glycoprotein in which chondroitinsulfuric acid is the prosthetic group.

chon″dro·myx·o·hem·an″gi·o·end″o·the″li·o·sar·co′ma. A malignant mesenchymoma.

chon″dro·myx·o′ma [*chondros;* G. *myxa*, mucus; *-ōma*, tumor]. A chondroma with myxomatous elements.

chon″dro·myx″o·sar·co′ma [*chondros; myxa;* G. *sarkōma*, fleshy excrescence]. See *myxochondrosarcoma.*

chon″dro·os″te·o·dys′tro·phy. A dwarfism of unknown cause, often familial, and usually not apparent until the child begins to walk or even later. It is characterized by flattening of the vertebrae, kyphosis, progressive changes in the head of the femur and the acetabulum, and, to a variable extent, deformities of all bones except those of the skull and face. Intelligence is usually not affected Also called *Morquio-Brailsford disease, familial osseous dystrophy, eccentro-osteochondrodysplasia, osteochondrodystrophia deformans.* Also see *gargoylism.*

chon″dro-os″te·o′ma. 1. Osteochondroma. 2. Exostosis.

chon″dro-os″te·o·sar·co′ma. See *osteosarcoma.*

chon·drop′a·thy (kon·drop′uth·ee) [*chondros;* G. *pathos*, disease]. Any disease involving cartilage only.

chon″dro·pha·ryn′ge·us. Pertaining to the cartilaginous tip of the hyoid bone and pharynx.

chon″dro·pha·ryn′ge·us mus′cle. A portion of the middle constrictor of the pharynx.

chon′dro·plast (kon′dro·plast). See *chondroblast.*

chon′dro·plas″ty [*chondros;* G. *plassein*, to form]. Plastic operation on cartilage.

chon″dro·po·ro′sis [*chondros;* G. *poros*, a passage; *-ōsis*, condition]. Thinning of cartilage by the enlargement of its lacuna; occurs preceding the process of endochondral ossification.

chon″dro·pro′te·in [*chondros;* G. *prōteios*, of the first quality]. A protein occurring normally in cartilage.

chon·dros′a·mine. 2-Amino-D-galactose; CHO.-HCNH$_2$.HOCH.HOCH.HCOH.CH$_2$OH, a structural unit of chondroitinsulfuric acid. Syn., *galactosamine.*

chon″dro·sar·co′ma [*chondros;* G. *sarkōma*, fleshy excrescence]. A malignant tumor of cartilage; it may occur as a central or peripheral tumor of bone.

c. myxomatodes. See *myxochondrosarcoma.*

chon′dro·sin. A disaccharide, representing a molecule each of glucuronic acid and chondrosamine, produced by the hydrolysis of chondroitinsulfuric acid.

chon·dro′sis [*chondros;* G. *-ōsis*, condition]. Formation of cartilage.

chon′dro·some (kon′dro·sohm). See *mitochondria.*

chon″dro·ster′nal [*chondros;* G. *sternon*, breast]. Pertaining to the costal cartilages and to the sternum.

chon′dro·tome [*chondros;* G. *tomos*, cutting]. An instrument for cutting cartilage.

chon·drot′o·my (kon·drot′o·mee) [*chondros;* G. *tomē*, a cutting]. *In surgery*, the division of a cartilage.

Chon′drus (kon′drus) [*chondros*]. Irish moss; a small genus of red algae of the Gigartinaceae.

C. crispus. The dried, bleached plant of the algae; yields carrageenin, a mucilaginous principle, proteins, and salts of iodine, chlorine, and bromine. It is demulcent and somewhat nutrient; used as an emulsifying agent and as a vehicle in lotions and jellies.

Chopart, François [*French surgeon*, 1743–95]. Remembered for his amputation of the foot, consisting of a disarticulation of the tarsal bones, leaving only the talus and calcaneus (1792). The operation, now obsolete, still bears his name. The mediotarsal articulation has been called *Chopart's joint.*

Chopra's test. See antimony *test* for kala-azar.

chor′da (kor′duh) [L., from G. *chordē*, string]. 1. A cord, tendon, or nerve filament. 2. The notochord; chorda dorsalis. —**chordal, chordate,** *adj.*

chordae Willisii. Fibrous bands crossing through the dural sinuses.

c. gubernaculum. That part of the genital ligament which develops in the inguinal crest and adjacent body wall. It forms a part of the gubernaculum testis in the male, and a part of the round ligament of the uterus in the female.

c. obliqua. The oblique ligament of the superior radioulnar articulation.

c. saliva. Saliva produced by stimulation of the chorda tympani nerve.

c. tendinea. Any one of the tendons of the papillary muscles of the ventricles of the heart, attached to the atrioventricular valves.

c. tympani. A nerve which originates from the facial, traverses the tympanic cavity, and joins the lingual branch of the mandibular nerve. See Table of Nerves in the Appendix. See Plate 15.

chor″da·blas′to·pore [*chordē;* G. *blastos*, germ; *poros*, passage]. A term applied to the primitive pit to indicate its supposed homology to a blastopore.

chor″da·mes′o·blast (kor″duh·mez′o·blast, ·mee′so·blast) [*chordē;* G. *mesos*, middle; *blastos*]. The middle germ layer before segregation into notochord and mesoblast.

chor″da·mes′o·derm (kor″duh·mez′o·durm, ·mee′so·durm) [*chordē; mesos;* G. *derma*, skin]. The embryonic area in a blastula or early gastrula destined to form the notochord and mesoderm. It occupies the region of the dorsal blastoporic lip and is thus the organizer.

Chor·da′ta (kor·day′tuh, ·dah′tuh) [*chordē*]. A phylum of the animal kingdom whose members are characterized by having at some stage in their development a notochord, a tubular central nervous system lying dorsal to the notochord, and lateral clefts in the walls of the pharynx. **—chor′date,** *n.*

chor′date [*chordē*]. Possessing a notochord; belonging or pertaining to the phylum, Chordata.

chor·dee′ (kor·dee′) [*chordē*]. A curvature of the penis with concavity downward; an accompaniment of hypospadias, occasionally caused by inflammation and infection of the urethra.

chord″en·ceph′a·lon. The portion of the central nervous system of vertebrates whose development is induced by the notochord; the mesencephalon, rhombencephalon, and spinal cord; it is segmental and divided into alar and basal plates. Also see *acrencephalon.*

chor·di′tis [*chordē*; G. *-itis*, inflammation]. 1. Inflammation of a spermatic cord. 2. Inflammation of a vocal fold. Also called *c. vocalis.*

c. fibrinosa. Old term for acute laryngitis with deposition of fibrin on the vocal folds.

c. nodosa. See singer's *node.*

c. tuberosa. See singer's *node.*

chor″do·car″ci·no′ma. See *chordoma.*

chor″do·ep″i·the″li·o′ma. See *chordoma.*

chor·do′ma [*chordē;* G. *-ōma*, tumor]. A tumor, often invasive but only rarely metastasizing, derived from persistent remnants of notochord; may be situated at the sacrococcygeal region, at the base of the brain (sometimes in sella turcica), and, rarely, in the cervical vertebral canal. Microscopically, it resembles hyaline cartilage, but is alveolated; often has intercellular mucoid; and may contain the so-called physaliphora cells, large globular cells with vesicular cytoplasm. Also called *acrochordoma, chordocarcinoma, chordoepithelioma, chordoid tumor, ecchondrosis physaliphora.*

chor·dot′o·my [*chordē;* G. *tomē*, a cutting]. Surgical division of certain tracts of the spinal cord, e.g. the lateral spinothalamic tract for relief of pain.

cho·re′a (ko·ree′uh) [G. *choreia*, dance]. A nervous disorder, characterized by irregular and involuntary action of the muscles of the extremities and the face; seen in many conditions as part of a syndrome following an infection. It is also a disease entity, and as such is identical with *Sydenham's chorea, St. Vitus' dance, choromania, dancing chorea,* or *chorea minor.* **—choreal, choreic, choreat′ic,** *adj.*

Bergeron's c. See Etienne Jules *Bergeron.*

c. gravidarum. Intractable chorea occurring during pregnancy, toward its close sometimes aggravated and attended with fever.

c. insaniens. Maniacal chorea; a severe form usually seen in pregnant women. It is associated with mania and generally ends fatally.

c. minor. Chorea.

chronic progressive hereditary c. See George *Huntington.*

chronic progressive nonhereditary c. A form of chorea in which the symptoms become progressively more severe; however, the patient shows no hereditary traits. It may or may not be accompanied by mental deterioration.

congenital c. Chorea due to birth palsy.

dancing c. See *chorea.*

Dubini's c. See Angelo *Dubini.*

electric c. See Etienne Jules *Bergeron*, Angelo *Dubini.*

essential c. That occurring independently and not as a symptom of some other disease.

general c. A form of chorea in which all or almost all of the voluntary muscles are subject to irregular contractions.

hereditary c. See George *Huntington.*

Huntington's c. See George *Huntington.*

imitative c. Choreic movements developed in children from association with choreic subjects.

posthemiplegic c. A form of involuntary movement seen in patients after an attack of hemiplegia. Also called *postparalytic c., athetosis.*

senile c. That occurring in old age, due to vascular lesions of the corpus striatum.

Sydenham's c. See *chorea.*

cho·re′i·form [*choreia*; L. *forma*, form]. Resembling chorea.

cho″re·o·ath′e·toid (kor″ee·o·ath′i·toyd) [*choreia;* G. *athetos*, not fixed; *eidos*, form]. Referring to both chorea and athetosis, as in the involuntary movements seen in both chorea and athetosis.

cho″re·o·ath″e·to′sis [*choreia; athetos;* G. *-ōsis*, condition]. A condition characterized by both choreiform and athetoid movements.

cho″ri·o·ad″e·no′ma (kor″ee·o·ad″i·no′muh) [G. *chorion*, skin; *adēn*, gland; *-ōma*, tumor]. A tumor intermediate in malignancy between hydatidiform mole and choriocarcinoma: also called *malignant hydatidiform mole, destructive* or *invasive mole, c. destruens, deciduoma malignum.*

cho″ri·o·al″lan·to′ic [*chorion;* G. *allas*, sausage]. Pertaining to the chorion and to allantois or to the chorioallantois. See *placenta.*

cho″ri·o·al·lan′to·is (kor″ee·o·a·lan′to·iss, ·a·lan′-toyss) [*chorion; allas*]. The membrane formed by the union of chorion and allantois in birds and certain mammals and vascularized by the allantoic blood vessels. That of chicks is used for the culture of viruses in the preparation of vaccines.

cho″ri·o·an″gi·op′a·gus [*chorion;* G. *aggeion*, vessel; *pagos*, that which is fixed]. One of identical (monochorionic) twins. Also called *uniovular twin.*

c. parasiticus. A placental parasitic twin, or omphalosite.

chor″i·o·blas·to′sis [*chorion;* G. *blastos*, offspring; *-ōsis*, condition]. Abnormal proliferation of cells of the chorion.

cho″ri·o·cap″il·la′ris [*chorion;* L. *capillaris*, from *capillus*, hair]. Network of capillaries over the inner portion of the choroid coat of the eye.

cho″ri·o·car″ci·no·ma. A highly malignant tumor composed of cytotrophoblast and syncytial trophoblast partially in villuslike arrangement; it is found most commonly in the uterus and testis, and more rarely in an ovary. Also called *syncytial carcinoma, chorioma (ectodermale), chorioepithelioma, chorionic carcinoma, trophoblastoma, epithelioma chorioepidermale.*

cho′ri·o·cele (kor′ee·o·seel) [*chorion;* G. *kēlē*, hernia]. A hernial protrusion of the choroid coat of the eye.

cho″ri·o·ep″i·the″li·o′ma. See *choriocarcinoma.*

cho″ri·o·gen′e·sis [*chorion;* G. *genesis*, production]. The development of the chorion.

cho′ri·oid-. For words beginning with *chorioid-* see words beginning *choroid-.*

cho″ri·o′ma [*chorion;* G. *-ōma*, tumor]. See *choriocarcinoma;* also see *chorioadenoma*, hydatidiform *mole.*

cho″ri·o·men″in·gi′tis [*chorion;* G. *mēnigx*, membrane; *-itis*, inflammation]. A nonpurulent meningitis, characterized by involvement of arachnoid membrane and choroid plexus.

lymphocytic c. A rare form of acute virus meningitis, occurring in the absence of any evident focal or general cause of infection; characterized clinically by the rapid onset of symptoms of meningeal irritation, pleocytosis in the cerebrospinal fluid, and a short, benign course with recovery. Syn., *acute aseptic meningitis*. Also called *acute benign lymphocytic meningitis, acute lymphocytic c., benign lymphocytic c., epidemic serous meningitis*.

cho′ri·on (kor′ee·on) [G., skin, membrane that encloses the fetus]. The outermost of the fetal membranes, consisting of an outer trophoblastic epithelium lined internally by extraembryonic mesoderm. Its villous portion, vascularized by allantoic blood vessels, forms the fetal part of the placenta. Also called *serosa*. —**chorial, chorion′ic,** *adj.*

c. allantoideum. See *allantochorion.*

c. frondosum. (a) The villous part of the chorion which forms the fetal placenta. (b) The entire chorion until the third month of development, when the chorion laeve develops. Also called *c. villosum.*

c. laeve. The smooth membranous part of the chorion devoid of villi. Also called *c. avillosum.*

c. omphaloideum. See *omphalochorion.*

shaggy c. Old term for the chorion frondosum.

smooth c. Old term for the chorion laeve.

cho″ri·on·ep″i·the″li·o′ma. Choriocarcinoma.

cho″ri·o·ni′tis (kor″ee·o·nigh′tis) [*chorion;* G. *-itis,* inflammation]. Scleroderma.

cho″ri·o·ret′i·nal [*chorion;* ML. *retina,* from L. *rete,* net]. Pertaining to the choroid and retina.

cho″ri·o·ret″i·ni′tis [*chorion; retina;* G. *-itis,* inflammation]. Inflammation of the choroid and retina.

cho″ri·o·ret″in·op′a·thy [*chorion;* L. *rete,* net; G. *pathos,* disease]. Disease involving both the choroid and retina.

chor′i·sis (kor′i·sis) [G., separation]. *In botany,* the splitting of an organ into parts, each of which forms a perfect organ.

cho·ris″to·blas·to′ma (ko·ris″to·blas·to′muh) [G. *chōristos,* separable; *blastos,* germ; *-ōma,* tumor]. A true tumor originating in a choristoma.

cho″ri·sto′ma (kor″i·sto′ma) [*chōristos; -ōma*]. An embryonal fault of development whereby cell groups of an organ are included in a neighboring organ, as the inclusion of adrenal cells in the renal cortex.

cho′roid (kor′oyd) [G. *chorion,* skin; *eidos,* form]. Vascular tunic of the eye, continuous with the iris in front, and lying between the sclera and the retina; the choroid membrane. See Plate 19.

cho′roid, choroi′dal. Related to or designating delicate vascular membranes or structures, as the choroid plexus.

cho″roid·e·re′mi·a [*chorion; eidos;* G. *erēmia,* absence]. Absence of the choroid.

cho″roid·i′tis [*chorion; eidos;* G. *-itis,* inflammation]. Inflammation of the choroid coat of the eye. It may be *anterior,* the foci of exudation being at the periphery of the choroid; *central,* the exudate being in the region of the macula lutea; *diffuse* or *disseminated,* characterized by numerous round or irregular spots scattered over the fundus; *exudative* or *nonsuppurative,* when there are isolated foci of inflammation scattered over the choroid; *metastatic,* when due to embolism; or *suppurative,* when proceeding to suppuration.

c. guttata. Familial degeneration of the macula combined with characteristically grouped hyaline bodies. Also called *Tay's c.*

cho·roi′do- (ko·roy′do-), **choroid-** [G. *choroeidēs,* choroid]. A combining form signifying *choroid.*

cho·roi″do·cy·cli′tis (ko·roy″do·sick·ligh′tis, ·sigh-kligh′tis) [*choroeidēs;* G. *kyklos,* circle; *-itis,* inflammation]. Inflammation of the choroid and of the ciliary body.

cho·roi″do·i·ri′tis (ko·roy″do·eye·rye′tis, ·i·rye′tis) [*choroeidēs;* G. *iris,* rainbow; *-itis*]. Inflammation of the choroid and the iris. See *uveitis.*

cho·roi″do·ret″i·ni′tis [*choroeidēs;* L. *rete,* net; *-itis*]. Inflammation of the choroid and retina.

cho″ro·ma′ni·a (kor″o·may′nee·uh). Old term for chorea.

choy, choy′a. See *chay.*

chre″ma·to·pho′bi·a [G. *chrēmata* (pl.), money; *phobos,* fear]. Morbid fear of money.

Christian, Henry Asbury (1876–1951). American clinician who described a rare disease of childhood (1919), noted earlier by Alfred Hand (1893) and Arthur Schüller (1915). See Hand-Schüller-Christian *disease.* He also described nodular nonsuppurative *panniculitis,* which is now named for him and Frederick P. Weber.

Chris′tian Sci′ence. A religious sect and system of healing through prayer and the triumph of mind over matter; founded by Mary Baker Eddy. Syn., *Eddyism.*

Christison, Robert [*Scottish physician and pharmacologist,* 1797–1882]. Remembered as a great toxicologist. Associated with the early study of leukemia (1845).

Christ′mas dis·ease′, fac′tor. See under *disease* and *factor.*

chro·maf′fin (kro·maf′in, kro′muh·fin) [G. *chrōma,* color; L. *affinis,* having affinity for]. Staining deeply with chromium salts; used of cells of the adrenal medulla or paraganglions which have an affinity for chromium and its salts.

chro·maf′fin·o·blas·to′ma. See *pheochromoblastoma.*

chro″maf·fi·no′ma. See *pheochromocytoma.*

malignant c. See *pheochromoblastoma.*

chro·maf″fi·nop′a·thy (kro·maf″i·nop′uth·ee, kro″muh·fi·) [*chrōma; affinis;* G. *pathos,* disease]. Any diseased or pathologic condition in chromaffin tissue (in the adrenals or elsewhere).

chro·mal′um. Chrome alum.

chro′ma·phil [G. *chroma,* color, and *philein,* to love]. A cell taking a deep stain: sometimes spelled *chromophil.*

chro′ma·phobe [G. *chroma,* color, and *phobos,* fear]. A cell which does not easily stain: sometimes spelled *chromophobe.*

chro·ma′si·a (kro·may′zhuh, ·zee·uh) [*chrōma*]. Color effect produced by chromatic aberration in the functioning of lenses.

-chro·ma′si·a [*chrōma*]. Combining form meaning *condition of pigmentation* or *of staining.*

chromat-. See *chromato-.*

chro′mate. Any salt of chromic acid.

chro″ma·te·lop′si·a, chro″ma·te·lop′sis [*chrōma;* G. *atelēs,* imperfect; *opsis,* sight]. Color blindness. Syn., *chromatopseudopsis.*

chro·mat′ic [G. *chrōmatikos,* relating to color]. Relating to or possessing color.

chro·mat′ic·ness. A characteristic of color consisting of hue and saturation taken together; it refers to the quality of color rather than to its intensity.

chro′ma·tid [*chrōma*]. One of the two bodies, sister chromosomes, resulting from the longitudinal splitting of a chromosome, in preparation for mitosis; especially one of the four parts of a tetrad, formed by the longitudinal splitting of synaptic mates, in preparation for miosis.

chro′ma·tin [*chrōma*]. The protoplasmic substance in the nuclei of cells which is readily stainable, as contrasted with the achromatic constituents which include the nuclear membrane, linin network, and nuclear sap. *Basichromatin* stains with basic dyes; *oxychromatin* with acid dyes. See Plate 28.

chro′ma·to-, chromat- [*chrōma*]. A combining form denoting *color, chromatin, pigment,* or *pigmentation.* Also see *chromo-.*

chro″ma·to·der″ma·to′sis, chro″mo·der″ma·to′sis [*chrōma;* G. *derma,* skin; *-ōsis,* condition]. A skin disease characterized by discoloration of the surface.

chro″ma·to·dys·o′pi·a [*chrōma;* G. *dys-,* bad; *opsis,* vision]. Color blindness.

chro″ma·tog′e·nous (kro″muh·todj′i·nus) [*chrōma;* G. *genesthai,* from *gignesthai,* to be produced]. Producing color.

chro·mat′o·gram. *In chromatography,* the porous solid matrix (column, paper) after the separation procedure has been applied and the matrix treated with a suitable developing agent or agents to indicate the location(s) of the separated components of the mixture submitted to chromatographic treatment.

chro″ma·tog′ra·phy [*chrōma;* G. *graphein,* to write]. The procedure by which a mixture of substances is separated by fractional extraction or adsorption or ion exchange on a porous solid (as a column of aluminum oxide, or filter paper) by means of flowing solvents, especially by the process described under *partition chromatography. Likmisis* has been suggested as a more rational name for chromatography. —**chromat′o-graph,** *v.;* **chromatograph′ic,** *adj.*

paper c. Chromatography in which paper strips or sheets are employed as the porous solid supporting medium; commonly two immiscible solvents are used, as described under *partition chromatography.* Minute quantities of material may be separated by this process.

partition c. The separation of substances based on countercurrent partition between two immiscible solvents: one nonmoving solvent is held in the interstices of a column of inert matrix (starch, cellulose, silica); the other, moving, solvent passes down the column. Each substance moves with the second solvent at a unique rate (R_F) depending on its partition coefficient.

chro″ma·tol′o·gy [*chrōma;* G. *logos,* word]. The science of colors.

chro″ma·tol′y·sis [*chrōma;* G. *lysis,* a loosing]. Disintegration and disappearance of the Nissl granules from nerve cells. —**chromatolyt′ic,** *adj.*

chro·mat′o·mere [*chrōma;* G. *meros,* part]. The part or parts of a platelet colored brightly with stains of the Romanovsky type: also called *chromomere.*

chro″ma·tom′e·ter [*chrōma;* G. *metron,* a measure]. An instrument for measuring color perception or the intensity of colors.

chro″ma·tom′e·try, chro·mom′e·try [*chrōma; metron*]. The measurement of degree of color or of color perception.

chro″ma·top′a·thy, chro″ma·to·path′i·a [*chrōma;* G. *pathos,* disease]. Any pigmentary skin disease.

chro′ma·to·phil [*chrōma;* G. *philein,* to love]. Chromophil.

chro″ma·to·pho′bi·a. See *chromophobia.*

chro′ma·to·phore″ (kro′muh·to·for″, kro·mat′o-for) [*chrōma;* G. *phoros,* bearing]. 1. *In botany,* a colored plastid. 2. *In zoology,* a cell containing pigment granules. Syn., *chromatoplast.*

chro″ma·to·phor·o′ma (kro″muh·to·fo·ro′muh, kro·mat″o·). See *melanoma.*

chro″ma·toph′o·rous [*chrōma; phoros*]. Containing pigment or pigment cells.

chro′ma·to·plasm (kro′muh·to·plaz″um, kro-mat′o·) [*chrōma;* G. *plasma,* anything formed]. The substance of the chromatophores as distinguished from the other cell substances, such as nucleoplasm, cytoplasm, metaplasm.

chro′ma·to·plast (kro′muh·to·plast, kro·mat′o·). See *chromatophore.*

chro″ma·to·pseu·dop′sis. See *chromatelopsia.*

chro″ma·top′si·a, chro′ma·top·sy [*chrōma;* G. *opsis,* vision]. A disorder of vision in which color impressions arise subjectively. It may be due to disturbance of the optic centers, or to drugs, especially santonin. Also called *chromopsia.*

chro″ma·top·tom′e·try [*chrōma;* G. *optikos,* pertaining to sight; *metron,* measure]. Testing of the sensibility of the eye with respect to color perception.

chro″ma·to′sis [*chrōma;* G. *-ōsis,* condition]. 1. Pigmentation. 2. A pathologic process or pigmentary disease consisting in a deposit of coloring matter in a locality where it is usually not present, or in excessive quantity in regions where pigment normally exists.

chrome. A name occasionally given to the element chromium or to one of its ores or compounds.

c. alum. $CrK(SO_4)_2.12H_2O$. Chromium potassium sulfate.

c. alum, ammonium. $CrNH_4(SO_4)_2.12H_2O$. Chromium ammonium sulfate.

c. green. Cr_2O_3. Chromic oxide, a green pigment. A mixture of chrome yellow and Prussian blue is also known by this name.

c. red. $PbO.PbCrO_4$. Basic lead chromate, used as a pigment.

c. yellow. $PbCrO_4$. Lead chromate, used as a pigment.

1,2-chro′mene. 1,2-Benzopyran, the parent substance of many plant pigments.

chrom″es·the′si·a, chrom″aes·the′si·a (krohm″-ess·thee′zhuh, ·zee·uh) [*chrōma;* G. *aisthēsis,* sensation]. The association of colors with words, letters, and sounds.

chrom″hi·dro′sis (krohm″hi·dro′sis, ·high·dro′sis) [*chrōma;* G. *hidrōsis,* sweating]. A rare condition in which the sweat is colored.

chro′mic. See under *chromium.*

chro′mic ac′id. Chromium trioxide.

chro′mi·cize [*chrōma*]. Impregnate with chromic acid or a chromium salt.

chro·mid′i·um (pl. *chromidia*) [*chrōma*]. One of the chromatic granules of nuclear substance found in the cytoplasm.

chro′mi·um [*chrōma*]. Cr = 52.01. A hard, bright, silvery metal; largely used as a protective plating for other metals and in the manufacture of alloys characterized by strength and resistance to corrosion. It forms *chromous* and *chromic* salts, wherein its valence is two and three respectively.

c. trioxide (*chromii trioxidum*). CrO_3. Dark, purplish red crystals, deliquescent, soluble in 0.6 part of water. In 5% solution it is astringent; in stronger solutions, caustic. It is used in dentistry in 2–5% solutions in the treatment of oral infections, especially Vincent's angina. Also called *chromic anhydride.* Syn., *chromic acid.*

chro′mo-, chrom- [*chrōma*]. A combining form denoting *color, pigment, pigmentation,* or *chromium.*

Chro″mo·bac·te′ri·um [*chrōma;* G. *baktērion,* little staff]. A genus of nonpathogenic bacteria of the Rhizobiaceae including aerobic forms which produce a violet, chromoparic pigment, soluble in alcohol but not in chloroform. The antibiotic substance chlororaphin is also obtained from this genus.

C. iodinum. The organism which elaborates the antibiotic iodinin.

C. violaceum. An organism which elaborates the antibiotic violacein.

chro′mo·blast [*chrōma;* G. *blastos*, germ]. Chromatophore.

chro″mo·blas″to·my·co′sis, chro″mo·my·co′sis (kro″mo·blas″to·migh·ko′sis) [*chrōma; blastos;* G. *mykēs*, fungus; *-ōsis*, condition]. A granulomatous skin disease, caused by one of several fungi, usually *Hormodendrum pedrosoi;* characterized by warty nodules which may ulcerate. The lesions are usually found on the lower extremities. A number of cases have been reported in this country, but the disease occurs more frequently in South America. Syn., *dermatitis verrucosa.*

chro′mo·cen″ter [*chrōma;* L. *centrum*]. A structural peculiarity of the salivary gland chromosomes in *Drosophila;* the fused mass of heterochromatin of all the chromosomes with six armlike extensions of euchromatin.

chro″mo·crin′i·a [*chrōma;* G. *krinein*, to separate]. The secretion or excretion of colored material.

chro″mo·cys·tos′co·py [*chrōma;* G. *kystis*, bladder; *skopein*, to examine]. Cystoscopy and inspection of the orifices of the ureters after the administration of a substance that will stain the urine.

chro′mo·cyte [*chrōma;* G. *kytos*, cell]. Any colored cell.

chro″mo·dac″ry·or·rhe′a. The flow of colored tears from the Harderian glands in rats. This oily, thick secretion contains large amounts of porphyrin resulting in "blood-caked whiskers."

chro″mo·der″ma·to′sis. See *chromatodermatosis.*

chro′mo·gen [*chrōma;* G. *genesthai*, from *gignesthai*, to be produced]. Any substance which, under suitable conditions, is capable of producing color. See *chromophore.*

chro″mo·gen′e·sis [*chrōma;* G. *genesis*, production]. The production of pigments or coloring matter, as by bacterial action. —**chromogenic,** *adj.*

chro″mo·lip′oid. See *lipochrome.*

chro′mo·mere [*chrōma;* G. *meros*, a part]. 1. One of the beadlike chromatin granules, arranged in a linear series in a chromosome. 2. Chromatomere.

chro·mom′e·try. See *chromatometry.*

chro″mo·my·co′sis (kro″mo·migh·ko′sis). See *chromoblastomycosis.*

chro″mo·ne′ma (pl. *chromonemata*) [*chrōma;* G. *nēma*, thread]. The fine chromatin thread, consisting of chromomeres and connectives, which constitutes the prophase chromosome.

chro″mo·nu′cle·ic ac′id. See *desoxyribonucleic acid.*

chro″mo·par′ic, chro·mop′a·rous [*chrōma;* L. *parere*, to produce]. Concerning excretion of pigment formed within cells into the surrounding medium.

chro′mo·phane [*chrōma;* G. *phainein*, to appear]. The pigment of the inner segments of the retinal cones of certain animals. There are at least three varieties: chlorophane, rhodophane, xanthophane.

chro′mo·phil. See *chromaphil.* —**chromoph′ilous,** *adj.*

chro′mo·phobe. 1. See *chromaphobe.* 2. A chromophobe cell of the adenohypophysis. See under *cell.*

chro″mo·pho′bi·a, chro″ma·to·pho′bi·a [*chrōma;* G. *phobos*, fear]. 1. Abnormal fear of colors. 2. Excessive dislike of certain colors. 3. *In histology*, staining little or not at all, said of intracellular granules or of certain cells, as the chromophobe cells of the adenohypophysis. —**chro′mophobe,** *adj., n.*

chro″mo·pho′bic (kro″mo·fo′bick, ·fob′ick) [*chrōma; phobos*]. Not stainable; not readily absorbing color.

chro′mo·phore [*chrōma;* G. *phoros*, bearing]. An atom or group of atoms or electrons in a molecule which is chiefly responsible for an absorption band.

chro″mo·phor′ic, chro·moph′o·rous [*chrōma; phoros*]. Bearing color: applied to cells, such as bacteria, which produce pigments and retain them within the cell. Also called *parachromophoric.*

chro′mo·phose (kro″mo·foze) [*chrōma;* G. *phōs*, light]. A subjective sensation of color.

chro″mo·phy·to′sis (kro″mo·figh·to′sis). See *pityriasis* versicolor.

chro′mo·plasm [*chrōma;* G. *plasma*, anything formed]. The chromatin network of a nucleus.

chro′mo·plast, chro″mo·plas′tid [*chrōma;* G. *plassein*, to form]. Any pigment-producing plastid other than a chloroplast. See *chromatophore.*

chro″mo·pro′te·in [*chrōma;* G. *prōteios*, of the first quality]. Any protein containing a chromophoric group, such as hematin.

chro·mop′si·a. Chromatopsia.

chro″mop·tom′e·ter [*chrōma;* G. *optikos*, pertaining to sight; *metron*, a measure]. An instrument for determining the extent of development of color vision. —**chromoptometry,** *n.*

chro·mos′co·py [*chrōma;* G. *skopein*, to examine]. The determination of the color of objects.

chro′mo·some (kro′mo·sohm) [*chrōma;* G. *sōma*, body]. Any one of the separate, deeply staining bodies, commonly rod-, J-, or V-shaped, which arise from the nuclear network during mitosis, and which split longitudinally in the course of that process. They carry the hereditary factors (genes), and are present in constant number in each species. In man, there are 48 in each cell, except in the mature ovum and sperm where the number is halved. A complete set of 24 is inherited from each parent. —**chromoso′mal,** *adj.*

accessory c. An X chromosome.

bivalent c. A pair of chromosomes, one maternal and the other paternal, temporarily united in the process of synapsis.

heterochromosome. An allosome.

homologous chromosomes. Chromosomes that have like gene loci in the same sequence; in man there are 23 pairs of homologous chromosomes; one member of each pair is derived from the mother and one from the father.

idiochromosome. A sex chromosome.

sex c. See *sex chromosome.*

X c. A sex-determining factor in both ovum and sperm. Ova fertilized by spermatozoa having the X chromosome give rise to female offspring.

Y c. A sex-determining factor in the sperm giving rise to male offspring.

chro″mo·trich″o·my·co′sis (·trick″o·migh·ko′sis, ·try″ko·). See *trichomycosis* axillaris.

chro″mo·tro′pic ac′id. $C_{10}H_8O_8S_2.2H_2O$; 4,5-dihydroxy-2,7-naphthalenedisulfonic acid, occurring as white needles, soluble in water: used as a reagent for formaldehyde.

chro′mous. See under *chromium.*

chro′nax·ie, chro′nax·y [G. *chronos*, time; *axia*, value]. The duration of time that a current of twice the rheobasic (galvanic threshold) intensity must flow in order to excite the tissue being tested. Chronaxie is related to irritability and is used in testing for irritability changes in nerve and muscle.

chron″ax·im′e·ter [*chronos; axia;* G. *metron*, a measure]. A device for measuring chronaxie.

chron′ic [*chronos*]. Long-continued; of long duration; opposed to *acute.* —**chronic′ity,** *n.*

chron′o-, chron- [*chronos*]. A combining form denoting *time.*

chron′o·graph [*chronos;* G. *graphein*, to write]. Instrument for recording small intervals of time in physiologic and psychophysical experiments.

chro·nom′e·try [*chronos;* G. *metron*, a measure]. The measuring of time.

mental c. Study of mental processes in relation to time.

chron″o·pho′bi·a [*chronos;* G. *phobos*, fear]. A morbid fear of time.

chron′o·scope [*chronos;* G. *skopein*, to examine]. An instrument for measuring short intervals of time.

chron″o·trop′ic [*chronos;* G. *tropos*, a turn]. Term used to describe the cardiac-slowing effect of impulses in certain fibers of the vagus nerve.

chrys′a·lis [L. *chrysallis*, gold-colored pupa of butterflies]. The pupa of an insect, especially during the stage in which it is enclosed in a cocoon.

chrys″a·ro′bin [G. *chrysos*, gold; Pg. *araroba*, Goa powder] (*chrysarobinum*). A mixture of neutral principles obtained from Goa powder, a substance deposited in the wood of *Andira Araroba*, a Brazilian tree. It is a brown to orange-yellow powder; chemically, it is largely a complex mixture of reduction products of chrysophanic acid, emodin, and the methyl ether of the latter. Locally, it is useful in psoriasis, but stains the skin a dark yellowish brown color.

c. ointment (*unguentum chrysarobini*). Contains chrysarobin 6 Gm., chloroform 7 Gm., yellow ointment 87 Gm.

chry′sa·zin. 1,8-Dihydroxyanthraquinone or danthron, a laxative and cathartic.

chry′sene (cry′seen, kris′een, kri·seen′). A carcinogenic compound obtained by dehydrogenation from cholesterol.

chry·si′a·sis [*chrysos;* NL. *-iasis*, condition]. A permanent pigmentation of the skin caused by the parenteral use of gold preparations; may be reticular in type, but is usually patchy; exaggerated by exposure to sunlight. Syn., *chrysoderma.*

chrys′o-, chrys- [*chrysos*]. A combining form signifying *gold, golden yellow*, or *yellow.*

chrys″o·cy″a·no′sis [*chrysos;* G. *kyanos*, blue; *-ōsis*, condition]. Pigmentation of the skin resulting from the injection or absorption of a gold salt.

chrys″o·der′ma. Chrysiasis.

chrys·oi′din Y. $C_6H_5N{:}N.C_6H_3(NH_2)_2.HCl$. 2,4-Diaminoazobenzene hydrochloride. A brown dye used in some procedures as a substitute for Bismarck brown Y.

Chrys″o·my′ia (kris″o·migh′yuh, ·migh′ee·uh) [*chrysos;* G. *myia*, fly]. A genus of blowflies.

C. bezziana. A species of flies which produces wound myiasis; found in India, Africa, and the Philippines.

chrys′o·phan [*chrysos;* G. *phainein*, to appear]. A glycoside found in rhubarb.

chrys″o·phan′ic ac′id. See *chrysophanol.*

chrys″o·phan′ol. $C_{15}H_{10}O_4$. 1,8-Dihydroxy-3-methylanthraquinone; a constituent of rhubarb, aloes, cascara, of species of *Rhamnus*, and of chrysarobin. Syn., *chrysophanic acid.*

Chry′sops [G. *chrysōps*, gold-colored]. A genus of small tabanid, biting flies, abundant in temperate and tropical America; certain species transmit diseases to man and animals. **C. discalis,** the western deer fly, transfers *Pasteurella tularensis*, which causes tularemia. **C. silacea** and **C. dimidiata** are intermediate hosts of *Loa loa.*

chry″so·ther′a·py. Therapy by the use of compounds of gold.

chrys″o·tox′in [G. *chrysos*, gold; *toxikon*, poison]. A constituent of ergot consisting of a small amount of ergotoxine, with inactive, yellow coloring matter.

chthon″o·pha′gi·a (thon″o·fay′juh, ·jee·uh), **chtho·noph′a·gy** (tho·nof′uh·jee) [G. *chthōn*, earth; *phagein*, to eat]. Dirt eating; geophagy.

CHU Centigrade heat unit.

chur′rus. See *cannabis.*

Chutro, Pedro [*Argentinian surgeon*, 1880–1937]. Renowned internationally for his contributions to surgery and orthopedic surgery, including the development of an amputation stump and a modification of Finochetto's stirrup. Originated a bone graft called *Chutro's bone graft.*

Chvostek's sign. See under *sign.*

chy·lae′mi·a (kigh·lee′mee·uh). See *chylemia.*

chyl·an″gi·o′ma (kigh·lan″jee·o′muh, kyle″an·) [G. *chylos*, juice; *aggeion*, vessel; *-ōma*, tumor]. 1. Retention of chyle in lymphatic vessels with dilatation of the latter. 2. A lymphangioma containing chyle.

chyle (kyle) [*chylos*]. A milk-white emulsion of fat globules in lymph formed in the small intestine during digestion. —**chy′lous,** *adj.*

chy·le′mi·a [*chylos;* G. *haima*, blood]. Presence of chyle in the blood.

chy″li·dro′sis (kigh″li·dro′sis, kigh″ligh·) [*chylos;* G. *hidrōsis*, sweating]. Milkiness of the sweat.

chy′lo- (kigh′lo-), **chyl-** [*chylos*]. A combining form denoting *connection with*, or *relation to, chyle.*

chy′lo·cele [*chylos;* G. *kēlē*, tumor]. Accumulation of fatty lymph in the tunica vaginalis of the testis; seen especially as a result of rupture of lymphatics in elephantiasis.

chy″lo·der′ma [*chylos;* G. *derma*, skin]. Cutaneous elephantiasis, with accumulation of lymph in the thickened skin and in the enlarged lymphatic vessels.

chy′loid (kigh′loyd) [*chylos;* G. *eidos*, form]. Resembling chyle.

chy″lo·me″di·as·ti′num (kigh″lo·mee″dee·ass·tye′num). See *chylothorax.*

chy″lo·mi′crons [*chylos;* G. *mikros*, small]. Extremely small particles of fat (0.5–1.0 μ).

chy″lor·rhe′a [*chylos;* G. *rhoia*, flow]. 1. An excessive flow of chyle. 2. A diarrhea characterized by a milky color of the feces.

chy″lo·tho′rax [*chylos;* G. *thōrax*, thorax]. An accumulation of chyle or a milky fluid in the pleural cavity, the turbid appearance being due to fat droplets.

chy·lu′ri·a (kigh·lew′ree·uh) [*chylos;* G. *ouron*, urine]. The presence of chyle or lymph in the urine, usually due to a fistulous communication between the urinary and lymphatic tracts or to lymphatic obstruction.

chyme (kime) [G. *chymos*, juice]. Viscid, fluid contents of the stomach consisting of food which has undergone gastric digestion, and has not yet passed into the duodenum. —**chy′mous,** *adj.*

chy′mo·sin (kigh′mo·sin) [*chymos*]. Rennin; the rennet enzyme.

chy″mo·sin′o·gen [*chymos;* G. *genesthai*, from *gignesthai*, to be produced]. The precursor of chymosin or rennin.

chy″mo·tryp′sin (kigh″mo·trip′sin) [*chymos;* G. *tryein*, to rub down, digest; *pepsis*, a cooking]. A proteolytic enzyme found in the intestine and formed from the chymotrypsinogen of the pancreatic juice by the action of trypsin. It acts simultaneously with trypsin to hydrolyze proteins and protein digestion products to polypeptides and amino acids.

chy″mo·tryp·sin′o·gen [*chymos; tryein; pepsis;* G. *genesthai*, from *gignesthai*, to be produced]. An enzyme occurring in the pancreas and giving rise to chymotrypsin.

C. I. Color index. See under *index.*

ci·bis′o·tome (sigh·bis′o·tome, si·bis′·) [G. *kibisis*, pouch; *tomos*, cutting]. An instrument for opening the capsule of the lens.

ci″bo·pho′bi·a [L. *cibus*, food; G. *phobos*, fear]. Morbid aversion to food.

cic″a·tric′u·la [L. *cicatrix*, scar]. A little scar.

cic′a·trix, ci·ca′trix (pl. *cicatrices*) [L., scar]. A scar. The connective tissue which replaces a localized loss of substance. It is usually white and glistening when old, red or purple when newly developed. —**cicatri′cial** (sick″uh·trish′ul), *adj.;* **cicatriza′tion,** *n.;* **cic′atrize,** *v.*

hypertrophic c. See *keloid.*

ci·cat′ri·zant (si·cat′ri·zunt) [*cicatrix*]. A medicine that aids the formation of a cicatrix. —**ci·cat′rizant,** *adj.*

cic′er·ism. An animal disease produced experimentally that corresponds to human lathyrism; it is due to toxic action of certain legumes.

Ci·cu′ta (si·cue′tuh, sigh·cue′tuh) [L., hemlock]. A genus of the Umbelliferae.

C. maculata. Water hemlock, a poisonous plant of North America.

C. virosa. A poisonous species of northern Europe; has been applied externally in rheumatism.

cic′u·tine (sick′yoo·teen, ·tin) [L. *cicuta*, hemlock]. A liquid alkaloid from *Cicuta virosa;* has been stated to be identical with coniine.

cic′u·tism [*cicuta*]. Poisoning with water hemlock, *Cicuta virosa.* It is marked by epileptiform convulsions, dilatation of the pupils, cyanosis of the face, and coma.

cic″u·tox′in [*cicuta;* G. *toxikon*, poison]. The nonnitrogenous poisonous principle of *Cicuta virosa.* Its actions are similar to those of picrotoxin.

cignolin. A trade-mark for anthralin.

cili-. See *cilio-.*

cil′i·a [plural of L. *cilium*, eyelid]. 1. The eyelashes. 2. The threadlike cytoplasmic processes of cells which beat rhythmically, thereby causing the locomotion of certain aquatic organisms or propelling fluids over surfaces covered by ciliated cells. —**ciliary, ciliated,** *adj.*

cil″i·ar′i·scope (sil″ee·ar′i·scope, ·air′i·scope, sigh″lee·) [L. *cilium*, eyelid; G. *skopein*, to examine]. An instrument (essentially a prism) for examining the ciliary region of the eye.

cil″i·ar·ot′o·my (sil″ee·ur·ot′o·mee, sigh″lee·) [*cilium;* G. *tomē*, a cutting]. Surgical section of the ciliary zone for glaucoma.

Cil″i·a′ta [*cilium*]. A class of Protozoa characterized by the presence of cilia. The only important human ciliate is the intestinal parasite *Balantidium coli.*

cil″i·ate′. An organism possessing cilia.

cil′i·o-, cili- [*cilium*]. 1. *In zoology*, a combining form denoting *having* or *like cilia.* 2. *In anatomy*, a combining form signifying *ciliary.* 3. *In surgery*, a combining form denoting *the ciliary margin* or *nerves.*

cil″i·o·scle′ral [*cilium;* G. *sklēros*, hard]. Pertaining to the ciliary body and the sclera.

cil′i·um. Singular of *cilia.*

cil·lo′sis [*cilium;* G. *-ōsis*, condition]. A spasmodic trembling of the eyelid. —**cillot′ic,** *adj.*

Ci′mex [L., bug]. A genus of insects of the family Cimicidae; bedbug. It can be infected (a) with *Pasteurella tularensis* and can transmit the infection to mice, (b) with other bacteria, and (c) with *Trypanosoma cruzi.*

C. hemipterus. An important bloodsucking species parasitic to man; the Oriental bedbug.

C. lectularius. The common bedbug.

C. rotundatus. Synonym for *C. hemipterus.*

ci″mi·ci′dine. $C_{23}H_{28}N_2O_5$; an insecticidal alkaloid present in the Mexican plant *Haplophyton cimicidum.* See also *haplophytine.*

cim″i·cif′u·ga [*cimex;* L. *fugare*, to drive away]. The dried rhizome and roots of *Cimicifuga racemosa;* cohosh bugbane. It contains 15–20% of cimicifugin, or macrotin, a resin. There is no evidence of therapeutic usefulness, but the drug is occasionally used in chronic rheumatism, chorea, and tinnitus. Also called *black cohosh.*

cim″i·cif′u·gin. The resin from cimicifuga.

cinaphyl. Trade-mark for *theophylline sodium glycinate.*

cin·cham′i·dine (sin·kam′i·deen, ·din). An alkaloid found in various cinchona species. Also called *hydrocinchonidine, dihydrocinchonidine.*

cin′cho·caine hy″dro·chlo′ride. British Pharmacopoeia title for the local anesthetic substance *dibucaine hydrochloride.* See *nupercaine hydrochloride.*

cin·cho′na (sin·ko′nuh) [after Countess *Chinchon*, 17th century]. The dried bark of the stem or of the root of *Cinchona succirubra* or its hybrids, known in commerce as red cinchona, or of *Cinchona ledgeriana, Cinchona calisaya*, or hybrids of these with other species of *Cinchona*, known in commerce as calisaya bark or as yellow cinchona. The trees are natives of South America. Cinchona contains not less than 5% of alkaloids, of which there are more than 20, the most important being quinine, quinidine, cinchonine, and cinchonidine. Cinchona has the physiologic action and therapeutic uses of its chief alkaloid, quinine. It is also an astringent, bitter, and stomachic tonic. Dose, 0.6–4.0 Gm. (10–60 gr.). Also called *Peruvian bark, Jesuit's bark.* —**cinchon′ic,** *adj.;* **cinchoniza′tion,** *n.;* **cin′chonize,** *v.*

compound c. tincture (*tinctura cinchonae composita*). Cinchona 10, bitter orange peel 8, serpentaria 2, in 100 cc. A bitter tonic. Dose, 4–8 cc. (1–2 dr.).

cin″chon·am′ine (sin″kon·am′een, ·in, sin·kon′uh·meen, ·min). An alkaloid of cuprea bark.

cin·chon′i·cine (sin·kon′i·seen, ·sin). $C_{19}H_{22}ON_2$. A rearrangement product derived from cinchonine.

cin·chon′i·dine (sin·kon′i·deen, ·din). $C_{19}H_{22}ON_2$. An alkaloid derived from cinchona. It is a crystalline substance resembling quinine in general properties.

c. bisulfate. $C_{19}H_{22}ON_2.H_2SO_4.5H_2O$. Prisms soluble in water and alcohol. Also called *c. disulfate, acid c. sulfate.*

c. salicylate. Used for rheumatism. Dose, 1.0–1.3 Gm. (15–20 gr.).

c. sulfate (*cinchonidinae sulfas*). $(C_{19}H_{22}ON_2)_2.H_2SO_4.3H_2O$. Less bitter than quinine, and valuable as an antipyretic. Dose, 0.065–1.3 Gm. (1–20 gr.) or more.

c. tannate. A tasteless, yellow, amorphous powder, soluble in alcohol; used in intermittent fevers.

cin′cho·nine (sin′ko·neen, ·nin). $C_{19}H_{22}ON_2$. An alkaloid derived from cinchona. It is a colorless, crystalline body, similar to quinine in therapeutic effects, but less active.

c. bisulfate. $C_{19}H_{22}ON_2.H_2SO_44H_2O$; a dosage form of cinchonine.

c. hydrochloride. $C_{19}H_{22}ON_2.HCl.2H_2O$; a dosage form of cinchonine.

c. iodosulfate. See *antiseptol.*

c. salicylate. Used in rheumatism in malarial regions. Dose, 0.32–1.3 Gm. (5–20 gr.).

c. sulfate (*cinchoninae sulfas*). $(C_{19}H_{22}ON_2)_2.H_2SO_4.2H_2O$; a dosage form of cinchonine.

c. tannate. Yellow powder, soluble in alcohol; a dosage form of cinchonine.

cin′cho·nism (sin′ko·niz·um) [*Chinchon*]. The systemic effect of cinchona or its alkaloids when given in full doses. The symptoms produced are a ringing in the ears, deafness, headache, giddiness, dimness of sight, and a weakening of the heart's action.

cin′cho·phen (sin′ko·fen) (*cinchophenum*). Phenylcinchoninic acid, or phenylquinoline-carboxylic acid, $C_9H_5C.C_6H_5.COOH$; a white powder, almost insoluble in cold water. It increases the elimination of uric acid and is used in treating rheumatism; it may produce toxic effects. Dose, 0.3–0.6 Gm. (5–10 gr.). Repeated administration of cinchophen may produce acute hepatitis which is usually fatal.

c. hydrochloride. The salt obtained by the interaction of cinchophen and hydrochloric acid. See *chloroxyl*.

cin″cho·tan′nic ac′id (sin″ko·tan′ick). Cinchotannin.

cin″cho·tan′nin. The characteristic tannin of cinchona; it exists as a glycoside. Syn., *cinchotannic acid, quinotannic acid*.

cin′e- [G. *kinēma*, movement]. For words beginning with *cine-* not found here, see words beginning with *kine-*.

cin″e·flu″o·rog′ra·phy. The motion-picture recording of fluoroscopic images. The camera shutter must be synchronized with the peak of the flash of the x-ray tube. Cerebral angiography by this method permits the recording of the flow of the contrast medium. Mechanisms of speech and swallowing have been studied by this method.

cin′e·ol. See *eucalyptol*.

ci·ne′re·a [L. *cinereus*, ash-colored]. Gray matter of the brain or spinal cord.

ala c. The area in the floor of the fourth ventricle overlying the dorsal sensory vagal nucleus.

lamina c. A thin layer of gray substance extending backward above the optic commissure from the termination of the corpus callosum to the tuber cinereum.

cin″e·roent″gen·og′ra·phy (sin″i·rent″ghin·og′-ruh·fee) [G. *kinēma*, movement; Wilhelm Konrad *Röntgen;* G. *graphein*, to write]. Motion-picture roentgenography of internal organs.

cin′gule. See *cingulum*.

cin″gu·lec′to·my [*cingulum;* G. *tomē*, a cutting]. Surgical removal of the cingulate gyrus. It is sometimes used in the control of psychotic reactions.

cin″gu·lo·trac′to·my. The surgical incision of the projections of the cingulate gyrus to the thalamus. It is used rarely, in control of psychotic reactions.

cin′gu·lum [L., girdle]. 1. A girdle or zone; the waist. 2. Herpes zoster or shingles. 3. A bundle of association fibers running in the callosal gyrus of the brain from the anterior perforated substance to the hippocampal gyrus. 4. The lingual lobe of incisor teeth, notably of the superior laterals, and canines; a bandlike ridge rising crownwise from the cervix and often accentuated to a blunt point or a rudimentary cusp.

c. extremitatis inferioris. The pelvic girdle.

c. extremitatis superioris. The shoulder girdle.

Ciniselli, Luigi [*Italian surgeon*, 1803–78]. Remembered for his treatment of aneurysm by galvanopuncture to secure clot formation; now obsolete.

cin″na·mal′de·hyde. Cinnamic aldehyde, C_6H_5-CH:CH.CHO, the chief constituent of cinnamon oil and prepared synthetically. A flavoring agent.

cin·nam′e·in, cin″na·me′in [G. *kinnamon*, prob. of Malay origin]. Benzyl cinnamate; a constituent of Peruvian and tolu balsams.

cin′na·mene (sin′uh·meen, sin·am′een). See *styrol*.

cin·nam′ic ac′id (si·nam′ick, sin′uh·mick), **cin″-na·myl′ic ac′id.** $C_6H_5CH:CHCOOH$. An acid occurring in Peruvian and tolu balsams, in storax, and in some benzoin resins. It has been used in treating tuberculosis.

cin·nam′ic al′co·hol. $C_6H_5CH:CH.CH_2OH$. Yellowish needles or crystalline masses; soluble in alcohol, ether, water, glycerin, and benzin. Also called *cinnamylic alcohol, styrylic alcohol, styrone crystals*.

cin·nam′ic al′de·hyde. Cinnamaldehyde.

cin′na·mon [G. *kinnamōmon*, cassia]. The dried bark of several species of *Cinnamomum*, native to Ceylon and China, the latter variety being known in commerce under the name of *cassia*. *C. loureirii*, Saigon cinnamon, and *C. zeylanicum*, Ceylon cinnamon, are commonly used. Its properties are due to a volatile oil. It is used as a carminative and aromatic stimulant, and as a spice. —**cin-nam′ic,** *adj*.

c. oil. The volatile oil obtained from the leaves and twigs of *C. cassia*. Its chief constituent is cinnamic aldehyde.

c. tincture. 20% of powdered Saigon cinnamon in glycerin, alcohol, and water. Dose, 1 cc. (15 min.).

cin″na·myl′ic ac′id. See *cinnamic acid*.

Ciocalteu's reagent. See Folin-Ciocalteu's *reagent*.

cir′ci·nate (sur′si·nayt) [L. *circinare*, to make round]. Having a circular outline or a ring formation.

cir′cle [L. *circulus*, circle]. 1. A ring; a line, every point on which is equidistant from a point called the center. 2. A ringlike anastomosis of arteries or veins.

c. of diffusion. The imperfect image formed by incomplete focalization, the position of the true focus not having been reached by some of the rays of light, or else having been passed.

c. of Willis. The arterial anastomosis at the base of the brain, formed in front by the anterior communicating artery joining together the anterior cerebral arteries; laterally, by the internal carotids and the posterior communicating arteries joining them with the posterior cerebral arteries; behind, by the posterior cerebral arteries branching from the basilar.

greater arterial c. of the iris. One around the circumference of the iris.

lesser arterial c. of the iris. An arterial circle around the free margin of the iris.

vascular c. of the optic nerve. An arterial circle close to the exit of the optic nerve from the eyeball. Formerly called *c. of Haller*.

venous c. of the mammary gland. An anastomosis of veins around the nipple.

circoid. Misspelling for *cirsoid*.

cir′cuit [L. *circumire*, to go around]. 1. The course of an electric current. 2. The path of a circulating fluid in a system of tubes. 3. The path of nerve impulses in reflex arcs.

Geiger-Müller counting c. An amplifier and accessories which make visible or audible, or in other ways record, the pulses from a Geiger-Müller tube.

cir′cu·lar [L. *circularis*, from *circulus*, circle]. 1. Ring-shaped. 2. Pertaining to a circle. 3. Marked by alternations of despondency and excitation, as circular insanity.

cir″cu·la′tion [L. *circulatio*, from *circulus*]. Passage in a circuit, as the circulation of the blood. See Plates 5, 8. —**cir′culatory,** *adj*.

allantoic c. See umbilical *c*.

chorionic c. See umbilical *c*.

collateral c. That established for an organ or a part through anastomotic communicating channels, when the original direct blood supply is obstructed or abolished.

coronary c. The circulation of the blood through the muscular walls of the heart.

fetal c. That of the fetus, including the circulation through the placenta and the umbilical cord. See Plate 6.

greater c. See systemic *c.*
hypophysioportal c. The passage of blood from superior hypophyseal arteries through capillary clusters in the median eminence and the neural stalk through a second capillary bed in the adenohypophysis.
intervillous c. The circulation of maternal blood in the intervillous spaces of the placenta.
lesser c. See pulmonary *c.*
omphalomesenteric c. See vitelline *c.*
placental c. (a) The umbilical circulation. (b) The intervillous circulation.
portal c. The passage of blood by a vein from one capillary bed to a second independent set of capillaries; specifically, the passage of the blood from the capillaries of the gastrointestinal tract and red pulp of the spleen into the sinusoids of the liver.
pulmonary c. The circulation of blood through the lungs by means of the pulmonary artery and veins, for the purpose of oxygenation and purification. Also called *lesser c.*
systemic c. The general circulation, as distinct from the pulmonary circulation. See Plates 7, 9. Also called *greater c.*
umbilical c. The circulation in the umbilical vessels between fetus and placenta.
vitelline c. The circulation between embryo and yolk sac via the vitelline or omphalomesenteric vessels.

cir″cu·la′tion time. The rate of blood flow; the time required for blood to flow from arm to lung or arm to tongue, etc.

cir′cu·la·to″ry fail′ure. Failure of the circulatory system to deliver sufficient blood to the tissues for their metabolic needs; due either to cardiac failure or to peripheral circulatory failure.
peripheral c. f. See *shock,* 1.

cir′cu·lin. An antibiotic substance derived from cultures of *Bacillus circulans,* being a basic peptide. It is active, both in vitro and in experimental animals, against a number of bacteria.

cir′cu·lus [L.]. Circle.
c. arteriosus Willisi. Circle of Willis.

cir′cum- [L., around]. A prefix meaning *around, about, on all sides.*

cir″cum·a′nal [*circum;* L. *anus,* anus]. Periproctal; surrounding the anus.

cir″cum·ar·tic′u·lar [*circum;* L. *articulus,* joint]. Around a joint.

cir″cum·ci′sion (sur″kum·sizh′un) [L. *circumcisum,* from *circumcidere,* to cut around]. The removal of the foreskin; excision of the prepuce.
pharonic c. See *infibulation.*

cir″cum·cor′ne·al [*circum;* L. *corneus,* horny]. Around or about the cornea.

cir″cum·duc′tion [L. *circumducere,* to lead around]. The movement of a limb in such a manner that its distal part describes a circle, the proximal end being fixed.

cir′cum·flex [L. *circumflectere,* to bend about]. Winding around; designating a number of arteries, veins, and nerves which have a winding course.

cir′cum·flex. The axillary nerve. See Table of Nerves in the Appendix.

cir″cum·in′su·lar [L. *circum,* around; *insula,* island]. Surrounding the insula of the cerebral cortex.

cir″cum·len′tal [*circum;* L. *lens,* lentil]. Surrounding a lens.

cir″cum·nu′cle·ar [*circum;* L. *nucleus,* kernel]. Surrounding a nucleus.

cir″cum·o′ral [*circum;* L. *os,* mouth]. Surrounding the mouth.

cir″cum·po″lar·i·za′tion [*circum;* L. *polus,* pole]. The rotation of a ray of polarized light.

cir″cum·scribed′. Enclosed within narrow limits by an encircling boundary.

cir″cum·stan″ti·al′i·ty [L. *circumstantia,* from *circum, stare,* to stand]. *In psychiatry,* indulging in many irrelevant and unnecessary details when answering a simple question; usually observed in mania.

cir″cum·val′late [L. *circumvallare,* to surround with a wall]. Surrounded by a trench, as the vallate papillae of the tongue.

cir″cum·vas′cu·lar [L. *circum,* around; *vasculum,* small vessel]. Surrounding a blood vessel, or other vessel; perivascular.

cir′cus move′ment. An excitation wave that reenters excitable tissues and continues to circulate; believed to be the mechanism responsible for the continuance of atrial and ventricular contraction.

cir·rho′sis (si·ro′sis) [G. *kirrhos,* orange-tawny; *-ōsis,* condition]. 1. A chronic, progressive disease of the liver, essentially inflammatory; characterized by proliferation of connective tissue, degeneration and death of parenchymal cells, regeneration of parenchymal cells, and distortion of architectural pattern. Liver may be enlarged or much reduced in size. 2. Sometimes used to mean interstitial inflammation of other organs, as pulmonary cirrhosis, interstitial pneumonia. —**cirrhot′ic,** *adj.*
alcoholic c. See Laennec's *c.*
atrophic c. See Laennec's *c.*
biliary c. The result of extrahepatic or intrahepatic obstruction of biliary passages, the liver being stained by accumulated bile.
capsular pseudo-c. Fibrous thickening of capsule with extension into subjacent liver.
cardiac c. Progressive fibrosis of central lobular structures as well as of portal spaces, the result of prolonged passive hyperemia often of cardiac origin. Also called *congestive c.*
central c. Cardiac *c.*
cholangiolitic c. A form of biliary cirrhosis involving the smaller intrahepatic bile ducts, accompanied by fibrosis and inflammation: also called *Hanot's c.*
cholangitic c. A form of biliary cirrhosis involving the larger intrahepatic bile ducts, accompanied by fibrosis and inflammation.
cholostatic c. A form of biliary cirrhosis caused by extrahepatic bile-duct obstruction and not accompanied by secondary inflammation.
coarse nodular c. See postnecrotic *c.*
congestive c. Cardiac *c.*
diffuse nodular c. See Laennec's *c.*
extrahepatic obstructive c. Biliary *c.*
fatty c. Usually of Laennec's type, accompanied by extensive infiltration of fat.
Hanot's c. See cholangiolitic *c.*
hypertrophic c. Enlargement with intralobular fibrosis, accompanied by icterus, but without ascites. Also called *Charcot's c., Hanot's c.*
infectious c. Usually of Laennec's type in which bacteria are present; there is no conclusive proof that the bacteria cause the disease.
insular c. Laennec's *c.*
intrahepatic obstructive c. Biliary *c.*
juvenile c. Usually of Laennec's type, due to congenital syphilis, congenital atresia or malformation of bile ducts (obstructive biliary); perhaps to erythroblastosis foetalis or to unknown cause.
Laennec's c. A type formerly thought to be due to excessive use of alcohol; now known to be due to the associated nutritional disturbances. The liver is slightly nodular, with fibrosis especially in the portal spaces; characterized by degeneration and regeneration of the hepatic parenchymal cells, often accompanied by ascites, esophageal varices,

and ultimately icterus. Syn., *alcoholic c., atrophic c., diffuse nodular c.*

monolobular c. Laennec's cirrhosis in which a single lobule is surrounded by fibrotic portal spaces.

multilobular c. A term used in contrast to *monolobular;* Laennec's cirrhosis in which several lobules are surrounded by fibrotic portal spaces: the usual form of the disease.

pericholangiolitic c. Xanthomatous *c.*

pigmentary c. Morphologically like Laennec's cirrhosis. May be hemosiderotic with marked deposit of hemosiderin, or hemochromototic with marked deposit of hemosiderin and also of hemofuscin.

pipe-stem c. A zooparasitic cirrhosis caused by deposition of the ova of *Schistosoma mansoni* in the portal spaces with reactive fibrosis and granulomatous inflammation.

portal c. Laennec's *c.*

postnecrotic c. Cirrhosis, usually due to toxic agents or viral hepatitis, characterized by necrosis of liver cells, regenerating nodules of hepatic tissue, the presence of large bands of connective tissue which course irregularly through the liver, and, in some areas, preservation of the normal hepatic architecture. Intermediate forms between postnecrotic cirrhosis and Laennec's cirrhosis exist, and may be difficult to distinguish. Also called *subacute* or *acute yellow atrophy, multiple nodular hyperplasia, coarse nodular cirrhosis, toxic nodular cirrhosis, postnecrotic scarring.*

syphilitic c. (a) Syphilitic nodular cirrhosis (hepar lobatum) in which gummas or their scars lead to irregularly disposed retractions of outer surface. (b) Packet liver, in which the cross section shows interlaced thin bands of connective tissue with relatively normal lobular structures within the network.

toxic c. See postnecrotic *c.*

toxic nodular c. See postnecrotic *c.*

tuberculous c. Secondary to tuberculosis of liver or other viscera. *Rare.*

xanthomatous c. A part of disseminated xanthomatosis; scarring of biliary passages leading to an intrahepatic biliary cirrhosis. Syn., *pericholangiolitic c.*

zooparasitic c. The result of animal parasites or their ova, such as *Schistosoma* within the liver.

cir′rus [L., lock of hair]. *In zoology,* a slender, flexible appendage, such as the hairlike appendages on worms and insects, especially the protruding male genital organ of Cestodes.

cir·sec′to·my (sur·seck′to·mee) [G. *kirsos,* enlargement of a vein; *ektomē,* excision]. Excision of a portion of a varicose vein.

cir′soid (sur′soyd) [*kirsos;* G. *eidos,* form]. Resembling a varix or dilated vein: often misspelled *circoid.*

cir·som′pha·los [*kirsos;* G. *omphalos,* navel]. A varicose condition about the umbilicus.

cir″soph·thal′mi·a [*kirsos;* G. *ophthalmia,* ophthalmia]. 1. Ophthalmia, with an apparent varicose condition of the conjunctival vessels. 2. Corneal staphyloma, with an appearance of varicosity of the surface.

cir·sot′o·my [*kirsos;* G. *tomē,* a cutting]. Excision of a varix.

c.i.s. Central inhibitory state.

cis- [L., on this side]. A prefix denoting *on this side, on the same side, since, following.*

cis′sa [G. *kissa,* craving for strange food]. A craving for strange and unnatural articles of food. See *pica.*

cis·sam′pe·line (si·sam′puh·leen, ·lin). An alkaloid from pareira root. See *bebeerine.*

Cis·sam′pe·los [G. *kissos,* ivy; *ampelos,* vine]. A genus of climbing plants of the Menispermaceae. **C. pareira** of tropical America, false pareira, has been used as a tonic and diuretic.

cis′tern [L. *cisterna,* cistern]. 1. A reservoir. 2. A large, subarachnoid space.

basal c. The subarachnoid space at the base of the brain, divided by the optic chiasma into the cistern of the chiasma and the interpeduncular cistern.

cerebellomedullary c. The cisterna magna.

c. of corpus callosum. The subarachnoid space between the arachnoid, which is in contact with the inferior border of the falx cerebri, and the corpus callosum.

c. of Sylvian fissure. The subarachnoid space at the temporal pole, formed by the piarachnoid stretching across the stem of the Sylvian fissure to the orbital surface of the frontal lobe.

c. of the chiasma. That part of the basal cistern below and in front of the optic chiasma.

c. of the great cerebral vein. That containing the great cerebral vein, formed by the arachnoid stretching over the transverse cerebral fissure from the splenium of the corpus callosum to the superior surface of the cerebellum. Formerly called *superior c.*

c. of the lateral cerebral fossa. The subarachnoid space of the lateral fossa of the cerebrum, formed by the arachnoid stretching over the lateral cerebral fissure.

interpeduncular c. That part of the basal cistern in the interpeduncular fossa posterior to the optic chiasma.

pontine c. That ventral to the pons.

superior c. See *c.* of the great cerebral vein.

cis·ter′na [L.]. 1. Cistern. 2. The cisterna chyli, the saclike beginning of the thoracic duct opposite the twelfth thoracic vertebra.

c. ambiens. Old term for cistern of the great cerebral vein.

c. magna. A large cistern formed by the arachnoid stretching across from the inferior surface of the cerebellum to the dorsal surface of the medulla oblongata. Syn., *cerebellomedullary cistern.*

c. perilymphatica. That portion of the vestibule of the ear lying just within the oval window and filled with perilymph which communicates with the subarachnoid spaces via the cochlear aqueduct.

cis·ves′ti·tism [L. *cis,* on this side; *vestire,* to clothe]. The act of dressing in clothes not suitable to the age, occupation, or position of the wearer, but of his own sex.

cit″ra·con′ic ac′id. $COOH.C.(CH_3):CH.COOH$; methylmaleic acid, a crystalline acid obtained on heating citric acid. Syn., *pyrocitric acid.*

cit′ral. An aldehyde, $C_9H_{15}CHO$, found in the oils of lemon, lemon grass, orange, and others. It is a yellow liquid of strong lemon odor used as a flavor. Syn., *geranial.*

cit′ra·min. See *helmitol.*

cit′rate. Any salt of citric acid.

cit′ric ac′id (*acidum citricum*). $H_3C_6H_5O_7.H_2O$. A tribasic acid occurring in the juice of many fruits. It is a normal constituent of whole cow's milk. Commercially, it is obtained from the lemon, lime, and bergamot or produced by the controlled fermentation of carbohydrates. Translucent crystals or a white, crystalline, odorless powder of acid taste; soluble in 0.5 part of water or in 2 parts of alcohol. It is used in refrigerant and diuretic beverages and as an acid flavor. It is oxidized in the body and eliminated as carbon dioxide.

cit′rin. A crystalline substance, said to be a mixture of hesperidin, quercitrin, and eriodictyol glycoside, isolated from lemon juice. It combats the increased permeability of capillary walls, such as occurs in scurvy and certain other diseases. Syn., *vitamin P.* See Table of Vitamins in the Appendix.

cit′rine oint′ment (sit′reen, ·rin). Ointment of mercuric nitrate.

cit′ri·nin. A quinone of the formula $C_{13}H_{14}O_5$, isolated from *Penicillium citrinum* and *Aspergillus candidus;* an antibiotic of limited bacteriostatic action against Gram-positive bacteria. It occurs in lemon-yellow crystals, soluble in water and alcohol.

cit″ro·gen′ase. An enzyme, present in muscle, capable of catalyzing condensation of acetoacetic acid and higher β-ketoacids with oxaloacetic acid to form citric acid or other tricarboxylic acids, as *cis*-aconitic and isocitric acids.

cit′ron [L. *citrus*, from G. *kedros*, cedar]. The tree, *Citrus medica*, or its fruit. The fruit rind is used in conserves.

cit″ron·el′lal. $C_{10}H_{18}O$. An aldehyde occurring in many essential oils, including citronella oil.

cit″ron·el′la oil. A yellowish green liquid of characteristic odor and pungent taste obtained chiefly from the sweet-scented grass *Cymbopogon nardus* or citronella grass. It consists largely of geraniol and citronellal; its insect-repelling property has been attributed to methylheptenone.

ci·trul′lin. A resinoid from *Citrullus colocynthis.* It is a cathartic used in veterinary practice.

ci·trul′line. $NH_2.CONH(CH_2)_3CH(NH_2).COOH$; an amino acid, first isolated from watermelon, believed to be involved in the formation, in the liver, of urea from ammonia and carbon dioxide; it is an intermediate between ornithine and arginine, two other amino acids involved in producing urea.

Cit′rus [L.]. A genus of trees of the Rutaceae. From this genus come the orange, lemon, citron, lime, and bergamot.

cit·to′sis [G. *kitta*, craving for strange food; *-ōsis*, condition]. Pica; a longing for strange or improper food.

Civiale, Jean [*French surgeon*, 1792–1867]. Known in his time for his operation of internal urethrotomy by the use of a special urethrotome he devised. Described his operation of litholapaxy or crushing a stone within the urinary bladder (1826). Responsible for putting litholapaxy on a sound basis in Europe.

Civinini, Filippo [*Italian anatomist*, 1805–44]. Remembered for his anatomic and pathologic studies. He described a small process on the lateral pterygoid plate, called *Civinini's spine.*

Cl Chemical symbol for chlorine.

Cl. Abbreviation for *Clostridium.*

cl, cl. Centiliter.

Clado, Spiro [*French gynecologist*, 1856–1905]. Described the suspensory ligament of the ovary, called *Clado's band.*

Cla·do′ni·a (kla·do′nee·uh, klay·do′·) [G. *klados*, branch]. A genus of lichens.

C. rangiferina. Reindeer moss; used as food in famine seasons. When distilled, it affords an alcoholic spirit.

Clad″o·spor′i·um wer′neck·i. A pleomorphic yeastlike and filamentous dark-colored fungus colony, which is the causative agent of tinea nigra.

clair·voy′ance [F. *clair*, clear; *voir*, to see]. The direct awareness, with no help from sense impressions, of events taking place in the outside world.

clamp [LG. or D. *klamp*]. An instrument for holding and compressing vessels or hollow organs to prevent hemorrhage or the escape of contents during the progress of an operation, as a **pedicle clamp** for grasping and holding a pedicle during removal of an organ or a tumor, or a **stomach clamp** for securing an entire segment of the stomach. Also see *clip, forceps.*

(Gaylor) cervical punch biopsy c. An instrument for the performance of biopsy of the cervix of the uterus.

clang as·so″ci·a′tion. A symptom observed in the manic phase of manic-depressive psychosis in which resonant sounds bring to mind certain words or ideas.

clap [OF. *clappoir*]. Gonorrhea.

clap′ping. *In massage*, percussion movements in which the cupped palms are brought down alternately in a rapid succession of blows. The movement of the hands is chiefly from the wrist.

cla·rif′i·cant [L. *clarificare*, from *clarus*, clear; *facere*, to make]. An agent used to make a turbid liquid clear.

clar″i·fi·ca′tion [L. *clarificatio*, from *clarus*, *facere*]. The operation of removing the turbidity of a liquid or a naturally transparent substance. It may be accomplished by allowing the suspended matter to subside; by the addition of a clarificant or substance that precipitates suspended matters; or by moderate heating. **—clar′ifying,** *adj.*; **clar′ify,** *v.*

Clark, Alonzo [*American physician*, 1807–87]. Known for his sign: obliteration of liver dullness, due to tympanites in beginning peritonitis.

Clark, Charles Patton [*American physician*, 1879–1951]. With F. B. Kingsbury, introduced permanent albumin standards, called *Kingsbury-Clark albumin standards.* See under *Kingsbury.*

Clark, Leon Pierce [*American psychiatrist*, 1878–1933]. Described infantile cerebral paralysis, called *Clark's paralysis.*

Clark-Collip method. See Kramer-Tisdall *method.*

Clarke, Jacob Augustus Lockhart (1817–1880). English physician, known for his studies of the spinal cord and the demonstration of the intermediolateral cell column and of the dorsal nucleus, called *dorsal nucleus of Clarke* or *Clarke's column.* He gave the first complete description of *syringomyelia* (1868), and also introduced the method of mounting cleared sections in Canada balsam, which was a major advance in histological technique.

Clarke, John [*English physician*, 1761–1815]. Remembered for his early account of infantile tetany and for his description of laryngismus stridulus (1815).

Clarke-Hadfield syndrome. Pancreatic infantilism. See *Hadfield.*

clas·mat′o·cyte (klaz·mat′o·sight, klass·mat′·) [G. *klasma*, fragment; *kytos*, cell]. 1. Old term for macrophage of connective tissue. 2. A monocyte.

clas″mo·cy·to′ma. See reticulum-cell *sarcoma.*

clas′tic [G. *klastos*, broken in pieces]. Breaking up into fragments; causing division.

Claude, Henri Charles Jules (1869–1945). French psychiatrist who described a syndrome due to a lesion in the central portion of one red nucleus, characterized by contralateral cerebellar ataxia and hemichorea and ipsilateral paralysis of the area innervated by the third cranial nerve.

clau″di·ca′tion [L. *claudicatio*, from *claudicare*, to limp]. Lameness.

intermittent c. Cramplike pains and weakness in the legs, particularly the calves; induced by walking and relieved by rest; associated with excessive smoking, vascular spasm, and arteriosclerosis. Syn., *angina cruris, dysbasia intermittens angiosclerotica.*

intermittent spinal c. Intermittent progressive weakness of the legs without pain, presumably caused by decreased circulation in the spinal cord.

venous c. Lameness due to venous stasis. Also called *angiosclerotic paroxysmal myasthenia.*

Claudius, Friedrich Matthias [*German anatomist,* 1822–69]. Remembered for his description of the polyhedral cells of the cochlear duct. Described the ovarian fossa.

claus″tro·phil′i·a [L. *claustrum,* a confined place, lock, bar; G. *philein,* to love]. A morbid desire to be shut up in a confined space.

claus″tro·pho′bi·a [*claustrum;* G. *phobos,* fear]. Morbid fear of being in a room or a confined space.

claus′trum [L.]. A barrier, as a membrane partially closing an opening, or one bearing a resemblance to a barrier, as the layer of gray matter between the insula of the cerebral cortex and the lenticular nucleus. —**claustral,** *adj.*

clau·su′ra. Atresia.

cla′va (pl. *clavae*) [L., a club]. One of the two ovoid eminences in the caudal end of the fourth ventricle, representing continuations of the fasciculus gracilis. Subjacent to the clava is the gracilis nucleus. The clava was formerly called *eminentia clavae.* —**claval,** *adj.*

clav′a·cin. An antibiotic substance produced in cultures of several different fungi; it is identical with *clavatin, claviformin,* and *patulin.*

cla′vate [*clava*]. Club-shaped.

clav′a·tin. Clavacin.

clav″e·li·za′tion (klav″uh·li·zay′shun, ·lye·zay′-shun) [F. *clavelée,* sheep pox]. Inoculation with sheep-pox virus. Also called *ovination.*

Clav′i·ceps [L. *clava,* club; *caput,* head]. A genus of fungi.

C. purpurea. The fungus producing the ergot of rye.

clav′i·cle (klav′i·kul) [L. *clavicula,* a small key]. A bone of the shoulder girdle articulating medially with the sternum and laterally with the acromion of the scapula; the collarbone. See Plates 1, 13. See Table of Bones in the Appendix. —**clavic′ular,** *adj.*

clav″i·cot′o·my [*clavicula;* G. *tomē,* a cutting]. Surgical section of the clavicle.

cla·vic′u·late [*clavicula*]. 1. Having a clavicle. 2. Wrinkled; corrugated.

cla·vic″u·lec′to·my [*clavicula;* G. *ektomē,* excision]. Surgical removal of the clavicle. The operation is indicated in cases of thyroid cancer, osteomyelitis of the clavicle, and limitation of arm motion where the shoulder joint has become fused.

clav″i·for′min. Clavacin.

cla′vine (clay′veen, ·vin). Inactive mixture of ergot constituents, consisting of nearly equal parts of leucine, isoleucine, and valine.

cla′vus [L., nail, corn]. 1. A cone-shaped, circumscribed hyperplasia of the horny layer of the epidermis, in which there is an ingrowth as well as an outgrowth of horny substance forming epidermal thickenings, chiefly about the toes; caused by friction or pressure. 2. *In psychiatry,* a severe pain in the head described as the sensation of a nail being driven into the head.

hard c. A dense and callous hypertrophy at points of pressure on the toes.

soft c. That type which develops on opposing surfaces of the toes. It is soft as a result of heat and moisture.

claw′foot″ [AS. *clawu;* fōt]. A foot having an abnormally high longitudinal arch, a depression of the metatarsal arch, and dorsal contractures of the toes. It exists in two forms: that in which the outstanding deformity is an exaggeration of the longitudinal arch, and that in which the exaggeration of the longitudinal arch is associated with contraction of the plantar fascia and limitation of dorsiflexion at the ankle. Also called *hollow foot, contracted foot, pes cavus, nondeforming clubfoot.*

claw′hand″ [*clawu;* AS. *hand*]. An acquired deformity of the hand. In the extreme type, due to a paralysis of the ulnar and median nerves, it is characterized by extension of the thumb, hyperextension and abduction of the proximal phalanges of the fingers, and flexion of the other phalanges. Lesser degrees of the deformity result from paralysis of the ulnar or median nerve separately.

Claybrook's sign. See under *sign.*

Clayton gas. See under *gas.*

clear′ance [ME. *cler,* from L. *clarus,* clear]. 1. The complete removal of a substance from the blood by the kidneys. 2. A test of renal function. See under *test.*

clear′ing of cas′u·al·ties. *In military medicine,* the process of disposing of casualties by sorting, returning to duty those who are fit and transferring all others to a medical unit of a higher echelon.

clear′ing sta′tion. A divisional medical unit operating in war, set up with or without shelter, for emergency treatment, including medical record. It is charged with rapid disposal of army casualties either by return to duty or by evacuation.

cleav′age [AS. *clēofan*]. 1. The linear clefts in the skin indicating the general direction of the fibers. They govern to a certain extent the arrangement of the lesions in skin diseases. The **lines of cleavage** run, for the most part, obliquely to the axis of the trunk, sloping from the spine downward and forward; in the limbs, they are mostly transverse to the longitudinal axis. See also Carl von *Langer.* 2. Cell division, especially of the zygote and blastomeres. Syn., *segmentation.* 3. An early stage of the process of development between fertilization and the blastula, when the embryo consists of a mass of dividing cells, the blastomeres.

adequal c. Cleavage producing almost equal blastomeres.

bilateral c. Cleavage in a single plane producing equal halves.

determinate c. Cleavage producing blastomeres, each of which is destined to form some particular part or structure. Also called *mosaic c.*

discoidal c. Meroblastic cleavage limited to the germinal disk, as in telolecithal avian ova.

equal c. That producing blastomeres of equal size.

equatorial c. Cleavage at right angles to the ovum axis, frequently the third cleavage plane.

holoblastic c. Total cleavage of the ovum.

indeterminate c. That producing blastomeres having similar developmental potencies, each of which can produce a whole embryo. Also called *regulative c.*

meridional c. Vertical cleavage in a plane through the egg axis.

meroblastic c. That restricted to the cytoplasmic part of a yolk-laden ovum; also known as *partial c.*

superficial c. Meroblastic cleavage restricted to the peripheral cytoplasm, as in the centrolecithal insect ovum.

unequal c. That producing blastomeres of unequal size.

cleft [ME. *clift*]. A fissure.

branchial c. (a) One of the slitlike openings between the gills, as in fishes. (b) See visceral *c.*

c. cheek. Transverse facial cleft. Syn., *macrostomia.*

c. foot. Division of the foot due to absence of one or more digits and the corresponding metatarsal(s).

c. hand. Division of the hand due to absence of one or more digits and the corresponding metacarpal(s).

c. lip. See *harelip.*

c. of Schmidt-Lantermann. See *incisure* of Schmidt-Lantermann.

c. palate. A congenital defect, due to failure of fusion of embryonic facial processes resulting in a fissure through the palate. This may be *complete,* extending through both hard and soft palates into the nose, or any degree of *incomplete,* or *partial,* cleft. Often associated with harelip.

coelomic c. The fissure in the lateral mesoderm which forms the coelomic cavity and divides the mesoderm into somatic and visceral layers.

facial c. An embryonic fissure between facial processes; the facial anomaly produced by failure of these processes to fuse. A **median facial cleft** (median harelip, median fissure) is one between the mandibular or the median nasal processes which may involve both mandible and maxilla or only one; an **oblique facial cleft,** one between the maxillary and frontonasal processes; a **transverse facial cleft,** a fissure at the angle of the mouth causing macrostomia.

genal c. Cleft cheek; transverse facial cleft: also called *genal fissure;* formerly called *genal coloboma.*

internatal c. That of the buttocks, in which is the anus.

Maurer's c. See under *dot.*

Stillman's c. A cleft in the gingival margin associated with periodontal disease.

visceral c. An embryonic fissure between the visceral arches, produced by rupture of the closing plate between a pharyngeal pouch and its corresponding external branchial groove.

cleft. Divided.

clei′do- (kly′do-), **cleid-** [G. *kleis,* clavicle]. A combining form denoting *the clavicle,* or *pertaining to the clavicle.*

clei″do·cos′tal [*kleis;* L. *costa,* rib]. Pertaining to the ribs and the clavicle.

clei″do·cra′ni·al. Referring to the clavicle and the cranium, as cleidocranial dysostosis.

clei″do·hu′mer·al. Relating to the clavicle and the humerus.

clei″do·hy′oid [*kleis;* G. *hyoeidēs,* shaped like the letter upsilon]. Relating to clavicle and hyoid.

clei′do·ic [G. *kleidoun,* to lock up, from *kleis*]. Isolated from the environment.

clei″do·mas′toid [*kleis;* G. *mastoeidēs,* like a breast]. Pertaining to the clavicle and to the mastoid process.

clei″do-oc·cip′i·tal (kly″do-ock·sip′i·tul). Relating to the clavicle and occiput.

c. muscle. A variable portion of the sternocleidomastoid extending from the occipital bone to the clavicle.

clei″do·scap′u·lar [*kleis;* L. *scapula,* shoulder blade]. Relating to the clavicle and the scapula.

clei″do·ster′nal [*kleis;* G. *sternon,* breast]. Pertaining to the clavicle and the sternum.

clei·dot′o·my [*kleis;* G. *tomē,* a cutting]. *In obstetrics,* section of the clavicles when the shoulders of the fetus are too broad to pass; an operation performed when the head is delivered, and the child dead.

clei″thro·pho′bi·a (kly″thro·fo′bee·uh) [G. *kleithron,* a bar; *phobos,* fear]. Morbid fear of being locked in.

cle′oid [AS. *clēa,* claw; G. *eidos,* form]. A clawlike instrument used by dentists in excavating cavities in the teeth.

clep″to·ma′ni·a. See *kleptomania.*

clep″to·pho′bi·a. See *kleptophobia.*

Clérambault, Gatian de [*French psychiatrist,* 1872–1934]. Described a state in which the subject feels that his mind is being controlled by another person or an outside influence; called *Clérambault-Kandinsky complex.*

Clevenger, Shobal Vail [*American neurologist,* 1843–1920]. Remembered for his description of the inferior temporal sulcus of the cerebral hemisphere, which extends from the occipital pole almost to the temporal pole of the temporal lobe.

cli′er, cly′er [D. *klier,* gland]. A scrofulous tumor in cattle, produced by tuberculous infection.

cli″ma·co·pho′bi·a [G. *klimax,* ladder, staircase; *phobos,* fear]. A morbid fear of staircases.

cli·mac′ter·ic (klye·mack′tur·ick, kly″mack·terr′·ick) [G. *klimaktēr,* rung of a ladder]. A period of life at which the system was believed to undergo marked changes. These periods were thought to occur every seven years. The word is now generally applied to the menopause.

male c. A condition presumably due to loss of testicular function, associated with an elevated urinary excretion of gonadotropins and symptoms such as loss of sexual desire and potency, hot flashes, and vasomotor instability: rarely seen clinically.

cli′mate [G. *klima,* slope, region]. The sum of those conditions in any region or country that relate to the air, the temperature, moisture, sunshine, and winds, especially in so far as they concern the health or comfort of mankind. —**climat′ic,** *adj.*

cli·mat′ic food and cloth′ing lab′o·ra·to″ry. A research and experimental development laboratory under the supervision of the Quartermaster General of the Army for the dual purpose of studying the physiologic effect of climatic variables (temperature and humidity) on military personnel and the development of food and clothing apposite to varied global climatic conditions.

cli′ma·to- [*klima*]. A combining form denoting *climate.*

cli″ma·tol′o·gy [*klima;* G. *logos,* word]. *In medicine,* the study of climate in relation to health and disease.

cli″ma·to·ther′a·py [*klima;* G. *therapeia,* treatment]. The treatment of disease by means of a suitable climate.

cli′max [G. *klimax,* ladder]. 1. The height of a disease; period of greatest intensity. 2. The sexual orgasm.

clin-. See *clino-.*

clin′ic [G. *klinē,* bed]. 1. Medical instruction given at the bedside, or in the presence of the patient whose symptoms are studied and whose treatment is considered. 2. A place where such instruction is given. 3. A gathering of instructors, students, and patients for the study and treatment of disease. 4. A place where medical care is given to ambulant patients who live at home.

clin′i·cal [*klinē*]. 1. Relating to bedside treatment or to a clinic. 2. Pertaining to the symptoms and course of a disease as observed by the physician, in opposition to the anatomic changes found by the pathologist.

clin′i·cal rec′ord. A group of forms used by a hospital to record a patient's medical history. It covers the results of physical examination, laboratory findings (including x-ray interpretations), admission diagnosis, progress of the disease, medications used, consultations, operations performed, and final diagnosis and disposition.

cli·ni′cian [*klinē*]. 1. A physician whose opinions, teachings, and treatment are based upon experience at the bedside. 2. A clinical instructor. 3. One who practices medicine.

clin′i·co- [G. *klinikos,* of a bed]. *In medicine,* a combining form denoting *clinical.*

clin″i·co·hem″a·to·log′ic (klin″i·ko·hem″uh·to·lodj′ik, ·hee″muh·to·lodj′ik) [*klinikos;* G. *haima,* blood; *logos*, word]. Relating to both clinical and blood problems.

clin″i·co·pa·thol′o·gy [*klinikos;* G. *pathos*, disease; *logos*]. The study of disease in the living patient; applied particularly to the study of the blood, urine, feces, and other secretions and excretions and to parts of the body, such as tumors, removed for examination.

clin″i·co·ra″di·o·log′ic. See *clinicoroentgenologic.*

clin″i·co·roent″gen·o·log′ic (klin″i·ko·rent″ghin-o·lodj′ick) [*klinikos; Röntgen; logos*]. Pertaining to the correlation between clinical and roentgenologic subjects. Syn., *clinicoradiologic.*

cli′no-, clin- [G. *klinein*, to incline]. A combining form denoting *inclination* or *declination.*

cli″no·ceph′a·lus [*klinein;* G. *kephalē*, head]. An individual having a clinocephalic skull.

cli″no·ceph′a·ly, cli″no·ceph′a·lism [*klinein; kephalē*]. A congenital defect of the skull in which the upper surface is concave or saddle-shaped. **—clinocephal′ic, clinocephalous,** *adj.*

cli″no·dac′ty·ly, cli″no·dac′tyl·ism [*klinein;* G. *daktylos*, finger]. A congenital defect consisting of abnormal deflection of fingers or toes. **—clinodactylous,** *adj.*

cli′noid [G. *klinē*, bed; *eidos*, form]. Resembling a bed, as the clinoid processes.

cli·nom′e·ter (klye·nom′i·tur, kli·nom′·) [G. *klinein*, to incline; *metron*, a measure]. An apparatus for measuring the rotational capacity of the ocular muscles.

cli′no·scope [*klinein;* G. *skopein*, to examine]. An instrument for measuring the torsion of the eyes when gazing at a fixed object with the axes of vision presumably parallel.

clip [AS. *clyppan*, to embrace]. *In surgery*, a device or appliance that grips skin or other tissue to secure apposition or to control hemorrhage. Also see *clamp, forceps.*

dura c. A thin wire suture applied by a special forceps to check hemorrhage in brain operations. Also called *brain c.*

skin c. A band of malleable metal with pointed ends, held in a magazine and applied by a special forceps to the apposed edges of a skin wound; a more rapid method of closure than the use of sutures. Also called *Michel c., wound c.*

clis″e·om′e·ter (kliss″ee·om′i·tur, kliz″ee·) [G. *klisis*, inclination; *metron*, a measure]. An instrument for measuring the degree of inclination of the pelvic axis.

clit′i·on [G. *klitys*, slope]. A point located where the median sagittal plane meets the center of the uppermost margin of the dorsum sellae.

clit″o·ral′gi·a (klit″o·ral′juh, ·jee·uh, kly″to·) [G. *kleitoris*, clitoris; *algos*, pain]. Pain referred to the clitoris.

clit″o·ri·daux′e (klit″o·ri·dawk′see, kly″to·ri·) [*kleitoris;* G. *auxē*, increase]. Hypertrophy of the clitoris. *Obs.*

clit″o·ri·dec′to·my [*kleitoris;* G. *ektomē*, excision]. Excision of the clitoris.

clit″o·ri·di′tis [*kleitoris;* G. *-itis*, inflammation]. Inflammation of the clitoris.

clit″o·ri·dot′o·my [*kleitoris;* G. *tomē*, a cutting]. Incision of the clitoris.

clit′o·ris (klit′o·ris, kly′to·ris) [*kleitoris*]. In the female the homolog of the penis, attached to the ischiopubic rami by two crura, which meet in front of the pubic symphysis to form the body, or corpus. It possesses erectility. See Plate 41. **—clitorid′ean,** *adj.*

clit′o·rism (klit′o·riz·um, kly′to·) [*kleitoris*]. 1. Enlargement or hypertrophy of the clitoris. 2. Tribadism. 3. A condition of painful and persistent erection of the clitoris; analogous to priapism in the male.

clit″o·ri′tis (klit″o·rye′tis, kly″to·) [*kleitoris;* G. *-itis*, inflammation]. Inflammation of the clitoris.

clit″o·ro·ma′ni·a (klit″o·ro·may′nee·uh, kly″to·ro·) [*kleitoris;* G. *mania*, madness]. Nymphomania.

clit″o·rot′o·my. See *clitoridotomy.*

clit″or·rha′gi·a [*kleitoris;* G. *rhegnynai*, to burst forth]. Hemorrhage from the clitoris.

cli′vus [L., a slope]. 1. A slope. 2. The slanting surface of the body of the sphenoid bone between the sella turcica and basilar process of occipital bone.

c. monticuli. Old term for declivus cerebelli, the declive of the cerebellum.

clo. *In aviation medicine*, an arbitrary unit of thermal insulation, used in expressing the thermal insulation value of clothing. A suit of clothing has a thermal insulation value of one clo when it will maintain in comfort a resting-sitting human adult male whose metabolic rate is approximately 50 kilogram calories per square meter of body surface per hour, when the environmental temperature is 70° F. In terms of absolute thermal insulation units, one clo is 0.18° C. per square meter kilogram calorie per hour.

clo·a′ca [L., sewer]. 1. In the early embryo, the entodermal chamber common to hindgut and allantois; later, to hindgut and urogenital duct or sinus. 2. In Anamniota, Sauropsida, and aplacental mammals, a common chamber for rectum and urogenital orifices. **—cloacal,** *adj.*

congenital c. A malformation in which the rectum opens into the genitourinary tract.

ectodermal c. That part of the cloaca derived from the proctodeal invagination after rupture of the cloacal membrane.

entodermal c. That part of the cloaca derived from the caudal end of the hindgut.

external c. See ectodermal *c.*

persistent c. The result of failure of the urorectal septum to develop, leaving a common chamber for rectum and urogenital system. See cloacal *duct.*

urogenital c. An abnormal common opening of the urethra and vagina due to a defective urethrovaginal septum.

vesicorectovaginal c. A cavity in the pelvis into which rectum, urinary bladder, and vagina all open; it may be congenital or due to trauma, infections, tumors, or irradiation damage.

clo·as′ma (klo·az′muh). See *chloasma.*

Cloetta, Max (1868–1940). Swiss pharmacologist, who isolated digalen, a soluble preparation of digitalis suitable for injection.

clone [G. *klōn*, twig]. A group of individuals of like genetic constitution obtained by asexual reproduction from a single original individual. Reproduction may occur by continued fission, as in protozoa; by continued budding, as in hydras; or by propagation from cuttings, as in plants. See *pure line.*

clon″i·co·ton′ic [G. *klonos*, violent, confused motion; G. *tonikos*, from *tonos*, tension]. Clonic and tonic at the same time; said of certain muscular spasms.

clon′ism (klon′iz·um, klo′niz·um), **clo·nis′mus** (klo·niss′mus, ·niz′mus) [*klonos*]. The condition of suffering from a succession of clonic spasms. See *clonus.*

clon′o·graph [*klonos;* G. *graphein*, to write]. An apparatus for recording the spasmodic movements of the head, extremities, lower jaw, trunk, and the tendon reflexes.

clo″nor·chi′a·sis (klo″nor·kigh′uh·sis, klon″or·kee·ay′sis), **clo″nor·chi·o′sis** (klo″nor·kee·o′sis, klon″or·) [G. *klōn*, branch; *orchis*, testis; NL. *-iasis*; G. *-ōsis*, condition]. Condition due to the presence of *Clonorchis sinensis* in the bile ducts, causing marked dilatation, proliferation of the biliary epithelium, and atrophy of the liver cells; characterized by edema, diarrhea, and hepatomegaly in moderate cases, and cirrhosis, anasarca, and cachexia in severe cases.

Clo·nor′chis (klo·nor′kis, klon·or′kis) [*klōn; orchis*]. A genus of flukes indigenous to the Orient.

C. sinensis. The most common of the liver flukes, having as definitive hosts man or other mammals.

clon′o·spasm [G. *klonos*, violent, confused motion; *spasmos*, spasm]. A clonic spasm.

clo′nus (klo′nus, klon′us) [*klonos*]. A series of movements characterized by alternate contractions and relaxations; a clonic spasm. Involuntary, reflex, irregular contractions of muscles when put suddenly upon the stretch. According to the part affected, the phenomenon is spoken of as ankle clonus, wrist clonus, etc. —**clon′ic,** *adj.;* **clonic′ity,** *n.*

Cloquet, Jules Germain [*French anatomist*, 1790–1883]. Known for his research into the cause of ventral hernia (1819) and for his *Human Anatomy* in several volumes (1821–31). The hyaloid canal was formerly named for him.

clorarsen. Trade-mark for dichlorophenarsine hydrochloride.

Clos·trid′i·um (klos·trid′ee·um, klo·strid′·) [dim. from G. *klōstēr*, spindle]. A genus of anaerobic spore-bearing bacteria of ovoid, spindle, or club shape; widely distributed in nature. See Table of the Most Common Microorganisms Pathogenic to Man in the Appendix. —**clostridial,** *adj.*

Cl. botulinum. A species which produces a very powerful toxin in food. The disease is a toxemia; the organism is not invasive but produces its toxin outside the body.

Cl. botulinum A. A type species found predominantly in the Rocky Mountain and Pacific Coast states and in English soils; produces botulism in man and limberneck in chickens.

Cl. botulinum B. This type is found most commonly in the Mississippi Valley, Great Lakes region, and Atlantic Coast states. It produces botulism in man and limberneck in chickens.

Cl. botulinum Cα. A toxin-producing form which produces a paralytic condition in chickens and botulism in wild ducks.

Cl. botulinum Cβ. This type species produces a forage poisoning of cattle in Australia.

Cl. botulinum D. A species producing lamziekte in African cattle.

Cl. botulinum E. A species which causes botulism; was isolated from fish.

Cl. chauvei. Synonym for *Cl. feseri.*

Cl. feseri. That species which is the principal cause of blackleg in cattle. It has not proved responsible for any human infection. Also called *Cl. chauvei.*

Cl. histolyticum. A species of *Clostridium*, Gram-positive, anaerobic, which is saccharolytic and proteolytic, and forms terminal oval spores.

Cl. novyi. This species is important in gas gangrene; also produces a strong soluble toxin.

Cl. oedematiens. Syn. for *Clostridium novyi.*

Cl. parabotulinum equi. Synonym for *Clostridium botulinum D.*

Cl. perfringens. A species of plump, nonmotile, Gram-positive rods of varying length, occurring in chains and singly. This organism produces a variety of toxins and is the most important cause of gas gangrene. It has also been found to be the cause of dysentery of sheep. It has been divided into types by Wilsdon as follows: **Type A,** the principal cause of gas gangrene in man; **Type B,** the lamb dysentery bacillus; **Type C,** the "struck" bacillus of sheep; **Type D,** the bacillus of enterotoxemia of sheep. Syn., *Cl. welchii.*

Cl. septicum. Species found in gas gangrene but not so frequently as some of the other anaerobic bacilli. It is also responsible for some cases of blackleg in cattle.

Cl. sporogenes. A species frequently found in deep wounds; it is generally agreed to be nonpathogenic but is the cause of the foul odor of such wounds.

Cl. tetani. The species which causes tetanus. It is characterized by spherical terminal spores and the production of tetanus toxin, a potent exotoxin.

Cl. welchii. See *Cl. perfringens.*

clo′sure [L. *clausura*, a lock, from *claudere*, to close]. 1. The act of completing or closing an electric circuit. Abbreviated, C. 2. The closing of a wound by suture.

clot [AS. *clott*]. 1. A semisolid coagulum of blood or lymph. 2. Coagulate.

blood c. See under *blood.*

chicken-fat c. That type formed after death, consisting of a light yellow, edematous, and fibrinous clot in its upper portion, and an accumulation of erythrocytes in its dependent portion.

currant-jelly c. A red, gelatinous blood clot formed quickly after death, which contains all of the elements of blood.

clot re·trac′tion. The contraction or shrinkage of a blood clot resulting in the extrusion of serum. Clot retraction does not occur in severe thrombocytopenia or some cases of thrombasthenia.

c. r. time. The length of time required for the appearance or completion of clot retraction, as determined by one of numerous methods.

clot′ting time. The length of time required for shed blood to coagulate. For the accurate measurement of clotting time, the blood must be obtained with minimal contamination with tissue fluids, preferably by venepuncture. Clotting time must always be referred to a normal standard for the particular conditions under which the test is performed. Syn., *coagulation time.* Also see *bleeding time, clot retraction time, prothrombin time.*

clove [OF. *clou*, from L. *clavis*, nail]. The dried flower bud of *Eugenia caryophyllata.* It yields not less than 16 cc. of volatile oil from 100 Gm. of drug; it also contains caryophyllin, a lactone. Clove is stimulant; it is occasionally used in nausea and vomiting and to correct flatulence. Dose, 0.32–0.65 Gm. (5–10 gr.).

c. oil (*oleum caryophylli*). The volatile oil distilled with steam from clove. It contains not less than 82% by volume of eugenol. It is a local anesthetic, a powerful germicide, and a local irritant. It is occasionally used internally in treating flatulent colic; externally, it is a favorite remedy for toothache. Dose, 0.12–0.4 cc. (2–6 min.).

clown′ism [akin to Icel. *klunni*, a clumsy fellow]. That stage of hysteroepilepsy in which there is an emotional display with a series of grotesque contortions.

CLSH Abbreviation for *corpus luteum-stimulating hormone.* See *luteinizing hormone.*

club′foot″ [ON. *klubba;* AS. *fōt*]. A congenital malformation, either single or bilateral, in which the forefoot is inverted and rotated, accompanied by shortening of the Achilles tendon and contracture of the plantar fascia. Also see *talipes.*

club′hand. A congenital deformity of the hand characterized by one of the following distortions: (a) palmar displacement with or without radial or ulnar deviation; (b) dorsal displacement with or without radial or ulnar deviation. The deformity may be due to contracture of ligaments and muscles, or it may be caused by defective development of the radius, ulna, or carpal bones. The most common form of clubhand is caused by defective development of the radius producing radial and palmar distortion.

clump′ing. See *agglutination.*

clu′ne·al [L. *clunis,* buttock]. Pertaining to the buttock.

clu·pan″o·don′ic ac′id. An unsaturated fatty acid occurring in certain fish oils; the formula has been reported as $C_{18}H_{28}O_2$ and also as $C_{22}H_{34}O_2$.

clu′pe·ine (kloo′pee·een, ·in). $C_{30}H_{57}N_{17}O_6 + 4H_2O$. A protamine from the herring. Syn., *salmine.*

Clu′si·a (kloo′shuh, ·see·uh) [L., after Charles de *Lécluse,* French botanist, 1526–1609]. A genus of plants of the Guttiferae, many species of which yield a gum resin called West Indian balsam. **C. rosea** yields a cathartic gum resin similar to gamboge.

Clute, Howard Merrill [*American surgeon,* 1890–1946]. Known for his incision for repair of diaphragmatic hernia, extending from below the umbilicus upward to the left costal margin, thence deflected across the fused costal cartilages of the sixth, seventh, and eighth ribs. The rectus muscle is cut across and cartilages are divided as necessary to give adequate access; called *Clute's incision.*

clut′ter·ing. Confused speech containing jumbled words and meaningless sounds.

Clutton, Henry Hugh [*English surgeon,* 1850–1909]. Known for his description of symmetrical synovitis, associated with prenatal syphilis. See syphilitic *arthritis.*

cly′ers. See *actinomycosis.*

cly′sis [G. *klysis,* a drenching by clyster]. Administration of an enema; cleansing by means of an enema.

Cm Symbol for curium.

cm, cm. Centimeter.

cne′mis [G. *knēmē,* tibia]. The shin or tibia. —**cnemic,** *adj.*

cni′cin (nigh′sin). $C_{42}H_{56}O_{15}$. A crystalline bitter substance found in *Cnicus benedictus,* blessed thistle.

C.N.S. Central nervous system.

Co Symbol for cobalt.

co″a·cer′vate (ko″a·sur′vayt, ko·ass′ur·vayt) [L. *coacervare,* to heap together]. The product formed when two hydrophilic colloids of opposite sign are mixed and form a stable particle which may form a separate phase. —**coacerva′tion,** *n.*

co″ad·ap·ta′tion [L. *cum,* together with; *adaptare,* to adapt]. The correlated variation in two mutually dependent organs.

co·ag′u·la. Plural of coagulum.

co·ag′u·lant [L. *coagulare,* to cause a fluid to curdle]. Causing the formation of a clot or coagulum. —**coag′ulable,** *adj.;* **coag′ulant,** *n.*

co·ag′u·lase (ko·ag′yoo·lace, ·laze) [*coagulare*]. An enzyme, produced by certain of the micrococci, particularly *Micrococcus pyogenes* var. *aurens,* which brings about the coagulation in human sera of fibrin, thus forming a sort of capsule protecting them against phagocytosis. There is a definite correlation between the ability to produce this substance and pathogenicity.

co·ag′u·late [*coagulare*]. 1. Curdle; clot. 2. Cause to change from a fluid state to a compact, jellylike mass; solidify.

co·ag″u·la′tion [L. *coagulatio,* from *coagulare*]. 1. The formation of a coagulum or clot, as in blood or in milk. 2. A clot. —**coag′ulated, coag′ulative,** *adj.*

co·ag″u·la′tion time. See *clotting time.*

co·ag′u·lin. See *precipitin.*

co·ag′u·lum (pl. *coagula*) [L.]. A clot; a curd; a coagulated mass.

Coakley, Cornelius Godfrey [*American laryngologist,* 1862–1934]. Remembered for his operation for the relief of frontal sinusitis, the anterior wall being removed and the sinus partially obliterated along with the nasofrontal duct by curettage, the cavity being allowed to heal by granulation.

co″a·les′cence [L. *coalescere,* to grow together]. The union of two or more parts or things previously separate. —**coalescent,** *adj.*

coal tar (*pix carbonis*). A by-product in the destructive distillation of coal; a black, viscid fluid, of a characteristic and disagreeable odor. Its composition is extremely complex, and many constituents may be separated from it by fractional distillation. Among the products obtained from coal tar are anthracene, benzene, naphtha, creosote, phenol, pitch, etc. From the basic oil of coal tar are manufactured the aniline or coal-tar colors or dyes. It is employed locally to relieve itching and in the treatment of certain skin diseases.

c. t. ointment (*unguentum picis carbonis*). One containing coal tar in a base of zinc oxide paste.

c. t. remedies. Synthetic preparations from coal tar or its derivatives.

c. t. solution (*liquor picis carbonis*). Coal tar, 20%, in alcohol, stabilized with polysorbate 80. It is used in treatment of skin diseases. A chloroformic solution of coal tar containing 5% of coal tar is sometimes employed.

co″ap·ta′tion [L. *cum,* with; *aptare,* to fit]. The proper union or adjustment of the ends of a fractured bone or the lips of a wound. —**co·apt′,** *v.*

co·arc′tate [L. *coarctare,* to press together]. Crowded together.

co″arc·ta′tion [L. *coarctatio,* from *coarctare*]. A compression of the walls of a vessel or canal, narrowing or closing the lumen; reduction of the normal or previous volume, as of the aorta; shriveling and consequent detachment, as of the retina. A stricture.

co″arc·tot′o·my [*coarctare;* G. *tomē,* a cutting]. The cutting of a stricture.

co″ar·tic″u·la′tion [L. *coarticulare,* to cause to articulate]. A synarthrosis.

coat [OF. *cote,* of Teutonic origin]. A cover or membrane covering a part or substance.

buffy c. The upper fibrinous layer of a clot of coagulated blood; characterized by a pale color, due to absence of erythrocytes.

internal elastic c. The internal elastic membrane of the tunica intima of an artery.

middle c. The tunica media of a vessel.

subendothelial c. The subendothelial layer of the tunica intima of the heart and vessels.

uveal c. The uvea.

vaginal c. (a) The fibrous capsule of the eyeball. (b) The vaginal coat of the testis.

coat′ing [*cote*]. A covering or layer of a substance, as of a wound or the tongue.

c. of pills. A covering of various substances to conceal the taste in swallowing.

c. of tongue. A condition of the tongue indicative of abnormality of the digestive tract.

enteric c. A coating for pills or tablets or capsules, intended as a protection against solutions found in the stomach, but dissolving in the intestines.

Coats, George [*English ophthalmologist,* 1876–1915]. Remembered for his description (1908) of retinitis exudativa, called *Coats's disease.*

co·bal′a·min. 1. Generic name for members of the vitamin-B_{12} family; specific members are identified through the use of prefixes, as cyanocobalamin, hydroxocobalamin, etc. 2. That portion of the molecule of crystalline vitamin B_{12} (cyanocobalamin), exclusive of the cyano group, occurring in all vitamin-B_{12} analogs.

co'balt (ko'bawlt) [Ger. *kobold*, goblin]. Co = 58.94. A hard, gray, ductile metal used in alloys. It is a component of cyanocobalamin; lack of the element may result in anemia. It appears that it effects more complete utilization of iron in hemoglobin synthesis. Polycythemia has been produced in animals by administration of cobalt. Larger doses of soluble salts are emetic, due to a local irritant effect.

c. chloride. $CoCl_2.6H_2O$; cobaltous chloride, dark-red crystals, freely soluble in water. Its administration to man has been reported to produce a favorable reticulocyte response, with rises in red-cell, hemoglobin, and hematocrit values, in some anemic patients.

co'balt-60. A radioactive isotope of cobalt, produced by irradiating cobalt in an atomic pile. The radiation is employed in the treatment of cancer. This isotope, of atomic weight 60, has a half-life of about 5 years and emits beta and gamma rays.

Cobbold, Thomas Spencer [*English parasitologist*, 1826–86]. Distinguished helminthologist. Said to have named *Filaria bancrofti* (1877), now classified as *Wuchereria bancrofti*, and a number of other intestinal parasites.

cobefrin hydrochloride. Trade-mark for 3,4-dihydroxyphenylpropanolamine hydrochloride; $(OH)_2C_6H_3.CHOH.CH(NH_2).CH_3HCl$; a vasoconstrictor.

cobione. Trade-mark for crystalline vitamin B_{12}.

Co'bra [Pg., serpent, from L. *coluber*, serpent]. Any one of a species of snakes of the genus *Naja*.

co'bra lec'i·thid (ko'bruh less'i·thid). A combination of cobra venom and lecithin which is actively hemolytic. The hemolytic product is regarded by some as a venom-free lecithin derivative and termed *cobra lecithinase*.

co"bra·ly'sin (ko"bruh·lye'sin, ko·bral'i·sin) [Pg. *cobra de capello*, serpent of the hood; G. *lysis*, a loosing]. The hemolytic toxin of cobra venom. It is destroyed by heat and neutralized by antivenin.

co'ca [Sp., from Quechua *coca*]. The leaves of *Erythroxylon coca*, *E. truxillense*, or *E. novogranatense*, containing cocaine and other alkaloids.

co·caine' (ko·kayn', ko'kayn, ko'kuh·een, ·in) (*cocaina*). $C_{17}H_{21}NO_4$; methylbenzoylecgonine; an alkaloid obtained from the leaves of *Erythroxylon coca* and other species of *Erythroxylon;* occurs as colorless to white crystals, or as a white, crystalline powder; 1 Gm. dissolves in about 600 cc. of water, in 7 cc. of alcohol, in 12 cc. of olive oil, and in from 80–100 cc. of liquid petrolatum. For most purposes the hydrochloride is preferred to the base. The base is used in ointments and oily solution because of its greater solubility in fatty substances. —**cocainist,** *n.;* **cocainize,** *v.*

c. bug. Itching, crawling, and sticking skin sensations experienced in cocaine poisoning.

c. hydrochloride (*cocainae hydrochloridum*). $C_{17}H_{21}NO_4.HCl$. The hydrochloride of the alkaloid cocaine; occurs as colorless crystals, or as a white, crystalline powder; 1 Gm. dissolves in 0.5 cc. of water and in 3.5 cc. of alcohol. Locally cocaine is a paralyzant to the peripheral ends of the sensory nerves, to a lesser degree to the motor nerves, and stimulating to the muscular coats of the blood vessels. Systemically it is a stimulant to all parts of the central nervous system including the brain, spinal cord, and the medulla. The most important use of cocaine is as a local application to mucous membranes, either for the purpose of contracting blood vessels or of lessening sensation. Its continued use internally causes addiction.

c. nitrate. $C_{17}H_{21}NO_4.HNO_3$; a salt, similar to cocaine hydrochloride, useful in formulations in which chloride ion may provide chemical incompatibility (as with silver salts).

co·cain'ism (ko·kayn'iz·um, ko'kayn·iz·um, ko·kay'in·iz·um) [*coca*]. The cocaine habit.

co·cain"o·ma'ni·a (ko·kayn"o·may'nee·uh, ko"-kayn·o·, ko·kay"in·o·) [*coca;* G. *mania*, madness]. The habit of using cocaine; properly, mental derangement due to the cocaine habit. —**cocainomaniac,** *n.*

co"car·box'yl·ase. Thiamine pyrophosphate, the coenzyme or prosthetic component of carboxylase, an enzyme catalyzing decarboxylation of various α-keto acids, as pyruvic and α-ketoglutaric.

co"car·cin'o·gen [L. *cum*, with; G. *karkinos*, crab; *genesthai*, from *gignesthai*, to be produced]. A noncarcinogenic agent which augments the carcinogenic process.

cocc-. See *cocco-*.

coc'ci (cock'see). Plural of coccus.

Coc·cid'i·a (cock·sid'ee·uh) [NL. *coccidium*, dim. from G. *kokkos*, berry]. An order or group of cell parasites of the class Sporozoa; found in vertebrates and invertebrates; common in lower animals, rare in man.

coc·cid'i·a. Plural of coccidium.

coc·cid'i·al [*coccidium*]. Relating to, or caused by, coccidia.

Coc·cid"i·oi'des (cock·sid"ee·oy'deez, ·o'i·deez) [*coccidium;* G. *eidos*, form]. A genus of parasitic yeastlike fungi.

C. immitis. The causative agent of coccidioidomycosis, an infectious, systemic, suppurative, and granulomatous disease. The organism is spheroid, nonbudding, and endosporulating in the tissues; it produces branching, septate, aerial hyphae and arthrospores in culture.

coc·cid"i·oi'din (cock·sid"ee·oy'din, cock"sid·) [*coccidium; eidos*]. An extract of *Coccidioides immitis* used in testing for infection by this parasite.

coc·cid"i·oi"do·my·co'sis (cock·sid"ee·oy"do-migh·ko'sis) [*coccidium; eidos;* G. *mykēs*, fungus; *-ōsis*, condition]. A disease caused by inhalation of spores of *Coccidioides immitis*, causing pulmonary symptoms and later cutaneous nodules. Syn., *desert fever*, *San Joaquin Valley fever*.

primary c. A benign, self-limited, acute, respiratory infection.

progressive c. A chronic, often severe and fatal infection involving viscera, bones, and skin. Syn., *coccidioidal granuloma*.

coc·cid"i·oi·do'sis. Coccidioidomycosis.

coc·cid"i·o'sis [*coccidium; -ōsis*]. Group of symptoms produced by the presence of coccidia in the body. The pathogenicity of coccidia in humans is questionable.

coc·cid'i·um (cock·sid'ee·um) (pl. *coccidia*) [NL., dim. from G. *kokkos*, berry]. Any one of the order Coccidia.

coc'co-, cocc- [*kokkos*]. A combining form meaning *a grain, seed*, or *berry*.

coc"co·ba·cil'lus [*kokkos;* L. *bacillus*, small staff]. A short, thick, oval bacillus; in appearance, midway between the coccus and the bacillus.

Coccobacillus foetidus ozaenae. Old term for *Salmonella foetida*.

coc·cog'e·nous (cock·odj'i·nus) [*kokkos;* G. *genesthai*, from *gignesthai*, to be produced]. Produced by cocci.

coc'cu·lin. Picrotoxin.

coc'cu·lus [L., dim. from G. *kokkos*, berry]. The dried fruit of *Anamirta cocculus;* fishberry; a convulsant poison which has been used externally against pediculi. See *picrotoxin*.

coc'cus (pl. *cocci*) [*kokkos*]. 1. A bacterium whose greatest diameter is not more than twice its shortest. 2. Latin name for cochineal. —**coccal, coccoid,** *adj.*

coc″cy·al′gi·a (cock″see·al′juh, ·jee·uh). See *coccygodynia.*

coc″cy·ceph′a·lus [G. *kokkyx,* cuckoo; *kephalē,* head]. A monster with a beaked process for a head. —**coccycephalous,** *adj.*

coc″cy·dyn′i·a. See *coccygodynia.*

coc″cy·ge′al neu·ral′gi·a. See *coccygodynia.*

coc″cy·gec′to·my (cock″si·jeck′to·mee) [*kokkyx;* G. *ektomē,* excision]. Surgical excision of the coccyx.

coc″cy·ge″o·fem·o·ral′is. Pertaining to the coccyx and femur.

coc″cy·ge″o·fem·o·ral′is mus′cle. A variant of the gluteus maximus muscle extending from the coccyx to the linea aspera of the femur or from the sacrotuberous ligament to the fascia of the thigh.

coc·cyg′e·us (cock·sidj′ee·us) [*kokkyx*]. One of the pelvic muscles. See Table of Muscles in the Appendix. —**coccygeal,** *adj.*

c. dorsalis muscle. The posterior sacrococcygeus muscle.

c. ventralis muscle. The anterior sacrococcygeus muscle.

coc″cy·go·dyn′i·a [*kokkyx;* G. *odynē,* pain]. Pain in the region of the coccyx. Syn., *coccygeal neuralgia.*

coc′cyx (cock′sicks) [*kokkyx*]. The last bone of the vertebral column, formed by the union of 4 rudimentary vertebrae. See Plates 1, 14, 41. See Table of Bones in the Appendix. —**coccyg′eal,** *adj.*

coch″i·neal′ (kotch″i·neel′, kotch′i·neel) [L. *coccineus,* scarlet] (*coccus*). The dried female insects, *Coccus cacti,* enclosing the young larvae. Upon extracting the insects with an aqueous solution containing alum, a dark purplish solution representing an aluminum lake of the coloring principle carminic acid is obtained; the solution sometimes is used for coloring medicinal preparations.

coch′le·a (cock′lee·uh) [L., snail, from G. *kochlos,* shellfish]. A cavity of the internal ear resembling a snail shell; it contains the essential organs of hearing. It describes two and one-half turns about a central pillar called the modiolus or columella, forming the spiral canal, which is about one and one-half inches in length. Also see *ear.* See Plate 20. —**cochlear,** *adj.*

membranous c. The cochlear duct.

osseous c. The osseous cochlear canal.

coch′le·ar nerve. See under *nerve.*

coch″le·o·ves·tib′u·lar (cock″lee·o·) [*kochlos;* L. *vestibulum,* vestibule]. Pertaining to the cochlea and vestibule of the ear.

Coch″li·o·my′ia (cock″lee·o·my′yuh) [*kochlos;* G. *myia,* fly]. A genus of flies of the Calliphoridae.

C. americana. Synonym for *C. hominovorax.*

C. hominovorax. An obligate parasite of warm-blooded animals of tropical and subtropical regions of the Western Hemisphere. The ova are deposited on unbroken living tissue and the larvae, hatched in less than a half day, enter the skin and produce suppurative lesions. Syn., *C. americana.*

C. macellaria. The American screwworm fly; a species whose larvae feed on dead or moribund tissue of cattle, horses, and sheep.

co″cil·la′na (ko″si·lay′nuh, ·lan′uh, ko″see·yah′nuh, ·lah′nuh). The bark of the tree *Guarea rusbyi.* A nauseating expectorant.

Cock, Edward [*English surgeon,* 1805–92]. Devised his operation for external urethrotomy by opening the urethra, without a guide, behind the stricture in the midline of the perineum.

Cockcroft, John D. (1897–). British physicist, known for his extensive research in nuclear physics. With E. T. S. Walton, he received the Nobel prize in physics in 1951 for his pioneer work in atom-smashing.

cock′roach″. See *Blatella, Blatta, Periplaneta.*

co′co. See *yaws.*

co′coa, co′co. See *cacao, Theobroma.*

co·con′scious. See *foreconscious.*

coc″to·pre·cip′i·tin [L. *coctum,* from *coquere,* to cook; *praecipitare,* to cast down]. A precipitin produced in an animal by immunization with a boiled antigen, such as serum protein.

coc″to·sta′bile (cock″to·stay′bil, ·bile, ·stab′il), **coc″to·sta′ble** [*coctum;* L. *stabilis,* stable]. Able to withstand the temperature of boiling water without change.

cod. The common cod, *Gadus morrhua,* which furnishes cod-liver oil.

co″de·car·box′yl·ase. Pyridoxal phosphate; the prosthetic component of the enzyme carboxylase which catalyzes decarboxylation of L-amino acids, as well as of certain transaminating enzymes, in which latter case it is commonly referred to as *cotransaminase.*

co″de·hy′drase. See *coenzyme I* and *II.*

co″de·hy′dro·gen·ase. See *coenzyme I* and *II.*

co·de′ia. See *codeine.*

co′de·ine (ko′dee·een, ·in, ko′deen, ko·dee′in) [G. *kōdeia,* poppy head]. A white, crystalline alkaloid of opium, $C_{18}H_{21}O_3N.H_2O$, resembling morphine in action, but weaker; an analgesic and respiratory sedative. Dose, 0.008–0.13 Gm. (⅛–2 gr.). Syn., *codeia, methylmorphine.*

c. phosphate (*codeinae phosphas*). $C_{18}H_{21}NO_3.H_3PO_4.1\frac{1}{2}H_2O$; the most soluble salt of codeine, 1 Gm. dissolving in 2.5 cc. of water.

c. sulfate (*codeinae sulfas*). $(C_{18}H_{21}NO_3)_2.H_2SO_4.5H_2O$; 1 Gm. dissolves in 30 cc of water.

Codivilla, Alessandro [*Italian surgeon,* 1851–1913]. Known for his contributions to the knowledge of orthopedic surgery and for his development of technics for the transplantation of tendons in the treatment of infantile paralysis.

cod-liv′er oil (*oleum morrhuae*). The partially destearinated fixed oil obtained from fresh livers of *Gadus morrhua* and other species of the family Gadidae. Cod-liver oil is required to contain in each gram not less than 850 units of vitamin A and not less than 85 units of vitamin D; flavoring with not more than 1% of any one or any mixture of flavoring substances is permitted. The oil is useful in treating diseases of the bone, various forms of tuberculosis, and many types of general malnutrition. Two different emulsions of the oil are recognized: *cod-liver oil emulsion* (50% oil); *cod-liver oil emulsion with malt* (30% oil, 55% malt extract). The U.S.P. also recognizes *non-destearinated cod-liver oil* (*oleum morrhuae non-destearinatum*) of the same vitamin potency as cod-liver oil; the former oil is used chiefly for administration to animals. Cod-liver oil is also used locally in the treatment of burns and wounds. Dose of the oil, 4–15 cc. (1–4 fluidrachms).

co′dol. Retinol.

Codronchi, Giovanni Battista [*Italian physician,* 1547–1628]. Author of the earliest important work on legal medicine (1597). Wrote in the same year a treatise on diseases of the larynx, the earliest work extant devoted entirely to that field.

co″ef·fi′cient [L. *cum,* together; *efficere,* to accomplish]. Multiplier; figure indicating the degree of physical or chemical alteration characteristic of a given substance under stated conditions.

absorption c. In the law of absorption for homogeneous radiations, $I_d = I_o e^{-\mu d}$, where I_o is the intensity of the radiation beam falling on an absorber of the thickness *d; e,* the base of the natural system of logarithms; I_d, the intensity of the beam after it emerges from the absorber; and μ, the **linear absorption coefficient.** μ divided by the density of the absorber is called the **mass absorption coefficient.**

activity c. *In physical chemistry*, the thermodynamic behavior of a substance. It is a measure of how the behavior of a given substance differs from its theoretical or ideal behavior.

Bunsen absorption c. Quantitative expression of gas solubility; ratio of the volume which would be occupied by the dissolved gas at standard conditions to the volume of the solvent under the experimental conditions.

Bunsen solubility c. The volume of a gas, measured at 0° C. and one atmosphere pressure, dissolved by a unit volume of liquid when the liquid is equilibrated with the gas under one atmosphere of pressure at a specified temperature.

c. of correlation. A measure of the degree of association between two characteristics in a series of observations. Its value ranges from −1, representing perfect negative correlation, to +1, representing perfect positive correlation.

c. of fecundity. The number of conceptions per 1000 women-years of exposure to risk of conception, both taken after two years of married life.

c. of light extinction. Amount of light of a specific wavelength absorbed by a 1.0% solution of a substance in a layer 1.0 cm. thick.

c. of solubility of a gas. The amount of a gas which is dissolved at a given temperature in 1 cc. of a liquid, when the pressure of gas on the liquid is 760 mm. Hg.

c. of variation. The standard deviation of a series of observations expressed as a per cent of the mean of the series.

frictional c. The frictional coefficient for a particle moving through a medium is an indication of the viscous force opposing the motion of the particle and is mathematically represented as the ratio of the opposing force to the velocity.

isotonic c. The lowest degree of concentration of a solution of a salt in which laking of blood does not occur.

olfactory c. The minimum number of cubic centimeters of air saturated with a given odor that must enter the nostrils for the odor to be perceived.

osmotic c. Osmotic coefficient (g) in the ratio of the observed osmotic pressure to that of the ideal osmotic pressure. It may also be obtained from freezing-point depression, boiling-point elevation, and vapor-pressure depression of solvents.

Ostwald solubility c. Ratio of the volume which would be occupied by the dissolved gas in the gaseous state at standard conditions to the volume of the solvent under the experimental conditions.

respiratory c. See respiratory *quotient.*

temperature c. A quantitative expression of the effect of an increase in temperature on any chemical or physical process or reaction.

urotoxic c. The number of urotoxic units per kilogram of a body weight excreted in twenty-four hours.

-coele, -cele (-seel) [G. *koilia*, cavity]. A combining form denoting *a chamber*, *ventricle*, or *a normal cavity of the body.*

coe·len′ter·on (see·len′tur·on) [G. *koilos*, hollow; *enteron*, intestine]. 1. The entodermal gut cavity in diploblastic animals. 2. An archenteron.

coe′li·o- (see′lee·o-), **coe′li-** (see′lee-), **ce′li·o-, ce′li-** [G. *koilia*, cavity]. A combining form denoting *abdomen* or *belly.*

coe′lom, ce′lom (see′lum), **coe·lom′** [G. *koilōma*, cavity]. The embryonic body cavity formed in the lateral mesoderm, which subsequently becomes divided into pericardial, pleural, and peritoneal cavities in developing mammals. —**coelom′ic,** *adj.*

extraembryonic c. The cavity in the extraembryonic mesoderm; between chorionic mesoderm on one hand and the mesoderm of the amnion and yolk sac on the other. It is continuous with the embryonic coelom in the region of the umbilicus, and is obliterated by the growth of the amnion.

coe·los′chi·sis, ce·los′chi·sis (see·los′ki·sis). See *gastroschisis.*

coe″nes·the′si·a (see″ness·thee′zhuh, ·zee·uh, sen″-ess·), **coe″nes·the′sis.** See *cenesthesia.*

coe′no·cyte, ce′no·cyte (see′no·sight, sen′o·) [G. *koinos*, common; *kytos*, cell]. A multinucleate mass of protoplasm which has arisen as a result of nuclear division but without cytoplasmic division; seen in the vegetative bodies of some algae and fungi, as the plasmodium of slime molds (Uryxomycetes). —**coenocyt′ic,** *adj.*

co·en′zyme [L. *cum*, with; G. *en*, in; *zymē*, leaven]. A substance associated with and activating an enzyme; prosthetic group of an enzyme. A coenzyme can be separated from an enzyme by dialysis.

c. A. A derivative of pantothenic acid which in the presence of a suitable enzyme can accept an acetyl group, as from pyruvic acid, and transfer it to other substances.

c. I. A nucleotide composed of two molecules each of D-ribose and phosphoric acid, and one molecule each of adenine and nicotinic acid amide. It is the coenzyme for many dehydrogenases, taking up two hydrogen atoms to form dihydro coenzyme I. Occurs chiefly in yeast. Syn., *codehydrase I*, *codehydrogenase I*, *cozymase*, *diphosphopyridine nucleotide.*

c. II. A nucleotide composed of one molecule each of adenine and nicotinic acid amide, two molecules of D-ribose, and three molecules of phosphoric acid. It functions in a manner similar to coenzyme I. Syn., *codehydrase II*, *codehydrogenase II*, *triphosphopyridine nucleotide*, *Warburg's yellow enzyme coferment.*

c. R. Biotin.

coeur en sab′ot′ (kur on sab′o′) [Fr., heart like a boot]. The boot-shaped radiologic shadow of the heart seen in the tetralogy of Fallot.

co′fac·tor. *In bacteriology*, any amino acid which must be present in the medium to activate phage to adsorb to host bacteria.

co·fer′ment. Coenzyme.

cof′fee [Ar. *qahwah*, wine, coffee]. The dried and roasted ripe seeds of various species of *Coffea*, including *C. arabica*, *C. liberica*, and *C. robusta*. An infusion is stimulant due to its content of caffeine and, possibly, a volatile oil, caffeol; it is sometimes administered rectally in narcotic poisoning.

cof′fer dam. Rubber dam.

Coffey, Robert Calvin [*American surgeon*, 1869–1933]. Widely known for his operation of implantation of the ureters into the rectum, in which they are made to enter the lumen of the sigmoid flexure obliquely through the muscular and submucous layers, a valvelike action being obtained with minimal danger of infection. Called *ureterosigmoidostomy.*

cof′fin [OF. *cofin*, basket, from G. *kophinos*]. 1. A case for holding a dead body. 2. *In veterinary medicine*, the hollow portion of a horse's hoof.

cof′fin joint. Joint of the horse next above the coffin bone; the distal interphalangeal joint.

cofron. A trade-mark for hematinic preparations containing copper and iron and, in some, liver concentrate.

Coghill, George Ellett (1872–1941). American anatomist, known for his extensive studies of the relationships between the progressive differentiation of bodily structure and the overt behavioral patterns of that structure; in his studies on the salamander he showed that efficient movement occurs prior to development of reflex mechanisms.

cog·ni′tion. *In psychology,* the conscious faculty or process of knowing, of becoming, or being aware of thoughts or perceptions, as contrasted with *affectation* and *conation.*

cog′wheel″. See cogwheel *rigidity.*

co·hab″i·ta′tion [L. *cum,* with; *habitare,* to dwell]. The living together of a man and woman as husband and wife, with or without legal marriage.

co·her′ence [L. *cohaerentia,* from *cohaerere,* to stick together]. Reasonable connectedness of thought shown in speech or writing.

co·he′sion [L. *cohaesum,* from *cohaerere*]. The attractive force between the same kind of molecules, that is, the force which holds the molecules of a substance together. —**cohesive,** *adj.*

Cohn, Ferdinand Julius [*German bacteriologist,* 1828–98]. Remembered for his discovery of the ability of bacteria to form spores and of their multiplication by fission. Classified bacteria morphologically (1876).

Cohn, Hermann Ludwig [*German ophthalmologist,* 1838–1906]. Known for his promotion of hygiene in schools, especially for his advocacy of routine examination of the eyes of school children (1883). Developed a test for color perception by the use of colored skeins.

Cohn method. See Corper and Cohn *method.*

Cohnheim, Julius Friedrich [*German pathologist,* 1839–84]. Pupil of Virchow, and leading experimental pathologist of his time. Revolutionized the teaching of pathology; his textbook was standard in the nineteenth century. Studied sugar-forming ferments (1863). Investigated inflammation and suppuration (1867–73), showing that inflammation is characterized by the accumulation of leukocytes, which migrate through the capillary walls. Produced experimental tuberculosis in rabbits (1877). The experimental salt frog, a living frog whose blood has been replaced with physiological salt solution, is called *Cohnheim's frog.* Among other things, certain cancer cells, the small polygonal areas in transverse sections of muscle fibers, the end arteries without branches, and the theory that all true tumors are due to faulty embryonal development have been known by Cohnheim's name. See Cohnheim *theory.*

co′hosh, co·hosh′ [*Algonquian*]. An American Indian name for several medicinal plants.

blue c. Common name for *Caulophyllum thalictroides.*

c. bugbane. *Cimicifuga racemosa.*

coil [L. *colligere,* to gather]. A spiral formed by winding.

induction c. Rolls of wire used to transform a current of low potential into a current of high potential by electric induction.

primary c. The inner coil of an induction apparatus.

resistance c. A coil of wire of known electric resistance, used for estimating resistance.

secondary c. The outer coil of fine insulated wire in an induction apparatus.

Coindet, Jean François [*French physician,* 1774–1834]. Remembered as probably the first to use iodine internally in the treatment of goiter (1820).

coi′no·site (koy′no·sight, ko·in′o·), **ce′no·site** (see′no·sight, sen′o·) [G. *koinos,* common; *sitos,* food]. An animal parasite capable of separating itself from its host at will; a free, commensal organism.

co·i′tion (ko·ish′un) [L. *coire,* to come together]. Coitus.

co″i·to·pho′bi·a [L. *coitus,* coitus; G. *phobos,* fear]. Morbid dread of coitus.

co′i·tus [L., from *coire,* to come together]. The act of sexual connection; copulation.

c. interruptus. Sexual intercourse in which the penis is withdrawn and the semen discharged externally to the vagina. Also called *c. incompletus, c. reservatus.*

co′ko. Infrequent spelling of coco. See *yaws.*

col-. See *colo-.*

co′la nut. See *kola.*

co·la′tion [L. *colare,* to strain]. The operation of straining.

col″a·to′ri·um (kol″uh·tor′ee·um, ko″luh·) [*colare*]. *In pharmacy,* a sieve, colander, or strainer.

col′a·ture (kol′uh·choor, ko′luh·) [L. *colatura,* that which has been strained]. 1. *In pharmacy,* a liquid that has been subjected to colation. 2. Colation.

col″chi·ci′na (kol″chi·see′nuh, ·sigh′nuh) [L. *colchicum,* a plant with a poisonous root]. Colchicine.

col′chi·cine (kol′chi·seen, ·sin, kol′ki·) (*colchicina*). $C_{22}H_{25}O_6N$. An alkaloid of colchicum; a pale, brownish yellow, exceedingly bitter powder, freely soluble in water. Employed in the treatment of gout. It is a very active poison. Dose, 0.4–0.6 mg. (1/150–1/100 gr.). It speeds up the evolutionary processes in plants by doubling chromosome numbers.

c. salicylate. A yellow, amorphous powder, soluble in water. Dose, as for colchicine.

col″chi·cin″i·za′tion [L. *colchicum,* a plant with a poisonous root]. Treatment with colchicine.

col′chi·cum (kol′chi·kum, kol′ki·kum) [L., from G. *kolchikon*]. Meadow crocus; the corm and seed of *Colchicum autumnale,* the properties of which are due to an alkaloid, colchicine. It is an emetic, diuretic, diaphoretic, and drastic cathartic. It is valuable in acute gout and in some forms of rheumatism. Dose of the powdered corm (*colchici cormus*), 0.13–0.52 Gm. (2–8 gr.); of the powdered seeds (*colchici semen*), 0.065–0.32 Gm. (1–5 gr.).

c. seed fluidextract (*fluidextractum colchici seminis*). Contains 0.4–0.5% (w/v) of colchicine. Dose, 0.2 cc (3 min.).

c. seed tincture (*tinctura colchici seminis*). Contains 0.04–0.05% (w/v) of colchicine. Dose, 2 cc. (30 min.).

cold [AS. *kald*]. 1. The comparative lack of heat. Cold in the form of baths or ice packs is used therapeutically to lower fever, stop convulsions, or allay irritation and inflammation. 2. See *common cold.*

cold′-blood′ed. Poikilothermic; without ability to regulate the body temperature; said of fishes, reptiles, and amphibians whose temperatures correspond to that of the environment.

cold cream. A type of cosmetic cream of varying composition; sometimes, the official rose water ointment (U.S.P.).

cold′sore. See *herpes facialis.*

Cole, Warren Henry [*American surgeon,* 1898–]. Known for his part in the development of cholecystography (1924), called *Graham-Cole test.*

co·lec′to·my [G. *kolon,* colon; *ektōme,* excision]. Excision of all or a portion of the colon.

co″le·i′tis (ko″lee·eye′tis, kol″ee·) [G. *koleos,* sheath; *-itis,* inflammation]. Vaginitis. *Obs.*

Coleman diet. See under *diet.*

co′le·o- (ko′lee·o-, kol′ee·o-), **cole-** (ko′lee-, kol′ee-) [*koleos*]. A combining form denoting *a sheath.*

co′le·o·cele″ (ko′lee·o·seel″, kol′ee·o·) [*koleos;* G. *kēlē*, tumor]. Vaginal tumor or hernia.

co″le·o·cys·ti′tis [*koleos;* G. *kystis*, bladder; *-itis*, inflammation]. Inflammation of vagina and urinary bladder.

Co″le·op′ter·a (ko″lee·op′tur·uh, kol″ee·) [G. *koleopteros*, sheath-winged]. An order of insects which includes species of carnivorous and herbivorous beetles. —**coleop′terous,** *adj.*

co″le·op·to′sis [G. *koleos*, sheath; *ptōsis*, a falling]. Prolapse of the vaginal wall.

co″le·ot′o·my [*koleos;* G. *tomē*, a cutting]. A cutting operation upon the vagina; colpotomy.

co′les (ko′leez) [L.]. The penis.

c. femininus. The clitoris.

Coley, William Bradley [*American surgeon*, 1862–1936]. Remembered especially for his use of erysipelas and prodigiosus toxins, *Coley's fluid*, in the treatment of sarcoma (1891).

co″li·bac″il·le′mi·a (ko″li·bas″i·lee′mee·uh) [G. *kolon*, colon; L. *bacillus*, small staff; G. *haima*, blood]. Presence of *Escherichia coli* in the blood.

co″li·bac″il·lo′sis (·bas″i·lo′sis) [*kolon; bacillus;* G. *-ōsis*, condition]. Infection with *Escherichia coli.*

co″li·bac″il·lu′ri·a (·bas″i·lew′ree·uh) [*kolon; bacillus;* G. *ouron*, urine]. Presence of *Escherichia coli* in the urine.

co″li·ba·cil′lus [*kolon; bacillus*]. The colon bacillus, *Escherichia coli.*

col′ic [G. *kōlikos*, suffering in the colon]. Pertaining to the colon.

col′ic. Paroxysmal abdominal pain due to smooth-muscle spasm. A symptom of many different conditions; inflammatory, as that associated with appendicitis; obstructive, as that due to calculi in biliary or urethral passages; toxic, as in lead poisoning; overdistention from overeating or air swallowing; or due to emotional factors such as those associated with nervous indigestion. —**col′icky,** *adj.*

co′li·ca [*kōlikos*]. Colic artery.

col′i·cine. An antibiotic substance isolated from cultures of a strain of *Escherichia coli.*

col′i·form (kol′i·form, ko′li·form) [L. *colum*, a sieve; *forma*, form]. 1. Sievelike; ethmoid; cribriform. 2. Pertaining to or resembling the colon-aerogenes group: a group of nonspore-forming, Gram-negative, lactose-fermenting, aerobic bacilli; the demonstration of such organisms in water is accepted as presumptive evidence of fecal contamination. The coliform or colon-aerogenes group of bacteria includes members of the *Escherichia* and *Aerobacter* genera.

co′li group (ko′lye). Colon-aerogenes group. See *coliform.*

col′i·phage. A bacteriophage of *Escherichia coli.*

co″li·stat′in. An antibiotic substance, having bacteriostatic action against *Escherichia coli*, derived from an aerobic sporulating bacillus isolated from soil.

co·li′tis [G. *kolon*, colon; *-itis*, inflammation]. Inflammation of the colon.

acute c. That seen with acute infections or irritations; characterized by diarrhea. Also called *simple c.*

amebic c. An infectious disease due to infestation of the colon with *Endamoeba histolytica.*

balantidial c. That due to infestation by *Balantidium coli;* characterized by diarrhea and dysentery. Also called *balantidiasis.*

mucous c. A chronic affection of the mucous membrane of the colon; characterized by colicky pain, constipation, or diarrhea, and the passage of mucous or membranous threads or masses. Also called *chronic exudative enteritis, croupous c., desquamative c., diphtheritic c., follicular c., intestinal c., membranous c., mucomembranous c., plastic c.*

c. polyposa. That in which the mucosa between the masses of ulcers becomes swollen, thus projecting from the surface in polyplike masses: frequently associated with ulcerative colitis.

spastic c. That associated with an increased tonus of the colon.

ulcerative c. An idiopathic, nonspecific, inflammatory disease of the colon; characterized by friability and ulceration of the mucosa. It is generally considered to be a psychophysiologic, autonomic, and visceral disorder.

co″li·u′ri·a [*kolon;* G. *ouron*, urine]. Colibacilluria.

col′la·cin [G. *kolla*, glue; *eidos*, form]. A substance found in colloid degeneration of the skin.

col′la·gen [*kolla;* G. *genesthai*, from *gignesthai*, to be produced]. The albuminoid substance of the white fibers of connective tissues, cartilage, and bone. It is converted into gelatin by boiling. —**collagen′ic, collag′enous,** *adj.*

col′la·ge·nase [*kolla; genesthai*]. A proteolytic enzyme which hydrolyzes collagen; one of the major exotoxins of *Clostridium perfringens type A.* It attacks the collagen of subcutaneous tissues and muscles and thus facilitates the spread of gas gangrene. Probably synonymous with *bursting factor.* Also called *kappa toxin.*

col″la·gen′o·sis. A disease of adults characterized by congestive heart failure associated with necrosis of endocardium, formation of mural thrombi, and fibrosis. No coronary artery disease or other change that explains the endocardial damage has been identified.

col·lapse′ [L. *collapsus*, from *collabi*, to fall together]. 1. Extreme depression, exhaustion, or prostration; from failure of circulation, as in shock, hemorrhage, or vasomotor disturbance. 2. An abnormal sagging of an organ or falling together of its walls.

lung c. Decreased volume of any portion of a lung, with decrease or absence of its air content, due to any cause. See *atelectasis.*

massive c. The airless state of an entire lung, usually due to bronchial occlusion by accumulated secretions; often follows a surgical operation. Also called *massive atelectasis.*

col′lar·bone″ [L. *collum*, neck; AS. *bān*]. The clavicle.

col·lar·ette′. A ring or collar of scales, a rudiment of a blister.

col·lat′er·al [L. *cum*, together; *lateralis*, lateral]. Accessory or secondary; not direct or immediate.

col·lat′er·al. One of the first branches of an axon of a nerve cell passing at a right angle.

col·lec′tor. *In bronchoesophagology*, an instrument, variously modified, used to collect secretions for bacteriological and cytological examination.

Colles, Abraham [*Irish surgeon*, 1773–1843]. Celebrated for his elaboration of the law, a result of observation, that a child with congenital syphilis, whose mother has no clinical evidence of the disease, does not infect the mother (1837); called *Colles' law, Baumès' law.* Tied the subclavian artery (1811). Described the fracture at the carpal end of the radius with characteristic deformity (silver-fork); known as *Colles' fracture* (1814). See also under *fascia* and *ligament.*

Collet, Frédéric-Justin [*French otolaryngologist*, 1870–]. Known for his description of the syndrome following fracture of the floor of the posterior fossa of the skull: paralysis of the ninth, tenth, eleventh, and twelfth cranial nerves.

col·lic″u·li′tis [L. *colliculus*, a little hill; G. *-itis*, inflammation]. Inflammation of the colliculus seminalis. *Obs.*

col·lic′u·lus [L.]. A small eminence.

c. abducentis. See facial *c.*

c. cartilaginis arytaenoideae. A small eminence found on the ventral (anterior) margin and ventrolateral surface of the arytenoid cartilage.

c. seminalis. An elevation of the posterior wall of the prostatic portion of the urethra; on it opens the prostatic utricle; the ejaculatory ducts and numerous ducts of the prostate gland open on either side into the prostatic sinus. Formerly called *verumontanum.*

c. urethralis. Colliculus seminalis. *Obs.*

facial c. One of a pair of rounded eminences in the floor of the fourth ventricle; caused by the genu of the facial nerve passing around the nucleus of the abducens nerve. Formerly called *eminentia facialis, eminentia teres.* Syn., *c abducentis.*

inferior c. One of the posterior pair of rounded eminences arising from the dorsal portion of the mesencephalon. It contains centers for reflexes in response to sound. Also called *inferior quadrigeminal body.*

superior c. One of the anterior pair of rounded eminences arising from the dorsal portion of the mesencephalon. It contains centers for reflexes in response to visual stimuli. Also called *superior quadrigeminal body.*

col′li·dine (kol′i·deen, ·din). Any of three derivatives of pyridine of the composition $C_8H_{11}N$: *alpha collidine* is 4-ethyl-2-methylpyridine; *beta collidine* is 3-ethyl-4-methylpyridine; *gamma collidine* is 2,4,6-trimethylpyridine. All are liquids obtained from coal tar.

Collier, James Stansfield (1870–1935). English physician who gave the first complete description of subacute combined degeneration of the spinal cord and its relation to pernicious anemia. See under *degeneration.*

col′li·ga″tive. *In physical chemistry,* referring to those properties of matter that depend on the number of molecules but do not depend on their chemical nature, as for example the pressure of a volume of a (perfect) gas.

col′li·ma″tor [L. *collimare,* false reading for *collineare,* to aim]. 1. The diaphragm of a spectroscope, the purpose of which is to provide a beam of parallel rays of light by means of a small slit at the focus of its lens. 2. A fixed telescope for adjusting the optical axis of an instrument, as a photomicrographic camera.

col·lin′e·ar [L. *cum,* with; *linea,* line]. *In optics,* lying in the same straight line.

Col″lin·so′ni·a [L., after Peter *Collinson,* English botanist, 1694–1768]. A genus of Lamiaceae, the mint family.

C. canadensis. Stoneroot; healall; a coarse plant with a disagreeable smell; has been used as a tonic, diuretic, and diaphoretic.

Collip, James Bertram [*Canadian physician and biochemist,* 1892–]. With F. G. Banting, C. H. Best, W. R. Campbell, and A. A. Fletcher, first used insulin in the treatment of diabetes (1922). Improved insulin (1923). Isolated parathormone, the active principle of the parathyroids (1925). Introduced a dosage unit of parathyroid extract; see Collip *unit.* Discovered the anterior pituitary-like factor (A.P.L. factor), which he showed to be an ovary-stimulating hormone of the placenta (1930). With E. P. Clark, modified the Kramer-Tisdall method for serum calcium; see under *method.*

col″li·qua′tion [L. *cum,* with; *liquare,* to melt]. The breakdown of tissue, usually necrotic, so that it becomes liquefied.

reticular c. One characteristic of cutaneous vesicles due to viruses. The cytoplasm of adjoining cells, after becoming edematous and granular, partially coalesces and disintegrates. The residual cytoplasm forms reticulated septa between intraepidermal collections of fluid or septa.

col·liq′ua·tive [*cum; liquare*]. Profuse or excessive; marked by excessive fluid discharges.

col·li′sion [L. *collisio,* from *collidere,* to strike together]. 1. A violent meeting. 2. A complication in twin pregnancy which occurs occasionally when the twins are small and when their presenting parts attempt to enter the superior strait at the same time.

Compton c. See scattering *c.*

photoelectric c. Impact of a photon with an electron in an atom, whereby the photon gives up all of its energy, removes the electron from its place, and imparts a high velocity to the electron.

scattering c. Impact of a photon with an electron in an atom, whereby the photon gives up only a part of its energy to set the electron in motion and travels on in a different direction with reduced energy. Also called *Compton c.*

col·li′tis. See *trigonitis.*

col·lo′di·on [G. *kollōdēs,* glutinous] (*collodium*). A dressing for wounds made by dissolving pyroxylin in ether and alcohol. See *pyroxylin.*

flexible c. (*collodium flexile*). Collodion with the addition of castor oil and camphor.

salicylic c. (*collodium salicylicum*). Contains salicylic acid, 10 Gm.; flexible collodion, a sufficient quantity to make 100 cc. Used as a means of applying salicylic acid for its keratolytic effect, especially in the treatment of corns.

styptic c. (*collodium stypticum*). Contains tannic acid, 16 Gm.; flexible collodion, a sufficient quantity to make 100 cc. Intended as an application for wounds in order to stop the bleeding.

col·lo′di·um. See *collodion.*

col′loid [G. *kolla,* glue; *eidos,* form]. 1. A state of subdivision of matter in which the individual particles are of submicroscopic size and consist either of single large molecules, as of proteins, or aggregates of smaller molecules; such particles, collectively referred to as the disperse phase, occur more or less uniformly distributed in a dispersion medium. The dimension of a colloid particle, arbitrarily fixed, is between 1 and 100 millimicrons (mμ). 2. A substance in the colloid state. 3. The clear, gelatinous, eosinophilic, stored secretion of the thyroid gland; also other collections of gelatinous material, as colloid carcinoma or the secretion of the intermediate lobe of the hypophysis. **—colloi′dal,** *adj.*

hydrophilic c. One capable of combining with, or attracting to it, water to form a stable dispersion.

hydrophobic c. One incapable of combining with, or attracting to it, water.

irreversible c. One which, on being precipitated or otherwise separated from its dispersion medium, cannot be restored to its original state merely by adding the dispersion medium.

lyophilic c. One capable of combining with, or attracting to it, the dispersion medium.

lyophobic c. One incapable of combining with, or attracting to it, the dispersion medium.

protective c. A lyophilic colloid which, when added to a lyophobic colloid, confers upon the latter the stability of the former.

reversible c. One which, on being precipitated or otherwise separated from its dispersion medium, can be restored to its original state merely by adding the dispersion medium.

col·loi″do·cla′sis [*kolla; eidos;* G. *klasis,* a breaking]. A breaking up of the physical equilibrium of the colloids in the living body, producing anaphylactoid shock. Attributed to entrance into the blood stream of unchanged (undigested) colloids. *Obs.*

col·loi″do·pex′y. The phagocytosis of colloidal particles.

col″loid·oph′a·gy. Invasion and ingestion of colloid by macrophages, as in the thyroid gland.

col″lo·ne′ma (pl. *collonemata*) [*kolla*]. A lipoma with extensive mucoid degeneration.

col′lum [L.]. Neck.

c. anatomicum humeri [BNA]. The anatomical neck of the humerus.

c. chirurgicum humeri [BNA]. The surgical neck of the humerus.

c. distortum. Torticollis.

c. femoris [BNA]. The neck of the femur.

c. vesicae felleae [BNA]. The neck of the gallbladder.

col″lu·na′ri·um. A solution intended to be used in the nose.

col″lu·to′ri·um. A solution intended to be used as a mouthwash: also called *collutory.*

col·lyr′i·um (pl. *collyriums, collyria*) [G. *kollyrion*, poultice]. A preparation for local application to the eye, usually a wash or lotion.

col′ma·scope. An instrument for determining strains in optical lenses by the transmission of polarized light.

co′lo- (ko′lo-, kol′o-), **col-** [G. *kolon*, colon]. A combining form denoting *the colon.*

col″o·bo′ma [G. *kolobōma*, from *koloboun*, to mutilate]. Any congenital, pathologic, or operative defect, especially of the eye; it occurs most commonly in the iris, ciliary body, or choroid, usually as a cleft placed inferiorly. May be a congenital fissure of the eyelid, usually the upper.

atypical c. One located other than inferiorly in any part of the eye.

c. auris. A developmental malformation of the external ear caused by defect of the hyomandibular groove with resulting cleft between tragus and antitragus.

bridge c. A form affecting the iris, in which the cleft is separated from the pupil by a bridging strand of iris or by persistent pupillary membrane.

c. of the optic nerve. One caused by partial closure or nonclosure of the fetal fissure of the optic stalk.

c. of the retina. One caused by partial closure or nonclosure of the fetal fissure of the optic cup.

facial c. See facial *cleft.*

genal c. Old term for transverse facial *cleft.*

macular c. See macular *dysplasia.*

co″lo·ce·cos′to·my. See *cecocolostomy.*

co″lo·co·los′to·my [G. *kolon*, colon; *kolon; stoma*, mouth]. An anastomosis between two noncontinuous segments of the colon in order to short-circuit the lumen around inoperable obstructing tumors or to prepare for later resection.

col′o·cynth [G. *kolokynthis*] (*colocynthis*). The dried pulp of the unripe but full-grown fruit of *Citrullus colocynthis.* Its cathartic action is due to an alkaloid and one or more other principles. The colocynthin of earlier investigators is a mixture of the alkaloid and an alcohol, citrullol. Colocynth is a powerful purgative. Dose, 0.065–0.32 Gm. (1–5 gr.).

c. extract (*extractum colocynthidis*). One part represents four parts of colocynth. Dose, as a laxative, 0.065–0.13 Gm. (1–2 gr.)., as a purgative, 0.32–0.65 Gm. (5–10 gr.).

compound c. and jalap pills (*pilulae colocynthidis et jalapae*). Better known as vegetable cathartic pills; contain compound colocynth extract, hyoscyamus extract, jalap resin, leptandra extract, and podophyllum resin. The compound cathartic pills contain compound colocynth extract, mild mercurous chloride, jalap resin, and gamboge.

compound c. extract (*extractum colocynthidis compositum*). Colocynth extract 16, ipomea resin 14, aloe 65, cardamom seed 5. Is less drastic than colocynth. Dose, 0.065–0.13 Gm. (1–2 gr.).

col″o·cyn′thin. A mixture of certain active constituents of colocynth. See *colocynth.*

co·logne′ wa′ter. Perfumed spirit.

co″lo·hep′a·to·pex″y (ko″lo·hep′uh·to·peck″see, kol″o·) [G. *kolon*, colon; *hēpar*, liver; *pēxis*, fixing]. Fixation of the colon to the liver to form adhesions. *Obs.*

Colombo, Matteo Realdo (Realdus Columbus) [*Italian anatomist*, ca. 1516–ca. 1559]. Successor of Vesalius at Padua. Sometimes credited with the discovery of the pulmonary circulation, although it is probable that, in his excellent description (1559), he plagiarized the work of Servetus, whose book had been burned in 1553.

co′lon [G. *kolon*, colon]. The part of the large intestine beginning at the cecum and terminating at the end of the sigmoid flexure. In the various parts of its course it is known as **ascending c., transverse c., descending c.,** and **sigmoid c.** The last is sometimes divided into the **iliac c.** and the **pelvic c.** See Plates 8, 10, 13, 14. —**col′ic, colon′ic,** *adj.*

giant c. See *megacolon.*

redundant c. One with congenitally increased length, causing looping or reduplication; commonly associated with constipation.

col′o·ny [L. *colonia*, colony]. *In bacteriology*, a group or mass of microorganisms in a culture, derived from a single cell. Variations in bacterial structure or antigenic composition are often expressed in colonial appearance (e.g. smooth, rough, dwarf).

dwarf (D) c. A bacterial colony whose organisms have poorly developed enzyme systems, grow slowly, have little or no virulence, and revert slowly to the original type: frequently isolated from bacterial populations exposed to antibiotics.

glossy c. Originally, a smooth colony of streptococci; now commonly a colony of streptococci devoid of M substance.

gonidial (G) c. Bacterial colony whose organisms are composed of minute coccoid and bacillary forms which pass through filters retaining ordinary bacteria. Syn., *Hadley type c.*

Hadley type c. Gonidial *c.*

intermediate c. A bacterial colony which is intermediate between the typical smooth **(S)** and rough **(R)** forms, and designated according to the resemblance to the S or R form, **Sr, SR,** or **sR.**

matt (M) c. As originally introduced, a rough colony of streptococci: now commonly a colony of streptococci rich in M substance.

mucoid (M) c. A glistening smooth colony with gummy or viscid consistency: often associated with the production of definite capsules or abundant slime-layer material.

rough (R) c. A flat nonglistening colony with irregular surfaces and edges.

smooth (S) c. A raised colony with regular edges and a homogenous-appearing surface.

col′o·ny coun′ter. A device for counting bacterial colonies; usually consists of an illuminated transparent plate, divided into spaces of known area, over which a Petri dish containing the colonies is placed.

col′o·pex″y (kol′o·peck″see, ko′lo·) [G. *kolon*, colon; *pēxis*, a fixing]. Suturing of the sigmoid flexure to the abdominal wall. *Obs.*

co·loph′o·ny. Rosin.

col″o·proc·tos′to·my [*kolon;* G. *prōktos*, anus;

stoma, mouth]. Formation of a new passage between the colon and the rectum.

col″op·to′sis (kol″op·to′sis, ko″lop·), **col″op·to′si·a** (kol″op·to′shuh, ·see·uh, ·zhuh, ·zee·uh) [*kolon;* G. *ptōsis*, a falling]. Prolapse or displacement of the colon.

col′or [L.]. 1. A visual sensation due to radiated or reflected light. 2. Tint or hue; that quality of an object perceptible to sight alone. 3. A pigment.

complementary colors. Two colors which, when combined, produce white.

confusion c. A color which appears the same as another to a colorblind person.

primary colors. (a) *In painting*, those whose various combinations make all other colors; red, yellow, and blue; or, more loosely, a classification of distinct color sensations to which other shades or tints may be referred, as green, light or dark. (b) *In psychology*, red, yellow-green, and blue.

col′or·blind″ness. Inability to perceive one or more, rarely all, colors; achromatopsia. See Ishihara's *test* for colorblindness. Also spelled *color blindness.*

amnesic c. A form of aphasia in which colors are seen normally, but the names cannot be recalled.

partial c. A form characterized by a decrease or loss of perception of one of the three basic hues. Red-green colorblindness is the most common type. Forms of partial colorblindness are: *protanopia, partial protanopia, deuteranopia, partial deuteranopia, tritanopia.*

total c. The complete inability to distinguish different hues and saturations. Brightness perception is normal; the world is seen as shades of gray. Syn., *monochromatism.*

col″o·rec·tos′to·my (kol″o·reck·tos′to·mee, ko″lo-reck·) [G. *kolon*, colon; L. *rectus*, straight; G. *stoma*, mouth]. *In surgery*, the establishment of a new passage between the colon and the rectum.

col′or gus·ta′tion. Pseudogeusesthesia.

col′or hear′ing. The excitation of the visual center for color through the auditory nerve.

col″or·im′e·ter (kul″o·rim′i·tur) [L. *color*, color; G. *metron*, a measure]. An instrument for determining color intensity, as for measuring the proportion of hemoglobin in blood. Also see *photoelectric colorimeter.* —**colorimet′ric,** *adj.*

Dare c. An instrument used in hemoglobinometry. A film of whole blood is arranged between two glass plates and compared with a tinted wedge.

col″or·im′e·try. The science of determining colors; specifically chemical analysis by the use of a colorimeter.

capillary tube c. Colorimetry employing capillary tubes in which reagents are placed, mixed, and read colorimetrically.

col′or in′dex. See under *index.*

co·lor′rha·phy [G. *kolon*, colon; *rhaphē*, suture]. Suture of the colon.

co″lo·sig″moid·os′to·my [*kolon;* G. *sigmoeidēs*, shaped like the letter sigma; *stoma*, mouth]. Formation of an anastomosis between the sigmoid and some other part of the colon.

co·los′to·my [*kolon; stoma*]. The formation of an artificial anus in the anterior abdominal wall or loin. The opening into the colon may be anywhere depending on the location of the diseased condition, as cecostomy, sigmoidostomy, etc.

col″os·tra′tion [L. *colostratio*, from *colostrum*, the first milk after delivery]. Diarrhea of infants caused by colostrum.

co·los″tror·rhe′a [*colostrum;* G. *rhoia*, flow]. Profuse discharge of colostrum.

co·los′trum [L.]. The first milk from the mother's breasts after the birth of the child. It is laxative, and assists in the expulsion of the meconium. Contains greater quantities of lactalbumin and lactoprotein than later milk.

co·lot′o·my [G. *kolon*, colon; *tomē*, a cutting]. Incision of the colon; may be abdominal, lateral, lumbar, or iliac, according to the region of entrance.

colp-. See *colpo-.*

col·pal′gi·a (kol·pal′juh, ·jee·uh) [G. *kolpos*, vagina; *algos*, pain]. Vaginal pain or neuralgia.

col″pa·tre′si·a (kol″pa·tree′zhuh, ·zee·uh, ·shuh, ·see·uh) [*kolpos;* G. *atrētos*, not perforated]. Occlusion or atresia of the vagina.

col″pec·ta′si·a (kol″peck·tay′zhuh, ·zee·uh, ·shuh, ·see·uh) [*kolpos;* G. *ektasis*, a stretching out]. Vaginal dilatation.

col·pec′to·my [*kolpos;* G. *ektomē*, excision]. Excision of the vagina.

col″pe·de′ma [*kolpos;* G. *oidēma*, swelling]. Edema of the vagina.

col″peu·ryn′ter (kol″pew·rin′tur) [*kolpos;*. G *eurynein*, to make wide]. An inflatable bag or sac used for dilating the vagina. *Rare.*

col″peu·rys′is (kol″pew·ris′is, kol·pew′ris·is) [*kolpos; eurynein*]. Dilatation of the vagina, especially that effected by means of the colpeurynter. *Rare.*

col·pi′tis [*kolpos;* G. *-itis*, inflammation]. Inflammation of the vagina.

emphysematous c. See emphysematous *vaginitis.*

col′po-, colp- [*kolpos*]. A combining form denoting *connection with* or *relation to the vagina.*

col′po·cele [*kolpos;* G. *kēlē*, hernia]. Hernia or tumor in the vagina.

col″po·clei′sis (kol″po·kly′sis) [*kolpos;* G. *kleisis*, a closure]. Closure of the vagina by suturing.

col″po·hy″per·pla′si·a cys′ti·ca. See emphysematous *vaginitis.*

col″po·per″i·ne′o·plas″ty [*kolpos;* G. *perinaios*, space between the anus and the scrotum; *plassein*, to form]. Plastic surgery of the perineum and vagina.

col″po·per″i·ne·or′rha·phy [*kolpos; perinaios;* G. *rhaphē*, a suture]. Suture of a cut or lacerated vagina and perineum.

col′po·pex″y [*kolpos;* G. *pēxis*, a fixing]. Fixation of the vagina by suturing it to a surrounding structure.

col′po·plas″ty [*kolpos;* G. *plassein*, to form]. Plastic repair of the vagina.

col·por′rha·phy [*kolpos;* G. *rhaphē,* a suture]. Suture of the vagina for repair.

col″por·rhex′is (kol″po·reck′sis) [*kolpos;* G. *rhēxis*, a breaking]. Traumatic separation of the cervix of the uterus from its vaginal attachments. *Rare.*

col′po·scope [*kolpos;* G. *skopein*, to examine]. An instrument for the visual examination of the vagina and cervix; a vaginal speculum. —**colposcop′ic,** *adj.*; **colpos′copy,** *n.*

col·pot′o·my [*kolpos;* G. *tomē*, a cutting]. Surgical incision of the vagina.

col·sul′a·nyde″. See *sulfanilamide.*

colts′foot″ [AS. *colt; fōt*]. An herb, *Tussilago farfara*, of the aster family; its leaves are used as a demulcent and bitter, and sometimes as a domestic remedy for chronic cough.

co·lum′bin. A bitter principle found in calumba.

co·lum′bi·um [NL., from *Columbia*]. Cb = 92.91. Chemical element No. 41, now known as niobium.

Columbus, Realdus. See *Colombo.*

col″u·mel′la [L., small column]. 1. The septum of the nasal vestibule, the medial boundary of the nostrils. 2. The modiolus or central axis of the cochlea of the human ear. 3. A bone in birds which takes the place of the ossicles of the ear in man.

col′umn [L. *columna*, column]. A supporting pillar;

a pillar-shaped structure. —**colum′nar,** *adj.*

Clarke's c. See dorsal *nucleus* of Clarke.

c. of Burdach. Fasciculus cuneatus.

c. of the fornix. One of the two anterior, arched pillars of the fornix, terminating in the mammillary bodies. Also called *columna fornicis.*

columns of the gray matter. Divisions of the longitudinal column of gray matter in the spinal cord; usually classified as the **anterior column,** the **lateral column,** and the **posterior column.** Also called *cornua of the gray matter* or *horns.*

columns of the vagina. Two median, longitudinal ridges formed by the rugae of the vagina. That of the anterior wall is the **anterior column of the vagina;** that of the posterior wall, the **posterior column of the vagina.**

enamel c. See enamel *prism.*

fundamental c. See *fasciculus proprius.*

intermediolateral cell c. A division of the lateral gray column of the spinal cord, extending from the thoracic region to the upper lumbar segments, and composed of small neurons whose axons form preganglionic sympathetic fibers.

rectal c. One of the vertical folds of the mucous membrane of the upper part of the anal canal. Also called *anal c., c. of Morgagni.*

renal c. That part of the cortical substance of the kidney between the sides of any two pyramids. Also called *c. of Bertin, interpyramidal cortex.*

spinal c. See vertebral *c.*

vertebral c. The flexible, supporting column of the body made up of vertebrae separated by intervertebral disks and bound together by ligaments. Syn., *spinal c.* Also called *backbone.*

co·lum′na (pl. *columnae*) [L.]. Column.

columnae carneae. Trabeculae carneae.

columnae griseae. Columns of the gray matter. See under *column.*

columnae rugarum. Columns of the vagina. See under *column.*

c. nasi. Columella.

col′umn·ing, col″um·ni·za′tion [*columna*]. The placing of vaginal tampons to support a prolapsed uterus.

co′ma [G. *kōma*, deep sleep]. 1. Unconsciousness from which the patient cannot be aroused. It may be due to ingested poison such as opiates or alcohol; to a poison developed in the body, as in uremia or overwhelming toxemias; to profound disturbances of the acid-base balance, as in diabetic acidosis; or to brain injury, trauma, apoplexy, or tumor. 2. *In ophthalmology,* spherical aberration in oblique incidence.

c. vigil. A comatose condition in which the patient lies with eyes open but is unconscious.

hepatic c. A state of unconsciousness seen in patients severely ill with hepatic disease. The term has been used loosely to include the precomatose state. See *cholemia.*

hypochloremic c. That due to reduced blood chloride.

com′a·tose (kom′uh·toce, ·toze, ko′muh·) [*kōma*]. In a condition of coma.

Combe, James Scarfe [*Scottish physician,* 1796–1883]. Gave first description of pernicious anemia (1822–24), antedating Thomas Addison.

combevita. Trade-mark for capsules containing B vitamins together with B-complex factors from liver.

combex. Trade-mark for preparations containing B vitamins.

comb′ing. The radial arrangement of elongated cells around vessels or vascular spaces, seen particularly in spindle-cell sarcomas.

Comby, Jules [*French pediatrist,* 1853–1947]. Remembered for the sign, stomatitis of the buccal mucous membrane, said to be diagnostic of measles; called *Comby's sign.*

com′e·do, co·me′do (pl. *comedos, comedones*) [L., a glutton]. A collection of sebaceous material and dead cells retained in the hair follicle and excretory duct of the sebaceous gland, the surface covered with a dark crust due to hyperkeratosis at the follicular orifice. It is the primary lesion of acne vulgaris; usually found over the face, chest, and back, and more commonly during adolescence. Syn., *blackhead.*

com″e·do-car″ci·no′ma. A type of adenocarcinoma of the breast in which the ducts are filled with cells which, when expressed from the cut surface, resemble comedos. It may be slow to grow and noninfiltrating or, more rarely, rapid in growth and infiltrating.

com″e·do′nes (kom″i·do′neez). Plural of comedo, formerly used.

co′mes (ko′meez) [L., companion]. *In anatomy,* an artery which accompanies a nerve, or a vein which accompanies an artery. See Table of Arteries in the Appendix.

com′frey (kum′free, kom′free) [OF. *confirie*]. A plant of the genus *Symphytum;* the root of the common comfrey, *S. officinale,* has been used as a demulcent, slightly astringent, and bitter drug, and was a common ingredient of domestic cough mixtures.

com·men′sal·ism [L. *cum,* with; *mensa,* table]. A more or less intimate association between organisms of different species, without injury to either organism and with some benefit, such as nourishment and protection, to one or both; as the association of the small crab and the oyster in whose shell it lives; symbiosis. —**commensal,** *n.*

com′mi·nute [L. *comminuere,* to crumble to pieces]. 1. *In chemistry,* pulverize; divide into fine particles. 2. *In surgery,* fracture a bone so that it is shattered into several pieces. —**comminute, comminuted,** *adj.;* **comminu′tion,** *n.*

Com·miph′o·ra [G. *kommi,* gum; *phoros,* bearing]. A genus of shrubs and trees of the Burseraceae, found in Africa and the East Indies. Various species yield myrrh and bdellium. **C. meccanensis** yields Gilead or Mecca balsam.

com″mis·su′ra (kom″i·shoor′uh) [L., a joining together]. Commissure.

c. fornicis. See hippocampal *commissure.*

c. mollis. See *massa intermedia.*

com′mis·sure [L. *commissura,* a joining together]. 1. Strands of nerve fibers uniting like structures in the two sides of the brain or spinal cord. 2. The point of union of such structures as the lips, eyelids, labia majora, or cardiac valves. —**commis′sural,** *adj.*

anterior c. A rounded cord of nerve fibers placed in front of the columns of the fornix, joining the olfactory bulbs and the pyriform areas of the two cerebral hemispheres. See Plate 18.

anterior white c. of the spinal cord. A layer of fibers separating the anterior gray commissure from the bottom of the anterior median fissure.

Ganser's c. See anterior hypothalamic *decussation.*

gray c. of the spinal cord. The transverse band of gray matter connecting the masses of gray matter of the two halves of the spinal cord. It is divided by the central canal into the **anterior gray commissure** and the **posterior gray commissure.**

Gudden's c. One joining the two medial geniculate bodies; its fibers run with the optic tracts. Syn., *ventral supraoptic decussation.*

habenular c. Fibers joining one habenular nucleus to the other. See Plate 18.

hippocampal c. The transverse part of the fornix, uniting the crura: formerly called *psalterium, lyra Davidi.* Syn., *commissura fornicis.*

Meynert's c. A tract of nerve fibers crossing dorsally to the medial half of the chiasm from the tuber cinereum to the opposite side; it is probably connected with the subthalamus.

middle c. Old term for massa intermedia.

posterior c. A transverse band of nerve fibers crossing dorsal to the opening of the cerebral aqueduct into the third ventricle. See Plate 18.

posterior white c. of the spinal cord. A band of fibers separating the gray commissure from the bottom of the posterior median fissure.

com″mis·sur·ot′o·my [*commissura; tomē,* a cutting]. The surgical section of any commissure.

mitral c. An operation for the relief of mitral stenosis, commonly a valvulotomy.

com·mit′ment [L. *committere,* to commit]. *In legal medicine,* an act consigning a patient to an institution.

com′mon cold. A mild acute respiratory virus infection of short duration, characterized by chilly sensations, sneezing, watering of the eyes, nasal discharge, cough, and, occasionally, fever. It is endemic and contagious. Susceptibility is universal and immunity is only temporary. Very rarely the disease is followed by purulent sinusitis, pneumonia, or other complications due to such pathogenic bacteria as pneumococci, streptococci, *Micrococcus pyogenes,* or influenza bacilli. See also acute respiratory *disease.*

com·mo′ti·o (kuh·mo′shee·o) [L., commotion]. A concussion, commotion, or shock.

c. cerebri. Concussion of the brain.

c. retinae. Concussion or paralysis of the retina from a blow on or near the eye. It is characterized by sudden blindness, but there is little or no ophthalmoscopic evidence of any lesion. The sight is usually regained, and its loss is supposedly due to disturbance of the retinal elements.

c. spinalis. Railway spine.

com·mu′ni·ca·ble [L. *communicare,* to divide something with one]. Transmissible from one person to another.

com·mu′ni·cans (ko·mew′ni·kanz) [*communicare*]. Communicating; connecting.

comp. *Compositus;* compound.

com·pan′ion·ate mar′riage. Form of marriage for sexual companionship without legal obligation, economic responsibility, or desire for children.

com′pa·ny aid man. A medical department soldier attached to a company of combat troops, whose principal duties are to administer emergency treatment to casualties, to examine and tag the dead, and to instruct the walking wounded as to location of the nearest aid station.

com·par′a·scope [L. *comparare,* to compare; G. *skopein,* to examine]. An apparatus attached to two microscopes for the simultaneous comparison of two different specimens.

com·pat″i·bil′i·ty [L. *compati,* to suffer with one]. 1. Congruity; the power of a medicine or a substance in a medicine to mix with another without deleterious chemical change or loss of therapeutic power. 2. *In blood grouping,* (a) in vitro, no interaction between two bloods; (b) in vivo, no reaction whatsoever from the injection of a blood found to be compatible by laboratory tests. —**compat′ible,** *adj.*

compenamine. Trade-mark for certain preparations of L-ephenamine penicillin G, having long duration of action and reduced incidence of allergic reactions.

com″pen·sa′tion [L. *compensare,* to balance against]. 1. The act of making good a deficiency; the state of counterbalancing a functional or structural defect. 2. *In psychopathology,* a psychic phenomenon in which strong feelings of guilt or inferiority prompt excessive defensive reactions. —**com′pensating, compen′satory,** *adj.*

com·pen′sa·to″ry pause. *In cardiology,* any pause which, immediately following a premature beat, compensates by its length for the prematurity of the beat.

com′pe·tence [L. *competere,* to be qualified]. *In embryology,* the ability to react to a developmental stimulus; a state of reactivity or unstable equilibrium necessary for induction to occur. See *potency, determination.*

com·plaint′ [OF. *complainte*]. Lay term for disease or ailment. See also *presenting complaints.*

com′ple·ment [L. *complementum,* from *complere,* to complete]. A complex substance resembling a ferment; formed in the blood, plasma, or serum of animals; has the capacity, in cooperation with antibody and cellular elements, to destroy a variety of pathogenic organisms and other foreign substances. The common functions of complement are: bacteriolysis, bactericidal action, hemolysis, and acceleration of opsonic actions. Complement (C′) may be fractionated into four components, indicated by C′1, C′2, C′3, and C′4. Syn., *addiment, alexin, cytase.*

fixation of c. See under *fixation.*

com″ple·men′tal, com″ple·men′ta·ry [*complementum*]. Supplying a deficiency.

com″ple·men′ta·ry. See *complemental.*

com″ple·men′toid [*complementum;* G. *eidos,* form]. A complement which through the agency of heat has lost its capacity for causing lysis but still retains its binding property with the amboceptor.

com″ple·men′to·phil [*complementum;* G. *philein,* to love]. According to Ehrlich, the haptophore group of the intermediary body (amboceptor) by means of which it combines with the complement.

com′plex [L. *complexus,* an encircling]. 1. *In psychoanalysis,* a group of ideas with strong emotional tone, which have been transferred by the conscious mind into the unconscious, and from there influence the personality. 2. A combination of symptoms or related factors, as a symptom complex or syndrome; complexus.

aberrant c. An electrocardiographic deflection of ventricular origin, which varies from the normal. Syn., *anomalous c.*

anomalous c. See aberrant *c.*

anxiety c. A symptom of a neurosis, marked by fear and apprehension, especially with regard to beginning any task, or to impending accident, castration, infection, and the like.

castration c. Castration anxiety occurring after childhood, associated primarily with fear of loss of the genital, especially the male, organ; by extension, the symptoms of the fear of the loss of any pleasure-giving body part (or excretion) or of even the fear that every pleasure will be followed by loss and pain.

caudal pharyngeal c. Ultimobranchial body.

Eisenmenger's c. An anomaly of the heart consisting of a defect in the interventricular septum, dextroposition of the aorta, and hypertrophy of the right ventricle. Unlike the tetralogy of Fallot, the pulmonary artery has a normal or greater than normal diameter.

Electra c. The female analog of the Oedipus complex.

Lutembacher's c. A type of heart disease in which mitral stenosis is associated with patency of the interatrial septum: described by René Lutembacher (1916).

neuroinsular c. See *neuroinsular complex.*

Oedipus c. A carry-over into adult life of a son's childhood sexual desire for his mother, usually accompanied by hostility toward, or envy of, the position of his father. According to Freud, every male child experiences this Oedipus situation.

persecution c. See *paranoia.*

QRS c. of electrocardiography. The depolarization complex of the ventricular musculature. It consists usually of a downward deflection (Q wave), an upward (R wave), and a downward (S wave) deflection.

triple symptom c. of Behcet. See Behcet's *syndrome.*

com·plex′ion [L. *complexio,* combination]. Color and appearance of the skin of the face.

com·plex′us. Old term for the *semispinalis capitis muscle.*

com″pli·ca′tion [L. *complicare,* to fold together]. *In medicine,* an accidental condition or second disease occurring in the course of a primary disease. —**com′plicated,** *adj.*

com·po′nent [L. *componere,* to put together]. Constituent part.

c. A. Factor in the prothrombin complex which is adsorbable by tricalcium phosphate and requires vitamin K for its synthesis; its lack causes a type of hypoprothrombinemia.

d c. See *dysplasia,* 2.

g c. See *gynandromorphy.*

nerve c. The group of fibers in a nerve having similar functions, as the sensory and motor components of a mixed nerve.

plasma thromboplastin c. See under *plasma.*

t c. In the *somatotype,* the textural quality of the body, expressed numerically. Psychologically, it is the esthetic impression made by the individual's physique.

com″po·si′tion [L. *compositio,* a putting together]. 1. The constitution of a mixture. 2. The kind and number of atoms which are contained in the molecule of a compound.

com·po′si·tus [L., from *componere,* to put together]. Compound.

com′pos men′tis [L.]. Of sound mind.

com′pound [L. *componere,* to put together]. A substance composed of two or more elements chemically combined in definite proportion. Abbreviated, comp. —**compound′ing,** *n.;* **compound′,** *v.t.*

carbamino c. A type of compound formed by the combination of carbon dioxide with a free amino group in an amino acid or a protein. Carbhemoglobin, which plays an important role in carbon dioxide transport by the blood, is a carbamino compound formed by the combination of hemoglobin and carbon dioxide.

carbocyclic c. One having a ring or closed chain structure in which the atoms that are linked are all carbon.

closed chain organic c. An organic compound in which the carbon atoms are arranged or linked so as to form a closed chain or ring.

c. A (Kendall's). Dehydrocorticosterone.

c. B (Kendall's). Corticosterone.

c. C (Kendall's). Allopregnane-$3\alpha,11\beta,17\alpha,21$-tetrol-20-one, a steroidal constituent of the adrenal cortex.

c. D (Kendall's). Allopregnane-$3\beta,11\beta,17\alpha,20\beta$,-21-pentol, a steroidal constituent of adrenal cortex.

c. E (Kendall's). Cortisone.

c. F (Kendall's). Hydrocortisone.

c. F (Wintersteiner's). Cortisone.

c. Fa6 (Reichstein's). Cortisone.

c. G-11. Hexachlorophene.

c. Q (Reichstein's). Deoxycorticosterone (11-deoxycorticosterone, cortexone).

c. S (Reichstein's). 11-Deoxy-17-hydroxycorticosterone.

c. 1080. See *sodium fluoroacetate.*

cyclic c. *In chemistry,* an organic compound belonging to the closed chain series.

fatty c. Any aliphatic compound.

heterocyclic c. One having a ring or closed chain structure in which the atoms that are linked are of two or more different elements.

homocyclic c. One having a ring or closed chain structure in which the atoms that are linked are all the same, usually carbon.

open chain organic c. An organic compound in which the carbon atoms are arranged or linked to form an open chain.

organic c. Any chemical compound containing carbon.

quaternary ammonium compounds. Products wherein the hydrogen atoms of the ammonium radical, NH_4, have been replaced by organic groups. Certain of these compounds possess antibacterial and detergent properties; they are sometimes referred to as cationic detergents.

ring c. One in which the atoms form a ring or closed chain.

tagged compounds. Chemical elements, such as isotopes, which, bound in organic forms, can be traced in their transformation within the body.

com′press [L. *compressus,* from *comprimere,* to press together]. A folded cloth or pad of other soft material, wet or dry, applied firmly to a part for the relief of inflammation or the prevention of hemorrhage.

cold c. One moistened with cold or ice water.

cribriform c. A compress with holes for drainage or a hole for observation of the skin beneath. Also called *fenestration c.*

graduated c. A compress with folds of varying size, thick in the center and thinner toward the periphery.

hot c. One moistened with warm or hot water.

pressure c. One which is held in place with a bandage in order to produce pressure on the wound and prevent oozing.

com·pressed′-air′ ill′ness. See caisson *disease.*

com·pres′sion [*compressus*]. 1. The state of being compressed. 2. The act of pressing or squeezing together.

cerebral c. Compression of the brain by any space-taking, intracranial lesion such as tumors, hemorrhage, etc.

c. atelectasis. See *atelectasis.*

c. fracture. See under *fracture.*

digital c. Compression of an artery by the fingers.

com·pres′sor [*compressus*]. 1. An instrument for compressing an artery or other part. 2. A muscle having a compressing function. See Table of Muscles in the Appendix.

c. bulbi proprius muscle. That portion of the bulbocavernous muscle in the male which ensheathes the bulb of the corpus cavernosum urethrae.

c. hemisphericum bulbi muscle. A portion of the bulbocavernosus muscle in the male underlying the compressor bulbi proprius and ensheathing the bulb of the corpus cavernosum urethrae and proximal part of the penile urethra.

c. labii muscle. A portion of the orbicularis oris muscle.

c. naris. The nasalis muscle.

c. nasi. Old term for *nasalis muscle.*

c. radicis penis. A portion of the bulbocavernosus muscle in the male passing around the root of the penis.

c. urethrae. Old term for the sphincter of the membranous urethra.

c. vaginae. Old term for the sphincter of the vagina.

c. venae dorsalis. A variable portion of the bulbocavernosus muscle which unites with its fellow of the opposite side in a tendon which passes over the dorsal vein of the penis.

Compton, Arthur Holly [*American physicist*, 1892–1954]. Widely known for his investigations of the earth's rotation and his discovery of the change in wavelength of scattered x rays; this latter phenomenon is known as the *Compton effect*. Also see scattering *collision*. Nobel laureate (1927).

com·pul′sion [L. *compulsio*, from *compellere*, to compel]. An act performed on irresistible impulse. *In psychiatry*, it is an act performed against the conscious will of the individual at the time it is performed, and usually stems from an obsession.

repetition c. A tendency in the unconscious part of the mind to recreate a previously experienced state of affairs in actions or feelings or both. The individual may or may not be aware of the tendency.

com·pul′sive per″son·al′i·ty. See under *personality*.

co′mus [G. *komē*, luminous tail of a comet]. A crescentic patch of yellow near the optic disk; seen in high myopia.

con- [L., with]. 1. A prefix meaning *with, together*. 2. *In chemistry*, a prefix denoting *a substance found with a substance*.

co·na′ri·um [G. *kōnos*, cone]. Old term for pineal *body*.

co·na′tion [L. *conari*, to try]. The exertive power of the mind, including will and desire; a special act or exercise of the exertive power.

Concato, Luigi Maria [*Italian physician*, 1825–82]. Remembered for his excellent description of tuberculous inflammation of serous membranes, especially of polyserositis of the pericardium, pleura, and peritoneum in the absence of valvular disease (1881).

con′cave [L. *concavus*, hollow, vaulted]. Possessing a curved, depressed surface; opposed to *convex*. —**concav′ity,** *n.*

con·ceive′ [L. *concipere*, to take in]. Become pregnant.

con·cen·tra′tion [L. *con*, with; G. *kentron*, center]. A measure for the composition of solutions. Various systems of notation are in use. The most common are: grams of solute per 100 grams of solution (weight per cent) or per 100 milliliters of solution (weight volume per cent), and mole of solute per liter of solution (molarity).

mean corpuscular hemoglobin c. An index obtained by dividing the hemoglobin in g. per cent by the volume in packed cells in ml. per cent.

threshold c. The molecular concentration of a substance which produces a minimum response when an end organ is stimulated.

con·cen′tric [L. *con-*, with; G. *kentron*, center]. Having a common center.

con·cep′tion [L. *conceptus*, from *concipere*]. 1. The fecundation of the ovum by the spermatozoon, occurring in the human female usually about the twelfth to fifteenth day after the first day of menstrual flow. 2. The power or act of mentally forming ideas, especially abstract ideas. —**conceptive,** *adj.*

imperative c. Old term for obsession.

con·cep′tus [*conceptus*]. That which is conceived; a fetus.

con′cha (kong′kuh) (pl. *conchae*) [G. *kogchē*, mussel]. 1. A shell; a shell-like organ, as the hollow part of the external ear. 2. Any one of the three nasal conchae; a medial projection of thin bone from the lateral wall of the nasal cavity, covered by mucous membrane and designated by position as superior, middle, or inferior. Also called *turbinate bone*. See Plate 12. See Table of Bones in the Appendix. —**conchal,** *adj.*

c. sphenoidalis. A thin bony plate forming one lateral half of the anterior and inferior surface of the body of the sphenoid. Each originally forms as a hollow ossicle containing the rudiment of a sphenoidal sinus. In the adult skull the concha becomes fused with the remainder of the sphenoid and with the ethmoid and palatine bones. Also called *ossicle of Bertin*.

con′chi·nine (kong′ki·neen, ·nin). See *quinidine*.

con·chi′tis (kong·kigh′tis) [*kogchē;* G. *-itis*, inflammation]. Inflammation of a concha.

con′cho·tome (kong′ko·tohm) [*kogchē;* G. *tomos*, cutting]. An instrument for the surgical removal of the turbinate bones.

con·com′i·tant [L. *concomitari*, to accompany]. Accompanying.

con′cre·ment [L. *concrementum*, from *concrescere*, to grow together]. Concretion.

con·cres′cence [*concrescere*]. 1. A growing together of the roots of two teeth. 2. A process by which the formative embryonic cells of the germ ring converge and fuse at the blastopore to form the axial part of the embryo during gastrulation. Syn., *convergence*.

con·cre′tio cor′dis [*concrescere;* L. *cor*, heart]. See adhesive *pericarditis*.

con·cre′tion [*concrescere*]. 1. A calculus. 2. Union of parts normally separate, as the fingers. 3. *In dentistry*, a deposit.

prostatic c. See *amyloid bodies* under *body*.

con·cus′sion [L. *concussio*, concussion]. Shock; the state of being shaken; a severe shaking or jarring of a part; also, the morbid state resulting from such a jarring.

air c. Aerial compression generated at the moment of detonation of a high explosive. See *blast*.

c. of conjunctiva. Injury to the conjunctiva by a blow.

c. of the brain. A condition produced by a fall or blow on the head, and marked by unconsciousness, feeble pulse, cold skin, pallor, at times the involuntary discharge of feces and urine; this is followed by partial stupor, vomiting, headache, and eventual recovery. In severe cases, inflammation of the brain or a condition of feeblemindedness may follow.

c. of the labyrinth. Deafness and tinnitus from a blow or an explosion.

c. of the spinal cord. A condition caused by severe shock of the spinal column, with or without appreciable lesion of the cord. It leads to functional disturbances analogous to railway spine.

con″den·sa′tion [L. *condensare*, to condense]. 1. Making more compact or dense. 2. The changing of a gaseous substance to a liquid, or a liquid to a solid. 3. *In chemistry*, the union of two or more molecules by the linking of carbon atoms and the formation of more complex carbon chains. 4. The pathologic hardening, with or without contraction, of a soft organ or tissue. 5. *In dentistry*, the compression of gold pellets in building a gold-foil filling. 6. *In psychopathology*, a psychic mechanism whereby one idea becomes the symbolic expression of many incompatible, repressed ideas; the meaning of this symbol may not be clear to the conscious mind or to others.

con·dens′er [*condensare*]. 1. A lens or combination

of lenses used in microscopy for gathering and concentrating rays of light. 2. An apparatus for condensing gases. 3. An apparatus for the accumulation of electricity. 4. *In dentistry,* one of a number of instruments with a blunt serrated end, used to compress and pack amalgam or gold-foil filling materials. Syn., *plugger.*

Abbe's c. See Ernst *Abbe.*

current c. An apparatus for collecting the extra currents generated by an induction machine in operation; it combines these currents to form one of opposite direction to that of the battery current, and this, upon being transmitted to the core, demagnetizes it and thus increases the rapidity of the interruption and the strength of the induced current.

dark-field c. An apparatus attached to a microscope which reflects light through the microscopic field illuminating the object only, the surrounding field remaining unilluminated.

con·di'tion·ing [L. *conditio,* condition]. 1. *In psychology,* the process of attaching a new stimulus to an old response or a new response to an old stimulus. 2. The development of better physiologic condition through physical exercise.

con'dom [perhaps from *Conton,* English physician, 18th century, said to be the inventor]. A sheath worn over the penis during copulation for preventing conception or infection.

con·duct"i·bil'i·ty [L. *conducere,* to conduct]. 1. Capacity for being conducted. 2. Conductivity; conducting power.

centrifugal c. The power of carrying centrifugal impulses from the nervous centers to the periphery.

centripetal c. The power of conducting centripetal impulses from the periphery to the nervous centers.

con·duc'tion [L. *conductio,* from *conducere*]. The passage or transfer of electrons, heat, or sound waves through suitable media, or of nerve and muscle impulses through those tissues. **—conductiv'ity,** *n.*

aerotympanal c. Passage of sound vibrations from the external auditory meatus to the internal ear by air of the middle ear and by the tympanic membrane and ossicles. Also called *air c.*

air c. (a) Transmission of sound stimuli to the eardrum through the external auditory canal. (b) A test for hearing, using a watch or tuning forks at various distances from the ear. Abbreviated, A. C.

antidromic c. A conduction in the reverse direction from the normal.

bone c. Transmission of sound vibrations to the internal ear via the bones of the skull.

decremental c. A conduction in which the intensity of the impulse decreases progressively.

reflex c. The passage of a nerve impulse from the afferent to the efferent components of the reflex arc.

saltatory c. The passage of the action potential along peripheral axons which involves the serial excitation of the nodes of Ranvier by local circuits without significant activation of internodal segments. In the central nervous system, structures similar to nodes of Ranvier may exist; if so, there is possibility that this type of conduction occurs there as well. Syn., *saltatory transmission.*

con·duc'tor [*conducere*]. 1. A body or substance that transmits energy by direct molecular transfer; applied to carriers of heat, electric currents, and sound. 2. An instrument serving as a guide for the surgeon's knife.

con"du·pli·ca'to cor'po·re (kon"dew·pli·kay'to kor'po·ree) [L.]. With the body doubled on itself, said of a position of the fetus.

con"du·ran'gin (kon"dew·ran'jin, ·rang'ghin). A mixture of glycosides from condurango bark, occurring as amorphous yellow powder of an aromatic bitter taste, soluble in water, alcohol, and chloroform. Formerly used as a stomachic and astringent in chronic dyspepsia.

con"du·ran'go. The dried bark of *Marsdenia cundurango.* A bitter and astringent stomachic. Has been used in gastric carcinoma but has no specific effect.

con"dy·lar·thro'sis [G. *kondylos,* knuckle; *arthrōsis,* from *arthron,* joint; *-ōsis,* condition]. Old term for condyloid articulation or ellipsoid joint.

con'dyle (kon'dyle, ·dil) [*kondylos*]. Any rounded eminence such as occurs in the joints of many of the bones, especially the femur, humerus, and mandible. Deviations of the mandibular condyles forward, backward, upward, downward, and toward the right and left are referred to respectively as *procondylism, retrocondylism, supracondylism, infracondylism, dextrocondylism,* and *levocondylism.* **—condylar,** *adj.*

con"dy·lec'to·my [*kondylos;* G. *ektomē,* excision]. Excision of a condyle.

con·dyl'i·on [G. *kondylion,* dim. of *kondylos*]. A point either at the medial or the lateral tip of a condyle of the mandible.

con'dy·lo-, condyl- [*kondylos*]. A combining form denoting a *knuckle, joint,* or *knob.*

con'dy·loid [*kondylos;* G. *eidos,* form]. Resembling or pertaining to a condyle.

con"dy·lo'ma (plural *condylomas, condylomata*) [G. *kondylōma,* knob]. A wartlike growth or tumor, usually near the anus or pudendum. **—condylom'atous,** *adj.*

c. acuminatum. The pointed condyloma or wart of the genital organs of nonsyphilitic origin. Syn., *verruca acuminata.*

c. latum. A moist, syphilitic papule occurring where two surfaces of skin come in opposition, often warty and vegetative, very communicable, and usually teeming with *Treponema pallidum.* Syn., *moist papule.*

syphilitic c. See *c.* latum.

con"dy·lot'o·my [*kondylos;* G. *tomē,* a cutting]. Osteotomy; division through the condyles of a bone.

cone [G. *kōnos,* cone]. 1. A solid body having a circle for its base and terminating in a point. 2. The mechanical element of the tooth crown. 3. One of the light-receptive, flask-shaped cells which, with the associated rods, forms an outer layer, the neuroepithelial layer of the retina. Also called *retinal c.* 4. Conus. **—con'ical, co'noid,** *adj.*

antipodal c. The cone of astral rays opposite the achromatic fibrils in mitosis.

cell c. See *pearl.*

c. of light. The triangular reflection from the normal tympanic membrane; also the bundle of light rays entering the pupil and forming the retinal image.

ectoplacental c. The thickened trophoblast of the early blastocyst of rodents, which forms the fetal placenta.

ether c. An apparatus used in the administration of ether.

graduated c. A cone-shaped body used for measuring the size of orifices of vessels, etc., especially in post-mortem examinations.

sarcoplasmic c. One of the conical masses of sarcoplasm at either end of the nucleus of a smooth muscle cell or of a cardiac muscle fiber.

vascular c. Lobule of the epididymis.

cone'nose" [*kōnos;* AS. *nosu*]. Any bloodsucking bug of the Triatomidae.

conestron. Trade-mark for a preparation of naturally occurring, water-soluble, conjugated estrogens of equine origin.

con·fab″u·la′tion [L. *confabulatio*, a discoursing together]. The fabrication of ready answers and fluent recitals of fictitious occurrences; generally, a component of the amnestic *syndrome*.

con·fec′tion [L. *confectio*, a composing]. *In pharmacy*, a soft mass of sugar and water, or of honey; used as an excipient with a prescribed medicinal substance. Syn., *electuary*. Also called *conserve*.

con·fer′tus [L., from *confercire*, to cram together]. Pressed together, dense, crowded; applied to cutaneous eruptions.

con·fine′ment [L. *confinium*, common boundary]. Lying-in; giving birth to a child; accouchement.

con′flict [L. *conflictus*, from *confligere*, to strike together]. *In psychiatry*, the clash of pure instinct with various psychic forces in its attempt to discharge its energies without modification, or between opposing forces within the psyche, as wishes.

con′flu·ence [L. *confluere*, to flow together]. A flowing together; a uniting, as of neighboring pustules.

con′flu·ens si′nu·um (kon′floo·enz sin′yoo·um) [BNA]. Confluence of the sinuses; the dilated junction of the superior sagittal, the straight, the occipital, and the transverse sinuses of the dura mater: formerly called *torcular Herophili*. See Plate 17.

con′flu·ent [*confluere*]. 1. Running together; the opposite of *discrete*. 2. *In anatomy*, coalesced or blended; applied to two or more bones originally separate, but subsequently formed into one.

con·fo′cal [L. *con-*, with; *focus*, hearth]. Having the same focus. See *parfocal*.

con″fron·ta′tion [*con;* L. *frons*, face]. A method for measuring visual fields in which the patient sits on the same level three feet from the examiner and fixes with one eye on the examiner's corresponding eye. The examiner then raises his hands until he just sees them. Any movement at this point should be perceived readily by the patient.

con·fu′sion [L. *confusio*, from *confundere*, to mix together]. 1. State of mental bewilderment. 2. A mixing or confounding.

con·fu′sion col′ors. A set of colors so chosen that they cannot be distinguished by one who is color-blind.

con·fu′sion let′ters. Test type letters, such as C, G, O, or F, P, T, liable to be mistaken for one another.

cong. *Congius;* a gallon.

con″ge·la′tion [L. *congelatio*, a congealing]. 1. Freezing; frostbite; intense cold or its effect on the animal economy or any organ or part. 2. Coagulation.

con′ge·ner [L., of the same race or kind]. 1. A person, animal, plant, part, or thing allied by origin, nature, or function to another. 2. A congenerous muscle. —**congener′ic, congen′erous,** *adj.*

con·gen′i·tal [L. *congenitus*, born together with]. Existing at birth.

con·ges′tion [L. *congestio*, from *congerere*, to heap up]. An abnormal collection of blood in a part or organ; hyperemia. —**congested, congestive,** *adj.*

passive c. Hyperemia of a part as the result of deficiency in the return of venous blood.

pleuropulmonary c. Congestion of the lungs marked by symptoms similar to those of pleurisy. Also called *pulmonary c., Potain's type of c.*

con′gi·us [L., gallon]. A term frequently employed in the apothecaries' measure meaning a gallon. Abbreviated, C, C., c, c., cong.

con·glo′bate [L. *conglobare*, to gather into a ball]. Forming a rounded mass.

con·glom′er·ate [L. *conglomerare*, to crowd together]. Massed together; aggregated. —**conglom′erate, conglomera′tion,** *n.*

con·glu′tin [L. *conglutinare*, to glue together]. A simple protein of the globulin type; found in lupines, almonds, beans, and seeds of various leguminous plants.

con·glu′ti·nant [*conglutinare*]. Adhesive; promoting union, as of the edges of a wound.

con·glu″ti·na′tion [*conglutinare*]. Abnormal union of two contiguous surfaces or bodies. See also *conglutinin.*

con·glu′ti·nin [L. *conglutinare*, to glue together]. A nonspecific substance in the serums of certain animal species; it causes or aids in the agglomeration or lysis of certain cells or particles previously sensitized with antiserum and complement. Commonly found in bovine serums.

Con′go red (C.C.). An acid aniline dye of the azo group; used as a histologic stain and as an indicator, usually in 0.1% aqueous solution, for estimating free mineral acids, especially in the presence of organic acids. It is also used to test for amyloidosis, in the determination of plasma and blood volumes, and as a cytoplasmic stain. Also called *Congo; cotton red A, B,* or *C; direct red C, R,* or *Y.*

con′gress [L. *congressus*, a coming together]. 1. An assemblage for deliberative purpose. 2. A coming together.

sexual c. Coitus, or sexual intercourse.

con·hy′drine (kon·high′dreen, ·drin). A crystalline alkaloid, $C_8H_{17}ON$; obtained from conium.

co·nic′e·ine (ko·niss′ee·een, ·in, kon·i·see′in, ko′niseen). A liquid alkaloid, $C_8H_{15}N$, in conium.

co·nid′i·o-, co·nid′i- [G. *konis*, dust]. A combining form denoting *conidium.*

co·nid′i·o·phore″ [*konis;* G. *phoros*, bearing]. The mycelial thread of a fungus which bears conidia.

co·nid′i·o·spore″ [*konis;* G. *sporos*, seed]. A conidium.

co·nid′i·um (pl. *conidia*) [*konis*]. An asexual spore cut from the end of a fungus filament. —**conidial,** *adj.*

co′ni·ine (ko′nee·een, ·in, ko′neen). $C_8H_{17}N$. The most important of the five alkaloids of conium; it is a liquid but forms crystalline salts.

c. hydrobromide. $C_8H_{17}N.HBr$. Soluble in water; has been used in spasmodic disorders.

c. hydrochloride. $C_8H_{17}N.HCl$. Formerly employed like coniine hydrobromide.

co′ni·ism [G. *kōneion*, hemlock]. Poisoning by conium. It begins with paralysis of the legs and extends to the arms and respiratory muscles, leading to unconsciousness and death.

co′ni·o-, co′ni- [G. *konis*, dust]. A combining form signifying *dust.*

co″ni·om′e·ter. See *konimeter.*

co″ni·o′sis [*konis;* G. *-ōsis*, condition]. A disease or morbid condition due to inhalation of dust.

co″ni·o·spor″i·o′sis. Acute pneumonitis from inhalation of spores of the fungus *Coniosporium corticale.*

co′ni·um [G. *kōneion*, hemlock]. Poison hemlock, *Conium maculatum*, the fruit and leaves of which were formerly official. Both parts of the plant contain the alkaloids coniine, methyl-coniine, conhydrine, pseudoconhydrine, and coniceine, to which the activity of conium is due. Conium produces motor paralysis without loss of sensation or consciousness; toxic dose causes death by paralysis of the organs of respiration. It has been used in the treatment of spasmodic disorders; the fluidextract and the salt coniine hydrobromide were popular dosage forms.

con″i·za′tion [G. *kōnos*, cone]. Excision, or reaming out, as of a diseased endocervix by means of a fine, high-frequency current.

con″ju·ga′ta ve′ra [L.]. The true conjugate. The distance from the middle of the sacral promontory to the upper margin of the symphysis pubis.

con′ju·gate [L. *conjugare*, to yoke together]. 1. The anteroposterior diameter of the inlet of the pelvis, the plane of the inlet being regarded as an ellipse. 2. Any diameter of the pelvic inlet.

obstetric c. The minimum anteroposterior diameter of the pelvic inlet; usually a little shorter than conjugata vera.

true c. Conjugata vera.

con′ju·gate. Yoked or coupled.

con″ju·ga′tion [*conjugare*]. 1. The process in lower organisms, analogous to fertilization, involving the fusion of gametes or the temporary union of individuals with exchange of nuclear material. 2. *In biochemistry*, the reaction by which an organic compound foreign to the body combines with a substance naturally available in the body to produce the elimination form of the foreign compound.

con″junc·ti′va [L. *conjunctivus*, serving to connect]. The mucous membrane covering the anterior portion of the globe of the eye, reflected upon the lids and extending to their free edges. Its parts are called palpebral and bulbar or ocular. —**conjunctival,** *adj*.

bulbar c. That covering the anterior third of the eyeball, from the retrotarsal fold to the margin of the cornea. Also called *ocular c.*

palpebral c. The conjunctiva of the eyelid.

con·junc″ti·vi′tis [*conjunctivus;* G. *-itis*, inflammation]. Inflammation of the conjunctiva

actinic c. A form caused by repeated flashes of bright light or ultraviolet radiation, characterized by erythema and edema of the conjunctivae: commonly seen in welders.

acute contagious c. Pinkeye.

allergic c. Characterized by mild irritation and more or less abundant mucus; accompanies other symptoms of hay fever, but frequently occurs without rhinitis.

catarrhal c. The most common form, usually mild, resulting from cold or irritation. Also called *acute catarrhal c.*

chronic c. Any conjunctivitis which has become chronic; specifically, chronic catarrhal conjunctivitis in which there is usually an infective element and also an irritative element.

c. atrophicans diffusa. A rare complication of poikiloderma vasculare atrophicans, in which the conjunctiva becomes milky and clouded.

c. catarrhalis aestiva. See vernal *c.*

c. granulosa. See *trachoma.*

c. medicamentosa. Conjunctivitis caused by a drug, usually by direct contact.

diphtheritic c. A specific purulent inflammation of the conjunctiva due to the *Corynebacterium diphtheriae.*

divers′ c. See inclusion *c.*

eczematous c. See phlyctenular *c.*

Egyptian c. See *trachoma.*

follicular c. A form characterized by numerous round, pinkish bodies found in the retrotarsal fold.

gonorrheal c. A severe form of purulent conjunctivitis caused by infection with gonococci.

hemorrhagic c. See *pinkeye.*

hypertrophic c. Chronic catarrhal conjunctivitis attended with enlargement of the conjunctival papillae.

inclusion c. An acute purulent conjunctivitis, caused by a virus of large particle size (*Chlamydozoon oculogenitale*), and having a different clinical appearance in the neonate than in the adult. It is transmitted to the infant from the mother's genital tract during birth, and characterized by swelling and redness of the lids, purulent discharge, and chemosis, involving both eyes. In the adult the condition is often acquired in swimming pools; it is less severe, shows less discharge, but larger papillae and preauricular adenopathy, frequently involving one eye only. Clinical diagnosis is confirmed in both instances by finding of epithelial-cell inclusion bodies in conjunctival scrapings. Also called *swimming-pool c., swimmer's c., divers' c., inclusion blennorrhea, paratrachoma.*

infectious c. A conjunctivitis caused by bacteria, viruses, or fungi, which may or may not be contagious.

klieg c. A condition caused by ultraviolet rays from klieg lights used in motion-picture studios. Also called *klieg eyes.*

lithiasis c. Irritation of the conjunctiva due to deposition of calcareous matter in the tissue of the palpebral conjunctiva.

phlyctenular c. A nodular affection occurring, characteristically in children who show some metabolic defect or tuberculin sensitivity, as an allergic response by the conjunctiva or cornea to the endogenous toxin or allergen. Also called *eczematous c., phlyctenular, scrofulous,* or *strumous ophthalmia.* Also see *phlyctenular keratitis.*

purulent c. Conjunctivitis characterized by a thick, creamy discharge.

scrofulus c. See phlyctenular *c.*

spring c. See vernal *c.*

subacute c. Redness and thickening of the conjunctiva, largely confined to the conjunctiva of the lids and fornixes, a scanty secretion of mucus, with some pus corpuscles, due to the presence of a bacillus.

swimmers′ c. See inclusion *c.*

swimming-pool c. See inclusion *c.*

trachomatous c. Conjunctivitis associated with trachoma, characterized by a subepithelial cellular infiltration with a follicular distribution. See also *trachoma.*

vernal c. A form recurring each spring or summer and disappearing with frost. Syn., *c. catarrhalis aestiva.* Also called *spring catarrh, spring c.*

con·junc″tiv·o′ma [*conjunctivus;* G. *-ōma*, tumor]. A tumor consisting of conjunctival tissue; it occurs on the eyelid.

con″junc·tiv′o·plas″ty [*conjunctivus;* G. *plassein*, to form]. Plastic surgery of the conjunctiva.

Conn's technic for soil bacteria. See under *stain.*

Connell, Frank Gregory [*American surgeon*, 1875–]. Introduced a type of suture in enterorrhaphy, using only one row of inverting through-and-through stitches.

co′no-, con- [G. *kōnos*, cone]. A combining form denoting *cone.*

Conolly, John [*Irish physician in England*, 1794–1866]. Remembered for his championship of the no-restraint system for the humane treatment of the insane in England (1839).

co″no·my·oi′din (ko″no·migh·oy′din, ·my′oy·din) [*kōnos;* G. *mys*, muscle; *eidos*, form]. A contractile protoplasmic material found in the cones of the retina.

Co″no·rhi′nus [*kōnos;* G. *rhis*, nose]. Synonym for *Panstrongylus.*

con·quin′a·mine (kon·kwin′uh·meen, ·min). An alkaloid of cuprea bark.

Conradi, Andrew Christian [*Norwegian physician*, 1809–69]. Remembered for his description of a line drawn from the base of the xiphoid process to the point of the apex beat of the heart, marking the upper limit of percussion dullness of the left lobe of the liver.

con″san·guin′i·ty [L. *consanguinitas*, blood relationship]. The relationship arising from common parentage; blood relationship. —**consanguineous,** *adj*.

con′scious·ness [L. *conscius*, knowing something in one's self]. State of being aware of one's own existence, of one's own mental states, and of the impressions made upon one's senses; ability to take cognizance of sensations. —**conscious,** *adj*.

double c. That morbid condition in which there are two separate and alternating states of mental consciousness, in either one of which the events that have occurred in the other state are not remembered by the patient.

con·sen′su·al (kon·sen′shoo·ul) [L. *consensus*, agreement]. Pertaining to involuntary excitation by stimulation; especially, the constriction of both pupils when the retina of one eye is stimulated.

con·sent′ [L. *consentire*, to consent]. *In legal medicine*, willing participation in unnatural or illegal intercourse.

con·serv′a·tive [L. *conservare*, to retain]. Aiming at the preservation and restoration of injured parts; as conservative surgery or dentistry.

con·sist′ence [L. *consistere*, to stand still]. Degree of density or hardness.

con·sol′i·dant [L. *consolidare*, to make firm]. Tending to heal or promoting the healing of wounds or fractures; favoring cicatrization. —**consol′idant,** *n*.

con·sol″i·da′tion [*consolidare*]. Process of becoming firm or solid, as a lung in pneumonia.

con·sper′gent. A dusting powder, such as starch or lycopodium, often used on pills or suppositories to prevent their sticking to each other.

con′stant [L. *constare*, to stand firm]. Fixed, not changing.

constant. 1. *In physics*, a property which remains numerically the same, and which may serve as a unit of measurement. 2. *In mathematics*, a quantity, having a definite and fixed value in a certain stage of investigation; an **absolute constant** retains the same value under all circumstances.

decay c. of radioactive substances. The percentage of atoms of any radioactive substance that will disintegrate per unit of time. In any measurable quantity of radon 16.6% of the atoms present will change within 24 hours. Thus, when the decay rate (per hour, per day, or per year) of a given radioactive substance is known, the amount that will be present at a future time can be calculated from the amount on hand by means of the formula

$$Q = Q_o e^{-kt}$$

where Q_o is the amount at the present time, Q the amount at a future time t days hence, k the decay constant per day, and e a constant (the base of natural logarithms).

dielectric c. *In electricity*, inductivity; specific inductive capacity.

disintegration c. See decay *constant* of radioactive substances.

dissociation c. The equilibrium constant (K) pertaining to a reversible reaction in which a compound breaks up into two or more products.

equilibrium c. The constant, designated K, pertaining to a reversible chemical reaction; the product of the concentrations or activities of the reaction products divided by the product of the concentrations or activities of the reactants, each concentration or activity term being raised to the power of the number of molecules (or ions) involved in the reaction.

Michaelis c. The substrate concentration, in moles per liter, at which an enzymatic reaction proceeds at one-half the maximum rate. It is designated K_m and is a measure of the affinity of an enzyme for its substrate.

quantum c. Symbol, *h*. Numerical value is 6.55×10^{-27} erg-sec. Also called *Planck's c*.

Constantinus Africanus (Constantine) [*Carthaginian monk and physician in Italy*, 1015–87]. Exercised a profound influence on European medicine by his writings and translations of Greek, Arabic, and Jewish writers.

con″stel·la′tion [L. *constellatio*, a collection of stars]. *In psychiatry*, a group of allied thoughts held together by a common emotional experience around a nuclear idea.

con″sti·pa′tion [L. *constipatio*, from *constipare*, to press closely together]. A condition in which the bowels are evacuated at long intervals or with difficulty; costiveness.

atonic c. That due to decreased tonus of the colon.

spastic c. That due to increased tonus of the colon.

con″sti·tu′tion [L. *constitutio*, from *constituere*, to fix]. 1. Genotype. 2. *In medicine*, the total individuality of the person, including his inherited qualities and the cumulative effects of his reactions to all the environmental factors which influenced his physical and emotional development.

allergic c. The inherited tendency to develop allergy.

lymphatic c. See *lymphatism*.

con·stric′tor [L. *constrictum*, from *constringere*, to bind together]. Any muscle that contracts or tightens any part of the body. See Table of Muscles in the Appendix.

c. muscles of pharynx. There are three of these: the superior, middle, and inferior. See Table of Muscles in the Appendix.

c. radicis penis. A portion of the bulbocavernosus muscle, a few fibers encircling the root of the penis.

c. vaginae. A portion of the deep transverse perineal muscle in the female.

con·sult′ant [L. *consultare*, to take counsel]. A consulting physician; one summoned by the physician in attendance to give counsel in a case.

con″sul·ta′tion [*consultare*]. A deliberation between two or more physicians concerning the diagnosis and the proper method of treatment in a case.

con·sump′tion [L. *consumptio*, from *consumere*, to consume]. An old term, formerly used to designate progressive tuberculosis. —**consumptive,** *adj*.

galloping c. Popular term for a rapidly fatal form of pulmonary tuberculosis. Also called *florid phthisis*.

potter's c. Silicosis.

con′tact [L. *contactum*, from *contingere*, to touch]. 1. Direct or indirect exposure to a source of infection usually to a person affected with a contagious disease. 2. A person who has been exposed to a contagious disease. —**contac′tile, contac′tual,** *adj*.

absence of c. *In dentistry*, a condition in which the proximal surfaces have been ground or worn away so that they do not touch; also occurs when a tooth has become malposed or has erupted in malposition; diastema.

adequate c. *In epidemiology*, that degree of contact between one person and another, such that if the first person is infectious and the other is susceptible, the latter will become infected.

complete c. The touching of the entire proximal surfaces of two neighboring teeth. May be produced naturally through mastication or artificially by grinding.

proximal c. The touching of the adjacent surfaces of two teeth.

con·tac′tant [*contactum*]. Any one of the thousands of substances (allergens) which produce manifestations of hypersensitivity by means of direct contact with the skin or the mucosa.

con′tact bed. A large open basin containing a layer of coke or cinders, used for purifying sewage. The sewage is brought into contact with bacteria, which set up rapid decomposition and destruction of the organic matter. Also see *septic tank*.

con·ta′gion [L. *contagio*, from *contingere*, to touch]. 1. The process whereby disease spreads from one person to another, by direct or indirect human contact or by an intermediate agency. 2. The germ or virus which causes a communicable disease. —**contagious,** *adj.;* **contagiousness,** *n.*

con·tam″i·na′tion [L. *contaminare*, to bring into contact, defile]. 1. Soiling with bacteria. 2. *In psychology*, the fusion of words (Freud). 3. *In radiobiology*, the presence of radioactive material in an area where it is unwanted or harmful. —**contam′inating,** *adj., n.;* **contam′inant,** *n.;* **contam′inate,** *v.t.*

conteben. A trade-mark for *amithiozone*.

con″tem·pla′ti·o (kon″tem·play′shee·o) [L., a viewing]. Ecstasy.

con·tem′pla·tive [L. *contemplari*, to contemplate]. *In psychopathology*, a sexual pervert who induces an orgasm through phantasy.

con′tent [L. *contentum*, from *continere*, to contain]. That which is contained; especially in psychology, **latent content** refers to that part of a dream which is symbolic, disguised, or hidden; **manifest content** refers to the form or outer appearance of a dream.

con·tig′u·ous [L. *contiguus*, bordering upon]. In contact, or adjacent.

con′ti·nence [L. *continentia*, from *continere*, to hold back, refrain]. Self-restraint, especially in regard to sexual intercourse. —**continent,** *adj.*

con·tin′gen·cy ta′ble. A two-way frequency table showing the frequency of occurrence of classifications of one variable for specified classification of the other variable; a cross-classification table.

con·tor′tion [L. *contortio*, from *contorquere*, to twist]. A twisting or writhing, as of the body.

con′tour [F., from L. *cum*, with; *tornare*, to turn]. The line or contour that bounds, defines, or terminates a figure.

con′tour. *In operative dentistry*, to effect the restoration of lost parts of teeth by building them up with gold, etc.

con′toured [*contour*]. Having an irregular but smoothly undulating surface, like that of a relief map; said of a bacterial culture.

con′tra- [L., against]. A prefix meaning *against, contrary*, or *in opposition*.

con′tra-an′gles. Two or more bends in the shaft or shank of an instrument which place the distal or working end in line with the axis of the handle or proximal end.

con″tra·cep′tion [*contra;* L. *conceptio*, conception]. Prevention of conception.

con″tra·cep′tive [*contra; conceptio*]. An agent which prevents conception, such as medicated jelly in the vagina, the condom or thin rubber sheath for the penis, the cervical pessary or soft rubber diaphragm to cover the mouth of the uterus. —**contracep′tive,** *adj.*

con·tract′ [L. *contractum*, from *contrahere*, to draw together]. 1. Draw the parts together; shrink. 2. Acquire by contagion or infection.

con·trac′tile (kon·track′tile, ·til) [*contractum*]. Having the power or tendency to contract.

con″trac·til′i·ty [*contractum*]. The property of shortening upon the application of a stimulus.

faradic c. Ability to contract in response to induction shocks.

galvanic c. Ability to contract in response to galvanic or direct currents.

idiomuscular c. Localized unpropagated contractions that are peculiar to degenerated muscles.

neuromuscular c. Normal contractility as distinguished from idiomuscular contractility.

con·trac′tion [*contractum*]. Shortening, especially of the fibers of muscle tissue. Abbreviated, C.

aerobic c. A phase of muscular contraction in which oxygen is utilized.

allasotonic c. Contraction of muscle against a variable tension.

anaerobic c. A phase of muscular contraction utilizing no oxygen.

anodal closure c. The contraction resulting from excitation with galvanic current upon closing the circuit with the anode, the stigmatic testing electrode. Abbreviated, ACC, AnCC.

anodal opening c. The contraction resulting from excitation with galvanic current upon opening the circuit with the anode, the stigmatic testing electrode. Abbreviated, AOC, AnOC.

auxotonic c. Contraction of muscle against increasing tension.

Braxton Hicks c. A painless, intermittent uterine contraction occurring throughout pregnancy; valuable but not conclusive in diagnosing pregnancy.

cathodal closure c. The contraction resulting from excitation with galvanic current upon closing the circuit with the cathode, the stigmatic testing electrode. Abbreviated, CaCC, CCC.

cathodal opening c. The contraction resulting from excitation with galvanic current upon opening the circuit with the cathode, the stigmatic testing electrode. Abbreviated, CaOC.

clonic c. Alternate muscular contraction and relaxation.

c. remainder. Residual contraction persisting in a muscle after withdrawal of the stimulus.

fibrillary c. Incoordinate contraction of different muscle fibers in a muscle.

fractionate c. Contraction of fractions of syncytial heart muscle.

front tap c. Contraction of the gastrocnemius muscle when the muscles of the front of the leg are tapped.

hourglass c. A contraction of an organ, as the stomach or uterus, at the middle.

hunger contractions. Peristaltic movements of the stomach caused by emptiness. They extend from the lower esophagus to the duodenum.

idiomuscular c. Maintained local shortening resulting from a single direct stimulus; more correctly called a contracture.

isometric c. (a) One showing mainly the changes in tension in a muscle, without any marked shortening. (b) Contraction of the heart, with all valves closed.

isotonic c. Contraction of a muscle, its tension remaining the same throughout the act.

myoclonic c. The convulsive spasmodic contraction of a muscle.

premature c. Extrasystole.

tetanic c. *In obstetrics*, a state of continued

contraction of the uterine muscle; occurs in prolonged labors, usually in the second stage. Results from a pathologic retraction ring. Abbreviated, Te.

tonic c. See tonic *spasm.*

vermicular c. Peristaltic contraction.

con′tract prac′tice. Partial or complete medical service furnished to an individual, or a group of individuals, by a physician, or a group of physicians, for compensation that has been mutually agreed upon.

con·trac′ture [L. *contractura,* from *contrahere,* to draw together]. 1. Shortening, as of muscle or scar tissue, producing distortion or deformity. 2. Retarded relaxation of muscle, as when it is injected with veratrin.

congenital c. Deformity resulting from contractures originating in utero.

Dupuytren's c. A painless, chronic contracture of the hand, marked by thickening of the digital processes and of the palmar fascia, and flexion of the fingers, especially of the third and fourth, upon the palm. The disease is of uncertain etiology, and affects chiefly adult males.

fatigue c. A form of myotatic contracture.

functional c. See hypertonic *c.*

hypertonic c. That due to continuous discharge of nervous impulses; disappears during sleep or anesthesia. Seen in spastic paralysis.

idiomuscular c. Persistent local shortening due to a mechanical blow on muscle.

ischemic c. Shortening of muscle due to interference with the blood supply. Also called *Volkmann's c.*

myostatic c. Assumption of shortened length after fixation in cast or tendon section with innervation intact.

myotatic c. That occurring in a degenerating muscle when tapped or suddenly stretched; may also occur when a fatigued muscle is struck.

organic c. One that persists even when the person is unconscious.

Tiegel's c. One continuing after cessation of stimulation, observed in isolated muscle preparations to which supramaximal stimuli are applied successively until the base line of the twitch is kept at a steady level.

con″tra·fis·su′ra (kon″truh·fi·shoor′uh) [L. *contra,* opposite to; *fissura,* fissure]. Cranial fissure or fracture produced by a blow upon the skull at a point distant from, or opposite to, the lesion.

con″tra·in″di·ca′tion, con″tra·in′di·cant [*contra;* L. *indicare,* to indicate]. A symptom, indication, or condition in which a remedy or a method of treatment is inadvisable.

con″tra·lat′er·al [*contra;* L. *lateralis,* from *latus,* side]. Opposite; acting in unison with a similar part on the opposite side of the body.

con″tra·stim′u·lant [*contra;* L. *stimulare,* to goad]. Counteracting the effect of a stimulus; depressing; sedative. —**contrastim′ulant, contrastimulus,** *n.*

con″tre·coup′ (kawn″truh·koo′. *See* Notes § 35) [F.]. Counterstroke; injury of a part opposite to that struck, due to transmission of the shock, especially when the force is exerted against an organ or part containing fluid, as the skull, stomach, intestine, or urinary bladder. See coup-contrecoup *injury.*

con″trec·ta′tion [L. *contrectatio,* from *contrectare,* to touch]. 1. The impulse to approach and caress a person of the opposite sex. 2. Foreplay preparatory to coition.

con·trol′ [F. *contrôler,* from *contre,* counter; *rôle,* roll]. A standard by which to check observations, and insure the validity of their results. May refer to a **control animal** (one used experimentally) or to a **control experiment.**

Diack c. A sterilization detector consisting of a tablet of chemical materials contained in a hermetically sealed glass tube; when placed with a load in a steam sterilizer, the detector indicates adequate conditions for sterilization by melting, fusing, and changing its shape.

con·trol′ ex·per′i·ment. One used to check or verify other experiments, using conditions identical except for one factor.

con·trude′ [L. *contrudere,* to thrust, push, crowd]. Crowd together, as to crowd the teeth into an abnormal lingual curve on any part of the line of the dental arch. *Obs.*

con·tu′sion [L. *contusio,* from *contundere,* to crush]. A bruise; an injury in which the skin is not broken. —**contuse′,** *v.*

co′nus (pl. *coni*) [G. *kōnos,* cone]. 1. A cone. 2. A crescentic patch of atrophic choroid tissue near the optic papilla, most common in myopia.

c. arteriosus. The cone-shaped eminence of the right ventricle of the heart, from which the pulmonary artery arises. See Plate 5.

c. elasticus. The elastic upper part of the cricothyroid membrane.

c. medullaris. The conelike termination of the spinal cord, the pia mater of which continues as the filum terminale.

c. terminalis. See *c.* medullaris.

c. tubulosi. Old term for a renal pyramid.

con″va·les′cence [L. *convalescere,* to recover from a disease]. 1. The restoration of health after disease. 2. The time spent in recovery. —**convalescent,** *adj., n.*

con·val″la·mar′in (kon·val″uh·mair′in, kon″vuh·lam′ur·in). 1. A glycoside obtained from *Convallaria majalis.* It is used as a cardiac stimulant but is said to be of no great value. 2. A mixture of the glycosides of convallaria used as an uncertain cardiac stimulant.

con″val·la′ri·a [L. *convallis,* valley]. The dried rhizome and roots of *Convallaria majalis,* the lily of the valley. Its properties are due to convallarin, $C_{34}H_{62}O_{11}$, convallamarin, $C_{23}H_{44}O_{12}$, and convallatoxin, all glycosides which give an unreliable digitalislike action.

con″val·lar′in (kon″vuh·lair′in, kon·val′uh·rin). A crystalline purgative glycoside derived from *Convallaria majalis.*

con·val″la·tox′in. A glycoside derived from *Convallaria majalis.*

con·vec′tion [L. *convectio,* from *convehere,* to carry together]. A transmission or carrying, as of heat.

con·ver′gence [L. *convergere,* to incline together]. 1. Inclination or direction toward a common point, center, or focus, as of the axes of vision upon the near point. 2. Concrescence. 3. Coming together of a group of afferent nerves upon a motoneuron of the ventral horn of the spinal cord. —**convergent,** *adj.*

con·ver′sion [L. *conversio,* from *convertere,* to turn around]. 1. *In psychiatry,* a mental defense mechanism whereby unconscious emotional conflict is transformed into physical disability. The affected part always has symbolic meaning pertinent to the nature of the conflict in contrast to the physiologic responses to strong emotion, which are without symbolic meaning. See conversion *reaction.* 2. *In obstetrics,* an alteration in the presentation of the fetus to facilitate delivery.

con·ver′tin. A highly stable blood factor required for the optimal conversion of prothrombin to thrombin by thromboplastin. It is believed variously to be activated by thromboplastin from a precursor, or to be a combination of thromboplastin with the precursor. Syn., *serum prothrombin conversion accelerator (SPCA), cothromboplastin, stable prothrombin conversion accelerator, stable component, proconvertin-convertin, factor VII.*

con·vex' [L. *convexus*, convex]. Rounded, as a swelling of round or spherical form on the external surface; gibbous; opposed to concave. —**convex'-ity,** *n.*

con·vex'o-con'cave. Having one convex and one concave surface.

con·vex'o-con'vex. Having two convex surfaces; biconvex, as a lens.

con'vo·lu"ted [L. *convolutum*, from *convolvere*, to roll together]. Folded in curves or contorted windings; coiled, as tubules.

con"vo·lu'tion [*convolutum*]. A fold, twist, or coil of any organ, especially any one of the prominent convex parts of the brain, separated from each other by depressions or sulci. See *gyrus.*

con·vol'vu·lin. $C_{31}H_{50}O_{16}$. A glycosidal resin, one of the chief constituents of the roots of jalap (*Exogonium purga*).

con·vul'sant [L. *convulsum*, from *convellere*, to shake]. A medicine that causes convulsions.

con·vul'sion [L. *convulsio*, from *convellere*]. An involuntary general paroxysm of muscular contraction. It is either tonic (without relaxation) or clonic (having alternate contractions of opposite groups of muscles). —**convulsive,** *adj.*, **convulsionary, convulsivant,** *n.*

audiogenic c. One induced by acoustic stimuli, such as the sound of a whistle. Also called *audio-epileptic seizure.* See reflex *epilepsy.*

epileptiform c. One characterized by total loss of consciousness.

febrile c. A convulsion accompanying fever, usually in children, but not necessarily caused by fever.

hysterical c. One due to hysteria; consciousness is only apparently lost.

infantile c. One due to a number of causes, such as rickets, exhaustion, cerebral birth injury; sometimes called screaming fits.

local c. One affecting one muscle, member, or part of a member.

mimetic c. A facial convulsion.

oscillating c. One in which the separate fibers of a muscle are affected successively and not simultaneously. Also called *oscillatory c.*

puerperal c. See *eclampsia.*

salaam c. Salaam spasm.

suffocative c. Laryngismus stridulus.

tetanic c. General tonic convulsions without loss of consciousness.

tonic c. See tonic *spasm.*

toxic c. One due to the action of some toxic agent upon the nervous system.

traumatic c. One due to brain injury.

uremic c. One that occurs in kidney disease due to retention in the blood of matter that should be eliminated by the kidney.

Cooke-Ponder method. See under *method.*

Cooley, Thomas Benton [*American physician*, 1871–1945]. Known for his description, with E. R. Witwer and O. P. Lee, of familial erythroblastic anemia occurring in Mediterranean peoples (1927). Known as *Cooley's anemia.* See *thalassemia.*

Coolidge, William David [*American physical chemist*, 1873–]. Known for his many contributions to the knowledge of physical chemistry and electricity, and for his invention of a highly evacuated x-ray tube, equipped with a hot filament cathode and tungsten anode, called *Coolidge tube.*

Cooper, Astley Paston [*English surgeon and anatomist*, 1768–1841]. Made outstanding contributions to the knowledge of hernia. He ligated the carotid artery (1805) and the external iliac artery (1808) for aneurysm, and attempted ligation of the abdominal aorta (1817). Described deafness due to obstruction of the auditory tube (1801), and also the anatomy of the thymus (1832). Drew attention to a tumor of the breast (1829), called *Cooper's tumor.* His name has been given to an ointment containing arsenic, to the fascia transversalis, the cellular layer beneath the dartos, the fibrous processes in the mammary gland, an irritable testis, and numerous operations which he performed. For *Cooper's method* for the reduction of a dislocated humerus, see *White's method* under Charles *White.*

Coopernail, George Peter [*American physician*, 1876–]. Described ecchymosis of the perineum and parts adjacent as indicative of fracture of the pelvis.

co·or"di·na'tion [L. *cum*, together with; *ordinare*, to regulate]. 1. The harmonious activity and proper sequence of those parts that cooperate in the performance of any function. 2. *In neurology*, the combination of nervous impulses in motor centers to insure cooperation of the appropriate muscles in a reaction.

coot'ie. The body louse: slang.

co"pa·hu'vic ac'id, co·pai'vic ac'id (ko·pay'vick, ko·py'vick). $C_{20}H_{30}O_2$. An almost colorless, crystalline substance obtained from copaiba. Sometimes called *copaibic acid.*

co·pai'ba (ko·pay'buh, ko·py'buh) [Sp. and Pg., of Tupian origin]. Balsam of copaiba. The oleoresin of *Copaifera* species (Leguminosae), native to South America. Has been used as stimulant, diuretic, diaphoretic, and expectorant; formerly was used in gonorrhea. See copaiba *mixture.*

co·pai'vic ac'id (ko·pay'vick, ko·py'vick). See *copahuvic acid.*

co'pal. Any of various resins obtained from certain trees of the Leguminosae, Dipterocarpaceae, and Coniferae, some of which may be used to prepare dental cavity varnishes.

copavin. Trade-mark for a capsule or tablet preparation containing codeine sulfate and papaverine hydrochloride.

co'pe·pod [G. *kōpē*, oar; *pous*, foot]. A small freshwater or salt-water crustacean. Some copepods are intermediate hosts to worms parasitic in man.

cop"i·o'pi·a (kop"ee·o'pee·uh, ko"pee·) [G. *kopos*, toil and trouble; *ōps*, eye]. Eyestrain; weariness of the eyes; asthenopia.

Cop'lin jar. A boxlike glass vessel with perpendicular grooves for holding microscopic slides apart during staining.

cop"o·dys·ki·ne'si·a (kop"o·dis·ki·nee'shuh, ·see·uh, ·zhuh, ·zee·uh, kop"o·dis·kigh·nee'·, ko"-po·) [*kopos;* G. *dys-*, hard; *kinēsis*, motion]. Occupational or occupation neurosis.

co"po·lym"er·i·za'tion. A polymerization which involves two or more distinct molecular species.

cop'per [AS. *coper*, ultimately from G. *Kypros*, Cyprus, famous in ancient times for its copper mines] (*cuprum*). Cu = 63.54. A reddish brown, malleable metal, various salts of which are used in medicine. In toxic doses they are gastrointestinal irritants. In therapeutic doses they are used as astringents in inflammation of mucous membranes. They are also employed as emetics, and, externally, as caustics. In certain nutritional anemias, particularly in infants, copper appears to enhance absorption of iron.

black c. oxide. CuO; a brownish black, amorphous powder. Formerly used as taeniafuge. Externally it was used as ointment in the treatment of chronic glandular induration. Syn., *c. monoxide.*

c. acetate. $Cu(C_2H_3O_2)_2$. Used in pulmonary diseases and locally as an astringent and fungicide.

c. acetoarsenite. Paris green, used as a pigment and an insecticide.

c. amalgam. A metallic filling material composed of copper and mercury.

c. arsenite. Approximately $CuHAsO_3$; formerly used as an intestinal antiseptic; also recommended for anemia.

c. chloride. $CuCl_2.2H_2O$, green crystals, very soluble in water. Occasionally used in place of copper sulfate.

c. citrate. The cupric salt, containing 34–36% of copper; occurs as a green or bluish green, crystalline powder, slightly soluble in water. It possesses the astringent and antiseptic properties of copper salts and has been used in the treatment of conjunctivitis and trachoma.

c. lactate. $Cu(C_3H_5O_3)_2.2H_2O$, greenish blue crystals, soluble in water. Employed as a tonic, also as an injection in strumous and other buboes.

c. monoxide. See black *c.* oxide.

c. nose. See *acne* rosacea.

c. nucleinate. A compound of nuclein and copper containing 6% of copper; it occurs as a fine powder and is used in chronic conjunctivitis. Also called *cuprol.*

c. oleate. $Cu(C_{18}H_{33}O_2)_2$, a compound of 10% copper oxide dissolved in oleic acid, forming a greenish blue, granular powder, soluble in ether. Applied to indolent ulcers as a 10–20% ointment.

c. phenolsulfonate. $(C_6H_4.OH.SO_3)_2Cu.6H_2O$, blue crystals, soluble in water. Has been used in the treatment of diarrhea, and locally as a styptic, hemostatic, and antiseptic. Syn., *sulfocarbolate.*

c. sulfate (*cupri sulfas*). $CuSO_4.5H_2O$, occurring as blue crystals or powder, soluble in water, valuable as an emetic, tonic, and astringent. Dose, as an emetic, 0.13–0.32 Gm. (2–5 gr.); as a tonic, 10–30 mg. (1/6–1/2 gr.).

c. sulfocarbolate. See *c.* phenolsulfonate.

c. undecylenate. $[CH_2{:}CH(CH_2)_8COO]_2Cu$. Used locally as a fungicide.

cop′per·as (cop′ur·us) [OF. *couperose*]. Ferrous sulfate.

cop′per·head″. See *Agkistrodon mokasen.*

Coppet, Louis Cas de [*French physicist,* 1841–1911]. Stated the law that solutions with the same freezing point are equimolecular.

co″pre·cip″i·ta′tion [L. *cum,* with; *praecipitatio,* precipitation]. The precipitation of a contaminant with a desired precipitate even though the solubility constant of the contaminant has not been exceeded. This phenomenon is usually due to adsorption.

cop·rem′e·sis [G. *kopros,* excrement; *emesis,* vomiting]. Vomiting of fecal matter.

cop′ro-, copr- [*kopros*]. A combining form meaning *feces* or *dung.*

cop·roc′tic [*kopros*]. Relating to feces; fecal.

cop″ro·lag′ni·a [*kopros;* G. *lagneia,* coition]. Sexual perversion in which pleasure is obtained from the idea, sight, or handling of feces.

cop″ro·la′li·a [*kopros;* G. *lalia,* talk]. Repetitious reference to feces and fecal subjects.

cop′ro·lith [*kopros;* G. *lithos,* stone]. A hard mass of fecal matter in the bowels.

cop·roph′a·gy [*kopros;* G. *phagein,* to eat]. Eating of feces; a symptom occasionally seen in severe psychoses. —**coprophagous,** *adj.*

cop″ro·phe′mi·a [*kopros;* G. *phēmis,* speech]. Obscene speech.

cop″ro·phil′i·a [*kopros;* G. *philein,* to love]. An abnormal interest in fecal matter, seen in certain mental patients.

cop·roph′i·lous [*kopros; philein*]. Growing upon fecal matter; said of certain bacteria.

cop″ro·pho′bi·a [*kopros;* G. *phobos,* fear]. A morbid fear of fecal matter.

cop″ro·phra′si·a (cop″ro·fray′zhuh, ·zee·uh) [*kopros;* G. *phrasis,* speech]. The abnormal interjection of obscene words into speech.

cop″ro·por′phy·rin [*kopros;* G. *porphyra,* purple]. Any of four isomeric, metal-free porphyrins, characterized by having four methyl groups and four propionic acid residues ($—CH_2CH_2COOH$) as substituent groups: first isolated from feces in congenital porphyria. One or more coproporphyrins occur also in normal urine, and, in larger amounts, in urine in certain diseased states, and also following administration of certain drugs.

cop″ro·por″phy·ri·nu′ri·a. The excretion of an abnormal amount of coproporphyrin in urine.

cop′ro·stane. $C_{27}H_{48}$; a steroid hydrocarbon isomeric with cholestane, differing from the latter in the manner of juncture of two of the component rings (the A and B rings). Syn., *pseudocholestane.*

cop·ros′tan·ol. Coprosterol.

cop·ros′ter·ol [*kopros;* G. *stereos,* stiff]. $C_{27}H_{47}OH$. A sterol found in the lower intestine and excreted in feces; while it is apparently derived from cholesterol, it is structurally related to coprostane rather than to cholestane. Syn., *coprostanol.*

cop″ro·zo′ic [*kopros;* G. *zōikos,* of animals]. Living in feces, as protozoans found in fecal matter outside the body but not in the intestine.

cop′tine (cop′teen, ·tin). A colorless alkaloid of goldthread. See *Coptis groenlandica.*

Cop′tis [G. *koptein,* to cut]. A genus of herbs of the Ranunculaceae, the crowfoot family.

C. groenlandica. Goldthread; the plant is a simple bitter tonic containing coptine and berberine.

cop′u·la [L., a band, tie]. 1. A median swelling of the pharyngeal floor uniting the hyoid arches in the embryo, the future root of the tongue. 2. Old term for body of the hyoid.

cop″u·la′tion [L. *copulare,* to bind together]. The sexual union of male and female.

co·quilles′ (ko·keel′) [F., from G. *kogchos,* shell]. A variety of dark eyeglasses curved like shells.

cor [L.]. The heart.

c. biauriculare. See *c.* triloculare biatrium.

c. biloculare. A malformation of the heart in which there is only one atrium and one ventricle.

c. biventriculare. See *c.* triloculare biventriculare.

c. bovinum [L. cow heart]. See bovine *heart.*

c. pseudotriloculare. A malformation of the heart in which there are three functioning chambers, the fourth being rudimentary or absent.

c. pulmonale. A state of hypertension in the pulmonary artery with right ventricular strain and eventual right ventricular hypertrophy; it may be due to any condition that obstructs the pulmonary circulation.

c. triloculare biatrium. A rare anomaly consisting of complete absence of the ventricular septum; there are two atria and one ventricle. Also called *c. biauriculare.*

c. triloculare biventriculare. A serious defect of the upper part of the septum occasionally seen in adults. There are two ventricles, but only one atrium. Also called *c. biventriculare, c. triloculare monatriatum.*

c. villosum. Fibrinous pericarditis in which some of the fibrin projects from the surface in villous-like processes.

cor″a·cid′i·um [G. diminutive of *korax*, hooklet]. The ciliated larval stage of the fish tapeworm, *Diphyllobothrium latum*.

cor′a·co- [G. *korax*, crow]. A combining form denoting *pertaining to the coracoid process*.

cor″a·co·a·cro′mi·al [*korax;* G. *akron*, extremity; *ōmos*, shoulder]. Relating to the coracoid and the acromion processes.

cor″a·co·bra″chi·a′lis (kor″uh·ko·bray″kee·ay′-liss, ·brack″ee·ay′liss) [*korax;* L. *brachialis*, from *brachium*, arm]. A muscle of the upper and medial part of the arm, arising from the coracoid process of the scapula. See Table of Muscles in the Appendix.

c. brevis. A variable part of the coracobrachialis muscle.

c. superior. Same as *c. brevis*.

cor″a·co·cla·vic′u·lar [*korax;* L. *clavicula*, small key]. Relating to the coracoid process of the scapula and the clavicle.

cor″a·co·hu′mer·al [*korax;* L. *humerus*, upper bone of the arm]. Relating to the coracoid process of the scapula and the humerus.

cor′a·coid [G. *korakoeidēs*, like a crow]. Having the shape of a crow's beak.

cor′a·coid. The coracoid process of the scapula. See Plate 1.

cor′al·lin. Rosolic acid.

coramine. A trade-mark for nikethamide, the product supplied as a 25% solution.

cor·chor′ge·nin. $C_{23}H_{32}O_6$; a cardioactive aglycone isolated from seeds of *Corchorus olitorius*, from which jute is obtained and which is also used as a potherb. In cats corchorgenin is more potent than either strophanthidin or corchortoxin, which are isomeric with it.

cor″chor·tox′in. $C_{23}H_{32}O_6$; a cardioactive aglycone isolated from seeds of *Corchorus capsularis*, from which jute is obtained; it is isomeric with corchorgenin and strophanthidin.

cord [G. *chordē*, string]. 1. Any stringlike body. 2. The long, cylindrical structure bearing the umbilical arteries and vein and connecting the placenta and the fetus. Also called *umbilical c.* See Plates 6, 41. 3. A column of cells.

cortical cords. The secondary cordlike invaginations of the germinal epithelium of the embryonic gonad that differentiate into primary follicles and oogonia. Also called *ovarian cords, ovigerous cords, secondary cords*.

enamel c. In developing enamel organs, a transitory, centrally placed column of cells extending from inner to outer enamel epithelium; it later becomes part of the stellate reticulum.

epithelial c. See epithelial *rest*.

false vocal c. Ventricular fold.

genital c. A mesenchymal shelf bridging the coelom, produced by fusion of the caudal part of the urogenital folds. It contains the vertical part of the Müllerian and the Wolffian ducts, fuses with the urinary bladder in the male, and is the primordium of the broad ligament and the uterine walls in the female.

hepatic cords. The anastomosing columns of liver cells separated by the hepatic sinusoids. Also called *liver cords*.

medullary cords. (a) The primary invaginations of the germinal epithelium of the embryonic gonad that differentiate into rete testis and seminiferous tubules or into rete ovarii. Also called *primary cords, testis cords*. (b) The cords of dense, lymphatic tissue separated by sinuses in the medulla of a lymph node.

nephrogenic c. The longitudinal, cordlike mass of mesenchyme derived from the mesomere or nephrostomal plate of the mesoderm, from which develop the functional parts of the pronephros, mesonephros, and metanephros.

red pulp cords. The anastomosing, cordlike columns of reticular connective tissue separating the venous sinuses of the spleen; the splenic red pulp. Also called *Billroth's cords*.

rete cords. The deep, anastomosing region of the medullary cords (a) that forms the rete testis or the rete ovarii.

sex cords. The cordlike epithelial masses that invaginate from the germinal epithelium of the gonad and form the seminiferous tubules and rete testis, or the primary follicles of the ovary and the rete ovarii.

spermatic c. That extending from the testis to the abdominal inguinal ring and consisting of the ductus deferens, the vessels and nerves of the testis and of the epididymis, and the accompanying connective tissue. See Plate 4.

spinal c. That part of the central nervous system contained within the vertebral canal and extending from the medulla oblongata at the level of the foramen magnum to the filum terminale at the level of the first or second lumbar vertebra. See Plate 16.

tendinous c. Chorda tendinea.

true vocal c. Vocal *fold*.

umbilical c. See *cord*, 2.

cor·dec′to·my [*chordē;* G. *ektomē*, excision]. Excision of a cord, as removal of a vocal fold. Also called *chordotomy*.

cor′dial. 1. A preparation which supposedly stimulates the heart and is invigorating. 2. A pleasantly flavored alcoholic liqueur which supposedly aids digestion.

cor′di·form [L. *cor*, heart; *forma*, shape]. Cordate; shaped like a heart.

cor·di′tis [G. *chordē*, cord; *-itis*, inflammation]. Inflammation of the spermatic cord; funiculitis.

c. nodosa. A lesion in the larynx, particularly of the vocal cords, commonly found in singers, public speakers, and those working around irritating gases. The cords become covered with small grayish nodules. Also called *vocal nodes*.

cor′do·pex″y [*chordē;* G. *pēxis*, a fixing]. The operation of suturing a vocal fold to a new support to relieve the stenosis resulting from bilateral abductor paralysis.

cor·dot′o·my. See *chordotomy*.

Cordus, Euricius [*German physician and botanist*, 1486–1535]. Remembered for his important early account of sweating sickness or miliary fever (1529). The father of Valerius Cordus.

Cordus, Valerius [*German physician and pharmacologist*, 1515–44]. Published the earliest real pharmacopoeia (1535). Said to have been the discoverer of sulfuric ether (1540).

Cor″dy·lo′bi·a [G. *kordylē*, club; *lobos*, lobe]. A genus of African blowflies.

C. anthropophaga. The tumbu fly; a species whose first-stage larvae penetrate the skin of mammals and produce boil-like lesions.

cor″e·cli′sis [G. *korē*, pupil; *kleisis*, a closing]. Pathologic closure or obliteration of the pupil.

cor·ec′ta·sis [*korē;* G. *ektasis*, a stretching]. Dilatation of the pupil.

cor·ec′tome [*korē;* G. *ektomē*, excision]. An instrument used in iridectomy.

cor″ec·to′pi·a [*korē;* G. *ektopos*, away from a place]. Anomalous position of the pupil; displacement of the pupil.

cor″e·di·al′y·sis (kor″i·dye·al′i·sis) [*korē;* G. *dialysis*, separating]. Production of an artificial pupil at the ciliary border of the iris.

cor″e·di·as′ta·sis (·dye·ass′tuh·sis) [*korē;* G. *diastasis*, separation, distention]. Dilatation of the pupil.

co″re·duc′tase (ko″ri·duck′tace, ·taze). See *coenzyme I.*

co·rel′y·sis [*korē;* G. *lysis,* a loosing]. The detachment of iritic adhesions to the lens or cornea.

cor″e·mor′pho·sis [*korē;* G. *morphōsis,* a bringing into shape]. The operation for establishing an artificial pupil.

cor″en·cli′sis [*korē;* G. *egklisis,* inclination]. The formation of a new pupil by displacement, the iris being drawn aside and in part excised.

cor″e·om′e·ter [*korē;* G. *metron,* a measure]. An instrument for measuring the pupil of the eye. —**coreometry,** *n.*

cor″e·on′ci·on [*korē;* G. *ogkos,* barb]. A double-hooked iris forceps.

cor′e·plas″ty [*korē;* G. *plassein,* to form]. Any operation for forming an artificial pupil.

cor″e·ste·no′ma [*korē;* G. *stenōma,* a narrow place]. A narrowing of the pupil.

cor″e·to·me″di·al′y·sis (kor″i·to·mee″dye·al′i·sis). Iridectomy.

Cori, Carl Ferdinand [*American physiologist, pharmacologist, and biochemist,* 1896–]. With G. T. Cori, studied carbohydrate metabolism of the animal body. Their work resulted in the isolation of glucose-1-phosphate, which is known as the *Cori ester.* They described the anaerobic enzymatic synthesis and breakdown of glycogen with intermediate phosphate esters and the final breakdown product, lactic acid; called the *Cori cycle.* Also known for his work on malignant tumors. Nobel laureate with G. T. Cori and B. A. Houssay (1947).

Cori, Gerty Theresa [*American biochemist,* 1896–]. Collaborated with C. F. Cori in the study of carbohydrate metabolism, including the isolation and mode of action of enzymes involved in intermediate phosphorylation in the *Cori cycle.* Also studied the effect of thyroid on temperature regulation and the mechanism of insulin and epinephrine action. Nobel laureate with C. F. Cori and B. A. Houssay (1947).

co″ri·a·myr′tin [L. *corium,* leather; *myrtus,* myrtle]. A convulsant glycoside obtained from the fruit of *Coriaria myrtifolia.*

co″ri·an′der [G. *koriannon,* coriander]. Coriander seed. The dried ripe fruit of *Coriandrum sativum,* (Umbelliferae). An aromatic, carminative, and stimulant, used mainly to give flavor to other remedies and as a corrective to griping purgatives.

c. oil. The volatile oil, containing chiefly *d*-linaloöl (coriandrol). Dose, 0.1 cc. (1½ min.).

co″ri·an′drol. $C_{10}H_{18}O$. The chief constituent of coriander oil; *d*-linaloöl. See under *linaloöl.*

Co″ri·a′ri·a [L. *corium,* leather]. A genus of poisonous shrubs of a wide geographic distribution.

C. myrtifolia. Used in dyeing and tanning; has poisonous berries and shoots.

C. ruscifolia. A variety found in New Zealand; the seeds and shoots afford what is called toot-poison, a delirifacient.

co′ri·um [L.]. The deep layer of the skin. Syn., *cutis vera, derma.*

corn [L. *cornu,* horn]. A lay term for clavus.

cor′ne·a [L. *corneus,* horny]. The transparent anterior portion of the eyeball, its area occupying about one-sixth the circumference of the globe. It is continuous with the sclera, and is nourished from the looped blood vessels at its peripheral border. See Plate 19. —**corneal,** *adj.*

conical c. See *keratoconus.*

transplantation of c. Operation of engrafting a section of transparent cornea into the space of an excised central portion of an opaque human cornea.

Cornell, Ethel Letitia (1892–). American psychologist, who, with W. W. Coxe, developed a nonverbal test of intelligence to be used as a supplement to the Binet test or alone in cases with speech or language difficulty: called *Cornell-Coxe Performance Ability Scale.*

Cornell unit of riboflavin. See under *unit.*

cor′ne·o- [L. *corneus,* horny]. A combining form denoting *cornea* or *corneal.*

cor″ne·o·bleph′a·ron [*corneus;* G. *blepharon,* eyelid]. Adhesion of the surface of the eyelid to the cornea.

cor″ne·o·scle′ra [*corneus;* G. *sklēros,* hard]. The sclera and the cornea considered as forming one tunic. —**corneoscleral,** *adj.*

cor′ne·ous [*corneus*]. Horny or hornlike.

Corner, George Washington (1889–). American anatomist, known for his discovery, with W. M. Allen, of the corpus luteum hormone, progesterone (1928), and for his studies on the reproductive cycle of the rhesus monkey (1923–1945).

cor′ne·um [L. *corneus,* horny]. The stratum corneum or horny layer of the epidermis.

cor·nic′u·late [L. *corniculatus,* in the form of a horn]. Furnished with horns or horn-shaped appendages.

cor·nic′u·lum [L., little horn]. A small cornu or hornlike process.

c. laryngis. Old term for corniculate cartilage.

cor″ni·fi·ca′tion [L. *cornu,* horn; *facere,* to make]. The degenerative process by which the cells of a stratified squamous epithelium are converted into dead, horny squames as in the epidermis and such epidermal derivatives as hair, nails, feathers. Syn., *keratinization, hornification.* —**cor′nified,** *adj.*

Corning, James Leonard [*American neurologist,* 1855–1923]. Remembered for his introduction of spinal anesthesia (1885).

cor′nu (pl. *cornua*) [L.]. A horn; a horn-shaped process or excrescence. —**cornual,** *adj.*

c. Ammonis. Old term for hippocampus.

cornua of the falciform margin. Medial prolongations of the falciform margin of the fossa ovalis in the fascia lata. The **superior cornu of the falciform margin** is the upper one; the **inferior cornu of the falciform margin,** the lower.

cornua of the gray matter. Columns of the gray matter. See under *column.*

cornua of the hyoid bone. Segments of the hyoid bone. The **greater cornu** projects backward from the lateral border of the body; the **lesser cornu** projects upward from the angle of junction of the body and the greater cornu.

cornua of the lateral ventricle. Prolongations of the lateral ventricle of the cerebral hemisphere. The **anterior cornu** is that extending into the frontal lobe; the **inferior cornu,** that extending into the temporal lobe; and the **posterior cornu,** that extending into the occipital lobe. See Plate 17.

cornua of the thyroid cartilage. Processes of the thyroid cartilage; prolongations of its posterior border upward as the **superior cornu of the thyroid cartilage,** and downward as the **inferior cornu of the thyroid cartilage.**

c. cutaneum. A corneous excrescence, varying in size and shape, occurring most frequently on the face and scalp and occasionally on the glans penis and scrotum. Considered a precancerous lesion. Syn., *cutaneous horn.*

c. of the coccyx. Either of the paired, large superior articular processes of the first coccygeal vertebra, articulating with the cornu of the sacrum.

c. of the sacrum. Either of the paired inferior articular processes of the fifth sacral vertebra.

c. of the uterus. The lateral prolongation of the uterine cavity into which an oviduct opens.

dorsal c. The posterior column of gray matter of the spinal cord.

lateral c. The lateral column of gray matter of the spinal cord.

ventral c. The anterior column of gray matter of the spinal cord.

cor'nus [L.]. The bark of the root of *Cornus florida*, the flowering dogwood, containing bitter crystalline principles, cornin, tannin, etc.

cor·nu'tine (korn·yoo'teen, ·tin, korn'yoo·). An alkaloidal degradation product of ergotinine.

cor″o·cli'sis, cor″o·clei'sis. See *coreclisis*.

co·rom'e·ter. See *coreometer*.

co·ro'na [L., from G. *korōnē*, crown]. 1. A crown. 2. The corona radiata. —**coronal,** *adj.*

c. capitis. The crown of the head; the top of the head.

c. ciliaris. Old term for the ciliary zonule.

c. dentis. The crown of a tooth.

c. glandis. The posterior border of the glans penis.

c. radiata. (a) A radiating mass of white nerve fibers ascending from the internal capsule to the cerebral cortex. (b) A zone of follicular cells circumjacent to the zona pellucida of the ovum, which persists for some time after ovulation.

c. seborrheica. A clinical entity occurring in dermatitis seborrheica; marked by the formation of crusts at the hairline.

cor″o·na'le (kor″o·nah'lee) [L. *coronalis*, pertaining to a crown]. 1. The frontal bone. *Obs.* 2. The point on the coronal suture intersected by the greatest frontal diameter.

cor'o·nar″y (korr'o·nerr″ee) [L. *coronarius*, of a wreath]. A term applied to vessels, nerves, or attachments that encircle a part or an organ.

co·ro'ne (ko·ro'nee) [L. *corona*, crown]. The coronoid process of the mandible.

cor'o·ner [*corona*]. An officer who inquires by authority of the law into the causes of sudden or violent deaths.

cor'o·net [OF. *coronete*, dim. of *corone*, crown, from L. *corona*]. 1. *In biology*, a crowning circle of hairs. 2. *In veterinary surgery*, the lowest part of the pastern at its junction with the hoof. Also called *coronamen*.

co·ro'ni·on [*corona*]. The point at the tip of the coronoid process of the mandible. If the tip is divided into two, the measuring point is to be located on the anterior division.

cor″o·ni'tis [*corona;* G. *-itis*, inflammation]. Inflammation of the coronet of the horse's hoof.

co·ro″no·bas'i·lar (ko·ro″no·bas'i·lur, kor″o·no·) [*corona;* G. *basis*, base]. Relating to the coronal suture and the basilar aspect of the head.

co·ro″no·fa'cial [*corona;* L. *facies*, face]. Relating to the crown of the head and to the face.

cor'o·noid [*corona;* G. *eidos*, form]. Shaped like a crown, as the coronoid process of the ulna or of the mandible.

cor″o·pa·rel'cy·sis (kor″o·pa·rel'si·sis) [G. *korē*, pupil; *parelkysis*, from *parelkein*, to draw aside]. Displacing the pupil to remedy partial opacity of the cornea by bringing it opposite a transparent part.

co·roph'thi·sis [*korē;* G. *phthisis*, a wasting away]. Habitual or permanent contraction of the pupil due to a wasting disease of the eye. *Rare.*

co·ros'co·py. Retinoscopy.

Corper and Cohn method. See under *method*.

cor'po·ra. Plural of corpus.

cor'po·rin. Progesterone.

corpse [L. *corpus*, body]. A cadaver.

corps ronds (kor ronh. See NOTES §35). The large round dyskeratotic cells in the upper epidermis, found in Darier's disease and familial benign chronic pemphigus: originally called *psorosperms*.

cor'pu·lent [L. *corpulentus*, fat]. Excessively fat; obese. —**corpulence, corpulency,** *n.*

cor'pus (pl. *corpora*) [L.]. Body. —**corpo'real,** *adj.*

corpora amylacea. See *amyloid bodies* under *body*.

corpora arenacea. Psammoma bodies in the pineal body; brain sand.

corpora cavernosa. Cylindrical bodies of erectile tissue; the basic structures of the penis and clitoris. The two **corpora cavernosa clitoridis** form the crura and body of the clitoris; they are analogous to the two **corpora cavernosa penis** which form the crura of the penis, and, together with the **corpus cavernosum urethrae** which surrounds the male urethra, form the body of the penis. See Plate 44.

corpora quadrigemina. The inferior and superior colliculi collectively. See Plate 18.

c. adiposum buccae. See sucking *pad*.

c. adiposum orbitae. The fat body of the orbital cavity; fatty connective tissue filling the space between the eyeball, optic nerve, ocular muscles, and lacrimal glands, and supporting the orbital vessels and nerves.

c. albicans. The white, fibrous scar in an ovary; it is produced by the degeneration of a corpus luteum. Syn., *c. candicans*.

c. arantii. Fibrocartilaginous nodules in the center of the free edge of each of the cusps of the aortic and pulmonary semilunar valves.

c. callosum. The great transverse commissure connecting the cerebral hemispheres; a broad, arched band of white matter at the bottom of the longitudinal fissure of the cerebrum. See Plate 18.

c. candicans. See *c. albicans*.

c. cerebelli. The cerebellum exclusive of the flocculonodular lobe.

c. ciliare. The ciliary *body*.

c. fibrosum. The scarlike structure in the ovary which represents the end result of an atretic follicle. It has a small central cicatrix surrounded by a narrow zone of hyalinized tissue, and is usually smaller than the corpus albicans.

c. geniculatum. See geniculate *body*.

c. hemorrhagicum. A collapsed Graafian follicle containing blood: an early phase of a corpus luteum.

c. luteum. The yellow endocrine body formed in the ovary in the site of a ruptured Graafian follicle. The large **corpus luteum of pregnancy** is called a **true corpus luteum;** the smaller **corpus luteum of menstruation** is called a **false corpus luteum.** See Plate 41.

c. Luysii. See subthalamic *nucleus*.

c. mammillare. See mammillary *body*.

c. pontobulbare. A nuclear mass caudal to the dorsal cochlear nucleus, receiving fibers from the pons and sending fibers to the cerebellum.

c. spongiosum. The corpus cavernosum urethrae.

c. striatum. The caudate and lenticular nuclei together with the internal capsule which separates them.

c. uteri. The body of the uterus.

cor'pus·cle (kor'pus·ul, kor'pus″ul) [L. *corpusculum*, small body]. 1. A small rounded body. 2. An encapsulated sensory nerve end-organ. 3. Old term for cell, especially a blood cell. —**corpus'cular,** *adj.*

articular c. A tactile corpuscle in a joint capsule.

blood corpuscles. See *erythrocyte, leukocyte*.

bone c. Old term for osteocyte.

cancroid c. An epithelial pearl of a squamous-cell epithelioma or carcinoma.

cartilage c. Old term for chondrocyte.

chyle c. Any floating cell of the chyle.

colostrum c. One of the phagocytic cells of the mammary glands, found in the colostrum, containing fat globules. These corpuscles are present for the first two weeks after parturition and may again appear when the milk is diminishing. After the third day, the globules are freed by the bursting of cells, to form the true milk. Also called *colostrum body.*

conjunctival c. An encapsulated tactile nerve ending in the conjunctiva.

corneal c. A fibroblast of the substantia propria of the cornea.

genital c. A complex form of Krause's corpuscle in the skin of the external genitalia and of the nipple: also called *Dogiel's c., genital c. of Dogiel.*

ghost c. A hemolyzed erythrocyte. Also called *phantom c.*

Golgi's c. One of the small fusiform bodies resembling Pacinian corpuscles, found in tendons at the junction with a muscle. Also called *organ of Golgi.*

Golgi-Mazzoni's c. See Mazzoni's *c.*

Grandry-Merkel's c. See tactile *disk.*

Hassall's c. See thymic *c.*

Krause's c. One of the spheroid nerve corpuscles resembling Pacinian corpuscles, but having a more delicate capsule; found especially in the conjunctiva, the mucosa of the tongue, and in the external genitalia, and believed to be cold receptors. Also called *Krause's end bulb.*

lamellar c. See Pacinian *c.*

lymph c. Old term for lymphocyte.

Malpighian c. (a) See renal *c.* (b) A lymph nodule of the spleen.

Mazzoni's c. A sensory nerve ending similar to Krause's corpuscle.

Meissner's c. An ovoid corpuscle connected with one or more myelinated nerve fibers which lose their sheaths as they enter a surrounding capsule, make several spiral turns, and break up into a complex network of branches. Found, especially, in the papillae of the volar surfaces of the fingers and toes.

Merkel's c. See tactile *disk.*

milk c. (a) The detached, fat-drop filled, distal portion of a glandular cell of the mammary gland, constricted off from the rest of the cell body in apocrine secretion. It breaks down, freeing milk globules. (b) See milk *globule.*

Pacinian c. A large, elliptical corpuscle made up of many concentric lamellas of connective tissue around a core containing the termination of a nerve fiber. Found in the deeper layers of the skin, under mucous membranes, in association with tendons, intermuscular septums, periosteum, and serous membranes. Also called *lamellar c., c. of Vater-Pacini.*

pessary c. See target *cell.*

red c. See *erythrocyte.*

renal c. The glomerulus together with its glomerular capsule in the cortex of the kidney: formerly called *Malpighian c., Malpighian body.*

Ruffini's c. See under *Ruffini.*

salivary c. A leukocyte in the saliva.

splenic c. A lymph nodule of the spleen: formerly called *Malpighian c., Malpighian body.*

tactile c. Any encapsulated nerve end-organ or end-bulb having to do with the sense of touch. Also called *touch c.*

taste c. See taste *bud.*

terminal c. An encapsulated sensory nerve ending.

thymic c. A characteristic, rounded, acidophil body in the medulla of the thymus; composed of hyalinized cells concentrically arranged about a core which is occasionally calcified: also called *Hassall's body, Hassall's c.*

touch c. See tactile *c.*

Vater-Pacini c. See Pacinian *c.*

white c. See *leukocyte.*

cor·pus'cu·lum (pl. *corpuscula*) [L.]. A little body; a corpuscle.

c. articulare mobile. See *arthrolith.*

corpus delecti. [L. the body of the crime]. The existing facts necessary to establish proof that a crime has been committed.

cor·rec'tion [L. *correctum,* from *corrigere,* to correct]. Rectification of any abnormality, as a refractive or muscular defect, or of any undesirable quality, as in a medicine.

cor·rec'tive [*correctum*]. 1. Modifying favorably. 2. A substance used to modify or make more pleasant the action of the principal ingredients of a prescription.

cor"re·la'tion [L. *cum,* with; *relatio,* a bringing back]. 1. *In biometry,* the degree of association between two characteristics in a series of observations, usually expressed as the coefficient of correlation. 2. *In neurology,* the combination of nervous impulses in sensory centers resulting in adaptive reactions.

curvilinear c. A nonlinear relationship between two variables; a correlation in which the regression equation cannot be expressed by a straight line.

cor"re·spond'ence [F. *correspondre*]. The adaptation of things to each other.

abnormal retinal c. A condition found in concomitant strabismus, in which the retinal image formed at the macula of the fixing eye is associated with the image formed at the extramacular area of the retina of the squinting eye. Also called *binocular false projection, retinal incongruity.*

normal retinal c. The normal condition in which the retinal image formed at the macula of one eye is associated with that formed at the macula of the other eye.

retinal c. The relation in the two eyes of the retinal areas at which associated retinal images are formed.

Corrigan, Dominic John [*Irish physician,* 1802–80]. Eminent clinician of the Irish school of medicine who described aortic insufficiency, using the term water-hammer pulse; also called *Corrigan pulse.* Recognized that heart hypertrophy in aortic disease is a compensatory condition and not a disease in itself (1832). His name was formerly associated with other conditions connected with respiration and pulsation in aortic disease and also with a cautery iron called *Corrigan's button.*

cor·ro'sion [L. *corrosum,* from *corrodere,* to gnaw to pieces]. Process of eating away or the resulting state. —**cor·ro'sive,** *adj.*

c. preparation. One in which the vessels, ducts, or cavities of organs are filled by a fluid that will harden and preserve the shape of the vessel or cavity after the organ itself is corroded, digested, or destroyed.

cor·ro'sive [*corrosum*]. A substance that destroys organic tissue either by direct chemical means or by causing inflammation and suppuration.

cor·ro'sive sub'li·mate. See *mercury* bichloride.

cor'ru·ga"tor [L. *corrugare,* to wrinkle]. That which wrinkles, as the corrugator supercilii muscle. See Table of Muscles in the Appendix.

c. cutis ani. That of the anal orifice.

c. supercilii. That of the eyebrows.

cor'set [OF., dim. of *cors*, body]. *In surgery*, a removable appliance embracing the trunk from pelvis to chest; used for correction of deformities, for support of injured bones and muscles of spine or thorax, or in control of ventral hernia, etc. Also called *surgical c.*

cortalex. Trade-mark for tablets containing adrenal cortex and ascorbic acid.

cortate. Trade-mark for *deoxycorticosterone acetate.*

cortef. A trade-mark for *hydrocortisone.*

cor'tex (pl. *cortices*) [L., bark]. 1. The bark of an exogenous plant. 2. The external gray layer of the brain; cerebral cortex. Areas of the cortex are differentiated histologically by cell patterns. 3. The peripheral portion of an organ, situated just beneath the capsule. —**cortical,** *adj.*

adrenal c. See *adrenal cortex.*

agranular c. Cortex of the cerebrum which lacks a definite fourth cell layer, typical of areas in the frontal lobe.

c. cerebri. See *cortex*, 3.

eulaminate c. The typical six-layered cerebral cortex, distinguished from other areas of the isocortex, like the agranular cortex, which lacks a definite fourth layer, and the koniocortex, which has a dense inner granular layer, and small granular cells throughout: also called *eulaminate area.*

fetal c. of the adrenals. See androgenic *zone.*

heterogenetic c. See *allocortex.*

heterotypical c. See *allocortex.*

homogenetic c. See *isocortex.*

homotypical c. See *isocortex.*

limitrophic c. Limitrophic zone.

lipo-adrenal c. A proprietary preparation of adrenal cortical hormones dissolved in cottonseed oil.

visuopsychic c. See visuopsychic *area.*

visuosensory c. See visuosensory *area.*

Corti, Alfonso [*Italian anatomist*, 1822–88]. Made important studies of the anatomy of the eye and ear, particularly of the retina and the cochlea. Described the sensory part of the cochlear duct, the end-organ of hearing or *organ of Corti.* The *rods of Corti* are the columnar cells lining the *tunnel of Corti.* See under *tunnel.*

cor'ti·cate [L. *corticatus*, covered with a bark]. Having a bark or cortex.

cor'ti·ces. Plural of cortex.

cor"ti·cif'u·gal [L. *cortex*, bark; *fugere*, to flee]. Conducting away from the cortex.

cor"ti·cip'e·tal [*cortex;* L. *petere*, to seek]. Conducting toward the cortex.

cor'ti·co- [*cortex*]. A combining form denoting *cortex* or *cortical.*

cor'ti·coid. See *corticosteroid.*

cor"ti·co·pon"to·cer·e·bel'lar [*cortex;* L. *pons*, bridge; *cerebellum*, small brain]. Connecting the cerebral cortex with the cerebellum by way of the pons, as the corticopontocerebellar pathway.

cor"ti·co·spi'nal [*cortex;* L. *spinalis*, belonging to the spine]. Pertaining to the brain cortex and the spinal cord.

cor"ti·cos'ter·oid. Any steroid which has certain chemical or biological properties characteristic of the hormones secreted by the adrenal cortex. Syn., *corticoid.*

urinary c. Any corticosteroid found in the urine.

cor"ti·cos'te·rone. $C_{21}H_{30}O_4$; Δ^4-pregnene-3,20-dione-11,21-diol, a steroid hormone occurring in the adrenal cortex. It influences carbohydrate and electrolyte metabolism and muscular efficiency, and protects against stress. It is not as potent as deoxycorticosterone in maintaining life in adrenalectomized animals. Syn., *Kendall's compound B.* See Table of Hormones in the Appendix.

cor"ti·co·stri'ate [*cortex;* L. *striare*, to furnish with furrows or channels]. Pertaining to nerve fibers arising in the cerebral cortex and terminating in the corpus striatum.

cor"ti·co·tro'phin. World Health Organization designation for *corticotropin.*

cor"ti·co·tro'pin. The preferred generic name, as contrasted with *corticotrophin* (see definitions for *-tropic* and *-trophic* for difference in meaning), of a hormonal preparation having adrenocorticotropic activity derived from the adenohypophysis of certain domesticated animals. Also called *corticotropic hormone, pituitary adrenocorticotropic hormone, ACTH.* See *acthar, adrenocorticotropin.* —**corticotro'pic,** *adj.*

cor"ti·lac'tin [*cortex;* L. *lac*, milk]. An extract of the adrenal cortex alleged to increase lactation.

cor'tin [*cortex*]. An extract of adrenal cortex; contains several hormones; is life-sustaining in bilaterally adrenalectomized animals; also of value in treating adrenal cortical hypofunction.

cortinoral. Trade-mark for a lipid fraction of adrenal cortex extract offered in capsule form.

cor'ti·sol. See *hydrocortisone.*

cor'ti·sone. A constituent of adrenal cortical extract, 17-hydroxy-11-dehydrocorticosterone, $C_{21}H_{28}O_5$, produced commercially by one or another of several methods of synthesis. In the adrenalectomized animal, administration of cortisone maintains life and resistance to various forms of stress which otherwise would be lethal. Therapeutic doses produce in the normal human being a variety of physiological effects, including depression of the function of the adrenal cortex and inhibition of production of pituitary adrenocorticotropic hormone. Cortisone is indicated chiefly for substitution therapy in frank adrenal insufficiency and in certain acute conditions, notably in the so-called collagen diseases, in which the period of treatment is not long enough to incur the metabolic effects of protracted therapy. Syn., *Kendall's compound E, Wintersteiner's compound F, Reichstein's substance Fa.* See *cortogen, cortone.*

c. acetate. The monoacetate ester of cortisone, $C_{23}H_{30}O_6$; a crystalline substance, practically insoluble in water: the form in which cortisone is used therapeutically.

cortogen. A trade-mark for *cortisone.*

cortone. A trade-mark for *cortisone.*

cortril. A trade-mark for hydrocortisone or 17-hydroxycorticosterone, the substance being supplied in free alcohol and acetate forms.

cor"us·ca'tion [L. *coruscare*, to glitter]. The subjective sensation of light flashes.

Corvisart, Lucien [*French physician*, b. 1824]. Did research on pancreatic digestion (1857–63) and described infantile tetany (1852).

Corvisart des Marets, Jean Nicolas [*French clinician*, 1755–1821]. Eminent cardiologist, said to have founded cardiac symptomatology. Described the mechanics of heart failure and the dyspnea of effort (1806).

corvotone. Trade-mark for *nikethamide.*

cor'vus [L., raven]. Fellator.

co·ryd'a·line. An alkaloid from *Corydalis tuberosa.*

co·ryd'a·lis [G. *korydallis*, crested lark]. The tuber of *Dicentra canadensis*, squirrel corn, or of *D. cucullaria*, Dutchman's-breeches, containing several alkaloids, of which corydaline, isocorydine, and protopine are the most important. Corydalis has been used as a tonic and alterative.

cor'y·dine (kor'i·deen, ·din). An amorphous alkaloid from *Corydalis tuberosa.*

coryfin. Trade-mark for ethyl glycolic acid ester of menthol, a local analgesic and astringent.

cor″y·loph′il·line (kor″i·lof′i·leen, ·lin). An antibiotic identical with *Escherichia coli* factor, mycoin, notatin, penatin, and penicillin-B.

cor·ym′bi·form [L. *corymbus*, a cluster]. *In syphilology*, a form of syphilid in which a large lenticular papule is in the center of an irregular group of papules.

Co·ry″ne·bac·te′ri·um [G. *korynē*, club; *baktērion*, little staff]. A genus of slender, aerobic, nonmotile, nonsporeforming, Gram-positive bacteria of which **C. diphtheriae** is the type species; varying from slightly curved to club-shaped and branching forms; showing irregular staining. This genus includes a large group of diphtheroid bacilli, such as **C. acnes,** and **C. pyogenes,** mainly saprophytic and morphologically similar to *C. diphtheriae;* found in normal tissues and secretions as well as in pathologic conditions; probably not causative.

C. diphtheriae. The causative organism of diphtheria; the varieties *gravis* and *mitis* have been described; produces both an exotoxin and an endotoxin: formerly called *Bacillus diphtheriae.* See Plate 30.

C. hofmannii. Syn. for *C. pseudodiphtheriticum.*

C. pseudodiphtheriticum. A species with morphology similar to *C. diphtheriae*, but nonpathogenic, having its habitat in normal throats. Also called *Hofmann's bacillus.*

C. xerose. A form found in chronic conjunctivitis and also in normal eyes.

co·ry′za. Inflammation of the mucous membranes of the nose, usually marked by sneezing, discharge of watery mucus, and also watering of the eyes: sometimes used synonymously with *common cold.*

allergic c. Coryza occurring in an allergic person and due to exposure to an agent to which he is hypersensitive.

bacterial c. A cold in the head due to bacteria of which the patient is host.

pollen c. See *hay fever.*

cosanyl. Trade-mark for a compound syrup of cocillana used as a cough sedative.

cos·met′ic [G. *kosmētikos*, skilled in ordering, from *kosmos*, order]. A preparation applied to the skin or its appendages to alter its appearance, to protect it, to beautify, or to promote attractiveness.

cos·met′ic. Pertaining to any plastic operation on the external surfaces or configuration of a part of the body to improve the appearance of the patient, e.g., rhinoplasty.

cos′mo·tron. An apparatus for accelerating protons in the billion electron volt range. The accelerated protons are employed in studying the reactions of various atomic nuclei when bombarded with the particles.

cos′ta (pl. *costae*) [L.]. A rib. —**costal,** *adj.*

costae fluctuantes. Floating ribs.

costae spuriae. False ribs.

costae verae. True ribs.

cos·tal′gi·a [*costa;* G. *algos*, pain]. Intercostal neuralgia; pain in the ribs.

cos·tal′is. Of or pertaining to the ribs. See Table of Muscles in the Appendix.

cos′tate [*costa*]. Ribbed; furnished with ribs or connecting structures.

Coste, Jean Jacques Marie Cyprien Victor [*French embryologist*, 1807–73]. Known for discovery of the germinal spot of the animal egg (1837).

cos·tec′to·my [L. *costa*, rib; G. *ektomē*, excision]. Excision of a rib or a part of one.

Costen, James Bray [*American otolaryngologist*, 1895–]. Known for his description of a group of pain symptoms associated with destruction of the temporomandibular joint, due to loss of molar support in occlusion of the jaws. Pain is referred to the occiput, eye, nasal sinuses, the tongue, and lateral pharyngeal wall. There may be painful spasm of the muscles of mastication, interfering with normal opening of the mouth. Called *temporomandibular syndrome, Costen's syndrome complex.*

cos″ti·car′ti·lage [L. *costa*, rib; *cartilago*, cartilage]. A costal cartilage.

cos′ti·form [*costa;* L. *forma*, shape]. Rib-shaped.

cos′tive [OF. *costivé*, from L. *constipare*, to press together]. Constipated. —**costiveness,** *n.*

cos′to- [L. *costa*, rib]. A combining form denoting *a rib* or *costa.*

cos″to·car′ti·lage. A costal cartilage.

cos″to·cer″vi·cal′is. Of or pertaining to the ribs and neck. See Table of Muscles in the Appendix.

cos″to·chon′dral (kos″to·kon′drul) [*costa;* G. *chondros*, cartilage]. Pertaining to the ribs and their cartilages.

cos″to·cla·vic′u·lar [*costa;* L. *clavicula*, small key]. Pertaining to the ribs and the clavicle.

cos″to·cor′a·coid [*costa;* G. *korakoeidēs*, like a crow]. Pertaining to the ribs and the coracoid process.

c. muscle. A variable muscle arising from one or more ribs and inserted into the coracoid process.

cos″to·phren′ic [*costa;* phrēn, phrenŏs, the diaphragm]. Pertaining to the ribs and the diaphragm.

cos″to·scap′u·lar. Of or pertaining to the ribs and the scapula. Syn., *scapulocostal.*

cos′to·tome [*costa;* G. *tomos*, cutting]. Heavy curved shears or forceps with a hooked limb against which the knife blade acts; used for rib resection.

guillotine c. One specially designed for removal of the first rib in thoracic surgery. Also called *Lilienthal's c.*

cos·tot′o·my [*costa;* G. *tomē*, a cutting]. Division of a rib.

cos″to·trans·verse′ (kos″to·trans·vurs′, ·tranz·vurs′) [*costa;* L. *transversus*, transverse]. Pertaining to a rib and the transverse process of a vertebra; applied to the joint between them and to the ligaments joining them. See Table of Joints and Ligaments in the Appendix.

cos″to·trans″ver·sec′to·my (·trans″vur·seck′to·mee, ·tranz″vur·) [*costa; transversus;* G. *ektomē*, excision]. Excision of part of a rib and a transverse vertebral process.

cos″to·ver′te·bral [*costa;* L. *vertebra*, vertebra]. Pertaining to a rib and the vertebral column; applied to the joints between them.

cos″to·xiph′oid (kos″to·zif′oyd) [*costa;* G. *xiphos*, sword; *eidos*, form]. Relating to the ribs and the xiphoid cartilage.

cot [Hind. *khāt*, from Skr. *khatvā*]. A small bed.

cot [AS. *cot*]. The finger of a glove, or other covering to protect a finger.

co·tar′nine (ko·tahr′neen, ·nin) [from *narcotine*, by transposition of letters]. $C_{12}H_{15}NO_4$. An oxidation product of narcotine.

c. chloride. Small yellow crystals, soluble in water and alcohol; has been used in uterine hemorrhage and hemoptysis. See *stypticin.*

co·throm″bo·plas′tin. See *convertin.*

cotinazin. Trade-mark for a brand of isoniazid, an antituberculosis drug having the composition of isonicotinic acid hydrazide.

co′to [Tupi *cotó-cotó*]. Coto bark; the bark of a tree native to Bolivia, *Aniba coto.* It contains a bitter principle, cotoin, $C_{22}H_{18}O_6$, irritant to the skin and mucous membranes. It has been used in treatment of diarrhea and for the night sweats of pulmonary tuberculosis.

co′to·in, co·to′in. $C_{14}H_{12}O_4$. A crystalline principle from coto. Has been used in the same manner as coto.

co″trans·am′i·nase. Pyridoxal phosphate, the prosthetic component of certain transaminating enzymes, as well as of the enzyme carboxylase which catalyzes decarboxylation of L-amino acids, in which latter case it is commonly referred to as *codecarboxylase*.

Cotton, Frederick Jay [*American surgeon*, 1869–1938]. An authority on fractures, especially those of the forearm and wrist. He devised a position which received his name for treatment of fractures of the lower end of the radius, in which the wrist is immobilized in slight flexion with the hand everted on the forearm.

cot′ton [OF. *coton*, from Ar. *qutun*, cotton]. The hairs of the seed of cultivated varieties of *Gossypium herbaceum* or of other species of *Gossypium*.

absorbent c. Cotton so prepared that it readily absorbs water.

c.-oil. See cottonseed *oil*.

c.-root bark. See under *Gossypium*.

cottonseed oil. See under *oil*.

c. wool. Raw cotton.

guncotton. See *pyroxylin*.

styptic c. Cotton saturated with a styptic substance.

Cotugno, Domenico (Cotunnius) [*Italian anatomist*, 1736–1822]. Widely known as the first to describe the cerebrospinal fluid (1764). Investigated the structure and function of the internal ear and discovered the aqueducts of the internal ear (1761). Described sciatica and nervous arthritis (1764), *Cotugno's disease*. The endolymphatic space of the internal ear has received his name.

Cotunnius. See *Cotugno*.

cot″y·le′don [G. *kotylēdōn*, any cup-shaped hollow]. 1. Any one of the groups of villi separated by smooth chorion characteristic of the ruminant semiplacenta. 2. Any one of the rounded lobules bounded by placental septums into which the uterine surface of a discoid placenta is divided. 3. Any plant of the genus *Cotyledon*. 4. The primary or seed leaf in the phanerogamic embryo.

cot′y·loid [G. *kotyloeidēs*, cup-shaped]. Cup-shaped.

cot′y·loid. The cotyloid bone. The center of ossification appearing in the triradiate cartilage of the acetabulum between the pubis and ilium: also called *acetabular bone*.

couch grass. See *Triticum*.

Coué, Émile [*French pharmacist*, 1857–1926]. Known in his day for his experiments with autosuggestion, also called *Coué's treatment*. Said to have coined the term autosuggestion.

cough [ME. *coughen*]. A sudden, violent expulsion of air after deep inspiration and closure of the glottis.

chin c. Whooping cough.

dry c. That unattended by expectoration.

ear c. One excited reflexly from some irritation of the ear.

moist c. One with free expectoration.

pleuritic c. The dry, short, frequent cough of pleurisy, pneumonia, and pulmonary tuberculosis, which accompanies the pain and friction sounds of pleurisy and disappears with effusion or when bronchitis supervenes.

productive c. One in which mucus or exudate is raised by coughing.

reflex c. One produced by irritation of a remote organ.

stomach c. See reflex *c*.

tooth c. A reflex cough associated with difficult dentition.

uterine c. A reflex cough occurring in sufferers from genital diseases; due to irritation of the uterovaginal fibers of the hypogastric plexus supplying the fornix vaginae and cervix uteri, and the nerves and ganglions supplying the fundus uteri and ovaries.

whooping c. See *whooping cough*.

winter c. A short troublesome cough of old people due to chronic bronchitis and recurring every winter.

cou·lomb′ (kōō·lom′, kōō′lom) [after Charles Augustin de *Coulomb*, French physicist, 1736–1806]. The unit of electric quantity; the quantity of electricity transferred by a current of 1 ampere in 1 second.

cou′ma·rin (kōō′muh·rin) [Tupi *cumarú*, tonka-bean tree]. $C_6H_4(CH)_2OCO$. The lactone of orthohydroxycinnamic acid; found widely distributed in the vegetable kingdom, especially in tonka bean, and also prepared synthetically. It has been used for its odorous quality, as in imitation vanilla extracts, and for concealing odors. As continued ingestion may tend to produce hemorrhage, its use as a food flavor has been prohibited.

cou·min′gine (koo·min′jeen, ·jin). An alkaloid, $C_{28}H_{45}NO_6$, having a digitalislike action; obtained from *Erythrophleum couminga*.

Councilman, William Thomas [*American pathologist*, 1854–1933]. Known for his investigation, with Henry Amadée Lafleur, of amebic dysentery, a term they coined (1890). A genus of amebas is called *Councilmania*.

count [L. *computare*, to reckon]. The number obtained by reckoning the units of a series or collection, as blood count, the number of blood cells per unit volume of blood.

Addis c. The number of cells found in 10 cc. of a 12-hr. specimen of urine.

differential white c. The number of each variety of leukocytes in a count of 100 leukocytes. Syn., *differential blood count*.

direct platelet c. Using the red cell pipet, platelet diluting fluid is drawn to the 1 mark, blood from a fresh puncture wound is quickly drawn to the 0.5 mark, and diluting fluid then drawn to the 101 mark. The pipet is shaken for two minutes and the platelets counted on the counting chamber by the method used for erythrocytes. Normal ranges are 250,000 to 350,000 per cubic millimeter.

parasite c. The number of parasites infecting a certain volume of blood. This has been used in trypanosomiasis and malaria. It is considered to be unreliable in the latter since there may be no organisms in the peripheral blood at certain times in the course of the disease. See parasite *index*.

total white c. The number of leukocytes in one cubic millimeter of blood.

count′er. See *Geiger-Müller counter; scintillation counter*.

coun″ter·ac′tion [L. *contra*, against; *actum*, from *agere*, to act]. Action of a drug or agent opposed to that of some other drug or agent.

coun′ter-die. See *die*.

coun′ter·ex·ten″sion [*contra;* L. *extensio*, from *extendere*, to extend]. Traction made in a direction opposite to that in which traction is made by another force.

coun″ter·fis′sure. Contrafissura.

coun″ter·in·di·ca′tion. Contraindication.

coun″ter·ir′ri·tant [*contra;* L. *irritare*, to irritate]. An agent which produces an inflammation of the skin for the relief of a more deep-seated inflammation. —**counterirrita′tion,** *n.*

coun′ter·o″pen·ing [*contra;* AS. *open*]. A second incision into an abscess or cavity, made opposite to the first, for purposes of drainage.

coun′ter·poi″son [*contra;* L. *potio,* drink]. A poison which counteracts another poison.

coun′ter·pres″sure [*contra;* L. *pressura,* from *premere,* to press]. Manipulation to counterbalance pressure by exercising force in the opposite direction.

coun′ter·punc″ture. A counteropening.

coun′ter·shock″. A phase of the alarm reaction or first phase of the general adaptation syndrome.

coun′ter·stain [*contra;* abbrev. from *distain,* L. *dis-,* away, *tingere,* to color]. 1. A second stain used for contrast to color the parts of tissues not affected by the first stain. 2. Apply a counterstain.

coun′ter·stroke. Contrecoup.

coun′ter·trac″tion [*contra;* L. *tractum,* from *trahere,* to pull]. *In surgery,* a traction which offsets another, as in reducing fractures. See *counterextension.*

coun′ter·trans·fer′ence. *In psychiatry,* the unconscious attitudes and primitive feelings of the analyst toward his patient in response to displacement of repressed inclinations from patient to analyst (*transference*). This may impair psychotherapy.

cou′ple [L. *copula,* band]. Among the lower animals, to copulate.

Courvoisier, Ludwig George [*French surgeon,* 1843–1918]. Remembered for his laws: Malignant disease of the pancreas is to be suspected in the great majority of cases when there is enlargement of the gallbladder without biliary colic, but with increasing jaundice, in a middle-aged person. In obstruction of the common bile duct by gallstones, the gallbladder usually is contracted; in obstruction from other causes, it generally is dilated. With von Hacker, he devised an operation to relieve pyloric obstruction by posterior gastroenterostomy through an opening in the mesocolon.

Coutard, Henri [*French radiologist in the United States,* 1876–1950]. Known for his technic for the treatment of cancer of the larynx by radiotherapy (1921).

Couvelaire uterus. See under *uterus.*

co·va′lence. A bond between two atoms in which both of the atoms concerned contribute the electron or electrons; normal covalence. —**cova′lent,** *adj.*

coordinate c. That type of bond between two atoms in which one of the two atoms concerned contributes both electrons; dative covalence.

cov′er glass. *In microscopy,* the thin slip of glass covering the object mounted on the slide.

covermark. Trade name for a pigmented cosmetic used to cover skin blemishes; various shades are used to match different skins.

Cowie's test. See guaiac *test.*

Cowling's rule. To determine the dosage of medicines for children, the age of the child at the next birthday is used as the numerator and 24 as the denominator; the result is the appropriate fraction of the dose for adults.

Cowper, William [*English surgeon,* 1666–1709]. Remembered for his description of the bulbourethral glands (1697), also called *Cowper's glands, Méry's glands.* Gave a classic description of aortic insufficiency (1706). That part of the fascia lata attached to the pubic crest is known as *Cowper's ligament.*

cow″per·i′tis [*Cowper;* G. *-itis,* inflammation]. Inflammation of the bulbourethral glands (glands of Cowper), usually gonorrheal in origin.

cow′pox″. Vaccinia.

Cox, Herald Rea [1907–]. American bacteriologist who developed the Cox yolk-sac method of cultivating Rickettsiae in high concentration, which is of great value in the preparation of vaccines against typhus fever, Rocky Mountain spotted fever, and other rickettsial diseases. He was the first to isolate Q fever organisms in the United States from infected wood ticks; these organisms have been placed in a new genus, *Coxiella burnetii,* of the family Rickettsiaceae.

cox′a (pl. *coxae*) [L.]. The hip or hip joint. See Table of Bones in the Appendix.

c. magna. Enlargement of the hip due to degenerative joint disease of the head and neck of the femur.

c. plana. Osteochondritis deformans juvenilis.

c. valga. A condition, the reverse of coxa vara, in which the angle between the neck and the shaft of the femur is increased above 140 degrees.

c. vara. A condition in which the neck of the femur is bent downward sufficiently to cause symptoms; this bending may reach such an extent that the neck forms, with the shaft, a right angle or less, instead of the normal angle of 120–140 degrees.

malum coxae senile. Degenerative joint disease of the hip.

cox·al′gi·a, cox′al″gy [*coxa;* G. *algos,* pain]. Literally, pain in the hip joint, but generally used synonymously with hip disease. —**coxalgic,** *adj.*

cox′al″gy. See *coxalgia.*

cox″ar·thri′tis. See *coxitis.*

cox″ar·throc′a·ce (cocks″ahr·throck′uh·see) [*coxa;* G. *arthron,* joint; *kakē,* badness]. A fungoid inflammation of the hip joint.

Coxe, Warren Winfred [*American psychologist,* 1886–]. With E. L. Cornell, developed a nonverbal test of intelligence to supplement the Binet test or to be used alone in cases with speech or language difficulty: called the *Cornell-Coxe Performance Ability Scale.*

Cox″i·el′la bur·net·i. A genus of the family Rickettsiaceae, which is the causative agent of Q fever: so-called after Herald Rea Cox. On smear it appears intracellularly and occasionally extracellularly. The organism is filtrable and has no cross immunity with the other rickettsiae.

cox·i′tis [L. *coxa,* hip; G. *-itis,* inflammation]. Inflammation of the hip joint.

c. cotyloidea. That confined principally to the acetabulum.

senile c. A rheumatoid disease of the hip joint occurring in old people; marked by pain, stiffness, and wasting, with no tendency to suppuration.

cox″o·dyn′i·a. See *coxalgia.*

Cox·sa′ck·ie virus. See under *virus.*

co·zy′mase [L. *con-,* together; G. *zymē,* leaven; *-ase,* enzyme]. Coenzyme I.

C.P. Chemically pure.

cps, c.p.s. Cycles per second.

Cr Chemical symbol for chromium.

crab yaws. See under *yaws.*

cracked′-pot sound. A peculiar sound, elicited by percussion over a pulmonary cavity communicating with a bronchus.

cra′dle [AS. *cradel*]. A frame of wicker, wood, or wire, used to prevent the bedclothes from coming in contact with a fractured or injured part.

Craig, Charles Franklin [*American pathologist,* 1872–]. Known for his researches in parasitology, for his studies of the malarial plasmodium (1899–1907), for his investigation, with P. M. Ashburn, of the cause of dengue, proving the organism to be a filtrable virus (1907), and for his complement-fixation method for the diagnosis of *Endamoeba histolytica,* using a suspension of artificially cultured endamebas as antigen.

cramp [OF. *crampe,* from MD. *crampe*]. 1. Painful, involuntary contraction of a muscle, such as occurs in swimmers. 2. Any cramplike pain, as of the intestine. 3. Spasm of certain muscles, which may be intermittent, as in tetany, or occupational, resulting from their excessive use. 4. *In gynecology,* a colloquial term for dysmenorrhea.

heat cramps. Pain in the muscles, with nausea and vomiting; occurring during hard work in a hot environment; due to loss of salt through perspiration. Also called *miner's c., stoker's c.*

reader's c. A spasm of the ocular muscles following prolonged reading.

telegrapher's c. See *fatigue spasms* under *spasm.*

writer's c. An occupational neurosis occurring in those who write constantly with a pen or pencil; characterized by painful spasm of the muscles of the forearm, hand, and fingers; now seen infrequently.

Crandall's test. See Cherry and Crandall's *test.*

cra″ni·ec′to·my [G. *kranion,* skull; G. *ektomē,* excision]. Surgical removal of strips or pieces of the cranial bones.

cra′ni·o- [*kranion*]. A combining form denoting *the cranium, the fetal head, cranial.*

cra′ni·o·cele. See *encephalocele.*

cra″ni·o·cer′vi·cal [*kranion;* L. *cervix,* neck]. Relating to the cranium and the neck.

cra″ni·oc′la·sis, cra′ni·o·clas″ty [*kranion;* G. *klasis,* a breaking]. Operation of breaking the fetal cranium by means of the cranioclast.

cra′ni·o·clast [*kranion;* G. *klan,* to break]. Heavy forceps for crushing the fetal head.

cra″ni·o·clei″do·dys·os·to′sis (kray″nee·o·kly″-do·dis·os·to′sis) [*kranion;* G. *kleis,* clavicle; *dys-,* bad; *osteon,* bone; *-ōsis,* condition]. Congenital defect of the clavicle associated with imperfect ossification of the bones of the cranium, and frequently with other anatomical errors.

cra″ni·o·did′y·mus. See *craniopagus.*

cra″ni·o·fa′cial [*kranion;* L. *facies,* face]. Relating to the cranium and the face.

cra″ni·o·fe·nes′tri·a [Gr. *kranion,* skull; L. *fenestra,* window]. Congenital bony defect involving the total thickness of the skull. See *lacuna skull.*

cra′ni·o·graph [*kranion;* G. *graphein,* to write]. Instrument for recording the outlines of the skull.

cra″ni·og′ra·phy [*kranion; graphein*]. That part of craniology which describes the skull and its parts.

cra″ni·o·la·cu′ni·a [*kranion;* L. *lacuna,* hole]. A rare condition of the vault of the fetal and infant skull, characterized by areas of secondary resorption of bone on the internal surface; associated with spina bifida, meningocele, and intracranial pressure.

cra″ni·ol′o·gy [*kranion;* G. *logos,* word]. The scientific study of the cranium, comprising *craniography* and *craniometry.*

cra″ni·om′e·ter [*kranion;* G. *metron,* a measure]. A caliper used for measuring the dimensions of the skull.

cra″ni·o·met′ric point. Any one of the points on the skull used in craniometry. For the main craniometric points, see *acanthion,* alveolar *point, antinion, apex, asterion, auriculare, basion,* Bolton *point, bregma, clition, condylion, coronion, crotaphion, dacryon, entomion, fronto-temporale, gamma, genion, glabella, gnathion, gonion, hormion, infratemporale, inion, jugal* point, *lacrimale, lambda, maxillo-frontale, metopion, nasion, nasospinale, obelion, ophryon, opisthion, opisthocranion, orale, orbitale, porion, prosthion, pterion, rhinion, sphenion, staphylion, staurion, stephanion, symphysion, tylion, vertex, zygion, zygomaxillare.*

cra″ni·om′e·try [*kranion; metron*]. The science and technic of measuring the skull in order to establish exact, comparable, metric records for use in the comparative study of physical types, variation, and individual peculiarities in the skulls of man and the other primates. —**craniomet′ric,** *adj.*

cra″ni·op′a·gus. [*kranion;* G. *pagos,* fixation]. Conjoined twins united by their heads. Syn., *cephalopagus.* —**craniop′agous,** *adj.;* **craniop′-agy,** *n.*

c. frontalis. Conjoined twins united at the foreheads. Syn., *metopagus.*

c. occipitalis. Conjoined twins united in the occipital region. See Plate 25.

c. parasiticus. A parasitic individual or its parts attached cranially.

c. parietalis. Conjoined twins united in the parietal region. Syn., *cephalopagus parietalis.*

cra″ni·op′a·thy [*kranion;* G. *pathos,* disease]. Any disease of the head.

metabolic c. A condition marked by hyperostosis frontalis interna, obesity, and headache. Occurs most often in women past the menopause, may be hereditary. Also called *Stewart-Morel syndrome, Morgagni's syndrome.*

cra″ni·o·pha·ryn′ge·al (·fa·rin′jul, ·jee·ul, ·far″-in·jee′ul) [*kranion;* G. *pharygx,* throat]. Relating to the cranium and the pharynx.

cra″ni·o·pha·ryn″gi·o′ma. A tumor, usually occurring in children, derived from the epithelium of the embryonal craniopharyngeal canal. The **intrasellar type** arises from cells dispersed in the adenohypophysis; the **suprasellar type,** from cells in the infundibulum above the sella turcica. There are benign and malignant forms, which may be solid, cystic, or papillomatous. The cystic forms are also called *Rathke's pouch cyst, hypophyseal cyst.*

adamantinomatoid c. Ameloblastoma found in the pituitary gland: it is probably derived from Rathke's pouch.

cra′ni·o·plas″ty [*kranion;* G. *plassein,* to form]. Surgical correction of defects in the cranial bones, usually by implants of metal, plastic material, or bone.

cra″ni·o·rha·chis′chi·sis, cra″ni·or·rha·chis′-chi·sis (kray″nee·o·ra·kiss′ki·sis) [*kranion;* G. *rhachis,* spine; *schisis,* cleavage]. Congenital fissure of the cranium and vertebral column.

cra″ni·o·sa′cral. Relating to cranium and sacrum, as the craniosacral autonomic nervous system. See *outflow.*

cra″ni·os′chi·sis (kray″nee·os′ki·sis) [*kranion; schisis*]. Congenital fissure of the cranium.

cra″ni·o·spi′nal [*kranion;* L. *spina,* spine]. Pertaining to the cranium and the vertebral column.

cra′ni·o·stat″ [*kranion;* G. *statos,* standing still]. A device for holding the skull during craniometric study.

cra″ni·o·ste·no′sis [*kranion;* G. *stenōsis,* a being straitened]. Premature closing of the cranial sutures, resulting in a small skull.

cra″ni·os′to·sis (kray″nee·os′to·sis, ·os·to′sis) [*kranion;* G. *osteon,* bone; *-ōsis,* condition]. Premature ossification of the cranial sutures.

cra″ni·o·syn″os·to′sis. Premature closure of the sutures of cranial bones.

cra″ni·o·ta′bes (kray″nee·o·tay′beez) [*kranion;* L. *tabes,* a wasting away]. A change of the cranial bones occurring in infancy, with the formation of small, shallow, conical pits in the bone substance It results from rickets, syphilis, or marasmus. —**craniotabet′ic,** *adj.*

cra′ni·o·tome [*kranion;* G. *tomos,* cutting]. Instrument used in craniotomy.

cra″ni·ot′o·my [*kranion;* G. *tomē,* a cutting]. 1. Operation of reducing the size of the fetal head by cutting or breaking when delivery is otherwise impossible. 2. Excision of a part of the skull.

linear c. Craniectomy.

cra″ni·o·trac′tor [*kranion;* L. *tractum,* from *trahere,* to drag]. A cranioclast designed to be used as a tractor.

cra″ni·o·trip′so·tome [*kranion;* G. *tripsis,* a rubbing; *tomos,* cutting]. Instrument for performing cranioclasis. *Rare.*

cra″ni·o·tym·pan′ic [*kranion;* G. *tympanon,* drum]. Pertaining to the skull and the tympanum.

cra′ni·um [*kranion*]. The part of the skull that contains the brain, its membranes and vessels. See *skull.* See Table of Bones in the Appendix. —**cranial,** *adj.;* **craniad,** *adv.*

cerebral c. That portion of the skull containing the brain; the brain case; neurocranium.

c. bifidum. A hernial protrusion of the meninges through a cranial defect; the hernial sac contains cerebrospinal fluid and often elements of nervous tissue.

visceral c. The bones of the face.

cran′ter (pl. *cranteres*) [G., wisdom tooth, from *krainein,* to complete]. A wisdom tooth or third molar, the eruption of which theoretically perfects the dental arch.

crap′u·lent, crap′u·lous [L. *crapulentus,* very much intoxicated]. Marked by excess in eating and drinking.

cra·quel·é′ [Fr., cracked]. *In dermatology,* scaling, which is cracked in appearance, as in craquelé glassware.

cra″ter·i·za′tion (*of bone*) [L. *crater,* bowl]. The removal of a piece of bone, leaving a crater, as in operations for osteomyelitis.

cra·vat′ [F. *cravate,* from *Cravate,* a Croatian]. A bandage of triangular shape, used as a temporary dressing for a wound or fracture.

craw′-craw″. Itching; any pruritic dermatitis in the tropics, often followed by a pyoderma. The **craw-craw of O'Neil** is due to *Onchocerca volvulus.* Also spelled *kro-kro.*

cream [OF. *cresme,* from G. *chrisma,* an anointing]. The part of milk rich in butterfat.

creamalin. Trade-mark for an aluminum hydroxide gel used in gastric hyperacidity and as an adjunct in the treatment of peptic ulcer.

cream of tar′tar. Potassium bitartrate, $KHC_4H_4O_6$; it is diuretic and aperient.

crease [E. *creast,* variant of *crest,* from L. *crista,* crest]. An indentation made by folding.

gluteofemoral c. One which bounds the buttock below, corresponding nearly to the lower edge of the gluteus maximus muscle. Also called *iliofemoral c.*

cre′a·tine (kree′uh·teen, ·tin) [G. *kreas,* flesh]. $NH{:}C(NH_2)N(CH_3)CH_2COOH$; ($\alpha$-methylguanido)acetic acid or N-methyl-N-guanylglycine, an amino acid present in animal tissues, particularly muscle. Creatine reversibly combines with phosphate to form phosphocreatine, an important compound in the anaerobic phase of muscular contraction. See Table of Normal Values of Blood Constituents in the Appendix.

c. phosphate. Phosphocreatine.

dehydrated c. Creatinine.

cre″a·ti·ne′mi·a [*kreas;* G. *haima,* blood]. An excess of creatine in the blood.

cre″a·tine·phos·phor′ic ac′id (kree″uh·teen·, ·tin·). See *phosphocreatine.*

cre·at′i·nine (kree·at′i·neen, ·nin) [*kreas*]. $NH{:}C(NH)N(CH_3)CH_2CO$; a normal constituent of blood and urine, and a waste product of creatine, excreted in the urine at a constant rate. The normal daily excretion of creatinine independent of diet is about 1.25 Gm. per 24 hours; this value is the **creatinine coefficient.** See Table of Normal Values of Blood Constituents in the Appendix.

cre″a·ti·nu′ri·a [*kreas;* G. *ouron,* urine]. 1. The occurrence of creatine in the urine. 2. The occurrence of increased amounts of creatine in the urine.

cre″a·tor·rhe′a [*kreas;* G. *rhoia,* flow]. Increased amounts of nitrogen in the stool, characteristic of pancreatic insufficiency, but also occurring in excessive diarrhea, as is also ulcerative colitis; it is usually manifested by undigested muscle fibers in the stool.

Credé, Carl Caecil Benno [*German surgeon,* 1847–1929]. Remembered for his introduction of colloidal silver into surgery, called *Credé's treatment, Credé's argentum.*

Credé, Karl Siegmund Franz [*German gynecologist,* 1819–92]. Widely known for his description and development of manual expression of the placenta by grasping the uterus firmly through the abdominal walls, kneading it, and pressing downward to stimulate contraction (1854); called *Credé's method.* Introduced a prophylactic method against ophthalmia neonatorum, using a 1% or 2% silver nitrate solution instilled into the eyes of newborn infants (1884). Devised an incubator for the prematurely born, called *Credé incubator.*

creek dots. Small, shining dots, of unknown nature and often hereditary, occurring at times in the retina anterior to the retinal vessels.

creep′ing e·rup′tion. See *larva migrans.*

cre·mas′ter (kree·mass′tur) [G., suspender]. The muscle that draws up the testis. See Table of Muscles in the Appendix. —**cremaster′ic,** *adj.*

cre·ma′tion [L. *crematio,* from *cremare,* to burn]. Destruction of a dead body by burning, as distinguished from interment. —**cre′mate,** *v.*

cre′ma·to″ry [*cremare*]. 1. Establishment for burning the bodies of the dead. 2. Incinerator.

crem″no·pho′bi·a [G. *krēmnos,* crag; *phobos,* fear]. A morbid fear of precipices.

cremo-carbonates. Trade-mark of a product containing magnesium carbonate, bismuth subnitrate, calcium carbonate, and chloroform in aqueous dispersion medium.

cre′na [L., a notch]. A notch, especially as seen on the sutural margins of the cranial bones.

cre′nate, cre′nat·ed (kree′nay·tid) [L. *crena,* a notch]. 1. Notched or scalloped. 2. *In botany,* having rounded scalloped edges, as certain leaves.

cre·na′tion (kree·nay′shun) [*crena*]. A notched or cogwheel-like appearance of shrunken erythrocytes: seen when they are exposed to the air or to strong saline solutions.

Cren′o·thrix (kren′o·thricks, kree′no·) [G. *krēnē,* a spring; *thrix,* hair]. A genus of bacteria of the family Crenothrichaceae.

C. polyspora. A species of iron bacteria found growing in the conduits of public water supplies; causes stoppage.

creolin. A proprietary disinfectant of high germicidal strength combined with low toxicity; distilled and prepared from highly refined coal tar oils.

cre′o·sol. $C_8H_{10}O_2$. 4-Hydroxy-3-methoxy-methylbenzene, one of the principal phenols contained in creosote. It is a colorless, oily liquid of an agreeable odor and a burning taste, boiling at 220° C.

creosotal. A trade-mark for creosote carbonate.

cre′o·sote [G. *kreas,* flesh; *sōzein,* to save] (*creosotum*). A mixture of phenols obtained by the distillation of wood tar, preferably that from the beech, *Fagus sylvatica;* it is an inflammable, oily liquid. Creosote is antiseptic, astringent, styptic, anesthetic, and escharotic. Used in pulmonary tuberculosis. Dose, 0.3–0.6 cc. (5–10 min.).

beechwood c. That obtained from beechwood.

c. carbonate (*creosoti carbonas*). A mixture of

the carbonates of various constituents of creosote. Dose, 0.3–2.0 cc. (5–30 min.). Syn., *creosotal.*

c. iodide. A brownish powder containing 25% iodine; used as an expectorant and gastrointestinal antiseptic. Dose, 0.016–0.032 Gm. (¼–½ gr.).

c. phenylpropionate. An oily liquid containing 50% creosote; has the effects of creosote. Dose, 0.3–0.6 cc. (5–10 min.). See *proposote.*

c. valerate. A mixture of the valerates of various constituents of creosote. Dose, 0.2–0.6 cc. (3–10 min.).

cre″o·tox′in. See *kreotoxin.*

cre″o·tox′ism. See *kreotoxism.*

crep″i·ta′ti·o (krep″i·tay′shee·o), **crep″i·ta′tion, crep′i·tus** [L. *crepitare*, to creak, crackle, rattle]. 1. The grating of fractured bones. 2. The crackling of the joints. 3. The noise produced by pressure upon tissues containing an abnormal amount of air or gas, as in cellular emphysema. 4. The sound heard at the end of inspiration in the first stage of croupous pneumonia. It closely resembles the sound produced by rubbing the hair between the fingers held close to the ear. —**crep′itant,** *adj.*

cresatin. Trade-mark for *m*-cresylacetate, an antiseptic and analgesic compound useful in treating affections of the nose, throat, and ear.

cres′cent [L. *crescere*, to grow]. Sickle-shaped or shaped like the new moon.

cres′cent. A male or female gametocyte of the *Plasmodium falciparum* which is infectious for Anopheles mosquitoes. The most characteristic diagnostic form of malignant tertian parasites. —**crescen′tic,** *adj.*

crescents of the spinal cord. The lateral gray bands of the spinal cord as seen in traverse section.

gray c. One lateral half of the gray matter of the spinal cord.

myopic c. A yellowish white crescentic area about the optic disk due to atrophy or breaking away of the choroid and exposure of the sclerotic.

serous c. A group of serous cells arranged caplike at the distal end of a mucous acinus in a mixed gland. Also called *c. of Giannuzzi, demilune of Heidenhain.*

cre′sol. $CH_3.C_6H_4.OH$. A mixture of isomeric cresols obtained from coal tar. A colorless, brownish, or pinkish liquid of phenol-like odor; soluble in 50 volumes of water and miscible with alcohol. It is used chiefly as a surgical disinfectant, usually in the form of **saponated cresol solution** (*liquor cresolis saponatus*) which contains 50% of cresol. It is superior to phenol both as an antiseptic and as a germicide. Syn., *cresylic acid.*

cresolin. A proprietary preparation used as a disinfectant.

cre″sol·sul·fu′ric ac′id. $C_7H_7O.CO_2.OH$. An acid occurring in urine in small amounts.

cre·sot′ic ac′id (kree·sot′ick, ·so′tick), **cres″o·tin′ic ac′id.** $CH_3.C_6H_3.OH.COOH$. Hydroxytoluic acid, methylhydroxybenzoic acid. Any one of 10 isomers having this formula. Three of them, the methyl derivatives of ortho-hydroxybenzoic or salicylic acid, have been used medicinally in the form of sodium salts for the same purposes as the salicylates.

cres″o·tin′ic ac′id. See *cresotic acid.*

crest [L. *crista*]. A ridge or linear prominence, especially of bone. Also see *crista.*

alveolar c. The rim of a socket for the root of a tooth in the alveolar process. Syn., *limbus alveolaris.*

buccinator c. A ridge in the groove on the anterior surface of the coronoid process of the mandible, giving origin to fibers of the buccinator muscle.

bulboatrial c. A ridge on the internal surface of the embryonic heart corresponding to the external bulboatrial groove; earlier, the bulboventricular crest.

bulboventricular c. A ridge on the internal surface of the embryonic ventricles corresponding to the external bulboventricular sulcus. It later becomes the bulboatrial crest. Also called *septum interventriculare primum.*

conchal c. That on the medial surface of the maxilla and the palate bone, for articulation with the inferior concha. Syn., *turbinate c.*

c. of the head of the rib. One separating the articular surface of the head of a rib into two parts. Also called *crista capituli costae* [BNA].

c. of the neck of the rib. That on the superior border of the neck of a rib. Also called *crista colli costae.* [BNA].

ethmoidal c. (a) An oblique ridge on the medial surface of the frontal process of the maxilla. Its posterior end articulates with the middle nasal concha; its anterior part is known as the agger nasi. (b) The superior ridge of the medial surface of the palatine bone, articulating with the middle nasal concha.

external occipital c. A vertical ridge on the outer surface of the occipital bone, extending from the occipital protuberance to the foramen magnum. Syn., *median nuchal line.*

frontal c. A vertical ridge along the middle line of the internal surface of the frontal bone.

ganglionic c. See neural *c.*

iliac c. The thickened and expanded upper border of the ilium. See Plate 13.

incisor c. The forward prolongation of the nasal crest of the maxilla, terminating in the anterior nasal spine; the cartilage of the nasal septum rests upon it.

infratemporal c. One on the outer aspect of the great wing of the sphenoid and separating the part of the bone which partly forms the temporal fossa from that which aids in forming the zygomatic fossa.

infundibuloventricular c. See supraventricular *c.*

inguinal c. A prominence on the ventrolateral abdominal wall in the embryo within which develops a part of the chorda gubernaculi. Its base marks the site of the internal opening of the inguinal canal.

internal occipital c. That on the inner surface of the occipital bone, from the internal occipital protuberance to the foramen magnum.

intertrochanteric c. That between the greater and lesser trochanters of the femur.

lacrimal c. A vertical ridge dividing the lateral surface of the lacrimal bone into two parts. *O.T.* Also called *posterior lacrimal c.* [BNA].

nasal c. (a) That on the medial border of the palatal process of the maxilla, articulating with the vomer. (b) That on the medial border of the palatine bone, articulating with the vomer. (c) That on the internal border of the nasal bone and forming part of the septum of the nose.

neural c. A band of ectodermal cells on either side of the neural tube which is the primordium of the cranial and spinal ganglions. Syn., *ganglionic c.*

obturator c. A bony ridge running from the pubic tubercle to the acetabular notch.

pubic c. A crest extending from the pubic tubercle to the medial extremity of the pubis.

sacral c. A series of eminences forming a median longitudinal ridge on the posterior surface of the sacrum.

sphenoid c. A thin ridge of bone in the median line of the anterior surface of the body of the sphenoid bone.

spiral c. A ridge on the upper border of the spiral lamina of the cochlea.

superficial epidermal crests. The external ridges of the epithelium of the skin.

supinator c. A bony ridge on the upper lateral margin of the shaft of the ulna for the origin of the supinator muscle.

supramastoid c. A bony ridge on the squamous part of the temporal bone behind the external auditory meatus.

supraventricular c. A ridge on the inner wall of the right ventricle delimiting the conus arteriosus, a remnant of the bulboatrial crest. Syn., *infundibuloventricular c.*

terminal c. The crista terminalis.

tibial c. The prominent border or ridge on the front of the tibia; the shin.

turbinate c. The conchal crest.

urethral c. A longitudinal ridge of mucous membrane on the posterior wall of the prostatic portion of the male urethra.

zygomatic c. The anterior border of the great wing of the sphenoid; it articulates with the zygomatic bone and separates the orbital from the temporal surface.

m-cres″yl·ac′e·tate. $CH_3.C_6H_4.O.CH_3CO$; a colorless, oily liquid, practically insoluble in water. It possesses antiseptic and analgesic properties useful in treating certain affections of the nose, throat, and ear. Sometimes written *metacresylacetate.* See *cresatin.*

cres′yl·ate. Any compound of cresol with a metallic radical.

cres′yl blue. See *brilliant cresyl blue.*

cre·syl′ic ac′id. Cresol.

cres′yl vi′o·let (kress′il, kree′sil) (C.C.). A basic dye of the oxazine group, having strongly metachromatic properties; used for staining nervous tissue and fresh tumor tissue. Also called *cresylecht violet, cresyl fast violet.*

cre′ta [L., Cretan earth, chalk, white clay]. Chalk. Native calcium carbonate. —**creta′ceous,** *adj.*

cre′tin·ism [F. *crétin,* from L. *Christianus,* Christian]. A condition originating in fetal life or early infancy, due to severe thyroid deficiency; characterized by stunting of physical and mental development. Typically, the large tongue protrudes, the subcutaneous tissue is thickened, the skin is dry, the abdomen protrudes, the mentality is of idiot grade, and the stature is dwarfish. Commonest in regions where endemic goiter is severe; elsewhere it occurs sporadically. —**cretinous,** *adj.;* **cretinoid,** *adj., n.;* **cretin,** *n.*

acquired c. Myxedema. Also called *adult c.*

crev′ice [OF. *crevace,* from L. *crepare,* to crack]. A narrow opening in a tooth, due to a fissure or crack.

gingival c. Old term for gingival sulcus.

crib′bing [AS. *cribb*]. 1. Air swallowing; aerophagia. 2. *In veterinary medicine,* the repeated biting of the crib or manger by horses, resulting in a peculiar wearing of the incisor teeth.

crib′rate [L. *cribrum,* sieve]. Perforated, sievelike, cribriform.

crib′ri·form [*cribrum;* L. *forma,* shape]. Perforated like a sieve.

crib′rose [*cribrum*]. *In biology,* sievelike.

Cri·ce′tus [NL.; Slavic in origin]. A genus of hamsters including the European variety, **C. cricetus,** and the golden hamster, **C. auratus.** See *hamster.*

Crichton-Browne's sign. See under *sign.*

crick. Any painful spasmodic affection, as of the back or neck.

cri″co·ar″y·te′noid (cry″ko·ar″i·tee′noyd, ·ar·it′i-noyd) [G. *krikos,* ring; *arytaina,* pitcher; *eidos,* form]. One of two muscles attached to the cricoid and arytenoid cartilages. See Table of Muscles in the Appendix. —**cricoaryte′noid,** *adj.*

cri′coid [*krikos; eidos*]. Ring-shaped.

cri′coid. The signet-ring-shaped cartilage of the larynx.

cri″coi·dec′to·my [*krikos; eidos;* G. *ektomē,* excision]. The excision of the cricoid cartilage.

cri″co·pha·ryn′ge·al (cry″ko·fa·rin′jul, ·jee·ul, ·far″in·jee′ul) [*krikos;* G. *pharygx,* throat]. Relating to the cricoid cartilage and to the pharynx.

cri″co·phar·yn′ge·us. A portion of the inferior constrictor muscle of the pharynx attached to the cricoid cartilage.

cri″co·thy′roid [*krikos; thyreoeidēs,* shield-shaped]. Pertaining to the cricoid and thyroid cartilages.

cri″co·thy′roid. The muscle, attached to the cricoid and thyroid cartilages, which tenses the vocal folds.

cri·cot′o·my (cry·kot′o·mee) [*krikos;* G. *tomē,* a cutting]. Cutting of the cricoid cartilage.

cri″co·tra′che·al (cry″ko·tray′kee·ul) [*krikos;* G. *trachys,* rough]. Relating to the cricoid cartilage and to the trachea.

cri″co·tra″che·ot′o·my (·tray″kee·ot′o·mee) [*krikos; trachys;* G. *tomē,* a cutting]. Tracheotomy through the cricoid cartilage. *Rare.*

Crile, George Washington [*American surgeon,* 1864–1943]. One of the illustrious surgeons of his time. Widely known for his many ingenious contributions to surgery. Made experimental study of surgical shock (1897). Studied blood pressure in surgery (1903) and transfusion in shock (1909). Reported theory of shock (1913), called *Crile's theory.* Also developed blocking of nerve trunks in operations, using local anesthesia (block anesthesia) (1901).

crim″i·nol′o·gy [L. *crimen,* crime; G. *logos,* word]. The study of crime and of criminals; criminal anthropology.

crimp′er [D. and LG. *krimpen*]. Instrument for making more or less permanent folds in some material, as **foil crimpers,** which fold foil for tooth fillings.

crin″o·gen′ic [G. *krinein,* to separate; *genesthai,* from *gignesthai,* to be produced]. Stimulating the production of secretions.

cri′nose (cry′noce, crin′oce) [L. *crinis,* hair]. Hairy. —**crinos′ity,** *n.*

crise de de·glob″u·li·sa′tion. An episode of indefinite etiology, occurring in hereditary spherocytosis, characterized by fever, lassitude, palpitation, and shortness of breath, violent abdominal pain, vomiting, and anorexia. The blood count shows a pancytopenia and reduction in number of reticulocytes.

cri′sis [G. *krisis,* turning point, from *krinein,* to decide]. 1. A turning point, as that of a disease or fever; especially, the sudden favorable termination of the acute symptoms of an infectious disease. 2. Paroxysmal disturbance of function accompanied with pain. —**crit′ical,** *adj.*

anaphylactoid c. Anaphylactoid shock.

anxiety c. Anxiety attack.

cardiac c. A paroxysm of cardiac distress or disordered action.

clitoris c. A paroxysm of sexual excitement occurring in women suffering from tabes dorsalis.

Dietl's c. Severe nephralgia, chills, nausea, vomiting, and collapse resulting from angulation of a ureter of a floating kidney.

enteralgic c. A paroxysm of pain in the lower part of the abdomen occurring in tabes dorsalis.

gastric crises. Attacks of intense, paroxysmal pain in the abdomen, often attended with vomiting. They occur in tabes dorsalis.

glaucomatocyclitic c. Recurrent self-limited, usually unilateral, attacks of ocular hypertension with keratitic precipitates and moderate aqueous flare.

hemic c. The crisis in a fever marked by increase in the number of blood platelets.

hemoclastic c. A condition occurring during anaphylactic shock; characterized by temporary leukopenia, relative lymphocytosis, erythrocyte destruction, altered blood coagulability, and fall in blood pressure. Seen in those who have poor liver function.

hemolytic c. A sudden change in the patient's condition due to rapid erythrocyte destruction.

laryngeal c. See vagal *c.*

nephralgic c. A ureteral paroxysm of pain observed in tabes dorsalis.

oculogyric crises. Recurrent attacks of tonic conjugate deviation of the eyes, usually upward, lasting from a few seconds to an hour or more; a sequel of lethargic encephalitis.

rectal c. Paroxysmal rectalgia occurring in tabes dorsalis and in diabetes.

spastic vasoconstrictive c. One characterized by increased distress on lying down, pain, tympanites, and a marked and sudden increase of arterial hypertension.

tabetic c. Paroxysmal pain occurring in the course of tabes dorsalis.

vagal c. A paroxysmal alteration of pulse and respiration which may progress to apnea and syncope; due to spasm of the laryngeal muscles.

vesical c. Paroxysmal attack of bladder pain, with difficulty in urination, seen in tabes dorsalis.

Crisp's aneurysm. Aneurysm of the splenic artery.

cris·pa′tion [L. *crispare*, to put into a tremulous motion, brandish, wave]. 1. A puckering; contracture. Syn., *crispatura.* 2. A slight involuntary quivering of the muscles, usually uncomfortable.

cris″pa·tu′ra [*crispare*]. A puckering; contracture.

c. tendinum. Dupuytren's contracture.

cris′ta [L., crest]. Crest. —**cristate,** *adj.*

c. ampullaris. An elevation projecting into the lumen of the ampulla of the ear containing the sensory end-organ. Also called *c. acoustica.*

c. cutis. See *superficial epidermal crests* under *crest.*

c. dividens. The upper margin of the fetal foramen ovale that separates the inferior caval stream of blood into two portions.

c. falciformis. A crest dividing the macula cribrosa into a smaller superior one and a larger inferior one.

c. galli. The superior triangular process of the ethmoid bone, so called because it is shaped like a cock's comb.

c. septo marginalis. The moderator band of the heart when it appears as a prominent ridge.

c. terminalis. A crest on the wall of the right atrium derived from the cephalic part of the right valve of the sinus venosus; a point of attachment for the pectinate muscles of the right atrium.

c. urethralis. The urethral crest.

crit. *In nuclear technology,* the mass of a fissionable material which, under a given set of conditions, is critical.

Critchett, George [*English ophthalmologist,* 1817–82]. Remembered for his improvements in the treatment of glaucoma. Devised an operation for the relief of strabismus. Introduced operations for enucleation of the eye, for keratoconus, for staphyloma, and for epiphora, all bearing his name.

Cri·thid′i·a [G. *krithidion*, dim. of *krithidē*, barley]. A genus of protozoan parasites of the Trypanosomidae; occur only in invertebrate hosts.

crit′i·cal. *In nuclear technology,* of or pertaining to the state of a fissionable material in which it is capable of sustaining, at constant level, a chain reaction.

cro′cus [G. *krokos*, saffron]. Saffron; the stigma of the flowers of *Crocus sativus.* It has been used as an aromatic stimulant, emmenagogue, and antispasmodic. Dose, 0.3–1.5 Gm. (5–20 gr.).

Crohn, Burrill Bernard [*American physician,* 1884–]. Known for his description (with Leon Ginzburg and Gordon D. Oppenheimer) of regional ileitis (1932), called *Crohn's disease.*

croleum. Trade name for an emulsified emollient base suitable for use as a vehicle for topical drugs.

Crooke's change. Hyalinization and degranulation of beta cells of the adenohypophysis in some cases of basophilic adenoma: so called after Arthur Carleton Crooke, English endocrinologist (1905–).

Crookes tube. See under *tube.*

cross [L. *crux*, cross]. 1. *In biology,* a crossbreed in plants, the result of cross-fertilization. 2. A structure in which parts cross each other.

occipital c. See internal occipital *protuberance.*

crossed [*crux*]. 1. Having the shape of a cross. 2. Affecting alternate sides of the body.

cross′ing o′ver. An exchange of blocks of genes between homologous chromosomes during synapsis.

cross match′ing. A test to establish blood compatibility before transfusion, introduced by Ludvig Hektoen. In the **major cross match,** the prospective recipient's serum is mixed with the donor's cells. In the **minor cross match,** the donor's serum is mixed with the prospective recipient's cells. If agglutination (or hemolysis) does not occur in either test, the bloods are considered compatible, and the donor's blood may be used. Also see *blood groups.*

cross sec′tion. A slice of or cut through an object made in a plane perpendicular to its longest axis.

cross′way″ [*crux;* AS. *weg*]. A term sometimes applied to the crossing of two nerve paths. See *chiasma.*

Cro·tal′i·dae (kro·tal′i·dee) [G. *krotalon*, rattle]. Pit vipers; a family of venomous snakes differing from Viperidae (true vipers) in possessing a sensory pit situated between the eye and nostril. Found commonly in the Americas, southeastern Asia, and the East Indies, but unknown in Australia, Africa, and western Europe.

crot′a·line (krot′uh·leen, ·lin, kro′tuh·) [*krotalon*]. 1. A protein found in the venom of rattlesnakes. 2. A preparation of venom from the rattlesnakes, *Crotalus horridus* and *C. adamanteus,* which has been used in subcutaneous injection for immunization against snake bites and for the treatment of epilepsy.

Crot′a·lus (krot′uh·lus, kro′tuh·lus) [*krotalon*]. A genus of the Crotalidae possessing neurotoxic venom; the rattlesnakes. Thirteen species are found in the United States, including **C. adamanteus,** the Florida diamondback rattlesnake, found along the Gulf coastal regions; **C. atrox,** the Texas rattler or western diamondback; **C. confluentus,** the prairie rattlesnake; **C. exsul,** red rattler; **C. horridus,** timber rattler; **C. oreganus,** Pacific rattler; etc. **C. durissus durissus** is found in Central America and **C. durissus terrificus** in South America.

cro·tam′i·ton. Generic name for N-ethyl-*o*-crotonotoluidide, used as a scabicide and antipruritic. See *eurax.*

cro·taph′i·on [G. *krotaphos*, side of the forehead]. The point at the posterior extremity of the sphenoparietal suture.

crotch. The angle formed by the junction of the inner sides of the thighs and the trunk.

crotch′et [OF. *crochet*, from *croc*, hook]. A hook used in extracting the fetus after craniotomy.

cro′tin. A mixture of toxic albuminoids contained in croton seeds. It is a protoplasmic poison.

Cro′ton [G. *krotōn*, tick]. A genus of plants of the Euphorbiaceae.

C. eluteria. Yields cascarilla.

C. tiglium. Yields croton oil. See under *oil*.

cro″ton·al′de·hyde. $CH_3CH{:}CHCHO$. A colorless, pungent liquid; used as a component of tear gas and as an intermediate in chemical syntheses.

cro′ton chlo′ral hy′drate. See *butyl*-chloral hydrate.

cro′ton·ism [*krotōn*]. Poisoning by croton oil; a condition marked by hemorrhagic gastroenteritis.

cro·tox′in. A neurotoxin from the venom of the rattlesnake *Crotalus durissus terrificus*.

croup (krōōp) [probably imitative]. A condition of the larynx seen in children; characterized by a harsh, brassy cough and crowing, difficult respiration. It may be due to edema, inflammation with or without exudate or membrane formation, or spasm. —**croup′ous,** *adj.*, **croup′y,** *adj.*

artificial c. Posttraumatic membranous laryngitis.

catarrhal c. Usually occurs at night, during the course of an upper respiratory infection.

diphtheritic c. Laryngeal diphtheria.

false c. Laryngismus stridulus.

membranous c. Laryngeal diphtheria.

spasmodic c. Laryngismus stridulus.

true c. Laryngeal diphtheria.

uterine c. Inflammation of the endometrium with membrane formation. *Obs.*

croup′ine (krōōp′een, ·in) [*croup*]. Laryngismus stridulus.

croup ket′tle. A small boiler with an attached inhaling tube. Water or medicament is placed in the receptacle, heated, and the steam inhaled or allowed to escape to humidify the air in the room.

Crouzon, Octave [*French neurologist*, 1874–1938]. Known for his description of craniofacial dysostosis or hypertelorism (1912), also called *Crouzon's disease*.

Crowe, Samuel James [*American physician*, 1883–]. Known for his important experimental work, with Harvey Cushing and John Homans, on the pituitary and its relation to the reproductive system (1910). See also Crowe's *sign*.

crown [L. *corona*, crown]. Corona; the top part of anything; any structure like a crown.

anatomic c. That portion of a tooth covered with enamel.

artificial c. A metallic, porcelain, or plastic substitute which replaces all or part of the crown of a tooth.

clinical c. That portion of a tooth above the gingival attachment.

collar c. A collarlike device to hold an artificial tooth to a natural root.

c. of a tooth. That part covered with enamel.

c.-setting. The operation of joining an artificial crown to the root of a natural tooth.

jacket c. An artificial restoration of the crown of a tooth; consists of a covering of metal, porcelain, or acrylic.

pivot c. *In dentistry*, a tooth crown of porcelain or other material, attached to the root by means of a pin or post.

crown′work″. *In dentistry*, the adaptation of an artificial crown of gold, porcelain, or acrylic on the cervical portion of the natural root of a tooth.

Cruce. See *Della Croce*.

cru′cial [L. *crux*, a cross]. Resembling or pertaining to a cross, as a crucial incision.

cru′ci·ate. Resembling a cross; cross-shaped.

cru′ci·ble [ML. *crucibulum*, earthen pot]. Vessel of clay or other suitable material used in melting substances which require a high degree of heat.

cru′ci·form [L. *crux*, a cross; *forma*, shape]. Crucial; shaped like a cross.

Cruikshank, William Cumberland [*English surgeon*, 1745–1800]. Remembered for his demonstration that carbon dioxide is given off by the skin (1779). Contributed to knowledge of the lymphatic system (1786). Made experimental study of impregnation in the rabbit (1797).

crup′per [OF. *cropiere*]. 1. The buttocks of a horse. 2. The sacrococcygeal region in the horse. 3. The base of the tail in mammals.

cru′re·us. The vastus intermedius muscle.

crus (pl. *crura*) [L., leg]. A term applied to certain parts of the body, from their resemblance to legs or roots. —**cru′ral,** *adj.*

crura of the incus. The two main processes of the incus. The **short crus** projects into the fossa of the incus; the **long crus** articulates with the head of the stapes.

crura of the stapes. Anterior and posterior processes which connect the base and head of the stapes.

c. commune. One common to two structures, as that between the superior and posterior semicircular canals.

c. of the anthelix. Either of the two limbs of the bifurcation of the anthelix.

c. of the cerebellum. Any one of the cerebellar peduncles.

c. of the cerebrum. Either of the two peduncles connecting the cerebrum with the pons: also called *crus cerebri, basis pedunculi, cerebral peduncle*.

c. of the clitoris. Homolog of the crus of the penis.

c. of the diaphragm. Either of the two fibromuscular bands arising in front of the vertebrae and inserted into the central tendon of the diaphragm.

c. of the fornix. See *column* of the fornix.

c. of the helix. The curved root of the helix above the external auditory meatus.

c. of the penis. The posterior part of either corpus cavernosum penis, attached to the pubic arch.

c. pedunculi. The basis pedunculi. See *c.* of the cerebrum.

crush [OF. *cruisir*]. To press or squeeze between two unyielding bodies. —**crush,** *n.*

crust [L. *crusta*, crust]. A covering; especially, a dried exudate on the skin.

milk c. See under *milk*.

crus′ta [L.]. A thin layer; crust.

c. adamantina dentium. Dental enamel. *Obs.*

c. lactea. Seborrhea of the scalp in infants.

c. petrosa. Dental cementum.

Crus·ta′ce·a [L. *crusta*, crust]. A class of arthropods including the lobsters, crabs, shrimps, barnacles, and sow bugs.

crutch [AS. *crycc*]. A staff used as a support in walking, having a concave, padded crosspiece to fit the axilla, and a grip for the hand.

Canadian c. An adjustable hand crutch with a tripod or quadripod base: also called *Toronto c.*

hand c. A crutchlike support in which the weight of the body is partially borne by the hand and arm instead of by the axilla. The device is used in training the individual to use an artificial leg or legs after the usual crutch stage of training is ended.

perineal c. A support or brace attached to an operating table to hold a patient in certain positions.

Toronto c. See Canadian *c.*

Crutchfield, William Gayle [*American neurosurgeon*, 1900–]. Invented traction tongs, called *Crutchfield tongs*, for use in the treatment of fracture dislocations of the cervical spine.

Cruveilhier, Jean [*French pathologist*, 1791–1874]. Internationally known for his *Human Pathological Anatomy* (1829–42), one of the greatest works of its kind. Described multiple sclerosis. Described progressive myelopathic muscular atrophy, called *Cruveilhier's disease*, *Duchenne-Aran muscular atrophy*. Gave early description of hypertrophic pyloric stenosis and ulcer of the stomach, to both of which his name was applied. Congenital cirrhosis of the liver is known as *Cruveilhier-Baumgarten cirrhosis*. See also Cruveilhier's *sign*.

Cruz, Osvaldo Gonçalves [*Brazilian bacteriologist*, 1872–1917]. Reformed the Brazilian public health service. American trypanosomiasis, caused by the *Trypanosoma cruzi*, is called *Cruz's disease*, *Chagas' disease*.

cry [OF. *crier*, from L. *quiritare*, to wail]. The utterance of an inarticulate vocal sound, or the sound so uttered; the sound of the voice in lamentation.

cry-. See *cryo-*.

cry″al·ge′si·a (cry″al·jee′zee·uh, ·see·uh) [G. *kryos*, icy cold; *algēsis*, sense of pain]. Pain from the application of cold.

cry·an″es·the′si·a (cry·an″ess·thee′zhuh, ·zee·uh) [*kryos;* G. *anaisthēsia*, lack of sensation]. Loss of sensation or perception of cold.

cry″es·the′si·a (cry″ess·thee′zhuh, ·zee·uh) [*kryos;* G. *aisthēsis*, sensation]. 1. Temperature sense for cold. 2. Sensitiveness to cold.

cry″mo·dyn′i·a (cry″mo·din′ee·uh, ·dye′nee·uh) [G. *krymos*, frost; *odynē*, pain]. Cryalgesia; pain coming on in cold or damp weather.

cry″mo·phil′ic [*krymos;* G. *philein*, to love]. Psychrophilic.

cry′o-, cry- [G. *kryos*, icy cold]. A combining form meaning *cold* or *freezing*.

cry″o·cau′ter·y [*kryos;* G. *kautērion*, branding iron]. The destruction of tissues by application of extreme cold which causes an obliterative thrombosis; used especially in removing moles.

cry′o·chem (cry′o·kem) [*kryos;* G. *chymos*, juice]. A desiccation procedure involving rapid freezing of the material to be dried followed by evaporation of the moisture from the frozen state with the aid of a regenerable desiccant.

cry″o·glob′u·lin. A globulin, abnormally present in blood serum, which coagulates on cooling.

cry″o·glob″u·li·ne′mi·a. An abnormal condition in which blood serum contains cold-coagulable globulin (cryoglobulin): observed in multiple myeloma and also in certain other pathological conditions.

cry·om′e·ter (crye·om′i·tur) [*kryos;* G. *metron*, a measure]. Thermometer for measuring low temperatures.

cry″o·pro′te·in [*kryos;* G. *prōteios*, of first rank]. See *cryoglobulin*.

cry′o·scope [*kryos;* G. *skopein*, to examine]. Device for determining the freezing point of a liquid.

cry′o·stat [*kryos;* G. *statos*, standing]. Any device for maintaining very low temperatures: specifically, a refrigerator that operates by compressing, regeneratively cooling, and then expanding helium gas until part of the gas becomes liquid; it can cool contents to −45° F.

cry″o·ther′a·py [*kryos;* G. *therapeia*, treatment]. A form of therapy which consists of local or general refrigeration.

crypt [G. *kryptos*, hidden]. 1. A small sac or follicle. 2. A glandular cavity.

anal c. One of the small cul-de-sacs between the rectal columns. Syn., *rectal sinus*.

crypts of Lieberkühn. Simple tubular intestinal glands. Also called *Lieberkühn's glands*.

crypts of the tongue. Pits in the mucous membrane of the pharyngeal part of the tongue, surrounded by the lymphatic tissue of the lingual tonsils. They often serve also as excretory ducts of the mucous glands of this region.

dental c. The space filled by the dental sac and a developing tooth.

enamel c. See enamel *niche*.

multilocular c. (a) A simple gland with pouched or sacculated walls. (b) The lobule of a racemose gland.

sebaceous crypts. The sebaceous glands.

synoviparous crypts. Extensions of the synovial membranes sometimes perforating an articular capsule and occasionally becoming shut off from its main sac.

tonsillar c. A deep epithelium-lined invagination in the palatine or lingual tonsils.

cryp″tag·glu′tin·oid. An antibody against erythrocytes which combines specifically with the cells but does not agglutinate them in saline and does not give a positive blocking test: sometimes called *third-order antibody*, *agglutinin*.

cryp″tam·ne′si·a (krip″tam·nee′zhuh, ·zee·uh). See *cryptomnesia*.

crypt″an·am·ne′si·a (kript″an·am·nee′zhuh, ·zee·uh) [*kryptos;* G. *anamnēsis*, a calling to mind]. Subconscious memory.

cryp·ti′tis [*kryptos;* G. *-itis*, inflammation]. Inflammation of a crypt, or of crypts.

urethral c. Inflammation of the mucous glands of the urethra.

cryp′to-, crypt- [*kryptos*]. A combining form meaning *hidden, covered, secret*.

cryp″to·ceph′a·lus [*kryptos;* G. *kephalē*, head]. A parasitic conjoined twin with an imperfectly formed and concealed head.

cryp″to·coc·co′sis [*kryptos;* G. *kokkos*, grain; *-ōsis*, condition]. A subacute or chronic infection caused by the yeast *Cryptococcus histolyticus*. The infection may involve the lungs or skin, producing ulcers containing myxomatous exudates, but has a predilection for the meninges and the brain. Also called *torulosis*, *European blastomycosis*, *Busse-Buschke's disease*.

Cryp″to·coc′cus [*kryptos; kokkos*]. A genus of true yeast whose species are pathogenic.

C. histolyticus. The causative organism of cryptococcosis: also called *C. neoformans*, *Torula histolytica*, *Torulopsis neoformans*.

cryp″to·did′y·mus [*kryptos;* G. *didymos*, twin]. A form of duplicity in which a fetus (or fetal part) is included within the body of an individual. Syn., *fetus in fetu*.

cryp′to·gam [*kryptos;* G. *gamos*, marriage]. *In botany*, one of the Cryptogamia, a division of the vegetable kingdom comprising all plants without flowers or seeds, as the algae, fungi, mosses, and ferns. —**cryptog′amous,** *adj*.

cryp″to·gen′ic [*kryptos;* G. *genesthai*, from *gignesthai*, to be produced]. Of unknown or obscure cause; the opposite of *phanerogenic*.

cryp″to·grand′o·side. Either of two digitalislike glycosides, designated *cryptograndoside A* and *cryptograndoside B*, occurring in *Cryptostegia grandiflora*, commonly known as the rubber vine; the glycosides are cardioactive.

cryp′to·lith [*kryptos;* G. *lithos*, stone]. A concretion or calculus formed within a crypt, as in the tonsil.

cryp″to·men″or·rhe′a, cryp″to·men″or·rhoe′a (krip″to·men″o·ree′uh) [*kryptos;* G. *mēn*, month; *rhoia*, flow]. A condition in which there is menstrual flow from the uterus, the external escape of which is prevented by an obstruction in the lower genital canal, usually an imperforate hymen.

cryp″to·mer″o·rha·chis′chi·sis (·ra·kiss′ki·sis) [*kryptos;* G. *meros*, a part; *rhachis*, spine; *schisis*, cleavage]. Spina bifida occulta; a variety with bony deficiency but no rachicele.

cryp″tom·ne′si·a (krip″tom·nee′zhuh, ·zee·uh), **cryp″tam·ne′si·a** [*kryptos;* G. *amnēsia*, forgetfulness]. Subconscious memory; the recall to mind of a forgotten episode which seems entirely new to the patient, and not a part of his past experiences.

cryp″to·phan′ic ac′id. $C_{10}H_{18}N_2O_{10}$. An acid said to exist in urine.

cryp″toph·thal′mos [*kryptos;* G. *ophthalmos*, eye]. 1. Congenital union of the eyelids, usually over imperfect eyes: also *cryptophthalmus*, *cryptophthalmia*. 2. A person who has congenital union of the eyelids.

cryp′to·pine (krip′to·peen, ·pin). One of the minor alkaloids of opium; colorless and odorless.

cryp·top′or·ous [*kryptos;* G. *poros*, opening]. Having hidden or obscure pores.

crypt″or·chid·ec′to·my (krip″tor·kid·eck′to·mee) [*kryptos;* G. *orchis*, testis; *ektomē*, excision]. Removal of an undescended testis.

crypt·or′chid·ism. Cryptorchism.

crypt″or·chid″o·pex·y (krip″tor·kid′o·peck·see) [*kryptos; orchis;* G. *pēxis*, a fixing]. Fixation, within the scrotum, of an undescended testis.

crypt·or′chism (kript·or′kiz·um) [*kryptos; orchis*]. A developmental defect in which the testes fail to descend, and remain within the abdomen or inguinal canal. —**cryptorchid, cryptorchis,** *n.*

cryp″to·xan′thin (krip″to·zan′thin). A yellow pigment of the carotenoid group of chemical compounds, which is found in yellow corn and certain other natural sources, and which acts like vitamin A in the body.

cryp″to·zo′ite [*kryptos;* G. *zōion*, living being]. The exoerythrocytic stage of malarial parasites which are found in the cells of the skin and viscera before gaining access to the erythrocytes.

cryp·toz′y·gous [*kryptos;* G. *zygon*, yoke]. Having a wide skull and a narrow face, so that the zygomatic arches are not visible when the skull is viewed from above.

crys′tal [G. *krystallos*, rock-crystal]. *In chemistry*, a substance that assumes a definite geometric form.

asthma crystals. Charcot-Leyden crystals.

bismuth suboxide crystals. Those commonly found in feces after the administration of bismuth.

Böttcher's crystals. Spermin crystals.

calcium bilirubinate crystals. Those found in feces occasionally, especially in cases of cholelithiasis.

Charcot-Leyden crystals. Colorless, pointed, often needlelike crystals occurring in the sputum in bronchial asthma and in the feces in amebic colitis and other ulcerative diseases of the colon. Also called *asthma crystals*.

cockle-burr crystals. Dark yellow or brown crystals of ammonium urate occurring in alkaline urine.

coffin-lid crystals. Those of ammonium magnesium phosphate, triple phosphate, occurring in alkaline urine.

dumbbell crystals. Those of calcium oxalate or uric acid occurring in acid urine or those of calcium carbonate, in alkaline urine.

hematoidin crystals. Yellowish or brown, needlelike or rhombic crystals which may occur in the feces after hemorrhage in the gastrointestinal tract. Formerly called *Virchow's crystals*.

hemin crystals. Reddish brown, microscopic, prismatic crystals of hemin obtained by heating blood with glacial acetic acid and salt. Formerly called *Teichmann's crystals*.

osazone crystals. Yellow crystals of characteristic shape formed by the different sugars when they are combined with phenylhydrazine.

spermin crystals. A combination of phosphoric acid with a base, spermin ($C_5H_{14}N_2$), forming long, monoclinic, prismlike crystals with curved edges found in semen after drying it or allowing it to stand. A strong solution of iodine and potassium iodide stains them a deep brown or violet. Also called *Böttcher's crystals*.

Teichmann's crystals. See *hemin crystals* under *crystal*.

triple phosphate crystals. Coffin-lid or feathery crystals of ammonium magnesium phosphate occurring in alkaline urine.

Virchow's crystals. See *hematoidin crystals* under *crystal*.

whetstone c. One type of uric acid crystal found in acid urine.

crys″tal·bu′min. An albuminous substance found in the crystalline lens.

crys″tal·fi′brin. An albuminous body obtained by treating crystalline lens with hydrochloric acid.

crys′tal·lin. 1. The globulin of the crystalline lens. 2. A solution of pyroxylin in methanol and amyl acetate resembling collodion.

crys′tal·line (kris′tuh·lin, ·lyne) [G. *krystallos*, rock-crystal]. Like a crystal.

crys″tal·li′tis [*krystallos;* G. *-itis*, inflammation]. Phacitis.

crys″tal·li·za′tion [*krystallos*]. The process by which the molecules of a substance arrange themselves in geometric forms when passing from a gaseous or a liquid state to a solid state.

crys″tal·log′ra·phy [*krystallos;* G. *graphein*, to write]. The science of crystals, their formation, structure and classification.

crys′tal·loid [*krystallos;* G. *eidos*, form]. Having a crystal-like nature, as distinguished from colloid.

crys″tal·lo·mag′net·ism [*krystallos;* G. *Magnētis lithos*, magnet]. The property common to certain crystals of orienting themselves in a magnetic field.

crys″tal·lo·pho′bi·a [*krystallos;* G. *phobos*, fear]. A morbid fear of glass.

crys′tal·lose. Sodium saccharinate.

crys″tal·lu′ri·a [*krystallos;* G. *ouron*, urine]. The presence of crystals in the urine; often a normal condition but of importance when the crystals are of the sulfa drugs since the crystals may form in the kidney tubules and cause blocking.

crys′tal vi′o·let (C.C.). A basic dye of the triphenylmethane group, hexamethyl pararosaniline. A constituent of all the bluer shades of methyl violet and gentian violet; may be used in nearly all procedures calling for gentian violet, being of more constant composition than gentian violet. Also called *hexamethyl violet, methyl violet 10B, gentian violet*.

crysticillin. A trade-mark for *penicillin G procaine*.

crystoids anthelmintic. Trade-mark for hexylresorcinol in pill form.

Cs Symbol for cesium.

c/s Cycles per second.

CSF Abbreviation for cerebrospinal fluid.

CTAB Trade-mark for cetyltrimethylammonium bromide or cetrimide.

Cten″o·ce·phal′i·des (ten″o·si·fal′i·deez, tee″no·) [G. *kteis*, comb; *kephalē*, head]. A genus of fleas which are cosmopolitan in distribution. The species **Ct. canis,** the dog flea, and **Ct. felis,** the cat flea, while they infest primarily dogs and cats, may attack man and other mammals. Members of this genus also serve as intermediate hosts of the *Dipylidium caninum*.

Cten·op′syl·lus seg′nis (ten·op′sil·lus seg′nis) [*kteis;* G. *psylla,* flea; L. *segnis,* lazy]. The rodent flea.

C three, C₃. In the system of population classification in England, referring to that part of the population consisting of individuals exhibiting imperfect mental or physical development.

Cu Chemical symbol for copper.

cu′beb [Ar. *kabābah*]. The dried, unripe, nearly full-grown fruit of *Piper cubeba,* cultivated in Java and the West Indies. Its properties are due to a volatile oil containing terpenes, a sesquiterpene hydrate, $C_{15}H_{24}$, and an organic acid. It has been used as a diuretic, urinary antiseptic, and expectorant. Formerly used in cigarettes for respiratory catarrh.

c. oleoresin. Obtained by extraction of cubeb with alcohol, followed by evaporation of the solvent. It is a dosage form of cubeb now little used.

cu·beb′ic ac′id. An acid substance of uncertain composition obtained from cubeb berries; formerly used as a diuretic.

cu′be·bin. $C_{20}H_{20}O_6$. A bitter, crystalline substance obtained from cubeb.

cu′beb·ism [*kabābah*]. Poisoning by cubeb; marked by acute gastroenteritis.

cu′bi·form [G. *kybos,* cube; L. *forma,* shape]. Cuboid.

cu′bi·tus [L.]. The forearm; elbow: old term for *ulna.* —**cubital,** *adj.*

c. valgus. A decrease in the normal carrying angle of the arm.

c. varus. An increase in the normal carrying angle of the arm.

cu′bo- [G. *kybos,* cube]. A combining form denoting *a cube* or *cubital.*

cu′boid [*kybos;* G. *eidos,* form]. Resembling a cube.

cu′boid. That bone of the tarsus between the calcaneus and the fourth and fifth metatarsals. —**cuboid′al,** *adj.*

cu·boi′de·o-. See *cubo-.*

cu·boi″de·o·na·vic′u·lar [BNA] [G. *kyboeidēs,* like a cube; L. *navicula,* small boat]. Pertaining to the cuboid and the navicular bones, as in cuboideonavicular joint and ligaments. See Table of Joints and Ligaments in the Appendix.

cu′cum·ber shin. Curvature of the tibia with the convexity forward.

Cu′cu·mis [L., cucumber]. A genus of plants of the Cucurbitaceae.

C. melo. Muskmelon.

C. myriocarpus. Yields cacur; used by the Kaffirs as an emetic.

C. sativus. Cucumber; the juice of the fruit has been used in skin diseases and as a cosmetic.

Cu·cur′bi·ta [L., gourd]. A genus of plants of the Cucurbitaceae. Several species, such as **C. pepo,** the pumpkin, yield seeds that have been used as anthelmintics.

cud′bear [after *Cuthbert* Gordon]. A powder prepared from species of *Roccella, Lecanora,* or other lichens; it is used as a red coloring agent for pharmaceutical preparations, generally in the form of 10% tincture.

Cuignet, Ferdinand Louis Joseph [*French ophthalmologist,* b. 1823]. Introduced retinoscopy (1873), called *Cuignet's test.*

cui·rass′ (kwee·rass′, kwee′rass) [F. *cuirasse,* from L. *coriaceus,* made of leather]. A close-fitting or immovable bandage for the front of the chest.

c. cancer. See *cancer* en cuirasse.

tabetic c. An anesthetic area encircling the chest in tabetic patients.

cul′-de-sac′ (kul′-di-sack′, -sahk′, kōōl′-, kood-sahk′. *See* Notes §§ 29, 35) [F.]. 1. A closed or blind pouch or sac. 2. The rectouterine pouch; the prolongation of the peritoneal cavity between the anterior surface of the rectum and the posterior surface of the uterus. Also called *pouch of Douglas.*

cul″do·cen·te′sis. Removal of intraperitoneal fluid material (transudate, exudate, or blood) via the vagina and the rectouterine pouch (cul-de-sac). This may be bone by aspiration or incision.

cul′do·scope [perhaps from *cul-de-sac;* G. *skopein,* to examine]. An instrument for the visualization of the female internal genitalia and pelvic tissues, entering via the vagina and a perforation into the cul-de-sac. —**culdos′copy,** *n.*

cul″dot′o·my [*cul-de-sac;* G. *tomē,* a cutting]. A surgical incision through the cul-de-sac.

Cu′lex [L., a gnat]. A genus of mosquitoes which are vectors of disease.

C. fatigans. The most important intermediate host of *Wuchereria bancrofti.*

C. pipiens. This species is known as the common house mosquito and is found in temperate regions; of medical importance as a vector of filariasis.

C. quinquefasciatus. A mosquito which is the most common vector of *Wuchereria bancrofti.* Also called *C. fatigans.*

Cu·lic′i·dae (cue·liss′i·dee) [*culex*]. A family of insects belonging to the Diptera.

cu′li·cide [*culex;* L. *caedere,* to kill]. Any agent which destroys mosquitoes.

cu·lic′i·fuge [*culex;* L. *fugere,* to flee]. An agent to drive away mosquitoes.

Cu″li·ci′nae (cue″li·sigh′nee) [*culex*]. A subfamily of the Culicidae; contains all species of mosquitoes of medical significance, which are important as vectors of filariasis, malaria, hemoglobinuric fever, dengue, and yellow fever.

Cu″li·coi′des (cue″li·koy′deez) [*culex;* G. *eidos,* form]. A genus of flies, several species of which serve as intermediate hosts of filarial parasites. **C. austeni** and **C. grahami** are species which transmit the filarial worm, *Acanthocheilonema perstans;* **C. furens** has been found to transmit *Mansonella ozzardi.*

Cullen, Thomas Stephen [*American gynecologist,* 1868–1953]. Known for his studies of hyperplasia of the endometrium and for his investigations of cancer of the uterus. Remembered for his description of the sign of a ruptured ectopic pregnancy: a bluish discoloration of the skin about the umbilicus; called *Cullen's sign.*

Cullen, William [*Scottish physician,* 1710–90]. One of the great teachers of Edinburgh and Glasgow, he was among the first in Great Britain to give clinical lectures. Wrote on fevers, neuroses, and cachexias. Therapeutics in the British Isles was established as a medical science largely through his efforts.

cul′men [L., summit]. The superior portion of the monticulus of the vermis of the cerebellum.

cult [L. *cultus,* care]. Any spurious or unorthodox system of healing, usually based on the belief that all disease is due to a single underlying cause and can be cured by some simple treatment.

cul″ti·va′tion [*cultus*]. Successive transferring of organisms to different mediums favorable to growth. See *culture.*

cul′ture [L. *cultura,* from *colere,* to till]. 1. Growth of microorganisms on artificial mediums. 2. Act of cultivating microorganisms on artificial mediums. 3. A group of microorganisms grown in an artificial medium.

blood c. See under *blood.*

c. medium. A substance used for cultivating bacteria. Culture mediums are either liquid or solid, bouillon and milk being the important liquid mediums, and gelatin, agar, blood serum, and potato the principal solid mediums.

hanging-drop c. A culture in which the microorganism is inoculated into a drop of fluid on a cover glass and the latter is inverted over a glass slide having a central concavity.

mixed c. A culture containing more than one defined species of microorganism.

needle c. See stab *c.*

plate c. A culture of bacteria on a medium spread upon a flat plate or in a Petri dish.

pure c. A culture of a single microorganism.

slant c. One made on the slanting surface of a medium, to get a greater surface for growth.

stab c. One in which the medium is inoculated by means of a needle bearing the microorganisms, which is inserted deeply into the medium.

thrust c. Stab culture.

tissue c. The growing of tissue cells in artificial mediums.

cu'ma·rin. See *coumarin.*

cu'mene. C_9H_{12}. Cumol; isopropyl benzene. A hydrocarbon occurring in pine tar, petroleum, and some volatile oils.

cumertilin. Trade-mark for a mercurial diuretic preparation containing 8-(2′-methoxy-3′-hydroxymercuripropyl)coumarin-3-carboxylic acid (known as *mercumallylic acid*) and theophylline, the combination being designated by the generic name *mercumatilin.*

c. sodium. Trade-mark for a preparation containing the sodium salt of the mercurial compound described in the preceding and theophylline, the combination being designated by the generic name *mercumatilin sodium.*

cum'in, cu'min [Ar. *kammūn*]. An umbelliferous plant, *Cuminum cyminum*, native in Egypt and Syria. The fruit has been used as a flavoring agent and carminative. Its active principle is a volatile oil containing cuminaldehyde (cuminal). —**cu'mic,** *adj.*

cu'mol. Cumene.

cumopyran. Trade-marked name for *cyclocumarol.*

cu'mu·la"tive [L. *cumulare*, to heap up, increase]. Increasing; adding to.

cu'mu·lus [L., pile]. A heap or mound.

c. oophorus. The mass of follicular cells surrounding the ovum and protruding into the liquid-filled cavity of a Graafian follicle. Syn., *discus proligerus.*

c. ovigerus. Cumulus oophorus. *Obs.*

c. proligerus. Old term for *cumulus oophorus.*

cu'ne·ate [L. *cuneus*, wedge]. Wedge-shaped, as cuneate fasciculus, a fiber tract in the posterior funiculus of the spinal cord.

cu·ne'i·form, cu'ne·i·form [*cuneus;* L. *forma*, form]. Wedge-shaped; cuneate.

cu'ne·i·form. 1. Any of three tarsal bones. See Table of Bones in the Appendix. 2. Old term for *triquetrum.*

cu'ne·o- [*cuneus*]. A combining form meaning *a wedge* and denoting *cuneiform.*

cu"ne·o·cu'boid [*cuneus;* G. *kyboeidēs*, like a cube]. Pertaining to the cuneiform and cuboid bones, as the cuneocuboid joint and ligaments. See Table of Joints and Ligaments in the Appendix.

cu"ne·o·na·vic'u·lar [*cuneus;* L. *navicula*, small boat]. Pertaining to the cuneiform and the navicular bones, as the cuneonavicular joints and ligaments. See Table of Joints and Ligaments in the Appendix.

cu"ne·o·scaph'oid [*cuneus;* G. *skaphē*, boat]. Old term for cuneonavicular.

cu'ne·us [L.]. A wedge-shaped convolution on the medial aspect of the occipital lobe between the parieto-occipital and calcarine fissures. Also called *cuneate lobule, gyrus c.* —**cuneate,** *adj.*

cu·nic'u·lar [L. *cuniculum*, a passage under ground, canal, from *cuniculus*, rabbit]. Furrowed.

cu·nic'u·lus [L.]. The burrow of the itch mite.

cun'jah. See *cannabis.*

cun"ni·lin'gus [L. *cunnus*, vulva; *linguere*, to lick]. An abnormal sexual practice consisting of the licking of the vulva. —**cunnilinguist,** *n.*

cun'nus [L.]. The vulva.

cu'o·rin. $C_{71}H_{125}O_{21}NP_2$. A phospholipid which has been isolated from heart muscles.

cup [AS. *cuppe*, from L. *cupa*, tub, cask]. A drinking vessel.

dry c. A cup for drawing the blood to the surface.

favus c. A depression in a favus scale surrounding a hair.

feeding c. A cup used for feeding anyone incapable of self-feeding.

glaucomatous c. A deep depression in the optic disk seen in cases of glaucoma.

optic c. The double-walled cup formed by invagination of the optic vesicle which differentiates into pigmented and sensory layers of the retina.

physiologic c. The normal concavity of the optic disk.

quassia c. One made of quassia wood, which is filled with water and allowed to stand, the water acquiring the bitter taste of the quassia.

retinal c. Excavation of the optic disk.

suction c. A cupping glass.

wet c. A cup for abstracting blood through incisions in the skin.

cup. To bleed. See *cupping.*

cu'po·la [L. *cupula*, little tub]. A dome-shaped structure. See *diaphragm*, 4.

cupped [L. *cupa*, tub, cask]. Having the upper surface depressed; applied to the coagulum of blood after phlebotomy.

cup'ping [*cupa*]. 1. A method of bloodletting by means of the application of cupping glasses to the surface of the body. 2. Formation of a cuplike depression.

c. glass. A small bell-shaped glass capable of holding three to four ounces, in which the air is rarefied by heat or by exhaustion; the glass is applied to the skin, either with or without scarification of the latter.

dry c. A form of counterirritation in which the blood is drawn to the surface by means of a cup. This was used mainly in inflammatory affections of the lung.

wet c. The abstraction of blood after scarification.

cu"pram·mo'ni·a. A solution of cupric hydroxide in ammonia water used as a solvent for cellulose.

cu'pre·a bark. The bark of certain species of *Remijia*. It was at one time used as a substitute for cinchona bark; contains homoquinine and certain related alkaloids.

cu'pre·ine (cue'pree·een, ·in). An alkaloid, $C_{19}H_{22}O_2N_2.2H_2O$, derived from cuprea bark.

cuprex. A proprietary solution of a copper compound for use in treatment of pediculosis.

cu'pric [L. *cuprum*, copper, from *Cyprus*, renowned for its copper mines]. Containing copper as a bivalent element. See *copper.*

cu'prous [*cuprum*]. Containing copper as a univalent element. See *copper.*

cu'prum. See *copper.*

cu'pu·la [L., a little tub]. 1. A cup-shaped structure. 2. A colorless substance on the crista ampullaris that coagulates and becomes visible upon applying fixing fluids.

c. of the cochlea. The apex of the osseous cochlea.

c. of the diaphragm. The right or left dome of the diaphragm.

c. of the pleura. That part of the pleura covering the apex of the lung in the root of the neck.

cu″pu·lom′e·try. The picking up of electrical potentials at the cupula (apex) of the cochlea caused by an auditory stimulus. It is used only in experimental acoustic physiology.

cur′age (cure′idj, cue·rahzh′) [F. *curer*, to cleanse]. 1. Curettage; cleansing of the eye or of an ulcerated or carious surface. 2. A term used by some authorities for clearing the uterine cavity by means of the finger, as distinguished from the use of the curet. *Obs.*

cu·ran′gin (cue·ran′jin). $C_{48}H_{77}O_{20}$. A glycoside obtained from *Curanga amara* (Scrophulariaceae). It is used as a febrifuge and vermifuge in India.

cu·ra′re (cue·rah′ree) [Tupian]. A drug of uncertain and variable composition prepared from several species of *Strychnos* and *Chondodendron* plants. Curare from *Chondodendron tomentosum*, currently of chief medical interest, owes its characteristic action to the quaternary base *d*-tubocurarine, which paralyzes the skeletal muscles by a selective blocking of the neuromuscular junction and prevents response to nerve impulses and acetylcholine. Curare does not produce tissue injury except as a result of anoxia due to unrelieved respiratory paralysis. Used to control convulsions and muscular spasms, particularly in the treatment of certain neurologic disorders; also used to relax the skeletal muscles during anesthesia. In South America and elsewhere it is used as an arrow poison. —**cu′rarize,** *v.*

cu·ra″ri·mi·met′ic. Referring, or pertaining to, the action, similar to that of curare, of an agent that inhibits, at the neuromuscular junction, transmission of an impulse from a nerve to the skeletal muscle fibers that it innervates.

cu·ra′rine (cue·rah′reen, ·rin, cure′uh·). An alkaloid isolated from a curare by Boehm (1898); now called *d-tubocurarine*.

cu″ra·ri·za′tion [*curare*]. The subjection to the full influence of curare. Voice and power of motion are generally abolished, but not sensibility to pain.

spontaneous c. Conditions of autointoxication occasioned by the paralyzing influence of toxic substances upon the circulation and upon the end-plates of the neuromuscular system; produced in the body by the tetanization of the muscles.

cu′ra·tive [L. *curare*, to heal]. Having a healing tendency.

cur′cu·ma [NL., from Ar. *kurkum*]. Turmeric. The rhizome of *Curcuma longa*, of India, a plant of the Zingiberaceae, with properties similar to ginger. It contains a yellow coloring matter, curcumin, and is occasionally employed as a yellow dye in pharmacy to color ointments and other preparations. *In chemistry*, its solution in alcohol is used as a test for alkalies, which turn it brown. Paper treated with an alcoholic solution (turmeric paper) may be used instead. Curcuma contains about 5% volatile oil and is used also as a condiment.

cur′cu·min. The crystalline coloring matter of curcuma, $C_{21}H_{20}O_6$. Used as an indicator and dye. Gives a brownish red color with alkalies and a light yellow color with acids.

curd [ME.]. The coagulum that separates from milk on the addition of rennin or acids.

cure [L. *cura*, care]. 1. The successful treatment of an illness or a wound. 2. Special treatment for a disease or an invalid. —**cure,** *v.*

cu·ret′ [F., from *curer*, to cleanse]. An instrument, shaped like a spoon or scoop, for scraping away exuberant or dead tissue. —**curet′,** *v.*

suction c. A small hollow tube with a cutting window to which suction may be applied; used for obtaining endometrial biopsy.

cu·ret′tage (cue·ret′idj, cure″i·tahzh′) [F.]. *In surgery*, scraping of the interior of a cavity with a curet, or by the finger.

Curie, Marie Sklodowska [*Polish-French chemist*, 1867–1934]. Internationally renowned for her discovery of radium (with her husband, Pierre Curie) and for her continued investigation of the nature of radium and radioactive substances. Received Nobel award jointly with Pierre Curie and A. H. Becquerel (1903) and the undivided award (1911).

Curie, Pierre [*French chemist*, 1859–1906]. Famed internationally (with Marie Curie) for his discovery and isolation of radium from pitchblende (1898). Received Nobel prize with Marie Curie and A. H. Becquerel (1903).

cu′rie (cure′ee, koor′ee, cue·ree′) [after Marie and Pierre *Curie*]. 1. Formerly, the amount of radon in equilibrium with one gram of radium. 2. That quantity of any radioactive species (radioisotope) undergoing exactly 3.700×10^{10} disintegrations per second.

cu′rie·gram (cure′ee·gram, koor′ee·gram) [*Curie*; G. *gramma*, letter]. A photographic print made by radium rays, similar to a roentgenogram.

cu′rine (cure′een, ·in). An alkaloid obtained from a kind of curare.

cu′ri·um [*Curie*]. Chemical element No. 96, symbol Cm, produced artificially.

curled [ME. *curlen*]. Occurring in parallel chains of wavy strands, as the colonies of anthrax bacillus.

Curling, Thomas Blizard [*English surgeon*, 1811–88]. Known for his description of acute ulceration of the duodenum due to burns (1842), called *Curling's ulcer*. Was the first to note accurately the clinical aspect of cretinism, suggesting thyroid deficiency as the probable cause (1850).

cur′rent [L. *currere*, to run]. 1. The flow of electricity (electrons) through a circuit; also the rate of this flow. 2. The movement or flow of a liquid or gas, as of blood in vessels, or of air through the respiratory passages.

action c. The electric current accompanying activity of any reacting tissue.

alternating c. A current which changes its direction a number of times per second. Abbreviated, A. C.

anelectrotonic c. That produced around the anode on passage of a constant current through a nerve.

angular c. One with its wave form inclined at some angle.

ascending c. The current formed by placing the positive electrode upon the periphery of a nerve and the negative higher up on the trunk of the nerve, or on the surface over the nerve center in the spinal cord.

axial c. The column of erythrocytes which, by reason of the weight of the cells, occupies the center or axis of the blood stream. Also called *axial stream*.

battery c. See galvanic *c.*

branch c. See derived *c.*

catelectrotonic c. That produced around the cathode on passage of a constant current through a nerve.

continuous c. A current passing through a circuit in one direction.

convection c. A current of a liquid or gas heated to a temperature above that of the surrounding medium; it rises to the surface because of its lesser density, and thus the entire fluid or gas circulates until it acquires the same temperature.

c. of injury. See *injury potential.*

D'Arsonval c. A high-frequency oscillating current used in electrotherapy; it is of low voltage and high amperage.
demarcation c. Electric current that flows toward the depolarized surface of injured tissue from the polarized surface of adjacent intact tissue.
derived c. A current drawn off by a derivation wire from the main current.
descending c. One passing through a nerve centrifugally, the anode being placed proximally, the cathode distally.
direct c. An electric current which flows continuously in one direction, in contradistinction to an alternating current. Abbreviated D.C.
eye c. The normal electric current that passes from the cornea to the optic nerve under the stimulus of light.
faradic c. A current produced by an induction coil.
galvanic c. A direct current from a galvanic battery.
high-frequency c. A rapidly alternating electric current. See D'Arsonval *c.*, Oudin *c.*, Tesla *c.*
induced c. See secondary *c.*
induction c. Current produced in a coil of insulated wire by a changing magnetic field of force surrounding the coil.
interaxonal c. The stimulation or modification of excitability produced in one group of nerve fibers by the action potential of another group.
interrupted c. A current that is alternately opened and closed.
ionization c. A current produced in an ionized gas by an electric field.
labile c. That applied with one or both electrodes moving over the surface.
magnetoelectric c. A faradic current generated by a magnet.
monophasic action c. Action current derived from leads, one of which is on live active tissue and the other on a killed portion; records the electric change accompanying a response in one direction only.
Oudin c. A high-frequency current from only one pole or terminal, used in electrotherapy.
primary c. A current which, on opening and closing, produces an induced current in an adjacent coil.
reversed c. That produced by changing the poles.
secondary c. Momentary current produced in a coil of insulated wire, introduced within the field of another coil, when the circuit is made or broken in the latter.
sinuous c. One with a curved wave form.
sinusoidal c. A symmetrical alternating current, the rise and fall of which describes a sine curve.
stabile c. A current applied with both electrodes in a fixed position.
static c. Direct current from a static machine.
Tesla c. A high-frequency oscillating current used in electrotherapy; it is of medium voltage.
uniform c. An electric current which retains the same strength throughout its application.
voltaic c. See galvanic *c.*

Curschmann, Heinrich [*German physician*, 1846–1910]. Remembered for his description of the spiral threads of mucin contained in the small pellets expectorated in asthmatic paroxysm, called *Curschmann's spirals.*

cur'va·tor coc·cyg'e·us. Alternate term for the anterior sacrococcygeus muscle.

cur'va·ture [L. *curvatura*, from *curvare*, to bend]. A bending or curving. See *curve.*
angular c. The deformity resulting from tuberculosis of the vertebrae: also called *Pott's c.*
anterior c. See *kyphosis.*
compensatory c. In spinal curvature, a secondary curve, occurring as the result of the efforts of the trunk to maintain its upright position.
c. of the microscopic field. An aberration of the optical system which causes the image of a plane object to be curved.
c. of the spine. Bending of the vertebral column. See *kyphosis; lordosis; scoliosis.*
gingival c. A curve of the line of attachment of the gingival tissue at the cervix of a tooth.
lateral c. Scoliosis.

curve [L. *curvus*, curved]. 1. A bending or flexure; a curvature. 2. *In biometry*, a line, usually curved which in a graphic representation indicates the relationship between an independent and a dependent variable.
absorption c. *In radiobiology*, a curve showing variation in absorption of radiation as a function of wavelength.
alignment c. The line of the dental arch; one following the mesiodistal diameters of the teeth in correct position.
audiometric c. An audiogram.
base c. *In optics*, the standard curve on the back of a toric lens. The front surface is so ground that, in combination with the base curve, the desired optical strength is obtained.
camel c. Humpback curve used frequently to designate two successive clinical attacks of an acute infectious disease separated by a relatively brief symptomless interval, as the viremia and the major phase of acute anterior poliomyelitis.
decay c. *In radiobiology*, a curve showing the percentage of radioactive substance remaining as a function of time.
diphasic c. An electric curve consisting of two phases which are opposite in sign.
dose-effect c. *In radiology*, a curve relating the radiation dosage to the biological effects produced.
electrocardiographic c. Electrocardiogram.
photopic dominator c. A curve plotted from determinations of the sensitivity of elements from the light-adapted eye of animals with cones and also from the dark-adapted eyes of animals having only cones with its maximum at 0.560μ.
pressure c. A recording of pressure variations; particularly, that of pressure variations in a given heart chamber or blood vessel during the cardiac cycle.
Price-Jones c. See *Price-Jones.*
saddleback temperature c. A temperature curve characterized by a fever followed by a remission and a second bout of fever. Occurs in seven-day fever, dengue, and Rift Valley fever.
temperature c. A graphic curve showing variations in temperature for a given period.
transmission c. *In radiology*, a curve showing variation in dosage rate as a function of thickness of the absorbing material.
volume c. A recording of volume variations; particularly, that of ventricular volume during the cardiac cycle.

curve' fit"ting. *In biometry*, the process of determining the mathematical equation which best expresses the relationship between two variables. See *fit.*

cus·cam'i·dine (cuss·kam'i·deen, ·din). An amorphous minor alkaloid found in cusco bark.

cus'ca·mine (cuss'kuh·meen, ·min, cuss·kam'in). A crystalline minor alkaloid that is found in cusco bark.

cus'co bark. The bark of *Cinchona pelletierana* (Rubiaceae), yielding several minor alkaloids of the quinoline group.

cus·con'i·dine (cuss·kon'i·deen, ·din). An alkaloid found in cusco bark.

cus′co·nine (cuss′ko·neen, ·nin). $C_{23}H_{26}N_2O_4$.-$2H_2O$. A crystalline alkaloid found in cusco bark.

Cushing, Harvey Williams [*American surgeon*, 1869–1939]. The world's leading neurosurgeon of his time. Introduced an operation of excision of the semilunar ganglion, making the approach below the middle meningeal artery (1900). Operated successfully in intracranial hemorrhage of the newborn (1905). Established cerebral hernia as a means of decompression in inaccessible brain tumors (1905). Investigated tumors of the pituitary (1906). With Crowe and Homans, studied the relationship between the pituitary and the reproductive system, performing experimental hypophysectomy (1910). Devised operative technics for intracranial tumors (1932). His operation of anastomosis of the spinal accessory and facial nerves was devised for the relief of facial paralysis. *Cushing's incision* in subtentorial craniotomy extends in a curve, convex toward the vertex, across the lower occiput from a point near the mastoid process to a corresponding point on the other side, this line being joined by an incision beginning over the seventh cervical vertebra and extending upward; also called *crossbow incision.* He described a clinical condition now called *Cushing's syndrome* and ascribed by him to pituitary basophilism which is called *Cushing's disease. Cushing's law* states that an increase of intracranial tension causes an increase in blood pressure; the blood pressure remains somewhat higher than the intracranial pressure, thus ensuring continuous cerebral circulation. With Percival Bailey he put forth a scheme for the development of the cells of the nervous system in which the medullary epithelium gives rise to primitive spongioblasts, medulloblasts, and apolar neuroblasts from which all the cells of the nervous system arise.

Cushing, Hayward Warren [*American surgeon*, 1854–1934]. Remembered for his early successful work on the operative relief of hypospadias and epispadias. His suture is a right-angled continuous catgut stitch, the needle entering and leaving the tissues along a line parallel with the incision, each stitch crossing the line of incision to the other side. With each insertion of the needle, the new point of entrance is opposite the point of exit of the suture just completed. When drawn tight, the suture becomes nearly invisible. Adapted principally to intestinal and gastric surgery.

cush′ion [OF. *cossin*, from L. *culcita*, cushion]. *In anatomy*, an aggregate of adipose and fibrous tissue relieving pressure upon tissues lying beneath.

coronary c. The matrix of the upper edge of the hoofs in solipeds.

c. of the epiglottis. The tubercle of the epiglottis, a median elevation within the vestibule of the larynx.

endocardial c. Either of two masses of embryonic connective tissue concerned with the development of the atrioventricular canals and valves.

Passavant's c. The bulging of the posterior pharyngeal wall produced by the contraction of the overlapping superior and middle constrictors of the pharynx. Also called *Passavant's bar.*

plantar c. In solipeds, a cuneiform fibrous body lying between the plantar part of the hoof and the perforans tendon.

sucking c. Fatty pads found on the buccinator muscles in young infants.

Cushny, Arthur Robertson [*Scottish physician and pharmacologist*, 1866–1926]. With Edmunds, first recognized auricular fibrillation in man (1901). Investigated the pathology of heart disease, and made important studies of digitalis. Developed Ludwig's filtration theory of urine formation.

cusp [L. *cuspis*, pointed end]. 1. A pointed or rounded eminence on or near the masticating surface of a tooth; designed to occlude in the sulcus of a tooth or between two teeth of the opposite dental arch. 2. One of the pointed flaps or leaflets making up a heart valve. —**cus′pate, cus′pated,** *adj.*

cus′pid [*cuspis*]. A cuspid tooth; a canine tooth. See under *tooth.* —**cuspidal, cuspidate, cuspidated,** *adj.*

cus′so (kŏŏss′o, kuss′o). See *brayera.*

Custer's method. See under *stain.*

cu·ta″ne·o·mu·co′sal [L. *cutis*, skin; *mucosus*, mucous]. Pertaining to the junction between skin and mucous membrane, as cutaneomucosal boundary. More properly called *mucocutaneous.*

cu·ta′ne·ous [*cutis*]. Pertaining to the skin.

cute. See *pinta.*

Cu″te·re′bra [*cutis;* L. *terebra*, borer]. A genus of botflies, which attack especially rabbits and other rodents; the rodent botfly.

Cu″te·re′bri·dae (cue″ti·ree′bri·dee) [*cutis; terebra*]. A family of the Diptera, related to the botfly group. The important genera are *Cuterebra* and *Dermatobia.*

cu′ti- [*cutis*]. A combining form meaning *skin.*

cu′ti·cle [L. *cuticula*, dim. of *cutis*]. 1. A horny or chitinous, sometimes calcified, layer formed by and covering an epithelium. 2. Popular term for epidermis. —**cutic′ular,** *adj.;* **cuticulariza′tion,** *n.*

enamel c. (a) The *primary* enamel cuticle is the transitory remnants of the enamel organ and oral epithelium covering the enamel of a tooth after eruption. Also called *Nasmyth's membrane.* (b) The *secondary* enamel cuticle is a keratinized pellicle found between the gingival epithelium and the surface of a tooth. Also called *Gottlieb's c.*

hair c. The outermost layer of cells of a hair shaft.

root sheath c. The layer of cells lining the inner (epithelial) root sheath of a hair follicle.

cu′ti·col″or [*cutis;* L. *color*, color]. Simulating the color of the skin; said of various ointments and powders used in the treatment of skin diseases.

cu·tic′u·la. Cuticle.

cu″ti·fi·ca′tion [*cutis;* L. *facere*, to make]. Formation of skin.

cu′tin [*cutis*]. A waxlike substance found over most of the aerial parts of vascular plants. It serves to protect the underlying cells from too rapid loss of moisture.

cu″ti·re·ac′tion [*cutis;* cf. F. *réaction*]. A local skin reaction following the inoculation with or the application of extracts of pathogenic organisms.

cu′tis [L.]. The skin.

aurantiasis c. A golden-yellow discoloration of the skin, caused by eating an excessive amount of certain yellow vegetables or fruits, such as carrots, oranges, squash. It disappears quickly with no aftereffects when these foods are avoided. Also called *carotenoid pigmentation, carotenosis cutis.*

c. anserina. See goose *flesh.*

c. hyperelastica. A rare disorder, usually congenital or familial, characterized by hyperelasticity of the skin, fragility of the skin and blood vessels, hyperlaxity of the joints, pseudotumors following trauma, and subcutaneous nodules. The skin may be stretched out like rubber and snaps back with equal resiliency. Also called *Danlos syndrome, India rubber skin.*

c. laxa. See *dermatolysis.*

c. marmorata. Blue or purple mottling of the skin; seen in certain young persons on exposure of the skin to cold air. Also called *livedo reticularis.*

c. pendula. See *dermatolysis.*

c. rhomboidalis nuchae. The furrowed, leathery skin of the neck of old persons.

c. testacea. A variety of seborrhea in which the trunk and extensor surfaces of the extremities are covered with large, thick plates of greasy, inspissated sebum, usually greenish or blackish, from accumulation of dirt upon them.

c. unctuosa. Seborrhea.

c. vera. The corium, or derma.

c. verticis gyrata. Hypertrophy and looseness of the skin, with a tendency to hang in folds, with resulting appearance suggesting the convolutions of the cerebrum.

cu′ti·sec″tor, cu″ti·sec′tor [*cutis;* L. *sector,* cutter]. An instrument for taking small sections of skin from the living subject. Also called *biopsy punch.*

cu·ti′tis. Dermatitis.

cu″ti·za′tion [*cutis*]. Transformation of an exposed mucous membrane into corium at the mucocutaneous margins.

Cutler-Power-Wilder test. See under *test.*

Cutting's colloidal mastic test. See mastic *test.*

cu·vette′ [F. *cuve,* a tub]. 1. The absorption cell for spectrophotometry. 2. A small transparent tube or vessel, used in colorimetric determinations.

Cuvier, Georges Léopold Chrétien Frédéric Dagobert [*French scientist,* 1769–1832]. Remembered for his work on comparative anatomy (1800–05). One of the founders of modern morphology. Made a lifetime study of living and fossil animals and developed the science of paleontology. Formerly, the two short vessels opening into the common trunk of the omphalomesenteric veins in the embryo, the right becoming later the superior vena cava, were called *Cuvier's canals.* The two common cardinal veins are known as the *ducts of Cuvier.*

Cy Symbol for cyclonium.

cy″an·am′ide (sigh″uh·nam′ide, ·id, sigh·an′uh·mide, ·mid). 1. HN:C:NH. Colorless deliquescent crystals. 2. Calcium cyanamide.

cy′a·nate. The univalent radical, —C⁝N:O.

cy″an·eph″i·dro′sis [G. *kyanos,* blue; *ephidrōsis,* superficial perspiration]. Blue sweat.

cyan-hematin. A pigment used in hemoglobinometry. It is produced by the action of acid and cyanide on hemoglobin or the heme pigments.

cy″an·he″mo·glo′bin (sigh″an·hee″mo·glo′bin, ·hem″o·glo′bin) [*kyanos;* G. *haima,* blood; L. *globus,* globe]. A compound of hydrocyanic acid with hemoglobin formed in cases of poisoning with this acid. It gives the blood a bright red color.

cy″an·hi·dro′sis. Cyanephidrosis.

cy·an′ic ac′id (sigh·an′ick). HCNO. A poisonous liquid, stable only at low temperatures.

cy′a·nide. The univalent radical —CN; any compound containing this radical, as potassium cyanide, KCN.

cy″an·met″he·mo·glo′bin. A relatively nontoxic compound formed by the combination of cyanide and methemoglobin. One basis for the treatment of cyanide poisoning is the administration of a drug, such as sodium nitrite or methylene blue, which forms methemoglobin. The methemoglobin in turn combines with the cyanide and detoxifies it, thereby preventing it from combining with cytochrome oxidase and thus blocking intracellular oxidations.

cy′a·no-, cyan- [*kyanos*]. 1. A combining form meaning *dark blue.* 2. *In chemistry,* a combining form denoting *the presence of the cyanogen group.*

cy″a·no·chroi′a [*kyanos;* G. *chroia,* color]. Cyanosis.

cy·an″o·co·bal′a·min. Crystalline vitamin B_{12}, a cobalt-containing substance usually produced by the growth of suitable microbial substances, or obtained from liver; it occurs as dark red crystals or powder, and appears to be identical with the antianemia factor of liver.

cy″a·no·der′ma [*kyanos;* G. *derma,* skin]. Cyanosis.

cy·an′o·gen (sigh·an′o·jen) [*kyanos;* G. *genesthai,* from *gignesthai,* to be produced]. 1. NC.CN. A colorless toxic gas having the odor of bitter almonds. 2. The radical —CN. See *cyanide.*

c. bromide. CNBr, white crystals volatile at room temperature. It causes lacrimation, and is used as a reagent for nicotinic acid, with which it produces a yellow color.

c. chloride. CNCl, a colorless, volatile liquid used to kill vermin; it is lacrimatory.

c. iodide. CNI, colorless crystals used as preservative in taxidermy.

cy′a·nol. See *aniline.*

cy·an′o·phil (sigh·an′o·fil, sigh′uh·no·fil″) [*kyanos;* G. *philein,* to love]. The blue-staining nuclear substance of cells of plants and animals. —**cyanophil′ic, cyanoph′ilous,** *adj.*

cy·an′o·phil. Having a special affinity for a blue dye.

cy·an′o·phose (sigh·an′o·foze, sigh′uh·no·foze″) [*kyanos;* G. *phōs,* light]. A blue phose.

cy″a·no′pi·a, cy″a·nop′si·a [*kyanos;* G. *ōps,* eye]. A perverted state of the vision rendering all objects blue.

cy″a·nop′sin. A visual pigment synthesized by combining chicken cone opsin (photopsin) with retinene$_2$; it would be expected to occur in any retina containing vitamin A_2 or retinene$_2$ and cone opsin.

cy′a·nosed (sigh′uh·nosed) [*kyanos;* G. *-ōsis,* condition]. Affected with cyanosis.

cy″a·no′sis [*kyanos; -ōsis*]. A bluish tinge in the color of mucous membranes and skin, due to the presence of excessive amounts of reduced hemoglobin in capillaries, less frequently to the presence of methemoglobin. Certain drugs, such as the sulfonamides, may cause cyanosis. —**cyanot′ic,** *adj.*

compression c. Severe cyanosis of the head, neck, and upper arm when the superior vena cava is compressed, as in severe, prolonged compression of the chest: also called *traumatic c.*

congenital c. Cyanosis due to a congenital lesion of the heart or of the great vessels.

delayed c. See tardive *c.*

enterogenous c. Methemoglobinemia.

local c. Bluish discoloration of a part of the body.

tardive c. That due to arteriovenous shunt which is terminal or transient, resulting in venous blood entering the systemic circulation in patent ductus arteriosus, or localized defects of aortic, atrial, and interventricular septums. Syn., *delayed c.*

traumatic c. See compression *c.*

cy″a·nu′ric ac′id. (OH)C:N.C(OH):N.C(OH):N; a heterocyclic compound formed when urea is heated, three molecules of the latter producing a molecule of the acid, along with three molecules of ammonia.

cy·as′ma (sigh·az′muh) (pl. *cyasmata*) [G. *kyein,* to be pregnant]. The peculiar pigmentation sometimes seen upon pregnant women.

cy″ber·net′ics [*kybernetēs,* helmsman]. The science dealing with communication and communication-control theory as applied to mechanical devices and animals, and including the study of servomechanisms, i.e., feed-back mechanisms.

cycl-. See *cyclo.*

cyc′la·mate cal′ci·um. Generic name for calcium

cyclohexylsulfamate dihydrate; $(C_6H_{11}.NHSO_3)_2$-$Ca.2H_2O$; a synthetic, heat-stable sweetening agent used as a non-nutritive substitute for sucrose by persons on low-sodium diets. See *sucaryl calcium.*

cyc'la·mate so'di·um. Generic name for sodium cyclohexylsulfamate, $C_6H_{11}NHSO_3Na$, a synthetic, heat-stable, sweetening agent used as a non-nutritive substitute for sucrose. See *sucaryl sodium.*

cyc'la·men. A saponin; the active principle of the tuber of *Cyclamen europaeum.*

cy'cle [G. *kyklos,* circle]. A regular series of changes which involve a return to the original state or condition, and repetition; a succession of events or symptoms.

cardiac c. The complete series of events occurring in the heart during systole and diastole of all of its chambers up to the return to the beginning point.

cardiaco-vascular c. The circuit of the blood through the organism.

citric acid c. See Krebs *c.*

Cori c. A series of enzymatic reactions which purport to show the mode of conversion of lactic acid (formed during muscular activity from glycogen) to glucose in the liver, and its subsequent anabolism to glycogen in muscle.

c. of generation. Haeckel's term for the successive changes through which an individual passes from its birth to the period when it is capable of reproducing its kind.

c. of Golgi. See endogenous *c.*

c. of Ross. See exogenous *c.*

endogenous c. That phase of development of the *Plasmodium malariae* or other parasite which occurs in the vertebrate host, man. Also called *c. of Golgi.*

endometrial c. The periodically recurring series of changes in the uterine mucosa associated with menstruation and the intermenstrual interval in primates: e.g., menstruating endometrium to interval endometrium to secretory endometrium to premenstrual endometrium.

estrous c. The periodically recurring series of changes in uterus, ovaries, and accessory sexual structures associated with estrus and diestrus in lower mammals. See Plate 41.

exogenous c. That phase of development of the *Plasmodium malariae* or other parasite which occurs in the invertebrate host, the mosquito. Also called *c. of Ross.*

gastric c. A progression of peristaltic waves over the active stomach. They last about twenty seconds.

genesial c. The period between puberty and the menopause.

Krebs c. A series of enzymatic reactions originally described by H. A. Krebs as occurring in pigeon breast muscle and now believed to occur, in a modified form, in most living cells of aerobic organisms. It aims to define a cycle of reactions whereby the pyruvate (or a two-carbon derivative thereof), formed during the anaerobic phase of carbohydrate oxidation, is converted to carbon dioxide and water. As intermediates of the Krebs cycle are also formed in the oxidation of fatty acids and amino acids, it is thought to be the final common path for the burning of all foodstuffs to carbon dioxide and water. Syn., *citric acid c., tricarboxylic acid c.*

life c. Life history, including metamorphoses, hosts, habitats, and modes of reproduction.

menstrual c. The periodically recurring series of changes in the uterus, ovaries, and accessory sexual structures associated with menstruation and the intermenstrual periods in primates. See also endometrial *c.*

Meyerhof c. A series of enzymatic reactions which have been shown to occur in a variety of animal, plant, and microbial tissues, whereby glucose (or glycogen or starch) is converted to pyruvic acid. This conversion may occur anaerobically, and then lactic acid or ethanol and carbon dioxide are the end products; aerobically the pyruvate is further oxidized by the Krebs cycle or other mechanisms. The entire series of reactions is reversible. At present the Meyerhof cycle is believed to be the main pathway of the catabolism and of the anabolism of carbohydrate. Also called *Emden-Meyerhof scheme, Emden-Meyerhof-Parnas scheme.*

tricarboxylic acid c. See Krebs *c.*

cy·clec'to·my (sigh·kleck'to·mee, sick·leck'·) [*kyklos;* G. *ektomē,* excision]. Excision of part of the ciliary body.

cy"clen·ceph'a·lus (sigh"klen·sef'uh·lus, sick"-len·) [*kyklos;* G. *egkephalos,* brain]. A monster showing cyclencephaly.

cy"clen·ceph'a·ly [*kyklos; egkephalos*]. A monstrosity consisting of fusion or failure of formation of the cerebral hemispheres.

cy'clic (sigh'klick, sick'lick) [G. *kyklikos,* circular]. 1. Having cycles or periods of exacerbation or change; intermittent. 2. Having a self-limited course, as certain diseases. 3. *In chemistry,* referring or pertaining to compounds which have a closed-chain or ring structure.

cy"cli·cot'o·my (sigh"kli·cot'o·mee, sick"li·) [G. *kyklos,* circle; *tomē,* a cutting]. Cyclotomy.

cy·cli'tis (sigh·kly'tis, sick·lye'tis) [*kyklos;* G. *-itis,* inflammation]. Inflammation of the ciliary body, manifested by a zone of congestion in the sclerotic coat surrounding the cornea. It may be serous, plastic, or suppurative.

cy'clo- (sigh'klo-, sick'lo-), **cycl-** [*kyklos*]. A combining form meaning *circular, a cycle,* or *pertaining to the ciliary body.*

cy"clo·bar'bi·tal. Cyclohexenylethylbarbituric acid, a rapidly eliminated sedative used in insomnia. Dose, 0.1–0.4 Gm. (1½–6 gr.). See *phanodorn.*

cyclobis. Trade-mark for a 10% solution of bismuth camphenilanate used in the treatment of syphilis.

cy"clo·ceph'a·lus [*kyklos;* G. *kephalē,* head]. A congenital monster showing cyclocephaly.

cy"clo·ceph'a·ly [*kyklos; kephalē*]. A type of cyclopia in which there is more or less complete absence of the olfactory organs, and intimate union of rudimentary eyes, situated in a single orbit.

cy"clo·cho"roid·i'tis (sigh"klo·kor"oy·dye'tis, sick"lo·) [*kyklos;* G. *chorioeidēs,* choroid; *-itis,* inflammation]. Combined inflammation of the ciliary body and the choroid.

cy"clo·cu'ma·rol, cyc"lo·cu'ma·rol. 3,4-(2'-Methyl-2'-methoxy-4'phenyl)dihydropyrano-coumarin, an anticoagulant. See *cumopyran.*

cy"clo·di·al'y·sis (·dye·al'i·sis) [*kyklos;* G. *dialysis,* a separating]. Detaching the ciliary body from the sclera in order to effect reduction of intraocular tension in certain cases of glaucoma, especially in aphakia.

cy"clo·di'a·ther·my [*kyklos;* G. *dia,* through; *thermē,* heat]. Destruction, by diathermy, of the ciliary body.

cy·clog'e·ny (sigh·klodj'i·nee) [*kyklos;* G. *genesthai,* from *gignesthai,* to be produced]. The life cycle or development of a microorganism, from its lowest stage to its highest and back to its basal state.

cy"clo·hex'ane. C_6H_{12}; a saturated, cyclic, liquid hydrocarbon, representing a closed chain of six methylene (CH_2) groups; it occurs in some petroleums.

cy″clo·hex′a·nol. $C_6H_{11}OH$; hexahydrophenol, a widely used solvent of narcoticlike action and capable of damaging the liver and kidney.

cy″clo·hex′a·none. $C_6H_{10}O$; the ketone resulting from oxidation of cyclohexanol; it is an oily liquid extensively used as a solvent. Its vapor may be harmful.

cy′cloid [*kyklos;* G. *eidos*, form]. *In psychiatry*, pertaining to a type of personality characterized by alternating periods of well-being and mild depression.

cy′clol [*cy*clization + en*ol*ization]. A hypothetical protein structure in which an open polypeptide chain undergoes cyclization and enolization at the peptide linkage.

cy″clo·mas·top′a·thy. See mammary *dysplasia.*

cy·clo′ni·um. Cy. A name given to a synthetic form of element 61, now called *promethium.* See also *florentium, illinium.*

cyclopal. A trade-mark for the sedative and hypnotic substance cyclopentenylallylbarbituric acid.

cyclopal sodium. Trade-mark for a brand of the monosodium salt of cyclopentenylallylbarbituric acid, a sedative and hypnotic.

cy″clo·pen′tane. $CH_2.CH_2.CH_2.CH_2.CH_2$; a liquid hydrocarbon found in petroleum. It represents one of the four structural units or rings of cyclopentenophenanthrene.

cy″clo·pen·te′no·phen·an′threne. $C_{17}H_{24}$. A hydrocarbon representing the fusion of three benzene rings and one cyclopentane ring which is considered the basic structure of sterols and steroids.

cy″clo·pen·ten′yl·al·lyl·bar″bi·tu′ric ac′id. See *cyclopal.*

cy″clo·phor′ase. An enzyme catalyzing oxidation of members of the Krebs cycle.

cy″clo·pho′ri·a [*kyklos;* G. *phoros*, bearing]. An insufficiency of the oblique muscles of the eye, giving the eyes a tendency to roll outward or inward, so that the naturally vertical meridians would diverge at either the upper or lower extremities.

cy·clo′pi·a (sigh·klo′pee·uh) [*kyklos;* G. *ōps*, eye]. A large group of terata; characterized externally by fusion of the orbits and various degrees of fusion of the eyes; internally by severe defects of the facial skeleton and brain. A proboscis may or may not be present. Syn., *synopsia, synophthalmia.*

cy″clo·ple′gi·a [*kyklos;* G. *plēgē*, stroke]. Paralysis of ciliary muscle of the eye. —**cycloplegic,** *adj.*

cy″clo·pro′pane. C_3H_6. A saturated cyclic hydrocarbon gas having an odor of petroleum benzin. Is a potent but relatively nonirritating and nontoxic inhalation anesthetic which can be administered with a high concentration of oxygen.

cy″clo·pro′pyl meth′yl e′ther. $CH_2.CH_2.CH.O.$-CH_3; a volatile liquid which has been used as a general anesthetic and as an insecticide. Syn., *cyprome ether.*

Cy′clops [G. *Kyklōps*, round-eyed]. A genus of minute crustaceans having a large, median eye; widely distributed throughout fresh and salt waters but found most commonly in still water. Species of *Cyclops* have been found to be intermediate hosts of *Dracunculus medinensis, Diphyllobothrium latum, Drepanidotaenia lanceolata,* and *Gnathostoma spinigerum.*

cy′clops [*kyklōps*]. A monster with a congenital fusion of the two eyes into one.

cy′clo·scope [G. *kyklos*, circle; *skopein*, to examine]. 1. An instrument for determining the width of the field of vision. 2. A machine for measuring rotation velocity.

cy″clo·ser′ine. A broad-spectrum antibiotic substance, isolated from cultures of a *Streptomyces* species, showing therapeutic promise in treatment of human tuberculosis and genitourinary infections. See *seromycin.*

cy·clo′sis (sigh·klo′sis) [G. *kyklōsis*, a surrounding]. Streaming of protoplasm; occurs in certain plant cells.

cy′clo·stage [G. *kyklos*, circle; L. *stare*, to stand]. A stage in the development of bacteria characterized by coccal and coccoid elements; it represents gonidial forms. If favorable growth conditions continue, these bodies may, by division, return to the higher, or original, stage.

cy″clo·thy′mic per·son·al′i·ty. [*kyklos;* G. *thymos*, mind]. *In psychiatry*, a disposition marked by alternations of mood between elation and depression stimulated apparently by internal factors rather than external events; it may be hypomanic, depressed, or alternating. Also called *cyclothymosis.* —**cyclothymic,** *adj., n.;* **cyclothymiac, cy′clothyme, cyclothy′mia,** *n.*

cy·clo′ti·a (sigh·klo′shuh, ·shee·uh) [*kyklos;* G. *ous*, ear]. Cyclopia associated with more or less complete absence of the lower jaw (agnathia) and approximation or fusion of the ears (synotia).

cy′clo·tome [*kyklos;* G. *tomos*, cutting]. A knife used in cyclotomy.

cy·clot′o·my (sigh·clot′o·mee, si·clot′·) [*kyklos;* G. *tomē*, a cutting]. An operation for the relief of glaucoma, consisting of an incision through the ciliary body.

cy′clo·tron [*kyklos;* ēlek*tron*, amber]. A device for imparting high speeds to protons or deuterons by a combination of a constant powerful magnet and an alternating high-frequency charge. These high-speed particles can be directed to a target in order to produce neutrons, or they can be made to bombard various substances in order to make them artificially radioactive.

cy″clo·tro′pi·a [*kyklos;* G. *trepein*, to turn]. Permanent or essential cyclophoria.

cy·clo′tus (sigh·klo′tus). A monster with cyclotia.

cy′cri·mine hy″dro·chlo′ride. Generic name for 1-phenyl-1-cyclopentyl-3-piperidino-1-propanol hydrochloride, a drug used in the symptomatic treatment of parkinsonism. See *pagitane hydrochloride.*

cy·do′ni·um (sigh·do′nee·um) [L. *cydonia*, quince]. Quince seed. The seeds of *Cydonia oblonga;* employed mainly for the bland demulcent mucilage contained in the covering.

cy″e·si·og·no′sis [G. *kyēsis*, conception; *gnōsis*, knowledge]. Diagnosis of pregnancy.

cy·e″si·ol′o·gy (sigh·ee″see·ol′o·jee) [*kyēsis;* G. *logos*, word]. The science of gestation in its medical aspects.

cy·e′sis (sigh·ee′sis) [*kyēsis*]. Pregnancy.

Cyl. Cylinder; cylindrical lens.

cyl′in·der [G. *kylindros*, cylinder]. 1. An elongated body of the same transverse diameter throughout and circular on transverse section. 2. A cylindrical cast. 3. A cylindrical lens. Abbreviated, C., Cyl. —**cylin′dric, cylin′drical,** *adj.*

axis c. See *axon.*

Bence Jones's cylinders. Long, cylindrical formations derived from the seminiferous tubules, sometimes seen in the urine.

crossed cylinders. Two cylindrical lenses placed in apposition to each other with their axes at right angles; used by oculists to determine the strength and the axis of astigmatism.

cy·lin′dri·form [*kylindros;* L. *forma*, shape]. Shaped like a cylinder.

cy·lin′dro-, cylindr- [*kylindros*]. A combining form denoting *cylindrical*.

cyl′in·droid [*kylindros;* G. *eidos*, form]. Resembling a cylinder or tube; i.e., resembling a cylinder with elliptic right sections.

cyl′in·droids. 1. Certain bodies sometimes seen on microscopic examination of urine, which resemble hyaline casts but differ by tapering to a slender tail. They are seen most frequently along with hyaline casts, especially in cases of circulatory failure and inflammation of the kidney. 2. Microscopic mucous threads seen in normal urines: erroneous usage.

cyl″in·dro′ma [*kylindros;* G. *-ōma*, tumor]. Any neoplasm characterized by cylinders of hyaline or hyaline connective tissue containing the epithelial tumor. Two types occur: **cylindromas of the mucous membrane,** which are carcinomas, recur frequently, and often metastasize terminally; and **cutaneous cylindromas,** which are nevoid in their growth, benign, and characterized by single or multiple round growths located in the scalp or about the face or upper chest. The cutaneous tumors may cover the entire scalp like a turban. Transitions to or association with trichoepithelioma and syringoma occur. Also called *nevus epitheliomato-cylindromatosus, turban tumor, Spiegler's tumor, sarcoma capitis, endothelioma capitis.*

c. of bronchus. See *adenoma* of bronchus.

cyl″in·dro′sis [*kylindros;* G. *-ōsis*, condition]. A type of articulation which is produced by the approximation of bones on the sides of a cleft or groove in such a manner as to form a tube or canal which contains blood vessels, nerves, or a duct, as the infraorbital fissure.

cyl″in·dru′ri·a [*kylindros;* G. *ouron*, urine]. The presence of casts in the urine.

cyl″lo·so′ma [G. *kyllos*, lame; *sōma*, body]. A variety of abdominal fissure (gastroschisis) in which a lateral eventration occupies principally the lower portion of the abdomen, with absence or imperfect development of the lower extremity on that side.

cyl″lo·so′mus [*kyllos; sōma*]. A monster with an eventration in the side of the lower abdominal region and imperfect development of the corresponding leg.

cy·mar′in. A glycoside, $C_{30}H_{44}O_9$, from apocynum. On hydrolysis it yields a sugar, cymarose, and strophanthidin. It is used as a cardiac tonic and diuretic. Dose, 0.3 mg. (1/200 gr.) orally, repeated until 1–2 mg. are given daily; 0.5–1.0 mg. (1/130–1/60 gr.) intravenously or intramuscularly daily. Syn., *new apocynamarin.*

cy·mar′ose. $C_7H_{14}O_4$; the sugar resulting when certain cardioactive glycosides, as cymarin, undergo hydrolysis; it is a 3-methyl ester of digitoxose.

cym′ba [G. *kymbē*, boat]. *In biology*, a boat-shaped sponge spicule.

c. conchae. The upper part of the concha of the ear, above the root of the helix. *O.T.*

cym′bi·form [*kymbē;* L. *forma*, shape]. *In biology*, boat-shaped.

cym′bo- [*kymbē*]. A combining form denoting *cymbiform, boat-shaped.*

cym″bo·ceph′a·ly [*kymbē;* G. *kephalē*, head]. The condition of having a boat-shaped head. See *scaphocephaly.* —**cymbocephal′ic, cymbocephalous,** *adj.*

cy′mene [Ar. *kammūn*]. $C_{10}H_{14}$. 1-Methyl-4-isopropylbenzene, a hydrocarbon that occurs in Roman caraway, thyme, Monarda, and other volatile oils. Syn., *cymol.* —**cymic,** *adj.*

cy′me·nyl. Cymyl; the radical $C_{10}H_{13}$– derived from cymene.

cy′mol. Cymene.

cy′myl. Cymenyl.

cy·nan′che (si·nang′kee, sigh·nang′kee) [G. *kyōn*, dog; *agchein*, to strangle]. An old name for any acute affection of the throat in which the patient struggles for breath. *Obs.*

cy·nan′thro·py (si·nan′thro·pee, sigh·nan′·), **cyn″an·thro′pi·a** [*kyōn;* G. *anthrōpos*, man]. A mania in which the patient believes himself to be a dog and imitates the actions of one.

cyn″i·a′tri·a (sin″ee·ay′tree·uh, ·at′ree·uh, si·nigh″uh·try′uh, sin″ee·uh·tree′uh) [*kyōn;* G. *iatreia*, treatment]. That branch of veterinary medicine dealing with diseases of dogs and their treatment.

cyn′ic [G. *kynikos*, doglike]. Doglike, as a cynic spasm.

cyn′o- (sin′o-, sigh′no-), **cyn-** [*kyōn*]. A combining form denoting *dog.*

cyn″o·ceph′a·lous [*kyōn;* G. *kephalē*, head]. With the head shaped like a dog's.

cyn″o·don′tes (sin″o·don′teez, sigh″no·) [*kyōn;* G. *odous*, tooth]. The canine teeth, so called from their resemblance to the grasping teeth of a dog.

Cyn″o·glos′sum (sin″o·glos′um, sigh″no·) [*kyōn;* G. *glōssa*, tongue]. A genus of plants of the Boraginaceae. The powdered herb, **C. officinale,** common hound's-tongue, has been used as a demulcent and sedative.

cyn″o·lys′sa [*kyōn;* G. *lyssa*, rage]. Hydrophobia; rabies.

cyn″o·pho′bi·a (sin″o·fo′bee·uh, sigh″no·) [*kyōn;* G. *phobos*, fear]. 1. Morbid fear of dogs. 2. A psychotic reaction reproducing the symptoms of rabies.

cyn″o·rex′i·a. Bulimia.

cyn″u·ren′ic ac′id. A crystalline acid found in dog's urine. It is a decomposition product of proteins.

cyn′u·rin. A base derived from cynurenic acid.

Cyon, Élie de [*Russian physiologist*, 1843–1912]. Remembered for his discovery, with K. F. W. Ludwig, of the vasomotor reflexes (1866).

cy″o·pho′ri·a [G. *kyos*, fetus; *phoros*, bearing]. Pregnancy; gestation.

cy·oph′o·rin (sigh·off′o·rin). Gravidin; kyestein.

cy·ot′ro·phy (sigh·ot′ro·fee) [*kyos;* G. *trophē*, nourishment]. Nutrition of the fetus.

Cy·pe′rus (sigh·peer′us, sigh′pur·us) [G. *kypeiron*, galingale]. A genus of sedges.

C. articulatus. Jointed flat sedge; a species of South America, whose root is reputedly antiemetic and tonic.

cy·prid″o·pho′bi·a (si·prid″o·fo′bee·uh, sigh″prid·o·) [G. *Kypris*, Aphrodite; *phobos*, fear]. A morbid fear of acquiring a venereal disease.

cyp″ri·pe′di·um [*Kypris;* G. *podion*, slipper]. Lady-slipper. The dried rhizome and roots of *Cypripedium calceolus* (*pubescens*). It contains a volatile oil, resins, tannin, etc. Has been used as an antispasmodic and stimulant tonic.

cy′prome e′ther. Cyclopropyl methyl ethyl.

cyren. Trade name for a brand of diethylstilbestrol.

cyr′to- (sur′to-) [G. *kyrtos*, curved]. A combining form meaning *curved* or *convex*, as in cyrtometer.

cyr″to·ceph′a·lus [*kyrtos;* G. *kephalē*, head]. A person having a skull which is deformed or distorted in some manner.

cyr″to·cor′y·phus [*kyrtos;* G. *koryphē*, crown of the head]. A person having a skull with parietal bones markedly convex in the midsagittal plane. The absolute convexity is measured by the parietal angle of 122°–131°.

cyr′to·graph [*kyrtos;* G. *graphein*, to write]. An instrument used to measure and record the curves of the chest and head.

cyr′toid (sur′toyd) [*kyrtos;* G. *eidos,* form]. Resembling a hump or swelling.

cyr·tom′e·ter [*kyrtos;* G. *metron,* a measure]. An instrument for measuring or delineating the curves of parts of the body. Used to demonstrate the dilation and deformation of the chest in certain diseases, or to measure the shape and size of the head. —**cyrtometry,** *n.*

cyr″to·me·to′pus [*kyrtos;* G. *metōpon,* forehead]. A skull with a highly convex frontal bone, or a frontal angle of 120°–130.5°.

cyr″to·pis″tho·cra′ni·us [*kyrtos;* G. *opisthokranion,* the back part of the skull]. A skull with a very convex occipital bone, or with an occipital angle of 117°–139.9°.

cyr·to′sis [*kyrtos;* G. *-ōsis,* condition]. A curvature or deformity, especially of the vertebral column: more commonly known as kyphosis.

cyr″tu·ran′us (surt″yoo·ran′us, ·ray′nus) [*kyrtos;* G. *ouranos,* roof of the mouth]. A skull with a palate highly arched longitudinally, or with a uranal angle of 132°–147.5°.

cyst [G. *kystis,* bladder]. A sac with a distinct wall, containing fluid or other material. May be a normal or a pathologic structure.

adventitious c. One enclosing a foreign body or substance.

air c. One containing air.

allantoic c. Cystic dilatation of the urachus.

amniotic c. An uncommon placental cyst formed by adhesions of amniotic folds.

apoplectic c. A sac containing the remnants of blood extravasated in cerebral hemorrhage.

atheromatous c. Derived from distention of sebaceous glands and ducts and filled with greasy or cheesy semisolid material; occasionally applied to cystic masses of atheromatous material in the walls of the arteries.

Baker's c. See popliteal *bursitis.*

Bartholin c. A cyst resulting from chronic bartholinitis, containing a clear fluid which replaces the suppurative exudate.

blood c. One filled with degenerated blood following a hematoma.

blue dome c. See cystic *disease* of breast.

bone c. A tumor distending and thinning bone, filled with serum or bloody fluid; an osteogenic sarcoma.

branchial, branchiogenic c. One due to anomalous development of the embryonal visceral pouches or grooves. Also called *branchial cleft c., branchial inclusion c., cervical c.*

bronchogenic, bronchial c. A thin-walled cyst near the bifurcation of the trachea, lined by pseudostratified ciliated columnar epithelium. Cysts of this type may produce signs of tracheobronchial obstruction early in life. Also called *ciliated epithelial c., reduplication c. of respiratory tract.*

carinal c. A bronchogenic cyst attached at the ridge demarcating the trachea from its bifurcation (carina) and often to the anterior esophageal wall; it may lead to death in infancy due to tracheobronchial compression.

cervical c. A closed, epithelial sac in the neck arising by retention of a branchial groove, of a pharyngeal pouch, or of the cervical sinus. Also called *branchial c., branchiogenic c.*

chocolate c. (a) Any cyst filled with degenerated blood. (b) The lesion characteristic of endometriosis.

chorionic c. An uncommon cyst of the placenta, arising in the chorionic plate, usually near the umbilical cord bulging toward the fetus. Histologically, it is lined by cells of trophoblastic origin.

chylous c. One found in lymphatics, containing chyle.

ciliated columnar c. See thymic *c.*

ciliated epithelial c. See bronchogenic, bronchial *c.*

colloid c. One containing a hyaline material resembling the colloid of the thyroid gland.

colloid c. of choroid plexus. A thin-walled cyst located on the anterior part of the third ventricle. It produces hydrocephalic disturbances consisting of increasing intracranial pressure, sudden coma, and organic dementia. Headache is also present and is often affected by changes in posture. Treatment consists of surgical removal of the cyst.

compound c. See multilocular *c.*

conjunctival c. A rare congenital cyst occurring near the corneal margin.

corpus albicans c. A cystic corpus luteum remnant.

corpus luteum c. Cystic distention of a corpus luteum. Also called *luteal c., lutein c.*

Cowper's c. A retention cyst of the bulbourethral glands.

c. of broad ligament. One developing within the broad ligament; derived from embryonal tubules in the ligament or from cysts of adherent ovary: also called *epoophoral c., fimbrial c., junctional c., Kobelt's c., paratubal c., parovarian c., perisalpingial c., Wolffian c.*

c. of joint capsule. A ganglion, 2.

c. of semilunar cartilage. A ganglion, 2.

daughter c. A satellite cyst in or near larger cysts.

dentigerous c. One originating in the enamel organ of a developing tooth. Syn., *follicular c.*

dermoid c. See *teratoma.*

distention c. A collection of fluid in a serous cavity.

Dubois c. See thymic *c.*

echinococcus c. (a) A cyst formed by growth of the larval form of *Echinococcus granulosus,* usually in the liver. (b) The cysticercus stage of the life cycle of *Echinococcus granulosus.*

ectopic endometrial c. See *endometriosis.*

endocardial blood c. Small, circumscribed, nodular, dark-red, cystlike lesions usually seen on the atrial surface of the mitral and tricuspid valves, occurring frequently in newborn infants, occasionally in children, and rarely in adults.

endometrial implantation c. See chocolate *c.,* (b).

endothelial-lined c. See pericardial *c.*

enteric c. See gastroenteric *c.*

enterogenous c. See gastroenteric *c.*

epidermal c. Cystic lesion in the epidermis; seen in pemphigus and other bullous disorders.

epidermoid c. A cyst lined by stratified squamous epithelium without associated cutaneous glands.

epithelial c. A cyst of epithelial origin.

epoophoral c. See *c.* of broad ligament.

esophageal c. One, most often found in adults, in the lower half of the esophagus between the muscle layers of the esophageal wall. Histologically, it is lined with ciliated cuboidal and occasional groups of squamous cells.

extravasation c. A cyst formed by encapsulation of extravasated fluid, usually blood, as a hematoma.

fibrosed c. Any nonspecific cyst in which the usual structures have been partially replaced by connective tissue.

fibrous-walled c. (a) One developing in connective tissue such as a ganglion, 2. (b) One in which the epithelial lining has been destroyed leaving a fibrous wall.

fimbrial c. See *c.* of broad ligament.

follicular c. (a) A cyst due to retention of secretion in a follicular space, as in the ovary. (b) A dentigerous cyst.
Gartner's c. Localized cystic dilatation of Gartner's duct.
gas c. One containing gas, such as gas from the intestinal canal.
gastroenteric c. An intrathoracic cyst, usually found in the posterior mediastinum near the pulmonary hilus, usually producing symptoms at an early age, and frequently accompanied by associated congenital anomalies and intestinal diverticula. Histologically, the cyst wall may resemble either that of the stomach or of the intestine, respectively also called *gastric c.*, *gastrogenic c.*, *mediastinal c. of gastric origin*, *accessory stomach*, or *enteric c.*, *enterogenous c.*, *enterocystoma*, *mediastinal c. of enteric origin.*
germinal inclusion c. One located near the surface of an ovary, arising from inclusions of germinal epithelium.
glandular proliferous cysts. See *cystosarcoma phylloides.*
globulomaxillary c. Cystic embryonal inclusions in the alveolar process between upper lateral incisor and canine teeth.
hairy c. See *teratoma.*
hemorrhagic c. See extravasation *c.*
hidradenocytic c. A benign cyst, sometimes occurring in the breast, lined by hidradenocytes and derived from a sweat or apocrine gland.
hilar c. A bronchogenic cyst attached to one of the main or lobar bronchi, most commonly seen in older children or adults.
hydatid c. See echinococcus *c.*
hypophyseal c. See Rathke's pouch *c.*
inclusion c. A cyst due to embryonal or traumatic implantation of epithelium into another structure, as an epidermoid cyst.
intraligamentous c. See *c.* of broad ligament.
involutional c. Cystic dilatation of glands or ducts during the course of involution of a gland, as in the mammary gland in abnormal involution.
junctional c. See *c.* of broad ligament.
Kobelt's c. See *c.* of broad ligament.
luteal, lutein c. See corpus luteum *c.*
malignant hemorrhagic bone c. See *osteosarcoma.*
median maxillary c. Cystic dilatation of embryonal inclusions in the incisive fossa, (b), between the roots of the central incisors. Syn., *nasopalatine c.*
mediastinal c. of enteric origin. See gastroenteric *c.*
mediastinal c. of gastric origin. See gastroenteric *c.*
Meibomian c. See *chalazion.*
mixed c. See *teratoma.*
Morgagnian c. A vesicle derived from the paramesonephric duct attached to the oviduct or head of the epididymis.
mucoid c. An encapsulated mass of mucoid material produced by mucoid degeneration of mesodermal tissues. Also see pseudomucinous *cystadenoma.*
mucous c. A retention cyst of a gland, containing a secretion rich in mucin. Also called *mucinous c.*
Müllerian duct c. A congenital cyst arising from vestiges of the Müllerian ducts, usually quite large, and always situated in the midline. Such cysts occur in an area between the lobes of a normal prostate.
multilocular c. One with several more or less separate compartments.
Nabothian c. Cystic distention of the mucous (Nabothian) glands of the uterine cervix. Syn., *Nabothian follicle.*
nasopalatine c. A cyst occurring in the incisive canal or at its oral orifice.
neural c. One occurring in the brain or the spinal cord.
nevoid c. A cyst whose walls contain a congeries of blood vessels.
odontogenic c. A cyst originating in tissues associated with teeth; of two main types. See dentigerous *c.*; radicular *c.*
pancreatic c. A retention or a congenital cyst in the pancreas.
papillary c. of ovary. See serous *cystadenoma.*
papillary serous c. See serous *cystadenoma.*
paraesophageal c. A bronchogenic cyst intimately connected with the esophageal wall, containing cartilage, and usually filled with a mucoid material and desquamated epithelial cells.
paraphyseal c. A cyst of undetermined origin projecting into the third ventricle of the brain.
parasitic c. One formed by larval stages or cysticerci of animal parasites.
paratracheal c. A bronchogenic cyst attached to the tracheal wall.
paratubal c. See *c.* of broad ligament.
parovarian c. See *c.* of broad ligament.
periapical c. See radicular *c.*
pericardial c. A cyst adherent to the parietal pericardium, having a thin fibrous wall and lined by flattened endothelial or "mesothelial" cells: also called *endothelial-lined c.*, *pericardial celomic c.*, *"spring water c."*
pericoronal c. See dentigerous *c.*
periodontal c. See radicular *c.*
perisalpingial c. See *c.* of broad ligament.
pilonidal c. Cystic distention of a congenital tract, opening on the skin of the sacrococcygeal region; lined by stratified squamous epithelium, often contains hairs and the products of bacterial contamination; it may extend as deeply as the spinal dura. Syn., *sacrococcygeal c.*
proliferative c. One in which the lining epithelium proliferates and produces projections from the inner surface of the cyst.
proligerous c. Cyst formation in an adenocarcinoma.
pseudomucinous c. See pseudomucinous *cystadenoma.*
pyelogenic c. See calyceal *diverticulum.*
radicular c. One arising from a granuloma of the root of a tooth: also called periapical *c.*
Rathke's pouch c. Cystic distention of the remnants of Rathke's pouch. Also see *craniopharyngioma.*
reduplication c. of the respiratory tract. See bronchogenic *c.*; bronchial *c.*
retention c. A cyst due to obstruction of outflow of secretion from a gland.
sacral perineurial c. One found on the posterior sacral or coccygeal nerves or nerve roots in the extradural portion of the cauda. It arises as an outpouching between the arachnoid and the perineurium and may produce such symptoms as urinary retention, low backache, and hypalgesia of the lower extremities.
sacrococcygeal c. See pilonidal *c.*
salivary duct c. A cyst caused by obstruction of a salivary duct and retention of the secretion of the gland.
Sampson's c. See *endometriosis.*
sanguineous c. One containing blood-stained fluid.
sebaceous c. A retention cyst of a sebaceous gland.
secondary c. A cyst within a cyst.

seminal c. A cyst of the epididymis or the spermatic cord containing semen.
septal c. A cyst of the septum pellucidum.
simple serous c. See serous *cystadenoma.*
"spring water" c. See pericardial *c.*
sterile c. An echinococcus cyst in which the larvae of the worm have died.
sublingual c. See *ranula.*
suprasellar c. A cyst of the stalk of the hypophysis, above the sella turcica.
synovial c. One lined by synovia, as in joints or bursae. Also see *ganglion,* 2.
teratoid, teratomatous c. See *teratoma.*
thecal c. Localized distention of a tendon sheath, often called ganglion.
theca-lutein c. A cyst due to distention of the corpus luteum but with well-developed theca in the wall. See *thecoma.*
thymic c. A cyst, usually small and embedded in the thymus, which may be lined by flattened or ciliated columnar cells: also called *Dubois c.*
thyroglossal c. Cystic distention of the remnants of the thyroglossal duct, filled with secretion of lining epithelial cells.
tubo-ovarian c. A cyst involving an ovary and its oviduct.
umbilical c. See vitello-intestinal *c.*
unilocular c. One with but a single cavity.
urinary c. A retention cyst in the kidney.
vitello-intestinal c. Localized cystic dilatation of a part of the persistent vitelline duct.
Wolffian c. See *c.* of broad ligament.

cyst-. See *cysto-.*

cyst·ad″e·no·car″ci·no′ma. Cystic adenocarcinoma. Sometimes called *cystocarcinoma.*
papillary c. See serous *c.*
papillary c. of thyroid. See under *adenocarcinoma.*
pseudomucinous c. An ovarian tumor, the malignant variant of the pseudomucinous cystadenoma: also called *mucinous c., pseudomucinous papillary c., mucoid adenocarcinoma, mucinous carcinoma, pseudomucinous carcinoma* or *cystocarcinoma, carcinomatous pseudomucinous cystoma.*
serous c. An ovarian tumor, the malignant variant of the serous cystadenoma: also called *papillary c., papillary serous carcinoma, carcinomatous serous cystoma.*

cyst″ad·e·no′ma [*kystis;* G. *adēn,* gland; *-ōma,* tumor]. An adenoma containing cysts.
c. adamantinum. Cystic adamantinoma.
c. cylindrocellulare celloides ovarii. See pseudomucinous *cystadenoma.*
c. papilliferum. An adenoma containing cysts with papillae on the inner aspect of the cyst walls.
c. of thyroid. See papillary *adenoma* of thyroid.
gelatinous c. See pseudomucinous *c.*
mucinous, mucous c. See pseudomucinous *c.*
papillary c. lymphomatosum. See Warthin's *tumor.*
pseudomucinous c. A common tumor of the ovary, uni- or multilocular, lined with columnar secretory epithelium. It may attain great size, and may rupture, leading to pseudomyxoma peritonaei. It has a marked tendency to undergo malignant transformation. Also called *c. cylindrocellulare celloides ovarii, gelatinous c., mucinous c., mucous c., mucinous papillary c., pseudomyxomatous c., pseudomucinous adenofibroma, pseudomucinous (solid) adenoma, pseudomucinous tubular adenoma, pseudosolid adenoma of ovary, mucoid cyst, multilocular cyst of ovary, pseudomucinous cyst, colloid ovarian cystoma, cystoma ovarii pseudomucinosum, microcystic pseudomucinous cystoma, pseudocolloid ovarian cystoma, pseudomucinous racemose cystoma, ovarian pseudomyxoma, pseudomucinous papilloma, colloid ovarian tumor, parvilocular pseudomucinous tumor, pseudocolloid ovarian tumor.*
pseudomyxomatous c. See pseudomucinous *c.*
serous c. Cystic tumor of the ovary, often intraligamentous, not infrequently bilateral. It is lined by a single layer of low, cuboidal epithelium with centrally placed nuclei and is commonly ciliated. On the basis of certain structural differences, it is sometimes subdivided into **simple serous cyst** (no papillae), **papillary serous cyst** (some luminal papillae and psammoma bodies), and *serous cystadenoma* proper, with numerous papillae and epithelial cells in the stroma. There is a marked tendency toward malignant transformation. Also called *papillary c. of ovary, papillary adenoma of ovary, serous cystoma, endosalpingioma, papillocystoma, psammomatous papilloma.*

cyst″ad·e·no·sar·co′ma [*kystis; adēn;* G. *sarkōma,* fleshy excrescence]. Combined cystadenoma and sarcoma. See *cystosarcoma* phylloides.

cys·tal′gi·a [*kystis;* G. *algos,* pain]. Pain in the urinary bladder. *Obs.*

cys″ta·thi′o·nine. A mixed thio ether, COOH.-CH(NH_2).CH_2.CH_2.S.CH_2.CH(NH_2).COOH, formed from homocysteine and serine as an intermediate in the conversion of methionine to cysteine.

cyst″ec·ta′si·a (sis″teck·tay′zhuh, ·zee·uh, ·shuh, ·see·uh), **cys·tec′ta·sy** [*kystis;* G. *ektasis,* extension]. Dilatation of a bladder.

cys·tec′to·my [*kystis;* G. *ektomē,* excision]. 1. Excision of the gallbladder, or part of the urinary bladder. 2. Removal of a cyst.

cys·te′ic ac′id. COOH.CH(NH_2).CH_2.SO_3H; a crystalline acid obtained by the oxidation of cysteine or cystine.

cys′te·ine (sis′tee·een, ·in, sis·tee′in). 2-Amino-3-mercaptopropanoic acid; HS.CH_2.CH(NH_2).-COOH, obtained by reduction of cystine and important as a constituent of many proteins; a crystalline powder, soluble in water.

cys″te·in′yl. The univalent radical, $HSCH_2CH$-(NH_2)CO—, of the amino acid *cysteine.*

cyst′ic [*kystis*]. 1. Pertaining to or resembling a cyst. 2. Pertaining to the urinary bladder or to the gallbladder.

cys″ti·cer′coid [*kystis;* G. *kerkos,* tail; *eidos,* form]. A larval tapeworm, differing from the cysticercus in that it has a slightly developed bladder and a solid posterior; a stage in the life cycle of *Hymenolepis nana.*

cys″ti·cer·co′sis [*kystis; kerkos;* G. *-ōsis,* condition]. Infestation by cysticerci (the larval stage of *Taenia*) accompanied by muscular pain, general muscular weakness, fatigue, loss of weight, and nervousness; in severe cases, where the infestation is general and the brain is invaded, general paralysis, epileptic attacks, and convulsions.

cys″ti·cer′cus (pl. *cysticerci*) [*kystis; kerkos*]. The larval tapeworm; develops in man after ingestion of the ova of *Taenia solium* or *T. saginata.* The ova infestive to man develop only into the larval forms, complete development failing to take place.
c. cellulosae. See *Taenia solium.*

cys′ti·form [*kystis;* L. *forma,* shape]. Encysted, cystomorphous.

cys′tine (sis′teen, ·tin) [*kystis*]. [S.CH_2.$CHNH_2$.-COOH]$_2$. Di-(α-amino-β-thiopropionic) acid. An amino acid component of many proteins, especially keratin. It may be reduced to cysteine. Syn., *dicysteine.*

cys″ti·ne′mi·a [*kystis;* G. *haima,* blood]. The occurrence of cystine in the blood.

cys″ti·no′sis. A condition, generally considered to be a congenital metabolic disorder of sulfur-containing amino acids, usually cystine, characterized by deposits of cystine crystals in the body organs; it may be accompanied by aminoaciduria.

cys″ti·nu′ri·a [*kystis;* G. *ouron*, urine]. The presence of cystine crystals in the urine. This may occur in cystinosis or in some forms of renal dwarfism.

cys·ti′tis [*kystis;* G. *-itis*, inflammation]. Inflammation of the urinary bladder, involving principally the mucosa and submucosa. It may be of bacterial or other origin, and may be acute and self-limited or chronic.

allergic c. A nonspecific type of inflammation of the urinary bladder, characterized by discrete or diffuse areas of hyperemia and edema, often without pus or bacteria in the urine, and apparently due to a local sensitivity reaction to a certain antigen or antigens.

bullous c. An inflammation of the urinary bladder with pale, edematous polypoid projections of the mucous membrane: also called *bullous edema.*

chemical c. Inflammation, usually acute, of the mucosa and submucosa of the urinary bladder which, in contrast to bacterial invasion of the organ, is secondary to either local or systemic chemical trauma.

chronic glandular c. An unusual type of nonspecific chronic inflammation of the urinary bladder characterized by papillary or bleblike projections on the vesical mucosa, chiefly in the region of the trigone and lower segments of the vesical wall. Microscopically these projections consist of tracts of stratified columnar epithelium with mucus-secreting or goblet cells. The condition apparently is secondary to chronic infection and metaplasia of the vesical epithelium.

c. cystica. A type of nonspecific chronic inflammation of the urinary bladder characterized by the presence of minute translucent vesicles, usually with clear homogeneous mucoid contents scattered over the surface of the vesical mucosa.

c. emphysematosa. One in which cystic spaces in the urinary bladder wall are filled with gas; this may result from bacterial fermentation of sugar in the urine, as in diabetes or after glucose infusion.

c. follicularis. One in which there are lymphoid nodules or masses of lymphoid cells beneath the epithelium.

c. glandularis. A chronic form, of unknown cause, in which mucus-secreting glands are seen microscopically.

gangrenous c. An acute, severe, diffuse inflammation of the urinary bladder, involving principally the mucosa and submucosa, characterized by gross suppuration, necrosis, and gangrene of the involved tissues.

granulomatous c. A type in which the urinary bladder has been affected by a granulomatous reaction, commonly tuberculosis.

incrusted c. A chronic inflammation of the urinary bladder in which crystalline material is deposited on the vesical wall: also called *alkaline incrusted c.* because of the constant alkalinity of the urine.

interstitial c. A chronic form in which the inflammation is principally in the subepithelial connective tissue and extends in variable degree into the deeper tissues. Ulcers frequently accompany the process and are known as *Hunner's ulcer* or *elusive ulcer.*

irradiation c. Inflammation of the urinary bladder, usually in females, following roentgen-ray, radium, or other isotopic therapy of the pelvic organs.

schistosomal c. A granulomatous cystitis caused by the ova of *Schistosoma hematobium.*

cys·tit′o·my [*kystis;* G. *tomē*, a cutting]. 1. Incision into the capsule of the lens of the eye; capsulotomy. 2. Incision into the urinary bladder or gallbladder; cystotomy.

cys′to-, cyst- [*kystis*]. A combining form denoting *likeness to* or *connection with a bladder* or *cyst.*

cys″to·bu·bon′o·cele [*kystis;* G. *boubōn*, groin; *kēlē*, hernia]. Hernia of the urinary bladder through the inguinal ring. *Obs.*

cys″to·car″ci·no′ma. Cystadenocarcinoma.

cys′to·cele [*kystis; kēlē*]. Herniation of the urinary bladder into the vagina.

cys″to·co·los′to·my. See *cholecystocolostomy.*

cys″to·dyn′i·a [*kystis;* G. *odynē*, pain]. Old term for cystalgia.

cys″to·fi·bro′ma pap″il·lar′e. See *cystosarcoma phylloides.*

cys″to·gen′e·sis, cys″to·gen′i·a [*kystis;* G. *genesis*, production]. The formation or genesis of cysts.

cys′to·gram [*kystis;* G. *gramma*, letter]. Radiograph of the urinary bladder made after the injection of a contrast medium, either of a greater or lesser density than the surrounding soft tissues.

cys·tog′ra·phy [*kystis;* G. *graphein*, to write]. Radiography of the urinary bladder after the injection of a radiopaque medium. —**cysto·graph′ic,** *adj.*

cyst′oid [*kystis;* G. *eidos*, form]. 1. Having the form or appearance of a bladder or cyst. 2. Composed of a collection of cysts. 3. A pseudocyst.

cys″to·lith·ec′to·my [*kystis;* G. *lithos*, stone; *ektomē*, excision]. Old term for cystolithotomy.

cys″to·li·thi′a·sis [*kystis; lithos;* NL. *-iasis*, condition]. Calculus in the urinary bladder.

cys″to·li·thot′o·my [*kystis; lithos;* G. *tomē*, a cutting]. The removal of a calculus from the urinary bladder, by surgical excision.

cys·to′ma [*kystis;* G. *-ōma*, tumor]. A cystic mass, especially in or near the ovary; may be either neoplastic, inflammatory, or due to retention.

carcinomatous pseudomucinous c. See pseudomucinous *cystadenocarcinoma.*

carcinomatous serous c. See serous *cystoadenocarcinoma.*

colloid ovarian c. See pseudomucinous *cystadenoma.*

c. ovarii pseudomucinosum. See pseudomucinous *cystadenoma.*

mesonephric c. A cyst, probably of mesonephric origin, at the hilus of the ovary.

microcystic pseudomucinous c. See pseudomucinous *cystadenoma.*

parovarian c. Dilation and sometimes proliferation of the tubules of epoophoron, a remnant of the mesonephros, situated in the mesosalpinx.

pseudocolloid ovarian c. See pseudomucinous *cystadenoma.*

pseudomucinous racemose c. See pseudomucinous *cystadenoma.*

serous c. See serous *cystadenoma.*

simple c. Dilated ovarian follicles with associated proliferation suggestive of neoplasia.

tubo-ovarian c. A cyst formation which may occur when an ovarian cyst communicates with a fused oviduct.

cys·tom′e·ter [*kystis;* G. *metron*, a measure]. An instrument used to determine vesical pressure under standard conditions. —**cystometry,** *n.*

cys″to·met′ro·gram [*kystis; metron;* G. *gramma*, letter]. Graphic demonstration of intravesical pressure under various conditions, as determined by cystometry.

cys″to·mor′phous [*kystis;* G. *morphē*, form]. Having the structure of, or resembling, a cyst or bladder.

cys′to·pex″y [*kystis;* G. *pēxis*, a fixing]. Surgical fixation of the urinary bladder, or a portion of it, in a new location.

cys″to·pho·tog′ra·phy [*kystis;* G. *phōs*, light; *graphein*, to write]. Photographing the interior of the urinary bladder for diagnostic purposes.

cys′to·plas″ty [*kystis;* G. *plassein*, to mold]. Plastic operation upon the urinary bladder.

cys″to·pros·ta·tec′to·my. Surgical excision of the urinary bladder and the prostate.

cys″to·py″e·li′tis [*kystis;* G. *pyelos*, trough; *-itis*, inflammation]. Inflammation of the urinary bladder and the pelvis of the kidney.

cys″to·py″e·lo·ne·phri′tis [*kystis; pyelos;* G. *nephros*, kidney; *-itis*]. Cystopyelitis plus involvement of the kidney.

cys·tor′rha·phy [*kystis;* G. *rhaphē*, a suture]. Suture of the urinary bladder.

cys″to·sar·co′ma [*kystis;* G. *sarkōma*, fleshy excrescence]. Term introduced by Johannes Müller (1838) to describe a fleshy mass, then called sarcoma, which contained cysts.

c. phylloides, c. phyllodes. A tumor of the mammary gland, which grows slowly but may attain great size, with nodular proliferation of connective tissue and lesser adenomatous proliferation. It probably develops from preexisting adenofibroma, but is rarely malignant. Variously called *c. artaresceus, c. (polyposum) intracanaliculare, c. papillare, c. proliferum, c. simplex, gelatinous c.; adenocystosarcoma, adenoma pseudosarcomatodes, Brodie's serocystic disease of breast, Brodie's tumor, cystadenosarcoma, cystofibroma papillare, giant fibroadenoma of breast, fibromyxosarcoma of breast, fibrosarcoma of breast, giant intracanalicular fibroadenomyxoma, giant mammary myxoma, intracanalicular myxoma, myxosarcoma of breast, pseudosarcoma of breast, intracanalicular sarcoma, serocystic sarcoma, periductal sarcoma, mixed tumor of breast, tuberous cystic tumor of breast.*

cys′to·scope [*kystis;* G. *skopein*, to examine]. An instrument used in diagnosis and treatment of lesions of the urinary bladder, ureter, and kidney. It consists of an outer sheath bearing the lighting system, a well-fitted obturator, space for the visual system, and room for the passage of operative devices to be used under visual control.

cys·tos′co·py [*kystis; skopein*]. The procedure of using the cystoscope.

cys·tos″te·a·to′ma [*kystis;* G. *stear*, fat; *-ōma*, tumor]. A sebaceous cyst.

cys·tos′to·my [*kystis;* G. *stoma*, mouth]. The formation of a fistulous opening in the urinary bladder wall.

cys′to·tome [*kystis;* G. *tomos*, cutting]. 1. A knife used in cystotomy. 2. A knife used in rupturing the capsule of the lens in cataract operations.

cys·tot′o·my [*kystis;* G. *tomē*, a cutting]. Incision of the urinary bladder.

cys″to·u·re′thro·gram [*kystis;* G. *ourēthra*, urethra; *gramma*, letter]. A radiograph of the urinary bladder and urethra, made following injection of an opaque contrast medium.

cys″to·u″re·throg′ra·phy [*kystis; ourēthra;* G. *graphein*, to write]. Radiography of urinary bladder and urethra. —**cystourethrograph′ic,** *adj.*

cys″to·u·re′thro·scope [*kystis; ourēthra;* G. *skopein*, to examine]. An instrument for inspecting the urinary bladder and posterior urethra.

cys′tyl. The divalent radical, —COCH(NH_2)CH_2-$SSCH_2CH(NH_2)CO$—, of the amino acid *cystine.*

cy′tase (sigh′tace, ·taze). Metchnikoff's name for complement.

cy·tas′ter (sigh·tas′tur, sigh′tas·tur) [G. *kytos*, cell; *astēr*, star]. 1. The same as aster, the starlike system of cytoplasmic radiations surrounding the central body during mitosis. 2. Especially, an accessory aster, not associated with chromosomes, appearing under certain experimental treatment.

-cyte (-sight) [*kytos*]. A suffix denoting *a cell.*

cyth″e·mo·ly′sis (sith″uh·mo·lye′sis, sigh″thuh·mol′i·sis, sigh″tuh·) [*kytos;* G. *haima*, blood; *lysis*, a loosing]. Dissolution of erythrocytes and leukocytes.

cyth″er·o·ma′ni·a [G. *Kythereia*, Cytherea; *mania*, madness]. Nymphomania.

cyt′i·dine. A nucleoside containing cytosine and D-ribose; it is obtained by hydrolysis of cytidylic acid.

cyt″i·dyl′ic ac′id. A nucleotide composed of cytosine, D-ribose, and phosphoric acid.

cyt′i·sine (sit′i·seen, ·sin). $C_{11}H_{14}ON_2$. A poisonous alkaloid from *Laburnum anagyroides*, goldenchain laburnum, from baptisia and other plants. It stimulates, then paralyzes, autonomic ganglions. In large doses may produce convulsions and death by asphyxiation. Syn., *baptitoxine, sophorine, ulexine.*

cy′to-, cyt- [*kytos*]. A combining form denoting *connection with, relation to,* or *derivation from a cell, cells,* or *cytoplasm.*

cy″to·ar″chi·tec·ton′ic [*kytos;* L. *architectura*]. Pertaining to the cellular arrangement of a region, tissue, or organ.

cy″to·ar′chi·tec″ture [*kytos; architectura*]. The cell pattern typical of a region, as of an area of the cerebral cortex.

cy′to·blast [*kytos;* G. *blastos*, germ]. 1. Schleiden's term for the nucleus of a cell. 2. One of the hypothetical ultimate vital units of the cell. *Obs.*

cy″to·blas·te′ma [*kytos;* G. *blastēma*, offshoot]. The hypothetical formative material from which cells arise. See *blastema.*

cy″to·cen′trum. Centrosome.

cy″to·chem′ism (sigh″to·kem′iz·um) [*kytos;* G. *chymos*, juice]. The reaction of the living cell to chemical reagents, antitoxins, etc.

cy″to·chem′is·try [*kytos; chymos*]. That science dealing with the chemical constitution of cells and cell constituents.

cy′to·chrome [*kytos;* G. *chrōma*, color]. 1. A nerve cell which has only a small amount of cytoplasm and no Nissl bodies. 2. A mixture of three chromogens (cytochromes A, B, and C) widely distributed in animal tissues, and found also in yeast; the prosthetic group of cytochrome C is practically identical with that of hemoglobin. Cytochrome C functions as a reversible oxidation-reduction carrier, its iron atom being alternately oxidized and reduced, and is intimately concerned with cell respiration.

c. oxidase. An iron-containing oxidase which oxidizes the reduced form of cytochrome C so that the latter may again function as an oxidizing agent (hydrogen acceptor).

c. reductase. One or more enzymes, of the flavoprotein type, which serve as hydrogen acceptors and then react with cytochrome C to reduce it.

cy″to·chy·le′ma (sigh″to·kigh·lee′muh) [*kytos;* G. *chylos*, juice]. The interreticular portion of protoplasm; cell juice.

cy′to·cide [*kytos;* L. *caedere*, to kill]. An agent that is destructive to cells. —**cytoci′dal,** *adj.*

cy·toc′la·sis (sigh·tock′luh·sis, sigh″to·clay′sis) [*kytos;* G. *klasis*, a breaking]. Cell necrosis. —**cytoclas′tic,** *adj.*

cy″to·crin′i·a [G. *kytos*, from a cell; *krinein*, to separate]. The transfer of pigment from melanoblasts to other cells, melanin from basal to intermediate cells of the epidermis in sunburn.

cy′tode [*kytos;* G. *eidos*, form]. Haeckel's hypothetical simplest form of cell, without nucleus or nucleolus.

cy″to·den′drite. Lenhossék's term for a dendrite.

cy′to·derm [*kytos;* G. *derma*, skin]. *In botany*, a cell wall.

cy″to·di″ag·no′sis [*kytos;* G. *diagnōsis*, a deciding]. The determination of the nature of a pathogenic liquid by the study of the cells it contains. See *cytological cancer techniques.*

cy″to·di·er′e·sis (sigh″to·dye·err′i·sis). See *cytokinesis.*

cy″to·dis′tal [*kytos;* L. *distare*, to be distant]. Of or pertaining to that portion of a nerve fiber farthest removed from its cyton.

cy′to·gene [*kytos;* G. *genesthai*, from *gignesthai*, to be produced]. Any self-reproducing particle of the cytoplasm which is a direct product of the genes of the nucleus.

cy″to·gen′e·sis [*kytos;* G. *genesis*, production]. The genesis and differentiation of the cell. **—cytogenet′ic,** *adj.*

cy·tog′e·ny (sigh·todj′i·nee) [*kytos;* G. *genesthai*, from *gignesthai*, to be produced]. Cytogenesis. **—cytogenous, cytogen′ic,** *adj.*

cy″to·glob′u·lin [*kytos;* L. *globulus*, little ball]. A protein obtained from leukocytes and lymph nodes in the form of a white soluble powder.

cy′toid [*kytos;* G. *eidos*, form]. Resembling a cell.

cy″to·ki·ne′sis (sigh″to·ki·nee′sis, ·kigh·nee′sis) [*kytos;* G. *kinēsis*, motion]. The changes in the cytoplasm during cell division. Syn., *cytodieresis.*

cy·tol′er·gy (sigh·tol′ur·jee) [*kytos;* G. *ergon*, work]. Cell activity.

cy″to·log′i·cal can′cer tech·niques′. Procedures in which cells are obtained by aspirations, washings, smears, or scrapings. After fixation and staining, the cells are studied for malignancy on the basis of nuclear and cytoplasmic changes, and changes of the cell as a whole.

cy·tol′o·gy (sigh·tol′o·jee) [*kytos;* G. *logos*, word]. The subdivision of biology which deals with cells. **—cytolog′ic,** *adj.;* **cytologist,** *n.*

exfoliative c. The study of cells desquamated from tissues.

cy″to·ly′sin (sigh″to·lye′sin, sigh·tol′i·sin) [*kytos;* G. *lysis*, a loosing]. An antibody produced by injection of foreign cells, which causes dissolution of cells. May be specific or nonspecific.

cy·tol′y·sis [*kytos; lysis*]. The disintegration or dissolution of cells. **—cytolyt′ic,** *adj.*

-cy·to′ma (-sigh·to′muh) [*kytos;* G. *-ōma*, tumor]. Suffix meaning *a neoplasm made up of cells.*

cy·tom′e·ter (sigh·tom′i·tur) [*kytos;* G. *metron*, a measure]. A device for counting cells, especially blood cells. Also see *hemocytometer.* **—cytom′etry,** *n.;* **cytomet′ric,** *adj.*

cy″to·mi′cro·some [*kytos;* G. *mikros*, small; *sōma*, body]. 1. Any small granule in the cytoplasm. 2. A mitochondrion.

cy″to·mi′tome (sigh″to·my′tome, sigh·tom′i·tome) [*kytos;* G. *mitos*, thread]. The fibrillar part of cytoplasm; the cytoreticulum. See *mitome.*

cy″to·mor′pho·sis (sigh″to·mor′fo·sis, ·mor·fo′sis) [*kytos;* G. *morphōsis*, a bringing into shape]. All the structural alterations which cells or successive generations of cells undergo from the earliest undifferentiated stage to their final destruction.

cy″to·my·co′sis (sigh″to·migh·ko′sis). See *histoplasmosis.*

cy′ton [*kytos*]. 1. A cell. 2. A nerve cell exclusive of its processes.

cy″to·path·o·gen′ic. Pertaining to the destruction of cells (in tissue culture) by a transmissible agent, such as a virus.

cy″to·pa·thol′o·gy [*kytos;* G. *pathos*, disease; *logos*, word]. The branch of pathology concerned with alterations within cells.

cy·top′a·thy (sigh·top′uth·ee) [*kytos; pathos*]. Disease of the living cell.

cy·toph′a·gy (sigh·tof′uh·jee) [*kytos;* G. *phagein*, to eat]. The englobing of cells by other cells. Syn., *phagocytosis.* **—cytophagous,** *adj.*

cy″to·pe′ni·a [*kytos;* G. *penia*, want]. A cell count less than normal. See *leukopenia, anemia, thrombocytopenia, pancytopenia.*

cy′to·phil [*kytos;* G. *philein*, to love]. A chemical group, like those of antibodies, capable of combining with the receptor of a cell.

cy″to·phys″i·ol′o·gy [*kytos;* G. *physis*, growth; *logos*, word]. The physiology of a cell unit.

cy′to·plasm (sigh′to·plaz·um) [*kytos;* G. *plasma*, from *plassein*, to mold]. The protoplasm of a cell other than that of the nucleus, as opposed to *nucleoplasm.* **—cytoplas′mic,** *adj.*

cy″to·plas′tin [*kytos; plassein*]. The plastin of cytoplasm.

cy″to·poi·e′sis [*kytos;* G. *poiēsis*, a making]. The formation and development of a cell.

cy″to·prox′i·mal [*kytos;* L. *proximare*, to draw near]. Denoting that portion of a nerve fiber near its cyton.

cy″to·re·tic′u·lum [*kytos;* L. *reticulum*, a little net]. 1. The network of cells in reticular tissue. 2. Cytomitome. See *mitome.*

cy″to·ryc′tes [*kytos;* G. *oryktēs*, a digger]. Old term for inclusion body. Used originally as the genus name for inclusion bodies in virus diseases under the false assumption that these bodies were protozoan parasites.

cy·tos′co·py (sigh·tos′ko·pee) [*kytos;* G. *skopein*, to examine]. Cytodiagnosis. **—cytoscop′ic,** *adj.*

cy″to·sid′er·in. Any of a group of iron-containing lipid pigments found in various tissues.

cy′to·sine (sigh′to·seen, ·sin). $C_4H_5ON_3$. 2-Oxy-6-amino-pyrimidine. A pyrimidine base found in nucleic acid.

cy″to·skel′e·ton [*kytos;* G. *skeleton*, a dried body]. The structural framework of a cell, probably consisting of proteins which precipitate as fibers.

cy′to·some [*kytos;* G. *sōma*, body]. A cell body exclusive of the nucleus.

cy″to·spon′gi·um (sigh″to·spun′jee·um, ·spon′jee·um) [*kytos;* G. *spoggos*, sponge]. The fibrillar protein network of the cytoplasm.

cy′tost [*kytos*]. A substance, not a histamine, which is secreted by injured cells and is capable of modifying cellular activity.

cy″to·ste″a·to·ne·cro′sis. See *adiponecrosis neonatorum.*

cy′to·stome [*kytos;* G. *stoma*, mouth]. The oral aperture of a unicellular organism.

cy″to·tax′is [*kytos;* G. *taxis*, arrangement]. The movement of cells toward or away from a stimulus. **—cytotac′tic,** *adj.*

cy·toth′e·sis (sigh·toth′i·sis, sigh″to·theess′is) [*kytos;* G. *thesis*, a placing]. Cell repair.

cy″to·tox′in [*kytos;* G. *toxikon*, poison]. A serum, natural or immune, capable of injuring certain cells without lysis (a toxic action). **—cytotoxic,** *adj.*

cy″to·troph′o·blast (·trof′o·blast, ·tro′fo·blast) [*kytos;* G. *trophē*, nourishment; *blastos*, germ]. The inner, cellular layer of the trophoblast, covering the chorion and the chorionic villi during the first half of pregnancy. Also called *Langhans' layer.*

cy·tot′ro·phy [*kytos; trophē*]. Growth of the cell and sustentation of cell life.

cy·tot′ro·pism (sigh·tot′ro·piz·um) [*kytos;* G. *tropē*, a turning]. The tendency of cells to move toward or away from a stimulus. —**cytotrop′ic,** *adj.*

cy″to·zo′on [*kytos;* G. *zōion*, animal]. A protozoan, intracellular parasite.

cy′to·zyme [*kytos; zymē*, leaven]. A substance in various tissues, capable of activating thrombin, the fibrin ferment. Also see *thrombokinase.*

Czermak, Johann Nepomuk [*Bohemian physiologist*, 1828–73]. Discovered that pressure on a point in the inferior carotid triangle of the neck causes a slower heart beat (1865). Explored the nasopharynx with small mirrors (1859). Said to have been first to demonstrate the value of the laryngoscope in clinical diagnosis, although Türck used the instrument in the same year (1858).

Czerny, Adalbert [*German pediatrician*, 1863–1941]. Remembered for his concept of the exudative diathesis (1907), which plays a part in the pathogenesis of children's diseases.

Czerny, Vincenz [*German surgeon*, 1842–1916]. Known for being the first to perform total hysterectomy by the vaginal route (1879). Introduced the operation of enucleation of uterine fibroids by the vaginal route (1881). His suture of the intestine is a modification of Lembert's; first placing an inner row of interrupted sutures passing through the mucous coat of the bowel, he then secured the cut edges of the muscular and serous coats; called *Czerny's suture.* His name is also associated with operations for tonsillar tumors and for the radical cure of inguinal hernia.

D

D Deuterium.

2,4-D Dichlorophenoxyacetic acid.

D- *In chemistry*, a prefix, written as a small capital letter, used to indicate the structural configuration of a particular asymmetric carbon atom, with reference to the standard substance D-glyceraldehyde, so designated because its asymmetric carbon atom has the configuration represented by HC.OH rather than by HO.CH, which is the configuration of the asymmetric carbon atom in L-glyceraldehyde. When more than one asymmetric carbon atom is present in a compound, the configuration of the atom which is assigned the highest number in the case of carbohydrates, or the lowest number in the case of amino acids, determines whether the compound is designated as D- or L-. In D-amino acids the configuration of the relevant asymmetric carbon atom is represented as $HC.NH_2$, while that of L-amino acids is represented as $H_2N.CH$. When the prefix is used according to current rules of nomenclature, there is no correlation between the configuration represented by D- and the optical activity of the compound. If it is desired to indicate optical activity the symbol +, signifying *dextrorotation*, or −, signifying *levorotation*, may also be used, as **D(+)-** or **D(−)-.** In cases where it is not apparent if the numbering of the carbon atoms of a compound follows the rule for carbohydrates or that for amino acids, the prefix may be modified to $\mathbf{D_g}$**-** or $\mathbf{D_s}$**-,** the former indicating that the rule for carbohydrates is used, while the latter signifies that the rule for amino acids is used; the subscripts g and s refer to the carbohydrate glyceraldehyde and to the amino acid serine, respectively.

D., d. Abbreviation for da (L. give), day, days, dead, density, detur (L. let it be given) dexter, died, diopter, dose, duration.

d Deuteron.

d- 1. *In chemistry*, an abbreviation for *dextrorotatory*, referring to the direction in which the plane of polarized light is rotated by a substance: this usage not to be confused with the following. 2. *In chemistry*, a prefix formerly used to indicate the structural configuration of a particular asymmetric carbon atom in a compound, in the manner that the small capital letter D- is now used.

da·boi′a, da·boy′a (da·boy′uh, dab′oy·uh). See *Vipera russellii.*

Da Costa, Jacob Mendes [*American surgeon*, 1833–1900]. Remembered as a distinguished clinician and teacher who gave one of the first adequate descriptions of irritable heart (1871), a condition known later as neurocirculatory asthenia. See under *asthenia.* Also called *Da Costa's syndrome, soldier's heart, effort syndrome.*

dac′ry-. See *dacryo-.*

dac″ry·ad″e·no·scir′rhus (dack″ree·ad″i·no-skirr′us) [G. *dakryon*, tear; *adēn*, gland; *skirros*, hard]. An indurated tumor of the lacrimal gland.

dac″ry·ag″o·ga·tre′si·a (dack″ree·ag″o·ga·tree′-zhuh, ·shuh, ·zee·uh, ·see·uh) [*dakryon;* G. *agōgos*, leading; *a-*, not; *trēsis*, a boring]. Obstruction of a tear duct.

dac′ry·a·gogue (dack′ree·uh·gog), **dac′ry·a·gog** [*dakryon; agōgos*]. An agent causing a flow of tears. Syn., *lacrimator.* —**dac′ryagogue,** *adj.*

dac″ry·ge·lo′sis [*dakryon;* G. *gelōs*, laughter; *-ōsis*, condition]. A condition marked by alternate weeping and laughing. *Obs.*

dac′ry·o-, dac′ry- [*dakryon*]. Combining form meaning *a tear*, or denoting *relation to tears* or *to the lacrimal apparatus.*

dac″ry·o·ad″e·nal′gi·a [*dakryon;* G. *adēn*, gland; *algos*, pain]. Pain in a lacrimal gland.

dac″ry·o·ad″e·nec′to·my [*dakryon; adēn;* G. *ektomē*, excision]. Excision of a lacrimal gland.

dac″ry·o·ad″e·ni′tis [*dakryon; adēn;* G. *-itis*, inflammation]. Inflammation of a lacrimal gland. Syn., *lacrimal adenitis.*

dac″ry·o·blen″nor·rhe′a [*dakryon;* G. *blennos*, mucus; *rhoia*, flow]. Chronic inflammation of and discharge of mucus from the lacrimal sac.

dac′ry·o·cyst″ [*dakryon;* G. *kystis*, bladder]. Old term for the lacrimal sac.

dac″ry·o·cys·tec′to·my [*dakryon; kystis;* G. *ektomē*, excision]. Excision of any part of the lacrimal sac.

dac″ry·o·cys·ti′tis [*dakryon; kystis;* G. *-itis*, inflammation]. Inflammation of the lacrimal sac. Syn., *dacrocystoblennorrhea.*

blennorrheal d. Purulent inflammation of the lacrimal sac. Syn., *dacryocystoblennorrhea.*

phlegmonous d. Inflammation of the tissues composing the lacrimal sac and of the surrounding soft parts.

dac″ry·o·cys″to·blen′nor·rhea. Blennorrheal *dacryocystitis.*

dac″ry·o·cys′to·cele [*dakryon; kystis;* G. *kēlē,* hernia]. Protrusion of a lacrimal sac. Also called *dacryocele.*

dac″ry·o·cys″top·to′sis [*dakryon; kystis;* G. *ptōsis,* a falling]. Prolapse or downward displacement of a lacrimal sac.

dac″ry·o·cys″to·rhi·nos′to·my (dack″ree·o·sis″-to·rye·nos′to·mee) [*dakryon; kystis;* G. *rhis,* nose; *stoma,* mouth]. An operation to restore drainage into the nose from the lacrimal sac when the nasolacrimal duct is obliterated.

dac″ry·o·cys·tos′to·my [*dakryon; kystis; stoma*]. Incision into the lacrimal sac, particularly to promote drainage.

dac″ry·o·cys′to·tome [*dakryon; kystis;* G. *tomos,* cutting]. Instrument for dividing strictures of the lacrimal passages.

dac″ry·o·cys·tot′o·my [*dakryon; kystis;* G. *tomē,* a cutting]. Incision of the lacrimal sac.

dac′ry·o·lin [*dakryon*]. The albuminous material in tears.

dac′ry·o·lith″, dac′ry·o·lite″ [*dakryon;* G. *lithos,* stone]. A calcareous concretion in the lacrimal passages.

dac″ry·o·li·thi′a·sis [*dakryon; lithos;* NL. *-iasis,* condition]. The formation and presence of dacryoliths.

dac″ry·o′ma [*dakryon;* G. *-ōma,* tumor]. 1. A lacrimal tumor. 2. Obstruction of the lacrimal puncta, causing epiphora.

dac′ry·on [*dakryon*]. The point where the frontomaxillary, the lacrimomaxillary, and the frontolacrimal sutures meet.

dac′ry·ops [*dakryon;* G. *ōps,* eye]. 1. Watery eye. 2. A cyst of an excretory duct of a lacrimal gland. *Rare.*

dac″ry·op·to′sis [*dakryon;* G. *ptōsis,* a falling]. See *dacryocystoptosis.*

dac″ry·or·rhe′a [*dakryon;* G. *rhoia,* flow]. An excessive flow of tears.

dac″ry·o·so″le·ni′tis [*dakryon;* G. *sōlēn,* pipe; *-itis,* inflammation]. Inflammation of the lacrimal drainage system.

dac″ry·o·ste·no′sis [*dakryon;* G. *stenōsis,* a being straitened]. Stenosis or stricture of the lacrimal drainage system.

dac″ry·o·syr′inx (dack″ree·o·sirr′inks) [*dakryon;* G. *syrigx,* pipe]. 1. A lacrimal fistula. 2. A syringe for use in the lacrimal ducts.

dac′tyl [G. *daktylos,* finger]. *In zoology,* a digit; a finger or a toe. —**dactylar, dactylate,** *adj.*

dac″ty·lif′er·ous [*daktylos;* L. *ferre,* to bear]. Having fingers or fingerlike parts, organs, or appendages.

dac·tyl′i·on. Syndactyly.

dac″ty·li′tis [*daktylos;* G. *-itis,* inflammation]. Inflammation of a finger or a toe.

d. syphilitica. A rare tertiary syphilitic affection of the fingers or toes, consisting of a gummatous infiltration of the subcutaneous connective tissue and of the fibrous portions of the joints and bones.

tuberculous d. Spina ventosa.

dac′ty·lo-, dactyl- [*daktylos*]. A combining form meaning *finger, toe,* or *digit.*

dac′ty·lo·gram″, dac·tyl′o·gram″ [*daktylos;* G. *gramma,* letter]. A fingerprint, generally used for purposes of identification.

dac″ty·lol′y·sis spon·ta′ne·a. Ainhum.

dac″ty·lo·meg′a·ly [*daktylos;* G. *megas,* large]. A condition in which one or more of the fingers or toes is abnormally large.

dac″ty·lo·sym′phy·sis [*daktylos;* G. *symphysis,* a growing together]. Syndactyly.

dac′ty·lus [*daktylos*]. 1. A finger or toe. 2. A toe, in opposition to *digitus,* a finger.

Dae·mon′o·rops (dee·mon′o·rops) [G. *daimōn,* devil; *rhōps,* shrub]. A genus of plants of the Palmae. The resin prepared from the scale of the fruit of **D. draco,** and other species of palms native to the East Indies, constitutes dragon's blood.

dagenan. Trade-mark for a brand of sulfapyridine.

Dahl′ia (dahl′yuh, dal′yuh, dayl′yuh) [after A. *Dahl,* Swedish botanist]. A genus of the Compositae whose tuberous roots yield inulin.

dahl′ia pa′per. A purple test paper made from species of *Dahlia.* Acids change its color to red; alkalies, to green.

dahl′ia vi′o·let. See *methylrosaniline chloride.*

dah′lin. Inulin.

dahl′lite. The compound $CaCO_3.2Ca_3(PO_4)_2$, said to be the chief inorganic constituent of bones and teeth.

Dakin, Henry Drysdale [*English chemist in the United States,* 1880–1952]. With Carrel, developed a method of treating open wounds by irrigation with a solution of chlorinated soda and sodium bicarbonate; called *Carrel-Dakin treatment.* See also diluted *sodium* hypochlorite solution, called *modified Dakin's solution.*

dak′ry·on. Dacryon.

dak′ry·ops. Dacryops.

Dale, Henry Hallett [*English physiologist,* 1875–]. With George Barger and Francis Howard Carr, isolated ergotoxine (1906). Made studies of pituitrin (1909); of histamine, with Patrick Playfair Laidlaw (1910) and Alfred Newton Richards (1918–19); of histamine shock, with Laidlaw (1919). With Harold Ward Dudley, isolated acetylcholine from the spleens of animals (1929). Nobel laureate with O. Loewi (1936). See also Schultz-Dale *test.*

Dalton, John [*English chemist and physicist,* 1766–1844]. Developed the atomic theory. Discovered *Dalton's laws:* (1) The pressure of a mixture of gases equals the sum of the partial pressures of the constituent gases. (2) So long as no chemical change occurs, each gas in a mixture of gases is absorbed by a given volume of solvent in proportion not to the total pressure of the mixture but to the partial pressure of that gas.

Dal′ton·ism (dawl′tun·iz·um, dal′tun·) [after John *Dalton*]. Colorblindness.

dalyde. Trade-mark for 3,5-dibromosalicylaldehyde, $C_7H_4Br_2O_2$: used as a fungicide and antiseptic for certain infections of the ear.

dam [ME.]. *In dentistry* or *surgery,* a thin sheet of rubber used to keep fluids away from a part; also, a piece of dam used as a drain.

Dam, Henrik Carl Peter (1893–). Danish biochemist, known for his researches in the biochemistry of sterols, fats, and the vitamins K and E; Nobel prize winner in physiology and medicine with Edward A. Doisy (1943). See also Dam *unit.*

da″mal·u′ric ac′id (day″mul·yoor′ick, dam″ul·). $C_7H_{12}O_2$. An acid found in human urine.

dam″i·an′a (dam″ee·an′uh, ·ay′nuh, dah″mee·ah′-nuh) [Sp., of Mex. Ind. origin]. The dried leaves of *Turnera diffusa,* found in Mexico and Lower California; contains volatile oil, resins, tannin, and bitter principle. Formerly used as a stimulant and laxative, and by the laity as an aphrodisiac.

dam′mar, dam′ar [Malay *damar*]. A resinous exudate from *Shorea wiesneri* (Dipterocarpaceae) and other related genera. Contains gum dammar, dammar resins, volatile oil, and bitter principle.

A solution of dammar is a mounting medium used in microscopy. Also called *dammara.*

Damoiseau, Louis Hyacinthe Céleste [*French physician,* 1815–91]. Remembered for his description of an S-shaped curved line showing the upper limit of a pleuritic effusion of the chest. Called *Damoiseau's curve, Ellis' curve;* see under Calvin *Ellis.*

Dana, Charles Loomis [*American neurologist,* 1852–1935]. Known for his contributions to the study of surgery of the spinal nerves and nerve roots. Made many contributions to public health knowledge and to medical history. The operation of section of the posterior spinal nerve roots for the relief of spastic paralysis once bore his name. Subacute combined degeneration of the spinal cord is known as *Putnam-Dana syndrome.*

Dance's sign. See under *sign.*

D and C *D*ilatation of the cervix and *c*urettage of the cavity of the uterus: used as a diagnostic and therapeutic procedure in obstetrics and gynecology.

dan′de·li″on. See *taraxacum.*

dan′der [E. dial. *dan,* scurf]. Scales of the hairy skin of any animal; dandruff. May act as an allergen, dog, cat, and horse dander being the most common.

dan′druff [apparently from *dander,* dandruff; ON. *hrufa,* crust]. Scales formed upon the scalp in seborrhea; dander.

Dandy, Walter Edward (1886–1946). American surgeon who introduced ventriculography and pneumoencephalography as an aid in the diagnosis of cerebral disease, and devised numerous neurologic procedures, including operations for ruptured intervertebral disk.

Daniell, John Frederic [*English physicist and chemist,* 1790–1845]. Inventor of the metallic zinc and copper electrical cell known frequently by his name.

Danielssen, Daniel Cornelius [*Norwegian physician,* 1815–94]. With C. W. Boeck, described leprosy (1847), called *Danielssen-Boeck disease.* Regarded as the inaugurator of the modern treatment of leprosy.

Danlos, Henri Alexandre [*French dermatologist,* 1844–1912]. First to use radium in the treatment of lupus, with P. Bloch (1901). Described the *Ehlers-Danlos syndrome* (1908); see under *syndrome.*

dan′thron. $C_{14}H_8O_4$; 1,8-dihydroxyanthraquinone; an orange-colored powder, practically insoluble in water; it is laxative and cathartic, being used especially in veterinary practice. Syn., *chrysazin.* See *istizin.*

D'Antoni stain. See under *stain.*

Danysz, Jean [*Polish pathologist in France,* 1860–1928]. Remembered for his early studies of the value of radium in malignant disease; for his description of the bacillus *Salmonella typhimurium* which he isolated (1900); and for his description of the *Danysz phenomenon;* when toxin is added to antitoxin in an equal amount at once, the mixture is nontoxic; if added at intervals in fractions, the final mixture is generally toxic.

Danzer and Hooker's method. See under *method.*

Daph′ne (daf′nee) [G., laurel]. A genus of shrubs of the mezereon family; some species are used medicinally. See *mezereum.*

daph′ne·tin, daph·ne′tin. $C_9H_6O_4$. Dihydroxycoumarin, obtained by hydrolysis of the glycoside daphnin or by synthetic methods.

daph′nin. $C_{15}H_{16}O_9 + 2H_2O$. A glycoside from the bark of some species of *Daphne.*

daraprim. Trade-mark for the antimalarial substance *pyrimethamine.*

Darier, Jean Ferdinand [*French dermatologist* 1856–1938]. Described dermatofibrosarcoma, a tumor of the skin occurring singly or as multiple nodules, with a wide variation in malignancy; called *Darier-Roussy sarcoid.* Described keratosis follicularis (1889), known as *Darier's disease.* Made many contributions to the knowledge of cutaneous tuberculosis (1896), and described acanthosis nigricans (1893).

dark′-field″ il·lu″mi·na′tion, dark′-ground″ il·lu″mi·na′tion. See under *illumination.*

Darkshevich, Liverii Osipovich [*Russian neurologist,* 1858–1925]. Described the nerve fibers extending from the optic tract to the habenula. See also *nucleus* of Darkshevich.

Darling, Samuel Taylor [*American physician,* 1872–1925]. Known for his description of histoplasmosis, a disease caused by *Histoplasma capsulatum;* called *Darling's histoplasmosis.*

Darnall, Carl Roger [*American Army medical officer,* 1868–1941]. Discoverer of a practical means of water purification in the field by means of sodium hypochlorite; called *Darnall's method.*

dar″son·val″i·za′tion. See *arsonvalization.*

darstine bromide. Trade-marked name for 1-(3-hydroxy-5-methyl-4-phenylhexyl)-1-methylpiperidinium bromide or mepiperphenidol bromide, a visceral anticholinergic agent.

dar′tos [G., flayed]. The thin layer of smooth muscle in the subcutaneous tissue of the scrotum.

dar′trous [F. *dartre,* eruption, dandruff]. Of the nature of herpes; herpetic.

darvisul. Trade-mark for phenosulfazole.

Darwin, Charles Robert [*English naturalist,* 1809–82]. One of the great thinkers of all time; author of *On the Origin of Species* (1859) and *The Descent of Man* (1871). The word *Darwinism* denotes adherence to his theory of evolution by natural selection. He described the tuberculum auriculae, called *Darwin's tubercle,* which he considered evidence of the simian connections of the human species. See under *tubercle.*

Dattner-Thomas concept. A theory concerning the treatment of neurosyphilis. If, after treatment, cell count and total protein content of the cerebrospinal fluid become normal, treatment may be discontinued. If the cell count and protein content do not reach a constant normal level, treatment must be continued. Evidence of clinical improvement on the part of the patient is not considered.

Da·tu′ra [Skr. *dhattūra*]. A genus of Solanaceae. Stramonium is produced by the **D. stramonium.** Alkaloids of the solanaceous group, chiefly scopolamine, hyoscyamine, and atropine, are yielded by several species of *Datura.*

da·tu′rine (dat·yoor′een, ·in, dat′yoo·reen, ·rin). $C_{17}H_{23}NO_3$. A poisonous alkaloid from *Datura stramonium,* identical with hyoscyamine and isomeric with atropine.

dat′u·rism, da·tu′rism [*dhattūra*]. Stramonium poisoning.

Daubenton, Louis Jean Marie [*French physician and naturalist,* 1716–99]. Remembered for his description of the line passing through the points opisthion and orbitale, or orbitale projected upon the midsagittal plane, known as *Daubenton's line;* the plane of the foramen magnum, passing through the points basion and opisthion, called *Daubenton's plane;* and the occipital angle formed by the intersection of Daubenton's line with Daubenton's plane at opisthion, called *Daubenton's angle.*

Dau′cus (daw′kus) [G. *daukos,* carrot]. A genus of plants of the Umbelliferae.

D. carota. The wild carrot. The root of the cultivated plant contains sugar, starch, pectin, malic acid, albumin, a volatile oil, and a crystalline coloring matter (carotene). The aromatic seeds (fruit) have been used by the laity as a diuretic and anthelmintic for threadworms.

dau′er·schlaf″ (dow′er·shlahf″) [Ger. *Dauer*, duration; *Schlaf*, sleep]. Prolonged, induced sleep therapy.

daught′er. *In radiochemistry*, a radioactive or stable nuclide resulting from the disintegration of a radioactive nuclide, called the *parent*.

Davaine, Casimir Joseph [*French physician*, 1812–82]. Studied entozoa and verminous diseases (1860). Cultivated the *Bacillus anthracis*, called *Davaine body*, and transmitted the disease from one animal to another (1863). Demonstrated that anthrax is caused by a specific microorganism, and thus was among the first to give proof of the germ theory of disease.

Da·vai′ne·a (da·vay′nee·uh) [after C. J. *Davaine*]. A genus of cestode worms.

D. formosana. Synonym for *Raillietina celebensis*.

D· madagascariensis. (a) Synonym for *Raillietina madagascariensis*. (b) Synonym for *Raillietina quitensis*.

David, Jean Pierre [*French physician*, 1737–84]. Remembered for his excellent description of tuberculosis of the spine (1779), in which he is said to have excelled Pott, who described the disease in the same year and for whom it was named.

David, Vernon Cyrenius (1882–). American surgeon, who described operations for repair of rectovaginal fistula, and for anal incontinence. He developed one of the first means of measured transfusion of blood, and contributed to the study of lymphatic spread of carcinoma of the large intestine.

Davidsohn, Hermann [*German physician*, 1842–1911]. Known for his technic of illuminating a pupil by placing an electric light in the mouth. His sign of a tumor or fluid of the maxillary sinus is a lessening of the pupillary illumination on the suspected side; known as *Davidsohn's sign*.

Davidsohn's tests. See under *test*.

Daviel, Jacques [*French ophthalmologist*, 1693–1762]. Considered the outstanding ophthalmologist of his period. Originated the modern method of treating cataract by extraction of the lens (1748).

Davis, John Staige [*American surgeon*, 1872–1946]. Widely known for his ingenuity in plastic surgery, especially of the face. Devised a number of methods for the repair of facial defects. The *Davis graft* is a thick pinch graft.

Davis, Nathan Smith [*American physician*, 1817–1904]. An outstanding leader in American medicine. Assisted in organizing the American Medical Association (1846) and edited the journal of the Association (1883–89). Widely known for his *History of Medical Education and Institutions in the United States* (1851).

Davy, Edmund William [*Irish physician*, 1826–99]. Remembered for his discovery of a test for phenol in which molybdic acid in concentrated sulfuric acid is added to the solution to be tested, a positive reaction being a yellowish brown coloration passing to a deep purple.

Davy, Humphry [*English chemist and physicist*, 1778–1829]. Widely known for his contributions to science, especially to industrial hygiene by the invention of a coal miner's safety lamp (1815) which revolutionized mining methods and saved many lives. Discovered the anesthetic properties of nitrous oxide and suggested its use in surgery as early as 1800.

Dawson, James Walker (1870–1927). English neuropathologist, known for his work on disseminated sclerosis, osteitis fibrosa, and pigmented tumors (melanomas).

Day, Kenneth Mosier [*American otolaryngologist*, 1896–]. The operation which bears his name consists of destroying the function of a labyrinth by electrocoagulation. It is used in the treatment of hydrops of the labyrinth, a form of Ménière's disease.

day blind′ness. Hemeralopia. Also see under *blindness*.

day′mare″ [AS. *daeg; mara*, incubus]. A state of temporary distress and terror resembling nightmare which comes on when the patient is awake. *Obs.*

day rods. Elements of the fovea postulated to be of the nature of rods and to depend on visual purple for their photochemical properties though unable to accumulate it in sufficient quantity to subserve twilight vision.

DBE $(C_2H_5O.C_6H_4)_2.C{:}C(Br)C_6H_5$. αα-Di-(*p*-ethoxyphenyl)-β-phenyl bromoethylene; a synthetic estrogen absorbed from the alimentary tract but differing from other orally active estrogens in having a prolonged action because of its storage in the fatty tissues of the body.

D. C. Doctor of Chiropractic, direct current, Dental Corps.

DDD Dichlorodiphenyldichloroethane; more specifically 1,1-dichloro-2,2-bis (*p*-chlorophenyl) ethane; an insecticide similar to DDT.

D.D.O. Doctor of Dental Orthopedics (orthodontics). British.

D. D. S. Doctor of Dental Surgery.

DDT 1,1,1,-Trichloro-2,2-bis (*p*-chlorophenyl) ethane, an insecticide the medicinal grade of which is called *chlorophenothane*.

de- [L.]. A prefix denoting *down, away from; separation, off, away; intensification, completely, quite;* or *the reversing* or *undoing* of an action, *depriving* or *ridding of*, or *freeing from*.

de·ac″ti·va′tion [L. *de-*, indicating reversing of an action; *actum*, from *agere*, to act]. 1. Process of becoming inactive or of making inactive. 2. Loss of radioactivity.

dead [AS. *dēad*]. Without life; destitute of life.

dead′ly night′shade. Belladonna.

dead time. The time interval, after recording a count, during which a Geiger counter tube and its circuit are completely insensitive and thus incapable of detecting other ionizing events.

deaf′ened. Rendered deaf after previously having heard normally, especially after having learned to comprehend and produce speech.

de·af″fer·en·ta′tion [L. *de-*, indicating separation; *afferre*, to carry to]. The process of interrupting afferent nerve (sensory) fibers.

deaf′-mu′tism. Inability to speak, due to congenital deafness or loss of hearing before establishment of speech. —**deaf-mute,** *n.*

deaf′ness [AS. *dēaf*]. Loss, lack, or impairment of the sense of hearing. It may be due to disease of the external auditory canal, the middle ear, the internal ear, the auditory nerve, or the brain. —**deaf,** *adj.*

adventitious d. Loss of hearing after speech is established.

aviator's d. A nerve type of deafness, temporary or permanent, found in a moderate percentage of fliers; audiogram studies usually show marked depression of hearing in the 2000–5000 cycles per second range.

bass d. Deafness to certain bass notes, while higher notes are heard.

boilermakers' d. Deafness resulting from working among loud noises; characterized by inability to hear ordinary conversation in conditions of quiet, but an increase in hearing power in the midst of noise; paracusia Willisii.

central d. See cerebral *d.*

cerebral d. That due to a brain lesion.

clang d. A defect of hearing in which sounds are heard, but their more delicate qualities are not perceived.

conduction d. Deafness due to disease or a defect of the external or middle ear, or both, frequently caused by a lesion of the tympanic membrane, or of the ossicles.

cortical d. That due to disease of the cortical hearing centers.

mind d. Inability to comprehend sounds heard, due to injury of the auditory center; auditory aphasia. Also called *psychic d.*

perception d. Deafness caused by a lesion of the internal ear or of the cochlear nerve.

psychogenic d. Any deafness that has 50% or more of a psychic factor. Persons so affected do not know they can hear better than they manifest. Must be distinguished from malingering deafness.

speech d. A variety of mind deafness in which the faculty of repeating and writing after dictation is retained.

tone d. Sensory amusia; a form of mind deafness.

word d. Inability to understand words, although they are heard; a form of mind deafness.

de·al′bate [L. *dealbare*, to whitewash]. *In biology*, coated with a fine white down or powder.

de·al″co·hol″i·za′tion [L. *de-*, indicating separation; Ar. *al-kuhl*, powder]. *In microscopy*, the removal of alcohol from an object or compound.

de·al″ler·gi·za′tion [*de-;* G. *allos*, other; *ergon*, work]. The neutralization or inactivation of antibodies by any therapeutic means.

de·am′i·dase (dee·am′i·dace, ·daze). An enzyme that catalyzes oxidative deamination of purines and pyrimidines. —**deamidiza′tion,** *n.*

de·am′i·nase (dee·am′i·nace, ·naze). An enzyme which catalyzes the splitting off of an amino group from an organic compound. See Table of Enzymes in the Appendix.

de·am″i·na′tion. The process of removal of an amino (NH_2) group from an organic compound, particularly from an amino acid. This may be accomplished by reduction, in which case the $CHNH_2$ group of the amino acid is changed to CH_2, by hydrolysis, when $CHNH_2$ is converted to CHOH, or by oxidation, when $CHNH_2$ is transformed to CO; these are designated, respectively, *reductive deamination, hydrolytic deamination, oxidative deamination.* —**deaminiza′tion,** *n.;* **deam′inize,** *v.*

Dean's method. See Wiggers and Dean *method.*

de·an″es·the′si·ant (dee·an″ess·thee′zhunt, ·zee-unt) [*de-;* G. *anaisthēsia*, lack of sensation]. Any means of arousing a patient from a state of anesthesia.

de″a·qua′tion [*de-;* L. *aqua*, water]. Act or process of removing water from a substance; dehydration.

death [AS. *dēath*]. The cessation of life, beyond the possibility of resuscitation. Syn., *abiosis.*

local d. Death of one part of the body.

molecular d. Death of individual cells; ulceration.

muscular d. A state in which the muscles no longer react to stimuli.

serum d. Sudden death occurring in a sensitized person during the intravenous injection of serum.

somatic d. Death of the whole organism.

thymic d. Sudden death assumed to be due to enlargement of the thymus gland.

death cer·tif′i·cate. A form, usually required by law, for recording the event of death, its time, place, cause, the name and age of decedent, and other pertinent data.

standard d. c. The form recommended by the United States Bureau of the Census and in common usage in the United States.

death rate. The proportion of deaths in a given year to the total population, known as the **crude death rate. Specific death rates** are figured on the basis of the number of deaths reported in a given group; specific for age, race, sex, or cause, or for a combination of these variables.

death rat′tle. A gurgling sound heard in dying persons, due to the passage of the air through fluid in the trachea.

death reg″is·tra′tion a′re·a. That territory from which the United States Bureau of the Census collects death records. Since 1933, this has been the entire United States.

death strug′gle. The semiconvulsive twitches often occurring before death.

Deaver, John Blair [*American surgeon*, 1855–1931]. Author of many works on surgery, among which his *Surgical Anatomy of the Human Body* is especially noteworthy. *Deaver's incision* is made through the sheath of the right rectus, and extends from the costal margin to below the level of the umbilicus.

De·bar″y·o·my′ces ne″o·form′ans (di·bar″ee·o-my′seez nee″o·form′anz). Synonym for *Cryptococcus histolyticus.*

de·bil′i·tant [L. *debilitare*, to weaken]. Weakening. —**debil′itant,** *n.*

de·bil′i·ty [L. *debilis*, weak]. Weakness; asthenia.

nervous d. Neurasthenia.

Debove, Maurice Georges [*French physician*, 1845–1920]. Remembered for his description of splenomegaly, known also as *Debove's disease*, and for his description of the basement membrane of the tracheal and bronchial mucosa and the mucosa of the intestinal tract.

de·bride′ment′ (de·breed′mahn′; de·breed′ment) [F.]. *In surgery*, removal from a wound of foreign material and devitalized tissue.

de·bris′ (deh·bree′, day·bree′, deb′ree, day′bree) [F., from OF. *debrisier*, to break]. *In dentistry*, soft foreign material loosely attached to the surface of a tooth, as the refuse from the drilling of a cavity.

epithelial d. (of Malassez). See epithelial *rest.*

dec′a-, dec- [G. *deka*, ten]. A prefix denoting *ten.*

dec′a·gram [*deka;* G. *gramma*, a small weight]. A metric measure of weight equal to 10 grams.

de·cal″ci·fi·ca′tion (dee·kal″si·fi·kay′shun) [L. *de-*, indicating separation; *calx*, lime; *facere*, to make]. Withdrawal or removal by acid of the mineral salts of bone or other calcified substance. See *demineralization.* —**decal′cify,** *v.*

dec′a·li″ter (deck′uh·lee″tur) [G. *deka*, ten; *litra*, pound]. A metric measure of volume equal to 10 liters.

dec′a·me″ter [*deka;* G. *metron*, a measure]. A metric measure of length equal to 10 meters.

dec″a·me·tho′ni·um. One of a homologous series of polymethylene bis(trimethylammonium) ions, of the general formula $(CH_3)_3N^+(CH_2)_nN^+(CH_3)_3$, in which n is 10; it possesses powerful skeletal muscle relaxant action through blocking of motor impulses at the myoneural junction. It is used clinically in the form of one of its salts, usually the bromide.

d. bro′mide. $(CH_3)_3N(Br)(CH_2)_{10}N(Br)(CH_3)_3$; decamethylene bis(trimethylammonium bromide); a white, crystalline powder, soluble in water, and possessing potent curarelike action. See *syncurine.*

de·can″cel·la′tion (deecan″suh··lay′shun) [*de-;* L.

cancelli, a lattice]. The removal of cancellous bone either for use as bone chips in grafting operations or for correcting deformity.

dec'ane. $C_{10}H_{22}$. A hydrocarbon of the paraffin series.

dec'a·nor·mal [*deka;* L. *norma*, rule]. Having 10 times the strength of the normal; said of solutions.

de·cant' [ML. *decanthare*, to pour from the edge of a vessel]. Gently pour off a liquor or solution without disturbing the sediment. —**decanta'tion,** *n.*

de·cap"i·ta'tion (dee·cap"i·tay'shun) [L. *de-*, indicating separation; *caput*, head]. Beheading; removal of the head of a person, a fetus, or a bone; decollation. —**decap'itate,** *v.*

de·cap'i·ta"tor (dee·cap'i·tay"tur) [*de-; caput*]. Instrument used in performing decapitation in embryotomy.

decapryn succinate. Trade-marked name for the antihistaminic substance *doxylamine succinate.*

de·cap"su·la'tion (dee·cap"suh·lay'shun, ·cap"sue·lay'shun) [*de-;* L. *capsula*, little box]. Removal of a capsule or enveloping membrane, as the capsule of a kidney.

de·car'bon·ate (dee·kahr'bun·ate) [*de-;* L. *carbo*, coal]. Deprive of carbon dioxide or carbonic acid. —**decarbonated,** *adj.*

de·car"bon·i·za'tion (dee·kahr"bun·i·zay'shun, ·eye·zay'shun) [*de-; carbo*]. Removal of carbon. —**decar'bonize,** *v.*

de"car·box'yl·ase. See *carboxylase.*

de"car·box"y·la'tion, de"car·box"yl·i·za'tion. The splitting off of one or more molecules of carbon dioxide from organic acids, especially amino acids. —**decarbox'ylate,** *v.*

de·ca·thec'tion. *In psychiatry*, the process of dissolving or removing a specific or ambivalent affect directed toward a thing or person.

dec"a·vi'ta·min. A U.S. Pharmacopeia formulation of vitamins, containing not less than 1.5 mg. (5000 U.S.P. Units) of vitamin A, 10 micrograms (400 U.S.P. Units) of vitamin D, 75 mg. of ascorbic acid, 5 mg. of calcium pantothenate, 5 mcg. of cyanocobalamin, 2 mg. of folic acid, 20 mg. of nicotinamide, 2 mg. of pyridoxine hydrochloride, 3 mg. of riboflavin, 3 mg. of thiamine hydrochloride or thiamine mononitrate. One capsule or tablet supplies the recommended daily requirement of the vitamins contained therein.

de·cay' [L. *de*, down; *cadere*, to fall]. 1. *In bacteriology*, the progressive chemical decomposition of organic matter in the presence of atmospheric oxygen; due generally to aerobic bacteria. 2. Decline in health or strength. 3. Senility. 4. Dental caries: lay term.

radioactive d. The disappearance of an element because of its radioactive disintegration; the sum total of the processes by which unstable nuclear configurations are spontaneously converted into stable ones. The term as distinguished from radioactivity usually implies the statistical laws which govern these processes.

de'cem- [L., ten]. A combining form meaning *ten.*

de·cen'tered (dee·sen'turd) [L. *de-*, indicating separation; G. *kentron*, center]. Out of common center; said of a lens in which the visual axis and the axis of the lens do not coincide. —**decentra'tion,** *n.*

de·cer"e·bel·la'tion (dee·serr"i·buh·lay'shun) [*de-;* L. *cerebellum*, small brain]. The experimental removal of the cerebellum for the study of cerebellar functions.

de·cer"e·bra'tion (dee·serr"i·bray'shun) [*de-;* L. *cerebrum*, brain]. Removal of the brain in physiologic experiments. —**decer'ebrated,** *adj.;* **decer'ebrate,** *adj., v.t.;* **decer'ebrize,** *v.t.*

deceresol OT. Trade-mark for dioctyl sodium sulfosuccinate, used as a wetting agent.

de·chlo"ri·da'tion (dee·klor"i·day'shun) [*de-;* G. *chlōros*, pale-green]. Reduction of the quantity of chlorides in the body by the removal of salt from the diet.

de·chlo"ru·ra'tion (dee·klor"oo·ray'shun) [*de-; chlōros;* G. *ouron*, urine]. Reduction of the amount of chlorides excreted in the urine.

decholin. Trade-mark for dehydrocholic acid.

dec'i- (dess'i-) [L. *decimus*, tenth]. A combining form meaning *tenth;* used in the metric system to indicate *a measure one-tenth as large as the unit.*

dec'i·bel [*decimus; bel*, after A. G. *Bell*, inventor of the telephone]. A tenth of a bel. Abbreviated db.

de·cid'u·a (pl. *deciduae*) [L. *deciduus*, a falling off]. The mucous membrane (endometrium) of the uterus, especially that part subject to special modification in preparation for and during pregnancy and which is cast off at parturition and menstruation. Also called *membrana d., tunica d.* —**decidual,** *adj.*

d. basalis. That part of the endometrium between the chorionic vesicle and the myometrium that forms the maternal part of the placenta. Also called *d. serotina.*

d. capsularis. That part of the endometrium between the chorionic vesicle and the uterine lumen; the outer investing envelope of the fetus. Also called *d. reflexa.*

d. marginalis. That part of the endometrium at the junction of the decidua basalis, decidua parietalis, and decidua capsularis.

d. menstrualis. The outer layer of the uterine mucosa which is shed during menstruation.

d. parietalis. The endometrium exclusive of the region occupied by the embryo. Also called *d. vera.*

d. reflexa. See *d.* capsularis.

d. serotina. See *d.* basalis.

d. vera. See *d.* parietalis.

de·cid'u·ate [*deciduus*]. 1. Having, or characterized by, a decidua. 2. Formed in part from the decidua.

de·cid"u·a'tion [*deciduus*]. Act or process of dropping off or shedding.

de·cid"u·i'tis [*deciduus;* G. *-itis*, inflammation]. An acute inflammation of the decidua, frequently the result of attempts to induce abortion.

de·cid"u·o'ma [*deciduus;* G. *-ōma*, tumor]. 1. Decidual tissue produced in the uterus by mechanical or other methods in the absence of an embryo, so named by its discoverer, Leo Loeb (1908). 2. An intrauterine tumor containing decidual relics, and believed to arise from some hyperplasia of a retained portion of the decidua. —**deciduomal,** *adj.*

d. malignum. O.T. for *chorioadenoma.*

de·cid"u·o'sis. A condition in which decidual tissue develops in an ectopic site, such as vagina or cervix of the uterus.

de·cid'u·ous [*deciduus*]. Falling off or shed at maturity.

dec'i·gram (dess'i·gram) [L. *decimus*, tenth; G. *gramma*, scruple]. One-tenth of a gram.

dec'i·li"ter (dess'i·lee"tur) [*decimus;* G. *litra*, pound]. One-tenth of a liter.

dec'i·me"ter (dess'i·mee"tur) [*decimus;* G. *metron*, a measure]. One-tenth of a meter.

dec"i·nor'mal (dess"i·nor'mul) [*decimus;* L. *norma*, rule]. Having one-tenth the strength of the normal.

de·cip'a·ra [L. *decem*, ten; *parere*, to bring forth]. A woman who has borne ten children.

de·clive' [L. *declivis*, sloping]. A lower or descending part.

d. of the cerebellum. The first portion of the vermis behind the primary fissure, which with the culmen makes the monticulus: also called *d. of monticulus.*

de·coc′tion [L. *decoctio*, a boiling down]. *In pharmacology*, a liquid preparation obtained by boiling medicinal vegetable substances in water.

de″col·la′tion. Decapitation.

de′col·la″tor (dee′kuh·lay″tur, dee·kol′ay·tur) [L. *decollare*, to behead]. Instrument used for fetal decapitation.

de·col′or·ant (dee·kul′ur·unt) [L. *decolorare*, to deprive of its natural color]. An agent for the altering or removal of color. —**decol′orant,** *adj.;* **decoloriza′tion,** *n.;* **decolorize,** *v.*

de·com″pen·sa′tion (dee·kom″pen·say′shun) [L. *de-*, indicating reversing; *compensare*, to compensate]. Failure of compensation, as of the circulation or of the heart.

cardiac d. See *cardiac failure.*

de″com·po·si′tion [L. *de-*, indicating separation; *compositio*, from *componere*, to put together]. 1. The separation of the component principles of a body. 2. Putrefaction. —**decompose′,** *v.t., v.i.*

double d. The mutual reaction of two substances upon each other with formation of new substances; metathesis.

de″com·pres′sion [*de-;* L. *compressus*, from *comprimere*, to compress]. The removal of compression or pressure; particularly, various technics for reducing intracranial pressure, or for preventing caisson disease in divers and caisson workers.

cranial d. Surgical reduction of increased intracranial pressure.

d. chamber. *In aviation medicine*, an apparatus for the reduction of barometric pressure, used to study the biological effects of high-altitude flying and to evaluate the endurance of flight personnel.

d. sickness. See *aeroembolism.*

explosive d. *In aviation medicine*, a reduction of barometric pressure which is so rapid as to cause expansion of the involved gases in an explosive manner.

intestinal d. Release of pressure by means of suction through a tube inserted into the intestine, usually by way of the nose.

intracranial d. See cranial *d.*

orbital d. Cranial decompression by an approach in the orbital region.

suboccipital d. Cranial decompression by an approach in the occipital region.

subtemporal d. Cranial decompression by an approach in the temporal region.

surgical d. Any operative method to relieve excessive pressure, as in a body cavity, or the gastrointestinal tract.

de″con·ges′tive [*de-;* L. *congerere*, to bring together]. Relieving congestion.

de″con·tam″i·na′tion [*de-;* L. *contaminare*, to contaminate]. The process of making any object or area safe for unprotected personnel by making harmless chemical or biological agents, or by removing or blanketing radiological agents. —**decontam′inate,** *v.*

de·cor″ti·ca′tion [L. *decorticare*, to deprive of the bark]. 1. Stripping of the bark or husk of a plant. 2. Removal of the cortex or external covering from any organ or structure, as the removal of portions of the cortical substance of the brain from the summits of the gyri; decapsulation.

pulmonary d. Pleurectomy.

de″cu·ba′tion [*de-;* L. *cubare*, to recline]. The period in the recovery from an infectious disease beginning with the disappearance of the symptoms and lasting until the final exit of the microorganisms from the body. *Obs.*

de·cu′bi·tus [L., from *decumbere*, to lie down]. 1. The recumbent or horizontal posture. 2. Decubitus ulcer; a bedsore. —**decubital,** *adj.*

acute d. A form of bedsore due to cerebral lesions.

decurvon. Trade name for a pectin insulin which has the advantage of being slowly absorbed, possibly due to the high viscosity of the solution.

de·cus′sate, dec′us·sate [L. *decussare*, to divide crosswise in the form of an X]. Intersect; cross.

de″cus·sa′ti·o (dee″kuh·say′shee·o, deck″uh·). Decussation.

de″cus·sa′tion (dee″kuh·say′shun, deck″uh·) [L. *decussatio*, from *decussare*]. A chiasma or X-shaped crossing, especially of symmetrical parts, as of nerve fibers uniting unlike structures in the two sides of the brain or spinal cord.

anterior hypothalamic d. A bundle of nerve fibers dorsal to Meynert's commissure, which in part consists of pallidohypothalamic fibers and in part connects the hypothalamic regions of the two sides: also called *Ganser's commissure.*

d. of Forel. See ventral tegmental *d.*

d. of the brachia conjunctiva. Crossing of fibers from the dentate nucleus of each side to the opposite red nucleus.

d. of the lemnisci. Decussation of the medial lemnisci and associated fiber tracts.

d. of the optic nerve. The optic chiasma.

dorsal supraoptic d. See Meynert's *commissure.*

dorsal tegmental d. That of the tectospinal tracts; it is situated in the midbrain between the red nuclei and dorsal to them.

fountain d. Old term for either the dorsal or the ventral tegmental decussation.

posterior hypothalamic d. A small bundle of nerve fibers which arise in the globus pallidus and cross to the contralateral subthalamic nucleus or reticular formation. Syn., *supramammillary d.*

pyramidal d. The oblique crossing in the medulla oblongata of the corticospinal tracts (pyramidal tracts, O.T.) from the opposite sides of the anterior median fissure.

sensory d. The superior pyramidal decussation.

supramammillary d. See posterior hypothalamic *d.*

trochlear d. That of the trochlear nerves on the upper surface of the anterior medullary velum.

ventral supraoptic d. See Gudden's *commissure.*

ventral tegmental d. That of the rubrospinal tracts in the midbrain. Formerly called *d. of Forel.*

de″den·ti′tion (dee″den·tish′un) [L. *de-*, indicating separation; *dens*, tooth]. Loss of teeth, especially in old age as a result of atrophy of the alveoli.

de″dif·fer·en″ti·a′tion [*de-;* L. *differentia*, difference]. Loss of differentiation; a process of giving up specific characters and returning to a more generalized morphologic state.

Deen, Izaak Abrahamszoon van [*Dutch physiologist*, 1804–69]. Introduced a test to determine the presence of blood in any secretion or excretion. The reacting agents, which consist of tincture of guaiac and turpentine, produce a blue color if blood is present. Called *van Deen's test.*

deep [AS. *dēop*]. Not superficial.

deep sen″si·bil′i·ty. Perception of pressure, tension, and pain in the muscles, joints, tendons, and deep layers of the skin, as contrasted with sensations derived from the superficial layers of the skin.

deer fly. *Chrysops discalis*, the vector of tularemia. Most common in western U.S.A.

Dees, John Essary [*American urologist*, 1910–]. Known for his pyelolithotomy in which the stones are enmeshed in an artificial fibrin coagulum and withdrawn from the kidney pelvis as the clot is removed; called *Dees's operation.*

Deetjen, Hermann [*German physician*, 1867–1915].

Described the blood platelets which once were called *Deetjen's bodies.*

def An abbreviation applied to the quantitative estimate of dental caries in deciduous teeth. The letters stand for the number of *d*ecayed teeth, teeth to be *e*xtracted, and *f*illed teeth, respectively.

def″e·ca′tion [L. *defaecare*, to cleanse from dregs]. Evacuation of the bowels.

de·fect′, de′fect [L. *defectus*, a failure]. A lack or failure; absence of any part or organ; absence or failure of a normal function.

de″fem·i·na′tion [L. *de-*, indicating separation; *femina*, woman]. The loss or diminution of female characteristics.

de·fense′ mech′a·nism. A psychic device for guarding oneself against blame, guilt, anxiety, and unpleasant or disagreeable memories or experiences, or for concealing unacceptable desires, feelings, and beliefs; an unconscious attempt at self-justification and the maintenance of self-esteem. Rationalization is a common defense mechanism. Syn., *defense reaction.*

de·fense′ re·ac′tion. Defense mechanism.

def′er·ent [L. *deferre*, to carry away]. 1. Carrying away or down; efferent. 2. Pertaining to the ductus deferens.

def″er·en′tial [*deferre*]. Pertaining to the ductus deferens.

def″er·en″ti·o·ves′i·cal (def″ur·en″shee·o·) [*deferre;* L. *vesica*, bladder]. Pertaining to both the ductus deferens and the urinary bladder.

def″er·en·ti′tis [*deferre;* G. *-itis*, inflammation]. Inflammation of the ductus deferens.

de″fer·ves′cence [L. *defervescere*, to cease boiling]. Disappearance of fever.

de·fib″ril·la′tion. The arrest of fibrillation, usually that of the cardiac ventricles. An intense alternating current is briefly passed through the heart muscle throwing it into a refractory state. The quiescent myocardium allows the normal sinus impulse to resume rhythmic control of contraction. —**defibrillate,** *v.*

de·fib″ril·la′tor. An apparatus for defibrillating the ventricles of the heart, usually consisting of a source of alternating current and devices for controlling the intensity and duration of application of this current, together with appropriate electrodes for passing this current through the heart muscle.

de·fi″bri·na′tion (dee·figh″bri·nay′shun) [L. *de-*, indicating separation; *fibra*, fiber]. Removal of fibrin from blood or lymph.

def″i·ni′tion [L. *definitio*, from *definire*, to bound by limits]. *In optics*, the power of a magnifying lens to show clear outlines of the object examined, free from aberration or distortion.

def″la·gra′tion [L. *deflagrare*, to be consumed]. A sudden, violent combustion.

de·flec′tion [L. *deflectere*, to turn aside]. A turning, or state of being turned, aside.

extrinsic deflections. Deflections of the galvanometer string in direct leads which are derived from active muscle other than that immediately under the contacts.

intrinsic deflections. Deflections of the galvanometer string in direct leads which are derived from active muscle immediately under the contacts.

intrinsicoid d. The position of the QRS complex of a precordial lead indicating the time at which depolarization of the subjacent myocardium is complete.

QRS group of deflections. The initial deflections of the ventricular electrocardiogram; they correspond to the spread of the excitation wave in the ventricles (depolarization). Included in this group are: **notched QRS,** with spikes on one or the other of the limbs; **slurred QRS,** in which there is a distinct local thickening of one of the limbs or peak of the wave; and **splintered QRS,** having a wave with two or more apexes.

def″lo·ra′tion [L. *defloratio*, a plucking of flowers]. Loss of the physical sexual characteristics which in woman indicate virginity, usually regarded as typified by the rupture of the hymen at the first intercourse. The surgical removal or piercing of the hymen is not considered as defloration.

de″flo·res′cence [L. *deflorescere*, to drop its blossoms, fade]. Disappearance of the eruption of an exanthematous disease.

de·flu′vi·um cap·il·lo′rum. See *alopecia.*

de·flu′vi·um un′gui·um (ung′gwee·um). Complete loss of nails.

de·form′i·ty [L. *deformis*, misshapen]. 1. The state of being misshapen. 2. Marked deviation from the normal in size or shape of the body or of a part. —**deforming,** *adj.;* **deforma′tion,** *n.*

anterior d. Lordosis.

gunstock d. One following fracture of either condyle of the humerus in which the long axis of the fully extended forearm deviates outwardly from the arm.

Madelung's d. A congenital or developmental deformity of the wrist characterized by volar angulation of the distal end of the radius and dorsal dislocation of the head of the ulna.

seal-fin d. Ulnar deviation of the fingers, seen in rheumatoid arthritis.

silver-fork d. Displacement of the wrist, seen in Colles' fracture.

Sprengel's d. Congenital elevation of the scapula.

de·fuse′ (dee·fewz′) [L. *defusum*, from *defundere*, to pour out]. *In psychoanalysis*, to separate two primal instincts.

degalol. Trade-mark for desoxycholic acid.

de·gan′gli·on·ate (dee·gang′glee·un·ate) [L. *de-*, indicating separation; G. *gagglion*, knot]. Remove a ganglion or ganglions.

de·gas′sing [*de-; gas*, suggested by G. *chaos*, chaos]. The freeing of an area from toxic gas. —**degas′,** *v.*

de·gen′er·a·cy [L. *degenerare*, to depart from its race or kind]. A state marked by the deterioration of the mind and body. —**degen′erate,** *n.*

criminal d. That characterized by a tendency to commit criminal acts, especially sexual crimes.

de·gen′er·ate [*degenerare*]. To undergo the retrogressive changes of degeneration; to deteriorate in mental or psychic characters.

de″gen·er·a′tion [*degenerare*]. 1. A retrogressive, pathologic process in cells in which the cytoplasm undergoes deterioration and the nucleus is preserved. 2. A retrogressive process including even the death of nerves, axons, or tracts of the central nervous system. 3. Deterioration of mentality. —**degen′erative,** *adj.*

albuminous d. Cloudy swelling.

amyloid d. Formation and deposit of amyloid in tissues and organs; waxy or lardaceous degeneration. See also secondary *amyloidosis.*

ascending d. Degeneration of the myelin sheath and axons of sensory tracts progressing cranially from the point of injury.

atheromatous d. A retrogressive change, with the deposition of lipids in the degenerated tissue; observed especially in the hyalinized connective tissue of arteriosclerosis.

ballooning d. A morphologic phenomena leading to vesiculation in virus infections and characterized by marked intracytoplasmic edema and vacuolization.

basophilic d. (a) See mucoid *d.* (b) Basophilic stippling of erythrocytes such as occurs in lead poisoning.
calcareous d. Not a true degeneration, but rather a deposit of calcareous material in degenerate or necrotic tissue.
caseous d. See *caseation.*
cerebellofugal d. Progressive degeneration of the dentate nucleus and the superior cerebellar peduncles, manifested as ataxia, asthenia, and intention tremor. Syn., *progressive cerebellar asynergy* or *dyssynergy.*
cerebromacular d. Amaurotic familial idiocy.
colloid d. Abnormal production of colloid, as in the thyroid gland.
cortical d. See general *paresis.*
cystic d. Any form of degeneration with cyst formation.
cystoid d. of retina. A condition in which cystic spaces are found in the retina. When it occurs at the periphery of the retina, the condition is also called *Blessig-Ivanov cystoid d. of retina.*
descending d. Deterioration of myelin sheath and axons of descending tracts progressing caudally from the point of injury.
disciform d. Degeneration of Bruch's membrane of the choroid in the region of the macula lutea with the deposition of connective tissue under this membrane.
fascicular d. Degeneration, usually with necrosis, in fascicles of muscle supplied by diseased or interrupted motor neurons.
fatty d. A deteriorative process in which the cytoplasm of the cell contains microscopically visible, small droplets of fat, accompanied by other lipids. The fat is derived partly from lipids and proteins of the cell and partly from transported fat.
fibrinoid d. A form of degeneration in which the tissue involved is converted to a homogeneous or granular acellular mass with bright acidophilic staining reaction resembling that of fibrin.
fibrofatty d. of placenta. Fatty necrosis of placenta, usually the result of infarction.
fibroid d. Sometimes used to indicate a localized fibrosis.
glycogenic d. A form of degenerative change resulting from excess deposition of glycogen within cells.
granular d. Cloudy swelling. See *basophilia.*
hepatolenticular d. A motion dyskinesia resulting from degenerative changes in the lenticular nucleus with associated similar changes in the remaining parts of the basal ganglia, thalamus, cerebellum, and other regions of the central nervous system. Associated with the neurological manifestations are postnecrotic cirrhosis and a characteristic circumcorneal pigmentation of the limbus (*Kayser-Fleischer ring*). Aminoaciduria is present; copper content is elevated in the tissues, depressed in serum, and increased in urine. This condition, first described by S. A. K. Wilson (1912), is inherited as an autosomal recessive. Also called *progressive lenticular d., Wilson's disease.*
hyaline d. A form in which there is produced a clear, structureless or homogeneous, translucent change in tissues or cells.
hydropic d. Cellular degeneration with imbibition of so much water into the cytoplasm that microscopically visible droplets of water are formed.
keratinous d. See *keratinization,* 1.
lardaceous d. Amyloid degeneration. Also see *amyloidosis.*
liquefactive d. See liquefactive *necrosis.*
mucinous d. Mucous *d.*
mucoid d. A retrogressive change in mesodermal tissues in which mucoid is produced.
mucous d. Degeneration of epithelial cells or structures associated with abnormal production of mucus.
myelin d. A deterioration or necrosis of myelin sheaths of nerves.
myxomatous d. See mucoid *d.*
Nissl d. Degeneration of ganglion cells.
parenchymatous d. Cloudy swelling.
pigmentary d. A retrogressive change, especially in nerve cells, with abnormal deposit of pigmentary substances.
primary d. Degeneration of nerves at the point of injury or disease: also called *axon reaction, primary reaction of Nissl.*
progressive lenticular d. See hepatolenticular *d.*
red d. Red discoloration of fibromyoma due to degeneration, necrosis, and edema of the neoplasm.
reticular d. A process in which intracellular edema of the epidermis causes rupture of the cells with formation of multilocular bullae.
secondary d. Ascending or descending degeneration of nerves or tracts. Also called *Wallerian d.*
subacute combined d. of spinal cord. Combined degeneration of posterior and lateral columns of the spinal cord, with relatively little gliosis, such as occurs in pernicious anemia: also called *funicular myelitis, funicular myelosis, neuroanemia, Putnam-Dana syndrome, Putnam's type of sclerosis.* Syn., *combined system disease, dorsolateral* or *posterolateral sclerosis, subacute combined sclerosis, subacute combined system disease.*
traumatic d. The degeneration of the ends of nerves at the point of section, extending to the nearest node of Ranvier, after which fatty degeneration occurs.
vitreous d. Hyaline degeneration.
Wallerian d. Usually applied to degenerations as described under ascending and descending degenerations; due to interruption of nerve fibers.
waxy d. See *amyloid degeneration.* This term has also been used as a synonym for Zenker's hyaline *necrosis.*
Zenker's hyaline d. See under *necrosis.*

de·gen″i·tal′i·ty (dee·jen″i·tal′i·tee) [L. *de-*, indicating separation; *genitalis*, genital]. *In psychoanalysis*, a condition wherein genital instincts are expressed through activities of a nongenital character.

de″glu·ti′tion (dee″gloo·tish′un, deg″loo·) [L. *deglutire*, to swallow down]. The act of swallowing. —**deglu′titive, deglu′titory,** *adj.*

deg″ra·da′tion [*de-;* L. *gradus*, step]. The conversion of one organic compound to another containing a smaller number of carbon atoms.

de·grease′ (dee·grees′, ·greez′) [*de-;* OF. *gresse*, from L. *crassus*, fat]. Remove fat, as from bones in the preparation of skeletons.

de·gree′ [ME. *degre*, from L. *de-*, down; *gradus*, step]. 1. A position in a graded series. 2. One of the units or intervals of a thermometric or other scale. 3. The unit for measuring arcs or angles. One degree is $\frac{1}{360}$ of a circle. A right angle is 90° or one quarter of a circle. 4. A rank or title conferred by a college or university in recognition of attainment. 5. *In law*, the relative amount of guilt. 6. One remove in the direct line of descent; one remove in the chain of relationship, as a cousin of fourth degree.

de·gree′ of free′dom. 1. *In mechanics*, any of the ways in which a point, body, or system may change or move. 2. *In physical chemistry*, a system's capacity for variation due to the variability of one of its factors. 3. *In biometry,* the number of independent values in a statistical table.

de″gus·ta′tion [L. *degustare,* to taste]. Act of tasting.

Dehio, Karl Konstantinovich [*Russian physician,* 1851–1927]. *Dehio's test* is a method of ascertaining the cause of bradycardia. If a hypodermic dose of atropine gives relief, the condition is of vagus nerve origin; if not, it is due to pathologic change in the heart muscle.

de·his′cence [L. *dehiscere,* to gape]. 1. The act of splitting open. 2. A defect in the boundary of a bony canal or cavity.

de·hy′drase (dee·high′drace). See *dehydrogenase.*

de″hy·dra′tion (dee″high·dray′shun) [L. *de-,* indicating separation; G. *hydōr,* water]. The removal of water, as from the body or a tissue. —**dehy′drate,** *v.*

dehydrite. A trade-mark for anhydrous magnesium perchlorate, used in various chemical procedures for absorption of water.

de·hy′dro-, dehydr- [*de-; hydōr*]. *In chemistry,* a combining form signifying *dehydrated* or *dehydrogenated.*

de·hy″dro·an·dros′ter·one. Old term for dehydroisoandrosterone.

de·hy″dro·a·scor′bic ac′id. The relatively inactive acid resulting from elimination of two hydrogen atoms from ascorbic acid when the latter is oxidized by air or other agents.

7-de·hy″dro·cho·les′ter·ol (·ko·less′tur·ole, ·ol, ·awl). A provitamin of animal origin in the skin of man, in milk, and elsewhere, which upon irradiation with ultraviolet rays becomes vitamin D_3.

de·hy″dro·cho′lic ac′id (dee·high″dro·ko′lick, ·kol′ick). $C_{24}H_{37}O_5$. 3,7,12-Triketocholanic acid. The acid resulting when the three hydroxyl groups of cholic acid are oxidized to keto groups. Both the acid and its sodium salt are used for their hydrocholeretic and choleretic effects. Dose of the acid, 0.25–0.5 Gm. (4–8 gr.), two or three times daily for four to six weeks. See *cholan-DH, cholic acid,* 1; *decholin, procholon.*

de·hy″dro·cor″ti·cos′te·rone. $C_{21}H_{28}O_4$; 11-dehydrocorticosterone or Δ^4-pregnene-21-ol-3,11,20-trione; a steroid occurring in the adrenal cortex and possessing biologic activity similar to that of corticosterone. Syn., *Kendall's Compound A.* See Table of Hormones in the Appendix.

de·hy″dro·ep″i·an·dros′ter·one. Dehydroisoandrosterone.

de·hy′dro·gen·ase. An enzyme which catalyzes the oxidation of a specific substrate by removal of hydrogen. Some dehydrogenases (aerobic) can transfer hydrogen directly to gaseous oxygen, whereas other dehydrogenases (anaerobic) require a hydrogen acceptor. Also called *dehydrase.*

alcohol d. An enzyme occurring in yeast; capable of reversibly oxidizing ethanol to acetaldehyde. Coenzyme I is required, and other aliphatic alcohols of low molecular weight are likewise oxidized. A similar but not identical enzyme is found in animal tissues, particularly in liver. Syn., *alcoholase.*

1,3-diphosphoglyceric aldehyde d. The enzyme by which 1,3-diphosphoglyceric aldehyde is oxidized to 1,3-diphosphoglyceric acid, in the presence of coenzyme I.

glucose d. The enzyme that dehydrogenates D-glucose to D-gluconic acid in the presence of a hydrogen acceptor.

glutamic acid d. The enzyme that converts L (+) glutamic acid into α-ketoglutaric acid in the presence of coenzyme II.

glycerophosphate d. One of the two enzymes that dehydrogenate glycerophosphate to form 3-phosphoglyceric aldehyde; only one requires coenzyme I, the other transferring hydrogen to cytochrome C.

β-hydroxybutyric d. The enzyme that removes hydrogen from L-β-hydroxybutyric acid to form acetoacetic acid, in the presence of coenzyme I.

isocitric d. The enzyme that, in the presence of coenzyme II, converts L-isocitric acid to oxalosuccinic acid.

lactic d. The enzyme that dehydrogenates lactic acid to form pyruvic acid.

malic d. The enzyme that removes hydrogen from L(−) malic acid in the presence of coenzyme I, to form oxalacetic acid.

phosphogluconic d. The enzyme that oxidizes phosphogluconic acid in the presence of coenzyme II.

Robison ester d. The enzyme that converts the Robison ester to phosphohexonic acid in the presence of coenzyme II.

succinic d. The enzyme that dehydrogenates succinic acid to fumaric acid in the presence of a hydrogen acceptor.

de·hy′dro·gen·ize, de·hy′dro·gen·ate. Remove hydrogen from. —**dehydrogeniza′tion, dehydrogena′tion,** *n.*

de·hy″dro·i″so·an·dros′ter·one. $C_{19}H_{28}O_2$; 3(β)-hydroxy-17-keto-5:6-androstene; an androgenic steroid found in the urine of men and women. Syn., *dehydroepiandrosterone.*

de·hy″dro·stil·bes′trol. See *dienestrol.*

de·i′on·iz″er. An apparatus, charged with suitable ion exchanging and removing substances, which effects removal of ionic constituents from liquids, notably from water. —**dei′onize,** *v.*

Deiters, Otto Friedrich Karl [*German physician and anatomist,* 1834–63]. Known for his description of the branched flattened cells of the neuroglia, called astrocytes; his study of the cylindricoconical cells resting upon the basilar membrane of the organ of Corti and supporting the hair cells, called *Deiter's cells;* his description of the lateral vestibular nucleus, which once bore his name; his description of the neuraxon, proving that each nerve cell is equipped with an axis cylinder or nerve-fiber process.

dé″jà″ vu′ [F., already seen]. A feeling of familiarity; a dream state in which experiences seem to have occurred before. A symptom found in tumors or other lesions of the temporal lobe of the brain. Syn., *dreamy state epilepsy.*

de·jec′tion [L. *dejectio,* a throwing down]. 1. Depression, lowness of spirits. 2. Discharge of fecal matter; defecation. 3. Feces; excrement.

Dejerine, Joseph Jules [*French neurologist,* 1849–1917]. Justly famed as one of the greatest European neurologists of his time. With Sottas, gave the first description of progressive hypertrophic interstitial neuropathy (1893), called *Dejerine-Sottas disease, neuropathy.* With Roussy he described the thalamic syndrome (1906), called *Dejerine-Roussy syndrome;* he also described tabes of the nervous system (1887), and is credited with distinguishing types involving the peripheral or central nervous system. He wrote on tabetic muscular atrophies, the parietal lobe syndrome, and many other subjects, and demonstrated that certain aphasias may occur as the result of lesions of the supramarginal and angular gyri. Fascioscapulohumeral atrophy is known as *Landouzy-Dejerine atrophy.*

Dejerine-Klumpke, Augusta [*French neurologist,* 1859–1927]. Wife of Joseph Dejerine, and famous in her own right for her researches in many fields of neurology and, especially, for her contributions to the knowledge of lead paralysis. Gave the first adequate description of the paralysis and atrophy following lesion of the brachial plexus and the eighth cervical and first thoracic nerves, known as *Klumpke's paralysis* (1885).

Dekkers, Frederik [*Dutch physician*, 1648–1720]. Remembered as an early contributor to the knowledge of clinical pathology. Discovered the presence of albumin in urine (1673) by boiling the specimen with acetic acid.

delacillin. Trade-mark for an injectable preparation of penicillin calcium in peanut oil and beeswax.

de″lac·ta′tion [L. *de-*, indicating reversing; *lactare*, to give suck]. 1. Weaning. 2. Cessation of lactation.

Delafield's hematoxylin. See under *stain*.

de·lam″i·na′tion (dee·lam″i·nay′shun) [L. *de-*, indicating separation; *lamina*, a plate]. Separation or splitting into layers, as in the dividing of cells to form new layers.

delapan. Trade name for a pollen extract for subcutaneous or intradermal use for hyposensitization to the contained pollens.

Delbet, Paul [*French surgeon*, 1866–1924]. Remembered for his sign that, in a patient with aneurysm of the main artery of a limb, nutrition of the distal portion shows the status of circulation.

de le Boë. See Franciscus *Sylvius*.

De Lee, Joseph Bolivar [*American obstetrician*, 1869–1942]. Known for his contributions in the field of operative obstetrics and modern maternity care and for his textbook, *Principles and Practice of Obstetrics*.

Del′hi boil (del′hee, del′ee). See *oriental sore*.

Delille, Arthur [*French physician*, 1876–1950]. Known for his description, with Rénon, of the syndrome of dyspituitarism, characterized by lowered blood pressure, tachycardia, oliguria, insomnia, and hyperhidrosis (1908); called *Rénon-Delille syndrome*.

De Lima's operation. See transmaxillary *ethmoidectomy*.

de·lim″i·ta′tion [L. *delimitare*, to mark out]. The fixing of limits or boundaries.

de·lim′it·ed. Marked by bounds; having a line or lines of demarcation.

de·lin′quen·cy [L. *delinquere*, to do wrong]. 1. An offense or violation, especially that committed by a minor, as truancy, vandalism, lying, stealing, overt sex practices. 2. The tendency to commit delinquencies; the committing of such offenses.

de″lip·i·da′tion. Removal of lipids by fat solvents from a tissue or microscopic sections.

del″i·ques′cence [L. *deliquescere*, to melt away]. Process of liquefaction by absorption of water from the atmosphere, or the resultant state. —**deliquescent,** *adj.*; **deliquesce,** *v.*

de·liq′ui·um (di·lick′wee·um) [L., defect]. 1. Fainting or syncope. *Obs.* 2. Mental impairment. *Rare.*

d. animi. Syncope.

de·lir″i·fa′cient (di·lirr″i·fay′shunt, ·shee·unt) [L. *delirium*, delirium; *facere*, to cause]. Producing delirium. Syn., *deliriant*.

de·lir′i·um [L.]. A condition of mental excitement, confusion, and clouded sensorium, usually with hallucinations, illusions, and delusions; precipitated by toxic factors in diseases or drugs. —**delirious,** *adj.*

abstinence d. That occurring upon withdrawal of alcohol or of a drug from one addicted to it.

acute d. That form marked by convulsions and occasionally death.

alcoholic d. See *d.* tremens.

asthenic d. See exhaustion *d.*

collapse d. Delirium produced by physical collapse.

d. cordis. Fibrillation of the heart, usually atrial.

d. grandiosum. That in which the individual has greatly exaggerated ideas of his own importance or possessions; megalomania.

d. mite. See quiet *d.*

d. nervosum. That following severe surgical operations or injuries, or that associated with organic brain disease.

d. tremens. A delirious state marked by distressing delusions, illusions, hallucinations, constant tremor, fumbling movements of the hands, insomnia, and great exhaustion. Usually associated with alcoholic poisoning, but may appear in acute inflammatory brain diseases, arteriosclerosis, or senile encephalopathy, or in schizophrenia or manic-depressive psychoses. Syn., *alcoholic d.*

emotional d. That in which the state of mind is such that the individual will accept a false idea without qualifications.

exhaustion d. That brought about by fatigue and extreme lowering of psychologic tension. Syn., *asthenic d.*

oneiric d. Dream delirium; one occurring at night, made up of parts of dreams which vary uninterruptedly and may continue after the patient wakes.

quiet d. A mental condition marked by delirious, scarcely audible mumbling. Syn., *d. mite.*

traumatic d. Acute delirium resulting from head or brain injury.

de·liv′er·y [OF. *delivrer*, from LL. *deliberare*, to set free]. 1. Liberation; release. 2. Parturition; expulsion or extraction of a fetus and its membranes. See Plate 42. 3. Removal of a part, as a lens in cataract extraction, or of a tumor. —**deliver,** *v.*

post-mortem d. Extraction of the fetus after the death of the mother.

premature d. Expulsion of the fetus after the twenty-eighth week and before term.

Della Croce, Giovanni Andrea (Cruce) [*Italian physician*, 1514–75]. Celebrated as the author of works on surgery, in which he paid special attention to operations upon the head and skull by trephining. His works are well illustrated and contain many details of early operating room technic.

de″lo·mor′phous (dee″lo·mor′fus, del″o·) [G. *dēlos*, conspicuous; *morphē*, form]. Having a conspicuous form, as a delomorphous cell, the acid-secreting parietal cell of the fundic glands.

Delorme, Edmond [*French surgeon*, 1847–1929]. Remembered for his work on pulmonary and thoracic surgery and, especially, for his operation, now rarely used, of decortication of the lung for chronic empyema (1894), called *Fowler-Delorme operation*. Also devised an operation for the relief of chronic constrictive pericarditis, in which a portion of the pericardium is excised. See also *Rehn-Delorme operation* under *Rehn*.

de·louse′ (dee·louse′, ·louze′) [L. *de-*, indicating separation; ME. *lous*]. Free from lice; destroy lice. —**delous′ing,** *n.*

Delpech, Jacques Matthieu [*French orthopedic surgeon*, 1777–1832]. Known as one of the few deserving of the name orthopedist in his day. One of the first to practice subcutaneous division of the Achilles tendon in the treatment of clubfoot (1816). Established the tuberculous origin of Pott's disease.

del′phi·nin. A glycosidal dyestuff obtained from the flowers of *Delphinium consolida*.

del′phi·nine (del′fi·neen, ·nin). An alkaloid obtained from *Delphinium staphisagria* or stavesacre larkspur.

Del·phin′i·um [G. *delphis*, dolphin]. A genus of plants of the Ranunculaceae; the larkspurs.

D. ajacis. The dried, ripe seeds of this species (source of the crystalline alkaloids ajacine and ajaconine) possess an aconitelike toxicity. The tincture and acetic tincture (larkspur lotion) are used externally to destroy lice.

D. consolida. Source of delphinin.

D. staphisagria. Stavesacre; staphisagria.

del″phi·noi′dine (del″fi·noy′deen, ·din). $C_{22}H_{35}O_6N$. An amorphous alkaloid found in *Delphinium staphisagria.*

del′phi·sine (del′fi·seen, ·sin). An alkaloid from *Delphinium staphisagria* or stavesacre larkspur.

del′ta. 1. The fourth letter of the Greek alphabet (Δ, δ), used as a symbol in various ways, as: (a) *in chemistry,* (δ) the fourth carbon atom starting with the one bearing the characteristic functional group, or in some cases with the adjacent atom; (Δ with superscripts) double bond; (Δ) coefficient of diffusion; (Δ) freezing point lowering; (b) *in mathematics,* (Δ) increment. 2. See delta *rhythm.*

deltalin. Trade-mark for a brand of synthetic vitamin D_2.

del′toid [G. *delta,* fourth letter of the Greek alphabet; *eidos,* form]. Shaped like a Δ (capital delta), as the deltoid ligament of the ankle joint.

del′toid. The large, thick, delta-shaped muscle covering the shoulder joint. See Table of Muscles in the Appendix.

deltra. Trade-mark for *prednisone.*

de·lu′sion [L. *delusio,* from *deludere,* to deceive]. A belief maintained in the face of incontrovertible evidence to the contrary.

delvinal sodium. Trade-mark for sodium ethyl (1-methyl-1-butenyl) barbiturate, a rapidly acting sedative and hypnotic.

de″mar·ca′tion [L. *de-,* indicating separation; *marcar,* to mark, of Teutonic origin]. Separation, establishing of limits.

d. potential. See *injury potential.*

line of d. A line forming at the edge of a gangrenous area and marking the limit of the process.

De·ma′ti·um. See *Pullularia.*

de·ment′ed [L. *demens,* out of one's mind]. Deprived of reason. —**dement′,** *n., v.*

de·men′ti·a [L., the being out of one's mind]. Deterioration or loss of the intellectual faculties, the reasoning power, the memory, and the will; characterized by confusion, disorientation, apathy, and stupor of varying degrees.

alcoholic d. A dementia more prolonged but less intense than delirium tremens, occurring in late stages of chronic alcoholism.

apoplectic d. Dementia due to cerebral hemorrhage or to softening of brain tissue from other causes.

circular d. That characterized by alternating phases of excitement and depression.

d. agitata. Old term for a form distinguished by great excitement, motor activity, and continuous hallucinations; seen in patients with schizophrenia.

d. paralytica. See general *paresis.*

d. paranoides. Old term for the paranoid form of schizophrenia.

d. precox. The name given by Kraepelin to a form of insanity occurring during adolescence or early adulthood; was formerly thought to be a single psychotic disease, but is now known to be a group of heterogeneous psychoses. Four types are recognized—simple, hebephrenic, paranoid, and catatonic. Now more properly called schizophrenic *reactions.*

epileptic d. Mental deterioration in an epileptic person.

presenile d. Senium precox. See also presenile *sclerosis.*

primary d. Old term for simple dementia precox.

secondary d. Old term for dementia supposedly following an acute attack of dementia; a form of dementia precox not now recognized.

senile d. The progressive cerebral manifestation of deterioration associated with old age. A less intense mental involvement than senile psychosis.

traumatic d. That due directly or indirectly to an injury, usually of the head.

demerol hydrochloride. Trade-mark for a brand of meperidine hydrochloride.

de·meth″yl·a′tion. The removal of one or more methyl (—CH_3) groups from a compound.

dem′i- [F., from L. *dimidius,* half]. A prefix signifying *half.*

dem″i·fac′et (dem″ee·fass′it) [*dimidius;* F. *facette*]. One-half of an articulation surface adapted to articulate with two bones.

dem′i·lune [*demi-;* L. *luna,* moon]. A crescent-shaped aggregation of serous cells capping mucous cells in mixed glands: also called *serous crescent, demilune of Gianuzzi.*

dem″i·mon·stros′i·ty [*dimidius;* L. *monstrum,* monster]. A variety of congenital deformity that does not give rise to appreciable disorder of function. See *hemiterata.*

de·min″er·al·i·za′tion (dee·min″ur·ul·i·zay′shun, ·eye·zay′shun) [L. *de-,* indicating separation; ML. *mineralis,* from *minera,* ore mine]. Loss of mineral salts from the body, as from the bones.

coefficient of d. The quantity of mineral matter as compared with the total solids in the urine.

dem″i·pen′ni·form [*dimidius;* L. *penna,* wing; *forma,* shape]. Applied to structures or organs which have one of two margins wing-shaped.

de′mo-, dem- [G. *dēmos,* deme, populace]. A combining form denoting *populace.*

Democritus of Abdera [*Greek philosopher,* ca. 460–370 B.C.]. Noted for developing the atomic theory. Studied the anatomy of the chameleon and the causes of epidemic diseases.

Dem′o·dex (dem′o·decks, dee′mo·) [G. *dēmos,* fat; *dēx,* worm]. A genus of parasitic mites.

D. folliculorum. Species of mites which are parasites of the sebaceous glands and hair follicles. These parasites rarely cause discomfort, but when unusually numerous may cause a chronic erythema, with scaling of the epidermis, accompanied by burning sensations.

de·mog′ra·phy (dee·mog′ruh·fee) [G. *dēmos,* deme; *graphein,* to write]. The science of peoples collectively considered; social science, including that of vital statistics.

dynamic d. A study of the activities of human communities, their rise, progress, and fall.

de·mon′mi·a (dee·mon′mee·uh). See *demonomania.*

de′mon·o-, de′mon- [G. *daimōn,* demon]. A combining form signifying *demon.*

de″mon·ol′a·try [*daimōn;* G. *latreia,* service]. Worship of a demon or spirit.

de″mon·o·ma′ni·a [*daimōn;* G. *mania,* madness]. A form of madness in which a person imagines himself possessed of a devil. —**demonomaniac,** *n.*

de″mon·op′a·thy [*daimōn;* G. *pathos,* disease]. Demonomania.

de″mon·o·pho′bi·a [*daimōn;* G. *phobos,* fear]. Morbid fear of devils and demons.

de·mor″phin·i·za′tion (dee·mor″fin·i·zay′shun, ·eye·zay′shun) [L. *de-,* indicating separation; G. *Morpheus,* god of dreams, from *morphē,* form, because he calls up forms before the sleeper]. Treatment of morphinism by gradual withdrawal of the drug.

Demours, Antoine Pierre [*French ophthalmologist.*

1702–95]. Described the posterior elastic lamina of the cornea; called *Demours' membrane.* See Descemet's *membrane.*

de·mul'cent [L. *demulcere,* to stroke down]. Soothing; allaying irritation of surfaces, especially mucous membranes.

de·mul'cent. A soothing substance, particularly a slippery, mucilaginous liquid.

de Mussy's point. See *Guénau de Mussy.*

de·my'e·lin·ate [L. *de-,* indicating separation; G. *myelos,* marrow]. Remove or destroy the myelin sheath of nerves or nerve tracts.

de·nar'co·tized (dee·nahr'ko·tized) [*de-;* G. *narkōtikos,* from *narkē,* numbness]. 1. Deprived of narcotizing qualities. 2. Deprived of narcotine, said of opium.

de·na'tur·ant. 1. A substance added to another to make the latter unfit for certain uses, as when methyl alcohol is added to ethyl alcohol for the purpose of preventing beverage use of the ethyl alcohol. 2. *In nuclear science,* a nonfissionable isotope, which, when added to fissionable material, makes the latter unsuited for use in atomic weapons without considerable processing.

de·na"tur·a'tion. See *denaturization.*

de·na'tured [*de-;* L. *natura,* nature]. Changed, made different from normal.

de·na'tured al'co·hol. Alcohol into which some other substance has been introduced, rendering it unfit for drinking but still useful for other purposes.

de·na"tur·i·za'tion (dee·nay"chur·i·zay'shun, ·eye·zay'shun) [*de-; natura*]. Alteration in the characteristics of an organic substance, especially a protein, by physical or chemical action.

Den"dr·as'pis [*dendron;* G. *aspis,* asp]. Genus of snakes of the Elapidae found in Africa, south of the Sahara. This snake is slender and may be seven feet in length. It possesses a powerful neurotoxic venom.

D. angusticeps. The common mamba.

den'drite [G. *dendron,* tree]. The process of a neuron which carries the nerve impulse to the cell body. It is usually branched, like a tree. Syn., *dendron.*

den·drit'ic, den'droid. Branching in treelike or rootlike fashion; arborescent.

den'dron. See *dendrite.*

den"dro·phag"o·cy·to'sis. The phagocytic action of abnormal microglia cells in cases of brain injury. They envelop and remove the degenerating expansions of the fibrous astrocytes.

den"dro·phil'i·a [*dendron;* G. *philein,* to love]. *In psychiatry,* love of trees; a sexual attraction to trees.

Deneke, Theodor Karl August (1860–). German bacteriologist and internist, remembered for his description of a bacterium, *Vibrio tyrogenus,* resembling the bacillus of Asiatic cholera. Called *Deneke's spirillum.*

de·ner'va·ted (dee·nur'vay·tid) [L. *de-,* indicating separation; *nervus,* nerve]. Having the nerve supply interfered with, or the nerve removed.

de"ner·va'tion [*de-; nervus*]. 1. Sectioning or removal of a nerve to interrupt the nerve supply to a part. 2. *In veterinary medicine,* the cutting off of the nerve supply to the lower leg and foot to relieve certain types of lameness in the horse.

den'gue (deng'ghee, deng'gay) [West Indian Sp., after Sp. *dengue,* prudery]. An acute, infectious, endemic, and epidemic disease; caused by a filtrable virus transmitted by mosquitoes, especially by the *Aëdes aegypti.* Dengue is characterized by a febrile paroxysm, severe pains in the bones and muscles, and swelling, reddening, and pain of the joints. At times there is a cutaneous eruption. The period of incubation is from three to five days, and the invasion is sudden. The high fever (106° F.) lasts for three or four days and subsides for an interval, then is followed by a second paroxysm. Convalescence is slow and complications are rare. The disease is widespread throughout the tropics and the subtropics. Also called *breakbone fever, dandy fever.*

Mediterranean d. Pappataci fever.

de·ni'al. *In psychiatry,* the unconscious psychic mechanism or process whereby an observation is denied or refused recognition in order to avoid anxiety or pain; the simplest and commonest form of the ego defense mechanisms, and a part of many normal phenomena, as in the phantasies of children who deny the realities of their own lives to enjoy play.

den"i·da'tion (den"i·day'shun, dee"nigh·) [*de-;* L. *nidus,* nest]. Disintegration and ejection of the superficial part of the uterine mucosa.

Denigès, Georges [*French biochemist,* 1859–1935]. Introduced a test for formaldehyde in milk: Dilute hydrochloric acid and fuchsin, sodium bisulfite, and sulfuric acid in distilled water are added to the suspected milk; a violet color indicates a positive reaction.

den"i·gra'tion (den"i·gray'shun, dee"nigh·) [L. *denigrare,* to blacken utterly]. Act or process of rendering black; the state of having become black.

Denis, Jean Baptiste [*French physician,* d. 1704]. Performed the first recorded transfusion of blood into a human being (1667), using the blood of a lamb. Transfused human blood later in the same year without success.

Denis, Willey Glover [*American biochemist,* 1879–]. Both alone and with others, he originated many methods which bear his name, as the *Denis method* for serum magnesium, *Folin and Denis' method* for phenols, *Folin and Denis' method* for Bence Jones protein, and the *Folin, Cannon, and Denis' method* for epinephrine. Also see uric acid *reagent* of Folin and Denis.

de·ni'tri·fy (dee·nigh'tri·figh). Remove nitrogen.

de·ni"tro·gen·a'tion. A procedure by which one removes nitrogen from his body by breathing nitrogen-free gas.

Denonvilliers, Charles Pierre [*French surgeon,* 1808–72]. Known for his description of the rectovesical fascia between the prostate and the rectum, and for his contributions to plastic surgery. Devised an operation for reconstruction of the upper lip, using two full-thickness grafts raised from the cheeks and sutured in the midline, and one for restoration of the nose, using a triangular flap raised from the side of the nose above the defective ala, with the pedicle of the flap inward.

dens (denz) (pl. *dentes*) [L.]. 1. A tooth. 2. The toothlike process on the body of the axis, going through the front part of the ring of the atlas.

d. acutus. An incisor tooth.

d. adultus. A tooth of second dentition.

d. adversus. An incisor tooth.

d. angularis. A canine or cuspid tooth.

d. bicuspidatus. A premolar or bicuspid tooth.

d. caninus. A canine or cuspid tooth.

d. cariosus. A carious tooth.

d. columellaris. A molar tooth.

d. cuspidatus. A canine or cuspid tooth.

d. exsertus. A tooth which projects or is in front of the dental arch; applied more particularly to the canines.

d. incisor. An incisor tooth.

d. lacteus. A milk, temporary, or deciduous tooth.

d. molaris. A molar tooth.

d. primoris. An incisor tooth; so called because it occupies the front or anterior part of the dental arch.

d. sapientia. A wisdom tooth; a name given to the third molar tooth of each half of each jaw.

d. serotinus. A wisdom tooth.

d. tomici. An incisor tooth.

den·sim′e·ter [L. *densus*, dense; G. *metron*, a measure]. An appliance for ascertaining the specific gravity of a liquid. Syn., *hydrometer*. —**densimet′ric,** *adj.*

dens′ in den′te (denz′ in den′tee). An abnormality of development in which the enamel organ has invaginated within the pulp chamber, producing a deposition of enamel within the tooth.

den″sit·om′e·ter. 1. An instrument utilizing the photoelectric principle for measuring the opacity of exposed and processed photographic film. 2. See *densimeter*.

den′si·ty [*densus*]. Closeness of any space distribution; for example, **electron density** signifies the number of electrons per unit volume. Abbreviated, d.

absolute d. (a) The ratio of the mass of a substance to its volume. See specific *gravity*. (b) The light-absorbing power of the silver image in photographic materials.

photographic d. A measure of the opacity of an exposed film, the greater the exposure, the greater the photographic density.

den′so·gram [*densus;* G. *graphein*, to write]. A record of the changes in cardiac density during the cardiac cycle made with the electrokymographic lead completely covered by the heart shadow.

dent-. See *denti-*.

den·tag′ra (den·tag′ruh, den′tag·ruh, den·tay′-gruh) [L. *dens*, tooth; G. *agra*, a catching]. 1. Toothache. *Obs.* 2. A tooth forceps.

den′tal [*dens*]. Pertaining to the teeth.

den′tal en′gine. *In dentistry*, the apparatus used to operate rotating, cutting, or polishing devices such as burs, abrasive disks or wheels, and brushes. These interchangeable parts are held in a handpiece which is connected by a flexible arm to a controlled driving mechanism, usually an electric motor.

den′tal floss. A soft thread, usually flat and waxed; used to clean interdental spaces and tooth surfaces.

den·tal′gi·a [*dens;* G. *algos*, pain]. Toothache. *Obs.*

den′tal hy′gien·ist. A person trained and licensed in the technique of mechanically removing calcareous deposits and stains from the teeth.

den′tal i·den″ti·fi·ca′tion rec′ord. *In U.S. Army medicine*, an official form for recording every characteristic of the condition of a soldier's teeth: used as a means of identification if injuries causing death result in the destruction of other features of the soldier.

dentalone. Trade-mark for chlorobutanol dissolved in essential oils; used as an analgesic and antiseptic.

den′tal serv′ice. 1. That part of the U.S. Army Medical Service staff that provides dental care for military personnel. 2. The detection, treatment, and prevention of dental diseases as part of the medical service provided for military personnel.

den′ta·phone. See *dentiphone*.

den·tar′pa·ga [*dens;* G. *harpagē*, hook]. Instrument for the extraction of teeth. *Obs.*

den′tar·y [dens]. 1. A bone found chiefly in fishes, regarded as a phylogenetic component of the mammalian mandible. 2. Dental: incorrect use.

den′tate [L. *dentatus*, toothed]. 1. Having teeth or toothlike projections; *in botany*, having a toothed or serrated edge. 2. Having a scalloped edge, as the dentate ligament, which has about 21 pairs of dentations or pointed processes. —**denta′tion,** *n.*

den·ta′tum (den·tay′tum, ·tah′tum) [*dentatus*]. The dentate nucleus of the cerebellum.

den″te·la′tion [L. *dens*, tooth]. The state of having toothlike processes.

den′tes (den′teez). Plural of dens.

den′ti-, dent- [*dens*]. A combining form meaning *tooth* or *dental*.

den′ti·a pre′cox [L.]. The presence of erupted teeth at birth.

den″ti·a·ski′a·scope [*dens;* G. *skia*, shadow; *skopein*, to examine]. Instrument for examining the teeth and alveoli. It consists of a small fluorescent screen within an aluminum case, so situated that the screen image is reflected upon a mirror which the operator sees through a tube.

den′ti·cle [L. *denticulus*, a small tooth]. 1. A small tooth or projecting point. 2. A deposit of dentin-like or calcareous material within the pulp of the tooth, associated with degenerative or retrogressive changes of the pulp; pulpstone: also called *nodular calcification*.

den·tic′u·late [*denticulus*]. Having minute dentations; furnished with small teeth or notches.

den″ti·fi·ca′tion [L. *dens*, tooth; *facere*, to make]. Formation of teeth; dentition.

den′ti·form [*dens;* L. *forma*, shape]. Odontoid; tooth-shaped.

den′ti·frice (den′ti·friss) [L. *dentifricium*, from *dens; fricare*, to rub]. A substance or preparation used to aid the mechanical cleaning of the teeth.

den·tig′er·ous (den·tidj′ur·us) [*dens;* L. *gerere*, to carry]. Bearing or containing teeth.

den′ti·lave [*dens;* L. *lavare*, to wash]. A mouthwash or toothwash.

den′tin (den′tin, ·teen), **den′tine** [*dens*]. The calcified tissue which forms the major part of a tooth. Dentin is related to bone but differs from it in the absence of included cells. It is covered by the enamel over the crown of the tooth, by the cementum over the roots, and itself surrounds the pulp chamber and root canals which contain the dental pulp. Syn., *substantia eburnea, ivory, ebur*. —**dentinal,** *adj.*

adventitious d. See secondary *d.*

circumpulpar d. The major part of the dentin which lies next the pulp.

cover d. See mantle *d.*

hereditary opalescent d. See *dentinogenesis imperfecta*.

interglobular d. A small region of poorly calcified dentin found along the course of the incremental lines.

irregular d. See secondary *d.*

mantle d. The thin superficial layer of dentin.

secondary d. The dentin of repair; that which is deposited on the walls of the pulp chamber by the dental pulp in response to loss of tooth substance.

vitreous d. A variety of dentin with but few dentinal tubules. Syn., *vitreodentin*.

den′tine. See *dentin*.

den·tin″i·fi·ca′tion [*dens;* L. *facere*, to make]. See *dentinogenesis*.

den″ti·no·blas·to′ma. A benign odontogenic tumor made up of poorly developed dentin.

den″ti·no·ce·men′tal [*dens;* L. *caementum*, a rough stone]. Relating to the dentin and cementum of a tooth.

den″ti·no·gen′e·sis [*dens;* G. *genesis*, production]. The formation of dentin: also called *dentinification*.

d. imperfecta. A hereditary disease of the teeth, sometimes associated with skeletal disorders, in which the dentin is irregularly arranged and hypocalcific. The size of the pulp chamber is progressively reduced, even to obliteration. The crown appears opalescent bluish gray. Syn. *hereditary opalescent dentin.*

den′ti·noid [*dens;* G. *eidos,* form]. A calcified structure having some but not all of the characteristics of dentin.

den″ti·no′ma [*dens;* G. *-ōma,* tumor]. A benign odontogenic tumor made up of dentin.

den″ti·nos′te·oid [*dens;* G. *osteon,* bone; *eidos*]. A hard, calcified structure having some of the histologic appearance of both dentin and bone.

den·tip′a·rous [*dens;* L. *parere,* to bring forth]. Pertaining to the production of teeth.

den′ti·phone [*dens;* G. *phōnē,* sound]. A form of audiphone in which the vibrating disk is attached to or held in contact with the teeth, and is thus used to carry vibrations through the bony structures to the auditory nerves.

den′tist [*dens*]. One who practices dentistry.

den′tis·try [*dens*]. That department of medicine concerned with the prevention, diagnosis, and treatment of diseases of the teeth and adjacent tissues, and the restoration of missing dental and oral structures.

aviation d. That branch of dentistry concerned with the oral care of those who fly at high altitudes.

operative d. The branch of dentistry concerned with actual operations upon the natural teeth or the soft tissues of the oral cavity, as distinguished from those operations performed in the dental laboratory.

preventive d. The branch of dental science dealing with prevention of dental diseases by prophylactic and educational methods.

prosthetic d. That branch of dentistry which deals with the replacement of missing teeth or oral tissues by artificial means. Syn., *prosthodontics.*

den·ti′tion [L. *dentitio,* from *dens*]. 1. The process of teething; the eruption of the teeth through the alveolar ridge. 2. The character and arrangement of the teeth of an individual or species.

accessional d. The eruption of those teeth which are not preceded by deciduous teeth; in man, the permanent molars.

deciduous d. Primary *d.*

permanent d. Secondary *d.*

postpermanent d. See third *d.*

primary d. (a) The eruption of the deciduous teeth, numbering 20 in man. (b) The deciduous teeth. Syn., *deciduous d.* See also under *tooth.*

secondary d. (a) The eruption of the adult teeth, numbering 32 in man. (b) The permanent teeth. Syn., *permanent d.* See also under *tooth.*

third d. Eruption of teeth subsequent to loss of teeth of the permanent (secondary) dentition; the postpermanent dentition. Though multiple cases have been reported in man, there is no certain evidence which will rule out delayed eruption of teeth of the permanent dentition or eruption of supernumerary teeth in the approximate position of lost permanent teeth.

den′to- [*dens*]. Combining form meaning *dental, pertaining to dentistry.*

den″to·al·ve′o·lar [*dens;* L. *alveolus,* small hollow]. Pertaining to the alveolus of a tooth.

den″to·al″ve·o·li′tis. Periodontal disease of an inflammatory nature. *Obs.*

den″to·fa′cial (den″to·fay′shul) [*dens;* L. *facies,* face]. Pertaining to both the teeth and the face.

den·tog′ra·phy [*dens;* G. *graphein,* to write]. A description of teeth.

den′toid [*dens;* G. *eidos,* form]. Toothlike.

den″to·le′gal. Pertaining to dental jurisprudence.

den·ton′o·my. Classification of the teeth.

den′ture [*dens*]. The natural or artificial teeth of an individual, considered as a unit.

artificial d. A dental prosthesis that replaces missing teeth.

full d. One that replaces all of the teeth in an edentulous jaw.

partial artificial d. A replacement of less than the full number of teeth in either arch; a removable appliance is used, which is attached to the adjoining natural teeth.

de·nu′cle·a″ted (dee·new′klee·ay″tid) [L. *de-,* indicating separation; *nucleus,* kernel]. Deprived of a nucleus.

de·nude′ [L. *denudare,* to denude]. To deprive of covering; to strip, lay bare: said also of the root of a tooth. —**denuda′tion,** *n.*

de·ob′stru·ent [*de-;* L. *obstruere,* to obstruct]. Any agent or drug which removes an obstruction or obstructive material, as in the alimentary canal.

de″o′dor·ant [*de-;* L. *odorare,* to give a smell to a thing]. A substance that removes or conceals offensive odors. —**deo′dorant,** *adj.;* **deodorize,** *v.*

de″o·ral′i·ty [*de-;* L. *os,* mouth]. *In psychoanalysis,* the shifting of instinctual activity away from gratification through oral expression.

de·or″sum·duc′tion [L. *deorsum,* downward; *ducere,* to lead]. A turning downward of a part.

de·or″sum·ver′gence [*deorsum;* L. *vergere,* to turn]. A downward inclination, as of the eyes.

de·os″si·fi·ca′tion [*de-;* L. *os,* bone; *facere,* to make]. The absorption of bony material; the deprivation of the bony character of any part.

de·ox′y-, des·ox′y-. *In chemistry,* a combining form signifying loss of oxygen from a compound, frequently by replacement of a hydroxyl group by a hydrogen atom.

de·ox″y·cho′lic ac′id (dee·ock″si·ko′lick, ·kol′ick). Desoxycholic acid.

de·ox″y·cor′tone ac′e·tate. British Pharmacopoeia title for desoxycorticosterone acetate.

de·ox″y·cos′tone ac′e·tate. Desoxycorticosterone acetate.

de·ox″y·gen·a′tion [*de-;* G. *oxys,* sharp; *genesthai,* from *gignesthai,* to be produced]. The process of removing oxygen from a compound.

dep. *Depuratus;* purified.

De·part′ment of Health, Ed·u·ca′tion and Wel′fare″. A department of the U. S. government, created by Congress in 1953 and headed by a cabinet officer. It administers the Public Health Service and the Commissions of Food and Drugs, Education, and Social Security.

de·per″son·al·i·za′tion (dee·pur″sun·ul·i·zay′shun, ·eye·zay′shun) [*de-;* L. *personalis,* from *persona,* person]. Loss of the sense of one's own reality or identity. *In psychopathology,* a subjective feeling of estrangement or unreality within the personality. The subject feels changed and not himself; his feelings seem dead. Other people and objects often seem unreal; see *derealization.* Current events may seem to have happened before; see *déjà vu.* In a mild form depersonalization is a common occurrence; in severe forms, it is a finding in various neuroses, depressive states, and beginning schizophrenia. It is considered to be a pathological defense mechanism aimed at protecting the individual from severe outer or inner trauma on the basis that what is seen is unreal and hence not to be feared, or, that being not oneself, one's observations are not to be regarded as true, or accordingly, dangerous.

de·pig″men·ta′tion (dee·pig″men·tay′shun) [*de-;* L. *pigmentum,* pigment]. 1. The removal of natural pigments from the skin. 2. The removal of pigments from microscopic preparations by the action of weak preparations of bleaching or oxidizing solutions.

dep′i·late [L. *depilare*, to pull out the hair]. To remove hair. —**depil′atory,** *adj., n.;* **depila′tion,** *n.*

dep′i·lous [L. *depilis*, without hair]. Hairless.

de·ple′tion [L. *deplere*, to empty]. 1. The act of diminishing the quantity of fluid in the body or in a part, especially by bleeding. 2. The condition of the system produced by the excessive loss of blood or other fluids; reduction of strength; exhaustion. —**deplete′,** *v.t.*

de″plu·ma′tion [L. *de-*, indicating separation; *plumare*, to cover with feathers]. Loss of the eyelashes. *Rare.*

depo-cer-o-cillin. Trade-mark for chloroprocaine penicillin O, a long-acting penicillin preparation especially useful for patients sensitive to penicillin G.

depo-heparin sodium. Trade-marked name for an injectable preparation of heparin sodium, characterized by prolonged effect of the latter, achieved through combination with gelatin and dextrose.

de·po″lar·i·za′tion (dee·po″lur·i·zay′shun, ·eye-zay′shun) [*de-;* L. *polus*, pole]. The neutralization of polarity; the breaking down of polarized semipermeable membranes, as in nerve or muscle cells in the conduction of impulses.

de″po·lym′er·ase (dee″po·lim′ur·ace, dee·pol′i-mur·ace). One of a group of enzymes which depolymerize high molecular weight plant and animal nucleic acids, forming mononucleotides without the liberation of phosphoric acid.

de·pol″y·mer·i·za′tion. The cleavage, by various means, of a polymer of high molecular weight into simpler units of the same composition. —**depolymerize,** *v.*

de·pos′it [L. *depositum*, from *deponere*, to set down]. A sediment; a collection of morbid particles in a body.

dental d. Hard or soft material adherent to the surface of a tooth.

de′pot. *In physiology,* the site of accumulation, deposit, or storage of body products not immediately or actively involved in metabolic processes, such as a fat depot.

medical d. (dep′po). An installation of the defense department for concentrating, storing, and issuing medical supplies.

de·pres′sant [L. *depressum*, from *deprimere*, to depress]. A medicine that diminishes functional activity. —**depres′sant,** *adj.*

de·pres′sion [L. *depressio*, from *depressum*]. 1. A hollow or fossa. 2. Inward displacement of a part, as of the skull. 3. Lowering of vital functions under the action of some depressing agent. 4. *In psychopathology,* an emotional state of dejection usually associated with manic-depressive psychosis. Mild depression with anxiety and hypochondria is frequently seen in youth of both sexes (**adolescent depression**) and often occurs whenever the adult sex problem becomes acute, as after engagement or marriage. Depression may also occur as a result of an external situation, being relieved when the external situation is removed (**reactive depression**). See *melancholia.* —**depressed, depressive,** *adj.*

cryptic d. The state of mental depression characterized by sense of guilt, psychomotor retardation, and diurnal variation, patient being most depressed in the morning. It is often accompanied by headache, cardiovascular disturbances, reduction of sexual function, fatigue, and insomnia.

Leao's spreading d. A marked enduring reduction of the "spontaneous" electrical activity of the cerebral cortex, following repeated local stimulation of any area, and spreading slowly from the region stimulated to involve successively more distant parts of the cerebral cortex.

de·pres′sor [*depressum*]. 1. A muscle, instrument, or apparatus that depresses. 2. A nerve, stimulation of which lowers arterial blood pressure by reflex vasodilatation and by slowing the heart, as the depressor nerve.

d. alae nasi. That which depresses the alae of the nose.

d. anguli oris. The triangularis muscle.

d. epiglottidis. Certain fibers of the thyroepiglottic muscle.

d. labii inferioris. The quadratus labii inferioris muscle.

d. septi nasi. A portion of the depressor alae nasi.

tongue d. A spatula for pushing down the tongue during the examination of the mouth and throat.

depropanex. Trade-mark for a deproteinated pancreatic extract used intramuscularly as a vasodilator.

dep′side. Any of a class of compounds characterized by an ester type of union of two or more molecules of phenolic acids, in which the phenolic hydroxyl of one molecule interacts with the carboxyl of another molecule in a manner similar to the combination of amino acids to form peptides. Certain tannins are naturally occurring depsides.

depth [akin to D. *diepte*]. Measurement of distance from top to bottom or from front to back; deepness.

focal d. The power of a lens to give clear images of objects at different distances from it. Also called *field d.*

de·pu″li·za′tion (dee·pew″li·zay′shun, ·lye·zay′-shun) [L. *de-*, indicating separation; *pulex*, a flea]. The destruction or removal of fleas, as from infested animals or premises.

der″a·del′phus [G. *derē*, neck; *adelphos*, brother]. A monocephalic dual monster, with the body fused above the umbilicus, and with four lower extremities and three or four upper. Syn., *cephalothoracopagus.*

der″an·en″ce·pha′li·a [*derē;* G. *a-*, not; *egkephalos*, brain]. Teratism marked by absence of the head and brain, while the neck is present.

de·range′ment [F.]. Disorder of intellect; insanity.

internal d. of the knee. A condition of abnormal joint mobility with painful symptoms, usually due to injury to the medial semilunar cartilage.

deratol. A proprietary capsule containing vitamin D_2.

Dercum, Francis Xavier [*American neurologist,* 1856–1931]. Known for his description of adiposis dolorosa (1888), called *Dercum's disease.*

de·re″al·i·za′tion. *In psychiatry,* a subjective feeling that other people or objects are unreal, changed or changing, or strange in their particular characteristics and configuration: often accompanies *depersonalization.*

de′re·ism [L. *de-*, indicating separation; *res*, thing]. *In psychiatry,* a mental state in which the subject is lost in phantasy, showing no interest in external experiences or reality; autism. —**dereis′tic,** *adj.*

der″en·ceph′a·lus [G. *derē*, neck; *egkephalos*, brain]. A monster showing derencephaly.

der″en·ceph′a·ly [*derē; egkephalos*]. A monstrosity consisting of rudimentary development of the bones in the cranial vault and a markedly defective brain, which rests in the bifid upper cervical vertebrae; the posterior portion of the occiput is absent. A variety of anencephaly.—**derencephalous,** *adj.*

der'ic [G. *deros*, skin]. External; pertaining to the skin.

deriphyllin. Trade-mark for theophylline diethanolamine.

der"i·va'tion [L. *derivatio*, from *derivare*, to turn aside]. The deflection of blood from one part of the body to another, as by counterirritation; formerly thought to relieve inflammatory congestion. *Obs.*

de·riv'a·tive [*derivare*]. 1. An agent that produces derivation. 2. A substance derived from another substance. —**deriv'ative,** *adj.*

derm-. See *dermato-*.

-derm [G. *derma*, skin]. Suffix signifying *skin, integument*, or *covering*.

der'ma, derm [*derma*]. The layer of the skin between the epidermis and subcutaneous tissue; the connective tissue of the corium. Syn., *corium, cutis vera, dermis.* —**dermal, dermic,** *adj.*

der'ma-. See *dermato-*.

-der'ma [G.]. A combining form denoting *a type of skin, a type of skin disease*, or *a genus characterized by a type of skin.*

Der"ma·cen'tor [*derma;* G. *kentōr*, goader]. A genus of ticks some species of which are vectors of disease.

D. andersoni. The wood tick; medically, it is the most important North American species, transmitting Rocky Mountain spotted fever and tularemia as well as producing tick paralysis.

D. variabilis. A species widely distributed in North America which has as its principal host the dog, although man and other mammals may be attacked.

Der"ma·cen·trox'e·nus. A genus of rickettsia pathogenic for man, transmitted by ticks and, in rickettsialpox, by mites. On smear from yolk-sac films, the organisms appear to be located within both the nucleus and the cytoplasm. The species of the genus are the causative agents of the spotted fever group.

D. akari. The species of *Dermacentroxenus* which is the causative agent of rickettsialpox. Syn. *Rickettsia akari.*

D. pediculi. The species which is the causative agent of trench fever: also called *Rickettsia pediculi, R. wolhynica, R. quintana, R. weigli.*

D. rickettsi. The species which is the causative agent of the North American (Rocky Mountain) and South American (Brazilian and Colombian) spotted fevers.

D. rickettsi conori. The variety of *D. rickettsi* which is the causative agent of the tick-bite fevers of Africa: also called *Dermacentroxenus conori, Rickettsia conori.*

der'ma·drome. Any skin manifestation of an internal disorder; the cutaneous part of a syndrome.

der"ma·my·i'a·sis lin"e·ar'is mi'grans oes·tro'sa (dur"muh·migh·eye'uh·sis lin"ee·air'iss my'granz ess·tro'suh). See *larva migrans.*

der·man'a·plas"ty [*derma;* G. *anaplassein*, to form anew]. Skin grafting.

Der"ma·nys'sus [*derma;* G. *nyssein*, to prick]. A genus of itch mites.

D. avium, D. gallinae. A species which is a serious pest of poultry and sometimes attacks man.

der"ma·tag'ra (dur"muh·tag'ruh, ·tay'gruh). [*derma;* G. *agra*, a catching]. 1. Pellagra. 2. Dermatalgia.

der"ma·tal'gi·a [*derma;* G. *algos*, pain]. Pain, burning, and other sensations of the skin, unaccompanied by any structural change; probably caused by some nervous disease or reflex influence.

der"ma·ta·neu'ri·a [*derma;* G. *a-*, not; *neuron*, nerve]. Derangement of the nerve supply of the skin, causing any disturbance of sensation.

der"mat·he'mi·a (dur"mat·hee'mee·uh, dur"muh·tee'mee·uh) [*derma;* G. *haima*, blood]. A congestion of the skin. Also called *dermaemia, dermohemia.*

der'ma·therm [*derma;* G. *thermē*, heat]. An instrument, made up of differential thermocouples, used to measure skin temperature. The apparatus consists of two sensitive thermopiles in parallel with a millivoltmeter, with one thermopile maintained at a constant known temperature and the other applied to the skin. The reading in degrees on the millivoltmeter added to or subtracted from the constant gives the skin temperature.

der·mat'ic [*derma*]. Relating to the skin.

der·mat'ic. A remedy for diseases of the skin.

der"ma·ti'tis [*derma;* G. *-itis*, inflammation]. An inflammation of the skin.

allergic d. Dermatitis due to the action of an allergen upon sensitized tissues; it may be atopic dermatitis or contact dermatitis.

atabrine d. A distinctive drug eruption characterized by lichenoid lichen-planus-like papules. In some an eczematoid dermatitis is produced by the drug.

atopic d. That due to sensitization to substances by ingestion or inhalation. There is usually a familial history of some type of allergy.

"autosensitization" d. A generalized eczematoid reaction, most often considered to represent a spread from stasis dermatitis on the theory that the absorption of products from the stasis eczema causes an eczematoid reaction at distant sites.

berlock d. A brownish pigmentation seen on skin exposed to sun after the use of cologne.

blastomycetic d. A skin disease caused by one of the several yeastlike fungi.

carcinomatous d. An inflammation of the skin associated with a carcinoma. Also see inflammatory *carcinoma.*

caterpillar d. A form due to the highly irritating hairs of the larvae of certain Lepidoptera, characterized first by erythematous macules and then by wheals. Syn., *caterpillar urticaria.*

cercarial d. See schistosome *d.*

clam diggers' d. A form of contact dermatitis which has been observed in clam diggers working without protective clothing.

contact d. A dermatitis resulting either from the primary irritant effect of a substance or more frequently from the sensitization to a substance coming in contact with the skin: also called *d. venenata.*

contagious pustular d. A virus disease of sheep and goats characterized by formation of vesicles on the skin of the legs, nostrils, and eyelids, the vesicles being rapidly transformed into pustules. The disease may be transmitted to man, and is then called *orf.*

d. actinica. That due to the action of actinic rays, from sunlight or artificial ultraviolet radiation.

d. calorica. That due to burns and scalds.

d. coccidioides. Valley fever; coccidioidomycosis.

d. congelationis. See *frostbite.*

d. continuée. See *d.* repens.

d. contusiformis. Erythema nodosum.

d. dysmenorrheica. An eruption seen during the menstrual period in women having dysmenorrhea. Wheals, vesicles, or erythematous areas are seen over the body. Many eruptions are exaggerated during the menses. Also called *catamenial d.*

d. escharotica. A severe ulcerative type due to exposure to escharotic agents.

d. exfoliativa neonatorum. An acute or chronic inflammation in infants, in which the epidermis is shed more or less freely in large or small scales: first described by Ritter von Rittershain (1870). In a distinct form in adults, **d. exfoliativa** occurs in pityriasis rubra.

d. exsiccans palmaris. A scarring tylotic eczema of the hands which may lead to contracture of the fingers, most frequent in women in Formosa: also called *Formosa eczema.*

d. factitia. An eruption induced by the patient; varies from simple erythema to gangrene. Usually produced by some irritant in neurotic or hysterical subjects. Also called *feigned eruptions, d. autofactitia, hysterical dermatoneuroses.*

d. gangrenosa. Sphaceloderma; gangrenous inflammation of the skin.

d. gangrenosa infantum. A form of ecthyma marked by brown discolorations of the skin, usually surrounded by a halo; the center of these efflorescences rapidly becomes necrotic. Due to *Pseudomonas aeruginosa.*

d. herpetiformis. An inflammatory, recurring skin disease of a herpetic character, the various lesions showing a tendency to group. It is protean, appearing as erythema, vesicles, blebs, and pustules; associated with intense itching and burning. Also called *Duhring's disease.*

d. hiemalis. A recurrent inflammation of the skin, associated with cold weather and allied to the erythemas.

d. hypostatica. One occurring in an area of poor blood supply, usually the lower legs.

d. medicamentosa. Eruptions due to the action of certain drugs.

d. nodularis necrotica. An entity of indetermined etiology, described by Werther in 1910, characterized by a polymorphous eruption of vesicles, pustules, hemorrhagic papules, nodules, ulcers, plaques and their sequels, scars and hyperpigmentation.

d. papillaris capillitii. See *folliculitis keloidis.*

d. repens. A subacute peripherally spreading dermatitis due to *Micrococcus pyogenes* (staphyloderma) usually following minor injuries, and commencing almost exclusively on the distal part of the upper extremity, marked by vesicles or pustules which dry and crust.

d. rhus. Contact dermatitis due to poison ivy or poison oak.

d. seborrheica. An acute inflammatory form, occurring usually on oily skin in areas having large sebaceous glands; characterized by dry, moist, or greasy scales and by crusted yellowish patches, remissions, exacerbations, and itching. Syn., *eczema seborrheicum, seborrhea sicca.*

d. traumatica. That resulting from traumatism.

d. vegetans. Elevated, vegetating lesions covered with crusts; very prone to bleeding and believed to be due to some infection.

d. venenata. See contact *d.*

d. verrucosa. Chromoblastomycosis.

eczematoid d. See eczematoid *reaction.*

extrinsic allergic d. That caused by any external substance capable of penetrating the epidermis, such as that caused by contact with poison ivy.

flexural d. Atopic dermatitis seen primarily in infants and children on the face, anterior neck, antecubital and popliteal spaces, and other flexural areas.

follicular hyperkeratotic papular d. See *phrynoderma.*

hairdresser's d. Contact dermatitis due to the irritating effects of the reducing agents or sensitization to the gums and resins used in cold waving.

hop d. A contact dermatitis due to fresh hop oil, seen in hop pickers.

infectious eczematoid d. A low-grade skin infection; produces oozing, erythematous patches.

intrinsic d. That caused by ingested substances: most common in infants and young children, and may accompany asthma, allergic rhinitis, or urticaria. A hereditary predisposition is involved.

nummular d. See *eczema nummularis.*

pigmented purpuric lichenoid d. A form of capillaritis usually of the lower extremities, though the upper extremities and trunk may be involved, characterized by elevated papules which become purpuric or telangiectatic or pigmented in varying shades. Its course is chronic, leading to lichenification. Syn., *Gougerot-Blum disease.*

roentgen d. That due to prolonged exposure to roentgen rays, or radium. Also called *radium d., x-ray d.*

schistosome d. One caused by the penetration of the cercariae of schistosomes into the dermis, causing itching and wheal formation: also called *swimmer's itch, dew itch, cowlot itch.* Syn., *cercarial d.*

seborrheic d. See *d.* seborrheica.

solar d. A general term for skin eruptions caused by exposure to the sun, excluding sunburn; it may be plaquelike, eczematous, papular, or erythematous.

stasis d. Chronic eczematoid reaction of the skin of the legs, due to vascular stasis.

vegetative d. See *d.* vegetans.

verrucose mycotic d. Blastomycosis.

der′ma·to-, dermat- [*derma*]. A combining form meaning *skin* or *hide.*

Der″ma·to′bi·a [*derma;* G. *bios,* life]. A genus of botflies whose larvae are obligatory sarcobionts, producing cutaneous myiasis in many animals.

D. hominis. A species found in tropical America, causing dermal myiasis in man. The eggs are deposited by the adult female on the skin of the host. Upon emergence, the larva burrows into the skin, producing a swelling very much like an ordinary boil.

der″ma·to·bi′a·sis [*derma; bios;* NL. *-iasis,* condition]. Infection with *Dermatobia.*

der″ma·to·cel″lu·li′tis [*derma;* L. *cellula,* small storeroom; G. *-itis,* inflammation]. Acute inflammation of the skin and subcutaneous tissue.

der″ma·to·cha·la′sis [*derma;* G. *chalaō,* to become slack]. Diffuse relaxation of the skin, with associated folding and excess of elastic and collagenous fibers.

der″ma·to·co″ni·o′sis, der″ma·to·ko″ni·o′sis [*derma;* G. *konia,* dust; *-ōsis,* condition]. Any skin disease due to dust.

der′ma·to·cyst″ [*derma;* G. *kystis,* bladder]. A cyst of the skin.

der″ma·to·dyn′i·a. See *dermatalgia.*

der″ma·to·fi·bro′ma. Firm, single, or multiple slowly growing nodules, reddish, yellow, or bluish-black, found most commonly on the extremities in adults. Histologically, the nodules are composed chiefly of fibroblasts. Those containing additionally a variable number of histiocytes are called *histiocytomas.* Also called *d. lenticulare, fibroma durum, fibroma simplex, fibrome en pastille, nodular subepidermal fibrosis, noduli cutanei, sclerosing hemangioma.*

der″ma·to·fi″bro·sar·co′ma pro·tu′ber·ans. A local sclerotic protruding dermal neoplasm of low-grade malignancy which tends to recur repeatedly after inadequate excision. The majority of the tumors are located along or near the mammary ridge.

der″ma·to·glyph′ics [*derma;* G. *glyphein,* to carve]. Study of skin-pattern lines and whorls of the hands and feet; used for identification purposes. These patterns are individually characteristic and do not change during a person's lifetime.

der"ma·to·graph'ism. See *dermographia.*

der"ma·tog'ra·phy [*derma;* G. *graphein,* to write]. 1. A description of the skin. 2. Dermographia.

der"ma·to·het'er·o·plas"ty. See *graft.*

der"ma·to·ko"ni·o'sis. See *dermatoconiosis.*

der'ma·tol. Bismuth subgallate.

der"ma·tol'o·gist [*derma;* G. *logos,* word]. A skin specialist: a physician who makes a special study of diseases of the skin.

der"ma·tol'o·gy [*derma; logos*]. Science of the skin, its structure, functions, diseases, and their treatment. —**dermatolog'ic, dermatolog'ical,** *adj.*

der"ma·tol'y·sis [*derma;* G. *lysis,* a loosing]. 1. Abnormal laxation of the skin, usually congenital, producing folds. 2. Fibromas of the skin with masses of pendulous skin. Also called *chalazodermia, cutis pendula, fibroma pendulum, lax skin.*

der'ma·tome [*derma;* G. *tomos,* cutting]. 1. The areas of the skin supplied with sensory fibers from a single spiral nerve. 2. An instrument for cutting skin, as in grafting. 3. The lateral part of an embryonic somite; cutis plate. —**dermatom'ic,** *adj.*

der"ma·to·my'ces (·migh'seez) [*derma;* G. *mykēs,* fungus]. Dermatophyte.

der"ma·to·my'cete. Dermatophyte.

der"ma·to·my·co'sis (·migh·ko'sis) [*derma; mykēs;* G. *-ōsis,* condition]. Any skin disease caused by a vegetable parasite; a fungus infection of the skin.

der"ma·to·my·o'ma (·migh·o'muh) [*derma;* G. *mys,* muscle; *-ōma,* tumor]. Myoma located in the skin.

der"ma·to·my"o·si'tis [*derma; mys;* G. *-itis,* inflammation]. Degenerative changes of skin and muscles causing weakness and pain; the condition may be extensive or minimal, the cutaneous reaction may be severe with edema and erythema or completely absent. Myoglobinuria may occur. Also called *pseudotrichonosis.*

der"ma·to·neu·rol'o·gy [*derma;* G. *neuron,* nerve; *logos,* word]. Study of the nerves of the skin.

der"ma·to·neu·ro'sis [*derma; neuron;* G. *-ōsis,* condition]. A skin disease of nervous origin.

hysterical d. A self-produced eruption in a hysterical person.

der"ma·to·pa·thol'o·gy [*derma;* G. *pathos,* disease; *logos,* word]. Pathology of the skin.

der"ma·to·path"o·pho'bi·a [*derma; pathos;* G. *phobos,* fear]. Morbid fear of having a skin disease.

der"ma·top'a·thy [*derma; pathos*]. Any skin disease. —**dermatopath'ic,** *adj.*

der"ma·to·phi·li'a·sis [*derma;* G. *philein,* to love; NL. *-iasis,* condition]. Infestation by the chigoe flea, *Tunga penetrans.*

Der"ma·toph'i·lus pen'e·trans (pen'i·tranz). Synonym for *Tunga penetrans.*

der'ma·to·phyte" [*derma;* G. *phyton,* a plant]. One of a group of fungi which invade the superficial skin. The dermatophytes are now divided into three genera—*Microsporum, Epidermophyton,* and *Trichophyton* (Emmons' classification based on differences in morphologic features). Formerly, they were classified according to the type of lesion from which they were isolated, without regard to the form or structure of the organisms. Also spelled *dermophyte.* Syn., *dermatomycyte.*

der"ma·toph'y·tid [*derma; phyton*]. A rash associated with a skin disease caused by a vegetable parasite.

der"ma·to·phy·to'sis (·figh·to'sis) [*derma; phyton;* G. *-ōsis,* condition]. A skin eruption characterized by the formation of small vesicles on the hands and feet, especially between the toes, with cracking and scaling. There is sometimes secondary infection. The cause may be any one of the dermatophytes. Syn., *ringworm, athlete's foot.*

der'ma·to·plas"ty [*derma;* G. *plassein,* to form]. A plastic operation on the skin whereby skin losses or defects are replaced by skin flaps or grafts.

der"ma·to·pol"y·neu·ri'tis. See *erythredema polyneuropathy.*

der"ma·tor·rha'gi·a [*derma;* G. *rhēgnynai,* to burst forth]. Skin hemorrhage.

der"ma·to·scle·ro'sis. See *scleroderma.*

der"ma·tos'co·py [*derma;* G. *skopein,* to examine]. Examination of the skin; particularly, microscopical examination of the superficial capillaries of the skin.

der"ma·to'sis (pl. *dermatoses*) [*derma;* G. *-ōsis,* condition]. Any disease of the skin. See also *dermatitis.*

actinic d. A dermatosis due to exposure to sunlight. It may be urticarial, papular, or eczematous.

allergic d. See allergic *dermatitis.*

bullous d. A condition of the skin marked by bullae, as in erythema multiforme, dermatitis herpetiformis, and pemphigus.

cholinogenic d. A dermatosis, usually urticarial or erythematous, produced by efferent cholinergic impulses via the autonomic nervous system.

d. papulosa nigra. An eruption commonly seen in Negroes, usually on the face, consisting of many tiny tumors of the skin; probably nevoid in origin.

occupational d. One that results from chemicals or irritations resulting from the nature of an occupation.

postvaccinal d. A dermatosis following vaccination, marked by lesions similar to those of urticaria pigmentosa except that desquamation is present and dermographia is absent.

precancerous d. A skin disorder that sometimes develops into a malignant skin lesion.

progressive pigmentary d. A reddish, purpuric, papular eruption; it is seen principally on the legs and is progressive in character. Also called *Schamberg's disease.*

stress d. 1. A grouping of morphologically different cutaneous diseases which supposedly have a twofold origin: the variable emotional or psychic factors and the suppression of the pituitary-adrenal mechanism of resistance. 2. Psychocutaneous reaction. Examples are alopecia areata, lichen planus, and psoriasis.

der'ma·to·some" [*derma;* G. *sōma,* body]. A thickening or knot in the equatorial region of each spindle fiber in the process of cell division.

der"ma·to·stom"a·ti'tis (·stom"uh·tye'tis, ·sto"muh·tye'tis) [*derma;* G. *stoma,* mouth; *-itis,* inflammation]. A severe form of erythema multiforme. See Stevens-Johnson *syndrome.*

der"ma·to·ther'a·py [*derma;* G. *therapeia,* treatment]. Treatment of cutaneous affections.

der"ma·to·thla'si·a (dur"muh·to·thlay'zhuh, ·zee·uh) [*derma;* G. *thlasis,* a bruising]. A morbid state marked by an uncontrollable impulse to pinch or rub the skin.

der"ma·tot'o·my [*derma;* G. *tomē,* a cutting]. Anatomy or dissection of the skin.

der"ma·to·zo'on (pl. *dermatozoa*). Any animal parasite of the skin.

der"ma·to·zo"on·o'sis. Any pathologic condition due to a dermatozoon.

der'mis. Derma.

der·mi'tis. Dermatitis.

der'mo-, derm-, der'ma-. See *dermato-.*

der'mo·blast [*derma;* G. *blastos,* germ]. That part of the mesoderm which develops into the corium.

der″mo·cy′ma (dur″mo·sigh′muh), **der″mo·cy′mus** [*derma;* G. *kyma*, fetus]. A type of cryptodidymus in which the parasitic twin is in the body wall of the host.

der″mo·ep″i·der′mal [*derma;* G. *epiderma*, outer skin]. Pertaining to both the superficial and the deeper layers of the skin; said of skin grafts.

der″mo·graph′i·a (dur″mo·graf′ee·uh, ·gray′fee·uh), **der·mog′ra·phy** [*derma;* G. *graphein*, to write]. A condition in which the skin is peculiarly susceptible to irritation; characterized by elevations or wheals caused by tracing the fingernail or a blunt instrument over the skin. May or may not be accompanied by urticaria. Also called *dermographism, autographism, urticaria factitia.* —**dermograph′ic,** *adj.*

d. alba. A white line which briefly precedes the development of the initial reddening along the line of scratch as observed in the triple response.

d. rubra. The red line of the triple response.

der′moid [*derma;* G. *eidos*, form]. Resembling skin.

der′moid. A teratoma.

der″moid·ec′to·my [*derma; eidos;* G. *ektomē*, excision]. Excision of a dermoid cyst.

der″mo·la′bi·al [*derma;* L. *labia*, lip]. Having relation to the skin and the lips.

der·mop′a·thy [*derma;* G. *pathos*, disease]. Any skin disease. *Rare.*

der″mo·phle·bi′tis [*derma;* G. *phleps*, vein; *-itis*, inflammation]. Inflammation of the cutaneous veins.

der″mo·phyte′. Variant spelling for *dermatophyte.*

der″mo·skel′e·ton [*derma;* G. *skeletos*, dried up]. The exoskeleton, 2.

der″mo·ste·no′sis [*derma;* G. *stenōsis*, a being straitened]. A tightening of the skin, due to swelling or to disease.

der″mos·to′sis [*derma;* G. *osteon*, bone; *-ōsis*, condition]. Ossification occurring in the corium.

der″mo·syn″o·vi′tis (·sin″o·vy′tis, ·sigh″no·vy′tis) [*derma;* NL. *synovia*, of obscure origin; G. *-itis*, inflammation]. Inflammation of a subcutaneous bursa together with the adjacent skin.

der″mo·syph″i·lop′a·thy [*derma;* NL. *syphilis;* G. *pathos*, disease]. A syphilitic skin disease.

der″mo·ty′pho. See *typhus.*

der′o-, der- [G. *derē*, neck]. A combining form denoting *the neck.*

der″o·did′y·mus [*derē;* G. *didymos*, double]. A monster with a single body, two necks and heads, and two upper and lower extremities. Other rudimentary limbs are occasionally present. Syn., *dicephalus.*

de·rom′e·lus [*derē;* G. *melos*, limb]. A monster having an accessory limb attached to the neck or jaw.

der′rid. A highly toxic resin from *Derris elliptica*, a leguminous plant of Malaya; used in Borneo as an arrow poison.

des- [L. *de-, dis-*, through the French]. A prefix denoting the *reversing* or *undoing* of an action, *depriving* or *ridding of*, or *freeing from;* used before vowels, especially in chemistry. Also see *de-*.

des′am·i·dase. An amidase.

des″an·i·ma′ni·a [L. *de-*, meaning separation; *animus*, mind; G. *mania*, madness]. Psychosis associated with mental deficiency. *Obs.*

de·sat″u·ra′tion (dee·satch″uh·ray′shun) [*de-*, L. *saturatio*, from *saturare*, to fill]. Conversion of a saturated compound, such as stearin, into an unsaturated compound, such as olein, by the removal of hydrogen.

Desault, Pierre Joseph [*French surgeon*, 1744–95]. One of the founders of modern vascular surgery; developed the technic of ligating blood vessels for aneurysm (published 1801). Made many contributions to the knowledge of fractures and dislocations. Described various splints and dressings.

Descartes, René (Cartesius) [*French philosopher, mathematician, and anatomist*, 1596–1650]. His book *De L'Homme*, posthumously published (1664), is believed to be the first general text in the field of physiology. He has been called the inventor of analytic geometry. A number of rules, laws, and signs, mostly in the field of higher algebra, have received his name.

Descemet's membrane. See under *membrane.*

des″ce·me·ti′tis [after Jean *Descemet*, French anatomist, 1732–1810; G. *-itis*, inflammation]. Inflammation of Descemet's membrane; keratitis punctata.

des″ce·met′o·cele [*Descemet;* G. *kēlē*, hernia]. Hernia of Descemet's membrane.

de·scend′ens (di·send′enz) [L. *descendere*, to descend]. Downward.

d. cervicis. A loop of nerve fibers derived from the second and third cervical nerves which help form the ansa hypoglossi. See Table of Nerves in the Appendix.

d. hypoglossi. A branch of the hypoglossal nerve, which forms, with the descending cervical nerve, the ansa hypoglossi. The fibers come from the first and second cervical nerves and not from the hypoglossal nucleus. See Table of Nerves in the Appendix.

de·scen′sus (di·sen′sus) [L.]. A descent, fall, prolapse.

d. uteri. Prolapse of the uterus.

d. ventriculi. See *gastroptosis.*

de·scent′ [L. *descendere*, to descend]. Derivation from an ancestor, especially in regard to evolutionary origin.

desenex. Trade-mark for a fungicidal ointment or powder that contains undecylenic acid and zinc undecylenate.

de·sen″si·ti·za′tion (dee·sen″si·ti·zay′shun, ·tigh·zay′shun) [L. *de-*, indicating separation; ML. *sensitivus*, from *sentire*, to feel]. 1. A condition of insusceptibility to infection or an allergen, established in experimental animals by the injection of an antigen which produces sensitization or an anaphylactic reaction. After recovery, a second injection of the antigen is made, bringing about no reaction, thus producing desensitization. Also called *hyposensitization.* See also *antianaphylaxis.* 2. *In psychiatry*, the alleviation or removal of a mental complex. —**desen′sitize,** *v.*

des′ert sore. See *veldt sore.*

de·sex″u·al′i·ty (dee·seck″shoo·al′i·tee) [*de-;* L. *sexualis*, from *sexus*, sex]. A state in which a sexual impulse is deprived of its sexual quality by being diverted into other activities, as in sublimation.

de·sex″u·al·i·za′tion (dee·seck″shoo·ul·i·zay′shun, ·eye·zay′shun) [*de-; sexualis*]. Depriving an individual of his sexual powers.

Deshler's salve. See compound *rosin* cerate.

des′ic·cant [L. *desiccare*, to dry up]. A drying medicine or application. —**des′iccant,** *adj.*

des″ic·ca′tion [*desiccare*]. Process of drying up.

des′ic·ca″tor [*desiccare*]. A vessel containing some strongly hygroscopic substance, such as calcium chloride or sulfuric acid, used to absorb the moisture from any substance placed therein or to maintain it in a moisture-free state.

desicol. Trade-mark for proprietary choleretic and cholagogue consisting of desiccated whole bile in capsule form.

desivac. A process of drying substances which involves quick freezing followed by dehydration under vacuum while in the frozen state. See *lyophilization.*

des·lan′o·side. $C_{47}H_{74}O_{19}$; the desacetyl derivative of lanatoside C, a cardiotonic glycoside.

Desmarres, Louis Auguste (1810–1882). French ophthalmologist, remembered for his writings on ophthalmology. He devised an operation for pterygium (1850), is said to have introduced iridectomy in France, and described a dacryolith, known by his name, and also invented an ophthalmoscope.

des″mi·o·gnath′us (dess″mee·o·nath′us) [G. *desmios*, binding; *gnathos*, jaw]. A monster with a supplementary parasitic head joined to the lower jaw or neck by means of a ligamentous or muscular attachment. Also called *dicephalus parasiticus*.

des·mi′tis (dess·my′tis, dez·my′tis) [G. *desmos*, band; *-itis*, inflammation]. Inflammation of a ligament. *Obs.*

des′mo- (dess′mo-, dez′mo-), **desm-** [*desmos*]. Combining form meaning *bond, ligament,* or *fastening.*

des″mo·cra′ni·um [*desmos;* G. *kranion*, skull]. The mesenchymal or membranous anlage of the neurocranium from which the chondrocranium develops.

des′mo·cyte [*desmos;* G. *kytos*, cell]. Any kind of supporting tissue cell.

des″mo·gly′co·gen. The bound glycogen of tissues, representing a combination of glycogen with protein; heating the tissue with a solution of alkali releases the glycogen.

des′moid [*desmos;* G. *eidos*, form]. Like a ligament; fibrous.

des′mo·lase. Any of a group of enzymes which catalyze rupture of atomic linkages that are not cleaved through hydrolysis, such as the bonds in the carbon chain of D-glucose.

des′mone. A general term for growth-promoting substances, theoretically present in all cells.

des″mo·pla′si·a [G. *desmo-*, ligament; *plassein*, to form]. 1. The formation and proliferation of connective tissue, especially fibrous connective tissue; frequently, prominent proliferation of connective tissue in the growth of tumors. 2. The formation of adhesions. —**desmoplas′tic,** *adj.*

des′mo·some. A thickening in the middle of an intercellular bridge in epidermis.

des·mot′o·my [*desmos;* G. *tomē*, a cutting]. Incision of a ligament.

Desnos, Louis Joseph [*French physician,* 1828–93]. Remembered for his description of splenization in lobar pneumonia; called *splenopneumonia, Desnos' pneumonia, Grancher's pneumonia.*

des′o·gen. A mixture of the methosulfates of a group of trimethylammonium bases; it is used as a disinfectant.

des″o·mor′phine. Dihydrodesoxymorphine-D; $C_{17}H_{21}NO_2$; a morphine derivative reported to be powerfully analgesic but to have greater addiction liability than morphine.

de·sorp′tion. The process of removing adsorbed matter from an adsorbent: the reverse of the process of adsorption.

11-des·ox″o·cor′ti·sone. 11-Desoxy-17-hydroxycorticosterone.

des·ox′y-. See *deoxy-.*

des·ox″y·cho′lic ac′id (dess·ock″si·ko′lick, ·kol′ick), **de·ox″y·cho′lic ac′id.** $C_{24}H_{40}O_4$. 3,12-Dihydrocholanic acid. One of the unconjugated bile acids; in bile it is largely conjugated, with glycine or taurine, to form glycodesoxycholate and taurodesoxycholate salts.

des·ox″y·cor″ti·cos′te·rone [L. *de-*, indicating separation; G. *oxys*, sharp; L. *cortex*, bark; G. *steros*, stiff]. $C_{21}H_{30}O_3$; 11-desoxycorticosterone or Δ^4-pregnene-3,20-dione-21-ol; a steroid hormone occurring in the adrenal cortex and capable of maintaining the life of an adrenalectomized animal. In man it causes an increase in retention of sodium ion and water, and an increase in excretion of potassium ion; it has no demonstrable effect on protein or carbohydrate metabolism. It is of great value in the management of adrenal insufficiency, being administered by subcutaneous or intramuscular injection, or by subcutaneous implantation of pellets; therapy may have to be supplemented with other adrenal cortex hormones. Also called *compound Q* (*Reichstein's*). See Table of Hormones in the Appendix.

d. acetate (*desoxycorticosteroni acetas*). The acetate ester of desoxycorticosterone and the form in which the latter hormone is used clinically. Syn., *deoxycortone acetate, deoxycostone acetate.* See *cortate, doca, percorten.*

des·ox″y·cor′ti·sone. 1. 11-Desoxycortisone. See *11-desoxy-17-hydroxycorticosterone.* 2. 11-Keto-17-hydroxyprogesterone; gluconeogenic steroid studied in relation to rheumatoid arthritis: also called *21-desoxycortisone.*

11-d. 11-Desoxy-17-hydroxycorticosterone.

des·ox″y·e·phed′rine. Methamphetamine.

d. hydrochloride. Methamphetamine hydrochloride.

des·ox″y·eph″e·dro′ni·um sul″fa·thi′a·zole. A combination of desoxyephedrine and sulfathiazole which provides vasoconstrictor and antiseptic properties for intranasal use.

11-des·ox′y-17-hy·drox″y·cor·ti·cos′ter·one. $C_{21}H_{30}O_4$; a steroid of the adrenal cortex which influences sodium and potassium metabolism and increases blood pressure and water turnover: also called *Reichstein's Compound S, 11-desoxycortisone, 11-desoxocortisone.* See Table of Hormones in the Appendix.

des″ox·y·man′nose. The monosaccharide HCO.-HCOH.HCOH.HOCH.HOCH.CH_3; more specifically 6-desoxy-L-mannose; a component of many glycosides and of various disaccharides and trisaccharides.

desoxyn hydrochloride. Trade-marked name for methamphetamine hydrochloride, a sympathomimetic agent.

des·ox″y·pen′tose. Any pentose which contains less oxygen, commonly one atom, than its parent sugar. Biochemically the most important desoxypentose is desoxyribose, in consequence of which the two terms are sometimes used synonymously. Also written *deoxypentose.*

des·ox″y·pen″tose·nu·cle′ic ac′id. A nucleic acid containing a desoxypentose as the sugar component. Since the desoxypentose is commonly, if not exclusively, desoxyribose, the terms *desoxypentosenucleic acid* and *desoxyribonucleic acid* are often used synonymously. Also written *deoxypentosenucleic acid.*

des′ox″y·py″ri·dox′ine. $C_8H_{11}NO_2$; 2,4-dimethyl-3-hydroxy-5-hydroxymethylpyridine; a synthetic antimetabolite which antagonizes the action of pyridoxine in animals and bacteria.

des·ox″y·ri″bo·nu′cle·ase. Streptodornase. Sometimes abbreviated, DNASE.

streptococcal d. Streptodornase.

des·ox″y·ri″bo·nu′cle·ic ac′id. A type of nucleic acid, first isolated from animal cells but found also in plant cells, occurring in the nuclei; it contains phosphoric acid, D-2-desoxyribose, adenine, guanine, cytosine, and thymine. The exact composition may vary in different animal species; also, the substance from normal cells appears to differ from that of cancer cells. Also called *desoxyribose nucleic acid, thymus nucleic acid, thymo-*

nucleic acid, chromonucleic acid. Formerly erroneously called *animal nucleic acid.* Abbreviated, DNA

des″ox·y·ri′bose. CHO.HCH.HCOH.HCOH.CH_2-OH; 2-desoxyribose; a pentose found in nearly all cells, particularly in the form of desoxyribonucleic acid: also written *deoxyribose.*

des·ox′y-su″gar. A sugar containing one atom of oxygen less than the sugar from which it is derived.

de·spe″ci·a′tion (dee·spee″shee·ay′shun) [*de-;* L. *species,* species]. Change in properties characteristic of the species, as alteration of antigenic properties by digestion with taka-diastase. —**de-spe′ciated,** *adj.*

D'Espine's sign. See under *sign.*

des″qua·ma′tion [L. *desquamare,* to scale off]. Shedding; a peeling and casting off, as of the superficial epithelium, mucous membranes, renal tubules, and the skin. The horny layer of the epidermis is constantly shed as a normal physiologic process. In disease, an exaggerated process (**desquamatio insensibilis**) produces various-sized flakes and scales. Desquamation of newborn infants (**desquamatio neonatorum**) takes place during the first week of life. —**desquam′ative,** *adj.;* **des′quamate,** *v.*

des·sert′spoon″. A spoon of medium size, equal to approximately 2 fluidrachms or 8 cc.

des·thi′o-. *In chemistry,* a combining form signifying loss of sulfur from a compound.

des″thi·o·bi′o·tin. Methyl 4-methyl-5-imidazolidone-2-caproate. A substance used experimentally as a growth stimulant for yeast. It has been postulated that it is converted by the growing yeast cell into biotin, the normal growth-promoting agent. For certain other organisms, it is not a satisfactory substitute for biotin.

de·stru′do [L. *destruere,* to destroy; *-do* as in *libido*]. *In psychopathology,* the basic energy that is associated with the destructive or death instinct.

de·sul′fu·rase (dee·sul′few·race, ·sul′fur·ace). An enzyme causing the removal of sulfur from organic compounds.

det. *Detur;* let it be given.

de·tach′ment. Separation; the act of unfastening a structure from its support.

retinal d. See detachment of *retina.*

de·tec′tor cray′on. A chalklike crayon composed of a material which changes color on contact with liquid blister gas or concentrated blister-gas vapors.

de·tec′tor paint. Paint used as a detector for liquid blister-gas spray or drops, subject to certain limitations. Surfaces painted with detector paint change color wherever drops or splashes of blister gas strike.

de·tec′tor pa′per. Paper coated on one side with detector paint, used to detect liquid blister gas. It changes color wherever drops of blister gas strike it.

de·ter′gent [L. *detergere,* to wipe off]. A drug, compound, or solution used for cleansing wounds, ulcers, etc. —**deter′gent,** *adj.*

de·ter′mi·nant [L. *determinare,* to limit, determine]. *In biology,* a hypothetical unit of the germ plasm which, according to Weismann's theory of heredity, determines the final fate of the cell or the part which receives it during development.

de·ter″mi·na′tion [*determinare*]. 1. Tendency of the blood to collect in a part. 2. Fixation of the embryologic fate of a tissue or a part of an embryo by an evocator or other agent. 3. The performance of any measurement, as of length, mass, quantitative composition of a substance, etc.

sex d. Determination of the sex of an embryo at fertilization by the complement of sex chromosomes.

Detmold, William [*American surgeon,* 1808–94]. Performed the first operation on record in which a lateral ventricle was opened for the evacuation of a brain abscess (1850).

de·tor′sion [L. *detorsum,* from *detorquere,* to turn aside]. The correction of a torsion, as the twisting of a spermatic cord or ureter.

de·tox″i·ca′tion [L. *de,* from, away; G. *toxicon,* poison]. The process, usually consisting of a series of reactions, by which a substance foreign to the body is changed to a compound or compounds more readily excretable; the latter are not necessarily nontoxic. Syn., *detoxification.* —**detox′-icant,** *adj.;* **detox′icate,** *v.*

de·tox′i·fy (dee·tock′si·figh) [*de-; toxikon;* L. *facere,* to make]. Detoxicate. —**detoxifica′tion,** *n.*

Detre, Lászlo [*Hungarian pathologist,* 1875–1939]. Independently of Wassermann, though at almost the same time, he developed a nearly identical test for syphilis. Discovered a skin reaction, called *Detre's cutireaction,* indicating the presence of tuberculosis.

de·tri′tion (di·trish′un) [L. *detritum,* from *deterere,* to wear away]. Wearing away by abrasion.

de·tri′tus [*deterere*]. 1. Waste matter from disintegration. 2. *In dentistry,* waste material adherent to a tooth, or disintegrated tooth substance.

de″trun·ca′tion [L. *detruncare,* to cut off, behead]. Decapitation, especially of the fetus.

de·tru′sion [L. *detrusum,* from *detrudere,* to thrust down]. An ejection or expulsion; thrusting down or out.

de·tru′sor. A muscle that detrudes or thrusts down or out.

d. u·ri′nae. The smooth muscle of the urinary bladder which acts in emptying the viscus. O.T.

d. ves′i·cae. The smooth muscle in the wall of the urinary bladder which contracts the bladder and expels the urine: applied to all the muscle layers, since all are involved in the contraction. Also called *detrusor urinae.* O.T.

de″tu·mes′cence [L. *detumescere,* to cease swelling]. 1. Subsidence of any swelling. 2. Subsidence of the erectile sexual organs following orgasm.

deu″ter·a·nom′a·ly. See partial *deuteranopia.*

deu″ter·a·no′pi·a (dew″tur·uh·no′pee·uh) [G. *deuteros,* second; *a-,* not; *ōps,* eye]. Inadequate green vision; red-sightedness.

partial d. Decreased ability to perceive green. Syn., *deuteranomaly.*

deu″ter·a′tion. The process of introducing into a chemical compound one or more atoms of the hydrogen isotope deuterium in place of a like number of atoms of ordinary hydrogen (protium) commonly existing in the compound.

deu·ter′i·um (dew·teer′ee·um). Heavy hydrogen. The isotope of hydrogen of atomic weight approximately 2.0, symbol H^2, H^b, or D. It constitutes approximately 1 part in 6000 of ordinary hydrogen. See heavy *water.* Abbreviated, D.

d. oxide. Water of composition D_2O. Syn., *heavy water.*

deu′ter·o- (dew′tur·o-), **deuter-** (dew′tur-) [*deuteros*]. A combining form meaning *second* or *secondary.*

deu″ter·o·gen′ic [*deuteros;* G. *genesthai,* from *gignesthai,* to be produced]. Of secondary origin.

deu′ter·on. The nucleus of a heavy hydrogen atom.

deu′ter·o·plasm′ [*deuteros;* G. *plasma,* anything formed or molded]. 1. The passive or lifeless components of cytoplasm, especially reserve foodstuffs such as yolk. 2. The store of nutrient material in the ovum. Also called *deutoplasm.* Syn., *food yolk.*

deu″ter·o·pro′te·ose [*deuteros;* G. *prōteios,* holding first place]. A secondary proteose; a soluble product of proteolysis.

deu″ter·os′to·ma [*deuteros;* G. *stoma,* mouth]. A second mouth not formed from the blastopore; found in certain worms.

deu″ter·o·tox′in [*deuteros;* G. *toxikon,* poison]. One of the second group into which Ehrlich classified toxins, according to the avidity with which they combine with antitoxins, deuterotoxin having less affinity than has prototoxin and more than tritotoxin.

deu·tom′er·ite [*deuteros;* G. *meros,* part]. The second (posterior) cell of a cephaline gregarine.

deu′ton. Deuteron.

deu′to·plasm. See *deuteroplasm.*

deu″to·plas·mol′y·sis (dew″to·plaz·mol′i·sis) [*deuteros; plasma;* G. *lysis,* a loosing]. In cleavage, the elimination of the yolk from the blastomeres of mammals, especially marsupials.

deu″to·sco′lex [*deuteros;* G. *skōlēx,* worm]. *In biology,* a secondary or daughter cyst or bladder worm derived from a scolex or primary bladder worm.

Deutschländer, Carl Ernst Wilhelm [*German surgeon,* 1872–1942]. Known for his description of march fracture in soldiers, a fracture of the metatarsal bones without obvious trauma; also called *march foot, Deutschländer's disease.*

devegan. Trade-mark for a product containing acetarsone, boric acid, and hydrolyzed carbohydrates: used in the treatment of *Trichomonas vaginalis* infection.

de·vel′op·ment [F. *développer*]. *In biology,* the series of events occurring in an organism during the change from the fertilized egg to the adult stage.

arrested d. Failure of an organism to carry out its normal evolution, stopping at an initial or intermediate stage of the process.

postnatal d. That portion of the development occurring after birth. See Plate 23.

prenatal d. That portion of development occurring before birth. See Plate 23.

Deventer, Hendrik van [*Dutch obstetrician,* 1651–1724]. Because of his observations concerning the placental membranes and his study of the female pelvis (1701), he has been called the father of modern midwifery. Described a simple, nonrachitic pelvis, flattened anteroposteriorly, which once bore his name. The oblique diameter of the pelvis is called *Deventer's diameter.*

Devergie, Marie Guillaume Alphonse [*French dermatologist,* 1798–1879]. Remembered for his description of pityriasis rubra pilaris which was long known as *Devergie's disease.* Was the first to demonstrate the fungous origin of tinea cruris.

de″vi·a′tion [L. *deviare,* to turn from the straight road]. 1. Turning from a regular course, standard, or position; deflection. 2. *In optics,* the inability of the two eyes to fix upon an object at the same time; squint; strabismus. When the healthy eye is fixed upon the object, the squinting eye is unable to fix and consequently deviates; this is known as **primary deviation.** When the squint-eye is the one fixed, there is a corresponding deviation of the healthy eye, known as **secondary deviation.**

average d. See mean *d.*

axis d. *In electrocardiography,* a term indicating that the mean electric axis is beyond the normal limits (0°–90°), but without other electrocardiographic abnormalities. Due to variations in the position of the heart. See left axis *d.*; right axis *d.*

conjugate d. The forced and persistent turning of the eyes and head toward one side; observed with some lesions of the cerebrum.

left axis d. That in which the mean electric axis is less than 0°. This is so when the algebraic sum of the QRS deflections is positive in lead I and negative in lead III or in II and III depending upon whether the degree of left axis deviation is slight or marked. Also called *left axis shift.*

mean d. The arithmetic average of the differences between each observation in a series and the mean of the series, disregarding the sign of the differences.

normal equivalent d. In biological assay, conversion of a percentage response (e.g. of cases which responded to a certain dose) into the deviation on the normal frequency curve to which the percentage is equivalent: used to obtain a linear relation between log dose and percentage response. Abbreviated, N.E.D.

right axis d. That in which the mean electric axis is greater than 90°. This occurs when the algebraic sum of the initial ventricular deflections in lead I is negative. In leads II and III this value may be positive, negative in lead II, and positive in lead III, or negative in both, depending on the degree of right axis deviation. Also called *right axis shift.*

standard d. See *standard deviation.*

Devic, Eugène [*French physician,* d. 1930]. Known for his description of neuromyelitis optica, called *Devic's disease.*

Devine, Hugh Berchmans (1878–). Australian surgeon who devised an operation on the defunctioned distal colon, and devised the application of spur to ileocolic (1931) and to ileorectal (1948) anastomoses. He introduced synchronous resection of rectal growths into England (1937).

de″vi·om′e·ter [L. *devius,* out of the way; G. *metron,* a measure]. A variety of strabometer.

de·vi′tal·ize (dee·vy′tul·ize) [L. *de-,* meaning depriving of; *vitalis,* vital]. Destroy vitality. —**devitaliza′tion,** *n.*

dev″o·lu′tion [L. *devolutum,* from *devolvere,* to roll down]. 1. The reverse of evolution; involution. 2. Catabolism. 3. Degeneration.

Dew, James Harvie [*American physician,* 1843–1914]. Codeviser of a method for artificial respiration of infants known as the *Byrd-Dew method.*

dew′claw″. The more or less vestigial first digit of the hind foot of some animals, especially dogs.

dew′lap″ [ME. *dewlappe*]. A longitudinal fold of skin extending downward from the neck and between the forelegs of bovine animals.

dexamyl. Trade-mark for certain preparations containing dexedrine sulfate and amobarbital.

dexedrine. A trade-mark for the dextrorotatory isomer of amphetamine.

d. sulfate. *d*-Amphetamine sulfate. A sympathomimetic agent and central stimulant more powerful than the racemic mixture known as amphetamine sulfate. Dose, 2.5–5.0 mg. (1/24–1/12 gr.) daily. See *amphetamine.*

dexoval hydrochloride. A trade-marked name for *methamphetamine hydrochloride.*

dex′ter [L.]. Right; upon the right side. Abbreviated, d.

dex′trad [*dexter;* L. *ad,* to, toward]. Toward the right side.

dex′tral [*dexter*]. Pertaining to the right side; right-handed.

dex·tral′i·ty [*dexter*]. Condition in which the right side of the body is more efficient than the left; right-handedness.

dex″tra·li·za′tion. Development of the control of sensorimotor skill from a dominant area on the left side of the cerebral cortex in right-handed individuals. See *sinistration*, 2.

dex′tran. A water-soluble, high molecular weight polymer of glucose produced by the action of *Leuconostoc mesenteroides* on sucrose. A purified form, having an average molecular weight of 75,000, is used in 6% concentration in isotonic sodium chloride solution to expand plasma volume and maintain blood pressure in emergency treatment of hemorrhagic and traumatic shock; such a solution is approximately osmotically equivalent to serum album. See *expandex, gentran, plavolex.*

dex″tran·su′crase. The enzyme responsible for the conversion of sucrose into dextran.

dex·trau′ral [*dexter;* L. *auris,* ear]. Right-eared; pertaining to the right ear.

dextri-maltose. Trade-mark for a preparation of maltose and dextrins obtained by enzymic action of barley malt on corn flour. The product is used as a carbohydrate modifier in milk formulations for infants.

dex′trin. $(C_6H_{10}O_5)_n.xH_2O$. A white or yellow, amorphous powder, dextrorotatory. It is produced by the incomplete hydrolysis of starch. Used as an emulsifying, protective, and thickening agent.

animal d. Glycogen.

dex″tri·nu′ri·a [*dexter;* G. *ouron,* urine]. Presence of dextrin in the urine.

dex′tro- [*dexter*]. A combining form meaning *toward, of,* or *pertaining to the right.*

dex″tro·car′di·a [*dexter;* G. *kardia,* heart]. Transposition of the heart to the right side of the thorax. Also called *dexiocardia.* —**dextrocardial,** *adj.*

dex″tro·car′di·o·gram″ [*dexter; kardia;* G. *gramma,* letter]. That component of the normal electrocardiogram or bicardiogram for which the right ventricle is responsible.

dex″tro·cer′e·bral [*dexter;* L. *cerebrum,* brain]. Located in the right cerebral hemisphere.

dex″tro·com′pound [*dexter;* L. *componere,* to put together]. *In chemistry,* a compound body which causes a ray of polarized light to rotate to the right; a dextrorotatory compound.

dex″tro·con′dyl·ism [*dexter;* G. *kondylos,* knuckle]. Deviation of the mandibular condyles toward the right.

dex·troc′u·lar [*dexter;* L. *oculus,* eye]. Right-eyed; using the right eye in preference to the left. —**dextrocular′ity,** *n.*

dex″tro·duc′tion [*dexter;* L. *ducere,* to lead]. Movement of the visual axis toward the right.

dex″tro·glu′cose. Dextrose.

dex′tro·gram. See *dextrocardiogram.*

dex″tro·gy′rate. Dextrorotatory.

dex″tro·man′u·al [*dexter;* L. *manus,* hand]. Right-handed. —**dextromanual′ity,** *n.*

dex″tro·pe′dal, dex·trop′e·dal [*dexter;* L. *pes,* foot]. Right-footed.

dex″tro·pho′bi·a [*dexter;* G. *phobos,* fear]. Morbid fear of objects on the right side of the body.

dex″tro·pho′ri·a [*dexter;* G. *phoros,* bearing]. A tending of the visual lines to the right.

dex″tro·po·si′tion of heart. Displacement of the heart toward the right or into the right half of the thorax.

dex″tro·ro′ta·to″ry [*dexter;* L. *rotare,* to whirl about]. Turning the rays of light to the right.

dex′trose (decks′troce, ·troze) (*dextrosum*). $C_6H_{12}O_6.H_2O$. A dextrorotatory monosaccharide occurring as a white, crystalline powder; odorless and sweet; soluble in about one part of water. It is usually prepared by the hydrolysis of starch. An essential constituent of blood, being not only a source of energy but also a necessity for the complete combustion of fats. Liver glycogen is manufactured from the dextrose of the blood. It is administered intravenously for its food value; in isotonic solution to increase the blood volume; and in highly concentrated solution for its strengthening effect on the heart muscle or to withdraw fluid from surrounding tissues into the blood vessels. See *glucose.* Syn., *dextroglucose, grape sugar, starch sugar.* Also called D-*glucose.*

dex″tro·sin′is·tral (decks″tro·sin′is·trul, ·sin·iss′-trul) [*dexter;* L. *sinister,* left]. Extending from right to left.

dex″tro·su′ri·a [*dexter;* G. *ouron,* urine]. Presence of dextrose in the urine.

dex″tro·tar·tar′ic ac′id (deck″stro·tahr·tar′ick, ·tahr·tahr′ick). Tartaric acid.

dex″tro·tor′sion [*dexter;* L. *torsio,* from *torquere,* to twist]. A twisting to the right.

dex″tro·ver′sion (decks″tro·vur′zhun, ·vur′shun) [*dexter;* L. *vertere,* to turn]. Version to the right side.

D-forms. 1. Dwarf forms, said of organisms appearing in pure cultures. 2. Diphtheroid forms.

DFP Abbreviation for diisopropyl fluorophosphate.

D-glucose. See *dextrose.*

DHE-45. A trade designation for dihydroergotamine.

d'Herelle, Felix Hubert [*Canadian physician and bacteriologist in U.S.S.R.,* 1873–1949]. Described bacteriophage (1917), also called *d'Herelle phenomenon, Twort-d'Herelle phenomenon.*

dho′bie itch (do′bee). See *tinea* cruris.

dhur′rin, dur′rin (dew′rin, durr′in). A glycoside from various species of *Sorghum.* On hydrolysis, it yields glucose, hydrocyanic acid, and *p*-hydroxybenzaldehyde.

di- (dye-, *even when unstressed*). See *dis-.*

di′a-, di- [G. *dia,* through]. A prefix denoting *through, between, apart, asunder,* or *across.*

di″a·be′tes (dye″uh·bee′teez, ·bee′tiss) [G. *diabētēs,* from *diabainein,* to pass through]. A disease characterized by the habitual discharge of an excessive quantity of urine and by excessive thirst; used without qualification, the word means diabetes mellitus. —**diabet′ic,** *adj.*

alloxan d. An experimental diabetes. See *alloxan diabetes.*

amino d. A congenital disorder characterized by excessive quantities of amino acids, glucose, and phosphate in the urine, resulting from deficient resorption in the proximal convoluted tubule of the kidney; cytinosis may occur: also called *de Toni-Fanconi syndrome.* When associated with deficient ammonia formation, it is also called *Debré-de Toni-Fanconi syndrome.*

biliary d. Hypertrophic cirrhosis of the liver with icterus.

bronze d. Diabetes mellitus associated with hemochromatosis.

d. decipiens. Diabetic glycosuria, without other evidence of diabetes.

d. insipidus. A disease due to a disorder of the hypothalamus, either congenital or following injury or infection; characterized by the passage of a large quantity of urine of low specific gravity, associated with intense thirst and dehydration; relieved by extracts of the posterior pituitary lobe. Formerly called *neuropituitary syndrome.*

d. mellitus. An inheritable, constitutional disease of unknown cause, characterized by the failure of the body tissues to oxidize carbohydrate at a normal rate. The metabolic disturbance, which has as its most important factor a deficiency of insulin, manifests itself in an excess of sugar in the blood (hyperglycemia), presence of sugar in the urine (glycosuria), and, in more advanced stages, acidosis (ketosis), and coma, with symptoms of intense thirst and hunger, weakness, and loss of weight. The disease may be further attended in later life by degenerative changes such as arteriosclerosis, cataract, neuritis.

experimental d. Diabetes mellitus produced in animals by various methods, such as puncture of the diabetic center, pancreatectomy, injection of extracts of the anterior pituitary or of alloxan.

galactose d. See *galactosemia.*

meta d. Permanent diabetes in man, secondary to overstimulation of the pituitary, adrenal cortex, or the thyroid (respectively *metahypophyseal d., metaadrenal d., metathyroid d.*).

nephrogenic d. insipidus. Diabetes insipidus which is not responsive to the antidiuretic hormone. This is presumed to be the result of a lack of end-organ response, i.e., the renal tubule. More common in males, it has a high familial incidence.

pancreatic d. A variety of diabetes mellitus dependent upon disease of the pancreas.

pitressin resistant d. insipidus. See nephrogenic *d.* insipidus.

piqûre d. Old term for artificial *glycosuria.*

renal amino acid d. See amino *d.*

renal d. See renal *glycosuria.*

di″a·bet′ic [*diabainein*]. A person suffering from diabetes.

di″a·be″to·gen′ic (dye″uh·bee″to·jen′ick, dye″uh-bet″o·) [*diabainein;* G. *genesthai*, from *gignesthai*, to be produced]. Causing diabetes.

di″a·be·tog′e·nous (dye″uh·bi·todj′i·nus) [*diabainein; genesthai*]. Produced by diabetes.

di″a·be″to·pho′bi·a [*diabainein;* G. *phobos*, fear]. Morbid fear of becoming a diabetic.

di·ab′o·lep″sy [G. *diabolos*, devil; *lēpsis*, seizure]. Diabolical seizure or possession; delusion of supernatural possession. —**diabolep′tic,** *n.*

di″a·ce·te′mi·a [G. *dis*, twice; L. *acetum*, vinegar; G. *haima*, blood]. Presence of diacetic acid (acetoacetic acid) in the blood.

di″a·ce′tic ac′id (dye″uh·see′tick, ·set′ick). Acetoacetic acid.

di·ac′e·tin (dye·ass′i·tin, dye″uh·see′tin). $C_3H_5(OH)(OOC.CH_3)_2$. Glyceryl diacetate; a liquid derivative of glycerin with a bitter taste. Soluble in water, alcohol, or ether.

di·ac″e·tu′ri·a (dye·ass″i·tew′ree·uh), **di·ac″e·to-nu′ri·a** (dye·ass″i·to·new′ree·uh) [*dis; acetum;* G. *ouron*, urine)]. Presence of diacetic acid (acetoacetic acid) in the urine.

di·ac″e·tyl·mor′phine (dye·ass″i·til·mor′feen, ·fin, ·mor·feen′). Heroin.

di·ac″e·tyl·tan′nin. Acetyltannic acid.

di·ac′la·sis (dye·ack′luh·sis, dye″uh·clay′sis), **di″-a·cla′si·a** (dye″uh·clay′zhuh, ·shuh, ·zee·uh, ·see·uh) [G. *diaklasis*, a breaking up]. 1. Refraction. 2. A fracture produced intentionally. —**diaclas′tic,** *adj.*

di′a·clast [G. *diaklan*, to break in twain]. Instrument for breaking the fetal head.

di·ac″o·la′tion [G. *dia*, through; L. *colare*, to strain]. A method of drug extraction involving percolation of a suitable solvent through long narrow columns packed with the drug.

di″a·crit′ic, di″a·crit′i·cal [G. *diakritikos*, separative]. Diagnostic, distinctive.

di″ac·tin′ic [G. *dia*, through; *aktis*, ray]. Capable of transmitting actinic rays.

diactol. A proprietary capsule containing vitamin D_2.

di′ad [G. *dis*, twice; G. *-as*, fem. suffix denoting an aggregate]. 1. An element or radical having a valence of two. 2. A bivalent chromosome resulting from synapse, 2. —**di′ad,** *adj.*

di′a·derm [G. *dia*, through, originally dividing into two parts; *derma*, skin]. A two-layered blastoderm composed of ectoderm and entoderm. *O.T.*

di·ad″o·cho·ki·ne′si·a (dye·ad″o·ko·ki·nee′shuh, ·see·uh, ·zhuh, ·zee·uh, ·kigh·nee′·), **di·ad″o·cho-ki·ne′sis** (dye·ad″o·ko·ki·nee′sis, ·kigh·nee′sis), **di·ad″o·ko·ki·ne′si·a, di·ad″o·ko·ki·ne′sis.** [G. *diadochos*, succeeding; *kinēsis*, motion]. The normal power of performing alternating movements in rapid succession.

di″ag·nos′a·ble. Capable of being diagnosed.

di″ag·no′sis [G., a deciding].1. The art or the act of determining the nature of a disease. 2. The decision reached. —**diagnose′,** *v.*

anatomic d. (a) A diagnosis based upon the recognition of definite anatomic alterations lying back of the phenomena. (b) A postmortem diagnosis.

clinical d. One based upon the history and physical examination of the patient: used frequently in reference to diseases (processes) for which no diagnostic or laboratory tests are available.

deductive d. A diagnosis made by a physician after a consideration of all the manifestations of the disease, and after forming a conception of the disorder in terms of physiology, hence of the anatomic localization of the lesion, and, finally, by inference, of the pathologic process and its etiology.

d. by exclusion. The recognition of a disease by excluding all other known conditions.

differential d. The distinguishing between two diseases of similar character by comparing their symptoms.

laboratory d. One arrived at from the results of tests on and examination of various tissues and excretions.

microscopical d. That made by means of microscopical examination of tissues or specimens.

pathologic d. One based on the study of the structural lesions present.

physical d. The determination of disease by inspection, palpation, percussion, or auscultation.

quick-section d. A rapid histological diagnosis during a surgical operation, of a specimen removed for study, and prepared for microscopy by frozen section.

Rorschach d. See Rorschach *test.*

topographic d. One determined by the location of a lesion.

di″ag·nos′tic [G. *diagnōstikos*, able to distinguish]. Pertaining to or serving as evidence in diagnosis.

di″ag·nos·ti′cian [*diagnōstikos*]. One skilled in making diagnoses.

di″a·ki·ne′sis (dye″uh·ki·nee′sis, ·kigh·nee′sis) [G. *dia*, through; *kinēsis*, motion]. A stage in miosis during which the tetrads take on definitive form preceding the disappearance of the nuclear membrane.

dial. A trade-mark for *diallylbarbituric acid.*

di·al″kyl′a·mine. See *alkylamine.*

di·al″lyl·bar″bi·tur′ic ac′id. $(CH_2{:}CHCH_2)_2$-C.CO.NH.CO.NH.CO; a white, crystalline powder, slightly soluble in water; it is sedative and hypnotic, being characterized by intermediate duration of action. See *dial.*

di·al′y·sate (dye·al′i·sayt). See *dialyzate.*

di·al′y·sis (dye·al′i·sis) [G., a separating]. Separation of substances from one another in solution by taking advantage of their differing diffusibility through porous membranes. —**dialyt′ic, di′-alyzable,** *adj.;* **di′alyze,** *v.*

di·al′y·zate, di·al′y·sate [*dialysis*]. The portion of the liquid which passes through the membrane in dialysis, and contains the crystalloids in solution.

di′a·ly″zer [*dialysis*]. Apparatus for effecting dialysis; also the porous septum or diaphragm of such an apparatus.

di″a·mag·net′ic. Of, pertaining, or referring to a weakly magnetic substance, having a magnetic permeability less than unity, which is repelled by a magnet. —**di″a·mag′net·ism,** *n.*

di′a·mer-sul·fon′a·mides. The generic name for a mixture of equal weights of sulfadiazine and sulfamerazine.

di·am′e·ter [G. *diametros*, from *diametrein*, to measure through]. A straight line joining opposite points of a body or figure and passing through its center.

anteroposterior d. of the pelvic inlet. That which joins the sacrovertebral angle and pubic symphysis. See internal conjugate *d.*, external conjugate *d.*

anteroposterior d. of the pelvic outlet. That between the lower margin of the symphysis pubis and the tip of the sacrum or the tip of the coccyx. Syn., *sacropubic d.*, *coccygeopubic d.*

anterotransverse d. That joining the tips of the greater wings of the sphenoid. Syn., *temporal d.*

biparietal d. That joining the parietal eminences.

bispinous d. That joining the spines of the ischia.

bitemporal d. That joining the extremities of the coronal suture.

coccygeopubic d. See anteroposterior *d.* of the pelvic outlet.

conjugate d. Any of a number of diameters of the pelvis; especially, the anteroposterior diameter of the pelvic inlet.

craniometric d. A line connecting two corresponding points on opposite surfaces of the cranium.

dental d. That of the crown of a tooth joining the buccal and lingual surfaces, that is, the buccolingual diameter.

diagonal conjugate d. That connecting the sacrovertebral angle and the subpubic ligament.

external conjugate d. That connecting the depression above the spine of the first sacral vertebra and the middle of the upper border of the symphysis pubis. Also called *Baudeloque's d.*

fetal cranial diameters. Those including the biparietal, bitemporal, occipitofrontal, occipitomental, and suboccipitobregmatic diameters.

inferior longitudinal d. See sagittal *d.*

intercristal d. That joining the middle points of the iliac crests.

internal conjugate d. That connecting the sacrovertebral angle and the most prominent portion of the posterior aspect of the symphysis pubis. Also called *true conjugate d.*, *conjugata vera*, *anatomic conjugate d.*

interspinous d. That connecting the anterior superior iliac spines.

mean cell d. A measurement of cell size usually calculated by the Price-Jones method. This is valuable in the diagnosis of macrocytosis and in following the course of treatment in pernicious anemia. See also Cecil *Price-Jones.*

mentoparietal d. That joining the chin and the vertex.

oblique d. of the pelvic inlet. That joining the iliopectineal eminence to the sacroiliac articulation on the opposite side.

occipitofrontal d. That joining the root of the nose and the most prominent point of the occiput.

occipitomental d. That joining the occipital protuberance and the chin.

parietal d. See posterotransverse *d.*

pelvic d. Any one of the diameters of the pelvis.

posterotransverse d. That joining the parietal eminences.

pubotuberous d. An external diameter extending perpendicularly from the tuberosity of the ischium to the superior ramus of the pubis.

sacropubic d. See anteroposterior *d.* of the pelvic outlet.

sagittal d. That joining the glabella and the external occipital protuberance. Syn., *inferior longitudinal d.*

suboccipitobregmatic d. That joining the center of the anterior fontanel to the under surface of the occipital bone.

superior sagittal d. That joining the middle of the crest of the frontal bone to the external occipital protuberance.

temporal d. See anterotransverse *d.*

trachelobregmatic d. That joining the center of the anterior fontanel and the junction of the neck and floor of the mouth.

transverse d. of the pelvic inlet. That connecting the two most widely separated points of the pelvic inlet.

transverse d. of the pelvic outlet. That between the two ischial tuberosities. Also called *biischial d.*, *biischiatic d.*, *bituberal d.*, *intertuberal d.*

vertical d. That joining the foramen magnum and vertex.

vertical d. of the cranium. An imaginary line from the basion to the bregma.

di·am′i·dine (dye·am′i·deen, ·din). Any compound consisting of two amidine groups, $NH{:}C(NH_2)$—, linked together by a hydrocarbon chain. Certain ones, of related chemical structure, have been found to possess, in varying degrees, trypanocidal and antibacterial activity. See *pentamidine*, *phenamidine*, *propamidine*, *stilbamidine.*

di″a·mine′ (dye″uh·meen′, dye′uh·meen, ·min, dye·am′in). An amine formed by replacing hydrogen in two molecules of ammonia by a hydrocarbon radical. See *amine.*

d. oxidase. See *histaminase.*

di″a·mi″no·di·phen″yl·sul′fone (·dye·fen″il·sul′fohn, ·dye·fee″nil·sul′fohn). $NH_2.C_6H_4.SO_2.C_6H_4.NH_2$. A drug of the sulfonamide group especially effective against streptococci.

di″a·mi″no·phe′nol hy″dro·chlo′ride. See *amidol.*

di″a·mi″no·pu′rine. $C_5H_6N_6$; 2,6-diaminopurine or 2-aminoadenine, a compound selectively injurious to certain neoplastic cells in animals, and under investigation found to be a possible chemotherapeutic agent in human neoplastic diseases.

di″a·mi·nu′ri·a [diamine; *ouron*, urine]. Presence of diamine compounds in the urine.

Diamond's method. See Wallace and Diamond's *method.*

di″a·mor′phine hy″dro·chlo′ride (dye″uh·mor′feen, ·fin). Former British Pharmacopoeia title for heroin hydrochloride.

diamox. Trade-mark for 2-acetylamino-1,3,4-thiadiazole-5-sulfonamide;

$$CH_3CO.NH.\underbrace{C{:}N.N{:}C}_{S}.SO_2NH_2$$

having the generic name *acetazoleamide.* The substance, when administered orally, is a powerful inhibitor of renal carbonic anhydrase, thereby inducing alkalinization of urine and increasing excretion of sodium and bicarbonate ions, with enhancement of diuresis. It is used clinically for treating edema of congestive heart failure.

di·am′tha·zole di·hy″dro·chlo′ride. Generic name for 6-(β-diethylaminoethoxy)-2-dimethylaminobenzothiazole dihydrochloride, a water-soluble antifungal agent suitable for topical treatment of superficial fungous infections. See *asterol dihydrochloride.*

diaparene chloride. Trade-marked name for methylbenzethonium chloride, a quaternary ammonium salt used for bacteriostasis of urea-splitting organisms involved in diaper dermatitis.

di″a·pa′son (dye″uh·pay′zun, ·sun) [G. *diapasōn*, concord of the first and last notes, octave]. A tuning fork; used in the diagnosis of diseases of the ear, especially in determining the presence and extent of deafness.

di″a·pe·de′sis [G. *dia*, through; *pēdēsis*, a leaping]. Passage of blood cells, especially erythrocytes, through the unruptured vessel walls into the tissues. —**diapedet′ic,** *adj.*

di′a·phane [G. *diaphainein*, to show through]. 1. The transparent investing membrane of an organ or cell. 2. A small electric lamp used in transillumination. 3. A commercial mounting medium for histologic sections.

di·aph″a·nom′e·ter [*diaphainein;* G. *metron*, a measure]. Instrument for measuring the transparency of gases, liquids, or solids.

di·aph′a·no·scope (dye·af′uh·no·scope, dye″uh-fan′o·) [*diaphainein;* G. *skopein*, to examine]. Device for lighting an interior body cavity so as to render it visible from the exterior. —**diaphanos′copy,** *n.*

di·aph″e·met′ric (dye·af″i·met′rick, dye″uh·fi·) [G. *dia*, through; *haphē*, touch; *metron*, a measure]. Pertaining to measurements of tactile sensibility.

di″a·phe′nol. Vapors of chlorine dioxide passed into ice-cold 50% acetic acid: used for softening chitin.

di·aph′o·rase. The enzyme which catalyzes the oxidation of reduced coenzyme I.

di″a·pho·re′sis [G., perspiration, from *diaphorein*, to carry through]. Perspiration, especially perceptible perspiration.

di″a·pho·ret′ic [*diaphorēsis*]. Causing an increase of perspiration.

di″a·pho·ret′ic. A medicine that induces diaphoresis.

di′a·phragm (dye′uh·fram) [G. *diaphragma*, partition, diaphragm]. 1. *In anatomy*, a musculotendinous partition; especially that partition muscular at the circumference and tendinous at the center, which separates the thorax and abdomen and is the chief muscle of respiration and expulsion. See Table of Muscles in the Appendix. See Plates 13, 14. 2. A thin septum such as is used in dialysis. 3. *In microscopy*, an aperture placed between the mirror and object to regulate the amount of light that is to pass through the object. 4. A contraceptive device worn during copulation over the external cervical os for preventing conception or infection; it is usually dome-shaped and of thin rubber or plastic material. —**di″a·phrag·mat′ic,** *adj.*

Bucky's d. *In roentgenography*, a moving grid of alternate thin strips of lead and wood which permits only radiation traveling in the direction of the x-ray beam to strike the photographic film, thus producing pictures with sharper contrast.

central stop d. *In microscopy*, a diaphragm having a circular slit just within its margin, the center remaining opaque.

compression d. A device generally used in conjunction with fluoroscopy, particularly of the gastrointestinal tract. The compression device often delineates the mucosal pattern which may not be visualized when a barium-filled viscus is x-rayed or fluoroscoped without external pressure on the patient's body.

condensing d. A diaphragm containing lenses for converging the light rays.

cylindrical d. *In microscopy*, a piece of substage apparatus fitted with perforated stops, each allowing a different amount of light to pass.

d. opening. The opening in the disk or apparatus of a microscope through which the rays of light pass.

d. of the sella. The circular layer of dura mater which forms the roof of the hypophyseal fossa; its center is pierced by the stalk of the pituitary gland.

graduating d. One which allows a concentric increase or diminution of light.

iris d. A device for changing or regulating the amount of light directed upon an object under the microscope.

oral d. That formed by the mylohyoid and hyoglossus muscles, separating the sublingual from the submaxillary region.

pelvic d. That formed by the levator ani and the coccygeus muscles; the concave floor of the pelvis, separating it from the perineum.

Potter-Bucky d. See Bucky's *d.*

urogenital d. That stretching across the pubic arch, formed by the deep transverse perineal and the sphincter urethrae muscles. Also called *trigoneum urogenitale, triangular ligament.*

di″a·phrag′ma. Diaphragm.

di″a·phrag·mat′o·cele (dye″uh·frag·mat′o·seel) [*diaphragma;* G. *kēlē*, hernia]. Hernia through the diaphragm.

di″a·phrag·mi′tis [*diaphragma;* G. *-itis*, inflammation]. Inflammation of the diaphragm. *Rare.*

di″aph·y·sec′to·my (dye″af·i·seck′to·mee, ·zeck′-to·mee) [G. *diaphysis*, a growing through; *ektomē*, excision]. Excision of a portion of the shaft of a long bone.

di·aph′y·sis (pl. *diaphyses*). The shaft of a long bone. —**diaphys′eal, diaphys′ial,** *adj.*

di·ap′la·sis [G., a putting into shape]. Reduction of a dislocation or of a fracture.

di″a·poph′y·sis [G. *dia*, through; *apophysis*, side-shoot, process of a bone]. The superior or articular part of a transverse process of a vertebra. —**diapophys′ial,** *adj.*

di″a·rhe′mi·a, di″ar·rhae′mi·a (dye″uh·ree′-mee·uh). See sanguineous *ascites.*

di″ar·rhe′a, di″ar·rhoe′a [G. *diarrhoia*, a flowing through]. A common symptom of gastrointestinal disease; characterized by increased frequency and more or less fluid consistency of the stools; may be due to various causes from acute infections to psychogenic factors. Also see *dysentery.* —**diarrhe′al,** *adj.*

acute d. Characterized by the sudden onset of frequent liquid stools usually with constitutional symptoms of weakness and pain and often with fever and vomiting; may be of infectious origin (as bacillary dysentery) or noninfectious origin (as arsenic poisoning).

choleraic d. Old term for a severe, acute type with serous stools, vomiting, and collapse; so called because of its resemblance to cholera.

chronic d. That characterized by frequent stools over an extended period of time, occurring as a manifestation of an intestinal lesion or of a constitutional disease.

Cochin-China d. Sprue.

epidemic d. of the newborn. A form, seen in newborns in hospital nurseries, which occurs as an epidemic and is of unknown origin.

fermentative d. That associated with fermentation of the intestinal contents.

green d. A form of infantile diarrhea, characterized by the passage of green stools.

hill d. A form occurring in the hill country of India; may be due to low atmospheric pressure.

infantile d. An acute form seen in infants, most

frequently during the summer; due primarily to damage of the intestinal mucosa by infection. Many organisms have been thought to be causative. Seen most frequently in artificially fed infants, and associated with poor hygiene. The cholera infantum of older writers.

inflammatory d. A general term for diarrhea caused by poisons or infections which induce local inflammation of the intestinal mucosa.

lienteric d. That due to achylia gastrica.

membranous d. A form characterized by severe acute inflammation of the mucosa with membrane formation.

mucous d. Mucous colitis.

nervous d. That due to disturbances of the autonomic nervous system.

pancreatic d. A persistent form, due to absence of pancreatic digestive enzymes; characterized by the passage of large, greasy stools having a high fat and nitrogen content.

parenteral d. That due to infections outside of the intestinal tract.

putrefactive d. That associated with putrefaction of the intestinal contents.

summer d. An acute form seen during the intense heat of summer; usually caused by bacterial contamination of poorly refrigerated food.

summer d. of children. See infantile *d.*

white d. of chicks. A disease of chicks caused by *Salmonella pullorum.*

di″ar·rhoe′a (dye″uh·ree′uh). See *diarrhea.*

diarsenol. A brand of arsphenamine.

di·ar′thric [G. *dis*, twice; *arthron*, joint]. Relating to two joints.

di″ar·thro′sis [G., articulation]. A freely movable articulation. See *articulation.* —**diarthrodial,** *adj.*

di″ar·tic′u·lar [G. *dis*, twice; L. *articulus*, joint]. Diarthric.

di·as′chi·sis (dye·ass′ki·sis) [G., division]. An inhibition of function in a region of the nervous system, due to a localized injury in another region with which it is connected by fiber tracts.

di″a·schis′tic (dye″uh·skis′tick, ·shis′tick) [G. *dia*, through; *schizein*, to cleave]. Splitting transversely, applied to bivalent or tetrad elements.

di′a·scope [*dia;* G. *skopein*, to examine]. Device consisting of a thin piece of glass, used to press against the skin so that superficial lesions may be observed. —**dias′copy,** *n.*

diasone sodium. Trade-marked name for sulfoxone sodium, a substance introduced for treatment of tuberculosis but not found clinically satisfactory, although later found useful in the treatment of leprosy.

di″a·stal′sis [G., from *dia; stalsis*, a checking]. The downward moving wave of contraction, occurring in the small intestine during digestion.

di′a·stase [G. *diastasis*, a separation]. An enzyme from malt which converts starch to maltose by hydrolysis; vegetable amylase. Also called *vegetable d.*

animal d. Any of the amylolytic enzymes of animals, such as ptyalin, amylopsin, etc.

pancreatic d. Amylopsin.

salivary d. Ptyalin.

taka-diastase. Trade-mark for a powdered vegetable diastase, obtained by the action of *Aspergillus oryzae* on wheat bran; it is capable of liquefying 450 times its weight of starch in 10 minutes. Used in cases of faulty starch digestion.

di″a·sta′sic, di″a·stas′ic. See *diastatic.*

di·as′ta·sis [G.]. 1. Any simple separation of parts normally joined together, as the separation of an epiphysis from the body of a bone without true fracture, or the dislocation of an amphiarthrosis. 2. The final phase of diastole in which ventricular filling is reduced to the minimum.

d. recti abdominis. Separation in the median line of the two rectus abdominis muscles, usually from repeated childbirth.

di″a·stat′ic, di″a·sta′sic (dye″uh·stay′sick, ·stass′ick) [*diastasis*]. 1. Pertaining to diastasis. 2. Pertaining to a diastase.

di″a·ste′ma [G. *diastēma*, interval, separation]. 1. A cleft or fissure, especially if congenital. 2. *In dentistry*, an abnormal space between the teeth.

di″a·stem″a·to·my·e′li·a (dye″uh·stem″uh·to·migh·ee′lee·uh, dye″uh·stee″muh·to·) [*diastēma;* G. *myelos*, marrow]. A congenital, more or less complete doubling of the spinal cord associated with the formation of a bony or cartilaginous septum from the posterior wall of the vertebral canal, usually in spina bifida. Syn., *diplomyelia.*

di″as′ter [G. *di-*, twice; *astēr*, star]. Old term for *amphiaster.*

di″a·ster″e·o·i′so·mer. One of the isomeric forms of a compound, containing asymmetric carbon atoms, which when compared with another isomer of the same compound differs in the spatial distribution of its component atoms and groups of atoms in such manner as not to have a mirror-image relationship with the other isomer. In contrast to enantiomorphs diastereoisomers possess different physical properties. —**di″a·ster″e·o·i″so·mer′ic,** *adj.;* **di″a·ster″e·o·i·som′er·ism,** *n.*

di·as′to·le (dye·ass′to·lee) [G. *diastolē*, a drawing asunder]. The rhythmic period of relaxation and dilatation of a chamber of the heart during which it fills with blood; used alone the word means ventricular diastole. —**diastol′ic,** *adj.*

atrial d. The dilatation of the cardiac atria.

ventricular d. That of the cardiac ventricles.

di″a·tax′i·a [G. *dis*, twice; *ataxia*, disorder]. Bilateral ataxia, as opposed to *hemiataxia.*

di″a·ther′ma·nous. Allowing passage of heat rays.

di″a·ther′mi·a. See *diathermy.*

di″a·ther′mic. 1. Pertaining to the ability of a substance to permit passage of heat rays. 2. Of, or pertaining to, diathermy.

di″a·ther″mo·co·ag″u·la′tion [G. *dia*, through; *thermē*, heat; L. *coagulare*, to cause a fluid to coagulate]. Coagulation secured by the use of a high-frequency electrosurgical knife.

di″a·ther·mom′e·ter [*dia; thermē;* G. *metron*, a measure]. *In physics*, an instrument for measuring the heat-conducting capacity of substances.

di′a·ther″my (dye′uh·thur″mee, dye″uh·thur′mee), **di″a·ther′mi·a** [*dia; thermē*]. 1. The therapeutic use of an oscillating electric current of high frequency to produce local heat in the body tissues below the surface. 2. The electric current so used. 3. The machine producing it. —**diather′mal,** *adj.;* **diather′mize,** *v.*

conventional d. The use of a current of moderately high frequency, 500–3000 kilocycles per second, at wave lengths of 600–100 meters.

medical d. That form in which the tissues are heated to a point less than destructive temperature.

short-wave d. That form making use of a current of extremely high frequency, 10,000–100,000 kilocycles per second, at wave lengths of 30 to 3 meters.

di·ath′e·sis [G., a placing in order]. Constitution; hereditary influence. A state or condition of the body or a combination of attributes in one individual causing a susceptibility to disease. —**diathet′ic,** *adj.*

exudative d. A condition formerly recognized in children, associated with an irritable skin and chafing, intertrigo, seborrhea, eczema, and hypersusceptibility to external irritants of the skin and mucous membranes. There are also frequent respiratory infections with resulting lymphoid hyperplasia.

hemorrhagic d. An abnormal bleeding tendency as in hemophilia, purpura, scurvy, or vitamin-K deficiency.

hereditary hemorrhagic d. A rare, familial, nonthrombocytopenic hemorrhagic disorder that can affect both sexes. It is characterized by prolonged bleeding time but by normal clotting time and clot retraction. The condition has been ascribed to abnormal capillaries, defective thromboplastin, or both. Syn., *hereditary pseudohemophilia, hereditary hemorrhagic thrombasthenia, constitutional thrombopathy.*

hypersthenic gastric d. A constitutional type in which the individual has a short, high stomach associated with rapid peristalsis and evacuation. The theory that such persons have a strong tendency toward developing duodenal ulcers is unsubstantiated.

hyposthenic gastric d. The constitution of an individual with a long, low, hook-shaped stomach, associated with slow peristalsis and evacuation. The claim that such individuals tend to develop gastric ulcers is unsupported.

ulcer d. Susceptibility to ulcer formation.

uratic d. A condition in which there is a tendency to the deposition of urates in the joints and elsewhere; gout.

di′a·tom (dye′uh·tom, ·tome) [G. *diatomos*, cut in two]. Any of the Diatomaceae, a small family of microscopic, unicellular algae having a cell wall of silica, the skeleton persisting after death of the organism.

di″a·to·ma′ceous earth. A sedimentary rock composed of the empty shells of diatoms and other Protophyta; used as an absorbent, a filtration aid, and an insulating material. See also diatomaceous earth *pneumoconiosis.*

di″a·tom′ic [*diatomos*]. 1. Consisting of two atoms: commonly referring to a molecule. 2. Containing two replaceable univalent atoms or radicals. 3. Bivalent.

diatrin hydrochloride. Trade-marked name for the antihistaminic substance *methaphenilene hydrochloride.*

diatussin. A proprietary expectorant prepared from *Drosera rotundifolia* and *Thymus vulgaris.*

Diaz de Isla, Rodrigo Ruiz [*Spanish surgeon*, 1462–1542]. Said to have been the first to describe syphilis, which he observed in members of Columbus' crew (1493); hence the belief that the disease was of New World origin.

di′a·zine. 1. A heterocyclic compound having the formula $C_4H_4N_2$, containing two nitrogen and four carbon atoms in the ring. Three isomers are possible, distinguished as 1,2-diazine, 1,3-diazine, and 1,4-diazine, and commonly known as *pyridazine, pyrimidine,* and *pyrazine,* respectively. 2. Any derivative of any of the compounds in 1.

di·az′o- (dye·az′o-, dye·ay′zo-), **diaz-** [G. *dis*, twice; *a-*, not; *zōē*, life]. *In chemistry,* a combining form indicating the presence in a compound of a group involving two nitrogen atoms, usually arranged in the form of R—N=N—, where R is an aryl group. —**diazo,** *adj.*

di″a·zo′ni·um com′pound. A diazo compound, so called to emphasize its resemblance to ammonium compounds, presumably through formation of an R—N≡N group, rather than the isomeric R—N=N— group.

di·az″o·ti·za′tion. The process of converting certain compounds, notably aromatic amines, to their respective diazo derivatives, commonly by reaction with nitrous acid. —**diaz′otize,** *v.*

di·ba′sic (dye·bay′sick) [*dis;* G. *basis*, foundation]. Of a salt, containing two atoms of a monobasic element or radical; of an acid, having two replaceable hydrogen atoms.

di·ben″a·mine′. $(C_6H_5CH_2)_2NCH_2CH_2Cl$. N,N-Dibenzyl-beta-chloroethylamine, the hydrochloride of which has been employed experimentally as a sympatholytic and adrenolytic agent.

di″ben·zan′thra·cene. 1,2,5,6-*Di*benzanthracene. A polycyclic hydrocarbon, $C_{22}H_{14}$. A carcinogen; said to be the first pure chemical found experimentally to produce cancer in an animal.

dibenzyline. Trade-mark for N-phenoxyisopropyl-N-benzyl-β-chloroethylamine, known also by the generic name *phenoxybenzamine hydrochloride,* an adrenergic blocking agent useful in the treatment of peripheral vascular diseases and possibly in certain types of hypertension.

di·both″ri·o·ceph″a·li′a·sis. Old term for diphyllobothriasis.

Di·both″ri·o·ceph′a·lus. Synonym for *Diphyllobothrium.*

dibromin. Trade-mark for dibromobarbituric acid, a surgical disinfectant and germicide in 1:1,000 to 1:10,000 solution.

di·bro″mo·bar″bi·tu′ric ac′id. See *dibromin.*

di·bu′caine hy″dro·chlo′ride (dye·bew′cane). $C_{20}H_{29}N_3O_2.HCl$; 2-butoxy-N-(2-diethylaminoethyl) cinchoninamide hydrochloride, occurring as white crystals or powder, freely soluble in water. It is a local anesthetic which acts like cocaine hydrochloride when applied to mucous surfaces, and like procaine or cocaine hydrochloride when injected. Syn., *cinchocaine hydrochloride.* See *nupercaine hydrochloride.*

dibuline sulfate. Trade-marked name for *dibutoline sulfate.*

di·bu′to·line sul′fate. Generic name for the bis [(dibutylcarbamate) of ethyl (2-hydroxyethyl)-dimethylammonium] sulfate, having clinically useful spasmolytic, mydriatic, and cycloplegic actions. See *dibuline sulfate.*

di·cal′ci·um. Containing two atoms of calcium in each molecule.

d. phosphate. See dibasic *calcium* phosphate.

di·car″box·yl′ic ac′id. An organic compound with two —COOH groups.

di·cen′trine (dye·sen′treen, ·trin). $C_{20}H_{21}O_4N$. A toxic alkaloid from species of *Dicentra.*

di·ceph′a·lism, di·ceph′a·ly [G. *dis*, twice; *kephalē*, head]. The condition of having two heads.

di·ceph′a·lus [*dis; kephalē*]. A monster with two heads. See Plate 25. —**dicephalous,** *adj.*

d. diauchenos. An individual with two heads and two more or less separate necks.

d. monauchenos. An individual with two heads on a single neck.

d. parasiticus. An individual having a more or less incomplete parasitic head attached to the normal head or neck.

d. tetrabrachius. Conjoined twins single below the umbilicus, with two more or less separate thoraces, four arms, two heads, and two necks.

d. tribrachius. Conjoined twins single below the umbilicus; thoraces more or less double, with three arms, two necks, and two heads.

di·ceph′a·ly. See *dicephalism.*

di·chei′lus, di·chi′lus (dye·kigh′lus) [*dis;* G. *cheilos*, lip]. Double lip; due to a fold of mucous membrane giving the appearance of duplicity.

di·chi′lus. See *dicheilus.*

di·chi′rus (dye·kigh′rus) [*dis;* G. *cheir*, hand]. Partial or complete duplication of the hand.

di″chlor·a·mine′. Dichloramine-T.

di″chlor·a·mine′-T (dye″klor·uh·meen′, ·am′in, ·klor′uh·meen, ·min) $CH_3.C_6H_4.SO_2NCl_2$; p-toluenesulfondichloramide; a pale-yellow, crystalline powder with the odor of chlorine, almost insoluble in water, soluble in eucalyptol and chlorinated paraffin. It gradually decomposes on exposure to air, releasing chlorine. A surgical antiseptic in 2–10% oil solution. Syn., *dichloramine.* See *chloramine-T.*

dichlor-mapharsen. Trade-mark for a mixture containing dichlorophenarsine hydrochloride as the active ingredient.

di·chlo″ro·a·ce′tic ac′id. $CHCl_2.COOH$. A colorless liquid at ordinary temperatures, crystallizing at lower temperatures; soluble in water and alcohol. Used as an escharotic.

di·chlo″ro·di·eth″yl·sul′fide (·dye·eth″il·sul′fide, ·fid). $(C_2H_4Cl)_2S$. Mustard gas. A vesicant in chemical warfare. A heavy, somewhat volatile fluid with an odor resembling mustard. Produces severe vesication and slowly healing, painful ulcers.

di·chlo′ro-di·flu″o·ro·meth′ane (dye·klor′o-dye-flōō″o·ro·meth′ane). CCl_2F_2. A noninflammable gas of low toxicity used as a refrigerant. See *freon-12.*

di·chlo″ro·di·phen′yl tri·chlo″ro·eth′ane (dye-klor″o·dye·fen′il try·klor″o·eth′ane, ·dye·fee′nil). See *DDT.*

sym.-di·chlo″ro·eth′yl·ene. Acetylene dichloride.

di·chlo″ro·phen′ar·sine hy″dro·chlo′ride (dye-klor″o·fen′ahr·seen, ·sin, ·fen·ahr′sin). 3-Amino-4-hydroxy-phenyl-dichlorarsine hydrochloride, $C_6H_6AsCl_2NO.HCl$. A white, odorless powder used as an antisyphilitic. It is supplied as a mixture with buffering agents to render its solution suitable for intravenous use. Dose, 30–60 mg. (½–1 gr.) at intervals of 4–5 days. See *clorarsen, dichlor-mapharsen.*

di·chlo″ro·phe′nol-in″do·phe′nol so′di·um. Sodium 2,6-dichlorophenol-indophenol. $O:C_6H_2-Cl_2:N.C_6H_4ONa$. Dark-green powder, soluble in water and alcohol; used in analytical determination of ascorbic acid.

di·chlo″ro·phen·ox″y·a·ce′tic ac′id. 2,4-Dichlorophenoxyacetic acid; substance regulating plant growth; also found to be an effective herbicide. Abbreviated, 2,4-D.

di·cho′ri·al (dye·kor′ee·ul) [*dis;* G. *chorion,* skin]. Having two chorions.

di·chot′o·mize (dye·cot′o·mize) [G. *dichotomein,* to cut in twain]. Divide a distribution, variable, or series into two parts according to a specified classification, as persons with or without a known disease or characteristic.

di·chot′o·my [*dichotomein*]. 1. Division into two equal branches. 2. The type of branching of plants in which there are repeated equal divisions of the stem.

di·chro′ic [G. *dis,* twice; *chroia,* color]. Having or showing two colors; applied to doubly refracting crystals which show different colors when viewed from different directions; or to solutions that show different colors in varying degrees of concentration. —**di′chroism,** *n.*

di·chro′ine. Any of three isomeric alkaloids, designated α-dichroine, β-dichroine, and γ-dichroine, isolated from *Dichroa febrifuga,* which is the probable source of the Chinese antimalarial drug *ch′ang shan.* α-Dichroine is probably identical with isofebrifugine, while β-dichroine and γ-dichroine appear to be crystalline modifications of febrifugine.

di·chro′ma·sy, di″chro·ma′si·a (dye″kro·may′-zhuh, ·zee·uh). See *dichromatism.*

di′chro·mat, di′chro·mate [*dis;* G. *chrōma,* color]. A person affected with dichromatopsia. —**dichromat′ic,** *n.*

di·chro′mate. Any salt characterized by the presence of the $Cr_2O_7^{=}$ anion: also called *bichromate.*

di″chro·mat′ic [*dis; chrōma*]. 1. *In biology,* exhibiting two colors, regardless of sex or age. 2. *In psychology,* pertaining to that form of color blindness in which only two of the fundamental colors can be seen.

di·chro′ma·tism. A condition in which an individual can perceive only two of the three basic hues (red, green, and blue). See *protanopia, deuteranopia, tritanopia.*

di·chro″ma·top′si·a [*dis; chrōma;* G. *opsis,* vision]. See *dichromatism.*

di·chro′mic [*dis; chrōma*]. 1. Marked by two colors. 2. Containing two atoms of chromium.

di′chro·mism, di·chro′mism [*dis; chrōma*]. Dichroism; the state of being dichroic.

di·chro′mo·phil [*dis; chrōma;* G. *philein,* to love]. Characterizing a tissue or cell which takes both an acid and a basic stain.

di″chro·moph′i·lism [*dis; chrōma; philein*]. Capacity for double staining. —**dichro′mophil, dichro′mophile,** *adj.*

di·cin′cho·nine (dye·sin′ko·neen, ·nin, dye″sin-ko′nin). An alkaloid of cinchona bark.

Dick, George Frederick (1881–). American physician, who, with his wife, Gladys Rowena Henry Dick, isolated the erythrogenic (Dick) toxin and originated (1924) a test for individual susceptibility to scarlet fever (see Dick *test*) and with her prepared curative antitoxin and a method of immunizing against the disease.

Dick, Gladys Rowena Henry (1881–). American physician, known for her work on scarlet fever with her husband. See George Frederick *Dick.*

di″cli·dot′o·my. Valvotomy.

dicodid bitartrate. Trade-marked name for *dihydrocodeinone bitartrate.*

di′co·phane. A name sometimes applied to the medicinal grade of DDT. Syn., *chlorophenothane.*

di·co′ri·a. See *diplocoria.*

di·cou′ma·rin (dye·kōō′muh·rin). Bishydroxy-coumarin.

dicoumarol. British Pharmacopoeia title for *bishydroxycoumarin.*

Di″cro·coe′li·um (dye″kro·see′lee·um, dick″ro·) [G. *dikroos,* forked; *koilia,* belly]. A genus of trematodes.

D. dendriticum. A species of flukes which has as its definitive host sheep and other herbivorous animals, with some cases of human infestation reported.

di·crot′ic notch. A notch in the descending limb of the pulse of a peripheral artery, as recorded in a pulse tracing.

di′cro·tism [G. *dikrotos,* double-beating]. A condition of the pulse in which with every wave there is given to the finger of the examiner the sensation of two beats; occurs in fever and after inhalation of amyl nitrite. —**dicrot′ic,** *adj.*

dic′ty·o·cyte [G. *dictyon,* network; *kytos,* cell]. A cell associated with hyperplastic reticulum and excessive proliferation of reticulin fibrils; it is polyhedral and medium-sized with a neutrophilic cytoplasm, and has a large nucleus rich in basichromatin and with a prominent nucleolus.

dic″ty·o·cy·to′ma [*dictyon; kytos;* G. *-ōma,* tumor]. A type of reticulosarcoma in which the dictyocyte is the common cell.

dic″ty·o·ki·ne′sis [G. *diktyon,* net; *kinēsis,* motion]. Division of the Golgi apparatus in karyokinesis.

dicumarol. A collective trade-mark for *bishydroxycoumarin.*

di·cy′clo·mine hy″dro·chlo′ride. Generic name for diethylaminocarbethoxybicyclohexyl hydrochloride; $C_{19}H_{35}NO_2.HCl$; a smooth muscle antispasmodic supplied under the trade-marked name *bentyl hydrochloride.*

di·cys′te·ine. Cystine.

di·dac′tic (dye·dack′tick, di·dack′tick) [G. *didaktos*, from *didaskein*, to teach]. *In medicine*, pertaining to teaching by lectures and textbooks, as opposed to instruction by the clinical method.

di·dac′tyl·ism (dye·dack′til·iz·um) [G. *dis*, twice; *daktylos*, finger]. The congenital condition in which there are but two digits on a hand or foot. See *bidactyly.*

di·del′phic [*dis;* G. *delphys*, womb]. Having a double uterus.

Didot, Alphonse [*Belgian surgeon*, nineteenth century]. Remembered for his description of a standard operation for webbed fingers, in which a dorsal flap is moved from one finger and a volar flap from the other (1849); called *Didot's operation.*

did·y·mi′tis. Orchitis.

did′y·mous [G. *didymos*, twin]. Growing in pairs; arranged in a pair, or in pairs.

did′y·mus [*didymos*]. 1. A twin. 2. A double monstrosity. 3. A testis.

die [OF. *de*, from L. *datus*, given]. An exact reproduction in metal of any object or cast. Used in dentistry for the swaging of prosthetic appliances; referred to as the **male die,** and is usually made of zinc or Babbitt metal. The **counter-die** is the product of casting a lower fusing metal, lead, or an alloy to fit in opposition to the die. This is known as the **female die.** Prosthetic appliances are constructed by swaging a metal plate between the die and the counter-die.

die [ME. *dien*]. Cease to live; expire.

Dieffenbach, Johann Friedrich [*German surgeon*, 1792–1847]. An early worker in the fields of plastic and orthopedic surgery; succeeded in skin grafting and in treating clubfoot by tenotomy (1829–34). First to treat strabismus successfully by myotomy (1842), which operation later was abandoned because of unsatisfactory end results.

di·el′drin. The assigned common name for an insecticide containing not less than 85% of 1,2,3,4,-10,10-hexachloro-6,7-epoxy-1,4,4a,5,6,7,8,8a-octahydro-1,4,5,8-dimethanonaphthalene, a crystalline solid, soluble in many organic solvents but insoluble in water.

di″e·lec·trol′y·sis [G. *dia*, through; *ēlektron*, amber; *lysis*, a loosing]. Electrolysis of a compound, the current passing through a diseased portion of the body and carrying one of the elements of the compound with it.

Diels, Otto (1876–). German chemist, known for his research in the field of organic chemistry. In 1950 he shared the Nobel prize in chemistry with Kurt Alder for the development of the **Diels-Alder reaction,** a simple, practical, and inexpensive method for making ring compounds from such chain compounds as butadiene, chloroprene, and other similar rubber ingredients, by forcing them to combine with maleic anhydride.

di·em′bry·o·ny [G. *dis*, twice; *embryon*, embryo]. The formation or production of two embryos from a single ovum, twinning.

di″en·ceph′a·lon [G. *dia*, through; *egkephalos*, brain]. That part of the brain between the telencephalon and the mesencephalon. It includes the thalami and most of the third ventricle. Syn., *betweenbrain, interbrain.* —**diencephal′ic,** *adj.*

di″en·es′trol. $HO.C_6H_4.C(:CHCH_3)_2.C.C_6H_4.OH$.-3,4-Bis(*p*-hydroxyphenyl)-2,4-hexadiene; white crystals, practically insoluble in water. It is a synthetic estrogen, said to be more powerful than diethylstilbestrol and to be less toxic. The British Pharmacopoeia official name is *dienœstrol.* Syn., *dehydrostilbestrol.* See *restrol.*

Di·en″ta·moe′ba (dye·en″tuh·mee′buh) [G. *dis*, twice; *endon*, within; *amoibē*, change]. A genus of parasitic protozoa having two nuclei.

D. fragilis. A species of nonpathogenic intestinal amebas found in the colon of man.

di·es′trum, di·oes′trum (dye·ess′trum), **di·es′trus, di·oes′trus** (dye·ess′trus) [*dis;* G. *oistros*, gadfly, frenzy]. The period of quiescence or sexual rest of a polyestrous animal; the longest stage of the estrous cycle in which there is a gradual reconstitution of the uterine mucosa or endometrium in preparation for the reception of a fertilized ovum. —**diestrous,** *adj.*

di′et [G. *diaita*, manner of living]. 1. Food and drink regularly consumed. 2. Food prescribed, regulated, or restricted as to kind and amount, for therapeutic or other purposes. —**dietet′ic,** *adj.;* **dietist,** *n.*

acid-ash d. One used to lower the pH of the urine.

alkaline-ash d. One used to raise the pH of the urine.

bland d. One free of stimulating or irritating ingredients.

Coleman d. A high-caloric, largely liquid diet introduced by Coleman for the treatment of typhoid fever.

diabetic d. One used in the treatment of diabetes, usually containing weighed or measured amounts of carbohydrate, protein, and fat.

elimination d. A severely restricted diet designed to demonstrate to what foods, if any, a patient reacts allergically.

gout d. A low-purine, more or less low-protein diet used in gout.

high-caloric d. One containing a large number (3,000–5,000) of calories.

high-protein d. One containing a large amount of protein, used especially in anemia, hypoproteinemia, and obesity.

high-vitamin d. One rich in vitamins, used in vitamin-deficiency diseases, anemia, hyperthyroidism, tuberculosis, etc. It is often combined with a high-caloric diet.

Karell d. A restricted-fluid, low-salt regimen at one time much used in cases with edema, especially when due to myocardial failure.

Kempner rice d. A rigid diet of rice, fruit, and sugar, with no additional salt, and averaging about 2000 calories per day: used in the treatment of hypertension.

ketogenic d. One in which fat is high in relation to carbohydrate, so that ketosis is produced; it was formerly used in the treatment of epilepsy and urinary-tract infections.

Lenhartz d. A low-caloric regimen for the treatment of gastrointestinal ulcer; it consists chiefly of milk and eggs.

low-caloric d. One containing a small number (600–1500) of calories.

low-salt d. One low in its content of sodium salt; once widely used in the treatment of hypertension, this diet has been used chiefly in cases of edema.

Meulengracht d. One especially recommended for patients with bleeding peptic ulcer; it includes liberal amounts of food.

Minot-Murphy d. A diet high in protein, purines, and iron, the chief constituent of which is liver; used in the treatment of pernicious anemia.

necrogenic yeast d. A diet which contains only 7% protein and no tocopherol. The yeast used lacks cystine and methionine.

obesity d. A low-caloric diet, used to reduce weight; also called *reducing diet.*

Rowe diets. A regimen of elimination diets.

salt-free d. A term used erroneously to describe diets low in sodium chloride. A diet without added salt will contain approximately 3–5 Gm. of NaCl; when salt is not used in cooking, 2–3 Gm.; using only foods containing a minimum of salt may bring the total down to 0.5–1.0 Gm.

Schmidt d. Diet used to study fat metabolism in suspected cases of sprue.

S.H.G. d. Sauerbruch, Herrmannsdorfer, Gerson diet; used in the treatment of tuberculosis; characterized chiefly by the exclusion of sodium chloride from the diet.

Sippy d. One used in the treatment of gastric and duodenal ulcer; it combines alkalies with neutralizing foods.

soft d. One consisting of easily consumed, easily digested foods.

di′et. 1. To take food according to a regimen. 2. To cause to take food according to a regimen.

di′e·tar″y [*diaita*]. 1. A rule of diet. 2. A treatise describing such rule or rules. 3. A fixed allowance of food.

di″e·tet′ics [*diaitētikos*, of diet]. The science of the systematic regulation of the diet for hygienic or therapeutic purposes.

di·eth′a·zine. British generic name for 10-(β-diethylaminoethyl)-phenothiazine, a drug possessing atropinelike actions. The hydrochloride is supplied under the trade-marked name *diparcol.*

Diethelm's method. See under *method.*

di″e·thox′in. See under *intracaine.*

di·eth″yl·a·mine′ (dye·eth″il·uh·meen′, ·am′een, ·am′in, dye″eh·thil′uh·meen, ·min). $(C_2H_5)_2NH$. A colorless liquid which is found in putrefying fish.

di·eth″yl·bar″bi·tu′ric ac′id. Barbital.

di·eth″yl·car·bam′a·zine ci′trate. $C_{10}H_{21}N_3O.C_6H_8O_7$; 1-diethylcarbamyl-4-methylpiperazine dihydrogen citrate; a white, crystalline powder, very soluble in water. It is effective in treating wuchereriasis, loiasis, ascariasis, and onchocerciasis. See *hetrazan.*

di·eth″yl·ene·di″a·mine′ (dye·eth″il·een·dye″uh-meen′, ·dye·am′in). See *piperazine.*

di·eth′yl·ene gly′col mon″o·eth′yl e′ther. See *carbitol*, 1.

di·eth′yl·ene ox′ide. Dioxane.

di·eth′yl e′ther. Ether, 3.

di·eth″yl·mal″o·nyl·u·re′a. Barbital.

N,N-di·eth″yl·nic″o·tin·am′ide. Nikethamide.

di·eth″yl·stil·bes′trol (*diethylstilbestrol*). $HO.C_6H_4.(C_2H_5)C:C(C_2H_5).C_6H_4OH$; α,β-diethyl-4,4′-stilbenediol; occurs as a white, crystalline powder; insoluble in water but soluble in most organic solvents. Diethylstilbestrol is a synthetic compound possessing strong estrogenic properties, but does not have the steroid structure. It is used as a substitute for the natural hormones of this type. It is more readily absorbed from the alimentary canal than most of the natural hormones and hence is suitable for oral use. It is marketed under various trade-marks as *neo-oestranol I*, *cyren*, *stilrone*, *estrobene.* Dose, 0.5–2.0 mg. ($\frac{1}{120}$–$\frac{1}{30}$ gr.). Syn. *stilbestrol*, *stilboestrol.*

d. dipropionate. Diethylstilbestrol in which both phenolic groups are esterified with propionic acid. When administered intramuscularly in oil, reactions such as nausea and vomiting are less frequent than with free diethylstilbestrol. The dipropionate is relatively slowly absorbed.

di″e·ti′tian, di″e·ti′cian [G. *diaita*, manner of living]. An individual trained in the scientific management of the meals of an individual or a group of individuals; in institutions, one who arranges diet programs for purposes of adequate nutrition of the well and therapeutic nutrition of the sick; one trained in the science of dietetics.

chief d. An officer in the U. S. Women's Medical Specialist Corps who acts as an advisor to the commanding officer of a medical installation and is responsible for the supervision of the activities of dietitians and other personnel under her jurisdiction and of training programs as indicated.

Dietl, Józef (1804–78). Polish physician who described a symptom complex due to angulation of a ureter. See Dietl's *crisis.*

di″e·to·ther′a·py [*diaita;* G. *therapeia*, treatment]. That branch of dietetics which has to do with the use of food for therapeutic purposes.

Dieulafoy, Georges [*French physician*, 1839–1911]. Devised an apparatus used to evacuate pleural effusion: a glass cylinder or syringe with piston and two-way cock for cannula and trochar. Described a type of gastric erosion which complicates pneumonia; called *Dieulafoy's ulcer.*

dif″fer·en′tial [L. *differentia*, difference]. Pertaining to or creating a difference.

dif″fer·en″ti·a′tion [*differentia*]. 1. The act or process of distinguishing or making different. 2. An increase in complexity and organization of cells and tissues during development.

auxanodifferentiation. The differentiation of specific function in organs at the time when they are assuming adult proportions and structure.

dependent d. The differentiation of a tissue partly as a response to an inductor or factor external to itself. Also called *correlative d.*

functional d. Differentiation which arises as a result of function. Also called *corporative d.*

histodifferentiation. The differentiation of cell groups into tissues having characteristic cytologic and histologic appearances.

invisible d. Differentiation which is determined but not yet apparent microscopically. Also called *chemodifferentiation.*

regional d. The appearance of regional differences within an individuation field.

self-d. The differentiation of a tissue, even when isolated, solely as a result of intrinsic factors after determination.

dif′flu·ence (dif′loo·unss) [L. *diffluere*, to flow in different directions]. Fluidity.

dif·frac′tion [L. *diffractum*, from *diffringere*, to break in pieces]. The separation of light into component parts by means of prisms, parallel bars in a grating, or layers of atoms in a crystal; thus producing interference phenomena such as lines, bands, or spot patterns.

x-ray d. When x-rays are passed through crystals they are diffracted in a manner similar to light rays passed through a ruled diffraction grating. A study of the diffraction of x-rays gives information on the crystal structure.

dif·fus′ate (di·few′zayt, dif′yoo·sayt, ·zayt). Dialyzate.

dif·fuse′ (di·fews′) [L. *diffusum*, from *diffundere*, to spread by pouring]. Scattered; not limited to one tissue or spot; opposed to *localized.*

dif·fus″i·bil′i·ty (di·few″zi·bil′i·tee) [*diffusum*]. Capacity for being diffused. —**diffus′ible,** *adj.*

d. of gases. Dalton's term for that property by which two or more gases, which have no chemical action upon each other, in an enclosed space expand as if the space were occupied by one gas alone; the pressures of the mixture being equal to the sum of the pressures of the combined gases.

diffusin. Trade-mark for a form of lyophilized hyaluronidase.

dif·fu″si·om′e·ter (di·few″zee·om′i·tur) [*diffusum;*

G. *metron*, a measure]. A device for estimating the diffusion of gases or liquids.

dif·fu′sion [*diffusum*]. 1. A spreading-out. 2. Dialysis. 3. *In optics*, the diversion of an appreciable fraction of energy of any one incident light ray into more than a few directions.

di·fla′vine (dye·flay′veen, ·vin, ·flav′een, ·in). 2,7-Diaminoacridine hydrochloride; an antiseptic related to proflavine and approximately as efficient.

di·flu″o·ro·di·phen′yl (dye·flew″or·o·dye·fen′il, ·fee′nil). $(C_6H_4F)_2$. A white powder; insoluble in water, soluble in alcohol or ether. See *antitussin*.

digalen. Trade-mark for a product which represents the cardioactive principles of digitalis as isolated by Cloetta.

di·gal′lic ac′id. Tannic acid.

di·gas′tric [G. *dis*, twice; *gastēr*, belly]. Having two bellies; said of a muscle having a fleshy part at each end and a tendinous portion in the middle.

di·gas′tric. The digastric muscle. See Table of Muscles in the Appendix.

Di″ge·ne′a [*dis;* G. *genos*, offspring]. A subclass of the Trematoda, which in their life cycle exhibit alternation of generations and alternation of hosts. It includes all the species of flatworms parasitic in man, such as the liver flukes. —**dige′neous,** *adj*.

di·gen′e·sis [*dis;* G. *genesis*, generation]. Alternation of generations.

di″ge·net′ic [*dis; genesis*]. 1. Relating to alternation of generations. 2. Referring to the Digenetica.

Di″gen·et′ic·a. Digenea. —**digenetic,** *adj*.

di·gen′ic (dye·jen′ick) [*dis;* G. *genesthai*, from *gignesthai*, to be produced]. 1. Referring to a genetic constitution of nondiploid organisms, which contains two different genes for any given locus. 2. Referring to hereditary characters which are determined by two different genes.

di·gest′ant (di·jest′unt, dye·jest′unt) [L. *digestum*, from *digerere*, to separate, distribute]. Concerning or promoting digestion.

di·gest′ant. An agent that promotes digestion.

di·gest′er (di·jest′ur, dye·jest′ur) [*digerere*]. An apparatus used to subject substances to high temperature and pressure in order to decompose, soften, or cook them; autoclave.

di·ges′tine (di·jes′teen, ·tin) [*digerere*]. An agent that promotes digestion. —**diges′tine,** *adj*.

di·ges′tion (di·jes′chun, dye·jes′chun) [L. *digestio*, from *digerere*, to separate]. 1. The act or process of converting food into assimilable form. 2. The softening of substances by moisture and heat. 3. The disintegration of materials by strong chemical agents. —**digest′ible,** *adj.;* **digestibil′ity,** *n.*, **digest′,** *v.t., v.i.*

artificial d. Digestion carried on outside of the body.

gastric d. Digestion by the action of the gastric juice.

intestinal d. Digestion by the action of the intestinal juices, including the action of the bile and the pancreatic fluid.

pancreatic d. Digestion by the action of the pancreatic juice.

peptic d. See gastric *d.*

primary d. Gastrointestinal digestion.

salivary d. Digestion by the saliva.

secondary d. The assimilation by body cells of appropriate pabulum.

Dighton syndrome. See Adair-Dighton *syndrome*.

dig′i- (didj′i-) [L. *digitalis*, pertaining to a finger]. A combining form signifying *digitalis*.

digifolin. A proprietary preparation of digitalis said to represent the therapeutically valuable constituents of digitalis.

digiglusin. Trade-mark for a product containing digitalis glycosides.

digilanid. Trade-mark for a mixture of the cardioactive glycosides from the leaves of *Digitalis lanata* in the approximate proportion in which they occur in the crude drug. The respective glycosides are known as digilanid A, B, and C, or lanatoside A, B, and C. See *digoxin*.

diginutin. Trade-mark for a product containing digitalis glycosides.

digipoten. A proprietary preparation containing the digitalis glycosides in soluble form. It is said to be of the same strength as digitalis leaf.

dig′it (didj′it) [L. *digitus*, finger]. A finger or toe. Also see *digitus*. —**digital,** *adj*.

dig″i·ta′le·in (didj″i·tay′lee·in, ·tal′ee·in). A term used to designate a mixture of active and inactive glycosides of digitalis.

dig″i·ta′lin (didj″i·tal′in, didj′i·tuh·lin) [L. *digitalis*, pertaining to a finger]. The original *Digitalinum verum* of Schmiedeberg and Kiliani; a mixture of amorphous alcohol-soluble glycosides from the seeds of *Digitalis purpurea*.

crystallized d. Digitoxin. Also called *Nativelle d.*

French d. A yellowish, odorless, bitter powder; said to consist of digitalin, digitonin, and digitoxin. Also called *chloroformic d.*, *Homolle's amorphous d.*, *insoluble d.*

German d. A white or yellowish powder said to consist of a mixture of glycosides, chiefly digitonin.

soluble d. See German *d.*

dig″i·tal′is (didj″i·tal′is, ·tay′lis, ·tah′lis) [L.]. Common foxglove. The dried leaf of *Digitalis purpurea*, introduced into medicine by Doctor Withering, of Shropshire, England, in 1785. Its activity is due to a number of glycosides, notably digitoxin. Digitalis is a powerful cardiac stimulant, increasing contractility of heart muscle, but lengthened refractory period and diminished heart size frequently follow. It also acts indirectly as a diuretic. Employed mainly in diseases of the heart where compensation is lost. A standardized preparation, powdered digitalis should be employed medicinally. *Digitalis lanata* is the European species from which digoxin and other cardioactive glycosides are derived. See *digilanid*.

d. infusion. Represents powdered digitalis, 1.5 Gm.; alcohol, 10 cc.; cinnamon spirit, 0.5 cc.; distilled water, to 100 cc. Dose, 4–12 cc. (1–3 fluidrachms).

d. injection. A sterile solution of one or more of the glycosides of digitalis in water for injection.

d. tincture. Represents in each cc. the activity of 1 U.S.P. Digitalis Unit. Dose, 0.3–1.8 cc. (5–30 min.).

d. unit. The activity of 0.1 Gm. of U.S.P. Digitalis Reference Standard, as determined by biological assay on the cat.

powdered d. The leaf reduced to powder and standardized to contain 1 U.S.P. Digitalis Unit in each 0.1 Gm.

dig″i·tal·i·za′tion (didj″i·tul·i·zay′shun, ·eye·zay′shun) [*digitalis*]. Administration of digitalis in sufficient amount by any of several types of dosage schedules to build up the concentration of digitalis glycosides in the body of a patient. In this way therapeutic effects are attained and thereafter only a maintenance dose is required. —**dig″italize′,** *v.*

dig″i·ta′lose (didj″i·tay′loce, didj′i·tuh·loce). A methyl pentose; one of the sugars obtained in the hydrolysis of certain digitalis glycosides.

digitan. A proprietary preparation consisting of the active principles of the digitalis leaf, free of digitonin and most of the inactive substances.

dig″i·ta′tion [L. *digitatus*, having fingers]. A fingerlike process, or a succession of such processes, especially that of a muscle attachment.

dig′i·ti·form″ [L. *digitus*, finger; *forma*, form]. Finger-shaped.

dig″i·to·gen′in (didj″i·to·jen′in, ·todj′uh·nin). The aglycone of digitonin.

digitol. Trade-mark of a fat-free digitalis tincture.

dig″i·to′nin. $C_{54}H_{92}O_{28}$. A glycoside from digitalis, lacking in typical digitalis action and reputedly irritant.

dig″i·tox″i·gen′in. $C_{23}H_{34}O_4$; the aglycone formed by the removal of three molecules of the sugar, digitoxose, from digitoxin; also the aglycone of lanatoside A.

dig″i·tox′in. $C_{41}H_{64}O_{13}$. The principal active glycoside of digitalis, introduced as Digitaline Nativelle; it occurs in crystals which are practically insoluble in water. The action is like that of digitalis, 0.1 mg. digitoxin being therapeutically equivalent to about 0.1 Gm. digitalis. Syn., *digitoxoside*. See *unidigin*.

dig″i·tox′ose. $C_6H_{12}O_4$. The sugar resulting when certain digitalis glycosides, notably digitoxin, gitoxin, and gitalin, are hydrolyzed.

dig″i·tox′o·side. International Pharmacopoeia name for *digitoxin*.

dig′i·tus (didj′i·tus) [L.]. A finger or toe; digit.

d. annularis. The ring finger.

d. minimus. Old term for the little finger.

d. quintus. The little finger or toe.

di·glos′si·a (dye·glos′ee·uh) [G. *dis*, twice; *glōssa*, tongue]. A form of schistoglossia in which the lateral lingual swellings fail to fuse, producing a bifid tongue.

di·glos′sus [*dis; glōssa*]. A person showing diglossia.

di·glu·ta·thi′one. The known oxidized form of glutathione in which two molecules of the reduced form are united by loss of two hydrogen atoms.

di·gnath′us (dye·nath′us) [*dis;* G. *gnathos*, jaw]. A monster with two lower jaws.

di·gox″i·gen′in. $C_{23}H_{34}O_5$; the aglycone of digoxin and of lanatoside C.

di·gox′in (dye·gock′sin, didj·ock′sin). $C_{41}H_{64}O_{14}$; a cardiotonic secondary glycoside derived from lanatoside C, one of the glycosides of *Digitalis lanata*. On hydrolysis it yields the aglycone digoxigenin and three molecules of digitoxose.

di·hy′brid (dye·high′brid, dye′high·brid) [*dis;* G. *hybris*, outrage]. The offspring of parents differing in two characters.

di-hydranol. Trade-mark for heptylresorcinol.

di·hy′drate. A compound containing two molecules of water.

di·hy′dric. Containing two hydroxyl groups in the molecule.

di·hy″dro·cho·les′ter·ol. Cholestanol, 1.

di·hy″dro·co′de·i·none. $C_{18}H_{21}NO_3$; an alkaloid, isomeric with codeine, which may be prepared by a catalytic rearrangement of codeine or from the opium alkaloid thebaine. Its action is similar to that of codeine, but it is more active and more addicting; it is used primarily as an antitussive, though it has no clear-cut advantage for this purpose.

d. bitartrate. $C_{18}H_{21}NO_3.C_4H_6O_6.2\frac{1}{2}H_2O$, occurring as white crystals or crystalline powder, soluble in water. It is the form in which dihydrocodeinone is commonly used as an antitussive. Usual dose, 10 mg. (1/6 gr.). See *dicodid bitartrate, hycodan bitartrate*.

di·hy″dro·co·en′zyme I. The reduced form of coenzyme I resulting when the latter accepts two hydrogen atoms, these saturating the double bond of the pyridine nitrogen atom of the nicotinic acid amide component of coenzyme I. Abbreviated, DPN.2H, when the coenzyme is referred to as *diphosphopyridine nucleotide* (DPN).

di·hy″dro·co·en′zyme II. The reduced form of coenzyme II resulting when the latter accepts two hydrogen atoms, these saturating the double bond of the pyridine nitrogen atom of the nicotinic acid amide component of coenzyme II. Abbreviated TPN.2H, when the coenzyme is referred to as *triphosphopyridine nucleotide* (TPN).

di·hy″dro·di·eth″yl·stil·bes′trol. See *hexestrol*.

di·hy″dro·er″go·cor′nine. A hydrogenated derivative of the ergot alkaloid ergocornine. See *hydergine*.

di·hy″dro·er″go·cris′tine. A hydrogenated derivative of the ergot alkaloid ergocristine. See *hydergine*.

di·hy″dro·er″go·cryp′tine. A hydrogenated derivative of the ergot alkaloid ergocryptine. See *hydergine*.

di·hy″dro·er·got′a·mine. A derivative of ergotamine, employed intramuscularly in the treatment of migraine. It is less toxic than ergotamine and has no uterine effect. See *DHE-45*.

di·hy″dro·e·ryth′roi·dine (dye·high″dro·i·rith′·roy·deen, ·din). $C_{16}H_{21}NO_3$. The hydrogenated derivative of erythroidine; the dihydro-β-erythroidine has pronounced curarelike activity.

di·hy′drol. An associated form of water having the composition $(H_2O)_2$.

di·hy″dro·mor′phi·none hy″dro·chlo′ride (*dihydromorphinoni hydrochloridum*). $C_{17}H_{19}O_3N$.-HCl. An alkaloid prepared by the hydrogenation of morphine; a white, odorless crystalline powder soluble in 3 parts of water. A respiratory sedative and analgesic considerably more powerful than morphine. Dose, oral, 2.5 mg. (1/24 gr.); hypodermic, 2 mg. (1/32 gr.). See *dilaudid hydrochloride*.

di·hy″dro·strep″to·my′cin. A derivative of streptomycin having the antibacterial action of, and used clinically like, streptomycin. It is available as the sulfate, for intramuscular use, and is toxic to the eighth cranial nerve.

di·hy″dro·ta·chys′te·rol (dye·high″dro·ta·kiss′·tuh·role, ·rol, ·rawl, ·tack″i·steer′ole, ·ol, ·awl). A synthetic steroid derived from ergosterol; possesses some of the biologic properties of vitamin D and some of those of the parathyroid hormone. It produces hypercalcemia and increased urinary excretion of phosphorus. Useful in treating hypoparathyroidism. See *A.T. 10, hytakerol*.

di″hy·dro·the′e·lin (dye″high·dro·thee′uh·lin, thee′lin). Estradiol.

di″hy·drox″y·a·ce′tic ac′id (dye″high·drock″see·a·see′tick, ·a·set′ick). Glyoxylic acid.

di″hy·drox″y·ac′e·tone (dye″high·drock″see·ass′·i·tone). $CH_2OH.CO.CH_2OH$; a simple ketose sugar derivable from glycerin or dextrose.

d. phosphate. Dihydroxyacetonephosphoric acid.

di″hy·drox″y·a·cet·one·phos·phor′ic ac′id. CH_2-$OH.CO.CH_2OPO(OH)_2$; a phosphoric acid ester of dihydroxyacetone, produced as an intermediate substance in the conversion of glycogen to lactic acid during muscular contraction. Syn., *dihydroxyacetone phosphate*.

di″hy·drox″y·a·lu′mi·num a·mi″no·ac′e·tate. A basic aluminum salt of aminoacetic acid, principally $NH_2CH_2COOAl(OH)_2$, containing also small amounts of aluminum hydroxide and aminoacetic acid; it is a white, odorless powder, insoluble in water. It acts as a gastric antacid and is useful for control of hyperacidity in the management of peptic ulcer. Dose, 0.5–1 Gm. (8–15 gr.). See *alglyn, aspogen, alzinox, doraxamin, robalate*.

di″hy·drox″y·an′thra·nol. $C_{14}H_7(OH)_3$. Anthrarobin. See also *anthralin*.

m-di″hy·drox″y·ben′zene. Resorcinol.

2,5-di″hy·drox″y·ben′zyl al′co·hol. Gentisyl alcohol, $C_7H_8O_3$, obtained from ethereal mother liquors as a metabolic product of *Penicillium patulum* Bainier. It has slight antibacterial activity.

di″hy·drox″y·cin·nam′ic ac′id. Caffeic acid.

di″hy·drox″y-es′trin. Estradiol.

di″hy·drox″y·phen·yl·al′a·nine. $(OH)_2.C_6H_3.CH_2.CH(NH_2).COOH$; the 3,4-dihydroxyphenylalanine, formed by oxidation of tyrosine; it is converted by a series of biochemical transformations, utilizing the enzyme dopa oxidase, to high-molecular-weight, black pigments known as melanins. Syn., *dopa.*

di″hy·drox″y·pro′pane. Propylene glycol.

di″hy·drox″y·pro′pyl bis′muth·ate (dye″high-drock″see·pro′pil biz′muth·ate, ·bis′muth·ate, ·mew·thate). $C_3H_5(OH)_2BiO_3$. An oral antisyphilitic. Dose, 50–100 mg. (¾–1½ gr.) t.i.d.

di″hy·drox″y·tol′u·ene. Orcin.

di″i·o″do·an′i·line (dye″eye·o″do·an′i·leen, ·lin). $C_6H_3NH_2I_2$. Brown crystals used as antiseptic in skin diseases.

di″i·o′do·form. $I_2C{:}CI_2$. Ethylene tetraiodide. Light yellow crystals which darken on exposure to light. An antiseptic similar to iodoform used as dusting powder or in ointment.

di″i·o″do·hy·drox″y·pro′pane (dye″eye·o″do-high·drock″see·pro′pane). See *iothion.*

di″i·o″do·hy·drox′y·quin. U.S.P. XV official title for 5,7-diiodo-8-quinolinol; $C_9H_5I_2NO$; a colorless or light yellowish to tan, microcrystalline powder, almost insoluble in water. It is used as an antiprotozoan agent in intestinal amebiasis and in the treatment of *Trichomonas hominis* (*intestinalis*) infections. Dose, 0.4–2 Gm. (6–30 gr.) daily. Also called *diiodohydroxyquinoline.* See *diodoquin, yodoxin.*

di″i·o″do·hy·drox″y·quin′o·line. Diiodohydroxyquin.

di″i·o″do·sal″i·cyl′ic ac′id. $C_6H_2.I_2.OH.COOH$. A yellowish, crystalline powder which has been used as an antipyretic and analgesic.

di″i·o″do·thy′ro·nine (dye″eye·o″do·thigh′ro-neen, ·nin, ·thigh·ro′nin). $C_{15}H_{13}I_2NO_4$; a substance obtained as an intermediate product in the manufacture of synthetic thyroxin. It has been used like the latter. Dose, 50–75 mg. (¾–1¼ gr.) orally.

di″i·o″do·ty′ro·sine (dye″eye·o″do·tye′ro·seen, ·sin). $I_2(OH).C_6H_2.CH_2.CH(NH_2).COOH$; 3,5-diiodotyrosine; a constituent of thyroglobulin; thyroxin is apparently formed from two molecules of diiodotyrosine by oxidative condensation. Syn., *iodogorgoic acid.* See Table of Hormones in the Appendix.

di·i″so·pro′pyl flu″o·ro·phos′phate. $[(CH_3)_2CH.O]_2FPO$; a colorless, oily liquid, sparingly soluble in water but hydrolyzing rapidly; miscible with oils. It is a powerful inhibitor of cholinesterase, produces marked and prolonged miosis, and is used in the treatment of glaucoma. It is highly toxic. Abbreviated, DFP. Syn., *isoflurophate.* See *floropryl.*

di·kar′y·on [G. *dis*, twice; *karyon*, kernel]. A phase or stage in the growth of the mycelium of many fungi in which the cells each have two haploid nuclei.

di·ke″to·pi·per′a·zine. Any of a class of heterocyclic compounds formed from two molecules of the same or different amino acids by condensation of the carboxyl group of each with the amino group of the other; the compounds may be considered to be derivatives of piperazine.

dik″ty·o′ma. See *neuroepithelioma.*

di·lac″er·a′tion (dye·lass″uh·ray′shun, dye″-lass·uh·, di·lass″uh·) [L. *dilaceratio*, from *dilacerare*, to tear apart]. 1. Act of tearing apart; being torn in pieces. *Obs.* 2. *In dentistry,* a partial alteration of the position of the formative organ during development, resulting in teeth with sharp angulation of the root and crown.

dilantin sodium. A trade-mark for diphenylhydantoin sodium, an anticonvulsant in the treatment of epilepsy. See *diphenylhydantoin sodium.*

dil″a·tan′cy. A form of thixotropy in which a viscous suspension changes to a solid under the influence of pressure.

dil″a·ta′tion (dil″uh·tay′shun, dye″luh·) [L. *dilatatio*, from *dilatare*, to spread out]. 1. The state of being stretched. 2. Enlargement, as of a hollow part or organ.

congenital d. of the colon. Megacolon due to a congenital defect in innervation. Also called *Hirschsprung's disease.*

digital d. Dilatation of a body cavity or orifice by means of one or more fingers.

d. of heart. An increase in the size of one or more of the cavities of the heart, arising from a relaxation or weakening of the heart muscle. It is associated with evidences of failure of circulation, resulting in congestion of the lungs and other viscera.

d. of stomach. Increase in size of the stomach from relaxation of the walls and expansion with gas or liquid.

hydrostatic d. Dilatation of a cavity or part by an introduced elastic bag which is subsequently distended with water.

di·la′tion (dye·lay′shun, di·lay′shun) [*dilatare*]. The act of stretching or dilating, as contrasted with dilatation, which is the state of being stretched. The two words are often used synonymously.

di′la·tor (dye′lay·tur, dye·lay′tur, di·lay′tur) [*dilatare*]. 1. An instrument for stretching or enlarging a cavity or opening. 2. A dilating muscle.

d. naris. A dilating muscle of the nostril. See Table of Muscles in the Appendix.

d. pupillae. The set of radiating involuntary muscle fibers in the iris, dilating the pupil. Also called *d. iridis.* See Table of Muscles in the Appendix.

d. tubae. Variant term for tensor veli palatini. See Table of Muscles in the Appendix.

dilaudid hydrochloride. Trade-mark for dihydromorphinone hydrochloride.

di·lec′a·nus (dye·leck′uh·nus). Dipygus.

dill. See *anethum.*

dil′u·ent [L. *diluere*, to wash away]. 1. Agent that dilutes the strength of a solution or mixture. 2. Medication which dilutes any one of the body fluids. —**dil′uent,** *adj.*

di·lute′ (di·lute′, dye·lute′) [*diluere*]. Make weaker and thinner by the addition of liquid, especially water; or thin and dissolve.

di·lu′ted al′co·hol (*alcohol dilutum*). Contains 41–42% by weight, or 48.4–49.5% by volume at 15.56° C., of C_2H_5OH.

di·lu′tion [*diluere*]. 1. Process of adding a neutral fluid to some other fluid or substance, in order to diminish the qualities of the latter. 2. A diluted substance; the result of a diluting process.

Di·mas″tig·a·moe′ba (dye·mass″tig·uh·mee′buh) [G. *dis*, twice; *mastix*, whip; *amoibē*, change]. A genus of free-living, coprozoic amebas. The species **D. gruberi** has been found in decaying feces by various observers.

dimazon. A trade-mark for diacetylaminoazotoluene, $CH_3.C_6H_4.N{:}N.C_6H_3(CH_3).N(CH_3.CO)_2$, a compound related to scarlet red, and used as a dusting powder with talc or as a 2% ointment to promote epithelial growth in the treatment of burns, wounds, chronic ulcers, etc.

di·meg'a·ly [*dis;* G. *megas*, large]. The condition of having two sizes: applied to spermatozoa.

dimenformon. Trade-mark of a brand of estradiol.

di"men·hy'dri·nate. Generic name for the drug supplied under the trade-marked name *dramamine.*

di·men'sion. A measurable extent.

vertical d. *In dentistry,* the distance between the upper and lower jaws when the teeth, artificial dentures, or other devices are in centric relation or in the position of rest.

di'mer. The compound resulting from combination of two molecules of the same substance and having twice the molecular weight of the single molecule or monomer.

di"mer·cap'rol. BAL.

di"mer·cap"to·pro'pan·ol. BAL.

dim'er·ous [*dis;* G. *meros*, part]. Consisting of two parts; used especially to describe two-parted tarsi of certain insects.

di·meth'yl- [*dis;* G. *methys*, wine; *hylē*, material]. A combining form denoting *the presence of two methyl groups.*

di·meth'yl ac'e·tal (dye·meth'il ass'i·tal). CH_3.-$CH(OCH_3)_2$. A colorless liquid used as an anesthetic alone or combined with chloroform.

di·meth'yl·a·mi"no-az"o·ben'zene (dye·meth'-il·uh·mee"no-az"o·ben'zeen, -ay"zo·ben'zeen, dye-meth'il·am"i·no-). $C_{14}H_{15}N_3$. Yellow leaflets used for coloring fats and butter and as an indicator for acid-base titrations. Syn., *butter yellow, methyl yellow.*

di·meth"yl·a·mi"no·eth'yl-ben"zyl·an'i·line (dye·meth"il·uh·mee"no·eth'il-ben"zil·an'i·leen, ·lin, dye·meth"il·am"i·no·). $C_{17}H_{22}N_2$. A synthetic substance shown to be antagonistic to histamine when injected into guinea pigs or rats simultaneously with the latter substance.

dimethylane. Trade-mark for 2,2-diisopropyl-4-hydroxymethyl-1,3-dioxolane, a relaxant drug useful in controlling anxiety states.

di·meth"yl·ar·sin'ic ac'id. $(CH_3)_2AsO.OH$. A deliquescent, crystalline solid; soluble in water. Usually employed in the form of sodium cacodylate. Syn., *cacodylic acid.*

di·meth"yl·ben'zene. Xylene.

di·meth"yl·car'bi·nol. Isopropyl alcohol.

di·meth"yl·di·sul"fa·nil'a·mide (dye·meth"il-dye·sul"fuh·nil'uh·mide, ·mid). $NH_2.C_6H_4.SO_2$.-$NH.C_6H_4.SO_2N(CH_3)_2$. A compound similar to sulfanilamide but used chiefly in the treatment of gonorrhea. Dose, 0.5–1 Gm. (8–15 gr.). See *uleron.*

di·meth"yl·gly·ox'ine. $(CH_3.C:N.OH)_2$; a white crystalline powder, used as a reagent for the detection and determination of nickel.

di·meth"yl·ke'tone. Acetone.

di·meth"yl·pro"pi·o·the'tin. $(CH_3)_2S^+CH_2CH_2$-COO^-; a compound analogous to betaine, isolated from a marine alga. It is an active donor of methyl groups.

di·meth'yl sul'fate. $(CH_3)_2SO_4$. A colorless liquid used as a methylating agent in chemical syntheses. It is a strong caustic and its vapor is powerfully irritant to the respiratory tract.

di·meth"yl·the'tin. $(CH_3)_2S^+CH_2COO^-$; a compound analogous to betaine; an active donor of methyl groups.

di·meth"yl·tu"bo·cu·ra'rine i'o·dide. The iodide of the dimethyl ether of *d*-tubocurarine, possessing the curare action of the parent substance but less prone to cause respiratory paralysis and of longer duration of action: used to produce muscle relaxation in surgery. See *metubine iodide.*

di·meth"yl·xan'thine (dye·meth"il·zan'theen, ·thin). 1. Theobromine (3,7-dimethylxanthine). 2. Theophylline (1,3-dimethylxanthine).

di·me'tri·a [*dis;* G. *mētra*, womb]. Condition in which the uterus is a double organ. Also called *uterus duplex.*

dimol. Trade name of an intestinal antiseptic composed principally of dimethyl-methoxy-phenol.

di·mor'phism [*dis;* G. *morphē*, form]. Property of existing in two distinct structural forms. —**dimorphous,** *adj.*

dim'ple [ME. *dympull*]. A slight depression.

postanal d. See coccygeal *fovea.*

sacral d. See coccygeal *fovea.*

dimp'ling [*dympull*]. An abnormal skin depression from retraction occurring in subcutaneous carcinomas.

dinacrin. Trade-mark for a brand of isoniazid, an antituberculosis drug having the composition of isonicotinic acid hydrazide.

di-*n*-bu"tyl·car"ba·myl·cho'line sul'fate (·car"-bah·mil·ko'leen, ·lin). A mydriatic and cycloplegic drug administered by instillation of one drop of a 7.5% solution into the conjunctival sac.

di·neu'ric (dye·new'rick) [G. *dis*, twice; *neuron*, nerve]. Provided with two axons; said of a nerve cell.

di·neu'tron. An atomic nuclear particle of neutral electric charge and twice the weight of the ordinary neutron.

din'ic, din'i·cal [G. *dinos*, a whirling]. Pertaining to or relieving vertigo.

di·ni"tro·ben'zene (meta-). $C_6H_4(NO_2)_2$. A yellow, crystalline substance, sparingly soluble in water, soluble in alcohol; used in chemical manufacturing.

di·ni'tro-or'tho-cre'sol. $C_7H_6O_5N_2$. Yellow crystals used with considerable danger to increase the metabolic rate in obesity.

di·ni"tro·phe'nol. $C_6H_3(NO_2)_2OH$. A potent but extremely dangerous stimulant to metabolism. Symptoms of toxic effects are fever and profuse sweating. Skin eruptions, acute hepatitis, agranulocytosis, and cataracts have been known to follow its use.

di·ni"tro·phen"yl·hy'dra·zine (dye·nigh"tro-fen"il·high'druh·zeen, ·zin, dye·nigh"tro·fee"nil·). $C_6H_3(NO_2)_2NH.NH_2$. Red, crystalline powder soluble in dilute acids. Used in identification and analysis of aldehydes and ketones.

di·nu'cle·o·tide. A nucleotide which upon hydrolysis yields two molecules of mononucleotide, which may be identical or different.

di'nus [*dinos*]. Vertigo or dizziness.

Diocles of Carystos [*Greek physician,* fl. 350 B.C.]. One of the greatest ancient physicians after Hippocrates.

di'o·coele (dye'o·seel). Lumen of the diencephalon, especially in the embryo; it forms part of the third ventricle in the adult.

Di·oc"to·phy'ma [G. *diogkoin*, to distend, blow out; *phyma*, tubercle]. A genus of large nematodes of the superfamily Dioctophymoidea.

D. renale. A species of kidney worms which occasionally infest man.

di·oc'tyl so'di·um sul"fo·suc'ci·nate (sul"fo-suck'sin·ate) (*dioctylis sulfosuccinas sodicum*). $C_{20}H_{37}O_7SNa$. A white, waxlike, plastic solid, soluble in 70 parts of water; employed as a wetting agent in the formulation of lotions, creams, ointments, and shampoos. See *aerosol OT dry, deceresol OT.*

di'o·done in·jec'tion. Iodopyracet injection. See *diodrast.*

diodoquin. Trade-mark for diiodohydroxyquin.

diodrast. Trade-mark for the diethanolamine salt of 3,5-diiodo-4-pyridone-N-acetic acid, the active, but unisolated, ingredient of iodopyracet injection, a radiopaque medium. See *diodone injection.*

di·oes′trum (dye·ess′trum). See *diestrum.*

di·oes′trus (dye·ess′trus). See *diestrum.*

dioloxol. A trade-mark for *mephenesin.*

di′o·nin. Ethylmorphine hydrochloride (*aethylmorphinae hydrochloridum*). $C_{19}H_{23}O_3N.HCl.-2H_2O$. A white or faintly yellow, microcrystalline powder, soluble in 10 parts of water. An analgesic and hypnotic, somewhat more powerful than codeine, to which it is closely related chemically; a cough sedative; a local lymphagogue in 1–10% solution in various inflammations of the eye. Dose, 8–65 mg. (⅛–1 gr.).

di′o·nism. Homosexuality.

di″op·sim′e·ter [G. *diopsis*, a view through; *metron*, a measure]. An instrument for determining the visual field.

di·op′ter (dye·op′tur) [G., one who sees through, scout]. Unit of measurement of the refractive power of an optic lens. It is the refractive power of a lens having a focal distance of one meter. Abbreviated, d. —**diopter′ic, dioptral,** *adj.*

prism d. A unit of prismatic refractive power; the refractive power of a prism that deflects a ray of light 1 cm. on a tangent plane situated at a distance of 1 meter.

diopterin. A trade-mark for sodium pteroyldiglutamate, a derivative of folic (pteroylglutamic) acid which is being investigated for possible usefulness as an adjunct in the treatment of malignancy.

di″op·tom′e·ter [G. *diopsis*, a view through; *metron*]. Instrument for determining ocular refraction. Syn., *optometer.* —**dioptometry,** *n.*

di·op′tric [G. *dioptēr*, one who sees through]. Pertaining to transmitted and refracted light.

di·op tric. A diopter.

di·op′trics [G. *dioptrikos*, of the science of dioptrics]. The branch of optics treating of the refraction of light by transparent media, especially by the media of the eye.

di″op·trom′e·ter. See *dioptometer.*

di·op′try. See *diopter.*

di″or·tho′sis [G., a making straight]. Surgical correction of a deformity, or repair of an injury done to a limb; diaplasis. —**diorthot′ic,** *adj.*

di″os·co′re·a [*Dioscorides*, Greek herbalist]. Wild yam root. The dried rhizome of *Dioscorea villosa*, a creeping plant, indigenous to the eastern United States. It yields an acrid resin and a saponinlike principle; has been used as an expectorant, diuretic, and antispasmodic.

Dioscorides, Pedanios [*Cilician botanist and military surgeon*, fl. 54–68]. Considered the founder of materia medica. His work, describing more than 600 plants and plant remedies, is accepted as the authoritative source of information on the materia medica of ancient times.

di·os′co·rine (dye·os′ko·reen, ·rin). $C_{13}H_{19}O_2N$. An alkaloid obtained from the tubers of *Dioscorea hirsuta*. A bitter and toxic alkaloid resembling picrotoxin. It produces paralysis of the central nervous system.

di′ose (dye′oce, ·oze) [G. *dis*, twice; *-ose*, chemical suffix]. A monosaccharide containing only two carbon atoms; it is the simplest form of sugar.

di″os·gen′in. $C_{27}H_{42}O_3$; a steroid aglycone obtained from a saponin in *Dioscorea tokoro* and other sources; it is of interest as a starting compound in the synthesis of cortisone, progesterone, and possibly other hormones.

di·os′min (dye·oz′min, ·os′min). A glycoside found in buchu leaves and other Rutaceae. A white, tasteless, crystalline powder related chemically to hesperidin. Syn., *barosmin.*

di″os·phe′nol. A crystalline substance which deposits from chilled oil of buchu leaves. Also called *Barosma camphor.*

Di·os′py·ros [G. *Dios*, of Zeus; *pyros*, wheat]. A genus of trees of the Styraceae. The bark of **D. virginiana,** the persimmon tree of the United States, is astringent and bitter and has been used in diarrhea, intermittent fever, and uterine hemorrhage.

diothane hydrochloride. Trade-mark for piperidinopropanediol-di-phenylurethane hydrochloride, a local anesthetic for mucous membranes in 1% solution. See *diperodon hydrochloride.*

di·o′tic (dye·o′tick, ·ot′ick) [*dis;* G. *ous*, ear]. Binaural; pertaining to both ears.

di·ox′ane, di·ox′an. 1,4-Diethylene dioxide, $(CH_2CH_2)_2O_2$, a colorless liquid miscible with water and many organic solvents. Employed as a solvent, and a dehydrating agent in the process of paraffin-embedding in histologic technic.

di·ox′ide. A molecule containing two atoms of oxygen and one of a base.

dioxogen. Trade-mark for a solution of hydrogen peroxide.

di·ox″y·an′thra·nol. Dihydroxyanthranol.

di·ox″y·ben′zene. See *hydroquinone.*

di·ox′y·line. Generic name for 6,7-dimethoxy-1-(4′-ethoxy-3′-methoxybenzyl)-3-methyl isoquinoline, a synthetic analog of papaverine, possessing vasodilative action useful in effecting relief of vasospasm. The drug is supplied as the phosphate salt, under the trade-marked name *paveril phosphate.*

di·ox″y·tol′u·ene. Orcin.

dip [ME. *dippen*]. 1. Preparation for the destruction of skin parasites in animals. 2. A sudden drop, or downward inclination, as in the audiometric curve. —**dip,** *v.*

4000-cycle d. A marked dip in the audiometric curve at the 4000-cycle area. Loss of acuity in this area, the most vulnerable in the human hearing, may be due to congenital lesion or to auditory trauma.

di-paralene hydrochloride. A trade-marked name for *chlorcyclizine hydrochloride*, an antihistaminic compound.

diparcol. Trade-mark for 10-(β-diethylaminoethyl)-phenothiazine hydrochloride, a drug possessing atropinelike actions. See *diethazine.*

di·pep′ti·dase. The enzyme which splits dipeptides to amino acids.

di·pep′tide. A chemical combination of two molecules of amino acids obtained by condensation of the acids or by hydrolysis of proteins.

di·per′o·don hy″dro·chlo′ride. Generic name for the local anesthetic substance available under the trade-marked name *diothane hydrochloride.*

di·phal′lus [G. *dis*, twice; *phallos*, phallus]. 1. Partial or complete doubling of the penis or clitoris. 2. An individual with such a condition. —**diphal′lic,** *adj.*

di·phen′an. $C_6H_5CH_2.C_6H_4O.CONH_2$; para-benzylphenylcarbamate, a white powder, almost insoluble in water: employed in the treatment of oxyuriasis.

di″phen·hy′dra·mine hy″dro·chlo′ride (dye″fen·high′druh·meen, ·min). Generic name for 2-(benzhydryloxy)-N,N-dimethylethylamine hydrochloride; $C_{17}H_{21}NO.HCl$; an antihistaminic substance supplied under the trade-marked name *benadryl hydrochloride.*

di·phen″yl·a·mine′ (dye·fen″il·uh·meen′, ·am′een). $(C_6H_5)_2NH$: used as a reagent for nitrates, chlorates, and other oxidizing substances with which, in the presence of sulfuric acid, it gives a blue color.

di·phen″yl·a·mine″chlo·ro·ar′sine (dye·fen″il-uh·meen″klo·ro·ahr′seen, ·sin, dye·fee″nil·). $(C_6H_4)_2NH.AsCl$. Adamsite, a sternutator used in chemical warfare. See war *gas*.

di·phen″yl·car′ba·zide. $C_{13}H_{14}ON_4$; an organic compound used for determination of chloride and the detection of iron, mercury, and other metals.

di·phen″yl·chlo″ro·ar′sine. $(C_6H_5)_2AsCl$. A solid used as a sternutator in World War I.

di·phen″yl·cy″a·no·ar′sine. $(C_6H_5)_2AsCN$; a toxic agent proposed for use in chemical warfare.

di·phen″yl·hy·dan′to·in so′di·um (dye·fen″il-high·dan′to·in, ·high·dan′toyn, dye·fee″nil·) (*diphenylhydantoinum sodicum*).

$$(C_6H_5)_2\overline{C.NH.C.ONa(:N)CO}.$$

A white powder, soluble in water. An anticonvulsant particularly useful in grand mal seizures and automatisms; it does not produce undesirable lethargy. Dose, 0.06–0.12 Gm. (1–2 gr.). See *dilantin sodium*. Syn., *phenytoin sodium*.

di·pho′ni·a [*dis;* G. *phōnē*, sound]. The production of two distinct tones during speech; double voice.

di·phos′gene. $ClCOOCCl_3$, a gas similar in its effects to phosgene.

di·phos″pho·gly·cer′ic ac′id. $CH_2OPO(OH)_2.CHOH.C(O)\sim PO(OH)_2$; 1,3-diphosphoglyceric acid; an ester of glyceric acid with two molecules of phosphoric acid characterized by a high-energy phosphate bond. It is an important intermediate in the breakdown of carbohydrate in tissue; its high-energy phosphate group is believed to be transferred from adenosinediphosphate to adenosinetriphosphate, the latter supplying energy required for physiological processes.

di·phos″pho·gly·cer′ic al′de·hyde. $CH_2OPO(OH)_2.CHOH.C(H)(OH)PO(OH)_2$; 1,3-diphosphoglyceric aldehyde; an ester of the hydrate form of glyceric aldehyde with two molecules of phosphoric acid. It is an important intermediate in the breakdown of carbohydrate in tissue; in the presence of coenzyme I it is oxidized to diphosphoglyceric acid, the dihydrocoenzyme I formed in this reaction subsequently reacting with pyruvic acid to produce lactic acid while regenerating the coenzyme I. Also called *diphosphoglyceraldehyde*.

di·phos″pho·pyr′i·dine nu′cle·o·tide (dye·fos″-fo·pirr′i·deen, ·din). Coenzyme I; cozymase; a nucleotide made up of adenine, nicotinamide, ribose, and phosphoric acid. It is a coenzyme for numerous dehydrogenase reactions. Abbreviated, DPN

di·phos″pho·thi′a·mine. Thiamine pyrophosphate; cocarboxylase. Abbreviated, DPT.

diph·the′ri·a [G. *diphthera*, leather, membrane]. An acute, communicable disease caused by the *Corynebacterium diphtheriae* (Klebs-Loeffler bacillus); characterized by the formation of a false, adherent membrane on mucous membranes, usually of the pharynx, larynx, and trachea, and rarely of the conjunctiva and vagina. Locally, the disease produces pain, swelling, and obstruction; systemically, the toxin causes fever, prostration, cardiac damage, in some cases paralysis, and often death. —**diphtherit′ic, diphther′ic,** *adj.*

bull neck d. A condition in which edema of the anterior and lateral parts of the neck occurs in addition to swelling of the regional lymph nodes; it accompanies cases of severe faucial or nasopharyngeal diphtheria.

cutaneous d. An acute infection of the skin by *Corynebacterium diphtheriae*, manifested by a variety of cutaneous lesions, and sometimes followed by the systemic manifestations of diphtheria, due to absorption of the toxin. Rarely primary, the infection is usually secondary to autoinoculation, through contact with a carrier or through fomites.

d. antitoxin (*antitoxinum diphthericum*). Blood serum from a horse or other animal immunized against diphtheria toxin. A concentrated and refined serum (*serum anti-diphthericum purificatum*) is prepared by precipitating the various protein fractions and retaining the antibody-containing globulins. The antiserum is an aqueous solution of the globulins with a transparent or slightly opalescent quality. Average dose, prophylactic, 1000–1500 u.; therapeutic, 10,000 u. and over.

d. toxin. A toxalbumin produced by *Corynebacterium diphtheriae;* it is destroyed by a temperature over 60° C. and is capable of causing in susceptible animals the same phenomena induced by inoculation with the living bacilli.

d. toxin-antitoxin. A mixture of toxin and antitoxin used to produce active immunity against diphtheria; now superseded by toxoid.

d. toxoid. A detoxified diphtheria toxin used to produce active immunity against diphtheria. It has the advantage over toxin-antitoxin of not producing sensitivity to serum.

labial d. Localization of diphtheria to the outer two-third of the lips, with membrane formation, reported as a complication of cheilosis and fissures due to riboflavin deficiency.

surgical d. Formation of a diphtheritic membrane on the surface of a wound; cutaneous *d.*

diph·the′ri·a·phor [*diphthera;* G. *phoros*, bearing]. A diphtheria carrier.

diph′the·rin. Diphtheria toxin. See *diphtheria.*

diph″the·ri·ol′y·sin (dif″thi·ree·ol′i·sin, dif·theer″-ee·o·lye′sin) [*diphthera;* G. *lysis*, a loosing]. A lysin having a specific action on diphtheria toxin.

diph″the·ri′tis [*diphthera;* G. *-itis*, inflammation]. Infection with the *Corynebacterium diphtheriae.* —**diphtherit′ic,** *adj.*

diph′the·roid [*diphthera;* G. *eidos*, form]. Resembling diphtheria or the diphtheria bacteria.

diph′the·roid. 1. Any bacterium resembling the diphtheria bacteria, though not producing diphtheria toxin. 2. Any pseudomembranous formation not due to *Corynebacterium diphtheriae.*

diph″the·ro·tox′in. Diphtheria toxin.

diph·thon′gi·a [G. *dis*, twice; *phthoggos*, voice]. Production of a double tone of the voice; due to incomplete unilateral paralysis of the recurrent laryngeal nerve, or to some lesion of the vocal folds which causes each to produce its own sound.

diph″y·gen′ic [G. *diphyēs*, of double form; *genesthai*, from *gignesthai*, to be produced]. *In zoology*, characterized by or having two types of development.

di·phyl″lo·both·ri′a·sis [G. *dis*, twice; *phyllon*, leaf; *bothrion*, little trench; NL. *-iasis*, condition]. Infestation with *Diphyllobothrium latum.*

Di·phyl″lo·both′ri·um [*dis; phyllon; bothrion*]. A genus of tapeworms, formerly called *Dibothriocephalus.*

D. erinacei. A species of which only the larval stage is found in man, the adult worm being found only in dogs and cats.

D. latum. The fish tapeworm, a large tapeworm found in the intestine. The head has two suckers or bothria. The adult worm ranges from 3 to 10 meters in length, and may have over 4000 proglottids. The definitive hosts are man, dog, and cat. The first intermediate hosts are fresh-water copepods, and the secondary intermediate hosts are various fresh-water fishes. Infestation in man may cause disorders of the nervous and digestive systems, malnutrition, and anemia.

di·phy′o·dont″ [G. *diphyēs*, of double form; *odous*, tooth]. Having two sets of teeth, as the deciduous teeth and the permanent teeth.

dip″i·cryl′a·mine. $C_{12}H_5O_{12}N_7$; an organic compound used for Carere-Comes Siena orange method for potassium. Syn., *hexanitrodiphenylamine.*

dip″la·cu′sis [G. *diploos*, double; *akousis*, hearing]. Hearing of the same sound differently by the two ears.

d. binauralis. Perception of a single tone as having a higher fundamental pitch in one ear than in the other.

d. uniauralis. Hearing of two tones by one ear when only one tone is produced.

di″plas·mat′ic (dye″plaz·mat′ick) [G. *dis*, twice; *plasma*, anything formed or molded]. Containing matter other than protoplasm; said of cells.

di·plas′tic [*dis; plasma*]. Containing two substances; said of the constitution of some cells.

di·ple′gi·a [*dis;* G. *plēgē*, a stroke]. Paralysis of similar parts on the two sides of the body. —**diple′gic,** *adj.*

cerebellar d. Hereditary cerebellar ataxia associated with some degree of pyramidal paresis.

spastic d. Spastic paralysis of the legs; due to organic changes in the infantile brain, such as diffuse degeneration or atrophic lobar sclerosis, malformations or developmental defects, and microscopic cellular alterations. This disorder is sometimes associated with convulsions and mental deficiency.

dip′lo-, dipl- [G. *diploos*, double]. A combining form signifying *two, twice, twofold, double, twin*, etc.

dip″lo·al·bu″mi·nu′ri·a [*diploos;* L. *albus*, white; G. *ouron*, urine]. The coexistence or alternation of physiologic and pathologic albuminuria in the same subject.

dip″lo·ba·cil′lus [*diploos;* L. *bacillus*, small staff]. A pair of bacilli, joined end to end, as the result of incomplete fission.

dip″lo·blas′tic [*diploos;* G. *blastos*, germ]. Having two germ layers, ectoderm and entoderm.

dip″lo·car′di·ac [*diploos;* G. *kardia*, heart]. Having a double heart, or one in which the two sides are more or less separate, as in birds and mammals.

dip″lo·ce·pha′li·a, dip″lo·ceph′a·ly [*diploos;* G. *kephalē*, head]. Dicephaly. *Obs.*

dip″lo·ceph′a·lus [*diploos; kephalē*]. A monster with two heads. —**diploceph′alous,** *adj.*

dip″lo·coc′cin (dip″lo·cock′sin). An antibiotic substance obtained from cultures of certain streptococci.

dip″lo·coc′coid [*diploos;* G. *kokkos*, grain; *eidos*, form]. Resembling a diplococcus.

Dip″lo·coc′cus [*diploos; kokkos*]. A genus of bacteria of the family Lactobacteriaceae of the tribe Streptococceae.

D. gonorrhoeae. Synonym for *Neisseria gonorrhoeae.*

D. intracellularis meningitidis. See *Neisseria meningitidis.*

D. pneumoniae. A species that is oval or spherical, typically paired, encapsulated, nonmotile, and usually Gram-positive. It has been subdivided into types, of which 31 are recognized at present, but at least 55 have been described. It is one of the causes of pneumonia, especially lobar, but may also cause other infectious diseases, as meningitis, otitis media, pericarditis, and arthritis. Formerly called *pneumococcus.*

dip″lo·coc′cus [*diploos; kokkos*]. A micrococcus that occurs in groups of two, such as the pneumococcus.

dip″lo·co′ri·a [*diploos;* G. *korē*, pupil]. Double pupil.

dip′lo·ë (dip′lo·ee) [G. *diploē*, fold]. The cancellous bone between the outer and inner tables of the bones of the skull. —**diplo′ic, diploet′ic,** *adj.*

dip″lo·gen′e·sis [G. *diploos*, double; *genesis*, production]. Development of a double or twin monstrosity.

Dip″lo·go·nop′o·rus [*diploos;* G. *gonē*, offspring; *poros*, pore]. A genus of cestodes or tapeworms.

D. grandis. A species normally infesting whales and seals, with man accidentally infested by the ingestion of salt-water fishes, the second intermediate hosts.

dip·lo′i·cin. An antibiotic substance produced by the lichen *Buellia canescens.*

dip′loid [*diploos;* G. *eidos*, form]. Having double the haploid or gametic number of chromosomes.

dip″lo·kar′y·on [*diploos;* G. *karyon*, kernel]. A nucleus with twice the diploid number of chromosomes. *Obs.*

dip′lo·mate. One who has received a diploma. *In medicine*, a holder of a certificate of the National Board of Medical examiners, or a person who has been certified as a specialist by one of the American specialty boards, like the American Board of Surgery.

dip″lo·mel″li·tu′ri·a [*diploos;* G. *meli*, honey; *ouron*, urine]. Coexistence or alternation of diabetic and nondiabetic glycosuria in the same subject.

dip″lo·my′cin. An antibiotic substance elaborated by a *Diplococcus* species; it has been reported to produce promising results in pulmonary tuberculosis.

dip″lo·my·e′li·a (dip″lo·migh·ee′lee·uh) [*diploos;* G. *myelos*, marrow]. See *diastematomyelia.*

dip″lo·ne′ma [*diploos;* G. *nēma*, thread]. The chromosomes in the diplotene stage.

dip″lo·neu′ral (dip″lo·new′rul) [*diploos;* G. *neuron*, nerve]. Pertaining to a muscle supplied by two nerves from different sources.

di·plop′a·gus (di·plop′uh·gus) [*diploos;* G. *pagos*, that which is fixed]. A double monster consisting of conjoined twins equally developed but having one or more vital organs in common.

di·plo′pi·a (di·plo′pee·uh) [*diploos;* G. *opsis*, vision]. Double vision, one object being seen as two. —**diplop′ic,** *adj.*

binocular d. The most common type; due to a derangement of muscular balance of the two eyes; the images of an object are thrown upon nonidentical points of the retina.

crossed d. The result of divergent strabismus; the false image of the right eye appears upon the left side, and that of the left eye upon the right side. Also called *heteronymous d.*

homonymous d. The reverse of crossed diplopia; found in convergent strabismus. Also called *direct d.*

introspective d. Formation of images on noncorresponding retinal points, giving a perception of depth and perspective. Also called *physiologic d.*

monocular d. Diplopia with a single eye; usually due to hysteria, to double pupil, or to beginning cataract.

temporal d. See homonymous *d.*

dip″lo·pi·om′e·ter [*diploos; opsis;* G. *metron*, a measure]. Instrument for measuring the degree of diplopia.

dip′lo·sal. A trade-mark for *salicylsalicylic acid.*

dip′lo·scope [*diploos;* G. *skopein*, to examine]. Instrument for the investigation of binocular vision.

di·plo′sis [*diploos;* G. *-ōsis*, condition]. The establishment of the full double number of chromosomes by fusion of two haploid sets in fertilization.

dip′lo·some [*diploos;* G. *sōma*, body]. The pair of centrioles commonly found in certain cells.

Dip″lo·strep″to·coc′cus [*diploos;* G. *streptos,* curved; *kokkos,* berry]. Streptococcus.

dip′lo·tene [*diploos;* G. *tainia,* ribbon]. Applied to a stage of miosis in which the chromatin threads of the spireme are distinctly double.

di·po′lar (dye·po′lur). Bipolar.

di′pole″ [G. *dis,* twice; *polos,* pole]. 1. A particle or object bearing opposite charges. 2. A pair of electric charges, positive and negative, situated near each other in a conducting medium. Syn., *doublet.*

di′pole mo′ment. The measure of the electric asymmetry of a molecule. It is equal to the product of the ionic charges and their spatial separation.

Dippel's oil [for Johann Conrad *Dippel,* German alchemist, 1673–1734]. Bone *oil.*

dip′ping [AS. *dyppan*]. 1. Palpating the liver by quick depression of the abdomen. 2. *In veterinary medicine,* the act of submerging an animal for the application of a dip.

dip′pol·dism [after *Dippold,* German schoolteacher tried and convicted of manslaughter]. Flogging of children, especially school children.

dip″ro·so′pi·a (dip″ro·so′pee·uh, dye″pro·), **di·pros′o·py** (dye·pros′o·pee) [G. *dis,* twice; *prosōpon,* face]. *In teratology,* duplication of the face.

di·pro′so·pus (dye·pro′so·pus, dye″pro·so′pus) [*dis; prosōpon*]. A monster characterized by a duplicity of the face. Such monsters occur with all degrees of duplicity, as the **diprosopus dirrhinus** (a monster with a double nose) and the **diprosopus tetrotus** (one with four ears) (see Plate 25), and grade into dicephaly.

d. parasiticus. An individual with doubling of the face, one face being markedly smaller or less well formed.

dip·set′ic [G. *dipsētikos,* thirsty]. Causing or attended with thirst. *Rare.*

dip″so·ma′ni·a [G. *dipsa,* thirst; *mania,* madness]. Recurrent periodic compulsion to excessive drinking of alcoholic beverages. —**dipsoma′niac,** *n.*

dip″so·pho′bi·a [*dipsa;* G. *phobos,* fear]. A morbid fear of drinking.

dip″sor·rhex′i·a. See chronic *alcoholism.*

dip″so·ther′a·py [*dipsa;* G. *therapeia,* treatment]. Treatment of certain diseases by reducing the amount of fluid allowed the patient.

Dip′ter·a [G. *dipteros,* from *dis,* twice; *pteron,* wing]. An order of two-winged insects; includes mosquitoes, flies, midges.

Dip″ter·o·car′pus [*dipteros;* G. *karpos,* fruit]. A genus of trees, chiefly found in southern Asia, some of which furnish gurjun balsam.

dip′ter·ous [*dipteros*]. *In biology,* having two wings or winglike processes.

di′pus [G. *dis,* twice; *pous,* foot]. Bifid foot.

di′pus. Having two feet.

di·py′gus, dip′y·gus [*dis;* G. *pygē,* rump]. A monster with more or less duplication of the pelvis and lower parts of the back. Syn., *dilecanus.*

d. parasiticus. A monster having attached to its abdomen a more or less complete parasitic body. See Plate 25.

d. tetrapus. A dipygus with four legs.

d. tripus. A dipygus with three legs.

dip″y·lid·i′a·sis [G. *dipylos,* double-gated; NL. *-iasis,* condition]. A disease due to the *Dipylidium caninum,* the common tapeworm of dogs.

Di″py·lid′i·um (dye″pye·lid′ee·um) [*dipylos*]. A genus of tapeworms.

D. caninum. A species of which the dog and cat are definitive hosts, and man is an occasional host; these worms vary from 20–40 cm. in length. Fleas are the host of the larval stage.

di·rec′tor [L. *directum,* from *dirigere,* to send in a straight line]. Anything that guides or directs.

grooved d. An instrument grooved to guide the knife in surgical operations.

di·rhi′nus, di·rhy′nus. See *dirrhinus, dirrhynus.*

Di″ro·fi·la′ri·a [L. *dirus,* cruel; *filum,* thread]. A genus of filarial worms. Members of the species **D. immitis, D. magalhaesi,** and **D. repens** are parasites of dogs.

D. conjunctivae. A species of filarial worms reported in many areas of the Mediterranean basin and found in such diverse sites as the eyelids, conjunctiva, lips, and gastrosplenic ligament; considered by some authorities to be identical with *Filaria conjunctivae* and *F. palpebralis.*

dir·rhi′nus, dir·rhy′nus [G. *dis,* twice; *rhis,* nose]. Partial or complete doubling of the nose; mild degree of diprosopia: also sometimes spelled *dirhinus, dirhynus.*

dirt eat′ing. See *chthonophagia; geophagy.*

dis-, di- [G., twice]. A prefix signifying *two, twice,* or *double.*

dis- [L., asunder, in pieces, apart, in two, in different directions]. A prefix meaning *separation, the opposite of, reversal.*

di·sac′cha·ride (dye·sack′uh·ride, ·rid), **di·sac′cha·rid** (dye·sack′uh·rid). A carbohydrate formed by the condensation of two monosaccharide molecules.

dis·ag″gre·ga′tion [L. *dis-,* indicating separation; *aggregare,* to add to]. 1. A state of perpetual distraction which prevents an individual from entertaining any idea other than the one which dominates or occupies his mind, as in obsessive, ruminative states. 2. In hysteria, an inability to coordinate various new sensations and to connect them with visual impressions.

dis″ar·tic″u·la′tion [*dis-;* L. *articulatio,* putting forth of new joints]. Separation at a joint; amputation at a joint.

dis″as·so″ci·a′tion. The separation of a substance, initially present in a more complex state of organization, into its simpler parts, as when water in the form of $(H_2O)_2$ or $(H_3O)_3$ disassociates to single molecules of H_2O.

dis·az′o-, dis·a′zo-. *In chemistry.* a combining form indicating the presence in a compound of two azo (—N=N—) groups. —**disazo,** *adj.*

disc. See *disk.*

dis·charge′ [OF. *deschargier*]. 1. An emission, unloading, evacuation, or secretion. 2. That which is emitted. 3. *In electricity,* a setting free or escape of stored-up energy; the equalization of differences of potential between the poles of a condenser or other source of electricity by connecting or nearly connecting them with a conductor.

dis·charge′. To emit; to unload.

dis·charg′ing [*deschargier*]. Unloading; flowing out, as pus.

dis·cis′sion (di·sish′un, ·sizh′un) [L. *discissum,* from *discindere,* to tear]. 1. State of being torn apart. 2. *In eye surgery,* an operation for soft cataract in which the capsule is lacerated a number of times to allow the lens substance to be absorbed.

disc·i′tis (disk·eye′tis) [G. *diskos,* disk; *-itis,* inflammation]. Inflammation of a disk, especially of an intervertebral or articular disk.

dis′co-, disc- [*diskos*]. A combining form denoting *connection with,* or *resemblance to, a disk.*

dis″co·blas′tu·la [*diskos;* G. *blastos,* sprout]. A blastula produced by meroblastic, discoidal cleavage.

dis″co·gas′tru·la [*diskos;* G. *gastēr,* stomach]. The modified type of gastrula produced by meroblastic, discoidal cleavage of telolecithal ova.

disc′o·gram, disk′o·gram. A radiograph of an intervertebral disc after the injection of a water-soluble radiopaque substance into the disc proper. —**discog′raphy,** *n.*

dis′coid, dis″coid′al [*diskos;* G. *eidos,* form]. Shaped like a disk.

dis′coid. *In dentistry,* an excavator having a blade in the form of a disk.

dis·col″or·a′tion [L. *dis-,* indicating separation; *colorare,* to color]. Change in or loss of the natural color of a part.

dis″com·po·si′tion. A process by which an atom is dislodged from its position in a crystal lattice by direct nuclear collision.

Dis″co·my′ces (dis″ko·my′seez) [*diskos;* G. *mykēs,* fungus]. A name proposed and used to a minor extent for a genus of actinomycetes.

D. bovis. Synonym for *Actinomyces bovis.*

D. madurae. Synonym for *Nocardia madurae.*

D. minutissimus. Synonym for *Nocardia minutissima.*

D. tenuis. Synonym for *Nocardia tenuis.*

dis·coph′o·rous [*diskos;* G. *phoros,* bearing]. Furnished with a disklike organ or part.

dis″co·pla·cen′ta [*diskos;* L. *placenta,* cake]. A discoid placenta.

dis·co′ri·a. See *dyscoria.*

dis·crete′ [*discretus,* from L. *discernere,* to separate]. Not running together; separate; opposed to *confluent.*

dis·crim″i·na′tion [L. *discriminare,* to discriminate]. The act of distinguishing or differentiating.

one-point d. The act of distinguishing by localization a point of pressure on the surface of the skin.

tonal d. The act of distinguishing tone values. This function is located in the cochlea.

two-point d. The act of differentiating or identifying two points of pressure on the surface of the skin. The normal ability for this is proportional to the distance between the points.

dis′cus [G. *diskos,* disk]. A disk.

d. articularis. Interarticular fibrocartilage.

d. proligerus. The cumulus oophorus.

dis·cu′tient [L. *discutere,* to disperse]. A remedy which causes dispersion or disappearance, as of a swelling. —**discu′tient,** *adj.*

dis·ease′ [L. *dis-,* indicating separation; OF. *aise,* ease]. 1. The failure of the adaptive mechanisms of an organism to counteract adequately the stimuli or stresses to which it is subject, resulting in a disturbance in function or structure of any part, organ, or system of the body. A reaction to injury; sickness, or illness. 2. A specific entity which is the sum total of the numerous expressions of one or more pathological processes. The cause of a disease entity is represented by the cause of the basic pathological process in combination with important secondary causative factors. For any disease not listed here, see the specific name in alphabetical place and under *syndrome.*

aaa d. See *aaa disease.*

abiotrophic d. See *abiotrophy.*

acute d. One marked by rapid onset and short course.

acute respiratory d. Term applied by the Commission on Acute Respiratory Diseases to an acute febrile respiratory infection which occurs epidemically in military recruits, particularly during the winter months. Fever and constitutional symptoms predominate over respiratory symptoms of irritated or sore throat and cough. In contrast to the common cold, coryzal symptoms are not prominent. The disease has been transmitted to man with filtered secretions of the respiratory tract, and is presumably due to a specific virus. Immunity develops after infection. The infection is similar to influenza or grippe, but is not caused by the known influenza viruses. The duration of the illness is approximately one week. See also *common cold.*

Adams-Stokes d. Cerebral syncope with bradycardia.

adaptation d. See *adaptation disease.*

Addison's d. A condition brought about by hypofunction or dysfunction of the suprarenal glands; adrenal insufficiency. It is characterized by extreme emaciation, anemia, and deep bronzing of the skin, ending in death. The name also was applied formerly to pernicious anemia.

adenocystic d. See *adenosis of breast.*

air sac d. (*of poultry*). A disease of the respiratory system of chickens characterized by respiratory rales, slow rate of spread, and a protracted course. The etiologic agent is thought to belong to the pleuropneumonia group of bacteria.

Albers-Schönberg d. Osteopetrosis.

Albert's d. Achillodynia.

alkali d. Selenium poisoning.

Alzheimer's d. See presenile *sclerosis.*

amyloid d. See *amyloidosis.*

anserine d. A wasting of the muscles of the extremities, causing the tendons to be unduly prominent, suggesting the appearance of a goose's foot.

arc-welder's d. Benign pneumonoconiosis caused by inhalation of fine particles of iron oxide which eventually form aggregates in the lymphatics of the lung without producing pulmonary fibrosis: a form of *siderosis.* It is commonly seen in persons engaged in electric arc welding.

attic d. Chronic suppurative inflammation of the attic of the tympanic cavity.

Aujeszky's d. Infectious bulbar paralysis.

Australian X d. An epidemic virus encephalitis, prevalent in children; first appeared in Australia in 1917; it resembles poliomyelitis, and can be transmitted to some animals. It is thought to be related to, or identical with, Japanese B encephalitis.

Ayerza's d. A syndrome of chronic cyanosis, dyspnea, and sclerosis of the pulmonary artery.

Babinski-Froehlich d. See adiposogenital *dystrophy.*

bagasse d. See *bagassosis.*

Bang's d. Infectious abortion of cattle.

Banti's d. Chronic congestive splenomegaly. Also see Guido *Banti.*

Barcoo d. See *veldt sore.*

Barlow's d. Infantile scurvy.

Basedow's d. Exophthalmic goiter.

Batten-Mayou's d. The juvenile form of amaurotic familial idiocy, (c).

Bazin's d. See *erythema induratum.*

beetle d. Scarabiasis. A condition in which dung beetles are present in the intestinal tract. It occurs usually in children and produces symptoms of failing health such as anorexia, dysentery, and emaciation.

Behcet's d. Behcet's *syndrome.*

Bekhterev's d. Chronic arthritis of unknown etiology, with progressive deformity, stiffness, and bony fusion of vertebrae.

Bell's d. Neuropathy of the facial nerve.

Bernhardt's d. Abnormal sensations, especially of numbness, with hyperesthesia and pain on exertion, in the region supplied by the lateral cutaneous nerve of the thigh.

Besnier-Boeck-Schaumann d. Sarcoidosis.

Biermer's d. See pernicious *anemia.*

black d. An acute infectious disease of sheep. The most characteristic lesion is necrosis of the liver and extensive hemorrhages on the inner surface of the hide. The causative agent, *Clos-*

tridium novyi, Type B, multiplies in areas of the liver previously damaged by the liver fluke. This disease is prevalent in all areas where the liver fluke occurs.

blue d. Rocky Mountain spotted fever.

Bornholm d. Epidemic pleurodynia.

Bouillaud's d. See *rheumatic fever*.

Bourneville's d. See tuberous *sclerosis*.

Bowen's d. A disease involving the skin and sometimes the mucous membranes; may be a precancerous dyskeratotic process or a superficial epithelioma with lateral intraepithelial spread. Marked by reddish papules covered with a thickened horny layer.

Bright's d. Chronic nephritis.

Brill's d. See recrudescent *typhus*. Also see Nathan E. *Brill*.

Brill-Symmers d. See follicular *lymphoma*.

Buaki d. An avitaminosis due to lack of vitamin B, characterized by edema and depigmentation of the skin, the latter mostly on the face. The hair loses its luster and natural curl.

Buerger's d. Thromboangiitis obliterans, a chronic arteritis and phlebitis of the extremities, with thrombotic occlusion leading to gangrene; generally affects portions of the toes and feet.

Buschke's d. See *scleredema adultorum*.

Busquet's d. Periostitis resulting in dorsal metatarsal exostoses.

Busse-Buschke's d. Cryptococcosis.

caisson d. A condition caused by a too rapid return from high to normal (sea level) atmospheric pressure; affects tunnel and caisson workers, divers, and others who work under high atmospheric pressure; due to the formation of nitrogen bubbles in the blood and body tissues. Symptoms vary with the location of the bubbles and include pain in the abdomen, joints, and extremities, vertigo, various sensory or motor disturbances, itching of the skin, asphyxia, collapse, and unconsciousness. Prompt treatment usually assures recovery. Syn., *aeremia, bends, compressed-air illness, diver's neurosis.* Also see *aeroembolism*, cutaneous gaseous *embolism*.

California d. See *coccidioidomycosis*.

Calvé's d. Osteochondrosis involving primary growth centers of vertebral bodies.

Carrión's d. Bartonellosis. See also *verruca peruviana* and Oroya *fever*.

Castellani's d. See *bronchospirochetosis*.

cat-scratch d. See cat-scratch *fever*.

cave d. An apparently infectious disease of unknown etiology, so named because it was observed in persons who had spent several hours in a cave. The onset is abrupt, with epistaxis, headache, high fever, and squeezing chest pain. X-rays show pathologic changes of the lung.

celiac d. An idiopathic form of celiac syndrome seen in infants and young children in which recovery usually eventuates. The patient presents marked abdominal distention, malnutrition, and characteristic stools. Also called *Gee's d., Gee-Herter d., Gee-Thaysen d., Heubner-Herter d., chronic intestinal indigestion* or *insufficiency, chronic jejunoileal insufficiency, Herter's infantilism, intestinal infantilism, indigenous sprue, chronic idiopathic steatorrhea.*

Chagas' d. American trypanosomiasis.

Charcot-Marie-Tooth d. Progressive, familial, neuropathic muscular atrophy, characterized by weakness and atrophy of the peroneal muscles. This is accompanied by diminution of proprioceptive and cutaneous sensation and loss of deep reflexes. Talipes cavus frequently is present. Syn., *peroneal muscular atrophy, neuritic muscular atrophy.*

Chauffard-Still's d. See Augustus R. *Felty*.

Chiari's d. Obliterating endarteritis of the liver.

Christian-Weber d. Nodular, nonsuppurative panniculitis.

Christmas d. A hemophilialike disease due to a deficiency of the Christmas factor; PTC deficiency.

chronic d. One which is slow in its course and of long duration.

coal miner's d. See *anthracosilicosis*.

cobalt deficiency d. (*of ruminants*). A deficiency disease due to lack of cobalt in the forage. Cobalt is thought to be important in the synthesis of B_{12} in the rumen.

collagen diseases. Diseases characterized by widespread alterations of connective tissue, as rheumatic fever, rheumatoid arthritis, polyarteritis, acute disseminated lupus erythematosus, generalized scleroderma, or dermatomyositis: a clinically useful term.

comb d. Favus of fowls; a contagious skin disease of chickens, chiefly affecting the comb.

combined system d. See subacute combined *degeneration* of spinal cord.

communicable d. One which is readily transmitted from person to person by direct contact or through the agency of a vector.

complicating d. A secondary or independent disease superimposed upon one already existing. Syn., *intercurrent d.*

Concato's d. See *polyserositis*.

congenital d. One acquired in utero, and therefore present at birth.

congenital polycystic d. A hereditary disease in which parenchyma of the kidney and less frequently that of the liver and pancreas are replaced to a variable extent by multiple cysts.

constitutional d. (a) An inherent disease, owing to the individual's inherited genotypic characteristics. (b) A general disease involving the entire body, as contrasted to local disease confined to one part.

contagious d. A disease transmitted by direct contact with an affected person or with his secretions.

Cooley's d. Thalassemia.

cornstalk d. A disease of cattle and horses, resembling hemorrhagic septicemia.

Coxsackie d. A condition characterized by a group of clinical syndromes, as yet only partially established, related to infection with the Coxsackie viruses, and presenting the manifestations of such illnesses as poliomyelitis, aseptic meningitis, epidemic pleurodynia, and herpangina: a tentative designation.

Cruveilhier's d. See progressive spinal muscular *atrophy*.

Cushing's d. See pituitary *basophilism*.

cutaneous caisson d. See cutaneous gaseous *embolism*.

cystic d. of breast. A condition affecting women, usually near or at the menopause, characterized by the rapid development in the involuting breast of one or more fairly large cysts which can sometimes be transilluminated. At operation the cysts often show a thin blue dome and contain serous fluid. The bilateral polycystic form is also called *Reclus' disease.*

cystine d. Disturbance of amino-acid metabolism, probably faulty disintegration of these acids due to a recessive hereditary factor. It is characterized by aminoaciduria, dwarfism, albuminuria, polyuria, glycosuria, phosphaturia, presence of abnormal amounts of ammonia in the urine, or alkaline urine, skeletal changes suggesting rickets, hypophosphatemia, hypercholesterolemia, low alkali reserve, glycolability, and thermolability. Treatment is dietary: low-protein, alkaline ash, with high carbohydrate and fat.

cytomegalic inclusion d. A rare systemic disease characterized by the presence of intranuclear and intracytoplasmic inclusion bodies in the markedly enlarged cells of many organs: usually observed in infants and children and thought to be due to viral infection.

Darier's d. See *keratosis follicularis.*

Darling's d. Histoplasmosis.

David's d. A rare hemorrhagic disorder found exclusively in women, characterized by bleeding from mucous membranes, marked purpura, or both; it is probably due to ovarian hormone deficiency.

de Beurmann-Gougerot d. See *sporotrichosis.*

deficiency d. One resulting from the lack of a necessary dietary constituent, as minerals, vitamins, or fatty acids.

degenerative d. A general wearing-out process, in which no specific deficiency is recognized; common in old age.

degenerative joint d. A chronic joint disease of unknown cause, characterized by progressive loss of joint cartilage, condensation of subchondral bone, and in the advanced phase, spur formation. Early symptoms include some stiffness and pain about the joint, which characteristically are relieved by rest. Physical signs are joint crepitus and changes in the size and shape of the bones. Limitation of motion is due to bony deformity, never to bony ankylosis. Syn., *degenerative, hypertrophic,* or *senescent arthritis, arthritis deformans, osteoarthritis.*

demyelinating d. One of a large group of diseases of the nervous system which possess, as a common pathologic feature, foci in which the myelin sheaths of the nerve fibers are destroyed.

Dercum's d. Adiposis dolorosa.

diffused d. One which involves several tracts of the spinal cord.

DiGuglielmo's d. Acute erythremia.

Duchenne-Aran d. Progressive myelopathic muscular atrophy.

Duhring's d. See *dermatitis herpetiformis.*

Durand-Nicolas-Favre d. Venereal lymphogranuloma.

Durand's d. A febrile disease, occurring in North Africa, during the course of which a local cutaneous lesion develops accompanied by viremia, presence of virus in the cerebrospinal fluid, cough, vomiting, and lethargy. Recovery ensues after six to eight days with the development of complement-fixing antibodies in the serum.

dust d. See *pneumonoconiosis.*

Eale's d. Retinal periphlebitis associated with recurring vitreous hemorrhages; it is perhaps tuberculous in origin.

Ebstein's d. Congenital downward displacement of the tricuspid atrioventricular ring, usually associated with congenital hyperplasia of the right ventricle and patent foramen ovale.

Economo's d. See lethargic *encephalitis.*

Eddowe's d. See *osteogenesis imperfecta.*

endemic d. One which occurs continuously or repeatedly at the same season in a certain locality.

Engelmann's d. A rare disease of bone characterized by symmetrical fusiform enlargement and sclerosis of the shafts of the main long bones, usually associated with changes in the skull bones: also called *progressive diaphyseal dysplasia, osteopathia hyperostotica (scleroticans) multiplex infantalis.*

Engel-Recklinghausen's d. See *osteitis fibrosa cystica.*

epidemic d. One attacking a large number of people in one region at the same time.

Erb-Charcot d. Syphilitic spastic spinal paralysis.

familial d. One occurring in several members of the same family. Often restricted to mean several members of the same generation, in contrast to hereditary disease.

Favre d. Venereal lymphogranuloma.

Fete-Riga's d. Cachetic aphthae.

fibrocytic d. (*of breast*). See cystic *d.* of breast.

fifth d. See *erythema* infectiosum.

fishskin d. See *ichthyosis.*

Flajani's d. Exophthalmic goiter.

flint d. See *chalicosis.*

foot-and-mouth d. An acute febrile disease due to a filtrable virus; causes a vesicular eruption of the mucous membranes of the nose and mouth and the skin of the feet. It is contagious to ruminants and pigs and is often transmitted to other domestic animals as well as to man. Syn., *epidemic stomatitis, epizootic stomatitis.*

Fordyce's d. See John A. *Fordyce.*

fourth d. A syndrome occurring in childhood, characterized by an acute, reddish exanthema extending over the entire body, with the exception of the face, and followed by desquamation. It resembles scarlatina, but runs a mild course. The etiology is unknown.

fourth venereal d. Venereal lymphogranuloma.

Fox-Fordyce d. A chronic, itching, papular eruption, seen about the areola, the pubic area, the axillas; probably due to a disorder of the apocrine sweat glands. More common in women.

Freiberg's d. See Köhler's *d.*, (2).

Frei's d. See venereal *lymphogranuloma.*

Friedreich's d. Paramyoclonus multiplex.

functional d. One in which no definite cause or no demonstrable pathologic lesion can be discovered.

Gaisböck's d. See *polycythemia hypertonica.*

Gamna's d. See *splenogranulomatosis siderotica.*

Gaucher's d. A rare and frequently familial disease involving principally the reticuloendothelial system, and occurring in an acute infantile form and a more chronic adult form. It is characterized by enlargement of the spleen, bronzing of the skin, anemia, and, in children, by neurological symptoms. The cells of the lesion contain lipids of the cerebroside class. Also called *cerebroside lipoidosis, familial splenic anemia.* See also Gaucher *cells.*

Gee-Herter d. See celiac *disease.*

Gee's d. Celiac disease.

Gee-Thaysen d. See celiac *d.*

Gilchrist's d. See North American *blastomycosis.*

glycogen d. See *glycogenosis.*

Gougerot's d. 1. Sporotrichosis. 2. Gougerot's trisymptomatic disease. See nodular dermal *allergid.*

Gougerout-Blum d. A form of capillaritis, known as pigmented purpuric lichenoid *dermatitis,* seen principally in the lower extremities.

Graves's d. Exophthalmic goiter.

Guillain-Barré d. Guillain-Barré *syndrome.*

Gull and Sutton's d. Generalized *arteriosclerosis.*

Habermann's d. See *pityriasis lichenoides et varioliformis acuta.*

Hailey-Hailey d. See familial benign *pemphigus.*

Hammond's d. See *athetosis.*

Hand-Schüller-Christian d. A syndrome of childhood, insidious in onset and progressive, characterized by exophthalmos, diabetes insipidus, and softened areas in the bones, particularly in femurs and those of the skull, shoulder, and pelvic girdle. Pathologically the changes are due to lipoidosis of the xanthoma type. Both eosinophilic granuloma and Letterer-Siwe disease have been considered by some to be special manifestations of this disease. Syn. *lipoid granulomatosis.*

Hanot's d. Hypertrophic cirrhosis of the liver.

Hansen's d. Leprosy.

Hashimoto's d. See *struma lymphomatosa.*

Haxthausen's d. See *keratoderma climactericum.*

heart d. See *heart* disease.

heartwater d. A disease of ruminants seen in South Africa; due to *Rickettsia ruminantium* and transmitted by ticks. Resembles rickettsia infections in humans except for the large effusions in the serous cavities. There is a very high mortality.

Heberden's d. The condition associated with bony enlargement about the terminal phalangeal joints.

Hebra's d. See *pityriasis rubra, erythema multiforme exudativum.*

Heine-Medin d. See acute anterior *poliomyelitis.*

hemorrhagic d. Disease in which pathologic hemorrhage occurs, due to a disturbance in blood coagulation or to increased permeability of the walls of the blood vessels.

hemorrhagic d. of the newborn. A disease occurring in the first two weeks of life, usually between the second and fifth day; marked by spontaneous bleeding in any body tissues. Due to hypoprothrombinemia, resulting from a vitamin-K deficiency in the mother. Also called *hemophilia neonatorum.*

hereditary d. One transmitted from the parent to his offspring through the genes. May be dominant, recessive, or sex-linked.

Heubner-Herter d. See celiac *d.*

Hippel-Lindau d. See Arvid *Lindau.*

Hirschsprung's d. See *megacolon.*

hock d. *In veterinary medicine*, perosis, a deficiency disease characterized by the occurrence of deformed legs. Has been observed frequently in chicks fed on synthetic diets. The factor essential to prevent this disease in chicks so far has not been identified. Also called *slipped tendon.*

Hodgkin's d. A form of lymphoma of unknown cause, with manifold clinical manifestations terminating fatally, in which the histologic picture of the lymph nodes is characterized by pleomorphism, including besides adult lymphocytes, neutrophils, eosinophils, fibroblasts, and Reed-Sternberg cells. It is sometimes subdivided on the basis of the pathologic findings into three forms: (1) *Hodgkin's granuloma*, the most common and most protean in its clinical manifestations; (2) *Hodgkin's paragranuloma*, a comparatively benign form largely confined to the lymph nodes and exhibiting only limited systemic involvement; (3) *Hodgkin's sarcoma*, a highly malignant form of short duration. These three forms, which are probably different stages of this disease, may be difficult to distinguish, and generally, the less malignant forms mutate to the more malignant. Also called *scirrhous lymphoblastoma, granulomatous lymphoma, Hodgkin's lymphoreticuloma, pleomorphic lymphosarcoma.*

Holla d. Epidemic hemolytic jaundice.

hookworm d. See *ancylostomiasis.*

Hopf's d. See *acrokeratosis verruciformis.*

hunger d. See *hyperinsulinism.*

Huntington's d. See George *Huntington.*

Hurler's d. See *lipochondrodystrophy.*

hyaline d. of the newborn. A disease of unknown cause occurring during the first few days of the neonatal period, characterized by respiratory distress and frequently cyanosis. Diagnosis is made microscopically, a hyalinelike membrane being found lining many of the alveoli and alveolar ducts.

hypertensive vascular d. See *hypertensive vascular disease.*

idiopathic d. One in which no causative factor is recognized.

inclusion d. See cytomegalic inclusion *d.*

infectious d. One due to invasion of the body by pathogenic organisms.

intercurrent d. See complicating *d.*

Jaffé-Lichtenstein d. Fibrous dysplasia of the bones of the vertebral column.

Johne's d. A chronic enteritis of cattle, sheep, and deer, caused by *Mycobacterium paratuberculosis* and characterized by intermittent diarrhea and progressive emaciation without fever. Gross thickening of the mucosa of the small intestine and enlargement of the mesenteric lymph nodes without ulceration may occur.

Jüngling's d. See *osteitis* cystica of Jüngling.

kakke d. See *beriberi.*

Kaposi's d. Xeroderma pigmentosum.

Kienböck's d. Osteochondrosis of the lunate bone.

Kimmelstiel-Wilson d. See *intercapillary glomerulosclerosis.*

Köhler's d. Osteochondrosis: (1) of the navicular bone, formerly called *tarsal scaphoiditis;* (2) of a metatarsal head, usually the second, also called *Freiberg's disease.*

König's d. Osteochondritis dissecans.

Kufs' d. A late juvenile form of amaurotic familial idiocy.

Kümmel's d. Progressive collapse of a vertebral body following an injury. Possibly due to avascular necrosis.

Larsen-Johansson d. A rare form of *osteochondrosis* involving an accessory center of ossification in the patella: also called *Sinding-Larsen d.*

Legg-Calvé-Perthes d. See *osteochondritis deformans juvenilis.*

Leiner's d. See *erythroderma desquamativa.*

Léri's d. See *pleonosteosis.*

Letterer-Siwe d. A fatal disease of infancy and childhood, of unknown cause, characterized by hyperplasia of the reticuloendothelial system without lipoid storage. Manifestations include enlargement of spleen, liver, and lymph nodes, osseous defects, and involvement of the bone marrow resulting in secondary anemia. Cutaneous eruptions and purpura are frequently present. Also called *nonlipid reticuloendotheliosis, nonlipid histiocytosis.*

Lewandowsky's d. A rosacealike tuberculid.

Libman-Sacks d. See atypical verrucous *endocarditis.*

Lindau's d. See Arvid *Lindau.*

lipoid storage diseases. A group of rare diseases characterized by an accumulation of large, lipid-containing histiocytes throughout the reticuloendothelial system. They occur primarily in childhood. Included in this group are Gaucher's *d.*, Hand-Schüller-Christian *d.*, Niemann-Pick's *d.*, the infantile form of *amaurotic familial idiocy*, and *lipochondrodystrophy*. See also reticuloendothelial *granulomatosis.*

Little's d. See William John *Little.*

Lobstein's d. See *osteogenesis imperfecta.*

loco d. See *loco disease.*

Looser-Milkman's d. See Milkman's *syndrome.*

Lutembacher's d. The pathologic condition where there is an atrial septal defect in association with mitral stenosis.

Majocchi d. See *purpura annularis telangiectodes.*

malignant d. (a) Cancer. (b) Any disease in a

particularly violent form, threatening to produce death in a short time.

Marie's d. Rheumatic spondylitis involving the spine only, or invading the shoulders and hips (Strümpell-Marie type).

Mediterranean d. See *thalassemia.*

Ménière's d. See Ménière's *syndrome.*

Milkman's d. See Milkman's *syndrome.*

Mitchell's d. Erythromelalgia.

Moeller-Barlow d. Infantile *scurvy.*

Monge's d. Chronic mountain *sickness.*

Morquio-Brailsford d. See chondroosteodystrophy.

mosaic d. Virus disease of plants.

Newcastle d. An acute virus disease of fowls characterized by pneumonia and encephalomyelitis. This virus can cause mild conjunctivitis in man. Syn., *avian pneumoencephalitis, avian pseudoplague, Philippine fowl disease.*

Niemann-Pick d. An acute systemic disorder, affecting chiefly female Jewish infants; marked by slight anemia, enlargement of the liver, spleen, and lymph nodes, and by mental retardation; death regularly occurs before the child is two years old. Amaurotic familial idiocy is closely associated. Syn., *lipoid histiocytosis.*

nodule d. A disease of ruminants, characterized by nodules in the mucous membranes of the intestine; the nodules contain the larval form of species of *Oesophagostomum.*

occupational d. One arising from the particular toxic substances, characteristic hazards, or frequently repeated mechanical operations of a particular industry or trade.

Ollier's d. Dyschondroplasia.

organic d. One associated with recognizable structural changes in the organs or tissues of the body.

Osgood-Schlatter d. Osteochondrosis of the tuberosity of the tibia.

Osler-Rendu-Weber d. See hereditary hemorrhagic *telangiectasis.*

Osler-Vaquez d. See primary *polycythemia.*

overeating d. Infectious enterotoxemia of sheep.

Owren's d. Parahemophilia.

Paget's d. Osteitis deformans, a disease of the skeleton of unknown cause, characterized by slowly spreading changes in one or more bones, primarily the pelvis, long bones, and sometimes the skull bones, and consisting of decalcification coupled with hyperostosis. Later the marrow spaces in transformed bone are more or less filled with vascular fibrous tissue. Deformities, limitations of joint movement, and sometimes fractures accompany the progress of the disease, which affects principally males after middleage.

Paget's d. of nipple. A carcinoma involving the nipple or areola and the larger ducts, characterized by malignant cells, some of which are large and have clear cytoplasm (Paget's cells): also called *morbus Pageti papillae, carcinoma of nipple, intraepithelial carcinoma of nipple, Paget's cancer.*

pandemic d. One epidemic over a large area, as an entire country or several countries.

pararheumatic d. See *collagen diseases* under *disease.*

parasitic d. One due to invasion of the body by animal or vegetable parasites.

Parkinson's d. Parkinsonism.

Parry's d. Exophthalmic goiter.

Pel-Ebstein's d. Pseudoleukemia; multiple lymphadenoma.

periodic d. One occurring at regular intervals or at the same season of the year.

periodontal d. One affecting the periodontium.

Peyronie's d. A condition of unknown etiology characterized by the development of plaques or masses of dense fibrous tissue in the fascia about the corpora cavernosa of the penis, resulting in deformity of the penis. Syn., *cavernitis, penile strabismus.*

Philippine fowl d. See Newcastle *d.*

Pick's d. (a) Circumscribed cerebral *atrophy:* named for Arnold *Pick.* (b) Potyserositis: for Friedel *Pick.*

pilonidal d. An inclusive term for pilonidal sinus, pilonidal cyst, and combined cyst and sinus.

pink d. See *erythredema polyneuropathy.*

pneumatic hammer d. See traumatic vasospastic *syndrome.*

pock diseases. A group of dermatotropic virus diseases characterized clinically by vesicles, pustules, and crusting, and pathologically by "balloon degeneration" and necrosis of epidermis. Among the diseases are varicella, variola, herpes simplex, and herpes zoster.

porcupine d. See *ichthyosis.*

Pott's d. Tuberculosis of the spine.

PTC-deficiency d. A rare condition caused by the absence of plasma thromboplastin component and manifested by regularly recurring hemorrhagic episodes. It may be controlled by the administration of PTC or by blood transfusions.

pullorum d. An acute, highly contagious disease of young chicks caused by *Salmonella pullorum* and producing a characteristic white diarrhea. Also called *bacillary white diarrhea.*

pulpy kidney d. A disease of lambs, which has been reported in New Zealand and Wales, characterized by severe kidney degeneration. It is caused by *Clostridium perfringens,* Type D.

pulseless d. A disease characterized by absence of radial pulse, syncopal attacks, and arteriovenous anastomoses in the peripapillary region of the retina, visual disturbances, and cataracts. It is believed to be due to sclerosis of subclavian and carotid arteries secondary to panarteritis of unknown cause. Syn., *Takayasu's d.*

pyramidal d. Periostitis of the pyramidal process of the os pedis in the horse.

Quincke's d. Angioneurotic edema.

ragpicker's d. Anthrax. Also called *ragsorter's d.*

rat-bite d. See rat-bite *fever.*

Raynaud's d. See Raynaud's *syndrome.*

Réclus' d. See *cystic d. of breast.*

rheumatic brain d. See rheumatic *encephalopathy.*

rheumatic diseases. Those conditions in which pain and stiffness of some portion of the musculoskeletal system, usually articular or periarticular regions, are outstanding symptoms. See *rheumatism.*

Rhodesian cattle d. A piroplasmotic disease transmitted by ticks of the genus *Rhipicephalus.*

rickettsia d. Any disease caused by rickettsia. The most important groups are the typhus fever group, caused by *Rickettsia prowazekii;* the Rocky Mountain spotted fever group, caused by *R. rickettsii;* the scrub typhus group, caused by *R. tsutsugamushi;* and the Q fever group, caused by *Coxiella burnetii.*

Riga's d. Cachectic aphthae: also called *Fete-Riga's d.*

Ritter's d. See *dermatitis exfoliativa neonatorum.*

rolling d. A syndrome in mice associated with a pleuropneumonialike organism (L_5). A condition characterized by lateral rolling of the body and pathologically by an intense polymorphonuclear leukocyte reaction in the brain, also by neurolysis and, in some cases, by acute hydrocephaly.

rose d. Swine erysipelas.

Roth's d. Meralgia paresthetica.

sacroiliac d. An inflammation of the sacroiliac

joint, characterized by pain and tenderness over the joint, and thought to produce sciatica.

salivary gland d. A virus disease of guinea pigs and possibly man; characterized by the presence of cellular inclusion bodies. When naturally acquired, it apparently gives rise to no symptoms.

sandworm d. See *larva migrans.*

sartian d. Obsolete term for *oriental sore.*

Schamberg's d. See progressive pigmentary *dermatosis.*

Schenck's d. See *sporotrichosis.*

Scheuermann's d. Osteochondrosis involving the secondary growth centers of vertebral bodies.

Schilder's d. See *encephalitis periaxialis diffusa.*

Schimmelbusch's d. See *adenosis* of breast.

Schönlein's d. See Schönlein's *purpura.*

Schüller-Christian d. See Hand-Schüller-Christian *d.*

septic d. One due to the presence and multiplication of pyogenic or putrefactive organisms in the body.

Shaver's d. Bauxite fibrosis.

shimamushi d. See tsutsugamushi *d.*

sickle-cell-thalassemia d. See *microdrepanocytic disease.*

Simmonds' d. See hypopituitary *cachexia.*

Sinding-Larsen d. See Larsen-Johansson *d.*

sponge-gatherer's d. A disease of divers due to a secretion of a species of *Actinia* found in waters where sponges grow. At the point of contact upon the body, the viscid excretion causes a swelling and intense itching, followed by a papule surrounded by a zone of redness which later becomes black and gangrenous and forms a deep ulcer.

sporadic d. One occurring only occasionally and in single cases.

Steinert's d. See muscular *dystrophy.*

Stevens-Johnson d. See *erythema multiforme.*

Still's d. A type of chronic, infectious polyarthritis occurring in children. In the later stages, splenomegaly and glandular enlargement appear.

stomach worm d. Strongyliasis of cattle.

storage d. One characterized by excess deposition of exogenous or endogenous substances within the body.

Sturge-Weber-Dimitri d. See nevoid *amentia.*

Stuttgart d. A hemorrhagic, infectious gastroenteritis of dogs; characterized by loss of appetite, vomiting, weakness, anorexia, diarrhea, low temperature, and ulcerative stomatitis. Death occurs in the majority of cases. Syn., *canine typhus.* The etiological agent is *heptospira canicola.*

subacute combined system d. See subacute combined *degeneration* of spinal cord.

subacute d. One which is more prolonged and less active than an acute disease.

Sulzberger-Garbe d. A disease, thought to be a neurodermatitis, characterized by discoid, lichenoid, and eczematoid dermatitis.

Sutton's d. (a) Leukoderma acquisitum centrifugum. (b) Periadenitis mucosa necrotica recurrens.

sweet clover d. A hemorrhagic disease observed in animals after eating spoiled sweet clover; due to a toxic substance (dicoumarin) which lowers the fibrinogen content of the blood plasma.

swineherd's d. Pseudotyphoid meningitis. An acute febrile disease transmitted from swine to man by the hog louse; due to a virus.

systemic d. Any disease affecting the whole body.

tanner's d. Anthrax.

Tay-Sachs d. Amaurotic familial idiocy.

teart d. Molybdenosis or chronic molybdenum poisoning, applied especially to the condition as seen in cattle.

Thomsen's d. See *myotonia congenita.*

tsutsugamushi d. A disease occurring in Japan Formosa, and islands of the South Pacific; caused by *Rickettsia tsutsugamushi* and transmitted to man by the bite of the larval forms of a species of *Trombicula;* characterized by headache, fever, and a rash. Also called *scrub typhus, Queensland coastal fever, Malayan typhus, Sumatran mite typhus, Japanese river fever.*

tunnel d. (a) See caisson *d.* (b) Ancylostomiasis.

vagabond's d. See *pediculosis* corporis.

vagrant's d. A discoloration of the skin occurring especially in elderly persons who are uncleanly and infested with pediculi over a long period.

Vaquez's d. See primary *polycythemia.*

venereal diseases. Gonorrhea, syphilis, chancroid, granuloma inguinale, and venereal lymphogranuloma. Abbreviated, VD, V.D., vd, v.d.

Vincent's d. See necrotizing ulcerative *gingivitis;* see also Vincent's *angina,* Vincent's *stomatitis.*

von Gierke's d. Glycogenosis.

von Hippel's d. Angiomatosis retinae. See also *Hippel-Lindau d.* under Arvid *Lindau.*

von Jaksch's d. Infantile pseudoleukemic anemia.

von Recklinghausen's d. See *neurofibromatosis.*

Waldenström's d. See *osteochondritis deformans juvenilis.*

Weil's d. Spirochetal jaundice.

Whipple d. Intestinal lipodystrophy.

white-spot d. A special form of scleroderma.

Wilson's d. See hepatolenticular *degeneration.*

woolsorter's d. Anthrax.

dis″en·gage′ment [F. *désengager*]. Emergence from a confined state; especially the emergence of the head of the fetus from the vagina during parturition.

diseptal. Trade name for dimethyldisulfanilamide. Used chiefly in gonorrhea or as ointment in the treatment of infected wounds. Dose, 0.5–1.0 Gm. (8–15 gr.) t.i.d. Also called *uleron* and *uliron.*

dis·e″qui·lib′ri·um [L. *dis-*, indicating separation; *aequilibrium*, equilibrium]. Lack or loss of balance. Syn., *instability.*

dis″ger·min·o′ma. See *dysgerminoma.*

dis″gre·ga′tion [L. *disgregare*, to separate]. Dispersion; separation, as of molecules or cells.

dis″in·fect′ant [F. *désinfecter*]. An agent which destroys or inhibits the microorganisms causing disease.

complete d. One that destroys the spores as well as the vegetating cells.

incomplete d. One that destroys the vegetating cells but not the spores.

dis″in·fec′tion [*désinfecter*]. The destruction or removal of pathogenic organisms, especially by means of chemical substances. —**disinfect′,** *v.t.*

concurrent d. Prompt disinfection and disposal of infective material continuously throughout the course of a disease.

steam d. The destruction of pathogenic bacteria by application of live steam under pressure. Moist heat is regarded as a more effective germicide than dry heat.

terminal d. Disinfection and disposal of infectious material after the termination of a disease.

dis·in″fes·ta′tion [L. *dis-*, indicating separation; *infestare*, to infest]. Extermination of insects or animal parasites; delousing.

dis·in″hi·bi′tion. Revival of an extinguished conditioned response by an unconditioned stimulus.

dis·in′te·grate [*dis-;* L. *integrare*, to renew]. Break up or decompose.

dis·in″te·gra′tion. The process of breaking up or decomposing.

dis″in·vag″i·na′tion (dis″in·vadj″i·nay′shun)

[*dis-;* L. *in,* in; *vagina,* sheath]. The reduction or relief of an invagination.

dis·joint′ [OF. *desjoint,* from *desjoindre*]. Disarticulate; separate, as bones from their natural relations.

disk, disc [G. *diskos,* disk, quoit]. A circular, platelike organ or structure. *Disc* is more commonly used in biology, especially zoology; *disk* is more commonly used in chemistry.

anisotropic d. The doubly refractive, dark, broad disk of a myofibril of a striated muscle fiber. Abbreviated, A d, Q d.

articular d. One of fibrocartilage, dividing the joint cavity of certain joints.

blood d. Old term for erythrocyte.

choked d. Papilledema.

cupped d. Excavation of the optic disk, normally present in slight degree, but pathologic if excessive.

embryonic d. In mammals, the central, round, or oval area of the bilaminar blastodisk in which the primitive streak arises and from which the embryo proper develops. Also called *area germinativa, area embryonalis, embryonic blastoderm.*

epiphyseal d. Epiphyseal plate.

equatorial d. See equatorial *plate.*

germinal d. The protoplasmic area in the eggs of reptiles, birds, and lower animals which becomes the blastoderm, in the center of which arises the definitive embryo. In placental mammals, the germinal disk is synonymous with the inner cell mass, which becomes the embryonic disk, while the rest of the blastocyst becomes amnion, yolk sac, and trophoblast.

Hensen's d. The clear zone which appears in the middle of the anisotropic disk of a contracting myofibril. Abbreviated, H d.

herniated d. An intervertebral disk in which the nucleus pulposus has protruded through the surrounding fibrocartilage, forming a small hernial sac.

intercalated d. One of the irreversible contraction bands of a cardiac muscle fiber.

intermediate d. The thin, dark, doubly refractive disk in the middle of the isotropic disk. It is not confined to a single myofibril; it passes through the entire diameter of a striated muscle fiber. Abbreviated, Z d. Also called *Krause's membrane.*

intervertebral disks. The mass of fibrocartilage between adjacent surfaces of most of the vertebrae.

isotropic d. The singly refractive, light, broad disk of a myofibril of a striated muscle fiber. Abbreviated, I d., J d.

M d. A line in the middle of Hensen's disk in insect muscle.

Merkel's d. See tactile *d.*

Miller d. Ocular micrometer disk containing two squares whose areas have a 1:9 ratio; used in making reticulocyte counts: also called *Miller ocular d.*

nuclear d. See equatorial *plate.*

optic d. The circular area in the retina that is the site of the convergence of fibers from the ganglion cells of the retina to form the optic nerve. Syn., *optic papilla.*

ovigerous d. See *cumulus* oophorus.

Plácido's d. See *keratoscope.*

Q d. The anisotropic or dark disk or band of a striated myofibril.

ruptured d. An intervertebral disk whose nucleus pulposus has broken through the surrounding fibrocartilage into the spinal canal.

sarcous d. Old term for anisotropic disk.

stenopeic d. A lens allowing the passage of light rays only through a straight narrow slit; used for testing astigmatism.

strobic disks. Those drawn with concentric circles to produce an illusory impression of revolving.

tactile d. A terminal widening of an axon in contact with a specialized epithelial cell in the epidermis; a receptor for touch. Also called *Grandry-Merkel's corpuscle, Merkel's tactile d., Merkel's d.* or *corpuscle, tactile meniscus.*

vitelline d. See *cumulus* oophorus.

Z d. The thin membrane which bisects the isotropic disk in a relaxed muscle fiber and forms the boundary of a sarcomere. Syn., *Z band, Z line, intermediate d.* Also called *Krause's membrane, Dobie's line, telophragma.* See also Z, 2.

disk′o·gram. See *discogram.*

dis″lo·ca′tion [L. *dis-,* indicating separation; *locare,* to place]. The displacement of one or more bones of a joint or of any organ from the original position. See *diastasis, displacement, subluxation.* See Plates 37, 38. Syn., *luxation.* —**dis′located,** *adj.;* **dis′locate,** *v.t.*

complete d. One in which there is complete separation of the joint surfaces.

compound d. One in which there is a communication with the joint from outside, through an external wound.

congenital d. One existing from birth.

d. of lens. A displacement of the crystalline lens of the eye.

diverging d. A dislocation of the radius and ulna at the wrist, involving rupture of the annular ligament.

double d. One in which there are two similar joint dislocations, on opposite sides of the body.

fracture d. One in which there is a fracture accompanying the dislocation.

habitual d. One in which there are frequently relapsing dislocations of a particular joint, as the shoulder. Also called *recurrent d., relapsing d.*

incomplete d. One in which there has been only a partial separation of the joint surfaces; subluxation.

intrauterine d. One which occurs during fetal life.

old d. See unreduced *d.*

paralytic d. One resulting from flaccid paralysis of the muscles and muscular atrophy.

partial d. See incomplete *d.*

pathologic d. One resulting from joint disease with destruction of tissue, or from paralysis.

traumatic d. A dislocation as a result of violence.

unreduced d. One in which the dislocated bone has not been replaced in normal position. Syn., *old d.*

dis·mem′ber [*dis-;* L. *membrum,* member]. Amputate an extremity or a major portion thereof. —**dismemberment,** *n.*

dis″mu·ta′tion. *In chemistry,* a reaction in which two molecules of the same compound interact to yield one oxidized and one reduced product.

dis″oc·clude′ [*dis-;* L. *occludere,* to close up]. Grind or level a tooth surface so that it will fail to touch the opposing tooth in the other jaw during mastication.

di·so′ma (dye·so′muh), **di·so′mus** (dye·so′mus) (pl. *disomata, disomi*) [G. *dis,* twice; *sōma,* body]. A monster having two trunks. In some classifications the term is used to cover all monochorionic twinning.

dis·ord′er. A disturbance or derangement of physical or mental health or functions. Also see *disease, reaction, syndrome.* For specific psychiatric disorders, see under the qualifying adjective.

dis·or″gan·i·za′tion [L. *dis-;* denoting negation; G. *organon*, organ]. Act of deranging or the state of abnormal structure.

dis·o″ri·en·ta′tion [*dis-;* L. *oriens*, east]. Loss of normal relationship to one's surroundings; particularly the inability to comprehend time, place, and people, such as occurs in organic brain disease.

dis′pa·rate [L. *dispar*, dissimilar]. Not alike; unequal or unmated.

dis″pa·reu′ni·a (dis″puh·roo′nee·uh). See *dyspareunia.*

dis·par′i·ty [*dispar*]. Difference; inequality.

dis·pen′sa·ry [L. *dispensare*, to distribute by weight]. 1. A place where medicine or medical aid is given free or at low cost to ambulatory patients. 2. In a place of business, a medical office provided by the owner to serve sick or injured employees. 3. *In military medicine*, a medical treatment facility primarily intended to provide examination and treatment for ambulatory patients, to make necessary arrangements for the transfer of patients requiring bed care, and to provide first aid for emergency cases.

general d. *In military medicine*, a medical treatment facility which provides medical and dental care, but not hospitalization, for military personnel and their dependents not having access to hospital facilities of a post, camp, or station. They are usually located in large cities or military districts.

veterinary d. *In U.S. Army medicine*, an establishment providing for the care and treatment of animals not requiring hospitalization.

dis·pen′sa·to″ry [*dispensare*]. A book containing a systematic discussion of medicinal agents, including origin, preparation, description, use, and mode of action.

dis·pense′ [*dispensare*]. Prepare and distribute medicines for the sick.

di·sper′mine (dye·spur′meen, ·min). Piperazine.

di′sper″my, di·sper′my [G. *dis*, twice; *sperma*, seed]. Entrance of two spermatozoa into an ovum.

dis·per′sion [L. *dispersio*, from *dispergere*, to scatter on all sides]. Act of scattering; any scattering of light, as that passed through ground glass.

chromatic d. *In physics*, splitting of a beam of white light into different wave lengths or frequencies, and consequently into different colors.

dis·pers′oid [*dispersio;* G. *eidos*, form]. A colloid or finely divided substance.

dis·place′ment [F. *déplacement*]. 1. Removal from the normal position; dislocation, luxation; dystopia. 2. *In pharmacy*, a process occurring in percolation. 3. *In chemistry*, a change in which one element is removed by another element. 4. *In psychopathology*, the discharge of emotional tension arising out of a repressed feeling, as of guilt or inadequacy, through an unrelated, trivial act or conscious expression. The original intolerable situation or experience is thereby barred from entering the consciousness.

fish-hook d. A term referring to a vertical type of stomach, not an actual displacement; an orthotonic stomach.

hip d. See congenital *dislocation.*

toe d. Overlapping toes.

uterine d. Any change in position of the uterus from the accepted normal. See *anteversion, prolapse, retroversion.*

dis″po·si′tion [L. *dispositio*, from *disponere*, to arrange]. A tendency to acquire a certain disease; a peculiar predisposing factor, partly or wholly dependent upon heritable factors.

dis·rup′tive [L. *disruptum*, from *disrumpere*, to burst asunder]. Bursting; rending.

dis·sect′ [L. *dissecare*, to cut in pieces]. Cut tissues apart carefully and slowly, in order to allow study of the relations of parts.

dis·sec′tion [*dissecare*]. The cutting of tissues of the body for purposes of study.

dis·sec′tor [*dissecare*]. 1. One who makes a dissection. 2. Handbook or manual of anatomy and instructions for use in dissection.

dis·sem″i·na′tion [L. *disseminare*, to scatter seed, to spread abroad]. The scattering or dispersion of disease or disease germs. —**dissem′inated,** *adj.*

dis·sim″u·la′tion [L. *dissimulare*, to dissemble]. Act of feigning, disguising, or malingering.

dis·so″ci·a′tion [L. *dissociare*, to separate from fellowship]. 1. Separation; especially of a chemical compound into ions. 2. *In cardiology*, completely independent action of atria and ventricles; heart block. 3. *In psychology*, the segregation from consciousness of certain components of mental processes, which then function independently; the separation of ideas from their natural and appropriate affects or feelings. 4. *In bacteriology*, a change in colony form, often occurring in a new environment, and associated with modified growth or virulence. —**disso′ciant,** *adj., n.*

albuminocytologic d. Elevated protein in cerebrospinal fluid without corresponding rise in cell count, characteristic of the Guillain-Barré syndrome.

atrioventricular d. with interference. That condition in which there is a unidirectional block which prevents impulses from passing from the atrioventricular node back to the atria. This block is exhibited by a series of ventricular beats, representing responses to the atrioventricular node, and a premature ventricular beat, representing a response to the sinus node.

dis·so′ci·a·tive re·ac′tion. See under *reaction.*

dis·sog′e·ny (di·sodj′i·nee) [G. *dissos*, double; *genesthai*, from *gignesthai*, to be produced]. *In zoology*, having two periods of sexual maturity; one as a larva and one as an adult.

dis″so·lu′tion [L. *dissolutio*, from *dissolvere*, to separate]. 1. Separation of a body or compound into its parts. 2. Death; decomposition.

dis·solve′ [*dissolvere*]. To make a solution of; become a solution. —**dis·sol′vent,** *adj., n.*

dis′tad [L. *distare*, to be distant; *ad*, to]. Toward the periphery; in a distal direction.

dis′tal [*distare*]. 1. Extreme; at the greatest distance from a central point; peripheral. 2. *In dentistry*, referring to a position which lies away from the sagittal plane along the curve of a dental arch. See *mesial.* —**distad, distally,** *adv.*

dis′tance [L. *distantia*, distance]. The measure of space between two objects.

focal d. The distance between the center of a lens and its focus.

hearing d. The distance at which a certain sound can be heard.

hyperfocal d. *In photography*, the nearest point to a lens at which objects will appear sharp in the image space when the lens is focused for objects at an infinite distance.

infinite d. *In optics*, a distance of 20 feet or more, so established because the rays from an object at that distance to the lens of the eye are practically parallel.

working d. In the microscope, the distance from the front lens of an objective to the object, when the objective is correctly focused.

dis·tem′per [L. *dis-*, denoting negation; *temperare*, to mingle properly]. The common name applied to certain infectious diseases of animals.

canine d. That form occurring in young dogs, caused by a filtrable virus.

equine d. See *strangles.*

dis·ten′tion [L. *distentio*, from *distendere*, to stretch]. A state of dilatation.

dis·tich′i·a (dis·tick′ee·uh), **dis″ti·chi′a·sis** (dis″-ti·kigh′uh·sis) [G. *dis*, twice; *stichos*, row]. The presence of a row of cilia at the inner lid border, which turn in and rub on the cornea. This row of cilia is additional to the two or three rows arising at the outer lid border.

dis′til·land [L. *distillare*, to distill]. The substance being distilled.

dis′til·late [*distillare*]. The condensate obtained by distillation.

dis″til·la′tion [L. *distillatio*, from *distillare*]. Process of vaporization and subsequent condensation; it is used principally to separate liquids from non-volatile substances. —**distill′**, *v.t.*, *v.i.*

destructive d. Decomposition of complex organic substances by heat and distillation of the products.

fractional d. Separation of a liquid into its components by means of gradually increasing temperature, the different products being vaporized in the order of their respective boiling points.

molecular d. Distillation which permits the transfer of a molecule from the distilling to the condensing surface without suffering a collision with another molecule. It usually requires a very high vacuum and close proximity of the two surfaces.

dis′to-, dist- [L. *distare*, to be distant]. A combining form signifying *posterior, distant from the center.*

dis″to·buc′cal [*distare;* L. *bucca*, cheek]. Relating to the distal and buccal surfaces of the premolar and molar teeth.

dis″to·buc″co·oc·clu′sal [*distare; bucca;* L. *occludere*, to close up]. Relating to the distal, buccal, and occlusal surfaces of a tooth.

dis″to·oc·clu′sal [*distare; occludere*]. Relating to the distal and occlusal surfaces of premolar and molar teeth.

dis″to·clu′sion [*distare; occludere*]. Malocclusion of the teeth in which those of the lower jaw are displaced backward in relation to the upper teeth.

dis″to·la′bi·al [*distare;* L. *labia*, lip]. Relating to the distal and labial surfaces of incisors and canines.

dis″to·lin′gual [*distare;* L. *lingua*, tongue]. Relating to the distal and lingual surfaces of all teeth.

dis″to·lin″guo·oc·clu′sal [*distare; lingua;* L.*occludere*, to close up]. Pertaining to the distal, lingual, and occlusal surfaces of a tooth.

Dis′to·ma, Dis′to·mum [G. *dis*, twice, *stoma*, mouth]. Old name for a genus of trematode worms.

D. haematobium. Synonym for *Schistosoma haematobium.*

D. hepaticum. Synonym for *Fasciola hepatica.*

Di·sto′ma·ta [*dis; stoma*]. A suborder of the Trematoda or flukes.

di·sto′mi·a (dye·sto′mee·uh) [*dis; stoma*]. Congenital duplication of the mouth.

dis″to·mi′a·sis [*dis; stoma;* NL. *-iasis*, condition]. Infestation with flukes.

dis″to·mo′lar [*distare;* L. *molaris*, from *mola*, mill]. A supernumerary tooth distal to a third molar, hence in the position of a fourth molar.

d. tubercle. An accessory lobe with one or two cusps on the distolingual side of a third molar, believed to represent a rudimentary distomolar.

Dis′to·mum. See *Distoma.*

di·sto′mus (dye·sto′mus, di·sto′mus) [*dis; stoma*]. An individual with partial or complete duplicity of the mouth.

dis·tor′tion [L. *distortio*, from *distorquere*, to twist]. 1. A twisted or bent shape; deformity or malformation, acquired or congenital. 2. A writhing or twisting motion, as of the face. 3. *In optics*, a form of aberration in which objects viewed through certain lenses appear changed in shape but not broken in continuity. 4. *In psychoanalysis*, the adaptive alteration of an idea to conform with the subject's wishes or prejudices.

dis″to·ver′sion [L. *distare*, to be distant; *versum*, from *vertere*, to turn]. Tilting of a tooth so that the crown moves distally.

dis″tri·bu′tion [L. *distributio*, from *distribuere*, to distribute]. *In anatomy*, the branching of a nerve or artery, and the arrangement of its branches within those parts that it supplies.

dis″tri·chi′a·sis (dis″tri·kigh′uh·sis) [G. *dis*, twice; *thrix*, hair; NL. *-iasis*, condition]. Two hairs growing from a single follicle.

dis′trix [*dis; thrix*]. Splitting of the distal ends of the hair.

di·sul′fide (dye·sul′fide, ·fid). Bisulfide.

di′ta bark (dee′tuh). The bark of *Alstonia scholaris*, native to the Philippine Islands; alstonia. It has been employed as a bitter tonic, antiperiodic, and antimalarial.

dit′a·ine (dit′uh·een, ·in). $C_{22}H_{28}N_2O_4$. Echitamine. An alkaloid from *Alstonia.*

dit′a·mine (dit′uh·meen, ·min, dit·am′in). $C_{16}H_{19}O_2N$. An alkaloid found in *Alstonia.*

di·ter′pene. Any of the terpene hydrocarbons having the formula $C_{20}H_{32}$, or $(C_5H_8)_4$.

di·thi″o·bi″u·ret′ (dye·thigh″o·buy″yoo·ret′). $NH_2.CS.NH.CS.NH_2$. A substance which has been used experimentally to produce a reversible paralysis of motor function in animals.

di·thi″o·pro′pa·nol-1. Dimercaprol (see BAL).

di′thi·zone. Diphenyl-thiocarbazone, a reagent used as a sensitive test for heavy metals, particularly lead.

di′thra·nol. British Pharmacopoeia name for 1,8-dihydroxyanthranol, used locally in the treatment of skin diseases. See *anthralin, cignolin.*

di·thy″mol·di·i′o·dide. Thymol iodide.

dit′o·kous, dit′o·cous [*dis;* G. *tokos*, offspring]. 1. Producing two young at a birth. 2. Producing young of two kinds, as some worms.

Dittel, Leopold [*Austrian surgeon*, 1815–98]. Remembered for his advocacy of the removal of the median bar of the prostate for urinary obstruction (1880).

Dittrich, Franz [*German physician*, 1815–59]. Described small, dirty-white or yellowish masses, found in cases of bronchiectasis and in pulmonary abscess, which were called *Dittrich's plugs.* They are now not regarded as pathognomonic.

ditubin. Trade-mark for a brand of isoniazid; an antituberculosis drug having the composition of isonicotinic acid hydrazide.

di·u′re·ide [*dis;* G. *ouron*, urine]. 1. A derivative of urea in which a hydrogen of both NH_2 groups is replaced by an acyl radical. 2. An acyl derivative of urea containing residues of two urea molecules.

di″u·re′sis [G. *diourein*, to pass urine]. Increased excretion of urine. —**diuret′ic,** *adj.*

di″u·ret′ic [G. *diourētikos*, diuretic]. Agent that increases the volume of urine.

acidifying d. Substance that produces diuresis because of its acid-forming properties in the body.

cardiac d. Substance, such as digitalis, which produces diuresis by increasing the efficiency of the heart in patients with cardiac edema.

mercurial d. An organic mercurial compound, which acts primarily by reducing tubular reabsorption of water.

osmotic d. A substance producing diuresis because of the osmotic effect of the unabsorbed fraction in the renal tubules with resulting loss of water.

saline d. A salt which produces diuresis because of its osmotic effect in the tubules.

diuretin. Trade-mark for a brand of theobromine with sodium salicylate.

di·ur′nule [L. *diurnus*, of the day]. A medicinal product that contains the full quantity of a drug to be administered in 24 hours.

di″va·ga′tion [L. *divagari*, to wander about]. Rambling speech and thought.

di·va′lent (dye·vay′lunt, dye′vay·lunt, div′uh·lunt) [G. *dis*, twice; L. *valere*, to have power]. 1. Bivalent. 2. Having the ability to exist in two valence states.

di·var″i·ca′tion [L. *divaricare*, to spread asunder]. Separation, divergence.

di·var″i·ca′ti·o pal″pe·bra′rum (dye·var″i·kay′-shee·o) [L.]. Synonym of *ectropion*.

di·ver′gence (dye·vur′junss, di·vur′junss) [L. *dis-*, denoting separation; *vergere*, to bend]. *In ophthalmology*, the abduction of both eyes simultaneously, or of one eye when the other is fixed. —**divergent,** *adj*.

di′ver's ear. An inflammation of the middle ear and auditory tube; caused by sudden changes in atmospheric pressure that may occur during a diver's ascent or descent: seen in caisson disease. Similar to aerootitis media.

di′ver's neu·ro′sis. See caisson *disease*.

di″ver·tic′u·lar [L. *diverticulum*, a bypath, from *divertere*, to turn away]. Relating to or arising from a diverticulum.

di″ver·tic″u·lec′to·my [*diverticulum*; G. *ektomē*, excision]. Surgical removal of a diverticulum.

di″ver·tic″u·li′tis [*diverticulum*; G. *-itis*, inflammation]. Inflammation of a diverticulum.

di″ver·tic″u·lo′sis [*diverticulum*; G. *-ōsis*, condition]. Presence of many diverticula of the intestine.

d. of fallopian tube. See isthmic nodular *salpingitis*.

di″ver·tic′u·lum (pl. *diverticula*) [L.]. A pouch or sac springing from a hollow organ or structure; may be congenital or acquired.

allantoic d. The endodermal diverticulum from the cloaca into the extraembryonic coelom in most amniotes, or into the body stalk in primates, which forms the epithelial lining of the allantois. Also called *allantoenteric d.*

bladder d. See vesical *d.*

calyceal d. A rare unsymptomatic renal alteration, usually discovered only incidentally on pyelography, in which there is a dilatation of a calyx due to obstruction in the infundibulum: also called *hydrocalycosis, pyelogenic cyst.*

cervical d. An incomplete fistula in the cervical region, derived from a pharyngeal pouch (internal) or a visceral groove (external).

congenital d. One present at birth; the most common varieties are the esophageal diverticulum, intestinal diverticulum, and the diverticulum ilei.

d. ilei. The persistent proximal end of the yolk stalk. Also called *Meckel's d.*

esophageal d. A saclike protrusion of a part of the wall of the esophagus or of the pharynx just above the esophageal opening. See pulsion *d.*, traction *d.*

eustachian d. A small abnormal pouching of the lower portion of the auditory tube.

false d. One involving the large intestine, having only mucosal and serosal coats and lacking the muscular coat present in true diverticula.

gastric d. A pouching of the stomach generally seen near the pylorus in connection with duodenal or gastric ulcer.

giant d. A congenital enteric cyst or duplication of a portion of the ileum, jejunum, duodenum, or occasionally the stomach; the cyst has a common wall with the gastrointestinal tract.

hepatic d. The primordium of the liver, gallbladder, and their ducts. Also called *hepatic gutter*.

intestinal d. A sacculation of the intestinal wall.

Meckel's d. See *d.* ilei.

Nuck's d. The homolog in the female of the vaginal process of the peritoneum. Syn., *canal of Nuck.*

pancreatic d. One of two (dorsal and ventral) from the duodenum or hepatic diverticulum that form the pancreas and its ducts.

pharyngeal d. See pulsion *d.*, traction *d.*

pressure d. See pulsion *d.*

pulsion d. A thin-walled sac in the posterior wall of the laryngopharynx opposite the cricoid cartilage just above the esophageal opening: also called *Zenker d.*

synovial d. An abnormal pouch found in a large joint, such as the knee.

thyroid d. An evagination of the ventral floor of the pharynx between the first and second visceral arches which is the primordium of the thyroid gland. The site is marked by the cecal foramen.

traction d. A circumscribed sacculation of the esophagus due to the pull of adhesions.

ureteral d. A chronic localized bulging of the ureter, usually the result of obstruction; generally associated with hydronephrosis.

vesical d. One occurring in the urinary bladder, usually in males over 60 and generally secondary to urinary obstruction.

Zenker d. See pulsion *d.*

div′i-div′i [Sp.]. *Caesalpinia coriaria*, a tree of South America whose seed pods yield tannic and gallic acids: used as an astringent and in tanning.

di·vi′nyl e′ther (dye·vy′nil). $(CH_2{:}CH)_2O$. A highly volatile, unsaturated ether used as an inhalation anesthetic for short operations. Syn., *divinyl oxide, vinyl ether*. See *vinethene*.

di·vi′nyl ox′ide. See *divinyl ether*.

di·vi′sion [L. *divisio*, from *dividere*, to divide]. Act or process of dividing into parts.

cell d. Cytokinesis.

equational d. A nuclear division in which daughter chromosomes separate from each other, as in ordinary somatic cell division; applied especially to the second meiotic division in contrast with the reduction division in which maternal and paternal homologous chromosomes disjoin.

mitotic d. Mitosis.

nuclear d. Mitosis.

reduction d. Meiosis.

di·vul′sion (dye·vul′shun) [L. *divulsio*, from *divellere*, to tear asunder]. A tearing apart. —**divulse′**, *v.t.*

di·vul′sor (dye·vul′sur, di·vul′sur) [*divellere*]. Instrument for the forcible dilatation of a part or of stricture in any organ.

di·wa·kwad′i. See *witkop*.

di″zy·got′ic (dye″zye·got′ick) [G. *dis*, twice; G. *zygōtos*, yoked]. Developed from two fertilized eggs at a single birth, as fraternal twins.

diz′zi·ness [AS. *dyzig*]. An unpleasant sensation of disturbed relations to surrounding objects in space; giddiness. See also *vertigo*. —**dizzy,** *adj*.

dl *In organic chemistry*, a racemic mixture containing both dextrorotatory and levorotatory forms of an organic compound.

D.M.D. Doctor of Dental Medicine: equivalent to the more common *D.D.S.*

DMF An abbreviation for *d*ecayed, *m*issing, and *f*illed teeth: applied to the quantitative estimate of dental caries in permanent teeth.

DNA Abbreviation for *desoxyribonucleic acid.*

DNASE Desoxyribonuclease.

Dobell's solution. See compound *sodium* borate solution.

Dobie, William Murray [*English anatomist,* 1828–1915]. Remembered eponymically in such terms as *Dobie's globule,* a small, round body in the middle of the transparent disk of a muscular fibril; *Dobie's layer,* a dark line in the center of a light band of striated muscle fiber, defining the sarcomere.

doca. Trade-mark for desoxycorticosterone acetate.

Dochez, Alphonse Raymond [*American physician,* 1882–]. Known for his researches on scarlet fever and its toxins; investigated the importance of *Streptococcus hemolyticus* in scarlet fever (1924); obtained a scarlet fever serum, *Dochez's serum,* by immunization of horses.

doch·mi′a·sis. Old term for ancylostomiasis.

doc′tor [L., from *docere,* to teach]. 1. One licensed, usually after special study, and qualifying by examination, to practice medicine, dentistry, or veterinary medicine. 2. Recipient of an academic title signifying competence in a special branch of learning.

doc′tor. To treat medically. *Colloq.*

do′dec·a-, dodec- [G. *dōdeka,* twelve]. A prefix denoting *twelve.*

do·dec′yl. The organic chemical radical CH_3-$(CH_2)_{10}CH_2$—.

Döderlein, Albert Siegmund Gustav [*German obstetrician,* 1860–1941]. Remembered for his classic study of vaginal secretions in relation to puerperal fever (1892). *Döderlein's bacillus,* once thought to be of pathologic importance, now is known as a normal inhabitant of the vagina.

Dodoens, Rembert (Dodonaeus) [*Belgian botanist and physician,* 1517–85]. An eminent botanist, he is remembered as author of *Cruydeboeck* (1554). He made many observations on the pathology of diseases of the lungs.

Doehle, Karl Gottfried Paul [*German pathologist,* 1855–1928]. Described a type of aortitis (1885), now known to be syphilitic, called *Doehle-Heller aortitis, Welch's aortitis.* Described small, irregularly staining masses, called *Doehle's inclusion bodies,* found in the cytoplasm of neutrophil leukocytes. These once were thought to be the causative organisms in scarlet fever.

Doellinger, Johann Ignaz Josef [*German physician,* 1770–1841]. Remembered for his description of a thickening of Descemet's membrane, forming a ring about the cornea, called *Doellinger's ring.*

Doerfler-Stewart test. See under *test.*

Dogiel, Alexander Stanislavovich (1852–1922). Russian neurohistologist, known for his description of the spinal ganglia of man and other mammals, and his classification of the neuron types in spinal, sympathetic, cardiac, and intestinal ganglia (1899).

Dogiel, Jan [*Russian physiologist,* 1830–1905]. Remembered as the inventor of the stromuhr, a device for measuring the velocity of blood in circulation (1867).

dog′wood″. See *cornus.*

doigts en lorgnette. See opera-glass *hand.*

Doisy, Edward Adelbert (1893–). American physiologist and biochemist, known for his work on sex hormones and vitamin K. He collaborated with Edgar Allen on the ovarian hormone (1923); with Sidney Allen Thayer and Clement D. Veler isolated estrone (1929); with Thayer and Donald William MacCorquodale isolated estradiol from ovaries (1936). He was Nobel laureate with Henrik Dam in 1943 for work on Vitamin K. See mouse *unit,* which is also called the *Thayer-Doisy unit.*

doi″sy·nol′ic ac′id [named for E. A. *Doisy*]. $C_{18}H_{24}O_3$; 1-ethyl-7-hydroxy-2-methyl-1,2,3,4,4a,-9,10,10a-octahydrophenanthrene-2-carboxylic acid, obtained from estrone by rupture of its cyclopentane ring with alkali; it possesses high estrogenic activity.

do·lan′tin. Meperidine hydrochloride.

Dolbeau, Henri Ferdinand [*French surgeon,* 1830–77]. Remembered for his description of an operation for lithotomy in which a median incision was made in the urethra, the stone being crushed in the urinary bladder with a lithotrite, followed by evacuation of debris.

dol′i·cho- (dol′i·ko-), **dol′ich-** (dol′ick-) [G. *dolichos,* long]. A combining form meaning *long, narrow.*

dol″i·cho·ceph′a·lus [*dolichos;* G. *kephalē,* head]. A dolichocephalic or long-headed person.

dol″i·cho·ceph′a·ly [*dolichos; kephalē*]. The condition in which the length-breadth index of the head is 75.9 or less, indicating that the head is much longer than it is broad. **—dolichocephal′ic, dolichocephalous,** *adj.*

dol″i·cho·cham″ae·cra′ni·al [*dolichos;* G. *chamai,* on the ground; *kranion,* skull]. *In craniometry,* a condition in which a long skull is also markedly low-vaulted, i.e., having a length-breadth index of 74.9 or less and a length-height index of 69.9 or less.

dol″i·choc·ne′mic [*dolichos;* G. *knēmē,* leg]. Designating a tibia with a tibiofemoral index of 83 or more, indicating that it is relatively long as compared with the femur.

dol″i·cho·co′lon. An abnormally long colon.

dol″i·cho·de′rus (dol″i·ko·deer′us, ·kod′ur·us) [*dolichos;* G. *derē,* neck]. A person having a disproportionately long neck.

dol″i·cho·eu″ro·mes″o·ceph′a·lus (dol″i·ko-yoor″o·mez″o·sef′uh·lus) [*dolichos;* G. *eurys,* wide; *mesos,* middle; *kephalē,* head]. A person having a long skull which is markedly broad in the temporal region.

dol″i·cho·eu″ro-o·pis″tho·ceph′a·lus [*dolichos; eurys;* G. *opisthen,* behind; *kephalē*]. A person having a long skull that is very broad in the occipital region.

dol″i·cho·eu″ro·pro·ceph′a·lus [*dolichos; eurys;* G. *pro,* before; *kephalē*]. A person having a long skull that is very broad in the frontal region.

dol″i·cho·fa′cial [*dolichos;* L. *facies,* face]. Having an unusually long face.

dol″i·cho·hi·er′ic (dol″i·ko·high·err′ick) [*dolichos;* G. *hieros,* sacred]. Designating a sacrum with a length-breadth index of 99.9 or less, indicating that it is relatively long and narrow.

dol″i·cho·ker′kic [*dolichos;* G. *kerkis,* shuttle]. Designating a radius with a humero-radial index of 80 or more, indicating that it is relatively long as compared with the humerus.

dol″i·cho·lep″to·ceph′a·lus [*dolichos;* G. *leptos,* thin; *kephalē,* head]. A person whose skull, in addition to being long, is also high and narrow.

dol″i·cho·mor′phic [*dolichos;* G. *morphē,* form]. Marked by a long or narrow form or build.

dol″i·cho·pel′lic, dol″i·cho·pel′vic [*dolichos;* G. *pellis,* bowl; L. *pelvis,* basin]. Designating a pelvis the pelvic index of which is 95.0 or more.

dol″i·cho·plat″y·ceph′a·lus [*dolichos;* G. *platys,* broad; *kephalē,*head]. A person having a long skull which is also unusually broad.

dol′i·chor·rhine (dol′i·kor·een) [*dolichos;* G. *rhis,* nose]. Having a long nose.

Dol′i·chos (dol′i·koss) [G.]. A genus of tropical herbs and woody vines of the pea family (Fabaceae), bearing seed pods covered with stinging hairs.

dol″i·cho·sten″o·me′li·a. See *arachnodactyly.*

dol″i·cho·u·ran′ic [*dolichos;* G. *ouranos,* vault, palate]. Having a long palatal alveolar arch, with a palato-maxillary index of 109.9 or less.

Dolin's method. See Fishberg and Dolin's *method.*

Dolman test. See Howard-Dolman depth perception *test.*

dolophine hydrochloride. A trade-marked name for *methadone hydrochloride.*

do′lor (pl. *dolores*) [L.]. Pain.

dolores praesagientes. Fleeting, false pains occurring a few days before the onset of labor.

do·lor′es (do·lor′eez). Plural of dolor.

do″lo·rim′e·ter [*dolor;* G. *metron,* a measure]. A device for measuring sensitivity to pain and the degree of pain experienced in any nerve irritation caused by disease.

dol″or·o·gen′ic (dol″or·o·, do″lor·o·) [*dolor;* G. *genesthai,* from *gignesthai,* to be produced]. Possessing the quality of pain; causing or arousing pain.

Domagk, Gerhard (1895–). German pharmacologist; Nobel prize winner in medicine (1939) for his work on sulfonamides. He introduced prontosil, the first of the sulfonamides, as a therapeutic agent.

do″ma·to·pho′bi·a [G. *dōma,* house; *phobos,* fear]. Morbid fear of being in a house; a variety of claustrophobia.

dom′in·ance. The state of being dominant.

cerebral d. The tendency for one cerebral hemisphere, usually the left, to be better developed in certain functions, especially speech and handedness.

dom′i·nant [L. *dominari,* to rule]. *In biology,* a characteristic of one of the parents of a hybrid which is present in the offspring, the contrasting recessive characteristic of the other parent being absent. See *Mendel's law,* under Gregor Johann *Mendel.* —**dom′inant,** *adj.*

dom′i·na·tor. Receptive sense organ in light-adapted eyes representing the preponderant type, occurring in broad spectral response curves or absorption bands, having their maximum in the region of 5600 angstroms; it is regarded as responsible for the sensation of luminosity. See *modulator.*

Dominici stain. See under *stain.*

Donald, Archibald [*English surgeon and gynecologist,* 1860–1919]. Devised an operation for uterine prolapse in which he performed an extensive colporrhaphy with amputation of the cervix (1908). *Donald's operation* was later modified by W. E. Fothergill, *q.v.*

Donaldson's method. See under *stain.*

Donath, Willem Frederik [*Dutch physician and biochemist,* 1889–]. Known for his investigations in vitamins and, especially, for his isolation of vitamin B_1 with Barend Jansen (1926).

Donath-Landsteiner phenomenon. See Donath-Landsteiner *test* under *test.*

don′a·tism [after *Donato,* professional name of Alfred d'Hont, 1845–1900, the Belgian "magnetizer"]. A form of hypnosis based on imitation.

Donders, Frans Cornelis [*Dutch physician and ophthalmologist,* 1818–89]. Known for his studies of astigmatism and of physiologic optics. Defined aphakia and hypermetropia (1864). Said to have been the first to measure the reaction time in a mental process (1868). Author of a classic paper on the physiology of speech (1870). Discovered a law of rotation of the eyeball (1847), called *Donders' law.* His name has been given to simple glaucoma, and the rainbowlike rings observed in glaucoma are called *Donders' rings.*

do″nee′ [L. *donare,* to donate]. The patient who receives transfused blood or other tissues, as skin, bone, or cartilage.

Donnan, Frederick George [*English physical chemist,* 1870–]. Known for his researches in ionic equilibrium across a membrane impermeable to an ion. The *Donnan equilibrium theory* states, in the case of univalent ions, that the product of the concentrations of diffusible ions on one side of the membrane is equal to the product of the concentrations of such ions on the other side of the membrane.

Donné, Alfred [*French physician,* 1801–78]. Credited with having first described the blood platelets as a third blood particle (1842). Described *Trichomonas vaginalis,* which he thought was the causative agent of gonorrhea. Gave the first modern description of living organisms in pathologic conditions. Studied cast-off cells or corpuscles that had undergone fatty degeneration, characteristic of colostrum; called *Donné's corpuscles.* Devised a test for pus in urine. See Donné's *test.*

do′nor [*donare*]. A person who gives blood for transfusion to another, or other tissues, as skin, bone, or cartilage for grafting.

universal d. One whose blood is of group O; one whose erythrocytes are not agglutinated by the blood of anyone.

Donovan, Edward [*Irish chemist,* 1798–1837]. Remembered as the inventor of a solution of arsenic and mercuric iodides used in chronic diseases of the skin and joints.

Donovan bodies. See *granuloma inguinale* and *Donovania granulomatis.*

Don·o″van′i·a gran″u·lo′ma·tis. The bacterium causing granuloma inguinale; it is gram-negative, nonmotile, and grows in chick embryos but not on ordinary media. With Wright's stain blue cells with pink capsules (*Donovan bodies*) can be demonstrated histologically. Also called *Klebsiella granulomatis.*

do′pa. Dihydroxyphenylalanine.

d. reaction. See under *reaction.*

do′pa ox′i·dase, do′pase. An enzyme of the skin that catalyzes the oxidation of dihydroxyphenylalanine (dopa) to melanin. This enzyme plays an important role in skin pigmentation; the melanin pigment is formed in the basal cells of the epidermis. For a histologic test for this enzyme, see *dopa reaction* under *stain.*

dope [D. *doop,* a dripping]. Any drug administered to stimulate or to stupefy, temporarily, or taken habitually.

d. fiend. One addicted to the use of a drug.

dope. To administer or habitually take a narcotic drug.

Doppler, Christian Johann [*Austrian physicist and mathematician,* 1803–53]. Observed that when the source of light or sound is moving rapidly, the wavelength appears to decrease as the object approaches the observer, or to increase as the object recedes; the pitch of sound becomes higher or lower. This is called *Doppler's principle, phenomenon, effect.*

do″ra·pho′bi·a [G. *dora,* skin, hide; *phobos,* fear]. Morbid fear of touching the skin or fur of animals.

doraxamin. A trade-mark for preparations containing the gastric antacid substance, dihydroxyaluminum aminoacetate.

Dorello's canal. See under *canal.*

dor′mant. Literally, sleeping; hence, concealed; potential. Syn., *latent.*

dormison. Trade-mark for *methylparafynol,* a hypnotic.

Dorner's spore stain. See under *stain.*

Dorrance, George Morris [*American surgeon,* 1877–1949]. Known for his description of an operation devised by him for the repair of the soft palate, called *Dorrance's operation.*

dor′sa. Plural of dorsum.

dor'sad [L. *dorsum*, back; *ad*, to]. Toward the dorsal aspect.

dor'sal [L. *dorsualis*, from *dorsum*]. Pertaining to the back or to the posterior part of an organ.

dor·sal'gi·a [*dorsum;* G. *algos*, pain]. Pain in the back.

dor·sa'lis (dor·sah'lis, dor·say'lis). Dorsal.

dor·sa'lis pe'dis (pee'diss, ped'iss) [L.]. The main artery of the dorsum of the foot. See Table of Arteries in the Appendix.

dorsaphyllin. Trade-mark for *theophylline sodium glycinate.*

dor'si- [*dorsum*]. A combining form meaning *of* or *on the back.*

dor"si·flex'ion (dor"si·fleck'shun) [*dorsum;* L. *flectere*, to bend]. Bending the foot toward the dorsum, or upper surface of the foot; opposed to *plantar flexion.* If used with reference to the toes, same as extension or straightening.

dor"si·ven'tral [*dorsum;* L. *venter*, belly]. Old term for posteroanterior, as used in x-ray positioning.

dor'so- [*dorsum*]. A combining form denoting *the back, dorsal,* or *dorsally.*

dor"so·an·te'ri·or [*dorsum;* L. *anterior*, foremost]. Applied to a fetus having its back toward the ventral aspect of the mother.

dor"so·ceph'al·ad [*dorsum;* G. *kephalē*, head; L. *ad*, toward]. Toward the dorsal aspect of the head.

dor"so·ep"i·tro·chle·a'ris. A rare muscle found in the posterior part of the axilla, extending from the tendon of the latissimus dorsi muscle to neighboring structures. Sometimes called levator of tendon of latissimus dorsi muscle.

dor"so·lat'er·al [*dorsum;* L. *lateralis*, from *latus*, side]. Relating to the back and the side.

dor"so·lum'bar. Relating to the back and lumbar regions. Syn., *lumbodorsal.*

dor"so·me'di·an [*dorsum;* L. *medius*, middle]. Situated in or relating to the middle region of the back.

dor"so·na'sal (dor"so·nay'zul) [*dorsum;* L. *nasus*, nose]. Referring to the bridge of the nose.

dor"so·pos·te'ri·or [*dorsum;* L. *posterior*, behind]. Applied to the position of a fetus having its back toward the dorsal aspect of the mother.

dor"so·ra'di·al [*dorsum;* L. *radius*, radius]. Relating to or situated upon the dorsal aspect and radial border of the hand, finger, or forearm.

dor"so·ul'nar [*dorsum;* L. *ulna*, elbow]. Relating to or situated upon the dorsal aspect and ulnar border of the arm, hand, or finger.

dor"so·ven'tral [*dorsum;* L. *venter*, belly]. Pertaining to the dorsal and ventral regions; extending in a direction from the dorsal surface toward the ventral. Syn., *posteroanterior.*

dor'sum (pl. *dorsa*) [L.]. 1. The back. 2. Any part corresponding to the back, as the dorsum of the foot or hand.

d. nasi. The anterior border of the external nose, from the root to the apex.

d. sellae. A square-shaped plate of bone forming the posterior boundary of the sella turcica.

doryl. Trade-mark for *carbachol.*

do'sage [G. *dosis*, a giving]. The proper amount of a medicine or other agent for a given case or condition.

electric d. The regulation of the strength of an electric current for therapeutic purposes.

radiation d. The quantity of radiation absorbed by exposed personnel; the product of radiation intensity and time measured in roentgens. See median lethal *dose.*

dose [*dosis*]. 1. The measured portion of medicine to be taken at one time. Abbreviated, d. Doses in this book are stated in the metric system followed, in parentheses, by the approximate equivalent in the apothecaries' system. 2. *In radiology*, the measure, expressed in number of roentgens, of a property of x-rays at a particular place, whether in air, tissue, or other material, or even in a vacuum; exposure.

air d. (a) Roentgen dose delivered at a point in free air. (b) The number of roentgens in the air at the center of the field employed in treatment with roentgen rays.

average d. One which may be expected ordinarily to produce the therapeutic effect for which the ingredient or preparation is most commonly employed.

booster d. That portion of an immunizing agent given at a later period to stimulate effects of a previous dose of the same agent. Also see *immunization.*

cumulative d. *In radiology*, a total dose delivered in fractions over a period of time.

daily d. The total amount to be administered in 24 hours.

depth d. The number of roentgens within the body at a specified depth below the surface field of roentgen irradiation.

erythema d. That quantity of radiation which, when delivered at a single sitting, will produce in at least 95 per cent of cases a definite reddening of the skin within one week after irradiation, followed by subsequent bronzing without permanent injury to the skin.

exit d. The dose of radiation at the surface of the body opposite to that on which the beam is incident.

field d. The total number of roentgens which affect the skin during treatment with roentgen rays.

integral d. *In radiology*, the total energy absorbed by a patient during exposure to radiation. Syn., *volume dose.*

LD 50 d. See median lethal *d.*

LD 100 d. See total lethal *d.*

lethal d. A dose sufficient to kill. Abbreviated, LD.

maximum d. The largest dose consistent with safety.

median lethal d. That dose of an injurious agent (drug, virus, radiation) given to a population of animals or man, such that 50 per cent will die within a specific time period. Abbreviated, LD 50 d.

minimum d. The smallest quantity of a medicine that will produce physiologic effects.

minimum lethal d. (a) That amount of an injurious agent (drug, virus, radiation) which is the average of the smallest dose that kills and the largest dose that fails to kill, when each of a series of animals is given a different dose under controlled conditions. Because of its general lack of accuracy, this measurement has been largely abandoned in favor of *median lethal dose.* Abbreviated, MLD. (b) Formerly the quantity of a toxin which will kill a guinea pig of 250 gr. weight in from 4 to 5 days.

percentage depth d. *In radiology*, an amount of radiation delivered at a specific depth in tissue, expressed as a percentage of the dosage to the skin.

permissible d. *In radiology*, the amount of radiation an individual may receive during a specific period with no expectation of harmful effects: also called *tolerance d.*

radiation d. The amount of energy absorbed in the form of ionization and excitation per unit of tissue measured in ergs per gram.

skin d. The number of roentgens on the surface of the skin at the center of the field of treatment; the sum of the air dose and the back scatter from underlying tissues.

skin erythema d. The amount of x-ray radiation which will redden the normal skin. Abbreviated, SED.

threshold d. *In therapeutics*, the minimum dose that will produce a given response.

tissue d. The number of roentgens of radioactive substances at specified points in the tissues of the body.

tolerance d. See permissible *d.*

total lethal d. That dose of an injurious agent (drug, virus, radiation) given to a population of animals or man, such that 100 per cent die within a given time period. Abbreviated LD 100 d.

volume d. See integral *d.*

do·sim′e·ter, do·sem′e·ter [*dosis;* G. *metron*, a measure]. *In radiology*, an instrument for measuring, usually by ionization methods, exposure to x-rays or to radioactive emanations.

integrating d. One utilizing a thimble ionization chamber in which the ionization current is amplified and indicated on a meter.

do·sim′e·try [*dosis; metron*]. 1. Accurate determination of medicinal doses. 2. A system of therapeutics consisting in the use of only a few drugs, mainly alkaloids, in the form of granules administered according to certain fixed rules. 3. Measurement of exposures or doses of x-rays. —**dosimet′ric,** *adj.*

photographic d. The determination of personnel radiation dosage by use of photographic film. See *film badge.*

dot. A minute intracellular granule with special staining characteristics.

Maurer's dots. Small bodies, stained red with Leishman's stain, seen in erythrocytes infected by *Plasmodium falciparum.* See Maurer's *clefts.*

doub′let (dub′lit) [L. *duplus*, double]. 1. *In optics*, a combination of two lenses of different focal length. 2. *In electricity*, a dipole.

douche (dōōsh) [F., from L. *ductio*, from *ducere*, to conduct (water)]. 1. A stream of water or air directed against the body or into a body cavity. *In physiotherapy*, douches are commonly used on the body surface for their stimulating effect. They may be hot, cold, or alternating. 2. *In gynecology*, lavage of the vagina; used for cleansing or for the application of heat or medication to the parts.

Douglas, Beverly [*American plastic surgeon*, 1891–]. Introduced the sieve graft, which sometimes is known by his name. See under *graft.*

Douglas, Claude Gordon [*English physiologist*, 1882–]. Known for his researches on respiration. Studied breathing at high altitudes (1910), and, with John Scott Haldane, Yandell Henderson, and Edward Christian Schneider, investigated the effects of atmospheric pressure at high altitudes (1911). Invented a rubber bag, to be supported on the shoulder, for capturing expired air in experiments with ambulatory subjects (1911); called the *Douglas bag.* With Haldane and Johannes Christiansen, made a study of carbon dioxide in the blood (1914); also with Haldane, he studied cardiac output in man during muscular exercise (1922). Since 1936 he has devoted attention to respiratory metabolism during muscular exercise.

Douglas, James [*Scottish anatomist and obstetrician*, 1675–1742]. Well known in his time for his writings on comparative myology (1707), for making the first attempt at a systematic medical bibliography (1715), and for his description of the peritoneum (1730). Remembered especially for his description of the rectouterine pouch, also called the *pouch of Douglas, cul-de-sac.* Described a pelvic abscess of the cul-de-sac; formerly called *Douglas' abscess.*

Douglas, John Cuppage [*Irish obstetrician*, 1777–1850]. Described spontaneous version sometimes occurring in transverse presentations, called *Douglas' version.*

doug″la·si′tis (dug″luh·sigh′tis) [after James *Douglas;* G. *-itis*, inflammation]. Inflammation of the rectouterine cul-de-sac (pouch of Douglas).

dou·rine′ (doo·reen′, doo′reen) [F., perhaps from Ar. *darin*, filthy]. A contagious venereal disease of horses, the prominent signs and symptoms consisting of inflammation of the genital organs and lymph nodes, and paralysis of the hind legs. The exciting cause is believed to be the *Trypanosoma equiperdum.*

Dover's powder. Ipecac and opium powder.

Dover's p. syrup. Ipecac and opium syrup.

Dover's p. tincture. Ipecac and opium tincture.

dow′el [ME. *dowle*]. *In dentistry*, a metallic pin inserted into a prepared root canal of a tooth in order to attach an artificial crown.

Downey, Hal [*American hematologist*, 1877–]. Known for his neounitarian theory of the origin of blood cells. The theory states that all blood cells are derived from stem cells which are identical and originate in reticuloendothelial cells.

doxyfed hydrochloride. Trade-marked name for *metamphetamine hydrochloride.*

dox″yl·a·mine′ suc′cin·ate. Generic name for the antihistaminic substance 2-[α-(2-dimethylaminoethoxy)-α-methylbenzyl] pyridine succinate; $C_{17}H_{22}N_2O.C_4H_6O_4$; marketed under the trade-marked name *decapryn succinate.*

Doyen, Eugène Louis [*French surgeon*, 1859–1916]. Described an operation for rapid exposure of the heart through a U-shaped incision over the costal cartilages, and a panhysterectomy by the abdominal route. His operation for pericardial paracentesis through a vertical median incision and perforation of the sternum with a trephine is known as *Doyen's operation.*

DPN Abbreviation for *diphosphopyridine nucleotide.* See *coenzyme I.*

DPN.2H Abbreviation for the reduced form of diphosphopyridine nucleotide or *dihydrocoenzyme I.*

DPT Abbreviation for *diphosphothiamine* (cocarboxylase).

dr, dr. Drachm.

drachm (dram), **dram** [G. *drachmē*, as much as one can hold in the hand]. The eighth part of the apothecary's ounce. (Symbol, ʒ.) Also, less commonly, the sixteenth part of the avoirdupois ounce. Abbreviated, dr, dr.

fluidrachm. The eighth part of a fluidounce Symbol, fʒ.

drac″on·ti′a·sis. Dracunculosis.

dra·con″ti·so′mus [G. *drakontion*, little dragon; *sōma*, body]. Median cleft of abdomen and thorax, with twisted vertebral column and flaring ribs.

dra·cun″cu·li′a·sis [L. *dracunculus*, small dragon; NL. *-iasis*, condition]. Infestation with *Dracunculus medinensis.* See also *dracunculosis.*

dra·cun″cu·lo′sis [*dracunculus;* G. *-ōsis*, condition]. A morbid condition caused by infestation with the nematode parasite *Dracunculus medinensis;* characterized by abscesses produced in the leg muscles by the gravid female worm; found in Africa, India, and Brazil; dracontiasis. Also called *Guinea worm infestation.*

Dra·cun′cu·lus [L.]. A genus of threadworms belonging to the superfamily Dracunculoidea.

D. medinensis. A species of filarial worms of which certain species of *Cyclops* are the intermediate hosts and man is a definitive host. Human infestation is caused by drinking raw water containing infested *Cyclops.* Syn., *guinea worm.*

draft, draught [AS. *dragan*, to draw]. 1. A current

of air. 2. A quantity of liquid, usually medicine, taken at one swallow.

black d. Infusion of senna with magnesium sulfate.

dra·gee′ (drah·zhay′) [F.]. A sugar-coated pill.

drag′on's blood. Any of several resinous secretions, characterized by a dark red color, obtained from the scale of the fruits of various species of *Daemonorops*. It is used as a coloring agent.

Dragstedt, Lester Reynold (1893–). American surgeon, who introduced an operation for the relief of peptic ulcer by transthoracic supradiaphragmatic division of the vagus nerves. Subsequently he devised a method for sectioning the vagus nerves above the diaphragm by an abdominal operation: called *Dragstedt's operation.* He introduced the accordion *graft,* and with John van Prohaska and Herman Paul Harms (1936) discovered *lipocaic.*

drain [AS. *drēhnigean*]. A material, such as gauze, rubber tubing, rubber tissue, or twisted suture material, which affords a channel of exit for the discharge from a wound or cavity.

capillary d. One of horsehair or silkworm gut used to keep a wound open for a short period.

cigarette d. A drain of gauze surrounded by rubber tissue, rubber dam, or split rubber tubing. Also called *Penrose d., Penrose latex nasogastric tube.*

lamp chimney d. A tubular drain of large caliber glass or metal, anchored over selected areas within the abdomen and adapted to gastric, colonic, and urinary bladder surgery.

Mikulicz d. A large gauze tampon formed by placing continuous or cut strips upon a square which lines the interior of the wound, the strip ends remaining outside.

Penrose d. See cigarette *d.*

sump d. An aspirating tubular drain of rubber, plastic, glass, etc, sometimes with lateral openings and fishtail ends.

drain. *In surgery,* to procure the discharge or evacuation of fluid from a cavity by operation, tapping, or otherwise.

drain′age [*drēhnigean*]. The method of draining; also, the fluid drained off. See *drain.*

basal d. Removal of cerebrospinal fluid from the cisterna magna.

continuous d. Constant emptying of a viscus, usually the urinary bladder by a retained catheter or tube.

negative pressure d. A closed system for draining an empyema cavity.

postural d. Removal of bronchial secretions or of the contents of a lung abscess by placing the patient head downward.

Drake, Daniel [*American physician,* 1785–1852]. Outstanding figure in the annals of American medicine in the Middle West. Remembered especially for his book on the diseases of the interior valley of North America (1850–55).

dram. Drachm.

dramamine. Trade-mark for dimenhydrinate, the 8-chlorotheophyllinate of diphenhydramine, useful in motion sickness.

dram′a·tism [G. *drama,* deed, act]. Stilted and lofty speech or behavior, observed in the insane.

Dransart, Henri Narcisse [*French ophthalmologist,* 1847–1930]. Remembered for an operation for ptosis in which the orbicularis and levator fascia are buried, using absorbable sutures.

drape [F. *drap,* cloth]. Arrange sterile linen about a part preparatory to operation or examination.

drap″e·to·ma′ni·a [G. *drapetēs,* runaway; *mania,* madness]. A morbid desire to wander from home; dromomania.

draught. See *draft.*

draw [AS. *dragan*]. 1. Cause to soften and discharge, said of a poultice. 2. *In dentistry,* pull; remove a tooth from its socket.

draw′-sheet″. A narrow sheet, covering a rubber sheet, across the bed under the patient's buttocks; can easily be withdrawn and replaced if soiled.

dread [AS. *drǣdan*]. Extreme fear or apprehension.

dream [ME.]. An involuntary series of images, emotions, and thoughts occurring in the mind during sleep or during abstracted imagining. According to Freud, a dream is a vehicle which conveys impulses from the unconscious to the conscious levels of mind. **—dream′y,** *adj.*

day d. Idle reverie.

waking d. An illusion or hallucination.

wet d. Seminal emission during sleep, generally accompanying an erotic dream.

dream. To experience images and trains of thought during sleep, or as if asleep; to have a dream.

drench [AS. *drencan,* to give a drink]. *In veterinary medicine,* a draft of medicine administered to an animal. **—drench,** *v.*

drep′a·no·cyte (drep′uh·no·sight, dri·pan′o·sight) [G. *drepanē,* sickle; *kytos,* cell]. A crescent-shaped cell; a sickle cell.

drep″a·no·cy·the′mi·a. See sickle-cell *anemia.*

drep″a·no·cy·to′sis (drep″uh·no·sigh·to′sis, dri·pan″o·). Presence of sickle cells (drepanocytes) in blood. See also sickle-cell *anemia.*

Dresbach, Melvin [*American physician,* 1874–1946]. Known for his description of elliptocytes. Sickle-cell anemia is sometimes erroneously called *Dresbach's syndrome.*

dress′er [OF. *dresser,* to arrange, from L. *dirigere,* to direct]. An attendant in British hospitals, usually a medical student, whose special duty is to dress and bandage wounds.

dress′ing [*dresser*]. 1. Application of various materials for protecting a wound and favoring its healing. 2. Material so applied.

drib′ble [AS. *dryppan*]. 1. Drool. 2. Void in drops, as urine from a distended or paralyzed bladder.

drierite. A trade-mark for anhydrous calcium sulfate, a dehydrating agent.

drift. *In dentistry,* movement of teeth from their normal position in the dental arch.

mesial d. The tendency of teeth in proximal contact to move toward the midline as their contact-points become worn.

drill [D. *drillen,* to bore]. Cutting instrument for boring holes in tooth or bone by rotary motion.

Drinker, Philip [*American industrial hygienist,* 1894–]. Invented the iron lung or *Drinker respirator;* see under *respirator.* Invented a negative-pressure cabinet for maintaining respiration in the newborn. See also *Drinker's method* under *artificial respiration;* Drinker-Collins *resuscitation.*

drip [AS. *dryppan*]. The continuous slow introduction of fluid containing nutrients or drugs. **—drip,** *v.*

drisdol. Trade-mark for vitamin D_2 or calciferol.

driv′el·ing [AS. *dreflian*]. 1. An involuntary flow of the saliva, as in old age, infancy, idiocy, and mental stupor. 2. Talking, as in senile weakness of the mind, idiocy, and mental stupor.

dri′ving. *In electroencephalography,* the appearance of a certain frequency (cycles per second) in the electroencephalogram as a result of sensory stimulation at that frequency.

dro·car′bil. $C_{16}H_{23}AsN_2O_7$; the acetarsone salt of arecoline, a nearly white or slightly yellow powder, freely soluble in water; it is used as a veterinary anthelmintic. See *nemural.*

drom′o·graph, dro′mo·graph [G. *dromos,* course; *graphein,* to write]. Instrument for registering the velocity of the blood current.

drom″o·ma′ni·a (drom′o·may′nee·uh, dro″mo·) [*dromos;* G. *mania,* madness]. An insane desire to wander; vagabondage.

drom″o·pho′bi·a (drom″o·fo′bee·uh, dro″mo·) [*dromos;* G. *phobos,* fear]. Morbid fear of walking or roaming about.

dromoran hydrobromide. Trade-marked name for *racemorphan hydrobromide* (formerly *methorphinan hydrobromide*), a potent synthetic analgesic related chemically and pharmacologically to morphine.

drop [AS. *dropa*]. 1. A minute mass of liquid which in falling or in hanging from a surface forms a spheroid. 2. The falling of a part, as from paralysis.

ankle d. See toe *d.*

d. hand. See wrist *d.*

d. heart. See *cardioptosis.*

ear drops. Liquid medication instilled by drops into the external auditory meatus.

foot d. See toe *d.*

toe d. Inability to dorsiflex the foot; generally due to paralysis of the dorsiflexor muscles of the foot and toes, or to severance of a tendon.

wrist d. Inability to extend the hand; due to paralysis of the extensor muscles of the hand and fingers, or to severance of a tendon.

drop′let [*dropa*]. A minute particle of moisture expelled by talking, sneezing, or, coughing, which may carry infectious microorganisms from one individual to another.

drop′per [*dropa*]. A bottle, tube, or pipet, fitted for the emission of a liquid drop by drop.

drop′sy [G. *hydrōps,* from *hydōr,* water]. An infiltration of the tissues with diluted lymph, or the collection of such lymph in the body cavities; anasarca. —**dropsical,** *adj.*

abdominal d. Old term for ascites.

cachectic d. That occurring in cachexia; it is due to a decrease of the plasma proteins.

cardiac d. Edema due to congestive heart failure.

d. of brain. Hydrocephaly.

d. of pericardium. Hydropericardium.

encysted d. of peritoneum. Ascites saccatus.

epidemic d. A noninfectious disease occurring in India which is characterized by gastroenteric upsets, edema, decreased pigmentation in certain areas of the skin, and cardiac dysfunction. The exact etiology is unknown, but it probably is associated with foods and mustard oil.

famine d. Nutritional edema; war edema. A form of edema occurring in individuals suffering from protein deprivation, either as the result of disease, or from inadequate intake.

general d. (a) Dropsy of one or more of the large serous sacs of the body combined with anasarca. (b) Superficial dropsy when it affects the trunk and arms as well as the legs.

mechanical d. That due to mechanical obstruction of the veins or lymphatics.

renal d. Anasarca due to disease of the kidneys.

dros′er·in [G. *droseros,* dewy]. A ferment resembling pepsin and found in the digestive secretions of insectivorous plants.

Dro·soph′i·la [G. *drosos,* dew; *philein,* to love]. A genus of Diptera containing the common fruit flies.

D. melanogaster. The best known species because of its extensive use in genetic analysis.

drug [ME. *drogge*]. A substance used as a medicine.

crude d. An unrefined drug containing its entire ingredients from which the active principles are derived; commonly, the dried leaves, bark, or rhizome of a plant containing therapeutically active principles.

drug′gist [*drogge*]. A dealer in medicines.

drum [D. *trom*]. The tympanic membrane; eardrum.

drunk′en·ness [AS. *drincan*]. Intoxication; usually produced by drinking alcoholic liquor.

ether d. That produced by drinking ether.

punch d. A condition simulating drunkenness due to hemorrhagic encephalitis caused by blows to the head, as in boxing.

drunk·om′e·ter. See breath alcohol *method.*

drupe [G. *dryppa,* olive]. A fruit which has a thin epicarp, a fleshy mesocarp, and a stony endocarp which encloses a seed, as the plum or peach.

dru′sen (*See* NOTES § 35) [Ger. *Druse,* ore, crystal]. A term sometimes applied to the inflammatory thickenings of the choroid coat of the eye near Descemet's membrane. Often confused with the plural of the German word meaning gland.

Dry·op′ter·is (dry·op′tur·iss) [G. *drys,* oak; *pteris,* fern]. A large genus of medium-sized ferns of the Polypodiaceae; woodfern.

D. Filix-mas. European aspidium or male fern, the rhizome and stipes of which are a source of aspidium oleoresin.

D. marginalis. American aspidium or marginal fern, the rhizome and stipes of which are a source of aspidium oleoresin.

Drysdale, Thomas Murray [*American gynecologist,* 1831–1904]. Remembered for his description of certain bodies discovered in the contents of an ovarian cyst, possibly of pathognomonic significance, called *Drysdale's ovarian corpuscles.*

D. Sc., D. S. Doctor of Science.

D.t. Duration tetany.

du″al·is′tic the′o·ry. The theory that the lymphoblast of lymphatic tissue and the myeloblast of myeloid tissue are stem cells having entirely different potencies in hemopoiesis.

Duane, Alexander [*American ophthalmologist,* 1858–1926]. Remembered for his invention of various devices used in ophthalmology. He described his syndrome as fibrosis and paralysis of the external rectus muscle, so that rotation of the eye is impossible; there is retraction of the eyeball with narrowing of the palpebral fissure.

Dubini, Angelo [*Italian physician,* 1813–1902]. Remembered for his description of the myoclonic form of epidemic encephalitis affecting all ages; a fatal form of electric chorea (1846), also called *Dubini's disease.* Described the hookworm as a cause of ancylostomiasis.

Du Bois, Eugene Floyd [*American physiologist,* 1882–]. Known for his work on basal metabolism in health and disease (1924), and for his later studies of nutrition. His basal metabolism standards are expressed in tabular form as calories per square meter per hour. They were derived by measurement of the metabolic rates of many normal individuals of all ages and both sexes, and are stated by age groups for each sex. Called *Du Bois standards; Aub-Du Bois standards.*

Dubois, Jacques. See Jacobus *Sylvius.*

Dubois, Marie Eugene François Thomas [*Dutch anatomist and paleontologist,* 1858–1941]. Noted for his discovery of the prehistoric Java man, *Pithecanthropus erectus* (1891).

Du Bois, Paul [*French obstetrician,* 1795–1871]. Remembered for his description of the multiple necrotic foci found in the thymus of infants with hereditary syphilis, called *Du Bois' abscess.* Described the severe vomiting of pregnancy (1852).

Du Bois-Reymond, Emil Heinrich [*German physiologist,* 1818–96]. Internationally known for his researches in medical electricity. Described electrotonus (1843). Regarded as the founder of modern electrophysiology. Was the first to describe physiologic tetanus. His induction apparatus was an adjustable device provided with primary and secondary coils, and was used to stimulate tissue by controlled induction shock.

Du·boi′si·a [after F. N. *Dubois*, French botanist]. A genus of Far Eastern tropical plants, certain members of which contain scopolamine, hyoscyamine, and related alkaloids, while others contain nicotine and associated alkaloids.

du·boi′sine. Old term for an alkaloid, identified as hyoscyamine, or a mixture of alkaloids, including hyoscyamine and scopolamine, from certain species of *Duboisia*, especially *D. myoporoides*.

Dubos, René Jules [*French bacteriologist in the U.S.A.*, 1901–]. Discovered tyrothricin and gramicidin (1939). Cultivated tubercle bacilli by a quick method called *Dubos' method.*

Duboscq, Jules [*French optician*, 1817–86]. Remembered for his invention of an optical instrument for comparing and matching colors of solutions, called *Duboscq's colorimeter.*

Duchenne (de Boulogne), Guillaume Benjamin Amand (1806–75). French neurologist; founder of electrotherapy. He used faradism as early as 1830, and made important studies of electrophysiology (1855). He described progressive spinal muscular atrophy (1849), called *Duchenne-Aran muscular atrophy, Cruveilhier's disease*, and gave a classic description of tabes dorsalis (1859), which sometimes is called *Duchenne's disease;* also gave the first description of chronic progressive bulbar paralysis (1860), called *Duchenne's paralysis.* He studied the mechanism of facial expressions of emotion (1862). Progressive muscular dystrophy with pseudohypertrophy, described by Greisinger in 1865, by Duchenne in 1868, and by Erb in 1884, is known as *Duchenne-Greisinger disease, Erb's paralysis, dystrophy.* Partial paralysis of the brachial plexus, due to laceration at birth, is called *Erb-Duchenne paralysis, Erb's palsy.* He also introduced the technique of examining small bits of muscle taken from living patients (1868), now known as *biopsy*, 2.

duck′er·ing [after G. F. *Duckering*]. A method of disinfecting hair and wool, employed against the *Bacillus anthracis. Rare.*

duck heart. Enlargement of the left ventricle as a result of aortic insufficiency, giving the heart a duck-shaped configuration in its fluoroscopic and radiographic appearance. Also called *wooden-shoe heart.*

Ducrey's bacillus. See *Hemophilus ducreyi* under *Hemophilus.*

duct [L. *ductus*, from *ducere*, to lead]. 1. A tube or channel, especially one for conveying the secretions of a gland. 2. A small enclosed channel conducting any fluid, as the cochlear duct.

accessory pancreatic d. The proximal part of the dorsal pancreatic duct that usually persists. Also called *d. of Santorini.*

allantoic d. The proximal part of the allantois opening into the cloaca. Also called *allantoenteric d.*

alveolar d. One of the air passages in the lung branching from a respiratory bronchiole and leading to alveolar sacs.

archinephric d. See pronephric *d.*

Bartholin's d. (a) The duct of a major vestibular gland at the vaginal introitus. (b) The duct of the major sublingual gland. *Obs.*

bile d. A general term for the cystic, hepatic, or common duct or any of the small ducts of the liver connecting with the hepatic duct. Also called *biliary d.*

brachial d. The tubular second or fourth visceral grooves opening into the cervical sinus of the embryo.

cervical d. The temporary, external duct of the cervical vesicle formed as the cervical sinus is closed over by the opercular fold of the hyoid arch.

cloacal d. The caudal part of the cloaca before the urorectal septum completely divides rectum and urogenital sinus. Also called *Reichel's d.*

cochlear d. The ductus cochlearis; the endolymph-filled, triangular (in cross-section) canal between the scala tympani and scala vestibuli; it contains the organ of Corti. Syn., *membranous cochlea, membranous cochlear canal.* Formerly called *scala media.* See Plate 20.

common bile d. The duct formed by the union of the cystic and the hepatic ducts. Syn., *ductus choledochus.*

common pharyngobranchial d. The medial part of the fourth pharyngeal pouch forming a common duct for the ultimobranchial body (fifth pouch) and the lateral part of the fourth pouch.

cystic d. The duct of the gallbladder. See Plate 13.

deferent d. See *ductus* deferens.

dorsal pancreatic d. That of the embryonic dorsal pancreas.

d. of Bellini. Papillary *d.*

d. of Cuvier. One of the two common cardinal veins.

d. of Stensen (Steno). See parotid *d.*

d. of the epididymis. See epididymal *d.*

d. of the testis. That made up of the epididymal duct, the ductus deferens, and the ejaculatory duct.

efferent d. See efferent *ductule.*

ejaculatory d. The terminal part of the ductus deferens after junction with the duct of a seminal vesicle, embedded in the prostate gland and opening into the urethra on the colliculus seminalis. See Plate 44.

endolymphatic d. (a) The duct which unites the endolymphatic sac with the utriculosaccular duct: also called *otic d.* (b) *In embryology*, a dorsomedian diverticulum of the otocyst, the anlage of the endolymphatic sac.

epididymal d. The highly convoluted part of the duct of the testis which forms the main mass of the epididymis. Syn., *d. of the epididymis, ductus epididymidis.*

excretory d. A duct, lined by nonsecretory epithelium, which is solely conductive.

frontonasal d. See nasofrontal *d.*

galactophorous d. Old term for lactiferous duct.

Gartner's d. A persistent remnant of the mesonephric duct in the female. Syn., *longitudinal d. of the epoöphoron.*

hepatic d. The common duct formed by the union of the left hepatic duct which drains the left and caudate lobes of the liver and the right hepatic duct which drains the right and quadrate lobes of the liver. Also called *common hepatic d.* See Plate 13.

hepatocystic d. A bile duct connected directly with the gallbladder.

hepatopancreatic d. The terminal part of the embryonic common bile duct which also drains the ventral pancreas.

intercalated d. The narrow portion of the intralobular ducts of the pancreas, or the parotid or submaxillary glands.

lacrimal d. A tube in each eyelid extending from the punctum lacrimale to the vasolacrimal sac: also called *lacrimal canaliculus.*

lacrimonasal d. See nasolacrimal *d.*

lactiferous d. One of the excretory ducts of the mammary gland, opening on the nipple. Also called *milk d.* See Plate 43.

longitudinal d. of the epoophoron. See Gartner's *d.*

Luschka's d. One of the aberrant bile ducts

found in the wall of the gallbladder. It may connect with a bile duct, but never with the lumen of the gallbladder.

mesonephric d. The duct of the mesonephros or embryonic kidney. It becomes the excretory duct of the testis and gives rise to the ureteric bud in both sexes. Syn., *Wolffian d.*

metanephric d. The ureter.

milk d. See lactiferous *d.*

Müllerian d. The paramesonephric duct: also called *Müller's d.*

nasofrontal d. That between the frontal sinus and the middle meatus of the nose. Also called *frontonasal d.*

nasolacrimal d. The membranous duct lodged within the nasolacrimal canal; it gives passage to the tears from the lacrimal sac to the inferior meatus of the nose. See Plates 12, 19.

nasopalatine d. A duct or canal between the embryonic oral and nasal cavities formed at the site of fusion of the palatine process of the maxillary process of the embryo with the primitive palate. Rarely patent in adults; usually represented by vestigial cords, blind tubes, or cysts.

omphalomesenteric d. The vitelline duct.

otic d. See endolymphatic *d.*

pancreatic d. The main duct of the pancreas formed from the dorsal and ventral pancreatic ducts of the embryo. Also called *d. of Wirsung.*

papillary d. Any one of the largest collecting tubules of the kidney, opening into the minor calyxes of the renal pelvis: also called *duct of Bellini.*

paramesonephric d. An embryonic genital duct. In the female, the anlage of the oviducts, uterus, and vagina; in the male, it degenerates, leaving the appendix testis. Syn., *Müllerian d.*

paraurethral d. That of a paraurethral gland. Formerly called *Skene's duct.*

parotid d. That of the parotid gland. It passes horizontally across the lateral surface of the masseter muscle, pierces the buccinator muscle, and opens into the oral vestibule opposite the second upper molar tooth. Also called *Stensen's d., d. of Steno, Stenonian d.*

perilymphatic d. Aqueduct of the cochlea; a minute canal uniting the scala tympani with the subarachnoid space: also called *periotic d.*

periotic d. See perilymphatic *d.*

pharyngobranchial d. The narrow medial part of a pharyngeal pouch.

pleuropericardial d. The opening in the pleuropericardial membrane temporarily connecting the embryonic pleural and pericardial cavities. Also called *pleuropericardial canal.*

pleuroperitoneal d. The opening in the pleuroperitoneal membrane temporarily connecting the embryonic pleural and peritoneal cavities. Also called *pleuroperitoneal canal.*

primary genital ducts. The mesonephric and paramesonephric ducts.

pronephric d. That of the pronephros. It becomes the functional mesonephric duct. Syn., *archinephric d.*

prostatic d. Any one of the ducts conveying the secretion of the prostate into the urethra. See Plate 44.

right lymphatic d. The common lymph trunk receiving the right jugular, subclavian, and bronchomediastinal trunks, and emptying into the right subclavian vein at its junction with the right internal jugular vein.

salivary d. That of a salivary gland.

semicircular ducts. The membranous semicircular canals.

seminal d. The duct of the testis, especially the ductus deferens and the ejaculatory duct. Syn., *spermatic d.*

spermatic d. The seminal duct.

Stensen's d. See parotid *d.*

sublingual ducts. Those of the sublingual gland opening into the oral cavity. Some unite to form the **major sublingual duct.** Others, the **minor sublingual ducts,** open on the sublingual plica.

submaxillary d. That of the submaxillary gland receiving the major sublingual duct and emptying into the oral cavity at the side of the frenulum of the tongue. Also called *Wharton's d.*

thoracic d. The common lymph trunk beginning in the cisterna chyli, passing upward, and emptying into the left subclavian vein at its junction with the left internal jugular vein.

thymopharyngeal d. The third pharyngobranchial duct which may elongate and persist between thymus and pharynx.

thyrocervical d. The fourth branchial duct.

thyroglossal d. A slender temporary duct connecting the thyroid anlage with the surface of the tongue.

thyropharyngeal d. The fourth pharyngobranchial duct.

umbilical d. Old term for vitelline duct.

urogenital d. (a) The male urethra from the orifices of the ejaculatory ducts to the fossa navicularis. (b) In certain vertebrates, the mesonephric duct. (c) See urogenital *sinus.*

utricular d. The utriculosaccular *d.*

utriculosaccular d. A membranous tube uniting the utricle and the saccule; from it arises the endolymphatic duct.

vitelline d. The constricted part of the yolk sac opening into the midgut in the region of the future ileum. Syn., *omphalomesenteric d.* Formerly called *umbilical duct.*

Wharton's d. See submaxillary *d.*

Wolffian d. The mesonephric duct. Also spelled *wolffian d.*

duct'less [*ductus;* AS. *lēas*, free from]. Having no excretory duct, as the ductless glands.

duct'ule [dim. from *ductus*]. A small duct.

aberrant ductules. Blindly ending epithelial tubules associated with the epididymis; the ductuli aberrantes superiores and inferiores.

efferent d. Any one of eight to fifteen coiled ducts which connect the rete testis with the duct of the epididymis and form the head of the epididymis; derived from paragenital mesonephric tubules. Syn., *lobule of the epididymis, vascular cone, efferent duct.*

duc'tu·lus (pl. *ductuli*) [dim. from *ductus*]. A small duct. Also see *ductule.*

ductuli aberrantes inferiores. Vestigial remains of caudal mesonephric tubules attached to the lower part of the duct of the epididymis.

ductuli aberrantes superiores. Vestigial remains of caudal mesonephric tubules and duct; usually the first two epigenital tubules; appendix epididymidis.

ductuli transversi. That part of the epoöphoron consisting of the vestigial remains of paragenital mesonephric tubules.

d. alveolaris. See alveolar *duct.*

duc'tus (pl. *ductūs*) [L.]. Duct.

d. arteriosus. The distal half of the left sixth aortic arch forming a fetal blood shunt between the pulmonary artery and the aorta. **Patent d. arteriosus** refers to the congenital anomaly in which there is a persistence of this fetal blood shunt indefinitely after birth. Also called *Botallo's duct, duct of Botal.* See Plate 6.

d. arteriosus bilateral. A developmental anomaly in which the right sixth aortic arch persists entirely or in part.

d. caroticus. That part of the embryonic dorsal aortae between the third and fourth aortic arches which normally disappears early in development.

d. choledochus. The common bile duct.

d. cochlearis. The cochlear duct.

d. deferens. That portion of the excretory duct system of the testis which runs from the epididymal duct to the ejaculatory duct. Syn., *vas deferens.* Also called *deferent duct.* See Plate 44.

d. endolymphaticus. Endolymphatic duct.

d. epididymidis. Epididymal duct.

d. perilymphaticus. Aqueduct of the cochlea.

d. reuniens. A membranous tube in the inner ear uniting the saccule with the cochlear duct; it contains endolymph. Also called *Hensen's canal.*

d. venosus. A venous channel of the embryonic liver shunting blood from the left umbilical vein to the enlarging right sinus venosus of the heart. Also called *duct of Arantius.*

Duddell, Benedict [*English ophthalmologist,* eighteenth century]. Wrote on diseases of the fibrous coats of the eye (1729). Described the posterior elastic lamina, which sometimes is known as *Duddell's membrane.*

Dudley, Emilius Clark [*American gynecologist,* 1850–1928]. Known for his operation for retroversion of the uterus, in which a strip is denuded from the anterior surface of the uterus; this is followed by the removal of other strips along the inner side of each round ligament, the three denuded areas being sutured together. Devised an operation for painful menstruation in which the uterine cervix is split posteriorly and sutured to provide a permanently widened internal os.

Dudley, Harold Ward [*English physiologist and biochemist,* 1887–1935]. With Henry Hallett Dale (1929), isolated acetylcholine from the spleens of animals. With John Chassar Moir, isolated ergometrine (1935), now called ergonovine.

Dugas, Louis Alexander [*American surgeon,* 1806–84]. Remembered for his test for dislocation of the shoulder; the elbow cannot be made to touch the side of the chest when the hand of the affected side is placed on the opposite shoulder.

Duhring, Louis Adolphus [*American dermatologist,* 1845–1913]. Known for his description of dermatitis herpetiformis, called *Duhring's disease.*

Dührssen, Alfred [*German gynecologist,* 1862–1933]. Remembered for his description of an operation to correct displacement of the uterus by vaginal fixation. Credited with being the first to perform vaginal Cesarean section (1895). *Dührssen's incisions* are incisions of the cervix to facilitate delivery.

du·ip′a·ra [L. *duo,* two; *parere,* to bear]. A woman who has borne two children.

Duke's test. See under *test.*

Duke-Elder's device. See *stenopeic.*

Dukes, Clement [*English physician,* 1845–1925]. Known for his description of acute infectious erythema, which he distinguished from measles, rubella, and scarlet fever. Its existence as a separate entity is open to doubt. Called *fourth disease, Dukes's disease, Filatov-Dukes disease.*

dul″ca·ma′ra (dul″kuh·mair′uh, ·mah′ruh) [L. *dulcis,* sweet; *amarus,* bitter]. The dried stems of *Solanum dulcamara,* bitter nightshade, containing an alkaloid, solanine. In overdoses it causes nausea, emesis, and convulsive muscular movements; has been employed in psoriasis and similar skin diseases.

dul″ca·ma′rin [*dulcis; amarus*]. $C_{22}H_{34}O_{10}$. A yellow, amorphous glycoside found in dulcamara.

dul′cin. $C_9H_{12}O_2N_2$; *p*-phenetolcarbamide; 4-ethoxyphenylurea; it occurs as white, lustrous needles and is soluble in water and alcohol. It is about 250 times as sweet as cane sugar and has been suggested as a substitute for saccharin. See *sucrol, valzin.*

dul′cite (dul′sight, ·sit). Dulcitol.

dul′ci·tol. $C_6H_{14}O_6$. Sugar from *Melampyrum nemorosum* and other plants.

dul′cose. Dulcitol.

dull [ME. *dul*]. 1. Slow of perception. 2. Not resonant on percussion; may be normal as over the heart or pathologic as over an area of pulmonary consolidation. 3. Not bright in appearance. 4. Not sharp; blunt. —**dull′ness,** *n.*

dumb [AS.]. Unable to utter articular speech. —**dumb′ness,** *n.*

dumb mad′ness. Dumb rabies. See *rabies.*

dum′my [AS. *dumb*]. A substitute for a natural tooth; pontic.

Dunant, Jean Henri [*Swiss philanthropist,* 1828–1910]. Aroused public opinion with his account (1863) of the battlefield of Solferino (1859). Organized the first Geneva Convention (1864) which founded the International Red Cross Society.

Dunbar's serum. See *pollantin.*

Duncan, James Matthews [*Scottish gynecologist* 1826–90]. Remembered for his description of the folds in the loose peritoneal covering of the uterus seen immediately after delivery, called *Duncan's folds.* Described a manner of presentation of the placenta at the outlet by one margin, the maternal surface usually being delivered first; known as *Duncan's position.*

Dun·ferm′line scale (dun·furm′lyne, ·lin, dun′-furm·) [after *Dunfermline,* Scotland, where it was developed]. A scheme for classifying children, according to their state of nutrition, into four grades: (1) superior; (2) fair; (3) requiring supervision; (4) requiring medical treatment.

Dunglison, Robley [*American physiologist,* 1798–1869]. Gave earliest known description of chronic hereditary chorea (1842). Author of the first comprehensive medical dictionary in America (1833) and of several texts on physiology and medical practice.

Dunham, Edward Kellogg [*American pathologist,* 1860–1922]. Known as the inventor of a solution of 1% of peptone and 0.5% of sodium chloride in distilled water, used as a culture medium for bacteria as a preliminary step in ascertaining indol formation.

du′o- [L.]. A combining form meaning *two.*

du″o·crin′in (dew″o·krin′in, dew·ock′rin·in). The hormone, released by the intestinal mucosa when certain foodstuffs are in contact with it, which stimulates the duodenal glands of Brunner to secrete.

du″o·de·nec′ta·sis [L. *duodeni,* twelve, from the length of the duodenum—about twelve fingers' breadth; G. *ektasis,* a stretching out]. Chronic dilatation of the duodenum.

du″o·de·nec′to·my [*duodeni;* G. *ektomē,* excision]. Excision of part of the duodenum.

duodenin. Trade-mark for a preparation containing secretin and enterokinase.

du″o·de·ni′tis [*duodeni;* G. *-itis,* inflammation]. Inflammation of the duodenum.

du″o·de′no- (dew″o·dee′no-, ·den′o-, dew·od′i·no-), **duoden-** [*duodeni*]. A combining form meaning *related to* or *connected with the duodenum.*

du″o·de″no·chol″an·gi′tis (·kol″an·jy′tis, ·ko″-lan·jy′tis) [*duodeni;* G. *cholē,* bile; *aggeion,* vessel;

-itis, inflammation]. Inflammation of the duodenum and the common bile duct about the ampulla.

du″o·de″no·chol″e·cys·tos′to·my (·kol″i·sis·tos′-to·mee, ·ko″li·) [*duodeni; cholē;* G. *kystis*, bladder; *stoma*, mouth]. The formation of an anastomosis between the duodenum and gallbladder.

du″o·de″no·cho·led″o·chot′o·my (·ko·led″o-cot′o·mee, ·ko″led·o·) [*duodeni; cholē;* G. *dochos*, able to hold; *tomē*, a cutting]. A modification of choledochotomy by incising the duodenum in order to approach the common duct.

du″o·de″no·col′ic [*duodeni;* G. *kolon*, colon]. Relating to the duodenum and the colon, as a duodenocolic fistula.

du″o·de″no·cys·tos′to·my [*duodeni;* G. *kystis*, bladder; *stoma*, mouth]. Duodenocholecystostomy.

du″o·de″no·en″ter·os′to·my [*duodeni;* G. *enteron*, intestine; *stoma*]. Surgical formation of a passage between the duodenum and another part of the intestine.

du″o·de′no·gram (dew″o·dee′no·gram, dew·od′-i·no·) [*duodeni;* G. *gramma*, letter]. A roentgenogram of the duodenum.

du″o·de″no·he·pat′ic [*duodeni;* G. *hēpar*, liver]. Pertaining to the duodenum and the liver, as the duodenohepatic ligament.

du″o·de″no·il″e·os′to·my [*duodeni;* G. *eilein*, to roll; *stoma*, mouth]. The formation of a passage between the duodenum and the ileum.

du″o·de″no·jej″u·nos′to·my (dew″o·dee ″no·, ·jedj″yoo·nos′to·mee, dew″o·den″o·, dew·od″i·no·) [*duodeni;* L. *jejunus*, empty; *stoma*]. Surgical anastomosis of the duodenum to the jejunum.

du″o·de″no·pan″cre·a·tec′to·my [*duodeni;* G. *pagkreas*, pancreas; *ektomē*, excision]. The operative excision of a portion of the duodenum together with the head of the pancreas. Syn., *pancreatoduodenectomy.*

du″o·de′no·plas″ty [*duodeni;* G. *plassein*, to form, mold]. A reparative operation upon some portion of the duodenum. See *pyloroplasty.*

du·o·de″no·py″lo·rec′to·my. Resection of a portion of the duodenum and the pylorus.

du″o·de·nor′rha·phy [*duodeni;* G. *rhaphē*, suture]. The suture and repair of the duodenum after incision, as for the closure of a ruptured duodenal ulcer.

du″o·de·nos′co·py [*duodeni;* G. *skopein*, to examine]. Inspection and visual examination of the duodenum by instrumental means.

du″o·de·nos′to·my [*duodeni;* G. *stoma*, mouth]. The formation, temporarily, of a duodenal fistula by surgical procedure.

du″o·de·not′o·my [*duodeni;* G. *tomē*, a cutting]. Surgical incision of the duodenum.

du″o·de′num, du·od′e·num [*duodeni*]. The first part of the small intestine, beginning at the pylorus. It is from eight to ten inches long and is the most fixed part of the small intestine; consists of superior, descending, and inferior portions, and contains the openings of the pancreatic duct or ducts and the common bile duct. See Plates 10, 13. —**duodenal,** *adj.*

giant d. An enormously enlarged duodenum, similar to that seen in congenital megacolon.

inversed d. A congenital abnormality associated with acute angulation and dilatation.

mobile d. A movable condition of the duodenum.

du″o·pa·ren′tal [L. *duo*, two; *parens*, parent]. Derived from two sexual elements.

duotal. A trade-mark for guaiacol carbonate.

Duplay, Emanuel Simon [*French surgeon*, 1836–1924]. Remembered for his contributions to reconstructive surgery of the urethra. Devised an operation for epispadias, forming a new urethra at the expense of the corpora cavernosa; he also devised an operation for hypospadias, in three stages, and described subdeltoid bursitis.

du′pli·ca″ture [L. *duplicare*, to double]. A fold, as a membrane folding upon itself.

du″pli·ca′tus cru″ci·a′ta [L.]. Experimentally produced double monsters obtained by grafting on inversion of the two-celled stage in amphibia.

du·plic′i·tas (dew·pliss′i·tus) [L., a being double]. A monstrosity with duplication of either the cephalic or pelvic end, or both. See Plate 25.

d. cru″ci·a′ta. A rare form of conjoined twins in which there is superior and inferior duplicity, the long axes of the bodies forming a cross.

du·plic′i·ty (dew·pliss′i·tee) [*duplicitas*]. *In teratology*, the condition of being double; duplexity.

du·plic′i·ty the′o·ry. A theory of vision that the retinal rods are stimulated by differing intensities of light, the cones only by differing wave lengths.

duponol C. Trade-mark for a U.S.P. grade of sodium lauryl sulfate.

Dupuytren, Guillaume [*French surgeon*, 1777–1835]. Greatest of the early vascular surgeons. First to excise the lower jaw with success (1812). Ligated the external iliac artery (1815) and the subclavian artery (1819). Described fracture of the lower end of the fibula with displacement (1819); called *Dupuytren's fracture.* Divided the sternocleidomastoid muscle subcutaneously for torticollis (1822). Gave the first adequate description of congenital dislocation of the hip (1826). Devised an operation, in which he used his enterotome, for making an artificial anus (1828). Described an abscess of the right iliac fossa (1829). Classified burns (1832), and wrote a treatise on war wounds (1834). See also Dupuytren's *contracture.*

Duquesnel's aconitine. See *aconitine* nitrate.

du′ra. The dura mater: abbreviated terminology.

duracaine [L. *durare*, to endure; *cocaine*]. Trademark for a local anesthetic that contains procaine as the analgesic principle; the substance is used for spinal anesthesia.

duracillin. Trade-mark for certain preparations containing procaine penicillin G.

duralumin [L. *durus*, hard; *alumen*, alum]. A noncorroding alloy of aluminum and copper, used in surgical splints and appliances.

du′ra ma′ter [L., hard mother]. The fibrous membrane forming the outermost covering of the brain and spinal cord. Syn., *dura.* —**dural,** *adj.*

Duran-Reynals, Francisco [*American physician and bacteriologist*, 1899–]. Known for his research on cancer. Reported (1928) that vaccinal virus infection of rabbits was aggravated when extracts of rabbit, guinea pig, and rat testis were injected into the skin along with the virus, the effect being produced in the tissues of the host, not in the virus. Today the term *Duran-Reynals' spreading factors* is used to include various substances with the common property of increasing the permeability of connective tissue. Certain bacteria have been known to secrete a spreading factor known as hyaluronidase.

Durand, J. [*French physician*, contemporary]. With Maurice Favre and Joseph Nicolas, gave the first satisfactory description of venereal lymphogranuloma (1913), called *Durand-Nicolas-Favre disease, Frei's disease, fourth venereal disease.*

Durante, Francesco [*Italian surgeon*, 1844–1934]. Remembered for his important studies on the surgery of tumors and tuberculosis. Is credited with introducing the osteoplastic flap used in cranial surgery.

du′ra·plas″ty [*durus;* G. *plassein,* to form, mold]. Repair of defects in the dura mater.

durch″wan′der·ungs·per″i·to·ni′tis (doorkh″-von′dur·oongs·) [Ger., wandering through]. Peritonitis thought to be due to bacteria wandering through the intestinal wall to the peritoneum even though the mucosa is not ulcerated. The organisms may be carried by phagocytes to the peritoneal surface, where they then destroy the phagocytes and multiply.

Dürer, Albrecht [*German illustrator and engraver,* 1471–1528]. One of the world's great artists, supreme in his field. Of enduring medical interest is his work on the proportions of the human body (1528). His woodcuts are among the finest of early medical illustrations.

Durham, Herbert Edward [*English bacteriologist,* 1866–1945]. With Max von Gruber, discovered specific agglutination (1896), the basis of the Widal test for typhoid. See under *test.* Also called *Gruber-Durham reaction, Gruber-Widal reaction.* Devised a glass tube used to detect gas formation in bacterial cultures; called *Durham's fermentation tube.*

du·ri′tis [*durus;* G. *-itis,* inflammation]. Inflammation of the dura mater; pachymeningitis.

du″ro·ar″ach·ni′tis (dew″ro·ar″ak·nigh′tis) [*durus;* G. *arachnē,* spider; *-itis*]. Inflammation of the dura mater and arachnoid membrane.

du″ro·sar·co′ma. See *meningioma.*

Duroziez, Paul Louis [*French physician,* 1826–97]. First to describe congenital mitral stenosis (1877), called *Duroziez's disease.* See also Duroziez's *murmur* or *sign.*

Dusser de Barenne, Johannes Gregorius (1885–1940). Dutch physiologist who introduced the technique of local application of strychnine to the cerebral cortex, thereby greatly advancing physiological neuronography; he also demonstrated for the first time the major functional subdivisions of the sensory cortex in the rhesus monkey (1924).

dust count. The number of particles of dust in a given atmosphere, usually expressed as the number of particles less than 10μ in diameter per cu. ft. of air when counted by the light field method. Used chiefly in evaluation of silicosis hazards in industry.

Dutrochet, René Joachim Henri [*French physiologist,* 1776–1847]. Gave the first clear account of osmosis, and originated the terms exosmosis and endosmosis (1827).

Dutton, Joseph Everett [*English physician,* 1874–1905]. Gave the name *Trypanosoma gambiense* (for Gambia in West Africa) to the causative agent of mid-African sleeping sickness (1901). Trypanosomiasis sometimes is called *Dutton's disease.* With J. L. Todd, showed that relapsing fever is caused by a spirochete, *Borrelia duttonii* (1905).

Duval's bacillus. See *Shigella sonnei.*

Duverney, Joseph Guichard [*French anatomist,* 1648–1730]. Remembered for writing the first satisfactory scientific account of the anatomy, function, and diseases of the ear (1683).

d.v. Double vibration.

D. V. M. Doctor of Veterinary Medicine.

D. V. M. S. Doctor of Veterinary Medicine and Surgery.

D. V. S. 1. Doctor of Veterinary Science. 2. Doctor of Veterinary Surgery.

dwarf [AS. *dweorge*]. A diminutive human being. —**dwarf,** *adj.*

achondroplastic d. See *achondroplasia.*

asexual d. One with deficient sexual development.

chondrodystrophic d. One due to fetal chondrodystrophia; achondroplastic dwarf. See *achondroplasia.*

cretin d. One due to thyroid deficiency; a cretin.

diabetic d. One with retarded growth due to diabetes.

hypoplastic d. See normal *d.*

infantile d. See *infantilism.*

micromelic d. One with very small limbs.

normal d. One abnormal only in size. Also called *hypoplastic d.*

ovarian d. One due to absence of the ovaries. The person is not a true dwarf but is undersized and seldom over 54 inches in height; the external genitalia are undeveloped; premature aging is said to be common.

phocomelic d. One with abnormally short diaphyses.

physiologic d. A normal dwarf.

pituitary d. One due to deficiency of pituitary growth hormone.

primordial d. A normal dwarf.

rachitic d. One due to severe rickets.

renal d. One due to renal osteodystrophy.

sexual d. One with normal sexual development.

true d. One with general underdevelopment, characterized by delayed ossification of the epiphyses.

dwarf. 1. To prevent normal growth. 2. To become small or dwarfed.

dwarf′ism. Abnormal underdevelopment of the body; the condition of being dwarfed.

nephrotic glycosuric d. A form of renal dwarfism. See Debré-deToni-Fanconi *syndrome.*

ovarian d. See Turner's *syndrome.*

panhypopituitary d. Dwarfism characterized additionally by the metabolic defects of hypopituitarism.

primordial d. Dwarfism resulting from a deficiency in growth hormone without a deficiency in the other adenohypophyseal hormones.

renal d. Dwarfism resulting from several types of chronic renal disease in children, as in congenital malformations of the kidney, chronic nephritis, renal tubular acidosis, and the Debré-deToni-Fanconi syndrome.

thyroid d. See *cretinism.*

dwt, dwt. Abbreviation for pennyweight.

Dy Chemical symbol for dysprosium.

dy′ad [G. *dyas,* the number two]. 1. A pair or a couple. 2. One of the groups of paired chromosomes formed by the division of a tetrad in miosis. 3. *In chemistry,* a divalent element or radical.

dye [AS. *dēag*]. A coloring matter, generally used in solution. Certain dyes are used medicinally as antiseptics, as chemotherapeutic agents, or for special effects on tissue cells. —**dye,** *v.*

azo dyes. A group of synthetic organic dyes derivable from azobenzene, containing the chromophore —N=N—.

disazo d. A dye containing two —N=N— groups.

monoazo d. A dye containing one —N=N— group.

supravital d. See *supravital staining.*

vital d. A dye suitable for staining living tissues.

zinc-leuco d. A highly specific dye for hemoglobin made by dissolving acid fuchsin, acid violet, or patent blue, in 2% acetic acid, and decolorizing by boiling with a few grains of zinc dust.

dye′stuff″. See *dye.*

dymixal. Trade-mark for preparations, employed in the treatment of burns, that contain the dyes crystal violet, brilliant green, and acriflavine.

-dymus [G. *didymos,* twin]. Suffix signifying superior duplicity in conjoined twins: used by I. Geoffroy St. Hilaire.

dy·nam′e·ter (dye·nam′i·tur, di·nam′·). See *dynamometer.*

dy·nam′ic (dye·nam′ick, di·nam′ick) [G. *dynamikos,* powerful]. Pertaining to energy; sthenic; characterized by energy or great force.

dy·nam′ics [*dynamikos*]. The science which treats of matter in motion.

vital d. The science of the inherent power of an organism.

dy′na·mo [G. *dynamis,* power]. A machine for converting mechanical energy into electric energy by means of coils of insulated wire revolving through magnetic fields of force.

dy′na·mo- [*dynamis*]. A combining form denoting *power.*

dy″na·mo·gen′e·sis [*dynamis;* G. *genesis,* production]. The generation of power, force, or energy.

dy·nam′o·graph (dye·nam′o·graf, di·nam′·) [*dynamis;* G. *graphein,* to write]. An instrument designed to measure and record graphically muscular strength. —**dynamog′raphy,** *n.*

dy″na·mom′e·ter [*dynamis;* G. *metron,* a measure]. An instrument for the measurement of muscular strength, particularly of the hand, such as a spring balance.

dy·nam′o·neure (dye·nam′o·newr, di·nam′·) [*dynamis;* G. *neuron,* nerve]. A spinal motor neuron.

dy″na·moph′a·ny [*dynamis;* G. *phainein,* to show]. Any form of expression or discharge of psychic force.

dy·nam′o·scope (dye·nam′o·scope, di·nam′·) [*dynamis;* G. *skopein,* to examine]. An apparatus for auscultating the muscles.

dy′na·therm [*dynamis;* G. *thermē,* heat]. The apparatus used in diathermy.

dyne. That amount of force which, when acting continuously on a mass of one gram for one second, will accelerate the mass one centimeter per second.

dys- [G., prefix meaning hard, bad, unlucky]. 1. A prefix meaning *hard* or *ill;* used to signify *ill, bad, hard,* or *difficult.* 2. *In biology,* a prefix denoting *unlike.* 3. *In medicine,* a prefix denoting *difficult* or *painful; faulty* or *impaired;* or *abnormal* or *morbid.*

dys″a·cou′si·a (dis″uh·koo͞′zhuh, ·zee·uh, ·shuh, ·see·uh), **dys″a·cou′sis** (dis″uh·koo͞′sis), **dys″a·cu′si·a** (dis″uh·cue′zhuh, ·zee·uh, ·shuh, ·see·uh, dis″uh·koo͞′·), **dys″a·cous′ma** (dis″uh·koo͞z′muh) [*dys-;* G. *akouein,* to hear]. A condition in which pain or discomfort is caused by loud or even moderately loud noises.

dys·ad″ap·ta′tion [*dys-;* L. *adaptare,* to adjust]. Inability of the iris and retina to accommodate themselves to variable intensities of light.

dys″aes·the′si·a (dis″ess·thee′zhuh, ·zee·uh). See *dysesthesia.*

dys·an″ag·no′si·a [*dys-;* G. *anagnōsis,* reading]. Dyslexia.

dys·an″ti·graph′i·a (·graf′ee·uh, ·gray′fee·uh) [*dys-;* G. *antigraphon,* copy]. Inability to perform copy writing or to print.

dys·a′phi·a, dys·aph′i·a [*dys-;* G. *haphē,* touch]. Disordered sense of touch.

dys″ap·ta′tion. Dysadaptation.

dys″ar·te″ri·ot′o·ny [*dys-;* G. *artēria,* artery; *tonos,* tension]. Abnormal blood pressure.

dys·ar′thri·a [*dys-;* G. *arthron,* joint]. Impairment of articulation; stammering. —**dysar′thric,** *adj.*

dys″ar·thro′sis [*dys-;* *arthron;* G. *-ōsis,* condition]. 1. Deformity, dislocation, or disease of a joint. 2. A false joint. 3. Dysarthria.

dys·au″to·no′mi·a. Autonomic dysfunction of children, probably congenital, characterized by excessive sweating and salivation, skin blotching, and hypertension, as a response to anxiety. It is associated with defective lacrimation, bouts of cyclic vomiting, and usually mental retardation. Syn., *Riley-Day syndrome.*

dys′bar·ism. A condition of the body resulting from the existence of a pressure differential between the total ambient barometric pressure and the total pressures of dissolved and free gases within the body tissues, fluids, and cavities.

dys·ba′si·a (dis·bay′zhuh, ·shuh, ·zee·uh, ·see·uh) [*dys-;* G. *basis,* step]. Difficulty in walking.

d. intermittens angiosclerotica. Intermittent claudication due to arteriosclerosis of the lower extremities.

dys·bu′li·a [*dys-;* G. *boulē,* will]. Impairment of will power.

dys·chi′ri·a (dis·kigh′ree·uh) [*dys-;* G. *cheir,* hand]. Inability to tell which side of the body has been touched; partial allocheiria.

dys·chi′zi·a (dis·kigh′zhuh, ·zee·uh), **dys·che′zi·a** (dis·kee′zhuh, ·zee·uh) [*dys-;* G. *chezein,* to go to stool]. Painful or difficult defecation.

dys·chon″dro·pla′si·a (dis·kon″dro·play′zhuh, ·zee·uh, ·shuh, ·see·uh, dis″kon·dro·) [*dys-;* G. *chondros,* cartilage; *plassein,* to form]. A disease of unknown etiology, attacking the long bones and the metacarpal and phalangeal skeleton of the hand. It is characterized by cartilaginous tissue developing regularly but ossifying very slowly. Also called *Ollier's disease, skeletal enchondromatosis.*

dys′chro·a (dis′kro·uh, dis·kro′uh), **dys·chroi′a** [*dys-;* G. *chroia,* skin]. Discoloration of the skin; a bad complexion.

dys·chro″ma·to·der′mi·a, dys″chro·mo·der′mi·a. Dyschroa.

dys″chro·ma·top′si·a [*dys-;* G. *chrōma,* color; *opsis,* vision]. Partial colorblindness; difficulty in distinguishing colors. —**dyschro′matope,** *n.*

dys·chro′mi·a [*dys-;* *chrōma*]. Discoloration, especially of the skin.

dys″chro·mo·der′mi·a. See *dyschroa.*

dys′chro·nous [*dys-;* G. *chronos,* time]. Not agreeing as to time. —**dyschrona′tion,** *n.*

dys·co′ri·a [*dys-;* G. *korē,* pupil]. Abnormality of the form of the pupil.

dys·cra′si·a (dis·kray′zhuh, ·zee·uh, ·shuh, ·see·uh) [*dys-;* G. *krasis,* mixing]. An abnormal state of the body. —**dyscras′ic, dyscrat′ic,** *adj.*

blood d. Any abnormal condition of the formed elements of blood or of the constituents required for clotting: loose usage.

dys·cri′nism [*dys-;* G. *krinein,* to separate]. A condition of disordered function of the endocrine glands.

dys″di·ad″o·cho·ki·ne′si·a, dys″di·ad″o·ko·ki·ne′si·a (dis″dye·ad″o·ko·ki·nee′shuh, ·see·uh). [*dys-;* G. *diadochos,* succeeding; *kinēsis,* motion]. Impairment of the power to perform alternating movements in rapid succession, such as pronation and supination; a sign of cerebellar disease.

dys″e·coi′a [G. *dysēkoia,* deafness]. Deafness.

dys·em″bry·o′ma [*dys-;* G. *embryon,* embryo; *-ōma,* tumor]. Teratoma.

nephrogenic d. See Wilm's *tumor.*

dys·em″bry·o·pla′si·a (dis·em″bree·o·play′zhuh, ·zee·uh, ·shuh, ·see·uh) [*dys-;* *embryon;* G. *plassein,* to form]. A malformation which develops during embryonic life.

dys″e·me′si·a (dis″i·mee′zhuh, ·zee·uh), **dys·em′e·sis** [*dys-;* G. *emesia,* disposition to vomit]. Painful vomiting; retching.

dys·e′mi·a, dys·ae′mi·a (dis·ee′mee·uh) [*dys-;* G. *haima,* blood]. Any disease of the blood. *Obs.*

dys″en·do·cri·ni′a·sis, dys″en·do·cri·si′a·sis. Dysendocrinism.

dys″en·doc′rin·ism (dis″en·dock′rin·iz·um, dis-en′do·krin·iz·um) [*dys-;* G. *endon,* within; *krinein,* to separate]. Any abnormality in the function of the endocrine glands. —**dysen′docrine,** *adj.*

dys″en·te′ri·a. See *dysentery.*

dys′en·ter″y [G. *dysenteria,* from *dys-; enteron,* intestine]. Inflammation of the intestine, characterized by pain, rectal tenesmus, intense diarrhea with the frequent passage of small amounts of mucus and blood, and symptoms of toxemia. —**dysenter′ic,** *adj.*

amebic d. See amebic *colitis.*

bacillary d. An infectious disease which primarily involves the colon, caused by a species of the genus *Shigella.*

balantidial d. See balantidial *colitis.*

lamb d. An acute enteritis occurring among lambs chiefly along the English-Scottish border. The etiological agent is *Clostridium welchii,* Type B.

nonspecific d. A chronic ulcerative *colitis.*

schistosomal d. A type caused by *Schistosoma mansoni.* In the early stages there is congestion and edema with inflammatory polyp formation. During ova deposition there is mild diarrhea, low fever, abdominal discomfort, and often urticaria. There may be leukocytosis and usually eosinophilia, culminating in severe anemia.

Sonne d. One of the commonest forms of intestinal infection, caused by *Shigella sonnei,* found in hospital wards for babies and children.

dys″er·ga′si·a (dis″ur·gay′zhuh, ·zee·uh, ·shuh, ·see·uh) [*dys-;* G. *ergasia,* work]. *In psychobiology,* a mental disturbance due to toxic factors which are capable of producing delirium, such as uremia or alcohol.

dys″es·the′si·a, dys″aes·the′si·a (dis″ess·thee′-zhuh, ·zee·uh) [*dys-;* G. *aisthēsis,* sensation]. 1. Impairment of the senses, especially of the sense of touch. 2. Painfulness of any sensation not normally painful.

dys·func′tion [*dys-;* L. *functus,* from *fungi,* to perform]. Any abnormality or impairment of function, as of an organ.

constitutional hepatic d. A benign, often familial, disorder of bilirubin metabolism characterized by mild elevation of indirectly reacting bilirubin without the usual evidence for a hemolytic process. Otherwise, liver function tests are normal. Also called *hereditary nonhemolytic hyperbilirubinemia.*

dys″ga·lac′ti·a (dis″ga·lack′tee·uh, ·shee·uh) [*dys-;* G. *gala,* milk]. Loss or impairment of milk secretion.

dys·gen′ic [*dys-;* G. *genesthai,* from *gignesthai,* to be produced]. Detrimental to the hereditary constitution of the race; in contrast to *eugenic.*

dys″ger·mi·no′ma [*dys-;* L. *germen,* germ; G. *-ōma,* tumor]. A firm, elastic, usually well-encapsulated, solid tumor of the ovary, not disposed to metastasize. Occurs usually before 30 years of age, and microscopically resembles the embryonal carcinoma (seminoma) of the testis with lymphoid stroma. Also called *embryoma of ovary.* See also *seminoma.*

dys·geu′si·a (dis·jew′see·uh, ·zee·uh) [*dys-;* G. *geusis,* taste]. Morbidity or perversion of the sense of taste.

dys·glan′du·lar [*dys-;* L. *glans,* acorn]. Pertaining to any abnormality in the function of glands, particularly the glands of internal secretion.

dys·gnath′ic (dis·nath′ick, ·nay′thick) [*dys-;* G. *gnathos,* jaw]. Pertaining to jaws with improper development and in poor relation to each other.

dys·gno′si·a [*dys;* G. *gignoskein,* to know]. Disorder or distortion of gnostic function.

dys·gon′ic [*dys-;* G. *gonos,* seed]. Growing poorly; used of bacterial cultures.

dys·gram′ma·tism [*dys-;* G. *gramma,* letter]. Inability to make the proper use of words; a symptom of certain cerebral diseases; particularly diseases of the temporal lobe.

dys·graph′i·a (dis·graf′ee·uh, ·gray′fee·uh) [*dys-;* G. *graphein,* to write]. Impairment of the power of writing as a result of a brain lesion.

dys·hem″a·to·poi·et′ic (dis·hem″uh·to·, dis·hee″-muh·to·) [*dys-;* G. *haima,* blood; *poiein,* to make]. Pertaining to a disturbed formation of blood cells. —**dyshematopoie′sis,** *n.*

dys·hid′ri·a [*dys-;* G. *hidrōs,* sweat]. Old term for dyshidrosis.

dys″hi·dro′sis, dys″i·dro′sis [*dys-;* G. *hidrōsis,* sweating]. 1. Any disturbance in sweat production or excretion. 2. Pompholyx. —**dyshidros′i-form,** *adj.*

dys·in′su·lin·ism″. See *hypoglycemia.*

dys″ker·a·to′sis [*dys-;* G. *keras,* horn; *-ōsis,* condition]. A disturbance in the normal process of keratinization; occurs in many skin diseases, such as keratosis follicularis, certain precancerous lesions, etc. —**dyskeratot′ic,** *adj.*

dys″ki·ne′si·a (dis″ki·nee′shuh, ·see·uh, ·zhuh, ·zee·uh, dis″kigh·nee′·) [*dys-;* G. *kinēsis,* motion]. Impairment of the power of voluntary motion.

biliary d. A functional spasticity of the sphincter of Oddi.

dys·la′li·a, dys·lal′i·a [*dys-;* G. *lalein,* to talk]. Impairment of the power of speaking, due to a defect of the organs of speech.

dys·lex′i·a [*dys-;* G. *lexis,* speech]. Impairment of the ability to read.

dys·lo′gi·a [*dys-;* G. *logos,* word]. Difficulty in the expression of ideas by speech.

dys″ma·se′sis, dys″ma·se′si·a (dis″ma·see′-zee·uh) [*dys-;* G. *masēsis,* chewing]. Difficulty of mastication.

dys″men·or·rhe′a, dys″men·or·rhoe′a [*dys-;* G. *mēn,* month; *rhoia,* a flow]. Difficult or painful menstruation.

acquired d. See secondary *d.*

congenital d. See primary *d.*

congestive d. A form of painful menstruation due to an intense congestion of the pelvic viscera. Syn., *plethoric d., vascular d.*

d. intermenstrualis. Pain between the menses.

essential d. See primary *d.*

functional d. (a) That without anatomic or pathologic explanation. (b) That contributed to or caused by pelvic congestion from unsatisfied sexual stimulation.

inflammatory d. That due to inflammation.

mechanical d. That due to mechanical obstruction to the free escape of the menstrual fluid. Syn., *obstructive d.*

membranous d. That characterized by discharge of casts or shreds of uterine mucosa.

obstructive d. See mechanical *d.*

ovarian d. That form due to disease of the ovaries.

plethoric d. See congestive *d.*

primary d. That present from the menarche. Syn., *essential d., congenital d.*

psychogenic d. Menstrual pain of mental or psychic origin.

secondary d. That type associated with organic pelvic disease. Syn., *acquired d.*

spasmodic d. That due to sudden and severe uterine contraction.

tubal d. That form associated with disease of the oviduct.

uterine d. That type caused by uterine disease.

vaginal d. The type associated with disease of the vagina.

vascular d. See congestive *d.*

dys″mer·o·gen′e·sis [*dys-;* G. *meros*, part; *genesis*, production]. Cleavage resulting in unlike parts. —**dysmerogenet′ic,** *adj.*

dys·me′tri·a, dys·met′ri·a [*dys-;* G. *metron*, a measure]. Inability to control accurately the range of movement in muscular acts, as observed in cerebellar lesions.

dys·mim′i·a [*dys-;* G. *mimeia*, farce]. Impairment of the power to use signs and gestures as a means of expression; inability to imitate; caused by a disturbance in the innervation of the facial muscles.

dys·mne′si·a (dis·mnee′zhuh, ·zee·uh, dis·nee′·) [*dys-;* G. *mnēsis*, a remembering]. An impaired or defective memory.

dys·mor′phi·a [*dys-;* G. *morphē*, form]. Deformity. *Obs.*

dys·mor′phic. *In the somatotype*, badly formed, or of low primary t component.

dys·mor″pho·pho′bi·a [*dys-;* *morphē;* G. *phobos*, fear]. Morbid fear of deformity.

dys·no′mi·a [*dys-;* G. *onoma*, name]. Nominal aphasia.

dys″o·don·ti′a·sis (dis″o·don·ty′uh·sis, ·tee′uh·sis) [*dys-;* G. *odous*, tooth; NL. *-iasis*, condition]. Difficult or painful dentition.

dys·o′pi·a [*dys-;* G. *opsis*, vision]. Painful or defective vision.

dys″o·rex′·i·a [*dys-;* G. *orexis*, appetite]. A disordered or unnatural appetite.

dys·os′mi·a (dis·oz′mee·uh) [*dys-;* G. *osmē*, smell]. Impairment of the sense of smell.

dys″os·te·o·gen′e·sis. Dysostosis.

dys″os·to′sis [*dys-;* G. *osteon*, bone; *-ōsis*, condition]. Defective formation of bone.

cleidocranial d. A congenital complex consisting in incomplete ossification of the skull, malformation of the palatine arch, and more or less aplasia of the clavicles. Other bones may also be involved.

craniofacial d. Hypertelorism.

d. multiplex. See *gargoylism.*

mandibulofacial d. Hypoplasia of the facial bones, especially of the zygoma and the mandible. With this are associated a lateral downward sloping of the palpebral fissures, defects of the ear, macrostomia, and a peculiar fish-face appearance. It is presumed to be a sex-linked recessive trait. Also called *Teacher Collins syndrome.*

metaphyseal d. A very rare condition in which the roentgenographic appearance of the metaphyses is unique, being largely cartilaginous, irregularly cloudy, and impregnated with salts. Many metaphyses appear enlarged and the space between the epiphysis and the shafts is markedly widened.

dys·par″a·thy′roid·ism [*dys-;* G. *para*, near; *thyreoeidēs*, shield-shaped]. Any functional disorder of the parathyroid gland.

dys″pa·reu′ni·a (dis″puh·rōō′nee·uh) [*dys-;* G. *pareunos*, lying beside]. Painful or difficult intercourse.

psychologic d. That form of dyspareunia having an emotional basis with no anatomic or pathologic explanation.

dys·pep′si·a [*dys-;* G. *peptein*, *pessein*, to cook]. Disturbed digestion. —**dyspep′tic,** *adj.*

acid d. That attended with hyperacidity of the gastric juice.

anacidic d. That accompanied by lack of the normal acidity of the gastric juice.

bilious d. Intestinal dyspepsia due to impaired secretion of bile.

flatulent d. That marked by almost constant eructation of gas. Also called *gaseous d.*

gastric d. That confined to the stomach.

gastrointestinal d. That in which both the stomach and the intestine are concerned.

inflammatory d. That due to some form of gastritis.

intestinal d. That due to imperfect digestive action of the intestinal juices or a lack of tone in the muscular coat of the intestine.

muscular d. That due to atony of the muscular coat of the stomach or intestine.

nervous d. That characterized by gastric pains, precipitated by emotional states.

dys·pep′tic [*dys-;* *peptein*]. A person suffering from dyspepsia.

dys″per·i·stal′sis [*dys-;* G. *peristaltikos*, clasping and compressing]. Violent or abnormal peristalsis.

dys·pha′gi·a [*dys-;* G. *phagein*, to eat]. Difficulty in swallowing, or inability to swallow.

d. constricta. That due to stenosis of the pharynx or esophagus.

d. globosa. Globus hystericus.

d. lusoria. That caused by compression of the esophagus and trachea between the aorta and ductus arteriosus in the case of right-sided aortic arch, or between the two sides of the arch when it is double, or due to pressure on the esophagus by an anomalous right subclavian artery.

d. spastica. That due to hysterical spasm of the esophagus or pharynx.

sideropenic d. See Plummer-Vinson *syndrome.*

dys·pha′si·a (dis·fay′zhuh, ·zee·uh) [*dys-;* G. *phasis*, speech]. Difficulty in speaking or in understanding language; caused by a central lesion.

dys·phe′mi·a [*dys-;* G. *phēmē*, speech]. Stammering.

dys·pho′ni·a [*dys-;* G. *phōnē*, voice]. An impairment of the voice.

d. spastica. See spastic *aphonia.*

dys·pho′ri·a [*dys-;* G. *phoros*, bearing]. Impatience and restlessness; mental anxiety; fidgets. —**dysphor′ic,** *adj.*

dys·pho′ti·a [*dys-;* G. *phōs*, light]. Myopia.

dys·phra′si·a (dis·fray′zhuh, ·zee·uh) [*dys-;* G. *phrasis*, speech]. Imperfect speech due to impairment of mental power.

dys″pi·tu′i·ta·rism [*dys-;* L. *pituita*, phlegm]. A condition due to abnormal functioning of the pituitary gland.

dys·pla′si·a (dis·play′zhuh, ·zee·uh, ·shuh, ·see·uh) [*dys-;* G. *plassein*, to form]. 1. Abnormal development or growth. 2. In the *somatotype*, the extent to which an individual presents different components (somatotypes) in different bodily regions, expressed quantitatively by regarding the body as made up of a specific number of regions and somatotyping each. They may be endomorphic, mesomorphic, or ectomorphic. Also called *d-component.*

chondroectodermal d. A rare congenital disorder characterized by dyschondroplasia, ectodermal dyplasia, bilateral polydactyly, and polymetacarpalism, and sometimes congenital heart disease. Syn., *Ellis-van Creveld syndrome.*

d. epiphysialis multiplex. A rare congenital developmental error characterized by irregularities in the density and outline of several of the developing epiphyses, dwarfism, and short thick digits.

d. epiphysialis punctata. A rare congenital skeletal defect diagnosed by roentgenographic demonstration of multiple punctate epiphyseal calcific deposits. Other skeletal defects as shortening of limbs, and semiflexion and limitation of extension of the larger joints, bilateral congenital cataracts, and mild mental deficiency are frequently present. Also called *d. epiphysialis puncticularis, chondrodystrophia calcificans con-*

genita, chondrodystrophia fetalis calcarea or *hypoplastica, chondroangiopathia calcarea sen punctata, calcareous chondrodystrophy,* (*congenital*) *stippled epiphyses.*

d. epiphysialis puncticularis. See *d. epiphysialis punctata.*

familial metaphyseal d. An exceedingly rare condition marked by symmetrical enlargement of one or both ends of the shafts of long bones.

fibrous d. (*of bone*). A condition characterized by bone resorption, fibrosis of the marrow, irregular bone trabeculae replacing cancellous and cortical bone. It is often unilateral and segmental. When only one bone is affected, it is known as *monostotic fibrous d.;* if more than one, as *polyostotic fibrous d.* This latter is sometimes accompanied by segmental pigmentation. If precocious puberty is also present it is known as *Albright's syndrome,* and is seen mostly in girls. Also called *osteitis fibrosa disseminata, osteodystrophia fibrosa.*

hereditary anhidrotic ectodermal d. One of a very large group of primarily cutaneous congenital abnormalities, marked chiefly by deficient or absent sweat-gland function (anhidrosis), deficient development of the teeth (hypodontia), or their absence (anodontia), and by congenital alopecia.

macular d. An irregularly circular or oval defect of the macula, occurring in young children and causing a reduction in visual acuity.

mammary d. A group of common pathological conditions in the breasts of women during sexual maturity, due to endocrine imbalances. Included are *adenosis of breast, cystic disease of breast,* and *mastodynia.* Also called *cyclomastopathy;* formerly called *chronic cystic mastitis.*

monostotic fibrous d. See fibrous *d.*

neuroectodermal d. A congenital derangement of cerebral tissues associated with skin tumors, as tuberous sclerosis, Lindau's disease, and von Recklinghausen's neurofibromatosis.

periosteal d. See *osteogenesis imperfecta.*

polyostotic fibrous d. See fibrous *d.*

progressive diaphyseal d. See Engelmann's *disease.*

dysp·ne′a [*dys-;* G. *pnoia,* breath]. Difficult or labored breathing. —**dyspneal, dyspneic,** *adj.*

cardiac d. That due to cardiac failure.

renal d. That due to acidosis in uremia.

dys·pra′gi·a. Dyspraxia.

dys·prax′i·a [*dys-;* G. *praxis,* a doing]. Disordered or painful functioning of a part.

dys·pro′si·um (dis·pro′shee·um, ·see·um) [G. *dysprositos,* difficult of access]. Dy = 162.46. A rare earth metal.

dys′ra·phism [G. *dys-,* bad; *rhaphē,* seam]. Defective raphe formation; defective fusion. Syn., *araphia.*

prosencephalic d. Failure in closure of the embryonic prosencephalic vesicle.

spinal d. A general term for all manifestations of dysraphism in the dorsal midline whether cutaneous, vertebral, meningeal, or neural.

dys·rhyth′mi·a (dis·rith′mee·uh, dis·rith′·) [*dys-;* G. *rhythmos,* rhythm]. Disordered rhythm.

cerebral d. Any abnormal rhythm in brain waves, as revealed by the electroencephalogram. The waves may be too fast, too slow, or may alternate between the two types. Dysrhythmia is frequently associated with an epileptiform condition.

dys·se·ba′ci·a (dis·se·bay′she·ah). Plugging of the sebaceous glands, especially around the nose, mouth, and forehead, with a dry, yellowish material. It occurs in pellagra and other deficiencies of the vitamin-B complex. Also called *shark skin.*

dys″se·cre·to′sis [G. *dus,* faulty; L. *secretus,* separate out; G. *osis,* condition]. A condition in which there is faulty secretory activity of glands.

dys·sper′ma·tism, dys·sper′mi·a [*dys-;* G. *sperma,* seed]. 1. Difficulty of depositing the sperm within the vagina. 2. Occurrence of pain or discomfort in discharge of seminal fluid. 3. Any disturbance in the formation of normal sperms.

dys·sta′si·a (dis·stay′see·uh, ·zee·uh) [*dys-;* G. *stasis,* a standing]. Difficulty in standing. —**dysstat′ic,** *adj.*

dys·syn′er·gy. Asynergy.

progressive cerebellar d. See cerebellofugal *degeneration.*

dys·tax′i·a [*dys-;* G. *taxis,* arrangement]. Ataxia or partial ataxia.

d. agitans. Tremor due to irritation of the spinal cord. Also called *pseudoparalysis agitans.*

dys·tec′tic. *In physical chemistry,* characterizing the specific mixture of two or more substances which has the highest melting point of any mixture of the substances; it is the opposite of *eutectic.*

dys″tha·na′si·a (dis″thuh·nay′zhuh, ·zee·uh)[*dys-;* G. *thanatos,* death]. A slow and painful death.

dys·the′si·a (dis·thee′zhuh, ·zee·uh) [*dys-;* G. *thesis,* a setting]. Impatience; fretfulness; ill temper in the sick. —**dysthet′ic,** *adj.*

dys·thy′mi·a (dis·thigh′mee·uh, ·thim′ee·uh) [*dys-;* G. *thymos,* mind]. 1. Melancholia or mental perversion. 2. A state thought to be due to malfunction of the thymus during childhood.

dys·tith′i·a [*dys-;* G. *tittheia,* nursing]. Difficulty of nursing or inability to nurse at the breast.

dys·to′ci·a [*dys-;* G. *tokos,* birth]. Difficult labor. —**dystocic,** *adj.*

fetal d. Difficult labor due to abnormalities of position or size and shape of the fetus.

maternal d. Difficult labor due to deformities within the mother.

dys·to′ni·a [*dys-;* G. *tonos,* tension]. Disorder or lack of tonicity. —**dyston′ic,** *adj.*

d. musculorum deformans. A rare, progressive disease with a familial incidence, which affects children between 8 and 14 years of age. Tonic spasms and clonic contractions occur in the large muscles of the thigh and leg; the leg flexes, the toes flare; the forearm pronates; the abnormal tonus of the entire muscular system is so severe as to cause lordosis and scoliosis of the spine. Degenerative lesions are found chiefly in the corpus striatum. Also called *d. lenticularis, torsion d., torsion spasm.*

dys·to′pi·a [*dys-;* G. *topos,* place]. Displacement of any organ. —**dystop′ic,** *adj.*

dys′tro·phy, dys·tro′phi·a [*dys-;* G. *trophē,* nourishment]. 1. Defective nutrition. 2. Defective or abnormal development or degeneration. —**dystroph′ic,** *adj.*

adiposogenital d. Adiposity, retarded development of gonads, and occasionally diabetes insipidus; results from organically impaired function of the pituitary and hypothalamus. May be caused by craniopharyngioma, basilar meningitis, trauma, etc. Also called *adiposa dystrophia genitalis, Babinski-Froehlich syndrome, Froehlich's syndrome, neuropituitary syndrome.*

cleidocranial d. See cleidocranial *dysostosis.*

dystrophia mediana canaliformis. A rare form consisting of longitudinal grooves occupying the center of the nail from the lunula to the free edge; usually involves the thumb.

dystrophia myotonica. Muscular dystrophy.

dystrophia periostalis hyperplastica familiaris. A familial disorder characterized by early closure of cranial sutures and thickening of the clavicles and phalanges.

dystrophia unguium. An abnormality of the

finger or toe nails; of any degree, from simple longitudinal fissuring to complete absence.

endothelial d. A degenerative lesion of the cornea, with the formation of hyaline nodules on the posterior surface of Descemet's membrane. Passage of the aqueous into the cornea is frequently associated, causing bullae to form under the epithelium. This form is called *epithelial d.*

epithelial d. See endothelial *d.*

facioscapulohumeral d. See facioscapulohumeral *atrophy.*

familial corneal d. Degenerative changes in the anterior corneal layers, causing opacities; definitely hereditary, affecting adolescents and young adults. Syn., *lattice keratitis.*

familial osseous d. See *chondroosteodystrophy.*

fundus d. A disturbance, or usually genetic affection, involving initially the central area of the fundus of the eye and inducing atrophic changes that may become widespread.

juvenile progressive muscular d. A rare form beginning in childhood or early adolescence; affecting first the muscles of the shoulder girdle, lastly the face, forearms, hands, and legs. The muscles are hypertrophic early, later becoming atrophic.

Laurence-Moon-Biedl d. See Laurence-Moon-Biedl *syndrome.*

marginal d. A form of arcus senilis associated with degeneration of the cornea.

muscular d. A progressive, familial hereditary disorder, marked by atrophy and stiffness of the muscles, and observed when voluntary action is first attempted. Also called *dystrophia myotonica, myotonic dystrophy, myotonia dystrophica, Steinert's disease.*

myotonic d. Muscular dystrophy.

progressive muscular d. A primary wasting disease of muscles characterized by progressive muscular weakness; apparently due to peripheral rather than central nervous degeneration.

pseudohypertrophic muscular d. A progressive, familial disorder beginning in childhood; characterized by early hypertrophy and later atrophy of the muscles with lordosis, weakness, inability to rise from the ground, a waddling gait, and progressive helplessness. Also called *Erb's d.*

reflex (sympathetic) d. Causalgia. See also shoulder-hand *syndrome.*

dys·u′ri·a [*dys-;* G. *ouron,* urine]. Difficult or painful urination.

E

E Electromotive force.

E. 1. Abbreviation for eye, emmetropia. 2. An einstein, 6.06×10^{23} quanta.

$\mathbf{E_0}$ Symbol for electroaffinity.

e Symbol for an electron, as $H = H^+ + e$.

e- [L.]. A prefix denoting *without, out, out of, from.*

Eagle, Harry [*American pathologist,* 1905–]. Known for his flocculation test for syphilis, employing inactivated serum with antigen made of lecithin from beef heart, fortified with cholesterol and corn germ sterol, and for a complement-fixation test for syphilis. See Eagle *test.*

Eales, Henry [*English physician,* 1852–1913]. Known for his description of a condition characterized by repeated retinal and vitreous hemorrhages, called *Eales's disease.*

ear [AS. *ēare*]. The organ of hearing, consisting of the external ear, the middle ear, and the internal ear or labyrinth. The **external ear** is made up of an expanded portion, the pinna, and the external auditory canal. The **middle ear** consists of the tympanic cavity, with the auditory ossicles, the auditory tube, and the mastoid cells. The **internal ear** consists of the osseous and membranous labyrinths, which are separated from each other by a space containing the perilymph. The osseous labyrinth consists of three parts: the vestibule, the semicircular canals, and the cochlea. The semicircular canals are three in number: the superior, the posterior, and the lateral. The cochlea, so named from its resemblance to a snail-shell, is a cylindrical tube that winds around a central axis, the modiolus, which is perforated by canals for the passage of the cochlear nerves and blood vessels. The vestibule contains two small sacs, the utricle and the saccule, connected by the utriculosaccular duct. The saccule communicates through the ductus reuniens with the membranous cochlea. The membranous cochlea, or cochlear duct, contains the acoustic organ of the cochlea, the organ of Corti. See Plate 20.

aviator's e. See *barotitis media.*

cat e. A congenital deformity in which the upper posterior part of the (sometimes enlarged) helix is folded forward. In its most severe form the helix may meet and fuse with the tragus.

congenital deformity of e. See Darwin's *tubercle.*

flat e. A large, prominent ear, characterized by effacement of the ridges and grooves.

macacus e. One with a prominent auricular (Darwin's) tubercle.

pointed e. One with a satyr tubercle.

Stahl's e. See Friedrich Karl *Stahl.*

Wildermuth's e. See Hermann A. *Wildermuth.*

ear′ache″ [*ēare;* AS. *acan*]. Pain in the ear.

ear′drum″ [*ēare;* probably of D. or LG. origin, cf. D. *trom*]. The tympanic membrane.

ear dust. Otoconia or otoliths.

ear′plug″ [*ēare;* MD. *plugge*]. A device, usually made of rubber, plastic, or cotton kneaded with glycerin or petrolatum; to protect the ear, as from loud noises.

earth [AS. *eorthe*]. The soil.

diatomaceous e. Purified siliceous earth.

e. nuts. Peanuts.

e. wax. Ceresin.

fuller's e. A clay related to kaolin, and used similarly as an adsorbent and protective.

infusorial e. Purified siliceous earth.

purified siliceous e. (*terra silicea purificata*). A form of silica (SiO_2) consisting of the frustules and fragments of diatoms.

earth eat′ing. Geophagy.

ear′wax″ [AS. *ēare; weax*]. Cerumen.

Ebers, Georg Moritz [*German Egyptologist and novelist,* 1837–98]. Known for having discovered (1872) the oldest medical document in the world, a papyrus in hieratic script, containing a record of Egyptian medicine. Believed to date from about 1502 B.C. Called *Ebers Papyrus.*

E″ber·thel′la (ee″bur·thel′uh, ·tell′uh, ·tay′luh, ay″bur·) [L., after Karl Joseph *Eberth,* German pathologist, 1835–1926]. Old name for a genus of organisms now designated *Salmonella.*

E. typhosa. See *Salmonella typhosa.*

Ebner, Victor von [*Austrian histologist,* 1842–1925]. Remembered for his description of the serous glands opening into the trenches of the vallate papillae of the tongue, called *serous lingual glands, Ebner's glands.*

Ebstein, Wilhelm [*German physician,* 1836–1912]. Remembered for his description of hyaline degeneration of the epithelial cells of the renal tubules, sometimes occurring in diabetes mellitus (1881); this was once known as *Ebstein's disease.* Investigated pseudoleukemia, also called *multiple lymphadenoma, Pel-Ebstein's disease.* See also Pel-Ebstein *fever.*

e′bur [L., ivory]. A tissue similar to ivory in appearance or structure.

e. dentis. Dentin.

e″bur·na′tion [L. *eburneus,* of ivory]. An increase in the density of tooth or bone following some pathologic change. —**ebur′nated,** *adj.*

ec- [G. *ek,* from, out of]. A prefix meaning *out of.*

Ec·bal′li·um [G. *ekballein,* to throw out]. A genus of the Cucurbitaceae. See *elaterium.*

ec·bol′ic [G. *ekbolē,* a throwing out]. Producing abortion or accelerating labor. —**ecbol′ic,** *n.*

ec′bol·ine (eck′bo·leen, ·lin). An alkaloid of ergot.

ec·cen′tric [G. *ekkentros,* from *ek,* away from, *kentron,* circle]. Situated away from the center or median line.

ec·cen′tro-os″te·o·chon″dro·dys·pla′si·a. See *chondroosteodystrophy.*

ec·ceph″a·lo′sis (eck·sef″uh·lo′sis) [G. *ek,* out of; *kephalē,* head; *-ōsis,* condition]. Removal of the brain of the fetus to facilitate delivery. Syn., *cephalotomy, excerebration.*

ec″chon·dro′ma (eck″on·dro′muh) [*ek;* G. *chondros,* cartilage; *-ōma,* tumor]. A nodular outgrowth from cartilage at the junction of cartilage and bone; usually a hyperplasia (ecchondrosis) but may be neoplastic.

ec″chon·dro′sis (eck″on·dro′sis) [*ek; chondros;* G. *-ōsis,* condition]. A cartilaginous outgrowth.

e. physaliphora. See *chordoma.*

ec·chon′dro·tome (eh·kon′dro·tohm) [*ek; chondros;* G. *tomos,* cutting]. An instrument for the surgical removal of cartilaginous growths.

ec″chy·mo′sis (eck″i·mo′sis) [*ek;* G. *chymos,* juice; *-ōsis*]. An extravasation of blood into the subcutaneous tissues. It is marked by a purple discoloration of the skin, the color gradually changing to brown, green, and yellow. —**ecchymot′ic,** *adj.*

ec′crine. See *eccrine glands* under *gland.*

ec″cy·e′sis (eck″sigh·ee′sis) [*ek;* G. *kyēsis,* pregnancy]. Extrauterine gestation.

ec·dem′ic [G. *ekdēmos,* away from home]. Applied to diseases brought into a region from without; not endemic or epidemic.

ec·dem″o·ma′ni·a (eck·dem″o·may′nee·uh, eck-dee″mo·) [*ekdēmos;* G. *mania,* madness]. A morbid desire to wander. *Obs.*

ec′der·on [G. *ek,* out of; *deros,* skin]. The outermost or epithelial layer of the skin and mucous membranes; epidermis. —**ecderon′ic,** *adj.*

ec′dy·sis [G. *ekdysis,* a stripping]. Sloughing or casting off of the outer epidermis; desquamation.

ECG, EKG Electrocardiogram.

ec′go·nine (eck′go·neen, ·nin). $C_9H_{15}NO_3$; 3-hydroxy-2-tropanecarboxylic acid, the principal part of the cocaine molecule (which is benzoylmethylecgonine). Ecgonine may be obtained from cocaine by hydrolysis.

e·chid′nase (eh·kid′nace) [G. *echidna,* viper]. A phlogogenic principle found in snake venom.

e·chid′nin (eh·kid′nin) [*echidna*]. 1. Snake poison; the poison or venom of the viper and other similar snakes. 2. A nitrogenous and venomous principle found in poisonous secretion of various snakes.

Ech″id·noph′a·ga (eck″id·nof′uh·guh) [*echidna;* G. *phagein,* to eat]. A genus of fleas.

E. gallinacea. The species known as the sticktight or tropical hen flea, which attacks chickens in many parts of the world; may also become a human pest.

e·chid″no·tox′in (eh·kid″no·tock′sin) [*echidna;* G. *toxikon,* poison]. A principle of snake venom which produces a general reaction in the human body and has a powerful effect on the nervous system.

ech″i·na′ce·a (eck″i·nay′shuh, ·see·uh) [G. *echinos,* hedgehog, sea-urchin]. Cone flower. The dried rhizome and roots of *Echinacea pallida* and *E. angustifolia;* formerly used to treat ulcers, septicemia, etc.

e·chin′e·none (eh·kin′i·nohn, eh·kigh′ni·) [*echinos*]. A naturally occurring precursor of vitamin A derived from sea urchins.

e·chi′no- (eh·kigh′no-, eck′i·no-, eh·kin′o-), **echin-** [*echinos*]. A combining form usually denoting *spiny, bearing spines,* or *relation* or *resemblance to the sea urchins.*

e·chi′no·chrome [*echinos;* G. *chrōma,* color]. A respiratory pigment found in the Echinodermata.

e·chi″no·coc·ci′a·sis (·cock·sigh′uh·sis) [*echinos;* G. *kokkos,* berry; NL. *-iasis,* condition]. Infestation with cysticercus of the dog tapeworm.

e·chi″no·coc·co′sis [*echinos; kokkos;* G. *-ōsis,* condition]. Infestation of man with the *Echinococcus granulosus* in its larval or hydatid stage. Most important site of infestation is the liver, and secondly, the lungs.

E·chi″no·coc′cus [*echinos; kokkos*]. A genus of tapeworms.

E. granulosus. That species whose ova, when ingested by man or other intermediate hosts, develop into echinococcus cysts.

E·chi″no·der′ma·ta [*echinos;* G. *derma,* skin]. A phylum of marine animals including starfish, sea urchins, etc.

ech″i·nop′sine (eck″i·nop′seen, ·sin) [*echinos;* G. *ōps,* eye]. An alkaloid isolated from the fruits of *Echinops ritro* and other species of *Echinops.* It belongs to the strychnine group.

E·chi″no·rhyn′chus (·ring′kus, ·rin′kus) [*echinos;* G. *rhynchos,* snout]. Formerly a genus of acanthocephalan worms.

E. gigas. Synonym for *Macracanthorhynchus hirudinaceus.*

E. moniliformis. Synonym for *Moniliformis moniliformis.*

ech″i·no′sis (eck″i·no′sis). Crenation.

E·chi″no·sto′ma (eh·kigh″no·sto′muh, eck″i·no·, eh·kin″o·, eck″i·nos′to·muh) [*echinos;* G. *stoma,* mouth]. A genus of flukes parasitic in man, but of little pathologic importance.

Ech′is (eck′iss, ee′kiss) [G., viper]. A genus of vipers found in Africa, Arabia, and India.

E. carinatus. The saw-scaled viper, a small snake attaining one and one-half feet in length, possessing a hemotoxic venom.

e·chit′a·mine (eh·kit′uh·meen, ·min). See *ditaine.*

e·chit′e·nine (eh·kit′i·neen, ·nin). $C_{20}H_{27}NO_4$. An amorphous, brown alkaloid of dita bark.

ech′o [G. *ēchō,* echo]. A reverberated sound.

amphoric e. A vocal resonance in which the voice, when transmitted, sounds as if it were spoken into a narrow-necked bottle.

ech″o·a·cou′si·a (eck″o·a·kōō′zhuh, ·zee·uh, ·shuh, ·see·uh) [*ēchō;* G. *akousis,* hearing]. The subjective sensation of hearing echoes following sounds heard normally.

ech″o·graph′i·a (·graf′ee·uh, ·gray′fee·uh) [*ēchō;* G. *graphein,* to write]. A form of aphasia in which questions submitted to the patient are copied without ability to comprehend the inquiry; also, in writing, the last word or letter is repeated.

ech″o·kin·e′sis. See *echopraxia.*

ech″o·la′li·a [*ēchō;* G. *lalia,* talk]. The meaningless repetition of words spoken by others; commonly seen in the catatonic form of schizophrenia. Syn., *echophrasia.* —**echolal′ic,** *adj.*

ech″o·la′lus [*ēchō;* G. *lalos,* talkative]. A hypnotized person who repeats words heard without comprehension of their meaning.

ech″o·lo·ca′tion. See *catacoustics.*

ech·o′ma·tism (eh·ko′muh·tiz·um, eh·kom′uh·). See *echopraxia.*

ech″o·mim′i·a. See *echopraxia.*

ech″o·mo′tism. See *echopraxia.*

ech·op′a·thy (eck·op′uth·ee) [*ēchō;* G. *pathos,* disease]. *In psychiatry,* a morbid condition marked by the automatic and purposeless repetition of a word or sound heard or of an act seen. Also see *echolalia, echopraxia.*

ech·oph′o·ny [*ēchō;* G. *phōnē,* voice]. An echo of a vocal sound heard in auscultation of the chest.

ech″o·phot′o·ny [*ēchō;* G. *phōs,* light; *tonos,* tone]. The production of the sensation of color by the stimulus of aerial waves, or sound. See *phonism, photism.*

ech″o·phra′si·a (eck″o·fray′zhuh, ·zee·uh). See *echolalia.*

ech″o·prax′i·a [*ēchō;* G. *praxis,* a doing]. Automatic imitation by the patient of another person's movements or mannerisms; seen in the catatonic form of schizophrenia. Syn., *echokinesis, echomatism, echomimia, echomotism.*

echridine. A proprietary name for 4-(4′-ethylcyclohexylmethyl)pyridine, a compound of high fungistatic activity.

ech′u·gin (eck′yoo·jin). A crystalline glycoside from *Adenium boehmianum,* Apocynaceae. It is probably related to the digitalislike group of glycosides.

ec″i·o·ma′ni·a (eck″ee·o·may′nee·uh). See *ecomania.*

Eck, Nikolai Vladimirovich [*Russian physiologist,* b. 1847]. Reported on his experimental study of diseases of the liver and liver metabolism by means of an artificial communication made between the portal vein and inferior vena cava. Called *Eck's fistula.*

Ecker, Alexander [*German anatomist,* 1816–87]. Described the posterior occipital convolution of the brain, called *Ecker's convolution.*

Ecker's diluting fluid. Rees and Ecker's diluting fluid.

ec·la′bi·um [G. *ek,* out of; L. *labium,* lip]. Eversion of the lip.

ec·lamp′si·a [G. *eklampsis,* a shining forth]. 1. A convulsive or epileptiform seizure, usually of peripheral origin. 2. Specifically, a disease occurring during the latter half of pregnancy and characterized by an acute elevation of blood pressure, proteinuria, edema, and convulsions or coma. In the absence of convulsions or coma, the disease is referred to as *preeclampsia.* Preeclampsia and eclampsia collectively are referred to as *toxemia of pregnancy.* The cause is unknown, and the pathogenesis remains obscure; involved are sodium retention and diffuse vasospasm. —**eclamptic,** *adj.*

cerebral e. A form in which the irritation is presumed to originate in the brain; distinguished from eclampsia of pregnancy.

e. gravidarum. Eclampsia, 2.

e. nutans. A condition characterized by paroxysms, in which the head and upper part of the body are bowed forward several times in succession; the attacks are accompanied by disordered consciousness. It may be a form of psychomotor epilepsy. Syn., *salaam spasm* or *convulsion.*

e. rotans. Rotatory spasm of the head.

infantile e. A reflex convulsion of childhood associated with dentition, acute bowel disturbances, or cerebral congestion.

puerperal e. See *eclampsia,* 2.

uremic e. Convulsive seizures associated with suppression of urine.

ec·lamp′sism [*eklampsis*]. The preeclamptic toxemia of pregnancy which may lead to convulsions and coma; includes the preconvulsive prodromata, from true toxemia, nephritis, and vascular disease.

ec·lec′ti·cism [G. *eklektikos,* selective]. A system of medicine in which a group of physicians select, from various schools, what they consider to be the best doctrines or methods of treatment; special importance is attached to the development of indigenous plant remedies. —**eclectic,** *adj., n.*

ec′ly·sis [G. *eklysis,* release]. 1. Any loosening, as of the bowels. 2. A mild degree of syncope.

ec·mne′si·a (eck·nee′zhuh, ·zee·uh, eck·mnee′·) [G. *ek,* out of; *amnēsia,* forgetfulness]. Loss of memory for recent happenings, but a retention for a remote period.

e·col′o·gy [G. *oikos,* house; *logos,* word]. The study of the environmental relations of organisms.

e″co·ma′ni·a, ec″i·o·ma′ni·a (eck″ee·o·may′nee·uh) [*oikos;* G. *mania,* madness]. A psychosis marked by a domineering and haughty attitude toward members in the family, but an attitude of humility toward those in authority; domestic perversity.

Economo, Constantin von [*Austrian neurologist,* 1876–1931]. Known for giving the first adequate description of lethargic encephalitis (1917), called *von Economo's disease.*

e′co·site [*oikos;* G. *sitos,* food]. A microparasite whose host is immune to its action.

e·cos′tate (ee·kos′tayt) [L. *e,* without; *costa,* rib]. Without ribs. —**ecosta′tion,** *n.*

ec·pho′ri·a [G. *ekphoros,* carrying out]. The revival of a memory trace or engram, as by repetition of the original stimuli.

é″cra″seur′ (ay″krah″zur′. *See* Notes § 35) [F., from *écraser,* to crush]. An instrument used in veterinary surgery for the operation of castration, especially of stallions. It is armed with a chain or heavy wire loop which can be tightened until it cuts through the spermatic cord.

ECS Electroconvulsive shock.

ec′sta·sy [G. *ekstasis,* displacement]. A trancelike state with mental exaltation. —**ecstat′ic,** *adj.*

ECT Electroconvulsive therapy.

ec′tad [G. *ektos,* without; L. *ad,* to]. Outward.

ec′tal [*ektos*]. External; superficial.

ec·ta′si·a (eck·tay′zhuh, ·zee·uh, ·shuh, ·see·uh), **ec′ta·sis** [G. *ektasis,* a stretching out]. Dilatation of a tubular vessel. —**ectat′ic,** *adj.*

alveolar e. Ectatic emphysema.

diffuse arterial e. Cirsoid aneurysm.

e. ventriculi paradoxa. Hourglass stomach.

hypostatic e. Dilatation of a blood vessel, due to gravitational settling of the blood.

papillary e. Circumscribed dilatation of the capillaries, resulting in an elevated red spot on the skin.

senile e. Varices or dilated tufts of capillaries in the skin. Usually seen in older people as red or purplish areas on the trunk.

ec·ten′tal [G. *ektos,* without; *entos,* within]. Pertaining to the line of union between the ectoderm and the entoderm.

ect·eth′moid [*ektos;* G. *ēthmos,* sieve; *eidos,* form].

Either one of the lateral cellular masses of the ethmoid bone.

ec·thy′ma [G. *ekthyma*, pustule]. An inflammatory skin disease attended with an eruption of large, flat pustules that ulcerate and become crusted. They vary in size from a half to two centimeters in diameter, and are surrounded by a distinct inflammatory areola. The lesions as a rule appear on the legs and thighs, and occur in crops which persist for an indefinite period. See Plate 31.

contagious e. See contagious pustular *dermatitis*.

e. gangrenosum. Dermatitis gangrenosa infantum.

ec′to-, ect- [G. *ektos*, without]. A combining form signifying *without, upon the outer side.*

ec″to·bat′ic [*ektos;* G. *bainein*, to go]. Efferent; centrifugal; moving ectad or distad.

ec′to·blast [*ektos;* G. *blastos*, offspring]. 1. Old term for ectoderm. 2. Primitive ectoderm. 3. Improper spelling of *ectoplast.*

ec″to·car′di·a [*ektos;* G. *kardia*, heart]. An abnormal position of the heart. It may be outside the thoracic cavity (ectopia cordis) or misplaced within the thorax.

ec″to·cho·roi′de·a (eck″to·ko·roy′dee·uh) [*ektos;* G. *chorioeidēs*, from *chorion*, membrane, *eidos*, form]. The outer layer of the choroid.

ec″to·cor′ne·a [*ektos;* L. *corneus*, horny]. The outer layer of the cornea.

ec″to·cra′ni·al [*ektos;* G. *kranion*, skull]. Pertaining to the outside of the skull.

ec′to·derm [*ektos;* G. *derma*, skin]. The outermost of the three primary germ layers of the embryo. From it arise the epidermis, epithelial lining of stomodeum and proctodeum, and the neural tube, with all derivatives of these. —**ectoder′mal,** *adj.*

amniotic e. The internal epithelium of the amnion continuous with the epidermis of the embryo at the umbilicus.

basal e. That part of the trophoblast covering the eroded uterine surface of the placental sinuses, continuous with the tips of the chorionic villi; it partly disappears in late pregnancy.

epidermal e. That part of the ectoderm destined to form the epidermis. Syn., *epiblast.*

neural e. That part of the ectoderm destined to form the neural tube and neural crest. Syn., *neuroblast.*

primitive e. The undifferentiated external layer of a gastrula or of the bilaminar blastodisk. Syn., *ectoblast.* Also called *primary e.*

two-layered e. The epidermis of young embryos, consisting of a germinal layer and the epitrichium.

ec″to·der·mo′sis. Any disease entity of the ectoderm.

ec″to·der·mo′sis e″ro·siv′a plu″ri·or″i·fi·ci·a′lis. A form of erythema multiforme, usually limited to the extremities but may be accompanied by inflammation of the body orifices.

ec″to·en′zyme [*ektos;* G. *en*, in; *zymē*, leaven]. An extracellular enzyme; one which is excreted into the surrounding medium or tissue.

ec·tog′e·nous (eck·todj′i·nus) [*ektos;* G. *genesthai*, from *gignesthai*, to be produced]. Capable of growth outside of the body of its host; applied to bacteria and other parasites.

ec·tog′o·ny [*ektos;* G. *gonē*, offspring]. The influence of the developing zygote on the mother.

ec″to·men′inx [*ektos;* G. *mēnigx*, membrane]. The external part of the meninx primitiva, differentiating into dura mater and a more superficial part concerned with the formation of the chondrocranium and osteocranium.

ec′to·mere [*ektos;* G. *meros*, a part]. A blastomere destined to take part in forming the ectoderm.

ec″to·mes′o·derm [*ektos;* G. *mesos*, middle; *derma*, skin]. Mesoderm derived from the primary ectoderm of a bilaminar blastodisk or gastrula, in contrast to *endomesoderm.*

ec′to·morph. *In the somatotype*, an individual exhibiting relative predominance of ectomorphy.

ec′to·mor″phy [*ektos;* G. *morphē*, form]. Component III of the somatotype, representing relative predominance of linear and fragile body features; the skin or surface area, derived from ectoderm, is relatively great with respect to body mass. Ectomorphs appear to be more sensitive to their external environment. The counterpart on the behavioral level is cerebrotonia. —**ectomorph′ic,** *adj.*

-ec′to·my [G. *ektomē*, excision]. A combining form denoting *surgical removal.*

ec″to·pa′gi·a, ec·top′a·gy [G. *ektos*, without; *pagos*, that which is made firm]. The condition of being ectopagous; an ectopagous monstrosity.

ec·top′a·gus [*ektos; pagos*]. A monster consisting of conjoined twins united laterally at the thorax. —**ectopagous,** *adj.*

ec″to·par′a·site [*ektos;* G. *parasitos*, parasite]. A parasite that lives on the exterior of its host. —**ectoparasit′ic,** *adj.*

ec′to·phyte [*ektos;* G. *phyton*, plant]. An external parasitic plant growth; a vegetable parasite on the skin. —**ectophyt′ic,** *adj.*

ec·to′pi·a [G. *ektopos*, away from a place]. An abnormality of position of an organ or a part of the body; usually congenital. —**ectop′ic,** *adj.*

e. cordis. See *ectocardia.*

e. lentis. Malposition of the crystalline lens.

e. pupillae. See *corectopia.*

e. renis. See ectopic *kidney.*

e. testis. A rare, congenital anomaly in which the testis descends into an abnormal location, generally in the perineum or near the pubic bone.

vesical e. Exstrophy of the urinary bladder.

visceral e. A congenital hernia into the umbilical cord.

ec″to·pla·cen′ta [G. *ektos*, without; L. *placenta*, from G. *plakous*, flat cake]. The growing, functional part of the trophoblast that develops into the placenta, especially in rodents. Syn., *trophoderm.* —**ectoplacental,** *adj.*

ec′to·plasm [*ektos;* G. *plasma*, anything formed or molded]. The outer denser layer of cytoplasm of a cell or unicellular organism: also called *plasma membrane.* —**ectoplas′mic,** *adj.*

ec′to·plast. Ectoplasm.

ec″to·pot′o·my [G. *ektopos*, away from a place; *tomē*, a cutting]. Laparotomy for the removal of the contents of an extrauterine gestation sac.

ec′to·py. Ectopia.

ec″to·ret′i·na [G. *ektos*, without; L. *rete*, net]. The external and pigmentary layer of the retina.

ec′to·sarc [*ektos;* G. *sarx*, flesh]. The outer layer of a protozoan; ectoplasm.

ec′to·thrix [*ektos;* G. *thrix*, hair]. A type division of the genus *Trichophyton.*

Ec″to·tri·choph′y·ton (eck″to·trye·kof′i·ton) [*ektos; thrix;* G. *phyton*, plant]. A name sometimes given to the ectothrix type of the genus of fungi, *Trichophyton.*

ec″to·zo′on [*ektos;* G. *zōion*, living being]. An external animal parasite; ectoparasite.

ec′tro- [G. *ektrōsis*, miscarriage]. A combining form denoting *congenital absence.*

ec″tro·dac·tyl′i·a, ec″tro·dac′tyl·ism, ec″tro·dac′ty·ly [*ektrōsis;* G. *daktylos*, finger]. Congenital absence of any of the fingers or toes or parts of them.

ec·trog′e·ny (eck·trodj′i·nee) [*ektrōsis;* G. *genesthai*, from *gignesthai*, to be produced]. Loss or congenital absence of any part or organ. —**ectrogen′ic,** *adj.*

ec″tro·me′li·a, ec·trom′e·ly [*ektrōsis;* G. *melos,* limb]. Congenital absence or marked imperfection of one or more of the limbs.

infectious e. See *mousepox.*

ec·trom′e·lus [*ektrōsis; melos*]. An individual with one or more congenitally absent or imperfect limbs.

ec·tro′pi·on [G. *ek,* out of; *trepein,* to turn]. Eversion of a part, especially of an eyelid. —**ectropioniza′tion,** *n.;* **ectropionize,** *v.*

cicatrical e. Ectropion following trauma, in which scar tissue causes eversion of the lid.

paralytic e. Ectropion due to paralysis of the facial nerve.

senile e. Ectropion due to changes in the tissues of the lids as a result of age.

spastic e. Ectropion caused by spasm of the orbicularis.

ec·trop′o·dism [G. *ektrōsis,* miscarriage; *pous,* foot]. Congenital absence of a foot or feet.

ec″tro·syn·dac′ty·ly [*ektrōsis;* G. *syn,* together; *daktylos,* finger]. A developmental defect in which some of the digits are missing while others are fused.

ec·trot′ic [*ektrōsis*]. Tending to cut short; preventing the development of disease; abortive; abortifacient.

ec″ty·lot′ic [G. *ek,* out of; *tylos,* callus]. Removing warts or indurations.

ec′ze·ma (eck′si·muh, eg′zi·muh, eck′zi·muh) [G. *ekzema,* from *ekzein,* to boil over, break out]. Tetter; salt rheum. An acute or chronic, noncontagious, itching, inflammatory disease of the skin; usually characterized by irregular and varying combinations of edematous, vesicular, papular, pustular, scaling, thickened, or exudative lesions. The skin is reddened, the redness shading off into the surrounding unaffected parts. The cause is unknown. Eruptions of similar appearance due to such known causes as ingested drugs or local irritants are properly referred to as *dermatitis medicamentosa, contact dermatitis,* or *dermatitis venenata,* etc. —**eczem′atous, eczem′atoid,** *adj.*

atopic e. See atopic *dermatitis.*

camel-hair e. A contact dermatitis from hair of squirrels occurring in workers making camel-hair brushes.

e. erythematosum. The mildest form of eczema in which the skin is reddened and slightly swollen.

e. fissum. A form affecting the hands and skin over the articulations; characterized by deep, painful cracks or fissures.

e. herpeticum. A rare manifestation of primary herpes simplex infection which occurs in patients with eczema or neurodermatitis. Involving large areas of the eczematous skin, the grouped vesicles usually appear in crops over a period of several days; hence, it is similar to varicella. Fever may be high, but subsides during the second week, coincident with crust formation and healing of the skin lesions. See also Kaposi's varicelliform *eruption.*

e. hypertrophicum. A form characterized by permanent hypertrophy of the papillae of the skin, giving rise to general or limited warty outgrowths.

e. madidans. A form characterized by large, raw, weeping surfaces studded with red points. It follows eczema vesiculosum. Syn., *e. rubrum.*

e. marginatum. See *tinea* cruris.

e. nummularis. A distinctive eczema characterized by coin-sized marginated patches of eczematoid dermatitis favoring the extensor surfaces of the extremities below the elbows and the knees. In addition to allergic factors, nutritive and infective ones are involved. It is chronic and tends to relapse.

e. papulosum. A variety showing minute papules of deep-red color and firm consistence; accompanied by intense itching.

e. pustulosum. A stage characterized by the formation of pustules.

e. rubrum. See *e.* madidans.

e. seborrheicum. See *dermatitis* seborrrheica.

e. solare. That form due to irritation from the sun's rays; prickly heat.

e. squamosum. A variety characterized by the formation of adherent scales of shed epithelium.

e. sycomatosum. Pustular form occurring on the hairy parts and affecting the hair follicles. Also called *e. sycosiforme.*

e. tyloticum. Form occurring on the palms; attended with callosity.

e. vesiculosum. An eczema characterized by the presence of vesicles.

exudative e. An acute eczematous dermatitis with exudation of serum: also called *weeping eczema.*

Formosa e. See *dermatitis exsiccans palmaris.*

hyperkeratotic e. That type in which the stratum corneum is thickened.

infantile e. Cutaneous allergic (atopic) dermatitis seen in young children, usually due to foods, beverages, and other antigens, as the inhalants.

lichenoid e. That marked by acuminate papules on reddened and infiltrated bases, and accompanied by intense itching.

weeping e. See exudative *e.*

ec·zem′a·tid. An exudation dermatitis presumably caused by a circulating allergen.

ec·zem″a·ti·za′tion (eg·zem″uh·ti·zay′shun, ·tye·zay′shun, eck·sem″·, eck″si·mat·i·zay′shun) [*ekzema*]. A condition of the skin marked by persistent eczemalike lesions, due to continued injury from physical or chemical irritation.

ec·zem′a·toid re·ac′tion. A dermal and epidermal inflammatory response characterized by erythema, edema, vesiculation, and exudation in the acute stage, and in the chronic stage by erythema, edema, thickening (or lichenification) of the epidermis, and scaling.

ec·zem″a·to′sis [*ekzema;* G. *-ōsis,* condition]. Any eczematous skin disease.

Eddowes' disease. See *osteogenesis imperfecta.*

Ed′dy·ism [after Mary Baker Glover Patterson *Eddy,* American religious leader, 1821–1910]. Christian Science.

Edebohls, George Michael [*American surgeon,* 1853–1908]. Known for his contributions to the knowledge of surgery of the kidney. Made an attempt at a plastic operation for hydronephrosis (1886) and performed nephropexy (1893). The first to operate for the relief of chronic nephritis by renal decortication (1899), called *Edebohls' operation.* Described a position for vaginal operations called *Edebohls' position, Simon's position.* See Simon's *position.*

e·de′ma [G. *oidēma,* swelling]. Dropsy; excessive accumulation of fluid in the tissue spaces; due to disturbance in the mechanisms of fluid exchange. There may be decrease of osmotic pressure of the plasma from reduction in protein concentration, increased hydrostatic pressure in the capillaries due to cardiac failure, increased permeability of the capillary walls from injury or inflammation, or there may be obstruction of the lymph channels. —**edem′atous,** *adj.*

angioneurotic e. That marked by acute, transitory, localized swellings, usually about the face; the lesions resemble those of urticaria, but are larger and of less distribution. Some cases are hereditary, others seem to be due to food allergy. Syn., *angioedema, giant urticaria, giant e.* Also called *Quincke's disease.*

bullous e. See bullous *cystitis.*

cardiac e. That occurring in cardiac failure, due to increased venous pressure; most marked in dependent parts where hydrostatic pressure is the greatest.

cerebral e. Edema of the brain; due to toxic causes or nutritional or vitamin deficiencies. It is usually associated with delirium, convulsions, or coma.

congenital e. See hereditary *e.*, *e.* neonatorum.

e. neonatorum. That of the newborn, usually associated with severe erythroblastosis fetalis, but it may also occur without known cause.

endocrine e. Any edema of hormonal origin such as that associated with menstruation, pituitary tumor, deoxycorticosterone administration, and insulin therapy. They are probably primarily a result of salt retention.

giant e. See angioneurotic *e.*

heat e. Swelling of the hands and feet occurring in hot weather; due to increased blood volume and capillary dilatation. It is usually mild.

hereditary e. A chronic, hereditary process characterized by edema of the lower extremities, of unknown cause. The condition is ordinarily asymptomatic. Also called *Milroy's disease.*

inflammatory e. The swelling of inflammation. It results from increased permeability of the capillaries and thrombosis of the venules.

intercellular e. (of epidermis). See *spongiosis.*

lymphedema. That due to obstruction of lymph vessels; elephantiasis from filariasis.

malignant e. Inflammatory edema occurring in infections with gas bacilli.

nephrotic e. A type found in patients with chronic lipoid nephrosis or the nephrotic stage of glomerular nephritis, resulting from the loss of protein through proteinuria.

nutritional e. That occurring in starvation or in a poorly nourished state, due to an abnormally low plasma protein concentration of the blood.

periorbital e. That occurring in the unusually loose aveolar connective tissue of the lids and periorbital subcutaneous tissue.

pitting e. Edema of sufficient degree that the surface can be indented by pressure. Such indentation is temporary, lasting only several minutes after pressure is released.

pulmonary e. An effusion of fluid into the air sacs and interstitial tissue of the lungs.

e·den′tate [L. *edentare*, to render toothless, from *e*, out, *dens*, tooth]. 1. Without teeth. 2. Referring to the order of mammals Edentata. —**eden′tate,** *n.*

e·den′ti·a [*e; dens*]. Absence of the teeth, a condition congenital or acquired; anodontia.

e·den′tu·lous [*e; dens*]. Without teeth.

e·de′o-, e′de-, edo- [G. *aidoia*, genitals]. A combining form meaning *relating to the external genitals.* Most words from this stem are now obsolete.

e″de·ol′o·gy, ae″doe·ol′o·gy (ee″dee·ol′o·jee) [*aidoia;* G. *logos*, word]. The science of the organs of generation.

e·des′tan, e′des·tan [G. *edestos*, eatable]. A protein derivative of the class of proteins which is formed by the action of dilute acid or water on edestin.

e·des′tin, e′des·tin [*edestos*]. A globulin type of simple protein; obtained from the seeds of hemp.

ed′i·ble [L. *edibilis*, from *edere*, to eat]. Fit to eat.

Edinger, Ludwig (1855–1918). German neurologist known for his studies in neuroanatomy. He was the first to describe the ventral and dorsal spinocerebellar tracts and to distinguish between paleocerebrum and neocerebrum, and between paleocerebellum and neocerebellum, and also the first to describe a nucleus in the midbrain (1885), now known as the *Edinger-Westphal nucleus.*

ed′i·pism [after *Oedipus*, King of Thebes, who put out his own eyes because he unwittingly had killed his father]. Self-inflicted injury to the eyes. *Rare.*

Edkins, John Sydney [*English physician*, 1863–1940]. Discoverer of gastric secretin (1905).

Edmunds, Charles Wallis [*American physician*, 1873–1941]. Remembered for his association with Cushny in the recognition of atrial fibrillation in man (1901).

ed″o·ceph′al·us (ee″do·sef′uh·lus) [G. *aidoion*, genitals, penis; *kephalē*, head]. A type of otocephalus characterized by partially fused eyes in a single orbit (cyclopia), a proboscis above the fused orbit, no mouth, defective lower jaw, and synotia. —**edoceph′aly,** *n.*

ed″ro·phon′i·um chlo′ride. Generic name for the anticurare agent supplied under the trade-marked name *tensilon chloride.*

EDTAA Abbreviation for ethylenediaminetetraacetic acid.

EEG Electroencephalography, electroencephalogram, electroencephalograph.

ef·fect′. The result of any action.

Bezold-Brücke e. The perception of a given wavelength of light as different hues depending upon the amount of retinal illuminance. There are three wavelengths (478 mμ, 404 mμ, 573 mμ) which are always perceived as the same hue regardless of the amount of retinal illuminance.

detonator e. Excitatory effects at a synapse leading to a response (Eccles).

hypsochromic e. The shift of an absorption band to a higher frequency, caused by some external effect on the chromophore.

Wever-Bray e. See *Wever-Bray effect.*

ef·fec′tor [L., from *efficere*, to produce, accomplish]. A motor or secretory nerve ending in an organ, gland, or muscle, which is consequently called an effector organ; opposed to *receptor.*

ef′fer·ent [L. *efferre*, to carry away]. Carrying away, as efferent nerves, conveying impulses away from the central nervous system; or as efferent lymphatics, conveying lymph from the lymph nodes. Opposed to *afferent.*

ef″fer·ves′cence [L. *effervescere*, to foam up]. 1. The escape of a gas from a liquid; a bubbling. 2. In infectious diseases, that period following the prodrome; the onset or invasion of the disease.

ef″fer·ves′cent [*effervescere*]. Capable of producing effervescence.

ef″fleu·rage′ (ef″loo·rahzh′. *See* Notes § 35) [F.]. The stroking movement used in massage. It may be superficial, for producing reflex action, or deep, for actual emptying of the veins and lymphatic vessels.

ef″flo·res′cence [L. *efflorescere*, to bloom]. 1. The spontaneous conversion of a crystalline substance into powder by a loss of its water of crystallization. 2. The eruption of an exanthematous disease.

ef′flu·ent [L. *effluere*, to flow out]. 1. An outflow. 2. A fluid discharged from a basin or chamber for the treatment of sewage.

ef·flu′vi·um (pl. *effluvia*) [L., a flowing out]. Body odor; that which emanates from an animal body, especially an ill-smelling emanation.

ef·fuse′ (ef·yo͞oss′, ef·yo͞oz′) [L. *effusum*, from *effundere*, to pour out]. Of or pertaining to a type of growth produced by bacteria on solid mediums. The growth does not project above the surface, in contrast with the raised type of growth.

ef·fu′sion [*effundere*]. 1. A pouring-out of fluid, either serous, purulent, or bloody, into serous or other spaces. 2. The effused fluid.

pericardial e. An effusion into the pericardium.

peritoneal e. An effusion into the peritoneal cavity.
pleural e. An effusion into the pleural cavity.
serous e. An effusion of serum.
efocaine. Trade-mark for a long-acting local anesthetic and analgesic containing procaine base, procaine hydrochloride, and butyl *p*-aminobenzoate, dissolved in a mixture of polyethylene glycol-300, propylene glycol, and water. The preparation is administered by subcutaneous or intramuscular injection.
efroxine hydrochloride. Trade-marked name for *methamphetamine hydrochloride.*
e″ga·grop′i·lus [G. *aigagros,* goat; *pilos,* hair wrought into felt]. An intestinal concretion formed of hair; a hair ball.
Egas Moniz, Antonio Caetano de Abreu Freire (1874–). Portuguese neurologist who described frontal lobotomy (an operation which he named *prefrontal lobotomy*) in the treatment of certain mental disorders. He pioneered in angiography and obtained the first arteriograph in man. Nobel laureate, 1949, in medicine and physiology.
e·ger′sis (i·jur′sis, i·gur′sis) [G., an awaking]. Extreme wakefulness and alertness. —**egertic,** *adj.*
e·ges′ta (i·jes′tuh) [L. *egestum,* from *egerere,* to discharge]. The discharges of the intestines or other excretory organs.
egg. Ovum.
Eggleston, Cary [*American physician,* 1884–]. Known for advocating rapid digitalization of the heart by administering digitalis in large doses and at brief intervals.
egg′-white in′ju·ry. A syndrome developed in experimental rats fed on raw white of egg; characterized by dermatitis and emaciation resulting in death; caused by the presence of avidin in the white of egg which renders unavailable the biotin of the diet.
e·glan′du·lar, e·glan′du·lose [L. *e,* without; *glandulae,* glands, dim. of *glans,* acorn]. Without glands; aglandular.
e′go [L., I]. 1. *In psychology,* the self, regarded as a succession of mental states, or as the consciousness of the existence of the self as distinct from other selves. 2. In psychoanalytic theory, that part of the personality in conscious contact with reality.
e. restriction. See *restriction of ego.*
e″go·bron·choph′o·ny (ee″go·brong·kof′o·nee, ·bron kof′o·nee) [G. *aix, aigos,* goat; *brogchos,* trachea; *phōnē,* voice]. A combination of egophony and bronchophony.
e″go·cen′tric [L. *ego,* I; G. *kentron,* center]. Self-centered. —**egocentric′ity, egocentrism,** *n.*
e′go i·de′al. *In psychoanalysis,* the standard of perfection of the ego.
e″go·ma′ni·a [*ego;* G. *mania,* madness]. Abnormal self-esteem.
e·goph′o·ny [G. *aix, aigos,* goat; *phōnē,* voice]. A modification of bronchophony, in which the voice has a bleating character, like that of a goat. It is heard over a compressed lung, as above the level of fluid in hydrothorax.
Ehlers, Edvard Lauritz [*German dermatologist,* 1863–1937]. First to describe the syndrome of dermatolysis with chronic pseudotumors of the skin in the neighborhood of the joints (1901); called *Meekrin-Ehlers-Danlos syndrome.*
Ehrenritter, Johann [*Austrian anatomist,* d. 1790]. Described the jugular ganglion of the glossopharyngeal nerve, called *Ehrenritter's ganglion.*
Ehret, Heinrich [*German physician,* 1870–]. Known for his description of a traumatic neurosis following injury to the medial or inner aspect of the foot, in which there appear spasmodic contractures of the flexor muscles with functional paralysis of the peronei. Called *Ehret's paralysis.*
Ehrlich, Paul [*German bacteriologist and pathologist,* 1854–1915]. A pioneer in the fields of bacteriology, immunology, and chemotherapy. Developed the differential blood-count technic. Introduced methylene blue as a tissue stain (1881), and developed various staining technics. See *Ehrlich's stains,* under *stain.* Advanced his side-chain theory of immunity (1885); see under *theory.* Was the first to recognize aplastic anemia, and described inclusion bodies in erythrocytes seen in hemolytic anemias due to toxic agents (1892); see *Heinz-Ehrlich bodies* under *body.* His research on chemotherapy for experimental trypanosomiasis (1907) led to his discovery, with Hata, of arsphenamine, also called *salvarsan, Ehrlich's 606,* for the treatment of syphilis and yaws (1909); this marked the beginning of a new era in the treatment of bacterial diseases. Shared Nobel prize in physiology and medicine with Metchnikoff (1908). See also Ehrlich's *reagent,* Ehrlich's diazo *reagent,* Ehrlich's *test.*
Eichhorst, Hermann Ludwig [*Swiss physician,* 1849–1921]. Described interstitial neuritis, also called *Eichhorst's neuritis.*
Eichstedt, Carl Ferdinand [*German dermatologist,* 1816–92]. Remembered as the discoverer of *Malassezia furfur* in pityriasis versicolor, or *Eichstedt's disease.*
ei″co·nom′e·ter (eye″ko·nom′i·tur). See *aniseikometer.*
ei·det′ic im′age. An image (usually visual) so clear as to seem like an external or perceptual experience, but usually recognized as subjective. It is common in children, rare in later years.
ei′do·gen (eye′do·jen) [G. *eidos,* form; *genesthai,* from *gignesthai,* to be produced]. A chemical substance having the power of modifying the form of an embryonic organ after induction has occurred; a second-grade inductor involved in regional differentiation about the neural axis. See *organizer.*
ei″dop·tom′e·try (eye″dop·tom′i·tree) [*eidos;* G. *optikos,* of sight; *metron,* a measure]. The estimation of the acuity of vision.
Eijkman, Christiaan (1858–1930). Dutch bacteriologist and physiologist; Nobel laureate in medicine and physiology in 1929 for his discovery of the cause of beriberi, eventually identified as vitamin-B_1 deficiency. He studied "tropical anemia," showing that it was not a separate disease but an anemia due to vitamin deficiency, and also studied the influence of climate on metabolism. He developed a test for the presence of the colon bacillus in water.
ei″ko·nom′e·ter, ei″co·nom′e·ter (eye″ko·nom′i·tur). See *aniseikometer.*
Ei·me′ri·a (eye·meer′ee·uh) [L., after Theodor *Eimer,* German zoologist, 1843–98]. A genus of protozoans living in the body fluids or tissues of vertebrates and invertebrates, and having a life cycle characterized by alternation of generations. Only one species, **E. gubleri,** is perhaps a parasite of man.
Einhorn, Max [*American physician,* 1862–]. Introduced gastrodiaphany, also known as *Einhorn's method* (1889). Drew attention to a functional disorder of secretion, achylia gastrica (1892).
Einstein, Albert [*American theoretical physicist,* 1879–1955]. Famous the world over for his theory of relativity, his formula for Brownian movement, and for his contributions to the quantum theory. Did much to prepare the theoretical ground for the development of atomic research. Nobel laureate in physics (1921).

ein'stein [*Einstein*]. A unit of energy (6.06 × 10^{23} quanta) analogous to the faraday (6.06 × 10^{23} electrons); the amount of radiation absorbed by a system to activate one gram molecule of matter. Abbreviated, E.

Einthoven, Willem [*Dutch physiologist,* 1860–1927]. Devised a galvanometer for use in electrocardiography; see string *galvanometer*, also called *Einthoven's galvanometer.* Nobel laureate (1924). See also *Einthoven's formulas* under *formula,* Einthoven's *triangle,* Einthoven's *law.*

ei″san·the′ma (eye″san·theem′uh, eye·san′thimuh). Enanthema.

Eiselsberg, Anton Freiherr von [*Austrian surgeon,* 1860–1939]. Remembered for his contributions to the knowledge of neurosurgery. Produced artificial tetany experimentally in animals by thyroidectomy (1892).

Eisenmenger's complex. See under *complex.*

ei′sen·zuck″er (eye′zun·zuck″ur). See saccharated *iron* oxide.

e·jac″u·la′tion [*ejaculatio*]. The ejection of the semen.

e·jac″u·la′tor u′rin·ae. Old term for the bulbocavernosus muscle in the male.

e·jec′ta [L. *ejectum,* from *eicere,* to cast out]. Materials cast out; excretions or excrementitious matter; dejecta.

e·jec′tion [L. *ejecaio,* from *eicere*]. 1. The act of casting out, as of excretions or of excrementitious matter. 2. That which is cast out.

systolic e. The discharge of blood by the ventricles into the pulmonary artery and aorta after a previous short phase of isometric contraction.

e·jec′tor. One who, or that which, casts out or expels.

saliva e. *In dentistry,* a suction tube for removing saliva from the mouth during dental operations: also called *dental pump.*

e′ka-. *In chemistry,* a combining form meaning *first,* used as a prefix to a recognized chemical element to designate provisionally a predicted but as yet undiscovered element which should adjoin the former in the same group of the periodic system.

e″ka-i′o·dine (ee″kuh-eye′o·deen, ·din, ay″kuh-). The provisional name of the element of atomic no. 85, adjoining iodine in the halogen group of the periodic classification of elements. The element is now called *astatine.*

EKG Abbreviation for electrocardiogram, from German *Elektrokardiogram.*

e·lab″o·ra′tion [L. *elaboratio,* from *elaborare,* to get clear]. *In physiology,* any anabolic process, such as the making of crude food into higher tissue products, or the formation of secretory products in gland cells.

el′a·cin [G. *elastēs,* from *elaunein,* to drive]. The product of degeneration of elastin.

el″ae·o·my·en′chy·sis (el″ee·o·migh·en′ki·sis, ee″lee·o·). See *eleomyenchysis.*

el″ae·op′tene (el″ee·op′teen). See *eleoptene.*

el″ae·o·sac′cha·ra (el″ee·o·sack′uh·ruh, ee″lee·o·). Oleosacchara.

el″a·id′ic ac′id. $CH_3(CH_2)_7CH{:}CH(CH_2)_7COOH$; a solid, unsaturated fatty acid, being the trans-stereoisomer of oleic acid and obtained by treating the latter with nitrous acid.

e·la′i·din [G. *elaia,* olive-tree]. A white, crystalline, fatty substance, produced by the action of nitric acid upon olein and isomeric with the latter.

E·lap′i·dae [G. *elops,* serpent]. A family of venomous snakes possessing short, erect, immovable front fangs; includes cobras, tiger snakes, death adders, kraits, etc. —**elapine,** *adj.*

e·las′tase. An enzyme which acts on elastin to render it soluble; it has been isolated from the pancreas.

e·las′tic [G. *elaunein,* to drive]. Returning to the original form after being stretched or compressed.

e·las′ti·ca [*elaunein*]. 1. Elastic. 2. The tunica elastica of a blood vessel.

lamina e. The elastic layer of the mucous membrane of the pharynx and respiratory tract.

e·las′tin [*elaunein*]. The albuminoid base of elastic tissue.

e·las′ti·nase (i·lass′ti·nace, ·naze). An enzyme that digests or hydrolyzes the protein elastin.

e·las′to·mer. A generic term for all substances having the properties of natural or synthetic rubber. —**elastomer′ic,** *adj.*

e·las·tom′e·ter. An instrument which measures the indentation of skin under graded pressures and its return to normal on removal of weights.

e·las′tose. A proteose obtained from elastin.

e·las·to′sis se·ni′lis [L.]. Degeneration of the elastic connective tissue of the skin in old age.

e·lat′er·in [G. *elatērios,* driving]. $C_{20}H_{28}O_5$; neutral principle from juice of the fruit of *Ecballium elaterium;* a powerful hydragogue cathartic.

el″a·te′ri·um [*elatērios*]. The dried sediment from the juice of the squirting cucumber, *Ecballium elaterium.* It is a powerful hydragogue cathartic. Elaterin is extracted from it with ether or chloroform.

el′bow [AS. *elboga*]. The junction of the arm and forearm; the bend of the arm. See Table of Joints and Ligaments in the Appendix.

tennis e. Inflammation of the olecranon bursa, or of a bursa over the head of the radius.

el′der. Sambucus.

el′drin. See *rutin.*

el″e·cam·pane′, el″e·cam′pane. Inula.

Electra complex. See under *complex.*

e·lec′tric al″ter·na′tion. Alternation in amplitude of the QRS waves of the electrocardiogram; a sign of cardiac fatigue. Of grave importance if the heart rate is slow.

e·lec′tric cur′rent tran′sient. The passage of an electric current through the body to study passive electrical characteristics of tissue.

e·lec″tric′i·ty [G. *ēlektron,* amber]. One of the basic quantities in nature, consisting of the fundamental particles, electron and proton. Electricity in rest and in motion can be produced by friction, by magnetism, and by chemical methods. —**elec′tric, elec′trical,** *adj.*

animal e. Free electricity in the body.

faradic e. That produced by induction.

franklinic e. Frictional or static electricity.

frictional e. That produced by friction.

galvanic e. That which is generated by chemical action in a galvanic battery.

induced e. That produced in a body by proximity to an electrified body.

magnetic e. That developed by moving a conductor through a magnetic field of force.

negative e. That characterized by an accumulation of electrons.

positive e. That characterized by a deficiency of electrons.

static e. Frictional electricity.

voltaic e. Galvanic electricity.

e·lec′tri·fy [*ēlektron*]. Make electric.

e·lec″tri·za′tion [*ēlektron*]. The application of electricity to the body.

intragastric e. Electrotherapy practiced by the introduction of an electrode into the stomach.

e·lec′tro- [*ēlektron*]. A combining form denoting *connection with electricity.*

e·lec″tro·af·fin′i·ty [*ēlektron;* L. *affinis,* related]. The force by which ions hold their electric charges. Symbol, E_0.

e·lec″tro·an″es·the′si·a (·an″ess·thee′zhuh,

·zee·uh) [*ēlektron;* G. *anaisthēsia,* lack of sensation]. Local anesthesia induced by an electric current.

e·lec″tro·bi·ol′o·gy [*ēlektron;* G. *bios,* life; *logos,* word]. The science of electric phenomena in the living organism, either those produced by the organism itself or by outside sources. —**electrobiolog′ic,** *adj.*

e·lec″tro·bi·os′co·py (i·leck″tro·buy·os′ko·pee) [*ēlektron; bios;* G. *skopein,* to examine]. The use of electricity to determine the existence of life.

e·lec″tro·cap″il·lar′i·ty [*ēlektron;* L. *capillaris,* from *capillus,* hair]. The effect of an electric current upon the interface between two liquids in a capillary; due to changes in the surface tension.

e·lec″tro·car′di·o·gram″ [*ēlektron;* G. *kardia,* heart; *gramma,* letter]. A graphic record, made by an electrocardiograph, of the electric potential differences due to cardiac action, taken from the body surfaces. A typical normal record shows P, Q, R, S, T, and U waves: the P wave is due to excitation of the atria; Q, R, and S, to excitation of the ventricles; T, to repolarization of ventricles; U is a diastolic wave of unknown origin. Electrocardiograms furnish important aid in the diagnosis and management of patients with heart disease. Abbreviated, ECG, EKG. Also see *interval, lead, wave.*

e·lec″tro·car′di·o·graph″ [*ēlektron; kardia;* G. *graphein,* to write]. An instrument for making a permanent record of small voltages, due to the beating heart, that exist between different parts of the body. —**electrocardiograph′ic,** *adj.*

e·lec′tro·car″di·og′ra·phy [*ēlektron; kardia; graphein*]. The specialty of recording and interpreting electrocardiograms. See also axis *deviation, interval, preponderance, vector* quantity, ventricular *hypertrophy,* ventricular *strain.*

pattern e. Certain types of abnormalities or combinations which occur with such constancy as to indicate a specific cause.

e·lec″tro·car″di·o·pho·nog′ra·phy [*ēlektron; kardia;* G. *phōnē,* sound; *graphein*]. The electric recording of the heart sounds.

e·lec″tro·ca·tal′y·sis [*ēlektron;* G. *katalysis,* dissolution]. Catalysis or chemical changes produced by the action of electricity.

e·lec″tro·cau′ter·y [*ēlektron;* G. *kautērion,* branding-iron]. Cauterization by means of a wire loop or needle heated by a direct galvanic current: also called *galvanocautery.*

e·lec″tro·chem′is·try [*ēlektron;* G. *chymos,* juice]. The science treating of the chemical changes produced by electricity.

e·lec″tro·chro″ma·tog′ra·phy. A generic term for resolution of mixtures by differential electrical migration from a narrow zone; it applies to such migration of all solutes and suspensoids, ions, and colloids.

e·lec″tro·co·ag″u·la′tion [*ēlektron;* L. *coagulare,* to cause a fluid to curdle]. The destruction or hardening of tissues by coagulation induced by the passage of high-frequency currents; surgical diathermy.

e·lec″tro·co′ma [*ēlektron;* G. *kōma,* deep sleep]. The coma induced by electroshock therapy. See under *therapy.*

e·lec″tro·con″duc·tiv′i·ty [*ēlektron;* L. *conducere,* to conduct]. Facility for transmitting electricity.

e·lec″tro·con″trac·til′i·ty [*ēlektron;* L. *contractum,* from *contrahere,* to contract]. Capacity of muscular tissue for contraction in response to electric stimulation.

e·lec″tro·cor·ti·cog′ra·phy [*ēlektron; cortex;* G. *graphein,* to write]. The process of recording the electric activity of the brain by electrodes placed directly on the cerebral cortex, providing a much higher voltage, greater accuracy, and more exact localization than electroencephalography. —**electrocor′ticogram,** *n.*

e·lec″tro·cor′tin. Aldosterone.

e·lec″tro·cu′tion [*ēlektron;* L. *exsecutum,* from *exsequi,* to follow to the end]. Execution by electricity.

e·lec″tro·cys′to·scope [*ēlektron;* G. *kystis,* bladder; *skopein,* to examine]. A cystoscope combined with an electric light. —**electrocystos′copy,** *n.*

e·lec′trode [*ēlektron;* G. *hodos,* way]. 1. A surface of contact between a metallic and a nonmetallic conductor. 2. One of the terminals of metal, salts, or electrolytes through which electricity is applied to, or taken from, the body or an electric device or instrument.

active e. A small one used for its exciting effect in a sharply localized area for stimulating muscles or nerves.

antimony e. An electrode made of antimony for determining hydrogen-ion concentration.

brush e. One consisting of a wire brush, used to apply faradic current over a large area of skin.

calomel e. One used as a standard, as in determining hydrogen-ion concentration, because it develops a constant potential.

depolarizing e. One with a larger resistance than that of the part of the body enclosed in the circuit.

dispersing e. A large electrode used in treatment or testing which has little or no localizing effect.

dropping-mercury e. An electrode providing for a steady release of droplets of mercury falling through an electrolyte into a pool of mercury.

exciting e. Active electrode.

glass e. An electrode used in determining the hydrogen-ion concentration which operates by means of the tendency for hydrogen ions to diffuse through a thin glass membrane in contact with dilute hydrochloric acid.

hydrogen e. One made of platinum saturated with hydrogen. Used in the determination of hydrogen-ion concentration.

indifferent e. Dispersing electrode.

localizing e. Active electrode.

negative e. The cathode.

positive e. The anode.

therapeutic e. Active electrode.

thimble e. A device for very rapid localization of motor points, in the form of a long, thin, flexible thimble to fit the palpating index finger.

e·lec′tro·dent. *In dentistry,* the negative electrode of a device used to test the vitality of the pulp of a tooth.

e·lec″tro·der′ma·tome. An electrically driven cutting instrument used for obtaining split skin grafts.

e·lec″tro·des″ic·ca′tion [*ēlektron;* L. *desiccare,* to dry up]. The diathermic destruction of small growths of the urinary bladder, skin, cervix, etc., by means of a single terminal electrode with a small sparking distance.

e·lec″tro·di″ag·no′sis [*ēlektron;* G. *diagnōsis,* a deciding]. Diagnosis by means of electric instruments. —**electrodiagnos′tic,** *adj.*

e·lec″tro·di·al′y·sis (i·leck″tro·dye·al′i·sis) [*ēlektron;* G. *dialysis,* a separating]. A method for rapidly removing electrolytes from colloids by dialysis of the colloidal sol while an electric current is being passed through it.

e·lec″tro·di′a·phane [*ēlektron;* G. *diaphainein,* to show through]. An apparatus for illumination of body cavities; a diaphanoscope. —**electrodiaph′any,** *n.*

e·lec″tro·dy·nam′ics (i·leck″tro·dye·nam′icks, ·di-nam′icks) [*ēlektron;* G. *dynamikos,* powerful]. The science of energy transformations as related to electric currents and their magnetic fields.

e·lec″tro·dy″na·mom′e·ter [*ēlektron;* G. *dynamis,* power; *metron,* a measure]. An instrument for measuring the magnitude of electric currents.

e·lec″tro·en·ceph′a·lo·gram″ [*ēlektron;* G. *egkephalos,* brain; *gramma,* letter]. A graphic record of the minute changes in electric potential associated with the activity of the cerebral cortex, as detected by electrodes applied to the surface of the scalp. Also see under *rhythm, wave.* Abbreviated, EEG.

e·lec″tro·en·ceph′a·lo·graph″ [*ēlektron; egkephalos;* G. *graphein,* to write]. An instrument for recording the electric activity of the brain. Abbreviated, EEG. —**electroencephalograph′ic,** *adj.*

e·lec″tro·en·ceph″a·log′ra·phy [*ēlektron; egkephalos; graphein*]. A method of recording graphically the electric activity of the brain, particularly the cerebral cortex, by means of electrodes attached to the scalp. Electroencephalography is used in the diagnosis of epilepsy, trauma, tumors, and degenerations of the brain. Abbreviated, EEG.

e·lec″tro·en″dos·mo′sis. Electroosmosis.

e·lec″tro·fit′ [*ēlektron;* AS. *fit,* of uncertain origin]. The convulsion induced by electroshock therapy. See under *therapy.*

e·lec″tro·form′. To form by the electrodeposition of metal in finished or semifinished form, as sheets or tubes or electrotypes.

e·lec″tro·gas′tro·graph. A graphic tracing of changes in electrical potential of the stomach, associated with muscular contraction. —**electrogas′trogram,** *n.*

e·lec″tro·gen′e·sis [*ēlektron;* G. *genesis,* production]. Production of electricity.

e·lec′tro·gram″. The graphic representation of electric events in living tissues; most commonly, an electrocardiogram or electroencephalogram. Also see *electrocorticogram, electromyogram, electroretinogram.* —**electrog′raphy,** *n.*

e·lec″tro·he″mo·sta′sis [*ēlektron;* G. *haima,* blood; *stasis,* a standing]. Arrest of hemorrhage by means of a high-frequency clamp, which causes desiccation of the tissue.

e·lec″tro·hys″ter·og′ra·phy [*ēlektron;* G. *hystera,* womb; *graphein,* to write]. The recording of electric action potentials of the uterus.

e·lec″tro·ki·net′ics (·ki·net′icks, ·kigh·net′icks) [*ēlektron;* G. *kinētikos,* of motion]. The science of electricity in motion. —**electrokinetic,** *adj.*

e·lec″tro·ky′mo·graph″ [*ēlektron;* G. *kyma,* wave; *graphein,* to write]. An apparatus that combines a photoelectric recording system with a fluoroscope so as to make possible the continuous recording of the movements of a shadow within the fluoroscopic field or of changes in density in that shadow: usually employed in studying the heart. Also called *fluorocardiograph.*

e·lec″tro·li·thot′ri·ty [*ēlektron;* G. *lithos,* stone; L. *tritum,* from *terere,* to grind]. Disintegration of a vesical calculus by means of electricity.

e·lec″trol′o·gy [*ēlektron;* G. *logos,* word]. The science of electricity.

e·lec″trol′y·sis [*ēlektron;* G. *lysis,* a loosing]. The decomposition of a chemical compound by a direct electric current. —**elec′trolyze,** *v.*

cupric e. Electrolysis in which a bulb of chemically pure copper is applied directly to the diseased area; the copper oxychloride generated acts as a germicide.

e·lec′tro·lyte [*ēlektron;* G. *lytos,* soluble]. A substance which in solution is capable of conducting an electric current, and is decomposed by it. —**electrolyt′ic,** *adj.*

amphoteric e. An electrolyte that can act as either an acid or a base.

e·lec′tro·ly″zer [*ēlektron;* G. *lysis,* a loosing]. An instrument for removing urethral strictures by electricity.

e·lec″tro·mag′net [*ēlektron;* G. *Magnētis lithos,* magnet]. A core of soft iron surrounded by a coil of wire. A current passing through the wire will make the iron temporarily magnetic.

e·lec″tro·mag·net′ics [*ēlektron; Magnētis lithos*]. 1. The production of magnetic force by means of electricity. 2. The science dealing with the relation of electricity to magnetism.

e·lec″tro·mas·sage′ [*ēlektron;* F., from G. *massein,* to knead]. The transmission of electricity through a kneading instrument; electric treatment combined with massage.

e·lec″trom′e·ter [*ēlektron;* G. *metron,* a measure]. A device for measuring differences in electric potential. —**electromet′ric,** *adj.*

string e. One consisting of a fine conducting string placed between two conducting plates. An electric field between the plates causes the string to be displaced if a potential is applied to it.

e·lec″tro·mo′tive [*ēlektron;* L. *motum,* from *movere,* to move]. Pertaining to or producing electric action, as an electromotive force.

e·lec″tro·my′o·gram [*ēlektron;* G. *mys,* muscle; *gramma,* letter]. 1. A record of the response of a muscle to an electric stimulation. 2. A record of eye movements during reading, obtained by measuring the potential difference between an electrode placed at the center of the forehead and one placed at the temple.

e·lec″tro·my·og′ra·phy (i·leck″tro·migh·og′ruh-fee) [*ēlektron; mys;* G. *graphein,* to write]. Production and study of the electromyogram. —**electromyograph′ic,** *adj.*

e·lec′tron [*ēlektron*]. Commonly the smallest particle of negative electricity, sometimes called *negatron* to distinguish it from a corresponding particle of positive charge called a *positron.* The mass of an electron at rest is 9.035×10^{-28} grams, or $\frac{1}{1845}$ that of a hydrogen atom. Its unit electric charge is 4.77×10^{-10} electrostatic units. Symbol, e. —**electron′ic,** *adj.*

k e. Either of the two electrons in the first shell or orbit surrounding the nucleus of an atom.

l e. An electron in the l or second shell surrounding the nucleus of an atom.

m e. An electron in the m or third shell surrounding the nucleus of an atom.

n e. An electron in the n or fourth shell surrounding the nucleus of an atom.

negative e. The ordinary electron, also called *negatron.*

o e. An electron in the o or fifth shell surrounding the nucleus of an atom.

p e. An electron in the p or sixth shell surrounding the nucleus of an atom.

positive e. An elementary particle having the mass of an ordinary electron but carrying a positive charge. Syn., *positron.*

q e. An electron in the q or seventh shell surrounding the nucleus of an atom.

recoil e. An electron removed from its place in an atom and set into motion by impact of a photon; as a result of the collision the photon gives up only part of its energy to the electron and proceeds along a new path. Also called *Compton electron.*

secondary e. Any photoelectron or recoil electron produced when roentgen rays strike an atom.

subvalence electrons. All the electrons of any atom other than those in the valence or planetary shell.

e·lec″tro·nar·co′sis [*ēlektron;* G. *narkōsis,* a benumbing]. Narcosis produced by the application of electric currents to the body.

e·lec"tro·neg'a·tive [*ēlektron;* L. *negativus*, negative]. Pertaining to or charged with negative electricity.

e·lec"tro·neg"a·tiv'i·ty. The power of an atom in a molecule to attract electrons to itself.

e·lec"tro·neu'ro·tone (i·leck"tro·new'ro·tohn) [*ēlektron;* G. *neuron*, nerve; *tonos*, a stretching]. An apparatus for applying massage by electricity.

e·lec'tron lens. An electric field used to focus a stream of electrons on a target.

e·lec'tron op'tics. See under *optics*.

e·lec'tron volt. A unit of energy equal to the energy acquired by an electron when it falls through a potential difference of one volt.

e·lec"tro·os·mo'sis [*ēlektron;* G. *ōsmos*, impulse]. The movement of a conducting liquid through a permeable membrane under the influence of a potential gradient; it is thought to be caused by the opposite electrification of the membrane and the liquid. Syn., *electroendosmosis*.

e·lec"tro·pa·thol'o·gy [*ēlektron;* G. *pathos*, disease; *logos*, word]. The study of morbid conditions produced by the passage of electric current through living tissues.

e·lec"tro·pho'bi·a [*ēlektron;* G. *phobos*, fear]. A morbid fear of electricity.

e·lec"tro·pho·re'sis [*ēlektron;* G. *phorēsis*, from *pherein*, to bear]. The migration of charged colloidal particles through the medium in which they are dispersed, when placed under the influence of an applied electric potential. Also called, though less preferably, *cataphoresis*. The process of ion transfer is sometimes erroneously called electrophoresis. **Microscopic electrophoresis** is a method adapted to the study of larger particles which may be seen by means of the microscope or the ultramicroscope. It has been used to great advantage in studying surface and immunologic phenomena in liquids. **Moving-boundary electrophoresis** is a method applicable to dissolved substances. Used in the study of biologic mixtures in their natural state. It separates, isolates, and defines the homogeneity of various components of the mixture. Also see Tiselius *apparatus*.

e·lec"troph'o·rus [*ēlektron;* G. *phoros*, bearing]. An instrument used to generate small quantities of static electricity by induction.

e·lec"tro·pho"to·ther'a·py [*ēlektron;* G. *phōs*, light; *therapeia*, treatment]. Therapeutic treatment by means of electric light.

e·lec"tro·phren'ic [*ēlektron;* G. *phrēn*, diaphragm]. Pertaining to electric stimulation of the phrenic nerves.

e·lec"tro·phys"i·ol'o·gy [*ēlektron;* G. *physis*, nature; *logos*, word]. The branch of physiology dealing with the relations of the body to electricity; the physiologic production of electric phenomena.

e·lec"tro·pos'i·tive [*ēlektron;* L. *positivus*, positive]. Pertaining to or charged with positive electricity.

e·lec"tro·punc'ture [*ēlektron;* L. *punctura*, pricking]. *In surgery*, the use of needles as electrodes.

e·lec"tro·py·rex'i·a (i·leck"tro·pye·reck'see·uh) [*ēlektron;* G. *pyressein*, to be feverish]. The production of high body temperatures by means of an electric current.

e·lec"tro·re·sec'tion [*ēlektron;* L. *resectio*, a cutting off]. Excision by means of electrocautery.

e·lec"tro·ret'i·no·gram [*ēlektron;* L. *rete*, net; G. *gramma*, letter]. A record of the electric variations of the retina; made by placing one electrode over the cornea, the other over some indifferent region. **E e.** The type of electroretinogram in which excitatory phenomena are predominant and associated by Ragnar Granit with activity of the rods. **I e.** The type of electroretinogram in which inhibitory phenomena are dominant and associated by Ragnar Granit with activity of the cones.

e·lec"tro·scis'sion (i leck"tro·sizh'un, ·sish'un, i·leck'tro·sizh"un, ·sish"un) [*ēlektron;* L. *scissio*, from *scindere*, to tear]. Cutting of tissues by an electrocautery knife.

e·lec'tro·scope [*ēlektron;* G. *skopein*, to examine]. An instrument for detecting the presence of static electricity and its relative amount, and for determining whether it is positive or negative.

e·lec"tro·sec'tion [*ēlektron;* L. *sectio*, from *secare*, to cut]. Tissue division by a knifelike electrode operated by a high-frequency machine.

e·lec"tro·shock' [*ēlektron;* F. *choquer*, to shock]. Shock produced by electricity. See electroshock *therapy*.

e·lec"tros·mo'sis. See *electroosmosis*.

e·lec'tro·sol [*ēlektron;* hydro*sol*, confused with Ger. *sole*, salt water]. A colloidal dispersion of a metal, electrically obtained.

e·lec'tro·some [*ēlektron;* G. *sōma*, body]. A chondriosome in the cytoplasm which is responsible for chemical action.

e·lec"tro·stat'ics [*ēlektron;* G. *statikos*, causing to stand]. The science of static electricity.

e·lec"tro·steth'o·phone [*ēlektron;* G. *stēthos*, breast; *phōnē*, voice]. An amplifying stethoscope which increases and transmits sounds by the use of electronic circuits.

e·lec"tro·stric'tion. The contraction of a solvent resulting from the development of an electrostatic field by a dissolved electrolyte.

e·lec"tro·sur'ger·y [*ēlektron;* G. *cheirourgia*, working by hand]. The use of electricity in surgery; surgical diathermy. —**electrosur'gical,** *adj.*

e·lec"tro·syn'the·sis [*ēlektron;* G. *synthesis*, a putting together]. Chemical combination caused by electricity.

e·lec"tro·tax'is [*ēlektron;* G. *taxis*, arrangement]. The attraction or repulsion of organisms or cells to electric charges.

e·lec"tro·thal'a·mo·gram. A record of the electrical activity of the thalamus, obtained by inserting small electrodes deep into the cerebral hemispheres.

e·lec"tro·tha·na'si·a (i·leck"tro·thuh·nay'zhuh, ·zee·uh) [*ēlektron;* G. *thanatos*, death]. Death due to electricity.

e·lec"tro·ther"a·peu'tics (i·leck"tro·therr"uh-pew'ticks) [*ēlektron;* G. *therapeutikos*, inclined to serve]. Electrotherapy.

e·lec"tro·ther'a·py [*ēlektron;* G. *therapeia*, treatment]. The use of electricity for therapeutic purposes.

e·lec'tro·therm [*ēlektron;* G. *thermē*, heat]. An apparatus which generates heat electrically; for application to the body surface to relieve pain. —**electrother'mal,** *adj.*, **electrother'my,** *n.*

e·lec'tro·tome [*ēlektron;* G. *tomos*, cutting]. A surgical electrocautery device using low current, high voltage, and high frequency, which has a loop for engaging the part to be excised. No coagulation of tissues is produced.

e·lec"tro·ton'ic ef·fect'. An altered condition of excitability of a nerve or muscle, produced when in the electrotonic state.

e·lec"trot'o·nus (i·leck"trot'o·nus, i·leck"tro·to'-nus) [*ēlektron;* G. *tonos*, a stretching]. The change of condition in a nerve or a muscle during the passage of a current of electricity. Also see *anelectrotonus*, *catelectrotonus*. —**electroton'ic,** *adj.*

e·lec"tro·tro'pism. Electrotaxis.

e·lec"tro·tur"bi·nom'e·ter. A small turbine placed into the arterial blood stream for the purpose of measuring blood flow; a flowmeter.

e·lec″tro·va′go·gram [*ēlektron;* L. *vagus*, wandering; G. *gramma*, letter]. A record of the electric changes occurring in the vagus nerve. Also called *vagogram.*

e·lec″tro·va′lence [*ēlektron;* L. *valere*, to be strong]. The number of planetary electrons that an atom tends to lose or accept by transfer in chemical reaction.

e·lec″tro·win′. To recover, as metals from their ores, by electrodeposition.

electrozone. A proprietary disinfectant fluid produced by the electrolysis of sea water.

e·lec′tu·ar″y (i·leck′choo·err″ee) [L. *electuarium*, from G. *ekleigma*, a medicine that melts in the mouth]. A medicinal substance formed into a soft or pasty mass by combination with sugar or honey and water.

e·le′i·din [G. *elaia*, olive tree]. The semifluid, acidophil material in the stratum lucidum of the epidermis.

el′e·ment [L. *elementum*, element]. 1. Any one of the ultimate parts of which anything is composed, as the cellular elements of a tissue. 2. *In chemistry*, any one of the 100 ultimate chemical entities of which matter now is believed to be composed. Each element is composed wholly of atoms of the same atomic number (having the same charge on their nuclei), although their atomic weights may differ due to differences in nuclear weight. See *isotope.* For elements listed by name, see Table of Elements in the Appendix.

amphoteric e. One whose oxide in aqueous solution has the ability to act either as an acid or as a base.

electronegative e. An element having a tendency to attract additional electrons.

electropositive e. An element having a tendency to part with electrons.

transuranic e. An element with an atomic number greater than that of uranium (92).

el′e·mi (el′i·mee) [Ar. *al-lāmi*]. A resinous exudation frequently derived from the *Canarium commune*, but other plants of the Burseraceae are also used. It contains a crystalline resin, elemin or amyrin. Its action is similar to that of the turpentines. Elemi has been used in plasters and ointments.

el″e·o′ma [G. *elaion*, olive oil; *-ōma*, tumor]. A pathologic swelling caused by the injection of an oil into the tissues.

el″e·om′e·ter [*elaion;* G. *metron*, a measure]. An apparatus for ascertaining the specific gravity of oil.

el″e·o·my·en′chy·sis (el″ee·o·migh·en′ki·sis, ee″-lee·o·) [*elaion;* G. *mys*, muscle; *egchysis*, a pouring in]. The intramuscular injection and congelation of oils in treatment of clonic local spasm.

el″e·op′tene [*elaion;* G. *ptēnos*, winged]. The permanent liquid portion of volatile oils, as distinguished from stearoptene. Syn., *oleoptene.*

el″e·phan·ti′a·sis [G. *elephas*, elephant; NL. *-iasis*, condition]. A chronic enlargement of the subcutaneous and cutaneous tissues as a result of lymphatic obstruction. In the form commonest in the tropics, the recurrent lymphangitis is caused by *Wuchereria bancrofti.* The legs and scrotum are most commonly affected. —**elephan′tiac, elephantias′ic,** *adj.*

congenital e. A rare anomaly due to maldevelopment of the lymphatic channels.

e. anaesthetica. Anesthetic leprosy.

e. arabum. Elephantiasis, presumably filarial, occurring in the Middle East.

e. asturiensis. Pellagra.

e. congenita cystica. A state of malformation marked by skeletal defects, general anasarca, and formation of cysts in the subcutaneous tissue.

e. dura. A variety of elephantiasis marked by density and sclerosis of the subcutaneous connective tissues. Also called *e. scirrhosa.*

e. filariensis. That due to infection with filaria, most commonly *Wuchereria bancrofti.*

e. graecorum. That in leprosy.

e. nervorum. See *e.* neuromatosa.

e. neuromatosa. Diffuse neurofibromas of skin, causing great thickening, and seen in neurofibromatosis. Similar hypertrophic changes may occur also in bone and parts of the gastrointestinal tract. Syn., *e. nervorum.*

e. nostras. That associated with, and perhaps due to, chronic erysipelas.

e. sclerosa. Scleroderma.

e·leu′ther·a bark. Cascarilla.

el′e·va″tor [L., from *elevare*, to raise]. An instrument for elevating or lifting a part, or for extracting the roots of teeth.

Elford membrane. See under *membrane.*

e·lim′i·nant [L. *eliminare*, to turn out of doors]. Promoting elimination.

e·lim″i·na′tion [*eliminare*]. The process of expelling or casting out; especially, the expelling of the waste products of the body.

e·lin·gua′tion (e·lin·gway′shun, e·ling·) [L. *elinguare*, to deprive of the tongue]. Surgical removal of the tongue.

e·lix′ir [G. *xēros*, dry]. A sweetened, aromatic solution, usually hydroalcoholic, commonly containing soluble medicaments, but sometimes not containing any medication: intended for use only as a flavor and/or vehicle.

adjuvant e. Glycyrrhiza elixir.

aromatic e. (*elixir aromaticum*). A tasteful vehicle prepared from compound orange spirit, syrup, and alcohol. It contains 22–24% of alcohol.

compound digestive e. Compound pepsin elixir.

iso-alcoholic e. (*elixir iso-alcoholicum*). An elixir of the particular alcohol concentration which is most suitable for the intended medicament. It is prepared by combining in suitable proportions a high-alcoholic elixir and a low-alcoholic elixir, the former containing 73–78% of alcohol, the latter from 8–10%. Also called *iso-elixir.*

red aromatic e. (*elixir aromaticum rubrum*). Aromatic elixir colored with cudbear tincture.

simple e. Aromatic elixir.

Elkin, Daniel Collier [*American surgeon*, 1893–]. Has contributed to the knowledge of cardiac surgery. Devised a method of suturing the wounded heart by means of a stay suture passed deep into the cardiac muscle. This controls bleeding until the edges of the wound are approximated, when the deep suture is removed. Called *Elkin's operation.*

elkosin. Trade-mark for the sulfonamide compound *sulfadimetine.*

el·lag′ic ac′id. $C_{14}H_6O_8$; a tetracyclic, polyhydroxy compound occurring free or combined in galls and in certain bezoars.

Elliot, George Thompson [*American dermatologist*, 1855–1931]. Introduced a paste made of bassorin, dextrin, glycerin, and water for use as a protective skin dressing.

Elliot, John Wheelock [*American surgeon*, 1852–1925]. Originated a position in which the patient is supine with his upper abdomen raised by a support under the back; known as *Elliot's position.*

Elliot, Robert Henry [*English ophthalmologist in India*, 1864–1936]. Remembered for his operation of sclerocorneal trephining for the relief of glaucoma; called *Elliot's operation.*

Elliott treatment. See under *treatment.*

el·lip′sin [G. *elleipsis*, ellipse]. The protein constituents of the cell responsible for maintaining its form and structure.

el·lip′soid [*elleipsis;* G. *eidos*, form]. *In histology*, a condensation of reticular fibers and reticuloendothelial cells around an arteriole situated in the red pulp of the spleen between venous sinuses. —**ellip′soid,** *adj.*

el·lip′to·cyte [*elleipsis;* G. *kytos*, cell]. An elliptic erythrocyte. Syn., *ovalocyte.*

el·lip″to·cy·to′sis (i·lip″to·sigh·to′sis) [*elleipsis; kytos;* G. *-ōsis*, condition]. A rare hereditary phenomenon seen in humans, characterized by the presence of an abnormal number of oval or elliptic erythrocytes in the blood: ovalocytosis: also called *oval-cell anemia.*

Ellis, Arthur William Mickle [*English physician*, 1883–]. With Homer Swift, described a method for the treatment of cerebrospinal syphilis. See Swift-Ellis *treatment.*

Ellis, Calvin [*American physician*, 1826–83]. Described a sign of resorption of a pleuritic exudate: the curved line of dullness follows a convex course at the upper border toward the head, the highest point being lateral in the midaxillary line; called *Ellis' curve, Damoiseau's curve.*

Ellis, Henry Havelock [*English psychologist*, 1859–1939]. Celebrated for his investigations of the psychology of sex.

elm. See *Ulmus.*

e·lon″ga′tion [L. *elongare*, to prolong]. 1. The process of lengthening. 2. A lengthened condition, as of the cervix of the uterus through hypertrophy.

Elsberg, Charles Albert [*American neurosurgeon*, 1871–1948]. Described a quantitative method of measuring olfactory excitation by administering specific volumes of odor-laden air.

el′u·ant [L. *eluere*, to wash out]. The solvent used in elution in chromatography. Also spelled *eluent.*

el′u·ate [*eluere*]. The extract obtained from elution in chromatography; it represents a solution of the formerly adsorbed substance in the eluant.

e·lu′tion [*eluere*]. The process for the extraction of the adsorbed substance from the solid adsorbing medium in chromatography.

e·lu″tri·a′tion [L. *elutriare*, to wash out]. A process whereby the coarser particles of an insoluble powder are separated from the finer by mixing the substance with a liquid and decanting the upper layer after the heavier particles have settled. A form of water-sifting.

Elvehjem, Conrad Arnold (1901–). American biochemist who worked on many of the B vitamins as well as trace elements in nutrition and the relation of vitamins to enzymes. See also Elvehjem and Kennedy's *method.*

Ely's table. A table giving the duration of pregnancy. See Table in the Appendix.

el′y·tro-, elytr- [G. *elytron*, sheath]. A combining form meaning *connection with*, or *relation to, the vagina*, as in *elytritis*, inflammation of the vagina.

e·ma″ci·a′tion [L. *emaciare*, to make lean]. The process of losing flesh so as to become extremely lean, or the resultant state; a wasted condition.

e·mac″u·la′tion [L. *emaculare*, to clear from spots]. The removal of freckles or other skin lesions, especially skin tumors.

em″a·na′tion [L. *emanatio*, from *emanare*, to spring out of]. 1. That which flows or is emitted from a substance; effluvium. 2. Gaseous, radioactive products formed by the loss of alpha particles from radium (radon), thorium X (thoron), and actinium X (actinon).

em″a·na·to′ri·um [*emanare*]. An institution where patients are treated by radioactive waters and the inhalation of radium emanations.

e·man″ci·pa′tion [L. *emancipatio*, from *emancipare*, to emancipate]. *In embryology*, the process whereby organ districts acquire a definite boundary when forming from the primitive individuation field; the appearance of the presumptive organ rudiment after determination.

em″a·no·ther′a·py [L. *emanare*, to spring out of; G. *therapeia*, treatment]. Treatment by radioactive emanations; mild radium therapy.

e·man′si·o (e·man′see·o, ·shee·o) [L., from *emanere*, to remain beyond]. A failing.

e. mensium. Delay in the first appearance of the menses.

e·mas″cu·la′tion [L. *emasculare*, to make impotent]. Castration; removal of the testes, or of the testes and penis.

Em″ba·do·mo′nas (em″buh·do·mo′nus, ·dom′o·nus) [G. *embadon*, by foot, by land; *monas*, unit]. A genus of protozoan flagellates.

E. intestinalis. A species found in the intestine of man.

em·balm′ing [OF. *embaumer*]. The treatment of a cadaver with antiseptic and preservative substances for burial or for dissection.

em·bed′ [L. *in*, in; AS. *bed*]. *In histology*, to surround a specimen with a substance, as paraffin or celloidin, to give support during the process of cutting it into sections for microscopic examination. —**embedding,** *n.*

Em·be′li·a. A genus of shrubs of the Myrsinaceae.

E. ribes. An Asiatic species; the berries contain embelin, an anthelmintic principle.

em·bel′ic ac′id. Embelin.

em′be·lin. 2,5-Dihydroxy-3-lauryl-*para*-benzoquinone, the taeniacidal principle of *Embelia ribes.* Syn., *embelic acid.*

em″bo·la′li·a. See *embololalia.*

em″bo·lec′to·my [G. *embolos*, plug; *ektomē*, excision]. Surgical removal of an embolus.

em″bo·le′mi·a [*embolos;* G. *haima*, blood]. Presence of emboli in the blood.

em·bol′ic [*embolos*]. 1. Relating to an embolus or an embolism. 2. Pushing or growing in.

em′bo·lism [G. *embolisma*, from *emballein*, to throw in]. The occlusion of a blood vessel by an embolus, causing various syndromes depending on the size of the vessel occluded, the part supplied, and the character of the embolus. Also see *embolus.*

air e. Large amounts of air in the blood stream, such as may gain entrance through wounds of the great veins in the neck, and, reaching the heart, cause cardiac arrest; small amounts are resorbed and cause no symptoms.

amniotic e. A rare type seen in the mother following delivery, in which there are multiple emboli containing material from the amniotic fluid widely disseminated, the clinical picture resembling that seen in fat embolism.

bone-marrow e. A type similar to fat embolism, resulting from bone injuries in which emboli of marrow get into the circulation.

cerebral e. The blocking of a cerebral vessel by any type of embolus gives rise to a syndrome resembling cerebral hemorrhage.

coronary artery e. The blocking of a coronary artery by an embolus is rare, and clinically gives rise to a syndrome similar to that seen in coronary thrombosis or spasm.

cutaneous gaseous e. The cutaneous manifestations of caisson disease: generalized or local pruritis, purple erysipeloid plaques, scarlatiniform rash, cyanosis and subcutaneous emphysema.

fat e. Multiple, widely disseminated droplets of fat resulting in emboli of parenchymatous organs and often causing death. The fat droplets may be liberated in a crushing injury of adipose tissue or bone, or may follow the injection of oily solutions. Also called *oil e.*

gas e. See caisson *disease;* cutaneous gaseous *e.*

infective e. The obstruction of blood vessels by infected emboli, resulting in multiple abscess formation: also called *septic e., bacterial e.*

paradoxical e. See under *embolus.*

peripheral artery e. The blocking of a large artery supplying a limb results in gangrene of the part supplied. If the embolism occurs in a smaller artery, collateral circulation will take over the function of the occluded vessel.

pulmonary e. Obstruction of a pulmonary artery by lodgement of an embolus.

retrograde e. Embolism in which the embolus has gone against the normal direction of the blood stream.

em″bo·lo·la′li·a, em″bo·la′li·a [G. *embolos,* plug; *lalia,* chat]. The insertion of meaningless words into speech, occurring in some aphasic and schizophrenic states.

em″bo·lo·phra′si·a (em″bo·lo·fray′zhuh, ·zee·uh). Embololalia.

em′bo·lus (pl. *emboli*) [*embolos*]. A bit of matter foreign to the blood stream—it may be blood clot, air, cancer or other tissue cells, fat, cardiac vegetations, clumps of bacteria, or a foreign body, such as a needle or bullet—which either gains entrance to the circulation from the individual's body or is carried by the blood stream until it lodges in a blood vessel and obstructs it, causing embolism. **—embol′iform, emboloid,** *adj.*

paradoxical e. One which originates in the venous system and crosses to the arterial side through a patent foramen ovale.

riding e. An embolus at the bifurcation of an artery, blocking both branches. Also called *saddle e., straddling e.*

em′bo·ly [G. *embolē,* a putting in]. The process of invagination by which a two-layered gastrula develops from a blastula.

em·bra′sure (em·bray′zhur, ·shur) [F. *embraser,* to widen an opening, of uncertain origin]. *In dentistry,* the space between the sloping proximal surfaces of the teeth. The opening may be toward the cheek (*buccal*), toward the lips (*labial*), or toward the tongue (*lingual*).

em″bro·ca′tion [G. *embrechein,* to wet]. 1. The application, especially by rubbing, of a liquid to a part of the body. 2. The liquid so applied; liniment.

em″bry·ec′to·my [G. *embryon,* embryo; *ektomē,* excision]. The surgical removal of an extrauterine embryo.

em′bry·o [*embryon*]. 1. A young organism in the early stage of development. 2. The product of conception up to the third month of pregnancy. See Plate 41. **—embry′onal, embryon′ic,** *adj.*

presomite e. An embryo from the time of fertilization until the appearance of the first somite, about 21 days.

previllous e. An embryo from the time of fertilization until the development of the chorionic villi.

somite e. An embryo during the period when somites are formed, approximately the twenty-first to the thirty-first days of development.

em′bry·o-, embry- [*embryon*]. A combining form signifying *fetus, embryo, embryonic.*

em′bry·o·blast″ [*embryon;* G. *blastos,* germ]. That part of the germ disk or inner cell mass from which the embryo proper develops.

em″bry·o·car′di·a [*embryon;* G. *kardia,* heart]. A morbid condition in which the heart sounds resemble those of the fetus, the first and second sounds being almost identical.

em″bry·o·chem′i·cal [*embryon;* G. *chymos,* juice]. Relating to the changes in the chemistry of the ovum or embryo.

em″bry·oc′to·ny [*embryon;* G. *kteinein,* to kill]. The killing of a fetus. **—embryocton′ic,** *adj.*

em″bry·og′e·ny (em″bree·odj′i·nee), **em″bry·o·gen′e·sis** [*embryon;* G. *genesthai,* from *gignesthai,* to be produced]. Embryology; the development of the embryo. **—embryogen′ic, embryogenet′ic,** *adj.*

em′bry·oid [*embryon;* G. *eidos,* form]. Resembling an embryo.

em″bry·o·lem′ma (pl. *embryolemmata*) [*embryon;* G. *lemma,* that which is peeled off]. Any one of the fetal or extraembryonic membranes.

em″bry·ol′o·gist [*embryon;* G. *logos,* word]. One skilled in the science of embryology.

em″bry·ol′o·gy [*embryon; logos*]. The science dealing with the embryo and its development. **—embryolog′ic, embryolog′ical,** *adj.*

chemical e. Investigation of development of an embryo on a physicochemical basis.

comparative e. Investigation and comparison of the embryology of different orders of animals or of plants, one with another.

descriptive e. A study of the separate and individual portions of the embryo.

experimental e. That which uses experimental methods to investigate the development of an embryo.

em″bry·o′ma [*embryon;* G. *-ōma,* tumor]. Old term for *teratoma.*

e. of kidney. See Wilms's *tumor.*

e. of ovary. See *dysgerminoma.*

e. of testis. See embryonal *carcinoma* of testis.

em″bry·o·mor′phous [*embryon;* G. *morphē,* shape]. Like an embryo or of embryonic origin.

em′bry·on [G.]. Embryo. *Rare.*

em′bry·o·nate [*embryon*]. Fecundated; containing an embryo.

em″bry·o·ni·za′tion [*embryon*]. Change of a cell or tissue to an embryonic form of structure.

em′bry·o·noid [*embryon;* G. *eidos,* form]. Embryoniform.

em″bry·o·plas′tic [*embryon;* G. *plassein,* to form]. Participating in the formation of the embryo.

em″bry·o·to′ci·a (em″bree·o·to′shee·uh, ·see·uh) [*embryon;* G. *tokos,* birth]. Abortion. *Obs.*

em′bry·o·tome″ [*embryon;* G. *tomos,* cutting]. An instrument for performing embryotomy.

em″bry·ot′o·my [*embryon;* G. *tomē,* a cutting]. Any mutilation of the fetus in the uterus to aid in its removal when natural delivery is impossible.

em″bry·o·tox′on [*embryon;* G. *toxon,* bow]. An opaque marginal ring in the cornea resembling arcus senilis; sometimes seen at birth.

em′bry·o·trophe, em′bry·o·troph [*embryon;* G. *trophē,* nourishment]. 1. The total nutriment, both histotrophe and hemotrophe, supplied to the embryo during pregnancy. 2. See *histotrophe,* 1. **—embryotroph′ic,** *adj.*

em″bry·ot′ro·phy [*embryon; trophe*]. The nutrition of the fetus.

em″bry·ul′ci·a (em″bree·ul′see·uh) [G. *embryoulkia,* from *embryon; helkein,* to draw]. Extraction of the fetus from the uterus by means of instruments.

em″bry·ul′cus [G. *embryoulkos,* hook]. A blunt hook, or obstetric forceps, used in performing embryulcia.

e·mer′gen·cy med′ic·al tag. *In U. S. Army medicine,* an individual medical record in the form of a tag, so designed that it can be attached to each casualty, and bearing certain identifying and administrative data with diagnosis and treatment administered: used by aid stations, collecting stations, and clearing stations.

e·mer'gen·cy the'o·ry. The concept that the major function of adrenal medulla is to liberate epinephrine in states of emergency so as to increase heart rate, raise blood pressure, reduce blood flow to viscera, and mobilize blood glucose, thereby creating optimal conditions for function of skeletal muscles.

em'e·sis [G., vomiting]. Vomiting.

em"e·ta·mine' (em"i·tuh·meen', i·met'uh·meen, ·min) [G. *emetos*, vomiting]. $C_{29}H_{36}N_2O_4$; an alkaloid occurring in small amounts in ipecac and obtainable from emetine by dehydrogenation.

e·met"a·tro'phi·a [*emetos;* G. *atrophia*, atrophy]. Atrophy or wasting away, due to persistent vomiting.

e·met'ic [G. *emetikos*, provoking sickness]. Having the power to induce vomiting.

e·met'ic. An agent causing emesis.

direct e. One acting directly on the stomach.

indirect e. One acting through the blood upon the vomiting center. Also called *systemic e.*

em'e·tine (em'i·teen, ·tin) [G. *emetos*, vomiting]. $C_{29}H_{40}N_2O_4$; the principal alkaloid of ipecac, and the methyl ether of cephaeline, from which it may be prepared by methylation: a white, amorphous powder, sparingly soluble in water. It is emetic, diaphoretic, and expectorant, but its chief utility is as an amebicide, being used in the form of emetine hydrochloride and emetine bismuth iodide.

e. bismuth iodide. A complex iodide of emetine and of bismuth, containing 25–30% emetine and 18–22.5% bismuth (British Pharmacopoeia); a reddish-orange powder, insoluble in water: used orally in the treatment of amebic dysentery. Dose, 60–200 mg. (1–3 gr.) daily.

e. hydrochloride. $C_{29}H_{40}N_2O_4.2HCl.xH_2O$; a white or very slightly yellowish, crystalline powder, freely soluble in water. Dose, subcutaneously, 30–60 mg. (½–1 gr.) daily for 5 to 10 days.

em'e·to-, emet- [*emetos*]. 1. A combining form denoting *vomiting.* 2. A combining form denoting an *emetic.*

em"e·to·ca·thar'sis [*emetos;* G. *katharsis*, cleansing]. Vomiting and purgation at the same time, or produced by a common agent.

em"e·to·ma'ni·a [*emetos;* G. *mania*, madness]. Morbid desire to vomit.

em"e·to·mor'phine (em"i·to·mor'feen, ·fin) [*emetos;* G. *Morpheus*, god of dreams, from *morphē*, form, because he calls up forms before the sleeper]. Apomorphine.

em"e·to·pho'bi·a [*emetos;* G. *phobos*, fear]. Morbid fear of vomiting.

emf, e.m.f. Electromotive force. E and E.M.F. are also used.

EMG *E*lectro*m*yo*g*raphy; *e*lectro*m*yo*g*ram.

e·mic'tion [L. *e*, out; *mictum*, from *mingere*, to urinate]. Urination.

e·mic'to·ry [*e; mingere*]. Diuretic. —**emic'tory,** *n.*

em"i·gra'tion [L. *emigratio*, from *emigrare*, to depart from a place]. The outward passage of wandering cells or leukocytes through the walls of a small blood vessel.

em'i·nence [L. *eminentia*, from *eminere*, to stand out, project]. A projecting, prominent part of an organ, especially a bone.

acoustic e. See acoustic *tubercle.*

arcuate e. A round protuberance on the anterior aspect of the petrosal portion of the temporal bone, marking the location of the superior semicircular canal.

articular e. [BR]. The articular tubercle of the zygomatic process of the temporal bone, forming the anterior boundary of the mandibular fossa.

canine e. A prominence on the outer side of the maxilla, corresponding to the root of the canine tooth.

collateral e. A ridge on the floor of the lateral ventricle, corresponding to the depth of the collateral fissure of the temporal lobe.

cruciate e. Ridges intersecting in the form of a cross on the internal surface of the squamous portion of the occipital bone.

e. of the concha. The posterior projection on the pinna corresponding to the concha.

e. of the scaphoid fossa. The elevation on the medial side of the auricle corresponding to the scaphoid fossa on the lateral side.

e. of the triangular fossa. The elevation on the medial side of the auricle corresponding to the triangular fossa on the lateral side.

facial e. See facial *colliculus.*

frontal e. One of two rounded elevations of the frontal bone above the superciliary ridges.

genital e. An elevation which is the anlage of the penis in the male or the clitoris in the female.

hypobranchial e. A median swelling of the floor of the pharynx between the tongue and the laryngotracheal groove that forms the epiglottis and the aryepiglottic folds.

hypoglossal e. See *trigone* of the hypoglossal nerve.

hypothenar e. An elevation on the ulnar side of the palm corresponding to the muscles of the little finger.

iliopectineal e. A ridge on the hipbone, marking the site of union of ilium and pubis. Syn., *iliopubic e.*

iliopubic e. Iliopectineal eminence.

intercondyloid e. The spinous process lying between the two articular facets on the superior articular surface of the tibia.

jugular e. The spinelike extremity of the jugular process of the occipital bone.

median e. A longitudinal ridge in the floor of the fourth ventricle, bounded by the median sulcus medially and the sulcus limitans laterally. It includes the facial colliculus and the trigone of the hypoglossal nerve.

median e. of the tuber cinereum. The enlarged upper end of the stalk of the neurohypophysis, attached to the tuber cinereum and forming a small part of the third ventricle; it contains capillary anastomoses between the superior hypophyseal arteries and the hypophysis.

parietal e. The rounded part of the parietal bone. This is sometimes bosselated, due to rickets.

pyramidal e. A bony projection on the posterior wall of the tympanic cavity, having an opening at its tip for the tendon and an elongated cavity for the body of the stapedius muscle.

radial e. of the wrist. A prominence composed of the tubercles of the navicular and the greater multangular bones.

supracondylar e. An epicondyle.

thenar e. A rounded elevation on the radial side of the palm corresponding to the muscles of the thumb.

ulnar e. of the wrist. A prominence made up of the pisiform bone and the hook of the hamate bone.

em"i·nen'ti·a (em"i·nen'shee·uh) [L.]. Eminence.

e. carpi radialis [BNA]. See radial *eminence* of the wrist.

e. carpi ulnaris [BNA]. See ulnar *eminence* of the wrist.

em'is·sar"y (em'i·serr"ee) [L. *emissarius*, from *emittere*, to send forth]. Any venous channel through the skull, connecting the venous sinuses with the diploic veins and veins of the scalp.

e·mis′sion [L. *emissio*, from *emittere*]. 1. An ejaculation, or sending forth. 2. A seminal discharge, voluntary or involuntary.

cold e. Emission of electrons from an unheated cathode under the influence of a very strong electric field: also called *field e.*

secondary e. Emission of electrons from a metal plate which is being bombarded by a stream of high energy (primary) electrons.

em·men′a·gogue (eh·men′uh·gog, eh·mee′nuh·) [G. *emmēna*, the menses; *agōgos*, leading]. An agent that stimulates the menstrual flow. —**emmenagog′ic,** *adj.*

direct e. One acting directly on the generative organs.

indirect e. One acting by relieving an underlying condition, such as anemia or constipation.

em·men′i·a (eh·men′ee·uh, ·mee′nee·uh) [*emmēna*]. The menses.

emmenin. Trade-mark for a placental estrogenic substance, composed mainly of estriol glycuronide.

em·men″i·op′a·thy (eh·men″ee·op′uth·ee, ·o′puth·ee, eh·mee″nee·) [*emmēna;* G. *pathos*, disease]. Any menstrual disorder.

em″me·nol′o·gy [*emmēna;* G. *logos*, word]. That branch of medicine that treats of menstruation.

Emmet, Thomas Addis [*American gynecologic surgeon*, 1828–1919]. Famed in his time for his investigations of sterility (1865), his operation of vaginal cystotomy (1872), called *Emmet's operation*, and his technic for repair of the cervix and perineum after labor (1883), called *Emmet's perineorrhaphy.*

em″me·tro′pi·a [G. *emmetros*, in measure; *ōps*, eye]. Normal or perfect vision. The condition in which parallel rays are focused exactly on the retina without effort of accommodation. Abbreviated, E. —**emmetrop′ic,** *adj.;* **em′metrope,** *n.*

Emmons, Chester Wilson (1900–). American mycologist who investigated mycoses of man and the fungi causing them, particularly the natural and induced mutations of these fungi, simplification of their classification, and their natural occurrence in animal reservoirs and soil.

em′o·din. $C_{15}H_{10}O_5$; 1,3,8-trihydroxy-6-methylanthraquinone; a product of hydrolysis or oxidation of glycosidal compounds found in rhubarb, cascara, and other plants: it has also been synthesized. It is an irritant cathartic, acting mainly on the large intestine.

em′o·din-L-rham′no·side. Frangulin.

e·mol′li·ent [L. *emollire*, to soften]. A substance used externally to soften the skin; or, internally, to soothe an irritated or inflamed surface. —**emol′lient,** *adj.*

e·mo″ti·o·met″a·bol′ic (i·mo″shee·o·) [L. *emotum*, from *emovere*, to stir up; G. *metabolikos*, changeable]. Modifying metabolism as a result of emotion.

e·mo″ti·o·mo′tor [*emotum;* L. *motor*, from *movere*, to move]. Of, pertaining to, or inducing some activity as a result of emotion.

e·mo″ti·o·mus′cu·lar [*emotum;* L. *musculus*, muscle]. Relating to muscular activity which is due to emotion.

e·mo′tion [*emotum*]. 1. A mental feeling or sentiment. 2. Strong feeling, often of an agitated nature, accompanied frequently by physical and psychic reactions, as changes in heart action, gastrointestinal and vasomotor disturbances. —**emotional,** *adj.*

e·mo″ti·o·vas′cu·lar (i·mo″shee·o·) [*emotum;* L. *vasculum*, small vessel]. Relating to some vascular change brought about by emotion.

em·pasm′ (em·paz′um, em′paz·um), **em·pas′ma** (em·paz′muh) [G. *empasma*, dusting-powder, from *empassein*, to sprinkle on]. A perfumed powder for dusting the person.

em′pa·thy [G. *empatheia*, passion]. *In psychology*, emotional identification with another's feelings.

em′phly·sis [G. *en*, in; *phlysis*, eruption]. Any vesicular or exanthematous eruption terminating in scales.

em·phrac′tic [G. *emphraktikos*, likely to obstruct]. Obstructive; closing the pores of the skin.

em·phrac′tic. Any agent that obstructs the function of an organ, especially the excretory function of the skin.

em·phrax′is [G., *stoppage*]. An obstruction, infarction, or congestion.

phrenic e. See *phrenicoexeresis.*

em″phy·se′ma (em″fi·see′muh, ·zee′muh, em″-figh·) [G., inflation, from *emphysan*, to blow in]. A condition in which there is overdistention of the air spaces in the lungs (**pulmonary** or **alveolar e.**), or in which there is abnormal presence of air or gas in the body tissues (**nonpulmonary e.**). Overinflation of the alveoli may be physiologic (functional) or pathologic. —**emphysem′atous,** *adj.*

acute bullous e. A fulminating form of obstructive pulmonary emphysema, in which the lungs become severely overinflated due to extreme inspiratory efforts and bronchial obstruction, as in acute tracheobronchitis, suffocation from gases or drowning, or bronchial and cardiac asthma. Syn., *acute vesicular e.*

aero e. See *aeroembolism.*

atrophic e. See senile *e.*

chronic pulmonary e. An obstructive type of pulmonary emphysema characterized by voluminous lungs following prolonged overinflation of the alveoli, with atrophic changes of the alveolar walls, which may thin out, rupture, or coalesce, and of the blood vessels supplying them: also called *hypertrophic e., essential e., substantial e., inspiratory e., expiratory e., functional e., structural e., irreversible e., large-lunged e., hypoxic e.*

compensatory e. Simple nonobstructive overdistention of lung segments or an entire lung in intrathoracic adaptation to collapse, destruction or removal of contiguous portions of lung or the opposite lung: also called *complementary e., ectatic e.*

cutaneous e. See subcutaneous *e.*

ectatic e. See complementary *e.*

hypertrophic e. See chronic pulmonary *e.*

interlobular e. See interstitial *e.*

interstitial e. Air in tissue spaces between alveoli or lobules, or under the pleura, following rupture of alveoli or small respiratory bronchioles. Seen most often in the newborn following vigorous artificial respiration, in young children following pertussis, and in adults following trauma to the chest.

mediastinal e. Accumulation of air in the tissues of the mediastinum, often by extension from the interstitial connective stroma of the lungs.

nonobstructive e. See postural *e.*

obstructive e. Overdistention of the lung due to partial obstruction of the air passages, which permits air to enter the alveoli but which resists expiration of the air.

postural e. Overdistention of the lungs in conformity to changes in the size of the thoracic cage, as in acromegaly and other deformities, or as in senile emphysema.

senile e. A nonobstructive pulmonary emphysema associated with atrophic and involutionary changes seen with aging. Alveolar overdistention is considered to be due not so much to atrophic changes of the alveolar walls, but primarily to changes in the thoracic spine and subsequent adaptation of the lungs to the size of the thorax. The lungs are usually of normal size or only slightly enlarged. Also called *small-lung e.*

subcutaneous e. The accumulation of air or gas in the connective-tissue spaces under the skin; due to trauma, or infection with a gas-producing organism.

substantive e. See chronic pulmonary *e.*

tissue e. See *aeroembolism*, caisson *disease.*

vesicular e. An obstructive emphysema, which may be acute bullous emphysema or the chronic pulmonary form.

em·pir′ic [G. *empeirikos*, experience]. Based on practical observation and not on scientific reasoning or education.

em·pir′ic. One who in practicing medicine relies solely on experience and experimentation; in modern usage, a quack, or charlatan. —**empirical,** *adj.*

em·pir′i·cism [*empeirikos*]. Dependence upon experience or observation.

empirin. Trade-mark for a brand of acetylsalicylic acid.

e. compound. Trade-mark for a tablet containing acetylsalicylic acid, acetophenetidin, and caffeine.

em·plas′trum. A plaster.

em″pros·thot′o·nos [G. *emprosthotonos*, from *emprosthen*, in front, *tonos*, a stretching]. Tonic muscular spasm in which the body and head are forcibly flexed forward.

em″pros·tho·zy·go′sis (em″pross·tho·zye·go′sis) [*emprosthen;* G. *zygōsis*, from *zygoun*, to join together]. The condition of conjoined twins in which the fusion is anterior.

em″py·e′ma (em″pye·ee′muh, em″pee·ee′muh) [G. *empyēma*, gathering, abscess]. A term used to indicate the presence of pus in a cavity, hollow organ, or space; such as the pleural cavity, the gallbladder, the maxillary sinus, or the pericardial cavity. —**empyemic, empyem′atous,** *adj.*

e. of necessity. One in which pus from the pleural cavity burrows to the outside, appearing as a tumor in an intercostal space or at the costal border.

pulsating e. One in which there is pulsation, transmitted from the heart, through the chest wall.

streptococcal e. A pleural empyema caused by streptococci and occurring most frequently during extensive epidemics of measles and influenza as a complication of the original disease.

tuberculous e. A pleural empyema caused by the tubercle bacillus.

em″py·e′sis [G., suppuration]. A pustular eruption, as smallpox; any disease characterized by phlegmonous vesicles gradually filling with purulent fluid.

em″py·reu·mat′ic (em″pye·rōō·mat′ick, em″pi·) [G. *empyreuein*, to set on fire]. Referring to any odorous substance produced by destructive distillation of organic material.

e·mul′si·fi″er [L. *emulsum*, from *emulgere*, to milk out]. An agent used to assist in the production of an emulsion.

e·mul′si·fy″ [*emulgere*]. Make into an emulsion. —**emulsifica′tion,** *n.*

e·mul′sin [*emulgere*]. An enzyme, found in bitter almonds and other seeds, which selectively catalyzes hydrolysis of β-glucoside linkages; thus, it effects hydrolysis of amygdalin to benzaldehyde, hydrocyanic acid, and glucose. Syn., *amygdalase, glucosidase.*

e·mul′sion [*emulgere*]. A product consisting of minute globules of one liquid dispersed throughout the body of a second liquid. The portion which exists as globules is known as the internal, dispersed, or discontinuous phase; the other liquid is the external or continuous phase or the dispersion medium.

e·mul′soid [*emulgere;* G. *eidos*, form]. A colloid system whose internal phase is liquid; a lyophilic colloid.

e·munc′to·ry [L. *emunctum*, from *emugere*, to wipe the nose]. Excretory.

en- [F., from L. *in*, in, into; G. *en*, in]. A prefix signifying *in, into.*

-en [AS. *-nian*]. A suffix meaning *to make, to render.*

-en [AS.]. An adjective suffix meaning *made of.*

en·am′el [OF. *esmail*, enamel]. The hard, calcified substance that covers the crown of a tooth.

e. drop. See *enameloma.*

e. navel. In developing enamel organs, a transitory slight depression in the outer enamel epithelium where it is joined by the enamel cord.

e. pearl. See *enameloma.*

mottled e. Imperfectly calcified or hypoplastic dental enamel that is the result of excessive ingestion of fluorides; chronic dental fluorosis.

en·am″e·lo·blas·to′ma. See *ameloblastoma.*

en·am″el·o′ma [*esmail;* G. *-ōma*, tumor]. A benign odontogenic tumor consisting of enamel. It commonly appears as a nodule attached to the root of a tooth, but may lie free in the periodontal membrane. Also called *enamel pearl, enamel drop.*

en″an·thal′de·hyde. See *heptaldehyde.*

en″an·the′ma, en·an′them [G. *en*, in; *anthēma*, efflorescence, pustule]. An eruption on a mucous membrane, or within the body; in distinction from *exanthema.* —**enanthem′atous,** *adj.*

en·an″ti·o·la′li·a [G. *enantios*, opposite; *lalia*, talk]. Talking contrariwise; a disturbance in mental and speech function which prompts ideas and words opposite to those presented as a stimulus.

en·an′ti·o·mer. Enantiomorph.

en·an′ti·o·morph″ [G. *enantios*, opposite; *morphē*, shape]. 1. *In chemistry*, one of a pair of isomeric substances with asymmetric structures that are mirror images of each other. In general, enantiomorphs possess identical chemical and physical properties, but usually differ in their reactions with other asymmetric molecules or in reactions catalyzed by asymmetric molecules, including enzymes. Under identical conditions they rotate the plane of polarized light to the same extent but in opposite directions. Syn., *enantiomer, optical antipode.* 2. Either of two forms of a crystal which possesses neither a plane nor a center of symmetry but which has a mirror-image resemblance to the other form; under identical conditions the two forms rotate the plane of polarized light to the same extent but in opposite directions. —**enantiomor′phic, enantiomor′phous,** *adj.*

en″ar·thro′sis [G., from *en; arthron*, joint; *-ōsis*, condition]. A ball-and-socket joint, like that of the hip. —**enarthrodial,** *adj.*

enbin emulsion. Trade-marked name for a preparation containing benzyl benzoate, chlorophenothane, and ethyl aminobenzoate: used for treatment of pediculosis and scabies.

en·can′this [*en;* G. *kanthos*, corner of the eye]. A neoplasm in the inner canthus of the eye.

en·cap″su·la′tion [*en;* L. *capsula*, small box]. The process of surrounding a part with a capsule.

en·cap′suled [*en; capsula*]. Enclosed in a capsule or sheath.

en·ceph″a·lal′gi·a [G. *egkephalos*, brain; *algos*, pain]. Pain in the head.

en·ceph″a·lat′ro·phy [*egkephalos;* G. *atrophia*, want of food]. Atrophy of the brain.

en·ceph″a·li′tis [*egkephalos;* G. *-itis*, inflammation]. Inflammation of the brain; may be a specific disease, or a sequela or complication of another disease. According to etiology, encephalitis can be classified as *actinomycotic, parasitic, trichinotic,* etc. —**encephalit′ic,** *adj.*

American e. See St. Louis *e.*

cat-scratch e. That resulting from contact with a cat; a rare form of cat-scratch disease. Diagnosis is based on positive skin test with cat-scratch antigen and absence of all other infectious agents.

chronic e. A term sometimes applied to postencephalitic paralysis agitans.

eastern equine e. See equine *e.*

e. periaxialis diffusa. A disease, primarily of children, due to extensive inflammation and early demyelination of the white matter in a cerebral hemisphere; characterized by marked loss of hearing, speech, and sight. Also called *Schilder's disease.*

epidemic e. Lethargic *e.;* the term is also used to refer to *Japanese e., equine e.,* and *Australian X disease.*

equine e. A viral disease affecting lower animals, as birds, horses, and mules, and usually transmitted to man by mosquitoes. Three causative viral strains are known: the eastern, western, and Venezuelan equine viruses. Diagnosis of the type of encephalitis rests on identification of the virus or on serologic reactions. Also called *(epizootic) equine encephalomyelitis.*

hemorrhagic e. That form of encephalitis with hemorrhagic foci.

herpetic e. A type of meningoencephalitis, characterized by large intranuclear inclusion bodies (Lipschütz bodies) in the brain, and diagnosed on the basis of isolation of the herpes simplex virus and serological reactions.

inclusion e. An unusually chronic form of encephalitis, involving the gray and white matter, in which large intranuclear inclusion bodies, resembling those of the herpes simplex virus, are found primarily in oligodendria and less frequently in nerve cells; relationship to herpetic *e.,* however, is not known. Convulsions and progressive mental deterioration may develop.

Japanese e. A type due to a virus and epidemic in Japan; affects older persons primarily and has a high mortality rate. Diagnosis rests on identification of the specific virus and serologic reactions. It may be related to Australian X disease. Also called *Japanese B e.* to distinguish it from *lethargic e.* (*Japanese A e.*), *Russian autumnal e.*

lead e. That due to lead poisoning and resembling acute toxic encephalitis.

lethargic e. A meningoencephalomyelitis of unknown cause, occurring chiefly during spring and winter, characterized by its diversity of signs and symptoms simulating any type of neurologic syndrome in different individuals or even at different stages of the disease. The symptoms often include sleepiness at first, from which stems the name given this entity by von Economo (1917). Other common symptoms are ophthalmoplegia, aberrant forms of hyperkinesia and parkinsonism, and also signs suggestive of psychoneurotic or neurotic reactions. Thought to be infectious, the disease has occurred in epidemics in the past. Microscopically, the lesions seen in the mesencephalon and diencephalon are more chronic and productive than those of known viral encephalitides. Syn., *type A e., epidemic e., von Economo's disease, sleeping sickness.*

lymphogranuloma venereum e. Encephalitis caused by the virus of venereal lymphogranuloma.

measles e. A postinfectious form, following measles.

mumps e. Encephalitis caused by the virus of mumps, during or after the swelling of the parotid gland, or without the usual clinical picture of mumps, and characterized by high lymphocyte count in the cerebrospinal fluid: to be distinguished from postinfectious *e.* due to mumps virus.

otogenic nonpurulent e. A type of encephalitis quite similar to brain abscess, characterized by abrupt onset, high fever, sensorium disturbance, headache, vomiting, convulsions, paralysis, and changes in the optic nerves. Prognosis is good.

postinfectious e. That occurring as a sequela of any one of a variety of infectious diseases, such as influenza, measles, and chickenpox. Also called *acute disseminated e., encephalomyelitis.*

postvaccinal e. An acute form following vaccination against smallpox or rabies.

Russian autumnal e. See Japanese *e.*

Russian Far East e. A viral disease of man occurring in the spring and early summer. Its vector is the wood tick, *Ixodes.* Its signs and symptoms are those of either meningoencephalitis or polioencephalitis depending on the location of the lesions in the central nervous system. Diagnosis rests on identification of the specific virus and serologic reactions. Also called *Russian spring-summer e., Russian forest spring e., Russian tick-borne e.*

St. Louis e. A viral meningoencephalomyelitis occurring during the summer and endemic and epidemic in the central and western United States, first reported in Illinois (1932) and in St. Louis (1933 and 1937). Symptoms are variable and diagnosis rests on identification of the virus and serologic reactions. Also called *American e.*

suppurative e. A type caused by pyogenic organisms and characterized by abscess formation. Also called *purulent* or *pyogenic e.*

syphilitic e. See *dementia* paralytica.

torula e. A rare form of meningoencephalitis caused by *Torula histolytica* and resembling tuberculous meningitis, cerebral tumor, or epidemic encephalitis. The primary lesion is usually in the lung and involves the brain secondarily.

toxic e. A commonly acute cerebral disturbance of unknown etiology, occurring chiefly in children; characterized clinically by delirium or coma and convulsions, cerebral palsies, and symptoms of meningeal irritation.

type-A e. Lethargic *e.*

type-B e. See Japanese *e.*

type-C e. See St. Louis *e.*

Venezuelan equine e. See equine *e.*

western equine e. See equine *e.*

en·ceph″a·li·to·gen′ic [*egkephalos; -itis;* G. *gignesthai,* from *gignesthai,* to be produced]. Producing, or capable of producing, encephalitis.

en·ceph′a·lo-, encephal- [*egkephalos*]. A combining form meaning *the encephalon* or *brain.*

en·ceph′a·lo·cele″ [*egkephalos;* G. *kēlē,* hernia]. Hernia of the brain through a congenital or traumatic opening in the cranium.

en·ceph″a·lo·dys·pla′si·a (en·sef″uh·lo·dis·play′-zhuh, ·zee·uh, ·shuh, ·see·uh) [*egkephalos;* G. *dys-,* bad; *plassein,* to form]. Maldevelopment of the tissues of the central nervous system.

en·ceph′a·lo·gram″ [*egkephalos;* G. *gramma,* letter]. A roentgenogram of the brain made in encephalography.

en·ceph″a·log′ra·phy [*egkephalos;* G. *graphein,* to write].Roentgenography of the brain following removal of cerebrospinal fluid, by lumbar or cisternal puncture, and its replacement by air or oxygen.

en·ceph′a·loid [*egkephalos;* G. *eidos,* form]. Resembling the brain or brain tissue.

en·ceph'a·loid. A cancer of soft, brainlike consistency.

en·ceph'a·lo·lith" [*egkephalos;* G. *lithos,* stone]. A calculus of the brain.

en·ceph"a·lol'o·gy [*egkephalos;* G. *logos,* word]. The study of the brain; the sum of the knowledge regarding the brain.

en·ceph"a·lo'ma [*egkephalos;* G. *-ōma,* tumor]. 1. A tumor of the brain. 2. Encephaloid carcinoma.

en·ceph"a·lo·ma·la'ci·a (en·sef"uh·lo·ma·lay'-shuh, ·see·uh) [*egkephalos;* G. *malakia,* softness]. A disease of the brain dependent upon a deficient blood supply; the symptoms vary according to the part affected, and consist of partial or complete loss of function. Depending upon the appearance, the softening is distinguished as red, yellow, or white.

en·ceph"a·lo·men"in·gi'tis. Meningoencephalitis.

en·ceph"a·lo·me·nin'go·cele [*egkephalos;* G. *mēnigx,* membrane; *kēlē,* hernia]. Hernia of the membranes and brain substance through an opening in the cranium.

en·ceph"a·lo·men"in·gop'a·thy [*egkephalos; mēnigx;* G. *pathos,* disease]. Disease of the brain and meninges.

en·ceph'a·lo·mere" [*egkephalos;* G. *meros,* part]. Any one of the succession of segments of the embryonic brain; a neuromere of the brain. —**encephalomer'ic,** *adj.*

en·ceph"a·lom'e·ter [*egkephalos;* G. *metron,* a measure]. An instrument for measuring the cranium, and locating certain regions of the brain.

en·ceph"a·lo·my"e·li'tis [*egkephalos;* G. *myelos,* marrow; *-itis,* inflammation]. Inflammation of the brain and spinal cord.

acute disseminated e. An acute disorder of the brain and spinal cord with variable symptoms, due to various causes, as vaccination or acute exanthema.

equine e. An epidemic virus disease of horses, the virus being transmitted by the mosquito; occasionally communicable to man.

ovine e. Louping-ill.

en·ceph"a·lo·my"e·lo·neu·rop'a·thy [*egkephalos; myelos;* G. *neuron,* nerve; *pathos,* disease]. Disease of the brain, spinal cord, and peripheral nervous system.

en·ceph"a·lo·my"e·lop'a·thy [*egkephalos; myelos; pathos*]. Any disease affecting both brain and spinal cord.

en·ceph"a·lo·my"e·lo·ra·dic"u·li'tis [*egkephalos; myelos;* L. *radicula,* small root; G. *-itis,* inflammation]. Any acute inflammatory disease of the entire nervous system, particularly the acral portion of the peripheral nerves, the spinal roots, the cord and the bulbar nuclei; symptoms include paresthesia and weakness in the distal parts of the extremities, absence of tendon reflexes, and facial diplegia. Essential in diagnosis is an albuminocytologic dissociation in the spinal fluid. See also Guillain-Barré *syndrome.*

en·ceph"a·lo·my"e·lo·ra·dic"u·lop'a·thy [*egkephalos; myelos; radicula;* G. *pathos,* disease]. Disease of the brain, spinal cord, and roots of the spinal nerves.

en·ceph"a·lo·my·el·o'sis. A generalized softening of brain and spinal cord in senile persons; encephalomalacia with myelomalacia.

en·ceph"a·lo·my"o·car·di'tis. An acute, nonfatal, febrile disease of man, often accompanied by pharyngitis, stiff neck, positive Kernig's sign, and hyperactive deep reflexes. Cardiac lesions have been observed only in experimental animals. It is caused by small viruses (Columbia SK, MM, EMC, and Mengo-encephalomyelitis agent); diagnosis rests on identification of the virus and serologic reactions.

en·ceph'a·lon [*egkephalos*]. The brain. —**encephal'ic,** *adj.*

en·ceph"a·lo·nar·co'sis [*egkephalos;* G. *narkōsis,* a benumbing]. Stupor from some brain lesion.

en·ceph"a·lop'a·thy [*egkephalos;* G. *pathos,* disease]. Any disease of the brain.

anoxic e. Degeneration of the brain resulting from oxygen deprivation, manifested as stupor, visual disturbances, convulsions, or cerebral excitement.

lead e. Neuronal degeneration and cerebral edema, apparently resulting from the presence of lead in the brain. It may occur so acutely that the usual findings of a lead line, hypochromic anemia, and basophilic stippling of erythrocytes do not appear.

rheumatic e. A chronic inflammatory reaction of the smaller arteries of the cerebral cortex following rheumatic disease: also called *Breutsch's disease.*

saturnine e. See lead *encephalitis.*

en·ceph"a·lo·punc'ture [*egkephalos;* L. *punctura,* puncture]. Puncture of the brain, especially of the cisterna.

en·ceph"a·lo·py·o'sis (en·sef"uh·lo·pye·o'sis) [*egkephalos;* G. *pyōsis,* suppuration]. Suppuration or abscess of the brain.

en·ceph"a·lo·ra·chid'i·an (·ra·kid'ee·un) [*egkephalos;* G. *rhachis,* spine]. Cerebrospinal.

en·ceph"a·lor·rha'gi·a [*egkephalos;* G. *rhēgnynai,* to burst]. Cerebral hemorrhage.

en·ceph"a·lo·scle·ro'sis [*egkephalos;* G. *sklērōsis,* hardening]. Hardening of the brain.

en·ceph'a·lo·scope [*egkephalos;* G. *skopein,* to examine]. An instrument for examining abscess cavities in the brain substance. —**encephalos'copy,** *n.*

en·ceph"a·lo·sep'sis [*egkephalos;* G. *sēpsis,* decay]. Sepsis of brain tissue.

en·ceph"a·lo'sis [*egkephalos;* G. *-ōsis,* condition]. Any degenerative disease of the brain.

criminogenic e. A syndrome in which sleep disturbances and social disorders or delinquency are associated.

en·ceph"a·lo·spi'nal [*egkephalos;* L. *spina,* spine]. Pertaining to the brain and to the spinal cord.

en·ceph'a·lo·tome [*egkephalos;* G. *tomos,* cutting]. 1. An instrument for dissecting the brain. 2. A surgical instrument for incising the brain. 3. A surgical instrument for destroying the brain of a fetus to facilitate delivery.

en·ceph"a·lot'o·my [*egkephalos;* G. *tomē,* a cutting]. 1. Surgical incision of the brain. 2. Operative destruction of the fetal brain to facilitate delivery 3. Dissection of the brain.

en·chon'dral. Contraction of *endochondral.*

en"chon·dro'ma (en"kon·dro'muh) [G. *en,* in; *chondros,* cartilage; *-ōma,* tumor]. A benign cartilaginous tumor, appearing usually as a single centrally located lesion within a bone, commonly one of the bones of the hand and sometimes a long limb bone or rib. Roentgenographically, the tumor produces a rarefaction in the affected bone; histologically, the cells are uniform, small, with single nuclei, and a matrix which is sometimes edematous or myxoid. Also called *central e., solitary e., endochondroma.* —**enchondrom'atous,** *adj.*

multiple enchondromata. See *dyschondroplasia.*

en·chon·dro·ma·to'sis. The infrequent occurrence of multiple enchondromas [enchondromata] in a single bone. Histologically, the lesions are more cellular than the enchondroma, and there is a marked tendency toward malignant change. Enchondromatosis associated with multiple cutaneous hemangiomas is known as *Mafucci's syndrome.* Also called *enchondrosis, multiple chondroma, multiple enchondromata.*

en·chon″dro·sar·co′ma (en·kon″dro·sahr·ko′-muh). See *chondrosarcoma.*

en″chon·dro′sis. See *enchondromatosis.*

en″chy·le′ma (en″kigh·lee′muh, en″ki·). Old term for hyaloplasm.

en·clit′ic [G. *egklitikos,* from *egklisis,* inclination]. Presenting obliquely; not synclitic; designating the inclination of the pelvic planes to those of the fetal head.

en″col·pi′tis. See *endocolpitis.*

en″co·pre′sis. Psychically caused incontinence of feces; soiling.

en·cra′ni·us [G. *en,* in; *kranion,* skull]. An episphenoid teratoid parasite which lies within the cranium of the autosite.

en·crus·ta′tion. See *incrustation.*

en″cy·e′sis (en″sigh·ee′sis) [G. *egkyēsis,* germination]. Pregnancy. *Obs.*

en″cys·ta′tion. See *encystment.*

en·cyst′ed [G. *en,* in; *kystis,* bladder]. Inclosed in a cyst or capsule.

en·cyst′ment [*en; kystis*]. The state of being enclosed in a cyst, or sac, or the process of forming a cyst. —**encysted,** *adj.*

en″da·del′phus [G. *endon,* within; *adelphos,* brother]. A monster which encloses a more or less complete individual within its own body.

En″da·moe′ba (en″duh·mee′buh) [*endon;* G. *amoibē,* change]. A genus of protozoan parasites which includes species parasitic in man: also spelled *Entamoeba.*

E. buccalis. Old term for *Endamoeba gingivalis.*

E. coli. A nonpathogenic species inhabiting the intestinal tract.

E. gingivalis. A species found in the mouth, about the gums, and in the tartar of the teeth.

E. histolytica. The etiologic agent of amebic, or tropical, dysentery. See Table of the Most Common Microorganisms Pathogenic to Man in the Appendix.

E. nana. See *Endolimax nana.*

en″da·me·bi′a·sis. See *amebiasis.*

en″dan·gi·i′tis, en″dan·ge·i′tis [*endon;* G. *aggeion,* vessel; *-itis,* inflammation]. Inflammation of the intima of a blood vessel; endarteritis or endophlebitis.

en″da·or·ti′tis [*endon;* G. *aortē,* aorta; *-itis*]. Inflammation of the intima of the aorta.

end′-ar″bor·i·za′tion. One of the small non-myelinated branches at the end of an axon: also called *end-branch.*

en″dar·ter·ec′to·my, en″dar·ter′i·ec·to·my [*endon;* G. *artēria,* artery; G. *tomē,* a cutting]. The surgical removal of an organized thrombus and the attached endothelium from a segment of an artery which has become thrombosed.

en″dar·te′ri·al [*endon;* G. *artēria,* artery]. Within an artery.

en″dar·te·ri′tis [*endon; artēria;* G. *-itis,* inflammation]. Inflammation of the inner coat of an artery: also spelled *endoarteritis.*

infectious e. An inflammatory lesion of an artery arising as the result of a septic embolus.

obliterating e. A form in which the production of new intimal connective tissue obliterates the lumen of a vessel.

verrucous e. Rheumatic arteritis sometimes affecting the coronary arteries. The lumen contains granular material, having the same structure and staining affinities as verrucae on valves in rheumatic endocarditis.

end·au′ral [*endon;* L. *auris,* ear]. Pertaining to the inner surface or part of the external auditory canal, as endaural approach for mastoidectomy.

end″ax·o·neu′ron [*endon;* G. *axōn,* axis; *neuron,* nerve]. A neuron whose nerve process does not leave the spinal cord; the endaxoneurons include the column cells and the internal cells. *Obs.*

end′brain″. See *telencephalon.*

end′-bulb″. 1. An end-foot, particularly one of the larger end-feet. 2. Krause's corpuscle.

en·dem′ic [G. *endēmos,* dwelling in a place, native]. Peculiar to a certain region; said of a disease which occurs more or less constantly in any locality.

end·ep″i·der′mis [G. *endon,* within; G. *epidermis,* outer skin]. The inner layer of the epidermis. *Obs.*

end″er·gon′ic [*endon;* G. *ergon,* work]. Of or pertaining to a chemical reaction in which the final products possess more free energy than the starting materials: usually associated with anabolism. This energy may be drawn from concomitant catabolism or from an external source.

en·der′mic [G. *en,* in; *derma,* skin]. Acting through the skin by absorption, as medication applied to the skin.

en″der·mo′sis [*en; derma;* G. *-ōsis,* condition]. 1. Administration of medicines through the skin, by rubbing. 2. Any herpetic affection of a mucosa.

Enders, John Franklin (1897–). American bacteriologist, who, with F. C. Robbins and T. H. Weller, shared the Nobel prize (1954) in physiology and medicine for their discovery of the ability of the poliomyelitis virus to grow in cultures of different tissues. He is also widely known for his work on mumps and the mumps virus, including a skin test for that disease.

end-feet. Small terminal enlargements of nerve fibers which are in contact with the dendrites or cell bodies of other nerve cells. The synaptic ending of a nerve fiber. Also called *boutons terminaux, end-bulbs.*

Endo, Shigeru [*Japanese bacteriologist and physician,* 1869–1937]. Produced a lactose agar medium, with sodium hydroxide, phenolphthalein, fuchsin, and sodium sulfite, formerly in general use in bacteriology.

en′do-, end- [G. *endon,* within]. A combining form signifying *within.*

en″do·ab·dom′i·nal [*endon;* L. *abdomen,* abdomen]. Within the abdomen; intraabdominal.

en″do·an″eu·rys·mor′rha·phy (en″do·an″yoor-iz·mor′uh·fee) [*endon;* G. *aneurysma,* aneurysm; *rhaphē,* suture]. The operation for aneurysm consisting of opening the sac and folding and suturing the walls of the aneurysm, thus leaving a lumen of approximately normal size.

en″do·an″gi·i′tis. Endangiitis.

en″do·a″or·ti′tis (en″do·ay″or·tye′tis). See *endaortitis.*

en″do·ar″te·ri′tis. See *endarteritis.*

en″do·bi·ot′ic (en″do·buy·ot′ick) [*endon;* G. *bios,* life]. Living in the tissues of the host.

en″do·bron′chi·al (en″do·brong′kee·ul, ·bron′-kee·ul) [*endon;* G. *brogchia,* bronchial tubes]. Within a bronchus.

en″do·car·di′tis [*endon;* G. *kardia,* heart]. Inflammation of the endocardium or lining membrane of the heart and its valves. The condition may be acute, subacute, or chronic. **Acute endocarditis** is either warty or ulcerative, the most frequent causes being rheumatism and the infectious diseases. The disease usually affects the valves of the left side of the heart and gives rise to a murmur, fever, dyspnea, and rapid pulse. **Chronic** or **sclerotic endocarditis** is a terminal process following the acute or recurrent rheumatic forms, or is a primary endocarditis due to gout, rheumatism, alcoholism, syphilis, and to other obscure causes, and usually is associated with general arteriosclerosis. Both the acute and the chronic forms give rise to insufficiency or obstruction of the valvular orifice, or to both combined. —**endocardit'ic,** *adj.*

acute bacterial e. A form due to invasion of bacteria such as streptococci, pneumococci, *Micrococcus pyogenes*, meningococci, gonococci, or the *Hemophilus influenzae*. Affects the valves more often than the mural endocardium. Usually vegetative in morphology but may be ulcerative. The symptoms resemble those of pyemia.

atypical verrucous e. A clinical and pathological entity of unknown cause, occurring frequently in systemic lupus erythematosus, generally involving the ventricular aspect of the valve cusps with flat extensions of finely granular verrucae upon the mural endocardium and with negative blood culture. Syn., *Libman-Sacks disease* or *syndrome.*

e. lenta. Subacute bacterial endocarditis.

infectious e. That due to infectious microorganisms, usually bacteria, but rarely other vegetable parasites.

pneumococcal e. See acute bacterial *e.*

rheumatic e. That which occurs in the course of, and following, rheumatic fever.

subacute bacterial e. A form which runs a somewhat prolonged course, usually due to alpha streptococcus (*S. viridans*). Syn., *e. lenta.*

tuberculous e. A rare type characterized by small vegetations, without typical tubercles, but in proved cases showing acid-fast baccilli.

verrucous e. A form which anatomically is characterized by the presence on the endocardium, usually valvular, of minute, pale-yellow, soft, sessile, loosely attached nodules made up principally of fibrin. Most common in rheumatic cardiac disease but may occur in septicemias.

en"do·car'di·um [*endon; kardia*]. The membrane lining the interior of the heart, consisting of endothelium and the subjacent connective tissue. See Plate 5. —**endocardial,** *adj.*

en"do·car'do·fi·bro'sis [*endon; kardia;* L. *fibra,* fiber; G. *-ōsis,* increase]. Endocardial fibrosis.

en'do·carp. The inner coat of a pericarp.

en"do·ce'li·ac [*endon;* G. *koilia,* cavity]. Within one of the body cavities.

en"do·cer'vi·cal [*endon;* L. *cervix,* neck]. Relating to the inside of the uterine cervix.

en"do·cer"vi·ci'tis [*endon; cervix;* G. *-itis,* inflammation]. Inflammation of the lining membrane of the cervix uteri.

en"do·cer'vix [*endon; cervix*]. The endometrium or mucous membrane of the cervix uteri.

en"do·chol'e·doch·al. Within the common bile duct.

en"do·chon'dral (en"do·kon'drul) [*endon;* G. *chondros,* cartilage]. Situated within a cartilage.

en"do·col·pi'tis [*endon;* G. *kolpos,* vagina; *-itis,* inflammation]. Mucous vaginitis.

en"do·cra·ni'tis [*endon;* G. *kranion,* skull; *-itis*]. Inflammation of the endocranium; pachymeningitis externa. *Obs.*

en"do·cra'ni·um [*endon; kranion*]. The inner lining of the skull; the dura mater. —**endocranial,** *adj.*

en'do·crine (en'do·kryne, ·krin) [*endon;* G. *krinein,* to separate]. Secreting internally. —**endocrin'ic,** *adj.*

en'do·crine. Any of the ductless glands, such as the adrenals, the thyroid, the pituitary, whose secretions pass directly into the blood stream. See under *gland.*

en"do·cri·nol'o·gy (en"do·kri·nol'o·jee, ·cry·nol'o·jee) [*endon; krinein;* G. *logos,* word]. The study of the internal secretions and the endocrine glands.

en"do·cri·nop'a·thy (·kri·nop'uth·ee, ·cry·nop'uth·ee) [*endon; krinein;* G. *pathos,* disease]. A disorder resulting from abnormality in one or more of the endocrine glands or their secretions.

en"do·crin"o·ther'a·py (en"do·krin"o·therr'uh·pee, [*endon; krinein;* G. *therapeia,* therapy]. Treatment of disease by the use of hormones secreted by the endocrine glands.

en·doc'ri·nous [*endon; krinein*]. Obsolete term for endocrine.

en"do·cy'ma [*endon;* G. *kyma,* fetus]. A type of cryptodidymus in which the parasitic twin is visceral in location.

en'do·cyst [*endon;* G. *kystis,* bladder]. The inner wall of a cyst.

en"do·cys·ti'tis. See *cystitis.*

en'do·derm. Entoderm.

en"do·der"ma·to·zo"o·no'sis. A skin disease in which the parasite burrows deeply into, and remains embedded within, the skin, as certain ascari and some oestridae larvae.

En"do·der·moph'y·ton [*endon;* G. *derma,* skin; *phyton,* plant]. Formerly a genus of the dermatophytes, now included in the genus *Trichophyton.*

en"do·der"mo·phy·to'sis (en"do·dur"mo·figh·to'sis]. See *tinea* imbricata.

en"do·don'tics. The branch of dentistry concerned with the treatment of pulpless teeth: also called *endodontia.*

en"do·don'tist. A dentist who specializes in endodontics.

en"do·en"ter·i'tis. See *enteritis.*

en"do·en'zyme [*endon;* G. *en,* in; *zymē,* leaven]. An intracellular enzyme, one which is not excreted but is retained in the originating cell.

en"do·er'gic. Endothermic.

en·dog'a·my [*endon;* G. *gamos,* marriage]. Conjugation between cells having the same chromatin ancestry.

en·dog'e·nous (en·dodj'i·nus) [*endon;* G. *genesthai,* from *gignesthai,* to be produced]. 1. Produced within; due to internal causes; applied to the formation of cells or of spores within the parent cell. 2. Relating to the metabolism of the nitrogenous elements of tissues. 3. *In psychology,* arising from within the body and directly affecting the nervous system, as a hereditary or constitutional disorder.

en·dog'e·ny (en·dodj'i·nee) [*endon; genesthai*]. *In biology,* growth from within; endogenous formation.

en"do·gna'thi·on (en"do·nayth'ee·on, ·nath'ee·on, en"dohg·) [*endon;* G. *gnathos,* jaw]. Albrecht's hypothetical mesial portion of the premaxilla, his lateral portion being the mesognathion.

en"do·go'ni·um [*endon;* G. *gonos,* offspring]. A gonidium formed inside a receptacle or parent cell. Also called *endogonidium.*

en"do·la·ryn'ge·al (en"do·la·rin'jul, ·jee·ul, ·lar"in·jee'ul) [*endon;* G. *larygx,* larynx]. Within the larynx.

En"do·li'max [*endon;* G. *leimax,* meadow]. A genus of protozoans of the family Amoebidae, parasitic in man, but nonpathogenic.

E. nana. A species of nonpathogenic amebas containing a characteristic single small nucleus in which the chromatin is clustered in a single, coarse, irregularly shaped karyosome; widely distributed in both temperate and tropical countries. Man is the common host, though these amebas are also found in the intestine of various species of monkeys. Formerly called *Entamoeba nana* and *Endolimax intestinalis.*

en'do·lymph [*endon;* L. *lympha,* water]. The fluid

of the membranous labyrinth of the ear. —**endolymphat′ic, endolym′phic,** *adj.*

en″do·lym·phan′gi·al, en″do·lym·phan′ge·al [*endon; lympha;* G. *aggeion,* vessel]. Situated or belonging within a lymph vessel.

en″do·ly′sin, en·dol′y·sin [*endon;* G. *lysis,* a loosing]. Obsolete term for *leucin.*

en″do·men′inx [*endon;* G. *mēnigx,* membrane]. The internal part of the meninx primitiva that differentiates into the pia mater and arachnoid membrane.

en″do·mes′o·derm [*endon;* G. *mesos,* middle; *derma,* skin]. Mesoderm derived from the primary entoderm of a bilaminar blastodisk or gastrula.

en″do·me·trec′to·my [*endon;* G. *mētra,* womb; *ektomē,* excision]. The extirpation of the entire mucosa of the uterus through the abdomen and incised uterus. *Obs.*

en″do·me″tri·o′ma. Endometriosis in which there is a discrete tumor mass.

en″do·me″tri·o′sis [*endon; mētra;* G. *-ōsis,* condition]. The presence of endometrial tissue in abnormal locations, including the uterine wall, ovaries, or extragenital sites: also called *Sampson's cyst.*

external e. Abnormal endometrial tissue outside or beneath the serosal surface of the uterus. The uterine serosa and myometrium may be involved from without.

internal e. That involving primarily the myometrium with diffuse involvement of the uterine wall; adenomyosis.

interstitial e. See stromal *e.*

stromal, stromatous e. A rare form, in which the ectopic tissue resembles the stroma of late proliferative endometrium: also called *interstitial e., stromal myosis, parathelioma, stromatosis, endolymphatic stromomyosis* or *fibromyosis.*

en″do·me·tri′tis [*endon; mētra;* G. *-itis,* inflammation]. Inflammation of the endometrium. Formerly a common clinical diagnosis; now, for the most part, a laboratory term.

cervical e. See *endocervicitis.*

decidual e. See *deciduitis.*

e. exfoliativa. See membranous *dysmenorrhea.*

gangrenous e. Rare gangrenous inflammation of the endometrium.

infectious granuloma e. Granulomatous inflammation of the endometrium which may be due to any of a particular group of disease processes which characteristically produce this type of response in tissues, such as tuberculosis, syphilis, and actinomycosis.

streptococcal e. Postpartum infection in which streptococci invade the uterus and produce lesions which have a peculiar foul odor. If secondary pulmonary abscesses occur, the patient's breath also has this same foul odor.

syncytial e. Excessive proliferation of the syncytial trophoblastic cells near the site of the placenta with invasion of the endometrium, decidua, and adjacent myometrium by these cells: called *syncytioma,* when localized into a tumorlike mass. Syn., *syncytial deciduitis.*

tuberculous e. That caused by the tubercle bacillus.

en″do·me′tri·um [*endon; mētra*]. The mucous membrane lining the uterus. —**endometrial,** *adj.*

isthmic e. That portion of the endometrium lying between the endocervix and fundus of the uterus, whose tubules are neither racemose nor secretory, and which does not show the cyclic changes characteristic of the rest of the endometrium.

en·dom′e·try [*endon;* G. *metron,* a measure]. The measurement of the interior of an organ or cavity.

en″do·mi·to′sis. The duplication of chromosomes without any accompanying spindle formation or cytokinesis.

en′do·morph. *In the somatotype,* an individual exhibiting relative predominance of endomorphy.

en′do·mor″phy [*endon;* G. *morphē,* form]. Component I of the somatotype, representing relative predominance of soft and round body features. In normal nutritional status, the abdominal viscera, whose functional elements are derived from entoderm, are prominent. Endomorphs tend to be fat. The counterpart on the behavioral level is viscerotonia. —**endomor′phic,** *adj.*

En″do·my′ces (en″do·migh′seez) [*endon;* G. *mykēs,* fungus]. An invalid name for a genus of fungi.

E. albicans. Synonym for *Candida albicans.*

E. capsulatus. Synonym for *Blastomyces dermatitidis.*

en″do·my″o·car·di′tis [*endon;* G. *mys,* muscle; *kardia,* heart; *-itis,* inflammation]. Inflammation of both endocardium and myocardium.

en″do·mys′i·um (en″do·miss′ee·um, ·miz′ee·um) [*endon; mys*]. The connective tissue between the fibers of a muscle bundle, or fasciculus. —**endomysial,** *adj.*

en″do·na′sal [*endon;* L. *nasus,* nose]. Within the nasal cavity, as endonasal approach in sinus drainage.

en″do·neu′ral [*endon;* G. *neuron,* nerve]. Relating to or situated in the interior of a nerve.

en″do·neu′ri·um [*endon; neuron*]. The delicate connective tissue holding together the fibers of a nerve bundle, or fasciculus. —**endoneurial,** *adj.*

en″do·nu·cle′o·lus [*endon;* L., dim. of *nucleus,* kernel]. A nonstaining area within a nucleus.

en″do·par′a·site [*endon;* G. *parasitos,* parasite]. A parasite living within its host. —**endoparasit′ic,** *adj.*

en″do·pep′ti·dase. Any of a group of enzymes, including pepsin and trypsin, capable of attacking both centrally located and terminal peptide bonds (Bergmann); a proteinase.

en″do·per″i·car·di′tis [*endon;* G. *perikardios,* around the heart; *-itis,* inflammation]. Inflammation of both endocardium and pericardium.

en″do·per″i·my″o·car·di′tis [*endon;* G. *peri,* around; *mys,* muscle; *kardia,* heart; *-itis*]. Inflammation of endocardium, pericardium, and myocardium.

en″do·phle·bi′tis [*endon;* G. *phlebs,* blood vessel; *-itis*]. Inflammation of the intima of a vein.

en·doph″thal·mi′tis [*endon;* G. *ophthalmos,* eye; *-itis*]. Inflammation of the internal tissues of the eyeball.

e. phacoanaphylactica. The anaphylactic sensitization of the human to his own lens protein by extracapsular cataract extraction. A second attempt at cataract extraction results in a sterile endophthalmitis.

suppurative e. Septic inflammation of the uveal tract with pus formation.

en′do·plasm [*endon;* G. *plasma,* anything formed]. The inner cytoplasm of a protozoon or of certain cells.

end or′gan. The expanded termination of a nerve fiber in muscle, skin, mucous membrane, or other structure.

en″do·sal·pin·gi·o′ma. See serous *cystadenoma.*

en″do·sal·pin·gi·o′sis. See isthmic nodular *salpingitis.*

en′do·scope [*endon;* G. *skopein,* to examine]. An instrument, equipped with an electric light or a system of lenses, used for the visual examination of the interior of a body cavity or viscus through its natural outlet. —**endoscop′ic,** *adj.;* **endos′copy,** *n.*

en″do·skel′e·ton [*endon;* G. *skeletos,* dried up]. The internal supporting structure of an animal; the vertebrate skeleton.

en″dos·mom′e·ter (en″dos·mom′i·tur, en″doz·) [*endon;* G. *ōsmos,* a pushing; *metron,* a measure]. An instrument for measuring endosmosis.

en″dos·mo′sis (en″dos·mo′sis, en″doz·), **en′dos·mose** (en′dos·moce, en′doz·) [*endon; ōsmos;* G. *-ōsis,* condition]. The passage of a liquid inward through a porous septum. —**endosmo′sic, endosmot′ic,** *adj.*

en′do·sperm [*endon;* G. *sperma,* seed]. *In biology,* the protein of a seed.

en′do·spore [*endon;* G. *sporos,* seed]. 1. A spore formed within the parent cell. 2. The inner coat of a spore.

en·dos″te·i′tis. See *endostitis.*

en·dos″te·o′ma, en″dos·to′ma [*endon;* G. *osteon,* bone; *-ōma,* tumor]. A tumor within a bone.

en·dos′te·um [*endon; osteon*]. The membranous layer of connective tissue lining the medullary cavity of a bone. —**endosteal,** *adj.*

en″dos·ti′tis [*endon; osteon;* G. *-itis,* inflammation]. Inflammation of the endosteum.

en″do·sto′mus. See *epignathus.*

en″dos·to′sis [*endon; osteon;* G. *-ōsis,* condition]. Ossification of a cartilage.

en″do·sub·til′y·sin. An antibiotic substance derived from *Bacillus subtilis;* it is active against *Staphylococcus aureus, Escherichia coli, Eberthella typhosa,* and *Mycobacterium tuberculosis.*

en″do·ten·din′e·um [*endon;* L. *tendere,* to stretch]. The delicate connective tissue between the fibers of a tendon bundle or fasciculus.

en″do·the″li·o·an″gi·i′tis [*endon;* G. *thēlē,* nipple; *aggeion,* vessel; *-itis,* inflammation]. A systemic infection similar to, and possibly the same as, lupus erythematosus, and marked by fever, arthritis, and angiitis.

en″do·the″li·o·cho′ri·al (·kor′ee·ul) [*endon; thēlē;* G. *chorion,* skin]. Pertaining to maternal endothelium and chorionic ectoderm, as endotheliochorial placenta.

en″do·the′li·o·cyte″. Old term for macrophage.

en″do·the′li·oid [*endon; thēlē;* G. *eidos,* form]. Resembling endothelium.

en″do·the″li·o·ly′sin (en″do·theel″ee·o·lye′sin, ·theel″ee·ol′i·sin) [*endon; thēlē;* G. *lysis,* a loosing]. A cytotoxin endowed with the capacity of dissolving endothelial cells. Syn., *hemorrhagin.*

en″do·the″li·o′ma [*endon; thēlē;* G. *-ōma,* tumor]. A group of tumors made up of large cells morphologically like endothelium and supposedly derived from cells lining blood vessels, lymphatics, and various serous spaces. The different forms vary as to malignant character, and may affect solid organs, such as lymph nodes, skin, etc., because of growth from vascular or tissue spaces.

diffuse e. of bone. See Ewing's *sarcoma.*

dural e. See *meningioma.*

e. capitis. See *cylindroma.*

e. of bone. See Ewing's *sarcoma.*

e. of lymph node. See reticulum-cell *sarcoma.*

e. of meninges. See *meningioma.*

perithelial e. See *hemangiopericytoma.*

en″do·the″li·o·ma·to′sis [*endon; thēlē; -ōma;* G. *-ōsis,* condition]. The presence of multiple endotheliomas.

en″do·the″li·o′sis [*endon; thēlē; -ōsis*]. Overgrowth of endothelium from unknown cause; better called nonthrombopenic purpura.

e. of meninges. See *meningioma.*

en″do·the″li·o·tox′in. See *endotheliolysin.*

en″do·the′li·um [*endon; thēlē*]. 1. The simple squamous epithelium lining the heart, blood vessels, and lymph vessels; vascular endothelium. 2. The mesodermally derived, simple, squamous epithelium lining any closed cavity in the body. *Obs.* —**endothelial,** *adj.*

en″do·ther′mic [*endon;* G. *thermē,* heat]. 1. *In chemistry,* relating to the absorption of heat. 2. Pertaining to endothermy. Syn., *endoergic.*

en′do·ther″my, en″do·ther′my. Diathermy.

en′do·thrix [*endon;* G. *thrix,* hair]. A type division of the genus *Trichophyton.*

en″do·tox″i·co′sis [*endon;* G. *toxikon,* poison; *-ōsis,* condition]. Poisoning by an endotoxin.

en″do·tox′in [*endon; toxikon*]. A toxin produced within a microorganism which does not diffuse out of the bacterial cell until the cell is disintegrated.

end-plate. 1. A complex hypolemmal terminal arborization of a motor nerve fiber in a bed of specialized sarcoplasm; it transmits nerve impulses to muscle. 2. The achromatic masses at the poles of the mitotic spindle of Protozoa.

end pleas′ure. *In psychoanalysis,* the pleasure accompanying sexual discharge or detumescence, brought about by a relief of the tension built up during the forepleasure.

end prod′uct. The final product formed by a series of reactions, as the end products of sugar metabolism.

-ene [cf. L. adj. suff. *-enus,* G. *-ēnos*]. *In chemistry,* a suffix used in the naming of certain hydrocarbons; specifically, indicates *the presence of one double bond.*

en′e·ma [G., injection]. A rectal injection for therapeutic, diagnostic, or nutritive purposes.

high e. An injection into the colon.

retention e. Liquid injected into the rectum, the expulsion of which is delayed voluntarily in order to liquefy the rectal contents or provide medication.

en″er·get′ics (en″ur·jet′icks) [G. *energētikos,* active]. The branch of physics dealing with energy and the laws and conditions governing its manifestations.

en″er·gom′e·ter [G. *energos,* at work; *metron,* a measure]. 1. Any apparatus for measuring energy. 2. One designed to measure the energy of pulse beats. —**energometry,** *n.*

en′er·gy [G. *energeia,* from *en,* in; *ergon,* work]. The capacity for doing work. All forms of energy are mutually convertible one into the other. The quantity of work done in the process of transfer is a measure of energy. Therefore, work units are commonly used as energy units.

free e. That portion of the total potential energy of a natural system available for the performance of work.

kinetic e. That part of the total energy of a body in motion which is due to its motion.

nuclear e. Energy released in reactions involving the nucleus of an atom, especially in quantities sufficient to be of interest in engineering or in astrophysics.

potential e. The power possessed by a body at rest, by virtue of its position, as the potential energy of a suspended weight. Also called *latent e.*

radiant e. Energy transmitted through electromagnetic radiation.

solar e. Energy derived directly from the sun.

en″er·va′tion [L. *enervatio,* from *enervare,* to take out the sinews, to weaken]. Weakness, lassitude, neurasthenia; reduction of strength.

en·gage′ment [F., from *en,* in; *gage,* pledge]. *In obstetrics,* the entrance of the presenting part of the fetus into the superior pelvic strait.

en·gas′tri·us [G. *en,* in; *gastēr,* belly]. A form of duplicity in which a parasitic fetus (or fetal parts) is included within the peritoneal cavity of its autosite.

Engelmann, Theodor Wilhelm [*German physiologist,* 1843–1909]. Described the narrow zone of transparent substance on each side of the intermediate or Z disk of the cross striae of the myofibril of a muscle fiber as a lateral disk (1893), called *Engelmann's disk. Obs.*

en·globe′ment [F. *englober,* to take in]. The absorption or engulfing of a substance by such a cell as a protozoon, leukocyte, or macrophage; phagocytosis. —**englob′ing,** *n.*

Engman, Martin Feeney [*American dermatologist,* 1869–]. Described infectious eczematoid dermatitis, a low-grade infection of the skin characterized by vesicles, pustules, and crusts with a scale about the edge. Often associated with drainage from some other infection such as a suppurating ear (1902). Called *Engman's disease.*

en·gorge′ment [F. *engorger,* to cram in]. Hyperemia; an excessive amount of blood in a part, usually with local edema. —**engorged′,** *adj.*

en′gram [G. *en,* in; *gramma,* letter]. The hypothetic impression or trace left upon neurons by psychic experiences; a latent memory picture.

engran. Trade-mark for an encapsulated multiple vitamin preparation.

en grappes (ahn grahp′. *See* NOTES § 35) [F.]. Grapelike; used of fungus spores in grapelike clusters.

en·hem′a·to·spore (en·hem′uh·to·spor, en·hee′-muh·to·), **en·he′mo·spore** (en·hee′mo·spor, en-hem′o·) [G. *en,* in; *haima,* blood; *sporos,* seed]. A spore of the malarial parasite produced within the human body; merozoite.

en·large′ment. Increase in size; broadening; expansion.

cervical e. Broadening of the spinal cord from the level of the third cervical to the second thoracic vertebra, maximal at the fifth cervical vertebra: also called *cervical intumescence.*

lumbar e. Broadening of the spinal cord starting at the level of the ninth and maximal at the level of the twelfth thoracic vertebra. Syn., *lumbar intumescence.*

en′ni·a·tine. A multiple antibiotic from *Fusarium orthoceras* var. *enniatinum;* it is active against several species of mycobacteria.

e′nol. *In chemistry,* of or designating the form of a compound when it contains the =C:C(OH)— group, as distinguished from that in which it contains the tautomeric =CH.CO— group, designated *keto.* The enol form is produced from the keto form by migration of a hydrogen atom from the carbon atom adjoining the carbonyl group of the keto form.

e′no·lase. The enzyme that converts 2-phosphoglyceric acid to phosphopyruvic acid.

e″nol·py·ru′vic ac′id. CH_2:COH.COOH; the enol form of pyruvic acid, presumably formed in certain metabolic reactions involving pyruvic acid.

en″oph·thal′mos [*en;* G. *ophthalmos,* eye]. Recession of the eyeball into the orbit.

en″o·si·ma′ni·a (en″o·si·may′nee·uh) [G. *enosis,* a shaking; *mania,* madness]. A mental disorder marked by extreme terror.

en″os·to′sis [G. *en,* in; *osteon,* bone; *-ōsis,* condition]. A bony ingrowth within the medullary canal of a bone.

en′si·form [L. *ensis,* sword; *forma,* shape]. Shaped like a sword, as the ensiform cartilage.

Enslin [*German army physician,* contemporary]. Remembered eponymically for his description of a syndrome including a tower skull and atrophy of the optic nerve (1904).

en·som′pha·lus [L. *ensis,* sword; G. *omphalos,* navel]. Conjoined twins (diplopagi) united by a band in the epigastric and lower sternal regions; Siamese twins. See *xiphopagus.* —**ensomphal′-ic,** *adj.*

en′stro·phe (en′stro·fee) [G. *enstrephein,* to turn in]. Inversion, as of the margin of an eyelid.

en″ta·cous′tic (en″tuh·kōōss′tick) [G. *entos,* within; *akoustikos,* of hearing]. Of or pertaining to subjective auditory sensations having their origin within the ear or in its vicinity.

en′tad [*entos;* L. *ad,* toward]. Inward.

en′tal [*entos*]. Internal.

en″ta·me·bi′a·sis. See *amebiasis.*

En″ta·moe′ba (en″tuh·mee′buh). Synonym for *Endamoeba.*

en·ta′si·a (en·tay′zhuh, ·zee·uh, ·shuh, ·see·uh), **en′ta·sis** [G. *entasis,* a straining]. A generic term for spasmodic muscular action; tonic spasm. —**entat′ic,** *adj.*

en·tel′e·chy (en·tel′i·kee) [G. *entelecheia,* complete reality, from *entelēs,* complete, *echein,* to have]. 1. The complete realization or expression of some principle. 2. A vital influence which guides living organisms in the right direction.

en′ter·al [G. *enteron,* intestine]. Intestinal.

en″ter·al′gi·a [*enteron;* G. *algos,* pain]. Pain in the intestine.

en″ter·ec′ta·sis [*enteron;* G. *ektasis,* extension]. Dilatation of some part of the small intestine.

en″ter·ec′to·my [*enteron;* G. *ektomē,* excision]. Excision of a part of the intestine.

en″ter·e·pip′lo·cele [*enteron;* G. *epiploon,* fold of the peritoneum; *kēlē,* hernia]. Hernia in which both the intestine and the omentum are involved.

en·ter′ic [*enteron*]. Pertaining to the intestine.

en·ter′i·coid [*enteron;* G. *eidos,* form]. Resembling typhoid fever.

en″ter·i′tis [*enteron;* G. *-itis,* inflammation]. Any intestinal tract inflammation, acute or chronic.

acute fibrinous e. An acute inflammatory process associated with desquamation and fibrin deposition on the mucosa; not a clinical entity but a pathologic classification: also called *membranous e.*

acute follicular e. An acute inflammation characterized by hyperplasia of the lymph nodules in the intestine; occurs commonly in children suffering from summer complaint or diarrhea.

chronic catarrhal e. A form due to passive hyperemia in which the mucosa is thickened and covered by mucus, and, in cases of long standing, is associated with atrophy.

membranous e. See acute fibrinous *e.*

regional e. See *ileitis.*

tuberculous e. A common complication of far-advanced or moderate cases of tuberculosis; inflammation of the alimentary canal due to the presence of tubercle bacilli which are swallowed with the sputum. Diarrhea, abdominal pain, anorexia, and loss of weight are the common symptoms.

en′ter·o-, enter- [*enteron*]. A combining form denoting *the intestine.*

en″ter·o·a·nas″to·mo′sis [*enteron;* G. *anastomōsis,* opening]. Intestinal anastomosis.

en·ter″o·an′thel·one. Anthelone derived from the mucosa of the small intestine.

En″ter·o·bac·te″ri·a′ce·ae (en″tur·o·back·teer″-ee·ay′see·ee) [*enteron;* G. *baktērion,* small staff]. A family of bacteria including many animal and some plant parasites, causing blight and soft rot; the five tribes are the Eschericheae, Erwineae, Serrateae, Proteae, and Salmonelleae.

en″ter·o·bi′a·sis [*enteron;* G. *bios,* life; NL. *-iasis,* condition]. Infestation of the small intestine, colon, and rectum with the *Enterobius vermicularis;* characterized by mild catarrhal inflammation of the intestinal mucosa, occasionally by secondary bacterial invasion, and, if the infection is very severe, obstruction of the intestine.

En″ter·o′bi·us [*enteron; bios*]. A genus of nematode parasites of man.

E. vermicularis. The pinworm or seatworm; the etiologic agent of enterobiasis in man.

en′ter·o·cele″ [*enteron;* G. *kēlē,* hernia]. A hernia containing a loop of intestine.

en″ter·o·cen·te′sis [*enteron;* G. *kentēsis,* a pricking]. Surgical puncture of the intestine.

en″ter·o·chro′maf·fin. See under *cell.*

en″ter·o′cin [*enteron;* G. *kinein,* to set in motion]. A proposed term for the active principle stimulating intestinal motility; the existence of such a hormone or principle is disputed.

en″ter·oc′ly·sis [*enteron;* G. *klysis,* a drenching]. Injection of a fluid preparation into the rectum for nutrient, medicinal, or cleansing purposes.

en″ter·o·coc′cus [*enteron;* G. *kokkos,* seed]. A group of *Streptococci,* normally found in the intestinal tract of man and other species, pathogenic when found elsewhere, as in urinary- and respiratory-tract diseases and in subacute bacterial endocarditis. All members elaborate group D C-substance.

en′ter·o·coele″ (en′tur·o·seel″) [*enteron;* G. *koilos,* hollow]. A coelom formed by evagination of the wall of the primitive gut. —**enterocoe′lic,** *adj.*

en″ter·o·co·lec′to·my [*enteron;* G. *kolon,* colon; *ektomē,* excision]. Resection of parts of both small intestine and colon.

en″ter·o·co·li′tis [*enteron; kolon;* G. *-itis,* inflammation]. Inflammation of small intestine and colon.

en″ter·o·co·los′to·my [*enteron; kolon;* G. *stoma,* mouth]. Operation for the formation of a communication between the small intestine and colon; enterocolic anastomosis.

en″ter·o·crin′in (en″tur·o·krin′in, en″tur·ock′-rin·in) [*enteron;* G. *krinein,* to separate]. A hormone produced by the intestinal mucosa which stimulates the glands of the small intestine. See Table of Hormones in the Appendix.

en′ter·o·cyst″ [*enteron;* G. *kystis,* bladder]. An intestinal cyst.

en″ter·o·cys′to·cele [*enteron; kystis;* G. *kēlē,* hernia]. Hernia involving urinary bladder and intestine.

en″ter·o·cys·to′ma. See gastroenteric *cyst.*

en″ter·o·cys·to·plas′ty. A surgical procedure wherein a loop of small bowel is anastomosed to the urinary bladder to increase its capacity.

en″ter·o·cys·tos′che·o·cele (en″tur·o·sis·tos′kee-o·seel) [*enteron; kystis;* G. *oscheon,* scrotum; *kēlē,* hernia]. A scrotal hernia containing both intestine and urinary bladder. *Obs.*

en″ter·o·en·ter′ic [*enteron; enteron*]. Involving two separate portions of the intestine.

en″ter·o·en″ter·os′to·my [*enteron; enteron;* G. *stoma,* mouth]. The surgical formation of a passage between two parts of the intestine.

en″ter·o·gas·tri′tis. Gastroenteritis.

en″ter·o·gas′tro·cele [*enteron;* G. *gastēr,* belly; *kēlē,* hernia]. A hernia containing the stomach and intestine or portions of them; ventral hernia.

en″ter·o·gas′trone [*enteron; gastēr*]. A hormone from the upper intestinal mucosa. It inhibits gastric motility and secretion. See Table of Hormones in the Appendix.

en″ter·og′e·nous (en″tur·odj′i·nus) [*enteron;* G. *genesthai,* from *gignesthai,* to be produced]. Originating in the intestine.

en′ter·o·graph″ [*enteron;* G. *graphein,* to write]. An apparatus which records graphically the movements of the intestine.

en″ter·o·ki′nase (en″tur·o·kigh′nace, ·naze, ·kin′-ace, ·aze). An enzyme present in the succus entericus which converts inactive trypsinogen into active trypsin.

en′ter·o·lith [*enteron;* G. *lithos,* stone]. A concretion formed in the intestine.

en″ter·o·li·thi′a·sis [*enteron; lithos;* NL. *-iasis,* condition]. The presence of calculi in the intestine.

en″ter·ol′o·gist. Old term for gastroenterologist.

en″ter·ol′o·gy. Old term for gastroenterology.

en″ter·ol′y·sis [*enteron;* G. *lysis,* a loosing]. Removal of adhesions binding the intestine.

en″ter·o·meg′a·ly. See *megacolon.*

en″ter·o·me′ro·cele [*enteron;* G. *mēros,* thigh; *kēlē,* hernia]. Femoral hernia involving intestine. *Obs.*

En″ter·o·mo′nas (en″tur·o·mo′nas, ·om′o·nas) [*enteron;* G. *monas,* unit]. A genus of intestinal flagellates of the family Cercomonadidae; contains only one species parasitic in man, **E. hominis.**

en″ter·o·my·co′sis (·migh·ko′sis) [*enteron;* G. *mykēs,* fungus; *-ōsis,* condition]. Intestinal mycosis.

en″ter·o·my′ia·sis (en″tur·o·migh′yuh·sis, ·migh-eye′uh·sis) [*enteron;* G. *myia,* fly; NL. *-iasis,* condition]. Disease due to the presence of the larvae of flies in the intestine.

en′ter·on [G., intestine]. The alimentary canal.

en″ter·op′a·thy [*enteron;* G. *pathos,* disease]. Any disease of the intestine.

en″ter·o·pex′y, en′ter·o·pex″y [*enteron;* G. *pēxis,* a fixing]. *In surgery,* the fixation of a portion of the intestine to the abdominal wall, for the relief of enteroptosis, splanchnoptosis, etc.

en′ter·o·plas″ty [*enteron;* G. *plassein,* to form]. A plastic operation upon the intestine. —**enteroplas′tic,** *adj.*

en″ter·o·ple′gi·a [*enteron;* G. *plēgē,* stroke]. Paralysis of the intestine.

en″ter·o·proc′ti·a (en″tur·o·prock′shee·uh) [*enteron;* G. *prōktos,* anus]. The existence of an artificial anus. *Obs.*

en″ter·op·to′sis [*enteron;* G. *ptōsis,* a falling]. Prolapse of the intestine. Syn., *visceroptosis.* —**enteroptot′ic,** *adj.*

en″ter·or·rha′gi·a [*enteron;* G. *rhēgnynai,* to burst]. Intestinal hemorrhage.

en″ter·or′rha·phy [*enteron;* G. *rhaphē,* suture]. Suture of the intestine.

circular e. The suturing of two completely divided sections of an intestine.

en″ter·or·rhe′a. Old term for diarrhea.

en″ter·or·rhex′is [*enteron;* G. *rhēxis,* a breaking]. Rupture of the intestine. *Obs.*

en′ter·o·scope [*enteron;* G. *skopein,* to examine]. An endoscope for examining the inside of the intestine.

en″ter·o·sep′sis [*enteron;* G. *sēpsis,* decay]. Intestinal toxemia or sepsis.

en′ter·o·spasm [*enteron;* G. *spasmos,* spasm]. Spasm of the intestine.

en″ter·o·sta′sis (en″tur·o·stay′sis, ·os′tuh·sis) [*enteron;* G. *stasis,* a standing]. Intestinal stasis; delay in the passage of the intestinal contents.

en″ter·o·ste·no′sis [*enteron;* G. *stenōsis,* a being straitened]. Stricture or narrowing of the intestinal canal.

en″ter·os′to·my [*enteron;* G. *stoma,* mouth]. The formation of an artificial opening into the intestine through the abdominal wall.

en′ter·o·tome [*enteron;* G. *tomos,* cutting]. An instrument for cutting open the intestine.

en″ter·ot′o·my [*enteron;* G. *tomē,* a cutting]. Incision of the intestine.

en″ter·o·tox·e′mi·a [*enteron;* G. *toxikon,* poison; *haima,* blood]. The presence in the blood stream of toxins produced in the intestine.

infectious e. of sheep. A toxemia of sheep occurring in Australia and in scattered parts of the

United States, thought to be caused by *Clostridium perfringens,* Type D. Syn., *overeating disease.*

en″ter·o·tox′in [*enteron;* G. *toxikon,* poison]. A toxin produced by the *Micrococcus pyogenes* var. *aureus* (*Staphylococcus aureus*) which gives rise to typical symptoms of food poisoning in man and the rhesus monkey (upon feeding), and in kittens (following intraperitoneal injection).

en″ter·o·zo′on [*enteron;* G. *zōion,* living being]. An animal parasite of the intestine.

en″the·o·ma′ni·a [G. *entheos,* full of the god; *mania,* madness]. A mania in which the patient believes himself to be inspired; religious insanity.

en′the·sis [G., a putting in]. The employment of metallic or other inorganic material to replace lost tissue.

en·thet′ic [G. *enthetikos,* fit for implanting]. 1. Pertaining to enthesis. 2. Exogenous.

en·ti′ris [G. *entos,* within; *iris,* iris]. The uvea of the iris, forming its inner and pigmentary layer.

en′to-, ent- [*entos*]. A combining form signifying *within, inner.*

en′to·blast [*entos;* G. *blastos,* germ]. The primitive entoderm; hypoblast.

en′to·cele [*entos;* G. *kēlē,* hernia]. Internal hernia.

en″to·cho·roid′e·a (en″to·ko·royd′ee·uh) [*entos;* G. *chorioeidēs,* choroid]. The inner lining of the choroid membrane of the eye, made up mainly of capillaries.

entocine. Trade-mark for a vaccine for immunization against the common cold.

en′to·cone [*entos;* G. *kōnos,* cone]. The posterior lingual cusp of a maxillary molar tooth.

en″to·co′nid [*entos; kōnos*]. The posterior lingual cusp of a mandibular molar tooth.

en′to·derm [*entos;* G. *derma,* skin]. The innermost of the three primary germ layers, which forms the lining of the gut, from pharynx to rectum, and its derivatives. Syn., *endoderm.* —**entoder′mal,** *adj.*

presumptive e. Tissue which is the primordium of the entoderm.

primitive e. The internal layer of the gastrula; the group of cells that segregate from the inner cell mass on the ventral surface of the primitive ectoderm and from which are derived the yolk sac and embryonic gut: also called *primary e.* Syn., *entoblast, hypoblast.*

yolk-sac e. The epithelial lining of the yolk sac, continuous with that of the gut.

en′to·mere [*entos;* G. *meros,* part]. A blastomere capable of forming entoderm.

en·to′mi·on [G. *entomē,* notch]. The point where the tip of the mastoid angle of the parietal bone fits into the parietal notch of the temporal bone.

en·to·mog′e·nous (en to·moj′e·nus). Originating with insects, their bites, or products; originating (growing) within an insect.

en″to·mol′o·gist [G. *entomos,* cut in pieces; *logos,* word]. A specialist in that department of zoology which deals with insects.

en″to·mol′o·gy [*entomos; logos*]. The study of insects.

en″to·mo·pho′bi·a [*entomos;* G. *phobos,* fear]. A morbid fear of insects.

ent″oph·thal′mi·a [G. *entos,* within; *ophthalmos,* eye]. Inflammation of the internal parts of the eyeball.

ent·op′tic [*entos;* G. *optikos,* of sight]. Pertaining to the internal parts of the eye.

ent″op·tos′co·py [*entos; optikos;* G. *skopein,* to examine]. Examination of the interior of the eye, or of the shadows within the eye. —**entoptoscop′ic,** *adj.*

en″to·ret′i·na [*entos;* L. *rete,* net]. The innermost portion of the retina, itself composed of five layers and an inner limiting membrane.

ent″os·to′sis, ent·os″te·o′sis [*entos;* G. *osteon,* bone; *-ōsis,* condition]. A benign growth of bone extending from the endosteal cortex into a medullary cavity; enostosis.

ent·o′tic (ent·o′tick, ·ot′ick) [*entos;* G. *ōtikos,* of the ear]. Pertaining to the internal ear.

en″to·zo′on [*entos;* G. *zōion,* living being]. An animal parasite living within another animal. —**entozoal,** *adj.*

en·train′ment. A condition in which a liquid boils at such a rapid rate as to carry droplets of liquid in the vapor.

en·tro′pi·on [G. *en,* in; *trepein,* to turn]. Inversion of the eyelid, so that the lashes rub against the globe of the eye. —**entropionize,** *v.t.*

cicatricial e. That due to scar tissue on the inner side of the lid; affects the upper lid most commonly.

senile e. That caused by relaxation of a portion of the orbicularis, resulting from senile changes.

spastic e. That caused by excessive contraction of the ciliary portion of the orbicularis muscle; occurring almost always in the lower lid.

trachomatous e. That due to trachomatous cicatrization of the conjunctiva.

en′tro·py [*en; trepein*]. That portion of the energy of a system, per degree of absolute temperature, which cannot be converted to work. All spontaneous changes—i.e., those occurring in nature—are accompanied by an increase in the entropy of the system.

en′ty·py [G. *entypē,* pattern]. A condition in which the trophoblastic layer remains uninterrupted over the inner cell mass of the blastocyst.

e·nu′cle·ate [L. *enucleare,* to take out the kernels]. Remove an organ or a tumor in its entirety, as an eye from its socket. —**enuclea′tion, enucleator,** *n.*

enule. Trade name applied to suppositories or medicated bougies.

en″u·re′sis [G. *enourein,* to make water in]. Incontinence of urine; more specifically and preferably, urinary incontinence in the absence of demonstrable organic causes at an age when urethral sphincter control may normally be expected; a habit disturbance. —**enuret′ic,** *adj., n.;* **enurese,** *v.*

diurnal e. The less common form, occurring in the daytime.

nocturnal e. That occurring at night during sleep.

en·vi′ron·ment [F. *environ,* about]. Those external conditions which surround, act upon, and influence an organism or its parts.

en″zo·ot′ic [G. *en,* in; *zōion,* living being]. Pertaining to a disease afflicting animals in a limited district; neither epizootic nor sporadic.

en′zyme (en′zime, ·zim) [*en;* G *zymē,* leaven]. A catalytic substance formed by living cells and having a specific action in promoting a chemical change. Syn., *ferment.* See Table of Enzymes in the Appendix. —**enzymat′ic, enzy′mic,** *adj.*

activation of enzymes. The means by which an enzyme that has little or no catalytic activity undergoes an increase in such activity; commonly, the presence of another substance, of diverse nature, is required.

amylolytic e. One hydrolyzing starch to dextrin and maltose, as ptyalin, pancreatic amylase.

autolytic e. That producing autolysis or digestion of the cell in which it exists, usually at the death of the cell.

bacterial e. That existing in, or produced by, bacteria.

coagulating e. One converting soluble proteins into insoluble products, as rennin, myosinase.

copper e. One of the copper-containing enzymes.

deaminating e. One splitting off —NH_2 groups; usually followed by a secondary oxidative reaction, as guanase, adenase.

decarboxylating e. That splitting CO_2 from organic acids, as carboxylase.

diastatic e. See amylolytic *e.*

digestive e. The enzyme concerned with digestion in the alimentary tract.

extracellular e. An enzyme which retains its activity when removed from the cell in which it is formed, or which normally exerts its activity at a site removed from the place of formation. Also called *unorganized ferment, lyoenzyme.*

glycolytic e. One capable of decomposing sugars, either by hydrolysis or by oxidation.

Haas e. A yellow enzyme that oxidizes coenzyme II, having the same action as that of Warburg's old yellow enzyme.

hydrolytic e. One capable of inducing hydrolytic reactions, as carbohydrase, esterase, protease, etc.

intracellular e. An enzyme which exerts its activity within the cell in which it is formed and which loses its activity when removed from the cell. Also called *organized ferment.*

iron e. One of the group of enzymes that contain iron in the prosthetic group.

iron-porphyrin-protein enzymes. Iron porphyrin proteins, with enzymatic function.

lipolytic e. One hydrolyzing fats to glycerol and fatty acids, as pancreatic lipase.

oxidizing e. That influencing oxidation reactions, as oxidase, dehydrogenase.

phosphorylating enzymes. Enzymes which catalyze the phosphorylation or dephosphorylation of compounds.

proteolytic e. Protease; an enzyme involved in the breaking down of protein, as pepsin, rennin, etc.

pyridinoprotein enzymes. See *phosphopyridine nucleotide.*

Q e. An enzyme from potato extracts which, in conjunction with potato phosphorylase, catalyzes conversion of glucose-1-phosphate to a branched-chain polysaccharide.

respiratory e. An enzyme concerned with the mechanism by which molecular oxygen produces oxidations in the living cell. Indophenol oxidase, cytochrome oxidase.

steatolytic e. See lipolytic *e.*

Warburg's old yellow e. The oxidative enzyme that removes hydrogen from coenzyme II and gives it to gaseous oxygen. Its prosthetic group is riboflavin-5-phosphate.

yellow e. Any one of 12 enzymes containing a specific protein combined with isoalloxazine mononucleotide or isoalloxazine-adenine dinucleotide, involved in certain biologic oxidations; sometimes called flavoprotein.

enzymol. Trade name for a liquid extract prepared from mucous membranes of animal stomachs: used as a solvent of necrotic and sloughing tissues.

en″zy·mol′o·gy (en″zye·mol′o·jee, en″zi·) [*en; zymē;* G. *logos,* word]. The science and study of enzymes and the chemical reactions they catalyze.

en″zy·mol′y·sis (en″zye·mol′i·sis, en″zi·) [*en; zymē;* G. *lysis,* a loosing]. A chemical change produced by enzyme action. —**enzymolyt′ic,** *adj.*

en″zy·mo′sis (en″zye·mo′sis, en″zi·). See *enzymolysis.*

e′on·ism [from Charles Geneviève Louis Auguste André Timothée, chevalier d'*Eon* de Beaumont, 1728–1810, French diplomatic agent]. The adoption of feminine habits, manners, and costume by a male. Also see *sexo-esthetic inversion, transvestitism.*

e′o·sin. $C_{20}H_8Br_4O_5$. Tetrabromofluorescein. A bronze-colored, crystalline powder; its aqueous solution is red with a green fluorescence. A bacteriologic stain and diagnostic reagent. Commercially several rose-colored fluorescein dyes of the xanthine series are called eosins: eosin Y, ethyl eosin, eosin B, phloxine, and rose bengal. See also under *stain.*

alcohol-soluble e. The potassium or sodium salt of the ethyl ester of tetrabromofluorescein. A moderately coarse, red powder; used as histologic stain. Also called *ethyl e.*

soluble e. The sodium salt of tetrabromofluorescein.

e″o·sin″o·pe′ni·a [G. *ēōs,* dawn; *penia,* poverty]. A decrease of the normal number of eosinophils in the peripheral blood. —**eosinope′nic,** *adj.*

e″o·sin′o·phil [*ēōs;* G. *philein,* to love]. Having an affinity for eosin or any acid stain.

e″o·sin′o·phil. One of the eosinophil leukocytes of the blood or connective tissues. See Plate 26. —**eosinophil′ic, eosinoph′ilous,** *adj.*

e″o·sin″o·phil′i·a [*ēōs; philein*]. An increase above the normal number of eosinophils in the circulating blood or in the tissues: also called *acidophilia, oxyphilia.*

tropical e. A condition of unknown cause, described in India and the South Pacific area, which presents a clinical picture similar to that of *Loeffler's syndrome,* and may be identical with it.

e·pac′tal [G. *epaktos,* brought in]. Intercalated, supernumerary.

e·pac′tal. An epactal bone, as the interparietal or Inca bone, or the sutural or Wormian bones.

epanutin. A British brand of diphenylhydantoin sodium.

ep″ar·te′ri·al [G. *epi,* on; *artēria,* artery]. Situated upon or above an artery; applied especially to the first branch of the right primary bronchus.

ep·ax′i·al [*epi;* L. *axis,* axis]. Situated above an axis.

ep·en′dy·ma [G. *ependyma,* upper garment]. The lining membrane of the cerebral ventricles and the central canal of the spinal cord. —**ependymal,** *adj.*

ep·en″dy·mi′tis [*ependyma;* G. *-itis,* inflammation]. Inflammation of the ependyma.

ep·en″dy·mo·blas·to′ma [*ependyma;* G. *blastos,* germ; *-ōma,* tumor]. A more malignant type of ependymoma, histologically showing no characteristic arrangement of cells and containing a large number of oligodendroglialike cells.

ep·en′dy·mo·cyte [*ependyma;* G. *kytos,* cell]. A cell lining the cavities of the brain; derived from embryonic epithelial cells.

ep·en″dy·mo′ma [*ependyma;* G. *-ōma,* tumor]. A glioma which originates in or near the ependyma and grows into a ventricle; histologically, the tumor may have an epithelial or papillary pattern, or there may be no characteristic arrangement; varying degrees of cellular differentiation occur in the ependymal cells, (b), varying with the degree of malignancy. Also called *blastoma ependymale, medulloepithelioma, spongioblastoma primitivum.*

ep·en″dy·mop′a·thy [*ependyma;* G. *pathos,* disease]. Disease of the ependyma.

eph″e·bo·gen′e·sis [G. *ephēbos,* one arrived at adolescence; *genesis,* production]. The spontaneous development of a male germ cell thought to cause chorionic carcinoma or teratoma of the testis.

E·phe′dra, Eph′e·dra [G. *ephedra,* a sitting upon]. A genus of shrubs of the Gnetaceae, from some species of which is obtained the alkaloid ephedrine.

Under the name *ma-huang*, species of *Ephedra* have been used in China for many years.

e·phed′rine (eh·fed′rin, ef′i·dreen, ·drin) (*ephedrina*). $C_6H_5CHOH.CH(CH_3).NH.CH_3$. An alkaloid obtained from *Ephedra equisetina*, *E. sinica*, and other species, or produced synthetically. It is anhydrous or contains up to one-half molecule of water of hydration. White crystals or granules slowly decomposed by light. Soluble in 20 parts of water or 0.2 part of alcohol; slowly soluble in liquid petrolatum. Aqueous solutions are alkaline. Its actions are similar to those of the chemically related epinephrine, but slower and longer lasting. Stimulant to the peripheral endings of the sympathetic nerves. Used in hay fever and asthma, urticaria, surgical shock and as a topical application to mucous membranes in congestions such as colds, etc. Dose, 15–50 mg. (¼–⅚ gr.).

e. hydrochloride (*ephedrinae hydrochloridum*). Fine, white, odorless crystals or powder soluble in 3 parts of water or 14 parts of alcohol. Dose, 15–60 mg. (¼–1 gr.).

e. sulfate (*ephedrinae sulfas*). Fine, white, odorless crystals or powder soluble in 1.2 parts of water or 95 parts of alcohol. Dose, 15–60 mg. (¼–1 gr.). Locally, solutions of 0.5–3.0% are used.

eph·e′lis (ef·ee′lis) (pl. *ephelides*) [G. *ephelis*, freckle, from *hēlios*, sun]. A freckle.

e·phem′er·al [G. *ephēmeros*, living but a day]. Temporary; applied to fevers that are of short duration.

***l*-e·phen′a·mine pen″i·cil′lin G.** Generic name for the antibiotic supplied under the trade-marked name compenamine.

ephetonin. A trade-mark for a racemic (optically inactive) form of ephedrine hydrochloride. It is used like ephedrine but is less active and also causes side reactions less frequently.

eph″i·dro′sis [G., superficial perspiration]. Excessive perspiration; hyperhidrosis.

e. cruenta. Bloody sweat.

e. tincta. Colored sweat; chromhidrosis.

ephynal. Trade-mark for a synthetic α-tocopherol, a substance having potent vitamin-E activity.

ep′i-, ep- [G. *epi*, on, upon]. 1. A prefix meaning *upon, beside, among, above, anterior, over, on the outside*. 2. *In chemistry*, a prefix denoting relation of some kind to a (specified) compound.

ep″i·a·gnath′us (ep″ee·a·nath′us, ·nayth′us, ep″ee·ag′nuth·us) [*epi*; G. *a-*, not; *gnathos*, jaw]. An individual with a deficient upper jaw.

ep′i·blast [*epi*; G. *blastos*, germ]. 1. The epidermal ectoderm after segregation of the neuroblast. 2. Old term for primitive ectoderm of blastula.

ep″i·bleph′a·ron [*epi*; G. *blepharon*, eyelid]. A congenital fold of skin on the lower eyelid, causing lashes to turn inward. *Rare.*

e·pib′o·ly [G. *epibolē*, a throwing on]. A process of overgrowth in gastrulation in telolecithal eggs, in which the blastoporal lips spread over the vegetal hemisphere of the gastrula. —**epibol′ic,** *adj.*

ep″i·bulb′ar [G. *epi*, on; L. *bulbus*, bulb]. Situated upon the globe of the eye.

ep″i·can′thus [*epi*; G. *kanthos*, corner of the eye]. A congenital anomaly in which a fold of skin covers the inner canthus and caruncle. Epicanthus is a racial characteristic of the Mongolian race, and is not uncommon in infants of other races in whom the nasal bone is underdeveloped.

ep″i·car′di·a [*epi*; G. *kardia*, heart]. The lower end of the esophagus, between the diaphragm and the stomach. —**epicardial,** *adj.*

ep″i·car′di·um [*epi*; *kardia*]. The visceral layer of the pericardium. See Plate 5. —**epicardial,** *adj.*

e·pic′a·rin, ep″i·car′in. An antiseptic and antiparasitic, chemically β-hydroxynaphthyl-*o*-hydroxy-*m*-toluic acid; used in the form of a 5–20% ointment or a 10% alcoholic solution in skin diseases.

ep′i·carp [G. *epikarpos*, from *epi*; *karpos*, fruit]. The outermost layer of the pericarp of a fruit.

ep″i·chor′dal (ep″i·kor′dul) [*epi*; G. *chordē*, chord]. Located above or dorsad of the notochord; applied especially to cerebral structures.

ep″i·cho′ri·al (ep″i·kor′ee·ul) [*epi*; G. *chorion*, membrane]. Located on the chorion.

ep″i·cho′ri·on (ep″i·ko′ree·on) [*epi*; *chorion*]. The decidua capsularis.

ep″i·col′ic [*epi*; G. *kolon*, colon]. Situated over the colon.

ep″i·co′mus [*epi*; G. *komē*, hair]. An individual (autosite) with a parasitic accessory head attached to its vertex. Syn., *craniopagus parasiticus*.

ep″i·con″dyl·al′gi·a [*epi*; G. *kondylos*, knuckle; *algos*, pain]. Pain in the vicinity of an epicondyle.

ep″i·con′dyle [*epi*; *kondylos*]. An eminence upon a bone above its condyle. —**epicondylar, epicondyl′ian, epicondyl′ic,** *adj.*

ep″i·con″dy·li′tis [*epi*; *kondylos*; G. *-itis*, inflammation]. Inflammation of an epicondyle, specifically, that of the humerus; often applied to synovitis of the radiohumeral articulation. Also called *radiohumeral bursitis, radiohumeral e.*

ep″i·cra′ni·o·tem″po·ral′is. A portion of the auricularis anterior muscle.

ep″i·cra′ni·um [*epi*; G. *kranion*, skull]. The structures covering the cranium.

ep″i·cra′ni·us [*epi*; *kranion*]. The occipitofrontalis muscle. See Table of Muscles in the Appendix.

ep″i·cri′sis [G. *epikrisis*, determination]. The disease phenomena succeeding crisis.

e·pic′ri·sis [*epikrisis*]. A critical summary or analysis of the record of a case or of a scientific article.

ep″i·crit′ic [G. *epikritikos*, determinative]. Pertaining to sensory nerve fibers which enable one to appreciate very fine distinctions of temperature and touch. These fibers are found in the skin and oral mucosa.

ep″i·cys·ti′tis [G. *epi*, on; *kystis*, bladder; *-itis*, inflammation]. Inflammation of the tissues about the urinary bladder.

ep″i·cys·tot′o·my [*epi*; *kystis*; G. *tomē*, a cutting]. Suprapubic incision of the urinary bladder. *Obs.*

ep′i·cyte [*epi*; G. *kytos*, cell]. 1. The cell wall. 2. A cell of epithelial tissue.

ep″i·dem′ic [G. *epidēmios*, among the people]. Unusual prevalence of a disease; ordinarily affecting large numbers or spreading over a wide area. An arbitrary standard of normal incidence is used to determine the presence of an epidemic. The number of cases occurring for the equivalent chronological period during the previous five years is used to determine the median. —**epidemic′ity** (ep″i·di·miss′i·tee), *n.*

ep″i·de″mi·ol′o·gist (ep″i·dee″mee·ol′o·jist, ep″i·dem″ee·) [*epidēmios*; G. *logos*, word]. One who has made a special study of epidemiology.

ep″i·de″mi·ol′o·gy [*epidēmios*; *logos*]. The study of occurrence and distribution of disease; usually restricted to epidemic and endemic, but sometimes broadened to include all types of disease. —**epidemiolog′ic,** *adj.*

ep′i·derm. See *epidermis*.

ep″i·der″ma·to·plas′ty (ep″i·dur″muh·to·plas′tee, ep″i·dur′muh·to·plas″tee, ep″i·dur·mat′o·plas·tee) [G. *epiderma*, epidermis; *plassein*, to mold]. Skin grafting by transplanting small pieces to denuded areas.

ep″i·der″ma·to′zo″on·o·sis [*epiderma*; G. *zōion*, animal; *-ōsis*, condition]. Any skin disease in which the parasite, such as the louse, remains on the surface of, and does not burrow into, the skin. Syn., *epizoonosis.*

ep″i·der″mi·dal·i·za′tion [*epiderma*]. The conversion of columnar into stratified squamous epithelium.

ep″i·der″mi·do′sis. See *epidermosis.*

ep″i·der′min. A fibrous protein isolated from skin, having an alpha-keratin structure.

ep″i·der′mis, ep′i·derm [*epiderma*]. The protective, epithelial outer layer of the skin apposed to the dermis or corium. —**epider′mal, epider′mic, epidermat′ic,** *adj.*

ep″i·der·mi′tis [*epiderma;* G. *-itis,* inflammation]. Inflammation of the outer layer of the skin.

ep″i·der″mi·za′tion [*epiderma*]. 1. The formation of epidermis. 2. Skin grafting.

ep″i·der′mo- [*epiderma*]. A combining form denoting *epidermis.*

ep″i·der″mo·dys·pla′si·a ver·ru″ci·for′mis (ep″-i·dur″mo·dis·play′zhuh verr·oo″si·for′miss, ·play′-zee·uh, ·play′shuh, ·play′see·uh). A congenital defect in which verrucous lesions occur on the hands, feet, face, or neck.

ep″i·der′moid [*epiderma;* G. *eidos,* form]. Resembling epidermis.

ep″i·der′moid. A neoplasm occurring as a cyst in the epidermis; containing keratin, hair, or any other parts arising from epidermis.

ep″i·der·mol′y·sis. The easy separation of various layers of skin, primarily of the epidermis from the corium. See Nikolsky's *sign.*

ep′i·der·mol′y·sis bul·lo′sa. A genodermatosis characterized by the development of vesicles and bullae on slight, or even without, trauma. It was described by Heinrich Koebner.

e. b. dystrophica. A condition in which bullae of skin form on slight trauma or without it, followed by scarring and atrophy. Nails become dystrophic and are sometimes destroyed. Oral mucosa may show bullae, infiltration, or patches of leukoplakia. There may be alopecia and electroencephalographic changes. There is linkage with acrodermatitis enteropathica.

e. b. hereditaria letalis. A rare form characterized by bullae which may contain lymph or blood. The nails are loosely attached and there are oral lesions. Death usually occurs before the third month.

e. b. simplex. The mild type; bullae form in early childhood; there is complete healing, tendency to remission at puberty, with none of the other symptoms which occur in the dystrophic type.

ep″i·der″mo·my·co′sis (·migh·ko′sis) [*epiderma;* G. *mykēs,* fungus; *-ōsis,* condition]. Any dermatitis caused by a fungus.

ep″i·der·moph′y·tid [*epiderma;* G. *phyton,* plant]. A secondary allergic skin eruption thought to occur when the fungus *Epidermophyton floccosum,* or its products, is carried through the blood stream to sensitized areas of the skin.

Ep″i·der·moph′y·ton (ep″i·dur·mof′i·ton, ep″i-dur″mo·figh′ton) [*epiderma; phyton*]. A genus of fungi of the dermatophyte group; contains but one recognized species. See Table of the Most Common Microorganisms in the Appendix.

E. floccosum. The single species of this genus, found in infections of the skin and nails, and especially of the groin. Syn., *Acrothecium floccosum.*

E. inguinale. Synonym for *E. floccosum.*

ep″i·der″mo·phy·to′sis (ep″i·dur″mo·figh·to′sis) [*epiderma; phyton;* G. *-ōsis,* condition]. Infection by the *Epidermophyton floccosum.* It has commonly been used to include any fungus infection of the feet producing scaliness and vesicles with pruritus.

ep″i·der″mo·pro′te·ase. A protease isolated from the epidermis.

ep″i·der·mo′sis [*epiderma; -ōsis*]. A collective name for anomalous growths of the skin of epithelial origin and type.

ep″i·did″y·mec′to·my [G. *epididymis,* from *epi,* on, *didymos,* testis; *ektomē,* excision]. Surgical removal of the epididymis.

ep″i·did′y·mis (pl. *epididymides*) [G.]. That portion of the seminal duct lying posterior to the testis and connected to it by the efferent ductules of the testis. See Plate 44. —**epididymal,** *adj.*

ep″i·did″y·mi′tis [*epididymis;* G. *-itis,* inflammation]. Inflammation of the epididymis.

ep″i·did′y·mo- [*epididymis*]. A combining form signifying *epididymis.*

ep″i·did′y·mo-or·chi′tis (ep″i·did′i·mo-or·kigh′-tis) [*epididymis;* G. *orchis,* testis; *-itis,* inflammation]. Inflammation of both the epididymis and testis.

ep″i·did″y·mot′o·my [*epididymis;* G. *tomē,* a cutting]. Making an incision into the epididymis.

ep″i·did″y·mo·vas·os′to·my (·vass·os′to·mee, ·vaz·) [*epididymis;* L. *vas,* vessel; G. *stoma,* mouth]. Surgical anastomosis of the ductus deferens with the epididymis.

ep″i·du′ral [G. *epi,* on; L. *durus,* hard]. Situated upon or over the dura.

ep″i·fas′ci·al (ep″i·fash′ee·ul, ·fash′ul) [*epi;* L. *fascia,* band]. Of, pertaining to, or on a fascia.

ep″i·fol·lic″u·li′tis [*epi;* L. *folliculus,* small bag; G. *-itis,* inflammation]. Inflammation of the hair follicles of the scalp.

ep″i·gas·tral′gi·a [*epi;* G. *gastēr,* belly; *algos,* pain]. Pain in the epigastrium.

ep″i·gas′tric [*epi; gastēr*]. Of or pertaining to the epigastrium.

ep″i·gas′tri·o·cele″. See *epigastrocele.*

ep″i·gas′tri·um [*epi; gastēr*]. The upper and middle part of the abdominal surface between the two hypochondriac regions; the epigastric region.

ep″i·gas′tri·us [*epi; gastēr*]. A form of double monster having a parasitic twin or part attached to the epigastric region of the other. Also called *thoracopagus parasiticus, epigastrius parasiticus.*

ep″i·gas′tro·cele, ep″i·gas′tri·o·cele″ [*epi; gastēr;* G. *kēlē,* hernia]. A hernia in the epigastric region.

ep″i·gen′e·sis [*epi;* G. *genesis,* production]. The theory that the fertilized egg gives rise to the organism by the progressive production of new parts, previously nonexistent as such in the egg's original structure. Distinguished from preformation. —**epigenet′ic,** *adj.*

ep″i·glot″ti·dec′to·my [*epi;* G. *glōttis,* glottis; *ektomē,* excision]. Excision of the epiglottis.

ep″i·glot′tis [*epi; glōttis*]. An elastic cartilage covered by mucous membrane forming that superior part of the larynx which guards the glottis during swallowing. See Plate 12. —**epiglottic,** *adj.*

ep″i·glot·ti′tis [*epi; glōttis;* G. *-itis,* inflammation]. Inflammation of the epiglottis.

e·pig′na·thus, ep″i·gnath′us [*epi;* G. *gnathos,* jaw]. A condition in which a mixed tumor, teratoma, or parasitic twin fetus (or part of a fetus) is attached to the base of the skull or to the jaws, usually to the hard palate.

ep″i·gua′nine (ep″i·gwah′neen, ·nin, ·gwan′een, ·in), **ep″i·gua′nin.** $C_6H_7ON_5$. Methyl guanine. A purine base found in human urine, especially during leukemia.

ep″i·hy′oid [*epi;* G. *hyoeidēs,* shaped like the letter upsilon]. Situated upon the hyoid bone.

ep″i·la·mel′lar (ep″i·luh·mel′ur, ·lam′i·lur) [*epi;* L.

lamella, small plate of metal]. Situated upon a basement membrane.

ep″i·la′tion [L. *e*, out; *pilus*, hair]. Removal of the hair by the roots by the use of forceps, chemical means, or roentgentherapy. —**ep′ilate,** *v.*

ep″i·lem′ma (pl. *epilemmata*) [G. *epi*, upon; *lemma*, that which is peeled off]. The perineurium of very small nerves. *Obs.*

ep′i·lep″sy, ep″i·lep′si·a [G. *epilēpsia*, a seizure]. A disorder of the brain characterized by a recurring excessive neuronal discharge, manifested by transient episodes of motor, sensory, or psychic dysfunction, with or without unconsciousness or convulsive movements. The seizure is associated with marked changes in recorded electrical brain activity. —**epilep′tic,** *adj., n.*

acousticomotor e. See reflex *e.*

adversive e. A seizure characterized by a turning of the head, eyes, and trunk in a single direction, until the entire body is twisted, usually caused by a lesion in one frontal lobe.

affective e. See psychic *e.*

akinetic e. A form in which there are seizures characterized by sudden loss of muscle tone and postural control, with nodding of the head, and falling. The electroencephalogram is not characteristic, and usually resembles that of petit mal epilepsy. Also called *atonic "drop" e.*

Amantea's reflex e. A form characterized by intense clonic movements, sometimes produced in experimental animals by applying strychnine to the motor areas of the cortex, after tactile stimulation of corresponding skin areas.

atonic "drop" e. See akinetic *e.*

autonomic e. That in which seizures are confined to the autonomic nervous system, predominantly the sympathetic portion. The visceromotor manifestations include pupillary changes, fluctuations of temperature, and cardiovascular, gastrointestinal, and pilomotor disturbances. Viscerosensory manifestations, such as the epigastric aura or sense of nausea, are sometimes also present. See also diencephalic autonomic *e.*

brain-stem e. See tonic postural *e.*

central e. Any epilepsy characterized by seizures in which the epileptogenic discharge originates in the higher integrating brain stem. Included are grand mal, petit mal, psychomotor epilepsy, and certain forms of automatism.

"centrencephalic" e. See central *e.*

cerebellar e. A term sometimes used for tonic postural epilepsy because the manifestations simulate those produced by cerebellar lesions, although the cerebellum is not involved.

continuous e. Epilepsy characterized by continuous muscular twitchings of some part of the body without loss or impairment of consciousness. Attributed to a brain infection. Also called *partial continuous epilepsy, Kozhevnikov's* (*Kojewnikoff's*) *e.*

cortical e. See Jacksonian *e.*

cryptogenic e. That for which no cause has been found. Syn., *idiopathic e.*

cursive e. A form manifested by seizures characterized by uncontrollable forward running of the patient who appears oblivious to any obstacles in his course: also called *running fits.*

decerebrate e. See tonic postural *e.*

diencephalic autonomic e. A form of autonomic epilepsy with sudden vasodilation, lacrimation, salivation, tachycardia, slowed respiration, and other signs of autonomic system disturbances. Gastrointestinal (viscerosensory) signs, however, are absent. It is usually caused by a lesion of the floor of the third ventricle.

dreamy state e. An illusional seizure consisting of a rather sudden alteration of the patient's own perceptions, as a sudden feeling of familiarity or strangeness in the environment; indicative of a lesion in the temporal lobes. Syn., *déjà vu.*

focal e. See Jacksonian *e.*

grand mal e. A complete epileptic seizure; characterized by sudden loss of consciousness, tonic convulsion, cyanosis, and dilated pupils, followed by a clonic spasm of all voluntary muscles, with the eyes rotated upward, the head extended, a frothing at the mouth, and, frequently, incontinence of urine. After the convulsion subsides, the patient is confused and then falls into a deep sleep. The electric rhythm or brain wave during a grand mal attack is one of increased rate and high voltage. Also called *epilepsia gravis.*

gustatory e. A convulsive seizure announced by an aura of peculiar taste; frequently characterized by smacking movements of the tongue and lips, usually indicative of an irritation of the cortex in the region of the hippocampal convolution.

hypothalamic e. See autonomic *e.*

hysterical e. A functional disorder in which the seizures occur in the presence of others; they are violent, marked by disorganized muscular movements, do not cause injury, and are abruptly terminated without the confusion and lethargy which usually occur in true epilepsy.

idiopathic e. A convulsive disorder not caused by a known or specific brain disease.

Jacksonian e. Spasmodic contractions in certain groups of muscles or paroxysmal paresthesias in certain skin areas; due to local disease of the cortex. May be limited to one side of the body with retention of consciousness or it may progress and become generalized with loss of consciousness. Syn., *focal e., cortical e.*

Kozhenikov e. See continuous *e.*

musicogenic e. See reflex *e.*

myoclonic petit mal e. Severe petit mal epilepsy in which the patient exhibits symmetrically bilateral jerks of the eyes, face, neck, limbs, or trunk muscles; its electroencephalogram is typical of petit mal, but also shows sporadic multiple spike-and-wave complexes.

myoclonus e. A degenerative disease characterized by recurrent fibrillary twitching of muscle fibers, associated with generalized convulsions and progressive impairment of mental functions; it may be identical with paramyoclonus multiplex.

nocturnal e. That in which the attacks occur during sleep.

opisthotonic e. See tonic postural *e.*

organic e. That due to a known brain disease, as contrasted with idiopathic epilepsy.

partial continuous e. See continuous *e.*

petit mal e. A form characterized by very short lapses of consciousness and by a sudden momentary pause in conversation or movement, the duration of which is rarely more than 30 seconds. Petit mal attacks are frequent in children, and may occur as often as 200 times a day, but rarely cause the patient to fall or to show muscular spasm. The brain wave disturbance is a very slow rate of three or four waves per second. Also called *epilepsia mitis, epilepsia vertiginosa.* See *pyknolepsy.*

photogenic, photic e. A form characterized by convulsive seizures induced by photic stimulation, i.e., flicker or intermittent light; the attacks are usually of the myoclonic type.

psychic e. A form in which the seizures are precipitated by an emotional or mental experience.

psychomotor e. That in which transient mental disturbances replace the typical convulsions. Syn., *epileptic equivalent.*

reflex e. A form characterized by convulsive seizures brought about by sensory stimuli such as music, sudden noise (*acousticomotor e.*), or an object of touch or sight, with electroencephalographic changes in the sensory projection area corresponding to the trigger zone.
sensory e. Various disturbances of sensation occurring in paroxysms that replace the epileptic convulsion.
spinal e. Clonic spasm of certain muscle groups of the lower extremities; seen in spastic paraplegia.
striate e. A form characterized by tonic seizures of one or both limbs, attributed to lesions of the corpus striatum. Syn., *subcortical e.*
sympathetic e. See autonomic *e.*
symptomatic e. A convulsive state in which a causative lesion or agent has been found.
tonic postural e. A form in which seizures are characterized by a rigid posture with arms and legs extended, hands pronated, and feet held in plantar flexion. The state may resemble decerebrate rigidity or opisthotonos. The focus of the discharge is localized in the brain stem.
toxemic e. That due to poisonous substances in the blood, as in uremia, or due to convulsant doses of drugs, such as strychnine, picrotoxin, metrazol, or camphor.
traumatic e. That form following the cicatrization of a laceration of the brain; it is clinically similar to Jacksonian epilepsy.
uncinate e. That characterized by an olfactory aura, as a recurring, pungent odor preceding the period of unconsciousness and muscle spasm. Usually caused by an irritation of the uncinate gyrus in the anterior-inferior portion of the temporal lobe.
vasomotor e. That in which extreme constriction of the arteries precedes the attacks, causing a dusky, cyanotic discoloration of the skin.
visceral e. See autonomic *e.*

ep″i·lep″to·gen′ic, ep″i·lep·tog′e·nous (ep″i-lep·todj′i·nus) [G. *epilēptos*, caught in anything; *genesthai*, from *gignesthai*, to be produced]. Producing epilepsy.

ep″i·lep′toid [*epilēptos;* G. *eidos*, form]. Resembling epilepsy.

ep″i·lep′toid. A person subject to nervous attacks of the general nature of epilepsy.

ep″i·loi′a. See tuberous *sclerosis.*

ep′i·mer [G. *epi*, on; *meros*, part]. Either of a pair of isomeric aldoses the configurations of which are identical except in the positions of H and OH attached to the number 2 carbon atom, i.e., the carbon atom next to the aldehyde group. D-Glucose and D-mannose, for example, are epimers. **—epimer′ic,** *adj.*

ep′i·mere. The dorsal portion of the mesothelial lining of the coelom of primitive chordates, forming skeletal musculature and contributing to derma and axial skeleton.

ep″i·my″o·car′di·um [*epi;* G. *mys*, muscle; *kardia*, heart]. The external part of the embryonic heart that develops into the epicardium and myocardium.

Ep′i·mys [*epi;* G. *mys*, mouse]. A genus of rats and mice of the family Muridae. **E. norvegicus** is the common ship rat; **E. rattus,** the plague rat of India.

ep″i·mys′i·um (ep″i-miz′ee·um, ·miss′ee·um) [*epi;* G. *mys*, muscle]. The sheath of connective tissue surrounding a muscle.

ep″i·neph′rine (ep″i·nef′reen, ·rin). $C_9H_{13}NO_3$; l-α-3,4-dihydroxyphenyl-β-methylaminoethanol; the chief hormone of the adrenal medulla, occurring as minute, colorless crystals that gradually acquire a brown color on exposure to light and air; it is sparingly soluble in water. It may be obtained by extraction from the gland or prepared synthetically. The physiologic actions of epinephrine are incompletely understood. It is sometimes used as a vasoconstrictor and cardiac stimulant in acute circulatory failure; as a local vasoconstrictor in hemorrhage and local congestion; to relax the bronchi in asthmatic paroxysms. The effect of local anesthetics is prolonged by its vasoconstrictor action. It causes uterine contractions. Dose, 0.3–1.0 cc. (5–15 min.) of a 1:1000 solution intravenously, intramuscularly, or subcutaneously. Its action is fleeting. For local application, 1:10,000 to 1:1000 solutions are used. Employed by inhalation in the form of a 1:100 solution. It is marketed under various names as *adrenalin, suprarenalin, adrenine,* and *suprarenin.* See Table of Hormones in the Appendix.
demethylated e. See *norepinephrine.*
e. bitartrate. $C_9H_{13}NO_3.C_4H_6O_6$, occurring as a white or grayish-white or light brownish-gray crystalline powder; 1 Gm. dissolves in about 3 cc. of water. This salt is well suited for preparation of solutions and ointments containing epinephrine, the products being more stable and less irritant than those made from hydrochloric acid solutions of epinephrine.
e. inhalation (*inhalatio epinephrinae*). A 1:100 solution of epinephrine in distilled water, prepared with the aid of hydrochloric acid. Dispersed in the form of a fine mist, it is employed as an inhalation to control bronchospasm. Dose, 0.5–1.0 cc. (8–15 min.), by inhalation.
e. injection (*injectio epinephrinae*). A solution of epinephrine, generally 1:1000, in water for injection, prepared with the aid of hydrochloric acid.
e. solution (*liquor epinephrinae*). A 1:1000 solution of epinephrine in distilled water, prepared with the aid of hydrochloric acid. For local application.
slow e. An epinephrine suspension in a vegetable oil; the action is thereby retarded and prolonged. A solution in an aqueous gelatin base is used similarly.

ep″i·neph″ri·ne′mi·a [*epi;* G. *nephros*, kidney; *haima*, blood]. The presence of epinephrine in the blood.

ep″i·ne·phri′tis [*epi; nephros;* G. *-itis*, inflammation]. Inflammation of a suprarenal capsule.

ep″i·neph′ros [*epi; nephros*]. Suprarenal gland. *Obs.*

ep″i·neu′ral [*epi;* G. *neuron*, nerve]. Attached to a neural arch.

ep″i·neu′ri·um [*epi; neuron*]. The connective-tissue sheath of a nerve trunk. **—epineurial,** *adj.*

epinine. Trade-mark of a product, dihydroxyphenyl-methylaminoethane, having a vasomotor effect similar to that of epinephrine, to which it is chemically related, but about one-tenth as powerful and more prolonged in its action.

ep″i·ot′ic (ep″ee·ot′ick, ·o′tick) [*epi;* G. *ōtikos*, of the ear]. Situated above or on the cartilage of the ear.

ep″i·pal′a·tum [*epi;* L. *palatum*, palate]. That variety of epignathus in which the parasitic fetus or fetal remnant is attached to the palate.

ep″i·pas′tic [G. *epipassein*, to sprinkle over]. Having the qualities of a dusting powder.

ep″i·pas′tic. A powder for use on the surface of the body, as talc.

ep″i·phar′ynx [G. *epi*, on; *pharygx*, pharynx]. The nasopharynx. **—epipharyn′geal,** *adj.*

ep″i·phe·nom′e·non [*epi;* G. *phainomenon*, from *phainesthai*, to appear]. An unusual or peculiar event or process in the course of a disease, not necessarily due to the same cause, for example, epituberculosis in lungs due to focal atelectasis or nontuberculous pneumonia.

e·piph'o·ra [G., from *epipherein*, to bring upon]. A persistent overflow of tears, due to excessive secretion or to impeded outflow.

ep"i·phy·lax'is (ep"i·figh·lack'sis, ·fi·lack'sis) [G. *epi*, on; *phylaxis*, a watching]. The reinforcing or increase of the defensive agencies of the body.

ep"i·phys"e·o·ne·cro'sis, ep"i·phys"i·o·ne·cro'sis [*epiphysis;* G. *necrosis*, mortification]. Aseptic necrosis involving the epiphysis of a long bone.

ep"i·phys"e·op'a·thy (ep"i·fizz"ee·op'uth·ee) [G. *epiphysis*, ongrowth; *pathos*, disease]. Any disorder of an epiphysis of a bone or of the pineal gland.

ep"i·phys"i·o·de'sis [*epiphysis;* G., *desis*, a binding together]. The surgical production of permanent or temporary arrest of epiphyseal growth.

ep"i·phys"i·ol'is·the'sis. The slipping of an epiphysis.

ep"i·phys"i·ol'y·sis, ep"i·phys"e·ol'y·sis (ep"i-fizz"ee·ol'i·sis) [*epiphysis;* G. *lysis*, a loosing]. The separation of an epiphysis from the shaft of a bone.

e·piph'y·sis [G.]. A portion of bone attached for a time to a bone by cartilage, but subsequently becoming consolidated with the principal bone. —**epiphys'eal,** *adj.*

e. cerebri. The pineal body.

slipping e. Displacement of the upper femoral epiphysis; of uncertain etiology. It occurs in children.

e·piph"y·si'tis [*epiphysis;* G. *-itis*, inflammation]. Inflammation of an epiphysis.

ep'i·phyte [G. *epi*, on; *phyton*, plant]. 1. A vegetable parasite growing on the exterior of the body. 2. A plant growing upon another plant, but deriving the moisture required for its development from the air.

ep"i·pi'al [*epi;* L. *pius*, tender]. Upon or above the pia mater.

ep"i·pleu'ral (ep"i·ploor'ul) [*epi;* G. *pleura*, rib]. 1. Relating to a pleurapophysis. 2. Located on the side of the thorax.

e·pip'lo·cele [G. *epiploon*, omentum; *kēlē*, hernia]. A hernia containing omentum only.

ep"i·plo·ec'to·my [*epiploon;* G. *ektomē*, excision]. Excision of the omentum.

e·pip"lo·en'ter·o·cele" [*epiploon;* G. *enteron*, intestine; *kēlē*, hernia]. A hernia containing both omentum and intestine.

e·pip"lom·phal'o·cele" (i·pip"lom·fal'o·seel", ep-ip·lom'ful·o·seel") [*epiploon;* G. *omphalos*, navel; *kēlē*]. Omphalocele containing omentum only.

e·pip'lo·on [G.]. The omentum; specifically, the great omentum. —**epiplo'ic,** *adj.*

e·pip'lo·pex"y [*epiploon;* G. *pēxis*, a fixing]. The operation of suturing the great omentum to the anterior abdominal wall, for the purpose of establishing a collateral venous circulation in cirrhosis of the liver.

ep"i·plor'rha·phy [*epiploon;* G. *rhaphē*, a suture]. Suture of the omentum.

ep"ip·ter'ic [G. *epi*, on; *pteron*, wing]. Near the pterion, as the Wormian bones.

ep"i·py'gus, e·pip'y·gus [*epi;* G. *pygē*, rump]. An individual with an accessory limb attached to the nates. Syn., *pygomelus.*

ep"i·scle'ra (ep"i·skleer'uh) [*epi;* G. *sklēros*, hard]. The loose connective tissue lying between the conjunctiva and the sclera.

ep"i·scle'ral [*epi; sklēros*]. 1. Situated on the outside of the sclerotic coat. 2. Relating to the episclera.

ep"i·scle·ri'tis [*epi; sklēros;* G. *-itis*, inflammation]. An inflammation of the subconjunctival tissues or of the sclera itself.

e·pi'si·o- (eh·pee'see·o-, eh·pis'ee·o-, eh·piz'ee·o-, ep"i·sigh'o-) [G. *epision*, pubic region]. A combining form indicating *relation to the vulva.*

e·pi"si·o·cli'si·a (·kly'see·uh, ·kliss'ee·uh) [*epision;* G. *kleisis*, a closing]. Surgical closure of the vulva.

e·pi"si·o·el"y·tror'rha·phy [*epision;* G. *elytron*, covering; *rhaphē*, a suture]. The operation of suturing a relaxed or lacerated perineum and narrowing the vagina.

e·pi"si·o·per"i·ne'o·plas"ty [*epision;* G. *perinaion*, space between the anus and scrotum; *plassein*, to form]. Surgical repair of the perineum and vestibule in the female.

e·pi"si·o·per"i·ne·or'rha·phy [*epision; perinaion;* G. *rhaphē*, a suture]. Surgical repair of lacerated vulva and perineum.

e·pi'si·o·plas"ty [*epision;* G. *plassein*, to mold]. A plastic operation upon the pubic region or the vulva.

e·pi"si·or·rha'gi·a [*epision;* G. *rhēgnynai*, to burst]. Hemorrhage from the vulva.

e·pi"si·or'rha·phy (eh·pee"see·or'uh·fee, eh·pis"-ee·, eh·piz"ee·, ep"i·sigh·) [*epision;* G. *rhaphē*, suture]. An operation for the repair of lacerations about the vulva.

e·pi"si·o·ste·no'sis [*epision;* G. *stenōsis*, a being straitened]. Contraction or narrowing of the vulva.

e·pi"si·ot'o·my (eh·pee"see·ot'o·mee, eh·pis"ee·, eh·piz"ee·, ep"i·sigh·) [*epision;* G. *tomē*, a cutting]. Medial or lateral incision of the vulva during childbirth, to avoid undue laceration.

ep'i·sode [G. *epeisodios*, coming in beside]. An event having a distinct effect on a person's life, or on the course of a disease.

psycholeptic e. A strikingly vivid mental experience in the life of a patient which he believes started his illness.

ep"i·spa'di·as (ep"i·spay'dee·us, ·spad'ee·us) [G. *epi*, on; *span*, to draw]. A congenital defect of the anterior urethra in which the canal terminates on the dorsum of the penis and posterior to its normal opening or, rarely, above the clitoris. —**epispadial,** *adj.;* **epispadiac,** *adj., n.*

female e. A congenital defect in which the urethra, usually dilated, opens between the divided halves of the clitoris, usually associated with absence of all, or at least the upper portion, of the labia minora and other developmental defects.

ep"i·spas'tic [*epi;* G. *spastikos*, drawing in]. Causing blisters.

ep"i·spas'tic. A blistering agent.

ep"i·sphe'noid [*epi;* G. *sphēnoeidēs*, wedge-shaped]. A parasitic fetus or fetal parts attached in the sphenoid region; one of the varieties of epignathus.

ep"i·spi'nal [*epi;* L. *spina*, spine]. 1. Upon the spinal column. 2. Upon the spinal cord. 3. Upon any spinelike structure.

ep"i·sta'sis [G., a stopping]. 1. A scum or film of substance floating on the surface of urine. 2. A checking or stoppage of a hemorrhage or other discharge.

ep"i·stat'ic [G. *epistatikos*, giving an impulse toward] *In genetics*, dominating or suppressing, as a gene which suppresses the effect of another mutant gene that affects the same part of the organism. —**epis'tasy,** *n.*

ep"i·stax'is [G., a dripping]. Bleeding from the nose.

ep"i·stern'um [G. *epi*, on, upon; *sternon*, breast]. A dermal bone or pair of bones ventral to the sternum of certain fishes and reptiles: formerly confused with the *prosternum.*

ep"i·stro'phe·us [BNA] [G., turning on a pivot]. Axis; the second cervical vertebra. See Table of Bones in the Appendix.

ep"i·sym'pus di'pus. An individual in which

the legs are rotated as in sympodia, but are united by a membrane only.

ep″i·ten·din′e·um [G. *epi*, on; L. *tendere*, to stretch]. The fibrous sheath surrounding a tendon.

ep″i·thal′a·mus [*epi;* G. *thalamos*, chamber]. The region of the diencephalon including the habenula, the pineal gland, and the posterior commissure.

ep″i·tha·lax′i·a [*epi;* G. *thēlē*, nipple; *allaxis*, a shedding]. Shedding of epithelial cells, especially in the lining of the intestine.

ep″i·the′li·a. Plural of epithelium.

ep″i·the′li·al rem·nant. See epithelial *rest.*

ep″i·the″li·o·cho′ri·al (ep″ith·ee″lee·o·kor′ee·ul) [*epi; thēlē;* G. *chorion*, skin]. Pertaining to the uterine epithelium and the chorionic ectoderm, as epitheliochorial placenta.

ep″i·the″li·o·ge·net′ic [*epi; thēlē;* G. *genesthai*, from *gignesthai*, to be produced]. Relating to, or caused by, epithelial proliferation.

ep″i·the′li·oid [*epi; thēlē*, G. *eidos*, form]. Resembling epithelium.

ep″i·the″li·o′ma [*epi; thēlē;* G. *-ōma*, tumor]. Any benign tumor derived from epithelium and composed largely of epithelial cells; formerly applied to epidermoid carcinoma. —**epitheliomatous,** *adj.*

adenoid basal-cell e. A variety of basal-cell *e.*

basal-cell e. A nevoid tumor of the epidermis or its appendages, characterized by masses of basal cells having a palisaded arrangement at the periphery, and found in skin of exposed parts, especially in elderly people. Two classes, undifferentiated and differentiated, are described; both types are only locally malignant, but in late stages may ulcerate. Also known as *basal-cell carcinoma, rodent ulcer.*

basal-squamous cell e. See basosquamous *carcinoma.*

calcifying e. (*of Malherbe*). A solitary, hard tumor of the lower derma or subcutaneous fat of skin, most commonly seen on the face and upper extremities, characterized histologically by the presence of so-called shadow cells and a variable number of their basophilic precursors, which resemble the cells of basal-cell epithelioma. Areas of keratinization are present, and calcification is a frequent though not constant feature.

e. adenoides cysticum. Trichoepithelioma.

e. basocellulare. See basal-cell *e.*

e. chorioepidermale. See *choriocarcinoma.*

e. contagiosum. *In veterinary medicine*, fowl pox.

hair matrix e. See keratotic basal-cell *e.*

intraepidermal e. Carcinoma in situ, of either the squamous-cell or basal-cell type.

keratotic basal-cell e. A basal-cell epithelioma that has differentiated towards hairs, thus producing keratin cysts.

multiple benign cystic e. See *trichoepithelioma.*

myxopleomorphic e. See mixed *tumor* of salivary gland type.

pigmented basal-cell e. Basal-cell epithelioma in which there is sufficient melanin to produce a brown or black papule. Clinically, it may be difficult to differentiate from a melanoma.

squamous-cell e. One made up of squamous cells.

ep″i·the″li·o·my·o′sis. See isthmic nodular *salpingitis.*

ep″i·the·li′tis [*epi; thēlē;* G. *-itis*, inflammation]. Inflammation and overgrowth of epithelium of a mucous membrane, due to an x-ray burn.

ep″i·the′li·um (pl. *epithelia*) [*epi; thēlē*]. A tissue composed of contiguous cells with a minimum of intercellular substance. It forms the epidermis and lines hollow organs and all passages of the respiratory, digestive, and genitourinary systems. Special types include **endothelium,** lining blood and lymph vessels; and **mesothelium,** lining body cavities. Epithelium is divided, according to the shape and arrangement of the cells, into columnar, cuboidal, and squamous; simple, pseudostratified, and stratified epithelium; according to function, into protective, sensory, and glandular or secreting. —**epithelial,** *adj.*

ciliated e. A form in which the cells bear vibratile filaments or cilia on their free extremities.

columnar e. Distinguished by elongated, prismatic, or columnar cells.

crevicular e. That lining the gingival sulcus.

cuboidal e. Distinguished by prismatic cells in which height and width are approximately equal.

germinal e. A region of the dorsal coelomic epithelium, lying between the dorsal mesentery and the mesonephros. It becomes the covering epithelium of the gonad when it arises from the genital ridge. Some believe that it gives rise to the germ cells. Also called *germ e.*

glandular e. An epithelium in which the cells are predominantly secretory in function.

heterotopic e. Intestinal epithelial cells, including goblet cells, found in the stomach.

laminated e. See stratified *e.*

Malpighian e. See mucous *e.*

mesenchymal e. The simple layer of squamous cells lining subdural, subarachnoid, and perilymphatic spaces, and the chambers of the eyeball.

mucous e. (a) The rete mucosum, or germinative layer of a stratified squamous epithelium, especially of the epidermis. (b) The entire embryonic epidermis with the exception of the epitrichium.

nerve e. See sensory *e.*

olfactory e. The sensory epithelium lining the olfactory region of the nasal cavity.

pavement e. Simple squamous epithelium.

pigmented e. Epithelial cells holding pigment granules.

protective e. That serving for protection, as the epidermis, as distinguished from that serving for secretion or sensation.

pseudostratified e. One in which all cells are seated on the basement membrane, but not all reach the free surface.

pyramidal e. Cuboidal or columnar epithelium, the cells of which are modified by pressure of surrounding cells to the form of truncated hexagonal pyramids, as in the acini or tubules of glands.

respiratory e. The pseudostratified, ciliated epithelium lining most of the respiratory tract.

rod e. Striated cells lining certain glands.

sensory e. Epithelium in which sensory cells combined with ordinary epithelial cells form the peripheral terminations of the nerves in the organs of sense.

simple e. One with only one layer of cells.

squamous e. The form in which the cells have been reduced to thin plates.

stratified e. A form in which the cells are arranged in distinct layers.

striated e. That consisting of striated cells.

subcapsular e. The epitheliumlike lining of the internal surface of the capsule of the nerve cells of spinal ganglions; satellite cells.

tabular e. Pavement epithelium.

tegumentary e. The epidermis.

tessellated e. Flattened epithelial cells joined at their edges. Also called *simple squamous e.*

transitional e. The epithelium of the urinary tract. The cells of this form vary in shape between squamous, when the epithelium is stretched, and columnar, when not stretched.

vascular e. Endothelium.

vibrating e. Ciliated epithelium.

ep″i·the″li·za′tion [*epi; thēlē*]. The growth of epithelium over a raw surface.

ep′i·them [G. *epithēma*, something put on]. Any local application, as a compress, fomentation, lotion, or poultice.

ep″i·to′nos, ep″i·to′nus [G. *epitonos*, on the stretch]. Anything exhibiting abnormal tension or tone, or stretched from one point to another. —**epiton′ic,** *adj.*

ep″i·trich′i·um (ep″i·trick′ee·um) [G. *epi*, on; *trichion*, small hair]. 1. The superficial layer of fetal epidermis, the remnant of which forms the cellular component of the vernix caseosa. Syn., *periderm.* 2. The superficial layers of squamous cells overlying a hair shaft in its canal before it breaks through the epidermis. —**epitrichial,** *adj.*

ep″i·troch′le·ar (ep″i·trock′lee·ur) [*epi;* L. *trochlea*, mechanical contrivance containing one or more pulleys]. Applied to a lymph node which lies above the trochlea of the elbow joint.

ep″i·troch″le·ar′is. The chondrohumeralis muscle.

ep″i·troch′le·o-ol″e·cra·no′nis. An occasional bundle of muscle running from the medial epicondyle of the humerus to the olecranon.

ep″i·tu·ber″cu·lo′sis [*epi;* L. *tuberculum*, small swelling; G. *-ōsis*, condition]. A pulmonary lesion occurring in tuberculin-positive children; characterized by a massive or lobar density in the x-ray films, paucity of clinical symptoms, and eventual complete resolution. Originally interpreted as nonspecific pneumonia modified by association with tuberculous infection, but no longer accepted as a single pathologic entity.

ep″i·tym′pa·num [*epi;* G. *tympanon*, kettledrum]. The attic of the middle ear, or tympanic cavity. —**epitympan′ic,** *adj.*

ep″i·zo′ic [*epi;* G. *zōion*, a living being]. Parasitic on the surface of the body.

ep″i·zo′i·cide [*epi; zōion;* L. *caedere*, to kill]. A drug or preparation that destroys external parasites.

ep″i·zo′on (pl. *epizoa*) [*epi; zōion*]. An animal parasite living upon the exterior of the body; ectozoon.

ep″i·zo″o·no′sis. Darier's term for *epidermatozoonosis.*

ep″i·zo·ot′ic [*epi; zōion*]. Attacking many animals of one kind in any region simultaneously; widely diffused and rapidly spreading.

ep″i·zo·ot′ic. A disease of animals which is widely prevalent in contiguous areas.

ep″o·nych′i·um (ep″o·nick′ee·um) [*epi;* G. *onyx*, nail]. 1. A horny condition of the epidermis from the second to the eighth month of fetal life, indicating the position of the future nail. 2. The horny layer (stratum corneum) of the nail fold attached to the nail plate at its margin.

ep′o·nym [G. *epōnymos*, given as a significant name]. A name formed or derived from that of a person known or assumed to be the first, or one of the first, to discover or describe a disease, symptom complex, theory, etc. Eponyms often honor persons who are proponents of systems and procedures, methods, surgical operations, etc., even though these are not original with the person so honored. —**eponym′ic, epon′ymous,** *adj.*

ep″o·oph′o·ron [G. *epi*, on; *ōiophoros*, bearing eggs]. A vestigial structure in the female; derived from paragenital mesonephric tubules, a part of the mesonephric duct, and perhaps the rete ovarii.

ep·ox′y-. *In chemistry*, a prefix indicating that two different atoms in a molecule, already otherwise linked, are joined by an atom of oxygen.

ep′ro·caine. A product, 2-diethylaminoethyl *p*-(3,4-dihydroxyphenacylamino) benzoate hydrochloride, which has been shown experimentally to raise blood pressure and produce anesthesia.

eprolin-S. A trade-mark for α-tocopherol.

EPS Exophthalmos-producing substance.

Ep′som salt. Magnesium sulfate.

Epstein, Alois [*German physician*, 1849–1918]. Described the small, slightly elevated, yellowish white masses seen on each side of the hard palate at birth; called *Epstein's pearls.*

ep·u′lis (pl. *epulides*) [*epi;* G. *oulon*, gum]. Any solitary tumorlike lesion developing from the periosteum of the maxilla or mandible, appearing clinically as a circumscribed swelling beneath the gums. It may be a true giant-cell tumor, a fibroma, or a reparative hyperplasia. —**ep′uloid,** *adj.*

e. of newborn. See granular-cell *myoblastoma.*

ep″u·lo·fi·bro′ma (ep″yoo·lo·figh·bro′muh) [*epi; oulon;* L. *fibra*, fiber; G. *-ōma*, tumor]. A fibroma of the gums.

equanil. A trade-mark for *meprobamate.*

e·qua′tion [L. *aequatio*, from *aequare*, to make equal]. A means of expressing equality between two parts.

allometric e. The power function, $y = bx^k$, to which many data in studies of relative growth conform. In this equation, y is a part, x the whole or another part of the organism, b and k are constants.

chemical e. An expression representing a chemical reaction.

e·qua′tor, ae·qua′tor [L., from *aequare*]. Any imaginary circle which divides a body into two equal and symmetrical parts in the manner of the equator of a sphere. —**equato′rial,** *adj.*

e. of a cell. The boundary of the plane through which division takes place.

e. of the eye. A line joining the four extremities of the transverse and the vertical axis of the eye; aequator bulbi oculi.

e. of the lens. The periphery of the crystalline lens between the two layers of the ciliary process; aequator lentis.

e′qui- [L. *aequus*, equal]. A prefix meaning *equally.*

e″qui·ax′i·al. Having equal axes.

Eq′ui·dae [L. *equus*, horse; G. *-idēs*, descendant]. A family of mammals having a single extant genus, *Equus*, which includes the horse, ass, and zebra.

e″qui·len′in, e·quil′e·nin. $C_{18}H_{18}O_2$. An estrogenic steroid hormone, chemically 3-hydroxy-17-keto-1,3,5,6,8-estrapentaene, occurring in the urine of pregnant mares; structurally it differs from estrone in containing two additional double bonds.

e″qui·li·bra′tion (ee″kwi·li·bray′shun, ·lye·bray′shun, i·kwil″i·bray′shun) [L. *aequilibrium*, equilibrium]. Maintenance of equilibrium.

e″qui·lib′ri·um [*aequilibrium*]. 1. A state of balance; a condition in which opposing forces equalize one another so that no movement occurs. 2. A well-balanced condition of mind or feeling.

acid-base e. See acid-base *balance.*

Donnan e. See membrane *e.* See also Frederick George *Donnan.*

fluid e. A state of balance between the water intake and the water loss in the body.

membrane e. A state of ionic balance created on opposite sides of a membrane which is impermeable to an ion. Also called *Donnan e.*

nitrogen e. A state of balance between the intake of nitrogen as proteins and its excretion, in urine, feces, sweat, etc. See *nitrogen* balance.

nutritive e. A condition of balance between the intake of a nutritive material and the excretion of the products of its metabolism.

radioactive e. A relationship between a radioactive substance and its parent substance, in which at any given moment the rate of disintegration of the former is equal to its rate of formation from the latter.

e′qui·lin (ee′kwi·lin, eck′wi·lin). $C_{18}H_{20}O_2$. An estrogenic steroid hormone, chemically 3-hydroxy-17-keto-1,3,5,7-estratetraene, occurring in the urine of pregnant mares; structurally it differs from estrone in containing one additional double bond.

e″qui·mo·lec′u·lar [L. *aequus*, equal; dim. from *moles*, mass]. 1. Containing or representing quantities of substances in the proportion of their molecular weights. 2. Containing or representing an equal number of molecules.

eq′uine (eck′wine) [L. *equinus* from *equus*, horse]. Of, pertaining to, or derived from a horse; horse-like.

e·quin′i·a. See *glanders*.

eq″ui·no·ca′vus (eck″wi·no·kay′vus, ee″kwi·no·, i·kwye″no·). See under *talipes*.

eq″ui·no·va′rus. See under *talipes*.

e·qui′nus. See under *talipes*.

eq″ui·se·to′sis (eck″wi·si·to′sis, ee″kwi·) [L. *equus*, horse; *saeta*, stiff hair; G. *-ōsis*, condition]. The poisoning of horses due to ingestion of horsetail (*Equisetum*).

Eq″ui·se′tum (eck″wi·see′tum, ee″kwi·) [*equus; saeta*]. A genus of cryptogamous plants, some of which have been shown to have a diuretic effect.

e·quiv′a·lent [L. *aequus*, equal; *valere*, to be strong]. Having an equal value.

e·quiv′a·lent. 1. That which is equal in value, size, weight, or in any other respect, to something else. 2. *In chemistry*, the weight of a substance which is chemically equal to 8 parts by weight of oxygen; the weight is commonly expressed in grams. The weight of a substance which combines with or replaces one gram atomic weight of hydrogen. Syn., *equivalent weight*.

abdominal convulsive e. Abdominal symptoms such as pain, vomiting, and distress, occurring paroxysmally, without intraabdominal causes, and thought to be, like epileptic convulsions, an expression of a cerebral seizure discharge. Such seizures are rare and diagnosis depends on electroencephalographic proof.

combustion e. The amount of heat obtained by burning one gram of fat or carbohydrate.

endosmotic e. The ratio obtained by dividing the amount of the replacing liquid in osmotic action by the amount replaced.

epileptic e. Attacks, such as automatic motor acts or fugue states, followed by amnesia, which are experienced by epileptic patients in place of or as equivalents of grand or petit mal attacks.

Joule's e. The number of units of work equivalent to a unit of heat, first experimentally determined by Joule; the mechanical equivalent of heat. Symbol, J.

lead e. The thickness of lead which absorbs radiation at the same rate as the material in question.

mechanical e. of heat. The mechanical energy required to raise the temperature of one gram of water one degree centigrade; it is 4.185×10^7 ergs per calorie (15°); Joule's equivalent.

psychic epileptic e. Mental disturbance or excitement which may take the place of epileptic attacks.

thermometric e. A change of 180 Fahrenheit degrees is equivalent to a change of 100 centigrade degrees and a change of 80 Réaumur degrees. See Tables of Thermometric Equivalents in the Appendix.

toxic e. The quantity of poison capable of killing, by intravenous injection, one kilogram of animal.

ventilatory e. The amount of air which must be inspired for the absorption of 100 ml. of oxygen.

Er Chemical symbol for erbium.

e·ra′sion (i·ray′zhun) [L. *erasum*, from *eradere*, to scrape off]. 1. Surgical removal of tissue by scraping. 2. Excision of a joint; arthrectomy.

Erasistratus [*Greek physician and anatomist in Egypt*, ca. 310–250 B.C.]. Pioneer physiologist and pathologist. Traced veins and arteries to the heart, and developed a reversed theory of circulation. Devised a catheter. Disputed the theory of humors; regarded the blood as a nourishing factor of the body and the pneuma as the vital substance. Said to have discovered and named the prostate gland.

Er″a·ty′rus. A genus of bugs of the Triatomidae.

E. cuspidatus. A species found in South America which has been incriminated in the transmission of American trypanosomiasis.

Erb, Wilhelm Heinrich [*German neurologist*, 1840–1921]. Pioneer in electrotherapy. Described partial paralysis of the brachial plexus, due to laceration at birth, called *Erb's palsy, paralysis, Erb-Duchenne paralysis.* Syphilitic spastic spinal paralysis is called *Erb's paralysis, Erb-Charcot disease.* Progressive muscular dystrophy with pseudohypertrophy is known as *Erb's paralysis, dystrophy, Duchenne-Greisinger disease.* Erb drew attention to myasthenia gravis, called *Erb-Goldflam disease.* In the same year as Westphal (1875) he discovered the diagnostic value in tabes dorsalis of absence of the patellar reflex; he is said to have introduced the term *tendon reflex.* See also Erb's *sign* of tetany.

Erben, Siegmund [*Austrian physician*, 1863–]. Described various phenomena, such as the temporary slowing of the pulse on bending forward or attempting to sit down, due to stimulation of the vagus nerve; the pain in sciatica which is increased by hyperflexion of the leg on the sound side, and the reduction of the temperature of the knee on the painful side in sciatica. Each of these is known as *Erben's phenomenon, reflex.*

er′bi·um [NL., from *Ytterby*, in Sweden]. Er = 167.2. A rare earth metal.

Erdmann, Hugo [*German chemist*, 1862–1910]. Introduced a reagent used in identifying alkaloids. It consists of a mixture of 10 drops of nitric acid in 20 cc. of sulfuric acid. Known as *Erdmann's reagent.*

e·rec′tile [L. *erectum*, from *erigere*, to erect]. Capable of being dilated or erected.

e·rec′tion [L. *erectio*, from *erigere*]. The enlarged state of erectile tissue when engorged with blood, as of the penis or clitoris. —**erect′,** *adj.*, *v.*

e·rec′tor [L. *erectum*, from *erigere*]. 1. A muscle that produces erection of a part. See Table of Muscles in the Appendix. 2. A prism attached to the eyepiece of a microscope for correcting the inversion of the image.

e. clitoridis. The ischiocavernosus muscle in the female.

e. penis. The ischiocavernosus muscle in the male.

e. pili. Old term for an arrector pili muscle.

e. spinae. Old term for sacrospinalis muscle.

er″e·mi·o·pho′bi·a [G. *ēremia*, rest; *phobos*, fear]. Morbid fear of stillness.

er″e·mo·pho′bi·a [G. *erēmos*, lonely, solitary; *phobos*]. 1. Morbid fear of being lonely. 2. Morbid fear of large, desolate places; agoraphobia.

e·rep′sin. An enzyme mixture produced by the intestinal mucosa, consisting of various peptidases which split peptones and proteoses into simpler products; it has no effect on native proteins.

er′e·thism [G. *erethismos*, irritation]. 1. An abnormal increase of nervous irritability. 2. Quick response to stimulus. —**erethis'mic, erethis'tic, erethit'ic,** *adj.*

e·reuth″o·pho'bi·a (i·rōōth″o·fo'bee·uh, err″-yooth·o·). See *erythrophobia.*

erg [G. *ergon,* work]. A unit of work, representing the work done in moving a body against the force of one dyne through a distance of one centimeter.

ergamine. Trade-mark for histamine.

er·ga'si·a (ur·gay'zhuh, ·zee·uh, ·shuh, ·see·uh) [G., work]. 1. *In psychobiology,* the sum total of the functions and reactions of an individual; the actions or responses which spring from the whole organism or personality. 2. A tendency toward work.

er·ga'si·a·try (ur·gay'see·uh·tree, ur″guh·sigh'uh-tree) [*ergasia;* G. *iatreia,* medical treatment]. Adolph Meyer's term for psychiatry.

er·ga″si·o·ma'ni·a (ur·gay″see·o·may'nee·uh, ur-gass″ee·o·) [*ergasia;* G. *mania,* madness]. An exaggerated desire for work of any kind; seen in the manic state of manic-depressive psychoses. *Rare.*

er·ga″si·o·pho'bi·a [*ergasia;* G. *phobos,* fear]. A morbid fear of work.

er″gas·the'ni·a [G. *ergon,* work; *astheneia,* weakness]. Weakness due to overwork.

er·gas'to·plasm. Indefinite collective term for basophil cytoplasmic substances.

er'go-, erg- [*ergon*]. A combining form denoting *work.*

ergoapiol. A proprietary remedy used as an emmenagogue.

er″go·ba'sine (ur″go·bay'seen, ·sin). Ergonovine.

er″go·ba'si·nine (ur″go·bay'si·neen, ·nin). Ergometrinine.

er″go·cal·cif'er·ol. The recently adopted designation for calciferol or vitamin D_2, prepared from ergosterol.

er″go·cor'nine. $C_{31}H_{39}N_5O_5$; a levorotatory alkaloid from ergot, isomeric with ergocorninine.

er″go·cor'ni·nine. The dextrorotatory isomer of ergocornine, occurring in ergot; physiologically, it is relatively inactive.

er″go·cris'tine (ur″go·kris'teen, ·tin). $C_{35}H_{39}N_5O_5$; a levorotatory alkaloid from ergot, isomeric with ergocristinine.

er″go·cris'ti·nine. The dextrorotatory isomer of ergocristine, occurring in ergot; physiologically, it is relatively inactive.

er″go·cryp'tine. $C_{32}H_{41}N_5O_5$; a levorotatory alkaloid from ergot, isomeric with ergocryptinine.

er″go·cryp'ti·nine. The dextrorotatory isomer of ergocryptine, occurring in ergot; physiologically, it is relatively inactive.

er'go·graph [*ergon;* G. *graphein,* to write]. An instrument which, by means of a weight or spring against which a muscle can be contracted, records the extent of movement of that muscle or the amount of work it is capable of doing.

ergoklonin. Trade-mark for a biologically standardized solution of ergot alkaloids.

er·gom'e·ter [*ergon;* G. *metron,* a measure]. An instrument which permits calculation of the work performed (weight multiplied by shortening) by a muscle or muscles over a period of time. One form of this instrument is the **ergometer bicycle,** a stationary bicycle on which the subject pedals against a measurable load.

er″go·met'rine (ur″go·met'reen, ·rin, ·mee'treen, ·trin). Ergonovine.

er″go·met'ri·nine (ur″go·met'ri·neen, ·nin). The dextrorotatory, relatively inactive isomer of ergonovine. Syn., *ergobasinine.*

er″go·no'vine (ur″go·no'veen, ·vin). $C_{19}H_{23}N_3O_2$. An alkaloid obtained from ergot. Discovered almost simultaneously by several investigators, it has been known as ergotocin, ergometrine, ergostetrine, and ergobasine. It causes rhythmic uterine contractions and is more prompt but less persistent in its action than other ergot alkaloids. A white or faintly yellow powder, affected by light.

e. maleate (*ergonovinae maleas*). $C_{19}H_{23}N_3O_2$.-$C_4H_4O_4$; the form in which ergonovine is commonly administered. Dose, oral, intramuscular, or subcutaneous, 0.2–0.5 mg. See *ergotrate.*

er″go·pho'bi·a [*ergon;* G. *phobos,* fear]. Morbid dread of work; ergasiophobia.

er'go·phore group. A chemical group which determines the specificity of an antibody.

er'go·plasm. See *archoplasm.*

er'go·sine (ur'go·seen, ·sin). An alkaloid, $C_{30}H_{37}O_5N_5$, of ergot, having physiologic activity similar to that of ergotoxine.

er·go'si·nine. The dextrorotatory isomer of ergosine, occurring in ergot; it is nearly devoid of physiologic activity.

er·gos'tan·ol. $C_{28}H_{49}OH$; a sterol having the structure of ergosterol but with all three double bonds of the latter saturated.

er·gos'ten·ol. Any of a group of sterols of the composition $C_{28}H_{47}OH$, differing from ergostanol in having one double bond, the position of which varies and thus characterizes the individual ergostenols.

er·gos'ter·in. Ergosterol.

er·gos'ter·ol. $C_{28}H_{43}OH$; ergosta-5:6,7:8,22:23-triene-3-ol; an unsaturated sterol occurring in ergot, yeast, and other fungi; it occurs in crystals, insoluble in water. It is provitamin D_2; on irradiation with ultraviolet light or activation with electrons, it is converted to vitamin D_2 (calciferol). Syn., *ergosterin.*

irradiated e. Vitamin D_2 or calciferol.

er″go·stet'rine (ur″go·stet'reen, ·rin). Ergonovine.

er'got [OF. *argot,* a spur] (*ergota*). The dried sclerotium of *Claviceps purpurea,* a fungus developed on rye plants. It contains at least five optically isomeric pairs of alkaloids; the levorotatory isomers are physiologically active, the dextrorotatory isomers nearly inactive. Ergot causes powerful uterine contractions, and is useful in menorrhagia and metrorrhagia and in preventing and checking postpartum hemorrhage. Its injudicious use during labor is exceedingly dangerous. Through its vasoconstrictor action, it is useful in cerebral or spinal congestion, in colliquative sweats, and in similar conditions where there are local passive congestions. It is a common allergen.

e. extract (*extractum ergotae*). Each gram is equivalent to 4 Gm. of ergot. Dose, 0.5 Gm. (8 gr.).

e. fluidextract (*fluidextractum ergotae*). A preparation which deteriorates rapidly under the influence of air and heat. Dose, 2–8 cc. (½–2 fluidrachms).

er·got'a·mine (ur·got'uh·meen, ·min, ur″guh·tam'-een, ·in). A levorotatory alkaloid, $C_{33}H_{35}O_5N_5$, from ergot, having activity qualitatively identical with that of ergotoxine but two-thirds as strong.

e. tartrate (*ergotaminae tartras*). White crystals used as uterine contractor and in migraine. Dose, oral, 1 mg. (1/60 gr.); subcutaneous, 0.25–0.5 mg. (1/240–1/120 gr.). See *gynergen.*

er″go·tam'in·ine. The dextrorotatory isomer of ergotamine; it is nearly devoid of therapeutic activity.

er″go·ther'a·py [G. *ergon,* work; *therapeia,* treatment]. Treatment of disease by physical work.

er″go·thi″o·ne'ine. See *thioneine.*

er'got·in. Ergot extract.

Bonjean's e. An aqueous ergot extract.

er·got'i·nine (ur·got'i·neen, ·nin). A dextrorotatory alkaloid, $C_{35}H_{39}O_5N_5$, discovered in ergot by Tanret in 1875. It is practically inert physiologically.

er′got·ism [OF. *argot*, spur]. The constitutional effects following the prolonged use of ergot, or of grain containing the fungus *Claviceps purpurea*. There are two types: a spasmodic form with contractions and cramps of the muscles, and a form characterized by dry gangrene.

er′got·ized [*argot*]. Affected by ergot as a result of treatment or poisoning, as wheat infested with the fungus of ergot.

er″go·to′cin. Ergonovine.

er″go·tox′ine (ur″go·tock′seen, ·sin). A crystalline alkaloidal substance, long believed to be a chemical individual, isolated from ergot and having pronounced physiological activity, now known to be a mixture of ergocristine, ergocornine, and ergocryptine.

ergotrate. Trade-mark for ergonovine maleate.

Erichsen, John Eric [*English surgeon*, 1818–96]. Described a train of symptoms following accidents, which may assume the form of traumatic hysteria, neurasthenia, hypochondriasis, or melancholia; called *railway spine, railway brain, Erichsen's disease.*

Erickson test. See Harrower-Erickson *test.*

e·ric′o·lin. A yellow, resinous, glycosidal substance obtained from uva-ursi and other sources. It has been reported to be impure arbutin.

er′i·gens. Pertaining to the sacral parasympathetic preganglionic nerve fibers.

E·rig′er·on (i·ridj′ur·on) [G., early-old]. A genus of the Compositae. Several species have been used in urinary diseases, diarrhea, and dysentery, in the form of an oil (erigeron oil), present to the extent of 0.2–0.4%. Syn., *fleabane.*

e″ri·o·dic′tin. $C_{21}H_{22}O_{10}$; the L-rhamnoside of eriodictyol, a constituent of citrin, isolated from citrus fruits.

e″ri·o·dic′ty·ol. $C_{15}H_{12}O_6$; 3′,4′,5,7-tetrahydroxyflavanone; a constituent of *Eriodictyon californicum* leaves. The L-rhamnoside of eriodictyol is known as *eriodictin.*

E″ri·o·dic′ty·on (eer″ee·o·dick′tee·on, err″ee·o·) [G. *erion*, wool; *diktyon*, net]. A genus of shrubs of the Hydrophyllaceae.

E. californicum. California yerba santa; mountain balm. The leaves of this California shrub have been used as an expectorant and in fluid preparations to mask the taste of bitter drugs.

er·i·om′e·ter. See *halometer.*

e·ris′o·phake. See *erysiphake.*

E·ris′ta·lis [NL.]. A genus of the Diptera of the Syrphidae; commonly called drone flies. The rat-tailed larvae of several species have been known to cause intestinal myiasis in man.

Erlanger, Joseph (1874–). American physiologist, who, with H. S. Gasser combined the amplifier with the cathode-ray oscillograph and studied the highly differentiated functions of the individual nerve fibers, concluding that each group of nerve fibers (A,B,C) had its own threshold of stimulation, conduction rate (alpha, beta, and gamma waves), and refractory period. Nobel laureate in medicine and physiology with Gasser (1944).

Erlenmeyer flask. See under *flask.*

Ermengem, Emile Pierre Marie van [*Belgian physician*, 1851–1932]. Discovered the *Bacillus botulinus* in cases of food poisoning (1897).

Ernst, Paul [*German pathologist*, 1859–1937]. Described, with Babes, metachromatic granules in bacteria, called *Babes-Ernst bodies.* See under *Babes.*

ernutin. A proprietary preparation of ergot.

E·ro′di·um [G. *erōidios*, heron]. A genus of herbs of the Geraniaceae.

E. cicutarium. Alfilaria; has been used as a substitute for hydrastis.

e·rog′e·nous (i·rodj′i·nus), **er″o·gen′ic** [G. *erōs*, love; *genesthai*, from *gignesthai*, to be produced]. Producing or stimulating the sexual appetite.

eros (ē′ros, er′os) [G. love]. *In psychoanalysis*, all the instinctive tendencies which lead the organism toward self-preservation: often used synonymously with *libido*. Also called *life instinct*, in contrast to *thanatos*, death instinct.

e·rose′ (i·rohss′) [L. *erosum*, from *erodere*, to gnaw away]. *In botany*, having a margin or border irregularly toothed.

e·ro′si·o in″ter·dig″i·ta′lis blas″to·my·ce′ti·ca (eh·ro′see·o in″tur·didj″i·tah′lis blas″to·migh·see′ti·kuh, ·set′i·kuh). A form of moniliasis which involves the webs of the fingers and particularly the third or fourth interdigital web. This disease is seen in laundresses and in others whose hands are exposed to the macerating effects of water and strong alkalies.

e·ro′sion [*erodere*]. Superficial destruction of a surface area by inflammation or trauma. —**erosive,** *adj.;* **erode′,** *v.*

dental e. A process, probably chemical, which results in the loss of calcified tissues at the neck of a tooth.

e. of cervix uteri. Destruction of the squamous epithelium of the vaginal cervix, the eroded area being covered by columnar cells.

e·rot′ic [G. *erōtikos*, amorous]. 1. Pertaining to the libido or sexual passion. 2. Moved by or arousing sexual desire. —**erot′ic,** *n.*

e·rot′i·ca [*erōtikos*]. Literature devoted to erotic themes; sexual literature.

er′o·tism, e·rot′i·cism [G. *erōs*, love]. 1. Sexual excitement or desire. 2. *In psychoanalysis*, any manifestation of the sexual instinct or love life.

anal e. Sexual excitement localized in the anal zone.

ego e. See *narcissism.*

muscle e. The association of the libido with muscular activity.

organ e. Sexual desire localized in an organ of the body.

er″o·to·gen′ic (err″o·to·jen′ick, i·ro″to·, i·rot″o·) [*erōs;* G. *genesthai*, from *gignesthai*, to be produced]. Causing, or originating from, erotic feelings.

er″o·to·ma′ni·a [*erōs;* G. *mania*, madness]. Morbid exaggeration of the affections, usually toward the opposite sex. Also called *eromania, eroticomania.* —**erotomaniac,** *n.*

er″o·top′a·thy [*erōs;* G. *pathos*, disease]. Any perversion of the sexual instinct. —**erotopath′ic,** *adj.;* **ero′topath,** *n.*

er″o·to·pho′bi·a [*erōs;* G. *phobos*, fear]. A morbid fear of love.

ertron. Trade-mark for a highly concentrated form of vitamin D in capsules.

e·ru′cic ac′id. $CH_3(CH_2)_7CH{:}CH(CH_2)_{11}COOH$. An unsaturated acid found in the glycerides of rape seed oil and mustard oil.

e″ruc·ta′tion (ee″ruck·tay′shun, err″uck·) [L. *eructatio*, from *eructare*, to belch forth]. Belching.

e·ru′ga·to″ry [L. *erugare*, to clear from wrinkles]. Tending to remove wrinkles.

e·rup′tion [L. *eruptio*, from *erumpere*, to break forth]. 1. Lesions on the skin, especially applied to those of the exanthematous diseases. 2. The appearance of a tooth through the gums.

creeping e. See *larva* migrans.

drug e. Dermatitis medicamentosa.

fixed e. A skin eruption in which the sensitivity

to certain circulating substances remains localized and fixed to certain areas; the term usually refers to *dermatitis medicamentosa.*

Kaposi's varicelliform e. A secondary infection of abnormal skin (usually atopic eczema) with the virus of herpes simplex and at times with vaccinia virus. See also *eczema herpeticum.*

miliary e. An eruption of little vesicles occurring in the course of febrile diseases.

ringed e. See *granuloma* annulare.

e·rup′tive [L. *eruptum,* from *erumpere*]. Attended by or producing an eruption, as an eruptive fever.

E·ryn′gi·um [G. *ēryggion,* of the eryngo]. A genus of plants of the Umbelliferae.

E. aquaticum. Button snakeroot eryngo; a species indigenous to the western prairies and southern barrens of the United States. The root is reputedly diaphoretic, expectorant, and emetic.

er″y·sip′e·las (err″i·sip′i·lus, irr″i·) [G.]. An acute, infectious disease due to *Streptococcus pyogenes;* characterized by a spreading inflammation of the skin and subcutaneous tissues, rarely of the mucous membranes. Sulfa drugs are very effective in treatment. —**erysipel′atous,** *adj.*

e. ambulans. See wandering *e.*

e. antitoxin. One prepared from animals immunized against the *Streptococcus pyogenes* of erysipelas; not so effective in treatment as the sulfa drugs.

e. bullosum. That attended with formation of bullae.

e. chronicum. A chronic or relapsing erysipelas leading to elephantiasis of the affected part.

e. diffusum. That in which the affected area is not sharply defined, the redness merging gradually with the color of the surrounding skin.

e. glabrum. That in which the skin is tightly stretched and has a smooth, shining appearance.

e. medicamentosum. A rash resembling erysipelas, but marked by rapid development, the absence of well-defined areas, and tenderness on pressure; produced by ingested drugs.

e. migrans. See wandering *e.*

e. perstans. A chronic, erysipelaslike condition of the face.

facial e. Erysipelas of the face; the most common form. After an initial chill, the temperature rises very high and there are severe symptoms of toxemia; there may be vomiting and delirium, and the disease may spread rapidly over a great part of the body. The affected area is swollen, itches, has a deep-red color and an elevated margin, and tends to heal centrally while spreading peripherally.

idiopathic e. That occurring without any visible wound.

phlegmonous e. A form of erysipelas in which there is abscess formation.

pustular e. A variety of erysipelas bullosum in which the bullae contain pus.

serpiginous e. A form which extends by involving neighboring parts of the skin.

spontaneous e. Idiopathic *e.*

surgical e. That occurring in the site of a wound. Also called *traumatic e.*

swine e. An infectious disease of hogs; caused by *Erysipelothrix rhusiopathiae;* occurring in acute, subacute, and chronic forms.

wandering e. A form in which the erysipelatous process successively disappears from one part of the body to appear subsequently in another part.

er″y·sip″e·lo·coc′cus [*erysipelas;* G. *kokkos,* berry]. *Streptococcus erysipelatis,* to which erysipelas is ascribed.

er″y·sip′e·loid [*erysipelas;* G. *eidos,* form]. An infection caused by *Erysipelothrix rhusiopathiae;* occurs on the hands of those who handle infected meat or fish. Characterized by circumscribed, multiple lesions of a red color; erythema is present in some cases.

Er″y·si·pel′o·thrix (err″i·si·pel′o·thricks, err″i-sip′i·lo·) [*erysipelas;* G. *thrix,* hair]. A genus of filamentous, branching bacteria of the family Corynebacteriaceae.

E. rhusiopathiae. The causative organism of swine erysipelas and of erysipeloid in man.

e·rys′i·phake [G. *erysis,* a drawing; *phakos,* lentil]. An instrument shaped like a small spoon, with blunt edges and a long handle, connected with an apparatus for producing a vacuum; used in an operation for cataract known as phacoerisis. Also spelled *erisophake.*

er″y·the′ma [G., redness]. A redness of the skin occurring in patches of variable size and shape. It can be caused by heat, certain drugs, ultraviolet rays, and ionizing radiation. —**erythem′atous** (err″ith·em′uh·tus, ·eem′uh·tus), *adj.*

butterfly e. Skin lesions on the malar eminences in pellagra, hyperemic and edematous at first; later they scale and leave a rough, red area.

choleraic e. Erythema multiforme occurring in cholera patients; affects chiefly the extremities; marked by bluish-red or livid papules.

cholinogenic e. Erythema of the skin produced by efferent cholinergic impulses via the autonomic nervous system.

epidemic arthritic e. An acute, infectious disease; characterized by abrupt onset with chills, fever, back and joint pains; after a few days a rubelliform or morbilliform eruption appears. Syn., *Haverhill fever.*

e. ab igne. An eruption of varying form and color, often with pigmentation; due to prolonged exposure to artificial heat; seen typically on the extremities of stokers.

e. annulare centrifugum. A rare disease characterized by gyrate, annular lesions, with hard, cordlike edges and peripheral enlargement.

e. brucellum. An eruption of papules, vesicles, and pustules; may occur on the arms of individuals coming in contact with cows affected with infectious abortion.

e. bullosum. The bullous type of erythema multiforme.

e. caloricum. Transitory redness of the skin induced by heat.

e. chronicum migrans. An afebrile erythema; appears as a single elevated ring, progressive at the border and healing at the center.

e. chronicum migrans Afzelius. A form of annular peripherally extending erythema progressing from the site of a bite, usually that of a tick.

e. circinatum. A form of erythema multiforme showing lesions with depressed centers and erythematous borders.

e. congestivum. Erythema with congestion of the skin.

e. diffusum. A form resembling scarlatina, with ill-defined outline, the red color of the affected skin merging gradually into that of the surrounding parts.

e. elevatum diutinum. A clinical variety of granuloma annulare; characterized by firm, painless nodules, which, discrete at first, later coalesce to form flat, raised plaques or nodular tumors.

e. endemicum. Pellegra.

e. epidemicum. Erythredema polyneuropathy.

e. figuratum perstans. A form of erythema multiforme with gyrate figures on the skin.

e. fugax. Transitory redness of the skin, possibly urticarial in nature.

e. gangrenosum. A feigned or self-induced eruption. Syn., *dermatitis factitia.*

e. gluteale. An eruption in the napkin or diaper area in children. Also called *Jacquet's e.*

e. gyratum persistens. An eruption characterized by persistent erythematous patches in annular, marginate, or gyrate forms. Syn., *erythema figuratum perstans.*

e. induratum. A chronic recurrent disorder; characterized by deep-seated nodosities and subsequent ulcerations; usually involves the skin of the legs of younger women; often tuberculous. Also called *Bazin's disease.* See Plate 32.

e. infectiosum. Fifth disease; a feebly infectious rash occurring in epidemics as a disease of early childhood; of unknown etiology.

e. intertrigo. Intertrigo; a hyperemia of the skin occurring where the folds of the integument come into contact. The epidermis may be abraded.

e. iris. A variety of erythema multiforme in which the skin lesions appear in variously colored, concentric rings.

e. marginatum. A type of erythema multiforme in which an elevated, well-defined band remains as a sequela of an erythematous patch.

e. migrans. See geographic *tongue.*

e. multiforme. An acute, inflammatory skin disease; characterized by reddish macules, papules, or tubercles; the lesions, varying in appearance, occur usually on neck, face, legs, and dorsal surfaces of hands, forearms, and feet; initial symptoms are often gastric distress and rheumatic pains. Ectodermosis erosiva pluriorificialis and Stevens-Johnson syndrome are clinical variants of erythema multiforme.

e. nodosum. An eruption, usually on the anterior surfaces of the legs below the knees, of pink to blue, tender nodules appearing in crops; more frequently seen in women; often associated with joint pains.

e. nuchae. Redness on the back of the neck seen in early infancy, lasting for a variable time.

e. of ninth day. A morbilliform or scarlatiniform eruption associated with constitutional disturbances; occurs about the ninth day following the administration of arsphenamine.

e. palmaris hereditarum. Condition described by J. E. Lane in which palms showed a bright-red color; considered as a nevus.

e. papulatum. Type of erythema multiforme in which lesions are nodular or papular.

e. paralyticum. Early stage of diffuse idiopathic atrophy of the skin.

e. pernio. A condition occurring, in cold weather only, on hands and feet of individuals with feeble circulation, or following frostbite. Syn., *pernio, chilblain.*

e. perstans. Persisting, recurring erythema; a group including erythema figuratum perstans, erythema annulare centrifugum, erythema simplex gyratum, erythema chronicum migrans.

e. punctatum. See *e.* scarlatiniforme.

e. scarlatiniforme. An eruption from different causes but simulating the rash of scarlet fever. Syn., *e. punctatum, scarlatinoid e.*

e. serpens. See *erysipeloid.*

e. simplex. A hyperemia showing various shades of redness, either diffuse or circumscribed. The symptomatic erythemas may be precursors of systemic disturbances or febrile disorders. Also called *e. hyperemicum.*

e. simplex gyratum. An eruption of circinate and gyrate lesions disappearing after a few days only to be succeeded by fresh outbursts.

e. solare. Sunburn.

e. traumaticum. Redness of the skin produced by trauma.

e. tuberculatum. A type of erythema multiforme in which the lesions are nodular in character.

e. urticans. A type of erythema multiforme in which the lesions are urticarial in appearance.

e. venenatum. Redness of the skin produced by external irritants.

e. vesiculosum. A type of erythema multiforme characterized by vesicles.

lepromatous e. necroticans. See Lucio *leprosy.*

nummular e. Discoid lesions of tinea corporis.

reticulate e. See *e.* ab igne.

scarlatinoid e. See *e.* scarlatiniforme.

symptomatic e. Redness of skin as a surface manifestation of an internal cause. A simple form is blushing.

tertiary circinate e. Skin lesions of pink to red color occurring as circular or oval patches with normal or pigmented centers, or in segments of circles which may form gyrate figures by coalescence; occurring several years after syphilitic infection. Also called *neurosyphilid, circinate syphilitic erythema.*

toxic e. Redness of the skin produced by toxic cause.

variolous e. The initial eruption of variola.

er″y·the′moid, er″y·the′ma·toid [*erythēma;* G. *eidos,* form]. Resembling erythema.

er″y·thral′gi·a. See *erythromelalgia.*

er″y·thras′ma (err″i·thraz′muh) [G. *erythros,* red]. A skin disease seen in the axillas or the inguinal or pubic regions. It forms reddish or brownish, sharply defined, slightly raised, desquamating patches which cause little or no inconvenience. It is due to the fungus *Nocardia minutissima.*

e·ryth″re·de′ma pol″y·neu·rop′a·thy (eh·rith″-ri·dee′muh pol″i·new·rop′uth·ee). A syndrome of uncertain cause, but possibly related to mercury poisoning, occurring in infancy and characterized by pink itching hands and feet, and marked vasomotor and emotional disturbances. There is profuse sweating, photophobia, irritability, tachycardia, and hypertension. Also called *pink disease, acrodynia, Selter's disease, Feer's disease, Swift's disease.*

er″y·thre′mi·a. 1. Erythrocytosis. 2. Primary polycythemia.

acute e. A rare acute disease of the blood-forming organs, characterized by uncontrolled proliferation of the cells of the erythrocytic series, corresponding to, and in later stages often accompanied by, leukemia (*erythroleukemia*). The hematologic picture shows erythrocyte precursors in all stages of maturation; clinically, there is hepatomegaly, splenomegaly, and hemorrhagic diathesis. Syn., *erythromyelosis, acute erythremic myelosis, DiGuglielmo's erythromyelosis* or *disease.*

chronic e. Thalassemia major.

high-altitude e. See chronic mountain *sickness.*

e·ryth′rin. 1. An antibiotic substance derived from animal tissues, apparently from erythrocytes. 2. A chromogen derived from *Roccella tinctoria* and other lichens.

Er″y·thri′na [*erythros*]. A genus of tropical and subtropical trees and shrubs, various species of which have long been used in folk medicine. The seeds of some species contain one or more alkaloids having curarelike action; of these beta-erythroidine and its derivative dihydro-β-erythroidine are potentially of clinical importance.

er′y·thrite (also pronounced e·ryth′rite). Erythritol.

e·ryth′ri·tol. $CH_2OH(CHOH)_2CH_2OH$; 1,2,3,4,-

butanetetrol; a polyhydric alcohol existing as several different optical isomers. The meso- isomer occurs in algae and fungi and is also obtained by synthesis; it occurs in crystals, is very soluble in water, and is about twice as sweet as sucrose. Syn., *erythrol, erythrite.*

e. tetranitrate. Erythrityl tetranitrate.

e·ryth′ri·tyl tet″ra·ni′trate. $C_4H_6(NO_3)_4$; the tetranitrate of erythritol; a vasodilator which gives its maximum effect in about 20 minutes and lasts for five or six hours. Syn., *erythritol tetranitrate, erythrol tetranitrate.*

e·ryth′ro-, er′yth·ro- [*erythros*]. A combining form signifying *red.*

e·ryth′ro·blast [*erythros;* G. *blastos*, germ]. *In hematology,* generally a nucleated precursor of the erythrocyte in which cytoplasmic basophilia is retained. Erythrocytes of the embryo are primitive erythroblasts, those in the fetal liver and in normal bone marrow are definitive erythroblasts. According to size and nuclear characteristics these cells can be divided into early and late forms. —**erythroblas′tic,** *adj.*

acidophilic e. See *normoblast,* 1.

basophilic e. An early *e.*

early e. The earliest form of erythroblast, preceded by the proerythroblast, which may retain nucleoli and which is generally larger than later forms: also called *basophilic e., basophilic* or *early normoblast.*

eosinophilic e. See *normoblast,* 1.

late e. An erythroblast characterized by a less vesicular and smaller nucleus, absence of nucleoli, and incipient cytoplasmic polychromatophilia indicating beginning hemoglobin synthesis. It is generally smaller than the early erythroblast, but larger than the normoblast. Also called *polychromatic e.* Also see *normoblast.*

mitroid e. A temporary type of secondary erythroblast in rat fetuses, shaped like a head wearing a cap.

orthochromatic e. See orthochromatic *normoblast.*

polychromatic e. See late *e.*

e·ryth″ro·blas·to′ma [*erythros; blastos;* G. *-ōma,* tumor]. A tumor of bone marrow which is composed of cells that resemble large erythroblasts.

e·ryth″ro·blas″to·pe′ni·a [*erythros; blastos;* G. *penia,* poverty]. A decrease in number of the erythroblasts in the bone marrow. It may be absolute, due to bone marrow aplasia or erythroid aplasia, or it may be relative, due to hyperplasia of other bone marrow elements. Also see aplastic *anemia.*

e·ryth″ro·blas·to′sis foe·tal′is (fee·tah′lis). A hemolytic anemia of the newborn, characterized by icterus and an increased number of nucleated red blood cells. Occurs when a mother is Rh negative and develops antibodies against the fetus, which is Rh positive.

e·ryth″ro·chlo·ro′pi·a, e·ryth″ro·chlor′o·py, e·ryth″ro·chlo·rop′si·a [*erythros;* G. *chlōros,* green; *ōps,* eye]. A form of subnormal color perception in which green and red are the only colors correctly distinguished.

erythrocin. A trade-mark for the antibiotic substance *erythromycin.*

e·ryth′ro·conte [*erythros;* G. *kontos,* pole]. One of the many fine azurophilic rods found in erythrocytes, and especially in stippled cells.

e·ryth″ro·cru·or′in. Any of the respiratory pigments found in the blood and tissue fluids of some invertebrates; it is an iron-porphyrin protein corresponding to hemoglobin in vertebrates.

e·ryth″ro·cy″a·no′sis [*erythros;* G. *kyanos,* blue; *-ōsis,* condition]. Irregular reddish-blue markings on the skin, usually reticular in arrangement; due to a circulatory disturbance of the skin.

e·ryth′ro·cyte [*erythros;* G. *kytos,* cell]. The nonnucleated and agranular cell of human blood whose oxygen-carrying pigment, hemoglobin, is responsible for the red color of fresh blood. The cell is generally disk-shaped and biconcave. Red blood cells or corpuscles normally are from 5 to 9 microns in diameter (mean 7.2 to 7.8μ), and 1 to 2 microns thick; they number around 5 million per cubic millimeter in the adult, usually slightly less in the female. It is the mature cell of the erythrocytic series. Also called *akaryocyte, erythroplastid, normocyte, rubricyte.* For abnormal forms see *macrocyte, microcyte, elliptocyte, poikilocyte, sickle cell, target cell, anisocytosis, spherocytosis.* See Plate 26. —**erythrocyt′ic,** *adj.*

crenated e. One with indented edges, due to withdrawal of fluid from the inside of the cell.

dichromatic e. One that is slightly immature; a slightly basophilic, nonnucleated erythrocyte.

immature e. See *reticulocyte.*

orthochromatic e. One that stains with acid stains only.

polychromatic e. One that does not stain evenly.

polychromatophilic e. An erythrocyte which contains variable amounts of basophilic staining material giving an appearance of polychromatophilia on Wright-Giemsa-stained blood films. Also see *reticulocyte.*

series e. Any cell of the blood and bone marrow which contains hemoglobin, or which will develop into a cell which contains hemoglobin.

young e. See *reticulocyte.*

e·ryth″ro·cy·the′mi·a (eh·rith″ro·sigh·thee′mee·uh, err″ith·ro·). 1. Erythrocytosis. 2. Primary polycythemia.

e·ryth″ro·cyt′ic se′ries. *In hemopoiesis,* the cells at progressive stages of development from a primitive cell to the mature erythrocyte. Concepts and terminology vary greatly. See under *proerythroblast, erythroblast* (early *e.,* late *e.*), *normoblast, reticulocyte, erythrocyte.* See also *rubriblast, prorubricyte, rubricyte, metarubricyte, prokaryocyte, karyocyte, metakaryocyte.*

e·ryth″ro·cy′to- [*erythros; kytos*]. A combining form signifying *erythrocyte.*

e·ryth″ro·cy′to·blast. See *erythroblast.*

e·ryth″ro·cy″to·ly′sin (·sigh″to·lye′sin, ·sigh·tol′i-sin) [*erythros; kytos;* G. *lysis,* a loosing]. An agent capable of producing erythrocytolysis; hemolysin.

e·ryth″ro·cy·tol′y·sis [*erythros; kytos; lysis*]. The plasmolysis of erythrocytes; the escape of soluble substances and the reduction of the volume of the corpuscle; hemolysis.

e·ryth″ro·cy·tom′e·ter (·sigh·tom′i·tur) [*erythros; kytos;* G. *metron,* a measure]. Hemocytometer. —**erythrocytometry,** *n.*

e·ryth″ro·cy′to-op′so·nin [*erythros; kytos;* G. *opsōnein,* to buy victuals]. A substance which is opsonic for erythrocytes.

e·ryth″ro·cy″to·poi·e′sis [*erythros; kytos;* G. *poiēsis,* production]. The formation or development of erythrocytes. Syn., *erythropoiesis.* See also *erythrocytic series.*

normoblastic e. Greater than normal numbers of normoblasts in erythrocytopoietic tissue.

megaloblastic e. The abnormal development of erythrocytes characteristically seen in deficiency of antianemia factor (erythrocyte maturation factor). The cells are larger and are precursors of the megalocytes of these deficiency syndromes. They are characterized by a discrepancy between nuclear and cytoplasmic maturation.

e·ryth″ro·cy″tor·rhex′is [*erythros; kytos;* G. *rhēxis,* a breaking]. Breaking up or fragmentation of the erythrocytes. Syn., *erythrorrhexis*.

e·ryth″ro·cy·tos′chi·sis (eh·rith″ro·sigh·tos′ki·sis, err″ith·ro·) [*erythros; kytos;* G. *schisis*, cleavage]. The fragmentation or splitting up of erythrocytes into disks resembling blood platelets.

e·ryth″ro·cy·to′sis (·sigh·to′sis) [*erythros; kytos;* G. *-ōsis*, increase]. 1. Increased erythrocyte count of more than two standard deviations above mean normal, as determined by the same method on the bloods of healthy persons of the patient's age and sex, and associated with increased total blood volume: also called *erythremia, erythrocythemia, polycythemia*. 2. An increase in the number of erythrocytes in the fetus and newborn.

anoxemic e. See secondary *polycythemia*.

e. megalosplenica. See primary *polycythemia*.

e·ryth″ro·de·gen′er·a·tive [*erythros;* L. *degenerare*, to degenerate]. Involving degenerative changes in the erythrocytes with increase in ploychromatic basophilic stippling.

e·ryth″ro·der′ma [*erythros;* G. *derma*, skin]. A dermatosis characterized by an abnormal redness of the skin; erythema: also spelled *erythrodermia*.

e. desquamativa. A generalized redness and scaly eruption seen in children. The nails, scalp, and intestinal tract are usually involved. May be fatal. Differentiated from dermatitis exfoliativa. Also called *Leiner's disease*.

e. ichthyosiforme congenitum. A type of congenital dermatosis in which there is a thickening and reddening of the skin, and a tendency to resemble lichen.

e. maculosa perstans. A plaquelike variety of psoriasis in which the areas involved are about one-half inch in diameter and without marked desquamation.

e. psoriaticum. Generalized psoriasis, with an increase in the inflammatory changes.

exfoliative e. A dermatosis having a scarlatiniform eruption lasting from six to eight weeks, with free desquamation. See *pityriasis* rubra.

e·ryth″ro·dex′trin. A dextrin formed by the partial hydrolysis of starch with acid or amylase. It yields a red color with iodine.

e·ryth″ro·gen′e·sis [*erythros;* G. *genesis*, production]. The formation of erythrocytes.

e·ryth′ro·gone, e·ryth″ro·go′ni·um. A basophilic leptochromatic precursor of an erythroblast or a megaloblast; a stem cell.

er′y·throid [*erythros;* G. *eidos*, form.] Reddish; of a red color: used of cells of the *erythrocytic series*.

e·ryth′roi·dine (eh·rith′roy·deen, ·din). An alkaloid, $C_{16}H_{19}NO_3$, obtained from species of *Erythrina*. It occurs in α- and β-varieties, both of which are crystalline compounds easily soluble in water or alcohol. It has a curarelike action of short duration. β-Erythroidine and its derivative dihydro-β-erythroidine are potentially useful because of their curarelike action.

er′y·throl. 1. Erythritol. 2. 3-Butene-1,2-diol; $CH_2OH.CHOH.CH{:}CH_2$.

e. tetranitrate. Erythrityl tetranitrate.

e·ryth″ro·leu·ke′mi·a. See *erythremia*.

e·ryth″ro·leu″ko·blas·to′sis (·lew″ko·blas·to′sis) [*erythros; leukos;* G. *blastos*, germ; *-ōsis*, increase]. Erythroblastosis foetalis with changes in leukocytes.

e·ryth″ro·leu·ko′sis (eh·rith″ro·lew·ko′sis, err″ith·ro·) [*erythros;* G. *leukōsis*, a whitening]. A condition characterized by an increase in the number of immature erythrocytes and leukocytes in the blood: also called *leukanemia, panmyelosis*.

er″y·throl′y·sin (err″i·throl′i·sin, eh·rith″ro·lye′sin). Erythrocytolysin; hemolysin.

er″y·throl′y·sis [*erythros;* G. *lysis*, a loosing]. Erythrocytolysis.

e·ryth″ro·me·lal′gi·a [*erythros;* G. *melos*, limb; *algos*, pain]. A cutaneous vasodilatation of the feet or, more rarely, of the hands; characterized by redness, mottling, changes in skin temperature, and neuralgic pains. It is thought to be an angioneurosis of the sympathetic system, of unknown etiology. Also called *acromelalgia, Mitchell's disease*.

e. of the head. See histamine *headache*.

e·ryth″ro·me′li·a [*erythros; melos*]. A condition of the extensor surfaces of the arms and legs; characterized by painless progressive redness of the skin; distinct from erythromelalgia.

er″y·throm′e·ter [*erythros;* G. *metron*, a measure]. Apparatus for measuring degrees of redness. *Rare*.

e·ryth″ro·my′cin. An antibiotic substance isolated from cultures of the red-pigment-producing organism *Streptomyces erythreus;* it is a basic compound having the empirical formula $C_{39}H_{73-75}NO_{13}$. Erythromycin is effective orally against many Gram-positive and some Gram-negative pathogens. See *erythrocin, ilotycin*.

e·ryth″ro·my″e·lo′sis. Acute erythremia.

er′y·thron. *In hematology*, a concept of the erythrocytes, their precursors, and the erythropoietic bone marrow, as one functional organ unit affected in a great variety of disorders.

e·ryth″ro·ne″o·cy·to′sis (·nee″o·sigh·to′sis) [*erythros;* G. *neos*, new; *kytos*, cell; *-ōsis*, condition]. The presence of regenerative forms of erythrocytes in the circulating blood.

Er″y·thro′ni·um [G. *erythronion*, from *erythros*]. A genus of plants of the Liliaceae.

E. americanum. A species indigenous to the United States; the dried plant is emetic in large doses.

e·ryth″ro·no·cla′si·a. Destruction of erythrocytes, not only in circulating blood, but also in the hematopoietic tissues.

er″y·thro·pe′ni·a [*erythros;* G. *penia*, poverty]. Deficiency in the number of erythrocytes.

e·ryth′ro·phage [*erythros;* G. *phagein*, to eat]. A phagocytic cell containing ingested erythrocytes. Syn., *macrophage, histiocyte*.

e·ryth″ro·pha′gi·a. See *erythrophagocytosis*.

e·ryth″ro·pha″go·cy·to′sis [*erythros; phagein; kytos; -ōsis*]. The ingestion of an erythrocyte by a phagocytic cell, such as a blood monocyte or a tissue macrophage.

e·ryth′ro·phil [*erythros;* G. *philein*, to love]. 1. Auerbach's term for the red-staining nuclear substance of cells. 2. Eosinophil; acidophil; having an affinity for a red dye. —**erythroph′ilous,** *adj*.

e·ryth″ro·phle′ine (eh·rith″ro·flee′een, ·in, err″ith·ro·, err″ith·rof′lee·een, ·in). An alkaloid from casca bark having a digitalislike action.

e·ryth″ro·phle′um [*erythros;* G. *phloios*, bark]. Casca bark.

e·ryth″ro·pho′bi·a [*erythros;* G. *phobos*, fear]. 1. Morbid intolerance or fear of red colors; may be associated with a fear of blood. 2. Fear of blushing. Syn., *ereuthophobia*.

e·ryth′ro·phose (eh·rith′ro·fohz, err′ith·ro·) [*erythros;* G. *phōs*, light]. A red phose.

er″y·thro′pi·a. See *erythropsia*.

e·ryth″ro·pla′si·a of Quey·rat′ (eh·rith″ro·play′zhuh uv kay·rah′, ·play′zee·uh, ·play′shuh, ·play′see·uh, err″ith·ro·. *See* NOTES §§ 29, 30, 35). A condition characterized by a circumscribed, erythematous, velvety lesion affecting mucocutaneous junctions or mucosa of the mouth, tongue, vulva, glans penis, or prepuce. Considered precancerous to squamous-cell carcinoma.

e·ryth″ro·plas′tid [*erythros;* G. *plassein,* to form]. See *erythrocyte.*

e·ryth″ro·poi·e′sis. See *erythrocytopoiesis.*

er″y·throp′si·a, er″y·thro′pi·a [*erythros;* G. *opsis,* vision]. An abnormality of vision in which all objects appear red; red vision.

er″y·throp′sin. Visual purple. See *rhodopsin.*

er″y·thror·rhex′is. See *erythrocytorrhexis.*

e·ryth″ro·sar·co′ma. An erythrocytic proliferation, with polycythemia, multiple metastatic lesions, and fatal termination.

er′y·throse. The tetrose sugar CHO.CHOH.-CHOH.CH_2OH, existing in D- and L- forms, variously obtained.

e·ryth′ro·sin (eh·rith′ro·sin, err″ith·ro′sin), **e·ryth′ro·sine** (eh·rith′ro·seen, ·sin, err″ith·ro′-seen, ·sin). A red dye; an iodine derivative of fluorescein.

e., yellowish. Di-iodofluorescein; a valuable counterstain after Delafield's hematoxylin or methylene blue. Also called *e. R* or *G, pyrosin J, dianthin G, iodoeosin G.*

e·ryth′ro·sin B (C.C.). Tetraiodofluorescein; used as a counterstain. Also called *bluish e., pyrosin B, eosin J, iodoeosin B, dianthin B.*

e·ryth′ro·sin BB (C.C.). See *phloxine.*

e·ryth″ro·sin′o·phil [*erythros;* G. *philein,* to love]. Easily stainable with erythrosin.

e·ryth·ro′sis. 1. Overproliferation of erythrocytopoietic tissue as found in polycythemia. 2. The unusual red skin color of individuals with polycythemia.

e·ryth″ro·sta′sis. The processes to which erythrocytes are subjected when denied free access to fresh plasma, resulting from stasis of the blood.

er″y·throx′y·lon. Coca.

e·ryth′ru·lose. The tetrose sugar CH_2OH.CO.-CHOH.CH_2OH, existing in D- and L- forms, variously obtained; the sugars are isomeric with the corresponding erythroses.

er″y·thru′ri·a [*erythros;* G. *ouron,* urine]. Passage of red urine.

Esbach's method. See under *method.*

Esbach's reagent. See under *reagent.*

es·cape′ [OF. *escaper*]. *In medicine,* leakage or outflow, as of nervous impulses.

vagal e. One or more spontaneous beats of the heart, occurring in spite of the fact that the function of the sinus node that normally initiates heart beats has been arrested by stimulation of the vagus nerve.

ventricular e. See *ventricular escape.*

es·cape′ mech′a·nism. A mode of adjustment to difficult and/or unpleasant situations by utilizing a means easier or pleasanter than that required for a permanent solution of the difficulty, often resulting in an evasion of responsibility

es′char (ess′kahr) [G. *eschara,* scab]. A dry slough, especially that produced by heat or a corrosive or caustic substance.

es″cha·rot′ic (ess″kuh·rot′ick) [*eschara*]. Caustic; producing a slough. —**escharo′sis,** *n.*

es·cha·rot′ic. A substance that produces an eschar; a caustic or corrosive.

eschatin. Trade-mark for an extract of the suprarenal cortex.

Esch″er·ich′i·a (esh″ur·ick′ee·uh) [NL., after Theodor *Escherich,* 1857–1911, German physician]. A genus of nonsporeforming, Gram-negative bacteria, widely distributed in nature.

E. coli. A normal inhabitant of the intestine of man and all vertebrates. It occasionally causes peritonitis and infections of the urinary tract. Formerly called *Bacillus coli.* Also called *colon bacillus.*

E. foetida. Old term for *Salmonella foetida.*

es″chro·la′li·a (ess″kro·lay′lee·uh). See *coprolalia.*

es·cor′cin. Escorcinol, $C_9H_8O_4$, prepared by the action of sodium amalgam on esculetin. A brown powder soluble in alkalies to give a green solution which quickly changes to red. One drop of a 10–20% aqueous solution is used in observation of corneal defects and lesions of the conjunctival epithelium; it imparts a red color to the lesions.

es″cu·le′tin, es·cu′le·tin. 6,7-Dihydroxycoumarin, $C_9H_6O_4$. A cleavage product of esculin.

es′cu·lin. A glycoside, $C_{15}H_{16}O_9.1\frac{1}{2}H_2O$, from the bark of the horse chestnut, *Aesculus hippocastanum.* Being fluorescent, it absorbs ultraviolet rays which are then gradually given off. It has been used as a protective against the sun and in heliotherapy.

es·cutch′eon [L. *scutum,* shield]. The pattern of the pubic hair growth which differs in men and women.

-ese [from *-ase,* diastase, from G. *diastasis,* separation]. *In biochemistry,* a suffix denoting *an enzyme which exerts a synthetic action.*

e·ser′a·mine. $C_{16}H_{25}N_4O_3$; an alkaloid from Calabar beans.

e·ser′i·dine (eh·serr′i·deen, ·din). An alkaloid, $C_{15}H_{21}O_3N_3$, found in Calabar beans. Syn., *geneserine.*

es′er·ine (ess′ur·een, ·in). Physostigmine.

eskadiazine. Trade-mark for an orange-flavored aqueous suspension of sulfadiazine.

Esmarch, Johann Friedrich August von [*German military surgeon,* 1823–1908]. Celebrated in surgical annals for his introduction of the first-aid packet for use on the battlefield (1869). Devised the widely used rubber bandage and tourniquet, a pure rubber elastic bandage about three inches in width, of great value in operations upon limbs where a bloodless field is desired. His name is associated also with a chloroform inhaler which consists of a drop bottle and a wire frame over which is stretched a double layer of gauze; adapted to the open method of ether inhalation. He devised a number of operations, including an amputation at the hip joint, which bore his name.

e·soph″a·gal′gi·a [G. *oisophagos,* gullet; *algos,* pain]. Pain in the esophagus.

e·soph″a·gec·ta′si·a (i·sof″uh·jeck·tay′zhuh, ·zee·uh, ·shuh, ·see·uh), **e·soph″a·gec·ta′sis** (i·sof″uh·jeck·tay′sis, ·jeck′tuh·sis) [*oisophagos;* G. *ektasis,* extension]. Idiopathic dilatation of the esophagus.

e·soph″a·gec′to·my [*oisophagos;* G. *ektomē,* excision]. Surgical resection of part of the esophagus.

e·soph″a·gec′to·py [*oisophagos;* G. *ektopos,* away from a place]. Displacement of the esophagus.

e·soph′a·gism, e·soph″a·gis′mus (i·sof″uh·jiz′-mus, ·jiss′mus). See *esophagospasm.*

e·soph″a·gi′tis [*oisophagos;* G. *-itis,* inflammation]. Inflammation of the esophagus.

e·soph′a·go-, oe·soph′a·go- (i·sof′uh·go-), **e·soph′a·g-, oe·soph′a·g-** [*oisophagos*]. A combining form denoting *relation to the esophagus.*

e·soph″a·go·du″o·de·nos′to·my (i·sof″uh·go-dew″o·di·nos′to·mee, ·dew·od″i·nos′to·mee). See *esophagoenterostomy.*

e·soph″a·go·en″ter·os′to·my [*oisophagos;* G. *enteron,* intestine; *stoma,* mouth]. Total gastrectomy, with suture of the cardiac end of the esophagus to the duodenum (**esophagoduodenostomy**) or to the jejunum (**esophagojejunostomy**).

e·soph″a·go·e·soph″a·gos′to·my [*oisophagos;* G. *stoma,* mouth]. The surgical reunion of the esophagus after removal of an intervening portion.

e·soph″a·go·gas·trec′to·my [*oisophagos;* G. *gastēr,* belly; *ektomē,* excision]. Excision of parts of the stomach and esophagus.

e·soph″a·go·gas′tro·plas″ty [*oisophagos; gastēr;* G. *plassein,* to form]. Surgical repair of the stomach and esophagus.

e·soph″a·go·gas′tro·scope [*oisophagos; gastēr;* G. *skopein,* to examine]. An instrument for examining the interior of the esophagus and the stomach. —**esophagogastros′copy,** *n.*

e·soph″a·go·gas·tros′to·my [*oisophagos; gastēr;* G. *stoma,* mouth]. The surgical establishment of an anastomosis between the esophagus and the stomach; may be performed by the abdominal route or by transpleural operation.

e·soph″a·go·je″ju·nos′to·my (i·sof″uh·go·jee″-jew·nos′to·mee, ·jedj″oo·nos′to·mee). See *esophagoenterostomy.*

e·soph″a·gom′e·ter [*oisophagos;* G. *metron,* a measure]. An instrument for measuring the esophagus.

e·soph″a·gop′a·thy [*oisophagos;* G. *pathos,* disease]. Any disease of the esophagus.

e·soph′a·go·plas″ty (i·sof′uh·go·plas″tee, i·sof″-uh·go·plas′tee, ee″so·fag′o·plas″tee) [*oisophagos;* G. *plassein,* to form]. Plastic surgery of the esophagus.

e·soph″a·gop·to′sis [*oisophagos;* G. *ptōsis,* a falling]. Prolapse of the esophagus.

e·soph′a·go·scope″ (i·sof′uh·go·scope″, ee″so-fag′o·) [*oisophagos;* G. *skopein,* to examine]. An electrically illuminated instrument for direct visualization of the interior of the esophagus. —**esophagos′copy,** *n.*

e·soph′a·go·spasm (i·sof′uh·go·spaz·um, ee″so-fag′o·) [*oisophagos;* G. *spasma,* spasm]. Spasmodic contraction of the esophagus.

e·soph″a·go·ste·no′sis [*oisophagos;* G. *stenōsis,* a being straitened]. Constriction of the esophagus.

e·soph″a·gos′to·ma [*oisophagos;* G. *stoma,* mouth]. An abnormal aperture or passage into the esophagus.

e·soph″a·gos″to·mi′a·sis [*oisophagos; stoma;* NL. *-iasis,* condition]. Infestation with *Œsophagostomum.*

e·soph″a·gos′to·my [*oisophagos; stoma*]. The formation of an artificial opening in the esophagus.

e. externa. The surgical opening of the esophagus from the surface of the neck; for the removal of foreign bodies.

e. interna. Incision of the esophagus from the inside by means of the esophagotome; for relief of stricture.

e″so·phag′o·tome (ee″so·fag′o·tohm, i·sof′uh·go-tohm″) [*oisophagos;* G. *tomos,* cutting]. Instrument devised for cutting into the esophagus.

e·soph″a·got′o·my [*oisophagos;* G. *tomē,* a cutting]. Opening of the esophagus by an incision.

e·soph′a·gus, oe·soph′a·gus [*oisophagos*]. The gullet; the musculomembranous canal, about nine inches in length, extending from the pharynx to the stomach. See Plate 12. —**esophag′eal,** *adj.*

e·soph′o·gram, e·soph′a·go·gram. Radiographic image of the esophagus, obtained by outlining its lumen with a radiopaque contrast material, such as barium sulfate suspension.

es″o·pho′ri·a [G. *esō,* within; *phoros,* bearing]. Form of heterophoria in which the visual lines tend inward.

es″o·tro′pi·a [*esō;* G. *tropē,* a turning]. Convergent concomitant strabismus; one eye fixes upon an object and the other deviates inward.

ESP Extrasensory perception.

es·pun′di·a. South American *leishmaniasis.*

Esquirol, Jean Étienne Dominique [*French psychiatrist,* 1772–1840]. Remembered for his influence on the care of the insane in France. Founded 10 asylums and contributed a classical study and description of paresis (1838).

ESR Erythrocyte sedimentation rate.

es′sence [L. *essentia,* essence]. 1. That which gives to anything its character or peculiar quality. 2. A solution of an essential oil in alcohol.

es·sen′tial [*essentia*]. 1. Pertaining to the essence of a substance. 2. Of diseases, idiopathic; occurring without a known cause.

Esser, Johannes Fredericus Samuel [*Dutch plastic surgeon,* 1877–1946]. Known for his ingenuity in devising reconstructive technics in plastic surgery, and especially for his epithelial inlay graft known as the *Esser inlay.* See inlay *graft.*

es′ter. A compound formed from an alcohol and an acid by elimination of water, as ethyl acetate, $CH_3CO.OC_2H_5$.

Harden-Young e. Fructose-1,6-diphosphate.

Neuberg e. Fructose-6-phosphate.

es′ter·ase (ess′tur·ace, ·aze). Any enzyme which catalyzes the hydrolysis of an ester into an alcohol and an acid. See Table of Enzymes in the Appendix.

acetylcholine e. An enzyme found in the blood which rapidly hydrolyzes any excess of acetylcholine to acetic acid and choline.

es·ter″i·fi·ca′tion. The process of converting an alcohol or an acid to an ester.

es·the′si·a (ess·thee′zhuh, ·zee·uh) [G. *aisthēsis,* feeling]. Capacity for perception, feeling, or sensation. Opposed to *anesthesia.*

es·the′si·o-, aes·the′si·o- (ess·thee′zee·o-, ·see·o-) [*aisthēsis*]. A combining form meaning *pertaining to the perceptive faculties.*

es·the″si·ol′o·gy [*aisthēsis;* G. *logos,* word]. The science of the senses and sensations.

es·the″si·om′e·ter [*aisthēsis;* G. *metron,* a measure]. An instrument for measuring tactile sensibility.

es·the″si·o·neu″ro·blas·to′ma. See *neuroepithelioma.*

es·the″si·o·neu″ro·ep″i·the·li·o′ma. See *neuroepithelioma.*

es·the″si·o·phys″i·ol′o·gy [*aisthēsis;* G. *physis,* nature; *logos*]. The physiology of sensation and the sense organs.

es·thet′ic [G. *aisthētikos,* perceptive]. Pertaining to the senses.

es″thi·om′e·ne (ess″thee·om′i·nee) [G. *esthiomenos,* from *esthiein,* to eat]. A term applied to the chronic ulcerative lesion of the vulva in venereal lymphogranuloma.

Estienne, Charles (Carolus Stephanus) [*French publisher and bookseller,* ca. 1504–64]. Remembered for his illustrated works on normal and pathologic anatomy, containing noteworthy plates of both the venous and the nervous systems (1545).

estinyl. Trade-mark for ethynyl estradiol.

es′ti·val, aes′ti·val (es′ti·vul, es·tye′vul) [L. *aestivus,* pertaining to summer]. Of, or belonging to, the summer.

es″ti·va′tion [L. *aestivare,* to pass the summer]. 1. The adaptation of certain animals to the conditions of summer, or the taking on of certain modifications, which enables them to survive a hot dry summer. 2. The dormant condition of an organism during the summer.

estivin. A proprietary liquid preparation of *Rosa gallica;* used to relieve congestion of the conjunctiva and nasal mucosa.

Estlander, Jakob August [*Finnish surgeon,* 1831–81]. Widely known for his radical surgical treatment of chronic empyema by resection of portions of several ribs to produce obliteration of the cavity; the precursor of modern thoracoplasty.

Devised also an operation for plastic repair of the upper lip.

es·tra·di'ol. $C_{18}H_{24}O_2$; 3,17-dihydroxy-1,3,5-estratriene; an estrogenic hormone secreted in the ovarian follicular fluid and placenta; it occurs in pregnancy urines. Two isomers exist; the active isomer was originally designated *alpha*-estradiol, the other *beta*-estradiol. Structural studies show that *alpha*-estradiol is actually 17β-estradiol, and that *beta*-estradiol is 17α-estradiol. Syn., *dihydrotheelin.* See Table of Hormones in the Appendix.

e. benzoate. Estradiol-3-benzoate, a white, crystalline powder, insoluble in water but sparingly soluble in vegetable oils. It is an intramuscular dosage form of estradiol.

e. dipropionate. Estradiol in which both hydroxyl groups are esterified with propionic acid. It is injected intramuscularly, and is claimed to maintain a more prolonged effect than any other estrogen.

ethinyl e., ethynyl e. $C_{20}H_{24}O_2$. An orally active, synthetic estrogen. See *estinyl, lynoral.*

es'trane. $C_{18}H_{30}$; the saturated parent hydrocarbon of estrone, estradiol, estratriol, and related estrogenic steroids.

es·tri'a·sis. Variant spelling for oestriasis.

es'trin. Old term for estrogen.

es'tri·ol (es'tree·ole, ·ol, ·awl, es'try·, es·try'·). $C_{18}H_{24}O_3$. A crystalline estrogenic hormone, 3,16,-17-trihydroxy-1,3,5-estratriene, from human pregnancy urine. Formerly called *theelol.* See Table of Hormones in the Appendix.

estrobene. Trade name for a brand of diethylstilbestrol.

es'tro·gen [G. *oistros,* gadfly; *genesthai,* from *gignesthai,* to be produced]. Any substance possessing the biologic activity of estrus-producing hormones, either occurring naturally or prepared synthetically. —**estrogen'ic,** *adj.*

es'trone. $C_{18}H_{22}O_2$. 3-Hydroxy-17-keto-1,3,5-estratriene. An estrogenic hormone present in the ovary, adrenal glands, placenta, and urine. Syn., *theelin, folliculin.* See Table of Hormones.

e. sulfate. A naturally occurring conjugated form of estrone, in which the hydroxyl group of the latter is esterified with sulfuric acid. The sodium salt of estrone sulfate is soluble in water, and is the principal estrogen in certain commercial products.

es"tru·a'tion, oes"tru·a'tion. Estrus.

es'trum, oes'trum. See *estrus.*

es'trus, oes'trus (es'trus) [*oistros*]. 1. Sexual desire in the lower animals; the mating period of animals, especially of the female; heat; rut. 2. The whole sequence of changes in the uterine mucosa of animals, corresponding to the various phases of ovarian activity. —**estrous, estrual,** *adj.*

es"tu·a'ri·um [L. *aestuarium,* from *aestus,* swell of the sea, boiling, heat]. A vapor bath.

etalate. Trade name for a sclerosing solution containing ethylamine oleate and benzyl alcohol.

etamon chloride. Trade-mark for tetraethylammonium chloride, $(C_2H_5)_4NCl$, available in solution for parenteral use. See *tetraethylammonium.*

é·tat' mar·bré' (ay·tah' mar·bray'). See *status marmoratus.*

eth'an·al. Formaldehyde.

eth'ane [G. *aithēr,* ether, the heaven]. C_2H_6. A saturated, gaseous hydrocarbon, $CH_3.CH_3$; found in natural and illuminating gas. Syn., *methylmethane.*

eth"ane·di·o'ic ac'id. Oxalic acid.

eth"a·no'ic ac'id. Acetic acid.

eth'a·nol. Ethyl alcohol.

eth"a·nol'a·mine. Cholamine.

eth'ene. Ethylene.

eth'e·noid. Resembling ethylene in containing a double bond.

eth'e·none. Ketene.

e'ther, ae'ther [*aithēr*]. 1. An all-pervading and permeating medium, formerly believed to exist and to transmit light and similar energy. 2. A compound formed hypothetically from H_2O by the substitution of two hydrocarbon radicals for the H. 3. Ethyl ether $(C_2H_5)_2O$; a thin, colorless, volatile, and highly inflammable liquid. The ether of the U.S.P. contains 96–98% by weight of $(C_2H_5)_2O$, the remainder consisting of alcohol and water; its specific gravity at 25° C. is 0.713–0.716. Its chief use is as an anesthetic. Also called *ethyl oxide, sulfuric ether, diethyl ether, diethyl oxide,* although the United States Pharmacopeia recognizes as *ethyl oxide* a less pure form of the substance for use as a solvent and other nonanesthetic purposes. —**ethe'real,** *adj.*

absolute e. Ether, 3, containing no alcohol or water.

anesthetic e. Ethyl ether. See *ether,* 3.

compound e. spirit. A solution containing 32.5% ethyl oxide, and 2.5% of ethereal oil, by volume, in alcohol. Used as an anodyne and antispasmodic. Also called *Hoffmann's anodyne.*

diethyl e. Ether, 3.

diethylene glycol monoethyl e. See *carbitol,* 1.

e. spirit. A solution containing 32.5% by volume of ethyl oxide in alcohol; used like compound ether spirit. Also called *Hoffmann's drops.*

ethyl e. See *ethyl* ether.

isopropenyl vinyl e. See *isopropenyl* vinyl ether.

nitrous e. See *nitrous* ether.

propenyl ethyl e. See *propenyl* ethyl ether.

propethylene e. See *propethylene* ether.

vinyl e. CH_2:CH.O.CH:CH_2. An inhalation anesthetic used for short operations. The recovery is usually quick and uneventful. Syn., *divinyl oxide, vinethene.*

e'ther·ide. A comprehensive term for any combination of formyl with a haloid.

e·ther"i·fi·ca'tion [*aithēr;* L. *facere,* to make]. The formation of an ether from an alcohol. —**ether'ify,** *v.t.*

e"ther·i·za'tion [*aithēr*]. The administration of ether to produce anesthesia. —**e'therize,** *v.t.*

eth'ics [G. *ethikos,* from *ethos,* custom, habit]. A system of moral principles.

medical e. Principles of medical conduct; duties a physician owes to himself, his profession, and his fellow men.

eth'i·dene. Ethylidene.

eth'ine. Ethyne or acetylene.

eth'i·nyl. Ethynyl.

17-eth·i·nyl"tes·tos'ter·one, 17-eth·y·nyl"tes·tos'ter·one. Anhydrohydroxyprogesterone or ethisterone.

e·thi'o·nine. $C_2H_5.S.(CH_2)_2.CHNH_2.COOH$; the ethyl homolog of methionine; it inhibits growth of experimental animals, presumably by interfering with the metabolism of methionine.

e·this'ter·one. Currently official title for *anhydrohydroxyprogesterone.*

eth'mo- [G. *ēthmos,* sieve]. A combining form signifying *ethmoid.*

eth"mo·ceph'a·lus [*ēthmos;* G. *kephalē,* head]. A variety of cebocephalus with a rudimentary nose similar to a proboscis, which terminates anteriorly in two imperfect nostrils or in a single opening.

eth"mo·fron'tal [*ēthmos;* L. *frons,* forehead]. Relating to the ethmoid and frontal bones.

eth'moid [*ēthmos;* G. *eidos,* form]. A bone of the base of the skull perforated for the olfactory nerves and forming the upper bony nose. See Plate 12.

See Table of Bones in the Appendix. —**ethmoid, ethmoi'dal,** *adj.*

eth"moid·ec'to·my [*ēthmos; eidos;* G. *ektomē,* excision]. Surgical removal of the ethmoid sinuses or part of the ethmoid bone.

transmaxillary e. Ethmoidectomy by incision through canine fossa and maxillary sinus, preserving the mucous membrane of the lateral nasal wall. Also called *De Lima operation.*

eth"moid·i'tis [*ēthmos; eidos;* G. *-itis,* inflammation]. Inflammation of the ethmoid bone or of the ethmoid sinuses.

eth"moid·ot'o·my [*ēthmos; eidos;* G. *tomē,* a cutting]. Incision of an ethmoid sinus.

eth"mo·lac'ri·mal [*ēthmos;* L. *lacrima,* tear]. Relating to the ethmoid and lacrimal bones.

eth"mo·max'il·lar"y (eth"mo·mack'si·lerr"ee) [*ēthmos;* L. *maxilla,* jaw]. Pertaining to the ethmoid and the maxillary bone.

eth"mo·na'sal [*ēthmos;* L. *nasus,* nose]. Pertaining to the ethmoid and the nasal bones.

eth"mo·tur'bi·nal [*ēthmos;* L. *turbo,* whirl]. Relating to the turbinal portions of the ethmoid bone, forming what are known as the superior and middle turbinates.

eth'nic [G *ethnos,* nation]. Pertaining to races, and peoples, and to their traits and customs.

eth·nog'ra·phy [*ethnos;* G. *graphein,* to write]. A branch of anthropology concerned with the geographic distribution of mankind and description of the physical types of races and peoples.

eth·nol'o·gy [*ethnos;* G. *logos,* word]. The study of mankind, including the origins of races and peoples, their distribution, and their classification according to physical types and linguistic families.

eth'o·caine hy"dro·chlo'ride. British Pharmacopoeia synonym for *procaine hydrochloride.*

ethocel. Trade-mark for *ethyl cellulose.*

eth"o·hex"a·di'ol. $CH_3CH_2CH_2CH(OH)CH(C_2H_5)CH_2OH$; 2-ethylhexane-1,3-diol, a colorless, oily liquid: used as an insect repellent and toxicant. Syn., *Rutgers 612.*

eth"o·pro'pa·zine hy"dro·chlo'ride. Approved British generic name for *profenamine hydrochloride.*

eth·ox'y. The radical C_2H_5O—.

eth·ox"y·caf'fe·ine (eth·ock"si·kaf'ee·in, ·een). $C_{10}H_{14}O_3N_4$. A white to yellowish crystalline powder formerly used as an analgesic and local anesthetic.

eth'yl. The monovalent radical, C_2H_5—.

e. acetate. $CH_3CO.OC_2H_5$. A colorless, pleasantly odorous liquid used chiefly as a solvent and in artificial fruit essences. Syn., *acetic ether.*

e. acetoacetate. See *acetoacetic ester.*

e. alcohol. See *alcohol,* 2.

e. aminobenzoate (*aethylis aminobenzoas*). $H_2N.C_6H_4.CO.OC_2H_5$. A white, crystalline powder soluble in 2500 parts of water, in 5 parts of alcohol, or in 30 to 50 parts of olive oil or expressed almond oil. It is a local anesthetic of low toxicity used chiefly in dusting powders and ointments. In suppositories it is of value in relieving the pain of hemorrhoids. Internally it is used in gastralgia and to stop vomiting due to gastric irritation. Dose, 0.2–0.5 Gm. (3–8 gr.). Syn., *benzocaine.* See *anesthesin.*

e. bromide. C_2H_5Br. A rapid and transient anesthetic more dangerous than ethyl chloride.

e. biscoumacetate. British generic name for *bis*-3,3'-(4-oxycoumarinyl)ethyl acetate, an anticoagulant. See *tromexan.*

e. carbamate (*aethylis carbamas*). $H_2N.CO.-OC_2H_5$. Colorless crystals or granular powder easily soluble in water or alcohol. A somnifacient of uncertain power. It has been employed successfully in treating myeloid and lymphatic leukemia, and has brought about disappearance of nodules of anaplastic undifferentiated cancer. Dose, 1–3 Gm. (15–45 gr.). It increases the solubility of quinine salts. Syn., *urethane.*

e. cellulose. The ethyl ether of cellulose, useful as a dispersing agent and to increase viscosity in aqueous systems. A 4–5% solution in a mixture of three parts of ether and one of alcohol has been suggested under the name ethyl collodion as a vehicle for many externally applied medicaments. See *ethocel.*

e. chaulmoograte (*aethylis chaulmoogras*). The ethyl esters of the mixed acids of chaulmoogra oil, chiefly chaulmoogric and hydnocarpic; used in leprosy. Dose, oral or intramuscular, 0.5–4.6 cc. (8–70 min.).

e. chloride (*aethylis chloridum*). $CH_3.CH_2Cl$. A colorless liquid boiling between 12° and 13° C. It acts as a local anesthetic of short duration through the superficial freezing produced by its rapid vaporization from the skin. It is occasionally used by inhalation as a rapid and fleeting general anesthetic, comparable to nitrous oxide but somewhat more dangerous.

e. chlorophyllide. The chief constituent of crystalline chlorophyll.

e. diacetate. Acetoacetic ester.

e. ether. Ether, 3.

e. formate. $HCOOC_2H_5$. A colorless liquid of aromatic odor used as a fumigant and larvicide and in organic syntheses.

e. green. See *brilliant green.*

e. iodide. $CH_3.CH_2I$. Colorless liquid which reddens with age. Has been used by inhalation in bronchial asthma, etc.

e. iodophenylundecylate. See *iophendylate injection.*

e. nitrite. $C_2H_5O.NO$. A pale yellow liquid of pleasant ethereal odor, boiling at 18° C. Syn., *nitrous ether.*

e. nitrite spirit (*spiritus aethylis nitritis*). An alcoholic solution of 3.5–4.5% of ethyl nitrite. A popular diaphoretic in mild fevers. Dose, 2–4 cc. (30–60 min.). Also called *spirit of nitrous ether, sweet spirit of niter.*

e. oxide. Ether, 3.

e. parahydroxybenzoate. A preservative.

e. salicylate. $HO.C_6H_4.COOC_2H_5$; a liquid, slightly soluble in water, miscible with alcohol; its odor resembles that of methyl salicylate, and the liquid is used similarly.

e. valerate. $CH_3(CH_2)_3COOC_2H_5$; a liquid which has been used as an antispasmodic and sedative in asthma.

e. vanillate. $C_6H_3.OCH_3.OH.COOC_2H_5$; ethyl 4-hydroxy-3-methoxybenzoate; the ethyl ester of vanillic acid. It is a fungicide and has been found useful in the treatment of histoplasmosis, being administered in 40% solution in olive oil by gavage. Not to be confused with *ethyl vanillin.*

e. vanillin. $CHO.C_6H_3.OC_2H_5.OH$; 3-ethoxy-4-hydroxybenzaldehyde, occurring as white or slightly yellowish crystals, sparingly soluble in water. It has a finer and more intense vanilla odor and taste than has vanillin, and is used as a flavor. Not to be confused with *ethyl vanillate.*

17-eth"yl·an'dro·stane. Allopregnane.

eth'yl·ate. A compound of ethyl alcohol in which the H of the hydroxyl is replaced by a base.

eth"yl·a'tion. The introduction of an ethyl group into a compound.

eth'yl·ene (*aethylenum*). Ethene, olefiant gas, C_2H_4. A colorless gas of slightly sweet odor and taste; used as an inhalation anesthetic. The ripening of certain fruits is hastened by its application.

e. glycol. $HOCH_2CH_2OH$. A colorless, viscid, hygroscopic liquid of sweet taste. It has been used in the manufacture of some pharmaceutical products intended only for external use. It is markedly toxic. Also called *glycol, ethylene alcohol.*

e. oxide. $(CH_2)_2O$. A colorless gas used as a fumigant, insecticide, and sterilizer of bacteriological media. See *carboxide.*

e. series. A group of hydrocarbons of the general formula, C_nH_{2n}, having one double bond. Also called *ethene, alkene series.*

e. tetraiodide. Diiodoform.

eth″yl·ene·di″a·mine′ (eth″i·leen·dye″uh·meen′, ·dye·am′in, ·dye′uh·meen, ·min). $H_2N.CH_2.CH_2.NH_2$. A colorless, strongly alkaline liquid of ammoniacal odor. It is used to increase the solubility of certain medicinal substances. See *aminophylline.*

e. dihydrochloride. A urine acidifier. Dose, 0.3–1.0 Gm. (5–15 gr.). See *chlor-ethamin.*

eth″yl·ene·di″a·mine·tet″ra·a·ce′tic acid. $(HOOC.CH_2)_2N.CH_2CH_2N(CH_2COOH)_2$; an amino acid, produced synthetically, occurring as a white, crystalline solid, slightly soluble in water. Water-soluble salts of the acid, such as tetrasodium ethylenediaminetetraacetate, are powerful chelating and sequestering agents, forming water-soluble complexes with many different cations in solution, thereby preventing such cations from exhibiting their characteristic chemical properties. Salts of ethylenediaminetetraacetic acid are used chiefly for their solubilizing and stabilizing actions; the disodium salt prevents coagulation of blood. Abbreviated, EDTAA. See *sequestrene, versene.*

eth″yl·e·phed′rine (eth″il·eh·fed′rin, ·ef′i·dreen, ·drin). *l*-N-Ethylephedrine hydrochloride or *l*-1-phenyl-2-methylethylaminopropan-1-ol hydrochloride. A white, odorless, crystalline compound having pharmacologic action and toxicity similar to *l*-ephedrine hydrochloride, except that its stimulating effect on the central nervous system is very slight. See *nethamine.*

eth′yl e′ther. Ether, 3.

eth″yl·hy″dro·cu′pre·ine (·high″dro·cue′pree·een, ·in). A synthetic derivative of cupreine; it is also chemically related to quinine and possesses the latter's antimalarial and anesthetic action. See *optochin.*

e. hydrochloride (*aethylhydrocupreinae hydrochloridum*), $C_{21}H_{28}N_2O_2.HCl$. A 1 or 2% solution is used in the eye and instilled into the conjunctival sac in pneumococcic infections of the eye. See *optochin.*

eth′yl·i·dene. The bivalent hydrocarbon radical $CH_3CH=$. Syn., *ethidene.*

eth″yl·mor′phine hy″dro·chlo′ride (eth″il·mor′feen, ·fin). A sedative used especially in diseases of the bronchi. Dose, 0.008–0.065 Gm. (⅛–1 gr.). Syn., *dionin.*

ethylnorsuprarenin hydrochloride. Trade name for an antiasthmatic; chemically, 1-(3,4-dihydroxyphenyl)-2-amino-1-butanol hydrochloride or ethylnorepinephrine hydrochloride.

eth′yl ox′ide. See under *ethyl.*

N-eth″yl·pi·per′i·dine. $C_5H_{10}NC_2H_5$. A compound used in a chemical assay for penicillin G.

eth″yl·stib′a·mine (eth″il·stib′uh·meen, ·min). Generic name for a pentavalent antimony complex consisting principally of the tetramer of *p*-aminobenzenestibonic acid, the dimer of *p*-acetylaminobenzenestibonic acid, antimonic acid, and diethylamine; a light yellow to yellow-brown powder, soluble in water: used in the treatment of kala-azar and other forms of leishmaniasis, also filariasis. See *neostibosan.*

eth′yl va·nil′late. See under *ethyl.*

eth′yl va·nil′lin. See under *ethyl.*

eth′yne. Acetylene.

eth′y·nyl, eth′i·nyl (eth′igh·nil). The radical $CH\vdots C—$.

e. estradiol. $C_{20}H_{24}O_2$; 17-ethynyl estradiol, produced synthetically from estrone. The ethynyl radical delays decomposition of the estradiol molecule in the stomach, intestine, and liver, so that the drug can be given orally; it is one of the most potent estrogens known. See *estinyl, eticylol, lynoral, oradiol, orestralyn.*

eticylol. A trade-mark for *ethynyl estradiol.*

e″ti·o·cho·lan′o·lone (ee″tee·o·ko·lan′o·loan). $C_{19}H_{30}O_2$. Etiocholane-3(α)-ol-17-one. A biologically inactive isomer of androsterone found in urine.

e″ti·o·la′tion [F. *étioler*, from L. *stipula*, stubble]. Pallor caused by the exclusion of light.

e″ti·ol′o·gy [G. *aitia*, cause; *logos*, word]. The science or study of the causes of disease, both direct and predisposing, and the mode of their operation; not synonymous with cause or pathogenesis of disease, but often loosely used to mean pathogenesis. **—etiolog′ic,** *adj.*

e″ti·o·path″o·gen′e·sis [*aitia;* G. *pathos*, disease; *genesis*, production]. The cause and course of development of a disease or lesion.

e″ti·o·por′phy·rin. Any of the four isomeric, metal-free porphyrins containing four methyl and four ethyl groups, in different positions, distinguished as etioporphyrins I, II, III, and IV. The particular spatial arrangements of the etioporphyrins provides the basis for classification of naturally occurring porphyrins.

Eu Chemical symbol for europium.

Eu″bac·te″ri·a′les (yoo″back·teer″ee·ay′leez) [G. *eu*, well; *baktērion*, little staff]. An order of bacteria, class Schizomycetes, including forms least differentiated and least specialized; the true bacteria. According to Bergey, suborder I, the Eubacteriineae, is composed of the following 13 families: Nitrobacteriaceae, Pseudomonadaceae, Azotobacteriaceae, Rhizobiaceae, Micrococcaceae Neisseriaceae, Lactobacteriaceae, Corynebacteriaceae, Achromobacteriaceae, Enterobacteriaceae, Parvobacteriaceae, Bacteriaceae, and Bacillaceae. Suborder II, the Caulobacteriineae, is composed of five families: Nevskiaceae, Gallionellaceae, Caulobacteriaceae, Siderocapsaceae, and Pasteuriaceae. Suborder III, the Rhodobacteriineae, is composed of three families: Thiorhodaceae, Athiorhodaceae, and Chlorobacteriaceae.

eu·caine′ hy″dro·chlo′ride (yoo·cane′, yoo·kay′in, yoo′kuh·een, ·in). $C_{15}H_{21}O_2N.HCl$. The hydrochloride of benzoyl vinyl-diacetone alkamine; crystalline powder, soluble in water. A local anesthetic introduced early as a substitute for cocaine but rarely used today. Also called *betaeucaine hydrochloride.*

eu″ca·lyp′tene (yoo″kuh·lip′teen). $C_{10}H_{16}$. A terpene derived from eucalyptol.

e. hydrochloride. Eucalypteol.

eu″ca·lyp′te·ol. $C_{10}H_{16}.2HCl$. Eucalyptene hydrochloride. Yellowish crystals; camphorlike odor. Formerly used like eucalyptol. Syn., *terpilene dihydrochloride.*

eu″ca·lyp′tol. $C_{10}H_{18}O$; cineol, eucalyptol; a constituent of the volatile oils of eucalyptus and cajeput; a mild local irritant; used in bronchitis, coryza, etc., and formerly as a vermifuge and antimalarial. Dose, 0.3 cc. (5 min.).

eu″ca·lyp′tus [G. *eu*, well; *kalyptos*, covered]. The leaf of *Eucalyptus globulus*, formerly used medicinally.

gum. The dried gummy exudate from *E.*

camaldulensis containing 46% kinotannic acid; formerly used as an astringent.

e. oil. A volatile oil from the leaves of *E. globulus* of Australia (cultivated in California); contains eucalyptol. Used as a stimulant antiseptic.

eu'ca·sin, eu·ca'sin. Ammonium caseinate. A soluble derivative of casein obtained by dissolving casein in dilute ammonium hydroxide. Has been used as a proprietary food product.

eu·cat'ro·pine hy"dro·chlo'ride (yoo·cat'ro·peen, ·pin) (*eucatropinae hydrochloridum*). $C_{17}H_{25}O_3N$.-HCl. A white, granular powder freely soluble in water; used in 5% solution as a mydriatic of brief duration. See *euphthalmine*.

eucerin. Trade-mark of a hydrophilic substance made from wool fat; used as an ointment base.

eu"chlor·hy'dri·a (yōō"klor·high'dree·uh, ·hid'·ree·uh) [*eu;* G *chlōros*, pale green; *hydōr*, water]. Presence of a normal amount of hydrochloric acid in the gastric juice.

eu·chol'i·a (yoo·kol'ee·uh, ·ko'lee·uh) [*eu;* G. *cholē*, bile]. Normal condition of the bile.

eu·chro'ma·tin [*eu;* G. *chrōma*, color]. 1. The deeply staining substance of the chromosomes, rich in nucleic acid, which is genetically active (contains the genes). 2. The substance of the euchromosomes, more usually called autosomes, in contrast to the substance of heterochromosomes. See *heterochromatin*. —**euchromat'ic,** *adj.*

eu·chro"ma·top'si·a [*eu; chrōma;* G. *opsis;* vision]. Capacity for correct recognition of colors.

eu·chro'mo·some. See *autosome*.

eu'co·dal. A synthetic, narcotic alkaloid, dihydrohydroxycodeinone hydrochloride, $C_{18}H_{21}O_4N$.-HCl. Used for pain and spasmodic cough, dose, 3–10 mg. (1/20–1/6 gr.); and as a miotic.

eu·cor'tism. Normal adrenal cortical function.

eucupin. Trade-mark for isoamylhydrocupreine, a local anesthetic.

eu"di·om'e·ter [G. *eudia*, fair weather; *metron*, a measure]. Instrument for the analysis and volumetric measure of gases. —**eudiometry,** *n.*

eu"es·the'si·a (yōō"ess·thee'zhuh, ·zee·uh) [G. *eu*, well; *aisthēsis*, sensation]. The sense of well-being; vigor and normal condition of the senses.

euflavine. Trade-mark for acriflavine.

eugallol. Trade-mark for a brand of pyrogallol monoacetate.

Eu·ge'ni·a [L., after Prince *Eugene* of Savoy, 1663–1736]. A genus of trees and shrubs of the Myrtaceae, mostly tropical.

E. caryophyllata. A species which yields cloves.

eu·gen'ics [G. *eugenēs*, well-born]. The applied science concerned with improving the genetic constitution of a stock or race: term usually limited now to man. **Positive eugenics** includes all those measures under social control which aim to increase the families of the better types; **negative eugenics,** those measures which aim to decrease the worse types. —**eugenic,** *adj.*

eu'ge·nol. 4-Allyl-2-methoxyphenol. A colorless or pale yellow liquid having a clove odor and spicy, pungent taste; obtained from clove oil and other sources. Used in dentistry as a local anesthetic and disinfectant in root canals; in ointments, as an anesthetic and antiseptic.

eu·glob'u·lin. True globulin. A globulin fraction soluble in distilled water and dilute salt solutions. Also see *pseudoglobulin*.

eu·gnath'ic (yoo·nath'ick, ·nay'thick) [G. *eu*, well; *gnathos*, jaw]. Pertaining to jaws that are well developed and in proper relation to each other.

eu·gon'ic [*eu;* G. *gonos*, offspring]. Growing luxuriantly; used to describe bacterial cultures.

eu·ker'a·tin. One of the two main groups of keratins. Eukeratins are insoluble in water, dilute alkali, and acids, are not digested by common proteolytic enzymes, and contain histidine, lysine, and arginine in the ratio of approximately 1:4:12.

eu"ki·ne'si·a (yōō"ki·nee'shuh) [*eu;* G. *kinēsis*, motion]. Normal power of movement.

eu'ko·dal. See *eucodal*.

Eulenburg, Albert [*German physician*, 1840–1917]. Described paramyotonia congenita, a spasm of the muscles of the neck, face, and throat of heredofamilial origin; called *Eulenburg's disease*.

eu·mor'phic. Well and normally formed; not misshapen.

Eu"my·ce'tes (yōō"migh·see'teez) [*eu;* G. *mykēs*, fungus]. A class of thallophytes containing all the true fungi.

eu·my'cin. An antibiotic substance derived from a strain of *Bacillus subtilis*. It is active against *Corynebacterium diphtheriae, Trichophyton mentagrophytes, Mycobacterium tuberculosis*, and other organisms.

eumydrin. Trade-mark for a brand of atropine methylnitrate.

eunarcon. Trade-mark for sodium 5-(2-bromoallyl)-5-isopropyl-1-methylbarbiturate, a rapidly acting narcotic used intravenously in surgical anesthesia.

eu·noi'a [G., goodwill]. Normal condition of mind and will.

eu'nuch (yōō'nuck) [G. *eunouchos*, guarding the couch]. One who has undergone complete loss of testicular function from castration, inflammation, or mechanical injury. If this occurs before puberty, it is associated with failure of development of secondary sex characters and typical changes in skeletal maturation, with increased height and span and disproportionate length of the lower extremities to trunk. —**eu'nuchism,** *n.*

eu'nuch·oid·ism (yōō'nuck·oyd·iz·um) [*eunouchos;* G. *eidos*, form]. A state in which there is hypogonadism or agonadism accompanied by alterations in the development of secondary sex characters and the skeleton, similar to those seen in true prepuberal eunuchs; it may be due to a primary gonadal defect or to inadequate stimulation by the adenohypophysis. —**eu'nuchoid,** *adj.*

idiopathic e. A type of eunuchoidism without enlargement of the mammary gland, in which the testes are similar in histological appearance to those of a prepuberal male. There is a normal to low level of urinary 17-ketosteroids.

pituitary e. A clinical condition in which a specific deficiency of adenohypophyseal gonadotropins results in sexual retardation. Syn., *pituitary hypogonadism*.

eu·on'y·mus [G. *euōnymos*, of good name]. The dried bark of *E. atropurpureus;* used as a cathartic. Dose, 0.3–1.0 Gm. (5–15 gr.). Syn., *wahoo bark*.

eu'pad. A mixture of equal parts of chlorinated lime and boric acid, for use in preparing eusol.

eu'pa·ral. A mixture of resins used as a mounting medium for histologic sections; it has a refractive index of 1.483. The colorless form lacks (the green form contains) a copper salt for intensification of hematoxylin stain.

Eu"pa·to'ri·um [G. *eupatorion*, agrimony]. A genus of composite-flowered plants. The leaves and flowering tops of *E. perfoliatum*, thoroughwort or boneset, are used, principally by the laity, as a bitter tonic, diaphoretic, and feeble emetic.

eu·pav'er·ine. $C_{19}H_{15}NO_4$.HCl; the hydrochloride of 3-methyl-6,7-methylenedioxy-1-piperonylisoquinoline, a synthetic homolog of papaverine. It is a smooth muscle antispasmodic.

eu·pho′ni·a [G. goodness of voice]. A normal, good, and clear condition of the voice.

Eu·phor′bi·a [G. *euphorbion*, spurge]. A genus of plants of the Euphorbiaceae. **E. corollata** and **E. ipecacuanhae,** the American species, were formerly employed in medicine because of their emetic and cathartic properties. **E. pilulifera** of South America and Australia is used in asthma and bronchitis. **E. resinifera** of Africa produces euphorbium.

Eu·phor″bi·a′ce·ae [*euphorbion*]. A plant family of herbs, shrubs, or trees.

eu·phor′bin. A constituent of euphorbium.

eu·phor′bi·um [*euphorbion*]. The dried resinous latex obtained from *Euphorbia resinifera.* It is strongly purgative and vesicant; now mainly employed in veterinary medicine.

eu·phor′bon. A constituent of euphorbium.

eu·pho′ri·a [G., sense of well-being]. *In psychology,* the exaggerated sense of well-being. —**euphor′ic,** *adj.*

euphthalmine. Trade-mark for eucatropine hydrochloride; a mydriatic.

eu·phys″i·o·log′ic. Of, pertaining to, or characterizing the normal range of function of an organism or part.

eu′ploid [G. *eu*, well; di*ploos*, twofold; *eidos*, form]. *In biology,* having an exact multiple of the basic haploid number of chromosomes. —**euploidy,** *n.*

eup·ne′a, eup·noe′a (yo͞op·nee′uh) [G. *eupnoia*, easiness of breathing]. Normal or easy respiration. *Obs.*

eu·por′phin. Apomorphine methylbromide.

eu·prax′i·a [G., from *eu; praxis*, a doing]. Normal and perfect performance of coordinated movements.

Eu·proc′tis chrys·or·rhe′a. The brown-tail moth which causes brown-tail rash.

eu·py′rene [*eu;* G. *pyrēn*, stone of a fruit]. Descriptive of the normal functional type of mature sperm cell. See *apyrene, oligopyrene.*

eu·qui′nine (yo͞o·kwye′nyne, ·kwin′een, ·in, yo͞o′-kwi·neen, ·nin). Quinine ethylcarbonate.

eurax. Trade-mark for crotamiton or N-ethyl-*o*-crotonotoluidide; $C_{13}H_{17}NO$: used as a scabicide and antipruritic.

euresol. Trade-mark for resorcinol monoacetate, used in certain skin diseases.

e. pro capillis. A proprietary perfumed resorcinol monoacetate for scalp lotions.

eu″ro·don′ti·a [G. *eurōs*, mold, dank decay; *odous*, tooth]. Dental caries. *Obs.*

eu″ro·pis″o·ceph′a·lus [G. *eurys*, broad; *opisō*, behind; *kephalē*, head]. A person whose head is unusually broad in the occipital region.

eu·ro′pi·um [*Europe*]. Eu = 152.0. A rare earth metal found in cerium minerals.

eu″ro·pro·ceph′a·lus [G. *eurys*, broad; *pro*, in front; *kephalē*, head]. A person whose head is unusually broad in the frontal region.

eu″ry·ce·phal′ic [G. *eurys*, broad; *kephalē*, head]. Designating a head that is unusually broad. Sometimes used to designate a brachycephalic head with a cephalic index of 81 to 85.4. Also *eurycephalous.*

eu″ry·chas′mus (yoor″i·kaz′mus) [*eurys;* G. *chasma*, chasm]. An individual with an unusually wide nasopharynx, with corresponding skull differences.

eu″ryc·ne′mic [*eurys;* G. *knēmē*, leg]. Referring to a cnemic index of 70 or above.

eu″ry·gnath′ism (yoor″i·nath′iz·um, yoo·rig′nuh-thiz·um) [*eurys;* G. *gnathos*, jaw]. A condition in which the jaws are unusually broad. —**eurygnath′ic, eurygnathous,** *adj.*

eu″ry·mer′ic [*eurys;* G. *meros*, part]. *In osteometry,* designating a femur that is nearly circular in cross section in the proximal portion of the shaft; having a platymeric index of 85.0 to 99.9.

eu′ry·on [*eurys*]. That point on either lateral surface of the skull which is located at the extremities of the greatest width of the skull.

eu″ry·ther′mal, eu″ry·ther′mic [*eurys;* G. *thermē*, heat]. Capable of tolerating a great range of temperature, as certain organisms.

eu′scope [G. *eu*, well; *skopein*, to examine]. A modified microscope which projects enlarged images of stereoscopic effect on a screen.

Eu·scor′pi·us [*eu;* G. *skorpios*, scorpion]. A genus of scorpions.

E. italicus. A poisonous black scorpion found in northern Africa and southern Europe.

eu′sol [*E*dinburgh *U*niversity *sol*ution]. A solutoin used as a wound antiseptic, prepared by the interaction of 12.5 Gm. each of chlorinated lime and boric acid in water to make 1 liter.

Eustacchio, Bartolommeo (**Eustachius**) [*Italian anatomist*, ca. 1520–74]. Described the *auditory* or *Eustachian tube;* see under *tube.* The bony portion of the tube was once known as the *Eustachian canal.* Eustacchio described the tensor tympani, and identified the chorda tympani as a nerve. He discovered the thoracic duct, and gave the first description of the suprarenal glands. The caval valve is also called the *Eustachian valve.* See also, Eustachian *catheter.*

eu·sta′chi·an, Eu·sta′chi·an (yoo·stay′kee·un, ·stay′shee·un, ·stay′shun) [after *Eustacchio*]. Pertaining to the eustachian or auditory tube.

Eu·stron′gy·lus gi′gas (yoo·stron′ji·lus jy′gas). Synonym for *Dioctophyma renale.*

eu·sys′to·le (yoo·sis′to·lee) [G. *eu*, well; *systolē*, contraction]. A normal contraction of the cardiac cavities.

eu·tec′tic [*eu;* G. *tēktos*, melted, from *tēkein*, to melt]. *In physical chemistry,* of, pertaining to, or designating the specific mixture of two or more substances which has the lowest melting point of any mixture of the substances.

e. mixture. Through common usage, any mixture which has a lower melting point than the individual constituents; more usually a mixture which softens or melts at room temperature.

eu″tha·na′si·a (yo͞o″thuh·nay′zhuh, ·zee·uh) [G., from *eu; thanatos*, death]. 1. An easy or calm death. 2. The painless killing of people who are suffering from an incurable or painful disease.

eu·then′ics [G. *euthenein*, to thrive]. The science which deals with the improvement of the human race by means of the betterment of living conditions. Also see *eugenics.* —**eu′thenist,** *n.*

Eu·the′ri·a [G. *eu*, well; *thērion*, beast]. The true placental mammals. —**eutherian,** *adj.*

eu·thy′roid·ism [*eu;* G. *thyreoeidēs*, shield-shaped]. Denoting normal thyroid function.

eu·to′ci·a (yoo·to′shee·uh, ·see·uh) [*eu;* G. *tokos*, childbirth]. Natural or easy childbirth; normal labor.

Eu″tri·at′o·ma (yo͞o″try·at′o·muh). A genus of bugs, some members of which transmit American trypanosomiasis.

e·vac′u·ant [L. *evacuare*, to empty out]. A medicine which empties an organ, especially the bowels; a purgative. —**evac′uant,** *adj.*

e·vac″u·a′tion [L. *evacuatio*, from *evacuare*]. 1. The voiding of any matter either by the natural passages of the body or by an artificial opening; specifically, defecation. 2. *In military medicine,* the withdrawal of sick and wounded personnel, or material, or both, as in **air evacuation.**

e·vac″u·a′tion of′fi·cer. The U. S. Army Medical Service officer in charge of the movement of patients through the Army Medical Service channels of evacuation.

e·vac″u·a′tion pol′i·cy. *In military medicine,* (a) the command decision, indicating the length in days of the maximum period of noneffectiveness that patients may be held within the command for treatment. Patients who, in the opinion of responsible medical officers, cannot be returned to duty status within the period prescribed are evacuated by the first available means, provided the travel involved will not aggravate their disabilities; (b) a command decision concerning the movement of civilians from the proximity of military operations for security and safety reasons, and involving the need to arrange for movement, reception, care, and control of such individuals.

e·vac′u·a″tor [*evacuare*]. An instrument for the removal of fluid or particles from the urinary bladder or intestine.

e·vag″i·na′tion (i·vadj″i·nay′shun) [L. *evaginare,* to unsheathe]. Outpouching.

ev″a·nes′cent [L. *evanescere,* to vanish away]. Unstable; tending to vanish quickly.

Evans, Herbert M. (1882–). American anatomist, known for many discoveries in biology and medicine, among which are vitamin E, the 48 chromosomes in man, and the growth hormone of the hypophysis. See also *Evans blue,* Evans blue *method.*

Evans blue. $C_{34}H_{24}N_6Na_4O_{14}S_4$; tetrasodium salt of 4,4′-bis[7-(1-amino-8-hydroxy-2,4-disulfo)-naphthylazo]-3,3′-bitolyl; a diazo dye, occurring as a bluish-green or brown iridescent powder, very soluble in water. It is used as an intravenous diagnostic agent for colorimetric determination of blood volume, cardiac output, and residual blood volume in the heart; when injected into the blood stream it combines with plasma albumin and leaves the circulation slowly. Syn., *T 1824.*

Eve, Frank Cecil [*English physician,* contemporary]. Invented a halometer for measuring the degree of angulation between the axial beam of light and the edge of a halo, a micrometer for determining the size of erythrocytes. See also *Eve's method* under *artificial respiration.*

e″ven·tra′tion [L. *e,* out; *venter,* belly]. Protrusion of the abdominal viscera through the abdominal wall, as in ventral hernia, to be distinguished from evisceration.

e. of the diaphragm. A condition where there is defective muscular action of the diaphragm, the left leaf being abnormally high, not moving through the normal excursion.

Eversbusch, Oscar [*German ophthalmologist,* 1855–1912]. Devised an operation for the relief of ptosis by shortening the levator palpebrae by infolding; called *Eversbusch's operation.*

e·ver′sion [L. *eversio,* from *evertere,* to turn out]. A turning outward. —**evert′,** *v.t.*

e. of the eyelid. (a) A method of folding the lid upon itself for the purpose of exposing the conjunctival surface or sulcus. (b) Ectropion.

ev′i·dence [L. *evidens,* clear]. *In legal medicine,* the means by which the existence or nonexistence of the truth or falsehood of an alleged fact is ascertained or made evident; proof, as of insanity.

circumstantial e. Evidence which is beyond actual demonstration, but upon which conclusions are based.

conclusive e. Evidence that admits of no doubt.

expert e. That given before a jury by an expert in any science, art, profession, or trade.

e′vil eye. An eye whose glance brings disease, bad luck, or death: still a living belief in many parts of the world. The delusion of being the victim of the evil eye is frequent among patients with the paranoid type of schizophrenic reaction. The Latin term *fascinum* is more common in psychiatric usage.

evipal. Trade-mark for hexobarbital, a rapidly acting barbiturate.

evipal sodium. Trade-mark for hexobarbital sodium.

ev″i·ra′tion (ev″i·ray′shun, ee″vi·) [L. *evirare,* to emasculate]. 1. Castration; emasculation. 2. A psychic process in which there is a deep and permanent assumption of feminine qualities, with corresponding loss of manly qualities. In contrast to *defemination.*

e·vis″cer·a′tion [L. *eviscerare,* to disembowel]. 1. Removal of the abdominal or thoracic viscera. 2. Protrusion of the viscera through an abdominal incision following an operation. 3. Removal of the contents of an organ, such as the eye.

e. of the eye. Removal of the contents of the globe, the sclera being left intact.

obstetric e. Removal of the abdominal or thoracic viscera of a fetus to permit delivery.

e·vis″cer·o·neu·rot′o·my (i·vis″ur·o·new·rot′o-mee) [*eviscerare;* G. *neuron,* nerve; *tomē,* a cutting]. Evisceration of the eye with division of the optic nerve.

ev″o·ca′tion (ev″o·kay′shun, ee″vo·) [L. *evocatio,* from *evocare,* to call forth]. That part of the morphogenic effect of an organizer which can be referred to the action of a single chemical substance, the evocator.

ev′o·ca″tor (ev′o·kay″tur, ee′vo·) [L., from *evocare*]. The chemical substance emitted by an organizer, which acts as all or part of a morphogenic stimulus. Syn., *morphogenic hormone.*

ev″o·lu′tion [L. *evolutio,* from *evolvere,* to roll out]. The view that present-day species of plants and animals have originated by descent with modification from preexisting species. The development has been through a series of progressive changes, leading from the simpler and more generalized to the complex and more specialized forms, although there has been some retrogression and degeneration, as in parasitic forms.

e·vul′sion [L. *evulsio,* from *evellere,* to pull out]. Forcible tearing or plucking away of a part. See *avulsion.*

Ewald, Carl Anton [*German physician,* 1845–1915]. Known for his studies of digestive disorders and of gastric secretion. Said to have introduced the use of flexible rubber tubing for the aspiration of stomach contents (1875). With Boas, introduced the test meal (1885).

Ewart, William [*English physician,* 1848–1929]. Called attention to numerous signs which indicate pericardial effusion. Of these the most important are the patch of dullness at the inner part of the left lung base, and the area of bronchial respiration below the tip of the left scapula, associated with egophony.

Ewing, James [*American pathologist,* 1866–1943]. Widely acclaimed for his evaluation of different varieties of tumors in a masterly work on neoplastic disease (1919). Described a form of bone sarcoma involving the shaft of the long bones. See Ewing's *sarcoma.*

ex- [L.]. A prefix denoting *beyond, from, off, out of, thoroughly,* or *without.*

ex·ac″er·ba′tion (eg·zass″ur·bay′shun, eck·sass″-ur·) [L. *exacerbatio,* from *exacerbare,* to irritate]. Increase in the manifestations of a disease.

ex″al·ta′tion [L. *exaltatio,* from *exaltare,* to exalt]. A mental state characterized by self-satisfaction, ecstatic joy, abnormal cheerfulness, optimism, or delusions of grandeur.

ex·am″i·na′tion [L. *examinatio,* from *examinare,* to examine]. Investigation for the purpose of diagnosis. Qualified as: bimanual, digital, oral, physical, etc.

physical e. Investigation to determine an individual's physical status. A final type consists of a complete physical and neuropsychiatric examination, including a detailed medical history, chest x-ray, serological test for syphilis, urinalysis (including microscopic), other tests as indicated, and pelvic examination in women examinees. Preliminary physical examination includes these procedures in order to give advanced information regarding the physical status of an individual; approval of an individual's physical status based on a preliminary examination is not binding. A screening physical examination includes a brief medical history, physical examination, and appropriate x-ray or other laboratory procedures of any particular system of the body suspected or found to be abnormal or defective. A supplemental physical examination consists of reexamination of any part of a final type, special tests, or special examination of any particular system of the body. It is performed when indicated, usually by a specialist in some particular field of medicine or surgery.

ex″an·the′ma, ex·an′them (pl. *exanthemas, exanthems*) [G., eruption]. 1. An eruption upon the skin. 2. Any eruptive fever such as measles or scarlet fever. **—exanthem′atous, exanthemat′ic,** *adj.*

e. subitum. A noncontagious roseola occurring in infants; roseola infantum.

vesicular e. An acute, febrile virus disease of swine characterized by the presence of vesicles on the nose, feet, and mucous membrane of the mouth.

ex·ar″te·ri′tis [L. *ex*, out; G. *artēria*, artery; *-itis*, inflammation]. Inflammation of the outer coat of an artery.

ex″ca·va′tion [L. *excavatio*, from *excavare*, to hollow out]. 1. A hollow or cavity, especially one with sharply defined edges. 2. Act or process of making hollow.

dental e. (a) The cavity prepared in a tooth, prior to filling or the insertion of an inlay. (b) The preparation of such a cavity.

e. of the optic disk. A cupping of the optic disk, which is more pronounced than the normal physiologic cupping, seen in glaucoma and certain other ophthalmic diseases.

rectouterine e. [BNA]. The rectouterine pouch; cul-de-sac.

rectovesical e. [BNA]. The rectovesical pouch.

vesicouterine e. See vesicouterine *pouch*.

ex′ca·va″tor [*excavare*]. 1. An instrument like a gouge or scoop used to scrape away tissue. 2. A dental instrument for removing decayed matter from a tooth cavity.

ex·cel′sin. A simple protein of the globulin type which occurs in Brazil nuts.

ex″ce·men·to′sis [L. *ex*, out; *caementum*, rough stone; G. *-ōsis*, condition]. Hypertrophy of the cementum of the teeth; hypercementosis.

ex·cer″e·bra′tion [*ex;* L. *cerebrum*, brain]. Removal of the fetal brain in the process of embryotomy.

ex·cip′i·ent [L. *excipere*, to take a thing to one's self]. Any substance combined with an active drug to give the latter an agreeable or convenient form.

ex·ci′sion (eck·sizh′un) [L. *excisio*, from *excidere*, to cut out]. The cutting out of a part; removal of a foreign body or growth from a part, organ, or tissue. **—excise′,** *v.*

e. of a wound. Clearing away all devitalized or infected tissue.

ex·cit″a·bil′i·ty (eck·sight″uh·bil′i·tee) [L. *excitabilis*, from *excitare*, to rouse up]. Readiness of response to a stimulus; irritability. **—excit′able,** *adj.*

ex·ci′tant (eck·sigh′tunt) [*excitare*]. An agent that stimulates the activity of an organ. **—exci′tant,** *adj.*

ex″ci·ta′tion (eck″sigh·tay′shun) [*excitare*]. 1. The act of stimulating or irritating an organ or tissue. 2. *In physics and chemistry*, the addition of energy to a system, thereby transforming it from its ground state to an excited state. Excitation of a nucleus, atom, or molecule can result from absorption of photons or from inelastic collisions with various atomic or nuclear particles. **—excit′ing,** *adj.;* **excite′,** *v.t.*

direct e. The stimulation of a muscle by placing an electrode on the muscle itself.

indirect e. The stimulation of a muscle through its nerves.

ex·clu′sion [L. *exclusio*, from *excludere*, to shut out]. 1. The process of extruding or shutting out. 2. A surgical operation by which part of an organ is disconnected from the rest, but not excised.

ex″coch·le·a′tion [L. *ex*, out of; *cochlea*, snail shell]. Removal by scraping.

ex·con′ju·gant [*ex;* L. *conjugare*, to join together]. A protozoon immediately after the separation following conjugation.

ex·co″ri·a′tion [L. *excoriare*, to strip of its skin]. Abrasion of a portion of the skin. **—exco′riate,** *v.*

neurotic e. Severe scratching of the skin due to psychogenic pruritis.

ex′cre·ment [L. *excrementum*, from *excernere*, to sift out]. An excreted substance; the feces. **—excrementi′tious,** *adj.*

ex·cres′cence [L. *excrescere*, to grow out]. Abnormal outgrowth upon the body.

cauliflower e. A tumor or other lesion with an irregular corrugated surface resembling a cauliflower.

Lambl's excrescences. Fine, hairlike proliferations of fibrous connective tissue in the region of the nodules of Arantius, usually on the aortic valve.

ex·cre′ta [L. *excretum*, from *excernere*, to sift out]. Waste material cast out or separated from an organism.

ex′cre·tin [*excernere*]. That fraction of secretin which stimulates pancreatic secretion. Also see *incretin*.

ex·cre′tion [*excernere*]. 1. The discharge of waste products. 2. The matter so discharged. **—ex′cretory,** *adj., n.;* **excrete′,** *v.t.*

ex″cre·to′lic ac′id. A fatty acid occurring in feces.

ex·cur′sion [L. *excursio*, from *excurrere*, to run out]. 1. A wandering from the usual course. 2. The extent of movement, as of the eyes from a central position, or of the chest during respiration.

lateral e. The sideways movement of the mandible causing the inclined planes of the opposing teeth to glide upon each other.

ex·cur′va·ture, ex″cur·va′tion [L. *ex*, out; *curvatio*, from *curvare*, to curve]. Outward curvature.

ex·cy″clo·pho′ri·a [G. *ex*, out; *kyklos*, circle; *phoros*, bearing]. A latent outward tilting of the upper pole of the eye. See *cyclophoria*.

ex·cy″clo·tro′pi·a [*ex; kyklos;* G. *tropē*, a turning]. A defect of vision in which the vertical median superior pole of the eye is turned outward.

ex″cys·ta′tion [*ex; kystis*, bladder]. The escape from a cyst by the bursting of the surrounding envelope; a stage in the life of an intestinal parasite which occurs after the parasite has been swallowed by the host.

ex′e·dens. *In dermatology*, progressively ulcerative.

ex″en·ce·pha′li·a (ecks″en·si·fay′lee·uh, ·fal′-ee·uh), **ex″en·ceph′a·ly** [*ex;* G. *egkephalos,* brain]. Cranioschisis and partial anencephalia, with encephalocele, or hydrencephalocele. —**exencephal′ic,** *adj.*

ex″en·ceph′a·lus [*ex; egkephalos*]. A monster showing exencephalia.

ex·en″ter·a′tion [L. *exenterare,* from G. *ex,* out of; *enteron,* intestine]. 1. Evisceration or surgical removal, as of the orbital contents. 2. Destruction of cells of an air sinus by removing the bony partitions and forming a single, large cavity, as of the cells of the petrous pyramid.

ex′er·cise [L. *exercitium,* from *exercere,* to work at]. Functional activity of the muscles; such activity when its purpose is the preservation or restoration of the health, or the development of physical prowess or athletic skill.

active e. Exercise due to the voluntary effort of the patient.

graduated resistance e. See progressive resistance *e.*

passive e. The moving of parts of the body by another without help or hindrance by the patient.

postural e. That designed to improve posture by correcting mild deformities.

progressive resistance e. An exercise to increase the power of a weakened muscle, or muscles, in which resistance to contraction is progressively increased as muscle power improves. In a **load-assisting exercise,** the load with which the patient performs the exercise serves as a counterbalance, i.e., helps the muscle; in a **load-resisting exercise,** the load resists the muscle. Syn., *graduated resistance e.*

setting-up e. That designed for routine use by normal persons.

underwater e. That done under water so that buoyancy makes movement easy enough for weakened muscles to control.

ex′er·cise gloves. Soft leather gloves used in graduated resistance exercises for patients who lack strength in the upper extremities. They eliminate hazards involved in using the bare hands.

ex·er′e·sis [G. *exairesis,* removal]. Surgical excision or extraction.

ex″er·gon′ic [*ex;* G. *ergon,* work]. Of, pertaining, or referring to a chemical reaction in which the end products possess less free energy than the starting materials: usually associated with catabolism.

ex″fe·ta′tion [L. *ex,* out; *fetus,* offspring]. Ectopic or extrauterine fetation.

ex·flag″el·la′tion (ecks·fladj″i·lay′shun) [*ex;* L. *flagellare,* to whip]. The formation of actively motile flagella in the microgametocyte, the male malarial parasite.

ex·fo″li·a′tion [L. *exfoliare,* to strip of leaves]. 1. The separation of bone or other tissue in thin layers; a superficial sequestrum. 2. A peeling and shedding of the horny layer of the skin. A normal process that may be exaggerated after an inflammation or as part of a skin disease. —**exfo′liative,** *adj.*

ex″ha·la′tion [L. *exhalatio,* from *exhalare,* to breathe out]. 1. The giving off or sending forth in the form of vapor; expiration. 2. That which is given forth as vapor; emanation.

ex·haust′er [L. *exhaurire,* to draw out]. Instrument for the removal of soft cataracts.

ex·haus′tion [L. *exhaustum,* from *exhaurire*]. 1. Loss of vital and nervous power from fatigue or protracted disease. 2. The pharmaceutical process of dissolving out one or more of the constituents of a crude drug by percolation or maceration.

e. from cold. The condition seen when the body is no longer able to compensate for exposure to cold; marked by fatigue, drowsiness, and coma.

heat e. See heat *prostration.*

ex″hi·bi′tion [L. *exhibitio,* from *exhibere,* to hold forth]. The administration of a remedy.

ex″hi·bi′tion·ism [*exhibere*]. 1. A sexual perversion in which pleasure is obtained by exposing the genitals. 2. *In psychoanalysis,* gratification of early sexual impulses in young children by physical activity, such as dancing. —**exhibitionist,** *n.*

ex·hil′a·rant [L. *exhilarare,* to make merry]. Exhilarating; causing a rise in spirits.

ex·hil′a·rant. An agent to enliven and cheer the mind. —**exhilara′tion,** *n.*

ex″hu·ma′tion [L. *ex,* out; *humus,* ground]. Removal from the ground after burial; disinterment. —**exhume′,** *v.*

ex′i·tus [L.]. 1. Exit; outlet. 2. Death.

Exner, Siegmund [*Austrian physiologist,* 1846–1926]. Described a layer of sensory fibers in the cerebral cortex near the surface, called *Exner's plexus.*

ex′o-, ex- [G., outside]. A prefix signifying *outside, outer layer, out of.*

ex″o·car′di·a [*exō;* G. *kardia,* heart]. Displacement of the heart.

ex″o·car′di·ac, ex″o·car′di·al [*exō; kardia*]. Originating or situated outside of the heart.

ex″o·cat″a·pho′ri·a [*exō;* G. *kata,* down; *pherein,* to bear]. Condition in which the visual axis turns outward and downward.

ex″oc·cip′i·tal (ecks″ock·sip′i·tul) [L. *ex,* out; *occiput,* back part of the head]. Lying to the side of the foramen magnum, as the exoccipital bone.

ex″o·cho′ri·on (eck″so·kor′ee·on) [G. *exō,* outside; *chorion,* skin]. External layer of the chorion.

ex″o·coe′lom (eck″so·see′lum) [*exō;* G. *koilos,* hollow]. That part of the coelom outside the embryo proper. Originally extensive, it becomes restricted to the proximal umbilical cord by the growth of the amnion. —**exocoelom′ic,** *adj.*

ex′o·crine (eck′so·kryne, ·krin, ·kreen) [*exō;* G. *krinein,* to separate]. Pertaining to glands which deliver their secretion or excretion to an epithelial surface, either directly or by means of ducts. Cf. *endocrine.*

ex″o·don′ti·a, ex″o·don′tics. The art and science of the extraction of teeth.

ex″o·don′tist [G. *ex,* out; *odous,* tooth]. One who specializes in tooth extraction.

ex″o·er′gic. Exothermic.

ex″o·e·ryth″ro·cyt′ic [G. *exō,* outside; *erythros,* red; *kytos,* cell]. Outside of erythrocytes; said of the development of some of the malaria plasmodia in the cells of the lymphatic system of birds.

ex·og′a·my [*exō;* G. *gamos,* marriage]. Union of gametes of different ancestry; outbreeding; cross-fertilization.

ex″o·gas′tru·la [*exō;* NL. dim. from G. *gastēr,* stomach]. An abnormal embryo with evagination of the primitive gut and absence of further development.

ex·og′e·nous (eck·sodj′i·nus), **ex″o·gen′ic, ex″o·ge·net′ic** [*exō;* G. *genesthai,* from *gignesthai,* to be produced]. 1. Due to an external cause; not arising within the organism. 2. *In physiology,* pertaining to those factors in the metabolism of nitrogenous substances obtained from food.

ex″o·hys′ter·o·pex″y [*exō;* G. *hystera,* uterus; *pēxis,* a fixing]. Fixation of the uterus in the abdominal wall outside the peritoneum.

ex″o·me·tri′tis. Parametritis.

ex·om′pha·los [G., from *ex,* out; *omphalos,* navel]. A prominence of the navel due to umbilical hernia; a congenital hernia into the umbilical cord.

ex″o·pep′ti·dase. Any of a group of enzymes, including aminopeptidases and carboxypeptidases, capable of acting only upon terminal peptide bonds.

ex″o·pho′ri·a [G. *exō*, outside; *pherein*, to bear]. A type of heterophoria in which the visual lines tend outward.

ex″oph·thal·mom′e·ter [G. *exophthalmos*, from *ex*, out; *ophthalmos*, eye; *metron*, a measure]. Instrument for measuring the degree of exophthalmos.

ex″oph·thal·mom′e·try [*exophthalmos; metron*]. Mean measurement of the anterior plane of the cornea from the external orbital rim.

ex″oph·thal′mos, ex″oph·thal′mus [*exophthalmos*]. Abnormal protrusion of the eyeball from the orbit. —**exophthalmic,** *adj.*

malignant e. Severe intractable exophthalmos arising in previously hyperthyroid individuals after thyroidectomy and thought to have the same cause as thyrotropic exophthalmos.

pituitary e. See thyrotropic *e.*

pulsating e. That characterized by a bruit and pulsation, due to an aneurysm that pushes the eye forward.

thyrotropic e. Exophthalmos associated with either a normal or a low metabolic rate. Asymmetric proptosis is common, often accompanied by chemosis, lid edema, and pareses of extraocular muscles, believed to be due to hypersecretion of a pituitary factor (exophthalmos-producing substance) associated with, but not identical to, thyrotropin. Syn., *pituitary e.*

ex″oph·thal′mos-pro·duc′ing sub′stance (EPS). A substance, considered to be distinct from thyroid-stimulating hormone (TSH), obtained from extracts of the anterior pituitary, which, in experimental animals, produces exophthalmos.

ex·or′bi·tism. Exophthalmos.

ex″o·skel′e·ton [G. *exō*, outside; *skeletos*, dried up]. 1. The usually chitinous external skeleton of invertebrates. 2. The bony or horny supporting structures in the skin of many vertebrates, such as fish scales, the carapace of a turtle.

ex″os·mom′e·ter (eck″sos·mom′i·tur, eck″soz·) [G. *ex*, out; *ōsmos*, impulse; *metron*, a measure]. Instrument for measuring the degree of exosmosis.

ex″os·mo′sis (eck″sos·mo′sis, eck″soz·), **ex′os·mose** (eck′sos·mohss, eck′soz·) [*ex; ōsmos;* G. *-ōsis*, condition]. Passage of a liquid outward through a porous membrane. —**exosmot′ic,** *adj.*

ex·os″to·sec′to·my [*ex;* G. *osteon*, bone; *ektomē*, excision]. Excision of an exostosis.

ex″os·to′sis (pl. *exostoses*) [*ex; osteon;* G. *-ōsis*, increase]. The most common benign tumor of bone, usually seen as a cartilage-capped bony growth protruding from the surface of long bones but also seen on flat bones, and thought to arise from periosteum with formation of anomalous foci of metaplastic cartilage. It appears in two forms: (1) **solitary exostosis,** also called *osteochondroma* or *chondro-osteoma*, thought to be a limited or abortive form of (2) **multiple hereditary exostoses,** the most common systematized congenital skeletal abnormality, revealing itself in childhood or adolescence. This form is also called *hereditary multiple cartilaginous exostoses*, *hereditary deforming chondrodysplasia*, *diaphyseal* or *metaphyseal aclasis*. —**exos′tosed, exostot′ic,** *adj.*

ex″o·ther′mic, ex″o·ther′mal [G. *exō*, outside; *thermē*, heat]. Relating to the giving out of energy, especially heat energy. Syn., *exoergic*.

ex″o·ther′mic. A substance formed with the liberation of heat.

ex″o·tox′in [*exō;* G. *toxikon*, poison]. A toxin which is excreted by a living microorganism and can afterwards be obtained in bacteria-free filtrates without death or disintegration of the microorganisms. —**exotoxic,** *adj.*

ex″o·tro′pi·a [*exō;* G. *trepein*, to turn]. Divergent concomitant strabismus; occurring when one eye fixes upon an object and the other deviates outward.

expandex. A trade-mark for the plasma-expanding and blood-pressure-maintaining substance *dextran*.

ex·pan′sive [L. *expansio*, from *expandere*, to spread apart]. 1. Comprehensive; wide-extending. 2. *In psychiatry*, characterized by megalomania, euphoria, talkativeness, overgenerosity, grandiosity. —**expansiveness,** *n.*

ex″pec·ta′tion of life. 1. *In biometry*, the average number of years lived by a group of individuals after reaching a given age, as determined by the mortality experience of a specific time and geographic area; mean afterlifetime. 2. Commonly, the probable number of years of survival for an individual of a given age.

ex·pec′to·rant [L. *expectorare*, to drive from the breast]. Promoting expectoration.

ex·pec′to·rant. A remedy that promotes or modifies expectoration.

ex·pec″to·ra′tion [*expectorare*]. 1. Ejection of material from the mouth. 2. The fluid or semifluid matter from the lungs and air passages expelled by coughing and spitting; sputum.

prune-juice e. A peculiar bloody sputum, of a dark purple color, resembling prune juice, occurring in pneumonia, gangrene, and in carcinoma of the lung.

ex·pel′ [L. *expellere*, to drive out]. Drive or force out, as the fetus, by means of muscular contractions.

ex·per′i·ment [L. *experimentum*, from *experiri*, to try]. A trial or test; a procedure undertaken to discover some unknown principle or effect, to test a hypothesis, or to illustrate a known principle or fact. —**experimen′tal,** *adj.*; **experimenta′tion,** *n.*

control e. See *control experiment*.

ex′pert [L. *expertum*, from *experiri*]. A person specially qualified in a certain subject, as a science or an art.

medical e. A physician particularly fitted by experience or special learning to render an authoritative opinion in medicolegal or diagnostic questions. —**expert′ness,** *n.*

ex″pi·ra′tion [L. *expirare*, to breathe out]. Act of breathing forth or expelling air from the lungs. —**expi′ratory,** *adj.*

ex·pire′ [*expirare*]. 1. Breathe out. 2. Die.

ex″plan·ta′tion [L. *explantare*, to pull up (a plant)]. Removal of living tissue from its habitat for cultivation in artificial mediums; tissue culture. —**explant′,** *v.*

ex·plode′ [L. *explodere*, to drive out by clapping]. 1. Burst violently and noisily because of sudden release of energy. 2. Cause to burst violently. 3. Discredit and reject, as a theory. 4. Break out suddenly, as an epidemic. —**explo′sive,** *adj.*; **explo′sion,** *n.*

ex″plo·ra′tion [L. *explorare*, to spy out]. The act of exploring for diagnostic purposes, through investigation of a part hidden from sight, by means of operation, by touch, by artificial light, or by instruments. —**explor′atory,** *adj.*

ex·plor′er [*explorare*]. A probe; an instrument for use in exploration.

ex·po′sure [OF. *exposer*, from L. *ex*, out, F. *poser*, to place]. 1. Act of exposing or laying open. 2. State of being open to some action or influence that may affect detrimentally, as cold or wet. 3. *In radiology,* dose.

acute e. *In radiology,* a short exposure to radiation.

chemical e. The product of gas concentration and time of exposure, commonly measured in milligram minutes per cubic meter of air. See median lethal gas *e.*

e. of person. *In legal medicine,* the exhibiting of the genitalia in public, before a person of the opposite sex. Also called *indecent exposure.* See *exhibitionism.*

median lethal gas e. The exposure to a war gas required to kill 50% of those exposed: commonly expressed as LCT 50. See chemical *e.*

ex·pres′sion [L. *expressio,* from *exprimere,* to press out]. 1. Act of pressing out. 2. The product of the act of pressing out.

e. of fetus. Pressure exerted upon the uterus through the abdominal walls to aid in the expulsion of the fetus.

ex″pres·siv′i·ty [L. *expressum,* from *exprimere*]. The degree to which a given gene manifests itself in the hereditary characteristic which it governs. Also see *penetrance.*

ex·pul′sion [L. *expulsio,* from *expellere,* to drive out]. 1. Act of forcing out. 2. Summary dismissal from membership. —**expulsive,** *adj.*

ex·san′gui·nate [L. *exsanguis,* deprived of blood]. Bloodless. —**exsanguine,** *adj.;* **exsanguina′tion, exsanguin′ity,** *n.*

ex·san′gui·nate. To drain of blood.

ex·sec′tion. See *excision.*

ex·sic′cant [L. *exsiccare,* to dry up]. Drying or absorbing moisture.

ex·sic′cant. A dusting powder.

ex″sic·ca′tion [L. *exsiccatio,* from *exsiccare*]. Act of drying; especially, depriving a crystalline body of its water of crystallization. —**exsic′cative,** *adj.*

ex′sic·ca″tor. Old term for desiccator.

ex′stro·phy [G. *ex,* out; *strephein,* to turn]. Eversion; the turning inside out of a part.

e. of bladder. A congenital malformation in which the lower anterior part of the abdominal wall, the anterior wall of the urinary bladder, and usually the symphysis pubis are wanting, and the posterior wall of the bladder is pressed through the opening.

ex″suf·fla′tion [L. *exsufflare,* to blow away]. Forced discharge of the breath.

ext. *Extractum;* extract.

ex·ten′sion [L. *extensio,* from *extendere,* to stretch out]. 1. A straightening out, especially the muscular movement by which a flexed limb is made straight. 2. Traction upon a fractured or dislocated limb. **Counterextension** is traction made on a part in a direction opposite to that in which traction is made by another force.

Buck's e. See Gurdon *Buck.*

ex·ten′sor [L., from *extendere*]. 1. A muscle which extends or stretches a limb or part, as opposed to a *flexor.* See Table of Muscles in the Appendix. 2. *In dermatology,* the extensor surfaces of an extremity.

e. carpi radialis accessorius. A variant part of the extensor carpi radialis brevis muscle which is inserted into the base of the first metacarpal, the base of the first phalanx of the thumb, or into the short abductor of the thumb.

e. carpi radialis brevior. Old name for extensor carpi radialis brevis muscle.

e. carpi radialis brevis. The short radial extensor of the wrist.

e. carpi radialis intermedius. A variant part of the extensor carpi radialis brevis muscle inserted into the base of the second or third metacarpal or both.

e. carpi radialis longior. The old name for extensor carpi radialis longus muscle.

e. carpi radialis longus. The long radial extensor of the wrist.

e. carpi ulnaris. The ulnar extensor of the wrist.

e. carpi ulnaris digiti quinti. A rare variant part of the extensor carpi ulnaris muscle inserted into the base of the proximal phalanx of the little finger.

e. coccygeus. An occasional slip of muscle arising from the lower posterior surface of the sacrum and the upper posterior surface of the coccyx and inserted into the lower part of the coccyx; a rudiment of the extensor of the caudal vertebrae of tailed animals.

e. communis pollicis et indicis. An occasional extra extensor arising from the dorsal surface of the ulna and the interosseous membrane and inserted into both thumb and index finger.

e. digiti annularis. A rare anomalous muscle arising from the dorsal surface of the distal end of the ulna and inserted into the ring finger; a variant of the extensor indicis proprius muscle.

e. digiti medii. A rare anomalous muscle arising from the dorsal surface of the distal end of the ulna and inserted into the middle finger; a variant of the extensor indicis proprius muscle.

e. digiti minimi proprius. The extensor digiti quinti proprius.

e. digiti quinti proprius. The extensor of the little finger.

e. digitorum. The BR name for extensor digitorum communis muscle.

e. digitorum brevis manus. Various rare anomalous muscle bands arising from the dorsal surface of the ulnar carpal bones and inserted into the usual extensor tendons of the fingers or into the metacarpals.

e. digitorum brevis pedis. The short extensor of the toes.

e. digitorum communis. The extensor of the fingers.

e. digitorum longus. The long extensor of the toes.

e. hallucis brevis. The part of extensor digitorum brevis muscle for the great toe.

e. hallucis longus. The long extensor of the great toe.

e. hallucis proprius. The extensor hallucis longus muscle.

e. indicis. The BR name for extensor indicis proprius muscle.

e. indicis proprius. The extensor of the index finger.

e. ossis metacarpi pollicis. Old name for abductor pollicis longus muscle.

e. ossis metatarsi hallucis. Old name for an occasional part of the extensor hallucis longus muscle inserted into the first metatarsal.

e. pollicis brevis. The short extensor of the thumb.

e. pollicis longus. The long extensor of the thumb.

e. primi internodii longus hallucis. Old name for an occasional part of the extensor hallucis longus muscle inserted into the proximal phalanx of the great toe.

e. primi internodii pollicis. Old name for extensor pollicis brevis muscle.

e. secundi internodii pollicis. Old name for extensor pollicis longus muscle.

ex·ten′sor thrust. Rapid reflex contraction of extensor muscles; occurs in the leg of a spinal animal when the bottom of the foot makes a firm contact with a solid surface.

ex·te″ri·or·i·za′tion [L. *exterior*, comp. of *exterus*, on the outside]. 1. *In psychiatry*, the act of objectivating one's interests; the turning of one's interests outward. 2. *In surgery*, the operation of marsupialization.

ex′tern [F. *externe*, L. *externus*, external]. A medical school student or graduate who helps with the care of patients but lives outside of the hospital.

ex·ter′nal [*externus*]. 1. Exterior, acting from without. 2. *In anatomy*, on or near the outside of the body; away from the center or middle line of the body. 3. Not essential, superficial. —**externad,** *adv.*

ex·ter′nal·ize [*externus*]. 1. *In psychology*, transform an idea or impression which is on the percipient's mind into a phantasm apparently outside him. 2. Refer to some outside source, as the voices heard by the subject of hallucinations.

ex′ter·o·cep″tor (eck′stur·o·sep″tur, eck″stur·o·sep′tur) [L. *exterus*, outward; *capere*, to take]. An end organ, in or near the skin or a mucous membrane, which receives stimuli from the external world.

ex″ter·o·fec′tive [*exterus;* L. *facere*, to make]. Pertaining to the voluntary nervous system (the central nervous system and the somatic nerves).

ex·tinc′tion [L. *extinctum*, from *extinguere*, to extinguish]. 1. The act of putting out or extinguishing; destruction. 2. *In psychology*, the disappearance of a conditioned reflex when excited repeatedly without reinforcement.

e. of mercury. The rubbing of mercury with lard or some other substance until the particles of mercury are no longer visible.

ex″tir·pa′tion [L. *exstirpare*, to pluck out by the stem or root]. Complete removal of a part or surgical destruction of a part.

Exton, William Gustav [*American physician*, 1876–1943]. Introduced a test for albumin, and, with A. R. Rose, a test for glucose tolerance. See under *test*. See also Exton's *method*, Exton's *reagents* under *reagent*.

Exton immiscible balance. Trade name for an instrument used to determine the specific gravity of urine when only small amounts are available, as in ureteral catheterization.

ex·tor′sion [L. *extorsio*, from *extorquere*, to twist out]. 1. Outward rotation of a part. 2. *In ophthalmology*, a turning outward of the vertical meridians.

ex′tra- [L.]. A prefix denoting *outside of, beyond the scope of*.

ex″tra·ar·tic′u·lar. Outside of a joint.

ex″tra·buc′cal [L. *extra*, outside of; *bucca*, cheek]. Outside of the mouth; extraoral.

ex″tra·bulb′ar [*extra;* G. *bolbos*, bulb]. Exterior to a bulb; specifically, exterior to the medulla oblongata.

ex″tra·cap′su·lar [*extra;* L. *capsula*, small box]. Outside a capsule; outside the capsular ligament of a joint.

ex″tra·car′pal [*extra;* G. *karpos*, wrist]. Exterior to the wrist bones.

ex″tra·cel′lu·lar [*extra;* L. *cellula*, little cell]. External to the cells of an organism.

ex″tra·cer′e·bral [*extra;* L. *cerebrum*, brain]. Outside of the brain, but within the cranial cavity.

ex″tra·cor·po′re·al [*extra;* L. *corporeus*, corporeal]. Outside of the body.

ex″tra·cor·pus′cu·lar (eck″struh·kor·pus′cue·lur) [*extra;* L. *corpusculum*, little body]. Outside of a corpuscle; especially, outside a blood cell or blood cells.

ex″tra·cra′ni·al [*extra;* G. *kranion*, skull]. Outside of the cranial cavity.

ex′tract [L. *extractum*, from *extrahere*, to draw out]. A pharmaceutical preparation obtained by dissolving the active constituents of a drug with a suitable menstruum, evaporating the solvent, and adjusting to prescribed standards, generally so that one part of the extract represents four to six parts of the drug. Abbreviated, ext. —**extract′,** *v.*

fluid e. See *fluidextract.*

liver e. A water-soluble, thermostable preparation of a fraction of mammalian livers used in the therapy of pernicious anemia.

pilular e. A soft extract suitable for molding into pills or incorporation in an ointment.

powdered e. A powder form of an extract, more suitable for encapsulation.

protein e. A protein substance dissolved out of materials such as foods or inhaled matter. Used in testing and treating allergic patients.

ex·trac′tion [*extractum*]. 1. The act of drawing out. 2. The process of making an extract.

e. of cataract. The surgical removal of a cataractous lens.

e. of tooth. The surgical removal of a tooth from its alveolus.

ex·trac′tive [*extractum*]. 1. That which is extracted. 2. An unidentified substance extracted in chemical analyses; as ether extractive, that material which is extracted with ether.

ex·trac′tor [*extractum*]. 1. An instrument or forceps for extracting bullets, sequestra, or foreign bodies. 2. *In dentistry*, an instrument for extracting the root of a tooth.

ex″tra·cyst′ic [L. *extra*, outside of; G. *kystis*, bladder]. Outside of a cyst, urinary bladder, or gallbladder.

ex″tra·du′ral [*extra;* L. *durus*, hard]. Situated outside of or upon the dura.

ex″tra·em″bry·on′ic [*extra;* G. *embryon*, embryo]. Situated outside, or not forming a part of, the embryo; e.g., the fetal membranes.

ex″tra·ep″i·phys′e·al (eck″struh·ep″i·fizz′ee·ul) [*extra;* G. *epiphysis*, excrescence]. Outside, or away from, an epiphysis.

ex″tra·e·ryth″ro·cyt′ic. See *exo-erythrocytic.*

ex″tra·e″so·phag′e·al (·ee″so·fadj′ee·ul, ·fay′jee·ul) [*extra;* G. *oisophagos*, gullet]. Immediately surrounding the esophagus, as the extraesophageal region of the mediastinum.

ex″tra·gen′i·tal [*extra;* L. *genitalis*, genital]. Situated outside of, or unrelated to, the genitals.

ex″tra·he·pat′ic [*extra;* G. *hēpar*, liver]. Not connected with the liver.

ex″tra·lig″a·men′tous [*extra;* L. *ligamentum*, a tie]. External to a ligament.

extralin. Trade-mark for a liver-stomach concentrate used orally in the treatment of pernicious anemia.

ex″tra·med′ul·lar″y (eck″struh·med′uh·lerr″ee, ·mi·dull′uh·ree) [*extra;* L. *medulla*, marrow]. 1. Situated or occurring outside the spinal cord or medulla oblongata. 2. Situated or occurring outside the bone marrow, as extramedullary hematopoiesis.

ex″tra·mu′ral [*extra;* L. *murus*, wall]. Outside the wall of an organ.

ex″tra·nu′cle·ar [*extra;* L. *nucleus*, nut]. Outside of the nucleus of a cell.

ex″tra·pa·ren′chy·mal (·pa·reng′ki·mul) [*extra;* G. *paregchyma*, anything poured in beside]. Outside of or unrelated to a parenchyma.

ex″tra·pel′vic [*extra;* L. *pelvis*, basin]. Situated or occurring outside of the pelvis.

ex″tra·per″i·ne′al [*extra;* G. *perinaion*, space

between the anus and scrotum]. Outside of or away from the perineum.

ex″tra·per″i·to·ne′al [*extra;* G. *peritonaion*, something stretched over, especially the membrane which contains the lower viscera]. External to the peritoneal cavity.

ex″tra·pla·cen′tal [*extra;* L. *placenta*, a cake]. Not connected with the placenta.

ex″tra·pros·tat′ic [*extra;* G. *prostatēs*, one who stands before]. Outside or away from the prostate.

ex″tra·py·ram′i·dal [*extra;* G. *pyramis*, pyramid]. Outside of the pyramidal tracts, applied to other descending pathways.

ex″tra·sen′sor·y [*extra;* L. *sensus*, sense]. 1. Of or pertaining to phenomena outside the realm normally perceived through the senses; not sensory. 2. Of or pertaining to certain capacities of perception unexplainable in relation to the senses. See *psi phenomena* under *phenomenon; extrasensory perception.*

ex″tra·sys′to·le (eck″struh·sis′to·lee) [*extra;* G. *systolē*, a drawing together]. A heartbeat occurring before its normal time in the rhythm of the heart and followed by a compensatory pause, due to abnormal or re-entry stimuli in various parts of the heart—atria, ventricles, atrioventricular bundle, and even the nodes themselves—and named from the origin of the stimuli, as ventricular extrasystole. Also called *premature beat, premature contraction.*

frustrane e. One faintly heard.

interpolated e. One of ventricular origin, occurring early in diastole and not disturbing the normal rhythm.

ex″tra·tu′bal [*extra;* L. *tubus*, tube]. Outside of a tube, as the uterine tube.

ex″tra·u′ter·ine (·yoo′tur·in, ·yne) [*extra;* L. *uterus*, womb]. Outside of the uterus.

ex″tra·vag′i·nal (·vadj′i·nul, ·va·jy′nul) [*extra;* L. *vagina*, sheath]. Outside of the vagina or any sheath.

ex·trav″a·sa′tion [*extra;* L. *vas*, vessel]. 1. Passing of a body fluid out of its proper place, as blood into surrounding tissues after rupture of a vessel, or urine after rupture of the bladder or urethra. 2. Material so discharged.

ex″tra·vas′cu·lar [*extra;* L. *vasculum*, small vessel]. Outside of a vessel.

ex″tra·ven·tric′u·lar [*extra;* L. *ventriculus*, stomach]. External to a ventricle.

ex′tra·vert. See *extrovert.*

ex″tra·vis′u·al [*extra;* L. *visualis*, from *visus*, a seeing]. Outside the limits of vision.

ex·trem′i·ty [L. *extremitas*, extremity]. The distal, or terminal, end of any part.

lower e. The hip, thigh, leg, ankle, and foot. See Plates 7, 9, 16.

upper e. The shoulder girdle, arm, forearm, wrist, and hand. See Plates 7, 9, 16.

ex·trin′sic [L. *extrinsecus*, on the outside]. Originating outside of a part.

ex″tro·gas″tru·la′tion. See *exogastrula.*

ex′tro·phy [G. *ex*, out; *trophē*, nourishment]. 1. Malformation of an organ. 2. Incorrect spelling of exstrophy.

ex′tro·vert, ex′tra·vert [L. *extra*, outside of; *vertere*, to turn]. One whose interests center in the outside world rather than in subjective activity.

ex′tro·vert, ex′tra·vert. To turn one's interests to external things rather than to oneself.

ex·tru′sion (ecks·troo′zhun) [L. *extrusum*, from *extrudere*, to drive out]. 1. A forcing out; expulsion. 2. *In dentistry*, extension of a tooth beyond the occlusal plane. —**extrude′,** *v.*

ex″tu·ba′tion [L. *ex*, out; *tubus*, tube]. The removal of a tube used for intubation.

ex′u·date [L. *exudare*, to sweat out]. The material that has passed through the walls of vessels into adjacent tissues or spaces in inflammation.

crevicular e. One from the gingival sulcus.

fibrinous e. One in which fibrin is the main solid constituent.

mucinous e. One containing mucin.

purulent e. An exudate containing a large proportion of pus.

sanguineous e. One containing visible blood. Also called *hemorrhagic e.*

serous e. One composed principally of serum.

ex″u·da′tion [*exudare*]. The passage of various constituents of the blood through the walls of vessels into adjacent tissues or spaces in inflammation. —**exu′dative,** *adj.;* **ex′udate,** *v.*

ex·u″vi·a′tion [L. *exuviae*, from *exuere*, to strip off]. The shedding of the deciduous teeth, or of epidermal structures.

eye [AS. *ēage*]. The organ of vision. It occupies the anterior part of the orbit, and is nearly spherical. It is composed of three concentric coats: the sclerotic and cornea; the choroid, ciliary body, and iris; and the retina. The sclerotic coat, or sclera, is an opaque, white, fibrous membrane, into the anterior part of which the transparent, nonvascular cornea is fitted. The choroid is a soft, vascular tissue which connects with the iris in front by means of a ciliary body. The iris is a colored, circular membrane with a central perforation, the pupil. The retina, the innermost of the three coats, is a delicate, transparent membrane containing the terminations of the optic nerve. The vitreous body, a firm, transparent jelly, constitutes about four-fifths of the volume of the eyeball. In front of the vitreous body is the crystalline lens, a slightly yellowish, transparent, biconvex disk. The space between the lens and the cornea is divided by the iris into two compartments, the anterior and posterior chambers, which contain the aqueous humor. Anteriorly, the eye is covered by conjunctiva; posteriorly, by a fibrous capsule (capsule of Tenon). The eyeball is moved by a group of muscles attached on the outer surface. Changes in the curvature of the lens are brought about by the ciliary muscle, while the size of the pupil is modified by the action of dilator and constrictor fibers in the iris. Abbreviated, E. See Plate 19.

alternating dominance of the eyes. Dominance of one eye at one time or for one function, alternating with that of the fellow for another time or function.

aphakic e. The eye deprived of its crystalline lens.

appendages of the e. The eyelids, brows, and lacrimal apparatus.

artificial e. Glass, celluloid, rubber, or plastic made to resemble the front of the eye, and worn in the socket to replace a lost organ, or over a blind eye, for cosmetic effect.

black e. See *ecchymosis.*

blue e. See habronemic *ophthalmomyiasis.*

bung e. See habronemic *ophthalmomyiasis.*

camp e. A syndrome characterized by a loss of visual acuity and the presence of a central scotoma; it was seen in inmates of concentration camps in World War II.

compound e. The organ of vision formed of several closely grouped, prismatic eyes (ommatidia) as in most arthropods.

cross-e. See *strabismus.*

dominant e. The eye which is unconsciously and preferentially chosen to guide decision and action.

equidominant eyes. Eyes having equal or divided dominance.

evil e. See *evil eye.*

exciting e. The originally injured or diseased eye in sympathetic ophthalmia.

fixing e. In strabismus, the eye which is directed toward the visual object.

gas e. A peculiar disease prevalent among the employees of the gas pumping stations in the natural gas regions of the United States. The eyes are inflamed, tender, and sensitive to light.

pineal e. The rudimentary median eye in some lizards. Also called *epiphyseal e.*

reversed dominance of the eyes. In a right-handed person, dominance of the left eye because of disease, operation, or ametropia of the right eye; in a left-handed person, dominance of the right eye.

schematic e. An apparatus representing an ideal or normal eye.

sticky e. An infection of the eye, caused most often by micrococci, sometimes seen in newborn infants.

sympathizing e. The noninjured eye that becomes involved in sympathetic ophthalmia.

eye'ball" [*ēage;* ME. *bal*]. The globe of the eye. See Plate 19.

eye'brow" [*ēage;* AS. *brū*]. The supercilium; the arch above the eye; the hair covering the arch.

eye'cells" [*ēage;* L. *cella,* cell]. Cup-shaped cells of porcelain, enameled black, to place over the eye after operations.

eye'cup" [*ēage;* AS. *cuppe,* from L. *cupa,* tub]. 1. The optic vesicle. 2. A small cup which fits over the eye; used for bathing the conjunctiva.

eye ground. The fundus of the eye; the internal aspect of the eye as seen through an ophthalmoscope.

eye'lash" [*ēage;* ME. *lasche*]. One of the stiff hairs growing on the margin of the eyelid; a cilium.

eye'lid" [*ēage;* AS. *hlid*]. One of the two protective coverings of the eyeball; a curtain of movable skin lined with conjunctiva, having the tarsus, glands, and cilia in the distal part, muscle in the proximal part. See Plate 19.

e. lag. See von Graefe's *sign.*

fused eyelids. (a) The normal fusion between the epithelia of the fetal eyelid folds, occurring about the ninth week and persisting until the seventh or eighth month. (b) A congenital anomaly caused by the failure of the two fetal eyelids to separate.

eye'piece" [*ēage;* OF. *pece,* of Celtic origin]. *In optics,* the ocular; the lens or combination of lenses of an optical instrument nearest the eye.

eye'point" [*ēage;* OF. *pointe,* from L. *pungere,* to prick]. The point above an ocular or simple microscope where the greatest number of emerging rays cross.

eye'spot" [*ēage;* ME.]. A pigmented spot in invertebrates, thought to stimulate reactions in response to light.

eye'strain" [*ēage;* OF. *estraindre,* from L. *stringere,* to draw tight]. Irritation and weariness of the eye as a result of excessive use or uncorrected defects of vision.

eye'tooth" [*ēage;* AS. *tōth*]. A canine tooth of the upper jaw.

eye'wash" [*ēage;* AS. *wascan*]. A medicated solution for the eye; a collyrium.

F

F Chemical symbol for fluorine.

F Symbol for luminous flux.

F. Abbreviation for Fahrenheit, field of vision, formula.

F_1 The first filial generation. The offspring of a given mating.

F_2 The second filial generation. The grandchildren of a given mating.

f-12. See under *freon.*

Fa Chemical symbol for francium.

fa·bel'la [dim. of L. *faba,* bean]. A sesamoid fibrocartilage or small bone occasionally developed in a head of the gastrocnemius muscle.

Faber, Knud Helge (1862–). Danish physician who described hypochromic anemia associated with achlorhydria. See achlorhydric *anemia.*

fa'bism, fa·bis'mus. Favism.

fab"ri·ca'tion. See *confabulation.*

Fabricius ab Aquapendente, Hieronymus (Girolamo Fabrizio) [*Italian anatomist and surgeon,* ca. 1537–1619]. Remembered especially for his researches in embryology. Made observations on the valves of the veins, although he is not credited with their discovery. Teacher of Harvey.

Fabricius Hildanus (Wilhelm Fabry) [*German surgeon,* 1560–1634]. Called the father of German surgery. Made the first known classification of burns (1607). Described a chest of medicines and surgical instruments for military use in the field.

Fabricus-Moller urine test. See under *test.*

Fabrizio. See *Fabricius ab Aquapendente.*

Fabry. See *Fabricius Hildanus.*

fab"u·la'tion. See *confabulation.*

F.A.C.D. Fellow of the American College of Dentists.

face [OF., from L. *facies,* form, face]. The anterior part of the head including forehead and jaws, but not the ears. See Table of Bones in the Appendix. —**fa'cial,** *adj.*

adenoid f. One showing the characteristic open-mouthed and stupid appearance associated with adenoid growths which interfere with nasal breathing.

bird f. One characterized by a receding chin and beaklike appearance of the nose; the result of mandibular hypoplasia (micrognathia).

bovine f. See *facies* bovina.

f. grippée. The pinched face observed in peritonitis.

frog f. A facial deformity due to growth of polyps or other tumors in the nasal cavities. A temporary condition of this kind may be due to orbital cellulitis or facial erysipelas.

Hippocratic f. See *facies* hippocratica.

mask f. A condition present in paralysis agitans; the facial muscles are fixed and do not react to emotions. Also called *Parkinsonian mask.*

masklike f. A face often seen in alcoholic multiple neuritis; expressionless and immobile between the eyes and lips, while the eyebrows, forehead, and lips may be moving freely.

moon f. Rounded, full facies characteristic of Cushing's syndrome.

scaphoid f. One that appears concave because

of weakly developed nasal and maxillary regions: also called *dishface.*

face bow. *In dentistry,* a device used to record the spatial relationship between the alveolar ridges and the mandibular joints.

fac′et (fass′it) [F. *facette,* little face]. A small plane surface, especially on a bone or a hard body; may be produced by wear, as a worn spot on the surface of a tooth.

fa′cial ar′ter·y. BR term and O.T. for *external maxillary artery.* See Table of Arteries in the Appendix.

fa′cial (seventh cranial) nerve. See Table of Nerves in the Appendix.

fa′ci·es (fay′shee·eez, fash′ee·eez) [L., face]. 1. The appearance of the face. 2. A surface.

f. abdominalis. The pinched, dehydrated facial mien of a person with marked gastrointestinal disturbance, often an accompaniment of generalized systemic disease.

f. articularis. An articular surface.

f. auricularis. Auricular surface.

f. bovina. Cow face, as may occur with ocular hypertelorism.

f. cerebralis. Cerebral surface.

f. costalis. Costal surface.

f. diaphragmatica. Diaphragmatic surface.

f. epileptica. Dull expression of the face with little emotional lability, seen in some epileptics.

f. frontalis. Frontal surface.

f. gastrica. Gastric surface.

f. hippocratica. An appearance of the face indicative of the rapid approach of death: the nose is pinched, the temples hollow, the eyes sunken, the ears leaden and cold, the lips relaxed, the skin livid.

f. intestinalis. Intestinal surface.

f. labialis. Labial or buccal surface.

f. lateralis. Lateral surface.

f. leontina. The lionlike face seen in lepers.

f. lingualis. Lingual surface.

f. malaris. Malar surface.

f. malleolaris. Malleolar surface.

f. maxillaris. Maxillary surface.

f. medialis. Medial surface.

f. mediastinalis. Mediastinal surface.

f. myopathica. A peculiar expression seen in some forms of myopathic muscular atrophy. It is characterized by imperfect movement of the facial muscles, sinking in of the cheeks, and drooping of the lower lip.

f. nasalis. Nasal surface.

f. orbitalis. Orbital surface.

f. ossea. Bony portion of the face.

f. palatina. Palatine surface.

f. parietalis. Parietal surface.

f. patellaris. Patellar surface.

f. pelvina. Pelvic surface.

f. renalis. Renal surface.

f. sphenomaxillaris. Temporal surface.

f. volaris. Volar surface.

hepatic f. The sharp, pinched features and yellowish skin seen in patients with chronic liver disorders.

fa·cil″i·ta′tion [L. *facilis,* easy]. 1. Increased ease in carrying out an action or function. 2. The furtherance of neural activities by conditioning or by previous or simultaneous stimulation.

fa′ci·o- [L. *facies,* face]. A combining form meaning *the face.*

F.A.C.P. Fellow of the American College of Physicians.

F.A.C.S. Fellow of the American College of Surgeons.

fac·ti′tious [L. *facticius,* from *facere,* to make]. Pertaining to a state or substance which is brought about or produced by means other than natural.

fac′tor [L., a maker]. 1. A circumstance, fact, or influence which tends to produce a result; a constituent. 2. *In biology,* a gene. 3. An essential or desirable element in diet.

accelerator f. Any factor which accelerates clotting; more specifically, any blood factor accelerating the conversion of prothrombin to thrombin; most specifically, proaccelerin or accelerin.

accessory food factors. Substances, present in foods, which are necessary to life, or for proper growth and development. See *vitamin.*

animal protein f. See *vitamin* B_{12}.

antialopecia f. Inositol.

antianemia f. See *vitamin* B_{12}.

anti-egg-white-injury f. Biotin.

anti-gray-hair f. Para-aminobenzoic acid.

antihemophilic f. A factor associated with human plasma globulin but deficient in hemophilic blood, required for the development of plasma thromboplastic activity. Syn., *plasma thromboplastinogen, globulin substance.*

anti-pernicious-anemia f. See *vitamin* B_{12}.

anti-pernicious-anemia liver f. See *vitamin* B_{12}.

antistiffness f. Fat-soluble vitamin, not known to be essential to man, found in green vegetables, raw cream, etc.; in experimental animals its lack produces inflammatory lesions of the fibrous connective tissue and influences phosphorus metabolism.

antixerotic f. Vitamin A.

Bittner milk f. See milk *f.*

bursting f. See *collagenase.*

CH f. A substance in liver extract that intervenes in the metabolic process to correct deficiencies of methionine or choline. It protects against lathyrism.

chick antidermatitis f. Pantothenic acid.

Christmas f. A component of plasma necessary for the development of plasma thromboplastic activity. Deficiency of the factor results in a hemophilialike disease (*Christmas disease*). Syn., *plasma thromboplastic component.*

chromotrichia f. Para-aminobenzoic acid.

citrovorum f. A factor necessary for the growth of the bacillus *Leuconostoc citrovorum.* It is a B-complex vitamin, apparently folinic acid, and has been used in the treatment of anemia and malnutrition. Syn., *folinic acid.*

diabetogenic f. Originally, the factor in crude anterior pituitary extract which was diabetogenic in dogs. Growth hormone is now known to be the major diabetogenic agent in crude pituitary extract.

erythrocyte aggregation f. A serum or plasma factor first discovered in cases of lupus erythematosus and demonstrable by cold conglutination tests.

erythrocyte-maturing f. See *vitamin* B_{12}.

Escherichia coli f. An antibiotic identical with corylophilline, mycoin, notatin, penatin, and penicillin-B.

external f. An external component of the environment of an organism, as heat, gravity, etc.

extrinsic f. See *vitamin* B_{12}.

f. V. See *proaccelerin.*

f. VI. See *accelerin.*

f. VII. See *convertin.*

fibrin f. A substance necessary for, and concerned in, the formation of fibrin, as fibrinogen and thrombin.

filtrate f. Pantothenic acid.

glycotrophic f. The factor from the adenohypophysis, which is capable of antagonizing the action of insulin.

growth f. A chemical constituent of the diet, the lack of which retards normal growth and development.

hyperglycemic f. Hyperglycemic-glycogenolytic factor. See *glucagon*.

hyperglycemic-glycogenolytic f. Glucagon. Abbreviated, HGF.

internal f. An internal component of the environment of an organism.

intrinsic f. A substance, produced by the stomach, which combines with the extrinsic factor (vitamin B_{12}) in food to yield an antianemic principle; lack of the intrinsic factor is believed to be a cause of pernicious anemia. Also called *intrinsic f. of Castle*.

Jarrell f. A dominant hereditary blood factor; in persons lacking it, the presence of the antibody may be related to the development of cancer in some cases.

kappa f. A cytoplasmic genic factor in paramecia, believed to be a desoxyribonucleoprotein. When this factor is transmitted to a susceptible paramecium through cytoplasmic conjugation, it causes cell death.

labile f. See *accelerin*.

Lactobacillus casei f. See *folic acid*.

Lactobacillus lactis Dorner f. Vitamin B_{12}; cyanocobalamin. Abbreviated, LLD factor.

lethal f. A gene which causes the death of the gamete or the zygote before development is completed.

lipotropic f. A substance that reduces the amount of liver fat; more specifically, choline or any compound, or compounds, which metabolically can give rise to choline. Syn., *lipotropia*.

LLD f. The Lactobacillus lactis Dorner *f.*

lytic f. Plasminogen: former usage.

maturation f. of liver. See *vitamin B_{12}*.

melanophore-stimulating f. A hormone or part of a hormone, *intermedin*, present in lower vertebrates, that effects the dispersion of pigment granules in the melanophores.

milk f. A filtrable, noncellular agent in the milk and tissues of certain strains of inbred mice; transmitted from the mother to the offspring by nursing. It seems to be an essential factor in the genesis of mammary cancer in these strains. Syn., *Bittner milk f.*

mouse antialopecia f. See *inositol*.

norite f. A bacterial growth factor adsorbable on certain types of charcoal (norite) and related to, or identical with, pteroylglutamic acid.

pellagra preventive f. Nicotinic acid. Abbreviated, PP factor.

Peters' f. Another name for vitamin B_5.

PP f. Pellagra preventive *f.*

reflection f. The ratio of reflected light from a surface to the incident light. Also called *coefficient of reflection*.

R f. Vitamin B_{11}.

Rh f. See *Rh factors*.

semilethal f. A gene which causes the death of the individual soon after development is completed or before reproductive age.

Simon's septic f. The phenomenon of the reduction or disappearance of eosinophils during infections in which neutrophilia occurs; it is now attributed to the action of adrenocortical hormones.

skin f. Biotin.

van't Hoff's f. A factor indicating the dissociation of an electrolyte in solution; a correction factor between theoretical figures based on concentration and experimental value of activity derived from measurements of osmotic pressure, freezing or boiling point.

V f. of the blood. A thermolabile factor found in blood, which is sensitive to alkali but not to acid; diffuses through parchment membranes and is necessary for the growth of *Hemophilus influenzae*.

Williams-Waterman f. Vitamin B_3.

Wills's f. A hematopoietic principle, present in certain crude liver extracts and in autolyzed yeast, effective in cases of macrocytic anemia that are unresponsive to Vitamin B_{12} and to highly refined liver extracts. It may be identical with folic acid.

Y f. See *pyridoxine*.

fac'ul·ta"tive [L. *facultas*, capability]. Voluntary; optional; having the power to do or not to do a thing.

FAD Flavin adenine dinucleotide.

fae'ces (fee'seez). See *feces*.

faex (fecks) [L.]. The dregs or sediment of any liquid; fecula.

f. medicinalis. Yeast.

fa'gar·ine (fay'gur·een, ·in, fag'ur·). The name applied to the three alkaloids of *Fagara coco*, a tree of Argentina; they are differentiated by the prefixes α, β, and γ. **Alpha-fagarine,** $C_{19}H_{23}NO_4$, has been used as a substitute for quinidine in restoring normal rhythm in atrial fibrillation.

Faget, Jean Charles [*French physician*, 1818–84]. Remembered for his description of an important sign in yellow fever, the fall in pulse rate with a rise in the temperature curve or its maintenance at the horizontal.

fag"o·py'rism, fag·op'y·rism [L. *fagus*, beech; G. *pyros*, wheat]. Photosensitization of the skin and mucous membranes, accompanied by convulsions; produced in white and piebald animals by feeding with the flowers or seed husks of the buckwheat plant (*Fagopyrum sagittatum*) or clovers and grasses containing flavin or carotin and xanthophyll.

Fahr, Karl Theodor [*German physician*, 1877–]. With Volhard, he described arteriolar nephrosclerosis and malignant nephrosclerosis, both of which are sometimes called *Fahr-Volhard's disease*. See also *Volhard's and Fahr's tests* under *test*.

Fahr. Fahrenheit scale or thermometer. Also abbreviated, F.

Fåhraeus, Robin [*Swedish pathologist*, 1888–]. Described his test for estimating the speed of settling of the red blood cells in a specimen of blood to which an anticoagulant has been added. Called *Fåhraeus' sedimentation test*.

Fahrenheit, Gabriel Daniel [*German physicist*, 1686–1736]. The inventor of the thermometer and scale bearing his name, in which the space between the freezing point of water (32°) and its boiling point (212°) is divided into 180 degrees.

Failla, Gioacchino (1891–). American radiological physicist, known for his research in measurement of x-rays and radium rays, and in the biological effects of radiations. He developed the small radon tube (gold radon seed) in 1924.

fail'ure. See *cardiac failure, circulatory failure, metabolic failure*.

coronary f. A mild form of acute coronary insufficiency with subendocardial ischemia, but without necrosis or infarction.

faint [OF., from *faindre*, to feign]. Weak; wanting strength; ready or about to swoon.

faint. A state of syncope or swooning.

faint. To swoon; suffer syncope.

faith cure. The system or practice of treating disease by religious faith and prayer.

fal′cate [L. *falcatus*, from *falx*, sickle]. Sickle-shaped.

fal′ci·form (fal′si·form) [*falx;* L. *forma*, shape]. Having the shape of a sickle.

fal′cu·la [L. *falcula*, small sickle]. The falx cerebelli.

fal′cu·lar [*falcula*]. 1. Sickle-shaped. 2. Pertaining to the falx cerebelli.

fal·lo′pi·an, Fal·lo′pi·an tube. See under *tube.*

Fallopius, Gabriel (Gabrielle Falloppia) [*Italian anatomist*, 1523–62]. Described ovaries, round ligaments of the uterus, and oviducts, called *fallopian* or *uterine tubes.* Gave the vagina and placenta their present names. Made a detailed study of the ear, being first to describe the semicircular canals. Was first to describe the facial canal, called the *fallopian aqueduct.*

Fallot, Etienne Louis Arthur [*French physician*, 1850–1911]. Described a type of congenital heart disease with dextroposition of the aorta, hypertrophy of the right ventricle, ventricular septal defect, and pulmonary stenosis or atresia. Called *tetralogy of Fallot.*

Falls's test. See colostrum *test.*

Falret, Jean Pierre [*French psychiatrist*, 1794–1870]. Described manic-depressive psychosis (1854), called *circular insanity, cyclic insanity.* A pioneer in French psychiatry, he was the precursor of Charcot.

false [L. *falsus*, from *fallere*, to deceive]. Not genuine; not real; imitating.

falx [L.]. A sickle-shaped structure. —**fal′cial,** *adj.*

f. aponeurotica. The conjoined tendon.

f. cerebelli. A sicklelike process of dura mater between the lobes of the cerebellum.

f. cerebri. The process of the dura mater separating the hemispheres of the cerebrum. See Plate 18.

f. inguinalis. See *f.* aponeurotica.

fa′mes (fay′meez) [L.]. Hunger.

fa·mil′ial [L. *familia*, household]. Of, pertaining to, or occurring among, the members of a family, as a familial disease.

fam′i·ly [*familia*]. 1. A group of closely related persons; parents and children; those descended from a common ancestor. 2. *In biology*, a classification group higher than a genus; the principal division of an order.

fa·nat′i·cism [L. *fanaticus*, pertaining to a temple]. Perversion and excess of the religious sentiment; unreasoning zeal in regard to any subject. Sometimes a manifestation of mental disease.

Fanconi, Guido [*Swiss pediatrician*, 1882–]. Described constitutional infantile anemia, resembling pernicious anemia, called *Fanconi's disease;* he also described (1934) fibrosis of the pancreas with bronchiectasis, and amino diabetes (1936), called *de Toni-Fanconi syndrome.*

fang [AS. *fōn*, to make fast]. 1. A sharp or pointed tooth; especially, the tooth of a wild beast or serpent. 2. The root of a tooth. *Obs.*

fan′go [It., mud]. Clay from the hot springs of Battaglio, Italy; used as a local application.

fan″go·ther′a·py [*fango;* G. *therapeia*, treatment]. Treatment with fango: used in arthritis or gout.

Fan′ni·a [G. *phanos*, conspicuous]. A genus of flies of the family Anthomyiidae. The species **F. canicularis,** the lesser house fly, and **F. scalaris,** the latrine fly, breed under unsanitary conditions; occasionally their larvae cause intestinal myiasis in man.

Fano, Giulio [*Italian physiologist*, 1856–1930]. Known for his studies of the physiology of the circulation and of the electric impulses of the heart, which contributed to the development of electrocardiography.

fan′ta·sy [G. *phantasia*, appearance, imagination]. 1. Imagination; the ability to form mental pictures of scenes, occurrences, or objects not actually present; fanciful, whimsical image making. 2. An image. Also see *phantasy.*

Farabeuf, Louis Hubert [*French anatomist and surgeon*, 1841–1910]. Described operations, each called *Farabeuf's operation*, for amputation of the forefinger and for disarticulation of the great toe. Also devised operations for amputation of the foot, of the arm at the elbow, and of the leg above the knee joint. Invented a bone-holding instrument for use in amputations. Described a triangle, called *Farabeuf's triangle*, formed in the upper part of the neck by the internal jugular vein, the common facial vein, and the hypoglossal nerve.

far′ad [after Michael *Faraday*]. The unit of electric capacitance; the capacitance of a capacitator that is charged to a potential of 1 volt by 1 coulomb of electricity.

Faraday, Michael [*English chemist and physicist*, 1791–1867]. Discovered electromagnetic induction. Stated *Faraday's laws* (a) of electrolysis: the weight of an ion deposited electrolytically is proportional to the strength of the current passing through the solution; (b) see *faraday.*

far′a·day [*Faraday*]. The quantity of electricity which will liberate one gram equivalent of an element in electrolysis. It equals 96,489 coulombs.

fa·rad′ic [*Faraday*]. Relating to induced rapidly alternating currents of electricity.

far″a·dim′e·ter [*Faraday;* G. *metron*, a measure]. An instrument for measuring the strength of an induced rapidly alternating electric current.

fa·rad″i·punc′ture [*Faraday;* L. *punctura*, puncture]. The application of faradic currents by means of needle electrodes thrust into the tissues.

far′a·dism [*Faraday*]. 1. Induced rapidly alternating currents. 2. Faradization.

far″a·di·za′tion [*Faraday*]. Faradism; the therapeutic application of induced rapidly alternating currents to a diseased part. —**far′adize,** *v.*

general f. The therapeutic application of the electric current to the organism as a whole.

far′a·do- [*Faraday*]. A combining form signifying *faradic.*

far″a·do·con″trac·til′i·ty [*Faraday;* L. *contrahere*, to contract]. Contractility in response to faradic stimulus.

far″a·do·mus′cu·lar [*Faraday;* L. *musculus*, muscle]. Pertaining to the reaction of a muscle when a faradic current is applied.

far″a·do·ther′a·py [*Faraday;* G. *therapeia*, treatment]. Therapeutic use of faradism; faradization.

farastan. The trade-mark for a compound of cinchophen and mono-iodo-cinchophen, used in the treatment of arthritis, neuritis, sciatica, and gout.

far′cy. Glanders.

far′del-bound″. Having a disease in which the omasum becomes static and the food dry and impacted; said of ruminants.

far″i·na′ceous [L. *farina*, flour]. Having the nature of or yielding flour; starchy; containing starch.

Farley, St. Clair, and Reisinger's method. See under *method.*

Farmer's method. See Farmer and Abt's *method*, Folin-Farmer *method.*

far′ne·sol. $C_{15}H_{26}O$; 3,7,11-trimethyl-2,6,10-dodecatrien-1-ol; an unsaturated liquid alcohol found in various volatile oils, also in Peruvian balsam and tolu balsam. It is used in perfumery to emphasize the odor of certain floral perfumes.

far′-point″. The most distant point at which an eye can see distinctly when accommodation is completely relaxed.

Farr, William [*English medical statistician*, 1807–83]. One of the founders of morbidity and mortality statistics. Showed that in a typical epidemic the incidence of the disease is represented by a curve rising at first sharply, then more gradually to a peak, and descending more rapidly than it rose at first; called *Farr's law*.

Farre, Arthur [*English gynecologist*, 1811–87]. Described the boundary line at the hilum of the ovary in the broad ligament, called *Farre's white line*.

far′ri·er·y [L. *ferrarius*, blacksmith]. The treatment of the diseases of the horse. *Obs.*

far′-sight″. Hypermetropia. —**farsight′edness,** *n.*

fas′ci·a (fash′ee·uh) (pl. *fasciae*) [L., band]. 1. The areolar tissue layers under the skin (superficial fascia), or between muscles and forming the sheaths of muscles, or investing other deep, definitive structures, as nerves and blood vessels (deep fascia). 2. A bandage. *Obs.* —**fascial,** *adj.*

Buck's f. The deep fascia of the penis.

Camper's f. The superficial, loose, fat-containing layer of the superficial fascia of the lower abdomen.

clavipectoral f. That portion of the deep fascia of the pectoral region which is attached above to the clavicle and coracoid process and which surrounds the subclavius and pectoralis minor muscles. The portion between the two muscles is also called the *costocoracoid membrane* or *ligament.*

Colles' f. The deep layer of the superficial perineal fascia.

Cooper's f. The cremasteric fascia.

cremasteric f. A thin covering of the spermatic cord, enclosing the fibers of the cremaster muscle.

cribriform f. The sievelike covering of the fossa ovalis of the thigh.

crural f. The deep fascia of the leg, extending from knee to ankle.

deep cervical f. That which invests the muscles of the neck and encloses the vessels and nerves. It consists of three fascial planes, one surrounding the trapezius and sternocleidomastoid muscles, a second surrounding the larynx, pharynx, and thyroid gland, and a third, the prevertebral fascia.

Denonvillier's f. That portion of the pelvic fascia between the anterior surface of the rectum and the seminal vesicles and prostate gland.

diaphragmatic f. That portion of the pelvic fascia which surrounds the pelvic diaphragm.

endopelvic f. The visceral portion of the pelvic fascia.

external spermatic f. The outer covering of the spermatic cord and testis, continuous with the aponeurosis of the external oblique muscle at the subcutaneous inguinal ring.

f. colli. See deep cervical *fascia*.

f. dentata. A serrated band of gray matter lying upon the medial side of the hippocampus of the cerebrum.

f. lata. The dense fascia surrounding the muscles of the thigh.

f. lunata. The deep fascia of the ischiorectal fossa.

Gerota's f. The renal fascia.

iliac f. The fascia covering the pelvic surface of the iliacus muscle.

infundibuliform f. See internal spermatic *f.*

intercolumnar f. (a) A fascia attached to the crura of the external abdominal ring. (b) That portion of the diaphragmatic fascia located between the two pubococcygeus muscles.

internal spermatic f. The inner covering of the spermatic cord and testis, continuous with the transversalis fascia at the abdominal inguinal ring.

ischiorectal f. That covering the perineal aspect of the levator ani muscle and filling the ischiorectal fossa.

lumbodorsal f. Variously described as the sheath of the sacrospinalis muscle alone, or the sheaths of the sacrospinalis and the quadratus lumborum muscles.

obturator f. The portion of the parietal pelvic fascia overlying the obturator internus muscle.

palpebral f. Fascia of the eyelids; orbital septum.

pectineal f. The portion of the fascia lata associated with the pectineus muscle: also called *pubic f.*

pectoral f. Deep fascia over the pectoralis major muscle on the anterior aspect of the thorax. Also called *pectoralis f.* See Plate 43.

pelvic f. A collective name for all of the fascia located within the pelvic cavity. It is usually divided into three portions: parietal, diaphragmatic, and endopelvic or visceral.

prevertebral f. The third layer of the deep cervical fascia; a band of connective tissue covering the front of the cervical vertebrae and the prevertebral muscles. It is attached to the esophagus and pharynx by loose connective tissue.

pubic f. See pectineal *f.*

renal f. The connective tissue investment of the kidney. There is an anterior and a posterior layer with the kidney and perirenal fat between. The two layers form a pocket; above, below, and laterally they are fused. Also called *Gerota's f.*

Scarpa's f. The deep, membranous layer of the superficial fascia of the lower abdomen.

Sibson's f. A domelike expansion of fascia strengthening the pleura over the apex of the lung, extending from the first rib to the transverse process of the seventh cervical vertebra.

transversalis f. That lying between the transversus abdominis muscle and the peritoneum.

triangular f. The reflected inguinal ligament.

Waldeyer's f. That portion of the pelvic fascia surrounding the distal end of each ureter.

fas′ci·cle (fass′i·kul). Fasciculus. —**fascic′ular,** *adj.*

fas·cic′u·la″ted (fa·sick′yoo·lay″tid) [L. *fasciculus*, small bundle]. United into bundles or fascicles.

fas·cic″u·la′tion (fa·sick″yoo·lay′shun) [*fasciculus*]. 1. An incoordinate contraction of skeletal muscle in which groups of muscle fibers innervated by the same neuron contract together. 2. The formation of fasciculi.

fas·cic′u·lus (fa·sick′yoo·lus) [L.]. 1. *In histology*, a bundle of nerve, muscle, or tendon fibers separated by connective tissue; as that of muscle fibers, by perimysium. 2. *In neurology*, a bundle or tract of nerve fibers presumably having common connections and functions. Also see *tract.* —**fascicular,** *adj.*

arcuate f. (*of the cerebrum*). Long association fibers that form a ventral part, connecting the superior and middle frontal convolutions with the temporal lobe, and a dorsal part (superior longitudinal fasciculus), connecting the upper and caudal portions of the frontal lobe with the occipital and parietal portions of the temporal lobe.

basal olfactory f. A diffuse system of nerve fibers that arise in the basal olfactory nuclei, pass beneath the head of the caudate nucleus, give terminal or collateral fibers to the tuber cinereum and mammillary body (olfactohypothalamic tract), and continue to the tegmentum of the midbrain (olfactotegmental tract), some reaching the medulla and spinal cord.

dorsal longitudinal f. A bundle of long association fibers in the cerebrum, connecting the frontal lobe with the occipital and temporal lobes.

f. cuneatus. The lateral part of the dorsal funiculus. Also called *Burdach's column.*

f. gracilis. The medial part of the dorsal funiculus of the spinal cord carrying proprioceptive impulses from the lower regions of the trunk and legs. Also called *Goll's column* or *tract.*

f. interfascicularis. Comma tract.

f. proprius. That which immediately surrounds the gray columns of the spinal cord, containing short ascending and descending correlation fibers. Syn., *ground bundle, fundamental column, spinospinal tract.*

f. retroflexus. A bundle of nerve fibers connecting the habenular nucleus with the interpeduncular nucleus of midbrain. It is concerned with olfactory impulses. Syn., *habenulopeduncular tract.* Also called *Meynert's bundle.*

f. solitarius. The tractus solitarius.

gyral f. See *association fibers* under *fiber.*

inferior longitudinal f. A bundle of long association fibers coursing horizontally in the lateral wall of the inferior and posterior horns of the lateral ventricle, extending from the occipital to the temporal lobe.

medial longitudinal f. One of two heavily medullated bundles close to the midline, just ventral to the central gray matter and extending from the upper spinal cord to the rostral end of the midbrain.

occipitofrontal f. A bundle of long association fibers extending from the cortex of the frontal lobe to the cortex of the occipital lobe.

occipitothalamic f. A bundle of nerve fibers connecting the thalamus with the occipital lobe.

spino-olivary f. See spino-olivary *tract.*

subcallosal f. A tract of long association fibers lying under the corpus callosum and connecting the frontal, parietal, and occipital lobes.

superior longitudinal f. See arcuate *f.*

uncinate f. of hemisphere. Long association fibers which lie immediately below the limen insulae and connect the orbital gyri with the hippocampal gyrus and temporal lobe and the frontal lobe with the occipital lobe.

fas″ci·ec′to·my (fash″ee·eck′to·mee, fass″ee·) [L. *fascia,* band; G. *ektomē,* excision]. Surgical excision of fascia; specifically, excision of strips from the lateral part of the fascia lata (iliotibial tract) for use in plastic surgery.

fas·ci′num [L. a spell, a bewitching]. 1. Literally, a spell, a bewitching; specifically, a spell cast by the evil eye: in modern Italian *fascino.* 2. Any amulet or charm worn to protect against the evil eye; frequently, a tiny image of a penis hung around the necks of children as a protective amulet against the evil eye and other forms of witchcraft.

fas′ci·o- (fash′ee·o-, fass′ee·o-) [L. *fascia,* band]. *In anatomy,* a combining form for *fascia.*

fas″ci·od′e·sis (fash″ee·od′i·sis, fass″ee·) [*fascia;* G. *desis,* a binding]. The operation of suturing a tendon to a fascia.

Fas·ci′o·la (fa·sigh′o·luh, fa·see′·) [L., small bandage]. A genus of trematodes; hermaphroditic flukes.

F. gigantica. A species related to *F. hepatica;* a natural parasite of cattle, sheep, and swine; human infestation has been reported from Indo-China, central Asia, Africa, and Hawaii, where it is the commonest cause of fascioliasis.

F. hepatica. A species which is a natural parasite of sheep and cattle and, occasionally, man.

fas·ci′o·la ci·ne′re·a. The dorsal continuation of the fascia dentata of the cerebrum.

fas″ci·o·li′a·sis [*fasciola;* NL. *-iasis,* condition]. Infestation with the *Fasciola hepatica;* normally occurs in sheep and other herbivorous animals, but man has served as an accidental host. The liver is usually the site of infestation. Also called *liver rot.*

Fas″ci·o·loi′des (fass″ee·o·loy′deez, fash″ee·o·) [*fasciola;* G. *eidos,* form]. A genus of digenetic trematodes.

F. magna. A species of flukes occurring in the liver, rarely the lungs, of cattle and other herbivores in North America and northern Europe.

fas″ci·o·lop·si′a·sis (fash″ee·o·lop·sigh′uh·sis, fass″ee·o·) [*fasciola;* G. *opsis,* appearance; NL. *-iasis,* condition]. Intestinal infestation of man and the hog by the *Fasciolopsis buski;* characterized by toxic diarrhea with visceral complications in severe cases.

Fas″ci·o·lop′sis [*fasciola; opsis*]. A genus of flukes parasitic in both man and the hog.

F. buski. Largest intestinal fluke of man; endemic only in the Orient; the causative organism of fasciolopsiasis.

fas′ci·o·plas″ty [L. *fascia,* band; G. *plassein,* to form]. Plastic surgery upon fascia.

fas″ci·or′rha·phy [*fascia;* G. *rhaphē,* a suture]. Suture of cut or lacerated fascia.

fas″ci·o·scap″u·lo·hu′mer·al. Involving the scapula, humerus, and adjacent fascia.

fas″ci·ot′o·my (fash″ee·ot′o·mee, fass″ee·) [*fascia;* G. *tomē,* a cutting]. Incision of a fascia.

fas·ci′tis (fass·eye′tis, fash·eye′tis) [*fascia;* G. *-itis,* inflammation]. Inflammation of a fascia.

plantar f. An inflammatory process, usually secondary to trauma or chronic strain, involving the plantar fascia, most commonly at its attachment to the calcaneus.

fast [AS. *faest*]. Resistant to the action of a drug or chemical, especially to the action of a stain.

fast green FCF (C.C.). An acid dye of the diamino triphenyl methane series; used as a counterstain.

fas·tig′i·um (fas·tidj′ee·um) [L., summit]. 1. The acme of a disease. 2. That portion of the cerebellum which forms an angle in the roof of the fourth ventricle between the anterior medullary velum and the tela choroidea.

fat [AS. *fǣtt*]. 1. Plump, corpulent. 2. Oily, greasy.

fat. 1. Any of a class of neutral organic compounds, mixtures of which form the natural fats. They are glyceryl esters of certain acids (in animal fat chiefly oleic, palmitic, and stearic). They are soluble in ether but not in water, are combustible, and on saponification yield glycerin. Fat is an energy-yielding foodstuff, one gram furnishing 9.3 Calories. 2. The chief component of the cell contents of adipose tissue; occurs also in other animal tissue to a lesser degree, and in plant cells. —**fat′ty,** *adj.*

brown f. See hibernating *gland.*

depot f. Fat occurring in certain regions like the abdominal wall or the buttocks, which are called fat depots.

fat′i·ga·ble [L. *fatigabilis,* from *fatigare,* to weary]. Susceptible to fatigue; easily tired. —**fatigableness, fatigabil′ity,** *n.*

fa·tigue′ [F., from L. *fatigare,* to tire]. 1. Exhaustion of strength; weariness from exertion. 2. Condition of cells or organs in which, through overactivity, the power or capacity to respond to stimulation is diminished or lost.

battle f. A neurotic or psychotic reaction developed in combat: formerly called *shellshock.*

flying f. A chronic psychosomatic disturbance developed by a flier after relatively long exposure to the stresses associated with flying, especially in combat flying: also called *operational f., pilot f.*

operational f. Flying *f.*

fa·tigue. 1. To induce a condition of fatigue in. 2. To become weary. 3. To suffer fatigue.

fa·tigue′-pos′tur·al par′a·dox. See scapulocostal *syndrome.*

fat′si·a [perhaps from Malagasy *fatsy*, spur]. The bark of the root of *Oplopanax horridus*, believed to contain a hypoglycemic principle. Also called *devil's club*.

fat′-sol′u·ble. Soluble in fats or fat-solvents; specifically, used with a letter to designate certain vitamins, as fat-soluble A.

fat′ty ac′id. See under *acid*.

fau′ces (faw′seez) [L., upper part of the throat]. The space surrounded by the soft palate, palatine arches, and base of the tongue. —**fau′cial,** *adj*.

Fauchard, Pierre [*French dentist*, 1678–1761]. Has been called the father of dentistry. Wrote a classic account of the dental science of his time. Was one of the founders of orthodontics, and the inventor of many prosthetic appliances. Described alveolar pyorrhea, called *Fauchard's disease*.

fau′na [L. *Faunus*, Roman god of animals and crops]. The entire animal life peculiar to any geographic area or geologic period.

Faust's method. See Faust's zinc sulfate centrifugal flotation *method*.

fa·vag′i·nous (fa·vadj′i·nus) [L. *favus*, a honeycomb]. Resembling favus; having a honeycombed surface. *Rare*.

fa·ve′o·late [dim. from *favus*]. Favose; honeycombed; alveolate.

fa·ve′o·lus [*favus*]. A pit or cell like that of the honeycomb. See *foveola*.

fa′vi·des (fay′vi·deez) [*favus*]. Allergic skin reactions to favus.

fa′vism (fay′viz·um, fah′viz·um) [L. *faba*, bean]. An acute hemolytic anemia, common in Sicily and Sardinia; caused by sensitivity to the broad bean, *Vicia faba*. May result from ingestion of the seeds or from inhalation of the pollen. Also called *fabism*, *fabismus*.

Fav″o·tri·choph′y·ton (fav″o·tri·kof′i·ton, ·trye-kof′i·ton) [L. *favus*, honeycomb; G. *thrix*, hair; *phyton*, plant]. Synonym for *Trichophyton*.

Favre, Maurice (1876–). French physician, who with J. Durand and Joseph Nicolas gave the first satisfactory description (1913) of venereal lymphogranuloma.

fa′vus (fay′vus, fah′vus) [L., honeycomb]. A parasitic skin disease due to the presence of the vegetable parasite, *Trichophyton schoenleini*, *T. violaceum*, or *Microsporum gypseum*. It is characterized by the presence of round, sulfur-yellow, cup-shaped crusts (**favus cups**) having a peculiar mousy odor. This crust formation, scutulum, is found on microscopic examination to contain the elements of the fungus. The disease affects the scalp most frequently, but may occur elsewhere. Syn., *tinea favosa*. See Plate 32.

Fayrer, Joseph [*English surgeon*, 1824–1907]. Known for his contributions to tropical medicine. Described the venomous snakes of India (1872).

Fazio, Eugenio [*Italian physician*, 1849–1902]. Described a type of progressive bulbar paralysis in early life, called *Fazio-Londe's atrophy*.

F.D.I. *Fédération Dentaire Internationale;* International Dental Federation.

Fe Chemical symbol for iron.

fear [AS. *fǣr*, danger]. An emotion marked by dread, apprehension, or alarm. An irrational and persistent fear is called a *phobia*.

fear re·ac′tion. A euphemism for a neurosis, particularly one developed in combat, in which anxiety is manifested by the conscious fear of a particular object or event.

fea′ture [L. *factura*, a making]. Any single part or lineament of a structure, as of the face.

feb′ri-. Combining form meaning *fever*.

feb′ri·cant [L. *febris*, fever]. Febrifacient.

feb″ri·fa′cient (feb″ri·fay′shunt) [*febris;* L. *facere*, to make]. Producing fever.

fe·brif′ic [*febris*]. Febrifacient.

feb′ri·fuge [*febris;* L. *fugare*, to make flee]. A substance which mitigates or reduces fever; an antipyretic. —**feb′rifuge,** *adj*.

feb″ri·fu′gine. An alkaloid, possessing antimalarial activity, isolated from *Dichroa febrifuga*, which is the probable source of the Chinese antimalarial drug *ch'ang shan*. Febrifugine may be identical with α-dichroine and β-dichroine from ch'ang shan.

fe′brile (fee′bril, ·bryle, feb′ril, ·ryle) [*febris*]. Pertaining to or characterized by fever.

feb″ri·pho′bi·a [*febris;* G. *phobos*, fear]. A morbid fear of fever; pyrexeophobia.

fe′ca·lith (fee′kuh·lith, feck′uh·) [L. *faex*, dregs; G. *lithos*, stone]. A concretion or calcified mass of fecal material; coprolith.

fe′cal·oid (fee′kuh·loyd, feck′uh·) [*faex;* G. *eidos*, form]. Resembling feces.

fe′ces, fae′ces (fee′seez) [*faex*]. The excretions of the bowels. The excretions from the intestine of unabsorbed food, indigestible matter, and intestinal secretions. —**fe′cal,** *adj*.

Fechner, Gustav Theodor [*German physicist and experimental psychologist*, 1801–87]. One of the founders of the science of psychophysics. See Fechner's *law*.

fec′u·la [L. *faecula*, dim. of *faex*]. 1. The starchy part of a seed. 2. The sediment subsiding from an infusion.

fec′u·lent [*faecula*]. 1. Having sediment. 2. Excrementitious.

fe″cun·da′tion (fee″kun·day′shun, feck″un·) [L. *fecundus*, fertile]. The act of fertilizing; fertilization. —**fe′cundate,** *v.t.*

artificial f. Artificial insemination.

fe·cun′di·ty [*fecundus*]. The innate potential reproductive capacity of the individual organism, as denoted by its ability to form and separate from the body mature germ cells. —**fe′cund,** *adj*.

Fede, Francesco [*Italian pediatrician*, 1832–1913]. Described an oral disease of infancy occurring during dentition and marked by induration of the frenulum of the tongue; called *sublingual granuloma of infancy*, *Fede's disease*, *Fede-Riga disease*.

fee″ble·mind′ed·ness. Mental deficiency.

feed′ing [AS. *fēdan*]. The taking or giving of food.

artificial f. (a) The introduction of food into the body by means of artificial devices. (b) The nourishing of an infant by any means other than breast milk.

extrabuccal f. The introduction of food into the system by channels other than the mouth; feeding by nutritive enema, by intravascular injection, or through gastric fistulas.

forced f. The administration of food against the will of the patient.

sham f. That in which the food is swallowed and then diverted to the exterior by fistula or other means.

feel′ing [AS. *fēlan*]. 1. The sense of touch. 2. A sensation, as a sensation of touch, bodily consciousness, temperature, pain. 3. An emotion or emotional state. 4. *In psychology*, any conscious process; consciousness, including sensation, thought, and emotion. —**feel,** *v*.

feel′ing. Of great sensibility; easily moved.

Feer, Emil (1864–). Swiss pediatrician who described erythredema polyneuropathy (1923), also called *Feer's disease*.

fee split′ting. A division of the consultant's fee between consultant and referring physician.

Fehleisen, Friedrich [*German physician in the United States*, 1854–1924]. Described the streptococcus of erysipelas (1883), called *Streptococcus pyogenes, Fehleisen's streptococcus.*

Fehling's reagent, test. See under *reagent, test.*

Feil, André [*French physician*, 1884–]. With Klippel, described congenital fusion of the cervical vertebrae. See Klippel-Feil *syndrome.*

fel [L.]. Bile.

f. bovis. Ox bile.

felamine. The trade-mark for a compound of cholic acid and methenamine employed as a cholagogue, and a biliary and urinary antiseptic.

fe'line [L. *felinus*, from *felis*, cat]. 1. Of, pertaining to, or derived from cats [genus *Felis*] or the family (Felidae) which includes cats, tigers, lions, leopards. 2. Catlike. —**fe'line,** *n.*

Felix test. See Weil-Felix *test.*

fel·la'ti·o (feh·lay'shee·o) [L. *fellare*, to suck]. An act of sexual perversion in which the penis is introduced into the mouth of another; friction by the lips or tongue produces the orgasm. Syn., *irrumation.*

fel"la·tor' (fel"uh·tor', fel'uh·tor, feh·lay'tur) [L., from *fellare*]. A male who takes the penis of another into his mouth.

fel"la·trice' (fel"uh·treess') [*fellare*]. A female who takes the penis into her mouth in fellatio.

fel'lic ac'id. $C_{23}H_{40}O_4$. An acid claimed to exist in human bile.

Fell-O'Dwyer method. See under *artificial respiration.*

fel'on [ME.]. A deep infection in the distal closed space on the palmar surface of a finger; it may progress to osteomyelitis of the distal phalanx.

felsol. The trade-mark for a mixture of antipyrine, iodopyrine, citrated caffeine, digitalin, strophanthin, and lobeline employed as an antiasthmatic.

Felty, Augustus Roi [*American physician*, 1895–]. Known for his description of a syndrome of rheumatoid arthritis in adults, characterized by lymphatic glandular enlargement with splenomegaly and liver enlargement, accompanied by anemia. Called *adult Still's disease, Chauffard-Still's disease, Felty's syndrome.*

fe'male [L. *femella*, dim. of *femina*, woman]. Pertaining to the sex which produces the ovum. Symbol, ○, ♀. (That of the male is □, ♂.)

fe'male. Denoting that part of a double-limbed instrument that receives the complementary part.

fem'i·nism [*femina*]. The presence in a male of various mental and physical approximations to the characters of the female sex. —**feminiza'tion,** *n.*

fem'or·al ar'ter·y. See Table of Arteries in the Appendix.

fem'or·al nerve. See Table of Nerves in the Appendix.

fem"o·ro·tib'i·al [L. *femur*, thigh; *tibia*, shinbone]. Relating to the femur and the tibia.

fe'mur (plural, *femora*) [L.]. 1. Thigh bone. See Table of Bones in the Appendix. 2. Old term for the thigh. See Plates 1, 2. —**fem'oral,** *adj.*

pilastered f. A femur with exaggerated backward concavity and prominent linea aspera.

fen'chone (fen'chone, ·kone). A ketone, $C_{10}H_{16}O$, which provides the characteristic bitter taste of some specimens of fennel oil. A levorotatory isomer occurs in thuja oil.

fe·nes'tra (pl. *fenestrae*) [L., window]. 1. *In anatomy*, a name given to two apertures of the medial wall of the middle ear; the **fenestra cochleae** (or **fenestra rotunda**) or round window and the **fenestra vestibuli** (or **fenestra ovalis**) or oval window. 2. An opening in a bandage or plaster splint for examination, drainage, etc. 3. The open space in the blade of a forceps. —**fenestral,** *adj.*

fen"es·tra'tion [*fenestra*]. 1. The presence of fenestrae or openings in a structure. 2. An operation to create a permanently mobile window in the lateral semicircular canal; used in cases of deafness caused by stapedial impediment of sound waves. Sometimes referred to as *Lempert operation.* —**fenes'trated,** *adj.*

Fenger, Christian [*American surgeon and pathologist*, 1840–1902]. Devised an operation for stricture of the upper end of the ureter, in which he employed the plastic methods applied for the relief of pyloric stenosis.

fen'nel [AS. *fenol*, from L. *faeniculum*, fennel] (*foeniculum*). The dried, ripe fruit of cultivated varieties of *Foeniculum vulgare;* contains 2% of volatile oil. It is used as a carminative.

f. oil. See under *oil.*

f. water. A saturated solution of the volatile oil of fennel; used as a vehicle.

fen'u·greek [L. *faenum Graecum*, Greek hay]. The *Trigonella foenum-graecum*, a leguminous plant whose seeds are used as a condiment and in preparing emollient applications.

Fenwick, Samuel [*English physician*, 1821–1902]. Remembered for his description of primary atrophy of the stomach, called *Fenwick's disease.*

feosol. A trade-mark for certain preparations of ferrous sulfate.

ferad. A trade-mark for certain preparations containing ferrous sulfate.

fer"-de-lance' (fair"-duh-lahns', -lans'. *See* NOTES § 35) [F., iron of a lance]. A large, venomous snake of Central America; the *Bothrops atrox.*

Féréol, Louis Henri Félix [*French physician*, 1825–91]. Described nodosities observed about the joints in acute articular rheumatism, called *Féréol's nodosities.* Drew attention to a paralysis of the medial rectus muscle occurring with that of the lateral rectus in the other eye, called *Féréol's ocular palsy, Féréol-Graux ocular palsy.*

fergon. A trade-mark for certain preparations containing ferrous gluconate.

Ferguson, Alexander Hugh [*Canadian surgeon*, 1853–1911]. Devised the operation bearing his name for the repair of inguinal hernia. A modification of Bassini's technic, it omits the transplantation of the spermatic cord. The conjoined tendon is sutured to the inguinal ligament, the external oblique muscle being closed over the canal.

Fergusson, William [*Scottish anatomist and surgeon*, 1808–77]. Has been called the founder of conservative surgery. Devised many operations, including one for harelip, lithotomy, and removal of the maxilla for malignant tumor. Described a number of amputations, including one of the foot and one of the leg at the hip joint.

fer'ment [L. *fermentum*, ferment]. A catalytic agent produced by, and associated with, a living organism (*organized ferment*), as distinguished from an enzyme which may be separated from the living organism (*unorganized ferment*). This distinction is no longer commonly made, having been replaced by intracellular and extracellular enzymes. See under *enzyme.*

fer"men·ta'tion [*fermentum*]. The decomposition of complex molecules under the influence of ferments or enzymes.

acetic f. The fermentation whereby weak alcoholic solutions are converted into vinegar.

alcoholic f. That resulting in the conversion of carbohydrates into alcohol.

ammoniacal f. That giving rise to ammoniacal gas and carbon dioxide, which combine to form ammonium carbonate.

butyric f. That resulting in the conversion of sugars, starches, milk, etc., into butyric acid.

caseous f. That resulting in the conversion of milk into cheese.

diastatic f. That resulting in the conversion of starch into glucose by the action of ptyalin, etc.

lactic f. That resulting in the souring of milk.

propionic f. That resulting in the production of propionic acid from carbohydrates.

viscous f. A fermentation characterized by the production of a gummy substance.

Fernel, Jean François [*French physician,* 1497–1558]. First to use the terms physiology (1552) and pathology (1554) in the modern sense. Gave the earliest clear descriptions of appendicitis and endocarditis.

fer′ra·ted [L. *ferratus,* from *ferrum,* iron]. Combined with iron; containing iron.

Ferraton, Louis [*French orthopedic surgeon,* contemporary]. Described snapping hip; called *Perrin-Ferraton's disease.* Also see under *Perrin.*

Ferrein, Antoine Aesculape [*French anatomist,* 1693–1769]. Described the small groups of straight tubules radiating from the boundary zone of the renal pyramids into the cortex, the medullary (cortical) rays; once called *Ferrein's pyramids.* Described the convoluted uriniferous tubules.

fer′ri- [*ferrum*]. A combining form indicating *ferric compounds, containing iron as a trivalent element.*

fer′ric [*ferrum*]. 1. Pertaining to or of the nature of iron. 2. Containing iron as a trivalent element.

f. alum. Ferric ammonium sulfate.

f. ammonium citrate (*ferri ammonii citras*). A complex salt containing 16.5 to 18.5% iron; it occurs in red scales or granules, or as a brownish yellow powder. Used as a nonastringent hematinic. Dose, 1 Gm. (15 gr.). Syn., *soluble ferric citrate.* Also called *iron and ammonium citrates.*

f. ammonium sulfate. $FeNH_4(SO_4)_2.12H_2O$. Formerly used for its astringent and styptic effects. Syn., *f. alum.*

f. ammonium tartrate. A salt of somewhat indefinite composition occurring in reddish-brown scales; formerly much used as a mild chalybeate.

f. cacodylate. Approximately $Fe\ [(CH_3)_2AsO_2]_3$, a yellowish, amorphous powder, soluble in water; has been used for treatment of leukemias, also in iron-deficiency states.

f. chloride. $FeCl_3$ + water. Astringent and styptic.

f. chloride solution (*liquor ferri chloridi*). An aqueous solution representing 10–11% of iron. Principal use is as a styptic and astringent. Dose, 0.06–0.3 cc. (1–5 min.).

f. chloride tincture (*tinctura ferri chloridi*). A hydroalcoholic solution representing about 4.5% of iron. An astringent and styptic. Occasionally used as a hematinic. Dose, 0.6–2.0 cc. (10–30 min.).

f. glycerophosphate (*ferri glycerophosphas*). $Fe_2[C_3H_5(OH)_2PO_4]_3$. Formerly used as a chalybeate.

f. hydroxide. Hydrated iron oxide, an antidote to arsenic.

f. hydroxide with magnesium oxide (*magma ferri hydroxidi*). An antidote to arsenic prepared by adding a suspension of magnesium oxide to a ferric sulfate solution.

f. hypophosphite (*ferri hypophosphis*). $Fe(H_2PO_2)_3$. Formerly used as a chalybeate.

f. pyrophosphate. Approximately $Fe_4(P_2O_7)_3.9H_2O$; a yellowish-white powder, insoluble in water, and lacking the astringency characteristic of iron salts. It is used in nutrition and medicinally as a source of iron. **Ferric pyrophosphate soluble** is ferric pyrophosphate rendered soluble by the inclusion of sodium citrate.

f. subsulfate solution (*liquor ferri subsulfatis*). Monsel's solution. A powerful styptic.

f. sulfate. $Fe_2(SO_4)_3$; a salt occurring as a grayish-white powder, very hygroscopic, slowly soluble in water, and forming an acid solution. It is largely used industrially.

green f. ammonium citrate (*ferri ammonii citras viridis*). A complex salt containing 14.5 to 16% iron, with a higher proportion of citric acid than in ferric ammonium citrate. It occurs in green scales, granules, or powder, and is the preferred form of the salt for intramuscular injection. Dose, 0.1 Gm. (1½ gr.). Also called *green iron and ammonium citrates.*

red f. oxide (*ferri oxidum rubrum*). A reddish brown powder used, along with yellow ferric oxide, to confer a flesh color to neocalamine.

saccharated f. oxide (*ferri oxidum saccharatum*). A mild chalybeate. Dose, 2 Gm. (30 gr.).

soluble f. citrate. See *ferric* ammonium citrate.

soluble f. phosphate (*ferri phosphas solubilis*). Mild chalybeate. Dose, 0.6–2.0 Gm. (10–30 gr.).

yellow f. oxide (*ferri oxidum flavum*). A hydrated ferric oxide occurring as a yellowish-orange powder. Used, along with red ferric oxide, to confer a flesh color to neocalamine.

fer″ri·cy′a·nide. A salt containing the trivalent $[Fe(CN)_6]$ anion.

Ferrier, David [*Scottish neurologist in England,* 1843–1928]. His study of the localization of cerebral functions (1876) has been called the foundation of present knowledge in this field.

fer′ri·heme. Heme in which the ferrous iron normally present is in the ferric (oxidized) state; the resulting higher valence imparts a positive charge which in alkaline solution attracts a hydroxyl ion, forming hematin, and in hydrochloric acid solution attracts a chloride ion, forming hemin.

fer″ri·he″mo·glo′bin. Methemoglobin, characterized by containing iron in the ferric state.

fer″ri·py′rin. See *ferropyrin.*

fer′ri·tin. An iron-protein complex occurring in tissues, probably being a storage form of iron. It is in many characteristics similar to hemosiderin. See *apoferritin.*

ferrivenin. Trade-mark for a preparation of saccharated iron oxide suitable for intravenous injection.

fer′ro- [*ferrum*]. A combining form generally used to indicate *a ferrous compound;* sometimes to designate *a substance containing metallic iron.*

fer″ro·cy′a·nide. A salt containing the divalent $[Fe(CN)_6]$ anion.

fer′ro·heme. Heme.

fer″ro·he″mo·glo′bin. Hemoglobin, in which the iron is normally in the ferrous state.

fer″ro·pro″to·por′phyr·in 9. Heme.

ferropyrin. Trade-mark for a hemostatic compound of antipyrine and ferric chloride. The substance is used for external bleeding either in the form of a dusting powder or a 15–20% solution.

fer″ro·ther′a·py [*ferrum;* G. *therapeia,* treatment]. Treatment of disease by the use of chalybeates.

fer′rous [*ferrum*]. Containing iron in divalent form.

f. bromide. $FeBr_2.2H_2O$; a reddish crystalline powder, hygroscopic and soluble in water. It occurs also with $6H_2O$ as bluish-green crystals, and has been used in chorea and tuberculous cervical adenitis.

f. chloride. $FeCl_2.4H_2O$; pale-green, deliquescent crystals or crystalline powder, soluble in acidulated water: used largely industrially.

citrated f. chloride (*ferri subchloridum citratum*). A mixture of ferrous chloride and citric acid, used as a hematinic. Dose, 0.2–0.3 Gm. (3–5 gr.).

exsiccated f. sulfate (*ferri sulfas exsiccatus*). A hematinic. Dose, 0.06–0.2 Gm. (1–3 gr.).

f. ascorbate. An iron salt possessing antiscorbutic properties. May be administered intravenously. Dose, 0.2 Gm. (3 gr.).

f. carbonate mass (*massa ferri carbonatis*). Vallet's mass. Contains 36–41% $FeCO_3$; a hematinic. Dose, 0.3–1.0 Gm. (5–15 gr.).

f. carbonate pills (*pillulae ferri carbonatis*). Blaud's pills. The official pill contains not less than 60 mg. of $FeCO_3$.

f. gluconate (*ferri gluconas*). $Fe(C_6H_{11}O_7)_2.2H_2O$. A yellowish-gray or pale, greenish-yellow powder containing not less than 11.5% Fe; soluble in water. Appears to be better tolerated than other iron salts. Dose, 0.3 Gm. (5 gr.).

f. iodide. $FeI_2.4H_2O$, occurring as almost black, very deliquescent masses, rapidly decomposing in air with liberation of iodine. It has been used in chronic tuberculosis, and is employed in veterinary medicine as a source of iron and iodine.

f. iodide pills (*pilulae ferri iodidi*). Blancard's pills; each pill contains one grain of ferrous iodide.

f. iodide syrup (*syrupus ferri iodidi*). Contains 6.5–7.5% of FeI_2. An alterative and chalybeate. Dose, 0.6–2.5 cc. (10–40 min.).

f. lactate. $Fe(C_3H_5O_3)_2.3H_2O$. A mild chalybeate. Dose, 0.06–1.3 Gm. (1–20 gr.).

f. sulfate (*ferri sulfas*). $FeSO_4.7H_2O$. Pale bluish green crystals or granules. An effective hematinic, used also as a deodorant. Dose, 0.13–0.3 Gm. (2–5 gr.).

saccharated f. carbonate (*ferri carbonas saccharatus*). Contains not less than 15% $FeCO_3$. Dose, 0.6–2.0 Gm. (10–30 gr.).

fer·ru·gi·na'tion. Deposition of iron in tissues.

fer·ru'gi·nous [L. *ferrugo*, iron rust]. 1. Chalybeate. 2. Having the color of iron rust.

fer'rum. See *iron.*

fer'tile [L. *fertilis*, fertile]. Prolific; fruitful. —**fertil'ity,** *n.*

fer·til'i·ty clin'ic. A clinic to help diagnose the causes for lack of reproduction and to assist reproductive ability: popularly known as *sterility clinic.*

fer"ti·li·za'tion [*fertilis*]. The act of making fruitful; impregnation; union of male and female gametes.

cross-f. *In biology*, the fertilization of the ovules of one species by the seed germs of another.

fer'ti·li·zin (fur'ti·lye·zin, fur·til'i·zin) [*fertilis*]. A colloidal substance in ripe ova, in certain species, which is capable of agglutinating and binding spermatozoa to the ova.

Fer'u·la (ferr'yoo·luh, ferr'oo·luh) [L., fennel-giant]. A genus of the family Umbelliferae whose genera and species yield asafetida, galbanum, and sumbul.

fe·ru'lic ac'id. $CH_3O.C_6H_3(OH)CH{:}CHCOOH$. Meta-methoxy-para-hydroxycinnamic acid; a constituent of asafetida.

fes'ter [ME. *festren*]. 1. Superimpose a suppuration on a lesion such as an ulcer. 2. Suppurate.

fes"ti·na'tion [L. *festinare*, to hasten]. An involuntary increase or hastening in gait, seen in paralysis agitans.

fes·toon' [F. *feston*, from It. *festa*, feast]. The papilliform interproximal gingiva which fills each buccal and lingual embrasure between the necks of adjacent teeth.

McCall's f. A thickening of the gingiva along its margin, usually due to traumatic occlusion or incorrect toothbrushing.

fe'tal·ism [L. *fetus*, offspring]. The presence or persistence of certain prenatal conditions in the body after birth.

fe·ta'tion [*fetus*]. 1. The formation of a fetus. 2. Pregnancy.

fe'ti·cide [*fetus;* L. *caedere*, to kill]. The killing of the fetus in the uterus.

fet'id (fet'id, fee'tid) [L. *fetere*, to stink]. Having a foul odor.

fe'tish, fe'tich (fee'tish, fet'ish) [Pg. *feitiço*, from L. *facticius*, artificial]. 1. Any material object thought to have magical power or to bring supernatural aid. 2. *In psychiatry*, a personalized inanimate object, love object, or any maneuver or body part which, through association, arouses erotic feelings. —**fetishism, fetishist,** *n.*

fet'lock [ME. *fetlak*]. That region of the leg of the horse extending from the lower extremity of the metacarpal or metatarsal bone to the pastern joint.

fe·tom'e·try (fee·tom'i·tree) [L. *fetus*, fetus; G. *metron*, a measure]. The measurement of the fetus, especially of its cranial diameters.

fe'tor, foe'tor (fee'tur, ·tor) [L., an offensive smell]. Stench.

f. ex ore. Bad breath.

f. hepaticus. A peculiar musty or sweetish odor of the breath occurring in the terminal stage of hepatocellular jaundice.

fe'tus, foe'tus (fee'tus) [L.]. The unborn offspring of viviparous mammals in the later stages of development. In man, from the end of the third month until birth. See Plate 41. —**fetal,** *adj.*

amorphous f. See *anideus.*

calcified f. See *lithopedion.*

cuspidate f. See *sympus.*

f. compressus. See *f.* papyraceus.

f. cylindricus. A malformed, abortive fetus with but little indication of head and extremities, being roughly cylindrical in form.

f. in fetu. Cryptodidymus.

f. papyraceus. A dead twin fetus which has been compressed by the growth of its living twin.

harlequin f. See *ichthyosis congenita.*

mermaid f. See *sympus.*

parasitic f. A more or less completely formed fetus which is attached to its autosite.

sirenoform f. See *sympus, sirenomelus.*

Feulgen reaction. See under *reaction.*

fe'ver [AS. *fēfer;* L. *febris*, fever]. 1. Elevation of the body temperature above the normal; in human beings, above 37° C. or 98.6° F. 2. A disease whose distinctive feature is elevation of body temperature. Syn., *pyrexia.* —**feverish,** *adj.*

abortus f. A form of brucellosis.

Aden f. Dengue.

algid pernicious f. A severe attack of malaria; characterized by collapse, extremely cold skin, and a tendency to fatal syncope.

American mountain f. Colorado tick *f.*

aphthous f. See foot-and-mouth *disease.*

artificial f. One purposefully produced for therapeutic benefit, as by the induction of malaria, by the injection of foreign protein, or by means of a fever cabinet.

Assam f. Kala-azar.

barbiero f. American trypanosomiasis.

Basra f. See *malaria.*

black f. See *Rocky Mountain spotted fever.*

blackwater f. See hemoglobinuric *f.*

boutonneuse f. An acute tick-bite fever of Africa and other regions of the Mediterranean basin, characterized by maculopapular eruptions on hands and feet, and a characteristic lesion (*tache noire*) at the site of the bite. Also called *exanthematous f., eruptive f., Marseilles f.*

brain f. Cerebrospinal meningitis.

Brazilian spotted f. São Paulo typhus. See *Rocky Mountain spotted fever.*

breakbone f. Dengue.

Brushy Creek f. See pretibial *f.*

Bull f. See *Rocky Mountain spotted fever.*

Bullis f. An acute disease, due to a rickettsialike agent, which occurred in an epidemic at Camp Bullis, Texas, in 1942.
bullous f. That which accompanies pemphigus.
Bwamba f. A mild febrile viral disease occurring in Uganda and characterized by headache, generalized pains, and conjunctivitis.
camp f. See classic epidemic *typhus*.
canebrake yellow f. See hemoglobinuric *f.*
canicola f. The disease caused in man by infection with *Leptospira canicola*.
canine yellow f. Nambi uvu.
catarrhal f. Old term for the common cold.
cat-scratch f. A self-limited disease clinically manifested by fever and generalized lymphadenitis, caused by a virus closely related to the viruses causing psittacosis and lymphogranuloma venereum. Diagnosis is confirmed by history of recent skin contact with a cat (bite, scratch) and by an intradermal skin test using material from an infected lymph node or bubo of a known case. Syn., *cat-scratch disease, benign lymphorcticulosis.*
cerebrospinal f. Cerebrospinal meningitis.
Charcot's intermittent f. A condition often accompanying common bile duct obstruction. It may be a sign of cholangitis or obstructive jaundice.
childbed f. See puerperal *f.*
Chitral f. Phlebotomus fever.
Colombian spotted f. Rocky Mountain spotted fever, occurring in Colombia, South America.
Colorado tick f. A nonexanthematous viral disease of man occurring in the western United States and transmitted by the tick, *Dermacentor andersoni*. Clinically the disease is characterized by short course and intermittent fever, variegated symptomatology, and usually leukopenia, but no specific pathologic findings are known. Diagnosis rests on serologic reactions. Also called *American mountain f., tick f.*
continued f. One which does not vary more than 1° or 2° F. during 24 hours.
dandy f. See *dengue*.
deer fly f. Tularemia.
dengue f. See *dengue*.
desert f. Coccidioidomycosis.
double quartan f. A form of malaria with a three-day cycle; paroxysms occurring on two successive days are followed by a one-day interval.
drug f. That resulting from the administration of a drug, often by sensitization, as the sulfonamides.
dumdum f. Visceral leishmaniasis; kala-azar.
East Coast f. A form of piroplasmosis in cattle which occurs chiefly in East and South Africa. Syn., *Rhodesian f.*
Eastern spotted f. Rocky Mountain spotted fever, occurring in the eastern United States.
elephantoid f. See filarial *f.*
English sweating f. A contagious malignant fever, also known as *ephemera maligna*, characterized by black or dark-colored sweat: of historical significance. Syn., *Anglicus sudor*.
enteric f. Typhoid.
entericoid f. See parenteric *f.*
epidemic catarrhal f. Influenza.
epidemic hemorrhagic f. An acute infectious disease of unknown cause, but probably viral, occurring in parts of Siberia, Manchuria, and Korea. It is characterized by fever, prostration, anorexia, vomiting, proteinuria, hemorrhagic manifestations, cardiovascular instability, and renal abnormalities resembling those of lower nephron nephrosis. Syn., *Far Eastern hemorrhagic f., hemorrhagic nephroso-nephritis, Manchurian f.*
equine biliary f. A form of piroplasmosis in horses, mules, donkeys; caused by the *Babesia equi* and transmitted by ticks.
eruptive f. See boutonneuse *f.*
essential f. One of unknown cause.
estivo-autumnal f. Malaria.
European typhus f. See classic epidemic *typhus*.
exanthematous f. See boutonneuse *f.*
famine f. See *relapsing fever*, classic epidemic *typhus*.
Far Eastern hemorrhagic f. See epidemic hemorrhagic *f.*
field f. Marsh *f.*
filarial f. A recurrent fever occurring irregularly at intervals of months or years in most forms of filariasis. Syn., *elephantoid f.*
five-day f. Dengue.
flood f. See tsutsugamushi *disease*.
Fort Bragg f. See pretibial *f.*
gaiter-pain f. Trench *f.*
Gibraltar f. Brucellosis.
gin f. Byssinosis.
glandular f. See infectious *mononucleosis*.
goat f. Brucellosis.
harvest f. A form of spirochetosis affecting field workers.
Haverhill f. See epidemic arthritic *erythema*.
hay f. See *hay fever*.
heartwater f. A disease of cattle, sheep, and goats caused by *Rickettsia* (*coudria*) *ruminatum*, transmitted by the tick, *Amblyomma hebraeum*. It occurs in South Africa, the Belgian Congo, and surrounding areas, and is characterized by hydropericardium.
hectic f. One recurring daily, with the highest temperature in the evening; accompanied by chills and sweats. It occurs frequently in tuberculosis.
hemoglobinuric f. A severe form of malaria, associated with hematuria; occurs mainly in endemic areas of malignant tertian malaria. Also called *blackwater f., canebrake yellow f.*
hepatic f. Catarrhal cholangitis.
herpetic f. One with chills, sore throat, and herpetic eruption on the face.
hospital f. See classic epidemic *typhus*.
icterohemorrhagic f. Spirochetal jaundice.
intermittent f. Malaria.
inundation f. Tsutsugamushi disease.
jail f. See classic epidemic *typhus*.
Japanese river f. Tsutsugamushi disease.
jungle yellow f. A form of yellow fever endemic in parts of Brazil; occurs in or near forested areas where the *Aëdes aegypti* has not been found.
kedani f. See tsutsugamushi *disease*.
Kenya typhus f. See tick-bite *fevers* of Africa.
malarial f. See *malaria*.
Malta f. Brucellosis.
Manchurian f. Epidemic hemorrhagic *f.*
Marseilles f. See boutonneuse *f.*
marsh f. The disease caused in man by *Leptospira grippotyphosa*. Syn., *field fever*.
Mediterranean f. Brucellosis.
melitococcic f. See *brucellosis*.
metal fume f. A febrile reaction following the inhalation of finely divided particles of metallic oxides. Also called *brass chills, brass founder's ague, metal ague, zinc chills, spelter shakes.*
miliary f. An acute, infectious disease; characterized by fever, profuse sweating, and a papular rash later forming pustules. Syn., *sweating sickness*.
milk f. (a) A misnomer for a fever during the puerperium, once thought to be due to a great accumulation of milk in the breasts, but now generally believed to be due to actual puerperal infection. (b) Parturient paresis.

Monday morning f. Byssinosis.
mountain f. See *Rocky Mountain spotted fever.*
North African tick-bite f. See tick-bite *fevers* of Africa.
Oroya f. The more malignant form of *bartonellosis* (Carrión's disease) endemic in the mountainous areas of northwestern South America, characterized by fever, macrocytic and hemolytic anemia, and having a rapid course which, when untreated, is highly fatal. The causative organism, *Bartonella bacilliformis,* can be demonstrated in the erythrocytes in a blood smear, as well as in the cytoplasm of vascular endothelium. The liver, spleen, and lymph nodes are frequently involved and may be markedly enlarged. Related etiologically and immunologically to verruca peruviana, it differs greatly in the clinical picture; but Oroya fever is frequently followed by verruca peruviana. Both diseases are associated with the name of Daniel A. Carrión, who first demonstrated their relationship.
Pahvant Valley f. Tularemia.
pappataci f. Phlebotomus fever.
papular f. A disease characterized by fever, papular eruption, and rheumatic pains.
paratyphoid f. Paratyphoid.
parenteric f. One resembling typhoid or paratyphoid, but due to a different organism.
parrot f. See *psittacosis.*
Pel-Ebstein f. Periodic hyperpyrexia, occasionally seen in Hodgkin's disease.
petechial f. See classic epidemic *typhus.*
phlebotomus f. An infectious viral disease transmitted by *Phlebotomus papatasii,* found in the Mediterranean area, British India, China, East Africa, and South America. It resembles dengue but is less severe and of shorter duration. Syn., *Chitral f., pappataci f., sandfly f., three-day f.*
polka f. Dengue.
pretibial f. A febrile disease caused by a species of *Leptospira,* and characterized by an erythematous rash in the pretibial region, frontal, postorbital, and lumbar aching, nausea, vomiting, leukopenia, and enlargement of the spleen. Also called *autumnal f., Fort Bragg f., Brushy Creek f.*
protein f. Artificial fever produced by the intravenous or intramuscular injection of a foreign protein.
puerperal f. Infection of the endometrium and septicemia following delivery. Also called *childbed f., puerperal sepsis.*
putrid f. Typhus.
Q f. An acute infection transmitted by *Coxiella burnetii,* characterized by pneumonitis, fever, nausea, and vomiting. The disease is of short duration, without mortality. Also called *quadrilateral f., Queensland f.*
quartan f. Malaria, with paroxysms every 72 hours.
Queensland coastal f. See tsutsugamushi *disease.*
Queensland f. See Q *f.*
quinine f. A disease marked by fever and skin eruption; occurs in persons exposed to quinine during its preparation.
rabbit f. Tularemia.
ragweed f. See *hay fever.*
railway f. See shipping *f.*
rat-bite f. A form which includes two distinct diseases contracted from the bite of infected rats or other animals. One caused by *Streptobacillus moniliformis* is identical with epidemic arthritic erythema. The other, due to a spirochete, *Spirillum minus,* is characterized by an indurated ulcer at the site of inoculation, remittent fever, and a purplish maculopapular rash. Also called *sodoku.*
recurrent f. See relapsing *f.*
red f. of Congo. See murine *typhus.*
relapsing f. Any of a group of specific infectious diseases caused by spirochetes, *Borrelia recurrentis* and *Borrelia duttonii* being most common, and transmitted to man by lice or ticks, characterized by acute onset, chills, fever, pain in the back and legs, splenomegaly, delirium, and sometimes convulsions: also called *famine f., remittent f., spirillum f., recurrent f.*
remittent f. A paroxysmal fever with exacerbations and remissions, but without intermissions. The term is sometimes used for relapsing *f.*
rheumatic f. See *rheumatic fever.*
Rhodesian f. See East Coast *f.*
Rift Valley f. An epizootic hepatitis of mild degree caused by a filtrable virus and of limited geographic distribution.
Rocky Mountain spotted f. See *Rocky Mountain spotted fever.*
rose f. See *hay fever.*
Salmonella f. A mild disease caused by a member of the genus *Salmonella;* similar to typhoid.
sandfly f. Phlebotomus fever.
San Joaquin Valley f. See *coccidioidomycosis.*
São Paulo f. São Paulo typhus, now known to be identical with Rocky Mountain spotted fever.
scarlet f. See *scarlet fever.*
septic f. One due to septicemia.
seven-day f. A disease similar to dengue, lasting about one week; due to the spirochete *Leptospira hebdomadis.*
ship f. See classic epidemic *typhus.*
shipping f. Hemorrhagic septicemia of cattle. It is an acute, occasionally subacute, septicemic disease caused by *Pasteurella boviseptica.*
shoddy f. A febrile disease with cough and dyspnea; seen in persons who work with shoddy.
South African tick-bite f. A tick-bite fever of Africa always accompanied by lymphadenopathy. Appearance of a rash is variable.
spirillum f. Relapsing fever.
spotted f. group. A group of rickettsial diseases caused by species of *Dermacentroxenus,* transmitted by ticks and mites, and having certain clinical features in common. In the United States the type disease is Rocky Mountain spotted fever. Others are the tick-bite fevers of Africa, Brazilian and Colombian spotted fevers, pinta fever (Choix) of Mexico, North Queensland tick typhus, rickettsialpox, maculatum disease, and probably some of the rickettsioses of India and Russia.
sthenic f. Old term for a fever with high temperature and delirium.
suppurative f. Old term for pyemia.
swamp f. of horses. Infectious anemia of horses.
swine f. Hog cholera.
symptomatic f. See traumatic *f.*
tertian f. A form of malaria due to *Plasmodium vivax,* which completes its life cycle in 48 hours. Chills recur every two days.
Texas f. An infectious disease of cattle; due to the parasite *Babesia bigemina,* which is transmitted by the cattle tick *Boöphilus annulatus,* and invades the red blood corpuscles. Characterized by high fever, hemoglobinuria, and enlargement of the spleen.
therapeutic f. See artificial *f.*
thermic f. Sunstroke.
three-day f. Phlebotomus fever.
threshing f. A form of pneumonoconiosis affecting threshers; characterized by headache, fever, and irritation of the respiratory tract.
tick f. Colorado tick *f.*

tick-bite fevers of Africa. Tick-borne typhus-like fevers belonging to the spotted fever group, caused by *Dermacentroxenus rickettsi conori* and characterized by a local lesion (*tache noire*) with black necrotic center appearing at the site of the tick bite and generally also by lymphadenopathy. Diagnosis rests on identification of serologic tests. The African tick-bite fevers, representing wide geographic distribution, include boutonneuse fever, Kenya typhus, Nigerian typhus, and South African and North African tick-bite fevers; their clinical features are similar and cross immunity between several of them has been established.
Tobia f. See *Rocky Mountain spotted fever.*
traumatic f. That following a wound or an injury. Syn., *symptomatic f.*
trench f. An acute infection lasting several days; caused by *Rickettsia quintana* and transmitted by the body louse. Syn., *Volhynia f.*
trypanosome f. Trypanosomiasis.
tsutsugamushi f. See tsutsugamushi *disease.*
typhoid f. See *typhoid.*
typhomalarial f. Malaria with typhoidlike symptoms.
typhus f. See classic epidemic *typhus.*
undulant f. Brucellosis.
urticarial f. That accompanying an urticarial rash.
uveoparotid f. A syndrome of uveitis, parotitis, and fever; of unknown origin: also called *Heerfordt's disease, Heerfordt's syndrome, uveoparotitis.* See also *sarcoidosis.*
vaccinal f. That following vaccination.
valley f. Coccidioidomycosis.
Volhynia f. See trench *f.*
war f. See classic epidemic *typhus.*
yellow f. An acute infectious disease of tropical and subtropical regions of America; caused by a filtrable virus disseminated by the *Aëdes aegypti* (*Stegomyia fasciata calopus*). After a period of incubation varying from a few hours to several days, the disease begins with a chill and pain in the head, back, and limbs. The temperature rises rapidly to from 103° to 105° F., vomiting occurs, the bowels are constipated, the urine scanty and albuminous. A remission follows, after which, in severe cases, the temperature rises to its original height, jaundice develops, and the vomited material becomes dark from the presence of blood (black vomit). Hemorrhages may occur from the intestinal mucous membrane. The disease is often fatal, death occurring in the typhoid state or from uremia.

F.F.P.S. Fellow of the Faculty of Physicians and Surgeons (Glasgow).

FFT Flicker fusion test; flicker fusion threshold.

fi'ant. Plural of fiat.

fi'at (pl. *fiant*) [L., pres. subj. of *fieri*, to be made]. Let there be made; used in the writing of prescriptions. Abbreviated, ft.

fi'ber, fi'bre [L. *fibra*, fiber]. A filamentary or threadlike structure. —**fibrous,** *adj.*
accelerating fibers. Sympathetic nerve fibers which convey impulses that hasten the rapidity and increase the force of the heartbeat. Also called *augmentor fibers.*
adrenergic fibers. Nerve fibers which liberate an adrenalinlike substance at their terminations; include most of the postganglionic fibers of the sympathetic nervous system.
arcuate f. One of a number of bow-shaped or arched nerve fibers in the brain; those on the ventral surface of the medulla are called **ventral external arcuate fibers,** others within the medulla are called **internal arcuate fibers.**
argentaffin f., argentophile f. See reticular *fibers.*
argyrophil fibers. See reticular *fibers.*
association fibers. White nerve fibers situated just beneath the cortical substance and connecting the adjacent cerebral gyri.
axial f. (a) The axis cylinder of a nerve fiber. (b) The central spiral filament, probably contractile, of the flagellum of the spermatozoon.
basilar fibers. Specialized connective-tissue fibers in the basilar membrane of the cochlea.
cerebellorubral f. A fiber of the brachium conjunctivum terminating in the red nucleus.
cerebellothalmic f. A fiber of the brachium conjunctivum terminating in the thalamus.
cholinergic fibers. Nerve fibers which liberate an acetylcholinelike substance at their terminations; include most of the motor nerves of the body except postganglionic sympathetics.
climbing fibers of cerebellum. Afferent fibers entering the cerebellar cortex from the white matter, probably through the brachium pontis, to synapse directly with the dendrites of the Purkinje cells.
collagenous fibers. The flexible, fibrillar, nonelastic, connective-tissue fibers which are the commonest type. They make up the main mass of such structures as the corium, fasciae, tendons, ligaments, aponeuroses, periostea, and capsules of organs, and form also the fibrillar, intercellular substance of bone and cartilage. Syn., *white fibers.*
collateral fibers. The delicate lateral branches of the axon of a neuron. Also called *paraxons.*
commissural fibers. Fibers joining an area of the cortex of one cerebral hemisphere to a similar area of the other.
cone f. One of the fibers of the retinal cones.
corticifugal f. Any nerve fiber carrying impulses away from the cerebral cortex to other centers.
corticopontile f. A fiber arising from the cortex of the frontal lobe and from the parietal, temporal, and portions of the occipital lobe, and descending uncrossed to the pontile nuclei: also called *corticopontine f., palliopontile f.*
corticorubral f. One going from the premotor frontal cortex to the red nucleus.
corticostriate fibers. Fibers transmitting impulses from the cerebral cortex to the corpus striatum; part of the extrapyramidal system.
corticothalamic fibers. Fibers transmitting impulses from the cerebral cortex to the thalamus. It is believed that they bring about thalamic receptivity to incoming impulses from the secondary sensory pathways.
dentinal fibers. The processes of odontoblasts in the dentinal tubules. Syn., *Tomes's fibers.*
dentinogenic fibers. The precollagenous fibers which pass between the odontoblasts into the dentine to form the fibrillar component of the dentinal matrix. Also called *Korff's fibers.*
elastic fibers. The nonfibrillar, branching, highly elastic fibers of fibroelastic connective tissue. They form also the fenestrated membranes of large arteries. Syn., *yellow fibers.*
enamel f. See enamel *prism.*
f. cell. Any cell elongated to a fiberlike appearance; for example, muscle cells are commonly referred to as muscle fibers.
fibers of Remak. Peripheral nonmedullated nerve fibers.
fibers of Sharpey. See perforating *fibers.*
fibroglia fibers. Tonofibrils intimately associated with fibroblasts. See *fibroglia.*
Korff's f. See dentinogenic *fibers,* osteogenic *fibers.*
lattice fibers. See reticular *fibers.*
lens fibers. The highly modified epithelial cells which form the main mass of the lens of the eye.
mossy fibers. Fibers entering the cerebellum

from the restiform body to synapse with the granule cell dendrites.

Müller's fibers. Modified neuroglia cells which traverse perpendicularly the layers of the retina, and connect the internal and external limiting membranes.

muscle f. The ultimate element of which muscular tissue is made up. Voluntary muscles consist of transversely striated fibers, involuntary muscles of spindle-shaped fibers or cells.

nerve f. The long process of a neuron, usually the axon. **Myelinated nerve fibers** have a thick layer of myelin surrounding the nerve fiber; **unmyelinated nerve fibers** contain very little myelin.

osteogenic fibers. The precollagenous fibers which pass between the osteoblasts during bone formation to form the fibrillar component of the bone matrix. Also called *Korff's fibers.*

pallidohypothalamic f. An efferent fiber from the globus pallidus to the anterior ventral and several medial thalamic nuclei.

palliopontile f. See corticopontile *f.*

perforating fibers. Collagenous fibers of a tendon, ligament, or periosteum buried in the matrix of subperiosteal bone. Also the similar fibers in the cementum of a tooth. Syn., *fibers of Sharpey, Sharpey's fibers.* Also called *penetrating fibers.*

precollagenous fibers. See reticular *fibers.*

projection fibers. Fibers joining the cerebral cortex to lower centers and vice versa.

Purkinje fibers. The modified cardiac muscle fibers of the conduction system of the heart: also called *Purkinje system.*

reticular fibers. The delicate, branching connective-tissue fibers forming the reticular framework of lymphatic tissue, myeloid tissue, the red pulp of the spleen, the finest stroma of many glands, and most basement membranes. They differ from collagenous fibers in their response to silver impregnation, in which they are blackened. Also called *argentaffin f., argentophile f., argyrophil f., lattice f., precollagenous f.*

rivet fibers. Protoplasmic processes on the basal surface of the columnar cells of stratified squamous epithelium.

secretory fibers. Centrifugal nerve fibers exciting secretion.

smooth muscle fibers. The straight, or slightly bent, elongated, spindle-shaped, nucleated cells, bearing more or less distinct longitudinal striations, which make up involuntary, or unstriped, muscles. Also called *involuntary fibers, nonstriated fibers, unstriated fibers, unstriped fibers.* See muscular *tissue.*

spindle fibers. See *achromatic fibrils* under *fibril.*

sustentacular fibers. A supporting connective tissue that unites the various layers of the retina.

sympathetic fibers. Sympathetic nerve fibers.

Tomes's fibers. Odontoblastic processes occupying the dentinal tubules: also called *dentinal fibers.*

vasoconstrictor fibers. Nerve fibers which, upon stimulation, produce constriction of blood vessels.

vasodilator fibers. Nerve fibers whose function is to dilate blood vessels.

white fibers. See *collagenous fibers* under *fiber.*

yellow fibers. See *elastic fibers* under *fiber.*

zonular fibers. The fibers of the ciliary zonule of Zinn.

Fibiger, Johannes (1867–1926). Danish bacteriologist who discovered *Spiroptera* carcinoma, supporting Virchow's theory that cancerous growths are due to chronic irritation. Nobel laureate in medicine and physiology (1926).

fi'bra. Fiber.

fi'bre. See *fiber.*

fi·bre'mi·a, fi·brae'mi·a (figh·bree'mee·uh) [*fibra;* G. *haima,* blood]. The presence of fibrin in the blood.

fi'bri·form [*fibra;* L. *forma,* form]. Shaped like a fiber.

fi'bril [*fibra*]. A component filament of a fiber, as of a muscle or of a nerve. Also called *fibrilla.* —**fibrillar, fibrillary,** *adj.*

achromatic fibrils. Fibrils of achromatic, nuclear, or cell substance forming lines which extend from pole to pole in a dividing nucleus, so as to form a spindle- or barrel-shaped figure.

chromatic fibrils. The threadlike fibrils consisting of the chromatin in a cell nucleus; nuclear fibrils.

dentinal f. One of the fibrils of the dentinal matrix. The term is sometimes erroneously used for dentinal fiber.

fi"bril·la'tion [*fibra*]. 1. The formation of fibrils. 2. A local quivering of muscular fibers. —**fi'brillated,** *adj.*

atrial f. A cardiac arrhythmia due to a disturbed spread of excitation through atrial musculature; generally believed to be due to waves of excitation circulating irregularly and continuously at rapid rates around a variable "ring" of muscle in the atria from where excitation of the rest of the atria and ventricles occurs, giving rise to an irregular, usually rapid, rate of ventricular excitation. Also called *auricular f.*

auricular f. Term clinically used for atrial *f.*

ventricular f. A cardiac arrhythmia characterized by an absolutely irregular spread of idioventricular excitation whose origin and spread are completely disordered, analogous to atrial fibrillation. It produces only limited, ineffectual, and irregular ventricular contractions and, being almost always irreversible in man, usually is fatal.

fi·bril"lo·gen'e·sis (figh·bril"o·jen'i·sis) [*fibra;* G. *genesis,* production]. The formation and development of fibrils, especially those of connective tissue.

fi'brin [*fibra*]. The fibrous insoluble protein, formed by the interaction of thrombin and fibrinogen, in the network of which blood corpuscles are enmeshed in the clotting of shed blood. —**fi'brinous,** *adj.*

f. ferment. Thrombin.

f. film. A pliable, elastic, translucent film of fibrin, prepared from human blood plasma; used in neurosurgery for the repair of dural defects and in the prevention of meningocerebral adhesions.

f. foam. A spongy material made from human fibrin which, when soaked in human thrombin, is a useful hemostatic agent in neurosurgery, in wounds of parenchymatous organs, and in cases of jaundice and hemophilia. It causes little tissue reaction and is absorbable.

gluten f. Vegetable fibrin; a brownish mass extracted from gluten.

fi"bri·ne'mi·a, fi"bri·nae'mi·a (figh"bri·nee'mee·uh) [*fibra;* G. *haima,* blood]. Fibremia.

fi'bri·no-, fi'brin- [*fibra*]. A combining form meaning *relating to fibrin.*

fi·brin'o·gen (figh·brin'o·jen) [*fibra;* G. *genesthai,* from *gignesthai,* to be produced]. A protein of the globulin class present in blood plasma and serous transudations; the soluble precursor of fibrin. See Table of Normal Values of Blood Constituents in the Appendix. —**fibrinogen'ic, fibrinog'enous** (figh"bri·nodj'i·nus), *adj.*

fi·brin"o·gen"o·pe'ni·a (figh·brin"o·jen"o·pee'nee·uh) [*fibra; genesthai;* G. *penia,* poverty]. Decrease in the fibrinogen of the blood plasma, often associated with hemorrhagic disorders of parturition, although other acquired and congenital cases are observed. Formerly called *fibrinopenia.*

fi′bri·noid [*fibra;* G. *eidos,* form]. The fibrinlike material of the placenta; produced by necrosis of the mucosa and trophoblast and by fibrin from maternal blood. It occurs as an incomplete layer in the chorion and decidua and as patches on the chorionic villi. Also called *stria.*

canalized f. The layered fibrinoid material having a striated or canalized appearance, found especially on the chorionic plate during the last half of pregnancy.

fi″brin·o·kin′ase. The activators of plasminogen, found in animal tissues.

fi″bri·no·ly′sin, fi″bri·nol′y·sin [*fibra;* G. *lysis,* a loosing]. Any enzyme which digests fibrin. Plasma contains a fibrinolysin, called *plasmin,* present as a precursor, which can be activated by streptokinase, staphylokinase, fibrinokinase, or certain organic solvents, including chloroform. The term was formerly applied to the bacterial products which activate plasminogen.

fi″brin·ol′y·sis [*fibra; lysis*]. 1. The slow digestion and solution of fibrin which occurs when a blood clot is allowed to stand aseptically in the serum in which it was formed; presumably due to the action of a proteolytic enzyme. 2. The hydrolysis of fibrin.

fi·brin″o·pe′ni·a (figh·brin″o·pee′nee·uh, figh″-brin·o·). See *fibrinogenopenia.*

fi′bro-, fibr- [*fibra*]. A combining form signifying *pertaining to fibers, relation to fibrous tissue or structure.*

fi″bro·ad″e·no′ma [*fibra;* G. *adēn,* gland; *-ōma,* tumor]. Benign adenomatous tumor containing variable amounts of connective tissue, which may vary from densely collagenous to myxoid: also called *adenofibroma, cystadenofibroma, fibroadenoma xanthomatodes, fibropapilloma, fetal fibroadenoma, myxofibroadenoma, pleomorphic fibroadenoma.*

giant f. of breast. See *cystosarcoma phylloides.*

intracanalicular f. (*of breast*). A benign breast tumor with proliferation of connective tissue causing distortion of the lumina of the glands and ducts in the tumor: also called *intracanalicular myxoma.*

periacinar f. See pericanalicular *f.* (*of breast*).

pericanalicular f. (*of breast*). A glandular type of benign breast tumor with large amounts of connective tissue which is often arranged concentrically around the multiplied ductules: also called *periacinar f.*

fi″bro·ad′i·pose [*fibra;* L. *adeps,* fat]. Both fibrous and fatty.

fi″bro·an″gi·o′ma [*fibra;* G. *aggeion,* vessel; *-ōma,* tumor]. A benign tumor composed of blood or lymph vessels, with abundant connective tissue.

fi″bro·a·re′o·lar [*fibra;* L. *areola,* small, open place]. Both fibrous and areolar. *Obs.*

fi′bro·blast [*fibra;* G. *blastos,* germ]. A stellate or spindle-shaped cell (rod-shaped, if seen on edge) with a large, oval, flattened nucleus and a thin layer of cytoplasm; found in fibrous tissue. Syn., *fibrocyte.* Also called *connective-tissue cell.*

fi″bro·blas′tic [*fibra; blastos*]. 1. Pertaining to fibroblasts. 2. Fibroplastic.

fi″bro·blas·to′ma [*fibra; blastos;* G. *-ōma,* tumor]. Term used for fibroma.

arachnoid f. Term used for meningioma.

meningeal f. See *meningioma.*

perineural f. See *neurilemmoma; neurofibroma.*

fi″bro·bron·chi′tis [*fibra;* G. *brogchos,* windpipe; *-itis,* inflammation]. Bronchitis with expectoration of fibrinous casts.

fi″bro·cal·car′e·ous (figh″bro·kal·kair′ee·us) [*fibra;* L. *calcarius,* pertaining to lime]. Both fibrous and calcareous, as a deposit of calcific material in tissues (occurring in fibromas or as the seat of fibrosis).

fi″bro·car″ci·no′ma [*fibra;* G. *karkinos,* crab; *-ōma,* tumor]. A carcinoma with fibrous elements.

fi″bro·car′ti·lage [*fibra;* L. *cartilago,* cartilage]. Dense, white, fibrous connective tissue in which the cells have formed small masses of cartilage between the fibers, and have impregnated the fibers with chondrin. —**fibrocartilag′inous** (figh″bro·kahr″ti·ladj′i·nus), *adj.*

fi″bro·cel′lu·lar [*fibra;* L. *cellula,* small store-room]. Both fibrous and cellular; fibroareolar.

fi″bro·chon·dro′ma (figh″bro·kon·dro′muh) [*fibra;* G. *chondros,* cartilage; *-ōma,* tumor]. A chondroma with a considerable amount of fibrous tissue.

fi″bro·chon·dro·os″te·o′ma. See *osteochondroma.*

fi″bro·cys·to′ma [*fibra;* G. *kystis,* bladder; *-ōma*]. A fibrous tumor accompanied by cystic degeneration.

fi′bro·cyte. Fibroblast.

fi″bro·dys·pla′si·a. See fibrous *dysplasia.*

fi″bro·e·las′tic [*fibra;* G. *elaunein,* to drive]. Applied to connective tissue in which interlacing collagenous fibers are interspersed by more or less strongly developed networks of elastic fibers.

fi″bro·e·las·to′sis [*fibra; elaunein;* G. *-ōsis,* condition]. See endocardial *fibrosis.*

fi″bro·en″chon·dro′ma (·en″kon·dro′muh) [*fibra;* G. *en,* in; *chrondros,* cartilage; *-ōma,* tumor]. An enchondroma containing fibrous elements.

fi″bro·en″do·the·li·o′ma of joint. See *synovioma.*

fibrogen. Trade-mark for a suspension of tissue fibrinogen and cephalin in a sodium chloride solution. Possesses thromboplastic activity, and is employed orally as a hemostatic.

fi·brog′li·a (figh·brog′lee·uh, fi·brog′·, figh·bro′-glee·uh, fi·bro′·) [*fibra;* G. *glia,* glue]. Old term for the ground substance of connective tissue. Tonofibrils associated with fibroblasts are called *fibroglia fibers.* See under *fiber.*

fi″bro·gli·o′ma (figh″bro·glye·o′muh) [*fibra; glia;* G. *-ōma,* tumor]. A glioma with a considerable amount of mesodermal fibrous tissue.

f. of nose. See heterotopic *glioma.*

fi′broid [*fibra;* G. *eidos,* form]. Composed of fibrous tissue; said of a tissue or structure which has become the seat of extensive fibrosis.

fi″broid·ec′to·my [*fibra; eidos;* G. *ektomē,* excision]. Removal of a uterine fibroid.

fi″bro·lam′i·nar [*fibra;* L. *lamina,* plate]. Relating to a fibrous layer, as fibrolaminar thrombus.

fi″bro·lei″o·my·o′ma. A leiomyoma containing a fibromatous component.

fi″bro·li·po′ma [*fibra;* G. *lipos,* fat; *-ōma,* tumor]. A lipoma with a considerable amount of fibrous tissue. —**fibrolipom′atous,** *adj.*

fi″bro·li·po·sar·co′ma. A liposarcoma with fibromatous component.

fibrolysin. Trade-mark for a thiosinamine and sodium salicylate solution used as a resolvent of cicatrices.

fi·bro′ma (figh·bro′muh) [*fibra; -ōma*]. A benign tumor composed principally of whorls of white fibrous connective tissue. —**fibrom′atous,** *adj.*

chondromyxoid f. of bone. A rare, peculiarly differentiated tumor of connective tissue, characterized cytologically by spindle-shaped cells in a myxoid intercellular matrix and in parts, as well as gross appearance, simulating cartilage.

endoneural f. See *neurofibroma.*

f. durum. A hard fibroma, firm because of large quantities of collagenous material in comparison with the number of cells; a dermatofibroma.

f. fungoides. See *mycosis* fungoides.

f. lipomatodes. See *xanthoma.*
f. molle. A soft fibroma, soft because cellular components are rich as compared with collagenous fibers; it is often pedunculated.
f. molluscum. See *neurofibromatosis.*
f. of nerve sheath. See *neurofibroma.*
f. simplex. See *dermatofibroma.*
nonosteogenic f. of bone. A common benign tumor of bone, exhibiting no osteogenic tendencies, usually found in the shaft of long bones, and histologically characterized by whorls of spindle-shaped connective-tissue cells. There are giant cells containing several nuclei, and lipid-laden cells.
odontogenic f. A benign odontogenic tumor formed from the mesenchymal derivatives of the tooth germ, which usually develops at the apex of a tooth.
ossifying f. of bone. A benign tumor of bone derived from bone-forming connective tissue, seen particularly in the vertebral column, which microscopically appears as vascularized connective tissue interspersed with fibrous bone trabeculae. Syn., *osteogenic f.*, *osteofibroma*, *fibrous osteoma.*
osteogenic f. Ossifying *f.*
papillary f. A superficial fibroma with papillary projections.
perineural f. See *neurofibroma.*

fi·bro′ma·toid (figh·bro′muh·toyd) [*fibra; -ōma;* G. *eidos,* form]. Resembling a fibroma.

fi·bro″ma·to′sis (figh·bro″muh·to′sis) [*fibra; -ōma;* G. *-ōsis,* condition]. The simultaneous occurrence of many fibromas.

fi″bro·mus′cu·lar [*fibra;* L. *musculus,* muscle]. Made up of connective tissue and muscle.

fi″bro·my·o′ma (·migh·o′muh) [*fibra;* G. *mys,* muscle; *-ōma,* tumor]. A myoma in which connective tissue is so intermingled with the muscle as to constitute a fibromatous component.
f. of uterus. See *leiomyoma.*

fi″bro·my″o·mec′to·my [*fibra; mys; -ōma;* G. *ektomē,* excision]. Excision of a fibromyoma.

fi″bro·my″o·si′tis. See *myositis.*

fi″bro·myx″o·en·do·the″li·o′ma [*fibra;* G. *myxa,* mucus; G. *endon,* within; G. *-ōma,* tumor]. See mixed *tumor* of salivary gland type.

fi″bro·myx″o·li·po′ma [*fibra;* G. *myxa,* mucus; *lipos,* fat; *-ōma*]. A mixed, fatty tumor with fibrous and myxomatous tissues.

fi″bro·myx·o′ma [*fibra; myxa; -ōma*]. A connective-tissue tumor composed of fibrous and myxomatous components.
f. of breast. See *cystosarcoma phylloides.*
f. of nerve sheath. See *neurofibroma.*

fi″bro·myx″o·sar·co′ma [*fibra; myxa;* G. *sarkōma,* fleshy excrescence]. A fibrosarcoma with mucoid degeneration; rarely, a combination of fibrosarcoma and myxosarcoma.
f. of breast. See *cystosarcoma phylloides.*

fi″bro·neu·ro′ma. See *neurofibroma.*

fi″bro-os″te·o·chon·dro′ma. See *osteochondroma.*

fi″bro-os·te·o′ma. An osteoma.

fi″bro-os″te·o·sar·co′ma. An osteosarcoma.

fi″bro·pla′si·a (figh″bro·play′zhuh, ·zee·uh, ·shuh, ·see·uh) [*fibra;* G. *plassein,* to form]. The growth of fibrous tissue, as in the second phase of wound healing. —**fibroplas′tic,** *adj.*
retrolental f. A blinding disease of the eye affecting premature infants with low birth weight: so-called because in the ultimate stage the contracture of organized fibrous tissue detaches the retina and occupies the pupillary area back of the lens.

fi′bro·plate [*fibra;* OF. *plate*]. A disk of interarticular fibrocartilage.

fi″bro·psam·mo′ma (·sam·o′muh) [*fibra;* G. *psammos,* sand; *-ōma,* tumor]. 1. A psammoma with a considerable amount of fibrosis. 2. A fibroma in which psammoma bodies are present.

fi″bro·pu′ru·lent [*fibra;* L. *purulentus,* purulent]. Consisting of pus containing flakes of fibrin.

fi″bro·sar·co′ma [*fibra;* G. *sarkōma,* fleshy excrescence]. Spindle-cell sarcoma, mature in type, with production of collagenous fibrils.
f. myxomatodes. See *fibromyxosarcoma.*
f. of breast. See *cystosarcoma phylloides.*
f. of nerve sheath. See malignant *schwannoma.*
f. ovarii mucocellulare carcinomatodes. See *Krukenberg tumor.*
f. phyllodes. See *cystosarcoma phylloides.*
odontogenic f. A malignant tumor derived from mesenchymal odontogenic tissues.

fi″bro·se′rous [*fibra;* L. *serum,* whey]. Composed of fibrous tissue with a serous surface.

fi·bro′sis (figh·bro′sis) [*fibra;* G. *-ōsis,* increase]. Growth of white fibrous connective tissue in an organ or part in excess of that naturally present. —**fibrot′ic,** *adj.*
arteriocapillary f. Fibrosis of small arteries and arterioles, with variable degrees of hyalinization and reduction in the size of the lumens. One of the manifestations of what is now called arteriolar sclerosis. Also called *arteriocapillary fibrosis of Gull and Sutton.*
bauxite f. A type of pulmonary fibrosis observed in the abrasive manufacturing industry among workers exposed to concentrated fumes of amorphous alumina and silica. Exact etiology has not been established. It is characterized by pulmonary insufficiency, diffuse roentgenologic changes, and the frequent occurrence of spontaneous pneumothorax. Fatal termination may occur within a period of months. Also called *Shaver's disease.*
cystic f. See pancreatic *f.*
endocardial f. Congenital thickening (hyperplasia) of the endocardium in infants' hearts, with or without valvular deformity. Syn., *endocardofibrosis, fibroelastosis, endocardial sclerosis.*
hepatolienal f. Intrahepatic obstruction to the portal flow as the result of a fibrosing factor operating during childhood, adolescence, and early adult life. There is no known etiological factor.
nodular f. Fibrosis in the form of small nodules.
pancreatic f. Congenital disease which may involve widespread change in the mucous glands of the entire body. Obstructive lesions of the pancreas with acinar atrophy and eventually marked fibrosis of the entire gland, causing pancreatic exocrine insufficiency and having the clinical appearance of the celiac syndrome comprise a prominent feature. There is also severe pulmonary disease, which may precede, accompany, or follow the symptoms of pancreatic insufficiency. Diagnosis is substantiated by the deficiency or absence of trypsin. Also called *cystic fibrosis of pancreas, congenital pancreatic* or *familial steatorrhea, chronic interstitial pancreatitis of infancy, mucosis, mucoviscidosis.*
pulmonary f. Proliferation of fibrous tissue in the lung.
replacement f. That which replaces destroyed tissues, in part or wholly.
silica f. A condition produced in dogs by the experimental injection of ground quartz into the hepatic portal vein. As a result, a marked collateral circulation to the intrahepatically obstructed portal circuit develops.

fi″bro·si′tis [*fibra;* G. *-itis,* inflammation]. (a) Inflammatory hyperplasia of the white fibrous tissue. (b) A form independent of gross anatomic disease of the structures involved; it may be *primary* or without demonstrable cause, or *secondary* to some form of arthritis, trauma, or other disease or abnormality. —**fibrosit'ic,** *adj.*

bursal f. Bursitis.

fascial f. See tendinous *f.*

f. ossificans progressiva. The multiple progressive form of myositis ossificans.

intramuscular f. Myositis.

periarticular f. That involving the joint capsule.

tendinous f. That involving the fibrous sheaths of tendons.

fi'brous [*fibra*]. Containing fibers; similar to fibers.

fib'u·la [L., clasp]. The slender bone at the outer part of the leg, articulating above with the tibia and below with the talus and tibia. See Plates 1, 2. See Table of Bones in the Appendix. —**fibular,** *adj.*

fib″u·lo·cal·ca'ne·al [*fibula;* L. *calcaneum,* heel]. Pertaining to or connecting the fibula and the calcaneus.

F.I.C. Fellow of the Institute of Chemistry.

fi'cin [L. *ficus,* fig]. A proteolytic enzyme from the fig-tree sap. It is an active *Ascaris* and *Trichuris* vermicide.

Fick, Adolf [*German physiologist,* 1829–1901]. Introduced a number of instruments used in the study of muscle and nerve physiology, including the myotonograph and the cosine lever (1864). He described a method, called *Fick's principle,* for determining cardiac output by gasometry: if the total quantity of oxygen consumed per minute is known, and also the oxygen content of both the arterial and the mixed venous blood, the output can be calculated by means of the following formula:

$$\frac{\text{Total oxygen consumption}}{\text{Arteriovenous oxygen difference}} \times 100 = \text{cardiac output}$$

fi·co'sis. See *sycosis.*

F.I.C.S. Fellow of the International College of Surgeons.

Fiedler, Carl Ludwig Alfred [*German physician,* 1835–1921]. Described spirochetal jaundice, called *Weil's disease, Fiedler's disease.* Described progressive myocardial failure caused by idiopathic, diffuse, nonsuppurative myocarditis, called *Fiedler's myocarditis.*

field [AS. *feld*]. 1. An open space or area. 2. A concept of development in which the whole and the parts of a structure or organism are dynamically interrelated, reacting to each other and to the environment. 3. A region of the embryo that is the anlage of some organ or part.

adversive fields. Regions of the cerebral cortex in which stimulation evokes a turning of the eyes, head, and trunk toward the opposite side.

auditory f. The area within which a given sound is audible to the ear.

deaf f. One of the small areas near the external auditory meatus in which the vibrating tuning fork is not heard.

electrical f. *In cardiology,* the electrical line of force in the body exerted by the heart currents. Abbreviated, EMF or E.M.F.

f. of fixation. *In optics,* the region bounded by the utmost limits of distinct or central vision, which the eye has under its direct control throughout its excursions when the head is not moved.

f. of microscope. The area within which objects can be seen through a microscope at one time.

f. of vision. The space visible to the patient when the eye is fixed steadily on an object in the direct line of vision. Abbreviated, F.

frontal adversive f. Adversive field of the frontal cerebral cortex.

individuation f. A term denoting the ability of an organizer to rearrange the regional structure of both itself and the adjacent tissue, to make the adjacent tissue part of a complete embryo.

magnetic f. The portion of space around a magnet in which its action can be felt.

nasal f. The anlage of the olfactory placode. Syn., *olfactory f., nasal area.*

occipital eye f. A region on the lateral aspect of the occipital portion of the cerebral cortex whose stimulation produces conjugate deviation of the eyes toward the opposite side.

olfactory f. See nasal *f.*

parietal adversive f. Adversive field of the parietal cerebral cortex.

field med'i·cal card. *In U. S. Army medicine,* a type of individual medical record, usually used by numbered hospitals and fixed dispensaries in oversea commands.

field med'i·cal rec'ord. *In U. S. Army medicine,* a field medical card and the field medical record jacket, with all the enclosed medical and clinical records.

fi·èvre' bou·ton·neuse' (fyev'ruh boo·taw·nehz'. *See* NOTES § 35). See boutonneuse *fever.*

fig [L. *ficus,* fig]. The fruit of *Ficus carica,* having nutritive and laxative qualities.

fig'ure [L. *figura,* form]. The visible form of anything; the outline of an organ or part.

achromatic f. The spindle and asters in mitosis or miosis.

chromatic f. The chromosomes or the pattern formed by the chromosomes in miosis or mitosis.

nuclear figures. The peculiar arrangement of the chromosomes during karyokinesis.

fig'wort. Any member of the botanical family Scrophulariaceae; specifically, the herb *Scrophularia nodosa* var. *marilandica,* formerly variously used medicinally.

fi'la. Plural of filum.

fi·la'ceous (fi·lay'shus, figh·lay'shus) [L. *filum,* thread]. Consisting of threads or threadlike fibers or parts. *Rare.*

fil'a·ment [F., from L. *filare,* to spin]. A small, threadlike structure. —**filamen'tous,** *adj.*

axial f. The central contractile fibril of a cilium or flagellum which arises from a centriole or blepharoplast.

spermatic f. The axial filament of a spermatozoon.

terminal f. The end piece or naked axial filament of the tail of a spermatozoon.

fil″a·men·ta'tion [*filare*]. Thread formation; a peculiar reaction observed when bacteria are grown in an immune serum. Long threads of bacteria occur. The reaction is shown by the typhoid and proteus bacilli. Also called *Pfaundler's reaction, thread reaction, Mandelbaum's reaction.*

fi'lar [L. *filum,* thread]. Filamentous.

fi·la'ri·a (pl. *filariae*) [*filum*]. A long filiform nematode which is a member of the superfamily Filarioidea. The adults may live in the circulatory or lymphatic systems, the connective tissues, or serous cavities of a vertebrate host. The larval forms, or microfilariae, are commonly found in the circulating blood or lymph spaces from which they are ingested by some form of blood-sucking arthropod. After a series of metamorphoses in the body of the arthropod, the larvae migrate to the proboscis as infestive forms. —**filar'ial,** *adj.*

blinding f. Onchocerciasis.

fil″a·ri'a·sis [*filum;* NL. *-iasis,* condition]. A diseased state due to the presence of filariae in the body.

f. bancrofti. Elephantiasis due to *Wuchereria bancrofti.*

Malayan f. Filariasis of man caused by *Wuchereria malayi*, occurring exclusively in the Far East (India, China, Celebes, New Guinea, etc.). It is frequently associated with elephantiasis of the upper extremities.

fi·lar′i·cide [*filum;* L. *caedere*, to kill]. A drug which destroys filariae. —**filarici′dal,** *adj.*

fi·lar′i·form [*filum;* L. *forma*, shape]. In the form of, or resembling, filariae.

Filatov, Nil Fedorovich [*Russian pediatrician*, 1846–1902]. Described infectious mononucleosis, calling it idiopathic adenitis (1885–87); this is also known as *Filatov's disease, Pfeiffer's disease.* Described a form of rubella with a scarlatiniform rash, under the name rubeola scarlatinosa (1887); its existence as a separate entity is open to doubt. Called *fourth disease, Filatov-Dukes disease.*

Filatov, Vladimir Petrovich [*Russian ophthalmologist*, 1875–]. Renowned for his operation of transplantation of the cornea, in which a protecting celluloid shield is passed into the anterior chamber, a disk of cornea removed, and a similar disk from the donor eye placed in the defect. The graft is secured in place by a conjunctival flap turned down from above.

fi·lic′ic ac′id (fi·liss′ick). The term applied to a mixture of related constituents found in aspidium, which appear to be derivatives of a methyl and a dimethyl phloroglucinol.

fil′i·cin. Filicic acid.

fil″i·cin′ic ac′id. 11-Dimethylcyclohexane-2,4,6-trione; a decomposition product of several constituents of aspidium.

fil′i·form [*filum; forma*]. Threadlike.

Filipowicz, Casimir [*Polish physician*, contemporary]. Described a yellowish discoloration of the palmar and plantar regions seen in typhoid fever, called *palmoplantar phenomenon, Filipowicz's sign.*

fil′i·punc″ture [*filum;* L. *punctura*, a puncture]. A method of treating aneurysm by inserting wire threads, hair, or the like to promote coagulation. *Obs.*

fil′let [*filum*]. 1. A loop for the purpose of making traction on the fetus. 2. Old term for *lemniscus.*

fill′ing [AS. *fyllan*]. 1. The material used in closing cavities in carious teeth. 2. The process of inserting, condensing, shaping, and finishing a filling substance.

contour f. *In dentistry*, a filling in which the material is so built out as to restore the lost portion of the crown of the tooth.

root canal f. The closure and filling of the prepared root canal from the apex to the coronal portion of the tooth with an impervious material to prevent subsequent infection.

temporary f. A substance, as cement or gutta percha, used in teeth as a filling which is to be replaced later by a permanent restoration.

film [AS. *filmen*]. 1. A pellicle or thin skin. 2. An opacity, as of the cornea. 3. *In microscopy*, a thin spread of blood, usually on a glass slide or coverslip.

film badge. A device containing enclosed photographic film, worn by personnel exposed to radiation to show dosage received. See photographic *dosimetry.*

fil′ter [F. *filtre*, from ML. *feltrum*, felt]. 1. An apparatus which separates one or more components of a mixture from the others. 2. A special part of a high-frequency circuit which suppresses certain frequencies of electric waves. 3. *In acoustics*, a device which suppresses certain frequencies of sound waves. 4. *In photography*, a colored glass or gelatin plate used in front of the photographic lens to alter the relative intensity of different wavelengths in the light beam.

Berkefeld f. An apparatus for sterilizing any liquid or solution by separating bacteria and spores by means of diatomaceous earth.

inherent f. One built into roentgen-ray tubes, consisting of tube wall, oil layer, and plastic layer.

Mandler f. The American modification of the German Berkefeld candle, made of kieselguhr, asbestos, and plaster of Paris, and used in the recovery and study of viruses.

Pasteur-Chamberland f. Unglazed porcelain filter, made of kaolin and sand, of graded porosities, L_1 to L_{13}, which permits the recovery of bacteria-free filtrates: used in the study of viruses.

pollen f. A means of removing pollen from the air; may either make the atmosphere pollen-free, as by means of a forced draft through various sized filters, or filter the respired air, as with a gauze mask worn over mouth and nose, or an adjustable device worn in the nostrils.

primary f. *In radiology*, a thin layer of any one of several materials used to absorb a greater percentage of low energy rays than of the high energy rays of a roentgen beam, thus producing a beam with greater penetrating power. Aluminum filters are used for superficial and medium work, copper or thoraeus filters for deep therapy, and lead or tin filters for supervoltage work.

secondary f. *In radiology*, a sheet of material of low atomic number relative to that of the primary filter, placed in the path of the filtered beam of radiation to remove the characteristic radiation of the primary filter.

Seitz f. A bacterial filter utilizing a matted asbestos filtering pad or disk, the unit being used with either vacuum or pressure.

Thoraeus f. A combination filter consisting of tin, copper, and aluminum, used in x-ray therapy.

ultraviolet f. One which passes ultraviolet radiation but which is relatively opaque to longer wave lengths.

virus f. A filter such as the Berkefeld, Chamberland, Seitz, and Mandler: used in the recovery and study of viruses. See individual filters.

Wood's f. See Robert William *Wood.*

fil′ter. To separate one or more components of a mixture from the others.

fil′ter aid. A substance added to a liquid to be filtered to assist filtration, generally through formation of a bed of the added material which functions as an auxiliary filter, preventing passage of particles which would otherwise either pass through or clog the primary filter.

fil′trate [*feltrum*]. The liquid that has passed through a filter.

fil·tra′tion [*feltrum*]. The operation of straining through a filter.

fil′trum (pl. *filtra*) [*feltrum*]. A filter or strainer.

f. ventriculi. A small vertical groove in the mucosa of the lateral wall of the larynx between the cuneiform and arytenoid cartilages: also called *Merkel's f.*

fi′lum (pl. *fila*) [L., thread]. Any threadlike or filamentous structure.

fila coronaria. Fibrous bands of the cardiac skeleton extending from the base of the medial cusp of the tricuspid valve to the aortic opening and right trigone.

fila olfactoria. The component fasciculi of the olfactory nerve before and during their passage through the cribriform plate of the ethmoid bone.

f. durae matris spinalis. The caudal tip of the filum terminale invested by the dura mater.

f. lateralis pontis. A fiber bundle running along the rostral border of the pons which may go to the cerebellum or connect the pons to the midbrain. Syn., *taenia pontis.*

f. terminale. The atrophic slender inferior end

of the spinal cord, the caudal part of which is mostly pia mater.

fim′bri·a [L., fringe]. 1. A fringe. 2. The fringelike process of the outer extremity of the uterine tube. 3. A flattened band of white fibers along the medial margin of the hippocampus, continuous with the crus of the fornix. Formerly called *f. cornu Ammonis.* —**fimbrial,** *adj.*

fim′bri·ate, fim′bri·a″ted [*fimbria*]. Fringed with slender processes which are larger than filaments; said of bacterial cultures and of the ostium of the uterine tube.

Findlay, Francis McRae [*American surgeon,* 1898–]. Known for his description of an original method of closure of a gastrojejunocolic fistula, called *Findlay's operation.*

fin′ger [AS.]. A digit of the hand.

baseball f. Luxation of a distal phalanx with rupture of the distal portion of the extensor tendon, resulting in a drop of the phalanx; caused by a baseball injury.

clubbed f. A finger, the terminal phalanx of which is short and broad, with an overhanging nail; seen in some cases of pulmonary and cardiac disease. Also called *Hippocratic f., chronic hypertrophic pulmonary osteoarthropathy, drumstick f.*

giant fingers. Macrodactylia.

hammer f. A congenital flexion deformity, usually of middle phalanx of middle finger.

lock f. A peculiar affection of the fingers in which they suddenly become fixed in a flexed position, due to the presence of a small fibrous growth in the sheath of a flexor tendon.

mallet f. A deformity marked by undue flexion of the last phalanx.

seal f. An infection occurring in Norway believed to be contracted from seals, characterized by the glistening appearance of the swollen finger; it is similar clinically to erysipeloid.

spatulate f. A particular type of broad finger, flattened at the tip.

spider fingers. See *arachnodactyly.*

springfinger. Condition in which there is an obstruction to flexion and extension of one or more fingers; due to injuries or inflammation of the tendinous sheaths.

trigger f. A condition in which flexion or extension of a finger is at first obstructed, but finally accomplished with a jerk or sweep. It is due to chronic tenosynovitis.

webbed fingers. Union of adjacent fingers by interdigital tissue; fingers fused at the lateral aspects. Syn., *syndactyly.*

fin′ger cot. A covering of rubber or other material to protect the finger or to prevent infection. Also called *finger stall.*

fin′ger·print″ [*finger;* ME. *printe*]. An impression of the cutaneous ridges of a finger tip. May be a direct pressure print or a rolled print, the latter recording the entire flexor and lateral aspects of the phalanx. See *dermatoglyphics.* —**fingerprinting,** *n.*

fin′ger stall. A rubber cap for a finger.

Finkeldey cells. See *Warthin-Finkeldey giant cells* under *cell.*

Finkelstein, Heinrich [*German pediatrist,* 1865–1942]. Devised an albumin milk preparation which has a low lactose and salts content and a high casein and fat content, known as *Finkelstein's albumin milk.*

Finkler, Dittmar [*German bacteriologist,* 1852–1912]. Isolated, with J. Prior, *Vibrio proteus* from human stools in acute gastroenteritis (1884). The spirillum also received the name *Finkler-Prior spirillum.*

Fin·lay′a [after Carlos *Finlay*]. A subgenus of *Aëdes* mosquitoes, members of which transmit yellow fever.

Finlay y de Barres, Carlos Juan [*Cuban biologist and physician,* 1833–1915]. Stated the theory, some years before this was proved by Reed and his associates, that yellow fever is transmitted to man by mosquitoes (1881).

Finney, John Miller Turpin [*American surgeon,* 1863–1942]. Eminent surgeon and teacher. Widely known for having introduced a special type of pyloric operation in which anastomosis of the first portion of the duodenum is made with the pyloric end of the stomach, employing the principles of the posterior gastroenterostomy technic and using a large, U-shaped incision in the pyloric and duodenal region; called *pyloroplasty, Finney's operation.*

Finochetti, Enrique [*Argentinian surgeon,* 1880–]. *Finochetti's stirrup* is an apparatus used for skeletal traction in leg fractures.

Finsen, Niels Ryberg [*Danish physician,* 1860–1904]. Proved the therapeutic value of actinic rays (1896); considered the father of modern phototherapy. See Finsen *light.* Advocated heliotherapy. Nobel laureate (1903).

Finsterer, Hans [*Austrian surgeon,* 1877–]. The *Hofmeister-Finsterer operation* is a modification of Pólya's operation of subtotal gastrectomy.

fire′damp″. An explosive mixture of methane and air.

first aid. Emergency treatment given to a casualty before regular medical or surgical care can be administered by trained individuals. —**first′-aid′,** *adj.;* **first-aid′er,** *n.*

first′-aid′ kit. A pouch, bag, or box containing sterilized dressings, adhesive plaster, iodine, bandages, and simple instruments; for use in giving first aid in an emergency.

first′-aid′ pack′et. A hermetically sealed, waterproof metal case containing emergency first-aid material. It is issued to each soldier of the U. S. Army, and is not to be opened until needed.

first in·ten′tion. See *healing* by first intention.

Fischer, Emil [*German chemist,* 1852–1919]. Made important contributions to the knowledge of animal and vegetable proteins. Synthesized purines, polypeptides, and various sugars. With von Mering, introduced the use of barbital. Nobel laureate (1902).

Fischer, Hans (1881–1945). German chemist, noted for his investigation of heme compounds, especially for his synthesis of hemin. Nobel laureate in chemistry (1930).

Fischer, Louis [*American physician,* 1864–1944]. Described a systolic murmur heard over the anterior fontanel or in the temporal region of infants with rickets. Also described a presystolic murmur in cases of adherent pericarditis in the absence of valvular disease.

Fishberg's test. See under *test.*

Fishberg and Dolin's method. See under *method.*

fish′ber″ry, See *cocculus.*

fis′sile. Fissionable.

fis′sion [L. *fissio,* from *findere,* to cleave]. 1. Any splitting or cleaving. 2. *In biology,* asexual reproduction by the division of the body into two or more parts, each of which grows into a complete organism. It is the common method of reproduction among the bacteria and protozoa. —**fis′sionable,** *adj.*

atomic f. The splitting of the nucleus of an atom by neutron bombardment into two main fragments. For example, the uranium isotope 235 can be split in two, barium and krypton resulting, with the release of a vast amount of energy. Also called *nuclear f.*

binary f. The division of first the nuclear material, then the cytoplasm into two equal parts; common in protozoa.

multiple f. A series of divisions of the nucleus followed by a division of the body into as many parts as there are nuclei.

nuclear f. Fission or splitting of the nucleus, the center of an atom. Also called *atomic f.*

uranium f. See atomic *f.*

fis·sip'a·rous [L. *fissum*, from *findere; parere*, to bring forth]. Propagating by fission.

fis'su·la. A small fissure.

f. ante fenestram. A channel, irregular in size and shape, extending from the vestibule of the inner ear from a point just anterior to the fenestra vestibuli toward the tympanum. There may or may not be an external opening. Also called *Cozzolino's zone.*

fis'sure [L. *fissura*, cleft]. A groove or cleft; applied to the clefts or grooves in various organs, as the skull, the brain, the liver, the spinal cord; also to cracks in the skin or linear ulcers in mucous membranes. When applied to the brain, the term is used for the deepest linear depressions, as the lateral cerebral fissure. Also see *sulcus.* —**fissured, fissural,** *adj.;* **fissura'tion,** *n.*

abdominal f. See *celosoma.*

anal f. A linear ulcer at the mucocutaneous junction of the anus, causing intense suffering on defecation.

anterior median f. A groove extending the entire length of the spinal cord in the midline anteriorly, and incompletely dividing it into two symmetrical parts.

ape f. A fissure of the human brain which corresponds with that present in an ape, as the lunate sulcus.

avulsion f. The separation of the tibial tuberosity, due to violent action of the patellar tendon.

basal f. See decidual *f.*

calcarine f. One on the medial aspect of the occipital lobe of the cerebrum, between the lingual gyrus and the cuneus.

callosomarginal f. See cingulate *sulcus.*

central f. See central *sulcus.*

choroid f. (a) The ventral fissure in the optic cup and the optic stalk of the embryo. Syn., *fetal f.* (b) The line of invagination of the tela choroidea of the lateral ventricles of the brain.

cingulate f. See cingulate *sulcus.*

collateral f. One on the medial aspect of the cerebrum, between the subcalcarine and subcollateral gyri, corresponding to the collateral eminence.

decidual f. One of the fissured spaces developing in the decidua basalis, parallel with the uterine wall, in the later months of pregnancy.

dentate f. Old term for hippocampal *f.*

fetal f. See choroid *f.*

f. of the gallbladder. See cystic *fossa.*

f. of the optic cup. That part of the choroid fissure of the embryonic eye located in the optic cup.

f. of the optic stalk. That part of the choroid fissure of the embryonic eye located in the optic stalk.

genal f. Genal cleft, (a).

genitovesical f. A groove, developing about the third fetal month, between the cranial end of the genital cord and the urinary bladder. It disappears in the male, but deepens in the female to form the vesicouterine excavation.

Glaserian f. Old term for petrotympanic *f.*

hippocampal f. That situated between the hippocampal gyrus and the fascia dentata.

inferior orbital f. That of the orbit which gives passage to the infraorbital blood vessels, and ascending branches from the sphenopalatine ganglion.

interarytenoid f. The narrow cleft between the embryonic arytenoid folds.

interhemispheric f. See longitudinal *f.* of the cerebrum.

lateral cerebral f. A deep fissure of the brain, beginning on the outer side of the anterior perforated space, and extending outward to the lateral surface of the hemisphere. It has two branches, a short vertical and a long horizontal, the latter separating the temporal from the frontal and parietal lobes. Also called *sylvian f.* See Plate 18.

lip f. Harelip.

longitudinal f. of the cerebrum. The deep fissure that divides the cerebrum into two hemispheres: also called interhemispheric *f.*

longitudinal f. of the liver. A fissure on the lower border of the liver, through which passes the round ligament.

palpebral f. The space between the eyelids extending from the outer to the inner canthus.

parieto-occipital f. A fissure on the medial aspect of the cerebral hemisphere, separating the parietal and occipital lobes.

petrosquamous f. The narrow cleft formed by incomplete fusion of the petrous and squamous portions of the temporal bone.

petrotympanic f. The narrow slit posterior to the mandibular fossa of the temporal bone, giving passage to the chorda tympani nerve: formerly called *Glaserian f.*

portal f. See transverse *f.* of the liver.

precentral f. A fissure in front of the central sulcus and parallel to it.

presylvian f. The anterior branch of the sylvian fissure.

primary f. A transverse fissure separating the anterior and posterior cerebellar lobes. Also called *fissura prima, sulcus primarius.*

pterygoid f. The gap at the inferior portion of the pterygoid fossa between the medial and lateral laminas.

pterygomaxillary f. A narrow gap between the lateral pterygoid plate and posterior portion of the maxilla leading into the pterygopalatine fossa: also called *sphenomaxillary f.*

rhinal f. A shallow groove separating the terminal archipallial part of the hippocampal gyrus from the rest of the temporal lobe.

Rolandic f. Old term for central sulcus.

sphenoidal f. The superior orbital *f.*

sphenomaxillary f. The pterygomaxillary *f.*

superior orbital f. The elongated opening between the small and the great wings of the sphenoid: also called *sphenoidal f.*

sylvian, Sylvian f. Lateral cerebral fissure.

transverse cerebral f. The space between the diencephalon and the cerebral hemispheres.

transverse f. of the liver. A fissure crossing transversely the lower surface of the right lobe of the liver. It transmits the portal vein, hepatic artery and nerves, and hepatic duct.

umbilical f. The anterior portion of the longitudinal fissure of the liver.

urogenital f. The cleft between the urogenital folds forming the aperture of the urogenital sinus.

ventral median f. See anterior median *f.*

fis'tu·la [L., tube]. An abnormal tube or canal formed by incomplete closure of a wound, abscess, disease process, or (congenitally) a part, and communicating between two hollow viscera, two surfaces, or a hollow viscus and a surface. It usually transmits some fluid, either pus or the secretions or contents of some organ, viscus, or body cavity. Fistulas opening from a viscus to the exterior of the body are named according to the viscus involved, as biliary, gastric, cecal, vesical. When the communication is between two organs, the names are combined, as esophagotracheal, gastrocolic, vesicovaginal, anorectal. —**fistular, fistulate, fistulous,** *adj.*

abdominal f. One opening through the abdominal wall and communicating with an abdominal viscus or space.

alveolar f. One communicating with a diseased alveolar process: more properly called *alveolar sinus.*

antral f. One communicating with an antrum or cavity in bone.

arteriovenous f. Arteriovenous aneurysm.

blind f. One having an opening at one end only; may be an internal or external opening or, more properly, a sinus.

bone f. One leading to an osteomyelitic process or to the site of an ostitis: more properly called *bone sinus.*

branchial f. Old term for lateral fistula of the neck.

bronchial f. (a) An abnormal tract communicating between the pleural cavity and a bronchus and generally closing when the empyema is healed. (b) An abnormal tract leading from a bronchus to a cutaneous opening, the result of gangrene or abscess of the lung.

bronchobiliary f. One communicating between a bronchus and the biliary tract, usually as a result of empyema or subphrenic hepatic abscess.

bronchocolic f. One communicating between a bronchus and the colon, usually as a result of empyema or subphrenic abscess.

bronchoesophageal f. One communicating with a bronchus and the esophagus.

cervical f. An open communication between the pharynx and the surface of the neck arising by retention of a visceral groove and pouch with perforation of their closing plate.

coccygeal f. See sacrococcygeal *f.*

craniosinus f. Cerebrospinal rhinorrhea; a condition in which there is leakage of cerebrospinal fluid into the nose, usually the result of a fracture of the posterior wall of the frontal sinus or the cribriform plate of the ethmoid, with an opening through the meninges.

Eck f. An experimental procedure of anastomosing the portal vein to the inferior vena cava, so that the portal blood by-passes the liver.

esophageal f. An abnormal tract of congenital origin, communicating between the esophagus and some portion of the skin through an external opening, or between esophagus and some viscus or organ through an internal opening. A similar fistula may result from trauma or disease.

external f. A fistula opening from some body cavity to the skin.

extrasphincteric f. A rectal or anal fistula external to the sphincter.

fecal f. An opening from an intestine through the abdominal wall to the skin, with discharge of intestinal contents; usually applied to openings from the ileum and colon.

f. auris congenita. A congenital, hereditary, narrow, usually blind pit opening at the crus of the helix.

gastric f. An abnormal tract from the stomach communicating through an external opening with the skin, or through an internal opening with some other viscus or organ.

gastrojejunal f. A fistula between the stomach and the jejunum: a condition following posterior gastroenterostomy which develops in about 10% of anastomotic ulcer patients. The symptoms include diarrhea, vomiting, and loss of weight. Diagnosis is confirmed by roentgenologic examination.

gastrojejunocolic f. One between stomach, jejunum, and transverse colon. It is an occasional complication arising in patients who have developed a marginal ulcer at the site of a gastrojejunostomy; later the ulcer perforates into the lumen of the colon.

horseshoe f. A semicircular fistulous tract in the perineum near the anus.

internal f. A fistula in which the openings are within the body without communication through the skin.

labial f. A minute fistulous tract or congenital pit near the vermilion border of the lower lip: more properly called *labial sinus.*

lacrimal f. A fistula communicating with a lacrimal duct.

lateral f. of the neck. A congenital fistula opening lateral to the midline, anywhere from the mandible to the sternum, and communicating with the pharynx, a cyst, a cell rest, or a duct; due to faulty closure of pharyngeal pouches or the thymopharyngeal duct, or to other developmental defects.

lymphatic f. A tract communicating through an external opening in the skin with a lymphatic vessel or duct, as the thoracic or right lymphatic, with discharge of chylous fluid and lymph.

Mann-Bollman f. A fistula of the small intestine produced in animal experimentation by suturing the proximal end of a loop of small intestine to the edges of the opening in the abdominal wall and anastomosing the distal end with the functioning intestine, thus preventing movement of material out through the skin by peristalsis; movement will be in the reverse direction.

median f. of the neck. A rare congenital fistula with its opening in the midline, due to imperfect closure of the cervical sinus.

pancreatic f. 1. An external opening from the pancreas to the skin of the abdominal wall following the drainage of a pancreatic cyst or other gastric or duodenal operation. 2. An internal opening from the pancreas to the jejunum, duodenum, stomach, or gallbladder, to overcome the formation of an external fistula.

pilonidal f. See pilonidal *cyst.*

pleuropulmonary f. One extending from the lung to an external opening on the skin. See bronchial *f.*

rectovaginal f. An opening between the vagina and the rectum.

rectovesical f. A congenital or acquired opening between the rectum and the urinary bladder.

sacrococcygeal f. One communicating with a dermoid cyst in the coccygeal region.

salivary f. One communicating with a salivary gland or its duct, usually the parotid, with discharge of saliva through an external opening in the skin.

scrotal f. One extending from some portion of the testis or epididymis to an external opening in the skin of the scrotum.

sigmoidovesical f. A fistula connecting the sigmoid flexure and urinary bladder.

Thiry's f. An experimental fistula produced in the dog to obtain secretions from the intestine.

thyroglossal f. A developmental abnormality, due to incomplete obliteration of the thyroglossal duct, resulting in a midline cervical fistula.

urinary f. An abnormal tract from any portion of the urinary system; discharges urine through an opening on the skin or into an organ, viscus, or cavity.

vesical f. An abnormal opening from the urinary bladder communicating externally with the skin or internally with another pelvic organ.

vesicoabdominal f. A fistula extending from the urinary bladder through the abdominal wall and opening externally onto the skin of the abdomen.

vesicouterovaginal f. An abnormal opening connecting the vagina, urinary bladder, and uterine cavity.

vesicovaginal f. An abnormal tract between the urinary bladder and the vagina.

fis″tu·lec′to·my [*fistula;* G. *ektomē*, excision]. The surgical excision of a fistula.

fis″tu·li·za′tion [*fistula*]. The development or formation of a fistula.

fis″tu·lo·en″ter·os′to·my [*fistula;* G. *enteron*, intestine; *stoma*, mouth]. *In surgery*, the establishment of anastomosis between a biliary fistula and the duodenum.

fis″tu·lot′o·my [*fistula;* G. *tomē*, a cutting]. Incision of a fistula.

fit [AS.]. 1. Any sudden paroxysm of a disease, especially an epileptic convulsion. 2. *In biometry*, the agreement of probable data with actual data; in a graphic representation, the way in which a curve of specified type approaches a given set of points in a plane.

running f. See cursive *epilepsy*.

uncinate f. See *uncinate fit*.

fit. *In biometry*, to adjust obtained data in such a way that it may be expressed by an equation or that the difference between it and the probable data is reduced. See *curve fitting*.

Fitz, Reginald Heber [*American physician*, 1843–1913]. Demonstrated the pathology and symptoms of inflammation of the vermiform appendix (1886); said to have introduced the term appendicitis. Made valuable contributions to the knowledge of acute pancreatitis (1889).

fix·a′tion [L. *fixum*, from *figere*, to fix]. 1. The act of fixing or making firm. 2. The operation of rendering fixed a displaced or floating organ by means of sutures. 3. *In microscopy*, fixing. 4. *In psychiatry*, the arrest of development of an emotion or desire at an immature level.

external skeletal f. *In dentistry and surgery*, a method of immobilizing bony fragments of fractures by the use of metal pin or screw devices applied externally; adapted especially to edentulous mouths.

field of f. See under *field*.

f. of complement. The entering of complement into combination with an antigen-antibody aggregate so that it is not available for subsequent reaction in the indicator systems of hemolysis or bacteriolysis. The basis of the Wassermann test and other serologic tests.

intramedullary f. A method of holding a fractured bone in proper alignment by means of a metal pin or nail in the marrow cavity. See also intramedullary *nail*.

nitrogen f. See *nitrogen fixation*.

fix′a·tive [*fixum*]. 1. Any substance used to fasten a microscopic section to a slide. 2. Any substance, like shellac, used to render a drawing or painting more permanent. 3. Any substance used to preserve tissues for microscopic study. See *fixing fluid*.

formol-corrosive f. Formol-sublimate *f.*

formol-sublimate f. An apparently stable mixture of 9 parts aqueous mercuric chloride (5.6%) with 1 part commercial formalin. It acts very rapidly. Also called *formol-corrosive f.*

Mayer's albumen f. Egg albumen dissolved in glycerine, used to make sections of tissues adhere to glass slides.

fixed. *In clinical medicine*, pertaining to a persistent, nongrowing lesion, or one recurring frequently at the same site: used particularly *in dermatology*, as fixed drug eruption.

fixed med′i·cal treat′ment fa·cil′i·ty. *In U. S. Army medicine*, a medical treatment facility designed to operate in the same location over a considerable period of time. Included are the following unnumbered or table of distribution medical treatment facilities: hospitals, infirmaries, and dispensaries; and the following numbered or table of organization and equipment medical treatment facilities: general hospitals, station hospitals, field hospitals, and dispensaries. See *nonfixed medical treatment facility*.

fix′ing [*fixum*]. The preparation of tissue for microscopical study by means of some agent that hardens it and preserves the form and arrangement of the cells.

fix′ing flu′id. A solution, or mixture of solutions, used to prepare tissues for microscopical study. Formalin, Zenker's fluid, and Regaud's fluid are the most widely used. Also see *fixation*.

Bouin's f. f. Saturated aqueous picric acid, 75 cc.; formalin, 25 cc.; acetic acid, 5 cc. The most generally useful of all the picric acid fixatives.

Carnoy's f. f. Absolute alcohol, 6 parts; chloroform, 3 parts; glacial acetic acid, 1 part. A quick fixative, used for many purposes.

Champy's f. f. 3% potassium bichromate, 7 parts; 1% chromic acid, 7 parts; 2% osmic acid, 4 parts. An excellent fixative for cytologic details.

Flemming's f. f. Weak: 0.25 Gm. chromic acid, 0.1 Gm. osmic acid, 0.1 cc. glacial acetic acid, in distilled water, 100 cc. Strong: 1% chromic acid, 15 cc.; 2% osmic acid, 4 cc.; glacial acetic acid, 1.0 cc. Now used more in biology than in medicine, largely for the study of chromosomes.

formalin. Trade-mark for a 37% aqueous solution of formaldehyde. The solution is the most generally useful of all fixing fluids.

formalin-ammonium bromide f. f. Formalin, 15 cc.; distilled water, 85 cc.; ammonium bromide, 2 Gm. A central nervous system fixative for Cajal's gold sublimate procedure.

Gendre's f. f. Saturated alcoholic picric acid, 8 vols.; formalin, 1.5 vols.; glacial acetic acid, 0.5 vol. Used for the fixation of glycogen in the liver.

Helly's f. f. See under Zenker's *f. f.*

Müller's f. f. Potassium bichromate, 2.0–2.5 Gm.; sodium sulfate, 1.0 Gm.; distilled water, 1.0 Gm. Used for hardening nervous tissue after preliminary fixation. Often used in conjunction with formalin to make other fixing fluids, such as Orth's and Regaud's. The sodium sulfate is often omitted.

Ohlmacher's f. f. Absolute alcohol, 32 cc.; chloroform, 6 cc.; glacial acetic acid, 2 cc. Just before use add $HgCl_2$. A fixative for animal tissue giving rapid fixation and good penetration.

Orth's f. f. To 9 parts of 2.0–2.5% aqueous potassium bichromate, add one part of 10.0% formalin on using.

osmic acid. The tetroxide of osmium; generally used in the 2% aqueous solution.

Regaud's f. f. 3% aqueous potassium bichromate, 20 cc.; formalin, 5 cc. A fixing fluid used for many purposes.

Schaudinn's f. f. (A) Cold-saturated aqueous $HgCl_2$, 66 cc.; alcohol 95%, 33 cc. (B) Glacial acetic acid, 1 cc. Mix (A) and (B) immediately before use. A general animal tissue fixative.

SUSA f. f. Mercuric chloride, 4.5 Gm.; sodium

chloride, 0.5 Gm.; distilled water, 80 cc.; formalin, 20 cc.; trichloroacetic acid, 4 cc.

Zenker's f. f. Potassium bichromate, 2.5 Gm.; mercuric chloride, 5.0 Gm.; distilled water, 100 cc.; glacial acetic acid, 5.0 cc. Used in numerous technics. The acetic acid is often omitted, or more frequently replaced by 5 cc. of formalin, thus forming **Helly's fixing fluid;** or by 10 cc. of formalin, thus making **Bensley's formalin-Zenker.**

F.K.Q.C.P. Fellow of the King and Queen's College of Physicians (of Ireland).

Fl Symbol for florentium.

fl. Fluid.

flac'cid (flack'sid) [L. *flaccus,* flabby]. Soft; flabby; relaxed. **—flaccid'ity,** *n.*

Flack, Martin William [*English physiologist,* 1882–1931]. With Arthur Keith, discovered the sinoatrial node, called *Flack's node, node of Keith and Flack.*

flag [ME. *flagge*]. Any one of several monocotyledonous plants having long, ensiform leaves.

sweet f. *Acorus calamus.* See *calamus.*

flagecidin. Trade-mark for the antibiotic substance *anisomycin.*

Flag"el·la'ta (fladj"uh·lay'tuh). Synonym for *Mastigophora.*

flag'el·late (fladj'uh·late) [L. *flagellare,* to whip]. A protozoon furnished with slender, whiplike processes.

flag"el·la'tion (fladj"uh·lay'shun) [L. *flagellatio,* from *flagellare*]. 1. Flogging or beating. 2. Beating or whipping as a means of producing sexual gratification. 3. Massage by strokes or blows.

fla·gel'li·form [L. *flagellum,* whip; *forma,* shape]. Having the form of a flagellum or whiplash.

flag"el·lo'sis (fladj"uh·lo'sis) [*flagellum;* G. *-ōsis,* condition]. Infection with flagellate protozoa.

fla·gel'lum [L.]. A whiplike process consisting of an axial filament enclosed in a thin cytoplasmic sheath; the organ of locomotion of sperm cells, and of certain bacteria and protozoa.

Flagg resuscitation. See under *resuscitation.*

Flajani, Giuseppe [*Italian surgeon and anatomist,* 1741–1808]. Said to have been the first to describe exophthalmic goiter, in which he noted cardiac disturbance (1802); called *Flajani's disease, Basedow's disease, Graves's disease, Parry's disease.*

flank [OF. *flanc*]. The fleshy or muscular part of an animal or a man between the ribs and the hip; the thigh of an animal; the outer side of the thigh, hip, and buttock of a human being.

flap [ME. *flappe*]. A partially detached portion of skin or other tissue, either accidentally formed, or created by the surgeon to be used as a graft to fill a defect or to improve contour. Flaps which are composed of special tissue, such as mucous membrane, conjunctiva, dura, wall of intestinal tract, omentum, muscle, etc., are named after the tissue contained, as muscle flap, etc. They may also be named according to the special purpose for which they are used, as a rhinoplastic flap, for repair of the nose. See also *graft.*

amputation f. A simple, broad-based flap which needs no advancement, and is shaped to provide proper contour of the part to be covered.

osteoplastic f. A flap of skin and underlying bone, commonly of scalp and skull, raised for the purpose of exploring the underlying structures.

pedicle f. A type which obtains its blood supply through a narrow base, or pedicle; used when length is required to fill a remote defect, or on a movable part which can be approximated to the donor site. The pedicle flap has many forms for specific purposes and therefore many named varieties. For instance, a pedicle flap which has the ends reversed to gain more distance is called an **advanced jump, caterpillar,** or **waltzing flap.** Long pedicle flaps are usually tubed or rolled on themselves, so the free edges are sutured together: such a **tubed flap** (rope graft) attached at both ends is a **bipedicled flap;** attached also in the center, it is a **bridge flap.** A flap raised and applied to a movable part, such as one from the abdominal wall applied to the hand, may be a **gauntlet, pocket,** or **tunnel flap.** A pedicle flap may include a large artery in its base; it is then called an **artery flap.** It may be lined with skin or mucous membrane, for repair of cheek or nose, or contain other tissue, as bone, cartilage, etc.; it is then called a **compound flap.**

sliding or **rotation f.** A simple flap which is rotated on a broad base to fill an adjacent defect.

z f. A means of lengthening a linear contracted scar by transposing two triangular flaps of skin, the sutured incision having a z shape.

flaps [*flappe*]. Swelling of the lips in horses.

flare [of uncertain origin]. An abnormal vasomotor reaction manifested by a prolonged, widespreading flush of the skin after a pointed instrument has been drawn heavily across it.

aqueous f. The Tyndall effect or light scattering of increased protein concentrations in the aqueous humor of the eye in inflammation of the anterior segment.

Flarer, Francesco [*Italian ophthalmologist,* 1791–1850]. Eminent ophthalmic surgeon; devised operations for trichiasis and entropion by ablation of the line of cilia.

flask [VL. *flasca,* wine bottle]. A glass or metal vessel having a narrow neck.

Carrel f. See Alexis *Carrel.*

Erlenmeyer f. A conical flask with a flat bottom.

Fenwall f. A flask having a heavy rubber cap with a central outlet fitted with a stainless steel secondary stopper: used for sterilizing fluids by steam.

Florence f. A round-bottomed flask used in distillation.

Lindbergh f. See Charles Augustus *Lindbergh.*

flat [ON. *flatr*]. Lying on one plane. **—flat'ness,** *n.*

flat. A percussion note that is low-pitched and without resonance.

Flatau, Edward [*Polish neurologist,* 1869–1932]. Observed that the greater the length of the fibers of the spinal cord, the nearer they are to the periphery; called *Flatau's law, law of the eccentric situation of long tracts.* Schilder's disease, or progressive subcortical encephalopathy, is sometimes called *Flatau-Schilder disease.*

flat'foot" [*flatr;* AS. *fōt*]. Pes planus; a depression of the plantar arch of varying degree. It may be congenital, or acquired as a result of loss of muscle tone often caused by ill-fitting shoes, incorrect walking habits, and/or standing long hours at certain occupations. The acquired form is usually associated with eversion.

spastic f. A planovalgus deformity of the foot associated with spasm of the peroneal muscles.

flat'sedge" [*flatr;* AS. *secg*]. A genus of plants of the family Cyperaceae. The root of the jointed flatsedge, *Cyperus articulatus,* is anthelmintic, aromatic, and stomachic.

flat'u·lence [F., from L. *flatus,* a blowing]. The presence of gas in the stomach and intestinal tract. **—flatulent,** *adj.*

fla'tus [L.]. Gas, especially gas or air in the gastrointestinal tract.

f. vaginalis. Expulsion of gas from the vagina.

flat'worm" [ON. *flatr;* AS. *wyrm*]. Any worm of the phylum Platyhelminthes.

fla·vac'i·din (fla·vass'i·din). See *flavicin.*

flav'a·cin. Flavicin.

flav′a·nol. See *flavonol.*

flav′a·tin. See *flavicin.*

flavaxin. A trade-mark for synthetic riboflavin.

fla·ve′do [L. *flavus*, yellow]. Yellowness of the skin.

fla″vi·an′ic ac′id. $HO.C_{10}H_4(NO_2)_2.SO_3H.3H_2O$; 2,4-dinitro-1-naphthol-7-sulfonic acid, occurring as light-yellow needles, freely soluble in water: employed as a precipitant for arginine, also histidine.

fla′vi·cid. A dye. The 3,7-dimethyl-8-amino-2-dimethylamino-10-methylacridinium chloride, a reddish brown powder, soluble in water. Used as a local germicide, in dilute solutions.

flav′i·cin (flav′i·sin, flay′vi·sin). An antibiotic substance from certain fungi. It is identical with aspergillin, flavacidin, flavatin, gigantic acid, and parasiticin.

flavicrine. Trade-mark for a thiazonium derivative of diamino-alkyl-acridine used intravenously as a urinary antiseptic.

fla′vin, flav′in. 1. One of a group of yellow pigments, derived from isoalloxazine, isolated from various plant and animal sources. 2. Quercetin.

f. ad′e·nine di·nu′cle·o·tide. $C_{27}H_{33}N_9O_{15}P_2$; a compound resulting from the condensation of a molecule each of riboflavin-5′-phosphate (flavin mononucleotide) and adenosine-5′-phosphate (adenine nucleotide), linkage being effected through the respective phosphoric acid residues. It is the prosthetic group of a number of flavoproteins, including D-amino acid oxidase. Abbreviated FAD. Syn., *isoalloxazine adenine dinucleotide, riboflavin adenine dinucleotide.*

f. mon″o·nu′cle·o·tide. Riboflavin-5′-phosphate. Abbreviated, FMN.

f. phos′phate. Riboflavin-5′-phosphate. Abbreviated, FP.

fla′vine (flay′veen, ·vin, flav′een, ·in). 1. Flavin. 2. Acriflavine.

fla′vo- [*flavus*]. 1. *In botany*, a combining form designating a *yellow* tint. 2. *In chemistry*, a combining form designating a series of complex *yellow* salts of cobalt.

Fla″vo·bac·te′ri·um [*flavus;* G. *baktērion*, little staff]. A genus of the Achromobacteriaceae whose species become orange-yellow in cultures.

fla″vo·ki′nase. An enzyme, obtained from yeast, that catalyzes the phosphorylation of riboflavin to riboflavin-5′-phosphate by adenosinetriphosphate.

fla′vone. 1. $C_{15}H_{10}O_2$. 2-Phenylbenzopyrone. 2. One of the yellow vegetable dye derivatives of flavone, 1.

fla′vo·noid. 1. A substance obtained from flavone, 1, or one of its derivatives. 2. Any of the flavone derivatives, including citrin, hesperetin, hesperidin, rutin, quercetin, and quercitrin, which may reduce capillary fragility in certain cases. —**fla′vonoid,** *adj.*

flav′o·nol (flav′o·nole, ·nol, ·nawl, flay′vo·). 1. $C_{15}H_{10}O_3$. 3-Hydroxyflavone. 2. One of a group of vegetable dyes, including the anthocyanins, derived from flavonol, 1. Also spelled *flavanol.*

fla′vo·none. $C_{15}H_{12}O_2$. 2,3-Dihydroflavone, derivatives of which include hesperetin and citrin.

fla″vo·pro′te·in [*flavus;* G. *prōteios*, of the first quality]. One of a group of conjugated proteins of the chromoprotein type which constitute the yellow enzymes. The prosthetic group in the known enzymes of this type is either a phosphoric acid ester of riboflavin or the latter combined with adenylic acid.

fla″vo·xan′thin. $C_{40}H_{56}O_3$; a carotenoid pigment often found in plants in minute amounts; it has no vitamin-A activity.

flaxedil. Trade-marked name for 1,2,3-*tris*(β-diethylaminoethoxy) benzene triethiodide, a powerful curariform substance.

flax′seed″ [AS. *fleax; sǣd*]. Linseed.

flea [AS. *flēa*]. 1. Any blood-sucking, laterally compressed, wingless insect of the order Siphonaptera. Fleas are of medical importance as hosts and transmitters of disease and their bites produce a form of dermatitis. 2. A stirring apparatus consisting of an iron-filled glass bead which is operated upon by a discontinuous electromagnetic field: useful in microtechniques.

cat f. See *Ctenocephalides felis.*

dog f. See *Ctenocephalides canis.*

human f. See *Pulex irritans.*

rat f. See *Xenopsylla cheopis.*

flea′bane″. See *Erigeron.*

Flechsig, Paul Emil (1847–1929). German neurologist, known for his studies of the myelogenesis of spinal cord and brain. He also mapped the motor and sensory areas of the cerebral cortex (1876). He described the dorsal spinocerebellar tract, called *Flechsig's tract*, and the septomarginal root zone, called *Flechsig's oval bundle.*

Fleischer, Richard [*German physician*, 1848–1909]. Described a sign of hepatolenticular degeneration. See Kayser-Fleischer *ring.*

Fleischmann, Friedrich Ludwig [*German physician*, fl. 1841]. Described a sublingual bursa, sometimes known as *Fleischmann's bursa.*

Fleitmann's test. See under *test.*

Fleming, Sir Alexander (1881–1955). Scottish bacteriologist who discovered that cultures of *Penicillium* inhibited the growth of certain bacteria (1928); hence the development of penicillin. He is known also for his work in immunology and chemotherapy. Nobel laureate with E. B. Chain and H. Florey (1945).

Flemming, Walther [*German anatomist*, 1843–1905]. Made early researches on cell division and karyokinesis (1882), and was first to describe the centrosome (1876). Described germinal centers, called *Flemming's germ centers.* See also Flemming's *fixing fluid.*

flesh [AS. *flǣsc*]. The soft tissues of the body, especially the muscles. —**flesh′y,** *adj.*

goose f. A rough condition of the skin, due to erection of the hairs; caused by cold or fear. Syn., *cutis anserina.*

proud f. See exuberant *granulation.*

Fletcher, Horace [*American dietitian*, 1849–1919]. Remembered for his investigation in dietetics. Advocated the thorough mastication of food taken in definite quantities and at regular intervals, combined with sipping of fluids. The term *Fletcherism* was once applied to the method he advised.

Fletcher, Robert [*American surgeon and bibliographer*, 1823–1912]. With Billings, founded the monthly *Index Medicus* (1879). Assisted Billings and later continued his work in directing the compilation of the *Index-Catalogue of the Library of the Surgeon General.*

flex [L. *flexum*, from *flectere*, to bend]. Bend.

flex″i·bil′i·tas ce′re·a (fleck″si·bil′i·tass seer′-ee·uh). The tendency of a cataleptic or catatonic patient to maintain with seemingly indifferent passivity any posture in which he is placed.

flex′i·ble [L. *flexibilis*, pliant]. Capable of being bent, without breaking; pliable. —**flexibil′ity,** *n.*

flex′ile (fleck′sill) [L. *flexilis*, pliant]. Easily bent.

flex·im′e·ter [L. *flexum*, from *flectere*, to bend; G. *metron*, a measure]. An instrument for measuring the amount of flexion possible in a joint.

flex′ion (fleck′shun) [L. *flexio*, a bending]. The act of bending; the condition of being bent.

Flexner, Abraham (1866–). American educator, widely known for his study, *Medical Education in the United States and Canada* (1910), made for the Carnegie Foundation for the Advancement of Teaching, and now commonly called the *Flexner report.* He reported on the 155 medical institutions then existing, and his study became a basic document in the reform and standardization of medical education and statutory requirements for physicians in these two countries.

Flexner, Simon [*American pathologist and bacteriologist,* 1863–1946]. Made many contributions to our knowledge of the transmission of infectious diseases. With William Henry Welch, made experimental studies of the action of diphtheria toxin (1891–92). Isolated *Shigella paradysenteriae,* called *Flexner's bacillus* (1900). This bacillus, at first incorrectly identified with *Shigella dysenteriae,* was found in tropical dysentery. It produces acid, indole, and endotoxin. With Noguchi, Flexner studied the effects of snake venom. Developed *Flexner's serum* for cerebrospinal meningitis (1907). With Paul A. Lewis, transmitted poliomyelitis to monkeys by means of cultures of a filtrable virus (1909). An experimentally transmissible carcinoma of the rat is called *Flexner-Jobling tumor.*

Flexner report. See Abraham *Flexner.*

flex'or (fleck'sur, ·sor) [L. *flexum,* from *flectere,* to bend]. A muscle that bends or flexes a limb or a part, as opposed to an *extensor.* See Table of Muscles in the Appendix.

f. accessorius. Old name for quadratus plantae muscle.

f. carpi radialis. The radial flexor of the wrist.

f. carpi radialis brevis. An anomalous muscle arising from the lateral or volar surface of the distal half of the radius and inserted into the carpus, metacarpus, or proximal phalanx of the index finger.

f. carpi ulnaris. The ulnar flexor of the wrist.

f. carpi ulnaris brevis. An anomalous muscle arising from the distal fourth of the volar surface of the ulna and inserted into the ulnar carpals or proximal end of fifth metacarpal.

f. digiti minimi. BR name for the flexor digiti quinti muscle.

f. digiti quinti brevis manus. A variable short flexor of the little finger.

f. digiti quinti pedis. The short flexor of the little toe.

f. digitorum accessorius. BR name for the quadratus plantae muscle.

f. digitorum brevis. The short flexor of the toes.

f. digitorum longus. The long flexor of the toes.

f. digitorum profundus. The deeper long flexor of the fingers.

f. digitorum sublimis. The more superficial long flexor of the fingers.

f. hallucis brevis. The short flexor of the great toe.

f. hallucis longus. The long flexor of the great toe.

f. ossis metacarpi pollicis. Old name for opponens pollicis muscle.

f. pollicis brevis. The short flexor of the thumb.

f. pollicis longus. The long flexor of the thumb.

flex'u·ous (fleck'shoo·us, flecks'yoo·us) [L. *flexuosus,* full of turns]. Curving in an undulant manner.

flex·u'ra (fleck·shoor'uh, fleck'shoor·uh). See *flexure.*

flex'ure (fleck'shur) [L. *flexura,* a bending]. A bend or fold. —**flex'ural,** *adj.*

caudal f. A flexure of the caudal end of the embryo.

cephalic f. See mesencephalic *f.*

cervical f. A flexure of the embryonic brain concave ventrally occurring at the junction of hindbrain and spinal cord. Also called *nuchal f., spinal f.*

cranial f. A flexure of the embryonic brain.

duodenojejunal f. The abrupt bend at the junction of the duodenum and jejunum.

hepatic f. An abrupt bend in the ascending colon to the right of the gallbladder.

mesencephalic f. A flexure of the embryonic brain concave ventrally occurring in the region of the midbrain. Syn., *cephalic f.*

perineal f. The second curve of the rectum; its concavity is directed posteriorly.

pontine f. A flexure of the embryonic brain concave dorsally occurring in the region of the myelencephalon.

sacral f. The curve of the rectum in front of the sacrum; its concavity is directed anteriorly.

sigmoid f. An S-shaped bend in the colon between the descending portion and the rectum.

splenic f. An abrupt turn of the colon beneath the lower end of the spleen, connecting the descending with the transverse colon.

flick'er [AS. *flicorian*]. A sensation of fluctuating vision; caused by a light of such slow intermittence that the visual impressions produced do not fuse.

flight of i·de'as. A condition in acute mania in which disconnected ideas and fancies flow rapidly through the mind. Also called *idea chase.*

Flint, Austin [*American physician,* 1812–86]. Eminent teacher who contributed to the knowledge of diseases of the heart and respiratory system. Said to have introduced the terms cavernous respiration and bronchovesicular respiration. See also Flint's *murmur.*

Flint, Austin (Junior) [*American physician,* 1836–1915]. Discovered coprosterol, formerly called stercorin, in human feces (1862). Made an important study of human output of nitrogen after exercise (1871), and described arterial and venous arches, called *Flint's arcade,* at the bases of the renal pyramids.

float'ing [AS. *flota,* ship]. Abnormal movability or situation of a structure, due to natural lack abnormal stretching, or destruction of its attachments.

float'ing kid'ney. See under *kidney.*

float'ing rib. See under *rib.*

floc"cil·la'tion (flock"si·lay'shun). See *carphology.*

floc"cu·la'tion (flock"yoo·lay'shun) [L. *floccus,* a flock of wool]. The coagulation or coalescence of finely divided or colloidal particles into larger particles which precipitate.

floc'cu·lent [*floccus*]. 1. Flaky, downy, or woolly, said of a liquid containing irregularly shaped particles. 2. Causing flocculation. —**floc'culent,** *n.*

floc'cu·lus [dim. of *floccus*]. A prominent lobe of the cerebellum situated behind and below the middle cerebellar peduncle on each side of the median fissure. See Plates 17, 18. —**floccular,** *adj.*

accessory f. The paraflocculus. *O.T.*

floor [AS. *flōr*]. The basal limit of any hollow organ or open space.

f. of the pelvis. The united mass of tissue forming the inferior boundary of the pelvis, consisting mainly of the levator ani muscles.

flo'ra [L. *Flora,* goddess of flowers]. The entire plant life of any geographic area or geologic period.

floraquin. A proprietary preparation of the substance known by the trade-marked name diodoquin (5,7-diiodo-8-hydroxyquinoline), lactose, dextrose, and boric acid. It is used in the treatment of vaginal infections.

Florence's reagent. See under *reagent.*

Florence's test. See under *test.*

Florentinus. See *Alderotti.*

flo·ren'ti·um. Fl. The name given by Rolla and Fernandez to element 61, which has been called *illinium* by Hopkins, and for synthetic forms of which the names *cyclonium* and *promethium* have been proposed. It is now called *promethium*.

flo'res (flor'eez) [L. *flos*, flower]. 1. The flowers or blossoms of a plant. 2. A flocculent or pulverulent form of certain substances after sublimation.

Florey, Howard W. (1898–). Australian pathologist in England, who, in association with E. B. Chain, discovered the chemotherapeutic value of penicillin. Nobel laureate in medicine and physiology with A. Fleming and E. B. Chain (1945).

flor'id [L. *floridus*, abounding with flowers]. Bright red in color.

floropryl. A trade-mark for *diisopropyl fluorophosphate* or *isoflurophate*.

Flosdorf, Earl William (1904–). American bacteriologist who developed a skin test for whooping cough, and with Stuart Mudd devised a method of dehydrating serums, plasma, bacterial suspensions, and other products by vacuum desiccation in the frozen state. They called the method *lyophilization*.

flo·ta'tion [F. *flotter*, to float]. *In colloid chemistry*, the process of separating the valuable constituents (minerals) of ores from the valueless gangue by agitation with water, a small proportion of an oil and a foaming agent, the mineral rising with the foam and the gangue sinking.

Flourens, Marie Jean Pierre [*French physiologist and anatomist*, 1794–1867]. In experiments with pigeons, found that removing the cerebrum caused a loss of cerebration, although the reflexes were not affected, whereas removal of the cerebellum caused a loss of equilibrium and coordination (1823). Later showed that injury to the semicircular canals affects equilibrium and coordination (1830). Demonstrated that integrity of the cerebral cortex is essential for vision (1824).

Flournoy, Thomas [*American physician*, 1877–]. With Charles Norris and A. M. Pappenheimer, reported discovery of a spirochete in an American case of relapsing fever (1906).

flow [AS. *flōwan*]. 1. The free discharge of a liquid, as the blood. 2. The menses.

cerebral blood f. The rate, in cubic centimeters per minute, at which blood flows through the brain, measured by the rate of diffusion of inert gases (N_2O, krypton) into the brain. Normal value of cerebral blood flow is 750 cc per minute.

intermenstrual f. See *metrorrhagia*, *polymenorrhea*.

streamline f. A flow in which particles in the axial stream move more rapidly than those in the periphery, as the blood cells in the capillaries.

flow. To menstruate profusely.

Flower, William Henry [*English anatomist*, 1831–99]. Described the nasomalar and dental indices; see *index* of Flower.

flow'ers [L. *flos*, flower]. 1. The blossoms of a plant. 2. A sublimated drug, usually sulfur. 3. The menses. *Obs.*

flow'er-spray. *In neurohistology*, an afferent nerve ending with extensive arborizations, found in the muscle spindles.

flow'me"ter [AS. *flōwan;* G. *metron*, a measure]. A physical device for measuring the rate of flow of a gas or liquid, as blood in the blood vessels; a stromuhr. Flowmeters may record the mean flow, as with bubble flowmeters, or with the thermostromuhr, which measures the blood flow by the difference in temperatures at two points in the blood stream. Flowmeters capable of registering the instantaneous rate of flow are the differential manometer, air expansion flowmeter, and electromagnetic flowmeter.

electromagnetic f. One in which changes in the flow of blood are measured through impedance to electromagnetic lines of force introduced across a stream. It has the great advantage that an intact blood vessel can be used.

Floyer, John [*English physician*, 1649–1734]. First to count the pulse with a watch, for which purpose he invented a watch dividing the minute. Wrote the first book on geriatrics (1724).

F.L.S. Fellow of the Linnean Society.

fluagel. Trade-mark for *aluminum hydroxide gel.*

Flückiger's nepaline. See British *aconitine.*

fluc"tu·a'tion [L. *fluctuare*, to move in the manner of waves]. 1. The wavelike motion produced when a body containing fluid is tapped between the fingers or hands. 2. A slight deviation from the average of the sort which gives rise to the continuous variability of the normal frequency curve.

Fluhmann's test. See under *test.*

flu'id [L. *fluidus*, from *fluere*, to flow]. 1. A substance whose molecules move freely upon one another. 2. Any liquid secretion of the body. Abbreviated, fl.

allantoic f. The fluid contents of the allantois.

amniotic f. The transparent, almost colorless, albuminous fluid contained within the amniotic sac surrounding the fetus.

cerebrospinal f. The fluid within the cerebral ventricles and between the arachnoid membrane and pia mater of the brain and spinal cord.

follicular f. The fluid filling the follicle or space about the developing ovum in the Graafian follicle.

intermicellar f. *In colloid chemistry*, a liquid medium in which the colloidal particles (micelles) are dispersed.

labyrinthine f. The perilymph.

otic f. See *endolymph.*

pericardial f. The fluid in the pericardial cavity.

periotic f. See *perilymph.*

pleural f. A film of fluid in the pleural cavity.

Rees and Ecker diluting f. A solution of 2 Gm sodium citrate and 8 Gm sucrose dissolved in about 75 cc water, to which is added 0.04 Gm ground brilliant cresyl blue; the mixture is brought up to 100 cc with water: used in counting platelets.

Rossman's f. See under Isadore *Rossman.*

seminal f. See *semen.*

serous f. Normal lymphatic fluid.

subarachnoid f. See cerebrospinal *f.*

synovial f. The clear fluid, resembling white of egg, found in various joints, bursae, and sheaths of tendons. An example of tissue fluid in general, being produced by dialysis from the plasma.

flu'id. Liquid or gaseous.

flu'id·ex'tract [*fluidus;* L. *extractum*, from *extrahere*, to draw out]. A hydroalcoholic solution of vegetable principles so made that each cc. contains the therapeutic constituents of 1 Gm. of the standardized drug which it represents. Maceration and percolation with suitable solvent are employed as the means of obtaining solution of the desired constituents. See *extract*, *diacolation.*

flu'id·glyc'er·ate (·gliss'ur·ate). A preparation containing about 50% of glycerin, but no alcohol, and of such strength that 1 cc. of the fluidglycerate represents 1 Gm. of the crude drug.

fluid level. *In radiology*, a roentgenographic line demarcating radiopaque liquid from radiolucent gas, as in the stomach.

fluid line. *In radiology*, a roentgenographic line demarcating the extent of a fluid effusion or inclusion; gas need not be present to demonstrate this line.

flu'id·ounce' [*fluidus;* L. *uncia*, twelfth part of a pound]. A liquid measure; 8 fluidrachms. Equivalent to approximately 29.57 cc. Symbol, f℥.

flu'i·drachm", flu'i·dram" (flōō'i·dram", floo"i-dram′) [*fluidus;* G. *drachmē,* drachm]. A liquid measure equal to one-eighth fluidounce, roughly equivalent to one teaspoonful. 60 minims = 1 fluidrachm. Symbol, fʒ.

fluke [AS. *flōc*]. A trematode worm of the order Digenea.

blood f. *Schistosoma haematobium, S. mansoni, S. japonicum.*

intestinal f. *Fasciolopsis buski, Heterophyes heterophyes, Metagonimus yokogawai.*

liver f. *Clonorchis sinensis, Fasciola hepatica, Opisthorchis felineus.*

lung f. *Paragonimus westermani.*

flu′mer·in. The disodium salt of hydroxymercurifluorescein; it is a powder, freely soluble in water, formerly used in treating syphilis.

flu′mi·na pi·lor′um. Regional hair tracts. Certain areas of the skin have the hairs so arranged that they point in a common direction.

flu′o- [L. *fluor,* from *fluere,* to flow]. *In chemistry,* a combining form indicating *the presence of fluorine.*

flu′or·chrome. A dye which fluoresces when irradiated with ultraviolet radiation.

flu′o·rene. $C_6H_4\langle CH_2 \rangle C_6H_4$. A solid hydrocarbon from coal tar employed in the synthesis of several dyes and medicinals.

flu″o·rene′a·mine (flōō″o·reen′uh·meen, ·min, flōō″o·reen″uh·meen′). An amine of fluorine; various derivatives produce experimental tumors. Syn., *aminofluorene.*

flu″o·res′ce·in. $C_{20}H_{12}O_5 + H_2O$; resorcinolphthalein, a condensation product of resorcinol and phthalic anhydride. It dissolves in alcohol to form a yellow solution with green fluorescence.

f. sodium (*fluoresceinum sodicum*). $C_{20}H_{10}O_5Na_2$, freely soluble in water. A 2% solution is employed in diagnosing corneal lesions and in the detection of minute foreign bodies in that tissue; it is suggested as a means of determining apparent death by injection of one gram; if circulation remains, the mucosae will be stained yellow within a few minutes. Syn., *soluble fluorescein, uranin.*

soluble f. See *f.* sodium.

flu″o·res′cence [*fluere*]. A property possessed by certain substances of radiating, when illuminated, a light of a different, usually greater, wavelength. —**fluorescent,** *adj.*

secondary f. The type of fluorescence found in nonfluorescent tissues which have been treated with fluorochromes.

flu″o·res′cin. $C_{20}H_{14}O_5$; a reduction product of fluorescein which readily oxidizes to the latter, occurring as a bright yellow powder, insoluble in water but soluble in alkaline solutions: used as a reagent.

flu′or·i·date. To add a fluoride to drinking water in such concentration that the incidence rate of caries will be diminished. —**fluorida′tion,** *n.*

flu′o·ride. A salt of hydrofluoric acid.

flu′o·ri·dize. To use a fluoride, especially as a therapeutic measure for the prevention of dental caries.

flu″o·ri·na′tion. The addition of fluorine in one of several compounds to water, especially to the water supply of a community as an aid in control of dental caries.

flu′o·rine (flōō′o·reen, ·rin). F = 19.00. A gaseous element belonging to the halogen group. Certain of its salts, the fluorides, have been used in goiter and in rheumatism. Fluorides may prevent dental caries but in excessive amounts in drinking water they may cause mottling of tooth enamel.

flu′o·rite. Native calcium fluoride, CaF_2; used as a source of fluorine compounds, as a flux, and in manufacture of certain lenses.

flu″o·ro·a·ce′tic ac′id. CH_2FCOOH; a crystalline substance, prepared synthetically, but occurring in *Dichapetalum* (*Chailletia*) *cymosum,* a poisonous South American plant. It is highly poisonous; the sodium salt is used as a water-soluble rodenticide.

flu″o·r·o·car′bon. Any compound composed only of carbon and fluorine, representing a corresponding hydrocarbon in which the hydrogen atoms have been replaced by fluorine. Fluorocarbons are characterized by extreme resistance to chemical action and stability at high temperatures.

flu″or·o·car″di·og′ra·phy. See *electrokymography.*

flu·or′o·chrome, fluor′o·chrome. One of a group of fluorescent substances which are absorbed by certain tissues not fluorescent in themselves.

flu·or′o·gen. Any of the particular groups or arrangements of atoms the presence of which in a compound is essential for development of fluorescence.

flu″or·og′ra·phy [*fluere;* G. *graphein,* to write]. A combination of fluoroscopy and photography whereby a photograph of small size is made of the fluoroscopic image. Used to reduce the cost of making large numbers of chest examinations for tuberculosis surveys. Also called *miniature fluorography.* —**fluorograph′ic,** *adj.*

flu″o·ro·pho·tom′e·try [*fluere;* G. *phōs,* light; *metron,* a measure]. The quantitative assay of fluorescent substances in solution. The exciting radiation of about 3650 Å wavelength is concentrated upon the substance under investigation and the intensity of fluorescence is compared, either visually or photoelectrically, against the fluorescence of a standard solution. —**fluorophotomet′ric,** *adj.*

flu′o·ro·scope [*fluere;* G. *skopein,* to examine]. The instrument used for examining the form and motion of the internal structures of the body by means of roentgen rays. It consists of a fluorescent screen composed of crystals of cadmium tungstate.

biplane f. One having two fluorescent screens and two x-ray tubes at right angles to each other for examination of foreign bodies, fractures, and other lesions in two planes.

flu″or·os′co·py. Examination of internal body structures by means of a fluoroscope.

function f. Estimation of pulmonary ventilatory ability with the fluoroscope by observing the motion of ribs and diaphragm and the emptying rate of lungs.

flu″o·ro′sis [*fluere;* G. *-ōsis,* increase]. 1. Poisoning by absorption of toxic amounts of fluorine. 2. A condition of generalized increased density of the skeleton, including dental fluorosis, resulting from prolonged ingestion of fluorides. In endemic areas, this may lead to rigidity of the spinal column, increased bone fragility, and other symptoms referable to bone and joint changes.

chronic dental f. Hypoplasia and discoloration of the teeth, resulting from the continued use, during the formative period of the tooth, of water containing toxic amounts of fluorine: commonly called *mottled enamel.*

flush [ME. *fluschen*]. 1. Blush, become suffused, as the cheeks; due to vasodilation of small arteries and arterioles especially when these vessels are hypotonic. Occurs in emotional states, hyperthyroidism, local inflammation, pyrexia, and in states of chronic malnutrition of the skin. 2. Cleanse a wound or cavity by a rapid flow of water. —**flush,** *n.*

flut′ter [AS. *floterian,* to float about]. Quick, irregular motion; agitation.

atrial f A cardiac irregularity closely resembling atrial fibrillation, consisting of regular but abnormal atrial contractions said to be caused by a wave of excitation and contraction constantly circulating, about 300 times per minute, around a fixed ring of muscle in the atria. The ventricles respond at a fraction of the atrial rate (usually about 150 per minute). Electrocardiograms indicate two types of atrial flutter: impure, in which the events are not accurately repeated from cycle to cycle; pure, in which the events are constant from cycle to cycle. Clinically often called *auricular f.*

auricular f. Clinical term used for atrial *f.*

diaphragmatic f. See under *tic.*

flu″vo·my′cin. An antibiotic substance produced by a strain of *Bacillus subtilis*, active, in vitro, against many Gram-positive and Gram-negative bacteria, also fungi, but does not appear to be active in vivo.

flux [L. *fluxus*, from *fluere*, to flow]. 1. An excessive flow of any of the excretions of the body, especially the feces. 2. *In chemistry*, material added to minerals or metals to promote fusion.

luminous f. Radiant flux applied to visible light; symbol, *F*.

radiant f. The rate of transfer of radiant energy; symbol, *P*.

fly [AS. *flӯge*]. Any insect of the order Diptera. Many insects not belonging to the Diptera are popularly called flies, such as dragonflies, caddis flies, Mayflies, butterflies, sawflies, gallflies, etc. Some insects belonging to the Diptera are not popularly known as flies, notably the mosquitoes.

black f. See *Simulium.*

blowfly. See *Calliphoridae.*

bluebottle f. See *Calliphoridae.*

botfly. See *Oestridae, Gastrophilidae, Cuterebridae.*

cheese f. See *Piophila.*

Columbacz f. See *Simulium.*

Congo-floor maggot f. See *Auchmeromyia luteola.*

crane f. A fly of the genus *Tipulidae.*

deer f. See *Chrysops.*

drone f. See *Eristalis.*

flesh f. See *Sarcophagidae.*

frit f. See *Oscinidae.*

gadfly. See *Tabanidae.*

green-bottle f. See *Calliphoridae.*

heel f. See *Hypoderma.*

horn f. See *Haematobia irritans.*

horsefly. See *Tabanidae.*

housefly. See *Muscidae.*

latrine f. See *Fannia.*

louse f. See *Hippoboscidae.*

mango f. See *Chrysops.*

moth f. See *Psychodidae.*

sand f. See *Phlebotomus.*

screwworm f. See *Calliphoridae, Sarcophagidae.*

soldier f. See *Hermetia.*

Spanish f. The beetle, *Lytta vesicatoria.*

stable f. See *Stomoxys.*

tsetse f. See *Glossina.*

tumbu f. See *Cordylobia anthropophaga.*

warble f. See *Oestridae.*

FMN Abbreviation for flavin mononucleotide (riboflavin-5′-phosphate).

Foà, Pio [*Italian pathologist*, 1848–1923]. Made important studies of the pneumococcus and of cytotoxic serums. Described a lymphocyte or monocyte, found in the guinea pig, containing one or more Kurlov bodies; called *Foà-Kurlov cell, Kurlov cell.*

foam [AS. *fām*]. *In physicochemistry*, a heterogeneous mixture of a gaseous phase, or finely divided gas bubbles suspended in a liquid.

fibrin f. See *fibrin* foam.

fo′cal length. The distance from the second principal point of a lens to a point on the axis where rays from an infinitely distant source converge to a common point or focus.

Fochier, Alphonse [*French gynecologist*, 1845–1903]. Described fixation abscess as one resulting from the injection of an irritant under the skin; formerly called *Fochier's abscess.*

fo′cus (pl. *foci*) [L., hearth]. 1. The principal seat of a disease. 2. The point (called **principal focus** or **real focus**) at which rays of light converge that pass through a convex lens or are reflected from a concave mirror. —**focal,** *adj.*

Assmann f. A small caseous lesion discovered roentgenologically and usually located in the subapical or infraclavicular region of the lung; it may represent the first sign of early infiltration in reinfection tuberculosis and tends to have a more severe prognosis than an apical lesion.

conjugate foci. Two interchangeable points at corresponding distances from a lens; the focal point of the image and the point of the object.

Elschnig's f. A black point in the fundus surrounded by a yellowish halo, usually associated with sclerosis of the choroidal vessels.

epileptogenic f. The exact location in the brain from which an epileptic discharge originates. In some cases it may be identified by the electrocephalogram or electrocorticogram.

Ghon's f. See Anton *Ghon.*

secondary f. The site of a secondary bacterial infection which in turn may become another center of dispersal.

Simon foci. Caseous nodules with a marked tendency to calcification, which develop in children in the apical portions of the lungs due to hematogenous spread of *Mycobacterium tuberculosis* after primary infection is established.

virtual f. The point at which divergent rays would meet if prolonged in a backward direction. Also called *negative f.*

Foderà, Michele [*Italian physician*, 1792–1848]. Credited with the discovery of the law of absorption or osmosis (1822), later demonstrated by Dutrochet.

Foerster, Otfrid [*German neurologist and surgeon*, 1873–1941]. With Hermann Küttner, described an operation of resection of the posterior spinal nerve roots for relief of spastic paralysis and tabetic incoordination; called *Foerster's operation.* With Wilder Penfield, devised an operation for traumatic epilepsy, in which the cerebral cortical scar is excised; called *Foerster-Penfield operation.* See also Foerster's cutaneous numeral *test.*

foe′tus (fee′tus). See *fetus.* —**foetal,** *adj.*

fog′ging [perhaps from Danish *fog*, spray]. 1. In repression treatment of esophoria, the reduction of vision to about 20/80 by combining prisms (varying with the muscular imbalance), bases in, with a convex sphere; the patient reads with these glasses for a half hour at night before retiring. 2. A method of refracting the eye by using a convex lens sufficiently strong to cause the eye to become artificially myopic and fog the vision. Astigmatism is then corrected by means of minus cylinders, after which the fog is removed by gradually reducing the convex lens. Generally used in adults or when cycloplegia might precipitate glaucoma.

fo′go sel·va′gem. An endemic bullous disease found in certain lowland areas of Brazil, believed to be an attenuated tropical form of pemphigus foliaceus.

foil [L. *folium*, leaf]. A thin sheet of metal, especially gold or tin.

Foix, Charles [*French neurologist*, 1882–1927]. Made detailed study of the vascular topography of the brain. Described a syndrome of complete unilateral paralysis of all nerve elements, motor and sensory as well as sympathetic but excluding the optic nerve, which enter the orbit; it is indicative of a lesion in the lateral wall of the cavernous sinus; called *Foix syndrome.* Described a second syndrome of cerebellar ataxia and hemichorea without ocular paralysis, due to a lesion in the red nucleus.

fold [AS. *fealdan*]. A plication or doubling of various parts of the body.

amniotic f. One of the folds of the blastoderm that unite over the embryo to form amnion and chorion in Sauropsida and many mammals. Also called *amnionic f.*

anterior malleolar f. A fold on the external surface of the tympanic membrane stretching from the malleolar prominence to the anterior portion of the tympanic sulcus of the temporal bone. It forms the lower anterior border of the pars flaccida.

aryepiglottic f. A fold of mucous membrane that extends from each arytenoid cartilage to the epiglottis.

bloodless f. of Treves. See ileocecal *f.*

body f. One of the various folds formed by the rapid growth of the embryonic area.

bulboventricular f. A transverse fold between the bulb of the heart and ventricle, which disappears when the proximal part of the bulb is incorporated into the right ventricle.

caudal genital f. See epigonal *f.*

caval f. See caval *mesentery.*

circular folds. The shelflike folds of the mucous membrane of the small intestine. Also called *valvulae conniventes, valves of Kerckring, plicae circulares.*

costocolic f. See phrenicocolic *ligament.*

cranial genital f. See progonal *f.*

epigastric f. A ridge of peritoneum covering the inferior epigastric vessels.

epigonal f. The caudal part of the genital ridge, in which the ovarian ligament or the upper part of the gubernaculum testis develops.

fimbriated f. A fold of mucous membrane having a fringed, free edge, on either side of the frenulum of the tongue.

f. of the urachus. See median umbilical *f.*

genital f. (a) A lateral swelling on either side of the cloacal membrane; produced by the growth of mesoderm. (b) Genital ridge. (c) See urethral *f.*

glossoepiglottic f. A fold separating the glossoepiglottic fossa into the two valleculae.

gluteal f. Crease between buttock and thigh.

gonadal f. That part of the genital ridge containing the gonad and mesorchium or mesovarium.

gubernacular f. A fold of peritoneum containing the lower part of the gubernaculum testis.

head f. A ventral fold formed by rapid growth of the head of the embryo over the embryonic disk, resulting in the formation of the foregut accompanied by anteroposterior reversal of the anterior part of the embryonic disk.

hypogastric f. See lateral umbilical *f.*

ileoappendicular f. See ileocecal *f.*

ileocecal f. A fold of peritoneum extending from the terminal part of the ileum to the cecum and to the mesentery of the vermiform appendix, or to the appendix itself. Also called *bloodless f. of Treves, ileoappendicular f., ileocolic f.*

ileocolic f. See ileocecal *f.*

inguinal f. A fold, developing on the urogenital ridge, which unites with the inguinal crest at the brim of the embryonic pelvis. The gubernaculum testis develops within these structures. Also called *plica inguinalis, inguinal fold of the mesonephros.*

lacrimal f. An inconstant, valvular fold of mucosa at the inferior meatus of the nasolacrimal duct. Also called *Hasner's valve.*

lateral nasal f. See lateral nasal *process.*

lateral umbilical f. A fold of peritoneum covering an obliterated hypogastric artery.

malleolar f. A small fold of the tympanic membrane extending outward from the projection produced by the lateral process of the malleus. There is an anterior and a posterior malleolar fold.

mammary f. See mammary *ridge.*

median nasal f. See median nasal *process.*

median umbilical f. A fold of peritoneum covering the urachus.

mesonephric f. A fold or swelling of the dorsal coelomic wall, created by the growth of the mesonephros, which bulges into the coelomic cavity.

neural f. One of the paired, longitudinal folds of the neural plate which unite in the midline to form the neural tube.

palmate folds. Radiating folds in the mucous membrane of the cervix of the uterus.

palpebral f. That formed by the reflection of the conjunctiva from the eyelids onto the eye. There are two folds, the superior and the inferior.

pharyngoepiglottic f. One of the paired folds of mucous membrane passing from the pharynx to the epiglottis.

posterior malleolar f. A fold on the external surface of the tympanic membrane stretching from the malleolar prominence to the posterior portion of the tympanic sulcus of the temporal bone. It forms the lower posterior border of the pars flaccida.

progonal f. The cephalic part of the genital ridge, in which develops the suspensory ligament of the ovary.

salpingopalatine f. A fold of mucous membrane extending from the torus tubarius to the palate.

salpingopharyngeal f. A vertical fold of mucous membrane extending from the torus tubarius to the pharynx.

semilunar f. A conjunctival fold in the inner canthus of the eye, the vestigial homolog of the nictitating membrane of Amphibia and Sauropsida.

sexual f. See genital *ridge.*

sublingual f. A fold of mucous membrane caused by the projection of the sublingual gland.

tail f. A fold formed by rapid growth of the caudal end of the embryo over the embryonic disk, resulting in the formation of hindgut and ventral body wall in this region.

transverse rectal folds. Large, semilunar folds projecting into the lumen of the first part of the rectum. Also called *Houston's valves.*

triangular f. A triangular membrane extending from the upper posterior portion of the glossopalatine arch backward and downward, until lost in the tissues at the base of the tongue.

urethral f. One of a pair of folds flanking the urethral groove on the caudal surface of the genital tubercle or phallus.

urogenital f. A fold or swelling of the dorsal coelomic wall containing the mesonephros and its duct and, later, the gonad and paramesonephric duct. Syn., *urogenital ridge.*

vascular f. A fold of peritoneum containing the spermatic vessels.

ventricular f. A fold of mucous membrane on either side of the larynx, enclosing the superior thyroarytenoid ligament. Also called *false vocal cord, plica ventricularis.*

vestigial f. of Marshall. See John *Marshall.*

vocal f. One of the two membranous bands extending from the thyroid cartilage to the arytenoid cartilage; their tension controls the pitch of the voice. Also called *true vocal cord, plica vocalis.*

Foley, Frederic Eugene Basil (1891–). American urologist who devised a procedure for relief of stricture at the ureteropelvic junction, the so-called *Foley (Y) plasty,* and the Foley lumbar ureterolithotomy operation; he also devised the Foley balloon *catheter.*

Foley's combined method. See under *stain.*

fo″li·a′ceous [L. *folium,* leaf]. Leaflike.

fo′lic ac′id. Pteroylglutamic acid, or N-[4-{[(2-amino-4-hydroxy-6-pteridyl)methyl]amino}benzoyl]glutamic acid; a substance occurring in green leaves, liver, and yeast, also produced by synthesis. It is essential for the growth of *Lactobacillus casei,* for synthesis of nucleic acid in the body, and also for growth, reproduction, tissue respiration, etc., probably through conversion to folinic acid, 2. It is employed clinically in treating certain types of macrocytic anemia. Also called *liver L. casei factor, vitamin B_c.* See *folvite.*

fo″lie′ (fo″lee′. *See* Notes § 35) [F.]. 1. A mental disorder or psychosis. 2. Old term for insanity.

f. à deux. A type of communicated psychosis involving two persons, one of whom has an essential psychosis. His control of and influence over the other person is so potent that the latter will simulate or accept the elements of the psychosis without question. Similar supposed syndromes are also called *communicated insanity, double insanity, induced insanity.*

Folin, Otto [*American biochemist,* 1867–1934]. Alone and with various co-workers, devised a number of useful biochemical technics. Especially notable are his colorimetric tests for the estimation of amino acids, blood gases, and alkaline reserve. See under *method, reagent, test.*

fo·li·ner′in, fo·lin′er·in. A glycoside from *Nerium oleander* which, on hydrolysis, yields gitoxigenin, the same steroid aglycone as is obtained from the digitalis glycoside, gitoxin. Syn., *oleandrin.*

fo·lin′ic ac′id. 1. A collective term for a group of factors, occurring in liver extracts and also obtained from pteroylglutamic acid by synthesis: essential for growth of *Leuconostoc citrovorum.* 2. $C_{20}H_{23}N_7O_7$; 5-formyl-5,6,7,8-tetrahydrofolic acid, the form in which folic acid probably exists and is active in tissues. It appears to be identical with principles variously referred to as *citrovorum factor* (abbreviated, CF) and *leucovorin.*

fo′li·um (pl. *folia*) [L.]. Any lamina or leaflet of gray matter, forming a part of the arbor vitae of the cerebellum.

f. cacuminis. A lobule on the upper surface of the vermis.

f. vermis. The terminal lobule in the superior surface of the vermis.

Folius. See Cecilio *Folli.*

follacro. The trade-mark for a preparation of estradiol-17-propionate, offered in ampuls containing a sesame oil solution of the hormone. Also see *estradiol.*

Folli, Cecilio (Folius) [*Italian anatomist,* 1615–60]. Discovered the anterior process of the malleus (1645). Called *Folian process, Rau's process.*

Folli, Francesco [*Italian physician,* 1624–85]. Accomplished blood transfusion by means of a silver tube inserted in the artery of the donor and a bone cannula inserted in the vein of the recipient, these being united by a tube made from the blood vessel of an animal (1654).

fol′li·cle [L. *folliculus,* small bag]. 1. Old term for a lymph nodule. 2. A small secretory cavity or sac, as an acinus or alveolus. —**follic′ular,** *adj.*

aggregate f. An aggregation of lymph nodules situated in the mucous membrane of the lower part of the small intestine, opposite the mesenteric attachment. Also called *Peyer's glands, Peyer's patches.*

atretic f. An involuted or degenerated ovarian follicle. Also called *corpus atreticum.*

dental f. The dental sac.

graafian, Graafian f. The mature ovarian follicle. Syn., *vesicular f.* See Plate 41.

growing f. Any stage in the maturation of an ovarian follicle between the primary follicle and the graafian follicle.

hair f. The tubular epithelial invagination containing the root of a hair.

lymph f. See lymph *nodule.*

Nabothian f. See Nabothian *cyst.*

ovarian f. An ovum and the epithelial follicular cells which surround it, lying in the cortex of the ovary.

palpebral follicles. The tarsal glands.

primary f. An ovarian follicle in which the ovum is surrounded by a single layer of follicular cells.

sebaceous f. A sebaceous gland of the skin.

solitary f. Old term for solitary lymphatic nodule.

vesicular f. See graafian *f.*

fol′li·clis [*folliculus*]. A tuberculid involving the extremities and at times the face. The histopathology is that of tuberculosis, and the lesions are papules or crusted pustules.

fol·lic′u·lin. See *estrone.*

fol·lic″u·li′tis [*folliculus;* G. *-itis,* inflammation]. Inflammation of a group of hair follicles.

agminate f. Inflammation of a set of hair follicles.

deep f. See *sycosis vulgaris.* See also *tinea barbae.*

f. abscedens et suffodiens. A rare scalp cellulitis with multiple follicular abscess formation.

f. barbae. Inflammation of the hair follicles of the beard; sycosis.

f. decalvans. Inflammatory disease of the hair follicles resulting in patches of baldness.

f. keloidis. A chronic skin disease affecting the nape of the neck and adjacent parts, characterized by minute red papules, which occasionally suppurate and are usually traversed by a hair. They unite to form hard white or reddish keloids. Also called *keloid acne, dermatitis papillaris capillitii.*

f. simplex. See superficial *f.*

f. ulerythematosa reticulata. An eruption over the face, especially the cheeks; characterized by small areas of atrophy separated by narrow ridges, producing a reticulated honeycomb appearance. Also called *atrophoderma vermicularis, acne vermoulante, atrophoderma reticulatum.*

pustular f. A pustular inflammation of the hair follicles, usually micrococcal.

superficial f. A type of pustular folliculitis in which the pustule is limited to the distal portion of the hair follicle: also called *f. simplex.*

fol·lic″u·lo′ma [*folliculus;* G. *-ōma,* tumor]. See feminizing *tumor* of ovary.

follutein. The trade-mark for a preparation of chorionic gonadotropin obtained from the urine of pregnant women.

fo″men·ta′tion [L. *fomentare,* to foment]. 1. The application of heat and moisture to a part to relieve pain or reduce inflammation. 2. The substance applied to a part to convey heat or moisture.

fo′mes (fo′meez, fom′eez) (pl. *fomites*) [L., tinder]. Any substance regarded as capable of transmitting contagious disease. *Obs.*

fo′mi·tes (fo′mi·teez, fom′i·). Plural of fomes.

Fon″se·cae′a (fon″si·see′uh) [L., after O. da *Fonseca,* contemporary Brazilian physician]. Name proposed by Negroni for a genus of fungi; synonym for *Hormodendrum.*

Fonseca's disease. See *chromoblastomycosis.*

fon·tac'to·scope. An instrument for ascertaining the radioactivity of waters and gases.

Fontana, Arturo [*Italian dermatologist,* 1873–1950]. See Fontana's *stain.*

Fontana, Felice [*Italian physiologist and naturalist,* 1720–1805]. Made an important experimental study of viper venom (1767). Said to have been the first to describe the renal tubules. See also *Fontana's spaces* under *space.*

fon"ta·nel', fon"ta·nelle' [F., dim. of *fontaine,* fountain]. A membranous space between the cranial bones in fetal life and infancy.

anterior f. That at the point of union of the frontal, sagittal, and coronal sutures. Closes during the second year. Also called *fonticulus major, fonticulus quadrangularis.*

great f. See anterior *f.*

lateral fontanels. Two membranous spaces, one in front between the parietal, frontal, great wing of the sphenoid, and temporal bones (the **anterior lateral** or **sphenoid fontanel**), and one behind between the parietal, occipital, and temporal bones (the **posterior lateral, mastoid, Casser's** or **Casserio's fontanel**). They usually close by three months after birth.

nasofrontal f. An abnormal one at the union of the nasal and frontal bones.

posterior f. That at the point of junction of lambdoid and sagittal sutures. Also called *fonticulus minor, fonticulus triangularis.*

sagittal f. One occasionally found in the sagittal suture, about midway between the anterior and posterior fontanels.

small f. See posterior *f.*

supraoccipital f. *In comparative embryology,* a cordate membranous space between the occipital cartilage and the more anterior parts of the cranium.

fon"ta·nelle'. Fontanel.

fon·tic'u·lus [L., a little fountain]. 1. Old term for suprasternal notch. 2. A small artificial ulcer or issue. 3. Fontanel.

food [AS. *fōda*]. Nutriment; any substance which, when taken into the body of an organism, may be used either to supply energy or to build tissue. Foods are organic substances classified in three groups: proteins, carbohydrates, and fats. All of these may occur in animal or vegetable substance.

Food and Drug Ad·min"is·tra'tion. An enforcement agency of the Federal Security Agency dealing with interstate commerce involving misbranding, false labeling, and adulteration of foods, insecticides, fungicides, drugs, cosmetics, and health devices.

food ball. A phytobezoar.

food yolk. See *deutoplasm.*

foot [AS. *fōt*]. 1. The terminal extremity of the leg. It consists of the tarsus, metatarsus, and phalanges or toes. 2. A measure of length equal to 12 inches, or 30.479 cm. Abbreviated, ft.

cleft f. A condition similar to cleft hand.

congenital deformity of the f. See *talipes.*

contracted f. Clawfoot.

f. cell. One of the branching parenchymatous cells of the pineal body.

frosted feet. See *chilblain.*

hollow f. Clawfoot.

immersion f. See *immersion foot.*

march f. See march *fracture.*

perivascular f. The expanded pedicle of a neuroglial cell process attaching it to a blood vessel.

shelter f. A condition resembling trench foot and immersion foot, but of less severity; it occurs in persons who are confined to cold and damp shelters; associated with some vitamin deficiency.

splay f. Flatfoot with extreme eversion of the forefoot and tarsus.

tabetic f. (a) An extension of the foot in preataxic tabes, observed when the patient is lying down. (b) An affection of the foot in the beginning of tabes, marked by numbness and formication, followed by hypertrophy of the head of the talus, navicular, cuneiform, and metatarsal bones.

trench f. A condition of the feet somewhat like frostbite; it occurs in those exposed in the trenches.

weak f. Chronic eversion of the foot, due usually to faulty walking habits associated with loss of muscular tone. Frequently confused with flatfoot.

foot-can'dle. The illumination received at a surface 1 foot from a standard lamp of 1 candlepower; 1 foot-candle = 1 lumen per square foot.

foot drop. A falling of the foot due to a paralysis of the dorsiflexors of the ankle.

foot'-pound'. A unit of energy; the work equal to that of raising a pound to the height of one foot. Abbreviated, ft.-lb.

foot'print" [*fōt;* ME. *printe,* from L. *premere,* to press]. An ink impression of the sole of the foot; used for identification of infants.

foot rot. A disease of cattle and sheep marked by a necrosis of the skin around the hoof.

foots. The bottom portion, sediment, or residue from certain crude liquids, as fixed animal or vegetable oils, obtained in a process of refining.

Foot's methods. See under *stain.*

fo·ra'men (pl. *foramens, foramina*) [L., an opening]. A perforation or opening, especially in a bone. —**foram'inal,** *adj.*

anterior ethmoid f. A canal between the ethmoid and frontal bones, giving passage to the nasal branch of the ophthalmic nerve and anterior ethmoid vessels.

anterior palatine f. Incisive *fossa,* (a): old term.

anterior sacral f. One of the eight (four on each side) on the anterior surface of the sacrum, connecting with the sacral canal, and giving passage to the anterior branches of the sacral nerves.

aortic f. See aortic *hiatus.*

apical f. The passage at the end of the root of a tooth for the vessels and nerves of the dental pulp.

cecal f. of the frontal bone. A small foramen formed by the frontal bone and the crista galli of the ethmoid, occasionally giving passage to a vein.

cecal f. of the medulla oblongata. One located in a depression at the termination of the anterior median fissure.

cecal f. of the tongue. One located in the posterior termination of the median raphe of the tongue at the apex of the terminal sulcus; the site of the former orifice of the thyroglossal duct.

common interclinoid f. A canal formed by an anomalous process connecting the anterior, middle, and posterior clinoid processes of the sphenoid bone.

condylar, condyloid f. See condylar *canals.*

cotyloid f. A notch in the acetabulum converted into a foramen by a ligament; it gives passage to vessels and nerves.

epiploic f. An aperture of the peritoneal cavity situated between the liver and the stomach, bounded in front by the portal vein, hepatic artery and common bile duct, behind by the inferior vena cava, below by the duodenum, and above by the liver. Formed by folds of the peritoneum, it establishes communication between the greater and lesser cavities of the peritoneum. Also called *f. of Winslow.*

esophageal f. See esophageal *hiatus.*

external auditory f. The lateral opening of the

external auditory canal; also called *porus acusticus externus*.

f. caecum. See cecal *f.* of the tongue.

f. caroticum externum. The outer or lateral opening of the carotid canal.

f. caroticum internum. The inner or medial opening of the carotid canal.

f. infrapiriforme. The passageway through the pelvic wall below the piriformis muscle where the inferior gluteal nerve and vessels leave the pelvic cavity; a subdivision of the greater sciatic foramen.

f. lacerum. An irregular aperture between the apex of the petrous portion of the temporal bone and the body and great wing of the sphenoid, and the basilar process of the occipital bone: also called *lacerated f.*

f. magnum. A large oval aperture centrally placed in the lower and anterior part of the occipital bone; it gives passage to the spinal cord and its membranes and venous plexuses, the spinal accessory nerves, and the vertebral arteries.

f. nasale. A small opening on the outer (facial) surface of the nasal bone which transmits a tributary to the anterior facial vein.

f. of Bochdalek. Either of two potentially weak areas of the diaphragm between the dorsal or lumbar portion and each costal portion. Either may be the site of a diaphragmatic hernia, but the condition is more common on the left.

f. of Huschke. See Emil *Huschke*.

f. of Key. A small opening in the roof of the fourth ventricle, allowing passage of cerebrospinal fluid into the subarachnoid space.

f. of Magendie. A posterior median foramen in the membranous roof of the fourth ventricle of the brain.

f. of Monro. The interventricular foramen.

f. of Morgagni. Either of two potentially weak areas of the diaphragm between the sternal portion and each costal portion. Either may be the site of a diaphragmatic hernia. Also called *parasternal orifice of the diaphragm.*

f. of Retzius. See *f.* of Key.

f. of Scarpa. A median incisive *f.* See incisive *f.*

f. of Stensen. A lateral incisive *f.* See incisive *f.*

f. of Vesalius. An inconstant foramen in the great wing of the sphenoid, situated between the foramen ovale and foramen rotundum, which when present transmits an emissary vein from the cavernous sinus.

f. of Winslow. See epiploic *f.*

f. ovale of the heart. A fetal opening between the two atria of the heart, situated at the lower posterior portion of the septum. Through this opening blood is shunted from the right atrium to the left atrium. In a **patent f. ovale** there is persistence of this fetal opening after birth, and the term usually refers to a *functional patency.* An *anatomical patency* can frequently be demonstrated at autopsy of individuals who displayed no signs of functional patency in life.

f. ovale of the sphenoid. An oval opening near the posterior margin of the great wing of the sphenoid, giving passage to the mandibular branch of the trigeminal nerve, the accessory meningeal artery, and occasionally the lesser superficial petrosal nerve.

f. ovale primum. See *f.* secundum.

f. palatinum majus. See greater palatine *f.*

f. palatinum minus. See lesser palatine *f.*

f. primum. The temporary interatrial opening bounded by the growing margins of the septum primum and the endocardial cushions. Also called *primitive interatrial f.*

f. rotundum. A round opening in the great wing of the sphenoid bone for the maxillary branch of the fifth nerve.

f. secundum. The secondary opening in the septum primum due to thinning and perforation of its cranial portion. Also called *f. ovale primum.*

foramens of Luschka. Openings, one in each lateral recess of the fourth ventricle, allowing passage of the cerebrospinal fluid into the subarachnoid space. The free ends of the choroid plexus project through them.

f. spinosum. A passage in the great wing of the sphenoid bone, near its posterior angle, giving passage to the middle meningeal artery and spinosus nerve.

f. suprapiriforme. The passageway through the pelvic wall above the piriformis muscle where the superior gluteal nerve and vessels leave the pelvic cavity; a subdivision of the greater sciatic foramen.

f. transversarium. A foramen in the transverse process of each of the upper six cervical vetrebrae, which transmits the vertebral artery and vein: also called *vertebrarterial f.*

f. venae cavae. The opening in the diaphragm for the transmission of the inferior vena cava.

f. venarum minimarum. Any one of the small openings into the right atrium of the heart, which are the orifices of the Thebesian veins.

f. venosum. Any small opening, especially on the surface of a bone, for the passage of a vein.

f. zygomaticofaciale. An opening on the outer aspect of the zygomatic bone for the passage of the zygomaticofacial nerve and accompanying vessels.

f. zygomaticoorbitale. An opening on the orbital surface of the zygomatic bone for the passage of the zygomatic branch of the maxillary nerve and accompanying vessels.

f. zygomaticotemporale. An opening on the temporal surface of the zygomatic bone for the passage of the zygomaticotemporal nerve.

greater palatine f. The lower opening of the greater palatine canal; it is formed on the medial side by a notch in the horizontal part of the palatine bone and on the lateral side by the adjacent part of the maxilla: also called *major palatine f., f. palatinum majus.*

incisive f. One of the two to four openings of the incisive canal or canals on the floor of the incisive fossa, (a). A pair in the midline, the **median incisive foramens** (*f. of Scarpa*), transmit the nasopalatine nerves from the anterior nasal floor to the anterior hard palate. A pair of **lateral incisive foramens** (*f. of Stensen*) transmit terminal branches of the greater palatine arteries from the palate to the floor of the nasal cavities.

infraorbital f. In the maxilla, the external aperture of the infraorbital canal; it gives passage to the infraorbital nerve and artery.

innominate f. See innominate *canaliculus.*

internal auditory f. One located in the petrous portion of the temporal bone; it gives passage to the auditory and facial nerves and vessels, and the internal auditory vessels.

interventricular f. Either one of the two foramens that connect the third ventricle with each lateral ventricle. Also called *f. of Monro.* See Plate 18.

intervertebral f. The aperture formed by the notches opposite to each other in the laminas of the adjacent vertebrae; a passage for the spinal nerves and vessels.

jugular f. The space formed by the jugular notches of the occipital and temporal bones, divided into two portions, the posterior portion giving passage to an internal jugular vein and the anterior portion giving passage to the ninth, tenth, and eleventh cranial nerves and the inferior petrosal sinus.

lacerated f. See *f.* lacerum.

lesser palatine f. The lower opening or openings of the lesser palatine canals on the lower surface of the palatine bone: also called *minor palatine f., f. palatinum minus.*

major palatine f. See greater palatine *f.*

mandibular f. The external aperture of the inferior dental or alveolar canal in the ramus of the mandible; it transmits the inferior dental or alveolar vessels and nerve to the lower jaw.

mastoid f. A small foramen behind the mastoid process; it transmits a small artery from the dura and a vein opening into the lateral sinus.

medullary f. See nutrient *f.*

mental f. The external aperture of the inferior dental canal in the mandible; it transmits the mental nerves and vessels to the skin of the face.

minor palatine f. See lesser palatine *f.*

nutrient f. The opening into the canal which gives passage to the blood vessels of the medullary cavity of a bone.

obturator f. The large oval opening between the ischium and the pubis, anterior, inferior, and medial to the acetabulum, partly closed in by a fibrous membrane; it gives passage to the obturator vessels and nerves.

olfactory foramens. Numerous foramens in the cribriform plate of the ethmoid, giving passage to the fila olfactoria of the olfactory nerves.

optic f. The canal at the apex of the orbit, the anterior termination of the optic groove, just beneath the lesser wing of the sphenoid bone; it gives passage to the optic nerve and ophthalmic artery.

palatine f. See greater palatine *f.*, lesser palatine *f.*

papillary f. The orifice of a papillary duct in a minor calyx of the kidney.

parietal f. That near the posterior superior angle of the parietal bone; inconstant. It gives passage to an emissary vein of the superior longitudinal sinus and occasionally a small branch of the occipital artery.

posterior sacral f. One of the eight (four on each side) on the posterior surface of the sacrum, external to the articular processes, and giving passage to the posterior branches of the sacral nerves.

posterior superior alveolar f. One of the two or more openings on the infratemporal surface of the maxilla which is the external orifice of a superior alveolar canal.

primitive interatrial f. See *f.* primum.

pterygoalar f. See *porus* crotaphitico-buccinatorius.

pterygospinous f. A foramen formed by the ossification of the pterygospinous ligament running between the lateral pterygoid lamina and the angular spine of the sphenoid bone.

quadrate f. A passage in the diaphragm for the inferior vena cava.

sciatic foramens. The **greater sciatic foramen** is the oval space between the sacrotuberous ligament and the innominate bone, conveying the piriformis muscle, the gluteal, sciatic, and pudendal vessels and nerves; the **lesser sciatic foramen** is the space included between the sacrotuberous and sacrospinous ligaments and the portion of the innominate bone between the spine and tuberosity of the ischium, giving passage to the internal obturator muscle and the internal pudendal vessels and pudendal nerves.

sphenopalatine f. The space between the sphenoid and orbital processes of the palate bone; it opens into the nasal cavity and gives passage to branches from the sphenopalatine ganglion and the sphenopalatine branch of the internal maxillary artery.

spurious jugular f. A foramen in the temporal bone of the embryo; it gives passage to a vein from the lateral sinus to the external jugular vein.

stylomastoid f. One between the styloid and mastoid processes of the temporal bone; the external aperture of the facial canal.

supraorbital f. A notch in the superior orbital margin at the junction of the middle with the inner third, sometimes converted into a foramen by a bony process or a ligamentous band; it gives passage to the supraorbital artery, veins, and nerve.

thyroid f. One in the ala of the thyroid cartilage.

transverse accessory foramens. Anomalous foramens in the transverse processes of the cervical vertebrae giving passage to an inconstant accessory vertebral artery.

vascular f. Any small opening, especially on the surface of a bone, for the passage of a blood vessel.

vertebral f. The space included between the body and arch of a vertebra, giving passage to the spinal cord and its appendages.

vertebrarterial f. Foramen transversarium.

fo·ra′mi·na. Plural of foramen.

for″a·min′u·lum [dim. of *foramen*]. A very small foramen. —**foraminulate,** *adj.*

force [OF., from L. *fortis,* strong]. 1. Strength, power; physical might, vigor. 2. That which initiates, changes, or arrests motion. 3. Binding power, validity. —**forced,** *adj.*

animal f. Muscular energy.

catabiotic f. The energy derived from the breakdown of food.

catalytic f. Chemical work initiated by a catalyst.

chemical f. That form of energy which holds atoms together in a molecule.

coercive f. The magnetic force required to remove the magnetic induction in a previously magnetized material.

electrical forces of the heart. Forces produced by electrical depolarization and repolarization of the myocardium.

electromotive f. The force which tends to alter the motion of electricity, measured in volts. Abbreviated, E, emf., e.m.f., E.M.F.

nerve f. The capacity of nerve tissue to conduct stimuli.

occlusal f. The force exerted upon opposing teeth when biting.

psychic f. Mental power or force generated by thinking; contrasted with physical force.

reserve f. Energy latent within an organism or part over and above that required for normal functions. Cardiac reserve is the latent force of the heart available to meet any additional burden placed on the circulation.

rest f. The cardiac energy expended in maintaining the circulation when the body is at rest.

vital f. The energy or power characteristic of living organisms.

for′ceps [L., pincers]. 1. A surgical instrument with two opposing blades or limbs; controlled by handles or by direct pressure on the blades. Used to grasp, compress, and hold tissue, a part of the body, needles, or other surgical material. 2. Fiber bundles in the brain resembling forceps. —**forcip′ial,** *adj.*

alligator f. A special type of forceps having long slender angulated handles designed to be used with such instruments as an operating cystoscope or proctoscope.

alveolar f. Dental forceps for biting into the alveolar processes.
anterior f. The U-shaped bundles from the radiation of the corpus callosum that are distributed to the frontal pole of the cerebral hemisphere. Syn., *f. minor.*
artery f. Any forceps used for seizing and compressing an artery; usually self-locking, with scissors handles. Frequently various types are named for individual surgeons who devised them, as Halstead, Jones, Kelly, Mayo-Ochsner. Syn., *hemostatic f.*
aural f. A delicate dressing forceps used in aural surgery.
axis-traction f. An obstetric forceps, the so-called high forceps instrument, equipped with a mechanism to permit rotation of the fetal head and traction in the line of the pelvic axis.
bone-cutting f. A double-jointed or single-jointed, powerful, heavy-bladed cutting forceps, with great power derived from the leverage exerted by the long handles. Syn., *rongeur f.*
bone-holding f. A forceps with heavy jaws and long handles, for use in holding bone during an operation. Syn., *lion-jawed f.*
Bruning's f. A forceps for biopsy in rectal disease.
bulldog f. Forceps with strong teeth and a clasp to prevent slipping.
bullet f. Instrument for extracting bullets.
crushing f. A forceps, usually in the form of a clamp, for crushing heavy tissues or pedicles prior to ligation.
dental f. Any one of a variety of forceps adapted for the extraction of teeth.
disk f. A type used in ophthalmic surgery.
dissecting f. Any of a variety of forceps used for dissection. They may have sharp, smooth, or notched points, may be curved or straight, or self-closing, and come in various sizes.
dressing f. A two-limbed, slender-bladed instrument or spring forceps, with blunt or serrated teeth; for use in surgical dressings.
epilating f. Special forceps used for removing the hairs of the lashes, eyebrows, or other areas where hair is not desired.
esophageal f. A special forceps for removing foreign bodies from the esophagus.
extracting f. Dental forceps.
f. major. See posterior *f.*
f. minor. See anterior *f.*
hemostatic f. See artery *f.*
high f. An obstetric forceps applied to the fetal head which has descended into the pelvic canal, when its greatest diameter is still above the superior strait.
lion-jawed f. See bone-holding *f.*
lithotomy f. A special type of forceps for removing a stone from the urinary bladder or ureter.
low f. An obstetric forceps applied to the fetal head when it is well within the lower portion of the pelvic canal.
mid f. An obstetric forceps applied when the presenting part is at, or immediately above, the ischial spines.
mosquito f. A delicate, sharp-pointed hemostat. Also called *Halsted's mosquito f.*
mouse-tooth f. A dressing forceps with interlocking fine teeth at the tips of the blades.
needle f. A needle holder.
obstetric f. A large, fenestrated, double-bladed traction forceps; the blades are demountable and are applied separately before interlocking at the handles, in order to fit the fetal head. Employed in difficult or delayed labor.
posterior f. The U-shaped bundles from the radiation of the corpus callosum that are distributed to the occipital pole of the cerebral hemisphere. Syn., *f. major.*
rib-cutting f. A type of forceps with one heavy semicircular cutting edge and one heavy hook-shaped blade designed to cut ribs and firm cartilages.
roller f. A forceps equipped with small rollers; used for compressing the eyelids in cases of trachoma.
rongeur f. Bone-cutting forceps.
sequestrum f. Forceps designed for removing spicules or sequestra of bone.
tenaculum f. A slender forceps with scissors handles and one or two long, overlapping teeth or hooks at the end of the blade; adapted especially for gynecologic surgery.
towel f. A snap, clamp, or forceps with sharp hooked ends which overlap; adapted to holding towels fast to the skin during operations. Also called *towel clamp, skin-holding f.*
volsella f. A type of tenaculum forceps.

Forchheimer, Frederick [*American physician,* 1853–1913]. Described a maculopapular, rose-red eruption on the soft palate and uvula, characteristic of rubella, in the absence of cutaneous eruption; called *Forchheimer's sign.*

for'ci·pate [*forceps*]. Shaped like a forceps.

for'ci·pres"sure [*forceps;* L. *pressura,* pressure]. Pressure exerted on a blood vessel by means of a forceps, to prevent hemorrhage.

Fordyce, John Addison [*American dermatologist,* 1858–1925]. Described a condition affecting the mucous membrane of the lips and buccal region and characterized by numerous yellowish-white, millet-sized granules due to the presence of sebaceous glands (1896); called *Fordyce's disease.* With G. H. Fox, described a rare disease, called *Fox-Fordyce disease,* affecting principally the axillas and characterized by an itching papular eruption (1902). This is thought to be due to dysfunction of the apocrine glands.

fore- [AS.]. A prefix signifying *before* (in time or place), *in front.*

fore'arm" [*fore;* AS. *arm*]. That part of the upper extremity between the wrist and the elbow.

fore'brain". See *prosencephalon.*

fore'con"scious [*fore;* L. *conscius,* knowing with another]. *In psychoanalysis,* that portion of the unconscious containing mental experiences which are not in the focus of immediate attention, but which may be recalled to consciousness.

fore'con"scious. Capable of being recalled into the conscious mind, although not in the realm of consciousness. Syn., *coconscious, preconscious.*

fore'fin"ger [*fore;* AS. *finger*]. The index finger.

fore'foot" [*fore;* AS. *fōt*]. Anterior part of the foot; from a clinical standpoint, that portion of the foot which includes the toes, metatarsal, cuneiform, and cuboid bones.

fore'gut. The cephalic part of the embryonic digestive tube that develops into pharynx, esophagas, stomach, part of the small intestine, liver, pancreas, and respiratory ducts.

fore'head [AS. *forhēafod*]. That part of the face above the eyes.

fore'kid"ney [*fore;* ME. *kydney*]. The pronephros.

Forel, Auguste Henri (1848–1931). Swiss neurologist, psychiatrist, and entomologist who contributed to the neuron doctrine (1887), made an important study of sexual problems (1905), and described the ventral tegmental decussation, formerly called *decussation of Forel.*

fore'milk" [*fore;* AS. *meoluc*]. Colostrum.

fo·ren'sic [L. *forensis,* of the forum]. Relating to a law court.

fore'pleas"ure. *In psychoanalysis*, the erotic pleasure, both physical and emotional, accompanied by a rise in tension, which precedes the culmination of the sexual act, or end pleasure.

fore'skin" [*fore;* ON. *skinn*]. The prepuce.

fore'wa"ters [*fore;* AS. *waeter*]. Hydrorrhea gravidarum.

Forlanini, Carlo [*Italian physician,* 1847–1918]. First to induce artificial pneumothorax in pulmonary tuberculosis (1892).

form [L. *forma,* form]. The configuration, shape, or particular appearance of living things or tissues, especially when modified under particular conditions.

stab f., staff f. See band *cell.*

form·al'de·hyde. Formic aldehyde or methanal, HCHO. A colorless gas obtained by the oxidation of methyl alcohol. It is soluble in water and in alcohol.

f. sodium sulfoxylate. $CH_2OHSO_2Na.2H_2O$. A white, crystalline, water-soluble compound, introduced as an antidote for poisoning by mercury bichloride. Syn., *sodium formaldehyde sulfoxylate, rongolite, formopone.* Also called *sodium sulfoxylate, formaldehyde hydrosulfite.*

f. solution (*liquor formaldehydi*). An aqueous solution containing not less than 37% by weight of formaldehyde. It is a powerful antiseptic. By means of oxidizing agents or heat, it may be converted into a gas for the disinfection of rooms and dwellings previously exposed to contagion.

para-f. $(CH_2O)_3$. A solid polymer of formaldehyde. On heating, a portion of it is converted to formaldehyde.

formalin. A trade-mark for a formaldehyde solution. See under *fixing fluid.*

form·am'ide, form'am·ide. 1. $HCONH_2$, the amide of formic acid. 2. A compound containing the HCONH— radical.

for'ma·mol. See *helmitol.*

for'mate, for'mi·ate. A salt of formic acid.

for·ma'tion [L. *formatio,* from *formare,* to form]. 1. The process of developing shape or structure. 2. That which is formed; a structure or arrangement.

reticular f. That in the central nervous system, consisting of small islands of gray matter separated by fine bundles of nerve fibers running in every direction; in the medulla oblongata, it fills the interspaces among the larger fiber tracts and nuclei. Also called *formatio reticularis.*

form'a·tive [*formare*]. 1. Relating to the process of development, as of tissue or of the embryo. 2. Forming, producing, originating.

for'ma·zan. A generic name for a deeply colored pigment obtained by reducing 2,3,5-triphenyltetrazolium chloride or certain other related tetrazolium salts by highly labile enzyme systems. The reaction is utilized in testing the ability of seeds to germinate; also, the extent of pigment production is sometimes employed in estimating the spread of carcinoma. The red pigment obtained when 2,3,5-triphenyltetrazolium chloride is used in such tests is specifically designated *2,3,5-triphenyl formazan.*

for'ma·zin. Formalazin; an insoluble, white, amorphous compound formed from hydrazine sulfate and hexamethylenetetramine. In gelatin suspension, it is used in making permanent albumin standards in the life insurance method for the determination of protein in urine.

forme fruste' (form froost'. *See* NOTES § 35). An incomplete or atypical form of a disease.

for'mi·ate. See *formate.*

for'mic [L. *formica,* ant]. Relating to, or derived from, ants; or pertaining to formic acid.

for'mic ac'id. 1. The anhydrous liquid HCOOH; a strong reducing agent, dangerously caustic to the skin. Syn., *methanoic acid.* 2. An aqueous solution containing 24–26% HCOOH; it is counterirritant and astringent.

for'mic al'de·hyde. Formaldehyde.

for"mi·ca'tion [L. *formicatio,* from *formica*]. Paresthesia; an abnormal sensation as of insects crawling in or upon the skin; a common symptom in diseases of the spinal cord and the peripheral nerves.

formin. A trade-mark for methenamine.

for"mo·cre'sol. A mixture of equal parts of formaldehyde solution and cresol, used in dentistry for treating putrescent pulps.

formohydrion. Trade-mark for a granular effervescent salt containing methenamine and sodium biphosphate. The salt is employed as a urinary acidifier and antiseptic.

for'mol. A solution of formaldehyde.

for"mo·ni'trile (for"mo·nigh'tril, ·treel, ·tryle). Hydrocyanic acid.

for'mo·pone. See *formaldehyde* sodium sulfoxylate.

for'mose. The mixture of sugar and sugarlike compounds formed by formaldehyde in alkaline solution.

for·mox'yl. Formyl.

for'mu·la [L., small pattern]. 1. A prescribed method. 2. The representation of a chemical compound by symbols. 3. A recipe or prescription. Abbreviated, F.

Arneth's f. See Joseph *Arneth.*

constitutional f. One that indicates the relation to each other of various radicals and atoms in a compound. It does not show the linkage of each atom.

dental f. One showing the number and arrangement of teeth.

Einthoven's formulas. Used for the determination of the mean electrical axis from the electrocardiogram (Leads I, II, III).

$$\tan a = \frac{2E_2 - E_1}{E_1\sqrt{3}}$$

$$\tan a = \frac{E_2 - E_3}{(E_2 - E_3)\sqrt{3}}$$

where a equals angle a and E_1, E_2, E_3 equal net of positive and negative deflection of QRS in leads I, II, and III.

empirical f. One that indicates only the constituents and their proportions in a molecule, as $C_6H_{12}O_6$, dextrose.

graphic f. See structural *f.*

official f. One given in an official publication.

officinal f. A pharmaceutical formula which, though not official, is commonly followed by pharmacists.

structural f. One which shows the arrangement and relation of every atom in a molecule. One in which the symbols are united by the bonds of affinity according to their valence, as H—O—H.

vertebral f. One used to indicate the number and arrangement of the vertebrae.

for'mu·lar"y (for'mew·lerr"ee) [*formula*]. A collection of formulas for making medicinal preparations.

for'myl. 1. HCO—, the radical of formic acid. Also called *formoxyl.* 2. The trivalent radical, HC≡.

f.-amide. See *formamide.*

f. bromide. Bromoform.

f. chloride. Chloroform. Also called *f. perchloride.*

f. iodide. Iodoform.

f. tribromide. Bromoform.

f. trichloride. Chloroform.

f. triiodide. Iodoform.

for′myl·ase. An enzyme, present in the liver of certain experimental animals, which effects hydrolysis of formylkynurenine to tryptophan.

for″myl·fo′lic ac′id. The formyl derivative (at the nitrogen atom of the *p*-aminobenzoyl component) of folic acid; it may be an intermediate in the biogenesis of folic acid. See also *rhizopterin.*

for″myl·for′mic ac′id. Glyoxylic acid.

for″myl·gly′cine. $NH_2.CH(CHO)COOH$; a postulated intermediate in the conversion of serine to glycine; it represents serine in which the CH_2OH group has been converted to CHO.

for″myl·ky·nur′e·nine. A compound resulting from oxidation of tryptophan in certain experimental animals; upon hydrolysis in the presence of formylase it is converted to kynurenine and formic acid.

for″myl·pter·o′ic ac′id. Rhizopterin.

for′ni·cate [L. *fornicatio*, from *fornicari*, to commit fornication]. Commit fornication.

for′ni·cate [L. *fornicatus*, from *fornix*, arch]. Arched.

for″ni·ca′tion [L. *fornicatio*, from *fornicari*, to commit fornication]. The illicit sexual intercourse of unmarried persons.

for′nix [L., arch]. 1. An arched body or surface; a concavity or cul-de-sac. 2. A nerve fiber that arises in the hippocampus and dentate gyrus and ends in the mammillary body (corticomammillary tract), habenular nucleus (corticohabenular tract), and septal and preoptic areas. See Plate 18. —**fornical,** *adj.*

f. of stomach. See *fundus ventriculi.*

f. of the conjunctiva. The cul-de-sac at the line where the bulbar conjunctiva is reflected upon the lid.

f. of the vagina. The vault of the vagina: the upper part of the vagina which surrounds the cervix of the uterus.

Forssman antigen. See under *antigen.*

forthane. Trade-mark for methylhexaneamine, a volatile amine employed for vasoconstrictor action on nasal mucosa.

Foshay's serum. See Foshay's *test.*

Foshay's test. See under *test.*

fos′sa (pl. *fossae*) [L., ditch]. A depression or pit.

acetabular f. A depression in the center of the acetabulum.

antecubital f. One in front of the elbow.

anterior cranial fossae. The most elevated in position of the three pairs (right and left) of fossae into which the internal base of the skull is divided. They lodge the frontal lobes of the brain and are formed by the orbital part of the frontal bone, the cribriform plate of the ethmoid bone, and the small wings of the sphenoid bone.

axillary f. The armpit.

canine f. A depression on the external surface of the maxilla, above and to the outer side of the socket of the canine tooth.

cecal f. A fold of peritoneum forming a pouch upon the surface of the right iliopsoas muscle, and extending to the apex of the cecum.

cerebellar fossae. Two shallow, concave recesses on the lower part of the inner surface of the occipital bone for the reception of the hemispheres of the cerebellum. Also called *inferior occipital fossae.*

cerebral fossae. Two shallow, concave recesses on the upper part of the internal surface of the occipital bone for the reception of the occipital lobes of the cerebrum. Also called *superior occipital fossae.*

condylar, condyloid f. Either of two small pits on the lower surface of the basilar part of the occipital bone, one situated behind each occipital condyle.

coronoid f. A depression in the humerus into which the apex of the coronoid process of the ulna fits in extreme flexion of the forearm.

costal fossae. The facets on the bodies of the vertebrae where articulation occurs with the heads of the ribs.

cranial f. Any of the three depressions, **anterior, middle,** and **posterior,** in the base of the skull.

cubital f. See antecubital *f.*

cystic f. A depression on the lower surface of the right lobe of the liver, in which the gallbladder is situated: also called *f. vesicae felleae.*

digastric f. (a) A deep groove on the inner aspect of the mastoid process marking the attachment of the posterior belly of the digastric muscle. (b) A depression on the inside of the mandible for the attachment of the anterior belly of the digastric muscle.

digital f. (a) A depression at the base of the inner surface of the greater trochanter of the femur. (b) A cul-de-sac in the serous membrane which separates the body of the epididymis from the testis. Also called *epididymal sinus.* (c) A depression on the posterior inferior end of the fibula.

duodenojejunal f. A pouch formed by a fold of peritoneum from the terminal portion of the duodenum blending with parietal peritoneum.

epigastric f. The midline infrasternal depression.

f. ductus venosi. A narrow groove on the posterior surface of the liver between the caudate and left lobes, occupied by the ductus venosus in fetal life and by the ligamentum venosum after birth.

f. innominata. A shallow depression between the ventricular and the aryepiglottic fold.

f. occipitalis. That portion of the posterior cranial fossa which is bounded by the inner surface of the occipital bone; it may be further subdivided into a superior occipital fossa lying above the groove for the transverse sinus and an inferior occipital fossa lying below the groove.

f. of the incus. That in the posterior wall of the tympanic cavity, for attachment of the short crus of the incus. Also called *fossa incudis.*

f. ovalis. (a) An oval fossa in the interatrial septum; its floor is derived from the embryonic septum primum, and its rim from the septum secundum. (b) An opening in the fascia lata of the thigh which gives passage to the great saphenous vein.

f. poplitea. See popliteal *space.*

f. venae cavae. A groove on the posterior surface of the liver between the caudate and right lobes occupied by the inferior vena cava.

f. vesicae felleae. See cystic *f.*

genital f. The embryonic urogenital groove bounded by the urethral folds and the urethral portion of the cloacal membrane.

glenoid f. Old term for mandibular fossa.

helical f. A furrow between the helix and antihelix.

hyaloid f. A depression in the anterior surface of the vitreous body for the crystalline lens.

hypophyseal f. A depression in the sphenoid bone lodging the hypophysis: also called *f. hypophyseos, pituitary f.*

ileocecal fossae. Peritoneal recesses in the region of the ileocecal junction.

iliac f. A wide depression on the internal surface of the ilium.

incisive f. (a) A bony pit behind the upper incisors into which the incisive canals open. (b) A depression on the maxilla at the origin of the depressor muscle of the nose. (c) A depression on the mandible at the origin of the mentalis muscle.

inferior duodenal f. A small pocket of peritoneum formed on the left of the terminal portion of

the duodenum by a triangular fold of peritoneum and having the opening directed upward.
infraclavicular f. The depression of the skin below the clavicle.
infraspinous f. The recess on the posterior surface of the scapula occupied by the infraspinatus muscle.
infratemporal f. An irregular space situated below and medial to the zygomatic arch, behind the maxilla and medial to the upper part of the ramus of the mandible: also called *zygomatic f.*
intercondyloid f. One on the back of the femur between the condyles.
interpeduncular f. A deep groove in the anterior surface of the midbrain.
intersigmoid f. See subsigmoid *f.*
intertrochanteric f. That located medial to the intertrochanteric crest of the femur.
ischiorectal f. The region on either side of the rectum, bounded laterally by the obturator internus muscle, medially by the levator ani and coccygeus muscles, and posteriorly by the gluteus maximus muscle.
jugular f. One between the carotid canal and the stylomastoid foramen, containing the superior bulb of the internal jugular vein.
lacrimal f. The depression in the frontal bone for the reception of the lacrimal gland.
lateral pharyngeal f. A depression in the lateral wall of the nasopharynx posterior to the opening of the auditory tube. Also called *pharyngeal recess, Rosenmueller's f.*
mandibular f. The fossa in the temporal bone that receives the condyle of the mandible.
mastoid f. That on the lateral surface of the temporal bone, behind the suprameatal spine.
middle fossae of the skull. One of the three pairs (right and left) of fossae into which the interior base of the cranium is divided; they are deeply concave on a much lower level than the anterior cranial fossae, and lodge the temporal lobes of the cerebrum.
nasal f. (a) Old term for nasal pit of the embryo. (b) Old term for nasal cavity.
navicular f. (a) The dilated portion of the urethra in the glans penis. (b) In the vulva, the depression between the posterior commissure and the fourchette.
navicular f. of the ear. Helical fossa.
olecranon f. One at the dorsal side of the distal end of the humerus, for the reception of the olecranon.
palatine f. The incisive fossa.
paracecal f. An infrequent peritoneal pouch behind and to one side of the cecum.
paraduodenal f. See paraduodenal *recess.*
pararectal f. A pouch of the peritoneum on either side of the rectum.
paravesical f. One on either side of the urinary bladder.
phrenicohepatic f. A pouch of the peritoneum between the left lateral ligament of the liver and the extremity of the left lobe.
pituitary f. The hypophyseal fossa.
postauditory f. A crescentic notch on the temporal bone separating the temporal ridge from the auditory plate.
posterior cranial fossae. The lowest in position of the three pairs (right and left) of the cranial fossae; they lodge the cerebellum, pons, and medulla oblongata. Each fossa is formed by the posterior surface of the petrous and inner surface of the mastoid portion of the temporal bone and the inner surface of the occipital bone below the horizontal limb of the confluence of the sinuses.
pterygoid f. The groove between the medial and lateral laminas of the pterygoid process of the sphenoid bone.
pterygopalatine f. The gap between the pterygoid process of the sphenoid bone and the maxilla and palatine bone: also called *sphenomaxillary f.*
radial f. The depression on the humerus above the capitulum which accommodates the head of the radius in extreme flexion of the forearm.
rectouterine f. The peritoneal pouch between rectum and uterus; the pouch, or cul-de-sac, of Douglas.
retroduodenal f. See retroduodenal *recess.*
rhomboid f. The diamond-shaped floor of the fourth ventricle of the brain.
Rosenmueller's f. See lateral pharyngeal *f.*
scaphoid f. (a) A depression in the base of the medial pterygoid plate of the sphenoid bone. (b) A furrow between the helix and antihelix of the auricle. Syn., *scapha.*
sigmoid f. See sigmoid *sulcus.*
sphenomaxillary f. See pterygopalatine *f.*
subarcuate f. An orifice situated in the newborn on the superior margin of the petrosal portion of the temporal bone, through which the vessels pass to the temporal bone. This opening disappears after birth and is represented in the adult by a depression beneath the arcuate eminence.
subauricular f. The depression just below the external ear.
subinguinal f. The depression of the anterior aspect of the thigh over the femoral triangle.
sublingual f. A depression on the internal surface of the mandible next to the sublingual gland.
submaxillary f. The oblong depression on the internal surface of the mandible, next to the submaxillary gland.
suborbital f. See canine *f.*
subscapular f. The ventral concave surface of the scapula.
subsigmoid f. A peritoneal recess at the apex of the attachment of the mesosigmoid: also called *intersigmoid f.*
sulciform f. A shallow furrow in the inner fore part of the cavity of the vestibule of the ear, behind the fovea hemielliptica and the fovea hemisphaerica, into which the vestibular aqueduct opens.
superior duodenal f. A small pocket of peritoneum formed on the left of the terminal portion of the duodenum by a triangular fold of peritoneum and having the opening directed downward.
supraclavicular f. The depression on either side of the neck above the clavicle.
supraspinous f. The triangular depression on the posterior surface of the scapula above the spine.
suprasternal f. The depression in the midline of the base of the neck above the upper border of the sternum and between the insertion of the sternal portions of the two sternocleidomastoid muscles. Also called *jugular notch.*
supratonsillar f. The upper recess of the tonsillar sinus between the faucial pillars and above the palatine tonsil; it is covered by a semilunar fold.
temporal f. The depression that lodges the temporal muscle.
tonsillar f. The depression between the glossopalatine and pharyngopalatine arches, in which the palatine tonsil is situated. It is approximately at the site of the second visceral pouch.
triangular f. The fossa of the anthelix.
trochanteric f. A hollow at the base of the inner surface of the greater trochanter of the femur.
trochlear f. A hollow in the frontal bone, below the internal angular process, furnishing attachment to the pulley of the superior oblique muscle.

umbilical f. A narrow groove on the visceral and anterior surfaces of the liver occupied by the falciform ligament and round ligament of the liver (the left umbilical vein of the fetus).

urachal f. The prevesical space.

zygomatic f. See infratemporal *f.*

fos·sette′ [F., dim. of *fosse*, canal, ditch]. 1. A dimple; a small depression. 2. A small, deep ulcer of the cornea.

fos′su·la [L., little ditch]. A small fossa; any one of the numerous slight depressions on the surface of the cerebrum.

f. post fenestram. A small inconstant outpouching from the vestibule into the otic capsule just posterior to the fenestra vestibuli.

f. rotunda. Fenestra cochleae, or round window of the ear.

f. tonsillaris. A crypt of the palatine tonsil.

Foster, Michael [*English physiologist*, 1836–1907]. One of the great teachers of physiology of modern times. Investigated the contractility of the heart. Wrote works on general physiology (1877) and the history of physiology (1901).

Fothergill, John [*English physician*, 1712–80]. Described an epidemic of either diphtheria or anginal scarlet fever, perhaps of both (1748); anginal scarlet fever is called *Fothergill's sore throat.* Called attention to the influence of weather on certain diseases. Gave the first clear account of migraine (1777). Described facial neuralgia, called *Fothergill's disease, trigeminal neuralgia, tic douloureux.*

Fothergill, William Edward [*English gynecologist*, 1865–1926]. Emphasized the importance of the parametrial tissue as a support for the uterus. Modified Donald's colporrhaphy by exposing the parametrium and suturing the right and left sides together. Called *Fothergill* or *Manchester operation.*

fou′a·din (fōō′uh·din, ·deen). See *fuadin.*

foun′der [OF. *fondrer*, to fall in]. 1. An acute gastroenteritis in cattle, horses, and sheep caused by the overeating of foods with a high caloric content. 2. Condition of lameness in horses.

found′ling [AS. *findan*]. An infant found after being abandoned by its parents.

four·chet′. 1. *In veterinary medicine*, foot rot. 2. Incorrect spelling for fourchette.

four-chette′ (foor·shet′) [F.]. 1. A fold of skin just inside the posterior commissure of the vulva. 2. A fork used in dividing the frenulum linguae.

Fourneau, Ernest François Auguste [*French chemist and pharmacologist*, 1872–1949]. Introduced amylocaine hydrochloride (1903) and suramin (1923).

Fourneau 309. See *suramin.*

Fournier, Jean Alfred [*French syphilologist*, 1832–1914]. Noted for his profound study of prenatal syphilis. Pointed out the syphilitic nature of the parasyphilitic diseases. Made important contributions to the knowledge of extragenital chancre (1897). Dome-shaped molars are called *Fournier's molars.* See under *molar.*

fo′ve·a [L., a small pit]. A small pit or depression; applied to many depressions in the body, but especially to the **fovea centralis** of the retina (the spot of most distinct vision), a small pit in the macula lutea in the visual axis. —**foveate,** *adj.*

coccygeal f. A persistent depression near the tip of the coccyx at the site of the terminal attachment of the embryonic neural tube to the dermis: also called *postanal dimple, f. sacrococcygea.*

costal f. A costal depression on a vertebra, a demifacet for the head of a rib.

f. articularis superior atlantis. Either of the superior articular surfaces of the atlas.

f. of the head of the femur. That giving attachment to the ligamentum teres femoris. Also called *f. capitis femoris.*

f. of the head of the radius. That for articulation with the capitulum of the humerus. Also called *f. capituli radii.*

f. of the pharynx. An anomalous depression in the median line of the pharynx.

f. palatina. See *foveola palatina.*

f. pterygoidea mandibulae. A small depression on the anterior aspect of the neck of the mandible where the external pterygoid muscle is inserted.

f. sublingualis mandibulae. A smooth shallow depression on the internal surface of the body of the mandible above the mylohyoid line for the sublingual gland: also called *sublingual fossa, sublingual pit.*

f. submaxillaris mandibulae. A smooth shallow depression on the internal surface of the body of the mandible below the mylohyoid line for the submaxillary gland: also called *submaxillary fossa, submaxillary pit.*

hemielliptical f. A small depression on the inner wall of the labyrinth. It is perforated for the passage of filaments of the auditory nerve.

hemispheric f. A depression in the roof of the bony labyrinth.

inferior f. That in the inferior part of the floor of the fourth ventricle, marking the end of the sulcus limitans.

lateral inguinal f. A depression in the anterior wall of the peritoneal cavity lateral to the epigastric fold.

medial inguinal f. A depression in the anterior wall of the peritoneal cavity between the lateral umbilical fold and the ridge made by the inferior epigastric vessels, the epigastric fold.

oblong f. A shallow depression on the external surface of an arytenoid cartilage.

superior f. That in the floor of the fourth ventricle near the facial colliculus, formed by the widening of the sulcus limitans.

supravesical f. A depression in the anterior wall of the peritoneal cavity between the medial and lateral umbilical folds.

triangular f. A deep depression on the external surface of an arytenoid cartilage.

trochlear f. A hollow in the orbital plate of the frontal bone for the trochlea of the superior oblique muscle.

fo·ve′o·la [dim. of *fovea*]. A small fovea or depression. —**foveolate,** *adj.*

f. palatina. One of a pair of small depressions in the mucous membrane at the boundary between hard and soft palate, into which several palatine glands open. Syn., *fovea palatina.*

gastric f. One of the pits or grooves in the mucous membrane of the stomach, which receive the secretions of the gastric glands.

granular f. Any one of the small pits in the cranial bones produced by the Pacchionian bodies.

triangular f. A triangular depression between the anterior pillars of the fornix, 2.

Foville, Achille Louis François [*French neurologist*, 1799–1878]. Remembered for his important contributions to neurology. Described a syndrome of conjugate ocular deviation palsy, with or without peripheral facial paralysis on one side and upper motor paralysis of the bulbar muscles and limbs on the opposite side, due to lesions of the pons (1858); called *crossed paralysis, Foville's syndrome* or *paralysis, unilateral* or *bilateral gaze paralysis.*

Fowler, George Ryerson [*American surgeon*, 1848–1906]. Credited with introducing thoracoplasty

(1893). Described an incision somewhat similar to the gridiron incision, but slightly nearer the median line, for appendectomy. Devised an operation, now rarely used, of decortication of the lung for chronic empyema; called *Fowler's* or *Fowler-Delorme operation.* See also Fowler's *position.*

Fowler, Thomas [*English physician,* 1736–1801]. Introduced *Fowler's solution.* See *potassium* arsenite solution.

Fox, George Henry [*American dermatologist,* 1846–1937]. With Fordyce, described a rare disease, called *Fox-Fordyce disease,* characterized by an itching papular eruption affecting principally the axillas (1902). This is thought to be due to dysfunction of the sweat glands.

Fox, William Tilbury [*English dermatologist,* 1836–79]. Internationally known for his many contributions to the knowledge of dermatology. Gave first description of impetigo contagiosa (1864), called *impetigo of Tilbury Fox.* Gave first description of dyshidrosis or pompholyx (1873). First to describe epidermolysis bullosa (1879), called *Goldscheider's disease* (1882). Gave first description of dermatitis herpetiformis (1880), also called *Duhring's disease.*

fox′glove″. See *digitalis.*

FP Abbreviation for flavin phosphate (riboflavin-5′-phosphate).

Fracastoro, Girolamo (Fracastorius) [*Italian pathologist,* 1483–1553]. Author of the famous medical poem, *Syphilis Sive Morbus Gallicus,* which included all the knowledge of the time regarding syphilis and gave the disease its name (1530). Recognized the origin of syphilis and suggested mercury treatment. Contributed greatly to the knowledge of infectious and contagious disease and suggested the germ theory of infection (1546). Has been described as the founder of scientific epidemiology. Gave the first authentic account of typhus (1546).

frac′tion·al [L. *fractio,* from *frangere,* to break]. 1. Pertaining to a fraction. 2. *In chemistry,* divided successively; applied to any one of the several processes for separating a mixture into its constituents through differences in solubility, boiling point, etc., such as fractional distillation, fractional sterilization, etc.

frac″tion·a′tion [*fractio*]. 1. *In chemistry,* the separation of a mixture into its constituents, as in fractional distillation. 2. *In microbiology,* the process of obtaining a pure culture by successive culturing of small portions of a colony. Also called *fractional cultivation.* 3. *In physiology,* the phenomenon whereby maximal stimulation of a given efferent nerve produces contraction of only a fraction of the fibers in the responding muscle.

fract′ure [L. *fractura,* fracture, from *frangere*]. The breaking of a bone or cartilage. See Plates 35, 36, 37.

articular f. A fracture entering into a joint.

avulsion f. The tearing off of a bony prominence, as a tuberosity, by the forcible pull of its tendinous or muscular attachments.

bumper f. A fracture of the leg from collision with the bumper of a motor car.

buttonhole f. See puncture *f.*

chip f. A minor fracture involving a bony process.

closed f. A simple fracture.

Colles' f. A fracture of the distal end of the radius within one inch of the articular surface; characterized by dorsal displacement of the distal fragment, radial and dorsal deviation of the wrist and hand, and disturbance of the radioulnar articulation. See Plate 35.

comminuted f. A fracture in which there is splintering or fragmentation of the bone.

complete f. One in which the continuity of the entire bone is destroyed.

complicated f. One associated with injury of the surrounding soft parts, which will complicate treatment and/or recovery.

compound f. One in which the point of fracture is in contact with the external surface of the body: also called *open f.*

compression f. One in which a surface of a bone is driven toward another bony surface: commonly found in vertebral bodies.

congenital f. See intrauterine *f.*

Cotton's f. See trimalleolar *f.*

dentate f. One in which the ends of the fragments are toothed and interlocked.

depressed f. A fracture of the skull in which the fractured part is depressed below the normal level.

double f. One in which there are two fractures in the same bone.

epicondylar f. One involving an epicondyle of one of the long bones.

epiphyseal f. One occurring along the epiphyseal line.

extracapsular f. A fracture near a joint but not entering within the joint capsule.

fatigue f. See march *f.*

fissured f. One in which there is an incomplete break; a crack or fissure extending into, but not through, a bone.

f. by contre-coup. A fracture of the skull caused by transmitted violence to the cranial vault, causing a break at a point distant from, and usually opposite, the site of trauma.

greenstick f. An incomplete fracture of a long bone, seen in children; the bone is bent but splintered only on the convex side.

gutter f. A form of depressed fracture of the skull with an elliptic depression; often caused by a missile.

impacted f. A fracture in which the harder cortical bone of one fragment has been driven into the softer cancellous bone of another fragment.

incomplete f. One which does not extend through the entire bone.

intracapsular f. One within the joint capsule.

intrauterine f. A fracture occurring during fetal life.

march f. Fracture of the metatarsal bones without obvious trauma, as a result of marching. Syn., *fatigue f., stress f.*

multiple f. Two or more fractures occurring in the same or different bones.

open f. See compound *f.*

pathologic f. One which occurs at the site of a local disease in a bone (as metastatic carcinoma) without external violence.

Pott's f. Fracture of the inferior tibiofibular joint; usually associated with a splitting off of the tip of the medial malleolus, rupture of the tibial collateral ligament, and outward displacement of the foot. See Plate 36.

puncture f. One in which there is a loss of bone without disruption of continuity, as a hole drilled through a bone by a projectile.

pyramidal facial f. A fracture of the face in which the upper jaw is completely separated from the rest of the skull. The break extends upward through each maxillary sinus to the ethmoid region and base of the nose, assuming a pyramidal shape with base upward.

silver-fork f. See Colles' *f.*

simple f. One in which there is no communication with the outside.

spontaneous f. One occurring without apparent trauma; occurs in cases of bone atrophy or other general diseases of the bone.

sprain f. A sprain, usually of the ankle joint, complicated by a fracture or chipping of the bone.
stellate f. One in which there are numerous fissures radiating from the central point of injury.
stress f. See march *f.*
subperiosteal f. One in which the overlying periosteum is intact.
supracondylar f. A fracture of the lower end of the humerus above the condyles. See Plate 35.
T f. A fracture of the end of a long bone, in the form of the letter T. Specifically, the intercondylar fracture of the lower end of the humerus, with splitting of the shaft.
trimalleolar f. A fracture in which the medial and lateral malleoli and the posterior lip of the tibia are fractured, usually associated with a posterior dislocation of the talus: also called *Cotton's f.*
ununited f. One in which, after the normal period, there is failure of union.

frac'ture box. A wooden case for immobilizing fractures of the leg.

frac'ture-dis"lo·ca'tion. See under *dislocation.*

frad'i·cin. An antibiotic substance isolated from cultures of *Streptomyces fradiae;* it is active against certain fungi.

Fraenkel, Albert [*German physician,* 1848–1916]. Showed the causal relation of the *Diplococcus pneumoniae* to pneumonia (1886). The organism had been isolated previously by both Pasteur and Sternberg.

frae'nu·lum (freen'yoo·lum, fren'yoo·lum). See *frenulum.*

frae'num (free'num). See *frenum.*

fra·gil'i·tas [L.]. Brittleness.
f. crinium. Atrophic condition of the hair in which the individual hairs split into numerous fibrils or break off.
f. ossium. Osteogenesis imperfecta.

fra·gil'i·ty [*fragilitas*]. Quality of being easily broken or destroyed. —**frag'ile,** *adj.*
capillary f. Weakness of the capillaries, as in purpura.
erythrocytic f. See osmotic *f.* and mechanical *f.*
mechanical f. The susceptibility to breakage of erythrocytes when mechanically agitated, as with glass beads in a flask. Also see under *test.*
osmotic f. The susceptibility to the lysis of the erythrocytes when placed in hypotonic saline solutions. Also see under *test.*

frag"men·ta'tion [L. *fragmentum,* a piece, from *frangere,* to break]. 1. Division into small portions. 2. Amitosis.

fragments of Spengler. See Carl *Spengler.*

fram·be'si·a (fram·bee'zhuh, ·zee·uh). See *yaws.*

fram·be'si·form. Of, pertaining to, or like frambesia: said especially of a cutaneous eruption simulating or identical to that of yaws.

Frame, Russell, and Wilhelmi's method. See under *method.*

Francis, Edward (1872–). American bacteriologist and physician, principal investigator of transmission of tularemia by insects among small animals to man. He discovered the essential requirement of cystine for the growth of *Pasteurella tularensis* (1923).

Francis, Thomas, Jr. [*American pathologist,* 1900–]. Introduced a skin test for the presence of antibody in pneumococcal pneumonia. See Francis *test.*

fran'ci·um [after *France*]. Element number 87, symbol Fr, isolated in 1939 by Perey; formerly called virginium.

Franco, Pierre [*French surgeon,* 1500–61]. Gave first description of an operation for strangulated hernia (1556) and performed first suprapubic cystotomy in the same year.

fran'gu·la [L. *frangere,* to break]. The bark of *Rhamnus frangula,* or glossy buckthorn. The fresh bark is strongly irritant and causes violent catharsis; when dried it is laxative. Dose, 1–2 Gm. (15–30 gr.). The dose of the fluidextract is 1 cc. (15 min.).

fran'gu·lin. $C_{21}H_{20}O_9$; 4,5,7-trihydroxy-2-methylanthraquinone-L-rhamnoside; a glycoside occurring in *Rhamnus* species. On hydrolysis it yields emodin and L-rhamnose. Syn., *avornin, emodin-L-rhamnoside, franguloside, rhamnoxanthin.*

fran'gu·lo·side. Frangulin.

frank. *In medicine,* actual, unmistakable, obvious: jargon.

Frank, Alfred Erich [*German physician,* 1884–]. Described essential thrombopenia (1915). Nonthrombopenic purpura is also called *Frank's capillary toxicosis.* Demonstrated the relationship of the posterior lobe of the pituitary body to diabetes insipidus (1912).

Frank, Fritz [*German gynecologist,* 1856–1923]. Described an operation of Cesarean section in which the uterus is drawn out of the abdomen before incising.

Frank, Johann Peter [*German physician,* 1745–1821]. Called one of the founders of the science of public health. First to differentiate between diabetes insipidus and diabetes mellitus.

Frank, Rudolph [*Austrian surgeon,* 1862–1913]. Devised an operation of gastrostomy equivalent to that described by Sabaneev. A cone of stomach is pulled through a high rectus incision and under the costal arch, passing through a skin tunnel, to be anchored. Called *Frank's operation, Sabaneev-Frank operation.*

Franke's method. See Benedict and Franke's *method.*

frank'in·cense [OF. *franc,* free; *encens,* incense]. An aromatic gum resin. See *olibanum.*

Franklin, Benjamin [*American scientist and statesman,* 1706–90]. Influenced American medicine by his gospel of fresh air and his modern views on "catching cold." Invented bifocal spectacles, called *Franklin's glasses.* Gave an account of the success of inoculation for smallpox in England and America (1759). His investigations of static electricity were of the first importance.

Frapolli, Francesco [*Italian physician,* d. ca. 1773]. Remembered for his description of pellagra, in which he gave the disease its name (1771).

Fraser, John [*English botanist,* 1750–1817]. Remembered for his discovery of the tonic properties of the root of the American calumba or *Frasera carolinensis.*

Fraser, Thomas Richard [*British pharmacologist,* 1841–1920]. Remembered for his introduction of *Strophanthus* as a medicine (1892). Did valuable work in immunization against cobra venom in India, leading to his production of antivenin (1895). With Alexander Crum Brown, was first to study the chemical constitution of drugs in relation to their physiologic action.

Fraunhofer's lines. See *absorption* bands.

frax'in. A glycoside, $C_{16}H_{18}O_{10}$, from the bark of the European ash, *Fraxinus excelsior;* it is diuretic.

Frazier, Charles Harrison [*American neurologist and surgeon,* 1870–1936]. With Spiller, introduced intracranial trigeminal neurotomy of the sensory root for the relief of trigeminal neuralgia (1901), called *Frazier's operation, Spiller's operation.* He made cordotomy a practical surgical procedure. *Frazier's needle* is a hollow needle to be inserted in the lateral ventricles of the brain when continuous drainage is desired.

F.R.C.P. Fellow of the Royal College of Physicians.

F.R.C.P.E. Fellow of the Royal College of Physicians of Edinburgh.

F.R.C.P.I. Fellow of the Royal College of Physicians of Ireland.

F.R.C.S. Fellow of the Royal College of Surgeons.

F.R.C.S.E. Fellow of the Royal College of Surgeons of Edinburgh.

F.R.C.S.I. Fellow of the Royal College of Surgeons of Ireland.

Fredet, Pierre [*French surgeon,* 1870–1946]. Distinguished for his original work on the relief of congenital pyloric stenosis by incision of the serosa and muscular layer to the mucosa without opening the duodenum. Called *Fredet-Ramstedt operation.*

free′mar″tin. An intersexual female calf, commonly sterile, twinborn with a male; produced by masculinization by sex hormones of the male twin when the placental circulations are partially fused.

free rad′i·cal. A non-ionic compound, highly reactive and of relatively short life, in which the central element is linked to an abnormal number of atoms or groups of atoms.

Frei, Wilhelm Siegmund [*German dermatologist,* 1885–1943]. Established a specific test for venereal lymphogranuloma (1925). This consists of an intradermal antigen injection prepared from material containing the virus, called *Frei test, Frei's reaction.* Venereal lymphogranuloma is known as *Frei's disease, Durand-Nicolas-Favre disease.*

Freiberg, Albert Henry [*American orthopedic surgeon,* 1868–1940]. Described osteochondrosis of the epiphysis of the head of the second metatarsal bone of adolescents, called *Freiberg's disease, Freiberg's infraction of metatarsal head, Köhler's disease.*

frem′i·tus [L., a resounding, murmuring noise]. A palpable vibration.

echinococcus f. The vibration felt over an echinococcus cyst.

friction f. The vibrations produced by the rubbing together of two dry surfaces.

rhonchal f. Vibrations produced by the passage of air through a large bronchial tube containing mucus.

tactile f. The vibratory sensation conveyed to the hand when applied to the chest of a person speaking.

tussive f. Thrill felt by the hand when applied to the chest of a person coughing.

vocal f. The sounds of the voice transmitted to the ear when applied to the chest of a person speaking.

Frenkel, Heinrich S. [*Swiss neurologist,* 1860–1931]. Devised a system of muscular exercises for the treatment of incoordination in tabes dorsalis in which the limbs are flexed and extended, abducted and adducted; this is followed by sitting and rising, then stepping forward and backward. Called *Frenkel's exercise treatment of ataxia* (1890). Described a sign of hypotony of the muscles of the lower extremities in tabes, called *Frenkel's sign.*

fre·not′o·my [L. *frenum,* curb; G. *tomē,* a cutting]. The cutting of any frenum, particularly of the frenulum of the tongue for tongue-tie.

fren′u·lum, frae′nu·lum (freen′yoo·lum, fren′·) [L., dim. of *frenum*]. A small frenum; a slight ridge on the upper part of the anterior medullary velum.

f. of Giacomini. A narrow band between the uncus and the fascia dentata. Also called *band of Giacomini.*

f. of the clitoris. Either of two folds of skin coming from the labia minora and being united under the glans of the clitoris.

f. of the ileocecal valve. The upper or lower lip of the ileocecal valve.

f. of the lips. One of the folds of mucous membrane in the median line uniting each lip to the corresponding gum.

f. of the prepuce. The fold on the lower surface of the glans penis connecting it with the prepuce.

f. of the pudendum. The fourchette.

f. of the tongue. The vertical fold of mucous membrane under the tongue.

f. of the velum. The thickened median portion of the anterior medullary velum.

f. valvulae coli. The fold at either extremity of the ileocecal valve where the upper and lower margins fuse.

fre′num, frae′num [L.]. A fold of integument or mucous membrane that checks or limits the movements of any organ. See *frenulum.* —**frenal,** *adj.*

fren′zy [G. *phrēn,* mind]. Violent mania.

freon. Trade-mark for a group of halogenated hydrocarbons containing one or more fluorine atoms; widely used as refrigerants and propellants for the dispersion of insecticidal mists.

freon-12. Trade-mark for dichlorodifluoromethane, CCl_2F_2, used as a refrigerant and propellant.

fre′quen·cy [L. *frequens,* crowded, frequent]. 1. Rate of occurrences of a periodic process. 2. *In biometry,* the ratio of the number of observations falling within a classification group to the total number of observations made.

audio f. Any one or all of the frequencies within the audible range.

electromagnetic f. The number of complete electromagnetic waves, or cycles, per second.

fusion f. The lowest frequency at which flashes of light produce on the retina the impression of a steady light rather than a flicker. Also called *critical fusion f.*

gene f. The ratio in which the members of a given gene pair, *A* and *a*, are present in the population, or the relative number in which the three types of individuals, *AA*, *Aa*, and *aa* occur in the population.

radio f. Any one or all of the frequencies above the audible range.

fre′quen·cy dis″tri·bu′tion. *In biometry,* a statistical table showing the frequency, or number, of observations (as test scores, ages, etc.) falling in each of certain classification groups or intervals (as 10–19, 20–29, etc.).

Frerichs, Friedrich Theodor von [*German pathologist and clinician,* 1819–85]. Discovered leucine and tyrosine in the urine in acute yellow atrophy of the liver (1855). Gave the first scientific description of multiple sclerosis (1849), and the first description of progressive lenticular degeneration (1861).

Freud, Sigmud (1856–1939). Austrian psychiatrist, who first suggested the use of cocaine as a surface analgesic. With J. Breuer, he is credited with the discovery of the unconscious mind. From his observations of neurosis, especially hysteria, he developed a system of psychology, first employed as a technique in the therapeutic management of psychoneurotic disorders, which he named *psychoanalysis* and which evolved into the *psychoanalytic theory.* Stressing the formative years of childhood, it approaches mental phenomena of the present by a study of the individual's past. By studying dreams, neurotic symptoms, slips of tongue, hypnotic phenomena, common errors, and the like, Freud demonstrated many unconscious mental forces. He introduced a hypothetical but useful division of the mind into the *id, ego,* and *superego;* the pleasure-pain principle; the phase or stage concept of child development (oral, anal, phallic, latent, and genital); the Oedipus complex; and many other concepts and their terminology now employed in psychiatry as well as by society at large. —**Freud′ian,** *adj.*

Freud′i·an (froyd′ee·un) [*Freud*]. One who adheres to Freud's school of psychoanalysis.

Freundlich, Herbert Max Finlay [*German physiological chemist,* 1880–1941]. Known for his description of an adsorption equation as one relating the amount of a solute adsorbed and its concentration; called *Freundlich's adsorption equation.*

Freyer, Peter Johnston [*English surgeon,* 1851–1921]. Did much to popularize the suprapubic prostatectomy. Although his claim to its origination (1900) was antedated by Fuller, the operation is still called *Freyer's operation.*

Frey's syndrome. See auriculotemporal *syndrome.*

F.R.F.P.S. Fellow of the Royal Faculty of Physicians and Surgeons.

F.R.F.P.S.G. Fellow of the Royal Faculty of Physicians and Surgeons of Glasgow.

fri′a·ble [L. *friare,* to break into small pieces]. Easily broken or crumbled.

Frick, George [*American ophthalmologist,* 1793–1870]. Remembered for his operation for entropion, a blepharoplasty in which a tongue-shaped flap is taken from the temple or cheek; called *Frick's operation.* Published first important textbook on ophthalmology in America (1823).

fric′tion [L. *frictio,* from *fricare,* to rub]. 1. The act of rubbing, as rubbing the body for stimulation of the skin. 2. The resistance offered to motion between two contacting bodies.

Friderichsen, Carl (1886–). Danish pediatrician, who described a syndrome, previously observed by R. Waterhouse, and now called *Waterhouse-Friderichsen syndrome.*

Friedemann and Graeser's method. See under *method.*

Friedländer, Carl [*German pathologist,* 1847–87]. First to describe thromboangiitis obliterans (1876). Isolated *Klebsiella pneumoniae* (1883), called *Friedländer's bacillus,* the causative agent of Friedländer pneumonia. He also described the large connective-tissue cells of the decidua, called *Friedländer's cells.*

Friedman, Maurice Harold (1903–). American physiologist who investigated the mechanisms of ovulation in the rabbit, and the physiology of the female reproductive tract. He is known for his test for pregnancy. See Friedman *test.*

Friedman test. See under *test.*

Friedmann, Max [*German neurologist,* 1858–1925]. Remembered for his description of relapsing spastic spinal paralysis and for his observations on postconcussion syndrome, which he attributed to a slowly developing encephalitis with acute exacerbations. See Friedmann's vasomotor *symptom complex.*

Friedreich, Nikolaus [*German neurologist,* 1825–82]. Described paramyoclonus multiplex (1881), called *Friedreich's disease.* First to describe a hereditary spinal sclerosis with impairment of speech, lateral curvature of the spine, and lower limb palsy (1863), called *Friedreich's ataxia.* Described a sign for cavitation of the lungs, in which there is a change in the percussion note during inspiration and expiration; called *Friedreich's sign.*

Friedrich, Paul Leopold [*German surgeon,* 1864–1916]. Described his operation, now obsolete, for lung collapse, in which he employed extrapleural thoracoplasty from the second to the ninth ribs, removing periosteum and muscle bundles; called *Friedrich-Brauer operation.*

fright [AS. *fryhto*]. Sudden and extreme fear.

precordial f. The precordial sensations of impending physical collapse experienced in the acute panic of an anxiety neurosis.

fri·gid′i·ty [L. *frigidus,* cold]. Coldness; absence of sexual desire in women, probably of psychic origin.

frig″o·ther′a·py [L. *frigus,* cold; G. *therapeia,* treatment]. The treatment of disease by cold.

fringe [OF., from L. *fimbria,* fringe]. One of a number of bands, light or dark, produced by the interference of light.

Frisch, Anton Ritter von [*Austrian surgeon and bacteriologist,* 1849–1917]. Known for his description of *Klebsiella rhinoscleromatis,* called *Frisch's bacillus,* found in cases of rhinoscleroma.

Fritsch, Gustav Theodor [*German neurologist,* 1838–1927]. Made experimental studies with Hitzig (1870) on electric stimulation of the cerebral cortex of the frontal lobe, proving the existence of a motor area.

Froehlich, Alfred [*Austrian neurologist and pharmacologist in the United States,* 1871–]. Gave a classic description of adiposogenital dystrophy (1901), also called *Froehlich's syndrome, Babinski-Froehlich's disease.*

frog [AS. *frogga*]. 1. A leaping amphibian of the genus *Rana;* it is tailless, smooth-skinned, and has webbed feet. 2. An elastic, horny pad, in the middle of the sole of a horse's hoof; it is triangular in shape and serves to separate the two bars.

Frohde's reagent. See under *reagent.*

Froin's syndrome. See loculation *syndrome.*

frôle″ment′ (frawl″mahn′. *See* Notes § 35) [F.]. A succession of slow, brushing movements in massage, done with the palmar surfaces of the fingers.

Froment's sign. See under *sign.*

Frommann, Carl [*German anatomist,* 1831–92]. Described the transverse striae or lines appearing in the axis cylinder of medullated nerve fibers after staining with silver nitrate, called *Frommann's lines.*

Frommel, Richard [*German gynecologist,* 1854–1912]. Described an operation for retrodisplacement of the uterus by shortening the uterosacral ligaments by the abdominal route, called *Frommel's operation.* Drew attention to the atrophy of the uterus sometimes occurring after prolonged lactation, called *Frommel's disease.*

front′ad (frun′tad, fron′tad) [L. *frons,* forehead; *ad,* toward]. Toward the frontal aspect.

fron′tal (frun′tul, fron′tul) [*frons*]. 1. Pertaining to the anterior part or aspect of an organ or body. 2. Belonging to the forehead. See Table of Bones in the Appendix.

fron·ta′lis (frun·tah′lis, ·tay′lis, ·tal′is) [*frons*]. The frontal portion of the epicranius muscle.

fron′tal nerve. See Table of Nerves in the Appendix.

fron′to- [*frons*]. *In anatomy* and *zoology,* combining form denoting *anterior position* or expressing *a relation with the forehead* or *frontal region.*

fron″to·ma′lar [*frons;* L. *mala,* cheek-bone]. Relating to the frontal and to the zygomatic bones.

fron″to·max′il·lar″y (fron″to·mack′si·lerr″ee) [*frons;* L. *maxilla,* jawbone]. Relating to the frontal bone and the maxilla.

fron″to·men′tal [*frons;* L. *mentum,* chin]. Running from the top of the forehead to the point of the chin or relating to the forehead and chin.

fron″to·na′sal [*frons;* L. *nasus,* nose]. Pertaining to the frontal and nasal bones, as frontonasal suture: also *nasofrontal.*

fron″to-oc·cip′i·tal (fron″to-ock·sip′i·tul) [*frons;* L. *occiput,* back part of the head]. Pertaining to the forehead and the occiput or to the frontal and occipital bones, as fronto-occipital muscle.

fron″to-tem″po·ra′le (fron″to-tem″po·rah′lee, ·ray′lee) (pl. *fronto-temporalia*) [*frons;* L. *tempus,* temple]. That point on the superior temporal line on the zygomatic process of the frontal bone which is located most anteriorly and medially. The two fronto-temporalia form the points of departure for measuring the least frontal diameter of the skull.

Froriep, August von [*German anatomist,* 1849–1917]. Described fibrous myositis, called *Froriep's induration.* See also Froriep's *ganglion.*

Frosch, Paul [*German physician,* 1860–1928]. With Loeffler, was first to discover a filtrable virus to be the cause of a disease of animals (foot and mouth disease, 1897).

frost′bite″ [AS. *frost; bītan*]. A condition similar to the lesions produced by burns, resulting from exposure to severe degrees of cold. The three stages of frostbite are marked by erythema, vesication, and necrosis, respectively. The parts most commonly affected are the ears, tip of the nose, fingers, and toes.

frost′-itch″ [*frost;* AS. *gicce*]. Pruritus hiemalis.

froth sta′bi·li″zer. Certain oils and chemicals which produce stable froths in water; they function best in the presence of finely divided solids.

frot″tage′ (fraw″tahzh′. *See* NOTES § 35) [F.]. 1. Massage, rubbing. 2. A form of sexual perversion in which orgasm is induced by rubbing against someone.

frot″teur′ (fraw″tur′. *See* NOTES § 35) [F.]. A sexual pervert who practices frottage.

fro′zen sec′tions. Histologic sections cut from frozen tissues or organs, as from those removed from the body during operation and examined immediately for possible malignancy.

F.R.S. Fellow of the Royal Society.

F.R.S.E. Fellow of the Royal Society of Edinburgh.

fruc″to·fu·ran′o·san. One of the polysaccharides of fructose.

fruc″to·fu′ran·ose. A fructose with a 2-5 butylene oxide or furanose ring.

fruc″to·fu·ran′o·side. A glycoside of fructofuranose.

fruc″to·py′ran·ose. A fructose with a 2-6 pyranose ring.

fruc′to·san. See *levulosan.*

fruc′tose [L. *fructus,* fruit]. Levulose.

fruc′tose-1,6-di·phos′phate. $C_6H_{14}O_{12}P_2$; D-fructose-1,6-diphosphoric acid; an ester formed from fructose-6-phosphate and adenosinetriphosphate in the presence of magnesium ion and phosphohexokinase; it is an intermediate in carbohydrate metabolism. Syn., *Harden-Young ester, hexosediphosphate.*

fruc′tose-1-phos′phate. $C_6H_{13}O_9P$; D-fructose-1-phosphoric acid, formed by the action of liver hexokinase upon fructose; presumably it is then converted to fructose-6-phosphate in the presence of phosphofructomutase.

fruc′tose-6-phos′phate. $C_6H_{13}O_9P$; D-fructose-6-phosphoric acid, present in animal tissues in equilibrium with glucose-6-phosphate, into which it may be reversibly converted in the presence of phosphohexose isomerase; it is an intermediate in carbohydrate metabolism. Syn., *fructose monophosphate, hexosemonophosphate, Neuberg ester.*

fruc′to·side. A glycoside which yields fructose (levulose) on hydrolysis.

fruc″to·su′ri·a [*fructus;* G. *ouron,* urine]. The presence of fructose in the urine; levulosuria.

fru·giv′o·rous (froo·jiv′o·rus, ·giv′o·rus) [L. *frux,* fruit; *vorare,* to devour]. Fruit-eating.

fruit [L. *fructus,* fruit]. The developed ovary of a plant, including the succulent, fleshy parts gathered about the same.

fruit sug′ar. Levulose.

fru″men·ta′ceous [L. *frumentum,* grain]. Belonging to or resembling grain.

fru·men′tum [L.]. Wheat or other grain.

spiritus frumenti. Whisky.

frus′trane [L. *frustra,* without effect]. Faintly heard, as a frustrane extrasystole.

frus·tra′tion [L. *frustratio,* from *frustrari,* to frustrate]. 1. The condition that results when an impulse to act or the completion of an act is blocked or thwarted, preventing the satisfaction of attainment. 2. The blocking or thwarting of an impulse.

frus′tule. The siliceous shell of a diatom, consisting of two overlapping valves.

FSH Abbreviation for follicle-stimulating *hormone.*

ft. 1. *In pharmacy,* fiat or fiant; let there be made. 2. Abbreviation for foot.

ft.-lb. Abbreviation for foot-pound.

fuadin. The trade-mark of sodium-antimony-bispyrocatechol-3,5-sodium disulfonate, employed in the treatment of granuloma inguinale and of schistosomiasis. See *stibophen.*

Fuchs, Alfred [*Bohemian neurologist in Austria,* 1870–1927]. With Robert Rosenthal, devised a chamber for cytologic counting other than blood counting. The *Fuchs-Rosenthal counting chamber,* which is 0.2 mm. deep, has triple lines marking 16 divisions 1 mm. square, and single lines dividing each of these squares into 16 smaller squares.

Fuchs, Ernst [*Austrian ophthalmologist,* 1851–1930]. Described peripheral optic nerve atrophy (1885), called *Fuchs's atrophy.* His textbook (1889) became a classic and was translated into many languages. A crescentic conus is known as *Fuchs's conus. Fuchs's black spot* is observed in choroidal changes in myopia.

Fuchs, Leonhard [*German botanist,* 1501–66]. Author of the most widely known herbal of the sixteenth century, the most extensive study of pharmacology of the time (1542). Described many varieties of American plants, including the *fuchsias,* whose name is derived from the author's.

fuch′sin (fŏŏk′sin, fōōk′sin). A red dyestuff occurring in two forms, acid and basic.

acid f. (a) A mixture of sodium and ammonium salts of rosaniline sulfonic acids; reddish brown crystals. (b) (C.C.) The disodium salt of rosaniline, or pararosaniline, trisulfonate, or a mixture of these; used as a biologic stain. Also called *acid magenta, acid rubin, fuchsin S, SN, SS, ST,* or *SIII.*

basic f. (C.C.). A dye, or group of dyes, of the triphenyl methane group; mixtures of the chlorides or acetates of pararosaniline and rosaniline and magenta II in varying proportions. Used as a bacterial stain and in general histologic work; a 0.06% aqueous solution of basic fuchsin (90% dye content) is employed. The lustrous green crystals are used as a germicide and granulating agent in skin diseases, generally in 1% strength. Also called *diamond fuchsin, magenta, aniline red, rubin.*

fuch·sin′o·phil (fŏŏk·sin′o·fil, fŏŏk·). Stainable with fuchsin.

fu′co·san. Polysaccharide yielding L-fucose, an aldohexose, upon hydrolysis. Occurs in the seaweed Japanese nori.

fu′cose. $C_6H_{12}O_5$; an aldose, terminating in a methyl group at the number 6 carbon atom, existing in D- and L-forms. D-Fucose is obtained by hydrolysis of convolvulin, jalapin, and other glycosides; L-fucose occurs in certain seaweeds. Syn., *6-desoxygalactose,* D-*galactomethylose, rhodeose* (D-*fucose*).

fu″co·ster′ol. $C_{29}H_{47}OH$; the typical sterol of the marine brown algae of the class Phaeophyceae.

fu″co·xan′thin. A carotenoid pigment found in fresh brown algae of the class Phaeophyceae.

fu′cus. The dried thallus of *Fucus vesiculosus* and other common brown algae of the rockweed group. It contains a small amount of combined iodine, and has been used in the treatment of obesity.

Fuerbringer, Paul [*German physician*, 1849–1930]. Remembered for his description of a sign of subphrenic abscess in which respiratory movement is transmitted to a needle inserted into the abscess, whereas in an abscess situated above the diaphragm, the inserted needle does not move; called *Fuerbringer's sign.*

Fuerstner, Carl [*German psychiatrist*, 1848–1906]. Described pseudospastic paralysis accompanied by tremor, called *Fuerstner's disease.*

fu·ga′cious [L. *fugax*, flying swiftly]. *In biology*, falling off, as the falling off or fading of petals after the full bloom of a flower.

-fuge (-fewdj) [L. *fugere*, to flee]. A combining form denoting *that which causes to flee*, or *drives away.*

fu′gi·tive [L. *fugitivus*, fugitive]. Wandering or transient, as a pain.

fugue (fewg) [L. *fuga*, a fleeing]. A state of amnesia of considerable duration, sometimes involving a flight from familiar surroundings. During the fugue, the patient appears to act in a conscious way and retains his mental faculties, but after recovery has no remembrance of the state.

fu′gu poi′son. A poison in the roe and other parts of certain fish of the *Tetrodon* genus, found in Japanese and other eastern Asiatic waters.

ful′gu·ra″ting, ful′gu·rant [L. *fulgurare*, to lighten]. Lightninglike; used to describe sudden excruciating pain.

ful″gu·ra′tion [L. *fulguratio*, from *fulgurare*]. Destruction of tissue, usually malignant tumors, by means of electric sparks.

fu·lig′i·nous (few·lidj′i·nus) [L. *fuliginosus*, full of soot]. Smokelike; very dark; soot-colored.

Fuller, Eugene [*American surgeon*, 1858–1930]. First to publish an account of the successful removal of both intravesical and intraurethral enlargements of the prostate by enucleation, using the suprapubic route (1895). Devised *Fuller's operation* for drainage of the seminal vesicles.

ful′mi·nant, ful′mi·na″ting [L. *fulminare*, to lighten]. Sudden, severe, and rapid in course.

Fulton, John Farquhar (1899–). American neurophysiologist, best known for his writings on the physiology of the nervous system, the history of medicine, and his biography of Harvey Cushing.

Fulton's stain. See *Schaeffer-Fulton modification of Wirtz method* under *stain.*

fu″ma·gil′lin. Generic name for an antibiotic substance produced by certain strains of *Aspergillus fumigatus*, occurring in light-yellow crystals, practically insoluble in water. It possesses an extremely narrow pathogenic spectrum, showing little or no activity as an antimicrobial or antifungal agent; it has specific activity against *Endameba histolytica*, and is used in treating acute intestinal amebiasis. See *fumidil.*

fu′ma·rase. An enzyme occurring in bacteria, molds, yeasts, higher plants, and animals, particularly in liver and muscle. It is a specific catalyst for the conversion of fumaric acid (plus water) to *l*-malic acid.

fu·mar′ate. A salt of fumaric acid.

Fu·ma″ri·a′ce·ae (few·mair″ee·ay′see·ee) [L. *fumus*, smoke]. A family of plants including the genera *Adlumia*, *Corydalis*, *Dicentra*, and *Fumaria;* by some authorities this family is ranked as a subfamily (Fumaroidae) of the Papaveraceae. Many alkaloids are found among the plants of the Fumariaceae.

fu·mar′ic ac′id. COOH.CH:CH.COOH. Trans-ethylene dicarboxylic acid. A dibasic acid, the trans-isomer of maleic acid. It occurs in *Fumaria officinalis* and in mammalian tissues as an intermediate in the metabolism of carbohydrate.

fu′ma·rine (few′muh·reen, ·rin). An alkaloid, $C_{20}H_{19}O_5N$, found in the opium poppy and other Papaveraceae, as well as in plants of the Fumariaceae. It is identical with protopine and macleyine.

fumidil. Trade-mark for the antibiotic substance *fumagillin.*

fu·mi·ga′cin. An antibiotic substance produced by different strains of *Aspergillus fumigatus*. It is identical with helvolic acid.

fu·mi·ga′tin. A maroon-colored, crystalline substance, 3-hydroxy-4-methoxy-2:5-toluquinone, $C_8H_8O_4$, isolated from cultures of *Aspergillus fumigatus*. It has antibacterial properties, but differs from fumigacin.

fu″mi·ga′tion [L. *fumigare*, to smoke]. Disinfection by exposure to the fumes of a vaporized disinfectant.

fu′ming [L. *fumus*, smoke]. Emitting smoke or vapor, as fuming nitric acid.

func′tion [L. *functio*, a performance, from *fungi*, to perform]. 1. The normal or special action of a part. 2. The chemical character, relationships, and general properties of a substance. —**func′tion,** *v.*

func′tion·al. *In psychiatry*, nonorganic.

fun′da·ment [L. *fundamentum*, foundation]. 1. The foundation or base. 2. The buttocks.

fun·dec′to·my. See *fundusectomy.*

fun′di·form [L. *funda*, a sling; *forma*, shape]. Shaped like a sling, or loop.

fun′dus (pl. *fundi*) [L., bottom]. The base of an organ; the part farthest removed from the opening of the organ. —**fundic,** *adj.*

central f. The area of the fundus of the eye that includes the macular and perimacular regions.

f. meatus acustici interni. The bottom or lateral end of the internal auditory canal.

f. oculi. The posterior portion of the interior of the eye. See Plate 19.

f. of the gallbladder. The wide, anterior end of the gallbladder.

f. uteri. That part of the uterus most remote from the cervix. See Plate 41.

f. ventriculi. The large, rounded cul-de-sac cephalad to the cardia of the stomach, when that organ is dilated: also called *fornix of the stomach.*

f. vesicae. The posterior part or base of the urinary bladder.

pepper-and-salt f. A fundus oculi in which yellowish-red, gray, and black spots are present in the choroid: often found in syphilis.

fun′du·scope [L. *fundus*, bottom; G. *skopein*, to examine]. An instrument for the visualization of the fundus of the eye.

fun″du·sec′to·my [L. *fundus*, base; G. *ektomē*, a cutting, excision]. Surgical removal of the fundus of an organ, as of the uterus; often the removal of a wedge-shaped portion of the fundus of the stomach. This operation, removing much of the parietal cell area, is used in the treatment of postoperative jejunal ulcer. Syn., *fundectomy.*

fun′gate (fung′gate, fun′gate) [L. *fungus*, mushroom]. Grow up rapidly, like a fungus, as certain pathologic growths.

fun′gi (fun′jye). Plural of fungus.

fun′gi·cide [*fungus;* L. *caedere*, to kill]. An agent that destroys fungi. —**fungici′dal,** *adj.*

fun′gi·form [*fungus;* L. *forma*, form]. Having the form of a mushroom, as the fungiform papillae of the tongue.

Fun'gi im"per·fec'ti (fun'jye im"pur·feck'tye). Fungi which lack a known sexual phase of reproduction in their life history.

fun"gin·ert'ness. Failure to support fungus growth because of absence of the necessary nutrients: to be distinguished from *fungistasis*. —**funginert',** *adj.*

fun"gi·sta'sis. The active prevention or hindrance of fungus growth by a chemical or physical agent: to be distinguished from *funginertness*.

fun"gi·stat'ic. Inhibiting or preventing the growth of fungi. —**fungistat'ic,** *n.*

fun'goid [*fungus;* G. *eidos,* form]. Resembling a fungus.

fun·gos'i·ty [*fungus*]. 1. A fungous excrescence. 2. Fungous quality.

fun'gus (pl. *fungi*) [L.]. 1. A low form of plant life, a division of the Thallophytes without chlorophyll. The chief classes of fungi are the Phycomycetes, Ascomycetes, Basidiomycetes, and Fungi imperfecti. Most of the pathogenic fungi belong to the last group. 2. A spongy morbid excrescence. For a list of the fungi pathogenic to man, see Table in the Appendix. —**fungous, fungal,** *adj.*

imperfect f. See *Fungi imperfecti.*

mosaic f. An artefact consisting of a deposition of cholesterol crystals deposited around the borders of epithelial cells.

ray f. Any fungus of the genera *Actinomyces* or *Nocardia;* asteroid bodies.

thread f. Any kind of *Trichophyton.*

fu'ni·cle [L. *funiculus,* dim. of *funis,* a cord]. A slender cord, a funiculus.

fu·nic"u·li'tis [*funiculus;* G. *-itis,* inflammation]. Inflammation of a funiculus, specifically, of the spermatic cord.

fu·nic'u·lus (plural *funiculi*) [L.]. 1. One of the three main divisions of white matter, which are named with reference to the gray matter of the cord as dorsal, lateral, and ventral. 2. Old term for fasciculus. 3. Old term for the umbilical or spermatic cord. —**funicular,** *adj.*

f. separans. A white ridge of thickened ependyma, separating the ala cinerea from the area postrema.

fu'nis [L.]. A cord, particularly the umbilical cord. —**funic,** *adj.*

Funk, Casimir [*American biochemist,* 1884–]. Pioneer in the study of vitamins. Credited with introducing the term vitamine, now called vitamin. In a study of multiple neuritis, induced in birds by a diet of polished rice, isolated a curative substance (vitamin B_1) found in rice polishings.

Funke, Otto [*German physician,* 1828–79]. Discovered hemoglobin (1851).

fun'nel [L. *fundere,* to pour]. A wide-mouthed, conical vessel ending in an open tube; for filling bottles or other containers, and as a support for filter papers.

mitral f. A funnellike deformation of the mitral valve; sometimes present in mitral stenosis.

muscular f. The space bounded by the four rectus muscles of the eye (the superior, inferior, lateral, and medial muscles), said to resemble a funnel.

vascular f. The opalescent central depression in the retinal disk.

fun'ny bone. The region behind the medial condyle of the humerus, crossed superficially by the ulnar nerve. Blows upon it give a painful tingling sensation to the cutaneous area supplied by the ulnar nerve.

fur [ME. *furre*]. 1. A coating of epithelial debris, as on the tongue. 2. The hairy coat of some animals. —**furred,** *adj.*

furacin. Trade-mark for nitrofurazone.

furadantin. Trade-mark for the antibacterial agent *nitrofurantoin.*

fur·al'de·hyde. See *furfural.*

fu'ran, fu'rane. CH:CH.CH:CH (ring closed through O). A constituent of wood tars; a colorless liquid, insoluble in water. Also called *furfuran, furfurane.*

2-fu"ran·car"box·yl'ic ac'id. Furoic acid.

fu'ran·ose. A sugar having a ring structure resembling that of furan.

fur'ca [L.]. A fork. —**furcal, furcate,** *adj.*

f. orbitalis. The orbital fork; one of the earliest signs of the orbit seen in the embryo; it is a mere trace of bifurcated bony tissue.

fur'cal·is. Old name for the fourth lumbar nerve.

fur'cu·la (pl. *furculae*) [L., a forked prop]. 1. A crescentic median elevation of the floor of the embryonic pharynx, at the level of the third and fourth visceral arches; differentiates into epiglottis and aryepiglottic folds. Also called *hypobranchial eminence.* 2. A forked process, especially the joined clavicles of a bird; wishbone.

fur'cu·lum [incorrect form of *furcula*]. A furcula; especially the wishbone.

fur'fur [L., bran]. Dandruff; a branny desquamation of the epidermis. —**furfura'ceous,** *adj.*

fur'fur·al. $C_4H_3O.CHO$. A liquid obtained by distillation of oat hulls and corn cobs with diluted sulfuric acid. Used as a solvent and reagent, and as an insecticide and fungicide. Also called *fural, furole, furaldehyde, furfuraldehyde.*

fur'fur·an, fur'fur·ane. Furan.

fur'fur·yl [*furfur;* G. *hylē,* material]. The monovalent radical C_5H_5O— derived from furfural.

fur'fur·yl al'co·hol. $C_5H_6O_2$; a poisonous liquid obtained from furfural, and also by steam distillation of roasted coffee bean: used as a solvent and in various syntheses.

fu'ri·bund [L. *furibundus,* raging]. Raging; maniacal; applied to certain insane patients. *Obs.*

furmethide iodide. Trade-marked name for furtrethonium iodide.

fu"ro·cu'ma·rine. A substance present in herbs and plants that modifies the light sensitivity of the skin and causes the appearance of irregularly shaped, erythematous, and slightly pigmented lesions in phytophotodermatosis.

fu·ro'ic ac'id. The acid resulting when the aldehyde group of furfural is oxidized to carboxyl; it occurs in crystals, soluble in water. The acid is sometimes employed for standardizing basic volumetric solutions. Also called *2-furoic acid, α-furoic acid.* Syn., *2-furancarboxylic acid, pyromucic acid.*

fu'ror [L.]. Madness; fury; a mania or maniacal attack.

f. amatorius. Excessive sexual desire. *Obs.*

f. genitalis. See *erotomania. Obs.*

paroxysmal f. Unprovoked attacks of intense anger occurring in patients with epileptic psychoses, not associated with convulsions. Also called *f. epilepticus.*

fu'ro·yl. The radical O.CH:CH.CH:C.CO— (ring closed from O to C) known as 2-furoyl, or the radical

CH:CH.O.CH:C.CO— (ring closed from first CH to C)

known as 3-furoyl.

fur'row [AS. *furh*]. A groove.

digital f. One of the transverse lines or furrows on the palmar surface of the fingers.

genital f. A groove appearing on the genital tubercle of the fetus at the end of the second month.

gluteal f. The groove between the nates.

interventricular furrows. Two longitudinal grooves separating the two ventricles of the heart.

fur″tre·tho′ni·um i′o·dide. Furfuryltrimethylammonium iodide, $C_8H_{14}INO$, a white to cream-colored crystalline powder, very soluble in water. A parasympathomimetic agent having a greater and more selective action on the urinary bladder than other cholinergic agents: used to encourage micturition. See *furmethide iodide.*

fu′run·cle (few′rung·kul, ·run·kul) [L. *furunculus,* boil, dim. of *fur,* thief]. A boil; a cutaneous abscess a few millimeters or less in size; usually the result of infection of a hair follicle or, more rarely, of ducts of cutaneous glands by pyogenic bacteria, especially by *Micrococcus aureus* (*Staphylococcus aureus*). —**furun′cular,** *adj.*

fu·run″cu·lo′sis [*furunculus;* G. *-ōsis,* increase]. A condition marked by affection with numerous furuncles, or in which new crops of furuncles follow repeatedly after healing of preceding crops.

f. orientalis. Obsolete term for cutaneous leishmaniasis.

fu·run′cu·lus. See *furuncle.*

fu′ryl. The radical O.CH:CH.CH:C—, known as *alpha*-furyl, or the radical O.CH:CH.C:CH, known as *beta*-furyl.

Fu·sa′ri·um (few·sair′ee·um, ·zair′ee·um) [L. *fusus,* spindle]. A genus of fungi, including species that may act as allergens, and that are pathogenic for plants. Produces verticillate conidiophores, which give rise to sickle-shaped, multiseptate conidia. The spores are airborne.

fus′cin (fuss′in, few′sin) [L. *fuscus,* dusky]. The brown melanin pigment of the retina.

fus′co cae·ru′li·us oph·thal″mo·max·il·la′ris of O′ta. An aberrant Mongolian spot.

fu″seau′ (few″zo′. *See* NOTES § 35) (pl. *fuseaux*) [F., spindle]. An oat-shaped spore which may be connected with mycelium or may be free; produced by fungi of the genus *Trichophyton.*

fu′sel oil. See under *oil.*

fu′si·ble (few′zi·bul) [L. *fusum,* from *fundere,* to pour]. Capable of being melted.

fu′si·form (few′zi·form, few′si·) [L. *fusus,* a spindle; *forma,* shape]. Spindle-shaped.

Fu″si·for′mis (few″zi·for′miss, few″si·) [*fusus; forma*]. Bacteria with the form of elongated spindles. There are aerobic and anaerobic types.

F. dentium. A bacillus found in Vincent's angina. Syn., *Fusobacterium plauti-vincenti.* Also called *fusiform bacillus.*

fu′sion [L. *fusio,* from *fundere,* to pour]. The process of melting; the act of uniting or cohering.

flicker f. threshold. See under *threshold.*

spinal f. The fusion of two or more vertebrae, for immobilization of the spinal column. Used in the treatment of spinal deformities, tuberculosis of the spine, and severe arthritis of the spine.

vulvar f. Cohesion of the labia minora occluding all or part of the vestibule; it may be congenital, but is more generally acquired following irritation. Also called *atresia vulva, synechia vulva, acquired gynetresia, vulvar atresia, agglutination of the vulva.*

Fu″so·bac·te′ri·um (few″zo·back·teer′ee·um, few″so·) [L. *fusus,* spindle; G. *baktērion,* little staff]. A genus of bacteria, including slender, Gram-negative, anaerobic, rectilinear, or incurving bacilli, which are frequently spindle-shaped and which stain irregularly. They are obligatory parasites of man and animals, and are found in necrotic areas, often in association with spirochetes.

F. plauti-vincenti. A species present in certain forms of gingivitis, in Vincent's angina, and in abscesses in the lungs and other organs. Also called *Fusiformis dentium.*

fu″so·cel′lu·lar [*fusus;* L. *cellula,* small storeroom]. Consisting of spindle-shaped cells, as spindle-cell sarcoma.

fu″so·spir″il·lo′sis. See Vincent's *angina.*

fu″so·spi″ro·che′tal (few″zo·spy″ro·kee′tul, few″so·) [*fusus;* G. *speira,* coil; *chaitē,* hair]. Pertaining to the association of fusiform bacteria and spirochetes.

fu″so·spi″ro·che·to′sis (few″zo·spy″ro·ki·to′sis, few″so·) [*fusus; speira; chaitē;* G. *-ōsis,* condition]. Infection characterized by the presence of fusiform bacilli and spirochetes. These organisms are present in certain forms of gingivitis, Vincent's angina, and in abscesses in the lungs and other organs.

Futaki, Kenzo [*Japanese physician,* 1873–]. Futaki and his colleagues, Takaki, Taniguchi, and Osumi, discovered the cause of rat-bite fever (sodoku) to be *Spirillum minus* (1916).

G

G 1. Gravitation constant or Newtonian constant. A constant in Newton's law of gravitation which gives the attraction f between two particles m_1 and m_2 at a distance r as

$$f = G\frac{m_1m_2}{r^2}$$

G is a constant whose value depends on the units in which f, m_1, m_2, and r are expressed. If f is given in dynes, m_1 and m_2 in grams, and r in centimeters, then G is 6.673×10^{-8} dyne cm.^{2}/gm.^{2} Also written g. 2. *In aviation,* the force of acceleration is expressed as the number of pounds of force per pound of mass of the pilot; G is one gravitational unit and equals one pound of force divided by one pound of mass. Greater accelerations are expressed in multiples of G. Blackout occurs above 7G in most pilots. 3. *In electrocardiography,* symbol for the ventricular gradient as projected on the frontal plane of the body: also written g, Ĝ, ĝ.

Ĝ See G, 3.

G. Gage.

G See G, 1 and G, 3.

ĝ Same as G, 3.

g. Gram(s); gage; G, 3.

g 1. Abbreviation for gram(s). 2. *In electrocardiography,* symbol for the ventricular gradient as projected on the frontal plane of the body: also written ĝ. 3. Abbreviation for gravity; one g represents the normal force of gravity; two g's, twice as much force, and so on.

Ga Chemical symbol for the element gallium.

Gabbett's stain. See under *stain.*

gad″o·lin′i·um [NL., after Johan *Gadolin,* Finnish chemist, 1760–1852]. Gd = 156.9. A rare earth metal discovered in 1880 by Marignac in gadolinite; because of its scarcity it is of scientific interest only.

Ga'dus [G. *gados*, a fish]. A genus of soft-finned fish.

G. morrhua. The common cod; a fish from the livers of which cod liver oil is obtained.

Gaebler's method. See Breh and Gaebler's *method.*

Gaertner, Gustav [*Austrian physician*, 1855–1937]. Devised an instrument for measuring the blood pressure by means of a heavy ring compressing the finger (1899), called *Gaertner's tonometer*.

Gaffky, Georg Theodor August [*German bacteriologist*, 1850–1918]. First to produce pure cultures of the typhoid bacillus; proved that the bacillus is the causative agent of the disease (1884). Devised a formula for the prognostic classification of specimens of sputum in tuberculosis. According to the *Gaffky scale* as modified by Lawrason Brown, specimens are graded as follows: (I) Less than five bacilli in the whole preparation. (II) No more than one bacillus on an average in each of many microscopical fields. (III) An average of one bacillus in each field. (IV) An average of two or three bacilli in each field. (V) An average of four to six bacilli in each field. (VI) An average of 7 to 12 bacilli in each field. (VII) An average of 13 to 25 bacilli in each field. (VIII) About 50 bacilli in each field. (IX) About 100 bacilli in each field.

Gaff'ky·a [*Gaffky*]. A genus of the Micrococcaceae.

G. tetragena. Synonym for *Micrococcus tetragenus.*

gag [imitative in origin]. An instrument placed between the teeth to prevent closure of the jaws.

gag. To retch; to cause to heave.

gage, gauge. An instrument for measuring the size of a structure, or the status of a process or phenomenon, as blood pressure.

Gaisböck, Felix [*Austrian physician*, 1868–]. Described polycythemia with hypertension; called *polycythemia hypertonica, Gaisböck's disease.*

gait [ON. *gata*]. The manner of walking.

ataxic g. A gait in which the foot is raised high, thrown forward, and brought down suddenly, the whole sole striking the ground at once; it is characteristic of lesions of the posterior column of the spinal cord. Syn., *tabetic g., hypotonic g.*

cerebellar g. A staggering, lurching gait, causing a zigzag line of travel.

cow g. A swaying movement due to knock-knee.

equine g. That seen in peroneal nerve paralysis. Because of foot drop, the leg must be raised high by flexing the thigh on the abdomen. Syn., *steppage g.*

festinating g. See *festination.*

frog g. The hopping gait of infantile paralysis.

hemiplegic g. That seen in partially paralyzed patients. There is a characteristic swing to the leg and dragging of the foot on the affected side, and the arm usually hangs stiffly.

hypotonic g. See ataxic *g.*

paraparetic g. That observed in chronic myelitis in which the steps are short and the feet are dragged, from inability to lift them.

paretic g. A gait in which the steps are short, the feet are dragged, and the legs are held more or less widely apart; as the disease progresses, there is uncertainty, shuffling, and staggering.

scissors g. That seen in congenital or acquired infantile paraplegia and in certain brain tumors. The gait is spastic and the legs are adducted.

spastic g. That seen in lesions of the spinal pyramidal tracts. The leg is extended at the knee and hip, the thigh adducted, and the heel raised; causes a stiff gait in which the foot is circumducted because it cannot be lifted.

staggering g. That resulting from central nervous system intoxication, or cerebellar or other severe diseases.

steppage g. See equine *g.*

tabetic g. See ataxic *g.*

waddling g. That of pseudohypertrophic muscular dystrophy, resembling the gait of a duck.

ga·lact'-, ga·lac'to- [G. *gala*, milk]. A combining form meaning *milk, milky fluid.*

ga·lac"ta·cra'si·a (ga·lack"tuh·kray'zhuh, ·zee·uh) [*gala;* G. *akrasia*, bad mixture]. Deficiency of or abnormality in mother's milk.

gal"ac·tae'mi·a (gal"ack·tee'mee·uh). See *galactemia.*

ga·lac'ta·gogue [*gala;* G. *agōgos*, leading]. An agent that induces or increases the secretion of milk: also called *galactopoietic.*

ga·lac'tan [*gala*]. Any polysaccharide composed of galactose units; on hydrolysis it yields galactose. The major part of gelose, the gelatinizing principle of agar, is a galactan. Syn., *galactosan.*

ga·lac'tase [*gala;* -*ase*, enzyme]. A soluble proteolytic enzyme present normally in milk.

gal"ac·te'mi·a, gal"ac·tae'mi·a (gal"ack·tee'mee·uh) [*gala;* G. *haima*, blood]. A milky state or appearance of the blood.

ga·lact"hi·dro'sis [*gala;* G. *hidrōsis*, sweating]. Sweating of a milklike fluid.

ga·lac'tic [*gala*]. Relating to or promoting the flow of milk.

ga·lac'tin [*gala*]. 1. An amorphous substance derived from milk. 2. Pituitary hormone stimulating lactation. See *prolactin.*

gal"ac·tis'chi·a (gal"ack·tiss'kee·uh) [*gala;* G. *ischein*, to check]. Suppression of the secretion of milk; galactoschesis.

ga·lac'to·blast [*gala;* G. *blastos*, germ]. Old term for colostrum corpuscle.

ga·lac'to·cele [*gala;* G. *kēlē*, tumor]. 1. A cystic tumor in the ducts of the breast. 2. Hydrocele with milky contents.

ga·lac"to·fla'vin. An analog of riboflavin in which D-galactose replaces D-ribose; it is a potent riboflavin antagonist.

ga·lac'to·gen [*gala; genesthai*, from *gignesthai*, to be produced]. A carbohydrate comparable to glycogen; has been prepared from the protein gland of the snail, *Helix pomatia.* It is hydrolyzed by dilute acids, forming galactose.

ga·lac'toid [*gala;* G. *eidos*, form]. Resembling milk.

ga·lac"to·ke"to·hep'tose. See *perseulose.*

ga·lac"to·lip'id. Any phosphorus-free, nitrogenous, fatty substance, containing also galactose, found in large amounts in the brain; on acid hydrolysis galactolipids yield galactose, sphingosine, and a fatty acid. Kerasin and phrenosin are galactolipids. Syn., *cerebroside, galactolipin.*

ga·lac"to·lip'in. Galactolipid.

gal"ac·to'ma. See *galactocele*, 1.

gal"ac·tom'e·ter [*gala;* G. *metron*, a measure]. 1. Graduated glass funnel for determining the fat in milk. 2. Instrument for determining the specific gravity of milk.

gal"ac·ton'ic ac'id. $C_6H_{12}O_7$. Pentahydroxyhexoic acid; a monobasic acid derived from galactose.

gal"ac·toph'a·gous [*gala;* G. *phagein*, to eat]. Subsisting on milk.

gal"ac·toph'ly·sis [*gala;* G. *phlysis*, a breaking out]. 1. A vesicular eruption containing a milklike fluid. 2. Crusta lactea.

ga·lac'to·phore [*gala;* G. *phoros*, bearing]. A lactiferous duct. —**galactoph'orous,** *adj.*

gal"ac·toph"o·ri'tis [*gala; phoros;* G. -*itis*, inflammation]. Inflammation of a lactiferous duct.

gal"ac·toph'thi·sis (gal"ack·tof'thi·sis, ga·lack"-tof·thigh'sis, ·theess'is) [*gala;* G. *phthisis*, a wasting away]. Old term for emaciation and debility due to excessive secretion of milk.

gal″ac·toph′y·gous [*gala;* G. *pheugein,* to avoid]. Arresting the secretion of milk.

ga·lac″to·poi·et′ic, ga·lac″to·po·et′ic [*gala;* G. *poiētikos,* from *poiein,* to make]. Pertaining to the formation and secretion of milk. —**galactopoiet′ic,** *n.*

ga·lac″to·py′ra [*gala;* G. *pyr,* fire]. Milk fever. See under *fever.* —**galactopyret′ic,** *adj.*

ga·lac″to·py′ra·nose. A pyranose-type, closed-chain form of galactose.

ga·lac″tor·rhe′a, ga·lac″tor·rhoe′a (ga·lack″to-ree′uh) [*gala;* G. *rhoia,* flow]. Excessive flow of milk.

ga·lac″to·sac·char′ic ac′id. D-Galactosaccharic acid or mucic acid.

ga·lac″tos·a·mine′. Galactose containing an amine group in 2-position, hence 2-amino-D-galactose. Syn., *chondrosamine.*

ga·lac′to·san. Galactan.

gal″ac·tos′che·sis (gal″ack·tos′ki·sis) [*gala;* G. *schesis,* retention]. Retention or suppression of milk.

ga·lac′to·scope [*gala;* G. *skopein,* to examine]. Instrument for determining the quality of milk.

ga·lac′tose (ga·lack′toce, ·toze). CHO.HCOH.-HOCH.HOCH.HCOH.CH_2OH; a D-type aldohexose obtained by hydrolysis of lactose, occurring also as a component of cerebrosides and of many oligosaccharides and polysaccharides; it exists in α- and β-forms. On oxidation it yields mucic acid. L-Galactose occurs in small amounts in certain polysaccharides, as the mucilage of agar and flaxseed.

gal·ac″to·se′mi·a. A congenital metabolic disorder in which there is an increased galactose level in the blood: also called *galactose diabetes.*

ga·lac″to·si′dase. See *lactase.*

ga·lac′to·side. A glycoside which, on hydrolysis, yields the sugar galactose and an aglycone.

gal″ac·to′sis [*gala;* G. *-ōsis,* condition]. The secretion of milk by the mammary glands.

gal″ac·tos′ta·sis, ga·lac″to·sta′si·a (ga·lack″to-stay′zee·uh, ·see·uh) [*gala;* G. *stasis,* a standing]. 1. Suppression of milk secretion. 2. An abnormal collection of milk in a breast.

ga·lac″to·su′ri·a [*gala;* G. *ouron,* urine]. Passage of urine containing galactose.

ga·lac″to·ther′a·py [*gala;* G. *therapeia,* treatment]. 1. The treatment of disease in suckling infants by the administration of drugs to the mother or wet nurse. 2. Milk cure. 3. Hypodermic use of milk to produce fever in fever therapy.

ga·lac″to·tox′i·con [*gala;* G. *toxikon,* poison]. The active agent or toxin present in poisonous milk.

ga·lac″to·tox′in [*gala; toxikon*]. A poisonous substance or ptomaine generated in milk by the growth of microorganisms.

ga·lac″to·tox′ism [*gala; toxikon*]. Milk poisoning.

gal″ac·tot′ro·phy [*gala;* G. *trophē,* nourishment]. Nourishing with milk only.

ga·lac″to·zy′mase (ga·lack″to·zy′mace, ·maze) [*gala;* G. *zymē,* leaven; *-ase,* enzyme]. A ferment found in milk; capable of liquefying starch.

gal″ac·tu′ri·a [*gala;* G. *ouron,* urine]. Milkiness of the urine; chyluria.

ga·lac″tu·ron′ic ac′id. The monobasic acid resulting from oxidation of the primary alcohol group of D-galactose to carboxyl; it is widely distributed as a constituent of pectins and many plant gums and mucilages.

gal′a·lith [*gala;* G. *lithos,* stone]. An absorbent material made of casein and formol.

ga·lan′ga, ga·lan′gal (ga·lang′gul, gal′ang·gul) [Per. *khalanjan*]. The rhizome of *Alpinia officinarum.* The active principles are a volatile oil and a resin; the actions are those of a stimulant aromatic with effects similar to those of ginger.

gal′ba·num [G. *chalbanē,* resinous juice of all-heal, from Heb. helbenāh]. A gum resin of *Ferula galbaniflua;* formerly used as a stimulant and expectorant and externally in plasters.

Galbiati, Gennaro [*Italian obstetrician,* 1776–1844]. Remembered for his use of symphysiotomy with double pelviotomy in cases of difficult birth; called *Galbiati's operation.* Also devised a special knife for dividing the tissues.

ga′le·a (gay′lee·uh, gal′ee·uh) (pl. *galeae*) [L., helmet]. 1. Any structure resembling a helmet. 2. A form of head bandage. 3. The aponeurotic portion of the occipitofrontal muscle, called the **galea aponeurotica.**

g. capitis. The thin sheath of cytoplasm covering the nucleus and acrosome of the sperm head.

gal″e·an′thro·py (gal″ee·an′thro·pee, gay″lee·) [G. *galeē,* weasel, polecat; *anthrōpos,* man]. A form of zoanthropy in which the patient believes himself to be transformed into a cat.

Galeazzi, Domenico Maria Gusmano (Galeati) [*Italian anatomist and physician,* 1686–1775]. Described short, simple, tubular glands in the intestinal mucosa (1731); called *Galeati's glands, Lieberkühn's glands, crypts of Lieberkühn.*

Ga·le′ga [G. *gala,* milk]. A genus of the Leguminosae.

G. officinalis. Goat's rue; formerly used mistakenly as a galactagogue. See *galegine.*

ga·le′gine (ga·lee′jeen, ·jin). An alkaloid, $C_6H_{13}N_3$, from *Galega officinalis,* or goat's rue. It is said to reduce blood sugar.

Galen, Claudius [*Mysian physician in Rome,* ca. 130–ca. 200]. One of the greatest figures in medical history. Galen is called the father of experimental physiology. He seems to have recognized cholera, rabies, malaria, and empyema as definite medical entities. Many parts of the body have been known by his name. See *venae Galeni* under *vena.* See also *Galen's four humors* under *humor.*

ga·le′na. Native lead sulfide.

Ga·len′ic (ga·len′ick, ·lee′nick), **Ga·len′i·cal** (ga-len′i·kul, ·lee′ni·kul) [*Galen*]. Relating to, or consistent with, the teachings of Galen.

Ga·len′i·cal [*Galen*]. Medicine prepared from plants, according to standard formulas, as contrasted with definite chemicals.

gal″e·o·phil′i·a [G. *galeē,* weasel, polecat; *philein,* to love]. Excessive love of cats.

gal″e·o·pho′bi·a [*galeē;* G. *phobos,* fear]. A morbid fear of cats. Also called *gatophobia, ailurophobia.*

gal″e·ro′pi·a, gal″e·rop′si·a [G. *galeros,* cheerful; *opsis,* appearance]. An abnormally clear and light appearance of objects due to some defect in the visual apparatus.

Galezowski, Xavier [*Ukrainian ophthalmologist,* 1832–1907]. Devised an operation for cataract, the incision being entirely within the cornea, the point of the knife dividing the capsule. Introduced a special type of operation for pterygium, turning the apex under the base, called *Galezowski's operation.* With Parinaud, described an infectious conjunctivitis transmissible from animals to man (1889), called *Parinaud's conjunctivitis, leptotrichosis of the conjunctiva.*

Galilei, Galileo [*Italian physicist and astronomer,* 1564–1642]. One of the founders of modern experimental science. Exercised great influence on the development of scientific medicine. Inventor of the hydrostatic balance and the telescope.

Gall, Franz Joseph [*German anatomist,* 1758–1828]. Made important contributions to the knowledge of cerebral anatomy. With Johann Caspar

Spurzheim, projected the theory of the localization of cerebral function (1810–19). Founder of the pseudoscience of phrenology.

gall (gawl) [AS. *geалla*]. The bile.

gall (gawl) [ME. *galle*, from L. *galla*, gall-nut]. A sore on the skin of a horse, caused by a saddle or harness.

gal·lac″e·to·phe·none′ (ga·lass″i·to·fi·nohn′, ·fee′-nohn). Trihydroxyacetophenone, $CH_3CO.C_6H_2(OH)_3$. White to brownish powder used as 10% ointment or solution in skin diseases. Also called *alizarin yellow C.*

gal′la·mine tri″eth·i′o·dide. Generic name for the curariform substance supplied under the trade-marked name *flaxedil* (triethiodide).

gall′blad″der (gawl′blad″ur) [AS. *gealla; blǣdre*]. A hollow, pear-shaped, musculomembranous organ, situated on the under surface of the right lobe of the liver, for the storage and concentration of bile and the secretion of mucus. See Plate 13.

sandpaper g. Roughness of the lining of the gallbladder, due to deposition of cholesterin crystals.

strawberry g. A benign papilloma or hyperplasia of the folds lining the organ. It is a soft, friable, reddish mass containing cholesterin crystals and fat, which may fill the entire gallbladder, the color and appearance giving it the name.

gal′le·in. $C_{20}H_{12}O_7$. Pyrogallolphthalein. An indicator; brownish yellow in acid, red in alkali.

gal′lic ac′id (*acidum gallicum*). $(OH)_3C_6H_2COOH.H_2O$. Trihydroxybenzoic acid, occurring in white to yellowish crystals; 1 Gm. dissolves in 87 cc. of water. Occasionally used for its astringent effect. Dose, 0.3–1.3 Gm. (5–20 gr.).

Gallie, William Edward [*Canadian surgeon*, 1882–]. With Le Mesurier, devised an original operation for the radical cure of inguinal hernia, using living fascial strips obtained from the thigh and passing them as running sutures through the aponeurotic layers of the oblique and transverse muscles to form a sort of basketwork. Called *Gallie's operation, Gallie and Le Mesurier's operation.* The strips are called *Gallie's transplant.*

gal′li·um [L. *Gallia*, Gaul]. Ga = 69.72. A gray-white metal which melts at 29.7° C. It is used in thermometers for measuring temperatures between 500° and 1000°, and for certain other special purposes.

gal′lo- [L. *galla*, gall-nut]. *In chemistry*, a combining form denoting *gallic acid.*

gal″lo·cy′a·nin. A basic oxazine dye; used in an aqueous solution with chrome alum as a stain for Nissl bodies; sometimes used as a nuclear stain.

gal′lon [OF. *jallon*, of obscure origin]. A standard unit of volumetric measurement. Capacity in the United States 231 cubic inches; four quarts. In the apothecaries' measure, the Latin equivalent, congius, abbreviated C., is frequently employed.

imperial g. In Great Britain, a capacity equivalent to 1.20094 U. S. gallons.

gal″lo·tan′nic ac′id. Tannic acid.

gall′stone″ (gawl′stone″) [AS. *gealla;* ME. *ston*]. A concretion formed in the gallbladder or the biliary ducts, composed, in varying amounts, of cholesterol, bilirubin, and other elements found in bile.

Galton, Francis [*English geneticist*, 1822–1911]. Considered the founder of eugenics. Suggested a hereditary basis for genius (1869). See Galton's *law* of filial regression. Invented *Galton's whistle* for testing the hearing of high tones. Was among the first to suggest the use of fingerprints for the identification of criminals (1892). See Galton system of *identification.*

galv. Galvanic; galvanized; galvanism.

Galvani, Luigi [*Italian physician and anatomist*, 1737–98]. In experiments with frog legs, he discovered the electric properties of animal tissue (1791).

gal·van′ic. Pertaining to galvanism. Abbreviated, galv.

gal′va·nism [*Galvani*]. Primary direct current electricity produced by chemical action, as opposed to that produced by heat, friction, or induction. Abbreviated, galv.

gal″va·ni·za′tion [*Galvani*]. The transmission of a direct current of low electromotive force through any part of the body for the purpose of diagnosing or treating disease. —**gal′vanize,** *v.*

gal′va·no- (gal′vuh·no-, gal·van′o-) [*Galvani*]. A combining form denoting *a galvanic* or *direct current of electricity; employing* or *produced by the galvanic current.*

gal″va·no·cau′ter·y. Electrocautery.

gal″va·no·con″trac·til′i·ty [*Galvani;* L. *contractus*, from *contrahere*, to contract]. The property of being contractile under stimulation by a direct galvanic current.

gal″va·no·far″a·di·za′tion [*Galvani;* Michael *Faraday*, English physicist]. The simultaneous use of direct galvanic currents and rapidly alternating faradic currents.

gal″va·nol′y·sis [*Galvani;* G. *lysis*, a loosing]. Old term for electrolysis.

gal″va·nom′e·ter [*Galvani;* G. *metron*, a measure]. An instrument for measuring relatively small electric currents.

aperiodic g. A galvanometer devoid of periodicity; one in which the indicator comes quickly to rest.

string g. A galvanometer for use in electrocardiography; the current is measured by lateral displacement of a wire carrying the current across a strong magnetic field. Also called *Einthoven's g.*

gal″va·no·mus′cu·lar [*Galvani;* L. *musculus*, muscle]. Denoting a reaction produced by the application of a direct galvanic current to a muscle.

gal′va·no·punc″ture. Electropuncture.

gal′va·no·scope″, gal·van′o·scope″ [*Galvani;* G. *skopein*, to examine]. An instrument for detecting the presence and direction of small direct or galvanic currents. —**galvanos′copy,** *n.*

gal″va·no·sur′ger·y [*Galvani;* OF. *surgerie*, contr. from G. *cheir*, hand; *ergon*, work]. The surgical use of direct or galvanic currents.

gal″va·no·tax′is. See *galvanotropism.*

gal″va·no·ther′a·py [*Galvani;* G. *therapeia*, treatment]. Treatment of disease through the use of direct or galvanic currents.

gal′va·no·ther″my (gal′vuh·no·thur″mee, gal-van′o·, gal″vuh·no·thur′mee, gal·van″o·) [*Galvani;* G. *thermē*, heat]. The production of heat by direct or galvanic currents.

gal″va·not′o·nus [*Galvani;* G. *tonos*, tension]. 1. Electrotonus. 2. The continued tetanus of a muscle between the make and break contraction of direct or galvanic current. —**galvanoton′ic,** *adj.*

gal″va·not′ro·pism [*Galvani;* G. *trepein*, to turn]. The turning movements of living structure or beings, under the influence of a direct current of electricity.

gal′vo. See brass founder's *ague.*

gal′ziek″te (gahl′zeek″tuh, gahl·zeek′tuh) [S. Afr. D. *gal*, gall; *ziekte*, sickness]. A South African cattle disease of infectious origin and febrile characteristics; spread by ticks.

gam″a·soi·do′sis. Infestation by Gamasidae (a family including the fowl mite).

gam′bir [Malay] (*gambir*). An aqueous extract from the twigs and leaves of *Uncaria gambir*. Gambir yields catechutannic acid and catechin. Used as an astringent and in dyeing and tanning.

gam·boge′ (gam·bohdj′, bōōdj′, ·bōōzh′) [*Cambodia*] (*cambogia*). The gum resin obtained from *Garcinia hanburyi*. It is a drastic, hydragogue cathartic; a constituent of compound mild mercurous chloride pills. Dose, 0.03–0.2 Gm. (½–3 gr.).

Gam·bu′si·a (gam·bew′zee·uh, ·see·uh) [Amer. Sp. *gambusina*, nothing]. A genus of top-feeding minnows, found in the southern United States and other warm climates. Their surface-feeding habits make them valuable in the destruction of mosquito larvae.

gam″e·tan′gi·um [G. *gamein*, to marry; *aggeion*, vessel]. A gamete-producing organ occurring especially in the lower plants.

gam′ete (gam′eet, ga·meet′, *the latter commonly in compounds*) [G. *gametē*, wife, *gametēs*, husband, from *gamein*, to marry]. A male or female reproductive cell capable of entering into union with another in the process of fertilization or of conjugation. In higher animals, these sex cells are the egg and sperm; in higher plants, the male gamete is part of the pollen grain, while the ovum is contained in the ovule. In lower forms, the gametes are frequently similar in appearance and their union is called conjugation. —**gamet′ic,** *adj*.

ga·me′to·cyte (ga·mee′to·sight, gam′i·to·sight) [*gamein;* G. *kytos*, cell]. A cell which by division produces gametes; a spermatocyte or oocyte. See Plates 27, 28, 29.

gam″e·to·gen′e·sis [*gamein;* G. *genesis*, production]. The origin and formation of gametes.

gam″e·tog′o·ny (gam″i·tog′o·nee) [*gamein;* G. *gonē*, seed]. A process of reproduction leading to the formation of gametocytes and gametes in the sexual phase of the life cycle in certain protozoa.

ga·me′to·phyte (ga·mee′to·fight, gam′i·to·fight) [*gamein;* G. *phyton*, plant]. A sexual, gamete-producing individual which alternates in the life history of plants with the asexual sporophyte. The leafy moss plant is a gametophyte, but the leafy fern plant is a sporophyte. In the seed plants, the male and female gametophytes are microscopic and are contained in the pollen grain and ovule, respectively.

gam′ic [G. *gamos*, marriage]. Sexual; applied especially to the members of the bisexual generation in such animals as aphids, in which there is a parthenogenetic-bisexual cycle.

gam′ma [G.]. 1. The third letter of the Greek alphabet (Γ, γ), equivalent to English g. For many terms beginning with gamma, see the specific noun. 2. *In chemistry*, microgram (one thousandth of a milligram). 3. *In photography*, the contrast of a negative or print, usually controlled by developing time, and expressed as a relationship between the density of the negative and the time of exposure.

g. roentgen. A unit of radium dosage such that the same amount of ionization in air is produced as by one roentgen unit of gamma rays: also called *gamma-ray roentgen*.

gam′ma·cism [*gamma*]. Guttural stammering; difficulty in pronouncing guttural consonants, especially hard g and k.

gammexane. Trade-mark for gamma-hexachlorocyclohexane, $C_6H_6Cl_6$, an insecticide more powerful than DDT and effective in the treatment of scabies. The chemical is also known as *666* and *benzene hexachloride*. See *lindane*.

Gamna nodules. See *siderotic nodules* under *nodule*.

Gamna spleen. See Gandy-Gamna *spleen*.

gam′o- [G. *gamos*, marriage]. 1. *In biology*, a combining form denoting *sexual union*. 2. *In botany*, a combining form signifying *union* or *fusion of parts*.

gam″o·ma′ni·a [*gamos;* G. *mania*, madness]. Insane desire for marriage.

gam′one. Hypothetical hormonelike substance present in gametes, concerned with fertilization.

gam″o·pet′al·ous [*gamos;* G. *petalon*, leaf]. *In biology*, sympetalous.

gam″o·pho′bi·a [*gamos;* G. *phobos*, fear]. A morbid fear of marriage.

gam″o·sep′al·ous [*gamos;* NL. *sepalum*, proposed by Necker from G. *skepē*, covering]. *In biology*, symsepalous.

Gandy-Gamna nodules. See *siderotic nodules* under *nodule*.

Gandy-Gamna spleen. See under *spleen*.

gan′gli·a″ted (gang′glee·ay″tid, gang′lee·), **gan′gli·on·a″ted** [G. *gagglion*, encysted tumor on a tendon]. Supplied with ganglions.

gan″gli·ec′to·my (gang″glee·eck′to·mee, gang″lee·). See *ganglionectomy*.

gan″gli·i′tis (gang″glee·eye′tis, gang″lee·). See *ganglionitis*.

gan′gli·o- (gang′glee·o-, gang′lee·o-) [*gagglion*]. A combining form meaning *ganglion*.

gan′gli·o·blast″ [*gagglion;* G. *blastos*, germ]. 1. An embryonic ganglion cell. 2. A neuroblast. *Obs.*

gan″gli·o·blas·to′ma. Ganglioneuroma.

g. of nose. See heterotopic *glioma*.

gan′gli·o·cyte″ [*gagglion;* G. *kytos*, cell]. A ganglion cell. *Obs.*

gan″gli·o·cy·to′ma. See *neuroastrocytoma*.

gan″gli·o·cyt″o·neu·ro′ma. See *ganglioneuroma*.

gan″gli·o·gli·o′ma. Neuroastrocytoma.

g. of nose. See heterotopic *glioma*.

gan′gli·oid (gang′glee·oyd, gang′lee·oyd) [*gagglion;* G. *eidos*, form]. Resembling a ganglion.

gan″gli·o′ma. See *ganglioneuroma*.

gan′gli·on (gang′glee·un, gang′lee·un) (pl. *ganglions, ganglia*) [G.]. 1. A group of nerve cell bodies, usually located outside of the brain and spinal cord, as the dorsal root ganglion of a spinal nerve. 2. A cystic, tumorlike localized lesion in a tendon sheath or joint capsule, especially of the hands, wrists, and feet, but also occasionally within other connective tissues. It is composed of stellate cells in a matrix of mucoid hyaluronic acid and reticular fibers. Also called *cystic tumor of tendon sheath, cyst of joint capsule, cyst of semilunar cartilage, weeping sinew*. —**gangliar, ganglion′ic,** *adj*.

accessory g. One of several vestigial ganglions associated with the embryonic dorsal roots of the vagus nerve; also with the hypoglossus in certain mammals.

acoustic g. The embryonic ganglionic mass which separates into cochlear and vestibular ganglions. Syn., *vestibulocochlear g.*

acousticofacial g. See acousticofacial *primordium*.

aorticorenal g. An outlying portion of the celiac ganglion, near the origin of each renal artery: also called *g. renale*.

Auerbach's ganglions. Nerve cell bodies in the myenteric plexus.

basal ganglions. An old term for the corpus striatum, or the corpus striatum and the thalamus considered together as the important subcortical centers.

Bidder's g. See Friedrich H. *Bidder*.

Bochdalek's g. A gangliform enlargement at the junction of the middle and anterior branches of the superior dental plexus; a pseudoganglion.

cardiac g. A ganglion of the superficial cardiac plexus, located between the aortic arch and the bifurcation of the pulmonary artery. Formerly called *Wrisberg's g.*

carotid g. A small enlargement sometimes found

in the internal carotid plexus inferior to the internal carotid artery.
celiac g. A collateral sympathetic ganglion lying in the celiac plexus near the origin of the celiac artery: formerly called *semilunar g.*
cervical g. (a) One of two or three ganglions on the sympathetic chain in the neck, named superior (see Plate 15), middle (sometimes absent), and inferior. (b) A ganglion of the craniosacral autonomic system, located at the uterine cervix: also called *Frankenhäuser's g.*
ciliary g. That at the back of the orbit; from it arise postganglionic parasympathetic fibers to the ciliary muscle and the constrictor muscle of the iris. See Plate 15.
Cloquet's g. A plexiform intermingling of fibers of the two nasopalatine nerves in the incisive canal. It is not a true ganglion.
coccygeal g. The terminal ganglion formed by the fusion of the caudal ends of the sympathetic trunks of both sides, situated in front of the coccyx. Syn., *g. impar.*
cochlear g. See spiral *g.*
collateral g. Any of the ganglia of the sympathetic nervous system located in the mesenteric nervous plexuses around the abdominal aorta and its larger visceral branches. Syn., *prevertebral g.*
dorsal root g. One of the sensory ganglions associated with the dorsal root of a spinal nerve.
Ehrenritter's g. See superior *g.*
enteric ganglions. Small ganglions of the myenteric and submucous plexuses of the intestine.
Frankenhäuser's g. See cervical *g.*, (b).
Froriep's g. A rudimentary or vestigial dorsal root ganglion of the hypoglossal nerve.
g. habenulae. Old term for habenular nucleus.
g. impar. See coccygeal *g.*
g. molle. Enlarged and engorged, but nonindurated lymph node found in African trypanosomiasis.
g. renale. See aorticorenal *g.*
gasserian, Gasserian g. See semilunar *g.*
geniculate g. The sensory ganglion of the nervus intermedius, lying in the genu of the facial nerve in the facial canal of the temporal bone.
inferior g. See petrosal *g.*
inferior mesenteric g. An outlying or collateral sympathetic ganglion lying in the inferior mesenteric plexus near the aorta at the origin of the inferior mesenteric artery. See Plate 15.
intermediate g. The middle cervical ganglion.
interpeduncular g. See interpeduncular *nucleus.*
jugular g. (a) The superior ganglion of the vagus nerve. (b) The superior ganglion of the glossopharyngeal nerve.
lateral chain g. Any ganglion of the sympathetic trunk.
lateral g. (a) In fishes and certain amphibians, a ganglion associated with cranial nerve VII and another with X, whose postganglionic fibers supply the lateral line organs. (b) *In comparative anatomy,* a ganglion of the sympathetic trunk.
lumbar g. Any of the ganglia of the lumbar sympathetic trunk.
Meckel's g. See sphenopalatine *g.*
nodose g. The lower ganglion of the vagus nerve.
otic g. That immediately below the foramen ovale of the sphenoid bone, medial to the mandibular nerve; from it arise postganglionic parasympathetic fibers to the parotid gland. See Plate 15.
paravertebral g. Any of the chain of sympathetic ganglia of the sympathetic trunks; according to location they are grouped into cervical, thoracic (dorsal), lumbar, and sacral.
pelvic g. The ganglion cells located in the pelvic nerve plexus.
peripheral g. See terminal *g.*
petrosal g. The inferior sensory ganglion of the glossopharyngeal nerve, located in a depression at the lower orifice of the jugular foramen: also called *Andersch's g., inferior g.*
phrenic g. One located at the junction of the right phrenic nerve with the phrenic plexus, which sends nerve fibers to the inferior vena cava, right adrenal gland, and the hepatic plexus.
posterior root g. See dorsal root *g.*
prevertebral g. See collateral *g.*
pterygopalatine g. The sphenopalatine *g.*
Remak's g. See Robert *Remak.*
Scarpa's g. See vestibular *g.*
semilunar g. (a) The large ganglion of the sensory root of the trigeminal nerve; from it arise the ophthalmic, maxillary, and mandibular divisions of the trigeminal nerve. Syn., *trigeminal g.* Also called *gasserian g.* See Plate 17. (b) Old term for *celiac g.*
sphenopalatine g. One in the pterygopalatine fossa near the sphenopalatine foramen; from it arise postganglionic parasympathetic fibers to the lacrimal gland and to the mucous membrane of the nose and palate. Also called *Meckel's g.* See Plate 15.
spinal g. One of the sensory ganglions associated with the dorsal roots of spinal nerves. Syn., *dorsal root g.*
spiral g. That of the cochlear nerve, lodged in the spiral canal of the modiolus.
splanchnic g. One located on the greater splanchnic nerve near the disk between the eleventh and twelfth thoracic vertebrae.
stellate g. That formed by the fusion of the inferior cervical and the first thoracic sympathetic ganglions. See Plate 15.
submaxillary g. A small fusiform ganglion lying on the hyoglossus muscle above the deep part of the submaxillary gland; from it arise postganglionic parasympathetic fibers to the submaxillary and sublingual glands. See Plate 15.
superior g. The superior ganglion of the glossopharyngeal nerve, located in the upper part of the jugular foramen: also called *Ehrenritter's g., jugular g., g. superius.*
superior mesenteric g. A collateral sympathetic ganglion lying in the superior mesenteric plexus near the origin of the superior mesenteric artery. See Plate 15.
sympathetic ganglions. The ganglions of the sympathetic nervous system, including those of the sympathetic trunk, the collateral, and the peripheral or terminal ganglions.
terminal g. One of the smaller, most peripheral, of the sympathetic ganglions: also called *peripheral g.*
thoracic g. One of the ganglions of the thoracic sympathetic trunk.
trigeminal g. See semilunar *g.*
tympanic g. A ganglion of the tympanic nerve lying on the promontory of the middle ear.
Valentin's g. A gangliform enlargement at the junction of the middle and posterior branches of the superior dental plexus; a pseudoganglion.
vestibular g. That of the vestibular nerve, located in the internal auditory meatus. Also called *Scarpa's g.*
vestibulocochlear g. See acoustic *g.*
Wrisberg's g. See cardiac *g.*
gan′gli·on·a″ted (gang′glee·un·ay″tid, gang′lee·). See *gangliated.*
gan″gli·on·ec′to·my [*gagglion;* G. *ektomē,* excision]. The surgical excision of a ganglion.

gan″gli·o·neu″ro·blas·to′ma. See *ganglioneuroma, neuroastrocytoma.*

gan″gli·o·neu″ro·cy·to′ma. See *ganglioneuroma.*

gan″gli·o·neu·ro′ma [*gagglion;* G. *neuron,* nerve; *-ōma,* tumor]. A tumor composed of sympathetic ganglion cells and large numbers of sheathed nerve fibers, principally located in the sympathetic ganglia and the adrenal medulla. Some are incompletely differentiated, showing some features of the sympathicoblastoma, and some may metastasize. The differentiated forms are variously also called *gangliocytoneuroma, ganglioma, ganglioneuroblastoma* (*sympathicum* or *simplex*); *ganglioneuroma telangiectatum cysticum; myelinated neuroma gangliocellulare, neurofibroma ganglionare, neuroganglioma myelinicum verum, neuroma gangliocellulare* (*amyelinicum, benignum*); *neuroma verum gangliosum amyelinicum, sympathicocytoma.* The partly differentiated forms are also called *gangliocytoma, ganglioneuroblastoma; immature, malignant, metastasizing,* or *mixed ganglioneuroma; neuroma gangliocellulare malignum, sympathetic neuroma.*

dumbbell g. See dumbbell *tumor.*

hourglass g. See dumbbell *tumor.*

gan″gli·o·ni′tis [*gagglion;* G. *-itis,* inflammation]. Inflammation of a ganglion.

gan″gli·o·schwan″no·spon″gi·o·blas·to′ma. See heterotopic *glioma.*

gan′gli·o·sides. Brain cerebrosides which contain a special fatty acid, called neuraminic acid, and which yield more than one equivalent of galactose.

gan″gli·o·sym·path″i·co·blas·to′ma. See *sympathicoblastoma.*

gan·go′sa [Sp., snuffling]. Destructive lesions of the nose and hard palate, sometimes more extensive, considered to be a tertiary stage of yaws: also called *rhinopharyngitis mutilans.*

gan′grene (gang′green, gang·green′) [G. *gaggraina,* gangrene]. 1. Mortification or death of a part; due to failure of the blood supply, to disease, or to injury. 2. The putrefactive changes in dead tissue.—**gangrenous,** *adj.*

amebic g. An extensive destruction of the skin surrounding a drainage wound, following removal of an amebic abscess of the liver.

arteriosclerotic g. Senile *g.*

carbolic acid g. See chemical *g.*

chemical g. That following burns from caustic or poisonous chemicals, as carbolic acid.

cutaneous g. Skin gangrene. See decubital *g.*

decubital g. A pressure gangrene of the skin and adjacent tissues; occurs in patients who are bedridden for long periods. Also called *decubitus.*

diabetic g. A moist type occurring in the course of diabetes mellitus; often the result of slight injuries.

direct g. That due to direct destruction of tissue from injury, pressure, burns, chemical action, etc.

dry g. Local death of a part which does not become infected and undergoes mummification. Seen commonly following blocking of blood supply, as that due to freezing or embolism.

Egyptian g. A characteristic, necrotizing lesion of the eyelids found in North Africa; it may be of viral origin and perhaps may be associated with necrotizing desert sore.

foudroyant g. Infectious, fulminating, or spreading gangrene.

fusospirochetal g. Gangrenous lesions, believed to be due to *Borrellia refringens* (spirochetes) and fusiform bacilli. They are seen in the oropharynx as a complication of Vincent's angina, following penetrating wounds involving the oropharynx, following human bites, or as a venereal infection, usually in males with redundant prepuce.

g. of the appendix. Necrosis of the appendix in appendicitis, with sloughing of the organ.

g. of the lung. A diffuse, putrefactive necrosis of the lung or of a lobe; due to anaerobic or other bacteria; usually a termination of lung abscess in a patient with low resistance.

gas g. A form occurring in massive wounds, where there is crushing and devitalization of tissue and contamination with earth. The organisms found are anaerobes, including *Clostridium perfringens* Type A and *Clostridium septicum.* It is marked by high fever, offensive, thin, purulent discharge from the wound, and the presence of gas bubbles in the tissues.

hospital g. An infectious type especially involving amputation stumps.

line of separation in g. The deepening groove of ulceration and granulation which gradually separates living and dead tissue.

moist g. Local death of a part which becomes infected, so that the signs and symptoms of infection are superimposed upon those of gangrene.

pudendal g. See *noma* pudendi.

senile g. A dry gangrene of the extremities; due to failure of the terminal circulation in elderly persons or those afflicted with arteriosclerosis. Also called *arteriosclerotic g., g. of the aged.*

symmetric g. See Raynaud's *disease.*

wet g. Moist *g.*

white g. Gangrene with anemia of the tissues.

gangue [F., from G. *gang,* metallic vein]. The earth or stone of an ore.

gan′ja, gan′jah [Hind.]. Gunjah. See *cannabis.*

gan′o·blast [G. *ganos,* brightness; *blastos,* germ]. An enamel-forming cell. Syn., *ameloblast.*

Ganser syndrome. See under *syndrome.*

Gant, Frederick James [*English surgeon,* 1825–1905]. Remembered for his introduction of subtrochanteric osteotomy of the femur for ankylosis of the hip joint with flexion and adduction. He divided the femur below the lesser trochanter and overcorrected the deformity in abduction, immobilizing the fracture until bony union occurred.

gantrisin. Trade-mark for 3,4-dimethyl-5-sulfanilamido-isoxazole, a sulfonamide characterized by high solubility in neutral or slightly acid body fluids. See *sulfisoxazole, sulphafurazole.*

gap [ON.]. Any break or opening.

auscultatory g. A zone of silence which occasionally occurs, for some unknown reason, in auscultatory determination of human arterial pressure while cuff pressure is declining.

cranial gaps. Occasional congenital fissures of the skull.

silent g. The interval occasionally noted in auscultatory blood-pressure estimations where no sound is heard even though no interruption is detected at the wrist.

sphere g. A spark gap between two polished spheres, connected in parallel to an x-ray tube. The length of the spark for spheres of a given diameter measures the voltage at the tube.

gapes. See *gapeworm.*

gape′worm″. A disease of young fowls; caused by the presence of a nematode worm, *Syngamus trachealis,* in the trachea.

gar′an·tose. Saccharin.

gar′bled (gahr′buld) [It. *garbellare,* from L. *cribrum,* sieve]. Applied to crude drugs which have been separated from worthless material and made ready for market. *Obs.*

Gar·cin′i·a [after Laurent *Garcin,* French botanist, 1683–1752]. A genus of the Guttiferae. **G. hanburyi,** the Siam gamboge tree, yields the gum oleoresin, gamboge. **G. mangostana** yields the palatable fruit called mangosteen.

Garel, Jean [*French physician*, 1852–1931]. Described *Garel's sign* of empyema of the maxillary sinus: when an electric bulb is placed in the oral cavity, the eye on the sound side perceives the light but the eye on the affected side does not.

gar′get (gahr′ghit) [ME., from L. *gurges*, whirlpool]. A progressive inflammation of the udder; usually applied to cattle.

gar′gle [F. *gargouiller*, to gargle]. A solution for rinsing the pharynx and nasopharynx.

gar′gle. To rinse the pharynx and nasopharynx.

gar′goyl·ism [L. *gurgulio*, gullet]. A congenital disease characterized by dwarfism, with short, kyphotic spinal column, short fingers, depression of bridge of the nose, and heavy ugly facies, stiffness of joints, cloudiness of cornea, hepatosplenomegaly, and mental deficiency. It may represent a form of lipoidosis. In contrast to *chondro-osteodystrophy*, the changes of the vertebral bodies and hip joints are quite distinct, and also there are changes of the bones of skull and face. Also called *Hurler's syndrome, dystostosis multiplex, lipochondrodystrophy.*

Garland's triangle. See under *triangle.*

gar′lic [AS. *gārlēac*]. The fresh bulb of *Allium sativum.* It contains a volatile oil consisting of allyl compounds of sulfur. It is sometimes used in pulmonary conditions, and in the dehydrated form, as a carminative.

Garré, Carl [*Swiss surgeon*, 1857–1928]. Described chronic sclerosing osteomyelitis with little suppuration, characterized by small areas of necrosis, called *Garré's disease, Garré's osteomyelitis.*

Garretson, James Edmund [*American dentist*, 1828–95]. Pioneer in oral and maxillary surgery and often called the father of oral surgery.

Garrison, Fielding H. (1870–1935). American medical librarian and historian, author of *An Introduction to the History of Medicine*, the standard English textbook of medical history. He was associated for many years with the *Index Medicus* and the Army Medical Library.

Garrod, Archibald Edward [*English physician and biochemist*, 1857–1936]. Showed that constitutional metabolic variations can produce such conditions as cystinuria, pentosuria, and alkaptonuria (1909). Devised *Garrod's test* for porphyrins in the urine. See under *test.*

gar·rot′ing (ga·ro′ting, ga·rot′ing) [Sp. *garrote*]. *In legal medicine*, forcible compression of a victim's neck from behind with intent to rob or kill.

Gärtner, August [*German bacteriologist*, 1848–1934]. Described the bacillus known as *Gärtner's bacillus*, now classified as *Salmonella enteritidis*, as a cause of food poisoning (1888).

Gartner's cyst. See under *cyst.*

Gartner's duct. See under *duct.*

gas [invented by van Helmont; suggested by G. *chaos*, chaos]. 1. The vaporous or airlike state of matter. A fluid which distributes itself uniformly throughout any space in which it is placed, regardless of its quantity. 2. Any combustible gas used as a source of light or heat. —**gas′eous,** *adj.*

asphyxiating g. Carbon monoxide.

blister g. *In military medicine*, a gas used for casualty effect; it injures the eyes and lungs and blisters the skin: formerly called *vesicant.*

choking g. *In military medicine*, a casualty gas which causes irritation and inflammation of the bronchial tubes and lungs. Phosgene is an example of this type of gas.

Clayton g. Sulfurous acid gas generated by means of the Clayton furnace, for disinfection and for destroying rats and other vermin.

laughing g. Nitrous oxide.

marsh g. Methane.

mustard g. $(C_2H_4Cl)_2S$. Dichlorodiethylsulfide. Syn., *yperite.*

nerve gases. A group of war gases having a rapid, profound, cumulative, and only slowly reversible effect on the central, peripheral, and parasympathetic nervous systems. They exert their effects by specifically inhibiting cholinesterase; treatment is primarily with atropine. They are derivatives of organic esters of phosphoric acid, and are not to be confused with hydrogen cyanide, carbon monoxide, and various fluorophosphates.

olefiant g. Ethylene.

persistent war g. *In military medicine*, one which is normally effective in the open at the point of dispersion more than 10 minutes, used against troop concentrations for casualty effect or on materiel and terrain to restrict use through threat of casualties. A moderately persistent war gas is normally effective in the open at the point of dispersion from 10 minutes to 12 hours.

sewer g. The mixture of gases and vapors which emanate from a sewer.

tear g. Substances used by civil authorities to produce physical discomfort without injury by causing inflammation of the mucous membranes of the eyes and nose, followed by lacrimation. Especially useful in dispersing mobs.

vomiting g. *In military medicine*, a chemical agent that causes coughing, sneezing, pain in nose and throat, nasal discharge, sometimes tears, often followed by headache and vomiting: formerly called *irritant smoke* or *sternutator.* Adamsite is an example of a vomiting gas.

war g. A chemical agent which, in field concentrations, produces a toxic or strongly irritant effect. May be a finely dispersed liquid or solid as well as a true gas. Based on physiologic action, five classes of war gases, or chemical warfare agents, are recognized. The *lacrimators* include chloroacetophenone and bromobenzylcyanide. The *sternutators* include diphenylchloroarsine and diphenylaminechloroarsine (adamsite). The *lung irritants* are chlorine, phosgene, and chloropicrin, the latter being lacrimatory and emetic as well. The *vesicants* include dichloro-diethylsulfide (mustard gas) and chlorovinyldichloroarsine (lewisite), which is also a lacrimator, lung irritant, and systemic poison. Other *systemic poisons* are hydrocyanic acid and carbon monoxide.

Gaskell, Walter Holbrook [*English physiologist and anatomist*, 1847–1914]. Made important studies of the innervation of the heart and of cardiac rhythm. Demonstrated that the preganglionic neurons originate in the central nervous system (1886). His work laid the histologic foundation for later investigations of the autonomic nervous system. The atrioventricular bundle is called *Gaskell's bridge, bundle of His.*

gas·om′e·ter [*gas;* G. *metron*, a measure]. A device for holding and measuring gas. See also *spirometer.* —**gasomet′ric,** *adj.*

Tissot g. See *Tissot spirometer.*

gasp [ON. *geispa*, to yawn]. To breathe spasmodically with open mouth.

Gasser, Herbert Spencer (1888–). American physiologist and medical administrator, one of the first to use amplifiers in physiology. He and J. Erlanger combined this instrument with the cathode-ray oscillograph and studied the highly differentiated functions of the individual nerve fibers. Nobel laureate in medicine and physiology with Erlanger (1944).

gas·ser′i·an, Gas·ser′i·an gan′gli·on. See semilunar *ganglion.*

gas′sing [*gas*, suggested by G. *chaos*, chaos]. 1. In warfare, the drenching of an area with poisonous gas. 2. The execution or attempted execution of a person by means of toxic gas. —**gassed,** *adj.*

-gas′ter [G. *gastēr*, belly]. 1. *In anatomy* and *biology*, a combining form denoting *part of* or *like a stomach.*

gas′ter·o-, gaster- [*gastēr*]. A combining form denoting *pertaining to the stomach.*

Gas″ter·oph′i·lus [*gastēr;* G. *philein*, to love]. A genus of botflies. The larvae are parasites of horses and occasionally infest the cutaneous and subcutaneous tissues in man.

G. hemorrhoidalis. A species which attacks the lower lip or jaw.

G. intestinalis. A species attacking the inner side of the legs and the sides of the abdomen. This species produces a cutaneous lesion in man, the hatched larvae causing an eruption similar to that produced by the *Ancylostoma braziliense.*

G. nasalis. The chin fly, which attacks the lower lip or jaw.

gastr-. See *gastro-.*

gas·tral′gi·a [*gastēr;* G. *algos*, pain]. Pain in the stomach.

gas″tral·go·ke·no′sis (gas″trul·go·keh·no′sis, gastral″go·) [*gastēr; algos;* G. *kenos*, empty; *-ōsis*, condition]. Pain due to emptiness of the stomach; relieved by taking food.

gas″tras·the′ni·a [*gastēr;* G. *astheneia*, want of strength]. Debility of the stomach. *Obs.*

gas″tra·tro′phi·a [*gastēr;* G. *atrophia*, want of food]. Atrophy of the stomach.

gas·trec′ta·sis [*gastēr;* G. *ektasis*, extension]. Dilatation of the stomach.

gas·trec′to·my [*gastēr;* G. *ektomē*, excision]. Excision of the whole or a part of the stomach.

gas′tric [*gastēr*]. Pertaining to the stomach.

gas′trin [*gastēr*]. A hormone, originating in the pyloric glands of the stomach, purported to excite secretion of the fundic cells.

gas·tri′tis [*gastēr;* G. *-itis*, inflammation]. Acute or chronic inflammation of the stomach. —**gastrit′ic,** *adj.*

atrophic g. A chronic form with atrophy of the mucous membrane.

cancer g. A diffuse subacute gastritis with atrophy of the gastric glands, considered to be a precancerous inflammation.

catarrhal g. A type, usually acute, with mucinous exudate.

corrosive g. An acute gastritis which is caused by corrosive poisons.

fibrinous g. An acute inflammation with a large amount of fibrin in the exudate. Also called *croupous g., diphtheritic g., membranous g., pseudomembranous g.*

hypertrophic g. A chronic form with increased thickness of mucosa, exaggerated granulation, and larger, more numerous rugae. Polyps may develop.

infectious g. Acute gastritis associated with infectious diseases such as measles, scarlet fever.

interstitial g. An uncommon, chronic gastritis; characterized by increase in thickness and density of the submucosa.

phlegmonous g. An extended form of acute, suppurative gastritis.

simple exogenous g. The acute type often associated with enteritis and characterized by vomiting, pain, and malaise; may be due to ingested food or to an infection.

suppurative g. Acute, purulent gastritis.

gas′tro-, gastr- [*gastēr*]. A combining form meaning *stomach* or *belly.*

gas″tro·a·ceph′a·lus [*gastēr;* G. *a-*, not; *kephalē*, head]. A monster having an acephalic abdominal parasite.

gas″tro·a·mor′phus [*gastēr; a-;* G. *morphē*, form]. A form of cryptodidymus in which fetal parts are included within the abdomen of the host. Syn., *endocyma.*

gas″tro·an·as″to·mo′sis [*gastēr;* G. *anastomōsis*, opening]. In hour-glass contraction, the formation of a communication between the two pouches of the stomach. Also called *gastrogastrostomy.*

gas′tro·cele [*gastēr;* G. *kēlē*, hernia]. A hernia of the stomach.

gas″troc·ne′mi·us [G. *gastroknēmia*, calf of the leg]. A muscle on the posterior aspect of the leg, arising by two heads from the posterior surfaces of the lateral and medial condyles of the femur, and inserted with the soleus muscle into the Achilles tendon, and through this into the back of the calcaneus.

gas′tro·coel (gas′tro·seel). Archenteron.

gas″tro·col′ic [*gastēr;* G. *kolon*, colon]. Pertaining to the stomach and the colon.

gas″tro·co·lot′o·my [*gastēr; kolon;* G. *tomē*, a cutting]. Incision into the stomach and colon.

gas″tro·col·pot′o·my [*gastēr;* G. *kolpos*, vagina; *tomē*]. The operation of Cesarean section in which the opening is made through the linea alba and continued into the upper part of the vagina. *Obs.*

gas″tro·di′a·phane [*gastēr;* G. *diaphainein*, to show through]. An electric apparatus for illuminating the interior of the stomach so that its outlines can be seen through the abdominal wall. —**gastrodiaph′any,** *n.*

gas″tro·di·aph″a·nos′co·py [*gastēr; diaphainein;* G. *skopein*, to examine]. The examination of the stomach by means of the diaphanoscope; gastrodiaphany.

gas″tro·did′y·mus [*gastēr;* G. *didymos*, twin]. A monster consisting of equal conjoined twins united at the epigastric region. Syn., *omphalopagus, omphalodidymus, anakatadidymus.*

gas″tro·dis·ci′a·sis (gas″tro·dis·kigh′uh·sis) [*gastēr;* G. *diskos*, disk; NL. *-iasis*, condition]. Infestation of the cecum by the *Gastrodiscoides hominis*, causing inflammation and producing diarrhea.

Gas″tro·dis·coid′es (gas″tro·dis·koy′deez) [*gastēr;* G. *diskoeidēs*, disk-shaped]. A genus of flukes of the family Gastrodiscidae.

G. hominis. A species which has as its natural host the hog; man serves as an accidental host.

Gas″tro·dis′cus hom′i·nis. Synonym for *Gastrodiscoides hominis.*

gas′tro·disk [*gastēr;* G. *diskos*, disk]. *In embryology*, the germinal disk.

gas″tro·du″o·de′nal (gas″tro·dew″o·dee′nul, ·dewod′i·nul) [*gastēr;* L. *duodeni*, twelve]. Pertaining to the stomach and the duodenum.

gas″tro·du″o·de·ni′tis [*gastēr; duodeni;* G. *-itis*, inflammation]. Inflammation of the stomach and duodenum.

gas″tro·du″o·de·nos′to·my [*gastēr; duodeni;* G. *stoma*, mouth]. Establishment of an anastomosis between stomach and duodenum.

gas″tro·en″ter·al′gi·a [*gastēr;* G. *enteron*, intestine; *algos*, pain]. Common but inexact term for pain in the stomach and intestine.

gas″tro·en′ter·ic. Pertaining to the stomach and the intestines; gastrointestinal.

gas″tro·en″ter·i′tis [*gastēr; enteron;* G. *-itis*, inflammation]. Inflammation of stomach and intestine.

acute nonbacterial g. An infectious, brief, self-limited viral disease of the digestive tract occurring most frequently in late fall and early winter. Clinical diagnosis is made after other diagnoses have been ruled out, and when two or more of the following major symptoms are present: fever, diarrhea, vomiting, and abdominal pain. It is **epidemic** if another member of the patient's family acquires one of the above four symptoms within ten days of the patient's recovery. Recent evidence suggests two types: an **afebrile type** caused by Marcy strain virus and characterized by frequent watery stools; a **febrile type** caused by FS strain virus in which constitutional symptoms are more severe but watery diarrhea is absent.

gas″tro·en″ter·o·a·nas″to·mo′sis [*gastēr; enteron;* G. *anastomōsis*, opening]. Anastomosis between the intestine and the stomach. See *gastroenterostomy, gastroduodenostomy, gastrojejunostomy.*

gas″tro·en″ter·ol′o·gist [*gastēr; enteron;* G. *logos*, word]. One who specializes in diseases of the stomach and intestine.

gas″tro·en″ter·ol′o·gy [*gastēr; enteron; logos*]. The study of the stomach and intestine and their diseases.

gas″tro·en″ter·op·to′sis. Sagging or prolapse of the stomach and intestines.

gas″tro·en″ter·os′to·my [*gastēr; enteron;* G. *stoma*, mouth]. The formation of a communication between the stomach and the small intestine, usually the jejunum. See *gastroduodenostomy, gastrojejunostomy.*

gas″tro·ep″i·plo′ic [*gastēr;* G. *epiploon*, fold]. Pertaining to the stomach and omentum, as the gastroepiploic artery. See Table of Arteries in the Appendix.

gas″tro·e·soph″a·gi′tis [*gastēr;* G. *oisophagos*, gullet; *-itis*, inflammation]. Combined inflammation of the stomach and the esophagus.

gas″tro·gas·tros′to·my [*gastēr; gastēr;* G. *stoma*, mouth]. The surgical anastomosis of one portion of the stomach with another.

gas″tro·ga″vage′ (gas″tro·gah″vahzh′) [*gastēr;* F., from *gaver*, to gorge]. Artificial feeding through an opening in the stomach wall; gavage.

gas′tro·graph [*gastēr;* G. *graphein*, to write]. An apparatus for registering the peristaltic movements of the stomach from the outside.

gas″tro·he·pat′ic [*gastēr;* G. *hēpar*, liver]. Relating to the stomach and liver, as the gastrohepatic ligament.

gas″tro·hy″per·ton′ic [*gastēr;* G. *hypertonos*, strained to the utmost]. Relating to morbid or excessive tonicity or irritability of the stomach.

gas″tro·hys″ter·ec′to·my [*gastēr;* G. *hystera*, womb; *ektomē*, excision]. Removal of the uterus through the abdominal wall; abdominal hysterectomy. *Obs.*

gas″tro·hys′ter·o·pex″y [*gastēr; hystera;* G. *pēxis*, a fixing]. Ventrofixation of the uterus by an operation. *Obs.*

gas″tro·hys″ter·ot′o·my [*gastēr; hystera;* G. *tomē*, a cutting]. Old term for high abdominal Cesarean section. *Obs.*

gas″tro·in·tes′ti·nal [*gastēr;* L. *intestinum*, intestine]. Pertaining to the stomach and intestine.

gas″tro·je·ju′nal [*gastēr;* L. *jejunus*, empty]. Pertaining to the stomach and to the jejunum, as gastrojejunal anastomosis.

gas″tro·je″ju·ni′tis (gas″tro·jee″jew·nigh′tis, ·jedj″oo·nigh′tis) [*gastēr; jejunus;* G. *-itis*, inflammation]. Inflammation of both the stomach and jejunum; may occur after gastrojejunostomy.

gas″tro·je″ju·nos′to·my (·jee″jew·nos′to·mee, ·jedj″oo·nos′to·mee) [*gastēr; jejunus;* G. *stoma*, opening]. The surgical anastomosis of the jejunum to the anterior or posterior wall of the stomach; gastroenterostomy.

gas″tro·lav′age (gas″tro·lav′idj, ·la·vahzh′) [*gastēr;* L. *lavare*, to wash]. Washing out of the stomach; gastric lavage.

gas″tro·li′e·nal (gas″tro·lye′i·nul, ·lee′i·nul). Incorrect form for gastrosplenic.

gas′tro·lith [*gastēr;* G. *lithos*, stone]. A calcareous formation in the stomach.

gas″tro·li·thi′a·sis [*gastēr; lithos;* NL. *-iasis*, condition]. A morbid condition associated with the formation of gastroliths.

gas·trol′o·gy [*gastēr;* G. *logos*, word]. The science of the stomach and its functions and diseases.

gas·trol′y·sis [*gastēr;* G. *lysis*, a loosing]. The breaking-up of adhesions between the stomach and adjacent organs.

gas″tro·ma·la′ci·a (gas″tro·ma·lay′shee·uh, ·see·uh) [*gastēr;* G. *malakia*, softness]. An abnormal softening of the walls of the stomach. *Obs.*

gas″tro·meg′a·ly [*gastēr;* G. *megas*, large]. Abnormal enlargement of the stomach.

gas·trom′e·lus [*gastēr;* G. *melos*, limb]. An individual with an accessory limb attached to the abdomen.

gas″tro·my·co′sis (gas″tro·migh·ko′sis) [*gastēr;* G. *mykēs*, fungus; *-ōsis*, condition]. Gastric disease due to fungi.

gas″tro·my·ot′o·my (gas″tro·migh·ot′o·mee) [*gastēr;* G. *mys*, muscle; *tomē*, a cutting]. Incision of the circular muscle fibers of the stomach. See *pyloromyotomy.*

gastron. A proprietary preparation representing the soluble contents of the gastric mucosa; used in gastric dysfunction.

gas″tro·par·a·si′tus [*gastēr;* G. *parasitos*, parasite]. A monster having a parasite attached to its abdomen.

gas·trop′a·thy [*gastēr;* G. *pathos*, disease]. Any disease or disorder of the stomach.

gas′tro·pex″y, gas″tro·pex′y [*gastēr;* G. *pēxis*, a fixing]. The fixation of a prolapsed stomach in its normal position by suturing it to the abdominal wall or other structure.

Gas″tro·phil′i·dae (gas″tro·fil′i·dee) [*gastēr;* G. *philein*, to love]. A family of the Diptera, whose larvae, known as bots, are parasitic in the stomach and intestine of horses and related animals. The principal genus is *Gasterophilus.*

gas″tro·pho′tor [*gastēr;* G. *phōs*, light]. A stomach camera which takes pictures of the inside of the stomach.

gas″tro·phren′ic. Pertaining to the stomach and diaphragm, as gastrophrenic ligament.

gas″tro·plas′ty, gas′tro·plas″ty [*gastēr;* G. *plassein*, to form]. Plastic operation on the stomach.

gas″tro·pli·ca′tion [*gastēr;* L. *plicare*, to fold]. An operation for relief of chronic dilatation of the stomach, consisting in suturing a large horizontal fold in the stomach wall; quilting of the stomach wall for redundancy due to chronic dilatation. See *gastroplasty, gastrorrhaphy.*

gas′tro·pore. See *blastopore.*

gas″trop·to′sis [*gastēr;* G. *ptōsis*, a falling]. Prolapse or downward displacement of the stomach.

gas″tro·py″lo·rec′to·my [*gastēr;* G. *pylōros*, gatekeeper; *ektomē*, excision]. Excision of the pyloric portion of the stomach; pylorectomy.

gas″tror·rha′gi·a [*gastēr;* G. *rhēgnynai*, to break forth]. Hemorrhage from the stomach.

gas·tror′rha·phy [*gastēr;* G. *rhaphē*, a suture]. Surgical repair of a stomach wound by infolding of the edges and employing repeated rows of sutures.

gas″tror·rhe′a [*gastēr;* G. *rhoia*, a flow]. Excessive secretion of gastric mucus or of gastric juice.

gas·tros′chi·sis (gas·tros′ki·sis) [*gastēr;* G. *schisis*, cleavage]. A congenital malformation in which the abdomen remains open.

gas′tro·scope [*gastēr;* G. *skopein*, to examine]. An instrument for examining the interior of the stomach. **—gastros′copy,** *n.*

gas′tro·spasm [*gastēr;* G. *spasmos*, spasm]. Stomach spasm.

gas″tro·splen′ic [*gastēr;* G. *splēn*, spleen]. Relating to the stomach and the spleen.

gas″tro·stax′is [*gastēr;* G. *staxis*, a dripping]. The oozing of blood from the mucous membrane of the stomach.

gas·tros′to·my [*gastēr;* G. *stoma*, mouth]. The establishing of a fistulous opening into the stomach, with an external opening in the skin; usually for artificial feeding.

gas″tro·tho·ra·cop′a·gus [*gastēr;* G. *thōrax*, thorax; *pagos*, that which is fixed]. A monster consisting of conjoined twins united at the abdomen and thorax.

gas·trot′o·my [*gastēr;* G. *tomē*, a cutting]. Incision into the stomach.

gas″tro·tox′in [*gastēr;* G. *toxikon*, poison]. A cytotoxin which has a specific action on the cells lining the stomach.

gas″tro·tym″pa·ni′tes (gas″tro·tim″puh·nigh′teez, ·nigh′tis) [*gastēr;* G. *tympanitēs*, from *tympanon*, drum]. Gaseous distention of the stomach.

gas′tru·la [NL. dim. from *gastēr*]. An embryo at that stage of its development when it consists of two cellular layers, the primary ectoderm and entoderm, and a primitive gut or archenteron opening externally through the blastopore. The simplest type is derived by the invagination of the spherical blastula, but this is greatly modified in the various animal groups. **—gastrula′tion,** *n.*

gas war′fare″. See *chemical warfare.*

Gatch, Willis Dew [*American surgeon*, 1878–]. Inventor of a surgical bed with adjustable frame and springs for raising and lowering the head and maintaining a semisitting position; called *Gatch bed.*

gat″o·phil′i·a [It. *gatto*, from LL. *catus*, cat; G. *philein*, to love]. Fondness for cats.

gat″o·pho′bi·a [*catus;* G. *phobos*, fear]. A morbid fear of cats.

-gat·tel [Indonesian, itch]. In Indonesia, suffix of names of plants, contact with which causes severe itching.

Gaucher, Philippe Charles Ernest [*French physician*, 1854–1918]. Described familial splenic anemia (1882), called *cerebroside lipoidosis, Gaucher's disease.* The characteristic cells are called *Gaucher's cells.*

gauge. See *gage.*

Gault's reflex. See under *reflex.*

gaul·the′ri·a [after Jean François *Gaultier*, Canadian physician and botanist, 1708–56]. The plant, *Gaultheria procumbens*, the leaves of which yield a volatile oil. Syn., *teaberry; wintergreen.*

g. oil. Contains 90% of methyl salicylate; used in acute rheumatism and as a local antiseptic and flavoring agent. Dose, 0.3–1.2 cc. (5–20 min.).

synthetic g. oil. See *methyl* salicylate.

gaul′ther·in. A glycoside obtained from the bark of the sweet birch, *Betula lenta*, and from wintergreen, *Gaultheria procumbens.* On enzymatic hydrolysis it yields methyl salicylate and primeverose; on acid hydrolysis the latter yields D-glucose and D-xylose.

gaul·ther′o·lin. Methyl salicylate.

gaunt′let [F. *gantelet*, dim. of *gant*, glove]. A bandage that covers the hand and fingers like a glove.

Gauss, Karl Friedrich [*German mathematician and optician*, 1777–1855]. Devised Gaussian points, addition and subtraction logarithms, and the probability curve.

gauze [F. *gaze*]. A thin, open-meshed cloth of varying degrees of fineness, used in surgical operations and for surgical dressings. When sterilized, it is called **aseptic gauze;** when packaged for use in the operating room, the individual folded pieces are called sponges.

ga″vage′ (gah″vahzh′) [F.]. The administration of liquid nourishment through the stomach tube.

Gavard, Hyacinthe [*French anatomist*, 1753–1802]. Described the oblique muscular fibers of the stomach wall, called *Gavard's muscle.*

Gay-Lussac, Joseph Louis [*French chemist and physicist*, 1778–1850]. Isolated boron and cyanogen. Studied the expansion of gases. *Gay-Lussac's law* states that the volumes of interacting gases and of the reaction products are in simple proportions that can be expressed in whole numbers.

g-component. See *gynandromorphy.*

Gd Chemical symbol for gadolinium.

Ge Chemical symbol for germanium.

Gee, Samuel Jones [*English pediatrician*, 1839–1911]. First to describe celiac disease (1888), a nontropical disease similar to if not identical with sprue; see under *disease.*

Gegenbaur, Carl [*German anatomist*, 1826–1903]. One of the first to study comparative anatomy in relation to evolution. Demonstrated that the vertebrate ovum is a single cell (1861). See *muscle of Gegenbaur.*

Gehuchten, Arthur van (1861–1914). Belgian neurologist, known for his studies of the central nervous system and his contributions to the neuron doctrine.

Geigel's reflex. See under *reflex.*

Geiger, Hans [*German physicist*, 1882–1945]. Made important studies of radioactivity. See Geiger-Müller counting *circuit*, Geiger-Müller *tube*, *Geiger-Müller counter.*

Geiger, Philipp Lorenz [*German pharmacologist*, 1785–1836]. Isolated atropine (1883) with Hermann Hesse.

Gei′ger-Mül′ler count′er. An instrument for the detection of individual ionizing particles; entry of a charged particle into the apparatus produces ionization and a momentary flow of current which is relayed to a counting device: also called *Geiger counter.*

Gei′ger re′gion. The voltage interval of a Geiger counter tube in which the charge transferred per isolated count is independent of the charge produced by the initial ionizing event.

Gei′ger thresh′old. The lowest voltage at which all pulses produced by an ionizing event in a Geiger counter tube are the same size regardless of the energy of the initial ionizing radiation.

gei·so′ma (guy·so′muh) [G. *geison*, cornice]. The eyebrows of the face, or the supraorbital ridges of the skull. Also called *geison.*

gei′son (guy′son). See *geisoma.*

Geissler tube. See *roentgen rays* under *ray.*

gel (jel). A colloidal system comprising a solid and a liquid phase which exists as a solid or semisolid mass.

inelastic g. One that loses its property of elasticity and pulverizes when dried, becoming amorphous.

irreversible g. One transformed from a sol, which cannot be reversed to a sol.

gel′a·sin. A preparation of agar-agar.

ge·las′mus (jeh·laz′mus, ·lass′mus), **ge·las′ma** (jeh·laz′muh, ·lass′muh) [G. *gelasma*, smile]. Insane or hysterical spasmodic laughter.

ge·lat″i·fi·ca′tion [L. *gelare*, to freeze; *facere*, to make]. The conversion of a substance into a jelly-like mass.

gel′a·tin [*gelare*] (*gelatinum*). The product obtained by the partial hydrolysis of collagen, derived from the skin, white connective tissue, and bones of animals. Gelatin derived from an acid-treated precursor exhibits an isoelectric point between pH 7 and pH 9, while gelatin derived from an alkali-treated precursor has an isoelectric point between pH 4.7 and 5.0. It occurs in sheets, flakes, shreds, or as a coarse or fine powder, insoluble in cold water but soluble in hot water. Gelatin is used in many pharmaceutical preparations, as an ingredient of bacteriologic culture mediums, and as a food. In medicine it finds some use in accelerating coagulation of blood by intravenous injection; it is of some interest as a possible blood substitute. —**gelat'inoid, gelat'inous,** *adj.*

glycerinated g. (*gelatinum glycerinatum*). A preparation of gelatin and glycerin, used as a vehicle for suppositories and bougies: also called *glycerin-jelly.*

medicated g. Gelatin disks or lamellas mixed with medicated substances. The gelatin lamellas of the British Pharmacopoeia contain small amounts of alkaloids, for introduction into the conjunctival sac. They are dissolved by the tears, and the effects of the alkaloids are thus obtained.

ossein g. A gelatin obtained by boiling bone.

ge·lat'i·nase. An enzyme liquefying gelatin. It is found in various molds and yeasts.

ge·lat'i·nize [*gelare*]. Convert into a jellylike mass.

ge·lat"i·no·lyt'ic [*gelare;* G. *lysis,* a loosing]. Dissolution or splitting up of gelatin.

ge·lat"i·no'sa. See *substantia* gelatinosa Rolandi.

gel·a'tion. 1. The change of a colloid from a sol to a gel. 2. Freezing.

gel'a·tose. A product of the hydrolysis of gelatin by acid, alkali, or enzyme.

geld (gheld) [ON. *geldr,* barren]. To castrate, as a horse; to emasculate.

geld'ing (gheld'ing) [*geldr*]. 1. Castration. 2. A castrated stallion.

gelfoam. Trade-mark for partly denatured gelatin, in the form of a powder or a light porous matrix, employed as a hemostatic agent, often in combination with thrombin.

Gélineau, Jean Baptiste Edouard [*French physician,* 1859–]. First to describe narcolepsy (1880), called *Gélineau's disease* or *syndrome, Gélineau-Redlich syndrome.*

Gellé, Marie Ernest [*French aural surgeon,* 1834–1923]. Described a hearing test, called *Gellé's test,* to detect complete or partial fixation of the stapes. A tuning fork is placed in contact with a rubber tube whose nozzle is inserted into the external auditory meatus. If the sound is diminished in intensity when air is compressed in the tube by pressure upon a connecting bulb, the test is positive, and the ear is normal.

gel'ose (jel'oce, jee'loce, jeh·loce'). 1. The gelatinizing principle of agar, being the calcium salt of a complex carbohydrate substance composed of galactose units. 2. A culture medium for bacteria. See *agar-agar.*

gel'o·sin (jel'o·sin, jeh·lo'sin). A mucilage from a Japanese alga.

ge·lot'o·lep"sy, gel'o·to·lep"sy [G. *gelōs,* laughter; *lēpsis,* a seizing]. A sudden loss of muscle tone during laughter, with a transitory loss of consciousness.

gel·sem'i·cine (jel·sem'i·seen, ·sin). An alkaloid from gelsemium.

gel·sem'i·dine. An alkaloid from gelsemium.

gel'se·mine (jel'si·meen, ·min). An alkaloid, $C_{20}H_{22}O_2N_2$, from gelsemium.

gel·sem'in·ine. An alkaloid from gelsemium.

gel·se'mi·um (jel·see'mee·um, ·sem'ee·um) [NL. from It. *gelsomino,* jessamine] (*gelsemium*). The dried rhizome and roots of *Gelsemium sempervirens,* used as an antispasmodic and antineuralgic. Dose, 0.03–0.13 Gm. (½–2 gr.). Also called *yellow jasmine root.*

ge·mel'lus [L., twin]. A name applied to certain paired muscles. See Table of Muscles in the Appendix.

gem'i·nate, gem'i·nous [L. *geminare,* to double]. 1. In pairs; coupled. 2. Double; become double. —**gemina'tion,** *n.*

gem"i·na'tion [L. *geminatio,* a doubling]. The formation of two teeth, separate or more or less fused, where only one tooth is normal.

gem'i·nous. See *geminate.*

ge·mis'to·cyte [Ger. *mästen,* to fatten; G. *kytos,* cell]. Anglicized form of Nissl's *gemästete Zellen* or plump astrocyte; a large, round cell with pale, acidophilic, homogeneous cytoplasm and eccentrically displaced nucleus, observed in certain neuropathological conditions, as in so-called gemistocytic astrocytoma. —**gemis'tocytic,** *adj.*

gem'ma [L., a bud]. An asexual, budlike body, either unicellular or multicellular.

gem·ma'tion [L. *gemmare,* to put forth buds]. Budding; a mode of reproduction seen in low forms of animal and vegetable life characterized by the formation of a small projection from the parent organism, which is constricted off and forms another organism.

gem'mule [L. *gemmula,* little bud]. 1. A small bud or gemma. 2. A term applied to the short thorny processes of the dendrites of pyramidal nerve cells.

gemonil. Trade-mark for metharbital, chemically 5,5-dimethyl-1-methylbarbituric acid; a barbituric acid derivative useful in treating epilepsy.

gen. See *gene.*

-gen [G. *genesthai,* from *gignesthai,* to be produced]. 1. *In chemistry,* a combining form denoting *a substance that produces* or *generates.* 2. *In biology,* a combining form denoting *a thing produced* or *generated.*

ge'na [L.]. The cheek. —**genal,** *adj.*

Gendre's fixing fluid. See under *fixing fluid.*

gene, gen [G. *genesthai,* from *gignesthai,* to be produced]. Any hereditary factor; the ultimate unit in the transmission of hereditary characteristics, regarded as an ultramicroscopic particle, capable of self-reproduction and imitation, which occupies a definite locus on a chromosome. Any known gene is a modifier of development and is regarded as a cellular physiologic agent which acts as a center of specific chemical activity.

gen'er·a. Plural of genus.

gen'er·al [L. *generalis,* of or belonging to a species, from *genus,* kind]. Common to a class; distributed through many parts; diffuse. —**generalize,** *v.t.*

gen"er·a'ti·o (jen"ur·ay'tee·o). See *generation.*

gen"er·a'tion [L. *generare,* to produce]. 1. The act or process of producing offspring. 2. A period extending from the birth of an individual to the birth of his offspring, in humans usually a third of a century. 3. The production of a gas or electric current. —**gen'erative,** *adj.;* **gen'erate,** *v.t.*

alternate g. See *alternation of generations.*

asexual g. Reproduction without sexual union; reproduction by fission or gemmation.

sexual g. Reproduction by the union of a male and a female gamete.

spontaneous g. See *abiogenesis.*

gen'er·a"tor [L., from *generare*]. 1. *In electricity,* a machine which transforms mechanical power into electric power. 2. *In radiology,* a machine which supplies the roentgen-ray tube with the electric energies necessary for the production of roentgen rays. 3. *In chemistry,* an apparatus for the formation of vapor or gas from a liquid or solid by heat or chemical action.

cascade g. A generator in which the transformers are arranged in a cascaded series with separate insulation for the production of high voltages. Used in supervoltage roentgen therapy.

electrostatic g. Apparatus for producing voltages up to several million volts by accumulating a small static charge on an insulated high-voltage metal collector.

supervoltage g. One that produces voltages over 250,000; used in the production of short-wave roentgen rays.

ge·ner′ic [L. *genus*, kind]. 1. Pertaining to a genus. 2. General.

gen·es′er·ine (jen·ess′ur·een, ·in). Eseridine.

ge·ne′si·al [G. *genesis*, production]. Old term for pertaining to generation.

ge·nes′ic (ji·ness′ick, ji·nee′sick) [*genesis*]. Of or relating to generation or to the genital organs.

ge·ne″si·ol′o·gy (ji·nee″see·ol′o·jee, ji·nee″zee·) [*genesis;* G. *logos*, word]. The science of reproduction or heredity.

gen′e·sis [G.]. The origin or generation of anything; the developmental evolution of a specific thing or type.

-gen′e·sis [G.]. A combining form signifying *origination, development, evolution of a thing* or *type.*

ge·net′ic [*genesis*]. 1. Pertaining to or having reference to origin, mode of production or development. 2. Pertaining to genetics. 3. Produced by genes.

ge·net′i·cist [*genesis*]. A specialist in genetics.

ge·net′ics [*genesis*]. The branch of biology which deals with the phenomena of heredity and variation. It seeks to understand the causes of the resemblances and differences between parents and progeny, and, by extension, between all organisms related to one another by descent.

ge·net″o·troph′ic. 1. Of or pertaining to genetics and nutrition. 2. Of, pertaining to, or descriptive of a disease caused by a high inherited demand for some nutrient which is not included in the consumed foods, e.g., some cases of alcoholism.

gen′e·tous [G. *genesthai*, from *gignesthai*, to be produced]. Old term for congenital.

Ge·ne′va con·ven′tion. An agreement signed by the European powers in Geneva, Switzerland, in 1864, guaranteeing humane treatment of the wounded and those caring for them in time of war. In July, 1906, a full revised convention was adopted in Geneva. In 1907, this was again revised at The Hague Peace Conference, and was adopted as Convention X.

Gengou, Octave [*French bacteriologist*, contemporary]. With Bordet, discovered the complement-fixation reaction, also called *Bordet-Gengou reaction* (1900), and described *Hemophilus pertussis*, called *Bordet-Gengou bacillus* (1906). See also *Bordet-Gengou medium* under *Bordet.*

ge′ni·al (jee′nee·ul, ji·nigh′ul) [G. *geneion*, chin]. Pertaining to the chin. Syn., *mental.*

ge·nic′u·lar [L. *geniculum*, little knee]. Pertaining to the knee joint, as the genicular artery. See Table of Arteries in the Appendix.

ge·nic′u·late, ge·nic′u·la″ted [L. *geniculare*, to bend the knee]. Abruptly bent.

ge·nic′u·lum [L.]. A small, kneelike structure; a sharp bend in any small organ.

gen′in (jen′in). See *aglycone.*

ge′ni·o- (jee′nee·o-, ji·nigh′o-) [G. *geneion*, chin]. *In anatomy*, a combining form meaning *chin.*

ge″ni·o·glos′sus [*geneion;* G. *glōssa*, tongue]. An extrinsic muscle of the tongue, arising from the superior genial tubercle of the mandible.

ge″ni·o·hy″o·glos′sus [*geneion;* G. *hyoeidēs*, Y-shaped; *glōssa*, tongue]. Old name for the genioglossus muscle.

ge″ni·o·hy′oid [*geneion; hyoeidēs*]. A muscle arising from the inferior genial tubercle of the mandible and inserted into the body of the hyoid.

ge′ni·on (jee′nee·on, ji·nigh′on) [*geneion*]. The point at the tip of the mental spine. If several spines are present, the point is located between these in the sagittal plane.

ge″ni·o·pha·ryn′ge·us [*geneion;* G. *pharygx*, throat]. A variant part of the genioglossus muscle, which blends with the superior constrictor of the pharynx.

ge′ni·o·plas″ty (jee′nee·o·plas″tee, ji·nigh′o·) [*geneion;* G. *plassein*, to form]. Plastic operation on the chin.

gen′i·tal [L. *genitalis*, from *gignere*, to produce]. Pertaining to the organs of generation or to reproduction.

gen″i·ta′li·a (jen″i·tay′lee·uh, ·tal′ee·uh) [*genitalis*]. The organs of generation. The male has two testes or seminal glands, with their excretory ducts, the prostate, the penis, and the urethra. (See Plate 44.) The female genitalia include the vulva, the vagina, the ovaries, the uterine tubes, and the uterus. (See Plate 41.)

indifferent g. The genitalia of the embryo before sexual differences are recognizable.

infantile g. The organs of generation of an infant; more commonly, underdevelopment to a marked degree of the chronologically adult organs of generation.

gen′i·ta·loid [*genitalis;* G. *eidos*, form]. Pertaining to the primordial germ cells, and indicating potentialities for either sex.

gen′i·tals. Genitalia: a common usage.

gen′i·to- [*genitalis*]. A combining form signifying *genital.*

gen″i·to·cru′ral [*genitalis;* L. *crus*, leg]. Pertaining to the genitalia and the leg.

gen″i·to·fem′o·ral [*genitalis;* L. *femur*, thigh]. Pertaining to the genitals and the thigh; genitocrural.

gen″i·to·u′ri·nar″y (jen″i·to·yoor′i·nerr″ee) [*genitalis;* L. *urina*, urine]. Relating to the genitalia and the urinary organs or functions.

gen′i·us [L., tutelar deity, from *gignere*, to produce]. 1. Distinctive character or inherent nature. 2. Unusual artistic or creative abiltiy; mental superiority.

g. epidemicus. The totality of conditions, atmospheric, cosmic, supernatural, etc., formerly regarded as most favorable to the prevalence of an endemic or of an epidemic disease. *Obs.*

g. morbi. The special or predominant feature of a disease.

Gennari, Francesco [*Italian anatomist*, ca. 1750–ca. 1795]. Described the single tangential striation of the cerebral cortex (1782); called *line, stria*, or *stripe of Gennari, Gennari's layer.*

gen′o·cide [G. *genos*, race; L. *caedere*, to kill]. The killing off of entire human groups, as homicide is the killing of an individual human being.

gen″o·der·ma·to′sis. Any congenital skin disease, as ichthyosis, pachyonychia congenita, epidermolysis bullosa, or phacomatoses.

ge′nome, ge′nom [G. *genesthai*, from *gignesthai*, to be produced; *-ōma*, group]. A complete set of the hereditary factors, such as is contained in a haploid set of chromosomes.

gen″o·mor′phine. The N-oxide of morphine, occurring in white crystals, slightly soluble in water. It has been proposed as a substitute for morphine, but causes true addiction.

gen″o·pho′bi·a [G. *genos*, sex; *phobos*, fear]. A morbid fear of sex.

genoscopolamine. Trade-mark for the N-oxide of scopolamine.

gen′o·type [G. *genesthai*, from *gignesthai*, to be produced; *typos*, impression]. 1. The hereditary constitution of an organism resulting from its particular combination of genes. 2. A class of individuals having the same genetic constitution.

—**genotyp′ic, genotyp′ical,** *adj.*

gen′tian [L. *gentiana*, from the Illyrian king *Gentius*]. 1. The common name for species of *Gentiana*. 2. The official gentian; the dried rhizome and roots of *Gentiana lutea*, containing the glycosides gentiopicrin and gentiin, as well as gentiomarin, gentisin (also called *gentianin* or *gentianic acid*), gentisic acid, and gentianose. Gentian is a bitter tonic.

compound g. tincture (*tinctura gentianae composita*). A tincture of gentian, bitter orange peel, and cardamom. Dose, 4–8 cc. (1–2 dr.).

g. violet. (a) A violet aniline dye; a mixture of the chlorides of methylated pararosanilines composed of pentamethyl and hexamethyl pararosaniline, or either of these compounds alone. It is a biologic stain having many histologic and cytologic applications, including its use in Gram's stain. (b) Methylrosaniline chloride.

glycerinated g. elixir (*elixir gentianae glycerinatum*). A useful vehicle.

gen″ti·an′ic ac′id (jen″shee·an′ick). See *gentianin.*

gen′tian·in. A constituent of gentian, chemically the 3-monomethyl ether of 1,3,7-trihydroxyflavone. Syn., *gentisin, gentianic acid.*

gen′tian·ose. A crystallizable trisaccharide from gentian root.

gen′ti·in (jen′shee·in). A glycosidal constituent of gentian.

gen″ti·o·bi′ose. A disaccharide, composed of two D-glucose units, resulting from hydrolysis of gentianose; it is also the disaccharide component of amygdalin.

gen″ti·o·mar′in. A glycosidal constituent of gentian.

gen″ti·o·pic′rin (jen″shee·o·pick′rin). A bitter, crystalline glycoside obtained from gentian.

gen·tis′ic ac′id. $C_6H_3(OH)_2COOH$; 2,5-dihydroxybenzoic acid; a constituent of gentian; it occurs in urine after ingestion of salicylates. The sodium salt has been recommended as an antirheumatic agent.

gen′ti·sin. Gentianin.

gen·tis′yl al′co·hol. 2,5-Dihydroxybenzyl alcohol. $C_7H_8O_3$. A substance of slight antibacterial activity obtained as a metabolic product of *Penicillium patulum.*

gentran. A trade-mark for the plasma-expanding and blood-pressure-maintaining substance *dextran.*

ge′nu (jeen′yōō, jen′yōō) (pl. *genua*) [L.]. 1. The knee. 2. Any structure like a knee, as the genu of the corpus callosum (see Plate 18) or the internal capsule. —**gen′ual,** *adj.*

g. capsulae internae. The portion of the internal capsule which, in cross sections, appears bent at an angle. It occurs where the capsule approaches the cavity of the lateral ventricle.

g. facialis. 1. The **internal genu** is the C-shaped curve of the intracranial part of the motor nerve root of the facial nerve around the nucleus of the abducens nerve; produced by a shift in the positions of the nuclei of both facial and abducens nerves late in development. 2. The **external genu** is the sharp bend of the facial nerve around the outer border of the vestibule of the inner ear. The geniculate ganglion is located at this bend.

g. recurvatum. The backward curvature of the knee joint.

g. valgum. Inward curving of the knee; knock-knee.

g. varum. Bowleg.

gen′u·clast, ge′nu·clast [*genu;* G. *klastos*, from *klainein*, to break]. An instrument for breaking adhesions of the knee joint. *Obs.*

gen″u·cu′bi·tal (jen″yōō·cue′bi·tul, jeen″yōō·) [*genu;* L. *cubitus*, elbow]. Relating to or supported by the knees and elbows.

gen″u·fa′cial (jen″yōō·fay′shul, jeen″yōō·) [*genu;* L. *facies*, face]. Relating to, or resting on, the knees and face.

gen″u·pec′tor·al [*genu;* L. *pectus*, chest]. Relating to the knee and the chest, as the knee-chest posture.

ge′nus (pl. *genera*) [L., race, kind]. A taxonomic group, next above a species and forming the principal subdivision of a family.

gen″y·chei′lo·plas″ty (jen″i·kigh′lo·plas″tee, jee″ni·) [G. *genys*, jaw; *cheilos*, lip; *plassein*, to form]. Plastic operation on both cheek and lip.

gen′y·o-, gen′y- [*genys*]. A combining form meaning *the under jaw.*

gen′y·plas″ty [*genys; plassein*]. Plastic operation on the lower jaw.

ge′o·din. An antibiotic substance isolated from cultures of *Aspergillus terreus;* it is active in vitro against a variety of bacteria.

Geoffroy Saint-Hilaire, Étienne [*French zoologist*, 1772–1844]. Teratologist. Father of Isidore Geoffroy Saint-Hilaire.

Geoffroy Saint-Hilaire, Isidore [*French zoologist*, 1805–61]. Classified human and animal monsters.

ge″o·med′i·cine [G. *gē*, earth; L. *medicina*, medicine]. The study of diseases from the standpoint of their geographic distribution.

ge″o·met′ric mean. The antilogarithm of the arithmetic mean of the logarithms of a series of observations.

ge·oph′a·gy, ge″o·pha′gi·a, ge·oph′a·gism [*gē;* G. *phagein*, to eat]. The practice of eating earth or clay; chthonophagia. —**geoph′agous,** *adj.*, **geoph′agist,** *n.*

Georgi, Walter [*German bacteriologist*, 1889–1920]. Introduced, with Hans Sachs, a precipitation test used in the diagnosis of syphilis; known as *Georgi-Sachs reaction.*

Georgi-Sachs test. See under *test.*

ge″o·tri·cho′sis (jee″o·tri·ko′sis, ·trye·ko′sis) [*gē;* G. *thrix*, hair; *-ōsis*, condition]. An infection caused by one or more species of the fungus *Geotrichum.* Lesions may occur in the mouth, intestinal tract, bronchi, and lungs.

Ge·ot′ri·chum. A genus of Fungi imperfecti (Link, 1809), characterized by abundant development of rectangular and rounded arthrospores and associated with bronchopulmonary and oral lesions. See *geotrichosis.*

ge·ot′ro·pism [*gē;* G. *trepein*, to turn]. *In biology*, the gravitational factor which in plants causes roots to grow downward toward the earth and shoots to grow up, and in some animals causes the climbing, swimming, or right-side-up orientation.

ge·phy″ro·pho′bi·a (ji·figh″ro·fo′bee·uh, jef″i·ro·) [G. *gephyra*, a bridge; *phobos*, fear]. A morbid fear of crossing a bridge.

Geraghty, John Timothy [*American urologist*, 1876–1924]. With L. G. Rowntree, devised the phenolsulfonphthalein test for kidney function (1910). With Rowntree and N. M. Keith, introduced a method of estimating the blood and plasma volume (1915); the method includes the intravenous injection of a dye. Reported a modification of Young's method of perineal prostatectomy (1922); called *Geraghty's method.*

ge·ral′bine. $C_{22}H_{33}NO_2$; an alkaloid isolated from *Veratrum album.*

ge·ra′ni·al. See *citral.*

ge·ra′ni·ol. $C_{10}H_{17}OH$. A colorless liquid of pleasant odor; the chief constituent of geranium oil or palmarosa oil; occurs also in rose oil, citronella oil, and others.

ge·ra′ni·um [G. *geranion*, geranium]. Cranesbill.

The rhizome of *Geranium maculatum*. An astringent due to its content of tannin.

ge·rat′ic [G. *gēras*, old age]. Pertaining to old age; gerontic.

ger″a·tol′o·gy [*gēras;* G. *logos*, word]. The scientific study of decadence and its phenomena.

Gerdy, Pierre Nicolas [*French surgeon*, 1797–1856]. Described the superficial transverse ligament of the fingers, a fibrous band bounding the distal margin of the palm; called *Gerdy's fibers*. Described an abnormal or supernumerary fontanel existing between the two parietal bones at the point at which the sagittal suture ceases to be serrated and becomes rectilinear; called *Gerdy's fontanel*.

Gerhard, William Wood [*American physician*, 1809–72]. Described tuberculous meningitis (1833). Credited with differentiating typhus from typhoid fever (1836).

Gerhardt, Carl Adolf Christian Jacob [*German physician*, 1833–1902]. Described erythromelalgia, called *Gerhardt's disease*. Studied paralysis of the vocal folds, noting the so-called cadaveric position of the folds when they are totally paralyzed. The *Gerhardt-Semon law* states that in certain central and peripheral lesions of the recurrent laryngeal nerve, the vocal folds lie midway between adduction and abduction. Gerhardt has been credited with the discovery of a number of clinical signs, among them the systolic heart sound heard between the mastoid process and the spinal column in aneurysm of the vertebral artery; incomplete filling of the jugular vein in thrombosis of the transverse cerebral sinus; absence of movement of the larynx in dyspnea, in aortic aneurysm. See also Gerhardt's *sign* of cavitation of the lungs, Gerhardt's *test*.

ger″i·a·tri′cian (jerr″ee·uh·trish′un, jeer″ee·uh·) [G. *gēras*, old age; *iatrikos*, healing]. One who specializes in the treatment of the diseases of old age. Also called *geriatrist*.

ger″i·at′rics (jerr″ee·at′ricks, jeer″ee·) [*gēras; iatrikos*]. That branch of medical science which is concerned with old age and its diseases.

ger″i·o·psy·cho′sis (jerr″ee·o·sigh·ko′sis) [*gēras;* G. *psychōsis*, from *psychē*, soul, *-ōsis*, condition]. Psychosis of old age.

Gerlach, Joseph von [*German histologist*, 1820–96]. Devised a tissue stain, a solution of ammoniated carmine and gelatin, called *Gerlach's stain*. Described a mass of lymphatic tissue in the lower portion of the auditory tube near the pharyngeal orifice; called *Gerlach's tubal tonsil*. Described a mucosal fold sometimes surrounding the orifice of the appendix; called *Gerlach's valve*.

Gerlier, Felix [*Swiss physician*, 1840–1914]. Known for his description of an endemic disease of Switzerland, of undetermined etiology, characterized by periodic attacks of severe vertigo with sudden flaccid paralysis of the neck muscles, the levator palpebrae, and occasionally the extraocular muscles and those of the throat and extremities; called *paralyzing vertigo, Gerlier's disease*. A similar disease, called kubisagari, has been observed in Japan.

germ [L. *germen*, sprout]. 1. A small bit of protoplasm capable of developing into a new individual, especially an egg, spore, or seed; any of the early stages in the development of an organism. 2. Any microorganism, especially any of the pathogenic bacteria. —**ger′minal,** *adj.*

dental g. The dental sac, enamel organ, and dental papilla regarded as a unit; comprising all the formative tissues of a tooth. Also called *tooth germ*.

hair g. The solid epithelial invagination of the germinal layer of the fetal epidermis that forms the primordium of the hair. Also called *hair column*.

germanin. See *suramin*.

ger·man′i·trine. $C_{39}H_{59}NO_{11}$; an ester alkaloid, hypotensively active, isolated from *Veratrum fimbriatum* Gray; on hydrolysis it yields germine and one mole each of acetic acid, tiglic acid, and methylethylacetic acid.

ger·ma′ni·um [L. *Germania*, Germany]. Ge = 72.60. A brittle, grayish white, metallic element.

g. dioxide. GeO_2. Has been claimed to stimulate the formation of red blood cells.

germ′bu·dine. An ester alkaloid isolated from *Veratrum viride;* on hydrolysis it yields germine.

ger′mer·ine. An ester alkaloid isolated from *Veratrum album;* on hydrolysis it yields germine, methylethylacetic acid, and methylethylglycolic acid.

ger′mi·cide [L. *germen*, sprout; *caedere*, to kill]. An agent that destroys germs. —**germici′dal,** *adj.*

ger′mi·dine. A highly active diester alkaloid isolated from *Veratrum viride;* on hydrolysis it yields germine, acetic acid, and 2-methylbutyric acid.

ger″mi·na′tion [L. *germinatio*, from *germinare*, to germinate]. The beginning of growth of a spore or seed.

ger′mi·na″tive [*germinare*]. Having the power to begin growth or to develop.

ger′mine. $C_{27}H_{43}NO_8$; a highly hydroxylated alkanolamine base, steroidal in character, various esters of which constitute certain of the alkaloids of *Veratrum viride* and *Veratrum album*. Germine is isomeric with cevine and protoverine, which are parent bases of other alkaloids in the veratrums. Under certain conditions germine may be isomerized to isogermine or pseudogermine.

ger·min′i·trine. $C_{39}H_{57}NO_{11}$; an ester alkaloid, hypotensively active, isolated from *Veratrum fimbriatum* Gray; on hydrolysis it yields germine and one mole each of acetic acid, tiglic acid, and angelic acid.

ger·mi·no′ma [L. *germen*, germ; G. *-ōma*, tumor]. A gonadal tumor. See *dysgerminoma, seminoma*.

pineal g. See *pinealoma*.

ger″mi·tet′rine B. A tetraester alkaloid isolated from *Veratrum album;* on hydrolysis it yields germine, two moles of acetic acid, and one mole each of 2-methylbutyric acid and 2,3-dihydroxy-2-methylbutyric acid.

ger′mi·trine. A triester alkaloid, hypotensively active, isolated from *Veratrum viride;* on hydrolysis it yields germine, and one mole each of acetic acid, 2-methylbutyric acid, and 2-hydroxy-2-methylbutyric (methylethylglycolic) acid.

germ track. The continuity of sexual cells observed through many generations.

ge·roc′o·my (ji·rock′o·mee, jerr′o·ko·mee), **ger″o·co′mi·a** (jerr″o·ko′mee·uh, jeer″o·) [G. *gerōn*, old man; *komein*, to care for]. The medical and hygienic care of old people. —**gerocom′ical,** *adj.*

ger″o·der′ma (jerr″o·dur′muh, jeer″o·) [*gerōn;* G. *derma*, skin]. The skin of old age, showing atrophy, loss of fat, loss of elasticity, etc.

ger″o·don′ti·a. Dentistry for the aged.

ger″o·ma·ras′mus (jerr″o·ma·raz′mus, jeer″o·) [*gerōn;* G. *marasmos*, a wasting]. Emaciation characteristic of extreme old age.

ger″o·mor′phism [*gerōn;* G. *morphē*, form]. The condition of appearing aged while still young.

ge·ron′tic, ge·ron′tal [*gerōn*]. Pertaining to decadence or old age. —**gerontism,** *n.*

ger″on·tol′o·gy (jerr″on·tol′o·jee, jeer″on·) [*gerōn;* G. *logos*, word]. Scientific study of the phenomena of old age.

ge·ron″to·phil′i·a [*gerōn;* G. *philein*, to love]. Love for old people.

ge·ron″to·pho′bi·a. Morbid fear of old age.

ge·ron″to·ther′a·py [*gerōn;* G. *therapeia,* treatment]. Treatment of the aging process.

ger″on·tox′on [*gerōn;* G. *toxon,* bow]. The arcus senilis.

Gerota, Dumitru (1867–1939). Rumanian surgeon who studied the lymphatic system by the injection method. The lymphatic drainage from the mammary glands through the abdominal lymphatics to the liver or subdiaphragmatic nodes by which breast cancer may spread is called *paramammary route of Gerota;* the renal fascia is called *Gerota's fascia,* the space enclosed by the renal fascia of the two sides, *Gerota's space.*

Gersh method. See Altmann-Gersh *method.*

Gerson diet. See S.H.G. *diet.*

Gerssdorff, Hans von [*German surgeon,* ca. 1456–1517]. Famous military surgeon. His classic *Feldtbuch* on the treatment of wounds contains the first known illustration of an amputation (1517).

Gerstmann, Josef (1887–). American neurologist and psychiatrist who described a complex disorder of cerebral function due to a lesion in the left angular and the adjoining area of the middle occipital gyri, giving rise to right-left disorientation, agraphia, acalculia, and hemianopsia, called *Gerstmann's syndrome.*

Gersuny, Robert [*Austrian surgeon,* 1844–1924]. Described his operation, now obsolete, for fecal incontinence in which the rectum is freed and twisted on its long axis and sutured in place: called *Gersuny's operation.*

Gesell, Arnold (1880–). American psychologist and pediatrician, known widely for his studies on the genesis of behavior and the growth and development of the infant and child.

Gesell developmental schedule. See under *test.*

Gesner, Conrad [*Swiss physician and naturalist,* 1516–65]. His *Historia Animalium* is considered one of the cornerstones of modern zoology. Compiled numerous bibliographies in various fields, and also a universal bibliography. Called the German Pliny and the father of bibliography.

ge·stalt′, Ge·stalt′ (gu·shtolt′) [Ger., form, shape]. Form; shape; the configuration of separate units into a pattern or shape which itself seems to function as a unit. See gestalt *psychology.*

ge·stalt′ist, Ge·stalt′ist (gu·shtol′tist). A psychologist of the gestalt school. See gestalt *psychology.*

ges·ta′tion [L. *gestatio,* from *gestare,* to carry]. Pregnancy.

abdominal g. The form of extrauterine gestation in which the product of conception is developed in the abdominal cavity.

double g. (a) Twin pregnancy. (b) The coexistence of uterine and extrauterine pregnancy.

ectopic g. See extrauterine *g.*

extrauterine g. Development of the ovum outside of the uterine cavity. See *pregnancy.*

ges·to′sis (pl. *gestoses*) [*gestare;* G. *-ōsis,* condition]. Any toxemic manifestation in pregnancy.

Getsowa adenoma. See under *adenoma.*

Getsowa, struma postbranchialis of. See under Getsowa *adenoma.*

geu″ma·pho′bi·a (gew″muh·fo′bee·uh) [G. *geuma,* taste; *phobos,* fear]. A morbid fear of taste.

-geu′si·a (-gew′see·uh, -jew′see·uh) [G. *geusis,* sense of taste]. A combining form denoting *a condition of the taste sense.*

ghat′ti gum. The gummy exudate from stems of *Anogeissus latifolia,* a tree of India and Ceylon. It forms a viscous mucilage, and may be used in certain pharmaceutical preparations in place of acacia. Syn., *Indian gum.*

Ghon, Anton [*Austrian pathologist,* 1866–1936]. Described the development of lesions in juvenile pulmonary tuberculosis. The primary lesion is called *Ghon's primary focus* or *lesion, Ghon tubercle.* The *Ghon complex,* also called *primary complex, Küss-Ghon focus,* comprises the Ghon tubercle plus the satellite lymph node involvement.

Giacomini, frenulum of. See under *frenulum.*

Giacosa, Piero [*Italian physician,* 1853–1928]. Remembered for his study of the transformation of nitrates in the body.

Giannuzzi, cells of. See *demilune cells* under *cell.*

gi′ant [G. *gigas,* giant]. A being or organism of abnormally large size.

gi′ant in″tra·can·al·ic′u·lar fi″bro·ad″e·no·myx·o′ma. See *cystosarcoma phylloides.*

gi′ant·ism. See *gigantism.*

Gi·ar′di·a [after Alfred *Giard,* 1846–1908, French biologist]. A genus of protozoan parasites.

G. lamblia. A species found in the small intestine of man. It is not a tissue invader and its pathogenicity is doubtful.

gi″ar·di′a·sis (jee″ahr·dye′uh·sis, jy″ahr·) [*Giard;* NL. *-iasis,* condition]. Presence of the *Giardia lamblia* in the small intestine of man. Although this protozoan is found in large numbers in chronic recurring diarrheas, its pathogenicity is doubtful.

Giauque, William Francis (1895–). American physical chemist, known for his extensive research on the third law of thermodynamics, low temperature calorimetry, and isotopes and band spectra. He originated the magnetic method of attaining temperatures below 1° absolute. In 1949 he received the Nobel prize in chemistry for his work in thermodynamics, especially for his investigations of the properties of substances at extremely low temperatures.

gib·bos′i·ty (ghi·bos′i·tee, ji·bos′i·tee) [L. *gibbus,* hunched]. The condition of being humpbacked.

gib′bous (ghib′us, jib′us) [*gibbus*]. Humpbacked; swollen, convex, or protuberant, especially on one side.

Gibbs, Josiah Willard [*American physicist,* 1839–1903]. A distinguished pupil of von Helmholtz. The *Gibbs-Helmholtz equation* for determining the amount of work of which a galvanic cell is capable is considered one of the first principles of physical and physiological chemistry. Gibbs applied the second law of thermodynamics (all energy flows or tends to flow from a state of concentration to a state of dissipation) to all physical and chemical phenomena. The *Gibbs adsorption law* states that a substance which lowers interfacial or surface tension of a dispersion medium will collect at the surface or interfaces, whereas substances which increase surface tension are more concentrated within the interior of the liquid. Also called *Gibbs-Thomson principle.*

Gibbs's test. See under *test.*

gib′bus (ghib′us, jib′us) [L. *gibbus,* hump]. A hump specifically the dorsal convexity seen in tuberculosis of the spine; Pott's disease.

Gibert, Camille Melchior [*French dermatologist,* 1797–1866]. First to show pityriasis rosea, also called *Gibert's disease,* to be a clinical entity (1860).

Gibson, George Alexander [*Scottish physician,* 1854–1913]. Remembered for his rule in the prognosis of lobar pneumonia. *Gibson's rule* states that if the systolic blood pressure in millimeters does not fall below the pulse rate, the prognosis for recovery is good, and vice versa.

Gibson, Kasson Church [*American dentist,* 1849–1925]. Remembered for the bandage he devised for holding in position the fragments in fracture of the mandible; called *Gibson's bandage.*

Gibson, Robert Banks [*American physiological chemist,* 1882–]. With Geneva E. Goodrich, devised a modification of van den Bergh's method for bile pigment. See van den Bergh's *method.*

gid (ghid) [AS. *gydig*, insane]. A chronic brain disease of sheep, less frequently of cattle; characterized by forced movements of circling, rolling. Caused by the larval form of the tapeworm, *Multiceps multiceps.*

gid′di·ness [*gydig*]. Dizziness; an unpleasant sensation of disturbed relation to surrounding objects in space; it differs from vertigo in that there is no experience of the external world or of the patient being in motion.

Giemsa, Gustav (1867–1948). German chemist, best known for devising Giemsa stain. Other contributions include his work on the chemotherapeutic effect of derivatives of quinine, arsenic, and bismuth; the control of rats on ships with a mixture of carbon dioxide, carbon monoxide, and nitrogen; and the control of mosquitoes with a mixture of formaldehyde and soap.

Giem′sa stain (gheem′suh, ·zuh, ghem′·) (C.C.). A neutral stain used in staining blood and as a general cytologic stain; the compound formed from eosin with one of the derivatives of methylene blue, such as azure II.

Gierke, Edgar von [*German pathologist*, 1877–1945]. Described glycogenosis, also called *von Gierke's disease.*

Gierke, Hans Paul Bernhard [*German anatomist*, 1847–86]. Described thymic corpuscles, also known as *Gierke's corpuscles, Hassall's corpuscles. Gierke's respiratory bundle* is the tractus solitarius.

Gifford, Harold [*American ophthalmologist*, 1858–1929]. Described a sign indicative of exophthalmic goiter. *Gifford's sign* consists of inability to evert the upper eyelid in early stages of the disease. Described *Gifford's reflex:* if the eyelids are held apart, the pupil contracts when the subject makes a strong effort to close the eye. Delimiting keratotomy is known as *Gifford's operation.*

gi·gan′tic ac′id (jye·gan′tick). An antibiotic substance from *Aspergillus giganteus;* identical with aspergillin, flavacidin, flavicin, flavatin, and parasiticin.

gi·gan′tism (jye·gan′tiz·um) [G. *gigas*, giant]. Abnormal size and tallness; a height in man in excess of 79 inches; due to an oversupply of growth hormone of the anterior pituitary before the fusion of the epiphyses, or to an enhanced ability of the body tissues to respond to growth stimuli. Gigantism may be *normal*, the type in which bodily proportions and sexual function are normal; or *eunuchoid*, the type in which there are eunuchoid proportions and sexual insufficiency; or *acromegalic*, the form in which features of acromegaly are superimposed on those of gigantism.

gi·gan′to·blast [*gigas;* G. *blastos*, germ]. A large nucleated erythroblast.

gi·gan″to·chro′mo·blast [*gigas;* G. *chrōma*, color; *blastos*]. A gigantoblast.

gi·gan′to·cyte [*gigas;* G. *kytos*, cell]. A large, nonnucleated red blood corpuscle.

Gigli, Leonardo [*Italian surgeon and gynecologist*, 1863–1908]. Described pubiotomy for contracted pelvis in cases of dystocia; called *Gigli's operation.* Devised a chain saw for dividing bone, originally for use in his operation, but later adopted for general surgical use; see Gigli's *saw.*

Gi′la mon′ster (hee′luh). *Heloderma suspectum.*

Gilbert, Augustin Nicolas [*French physician*, 1858–1927]. Described a sign observed in cirrhosis of the liver. *Gilbert's sign* is the fact that more urine is excreted in a given time during fasting than following a full meal.

Gilchrist's disease. See North American *blastomycosis.*

Giles, Carl Prausnitz (1876–). German bacteriologist and hygienist, born Carl Willy Prausnitz, but later changed his name legally to C. P. Giles. With Heinz Küstner, he produced local hypersensitivity in man by using injections of serum from a hypersensitive person (1921); this reaction is known as *Prausnitz-Küstner reaction* or *Prausnitz-Küstner test.*

Gilford, Hastings [*English physician*, 1861–1941]. Described progeria (1904), also called *Hutchinson-Gilford disease.*

gill (ghill) [ME. *gile*]. A respiratory organ of water-breathing animals.

gill (jill) [OF. *gille*]. One-fourth of a pint.

Gil·le′ni·a (ji·lee′nee·uh, ghi·) [L., after Arnold *Gille*, German botanist, seventeenth century]. A genus of rosaceous herbs, **G. trifoliata,** or bowmans root, and **G. stipulata,** or indian physic, having emetic power. Dose, 1.3–2.0 Gm. (20–30 gr.).

Gilles de la Tourette, Georges [*French neurologist*, 1857–1904]. Described motor incoordination associated with echolalia and coprolalia (1884); called *Gilles de la Tourette's disease.*

Gilliam, David Tod [*American gynecologist*, 1844–1923]. Known for his description of his operation for displacement of the uterus, in which a loop of each round ligament is drawn through the abdominal wall and fixed to the abdominal fascia.

Gillies, Harold Delf [*English surgeon*, 1882–]. Celebrated for his skill and invention in plastic surgery of the face. Devised an operation for ectropion, excising scar tissue and grafting the defect, and one for plastic repair in which a tubed pedicle flap is formed. Called *Gillies' operations.*

Gimbernat, Antonio de [*Spanish surgeon and anatomist*, 1734–1816]. Described *Gimbernat's operation* for strangulated femoral hernia. The lacunar ligament is also called *Gimbernat's ligament.*

gin′ger [G. *ziggiberis*] (*zingiber*). The dried rhizome of *Zingiber officinale*, containing not less than 4.5% of ether-soluble extractive and not less than 12% of cold water extractive. A carminative in dyspepsia and flatulent colic. Dose, 0.6–1.3 Gm. (10–20 gr.). See *zingerone.*

g. fluidextract (*fluidextractum zingiberis*). Dose, 0.3–1.0 cc. (5–15 min.).

g. oleoresin (*oleoresina zingiberis*). Used like ginger in a dose of 0.03–0.12 Gm. (½–2 gr.).

g. syrup (*syrupus zingiberis*). A stomachic and flavor. Dose, 4–15 cc. (1–4 fluidrachms).

wild g. See *asarum.*

gin′ger·ol. Zingerone.

gin′gi·va (pl. *gingivae*) [L., gum]. That part of the oral mucous membrane which surrounds the tooth distal to the alveolar crest. —**gingival,** (jin′ji·vul, jin·jy′vul) *adj.;* **gingivally,** *adv.*

attached g. That portion of the gingiva firmly attached to the tooth and to the periosteum of the alveolar crest.

free g. That portion of the gingiva which lies occlusally or incisally to the floor of the gingival sulcus. Syn., *marginal gingiva.*

marginal g. Free *g.*

gin″gi·val′gi·a [*gingiva;* G. *algos*, pain]. Neuralgia of the gums.

gin″gi·vec′to·my [*gingiva;* G. *ektomē*, excision]. Excision of a portion of the gums.

gin″gi·vi′tis [*gingiva;* G. *-itis*, inflammation]. Inflammation of the gingiva.

expulsive g. Osteoperiostitis of a tooth, which is gradually expelled from its socket.

interstitial g. An inflammation of the gums and alveolar processes preceding periodontoclasia.

necrotizing ulcerative g. An infection of the gums characterized in the acute form by necrosis of the gingival margins, pain, foul odor, and the formation of a gray pseudomembrane. A spirillum and fusiform bacillus are associated with this disease. Also called *trench mouth, Vincent's infection, Vincent's gingivitis, Vincent's periodontitis, ulceromembranous gingivitis.* See also Vincent's *angina,* Vincent's *stomatitis.*

pregnancy g. Changes in the gums seen most frequently during pregnancy; they are thought to be related to endocrine imbalance, since similar changes are also seen at puberty in both sexes; marked by bleeding, hypertrophy of interdental papillae, inflammation, and, occasionally, a tumorlike formation.

ulceromembranous g. See necrotizing ulcerative *g.*

Vincent's g. See necrotizing ulcerative *g.*

gin″gi·vo·glos·si′tis [*gingiva;* G. *glōssa,* tongue; *-itis*]. Inflammation of the gums and tongue; stomatitis.

gin″gi·vo′sis [*gingiva;* G. *-osis,* condition]. A disease of the gums of poorly nourished children, characterized by degenerative changes in the connective tissue and edema, and later by necrosis, ulceration, and recession.

gin″gi·vo·sto″ma·ti′tis (jin″ji·vo·sto″muh·tye′tis, ·stom″uh·tye′tis) [*gingiva;* G. *stoma,* mouth; *-itis*]. See *gingivitis.*

gin′gly·mus (jing′gli·mus, ghing′·) [G. *gigglymos,* hinge]. A hinge joint. —**ginglymoid,** *adj.*

gin′seng [Chin.]. The root of several species of *Panax.* It has no medicinal virtues other than those of a demulcent.

Giovannini, Sebastiano [*Italian dermatologist,* 1851–1920]. Described a rare nodular disease of the hair (1887), of fungus origin, called *Giovannini's disease.*

"gip′py tum′my." A diarrheal condition occurring in tropical and subtropical countries which probably is caused by one of the usual dysentery organisms but is precipitated by sudden chilling.

Giraldès, organ of. See *paradidymis.*

gir′dle [AS. *gyrdel*]. A band designed to go around the body; a structure resembling a circular belt or band.

pelvic g. The two hip bones united at the pubic symphysis; they support the trunk on the lower extremities.

shoulder g. The system of bones supporting the upper limbs or arms; it consists of the clavicles, scapulas, and, for some authorities, the manubrium of the sternum. Also called *pectoral girdle.*

Girdlestone, Gathorne Robert [*English surgeon.* 1881–1950]. Described an operation for radical drainage of a dangerously infected hip joint. A wedge of skin and muscle with the detached great trochanter is removed, exposing the upper portion of the joint capsule. The femoral head is removed and the joint saucerized. Called *Girdlestone's operation.*

Girdner, John Harvey [*American physician,* 1856–1933]. Devised an electrically operated apparatus, now obsolete, for the detection of bullets embedded in the tissues. Called *Girdner's probe.*

git′a·lin (jit′uh·lin, ji·tay′lin, ji·tal′in). $C_{35}H_{56}O_{12}$. A glycoside from digitalis leaves. It probably represents a hydrolytic product of a precursor actually present in the drug but decomposed during extraction. Small white rosettes, soluble in alcohol. On hydrolysis it yields two molecules of the sugar, digitoxose, $C_6H_{12}O_4$, and the steroid aglycone, gitaligenin, which is a hydrate of gitoxigenin. See *digitoxin, gitoxin.*

git″o·gen′in (jit″o·jen′in, ji·todj′i·nin). The steroid aglycone of gitonin.

git′o·nin (jit′o·nin, ji·to′nin). A saponin from *Digitalis purpurea.* On acid hydrolysis it yields the steroid aglycone gitogenin, galactose. and a pentose.

gi·tox″i·ge′nin (ji·tock″si·jee′nin, ·jen′in, ji·tock′·si·ji·nin). The steroid aglycone or sugar-free component of gitoxin and of lanatoside B.

gi·tox′in. $C_{41}H_{64}O_{14}$. One of the partially hydrolyzed glycosides obtained from both *Digitalis purpurea* and *Digitalis lanata;* on complete hydrolysis it yields the steroid aglycone gitoxigenin and three molecules of the sugar digitoxose.

git′ter·fa″sern. See *reticular fibers* under *fiber.*

Giuffrida-Ruggeri, Vincenzo [*Italian anthropologist,* 1872–1922]. Noted absence or incompleteness of the glenoid fossa, called *Giuffrida-Ruggeri's stigma.*

giz′zard (ghiz′urd) [L. *gigeria,* cooked entrails of poultry]. The strong muscular stomach of birds used for triturating the food.

Gl Chemical symbol for glucinum, an obsolete name for beryllium.

gla·bel′la [L. *glabellus,* dim. of *glaber,* smooth]. 1. The bony prominence on the frontal bone joining the supraorbital ridges. 2. A craniometric point found in the sagittal plane of the bony prominence joining the supraorbital ridges, usually the most anteriorly projecting portion of this region.

coccygeal g. A minute hairless area located in the coccygeal region at the vortex of the hair whorls. It may become a small pit, the foveola coccygea.

gla′brate [*glaber*]. Glabrous.

gla′brous [*glaber*]. Smooth; devoid of hairs.

gla′cial [L. *glacialis,* icy]. Icy; resembling ice in appearance, as glacial acetic or phosphoric acid.

glad″i·ol′ic ac′id. An antibiotic substance, isolated from cultures of *Penicillium gladioli;* it is active against some bacteria and has marked fungistatic properties.

glad″i·o′lus (glad″ee·o′lus, gla·dye′o·lus) [L., small sword]. The middle or second piece of the sternum. *O.T.*

glair′in [OF. *glaire,* white of egg]. A peculiar organic gelatinous substance found on the surface of some thermal waters.

glair′y [*glaire*]. Slimy; viscous; mucoid. Resembling the white of an egg.

gland [L. *glans,* an acorn]. 1. A cell, tissue, or organ which elaborates and discharges a substance which is used elsewhere in the body (secretion), or eliminated (excretion). 2. Acorn-shaped termination of the penis or clitoris; see *glans clitoridis; glans penis.* 3. Obsolete term for lymph node. —**glan′dular,** *adj.*

accessory g. A mass of glandular tissue separate from the main body of a gland of similar structure.

accessory parotid g. A small auxiliary parotid gland: also called *socia parotis.*

acid glands. Glands of the stomach which secrete acid. Syn., *fundic glands.*

acinotubular g. One with both tubular and saccular elements.

acinous g. One in which the secretory end-pieces have the form of an acinus.

adipose glands. Hibernating glands of certain mammals, containing pigmented multilocular fat cells (brown fat).

admaxillary g. The accessory parotid gland.

adrenal g. An endocrine gland located immediately above the superior pole of the kidney. It consists of two portions: a *cortex,* which elaborates steroid hormones, the adrenal cortical hormones, and a *medulla,* which elaborates epinephrine. Syn., *suprarenal g.* See Plates, 7, 8, 9, 14, 45.

aggregate g. Old term for aggregate lymphatic nodule. Also called *agminated g., Peyer's patch.*

Albarran's g. See subcervical *g.*

albuminous g. See serous *g.*
alveolar g. One in which the secretory end-pieces have the form of an alveolus.
anal g. Any gland of the anal region.
apocrine glands. Those in which part of the free end of the glandular cell is pinched off with the secretion, leaving the nuclei and most of the cytoplasm intact. Specifically, those sweat glands periodically producing a viscous milky sweat of a characteristic odor; they are larger, branched, and more deeply situated than the common eccrine sweat glands, and found in the axillary, mammary, anal, and genital areas. Their exact function is not known, but activity has been correlated with production of sex hormones.
areolar glands. Glands in the areola about the nipple in the female breast. They are intermediate in character between mammary glands and apocrine sweat glands. Syn., *Montgomery's glands.*
arytenoid glands. Mixed glands, found in large numbers along the posterior margin of the aryepiglottic fold in front of the arytenoid cartilages.
axillary glands. The axillary lymph nodes.
Bartholin's glands. The major vestibular glands.
Blandin's g. The anterior lingual gland, a mixed gland on the under surface of the tongue. Syn., *Nuhn's g.*
Bowman's glands. Serous glands found in the olfactory mucous membrane. Also called *olfactory glands.*
bronchial glands. (a) The mixed glands of the mucous membrane of the bronchi. (b) The chain of lymph nodes along the bronchi.
Brunner's glands. The duodenal glands.
buccal glands. The mixed glands of the mucous membrane of the cheek.
bulbourethral g. One of two compound tubular glands situated in the urogenital diaphragm, anterior to the prostate gland. Also called *Cowper's g.* See Plate 44.
cardiac glands. (a) Glands of the cardia of the stomach. (b) Branched tubular glands of the upper and lower cardiac patches of the esophagus.
carotid glands. See *carotid bodies* under *body.*
ceruminous glands. The sweat glands of the external auditory meatus which secrete the watery component of the cerumen.
cervical glands. The lymph nodes of the neck.
ciliary glands. Modified sweat glands of the eyelids. Also called *Moll's glands.*
circumanal glands. The anal glands.
Cloquet's g. See Rosenmueller's *g.*
closed g. A ductless or endocrine gland. *Obs.*
coccygeal g. See coccygeal *body.*
coil g. Old term for sweat gland.
compound g. A gland which has a branching system of ducts.
conglomerate glands. Acinous glands.
conjunctival glands. The accessory lacrimal glands. Also called *Krause's glands.*
convoluted g. Sweat gland.
Cowper's g. The bulbourethral gland.
cutaneous g. Any gland of the skin.
cytogenic g. A gland producing living cells, as the testis or ovary.
deep g. A gland which has its secreting portion deep to a mucous membrane, usually in the tunica submucosa.
ductless glands. Glands without ducts, secreting directly into the blood stream. See endocrine *g.*
duodenal glands. The deep mixed glands of the first part of the duodenum. Also called *Brunner's glands.*
Ebner's glands. The serous glands opening into the trenches of the vallate papillae of the tongue. Also called *von Ebner's glands.*
eccrine glands. The small sweat glands distributed all over the human body surface. Histologically, they are tubular coiled merocrine glands that secrete the clear aqueous sweat important for heat regulation and chemically different from apocrine sweat.
endocrine g. One secreting hormonal substance into the blood stream; a ductless gland. See *pancreas, parathyroid, pineal g., thyroid g.* See also *pituitary, suprarenal, thymus.* See Plate 45.
epithelial g. A group of glandular cells within an epithelial layer.
exocrine glands. Glands which secrete onto an epithelial surface.
Fraenkel's glands. Minute mixed glands immediately inferior to the vocal folds.
fundic glands. Those of the corpus and fundus of the stomach. Syn., *acid glands.*
gastric glands. Glands of the stomach, including the cardiac, fundic, and pyloric glands.
glands of Shambaugh. The epithelium along the outer wall of the cochlear duct, modified to resemble a glandular epithelium, which rests upon the stria vascularis.
Gley's glands. See Marcel Eugène Emile *Gley.*
hair glands. The sebaceous glands of hair follicles.
Harderian g. The lacrimal gland of the third eyelid in many mammals; vestigial in man.
Haversian glands. Fat lobules in some synovial fringes.
hemal g. See hemal *node.*
hemolymph g. See hemal *node.* Also called *hemal g.*
hibernating g. The brown fat of certain rodents, once believed concerned with hibernation.
holocrine g. One which forms its secretion by degeneration of its cells. Also called *holocrinous g.*
Home's g. See subtrigonal *g.*
incretory g. Endocrine gland.
interscapular g. The brown fat between the scapulas of certain rodents. See hibernating *g.*
interstitial g. (a) Mass of epithelioid cells in the medulla of the ovary of many lower animals. It is questionable whether or not it is present in women. The term has been applied to the hypertrophic theca cells about the periphery of follicles. (b) Cell-groups in the testis which secrete androgen; Leydig cells.
intraepithelial g. A small aggregation of mucous cells within an epithelial layer.
Krause's glands. Accessory lacrimal glands in the eyelids.
lacrimal g. The compound tubuloalveolar gland secreting the tears, situated in the orbit in a depression of the frontal bone. See Plate 19.
Lieberkühn's glands. The simple straight tubular glands of the intestinal mucous membrane.
Littré's glands. The small mucous glands of the male urethra. Formerly called *glands* or *lacunas of Morgagni.* Syn., *urethral glands.*
Luschka's glands. Aberrant bile ducts in the wall of the gallbladder. Also called *Luschka's ducts.*
lymph, lymphatic g. See *lymph* nodes.
mammary g. One which secretes milk. See Plate 43.
mandibular g. The submaxillary gland.
Meibomian glands. Tarsal glands.
merocrine g. One in which the secreting cells maintain their integrity in successive cycles of secretory activity. Also called *merocrinous g.*
mixed g. A gland containing both serous and mucous components, such as the submaxillary.
molar glands. A group of mixed (buccal) glands near the opening of the parotid duct.

Moll's glands. See *ciliary glands* under *gland.*
monkey g. Testis of a monkey once used as an implant in *Voronoff's operation.*
Montgomery's glands. The areolar glands.
Morgagni's g. See *Littré's glands* under *gland.*
mucous g. One which forms mucus: also called *muciparous g.*
myometrial g. A collection of cells appearing between the muscle cells of the rabbit's uterus about the middle of pregnancy.
Naboth's glands. The mucous glands of the external os of the cervix uteri.
Nuhn's glands. The anterior lingual glands. See Blandin's *g.*
oil g. Old term for sebaceous gland.
olfactory glands. See Bowman's *glands* under *gland.*
parathyroid g. See *parathyroid.*
paraurethral glands. Small vestigial glands opening into the posterior wall of the female urethra close to its orifice. The homolog of the distal prostatic glands of the male. Syn., *Skene's glands* or *tubules.*
parotid g. The salivary gland in front of and below the external ear. It is a compound racemose gland. Its duct is Stensen's duct. See Plate 3.
peptic glands. The fundic glands of the stomach.
perspiratory g. See sweat *g.*
pilous g. The sebaceous gland of a hair follicle.
pineal g. See pineal *body.*
pituitary g. See *pituitary.*
preen g. Uropygial *g.*
preputial glands. Sebaceous glands in the prepuce of the penis.
prostate g. See *prostate.*
pyloric glands. The glands of the mucous membrane of the pyloric portion of the stomach.
racemose g. A compound alveolar or tubuloalveolar gland.
retrolingual g. A large salivary gland in certain mammals other than man, the equivalent of the human sublingual gland.
Rivinus' g. The sublingual gland.
Rosenmueller's g. The large lymph node in the femoral canal. Syn., *Cloquet's g.*
saccular g. Same as alveolar gland.
salivary g. One that secretes saliva, as the parotid.
sebaceous g. One which secretes sebum, an unctuous material composed primarily of fat.
seminal g. Old term for a testis.
seromucinous g. See mixed *g.*
serous g. One which secretes a watery, albuminous fluid.
serous lingual g. See Ebner's *g.*
sexual g. Old term for a gonad.
simple g. (a) A gland which is entirely composed of secretory cells, without a differentiated ductile portion. (b) A gland with but one secretory endpiece and an unbranched duct.
Skene's glands. The paraurethral glands.
subcervical g. One of a group of small subsidiary prostatic glands which lie beneath the neck of the urinary bladder: also called *Albarran's g.*
sublingual g. A complex of small salivary glands situated in the sublingual fold on each side of the oral floor. See Plate 15.
submaxillary g. A large salivary gland situated below each lower jaw: also called *mandibular g., submandibular g.* See Plate 15.
subtrigonal g. One of a group of small subsidiary prostatic glands which lie beneath the mucosa of the trigone: also called *Home's g.* or *lobe.*
sudoriferous glands. The sweat glands.
sudoriparous glands. The sweat glands.
superficial g. One lying entirely within the limits of a mucous membrane.
suprarenal g. See adrenal *g.*
sweat g. One of the coiled tubular glands of the skin which secrete perspiration. See also *apocrine glands* and *eccrine glands* under *gland.*
target g. Any gland directly affected by the hormone of another gland.
tarsal glands. Sebaceous glands in the tarsal plates of the eyelids. Also called *Meibomian glands.*
thyroid g. One of the endocrine glands, lying in front of the trachea and consisting of two lateral lobes connected centrally by an isthmus. The organ is composed of follicles lined by epithelium, producing a colloid material. Hypertrophy of the gland (goiter) is sometimes associated with a peculiar disease known as exophthalmic goiter; hypofunction of the gland leads to cretinism or myxedema. See Plates 13, 45.
tubular g. A secreting gland, tubelike or cylindrical in shape.
tubuloalveolar g. One whose secretory endpieces are tubular and alveolar. To this group belong most of the larger exocrine glands. An obsolete term for this is *tubuloacinous gland.*
Tyson's glands. Sebaceous glands of the prepuce which secrete the smegma.
unicellular g. One consisting of a single cell.
urethral glands. Small, branched, tubular mucous glands in the mucous membrane of the urethra. Syn., *Littré's glands.*
uropygial g. A large bilobed sebaceous gland found dorsal to the last sacral vertebra of fowl. Its oily secretion reaches the surface of the skin by way of a short duct. Syn., *preen gland.*
uterine g. A gland of the endometrium.
vaginal g. One of the mucous glands found exceptionally in the mucous membrane of the fornix of the vagina.
vestibular glands. Glands of the vestibule of the vagina. They comprise the compound tubuloalveolar **major vestibular glands** (of Bartholin), one in each lateral wall, and the **minor vestibular glands,** which are several small branched tubular mucous glands around the urethral orifice.
Zeis's glands. The sebaceous glands associated with the cilia.

glan′ders [OF. *glandres*, glands, from *glans*]. A highly contagious acute or chronic disease of horses, mules, and asses; caused by *Malleomyces mallei.* It is communicable to dogs, goats, sheep, and man, but not to bovines. It is characterized by fever, inflammation of mucous membranes (especially of the nose), enlargement and hardening of the regional lymph nodes, formation of nodules which have a tendency to coalesce and then degenerate to form deep ulcers. In man the disease usually runs an acute febrile course and terminates fatally. Syn., *farcy, equinia.*

glans (glanz) [L.]. The conical body which forms the distal end of the clitoris (**glans clitoridis**) or of the penis (**glans penis**). See Plate 44.

Glaser, Hans Heinrich (Glaserius) [*Swiss anatomist,* 1629–75]. Described the petrotympanic fissure, called *Glaserian fissure.* Described the tympanic artery, called *Glaserian artery.*

glass [AS. *glaes*]. 1. A brittle, hard, transparent substance, consisting usually of the fused amorphous silicates of potassium and calcium, or sodium and calcium, with an excess of silica. 2. Any article made of glass.
crown g. A very hard glass; a silicate of sodium and calcium.
flint g. That composed of lead and potassium silicates.
soluble g. Potassium or sodium silicate, used as a substitute for plaster of Paris. Syn., *waterglass.*

glass'es [*glaes*]. The popular term for spectacles or eyeglasses.

bifocal g. Those that have a different refracting power in the upper part from that in the lower; the effect usually is produced by the superposition of segment lenses.

prismatic g. Those formed of prisms; used in insufficiency and paralysis of the ocular muscles.

trifocal g. Glasses or spectacles having three refractive powers to correct for distant, intermediate, and near vision.

glass'pox" [*glaes;* ME. *pokkes*]. Alastrim.

glass wool. White, silky threads obtained by the action of a powerful blast of air on a falling stream of molten glass; it is used in draining wounds and in filtering strong acids and alkalies: also called *slag wool.*

glass'y [*glaes*]. 1. Having the appearance of glass; vitreous; hyaline. 2. Expressionless; dull; lifeless.

Glauber's salt. See *sodium* sulfate.

glau·co'ma (glaw·ko'muh) [G. *glaukōma*, opacity of the crystalline lens]. A disease of the eye marked by heightened intraocular tension; results in hardness of the globe, excavation of the optic disk, restricted field of vision, corneal anesthesia, a colored halo seen surrounding artificial lights, and lessening of the visual power; it may lead to blindness.

absolute g. The completed glaucomatous process when the eyeball is exceedingly hard and totally blind.

acute g. The first (or the renewed) attack, with the characteristic and inflammatory symptoms.

auricular g. That associated with a great increase in the intralabyrinthine pressure.

congenital g. See infantile *g.*

hemorrhagic g. That associated with retinal hemorrhage. Also called *apoplectic g.*

infantile g. That affecting infants or children; due to a failure of development of Schlemm's canal and a consequent lack of normal drainage for the intraocular fluid. May be very mild with low tension, or may be clinically severe with a distention and stretching of the eye due to its increased fluid contents (buphthalmia or hydrophthalmos). Syn., *congenital g., intercalary staphyloma.*

malignant g. A grave form attended with violent pain and rapidly leading to blindness.

secondary g. That consequent upon other ocular diseases.

simple g. That chronic form occurring without inflammatory symptoms.

gleet [OF. *glete*]. The chronic stage of urethritis, characterized by a slight mucopurulent discharge. —**gleet'y,** *adj.*

Glénard, Frantz [*French physician,* 1848–1920]. Known for his observations on nervous dyspepsia, in which he described enteroptosis and gastroptosis (1885). Described the neurasthenic implications of enteroptosis (1886), called *Glénard's disease.*

gle"no·hu'mer·al [G. *glēnē*, socket of a joint, honeycomb; L. *humerus*, shoulder]. Pertaining to the glenoid cavity and the humerus, as the glenohumeral ligament.

gle'noid [G. *glēnoeidēs*, like a socket]. Having a shallow cavity; resembling a shallow cavity or socket.

gle'noid. The articular surface on the scapula for articulation with the head of the humerus.

Gle·nos'po·ra [*glēnē;* G. *sporos*, seed]. A genus of fungi of the class Fungi imperfecti, species of which have been isolated in cases of mycetoma.

Gley, Marcel Eugène Emile [*French physiologist,* 1857–1930]. Described the interstitial cells of the testis; called *Gley's cells, Leydig cells.* Described the parathyroids, showing that they are necessary for life (1891); called *Gley's glands, Sandström's bodies.*

gli'a [G. *glia*, glue]. The neuroglia. —**gli'al,** *adj.*

gli'a·cyte [*glia;* G. *kytos*, cell]. A neuroglia cell. *Obs.*

gli'a·din. A protein derived from gluten of wheat, rye, oats, and other grains. See American Classification of Proteins in the Appendix.

gli"o·bac·te'ri·a [*glia;* G. *baktērion*, little staff]. Bacteria embedded in a gelatinous matrix.

gli"o·blas·to'ma-as"tro·blas·to'ma. See *astroblastoma.*

gli"o·blas·to'ma i"so·morphe'. See *medulloblastoma.*

gli"o·blas·to'ma mul"ti·for'me. The most frequent glioma of the central nervous system, usually the brain, composed of a few normal astrocytes, and varying numbers of pleomorphic cells. Giant nuclei and multinucleated giant cells are common in contrast to the astrocytoma and astroblastoma. Also called *ameboid glioma, astrocytoma gigantocellulare, gliocarcinoma, gliofibrosarcoma, glioma sarcoides, gliosarcoma, spongioblastoma multiforme.* Syn., *astrocytoma, Grade 3* and *Grade 4.*

gli"o·blas·to'ma of ret'i·na. Neuroepithelioma of the retina.

gli"o·car"ci·no'ma. See *glioblastoma multiforme.*

gli"o·coc'cus [*glia;* G. *kokkos*, berry]. A micrococcus having a gelatinous envelope.

gli"o·fi"bro'sar·co'ma. See *glioblastoma multiforme.*

gli·o'ma (glye·o'muh) [*glia;* G. *-ōma*, tumor]. A tumor composed of cells and fibers representative of the special supporting tissue of the central nervous system, and derived from neuroglial cells or their antecedents; occurs principally in the brain, spinal cord, peripheral nerves, and adrenals. —**gliom'atous,** *adj.*

ameboid g. See *glioblastoma multiforme.*

astrocytic g. See *astrocytoma.*

extramedullary g. One arising in heterotopic glial tissue.

ganglion-cell g. See *astroblastoma.*

g. of retina. Neuroepithelioma of the retina.

g. sarcoides. See *glioblastoma multiforme.*

g. sarcomatoides. See *medulloblastoma.*

heterotopic g. A rare tumor composed largely of masses of fibrillar astrocytes and occasionally a few ganglion cells. Its more common site of origin is in the orbit outside of the optic nerve, but it also appears in the form of subcutaneous nodules over the bridge of the nose or as an intranasal polypoid growth. The latter is also called *nasal g., astroblastoma, astrocytoma, astroglioma, fibroglioma, ganglioblastoma, ganglioglioma of nose, ganglioschwannospongioblastoma.*

malignant peripheral g. See malignant *schwannoma.*

nasal g. See heterotopic *g.*

perineural g. See *neurilemmoma.*

peripheral g. See *neurilemmoma.*

retinal g. See *neuroepithelioma* of the retina.

gli"o·ma·to'sis. The proliferation of gliomas.

meningeal g. Widespread involvement of the subarachnoid space by cells originating in a glioma: also called *gliosarcoma of meninges, meningeal sarcomatosis.*

gli"o·neu"ro·blas"to'ma. See *neuroastrocytoma.*

gli"o·neu·ro'ma. See *neuroastrocytoma.*

gli"o·sar·co'ma. Glioblastoma multiforme.

g. of meninges. See meningeal *gliomatosis.*

gli·o'sis (glye·o'sis) [*glia;* G. *-ōsis*, condition]. Proliferation of neuroglia in the brain or spinal cord, as a replacement process or due to low-grade inflammation; may be diffuse or focal. **Gliosis of the spinal cord** is the earliest pathologic change in syringomyelia.

anisomorphous g. See heteromorphous *g.*

heteromorphous g. Gliosis in which the glial fibrils appear as a network. Syn., *anisomorphous g.*

isomorphous g. Gliosis in which the glial fibrils appear as parallel bundles.

gli′o·some [*glia;* G. *sōma*, body]. One of the small granules in the cytoplasm of neuroglial cells.

gli″o·tox′in [*glia;* G. *toxikon*, poison]. An antibiotic, $C_{13}H_{14}N_2O_4S_2$, obtained from cultures of *Trichoderma, Gliocladium*, and *Aspergillus fumigatus*. It is bacteriostatic toward certain Gram-positive and certain Gram-negative bacteria, and is sensitive to heat and oxygen.

Glisson, Francis [*English physician*, 1597–1677]. Gave a classic description of rickets (1650), called *Glisson's disease*, and the first clear description of the liver stroma, called *Glisson's capsule*, and its blood supply (1854). Invented an apparatus, called *Glisson's sling*, for use in the treatment of spinal deformities.

globe. *In ophthalmology*, the eyeball.

g. lag. See Kocher's *sign.*

glo′bin [L. *globus*, ball]. One of a class of proteins, histone in nature, obtained from the hemoglobins of various animal species. Globin is soluble in water, soluble in acids and alkalis, coagulable by heat.

glob″u·lar′e·tin, glob″u·la·re′tin. A hydrolysis product of globularin obtained by the action of dilute acids. A diuretic and purgative; has been used in gout.

glob″u·lar′in, glob′u·lar·in. A glycoside from the leaves of *Globularia alypum*. Its action upon the heart and nervous system is similar to that of caffeine, but it diminishes the quantity of the urine. Has been used in the treatment of gout, rheumatism, etc.

glob′ule [L. *globulus*, little ball, globule]. A small spherical droplet of fluid or semifluid material.

milk g. A fat drop in milk.

glob′u·li·cide″, glob·u′li·cide″ [*globulus;* L. *caedere*, to kill]. 1. Destructive of blood cells. 2. An agent that destroys blood cells. —**globulici′dal,** *adj.*

glob′u·lin [*globulus*]. A general name for a group of animal and plant proteins characterized by solubility in dilute salt solutions and differentiated from albumins by lesser solubility, more alkaline isoelectric points, larger molecular weight, faster sedimentation rates, and slower electrophoretic mobilities. **Alpha-, beta-, gamma-globulins** are fractions of serum globulin separated by electrophoresis. See *euglobulin, pseudoglobulin.* **Alpha-g.** contains certain sero-enzymes and hormones; **beta-g.** contains the blood group antibodies, prothrombin, and certain fractions of complement; **gamma-g.** includes most antibodies.

Ac g., accelerator g. A factor which accelerates the activation of purified prothrombin by thromboplastin. See *plasma accelerator globulin, serum accelerator globulin.*

antihemophilic g. See *thromboplastinogen.*

coagulation g. A substance derived from normal plasma that reduces the coagulation time of hemophilic blood: also called *fraction I.*

gamma-g. (human). A sterile, concentrated, and refined preparation of globulin, prepared from human blood and meeting certain requirements of electrophoretic mobility. It contains protective antibodies against certain bacterial and viral infections. Injection of the globulin preparation from pooled bloods may, under certain conditions, provide short-term passive immunity; hence it has been used in the prevention and treatment of measles, notably in cases of previously unexposed pregnant mothers, and against poliomyelitis in individuals risking exposure in an area where the disease is epidemic.

g. substance. See antihemophilic *factor, thromboplastinogen.*

g. X. An intracellular protein found in muscle tissue.

immune g. See gamma-*g.*

poliomyelitis immune g. See gamma-*g.*

serum g. The globulin fraction of blood serum. By definition, it is the fraction of serum protein precipitated by half-saturation with ammonium sulfate in contrast to the albumin fraction which is soluble in this salt concentration.

glob″u·li·nu′ri·a [*globulus;* G. *ouron*, urine]. The presence of globulin in the urine.

glob′u·lus (pl. *globuli*) [L.]. See *globule.*

glo′bus [L.]. A ball or globe.

g. hystericus. The choking sensation, or so-called lump in the throat, occurring in hysteria.

g. major epididymidis. The larger end or head of the epididymis, consisting largely of the efferent ductules. Syn., *caput epididymidis.*

g. minor epididymidis. The lower end of the epididymis. Syn., *cauda epididymidis.*

g. pallidus. The inner and lighter part of the lenticular nucleus of the corpus striatum.

gloe′a (glee′uh) [G. *gloia*, glue]. A mucuslike substance secreted about the spore heads of some fungi.

glo″man·gi·o′ma. See glomus *tumor.*

glome [L. *glomus*, ball]. 1. Glomerulus. 2. One of the two rounded prominences which form the backward prolongations of the frog of a horse's foot.

glom′er·ate [L. *glomerare*, to wind into a ball]. Rolled together like a ball of thread.

glom′er·ule. See glomus.

glo·mer″u·lo·ne·phri′tis [dim. from L. *glomus*, ball; G. *nephros*, kidney; *-itis*, inflammation]. A diffuse nonsuppurative inflammation of the kidneys, affecting the glomeruli primarily. Proliferative, degenerative, and exudative changes may occur. Classified as to duration, there are acute, subacute, chronic, and latent types, which may or may not represent progressive stages. Symptoms include hematuria, albuminuria, edema, hypertension, and also cardiac and cerebral involvement.

acute g. A form of glomerulonephritis occurring principally in (male) children and lasting up to three months. In the majority of cases, there is an antecedent or associated infection, usually of the upper respiratory tract. Streptococci *Group A, Type 12*, and to a lesser extent *Type 4*, have been most frequently implicated and an immunologic reaction postulated.

chronic g. A form of glomerulonephritis characterized clinically by its prolonged duration, hypertension, and progressive uremia. Pathologically there is progressive fibrosis and hyalinization of the glomeruli.

embolic g. See focal *g.*

focal g. A type usually seen in patients with subacute bacterial endocarditis, and which results from the lodging in glomerular tufts of minute emboli derived from the valve lesion. The emboli are scattered over the kidney, giving it a "flea-bitten" appearance. Resulting renal failure is rare. Also called *focal embolic g.*

focal nonembolic g. A type which is focal rather than diffuse, which may result from damage to the glomerular tuft capillaries by toxins from a distant site of infection, as minor acute upper respiratory infections.

membranous g. See lipoid *nephrosis.*

subacute g. A type of glomerulonephritis similar to chronic *g.*, but lasting only a few months.

glo·mer″u·lo·scle·ro′sis. See *intercapillary glomerulosclerosis.*

glo·mer′u·lus (pl. *glomeruli*) [*glomus*]. 1. A small rounded mass. 2. The tuft of capillary loops projecting into the lumen of a renal corpuscle. —**glomerular, glomerulose,** *adj.*

olfactory g. A group of nerve cells, a number of which are embedded in the olfactory bulb.

pancreatic glomeruli. The islets of the pancreas. *Obs.*

glo′mus (pl. *glomera*) [L.]. 1. A fold of the mesothelium arising near the base of the mesentery in the pronephros, and containing a ball of blood vessels. Also called *glomerule of the pronephros.* 2. The part of the choroid plexus of the lateral ventricle which covers the thalamus. Also called *glomus chorioideum.* —**glomic,** *adj.*

cutaneous g. See *g.* body.

g. aorticum. See *aortic bodies* under *body.*

g. body. An arteriovenous anastomosis which has a special arrangement of muscle and nerve tissue; usually present in the cutis and subcutis of fingers and toes: also called *cutaneous glomus.*

g. caroticum. Old term for the carotid body.

g. coccygeum. Old term for the coccygeal body.

g. jugulare. Any of a number of tiny masses of epithelioid tissue similar in structure to that of the carotid body. They are usually situated in the adventitia of the superior bulb of the internal jugular vein.

glon′o·in (glon′o·in, glo′no·in, glo·no′in) [from Gl = glyceryl; O = oxygen; N = nitrogen, in the formula $C_3H_5O_3(NO_2)_3$, in which C_3H_5 stands for glyceryl]. Glyceryl trinitrate or nitroglycerin.

glos′sa [G. *glōssa,* tongue]. The tongue. —**glossal,** *adj.*

-glos′sa [*glōssa*]. A combining form meaning *tongue.*

glos·sal′gi·a [*glōssa;* G. *algos,* pain]. Pain in the tongue.

glos·san′thrax [*glōssa;* G. *anthrax,* carbuncle]. Anthrax, or carbuncle, of the tongue.

glos·sec′to·my [*glōssa;* G. *ektomē,* excision]. Excision of the tongue.

Glos·si′na, Glos′si·na [*glōssa*]. A genus of blood-sucking flies, known as tsetse flies; confined to tropical and subtropical Africa. The species *G. fusca, G. palpalis,* and *G. morsitans* transmit the trypanosomes of sleeping sickness in man and of nagana and the souma disease of horses, cattle, and sheep.

glos·si′tis [*glōssa;* G. *-itis,* inflammation]. Inflammation of the tongue. —**glossit′ic,** *adj.*

acute g. Swelling of the tongue accompanied by high fever, salivation, pain referred to the ears.

chronic superficial g. A rare glossitis usually seen in adult females. There are smooth, red areas involving part or all of the dorsum of the tongue; contact with food may elicit a burning sensation. Syn., *glossodynia exfoliativa.*

median rhomboidal g. A diamond-shaped inflammatory patch on the tongue anterior to the vallate papillae.

Moeller's g. See chronic superficial *g.*

glos′so-, gloss- [*glōssa*]. A combining form meaning *tongue.*

glos′so·cele [*glōssa;* G. *kēlē,* tumor]. Swelling, or edema, of the tongue, with consequent extrusion of the organ.

glos″so·dy″na·mom′e·ter (glos″o·dye″nuh·mom′i·tur, ·din″uh·mom′i·tur) [*glōssa;* G. *dynamis,* power; *metron,* a measure]. An apparatus for measuring the capacity of the tongue to resist pressure.

glos″so·dyn′i·a [*glōssa;* G. *odynē,* pain]. Pain in the tongue.

g. exfoliativa. Chronic superficial glossitis.

glos″so·ep″i·glot′tic, glos″so·ep″i·glot·tid′e·an [*glōssa;* G. *epiglottis,* epiglottis]. Pertaining to both tongue and epiglottis.

glos′so·graph [*glōssa;* G. *graphein,* to write]. An instrument for registering the movements of the tongue in speech.

glos″so·hy′al, glos″so·hy′oid [*glōssa;* G. *hyoeidēs,* shaped like the letter upsilon]. Pertaining to the tongue and the hyoid bone.

glos″so·kin″es·thet′ic [*glōssa;* G. *kinein,* to move; *aisthēsis,* perception]. Relating to the motions of the tongue in speech.

glos″so·la′bi·al [*glōssa;* L. *labium,* lip]. Relating to the tongue and lips, as glossolabial paralysis.

glos″so·la′li·a (glos″o·lay′lee·uh, ·lal′ee·uh) [*glōssa;* G. *lalia,* talk]. Unintelligible jabbering; talk in a strange or unknown tongue; jargon.

glos·sol′o·gy [*glōssa;* G. *logos,* word]. 1. The study of the tongue and its diseases. 2. The definition and explanation of terms; nomenclature.

glos″so·man′ti·a (glos″o·man′tee·uh, ·man·tye′uh) [*glōssa;* G. *manteia,* divination]. Prognosis of a disease based on the appearance of the tongue. *Obs.*

glos″so·pal′a·tine (·pal′uh·tyne, ·tin) [*glōssa;* L. *palatum,* palate]. Relating to the tongue and the palate, as the glossopalatine arch, or anterior pillar of the fauces.

g. nerve. Variant term for the sensory root of the nervus intermedius.

glos″so·pal·a·ti′nus [*glōssa;* L. *palatum,* palate]. A muscle extending from the soft palate to the tongue in the glossopalatine arch.

glos·sop′a·thy [*glōssa;* G. *pathos,* disease]. Any disease of the tongue.

glos″so·pha·ryn′ge·al (glos″o·fa·rin′jee·ul, ·far″in·jee′ul) [*glōssa;* G. *pharygx,* throat]. Pertaining to tongue and pharynx, as glossopharyngeal nerve.

glos″so·pha·ryn′ge·us (·fa·rin′jee·us, ·far″in·jee′us) [*glōssa; pharygx*]. A portion of the superior constrictor muscle of the pharynx, attached to the tongue.

glos′so·plas″ty, glos″so·plas′ty [*glōssa;* G. *plassein,* to form]. Plastic surgery of the tongue.

glos″so·ple′gi·a [*glōssa;* G. *plēgē,* stroke]. Paralysis of the tongue.

glos″so·py·ro′sis (glos″o·pye·ro′sis) [*glōssa;* G. *pyr,* fire; *-ōsis,* condition]. A condition characterized by a burning sensation in the tongue.

glos·sor′rha·phy [*glōssa;* G. *rhaphē,* suture]. Surgical suturing of the tongue.

glos·sos′co·py [*glōssa;* G. *skopein,* to examine]. Diagnostic inspection of the tongue.

glos′so·spasm″ [*glōssa;* G. *spasmos,* spasm]. Spasm of the tongue.

glos·sot′o·my [*glōssa;* G. *tomē,* a cutting]. 1. The dissection of the tongue. 2. An incision of the tongue.

glos″so·trich′i·a (glos″o·trick′ee·uh) [*glōssa;* G. *thrix,* hair]. Hairy tongue.

glot′tic [G. *glōttis,* glottis]. Pertaining to the glottis.

glot′tis [G.]. The opening between the free margins of the vocal folds. —**glottal, glottid′ean,** *adj.*

glu′ca·gon, glu′ca·gone. A protein believed to be formed by alpha cells of the islets of Langerhans, and by some considered to serve a hormonal function, which causes glycogenolysis and hyperglycemia; it occurs in some, but not all, preparations of insulin. Also called *hyperglycemic factor, hyperglycemic-glycogenolytic factor* (abbreviated HGF), *glycogenolytic hormone.*

glu′case. The enzyme that converts starch into glucose. *Obs.*

glu′cide [G. *glykys,* sweet]. A group term for carbohydrates and glycosides. —**glucid′ic,** *adj.*

glu′cin. Sodium aminotriazinesulfonate, a substance resembling saccharin, but less sweet.

glu·ci′num. Beryllium; symbol, Gl. *Obs.*

glu′co-, gluc- [*glykys*]. 1. *In chemistry,* a combining form signifying *glucose.* 2. See *glyco-.*

glu″co·a·scor′bic ac′id.

CO.COH:COH.CH.HCOH.HCOH.CH_2OH;

D-glucoascorbic acid, a homolog of ascorbic acid; it has been claimed and denied that it has antivitamin-C activity.

glu″co·chlo′ral. See *chloralose.*

glu″co·cor′ti·coid. An adrenal cortex hormone which affects the metabolism of glucose; by extension, any related natural or synthetic substance which functions similarly.

glu″co·fu′ran·ose. A cyclic form of glucose having a furanose structure in which carbon atoms 1 and 4 are bridged by an oxygen atom.

glu′co·gen. See *glycogen.*

glu″co·he′mi·a, glu″co·hae′mi·a (glōō″ko·hee′-mee·uh). Old term for glycemia.

glu″co·ki′nase. An enzyme, present in liver, which in the course of glycogenesis catalyzes phosphorylation of D-glucose, by adenosinetriphosphate, to glucose-6-phosphate.

glu″co·kin′in. Vegetable insulin.

glu·col′y·sis. See *glycolysis.*

glu″co·ne″o·gen′e·sis [*glykys;* G. *neos,* new; *genesis,* production]. The formation of glucose by the liver from noncarbohydrate sources.

glu·con′ic ac′id. $CH_2OH(CHOH)_4COOH$. An acid resulting from the oxidation of dextrose and other sugars. Several of its salts, notably calcium gluconate and ferrous gluconate, are used medicinally.

glu″co·no·ki′nase. An enzyme, present in microorganisms adapted to growing on D-gluconic acid, which catalyzes phosphorylation of the acid, by adenosinetriphosphate, to 6-phosphogluconic acid.

glu″co·no·lac′tone. The ring structure of D-gluconic acid.

glucophylline. Trade-mark for an equimolecular mixture of theophylline and N-methylglucosamine, having the action and uses of aminophylline.

glu″co·pro′te·in. Old term for glycoprotein.

glu″co·py′ran·ose. A cyclic form of glucose having a pyranose structure in which carbon atoms 1 and 5 are bridged by an oxygen atom.

glu″co·sac·char′ic ac′id. D-Glucosaccharic acid, a dibasic acid resulting from oxidation of D-glucose. Syn., *saccharic acid,* 2.

glu″cos·a·mine′ (glōō″ko·suh·meen′, ·sam′in, glōō-ko′suh·meen, ·min). CHO.HC(NH_2).HOCH.-HCOH.HCOH.CH_2OH; an amino sugar derived from D-glucose; it is a structural component of chitin, chondroitin, and heparin, and occurs also in mucus, fungi, and lichens. Syn., *2-amino-D-glucose, chitosamine, glycosamine.*

glu′co·san. A polysaccharide which yields glucose upon hydrolysis.

glu·co′sa·zone (glōō·ko′suh·zone, ·kose′uh·zone, glōō″ko·say′zone). See *phenylglucosazone.*

glu″co·scil′lar·en A. A cardioactive glycoside present in the fraction of squill glycosides, identified by the trade-marked name *scillaren-B.*

glu″co·scil″li·phe′o·side. A cardioactive glycoside present in the fraction of squill glycosides identified by the trade-marked name *scillaren-B.*

glu′cose. 1. The crystalline monosaccharide dextrose, $C_6H_{12}O_6$, sometimes called *dextro*-glucose, but properly designated D-glucose. See *dextrose.* 2. A product obtained by the incomplete hydrolysis of starch, consisting chiefly of dextrose (D-glucose), dextrins, maltose, and water; being liquid, it is more correctly designated liquid glucose (*glucosum liquidum*). It is a colorless or yellowish, thick, syrupy liquid, odorless, possessing a sweet taste, and very soluble in water. Liquid glucose is employed for its food value, for its local dehydrating effect, for its diuretic action, and in various pharmaceutical and industrial manufacturing operations. See Table of Normal Values of Blood Constituents in the Appendix.

glu″cose-1-phos′phate. $CH_2OHCH(CHOH)_3CH$.-$OPO(OH)_2$ (ring O bridging). The postulated first product in the breakdown of glycogen; a hexosemonophosphate. See *glycophosphomutase.*

glu″cose-6-phos′phate. $(OH)_2OPOCH_2$-CH$(CHOH)_3$CHOH (ring O bridging). A product, resulting from a reversible change of glucose-1-phosphate, obtained in the breakdown of glycogen; a hexosemonophosphate. See *glycophosphomutase.*

glu′co·si·dase. 1. An enzyme which catalyzes the hydrolysis of glucosides. 2. Emulsin.

glu′co·side. 1. Any member of a series of compounds, usually of plant origin, that may be hydrolyzed into dextrose (D-glucose) and another principle; the latter is often referred to as an aglucone. 2. Any substance, commonly a plant principle, which on hydrolysis yields a sugar and another principle. Now called glycoside.

glu′co·sin. 1. Any one of a series of bases obtained by the action of ammonia on dextrose. 2. Trade name of a substitute for sugar.

glu′co·sone. CHO.CO.HOCH.HCOH.HCOH.-CH_2OH; a hydrolysis product of the osazone of D-glucose; a possible intermediate compound in the conversion of glucose to glucosamine.

gluco-sulfathiazole. Trade-mark for a solution of sulfathiazole with sodium lactate, potassium citrate, and glucose, intended for oral administration.

glu·co′sum. Glucose.

glu″co·su′ri·a. Old term for glycosuria.

glu·cu′ron·ate. A salt or ester of glucuronic acid.

conjugated g. A glucuronide.

glu″cu·ron′ic ac′id, gly″cu·ron′ic ac′id. CHO.-HCOH.HOCH.CHOH.CHOH.COOH; D-glucuronic acid; the acid resulting from oxidation of the CH_2OH of D-glucose to COOH; it is also part of the aldobionic acid component of the polysaccharides of certain gums and of Type 3 pneumococcus polysaccharide. It is an excretion product in animals, generally in the form of conjugates called *glucuronides.*

glu″cu·ron′i·dase, gly″cu·ron′i·dase. An enzyme which catalyzes hydrolysis of glucuronides.

glu·cu′ron·ide, gly·cu′ron·ide. A compound resulting from the interaction, commonly referred to as conjugation, of glucuronic acid with a phenol, an alcohol, or an acid containing a carboxyl group. In man many of the latter substances are excreted in the form of glucuronides. Also called *conjugated glucuronate.*

glue [OF. *glu,* from LL. *glus*]. An impure gelatin prepared by boiling the skin, hoofs, and horns of animals. It is adhesive, and is used to unite surfaces.

fish g. Isinglass, prepared from the swim-bladder of fishes.

Gluge, Gottlieb [*German histologist in Belgium,* 1812–98]. Described the compound granular cells, called *Gluge's cells* or *corpuscles,* occurring usually in nervous tissues undergoing fatty degeneration.

glu′side. See *saccharin.*

glu·tae′us (gloo·tee′us). See *gluteus.*

glu·tam′ic ac′id. COOH.$(CH_2)_2$.$CHNH_2$.COOH; 2-aminopentanedioic acid or α-aminoglutaric acid; an amino acid obtained by hydrolysis of various proteins. It has been used in treating muscular dystrophies. Syn., *glutaminic acid.*

g. a. hydrochloride. A water-soluble glutamic acid salt which releases hydrochloric acid in the stomach.

glu·tam′i·nase. The enzyme which catalyzes the conversion of glutamine to glutamic acid and ammonia.

glu′ta·mine (gloo′tuh·meen, ·min, gloo·tam′een, ·in). The monamide of glutamic acid, COOH.-$CHNH_2.CH_2.CH_2.CONH_2$; it is found in the juice of many plants and is essential to the development of certain bacteria.

glu″tam·in′ic ac′id. Glutamic acid.

glu·tam′i·nyl. The univalent radical, H_2NCO-$CH_2CH_2CH(NH_2)CO$—, of glutamine, the monamide of glutamic acid.

glu·tam′o·yl. The divalent radical, $—COCH_2CH_2$-$CH(NH_2)CO$—, of glutamic acid, an amino acid having two carboxyl groups.

glu·tam′yl. The univalent radical, $HOOCCH_2CH_2$-$CH(NH_2)CO$—, of glutamic acid, an amino acid having two carboxyl groups.

glu·tar′ic ac′id (gloo·tar′ick, ·tahr′ick). COOH-$(CH_2)_3COOH$; 1,3-propanedicarboxylic acid; a crystalline acid, soluble in water. It occurs in green sugar beets and in water extracts of crude wool, and is formed from lysine by liver homogenates of certain animals.

glu″ta·thi′one (gloo″tuh·thigh′ohn, ·thigh·ohn′). $HOOC.CH(NH_2).(CH_2)_2.CONH.CH(CH_2SH)$.-$CONH.CH_2.COOH$. A tripeptide widely distributed in plant and animal tissues. It is important in tissue oxidations, acting through the sulfhydryl group (—SH) with the formation of disulfide (—S—S—) linkages.

glu·te′al, glu′te·al [G. *gloutos*, buttock]. Pertaining to the buttocks.

glu′te·lin [L. *gluten*, glue]. A class of simple proteins occurring in seeds of cereals; soluble in dilute acids and alkalies, insoluble in neutral solutions, and coagulated by heat. See American Classification of Proteins in the Appendix.

glu′ten [L.]. A mixture of proteins found in the seeds of cereals. It confers the property of toughness to dough.

g. sulfate. A cream-colored solid prepared from wheat gluten, and suggested as a pharmaceutical vehicle and suspending agent. It absorbs up to 300 times its weight of water to form an almost clear gel.

glu′ten bread. Bread made from wheat flour from which all the starch has been removed; it is used as a substitute for ordinary bread in diabetes.

glu′te·nin [*gluten*]. A protein of wheat.

glu·te′us, glu·tae′us (gloo·tee′us) [G. *gloutos*, buttock]. One of the large muscles of the buttock, attached to the ilium and femur. See Table of Muscles in the Appendix.

g. maximus. The largest and most superficial gluteal muscle.

g. medius. The gluteal muscle lying between the gluteus maximus and gluteus minimus.

g. minimus. The smallest and deepest gluteal muscle.

small anterior g. An isolated slip of the gluteus minimus muscle, occasionally present along the anterior margin of the main muscle.

glu′tin. 1. A protein obtained from gelatin. 2. Vegetable casein.

glu″tin·os′in. An antibiotic substance isolated from cultures of *Metarrhizium glutinosum;* it inhibits, in vitro, a variety of bacteria.

glu′ti·nous [L. *gluten*, glue]. Viscid; gluelike.

glut′ton·y [L. *gluto*, glutton]. Abnormally excessive indulgence in eating.

gly′case (glye′case, ·kayz). Old term for maltase.

gly·ce′mi·a, gly·cae′mi·a (glye·see′mee·uh) [G. *glykys*, sweet; *haima*, blood]. The presence of glucose in the blood.

glyc″er·al′de·hyde. Glyceric aldehyde; the simplest aldose exhibiting optical activity, formed by mild oxidation of glycerin. It exists as CHO.-$HCOH.CH_2OH$, called D-glyceraldehyde, as $CHO.HOCH.CH_2OH$ (called L-glyceraldehyde), or as a racemic mixture of the two, designated DL-glyceraldehyde. The D- and L-forms are the configurational reference standards for carbohydrates. Glyceraldehyde and phosphoric acid derivatives of it are intermediates in certain biochemical reactions of carbohydrates.

gly·cer′ic ac′id. $CH_2OH.CHOH.COOH$; α,β-dihydroxypropionic acid or 2,3-dihydroxypropanoic acid, occurring in dextrorotatory and levorotatory forms, variously obtained, as by oxidation of glycerin; both forms are liquid and are miscible with water.

gly·cer′ic al′de·hyde. Glyceraldehyde.

glyc′er·i·dase. An enzyme catalyzing hydrolysis of glycerides. If the glyceride is also a lipid, the enzyme is more commonly called a *lipase.*

glyc′er·ide (gliss′ur·ide, ·id). An ester in which glycerin provides the alcohol radical. Fats are glycerides of certain long-chain organic acids.

glyc′er·in (gliss′ur·in) [G. *glykeros*, sweet]. 1. (*glycerinum*). Trihydroxypropane. $C_3H_5(OH)_3$. A clear, colorless, syrupy liquid of sweet taste, miscible with alcohol and water. It is obtained by the hydrolysis of fats, especially by their saponification in soap manufacture. It is used as a vehicle, an emollient, and, rectally, as a prompt laxative, particularly in the form of suppositories. Syn., *glycerol.* 2. British Pharmacopoeia name for a glycerite.

g. suppositories (*suppositoria glycerini*). Prepared from glycerin, sodium stearate, and water.

glyc′er·ite (gliss′ur·yte) [*glykeros*]. A solution of one or more medicinal substances in glycerin.

boroglycerin g. (*glyceritum boroglycerini*). A viscid, yellowish liquid prepared by heating together boric acid and glycerin. It is miscible in all proportions with water but is decidedly acid in reaction.

glyc″er·o·gel′a·tin (gliss″ur·o·jel′uh·tin) [*glykeros;* L. *gelare*, to freeze]. One of a class of pharmaceutical preparations composed of glycerin, gelatin, water, and one or more medicinal substances; they are soft solids, melting at body temperature, and can be applied to the skin or molded as suppositories.

glyc′er·ol (gliss′ur·ole, ·ol, ·awl). Glycerin.

glyc″er·ol·cho′line phos′phate. A postulated intermediate product in the hydrolysis of lecithin.

glyc″er·o·phos′pha·tase. An enzyme, found in pancreatic juice, and generally in cells capable of liberating phosphoric acid from glycerophosphoric acid and certain of its derivatives.

glyc″er·o·phos′phate. A salt of glycerophosphoric acid.

compound glycerophosphates elixir (*elixir glycerophosphatum compositum*). Contains the glycerophosphates of sodium, calcium, ferric iron, and manganese. Dose, 8 cc. (2 fluidrachms). Also called *compound glycerophosphates solution.*

glyc″er·o·phos·phor′ic ac′id. $CH_2OH.CHOH$.-$CH_2.O.PO(OH)_2$. A pale yellow, oily liquid, soluble in water. Its salts, especially calcium and sodium glycerophosphate, have been used in the mistaken belief that their phosphorus was more readily utilized than that of other compounds.

glyc′er·ose. An equilibrium mixture of the interconvertible isomers, glyceraldehyde and dihydroxyacetone, obtained by mild oxidation of glycerin.

glyc″er·ose-3-phos′phate. Glyceraldehyde-3-phosphoric acid, $CHO.CHOH.CH_2OPO(OH)_2$, an intermediate in a postulated cleavage of carbohydrates to form lactic acid.

glyc'er·yl (gliss'ur·il). The trivalent radical, C_3H_5, combined with fatty acids in fats and in animal and vegetable oils.

g. diacetate. Diacetin.

g. guaiacolate. Guaiacol glyceryl ether.

g. monostearate. $(C_{17}H_{35}COO)(OH)_2C_3H_5$; a white, waxlike solid, insoluble in water; it is employed as a stabilizing agent in various dermatologic preparations.

g. triacetate. $(CH_3COO)_3C_3H_5$; a colorless, somewhat oily liquid, soluble in water. It is used as a solvent, as for certain local antiseptics. Syn., *triacetin.*

g. tributyrate. Butyrin.

g. trinitrate. $C_3H_5(NO_3)_3$. A colorless, or pale yellow, volatile liquid used in the preparation of explosives. Physiologically, it possesses the actions of the nitrites; in medicinal doses it reduces blood pressure in 2–3 minutes, the effect lasting about half an hour. Dose, 0.3–1.2 mg. (1/200–1/50 gr.). Syn., *nitroglycerin, glonoin.*

g. trinitrate spirit (*spiritus glycerylis trinitratis*). A 1% alcoholic solution used as a rapid and fleeting vasodilator. Dose, 0.06–0.12 cc. (1–2 min.).

g. trinitrate tablets (*tabellae glycerylis trinitratis*). Administered sublingually. Dose of active ingredient, 0.3–1.2 mg. (1/200–1/50 gr.).

g. trioleate. Olein.

g. tripalmitate. Palmitin.

g. tristearate. Stearin.

gly'cin. A poisonous photonegative developer, *p*-hydroxyphenylaminoacetic acid.

gly'cin·ate. Any salt of aminoacetic acid (glycine).

gly'cine (glye'seen, ·sin, glye·seen'). Aminoacetic acid.

g. oxidase. An enzyme, present in liver and kidney, which catalyzes conversion of glycine to glyoxylic acid and ammonia; its prosthetic group is flavin adenine dinucleotide.

gly'ci·nin. The principal protein of the soybean.

Gly·ciph'a·gus do·mes'ti·cus. The mite causing grocer's itch.

gly'co-, glyc- [G. *glykys*, sweet]. A combining form meaning *sweet*, or denoting *glycerin.*

gly"co·bi·ar'sol. The official name for *bismuth glycolylarsanilate*, an intestinal amebicide.

gly"co·cho'late (glye"ko·ko'late, ·kol'ate). A salt of glycocholic acid.

gly"co·chol'ic ac'id. $C_{26}H_{43}O_6N$. An acid obtained by the conjugation of cholic acid with glycine; found in bile, especially of herbivorous animals.

gly'co·coll. Aminoacetic acid.

gly"co·cy"a·mine'. $COOHCH_2NH.C(:NH).NH_2$; guanidinoacetic acid; a product of interaction of aminoacetic acid (glycine) and arginine, which on transmethylation with methionine is converted to creatine: also called *guanidine-acetic acid;* incorrectly called *guanidoacetic acid.*

gly'co·gen. $(C_6H_{10}O_5)_n$. A carbohydrate found in the liver cells, in all tissues in the embryo, in the testes, muscles, leukocytes, fresh pus cells, cartilage, and other tissues. It is formed from carbohydrates and is stored in the liver, where it is converted, as the system requires, into sugar (glucose). It is also known as *animal starch.* Glycogen is soluble in water, is dextrorotatory, and is colored red by iodine.

gly'co·ge·nase" (glye'ko·ji·nace", glye"ko·ji·nace', glye·ko'ji·nace). An enzyme found in the liver, which hydrolyzes glycogen to maltose and dextrin.

gly"co·gen'e·sis [*glykys;* G. *genesis*, production]. Formation of sugar in the liver. —**glycogenet'ic, glycog'enous,** *adj.*

gly"co·gen'ic [*glykys;* G. *genesthai*, from *gignesthai*, to be produced]. Pertaining to glycogen or to glycogenesis.

gly"co·ge·nol'y·sis [*glykys;* G. *genesis*, production; *lysis*, a loosing]. The conversion of glycogen into glucose by hydrolysis.

gly"co·ge·no'sis [*glykys; genesis;* G. *-ōsis*, increase]. A disturbance of glycogen metabolism occurring in early infancy; characterized by abnormal deposit of glycogen, predominantly in the heart, which as a result becomes enlarged (cardiomegalia glycogenica). In the circumscribed form, glycogen is distributed focally in the heart, predominantly subendocardially (cardiomegalia glycogenica circumscripta). Other organs, as liver, kidney, and skeletal muscle, may also contain excessive glycogen deposits. Syn., *glycogen disease, von Gierke's disease.*

gly·cog'e·ny (glye·kodj'i·nee). See *glycogenesis.*

gly"co·he'mi·a, gly"co·hae'mi·a (gly"ko·hee'mee·uh). Old term for glycemia.

gly'col. 1. An aliphatic compound containing two hydroxyl groups. 2. Ethylene glycol.

gly'col al'de·hyde. $CHO.CH_2OH$; the simplest sugar; a diose. It may be an intermediate in the biochemical breakdown of certain sugars. Also called *glycolic aldehyde.*

gly·col'ic ac'id (glye·kol'ick). $CH_2OH.COOH$. Hydroxyacetic acid produced by the reduction of oxalic acid.

gly"co·lip'id. Any lipid which, on acid hydrolysis, yields a carbohydrate, an alcohol, and a fatty acid. Syn., *glycolipin.*

gly"co·lip'in. Glycolipid.

gly'co·lyl. 1. Properly, the univalent radical $CH_2OH.CO$—. 2. The bivalent radical $—CH_2CO—$.

gly·col'y·sis (glye·kol'i·sis) [*glykys;* G. *lysis*, a loosing]. The process of conversion of carbohydrate, in tissues, to pyruvic acid or lactic acid. Commonly it is considered to begin with hydrolysis of glycogen to glucose (glycogenolysis), which subsequently undergoes a series of chemical changes. —**glycolyt'ic,** *adj.*

gly"co·me·tab'o·lism [*glykys;* G. *metabolē*, change]. The metabolism of sugar in the body. —**glycometabol'ic,** *adj.*

gly"co·ne"o·gen'e·sis [*glykys;* G. *neos*, new; *genesis*, production]. The formation of carbohydrates from substances which are not carbohydrates, such as protein or fat.

gly'co·nin. Glycerite of egg yolk. An emulsifying agent prepared by mixing together 45 Gm. of strained egg yolk and 55 Gm. of glycerin.

gly"co·pe'ni·a [*glykys;* G. *penia*, poverty]. Tendency to hypoglycemia.

gly"co·pex'is [*glykys;* G. *pēxis*, a fixing]. The storing of glucose or glycogen.

gly"co·phil'i·a [*glykys;* G. *philein*, to love]. Tendency to hyperglycemia, after the ingestion of very little glucose.

gly"co·phos"pho·mu'tase. An enzyme which catalyzes the reaction glucose-1-phosphate ⇌ glucose-6-phosphate.

gly"co·pro'te·in [*glykys;* G. *prōteios*, of first rank]. One of a group of conjugated proteins which upon decomposition yield a protein and a carbohydrate, or derivatives of the same. See American Classification of Proteins in the Appendix. Syn., *mucoprotein.*

gly"co·pty'a·lism (gly"ko·ty'uh·liz·um) [*glykys;* G. *ptyalon*, saliva]. Excretion of glucose in the saliva.

gly"cor·rha'chi·a (gly"ko·ray'kee·uh, ·rack'ee·uh) [*glykys;* G. *rhachis*, spine]. Glucose in the cerebrospinal fluid.

gly"cor·rhe'a, gly"cor·rhoe'a (gly"ko·ree'uh)

[*glykys;* G. *rhoia,* a flow]. Discharge of sugar-containing fluid from the body.

gly″cos·a·mine′ (gly″ko·suh·meen′, ·sam′een, ·in, gly·ko′suh·meen, ·min). Glucosamine.

gly″co·se·cre′to·ry [*glykys;* L. *secretum,* from *secernere,* to separate]. Concerned in the secretion of glycogen.

gly″co·se′mi·a, **gly″co·sae′mi·a** (gly″ko·see′-mee·uh). See *glycemia.*

gly″co·si·al′i·a (gly″ko·sigh·al′ee·uh, ·ay′lee·uh) [*glykys;* G. *sialon,* saliva]. The presence of glucose in the saliva.

gly″co·si″a·lor·rhe′a [*glykys; sialon;* G. *rhoia,* flow]. Excessive salivary secretion containing glucose.

gly′co·side. Any plant principle which yields on hydrolysis a sugar and another substance designated as an aglycone. In order to indicate the specific sugar which is formed, a more descriptive term such as glucoside, galactoside, etc., may be used. Many glycosides are therapeutically valuable. See also *glucoside.* —**glycosi′dal, glycosid′ic,** *adj.*

gly″co·su′ri·a [*glykys;* G. *ouron,* urine]. The presence of sugar in the urine.

alimentary g. That due to excessive ingestion of carbohydrates.

anxiety g. A transitory form due to worry.

artificial g. Glycosuria resulting from puncture of the floor of the fourth ventricle in the inferior part of the medulla. Formerly called *traumatic g., piqûre diabetes.*

diabetic g. That resulting from diabetes mellitus.

renal g. An anomalous condition characterized by a low renal threshold for sugar together with a normal blood sugar level; of little or no pathologic significance. Erroneously called renal diabetes.

toxic g. That observed after poisoning by chloral, morphine, or curare, after the inhalation of chloroform or carbon monoxide, or after the ingestion of phlorhizin.

traumatic g. See artificial *g.*

gly″co·su′ric ac′id. Homogentisic acid.

glyco-thymoline. A proprietary liquid similar to alkaline aromatic solution.

glyc″u·re′sis (glick″yoo·ree′sis, gly″cue·) [*glykys;* G. *ourēsis,* a making water]. Excretion of sugar seen normally in the urine.

gly″cu·ron′ic ac′id. Glucuronic acid.

gly″cu·ron′i·dase. Glucuronidase.

gly·cu′ron·ide. Glucuronide.

gly″cu·ro·nu′ri·a [*glykys;* G. *ouron,* urine; *ouron*]. The presence of glucuronic acid in the urine.

gly′cyl. The univalent radical, $H_2NCH_2CO—$, of the amino acid glycine.

glyc″yr·rhe′tic ac′id (glis″ir·ree′tic). Glycyrrhetinic acid.

glyc″yr·rhe·tin′ic ac′id (glis″ir·ri·tin′ic). $C_{30}H_{46}O_4$; a pentacyclic terpene, obtained by hydrolysis of glycyrrhizic acid; its structure resembles that common to steroids. It possesses certain of the physiological actions of desoxycorticosterone. Syn., *glycyrrhetic acid.*

glyc″yr·rhi′za (glis″i·rye′zuh) [*glykys;* G. *rhiza,* root]. Licorice. The dried rhizome and roots of several varieties of *Glycyrrhiza glabra.* **Glycyrrhiza extract** and **pure glycyrrhiza extract** are used as diluents, excipients. **Glycyrrhiza fluidextract** is used as a vehicle. **Compound opium and glycyrrhiza mixture,** also called *brown mixture,* is administered in bronchitis. Dose, 4 cc. (1 fluidrachm). **Glycyrrhiza elixir** is used as a vehicle for disguising or obtunding the taste of bitter substances.

glyc″yr·rhi′zic ac′id (glis″i·rye′zick). A very sweet, crystalline glycoside, probably of the formula $C_{42}H_{62}O_{16}$, salts of which occur in glycyrrhiza; on hydrolysis it yields two molecules of glucuronic acid and one molecule of glycyrrhetinic acid. It appears to have certain of the physiological actions of desoxycorticosterone. Syn., *glycyrrhizin.*

glyc″yr·rhi′zin (glis″i·rye′zin). Glycyrrhizic acid.

ammoniated g. A sweet preparation consisting of an impure form of glycyrrhizin combined with ammonia.

glynazan. A trade-mark for *theophylline sodium glycinate.*

gly′o·din. Generic name for the fungicidal substance 2-heptadecyl-2-imidazoline acetate, also known as 2-heptadecylglyoxalidine acetate; $C_{22}H_{44}N_2O_2$; a light-orange crystalline compound.

gly·ox′al. OHC.CHO; a compound resulting from oxidation of acetaldehyde; it occurs as yellow crystals, polymerizing on standing or on contact with water, in which violent reaction takes place.

gly·ox′a·lase (glye·ock′suh·lace). An enzyme present in various body tissues which catalyzes the conversion of methyloglyoxal into lactic acid.

gly″ox·al′ic ac′id. Glyoxylic acid.

gly·ox′a·line (glye·ock′suh·leen, ·lin). Imidazole.

gly″ox·yl′ic ac′id. CHO.COOH; a constituent of various plant and animal tissues; it may be obtained by oxidative deamination of glycine but it may also serve as a precursor of glycine. It is used as a reagent for tryptophan (Hopkins-Cole reaction). Syn., *formylfornic acid, glyoxalic acid, oxoethanoic acid.*

glytheonate. Trade-mark for *theophylline sodium glycinate.*

Gm, Gm. Gram(s); gramme(s).

gm, gm. Gram(s); gramme(s).

Gmelin, Leopold [*German chemist and physiologist,* 1788–1853]. Made important studies of bile. See also Gmelin's *test.*

gnat [AS. *gnaet*]. Any one of various dipterous insects belonging to the suborder Nematocera. Mosquitoes, black flies, biting midges, and sand flies are included.

gnath-. See *gnatho-.*

gnath·al′gi·a (na·thal′juh, ·jee·uh) [G. *gnathos,* jaw; *algos,* pain]. Pain or neuralgia of the jaw.

gnath′ic (nath′ick, nay′thick) [*gnathos*]. Pertaining to the jaw.

gna′thi·on (nayth′ee·on, nath′·) [*gnathos*]. The most inferior point on the inferior border of the mandible, in the sagittal plane. Also called *menton.*

gnath·i′tis (na·thigh′tis) [*gnathos;* G. *-itis,* inflammation]. Inflammation of the jaw or cheek.

gnath′o- (nath′o-, nayth′o-), **gnath-** [*gnathos*]. A combining form signifying *the jaw.*

gnath″o·ceph′a·lus [*gnathos;* G. *kephalē,* head]. A monster lacking all parts of the head except large jaws.

gnath″o·dy″na·mom′e·ter (·dye″nuh·mom′i·tur, ·din″uh·mom′i·tur) [*gnathos;* G. *dynamis,* power; *metron,* a measure]. An instrument for recording the force exerted in closing the jaws.

gnath″o·dyn′i·a [*gnathos;* G. *odynē,* pain]. Pain in the jaw; gnathalgia.

gnath·op′a·gus par″a·sit′i·cus. See *epignathus.*

gnath′o·plas″ty [*gnathos;* G. *plassein,* to form]. Plastic surgery of the cheek or jaw.

gnath·os′chi·sis (na·thos′ki·sis) [*gnathos;* G. *schisis,* cleavage]. Cleft alveolar process.

Gnath·os′to·ma [*gnathos;* G. *stoma,* mouth]. A genus of nematode worms of the family Gnathostomatidae.

G. hispidum. A species infesting the stomach walls of hogs and sometimes of cattle in Europe, Asia, Africa, and Australia. Of little pathologic importance in man.

G. spinigerum. A species infesting the subcutaneous tissues and intestinal walls of domestic and wild felines, dogs, hogs, and mink, restricted geographically to India, Malaya, China, and Japan. Man serves as an accidental host in whom the parasites do not fully develop.

gnath″o·sto·mi′a·sis [*gnathos; stoma;* NL. *-iasis*, condition]. Infestation with *Gnathostoma spinigerum* larvae; deep burrows, boils, and abscesses in the skin are caused by this parasite.

gnos′co·pine (nos′ko·peen, ·pin). Racemic narcotine from opium.

gno′sis (no′sis) [G., knowledge]. The faculty of knowing in contradistinction to the function of feeling, in respect to any external stimulus.

gnos′tic (nos′tick) [G. *gnōstikos*, of knowing, from *gignōskein*]. Relating to discriminative or epicritic sensations in contradistinction to vital or protopathic sensations.

Go′a powder (go′uh). See *araroba.*

goat′pox″ [AS. *gat;* ME. *pokkes*]. An acute disease seen in goats; marked by a vesicular eruption.

Goblet. See *Gubler.*

gob′let cell. See under *cell.*

god′et. See *scutulum.*

Goethe, Johann Wolfgang von [*German comparative anatomist and poet,* 1749–1832]. Pioneer student of evolution. Coined the term morphology. Discovered the human intermaxillary bone (1831), called *Goethe's bone.*

Goetsch, Emil (1883–) American surgeon known for his description of the epinephrine hypersensitiveness test to differentiate hyperthyroidism from functional nervous disorders, tuberculosis, and asthma, in which the subject is given a subcutaneous injection of epinephrine hydrochloride. A positive reaction is characterized by an increase in blood pressure and pulse rates of at least 10 points with an exaggeration of the symptoms of hyperthyroidism lasting 1 to 1½ hours. The test is also called *Goetsch's test.*

goi′ter, goi′tre [OF. *goitron*, from L. *guttur*, throat]. Enlargement of the thyroid gland. Also see *struma.* —**goitrous,** *adj.*

aberrant g. That of a supernumerary thyroid gland. Also called *accessory g.*

acute g. One which develops rapidly.

adenomatous g. An asymmetric type due to isolated nodular masses of thyroid tissue (adenomas).

adolescent g. Diffuse enlargement of the thyroid in adolescents. Also called *juvenile g.*

benign metastasizing g. See follicular *carcinoma* of thyroid.

cabbage g. One produced experimentally by the feeding of cabbage to rabbits and other animals.

cancerous g. Carcinoma of the thyroid gland. Also called *carcinomatous g.*

colloid g. A diffuse, soft, sometimes large goiter in which many of the acinar spaces are distended with colloid.

congenital g. One present at birth.

cyanide g. A goiter produced experimentally by the administration of cyanide; associated with deficient use of the thyroid hormone by the tissues.

cystic g. One in which a cyst, or cysts, forms by the degeneration of tissue, as within preexisting adenomas.

diffuse g. A type in which the thyroid gland is diffusely enlarged, in contrast to adenomatous goiter.

endemic g. That occurring commonly in iodine-poor and mountainous areas.

exophthalmic g. A disease caused chiefly by overproduction of the thyroid hormone; characterized by goiter, tachycardia, nervous excitability, fine involuntary tremor, exophthalmos and other ocular signs, loss of weight, muscular weakness, and a tendency to intense, acute exacerbations called thyroid crises. There is excessive excretion of nitrogen and increased excretion of calcium, leading to osteoporosis and disturbance in carbohydrate metabolism. Also called *Basedow's disease, Flajani's disease, Graves's disease, hyperthyroidism, Parry's disease, thyrotoxicosis, toxic g.*

hyperplastic g. One characterized by an increased number of cells, particularly those lining the acini, with an accompanying increase in vascularity of the gland. Also called *parenchymatous g.*

intrathoracic g. A goiter which has a portion lying within the thoracic cavity.

lingual g. A tumor, composed of thyroid tissue, at the upper end of the original thyroglossal duct, near the foramen cecum of the tongue.

lymphadenoid g. See *struma lymphomatosa.*

malignant g. One which is the seat of carcinoma or sarcoma.

nodular g. See adenomatous *g.*

parenchymatous g. See hyperplastic *g.*

sarcomatous g. Sarcoma of the thyroid gland.

simple g. A diffuse goiter, either colloid or hyperplastic in type; usually unassociated with constitutional features.

sporadic g. Goiter which occurs in limited geographic areas.

sulfonamide g. That due to continued administration of one of the soluble sulfonamides.

thiocyanate g. One due to prolonged administration of a thiocyanate.

thiourylene g. One due to administration of a thiourylene compound; as thiourea, thiouracil, thiobarbital; associated with hyperplasia of the thyroid gland and thought to be due to prevention of synthesis of thyroglobulin.

toxic g. See exophthalmic *g.*

goi′tre. See *goiter.*

goi″tro·gen′ic [*goitron;* G. *genesthai*, from *gignesthai*, to be produced]. Producing goiter; as iodine-deficient diets or, experimentally, diets of cabbage and other brassica plants, the feeding of sulfonamides, drugs of the thiourea group, etc.

gold [AS.] (*aurum*). Au = 197.0. A yellow metal, easily malleable and ductile. Gold salts are used in rheumatoid arthritis and in various forms of tuberculosis. Toxic effects are numerous.

g. bromide. Gold tribromide, auric bromide, $AuBr_3$. Used in epilepsy and in whooping cough. Dose, 8–12 mg. (⅛–⅕ gr.).

g. leaf. Pure gold in very thin, transparent sheets of blue-green color.

g. sodium thiomalate.

$$\begin{array}{l} CH_2COONa \\ | \qquad\qquad .H_2O \\ AuSCHCOONa \end{array}$$

A white to yellowish-white powder, very soluble in water, used in the treatment of rheumatoid arthritis and lupus erythematosus. See *myochrysine.*

g. sodium thiopropanolsulfonate. See *allochrysine.*

g. sodium thiosulfate (*auri sodii thiosulfas*). Sodium aurothiosulfate. $Na_3Au(S_2O_3)_2.2H_2O$, occurring in white crystals, freely soluble in water, and used in rheumatoid arthritis and lupus erythematosus. See *sanocrysin.* Also see *triphal.*

g. thioglucose. Aurothioglucose.

g. trihydroxide. See *auric acid.*

Goldberger, Joseph [*American pathologist,* 1874–1929]. With J. F. Anderson, studied the experimental transmission of measles to monkeys (1911). Pioneered in the study of vitamins and of pellagra. With G. A. Wheeler, R. D. Lillie, and L. M. Rogers, discovered the pellagra-preventive factor, later identified as nicotinic acid.

Goldblatt, Harry [*American pathologist*, 1891–]. Author of a theory on the mechanism of hypertension; devised a clamp for gradual occlusion of arteries; called *Goldblatt clamp*. See experimental renal *hypertension*, Goldblatt *method*. With Louis Gross he invented the Autotechnicon (1929).

gold′en·rod″ [AS.]. The common name for several species of the genus *Solidago* of the Compositae. Their pollen produces hay fever.

Goldflam, Samuel Vulfovich [*Polish neurologist*, 1852–1932]. Remembered for his description of myasthenia gravis (1893), called *Erb-Goldflam disease*, *Hoppe-Goldflam symptom complex*.

Goldmann's test. See Baumann and Goldmann's *test*.

Goldscheider, Johannes Karl August Eugene Alfred [*German neurologist*, 1858–1935]. Made important studies of cutaneous sensation (1884–85). Described epidermolysis bullosa (1882), known as *Goldscheider's disease*.

Goldstein-Scheerer test. See under *test*.

gold′thread′. See *Coptis groenlandica*.

Goldthwait, Joel Ernest [*American orthopedic surgeon*, 1866–]. Introduced his operation for recurrent dislocation of the patella, in which an incision is made over the patella and patellar tendon and carried to a point over the medial condyle of the tibia. The tendon is split lengthwise, and the outer half is detached from the tibial tubercle, transplanted beneath the inner half, and sutured to the periosteum of the inner anterior surface of the tibia. Known as *Goldthwait's operation*.

Golgi, Camillo [*Italian histologist*, 1844–1926]. Introduced the use of silver nitrate for staining nerve cells; see *Golgi's silver method* under *stain*. Described the development of the quartan malarial parasite (1886) and distinguished it from the tertian (1889). See endogenous *cycle*, also called *cycle of Golgi*. Described the internal reticular apparatus, a network of fibers or canals of unknown significance, found in the cytoplasm of cells, called *Golgi apparatus, network, material*. These fibers or canals, which may take the form of rods, granules, or spheres, react selectively to osmic acid. See also *organ* of Golgi (also called *Golgi's corpuscle*); Golgi *cells;* Mazzoni's *corpuscle* (also called *Golgi-Mazzoni's corpuscle*). The acroblast is known as the *Golgi remnant*. Nobel laureate with Ramón y Cajal (1906).

gol″gi·o·kin·e′sis. The division of the Golgi apparatus during karyokinesis.

Goll, Friedrich [*Swiss anatomist*, 1829–1903]. Described the fasciculus gracilis (1860), also called *Goll's column* or *tract*. See also gracilis *nucleus;* formerly called *nucleus of Goll*.

Goltz, Friedrich Leopold [*German physiologist*, 1834–1902]. Known especially for his researches on the physiology of the nervous system. Made an experimental study of reflex actions, with frogs (1869) and decorticated dogs. See also static *theory*, called *Goltz's theory*.

Gombault, François Alexis Albert [*French physician*, 1844–1904]. Described the triangular area formed by the septomarginal tract in the sacral region of the spinal cord, at the dorsomedian angle of the dorsal funiculus. This was described also by Claudien Philippe, and is called *Gombault-Philippe's triangle*.

gom·phi′a·sis [G. *gomphios*, molar; NL. *-iasis*, condition]. Looseness of the teeth in their sockets; periodontosis. *Obs.*

gom·pho′sis [G. *gomphos*, bolt; *-ōsis*, condition]. A form of synarthrosis.

gon″a·cra′ti·a [G. *gonē*, seed; *akrateia*, incontinence]. Spermatorrhea. *Rare.*

gon′ad [*gonē*]. 1. A gland or organ producing gametes; a general term for ovary or testis. 2. The embryonic sex gland before morphologic identification as ovary or testis is possible. Also called *indifferent g.* —**gonadal,** *adj.*

female g. The ovary.

male g. The testis.

gon′ad·arch″e. The time when ovarian or testicular activity begins in the adolescent.

gon″a·dec′to·my [*gonē;* G. *ektomē*, excision]. Surgical removal of a gonad.

gon″a·do·cen′tric [*gonē;* G. *kentron*, center of a circle]. Relating to a focusing of the sex urge upon the genitals; a phase of sex development normally occurring in puberty.

gonadophysin. Trade-mark for a purified pituitary gonadotropin.

gon″a·do·ther′a·py [*gonē;* G. *therapeia*, treatment]. Treatment with gonadal extracts or hormones.

gonadothyn. Trade-mark for a purified pituitary gonadotropin.

gon″a·do·tro′phin. See *gonadotropin*.

gon″a·do·tro′pin [*gonē;* G. *-tropos*, turning]. A gonad-stimulating hormone. The principal sources are: (a) the anterior pituitary gland of various animal species; (b) the urine of pregnant women (chorionic gonadotropin); (c) the serum of pregnant mares (serum gonadotropin). Formerly written *gonadotrophin*. Syn., *gonadotropic substance*.

anterior pituitary g. The multiple gonadotropin produced by the anterior lobe of the pituitary gland, consisting of: (a) follicle-stimulating hormone (FSH, prolan A); (b) luteinizing hormone (LH, prolan B), which is also an interstitial-cell-stimulating hormone (ICSH).

chorionic g. The water-soluble gonadotropic substance, originating in chorionic tissue, obtained from the urine of pregnant women. It is recommended in treating cryptorchism, and has been used in treating hypogonadism in the adult, and in uterine bleeding of functional nature.

luteotropic g. See *luteotropin*.

serum g. The water-soluble follicle-stimulating substance, by some believed to originate in chorionic tissue, obtained from the serum of pregnant mares. It may be identical with the follicle-stimulating hormone obtained from the anterior lobe of the pituitary gland. It is used to supplement the action of estrogens in the treatment of delayed puberty and amenorrhea and hypomenorrhea, and also of acne vulgaris in the female.

gon′a·duct [*gonē;* L. *ductus*, a leading]. Duct of a gonad; oviduct or sperm duct.

go·nag′ra (go·nag′ruh, ·nay′gruh, gon′ag·ruh) [G. *gony*, knee; *agra*, a catching]. Gout of the knee joint.

go·nal′gi·a [*gony;* G. *algos*, pain]. Pain in the knee joint.

gon″an·gi·ec′to·my (gon″an·jee·eck′to·mee, go-nan″jee·) [G. *gonē*, seed; *aggeion*, vessel; *ektomē*, excision]. Excision of part of the ductus deferens.

gon″ar·thri′tis [G. *gony*, knee; *arthritis*, from *arthron*, joint, *-itis*, inflammation]. Inflammation of the knee joint.

gon″ar·throc′a·ce (gon″ahr·throck′uh·see) [*gony; arthron;* G. *kakos*, bad]. White swelling of the knee joint. *Obs.*

gon″ar·throt′o·my [*gony; arthron;* G. *tomē*, a cutting]. Incision into the knee joint.

go·nat′o·cele [*gony;* G. *kēlē*, tumor]. A swelling or tumor of the knee.

Gonda reflex. See under *reflex.*

gon′e·cyst, gon″e·cys′tis [G. *gonē*, seed; *kystis*, bladder]. A seminal vesicle. —**gonecys′tic,** *adj.*

gon″e·cys·ti′tis [*gonē; kystis*, G. *-itis*, inflammation]. Inflammation of the seminal vesicles.

gon″e·cys′to·lith [*gonē; kystis;* G. *lithos*, stone]. A concretion or calculus in a seminal vesicle.

gon″e·cys″to·py·o′sis [*gonē; kystis;* G. *pyōsis*, suppuration]. Suppuration of a seminal vesicle.

gon″e·poi·e′sis [*gonē;* G. *poiēsis*, production]. The formation of semen. —**gonepoiet′ic,** *adj.*

Gon″gy·lo·ne′ma (gon″ji·lo·nee′muh) [G. *goggylos*, round; *nēma*, thread]. A genus of nematode parasites of the family Spiruridae. The variously named species are usually grouped under the single species *G. pulchrum.*

G. pulchrum. A parasite found in the upper digestive tract of sheep, cattle, goats, hogs, and horses. In cases of accidental human infestation, the worm invades the buccal mucosa.

gon″gy·lo·ne·mi′a·sis (gon″ji·lo·nee·my′uh·sis) [*goggylos; nēma;* NL. *-iasis*, condition]. Infestation with *Gongylonema*, a genus of filarial nematodes.

gon′ic [*gonē*]. Pertaining to semen or to generation.

Gonin, Jules [*Swiss ophthalmologist*, 1870–1935]. Devised an operation of ignipuncture for detachment of the retina, in which he employed thermocauterization of the retinal fissure through an opening in the sclera (1927).

go″ni·o·chei·los′chi·sis (go″nee·o·kigh·los′ki·sis) [G. *gōnia*, angle; *cheilos*, lip; *schisis*, cleavage]. Transverse facial cleft; intermaxillary fissure; macrostomia; genal cleft.

go″ni·o·cra″ni·om′e·try [*gōnia;* G. *kranion*, skull; *metron*, a measure]. Measurement of the various angles of the skull.

go″ni·om′e·ter [*gōnia; metron*]. An instrument for measuring angles, as the angle of the mandible.

go′ni·on [*gōnia*]. A craniometric point, the tip of the angle of the mandible. —**go′nial,** *adj.*

go″ni·o·punc′ture. A filtering operation for congenital glaucoma achieved by puncturing the filtration angle with a goniotomy needle.

go′ni·o·scope [*gōnia;* G. *skopein*, to examine]. A special optical instrument for studying in detail the angle of the anterior chamber of the eye, and for testing ocular motility. —**gonios′copy,** *n.*

go·ni·ot′o·my [*gōnia;* G. *tomē*, a cutting]. An operation for glaucoma in which Schlemm's canal is opened under direct vision.

go·ni′tis [G. *gony*, knee; *-itis*, inflammation]. Inflammation of the knee joint.

go′ni·um (pl. *gonia*) [G. *gonē*, seed]. A general term for spermatogonium and oogonium.

gon′o·blast [*gonē;* G. *blastos*, germ]. Old term for germ cell.

gon″o·coc·ce′mi·a, gon″o·coc·cae′mi·a (gon″o-cock·see′mee·uh) [*gonē;* G. *kokkos*, grain; *haima*, blood]. The presence of gonococci in the blood.

gon″o·coc′ci (gon″o·cock′sigh). Plural of gonococcus.

gon″o·coc′cide. Any substance or agent having properties which destroy gonococci. Less desirable terms sometimes used are *gonocide, gonoccicide.* —**gonococ′cide,** *adj.*

gon″o·coc′cin (gon″o·cock′sin). A glycerin extract of gonococci, employed in testing for gonorrhea by the cutireaction. *Obs.*

gon″o·coc′cus (pl. *gonococci*) [*gonē; kokkos*]. The common name for the organism causing gonorrhea; *Neisseria gonorrhoeae.* —**gonococcal, gonococcic,** *adj.*

gon′o·cyte [*gonē;* G. *kytos*, cell]. A germ cell.

primary g. A primordial germ cell derived from endoderm and found in the germinal epithelium of the gonads.

secondary g. The definitive or functional germ cells derived from the germinal epithelium of the gonads, but not necessarily from a primary gonocyte.

go·nom′er·y [*gonē;* G. *meros*, part]. The independence of the pronuclei or their chromosomes in the zygote and the first few cleavage stages.

gon″or·rhe′a [G. *gonorroia*, from *gonē; rhoia*, flow]. A specific infectious inflammation of the mucous membrane of the urethra and adjacent cavities, due to the *Neisseria gonorrhoeae.* The disease is characterized by pain, burning urination, a profuse mucopurulent discharge, and may be accompanied by complications: prostatitis, periurethral abscess, epididymitis, cystitis, purulent conjunctivitis. It may also cause arthritis (gonorrheal rheumatism), endocarditis, and salpingitis. —**gonorrhe′al,** *adj.*

gon″y·ba′ti·a [G. *gony*, knee; *bainein*, to walk]. Walking upon the knees; a symptom in some paralytic and paretic cases.

gon″y·camp′sis [*gony;* G. *kampsis*, a bending]. Deformity of knee due to abnormal bending or curving.

gon′y·o·cele″. See *gonyoncus.*

gon″y·on′cus [*gony;* G. *ogkos*, a mass]. A tumor or swelling of the knee.

Goodell's sign. See under *sign.*

good′ness of fit. A measure of how accurately a particular mathematical formula fits a series of observations.

Goodpasture, Ernest William [*American pathologist*, 1886–]. Known for his investigation of viruses by means of chick embryos. This study led the way to the production of vaccines against fowlpox, smallpox, yellow fever, and typhus. See also *Goodpasture's stains* under *stain*, carbol-aniline fuchsin *stain.*

Goodrich method. See van den Bergh's *method* (Gibson and Goodrich modification).

goose flesh. Skin marked by prominence about the hair follicles. Results from contraction of the arrectores pilorum muscles: also called *goose skin, cutis anserina.*

Gor″di·a′ce·a [*Gordius*, who tied the Gordian knot]. A subclass of the Nematomorpha; the so-called hair snakes.

Gordon, Alfred (1874–). American neurologist who described a great-toe reflex elicited in diseases of the pyramidal tract, called Gordon's *reflex.*

Gordon, Mervyn Henry [*English bacteriologist*, 1872–]. Described a test for Hodgkin's disease. See Gordon's *test.*

Gorgas, William Crawford [*American Army surgeon*, 1854–1920]. As chief sanitary officer of the Panama Canal Commission (1904–13), directed the anti-yellow-fever and antimalaria campaign which made the construction of the Canal possible. Surgeon General of the Army during World War I.

gor′get (gor′jit) [OF. *gorgete*, dim. of *gorge*, throat]. A channeled instrument similar to a grooved director, formerly used much in lithotomy.

probe g. One whose tip is probe-pointed.

gorit. Trade name of a preparation of calcium peroxide.

go·ron′dou (go·ron′dōō). See *goundou.*

Gos·syp′i·um [L. *gossypion*, cotton-tree]. A genus of plants of the Malvaceae from which cotton and cotton-root bark are obtained.

gos′sy·pol. A phenolic compound sometimes found in the oil cake after expression of the oil from cottonseed. It has produced toxic symptoms in cattle fed such oil cake.

Gottlieb's cuticle. See enamel *cuticle.*

Gottschalk, Sigmund [*German surgeon,* 1860–1914]. Described an operation for displacement of the uterus. In *Gottschalk's operation,* the uterosacral ligaments are shortened by the vagalin route.

gouge [F., from LL. *gubia*]. A transversely curved chisel for cutting or removing bone or other hard structures.

Gougerot, Henri [*French physician,* 1881–]. With de Beurmann, described sporotrichosis (1906), which is known as *de Beurmann-Gougerot disease, Schenck's disease.* Nodular dermal allergid is known as *Gougerot's trisymptomatic disease.*

Goulard's extract. See *lead* subacetate solution.

Gould, Alfred Henry [*American surgeon,* 1872–1907]. Devised an interrupted mattress suture for intestinal repair, so applied as to evert the cut edges of the intestine. Called *Gould's suture.*

Gould, George Milbry [*American ophthalmologist and medical lexicographer,* 1848–1922]. Editor of various medical dictionaries from 1890 on. *Blakiston's New Gould Medical Dictionary* is based on *Gould's Medical Dictionary,* 5th edition, which was the sum of all his previous work. He described *Gould's bowed-head sign,* indicative of retinitis pigmentosa or other disease destroying the peripheral part of the retina: the subject walks with the head bowed in order to bring the image of the ground onto the functioning area of the retina.

Gouley, John Williams Severin [*American surgeon,* 1832–1920]. Invented a solid, curved steel instrument grooved on its inner aspect for passing over a guide inserted through a stricture into the urinary bladder, called *Gouley's catheter.*

goun′dou (gōōn′dōō). An exostosis of the face; probably a sequela of yaws, involving the nasal and adjacent bones to produce a projecting, tumorlike mass. Also called *anakhre, big nose, henpue.*

gout [OF. *goute,* from L. *gutta,* drop]. A constitutional hereditary condition of uric acid metabolism, associated with a high blood level and a decreased urinary excretion of uric acid often with fever and leukocytosis. There are sudden attacks of acute, painful arthritis which may last a few days to a few weeks, recurring at irregular intervals with complete remission between attacks. Usually one joint is involved, the great toe being the part most commonly affected. The joint involved may be hot, red, and tender, and the surrounding skin is shiny. Repeated attacks may result in deformity. —**gout′y,** *adj.*

abarticular g. That in which structures other than the joints are involved.

atypical g. That marked by unusual symptoms, affecting unusual portions of the body.

calcium g. See pathologic *calcification* (c).

chalk g. Circumscribed calcinosis.

guanine g. Pathologic accumulations of guanine.

latent g. Hyperuricemia without gouty symptoms; sometimes recognized in the relatives of gouty people.

rheumatic g. Rheumatoid arthritis. *Obs.*

tophaceous g. A condition associated with deposits of sodium urate (tophi) in the skin over the cartilage of the ear and about the fingernails and in the cartilages of the joints.

Gowers, William Richard [*English neurologist,* 1845–1915]. Described retinal changes in Bright's disease (1876). Invented the hemoglobinometer (1878). Described a tract of ascending anterolateral fibers in the spinal cord (1880); called *Gowers' column* or *tract.* Gave a notable description of epilepsy (1881). With V. A. H. Horsley, was first to remove a tumor of the spinal cord successfully (1888). Described distal myopathy (1902), a form of progressive muscular atrophy, called *distal myopathy of Gowers. Gowers' sign,* seen in tabes dorsalis, is an irregular contraction of the pupil in response to light. Paroxysmal vasovagal attacks constitute *Gowers' syndrome.* See also Gowers' *phenomenon.*

gr. Grain(s).

Graaf, Reinier [Regnier] de [*Dutch anatomist,* 1641–73]. Studied digestion and the anatomy of the genital organs. The efferent ductules are known as the *graafian vessels.* See also *graafian follicle* under *follicle.*

graaf′i·an, Graaf′i·an follicle. See under *follicle;* see *liquor* folliculi. See also Reinier de *Graaf.*

Grace, Arthur William [*American dermatologist,* 1894–]. With Florence H. Suskind, developed a standardized mouse-brain antigen for use in a test for venereal lymphogranuloma.

grac′i·lis (grass′i·lis) [L., slender]. A long, slender muscle on the medial aspect of the thigh. See Table of Muscles in the Appendix.

gra·da′tim [L.]. Gradually.

Gradenigo, Giuseppe [*Italian otolaryngologist,* 1859–1926]. Described the syndrome of intense pain in the temporoparietal region, with paralysis of the lateral rectus muscle of the eye associated with otitis media and mastoiditis, as indicative of extradural abscess involving the apex of the petrous bone. Called *Gradenigo's sign, syndrome.* Author of a monograph on the auricular manifestations of hysteria (1901).

gra′di·ent [L. *gradi,* to step]. 1. The rate of increase of a variable magnitude or the curve which represents it. 2. *In biology,* a system of relations within the organism, or a part of it, which involves progressively increasing or decreasing differences in respect to rate of growth, rate of metabolism, or of any other structural or functional property of the cells.

ventricular g. *In electrocardiography,* a term introduced by F. N. Wilson to express the electric effects produced by local variations in the excitatory process of the heart; determined by measurement of the areas of the ventricular deflections of the ECG in two simultaneous limb leads, an expression of those electric forces which appear when the sequence of repolarization differs from the sequence of depolarization. Symbol, G, g, $\hat{G}$, $\hat{\hat{g}}$.

grad′u·ate [L. *gradus,* step]. A vessel, usually of glass, marked with lines at different levels; used for measuring liquids.

grad′u·a″ted [*gradus*]. Divided into units by a series of lines, as a barometer, a graduate, a thermometer.

Graefe, Alfred Karl [*German ophthalmologist,* 1830–99]. Made an important study of pathologic movements of the eye (1858).

Graefe, Carl Ferdinand von [*German surgeon,* 1787–1840]. Has been called the father of modern plastic surgery. Devised an operation for the repair of cleft palate. Introduced improvements in the technic of rhinoplasty and in that of Cesarean section.

Graefe, Friedrich Wilhelm Ernst Albrecht von [*German ophthalmologist,* 1828–70]. Introduced iridectomy for the treatment of glaucoma, iritis, and iridochoroiditis. Devised an operation for strabismus. Was among the first to point out that impairment of vision or blindness accompanying cerebral disorders usually is due to optic neuritis (1860). By improving the technic of linear extraction (1865), reduced eye loss in operations for cataract. Gave a classic description of sympathetic ophthalmia (1866), and an important account of the symptomatology of ocular paralysis (1867). Described keratoconus (1868). See also von Graefe's *sign.*

Graeser's method. See Friedemann and Graeser's *method.*

graft [OF. *greffe*, from G. *graphein*, to write]. A portion of tissue, such as skin, periosteum, bone, fascia, or, rarely, an entire organ, used to replace a defect in the body. See *autograft, flap, heterograft, homograft, implantation, implants, transplant, transplantation, zoograft.*

accordion g. A full-thickness graft in which multiple slits are made so that the graft may be stretched to cover a large area: also called *Dragstedt g.*

arterial g. See arterial *bridge.*

autogenous g. See *autograft.*

autoplastic g. See *autograft.*

bone g. One composed of osseous tissue; may be cortical, cancellous, or medullary; used to repair bone defects, to afford support, or to supply osteogenic tissue.

bridging g. One which connects the cut ends of arteries, bones, nerves, etc., where there is loss of substance and the divided ends cannot be approximated.

cable g. *In neurosurgery*, the placing together of several sections of nerve to be transplanted, to bridge a gap in a nerve larger than the sections available for the grafting.

cartilage g. Cartilage autograft or homograft, commonly used for replacing damaged or destroyed cartilage, or to replace bone loss.

chorioallantoic g. A graft of tissue onto the chorioallantoic membrane of the hen's egg, which furnishes a favorable environment for growth. Also used for culturing viruses for the preparation of vaccines.

corneal g. Corneal tissue, usually human, transplanted into a defective cornea to provide a clear window.

derma-fat-fascia g. A tissue graft employing full-thickness skin, fat, and fascia.

dermic g. A skin graft.

fascial g. A strip of fascia lata or aponeurosis; used either for the repair of a defect in muscle or fascia, or for suturing.

fat g. A portion of fat, implanted to fill a hollow and improve a contour.

free g. A graft of any type of tissue which is cut free and transplanted to another area.

full-thickness g. A skin graft including all layers of the skin: also called *Krause-Wolfe g.*

heterogenous g. A heterograft.

heteroplastic g. See *heterograft.*

homogenous g. See *homograft.*

homologous g. See *homograft.*

homoplastic g. See *homograft.*

ileal g. *In urology*, the use of a loop of ileum to replace a part of the genitourinary tract, usually a ureter.

implantation g. See *implantation*, 1.

inlay g. One placed beneath the tissue, as a bone graft placed in the medullary cavity of a bone, or an Esser inlay beneath the skin or mucous membrane.

intermediate split g. A graft consisting of the epidermis, papillary layer, and reticular layer of intermediate thickness: also called *Blair-Brown g.*

isograft. See *homograft.*

mucosal g. A graft of oral mucous membrane or of conjunctiva to repair a defect.

muscle g. A portion of muscle sutured in place, for checking hemorrhage where a bleeding vessel cannot be secured.

nerve g. A portion of a nerve sutured in place to restore the continuity of a severed nerve trunk where apposition cannot be secured.

Ollier g. Intermediate split-skin *g.*

omental g. A portion of omentum transplanted to fill a defect or to check a hemorrhage, or placed over an intestinal suture line to prevent adhesions.

onlay g. A bone graft which is laid on the surface of a bone where bone substance has been lost and where conditions are unsuited to inlay grafts. Onlay grafts are fixed in place by vitallium screws.

osteoperiosteal g. One of bone and periosteum.

ovarian g. A portion of ovary implanted anywhere except in its normal bed, usually in the abdominal wall, for the preservation of the hormone production.

pedicle g. See pedicle *flap.*

periosteal g. One consisting entirely of periosteum and used for minor bone defects to promote healing or union. See bone *g.*

pinch g. A small, full-thickness graft lifted from the donor area by a needle and cut free with a razor. Many such small deep grafts are fitted together to cover the defect. Also called *implant pinch g. Braun g.*

rope g. A tubed pedicled flap.

sieve g. A large skin graft, with openings throughout, corresponding to skin islands left on the donor area: also called *Douglas g.*

skin g. A portion of skin, of any size or thickness, cut from a donor area and transferred to the recipient site where repair is needed.

split g. A free graft of skin using less than full thickness, varying from the very thin epidermal graft (Thiersch *g.*) to the intermediate split-skin graft (Ollier *g.*) and the thick-split graft: also called *split-skin g., split-thickness g.*

surface g. A graft applied anywhere on the surface of the body where part of the skin is missing.

tendon g. One of tendon to bridge a gap in a tendon. Also see tendon *transplantation.*

testis g. The grafting by implantation of an entire testis or portion to replace one lost or destroyed, for the production of hormones.

Thiersch g. A thin epidermal split *g.*

tunnel g. A skin graft with the epithelial side inward, introduced into tissues under a contracted scar, etc. The tunnel is split later, and the epithelial surface becomes superficial or is left in place to replace a part, such as the urethra.

zooplastic g. A graft of tissue obtained from an animal.

Graham, Evarts Ambrose (1883–). American surgeon who with W. H. Cole, introduced cholecystography (1924), also called *Graham-Cole test.* With J. J. Singer he successfully removed an entire lung for carcinoma (1933).

Graham, Roscoe Reid [*Canadian surgeon*, 1890–1948]. Described an operation, called *Graham's operation*, for closure of a perforated gastric or duodenal ulcer. Sutures are placed at the top, middle, and bottom of the perforation, and an omental plug is then sutured over the area.

Graham, Sylvester [*American reformer*, 1794–1851]. Popularized bread made from unbolted flour, called *graham flour.* Whole-wheat bread is also called *graham bread.*

Graham, Thomas [*Scottish chemist*, 1805–69]. Studied diffusion of gases, osmotic force, and dialysis. *Graham's law* states that the rates of diffusion of any two gases are inversely proportional to the square roots of their densities.

Graham Steell murmur. See under *murmur.*

grain [OF. from L. *granum*, grain]. 1. The seed or seedlike fruit of the cereal grasses. 2. A minute portion or particle, as of sand, or of starch. 3. A unit of weight of the troy, the avoirdupois, and the apothecaries' systems of weights. Abbreviated, gr.

grains of paradise (*grana paradisi*). The seed of *Aframomum melegueta*, a reedlike herb of Western Africa. Its pungency is due to an oily substance called paradol which is chemically related to gingerol. Used as a flavor and as a carminative chiefly in veterinary medicine.

grain'age [*granum*]. Weight expressed in grains or fractions of grains.

Gram, Hans Christian Joachim [*Danish bacteriologist*, 1853–1938]. Introduced a method for staining bacteria. See Gram's *stain, Gram-Weigert staining method, Lugol's solution* under *stain*.

gram, gramme [F. *gramme*, from G. *gramma*, letter, a small weight]. The basic unit of mass, and of weight, in the metric system, and one of the fundamental units of physical measurement; corresponds almost exactly to the weight of a milliliter, or cubic centimeter, of water at the temperature of maximum density. Abbreviated Gm, Gm., gm, gm., g, g.

gram″i·ci′din (gram″i·sigh′din, gram″i·sid′in, gramiss′i·din). A potent germ-killing chemical obtained from cultures of soil bacilli. It appears to be antibacterial chiefly to Gram-positive organisms.

gram″i·ci′din S. A heat-stable antibiotic obtained from *Bacillus brevis* and reported to be more effective than gramicidin against Gram-negative organisms but not less toxic. Its clinical use for application to infected wounds and for other local therapy has been recommended.

gram ion. That weight of an ion, in grams, equivalent to its atomic weight or to the sum of the atomic weights of its constituent atoms.

gramme. See *gram*.

gram′-me·ter, gram-me′ter [*gramma;* G. *metron*, a measure]. A unit of work, equal to the energy used in raising one gram to a height of one meter.

gram′mole. See *gram-molecule*.

gram-mol′e·cule. That weight of any substance, in grams, equivalent to its molecular weight. Syn., *grammole, mol, mole*.

Gram′-neg′a·tive. Remaining unstained by the Gram method.

Gram′-pos′i·tive. Holding the dye after being stained by the Gram method.

gra′na. Minute disks of chlorophyll in the stroma of plants.

gra·na′tum [L., having many seeds, pomegranate]. Pomegranate. The bark of the stem and root of *Punica granatum;* contains several alkaloids, notably pelletierine, $C_8H_{15}ON$. The chief use of pomegranate and its preparations has been as a taeniacide. Pelletierine salts usually are used now instead of bark. See *pelletierine tannate*.

Grancher, Jacques Joseph [*French physician*, 1843–1907]. Described hepatization of the lung in pneumonia; called *the hepatization stage of pneumonia, Desnos' pneumonia, Grancher's pneumonia*. The boarding out of children from tuberculous households is known as *Grancher's system*.

gran′di·ose [It. *grandioso*]. *In psychiatry*, characterized by a feeling of being important, wealthy, or influential, when there is no true basis for such feeling.

grand″ mal′ (grahn″ mahl′. *See* NOTES § 35) [F.]. A complete epileptic seizure; see under *epilepsy*.

gran″o·plas′ma (gran″o·plaz′muh) [L. *granum*, grain; G. *plasma*, anything formed]. Granular cytoplasm.

gran′u·la. Granule.

gran′u·lar lids. Trachoma.

gran′u·la″ted lids. Lay term for chronic blepharitis.

gran″u·la′tion [L. *granulum*, a small grain]. 1. The tiny red granules which are grossly visible in the base of an ulcer; made up of loops of newly formed capillaries and fibroblasts. 2. The process of formation of granulation tissue in or around a focus of inflammation. 3. The formation of granules. —**gran′ulated,** *adj.*

arachnoidal granulations. Prolongations of the arachnoid layer of the cerebral meninges through the dura mater into the superior sagittal sinus and into the parasinoidal sinuses: also called *arachnoid villi, Pacchionian bodies*.

exuberant g. An excess of granulation tissue in the base of an ulcer or in a healing wound. Also called *fungous g., proud flesh*.

g. tissue. The mixture of newly formed capillaries and fibroblasts in connection with inflammation, especially of exudative character, representing the early stages of healing. Followed by a growth into exudate or destroyed tissue, the process becomes one of organization. As it progresses to cicatrization by atrophy of blood vessels and maturation of connective tissue, inflammatory foci are cicatrized, or such foci or foreign bodies are encapsulated; on surfaces, especially serous, fibrous adhesions are formed; wounds are healed. See Plate 40.

gran′ule [*granulum*]. 1. A minute particle or mass. 2. A small, intracellular particle, usually staining selectively. 3. A small pill. —**granular,** *adj.*

acidophil granules. Those staining with acid dyes, especially eosin, acid fuchsin, or orange G.

alpha granules. Those of the alpha cells of the hypophysis or of the pancreatic islets.

Altmann's granules. Old term for mitochondria.

amphophil granules. Those staining with both acid and basic dyes.

azurophilic granules. Fine granules, azure-staining with a stain containing methylene azure; they are frequently, but inconstantly, present in the cytoplasm of lymphocytes and monocytes.

basal granules. Blepharoplast.

basophil granules. Those staining with basic dyes, especially those of the methylene blue series, or hematoxylin.

beta granules. Those of the beta cells of the hypophysis or pancreatic islets.

brain-sand granules of pineal body. See *corpora arenacea* under *corpus*.

chromophil granules. Small granules of chromophil substance in nerve cells; also called *Nissl bodies*.

cone granules. Those of the outer nuclear layer of the retina, connected externally with the cones of the ninth layer, and internally by a thick process which becomes bulbous (the cone foot); they terminate in fine fibers in the outer molecular layer. They are the nuclei of the cone cells. *Obs.*

delta granules. Those of the delta cells of the pancreatic islets.

Ehrlich-Heinz granules. See *Heinz-Ehrlich bodies* under *body*.

eosinophil granules. Those staining selectively with eosin, erythrosin, and similar dyes.

gamma granules. Those of the chromophobe cells of the hypophysis.

interstitial granules. Those occurring in the sarcoplasm of muscle.

metachromatic granules. (a) Granules which take on a color different from that of the dye used to stain them. (b) Those in bacteria which stain differently from the surrounding cytoplasm. Also called *metachromatic bodies*.

Much's granules. See Hans Christian R. *Much*.

neutrophil granules. Granules which take up simultaneously both a basic and an acid dye, assuming a combination tint.

Nissl's granules. Chromophil bodies of nerve cells.

oxyphil granules. Those staining with acid dyes.

pigment g. One of the minute structureless masses of which pigment consists.

sulfur g. A characteristic mass of hyphae found in cases of actinomycosis.

tannophil granules. Cell granules which stain specifically by various methods after mordanting with tannin.

yolk granules. The elements composing the yolk.

zymogen granules. Secretion antecedent granules in gland cells, particularly those of the pancreatic acini and of the chief cells of the stomach, which are precursors of the enzyme secretion.

gran′u·li·form″, gran·u′li·form″ [*granulum;* L. *forma,* form]. Resembling small grains.

gran′u·lo·blast″ [*granulum;* G. *blastos,* germ]. See *myeloblast.*

gran′u·lo·cyte″ [*granulum;* G. *kytos,* cell]. A mature granular leukocyte; a polymorphonuclear leukocyte, either eosinophilic, basophilic, or neutrophilic. Also called *polymorph, polymorphonuclear, eosinophil, basophil, neutrophil.* —**granulocyt′ic,** *adj.*

gran″u·lo·cyt′ic se′ries. The cells concerned in the development of the granular leukocytes (*basophil, eosinophil,* or *neutrophil*) from the primitive myeloblasts to the adult segmented cells. Other terms applied to this series are *myeloid, myelogenous, myelocyte* or *myelocytic,* and *leukocyte* or *leukocytic.* See *myeloblast, promyelocyte, myelocyte, metamyelocyte; band cell* and *segmented cell* under *cell.*

gran″u·lo·cy″to·pe′ni·a. Agranulocytosis.

gran″u·lo·cy″to·poi·e′sis [*granulum; kytos;* G. *poiēsis,* production]. The process of development of the granular leukocytes, occurring normally in the bone marrow. —**granulocytopoiet′ic,** *adj.*

gran′u·lo·fil″ [*granulum;* L. *filum,* thread]. See *reticulocyte.*

gran″u·lo′ma [*granulum;* G. *-ōma,* tumor]. A focalized nodule of inflammatory tissue in which the process of granulation is significant. —**granulom′atous,** *adj.*

amebic g. A massive, usually focal, involvement of the colon by *Endamoeba histolytica,* resulting in a chronic proliferative inflammation that may be clinically confused with carcinoma: also called *ameboma.*

apical g. See dental *g.*

coccidioidal g. Progressive coccidioidomycosis.

dental g. Localized nodule of organizing and cicatrizing inflammation in the dental alveolus, at or near the apex of a tooth; often contains islands of epithelium (epithelial rests).

eosinophilic g. A disease principally of childhood characterized by one or more foci of destruction of bones, and possibly related to Hand-Schüller-Christian disease and Letterer-Siwe disease. The granuloma contains lipids, mononuclear cells, giant cells, and a variable number of eosinophils: also called *eosinophilic xanthomatous g.* Syn., *solitary granuloma.*

g. annulare. A chronic, self-limiting disease of the skin, usually on the extremities; characterized by reddish nodules, arranged in a circle.

g. contagiosa. See *g.* inguinale.

g. faciale. Eosinophilic granuloma of the face, consisting of well-defined soft, purplish, patches of skin. Histologically there is a granulomatous infiltration into the dermis only, which contains many eosinophils and which has been divided into an early leukocytic and a late fibrotic stage.

g. fissuratum. Discoid mucous membrane tumor indented by a deep fissure and located in the labioalveolar sulcus of the mouth. Acanthotic epidermis, proliferation of connective tissue in the skin, and polymorphonuclear leukocyte infiltration are seen histologically.

g. fungoides. See *mycosis* fungoides.

g. inguinale. A chronic, often serpigenous, destructive ulceration of the external genitalia due to a Gram-negative rod, *Donovania granulomatis,* and exhibiting encapsulated forms in infected tissue, called Donovan bodies: also called *g. contagiosa, g. genitoinguinale, g. pudenda tropicum.*

g. pendulum. A granuloma pyogenicum which hangs by a stalk.

g. pudenda tropicum. See *g.* inguinale.

g. pyogenicum. Growth of capillaries from larger parent vessels, which forms lobulations and produces a growth somewhat like hyperplastic granulation tissue. It occurs spontaneously beneath an intact epidermis or mucosa without known cause. Also called *g. telangiectaticum.* Syn., *capillary hemangioma of granuloma type.*

g. tropicum. The third stage of nodule formation in yaws.

g. venereum. See venereal *lymphogranuloma.*

Hodgkin's g. See Hodgkin's *disease.*

infectious g. A disease, due to a specific microorganism, which in some stage exhibits the formation of a granuloma, as tuberculosis, syphilis, or leprosy.

lipophagic g. A granuloma with loss of fat in the surrounding tissue.

malignant g. The type of granuloma found in Hodgkin's disease.

Miescher's g. A nodule, seen histologically, and composed of polymorphous histiocytes, leukocytes, and lymphocytes, found in the subcutis in erythema nodosum.

paracoccidioidal g. A chronic granulomatous disease of the skin and mucous membranes which may involve the lymph nodes and viscera; it is usually fatal. The etiologic agent is *Blastomyces brasiliensis.* Syn., *paracoccidioidomycosis, South American blastomycosis.*

silicous g. See talcum-powder *g.*

solitary g. See eosinophilic *g.*

talcum-powder g. A granulomatous reaction to the talcum powder frequently used in surgical rubber gloves. Syn., *surgical glove talc g., talc g., silicous g., pseudosilicoticum.*

gran″u·lo″ma·to′sis [*granulum; -ōma;* G. *-ōsis,* increase]. A disease characterized by multiple granulomas.

allergic g. A form of polyarteritis nodosa in which allergic manifestations predominate; severe asthma is frequent and eosinophilia in peripheral blood is marked. Histologically there appear, in addition to the usual lesions of polyarteritis nodosa, extravascular granulomas, consisting of foci of central necrosis surrounded by histiocytes and giant cells within areas of inflammation rich in eosinophils.

g. disciformis chronica progressiva. A skin disorder similar to necrobiosis lipoidica but without lipid deposits.

lipoid g. See Hand-Schüller-Christian *disease.*

reticuloendothelial g. A group of rare diseases characterized by generalized reticuloendothelial hyperplasia with or without intracellular lipid deposition. Included in this group are Letterer-Siwe's disease, Hand-Schüller-Christian disease, and eosinophilic granuloma. Also see lipoid storage *diseases.*

gran″u·lo·pe′ni·a. See *agranulocytosis.*

gran′u·lo·plasm″ [*granulum;* G. *plasma,* anything formed]. Old term for granular cytoplasm.

gran″u·lo·plas′tic [*granulum;* G. *plassein,* to form]. Forming granules.

gran″u·lo·poi·e′sis [*granulum;* G. *poiēsis,* production]. The formation of granulocytes. —**granulopoiet′ic,** *adj.*

gran′u·lose (gran′yoo·loce, ·loze) [*granulum*]. The

inner and soluble portion of starch-granules; β-amylose.

gran″u·lo′sis ru′bra na′si (gran″yoo·lo′sis roo′-bruh nay′sigh). A rare disease seen in undernourished children, affecting the nose, cheeks, and chin; characterized by a diffuse redness, persistent hyperhidrosis, and small, red papules.

gra′num. See *grain.*

Granville, Joseph Mortimer [*English physician,* 1833–1900]. Devised *Granville's hammer,* an instrument for vibratory massage, used in the treatment of neuralgia.

graph [G. *graphein,* to write]. A representation of statistical data by means of points, lines, surfaces, or solids, their position being determined by a system of coordinates.

graph″es·the′si·a [*graphein;* G. *aisthēsis,* feeling]. The sense or sensation of recognizing numbers, figures, or letters which are traced on the skin.

Grapheus. See *Grassi.*

graph′ite [*graphein*]. Plumbago, or black lead; an impure allotropic form of carbon.

graph′o- [*graphein*]. A combining form denoting *pertaining to writing.*

graph·ol′o·gy [*graphein;* G. *logos,* word]. The study of the handwriting; may be used in diagnosing nervous disorders.

graph″o·ma′ni·a [*graphein;* G. *mania,* madness]. An insane desire to write. —**graphomaniac,** *n.*

graph″o·mo′tor [*graphein;* L. *motor,* from *movere,* to move]. Relating to graphic movements or to the movements concerned in writing.

graph″o·pho′bi·a [*graphein;* G. *phobos,* fear]. A morbid fear of writing.

graph″or·rhe′a [*graphein;* G. *rhoia,* flow]. *In psychiatry,* an uncontrollable desire to write, in which pages are covered with usually unconnected and meaningless words; an intermittent condition, most often seen in manic patients.

Graser, Ernst [*German surgeon,* 1860–1929]. Described false diverticulum of the sigmoid colon (1899), called *Graser's diverticulum.*

Grasset law. See *Landouzy-Grasset law* under *Landouzy.*

Grassi, Benevenuto (Grapheus, Grassus) [*Palestinian physician in Italy,* twelfth century]. His book on diseases of the eye was considered the classic text in this field for five centuries. This was also the first book on ophthalmology to appear in print (1474).

grass sick′ness. A disease of horses occurring mainly in Scotland. It is most common in June when the grass is most luxuriant. The etiology is still in doubt, but the cause is thought to be a virus similar to that causing poliomyelitis in man.

grass tet′a·ny. Lay term for a disease of cows which overeat on green fodder; probably caused by magnesium deficiency.

gra·ti′o·la [NL. dim. from L. *gratia,* grace]. Hedge-hyssop; a diuretic, cathartic, and emetic.

Gratiolet, Louis Pierre [*French anatomist and zoologist,* 1815–65]. Described the visual projection from the lateral geniculate body to the calcarine cortex. Called *optic* or *occipitothalamic radiation, Gratiolet's optic radiation.*

grat·tage′ (gra·tahzh′) [F.]. Brushing, scrubbing, or scraping; a method sometimes used in treatment of trachoma. A hard brush, as a toothbrush, is used to scrub the conjunctival surface of the eyelid in order to remove the granulations.

Graunt, John [*English haberdasher,* 1620–74]. Pioneer medical statistician. His analysis of the *Bills of Mortality* which were published at that time by various London parishes, and which listed deaths from all causes, probably was the first study of its kind (1662).

Graux, Gaston [*French physician,* nineteenth century]. Described paralysis of the medial rectus muscle of one eye occurring with that of the lateral rectus muscle of the other eye. Called *Féréol-Graux ocular palsy.*

grav′el [OF. *gravele,* dim. of *greve,* sandy shore]. A granular, sandlike material forming the substance of urinary calculi and often passed with the urine.

Graves, Robert James [*Irish physician,* 1797–1853]. One of the founders of the Irish school of medicine. Gave the first satisfactory account of exophthalmic goiter (1835), called *Graves's disease, Basedow's disease, Flajani's disease, Parry's disease.* Said to have discarded the then universal custom of starving fever patients.

grav′id [L. *gravidus,* heavy with child]. Pregnant; heavy with child, as the gravid uterus. Used also of other than human females when carrying young or eggs. —**gravid′ity,** *n.*

gra′vi·da [*gravidus*]. A pregnant woman.

grav′i·din. Kyestein.

grav″i·do·car′di·ac [*gravidus;* G. *kardia,* heart]. Relating to cardiac disorders due to pregnancy.

gra·vim′e·ter [L. *gravis,* heavy; G. *metron,* a measure]. An instrument used in determining the specific gravity of a substance, especially a hydrometer, aerometer, or urinometer. —**gravimet′ric,** *adj.;* **gravimetry,** *n.*

grav″i·stat′ic [*gravis;* G. *statikos,* causing to stand]. Due to gravitation, as gravistatic congestion.

grav″i·ta′tion [L. *gravitas,* heaviness]. The force by which bodies are drawn together.

g. constant. See under *G,* 1.

grav′i·ty [*gravitas*]. The effect of the attraction of the earth upon matter.

specific g. The measured mass of a substance compared with that of an equal volume of another taken as a standard. For gases, hydrogen or air may be the standard; for liquids and solids, distilled water at a specified temperature. Abbreviated, sp. g., sp. gr.

Grawitz, Paul Albert (1850–1932). German pathologist who investigated and hypothesized the origin of hypernephroma (1884), also called *Grawitz's tumor,* and now generally classified as a *clear-cell carcinoma.* He also described minute granules, called *Grawitz's granules,* which stain with basic dyes, and are seen in red blood cells in certain pathologic conditions.

Gray's stain. See under *stain.*

grease. See *grease-heel.*

grease′-heel″. An infection of the fetlock joint of a horse; characterized by cracking of the skin and an oily exudate.

Greenberg's method. See under *method.*

green blind′ness. Aglaucopsia; a variety of color blindness in which green is not distinguished: also called *green sightedness.*

gref′fo·tome [OF. *greffe,* from G. *graphein,* to write; *tomos,* cutting]. A knife for cutting surgical grafts. *Obs.*

Greg″a·ri′na [L. *gregarius,* from *grex,* a herd]. A genus of Sporozoa, parasitic in insects.

greg′a·rine (greg′uh·ryne, ·rin) [*gregarius*]. Any member of the genus *Gregarina.* —**greg′a·rine,** *adj.*

acephalic gregarines. Sporozoa with a single unsegmented mass of cytoplasm.

cephaline gregarines. Sporozoa in which the body is divided into two portions: the anterior protomerite, and the posterior deutomerite. Also called *dicystid g.*

gre·ga′ri·ous·ness [*gregarius*]. The herd instinct.

Gregersen's test. See under *test.*

Gregory's powder. See compound *rhubarb* powder.

Greig, David Middleton [*Scottish physician,* 1864–

1936]. Said to have been the first to describe hypertelorism as an entity (1924); called *ocular hypertelorism, Greig's hypertelorism.*

Grenacher's stain. See *borax carmine* under *stain.*

Griesinger, Wilhelm [*German neurologist,* 1817–68]. Made important contributions to the knowledge of mental disease (1845). Was among the first to abandon harsh measures in the control of psychotic patients. Described pseudohypertrophic progressive muscular dystrophy (1865), later described by Duchenne and Erb; called *Duchenne-Griesinger disease, Erb's paralysis* or *dystrophy.* Gave the first report of infantile splenic anemia (1866). Ancylostomiasis was once called *Griesinger's disease.* See also Griesinger's *sign.*

grif'fin claw. Clawhand.

Griffith's method. See under *method.*

grin·de'li·a [after David Hieronymus *Grindel,* German botanist in Latvia, 1776–1836] (*grindelia*). The leaves and flowering tops of *Grindelia camporum, G. humilis,* or *G. squarrosa.* It contains considerable amorphous resin. It has been used in bronchitis and asthma as stimulating expectorant and antispasmodic.

g. fluidextract (*fluidextractum grindeliae*). Diluted with an equal volume of water it has been used locally in rhus poisoning.

grip, grippe [F. *grippe*]. Old term for influenza.

gripes [AS. *gripan*]. A lay term for colic.

gris'e·in. An antibiotic substance isolated from cultures of *Streptomyces griseus;* it is active, in vitro, against a variety of bacteria but several susceptible organisms show rapid development of resistant strains.

gris"e·o·ful'vin. An antibiotic substance, isolated from *Penicillium griseofulvum* and other species of *Penicillium;* it is active against a number of fungi and some bacterial species.

gris'ic ac'id. An antibiotic substance isolated from cultures of species of *Basidiomycetes.*

Grisolle, Augustin [*French physician,* 1811–69]. Described *Grisolle's sign:* since the early eruption of smallpox is papular, it is palpable even when the skin is tightly stretched, and thus can be distinguished by touch from the eruptions of other exanthemas.

Gritti, Rocco [*Italian surgeon,* 1828–1920]. Devised an operation for amputation above the knee (1857). He made long anterior and short posterior flaps, the patellar tendon being preserved and raised with the flap. The articular portion of the patella was removed, and the femur divided through the condyles to provide anchorage for the patella on the lower end of the femur. The operation was modified by William Stokes the younger, who divided the femur above the condyles in order to make a better anchorage for the patella (1870). Called *Gritti's operation, Gritti-Stokes amputation.*

Grocco's sign. See under *sign.*

Grocco's triangle. See paravertebral *triangle.*

groin [ME. *grynde*]. The depression between the abdomen and thigh. Also called *inguinal region.* See Plate 4.

Grollman, Arthur (1901–). American physiologist who investigated the physiology of the heart and determined the cardiac output of normal and diseased hearts by the acetylene method (indirect method of Fick).

groove [MD. *groeve*]. An elongated depression. Also see *sulcus, furrow.* —**grooved,** *adj.*

alveolingual g. One between the tongue and the lower jaw.

atrioventricular g. The coronary sulcus.

auriculoventricular g. See atrioventricular *g.*

bicipital g. The deep groove on the anterior surface of the humerus, separating the greater and lesser tuberosities and containing the long tendon of the biceps. Syn., *intertubercular g.*

branchial g. The external groove or furrow between two embryonic visceral arches, lined by ectoderm. Syn., *visceral g.*

carotid g. That lodging the cavernous sinus and the internal carotid artery; it lies lateral to the sella turcica, from the foramen lacerum to the medial side of the anterior clinoid process.

cavernous g. The carotid groove.

chiasmatic g. A groove between the optic foramens, anterior to the tuberculum sellae.

costal g. A deep furrow lying along the lower border and inner surface of a rib, for lodgment of the intercostal vessels and nerve.

digastric g. A groove on the medial surface of the mastoid process, which serves for the origin of the digastric muscle. Also called *mastoid notch.*

Harrison's g. See Edward *Harrison.*

infraorbital g. A groove in the middle of the floor of the orbit, lodging the infraorbital nerve and vessels.

interatrial g. That separating the atria of the heart.

intertubercular g. See bicipital *g.*

interventricular g. External, longitudinal groove indicating the beginning of separation of right and left ventricles in the developing heart.

labial g. A groove, developing in the labial lamina by disintegration of its central cells, which deepens to form the vestibule of the oral cavity.

lacrimal g. See nasolacrimal *g.*

laryngotracheal g. A gutterlike groove of the floor of the embryonic pharynx, which is the anlage of the respiratory system.

lateral phallic g. A groove on either side of the phallus, separating it from the labioscrotal swellings.

medullary g. See neural *g.*

musculospiral g. One on the posterior aspect of the humerus, which lodges the radial nerve, formerly called the musculospiral nerve, and the deep, brachial vessels. Also called *radial g.*

mylohyoid g. A groove running obliquely downward and forward on the medial surface of the ramus of the mandible, below the lingula mandibulae; it lodges the mylohyoid vessels and nerve.

nasal g. One between the nasomedian and maxillary process on either side along the course of a bucconasal membrane.

nasolacrimal g. The groove or furrow between the embryonic maxillary and lateral nasal processes, the epithelium of which is said to form part of the lacrimal duct.

nasomaxillary g. See nasolacrimal *g.*

nasopalatine g. That on the vomer lodging the nasopalatine nerve and vessels.

neural g. A longitudinal groove between the neural folds of the embryo before the neural tube is completed.

obturator g. The furrow at the superior border of the obturator foramen, lodging the obturator vessels and nerves.

occipital g. That medial to the digastric groove, lodging the occipital artery.

olfactory g. That formed by the cribriform plate of the ethmoid, lodging the olfactory bulb.

optic g. See chiasmatic *g.*

peroneal g. One on the lateral aspect of the calcaneus, lodging the tendon of the peroneus longus.

pharyngeal g. See branchial *g.*

primitive g. The longitudinal groove in the primitive streak between the primitive folds.

pterygopalatine g. (a) One in the ventral aspect of the pterygoid process of the sphenoid. (b) A furrow on the vertical part of the palatine bone.

radial g. See musculospiral *g.*

rhombic g. One of the seven transverse furrows between the neuromeres of the rhombencephalon.

Schmorl's grooves. Those resulting from emphysematous inflation of those portions of the lungs which lie between the ribs.

sigmoid g. See sigmoid *sulcus.*

sphenobasilar g. The depression on the body of the sphenoid bone and the basilar portion of the occipital bone, upon which the pons rests. The sphenoid part is called the clivus. Also called *spheno-occipital g.*

subcostal g. See costal *g.*

tracheobronchial g. See laryngotracheal *g.*

urethral g. A groove on the caudal surface of the genital tubercle or phallus, bounded by the urethral folds and urethral membrane. Also called *urogenital g., genital fossa.*

urogenital g. See urethral *g.*

ventricular grooves. Two furrows, one on the anterior, one on the posterior surface of the heart; they indicate the interventricular septum.

vertebral g. That formed by the laminas of the vertebrae and the sides of the spinous processes; it lodges the deep muscles of the back.

visceral g. See branchial *g.*

Gross, Robert Edward [*American surgeon,* 1905–]. With John Perry Hubbard, reported an operation for patent ductus arteriosus. Transpleural ligation was performed by exposing the heart, entering the mediastinal pleura, and isolating the ductus, which was tied with a double silk ligature but left undivided.

Gross, Samuel David [*American surgeon,* 1805–84]. One of the outstanding surgeons of his time. Studied the character and treatment of intestinal wounds (1843). Formulated principles of treatment for foreign bodies in respiratory passages (1854).

Gross, Samuel Weissel [*American surgeon,* 1837–89]. Devised a urethrotome with which a stricture is divided from behind forward in internal urethrotomy.

ground sub'stance. The fluid, semifluid, or solid material, in the connective tissues, cartilage, and bone, which fills in part or all of the space between the cells and fibers. Syn., *matrix,* in the strict sense, see *matrix,* 3; *interstitial substance.*

group'ing. See *blood* groups.

growth [AS. *grōwan*]. 1. The increase in the amount of actively metabolic protoplasm, accompanied by an increase in cell number, or cell size, or both. In a broader sense, growth is the increase in the size of the organism or its parts, measured as an increase in weight, volume, or linear dimensions. See Plates 23, 24. 2. Any abnormal, localized increase in cells, such as a tumor, a neoplasm.

growth hor'mone. See under *hormone.*

Gruber, Josef [*Austrian otologist,* 1827–1900]. Invented an ear speculum, called *Gruber's speculum.* Devised *Gruber's test* of the hearing: when the sound of a tuning fork held near the ear becomes inaudible, a finger is inserted in the ear and the tuning fork is placed in contact with the finger; the sound should again become audible to the subject.

Gruber, Max von [*German bacteriologist,* 1853–1927]. With Durham, discovered specific agglutination (1896), the basis of the Widal test for typhoid. See under *test.* Also called *Gruber's reaction, Gruber-Durham* or *Gruber-Widal reaction.*

Gruber, Wenzel Leopold [*Bohemian anatomist in Russia,* 1814–90]. Described internal mesogastric hernia (1863), called *Gruber's hernia.* See *muscle* of Gruber.

Grübler stain. See panchrome *stain.*

Gruby, David [*French dermatologist,* 1810–98]. Described the fungi of favus as causative agents of the disease (1841). Gave the first description of *Trichophyton ectothrix* (1842). Discovered *Candida albicans* in thrush (1842). Described *Microsporum audouini* (1843) and discovered *Trichophyton tonsurans* (1844); tinea capitis is called *Gruby's disease.* Discovered trypanosomes in the frog (1843) and applied the name to Protozoa.

grume [L. *grumus,* a little heap]. A clot, as of blood; a thick and viscid fluid. —**gru'mous,** *adj.*

Grünfelder's reflex. See under *reflex.*

Grünwald stain. See May-Grünwald *stain.*

gru'tum. See *milium.*

Grynfeltt, Joseph Casimir [*French surgeon,* 1840–1913]. Described the triangular space through which lumbar hernia may occur. It is bounded above by the twelfth rib and lower border of the serratus posterior inferior, behind by the quadratus lumborum, and anteriorly by the posterior border of the internal oblique. Called *Grynfeltt's triangle.*

gry'o·chrome [G. *gry,* morsel; *chrōma,* color]. Old term for a nerve cell with a large amount of cytoplasm in which the chromophil substance tends to form threads.

gry·po'sis (grye·po'sis, gri·po'sis) [G. *grypōsis,* a crooking]. Curvature; especially abnormal curvature of the nails.

g stress. Structural and functional stress on the body of aviators who experience rapid changes in velocity and direction of flight.

G sub'stance. See under *substance.*

g suit. See *anti-g suit.*

gt. *Gutta,* drop.

gtt. *Guttae,* drops.

guac'e·tin (gwass'i·tin). See *guaiacetin.*

gua"cha·ma'ca (gwah"chuh·mah'kuh, gwah"chah-mah·kah') [Sp., from Cumanagoto *uatchamaca*]. The bark of the *Malouetia nitida* (Apocynaceae), used as a source of a type of curare.

gua'cin (gwah'sin, gway'sin, gwaw'sin) [Sp. *guaco,* prob. of Taino origin]. A bitter resin from guaco; it is diaphoretic, stimulant, and emetic.

gua'co (gwah'ko) [Sp.]. The plants *Mikania guaco* and other species of *Mikania* and *Aristolochia;* used in South America for snake-bites; formerly also used as an antirheumatic, antisyphilitic, and anthelmintic.

guai'ac (gwy'ack) [NL. *guaiacum,* from Taino *guayacan*] (*guaiacum*). The resin of the wood of *Guajacum officinale* or of *G. sanctum.* It contains guaiaconic acid, guaiaretic acid, guaiac yellow, guaiacene, guaiacol, and pyroguaiacin. It has been used in treatment of syphilis, chronic rheumatism, and gout.

ammoniated g. tincture (*tinctura guaiaci ammoniata*). A solution of the resin in aromatic ammonia spirit. Dose, 2–8 cc. (½–2 dr.).

g. tincture (*tinctura guaiaci*). A solution of the resin in alcohol. Dose, 2–8 cc. (½–2 dr.).

g. yellow. A coloring matter present in guaiac.

guai'a·cene (gwy'uh·seen). C_5H_8O. An oily, crystallizable liquid obtained from guaiac resin by dry distillation.

guai·ac'e·tin (gwye·ass'i·tin, gwye"uh·see'tin). Pyrocatechin monoacetate, $C_6H_4OH.OCH_2$-COOH. It was formerly used like guaiacol, in the treatment of tuberculosis.

guai'a·col (*guaiacol*). A liquid consisting principally of $C_6H_4(OH)(OCH_3)$ 1:2, usually obtained from wood creosote; or a solid, consisting almost entirely of $C_6H_4(OH)(OCH_3)$ 1:2, usually prepared synthetically. It is used internally chiefly as a stimulating expectorant in pulmonary tuberculosis and bronchitis; externally, it is employed for its anesthetic and antiseptic effects. Dose, 0.3–0.6 cc. (5–10 min.).

g. benzoate. $C_6H_5COO.C_6H_4.OCH_3$. A crystalline compound, almost insoluble in water, employed in pulmonary tuberculosis, cystitis, and as an intestinal antiseptic. Dose, 0.3–0.6 Gm. (5–10 gr.). See *benzosol.*

g. cacodylate. $C_6H_4(OH)(OCH_3)(CH_3)_2.AsO.OH$. A reddish white, crystalline mass; an oil solution of it has been employed hypodermically in tuberculosis.

g. carbonate (*guaiacolis carbonas*). $CO(OC_6H_4.OCH_3)_2$. Occurs in crystals which are insoluble in water; it is used as an expectorant, less irritant than guaiacol but also less effective. Dose, 0.6–1.2 Gm. (10–20 gr.). See *duotal.*

g. glyceryl ether. $CH_3O.C_6H_4.OC_3H_5(OH)_2$; a white, crystalline powder, soluble in 20 parts of water; it is used internally as an intestinal antiseptic and an expectorant; externally, it is applied as an ointment in rheumatism. Dose, 0.3–1.0 Gm. (5–20 gr.). Also called *glyceryl guaiacolate.* See *guaiamar, resyl.*

g. phosphate. $(C_6H_4.O.CH_3.O)_3PO$. A white, crystalline powder, insoluble in water; it has the therapeutic effects of guaiacol but is less effective.

g. salicylate. $C_6H_4.O.CH_3C_7H_5O_3$. A crystalline substance; it has been used in pulmonary tuberculosis and as an intestinal antiseptic.

guai″a·con′ic ac′id. $C_{20}H_{24}O_5$. An acid from guaiac.

guaiamar. A trade name for guaiacol glyceryl ester.

guai″a·ret′ic ac′id. $C_{20}H_{26}O_4$. An acid from guaiac.

gua′nase (gwah′nace, ·naze, gwan′ace, ·aze). An enzyme found in the pancreas, thymus, and adrenals; it converts guanine into xanthine.

guanatol hydrochloride. A trade-mark for chloroguanide hydrochloride.

gua·na·zo′lo. 5-Amino-7-hydroxy-1H-*v*-triazolo(*d*)-pyrimidine, a compound which inhibits certain types of tumor growth in experimental animals.

guan′i·dine (gwan′i·deen, ·din, gwah′ni·). Aminomethanamidine, $NH:C(NH_2)_2$, a normal product of protein metabolism found in the urine. It has been employed medicinally but appears to have injurious effects on the liver. Syn., *carbamidine, iminourea.* See Table of Normal Values of Blood Constituents in the Appendix.

g.-acetic acid. Glycocyamine.

guan″i·di·no·a·ce′tic ac′id. Glycocyamine.

gua′nine (gwah′neen, ·nin, gōō′uh·neen, ·nin, gwan′in, gōō·an′in). $C_5H_5N_5O$; 2-amino-6-oxypurine or 2-aminohypoxanthine; a nitrogenous base of the class of purines, being a component of ribonucleic and desoxyribonucleic acids; it is found in various tissues and in excreta.

gua′no (gwah′no) [Sp., from Quechua *huanu*, dung]. The excrement of sea fowl found on certain islands in the Pacific Ocean. It contains guanine and various other nitrogen bases, alkaline urates, and phosphates; was used externally in certain skin diseases.

gua′no·sine. $C_{10}H_{13}N_5O_5$; guanine riboside; a nucleoside containing guanine and ribose, occurring in plant and animal tissues. Syn., *vernine.*

gua·nyl′ic ac′id (gwa·nil′ick). A nucleotide obtained by the hydrolysis of nucleic acid. Contains guanine, a pentose sugar, and phosphoric acid.

gua″ra·na′ (gwah″rah·nah′, gwah·rah′nah) [Sp. and Pg., from Tupi]. A dried paste prepared from the seeds of *Paullinia cupana,* found in Brazil. It contains 4% of caffeine. It is astringent and stimulant.

gua·ra′nine (gwah·rah′neen, ·nin, gwah′ruh·). An alkaloid derived from guarana; at one time thought to be different from caffeine, but later shown to be identical with it.

guard [OF. *guarder*]. An appliance placed on a knife to prevent too deep an incision.

guar gum. The ground endosperms of *Cyanopsis tetragonolaba,* cultured in India as a livestock feed; it occurs as a light-gray powder, about 85% of which is soluble in water and consists of galactose and mannose. The gum is used, like starch, as a tablet-disintegrating material and to prepare mucilages.

Guarnieri, Giuseppe [*Italian pathologist,* 1856–1918]. Described the inclusion bodies observed in the lesions of vaccinia and smallpox; called *Guarnieri's bodies.*

gua′za (gwah′zuh, gwaz′uh). See *cannabis.*

gu″ber·nac′u·lum [L., helm, rudder]. A guiding structure.

chorda g. See under *chorda.*

g. dentis. A bundle of fibrous tissue connecting the tooth sac of a permanent tooth with the gum.

g. testis. A fibrous cord extending from the fetal testis to the scrotal swellings; it occupies the potential inguinal canal and guides the testis in its descent. See *chorda* gubernaculum.

Gubler, Adolphe (**Goblet**) [*French physician,* 1821–79]. Described alternate hemiplegia (1856), called *Gubler's paralysis, Weber-Gubler syndrome, Millard-Gubler paralysis* or *syndrome.* See under *Millard.*

Gudden, Bernhard Aloys von (1824–86). German neurologist who made important studies of the thalamus. He is known for his studies on the partial decussation of optic paths and his description of a commissure joining the medial geniculate bodies at the posterior portion of the optic chiasma; called *Gudden's commissure.* Drew attention to thalamic degeneration occurring when certain areas of the cerebral cortex are destroyed. This is a retrograde process involving the cells of specific thalamic nuclei after interruption of their axons, called *Gudden's atrophy.* He also observed that lesions of the cerebral cortex do not cause atrophy of the peripheral nerves; this is called *Gudden's law.*

Gudernatsch's test. See under *test.*

Guéneau de Mussy, Noël François Odon [*French physician,* 1813–85]. Described a point of referred pain accompanied by tenderness and hyperesthesia at the intersection of a downward extension of the sternal border and a line drawn through the tenth rib. Occurs in diaphragmatic pleurisy. Called *de Mussy's point, Guéneau de Mussy's point.*

Guenther von Andernach, Johann (**Guinterius Andernacus**) [*German physician,* 1487–1574]. The Wormian bones are sometimes called *Andernach's ossicles.*

Guérin, Alphonse François Marie [*French surgeon,* 1816–95]. Described the valve of the navicular fossa; see under *valve.* Called *Guérin's valve* or *fold. Guérin's sinus* is a diverticulum found behind the valve.

Guerreiro reaction. See Machado-Guerreiro *reaction.*

Guidi, Guido (**Vidus Vidius**) [*Italian physician and anatomist,* d. 1569]. Described the internal maxillary artery (1611), called the *Vidian artery.* The pterygoid canal is called the *Vidian canal,* and the nerve which passes through it is called the *Vidian nerve.*

Guillain, Georges [*French neurologist,* 1876–   ]. Described a diffuse, infectious disease of the nervous system. See Guillain-Barré *syndrome.*

guil′lo·tine (ghil′o·teen) [after Joseph Ignace *Guillotin,* French physician, 1738–1814]. A surgical instrument for excision of the tonsils or growths in the larynx. *Obs.*

guin'ea pig. A prolific rodent of the genus *Cavia*, of South American origin; widely domesticated and used experimentally in bacteriology and genetics.

Guin'ea worm. See *Dracunculus medinensis*.

Guin'ea worm in·fec'tion. See *dracunculosis*.

Guinterius Andernacus. See *G. von Andernach*.

guipsine. A proprietary preparation of mistletoe (*Viscum album*) for reducing hypertension.

Guist, Gustav [*German ophthalmologist*, contemporary]. Described his operation for detachment of the retina, in which he employed multiple trephining and chemical cauterization of the choroid (1931).

Guldberg-Waage law. See *law* of mass action.

Gull, William Withey [*English physician*, 1816–90]. One of the first to recognize the cause of myxedema; atrophy of the thyroid gland with myxedema is called *Gull's disease*. With H. G. Sutton, described arteriocapillary fibrosis; generalized arteriosclerosis has come to be known as *Gull and Sutton's disease*. The *Gull-Toynbee law* states that when otitis media extends to the brain, mastoiditis usually affects the cerebellum and the lateral sinuses, whereas inflammation of the tympanic roof usually affects the cerebrum.

gul'let. See *esophagus*.

Gullstrand, Allvar [*Swedish ophthalmologist*, 1862–1930]. Made an important study of dioptrics. Discovered the intracapsular mechanism of accommodation (1911). Introduced *Gullstrand's slit lamp*. Nobel laureate (1911). *Gullstrand's law* states that, when a patient turns his head while focusing his eyes on a distant object, if the reflected image on the cornea moves in the direction in which the head turns, this is always toward the weaker muscle.

gu·lon'ic ac'id. A sugar acid, $C_6H_{12}O_7$, representing gulose in which the CHO group has been oxidized to COOH; the acid occurs in D- and L- forms, corresponding to D- and L-gulose.

gu'lose. An aldohexose, $C_6H_{12}O_6$, synthetically produced; it occurs in D- and L- forms.

gum [AS. *gōma*, palate]. The mucous membrane and underlying connective tissue covering the alveolar processes and the necks of erupted teeth; the gingiva.

raspberry red gums. Inflamed tissue of a raspberry red color; occurs in one type of pregnancy gingivitis.

receding gums. See alveolar *pyorrhea*.

spongy g. Hyperplastic gingival tissue, associated with inflammation and other gingival swelling.

gum [L. *gummi*, G. *kommi*, gum, from the Egyptian]. A concrete vegetable juice exuded from many plants, insoluble in alcohol or ether, but swelling or dissolving in water into a viscid mass. The gums consist of glycosidal hexose-uronic acids, partly or wholly combined with calcium, potassium, or magnesium.

acacia g. Gum arabic. See *acacia*.

British g. Dextrin.

g. arabic. See *acacia*.

g. benjamin. See *benzoin*.

g. resin. A concrete vegetable juice insoluble in water, but soluble in organic solvents.

g. tragacanth. See *tragacanth*.

gum'boil". See alveolar *abscess*.

gum'ma [*gummi*]. The specific lesion of tertiary or late syphilis, which may occur in almost any tissue but is observed particularly in the brain, liver, and heart. Grossly, it is a well-defined mass a few millimeters to a centimeter or more in diameter, with a tendency to encapsulation and surrounding fibrosis, and with a gelatinous, hyalinized, necrotic center which has the elastic consistency of firm rubber or gum. Microscopically, the necrotic mass is surrounded by lymphocytes, epithelioid cells, and a few Langhans' giant cells. —**gummatous,** *adj*.

miliary g. A localized lesion of late syphilis differing from the usual gumma in its small size.

gum'mic ac'id. Arabin.

gun'cot"ton. See *pyroxylin*.

gun'jah. See *cannabis*.

Gunn, Robert Marcus [*English ophthalmologist*, 1850–1909]. Described the brilliant white dots seen with the ophthalmoscope above the macula lutea; called *Gunn's dots*. Described an anomalous, congenital maldistribution of cranial motor fibers causing ptosis of the upper eyelid, which can be activated only by an associated movement of the jaw; called *Gunn's syndrome*.

Gunning, Jan Willem [*Dutch chemist*, 1827–1901]. With C. Arnold, made an important modification of the Kjeldahl method for determining total nitrogen. See Arnold and Gunning's *method*.

Gunning, Thomas Brian [*American dentist*, 1813–89]. Invented an apparatus employed in caring for fractured jaws. *Gunning's splint* is made in one solid piece, resembling a double dental plate, with a frontal aperture for feeding purposes.

gur'ney, guer'ney. A stretcher with wheels for transporting a recumbent patient. Sometimes spelled *girney*.

Gurvich radiation. See mitogenetic *radiation*.

gus·ta'tion [L. *gustatio*, from *gustare*, to taste]. The sense of taste; the act of tasting.

gus'ta·to"ry [*gustare*]. Pertaining to the sense of taste.

gut [AS. plural *guttas*]. 1. The intestine. 2. The embryonic digestive tube, consisting of *foregut*, *midgut*, and *hindgut*. 3. Short term for catgut. Also see *suture*.

blind g. The cecum.

head-g. See *foregut*.

postanal g. A transient part of the hindgut caudal to the cloaca.

primary g. See *archenteron*.

primitive g. See *archenteron*.

tail g. See postanal *g*.

gut'ta (pl. *guttae*) [L.]. A drop. Abbreviated, gt.

gut'tae (gut'ee). Plural of gutta. Abbreviated, gtt.

gut'ta-per'cha. The latex of various trees of the family Sapotaceae. It is essentially a polymerized hydrocarbon of the general formula $(C_5H_8)_n$ with other resinous substances. Used to make splints, as a wound dressing, as an insulator, etc.

gut'tate [L. *gutta*, drop]. *In biology*, spotted as if by drops of something colored; resembling a drop.

gut·ta'tim [L.]. Drop by drop.

gut'ter [OF. *goutiere*, from L. *gutta*, drop]. A shallow groove.

gut'ter. To shape bone to eliminate dead spaces in the operation for chronic osteomyelitis. Syn., *saucerize*.

hepatic g. The anlage of the liver and gallbladder. See hepatic *diverticulum*.

gut'ti·form [*gutta*; L. *forma*, form]. Drop-shaped.

Guttmann, Paul [*German physician*, 1834–93]. Described a sign in exophthalmic goiter. *Guttmann's sign* is a thrill or bruit heard with a stethoscope over the thyroid.

gut"tu·ro·tet'a·ny [L. *guttur*, throat; G. *tetanos*, convulsive tension]. A stammering due to tetanoid spasm of the laryngeal muscles.

Gutzeit's test. See under *test*.

gu·va'cine (gew·vay'seen, ·sin, guh·vay'·, gew'·vuh·). Tetrahydronicotinic acid, $C_6H_9NO_2$. An alkaloid from seeds of *Areca catechu*, the areca nut or betelnut. Has been used as an anthelmintic but is stated to be inactive.

Guy de Chauliac [*French surgeon*, ca. 1300–ca.

1368]. His book covering the surgical practices of his time was the standard authority until the time of Paré.

Guy's method. See Leake and Guy's *method.*

Gwathmey, James Tayloe [*American surgeon,* 1863–1944]. Devised a method of producing general anesthesia by a rectal injection of liquid ether with olive oil or liquid petrolatum. Called *synergistic anesthesia, Gwathmey's method.*

gym·nas'tics [G. *gymnazein,* to exercise]. Systematic exercise for restoring or maintaining bodily health. —**gymnastic,** *adj.*

medical g. Systematic muscular movements designed to bring an ailing or feeble part back to normal.

ocular g. Regular muscular exercise of the eye by the use of prisms or other means to overcome muscular insufficiency.

Swedish g. A system of movements made by the patient against the resistance of an attendant.

gym·ne'mic ac'id (jim·nee'mick, ·nem'ick). $C_{32}H_{55}O_{12}$. A substance obtained from the leaves of *Gymnema sylvestre,* said to obtund certain taste sensations temporarily.

gym"no·pho'bi·a [G. *gymnos,* naked; *phobos,* fear]. A morbid fear of a naked person or a naked part of the body.

gym'no·spore [*gymnos;* G. *spora,* seed]. *In biology,* a naked spore.

gyn'ae- (jin'i-, jy'ni-). For words beginning with *gynae-,* see *gyne-.*

gy·nan'der (ji·nan'dur, jye·nan'dur) [G. *gynē,* woman; *anēr,* man]. A pseudohermaphrodite.

gy·nan'dri·a (ji·nan'dree·uh, jye·nan'dree·uh). See *gynandry.*

gy·nan'drism [*gynē; anēr*]. See feminine *pseudohermaphroditism.*

gy·nan"dro·blas·to'ma. A rare ovarian tumor, histologically characterized by elements resembling arrhenoblastoma and granulosa-cell tumor. Clinically, masculinizing effects are said to dominate, but excessive estrogen-induced bleeding has also been reported.

gy·nan'dro·morph [*gynē; anēr;* G. *morphē,* form]. A sex mosaic in which certain areas of the organism have male characters and others female characters due to genetic differences in the cells.

gy·nan"dro·mor'phism [*gynē; anēr; morphē*]. An abnormality in which the individual contains both genetically male and genetically female tissue.

gy·nan'dro·mor"phy [G. *gynē,* woman; *anēr,* man; *morphē,* form]. Bisexuality. In the *somatotype,* the degree or prominence of feminine characteristics in a male physique, or vice versa, expressed numerically as the *g-component.*

gy·nan'drous [*gynē; anēr*]. *In biology,* having the stamens and pistils more or less united.

gy·nan'dry, gy·nan'dri·a [*gynē; anēr*]. Feminine pseudohermaphroditism. —**gynandroid,** *adj., n.*

gy·nan'thro·pus [*gynē;* G. *anthrōpos,* man]. A gynander. See *pseudohermaphroditismus femininus. Obs.*

gyn"a·tre'si·a (jin"uh·tree'zhuh, ·zee·uh, ·shuh, ·see·uh) [*gynē;* G. *a-,* not; *trēsis,* perforation]. Imperforate condition of the vagina or, less commonly, of other areas of the female genital system; often, occlusion of any portion of the female genital system.

gy·ne'cic, gy·nae'cic (ji·nee'sick, ·ness'ick, jye·) [*gynē*]. Relating to women or the female sex.

gyn"e·co·gen'ic (jin"i·ko·jen'ick, guy"ni·ko·) [*gynē;* G. *genesthai,* from *gignesthai,* to be produced]. Causing or producing female characteristics; estrogenic.

gyn"e·cog'ra·phy. A roentgenologic method of visualization of the female internal genitalia by means of the injection of air or carbon dioxide intraperitoneally. The pelvic organs can then be visualized on the x-ray plate by contrast shadows.

combined g. Gynecography plus the injection of a contrast medium into the uterus and oviducts (hysterosalpingography).

gyn'e·coid (jin'i·koyd, jy'ni·, jin"i·koyd') [*gynē;* G. *eidos,* form]. Pertaining to or like a woman.

gyn"e·col'o·gist (jin"i·kol'o·jist, guy"ni·, jy"ni·) [*gynē;* G. *logos,* word]. One who practices gynecology.

gyn"e·col'o·gy (jin"i·kol'o·jee, guy"ni·, jy"ni·) [*gynē; logos*]. The science of the diseases of women, especially those affecting the sexual organs. —**gynecolog'ic, gynecolog'ical,** *adj.*

gyn"e·co·ma'ni·a (jin"i·ko·may'nee·uh, guy"ni·ko·, jy"ni·ko·) [*gynē;* G. *mania,* madness]. Satyriasis.

gyn"e·co·mas'ti·a [*gynē;* G. *mastos,* breast]. Enlargement of the mammary gland in the male, more frequently unilateral. Microscopically, there is multiplication of ducts and proliferation of lining epithelium; increase in amount of supporting connective tissue; infiltration of lymphocytes, plasma cells, large mononuclear cells, and, sometimes, polymorphonuclear leukocytes and eosinophils. The condition may accompany outspoken endocrine disorders, especially of the adrenals and of the testes, and neoplasms such as choriocarcinoma; may follow administration of estrogenic substances; or may have no apparent cause, appearing often in adolescence. **Anisogynecomastia** is unequal enlargement of the breasts. **Pseudogynecomastia** is enlargement of the breasts due to deposition of adipose tissue. Also called *gynecomazia, gynecomasty.*

gyn"e·cop'a·thy (jin"i·kop'uth·ee, guy"ni·, jy"ni·) [*gynē;* G. *pathos,* disease]. Any disease of, or peculiar to, women.

gyn"e·pho'bi·a (jin"i·fo'bee·uh, jy"ni·) [*gynē;* G. *phobos,* fear]. Morbid fear of the society of women.

gyn"e·phor'ic [*gynē;* G. *phoros,* bearing]. Pertaining to a mode of inheritance in which phenotypically normal heterozygous women transmit the recessive gene to some of their sons, as in sex-linked recessive characters (e.g., hemophilia).

gynergen. Trade-mark for ergotamine tartrate.

gyn"i·at'rics (jin"ee·at'ricks, ·ay'tricks, jy"nee·) [*gynē;* G. *iatrikos,* healing]. Treatment of the diseases of women.

gyn'o- (jin'o-, jy'no-), **gyn-** [*gynē*]. 1. A combining form denoting *woman.* 2. *In botany and medicine,* a combining form denoting *a female reproductive organ.*

gyn"o·car'dic ac'id. An acid from the oil of *Gynocardia odorata;* formerly used as an antisyphilitic and antirheumatic.

gyn"o·gam'one. A gamone present in an ovum.

gyn"o·gen'e·sis [*gynē;* G. *genesis,* production]. Development of the egg without the participation of the sperm nucleus, but after penetration of the egg by the sperm.

gyn·og'ra·phy. Contraction of *gynecography.*

gyn'o·plas·ty, gyn"o·plas'ty [*gynē;* G. *plassein,* to form]. Plastic surgery of the female genitals. —**gynoplas'tic,** *adj.*

gyp'sum. $CaSO_4.2H_2O$. Native calcium sulfate. Deprived of the major portion of its water of crystallization, it constitutes plaster of Paris.

gy·ra'tion (jye·ray'shun) [G. *gyros,* circle]. 1. A turning in a circle. 2. Old term for arrangement of gyri in the cerebral hemisphere. —**gy'rate,** *adj.*

Gy·rau'lus [*gyros*]. A genus of fresh-water snails.

G. saigonensis. A species of China and Formosa which serves as the intermediate host of the oriental fluke, ***Fasciolopsis buski.***

gyre. See *gyrus. Obs.*

gy·rec′to·my. The surgical excision of any gyrus of the brain.

frontal g. Surgical excision of a block of cortex, bilaterally, from the frontal lobes of the brain, as a treatment for certain mental illnesses: also called *bilateral subtotal ablation of frontal cortex.*

gyr″en·ceph′a·late (jirr″en·sef′uh·late, jy″ren·) [*gyros;* G. *egkephalos,* brain]. Having the surface of the brain convoluted.

gyr″en·ce·phal′ic. See *gyrencephalate.*

gyr″en·ceph′a·lous. See *gyrencephalate.*

gy′ro·mele [*gyros;* G. *melē,* a sort of cup]. A probe with a rotating center, fitted with various attachments for treating the stomach. *Obs.*

gy′rose [*gyros*]. Marked with curved or undulating lines.

gy′ro·spasm. See *spasmus nutans.*

gy′rus (pl. *gyri*) [L., from *gyros*]. A convolution on the surface of the cerebral hemisphere. See Plate 18. —**gyral,** *adj.*

angular g. A cerebral convolution which forms the posterior portion of the inferior parietal lobule and arches over the posterior end of the superior temporal sulcus.

annectant g. Any one of many short bridges of gray substance which may connect two neighboring gyri across the intervening fissure.

anterior central g. See ascending frontal *g.*

ascending frontal g. The cerebral convolution which lies between the precentral sulcus and the central sulcus and extends from the superomedial border of the hemisphere to the posterior ramus of the lateral fissure. Syn., *g. centralis anterior, precentral g., anterior central g.* See Plate 18.

ascending parietal g. The cerebral convolution which lies immediately posterior to the central sulcus and extends from the longitudinal fissure above to the posterior ramus of the lateral fissure below. Syn., *posterior central g., postcentral g., g. centralis posterior.* See Plate 18.

callosal g. The convolution which lies immediately above the corpus callosum on the medial aspect of each cerebral hemisphere. Syn., *g. cinguli.* Aso called *cingulate g., g. callosus.*

dentate g. A narrow band of gray matter extending downward and forward above the hippocampal gyrus but separated from it by the hippocampal fissure; anteriorly it is continued into the uncus. Also called *fascia dentata hippocampi.*

diagonal g. The posterior part of the anterior perforated substance which is relatively free from foramina and borders on the optic tract. Syn., *diagonal band of Broca.*

fusiform g. A long gyrus situated on the inferior aspect of the occipital and temporal lobes between the collateral fissure and the inferior temporal sulcus. Syn., *occipitotemporal g.*

gyri Andreae Retzii. Two or three inconstant, small, rudimentary gyri, which occupy the angle between the gyrus dentatus and the gyrus hippocampi immediately beneath the splenium of the corpus callosum.

gyri breves insulae. Three or four short gyri which make up the anterior part of the insula or island of Reil.

gyri profundi. Annectant gyri which connect two neighboring gyri across the bottom of the intervening fissure.

gyri transitivi. Annectant gyri which are located superficially on the surface of the brain.

g. ambiens. A lateral elevation of the upper concealed surface of the uncinate gyrus of the temporal lobe.

g. centralis anterior. See ascending frontal *g.*

g. centralis posterior. See ascending parietal *g.*

g. cinguli. See callosal *g.*

g. epicallosus. See supracallosal *g.*

g. fasciolaris. A small cylindrical strand of cortical substance situated between the gyrus dentatus (dentate gyrus) and fimbria in the fimbriodentate sulcus: also called *fasciola cinerea.*

g. fornicatus. A convolution on the medial surface of the brain, consisting of the gyrus cinguli, isthmus hippocampi, and gyrus hippocampi.

g. frontalis inferior. See supracallosal *g.*

g. frontalis medius. See supracallosal *g.*

g. frontalis superior. See supracallosal *g.*

g. hippocampi. A convolution between the hippocampal and the collateral fissures.

g. intralimbicus. A portion of the uncinate gyrus situated above the frenulum of Giacomini.

g. lingualis. See lingual *g.*

g. longus insulae. A long gyrus of the posterior part of the insula.

g. of Broca. The left inferior frontal gyrus; location of Broca's center for articulate speech.

g. rectus. A narrow strip of cortex medial to the olfactory sulcus on the inferior surface of the frontal lobe and continuous with the superior frontal gyrus on the medial surface. Syn., *straight g.*

g. rolandicus. A rare anomalous gyrus found in the presence of two central fissures in the brain.

g. semilunaris. A median elevation of the upper concealed surface of the uncinate gyrus of the temporal lobe.

g. subcallosus. See subcallosal *g.*

g. supracallosus. See supracallosal *g.*

Heschl's gyri. Transverse temporal *gyri.*

hippocampal g. A gyrus of the medial portion of the temporal lobe, continuous caudally with the gyrus cinguli above and the lingual gyrus below, and lying between the hippocampal fissure and the anterior part of the collateral fissure. Also called *g. hippocampi.*

inferior frontal g. The most inferior of the three frontal convolutions, situated in relation to the horizontal and ascending branches of the Sylvian fissure. Also called *g. frontalis inferior.* See Plate 18.

inferior temporal g. A convolution of the temporal lobe which lies below the middle temporal sulcus and extends around the inferolateral border onto the inferior surface of the temporal lobe, where it is limited by the inferior sulcus.

lingual g. A gyrus of the medial surface of the occipital lobe, lying between the calcarine fissure and the posterior part of the collateral fissure. Syn., *g. lingualis.*

marginal g. The medial part of the superior frontal gyrus, lying between the cingulate sulcus and the supero-medial margin of the hemisphere.

middle frontal g. A convolution of the frontal lobe lying below and parallel to the superior frontal gyrus and above the inferior frontal gyrus. Also called *g. frontalis medius.* See Plate 18.

middle temporal g. A convolution of the temporal lobe which lies between the superior and middle temporal sulci. See Plate 18.

occipital gyri. Two gyri, superior and inferior, on lateral aspect of occipital lobe. See Plate 18.

occipitotemporal g. See fusiform *g.*

orbital gyri. Four convolutions—the anterior, posterior, lateral, and medial orbital gyri—which compose the inferior surface of the frontal lobe.

parietal gyri. The postcentral, superior parietal, and inferior parietal convolutions which form the lateral aspect of the parietal lobe of the brain.

postcentral g. See ascending parietal *g.*

posterior central g. See ascending parietal *g.*

precentral g. See ascending frontal *g.*

sigmoid g. The S-shaped cerebral fold about and behind the cruciate fissure in carnivora.
straight g. See *g.* rectus.
subcalcarine g. A narrow convolution ventral to the cuneus and lying between the collateral and calcarine fissures.
subcallosal g. A convolution at the rostrum of the corpus callosum limited anteriorly by the posterior parolfactory sulcus.
subcollateral g. A convolution connecting the occipital and temporal lobes.
superior frontal g. A convolution of the frontal lobe situated between the dorsal margin of the hemisphere and the superior frontal sulcus, immediately above the middle frontal gyrus. Also called *g. frontalis superior.* See Plate 18.
superior temporal g. A convolution of the temporal lobe lying between the lateral cerebral fissure and superior temporal sulcus. See Plate 18.
supracallosal g. A thin layer of gray matter in contact with the upper surface of the corpus callosum and continuous laterally with the gray matter of the cingulate gyrus. Also called *g. epicallosus, indusium griseum, g. supracallosus.*
supramarginal g. A cerebral convolution which forms the anterior portion of the inferior parietal lobule and arches over the upturned end of the lateral cerebral fissure.
transverse temporal gyri. Two or three gyri which cross the upper surface of the superior temporal gyrus transversely. Syn., *Heschl's gyri.*
uncinate g. The recurved, hooklike end of the hippocampal gyrus. Also called *g. uncinatus, uncus.*

H

H 1. Chemical symbol for hydrogen. 2. *In electrocardiography,* symbol for the longitudinal anatomic axis of the heart as projected on the frontal plane: also written $\hat{H}$. 3. Abbreviation for henry.
$\hat{H}$ Same as H, 2.
H^+ Symbol for hydrogen ion.
H^1 Symbol for protium.
H^2, H^b Symbol for deuterium.
H^3 Symbol for tritium.
H. Abbreviation for hypermetropia.
h Symbol for quantum constant; henry.
h. Latin *hora,* hour; height; hundred.
Haab, Otto [*Swiss ophthalmologist,* 1850–1931]. Described the cerebral cortex reflex, called *Haab's reflex* and invented the powerful *Haab's magnet,* for removing metallic particles from the eyeball.
ha·be′na [L., rein, thong, strap]. Old term for frenum or bandage. —**habenar,** *adj.*
ha·ben′u·la [L., dim. of *habena,* small strip of diseased flesh which is cut out from the body]. 1. The stalk of the pineal body, attaching it to the thalamus. 2. A ribbonlike structure. —**habenular,** *adj.*
h. perforata. The upper surface of the tympanic lip of the spiral lamina, having a regular row of holes.
Haber, Fritz (1868–1934). German organic chemist, known for his work in electrochemistry and his synthesis of ammonia from the elements nitrogen and hydrogen. Nobel laureate in chemistry (1918).
hab′it [L. *habitus,* state]. 1. A behavior pattern fixed by repetition. 2. The body build, as associated with a disease or a predisposition thereto; as an **apoplectic habit,** said of a stocky, thick-necked, plethoric individual, presumably liable to apoplexy. Syn., *habitus.*
hab′i·tat [L. *habitare,* to dwell]. The natural home of an animal or vegetable species.
ha·bit″u·a′tion [L. *habituare,* to bring into a habit of body]. 1. A condition of tolerance to the effects of a drug or a poison, acquired by its continued use; marked by a psychic or emotional craving for it when the drug is withdrawn. 2. Drug addiction, especially a mild form in which withdrawal does not result in severe abstinence symptoms.
hab′i·tus. See *habit.*
ha·bu′ (ha·bōō′). See *Trimeresurus flavoviridis.*
Hacker, Viktor von [*German surgeon,* 1852–1933]. With Courvoisier, introduced an operation for pyloric obstruction, in which a posterior gastroenterostomy is performed through an opening in the mesocolon.
hack′ing [AS. *haeccan*]. Form of massage consisting of a succession of chopping strokes with the edge of the extended fingers or with the whole hand.
hack′ing cough. Lay term for a short, dry cough.
Haden method. See under *method.*
Haden-Hausser method. See under *method.*
ha″de·pho′bi·a [G. *Haidēs,* Hades; *phobos,* fear]. A morbid fear of hell.
Hadfield, Geoffrey [*English pathologist,* 1889–]. With Cecil Clarke, described pancreatic infantilism, called *Clarke-Hadfield syndrome.*
hae-. For words beginning with *hae-* not found here, see *he-.*
Haeckel, Ernst Heinrich Philipp August [*German biologist,* 1834–1919]. Made important studies of morphology and embryology. See *cycle* of generation, *cytode,* recapitulation *theory.*
Hae″ma·dip′sa (hee″muh·dip′suh, hem″uh·) [G. *haima,* blood; *dipsa,* thirst]. A genus of terrestrial leeches species of which produce external hirudiniasis. The most commonly encountered species is the **H. zeylanica.**
Hae″ma·gog′us (hee″muh·gog′us, ·go′gus, hem″-uh·) [*haima;* G. *agōgos,* leading]. A genus of mosquitoes, one species of which, **H. capricorni,** has been incriminated in the transmission of jungle yellow fever.
Hae·man′thus (hi·manth′us) [*haima;* G. *anthos,* flower]. Blood-lily. A genus of the Amaryllidaceae. **H. toxicarius** yields an alkaloid that has been found to produce effects similar to those of scopolamine.
Hae″ma·phy′sa·lis (hee″muh·figh′suh·lis, hem″-uh·) [*haima;* G. *physallis,* bladder]. A genus of ticks which includes the dog tick and the rabbit tick.
H. leporis-palustris. A species of ticks limited to rabbits as hosts, and known to be a reservoir of Rocky Mountain spotted fever virus in nature.
haem′a·tin (hem′uh·tin, hee′muh·tin). See *hematin.*
Haem″a·to′bi·a (hem″uh·to′bee·uh, hee″muh·) [*haima;* G. *bios,* life]. A genus of small flies of the family Muscidae, similar to the common stable fly but more slender.
H. irritans. A species known as the horn fly; a great pest of cattle; annoys man but seldom bites him.

Haem″a·to·ther′ma (hem″uh·to·thur′muh, hee″-muh·to·) [*haima;* G. *thermē*, heat]. The warm-blooded vertebrates; birds and mammals.

haem″a·to·ther′mal, haem″a·to·ther′mous, hem″a·to·ther′mal, hem″a·to·ther′mous [*haima; thermē*]. Warm-blooded; of or pertaining to the Haematotherma.

hae″mo·coe′lom (hee″mo·see′lum, hem″o·) [*haima;* G. *koilōma*, hollow]. The body cavity of the embryo which contains the heart. *Rare.*

Hae·mon′chus (hee·mong′kus). A genus of nematode worms infesting sheep and cattle.

H. contortus. A species parasitic to sheep and other herbivores throughout the world; occasionally infests man.

Hae″mo·pro′teus (hee″mo·prot′yooss, ·pro′-tee·us, hem″o·) [*haima;* G. *Prōteus*, sea-god who could change his shape readily]. A genus of intracellular parasites found in the red blood cells of birds. Observations on species of this genus helped explain exflagellation in the life cycle of malarial parasites.

Hae″mo·spo·rid′i·a (hee″mo·spo·rid′ee·uh, hem″o·) [*haima;* G. *spora*, seed]. An order of sporozoa which live for a part of their life cycle within the red blood cells of their hosts.

Haenel's sign. See under *sign.*

Haenel's variant. Progressive muscular atrophy affecting only the upper extremities.

Haeser, Heinrich [*German physician and medical historian,* 1811–84]. Introduced *Haeser's formula* for estimating the amount of solids in urine: the last two figures of the specific gravity are multiplied by 2.33 (*Haeser's coefficient*); the result is the approximate number of grams in 1000 cc. of urine.

Haff disease. Poisoning by a resin acid. The condition is manifested by muscular weakness, pains in the limbs, and myoglobinuria. The first cases were reported near Königsberg Haff, an arm of the Baltic Sea. These were found to be caused by eating fish affected by the waste products of a celluloid factory. The disease has also occurred in epidemic form in Sweden and Karelia. Inactivation of vitamin B_1 by a substance found in certain fish may be involved.

Haffkine, Waldemar Mordecai Wolff [*Russian bacteriologist,* 1860–1930]. Introduced a method of inoculation against cholera, using first an attenuated culture of *Vibrio comma* and later a virulent culture. Also introduced a vaccine for bubonic plague. A six-week-old culture of *Pasteurella pestis* is killed by heat, and 0.5% of carbolic acid is added. The use of *Haffkine's vaccines* is called *haffkinizing.*

haf′ni·um (haf′nee·um, hahf′nee·um) [*Hafnia*, L. name of Copenhagen]. Hf = 178.6. A rare earth element.

Hagedorn, Werner [*German surgeon,* 1831–94]. Devised a curved surgical cutting needle with flat sides, in graded sizes, called *Hagedorn needle.*

Hagedorn and Jensen's method. See under *method.*

Hagner, Francis Randall [*American surgeon,* 1873–1940]. Introduced a rubber bag for packing the cavity resulting from a suprapubic prostatectomy. The *Hagner bag* is distended by water through a rubber tube, thereby controlling urinary bladder hemorrhage. Surgical drainage of the epididymis in epididymitis following gonorrhea is called *Hagner's operation.*

Hague con·ven′tion. See *Geneva convention.*

Hahn, Eugen [*German surgeon,* 1841–1902]. Introduced nephropexy, in which sutures are passed through the fatty capsule of the kidney and the outer edges of the wound (1881). Devised operation of gastrostomy in which the stomach is brought out through the eighth intercostal space.

Hah′ne·mann·ism. Homeopathy.

Haidinger, Wilhelm Karl von [*Austrian mineralogist and geologist,* 1795–1871]. Described images, called *Haidinger's brushes,* seen after polarized light has been directed into the eye. These probably are accounted for by the double refractive action of the cone fibers around the fovea.

Haight, Cameron [*American surgeon,* 1901–]. Devised a type of anterior thoracoplasty combined with conventional posterior operative procedure; called *Haight's operation. Haight's method* consists of intratracheal and intrabronchial catheter aspiration in postoperative atelectasis.

haimased. A proprietary solution of sodium thiocyanate.

Haines's reagent. See under *reagent.*

Haines's test. See under *test.*

hair [AS. *hǣr*]. A keratinized filament growing from the skin of mammals; collectively, all the filaments covering the skin. Hair is a modified epidermal structure, consisting of a *shaft,* which is the hair itself, exclusive of its sheaths and papilla, and a *root.* The root is found in the **hair follicle,** an epithelial ingrowth into the corium and hypodermis, and is expanded at its lower end into the **hair bulb.** This caps the **hair papilla,** a portion of the corium which projects upward into the center of the bulb. The epithelial parts of a hair and its sheaths are developed from the **hair column,** an epithelial ingrowth. The space in this hair column through which the developing hair shaft grows toward the surface is known as the **hair canal.**

Hajek, Markus [*Austrian laryngologist,* 1861–1941]. Author of a classic work on the paranasal sinuses (1899). He devised an operation for the relief of frontal sinus disease, in which the anterior wall of the sinus is removed and the frontonasal canal enlarged, with removal of diseased tissue.

hal′a·kone [L. *halare*, to breathe; G. *kōnos*, cone]. A small cone of stiffened gauze, designed to fit the nostril; it is filled loosely with absorbent material which may be medicated, and through which inhaled air must pass.

ha·la′tion [G. *halōs*, circular threshing-floor; also, disk of the sun or moon]. Blurring of the visual image under a powerful direct light coming from a direction different from the line of vision.

halazone (*halazonum*). *p*-Sulfonedichloramidobenzoic acid, $C_6H_4(SO_2NCl_2)COOH$—1,4. A white, crystalline powder sparingly soluble in water; in strengths of 1:200,000 to 1:500,000, it sterilizes water. **Halazone tablets** contain 4 mg. of halazone, with sodium borate and sodium chloride. One or two tablets are used per liter of water.

Halban, Josef (1870–1937). Austrian gynecologist who introduced an operation for uterine prolapse in which he amputated the cervix, called *Halban's operation.*

Halberstaedter bodies. See *Prowazek-Halberstaedter bodies* under *body.*

Haldane, John Scott [*Scottish physiologist,* 1860–1936]. Made important contributions to the knowledge of the physiology of respiration. Invented the *Haldane chamber* or *apparatus* for analyzing respiratory gases (1892). With Claude Gordon Douglas, Yandell Henderson, and Edward Christian Schneider, studied the physiologic effects of atmospheric pressure at high altitudes (1911). With Johanne Christiansen and Douglas, made a study of carbon dioxide in the blood (1914). Introduced modern oxygen therapy (1917). See also *Haldane scale.*

Haldane scale. A standard for establishing hemoglobin levels in which 13.8 Gm. in 100 cc. of blood equals 100 per cent.

Hales, Stephen [*English clergyman and physiologist*, 1677–1761]. First to measure blood pressure; invented a manometer (1733), the precursor of modern apparatus for measuring blood pressure. Pioneer in the study of plant physiology. Invented a ventilator for use in ships, mines, etc.; called the originator of artificial ventilation.

half-life. The time during which half of any given amount of a radioactive substance will have undergone transmutation; a constant for any given radioactive isotope.

effective h.-l. *In radiobiology*, the half-life of a radioactive substance in a biological system; a combination of the radioactive half-life and biological alteration or excretion of the chemical substance.

half-val'ue lay'er. *In radiology*, an internationally accepted index of the quality of a roentgen-ray beam; a layer or thickness of an absorbing material, which reduces the intensity of a roentgen-ray beam or a gamma-ray beam of a radioactive substance to one-half of its original value. Also called *half-value thickness*.

hal'i·but-liv'er oil (*oleum hippoglossi*). The fixed oil from the livers of *Hippoglossus hippoglossus*. Each gram contains at least 60,000 U.S.P. units of vitamin A and at least 600 U.S.P. units of vitamin D. It has the advantage over cod-liver oil of a much smaller dose, but contains a smaller proportion of vitamin D.

hal'ide. A binary salt in which a halogen serves as anion.

ha·lis"ter·e'sis [G. *hals*, salt; *sterēsis*, deprivation]. The loss of lime salts from previously well-calcified bone. —**halisteret'ic,** *adj.*

hal'ite [*hals*]. Rock salt; a native sodium chloride occurring in extensive deposits.

hal"i·to'sis [L. *halitus*, breath; G. *-ōsis*, condition]. The state of having offensive breath. Syn., *bromopnea, fetor ex ore.*

hal'i·tus [L.]. A vapor, as that expired from the lung.

haliver oil. Trade-mark for a brand of halibut liver oil.

Hall, Maurice Crowther [*American physician*, 1881–1938]. Introduced the carbon tetrachloride treatment of ancylostomiasis (1921).

hal'la·chrome. 5,6-Dihydro-5,6-dioxo-2-indolinecarboxylic acid; an intermediate compound in the series of transformations by which tyrosine is converted, through the action of tyrosinase, to the black pigment, melanin.

Hallé, Adrien Joseph Marie Noël [*French physician*, 1859–1947]. Remembered for his description of a point on the surface of the abdomen. *Hallé's point* represents the level at which the ureter crosses the brim of the pelvis and can be palpated most easily.

Haller, Albrecht von [*Swiss physiologist, anatomist, botanist, and poet*, 1708–77]. Credited with establishing physiology as a special branch of science; in his *Elementa Physiologiae Corporis Humani* he organized the physiologic knowledge of his time (1757–66). Demonstrated experimentally that contractility is a specific property of muscle tissue. Made numerous contributions to descriptive anatomy. The constriction separating the ventricle from the arterial bulb in the fetal heart is called *Haller's isthmus*. The solid cord of cells formed when the canal of the vaginal process of the peritoneum closes is called *Haller's habenula;* this persists for some time after birth. The vascular circle of the optic nerve formerly was called the *circle of Haller*. Haller compiled extensive bibliographies of botany, anatomy, medicine, and surgery.

Hallervorden, Julius [*German neurologist*, 1882–]. With H. Spatz, described an extrapyramidal syndrome of athetosis, mental deterioration, and speech defect, beginning in childhood (1922), called *Hallervorden-Spatz syndrome.*

hal'lex. See *hallux.*

Hallion, Louis [*French physiologist and biologist*, 1862–1940]. *Hallion's law*, which no longer is accepted, states that extracts of an organ have a stimulating effect on that organ.

Hallopeau, François Henri [*French dermatologist*, 1842–1919]. Described acrodermatitis continua, called *Hallopeau's acrodermatitis.*

hal·lu"ci·na'tion [L. *hallucinari*, to wander in mind]. Perception without external stimulus, which may occur in every field of sensation: auditory, visual, olfactory, gustatory, and tactile (*haptic*). It is a sensation, implicitly felt by the individual to originate in or from an object in the external environment, but in reality arising within himself. Seen most often in psychotic reactions, hallucinations may also occur in response to certain drugs and toxic substances, and to mechanical irritation of certain brain areas as a part of organic disease. In healthy individuals, hallucinations may occur in hypnosis and in partial sleep states. In general, they are projections of deep needs and conflicts. —**hallu'cinative, hallu'cinatory,** *adj.*

extracampine h. One which occurs outside of the normal field of perception of the sense organ(s) involved, as seeing someone behind one's head.

haptic h. See tactile *h.*

hypnagogic h. One occurring while falling asleep; a normal phenomenon, usually a pseudohallucination, as the subject commonly realizes the unreal nature of the perception.

hypnopompic h. One occurring while waking from sleep; a normal phenomenon, usually a pseudohallucination.

Lilliputian h. A visual one in which all objects and persons appear diminutive, often seen in febrile or intoxicated states, and the manic-depressive reactions. Syn., *microptic h.*

psychomotor h. The vivid but unfounded sensation that a part or parts of the body are being manipulated or are moving.

sexual h. One of sexual excitement or experience, occurring most frequently in certain schizophrenic reactions and often associated with grotesque delusions in which nongenital parts of the body are sexualized.

tactile h. One of touching or being touched: also called *haptic h.*

teleologic h. One which fits into the delusional scheme of the patient, often directing him to carry out certain acts.

hal·lu"ci·no'sis [*hallucinari;* G. *-ōsis*, condition]. *In psychiatry*, the condition of being possessed by more or less persistent hallucinations.

hal'lux (pl. *halluxes*) [NL., from L. *hallex*]. The great toe. —**hallucal,** *adj.*

h. flexus. A condition allied to and perhaps identical with hammertoe, or flexion of the first phalanx of the great toe. The second phalanx is usually extended upon the first, and there is more or less rigidity of the metatarsophalangeal joint.

h. rigidus. A condition in which there is restriction in the range of motion in the first metatarsophalangeal joint; it is frequently secondary to degenerative joint disease.

h. valgus. A deformity of the great toe, in which the head of the first metatarsal deviates away from the second metatarsal and the phalanges are deviated toward the second toe, causing undue prominence of the metatarsophalangeal joint.

h. varus. A deformity of the great toe, in which the head of the first metatarsal deviates toward the second metatarsal and the phalanges are deviated away from the second toe.

hal″ma·to·gen′e·sis [G. *halma*, jump; *genesis*, production]. A sudden change of type from one generation to another.

hal′o- [G. *hals*, (masc.) salt, (fem.) sea]. 1. A combining form denoting *the sea, salt*. 2. *In chemistry*, a combining form signifying *of* or *pertaining to a salt* or denoting *the presence of a halogen*.

hal″o·chro′mism. The phenomenon of the development of color when certain colorless organic compounds, notably those containing a carbonyl group, are dissolved in acids.

hal′o·gen [G. *hals*, salt; *genesthai*, from *gignesthai*, to be produced]. Any one of the nonmetallic elements chlorine, iodine, bromine, and fluorine.

hal′oid [*hals;* G. *eidos*, form]. Resembling, or derived from, a halogen.

ha·lom′e·ter [G. *halōs*, threshing-floor, circle; *metron*, a measure]. An instrument for measuring the mean diameter of erythrocytes by the diffraction areas produced: also called *eriometer*.

Halsted, William Stewart [*American surgeon*, 1852–1922]. Introduced regional block anesthesia. Made a pioneer study of infiltration anesthesia (1885). Made many contributions to the development of surgical technic. Introduced an interrupted intestinal suture, called *Halsted's suture*. Devised an operation, similar to Bassini's, for the radical cure of inguinal hernia, and also one for radical amputation of the breast; each of these is called *Halsted's operation*. Introduced the use of sterile rubber gloves in surgery. Devised a metal band for use instead of a ligature for the occlusion of a large artery. *Halsted's mosquito forceps* is a delicate, sharp-pointed hemostat.

Haly, Jesu. See *Jesu Haly*.

Haly Abbas ('Ali ibn 'Abbās) [*Persian physician and surgeon*, d. 994]. Author of an encyclopedia of medicine which was regarded as authoritative for several centuries.

ham [AS.]. 1. The posterior portion of the thigh above the popliteal space and below the buttock. 2. The popliteal space. 3. Colloquial term for the buttock, hip, and thigh.

Ham″a·dry′as han′nah. Synonym for *Naja hannah*.

Ham″a·me′lis [G. *hamamēlis*, medlar]. A genus of small trees or shrubs.

H. virginiana. The witch hazel. Its dried leaf, **hamamelis leaf** (*hamamelidis folium*), is sometimes used in the form of the fluidextract as a mild astringent. Witch hazel extract, or **hamamelis water** (*aqua hamamelidis*), is used as an embrocation.

ham″a·me′lose. $CH_2OH.HOC(CHO).HCOH.-HCOH.CH_2OH$; an unusual hexose occurring in the bark of *Hamamelis virginiana*.

ha·mar′ti·a [G., fault]. A nodular or localized fault of embryonal development; cells and structures natural to the part are not in normal orderly arrangement, giving rise to a hamartoma.

ham·ar″to·blas·to′ma [G. *hamartanein*, to fail, err; *blastos*, germ; *-ōma*, tumor]. A neoplasm arising from a hamartoma.

h. of kidney. See Wilms's *tumor*.

ham″ar·to′ma [*hamartanein; -ōma*]. A nodular or tumorlike mass resulting from faulty embryonal development of cells and tissues natural to the part, as exemplified in vascular birthmarks (angiomas) and nevi. They are not true neoplasms but may undergo neoplastic transformation.

tubular h. of ovary. See adrenocorticoid *adenoma* of ovary.

ham″ar·to·pho′bi·a [*hamartanein;* G. *phobos*, fear]. A morbid fear of error or sin.

ha·ma′tum [L. *hamatus*, hooked]. The hamate bone; the most ulnar of the distal row of carpal bones. Formerly called *unciform bone*. See Table of Bones in the Appendix.

Hamberger, Georg Erhard [*German physician*, 1697–1755]. Described the mechanism of respiratory movement, recognizing the function of the external intercostal muscles as inspiratory and that of the internal intercostal muscles as expiratory.

Hamburger, Hartog Jakob [*Dutch physiologist*, 1859–1924]. Remembered for his studies of osmosis (1902–04). Described the chloride shift, which is called *Hamburger's phenomenon*.

Hamman, Louis Virgil [*American physician*, 1877–1946]. Described a crunching sound heard over the pericardium on auscultation, due to the presence of air between the anterior parietal pericardium and the thoracic cage, in cases of pneumomediastinum; called *Hamman's sign*.

Hammarsten, Olof [*Swedish physiologist*, 1841–1932]. Investigated the mechanism of blood coagulation (1875). Devised a test for globulin: to the neutral solution, powdered magnesium sulfate is added to the point of saturation; this precipitates the globulin, which can then be filtered and washed.

ham′mer [AS. *hamer*]. 1. *In anatomy*, the malleus. See Table of Bones in the Appendix. 2. An instrument for striking.

percussion h. A small hammer with a rubber head; used to tap the surface of the body to elicit sounds of diagnostic value. Syn., *plexor*.

reflex h. One used to elicit reflexes by tapping on muscles, nerves, and tendons.

Hammerschlag, Albert [*Austrian physician*, 1863–1935]. Devised a method for determining the specific gravity of blood. A drop of blood is suspended in a mixture of benzene and chloroform, and the specific gravity is then determined by means of a hydrometer. Called *Hammerschlag's method*.

ham′mer·toe″ [AS. *hamer;* ME. *too*]. A condition of the toe, usually the second, in which the proximal phalanx is extremely extended while the two distal phalanges are flexed.

Hammond, William Alexander [*American neurologist*, 1828–1900]. Described athetosis, called *Hammond's disease*. Founder of the Army Medical Museum.

ham′ster [Ger.]. A short-tailed rodent with large cheek pouches, belonging to the family Cricetidae. Found in Europe, western Asia, and Africa. It is susceptible to a variety of microorganisms, and is used for laboratory purposes.

ham′string″ [AS. *ham; streng*]. The tendon bounding the ham on the outer and inner side. See Table of Muscles in the Appendix.

inner h. The tendon of the semimembranosus and semitendinosus muscles.

outer h. The tendon of the biceps femoris muscle.

ham′string″. To cripple by cutting the hamstring tendons.

ham′u·lus [L., small hook]. A hook-shaped process, as of the hamate bone, of the medial plate of the pterygoid process of the sphenoid bone, and of the osseous cochlea at the cupula (h. laminae spiralis). —**ham′ular, ham′ulate,** *adj.*

Hanau, Arthur Nathan [*German pathologist*, 1858–1900]. First to make a successful transplantation of cancer in mammals (1889).

Hand, Alfred (1868–1949). American physician who described a rare disease, occurring in children, which he called polyuria and tuberculosis (1893). The syndrome was later described more accurately by Artur Schüller (1915) and H. A. Christian (1919). See Hand-Schüller-Christian *disease.*

hand [AS.]. The organ of prehension; composed of the carpus, metacarpus, and phalanges.

accoucheur's h. A characteristic cone-shaped deformity of the hand; seen in tetany with carpal spasm and muscular dystrophy. Also called *obstetrician's h.*

ape h. An unusual shape of the hand, resembling that of apes; caused by wasting pollex muscles, as in progressive muscular atrophy.

battledore h. The large hand seen in acromegaly.

claw h. A deformity resulting from paralysis of the ulnar and/or median nerve.

cleft h. A congenital deformity of the hand in which the cleft between adjacent fingers extends into the metacarpal region.

club h. See *clubhand.*

forceps h. One which has lost the three middle fingers.

ghoul h. A slowly developing depigmation of the palm with scattered areas of hyperpigmentation, and with thickened, dry, taut skin: thought to be due to tertiary yaws.

opera-glass h. Hand changes including shortening of fingers and/or wrists caused by bone resorption, increased range of motion, and skin redundancy; it may occur after generalized, longstanding, severe rheumatoid arthritis. Also called *mains en lorgnette, doigts en lorgnette.*

trailing h. In synchronous writing of both hands, that upon which the attention, visual or central, is not fixed.

hand'ed·ness [*hand*]. The tendency to use the right or left hand more frequently, according to cerebral dominance, preference, or habit.

Handley, William Sampson (1872–). English surgeon who stressed the importance of the lymphatic spread of mammary carcinoma to the surrounding tissues (1906).

Hanger's test. See cephalin-cholesterol flocculation *test.*

hang'nail" [corruption from *agnail,* AS. *angnaegl,* from *ang,* painful, *naegl,* nail]. A partly detached piece of skin of the nail fold, friction against which has caused inflammation.

Hanot, Victor Charles [*French physician,* 1844–96]. Described hypertrophic cirrhosis of the liver, called *Hanot's disease.*

Hansen, Gerhard Henrik Armauer [*Norwegian physician,* 1841–1912]. Discovered *Mycobacterium leprae* (1871), called *Hansen's bacillus.* In some classifications the preferred term for leprosy is *Hansen's disease.*

Han'sen·id. See tuberculoid *leprosy.*

Hanson, Samuel [*American obstetrician,* 1895–]. Devised an instrument for making internal pelvic measurements (1933). *Hanson's pelvimeter* consists of a vaginal and rectal blade; it is useful in determining the biischial and interischial diameters and the anteroposterior diameter at the outlet.

Hanus' method. See *iodine* value.

hap"a·lo·nych'i·a (hap"uh·lo·nick'ee·uh) [G. *hapalos,* soft; *onyx,* nail]. A condition in which the nails are soft, may fold, and split easily. They become atrophied due to defective nail production.

hapamine. Trade-mark for a product made from histamine and despeciated horse serum globulin; used subcutaneously in allergic conditions.

haph"al·ge'si·a (haf"al·jee'zee·uh, ·see·uh) [G. *haphē,* touch; *algos,* pain]. A sensation of pain experienced upon the mere touching of an object.

haph"e·pho'bi·a [*haphē; phobos,* fear]. A morbid fear of being touched.

hap'lo-, hapl- [G. *haploos,* single]. A combining form signifying *single, simple.*

hap'lo·dont [*haploos;* G. *odous,* tooth]. *In biology,* having or pertaining to molar teeth having simple or single crowns.

hap'loid [*haploos;* G. *eidos,* form]. Having the reduced number of chromosomes, as in mature germ cells, as distinguished from the diploid or full number of chromosomes in normal somatic cells.

hap"lo·phy'tine. $C_{27}H_{31}N_3O_5$; an insecticidal alkaloid present in the Mexican plant *Haplophyton cimicidum.* See also *cimicidine.*

ha·plo'pi·a [*haploos;* G. *ōps,* eye]. Single vision, as opposed to *diplopia.*

hap'lo·scope [*haploos;* G. *skopein,* to examine]. An instrument for measuring the visual axes.

mirror h. An instrument for observing the effects of varying degrees of convergence of the visual axels

hap'ten, hap'tene [G. *haptein,* to fasten]. A partia. antigen which reacts with a specific antibody in vitro only; when combined with a protein it may behave as a true antigen.

hap"te·pho'bi·a [G. *haptesthai,* to touch; *phobos,* fear]. Morbid fear of being touched.

hap'tics [G. *haptikos,* sensitive to touch]. The branch of psychology dealing with the tactile sense. —**haptic,** *adj.*

hap"to·dys·pho'ri·a [G. *haptesthai,* to touch; *dys-,* bad; *phoros,* bearing]. The disagreeable sensation aroused by touching certain objects, as velvet, a peach, or a russet apple.

hap"to·glo'bin. An α-globulin, with a probable molecular weight of about 120,000, occurring in normal blood serum to the extent of 1 to 2% of the total protein content. It appears to contain about 5% of carbohydrate, but no lipid.

hap'to·phore [*haptesthai; phoros*]. Ehrlich's term for the specific molecular group by which toxins or agglutinins become attached to antibodies or antigens.

Harder, Johann Jacob [*Swiss anatomist,* 1656–1711]. Described a racemose gland at the inner canthus of the eye in vertebrates, especially in those having a well-developed nictitating membrane; called *Harder's gland, Harderian gland.*

Hardisty's test. See Ruttan and Hardisty's *test.*

hard'ness. *In radiology,* the penetrating power of roentgen rays; increased hardness is associated with increased penetrating power, greater energy, and shorter wavelengths.

Hare, Edward Selleck [*English surgeon,* 1812–38]. Remembered for his description of a syndrome of pressure symptoms from irritation of the cervical and brachial plexuses. Called *Hare's syndrome.*

hare'lip" [AS. *hara; lippa*]. A cleft, or clefts, in the upper lip, so called from its resemblance to a hare's lip.

acquired h. A cleft in the lip, due to accidental means, giving the same appearance as congenital harelip.

congenital h. Congenital fissure of the upper lip, due to failure of fusion of embryonic facial processes, often associated with cleft palate. The fissure may be of varying degrees, from a notch at the vermilion border to complete separation between the median nasal process and the maxillary process, the cleft extending into the nostril.

double h. One in which there is a cleft on both sides of the upper lip. Also called *bilateral h.*

median h. See facial *cleft.*

single h. One in which the cleft occurs on one side only. Also called *unilateral h.*

hare's'-eye". See *lagophthalmos.*

Harger, Rolla Neil (1890–). American chemist and toxologist who invented an instrument called the *drunkometer*. See alcohol breath *method*. He also invented a viscosity-effusion meter. See under *meter*.

Harkins, Henry Nelson (1905–). American surgeon who, in cases of shock due to burns, advised the administration of 100 cc. of plasma for every point by which the hematocrit exceeds 45; called *Harkins' method*.

Harley, George [*English physician*, 1829–96]. Described paroxysmal hemoglobinuria (1865), called *Harley's disease*.

har'ma·line (hahr'muh·leen, ·lin). An alkaloid, $C_{13}H_{14}N_2O$, in wild rue, *Peganum harmala;* toxic to helminths and protozoa.

har'ma·lol. An alkaloid in wild rue, *Peganum harmala*.

har'mine (hahr'meen, ·min). $C_{13}H_{12}N_2O$. An alkaloid from wild rue; chemically identical with banisterine from *Banisteria caapi*. Used in encephalitis lethargica as a stimulant to the central nervous system.

har'mo·sones, har'mo·zones [G. *harmozein*, to govern]. Name applied by Gley to a class of hormones which influence growth.

har"pax·o·pho'bi·a [G. *harpax*, robber; *phobos*, fear]. Morbid fear of robbers.

Harrington, Francis Bishop [*American surgeon*, 1854–1914]. Remembered for his employment of a solution of mercury bichloride, hydrochloric acid, water, and alcohol. *Harrington's solution* was formerly in wide use for hand sterilization.

Harrington, Stuart William (1889–). American surgeon who devised a radical operation for the repair of diaphragmatic hernia, performing a temporary left phrenic nerve interruption by crushing the nerve.

Harris, Malcolm La Salle [*American surgeon*, 1862–1936]. Described a method of segregating urine from the right and left kidneys by using a double catheter in the urinary bladder and a lever in the rectum or vagina. The use of *Harris' segregator* is now obsolete.

Harris, S. Harry [*Australian surgeon*, 1880–1936]. Devised an operation for removal of the prostate by the suprapubic route, in which he repaired the urethra and controlled bleeding by suture.

Harris' hematoxylin. See under *stain*.

Harrison, Edward [*English physician*, 1766–1838]. Described a groove or sulcus extending from the xiphoid process laterally and corresponding to the attachment of the diaphragm. *Harrison's groove* is diagnostic in rickets.

Harrison, Ross Granville [*American biologist*, 1870–]. Known for his researches in embryology. Reported the growth of tissue in vitro (1907) and advanced the study of tissue cultures originated by Leo Loeb (1898). He also observed the outgrowth of nerve fibers from ganglion cells.

Harrison Act. The federal law regulating the possession, sale, purchase, and prescription of habit-forming drugs.

Harrower-Erickson test. See under *test*.

Hartley, Frank [*American surgeon*, 1856–1913]. Originator of an operation of intracranial neurectomy of the fifth nerve for the relief of facial neuralgia (1892). Called *Hartley-Krause operation*.

Hart"ma·nel'la. A genus of nonparasitic, free-living amebas. The species **H. hyalina** has been found in the feces of man.

Hartmann's fossa. A small infundibular fossa of the peritoneum near the mesoappendix.

Hartmann's pouch. A dilatation of the neck of the gallbladder.

harts'horn" [AS. *heort; horn*]. 1. Cornu cervi, the horn of a stag; formerly a source of ammonia, or hartshorn spirit. 2. A name popularly given to ammonia water, and sometimes applied to ammonium carbonate.

h. liniment. Ammonia liniment. A rubefacient.

Harvey, William [*English physiologist*, 1578–1657]. Discovered the mechanism of the circulation of the blood; his *Exercitatio de Motu Cordis et Sanguinis in Animalibus* (*Essay on the Motion of the Heart and Blood in Animals*), 1628, has been called the most important book in the history of medicine. Also made an important study of generation.

Harvie, John. English obstetrician of obscure dates, remembered as the author of a monograph in which he gave directions for expressing the placenta without violence (1767). In this he anticipated Credé by nearly 90 years.

Häser's coefficient. See under Heinrich *Haeser*.

Hashimoto's disease. See *struma* lymphomatosa.

Hashimoto's struma. See *struma* lymphomatosa.

hash'ish (hash'eesh, ·ish), **hash'eesh.** See *cannabis*.

Haskins test. See Osgood-Haskins *test*.

Hasner, Josef von [*Bohemian ophthalmologist*, 1819–92]. Described the lacrimal fold, also called *Hasner's valve*. Devised an operation for the repair of defects of the eyelid in which he raised a bifurcated pedicle flap.

Hassall's body. See thymic *corpuscle*.

Hassall's corpuscle. See thymic *corpuscle*.

Hasselbalch, Karl [*Danish biochemist and physician*, 1874–]. Did important research on the acid-base balance of the blood. See the *Henderson-Hasselbalch equation*, under Lawrence Joseph *Henderson*.

Hata, Sahachiro [*Japanese physician and bacteriologist*, 1873–1938]. With Ehrlich, discovered arsphenamine (1909). Was first to use arsphenamine in rat-bite fever (1912).

Haudek, Martin [*Austrian roentgenologist*, 1880–1931]. Drew attention to the characteristic niche of gastric ulcer (1910); called *Haudek's niche*.

haunch [OF. *hanche*]. Colloquial term for the part of the body which includes the hip and the buttock of one side.

Hausser method. See Haden-Hausser *method*.

haus'trum (haw'strum) (pl. *haustra*) [NL., from *haurire*, to draw]. One of the pouches or sacculations of the colon. —**haustral,** *adj*.

Haüy, Valentin [*French teacher of the blind*, 1745–1822]. Inaugurated systematic education of the blind, for whom he established a school in 1784. Introduced the use of embossed paper to enable the blind to read.

Haverhill fever. Epidemic arthritic erythema. An epidemic occurred in Haverhill, Mass., in 1926. See under *erythema*.

Havers, Clopton [*English anatomist*, d. 1702]. Made an important study of bone structure and growth (1691). See *Haversian canals* under *canal*. The concentric plates of bone which surround the canals are called the *Haversian systems*. The *Haversian glands* are fat lobules found in some synovial fringes.

hawk [imitative]. To clear the throat by a forcible expiration.

Hawkins, Caesar Henry [*English surgeon*, 1798–1884]. Described cicatricial hypertrophy resembling true keloid; called *Hawkins' keloid*.

Hawley, George Waller [*American orthopedic surgeon*, 1874–1940]. Devised a table for use in the operative treatment of fractures of the long bones, especially when traction and the application of plaster are contemplated.

Haworth, Walter Norman (1883–1949). English

chemist noted for his synthesis of vitamin C (ascorbic acid). Nobel laureate in chemistry (1937).

Hay's test. See under *test.*

Hayem, Georges [*French physician*, 1841–1933]. Contributed much to the development of modern hematology. Gave the hematoblast its name (1877). The achromacyte is also called *Hayem's corpuscle. Hayem's solution*, composed of sodium chloride, sodium sulfate, and mercuric chloride in water, is used as a diluting fluid in counting erythrocytes. Hayem gave a classic account of cirrhosis of the liver (1874). He described acquired hemolytic jaundice (1898), later described by Widal and Abrami; called *Hayem-Widal disease, Widal-Abrami's disease.*

hay fe'ver. An acute affection of the conjunctiva and upper air passages; due to a sensitivity to pollen. In common usage, the term refers to that produced by ragweed or biologically related pollens. May be caused by other allergens, as tree and flower pollens and atmospheric molds. That caused by grass pollen is known as *rose fever*. In a small percentage of cases, the etiologic factor is undetermined. Chief symptoms are coryza, sneezing, rhinorrhea, headache, and intense itching of the eyes and upper air passages. Also called *perennial h.f., perennial rhinitis, vasomotor rhinitis, allergic rhinitis, pollen coryza.*

Haygarth, John [*English physician*, 1740–1827]. Described the joint swellings in the fingers in arthritis deformans (1805); called *Haygarth's nodes* or *nodosities.*

Haynes, Irving Samuel [*American surgeon*, 1861–1946]. Advised operation in acute suppurative meningitis, in which he drained the cisterna magna; called *Haynes' operation.*

hazeline. Trade-mark for a preparation of *Hamamelis virginiana.*

hb Hemoglobin.

H d Hensen's disk.

h. d. *Hora decubitus*, at the hour of going to bed.

He Chemical symbol for helium.

Head, Henry [*English neurologist*, 1861–1940]. Described the role of the vagus nerve in respiration (1889). With Alfred Walter Campbell, described the pathology of herpes zoster, showing the disease to be an inflammation of the posterior nerve roots and spinal ganglions (1900). Made important contributions to the knowledge of the peripheral nerves. Studied the effects of injuries to the peripheral nerves, with James Sherren (1905) and with William Halse Rivers (1908); in the latter case Head was the subject of the experiment. Made a fundamental investigation of referred pain. Wrote a classic work on aphasia (1926).

head [AS. *hēafod*]. 1. The uppermost part of the body, containing the brain, organs of sight, smell, taste, hearing, and part of the organs of speech. See Plates 3, 8, 10, 11. 2. The top, beginning, or most prominent part of anything.

aftercoming h. The head of the fetus in a breech presentation.

apple h. The broad, thick skull of certain dwarfs.

floating h. A freely movable fetal head above the pelvic brim.

h. locking. The entanglement of the heads of twins at the time of birth.

scald h. Any crusting disease of the scalp. *Colloquial.*

steeple h. See *oxycephaly.*

sugar-loaf h. See *oxycephaly.*

tower h. See *oxycephaly.*

white h. See *witkop.*

head'ache" [*hēafod;* AS. *acan*]. Pain in the head. Syn., *cephalalgia.*

anoxic h. A generalized and sometimes throbbing headache caused by the extreme vasodilation of cerebral anoxia.

arterial h. A throbbing headache caused by the pulsating of dilated intracranial arteries.

bilious h. Migraine.

blind h. Migraine.

caffeine-withdrawal h. One caused by the abrupt withdrawal of caffeine after prolonged, excessive drinking of coffee. The headache is throbbing; nausea, rhinorrhea, and lethargy may also occur. It may be terminated by administering caffeine or benzedrine.

cervical myalgic h. Muscle-contraction *h.*

chronic indurative h. Muscle-contraction *h.*

cyclic h. That associated with menstruation.

drainage h. Frontotemporal or suboccipital headache resulting from withdrawal of cerebrospinal fluid. It is aggravated by jugular compression and relieved when the subject assumes the horizontal position. Also called *leakage h., puncture h.*

epinephrine h. A type of pressor headache of short duration in which there is throbbing pain in the frontotemporal region, following injection of epinephrine.

histamine h. A type of headache considered to be due to dilatation of the carotid vascular tree as the result of action by circulating histamine. It is characterized by abrupt onset, pain in the temple, neck, face, and one eye, lacrimation and congestion of the eye, stuffiness of the nostril, and swelling of the temporal vessels.

indurative h. See muscle-contraction *h.*

leakage h. See drainage *h.*

migrainous h. The headache of migraine.

muscle-contraction h. Any headache caused by painful contraction of the head and neck muscles, secondary to noxious stimulation elsewhere in the head, or associated with emotional tension or local muscle or nerve root injury. Terms such as indurative *h.*, nodular *h.*, rheumatic *h.*, and spastic *myalgia* usually refer to muscle-contraction headache associated with emotional tension.

nodular h. See muscle-contraction *h.*

ocular h. Pain in and about the head that results from organic disease or impaired function of the eye.

ophthalmic h. See ocular *h.*

overflow h. See spread *h.*

paraplegic h. A type of pressor headache of brief duration, seen in patients with partial or complete spinal cord transection, following painful stimuli from segments below the lesion; it is probably caused by distended intracranial arteries.

pheochromocytoma h. A transient type of pressor headache associated with paroxysmal hypertension resulting from pheochromocytoma.

posttraumatic h. The persistent and recurrent headache which often follows head injury.

pressor h. Any headache produced by sudden rise in systemic blood pressure, including paraplegic *h.*, epinephrine *h.*, pheochromocytoma *h.*

psychogenic h. Headache associated with tension, anxiety, or a basic personality disorder. Response to diagnostic tests and analgesics may be equivocal, but sedatives generally are effective. See muscle-contraction *h.*

puncture h. See drainage *h.*

rheumatic h. See muscle-contraction *h.*

sick h. Migraine.

spread h. A secondary headache caused by the spread of pain from anywhere in the head: also called *overflow h.*

traction h. Pain arising from traction on the dura mater, from whatever cause.

vascular dilatation h. Headache associated with or due to dilatation of intracranial arteries.

vasomotor h. See histamine *h.*

head'band" [*hēafod;* ME. *band*]. A strap for securing a mirror to the forehead.

heal'er [AS. *haēlan*]. 1. One who effects cures. 2. Colloquial term for a Christian Science practitioner. 3. One without formal medical education who claims to cure by some form of suggestion.

natural h. One supposed to possess personal magnetism capable of overcoming disease.

heal'ing [*haēlan*]. The process or act of getting well or of making whole; the restoration to normal, as in the closure of an ulcer or a wound, or the union of a broken bone. —**heal,** *v.t., v.i.*

h. by first intention. The primary union of a wound when the incised skin edges are approximated and so held and union takes place without the process of granulation.

h. by second intention. The process of wound closure where the edges remain separated; the wound becomes closed after granulation tissue has filled the cavity to the skin level so that epithelium can grow over the unhealed area.

mental h. Psychotherapy. Also called *spiritual h.*

health [AS. *haēlth*]. The state of dynamic equilibrium between the organism and its environment which maintains the structural and functional characteristics of the organism within the normal limits for the particular form of life (race, genus, species) and the particular phase of its life cycle. —**health'ful, health'y,** *adj.*

public h. The state of health of a population, as that of a state, nation, or a particular community.

health cer·tif'i·cate. A formal or official document signed by a physician, attesting to the state of health of the individual named therein.

health of'fi·cer. A quarantine officer or an officer of a board of health; an officer of sanitation.

health phys'ics. That branch of radiological physics dealing with the protection of personnel from harmful effects of ionizing radiation.

health so·ci'e·ty. An association which has for its objective the promotion of some phase of public health.

hear [AS. *hīeran*]. To perceive by the ear.

hear'ing [*hīeran*]. The special sense by which the sonorous vibrations of the air are communicated to the mind.

double h. Diplacusis.

h. loss. Impairment of an individual's hearing compared with the hearing of "normal" individuals; certain frequency ranges are especially considered.

residual h. In the measurement of hearing loss, the amount of hearing that a person retains irrespective of temporary reductions.

visual h. The understanding of speech by means of visual impulses. Also called *lip reading.*

hear'ing aid. An instrument that amplifies the intensity of sound waves for the benefit of those with impaired hearing.

air conduction h. a. An electric hearing aid, the transmitter of which fits into the ear canal.

bone conduction h. a. An electric hearing aid, the transmitter of which is held against the skin over the mastoid process.

carbon h. a. An electric hearing aid of the carbon granule transmitter type, as the telephone.

electric h. a. One getting its source of power from electricity.

fixed h. a. One that is permanently installed, as in a church, school, or theater.

mechanical h. a. One that amplifies the intensity of sound waves by some physical means other than electricity.

portable h. a. An electric hearing aid that can be carried with relative ease.

vacuum h. a. An electric hearing aid of the vacuum tube type, as a radio.

wearable h. a. One that can be worn on the person.

heart [AS. *heorte*]. A hollow, muscular organ, whose function is to pump the blood through the vessels. It is enveloped by the pericardium and consists of two symmetrical halves, a right atrium and ventricle and a left atrium and ventricle. The right atrioventricular orifice is guarded by the tricuspid valve; the left, by a valve with two leaflets, the mitral. These valves are broad and thin and consist of two layers of the lining membrane of the heart, the endocardium, separated by a slight amount of connective tissue. To support them, thin chordae tendineae join their free margins to the papillary muscles in the wall of the ventricle. The outlet of the right ventricle into the pulmonary artery, and of the left into the aorta, are guarded by the semilunar valves. See Plates 5, 7, 9, 13.

air in h. See *aerendocardia.*

apex of the h. The lowest and leftmost point of the heart represented by the left ventricle. It is usually described as being behind the fifth left intercostal space 8–9 cm (in the adult) from the midsternal line.

armored h. Chalky deposits on the pericardium, due to chronic inflammation.

athletic h. Generalized enlargement of the heart without disease of the valves, supposedly the result of excessive participation in sports.

base of h. The general area occupied by the roots of the great vessels and the portion of the wall of the heart between them.

beriberi h. Heart failure due to thiamin deficiency, characterized by no myocardial changes or hydropic degeneration.

bilocular h. A congenital defect in which there is a single atrium and a single ventricle with a common atrioventricular valve. It may also be one in which there is a nonfunctioning right ventricle and a gross defect in the atrial septum, creating a functionally bilocular heart. Syn., *biloculate h., cor biloculare.*

boat-shaped h. That caused by aortic disease.

bony h. One with calcareous patches on its walls.

bovine h. The markedly hypertrophied heart which develops as a result of aortic valvular disease. Also called *cor bovinum.*

chaotic h. action. Chaos created by the operation of multiple multifocal ectopic pacemakers, which may be atrial or ventricular. It is usually followed by fibrillation.

electrical position of the h. Direction of the mean spatial QRS vector. In the frontal plane, five basic electrical positions of the heart have been described: (1) vertical, (2) semivertical, (3) intermediate, (4) semihorizontal, (5) horizontal.

fatty h. A name given to two distinct pathologic conditions of the heart tissue. In the first, there is a true fatty degeneration of the cardiac muscular fibers; in the second, there is an increase in the quantity of subpericardial and intramyocardial fat, which is true fat infiltration.

fibroid h. Extensive fibrosis of myocardium, the fibrous tissue replacing numerous foci of necrosis.

glycogenic h. Deposits of glycogen in the heart muscles and consequent hypertrophy.

goiter h. A condition characterized by atrial fibrillation, cardiac enlargement, and congestive cardiac failure; due to thyrotoxicosis. Also called *thyroid h., thyrotoxic h.*

hairy h. The peculiar, shaggy appearance of the heart in acute fibrinous pericarditis, the deposited fibrin existing in long shreds. Also called *cor villosum, shaggy h.*

h. clot. Coagulation of blood in the cardiac cavity.

h. disease. The extrinsic form is caused by compression, angulation, and torsion of the heart, or by abnormally high pressure in either the systemic or pulmonary circulation; the intrinsic form by disease of the heart muscle, valves, or coronary arteries.

h. sac. The pericardium.

icing h. One whose entire surface is covered with a dense, thick, marble-white tissue.

irritable h. Neurocirculatory asthenia.

kyphotic h. Pulmono-cardiac strain and failure due to deformities of the thorax or spine.

left h. The part which furnishes blood to the systemic and coronary vessels.

low h. See *bathycardia.*

peripheral h. An obsolete term for the muscular coat of the blood vessels.

pseudotrilocular h. A heart having two atria with a defective interatrial septum and one ventricle.

pulmonary h. The effect of pulmonary hypertension on the right ventricle; caused by dilatation and failure of the left ventricle, mitral valve disease, massive pulmonary embolism, chronic pulmonary disease, severe chest deformity, or primary disease of the pulmonary arteries. It is acute or chronic. Also called *cor pulmonale.*

right h. The part which furnishes blood to the lungs.

skin h. The peripheral blood vessels.

soldier's h. Neurocirculatory asthenia.

tobacco h. A condition which is characterized by irregular action and palpitation; produced by excessive indulgence in tobacco.

villous h. See hairy *h.*

heart block. The cardiac mechanism resulting from defective transmission of impulses from atrium to ventricle. The first stage is that in which the P-R interval is prolonged; in the second stage, beats are dropped; in the third stage, the ventricular contractions are independent of the atrial.

arborization h. b. Heart block occurring in fibers of the Purkinje system. See also intraventricular *h. b.*

atrioventricular (AV) h. b. That in which conduction of the impulse between the atria and ventricles is slowed or impeded; three forms occur, first degree AV block (prolonged AV conduction); second degree (partial AV block); third degree (complete AV block).

bundle-branch h. b. The blocking produced by a localized lesion of a branch of the bundle of His, resulting in a difference in contraction time of the two ventricles, and producing a specific electrocardiographic pattern. See also intraventricular *h. b.*

complete h. b. The third stage of block, when the ventricles assume their own rhythm, about 30–40 beats per minute.

congenital h. b. That due to defective development of the conduction system.

entrance h. b. A term used in electrocardiography to describe the condition in which the automatic center in the ventricle is constantly operating and is not disturbed by outside stimuli. Also called *protective h. b.*

exit h. b. A term used in electrocardiography to describe the condition in which there is a local region of abnormal unidirectional block, which prevents some of the impulses generated by an ectopic pacemaker from passing on to the rest of the heart.

focal h. b. Altered intraventricular conduction due to focal injury of heart muscle.

incomplete h. b. The first stage of blocking, in which the conduction time is prolonged, recognized only by the electrocardiograph.

intraatrial h. b. A type which shows on the electrocardiographic record a broad, notched P wave of longer than normal duration.

intraventricular h. b. Any heart condition giving electrocardiograms with QRS interval of 0.12 seconds or more and not fitting the criteria of typical bundle-branch block. It includes arborization heart block, focal heart block, and prolonged QRS interval due to hypertrophy.

partial h. b. The second stage of blocking, in which beats are dropped, giving a 2:1, 3:1, 4:1, etc., AV ratio.

protective h. b. Entrance heart block.

sinoatrial h. b. A type in which the impulses originating in the sinoatrial node are partially or completely prevented from leaving it.

unidirectional h. b. A type in which the impulses will pass out of, but not into, the area of block.

heart'burn" [*heorte;* AS. *baernan*]. A burning sensation over the precordium or beneath the sternum; usually related to esophageal spasm. Gastric pyrosis.

heart fail'ure. See *cardiac failure, circulatory failure.*

heart mur'mur. An adventitious sound heard over the heart and sometimes transmitted to areas not directly over the cardiac dullness. These sounds are described according to intensity, pitch, quality, duration, and time of their occurrence in the cardiac cycle. Also see cardiac *murmur.*

heart rate. The number of heart beats per minute.

heart sounds. Those heard on auscultation over the heart. The first sound is deeper in pitch and longer than the second, and is attributed to ventricular systole and the closure of the AV valves. The second sound is higher pitched, short, and of snapping quality, and is attributed to closure of the semilunar valves. Heart sounds are described according to intensity, quality, duration, and time. Occasionally a faint third sound is heard, which is supposedly due to ventricular filling.

heart'wa"ter [*heorte;* AS. *waeter*]. Hemoglobinuria of sheep.

heart'worm" [*heorte;* AS. *wyrm*]. *Dirofilaria immitis.*

heat [AS. *hǣtu*]. 1. A form of kinetic energy communicable from one body to another by conduction, convection, or radiation; it is that form of molecular motion which is appreciated by a special thermal sense. 2. The periodic sexual excitement in animals.

atomic h. The specific heat of an atom of an element multiplied by its atomic weight.

h. capacity. The specific heat of a substance multiplied by its mass.

latent h. The quantity of heat necessary to convert a body into another state without changing its temperature.

mechanical equivalent of h. The mechanical energy which is required to produce a given amount of heat. One calorie is equivalent to 426.5 gram-meters, or 3.085 foot-pounds, of work.

molecular h. The molecular weight of a compound multiplied by its specific heat.

prickly h. See *miliaria.*

relaxation h. Heat evolved by muscle during relaxation.

specific h. The amount of heat required to raise the temperature of 1 Gm. of a substance 1° C.

Heath, Charles Joseph [*English otologist,* 1856–

1934]. Devised an operation for mastoid disease in which he removed the posterior osseous wall to a low level, a small portion of bone being left between the epitympanum and antrum; the posterior cartilaginous canal is then divided as in the radical operation. Called *Heath's operation.*

heat pros·tra'tion. A syndrome resulting from exposure to high temperatures, seen most frequently in infants and the aged; characterized by a moist, cold skin, poor circulation, a normal mouth and elevated rectal temperature, restlessness, and anxiety. Also called *heat exhaustion.*

heat stroke. See *sunstroke.*

heaves [AS. *hebban*]. A disease of horses, characterized by difficult and laborious respiration. Also called *broken wind.*

he"be·phre'ni·a (hee"bi·free'nee·uh, heb"i·) [G. *hēbē*, puberty; *phrēn*, mind]. A type of schizophrenia marked by silliness and mannerisms, often caricaturing certain adolescent behavior. See under *schizophrenic reaction.* —**hebephren'ic,** *n., adj.*

Heberden, William (Senior) [*English physician,* 1710–1801]. First to distinguish between chickenpox and smallpox (1767). Accurately described angina pectoris, so named by him (1768), and once called *Heberden's asthma, Rougnon-Heberden disease.* Described a degenerative disease producing nodular enlargement about the terminal joints of the fingers; called *Heberden's arthritis, Heberden's disease, Rosenbach's disease.* The swellings are called *Heberden's nodes.*

he·bet'ic [G. *hēbētikos*, youthful]. Relating to, or occurring at, puberty or adolescence.

heb'e·tude [L. *hebetare*, to dull]. Dullness of the special senses and intellect. —**hebetu'dinous,** *adj.*

he·bos"te·ot'o·my, he·bot'o·my. Old term for pubiotomy.

Hebra, Ferdinand von [*Austrian dermatologist,* 1816–80]. Has been called the founder of modern dermatology. Classified skin diseases according to pathologic anatomy (1845). Established the parasitic basis of many skin conditions. Described pityriasis rubra (1857), called *Hebra's pityriasis,* and tinea cruris (1860), called *Hebra's eczema.* Gave the first description of impetigo herpetiformis (1872). Erythema multiforme exudativum is known as *Hebra's disease.* See also compound *sulfur* ointment, also called *Hebra's itch ointment.*

hebulon. Trade-mark for an encapsulated hematinic containing liver extract, ferrous sulfate, and vitamin-B complex.

hec"a·ter·o·mer'ic, hec"a·ter·om'er·al, hec"a·to·mer'ic. [G. *hekateros*, each of two; *meros*, part]. Having processes which divide into two parts; as a neuron, with one process going to each side of the spinal cord.

Hecht-Schlaer night vision test. See under *test.*

Hecker, Karl von [*German obstetrician,* 1827–82]. *Hecker's law* states that in successive births, each child usually weighs from 150 to 200 Gm. more than its predecessor.

hec'tic [G. *hektikos*, habitual]. 1. Habitual. 2. Pertaining to or having hectic fever.

hec'tic. 1. Hectic fever; one suffering from hectic fever. 2. A hectic flush.

hec'to-, hect- [G. *hekaton*, hundred]. A combining form signifying *one hundred.*

hec'to·gram [*hekaton;* G. *gramma*, letter]. One hundred grams, or 1543.2349 grains. Abbreviated, hg.

hec'to·li"ter (heck'to·lee"tur) [*hekaton;* F. *litre*, from G. *litra*, a coin, pound]. One hundred liters; equal to 22 imperial or 26.4 United States gallons. Abbreviated, hl.

hec'to·me"ter [*hekaton;* G. *metron*, a measure]. One hundred meters, or 328 feet 1 inch. Abbreviated, hm.

he"de·o'ma (hee"dee·o'muh, hed"ee·) [NL., perhaps from G. *hēdys*, sweet; *osmē*, odor]. American pennyroyal. The leaves and tops of *Hedeoma pulegioides*, the medicinal properties of which are due to a volatile oil. It is carminative.

hed"er·ag'e·nin (hed"ur·adj'i·nin). A glycoside, $C_{31}H_{50}O_4$, obtained from English ivy, *Hedera helix.*

hed'er·in. A glycoside, $C_{41}H_{64}O_{11}$, from the fruit of the English ivy, *Hedera helix.*

he·do'ni·a [G. *hēdonē*, pleasure]. Abnormal cheerfulness; amenomania.

he'don·ism (hee'dun·iz·um, hed'un·iz·um) [*hēdonē*]. The pursuit of pleasure; the belief that acts should be directed toward the attainment of pleasure. Consequently, an unreasoning emphasis on pleasure or on some hobby or whim.

he"do·no·pho'bi·a [*hēdonē;* G. *phobos*, fear]. A morbid fear of pleasure.

heel [AS. *hēla*]. The hinder part of the foot.

big h. Epidemic enlargement of the calcaneus, a disease found on the west coast of Africa, on the coast of China, and notably in Formosa. It is marked by fever, pain, and enlargement of the heel. There are frequent remissions followed by recurrence. The etiology is unknown.

painful h. Tenderness of the heel, causing severe pain on walking; usually due to gonococcal infection or to bony spurs.

Heerfordt, Christian F. [*Danish ophthalmologist,* 1871–]. Described uveoparotid fever, called *Heerfordt's disease.* See also *sarcoidosis.*

Hefke-Turner sign. See obturator *sign.*

Hegar, Alfred [*German gynecologist,* 1830–1914]. Devised an operation for lacerated perineum: a triangular excision is made in the posterior wall of the vagina, and the muscles and fascia are sutured in the midline. Invented metal dilators in graduated sizes for stretching the cervix of the uterus; called *Hegar's dilators.* Softening of the lower segment of the uterus is called *Hegar's sign* of pregnancy in the early stages.

he·gem'o·ny [G. *hēgemonia*, a leading the way, rule]. Leadership, domination; as the supremacy of one function over a number of others.

Heidenhain, Martin [*German histologist,* 1864–1949]. See *Heidenhain's azocarmine* and *iron hematoxylin* (*Heidenhain's*), under *stain.*

Heidenhain, Rudolf Peter Heinrich [*German physiologist,* 1834–97]. Remembered for his important work on gastric motility. Investigated the effects of poisons on the submaxillary gland (1872). Formulated the secretion theory of renal function (1874). Described the "rodlets" in cells of the renal tubules; called *Heidenhain's rods* or *striae.* He also studied the nerve supply of glandular structures (1878). Described a denervated portion of the stomach with an exterior fistula, called *Heidenhain's pouch,* completely separated from the main organ. See also serous *crescent,* called *demilune of Heidenhain.*

Heim, Ernst Ludwig [*German physician,* 1747–1834]. Observed a sign of adherent pericardium: retraction of the intercostal spaces occurs with the cardiac systole. Called *Heim-Kreysig sign.*

Heine, Jacob von [*German orthopedist,* 1800–1879]. First to describe the deformities produced by acute anterior poliomyelitis (1840), sometimes called *Heine-Medin disease.* Differentiated the disease from other forms of paralysis. Made important contributions to the knowledge of congenital luxations (1842).

Heine, Leopold [*German ophthalmologist,* 1870–

1940]. Introduced cyclodialysis, called *Heine's operation.* Made important contributions to the development of modern contact lenses.

Heineke-Mikulicz operation. See *pylorotomy.*

Heinz, Robert [*German physician and pharmacologist,* 1865–1924]. Described refractile inclusion bodies seen in erythrocytes in hemolytic anemias due to toxic agents (1890), called *Heinz-Ehrlich bodies.* See under *body.*

Heisrath, Friedrich [*German ophthalmologist,* 1850–1904]. Devised his operation for the relief of trachoma by excision of the tarsal folds.

Heister, Lorenz [*German surgeon, anatomist, and botanist,* 1683–1758]. Described the spiral valve of the cystic duct; called *Heister's valve.* Described the sinus of the external jugular vein; this formerly was called *Heister's diverticulum.*

Hektoen, Ludvig [*American pathologist,* 1863–1951]. Known for his work in general pathology and immunology. Produced experimental cirrhosis of the liver. Contributed to the knowledge of carcinoma. With George J. Rukstinat, devised a test for the presence of spermatozoa; called *Hektoen-Rukstinat test.*

hel'co-, helc- [G. *helkos,* ulcer]. A combining form meaning *an ulcer.*

hel'coid, hel·cot'ic [*helkos*]. Resembling an ulcer; ulcerative.

hel·co'ma [*helkos*]. An ulcer. *Obs.*

hel·cot'ic. See *helcoid.*

he·len'a·lin. A toxic principle, $C_{15}H_{18}O_4$, from *Helenium autumnale* or wild sunflower. It is intensely irritant to mucous membranes and paralyzant to the heart and voluntary muscles. Proposed as a vermifuge and insecticide.

hel'e·nin. A stearoptene, $C_{15}H_{20}O_2$, from *Inula helenium.* A bactericide and anthelmintic. Dose, 10–20 mg. (1/6–1/3 gr.). Syn., *alantolactone.*

he·lex'in. Hederin.

he"li·an'thin, he"li·an'thine (hee"lee·an'thin, ·theen). Methyl orange, an acid-base indicator.

he·lic'i·form (hi·liss'i·form) [G. *helix,* spiral; L. *forma,* form]. Spiral; shaped like a snail shell.

hel'i·cin. $CHO.C_6H_4.O.C_6H_{11}O_5$; the D-glucoside of salicylaldehyde, obtained by oxidation of salicin: on hydrolysis it yields D-glucose and salicylaldehyde.

hel'i·cine (hell'i·sin, ·syne) [*helix*]. 1. Ascendingly spiral. 2. Pertaining to the helix.

hel'i·cis [*helix*]. A vestigial muscle associated with the helix of the external ear; a **h. major** and **h. minor** have been described.

hel'i·co-, helic- [*helix*]. A combining form meaning *spiral.*

hel'i·coid [*helix;* G. *eidos,* form]. Spiral; coiled like a snail shell.

hel"i·co·pep'sin [*helix;* G. *pepsis,* a cooking]. A proteolytic enzyme found in snails.

hel'i·co·pod, hel"i·co·po'di·a [*helix;* G. *pous,* foot]. Circumduction; movement of the leg in a lateral arc as it scrapes the floor; the gait seen in spastic hemiplegia.

hel"i·co·pro'te·in [*helix;* G. *prōteios,* of first rank]. A protein obtained from snails of the family Helicidae.

hel"i·co·ru'bin [*helix;* L. *ruber,* red]. A respiratory pigment found in the gut and liver of the snail.

hel"i·co·tre'ma [*helix;* G. *trēma,* perforation]. The opening connecting the scalae tympani and vestibuli of the spiral canal of the cochlea.

he"li·en·ceph"a·li'tis [G. *hēlios,* sun; *egkephalos,* brain; *-itis,* inflammation]. Encephalitis caused by exposure to the sun's rays.

he'li·o-, heli- [*hēlios*]. A combining form signifying *the sun.*

he'li·o·phage". See *chromatophore.*

he'li·o·phobe" [*hēlios;* G. *phobos,* fear]. One who is morbidly sensitive to the effects of the sun's rays.

he"li·o·pho'bi·a [*hēlios; phobos*]. Morbid fear of exposure to the sun's rays.

he'li·o·stat" [*hēlios;* G. *-statēs,* stationary]. A mirror moved by clockwork in such a manner as to reflect continuously the sun's rays on a given spot. —**heliostat'ic,** *adj.*

he"li·o·tax'is [*hēlios;* G. *taxis,* arrangement]. A form of taxis in which there is attraction toward (**positive heliotaxis**) or repulsion from (**negative heliotaxis**) the sun or sunlight.

he"li·o·ther'a·py [*hēlios;* G. *therapeia,* treatment]. The treatment of disease by exposure of the body to sunlight.

he"li·o·tro'pin (hee"lee·o·tro'pin, ·ot'ro·pin). Piperonal.

he"li·ot'ro·pism [*hēlios;* G. *trepein,* to turn]. *In biology,* that property of a plant or plant organ by virtue of which it bends toward or away from the sunlight. —**heliotrop'ic,** *adj.*

he'li·um [*hēlios*]. He = 4.003. A chemically inert, colorless, odorless, noninflammable, gaseous element, occurring in certain natural gases and in small amount in the atmosphere. Next to the lightest element known, it is used as a lifting gas in dirigibles and balloons. Mixed with oxygen, it forms an artificial air, useful when men are working under pressures of several atmospheres, as in tunnel construction. Being less soluble than nitrogen, less time is required for the adjustment of pressure without danger of bends. A similar mixture, being less dense than ordinary air, is useful in various types of dyspnea and in cases involving respiratory obstruction.

he'lix [G.]. The rounded, convex margin of the pinna of the ear.

Hel"ke·si·mas'tix [G. *helkein,* to drag; *mastix,* whip]. A genus of coprozoic flagellates.

H. faecicola. A species of free-living flagellates found in the feces of man.

hel'le·bore [G. *helleboros*]. A plant of the genus *Helleborus,* particularly *H. niger,* black hellebore. It has been used as a drastic purge. It contains the glycosides helleborein, helleborin, and hellebrin. Dose of the powdered root, as a purge, 0.13–0.2 Gm. (2–3 gr.).

American h. *Veratrum viride.*

false h. *Adonis vernalis.*

green h. *Veratrum viride.*

white h. *Veratrum album.*

hel"le·bo're·in. A poisonous glycoside, $C_{37}H_{56}O_{18}$, from *Helleborus niger* and *H. viridis.* It has a digitalislike action but is of doubtful practical value.

hel·leb'o·rin (heh·leb'o·rin, hell'i·bor·in). A poisonous glycoside, $C_{28}H_{36}O_6$, from *Helleborus niger* and *H. viridis.* Paralyzes the central nervous system.

hel'le·bo·rism [*helleboros*]. 1. The treatment of disease with hellebore. 2. The morbid condition induced by the free exhibition of hellebore.

hel'le·brin. A glycoside from *Helleborus niger* having an action resembling that of strophanthin.

Heller, Arnold [*German pathologist,* 1840–1913]. Established the role of syphilis in the causation of aortic aneurysm (1899). Syphilitic aortitis is known as *Doehle-Heller aortitis, Welch's aortitis.*

Heller's test. See under *test.*

Hellin's law. Twins occur in one of 80 pregnancies; triplets in one of 80^2, or 6,400; quadruplets in one of 80^3, or 512,000. A recent modification of this law states that in the United States, twins are to be expected in one of 88 pregnancies, triplets in one of 88^2, and quadruplets in one of 88^3 (Patten).

Helly's fixing fluid. See under Zenker's *fixing fluid.*

Helmholtz, Hermann Ludwig Ferdinand von (1821–1894). German physiologist and physicist. From his studies of muscular contraction, in which he showed that muscles are the chief source of animal heat, he developed and gave the mathematical formulation for the principle of the conservation of energy (1847). He measured the velocity of nerve impulses, and invented the ophthalmoscope (1851), which has been called the greatest event in ophthalmology. He developed Young's theory of color vision. See *Young-Helmholtz theory* under Thomas *Young.* He published a fundamental work on physiological optics (1856–66) and acoustics (1862). See Helmholtz's theory of *accommodation.* According to his resonance theory of hearing, the motion of the stapes produces vibrations in the perilymph, and thus produces secondary vibrations in the basilar membrane. He described the tympanum and the ossicles of the ear (1869). Important contributions were also made to thermodynamics, hydrodynamics, electrodynamics, and meteorological physics. He studied electrical oscillation and measured the velocity of propagation of electromagnetic induction. His student Hertz, to whom he gave the problem of measuring possible electrical waves, demonstrated electromagnetic waves and found that their velocity equaled that of light. Helmholtz also explained the principle of least action. The *Gibbs-Helmholtz equation* for determining the amount of work of which a galvanic cell is capable is considered one of the first principles of physical and physiological chemistry.

hel′minth [G. *helmins,* worm]. Originally any parasitic worm; now includes those wormlike animals, either parasitic or free-living, of the phyla Platyhelminthes and Nemathelminthes as well as members of the phylum Annelida. —**helmin′thic, helmin′thous, helmin′thoid,** *adj.*

hel·min′tha·gogue (hel·min′thuh·gog). See *anthelmintic.*

hel″min·them′e·sis [*helmins;* G. *emesis,* vomiting]. The vomiting of parasitic worms.

hel″min·thi′a·sis [*helmins;* NL. *-iasis,* condition]. The diseased condition produced by the presence of parasitic worms in the body.

h. elastica. Elastic tumors of the axilla and groin due to filarial worms.

hel′minth·ism. Helminthiasis.

hel·min′tho-, helminth- [*helmins*]. A combining form signifying *worm.*

hel″min·thol′o·gist. A specialist in the studies of helminths.

hel″min·thol′o·gy [*helmins;* G. *logos,* word]. The study of parasitic worms. —**helmintholog′ic,** *adj.*

hel″min·tho′ma [*helmins;* G. *-ōma,* tumor]. A tumor caused by the presence of a parasitic worm.

hel·min″tho·pho′bi·a [*helmins;* G. *phobos,* fear]. A morbid fear of worms or of becoming infested with worms.

helmitol. Trade-mark for a brand of citramin, chemically, methenamine anhydromethylene citrate, $C_7H_8O_7(CH_2)_6N_4$. The substance is a urinary antiseptic.

Helmont, Jean Baptiste van [*Flemish physiologist and chemist,* ca. 1577–1644]. One of the founders of biochemistry. Recognized the importance of ferments and gases in physiology. Is credited with coining the word "gas." Made important contributions to pharmacology, and did basic work in urinalysis.

he′lo- [G. *helos,* marshy ground]. A combining form meaning *a marsh.*

he′lo- [G. *hēlos,* nail]. A combining form meaning *nail.*

He″lo·der′ma [*hēlos;* G. *derma,* skin]. A genus of lizards composed of two species, which are said to be the only known species of venomous lizards.

H. horridum. A species found in Mexico.

H. suspectum. A species found in Arizona and New Mexico, known as the Gila monster.

he·lo′ma [*hēlos;* G. *-ōma,* tumor]. A corn or callosity occurring on the hand or foot. *Rare.*

he·lo′ni·as [G. *helos,* marsh]. The dried rhizome and roots of *Chamaelirium luteum,* a plant of the Liliaceae; used as a tonic and diuretic.

he·lot′o·my [G. *hēlos,* nail; *tomē,* a cutting]. The cutting of a corn; surgery upon a corn.

hel·vol′ic ac′id. An antibiotic substance, now known to be identical with fumigacin.

Helweg, Hans Kristian Saxtorph [*Danish psychiatrist,* 1847–1901]. Described a tract in the upper cervical segments; this is thought to arise in the inferior olive. Called *olivospinal tract* or *Helweg's bundle.*

hem-, haem-. See *hemo-.*

he′ma-, hae′ma- (hee′muh-, hem′uh-) [G. *haima,* blood]. For words beginning with *hema-, haema-* not found here, see *hemo-.*

He″ma·cha′tus (hee″muh·kay′tus). A genus of South African snakes of the Elapidae; known as the ringhals.

H. haemachatus. A species capable of ejecting or spitting its venom at its enemies. The venom is directed toward the eyes and causes intense pain and temporary blindness.

he′ma·chrome, hae′ma·chrome [*haima;* G. *chrōma,* color]. The coloring matter of the blood; heme.

he″ma·cy·tom′e·ter. See *hemocytometer.*

he″ma·cy″to·zo′on, hae″ma·cy″to·zo′on. See *hemocytozoon.*

he″ma·drom′o·graph, hae″ma·drom′o·graph. See *hemodromograph.*

he″ma·dro·mom′e·ter, hae″ma·dro·mom′e·ter. See *hemodromometer.*

he″ma·dy·nam′ics, hae″ma·dy·nam′ics (hee″-muh·dye·nam′icks, ·di·nam′icks, hem″uh·). See *hemodynamics.*

he″ma·dy″na·mom′e·ter, hae″ma·dy″na·mom′e·ter [*haima;* G. *dynamis,* power; *metron,* a measure]. An instrument for measuring the pressure of the blood within the arteries. —**hemadynamometry,** *n.*

he″mag·glu″ti·na′tion, hae″mag·glu″ti·na′tion [*haima;* L. *agglutinare,* to glue]. The clumping of red blood cells.

cold h. Phenomenon caused by the presence of cold agglutinin.

he″mag·glu′ti·nin, hae″mag·glu′ti·nin (hee″-muh·glue′ti·nin, hem″uh·) [*haima; agglutinare*]. A substance in normal blood serum which has the power to clump red blood cells.

cold h. See cold *agglutinin.*

hemagulen. Trade-mark for a brain thromboplastic suspension useful as a hemostatic agent by topical application.

he′mal, hae′mal [*haima*]. 1. Pertaining to the blood or the vascular system. 2. Pertaining to that part of the body containing the heart and major blood vessels.

he″ma·nal′y·sis [*haima;* G. *analysis,* a loosing]. Analysis of the blood.

he·man″gi·ec′ta·sis, he·man″gi·ec·ta′si·a (hee-man″jee·eck·tay′zhuh, ·zee·uh, ·shuh, ·see·uh, hem·an″·) [*haima;* G. *aggeion,* vessel; *ektasis,* extension]. Dilatation of blood vessels. —**hemangiectat′ic,** *adj.*

he·man″gi·o·blas·to′ma [*haima; aggeion;* G. *blastos,* shoot; *-ōma,* tumor]. An aggregation of blood vessels comprising a neoplastic disorder rather than a hamartoma. Most frequently found in the cerebellum, where it may be cystic. The brain, retina, pancreas, and kidneys may be involved.

he·man″gi·o·e·las″to·myx·o′ma. A mesenchymoma.

he·man″gi·o·en″do·the″li·o·blas·to′ma. See *hemangioendothelioma.*

he·man″gi·o·en″do·the″li·o′ma [*haima; aggeion;* G. *endon,* within; *thēlē,* nipple; *-ōma*]. A locally malignant single or multiple tumor arising from blood vessels, characterized by many atypical endothelial cells and the formation of anastomosing vascular tubes.

h. of bone. See Ewing's *sarcoma.*

he·man″gi·o·en″do·the″li·o·sar·co′ma. See *hemangioendothelioma.*

he·man″gi·o·lip·o′ma. A mesenchymoma.

he·man″gi·o′ma, hae·man″gi·o′ma (hee·man″-jee·o′muh, hem·an″·) [*haima; aggeion; -ōma*]. An angioma made up of blood vessels: also called *capillary angioma.*

capillary h. Vascular tumor composed solely of capillaries.

capillary h. of granuloma type. See *granuloma pyogenicum.*

cavernous h. Vascular tumor made up of widely dilated capillaries.

multiple hemorrhagic h. of Kaposi. See multiple idiopathic hemorrhagic *sarcoma.*

sclerosing h. See *dermatofibroma.*

venous h. Vascular tumor made up of vessels containing smooth muscle cells.

he·man″gi·o·my″o·li·po′ma. A mesenchymoma.

he·man″gi·o·per·i·cy·to′ma. An uncommon tumor, usually of skin and subcutaneous tissues, arising about capillaries. It resembles a glomus tumor but characteristically exhibits irregularly proliferating, closely packed pericytes about the vessels.

he·man″gi·o·sar·co′ma [*haima; aggeion;* G. *sarkōma,* fleshy excrescence]. See *hemangioendothelioma.*

he·man′thine (hi·man′theen, ·thin). An alkaloid from *Hemanthus coccineus;* it is poisonous, with the general properties of atropine.

he″ma·poph′y·sis (hee″muh·pof′i·sis, hem″uh·) [*haima;* G. *apophysis,* process]. That part of an ideal vertebra which forms the ventrolateral part of the hemal arch. In man, all the hemapophyses are detached; represented by the ribs.

he″mar·thro′sis, hae″mar·thro′sis (hee″mahr-thro′sis, hem″ahr·) [*haima;* G. *arthron,* joint; *-ōsis,* condition]. Extravasation of blood into a joint.

he″ma·te′in, hae″ma·te′in (hee″muh·tee′in, hem″uh·, hem·at′ee·in). $C_{16}H_{12}O_6$. The reddish brown substance obtained by oxidation of hematoxylin.

he″ma·tem′e·sis, hae″ma·tem′e·sis [*haima;* G. *emesis,* vomiting]. The vomiting of blood.

he″ma·ther′mous. See *haematothermal.*

he″mat·hi·dro′sis, hae″mat·hi·dro′sis (hee″-mat·hi·dro′sis, ·high·dro′sis, hem″at·) [*haima;* G. *hydrōsis,* sweating]. An excretion of blood or blood pigments through the glands of the skin.

he·mat′ic [*haima*]. Pertaining to, full of, or having the color of, blood.

he″ma·tim′e·ter, hae″ma·tim′e·ter. Hemocytometer. **—hematimetry,** *n.*

hem′a·tin. $C_{34}H_{32}N_4O_4FeOH$; the hydroxide of ferriheme, formed by treating hemin with alkali. In hematin the iron is in the ferric state. **—hematin′ic,** *adj.*

alkaline h. A pigment suitable for hemoglobinometry made by diluting blood with 0.1 normal sodium hydroxide.

hem″a·ti·ne′mi·a, haem″a·ti·ne′mi·a [*haima; haima*]. The presence of heme in the blood.

hem″a·tin′ic [*haima*]. An agent which tends to increase the hemoglobin content of the blood.

hem″a·tin·om′e·ter. See *hemoglobinometer.*

hem″a·ti·nu′ri·a. See *hemoglobinuria.*

hem′a·tite. Ferric oxide, Fe_2O_3, containing little water of hydration; red powder. See *iron* oxide.

hem′a·to-, haem′a·to- (hem′uh·to-, hee′muh·to-), **hemat-, haemat-** [*haima*]. A combining form signifying *of* or *pertaining to the blood.*

hem″a·to·aer·om′e·ter [*haima;* G. *aēr,* air; *metron,* a measure]. A device for recording the pressure of gases in the blood.

hem′a·to·blast″ [*haima;* G. *blastos,* germ]. An immature form of erythrocyte.

hem′a·to·cele″, haem′a·to·cele″ [*haima;* G. *kēlē,* tumor]. A tumor formed by the extravasation and collection of blood in a part, especially in the cavity of the tunica vaginalis testis or the pelvis.

hem″a·to·chy′lo·cele (hem″uh·to·kigh′lo·seel, hee″muh·to·) [*haima;* G. *chylos,* juice; *kēlē*]. A tumor formed by the extravasation and collection of chyle and blood in a part, especially in the tunica vaginalis testis. It is a complication of filariasis.

hem″a·to·chy·lu′ri·a (hem″uh·to·kigh·lew′ree·uh, hee″muh·to·) [*haima; chylos;* G. *ouron,* urine]. The presence of blood and chyle in the urine.

hem″a·to·col′pos [*haima;* G. *kolpos,* vagina]. A collection of blood within the vagina.

hem′a·to·crit″, haem′a·to·crit″ (hem′uh·to-krit″) [*haima;* G. *krinein,* to separate]. 1. A small centrifuge used to separate blood cells in clinical analysis. 2. The flat-bottomed graduated centrifuge tube in which the blood cells are separated: also called *h. tube.* 3. Hematocrit reading: common usage.

hem′a·to·crit″ read′ing. The percentage of the whole blood volume occupied by the blood cells after centrifugation in a special graduated tube.

hem″a·to·crys′tal·lin, haem″a·to·crys′tal·lin. See *hemoglobin.*

hem′a·to·cyst″, haem′a·to·cyst″ [*haima;* G. *kystis,* bladder]. A cyst containing blood.

hem′a·to·cyte″, haem′a·to·cyte″. See *hemocyte.*

hem″a·to·cy·tol′y·sis (hem″uh·to·sigh·tol′i·sis, hee″muh·to·) [*haima;* G. *kytos,* cell; *lysis,* a loosing]. Hemolysis; destruction of red blood cells with setting free of the contained hemoglobin.

hem″a·to·cy·tom′e·ter, haem″a·to·cy·tom′e·ter. See *hemocytometer.*

hem″a·to·cy″to·zo′on, haem″a·to·cy″to·zo′on. See *hemocytozoon.*

hem″a·to·dy·nam′ics, haem″a·to·dy·nam′ics (hem″uh·to·dye·nam′icks, ·di·nam′icks, hee″muh-to·). See *hemodynamics.*

hem″a·to·dy″na·mom′e·ter, haem″a·to·dy″-na·mom′e·ter. See *hemadynamometer.*

hem″a·to·dys·cra′si·a (·dis·kray′zhuh, ·zee·uh, ·shuh, ·see·uh) [*haima;* G. *dys-,* hard, bad, unlucky; *krasis,* mixing]. A diseased state of the blood.

hem″a·to·gen′e·sis, haem″a·to·gen′e·sis [*haima;* G. *genesis,* production]. Hematopoiesis; formation of the blood or blood cells. **—hematogenic, hematog′enous,** *adj.*

hem″a·to·glo′bin. See *hemoglobin.*

hem″a·to·hi·dro′sis, haem″a·to·hi·dro′sis (hem″uh·to·hi·dro′sis, ·high·dro′sis, hee″muh·to·). See *hemathidrosis.*

hem″a·to·his′tone. See *globin.*

he′ma·toi′din, hae″ma·toi′din. An iron-free pigment resulting from the decomposition of hemoglobin in tissues: probably a mixture of several related pigments.

hem′a·to·krit″, haem′a·to·krit. See *hematocrit.*

hem′a·to·lith″, haem′a·to·lith″ [*haima;* G. *lithos*, stone]. Hemolith.

he″ma·tol′o·gist (hee″muh·tol′o·jist, hem″uh·) [*haima;* G. *logos*, word]. One who specializes in the study of blood.

he″ma·tol′o·gy, hae″ma·tol′o·gy [*haima; logos*]. The science of the blood, its nature, functions, and diseases. —**hematolog′ic,** *adj.*

hem″a·to·lym″phan·gi·o′ma, haem″a·to·lym″phan·gi·o′ma [*haima;* L. *lympha*, water; G. *aggeion*, vessel; *-ōma*, tumor]. A tumor composed of blood vessels and lymph vessels.

hem″a·to·lym·phu′ri·a [*haima; lympha;* G. *ouron*, urine]. The discharge of urine containing lymph and blood. Sometimes occurs in filariasis.

he″ma·tol′y·sis (hee″muh·tol′i·sis, hem″uh·) [*haima;* G. *lysis*, a loosing]. Hemolysis; destruction of red blood cells with setting free of the contained hemoglobin.

he″ma·to′ma, hae″ma·to′ma (hee″muh·to′muh, hem″uh·to′muh) [*haima; -ōma*]. A focalized extravasation of blood, which soon clots to form a solid mass and readily becomes encapsulated by connective tissue. Of such a size as to constitute a visible, tumorlike swelling. May be due to traumatic injury or to other causes of rupture of blood vessels. May constitute a false aneurysm between artery and vein in so-called varicose aneurysm, a form of arteriovenous fistula.

chronic subdural h. A hematoma lying underneath the dura, or slightly adherent to it, usually resulting from head injury and giving rise to slowly progressive symptoms and signs of cerebral compression.

dissecting h. See dissecting *aneurysm.*

tuberous subchorial h. See tuberous *mole.*

hem″a·to·me″di·as·ti′num [*haima;* NL., from *medius*, middle]. An effusion of blood into the mediastinal spaces.

he″ma·tom′e·ter [*haima;* G. *metron*, a measure]. An instrument to estimate the properties or constituents of blood. —**hematometry,** *n.*

hem″a·to·me′tra, haem″a·to·me′tra [*haima;* G. *mētra*, womb]. An accumulation of blood or menstrual fluid in the uterus.

hem″a·to·my·e′li·a, haem″a·to·my·e′li·a (hem″uh·to·migh·ee′lee·uh, hee″muh·to·) [*haima;* G. *myelos*, marrow]. Hemorrhage into the spinal cord.

hem″a·to·my″e·li′tis, haem″a·to·my″e·li′tis [*haima; myelos;* G. *-itis*, inflammation]. An acute myelitis attended with an effusion of blood into the spinal cord.

he″ma·ton′ic, hae″ma·ton′ic (hee″muh·ton′ick, hem″uh·ton′ick) [*haima;* G. *tonikos*, from *tonos*, tension]. A blood tonic which increases the hemoglobin percentage of the blood.

hem″a·to·pa·thol′o·gy, haem″a·to·pa·thol′o·gy [*haima;* G. *pathos*, disease; *logos*, word]. The science treating of diseases of the blood.

he″ma·top′a·thy (hee″muh·top′uh·thee, hem″uh·) [*haima; pathos*]. Any disease of the blood.

hem″a·to·per″i·car′di·um, haem″a·to·per″i·car′di·um. See *hemopericardium.*

hem″a·to·per″i·to·ne′um, haem″a·to·per″i·to·ne′um. See *hemoperitoneum.*

hem′a·to·phage″, haem′a·to·phage″ (hem′uh·to·faydj″, hee′muh·to·). See *hemophage.*

hem″a·to·pha′gi·a, haem″a·to·pha′gi·a. See *hemophagia.*

hem″a·toph′a·gus [*haima;* G. *phagein*, to eat]. A bloodsucking insect. —**hematophagous,** *adj.*

hem″a·to·phil′i·a, haem″a·to·phil′i·a. See *hemophilia.*

hem″a·to·pho′bi·a. Hemophobia.

hem′a·to·phyte″, haem′a·to·phyte″ [*haima;* G. *phyton*, plant]. A vegetable organism, such as a bacterium, living in the blood.

hem″a·to·plas′tic, haem″a·to·plas′tic [*haima;* G. *plassein*, to form]. Blood-forming.

hem″a·to·poi·e′sis, haem″a·to·poi·e′sis [*haima;* G. *poiēsis*, production]. The formation of blood. —**hematopoiet′ic,** *adj.*

extramedullary h. See ectopic *myelopoiesis.*

hem″a·to·por·phy′ri·a, haem″a·to·por·phy′ri·a (hem″uh·to·por·figh′ree·uh, hee″muh·to·). See *porphyria.*

hem″a·to·por′phy·rin. $C_{34}H_{38}O_6N_4$. Iron-free heme. A porphyrin obtained in vitro by treating hemoglobin with sulfuric acid. It is closely related to the naturally occurring porphyrins.

hem″a·to·por″phy·ri·ne′mi·a, haem″a·to·por″phy·ri·ne′mi·a (hem″uh·to·por″fi·ri·nee′mee·uh, ·por″figh·ri·nee′mee·uh, hee″muh·to·) [*haima;* G. *porphyra*, purple-fish; *haima*]. Presence of hematoporphyrin in the blood.

hem″a·to·por″phy·ri·nu′ri·a, haem″a·to·por″phy·ri·nu′ri·a (hem″uh·to·por″fi·ri·new′ree·uh, ·por″figh·ri·new′ree·uh, hee″muh·to·) [*haima; porphyra;* G. *ouron*, urine]. The presence of hematoporphyrin in the urine.

hem″a·to·pre·cip′i·tin, haem″a·to·pre·cip′i·tin [*haima;* L. *praecipitare*, to precipitate]. A precipitin specific for blood.

hem″a·tor·rha′chis (hem″uh·to·ray′kis, hee″muh·to·, hem″uh·tor′uh·kis) [*haima;* G. *rhachis*, spine]. Hemorrhage into the spinal meninges producing irritative phenomena.

hem″a·tor·rhe′a [*haima;* G. *rhoia*, flow]. Copious or profuse hemorrhage.

hem″a·to·sal′pinx, haem″a·to·sal′pinx [*haima;* G. *salpigx*, trumpet]. A collection of blood in a uterine tube.

hem′a·to·scope [*haima;* G. *skopein*, to examine]. An instrument used in the spectroscopic examination of the blood, by means of which the thickness of the layer of the blood can be regulated.

hem′a·tose, haem′a·tose (hem′uh·toce, hee′muh·toce) [*haima*]. Full of blood.

hem″a·to·si·phon·i′a·sis. The polymorphous dermatitis, caused by the bite of *Hematosiphon inodora* (Duges), generally localized on the extremities and exposed parts of the body and accompanied by intense itching and systemic manifestations following secondary infection.

he″ma·to′sis (hee″muh·to′sis, hem″uh·) [*haima;* G. *-ōsis*, condition]. The process of the formation of blood; the arterialization of blood.

hem″a·to·so·nog′ra·phy. Quantitative study of blood clotting with an ultrasonic device.

hem″a·to·spec′tro·scope, haem″a·to·spec′tro·scope [*haima;* L. *spectrum*, image; G. *skopein*, to examine]. A spectroscope adapted to the study of the blood. —**hematospectros′copy,** *n.*

hem″a·to·sper′ma·to·cele″, haem″a·to·sper′ma·to·cele″ (hem″uh·to·spur′muh·to·seel″, ·spur·mat′o·seel, hee″muh·to·) [*haima;* G. *sperma*, seed; *kēlē*, tumor]. A spermatocele containing blood.

hem″a·to·sper′mi·a, haem″a·to·sper′mi·a [*haima; sperma*]. The discharge of bloody semen.

hem″a·to·stat′ic, haem″a·to·stat′ic. See *hemostatic.*

hem″a·to·ther′a·py, haem″a·to·ther′a·py. See *hemotherapy.*

hem″a·to·ther′mal. See *haematothermal.*

hem″a·to·tho′rax, haem″a·to·tho′rax. See *hemothorax.*

hem″a·to·tym′pa·num [*haima;* G. *tympanon*, drum]. Blood in the tympanic cavity.

he″ma·tox′y·lin (hee″muh·tock′si·lin, hem″uh·)

(C.C.). $C_{16}H_{14}O_6$. A colorless crystalline compound occurring in logwood. Upon oxidation, it is converted to hematein, the coloring matter of logwood. Used as a stain in microscopy.

chrome h. See under *stain*.

Delafield's h. See under *stain*.

Ehrlich's h. See under *stain*.

he″ma·tox′y·lon, hae″ma·tox′y·lon (hee″muh-tock′si·lon, hem″uh·) [*haima;* G. *xylon*, wood]. Logwood. The heartwood of *Haematoxylon campechianum;* contains tannic acid and a coloring principle, hematoxylin, and is a mild astringent.

hem″a·to·zo′on, haem″a·to·zo′on (pl. *hematozoa*) [*haima;* G. *zōion*, living being]. Any animal parasite living in the blood. —**hematozoal, hematozoic,** *adj.*

hem″a·tu′ri·a (hem″uh·tew′ree·uh, hee″muh·) [*haima;* G. *ouron*, urine]. The discharge of urine containing blood: often associated with diseases of the kidney.

false h. The passage of red urine, due to the ingestion of food or drugs containing red pigments.

heme (heem). $C_{34}H_{32}N_4O_4Fe$; the ferrous complex of protoporphyrin 9, constituting the prosthetic component of hemoglobin. If the iron of heme is oxidized to the ferric state, the higher valence of the iron imparts a positive charge which in alkaline solution attracts a hydroxyl ion, forming hematin, and in hydrochloric acid solution attracts a chloride ion, forming hemin. Heme combines with a variety of nitrogenous bases, forming hemochromogens; the cytochromes and hemoglobin are compounds of this type. Syn., *ferroheme, reduced heme, ferroprotoporphyrin 9.*

hem″er·a·lo′pi·a [G. *hēmera*, day; *alaos*, blind; *ōps*, eye]. Day blindness; frequently incorrectly used to describe the condition of reduced dark adaptation resulting temporarily from vitamin-A deficiency or permanently from retinitis pigmentosa or other peripheral retinal diseases. See also *night blindness.*

hem″er·a·pho′ni·a [*hēmera;* G. *phōnē*, voice]. Loss of voice during the day, and recovery of it at night; a hysterical symptom.

he″me·ryth′rin, hae″me·ryth′rin (hee″mi·rith′-rin, hem″i·, heh·merr′i·thrin). See *hemoerythrin.*

hem′i- [G. *hēmi-*, half]. 1. A prefix signifying *half.* 2. *In biology* and *medicine*, a prefix denoting either *the right* or *the left half of the body.* 3. *In chemistry,* a prefix denoting *a combining ratio of one-half.*

hem″i·a·blep′si·a. See *hemianopsia.*

hem″i·a·car′di·us [*hēmi-;* G. *a-*, not; *kardia*, heart]. A placental parasitic twin (omphalosite) in which the principal parts of a fetus are recognizable, with a more or less well-formed, rudimentary heart.

hem″i·a·ceph′a·lus [*hēmi-; a-;* G. *kephalē*, head]. Anencephalus.

hem″i·a·geu′si·a (hem″ee·ag·yoo′see·uh, hem″ee-a·jew′see·uh) [*hēmi-; a-;* G. *geusis*, sense of taste]. Loss or diminution of the sense of taste on one side of the tongue, usually caused by injury to the chorda tympani nerve.

hem″i·al′bu·mose [*hēmi-;* L. *albus*, white]. A product of the digestion of certain kinds of proteins. It is a normal constituent of bone marrow, and is found also in the urine of patients with osteomalacia. Also called *propeptone.*

hem″i·al·bu″mo·su′ri·a [*hēmi-; albus;* G. *ouron*, urine]. The presence of hemialbumose in the urine; propeptonuria.

hem″i·am″bly·o′pi·a. See *hemianopsia.*

hem″i·an″a·cu′si·a (hem″ee·an″uh·cue′zhuh, ·zee·uh, ·shuh, ·see·uh) [*hēmi-;* G. *a-*, not; *akousis*, hearing]. Deafness in one ear. *Obs.*

hem″i·an″al·ge′si·a (·an″al·jee′zee·uh, ·see·uh) [*hēmi-;* G. *analgēsia*, want of feeling]. Analgesia of one lateral half of the body and limbs.

hem″i·an″en·ceph′a·ly [*hēmi-; a-;* G. *egkephalos*, brain]. Anencephalia on one lateral half only.

hem″i·an″es·the′si·a (·an″ess·thee′zhuh, ·zee·uh) [*hēmi-;* G. *anaisthēsia*, lack of sensation]. Anesthesia of either lateral half of the body.

alternate h. That affecting one side of the head and the opposite side of the body.

cerebral h. That due to a lesion in the internal capsule or in the lenticular nucleus.

crossed h. See alternate *h.*

hysterical h. Hemianesthesia as a manifestation of hysteria.

hem″i·an·op′si·a [*hēmi-;* G. *a-*, not; *opsis*, vision]. Blindness in one half of the visual field; may be bilateral or unilateral. Also called *hemiopia, hemianopia.*

binasal h. Blindness on the nasal side of the visual field, usually due to disease of the outer sides of the optic commissure.

bitemporal h. Blindness on the temporal side of the visual field, due to disease of the central parts of the optic commissure.

heteronymous h. A general term for either binasal or bitemporal hemianopsia.

homonymous h. The form affecting the inner half of one field and the outer half of the other.

lateral h. A form in which the temporal half of one visual field and the nasal half of the other visual field are wanting; a vertical line through the center of vision sharply defines the defect. Syn., *vertical h.*

quadrantic h. Blindness in one quadrant; may be bitemporal or homonymous.

vertical h. See lateral *h.*

hem″i·a·tax′i·a [*hēmi-;* G. *ataxia*, disorder]. Ataxia affecting one side of the body.

hem″i·ath″e·to′sis [*hēmi-;* G. *athetos*, not fixed; *-ōsis*, condition]. Athetosis of one side of the body.

hem″i·at′ro·phy [*hēmi-;* G. *atrophia*, want of food]. Atrophy confined to one side of an organ or region of the body.

hem″i·bal·lis′mus, hem″i·bal′lism [*hēmi-;* G. *ballismos*, a jumping about]. A form of hemichorea, characterized by sudden, violent, spasmodic movements of the extremities of one side of the body. Caused by a destructive lesion of the subthalamic nucleus. The condition ceases suddenly if a true hemiplegia intervenes.

Hem·i·bi′a [G. *hēmibios*, half-alive]. A genus of operculate snails found only in the Far East. The species **H. hupensis** and **H. quadrasi** serve as intermediate hosts of *Schistosoma japonicum.*

he′mic, hae′mic (hee′mick, hem′ick) [G. *haima*, blood]. Pertaining to or developed by the blood.

hem″i·car′di·a [G. *hēmi-*, half; *cardia*, heart]. The presence of only a lateral half of the usual four-chambered heart.

hem″i·cel′lu·lose. A group of high molecular weight carbohydrates resembling cellulose but less complex.

hem″i·ceph′a·lus [*hēmi-;* G. *kephalē*, head]. A monster exhibiting hemicephaly.

hem″i·ceph′a·ly [*hēmi-; kephalē*]. A congenital anomaly with absence of cerebrum but with rudimentary cerebellum and basal ganglions; partial anencephalia.

hem″i·cho·re′a (hem″ee·kor·ee′uh) [*hēmi-;* G. *choreia*, dance]. A form of chorea in which the convulsive movements are confined to one side of the body.

hem″i·co·lec′to·my [*hēmi-;* G. *kolon*, colon; *ektomē*, excision]. Excision of a part of the colon.

hem″i·col′lin. An intermediate product, of indefinite composition, obtained on hydrolysis of gelatin.

hem″i·cra′ni·a [*hēmi-;* G. *kranion,* skull]. 1. Migraine. 2. Pain or headache on one side of the head only. 3. Partial anencephalia.

hem″i·cra″ni·o′sis [*hēmi-; kranion;* G. *-ōsis,* condition]. Enlargement of one half of the cranium or face.

hem″i·de·cor″ti·ca′tion. Removal of the cortex from one cerebral hemisphere.

hem″i·des′mus (hem″i·dez′mus, ·des′mus) [*hēmi-;* G. *desmos,* band]. Indian sarsaparilla. The dried root of *Hemidesmus indicus,* imported from India. It contains coumarin and a volatile oil consisting chiefly of 2-hydroxy-4-methoxy benzaldehyde. An infusion has been used as a diuretic.

hem″i·di′a·phragm [*hēmi-;* G. *diaphragma,* diaphragm]. 1. A lateral half of the diaphragm. 2. A half diaphragm, designating a diaphragm in which the muscle development is deficient on one side.

hem″i·dro′sis, haem″i·dro′sis. See *hemathidrosis.*

hem′i·dys″es·the′si·a [*hēmi-;* G. *dys,* bad; *aisthēsis,* feeling]. Dysesthesia involving one lateral half of the body.

hem″i·fa′cial [*hēmi-;* L. *facies,* form, face]. Pertaining to one lateral half of the face.

hem″i·glos·sec′to·my [*hēmi-;* G. *glōssa;* tongue; *ektomē,* excision]. Removal of one lateral half of the tongue.

hem″i·glos″so·ple′gi·a [*hēmi-; glōssa;* G. *plēgē,* stroke]. Unilateral paralysis of the tongue with relatively minor disturbances of motility; the tongue deviates toward the palsied side upon protrusion.

hem″i·gna′thi·a (hem″ee·nayth′ee·uh, hem″ee·nath′ee·uh) [*hēmi-;* G. *gnathos,* jaw]. Partial or complete absence of the lower jaw on one side. —**hemignath′us,** *n.*

hem″i·hy″pal·ge′si·a (hem″ee·high″pal·jee′zee·uh, ·see·uh) [*hēmi-;* G. *hypo,* under; *algēsis,* sense of pain]. Hypalgesia, or decreased sensitivity to pain, on one lateral half of the body.

hem″i·hy″per·es·the′si·a (·high″pur·ess·thee′·zhuh, ·zee·uh) [*hēmi-;* G. *hyper,* over; *aisthēsis,* perception]. Increased sensitivity on one lateral half of the body.

hem″i·hy″per·hi·dro′sis (·high″pur·hi·dro′sis, ·high″pur·high·dro′sis) [*hēmi-; hyper;* G. *hidrōsis,* sweating]. Excessive sweating on one side of the body.

hem″i·hy″per·to′ni·a [*hēmi-; hyper;* G. *tonos,* tone]. Increased muscular tonicity confined to one half of the body; may occur following apoplexy.

hem″i·hy·per′tro·phy [*hēmi-; hyper;* G. *trophē,* nourishment]. Hypertrophy of half of the body or unilateral hypertrophy of one or more bodily regions (e.g., the head, an arm).

hem″i·hy″pes·the′si·a (hem″ee·high″pes·thee′·zhuh, ·zee·uh) [*hēmi-;* G. *hypo,* under; *aisthēsis,* perception]. Decreased sensitivity in one lateral half of the body.

hem″i·hy″po·to′ni·a [*hēmi-; hypo;* G. *tonos,* tone]. Partial loss of tonicity of one side of the body.

hem″i·lab″y·rin·thec′to·my [*hēmi-;* G. *labyrinthos,* labyrinth; *ektomē,* excision]. Removal of one or more of the membranous semicircular canals while leaving the ampullated ends and the saccule.

hem″i·lam″i·nec′to·my [*hēmi-;* L. *lamina,* plate; *ektomē*]. Laminectomy in which laminas of only one side are removed.

hem″i·lar″yn·gec′to·my (hem″ee·lar″in·jeck′to·mee) [*hēmi-;* G. *larygx,* larynx; *ektomē*]. Extirpation of one lateral half of the larynx.

hem″i·man″di·bu·lec′to·my. The surgical removal of one lateral half of the mandible.

hem″i·me′lus [*hēmi-;* G. *melos,* limb]. An individual with incomplete or stunted extremities.

hem″i·me·tab′o·lous [*hēmi-;* G. *metabolē,* change]. Pertaining to a mode of insect metamorphosis in which the immature stage, known as a nymph, transforms into the adult without an intervening, quiescent, pupal stage; as in grasshoppers, crickets, roaches, the true bugs, Mayflies, stone flies, and dragonflies.

he′min. $C_{34}H_{32}N_4O_4FeCl$; the chloride of ferriheme, containing iron in the ferric state. It is formed by heating hemoglobin with glacial acetic acid in the presence of sodium chloride, reddish-brown crystals (Teichmann's crystals) being produced; this is the basis of a test for blood.

hem″i·ne·phrec′to·my [*hēmi-;* G. *nephros,* kidney; *ektomē,* excision]. Removal of part of a kidney.

hem″i·o′pi·a. Hemianopsia. —**hemiop′ic,** *adj.*

he·mip′a·gus [*hēmi-;* G. *pagos,* that which is fixed]. Conjoined twins united laterally by the thoraces and necks and in some cases also by the jaws. Syn., *prosopothoracopagus.*

hem″i·pal″a·to·la·ryn″go·ple′gi·a [*hēmi-;* L. *palatum,* palate; G. *larygx,* larynx; *plēgē,* stroke]. Paralysis of the muscles of the soft palate and larynx on one side.

hem″i·pa·re′sis, hem″i·par′e·sis [*hēmi-;* G. *paresis,* paralysis]. Paresis of one side of the body.

hem″i·pel·vect′o·my [*hēmi-;* L. *pelvis,* basin; G. *ektomē,* a cutting]. The surgical removal of an entire posterior extremity including the hipbone.

hem″i·pin′to. A unilateral distribution of the cutaneous eruption of pinta.

hem″i·ple′gi·a [*hēmi-;* G. *plēgē,* stroke]. Paralysis of one side of the body. —**hemipleg′ic,** *adj.*

alternate h. Paralysis of the facial muscles or tongue on one side of the body, and of the trunk and the extremities on the other side. Also called *crossed h., h. cruciata.*

capsular h. A hemiplegia due to a lesion in the internal capsule.

cerebral h. That resulting from a lesion of the brain.

congenital h. A spastic type due to a birth injury. Also called *infantile h.*

contralateral h. A paralysis of one side of the body due to a lesion of the opposite side of the brain.

crossed h. See alternate *h.*

facial h. Motor paralysis of one side of the face.

infantile h. Unilateral spastic paralysis of arm, leg, and face, caused by heterogeneous lesions of the contralateral cerebral hemisphere. Characteristically there is adduction at the shoulder, flexion at the elbow, pronation and flexion of the wrist, and sometimes equinovarus deformity of the foot. Choreoathetosis, epilepsy, or mental retardation may be present.

spastic h. A form characterized by rigidity of the affected extremities.

spinal h. One due to a lesion of the spinal cord.

He·mip′ter·a [*hēmi-;* G. *pteron,* wing]. An order of insects; the true bugs. Formerly the suborder Heteroptera of the order Hemiptera which also included the suborder Homoptera.

H. heteroptera. Formerly a suborder, now classified as the order Heteroptera.

hem″i·py″o·cy′a·nin. See under *pyo compounds.*

hem″i·ra·chis′chi·sis (hem″ee·ra·kis′ki·sis) [*hēmi-;* G. *rhachis,* spine; *schisis,* cleavage]. Incomplete spina bifida. See *spina* bifida occulta.

hem″i·scler·o·der′ma al′ter·nans. A skin disease characterized by indurated, and later degenerative, lesions, atrophy, and sclerosis, resulting in discoloration, pigmentation, or vitiligo, often accompanied by fibrosis and atrophy of the underlying muscles and atrophy of the underlying bones. It occurs in zones corresponding to the metameres, indicating a neurogenic influence.

hem″i·sco·to′sis [*hēmi-;* G. *skotōsis,* a darkening]. A dark spot in one half of the visual field.

hem″i·sec′tion [*hēmi-;* L. *sectum,* from *secare,* to cut]. Act of division into two lateral halves; bisection. —**hemisect′,** *v.t.*

h. of the spinal cord. A section of one lateral half of the spinal cord. See also Brown-Séquard's *paralysis.*

hem″i·so′mus [*hēmi-;* G. *sōma,* body]. An individual with one side of the body imperfectly developed.

hem′i·spasm [*hēmi-;* G. *spasmos,* spasm]. A spasm affecting only one side of the body.

hem′i·sphere [*hēmi-;* G. *sphaira,* ball]. The lateral half of the cerebrum or cerebellum.

dominant h. The cerebral hemisphere which controls certain motor activities, such as movements of speech; usually the left hemisphere in right-handed individuals.

hem″i·spher·ec′to·my [*hemi-;* G. *sphaira,* a ball; *ektomē,* a cutting]. Surgical excision of one cerebral hemisphere.

He·mis′po·ra [*hēmi-;* G. *spora,* seed]. A genus of fungi whose species are contaminants.

H. stellata. A species which has been found in osteoperiostitis, cold abscesses, and sporotrichoid lesions.

hem″i·spo·ro′sis [*hēmi-; spora;* G. *-ōsis,* condition]. Infection by *Hemispora.*

hem″i·syn·er′gi·a [*hēmi-;* G. *synergos,* working together]. Synergia on one lateral half of the body; due to asynergia on the opposite side.

hem″i·sys′to·le (hem″ee·sis′to·lee) [*hēmi-.;* G *systolē,* contraction]. Contraction of the left ventricle after every second atrial contraction so that for each two beats of the heart only one pulse beat is felt.

hem″i·ter′a·ta [*hēmi-;* G. *teras,* monster]. Individuals with malformations not grave enough to be called monstrous. —**hemiterat′ic,** *adj.*

hem″i·ter′pene. Any of a group of hydrocarbons of the general formula C_5H_8, as isoprene, related to terpenes.

hem″i·thy″roid·ec′to·my [*hēmi-;* G. *thyreoeidēs,* shield-shaped; *ektomē,* excision]. Removal of one lateral lobe of the thyroid gland.

hem″i·ver′te·bra [*hēmi-;* L. *vertebra,* vertebra]. A congenital anomaly of the spine in which one lateral half of a vertebra fails to develop, resulting in the absence of half of the vertebra.

hem″i·zo′na. See *herpes* zoster.

hem″i·zy′gote [*hēmi-;* G. *zygōtos,* yoked]. An individual with only one of a given pair of genes, as in the case of the sex-linked genes in the human male; or with only one of each of all the pairs of genes, as in the male bee. —**hemizygous,** *adj.*

hem′lock [AS. *hemlic*]. 1. An evergreen tree (genus *Tsuga*) of North America and Asia. 2. A large herb (*Conium maculata*) of the carrot family which yields coniine: also called **poison hemlock.** See *conium.*

he′mo-, hae′mo- (hee′mo-, hem′o-) [G. *haima,* blood]. A combining form signifying *of* or *pertaining to the blood.*

he″mo·al″ka·lim′e·ter, hae″mo·al″ka·lim′e·ter [*haima;* Ar. *al-qili,* ashes of saltwort; G. *metron,* a measure]. An apparatus for estimating the degree of alkalinity of the blood.

he″mo·bil″i·ru′bin (·bil″i·rōō′bin) [*haima;* L. *bilis,* bile; *ruber,* red]. 1. Bilirubin as it occurs normally in serum before passing through the hepatic cells. 2. The form of bilirubin present normally in blood serum, which is increased in amount in hemolytic jaundice. It gives a negative direct van den Bergh reaction, is determined quantitatively by the indirect reaction, and is extracted by chloroform. Also see *cholebilirubin.*

he′mo·blast, hae′mo·blast. A primitive blood cell. See stem *cell.*

he″mo·cho′ri·al (hee″mo·kor′ee·ul, hem″o·) [*haima;* G. *chorion,* chorion]. Pertaining to maternal blood and chorionic ectoderm.

he″mo·chro″ma·to′sis [*haima;* G. *chrōma,* color; *-ōsis,* condition]. A disease characterized by pigmentation of the skin, cirrhosis, and diabetes mellitus, accompanied by excessive deposition of iron-containing pigments in parenchymal tissues, particularly the liver and pancreas. The cutaneous pigmentation is due only in part to iron-containing pigments. —**hemochromatot′ic,** *adj.*

he″mo·chro′mo·gen. The compound formed by the union of heme with a nitrogen-containing substance, as a protein or base.

he″mo·chro·mom′e·ter, hae″mo·chro·mom′e·ter [*haima; chrōma;* G. *metron,* a measure]. Colorimeter; an instrument for estimating the amount of hemoglobin in the blood, by comparing a solution of the blood with a standard solution of picrocarminate of ammonium.

he″mo·cla′si·a, hae″mo·cla′si·a (hee″mo·klay′zhuh, ·zee·uh, hem″o·) **he″moc′la·sis, hae″moc′la·sis** [*haima;* G. *klasis,* a breaking]. Hemolysis; destruction of the erythrocytes. —**hemoclas′tic,** *adj.*

he″mo·con″cen·tra′tion, hae″mo·con″cen·tra′tion [*haima;* L. *con-,* together; *centrum,* center]. An increase in the concentration of blood cells resulting from the loss of plasma or water from the blood stream; anhydremia.

he″mo·co′ni·a, hae″mo·co′ni·a [*haima;* G. *konia,* dust]. Minute, colorless, highly refractive particles of fat found in the blood. Also called *blood dust, chylomicrons.*

he″mo·co″ni·o′sis, hae″mo·co″ni·o′sis [*haima; konia;* G. *-ōsis,* increase]. The condition of having an abnormal amount of hemoconia in the blood.

he″mo·cry·os′co·py, hae″mo·cry·os′co·py (hee″mo·krye·os′ko·pee, hem″o·) [*haima;* G. *kryos,* icy cold; *skopein,* to examine]. Determining the freezing point of the blood.

he″mo·cu′pre·in. A copper protein, having a molecular weight of about 35,000 and containing 2 atoms of copper per molecule, obtained from erythrocytes of several animals.

he″mo·cy′a·nin, hae″mo·cy′a·nin [*haima;* G. *kyanos,* blue]. A respiratory pigment which contains copper, found in the blood of certain invertebrates.

he′mo·cyte, hae′mo·cyte [*haima;* G. *kytos,* cell]. A blood cell.

he″mo·cy′to·blast, hae″mo·cy′to·blast [*haima; kytos;* G. *blastos,* germ]. 1. The cell considered by some to be the primitive stem cell, giving rise to all blood cells. Syn., *lymphoidocyte.* 2. In some terminologies, a large lymphocyte which, under certain conditions, may be a precursor of monocytes and granulocytes (Maximow). —**hemocytoblas′tic,** *adj.*

he″mo·cy″to·blas·to′ma. See stem-cell *leukemia.*

he″mo·cy″to·gen′e·sis, hae″mo·cy″to·gen′e·sis. Hematopoiesis.

he″mo·cy·tol′y·sis, hae″mo·cy·tol′y·sis (hee″mo·sigh·tol′i·sis, hem″o·) [*haima; kytos;* G. *lysis,* a loosing]. The dissolution of blood cells.

he″mo·cy·tom′e·ter, hae″mo·cy·tom′e·ter [*haima; kytos;* G. *metron,* a measure]. An instrument for estimating the number of blood cells. —**hemocytom′etry,** *n.*

he″mo·cy″to·poi·e′sis. Hematopoiesis.

he″mo·cy″to·zo′on, hae″mo·cy″to·zo′on [*haima; kytos;* G. *zōion,* living being]. A protozoan parasite inhabiting the red blood cells.

he·mo′di·a [G. *haimōdiaein,* to set the teeth on edge]. Hypersensitivity of the teeth.

he″mo·di″ag·no′sis, hae″mo·di″ag·no′sis [G. *haima,* blood; *diagnōsis,* a deciding]. Diagnosis by examination of the blood.

he″mo·di·al′y·sis. The process of exposing blood to a semipermeable membrane, thereby removing from it or adding to it diffusible materials, rate and direction being a function of the concentration gradient across that membrane.

he″mo·di′a·stase. The amylolytic enzyme of blood.

he″mo·di·lu′tion [*haima;* L. *diluere,* to dilute]. A condition of the blood in which the ratio of blood cells to plasma is reduced.

he″mo·drom′o·graph, hae″mo·drom′o·graph [*haima;* G. *dromos,* course; *graphein,* to write]. An instrument for registering small variations in the velocity of the blood stream.

he″mo·dro·mom′e·ter, hae″mo·dro·mom′e·ter [*haima; dromos;* G. *metron,* a measure]. An instrument for measuring the velocity of the blood current. —**hemodromom′etry,** *n.*

he″mo·dy·nam′ics, hae″mo·dy·nam′ics (hee″-mo·dye·nam′icks, ·di·nam′icks, hem″o·) [*haima;* G. *dynamis,* power]. The study of how the physical properties of the blood and its circulation through the vessels affect blood flow and pressure.

he″mo·dy″na·mom′e·ter, hae″mo·dy″na-mom′e·ter. See *hemadynamometer.*

he″mo·en″do·the′li·al [*haima;* G. *endon,* within; *thēlē,* nipple]. Pertaining to maternal blood and to the endothelium of the chorionic villi.

he″mo·e·ryth′rin, hae″mo·e·ryth′rin (hee″mo-eh·rith′rin, hem″o·, hem″o·err′i·thrin) [*haima;* G. *erythros,* red]. A red pigment found in the blood of worms and other invertebrates.

he″mo·flag′el·late, hae″mo·flag′el·late (hee″-mo·fladj′i·late, hem″o·) [*haima;* L. *flagellare,* to whip]. Any protozoan flagellate living in the blood of its host.

he″mo·fo′lin. An unidentified factor, essential for growth of *Leuconostoc citrovorum* but apparently not a folinic acid, produced by incubating hemopoietic tissue (human leukocytes or myeloid elements of bone marrow) with folic acid.

he″mo·fus′cin, hae″mo·fus′cin (hee″mo·fuss′in, hem″o·) [*haima;* L. *fuscus,* dark]. A yellow or brown pigment of unknown origin which gradually accumulates in smooth and cardiac muscle with age and is one of the two principal pigments of hemochromatosis. It contains no iron, but considerable sulfur, and has been suggested as being related to melanin.

he″mo·gen′e·sis, hae″mo·gen′e·sis. See *hematogenesis.*

hemo-genin. A proprietary multivitamin capsule with ferrous gluconate.

he″mo·glo′bin, hem″o·glo′bin [*haima;* L. *globus,* ball]. The respiratory pigment of erythrocytes, having the reversible property of taking up oxygen (**oxyhemoglobin, HbO$_2$**) or of releasing it (**reduced hemoglobin, Hb**), depending primarily on the oxygen tension of the medium surrounding it. At tensions of 100 mm Hg or more, hemoglobin is fully saturated with oxygen; at 50 mm Hg, oxygen is progressively more rapidly dissociated. Other factors affecting dissociation of oxyhemoglobin are temperature, electrolytes, and carbon dioxide tension (*Bohr effect*). Human hemoglobin consists of four heme molecules (iron-protoporphyrin) linked to the protein, *globin,* which is composed of complexly folded polypeptide chains. Globin may vary in its essential properties, resulting in definite normal and genetically determined abnormal types, which may be differentiated on biochemical, pathophysiological, and genetic bases; it may differ in the fetus and in the adult, and also in different animal species. The average molecular weight of hemoglobin is about 67,000. Hemoglobin combines with carbon monoxide to form the stable compound **carboxyhemoglobin.** Oxidation of the ferrous iron of hemoglobin to the ferric state produces **methemoglobin** (also called *ferrihemoglobin*). Abbreviated Hb. Syn., *ferrohemoglobin.* See Table of Normal Values of Blood Constituents and American Classification of Proteins, in the Appendix.

fetal (F) h. The type of hemoglobin present in amounts of 50%–90% at birth and gradually replaced by normal adult hemoglobin; it continues to be present, and may be produced, in small amounts normally after the third year of life. It is distinguished from all other types by its resistance to denaturation by alkali. See *one-minute denaturation value.* It is found in abnormally large amounts in sickle-cell anemia, thalassemia, and sometimes in hereditary spherocytosis, and in some acquired hematologic disorders, as leukemia, lymphoma, multiple myeloma, and aplastic anemia.

h. carbamate. Carbaminohemoglobin.

mean corpuscular h. See *MCH.*

mean corpuscular h. concentration. See *MCHC.*

normal adult (A) h. The type of hemoglobin found in normal adults, which moves as a single component in an electrophoretic field, is rapidly denatured by highly alkaline solutions, and contains two titratable sulfhydryl groups per molecule. It forms orthorhombic crystals. Specific A hemoglobin antibodies have been obtained.

sickle-cell (S) h. The type found in sickle-cell anemia, which moves more rapidly than normal adult (A) hemoglobin in the Tiselius apparatus at pH 6.1, and which contains three titratable sulfhydryl groups per molecule. In its reduced form, S hemoglobin is only one-hundredth times as soluble as oxy-S-hemoglobin, and, most importantly, the molecules line up in an orderly arrangement (tectoids) resulting in the sickled shape of the erythrocytes. In high concentration, S hemoglobin will gel. In sickle-cell anemia, S hemoglobin comprises 75% or more of total hemoglobin, the remainder being of the fetal (F) type; in the heterozygous condition, sickle-cell trait, type S comprises from 20% to 50%, the remainder being the normal adult (A) type of hemoglobin.

type C h. The hemoglobin which has the greatest motility of the types thus far observed in the electrophoretic field of the Tiselius apparatus at pH 6.1. It is found in a variant of sickle-cell anemia in combination with sickle-cell hemoglobin (type S), or with both the S type and the fetal hemoglobin (F type). It is also encountered in the heterozygous condition (A and C hemoglobin), the homozygous condition resulting in a hemolytic process, and in the C variant of thalassemia in combination with normal and fetal hemoglobin.

type D h. A rare type, resembling sickle-cell hemoglobin (S) in its electrophoretic mobility, but being more soluble. It is encountered in a rare variant of sickle-cell anemia (S and D hemoglobin).

type E h. A rare type, recently reported, and thought to occur frequently in Thailand, probably producing an anemia resembling thalassemia.

he″mo·glo″bi·ne′mi·a, hae″mo·glo″bi·ne′mi·a [*haima; globus; haima*]. A condition in which the hemoglobin is dissolved out of the red cells, and is held in solution in the serum.

he″mo·glo″bin·if′er·ous [*haima; globus*]. Yielding or carrying hemoglobin.

he″mo·glo″bi·nom′e·ter, hae″mo·glo″bi·nom′e·ter [*haima; globus;* G. *metron*, a measure]. An instrument for determining the hemoglobin concentration of the blood. —**hemoglobinometry,** *n.*

Newcomer h. A small colorimeter with colored glass standards.

Riecker-Dare h. One of the simplest of the more accurate clinical instruments based on comparison of a film of undiluted blood of uniform depth with a red glass plate of graduated intensity which has been suitably standardized.

he″mo·glo″bi·no·phil′ic, hae″mo·glo″bi·no·phil′ic. See *hemophilic*, 1.

he″mo·glo″bi·nu′ri·a [*haima; globus;* G. *ouron*, urine]. The presence of hemoglobin in the urine, due either to its solution out of the red cells or to disintegration of the red cells. —**hemoglobinuric,** *adj.*

epidemic h. Hemoglobinuria of the newborn; associated with jaundice, cyanosis, and nervous symptoms. Also called *Winckel's disease.*

march h. A paroxysmal hemoglobinuria noted in soldiers after strenuous marching.

paroxysmal h. A form characterized by repeated acute attacks of hemoglobinuria; it can occur in malaria. See paroxysmal cold *h.*, paroxysmal nocturnal *h.*

paroxysmal cold h. A rare disorder characterized by the sudden passage of hemoglobin in the urine following local or general exposure to cold, often considered a manifestation of syphilis.

paroxysmal nocturnal h. A rare disorder of insidious onset and chronic course characterized by hemolytic anemia and marked attacks of hemoglobinuria occurring chiefly at night. The defect lies with the erythrocytes which cannot tolerate lowering of the blood pH, such as occurs at night.

toxic h. That form due to poisoning.

he′mo·gram [*haima;* G. *gramma*, letter]. A differential count of the white cells to show the qualitative as well as the quantitative variations in the cells.

he″mo·his′ti·o·blast [*haima;* G. *histion*, web; *blastos*, germ]. The hypothetical reticuloendothelial cell from which all the cells of the blood are eventually differentiated; a stem cell.

he″mo·hy·per·ox′i·a. Any elevation of the oxygen tension of the blood above that normally existing at sea level.

he″mo·hy·pox′i·a. Any depression of the oxygen tension of the blood below that normally existing at sea level.

he″mo·ko′ni·a, hae″mo·ko′ni·a. See *hemoconia.*

he″mo·ko″ni·o′sis, hae″mo·ko″ni·o′sis. See *hemoconiosis.*

he′mo·lith [*haima;* G. *lithos*, stone]. A stone or concretion within the lumen of a blood vessel, or incorporated in the wall of a blood vessel, as in the pampiniform plexus in the aged.

he′mo·lymph, hae′mo·lymph [*haima;* L. *lympha*, water]. 1. Blood and lymph. 2. The circulating nutritive fluid of certain invertebrates.

he·mol′y·sin, hae·mol′y·sin (hee·mol′i·sin, hem·ol′·, hee″mo·lye′sin, hem″o·) [*haima;* G. *lysis*, a loosing]. A substance produced in the blood which frees hemoglobin from the red cells.

bacterial h. That formed by the action of bacteria.

cold h. See cold *agglutinin.*

immune h. One formed by the animal body in response to the injection of erythrocytes of another species.

he·mol′y·sis (hee·mol′i·sis, hem·ol′·) [*haima; lysis*]. The destruction of red blood cells and the resultant escape of hemoglobin. —**hemolyt′ic,** *adj.*

conditioned h. A phenomenon observed in hemagglutination tests for American trypanosomiasis in which red blood cells previously absorbed with a polysaccharide fraction of *Trypanosoma cruzi* are hemolyzed by contact with the serum of the same patient.

he·mol″y·to·poi·et′ic, hae·mol″y·to·poi·et′ic [*haima;* G. *lyein*, to loose; *poiein*, to make]. Relating to the process of blood destruction and blood making.

he′mo·lyze, hae′mo·lyze [*haima; lyein*]. Produce hemolysis. —**hemolyza′tion,** *n.*

he″mo·ma·nom′e·ter, hae″mo·ma·nom′e·ter [*haima;* G. *manos*, thin; *metron*, a measure]. A manometer used in estimating blood pressure.

he″mo·me″di·as·ti′num, hae″mo·me″di·as·ti′num. See *hematomediastinum.*

he·mom′e·ter, hae·mom′e·ter [*haima; metron*]. 1. Hemoglobinometer. 2. Hemadynamometer. —**hemometry,** *n.*

he″mo·me′tra, hae″mo·me′tra. See *hematometra.*

he″mo·my′e·lo·gram″ [*haima;* G. *myelos*, marrow; *gramma*, letter]. A differential count of the white blood cells.

he″mo·pa·thol′o·gy, hae″mo·pa·thol′o·gy [*haima;* G. *pathos*, disease; *logos*, word]. The science of the diseases of the blood.

he·mop′a·thy. Any disease of the blood.

hereditary h. Any hereditary disease of the blood, such as sickle-cell anemia, eosinophilia, hereditary spherocytosis, or disturbed hemoglobin metabolism: also called *familial hemopathy.*

he″mo·per″i·car′di·um, hae″mo·per″i·car′di·um [*haima;* G. *perikardios*, about the heart]. Blood in the pericardial sac. If abundant, cardiac tamponade may occur.

he″mo·per″i·to·ne′um, hae″mo·per″i·to·ne′um [*haima;* G. *peritonaion*, membrane which contains the lower viscera]. An effusion of blood into the peritoneal cavity.

he′mo·phage, hae′mo·phage (hee′mo·faydj, hem′o·faydj) [*haima;* G. *phagein*, to eat]. A phagocytic cell which destroys red blood cells. —**hemophag′ic, hemoph′agous,** *adj.*

he″mo·pha′gi·a, hae″mo·pha′gi·a [*haima; phagein*]. 1. Ingestion of blood as a therapeutic agent. 2. Feeding on the blood of another organism. 3. Phagocytosis of the red blood cells.

he′mo·phil [*haima;* G. *philein*, to love]. Denoting an organism growing preferably on blood mediums.

he″mo·phil′i·a (hee″mo·fill′ee·uh, hem″o·) [*haima; philein*]. A sex-linked, hereditary disease occurring only in males but transmitted by females. It is characterized by impaired blood coagulation, attributed by some to a deficiency in the plasma of effective thromboplastinogen. Sometimes called *hemophilia A;* formerly called *bluterkrankheit.*

h. B In some nomenclatures, this term refers to *Christmas disease.* See *plasma thromboplastin component.*

h. neonatorum. See hemorrhagic *disease* of the newborn.

he″mo·phil′i·ac [*haima; philein*]. One who is affected with hemophilia.

he″mo·phil′ic [*haima; philein*]. 1. *In biology*, pertaining to bacteria growing well in culture media containing hemoglobin. 2. Pertaining to hemophilia. 3. Pertaining to a hemophiliac.

he″mo·phil′oid. Hemophilialike: used to designate conditions clinically similar to hemophilia, but due to some other defect in the clotting mechanism. See Christmas *disease, PTA deficiency.*

He·moph′i·lus [*haima; philein*]. A genus of bacteria of the family Parvobacteriaceae.

H. aegyptius. The causative agent of acute contagious conjunctivitis: also called *Koch-Weeks bacillus.* Syn., *H. conjunctivitis.*

H. conjunctivitis. *H. aegyptius.*

H. ducreyi. A species of small, Gram-negative bacilli tending to grow in short chains; the cause of chancroid.

H. duplex. A species responsible for infections of the cornea and conjunctiva; pathogenic for the human eye only. Syn., *Moraxella lacunata.*

H. influenzae. Certain strains of this species produce conjunctivitis and influenzal meningitis and have a definite invasive power, but in respiratory infections commonly follow some other microorganism. Formerly called *Bacillus influenzae, Pfeiffer's bacillus.*

H. pertussis. This species is the causative agent of whooping cough: also called *Bordet-Gengou bacillus.*

H. suis. This species together with a filtrable virus produces swine influenza.

he″mo·pho′bi·a (hee″mo·fo′bee·uh, hem″o·), **hem″a·to·pho′bi·a** (hem″uh·to·fo′bee·uh, hee″-muh·to·) [*haima;* G. *phobos,* fear]. Morbid fear of the sight of blood.

he″moph·thal′mi·a, he″moph·thal′mos [*haima;* G. *ophthalmos,* eye]. Hemorrhage into the vitreous.

he″moph·thi′sis (hee″moff·thigh′sis, hem″off·, hee·moff′thi·sis) [*haima;* G. *phthisis,* a wasting away]. Anemia due to undue degeneration or inadequate formation of red blood cells.

he″mo·plas′tic, hae″mo·plas′tic. See *hematoplastic.*

he″mo·pleu′ra. See *hemothorax.*

he″mo·pneu″mo·tho′rax, hae″mo·pneu″mo·tho′rax (hee″mo·new″mo·thor′acks, hem″o·) [*haima;* G. *pneuma,* air; *thōrax,* chest]. A collection of air and blood within the pleural cavity.

he″mo·poi·e′sis, hae″mo·poi·e′sis. See *hematopoiesis.*

he″mo·poi′e·tin. Intrinsic factor. See under *factor.*

he″mo·por′phy·rin. See *porphyrin.*

he″mo·pre·cip′i·tin, hae″mo·pre·cip′i·tin. See *precipitin.*

hemo-protein. Trade-mark for a mixture of protein fractions of digested ox blood used in nonspecific protein therapy.

he·mop′ty·sis, hae·mop′ty·sis [*haima;* G. *ptysis,* spitting]. The spitting of blood from the larynx, trachea, bronchi, or lungs.

parasitic h. A disease caused by the fluke *Paragonimus westermani,* which lodges in the lungs. The diagnosis is made by finding the characteristic ova in the sputum.

he″mo·pyr′role, he″mo·pyr′rol. Any of several pyrrole derivatives formed by reduction of heme.

hem′or·rhage, haem′or·rhage (hem′o·ridj, hem′-ridj) [*haima;* G. *rhēgnynai,* to burst]. An escape of blood from the vessels, either by diapedesis through intact walls or by flow through ruptured walls. —**hemorrhag′ic** (hem″o·radj′ick), *adj.*

ante-partum h. Bleeding from the uterus before delivery.

autogenous h. One due to causes within the body; not traumatic.

capillary h. Oozing of blood from the capillaries.

cerebral h. Bleeding from blood vessels in the cerebrum, either traumatic or due to disease.

choroidal h. Bleeding of the vessels of the choroid of the eye, discoverable by ophthalmoscopic examination.

cyclic h. (a) Excessive menstruation. (b) Menstrual bleeding of ectopic endometrial implants, as in endometriosis.

external h. Hemorrhage that is visible to the eye by the escape of blood to the exterior of the body from a wound or ruptured tissue.

extradural h. Hemorrhage into the space outside of the dura mater.

internal h. Bleeding which is concealed by escape into a cavity, as the intestine, peritoneal cavity, or within the cranium.

petechial h. Hemorrhage in the form of petechiae, rounded spots.

post-partum h. Bleeding occurring shortly after childbirth.

primary h. One that immediately follows any traumatism.

secondary h. One that occurs some time after the traumatism.

splinter h. A subungual hemorrhage resembling a splinter under the nail; found in cases of subacute bacterial endocarditis.

subarachnoid h. Bleeding between the arachnoid and the pia mater of the brain.

subdural h. Hemorrhage between the dura mater and the pia arachnoid. It usually results from injury to the meningeal vessels on the inner side of the dura mater.

toxemic accidental h. Bleeding resulting from partial or complete, gradual or sudden, separation of the placenta which is normally implanted in a woman 28 weeks or more pregnant and whose catheter specimen urine contains albumin.

hem″or·rhag′ic ne·phro′so-ne·phri′tis. See epidemic hemorrhagic *fever.*

hem″or·rhag′in. See *endotheliolysin.*

hem″or·rhoi′dal, haem″or·rhoi′dal [*haima;* G. *rhein,* to flow]. 1. Pertaining to or affected with hemorrhoids. 2. Of or pertaining to blood vessels, nerves, etc., of the anus.

hem″or·rhoid·ec′to·my, haem″or·rhoid·ec′to·my [*haima; rhein;* G. *ektomē,* excision]. Surgical removal of hemorrhoids.

hem′or·rhoids [G. *haimorrois,* vein liable to discharge blood]. An enlarged and varicose condition of the veins of the lower portion of the rectum and the tissues about the anus. Syn., *piles.*

esophageal h. Varicose veins existing in the lower portion of the esophagus due to portal vein obstruction.

external h. Those outside of the sphincter ani.

internal h. Those within the anal orifice.

prolapsed h. Those in which the enlarged veins protrude through the anal sphincter.

thrombosed h. Those in which the blood within the varicosity has become thrombosed.

he″mo·sal′pinx, hae″mo·sal′pinx. See *hematosalpinx.*

he″mo·sid′er·in, hae″mo·sid′er·in [G. *haima,* blood; *sidēros,* iron]. An iron-protein complex occurring in tissues, probably a storage form of iron, and by many considered to be a product of the decomposition of hemoglobin. It is in many characteristics similar to ferritin.

he″mo·sid″er·i·nu′ri·a. Hemosiderin in urine, observed in association with hemoglobinemia, pernicious anemia, hemolytic anemia, and hemochromatosis.

he″mo·sid″er·o′sis, hae″mo·sid″er·o′sis. See *hemochromatosis.*

he″mo·sper′mi·a, hae″mo·sper′mi·a. See *hematospermia.*

he″mo·sta′si·a, hae″mo·sta′si·a (hee″mo·stay′-zhuh, ·zee·uh, ·shuh, ·see·uh, hem″o·), **he″mo-**

sta′sis, hae″mo·sta′sis [*haima;* G. *stasis,* a standing]. 1. Stagnation of the blood. 2. Arrest of a flow of blood. —**hemostat′ic, haemostat′ic,** *adj.*

he′mo·stat, hae′mo·stat [*haima;* G. *statikos,* causing to stand]. An agent or instrument which arrests the flow of blood.

he″mo·stat′ic, hae″mo·stat′ic [*haima; statikos*]. An agent that arrests hemorrhage. Syn., *hemostyptic.*

he″mo·styp′tic. See *hemostatic.*

he″mo·ta·chom′e·ter, hae″mo·ta·chom′e·ter (hee″mo·ta·kom′i·tur, hem″o·) [*haima;* G. *tachos,* speed; *metron,* a measure]. An instrument for measuring the rate of flow of blood. —**hemotachometry,** *n.*

he″mo·ther″a·peu′tics, hae″mo·ther″a·peu′tics. See *hemotherapy.*

he″mo·ther′a·py (hee″mo·therr′uh·pee, hem″o·) [*haima;* G. *therapeia,* treatment]. The treatment of disease by means of blood or blood derivatives.

he″mo·tho′rax, hae″mo·tho′rax [*haima;* G. *thōrax,* thorax]. An accumulation of blood in the pleural cavity. Syn., *hemopleura.*

he″mo·tox′in, hae″mo·tox′in [*haima;* G. *toxikon,* poison]. A cytotoxin capable of destroying red blood cells. —**hemotoxic,** *adj.*

he′mo·trophe, hae′mo·trophe (hee′mo·troaf, ·trof, hem′o·, hem·ot′ro·fee) [*haima;* G. *trophē,* nourishment]. All the nutritive substances supplied to the embryo from the maternal blood stream in viviparous animals having a deciduate placenta. —**hemotroph′ic,** *adj.*

he″mo·tym′pa·num [*haima;* G. *tympanon,* drum]. Blood in the tympanic cavity.

he″mo·zo′in [*haima;* G. *zōion,* living being]. A dark brown or red-brown pigment, seen within plasmodia, which has been formed from the disintegrated hemoglobin.

he″mo·zo′on, hae″mo·zo′on. See *hematozoon.*

hemp [AS. *henep*]. *Cannabis sativa;* the bast fiber is used for textile purposes.

black Indian h. Apocynum.

Canada h. Apocynum. Also called *Canadian h.*

Indian h. Cannabis.

hen′bane″. Hyoscyamus.

Hench, Philip (1896–). American physician known for his extensive research in the field of rheumatic diseases; in 1950 he shared the Nobel prize in medicine with E. C. Kendall and T. Reichstein for their discovery of cortisone and its properties.

Hench and Aldrich's test. See under *test.*

hen·dec′yl. The univalent organic radical CH_3-$(CH_2)_{10}$—. Syn., *undecyl.*

Henderson, Lawrence Joseph [*American biochemist,* 1879–1942]. Did important research on the acid-base balance of the blood. The *Henderson-Hasselbalch equation* expressing the pH of a buffered solution is based on the relative quantities of the acid and salt components of the buffer. In its usual application to the bicarbonate buffer system of the blood, the equation is:

$$pH = pK_1 + \log \frac{(BHCO_3)}{(H_2CO_3)}$$

Here pK_1 equals 6.1.

Henderson, Melvin Starkey [*American orthopedic surgeon,* 1883–]. Devised numerous orthopedic procedures, including a method of tendon suspension for habitual dislocation of the shoulder, in which he drilled through the acromion and the humeral head and utilized a section of peroneus longus tendon for anchorage. Called *Henderson's operation.*

Henderson, Yandell [*American physiologist,* 1873–1944]. Made important studies of respiration. With C. G. Douglas, J. S. Haldane, and E. C. Schneider, studied the physiologic effects of atmospheric pressure at high altitudes (1911). In *Henderson's test* for determining whether an individual was a good risk for anesthesia, ability to hold a breath for 30 seconds or more was considered normal, whereas failure to do so, in the absence of pulmonary or cardiac insufficiency, was taken as indicating acidosis and thus contraindicating anesthesia.

Henderson-Hasselbalch equation. See under Lawrence Joseph *Henderson.*

Henke, Philipp Jakob Wilhelm (1834–1896). German anatomist. The potential space between the spinal column and the pharynx is called *Henke's space. Henke's triangle* is an area of the lower abdomen between the lateral border of the rectus abdominis muscle and the fold of the groin.

Henle, Friedrich Gustav Jakob [*German anatomist,* 1809–85]. Made important contributions to histology; our knowledge of epithelial tissue is said to have begun with his work. He described the epithelium of the skin and of the intestines, and defined columnar and ciliated epithelium (1837). The hyaline formation of epithelial cells in the cornea is known as *Henle's warts.* He demonstrated the presence of smooth muscle in the walls of arterioles (1841). *Henle's fenestrated membrane* is one of the layers of elastic tissue in the media and intima of large arteries. The endoneurium is known as the *sheath of Henle.* The suprameatal spine is called *Henle's spine.* See also *layer* of Henle, *loop* of Henle. The ampulla of the ductus deferens formerly was called *Henle's ampulla.* See also *muscle* of Henle.

Henneberg reflex. See *Laehr-Henneberg hard palate reflex.*

Henoch, Eduard (1820–1910). German pediatrician who made many contributions to pediatrics. He described a form of nonthrombocytopenic purpura associated with gastrointestinal symptoms, called *Henoch's purpura,* and also a form of purpura, usually fatal, which he named purpura fulminans.

hen′pu·e. See *goundou.*

Henriques-Sørensen method for amino-acid nitrogen. See under *method.*

hen′ry [after Joseph Henry, American physicist, 1797–1878]. The unit of electric inductance; the inductance in a circuit such that an electromotive force of 1 volt is induced in the circuit by variation of an inducing current at the rate of 1 ampere per second.

Henry, William [*English chemist,* 1774–1836]. Discovered *Henry's law:* the amount of gas dissolved in a liquid is proportional to the pressure of the gas; hence, if the temperature is constant, the ratio of the concentrations of the gas in gaseous form and in solution is constant.

Henry's melano-flocculation test. See under *test.*

Henschen, Salomon Eberhard (1847–1930). Swedish pathologist. By astute clinical and gross-pathological observations he first proposed the existence of a cortical visual receptive area in the region of the calcarine fissure in the occipital lobe (Brodmann's area 17) and of visual association in the parastriate areas (18 and 19 of Brodmann).

Henseleit, Kurt [*German internist,* 1907–]. Described the ornithine cycle, also called *Krebs-Henseleit cycle.* See under *Krebs.* See also Krebs *cycle.*

Hensen, Victor [*German pathologist,* 1835–1924].

Described the ductus reuniens, also called *Hensen's duct* or *canal*. See also *cells* of Hensen, Hensen's *disk*, Hensen's *node*.

hep″ap·to′sis. See *hepatoptosis*.

he′par [G. *hēpar*, liver] 1. The liver. 2. An obsolete designation for a substance having the color of liver, generally a compound of sulfur, as *hepar sulfuris*.

h. lobatum. See syphilitic *cirrhosis*.

h. siccatum. The dried and powdered liver of swine freed from blood.

h. sulfuris. Sulfurated potash.

hep′a·rin, he′pa·rin [*hēpar*]. A substance or mixture of substances occurring in liver and other tissues, having the property of prolonging the clotting time of blood, presumably by preventing conversion of prothrombin to thrombin. It appears to be a polysulfuric acid ester of the glucoprotein mucoitin. By virtue of its anticoagulant action heparin is used as a substitute for citrate in blood transfusions, to prevent postoperative thrombosis and embolism, in treatment of thrombophlebitis, in vascular surgery, and for other conditions. —**heparinized,** *adj.*; **hep′arinize,** *v.*; **hep′arinoid,** *adj.*

h. sodium. A white or pale-colored amorphous powder; it is official and is used for preparing solutions for intravenous use; it must contain at least 100 U.S.P. Heparin Units per milligram.

hep″a·rin·e′mia. The presence of heparin in the circulating blood.

hep″a·rin′o·cyte. A cell which produces heparin: the term suggested for the mast cell.

hep″a·tal′gi·a [*hēpar*; G. *algos*, pain]. Neuralgic pain in the liver. —**hepatalgic,** *adj.*

hep″a·tec′to·my [*hēpar*; G. *ektomē*, excision]. Excision of the liver or of a part of it.

he·pat′ic [G. *hēpatikos*, of the liver]. Pertaining to the liver.

he·pat′ic. A hepatic medicine.

He·pat′i·ca [*hēpatikos*]. Liverwort; a genus of ranunculaceous plants. **H. triloba** and **H. acutiloba** formerly were employed in the treatment of hepatic, renal, and pulmonary complaints.

he·pat′ic ar′ter·y. See Table of Arteries in the Appendix.

he·pat′i·co- [*hēpatikos*]. A combining form for *hepatic*.

he·pat″i·co·du″o·de·nos′to·my [*hēpatikos*; L. *duodeni*, twelve; G. *stoma*, mouth]. Anastomosis between the hepatic duct and the duodenum.

he·pat″i·co·en″ter·os′to·my [*hēpatikos*; G. *enteron*, intestine; *stoma*]. The surgical establishment of communication between the hepatic duct and the intestine.

he·pat″i·co·gas·tros′to·my [*hēpatikos*; G. *gastēr*, stomach; *stoma*]. Anastomosis between the hepatic duct and the stomach.

he·pat″i·co·li·thot′o·my [*hēpatikos*; G. *lithos*, stone; *tomē*, a cutting]. Surgical removal of a biliary calculus from the liver or any of its ducts.

he·pat″i·co·pan″cre·at′ic [*hēpatikos*; G. *pagkreas*, pancreas]. Relating to the liver and the pancreas.

he·pat″i·cos′to·my [*hēpatikos*; G. *stoma*, mouth]. The formation of a fistula in the hepatic duct for the purpose of drainage.

he·pat″i·cot′o·my [*hēpatikos*; G. *tomē*, a cutting]. Incision into the hepatic duct.

he·pat′ic veins. See Table of Veins in the Appendix.

hep″a·tit′i·des (hep″uh·tit′i·deez) (pl. of *hepatitis*). A term denoting various inflammatory diseases of the liver.

hep″a·ti′tis [G. *hēpar*, liver; *-itis*, inflammation]. Inflammation of the liver.

amebic h. A diffuse inflammation of the liver due to *Endamoeba histolytica;* it may resolve or lead to hepatic abscess.

anicteric h. Hepatitis without demonstrable jaundice.

arsenical h. Hepatitis occurring in an individual exposed to arsenic. Many cases, formerly attributed to the use of antisyphilitic arsenical compounds, may in fact have been due to the virus of homologous serum hepatitis or infectious hepatitis.

chronic interstitial h. Cirrhosis of the liver.

epidemic h. See infectious *h.*

hemorrhagic h. A term applied to the lesions in the liver which often accompany eclampsia. Grossly, the liver is enlarged, showing foci of necrosis and of hemorrhage. Microscopically, the necrosis is usually peripheral in the lobule but may be widespread. The widened peripheral sinusoids may contain thrombi of agglutinated erythrocytes. Hemorrhage may be slight in the periphery of the lobule, more extensive in the lobule and, rarely, may constitute a hematoma. Exudation is absent or only slight; the lesion is not primarily or principally inflammatory.

homologous serum h. A form of viral hepatitis transmitted by the parenteral injection of the human blood or blood products contaminated with the causative agent. The term is sometimes used to designate specifically that form of the disease, due to specific strains of virus, called *SH virus* or *hepatitis virus B*, in which the incubation period is from 2 to 5 months, and transmission by nonparenteral routes is unusual. Also called *postvaccinal h.*, *homologous serum jaundice, syringe jaundice, inoculation jaundice, transfusion jaundice, late arsphenamine jaundice.*

infectious, infective h. A form of viral hepatitis probably transmitted by oral spread of the causative agent, and frequently epidemic in form; sometimes specifically, that form of the disease, due to specific strains of virus, called *IH virus* or *hepatitis virus A*, in which the incubation period is from two to seven weeks and transmission by parenteral routes is rare. This disorder must be distinguished from spirochetal jaundice (Weil's disease). Syn., *catarrhal jaundice, epidemic hepatitis, epidemic jaundice.*

interstitial h. A condition in which there are associated degeneration or necrosis of hepatic parenchymal cells and infiltration of lymphocytes, plasma cells, and large mononuclear cells, and sometimes polymorphonuclear leukocytes in the portal canals. Also called *acute nonsuppurative h.*

postvaccinal h. See homologous serum *h.*

syphilitic h. An inflammation of the liver usually seen in the latter stages of early syphilis. Also see syphilitic *cirrhosis*.

toxic h. Inflammation of the liver resulting from the action of toxic compounds. Examples of hepatotoxins include such diverse compounds as the chlorinated hydrocarbons, phosphorus, and alkaloids of the retrorsine type.

viral h. Any inflammation of liver due to viral infection, most commonly infectious *h.* and homologous serum *h.*

hep″a·ti·za′tion [*hēpar*]. The conversion of tissue into a liverlike substance, as of the lungs during pneumonia. **Red hepatization** refers to the gross appearance of the lungs during the first few days of consolidation in lobar pneumonia. **Gray hepatization** refers to their appearance just prior to resolution. —**hep′atized,** *adj.*

hep′a·to-, hepat- [*hēpar*]. A combining form denoting *the liver, hepatic.*

hep″a·to·cho·lan″gi·o·du″o·de·nos′to·my (hep″uh·to·ko·lan″jee·o·dew″o·di·nos′to·mee) [*hē-*

par; G. *cholē,* bile; *aggeion,* vessel; L. *duodeni,* twelve; G. *stoma,* mouth]. Establishment of communication by surgical means between the hepatic duct and the duodenum.

hep″a·to·cho·lan″gi·o·en″ter·os′to·my [*hēpar; cholē; aggeion,* G. *enteron,* intestine; *stoma*]. Anastomosis between the hepatic duct and some portion of the small intestine.

hep″a·to·cho·lan″gi·o·gas·tros′to·my [*hēpar; cholē; aggeion;* G. *gastēr,* stomach; *stoma*]. Anastomosis between the hepatic duct and stomach.

hep″a·to·cho·lan″gi·o·je″ju·nos′to·my (hep″-uh·to·ko·lan″jee·o·jee″jew·nos′to·mee, ·jedj″-oo·nos′to·mee) [*hēpar; cholē; aggeion;* L. *jejunus,* empty; *stoma*]. The surgical establishment of communication between the hepatic duct and the jejunum.

hep″a·to·col′ic [*hēpar;* G. *kolon,* colon]. Relating to the liver and the colon.

hep″a·to·cu′pre·in. A copper-containing protein, similar to hemocuprein, but isolated from liver.

hep″a·to·cyst′ic [*hēpar;* G. *kystis,* bladder]. Pertaining to the liver and the gallbladder.

hep″a·to·du″o·de′nal (hep″uh·to·dew″o·dee′nul, ·dew·od′i·nul) [*hēpar;* L. *duodeni,* twelve]. Relating to the liver and the duodenum.

hep″a·to·du″o·de·nos′to·my [*hēpar; duodeni;* G. *stoma,* mouth]. Old term for hepaticoduodenostomy.

hep″a·to·fla′vin. Riboflavin.

hep″a·to·gen′ic, hep″a·tog′en·ous (hep″uh-todj′i·nus) [*hēpar;* G. *genesthai,* from *gignesthai,* to be produced]. Produced by, or in, the liver.

hep′a·to·gram [*hēpar;* G. *gramma,* letter]. A graphic record of the liver pulse.

hep″a·tog′ra·phy [*hēpar;* G. *graphein,* to write]. Roentgenography of the liver.

hep″a·to·li·e′nal (hep″uh·to·lye·ee′nul, ·lye′i·nul) [*hēpar;* L. *lien,* spleen]. Pertaining to the liver and the spleen.

hep″a·to·li″en·og′ra·phy [*hēpar; lien;* G. *graphein,* to write]. Radiographic examination of the liver and spleen.

hep′a·to·lith [*hēpar;* G. *lithos,* stone]. A calculus in the biliary passages of the liver.

hep″a·to·lith·ec′to·my. Hepaticolithotomy.

hep″a·to·li·thi′a·sis [*hēpar; lithos;* NL. *-iasis,* condition]. A diseased condition characterized by the formation of gallstones in the biliary passages of the liver.

he·pat″o·ly′sin (hi·pat″o·lye′sin, hep″uh·tol′i·sin) [*hēpar;* G. *lysis,* a loosing]. A cytolysin acting especially on liver cells.

hep″a·to′ma [*hēpar;* G. *-ōma,* tumor]. A neoplasm, usually malignant, derived from and composed of cells resembling those of liver parenchyma. It is often multicentric and hence thought to be derived from nodular foci of regeneration. Syn., *liver-cell carcinoma.*

hep″a·to·meg′a·ly, hep″a·to·me·ga′li·a [*hēpar;* G. *megas,* large]. Enlargement of the liver.

hep″a·tom·phal′o·cele. See under umbilical *hernia.*

hep′a·to·pex″y [*hēpar;* G. *pēxis,* a fixing]. Surgical fixation of a movable, or ptosed, liver; usually by utilizing additional supportive power of the round and the falciform ligaments.

hep″a·top·to′sis (hep″uh·top·to′sis, hep″uh·to·to′-sis) [*hēpar;* G. *ptōsis,* a falling]. Abnormally low position of the liver in the abdomen, due to stretching of attachments to the diaphragm.

hep″a·to·re′nal [*hēpar;* L. *renalis,* of the kidneys]. Relating to both the liver and kidney.

hep″a·tor′rha·phy [*hēpar;* G. *rhaphē,* a suture]. Suturing of the liver following an injury or an operation.

hep″a·tor·rhex′is [*hēpar;* G. *rhēxis,* a breaking]. Rupture of the liver. *Obs.*

hep″a·tos′co·py [*hēpar;* G. *skopein,* to examine]. Inspection of the liver, as by laparotomy or peritoneoscopy.

hep″a·to′sis [*hēpar;* G. *-ōsis,* condition]. 1. Enlargement of the liver due to obstructive dilatation of intrahepatic biliary passages. 2. A degeneration or inflammation of the liver which cannot be clearly distinguished clinically.

hep″a·to·sple″no·meg′a·ly [*hēpar;* G. *splēn,* spleen; *megas,* large]. Enlargement of the liver and spleen.

hep″a·to·sple″nop′a·thy [*hēpar; splēn;* G. *pathos,* disease]. Any combination of disorders of the liver and spleen.

hep″a·to·ther′a·py [*hēpar;* G. *therapeia,* treatment]. Therapeutic use of liver or liver extract.

hep″a·tot′o·my [*hēpar;* G. *tomē,* a cutting]. Incision into the liver.

hep″a·to·tox′in [*hēpar;* G. *toxikon,* poison]. 1. An injurious substance, such as the chlorinated hydrocarbons, phosphorus, alkaloids of the retrorsine type, which acts especially on parenchymal cells of the liver. 2. A poisonous or deleterious product elaborated in the liver. —**hepatotox′ic,** *adj.*

hepicebrin. Trade-mark for a multivitamin product in capsules.

hepicoleum. Trade-mark for several preparations containing vitamins A and D.

hep·tal′de·hyde. Heptyl aldehyde. $CH_3(CH_2)_5$-CHO. Colorless liquid of aromatic odor. It has been used experimentally to induce certain retrogressive changes in tumors of animals. Syn., *enanthaldehyde.*

hep′tane. C_7H_{16}. *n*-Heptane. A liquid hydrocarbon of the paraffin series, contained in petroleum and also obtained by dry distillation from the resin of *Pinus sabiniana.* Used as a solvent and anesthetic.

hep′tose. Any member of the division of the monosaccharides containing seven carbon atoms.

heptuna. A proprietary hematinic consisting of ferrous sulfate with vitamins A, D, and vitamin-B complex in capsules.

hep′tyl. The univalent organic radical CH_3-$(CH_2)_6$—.

hep′tyl al′de·hyde. See *heptaldehyde.*

hep″tyl·res·or′ci·nol (hep″til·ri·zor′si·nole, ·nol, ·nawl). 2,4-Dihydroxyphenyl-*n*-heptane. A germicidal substance which has been used as an intestinal antiseptic.

her′a·path·ite, her·ap′a·thite [after William *Herapath,* English chemist, 1796–1868]. Quinine iodosulfate; platelike crystals of a pale olive-green by transmitted light, and a golden green to a reddish green by reflected light. Has strong polarizing ability.

herb (urb, hurb) [L. *herba,* grass]. 1. A plant without a woody stem. 2. A plant used for medicinal purposes or for its odor or flavor. —**herb′al,** *adj.*

her·ba′ceous [L. *herbaceus,* grassy]. *In biology,* applied to stems or other organs that have a tender, juicy consistence and perish at the close of the growing season; of the nature of herbs.

herb′al (hur′bul, ur′bul) [L. *herba,* grass]. A book on the medicinal virtues of herbs.

Herbert, Herbert [*English ophthalmic surgeon,* 1865–1942]. Devised an operation for glaucoma, in which he displaced a wedge-shaped flap of sclera, without completely excising it, in order to produce a filtering cicatrix.

her·biv′o·rous [L. *herba,* grass; *vorare,* to devour]. Living on vegetable food.

Herbst, Ernst Friedrich Gustav [*German anatomist,* 1803–93]. Described a type of sensory end organs, resembling Pacinian corpuscles, found in the mucous membrane of the tongue of the duck; called *Herbst's bodies* or *corpuscles.*

herd in'stinct. The fundamental psychic urge to identify oneself with a group and to function in the same manner as the group; group feeling.

he·red'i·ty [L. *hereditas,* heirship]. The inborn capacity of the organism to develop ancestral characteristics; it is dependent upon the constitution and organization of the cell or cells which form the starting point of the new individual. In biparental reproduction this starting point is the fertilized egg. —**hereditary,** *adj.*

her'e·do- [L. *heres,* heir]. *In medicine,* a combining form used for *hereditary.* Often used erroneously in the sense of congenital, as in heredosyphilis.

her"e·do·ak"i·ne'si·a (herr"i·do·ack"i·nee'shuh, ·see·uh, ·zhuh, ·zee·uh, herr"i·do·ack"eye·) [*heres;* G. *a-,* not; *kinēsis,* motion]. A rare, familial disease characterized by paroxysmal paralysis accompanied by severe pains in the extremities, a feeling of marked weakness, and an inability to carry out movements.

her"e·do·fa·mil'i·al [*heres;* L. *familia,* household]. Characterizing a disease or condition which occurs in more than one member of a family and is suspected of being inherited.

her"e·do·path'i·a a·tac'ti·a pol"y·neu·ri"ti·for'mis. A disease, seen most often in children of consanguineous marriages, manifested as appetite loss, ataxia, general weakness, muscular atrophy, weak to absent reflexes, dryness and desquamation of skin, progressive development of neurogenic deafness, atypical retinitis pigmentosa, and nyctalopia. Daylight vision, sensations, and intelligence are normal.

Hering, Heinrich Ewald [*German physiologist,* 1866–1948]. Described the carotid sinus reflex. See under *reflex.*

Hering, Karl Ewald Konstantin [*German physiologist,* 1834–1918]. Advanced a theory of color vision (1872). Devised a test for binocular vision. Described the connection between a hepatic cord and a bile duct, called *Hering's canal. Hering's law* states that the distinctness or purity of a sensation depends on the proportion of its intensity to the total intensities of all simultaneous sensations. See also Hering-Breuer *reflex, Traube-Hering waves* under *wave.*

her'it·age [L. *heres,* heir]. *In genetics,* the sum total of the genes or characteristics transmitted from parents to their children.

her·maph'ro·dite [G. *hermaphroditos,* a person partaking of the attributes of both sexes, from *Hermaphroditos,* son of Hermes and Aphrodite]. An individual showing hermaphroditism. See *pseudohermaphrodite.* —**hermaphrodit'ic,** *adj.*

her·maph'ro·dit·ism (hur·maf'ro·dye·tiz·um), **her·maph'ro·dism** [*Hermaphroditos*]. A condition characterized by the coexistence in an individual of ovarian and testicular tissue. It is rare in humans (Young admits only 20 human cases), but more common in lower forms. Pseudohermaphroditism is a more common condition.

bilateral h. That in which the individual has an ovary and testis on each side; seen in humans.

lateral h. The form of human hermaphroditism in which there is an ovary on one side and a testis on the other.

ovatesticular h. The rare form in which an ovatestis is present on one or both sides.

unilateral h. The form in which there is an ovary and testis on one side with either an ovary or a testis on the other.

Her·me'ti·a (hur·mee'shee·uh). A genus of the soldier fly family, Stratiomyiidae. The species **H. illucens** is an occasional cause of intestinal myiasis.

her·met'ic [G. *Hermēs,* Hermes]. Protected from exposure to air; airtight.

her'ni·a [L.]. The abnormal protrusion of an organ or a part through the containing wall of its cavity, beyond its normal confines. The term applies usually to the abdominal cavity and implies the existence of a covering or sac. Syn., *rupture.* Also see *prolapse.* See Plate 39. —**hernial,** *adj.*

abdominal h. See ventral *h.*

acquired h. A noncongenital form resulting from strain, weight lifting, or as the direct sequence of operation, muscular weakening, etc.

annular h. See umbilical *h.*

bladder h. The protrusion of any part of the urinary bladder through any opening in the abdominal wall. Syn., *cystic h., vesical h.*

cerebral h. A protrusion of the brain through an acquired opening in the skull, as a result of operation, injury, or disease. Syn., *h. of the brain.*

complete h. One in which the hernial sac and its contents have escaped through the opening; applied especially to inguinal hernias where the sac and its contents are to be found in the scrotum or labium majus.

concealed h. One which is not evident by ordinary manual examination.

congenital h. One in which the defect is present in fetal life and exists at birth. Examples of this form are inguinal hernias in which the processus vaginalis remains patent, leading to the early descent of intestine into the scrotum, and diaphragmatic hernias in which abdominal organs have passed into the thoracic cavity.

crural h. See femoral *h.*

cystic h. See bladder *h.*

diaphragmatic h. One which passes through the diaphragm into the thoracic cavity; may be congenital, acquired, or traumatic, and may contain the stomach, small intestine, and colon. Usually a false hernia.

direct h. An inguinal hernia in which the sac does not leave the abdominal cavity through the abdominal inguinal ring but through a defect in the floor of Hesselbach's triangle, between the inferior epigastric artery and the outer edge of the rectus muscle.

diverticulum h. A type of sliding hernia which contains a diverticulum of the urinary bladder; also hernia of an intestinal diverticulum.

duodenojejunal h. See retroperitoneal *h.*

epigastric h. A hernia in the linea alba, between the umbilicus and the xiphoid process, generally found in young adult males; the contents of the sac are usually extraperitoneal fat, lipomas, and, only rarely, bowel. Also called *properitoneal h., fatty h.*

false h. One which has no sac covering the hernial contents.

femoral h. That involving the femoral canal; the second most common hernia. Found more often in women, it is usually small and painless, often remaining unnoticed. The neck lies beneath the inguinal ligament and lateral to the tubercle of the pubic bone. Syn., *crural h.* See Plate 4.

foraminal h. (a) A so-called hernia of the medulla into the foramen magnum of the skull, from increased intracranial pressure. (b) A false hernia of a loop of bowel through the epiploic foramen.

funicular h. A variety of congenital, indirect hernia into the processus vaginalis which is closed below and open above.

h. of the brain. See cerebral *h.*

h. of the lungs. A rare, congenital anomaly associated with fissured chest, in which a portion of the lung protrudes through the opening, the swelling enlarging with each expiration.

h. of the nucleus pulposus. Protrusion of the substance of the intervertebral disk into the spinal canal, causing pressure upon the cord, nerves, or cauda equina.

hiatus h. A form of hernia through the esophageal hiatus; usually a small, intermittent hernia of a part of the stomach.

ileoappendicular h. See retroperitoneal *h.*

incarcerated h. A term applied either to an irreducible or to a strangulated hernia.

incisional h. One occurring from an operative or accidental incision, the predisposing factors being wound infection, prolonged drainage, or interference with nerve supply. Also called *postoperative h., posttraumatic h.*

incomplete h. An inguinal hernia in which the sac has not passed through the subcutaneous inguinal ring: also called *bubonocele.*

indirect h. An inguinal form which follows the spermatic cord into the scrotum or, in the female, the round ligament into the labium majus. The hernial sac leaves the abdomen through the internal abdominal ring, traverses the inguinal canal and passes through the external abdominal ring. See Plate 39. Syn., *lateral hernia, oblique hernia.*

industrial h. An incomplete inguinal hernia, or dilatation of the inguinal canal, producing signs and symptoms which make the subject a poor risk for employment in certain industries.

infantile h. A congenital, indirect, inguinal hernia in which the vaginal process is sealed high in the canal and remains open below. The sac then invaginates or passes behind the tunica vaginalis, so that two or three layers of peritoneum lie over the contents.

inguinal h. A hernia through the inguinal canal. This variety constitutes more than four-fifths of all hernias. See Plate 4.

inguinolabial h. An inguinal hernia which has descended into the labium majus.

intermuscular h. An interstitial hernia in which the sac lies between the muscles of the abdominal wall. Syn., *interparietal h.*

internal h. One occurring within the abdominal cavity; a sac of peritoneum, containing intraabdominal contents, protrudes through a normal or abnormal opening. It may be retroperitoneal or intraperitoneal.

interparietal h. See intermuscular *h.*

intersigmoid h. A hernia involving the prolapse of a loop of intestine into a subsigmoid fossa at the root of the mesosigmoid, left side.

interstitial h. A rare form of congenital hernia in which the sac leaves the inguinal canal and lies between layers of abdominal muscles; often associated with undescended testis.

intraperitoneal h. A type of false, internal hernia in which some of the intraabdominal contents pass through an anomalous opening in the mesentery, omentum, or broad ligaments.

iris h. Prolapse of the iris after iridectomy or following trauma.

irreducible h. A hernia which cannot be returned through the opening by manipulation; due to adhesions or blocking by fecal impaction, not by gaseous distention.

ischiadic h. See sciatic *h.*

ischiorectal h. See perineal *h.*

labial h. Complete, indirect inguinal hernia into the labium majus.

lateral h. See indirect *h.*

lumbar h. A hernia passing out of the abdomen through the lumbar triangle, resulting usually from operation, lumbar abscess, or injury.

masked h. A type of ventral hernia in which the hernial sac is situated within the abdominal wall.

mesenteric h. One in which a loop of intestine or a portion of omentum or other viscus has passed through an opening in the mesentery.

oblique h. See indirect *h.*

obturator h. A rare hernia through the upper part of the obturator foramen; occurs principally in women. Also called *pelvic h.*

omental h. A hernia which contains only omentum.

perineal h. A hernia passing through the pelvic diaphragm to appear as a rectal hernia, vaginal hernia, or bladder hernia: also called *ischiorectal h.*

postoperative h. See incisional *h.*

rectal h. A condition in which the small bowel, or other abdominal contents, protrudes through the rectovesical or rectouterine pouch, carrying the anterior rectal wall through the anus.

reducible h. One whose contents can be replaced through the hernial opening.

retroperitoneal h. Hernia into a recess of the peritoneum, as into a paraduodenal recess. Syn., *duodenojejunal h., ileoappendicular h.*

retrovesical h. A hernia behind the urinary bladder into the retrovesical space.

Richter's h. A form of enterocele in which only a part of the intestinal wall is situated within the hernial sac.

sciatic h. That through one of the sciatic notches. Also called *ischiadic h.*

scrotal h. Any hernia which is found within the scrotum. See complete *h.*, inguinal *h.*, sliding *h.* See Plate 39.

sliding h. A variety of indirect, irreducible inguinal hernia in which a section of a viscus, usually cecum or sigmoid colon, forms one wall of the sac; generally a large scrotal hernia.

Spigelian h. A ventral hernia occurring at the semilunar line.

strangulated h. A hernia involving intestine in which circulation of the blood and the fecal current are blocked. If unrelieved, it leads to ileus and necrosis of the intestine.

synovial h. The protrusion of the inner lining of a joint capsule through the outer portion of the capsule.

true h. One having a sac, usually of peritoneum, covering the hernial contents.

umbilical h. One occurring through the umbilical ring, either early in life (infantile) from imperfect closure, or later (acquired) from diastasis of the rectus abdominis muscles, obesity, or muscular weakness. Congenital midline defects lead to hernia into the umbilical cord, or omphalocele. If the liver is contained in the sac, it is called a *hepatomphalocele.* Syn., *annular h.*

vaginal h. A perineal hernia which follows the course of the vagina after leaving the abdomen, and which may enter the labium majus; resembles a labial inguinal hernia.

ventral h. A hernia of any part of the abdominal wall not involving the inguinal, femoral, or umbilical openings. It exists in three varieties: median, lateral, and postincisional. Syn., *abdominal h., epigastric h.*

vesical h. See bladder *h.*

her'ni·ate [*hernia*]. To form a hernia. —**herniated,** *adj.;* **hernia'tion,** *n.*

her'ni·o- [*hernia*]. A combining form used to mean *hernia.*

her'ni·o·plas"ty [*hernia;* G. *plassein,* to form]. Plastic operation for the radical cure of hernia.

her"ni·or'rha·phy [*hernia;* G. *rhaphē,* a suture]. Any operation which includes suturing for the repair of hernia.

her'ni·o·tome [*hernia;* G. *tomos,* cutting]. A special knife or curved bistoury, with a blunt end, sometimes used in operations for hernia.

her"ni·ot'o·my [*hernia;* G. *tomē,* a cutting]. An operation for the relief of irreducible hernia, by cutting through the neck of the sac. Often wrongly used to indicate hernioplasty.

her'o·in. Diacetylmorphine. $C_{21}H_{23}NO_5$. White, odorless, bitter, crystalline powder.

h. hydrochloride. $C_{21}H_{23}NO_5.HCl.H_2O$. White, odorless, bitter, crystalline powder soluble in two parts of water; a sedative and narcotic. Because of the pronounced danger of addiction, a federal law forbids the manufacture or importation of heroin or its salts in the U.S.A. See *diamorphine hydrochloride.*

her'o·in·ism [*heroin,* Ger. trade name]. Addiction to heroin; a very prevalent form of drug addiction.

Herophilus [*Bithynian surgeon and anatomist in Egypt,* 335–280 B.C.]. Has been called the father of anatomy. Systematically studied the anatomy of the brain and spinal cord. Described the ventricles of the brain, and also the spleen, the liver, and the genital organs. See *confluens* sinuum, formerly called *torcular Herophili.*

her·pan'gin·a. A mild disease probably caused by a virus of the Coxsackie group and characterized by fever, anorexia, dysphagia, and grayish-white papules or vesicles surrounded by a red areola on the pharynx, uvula, palate, and tonsils, or tongue.

her'pes (hur'peez) [G. *herpēs,* shingles, from *herpein,* to creep]. An acute inflammation of the skin or mucous membrane, characterized by the development of groups of vesicles on an inflammatory base. **—herpet'ic,** *adj.*

h. circinatus. Dermatitis herpetiformis.

h. corneae. See ocular *h.*

h. cornealis. See *h.* ophthalmicus.

h. desquamans. A type of endodermophytosis. See *tinea* imbricata.

h. facialis. A type of herpes simplex occurring on the face, usually about the lips. May also occur in the mouth and pharynx. Syn., *h. febrilis, h. labialis.* Also called *coldsore.*

h. febrilis. See *h.* facialis.

h. genitalis. See *h.* progenitalis.

h. gestationis. A type of dermatitis herpetiformis occurring during pregnancy.

h. iris. A form of erythema multiforme, characterized by vesicles growing in a ring. It is usually seen on the backs of the hands and feet.

h. labialis. See *h.* facialis.

h. ophthalmicus. Herpes zoster of the ophthalmic branch of the fifth cranial nerve: also called *h. cornealis.*

h. progenitalis. A form of herpes simplex in which vesicles from the size of a pin's head to the size of a small pea occur on the genitalia. Also called *h. praeputialis, h. genitalis.*

h. simplex. An acute disorder, characterized by groups of vesicles on an erythematous base. Commonly recurrent, and at times seen in the same place. Due to a virus.

h. tonsurans. See *tinea* capitis.

h. zoster. Herpes in which the lesions are distributed in relation to the course of a cutaneous nerve, and, as a rule, unilateral. They are often seen in the line of an intercostal nerve, but may follow in the course of any nerve. The outbreak of the eruption is often preceded and may be followed by severe neuralgic pain, referred to as *herpetic neuralgia.* It is a systemic infection, caused by a virus, and may be serious in elderly or debilitated persons. Syn., *shingles, zoster.* Also called *zona, hemizona, ignis sacer.*

h. zoster oticus. Aural herpes associated with facial paralysis and otalgia; due to disease of the seventh cranial nerve. Also called *Hunt's syndrome.*

ocular h. Infection of the lids, conjunctivae, or corneae by the virus of herpes simplex. It is characterized by groups of blisters on an erythematous, edematous base.

her·pet'ic neu·ral'gi·a. See *herpes zoster* under *herpes.*

her·pet'i·form [*herpēs;* L. *forma,* form]. Resembling herpes; having groups of vesicles.

her"pe·tol'o·gy [G. *herpeton,* reptile; *logos,* word]. The branch of zoology concerned with the structure, classification, and habits of reptiles.

Her"pe·tom'o·nas [*herpeton;* G. *monas,* unit]. A genus of the family Trypanosomidae; parasitic only in invertebrate hosts. **—herpetomonad,** *adj., n.*

her'que·in. An antibiotic substance obtained from cultures of *Penicillium herquei.*

Herrick, James Bryan [*American physician,* 1861–]. First to describe accurately the sickle-cell type of anemia (1910), sometimes spoken of as *Herrick's anemia.* Gave a classic description of coronary thrombosis (1912).

Herrmannsdorfer diet. See S.H.G. *diet.*

Herter, Christian Archibald [*American biochemist and pathologist,* 1865–1910]. Described infantilism due to a chronic intestinal disease similar to if not identical with sprue (1908). See celiac *disease.*

Herter-Foster method for indole. See under *method.*

Hertwig, Wilhelm August Oskar [*German embryologist,* 1849–1922]. Remembered for his description of the portion of the enamel organ which forms a mold for the root of a developing tooth; called *epithelial sheath of Hertwig.* Demonstrated the fact that the spermatozoon enters the ovum and that union of male and female pronuclei occurs.

Hertzian rays. See under *ray.*

Herxheimer, Karl [*German dermatologist,* 1861–1944]. Described spiral fibers found in the germinative layer of the epidermis; called *Herxheimer's fibers.* With K. Hartmann, described acrodermatitis atrophicans chronica (1902). See also Jarisch-Herxheimer *reaction.*

Herxheimer's technic for staining fat. See the various Sudan stains under *stain.*

Heryng, Théodor [*Polish laryngologist,* 1847–1925]. Described a solitary ulcer of the anterior fauces, of obscure origin, resembling a herpetic vesicle; called *Heryng's benign ulcer.* Described a sign indicating empyema of the maxillary sinus; *Heryng's sign* is an infraorbital shadow seen when an electric light is placed in the mouth.

herz'stoss' (hairts'shtoss') [Ger., heartbeat]. The widespread impact of the heart during systole against a large part of the entire precordium, seen especially in thin patients with cardiac hypertrophy, in contradistinction to the point of maximal impulse (*spitzenstoss*) seen normally.

Heschl's gyri. See under *gyrus.*

hes·per'e·tin. $C_{16}H_{14}O_6$; 3′,5,7-trihydroxy-4′-methoxyflavanone; the aglycone of hesperidin, obtained by hydrolysis of the latter or by synthesis. Certain derivatives may have a favorable effect in certain types of capillary fragility. See also *citrin.*

hes·per'i·din, hes'per·i'din. $C_{28}H_{34}O_{15}$; hesperetin-1-rhamnosido-D-glucoside, occurring in the rind of many citrus fruits; on hydrolysis it yields hesperetin, rhamnose, and D-glucose. It is a white, crystalline powder, practically insoluble in water. Pure hesperidin provides no protection against capillary fragility; certain water-soluble derivatives of it have such action, commonly attributed to vitamin P. See *citrin.*

Hess, Walter Rudolf (1881–). Swiss physiologist, who studied the control of the autonomic nervous system by the hypothalamus through his technique of applying pin-point electrical stimulation to specific areas in the brain. Nobel laureate in physiology and medicine (1949). He also contributed to knowledge of blood viscosity and strabismus (Hess screen, 1911).

Hesse, Hermann [*German pharmacologist,* nineteenth century]. Remembered for his isolation, with P. L. Geiger, of atropine (1833).

Hesselbach, Franz Caspar (1759–1816). German surgeon and anatomist. A complete femoral hernia and a direct inguinal hernia are each sometimes called *Hesselbach's hernia.* He also described the interfoveolar ligament, formerly called *Hesselbach's ligament.* See also Hesselbach's *triangle.*

het″er·a·del′phi·a. See *thoracoacephalus.*

het″er·a·del′phus [*heteros; adelphos*]. Thoracoacephalus. —**heteradelphous,** *adj.*

het″er·a·de′ni·a [*heteros;* G. *adēn,* gland]. Any abnormality in the formation or location of gland tissue. —**heteraden′ic,** *adj.*

het″er·a′li·us [*heteros; halios,* useless]. A double monster in which the parasite is only rudimentary, and with no direct connection with the umbilical cord of its host.

het″er·aux·e′sis [*heteros;* G. *auxēsis,* increase]. A type of allometry which deals with the relation of a part to the whole, or to another part, during the course of growth and development of the organism. Also see *allomorphosis.*

het″er·e′cious, het″er·oe′cious [*heteros;* G. *oikos,* house]. Parasitic upon different hosts at different stages of growth. —**heterecism,** *n.*

het″er·es·the′si·a (het″ur·ess·thee′zhuh, ·zee·uh) [*heteros;* G. *aisthēsis,* sensation]. A condition characterized by variations in the degree of response to a cutaneous stimulus as it passes from one point to another on the surface.

het′er·o-, heter- [*heteros*]. A combining form signifying *other, other than usual, different.*

het″er·o·ag·glu′ti·nin [*heteros;* L. *agglutinare,* to glue to]. An agglutinin in normal blood having the property of agglutinating foreign cells, including the blood corpuscles of other species of animals.

het″er·o·al′bu·mose. A variety of albumose soluble in salt solutions, insoluble in water, and precipitated by saturation with sodium chloride or magnesium sulfate.

het″er·o·al″bu·mo·su′ri·a [*heteros;* L. *albus,* white; G. *ouron,* urine]. Presence of heteroalbumose in the urine.

het″er·o·at′om. Any atom, linked in the ring of a heterocyclic compound, other than a carbon atom, as, for example, the nitrogen atom of pyridine, C_5H_5N.

het″er·o·aux′in. 3-Indoleacetic acid, $C_{10}H_9NO_2$. White, crystalline powder insoluble in water, soluble in alcohol. An activator of growth substance (auxin). Used experimentally as a plant growth stimulant.

het″er·o·aux′one (het″ur·o·awk′sohn). A growth-promoting substance. See *heteroauxin.*

het″er·o·blas′tic [*heteros;* G. *blastos,* germ]. Arising from tissue of a different kind.

het″er·o·cel′lu·lar [*heteros;* L. *cellula,* small storeroom]. Formed of cells of different kinds.

het″er·o·ceph′a·lus [*heteros;* G. *kephalē,* head]. A fetal monster with two heads of unequal size.

het″er·o·chro′ma·tin [*heteros;* G. *chrōma,* color]. Originally the substance of heterochromosomes; e.g., the Y chromosome. It has been extended to include any chromatin similarly characterized by an excessive amount of desoxyribose-type nucleoprotein, by a looser structure, and functionally by a more generalized metabolism other than the more specific action of genes in the euchromatin which gives the familiar Mendelian ratio. —**heterochromat′ic,** *adj.*

het″er·o·chro′mi·a [*heteros; chrōma*]. A difference in coloration in two parts of a structure, or in two structures that are normally alike, as the irises of the two eyes. —**heterochro′mous,** *adj.*

het″er·o·chro′mo·some [*heteros; chrōma;* G. *sōma,* body]. An allosome.

het″er·o·chro′ni·a [*heteros;* G. *chronos,* time]. 1. Variation in time relationships. 2. Departure from the typical sequence in the time of formation of organs or parts. 3. Difference in chronaxies of tissue elements functionally related, as between the chronaxie of a muscle and that of its nerve. —**heterochron′ic, heteroch′ronous,** *adj.*

het″er·o·cy′clic (het″ur·o·sigh′click, ·sick′lick). *In chemistry,* pertaining to compounds of the closed-chain or ring type in which the ring atoms are of two or more dissimilar elements. See *homocyclic.*

Het″er·od′er·a [*heteros;* G. *derē,* neck]. A genus of minute nematodes of the superfamily Anguillulinoidea.

H. radicicola. A species parasitic on the roots and stems of many edible plants. The ova are sometimes found in the feces of man and may be mistaken for hookworm eggs.

het″er·o·did′y·mus. See *heterodymus.*

het′er·o·dont″. *In biology,* having teeth of more than one shape, as does man. See also *homodont.*

het″er·o·dro′mi·a [*heteros;* G. *dromos,* course]. Better conduction in one than in the other direction in a nerve.

het″er·od′y·mus [*heteros;* G. *-dymos,* -fold]. A type of thoracopagus parasiticus in which the parasitic twin is represented by a head, neck, and thorax implanted in the thoracic or the epigastric wall of the host.

het″er·oe′cious. See *heterecious.*

het″er·o·er′o·tism [*heteros;* G. *erōs,* love]. The direction of the sexual desire toward another person or toward any object other than oneself. —**heteroerot′ic,** *adj.*

het″er·o·fer·men′ta·tive [*heteros;* L. *fermentum,* ferment]. Pertaining to the ability of certain bacteria, such as *Lactobacillus brevis, L. buchneri,* and *Leuconostoc dextranicum* to form lactic acid, ethyl alcohol, acetic acid, carbon dioxide, and glycerol from glucose, as well as mannitol from levulose. This reactivity sets aside these organisms as heterofermentative, in contrast to the *homofermentative* lactic acid bacteria which produce only lactic acid from glucose and other sugars.

het″er·o·ga·met′ic (het″ur·o·ga·met′ick, ·ga·mee′-tick) [*heteros;* G. *gamos,* marriage]. Referring to the production of two types of germ cells in regard to the sex chromosomes. The male, being XY in constitution, is the heterogametic sex.

het″er·og′a·my [*heteros; gamos*]. The conjugation of gametes of unlike size and structure, as in higher plants and animals.

het″er·o·ge′ne·ous [*heteros;* G. *genos,* race]. Differing in kind or nature; composed of different substances; not homogeneous. —**heterogene′ity,** *n.*

het″er·o·gen′e·sis [*heteros;* G. *genesis,* production]. Alternation of generations in the complete life cycle, especially the alternation of a dioecious generation with one or more parthenogenetic generations and sometimes with an alternation of hosts, as in many trematode parasites. —**heterogenet′ic,** *adj.*

het″er·o·gen′ic [*heteros;* G. *genesthai,* from *gignesthai,* to be produced]. Pertaining to polysomic or polyploid organisms which contain different alleles for any given locus; similar to the term *heterozygous*, used for diploid organisms.

het″er·og′e·nous [*heteros;* G. *genos*, race]. Of, relating to, or derived from a different species, as heterogenous graft.

het″er·og′o·ny [*heteros;* G. *gonos*, offspring]. An alternation of generations in which a generation of males and females is followed by a hermaphroditic generation.

het′er·o·graft″. A graft of tissue obtained from an animal of one species and transferred to the body of another animal of a different species: common contraction of *heterogenous graft.* Also called *heteroplastic graft.*

het″er·o·he″mag·glu′ti·nin (het″ur·o·hee″muh-glue′ti·nin, ·hem″uh·glue′ti·nin). See *heteroagglutinin.*

het″er·o·he·mol′y·sin (·hem·ol′i·sin, ·hee″mo-lye′sin, ·hem″o·lye′sin) [*heteros;* G. *haima*, blood; *lysis*, a loosing]. A hemolytic amboceptor, natural or developed by immunization, against the red cells of a species different from that used to obtain the amboceptor.

het″er·o·hyp·no′sis [*heteros;* G. *hypnos*, sleep; *-ōsis*, condition]. Hypnosis induced by another, as opposed to *autohypnosis.*

het′er·oid [*heteros;* G. *eidos*, form]. Formed diversely, as enclosed structures which differ from their investment.

het″er·o·i′on. A complex ion resulting from adsorption of a simple ion by a relatively large molecule, as by a protein.

het″er·o·in·tox′i·ca′tion [*heteros;* L. *in*, in; G. *toxikon*, poison]. Intoxication by a poison not produced within the body.

het″er·o·ki·ne′si·a (het″ur·o·ki·nee′shuh, ·see·uh, ·zhuh, ·zee·uh, het″ur·o·kigh·) [*heteros;* G. *kinēsis*, motion]. The execution of body movements which are opposite to those ordered.

het″er·o·ki·ne′sis. *In physiology*, movement resulting from external stimuli.

het″er·o·lac′tic. Pertaining to a type of sugar fermentation in which lactic acid and several other products, e.g., CO_2 and alcohol, are produced; ordinarily, fermentation by microorganisms.

het″er·o·la′li·a. Heterophemy.

het″er·o·lat′er·al [*heteros;* L. *lateralis*, from *latus*, side]. Pertaining to, or situated on, the opposite side.

het″er·ol′o·gy [*heteros;* G. *logos*, word]. Deviation from the normal in structure, organization, or time or manner of formation. —**heterol′ogous,** *adj.*

het″er·o·ly′sin (het″ur·o·lye′sin, het″ur·ol′i·sin). See *heterohemolysin.*

het″er·o·mer′ic [*heteros;* G. *meros*, part]. Applied to neurons originating in one lateral side of the spinal cord and sending processes to the other side.

het″er·om′er·ous [*heteros; meros*]. Pertaining to substances unlike in chemical composition.

het″er·o·met″a·pla′si·a (·met″uh·play′zhuh, ·zee·uh, ·shuh, ·see·uh) [*heteros;* G. *metaplassein*, to remodel]. The change in the character of a tissue after transplantation to another part of the body.

het″er·o·me·tro′pi·a [*heteros;* G. *metron*, a measure; *ōps*, eye]. The condition in which the refraction in the two eyes is dissimilar.

het″er·o·mor′phic [*heteros;* G. *morphē*, form]. 1. Differing in size or form as compared with the normal. 2. *In chemistry*, crystallizing in different forms. 3. *In zoology*, having different forms at different stages of the life history. 4. *In cytology*, unlike in form or size; applied to either chromosome of a synaptic pair of unlike chromosomes, as an X and a Y chromosome. —**heteromorphism,** *n.*

het″er·o·mor′pho·sis (het″ur·o·mor′fo·sis, ·mor-fo′sis) [*heteros;* G. *morphōsis*, a shaping]. *In biology*, the regeneration of an organ or part different from that normal to the site, as the production in certain Crustacea of an antennalike structure after the removal of an eye and its ganglion. See *homeosis.*

het″er·o·mor′phous [*heteros;* G. *morphē*, form]. Differing from the normal in form.

het″er·on′o·mous [*heteros;* G. *nomos*, law]. *In biology*, referring to the condition in which the metameres of a segmented animal are dissimilar.

het″er·on′y·mous [*heteros;* G. *onyma*, name]. *In optics*, relating to crossed images of an object seen double.

het″er·o·os′te·o·plas″ty [*heteros;* G. *osteon*, bone; *plassein*, to form]. The grafting, by operation, of bone taken from an animal. Also see *graft.*

het″er·op′a·gus [*heteros;* G. *pagos*, that which is fixed]. A type of thoracopagus parasiticus in which the parasite, although imperfectly developed, has a head and extremities. Syn., *epigastrius parasiticus.*

het″er·op′a·thy [*heteros;* G. *pathos*, disease]. Abnormal reaction to stimuli. —**heteropath′ic,** *adj.*

het″er·o·pha′si·a (het″ur·o·fay′zhuh, ·zee·uh). See *heterophemy.*

het′er·o·phe″my (het′ur·o·fee″mee, het″ur·off′i-mee), **het″er·o·phe′mi·a** [*heteros;* G. *phēmē*, speech]. The unconscious saying of one thing while another is intended; heterolalia; heterophasia.

het′er·o·phil [*heteros;* G. *philein*, to love]. Having an affinity for other than the usual, as a heterophil antigen.

het′er·o·phil. 1. The neutrophil of mammals or birds. 2. The polymorphonuclear leukocyte of mammals. Its granules may vary in size and staining reaction with the animal species.

het″er·o·pho′ni·a [*heteros;* G. *phōnē*, voice]. Abnormal quality or change of voice.

het″er·o·pho·ral′gi·a [*heteros;* G. *phoros*, bearing; *algos*, pain]. Pain caused by heterophoria.

het″er·o·pho′ri·a [*heteros; phoros*]. Any tendency of the eyes to turn away from the position correct for binocular vision; latent deviation. Actual deviation does not occur unless one eye is covered, as the desire for binocular vision is sufficient to overcome imbalance of the ocular muscles. In *esophoria*, the tendency is to deviate inward; in *exophoria*, outward; in *hyperphoria*, one eye tends to deviate upward; in *hyperesophoria*, upward and inward; in *hyperexophoria*, upward and outward.

het″er·o·phy·di′a·sis. See *heterophyiasis.*

Het″er·oph′y·es (het″ur·off′ee·eez) [*heteros;* G. *phyein*, to put forth]. A genus of trematode worms, found in Egypt and the Far East, which produces heterophyiasis in man.

H. heterophyes. A species which has as definitive hosts man, cats, dogs, foxes, hogs, and other fish-eating animals; as first intermediate hosts, the snails, and as the second intermediate hosts, mullet fish.

het″er·o·phy·i′a·sis (het″ur·o·figh·eye′uh·sis) [*heteros; phyein;* NL. *-iasis*, condition]. Infestation by any fluke of the family Heterophyidae, of which the species *Heterophyes heterophyes* and *Metagonimus yokogawai* are the most important and most common to man. The flukes inhabit the small intestine but may also pass into the muscles of the heart through the lymphatics.

het″er·o·pla′si·a (het″ur·o·play′zhuh, ·zee·uh, ·shuh, ·see·uh) [*heteros;* G. *plassein*, to form]. The formation of tissue abnormal in type or in location. —**heteroplas′tic,** *adj.*

het′er·o·plas″ty [*heteros; plassein*]. The operation

of grafting parts taken from another species. **—het″er·o·plas′tic,** *adj.*

het′er·o·ploid [*heteros;* G. *-ploos,* -fold; *eidos,* form]. Having a chromosome number that is not an exact multiple of the haploid number characteristic for the species. **—heteroploidy,** *n.*

het″er·o·pol″y·ac′id. Any of a large group of complex oxygen-containing acids, formed by condensation of at least two different types of acid anhydrides, such as the phosphomolybdic acids of the formulas $P_2O_5.24MoO_3.xH_2O$ and $P_2O_5.18MoO_3.xH_2O$, or the silicotungstic acids of the formulas $SiO_2.12WO_3.xH_2O$ and SiO_2.-$10WO_3.xH_2O$.

het″er·o·pro′so·pus (het″ur·o·pro′so·pus, ·pro·so′-pus) [*heteros;* G. *prosōpon,* face]. A diprosopus with three or four eyes and two ears.

het″er·o·pro′te·ose [*heteros;* G. *prōteios,* holding first place]. One of a group of hydrolytic products, intermediate in the conversion of proteins to peptones; formed during gastric digestion or by autolysis of tissue protein.

het″er·op′si·a [*heteros;* G. *opsis,* vision]. Inequality of vision in the two eyes.

Het″er·op′ter·a [*heteros;* G. *pteron,* wing]. The true bugs. Formerly a suborder of the order Hemiptera.

het″er·op′tics [*heteros;* G. *optikos,* of sight]. Perverted vision.

het″er·o·pyk·no′sis. A staining property of nuclei characterized by areas of heavier staining (**positive h.**) and areas of lighter staining (**negative h.**). **—heteropyknot′ic,** *adj.*

het″er·o·sac′cha·ride. A polysaccharide which yields, on hydrolysis, both sugars and nonsugars.

het′er·o·scope″ [*heteros;* G. *skopein,* to examine]. An instrument for the determination of the range of vision in strabismus. **—heteros′copy,** *n.*

het″er·o·sex″u·al′i·ty [*heteros;* L. *sexus,* sex]. Sexual feeling directed toward one of the opposite sex.

het′er·o·side″. A term proposed for a class of glycosides.

het″er·o′sis [*heteros;* G. *-ōsis,* increase]. The increased vigor and growth capacity exhibited frequently by first-generation hybrids.

het″er·o·sug·ges″ti·bil′i·ty [*heteros;* L. *suggestio,* from *suggerere,* to suggest]. The state of being susceptible to influence by another.

het″er·o·sug·ges′tion [*heteros; suggestio*]. Suggestion originating from a source outside of the individual's mind; suggestion by another.

het″er·o·tax′is, het″er·o·tax′i·a, het′er·o·tax″y [*heteros;* G. *taxis,* arrangement]. Anomalous position or transposition of organs. Also see *dextrocardia, situs inversus.*

het″er·o·to′ni·a [*heteros;* G. *tonos,* tension]. Variable tension.

het″er·o·to′pi·a [*heteros;* G. *topos,* place]. Displacement or deviation from natural position, as of an organ or a part; especially, congenital displacement of gray matter of the spinal cord into the white matter.

het″er·o·top′ic [*heteros; topos*]. Occurring in an abnormal location, as intestinal epithelial cells occurring in the gastric epithelium.

het″er·o·tox′in. A toxin introduced into, but formed outside of, the body.

het″er·o·trans·plan·ta′tion. Transplantation of a tissue or part from one species to another. **—heterotrans′plant,** *n.*

het′er·o·trophs [*heteros;* G. *trophē,* nourishment]. Bacteria, including all those pathogenic for man, which require for growth a source of carbon more complex than CO_2. Wide variation exists in respect to utilizable organic carbon sources and requirements for accessory growth factors.

het″er·o·troph′ic. Of or pertaining to heterotrophs.

het″er·o·tro′pi·a. See *strabismus.*

het″er·o·typ′ic, het″er·o·typ′i·cal [*heteros;* G. *typos,* pattern]. 1. Pertaining to the first division in miosis, as distinguished from the second, or regular, cell division. 2. Relating to a heterotypus.

het″er·o·ty′pus [*heteros; typos*]. A double monster in which the parasite hangs from the ventral wall of the autosite.

het″er·o·xan′thine (het″ur·o·zan′theen, ·thin). $C_6H_6O_2N_4$. Methyl xanthine; 7-methyl-2,6-diketo purine; a methylated purine, one of the xanthine bases.

het″er·ox′e·nous [*heteros;* G. *xenos,* host]. Infesting more than one kind of host during the life cycle. **—heteroxeny,** *n.*

het″er·o·zy·go′sis (het″ur·o·zye·go′sis) [*heteros;* G. *zygōsis,* a balancing]. The condition of having one or many pairs of genes in the heterozygous phase, which results from crossbreeding; opposed to *homozygosis,* which results from inbreeding.

het″er·o·zy′gote [*heteros;* G. *zygōtos,* yoked]. An individual having the two members of one or more pairs of genes dissimilar. **—heterozygous,** *adj.*

HETP. Hexaethyltetraphosphate.

hetrazan. Trade-mark for the basic component of diethylcarbamazine citrate.

Heubner, Otto Johann Leonhard [*German pediatrician,* 1843–1926]. Described syphilitic endarteritis of the cerebral arteries; called *Heubner's disease.* Isolated meningococci from cerebrospinal fluid (1896). With Rubner, determined the caloric requirements of infants. He also studied celiac disease.

Heuser's membrane. See exocoelomic *membrane.*

Hewson, William [*English surgeon,* 1739–74]. Remembered for his discovery that fibrinogen is responsible for the clotting of blood (1771). Studied the lymphatic system and divided the lymphatics into two groups, the superficial and the deep.

hexa-betalin. Trade-mark for a brand of pyridoxine hydrochloride.

hexabione hydrochloride. Trade-mark for a brand of pyridoxine hydrochloride.

hex″a·chlo″ro·cy″clo·hex′ane. $C_6H_6Cl_6$. More properly, gamma-hexachlorocyclohexane, commonly called *gammexane.*

hex″a·chlo′ro·phene. $HO.Cl_3C_6H.CH_2.C_6HCl_3$.-$OH$; bis-(2-hydroxy-3,5,6-trichlorophenyl)-methane, a germicide active in the presence of soap. Syn., *compound G-11.*

hex″a·chro′mic [G. *hex,* six; *chrōma,* color]. Capable of distinguishing only six of the seven spectrum colors, indigo not being distinguished.

hex′ad [*hex*]. An element the atom of which has a valence of six.

hex″a·dac′ty·lism [*hex;* G. *daktylos,* finger]. The state of having six fingers or toes.

hex″a·dec″a·no′ic ac′id. An exact chemical name, rarely used, for *palmitic acid.*

hex″a·dec″e·no′ic ac′id. The unsaturated acid $CH_3(CH_2)_6CH{:}CH(CH_2)_6COOH$, occurring as a component of the glycerides of some fats and oils.

hex″a·dec′yl. The univalent hydrocarbon radical $CH_3(CH_2)_{15}$—. Syn., *cetyl, palmityl.*

hex″a·di′e·nol. $CH_3.CH{:}CH.CH{:}CH.CH_2OH$. An amber-colored, semisolid substance insoluble in water but miscible with organic solvents and vegetable oils. A substance which causes sweating when applied locally to the skin. It is suggested as a sudorific and a diagnostic agent in localizing anhidrotic areas in the skin.

hex″a·eth″yl·tet″ra·phos′phate. $(C_2H_5)_6P_4O_{13}$-(?); a synthetic substance having the power to inhibit cholinesterase; it is probably a mixture of compounds, of which tetraethylpyrophosphate is the predominant and active constituent. It is used as an insecticide. Abbreviated HETP.

hex″a·gen′ic. Referring to genotypes of polysomic or polyploid organisms which contain six different alleles for any given locus.

hex″a·hy′dric. Containing six atoms of replaceable hydrogen.

hex″a·hy″dro·hem″a·to·por′phy·rin (heck″suh-high″dro·hem″uh·to·por′fi·rin, ·hee″muh·to·por′-fi·rin). A reduction product of hematin.

hex″a·hy·dro·phe′nol. Cyclohexanol.

hex″a·hy·drox″y·cy·clo·hex′ane. Inositol.

hex′al. Methenamine sulfosalicylate; $C_{13}H_{18}N_4O_6$-$S.H_2O$; a white, crystalline powder used as a urinary antiseptic. See *hexalet.*

hex·al′de·hyde. Hexanal.

hexalet. Trade-mark for methenamine sulfosalicylate. See *hexal.*

hexalin. Trade name for cyclohexanol, $C_6H_{11}OH$; a clear, viscous liquid used as solubilizer, homogenizer, and stabilizer for various liquid mixtures.

hex″a·me·tho′ni·um. One of a homologous series of polymethylene bis(trimethylammonium) ions, of the general formula $(CH_3)_3N^+(CH_2)_nN^+(CH_3)_3$, in which n is 6. It possesses potent ganglion-blocking action, effecting reduction in blood pressure. It is used clinically in the form of one of its salts, commonly the bromide or iodide. Syn., *C6.* See *bistrium bromide.*

hex″a·meth″yl·en·a·mine′ (heck″suh·meth″il-een·uh·meen′, ·am′een, ·in). Methenamine.

hex″a·meth″yl·ene·tet″ra·mine′ (·tet″ruh·meen′, ·tet·ram′een, ·in). Methenamine.

h. tetraiodide. See *siomine.*

hex″a·mine′. A former British Pharmacopoeia name for methenamine.

hex′a·nal. *n*-Hexaldehyde, $C_5H_{11}CHO$. A pleasantly odorous liquid; used in the preparation of dyes, perfumes, and other synthetics.

hex′ane. Any one of the isomeric liquid hydrocarbons, C_6H_{14}, of the paraffin series.

hex″ane·di·o′ic ac′id. Adipic acid.

hex″a·ni″tro·di·phen·yl′a·mine. See *dipicrylamine.*

hex″a·va′lent (heck″suh·vay′lunt, heck·sav′uh-lunt). Having a valence of six.

hex″a·vi′ta·min cap′sules or **tab′lets** (*capsulae hexavitaminarum; tabellae hexavitaminarum*). Each capsule or tablet contains not less than 5000 U.S.P. units of vitamin A, 400 U.S.P. units of vitamin D, 75 mg. of ascorbic acid, 2 mg. of thiamine hydrochloride, 3 mg. of riboflavin, and 20 mg. of nicotinamide.

hex′ene-ol. An alcohol, C_6H_9OH, useful as a protective covering for burns.

hexestrol. $HO.C_6H_4(C_2H_5)CH.CH(C_2H_5)$.-$C_6H_4.OH$; dihydrodiethylstilbestrol, a synthetic estrogen said to be more active than diethylstilbestrol.

hex′e·thal so′di·um. Generic name for sodium 5-ethyl-5-*n*-hexylbarbiturate, a sedative and hypnotic having short duration of action. See *ortal sodium.*

hexital. Trade-mark for a tablet containing hexestrol and phenobarbital.

hex″o·bar′bi·tal (heck″so·bahr′bi·tawl, ·tal). C_{12}-$H_{16}N_2O_3$; 5-(1-cyclohexenyl)-1,5-dimethylbarbituric acid, very slightly soluble in water; a rapidly acting barbiturate of low toxicity. Dose, 0.25–0.5 Gm. (4–8 gr.). Syn., *hexobarbitone.* See *evipal.*

h. sodium. $C_{12}H_{15}N_2NaO_3$; the monosodium derivative of hexobarbital which, because it is very soluble in water, may be administered intravenously: used to produce anesthesia of short duration. The dose must be individualized. Syn., *hexobarbitone sodium.* See *evipal sodium.*

hex″o·bar′bi·tone. British Pharmacopoeia name for hexobarbital.

h. sodium. British Pharmacopoeia name for hexobarbital sodium.

hexoestrol. Hexestrol.

hex″o·ki′nase, hex·ok′i·nase. The enzyme which catalyzes the transfer of phosphate from adenosinetriphosphate to glucose or fructose, forming glucose-6-phosphate or fructose-6-phosphate and adenosinediphosphate.

hex′one bas′es. Term applied to the diaminomonocarboxylic acids (arginine, lysine, and histidine) which contain six carbon atoms and are basic in reaction.

hex·os″a·mine′ (heck·sohss″uh·meen′, heck′sohss-uh·meen″, ·min″). $C_6H_{11}O_5.NH_2$. A primary amino-derivative of a hexose obtained on the hydrolysis of certain glycoproteins, mucins, heparin, chitin, etc.

hex′o·san. Any complex carbohydrate yielding a hexose on hydrolysis. Cellulose, starch, and glycogen are important hexosans.

hex′ose. $C_6H_{12}O_6$. Any monosaccharide which contains six carbon atoms in the molecule.

hex″ose·di·phos′phate (heck″sohss·dye·fos′fate). One of the hexosephosphates formed during the decomposition of glucose and glycogen in muscle-tissue metabolism.

hex″ose·mon″o·phos′phate. One of the hexosephosphates formed during the decomposition of glycogen in muscle-tissue action.

hex″ose·phos′phates. Any one of the phosphoric acid esters of a hexose, notably glucose, formed during the utilization of carbohydrates by mammalian tissues.

hex″u·ron′ic ac′id. The name originally given to the substance isolated from lemon juice and later identified as vitamin C.

hex′yl. The univalent radical, C_6H_{13}—.

hex″yl·res·or′cin·ol (heck″sil·ri·zor′sin·ole, ·ol, ·awl). $C_6H_{13}C_6H_3(OH)_2$. White, needle-shaped crystals of sharp taste, very slightly soluble in water, freely soluble in alcohol and fixed oils, becoming brown on exposure to light and air. Used as germicide, as urinary antiseptic, and as anthelmintic for hookworms and roundworms. Dose, 0.12–1.0 Gm. (2–15 gr.). See *caprokol, crystoids anthelmintic, S.T. 37.*

Hey, William [*English surgeon,* 1736–1819]. Described internal derangement of the knee joint; see under *derangement.* See also Hey's *amputation,* Hey's *saw.*

Heymans, Corneille (1892–). Belgian pharmacologist, who discovered the function of the carotid sinus and aortic mechanisms in the regulation of respiration and blood pressure. Nobel laureate in medicine and physiology (1938).

Hf Chemical symbol for hafnium.

Hg Chemical symbol for mercury (*hydrargyrum*).

hg. Hectogram.

HGF Hyperglycemic factor.

hi·a′tus (high·ay′tus) [L.]. A space or opening. —**hiatal,** *adj.*

adductor h. The hiatus tendineus adductorius [BNA]. The gap in the insertion of the adductor magnus; the point of transition between the femoral and popliteal vessels; the terminal opening of the adductor canal. Syn., *h. adductorius, h. tendineus.*

aortic h. An opening behind the diaphragm giving passage to the aorta: also called *aortic foramen.*

buccal h. Transverse facial cleft.

esophageal h. Passage through the diaphragm

for the esophagus: also called *esophageal foramen.*

facial h. See *h.* of the facial canal.

h. adductorius. The adductor hiatus.

h. of the facial canal. The opening which transmits the greater superficial petrosal nerve and the petrosal branch of the middle meningeal artery: also called *h. of Fallopius.*

h. of Fallopius. See *h. of the facial canal.*

h. of Schwalbe. A gap occasionally found in the pelvic fascia due to improper fusion of the obturator fascia with the tendinous arch (arcus tendineus).

h. tendineus. The adductor hiatus.

maxillary h. One on the inner aspect of the body of the maxilla, establishing communication between the nasal cavity and maxillary sinus.

pleuroperitoneal h. A small opening in the diaphragm between pleural and peritoneal cavities in the fetus.

sacral h. The lower or caudal opening of the sacral canal.

semilunar h. (a) A groove in the lateral wall of the middle meatus of the nasal cavity. The maxillary sinus and anterior ethmoid cells open into it. (b) An opening in the deep fascia of the arm for the passage of the basilic vein.

subarcuate h. A depression on the petrous part of the temporal bone lodging the flocculus.

Hibbs, Russell Aubra [*American orthopedist,* 1869–1932]. Devised an operation for ankylosis or fusion of the knee joint in tuberculosis. Also devised an operation, somewhat similar to Albee's, designed to eliminate motion in a diseased spine. The spinous processes, the laminas, and the lateral articulations are fused, and a cortical bone graft is inserted between the split spinous processes. Called *Hibbs's operation.*

hi″ber·na′tion [L. *hiberna,* winter quarters]. The dormant condition or winter sleep of certain animals.

hi″ber·no′ma. A rare subcutaneous tumor composed of large foamy cells, containing lipid-staining material, and having a lobulated arrangement simulating the appearance of the hibernating organs of certain animals. It usually grows slowly, may become very large, but is not known to become malignant.

hic′cup, hic′cough [probably imitative in origin]. A spasmodic contraction of the diaphragm causing inspiration, followed by a sudden closure of the glottis.

Hickman, Kenneth O. D. (1896–). American chemist, known for research in vitamin chemistry. He invented many high-vacuum processes. See Hickman molecular distillation *process.*

Hicks's sign. See under *sign.*

Hicks version. See Braxton Hicks *version.*

hid·rad″e·ni′tis [G. *hidrōs,* sweat; *adēn,* gland; *-itis,* inflammation]. Inflammation of the sweat glands: also spelled *hydradenitis.*

h. suppurativa. An inflammatory disease of the apocrine sweat glands, especially those of the axillas, characterized by painful red nodules, abscesses, and sinus tracts; partial remissions alternate with acute exacerbations. Syn., *hidrosadenitis axillaris.*

hid·rad″e·no·car″ci·no′ma. Sweat-gland tumor.

hid·rad′e·no·cyte (hid·rad′uh·no·site, high·drad′·). Cell found in certain cystic conditions of the breast; it resembles axillary apocrine sweat gland cells.

hid·rad″e·no′ma. A benign tumor, presumably derived from sweat glands, usually composed of solid islands of small basal cells, each group surrounded by hyaline connective tissue. See also *cylindroma.*

nodular h. See *myoepithelioma.*

papillary h. An infrequent benign tumor of the apocrine glands occurring most commonly on the labia majores and perineum of women.

hid′ro-, hidr- [G. *hidrōs,* sweat]. A combining form meaning *sweat.*

hid·ro′a (hid·ro′uh, high·dro′uh) [*hidrōs*]. Any dermal lesion associated with, or caused by, profuse sweating.

hid″ro·cys″ta·de·no′ma. See *hidrocystoma.*

hid″ro·cys·to′ma (hid″ro·sis·to′muh, high″dro·) [*hidrōs;* G. *kystis,* bladder; *-ōma,* tumor]. A group of clear vesicles, usually located around the eyes, composed of cystic sweat glands. Some cysts may contain small papillary projections. Also called *hidrocystadenoma.*

hid″ro·poi·e′sis (hid″ro·poy·ee′sis, high″dro·) [*hidrōs;* G. *poiēsis,* formation]. The formation of sweat. —**hidropoiet′ic,** *adj.*

hid″ror·rhe′a (hid″ro·ree′uh, high″dro·) [*hidrōs;* G. *rhoia,* flow]. Excessive flow of sweat.

hi″dros·ad″e·ni′tis (high″dro sad″i·nigh′tis, hid″-ro·) [*hidrōs;* G. *adēn,* gland; *-itis,* inflammation]. Inflammation of the sweat glands. Also called *hidradenitis, hydrosadenitis.*

h. axillaris. See *hidradenitis suppurativa.*

hid·ros′che·sis (hid·ros′ki·sis, high·dros′·) [*hidrōs;* G. *schesis,* retention]. Retention or suppression of the sweat.

hi·dro′sis (hi·dro′sis, high·dro′sis) [*hidrōs;* G. *-ōsis,* increase]. 1. The formation and excretion of sweat. 2. Abnormally profuse sweating. —**hi′drose,** *adj.*

hi·drot′ic (hi·drot′ick, high·drot′ick) [G. *hydrōtikos,* sudorific]. Diaphoretic or sudorific.

hi·drot′ic. A medicine that causes sweating.

hid″ro·to·path′ic [G. *hidrōs,* sweat; *pathos,* disease]. Relating to a morbid state of the perspiratory function.

hi″er·on′o·sus [G. *hieros,* sacred; *nosos,* disease]. Old term for epilepsy.

hi″er·o·pho′bi·a [*hieros;* G. *phobos,* fear]. A morbid fear of sacred things.

Highmore, Nathaniel [*English physician and anatomist,* 1613–85]. Described the maxillary sinus (1651), called the *antrum of Highmore.* Described the seminal ducts and the epididymis. The mediastinum testis formerly was called the *body of Highmore.*

high take-off. Colloquial term for unusual elevation—more than one millimeter—of the isoelectric line at origin; seen in electrocardiograms in cases of myocardial injury, infarction, trauma, and pericarditis.

hi′lar dance. Increased pulsations of pulmonary arteries in cases of widened pulmonary artery pulse pressure.

Hildanus. See *Fabricius Hildanus.*

Hildebrand method for hydrogen-ion concentration. See under *method.*

hi′li (high′lye). Plural of hilus.

Hill, Archibald Vivian (1886–). English biophysicist, who studied thermal changes in muscle and proved that oxygen is not used in the working phase of muscular activity, but in the recovery phase. He developed refined techniques to measure the course of heat production during a single contraction cycle. With Otto Meyerhof he was named Nobel laureate in medicine and physiology (1922).

Hill, Leonard Erskine [*English physiologist,* 1866–]. With Barnard, introduced a modification of the sphygmomanometer with a pressure gauge (1897). Made an important study of caisson disease (1912).

Hilliard's lupus. A form of lupus affecting the

hands and arms. The disease was named by Jonathan Hutchinson for a patient.

hill'ock [dim. of AS. *hyll*]. A slight prominence or elevation. Also see *colliculus.*

anal h. See anal *tubercle.*

auricular h. One of several small tubercles on the surface of the mandibular and hyoid arches, incorporated into the pinna of the external ear.

axon h. The region in a nerve cell, free from Nissl substance, from which the axon takes origin.

cloacal h. See genital *tubercle.*

Müller's h. An elevation on the dorsal wall of the embryonic urogenital sinus at the point of entrance of the Müllerian ducts. Also called *Müller's tubercle.*

seminal h. The colliculus seminalis.

Hilton, John [*English surgeon and anatomist,* 1804–78]. Author of a classic work, *On Rest and Pain* (1863). Advocated complete rest in surgical disorders. Suggested that symptoms are disordered reflexes. *Hilton's law* states that the nerve trunk supplying a joint also supplies the overlying skin and the muscles which move the joint.

hi'lum [L., a little thing]. Old term for hilus.

hi'lus (pl. *hili*) [*hilum*]. A pit, recess, or opening in an organ, usually for the entrance and exit of vessels or ducts. —**hilar,** *adj.*

hind"brain. See *rhombencephalon.*

hind'gut" [ME. *hind;* AS. plural *guttas*]. The caudal part of the embryonic digestive tube formed by the development of the tail fold.

Hines and Brown test. See cold pressor *test.*

Hinkle's pills. See under *pill.*

Hinton test. A macroscopic flocculation test for syphilis.

hip [AS. *hype*]. 1. The upper part of the thigh at its junction with the buttocks. See Plates 2, 4. 2. The hip joint. See Table of Joints and Ligaments in the Appendix. 3. The lateral prominence of the body at the level of the hip joint.

snapping h. An abnormality caused by the presence of a tendinous band on the surface of the gluteus maximus muscle. Certain movements of the hip cause this band to slip over the greater trochanter.

hip'bone', hip'bone" [*hype;* AS. *bān*]. The innominate bone or os coxae. See Table of Bones in the Appendix.

hip·pan'thro·py [G. *hippos,* horse; *anthrōpos,* man]. A delusional state in which the patient believes he is a horse. Also see *zoanthropy. Rare.*

Hippel, Arthur von [*German ophthalmologist,* 1841–1917]. Modern keratoplasty, in which a circular portion of the cornea extending down to Descemet's membrane is removed by means of a trephine, is based on the technic introduced by von Hippel.

Hippel, Eugen von [*German ophthalmologist,* 1867–1939]. Remembered for his description of angiomatosis retinae (1895), called *von Hippel's disease.* See also *von Hippel-Lindau's disease,* under *Lindau.*

Hip"pe·la'tes (hip"i·lay'teez) [G., driver of horses]. A genus of minute flies of the family Oscinidae.

H. flavipes. A species which transmits yaws and feeds on conjunctival exudates.

H. pusio. The American rye fly; a pest of both man and animals which feeds on drops of blood on the skin, open wounds, and mucous membranes; a factor in spreading conjunctivitis.

Hip"po·bos'ci·dae (hip"o·bos'i·dee) [G. *hippos,* horse; *boskein,* to feed]. A family of the Diptera which includes the louse flies and flat flies, blood-sucking ectoparasites of birds and mammals.

hip"po·cam'pus [G. *hippokampos,* monster with horse's body and fish's tail]. A curved elevation consisting largely of gray matter, in the floor of the inferior horn of the lateral ventricle. —**hippocampal,** *adj.*

Hippocrates [*Greek physician,* ca. 460–ca. 377 B.C.]. Called the father of medicine. Best known for his astute clinical descriptions of diseases. His voluminous works include discussions of epidemics, fevers, epilepsy, fractures, instruments for reduction, and climate and health. He knew the operations of trephining and paracentesis. He believed that the body tends to heal itself by natural processes, and that the role of the physician should be ancillary to that of nature. See also *facies* hippocratica; clubbed *finger,* also called *Hippocratic finger* or *nail.*

oath of H. An oath setting forth the duties of the physician to his patients, as follows: I swear by Apollo the physician, and Asclepios, and Health, and All-heal, and all the gods and goddesses, that, according to my ability and judgment, I will keep this Oath and this stipulation—to reckon him who taught me this Art equally dear to me as my parents, to share my substance with him, and relieve his necessities if required; to look upon his offspring in the same footing as my own brothers, and to teach them this art, if they shall wish to learn it, without fee or stipulation; and that by precept, lecture, and every other mode of instruction, I will impart a knowledge of the Art to my own sons, and those of my teachers, and to disciples bound by a stipulation and oath according to the law of medicine, but to none others. ¶ I will follow that system of regimen which, according to my ability and judgment, I consider for the benefit of my patients, and abstain from whatever is deleterious and mischievous. I will give no deadly medicine to any one if asked, nor suggest any such counsel; and in like manner I will not give to a woman a pessary to produce abortion. With purity and with holiness I will pass my life and practise my Art. ¶ I will not cut persons labouring under the stone, but will leave this to be done by men who are practitioners of this work. Into whatever houses I enter, I will go into them for the benefit of the sick, and will abstain from every voluntary act of mischief and corruption; and, further, from the seduction of females or males, of freemen and slaves. ¶ Whatever, in connexion with my professional practice, or not in connexion with it, I see or hear, in the life of men, which ought not to be spoken of abroad, I will not divulge, as reckoning that all such should be kept secret. While I continue to keep this Oath unviolated, may it be granted to me to enjoy life and the practice of the art, respected by all men, in all times! But should I trespass and violate this Oath, may the reverse be my lot!

hip'po·lith [G. *hippos,* horse; *lithos,* stone]. A calculus or bezoar found in the stomach of the horse.

Hip·pom'a·ne (hi·pom'uh·nee) [*hippos;* G. *mania,* madness]. A genus of euphorbiaceous trees.

H. mancinella. The manchineel tree of tropical America; extremely acrid and poisonous, even to the touch. Used locally in medicine, especially in skin diseases.

hip"po·myx·o'ma [*hippos;* G. *myxa,* discharge; *-ōma,* tumor]. The swelling attending glanders.

hippuran. Trade-mark for sodium ortho-iodohippurate, $C_6H_4I.CONH.CH_2COONa.2H_2O$, a radiopaque agent.

hip'pur·ase. See *hippuricase.*

hip·pu'ri·a [*hippos;* G. *ouron,* urine]. Excess of hippuric acid in the urine.

hip·pu'ric ac'id. $C_6H_5CONHCH_2COOH$. Benzoylaminoacetic acid; an acid found in high concentration in the urine of herbivorous animals and to a lesser extent in the urine of man; it is the detoxication product of benzoic acid. Syn., *urobenzoic acid.*

hip·pur′i·case. An enzyme found in kidney, liver, muscle, and pancreas which catalyzes the hydrolysis of hippuric acid to benzoic acid and glycine. The hippuricase occurring in liver and kidney probably exerts a synthetic, rather than a hydrolytic, action, detoxifying benzoic acid by the formation of hippuric acid. Syn., *hippurase, histozyme.*

hip′pus [*hippos*]. Spasmodic pupillary movement, independent of the action of light.

hip″ta·gen′ic ac′id. $C_3H_5NO_4$; a water-soluble crystalline substance, toxic to animals, obtained from *Hiptage benghalensis*, a plant native to India, and also from *Indigofera endecaphylla*, the trailing or creeping indigo, which is under investigation as a potential forage crop. The substance appears to be identical with β-nitropropionic acid, and would thus be the only aliphatic nitro compound isolated from natural sources.

Hirschberg, Julius [*German ophthalmologist*, 1843–1925]. Introduced the use of the electromagnet in ophthalmology (1885). Wrote an important history of ophthalmology and compiled a dictionary of the subject. In *Hirschberg's test* the degree of strabismus is estimated from the position of the corneal reflection of a candle flame or flashlight held one foot from the patient's eye. The examiner places his own eye near the light and looks just over it.

Hirschberg's reflex. See under *reflex.*

Hirschfeld, Ludwig Moritz [*Polish anatomist*, 1816–76]. An inconstant lingual branch of the facial nerve is sometimes called *Hirschfeld's nerve.*

Hirschsprung, Harald [*Danish physician*, 1830–1916]. Known for his description of congenital megacolon or congenital dilatation of the colon; known as *Hirschsprung's disease.* Contributed to the knowledge of congenital pyloric stenosis in infants.

Hirst, Barton Cooke [*American gynecologist*, 1861–1935]. Devised an operation for the relief of vaginismus: longitudinal incisions made on either side of the vulva and carried deep into the tissues are closed transversely, in order to enlarge the vaginal introitus. Called *Hirst's operation.*

hir′sute (hur′suit, hur·suit′) [L. *hirsutus*, rough, shaggy]. Shaggy; hairy.

hir·su′tic ac′id. Generic term for a series of substances, derived from the fungus *Stereum hirsutum*, certain of which have antibiotic activity.

hir·su′ti·es (hur·sue′shee·eez, ·tee·eez) [*hirsutus*]. Excessive growth of hair; hypertrichosis.

hir′sut·ism (hur′suit·iz·um, hur·suit′iz·um) [*hirsutus*]. A condition characterized by growth of hair in unusual places and in unusual amounts.

hir′u·din, hi·ru′din [L. *hirudo*, leech]. The active principle of a secretion derived from the buccal glands of leeches. It prevents the coagulation of blood.

Hir″u·din′e·a [*hirudo*]. A class of predatory or parasitic annelids; the leeches.

hir″u·di·ni′a·sis [*hirudo;* NL. *-iasis*, condition]. Infestation by leeches.

external h. That form produced by leeches of the genus *Haemadipsa*, which attach themselves to, and puncture the skin of humans. The leeches suck the blood and secrete an anticoagulating principle, hirudin.

internal h. A pathologic state caused by the ingestion of aquatic leeches of the genus *Limnatis*, or by their invasion of the genitourinary tract.

hi·ru′di·ni·cul″ture [*hirudo;* L. *cultura*, cultivation]. The artificial breeding of leeches.

Hi·ru′do [L.]. A genus of leeches of the class Hirudinea.

H. medicinalis. The medicinal leech; formerly extensively used for bloodletting.

His, Wilhelm (*Junior*) [*German physiologist*, 1863–1934]. Made important studies of the rhythmic action of the heart. Described the atrioventricular bundle, called *bundle of His, Gaskell's bridge.* The terminal cardiac sulcus on the surface of the right atrium is called *His's sulcus.* He also described trench fever, called *Werner-His disease.*

His, Wilhelm (*Senior*) (1831–1904). Swiss anatomist and embryologist, considered the founder of modern human embryology. The fetal thyroglossal duct, the perivascular spaces, the trabecular structure of the mammary gland, and many other structures formerly were known by his name. He showed that axons are outgrowths from primitive nerve cells, and introduced such terms as *dendrite, neuroblast*, and *spongioblast.*

Hiss, Philip Hanson [*American bacteriologist*, 1868–1913]. With F. F. Russell, described a type of *Shigella paradysenteriae*, also called *Hiss and Russell's Y bacillus.* See also *Hiss method* under *stain*, Hiss's *serum* water.

histadyl. A trade-mark for methapyrilene hydrochloride, a histamine-antagonizing agent.

his·tam′i·nase, his″tam·i·nase′. An enzyme, obtainable from extracts of kidney and intestinal mucosa, capable of inactivating histamine and other diamines; has been used in the treatment of anaphylactic shock, asthma, hay fever, serum sickness, and other allergic conditions which may be due to, or accompanied by, the liberation of histamine in the body. Syn., *diamine oxidase.*

his′ta·mine (hiss′tuh·meen, ·min). β-Imidoazolyl-4-ethylamine, $C_5H_9N_3$. An amine occurring as a decomposition product of histidine and prepared synthetically from that substance. It stimulates visceral muscles, dilates capillaries, stimulates salivary, pancreatic, and gastric secretions. Used in various allergies, in Ménière's disease, as a diagnostic agent in testing gastric secretion, and to contract the uterus. —**histamin′ic,** *adj.*

h. dihydrochloride. See *imido.*

h. phosphate (*histaminae phosphas*). Clear, colorless crystals soluble in 4 parts of water. Dose, 0.3–1.0 mg. ($\frac{1}{200}$–$\frac{1}{60}$ gr.) intravenously or subcutaneously. Also called *histamine acid phosphate.*

h. phosphate injection (*injectio histaminae phosphatis*). A 1:1000 solution. Dose, 0.3 cc. (5 min.).

his″ta·min·o·lyt′ic. Dissolving histamine.

his″ta·nox′i·a. See histotoxic *hypoxia.*

hist′ic [G. *histos*, web]. Relating to tissue. *Obs.*

his′ti·dase. An enzyme found only in the liver in higher animals. It is highly specific, acting only upon L-histidine, not upon D-histidine or other imidazole compounds, to open the imidazole ring with the formation of glutamic acid, formic acid, and ammonia.

his′ti·dine (hiss′ti·deen, ·din). $C_3H_3N_2.CH_2.CH(NH_2)COOH$. β-Imidazole-α-alanine, an amino acid resulting from the hydrolysis of many proteins. By elimination of a molecule of carbon dioxide it is converted to histamine.

h. decarboxylase. The enzyme which catalyzes decarboxylation of histidine to histamine.

h. hydrochloride. $C_6H_9N_3O_2.HCl$. White, crystalline powder freely soluble in water. Used in treatment of peptic ulcers. Dose, 5 cc. of 4 per cent solution intramuscularly daily. See *larostidin.*

his″ti·di·nu′ri·a. A state in which histidine is found in the urine, frequently occurring in women after the first month of pregnancy. Attributed to restricted activity of histidase in the liver.

his′ti·dyl. The univalent radical, $N_2C_3H_3CH_2CH(NH_2)CO$—, of the amino acid histidine.

his′ti·o-, histi- [G. *histion*, web]. A combining form meaning *a web, cloth, tissue.*

his′ti·o·cyte [*histion;* G. *kytos*, cell]. Fixed macrophage of the loose connective tissue. Histiocytes, in common with other cells belonging to the reticuloendothelial system, store electively certain dyes such as trypan blue or lithium carmine. Formerly called *resting wandering cell.*

his″ti·o·cy·to′ma (hiss″tee·o·sigh·to′muh) [*histion; kytos;* G. *-ōma*, tumor]. A tumor containing histiocytes. See *dermatofibroma.*

juvenile h. See *nevoxanthoendothelioma.*

his″ti·o·cy″to·sar·co′ma [*histion; kytos;* G. *sarkōma*, fleshy excrescence]. A tumor only slightly malignant, occurring in dermis especially; made up of large, mononuclear cells, supposed by some to be histiocytes. Others believe the cells to be fibrocytes and fibroblasts, and name the lesion a fibroma or fibrosarcoma.

his″ti·o·cy·to′sis (·sigh·to′sis) [*histion; kytos;* G. *-ōsis*, increase]. Proliferation of histiocytes, especially in lymph nodes and other organs of the hematopoietic system; sometimes occurs with lipoidosis.

lipoid h. See Niemann-Pick *disease.*

nonlipid h. See Letterer-Siwe *disease.*

his′ti·oid. Histoid.

his″ti·o·troph′ic [*histion;* G. *trophē*, nourishment]. Having a protective or anabolic influence on the energy of cells, as the histiotrophic functions of the autonomic nervous system.

his′to-, hist- [G. *histos*, web]. 1. A combining form meaning *loom, web.* 2. *In biology*, a combining form denoting *tissue.*

his′to·blast [*histos;* G. *blastos*, germ]. A cell engaged in the formation of tissue. *Obs.*

his″to·chem′is·try [*histos;* G. *chymos*, juice]. 1. The chemistry of the tissues of the body. 2. The study of microscopic localization and analysis of substances in cells and tissues. —**histochemical,** *adj.*

his′to·cyte. See *histiocyte.*

his″to·di·al′y·sis (hiss″to·dye·al′i·sis) [*histos;* G. *dialysis*, dissolution]. The dissolution of organic tissue.

his″to·flu″o·res′cence [*histos;* L. *fluere*, to flow]. Fluorescence of the tissues during x-ray treatment produced by the prior administration of fluorescing drugs.

his″to·gen′e·sis, his·tog′e·ny (hiss·todj′i·nee) [*histos;* G. *genesis*, production]. Differentiation of cells and cell products from their earliest appearance to the completion of a mature tissue. —**histogenet′ic,** *adj.*

his·tog′e·ny See *histogenesis.*

his·tog′ra·phy [*histos;* G. *graphein*, to write]. Description of the tissues.

his″to·hem′a·tin (hiss″to·hem′uh·tin, ·hee′muh·tin). Old term for cytochrome.

his′toid, his′ti·oid [*histos;* G. *eidos*, form]. 1. Resembling tissue. 2. Composed of only one kind of tissue.

his″to·ki·ne′sis (hiss″to·ki·nee′sis, ·kigh·nee′sis) [*histos;* G. *kinēsis*, motion]. Movement that takes place in the minute structural elements of the body.

his·tol′o·gist [*histos;* G. *logos*, word]. One who is learned in histology.

his·tol′o·gy [*histos; logos*]. The branch of biology which deals with the minute structure of tissues; microscopic anatomy. —**histolog′ic, histolog′ical,** *adj.;* **histolog′ically,** *adv.*

normal h. The study of healthy tissues.

pathologic h. The study of diseased tissue.

topographic h. The study of the minute structure of the organs and especially of their formation from the tissues.

his·tol′y·sis [*histos;* G. *lysis*, a loosing]. Disintegration and dissolution of organic tissue. —**histolyt′ic,** *adj.*

his·to′ma [*histos;* G. *-ōma*, tumor]. A tumor whose cells are typical of a tissue, such as a fibroma. Also called *histioma.*

his″to·met″a·plas′tic [*histos;* G. *metaplassein*, to remodel]. Causing the transformation of one tissue into another type. See *metaplasia.*

his″to·mor·phol′o·gy [*histos;* G. *morphē*, form; *logos*, word]. The morphology of the tissues of the body; histology.

his′tone, his′ton [*histos*]. Any one of a group of strongly basic proteins found in cell nuclei, such as thymus histone; soluble in water but insoluble in, or precipitated by, ammonium hydroxide, and coagulable by heat. See American Classification of Proteins in the Appendix.

his″to·neu·rol′o·gy. See *neurohistology.*

his·ton′o·my [*histos;* G. *nomos*, law]. The laws of the development and arrangement of organic tissue.

his″to·nu′ri·a [*histos;* G. *ouron*, urine]. The presence of histone in the urine.

his″to·pa·thol′o·gy [*histos;* G. *pathos*, disease; *logos*, word]. The study of minute changes in diseased tissue.

his″to·phys″i·ol′o·gy (hiss″to·fizz″ee·ol′o·jee) [*histos;* G. *physis*, nature; *logos*]. The science of tissue functions.

His″to·plas′ma [*histos;* G. *plasma*, anything formed]. A genus of parasitic fungi.

H. capsulatum. That species which is the causative agent of histoplasmosis; originally it was thought to be protozoan but now is established as a fungus. See *histoplasmin* and histoplasmin *test.*

his″to·plas′min. Extract of either the mycelial or yeast phase of *Histoplasma capsulatum*, used by intradermal injection to test for histoplasmosis. Many persons whose chest films show calcification, but who have been negative to tuberculin, have been reactors to histoplasmin.

his″to·plas·mo′sis (hiss″to·plaz·mo′sis) [*histos; plasma;* G. *-ōsis*, condition]. A fatal disease caused by the fungus *Histoplasma capsulatum.* It is characterized by fever, anemia, leukopenia, and emaciation. The infection primarily involves the reticuloendothelial system. Also called *Darling's h.* Syn., *cytomycosis.*

his′to·ry [G. *historia*, inquiry]. A written account of events; a record of past events; a narrative or story.

biologic h. The life story of any animal.

medical h. The account obtained from a patient as to his health, past and present, and the symptoms of his disease.

his″to·spec·tros′co·py. The application of spectroscopy to histochemistry.

emission h. The identification of certain elements in tissues by means of emission spectra, which are obtained by consuming in a high-frequency spark a chosen region of a tissue section.

roentgen absorption h. Quantitative estimation of elements in very small histological specimens by means of roentgen absorption spectra.

ultraviolet absorption h. Application of the quartz microscope to measurements of absorption spectra of cellular components in situ.

his″to·ther′a·py [G. *histos*, web; *therapeia*, treatment]. The remedial use of animal tissues.

his″to·throm′bin [*histos;* G. *thrombos,* clot]. A thrombin formed from connective tissue.

his′to·tome [*histos;* G. *tomos,* cutting]. An instrument for cutting tissue in preparation for microscopic study; a microtome.

his·tot′o·my [*histos;* G. *tomē,* a cutting]. 1. The dissection of tissues. 2. The cutting of thin sections of tissues; microtomy.

his″to·tox′ic [*histos;* G. *toxikon,* poison]. Designating a poisonous condition of the cells.

his′to·trip″sy [*histos;* G. *tripsis,* a rubbing]. The crushing of tissue by an ecraseur. *Rare.*

his′to·trophe, his′to·troph [*histos;* G. *trophē,* nourishment]. 1. In deciduate placentation, the temporary nutritive substances supplied from sources other than the circulating blood, such as glandular secretion, extravasated blood. Also called *embryotrophe.* 2. In nondeciduate placentation, the uterine secretion and transudates bathing the chorion and furnishing nutritive materials throughout gestation. Also called *uterine milk.* —**histotroph′ic,** *adj.*

his″to·zo′ic [*histos;* G. *zōion,* living being]. Living on or within the tissues; denoting certain protozoan parasites.

his′to·zyme. Hippuricase.

his′tri·o·nism [L. *histrio,* actor]. Dramatic action or attitude, as seen in some psychoses and psychoneuroses. —**histrion′ic,** *adj.*

Hitchcock's reagent. See Benedict and Hitchcock's uric acid *reagent.*

Hitschmann, Fritz [*German gynecologist,* 1870–1926]. With Ludwig Adler, described the cyclic change in the endometrium, and demonstrated histologically its normal nature (1908).

Hittorf method for ionic mobilities. See under *method.*

Hitzig, Eduard [*German neurologist and psychiatrist,* 1838–1907]. With G. T. Fritsch, made experimental studies of electric stimulation of the cerebral cortex in the frontal lobe, proving the existence of a motor area (1870). Accurately defined the limits of the cortical motor area in dogs and monkeys (1874).

hives. Urticaria.

hi-vi-tol. A proprietary product consisting of blended fish-liver oils, used as a source of vitamins A and D.

Hl. Latent hypermetropia.

hl. Hectoliter.

Hm. Manifest hypermetropia.

hm. Hectometer.

Ho Chemical symbol for holmium.

ho·ang·nan′ [Chin.]. A Chinese preparation obtained from the bark of *Strychnos malaccensis.* Its properties are due to a small percentage of strychnine. It has been used in the Orient as an alterative in syphilis, leprosy, and similar diseases.

hoar′hound″. See *marrubium.*

hoarse [ME. *hors*]. 1. Harsh, grating; used of sounds. 2. Having a harsh, discordant voice, resulting from an abnormal condition of the larynx or throat. —**hoarse′ness,** *n.*

hoar′y [AS. *hār*]. Gray or white with age; said of the hair. —**hoariness,** *n.*

hob′ble. 1. *In veterinary medicine,* a bond or shackle used to confine the foot of an animal. 2. Anything which restrains motion.

hob′ble. To have an uneven gait; to limp.

hob′nail″ liv′er. Colloquial term for more or less shrunken stage of Laennec's cirrhosis, in which nodules of parenchyma, a few millimeters in diameter and fairly uniform in size, project on the outer surface.

Hochberg-Melnick-Oser method for ascorbic acid. See under *method.*

Hochsinger, Karl [*Austrian pediatrician,* 1860–]. Described a sign suggestive of tetany, in which, if pressure is made on the inner side of the biceps muscle of the arm, the fist closes; called *Hochsinger's sign.*

hock [AS. *hōh,* heel]. The joint on the hind leg of a quadruped between the knee and the fetlock, corresponding to the ankle joint in man.

Hodge, Hugh Lenox [*American gynecologist and obstetrician,* 1796–1873]. Invented a type of obstetric forceps, called *Hodge's forceps,* and a pessary with a double curve, for the correction of uterine displacement.

Hodgen, John Thompson [*American surgeon,* 1826–82]. Invented a suspension splint resembling the Thomas splint. The *Hodgen splint* was once widely used in the treatment of fracture of the shaft of the femur.

Hodgkin, Thomas [*English physician,* 1798–1866]. Described aortic insufficiency several years before Corrigan. Contributed to the knowledge of the pathologic anatomy of membranes, and described a form of lymphoma (1832), sometimes subdivided on the basis of the pathologic findings into *Hodgkin's granuloma, paragranuloma,* and *sarcoma,* generally called *Hodgkin's disease.*

Hodgson, Joseph [*English physician,* 1788–1869]. Described a nonsacculated dilatation of the aortic arch (1815); called *Hodgson's disease.*

ho″do·pho′bi·a [G. *hodos,* road; *phobos,* fear]. Morbid fear of travel.

hoe [OF. *houe*]. 1. A scraping instrument used in operations for cleft palate. 2. *In dentistry,* an instrument used in cavity preparation.

Hoehne's sign. See under *sign.*

hof [Ger., courtyard]. *In hematology,* the little area between the lobes of a bilobed nucleus.

Hofbauer cell. See under *cell.*

Hoff, Jacobus Henricus van't [*Dutch physical chemist,* 1852–1911]. Known for his discoveries in pure physics and in stereochemistry. *Van't Hoff's law* states that in dilute solutions at a constant temperature, the osmotic pressure is in direct ratio to the concentration of the solution; if the concentration is constant, the osmotic pressure varies with the absolute temperature. See also van't Hoff's *factor* i. Nobel laureate (1901).

Hoffa, Albert [*German orthopedic surgeon,* 1859–1908]. Developed the open operation for the reduction of congenital dislocation of the hip (1890); he deepened the acetabulum and divided the muscles to secure reposition of the head of the femur. *Hoffa's operation* has been superseded by more modern methods. Traumatic solitary lipoma of the knee joint is known as *Hoffa's disease.*

Hoffmann, Erich (1868–). German dermatologist, who with Schaudinn, discovered *Treponema pallidum,* the causative agent of syphilis (1905).

Hoffmann, Friedrich [*German physician,* 1660–1742]. Author of an important treatise correlating physiology and pathology (1718). Recognized chlorosis as a clinical entity (1731). Ether spirit is called *Hoffmann's drops.* Compound ether spirit is known as *Hoffmann's anodyne.*

Hoffmann, Johann [*German neurologist,* 1857–1919]. Described hereditary familial spinal muscular atrophy, called *Hoffmann's atrophy, Hoffmann-Werdnig syndrome.* See *Werdnig.* See also Hoffmann's *phenomenon;* digital *reflex,* also called *Hoffmann's sign.*

Hoffmann, Moritz [*German anatomist,* 1622–98]. Credited with discovering the excretory duct of the pancreas in fowl (1642). This is said to have led to Wirsung's discovery of the duct in man in the same year. Called *Hoffmann's duct, duct of Wirsung.*

Hofmann's bacillus. *Corynebacterium pseudodiphtheriticum.*

Hofmeister, Franz [*Czechoslovakian physiological chemist*, 1850–1922]. Known for his researches on metabolism and in colloidal chemistry. See lyotropic *series*, also called *Hofmeister series.*

Hofmeister, Franz von [*German surgeon*, 1867–1926]. The *Hofmeister-Finsterer operation* is a modification of Pólya's operation of subtotal gastrectomy.

Hogben test. See frog *test.*

hog chol'er·a. See under *cholera.*

Högyes, Endre [*Hungarian physician*, 1847–1906]. Remembered for his introduction of the subcutaneous injection of a 1% rabies virus, diluted from 1:100 to 1:1,000, for the treatment of rabies; called *Högyes' treatment.*

Höjer method for vitamin C. See under *method.*

Hoke, Michael [*American orthopedic surgeon*, 1874–1944]. Known for his method of treating scoliosis by rib resection and a plaster jacket. Devised an operation for flatfoot in which he removed portions of the navicular and cuneiform bones and accomplished fusion of the joints, and also lengthened the Achilles tendon; called *Hoke's operation.*

holadin. Trade-mark for an extract of the pancreas used as a digestant.

ho·lan'dric [G. *holos*, whole; *anēr*, man]. Referring to genes carried by the Y chromosomes, or to characteristics inherited only through the paternal line.

Ho"lar·rhe'na an"ti-dys"en·ter'i·ca. An ancient Indian remedy for dysentery which has been found to have specific action in amebic dysentery. Also called *kurchi bark.*

holarsol. Trade-mark for dichlorophenarsine hydrochloride.

Holden, Luther (1815–1905). English surgeon known for his description of an indistinct crease in the anterior thigh lying over the site of attachment of Scarpa's fascia to the fascia lata.

hol"er·ga'si·a (hol"ur·gay'zhuh, ·zee·uh, ·shuh, ·see·uh) [G. *holos*, whole; *ergasia*, a working]. *In psychobiology,* a mental disorder which disrupts the entire structure of the personality; a major psychotic reaction, as schizophrenia.

hol'ism. A concept in modern biological thinking which states that for complex systems such as a cell or an organism the whole is greater than the sum of its parts from a functional point of view: also called *organicism.* —**holis'tic,** *adj.*

Holla disease [after *Holla*, a town in Norway]. Epidemic hemolytic jaundice.

hol'low·foot". See *talipes* cavus.

hol'low horn". See Texas *fever.*

Holmes, Oliver Wendell [*American physician and author*, 1804–94]. Recognized the contagiousness of puerperal fever (1842–43).

Holmes phenomenon. Rebound phenomenon.

Holmgren, Alarik Frithiof [*Swedish physiologist*, 1831–97]. Noted retinal action currents (1865). Investigated colorblindness as a cause of railroad accidents. See also the Holmgren *test* for color vision.

hol'mi·um (hole'mee·um, hol'mee·um) [L. *Holmia*, Stockholm]. Ho = 164.94. A rare earth element.

hol'o-, ho'lo- [G. *holos*, whole]. A combining form signifying *complete, entire.*

hol"o·a·car'di·us [*holos;* G. *a-*, not; *kardia*, heart]. A placental parasitic twin (omphalosite) which lacks a heart. Syn., *acardiacus, acardius.*

h. acephalus. One in which there is no head.

h. acormus. One in which there is little more than a head.

h. amorphus. One in which the parasite consists of a shapeless mass.

hol"o·a·cra'ni·a [*holos; a-;* G. *kranion*, skull]. Complete absence of the cranial vault, with partial or complete anencephaly.

hol"o·blas'tic [*holos;* G. *blastos*, germ]. Referring to an egg which divides completely into cells during cleavage.

holocaine hydrochloride. Trade name for the local anesthetic substance *phenacaine hydrochloride.*

hol"o·ce·phal'ic [*holos;* G. *kephalē*, head]. Pertaining to a monster deficient in certain parts but having the head complete.

hol'o·crine (hol'o·kryne, ·krin) [*holos;* G. *krinein*, to separate]. Designating a gland in which the secretion is formed by degeneration of the glandular cells. See *merocrine.*

hol"o·di"as·tol'ic [*holos;* G. *diastolē*, dilatation]. Relating to the entire diastole.

hol"o·en'zyme [*holos;* G. *en*, in; *zymē*, leaven]. The complete enzyme formed from the purely protein part, or apoenzyme, and the coenzyme.

hol"o·gas·tros'chi·sis (hol"o·gas·tros'ki·sis) [*holos;* G. *gastēr*, belly; *schisis*, a cleavage]. Fissure involving the entire length of the abdomen.

hol"o·gyn'ic (hol"o·jin'ick, ·jy'nick) [*holos;* G. *gynē*, woman]. Descriptive of a mode of inheritance in which a characteristic is transmitted only in the female line from mother to daughter generation after generation, as in the case of attached X chromosomes. Also see *holandric.*

hol"o·met"a·bol'ic, hol"o·me·tab'o·lous [*holos;* G. *metabolē*, change]. Pertaining to a mode of insect metamorphosis in which there is a quiescent pupal stage between the larva and the adult, as in beetles, moths, butterflies, midges, flies, ants, bees, and wasps.

hol"o·ra·chis'chi·sis (hol"o·ra·kis'ki·sis) [*holos;* G. *rhachis*, spine; *schisis*, a cleavage]. That type of spina bifida in which the entire spinal canal is open.

hol"o·sac'cha·ride. A polysaccharide which yields, on hydrolysis, only sugars. See *heterosaccharide.*

hol"o·so·mat'ic. Referring to the whole patient, in contrast to a local lesion.

hol"o·sys·tol'ic [*holos;* G. *systolē*, contraction]. Relating to the entire systole.

hol"o·zo'ic [*holos;* G. *zōikos*, of animals]. Having the characteristic animal type of nutrition which requires the ingestion of organic food materials.

Holt, Barnard Wight [*English surgeon*, 1816–94]. Remembered for his operation of rapid dilatation and rupture of a urethral stricture.

Holt, Luther Emmett [*American pediatrician and author*, 1855–1924]. Celebrated as medical writer and author of textbook on children's diseases. Proponent of modified milk, with pasteurization, in infant feeding. With W. H. Howell, isolated and named heparin (1918), which had been discovered by Howell's pupil, Jay McLean.

Holth, Sören [*Norwegian ophthalmic surgeon*, 1863–1937]. Introduced an operation of sclerectomy by means of a punch; called *Holth's operation.*

Holtz, Wilhelm [*German physicist*, 1836–1913]. Remembered for his invention of an early form of electrostatic generator for the production of high potentials; called the *Holtz machine.*

Holzmann, W. [*German physician*, contemporary]. With Much, claimed that the serum of a dementia precox patient inhibited hemolysis by cobra venom. This is called the *Much-Holzmann reaction.*

hom"a·lo·ceph'a·lus [G. *homalos*, level; *kephalē*, head]. An individual with a flat head.

hom"a·lo·cor'y·phus [*homalos;* G. *koryphē*, head]. A skull with a parietal angle of 132° to 141°, indicating a moderate degree of convexity of the parietal bone in the sagittal plane. The angle is formed by locating the point in the arch of the parietal bone that lies highest above the straight line which connects the points bregma and lambda, and then connecting this point with bregma and lambda, respectively. The angle included between these two lines is the parietal angle.

hom″a·lo·me·to′pus [*homalos;* G. *metōpon*, forehead]. A skull having a frontal angle between 130.5° and 141°.

hom″a·lo·pis″tho·cra′ni·us [*homalos;* G. *opisthen*, behind; *kranion*, skull]. A skull in which the angle formed by lines joining the external occipital protuberance and the occipital point, with the highest point of the skull, is 140° to 154°.

hom″a·lu·ra′nus [*homalos;* G. *ouranos*, vault]. A skull with an angle of the palatal arch of 147.5° to 164°, indicating a moderately flattened arching of the palate in the sagittal plane. The angle is formed by locating the point in the palatal arch that lies highest above the straight line which connects the inferior point of the premaxilla with the tip of the posterior nasal spine, and then connecting this point with the inferior point of the premaxilla and the tip of the posterior nasal spine, respectively. The angle included between these two lines is the angle of the palatal arch.

Homans, John [*American surgeon*, 1877–]. With S. J. Crowe and Harvey Cushing, made an experimental study of the pituitary and its relation to the reproductive system (1910). See also Homans' *sign* of thrombophlebitis.

hom′a·rine. A methylated picolinic acid, isomeric with trigonelline; has been isolated from mammalian urine.

hom·at′ro·pine (ho·mat′ro·peen, ·pin). $C_{16}H_{21}NO_3$. An alkaloid prepared from tropine and mandelic acid. It causes dilatation of the pupil and paralysis of accommodation, as does atropine, but its effects pass off more quickly, usually in two or three days.

h. hydrobromide (*homatropinae hydrobromidum*). $C_{16}H_{21}NO_3.HBr$; white crystals used as a mydriatic and in the night sweats of tuberculosis. Dose, 0.5–1 mg. (1/120–1/60 gr.). Application, 1% solution.

h. hydrochloride. $C_{16}H_{21}NO_3.HCl$. Used like the hydrobromide.

h. methylbromide. $C_{16}H_{21}NO_3.CH_3Br$. Used in treating gastrointestinal spasm and hyperchlorhydria. Dose, 2.5–5.0 mg. (1/24–1/12 gr.). See *mesopin, novatrin.*

hom·ax′i·al, hom″ax·o′ni·al [G. *homos*, one and the same, common; *axōn*, axis]. Having all axes equal.

Home, Everard (1756–1832). English surgeon who described the subtrigonal gland, a subsidiary lobe of the prostate, also called *Home's lobe* or *gland.*

ho′me·o-, ho′moe·o- [G. *homoios*, like, resembling]. A combining form meaning *like, similar.*

ho′me·o·chrome″ [*homoios;* G. *chrōma*, color]. Those special serous cells of salivary glands staining with mucin stains after fixation in a formalin-bichromate mixture. Also see *tropochrome.*

ho′me·o·graft″. See *homograft.*

ho″me·o·ki·ne′sis [*homoios;* G. *kinēsis*, motion]. A mitosis in which equal amounts of chromatin go to each daughter nucleus.

ho″me·o·mor′phous, ho″moe·o·mor′phous [*homoios;* G. *morphē*, form]. Like or similar in form and structure.

ho″me·o·path′ic al′co·hol. Ethyl alcohol of 87% strength; used in making attenuations.

ho″me·op′a·thy, ho″moe·op′a·thy [G. *homoios*, similar; *pathos*, disease]. A branch of medicine which deals with the investigation and application of the *simile phenomenon* or law of similars: *similia similibus curantur*, like is cured by like, i.e., the set of symptoms and signs a drug produces in healthy persons, when present as illness, may be brought back to normal by the same drug (*inverse reaction of drugs*). The significance of the simile phenomenon was known to Hippocrates, and was particularly expounded by Samuel Hahnemann (1755–1843), who coined the name *homeopathy.* Embodied in the homeopathic approach are (1) the testing of drugs on healthy human beings (called *proving*), (2) the giving of small doses of a drug (complete desensitization, active immunization), (3) the administration of not more than one drug at a time, and (4) treating not a single sign or symptom but the totality of signs and symptoms a patient presents (principle of *totality* of *symptoms*). —**homeopath′ic,** *adj.;* **ho′meopath, homeopathist,** *n.*

ho″me·o·pla′si·a, ho″moe·o·pla′si·a (ho″mee-o·play′zhuh, ·zee·uh, ·shuh, ·see·uh) [*homoios;* G. *plassein*, to form]. The growth of tissue resembling the normal tissue, or matrix, in its form and properties; also the tissue so formed. —**homeoplas′tic,** *adj.*

ho″me·o′sis, ho″moe·o′sis [*homoios;* G. *-ōsis*, condition]. The appearance of an organ or appendage not normal to its location, as a leg in place of a proboscis in a fly. —**homeot′ic,** *adj.*

ho″me·os′ta·sis [*homoios;* G. *stasis*, position]. The maintenance of steady states in the organism by coordinated physiologic processes. Thus all organ systems are integrated by automatic adjustments to keep within narrow limits disturbances excited by, or directly resulting from, changes in the surroundings of the organism. This concept, an extension of the *milieu intérieur* of Claude Bernard, was introduced by Walter B. Cannon (1926) and has come to be applied to psychological stability as well as physiological steadiness. —**homeostat′ic,** *adj.*

ho″me·o·ther′mal, ho·moi″o·ther′mal [*homoios;* G. *thermē*, heat]. Pertaining to animals that are warm-blooded, that maintain a uniform temperature despite variation in the surrounding temperature.

home′sick″ness [AS. *hām; sēoc*]. Nostalgia; an urgent desire to return to one's home. It may be accompanied by a morbid sluggishness of the functions of the various organs of the body, and may develop into depression and morbid anxiety.

ho″mi·chlo·pho′bi·a [G. *homichlē*, fog; *phobos*, fear]. A morbid fear of fog.

hom′i·cide [L. *homicida*, from *homo*, man, *caedere*, to kill]. 1. The killing of a fellow human being; by law, it may be justifiable, excusable, or felonious; felonious homicide is murder or manslaughter. 2. One who takes the life of another. —**homici′dal,** *adj.*

Ho′mo [L., man]. The genus, of the mammalian order Primates, whose single species, *H. sapiens*, includes all extant races of man.

ho′mo- (ho′mo-, hom′o-), **hom-** [G. *homos*, one and the same]. 1. A combining form denoting *common, like, same.* 2. *In chemistry*, a combining form designating *a homolog of a* (specified) *compound.*

ho″mo·a·rec′o·line (ho″mo·a·reck′o·leen, ·lin, ·a·ree′ko·leen, ·lin). $C_7H_{10}(C_2H_5)NO_2$. The ethyl ether of arecaidine. The hydrobromide, forming colorless soluble crystals, is used like arecoline.

ho″mo·bi′o·tin. A homolog of biotin containing an additional CH_2 group in the side chain; it is a potent antagonist of biotin toward some bacteria but is capable of replacing biotin in certain of its functions toward other organisms.

ho″mo·cen′tric (ho″mo·sen′trick, hom″o·), **ho″-mo·cen′tri·cal** [*homos;* G. *kentron,* center]. Concentric; having the same center. —**homocentrically,** *adv.*

ho″mo·cho′line. $(CH_3)_3N(OH)CH_2CH_2CH_2OH$; trimethyl-γ-hydroxypropyl-ammonium hydroxide, a homolog of choline.

ho′mo·chrome [*homos;* G. *chrōma,* color]. Referring to one of two types of serous cells of the salivary glands, which takes the same color as the stain.

ho″mo·chro″mo·i·som′er·ism. The phenomenon of two or more organic substances of different structure exhibiting similar absorption spectra in solution.

ho″mo·clad′ic [*homos;* G. *klados,* branch]. Referring to an anastomosis between twigs of the same artery.

ho″mo·cy′clic. *In chemistry,* pertaining to compounds of the closed-chain or ring type in which all the ring atoms are of the same element, usually carbon. See *carbocyclic, heterocyclic.*

ho″mo·cys′te·ine (ho″mo·sis′tee·een, ·in, ·sis-tee′in). $SH.(CH_2)_2.CHNH_2.COOH$. α-Amino-γ-thiol-*n*-butyric acid. A demethylated product of methionine. Capable of conversion to methionine in the animal body by a transmethylation reaction with choline, betaine, etc.

ho″mo·cys′tine (ho″mo·sis′teen, ·tin). $[—S.(CH_2)_2.CHNH_2.COOH]_2$. γ,γ′-Dithiobis (α-amino-butyric acid). The oxidized, disulfide form of homocysteine, analogous to cystine, the oxidized form of cysteine; a compound capable of replacing methionine in the diet provided choline is present. Apparently, choline acts as a methylating agent to transform homocystine to methionine.

ho′mo·dont, hom′o·dont [*homos;* G. *odous,* tooth]. *In biology,* having all the teeth alike, as the porpoises. See *heterodont.*

ho″mo·dy′na·my. Serial homology; the correspondence of parts arranged in series along the main axis of the body. —**homodynam′ic,** *adj.*

ho′moe·o-. See *homeo-.*

ho″mo·er′o·tism, ho″mo·e·rot′i·cism [*homos;* G. *erōs,* love]. The direction of the libido toward a member of the same sex; may find expression in homogenitality, homosexuality, or may be repressed. In true homoerotism, the erotic feeling is not sexual or genital, but is well sublimated and expressed in socially acceptable behavior. —**homoerot′ic,** *adj., n.*

ho″mo·fer·men′ta·tive [*homos;* L. *fermentum,* ferment]. Pertaining to the ability of certain bacteria to produce only lactic acid from glucose and other sugars. See *heterofermentative.*

ho″mo·ga·met′ic (ho″mo·ga·met′ick, ·ga·mee′-tick) [*homos;* G. *gamos,* marriage]. Referring to the production of one kind of germ cell in regard to the sex chromosomes. The female, being XX in constitution, is the homogametic sex.

ho·mog′e·nate [*homos;* G. *genesthai,* from *gignesthai,* to be produced]. A suspension of animal tissues that is ground in the all-glass "homogenizer" described by Potter and Elvehjem in 1936.

AIK homogenates. A homogenization medium of alkaline isotonic KCl, in which certain cellular elements are maintained intact.

ho″mo·ge′ne·ous (ho″mo·jee′nee·us, hom″o·) [*homos;* G. *genos,* race, kind]. Having the same nature or qualities; of uniform character in all parts. —**homogene′ity,** *n.*

ho″mo·gen′ic [*homos;* G. *genesthai,* from *gignesthai,* to be produced]. Referring to genotypes of polysomic or polyploid organisms which contain the same allele for any given locus; similar to the term homozygous, used for diploid organisms.

ho″mo·gen″i·tal′i·ty [*homos;* L. *genitalis,* genital]. A form of homoerotism in which the sexual impulses are given genital expression; that sexual perversion marked by genital relations between members of the same sex. —**homogen′ital,** *adj.*

ho″mo·ge″ni·za′tion (ho″mo·jee″ni·zay′shun, ho-modj″i·ni·zay′shun) [*homos;* G. *genos,* race, kind]. 1. The act or process of becoming homogeneous. 2. The production of a uniform suspension or emulsion from two or more normally immiscible substances.

ho·mog′e·ni·zer. See *viscolizer.*

Potter's h. All glass, consisting of a pestle which rotates inside a close-fitting ordinary pyrex test tube. Described by Potter and Elvehjem in 1936.

ho·mog′e·nous [*homos; genos*]. 1. Of, or derived from, an individual of a related or similar strain of the same species. 2. Of, or derived from another individual of the same species.

ho″mo·gen·tis′ic ac′id (ho″mo·jen·tiz′ick, ·jen-tiss′ick, hom″o·). $(OH)_2C_6H_3.CH_2.COOH$. Dihydroxyphenylacetic acid, a substance found in urine in alkaptonuria; it is an intermediate in the oxidation of tyrosine and phenylalanine. Formerly called *glycosuric acid.*

ho″mo·glan′du·lar [*homos;* L. *glans,* acorn]. Pertaining to the same gland.

ho′mo·graft. A tissue graft taken from a donor of the same species as the recipient: common contraction of *homogenous g.* Also called *homeograft, homologous g., homoplastic g., isograft.*

ho·moi′o-. See *homeo-.*

ho″mo·i·o·ther′mic. Referring to the ability of an organism to regulate physiologically the rate of heat production and heat loss so as to maintain itself at constant temperature. See also *poikilothermic.*

ho″mo·lac′tic. Pertaining to a type of sugar fermentation in which the only product is lactic acid: usually said of fermentation by microorganisms.

ho″mo·lat′er·al [*homos;* L. *lateralis,* of the side]. On, or of the same side. See *ipsilateral.*

Homolle's amorphous digitalin. See French *digitalin.*

ho·mol′o·gous [G. *homologos,* from *homos; logos,* word]. 1. Corresponding in structure, either directly or as referred to a fundamental type. 2. *In chemistry,* being of the same type or series; differing by a multiple, such as CH_2, or an arithmetic ratio in certain constituents. —**hom′-olog, hom′ologue, homology,** *n.*

ho·mon′o·mous [G. *homonomos,* from *homos; nomos,* law]. Referring to the condition in which the metameres of a segmented animal are similar. —**homonomy,** *n.*

ho″mo·mor′phic. Having similar structure without definite relation to bodily axes.

ho·mon′y·mous. 1. Having the same name. 2. *In ophthalmology,* referring to the same sides of the field of vision, as in homonymous hemianopsia.

ho′mo·plast, hom′o·plast [*homos;* G. *plassein,* to form]. *In biology,* a plastic compound of one tissue, as opposed to *alloplast.*

ho′mo·plas″ty, [*homos; plassein*]. Surgery using grafts from another individual of the same species. —**homoplas′tic,** *adj.*

ho·mo·po′lar. Covalent. See *covalence.*

Ho·mop′ter·a [*homos;* G. *pteron,* wing]. An order of insects; includes cicadas, plant lice, and scale insects. Formerly a suborder of the old order Hemiptera.

ho″mo·qui′nine (ho″mo·kwye′nine, ·kwi·neen′) A molecular compound of quinine and cupreine obtained from cuprea bark.

ho″mo·ser′ine. $HOH_2C.CH_2CH(NH_2)COOH$. An

amino acid formed in the breakdown of cystathionine to cysteine in animal tissues.

ho″mo·sex″u·al′i·ty [*homos;* L. *sexus*, sex]. 1. The state of being sexually attracted by members of one's own sex. 2. The state of being in love with one of the same sex. 3. *In psychoanalysis*, a form of homoerotism in which the interest is sexual but sublimated, not receiving genital expression. —**homosex′ual,** *adj.*, *n.*

ho″mo·sex′u·al pan′ic. An acute undifferentiated syndrome which comes as the climax of prolonged tension from unconscious homosexual conflicts or sometimes bisexual tendencies. The attack is characterized by a high degree of fear, paranoid ideas, great excitement, and a tendency towards disorganization. It may mark the onset of a schizophrenic reaction.

ho″mo·sul″fa·nil′a·mide. Marfanil.

ho″mo·ther′mic, ho″mo·ther′mal. Typically maintaining the temperature at a constant level: said of certain animals. See *animal heat.*

hom′o·tope. Any member of a particular group of elements in the periodic classification; thus, sodium is a homotope of lithium, potassium, rubidium, cesium, and francium.

ho″mo·trans″plan·ta′tion. Transplantation of tissue from one to another individual of the same species.

ho′mo·type, hom′o·type [*homos;* G. *typos*, impression]. A part corresponding to a part on the other lateral half of the body.

ho″mo·zy′gote [*homos;* G. *zygōtos*, yoked]. An individual in which the members of a given pair of genes are alike. —**homozygous** (ho″mo·zy′gus, ho·moz′i·gus), *adj.;* **homozygo′sis,** *n.*

ho·mun′cu·lus [L., little man]. 1. A little man with normal proportion of parts; a dwarf; a manikin. 2. The human fetus.

Hon·du′ras bark. Cascara amarga.

hon′ey. The saccharine secretion deposited in the honeycomb by the bee, *Apis mellifera;* the principal constituents are levulose and dextrose; it is used as a food and pharmaceutical excipient. 2. A preparation of honey with some medicinal substance. See *mel.*

hoof [AS. *hōf*]. The horny covering of the distal end of a digit in the ungulates. —**hoofed,** *adj.*

hook [AS. *hōc*]. A curved instrument for exerting traction.

blunt h. An instrument for exercising traction upon the fetus in an arrested breech presentation.

squint h. A right-angled or a curved instrument used in the operation for strabismus for exerting traction on tendons.

Hooker's method. See Danzer and Hooker's *method.*

hook′worm″ [*hōc;* AS. *wyrm*]. Any nematode belonging to the superfamily Strongyloidea, particularly the *Ancylostoma duodenale* and *Necator americanus.*

hook′worm″ dis·ease′. See *ancylostomiasis.*

hoove, hoov′en. See *hove.*

hop. See *humulus.*

Hope, James [*English physician*, 1801–41]. Made important contributions to the knowledge of diseases of the heart and blood vessels, especially valvular disease and aneurysm. Described an apical systolic murmur associated with mitral regurgitation; sometimes called *Hope's murmur.*

Hopkins, Frederick Gowland (1861–1947). English physiological chemist known for his work on the estimation of uric acid in urine. With Sydney William Cole, he isolated tryptophan (1901). He is credited with recognizing the significance of, and necessity for accessory factors in diet, now known as vitamins (1906) and demonstrated the growth-promoting effect of milk. His investigations largely gave impetus to vitamin research. With Walter Morley Fletcher, he made an important study of the production of lactic acid in muscular contraction (1907); he isolated glutathione (1922). Nobel laureate in medicine and physiology (1929).

Hopmann, Carl Melchior [*German rhinologist*, 1844–1925]. Described papillary hypertrophy of the nasal mucous membrane as presenting the appearance of a papilloma. Called *Hopmann's polyp.*

Hoppe, Johann Ignaz [*Swiss physiologist*, 1811–91]. Described myasthenia gravis, which sometimes is known as *Hoppe-Goldflam symptom complex.*

Hoppe-Seyler, Ernst Felix Immanuel [*German physiological chemist*, 1825–95]. Known especially for his research on the chemistry of the blood and his spectroscopic studies of hemoglobin. Was first to isolate hemoglobin in crystalline form.

hora [L.]. Hour; abbreviated, h.

h. decubitus. At the hour of going to bed; abbreviated, h. d.

h. somni. Bedtime; abbreviated, h. s.

hor′de·in [L. *hordeum*, barley]. A protein found in barley, the seed of *Hordeum sativum.*

hor′de·nine (hor′di·neen, ·nin, hor·dee′nin) [*hordeum*]. $C_{10}H_{15}NO$. An alkaloid from germinating barley. Has been used in diarrhea and dysentery, and as a heart tonic. Its action is similar to that of epinephrine.

hor·de′o·lum [L., sty, dim. of **hordeum**]. A sty; a furuncular inflammation of the connective tissue of the lids, near a hair follicle.

external h. A circumscribed, acute inflammation on the edge of the lid, produced by staphylococcus infection of one of the sebaceous glands of Zeis.

internal h. An infection of a tarsal (Meibomian) gland.

Hor′de·um. See *barley.*

hore′hound″. See *marrubium.*

ho·ris′ma·scope [G. *horisma*, boundary; *skopein*, to examine]. An instrument intended to facilitate the making of "ring" tests such as Heller's. If care is taken, there is no possibility of mixing the two solutions, and a definitely defined ring is easily obtained at the zone of contact. Also called *albumoscope.*

hor″me·pho′bi·a [G. *hormē*, assault, shock; *phobos*, fear]. Morbid fear of shock.

hor′mi·on [G. *hormē*, point of starting]. The point in the sagittal plane, between the alae of the vomer, where the vomer is attached to the body of the sphenoid bone.

Hor″mo·den′drum [G. *hormos*, chain; *dendron*, tree]. A genus of saprophytic fungi whose species act as common allergens. **H. compactum** and **H. pedrosoi** are pathogenic to man, and have been isolated from chromoblastomycosis.

hor′mone [G. *hormaein*, to excite]. A specific chemical product of an organ or of certain cells of an organ, transported by the blood or other body fluids, and having a specific regulatory effect upon cells remote from its origin. It may be considered an excitatory autacoid. For hormones listed by name, see Table of Hormones in the Appendix. —**hormo′nal, hormon′ic,** *adj.*

adenohypophyseal h. Any of the hormones produced by the adenohypophysis. The best established are: adrenocorticotropin, follicle-stimulating hormone, growth hormone, luteinizing hormone, prolactin, and thyrotropin.

adrenal medullary h. Epinephrine.

adrenocortical h. One of the steroid hormones of the adrenal cortex, which have one or more of the following biologic activities in adrenalectomized animals: maintenance of life; influence on carbohydrate, electrolyte, and protein metabolism; protection against stress; influence on muscular efficiency. Seven biologically active steroids have been isolated from the adrenal cortex.

adrenocorticotropic h. The adenohypophyseal hormone which stimulates the adrenal cortex: formerly spelled *adrenocorticotrophic h.* Syn., *adrenocorticotropic, corticotropin.*

adrenotrophic h. See adrenotropic *h.*

adrenotropic h. Adrenocorticotropin: formerly spelled *adrenotrophic h.*

anterior pituitary. h. See adenohypophyseal *h.*

antidiuretic h. A hormone of the posterior pituitary which increases the rate of water reabsorption in the distal convoluted tubules of the kidney, thereby diminishing water excretion and returning more water to plasma to combat plasma concentration.

chorionic gonadotropic h. Chorionic gonadotropin.

chromatophorotrophic h. See chromatophorotropic *h.*

chromatophorotropic h. Intermedin: formerly spelled *chromatophorotrophic h.*

corpus-luteum stimulating h. See luteinizing *h.*

cortical h. See adrenocortical *h.*

corticotrophic h. See corticotropic *h.*

corticotropic h. Adrenocorticotropin: formerly spelled *corticotrophic h.*

diabetogenic h. See diabetogenic *factor*, growth *h.*

embryonic h. See morphogenic *h.*

estrogenic h. A hormone, found principally in the ovary and also in the placenta, which stimulates the accessory sex structures and the secondary sex characteristics in the female; affects also the anterior pituitary. The production in pregnancy is greatly increased.

fat-metabolizing h. See ketogenic *h.*

follicle-stimulating h. An adenohypophyseal hormone which stimulates follicular growth in the ovary, and spermatogenesis in the testis: also called *follicle-ripening h., gametogenic h., pituitary A, gonadotropin.* Abbreviated FSH. Syn., *prolan-A, thylakentrin.*

gametogenic h. See follicle-stimulating *h.*

gastric h. See *gastrin.*

glycogenolytic h. Glucagon.

glycostatic h. Originally, the factor in crude anterior pituitary extract which increased muscle glycogen in fasting hypophysectomized animals. The metabolic actions which the term designates are now known to be induced by the growth hormone.

gonadotropic h. Any gonad-stimulating hormone. See *gonadotropin.*

growth h. 1. A hormone of the anterior pituitary which promotes growth. Syn., *somatotropic hormone, somatotropin.* 2. Any substance which promotes or stimulates an increase in the size of an organism, such as a plant, or of a part of an organism: also associated with a diabetogenic factor or hormone.

interstitial-cell stimulating h. See luteinizing *h.*

intestinal hormones. Those produced in the intestine: secretin and cholecystokinin.

ketogenic h. Originally, the factor in crude anterior pituitary extract which stimulated the rate of fatty acid metabolism. The metabolic actions which the term designates are now known to be induced by adrenocorticotropin and the growth hormone. Also called *fat-metabolizing h.*

lactation h. Prolactin.

lactogenic h. The adenohypophyseal hormone which stimulates lactation in the mammalian breast. Syn., *prolactin.*

luteinizing h. (LH). An adenohypophyseal hormone which stimulates both epithelial and interstitial cells in the ovary, where together with the follicle-stimulating hormone it induces follicular maturation and formation of corpora lutea. In the male, where it acts only on the interstitial cells of the testis, it is more appropriately called *interstitial-cell stimulating hormone* (ICSH). Also called *corpus-luteum stimulating hormone, metakentrin, pituitary B, gonadotropin.*

luteotropic h. A hormone of the anterior lobe of the pituitary which promotes lactation and is necessary for the maintenance of the corpus luteum: also called *lactation h., lactogenic h., prolactin.*

mammary-stimulating h. 1. See *prolactin.* 2. More appropriately, estrogen and progesterone, which induce proliferation of the ductile and acinous elements of the mammary glands respectively.

mammogenic h. 1. See *prolactin.* 2. Loosely, any hormone known to influence the mammary gland.

melanocyte-stimulating h. A substance found in the pituitary gland which causes darkening of human skin and nevi, formation of new pigmented nevi, and pigmentary changes in fish and amphibia, where it has been called *intermedin.* Formerly called *melanophore h., melanophore-dilating principle.* Abbreviated, MSH.

morphogenic h. The evocator, or chemical substance released by the primary organizer in development.

"N" h. The factor or factors in adrenocortical secretions having nitrogen-retaining, or protein-anabolic, as well as androgenic activity: also called *nitrogen h.*

neurohypophyseal h. Either of the hormones extracted from the neurohypophysis, antidiuretic hormone or oxytocin: thought to be the neurosecretory products of neural cells located in hypothalamic nuclei.

"nitrogen" h. See "N" *h.*

ovarian hormones. Two types of hormone are produced by the ovary: the follicular or estrogenic hormones, estradiol, estrone, and estrioll produce estrus in the spayed animal; the lutea, hormone, progesterone, is produced by the corpus luteum.

oxytocic h. See *oxytocin.*

pancreatic hormones. Those formed by the islets of the pancreas: insulin and lipocaic.

parathyroid h. Parathyrin.

placental h. Estrogenic hormone, chorionic gonadotropin.

posterior pituitary hormones. See neurohypophyseal *h.*

pregnant mare's serum h. (PMS). A placental hormone which has action similar to those of a combination of follicle-stimulating and luteinizing hormones of the adenohypophysis.

progestational h. The hormone, progesterone, which induces progestational changes of the uterine mucosa.

"S" h. The factor or factors in adrenocortical secretion having carbohydrate-regulatory activity: also called *glucocorticoid factor, sugar h.*

sex hormones. The gonadal hormones, estrogen and androgen, produced respectively by the ovary and testis, and the three hormones produced by the adenohypophysis: follicle-stimulating hormone (FSH), luteinizing hormone (LH), and prolactin.

somatotropic h. Growth hormone.

testicular hormones. Those elaborated by the testis; the best known is testosterone, a steroid which matures and maintains the male genitalia and the secondary sex characteristics.

thyroid h. Either iodothyroglobulin or one of its component chemical groups, the amino acid compound thyroxin. It accelerates the metabolism of all cells in the body, increasing oxygen consumption; stimulates growth, maturation, and differentiation of tissue; increases nervous irritability, muscular tonus, and circulation; and has a diuretic action. Without thyroid hormone, no cell in the body can function normally.

thyroid-stimulating h. Thyrotropic hormone. Abbreviated TSH.

thyrotrophic h. See thyrotropic *h.*

thyrotropic h. A hormone of the adenohypophysis which controls the status of the thyroid: formerly spelled *thyrotrophic h.* Syn., *thyroid-stimulating h.*

wound hormones. Substances which can stimulate growth by resumption of division in mature cells.

hor·mo″no·poi·e′sis (hor·mo″no·poy·ee′sis, hor″-mo·no·) [G. *hormaein*, to excite; *poiēsis*, a making]. The production of hormones. —**hormonopoiet′ic,** *adj.*

hor′mo·zone. One of the hormones which govern metabolism or maintain a stable fluid medium.

horn [AS.]. 1. A substance composed chiefly of keratin. 2. Cornu. —**horn′y,** *adj.*

cutaneous h. Cornu cutaneum.

dorsal h. The posterior column of gray matter in the spinal cord.

lateral h. The lateral column of gray matter in the spinal cord.

pulpal h. The extension of the dental pulp into a cusp of a tooth.

ventral h. The anterior column of gray matter in the spinal cord.

Horner, Johann Friedrich [*Swiss ophthalmologist*, 1831–86]. Described ptosis of the eyelid, due to section of the cervical sympathetic nerve fibers. *Horner's syndrome*, which may result from paralysis of the nerve fibers or from any lesion interrupting the cervical sympathetic chain, includes also constriction of the pupil and vasodilatation, and usually enophthalmos and absence of sweating on the affected side of the head and face. Also called *Bernard-Horner syndrome.*

Horner, William Edmonds (1793–1853). American anatomist who described the tensor tarsi muscle (1824) called *muscle of Horner*. He also described incisors with grooves due to a deficiency of enamel, which are called *Horner's teeth.*

horn″i·fi·ca′tion. Cornification.

ho·rop′ter [G. *horos*, limit; *optēr*, observer]. The sum of all the points seen singly by the two retinas while the fixation point remains stationary. —**horopter′ic,** *adj.*

Horowitz-Beadle method for choline. See under *method.*

hor·rip″i·la′tion [L. *horripilatio*, a bristling of the hair]. Old term for *piloerection.*

horse′foot″. See *talipes* equinus.

horse′pox″ [AS. *hors;* ME. *pokkes*]. A term loosely used to include such diseases of horses as pseudotuberculosis, contagious pustular stomatitis, or a vesicular exanthema.

horse′shoe′. A metal bow for the attachment of Steinmann pins and Kirschner wires.

horse′tail″. *Equisetum.*

Horsley, John Shelton [*American surgeon*, 1870–1946]. Widely known for his ingenuity in surgical technics. Introduced his operation of pyloroplasty or gastroduodenoplasty for the relief of duodenal ulcer. Incision is made into the pylorus anteriorly, longer on the gastric than on the duodenal side. The ends of the incision are brought together and sutured, after which the diamond-shaped opening is closed, bringing the line of incision at a right angle to its original direction.

Horsley, Victor Alexander Haden [*English surgeon*, 1857–1916]. Contributed to the development of neurosurgery and surgery of the endocrine glands. Made important studies of the thyroid gland and of the causal relationship of thyroid deficiency to myxedema and cretinism; produced experimental myxedema (1884). With Gowers, was first to remove a tumor of the spinal cord successfully (1888). Introduced a preparation of phenol, oil, and wax to prevent hemorrhage from the diploë in cranial operations; called *Horsley's putty* or *wax*. The *Horsley-Clarke apparatus*, named for Horsley and Robert Henry Clarke, is a stereotropic device for locating accurately a stimulus in the brain and brain stem; it is used in experimental studies of animals. See also Horsley's *sign* of middle meningeal hemorrhage.

Horton, Bayard Taylor [*American physician*, 1895–]. Described and studied histamine headache, called *Horton's syndrome.*

hos′pi·tal [L. *hospitalis*, relating to a guest]. A medical treatment facility primarily intended and appropriately staffed and equipped to provide diagnostic and therapeutic service in general medicine and surgery or in some circumscribed field or fields of restorative medical care, together with bed care, nursing, and dietetic service to patients requiring such care and treatment.

air evacuation h. *In the U.S. Army*, an Air Force hospital, at or near a terminus of the Military Air Transport Service, receiving patients evacuated by air from a forward area.

army h. New designation for a named station or general hospital in the Zone of the Interior (U.S.). Capacity varies depending on the type.

base h. An army hospital within the lines of communication, for receiving and caring for sick and wounded returned from field hospitals. *Obs.*

closed h. One closed to all physicians except those on its own staff.

contagious h. One restricted to the care of patients with communicable diseases. Syn., *isolation h.*

evacuation h. *In military medicine*, a mobile hospital or semimobile unit designed to provide facilities, as near the front as possible, for major medical and surgical procedures and for the preparation and sorting of casualties for extended evacuation to the rear.

field h. *In military medicine*, a hospital, usually under tentage, designed to function as a station hospital at isolated posts or airfields, but adaptable to support ground troops in combat. It is classified as a fixed hospital but it can be easily moved and even transported by air.

general h. (a) One in which many different types of patients are cared for; consists of various departments, as medicine, surgery, pediatrics, obstetrics, tuberculosis, and venereal, nervous, and mental diseases, all completely staffed. (b) *In military medicine*, a numbered fixed medical treatment facility especially staffed and equipped for observation, treatment, and disposition of patients requiring relatively long periods of hospitalization or highly specialized treatment: normally used in the communications zone.

governmental h. One supported and administered by a government subdivision; as a municipal, county, state, federal, army, navy, Public Health Service, or Veterans' Administration hospital.

isolation h. See contagious *h.*

maternity h. One restricted to the care of women during pregnancy and parturition.

mobile army surgical h. *In military medicine,* a mobile unit (60 beds) designed to provide early surgical treatment for nontransportable cases. It is designed for establishment with, or in the vicinity of, a division clearing station.

numbered h. *In military medicine,* a hospital designed for a theater of operations and to which an individual number is assigned. Numbered hospitals may be station hospitals, general hospitals, or other specific types, such as evacuation hospitals.

station h. *In U.S. Army medicine,* a fixed hospital established in or near a post, station, or military installation to give medical and dental care to military personnel.

surgical h. *In military medicine,* a mobile medical unit, attached to an army, that provides special facilities for giving immediate surgical aid to men wounded in combat.

unnumbered h. *In U.S. Army medicine,* a fixed hospital designed normally for operation in the continental United States or any of its possessions. All such hospitals are assigned names such as U.S. Army Hospital, Fort Belvoir, or in case of a general type hospital, Letterman Army Hospital.

veterinary h. 1. One for the care of animals. 2. *In military medicine,* a permanent animal hospital established at a military station and designed to serve only the needs of that hospital.

hos'pi·tal cen'ter. *In military medicine,* an aggregation of one or more general hospitals, often including schools, central laboratories, and utilities, all administered under the central authority of a commanding officer, generally an officer of the Medical Department of the army or navy.

hos'pi·tal corps'man. In the U.S. Navy, an enlisted man of the Medical Department.

hos"pit·al·i·za'tion. 1. Medical care and treatment at a hospital for serious cases or those needing care for a long time, as contrasted with emergency or first-aid treatment administered at a hospital. 2. The placing of a person under medical care in a hospital.

hos"pit·al·i·za'tion u'nit. *In military medicine,* a complete self-contained hospital unit able to function independently; one of three identical units that make up a field hospital.

mobile h. u. Any hospital installation whose organization and equipment permit ready movement under field or combat conditions.

hos'pi·tal plant. *In military medicine,* a permanent physical facility operated by a medical treatment facility in a theater of operations.

hos'pi·tal re·turns'. *In U.S. Army medicine,* persons who have been hospitalized, dropped from the rolls of their former unit or organization, carried on the Department of the U.S. Army detachment of patients, and are returning to duty through the replacement system.

hos'pi·tal ship. *In military medicine,* an unarmed ship, marked in accordance with the Geneva Conventions, staffed and equipped to provide hospitalization for the armed forces, and also used to evacuate casualties.

h. s. platoon. *In military medicine,* a unit assigned to cargo or transport ships with no special hospital facilities other than that on any transport to care for patients who may be evacuated on the ship as it returns to a port of debarkation.

hos'pi·tal train. *In military medicine,* a rail unit composed of one or more specially equipped railroad cars for the movement of sick and injured personnel and for the provision of emergency medical treatment en route.

hos'pi·tal trans'port. *In military medicine,* a transport provided with additional medical personnel and increased facilities for evacuation of casualties.

host [L. *hospes,* host]. 1. The organic body upon or in which parasites live. 2. The relatively normal twin to which a parasitic twin or part is attached.

alternate h. See intermediate *h.*

definitive h. One in which the sexual stages of the parasite develop.

intermediate h. One in which the parasite passes its larval or asexual stage.

reservoir h. Usually a vertebrate host which carries on the life cycle of the parasite by being infested when infestation in man is prevented by natural or artificial barriers.

hot. Highly radioactive. *Colloquial.*

hot atom. An atom which has high internal energy or high kinetic energy as a result of a nuclear process, such as neutron capture, beta decay, etc.

Hotchkiss, Lucius Wales [*American surgeon,* 1859–1926]. Devised an operation for the resection of carcinoma involving the jaw. A portion of the mandible and sometimes parts of the maxilla and hard palate were excised, and plastic repair of the cheek defect was made with tissue from the neck. Called *Hotchkiss operation.*

hot flash'es or **flush'es.** A sudden, recurring vasomotor phenomenon, generally associated with the menopause, which consists of a warm feeling spreading cephalically. It may be accompanied by a visible flush due to dilatation of the superficial vessels of the skin.

hot lab'or·a·tor"y. A laboratory designed for research with radioactive materials where the quantities of radioactive sources are so large (approximately 50 millicuries and more) that special facilities and precautions in handling are required.

Hot'ten·tot a'pron. An overgrowth of the labia minora, seen in the Hottentots.

hot'ten·tot·ism [S. Afr. D.]. An extreme form of stammering.

Hotz, Ferdinand Carl [*American ophthalmologist,* 1843–1909]. Devised an operation for the correction of entropion and trichiasis in which a considerable portion of the orbicularis oculi muscle was removed.

house'fly". See *Muscidae.*

house'maid's" knee. See prepatellar *bursitis.*

house phy·si'cian. A physician who lives in a hospital and is constantly available, as an intern.

house staff. The resident physicians and surgeons of a hospital. The term generally refers to those having the status of intern or resident.

house sur'geon. A surgeon who lives in a hospital and is constantly available.

Houssay, Bernardo Alberto [*Argentinian physiologist,* 1887–]. Known for his work in experimental physiology and endocrinology. The first to note amelioration of diabetes in the depancreatized animal after hypophysectomy and the diabetogenic action of anterior pituitary extract. An animal in which the pancreas and hypophysis both have been excised is known as the *Houssay animal.* Nobel laureate with G. T. and C. F. Cori (1947).

Houston's valves. See under *valve.*

hove, ho'ven. Distention of the stomach of a ruminant animal with gas. It is generally due to too much green food.

Howard's method. See under *artificial respiration.*

Howard test. See Howard-Dolman depth perception *test.*

Howe's ammoniacal silver nitrate. See ammoniacal silver nitrate *solution.*

Howell, William Henry [*American physiologist,* 1860–1945]. Made various important studies concerned with the blood, including studies of blood coagulation and of the formed elements of the blood. With L. Emmett Holt, isolated and named heparin (1918), which had been discovered by Howell's pupil, Jay McLean. *Howell's bodies* are nuclear bodies, probably detritus from the nuclei, found in erythrocytes; also called *Howell-Jolly bodies.* See also Howell's *method* of calculating blood coagulation time.

Howship, John [*English surgeon,* 1781–1841]. Described minute depressions or pits observed on the surface of bone undergoing resorption; called *Howship's lacunas.*

Hr blood fac'tors. See *blood groups.*

h. s. *Hora somni;* bedtime.

H-sub'stance. A substance similar to, if not identical with, histamine; believed to play a prominent role in the response of local blood vessels to tissue damage.

Ht. Total hypermetropia.

Hübener, Erich August [*German bacteriologist,* 1870–]. With Uhlenhuth, was first to describe *Salmonella paratyphi C* (1908). Described anomalous agglutination of human erythrocytes which had been acted upon by certain bacteria. This phenomenon, also described by Oluf Thomsen, is known as the *Hübener-Thomsen phenomenon.*

Huber's stain. See under *stain.*

Hubschmann's pseudaconitine. See British *aconitine.*

Huchard, Henri [*French physician,* 1844–1910]. Contributed to the knowledge of arteriosclerosis and hypertension. Called attention to the fact that diminution in pulse rate which occurs when the subject changes from the standing to the sitting position is much less in hypertensive than in normal individuals; called *Huchard's sign.* Excessive arterial tension was once called *Huchard's disease.*

Hucker's stain. See under *stain.*

Huddleson's test. See under *test.*

Hudson, W. H. [*American physician,* contemporary]. Designed a drill principally for use in opening the skull. *Hudson's bone drill* is operated by means of a holder similar to a carpenter's brace, and is provided with drills in graded sizes, so designed that the dura, when impinged on, is not injured.

hue. The quality of visual sensation which permits the observer to distinguish different wavelengths of light.

Hueck, Alexander Friedrich [*Estonian anatomist,* 1802–42]. Described the pectinate ligament of the iris, called *Hueck's ligament.*

Hughes reflex. See virile *reflex.*

Hughlings Jackson. See John Hughlings *Jackson.*

Huguier, Pierre Charles [*French gynecologist and surgeon,* 1804–74]. Made important studies of hysterectomy, of the treatment of ovarian cysts, and of amputation of the uterine cervix. Described a canal in the temporal bone, *Huguier's canal* which transmits the chorda tympani, the *iter chordae anterius.* Leiomyoma is also known as *Huguier's disease.*

Huhner, Max [*American surgeon and urologist,* 1873–1947]. Devised a test for sterility: one hour after coitus, the vagina of the female is aspirated and spermatozoa found therein are examined for motility.

Hulett and Bonner method. See under *method.*

hum [imitative in origin]. A low murmuring sound.

venous h. A continuous blowing or singing sound heard in the large veins of the neck in some cases of anemia. Also called *humming-top murmur.*

hu'man [L. *humanus,* human]. Of, pertaining to, or like mankind.

hu·man'o·scope [*humanus;* G. *skopein,* to examine]. A series of overlapping anatomic plates so arranged as to allow the examiner to study the relative sizes, shapes, and relationships of various parts of the body, as the pages are turned.

hu·mec'tant [L. *humectare,* to moisten]. Moistening; diluent.

hu·mec'tant. A diluent; a substance used to moisten.

hu"mer·o·ra'di·al [L. *humerus,* upper bone of the arm; *radius,* radius]. Pertaining to the humerus and the radius; applied to the joint between these two bones and to the ligaments joining them.

hu"mer·o·scap'u·lar [*humerus;* L. *scapula,* shoulder]. Pertaining to both the humerus and the scapula.

hu"mer·o·ul'nar [*humerus;* L. *ulna,* elbow]. Pertaining to the humerus and the ulna; applied to the joint between these two bones and to the ligaments joining them.

hu'mer·us (pl. *humeri*) [L.]. The bone of the upper arm, arm proper, or brachium. See Plates 1, 2. See Table of Bones in the Appendix. —**humeral,** *adj.*

hu'mic ac'id. A general term for any acid substance derived from humus.

hu·mic'o·lin. A weakly acidic antifungal substance produced by *Aspergillus humicola.*

hu·mid"i·fi·ca'tion. The process of moistening or humidifying air; specifically, in respiration, by moisture from mucous membranes.

hu·mid'i·ty [L. *humidus,* moist]. The state or quality of being moist; moisture; dampness. —**hu'mid,** *adj.*

absolute h. The percentage of water vapor in the air.

relative h. The amount of water vapor in the air as compared with the total amount the air would hold at a given temperature.

hu'min. 1. Any of several poorly defined substances, including humic acid, obtained from humus; the term is sometimes applied to humus itself. 2. A dark-colored substance or substances formed when proteins undergo acid hydrolysis, probably resulting by condensation of tryptophan with an aldehyde.

hu'mor [L., a liquid]. 1. Any fluid or semifluid part of the body. 2. *In old physiology,* one of the four cardinal body fluids, making up the four humors of Galen: the choleric, the melancholic, the phlegmatic, and the sanguine. They were said to determine a person's constitution, disposition, or temperament. 3. Disposition, temperament.

aqueous h. The aqueous.

crystalline h. The crystalline lens.

ocular h. Any one of the humors of the eye, the aqueous or vitreous, or the crystalline lens.

vitreous h. The vitreous body.

hu'mor·al [*humor*]. A term referring to the so-called humors of the body.

hu'mor·al·ism [*humor*]. An obsolete theory that disease was due to a disturbance of the humors or fluids of the body.

hump'back". See *kyphosis.*

Humphry, George Murray [*English surgeon,* 1820–96]. Devised an operation for excision of the condyle of the lower jaw; he exposed the condyle by reflecting a triangular flap upward, then sawed through the neck of the bone, and removed the condyle and lateral pterygoid plate. Called *Humphry's operation.*

hu′mu·lene. $C_{15}H_{24}$. A sesquiterpene contained in the volatile oil from hops.

hu′mu·lin. Lupulin.

hu′mu·lon, hu′mu·lone. $C_{21}H_{30}O_5$; an antibiotic constituent of humulus or hops. Syn., *α-lupulic acid.*

hu′mu·lus [ML.]. Hops. The dried strobile of *Humulus lupulus* bearing the glandular trichomes known as lupulin. Hops have been used as a calmative, stomachic, and tonic.

hu′mus [L., earth, ground]. A dark material in soil, consisting of decaying organic matter.

hunch′back″. Lay term for kyphosis.

hun′ger [AS. *hungor*]. A sensation of emptiness of the stomach, with a longing for food.

air h. Distressing dyspnea marked by deep, labored respiration, as in acidosis of diabetic coma. Also called *Kussmaul breathing.*

Hunner, Guy Le Roy (1868–). American gynecologic urologist, known for his description of interstitial cystitis with ulceration, called *Hunner's ulcer.*

Hunt, James Ramsay [*American neurologist,* 1874–1937]. Remembered for his many contributions to neurologic science. Described a syndrome of facial paralysis, earache, and herpes, appearing about the external auditory meatus, found when both motor and sensory fibers and the geniculate ganglion of the seventh cranial nerve are diseased; called *Hunt's syndrome.* Described neurotrophic atrophy of the small muscles of the hand, without sensory alteration; called *Hunt's atrophy.* See also striocerebellar *tremor,* also called *Hunt's tremor.*

Hunt's test. See opsonocytophagic *test.*

Hunter, John [*Scottish surgeon in England,* 1728–93]. Made important contributions to anatomy and physiology and to the development of experimental pathology. In an unsuccessful attempt to differentiate gonorrhea from syphilis, inoculated himself with what he thought was gonorrhea and acquired a syphilitic chancre (1767), called *Hunterian chancre.* Classified the teeth (1771). Described post-mortem digestion (1772). Performed proximal ligation of an artery at some distance from the aneurysm; this is called *Hunter's operation.* Described the descent of the testes and the structure of the placenta (1786). In a treatise on gunshot wounds, gave a classic description of inflammation (1794). See also adductor *canal,* also called *Hunter's canal.*

Hunter, William [*Scottish surgeon, obstetrician, and anatomist,* 1718–83]. Brother of John Hunter. Described arteriovenous aneurysm. Made an important study of the human gravid uterus (1774).

Hunter, William [*English physician,* 1861–1937]. Described glossitis in pernicious anemia; called *Hunter's glossitis.*

Hunter and Givens' modification of the Krüger-Schmid method. See under *method.*

Huntington, George [*American physician,* 1851–1916]. Remembered for his classic description of chronic progressive hereditary chorea. *Huntington's chorea* is characterized by irregular movements, disturbance of speech, and gradually increasing dementia.

Huntoon's stains. See under *stain.*

Huppert, Carl Hugo [*Bohemian physician,* 1832–1904]. Described multiple myeloma, called *Huppert's disease, Kahler's disease.* See under *Kahler.* See also Huppert's *test.*

Hurler, Gertrud [*German pediatrician,* contemporary]. Described lipochondrodystrophy, which is also called *Hurler's disease.*

Hürthle, Karl Wilhelm (1860–1945). German physiologist, known for his investigations on blood circulation and muscle structure. He also described an adenoma of the thyroid gland, composed of large cells, called *Hürthle cells,* with acidophilic cytoplasm and small nuclei.

Hurtley's test. See under *test.*

Huschke, Emil [*German anatomist,* 1797–1858]. An inconstant perforation of the tympanic portion of the temporal bone is called the *foramen of Huschke.*

Hutchinson, Jonathan [*English surgeon,* 1828–1913]. Described the notched or peg teeth seen in congenital syphilis (1861); called *Hutchinson's teeth.* Notched teeth, interstitial keratitis, and eighth nerve deafness comprise *Hutchinson's sign* or *triad,* diagnostic of congenital syphilis. Hutchinson performed the first successful operation for intussusception in an infant (1871). He described summer prurigo (1878), called *Hutchinson's prurigo,* and serpiginous angioma, called *Hutchinson's disease.* Generalized sarcoidosis is called *Hutchinson-Boeck disease.* Progeria is known as *Hutchinson-Gilford disease.*

Hutchison, Robert Grieve [*English physician,* 1871–1943]. Described suprarenal sarcoma in children (1907). This was accompanied by metastases in the skull and exophthalmos, and usually by discoloration about the eyes. Called *Hutchison's tumors.*

Huxham, John [*English physician,* 1692–1768]. Known for his *Essay on Fevers* (1739). Gave a classic description of diphtheria (1757), although he did not distinguish it from angina due to streptococcic infection. He also advocated the use of fruit and fruit juices for the prevention of scurvy.

Huxley, Thomas Henry [*English biologist,* 1825–95]. A leading advocate in his time of Darwin's theories. Made important contributions to comparative anatomy. See *layer* of Huxley.

Huygens, Christiaan [*Dutch physicist, mathematician, and astronomer,* 1629–95]. Postulated the wave theory of light. Improved telescopes and made important astronomic discoveries. See also Huygenian *ocular.*

hy′a·lin [G. *hyalos,* glass]. A clear, structureless, homogeneous, glassy material occurring normally in matrix of cartilage, vitreous body, colloid of thyroid gland, mucin, glycogen, jelly of Wharton; occurs pathologically in degenerations of connective tissue, epithelial cells, and in the form of mucinous and colloid degenerations, glycogen infiltration, etc. —**hyaline,** *adj.*

epithelial h. That produced by epithelial cells or resulting from degenerative change, usually in the form of intracytoplasmic droplets and seen in certain tumor cells, plasmacytes, and in various diseases of the liver and kidney.

mesenchymal h. A form of hyalin which results from degeneration or necrosis of nonepithelial tissue, usually of muscle, as in Zenker's hyaline necrosis, or of blood vessels.

Zenker's h. See Zenker's hyaline *necrosis.*

hy″a·lin·i·za′tion [*hyalos*]. Changes characterized by replacement or infiltration of tissues by an endogenous, amorphous, and frequently firm or hard material.

hy″a·lin·o′sis [G. *hyalos,* glass; *osis,* condition]. 1. Hyaline degeneration. 2. A condition produced experimentally in rats by the administration of desoxycortisone, after unilateral nephrectomy. Nephrosclerosis is produced, and a large number of the glomerular loops and afferent arterioles become hyalinized. Hyalinization is also seen beneath the endocardium and in many arteries.

hy″a·li·nu′ri·a [*hyalos;* G. *ouron,* urine]. Presence of hyalin or of hyaline casts in the urine.

hy″a·li′tis [*hyalos;* G. *-itis,* inflammation]. Inflammation of the vitreous body, or of the hyaloid membrane of the vitreous body.

hy′a·lo-, hyal- [*hyalos*]. 1. A combining form meaning *glass.* 2. A combining form signifying *of* or *pertaining to hyalin.*

hy″a·lo·cap″su·li′tis. Hyaloserositis of the capsule of the liver or spleen.

hy·al′o·gen (high·al′o·jen) [*hyalos;* G. *genesthai,* from *gignesthai,* to be produced]. 1. Insoluble substances resembling mucin, found in the walls of echinococcus cysts, the vitreous body, etc., and yielding hyalin on hydrolysis. 2. An albuminoid found in cartilage.

hy′a·loid [G. *hyaloeidēs,* glassy]. Transparent; glasslike.

hy″a·loid·i′tis. See *hyalitis.*

hy′a·lo·mere [*hyalos;* G, *meros,* part]. The clear part of the blood platelet after staining with stains of the Romanovsky type.

Hy″a·lom′ma [G. *hyalos,* glass; *omma,* eye]. A genus of ticks the males of which are characterized by submarginal eyes, ventral plates, and two protrusions from the tip of the abdomen which are capped with chitinous points. **H. aegyptium,** the most important species, is found on cattle and other large mammals in Africa, Asia, and south Europe.

hy″a·lo·mu′coid. A mucoid found in the fluid of the vitreous body.

hy″a·lo·nyx′is [*hyalos;* G. *nyxis,* a pricking]. Puncture of the vitreous body of the eye.

hy″a·lo·pho′bi·a. A morbid fear of glass.

hy′a·lo·plasm [*hyalos;* G. *plasma,* anything formed]. The fluid portion of the protoplasm. Also called *enchylema, interfilar mass, paraplasm, paramitome.*

hy″a·lo·se″ro·si′tis [*hyalos;* L. *serum,* watery part; G. *-itis,* inflammation]. Chronic inflammation of a serous membrane, observed principally in the capsule of the liver and of the spleen, with production of a thick layer of hyalinized, pearly gray, translucent connective tissue, said to resemble icing on a cake.

hy″a·lu·ron′ic ac′id. A viscous mucopolysaccharide occurring in connective tissues and in bacterial capsules.

hy″a·lu·ron′i·dase. An enzyme occurring in pathogenic bacteria, snake venoms, sperm, etc. It causes the breakdown of hyaluronic acid in protective polysaccharide barriers, promoting invasion of cells and tissues by the invading agent; it is a spreading factor. Hyaluronidase is used to promote the diffusion and absorption of various injected medicaments, also to increase protective urinary colloids in treatment and prevention of urinary calculi. See *alidase, wydase.* Syn., *invasin.*

hy′brid [L. *hibrida,* mongrel]. The offspring of parents belonging to different species, varieties, or genotypes. **—hybridism, hybrid′ity,** *n.*

hy″brid·i·za′tion [*hibrida*]. Crossbreeding.

hyclorite. Trade-mark for a solution of sodium hypochlorite, sodium chloride, and calcium hydroxide, containing 3.85% available chlorine.

hycodan bitartrate. Trade-marked name for dihydrocodeinone bitartrate: a cough sedative.

hy″dan·to′ic ac′id. $NH_2CONHCH_2COOH$. An acid resulting from the union of aminoacetic acid and carbamic acid which is an intermediary in the production of creatine in the body.

hy·dan′to·in (high·dan′to·in, high″dan·to′in). $\overline{NHCONHCOCH_2}$. Glycolyl urea. A crystalline substance derived from allantoin and related to urea.

hydase. Trade-mark for a brand of hyaluronidase.

hy·dat′id (high·dat′id) [G. *hydatis,* watery vesicle]. 1. A cyst formed in tissues due to growth of the larval stage of *Echinococcus granulosus* (dog tapeworm), containing a clear watery fluid, lined by an inner germinal cellular layer and an outer laminated layer of hyaline material. Formation of scolices in the germinal layer is followed by a deposit of pinched-off scolices and of hooklets in the fluid. 2. A cystic remnant of an embryonal structure. **—hydat′ic, hydatid′iform,** *adj.*

h. of Morgagni. A small, cystic remnant of the Müllerian duct attached by a fibrous stalk to the fimbriated end of the oviduct, or, in the male, to the head of the epididymis.

secondary h. Echinococcus cyst due to the rupture of another cyst and deposit of germinal cells and scolices in the neighborhood.

stalked h. The *h.* of Morgagni.

sterile hydatids. Echinococcus cysts in which the germinal layer, brood cysts, and scolices have disappeared; the so-called acephalocysts.

hy″da·tid′o·cele [*hydatis;* G. *kēlē,* hernia]. Scrotal hernia containing echinococcus cysts.

hy·dat″i·do′sis [*hydatis;* G. *-ōsis,* condition]. Multiple infection caused by echinococcus cysts.

Hyde, James Nevin [*American dermatologist,* 1840–1910]. Remembered for his description of prurigo nodularis, called *Hyde's disease.*

hydergine. Trade-mark for a mixture of the methanesulfonates of dihydroergocornine, dihydroergocristine, and dihydroergocryptine: used clinically to produce adrenergic blockade and peripheral vasodilatation, being administered intramuscularly.

hyd″no·car′pic ac′id. An acid, $C_{15}H_{27}COOH$, occurring as the glyceride in chaulmoogra oil.

hyd″no·car′pus oil. The British Pharmacopoeia name for the oil obtained by cold expression from fresh, ripe seeds of *Hydnocarpus Wightiana* Blume, but used by the National Formulary as a synonym for *chaulmoogra oil,* (IX) used in the treatment of leprosy.

hydracetin. Trade name for acetylphenylhydrazine.

hy·drac′id (high·dras′id). An acid containing no oxygen.

hy″dra·den·i′tis. See *hidradenitis.*

hy·drad″e·no′ma. Hidradenoma.

hy·drae′mi·a. See *hydremia.*

hy·dra″er·o·per″i·to·ne′um (high·dray″ur·o-perr″i·to·nee′um). See *hydropneumoperitoneum.*

hy′dra·gog, hy′dra·gogue [G. *hydōr,* water; *agōgos,* leading]. Causing the discharge of watery fluid.

hy′dra·gog, hy′dra·gogue. A purgative that causes copious liquid discharges.

hy·dral′a·zine hy″dro·chlo′ride. Generic name for 1-hydrazinophthalazine hydrochloride, an antihypertensive agent supplied under the trade-marked name *apresoline hydrochloride.*

hy·dram′ni·on. See *polyhydramnios.*

hy·dram′ni·os (high·dram′nee·os), **hy·dram′-ni·on.** See *polyhydramnios.*

hy·dran′ge·a (high·drain′juh, ·jee·uh, high·dran′·) [*hydōr;* G. *aggeion,* vessel]. The dried rhizome and roots of *Hydrangea arborescens;* contains a glycoside, hydrangin. Hydrangea has been used as a diuretic and antilithic. Dose, 2 Gm. (30 gr.).

hy·dran′gin (high·dran′jin) [*hydōr; aggeion*]. A crystalline glycoside from hydrangea.

hy″drar·gyr′i·a (high″drahr·jirr′ee·uh, ·jy′ree·uh), **hy″drar·gy·ri′a·sis, hy·drar′gy·rism** [G. *hydrargyros,* quicksilver]. Chronic mercurial poisoning.

hy″drar·gyr″o·pho′bi·a [*hydrargyros;* G. *phobos,* fear]. A morbid fear of mercurial medicines.

hy″drar·gyr″oph·thal′mi·a [*hydrargyros;* G. *ophthalmos,* eye]. Ophthalmia due to mercurial poisoning.

hy·drar′gy·rum (high·drahr′ji·rum). See *mercury.*

hy″drar·thro′sis [G. *hydōr*, water; *arthrōsis*, articulation]. An accumulation of fluid in a joint.

intermittent h. A condition characterized by acute regularly recurring effusions of fluid into the joint cavity.

hy′drase [*hydōr*]. An enzyme which removes or adds water to a substrate without hydrolyzing it. See Table of Enzymes in the Appendix.

hy·dras′tine (high·dras′teen, ·tin). An alkaloid, $C_{21}H_{21}NO_6$, from hydrastis; occasionally used, generally in the form of the hydrochloride, as an astringent, hemostatic, and uterine stimulant.

hy·dras′ti·nine (high·dras′ti·neen, ·nin). An oxidation product of hydrastine; sometimes used, in the form of the hydrochloride, in uterine hemorrhage as a stimulant and hemostatic.

hy·dras′tis [*hydōr*]. The rhizome and roots of *Hydrastis canadensis*, which contain the alkaloids *hydrastine*, *berberine*, and *canadine*. It is a hemostatic and astringent but is rarely employed. Syn., *yellow root*. Also called *goldenseal*.

hy′drate [*hydōr*]. 1. A compound containing water in chemical combination, water of hydration. 2. Hydroxide. *Obs.* —**hydrated,** *adj.*; **hydra′tion,** *n.*

hy·drau′lics [G. *hydraulis*, from *hydōr; aulos*, flute]. The science which deals with the mechanical properties of liquids.

hy′dra·zine (high′druh·zeen, ·zin). 1. $H_2N.NH_2$. Diamine; a colorless liquid, soluble in water, having a strong alkaline reaction. 2. One of a class of bodies derived from hydrazine by replacing one or more hydrogen atoms by a radical.

h. sulfate. $H_2N.NH_2.H_2SO_4$. Used in tests for blood; a reducing agent.

hy″dre·lat′ic [*hydōr;* G. *elaunein*, to drive]. Pertaining to the secretory effect of nerves upon glands, causing them to discharge the watery part of their secretion. Also called *hydrokinetic*.

hy·dre′mi·a, hy·drae′mi·a (high·dree′mee·uh) [*hydōr;* G. *haima*, blood]. A condition of the blood in which the fluid content is increased but the total amount of the blood does not increase proportionately. —**hydremic,** *adj.*

hy″dren·ceph′a·lo·cele [*hydōr;* G. *egkephalos*, brain; *kēlē*, hernia]. Protrusion through a defect in the cranium of a sac and brain substance in which a cystic cavity contains fluid.

hy″dren·ceph″a·lo·me·nin′go·cele [*hydōr; egkephalos;* G. *menigx*, membrane; *kēlē*]. A hernia through a cranial defect of meninges and brain substance, fluid filling the space between these.

hy·dri′a·try (high·dry′uh·tree, high′dree·at″ree). Hydrotherapy. *Obs.*

hy′dride. A compound containing hydrogen united to a more positive element or to a radical.

hy″dri·od′ic ac′id. The gas hydrogen iodide, HI, or an aqueous solution thereof. **Diluted hydriodic acid,** containing 10% HI, and **hydriodic acid syrup,** containing 1.4% HI, are sometimes used medicinally for the effects of iodide ion.

hy·dri′o·dide. An iodide formed by interaction of an organic nitrogenous base with hydriodic acid.

hy·dri′on (high·dry′on, high′dree·on). Hydrogen in the ionized form.

hydrionic. Trade-mark for glutamic acid hydrochloride used in hydrochloric acid therapy.

hy′dro-, hydr- [*hydōr*]. 1. A combining form meaning *water*. 2. *In chemistry*, a combining form denoting *the presence of hydrogen* or *the addition of hydrogen to a compound*. 3. *In medicine*, a combining form denoting *a disease characterized by an accumulation of water or other fluid in a bodily part*.

hy·dro′a (high·dro′uh, hid·ro′uh) [*hydōr;* G. *ōion*, egg]. Any skin disease characterized by vesicles or bullae.

h. herpetiforme. See *dermatitis* herpetiformis.

h. vacciniforme. A skin disease, occurring in the summer on the exposed parts, usually in young males. It is characterized by vesicles and crusted ulcers, and gradually disappears following puberty. Also called *h. aestivale, h. puerorum, summer prurigo*.

hy″dro·ab·do′men [*hydōr;* L. *abdomen*, belly]. Old term for ascites.

hy″dro·bil″i·ru′bin (high″dro·bil″i·roo′bin, ·buy″·li·roo′bin) [*hydōr;* L. *bilis*, bile; *ruber*, red]. A red pigment, a reduction product from bilirubin; probably the same as urobilin.

hy″dro·bro′mate. A hydrobromic acid salt; a hydrobromide.

hy″dro·bro′mic. Composed of hydrogen and bromine.

hy″dro·bro′mic ac′id. 1. Hydrogen bromide, HBr; a heavy, colorless gas with a pungent irritating odor. 2. An aqueous solution of HBr.

diluted h. a. An aqueous solution containing 10% of HBr; sometimes used for the same purpose as the bromides. Dose, 2–4 cc. (30–60 min.).

hy″dro·bro′mide. A bromide formed by interaction of an organic nitrogenous base with hydrobromic acid.

hy′dro·cal. A trade-mark for certain high-strength gypsum cements suitable for molding purposes.

hy″dro·ca′lix. Cystic dilatation of a renal calix, usually solitary.

hy″dro·cal″y·co′sis. See calyceal *diverticulum*.

hy″dro·car′bon. Any compound composed only of hydrogen and carbon.

saturated h. One that has the maximum number of hydrogen atoms; that is, without double or triple bonds between carbon atoms.

unsaturated h. One that has one or more double or triple bonds between carbon atoms.

hy′dro·cele [*hydōr;* G. *kēlē*, tumor]. An accumulation of fluid in the sac of the tunica vaginalis of the testis. In adults, the cause is unknown and the fluid is clear, slightly viscid, and contains 6–10% of solids, including proteins, salts, and sometimes cholesterol. See Plate 39.

congenital h. The presence of peritoneal fluid in the tunica vaginalis, due to failure of closure of the vaginal process.

encysted h. One which occupies a portion of the vaginal process with closure of the abdominal and scrotal ends.

h. hernialis. An accumulation of peritoneal fluid in a hernial sac, especially when hernia accompanies congenital or infantile hydrocele.

infantile h. Peritoneal fluid in the tunica vaginalis and the vaginal process, but with the process closed at the abdominal ring.

spermatic h. Accumulation of spermatic fluid in the tunica vaginalis of the testis; caused by the rupture of a spermatocele.

hy″dro·ce·lec′to·my [*hydōr; kēlē;* G. *ektomē*, excision]. Surgical removal of part of the tunica vaginalis for the cure of hydrocele.

hy″dro·ceph′a·lo·cele″ (high″dro·sef′uh·lo·seel″). See *hydrencephalocele*.

hy″dro·ceph′a·lus. 1. An individual with hydrocephaly. 2. Hydrocephaly.

hy″dro·ceph′a·ly [*hydōr;* G. *kephalē*, head]. An increase in the volume of cerebrospinal fluid within the skull. The term is commonly applied to distentions of the ventricular system by cerebrospinal fluid which cannot escape into the subarachnoid space, is blocked in the subarachnoid pathways, or cannot be absorbed into the venous system. Also called *hydrocephalus*. —**hydrocephal′ic,** *adj.*

communicating h. A form in which there is

normal communication between the ventricles and the subarachnoid space.

congenital h. A progressive form in infancy. Also called *chronic h., infantile h.*

external h. An increased accumulation of fluid in the subarachnoid space, or rarely, in the subdural space; usually a passive process due to atrophy of the brain.

internal h. That in which increased cerebrospinal fluid accumulates in the ventricular system as contrasted with external *h.* See obstructive *h.*

obstructive h. That caused by the blocking of the passage of cerebrospinal fluid from the brain ventricles, where it is produced, to the subarachnoid space where it is absorbed. Obstruction may occur at the interventricular foramens in the cerebral aqueduct, or at the foramens of Luschka in the roof of the fourth ventricle. Also called *noncommunicating h.*

hy″dro·chi′none (high″dro·kigh′nohn, ·kin′ohn). See *hydroquinone.*

hy″dro·chin″o·nu′ri·a (·kin″o·new′ree·uh) [*hydōr;* Sp. *quina,* cinchona bark; G. *ouron,* urine]. The presence in the urine of hydroquinone; due to ingestion of salol, resorcin, etc.

hy″dro·chlo′rate. An older name, incorrectly used, for salts formed by hydrochloric acid with certain organic nitrogenous bases, especially alkaloids.

hy″dro·chlo′ric ac′id. 1. Hydrogen chloride, HCl, a colorless gas of pungent odor which can be liquefied under pressure. 2. An aqueous solution containing 35% to 38% of HCl.

diluted h. a. An aqueous solution containing 10% of HCl; used in hydrochloric acid deficiency states. Dose, 0.6–4.0 cc. (10–60 min.).

hy″dro·chlo′ride. A chloride formed by interaction of an organic nitrogenous base with hydrochloric acid.

hy″dro·chol″er·e′sis (high″dro·kol″ur·ee′sis, ·ko″-lur·ee′sis) [G. *hydōr,* water; *cholē,* bile; *-ēsis,* denoting process of action]. Choleresis characterized by an increase of water output, or of a bile relatively low in specific gravity, viscosity, and content of total solids. —**hydrocholeret′ic,** *adj.*

hydrocholin. Trade-mark for a brand of dehydrocholic acid.

hy″dro·cin·chon′i·dine (high″dro·sin·kon′i·deen, ·din). An alkaloid, $C_{19}H_{24}NO_2$, from species of *Cinchona.* Syn., *cinchamidine.*

hy″dro·col′li·dine (high″dro·kol′i·deen, ·din). A highly poisonous ptomaine obtained from putrefying mackerel, horseflesh, and oxflesh.

hy″dro·col′loid. *In dentistry,* a type of impression material derived from marine kelp. It is introduced into the mouth as a viscous sol which is shortly converted into a rigid, insoluble gel. See *alginate.*

hy″dro·col′pos [*hydōr;* G. *kolpos,* vagina]. A vaginal retention cyst containing a watery fluid.

hy″dro·co′ni·on [*hydōr;* G. *konis,* dust]. An atomizer; a spraying apparatus.

hy″dro·con′qui·nine (high″dro·kon′kwi·neen, ·nin). Hydroquinidine.

hy″dro·cor′ti·sone. Generic name for 17-hydroxycorticosterone. See *cortril.*

h. acetate. Generic name for 17-hydroxycorticosterone-21-acetate. See *hydrocortone acetate.*

hydrocortone acetate. Trade-marked name for hydrocortisone acetate or 17-hydroxycorticosterone-21-acetate.

hy″dro·co·tar′nine (high″dro·ko·tahr′neen, ·nin). A crystalline alkaloid derived from narcotine and occurring in small amount in opium.

Hy″dro·cot′y·le. Pennywort; a genus of umbelliferous herbs, several species of which have been variously employed in therapeutics.

hy″dro·cu′pre·ine. $C_{19}H_{24}N_2O_2$. A reduction product of cupreine; employed in synthesis of ethylhydrocupreine and other similar medicinals.

hy″dro·cy·an′ic ac′id (high″dro·sigh·an′ick, high″-dro·see·an′ick). Hydrogen cyanide, HCN, boiling at 26° C.; used as a fumigant to rid vessels, buildings, orchards, etc. of vermin. It is a colorless, powerful, rapidly acting blood and nerve poison, having an odor of bitter almonds, which paralyzes and causes dizziness and coma. Syn., *prussic acid.*

diluted h. a. A 2% aqueous hydrogen cyanide solution; occasionally employed for its supposed antispasmodic or sedative action. Dose, 0.06–0.25 cc. (1–4 min.). Syn., *diluted prussic acid.*

hy″dro·cys·to′ma. See *hidrocystoma.*

hy″dro·dex′tran. A product of high-pressure catalytic hydrogenation of dextran, used similarly.

hy″dro·dip″so·ma′ni·a [*hydōr;* G. *dipsa,* thirst; *mania,* madness]. Periodic attacks of uncontrollable thirst; often seen in schizophrenia and epilepsy.

hy″dro·dy·nam′ics (high″dro·dye·nam′icks, ·di-nam′icks) [*hydōr;* G. *dynamis,* power]. That branch of mechanics which deals with liquids.

hy″dro·er·got′i·nine (·ur·got′i·neen, ·nin). A name given to ergotoxine before the latter was found to be a mixture of alkaloids.

hy″dro·flu·or′ic ac′id. 1. Hydrogen fluoride, HF; a highly corrosive, colorless gas. 2. An aqueous solution containing about 50% of HF; used for etching glass.

hy′dro·gel. A colloidal gel with water as the dispersion medium.

hy′dro·gen. H = 1.0080. A univalent, inflammable, gaseous element; the lightest element known. It occurs in water and in practically all organic compounds. It is used in various syntheses, as a reducing agent, for the hydrogenation of vegetable oils to form solid products, and in many other industrial applications. Three isotopes of hydrogen (namely, protium, deuterium, and tritium, having atomic masses of approximately one, two, and three, respectively) have been discovered.

arseniuretted h. Arsine. AsH_3.

heavy h. The hydrogen isotope of approximate mass two; deuterium. Its nucleus consists of a proton and a neutron. See heavy *water.*

h. acceptor. A substance which, on reduction, accepts hydrogen atoms from another substance called a hydrogen donor. See *coenzyme.*

h. arsenide. Arsine. AsH_3.

h. bond. See hydrogen *bond.*

h. bridge. Hydrogen bond.

h. bromide. HBr. A heavy, colorless gas with a pungent irritating odor. Also called *hydrobromic acid.*

h. chloride. HCl. A colorless gas of pungent odor; liquefied under pressure. Also called *hydrochloric acid.*

h. cyanide. Hydrocyanic acid.

h. dioxide. See *h.* peroxide.

h. donor. *In chemistry,* a chemical compound capable of transferring hydrogen atoms to another substance (hydrogen acceptor), thereby reducing the latter and oxidizing the donor.

h. fluoride. HF. A highly corrosive, colorless gas. An aqueous solution is used for etching glass. Also called *hydrofluoric acid.*

h. iodide. HI. A colorless gas. Also called *hydriodic acid.*

h. ion. The positively charged nucleus of the hydrogen atom, a proton. Acids are characterized by their ability to liberate hydrogen ions when in aqueous solution. Symbol, H^+. See *hydronium.*

h.-ion concentration. The number of gram ions

of hydrogen per liter of solution. See Table of Normal Values of Blood Constituents in the Appendix.

h. peroxide. H_2O_2, a colorless, caustic liquid, highly explosive in contact with oxidizable material.

h. peroxide solution (*liquor hydrogenii peroxidi*). A 3% aqueous solution used as antiseptic and germicide. One volume is capable of liberating approximately 10 volumes of oxygen. See *perhydrol.*

h. sulfide. H_2S. A colorless, highly toxic gas of unpleasant odor.

light h. Protium.

hy″dro·gen·a′tion. The process of combining with hydrogen.

hy″dro·gen·ly′ase. An enzyme, present in *Escherichia coli,* which catalyzes reversible decomposition of formic acid to molecular hydrogen and carbon dioxide, a reaction which appears to be associated with the anerobic decomposition, by extracts of *E. coli,* of pyruvic acid to acetic acid and formic acid.

hy″dro·glos′sa [G. *hydōr,* water; *glōssa,* tongue]. Ranula.

hy″dro·gym·nas′tics [*hydōr;* G. *gymnastikos,* skilled in athletic exercises]. Active exercises performed in water; the buoyancy thus obtained enables weakened muscles to move the limbs more easily.

hy″dro·hem″a·to·ne·phro′sis (high″dro·hem″uh-to·ni·fro′sis, high″dro·hee″muh·to·) [*hydōr;* G. *haima,* blood; *nephros,* kidney; *-ōsis,* condition]. The presence of blood and urine in a dilated renal pelvis.

hy″dro·ki·net′ic (high″dro·ki·net′ick, ·kigh·net′-ick) [*hydōr;* G. *kinētikos,* of motion]. Concerning or producing water transfer during glandular secretion; hydrelatic.

hy″dro·ki·net′ics [*hydōr; kinētikos*]. The science of the motion of liquids.

hy′drol [*hydōr*]. The single molecule of water, H_2O. Sometimes called *monohydrol.* See *dihydrol, trihydrol.*

hy″dro·lac·tom′e·ter [*hydōr;* L. *lac,* milk; G. *metron,* a measure]. An instrument used in estimating the percentage of water in milk.

hy′dro·lase (high′dro·lace, ·laze). An enzyme causing hydrolysis. See Table of Enzymes in the Appendix.

hy′dro·lin. Methyl hexalin, $CH_3C_6H_{10}OH$. A clear, viscous liquid used as a solubilizer, homogenizer, and stabilizer for various liquid mixtures. See also *hexalin.*

hy·drol′o·gy [*hydōr;* G. *logos,* word]. Knowledge of water in the widest sense.

hy·drol′y·sate. See *hydrolyzate.*

hy·drol′y·sis [*hydōr;* G. *lysis,* a loosing]. Any reaction with water, frequently of the type $AB + HOH \rightarrow AOH + HB$, the latter being the reverse reaction of neutralization. —**hydrolyt′ic,** *adj.;* **hy′-drolyze,** *v.*

hy′dro·lyst [*hydōr; lysis*]. A catalyst or enzyme causing hydrolysis.

hy′dro·lyte [*hydōr;* G. *lytos,* soluble]. The substance undergoing hydrolysis.

hy·drol′y·zate, hy·drol′y·sate [*hydōr;* G. *lysis,* a loosing]. The product of hydrolysis.

hy·dro′ma. See *hygroma.*

hy″dro·ma′ni·a [*hydōr;* G. *mania,* madness]. A maniacal desire for suicide by drowning. *Obs.*

hy″dro·mas·sage′. Massage by means of moving water.

hy′dro·mel [*hydōr;* G. *meli,* honey]. A mixture of honey and water, with or without a medicinal substance.

hy″dro·me·nin′go·cele [*hydōr;* G. *mēnigx,* membrane; *kēlē,* tumor]. 1. A cystic tumor of the meninges protruding through the skull. 2. A form of spina bifida in which the sac contains cerebrospinal fluid.

hy·drom′e·ter [*hydōr;* G. *metron,* a measure]. An instrument for determining the specific gravity of liquids. —**hydromet′ric,** *adj.;* **hydrometry,** *n.*

hy″dro·mi″cro·ceph′a·ly [*hydōr;* G. *mikros,* small; *kephalē,* head]. Microcephaly with increased cerebrospinal fluid.

hy″dro·my·e′li·a (high″dro·migh·ee′lee·uh) [*hydōr;* G. *myelos,* marrow]. A dilatation of the central canal of the spinal cord containing an increased quantity of cerebrospinal fluid.

acquired h. That due to tumors in the cerebellum or injuries to the spinal cord.

congenital h. Usually a diffuse dilatation of the canal with atrophy, mainly of the gray matter.

hy″dro·my′e·lo·cele″ [*hydōr; myelos;* G. *kēlē,* tumor]. 1. Excessive accumulation of fluid in the central canal of the spinal cord. 2. Hydromyelia.

hy″dro·my′rinx. Hydrotympanum.

hy″dro·ne·phro′sis [*hydōr;* G. *nephros,* kidney; *-ōsis,* condition]. A collection of urine in the distended pelvis of the kidney, from obstructed outflow. The pressure of the fluid in time causes atrophy of the kidney structure, and the whole organ is converted into a large cyst. —**hydronephrot′ic,** *adj.*

hy·dro′ni·um. The solvated hydrogen ion, $H^+(H_2O)$ or H_3O^+, considered to be present in aqueous solutions of all acids.

hy′dro·nol. $(HOH)_2$. A postulated form of water in the double molecule form, in which one of the molecules is resolved into H and OH, with increased chemical activity.

hy·drop′a·thy [*hydōr;* G. *pathos,* disease]. The internal and external use of water for the attempted cure of disease. —**hydropath′ic,** *adj.*

hy″dro·per″i·car·di′tis [*hydōr;* G. *perikardios,* about the heart; *-itis,* inflammation]. Pericarditis accompanied by serous effusion into the pericardium.

hy″dro·per″i·car′di·um [*hydōr; perikardios*]. A collection of a serous effusion in the pericardial cavity, resulting from passive congestion or lymphatic obstruction.

hy″dro·per′i·on [*hydōr;* G. *peri,* around; *ōion,* egg]. A seroalbuminous liquid existing between the decidua parietalis and the decidua capsularis.

hy″dro·per″i·to·ne′um [*hydōr;* G. *peritonaion,* peritoneum]. An accumulation of nonpurulent, watery fluid in the peritoneal cavity; ascites.

Hy·droph′i·dae (high·drof′i·dee) [*hydōr;* G. *ophis,* serpent]. A family of poisonous snakes, known as the sea snakes, which because of certain modifications are adapted to life in the sea. These snakes occur most abundantly in the seas of northern Australia and southern Asia; and although their venom is the most toxic known, bites are relatively rare.

hy′dro·phil, hy′dro·phile (high′dro·fill, ·file) [*hydōr;* G. *philein,* to love]. A substance, usually in the colloidal state, which is capable of combining with, or attracting, water. —**hydrophil′ic,** *adj.*

hy·droph′i·lism (high·drof′i·liz·um), **hy″dro-phil′i·a** [*hydōr; philein*]. The property of colloids, cells, and tissues to attract and hold water.

hy·droph′i·lous [*hydōr; philein*]. 1. *In botany,* applied to plants that are fertilized through the agency of water. 2. Absorbing water.

hy′dro·phobe [*hydōr;* G. *phobos,* fear]. 1. A substance, usually in the colloidal state, which lacks affinity for water. 2. One who has hydrophobia, 1. —**hydropho′bic,** *adj.*

hy″dro·pho′bi·a [*hydōr; phobos*]. 1. Morbid fear of water. 2. Rabies. —**hydrophobic,** *adj.*

hy″dro·pho″bo·pho′bi·a [*hydōr; phobos; phobos*]. An intense dread of hydrophobia; a condition sometimes producing a state simulating true hydrophobia; lyssophobia.

hy′dro·phone [*hydōr;* G. *phōnē*, voice]. An instrument used in auscultatory percussion, the sound being conveyed to the ear through a liquid column.

hy″droph·thal′mos, hy″droph·thal′mi·a, hy″droph·thal′mus [*hydōr;* G. *ophthalmos*, eye]. An increase in the fluid contents of the eye, causing the organ to become distended. Syn., *buphthalmia.* See infantile *glaucoma.*

hy′dro·plasm [*hydōr;* G. *plasma*, anything formed]. The fluid constituent of protoplasm. *Rare.*

hy″dro·pleu′ra. See *hydrothorax.*

hy″dro·pneu″ma·to′sis (high″dro·new″muh·to′-sis) [*hydōr;* G. *pneumatōsis*, inflation]. A collection of liquid and gas within the tissues.

hy″dro·pneu″mo·per″i·car′di·um [*hydōr;* G. *pneuma*, breath; *perikardios*, around the heart]. A collection of a serous effusion and gas in the pericardial sac.

hy″dro·pneu″mo·per″i·to·ne′um [*hydōr; pneuma;* G. *peritonaion*, peritoneum]. A collection of serum and gas within the peritoneal cavity.

hy″dro·pneu″mo·tho′rax [*hydōr; pneuma;* G. *thōrax*, chest]. The presence of serous fluid and gas in the pleural cavity.

hy′drops [G., dropsy]. Accumulation of the fluid of edema, or more rarely, of other watery fluids. —**hydrop′ic,** *adj.*

endolymphatic h. See Ménière's *syndrome.*

h. antri. Effusion of serous fluid into the maxillary sinus.

h. articulorum. Hydrarthrosis.

h. fetalis. Erythroblastosis foetalis.

h. gravidarum. Edema in pregnancy.

h. of the abdomen. Ascites.

h. of the gallbladder. Distention of the gallbladder by a clear, or slightly cloudy, somewhat mucinous, white or colorless thin fluid.

h. of the labyrinth. A condition of choked labyrinth caused by chronic high intracranial pressure as in brain tumor. Atrophy of end organs in the cochlea and maculas results.

hy″dro·py″o·ne·phro′sis [G. *hydōr*, water; *pyon*, pus; *nephros*, kidney; *-ōsis*, condition]. Distention of the pelvis of the kidney with urine and pus.

hy″dro·quin′i·dine (high″dro·kwin′i·deen, ·din). An alkaloid, $C_{20}H_{26}N_2O_2.2\frac{1}{2}H_2O$, in cinchona bark. Syn., *hydroconquinine.*

hy″dro·quin′ine (high″dro·kwin′een, ·in). $C_{20}H_{26}N_2O_2.H_2O$. An alkaloid obtained from cinchona, and frequently contaminating quinine. It is effective against malaria. Also called *dihydroquinine.*

hy″dro·quin′ol. Hydroquinone.

hy″dro·qui·none′ (high″dro·kwi·nohn′, ·kwin′ohn, ·kin′ohn). 1,4-$C_6H_4(OH)_2$. Para-dihydroxybenzene, an isomer of resorcinol and pyrocatechin, obtained synthetically and occurring also as a product of the decomposition of arbutin. A photographic developer; has been recommended as an antipyretic and antiseptic.

hy″dror·rhe′a [*hydōr;* G. *rhoia*, flow]. A flow of watery liquid.

h. gravidarum. A discharge of fluid from the vagina prior to parturition; often mistaken by the patient for amniotic fluid. The so-called fore-waters.

hy″dro·sal′pinx [*hydōr;* G. *salpigx*, trumpet]. A distention of a uterine tube with fluid.

hy″dro·sat′ur·nism [*hydōr;* L. *saturnus*, lead]. Lead poisoning that is caused by lead in water supply.

hy·dro′sis. See *hidrosis.*

hy′dro·sol. A colloid system in which water is the dispersion medium.

hy″dro·sol′u·ble [*hydōr;* L. *solutum*, from *solvere*, to loosen]. Soluble in water.

hydrosorb. Trade-mark for an ointment base capable of absorbing water.

hy″dro·sper′ma·to·cele″. See *spermatocele.*

hy″dro·sper′ma·to·cyst″. A hydrocele whose fluid contains spermatozoa. See *spermatocele.*

hy″dro·spi·rom′e·ter (high″dro·spy·rom′i·tur) [*hydōr;* L. *spirare*, to breathe; G. *metron*, a measure]. A spirometer in which a column of water acts as an index.

hy′dro·stat [*hydōr;* G. *statos*, standing]. An apparatus for preventing the spilling of the fluid of electric batteries.

hy″dro·stat′ics. That branch of hydrodynamics which treats of the properties of liquids in a state of equilibrium. —**hydrostatic,** *adj.*

hy″dro·sul·fu′ric ac′id. 1. Hydrogen sulfide, H_2S. 2. Dithionic acid, $H_2S_2O_6$. 3. An organic acid of the formula R.CS.SH.

hy″dro·sy·rin″go·my·e′li·a (·si·ring″go·migh·ee′-lee·uh) [*hydōr;* G. *syrigx*, tube; *myelos*, marrow]. Dilatation of the central canal of the spinal cord by watery effusion, accompanied by degeneration and the formation of cavities.

hy″dro·tax′is [*hydōr;* G. *taxis*, arrangement]. Response of organisms to stimulus of moisture. Also see *hydrotropism.*

hy″dro·ther″a·peu′tics (high″dro·therr″uh·pew′-ticks) [*hydōr;* G. *therapeutikos*, therapeutic]. Hydrotherapy.

hy″dro·ther′a·py [*hydōr;* G. *therapeia*, treatment]. The treatment of disease by means of water; hydrotherapeutics.

hy″dro·ther′mal [*hydōr;* G. *thermē*, heat]. Pertaining to warm water; said of springs.

hy″dro·thi′on. Hydrogen sulfide. *Obs.*

hy″dro·thi″o·nu′ri·a [*hydōr;* G. *theion*, brimstone; *ouron*, urine]. The presence of hydrogen sulfide in the urine.

hy″dro·tho′rax [*hydōr;* G. *thōrax*, chest]. A collection of serous fluid in the pleural space. —**hydrothorac′ic** (high″dro·thor·ass′ick), *adj.*

hy·dro′tis (high·dro′tis) [*hydōr;* G. *ous*, ear]. Dropsy of, or effusion into, the external ear, the middle ear, or the inner ear, seldom in combination.

hy·drot′ro·pism (high·drot′ro·piz·um, high″dro-tro′piz·um) [*hydōr;* G. *trepein*, to turn]. *In botany*, the tendency of a growing plant or organ to turn either away from, or toward, moisture.

hy·drot′ro·py [*hydōr; trepein*]. The power that certain substance have of making water-insoluble substances dissolve in water without any apparent chemical alteration of the dissolved substances, as, for example, the solubilizing action of bile salts on fatty acids. —**hydrotrop′ic,** *adj.*

hy″dro·tym′pa·num [*hydōr;* G. *tympanon*, drum]. Serous effusion into the cavity of the middle ear.

hy″dro-u·re′ter (high″dro·yoor·ee′tur, ·yoor′i·tur). Abnormal distention of the ureter with urine, usually due to partial obstruction.

hy′drous [*hydōr*]. Containing water.

hy·drox′ide (high·drock′side, ·sid). A compound formed by the union of a metal, or of an inorganic or organic radical, with one or more hydroxyl (OH) groups.

hy·drox′y- (high·drock′see-). *In chemistry*, a combining form indicating *the hydroxyl group —OH.*

p-hy·drox″y·ac″et·an′i·lid. *p*-Acetaminophenol.

hy·drox″y·a·ce′tic ac′id. Glycolic acid.

hy·drox″y·am·phet′a·mine hy″dro·bro′mide. $[HO.C_6H_4.CH_2CH(N^+H_3)CH_3]Br^-$; *p*-(2-aminopropyl)phenol hydrobromide; a white, crystalline powder, freely soluble in water; a sympathomimetic agent used as a mydriatic agent and nasal decongestant.

hy·drox″y·ap′a·tite. $3Ca_3(PO_4)_2.Ca(OH)_2$. The basic inorganic constituent of bone. In bone, the hydroxyl groups are partially substituted by other elements and radicals, such as fluoride, carbonate, etc.

hy·drox″y·as″per·gil′lic ac′id. An antibiotic substance, a hydroxy derivative of aspergillic acid, accompanying the latter and obtained from cultures of *Aspergillus flavus.*

hy·drox″y·ben′zene. Phenol.

hy·drox″y·ben·zo′ic ac′id. $C_6H_4.OH.COOH$; any of three isomeric acids, differing in the position of the OH and COOH groups, and distinguished by the prefixes *ortho-*, *meta-*, and *para-*. *Ortho*-hydroxybenzoic acid is salicylic acid; esters of *para*-hydroxybenzoic acid are used as preservatives against microbial action in various preparations.

β-hy·drox″y·bu·tyr′ic ac′id. $CH_3.CHOH.CH_2-COOH$. An organic acid that is an intermediary in fat metabolism. It is a member of a group of compounds called acetone bodies or ketone bodies. In ketosis, increased amounts of these compounds appear in the blood and in the urine.

17-hy·drox″y·cor″ti·cos′te·rone. $C_{21}H_{30}O_5$; 4-pregnen-11β,17α,21-triol-3,20-dione; a steroid hormone isolated from adrenal cortex and also prepared synthetically. It has the same metabolic and therapeutic effects as cortisone; its acetate has the advantage over cortisone acetate of causing less irritation and promoting more prolonged and intense local effect when injected into intraarticular spaces affected by rheumatoid arthritis and osteoarthritis. Syn., *hydrocortisone, Kendall's compound F, Reichstein's substance M.* See *cortril.*

17-h.-21-acetate. $C_{23}H_{32}O_6$; the 21-acetate ester of 17-hydroxycorticosterone, a white solid, practically insoluble in water. It is the usual dosage form of 17-hydroxycorticosterone. Syn., *hydrocortisone acetate.* See *hydrocortone acetate.*

17-hy·drox′y-11-de·hy″dro·cor″ti·cos′ter·one. Cortisone.

17-hy·drox″y-11-des·ox″y·cor″ti·cos′te·rone. $C_{21}H_{30}O_4$; a steroid hormone possessing adrenal cortical activity. See Table of Hormones.

hy·drox″y·eth′ane. A chemical name, rarely used, for ethyl alcohol.

hy·drox″y·eth″a·no′ic ac′id. An exact chemical name, rarely used, for glycolic acid.

hy·drox″y·eth″yl·ap″o·cu′pre·ine (high·drock″-see·eth″il·ap″o·cue′pree·een, ·in). A pneumococcide related chemically to ethylhydrocupreine.

hy·drox″y·glu·tam′ic ac′id. $COOH.CH_2.CHOH.-CHNH_2.COOH$; β-hydroxyglutamic acid, an amino acid originally thought to be a constituent of proteins but later found not to be present.

hy·drox′yl (high·drock′sil). The univalent radical OH, the combination of which with a basic element or radical forms a hydroxide.

hy·drox″yl·a·mine′. NH_2OH. A basic substance, known only in solution in water or in combination with acids.

hy·drox″y·ly′sine. Common name for the amino acid, α-ϵ-diamino-β-hydroxy-*n*-caproic acid, $CH_2-(NH_2)CH_2CH_2CH(OH)CH(NH_2)COOH$.

hy·drox″y·man·del′ic ac′id. $HO.C_6H_4.CH(OH).-COOH$. A substance found in the urine in cases of yellow atrophy of the liver.

hy·drox″y·pro′line (high·drock″see·pro′leen, ·lin). One of the natural amino acids,

$$NH.CH_2.CHOH.CH_2CH.COOH.$$

hy·drox″y·quin′o·line (·kwin′o·leen, ·lin). C_9H_7-NO; 8-hydroxyquinoline, produced synthetically; it occurs as a crystalline powder, almost insoluble in water but freely soluble in alcohol: used as an analytical reagent for metals, and also as a fungicide. Syn., *oxine, oxyquinoline, 8-quinolinone.*

h. citrate. $C_9H_7NO.C_6H_8O_7$; a yellow, crystalline powder, freely soluble in water; it has been used as an antiseptic. Syn., *oxyquinoline citrate.*

h. sulfate. $(C_9H_7NO)_2.H_2SO_4$; a yellow, crystalline powder, freely soluble in water; it has been used as an antiseptic. Syn., *oxyquinoline sulfate.* See *chinosol.*

hy·drox″y·stear′in sul′fate. A substance prepared by sulfating hydrogenated castor oil; it is a pale yellow-brown, semisoft, unctuous mass, dispersible in water: used in the formulation of hydrophilic ointment bases.

hy·drox″y·to·lu′ic ac′id. Cresotic acid.

hy·dru′ri·a (high·droor′ee·uh) [*hydōr;* G. *ouron,* urine]. The passage of large amounts of urine of low specific gravity, as in diabetes insipidus; polyuria. —**hydruric,** *adj.*

hy″e·tom′e·try [G. *hyetos,* rain; *metron,* a measure]. Measurement of the quantity of rainfall.

hyflavin. Trade-mark for a mixture of methylol derivatives of riboflavin, known collectively by the generic name *methylol riboflavin;* the substance possesses the activity of riboflavin and is recommended especially for parenteral therapy.

Hygeia. In Greek mythology, the goddess of health; daughter of Asclepios.

hy′giene [G. *hygieinos,* healthful]. The science that treats of the laws of health and the methods of their observation. —**hygien′ic,** *adj.*

industrial h. That branch concerned with the promotion of healthful conditions in industry, the prevention of occupational accidents and sickness, and measures for their emergency treatment.

mental h. That branch of hygiene dealing with the preservation of mental and emotional health.

hy′gi·en·ist [*hygieinos*]. One trained in the science of health; sometimes, specifically, a dental hygienist.

hy″gre·che′ma (high″gri·kee′muh) [G. *hygros,* moist; *ēchēma,* sound]. The peculiar sound produced by a liquid, as heard upon mediate or immediate auscultation. *Obs.*

hy′gric [*hygros*]. Pertaining or relating to moisture.

hy′grine (high′green, ·grin). $C_8H_{15}NO$; N-methyl-2-acetonylpyrrolidine, a liquid alkaloid occurring in the leaves of certain species of coca.

hy′gro-, hygr- [*hygros*]. A combining form denoting *moisture* or *humidity.*

hy″gro·ble·phar′ic [*hygros;* G. *blepharon,* eyelid]. Serving to moisten the eyelid.

hy·gro′ma [*hygros;* G. *-ēma,* tumor]. A cystic cavity derived from distended lymphatics and filled with lymph; a congenital malformation, most often seen in young children: also called *h. cysticum colli, cystic h., multiloculated h.* —**hygrom′atous,** *adj.*

acute traumatic subdural h. Collection of cerebrospinal fluid in the subdural space following trauma, apparently caused by tears in the arachnoid membrane near the villi. Symptoms include headache and depressed consciousness.

hy·grom′e·ter [*hygros;* G. *metron,* a measure]. An instrument for determining quantitatively the amount of moisture in the air. —**hygrometry,** *n.*

hy″gro·met′ric, hy″gro·met′ri·cal [*hygros; me-*

tron]. 1. Pertaining to hygrometry. 2. Readily absorbing water; hygroscopic. —**hygrometrically,** *adv.*

hy″gro·my′cin. A broad-spectrum antibiotic substance obtained from various strains of *Streptomyces hygroscopicus*. It is active, in vitro, against a variety of gram-positive and gram-negative bacteria, also against certain actinomycetes.

hy″gro·pho′bi·a [*hygros;* G. *phobos,* fear]. Morbid fear of liquids or of moisture.

hy′gro·scope [*hygros;* G. *skopein,* to examine]. An instrument for indicating the humidity of the atmosphere. —**hygros′copy,** *n.*

hy″gro·scop′ic [*hygros; skopein*]. 1. Pertaining to a hygroscope. 2. Sensitive to moisture; readily absorbing moisture.

hy″gro·sto′mi·a [*hygros;* G. *stoma,* mouth]. Chronic salivation.

hykinone. Trade-mark for 2-methyl-1,4-naphthoquinone-3-sodium sulfonate, a water-soluble product having vitamin-K activity. See *menadione.*

hy′lic [G. *hylē,* material]. Of or pertaining to matter; material.

hy′lo-, hyl- [*hylē*]. A combining form meaning *wood, material, substance, matter.*

hy″lo·pho′bi·a [G. *hylē,* forest; *phobos,* fear]. Morbid fear of forests.

hy″lo·trop′ic [G. *hylē,* material; *tropē,* a turn]. The capacity of a substance for changing its form without changing its composition.

hy″lo·zo′ism [*hylē;* G. *zōē,* life]. The theory that all matter is endowed with life.

hy′men [G., membrane]. A membranous partition partially blocking the orifice of the vagina. The opening may be of several forms, such as circular, crescentic, etc.; it may be multiple, entirely lacking, or imperforate. —**hymenal,** *adj.*

hy″me·nec′to·my [*hymēn;* G. *ektomē,* excision]. Excision of the hymen.

hy″me·ni′tis [*hymēn;* G. *-itis,* inflammation]. Inflammation of the hymen.

hy″me·no·le·pi′a·sis [*hymēn;* G. *lepis,* husk; NL. *-iasis,* condition]. Infestation of the intestine by members of the genus *Hymenolepis*. The disease is differentiated and described according to species: **hymenolepiasis nana** and **hymenolepiasis diminuta.**

Hy″me·nol″e·pid′i·dae (high″mi·nol″i·pid′i·dee) [*hymēn; lepis*]. A family of tapeworms (class Cestoda) of the phylum Platyhelminthes (flatworms).

Hy″me·nol′e·pis [*hymēn; lepis*]. A genus of tapeworms; any dwarf tapeworm.

H. diminuta. A species found commonly in rats and mice and occasionally in man.

H. nana. A species, cosmopolitan in distribution, which infests man; the smallest of the dwarf tapeworms.

hy″me·nol′o·gy [*hymēn;* G. *logos,* word]. The science of the nature, structure, functions, and diseases of the membranes. *Rare.*

Hy″me·nop′ter·a [*hymēn;* G. *pteron,* wing]. An order of insects which includes the bees, ants, wasps, sawflies, and gallflies. They are the most highly specialized group of invertebrates. —**hymenop′terous,** *adj.*

hy″me·nor′rha·phy [*hymēn;* G. *rhaphē,* a suture]. 1. Suture of the hymen to occlude the vagina. 2. Suture of any membrane.

hy·men′o·tome [*hymēn;* G. *tomos,* cutting]. A surgical instrument used for cutting membranes.

hy″me·not′o·my [*hymēn;* G. *tomē,* a cutting]. 1. Surgical incision of the hymen. 2. Dissection or anatomy of membranes.

hy′o-, hy- [G. *hyoeidēs,* shaped like the letter upsilon]. *In anatomy,* a combining form meaning *u,* indicating *connection with the hyoid bone* or *arch.*

hy″o·cho·lal′ic (high″o·ko·lal′ick, ·lay′lick) [G. *hys,* swine; *cholē,* bile; Ar. *al-kili,* ashes of saltwort]. Derived from pig's bile.

hy″o·ep″i·glot′tic, hy″o·ep″i·glot·tid′e·an [G. *hyoeidēs,* shaped like the letter upsilon; *epiglōttis,* epiglottis]. Relating to the hyoid bone and the epiglottis.

hy″o·glos′sal [*hyoeidēs;* G. *glōssa,* tongue]. 1. Pertaining to the hyoglossus. 2. Extending from the hyoid bone to the tongue.

hy″o·glos′sus [*hyoeidēs; glōssa*]. An extrinsic muscle of the tongue arising from the hyoid bone. See Table of Muscles in the Appendix.

hy′oid [*hyoeidēs*]. A bone between the root of the tongue and the larynx, supporting the tongue and giving attachment to some of its muscles. See Plate 45. See Table of Bones in the Appendix. —**hy′oid,** *adj.*

hy″o·man·dib′u·lar [*hyoeidēs;* L. *mandibula,* jaw]. Relating to the hyoid and mandibular arches of the embryo or to the groove and pouch between them.

hy″o·man·dib′u·lar. The upper cartilaginous or osseous element of the hyoid arch in fishes.

hy′os·cine (high′o·seen, ·sin). Scopolamine.

h. hydrobromide. Scopolamine hydrobromide.

hy″os·cy′a·mine (high″o·sigh′uh·meen, ·min). $C_{17}H_{23}NO_3$. An alkaloid occurring in many of the Solanaceae, notably belladonna, hyoscyamus, and stramonium. It is the levorotatory component of the racemic atropine, the pharmacologic activity of the latter being due largely to hyoscyamine.

h. hydrobromide. $C_{17}H_{23}NO_3.HBr.$: used as a parasympatholytic agent. Dose, 0.25–1.0 mg. ($\frac{1}{240}$–$\frac{1}{60}$ gr.).

h. sulfate. $(C_{17}H_{23}NO_3)_2.H_2SO_4$; use and dose, as of the hydrobromide.

hy″os·cy′a·mus [G. *hyoskyamos,* henbane] (*hyoscyamus*). Henbane. The dried leaf, with or without flowering tops, of *Hyoscyamus niger;* yields not less than 0.04% of alkaloids (hyoscyamine and scopolamine). Its therapeutic effects are similar to those of belladonna but are less intense because of lower alkaloid content; the presence of scopolamine imparts a central narcotic effect. It is uncertain in its action. Dose, 0.13–0.32 Gm. (2–5 gr.).

h. extract (*extractum hyoscyami*). Contains 0.135–0.175% alkaloids. Dose, 0.03–0.1 Gm. ($\frac{1}{2}$–$1\frac{1}{2}$ gr.).

h. tincture (*tinctura hyoscyami*). Contains 0.0034–0.0046% (w/v) alkaloids. Dose, 2–4 cc. (30–60 min.).

hy″o·sta·pe′di·al [G. *hyoeidēs; stapes,* stirrup]. Of or pertaining to the hyoid bar and the stapes, which are continuous in early embryological development.

hy″o·thy′roid. See *thyrohyoid.*

hy″o·ver″te·brot′o·my. *In veterinary medicine,* the operation of incising the guttural pouch.

hyp-. See *hypo-.*

hyp″a·cid′i·ty. See *hypoacidity.*

hyp″a·cu′si·a (hip″a·cue′zhuh, ·zee·uh, hip″a·kōō′·, high″pa·cue′), **hyp″a·cu′sis** (hip″a·cue′sis, hip″a·kōō′sis, high″pa·cue′sis, high″pa·kōō′sis) [G. *hypo,* under; *akousis,* hearing]. Impairment of hearing. Also called *hypoacusia.*

hyp″al·bu″min·e′mi·a. Hypalbuminosis.

hyp″al·bu″min·o′sis (hip″alb·yōō″min·o′sis, high″palb·yōō″min·) [*hypo;* L. *albus,* white; G. *-ōsis,* condition]. Diminution in the amount of albumin in the blood. Syn., *hypalbuminemia.*

hyp″al·ge′si·a (hip″al·jee′zee·uh, ·see·uh, high″·pal·) [*hypo;* G. *algēsis,* sense of pain]. Diminished sensitivity to pain. Also called *hypalgia.* —**hypalgesic,** *adj.*

hyp·am′ni·on (hip·am′nee·on, high·pam′·) [*hypo;* G. *amnion,* inner membrane around the fetus]. A small amount of amniotic fluid.

hy·pan″i·sog′na·thism (hi·pan″i·sog′nuth·iz·um, high·pan″i·) [G. *hypo,* under; *anisos,* unequal; *gnathos,* jaw]. *In biology,* the condition of having the upper teeth broader than the lower, with a lack of correspondence between the jaws. —**hypanisognathous,** *adj.*

hy·paph′o·rine (high·paf′o·reen, ·rin). $C_{14}H_{18}N_2O_2$; the betaine of tryptophan, occurring in various *Erythrina* species; it is a convulsive poison.

hy″par·te′ri·al (high″pahr·teer′ee·ul, hip″ahr·) [*hypo;* G. *artēria,* artery]. Situated beneath an artery; specifically applied to branches of the stem bronchi.

hy″pas·the′ni·a (high″pass·thee′nee·uh, hip″ass·) [*hypo;* G. *astheneia,* want of strength]. A slight loss of strength.

hy·pax′i·al (high·pack′see·ul, hip·ack′·) [*hypo;* L. *axis,* axis]. Situated beneath the vertebral column; ventral.

hy·paz″o·tu′ri·a. See *hypoazoturia.*

hy·pen″gy·o·pho′bi·a (high·pen″jee·o·fo′bee·uh) [G. *hypeggyos,* having given surety; *phobos,* fear]. Morbid fear of responsibility.

hy″pe·o·sin′o·phil, hy″pe·o·sin′o·phile [G. *hypo,* under; *ēōs,* dawn; *philein,* to love]. A histologic element which does not stain completely with eosin. —**hypeosin′ophil,** *adj.*

hy′per- [G. *hyper,* beyond, above, over]. 1. A prefix signifying *abnormal* or *excessive.* 2. *In anatomy* and *in zoology,* a prefix denoting *position above.*

hy″per·ab·duc′tion [*hyper;* L. *abductio,* from *abducere,* to lead away]. Excessive abduction of a limb or part. Syn., *superabduction.*

hy″per·ac′id [*hyper;* L. *acidus,* acid]. Excessively acid.

hy″per·ac″id·am·i·nu′ri·a [*hyper; acidus;* amino; G. *ouron,* urine]. The presence of an excessive amount of amino acids in the urine.

hy″per·a·cid′i·ty [*hyper; acidus*]. Excessive acidity.

hy″per·ac·tiv′i·ty [*hyper;* L. *activus,* active]. Excessive or abnormal activity.

hy″per·a·cu′i·ty [*hyper;* L. *acutus,* sharp]. Unusual sensory acuity or sharpness, especially of vision.

hy″per·a·cu′si·a (high″pur·a·cue′zhuh, ·zee·uh, ·shuh, ·see·uh, high″pur·a·kōō′·), **hy″per·a·cu′sis** (high″pur·a·cue′sis, ·a·kōō′sis) [*hyper;* G. *akousis,* hearing]. Abnormal acuteness of the sense of hearing; auditory hyperesthesia.

hy″per·ad″e·no′sis [*hyper;* G. *adēn,* gland; *-ōsis,* increase]. Enlargement of the lymph nodes.

hy″per·a·dre″nal·cor′ti·cal·ism. See *hyperadrenocorticism.*

hy″per·ad·re′nal·ism [*hyper;* L. *ad,* to; *renes,* kidneys]. A condition due to hyperfunction of the adrenal gland; marked by a tendency toward increased basal metabolism, decreased sugar tolerance, glycosuria, and adrenal hyperplasia; occurs chiefly in relation to adrenal cortical tumors.

hy″per·ad·re′ni·a [*hyper; ad; renes*]. Symptoms caused by overactivity of the adrenal gland.

hy″per·ad·re″no·cor′ti·cism. Hyperfunction of the adrenal cortex resulting in the overproduction of its hormones, resulting in Cushing's syndrome, or virilism or, rarely, feminism. It may be due to a primary abnormality in the adrenal cortex or secondary to pituitary hyperfunction. See also *hypercorticism.*

hy″per·ae′mi·a. See *hyperemia.*

hy″per·a″er·a′tion [*hyper;* G. *aēr,* air]. An excess of oxygen in the blood, such as occurs in voluntary accelerated respiration. Syn., *hyperventilation.*

hy″per·aes·the′si·a. See *hyperesthesia.*

hy″per·al·ge′si·a (high″pur·al·jee′zee·uh, ·see·uh) [*hyper;* G. *algēsis,* sense of pain]. Excessive sensitivity to pain. Also called *hyperalgia.* —**hyperalgesic,** *adj.*

hy″per·al″i·men·ta′tion [*hyper;* L. *alimentum,* nourishment]. Overfeeding; superalimentation.

hy″per·al″i·men·to′sis [*hyper; alimentum;* G. *-ōsis,* condition]. Any disease due to excessive eating.

hy″per·am″in·o·ac″id·u′ri·a. Abnormally high urinary excretion of amino acids.

hy″per·am·ne′si·a (high″pur·am·nee′zhuh, ·zee·uh). See *hypermnesia.*

hy″per·am″yl·a·se′mi·a (high″per·am″i·lay·see′mee·uh). Elevated serum amylase level.

hy″per·an″a·ki·ne′si·a (·an″uh·ki·nee′shuh, ·see·uh, ·zhuh, ·zee·uh, ·an″uh·kigh·nee′·) [*hyper;* G. *anakinēsis,* a swinging to and fro]. Excessive activity of a part.

h. ventriculi. Exaggerated activity of the gastric functions.

hy″per·a′phi·a [*hyper;* G. *haphē,* touch]. Excessive sensitivity to touch. —**hyperaph′ic,** *adj.*

hy″per·az″o·te′mi·a [*hyper;* G. *a-,* not; *zōē,* life; *haima,* blood]. The presence of an excessive amount of nitrogenous substances in the blood.

hy″per·az″o·tu′ri·a [*hyper; a-; zōē;* G. *ouron,* urine]. An excess of nitrogenous matter in the urine.

hy″per·bar′ic [*hyper;* G. *baros,* weight]. 1. Of greater weight, density or pressure. 2. Pertaining to an anesthetic solution of specific gravity greater than the spinal fluid.

hy″per·bar′ism. A condition resulting from an excess of the ambient gas pressure over that within the body tissues, fluids, and cavities.

hy″per·bil″i·ru″bi·ne′mi·a (·bil″i·rōō″bi·nee′mee·uh, ·buy″li·) [*hyper;* L. *bilis,* bile; *ruber,* red; G. *haima,* blood]. Excessive amount of bilirubin in the blood.

hereditary nonhemolytic h. See constitutional hepatic *dysfunction.*

physiologic h. A rare and benign form of jaundice, not due to increased hemolysis, obstruction of bile outflow, or histologically demonstrable disease of liver parenchyma, but due to some dysfunction in excretion of bilirubin by the liver, resulting in elevated blood levels of bilirubin. Syn., *constitutional h.* or *jaundice, familial* or *hereditary nonhemolytic jaundice.*

hy″per·brach″y·ceph′a·ly (high″pur·brack″i·sef′uh·lee) [*hyper;* G. *brachys,* short; *kephalē,* head]. Extreme brachycephaly; with a cephalic index over 85.5.

hy″per·bu′li·a [*hyper;* G. *boulē,* will]. Exaggerated willfulness.

hy″per·cal·ce′mi·a, hy″per·cal·cae′mi·a [*hyper;* L. *calx,* lime; G. *haima,* blood]. Excessive quantity of calcium in the blood. Syn., *calcemia.*

hy″per·cal·ci·nu′ri·a, hy″per·cal·ci·u′ri·a, hy″per·cal·cu′ri·a. An abnormally high level of calcium in the urine.

essential h. A high level of calcium in the urine in the absence of acidosis: also called *idiopathic h.*

idiopathic h. See essential *h.*

hy″per·cap′ni·a [*hyper;* G. *kapnos,* smoke]. Excessive amount of carbon dioxide in the blood, causing overactivity in the respiratory center: also called *hypercarbia.*

hy″per·car″o·te·ne′mi·a [*hyper;* L. *carota,* carrot; G. *haima,* blood]. Excessive carotenemia.

hy″per·ca·thar′sis [*hyper;* G. *katharsis,* a cleansing]. Excessive purgation of the bowels. —**hypercathartic,** *adj.*

hy″per·ca·thex′is [*hyper;* G. *kathexis,* retention]. Excessive concentration of the psychic energy upon a particular focus.

hy″per·ce″men·to′sis (high″pur·see″men·to′sis, ·sem″in·to′sis) [*hyper;* L. *caementum,* quarrystone; G. *-ōsis,* condition]. Excessive formation of cementum on the root of a tooth.

hy″per·ce″nes·the′si·a (·see″ness·thee′zhuh, ·zee·uh, ·sen″ess·) [*hyper;* G. *koinos,* common; *aisthēsis,* sensation]. A feeling of extreme well-being; euphoria.

hy″per·cham′aer·rhine [*hyper;* G. *chamai-,* low; *rhis,* nose]. 1. *In craniometry,* designating an apertura piriformis that is relatively very broad and short; having a nasal index of 58.0 or more. 2. *In somatometry,* designating a nose that is as broad as, or broader than, it is long; having a height-breadth index of 100.0 or more.

hy″per·chlo·re′mi·a, hy″per·chlo·rae′mi·a [*hyper;* G. *chlōros,* pale green; *haima,* blood]. An increase in the sodium chloride content of the blood.

hy″per·chlor·hy′dri·a (high″pur·klor·high′-dree·uh, ·hid′ree·uh) [*hyper; chlōros;* G. *hydōr,* water]. Excessive secretion of hydrochloric acid in the stomach; may be a manifestation of neuroticism.

hy″per·cho·les″ter·e′mi·a, hy″per·cho·les″-ter·ae′mi·a (·ko·les″tur·ee′mee·uh) [*hyper;* G. *cholē,* bile; *stereos,* stiff; *haima,* blood]. Excess of cholesterol in the blood, cells, or plasma.

hy″per·cho·les″ter·o·le′mi·a, hy″per·cho·les″-ter·o·lae′mi·a (·ko·les″tur·o·lee′mee·uh) [*hyper; cholē; stereos; haima*]. Hypercholesteremia.

hy″per·cho′li·a (high″pur·ko′lee·uh) [*hyper; cholē*]. Excessive secretion of bile.

hy″per·chro·mat′ic [*hyper;* G. *chrōma,* color]. 1. Pertaining to a cell or a portion of a cell which stains more intensely than is normal. 2. Pertaining to or describing the microscopic appearance of cells of the erythropoietic series, which is due not to increased concentration of hemoglobin, but to increased thickness of the cells. —**hyperchromas′ia,** *n.*

hy″per·chro′ma·tism [*hyper; chrōma*]. The excessive formation of the pigment of the skin.

hy″per·chro″ma·to′sis [*hyper; chrōma;* G. *-ōsis,* condition]. Excessive pigmentation, as of the skin.

hy″per·chro′mi·a. Hyperchromatism.

hy″per·chy′li·a (high″pur·kigh′lee·uh) [*hyper;* G. *chylos,* juice]. Excess of secretion; excessive formation of chyle.

hy″per·ci·ne′sis. See *hyperkinesia.*

hy″per·cor′ti·cism. A syndrome resulting from continued administration of cortisone (compound E), hydrocortisone (compound F), or adrenocorticotropic hormone (ACTH); symptoms and signs simulate those observed in Cushing's syndrome.

hy″per·cry″al·ge′si·a (·cry″al·jee′zee·uh, ·see·uh) [*hyper;* G. *kryos,* icy cold; *algēsis,* sense of pain]. Abnormal sensitivity to cold. Syn., *hypercryesthesia.*

hy″per·cry″es·the′si·a (cry″ess·thee′zhuh, ·zee·uh). See *hypercryalgesia.*

hy″per·dac·tyl′i·a. See *polydactyly.*

hy″per·di·crot′ic (high″pur·dye·krot′ick) [*hyper;* G. *dis,* twice; *krotos,* beat]. Referring to the dicrotic wave of the peripheral pulse which is increased in amplitude, so that it may be detected by palpation. —**hyperdi′crotism,** *n.*

hy″per·dis·ten′tion [*hyper;* L. *distentio,* from *distendere,* to stretch out]. Forcible or extreme distention.

hy″per·dy·na′mi·a (high″pur·dye·nay′mee·uh, ·di·nay′mee·uh, ·dye·nam′ee·uh) [*hyper;* G. *dynamis,* power]. Excessive strength or exaggeration of function, as of nerves or muscles. —**hyperdynam′ic,** *adj.*

hy″per·e·che′ma (high″pur·eh·kee′muh). [*hyper;* G. *ēchēma,* sound]. A normal sound abnormally exaggerated. *Obs.*

hy″per·em′e·sis [*hyper;* G. *emesis,* vomiting]. Excessive vomiting. —**hyperemet′ic,** *adj.*

h. gravidarum. Pernicious vomiting in pregnancy.

h. lactentium. Vomiting of nurslings.

hy″per·e′mi·a [*hyper;* G. *haima,* blood]. An increased content of blood in a part, with distention of the blood vessels. Hyperemia may be active, when due to active dilatation of blood vessels, or passive, when the drainage is hindered. **Active hyperemia** occurs in physiologic activity of glands or other organs and in inflammation. **Passive** or **venous hyperemia** occurs in congestive heart failure and in other conditions where veins are compressed or occluded. —**hyperemic,** *adj.*

neuroparalytic h. Hyperemia which is the result of interruption of stimuli through the vasoconstrictor nerves, as in Horner's syndrome.

peristatic h. See *peristasis.*

prestatic h. See *prestasis.*

hy″per·en·ceph′a·lus [*hyper;* G. *egkephalos,* brain]. A type of anencephalus in which the entire cranial vault above the level of the occipital protuberance is absent.

hy″per·e″o·sin″o·phil′i·a. Eosinophilia.

hy″per·eph″i·dro′sis. See *hyperhidrosis.*

hy″per·ep″i·thy′mi·a [*hyper;* G. *epithymia,* desire]. Exaggerated desire.

hy″per·e″qui·lib′ri·um [*hyper;* L. *aequilibrium,* equilibrium]. Excessive tendency to vertigo on rotary movement.

hy″per·er′gi·a [*hyper;* G. *ergon,* work]. Increased functional activity.

hy′per·er·gy [*hyper; ergon*]. An altered state of reactivity, in which the response is more marked than usual; hypersensitivity. It is one form of allergy or pathergy.

hy″per·es″o·pho′ri·a [*hyper;* G. *esō,* inward; *phoros,* bearing]. A form of heterophoria in which the visual axis tends to deviate upward and inward.

hy″per·es·the′si·a, hy″per·aes·the′si·a (high″-pur·ess·thee′zhuh, ·zee·uh) [*hyper;* G. *aisthēsis,* sensation]. Excessive sensibility. —**hyperesthet′ic,** *adj.*

hy″per·es′trin·ism, hy″per·es′tro·gen·ism. Excessive or prolonged secretion, or both, of the female estrogenic hormones.

hy″per·es″tro·ge·ne′mi·a. An excess of estrogens in the blood: also called *hyperestrinemia.*

hy″per·ex″o·pho′ri·a [*hyper;* G. *exō,* outside of; *phoros,* bearing]. A form of heterophoria in which the visual axis tends to deviate upward and outward.

hy″per·ex·ten′sion [*hyper;* L. *extensio,* from *extendere,* to stretch out]. Overextension of a limb or part for the correction of deformity or for the retention of fractured bones in proper position and alignment.

hy″per·flex′ion [*hyper;* L. *flexio,* a bending]. Overflexion of a limb or part of the body.

hy″per·func′tion [*hyper;* L. *functio,* from *fungi,* to perform]. Excessive function.

hy″per·gen′e·sis [*hyper;* G. *genesis,* production]. Excessive development or redundancy of the parts or organs of the body. —**hypergenet′ic,** *adj.*

hy″per·geu′si·a (high″pur·gew′see·uh, ·jew′see·uh) [*hyper;* G. *geusis,* taste]. Abnormal acuteness of the sense of taste.

hy″per·gi·gan″to·so′ma (high″pur·jye·gan″to·so′-muh) [*hyper;* G. *gigas,* giant; *sōma,* body]. Extraordinary gigantism. *Obs.*

hy″per·glob″u·li·ne′mi·a [*hyper;* L. *globulus,* little ball; G. *haima,* blood]. Increased amount of globulin in the blood plasma or serum.

hy″per·gly·ce′mi·a, hy″per·gly·cae′mi·a (·gly-see′mee·uh) [*hyper;* G. *glykys*, sweet; *haima*]. Excess of sugar in the blood.

hy″per·gly″co·ge·nol′y·sis [*hyper; glykys;* G. *genesthai*, from *gignesthai*, to be produced; *lysis*, a loosing]. Excessive glycogenolysis.

hy″per·gly″cor·rha′chi·a (·glye″ko·ray′kee·uh, ·rack′ee·uh) [*hyper; glykys;* G. *rhachis*, spine]. Excess of sugar in the cerebrospinal fluid.

hy″per·gly″co·su′ri·a [*hyper; glykys;* G. *ouron*, urine]. The presence of excessive amounts of sugar in the urine.

hy″per·gon′ad·ism [*hyper;* G. *gonē*, seed]. Excessive internal secretion of the sexual glands (testes or ovaries).

hy″per·go′ni·a [*hyper;* G. *gōnia*, angle]. Increase in size of the gonial angle.

hy″per·he·do′ni·a [*hyper;* G. *hēdonē*, pleasure]. 1. An excessive feeling of pleasure in the gratification of a desire. 2. Sexual erethism. Syn., *hyperhedonism.*

hy″per·he′don·ism (high″pur·hee′dun·iz·um, ·hed′un·iz·um). See *hyperhedonia.*

hy″per·hi·dro′sis (high″pur·hi·dro′sis, ·high·dro′-sis), **hy″per·i·dro′sis** [*hyper;* G. *hidrōsis*, sweating]. Excessive sweating; may be localized or generalized, chronic or acute; the sweat often accumulates in visible drops on the skin. Syn., *ephidrosis, sudatoria, polyhidrosis.*

gustatory h. The phenomenon of sweating over facial areas, particularly about the mouth and nose, accompanied by flushing of the involved areas, upon smelling or ingestion of spicy or acid foods, or some foods as chocolate. It may be caused even by the thought of these foods, and is found to varying degrees in most people. Also see auriculotemporal *syndrome.*

psychogenic h. Increased sweating due to psychogenic factors, most often on the palms, soles, axillas, and forehead.

hy″per·his″ta·mi·ne′mi·a [*hyper;* G. *histion*, web; Temple of Jupiter *Ammon*; *haima*, blood]. An increased amount of histamine in the blood.

hy″per·hor·mo′nal [*hyper;* G. *hormaein*, to excite]. Containing, or due to, excess of a hormone.

hy″per·in″o·se′mi·a [*hyper;* G. *is*, fiber; *haima*, blood]. An exaggerated tendency to the formation of fibrin in the blood.

hy″per·i·no′sis [*hyper; is;* G. *-ōsis*, condition]. Hyperinosemia; an exaggerated tendency to the formation of fibrin in the blood.

hy″per·in′su·lin·ism [*hyper;* L. *insula*, island]. The syndrome of spontaneous, intermittent, or continuous loss of consciousness, with or without convulsions, from excessive production of insulin by the pancreatic islands of Langerhans.

hy″per·in″vo·lu′tion [*hyper;* L. *involutum*, from *involvere*, to roll about]. A rapid return to less than normal size of an organ that has been enlarged, as of the uterus after delivery.

hy″per·i″so·ton′ic. See *hypertonic*, 2.

hy″per·ka·le′mi·a, hy″per·kal·i·e′mi·a [*hyper;* NL. *kalium*, potassium, from Ar. *qili;* G. *haima*, blood]. See *hyperpotassemia.*

hy″per·ker″a·tin·i·za′tion. See *hyperkeratosis.*

hy″per·ker″a·to′sis [*hyper;* G. *keras*, horn; *-ōsis*, condition]. 1. Hypertrophy of the cornea. 2. Hypertrophy of the horny layer of the skin, usually associated with hypertrophy of the granular and prickle-cell layers. —**hyperkeratot′ic,** *adj.*

congenital palmoplantar h. See *keratosis palmaris et plantaris.*

follicular h. That form of hyperkeratosis occurring about the openings of the hair follicles. It may be due to vitamin-A deficiency.

h. excentrica. Porokeratosis.

h. follicularis et parafollicularis. A rare disease starting as a follicular papule, becoming enlarged, yellow, and crusted. Lesions coalesce, forming plaques. Craters are formed as the plaques are removed.

h. lacunaris pharyngis. A condition characterized by numerous hard white masses sometimes developing into long horny spines, projecting from the nodules of the lymphatic ring about the pharynx.

h. linguae. See *black, hairy tongue* under *tongue.*

h. subungualis. That affecting the nail bed.

hy″per·ke″to·nu′ri·a. The presence of an excess of ketone in the urine.

hy″per·ki·ne′mi·a [*hyper;* G. *kinein*, to move; *haima*, blood]. A condition marked by a greater cardiac output of blood than normal.

hy″per·ki·ne′si·a (high″pur·ki·nee′shuh, ·see·uh, ·zhuh, ·zee·uh, high″pur·kigh·nee′·), **hy″per·ki·ne′sis** (high″pur·ki·nee′sis, ·kigh·nee′sis) [*hyper;* G. *kinēsis*, motion]. Excessive movement, as that associated with muscular spasm. —**hyperkinet′ic,** *adj.*

essential h. A condition seen in children, marked by excessive and sustained voluntary and involuntary movements; they are not, however, disorganized or dissociated as they are in the choreas and athetoses.

hy″per·lac·ta′tion [*hyper;* L. *lactare*, to give suck]. Excessive or prolonged secretion of milk.

hy″per·lep′tor·rhine [*hyper;* G. *leptos*, thin; *rhis*, nose]. *In somatometry,* designating a nose that is relatively very long and narrow, having a height-breadth index of 54.9 or less.

hy″per·ley′dig·ism (high·per·lye′dig·izm). Abnormally high secretion of the interstitial or Leydig cells, probably due to hypersecretion of pituitary gonadotropic (luteinizing) hormone, or, rarely, to tumor. In male children, this may result in precocious puberty and somatic development, but gives rise to no known clinical syndrome in the previously normal adult male.

hy″per·li·pe′mi·a [*hyper;* G. *lipos*, fat; *haima*, blood]. Excess of fat in the blood.

hy″per·li·thu′ri·a [*hyper; G. lithos*, stone; *ouron*, urine]. Excess of lithic acid in the urine.

hy″per·lo′gi·a (high″pur·lo′juh, ·jee·uh) [*hyper;* G. *logos*, word]. Excessive or maniacal loquacity.

hy″per·ma′ni·a [*hyper;* G. *mania*, madness]. An advanced maniacal state; a mania which has progressed beyond the acute stage. Marked by extreme excitation and acceleration of activity. —**hypermanic,** *adj., n.*

hy″per·mas′ti·a [*hyper;* G. *mastos*, breast]. Overgrowth of the mammary gland.

hy″per·ma·ture′ [*hyper;* L. *maturus*, ripe]. Overmature, overripe, as a cataract.

hy″per·meg″a·so′ma. See *hypergigantosoma.*

hy″per·men″or·rhe′a. Menorrhagia.

hy″per·me·tro′pi·a [*hyper;* G. *metron*, measure; *ōps*, eye]. The condition of the refractive media of the eye in which, with suspended accommodation, the focus of parallel rays of light is behind the retina. It is due to an abnormally short anteroposterior diameter of the eye or to a subnormal refractive power of the media. Abbreviated, H. Also called *hyperopia.* —**hypermetrop′ic,** *adj.;* **hypermet′rope,** *n.*

absolute h. That which cannot be corrected completely by accommodation, so that there is indistinct vision even for distance.

axial h. That due to abnormal shortness of the anteroposterior diameter of the eye, the refractive power being normal.

curvature h. A form often combined with astigmatism; due to changes in curvature of the cornea or lens.

facultative manifest h. That part of the manifest hypermetropia that can be concealed by the accommodation.

index h. That due to deficient refractive power in the media of the eye, as from sclerosis of the lens or decrease in sugar content during insulin reaction.

latent h. That part of the total hypermetropia that cannot be overcome by the accommodation, or the difference between the manifest and the total hypermetropia. Abbreviated, Hl.

manifest h. The amount of hypermetropia represented by the strongest convex lens which a person will accept without paralysis of the accommodation. Abbreviated, Hm.

relative h. A high hypermetropia in which distinct vision is possible only when excessive convergence is made.

total h. The entire hypermetropia, both latent and manifest. Abbreviated, Ht.

hy″per·mi″cro·so′ma [*hyper;* G. *mikros,* small; *sōma,* body]. Extreme dwarfism.

hy″per·mim′i·a (high″pur·mim′ee·uh) [*hyper;* G. *mimos,* actor, mime]. Excessive emotional expression or mimetic movement.

hy″perm·ne′si·a (high″purm·nee′zhuh, ·zee·uh), **hy″perm·ne′sis** [*hyper;* G. *mnēsis,* a remembering]. Increased retentiveness of memory.

hy″per·mo·til′i·ty [*hyper;* L. *movere,* to move]. Increased motility, as of the stomach or intestines.

hy″per·na·tre′mi·a (high″per·na·tree′mee·uh). Abnormally high sodium level in the blood.

hy″per·ne′a. Hyperpsychosis.

hy″per·neph′roid [*hyper;* G. *nephros,* kidney; *eidos,* form]. Resembling the adrenal gland.

hy″per·ne·phro′ma [*hyper; nephros;* G. *-ōma,* tumor]. Originally, Grawitz's term for a variety of tumors of the kidney, supposed to be derived from embryonal inclusions of adrenal in the kidney: now applied to clear-cell *carcinoma* of the kidney or other organs.

adrenal h. See cortical *adenoma.*

adrenal h. malignum. See cortical *carcinoma.*

hy″per·noi′a. Hyperpsychosis.

hy″per·nu·tri′tion. See *supernutrition.*

hy″per·on′to·morph [*hyper;* G. *ōn,* being; *morphē,* form]. *In constitutional medicine,* a person of a long, thin body type with short intestines. Also called *asthenic type, microsplanchnic type.*

hy″per·o·nych′i·a (high″pur·o·nick′ee·uh) [*hyper;* G. *onyx,* nail]. Hypertrophy of the nails.

hy″per·o′pi·a. See *hypermetropia.*

hy″per·o·rex′i·a. Bulimia.

hy″per·or′tho·gna″thy [*hyper;* G. *orthos,* straight; *gnathos,* jaw]. Excessive orthognathism: 1. The condition of having a profile angle of greater than 93°. 2. The condition of having an exceedingly low gnathic (alveolar) index. —**hyperorthognath′-ous,** *adj.*

hy″per·os′mi·a (high″pur·oz′mee·uh, ·oss′mee·uh) [*hyper;* G. *osmē,* smell]. An abnormally acute sense of smell.

hy″per·os″mo·lar′i·ty. Hypertonicity; *in medicine,* an osmotic pressure of a biological solution greater than that of normal plasma, usually due to hypernatremia.

hy″per·os″te·og′e·ny (·os″tee·odj′i·nee) [*hyper;* G. *osteon,* bone; *genesthai,* from *gignesthai,* to be produced]. Excessive development of bone.

hy″per·os·to′sis [*hyper; osteon;* G. *-ōsis,* condition]. Exostosis or hypertrophy of bony tissue. —**hyperostot′ic,** *adj.*

h. frontalis interna. A thickening of the inner table of the frontal bone, sometimes detected by roentgenologic examination; usually asymptomatic. It is more common in females and the aged. When symptomatic, it is called *Morgagni's syndrome.* See metabolic *craniopathy.*

infantile cortical h. A condition of unknown etiology occurring in infants, characterized by irritability associated with the appearance of tender swellings of soft tissues which overlie bones of the extremities, followed by roentgenographic signs of cortical hyperostosis: also called *Caffey's syndrome.*

hy″per·ox·e′mi·a [*hyper;* G. *oxys,* sharp; *haima,* blood]. Extreme acidity of the blood.

hy″per·ox″y·gen·a′tion [*hyper; oxys;* G. *genesthai,* from *gignesthai,* to be produced]. A condition of the blood in which it contains more than the normal amount of oxygen. It is caused by hyperventilation.

hy″per·par′a·site [*hyper;* G. *parasitos,* parasite]. A secondary parasite interfering with the development of a previously existing parasite. —**hyperparasitism,** *n.*

hy″per·par″a·thy′roid·ism [*hyper;* G. *para,* near; *thyreoeidēs,* shield-shaped]. A state produced by an increased functioning of the parathyroid glands, as osteitis fibrosa cystica and osteomalacia.

hy″per·path′i·a [*hyper;* G. *pathos,* disease]. A disagreeable or painful sensation in a region which is really hyperesthetic, observed in thalamic lesions.

hy″per·pep·sin′i·a [*hyper;* G. *pepsis,* a cooking]. Excessive secretion of pepsin in the stomach.

hy″per·per″i·stal′sis [*hyper;* G. *peristellein,* to wrap up]. An increase in the rate and depth of the peristaltic waves; nervous diarrhea.

hy·per·pha′gi·a. See *bulimia.*

hy″per·pha·lan′gism [*hyper;* G. *phalagx,* bone between two joints of the fingers and toes.] The presence of supernumerary phalanges.

hy″per·pho·ne′sis [*hyper;* G. *phōnēsis,* a sounding]. Increase of intensity of the percussion note.

hy″per·pho′ni·a [*hyper;* G. *phōnē,* voice]. Stammering or stuttering resulting from excessive irritability of the vocal muscles.

hy″per·pho′ri·a. See *heterophoria.*

hy″per·phos·pha·te′mi·a. Increased levels of inorganic phosphate in serum.

hy″per·phos″pha·tu′ri·a. See *phosphaturia.*

hy″per·pi·e′si·a (high″pur·pye·ee′zhuh, ·zee·uh, ·shuh, ·see·uh), **hy″per·pi·e′sis** [*hyper;* G. *piesis,* pressure]. Abnormally high blood pressure; especially, essential hypertension. —**hyperpiet′ic,** *adj.*

hy″per·pig″men·ta′tion [*hyper;* L. *pigmentum,* color]. Excessive or increased pigmentation.

periocular h. See *masque biliare.*

hy″per·pi·tu′i·ta·rism [*hyper;* L. *pituita,* phlegm]. Any one of a number of abnormal conditions resulting from overactivity of the cells of the anterior pituitary gland, such as acromegaly, gigantism.

hy″per·pla′si·a (high″pur·play′zhuh, ·zee·uh, ·shuh, ·see·uh) [*hyper;* G. *plasis,* a molding]. Excessive formation of tissue; an increase in the size of a tissue or organ owing to an increase in the number of cells. Syn., *numerical hypertrophy.* —**hyperplas′tic,** *adj.*

lipomelanotic reticular h. See lipomelanotic *reticulosis.*

multiple nodular h. See postnecrotic *cirrhosis.*

hy″per·plat″y·mer′ic [*hyper;* G. *platys,* broad; *mēros,* thigh]. *In osteometry,* designating a femur with an exaggerated anteroposterior compression of the proximal portion of the diaphysis; having a platymeric index of 74.9 or less.

hy″perp·ne′a [*hyper;* G. *pnoiē,* a breathing hard]. Increase in depth of inspiration.

hy″per·po·ro′sis [*hyper;* G. *pōrōsis,* uniting of fractured bones by a callus]. An excessive formation of callus in the reunion of fractured bones.

hy″per·pot″as·se′mi·a (high″per·pot·as·see′mee-uh). Abnormally high level of potassium in the blood: also called *hyperkalemia, hyperkaliemia.*

hy″per·pra′gi·a [*hyper;* G. *prattein,* to achieve, do]. An excess of thinking and feeling, commonly observed in the manic phase of manic-depressive psychoses. —**hyperprag′ic,** *adj.*

hy″per·prax′i·a [*hyper;* G. *praxis,* a doing]. The restlessness of movement characterizing certain forms of mania; hyperactivity.

hy″per·pres″by·o′pi·a (·prez″bee·o′pee·uh, ·press″bee·) [*hyper;* G. *presbys,* old man; *ōps,* eye]. Excessive presbyopia.

hy″per·pro″cho·re′sis (high″pur·pro″kor·ee′sis) [*hyper;* G. *prochōrēsis,* advance]. Excessive motor action of the stomach; hyperperistalsis.

hy″per·pro·sex′i·a [*hyper;* G. *prosexis,* application]. Marked attention to one subject, as, for example, one idea or symptom.

hy″per·pro″te·in·e′mi·a (high″per·pro″tee·in·ee′-mee·uh). Abnormally high blood protein level.

hy″per·psy·cho′sis (high″pur·sigh·ko′sis). Exaggerated mental activity. Syn., *hypernea. Obs.*

hy″per·py·rex′i·a (high″pur·pye·reck′see·uh) [*hyper;* G. *pyressein,* to be feverish]. Excessively high fever, as above 106° F. —**hyperpyret′ic,** *adj.*

hy″per·re·flex′i·a [*hyper;* L. *reflexus,* a bending back]. A condition in which reflexes are increased above normal; due to a variety of causes.

hy″per·res′o·nance [*hyper;* L. *resonare,* to resound]. Full resonance of a percussion note, which is slightly lower in pitch than normal resonance, and which possesses also a tympanitic element. It gives the impression of exaggeration of normal resonance. Heard chiefly in certain cases of pulmonary emphysema and of pneumothorax.

hy″per·sal″i·va′tion [*hyper;* L. *salivatio,* from *salivare,* to salivate]. Abnormally increased secretion of saliva.

hy″per·se·cre′tion [*hyper;* L. *secretum,* from *secernere,* to separate]. Excessive secretion.

hy″per·sen″si·tiv′i·ty [*hyper;* L. *sentire,* to feel]. The state of being abnormally sensitive or susceptible, as to the action of allergens. See *allergy.* —**hypersen′sitive,** *adj.*

atopic h. Atopy.

delayed h. A type in which the reactions to antigens are delayed, no relationship to circulating antibodies has been demonstrated, and any tissue is liable to injury after exposure to antigen. Certain drug reactions and contact dermatitides together with reactions of the tuberculin type are examples of this type.

immediate h. That type in which the hypersensitive response occurs quickly following exposure to antigens to which the animal is already sensitive. Circulating antibody is demonstrable in the blood stream; therefore, the sensitivity can be transferred from animal to animal. The allergic manifestations are confined to blood vessels, smooth muscle, and collagen. Some forms are serum sickness, anaphylaxis, Arthus phenomenon, and the atopic allergies.

tuberculin h. A specific delayed type of hypersensitivity (allergic reaction) to tuberculin: also called *tuberculin-type sensitivity.* See *Koch phenomenon* under Robert *Koch.*

hy″per·se″ques·tra′tion. Hypersplenism.

hy″per·som′ni·a [*hyper;* L. *somnus,* sleep]. Excessive sleepiness.

hy″per·sple′nism. An abnormal activity of the spleen, but generally not considered a disease entity. It is due to unknown causes, with reduction of one or more of the cellular elements of circulating blood, resulting in anemia, thrombocytopenia, or neutropenia, or a combination of these conditions. The bone marrow may be hyperplastic. Splenectomy may be helpful. Also called *hypersequestration.*

hy″per·ster″e·o·roent″gen·og′ra·phy (high″pur-sterr″ee·o·rent″ghin·og′ruh·fee, high″pur·steer″-ee·o·) [*hyper;* G. *stereos,* solid; *Röntgen;* G. *graphein,* to write]. Roentgenography with an increased distance between the homologous points, to provide better third-dimensional semblance in the stereogram.

hy″per·sthe′ni·a (high″pur·sthee′nee·uh, high″-pur·sthen′ee·uh) [*hyper;* G. *sthenos,* strength]. A condition of exalted strength or tone of the body. —**hypersthen′ic,** *adj.*

hy″per·sus·cep″ti·bil′i·ty. Hypersensitivity.

hy″per·syn′chro·ny [*hyper;* G. *sygchronein,* to be contemporary with]. Abnormally high potential waves of any frequency in an electroencephalogram.

hy″per·tel′or·ism [*hyper;* G. *tēle,* at a distance; *horismos,* marking out by boundaries]. Excessive width between two organs or parts; specifically, *ocular hypertelorism,* a deformity of the frontal region of the cranium, resulting in a low forehead and pronounced vertex, widened bridge of the nose, and hence increased distance between the eyes and divergent strabismus, often associated with mental deficiency marked by mental and physical retardation and resembling mongolism: also called *Grieg's h.,* Grieg's *disease.*

hy″per·ten′sin [*hyper;* L. *tensum,* from *tendere,* to stretch]. The pressor substance, a polypeptide, formed as the result of the interaction between an enzyme from the kidney, renin, and hypertensinogen, a globulin in the blood plasma. Syn., *angiotonin.*

hy″per·ten′sin·ase. An enzyme present in blood and tissues which destroys hypertensin. Syn., *angiotonase.*

hy″per·ten·sin′o·gen [*hyper; tensum;* G. *genesthai,* from *gignesthai,* to be produced]. A globulin in the blood plasma, the substrate upon which renin acts to produce hypertensin: also called *renin-activator, renin substrate.*

hy″per·ten′sion [*hyper;* L. *tensio,* a stretching]. Excessive tension, usually synonymous with high blood pressure; supertension. —**hypertensive,** *adj.;* **hypertensor,** *n.*

arterial h. Elevated blood pressure in the arterial side of the circulatory system.

benign h. That stage of essential hypertension which is very slowly progressive and not associated with any impairment of renal excretory function.

chronic h. A state of increased peripheral resistance to blood flow in which there is an increase in both systolic and diastolic pressure which has persisted for a sufficient period of time and with sufficient severity to have resulted in cardiac hypertrophy.

essential h. Common term for a clinical syndrome of unknown cause at first not associated with renal excretory functional disturbance, and characterized by a relatively sustained elevation in diastolic blood pressure usually accompanied by an increase in systolic pressure. Often it becomes associated with cardiac, cerebral, renal functional impairment, and vascular complications. Sometimes called "*primary*" *h.* Also see *hypertensive vascular disease.*

experimental renal h. Hypertension produced

in animals by constricting the main renal arteries, simulating the manifestations of human essential *h.* It was first described by H. Goldblatt (1934).

Goldblatt h. Experimental renal *h.*

malignant h. A fulminating progression of severe essential hypertension, with papilledema as a constant pathognomonic feature, and predominant cerebral and renal symptoms. Cause for the change is unknown. Death usually occurs within a few months from renal or cardiac failure or a cerebral vascular lesion.

orthostatic h. Hypertension which persists in the erect position.

portal h. Elevation of blood pressure in the portal vein above 100 mm. H_2O, considered to be due to obstruction of portal flow, extrahepatic, intrahepatic, or both. The obstruction may be congenital, but generally is acquired as part of a variety of diseases, especially cirrhosis or portal-vein thrombosis. When elevation of portal pressure rises to about 250 mm. H_2O or above, the primary clinical signs of hemorrhages from esophagogastric varices and splenomegaly become manifest.

"primary" h. See essential *h.*

renal h. Hypertension resulting from renal hemodynamic disturbance. Also see experimental renal *h.*

"secondary" h. Term sometimes used to designate hypertension of known organic origin.

senile h. Systolic elevation of blood pressure associated with arteriosclerosis, mainly of the aorta and of large arteries.

hy″per·ten′sive vas′cu·lar dis·ease′. A disease characterized by degenerative changes in the walls of arteries and arterioles, usually associated with chronic hypertension, but sometimes existing for a period of time without elevated blood pressure.

hy″per·the′li·a [*hyper;* G. *thēlē,* nipple]. The presence of supernumerary nipples.

hypertherm. Trade name for a cabinet designed for the production of therapeutic fever by means of heated and humidified air.

hy″per·ther″mal·ge′si·a (high″pur·thur″mal·jee′-zee·uh, ·see·uh) [*hyper;* G. *thermē,* heat; *algēsis,* sense of pain]. Abnormal sensitivity to heat.

hy″per·ther″mo·es·the′si·a (·thur″mo·ess·thee′-zhuh, ·zee·uh, ·shuh, ·see·uh). See *hyperthermalgesia.*

hy″per·ther′my, hy″per·ther′mi·a [*hyper; thermē*]. 1. An abnormally high fever; hyperpyrexia. 2. The treatment of disease by the induction of fever; this can be done by inoculation with malaria, by intravenous injection of foreign proteins, or by physical means.

hy″per·thy′mi·a [*hyper;* G. *thymos,* mind]. 1. Mental hyperesthesia; morbid oversensitiveness. 2. Vehement cruelty or foolhardiness as a symptom of mental disease. 3. Labile or unstable emotionality, as seen in some psychopathic personalities.

hy″per·thy′mism. See *hyperthymization.*

hy″per·thy″mi·za′tion [*hyper;* G. *thymos,* thymus]. Exaggerated activity of the thymus gland, with resulting toxic symptoms.

hy″per·thy′roid·ism [*hyper;* G. *thyreoeidēs,* shield-shaped]. An abnormal condition brought about by excessive functional activity of the thyroid gland.

hy″per·to′ni·a [*hyper;* G. *tonos,* tension]. Excess of muscular tonicity.

hy″per·ton′ic [*hyper; tonos*]. 1. Exceeding in strength or tension. 2. Referring to a solution whose osmotic pressure is greater than that of physiologic salt solution, or any other solution taken as a standard. —**hypertonic′ity,** *n.*

hy″per·tri·cho′sis (high″pur·tri·ko′sis), **hy″per-tri·chi′a·sis** (high″pur·tri·kigh′uh·sis) [*hyper;* G. *thrix,* hair; *-ōsis,* condition]. Excessive growth of normal hair; superfluous hair; abnormal hairiness. —**hypertrichot′ic,** *adj.*

hy·per′tro·phy, hy″per·tro′phi·a [*hyper;* G. *trophē,* nourishment]. An increase in size of an organ, independent of natural growth; due to enlargement or multiplication of its constituent cells; usually connotes accompanying increase in functional capacity. —**hypertroph′ic,** *adj.*

adaptive h. That which adapts an organ to increased functional requirements, as hypertrophy of the heart associated with valvular deformities or hypertension, hypertrophy of the urinary bladder in cases of enlarged prostate.

cardiac h. Hypertrophy of the heart. See concentric *h.* of the heart, eccentric *h.* of the heart.

cicatricial h. Overgrowth of connective tissue in a scar; increase in scar tissue.

compensatory h. That which follows destruction or injury in the opposite paired organ or in another part of the same organ.

concentric h. of the heart. An increase in the weight and volume of cardiac muscle, especially of the ventricles; accompanied by reduction in the volume of the chambers; probably due to rigor mortis rather than to a special form of cardiac hypertrophy.

eccentric h. of the heart. Hypertrophy accompanied by dilatation, beyond that usually seen in cardiac hypertrophy.

false h. An increase in size of an organ due to an increase in amount of tissue not associated with functional activity, such as connective tissue; a hyperplasia.

numerical h. That due to multiplication of component cells.

physiologic h. That due to natural physiologic rather than pathologic causes, as hypertrophy of the pregnant uterus.

simple h. That due to an increase in the size of the component cells rather than to their multiplication.

ventricular h. A term used in electrocardiography as either **right ventricular hypertrophy** (designating abnormal right axis deviation and QRS in the limb leads possibly over 0.10 sec.) or **left ventricular hypertrophy** (designating abnormal left axis deviation, QRS in the limb leads over 0.10 sec., T flat or inverted in lead I and at times T_2 similarly changed).

work h. Muscular hypertrophy due to increased work load; a form of adaptive *h.*

hy″per·tro′pi·a [*hyper;* G. *trepein,* to turn]. Vertical concomitant strabismus; one eye fixes upon an object and the other deviates upward.

hy″per·u·re′sis. See *polyuria.*

hy″per·u″ri·ce′mi·a. Abnormally high level of urates in the blood.

hy″per·vas′cu·lar [*hyper;* L. *vasculum,* small vessel]. Excessively vascular.

hy″per·veg′e·ta″tive (high″pur·vedj′i·tay″tiv) [*hyper;* L. *vegetus,* lively]. Referring to a constitutional body type in which visceral or nutritional function dominates the somatic or neuromuscular system. Syn., *brachymorphic, pyknic, megalosplanchnic.*

hy″per·ven″ti·la′tion [*hyper;* L. *ventilare,* to toss, from *ventus,* wind]. Hyperpnea or forced respiration; an increase in the quantity of air breathed (minute volume) as a result of an increase in the rate or depth of respiration, or both. Symptoms are those of hyperoxygenation of the blood and include tingling of the extremities and buzzing in the head, with occasional syncope.

involuntary h. Occurs in hysteria as a physiologic concomitant of fear or anger, or as a result of diffuse or focal encephalopathy.

hy″per·vi″ta·min·o′sis [*hyper;* vitamin; G. *-ōsis,* condition]. A condition due to the administration of toxic amounts of a vitamin.

hy″per·vo·le′mi·a [*hyper;* L. *volumen,* volume; G. *haima,* blood]. Blood volume greater than normal.

hyp″es·the′si·a, hyp″aes·the′si·a (hip″ess·thee′-zhuh, ·zee·uh, high″pess·) [G. *hypo,* under; *aisthēsis,* sensation]. Impairment of sensation; lessened tactile sensibility. —**hypesthesic, hypesthet′ic,** *adj.*

hy′pha (pl. *hyphae*) [G., web]. A filament which develops from the germ tube of a fungus. The **septate hyphae** are those divided into a chain of cells by cross walls forming at regular intervals. Those without cross walls, the **nonseptate hyphae,** allow an uninterrupted flow of protoplasm and are described as being coenocytic. —**hy′phal,** *adj.*

hyp″he·do′ni·a (hip″hi·do′nee·uh, hype″hi·do′-nee·uh) [G. *hypo,* under; *hēdonē,* pleasure]. Diminution of pleasure sensations in acts that normally give pleasure.

hy·phe′ma, hy·phae′ma (high·fee′muh) [*hypo;* G. *haima,* blood]. Blood in the anterior chamber of the eye.

hy·phe′mi·a (high·fee′mee·uh) [*hypo; haima*]. 1. Deficiency of blood. Also called *oligemia.* 2. Blood in the anterior chamber of the eye.

hyp″hi·dro′sis (hip″hi·dro′sis, hip″high·, hype″hi·) [*hypo;* G. *hidrōsis,* sweating]. Deficiency of perspiration.

Hy″pho·my·ce′tes (high″fo·migh·see′teez). See *Fungi imperfecti.*

hyp″i·no′sis [*hypo;* G. *is,* fiber; *-ōsis,* condition]. A deficiency of fibrin factors in the blood.

hyp″i·so·ton′ic (hip″i·so·ton′ick, high″pi·). See *hypotonic.*

hyp″na·gog′ic (hip″nuh·godj′ick) [G. *hypnos,* sleep; *agōgos,* leading]. Inducing sleep; pertaining to the inception of sleep. Applied to visions seen just preceding complete sleep.

hyp′na·gogue [*hypnos; agōgos*]. An hypnotic, 1.

hypnal. Trade-mark for antipyrine chloralhydrate; a white, crystalline powder, soluble in water; used as a hypnotic.

hyp·nal′gi·a [*hypnos;* G. *algos,* pain]. Pain occurring during sleep.

hyp′nic [G. *hypnikos,* producing sleep]. Pertaining to or inducing sleep.

hyp′nic. An agent that induces sleep.

hyp′no-, hypn- [G. *hypnos,* sleep]. A combining form meaning *sleep* or denoting *hypnotism.*

hyp″no·a·nal′y·sis [*hypnos;* G. *analysis,* a dissolving]. A form of psychotherapy combining certain psychoanalytic techniques with hypnosis.

hyp″no·gen′ic, hyp″no·ge·net′ic [*hypnos;* G. *genesthai,* from *gignesthai,* to be produced]. 1. Producing or inducing sleep. 2. Inducing hypnotism. —**hypnogen′esis,** *n.*

hyp′noid, hyp·noi′dal [*hypnos;* G. *eidos,* form]. Resembling sleep or hypnosis.

hyp′no·lep″sy [*hypnos;* G. *lēpsis,* a seizing]. Excessive or morbid sleepiness; narcolepsy.

hyp·nol′o·gy [*hypnos;* G. *logos,* word]. The science dealing with sleep or with hypnotism.

hyp″no·nar·co′sis [*hypnos;* G. *narkōsis,* a benumbing]. Deep sleep induced through hypnosis.

hyp″no·pho′bi·a [*hypnos;* G. *phobos,* fear]. Morbid dread of sleep or of falling asleep. —**hypnophobic,** *adj.;* **hyp′nophoby,** *n.*

hyp″no·phre·no′sis [*hypnos;* G. *phrenōsis,* from *phrēn,* mind, *-ōsis,* condition]. A general term for all forms of sleep disturbance.

hyp″no·pom′pic [*hypnos;* G. *pompē,* procession]. Pertaining to the state of awakening. Applied to visions seen at the moment of awakening from sleep or prior to complete awakening, as when a dream figure persists in waking life.

hyp″no·si·gen′e·sis [*hypnos;* G. *-ōsis,* condition; *genesis,* production]. Induction of hypnosis.

hyp·no′sis [*hypnos; -ōsis*]. A state of sleep or trance; induced artificially in a subject by means of verbal suggestion by the hypnotist or by the subject's concentration upon some object; characterized by extreme responsiveness to suggestions made by the hypnotist.

hyp″no·ther′a·py [*hypnos;* G. *therapeia,* treatment]. The treatment of disease by means of hypnotism.

hyp·not′ic [G. *hypnōtikos,* inclined to sleep]. 1. Inducing sleep. 2. Pertaining to hypnotism.

hyp·not′ic. 1. A remedy that causes sleep. 2. A person who is susceptible to hypnotism; one who is hypnotized.

hyp′no·tism [*hypnōtikos*]. 1. The act of inducing hypnosis. 2. The study of hypnosis. —**hypnotist,** *n.*

hyp′no·tize [*hypnōtikos*]. Bring into a state of hypnosis. —**hypnotiza′tion,** *n.*

hyp′no·toid [G. *hypnos,* sleep; *eidos,* form]. Resembling hypnotism.

hyp″no·tox′in [*hypnos;* G. *toxikon,* poison]. A hypothetical substance supposed to accumulate in the cerebrospinal fluid during the waking state, and credited with the power to produce sleep by stopping the activity of the cortical cells.

hy′po [G. *hypo,* under]. 1. Colloquial term for hypochondriasis; also for hypodermic syringe or medication. 2. Sodium thiosulfate.

hy′po- (high′po-, hip′o-), **hyp-** [*hypo*]. 1. A prefix denoting *deficiency* or *lack; below* or *beneath.* 2. A prefix indicating *acids and salts having the least number of atoms of oxygen in a series of compounds of the same elements.*

hy″po·a·cid′i·ty [*hypo;* L. *acidus,* sour]. Deficiency in acid constituents.

hy″po·ac·tiv′i·ty [*hypo;* L. *activus,* from *agere,* to do]. Diminished activity.

hy″po·ad·ren″al·i·ne′mi·a [*hypo;* L. *ad,* near; *renes,* kidneys; G. *haima,* blood]. A condition in which the adrenalin content of the blood is insufficient.

hy″po·ad·re′nal·ism [*hypo; ad; renes*]. Hypoadrenia.

hy″po·ad·re′ni·a [*hypo; ad; renes*]. Diminished activity of the adrenal glands. See *asthenocoria.*

hy″po·ag′na·thus [*hypo;* G. *a-,* not; *gnathos,* jaw]. An individual with no lower jaw.

hy″po·al″bu·min·e′mi·a. Abnormally low blood content of albumin.

hy″po·al″i·men·ta′tion [*hypo;* L. *alimentum,* food]. The state produced by insufficient or inadequate food.

hy″po·al·ler·gen′ic. Non-allergy-producing: a term applied to a preparation in which every possible care has been taken in formulation and production to insure minimum instance of allergic reactions.

hy″po·az″o·tu′ri·a [*hypo;* G. *a-,* not; *zōē,* life; *ouron,* urine]. A diminished amount of urea in the urine.

hy″po·bar′ic [*hypo;* G. *baros,* weight]. 1. Of less weight or pressure. 2. Pertaining to an anesthetic solution of specific gravity lower than the spinal fluid.

hy″po·bar′ism. A condition resulting from an excess of gas pressure within the body fluids, tissues, or cavities over the ambient gas pressure.

hy″po·ba·rop′a·thy. See chronic mountain *sickness.*

hy′po·blast [*hypo;* G. *blastos,* germ]. Old term for entoderm. —**hypoblas′tic,** *adj.*

hy″po·bran′chi·al (high″po·brang′kee·ul, hip″o·) [*hypo;* G. *bragchia,* gills]. A bone or cartilage located below or under the branchial or visceral arches. —**hypobran′chial,** *adj.*

hy″po·bro′mite [*hypo;* G. *brōmos,* bad smell]. A salt of hypobromous acid.

hy″po·bro′mous ac′id. HBrO. An unstable acid containing bromine having a positive valence number of one.

hy″po·bu′li·a [*hypo;* G. *boulē,* will]. Deficiency of will power.

hy″po·cal·ce′mi·a [*hypo;* L. *calx,* lime; G. *haima,* blood]. Condition in which there is a diminished amount of calcium in the blood.

hy″po·cal″ci·fi·ca′tion [*hypo;* L. *calx,* lime; *facere,* to make]. Reduction of the normal amount of mineral salts in calcified tissues, as bone, dentin, or dental enamel. —**hypocalcif′ic,** *adj.;* **hypocal′cify,** *v.*

hy″po·cap′ni·a. Subnormal concentration of CO_2 in the blood: also called *hypocarbia;* often incorrectly called *acapnia.*

hy″po·ca·thex′is [*hypo;* G. *kathexis,* a holding]. A lack of concentration of the psychic energy upon a particular object.

hy″po·ce′lom. See *hypocoelom.*

hy″po·chlo·re′mi·a, hy″po·chlo·rae′mi·a [*hypo;* G. *chlōros,* pale green; *haima,* blood]. Reduction in the amount of blood chlorides.

hy″po·chlor·hy′dri·a (high″po·klor·high′dree·uh, ·klor·hid′ree·uh, hip″o·) [*hypo; chlōros;* G. *hydōr,* water]. A condition in which there is a diminished amount of hydrochloric acid in the gastric juice.

hy″po·chlo′rite. Any salt of hypochlorous acid, HClO. The most important are those of calcium and sodium.

hy″po·chlo″ri·za′tion [*hypo; chlōros*]. Reduction in the intake of sodium chloride.

hy″po·chlo′rous ac′id. HClO. An unstable compound, known only in solution. It has disinfectant and bleaching properties and is used mostly in the form of its sodium and calcium compounds.

hy″po·chlor·u′ri·a [*hypo; chlōros;* G. *ouron,* urine]. A diminution in the amount of chlorides excreted in the urine.

hy″po·cho·les″ter·e′mi·a (·ko·les″tur·ee′mee·uh) [*hypo;* G. *cholē,* bile; *stereos,* stiff; *haima,* blood]. Decrease or deficiency of the cholesterol of the blood.

hy″po·chon′dri·a (high″po·kon′dree·uh, hip″o·). Hypochondriasis.

hy″po·chon′dri·ac [G. *hypochondriakos,* of the hypochondrium]. 1. Pertaining to the hypochondrium. 2. Affected with or caused by hypochondriasis.

hy″po·chon′dri·ac. A person who is affected with hypochondriasis.

hy″po·chon·dri′a·sis (high″po·kon·dry′uh·sis, hip″o·) [G. *hypochondrion,* soft part of the body below the costal cartilages and above the navel; NL. *-iasis,* condition]. A chronic condition in which the patient is morbidly concerned with his own health, and believes himself suffering from grave bodily diseases; traceable to some long-standing intrapsychic conflict. In true hypochondriasis, the symptoms are focused upon one organ.

hy″po·chon′dri·um (high″po·kon′dree·um, hip″o·) [*hypochondrion*]. The upper lateral region of the abdomen below the lower ribs.

hy″po·chor′dal (high″po·kor′dul, hip″o·) [G. *hypo,* under; *chordē,* chord]. Located below or ventral to the notochord.

hy″po·chro·mat′ic. Pertaining to or describing the microscopic appearance of cells of the erythropoietic series which show significant decrease in density of the characteristic hemoglobin color for the stained or unstained cell, due to either thinness of the cells or decreased concentration of hemoglobin, or both. —**hypochroma′sia, hypochro′matism,** *n.*

hy″po·chro′mic. Pertaining to a blood picture in which the erythrocytes have a mean corpuscular hemoglobin concentration (MCHC) or saturation index and usually a mean corpuscular hemoglobin (MCH) or color index more than two standard deviations below the mean normal, determined by the same method on bloods of healthy persons of the patient's age and sex group.

hy″po·chy′li·a (high″po·kigh′lee·uh, hip″o·) [*hypo;* G. *chylos,* juice]. Deficiency of chyle.

hy″po·ci·ne′si·a (·si·nee′shuh, ·see·uh, ·zhuh, ·zee·uh), **hy″po·ci·ne′sis.** See *hypokinesia.*

hy″po·coe′lom, hy″po·ce′lom (high″po·see′lum, hip″o·) [*hypo;* G. *koilōma,* hollow]. The ventral part of the coelom.

hy′po·cone [*hypo;* G. *kōnos,* cone]. The distolingual cusp of an upper molar tooth.

hy″po·con′id [*hypo; kōnos*]. The distobuccal cusp of a lower molar tooth.

hy″po·con′ule [*hypo;* dim. from *kōnos*]. The fifth, or distal, cusp of an upper molar tooth.

hy″po·con′u·lid [*hypo;* dim. from *kōnos*]. The fifth, or distal, cusp of a lower molar tooth.

hy″po·cy·clo′sis (high″po·sigh·klo′sis, hip″o·) [*hypo;* G. *kyklōsis,* from *kyklos,* circle]. Deficient accommodation.

ciliary h. That due to weakness of the ciliary muscle.

lenticular h. That due to lack of elasticity in the crystalline lens.

hy″po·cy·the′mi·a. Any deficiency of the formed elements of blood; usually *anemia.*

progressive h. See primary refractory *anemia.*

Hy″po·der′ma [*hypo;* G. *derma,* skin]. A genus of the Diptera, whose larvae, parasitic to cattle and occasionally to man, cause the cutaneous swellings known as warbles.

hy″po·der·mat′ic. See *hypodermic.*

hy″po·der″ma·toc′ly·sis. See *hypodermoclysis.*

hy″po·der·mi′a·sis [*hypo; derma;* NL. *-iasis,* condition]. A condition in which botfly larvae invade the subcutaneous tissue and produce a form of creeping eruption. See *warbles.*

hy″po·der′mic [*hypo; derma*]. 1. Pertaining to the region beneath the skin. 2. Placed or introduced beneath the skin.

hy″po·der′mic. 1. An injection under the skin. 2. Syringe used in hypodermic injection.

hy″po·der′mis [G., from *hypo, derma*]. The outermost layer of cells of invertebrates, which corresponds to the epidermis. It secretes the cuticular exoskeleton of arthropods, annelids, mollusks, and other forms.

hy″po·der·moc′ly·sis, hy″po·der″ma·toc′ly·sis [*hypo; derma;* G. *klysis,* a drenching]. The introduction into the subcutaneous tissues of large quantities of fluids, especially saline solution.

hy″po·der″mo·li·thi′a·sis. See circumscribed *calcinosis.*

hy″po·don′ti·a. Deficient development of the teeth.

hy″po·er′gy *hypo;* G. *ergon,* work]. A state of less than normal reactivity, in which the response is less marked than usual; hyposensitivity; one form of allergy or pathergy.

hy″po·es″o·pho′ri·a [*hypo;* G. *esō,* within; *phoros,* bearing]. A type of heterophoria in which the visual lines tend downward and inward.

hy″po·es′trin·ism. The state of deficient production of estrogen by the ovaries.

hy″po·ex″o·pho′ri·a [*hypo;* G. *exō,* without; *phoros*]. A type of heterophoria in which the visual lines tend downward and outward.

hy″po·fer·re′mi·a. Diminished, or abnormally low iron level in the blood.

hy″po·fi″brin·o·gen·e′mi·a. See *fibrinogenopenia.*

hy″po·func′tion [*hypo;* L. *functio,* from *fungi,* to perform]. Diminished function.

adrenal cortical h. See *adrenal cortical hypofunction.*

hy″po·gal·ac′ti·a. Decreased milk secretion.

hy″po·gas′tric [*hypo;* G. *gastēr,* belly]. Of or pertaining to the hypogastrium.

hy″po·gas′tri·um [*hypo;* G. *gastēr,* belly]. The lowest of the three median regions of the abdomen, above the symphysis pubis and below the umbilical region. Also called *hypogastric region.*

hy″po·gas″tro·did′y·mus [*hypo; gastēr;* G. *didymos,* twin]. Hypogastropagus.

hy″po·gas·trop′a·gus [*hypo; gastēr;* G. *pagos,* that which is fixed]. A monster consisting of conjoined twins united at the hypogastric region. Syn., *hypogastrodidymus.*

hy″po·gas·tros′chi·sis (high″po·gas·tros′ki·sis, hip″o·) [*hypo; gastēr;* G. *schisis,* a cleavage]. Abdominal fissure (gastroschisis) limited to the hypogastric region.

hy″po·gen′i·tal·ism [*hypo;* L. *genitalis,* genital]. Underdevelopment of the genital system. See also *eunuchoidism, hypogonadism.*

hy″po·geu′si·a (high″po·gew′see·uh, ·jew′see·uh, hip″o·) [*hypo;* G. *geusis,* taste]. Diminution in the sense of taste.

hy″po·glos′sal [*hypo;* G. *glōssa,* tongue]. Situated under the tongue.

hy″po·glos·si′tis [*hypo; glōssa;* G. *-itis,* inflammation]. Inflammation of the tissue under the tongue.

hy″po·glos′sus [*hypo; glōssa*]. The hypoglossal nerve.

hy″po·glot′tis, hy″po·glos′sis [G. *hypoglōttis,* under surface of the tongue]. The under part of the tongue.

hy″po·gly·ce′mi·a (·glye·see′mee·uh) [G. *hypo,* under; *glykys,* sweet; *haima,* blood]. The condition produced by a low level of glucose in the blood; due to excessive utilization of sugar or to interference with the formation of sugar in the liver. Symptoms, which usually appear when the blood sugar drops to 0.06–0.04%, are hunger, nervousness, profuse sweating, alternate pallor and flushing of the face, and vertigo. Also called *hypoglycemosis.* See *hyperinsulinism.*

hy″po·gly·ce·mo′sis [*hypo; glykys;* G. *-osis,* condition]. See *hypoglycemia.*

hy″po·gly″co·ge·nol′y·sis [*hypo; glykys;* G. *genesthai,* from *gignesthai,* to be produoed; *lysis,* a loosing]. Diminished glycogenolysis.

hy″po·gnath′ous (high″po·nath′us) [*hypo;* G. *gnathos,* jaw]. Having the lower jaw abnormally small.

hy″po·gnath′us (high″po·nath′us) [*hypo; gnathos*]. A monster having a parasite attached to the lower jaw. Syn., *paragnathus.*

hy″po·gon′ad·ism (high″po·gon′uh·diz·um, ·go′nuh·diz·um, hip″o·) [*hypo;* G. *gonē,* seed]. Diminished internal secretion of the testes or ovaries which may be due to a primary defect or secondary to insufficient stimulation by the adenohypophysis.

pituitary h. See pituitary *eunuchoidism.*

hy″po·gran″u·lo·cy·to′sis. Agranulocytosis.

hy″po·hi·dro′sis (high″po·hi·dro′sis, ·high·dro′sis, hip″o·) [*hypo;* G. *hidrōsis,* sweating]. Deficient perspiration.

hy″po·in′su·lin·ism [*hypo;* L. *insula,* island]. Old term for diabetes mellitus.

hy″po·i″so·ton′ic. See *hypotonic,* 2.

hy″po·kal·i·e′mi·a. Abnormally low serum potassium; hypopotassemia.

hy″po·ki·ne′si·a (·ki·nee′shuh, ·see·uh, ·zhuh, ·zee·uh, ·kigh·nee′·), **hy″po·ki·ne′sis** (·ki·nee′sis, ·kigh·nee′sis) [*hypo;* G. *kinēsis,* motion]. Abnormally decreased muscular movement. —**hypokinet′ic,** *adj.*

hy″po·lem′mal [*hypo;* G. *lemma,* rind, husk]. Lying under a sheath, as the motor end-plates under the sarcolemma or sheath of a muscle fiber.

hy″po·lep″si·o·ma′ni·a [*hypo;* G. *lēpsis,* a seizing; *mania,* madness]. A general term for all forms of monomania.

hy″po·ley′dig·ism. Retarded sexual development, or loss of some male sexual characteristics, as a result of a decrease or absence in the function of the interstitial (Leydig) cells of the testes.

hy″po·lo′gi·a [*hypo;* G. *logeia,* from *logos,* word]. Poverty of speech as a symptom of cerebral disease.

hy″po·mag″ne·se′mi·a [*hypo;* G. *Magnēsia lithos,* Magnesian stone; *haima,* blood]. A state of magnesium deficiency in the blood manifested by twitching and convulsions.

hy″po·ma′ni·a [*hypo;* G. *mania,* madness]. A slight maniacal state, in which the patient is easily distracted and clang associations occur, but no marked behavior differences are present; a less intense form of mania. —**hypomanic,** *adj.*

hy″po·mas′ti·a, hy″po·ma′zi·a [*hypo;* G. *mastos,* breast]. Abnormal smallness of the mammary glands.

hy″po·men″or·rhe′a. A deficient amount of menstrual flow at the regular period: to be distinguished from *oligomenorrhea.*

hy″po·mere [*hypo;* G. *meros,* part]. The ventral portion of the mesothelial lining of the coelom of primitive chordates, forming pleura, pericardium, and peritoneum.

hy″po·me·tab′o·lism [*hypo;* G. *metabolē,* change]. Metabolism below the normal rate.

hy″po·me·tro′pi·a [*hypo;* G. *metron,* a measure; *ōps,* eye]. Myopia.

hy″po·mi″cro·gnath′us (high″po·migh″kro·nath′us) [*hypo;* G. *mikros,* small; *gnathos,* jaw]. An individual having an abnormally small lower jaw.

hy″po·mi′cron [*hypo; mikros*]. A particle capable of being recognized by the ultramicroscope, but not by the ordinary microscope.

hy″po·mi″cro·so′ma (·migh″kro·so′muh, ·mick″ro·) [*hypo; mikros;* G. *sōma,* body]. The lowest stature which is not dwarfism.

hy″pom·ne′si·a (high″pom·nee′zhuh, ·zee·uh) [*hypo;* G. *mnēsis,* a remembering]. Weakened memory.

hy″po·mo·til′i·ty. Hypokinesia.

hy″po·nan″o·so′ma [*hypo;* G. *nanos,* dwarf; *sōma,* body]. Extreme dwarfishness.

hy″po·nat·re′mi·a (high″po·nat·ree′mee·uh). Abnormally low blood sodium level.

hy″po·no′ic [*hypo;* G. *nous,* mind]. Pertaining to that behavior which arises from unconscious processes.

hy″po·nych′i·um (high″po·nick′ee·um, hip″o·) [*hypo;* G. *onyx,* nail]. The thickened stratum corneum of the epidermis which lies under the free edge of a nail. —**hyponychial,** *adj.*

hy″po·os·to′sis [*hypo;* G. *osteon,* bone; *osis,* condition]. Hypoplasia of bone. —**hypoostot′ic,** *adj.*

hy″po·par″a·thy′roid·ism [*hypo;* G. *para,* near; *thyreoeidēs,* shield-shaped]. Insufficiency of the parathyroid gland, usually postoperative and rarely idiopathic, characterized by a well delineated pathologic state in which there is high serum phosphorus, low serum calcium, manifestations of tetany, usually an absence of calcium in the urine, and deposition of calcium in basal ganglia.

hy″po·per″me·a·bil′i·ty [*hypo;* L. *permeare,* to pervade]. A state in which membranes have reduced permeability for electrolytes, and other solutes, or colloids.

hy″po·pha·lan′gism [*hypo;* G. *phalagx,* bone between two joints of the fingers and toes]. Congenital absence of one or more phalanges in a finger or toe.

hy″po·phar″yn·gos′co·py [*hypo;* G. *pharygx,* pharynx; *skopein,* to examine]. Inspection of the laryngopharynx.

hy″po·phar′ynx [*hypo; pharygx*]. Old term for laryngopharynx.

hy″po·pho′ni·a [*hypo;* G. *phōnē,* voice]. Partial loss of voice owing to lack of coordination of the muscles concerned in voice production. *Rare.*

hy″po·pho′ri·a [*hypo;* G. *phoros,* bearing]. A tendency of the visual axis of one eye to deviate below that of the other.

hy″po·phos″pha·ta′sia [*hypo;* G. *phōsphoros,* light bringer]. Abnormally decreased phosphatase production.

hy″po·phos″pha·te′mi·a [*hypo;* G. *phōsphoros,* light-bringer; *haima,* blood]. Abnormally low concentration of phosphates in the blood serum.

hy″po·phos′phite. A salt of hypophosphorous acid.

compound hypophosphites syrup (*syrupus hypophosphitum compositus*). Contains the hypophosphites of calcium, potassium, sodium, ferric iron, and manganese. Dose, 8 cc. (2 fluidrachms).

hypophosphites syrup (*syrupus hypophosphitum*). Contains the hypophosphites of calcium, potassium, and sodium. Dose, 8 cc. (2 fluidrachms).

hy″po·phos′pho·rous ac′id (·fos′fo·rus, ·fos-for′us) (*acidum hypophosphorosum*). An aqueous solution containing 30–32% of HPH_2O_2. It is easily oxidized and, therefore, serves to prevent the oxidation of substances with which it may be combined.

hy″po·phre′ni·a [*hypo;* G. *phrēn,* mind]. Feeble-mindedness. **—hypophren′ic,** *adj., n.*

hy·poph″y·sec′to·my (high·pof″i·seck′to·mee, hi-pof″·) [G. *hypophysis,* undergrowth; *ektomē,* excision]. Surgical removal of the hypophysis cerebri, or pituitary body. **—hypophysectomize,** *v.*

hy·poph′y·sis, hy·poph′y·sis cer′e·bri (high-pof′i·sis). The pituitary gland or body. See Plates 17, 18, 45. **—hypophys′eal, hypophys′ial,** *adj.*

hy″po·pi·e′si·a (·pye·ee′zhuh, ·zee·uh, ·shuh, ·see·uh), **hy″po·pi·e′sis** (·pye·ee′sis, ·pye′i·sis) [*hypo;* G. *piesis,* pressure]. Subnormal arterial pressure.

hy″po·pin′e·al·ism (·pin′ee·ul·iz·um, ·pi·nee′ul-iz·um) [*hypo;* L. *pinea,* pine cone]. Hypothetical lessened secretion of the pineal gland.

hy″po·pi·tu′i·ta·rism [*hypo;* L. *pituita,* phlegm]. Deficient production of pituitary hormones, especially those of the adenohypophysis or with certain pituitary tumors. There may be impotence, sterility, amenorrhea, hypoglycemia, signs of adrenal cortical failure, hypometabolism, and a tendency of the tissues and viscera to shrink.

hy″po·pla′si·a (high″po·play′zhuh, ·zee·uh, ·shuh, ·see·uh, hip″o·), **hy′po·plas″ty** [*hypo;* G. *plassein.* to form]. Defective development of any tissue. **—hypoplas′tic,** *adj.*

hy·pop′nea [*hypo;* G. *pnoē,* breath]. Shallow breathing. It may accompany sleep, and is sometimes caused by poor posture, partial paralysis of the respiratory muscles, ankylosing spondylitis, or emphysema.

hy″po·pot″as·se′mi·a. Deficiency of potassium in the blood; hypokaliemia.

hy″po·prax′i·a [*hypo;* G. *praxis,* a doing]. Deficient activity; inactivity; listlessness.

hy″po·pro·sex′i·a [*hypo;* G. *prosexis,* application]. Inadequate attention; lack of the ability to give attention.

hy″po·pro″te·i·ne′mi·a [*hypo; protein;* G. *haima,* blood]. Abnormally low concentration of protein in whole blood or serum.

hy″po·pro·throm″bi·ne′mi·a [*hypo;* G. *pro,* before; *thrombos,* clot; *haima*]. Deficient supply of prothrombin in the blood.

hy″po·psel″a·phe′si·a (high″po·sel″uh·fee′zee·uh, ·see·uh, ·zhuh, ·shuh, hip″o·) [*hypo;* G. *psēlaphēsis,* a touching]. Diminution of sensitivity to tactile impressions.

hy″po·psy·cho′sis (high″po·sigh·ko′sis, hip″o·) [*hypo;* G. *psychōsis,* a giving life to]. Diminution or blunting of thought.

hy·po′py·on (high·po′pee·on, hi·po′·) [*hypo;* G. *pyon,* pus]. A collection of pus in the anterior chamber of the eye.

hy″po·que·bra′chine (·kwi·bray′keen, ·kin, ·kwi-brack′een, ·in). $C_{21}H_{26}N_2O_2$. An alkaloid of quebracho.

hy″po·sal″i·va′tion [*hypo;* L. *salivatio,* from *salivare,* to spit out]. Pathologically insufficient secretion of saliva; formerly called *xerostomia.*

hy″po·scle′ral [*hypo;* G. *sklēros,* hard]. Beneath the sclera.

hy″po·se·cre′tion [*hypo;* L. *secretum,* from *secernere,* to separate]. Diminished secretion.

hy″po·sen″si·tiv′i·ty [*hypo;* L. *sentire,* to feel]. A state of diminished sensitiveness, especially to external stimuli. **—hyposen′sitive,** *adj.;* **hyposen′sitiveness,** *n.*

hy″po·sen″si·ti·za′tion. See *desensitization,* 1.

hy·pos′mi·a (high·poz′mee·uh, hi·poz′·) [*hypo;* G. *osmē,* smell]. Diminution of the sense of smell.

hy″po·som′ni·a [*hypo;* L. *somnus,* sleep]. An insufficient number of hours of sleep.

hy″po·spa′di·ac [*hypo;* G. *span,* to draw]. 1. Pertaining to hypospadias.

hy″po·spa′di·ac. A person with hypospadias.

hy″po·spa′di·as [*hypo; span*]. 1. A congenital anomaly of the penis and urethra in which the urethra opens upon the ventral surface of the penis or in the perineum. 2. Term also used to denote a congenital malformation in which the urethra opens into the vagina.

balanitic h. The commonest form, in which the opening is at the site of the frenum, which is usually rudimentary or absent.

penile h. That in which the urethra opens ventrally at some point between the sulcus of the glans and penoscrotal junction.

penoscrotal h. A form in which the urethra opens at the junction of the penis and the scrotum.

perineal h. A form in which the urethra opens upon the perineum.

pseudovaginal h. A form in which the opening of the urethra is upon the perineum, and is funnel-like and wide open; this may be interpreted as a vagina and lead to confusion of sex. Also see *pseudohermaphroditism.*

hy″po·sper″ma·to·gen′e·sis [*hypo;* G. *sperma,* seed; *genesis,* production]. A decreased production of male germ cells, caused by such factors as diseased testes or hypoleydigism.

hy″pos·phre′si·a (high″pos·free′zhuh, ·zee·uh, ·shuh, ·see·uh, hip″os·) [*hypo;* G. *osphrēsis,* sense of smell]. Hyposmia.

hy′po·spray. A metallic device for administering injections subcutaneously; it operates on the principle that a stream of fluid ejected with high velocity through an orifice 75 to 80 microns in diameter and held against the skin, penetrates the skin without pain and usually without leaving a readily visible mark. Also called *jet injection.*

hy·pos′ta·sis (high·pos′ta·sis, hi·pos′·) [G., sediment]. 1. A deposit which forms at the bottom of a liquid; a sediment. 2. The formation of a sediment, especially the settling of blood in dependent parts of the body.

hy″po·stat′ic [G. *hypostatikos*, belonging to substance]. 1. Due to, or of the nature of, hypostasis. 2. *In genetics*, subject to being suppressed, as a gene whose effect is suppressed by another gene that affects the same part of the organism.

hy″pos·the′ni·a [G. *hypo*, under; *sthenos*, strength]. Weakness; subnormal strength. —**hypostheniant, hyposthen′ic,** *adj.*

hy·pos″the·nu′ri·a (high·poss″thi·new′ree·uh, hiposs″·) [*hypo; sthenos;* G. *ouron*, urine]. The secretion of urine of low specific gravity, due to the inability of the kidney to concentrate the urine adequately.

hy″po·sto′mi·a [*hypo;* G. *stoma*, mouth]. A form of microstomia in which the mouth is a vertical slit opening into a pharyngeal sac.

hy″po·sul′fite. A name, recommended to be abandoned, which has been applied to salts both of thiosulfuric acid and of hydrosulfurous acid.

hy″po·syn·er′gi·a [*hypo;* G. *synergia*, cooperation]. Defective coordination.

hy″po·tax′i·a [*hypo;* G. *taxis*, arrangement]. A condition of emotional rapport existing in the beginning of hypnosis between the subject and the hypnotizer.

hy″po·tax′is [G., subjection, submission]. Light, hypnotic sleep.

hy″po·tel′or·ism. Decrease in distance between two organs or parts; specifically, **ocular hypotelorism,** a rare craniofacial deformity possibly due to deficient development of the lesser wing of the sphenoid bone and premature closure of cranial sutures, characterized by marked microcephaly, slight oxycephaly, narrowing of the bridge of the nose, and hence decreased distance between the eyes and convergent strabismus; general physical and mental retardation accompany this condition, which may be regarded as the inverse of ocular hypertelorism.

hy″po·ten′sion [G. *hypo*, under; L. *tensio*, a stretching]. Diminished or abnormally low tension, usually synonymous with low blood pressure. —**hypotensive,** *adj.*

orthostatic h. A fall of blood pressure which occurs when the erect position is assumed.

postural h. That due to a sudden change from the horizontal to the upright position or from prolonged standing, causing dizziness, faintness, and sometimes syncope.

hy″po·ten′sor [*hypo;* L. *tensum*, from *tendere*, to stretch]. Any substance capable of lowering blood pressure. It implies a persistent effect, as opposed to the fleeting effect of a depressor.

hy″po·thal′a·mus [*hypo;* G. *thalamos*, chamber]. The region of the diencephalon forming the floor of the third ventricle, including neighboring, associated nuclei. It is divided into three regions: 1. *Anterior region* or *pars supraoptica*, which is superior to the optic chiasma. It includes *supraoptic* and *paraventricular nuclei* and a less differentiated nucleus which merges with the preoptic area called *anterior hypothalamic nucleus*. 2. *Middle region, pars tuberalis*, or *tuber cinereum*, including the *lateral hypothalamic* and *tuberal nuclei*, lateral to a sagittal plane passing through the anterior column of the fornix, the *dorsomedial, ventromedial*, and *posterior hypothalamic nuclei*, medial to the above plane. 3. *Caudal region, pars mammillaris*, or *mammillary bodies*, including *medial, lateral*, and *intercalated mammillary nuclei* and *premammillary* and *supramammillary nuclei*. —**hypothalam′ic,** *adj.*

hy″po·the′nar (high″po·thee′nur, high·poth′i·nur) [*hypo;* G. *thenar*, palm]. Designating the fleshy eminence on the ulnar side of the palm of the hand.

hy″po·therm″es·the′sia. Decreased temperature sensibility.

hy″po·ther′mi·a, hy′po·ther″my [*hypo;* G. *thermē*, heat]. Subnormal temperature of the body. —**hypother′mal,** *adj.*

hy·poth′e·sis [G., proposal]. 1. A supposition or conjecture put forth to account for known facts. 2. A theory accepted tentatively, as, for example,

Buergi's h. Drugs possessing identical pharmacological action summate their therapeutic effects when administered simultaneously; potentiation occurs only if the two agents have different pharmacological activity.

Kossel and Siegfried's protamine nucleus h., the theory that all proteins are built around a nucleus of the three amino acids, arginine, histidine, and lysine, and that arginine is the most important member of this triad.

Gesell's h. An explanation of the integration of breathing in terms of nervous integration electronically recorded.

lattice h. One which attributes the precipitation of antigen and antibody to the building up of a lattice or framework composed of alternating molecules of antigen and antibody.

mnemic h. See *mnemic hypothesis.*

orosin h. See *orosin hypothesis.*

hy″po·thy′mi·a [G. *hypo*, under; *thymos*, spirit]. Despondency; depression of spirits; a diminution in the intensity of emotions.

hy″po·thy′roid·ism [*hypo;* G. *thyreoeidēs*, shield-shaped]. A morbid condition due to deficiency of thyroid hormone; in advanced form expressed as cretinism or myxedema. In the mild form, a nonmyxedematous condition associated with basal metabolic rates approximating 20% below normal and, to a mild degree, with other characteristics of myxedema. Syn., *hypothyrosis.* Also see *cretinism, myxedema.*

primary h. That caused by primary loss of functioning thyroid tissue, such as surgical removal, infection, or atrophy.

secondary h. That due to inadequate stimulation of the thyroid.

hy″po·thy·ro′sis. Hypothyroidism.

hy″po·to′ni·a, hy·pot′o·ny [*hypo; tonos*]. Decrease of normal tonicity or tension; especially diminution of intraocular pressure.

hy″po·ton′ic [*hypo;* G. *tonos*, tension]. 1. Below the normal strength or tension. 2. Referring to a solution whose osmotic pressure is less than that of physiologic salt solution, or any other solution taken as standard. —**hypotonic′ity,** *n.*

hy″po·tri·cho′sis (high″po·tri·ko′sis, hip″o·). See *alopecia* congenitalis.

hy″po·tro′pi·a [*hypo;* G. *trepein*, to turn]. A form of strabismus in which one eye looks downward.

hy″po·tym′pan·um. That part of the tympanum lying below the level of the drum membrane. —**hypotympan′ic,** *adj.*

hy″po·veg′e·ta″tive (·vedj′i·tay″tiv) [*hypo;* L. *vegetare*, to enliven]. Referring to a human biotype in which purely somatic systems dominate over the visceral or nutritional organs; corresponds to the microsplanchnic or dolichomorphic body types.

hy″po·vi″ta·min·o′sis [*hypo; vitamin;* G. *-ōsis*,

condition]. A condition due to deficiency of one or more vitamins in the food.

hy″po·vo·le′mi·a [*hypo;* L. *volumen,* roll; G. *haima,* blood]. Low, or decreased, blood volume.

hy″po·xan′thine (high″po·zan′theen, ·thin, hip″o·). $C_5H_4N_4O$. 6-Oxypurine, 6-ketopurine. An intermediate product resulting when adenine, an amino purine formed by hydrolysis of nucleic acid, is transformed into uric acid and allantoin.

hy″po·xan·thyl′ic ac′id (·zan·thil′ick). Inosinic acid.

hy″pox·e′mi·a [*hypo;* G. *oxys,* sharp; *haima,* blood]. A condition of insufficient oxygen in the blood.

hy·pox′i·a (high·pock′see·uh, hi·pock′·) [*hypo;* G. *oxys,* sharp]. Oxygen want or deficiency; any state wherein a physiologically inadequate amount of oxygen is available to, or utilized by tissue, without respect to cause or degree. Clinically usually of mixed type, it is classified by physiologists according to etiology.

anemic h. Reduction in oxygen-carrying capacity of the blood due to decrease in functioning erythrocytes, as in anemia, hemorrhage, or carbon monoxide poisoning.

circulatory h. Stagnant *h.*

histotoxic h. Reduction in oxygen utilization due to interference in cellular metabolism by agents like cyanide which poison the respiratory enzymes, or through deficiency of a respiratory enzyme, as in certain infectious or deficiency diseases.

hypoxic h., hypoxemic h. Reduction in availability of oxygen to tissue due to a decrease in the partial pressure of oxygen ($_pO_2$) in the arterial blood, as in low oxygen tension in inspired air, interference with gas exchange in the lungs, and arteriovenous shunts.

stagnant h. Reduction in available oxygen due to slowed circulation of the blood, as in local or general circulatory failure. Syn., *circulatory h.*

hyprotigen. Trade-mark for certain preparations of protein hydrolyzate prepared from casein.

hyp″si·brach″y·ce·phal′ic (hip″si·brack″i·si·fal′·ick) [G. *hypsi,* on high; *brachys,* short; *kephalē,* head]. Having a skull which is high and broad.

hyp″si·ceph′a·ly [*hypsi; kephalē*]. The condition of a skull with a cranial index of over 75.1°.

hyp′si·conch″ (hip′si·konk″) [*hypsi;* G. *kogchē,* shell-like cavity]. *In craniometry,* designating an orbit that appears high because of an elongation of the supero-inferior diameter; having an orbital index of 85.0 or more.

hyp″si·sta·phyl′i·a [*hypsi;* G. *staphylē,* bunch of grapes, swollen uvula]. Condition in which the palatal arch is high and narrow. —**hypsistaphylic, hypsistaph′yline,** *adj.*

hyp″so·ceph′a·ly. See *hypsicephaly.*

hyp·so·chro′mic ef·fect′. The shift of an absorption band to a higher frequency, caused by some external effect on the chromophore.

hyp″so·pho′bi·a [G. *hypsos,* height; *phobos,* fear]. Morbid dread of being at a great height.

Hyrtl, Joseph [*Hungarian anatomist,* ca. 1810–94]. Author of various works on anatomy which were considered standard. Described an anastomosis sometimes found between the two hypoglossal nerves; called *Hyrtl's loop.*

hys′sop [G. *hyssōpos,* hyssop]. The leaves and tops of *Hyssopus officinalis,* an aromatic stimulant and carminative.

hys″ter·al′gi·a [G. *hystera,* womb; *algos,* pain]. Neuralgic pain in the uterus. —**hysteralgic,** *adj.*

hys″ter·ec′to·my [*hystera;* G. *ektomē,* excision]. Total or partial removal of the uterus. In **abdominal hysterectomy,** the removal is effected through an abdominal incision; in **vaginal hysterectomy,** through the vagina. In **supracervical hysterectomy** the cervix is not removed: also called *subtotal* or *supravaginal hysterectomy.*

cesarean h. A hysterectomy done immediately following a cesarean section.

hys″ter·e′sis [G. *hysterēsis,* deficiency]. 1. *In medicine,* a delayed reaction in the formation of gels, as the retraction of a blood clot after coagulation. 2. *In physics,* the retention of a magnetic state of iron in a changing magnetic field. 3. *In chemistry,* the lag of a chemical system in attaining equilibrium. 4. *In colloid chemistry,* the rehydration of a dried protein gel, the amount of water imbibed depending on the original water content of the gel.

hys″ter·eu·ryn′ter (hiss″tur·yoor·in′tur) [G. *hystera,* womb; *eurynein,* to make wide]. A metreurynter used for dilating the cervix uteri.

hys·te′ri·a (hiss·teer′ee·uh, hiss·terr′ee·uh) [*hystera*]. A psychoneurotic disorder, characterized by extreme emotionalism involving disturbances of the psychic, sensory, motor, vasomotor, and visceral functions. Frequently a result of repression of conflicts from the conscious mind. —**hyster′ic, hyster′ical,** *adj.;* **hyster′iac,** *n.*

anxiety h. The combination of an anxiety neurosis with hysteria.

conversion h. See conversion *reaction,* dissociation *reaction.*

major h. A hysteria marked by violent mental excitement and movements suggesting grand mal.

minor h. A mild form of hysteria, as in anorexia nervosa and globus hystericus.

hys·ter′i·cism [*hystera*]. The hysterical diathesis or temperament; proneness to great suggestibility and to the exhibition of hysterical symptoms. *Obs.*

hys·ter′ics [G. *hysterikos,* suffering in the womb, hysterical]. 1. Colloquial term for a hysterical attack. 2. A fit of laughing and crying, similar to that seen in hysteria.

hys·ter′i·form [G. *hystera,* womb; L. *forma,* form]. Resembling hysteria.

hys″ter·i′tis [*hystera;* G. *-itis,* inflammation]. Old term for metritis.

hys′ter·o-, hyster- [*hystera*]. A combining form denoting *connection with,* or *relation to, the uterus* or to *hysteria.*

hys″ter·o·bu·bon′o·cele [*hystera;* G. *boubōnokēlē,* inguinal hernia]. An inguinal hysterocele.

hys′ter·o·cele″ [*hystera;* G. *kēlē,* hernia]. A hernia containing all or part of the uterus.

hys″ter·o·clei′sis (hiss″tur·o·kly′sis) [*hystera;* G. *kleisis,* a closing]. The closure of the uterus by suturing the edges of the external os.

hys″ter·o·cys′tic [*hystera;* G. *kystis,* bladder]. Relating to the uterus and the urinary bladder.

hys″ter·o·cys″to·clei′sis (hiss″tur·o·sis″to·kly′sis) [*hystera; kystis;* G. *kleisis,* a closing]. Operation for relief of vesico-uterovaginal fistula, consisting in turning the cervix uteri into the urinary bladder and suturing it. Also called *Bozeman's operation. Obs.*

hys″ter·o·cys′to·pex″y. See *ventrovesicofixation.*

hys″ter·o·de″mon·op′a·thy [*hystera;* G. *daimōn,* spirit; *pathos,* disease]. Hysteria characterized by demonomania; frequently accompanied by self-reproach and motivated by a strong sense of guilt.

hys″ter·o·dyn′i·a [*hystera;* G. *odynē,* pain]. Pain in the uterus.

hys″ter·o·ep′i·lep″sy [*hystera;* G. *epilēpsia,* a seizure]. A type of hysteria associated with convulsions similar to epileptic convulsions.

hys″ter·o·fren′ic [*hystera;* L. *frenum,* curb]. Capable of checking an attack of hysteria.

hys″ter·og′e·ny (hiss″tur·odj′i·nee) [*hystera;* G.

genesthai, from *gignesthai*, to be produced]. The induction of the hysteric state or paroxysm. —**hysterogen'ic, hysterog'enous,** *adj.*

hys"ter·og'ra·phy [*hystera;* G. *graphein*, to write]. Roentgenologic examination of the uterus.

hys'ter·oid, hys"ter·oi'dal [*hystera;* G. *eidos*, form]. Resembling hysteria.

hys"ter·o·lap"a·rot'o·my [*hystera;* G. *lapara*, soft part of the body between the ribs and the hip; *tomē*, a cutting]. Abdominal hysterectomy.

hys'ter·o·lith [*hystera;* G. *lithos*, stone]. A calculus in the uterus.

hys"ter·o·li·thi'a·sis [*hystera; lithos;* NL. *-iasis*, condition]. The formation of a concretion in the uterus.

hys"ter·ol'o·gy [*hystera;* G. *logos*, word]. That branch of medical science dealing with the anatomy, physiology, and pathology of the uterus. *Obs.*

hys"ter·ol'y·sis [*hystera;* G. *lysis*, a loosing]. Severing the attachments or adhesions of the uterus.

hys"ter·o·ma'ni·a [*hystera;* G. *mania*, madness]. 1. A state or condition of psychomotor overactivity seen in hysteria. *Rare.* 2. Nymphomania. *Rare.*

hys"ter·om'e·ter [*hystera;* G. *metron*, a measure]. An instrument for measuring the length of the intrauterine cavity. —**hysterometry,** *n.*

hys"ter·o·my·o'ma (hiss"tur·o·migh·o'muh) [*hystera;* G. *mys*, muscle; *-ōma*, tumor]. Myoma of the uterus.

hys"ter·o·my"o·mec'to·my [*hystera; mys;* G. *ektomē*, excision]. Surgical removal of a fibroid tumor of the uterus.

hys"ter·o·my·ot'o·my (hiss"tur·o·migh·ot'o·mee) [*hystera; mys;* G. *tomē*, a cutting]. Incision into the uterus for removal of a solid tumor.

hys"ter·o-o"o·pho·rec'to·my. The surgical removal of the uterus and ovaries.

hys"ter·op'a·thy [*hystera;* G. *pathos*, disease]. Any disease or disorder of the uterus. —**hysteropath'ic,** *adj.*

hys'ter·o·pex"y [*hystera;* G. *pēxis*, a fixing]. Fixation of the uterus by a surgical operation to correct displacement.

hys"ter·o·phil'i·a [*hystera;* G. *philein*, to love]. A term applied to certain psychosomatic disturbances resembling hysteria, such as migraine, asthma, intestinal spasm, or occupational cramps.

hys"ter·o·plas'ty [*hystera;* G. *plassein*, to mold]. A plastic operation on the uterus.

hys"ter·op·to'sis [*hystera;* G. *ptōsis*, a falling]. Falling or inversion of the uterus.

hys"ter·or'rha·phy [*hystera;* G. *rhaphē*, a suture]. The closure of a uterine incision or rent by suture.

hys"ter·or·rhex'is [*hystera;* G. *rhēxis*, a bursting]. Rupture of the uterus.

hys"ter·o·sal"pin·gec'to·my (·sal"pin·jeck'to-mee) [*hystera;* G. *salpigx*, trumpet; *ektomē*, excision]. Excision of the uterus and oviducts.

hys"ter·o·sal"pin·gog'ra·phy [*hystera; salpigx;* G. *graphein*, to write]. Roentgenographic examination of the uterus and oviducts after injection of a radiopaque substance; metrosalpingography. See also combined *gynecography.*

hys"ter·o·sal·pin"go-o"o·pho·rec'to·my (-o"o-fo·reck'to·mee, -o"off·o·reck'to·mee). Excision of the uterus, oviducts, and ovaries.

hys"ter·o·sal·pin"go-o"o·the·cec'to·my (-o"o-thi·seck'to·mee). Hysterosalpingo-oophorectomy.

hys"ter·o·sal"pin·gos'to·my [*hystera; salpigx;* G. *stoma*, mouth]. The establishment of an anastomosis between an oviduct and the uterus.

hys'ter·o·scope" [*hystera;* G. *skopein*, to examine]. A uterine speculum, with a reflector. —**hysteros'copy,** *n.*

hys'ter·o·tome" [*hystera;* G. *tomos*, cutting]. An instrument for incising the uterus.

hys"ter·ot'o·my [*hystera;* G. *tomē*, a cutting]. 1. Incision of the uterus. 2. A Cesarean section.

hys"ter·o·tra"che·lec'to·my (·tray"ki·leck'to-mee, ·track"i·leck'to·mee) [*hystera;* G. *trachēlos*, neck; *ektomē*, excision]. Amputation of the cervix of the uterus.

hys"ter·o·tra'che·lo·plas"ty (·tray'ki·lo·plas"tee, ·track'i·lo·plas"tee) [*hystera; trachēlos;* G. *plassein*, to form]. Plastic surgery on the cervix of the uterus.

hys"ter·o·tra"che·lor'rha·phy [*hystera; trachēlos;* G. *rhaphē*, a suture]. A plastic operation for the restoration of a lacerated cervix uteri.

hys"ter·o·tra"che·lot'o·my [*hystera; trachēlos;* G. *tomē*, a cutting]. Surgical incision of the cervix uteri.

hys"ter·o·trau'ma·tism [*hystera;* G. *trauma*, wound]. Hysteric symptoms due to or following a severe injury.

hytakerol. A trade-mark for dihydrotachysterol.

hy'ther [G. *hydōr*, water; *thermē*, heat]. The effect of the atmospheric heat and humidity on an organism.

I

I The chemical symbol for iodine; symbol for permanent incisor.

I[131] Symbol for the radioactive isotope of iodine of atomic weight 131. See Table of Radioactive and Other Isotopes in Appendix.

i Symbol for deciduous incisor.

i Iso-; optically inactive.

I.A.D.R. International Association for Dental Research.

IALA International Auxiliary Language Association.

i·am"a·tol'o·gy. The science or study of remedies.

i·at'ro- (eye·at'ro-, eye·ay'tro-) [G. *iatros*, physician]. A combining form signifying *a relation to medicine or to physicians.*

i·at"ro·chem'is·try [*iatros;* G. *chymos*, juice]. 1. The application of chemistry to therapeutics; the treatment of disease by chemical means. 2. The theory developed in the seventeenth century that disease and its treatment are explicable on a chemical basis.

i·at"ro·gen'ic [*iatros;* G. *genesthai*, from *gignesthai*, to be produced]. Induced by a physician; referring to the effects of a physician's words or actions upon the patient.

i·at"ro·phys'ics [*iatros;* G. *physikos*, natural]. 1. The treatment of disease by physical measures. 2. The theory that disease and its treatment are explicable on a materialistic or physical basis. The materialistic explanation of disease applied especially to a seventeenth-century theory that sought to explain physiologic and therapeutic facts by means of the principles of physics.

iberin. Trade-mark for a multivitamin capsule containing ferric iron.

i. ferrous. Trade-mark for a multivitamin capsule containing ferrous iron.

ibn al-Haitham. See *Alhazen.*

ibn Rushd. See *Averroës.*

ibn Sinā. See *Avicenna.*

ibn Zuhr. See *Avenzoar.*

i″bo·ga′ine (eye″bo·gay′een, ·in, i·bo′gay·een, ·in). $C_{52}H_{66}O_2N_6$. An alkaloid from the roots of *Tabernanthe iboga*, a plant of the Congo. It is said to act as a stimulant like caffeine; in overdose, it produces hallucination and paralysis.

-ic [L. *-icus;* G. *-ikos*]. 1. A suffix signifying *of* or *pertaining to.* 2. *In chemistry,* a suffix denoting *the higher of two valencies assumed by an element* and, incidentally, in many cases, *a larger amount of oxygen.*

ice [ME. *is*]. Water in its solid state, which it assumes at a temperature of 0° C. or 32° F. It is used externally in the form of applications and internally both as a refrigerant and to combat nausea.

dry i. Carbon dioxide in its solid state; used as an escharotic for the destruction of warts, hairy moles, and vascular nevi.

Ice′land moss. See *Cetraria,* 2.

Ice′land spar. A crystalline form of calcium carbonate, having doubly refracting properties, and used in polariscopes.

ich′no·gram (ick′no·gram) [G. *ichnos,* track; *gramma,* letter]. *In legal medicine,* the record of a footprint.

i′chor (eye′kor, eye′kur) [G. *ichōr,* juice, serous discharge]. An acrid, thin discharge from an ulcer or wound. —**ichorous, ichoroid,** *adj.*

i″chor·rhe′a, i″chor·rhoe′a (eye″ko·ree′uh) [*ichōr;* G. *rhoia,* flow]. A copious flow of ichor.

i″chor·rhe′mi·a, i″chor·rhae′mi·a (eye″ko·ree′mee·uh) [*ichōr;* G. *haima,* blood]. The presence of purulent material in the blood.

ichovar. A proprietary, quick-drying varnish containing ichthyol, camphor, and charcoal. Used in skin diseases.

ich′tham·mol (ick′thuh·mole, ·mol, ·mawl) (*ichthammol*). A reddish-brown to brownish-black, viscid fluid of characteristic odor; obtained by the destructive distillation of certain bituminous schists, followed by sulfonation of the distillate and neutralization with ammonia. It is used as a weak antiseptic and stimulant in skin diseases, usually in ointment form; it has been occasionally used internally as expectorant.

i. ointment (*unguentum ichthammolis*). A 10% ointment.

ichthargan. Trade-mark for a combination of silver and ichthyolsulfonic acid containing 30% of silver; it has been used as an astringent, antiphlogistic, and bactericide.

ichthoform. Trade-mark for ichthyol formaldehyde: formerly used as an intestinal antiseptic, antiphlogistic, and vulnerary. Dose, 1–2 Gm. (15–30 gr.).

ich′thu·lin (ick′thew·lin). A variety of protein derived from fish eggs.

ich″thy·is′mus (ick″thee·iz′mus), **ich′thy·ism** (ick′thee·iz·um) [G. *ichthys,* fish]. Poisoning due to the absorption of mytilotoxin in mussels or from eating spoiled fish.

ichthymall. A trade-mark for ichthammol.

ichthynat. A trade-mark for ichthammol.

ich′thy·o- (ick′thee·o-), **ichthy-** [*ichthys*]. A combining form meaning *fish.*

ich″thy·o·col′la [G. *ichthyokolla,* fish-glue]. Isinglass; a gelatinous substance prepared from the air bladders of the sturgeon and other fish, occurring in horny, translucent, white sheets which form a jelly when combined with hot water. Used as a food, an adhesive, and a clarifying agent.

ich′thy·oid [G. *ichthys,* fish; *eidos,* form]. Resembling or shaped like a fish.

ichthyol. Trade-mark for a brand of ichthammol.

ich′thy·ol form·al′de·hyde. See *ichthoform.*

ich″thy·ol′o·gy [*ichthys;* G. *logos,* word]. The study of fishes.

ich″thy·ol·sul·fon′ic ac′id. $C_{28}H_{38}O_6S_3$. An acid produced from Tyrolean bituminous material by the action of sulfuric acid. When neutralized with ammonia, it forms a compound of the type of ichthammol.

ich″thy·oph′a·gous [*ichthys;* G. *phagein,* to eat]. Eating or subsisting on fish.

ich″thy·o·pho′bi·a [*ichthys;* G- *phobos,* fear]. A morbid fear of fish. —**ichthyopho′bic,** *adj.*

ich″thy·o′sis [*ichthys;* G. *-ōsis,* condition]. A genodermatosis characterized by a dry harsh skin with adherent scales. Involvement is most severe on the extensor surfaces of the extremities. Histologically, the epidermis shows hyperkeratosis, absence of the granular layer, and thinning, and in the dermis, follicular keratin plugs and atrophy of the skin appendages. Also called *fishskin disease, xeroderma.* —**ichthyot′ic,** *adj.*

i. congenita. A severe form occurring as an intrauterine modification of the skin. The infant at birth is usually a nonviable monstrosity or death occurs after a few days. Its skin resembles a cracked and brittle coat of armor. Also called *harlequin fetus, keratosis universalis congenita.*

i. follicularis. The genodermatosis with moderate ichthyosis and associated baldness, absence of eyebrows and eyelashes, "trachoma," and conjunctivitis.

i. hystrix. A disease characterized by warty growths, consisting of elongated and hypertrophied papillae covered by greatly thickened epidermis; a type of nevus.

i. simplex. The common form which develops in early life, characterized by large, finely corrugated, papery scales with deficient secretions of sebaceous glands and sometimes of the sweat glands. Also called *i. vulgaris.*

i. vulgaris. See *i.* simplex.

ich″thy·o·tox′i·con [*ichthys;* G. *toxikon,* poison]. 1. The toxin present in the serum of certain fishes, as in that of the eel. 2. A general term for the active agent in poisoning from eating fish.

ich″thy·o·tox′in [*ichthys; toxikon*]. The toxic constituent of eel serum, apparently related to one of the bile acids.

ich″thy·o·tox·is′mus (ick″thee·o·tock·siz′mus) [*ichthys; toxikon*]. Food poisoning produced by eating fish, raw or canned, which contains toxic substances of bacterial origin.

i′con [G. *eikōn,* image]. An image or model.

i″co·nog′ra·phy [*eikōn;* G. *graphein,* to write]. 1. Graphic or plastic representation or illustration. 2. History and theory of the technics and styles of illustration or representation.

i·con″o·lag′ny (eye·kon″o·lag′nee, eye·kon′o·lag″-nee) [*eikōn;* G. *lagneia,* the act of coition]. Sexual stimulation induced by the sight of statues or pictures.

i·con″o·ma′ni·a [*eikōn;* G. *mania,* madness]. A morbid interest in images.

ICSH Interstitial-cell-stimulating hormone, also known as the *luteinizing hormone,* occurring in the anterior pituitary gland.

ICT Insulin coma therapy.

ic·ter′ic [G. *ikteros,* jaundice]. Pertaining to or characterized by jaundice.

ic″ter·o·gen′ic, ic″ter·og′e·nous (ick″tur·odj′inus) [*ikteros;* G. *genesthai,* from *gignesthai,* to be produced]. Causing icterus.

ic′ter·oid [*ikteros;* G. *eidos,* form]. Resembling the color of, or having the nature of, jaundice.

ic′ter·us [*ikteros*]. Jaundice. —**icter′ic,** *adj.*

chronic familial i. See hereditary *spherocytosis.*

diffusion i. That due to the hepatic cells having lost their power of holding back the bile, which consequently diffuses into the fluids of the body.

familial hemolytic i. See hereditary *spherocytosis.*

i. febrilis. See spirochetal *jaundice.*

i. gravis. Acute yellow atrophy of the liver, a disease characterized by jaundice, marked nervous symptoms, diminution in size of the liver, and a rapid, fatal termination. The urine contains bile and crystals of leucine and tyrosine.

i. index. The index of the bilirubin content of the blood as expressed by comparison of the color of the serum with the color of a 1:10,000 potassium dichromate solution. The normal range is from 4 to 6. From 6 to 15 is the zone of latent jaundice, in which the blood holds an amount of bilirubin above the normal without spilling it over into the scleras or other tissues. With an icterus index above 15, clinical jaundice is present.

i. neonatorum. That which is sometimes observed in infants during the first few days after birth. The causes are various and range from physiologic jaundice, which has no aftereffects, through that of erythroblastosis foetalis and septic jaundice, to the severe jaundice due to absence of the bile ducts.

i. saturninus. Jaundice from lead poisoning.

nuclear i. See *kernicterus.*

ic′tus [L., blow]. 1. An acute apoplectic attack. 2. An epileptic attack with no aura and a sudden onset. *Obs.* —**ic′tal,** *adj.*

id [L., it]. *In psychoanalysis,* the primitive, preformed psychic force in the unconscious, which is the source of the instinctive energy necessary for self-preservation and propagation.

-id [G. *-is, -idos*]. A suffix pertaining to a sensitivity state of the skin, which reacts to bacterial, fungal, or other agents emanating from a distant focus of infection. The site of the -id reaction is almost always free of the allergen (except in some of the granulomatous infections) and relief is obtained by hyposensitization and by therapy of the infection or focus of the infection.

i·de′a [G., form]. 1. A mental impression or thought; a belief or object existing in the mind or thought. 2. *In psychology,* a mental representation of something not actually perceived.

autochthonous i. An idea which appears to the patient as a finished product, having originated in his unconscious.

compulsive i. One involving an irresistible urge for action.

fixed i. An unfounded, delusional idea which the patient refuses to relinquish even after its disproof, and which controls all his actions.

imperative i. One which the patient dislikes, but which persists in his consciousness and dominates his will; characteristic of the compulsive and ruminative ideas in psychasthenia.

ruminative i. One which is pondered repeatedly.

i·de″al·i·za′tion [L. *idealis,* from *idea*]. *In psychoanalysis,* a sexual overevaluation of the love object.

i·de′as of ref′er·ence. *In psychopathology,* a symptom complex, in which through the mechanism of projection the individual believes himself to be the object of ill will and evil intentions of those about him. All remarks overheard are taken egocentrically and interpreted as derogatory. The symptom is most commonly observed in various paranoid reactions, the paranoid type of schizophrenic reaction, and in manic-depressive reactions.

i″de·a′tion [*idea*]. The formation of a mental conception; the cerebral action by which, or in accord with which, an idea is formed. —**idea′tional,** *adj.*

i·den″ti·fi·ca′tion [F. *identifier,* from L. *idem,* the same]. 1. The classification, description, and registration of a specimen or a person by certain physical characteristics. 2. *In psychopathology,* a mental mechanism of defense in which one unconsciously assumes, on the basis of love or aggression, the characteristics of another.

anthropometric i. See Bertillon system of *i.*

Bertillon system of i. That method which uses those skeletal measurements which remain practically unchanged after adult life is reached. Syn., *anthropometric i.*

Galton system of i. That method based upon fingerprints. The records used are the printed impressions of the ten digits placed in definite order upon a card.

palm and sole system of i. An extension of the Galton system to include the palmar and plantar surfaces.

id′e·o- (id′ee·o-, eye′dee·o-) [G. *idea,* form]. A combining form meaning *idea.*

id″e·o·ge·net′ic [*idea;* G. *genesis,* production]. Relating to mental activity in which primary sense-impressions are employed in place of completed ideas.

id″e·o·glan′du·lar [*idea;* L. *glandula,* dim. of *glans,* acorn]. Relating to glandular activity as evoked by a mental concept.

id″e·ol′o·gy (id″ee·ol′o·jee, eye″dee·) [*idea;* G. *logos,* word]. The science of ideas.

id″e·o·me·tab′o·lism [*idea;* G. *metabolē,* change]. Metabolic processes induced by mental and emotional causes. —**ideometabol′ic,** *adj.*

id″e·o·mo′tor [*idea;* L. *motum,* from *movere,* to move]. Pertaining to nonvoluntary movement which results from some idea.

id″e·o·mus′cu·lar [*idea;* L. *musculus,* muscle]. Pertaining to nonvoluntary muscular movement produced by a mental concept.

id″e·o·pho′bi·a [*idea;* G. *phobos,* fear]. A morbid fear of ideas.

id′e·o·plas″ty [*idea;* G. *plassein,* to mold]. The process of making the subject's mind receptive to the suggestions of the hypnotizer. —**ideoplas′tic,** *adj.*

id″e·o·syn·chy′si·a (id″ee·o·sin·kigh′zee·uh, eye″-dee·o·), **id″e·o·syn′chy·sis** (·sing′ki·sis) [*idea;* G. *sygchysis,* a mixture]. Delirium. *Obs.*

id″e·o·vas′cu·lar [*idea;* L. *vasculum,* small vessel]. Relating to a vascular change resulting from an emotional impression.

id′i·o- [G. *idios,* one's own]. 1. A combining form meaning *one's own, separate, distinct.* 2. *In biochemistry* and *medicine,* a combining form meaning *self-produced.*

id′i·o·blast″. See *biophore.*

id″i·o·chro′mo·some [*idios;* G. *chrōma,* color; *sōma,* body]. A sex chromosome.

id″i·oc′ra·sy, id″i·o·cra′sis [G. *idiokrasia,* peculiar temperament]. Idiosyncrasy. —**idiocrat′ic,** *adj.*

id″i·oc·to′ni·a [G. *idios,* one's own; *ktonos,* murder]. Self-murder; suicide. *Obs.*

id′i·o·cy [G. *idiōtēs,* private person, ignoramus]. The lowest grade of mental deficiency, in which the subject's mental age is under 3 years and the I.Q. under 25; usually congenital, and accompanied by physical defects.

amaurotic familial i. See *amaurotic* familial idiocy.

hydrocephalic i. That due to hydrocephaly, whether congenital or acquired.

microcephalic i. That form associated with an abnormally small head.

Mongolian i. See *mongolism*.

moral i. That in which all feeling for or interest in others is entirely absent.

id″i·og′a·mist [G. *idios*, one's own; *gamos*, marriage]. One who is capable of coitus only with his marital partner or with a few women, and impotent with women in general.

id″i·o·gen′e·sis [*idios;* G. *genesis*, production]. Self-origin; referring to idiopathic diseases.

id″i·o·glos′si·a [*idios;* G. *glōssa*, tongue]. Any form of speech or utterance invented by an individual and unique with him, usually incomprehensible to others; in a very young child, a transition stage towards normal speech which may be understood by his parents and associates; in one in whom normal speech development may be expected, it often represents a psychopathological process. **—idioglot′tic,** *adj.*

id″i·o·hyp′no·tism [*idios;* G. *hypnos*, sleep]. Self-induced hypnotism.

id″i·ol′o·gism [*idios;* G. *logos*, word]. A form of utterance peculiar to any person, especially a speech defect.

id″i·o·me·tri′tis [*idios;* G. *mētra*, womb; *-itis*, inflammation]. Inflammation of the parenchymatous substance of the uterus. *Obs.*

id″i·o·mus′cu·lar [*idios;* L. *musculus*, muscle]. Referring to muscular tissue independent of any nerve stimulus.

id″i·o·neu·ro′sis [*idios;* G. *neuron*, nerve; *-ōsis*, condition]. A neurosis. *Obs.*

id″i·op′a·thy [*idios;* G. *pathos*, disease]. 1. A primary disease; one not a result of any other disease, but of spontaneous origin. 2. Disease for which no cause is known. **—idiopath′ic, idiopathet′ic,** *adj.*

id′i·o·plasm″ [*idios; plasma*, anything formed]. *In biology*, a hypothetic structural unit of the germ plasm, according to Weismann's theory. *Obs.*

id″i·o·psy·chol′o·gy [*idios;* G. *psychē*, soul; *logos*, word]. Psychology based upon introspective study of one's own mental acts.

id″i·o·re′flex [*idios;* L. *reflexum*, from *reflectere*, to bend back]. A reflex arising from a stimulus originating within the organ itself.

id″i·o·ret′i·nal [*idios;* L. *rete*, net]. Peculiar or proper to the retina.

id′i·o·some″, id′i·o·zome″ [*idios;* G. *soma*, body]. The central apparatus of an auxocyte, especially a spermatocyte, including the surrounding Golgi apparatus and mitochondria.

id′i·o·spasm [*idios;* G. *spasmos*, spasm]. A spasm confined to one part. **—idiospas′tic,** *adj.*

id″i·o·syn′cra·sy [G. *idiosygkrasia*, from *idios*, *sygkrasis*, a mingling together]. 1. Any special or peculiar characteristic or temperament by which a person differs from other persons. 2. A peculiarity of constitution that makes an individual react differently from most persons to drugs or treatments. **—idiosyncrat′ic,** *adj.*

id′i·ot. A person afflicted with idiocy.

i.-savant. An individual with general mental deficiency as measured by the intelligence quotient, but with some peculiar and isolated talent along special lines, such as music, mathematics, manual dexterity.

id″i·o·ven·tric′u·lar [*idios;* L. *ventriculus*, dim. of *venter*, belly]. Pertaining to the ventricle of the heart alone, and not affecting the atrium.

id′i·o·zome″. See *idiosome.*

id′i·tol. $CH_2OH.HCOH.HOCH.HCOH.HOCH.$-$CH_2OH$; L-iditol; an alcohol formed by reduction of the ketohexose L-sorbose.

idocol. Trade-mark for a colloidal iodine preparation containing 20% of iodine.

i·dol″o·ma′ni·a (eye·dol″o·may′nee·uh) [G. *eidōlon*, idol; *mania*, madness]. Exaggerated idolatry.

id′ose. A synthetic hexose sugar; isomeric with glucose.

i·dro′sis. Hidrosis.

i″ga·su′ric ac′id. An organic acid found in the seeds of nux vomica.

ig·na′ti·a [NL.]. St. Ignatius' bean. The seed of *Strychnos ignati;* contains the alkaloids strychnine and brucine. Its therapeutic effects are similar to those of nux vomica.

ig′ni·punc″ture [L. *ignis*, fire; *punctura*, a pricking]. Puncture with metal needles heated to either red or white heat.

ig·ni′tion (ig·nish′un) [*ignis*]. The process of heating solids until all volatile matter has been driven off. When performed in the presence of air, oxidizable matter such as carbon is burned.

Il Chemical symbol for illinium.

il″e·ec′to·my [G. *eilein*, to roll; *ektomē*, excision]. Excision of the ileum.

il″e·i′tis [*eilein;* G. *-itis*, inflammation]. Inflammation of the ileum. **—ileit′ic,** *adj.*

regional i. A chronic, nonspecific, granulomatous process frequently involving the terminal portion of the ileum, but occasionally extending into the colon or arising in the more proximal portions of the ileum. Also called *terminal i.*, *Crohn's disease.*

il′e·o- [*eilein*]. A combining form denoting *the ileum.*

il″e·o·ce·cos′to·my [*eilein;* L. *caecus*, blind; *stoma*, mouth]. The formation of an anastomosis between the cecum and the ileum.

il″e·o·ce′cum [*eilein; caecus*]. The ileum and the cecum regarded as one organ. **—ileocecal,** *adj.*

il″e·o·col′ic [*eilein;* G. *kolon*, colon]. Pertaining conjointly to the ileum and the colon.

il″e·o·co·li′tis [*eilein; kolon;* G. *-itis*, inflammation]. Inflammation of the ileum and the colon.

il·e·op′a·gus. See *iliopagus.*

il″e·o·co·los′to·my [*eilein; kolon;* G. *stoma*, mouth]. The establishment of an anastomosis between the ileum and the colon.

il″e·o·il″e·os′to·my [*eilein; eilein; stoma*]. The establishment of an anastomosis between two different parts of the ileum.

il″e·or′rha·phy [*eilein;* G. *rhaphē*, a suture]. Suture of the ileum.

il″e·o·sig″moid·os′to·my [*eilein;* G. *sigmoeidēs*, crescent-shaped; *stoma*, mouth]. The surgical formation of an anastomosis between the ileum and the sigmoid colon.

il″e·os′to·my [*eilein; stoma*]. The surgical formation of a fistula or artificial anus through the abdominal wall into the ileum.

il″e·ot′o·my [*eilein;* G. *tomē*, a cutting]. Surgical incision of the ileum.

Iletin. Trade-mark for a brand of insulin.

il′e·um [*eilein*]. The lower portion of the small intestine, extending from the jejunum to the large intestine. See Plate 13. **—il′eal, ileac,** *adj.*

il′e·us [G. *eileos*, intestinal obstruction]. Acute intestinal obstruction resulting from the interference of proper propulsion of intestinal contents, due either to functional or mechanical causes. The stasis of intestinal contents is followed by distention of the intestinal lumen and by systemic manifestations, as colicky pain, vomiting, dehydration, blood chemical changes, and toxemia. The condition may end fatally if not relieved.

acute duodenal i. Caused by obstruction of the lumen of the duodenum following operations or resulting from external pressure. Also called *arteriomesenteric i.; gastromesenteric i.*

adynamic i. Intestinal paresis thought to be due to hyperactive sympathetic influence, which follows almost all intraabdominal operations or other processes which supposedly cause splanchnic nerve irritation: also called *inhibitory i., paralytic i., reflex i., reflex inhibition i.*

decompensational i. A late phase in ileus in which the gut is so distended that the smooth muscle has lost its contractile properties.

dynamic i. Spastic *i.*

inhibitory i. See adynamic *i.*

mechanical i. Obstruction of the intestines by extrinsic pressure or internal blockage, due to a variety of causes.

meconium i. Intestinal obstruction caused by inspissation of the meconium, occurring in the newborn with cystic fibrosis of the pancreas.

metabolic i. Ileus resulting from interference with the function of the smooth muscles of the intestines, due to metabolic disturbances.

paralytic i. See adynamic *i.*

reflex i., reflex inhibition i. See adynamic *i.*

spastic i. Spastic contraction of a section of the bowel, usually the colon, causing obstruction. Syn., *dynamic i.*

il′i·a. Plural of ilium.

il′i·ac. Pertaining to the ilium.

i·li′a·cus. The portion of the iliopsoas muscle arising from the iliac fossa and sacrum.

i. minor. A variant of the iliacus muscle inserted into the capsule of the hip joint.

il″i·a·del′phus. See *iliopagus.*

il′i·o- [L. *ilium*, flank]. A combining form meaning *relating to the ilium; iliac.*

il″i·o·cap″su·lar′is. The iliacus minor muscle.

il″i·o·cap″su·lo·tro″chan·ter′i·cus. A variant of the iliacus minor muscle in which some fibers also insert into the lesser trochanter.

il″i·o·coc·cyg′e·al (il″ee·o·cock·sidj′ee·ul) [*ilium;* G. *kokkyx*, cuckoo]. Pertaining to the ilium and the coccyx, as the iliococcygeal muscle.

il″i·o·coc·cyg′e·us. The portion of the levator ani muscle overlying the obturator internus muscle.

il″i·o·cos·tal′is. The BR name for the iliocostalis lumborum muscle.

i. cervicis. That portion of the sacrospinalis muscle arising from the upper six ribs and inserted into the posterior tubercle of the transverse processes of the middle cervical vertebrae.

i. dorsi. That portion of the sacrospinalis muscle arising from the lower six ribs and inserted into the upper six ribs.

i. lumborum. That portion of the sacrospinalis muscle which arises from the lumbar vertebrae and adjacent area and is inserted into the lower six ribs.

il″i·o·cos″to·cer″vi·cal′is [*ilium;* L. *costa*, rib; *cervix*, neck]. A muscle composed of the iliocostalis cervicis and the iliocostalis dorsi. See Table of Muscles in the Appendix.

il″i·o·fem′o·ral [*ilium;* L. *femur*, thigh]. Pertaining conjointly to the ilium and the femur, as the iliofemoral ligament.

il″i·o·hy″po·gas′tric [*ilium;* G. *hypo*, under; *gastēr*, belly]. Pertaining conjointly to the ilium and the hypogastrium, as the iliohypogastric nerve. See Table of Nerves in the Appendix.

il″i·o·in′gui·nal [*ilium;* L. *inguen*, groin]. 1. Pertaining to the ilium and the groin. 2. Lying partly within the iliac and partly within the inguinal region, as the ilioinguinal nerve. See Table of Nerves in the Appendix.

il″i·op′a·gus [*ilium;* G. *pagos*, that which is fixed]. Conjoined twins united in the iliac region. Syn., *iliadelphus.*

il″i·o·par″a·si′tus [*ilium;* G. *parasitos*, parasite]. Parasitic, supernumerary limbs attached to one or both ilia.

il″i·o·pec·tin′e·al (il″ee·o·peck·tin′ee·ul, ·peck″ti-nee′ul) [*ilium;* L. *pecten*, comb, hair of the pubes]. Pertaining conjointly to the ilium and the pubis, as iliopectineal line.

il″i·o·pso′as (il″ee·o·so′us, il″ee·op′so·us) [*ilium;* G. *psoa*, muscles of the loins]. Pertaining conjointly to the ilium and the loin, as the iliopsoas muscle.

il″i·o·sac·ral′is. An occasional band of muscle ventral to the coccygeus, extending from the iliopectineal line to the lateral border of sacrum.

il″i·o·tho″ra·cop′a·gus [*ilium;* G. *thōrax*, thorax; *pagos*, that which is fixed]. Conjoined twins united laterally at their thoracic and iliac regions.

il″i·o·xi·phop′a·gus (il″ee·o·zi·fop′uh·gus) [*ilium;* G. *xiphos*, sword; *pagos*]. Conjoined twins united from the xiphoid to the iliac region.

il′i·um (pl. *ilia*) [L.]. 1. The flank. 2. The superior broad portion of the hipbone, a separate bone in the fetus. See Plates 1, 2, 14, and *coxae* in Table of Bones in the Appendix.

ill [ME.]. Not healthy; sick; indisposed.

il·laq″ue·a′tion (i·lack″wee·ay′shun, il″ack·) [L. *illaqueare*, to ensnare]. The correction of an ingrowing eyelash by drawing it with a loop through an opening in the lid. —**illaq′ueate,** *v.*

il″le·git′i·mate [L. *illegitimus*, unlawful]. 1. Not in accordance with statutory law. 2. Born out of wedlock; bastard. —**illegitimacy,** *n.*

il·lic′i·um (i·liss′ee·um) [L., that which entices] Star anise. The fruit of *Illicium verum;* yields a volatile oil consisting chiefly of anethol; may be used to prepare anise oil. The fruits known commercially as Japanese star anise are poisonous.

il″li·ni′tion (il″i·nish′un) [L. *illinire*, to besmear]. A rubbing in or on; inunction.

il·lin′i·um [from *Illinois*, *-ium*]. Il = 145 *ca.* A rare earth element, atomic number 61, reported in 1926 by B. S. Hopkins. Prior discovery has been claimed by Rolla and Fernandez, who named the element *florentium.* Both claims have been challenged, while other investigators have reported discovery of synthetic forms of element 61 and proposed the names *cyclonium* and *promethium.* It is now called *promethium*

ill′ness [ME.]. 1. The state of being ill or sick. 2. A malady; sickness; disease; disorder.

il·lu′mi·nance. That amount of light incident per unit area of a surface.

il·lu″mi·na′tion [L. *illuminare*, to make light]. 1. The lighting up or illuminating, as of a surface or cavity, in the examination of a patient. 2. The quantity of light thrown upon an object. 3. *In microscopy*, the type or direction of light thrown upon the object studied.

axial i. Illumination by light conveyed in the direction of the optical axis of the objective and ocular of the microscope.

central i. *In microscopy*, an illumination produced by the rays of light reflected from the mirror passing perpendicularly through the object.

critical i. That in which the image of a small source of light is focused exactly at the object on the stage of the microscope.

dark-field i. Illumination by which light enters the objective only if reflected, refracted, or scattered by the object, making it or its parts appear bright against a dark background. The central rays of light are obliterated by a central stop, in or below the condenser; a hollow cone of peripheral rays strikes the object obliquely from the side. Used especially for the examination of spirochetes.

dark-ground i. See dark-field *i.*

focal i. Light concentrated upon an object by means of a lens or mirror.

i. by transmitted light. *In microscopy,* the usual method of illuminating an object by sending a beam of light, concentrated by a substage condenser, through the object. If the beam is centered in the optical axis, the illumination is axial; if it strikes the objective at an angle to the optical axis, it is a form of oblique illumination.

Köhler's method of i. A method of microscopical illumination in which an image of the source is focused in the lower focal plane of the microscope condenser, and the condenser, in turn, focuses an image of the lamp lens in the object field.

oblique i. Illumination of an object by throwing light upon it, or through it, obliquely. Also called *lateral i.*

orthogonal i. The system of slit ultramicroscopical arrangement, the line of observation and the line of illumination being at right angles to each other.

vertical i. Microscopical illumination in which a beam of light is thrown on the object from above, or from the direction of observation. Also called *direct i.*

il·lu′mi·nism [*illuminare*]. A mental state in which the subject imagines that he converses with supernatural beings.

il·lu′sion [L., from *illudere,* to mock]. A false interpertation of a real sensation; a perception which misinterprets the object perceived. —**illusional,** *adj.*

il·lu′sor·y vis′u·al spread. Perseveration in space of a visual image; extension of part of a visual image outside its own boundaries.

ilotycin. A trade-mark for the antibiotic substance *erythromycin.*

I.M., i.m. Abbreviation for *intramuscular.*

im-. *In chemistry,* a prefix used to indicate the bivalent group NH.

i′ma [L. *imus,* lowest]. The lowest.

imadyl. Trade-mark for an unction containing histamine dihydrochloride in an absorbable base. Used in rheumatoid and arthritic conditions.

im′age [L. *imago,* image]. 1. A more or less accurate representation of an object. 2. The picture of an object formed by a lens; a collection of foci, each corresponding to a point in the object. 3. *In psychoanalysis,* see *imago,* 2. See also *afterimage.*

accidental i. See *afterimage.*

acoustic i. An idea of something which has been heard.

aerial i. A real image formed on a screen or any surface becomes an aerial image, existing in space.

body-i. *In psychiatry,* the concept which each person has of his own body as an object in and bound by space.

direct i. A picture obtained by rays that have not yet come to a focus. Also called *erect i.*

double i. The two images, known as true and false, which occur when one eye deviates, when the visual lines of the two eyes are not directed toward the same object.

false i. In diplopia, the image of the deviating eye; it is not on the macula, but is projected to a peripheral part of the retina.

inverted i. One turned upside down; the image on the retina is always inverted.

ocular i. That which reaches consciousness through the eye; determined by the dioptric image, also by the anatomic and physiologic modification imposed upon it before it reaches the brain.

parent i. See *imago,* 2.

Purkinje-Sanson images. A set of three images which may be seen reflected from the surface of the cornea, the anterior surface of the lens, and the posterior surface of the lens of the eye, respectively.

real i. One formed by the meeting of rays; an image formed of real foci.

retinal i. The image of external objects as focused on the retina.

true i. In diplopia, the image received by the undeviated eye, projected on the macula.

virtual i. One which can be seen only by looking through a lens or at a mirror; formed of diverging rays which are prolonged backward until they meet at a point. An image formed of virtual foci.

im·ag″i·na′tion [L. *imaginatio,* from *imaginari,* to imagine]. The picture-making power of the mind. The faculty by which one creates new ideas or mental pictures by means of separate data derived from experience, ideally revivified, extended, and combined in new forms.

i·ma′go [L., image]. 1. The adult, sexually mature stage of an insect. 2. *In psychoanalysis,* the childhood conception of the parent or of some loved person, which is carried into adulthood and retained in the unconscious. The term implies that the image is only partly based on reality.

im″a·pun′ga. A disease occurring to a limited extent among African cattle; closely related in pathology to African horse sickness.

im′a·zine. An organic compound containing the trivalent radical —C:N.CH:N—.

im·bal′ance [L. *in-,* not; *bilanx,* having two scales]. 1. Lack of balance. 2. Lack of muscular balance especially between the muscles of the eyes.

autonomic i. Lack of regulation of equilibrium particularly of the peripheral blood vessels; if severe enough may cause either hyperemia or ischemia. Also called *sympathetic imbalance, vasomotor instability.*

gene i. A chemical or morphologic change in the gene complex resulting in a modification of hereditary characteristics.

im′be·cile [L. *imbecillus,* weak, feeble]. One who is afflicted with imbecility.

im″be·cil′i·ty [*imbecillus*]. An intermediate grade of mental deficiency, in which the subject's mental age is between three and seven years and his I.Q. between 25 and 49.

im·bed′. See *embed, implantation,* 3.

im″bi·bi′tion (im″bi·bish′un) [L. *imbibere,* to drink in]. The absorption of liquid by a solid or a gel. —**imbibe′,** *v.*

imbicoll. Trade-mark for a bulk-producing mechanical laxative in granular form, consisting chiefly of a sterculia gum derivative.

im″bri·ca′tion [L. *imbricare,* to cover with tiles]. *In surgery,* closing wounds or covering deficiencies with tissue arranged in layers overlapping one another. —**im′bricated,** *adj.*

i. lines. The outcroppings of the incremental (Retzius) lines of the dental enamel upon the surface of the crown: also called *perikymaties.*

Imhotep. Ancient Egyptian physician (about 3000 B.C.); vizier and physician to King Zoser; later (about 500 B.C.) deified as a god of medicine, and as Imonthes the Greeks identified him with Asclepios.

im′id. See *imide.*

im″id·az′ole (im″id·az′ole, ·ay′zole, im″id·uh-zole′). NH.CH:N.CH:CH. A substance, readily synthesized, which is of interest because of the importance of a number of its derivatives, such as histamine, histidine, privine. Syn., *glyoxaline.*

im″id·az″ole·lac′tic ac′id. $C_3H_3N_2.CH_2.CHOH.$-

COOH; β-imidazolyllactic acid; a hydrolytic deamination product of histidine. It is partially effective as a dietary substitute for histidine.

im″id·az″ole·py·ru′vic ac′id. $C_3H_3N_2.CH_2.CO.$-COOH; β-imidazolylpyruvic acid; an intermediate product in the breakdown of histidine to glutamic acid, formic acid, and ammonia; it is produced by oxidative deamination of histidine.

im″id·az′o·lines. Derivatives of the compound, $NH.CH{:}N.CH_2.CH_2$. They show a variety of physiologic actions.

im″id·az′o·lyl. One of four univalent, isomeric radicals, $C_3H_3N_2$—, derived from imidazole.

im′ide, im′id. Any compound of the radical NH united to a divalent acid radical.

imido. Trade-mark for a brand of histamine dihydrochloride; a preparation used like histamine phosphate.

i·mi′do- (i·mee′do-, im′i·do-). *In chemistry*, a combining form denoting *imide*.

i·min′a·zole (i·min′uh·zole, i·mee′nuh·, im″i·nay′·). Imidazole.

i·mi′no- (i·mee′no-, im′i·no). *In chemistry*, a combining form designating the bivalent group NH when attached to or in nonacid radicals.

i·mi′no ac′id. An organic acid that contains the bivalent imino group (=NH). Imino acids are in some instances intermediaries in the metabolism of amino acids.

i·mi″no·glu·tar′ic ac′id. $COOH.CH_2.CH_2.C{:}$-$NH.COOH$; α-iminoglutaric acid, obtained by reduction of L-glutamic acid, the reaction being catalyzed by the enzyme glutamic dehydrogenase.

i·mi″no·u·re′a. Guanidine.

im″i·ta′tion [L. *imitari*, to imitate]. *In psychology*, the performance of an act as a result of seeing another person do the same thing; behaving in the manner in which another has been seen to behave.

morbid i. The occurrence of a convulsive or mental affection after observing a similar affection in another.

im″ma·ture′ [L. *immaturus*, not ripe]. Unripe; not yet adult or fully developed.

im·me′di·ate [L. *in-*, not; LL. *mediare*, to halve]. Direct; without the intervention of anything.

im·med′i·ca·ble [*in-;* L. *medicare*, to cure]. Characterizing that which does not yield to medicine or treatment; incurable.

im·mer′sion [L. *immersio*, from *immergere*, to plunge into]. The plunging of a body into a liquid.

homogeneous i. A fluid between the objective or condenser of a microscope, and the cover glass or slide, having about the same refractive and dispersive power as the glass.

im·mer′sion blast. See *blast injury*.

im·mer′sion foot. A serious and disabling condition of the feet due to prolonged immersion in sea water at 60° F. or lower, but not at freezing temperature. A condition similar to trench foot.

im·mer′sion lens. See under *lens*.

im·mer′sion oil. An oil, such as cedar, especially prepared to have a refractive index of 1.515 at 18° C.

im·mis′ci·ble [L. *in-*, not; *miscere*, to mix]. Not capable of being mixed.

im·mo″bi·li·za′tion [L. *immobilis*, immovable]. The act of rendering motionless, such as immobilization of a joint by means of splints in surgery.

im″mor·tal′i·ty [L. *immortalitas*, immortality]. *In psychiatry*, the belief or delusion that the person has always existed and will live forever; a delusion of timelessness.

im·mune′ [L. *immunis*, free from a public service]. Safe from attack; protected against a disease by an innate or an acquired immunity.

im·mu′ni·ty [*immunis*]. The condition of a living organism whereby it resists and overcomes infection.

acquired i. That obtained by a living organism as the result of active or passive immunity.

active i. That possessed by an organism as the result of disease or unrecognized infection, or that induced by immunization with bacteria or products of bacterial growth.

antiblastic i. One due to an antagonism for the development of microorganisms in tissues.

athreptic i. One caused by the failure of an infecting organism to find the necessary conditions for the production of infection.

herd i. Resistance of a group of animals to a specific infection from without.

individual i. The particular power of certain individuals to resist or overcome infection.

infection i. One due to the persistence of an infection, as in syphilis, the virus diseases, etc.

innate i. See native *i.*

local i. One confined to a given tissue or area of the body. Syn., *tissue i.*

native i. A constitutional attribute of individuals or various taxonomic groups of individuals, associated with a certain degree of resistance to a particular living or inanimate noxious agent. Among the important factors involved in this resistance are inflammation, humoral and tissue bacteriostatic and bactericidal agents, mechanical tissue barriers (epithelium), and endocrine balance. Environmental factors such as nutrition and climate may adversely or favorably modify this resistance. A strict demarcation between native and acquired immunity is not always possible. Syn., *innate i.*, *natural i.*, *natural resistance.*

nonspecific i. One produced by the introduction of microorganisms containing group antigens.

passive i. (a) That conferred through the parenteral injection of antibodies prepared in the lower animals or other human beings. (b) Immunity acquired by the child *in utero* by the placental transfer of antibodies from the mother.

racial i. Apparent differences in susceptibility among different races of the same species.

tissue i. See local *i.*

im″mu·ni·za′tion [*immunis*]. The act or process of rendering immune to a communicable disease. See booster *dose*. —**im′munize,** *v.*

i. register. 1. A form on which are recorded all immunizations or inoculations given to an individual. 2. Specifically, *in U.S. Army medicine*, the form given to a soldier.

im·mu′no- [*immunis*]. A combining form signifying *immune.*

im·mu″no·chem′is·try [*immunis;* G. *chymos*, juice]. That branch of science which deals with the chemical changes and phenomena of immunity; specifically, the chemistry of antigens, antibodies, and their reactions.

im·mu″no·gen′ic [*immunis;* G. *genesthai*, from *gignesthai*, to be produced]. Producing immunity.

im·mu′no-he″ma·tol′o·gy. A subdivision of both hematology and immunology which developed from immunology and genetics in relation to blood-cell antigens and their antibodies.

im″mu·nol′o·gist [*immunis;* G. *logos*, word]. A specialist in the science of immunity.

im″mu·nol′o·gy [*immunis; logos*]. That science which is concerned with the study of immunity. —**immunolog′ic,** *adj.*

im·mu″no·ther′a·py. See *serotherapy.*

im·mu″no·trans·fu′sion [*immunis;* L. *transfusio*, from *transfundere*, to pour off]. Transfusion with the blood of a donor previously rendered immune by repeated inoculations with a given agent.

im·pac′tion [L. *impactio*, from *impingere*]. 1. The state of being lodged and retained in a part or strait. 2. *In dentistry,* confinement of a tooth in the jaw so that its eruption is prevented. 3. *In surgery,* a condition in which a fragment of bone is firmly driven into another fragment of bone so that neither can move against the other. —**im·pact′ed,** *adj.*

im·pal′pa·ble [L. *in-*, not; *palpare*, to feel]. Not capable of being felt; imperceptible to the touch.

im′par [L., unequal]. Without a fellow; azygous.

im·par″i·dig′i·tate (im·par″i·didj′i·tayt) [*impar;* L. *digitatus*, having fingers]. Having an uneven number of fingers or toes.

im·passe′. *In psychoanalysis,* a stalemate in the therapeutic process with a breakdown in controlled emotional communication between patient and therapist.

im·pe′dance [L. *impedire*, to entangle the feet, impede]. The apparent resistance of a circuit to the flow of an alternating electric current.

im′pe·din [*impedire*]. An agent antagonistic to the antimicrobic powers of the body.

im·per′a·tive [L. *imperare*, to order]. Peremptory, absolute; compulsory; binding.

im″per·a·to′rin. $C_{16}H_{14}O_4$; a hydroxy-furocouramin ether from the rhizome of *Peucedanum ostruthium* (formerly *Imperatoria ostruthium*), identical with ammidin from *Ammi majus*.

im″per·cep′tion [L. *in-*, not; *perceptio*, from *percipere*, to perceive]. Defective perception.

im·per′fo·rate [*in-;* L. *perforare*, to bore through]. Without the normal opening. —**imperfora′tion,** *n.*

im·pe′ri·al green. Copper acetoarsenite; Paris green.

im·per′me·a·ble [*in-;* L. *permeare*, to pass through]. Not permitting a passage.

im·per′vi·ous [*in-;* L. *pervius*, passable]. Not permitting a passage, especially of fluids.

im″pe·tig″i·ni·za′tion (im″pi·tidj″i·ni·zay′shun, ·nigh·zay′shun) [L. *impetigo*, from *impetere*, to attack]. Lesions of impetigo occurring on a previous skin lesion.

im″pe·ti′go [L.]. An acute, inflammatory skin disease which may be circinate, bullous, gyrate, or furfuraceous in character. —**impetig′inous, impetig′inoid,** *adj.*

Bockhart's i. See *i.* follicularis.

bullous i. A type of impetigo characterized by bullae. It is seen usually in children, but also in adults with continued exposure to heat and humidity. The lesions develop particularly on the axillae, groins, intergluteal areas, arms, thighs, chest, and abdomen. Also called *tropical i.*, *i. neonatorum.*

i. circinata. A form characterized by a circle or semicircle of small vesicles or pustules; there are usually many such circles.

i. circumpilaris. See *i.* follicularis.

i. contagiosa. The highly contagious form of impetigo, due to *Micrococcus pyogenes* or *Streptococcus pyogenes*, characterized by vesicles, pustules, and crusts. It is commonly found on exposed parts of the body and heals without sequelae. Also called *i. vulgaris.* See Plate 31.

i. follicularis. A form of micrococcal (staphylococcal) infection of hair follicles characterized by vesicles 1 to 5 mm. in size at the pilosebaceous orifice, drying in about 5 days to form yellowish crusts: also called *Bockhart's i.* Syn., *i. circumpilaris.*

i. herpetiformis. A rare disease of the skin characterized by the formation of superficial miliary pustules that may be discrete but tend to form circular groups. Most cases of this disease have occurred in pregnant women; it is often fatal.

i. neonatorum. A form of bullous impetigo occurring in the newborn.

i. variolosa. That form occurring between the drying-up pustules of smallpox.

i. vulgaris. See *i.* contagiosa.

tropical i. See bullous *i.*

im·pin′ger (im·pin′jur) [L. *impingere*, to strike against]. An instrument for determining the number of dust particles in the air. A measured air sample is propelled through an underwater jet against a perpendicular plate. The dust is collected in the water, which is transferred to a shallow chamber in which the suspended particles can be counted under a microscope. Other instruments used for the same purpose are the jet dust counter, konimeter, and precipitator. Also see *dust count.*

im″plan·ta′tion [F. *implanter*, from L. *in*, in; *planta*, sprout]. 1. The act of setting in, as the transplantation of a tissue, tooth, duct, or organ from one place in the body to another, or from the body of one person to that of another, implying the placing of the tissue in depth, as distinguished from the placement of a surface graft. Tissue implants are sometimes used as guides or ladders for the restoration of damaged nerve trunks and tendons. 2. The placement within the body tissues of a substance, such as tantalum, vitallium, wire filigree, for restoration by mechanical means; as, for example, the closure of a bone defect or the repair of a ventral hernia. 3. The imbedding of the embryo into, or on, the endometrium. —**implant′,** *v,* **im′plant,** *n.*

i. of the bile ducts. The placement of the proximal end of the common or the hepatic duct into the wall of the duodenum, stomach, or jejunum for the cure of biliary fistula.

i. of the ureters. The transfer of the distal ends of the ureters into the intestine or the skin after cystectomy for malignant disease and in certain cases of exstrophy.

pellet i. Administration of hormone products by implantation of pellets of solid active material under the skin.

im′plants [*implanter*]. 1. Small tubes or needles which are radioactive, placed deep in tissues for therapeutic reasons. 2. Tissue grafts placed in depth. See *graft.*

basket implant. A fenestrated, lucite framework designed to be embedded in the eye socket after enucleation, for use as a prosthesis for an artificial eye.

im·pon′der·a·ble [L. *in-*, not; *pondus*, weight]. Incapable of being weighed; without weight.

im′po·tence, im′po·ten·cy [L. *impotentia*, from *impotens*, powerless]. Lack of power, especially inability for sexual intercourse in the man. Syn., *agonia, asynodia, invirility.* —**impotent,** *adj.*

functional i. Impotence due to a disturbance of the nervous mechanism of the sexual act.

organic i. Impotence due to some anatomic defect in the sexual organs; may occur in either male or female.

psychic i. That form of impotence which is due to some mental or emotional disturbance. Also called *cerebral i.*

im·preg′nate [L. *in*, in; *praegnans*, pregnant]. 1. Render pregnant. 2. Saturate or charge with. —**impregna′tion,** *n.*

im·pres′sion [L. *impressio*, from *imprimere*, to press into]. 1. A mark produced upon a surface by pressure. 2. *In dentistry,* a mold, usually of a jaw or its parts, from which a cast is made. Materials employed commonly include plaster of Paris, wax mixtures, and hydrocolloids.

basilar i. See *platybasia.*

digital impressions. Small, roundish pits on the inner surface of the bones of the skull.

maternal impressions. The effects formerly thought to be produced upon the fetus in the uterus by mental impressions of a vivid character received by the mother during pregnancy.

im·pro′cre·ant [L. *in-*, not; *procreare,* to beget]. Incapable of procreating; impotent. —**improcreance,** *n.*

im·pu′ber·al, im·pu′bic [*in-;* L. *pubes;* signs of manhood]. Destitute of hair on the pubes; not of adult age.

im′pulse [L. *impulsus,* a striking against, from *impellere*]. 1. A push or communicated force. 2. A sudden mental urge to an action. 3. *In neurophysiology,* nerve *i.*

cardiac i. The beat of the heart felt in the fifth intercostal space to the left of the sternum.

catabolic i. Generalized tissue breakdown in shock.

ectopic i. An impulse arising in any part of the heart other than the sinoatrial node.

enteroceptive impulses. Afferent nerve impulses which derive their stimulation from internal organs.

exteroceptive impulses. Afferent nerve impulses which derive their stimulation from external sources.

heterogenetic i. One depending for its origin upon abnormal processes in a muscle.

homogenetic i. An impulse depending for its origin upon normal processes in a muscle.

involuntary i. One not activated by the will of the person, as the cardiac impulse.

morbid i. A sudden, almost uncontrollable desire to do an unlawful act.

nerve i. A transient physicochemical change in the membrane of a nerve fiber which sweeps rapidly along the fiber to its termination, where it causes excitation of other nerves, muscle, or gland cells, depending on the connections and functions of the nerve.

voluntary i. One induced by will power.

im·pul′sion [L. *impulsio,* a pushing against, from *impellere*]. The act of driving or urging onward, either mentally or physically.

im·pu″ta·bil′i·ty [L. *imputare,* to bring into the reckoning]. *In legal medicine,* that degree of mental soundness which makes one responsible for his own acts.

I.M.S. Indian Medical Service (British India).

Imvic. A mnemonic designating four reactions (*I*ndole, *M*ethyl red, *V*oges-Proskauer, *C*itrate). *Escherichia coli* forms are indole and methyl red positive. They do not produce acetylmethylcarbinol and do not attack sodium citrate. Organisms classified as *Aerobacter aerogenes* are indole and methyl red negative, produce acetylmethylcarbinol, and attack sodium citrate. A symbol for *E. coli* becomes then $++--$, while the symbol for *Aerobacter aerogenes* is $--++$.

In Chemical symbol for indium.

in- [L. *in,* in]. A prefix signifying *into, within, in, toward, on.*

in- [L. *in-,* not]. A prefix denoting negation; *not, non-, un-.*

in-. See *ino-.*

-in [L. *-inus*]. 1. *In chemistry,* a termination applied to *neutral nitrogenous substances,* as proteins and bitter principles; *an ester,* as palmitin; *the names of glycosides* and *neutral principles.* Also see *-ine.* 2. A suffix to indicate an antigen, prefixed by the generic name of the organism from which the antigen is derived, as tuberculin, coccidioidin.

in″a·cid′i·ty [L. *in-,* not; *acidus,* sour]. Lack of acidity; applied to deficiency of hydrochloric acid in the gastric juice.

in·ac′ti·vate [*in-;* L. *activus,* active]. To render inactive; usually applied to fresh serum, heated at 56° C. for 30 minutes to destroy its complement.

Inada, Ryukichi [*Japanese bacteriologist and physician,* 1874–1950]. With R. Hoki, Y. Ido, H. Ito, and R. Kaneko, discovered *Leptospira icterohaemorrhagiae,* the causative agent of spirochetal jaundice, and demonstrated its presence in apparently healthy rats.

in·ad′e·qua·cy [L. *in-,* not; *adaequare,* to make equal to]. Insufficiency of function or capacity.

renal i. The condition in which the amount of urinary solids, and often the quantity of urine itself, is considerably diminished.

in·al″i·men′tal [*in-;* L. *alimentum,* nourishment]. Not nourishing; not suitable for food.

in·an′i·mate [*in-;* L. *animatus,* animate]. Not animate; dead; without life.

in″a·ni′tion (in″a·nish′un) [L. *inanire,* to empty]. A pathologic state of the body due to the lack of any foodstuff (including water) which is essential to the living organism.

in·ap′pe·tence [L. *in-,* not; *appetere,* to strive after]. Loss of appetite or desire.

in″ar·tic′u·late [*in-;* L. *articulare,* to divide into joints]. 1. Not jointed or articulated. 2. Not capable of arrangement into syllables, or of being understood, as certain vocal sounds.

in ar·tic′u·lo mor′tis [L.]. At the moment of death; in the act of dying.

in″as·sim′i·la·ble [*in-;* L. *assimilare,* to make like]. Incapable of being assimilated.

in′born″ [L. *in,* in; ME. *beren*]. A constitutional characteristic which is inherited or implanted during intrauterine life; innate; congenital.

in′breed″ing [*in;* ME. *breden*]. Any system of mating which gives a smaller number of ancestors than the maximum possible. The closest inbreeding is self-fertilization, as in plants, or brother-by-sister mating in animals.

In′ca bone. See *incarial bone.*

in·ca′nous [L. *incanus,* hoary]. Hoary white.

in·car″cer·a′tion [L. *in,* in; *carcer,* prison]. The abnormal imprisonment of a part, as in some forms of hernia. —**incar′cerated,** *adj.*

in·ca′ri·al bone. The interparietal bone; an anomaly in which the superior portion of the squama occipitalis is separated from the rest by a suture, or sutures: so-called because common in the ancient Incas. Also called *Inca bone.*

in·car′nant, in·car′na·tive [L. *incarnare,* to make flesh]. Flesh-forming; promoting granulation.

in·car′nant, in·car′na·tive. An agent which produces flesh or promotes granulation. —**incarna′tion,** *n.;* **incarn′,** *v.*

in′cest [L. *incestus,* unchaste]. Sexual intercourse between persons of such close relationship that their marriage is prohibited by law.

inch [ME. *inche,* from L. *uncia,* twelfth part]. The twelfth part of a foot; 2.54 cm.

in′ci·dence [L. *incidere,* to fall upon]. 1. The act or manner of falling upon; the way in which one body strikes another. 2. The amount or extent of occurrence, as of a disease.

angle of i. *In optics,* the angle at which a ray of light strikes a reflecting or refracting surface.

i. rate. The number of cases of a disease appearing per unit of population within a defined time interval.

line of i. The path of a ray or a projectile.

point of i. The point upon which a ray or projectile strikes a reflecting or refracting surface.
racial i. Incidence rate according to race.
in′ci·dent [*incidere*]. Falling upon.
in·cin″er·a′tion [L. *in*, in; *cinus*, ashes]. The process of heating organic substances until all organic matter is driven off and only the ash remains; cremation.
in·cip′i·ent [L. *incipere*, to begin]. Initial, commencing, as incipient tuberculosis. —**incipience, incipiency,** *n.*
in·ci′sal (in·sigh′zul) [L. *incisum*, from *incidere*, to incise]. Cutting; used of the cutting edge of incisor and canine teeth.
in·cised′ (in·sized′) [*incidere*]. Cut; made by cutting.
in·ci′sion (in·sizh′un) [L. *incisio*, from *incidere*]. 1. A cut or wound of the body tissue. It is named according to the location, as abdominal incision; the organ to be operated on, as appendiceal; the shape, as gridiron; the direction, as vertical, oblique; or, frequently, after the surgeon who first used it, as McBurney, Cushing. 2. The act of cutting.
buttonhole i. A small, straight cut made into an organ or cavity.
crucial i. Two cuts at right angles, made deep into the tissues, usually to insure free drainage.
exploratory i. One made for the purpose of diagnosis.
muscle-splitting i. One in which the muscles are split in the direction of their fibers in order to secure a better line of closure, as the McBurney incision.
paramedian i. That made to one side of the median line.
rectus i. One made through the rectus muscle or through its sheath.
in·ci′sive [*incidere*]. 1. Cutting. 2. Pertaining to the incisor teeth.
in·ci′sive. The intermaxillary bone.
in·ci·si′vus la′bi·i in″fer·i·or′is. A portion of the orbicularis oris muscle extending from the vicinity of the base of the lower canine tooth to the corner of the mouth.
in·ci·si′vus la′bi·i su″per·i·or′is. A portion of the orbicularis oris muscle extending from the vicinity of the base of the upper canine tooth to the corner of the mouth.
in·ci′sor [*incidere*]. A cutting tooth; one of the four front teeth of either jaw. —**inci′sor,** *adj.*
deciduous i. One of the eight incisors of the temporary (milk) dentition. Abbreviated, i.
permanent i. One of the eight teeth which replace the deciduous incisors in the permanent (adult) dentition. Abbreviated, I
in″ci·su′ra (in″sigh·sue′ruh, in″si·). Incisure.
in″ci·sur′ae he′li·cis. A vestigial band of muscle occasionally associated with the incisura of the helix of the external ear.
in·ci′sure (in·sigh′zhur, in·sizh′ur) [L. *incisura*, from *incidere*]. A slit or notch. Also see *notch.*
angular i. The transient notch in the lesser curvature of the stomach, formed during peristalsis near the gastric angle. Syn., *angular notch.*
cardiac i. See cardiac *notch.*
i. of Schmidt-Lantermann. One of the oblique partitions interrupting the myelin sheaths of each segment of a nerve fiber: also called *cleft* of Schmidt-Lantermann.
i. of the acetabulum. See acetabular *notch.*
i. of the cerebellum. One of the notches, anterior or posterior, separating the cerebellar hemispheres.
i. of the gallbladder. The cystic fossa.
i. of the tentorium. A deep notch in the tentorium of the cerebellum for the midbrain.
interarytenoid i. A small vertical notch between the corniculate cartilages and the apexes of the arytenoid cartilages of the two sides.
intertragic i. The notch between the tragus and antitragus.
pancreatic i. The pancreatic notch.
parietal i. Parietal notch.
radiologic i. Any indentation seen in an opaque meal radiograph of the stomach.
temporal i. A small fissure separating the uncus from the apex of the temporal lobe.
thyroid i. The thyroid notch.
tympanic i. See tympanic *notch.*
umbilical i. The umbilical notch.
in″cli·na′tion [L. *inclinatio*, a leaning]. 1. A propensity; a leaning. 2. The deviation of the long axis of a tooth from the vertical.
i. of the pelvis. In the erect position the angle which the plane of the pelvic inlet makes with the horizontal plane.
i. of uterus. Obliquity of the uterus.
in″cli·nom′e·ter [L. *inclinare*, to incline; G. *metron*, a measure]. A device for determining the diameter of the eye from the horizontal and vertical lines.
in″co·ag′u·la·ble [L. *in-*, not; *coagulare*, to cause a fluid to curdle]. Incapable of coagulation or curdling.
in″co·her′ence [*in-*; L. *cohaerere*, to stick together]. The quality of being incoherent; absence of connection of ideas or of language; incongruity or inconsequence of diction.
in″co·her′ent [*in-*; *cohaerere*]. Disconnected, illogical, inconsistent.
in″com·bus′ti·ble [*in-*; L. *combustum*, from *comburere*, to burn up]. Incapable of being burned.
in″com·pat′i·ble [*in-*; L. *compati*, to suffer with one]. Incapable of being used or put together because of resulting chemical change or of antagonistic qualities, as two drugs or two types of blood. —**incompatibil′ity,** *n.*
in″com·pen·sa′tion [*in-*; L. *compensatio*, from *compensare*, to weigh several things with one another]. Lack of compensation.
in·com′pe·tence [L. *incompetens*, insufficient]. 1. Insufficiency; inadequacy to perform the natural functions. 2. *In legal medicine*, incapacity; want of legal fitness, as the incompetence of a drunken man to drive a car. —**incompetent,** *adj.*
valvular i. The state or condition of failure of a heart valve to prevent regurgitation of blood; it is due to weakness or dilatation of the valve ring without the valve itself being deformed.
in·con′gru·ence. Incongruity.
in″con·gru′i·ty [L. *incongruus*, unsuitable]. Absence of agreement, correspondence, or needful harmony.
retinal i. Lack of correspondence in the situation of the percipient elements of the two retinas.
in·con′ti·nence [L. *incontinentia*, inability of retaining]. Inability to control the natural evacuations, as the feces or the urine; specifically, involuntary evacuation due to organic causes.
i. of pigment. Loss of melanin from the basal-cell layer of the epidermis due to injury, resulting in an aggregation of melanin in the upper corium, both inside and outside melanophores, seen in chronic inflammatory dermatoses as incontinentia pigmenti, lichen planus, lupus erythematosus, and others.
stress i. Involuntary loss of urine on effort, sudden movement, or rapid change of posture.
in·con·tin·en′ti·a pig·men′ti. Latin, literally, incontinence of pigment; a genodermatosis which is characterized by defective development of the skin and other organs of ectodermal origin, and by bone deformities. Inflammatory or bullous and

verrucous prodromes occur frequently before the final pigmented stage appears.

in″co·or″di·na′tion [L. *in-*, not; *cum*, together; *ordinare*, to regulate]. Inability to bring into common, harmonious movement or action, as inability to produce voluntary muscular movements in proper order or sequence.

in·cor″po·ra′tion [L. *incorporare*, to make into a body]. The process of intimately mixing the particles of different bodies into a practically homogeneous mass.

incotin. A proprietary analgesic ointment in a washable base.

in′cre·ment [L. *incrementum*, increase]. The amount of increase or growth in a given period of time. —**incremen′tal,** *adj.*

in′cre·tin. That fraction of secretin which, upon oral or intravenous administration, produces hypoglycemia and does not stimulate pancreatic secretion; obtained by treatment of secretin by pepsin. Also see *excretin.*

in·cre′tion [L. *in*, in; E. *secretion*, from L. *secernere*, to separate]. An internal secretion. —**in′cretory,** *adj.*

in″crus·ta′tion [L. *incrustare*, to cover with a coat]. The formation of a crust or hard coating, as from an exudate; scab, scale.

in″cu·ba′tion [L. *incubatio*, from *incubare*, to lie on, to hatch]. 1. The act or process of hatching or developing, as eggs or bacteria. 2. The phase of an infectious disease from the time of infection to the appearance of the first symptoms. 3. The process of culturing bacteria for qualitative or quantitative growth studies, as in microbiologic assays. 4. The process of maintaining mixtures of substances in suspension or solution at definite temperatures for varying periods of time for the study of enzyme action or other chemical reactions.

in′cu·ba″tor [L., from *incubare*]. 1. A small chamber with controlled temperature and humidity for the care of prematurely born infants. 2. A laboratory cabinet with controlled temperature for the cultivation of bacteria or for facilitating biologic tests. 3. A device for the artificial hatching of eggs.

in′cu·bus [L.]. 1. Nightmare. *Obs.* 2. A person or thing that oppresses like a nightmare. 3. A demon, said to have sexual intercourse with sleeping men or women, or to enter their bodies and thus direct and influence their behavior. *Obs.*

in″cu·dec′to·my [L. *incus*, anvil; G. *ektomē*, excision]. Surgical removal of the incus.

in″cu·do·mal′le·al [*incus;* L. *malleus*, hammer]. Relating to the incus and the malleus, as the ligaments joining these two ossicles.

in″cu·do·sta·pe′di·al [*incus;* LL. *stapes*, stirrup]. Relating to the incus and the stapes, as the ligaments joining these two ossicles.

in·cur′a·ble [L. *incurabilis*, without remedy]. Not curable.

in·cur′able. A person suffering from an incurable disease.

in′cus [L.]. The middle one of the chain of ossicles in the middle ear, so termed from its resemblance to an anvil. See Plate 20. See Table of Bones in the Appendix. —**incudal,** *adj.*

in·cy″clo·pho′ri·a [G. *en*, in; *kyklos*, circle; *phoros*, bearing]. A latent inward tilting of the upper pole of the eye. See *cyclophoria.*

in·cy″clo·tro′pi·a [*en; kyklos;* G. *trepein*, to turn]. A condition in which the vertical median superior pole of the eye is constantly turned inward.

in d. *In dies*, daily.

in″da·ga′tion [L. *indagare*, to trace out]. 1. Close investigation. 2. Digital examination.

indalone. Trade-mark for *butopyronoxyl.*

in′da·mine. A highly pigmented, usually blue or green, N-phenyl derivative of quinonediimine, obtained by oxidation of a *p*-diamine with an aromatic monoamine or phenol or condensation of *p*-nitroso-derivatives of tertiary amines with an amine in acid solution.

in·de′cent [L. *indecens*, unseemly]. Not decent; obscene.

in″de·ci′sion [L. *in-*, not; *decisio*, decision]. Morbid irresolution; want of firmness or of will; abulia. A symptom of early melancholia.

in″den·ta′tion [L. *in*, in; *dens*, tooth]. 1. A notch, dent, or depression. 2. A condition of being notched or serrated.

i. of the tongue. The notching of the borders of the tongue made by the teeth; seen after death.

in″de·pend′ent cu·ta′ne·ous gly″co·his·tech′i·a (glye″ko·hiss·teck′ee·uh). Rise in the skin sugar content alone without a corresponding increase in the blood sugar.

in′dex (pl. *indexes, indices*) [L., a pointer]. 1. The forefinger. 2. The ratio, or the formula expressing the ratio, of one dimension of a thing to another dimension. 3. *In craniometry*, the ratio of one dimension of the skull to another dimension, usually the length, which is taken as the standard and is represented by 100. The formula is

$$i = \frac{\text{breadth} \times 100}{\text{length}}$$

alpha i. *In electroencephalography*, the percentage of time during which the record shows alpha rhythm.

altitudinal i. See length-height *i.*

alveolar i. See gnathic *i.*

anesthetic i. On a body-weight basis, the volume of anesthetic agent required to produce respiratory arrest divided by the volume required to produce surgical anesthesia.

Arneth i. See Joseph *Arneth.*

atherogenic i. The ratio of the relationship between two major lipoprotein groups, S_f0–12 and S_f12–400: claimed to be a measure of coronary atherosclerosis.

Bazett i. Formula for correction for the rate of the heartbeat in measuring the Q-T interval in the electrocardiogram; $K = \frac{\text{Q-T interval}}{\sqrt{\text{cycle length}}}$, normal for K being 0.36–0.42.

cardiac i. Volume per minute of cardiac output per square meter of body surface area. Normal average 2.2 liters.

cephalic i. The ratio of the greatest width of the head, taken wherever it may be found in a horizontal plane perpendicular to the sagittal plane, × 100, to the greatest length, taken in the sagittal plane between glabella and opisthocranion. Its values are classified as:

dolichocephalic	x–75.9
mesocephalic	76.0–80.9
brachycephalic	81.0–85.4
hyperbrachycephalic	85.5–x

chemotherapeutic i. The relationship existing between the toxicity of a compound for the body and the toxicity for parasites. Kolmer represents it as follows:

$$\text{C.I.} = \frac{\text{maximal tolerated dose per kg. body wt.}}{\text{minimal curative dose per kg. body wt.}}$$

cnemic i. The ratio of the mediolateral (transverse) diameter of the diaphysis of the tibia (distance between the medial margin and the interosseous crest × 100) to the dorsoventral (sagittal) diameter (distance between the crista anterior and the facies posterior), both diameters taken at the level of the nutrient foramen. Values of the index are classified as:

platycnemic	x–64.9
mesocnemic	65.0–69.9
eurycnemic	70.0–x

color i. The amount of hemoglobin per cell relative to normal, obtained by the following formula:

$$C.I. = \frac{\text{per cent normal hemoglobin concentration}}{\text{per cent normal erythrocyte count}}.$$

Different workers use different normal values in this formula.

Cornell Medical Index. A medical history form, which can be checked by clerks, designed to save the physician's time: useful for large-volume work.

cranial i. The ratio of the greatest width of the cranium, taken wherever it may be found on the parietal bones or on the squama temporalis in a horizontal plane perpendicular to the sagittal plane, × 100, to the greatest length, taken in the sagittal plane between glabella and opisthocranion. Values of the index are classified as:

ultradolichocranial	x–64.9
hyperdolichocranial	65.0–69.9
dolichocranial	70.0–74.9
mesocranial	75.0–79.9
brachycranial	80.0–84.9
hyperbrachycranial	85.0–89.9
ultrabrachycranial	90.0–x

creatine i. Creatine tolerance; the ability of the body to retain ingested creatine, as measured under standard conditions. The percentage retained is low in hyperthyroidism and high in hypothyroidism and so may be used as an index of the level of thyroid function or of potency of administered thyroid substance.

dyspnea i. The ratio of the breathing response to mild exercise, walking ventilation (WV), in L/min. to maximum breathing capacity (MBC) in C/min.; a stress/capacity ratio.

facial i. The ratio of the height × 100 to the breadth of the facial part of the skull.

gnathic i. *In craniometry*, the ratio of the facial length (i.e., the distance between basion and prosthion) × 100, to the length of the cranial base (i.e., the distance between nasion and basion). Values of the index are classified as:

orthognathic	x–97.9
mesognathic	98.0–102.9
prognathic	103.0–x

height-breadth i. of the nose. *In somatometry*, the ratio of the width of the nose, taken between the two alaria, or the points of farthest lateral projection of the wings of the nose, to the height of the nose, taken between nasion and subnasale, × 100. Its values are classified as:

hyperleptorrhine	x–54.9
leptorrhine	55.0–69.9
mesorrhine	70.0–84.9
chamaerrhine	85.0–99.9
hyperchamaerrhine	100.0–x

hemolytic i. The ratio of urobilinogen excretion to total circulating hemoglobin. The normal ratio is 11–21 mg. per 100 Gm. Hb.

hieric i. The ratio of the width of the sacrum, taken between the tips of the greatest anterolateral extension of the facies auriculares, to the length, taken in the sagittal plane from the sacral promontory to the ventral edge of the apex, × 100. Values of the index are classified as:

dolichohieric (narrow sacrum)	x–99.9
subplatyhieric (moderately broad)	100.0–105.9
platyhieric (broad sacrum)	106.0–x

humeroradial i. The ratio of

$$\frac{\text{length of humerus} \times 100}{\text{length of radius}}.$$

hyperglycemia i.

$$\frac{\text{blood glucose after 2 hours} - \text{fasting level}}{\text{maximum level} - \text{fasting level}} \times 100.$$

The index is approximately zero for normal individuals. An index for evaluating the sugar-tolerance level.

i. of Flower. (a) The nasomalar index, which is

$$\frac{\text{nasomalar width} \times 100}{\text{biorbital breadth}}$$

(b) The dental index, which is

$$\frac{\text{dental length} \times 100}{\text{craniobasal length}}$$

i. of relative refraction. The ratio of the refractive index of a substance to the index of its surrounding medium.

inhibition i. The amount of an antimetabolite which is needed to overcome the biological effect of a unit weight of a metabolite; the index is a measure of the antagonism between metabolite and antimetabolite.

iodoacetate i. The ratio of the smallest amount of iodoacetate that, under constant conditions, prevents heat coagulation of serum to the total protein concentration of the serum. A low index occurs after major surgery, in some malignancies, and sometimes in other pathological states. Also called *Huggins test, Huggins-Miller-Jensen test.*

ischium-pubis i. The ratio $\frac{\text{length of pubis} \times 100}{\text{length of ischium}}$ by which the sex of an adult pelvis may be determined in most cases, the index being greater than 90 in the female, and less than 90 in the male.

length-height i. The ratio of the basion-bregma height of the skull to its greatest length × 100: also called *altitudinal i., height i.*

leukopenic i. An index depending on the capacity of certain substances to reduce the leukocytes after ingestion. The total count is made before and after taking the specific substance.

Meulengracht icteric i. See Meulengracht's *method.*

mitotic i. The number of dividing cells per thousand cells: used in the estimation of the rate of growth of a tissue.

nasal i. *In craniometry*, the ratio of the greatest width of the apertura piriformis wherever it is found, × 100, to the height of the nasal skeleton, which is the distance between nasion and nasospinale. Its values are classified as:

leptorrhine	x–46.9
mesorrhine	47.0–50.9
chamaerrhine	51.0–57.9
hyperchamaerrhine	58.0–x

opsonic i. The ratio of the phagocytic index of a patient's serum to that of pooled normal serum.

optical i. A constant applied to objectives for purposes of comparison, taking into account the focal length or magnifying power of the lens and also the numerical aperture.

orbital i. *In craniometry*, the ratio of the orbital height, taken at right angles to the orbital width between the upper and lower orbital margins, × 100, to the orbital width, taken between maxillofrontale and lateral margin of the orbit in such a manner that the line of the orbital width bisects the plane of the orbital entrance. Values of the index are classified as:

chamaeconch	x–75.9
mesoconch	76.0–84.9
hypsiconch	85.0–x

orbitonasal i. *In somatometry,* the ratio of the orbitonasal width, taken with a tape measure from the lateral margins of the orbits at the level of the lateral angles of the palpebral fissures, the tape measure passing over the lowest portion of the root of the nose, × 100, to the external orbital width, taken directly with a sliding or spreading caliper from the stated points. Values of the index are classified as:

platyopic	x–109.9
mesopic	110.0–112.9
prosopic	113.0–x

oscillometric i. Ratio of the oscillometric reading at the ankle to that at the wrist. Normal 0.75.
palatomaxillary i. One used to denote the various forms of the dental arch and palate; it is expressed by the formula

$$\frac{\text{palatomaxillary width} \times 100}{\text{palatomaxillary length}}$$

when the width is measured between the outer borders of the alveolar arch just above the middle of the second molar tooth, and the length measured from the alveolar point to the middle of a transverse line touching the posterior borders of the two maxillae.
parasite i. The percentage of individuals in a community showing parasites in the blood.
pelvic i. The relation of the anteroposterior to the transverse diameter of the pelvis.
pelvic-inlet i. That ratio of the sagittal diameter, or conjugata vera of the pelvic inlet, taken between the points where the sagittal plane cuts the sacral promontory and the posterior edge of the superior surface of the symphysis pubis, to the transverse diameter, taken between the points on the arcuate lines that lie farthest lateral from the midline, at right angles to the conjugata vera. When multiplied by 100, values of the index are classified as:

platypellic	x–89.9
mesatipellic	90.0–94.9
dolichopellic	95.0–x

phagocytic i. A figure characteristic for a serum, and denoting the average number of bacteria found per leukocyte after a mixture of the serum, a bacterial culture, and washed leukocytes have been incubated.
platymeric i. The ratio of the anteroposterior diameter of the proximal diaphysis of the femur × 100 to the transverse diameter taken parallel to the plane of the axis of the femoral neck at the level of the greatest width, from 2–5 cm. distal from the base of the trochanter minor. Diameters must be taken at right angles to each other. Values of the index are classified as:

hyperplatymeric	x–74.9
platymeric	75.0–84.9
eurymeric	85.0–99.9
stenomeric	100.0–x

Stenomeric femurs are regarded as pathologic.
refractive i. The refractive power of any substance as compared with air. It is the quotient of the angle of incidence divided by the angle of refraction of a ray passing through a substance. Symbol, n.
sacral i. The sacral breadth multiplied by 100, and divided by the sacral length.
saturation i. The amount of hemoglobin per unit volume of red cells relative to the normal. The normal is approximately 0.95.
Schilling i. See Victor *Schilling.*
Schneider's i. A test of general physical and circulatory efficiency, consisting of pulse and blood pressure observations under standard conditions of rest and exercise.
social adequacy i. The value assigned to one's bearing as evaluated by a new method suggested by J. H. Davis, R. H. Silverman, and T. E. Walsh.
stephano-zygomatic i. The ratio of the distance between the stephanion points × 100 to that between the zygomatic processes.
sweat chloride, sweating-rate i. A quotient which expresses sweat chloride concentration values relative to the rate of sweating; it may reflect the activity of certain adrenocortical hormones.
therapeutic i. The ratio of the toxicity (usually measured as the lethal dose) to the therapeutic dose.
thoracic i. The ratio of the anteroposterior diameter to the transverse, expressed in percentage.
transverse frontoparietal i. *In craniometry,* the ratio of the minimum frontal diameter, taken between the fronto-temporalia, × 100, to the greatest width of the cranium, taken wherever found on the parietal bones or on the squamous parts of the temporal bones, provided that the end-points of the line of greatest width lie in the same horizontal and frontal planes. Values of the index are classified as:

ultramicroseme	x–54.9
hypermicroseme	55.0–59.9
microseme	60.0–64.9
mesoseme	65.0–69.9
megaseme	70.0–74.9
hypermegaseme	75.0–79.9
ultrahypermegaseme	80.0–x

vertical i. The ratio of the vertical diameter of the skull to the maximum anteroposterior diameter, multiplied by 100.
volume i. The relation of the volume of the red corpuscles to their number.
xanthoproteic i. An approximate measure of the amount of phenolic substances present in blood; obtained by nitrating a protein-free serum filtrate, alkalizing with a strong base, and comparing the yellow color produced with an appropriate standard.

In'di·an gum. Any of several different gums, including sterculia gum and ghatti gum.

in'di·can. 1. Indoxyl glucoside, $C_{14}H_{17}NO_6.3H_2O$, occurring in indigo plants; upon hydrolysis and subsequent oxidation, it is converted to indigotin, the chief constituent of indigo. 2. Indoxyl potassium sulfate, $C_8H_6NSO_4K$, a substance occurring in urine and formed from indole.

in'di·cant [L. *indicare,* to indicate]. Serving as an index or as an indication.

in'di·cant. A fact or symptom that indicates a certain treatment.

in"di·ca·nu'ri·a [L. *indicum,* indigo; G. *ouron,* urine]. The presence of an excess of indican in the urine.

in"di·ca'tion [L. *indicare,* to indicate]. Any symptom, cause, or occurrence in a disease which points out its course of treatment.

in'di·ca"tor [L., from *indicare*]. *In chemistry,* a substance used to show by a color or other change when a reaction has taken place or a chemical affinity has been satisfied.

Clark and Lubs indicators. A sulfonephthalein series of indicators which are especially brilliant and reliable in hydrogen-ion concentration determinations.

radioactive phosphorus i. Indicator for the rate of formation of phospholipids.

in′di·ces. Plural of index.

in′di·co·phose (in′di·ko·foze) [L. *indicum*, indigo; G. *phōs*, light]. A blue-colored phose.

In″di·el′la. A genus of fungi of the class Fungi Imperfecti. It is one of several genera whose species cause mycetoma.

in di′es [L.]. Daily. Abbreviated, in d.

in·dif′fer·ent [L. *indifferens*, indifferent]. Neutral; undifferentiated or nonspecialized, as indifferent cells. —**indifferentism,** *n.*

in·dig′e·nous (in·didj′i·nus) [L. *indigena*, a native]. Native; originating or belonging to a certain locality or country.

in″di·ges′tion [L. *in-*, not; *digestio*, from *digerere*, to separate, digest]. Lack of digestion; imperfect digestion.

chronic intestinal i. See celiac *disease.*

early postprandial i. That immediately following eating, caused by a conscious increase of gastric motility rather than the normal unconscious gastric movements.

late postprandial i. That occurring one to two hours after eating.

in·dig″i·ta′tion (in·didj″i·tay′shun) [L. *indigitare*, to call upon, from *indiges*, native deity; confused with *digitus*, finger]. Invagination.

in″di·glu′cin. $C_6H_{10}O_6$. A yellow syrup, one of the decomposition products of indican.

in′di·go [L. *indicum*, indigo]. A blue pigment formed by the hydrolysis and oxidation of the indican contained in various species of *Indigofera* (*Indigofera tinctoria, I. anil, I. argentea*); the chief constituent of indigo is indigotin but there are also present varying amounts of the dyes indigo brown, indigo red, indigo yellow, etc.

i. blue. $C_{16}H_{10}N_2O_2$, indigotin.

i. carmine (C.C.). A blue dye, sodium or potassium indigotindisulfonate, very sensitive to oxidizing agents; used in urologic work and as a test for kidney function; as a coloring for foods, drugs, and cosmetics.

i. white. Indigogen; a substance obtained by the reduction of indigo blue.

in·dig′o·tin, in″di·go′tin. $C_{16}H_{10}N_2O_2$. The chief constituent of indigo. Also see *indican.*

in″di·go·u′ri·a [*indicum;* G. *ouron*, urine]. The presence of indigo in the urine; due to a decomposition of indican.

in″di·rect′ [L. *in-*, not; *directus*, straight]. Not direct; not in a direct line; acting through an intervening medium.

in′di·um [L. *indicum*, indigo]. In = 114.76. A rare metal. It is very soft, resembles lead in its properties, and is used in many alloys.

in″dol·ac″e·tu′ri·a (in″dol·ass″i·tew′ree·uh, in″-dohl·) [*indi*cum; E. phen*ol;* L. *acetum*, vinegar; G. *ouron*, urine]. Presence of indoleacetic acid in the urine; found in intestinal disturbances.

in′dole. C_8H_7N.2,3-benzopyrole; a substance formed from tryptophan during intestinal putrefaction and in certain bacterial cultures. It is responsible, in part, for the odor of feces. In intestinal obstruction it is converted into indican, which is eliminated in the urine.

in″dole·a·ce′tic ac′id. Indole-3-acetic acid, a bacterial decomposition product of tryptophan, found in the urine and feces. It possesses pronounced growth-promoting activity for leaves.

in′do·lent [L. *in-*, not; *dolens*, from *dolere*, to feel pain]. Sluggish; usually applied to slowness in healing, as an indolent ulcer, or to slow-growing nonpainful tumors.

in″dole·pro″pi·on′ic ac′id. The acid produced when tryptophan loses its NH_2 group.

in″dole·py·ru′vic ac′id. A product of tryptophan upon deamination of the α-amino group. Believed to be the first oxidative step in the breaking down of tryptophan.

in″dol·og′e·nous (in″do·lodj′i·nus). Producing indole.

in″do·lu′ri·a [L. *indi*cum, indigo; E. phen*ol;* G. *ouron*, urine]. The excretion of indole in the urine.

in″do·phe′nol (in″do·fee′nole, ·nol, ·nawl). Any of a series of dyes derived from quinone imine.

in″do·phe′nol ox′i·dase. An oxidizing enzyme, present in animal and plant tissues, which catalyzes formation of indophenol blue from dimethyl-*p*-phenylenediamine and α-naphthol when these are injected into tissue; it is identical with cytochrome oxidase.

in·dox′yl. C_8H_7ON. A yellow, crystalline substance in plants and animals. An oxidation product of indole and skatole, it is found in the urine among the products of intestinal putrefaction.

i. glucoside. See *indican,* 1.

i. potassium sulfate. Indican. $C_8H_6NSO_4K$. The potassium salt of indoxyl, conjugated with sulfuric acid; occurs in urine. Sometimes called *indoxyl sulfate.*

in·dox″yl·glu″cu·ron′ic ac′id. A product formed by the detoxification of indole. It is a combination of indoxyl and glucuronic acid.

in·dox″yl·og′e·nous (in·dock″si·lodj′i·nus) [L. *indicum*, indigo; G. *oxys*, sharp; *genesthai*, from *gignesthai*, to be produced]. Producing indoxyl.

in·dox″yl·sul·fu′ric ac′id. The substance resulting from conjugation of indoxyl, formed by oxidation of indole in the liver, with sulfuric acid, and eliminated in the urine as the potassium salt (indican).

in·dox″yl·u′ri·a [*indicum; oxys;* G. *ouron*, urine]. The presence of indoxyl in the urine.

in·duc′tion [L. *inductio*, from *inducere*, to lead into]. 1. The act of bringing on or causing. 2. The bringing about of an electric or magnetic state in a body by the proximity (without actual contact) of an electrified or magnetized body. 3. The period from first administration of the anesthetic until consciousness is lost and the patient is stabilized in the desired surgical plane of anesthesia. 4. *In embryology*, the specific morphogenetic effect brought about by the action of one tissue upon another, acting through organizers or evocators.

successive i. Facilitation of one reflex by its antagonistic reflex in rhythmic actions, as in stepping reflexes.

in·duc″to·py·rex′i·a (in·duck″to·pye·reck′see·uh) [*inducere;* G. *pyressein*, to be feverish]. Artificial fever produced by electromagnetic induction; a form of electrotherapy.

in″duc·to′ri·um [*inducere*]. *In physiology*, an instrument for the generation and administration of induction shocks; it consists of a primary and a secondary coil mounted on a stand.

in·duc′to·ther″my (in·duck′to·thur″mee, in-duck″to·thur′mee) [*inducere;* G. *thermē*, heat]. The application of energy to tissue through the agency of a high-frequency magnetic field. It is produced by means of a heavily insulated conductor wound into a coil of appropriate configuration and number of turns through which a high-frequency current is conducted from an oscillator. It is usually applied to local parts but may be used to produce general artificial fever.

in′du·lin. One of a group of dyes similar to the safranines, highly phenylated amino derivatives. The only important one in medicine is nigrosine. Also called *i. black.*

in″du·lin′o·phil, in″du·lin′o·phile. Staining with indulin or having an affinity for indulin. —**indulinophil′ic,** *adj.*

in″du·ra′tion [L. *indurare,* to harden]. 1. The hardening of a tissue or part, resulting from hyperemia, inflammation, or infiltration by neoplasm. 2. A hardened area of tissue. —**in′durated, in′durative,** *adj.*

black i. Fibrosis, especially of the lung, due to anthracosis.

brown i. Chronic, passive hyperemia of the lung, usually the result of left ventricular failure or mitral stenosis, with resultant fibrosis and pigmentation by hemosiderin. Histologically, heart-failure cells are seen in the alveoli. Also called *cardiac lung.*

gray i. More or less diffuse fibrosis of the lung in chronic interstitial pneumonitis.

red i. Fibrosis of the lung associated with deposit of red oxide of iron; marked passive hyperemia of the lung.

in·du′si·um (in·dew′zee·um) [L., an undergarment, from *induere,* to put on]. 1. A membranous covering. 2. A marginal layer of gray matter on the corpus callosum. Also called *i. griseum.*

-ine (-een, -in) [cf. L. *-inus*]. *In chemistry,* a termination indicating *a basic nitrogenous compound,* as morphine, purine; *a halogen,* as bromine. Also see *-in.*

in·e′bri·ant [L. *inebriare,* to make drunk]. Intoxicant; causing inebriation.

in·e′bri·ant. An agent that causes inebriation.

in·e″bri·a′tion [*inebriare*]. Intoxication.

in″e·bri′e·ty [*inebriare*]. Habitual drunkenness.

in·ef′fi·ca·cy [L. *inefficax,* ineffectual]. Failure to produce the desired effect.

in″e·nu′cle·a·ble [L. *in-,* not; *enucleare,* to take out the kernels]. Not removable by enucleation.

in·er′ti·a [L., inactivity]. 1. Dynamic opposition to acceleration, common to all forms of matter, including electrons and quanta. 2. Lack of activity, said of the uterus when in labor the contractions have diminished or ceased entirely. Also called *uterine i.* —**inert′,** *adj.*

in ex·tre′mis [L.]. At the end; at the last; at the point of death.

in′fant [L. *infans,* without speech, young child]. 1. A child, usually up to two years. 2. A minor; a person under legal age, according to common law, 21, though some states of the United States do not follow this rule. —**infancy,** *n.*

in·fan′ti·cide [*infans;* L. *caedere,* to kill]. 1. The murder of an infant. 2. The murderer of an infant.

in′fan·tile (in′fun·tile, ·til) [L. *infantilis,* of infants]. Pertaining to infancy; like an infant in actions.

in·fan′ti·lism [*infantilis*]. 1. The persistence of infantile or childish traits and characteristics into adolescent and adult life; the condition is marked by mental, physical, and sexual underdevelopment and sometimes dwarfish stature. Also called *ateliosis, Lorain syndrome.* 2. *In psychoanalysis,* the state of infancy prolonged into adult life.

angioplastic i. That caused by a deficiency of the vascular system.

cachectic i. That due to chronic infection or toxemia.

celiac i. That following celiac disease. Also called *intestinal i.*

dysthyroidal i. Infantilism resulting from impaired thyroid activity.

hepatic i. That form of infantilism associated with liver cirrhosis.

Herter's i. See celiac *disease.*

idiopathic i. Infantilism of unknown origin.

intestinal i. See celiac *disease.*

lymphatic i. That form associated with lymphatism. Also called *Paltauf's nanism.*

myxedematous i. The underdevelopment seen in cretinism, characterized by an infantile face, prominent lips and tongue, distended abdomen, rudimentary genitalia, arrested mental and emotional development, and delayed or absent second dentition.

pancreatic i. Arrested development associated with defective functioning of the pancreas: also called Clarke-Hadfield *syndrome.*

partial i. Arrested development limited to a single organ or part, or to a special area or system.

pituitary i. Dwarfism resulting from a lack of the growth-promoting and gonadotropic hormones of the pituitary gland.

regressive i. That which starts after the body has attained full growth. Also called *reversive i., tardy i.*

renal i. Arrested development resulting from deficiency of the urinary system.

sex i. Continuation of childish sex traits and development beyond puberty.

thyroid i. See *cretinism.*

toxemic i. Delayed development due to toxemia, especially of intestinal origin.

universal i. Generalized retarded physical development associated with absence of secondary sex characters.

in·farct′, in′farct [L. *infarcire,* to stuff into]. A region of necrosis of tissue due to complete interference with blood flow, usually the result of occlusion of the supplying artery or, rarely, to occlusion of the draining vein. If the region has a dual blood supply, hemorrhage without necrosis may result. In viscera, the infarct is generally of conical form, but in extremities it occupies the region supplied by the occluded artery (ischemic necrosis).

anemic i. See white *i.*

bland i. One free from infection.

cicatrized i. One in which the necrotic mass is replaced or encapsulated by fibrous tissue.

healed i. See cicatrized *i.*

hemorrhagic i. See red *i.*

infected i. One in which suppurative inflammation involves or surrounds the lesion, either because the embolus or thrombus causing the infarct contains pathogenic organisms, or because of infection implanted in the infarct, as in the lung.

marginal i. Zone of degeneration forming a yellowish white fibrous ring, found at term about the edge of the placenta.

myocardial i. One in the heart muscle.

pulmonary i. One in the lung. It usually results from an embolus due to phlebothrombosis of the deep vessels of the leg or thrombosis in a dilated right atrium.

recent i. One which shows no trace of cicatrization.

red i. One in which the necrotic focus is swollen, firm, and either bright or dark red, as the result of hemorrhage.

remote i. One in which shrinkage, or cicatrization, has begun or is advanced.

silent i. Myocardial infarct with no history of pain; pain is thought to be present but unnoticed because of other pathological conditions or high pain threshold.

systemic i. Any infarct other than one of the coronary or pulmonary circulation.

white i. One in which the hemorrhage is slight or the blood and blood pigments have been removed; that is, the infarct has become decolorized

in·farc′tion [*infarcire*]. The process leading to the development of an infarct. Immediately following vascular occlusion, there is successive occurrence of hyperemia, cloudy swelling, fatty degeneration, and necrosis. Necrotic tissue stimulates mild inflammation, which results in the formation of a cicatrix or capsule.

diaphragmatic myocardial i. Posterobasilar infarction. See myocardial *i.*

myocardial i. The process by which infarcts are produced in the cardiac muscle. These are usually found in the wall of the left ventricle and such terms as *posterobasilar*, *anterolateral*, *anterior*, *anteroseptal*, *posterior*, *posterolateral* all refer to the portion of the left ventricular wall involved.

in·fec′tion [L. *infectio*, infection]. 1. Implantation of an infective agent: in the strict sense, the presence of single-celled microorganisms (bacteria, rickettsiae, protozoa), viruses, or fungi in or on the body of a host; it is incorrectly but frequently used also for the invasion of a host by higher organisms, such as parasitic worms or insects (see *infestation*). 2. The communication of disease from one subject to another. 3. Communication of disease from one part of the body to another (autoinfection). —**infectious, infective,** *adj.;* **infect′,** *v.*

air-borne i. The transfer of infection from one individual to another without direct contact between them by means of droplets of moisture containing the causative agent. Also called *droplet i.*

atrium of i. Portal of entry of the infective agent.

concurrent i. Simultaneous existence of two or more forms of infection: also called *complex i.*, *mixed i.*, *multiple i.*

consecutive i. See secondary *i.*

cross i. A nonspecific term applied to any infection which a patient develops during hospitalization for another disorder.

focal i. One in which a bacterial disease process is limited to a definite area or focus, as in certain tissues, glands, or organs; not only may the local tissue be destroyed, but toxemia may result if the microorganism produces a soluble toxin.

food i. See food *poisoning*.

mixed i. See concurrent *i.*

multiple i. See concurrent *i.*

secondary i. Implantation of a new infection upon one already in existence.

synergistic i. A concurrent infection wherein two infectious agents exert a pathogenic effect of which either agent acting alone would be incapable; thus, swine influenza virus, causing mild respiratory disease, in association with *Hemophilus influenza suis* gives rise to highly fatal disease.

terminal i. An infection occurring late in the course of another disease, causing the death of the patient.

Vincent's i. See necrotizing ulcerative *gingivitis.*

in″fe·cun′di·ty [L. *infecundus*, unfruitful]. Sterility; barrenness.

in·fe′ri·or [L., lower]. Lower; applied to structures nearer the feet, as contrasted to superior, nearer the head.

in·fe″ri·or′i·ty [*inferior*]. A state or condition of being lower, inferior, less adequate, less well-developed or adapted; it may be organic or psychic.

feeling of i. *In psychology*, a morbid feeling of personal inadequacy; may result in timidity or submission, or, because of overcompensation, in selfish aggression. Also called *i. complex.*

in″fer·til′i·ty [L. *infertilis*, unfruitful]. Involuntary reduced reproductive ability: often incorrectly used synonymously with *sterility.*

in″fes·ta′tion [L. *infestatio*, from *infestare*, to infest]. The state or condition of being infested. The term is used with reference to the presence of animal parasites in or on the human or animal body. *In tropical medicine*, the presence of arthropod parasites (as insects, mites) on the body; also the presence of parasitic multicellular organisms such as roundworms, flatworms, and flukes, in or on the body of a host. Confusion with the use of the term *infection* has resulted from the fact that an infesting organism (e.g., louse) may transmit an infection (e.g., typhus). —**in·fest′,** *v.*

in·fib·u·la′tion [L. *infibulare*, to clasp or buckle together]. Act of clasping or fastening a ring, clasp, or frame to the genital organs to prevent copulation.

in·fil′trate [L. *in*, in; ML. *feltrum*, felt]. To pass into tissue spaces or cells, as fluids, cells, or other substances.

in′fil·trate. The material which has infiltrated.

corneal i. An opacity resulting from infiltration of fluids or cells or from scar tissue caused by such infiltration.

in″fil·tra′tion [*in; feltrum*]. 1. A process by which cells, fluid, or other substances pass into tissue spaces or into cells. The various substances may be natural to the part or cell, but in excess; or they may be foreign to the part or cell. 2. The material taking part in the process. 3. *In radiology*, the production in a part or organ of a change whereby radioluminescence is decreased.

amyloid i. Deposit in tissues of a hyaline material, probably a combination of protein and hexoses, with peculiar staining properties; in the gross specimen, Lugol's solution and dilute sulfuric acid give a dark brown or black coloration; in microscopic preparations, a red stain with metachromatic dyes such as aniline gentian violet, crystal violet, methyl green; also has a special affinity for Congo red in tissue sections.

calcareous i. Deposit of salts of calcium in degenerate or necrotic tissues.

cellular i. Exudation of cells into tissues in the course of acute, subacute, or chronic inflammation; migration or invasion of cells of neoplasms.

fat i. Deposit of neutral fats in tissues or cells as the result of transport.

glycogen i. Deposit of glycogen in cells in excessive amounts or in abnormal situation.

mineral i. Deposit of various kinds of minerals and their salts.

pigmentary i. Deposit of endogenous or exogenous pigments in tissues.

round-cell i. A general term used to indicate an infiltration by such cells as lymphocytes, plasma cells, and macrophages, without specifying cell type.

serous i. An excess of fluid in tissue spaces, a part of serous inflammation or of edema.

urinary i. Passage of urine into tissue spaces, as into tissues of the perineum following rupture of the urethra or the urinary bladder.

waxy i. See amyloid *i.*

in·fin′i·ty. *In optics*, a distance so great that light rays from a point source at that distance may be considered parallel.

in·firm′ [L. *infirmus*, not strong, weak]. Weak or feeble.

in·fir′ma·ry [*infirmus*]. 1. A hospital; an institution where ill and infirm persons are maintained during the period of treatment. 2. *In military medicine*, a medical treatment facility primarily intended to provide beds and treatment for patients from the local military command or from the immediate vicinity thereof, who are temporarily incapacitated for performance of duty because of relatively minor illness or injury with a favorable prognosis for early return to duty.

in·fir′mi·ty [*infirmus*]. 1. Weakness; feebleness. 2. A disease producing feebleness.

in″flam·ma′tion [L. *inflammatio*, from *inflammare*, to set on fire]. The reaction of the tissues to injury. The essential process, regardless of the causative agent, is characterized clinically by local heat, swelling, redness, and pain; pathologically, by primary vasoconstriction followed by vasodilatation, with slowing of the blood current, accumulation and emigration of leukocytes, exudation of fluid, and deposition of fibrin. Some authorities include under inflammation the process of repair, the production of new capillaries and fibroblasts, organization, and cicatrization. —**inflam′matory,** *adj.;* **inflame′,** *v.*

acute i. One in which the progress is rapid and the course is short.

allergic i. That which is excited by a localized, hyperactive response to an allergen to which the subject is hypersensitive. Also called *hyperergic i.*

alterative i. That in parenchymatous organs, such as the kidney, in which degeneration of parenchymal cells is accompanied by proliferation of cells of capillaries or of other origin, or by a slight amount of exudation. Also called *parenchymatous i.*

bacterial i. That caused by bacterial infection.

breast inflammations. See under *mastitis.*

catarrhal i. One affecting a mucous membrane, usually accompanied by excessive production of mucus.

chemical i. That caused by chemical means.

chronic i. One characterized by slow progression and long course; a progressive condition in contrast to an end stage of cicatrization.

croupous i. A fibrinous inflammation at, or below the level of, the larynx.

diphtheritic i. A fibrinous exudate due to infection with *Corynebacterium diphtheriae.* Syn., *pseudomembranous i.*, *pseudomembranous mucositis.*

exudative i. That in which exudation is the conspicuous feature.

fibrinous i. One in which the exudate is composed largely of fibrin.

gangrenous i. Severe inflammation complicated by secondary infection with putrefactive bacteria.

hemorrhagic i. Necrotic inflammation in which thrombosis of the blood vessels causes hemorrhage. Syn., *hemorrhagic mucositis.*

interstitial i. One in which the interstitial tissues show a slight or moderate exudation, principally by mononuclear cells, that has not proceeded to suppuration.

parenchymatous i. See alterative *i.*

productive i. One in which there is a considerable multiplication of fibroblasts. Also called *plastic i.*

pseudomembranous i. See diphtheritic *i.*

purulent i. One in which pus is formed. Also called *suppurative i.*

serous i. That in which the exudate is composed largely of serum.

subacute i. A form which has a somewhat longer progress and course than acute inflammation, with moderate proliferation of fibroblasts.

subchronic i. Inflammation of somewhat more rapid progress and course than chronic inflammation.

suppurative i. See purulent *i.*

in·fla′tion [L. *inflatio*, from *inflare*, to blow up]. Distention with air.

in·flec′tion, in·flex′ion [L. *inflectere*, to bend]. 1. A bending inward. 2. Modification of the pitch of the voice in speaking.

in″flo·res′cence [L. *in-*, in; *florescere*, to begin to blossom]. The structure and position of the flowering parts of a plant and their relation to each other.

in″flu·en′za [It., influence]. An epidemic disease, sometimes becoming pandemic; characterized by catarrhal inflammation of the mucous membrane of the respiratory tract, accompanied by a mucopurulent discharge, fever, pain in the muscles, and prostration. At times, symptoms are mainly referred to the nervous system. The cause is an influenza virus, the established immunological types being designated as A and B. Complications are common, pneumonia being the most frequent; pleurisy, otitis media, and neuritis also may appear.

abdominal i. That form which has abdominal symptoms, tympanites, diarrhea, pain, etc.

endemic i. That occurring during the winter season which is less severe than pandemic influenza.

equine i. An acute pantropic virus disease of horses which is characterized by inflammation of mucous membranes of the air passages and eyelids; frequently the tendons and subcutaneous tissues are inflamed as well.

swine i. A disease of swine caused by the associated effects of a filtrable virus and the *Hemophilus suis;* characterized by inflammation of the upper respiratory tract.

in·fold′ [L. *in*, in; AS. *faeldan*]. To enclose within folds, as in the plication of redundant stomach wall.

in′foot″ed. See *intoeing.*

in′fra- [L., below, under]. A prefix signifying *below* or *beneath*, *inferior*, or *within.*

in″fra·car′di·ac [*infra;* G. *kardia*, heart]. Situated below or beneath the heart.

in″fra·cla·vic′u·lar [*infra;* L. *clavicula*, little key]. Below the collarbone.

in″fra·cla·vic·u·lar′is. A rare muscle extending from above the clavicular part of the pectoralis major to the fascia over the deltoid muscle.

in″fra·con′dyl·ism [*infra;* G. *kondylos*, knuckle]. Downward deviation of the mandibular condyles.

in″fra·cos′tal. Old name for the subcostal muscle.

in·frac′tion [L. *in-*, not; *fractio*, a breaking in pieces]. Incomplete fracture of a bone.

in″fra·di″a·phrag·mat′ic [L. *infra*, below; G. *diaphragma*, partition]. Situated below the diaphragm.

in″fra·glenoid′ [*infra;* G. *glēnoeidēs*, like the socket of a joint]. Located below the glenoid cavity.

in″fra·glot′tic [*infra;* G. *glōttis*, glottis]. Below the glottis.

in″fra·hy′oid [*infra;* G. *hyoeidēs*, shaped like the letter upsilon]. Situated below the hyoid bone.

in″fra·oc·clu′sion [*infra;* L. *occlusum*, from *occludere*, to close up]. Failure of one or more teeth to reach the plane of occlusion.

in″fra·or′bit·al [*infra;* L. *orbita*, track]. Beneath or below the floor of the orbit.

in″fra·pa·tel′lar [*infra;* L. *patella*, small pan]. Below the patella.

in″fra·phys″i·o·log′ic. Of or having less than normal function; hypofunctional: said of an organ or part.

in″fra·pro′te·in. See *metaprotein.*

in″fra·red′ [*infra;* ME. *red*]. Beyond the red end of the spectrum. Pertaining to wavelengths of radiant energy longer than those of the red end of the visible spectrum and shorter than those of Hertzian waves.

in″fra·scap′u·lar [*infra;* L. *scapula*, shoulder blade]. Below the shoulder blade.

in″fra·spi·na′tus. A muscle arising from the infraspinous fossa of the scapula and inserted into the greater tubercle of the humerus.

in″fra·spi′nous [*infra;* L. *spina,* thorn]. Below the spine of the scapula.

in″fra·ster′nal [*infra;* G. *sternon,* chest]. Below the sternum.

in″fra·tem″po·ra′le (in″fruh·tem″po·rah′lee, ·ray′lee) [*infra;* L. *tempus,* temple of the head]. A craniometric point on the infratemporal crest of the greater wing of the sphenoid bone: used in measuring the least cranial breadth.

in″fra·ten·to′ri·al [*infra;* L. *tentorium,* tent]. Below the tentorium cerebelli, as increase of infratentorial pressure in the cranium.

in″fra·troch′le·ar. Below a trochlea, as the infratrochlear nerve situated below the trochlea of the superior oblique muscle of the eye.

in·fric′tion [L. *infrictio,* a rubbing]. The rubbing of a body surface with an ointment or liniment.

infron pediatric. Trade-mark for capsules containing 100,000 U.S.P. units of activated ergosterol; used in therapy of rickets.

in″fun·dib′u·li·form″ (in″fun·dib′yoo·li·form″, in″fun·dib·yōō′li·form″) [L. *infundibulum,* funnel; *forma,* form]. Funnel-shaped.

in″fun·dib·u·lo′ma. An uncommon tumor of the floor of the third ventricle, usually occurring in childhood, which histologically resembles the infundibulum of the hypophysis in its vascular pattern, pituicytes, and colloidal material.

in″fun·dib′u·lum [L.]. 1. A funnel-shaped passage or part. 2. The stalk of the neurohypophysis. —**infundibular,** *adj.*

cardiac i. That part of the right ventricle derived from the proximal part of the bulbus cordis of the embryonic heart; the anterosuperior part of the ventricle communicating with the pulmonary trunk.

ethmoidal i. A crescentic groove connecting the anterior ethmoid cells with the middle meatus of the nose.

i. of frontal sinus. See nasofrontal *duct.*

i. of the hypophysis. The stalk of the pituitary gland.

i. of uterine tube. The wide, funnel-shaped portion of the uterine tube at its fimbriated end.

infundin. Trade-mark for an aqueous extract of the posterior lobe of the pituitary gland.

in·fu′sion [L. *infusio,* from *infundere,* to pour into]. 1. The process of extracting the active principles of a substance by means of water, but without boiling. 2. The product of such a process. 3. The slow injection of a solution into a vein, into subcutaneous tissue, or into some other tissue of the body, from which it is absorbed into the blood stream, as, an intratibial infusion.

in″fu·so′ri·a (in″few·sor′ee·uh, ·zor′ee·uh) [*infundere*]. Formerly a class of Protozoa which is now called Ciliata.

in·ges′ta [L. *ingestum,* from *ingerere,* to put into]. Substances taken into the body, especially foods.

in·ges′tion [L. *ingestio,* from *ingerere*]. 1. The act of taking substances, especially food, into the body. 2. The process by which a cell takes up foreign matter, such as bacilli or smaller cells. —**ingestive,** *adj.*

in′glu·vin, in·glu′vin [L. *ingluvies,* crop, maw]. A preparation obtained from the gizzard of the domestic hen: formerly used in dyspepsia and nausea.

Ingrassia, Giovan Filippo [*Italian physician and anatomist,* 1510–80]. Distinguished chickenpox from scarlet fever. Described the stapes and the sphenoid bone. The lesser wings of the sphenoid bone are known as *Ingrassia's wings.*

in″gra·ves′cent [L. *ingravescere,* to become heavier]. Increasing in weight or in severity.

in·gre′di·ent [L. *ingredi,* to enter]. Any substance that enters into the formation of a compound or mixture.

in′guen (ing′gwen) [L.]. The groin.

in′gui·nal (ing′gwi·nul) [L. *inguinalis,* of the groin]. Pertaining to the inguinal region or groin.

in′gui·no- (ing′gwi·no-), **inguin-** [L. *inguen,* groin]. A combining form signifying *groin.*

in″gui·no·dyn′i·a (ing″gwi·no·din′ee·uh, ·dye′-nee·uh) [*inguen;* G. *odynē,* pain]. Pain in the groin. *Obs.*

in″gui·no·scro′tal [*inguen;* L. *scrotum,* scrotum]. Relating to the groin and the scrotum.

in·ha′lant [L. *inhalare,* to breathe at]. 1. One who inhales. 2. That which is inhaled, as a medicine. —**in·ha′lant, inhalent,** *adj.;* **inhaler,** *n.*

in″ha·la′tion [*inhalare*]. 1. The breathing in of air or other vapor. 2. A medicinal substance to be used by inhalation. —**inhale′,** *v.*

in′ha·la″tor, in″ha·la′tor [*inhalare*]. A device for facilitating the inhalation of a gas or spray. Used for providing oxygen or oxygen-carbon dioxide mixtures for respiration in resuscitation.

in·ha′ler [*inhalare*]. 1. An apparatus used for filtering air, etc., to protect the lungs against damp or cold air, dust, or gases. 2. Inhalator.

in·her′ent (in·heer′unt, in·herr′unt) [L. *inhaerere,* to adhere to]. Innate; natural to the organism.

in·her′it·ance [L. *in,* in; *hereditare,* to inherit]. 1. The acquisition of characteristics by transmission of germ plasm from ancestor to descendant. 2. The sum total of characteristics dependent upon the constitution of the fertilized ovum; also, the total set of genes in the fertilized ovum.

blending i. The apparent fusion in the progeny of the separate characteristics of the parents, now explained in Mendelian terms as dependent upon several pairs of genes.

collateral i. Term used to describe the appearance of characters in collateral members of a family, as when an uncle and a niece show the same character, inherited by the related individuals from a common ancestor.

cytoplasmic i. The acquisition of any trait which is causally dependent upon self-reproducing bodies in the nonnuclear constitution of the egg, as plastid implants.

maternal i. The acquisition of any characteristic that is causally dependent upon a peculiarity of the egg cytoplasm, which in turn is dependent upon genes in the nucleus, as dextral and sinistral coiling of snail shells.

in·her′it·ed [*in; hereditare*]. Derived from an ancestor.

in·hib′in. 1. A testicular hormone inhibiting the gonadotropic secretion of the anterior pituitary gland. 2. Antibacterial substance or substances in normal fresh human urine. 3. An antibiotic substance present in honey.

in″hi·bi′tion (in″hi·bish′un) [L. *inhibitio,* from *inhibere,* to restrain]. 1. The act of checking or restraining the action of an organ, cell, or chemical. 2. *In psychiatry,* an unconscious restraining of an instinctual impulse by an opposing impulse: generally synonymous with *repression,* but sometimes also used to cover *suppression.* —**inhib′itory,** *adj.;* **inhib′it,** *v.*

autogenous i. A reflex relaxation referred to the point of stimulation.

competitive i. *In physiology,* inhibition of the passage of an impulse through a neuron due to the dominance thereof by a stronger impulse.

Wedensky i. Phenomenon observed in a nerve-muscle preparation wherein a muscle moderately fatigued by previous stimuli fails to respond to rapid stimulation but still responds to slowly repeated stimuli.

in·hib'i·tor [*inhibere*]. 1. A substance which checks or stops a chemical action. 2. A neuron whose stimulation stops, or suppresses, the activity of the part it innervates, or of a neuron with which it synapses.

competitive i. A compound, similar in structure to a substrate or coenzyme, which competes with that substrate or coenzyme for active centers on the enzyme molecule.

specific i. In metabolic studies, a substance which inactivates particular enzymes.

in″i·en·ceph'a·lus [G. *inion*, occiput; *egkephalos*, brain]. A monster with occipital fissure of the cranium, with protrusion of brain substance, combined with rachischisis and retroflexion of the cervical spine. —**iniencephaly,** *n.*

in″i·od'·y·mus [*inion;* G. *-dymos*, -fold]. A monster exhibiting duplicity of the face, with four eyes, two noses, two mouths, and two, three, or four ears. Also called *diprosopus tetraophthalmus.*

in'i·on [G.]. The external protuberance of the occipital bone. See *craniometric point, craniometry.*

in″i·op'a·gus [*inion;* G. *pagos*, that which is fixed]. Conjoined twins united by their occiputs. Also called *craniopagus occipitalis, cephalopagus occipitalis.*

in'i·ops [*inion;* G. *ōps*, eye]. Conjoined twins with fused thoraxes and a single head which bears two opposite faces, one incomplete. Also called *cephalothoracopagus monosymmetros, syncephalus asymmetros, janus asymmetros, janiceps ateleus.*

in·i'tial [L. *initialis*, from *initium*, beginning]. Pertaining to the beginning of a process; primary.

in·ject' [L. *injectum*, from *inicere*, to throw in]. Introduce fluids into the skin, subcutaneous tissue, muscle, blood vessels, spinal canal, or any body cavity.

in·jec'tion [L. *injectio*, from *inicere*]. 1. The act of injecting or throwing in. 2. The substance injected. Classification is made according to the organ or region into which the injection is made, as urethral, intramuscular, subcutaneous, intravenous, vaginal injection, etc.

anatomic i. Filling the vessels of a cadaver or of an organ with preservative or coagulating solutions, for purposes of dissection.

coagulation i. Injection of coagulating solutions into the cavity of an aneurysm.

hypodermic i. Injection which is made into the subcutaneous connective tissue, by means of a syringe.

i. pneumonia. A condition of the lung somewhat resembling pneumonia following injections of Koch's tuberculin.

jet i. See *hypospray.*

nutrient i. Injection of nutrient fluids into the rectum or other cavity of the body.

opaque i. For anatomic or microscopic purposes, one made of plaster of Paris, tallow, vermilion and gelatin, lead acetate and potassium bichromate (yellow injection), india ink, or lead acetate and sodium carbonate (white).

repository i. One containing the therapeutic agent in slowly absorbable form so as to delay its absorption and prolong the effect.

transparent microscopic i. One made with carmine for red, potassium bichromate for yellow.

in'ju·ry [L. *iniuria*, injury]. *In medicine,* any stress upon a part or the whole of an organism that disrupts its structure or function, or both, to such a degree as to result in a pathologic process. An injury may be primarily somatic, due to physical, chemical, or biological causes, or it may be primarily psychic. The cause or causes may be unknown. Injury may be sudden or insidious, localized or generalized, primary or secondary, and the reaction of the organism, including its death or that of any of its parts, will depend upon the severity and extent of the injury as well as upon the capacity of the individual organism to cope with it. Thus injury, and not only the reaction thereto, is a dynamic process. Infection, trauma, deficiency states, degeneration, neoplastic growth, etc., may be considered specific types. Commonly the word *injury* is used in a limited sense as synonymous with injury by physical means.

abdominal i. Damage to the structures of the abdominal walls, with or without injury to the underlying viscera; it may involve injury to muscles, blood vessels, nerves, and peritoneum, resulting in hematomas, rupture of muscle fibers, concealed hemorrhage from injured blood vessels in the deep layers, and localized abscess. Peritonitis and occasionally ventral hernia may result. Also see internal *i.*

air-blast i. Injury to the viscera and to the central nervous system caused by rapid changes in the environmental pressure from air blast, as in bomb explosions.

antipersonnel mine i. Damage suffered by those engaged in military operations from the action of buried high explosives. Includes all varieties of high-explosive wounds, of which a large percentage involve the lower extremities only.

back i. Any injury to the muscles of the back or to the spinal column which gives rise to symptoms; includes sprains, concussions, and twists of the spine, and is frequently associated with lumbar pain which may be due to lesions of fascia, muscles, bones, or ligaments, or to specific ailments such as sacroiliac sprain or lumbosacral sprain, fracture-dislocation of the spine, fracture of a spinous process, or damage to an intervertebral disk.

birth i. See *birth injury.*

bladder i. (a) Damage to the urinary bladder through penetration of the abdominal wall, vagina, rectum, buttock, hernial sac, or by accidental injury during abdominal operation or hernioplasty. (b) Rupture of the urinary bladder, either intraperitoneal or extraperitoneal, from fracture of the pelvis, pressure or injury over a distended organ, or occasionally unrelieved retention in an atonic bladder. Extraperitoneal rupture results in extravasation of urine into the prevesical space.

blast i. See *blast injury.*

brain i. Damage to the brain; may be due to contusion and laceration, to disturbance of the cerebral circulation, to cerebral tumors, or in aviators to high velocity and acceleration. Cerebral injury results in edema of the brain, petechial hemorrhage, increased intracranial pressure, and other symptoms.

cauda equina i. A spinal injury from blows or falls, with marked sensory and motor symptoms of varying degree and distribution referred to the end of the spine.

cold i. Trauma from freezing of a body part, seen especially in aviation medicine.

coup-contrecoup i. Lesions produced in the brain as a result of the rebound of the brain against the inner surface of the skull on the same side on which the skull is hit by an external force. See also *contrecoup.*

decompression i. That due to a too rapid drop in atmospheric pressure; seen in caisson disease and aeroembolism.

egg-white i. See *egg-white injury.*
gallbladder i. Trauma of the gallbladder and its ducts from cholecystectomy; the common or hepatic ducts may be accidentally wounded, crushed, or divided; often followed by biliary fistula.
gunshot i. One from the penetration of any small-arms bullet, as from revolvers, pistols, rifles, machine guns, or shotguns.
high-explosive i. Damage to tissues from the action of high explosives, as shells, dynamite, or TNT; may be of all degrees of severity.
industrial i. Any injury due to one's employment in industry, as from tools, machinery, fumes, dust, or chemicals.
internal i. Damage from violence to the organs of the abdominal or thoracic cavity.
kidney i. See renal *i.*
latent tissue i. *In radiobiology,* injury which first becomes manifest at some time after exposure to radiation, usually a matter of days or weeks.
liver i. (a) Contusion or laceration of the liver, usually of the right lobe; may be due to crushing injuries, fractured ribs, gunshot wounds, stab wounds, or operations. (b) Necrosis of liver cells from poisoning and infectious disease, as from malaria or jaundice.
occupational i. Any injury which is brought about solely by an individual's occupation, whether it is industrial or otherwise.
parathyroid i. Damage to the parathyroid gland, resulting in tetany; it may occur during a thyroidectomy, especially when the posterior portion is removed, as in total thyroidectomy.
prostate i. That resulting from unskillful instrumentation, or rarely, from penetrating wounds or pelvic fracture.
radiation i. Localized injurious effects due to alpha or beta particles, gamma rays, and x-rays, which are not ordinarily associated with any systemic reaction, and most commonly due to prolonged and repeated exposure of a particular body area to radium or x-rays.
recurrent nerve i. Trauma or accidental division of the recurrent laryngeal nerve; may occur during a thyroidectomy, postoperatively from the formation of scar tissue, or as a pressure injury from a malignant growth; it results in paralysis of the intrinsic laryngeal muscles, and in the case of involvement of both nerves, in suffocative symptoms.
renal i. Damage of the kidney as a result of trauma, crushing, rib fractures, missiles, or muscular action; involves rupture, penetration, and tears of the ureter.
shell i. Damage due to shell explosions from artillery fire; due largely to bursting fragments and to secondary missiles set in motion by the burst. Also called *shell wound.*
traffic i. Any injury sustained in traffic, irrespective of whether the injured person is a passenger or a pedestrian.
ureteral i. That resulting from renal traumas, pelvic fractures, or accidental instrumental damage suffered during deep pelvic operations.
urethral i. Damage to any portion of the urethra, occurring during prostatectomy or from unskilled instrumentation or accidentally.
war i. Any wound or traumatism caused by small-arms or artillery fire, bomb burst, or other war weapons, incurred during battle action or during the disposition of military or naval forces in a theater of operations.

in'ju·ry cur'rent. Injury potential.

in'ju·ry po·ten'tial. A potential difference, measuring about 30–40 millivolts, between the injured and the uninjured portions of a damaged cell or tissue. Syn., *injury current, demarcation potential.*

in'-knee". Knock-knee. *Obs.*

in'lay" [L. *in,* in; ME. *leien*]. *In dentistry,* fillings which are first made and then cemented into a cavity.
bone i. A bone graft fitted into the two fragments and lying across a fracture or filling a gap between the fragments.

in'let [*in;* ME. *leten*]. The entrance to a cavity.
i. of the pelvis. The space within the brim of the pelvis; the superior pelvic strait.

in'nate, in·nate' [L. *innatus,* inborn]. Dependent upon the genetic constitution.

in"ner·va'tion [L. *in,* in; *nervus,* nerve]. 1. The distribution of nerves to a part. 2. The amount of nerve stimulation received by a part.
reciprocal i. The reciprocal effect of reflex excitation by antagonistic muscles, as extensors and flexors, by which the one set relaxes as the other contracts.

in'no·cent [L. *innocens,* from *in-,* not; *nocere,* to harm]. Benign; not malignant; not apparently harmful.

in·noc'u·ous [L. *innocuus,* harmless]. Not injurious; harmless.

in·nom'i·nate [L. *innominatus,* unnamed]. 1. Unnamed; unnamable, as innominate artery. 2. The irregular bone forming one side and anterior wall of the pelvic cavity, and composed of the ilium, ischium, and pubis; the hipbone.

in·nox'ious (i·nock'shus, in"nock'shus) [L. *innoxius,* harmless]. Innocuous.

in'o- (in'o-, eye'no-), **in-** [G. *is,* fiber]. A combining form denoting *fibrous tissue* or *fibrous components of a tumor.*

in'o·blast [*is;* G. *blastos,* germ]. Old term for fibroblast.

in"oc·ci·pit'i·a (in"ock·si·pit'ee·uh) [L. *in-,* not; *occiput,* back part of the head]. Deficiency of the occipital lobe of the brain.

in"o·chon·dri'tis (in"o·kon·dry'tis) [G. *is,* fiber; *chondros,* cartilage; *-itis,* inflammation]. Inflammation of fibrocartilage.

in·oc"u·la'tion [L. *inoculatio,* from *inoculare,* to ingraft a bud]. 1. The act of introducing the agent of a disease into an animal or plant; specifically, the intentional introduction of an organism for the purpose of producing a mild form of a disease which would be severe if spontaneously introduced. This is known as **preventive inoculation.** See *vaccination.* 2. *In bacteriology,* the planting of microorganisms in or on a culture medium.

in·oc'u·la"tor [L., an ingrafter]. One who or that which inoculates; an instrument used in inoculation.

in·oc'u·lum [L. *inoculare,* to ingraft a bud]. A small amount of bacteria-containing substance used to grow a culture of the bacteria or to infect an experimental animal.

in'o·cyte [G. *is,* fiber; *kytos,* cell]. Old term for fibrocyte, fibroblast.

in'o·gen [*is;* G. *genesthai,* from *gignesthai,* to be produced]. A term used for a hypothetical complex substance of high energy in muscle whose breakdown was thought to supply the energy for muscular contraction. *Obs.*

in·og'li·a (in·og'lee·uh, in·o'glee·uh) [*is;* G. *glia,* glue]. Old term for fibroglia.

in"o·kom'ma. See *sarcomere.*

in"o·lo'min. An antibiotic substance derived from the fungus *Inoloma traganum.*

in·op'er·a·ble [L. *in-,* not; *opera,* work]. Not to be operated upon; of or pertaining to a condition in which the prognosis is unfavorable if an operation is undertaken.

in″or·gan′ic [*in-;* G. *organikos*, serving as organs]. Not organic; not produced by animal or vegetable organisms.

in·os′cu·late [L. *in*, in; *osculare*, to supply with a mouth]. Unite by small openings; anastomose.

in·os″cu·la′tion [*in; osculare*]. The joining of blood vessels by direct communication.

in′ose. See *inositol.*

in″o·se′mi·a [G. *is*, fiber; *haima*, blood]. 1. An excess of fibrin in the blood. 2. The presence of inositol or muscle sugar in the blood.

in′o·sine (in′o·seen, ·sin, eye′no·). A compound occurring in muscle which is formed by the union of hypoxanthine and ribose. It is a decomposition product of the nucleotide, inosinic acid.

in″o·sin′ic ac′id (in″o·sin′ick, eye″no·). A nucleotide constituent of muscle, formed by deamination of adenylic acid; on hydrolysis with acid it yields hypoxanthine and D-ribose-5-phosphoric acid. Syn., *hypoxanthylic acid.*

in′o·site (in′o·sight). See *inositol.*

in·o′si·tol (in·o′si·tole, ·tol, ·tawl, in·oss′i·, in″o-sigh′·). $C_6H_6(OH)_6.2H_2O$. Hexahydroxycyclohexane; a sugarlike alcohol occurring in muscle tissue, brain, red blood cells, and the tissues of the eye; also in leaves and seeds of plants. It resembles the aliphatic polyhydric alcohols rhamnitol and sorbitol in many properties, and is essential for the growth of certain microorganisms and for the prevention of alopecia in mice. It is rarely found in urine. See Table of Vitamins in the Appendix.

in·o′si·tol·hex″a·phos·phor′ic ac′id. A compound of inositol in which all six hydroxyl groups have been esterified with phosphoric acid; it occurs in certain cereal grains. Syn., *phytic acid.*

in″o·si·tu′ri·a (in″o·sigh·tew′ree·uh, ·si·tew′-ree·uh), **in″o·su′ri·a** [*is;* G. *ouron*, urine]. The presence of inositol in the urine. *Rare.*

in″o·trop′ic [*is;* G. *trepein*, to turn]. Pertaining to influences which modify muscular contractility.

in′quest [L. *inquaesitus*, sought for]. *In legal medicine*, a judicial inquiry, as a coroner's inquest, for the purpose of determining the cause of death of one who has died by violence or in some unknown way.

in″qui·si′tion (in″kwi·zish′un) [L. *inquisitio*, from *inquirere*, to search for]. An inquiry, especially one into the sanity or lunacy of a person.

in·sal″i·va′tion [L. *in*, in; *salivare*, to salivate]. The mixture of the food with saliva during mastication. —**insal′ivate,** *v.*

in″sa·lu′bri·ous [L. *in-*, not; *salubris*, healthy]. Unhealthful; not wholesome.

in″sa·lu′bri·ty [*in-; salubris*]. Unwholesomeness or unhealthfulness, as of air or climate.

in·san′i·tar″y (in·san′i·terr″ee) [*in-;* L. *sanitas*, health]. Not sanitary; not in a proper condition as respects the preservation of health.

in·san″i·ta′tion [*in-; sanitas*]. Lack of proper sanitary conditions; defect of sanitation.

in·san′i·ty [L. *insanitas*, from *insanus*, insane]. 1. Loosely, any mental disorder or derangement. See *psychotic disorders.* 2. *In legal medicine*, a mental disorder of such severity that the individual is unable to manage his own affairs and fulfill his social duties or is dangerous to himself or others. —**insane′,** *adj.*

affective i. See affective-reaction *psychosis.*

alcoholic i. See alcoholic *psychosis.*

alternating i. See circular *i.*

circular i. That marked by alternating manic and depressive episodes. Syn., *alternating i.*

climacteric i. That occurring at or near the menopause.

communicated i. See *folie* á deux.

consecutive i. That following some disease or injury not of the brain.

cyclic i. See circular *i.*

delusional i. An acute condition in which delusions or hallucinations are the outstanding symptoms.

depressive i. Melancholia.

deuteropathic i. That caused by disorders of, or developmental changes in, organs other than the brain.

doubting i. A form of anxiety neurosis: also called *folie de doute.*

emotional i. See affective-reaction *psychosis.*

hysterical i. Severe hysteria resembling a psychosis. *Rare.*

ideal i. An old term embracing all the forms in which ideas dependent upon the senses are perverted.

imitative i. A form of folie á deux marked by mimicry of the insane characteristics of another.

imposed i. Delusional ideas imposed by one person upon another individual weaker than himself.

impulsive i. A form in which the patient possesses an uncontrollable desire to commit acts of violence.

intermittent i. Recurrent insanity.

melancholic i. Paranoid melancholia.

moral i. A form marked by perversion and depravity of the moral sense, apparently without impairment of the reasoning and intellectual faculties. *Rare.*

notional i. An old term which covered roughly the schizophrenias and psychoneurotic reactions of today.

periodic i. Manic-depressive psychosis.

pubescent i. Old term for hebephrenia.

puerperal i. Psychotic reaction in a woman at the time of childbirth.

recurrent i. That marked by a succession of many attacks.

senile i. That due to old age.

stuporous i. Old term for anergic stupor.

toxic i. An acute form due to systemic poisoning by certain drugs.

in·scrip′tion [L. *inscriptio*, from *inscribere*, to write on]. The body or main part of a prescription; contains the ingredients and amounts to be used.

in·scrip″ti·o′nes ten·din′e·ae (in·skrip″tee·o′-neez ten·din′ee·ee). Transverse, fibrous bands between segments of the rectus abdominis muscle.

in′sect [L. *insectum*, from *insecare*, to cut in]. A member of the class Insecta of the phylum Arthropoda. In the adult, the body is segmented and is divided into head, thorax, and abdomen; there are three pairs of legs and a single pair of antennae. Usually there are one pair or two pairs of wings, but sometimes none.

in·sec′ti·cide [*insectum;* L. *caedere*, to kill]. A substance that is destructive to insects.

in·sec′ti·fuge [*insectum;* L. *fugare*, to put to flight]. Any substance which repels insects.

in″se·cu′ri·ty [L. *in-*, not; *securitas*, freedom from care]. The state, feeling, or quality of being uncertain or unsafe; an attitude of apprehensiveness, as in respect to one's social status, circumstances, or safety.

in·sem″i·na′tion [L. *inseminare*, to implant]. 1. The planting of seed. 2. The introduction of semen into the vagina. 3. Impregnation.

artificial i. The instrumental injection of semen into the vagina or uterus to induce pregnancy.

in·sen′si·ble [L. *insensibilis*, insensible]. 1. Incapable of sensation or feeling; unconscious. 2. Incapable of being perceived or recognized by the senses. —**insensibil′ity,** *n.*

in·ser′tion [L. *inserere*, to ingraft]. 1. The act of setting or placing in. 2. That which is set in. 3. The point at which anything, as a muscle, is attached; the place or the mode of attachment of an organ to its support. The insertion of a muscle is contrasted with its origin as being the attachment to a relatively more movable part.

velamentous i. The attachment of the umbilical cord to the margin of the placenta.

in·sheathed′ (in·sheethd′, in·sheetht′) [L. *in*, in; AS. *scǣth*]. Enclosed, as within a sheath; invaginated; encysted.

in·sid′i·ous [L. *insidiosus*, deceitful]. Coming on gradually or almost imperceptibly, as a disease whose onset is gradual or inappreciable.

in′sight″ [L. *in*, in; AS. *gesiht*]. *In psychiatry*, the patient's ability to understand his symptoms and their origin and to know that they indicate abnormalities.

in·sip′id [L. *insipidus*, insipid]. Tasteless.

in si′tu (in sigh′tew) [L.]. In a given or natural position; undisturbed.

in″so·la′tion [L. *insolatio*, from *insolare*, to place in the sun]. 1. Exposure to the rays of the sun. 2. Treatment of disease by such exposure. 3. Sunstroke.

in·sol′u·ble [L. *in-*, not; *solubilis*, from *solvere*, to dissolve]. Incapable of dissolving in a liquid. —**insolubil′ity,** *n.*

in·som′ni·a [L., want of sleep]. Sleeplessness; disturbed sleep; a prolonged condition of inability to sleep.

in·spec′tion [L. *inspectio*, from *inspicere*, to look upon]. *In medicine*, the examination of the body or any part of it by the eye.

in″spi·ra′tion [L. *inspiratio*, from *inspirare*, to breathe into]. The drawing in of the breath; inhalation. —**inspire′,** *v.*

in′spi·ra″tor [*inspirare*]. An inhaler or respirator.

in·spi′ra·to″ry [*inspirare*]. Pertaining to the act of inspiration.

in″spi·rom′e·ter [*inspirare; G. metron*, a measure]. An instrument for measuring the amount of air inspired.

in·spis′sant [L. *in*, in; *spissare*, to thicken]. Tending to thicken; thickening, as of the bile or other fluids.

in·spis′sant. An agent that tends to increase the thickness of blood or other fluid.

in·spis′sate [*in; spissare*]. Make thick by evaporation or by absorption of fluid. —**inspissated,** *adj.*

in″sta·bil′i·ty [L. *instabilitas*, from *instabilis*, unsteady]. 1. Lack of firmness; insecurity of support or balance. 2. Lack of fixed purpose; inconstancy in opinions or beliefs.

in′stance [L. *instantia*, a being near or close upon]. *In psychoanalysis*, the dominance or perseverance of one level of mental function in comparison to others.

in′step [L. *in*, in; AS. *staepe*]. The arch on the medial side of the foot.

in″stil·la′tion [L. *instillare*, to pour in by drops]. The introduction of a liquid into a cavity drop by drop.

in′stil·la″tor [*instillare*]. An apparatus for introducing, by drops, a liquid into a cavity or space.

in′stinct [L. *instinctum*, from *instinguere*, to incite]. 1. A precise form of behavior in which there is an invariable association of a particular series of responses with specific stimuli; an unconditioned compound reflex. 2. *In psychoanalysis*, a primary tendency, as toward life, reproduction, and death.

death i. See *thanatos*.

life i. See *eros*.

in·stinc′tive [*instinctum*]. Prompted or determined by instinct; of the nature of instinct.

in′sti·tutes of med′i·cine. The fundamental principles of medicine, especially of physiology, pathology, therapeutics, and hygiene. *Obs.*

in′stru·ment [L. *instrumentum*, utensil]. A mechanical tool or implement. —**instrumen′tal,** *adj.*

stitching i. A surgical appliance consisting of a needle holder which utilizes all varieties of surgical needles, the suture material feeding from a continuous spool supply attached to the handle.

in″stru·men·ta′tion [*instrumentum*]. The use of instruments in treating a patient.

in″suf·fi′cien·cy [L. *in-*, not; *sufficere*, to suffice]. The state of being inadequate; incapacity to perform a normal function.

adrenal cortical i. Inadequate secretion by the adrenal cortex; it may be acute or chronic as in Addison's disease.

aortic i. Incompetent aortic valve action caused mainly by aortic cusp lesions, either rheumatic or syphilitic. Diagnostic symptoms consist of diastolic murmur and "water-hammer" pulse.

cardiac i. See *cardiac failure*.

chronic intestinal i. See celiac *disease*.

chronic jejuno-ileal i. See celiac *disease*.

coronary i. Incompetent heart action caused by restriction of blood supply to the myocardium and consequent lack of oxygen supply in that organ. It is characterized by anginal pains.

energetodynamic cardiac i. A disorder involving a disturbed metabolism of the myocardium. It is always a complication of some general disease.

i. of a muscle. Inability on the part of a muscle to contract sufficiently to produce the normal effect; applied especially to the eye muscles.

i. of the externi. A condition in which the contraction of the lateral muscles of the eye is weak and is overbalanced by that of the medial muscles, producing esophoria.

i. of the interni. Defective power on the part of the medial muscles, producing exophoria.

ovarian i. Deficiency of ovarian function, either primary or secondary, which can result in either amenorrhea, oligomenorrhea, or abnormal dysfunctional uterine bleeding: a clinical term.

pancreatic i. Absence of or reduced pancreatic secretion into the duodenum, and resultant poor digestion and absorption of fat, vitamins, nitrogen, and carbohydrates. It usually occurs after a prolonged disease of the pancreas.

renal i. Inadequate function of the kidney, characterized by its failure to remove urea from the blood at a normal rate.

respiratory i. Incompetence of the respiratory processes.

in″suf·fla′tion [L. *insufflare*, to breathe into]. The act of blowing into, as blowing a gas, powder, or vapor into one of the cavities of the body.

endopharyngeal i. A method of inducing anesthesia through a tube introduced through the mouth or nose to the back of the pharynx.

intratracheal i. Insufflation through a tracheal tube introduced into the larynx.

mouth-to-mouth i. The blowing of air into the mouth of a person, usually a newborn infant, to distend the lungs and counteract asphyxia.

perirenal i. *In roentgenography*, the injection of air or carbon dioxide into the perirenal tissue to outline the adrenal glands and kidneys.

tubal i. See Rubin *test*.

in′suf·fla″tor [*insufflare*]. An instrument used in insufflation.

in′su·la [L., island]. Portion of cortex overlying the corpus striatum; it lies hidden from view in the adult brain at the bottom of the lateral fissure. See Plate 17. —**insular,** *adj.*

insulated plastic boot. A high boot, consisting of an inner and outer sleeve with a filler of spun glass, used to increase blood flow to the lower extremities by conserving body heat and raising cutaneous temperature.

in'su·lin [*insula*]. The antidiabetic hormone arising from the beta cells of the islets of Langerhans of the pancreas. It is a protein which in monomeric form has a molecular weight of about 12,000, or possibly even 6,000; crystallizes in the form of twin rhombohedra in solutions slightly above its isoelectric point, provided the solutions contain salts of zinc, nickel, cadmium, or cobalt; is rich in sulfur with several constituent amino acids; is relatively stable in acid solution and readily hydrolyzed in alkaline solution. The United States Pharmacopeia Reference Standard is a crystalline sample of insulin containing 23 units per mg. Therefore, the unit corresponds to $\frac{1}{23}$ mg. of the United States Pharmacopeia Reference Standard insulin. It is inactive orally. Insulin, when injected parenterally in the diabetic organism, approximates normal ability to utilize sugars and fats; glycogen is deposited normally in the liver, and muscle glycogen may be increased; blood-sugar levels are reduced; glycosuria disappears; hyperlipemia and ketosis disappear; excessive destruction of protein is prevented, and the respiratory quotient rises. Its action may be modified greatly by various mechanisms, including pituitary, thyroid, and certain adrenal hormones. In normal animals or in man, insulin causes a reduction in blood-sugar levels. Large doses in the non-diabetic organism may reduce liver glycogen. —**insulinoid,** *adj.*

amorphous i. The form of insulin obtained in commercial processes in the absence of added zinc or certain other metal ions (see under *insulin*). In aqueous solution it is most effective usually between the second and the sixth hours after injection. It is marketed in strengths of 20, 40, 80, or 100 units per cc. Also called *regular i.*, *unmodified i.*

crystalline i. The crystalline product obtained when insulin is precipitated in the presence of added zinc ion. It contains 0.016 to 0.04 mg. of zinc per 100 units of insulin. The rapidity and duration of action are probably no different from that of amorphous insulin. It is considered advantageous in insulin-allergic patients.

globin i. with zinc. A preparation of insulin modified by the addition of globin (derived from the hemoglobin of beef blood) and zinc chloride; the commercial product is a solution, adjusted to a pH between 3.4 and 3.8, containing 40 or 80 U.S.P. units of insulin per cc. and from 3.6 to 4.0 mg. of globin for each 100 units of insulin. Its maximum effectiveness is between 8 and 16 hours after injection.

hexamine i. A combination of hexamethylenetetramine and insulin. Its effect is evident two to four hours after injection but has a sustained action rather comparable to protamine zinc insulin.

histone i. A preparation containing insulin and thymus histone which precipitates the insulin, the resulting suspension producing a prolonged hypoglycemic effect, as compared to amorphous or crystalline insulin solutions. Also combined with zinc as histone zinc insulin, comparable in action to protamine zinc insulin.

i. allergy. The tissue reaction to insulin which may be represented by varying degrees of local tissue reaction, urticaria, or anaphylaxis. Local reactions may be characterized by stinging, itching, soreness, heat, and induration about the site of injection. The reaction may depend upon the animal source of the insulin. Contamination or alteration of the proteins in solution must be considered. Similar reactions may be due to substances such as protamine in the mixture injected.

i. atrophy. Atrophy of the subcutaneous, chiefly fatty tissues about the site of injection of insulin. Such lesions are disfiguring but not dangerous. Also called *fat atrophy.*

i. hypertrophy. A painless, locally indurated, raised, rubbery area of fatty hypertrophy seen in some patients in an area repeatedly injected with insulin.

i. resistance. A condition in which insulin injected produces an unusually slight response. It varies from mild to severe degrees. Also called *i. insensitivity.*

i. sensitivity. A term used to describe the comparative degree of effectiveness of insulin. In juvenile diabetes the blood-sugar level is depressed quickly and markedly by relatively small doses. The opposite is commonly true in middle-aged and older patients.

i. shock. The reaction of the body to doses of insulin which produce hypoglycemia. Common symptoms are a sense of nervous agitation, weakness, trembling, sweating, speech difficulty, pallor, listlessness, negativism, unconsciousness; in severe attacks, convulsions, vomiting, diarrhea, and incontinence. Also called *i. reaction.*

i. tannate. A combination of tannic acid and insulin which precipitates at approximately pH 7. Its maximum effect occurs at about the fifth hour after injection.

i. tolerance. The relative degree of response of the body to insulin.

isophane i. A preparation of protamine and insulin in which the two substances are present in their combining proportion (isophane ratio), which is approximately 0.5 mg. of protamine for each 100 U.S.P. units of insulin. NPH insulin is an isophane insulin.

lente i. One of a series of protein-free injectable preparations of insulin, having varying duration of action, obtained by mixing proper proportions of crystalline, long-acting zinc insulin with amorphous, short-acting zinc insulin, the mixture being suspended in a phosphate-free, saline and acetate medium of pH 7.2.

NPH i. *N*eutral *P*rotamine *H*agedorn insulin; a preparation of isophane insulin developed by Hagedorn, consisting of crystals containing insulin, protamine, and zinc, suspended in a buffered medium of pH 7.1 to 7.4. It contains between 0.3 and 0.6 mg. of protamine for each 100 U.S.P. units of insulin, the two being present in isophane ratio. The injection contains 40 or 80 U.S.P. units of insulin in each cc. The average duration of action is somewhat longer than that of globin insulin but less than that of protamine zinc insulin.

pectin i. A slowly absorbed preparation of insulin in a viscous medium containing 4 to 5 per cent pectin and adjusted to pH 4.0 to 4.4. See *decurvon.*

protamine calcium i. A mixture of insulin and calcium salts in solution, formerly used in an attempt to prolong insulin action.

protamine i. A preparation of insulin combined with protamine, a protein prepared from the sperm of fishes of the trout family; the mixture by the gradual release of insulin produces a prolonged depressing effect upon blood-sugar levels. Its effect is evident between the third and sixth hours, is maximal from the twelfth to the eighteenth hours, and disappears almost completely about 24 hours after injection.

protamine zinc i. A preparation similar to protamine insulin; the commercial products are suspensions providing 40 or 80 U.S.P. units of insulin per cc. and containing 1.0 to 1.5 mg. of protamine and 0.20 to 0.25 mg. of zinc for each 100 units of insulin. Its action is longer than that of protamine insulin. The full cumulative effect of daily doses occurs in two or three days.

vegetable i. Any one of several noninsulin blood-sugar-depressing plant extracts, such as myrtillin which is made from the leaves of the blueberry plant, *Rehmannia glutinosa* extract, *Oplopanax horridus* (devil's-club) extract.

in″su·lin·e′mi·a [*insula;* G. *haima,* blood]. The presence of an abnormal, or dangerous, amount of insulin in the circulating blood.

in″su·lin·o′ma, in·su·lo′ma. See islet-cell *tumor.*

in′sult. Trauma or other stress to tissues or organs.

in″sus·cep″ti·bil′i·ty [L. *in-,* not; *susceptum,* from *suscipere,* to take up]. Absence of contagious quality; want of susceptibility.

in″te·gra′tion [L. *integrare,* to make whole]. 1. The process of unifying different elements into a single whole. 2. The combination of bodily activities to cooperate in the welfare of the whole organism. 3. *In neurology,* the impingement of impulses from various centers upon one final, common pathway, resulting in an adaptive response.

in·teg′u·ment [L., a covering]. A covering, especially the skin. —**integumen′tary,** *adj.*

fetal i. The fetal membranes. *Obs.*

in′tel·lect [L. *intellectus,* understanding]. The mind, the understanding, or the reasoning power.

in·tel′li·gence [L. *intellegentia,* intelligence]. 1. The understanding, intellect, or mind. 2. The ability to perceive qualities and attributes of the objective world, and to employ purposively a means toward the attainment of an end.

in·tel′li·gence quo′tient. A figure used to designate a person's intelligence; can be arrived at by dividing the mental age by the chronologic age (up to 16 years). The three grades of mental deficiency (idiocy, imbecility, and moronity) are marked by intelligence quotients of 69 or lower. Above 69, the classification is as follows: dull normal, 70–90; normal, 90–110; superior, 110–125; very superior, 125–140; and genius, 140 and above. Abbreviated, I.Q.

in·tem′per·ance [L. *intemperantia,* want of moderation]. Want of moderation; immoderate indulgence, especially in alcoholic beverages. —**intemperate,** *adj., n.*

in·tense′ [L. *intensus,* stretched]. 1. Extreme in degree; showing to a high degree the characteristic attribute. 2. Feeling deeply.

in·ten″si·fi·ca′tion [*intensus*]. The condition occurring in cutaneous sensory disturbances in which certain sensations are abnormally vivid.

in″ten·sim′e·ter (in″ten·sim′i·tur, in·ten′si·mee″-tur) [*intensus;* G. *metron,* a measure]. An instrument for measuring the intensity or dosage of x-rays.

in·ten′si·ty [*intensus*]. 1. The state or condition of being intense. 2. Amount or degree of strength or power. 3. *In radiology,* the amount of energy per unit time passing through a unit area perpendicular to the line of propagation.

i. of a magnetic field. At any point, the force per unit pole upon a free pole, placed at that point.

i. of an electric field. At any point, the force per unit charge upon a charged particle, placed at that point.

i. of x-rays. The dose of radiation in roentgens divided by the time required to deliver it.

luminous i. From a point source of light, the flux emitted per unit angle in a certain direction.

in·ten′tion [L. *intentio,* purpose]. 1. The end or purpose. 2. A process or manner of healing.

in′ter- [L., between]. A prefix signifying *between* or *among, mutual, intervening,* or *within.*

in″ter·ac·ces′so·ry (in″tur·ack·sess′o·ree) [*inter;* L. *accedere,* to add to]. Situated between accessory processes of the vertebrae.

in″ter·ac′i·nous (in″tur·ass′i·nus, **in″ter·ac′i·nar** (in″tur·ass′i·nur) [*inter;* L. *acinus,* berry]. Situated between acini.

in″ter·al·ve′o·lar (in″tur·al·vee′o·lur, ·al′vee·o·lur) [*inter;* L. *alveolus,* small hollow]. Between alveoli.

in″ter·ar″y·te·noid′e·us. A variant name for the combined oblique and transverse arytenoid muscles.

in″ter·a′tri·al (in″tur·ay′tree·ul, ·at′ree·ul) [*inter;* L. *atrium,* atrium]. Between the atria of the heart.

in′ter·brain″. See *diencephalon.*

in·ter′ca·la″ted [L. *intercalare,* to insert]. Placed or inserted between, as intercalated disks of cardiac muscle.

in″ter·cap′il·lar″y glo·mer″u·lo·scle·ro′sis (in″-tur·cap′i·lerr″ee). A lesion of the renal glomeruli which is accompanied by diabetes mellitus, renal edema, pronounced albuminuria, and sometimes hypertension and renal insufficiency. However, it occurs in diabetic persons without the associated phenomena mentioned and may occur in those without diabetes. Microscopically, the glomerular tufts show spherical, oval, or less well-defined foci of acellular, acidophilic, hyalinized tissue, with concentric argyrophilic laminas, situated between the capillaries. Said to be a more specific morphologic evidence of diabetes than is hyalinization of the islets of the pancreas. Syn, *Kimmelstiel-Wilson disease* or *syndrome.*

in″ter·car′pal [L. *inter,* between; G. *karpos,* wrist]. Between the carpal bones, as intercarpal ligaments. See Table of Joints and Ligaments in the Appendix.

in″ter·cav′ern·ous [*inter;* L. *caverna,* cavern]. Situated between the two cavernous sinuses, as the intercavernous sinuses.

in″ter·cel′lu·lar [*inter;* L. *cellula,* small storeroom]. Between cells, as intercellular substance of tissue.

in″ter·chon′dral (in″tur·kon′drul) [*inter;* G. *chondros,* cartilage]. Between cartilages.

in″ter·cli′noid [*inter;* G. *klinē,* bed; *eidos,* form]. Between the clinoid processes of the sphenoid bone.

in″ter·co·lum′nar [*inter;* L. *columna,* column]. Between pillars or columns.

in″ter·con′dy·lar, in″ter·con′dy·loid [*inter;* G. *kondylos,* knuckle]. Between condyles, as the intercondylar fossa, the notch between the condyles of the femur.

in″ter·con·ver′sion (*of protein, carbohydrate, and fat*). See Krebs *cycle.*

in″ter·cos′tal [*inter;* L. *costa,* rib]. Between the ribs, as intercostal spaces or muscles.

in″ter·cos″to·bra′chi·al. Associated with an intercostal space and the arm, as intercostobrachial nerve.

in″ter·coup′ler (in″tur·cup′lur) [*inter;* L. *copula,* band]. An apparatus used during the administration of an inflammable anesthetic to equalize the electric potential among anesthetist, patient, operating table, and anesthetic machine; designed to prevent explosions or fires due to static electricity.

in′ter·course [L. *intercursus,* from *intercurrere,* to run between]. Communication; intimate connection between persons.

sexual i. Sexual connection; coitus.

in″ter·cri″co·thy·rot′o·my (in″tur·cry″ko·thigh-rot′o·mee) [L. *inter*, between; G. *krikos*, ring; *thyreoeidēs*, shield-shaped; *tomē*, a cutting]. A cut into the larynx by transverse section of the crico-thyroid membrane.

in″ter·cris′tal [*inter;* L. *crista*, crest]. Between the surmounting ridges of a bone, organ, or process. Used particularly in intercristal diameter of the pelvis, the distance between the two iliac crests.

in″ter·cru′ral [*inter;* L. *crus*, leg]. Situated between the crura, particularly of the subcutaneous inguinal ring.

in″ter·cur′rent [*inter;* L. *currere*, to run]. Occurring or taking place between, as a disease arising or progressing during the existence of another disease in the same person.

in″ter·cusp′ing [*inter;* L. *cuspis*, pointed end]. *In dentistry*, the fitting together of the occlusal surfaces of opposing teeth.

in″ter·den′tal [*inter;* L. *dens*, tooth]. Located or placed between the teeth.

in″ter·den′ti·um (in″tur·den′shee·um) [*inter; dens*]. The space between any two of the teeth.

in″ter·dic′tion [L. *interdictio*, from *interdicere*, to prohibit]. *In legal medicine*, a judicial or voluntary restraint placed upon an insane person or one suspected of insanity, preventing him from the management of his own affairs or the affairs of others.

in″ter·dig″i·ta′tion (in″tur·didj″i·tay′shun) [L. *inter*, between; *digitus*, finger]. 1. The locking or dovetailing of similar parts, as the fingers of one hand with those of the other; or of the ends of the obliquus abdominis externus muscle with those of the serratus anterior. 2. *In dentistry*, in closure of the buccal teeth, the striking of the cusps of one denture fairly into the occluding sulci of the other denture.

in′ter·face. A surface which forms the boundary between two phases or systems.

in″ter·fere′ [*inter;* L. *ferire*, to strike]. In horses, to strike one hoof or the shoe of one hoof against the opposite leg or fetlock.

in″ter·fer′ence [*inter; ferire*]. 1. *In physics*, the mutual action of two beams of light, or of two series of sound vibrations, or, in general, of two series of any type of waves when they coincide or cross. 2. The mutual extinction of two excitation waves that meet in any portion of the heart.

dissociation i. See atrioventricular *dissociation* with interference.

in″ter·fer·om′e·ter (in″tur·feer·om′i·tur) [*inter; ferire;* G. *metron*, a measure]. An apparatus for the production and demonstration of interference fringes between two or more wave trains of light from the same area. It is chiefly used to compare wave lengths with a standard wave length, by means of interference fringes.

in″ter·fer·om′e·try (in″tur·feer·om′i·tree) [*inter; ferire; metron*]. Use of the interferometer to compare wave lengths with observable displacements of reflectors.

in″ter·fi′bril·lar (in″tur·figh′bril·ur, ·figh·bril′ur) [*inter;* dim. from L. *fibra*, fiber]. Situated between the fibrils of tissues, as interfibrillar substance.

in″ter·fol·lic′u·lar [*inter;* L. *folliculus*, small bag]. Between follicles.

in″ter·glob′u·lar [*inter;* L. *globulus*, little ball]. Situated between globules, as interglobular dentine.

in″ter·go′ni·al [*inter;* G. *gōnia*, corner]. Between the two gonia (angles of the lower jaw).

in·te′ri·or [L., inner]. Situated within, with reference to a cavity, part, or organ.

in″ter·kin·e′sis. A period in the life of a cell during which there is no mitotic activity: also called *interphase.*

in″ter·la′bi·al [L. *inter*, between; *labium*, lip]. Between the lips, or between the labia pudendi.

in″ter·la·mel′lar [*inter;* L. *lamella*, small plate of metal]. Between lamellas.

in″ter·lam′i·nar [*inter;* L. *lamina*, plate]. Situated between laminas.

In″ter·lin′gua (in″ter·ling′gwah). A linguistic system developed by the International Auxiliary Language Association (IALA) and proposed for use as a medium of international communication in science, technology, medicine, and other fields of science. The vocabulary includes all words common to English, French, Italian, Spanish, and Portuguese, with some German and Russian alternates.

in″ter·lo′bar [*inter;* G. *lobos*, lobe]. Situated between lobes, as interlobar pleurisy.

in″ter·lob′u·lar [*inter; lobos*]. Between lobules.

in″ter·mar′riage [*inter;* OF. *mariage*, from L. *maritare*]. 1. Marriage of blood relations. 2. Marriage between persons of different races.

in″ter·max′il·lar″y (in″tur·mack′si·lerr″ee) [*inter;* L. *maxilla*, jaw]. Between the maxillary bones.

in″ter·max′il·lar″y. The os incisivum, a small bone that receives the upper incisors, situated between the maxillary bones of the fetus. Also called *premaxilla.*

in″ter·me′din [L. *intermedius*, that which is between]. A hypophyseal substance influencing pigmentation and found in greatest concentration in the intermediate portion of the pituitary in certain animal species. A similar or identical principle active in man is now called *melanocyte-stimulating hormone* (MSH).

in″ter·me″di·o·lat′er·al [*intermedius;* L. *latus*, side]. Both lateral and intermediate, as the intermediolateral tract of the spinal cord, lying between the anterior and posterior gray columns.

in″ter·mem′bra·nous [L. *inter*, between; *membrana*, membrane]. Lying between membranes.

in″ter·me·nin′ge·al [*inter;* G. *mēnigx*, membrane]. Between the dura and the arachnoid, or between the latter and the pia, as intermeningeal hemorrhage.

in″ter·men′stru·al [*inter;* L. *menstrualis*, monthly]. Between menstrual periods.

in·ter′ment [L. *in*, in; *terra*, earth]. The burial of a body.

in″ter·mes″o·blas′tic [L. *inter*, between; G. *mesos*, middle; *blastos*, germ]. Between the layers or between the lateral plates of the mesoderm. *Obs.*

in″ter·met″a·mer′ic [*inter;* G. *meta*, between; *meros*, part]. Between two metameres, as the intermetameric or intersegmental ribs.

in″ter·mi·cel′lar flu′id. *In colloid chemistry,* a liquid medium in which the colloidal particles (micelles) are dispersed.

in″ter·mi·tot′ic. Pertaining to a period or stage during mitosis.

in″ter·mit′tent [L. *intermittere*, to leave off]. Occurring at intervals, as intermittent fever, intermittent insanity, intermittent pulse, intermittent sterilization.

in″ter·mu′ral [L. *inter*, between; *murus*, wall]. Situated between the walls of an organ.

in″ter·mus′cu·lar [*inter;* L. *musculus*, muscle]. Situated between muscles.

in′tern [F. *interne*]. A resident physician in a hospital, usually in his first year of service.

in·ter′nal [L. *internus*, internal]. Situated within or on the inside. —**internad,** *adv.*

in·ter′nal il′i·ac. The hypogastric artery.

in″ter·na′ri·al [L. *inter*, between; *nares*, nostrils]. Situated between the nostrils.

International Red Cross. The Swiss Red Cross. Also see *Red Cross Society.*

in″ter·neu′ron [*inter;* G. *neuron,* nerve]. A short neuron with its cell body in the dorsal horn of the spinal cord; one of the elements of a simple reflex arc. Also called *internuncial neuron, intercalated neuron.*

in″ter·neu′ro·nal [*inter; neuron*]. Between neurons.

in·ter′nist [L. *internus,* internal]. A physician who specializes in internal medicine.

in′ter·node″ [L. *inter,* between; *nodus,* knot]. The space between two nodes of a nerve fiber, as the internode between the nodes of Ranvier. Also called *internodal segment.* —**interno′dal,** *adj.*

in″ter·nun′ci·al (in″tur·nun′shul) [*inter;* L. *nuncius,* messenger]. Serving as a connecting or announcing medium, as internuncial neurons, nerve cells between two others in a nervous pathway.

in·ter′nus. See *internal.*

in″ter·o·cep′tor [L. *internus,* internal, perhaps by analogy with *externus; capere,* to take]. Any one of the end organs situated in the viscera which receive stimuli from visceral activities, such as digestion, excretion, circulation. Also called *visceroceptor.*

in″ter·o·fec′tive [*internus;* L. *facere,* to bring about]. Bringing about internal changes; the term applied by Cannon to the nerves of the autonomic nervous system.

in″ter·o·fec′tive sys′tem. That part of the nervous system that is concerned with the regulation of the internal environment of the body; essentially, equivalent to the autonomic nervous system.

in″ter·ol′i·var″y (in″tur·ol′i·verr″ee) [L. *inter,* between; *oliva,* olive]. Between the inferior olives.

in″ter·os′se·ous [*inter;* L. *os,* bone]. Between bones, as interosseous arteries, membranes, muscles, or ligaments.

in″ter·os′se·us [*inter; os*]. Interosseous muscle of the hand or foot, one of the small muscles inserting on the phalanges. See Table of Muscles in the Appendix.

in″ter·pal′pe·bral [*inter;* L. *palpebra,* eyelid]. Between the palpebrae, or eyelids.

in″ter·pa·ri′e·tal [*inter;* L. *paries,* wall]. Between walls; between the parietal bones, as interparietal suture; between parts of the parietal lobe, as interparietal fissure. Cf. *incarial bone.*

in″ter·pe·dun′cu·lar [*inter;* L. *pedunculus,* little foot]. Situated between the cerebral or cerebellar peduncles.

in″ter·pha·lan′ge·al [*inter;* G. *phalagx,* bone between two joints of the fingers and toes]. Between the phalanges of the fingers or toes. See Table of Joints and Ligaments in the Appendix.

in′ter·phase″. See *interkinesis.*

in″ter·prox′i·mal [*inter;* L. *proximus,* nearest]. *In dentistry,* between two adjacent teeth, as an interproximal space.

in″ter·prox′i·mate [*inter; proximus*]. Interproximal.

in″ter·pu′pil·la″ry dis′tance. The distance between the centers of the pupils of the two eyes.

interrenin. A trade-mark for a preparation of the adrenal cortex; in solution and capsule form.

in′ter·sex″ [*inter;* L. *sexus,* sex]. An individual whose constitution is intermediate between male and female, and who may be a true or a pseudohermaphrodite; a sex-intergrade. —**intersex′ual,** *adj.,* **intersexual′ity.** *n.*

in′ter·space″ [*inter;* L. *spatium,* space]. An interval between the ribs, or between the fibers or lobules of a tissue or organ.

in″ter·spi·nal′es. Variable small muscles running between adjacent spinous processes of the vertebrae.

in″ter·spi′nous [*inter;* L. *spina,* thorn]. Situated between spinous processes.

in·ter′sti·ces (in·tur′sti·siz) [L. *interstitium,* a place between]. Spaces or intervals; pores.

in″ter·sti′tial (in″tur·stish′ul) [*interstitium*]. 1. Situated between important parts; occupying the interspaces or interstices of a part. 2. Pertaining to the finest connective tissue of organs.

in″ter·sti″ti·o′ma (in″tur·stish″ee·o′ma). See interstitial-cell *tumor.*

in″ter·tar′sal [L. *inter,* between; G. *tarsos,* flat of the foot]. Located between adjacent tarsal bones.

in″ter·trans″ver·sal′es. Old name for the intertransversarii muscles.

in″ter·trans″ver·sa′ri·i (in″tur·trans″vur·sah′ree·ee) [*inter;* L. *transversus,* lying across]. Short bundles of muscular fibers extending between the transverse processes of contiguous vertebrae. They are sometimes divided into anterior and lateral. Also called *intertransversales.* See Table of Muscles in the Appendix.

in″ter·trans·verse′ (·trans·vurs′, ·tranz·) [*inter; transversus*]. Connecting the transverse processes of contiguous vertebrae.

in″ter·tri′go (in″tur·try′go, ·tree′go) [L., from *inter; tritum,* from *terere,* to rub]. An erythematous eruption of the skin produced by friction of adjacent parts. —**intertri′ginous,** *adj.*

in″ter·tro″chan·ter′ic (in″tur·tro″can·terr′ick) [*inter;* G. *trochantēr,* trochanter]. Between the trochanters.

in″ter·tu′bu·lar [*inter;* L. *tubulus,* small pipe]. Between tubes or tubules.

in′ter·val [L. *intervallum,* interval]. 1. The time intervening between two points of time. 2. The lapse of time between two recurrences of the same phenomenon. 3. The empty space between any two things or parts of the same thing.

a-c i. The time between the beginning of the a (presystolic) and the c (systolic) waves of the venous pulse, used to estimate atrioventricular conduction. It actually measures the time elapsing between the right atrial contraction and the onset of the left ventricular ejection: normally, two seconds or less.

A_s-V_s i. The interval between inception of atrial and ventricular contractions determined from cardiograms, pressure pulses, or volume curves of the heart.

cardioaortic i. The interval between the apex beat and the arterial pulse.

electrocardiographic i. 1. The duration of the waves (P, QRS, T) of an electrocardiogram. 2. The intervals between the waves (P-R, Q-T, R-R, ST-T, T-Q).

focal i. The distance between the anterior and posterior focal points.

isometric i. Period from the beginning of ventricular contraction to the beginning of ejection of blood: also called *presphygmic i.*

lucid i. *In psychiatry,* a transitory return of the normal mental faculties, seen in psychoses or delirious conditions.

P-Q i. The time interval from the beginning of the P wave to the beginning of the QRS complex of the electrocardiogram; the time taken for the activation process leaving the sinoauricular (SA) node to reach the ventricles.

P-R i. The time between the rise of the P wave and the Q wave, if present, or the R wave of a standard electrocardiogram; used to measure conduction time of impulses from the S-A node to the ventricles.

QRS i., Q-S i. The duration of the process of excitation of the ventricles, measured from the beginning of Q (or R) to the end of S on the electrocardiogram: usually 0.10 second or less.

Q-T i. The time from the beginning of the QRS complex to the end of the T wave. It measures the duration of electric systole. Bazett's formula is used to calculate the ideal Q-T interval for any rate: $QT = K\sqrt{C}$, where C = cycle length, K = 0.36 to 0.42.
R-R i. In the electrocardiogram, the time from one R wave to the next.
S-T i. The time between the end of the QRS complex and the end of the T wave. It represents the time between the completion of depolarization of the ventricles and their complete repolarization.

in″ter·vas′cu·lar [L. *inter*, between; *vasculum*, small vessel]. Located between vessels.

in″ter·ven·tric′u·lar [*inter;* L. *ventriculus*, belly]. Situated between ventricles, as interventricular septum.

in″ter·ver′te·bral [*inter;* L. *vertebra*, vertebra]. Between the vertebrae, as an intervertebral disk.

in″ter·vil′lous [*inter;* L. *villus*, tuft of hair]. Situated between villi.

in″ter·zo′nal [*inter;* G. *zōnē*, belt]. Between zones, applied to filaments between daughter cells in the telophase of mitosis.

in·tes′tine [L. *intestinum*, intestines]. The part of the digestive tube extending from the pylorus to the anus. It consists of the small and large intestine. The former is about 6¾ meters (20 feet) in length, and extends from the pylorus to its junction with the large intestine at the cecum. Three divisions are described—the duodenum, 22 cm. long, the jejunum, 2.2 meters long, and the ileum, 4 meters long. The large intestine is about 1.6 meters (5 feet) long, and consists of the cecum (with the vermiform appendix), the colon, and the rectum. The wall of the intestine is made up of four coats, mucous, submucous, muscular, and serous. Embedded in the wall are minute glands, and projecting from the surface, in the small intestine, are the villi. See Plates 13, 14. —**intestinal,** *adj.*

in″tes·ti′num [L.]. See *intestine.*
i. caecum. The cecum.
i. crassum. The large intestine.
i. ileum. The ileum.
i. jejunum. The jejunum.
i. rectum. The rectum.
i. tenue. The small intestine.
i. tenue mesenteriale. That portion of the small intestine which has a mesentery, namely the jejunum and ileum.

in′ti·ma [L. *intimus*, innermost]. The innermost of the three coats of a blood vessel. See Plate 6. —**intimal,** *adj.*

in′tine (in′tyne, ·tin) [G. *intus*, within]. The thin, inner coat of an endospore.

intocostrin. Trade-mark for a physiologically standardized curare extract or for its active component tubocurarine chloride; administered intravenously or intramuscularly. Used to produce relaxation of the voluntary muscles in the treatment of certain neurologic conditions. Also used to improve relaxation during anesthesia.

in′toe″ing [L. *in*, in; ME. *too*]. Pointing the toes inward in walking.

in·tol′er·ance [L. *intolerantia*, from *intolerans*, intolerant]. 1. Lack of capacity to endure, as intolerance of light or pain. 2. Sensitivity, as to a drug.

in·tort′er [L. *intortus*, from *intorquere*, to twist]. The muscle tilting the vertical meridian of the eye inward; the superior rectus muscle.

in·tox′i·cant [L. *in*, in; G. *toxikon*, poison]. Intoxicating; capable of producing intoxication or poisoning.

in·tox′i·cant. An agent capable of producing intoxication.

in·tox″i·ca′tion [*in; toxikon*]. 1. Poisoning, as by a drug, a serum, alcohol, or any poison. 2. State of being intoxicated, especially the acute condition produced by overindulgence in alcohol; drunkenness.
pathologic i. An alcoholic psychosis marked by unusual symptoms, as epileptiform seizures, confusion, illusions, anxiety, rage, violent criminal tendencies, and sometimes hallucinations; it is usually followed by amnesia for the episode. May occur in susceptible individuals after only a small amount of alcohol is consumed. Syn., *mania à potu.*
septic i. A form of poisoning resulting from absorption of products of putrefaction.
water i. A condition characterized by cramps, dizziness, headache, and vomiting; produced by the administration of large quantities of water with the resulting dilution of body salts. May occur in an experimental animal or in man, if certain diseases are present.

in″tox·im′e·ter (in″tok·sim′e·ter). See breath alcohol *method.*

in′tra- [L., within]. 1. A prefix signifying *within* or *into.* 2. *In anatomy*, a prefix denoting *situated within* a specified part.

in″tra·ab·dom′i·nal [*intra;* L. *abdomen*, belly]. Within the cavity of the abdomen, as intraabdominal pressure.

in″tra·ac′i·nar (in″truh·ass′i·nur) [*intra;* L. *acinus*, grape]. Situated or occurring within an acinus.

in″tra·ar·tic′u·lar [*intra;* L. *articulus*, joint]. Within a joint.

in″tra·a′tri·al [*intra;* L. *atrium*, atrium]. Within one of the atria of the heart.

intracaine. Trade-mark for β-diethylamino-ethyl-*p*-ethoxy-benzoate, also known as diethoxin, a local anesthetic.

in″tra·cap′su·lar [*intra;* L. *capsula*, small box]. Within the fibrous capsule of a joint, as intracapsular fracture.

in″tra·car″ti·lag′i·nous (·kahr″ti·ladj′i·nus) [*intra;* L. *cartilago*, cartilage]. Within a cartilage, as intracartilaginous ossification; endochondral.

in″tra·cav′i·ta·ry [*intra;* L. *cavitas* fr. *cavus*, hollow]. Within a cavity.

in″tra·cel′lu·lar [*intra;* L. *cellula*, small storeroom]. Within a cell.

in″tra·cra′ni·al [*intra;* G. *kranion*, skull]. Within the skull, as intracranial pressure.

in″tra·cu·ta′ne·ous [*intra;* L. *cutis*, skin]. Within the skin substance; applied to injection of substances into the skin.

in″tra·cys′tic [*intra;* G. *kystis*, bladder]. Situated or occurring within a cyst or bladder.

in″tra·der′mal, in″tra·der′mic [*intra;* G. *derma*, skin]. Within the skin.

in″tra·du′ral. Within the dura mater.

in″tra·fu′sal (in″truh·few′zul) [*intra;* L. *fusus*, spindle]. Pertaining to the striated muscular fibers contained in a muscle spindle.

in″tra·gem′mal (in″truh·jem′ul) [*intra;* L. *gemma*, bud]. Within a bud or a bulbous nerve end, as a taste bud of the tongue.

in″tra·ge·ner′ic. Within a genus.

in″tra·group′, in″tra·group′al [*intra;* It. *gruppo*, group]. Within a group.

in″tra·he·pat′ic [*intra;* G. *hēpar*, liver]. Within the liver.

in″tra·lo′bar [*intra;* G. *lobos*, lobe]. Within a lobe.

in″tra·lob′u·lar [*intra;* dim. from *lobos*]. Within a lobule, as an intralobular vein of the liver.

in″tra·lu′mi·nal [*intra;* L. *lumen*, light]. Within the lumen of a hollow or tubelike structure.

in″tra·med′ul·lar·y. 1. Within the substance of the spinal cord or medulla oblongata. 2. Within the substance of the bone marrow, as an intramedullary nail. 3. Within the substance of the adrenal medulla.

in″tra·mem′bra·nous [*intra;* L. *membrana,* skin]. Developed or taking place within a membrane, as intramembranous ossification.

in″tra·mu′ral [*intra;* L. *murus,* wall]. Within the substance of the walls of an organ, as intramural fibroid of the uterus.

in″tra·mus′cu·lar [*intra;* L. *musculus,* muscle]. Within the substance of a muscle, as intramuscular injection of drugs.

in″tra·na′sal (in″truh·nay′zul) [*intra;* L. *nasus,* nose]. Within the cavity of the nose.

in″tra·nu′cle·ar [*intra;* L. *nucleus,* kernel]. Within a nucleus.

in″tra·oc′u·lar [*intra;* L. *oculus,* eye]. Within the globe of the eye, as intraocular hemorrhage.

in″tra·o′ral [*intra;* L. *os,* mouth]. Within the mouth.

in″tra·or′bit·al [*intra;* L. *orbita,* orbit]. Within the orbit.

in″tra·pa·ri′e·tal [*intra;* L. *paries,* wall]. 1. Within the wall of an organ. 2. Within the parietal region of the cerebrum, as the intraparietal fissure. 3. Within the body wall.

in″tra·pel′vic [*intra;* L. *pelvis,* basin]. Within the pelvic cavity.

in″tra·per·i·to·ne′al [*intra;* G. *peritonaion,* membrane which contains the lower viscera]. Within the peritoneum, or peritoneal cavity, as intraperitoneal injection of drugs.

in″tra·pleu′ral (in″truh·ploor′ul) [*intra;* G. *pleura,* rib]. Within the pleural cavity.

in″tra·scro′tal [*intra;* L. *scrotum,* scrotum]. Within the scrotal sac.

in″tra·spi′nal [*intra;* L. *spina,* thorn]. Within the spinal canal, as intraspinal anesthesia.

in″tra·stro′mal [*intra;* G. *strōma,* mattress, bed]. Within the stroma of an organ, part, or tissue.

Intra-sul. Trade-mark for an aqueous preparation containing 1% of available sulfur and used in arthritis by intravenous or intramuscular injection.

in″tra·the′cal [*intra;* G. *thēkē,* a case]. Old term for intraspinal.

in″tra·tra′che·al (in″truh·tray′kee·ul) [*intra;* G. *trachys,* rough]. Within the trachea, as intratracheal insufflation through a tracheal tube introduced through the larynx.

in″tra·tu′bal [*intra;* L. *tubus,* pipe]. Within a tube; within a uterine tube.

in″tra·u·re′thral [*intra;* G. *ourēthra,* urethra]. Within the urethra.

in″tra·u′ter·ine (in″truh·yoo′tur·in, ·yoo′tuh-ryne) [*intra;* L. *uterus,* womb]. Within the uterus.

in″tra·vas′cu·lar [*intra;* L. *vasculum,* small vessel]. Within the blood vessels.

in″tra·ve′nous [*intra;* L. *vena,* vein]. Within, or into, the veins, as intravenous injection.

in″tra·ven·tric′u·lar [*intra;* L. *ventriculus,* belly]. Located, or occurring, within a ventricle.

in″tra·ves′i·cal [*intra;* L. *vesica,* bladder]. Within the urinary bladder.

in″tra·vi′tal [*intra;* L. *vita,* life]. Occurring during life, as intravital staining of cells.

in·trin′sic [L. *intrinsecus,* inward]. Inherent; situated within; peculiar to a part, as the intrinsic muscles of the larynx.

in′tro- [L. *intro,* inwardly]. A prefix signifying *within* or *into; inward.*

in″tro·ces′sion [L. *introcessum,* from *introcedere,* to go into]. A depression, as of a surface.

in′tro·fi·er. A liquid which, when not added in too great quantity, will help emulsification by lowering the interfacial tension.

in″tro·flex′ion [L. *intro,* inwardly; *flexio,* a bending]. A bending in; inward flexion. *Obs.*

in·tro′i·tus [L.]. An aperture or entrance, particularly the entrance to the vagina.

in″tro·jec′tion [L. *intro,* inwardly; *iacere,* to throw]. 1. A mechanism by which there is possible an absorption of parts of the environment or of the personality of others into one's own personality. 2. *In psychiatry* and *psychoanalysis,* the absorption into and toward oneself of concepts and feelings generated toward another person or object; an unconscious process. It is a partial form of identification (in which the person behaves like another person). Its effect in mental disorders is to motivate irrational behavior toward oneself, e.g., self-neglect or suicide arising from aggression stimulated by others, then introjected.

in″tro·mis′sion [L. *intromissum,* from *intromittere,* to send into]. Insertion, the act of putting in, the introduction of one body into another, as of the penis into the vagina.

in″tro·mit′tent [*intromittere*]. Conveying or allowing to pass into or within, as into a cavity; refers to the penis, which carries the semen into the vagina.

in″tro·spec′tion [L. *introspectum,* from *introspicere,* to look into]. The act of looking inward, as into one's own mind.

morbid i. The morbid habit of self-examination; irrational and obsessive dwelling upon one's own thoughts, feelings, impulses, fears, or conduct.

in″tro·sus·cep′tion. See *intussusception.*

in″tro·ver′sion (in″tro·vur′shun, ·zhun) [L. *introversus,* inward]. 1. A turning within, as a sinking within itself of the uterus. 2. *In psychopathology,* a turning inward of psychic energy in the form of introspection and subjective thinking.

in′tro·vert″ [L. *intro,* within; *vertere,* to turn]. One whose interests are directed inwardly upon himself and not toward the outside world.

in″tro·vert′. To turn one's interests to oneself rather than to external things.

in″tu·ba′tion [L. *in,* in; *tubus,* tube]. The introduction of a tube into a hollow organ to keep it open, especially into the larynx to insure the passage of air, in edema of the glottis or in the acute stage of diphtheria.

in′tu·ba″tor [*in; tubus*]. An instrument used for the introduction of an intubation tube.

in″tu·mes′cence [L. *intumescere,* to swell up]. 1. A swelling of any character whatever, as an increase of the volume of any organ or part of the body. 2. The process of becoming swollen. 3. *In neuroanatomy,* the cervical and lumbar enlargements. Syn., *tumescence.*

in″tus·sus·cep′tion [L. *intus,* within; *suscipere,* to receive]. The receiving of one part within another; especially, the invagination, slipping, or passage of one part of the intestine into another, occurring usually in young infants. Acute intussusception is characterized by the symptom complex of paroxysmal pain, vomiting, the presence of a sausage-shaped tumor in the lower abdomen, and the passage of blood and mucus per rectum.

agonal i. Single or multiple areas of intussusception, sometimes found in the small intestine at the time of death.

chronic i. One occurring gradually without acute symptoms.

colic i. One involving the colon only.

double i. One in which another area of bowel invaginates into an existing intussusception.

enteric i. One involving the small intestine only. Also called *ileal i.*

enterocolic i. Invagination of the ileum into the colon. See ileocecal *i.*, ileocolic *i.*

gastric i. One in which a jejunal loop may escape through a gastroenterostomy into the stomach.

ileocecal i. One which takes place at the ileocecal valve, the cecum as well as the ileum being invaginated into the colon.

ileocolic i. An intussusception of the ileum through the ileocecal valve, without invagination of the cecum.

multiple i. An enteric intussusception in which there are more than two areas of small intestine involved.

in″tus·sus·cep′tum [*intus; suscipere*]. In intussusception, the invaginated portion of intestine.

in″tus·sus·cip′i·ens (in″tus·suh·sip′ee·enz) [*intus; suscipere*]. In intussusception, the segment of the intestine receiving the other segment.

in′u·la [L., elecampane]. Elecampane. The root of *Inula helenium*, of the family Compositae. It contains a carbohydrate inulin, a volatile oil, and certain crystallizable principles. See *alantolactone*.

in′u·lase. An enzyme capable of converting inulin into levulose.

in′u·lin. $(C_6H_{10}O_5)_n$. A carbohydrate from many plants of the Compositae, yielding levulose on hydrolysis; white amorphous powder or granules, odorless, almost tasteless, and soluble in hot water: used to measure glomerular filtration rate (*inulin clearance*). After intravenous injection, it is not metabolized and is quantitatively excreted by the kidney by glomerular filtration only.

in·unc′tion [L. *inunctio*, from *inunguere*, to anoint]. 1. The act of rubbing an oily or fatty substance into the skin. 2. The substance used.

in u′te·ro [L.]. Within the uterus; not yet born.

in vac′u·o [L.]. In a vacuum; in a space from which most of the air has been exhausted.

in·vag″i·na′tion (in·vadj″i·nay′shun) [L. *in*, in; *vagina*, sheath]. 1. The act of ensheathing or becoming ensheathed. 2. The process of burrowing or infolding to form a hollow space within a previously solid structure, as the invagination of the nasal mucosa within a bone of the skull to form a paranasal sinus. 3. Intussusception. 4. *In embryology*, the infolding of a part of the wall of the blastula to form a gastrula. —**invag′inate,** *adj.*, *v.*

basilar i. See *platybasia*.

in′va·lid [L. *invalidus*, not strong]. 1. Not well. 2. One who is not well, especially one who is chronically ill or whose convalescence is slow. 3. Suitable or adapted for an invalid person, as invalid diet, invalid chair. —**invalidism,** *n.*

in·va′sin. See *hyaluronidase*.

in·va′sion [L. *invasio*, from *invadere*, to attack]. 1. That period in the course of disease, especially an infectious disease, immediately following inception or infection, and preceding prodromal signs and symptoms. 2. The process whereby bacteria or other microorganisms enter the body; subsequent multiplication of pathogens causes disease.

in·ver″mi·na′tion. Helminthiasis.

in·ver′sion (in·vur′shun, ·zhun) [L. *inversio*, from *invertere*, to turn upside down]. 1. The act of turning inward. 2. A turning upside down. 3. *In chemistry*, usually the change of a compound having optical activity into one or more other compounds conferring opposite optical activity on the product. Also the change of any compound into an isomeric form.

i. of bladder. A condition, occurring only in females, in which the urinary bladder is in part or completely pushed into the dilated urethra.

i. of the foot. A turning of the sole of the foot inward, so that the medial margin is elevated.

i. of uterus. A rare condition in which the fundus of the uterus is forced or pulled through the cervix and comes into close contact with, or protrudes through, the external os and even through the vagina.

sexo-esthetic i. The adoption of the habits, manners, and costume of the opposite sex. Also see *eonism, transvestitism*.

sexual i. *In psychiatry*, the direction of the sexual instinct toward one of the same sex; homosexuality.

in·ver′sive [*invertere*]. Applied to enzymes which convert sucrose into invert sugar.

in·vert′. To turn inward.

in′vert [*invertere*]. *In psychiatry*, a homosexual.

in·ver′tase (in·vur′tace, in′vur·taze). See *saccharase*.

in·ver′te·bral [L. *in-*, not; *vertebra*, joint]. Without a spinal column.

In·ver″te·bra′ta [*in-; vertebra*]. A division of the animal kingdom which includes all except the animals with a notochord.

in·ver′te·brate [*in-; vertebra*]. Without a spinal column; invertebral.

in·ver′te·brate. An animal without a notochord or vertebral column.

in·vert′in, in′vert·in. See *saccharase*.

in′ver·tose. See *invert sugar*.

in′vert sug′ar. A mixture of approximately equal parts of dextrose and levulose, obtained from the hydrolysis of sucrose. It is levorotatory, fermentable, and reduces Fehling's solution. Also called *invertose*.

in·vest′ing [L. *investire*, to clothe]. Enveloping, enclosing, embedding.

in·vest′ment [*investire*]. A sheath; a covering.

fibrous i. General term describing an outer sheath of connective tissue found about various organs outside the proper capsule of the organ.

in·vet′er·ate [L. *inveteratus*, of long standing]. Long established, chronic, resisting treatment.

in″vi·ril′i·ty [L. *in-*, not; *virilitas*, manhood]. Lack of virile power; male impotency.

in″vis·ca′tion [L. *in*, in; *viscare*, to besmear]. Insalivation.

in vit′ro [L.]. In glass; referring to a process or reaction carried out in a culture dish, test tube, etc., as opposed to *in vivo*.

in vi′vo [L.]. In the living organism: used in contrast to *in vitro*.

in″vo·lu′crum [L., that in which something is wrapped]. 1. The covering of a part. 2. New bone laid down by periosteum around a sequestrum in osteomyelitis.

in·vol′un·tar″y [L. *involuntarius*, involuntary]. Performed or acting independently of the will, as involuntary muscles of viscera.

in′vo·lute [L. *involutum*, from *involvere*, to roll upon]. *In biology*, rolled up, as the edges of certain leaves in the bud.

in″vo·lu′tion [L. *involutio*, from *involvere*]. 1. A turning or rolling inward. 2. The retrogressive change to their normal condition that certain organs undergo after fulfilling their functional purposes, as the uterus after pregnancy. 3. The period of regression or the process of decline or decay which occurs in the human constitution after middle life. —**involutional,** *adj.*

buccal i. The folding in of the ectoderm, which forms the stomodeum. *Obs.*

i. form. A form seen in microorganisms that have undergone degenerative changes as a result of unfavorable environment.

i. of the uterus. The return of the uterus to its normal weight and condition after childbirth.

senile i. Senile atrophy.

in′ward [AS. *inweard*]. Toward the inside or center.

iocamfen. Trade-mark of a liquid obtained by the interaction of iodine, phenol, and camphor; it contains about 7.25% of free iodine and is used as an antiseptic and fungicide.

iocapral. A proprietary tablet containing theobromine, mebaral, and calcium iodide di-triethanolamine. Used as a vasodilator, sedative, and antispasmodic.

iodalbin. Trade-mark for a compound of iodine and blood albumin; the substance is a brown powder containing about 21.5% of iodine and has been used where iodine therapy is indicated.

I·o″da·moe′ba (eye·o″duh·mee′buh, eye·od″uh·) [G. *ioeidēs,* violetlike; *amoibē,* change]. A genus of amebas.

I. bütschlii. A small, sluggish ameba which is nonpathogenic but is parasitic in the large intestine of man.

I. williamsi. Synonym for *I. bütschlii.*

i′o·date. Any salt of iodic acid.

iodeikon. A trade-mark for iodophthalein sodium, $C_{20}H_8O_4I_4Na_2$, used as a radiopaque medium.

iod-ethamin. Trade-mark for ethylenediamine dihydriodide, $C_2H_4(NH_2)_2.2HI$, used in iodine therapy.

iodex. A proprietary ointment containing iodine in organic combination with a fatty acid; also with methyl salicylate. Used for minor cuts, wounds, and abrasions.

i·od′ic ac′id (eye·od′ick). HIO_3. A crystalline powder, soluble in water. In 1 to 3% solution it has been employed in the treatment of trachoma and indolent corneal ulcers.

iodicin. Trade-mark for calcium iodoricinoleate used in iodine therapy.

i′o·dide. Any binary compound, such as a salt or ester, containing iodine having a negative valence of one.

i″o·dim′e·try [*ioeidēs;* G. *metron,* a measure]. Usually, volumetric analysis by titration with an iodine solution.

i′o·dine (eye′o·dyne, ·deen, ·din) [*ioeidēs*] (*iodum*). I = 126.91. A nonmetallic element occurring as gray-black plates or granules with metallic luster and characteristic odor. It is only sparingly soluble in water but more soluble in iodide solutions; soluble in 13 parts of alcohol or 80 parts of glycerin. A local irritant and germicide, generally applied for the latter purpose in the form of a 2 or 3% solution. An ointment or tincture is used for fungous infections. Iodine is a normal constituent of the thyroid gland and essential for its proper functioning. It is used as a preventive of simple goiter and in the treatment of exophthalmic goiter. In syphilis and tuberculosis it causes a breaking down of the local lesions, and in pleurisy, bronchitis, etc., it exerts a liquefying action on viscid secretions. For internal administration, preference is usually given to one of the iodides, although the strong iodine solution is sometimes employed. See Table of Normal Values of Blood Constituents in the Appendix.

i. antiseptic solution. Iodine tincture.

i. number. A measure of unsaturation of fatty acids: (*Hanus method*) the number of grams of iodine capable of being absorbed by 100 gm of a lipid. (*Schmidt-Nielsen method*) Unsaturated bonds of the lipid are saturated with excess bromine and the excess is determined iodometrically. (*Kretchmer-Holman-Burr method*) Same as Schmidt-Nielson method, using pyridine sulfate dibromide as the brominating agent.

i. ointment (*unguentum iodi*). An antiseptic and counterirritant; contains 4% each of iodine and potassium iodide.

i. pentoxide. I_2O_5. Iodic anhydride. White, crystalline powder used in determining carbon monoxide content of gases.

i. solution (*liquor iodi*). A solution of 20 Gm. iodine and 24 Gm. sodium iodide in distilled water to 1000 cc.

i. tincture (*tinctura iodi*). A solution of 20 Gm. iodine and 24 Gm. sodium iodide in diluted alcohol to 1000 cc.

i. value. See *i.* number.

phenolated i. solution (*liquor iodi phenolatus*). A solution prepared by exposing to sunlight until almost colorless a mixture of 15 cc. strong iodine solution, 6 cc. liquefied phenol, 165 cc. glycerin, and water to make 1000 cc. Also called *Boulton's solution, French mixture, carbolized i. solution.*

protein-bound i. (**PBI**). Iodine attached to protein; commonly, iodine bound to the protein fraction of the blood; in most instances, it reflects the level of circulating thyroid hormone.

strong i. solution (*liquor iodi fortis*). A solution of 50 Gm. iodine and 100 Gm. potassium iodide in distilled water to 1000 cc.; used for systemic effect of iodine. Dose, 0.12–0.3 cc. (2–5 min.) t.i.d. Also antidotal to many alkaloids. Also called *Lugol's solution, compound i. solution.*

strong i. tincture (*tinctura iodi fortis*). A solution of 70 Gm. iodine and 50 Gm. potassium iodide in 50 cc. distilled water and alcohol to 1000 cc.

i·od′i·nin (eye·od′i·nin). A purple-bronze antibiotic pigment produced by *Chromobacterium iodinum;* it is a di-N-oxide of dihydroxyphenazine. Iodinin inhibits the growth of streptococci, even in very dilute solutions.

i″o·din′o·phil, i″o·din′o·phile [*ioeidēs;* G. *philein,* to love]. 1. Having an affinity for iodine stain. 2. A histologic element staining readily with iodine. —**iodinophil′ic,** *adj.*

i″o·din″o·phil′i·a. See *iodophilia.*

iodipin. Trade-mark for an iodized vegetable oil. The substance is a yellowish brown liquid containing 0.54 Gm. of combined iodine per cc. Used as are the alkaline iodides or in 40% strength as a contrast medium in roentgen diagnosis.

i′o·dism [*ioeidēs*]. A condition arising from the prolonged use of iodine or iodine compounds; marked by frontal headache, coryza, ptyalism, and various skin eruptions, especially acne.

iodival. Trade-mark for alpha-monoiodoisovalerylcarbamide. The substance is used where iodine therapy is indicated.

i′o·dized [*ioeidēs*]. Impregnated with iodine. —**iodize,** *v.*

i·o′do- (eye·o′do-, eye′o·do-), **iod-** [*ioeidēs*]. *In chemistry,* a combining form signifying *iodine* or *an iodine compound.*

i·o″do·a·ce′tic ac′id. $CH_2I.COOH$; a compound of importance in experimental biochemistry because it has the ability to interfere with phosphorylating enzyme activity, thereby inhibiting absorption of glucose: generally employed in the form of a salt.

i·o″do·al″phi·on′ic ac′id. $C_6H_5.CH(COOH)CH_2.$-$C_6H_2I_2OH$; β-(4-hydroxy-3,5-diiodophenyl)-α-phenylpropionic acid, a white or faintly yellowish crystalline powder, insoluble in water. It is used orally as a contrast medium in cholecystography. Average dose, 3 Gm. (45 gr.). See *priodax.*

i·o″do·an″ti·py′rine (·an″ti·pye′reen, ·rin). See *iodopyrine.*

iodobismitol. Trade-mark for a solution of sodium iodobismuthite and sodium iodide with either benzocaine or saligenin. It has been used as an antisyphilitic.

iodo-casein. Trade-mark for a compound of iodine combined with milk casein. The substance is a yellowish brown powder, containing 18% of iodine. Used in iodine therapy.

i·o″do·chlor″hy·drox′y·quin. $C_9H_5C.INO$; 5-chloro-7-iodo-8-hydroxyquinoline; a brownish-yellow powder, practically insoluble in water. Introduced as a surgical dusting powder, it is now used for treating amebic dysentery; in combination with boric acid, lactic acid, zinc stearate, and lactose (compound iodochlorhydroxyquin powder) it is administered by intravaginal insufflation in treatment of *Trichomonas vaginalis* vaginitis. See *vioform*.

iodochlorol. Trade-mark for an iodized and chlorinated peanut oil used as a radiopaque medium.

i·o″do·der′ma [*ioeidēs;* G. *derma*, skin]. Skin eruptions due to iodine; generally used in reference to a pustular eruption caused by the ingestion of iodine compounds.

i·o′do·form (*iodoformum*). Triiodomethane, CHI_3. A yellow, finely crystalline powder having a peculiar, penetrating odor. It is readily soluble in chloroform and ether, less readily in alcohol, and only slightly in water. An antiseptic and anesthetic used as a local dressing to wounds and painful ulcers. Suppositories containing 0.3–0.6 Gm. are used in internal hemorrhoids.

i·o″do·gor·go′ic ac′id. Diiodotyrosine.

iodol. Trade-mark for tetraiodopyrrole; C_4HI_4N; a yellowish-gray powder which has been used as a surgical dusting powder.

i·o″do·meth′ane. Methyl iodide.

i″o·dom′e·try [*ioeidēs;* G. *metron*, a measure]. Usually, volumetric analysis for iodine present in, or liberated by, a compound. —**iodomet′ric,** *adj.*

i·o″do·pa·no′ic ac′id. Generic name for 3-(3-amino-2,4,6-triiodophenyl)-2-ethylpropanoic acid, a cholecystographic medium available under the trade-marked name *telepaque*. See *iopanoic acid*.

i·o″do·phe′nol. 1. $C_6H_4.OH.I$. Para-iodophenol; has been used as an antiseptic. 2. A solution of 20 parts of iodine in 76 parts of fused phenol with 4 parts of glycerin.

i·o′do·phil. See *iodinophil*.

i·o″do·phil′i·a [*ioeidēs;* G. *philein*, to love]. A pronounced affinity for iodine; the term is applied to the protoplasm of leukocytes in purulent conditions.

i·o″do·phthal′ein (eye·o″do·thal′een, ·fthal′een, ·ee·in, eye″o·do·). Tetraiodophenolphthalein. $C_{20}H_{10}I_4O_4$. A light yellow powder used externally as an antiseptic dusting powder. See *nosophen*.

soluble i. See *iodophthalein sodium*.

i·o″do·phthal′ein so′di·um (*iodophthaleinum sodicum*). $C_{20}H_8I_4O_4Na_2.3H_2O$. The disodium salt of tetraiodophenolphthalein; a pale, blue-violet powder, soluble in about 7 parts of water. It is employed to render the gallbladder opaque for roentgenologic examination. It may be administered intravenously or orally; the dose is to be adjusted to the weight of the patient. Syn., *soluble iodophthalein, tetiothalein sodium.* See *iodeikon*.

i″o·dop′sin [*ioeidēs;* G. *opsis*, vision]. Visual violet; a conjugated carotenoid protein found in the cones of the retina.

i·o″do·py′ra·cet in·jec′tion. Generic name for an injectable aqueous solution of the diethanolamine salt of 3,5-diiodo-4-pyridone-*N*-acetic acid; $C_5H_2I_2NOCH_2COONH_2(CH_2CH_2OH)_2$; a radiopaque medium. A 35% w/v solution is used for intravenous urography and retrograde pyelography, also for cholangiography, venography, and arteriography. A concentrated solution, 70% w/v, is used for cardioangiography. Syn., *diodone injection.* See *diodrast*.

i·o″do·py′rine (eye·o″do·pye′reen, ·rin, eye″o·do·). Iodoantipyrine. A chemical compound of iodine and antipyrine of the composition $C_{11}H_{11}IN_2O$. Formerly used as antipyretic.

i″o·do″so·ben·zo′ic ac′id. $C_6H_4.OI.COOH$. A colorless, crystalline compound which has been used as an antiseptic in the same manner as iodoform.

iodostarine. Trade-mark for an iodine addition product of tariric acid, derived from the fruit of a species of *Picramnia*. The product contains 47.5% iodine. A white, crystalline solid. Used where iodide therapy is indicated.

i·o″do·ther′a·py [*ioeidēs;* G. *therapeia*, treatment]. The treatment of disease by the use of iodine or its compounds.

i·o″do·thy′mol. See *aristol*.

i·o″do·thy′rine. Thyroiodine.

i″o·do·thy″ro·glob′u·lin [*ioeidēs;* G. *thyreos*, shield; L. *globulus*, little ball]. An iodine-containing globulin found in the thyroid gland.

i″o·dox″y·ben·zo′ic ac′id. $C_6H_4(IO_2)COOH$. A colorless, crystalline compound whose salts, notably the calcium compound, are used for antiarthritic and analgesic effects.

i″o·dox′yl. The official British Pharmacopoeia title for *sodium iodomethamate*. See *neo-iopax*.

i·om′e·ter (eye·om′i·tur) [G. *iōn*, from *ienai*, to go; *metron*, a measure]. A special type of monitor ionization chamber for the measurement of roentgen rays.

i′on [*iōn*]. An atom or group of atoms which, by a suitable application of energy (for example, through the action of roentgen or radium rays, or by the dissociation of a molecule) has lost or gained one or more orbital electrons and has thus become capable of conducting electricity.

dipolar i. Zwitterion.

i. exchange. The reversible exchange of ions in a solution with ions present in a solid material, called an *ion exchanger*. This consists of a matrix of insoluble material, which may be inorganic or organic, interspersed with cations and anions, certain of which may participate in the exchange process.

i. transfer. The migration of ionic medication through intact skin under the influence of a direct electric current: also called *iontophoresis*.

negative i. Anion.

positive i. Cation.

zwitter i. See *zwitterion*.

Ionescu, Toma [*Rumanian surgeon*, 1860–1926]. Known for his early studies of spinal anesthesia at a high level. Introduced an operation of cervical sympathectomy for angina pectoris (1916).

i·on′ic strength (eye·on′ick). Measure of the intensity of the electric field in a solution; half the sum of the activity of each ion in solution, multiplied by the square of its ionic charge.

i·o′ni·um (eye·o′nee·um) [G. *iōn*, from *ienai*, to go]. A radioactive element which emits alpha particles; an isotope of thorium and the direct parent of radium.

i″on·i·za′tion [*iōn*]. Electrolytic dissociation; the production of ions. —**i′onize,** *v.*

intermittent i. Further ionization of ions at a surface, occurring at the same time as neutralization of electrons at the surface.

specific i. *In radiobiology*, the number of ion pairs produced per unit length of path of radiation, e.g., per cm of air, or micron of tissue.

i″on·iz′ing e·vent′. Any occurrence of a process in which an ion or group of ions is produced, as by passage of alpha or beta particles or gamma rays, through a gas.

i″on·om′e·ter [*iōn;* G. *metron*, a measure]. An instrument for measuring x-ray dosages, based upon the production of ions in air by x-rays.

i″o·none′, i′o·none. A ketone, $C_{13}H_{20}O$, prepared from citral and used as a synthetic violet odor.

i·on′o·phose (eye·on′o·foze, eye′on·o·foze) [G. *ion*, violet; *phōs*, light]. A violet phose.

i·on″to·pho·re′sis (eye·on″to·fo·ree′sis) [G. *iōn*, from *ienai*, to go; *phorēsis*, from *phorein*, to bear].

1. The movement of charged particles through a fluid under the influence of an electric current. 2. *In medicine*, a method of introducing charged particles into the skin or other tissues by means of an electric current. It utilizes the principle that ions are repelled from an electrode of like charge.

i·on″to·quan·tim′e·ter (eye·on″to·kwon·tim′i-tur). See *ionometer*.

i″o·pa·no′ic ac′id. U.S.P. name for *iodopanoic acid*.

iopax. Trade-mark for sodium 2-oxy-5-iodopyrine-N-acetate, a water-soluble compound used as a contrast medium in radiology.

i″o·phen′dyl·ate in·jec′tion. U.S.P. name for a sterile mixture of isomers of ethyl iodophenylundecylate; $I.C_6H_4.CH(CH_3)CH_2(CH_2)_6CH_2$-$COOC_2H_5$, of uniform but unknown proportions; a colorless to pale yellow, viscous liquid, very slightly soluble in water: used as a radiopaque medium, particularly for study of the lumbar region. Syn., *ethyl iodophenylundecylate, ethyl iodophenylundecylate injection*. See *pantopaque*.

i″o·pho′bi·a [G. *ios*, poison; *phobos*, fear]. A morbid fear of poison.

i″o·pro′pane. See *iothion*.

iothion. Trade-mark for a brand of iopropane, chemically diiodohydroxypropane. The substance is a yellowish, oily liquid containing about 80% of iodine; used externally in oil solution or as an ointment for systemic effect of iodine.

ip′e·cac [from the Tupi] (*ipecacuanha*). The dried rhizome and roots of *Cephaëlis ipecacuanha*, known as Rio or Brazilian ipecac, or of *C. acuminata*, known as Cartagena, Nicaragua, or Panama ipecac. It yields not less than 2% of ether-soluble alkaloids, the most important from a therapeutic standpoint being emetine and cephaeline. Among other alkaloids present are psychotrine, O-methylpsychotrine, and emetamine. The action of ipecac depends on the dosage employed: emetic, 1–2 Gm. (15–30 gr.); nauseating expectorant and diaphoretic, 0.03–0.12 Gm. (½–2 gr.); stomachic, 16–32 mg. (¼–½ gr.).

i. and opium powder (*pulvis ipecacuanhae et opii*). A diaphoretic and sedative. Dose, 0.2–0.6 Gm. (3–10 gr.) preferably in conjunction with hot drinks. Syn., *Dover's powder*.

i. fluidextract (*fluidextractum ipecacuanhae*). Contains 2% of ether-soluble alkaloids. Dose, emetic, 1–2 cc. (15–30 min.); expectorant, 0.06–0.12 cc. (1–2 min.).

i. syrup (*syrupus ipecacuanhae*). The preferred form of administration for expectorant purposes. Dose, emetic, 15 cc. (4 fluidrachms); nauseating expectorant, 1–2 cc. (15–30 min.).

i. tincture (*tinctura ipecacuanhae*). Contains 0.2% of alkaloids. Dose, emetic, 8 cc. (2 fluidrachms); expectorant, 0.3–1.0 cc. (5–15 min.).

i. wine. The tincture is now used in place of this.

undulated i. The root of *Richardia scabra*, an adulterant of ipecac.

white i. The emetic root of *Ionidium ipecacuanhae;* an adulterant of ipecac.

wild i. The North American plant, *Euphorbia ipecacuanhae*. The root is emetic and cathartic.

ip′e·cine (ip′i·seen, ·sin). Emetine.

"I"-per·so′na. The sum of all the cortical or discriminative functions of the human brain which produce sentiment and partitive feeling, as contrasted with the primary instinctual and affective functions which motivate the organism as a whole.

Ipesandrine. Trade-mark for a liquid cough sedative containing opium alkaloids, emetine hydrochloride, and ephedrine hydrochloride.

Ip″o·me′a, Ip″o·moe′a (ip″o·mee′uh, eye″po·) [G. *ips*, woodworm; *homoios*, like]. The dried root of *Ipomoea orizabensis*, yielding not less than 15% of resins. Syn., *Mexican scammony, Orizaba jalap*.

i. resin. (*resina ipomoeae*). An active cathartic with a tendency toward griping. It consists largely of glycosides and methyl pentosides of jalapinolic acid, $C_{15}H_{30}(OH)COOH$, and its methyl ester. Dose, 0.13–0.32 Gm. (2–5 gr.).

ipral calcium. Trade-mark for probarbital calcium or calcium 5-ethyl-5-isopropyl barbiturate. The substance is used as a sedative and hypnotic.

ipral sodium. Trade-mark for probarbital sodium or sodium 5-ethyl-5-isopropyl barbiturate. The substance is used as a sedative and hypnotic.

i″pro·ni′a·zid. Generic name for the antituberculosis drug 1-isonicotinyl-2-isopropyl hydrazine. See *marsilid*.

ip″si·lat′er·al [L. *ipse*, self; *latus*, side]. Situated on the same side, as paralytic (or similar) symptoms which occur on the same side as the cerebral lesion causing them; homolateral.

IQ, I.Q. Intelligence quotient.

Ir Chemical symbol for iridium.

i·ral′gi·a (eye·ral′juh, ·jee·uh). See *iridalgia*.

i·ras″ci·bil′i·ty [L. *irasci*, to be angry]. The quality of being choleric, irritable, or of hasty temper. It is a frequent symptom in some psychoses and in neurasthenia.

ir″i·dad″e·no′sis (irr″i·dad″i·no′sis, eye″ri·) [G. *iris*, iris; *adēn*, gland; *-ōsis*, condition]. A lymphocytic affection of the iris.

i′ri·dal (eye′ri·dul, irr′i·dul), **i·rid′i·al** (eye·rid′ee·ul, i·rid′ee·ul), **i·rid′i·an** [*iris*]. Relating to the iris.

ir″i·dal′gi·a (irr″i·dal′juh, ·jee·uh, eye″ri·) [*iris;* G. *algos*, pain]. Pain referable to the iris.

ir″i·daux·e′sis [*iris;* G. *auxēsis*, increase]. Auxesis or tumefaction of the iris.

ir″i·da·vul′sion [*iris;* L. *avulsio*, a plucking off]. Surgical avulsion of the iris; iridoavulsion. Also see *iridectomy*.

ir″i·dec′tome [*iris;* G. *ek*, out; *tomos*, cutting]. A cutting instrument used in iridectomy.

ir″i·dec′to·mize [*iris;* G. *ektomē*, excision]. Excise a part of the iris; perform iridectomy.

ir″i·dec′to·my [*iris; ektomē*]. The cutting out of a part of the iris.

ir″i·dec·tro′pi·um [*iris;* G. *ektrepein*, to turn aside]. Eversion of a part of the iris.

ir″i·de′mi·a, ir″i·dae′mi·a (irr″i·dee′mee·uh, eye″ri·) [*iris;* G. *haima*, blood]. Hemorrhage of the iris.

ir″i·den·clei′sis (irr″i·den·klye′sis, eye″ri·). See under *iridotasis*.

ir″i·den·tro′pi·um [*iris;* G. *entrepein*, to turn in]. Inversion of a part of the iris.

i·rid″e·re′mi·a [*iris;* G. *erēmia*, absence]. Total or partial absence of the iris; aniridia.

ir′i·des (irr′i·deez, eye′ri·deez). Plural of iris.

ir″i·des′cence [*iris*]. A rainbowlike display of intermingling and changing colors, as in mother-of-pearl. —**iridescent,** *adj.*

i·rid′e·sis, ir″i·de′sis. See *iridotasis*.

ir″i·di″ag·no′sis. See *iridodiagnosis*.

i·rid′i·al (eye·rid′ee·ul, i·rid′·). See *iridal*.

i·rid′i·an (eye·rid′ee·un, i·rid′·). See *iridal*.

i·rid′ic (i·rid′ick, eye·rid′ick) [*iris*]. Pertaining to the iris.

i′ri·din (eye′ri·din, irr′i·din). 1. A precipitated extract of blue flag. See *Iris*. 2. A glycoside from the rhizome of *Iris florentina*.

i·rid′i·um (i·rid′ee·um, eye·rid′ee·um) [*iris*]. Ir = 192.2. An element of the platinum family; alloyed in small percentage with platinum, it confers rigidity upon the latter.

ir″i·di·za′tion (irr″i·di·zay′shun, ·dye·zay′shun, eye″ri·) [*iris*]. The appearance of an iridescent halo, seen by persons affected with glaucoma.

ir′i·do- (irr′i·do-, eye′ri·do-), **irid-** [*iris*]. A combining form denoting *the iris.*

ir″i·do·a·vul′sion [*iris;* L. *avulsio,* a plucking off]. Avulsion of the iris.

ir″i·do·cap″su·li′tis [*iris;* L. *capsula,* small box; G. *-itis,* inflammation]. Inflammation involving the iris and the capsule of the lens.

ir″i·do·cap″su·lot′o·my [*iris; capsula;* G. *tomē,* a cutting]. An incision through the iris and adherent secondary membrane to create a pupillary opening.

i·rid′o·cele (i·rid′o·seel, eye·rid′o·seel, irr′i·do·, eye′ri·do·) [*iris;* G. *kēlē,* hernia]. Protrusion of part of the iris through a wound or ulcer.

ir″i·do·cho″roid·i′tis (·ko″roy·dye′tis) [*iris;* G. *choroeidēs,* choroid; *-itis,* inflammation]. Inflammation of both the iris and the choroid of the eye.

ir″i·do·col″o·bo′ma [*iris;* G. *kolobōma,* the part taken away in mutilation]. A coloboma of the iris.

ir″i·do·cy·clec′to·my (·sigh·kleck′to·mee) [*iris;* G. *kyklos,* circle; *ektomē,* excision]. Excision of the iris and of the ciliary body.

ir″i·do·cy·cli′tis (irr″i·do·sigh·klye′tis, eye″ri·) [*iris; kyklos;* G. *-itis,* inflammation]. Inflammation of the iris and the ciliary body. Also see *iritis.*

ir″i·do·cy″clo·cho″roid·i′tis (·sigh″klo·ko″roy·dye′tis, ·sick″lo·ko″roy·dye′tis) [*iris; kyklos;* G. *choroeidēs,* choroid; *-itis*]. Combined inflammation of the iris, the ciliary body, and the choroid; uveitis.

ir″i·do·cys·tec′to·my [*iris;* G. *kystis,* bladder; *ektomē,* excision]. An operation for making a new pupil; the edge of the iris and the capsule are drawn out through an incision in the cornea and cut off.

ir′i·do·cyte″ [*iris;* G. *kytos,* cell]. A special cell in which an insoluble substance, guanine (2-amino-6-oxypurine) is deposited in crystalline form. Responsible for the beautiful iridescence of many fishes.

ir″i·dod′e·sis. See *iridotasis.*

ir″i·do·di″ag·no′sis [*iris;* G. *diagnōsis,* a deciding]. Diagnosis of disease in general from examination of the iris.

ir″i·do·di·al′y·sis (irr″i·do·dye·al′i·sis, eye″ri·) [*iris;* G. *dialysis,* a separating]. The separation of the iris from its attachments.

ir″i·do·di·la′tor (irr″i·do·dye·lay′tur, eye″ri·) [*iris;* L. *dilatare,* to dilate]. Causing dilatation of the pupil.

ir″i·do·do·ne′sis [*iris;* G. *donein,* to shake]. Tremulousness of the iris; hippus.

ir″i·do·ki·ne′si·a (·ki·nee′see·uh, ·zee·uh, ·kigh-nee′·), **ir″i·do·ki·ne′sis** (·ki·nee′sis, ·kigh·nee′-sis) [*iris;* G. *kinēsis,* movement]. Any movement of the iris, normal or otherwise, as in contracting and dilating the pupil.

ir″i·do·lep·tyn′sis [*iris;* G. *leptynsis,* attenuation]. Attenuation or atrophy of the iris.

ir″i·do·ma·la′ci·a (·ma·lay′shuh, ·see·uh) [*iris;* G. *malakia,* softness]. Morbid softening of the iris.

ir″i·do·mo′tor [*iris;* L. *motor,* from *movere,* to move]. Promoting the motion of the iris.

ir″i·don·co′sis [*iris;* G. *ogkōsis,* intumescence]. Thickening of the iris.

ir″i·don′cus [*iris;* G. *ogkos,* mass]. A tumor or swelling of the iris.

ir″i·do·pa·ral′y·sis [*iris;* G. *paralysis,* paralysis]. Paralysis of the iris; iridoplegia.

ir″i·do·pa·rel′ky·sis [*iris;* G. *parelkysis,* from *parelkein,* to draw aside]. An induced prolapse of the iris to effect displacement of the pupil.

ir″i·do·pa·re′sis (·pa·ree′sis, ·par′i·sis) [*iris;* G. *paresis,* a letting go]. A slight or partial paralysis of the smooth muscle of the iris.

ir″i·do·per″i·pha·ki′tis [*iris;* G. *peri,* around; *phakos,* lens; *-itis,* inflammation]. Inflammation of the iris and the anterior part of the capsule of the lens. *Obs.*

ir″i·do·plat′i·num [*iris;* Sp. *plata,* silver]. An alloy of iridium and platinum; used in making electrodes, etc.

ir″i·do·ple′gi·a [*iris;* G. *plēgē,* stroke]. Paralysis of the sphincter pupillae of the iris.

ir″i·dop·to′sis [*iris;* G. *ptōsis,* a falling]. Prolapse of the iris.

ir″i·do·pu′pil·lar″y (irr″i·do·pew′pi·lerr″ee, eye″ri·) [*iris;* L. *pupillaris,* from *pupilla,* pupil of the eye]. Pertaining to the iris and the pupil.

ir″i·do·rhex′is [*iris;* G. *rhēxis,* a breaking]. 1. Rupture of the iris. 2. The tearing away of the iris from its attachment.

ir″i·dos′chi·sis (irr″i·dos′ki·sis, eye″ri·), **ir″i·do·schis′ma** (irr″i·do·skiz′muh, eye″ri·do·) [*iris;* G. *schizein,* to cleave]. Coloboma of the iris; iridocoloboma.

ir″i·do·scle·rot′o·my [*iris;* G. *sklēros,* hard; *tomē,* a cutting]. Puncture of the sclera with division of the iris.

ir″i·do·ste·re′sis. See *irideremia.*

ir″i·dot′a·sis [*iris;* G. *tasis,* a stretching]. Stretching the iris, as in glaucoma; in place of iridotomy. The stretched iris is left in the wound, under the conjunctiva. If at the same time a piece of limbus is cut away to allow for better drainage of the aqueous into the areolar tissue of Tenon's capsule, the operation is called iridencleisis.

ir′i·do·tome [*iris;* G. *tomos,* cutting]. A cutting instrument employed in iridotomy.

ir″i·dot′o·my [*iris;* G. *tomē,* a cutting]. An incision into the iris.

ir″i·dot′ro·mos [*iris;* G. *tromos,* trembling]. Tremor of the iris. Also called *hippus.*

I′ris [G.]. A genus of plants of the Iridaceae. The dried rhizome of **Iris versicolor** (blue flag iris) has been used as a cathartic, emetic, and diuretic.

I. germanica florentina. Orris root iris. See *orris.*

i′ris (pl. *irises, irides*) [G.]. A colored, circular disk, part of the uvea of the eye, suspended in the aqueous humor from the ciliary body. Its posterior surface rests on the lens, hence it separates the anterior and posterior chambers. It is perforated by the adjustable pupil. It consists of a mass of loose, vascular connective tissue, the stroma, covered anteriorly by endothelium, posteriorly by heavily pigmented epithelium, the iridial part of the retina. Two sets of smooth muscle cells control the size of the pupil; one circularly arranged in the pupillary border, forms the sphincter pupillae; the other, radially arranged, is the dilator pupillae. The color is governed by the number of melanophores in the stroma. See Plate 19.

heterochromic i. A condition in which the two irides are of different color, or in which a portion of an iris is of different color from the remainder.

i. bombé. A condition in which the iris bulges forward at the periphery due to an accumulation of the intraocular fluid in the posterior chamber.

rubeosis of the i. Rubeosis iridis.

umbrella i. Synonym of *i. bombé.*

I′rish moss. See *Chondrus.*

i·ri′tis (eye·rye′tis, i·rye′tis) [*iris;* G. *-itis,* inflammation]. Inflammation of the iris; usually associated with inflammation of the ciliary body, and often used for iridocyclitis, —**irit′ic,** *adj.*

rheumatoid i. Inflammation of the iris of the eye in conjunction with rheumatic fever, rheumatoid arthritis, and other collagen diseases.

ir″i·to·ec′to·my (irr″i·to·eck′to·mee, eye″ri·to·) [*iris;* G. *ektomē*, excision]. The removal of a portion of the iris for occlusion of the pupil.

i·rit′o·my (i·rit′o·mee, eye·rit′o·mee). See *iridotomy.*

i′ron [AS. *īren*] (*ferrum*). Fe = 55.85. A silver-white or gray, hard, ductile, malleable metal. *In medicine*, iron is used as the powder (reduced iron) or in the form of one of its salts in the treatment of certain anemias, especially of the hypochromic type. Iron compounds are generally astringent and styptic. Iron forms two classes of salts: ferrous, in which it has a valence of two; and ferric, in which it has a valence of three. See *ferrous* and *ferric*. See Table of Normal Values of Blood Constituents in the Appendix.

alcoholized i. Finely powdered iron.

black i. oxide. A mixture of ferric and ferrous oxides, approximating the formula Fe_3O_4. Syn., *magnetic iron oxide*. Also called *magnetite.*

dialyzed i. Prepared by adding ammonia water to a concentrated ferric chloride solution and dialyzing the resulting solution until nearly free of ammonium salts. Contains about 3.5% iron.

dried i. sulfate. Exsiccated ferrous sulfate (*ferri sulfas exsiccatus*). Contains not less than 80% of $FeSO_4$. Dose, 0.06–0.2 Gm. (1–3 gr.).

i. adenylate. Ferrous adenylate, used in treatment of secondary anemias. See *ironyl.*

i. albuminate. Any one of a variety of preparations made from egg albumen and an iron compound. A chalybeate.

i. alum. Iron and ammonium sulfate.

i. and ammonium acetate solution (*liquor ferri et ammonii acetatis*). Contains 0.18% of iron. A hematinic and diuretic. Dose, 8–15 cc. (2–4 fluidrachms). Also called *Basham's mixture.*

i. and ammonium sulfate. $FeNH_4(SO_4)_2 \cdot 12H_2O$. An astringent.

i. and potassium tartrate. Ferric potassium tartrate; approximately $K(FeO)C_4H_4O_6 \cdot xH_2O$: a brown powder or red to reddish-brown scales, very soluble in water.

i. and quinine citrate (*ferri et quininae citras*). Contains 15% of anhydrous quinine and 13% of iron. Dose, 0.3–0.6 Gm. (5–10 gr.).

i. arsenate. Ferrous arsenate. $Fe_3(AsO_4)_2 \cdot 6H_2O$. It has been used for its arsenic content in chronic skin affections.

i. ascorbate. Ferrous ascorbate. A purple powder, soluble in water; used in anemia. It is claimed to be less toxic than other iron salts and to be readily absorbed. Dose, oral, 0.2 Gm. (3 gr.) t.i.d.; intravenous, 10 mg. (1⁄6 gr.) daily. Syn., *iron cevitamate.*

i. by hydrogen. Reduced iron.

i. cacodylate. Ferric cacodylate. Approximately $Fe[(CH_3)_2AsO_2]_3$. Used in chlorosis and other anemias. Dose, oral, 0.06–0.12 Gm. (1–2 gr.); subcutaneous, 10–30 mg. (1⁄6–1⁄2 gr.) in dilute solution.

i. cevitamate. See *i.* ascorbate.

i. chloride. Ferric chloride, $FeCl_3$.

i. gluconate. Ferrous gluconate. $[CH_2OH(CHOH)_4COO]_2Fe \cdot 2H_2O$. Well tolerated in hypochromic anemias. Dose, 0.3 Gm. (5 gr.).

i. glycerophosphate. Ferric glycerophosphate (*ferri glycerophosphas*). Dose, 0.3–1.0 Gm. (5–15 gr.).

i. hydroxide. Ferric hydroxide. $Fe(OH)_3$. When freshly precipitated, an antidote for arsenic.

i. iodide. Ferrous iodide. $FeI_2 \cdot 4H_2O$.

i. lactate. Ferrous lactate. $Fe(C_3H_5O_3)_2 \cdot 3H_2O$. A greenish white, crystalline powder used as chalybeate. Dose, 0.2–0.4 Gm. (3–6 gr.).

i. oxide. Ferric oxide. Fe_2O_3. Color varies from red to yellow depending on the degree of hydration. See *limonite, hematite.*

i. peptonate. Peptonized iron (*ferrum peptonatum*). Composed of iron oxide and peptone solubilized by sodium citrate. Contains 16–18% of iron. Dose, 0.3–1.0 Gm. (5–15 gr.).

i. perchloride. Ferric chloride. $FeCl_3$.

i. pheophytin. A chlorophyll derivative wherein the magnesium has been replaced by iron; it has been used in anemias.

i. sulfate. Ferrous sulfate (*ferri sulfas*). $FeSO_4 \cdot 7H_2O$. Bluish green crystals of saline, styptic taste. Used in hypochromic anemia. Dose, 0.13–0.32 Gm. (2–5 gr.). Syn., *green vitriol, copperas.*

i. tincture. See *ferric* chloride tincture.

magnetic i. oxide. See black *i.* oxide.

masked i. Organic compounds of iron, at one time thought to be preferable to the inorganic salts as a means of administering iron.

reduced i. (*ferrum reductum*). A fine, grayish black powder obtained by the action of hydrogen on ferric oxide or by other means: used as a chalybeate. Dose, 0.12–0.6 Gm. (2–10 gr.) several times daily. Also called *i. by hydrogen, Quévenne's i.*

saccharated i. carbonate. Saccharated ferrous carbonate (*ferri carbonas saccharatus*). Contains 15% of $FeCO_3$. A nonastringent chalybeate. Dose, 0.6–2.0 Gm. (10–30 gr.).

saccharated i. oxide. Saccharated ferric oxide (*ferri oxidum saccharatum*). Contains 3% of iron. A chalybeate. Dose, 2 Gm. (30 gr.). Also called *soluble ferric oxide, eisenzucker.*

soluble i. phosphate. Soluble ferric phosphate (*ferri phosphas solubilis*). A ferric phosphate rendered soluble by the presence of sodium citrate and containing 12–15% of iron. Dose, 0.6–2.0 Gm. (10–30 gr.).

soluble i. pyrophosphate. Soluble ferric pyrophosphate (*ferri pyrophosphas solubilis*). A ferric pyrophosphate rendered soluble by the presence of sodium citrate and containing from 10.5–12.5% of iron. Dose, 0.6–2.0 Gm. (10–30 gr.).

i·rone′ (eye·rohn′, eye′rohn). A cyclic ketone, $C_{14}H_{22}O$, which gives the characteristic odor to orris root.

i′ron lung. Lay term for a respirator which induces breathing in a patient with paralyzed respiratory muscles. The patient's chest expands and contracts alternately in response to changes in air pressure in the respirator which encloses the body up to the neck. Also called *Drinker respirator.*

Ironyl. Trade-mark for a ferrous adenylate solution used intramuscularly as a hematinic.

i·rot′o·my (eye·rot′o·mee). See *iridotomy.*

ir·pex′in. An antibiotic substance isolated from cultures of a species of the class Basidiomycetes.

ir·ra′di·ate [L. *irradiare*, to cast forth rays]. *In radiology*, to treat with radiation, either roentgen rays or radiation from radioactive isotopes.

ir·ra′di·a″ting [*irradiare*]. 1. Radiating from a center, as a pain arising from a definite focus of irritation. 2. Treating with roentgen or radium rays.

ir·ra″di·a′tion [*irradiare*]. Exposure to radiation of varying wavelengths, such as infrared, ultraviolet, roentgen rays, gamma rays.

intracavitary i. Irradiation by placement of a radioactive substance within a body cavity; e.g., irradiation treatment by means of inserting radium into the uterine cavity.

secondary corpuscular i. The interaction of x- or gamma rays and atoms of matter to produce high-speed electrons as the rays pass through matter.

Irradol-A. Trade-mark for a hematinic containing iron with vitamins A, B, and D.

ir·ra′tion·al (i·rash′un·ul) [L. *irrationalis*, without reason]. *In psychiatry*, outside the province of reason; said of mental behavior.

ir″re·du′ci·ble [L. *irredux*, that does not bring back]. Not reducible; not capable of being replaced in a normal position.

ir·reg″u·lar′i·ty [L. *in-*, not; *regularis*, from *regula*, rule]. *In medicine*, a deviation from a rhythmic activity.

i. of pulse. See *arrhythmia*.

phasic i. See *phasic irregularity*.

ir″re·sus′ci·ta·ble [*in-*; *resuscitare*, to raise up again, to revive]. Not capable of being resuscitated or revived; irrevivable.

ir″re·ver′si·ble [*in-*; L. *reversum*, from *reverti*, to return]. 1. Not capable of being reversed. 2. Irrecoverable; said of a stage of shock or nerve injury from which recovery cannot be achieved. —**irreversibil′ity,** *n.*

ir″ri·ga′tion [L. *irrigatio*, from *irrigare*, to conduct water to]. The act of washing out by a stream of water, as irrigation of the urinary bladder.

continuous i. A continuous stream of water washed over a surface to reduce or limit inflammation.

ir′ri·ga″tor, ir″ri·ga′tor [*irrigare*]. An apparatus, or device, for accomplishing the irrigation of a part, surface, or cavity.

ir″ri·ta·bil′i·ty [L. *irritabilis*, from *irritare*, to irritate]. 1. A condition or quality of being excitable; the power of responding to a stimulus. 2. A condition of morbid excitability of an organ or part, when it reacts excessively to a slight stimulation.

muscular i. The inherent capacity of a muscle to respond to stimuli by contraction.

myotatic i. That seen in a muscle in response to a mechanical stimulus, as stretching.

nervous i. The property of a nerve to respond to stimuli by conducting impulses.

ir′ri·ta·ble [*irritare*]. 1. Reacting to stimuli. 2. Easily excited; susceptible of irritation.

ir′ri·tant [*irritare*]. Causing or giving rise to irritation.

ir′ri·tant. An agent that induces irritation.

ir″ri·ta′tion [L. *irritatio*, from *irritare*]. 1. A condition of undue excitement or irritability. 2. The act of irritating or stimulating. 3. The stimulus necessary to the performance of a function.

spinal i. A form of neurasthenia characterized by pain in the back, tenderness along the spines of the vertebrae, fatigue on slight exertion, and, occasionally, numbness and tingling in the limbs.

sympathetic i. Irritation of an organ arising from irritation of another related organ, as sympathetic irritation of one eye from irritation of the other.

ir″ru·ma′tion. Fellatio.

Isaacs, Raphael [*American physician and hematologist*, 1891–   ]. Described small single refractive granules seen in erythrocytes in unstained and vitally stained moist preparations (1925). *Isaacs' refractive granules* occur in about 1 per cent of normal red blood cells. They are considered the final stage in the maturation of the cells.

isacen. Trade-mark for the diacetyl derivative of dihydroxyphenylisatin; a white, crystalline powder; used as a laxative.

i″sa·del′phi·a (eye″sa·del′fee·uh, iss″a·) [G. *isos*, equal; *adelphos*, brother]. Conjoined twins united by unimportant tissues; each body is normal in the development of all essential organs.

Isambert, Emile [*French physician*, 1827–76]. Remembered as an authoritative writer on laryngeal tuberculosis. Described tuberculous ulceration of the larynx and pharynx, also called *Isambert's disease*.

isarol. Trade-mark for a brand of ichthammol.

i′sa·tin. $C_8H_5NO_2$; 2,3-indolinedione, occurring in orange-colored crystals, soluble in boiling water. used as a reagent.

i″sa·tro″pyl·co·caine′ (eye″suh·tro″pil·ko·kayn′, ·ko·kay′in, ·ko′kay·in, iss″uh·). $C_{19}H_{23}NO_4$. An amorphous alkaloid from coca leaves. It has no anesthetic properties but is said to be an active cardiac poison. Also called *alpha-truxilline*.

i″saux·e′sis (eye″sawk·zee′sis, ·see′sis) [G. *isos*, equal; *auxēsis*, increase]. A type of relative growth in which a part grows at the same rate as the whole organism or another part.

is·che′mi·a (iss·kee′mee·uh) [G. *ischein*, to check; *haima*, blood]. Local diminution in the blood supply, due to obstruction of inflow of arterial blood; local anemia. This condition is seen in Raynaud's disease, in frostbite, in angina pectoris. —**ischemic,** *adj.*

is·che′sis (iss·kee′sis, iss′ki·sis) [*ischein*]. Retention of a discharge or secretion.

is″chi·ag′ra (iss″kee·ag′ruh, ·ay′gruh) [G. *ischion*, hip joint; *agra*, a catching]. Gout in the hip. *Obs.*

is″chi·al′gi·a [*ischion*; G. *algos*, pain]. Sciatica. —**ischialgic,** *adj.*

is″chi·a·ti′tis [*ischion*; G. *-itis*, inflammation]. Inflammation of the sciatic nerve.

is″chi·dro′sis (iss″ki·dro′sis) [G. *ischein*, to check; *hidrōsis*, sweating]. Suppression of the secretion of sweat. —**ischidrot′ic,** *adj.*

is′chi·o- (iss′kee·o-), **is′chi-** [G. *ischion*, hip joint]. A combining form denoting ***the ischium*** or ***the hip.***

is″chi·o·bul·bo′sus. A variable part of the bulbocavernosus muscle.

is″chi·o·cap′su·lar [*ischion*; L. *capsula*, small box]. Pertaining to the ischium and the fibrous capsule of the hip, as the ischiocapsular ligament of the hip joint.

is″chi·o·cav″er·no′sus [*ischion*; L. *caverna*, cavern]. A muscle arising from the ischium, encircling each crus of the penis or clitoris, and inserted into the upper surface of the crus. See Table of Muscles in the Appendix.

is″chi·o·cav′er·nous [*ischion*; *caverna*]. Pertaining to the ischium and one or both of the corpora cavernosa of the penis or clitoris.

is″chi·o·coc·cyg′e·al (iss″kee·o·cock·sidj′ee·ul) [*ischion*; G. *kokkyx*, cuckoo]. Pertaining to the ischium and the coccyx.

is″chi·o·coc·cyg′e·us (·cock·sidj′ee·us) [*ischion*; *kokkyx*]. The coccygeus muscle.

is″chi·o·did′y·mus [*ischion*; G. *didymos*, twin]. Conjoined twins united at the sacral or ischial region. Syn., *ischiopagus*.

is″chi·o·fe·mo·ra′lis. An occasional slip of the gluteus maximus muscle, attached to the ischial tuberosity.

is·chi·om′e·lus [*ischion*; G. *melos*, limb]. An individual with an accessory limb attached at the nates.

is″chi·o·my′e·li′tis (iss″kee·o·migh″uh·lye′tis) [*ischion*; G. *myelos*, marrow; *-itis*, inflammation]. Lumbar myelitis; osphyomyelitis.

is″chi·o·neu·ral′gi·a [*ischion*; G. *neuros*, nerve; *algos*, pain]. Old term for sciatica.

is·chi·op′a·gus [*ischion*; G. *pagos*, that which is fixed]. Conjoined twins united by their sacral or ischial regions. The **ischiopagus tetrapus** has four legs; the **ischiopagus tripus,** three. See Plate 25.

is·chi·op′a·gy [*ischion*; G. *pagē*, anything that fixes]. The monstrosity exhibited by the ischiopagus.

is″chi·o·pu′bi·cus. A variable part of the sphincter urethrae membranaceae muscle.

is″chi·o·pu″bi·ot′o·my (iss″kee·o·pew″bee·ot′o-mee) [*ischion;* L. *pubes*, private parts; G. *tomē*, a cutting]. Division of the ischial and pubic rami in otherwise impossible labor. *Obs.*

is″chi·o·pu′bis [*ischion; pubes*]. 1. The site of junction of the ischium and the pubis. 2. The ischium and pubis considered together. —**ischio-pu′bic,** *adj.*

is″chi·o·rec′tal [*ischion;* L. *rectus*, straight]. Pertaining to both the ischium and the rectum.

is′chi·um (iss′kee·um) (pl. *ischia*) [*ischion*]. The inferior part of the os innominatum; the bone upon which the body rests in sitting. See Plate 2, and *coxae* in Table of Bones in the Appendix. —**ischiad′ic, is′chial,** *adj.*

isch″no·pho′ni·a (isk″no·fo′nee·uh) [G. *ischnos*, feeble; *phōnē*, voice]. Stammering.

is′cho- (iss′ko-), **isch-** [G. *ischein*, to check]. *In medicine*, a combining form denoting *suppression, checking, stoppage*, or *deficiency*.

is″cho·ga·lac′ti·a (iss″ko·ga·lack′tee·uh, ·shee·uh) [*ischein;* G. *gala*, milk]. Suppression of the natural flow of milk.

is″cho·ga·lac′tic [*ischein; gala*]. Suppressing the natural flow of milk.

is″cho·ga·lac′tic. An agent which suppresses the flow of milk.

is″cho·gy′ri·a [*ischein;* G. *gyros*, circle]. A jagged appearance of the cerebral convolutions, produced by atrophy.

is″cho·me′ni·a [*ischein;* G. *mēn*, month]. Suppression of the menstrual flow.

is·chu′ri·a (isk·yoor′ee·uh) [*ischein;* G. *ouron*, urine]. Retention or suppression of the urine. See *anuria*. —**ischuret′ic,** *adj.*

I-sedrin. A proprietary solution containing ephedrine gluconate. Used as a vasoconstrictor in the upper respiratory passages. **I-sedrin compound** also contains merthiolate.

Ishihara, Shinobu (1879–). Japanese ophthalmologist who introduced a test for color vision. The subject is shown a series of cards, on each of which figures or winding lines composed of colored dots are printed on a field of dots of another color. The normal and the colorblind make different readings from the card; thus one can easily judge the color vision of the person tested.

i′sin·glass″ (eye′zing·glass″, eye′zin·). See *ichthyocolla*.

vegetable i. Obsolete term for agar, 2.

Isla. See *Diaz* de Isla.

is′land [AS. *igland*]. 1. An isolated structure; particularly, a group of cells differentiated from the surrounding tissue by staining or arrangement. 2. The insula of the cerebral hemisphere. Formerly called *i. of Reil*. See Plate 17.

blood i. One of the masses of condensed splanchnic mesenchyme in the wall of the yolk sac that gives rise to the primitive erythrocytes of the embryo and to the vascular plexus of the yolk sac.

i. of Langerhans. See *islet* of pancreas.

pancreatic i. See *islet* of pancreas.

tonal islands. See *tonal islands*.

is′let (eye′lit) [OF. *islette*]. A small island.

blood i. See blood *island*.

i. of pancreas. A small, irregular island of cell cords, found in the pancreas; it has no connection with the duct system, and is delimited from the acini by a reticular membrane. It is of an endocrine nature, as indicated by its great vascularity, and consists mainly of alpha and beta cells, the former secreting a hormone like lipocaic, and the latter secreting insulin. Syn., *island of Langerhans*.

-ism [G.*-isma, -ismos*]. Suffix indicating 1. Condition or disease from, as embol*ism*, alcohol*ism*. 2. Doctrine or practice of (often with a corresponding verb ending in *-ize* and noun ending in *-ist*), as Fletcher*ism*, hypnot*ism*.

i′so-, is- [G. *isos*, equal]. 1. A combining form denoting *equality, similarity, uniformity*, or *identity*. 2. *In bacteriology*, a combining form denoting *for* or *from different individuals of the same species*. 3. *In chemistry*, a combining form denoting *a compound isomeric with another*, or *a compound with a straight chain of carbon atoms at one end of which two methyl groups are attached*. Symbol, *i*.

i″so·ag·glu′ti·nin [*isos;* L. *agglutinare*, to glue]. An agglutinin which acts upon the red blood cells of members of the same species. Also called *isohemagglutinin*.

i″so·aj′ma·line. An alkaloid from *Rauwolfia serpentina*.

i″so·al·lox′a·zine (eye″so·a·lock′suh·zeen). 1. $C_{10}H_6N_4O_2$. The three-ring compound pyrimido [4,5-b] quinoxaline-2,4(3H,10H)-dione; an isomer of alloxazine. Derivatives of the compound are widely distributed in plants and animals and include such substances as riboflavin and the yellow enzymes; these substances are sometimes incorrectly named as derivatives of alloxazine. 2. A term loosely applied to derivatives of (1).

i″so·al·lox′a·zine ad′e·nine di·nu′cle·o·tide. Flavin adenine dinucleotide: sometimes incorrectly called *alloxazine adenine dinucleotide*.

i″so·al·lox′a·zine mon″o·nu′cle·o·tide″. Riboflavin-5′-phosphate: sometimes incorrectly called *alloxazine mononucleotide*.

i″so·am′yl ac′e·tate. $(CH_3)_2CH.CH_2.CH_2.COO.CH_3$; a colorless liquid having a pearlike odor and taste, soluble in 400 parts of water; it is used as a solvent. The technical product is known as *pear oil* or *banana oil*.

i″so·am′yl al′co·hol. $(CH_3)_2CH.CH_2.CH_2OH$; 3-methyl-1-butanol or fermentation amyl alcohol; a colorless liquid of disagreeable odor, soluble in 40 parts of water. It constitutes the major portion of fusel oil, which name is commonly applied to technical isoamyl alcohol.

i″so·am″yl·a·mine′ (eye″so·am″il·uh·meen′, ·am″-il·am′een, ·in). $C_5H_{11}.NH_2$. A ptomaine formed by the putrefaction of yeast.

i″so·an·dros′ter·one. $C_{19}H_{30}O_2$. 3(β)-Hydroxy-17-keto-androstane, an androgenic steroid found in the urine of men and women. See also *androsterone*.

i″so·an′ti·bod″ies [*isos;* G. *anti*, against; AS. *bodig*]. Antibodies, in certain members of a species, for cells of certain other members of the same species.

i″so·an′ti·gen [*isos; anti;* G. *genesthai*, from *gignesthai*, to be produced]. An antigen which is active only in serum of animals of the same species.

i′so·bar [*isos;* G. *baros*, weight]. 1. Any one of two or more atoms which have the same atomic mass but different atomic numbers. 2. A line drawn through points having equal barometric or manometric pressure. —**isobar′ic,** *adj.*

i″so·bes′tic point. *In applied spectroscopy*, the wavelength at which the absorbance of two substances, one of which can be converted into the other, is the same: sometimes written *isobastique point*.

i″so·bil″i·ru′bic ac′id. $C_{17}H_{24}N_2O_3$; a cleavage product obtained, along with the isomeric bilirubic acid, when bilirubin is reduced with hydriodic acid.

i″so·bor′nyl thi″o·cy″an·o·ac′e·tate. $C_{13}H_{19}NO_2S$; a yellow, oily liquid, practically insoluble in water; the technical grade, which contains 82% or more of isobornyl thiocyanoacetate, is used as a pediculicide and insecticide.

i″so·bu′tyl. The univalent hydrocarbon radical $(CH_3)_2CH.CH_2$—.

i″so·bu′tyl al′co·hol. $(CH_3)_2CH.CH_2OH$; a colorless, flammable liquid, soluble in 20 parts of water; it is produced by fermentation of carbohydrates and is a constituent of fusel oil. It is used as a solvent.

i″so·cel″lo·bi′ose [*isos;* L. *cella,* stall, chamber; *bis,* twice; *-ose,* chemical suffix]. A disaccharide formed during hydrolysis of cellulose.

i″so·cel′lu·lar [*isos;* L. *cellula,* small storeroom]. Composed of cells of the same size or character.

i″so·cho·les′ter·ol (eye″so·ko·less′tur·ole, ·ol). A substance isolated from wool fat; originally considered to be a sterol but now believed to consist of several complex terpene alcohols, including agnosterol and lanosterol.

i″so·cho′line (·ko′leen, ·lin, ·kol′een, ·in). $(CH_3)_3$-N(OH).CHOH.CH_3. An alkaloid, isomeric with choline, found in fungi of the genera *Amanita* and *Agaricus.* Syn., *amanitine.*

i′so·chore (eye′so·kor) [*isos;* G. *chōra,* space]. The plotted curve showing the relationship between the temperature and pressure of a gas at constant volume. —**isochor′ic,** *adj.*

i″so·chro·mat′ic [*isos;* G. *chrōma,* color]. Having the same color throughout.

i″so·chro·mat′o·phil, i″so·chro·mat′o·phile [*isos; chrōma;* G. *philein,* to love]. Denoting cells and tissues which are equally stained by the same dye.

i·soch′ro·nal (eye·sock′ro·nul, eye″so·kro′nul), **i·soch′ro·nous** (eye·sock′ro·nus) [*isos;* G. *chronos,* time]. Occurring at or occupying equal intervals of time. —**isochronism,** *n.*

i″so·chro′ni·a [*isos; chronos*]. The condition of normal nerve-impulse transference; the chronaxie of a muscle and that of its nerve are of the same order; supposedly essential for transmission of impulse from nerve to muscle.

i″so·cit′ric ac′id. COOH.CH_2.CH(COOH).-CHOH.COOH; an intermediate compound in the Krebs or tricarboxylic acid cycle by which metabolism of carbohydrate, fat, and protein is believed to occur.

i″so·co′ri·a [*isos;* G. *korē,* pupil]. Equality in diameter of the two pupils.

i″so·cor′tex [*isos;* L. *cortex,* bark]. Those parts of the cerebral cortex exhibiting the six characteristic layers or strata, each layer having certain predominant cells and histologic features common to all isocortical areas. Syn., *homogenetic cortex, homotypical cortex.*

i″so·cre·at′i·nine (eye″so·kree·at′i·neen, ·nin) [*isos;* G. *kreas,* flesh]. A substance of uncertain nature and questionable purity, isolated from fish muscle.

i″so·cy′a·nide. Any organic compound of the formula RNC, isomeric with but differing from RCN, which is a cyanide. On hydrolysis a cyanide (RCN) yields RCOOH and NH_3; an isocyanide (RNC) yields RNH_2 and HCOOH (formic acid). Syn., *carbylamine, isonitrile.*

i″so·cy·tol′y·sin (eye″so·sigh·tol′i·sin, ·sigh″to-lye′sin) [*isos;* G. *kytos,* cell; *lysis,* a loosing]. A cytolysin from the blood of an animal, capable of acting against the cells of other animals of the same species.

i″so·dac′ty·lism [*isos;* G. *daktylos,* finger]. The condition of having fingers or toes of equal length. —**isodactylous,** *adj.*

i″so·di″ag·no′sis [*isos;* G. *diagnōsis,* a deciding]. The diagnosis of a disease not apparent clinically by injecting the suspected individual's blood into a susceptible animal.

i″so·di′a·phere. One of two or more species of atoms which have the same difference between the numbers of neutrons and protons in their respective nuclei.

i′so·dont [*isos;* G. *odous,* tooth]. *In zoology,* having teeth of the same size and shape.

i″so·do′ses (·do′seez) [*isos;* G. *dosis,* a giving]. Surfaces of equal radiation intensities in irradiated tissue.

i″so·dul′ci·tol. Rhamnose.

i″so·dy·nam′ic (eye″so·dye·nam′ick, ·di·nam′ick) [*isos;* G. *dynamis,* power]. Having or generating equal amounts of force, as isodynamic foods. —**isodyna′mia,** *n.*

iso-efemist. A proprietary solution of ephedrine sulfate, chlorobutanol, and sodium chloride.

i″so·e·lec′tric [*isos;* G. *ēlektron,* amber]. Having the same electric properties throughout.

i. level. *In electrocardiography,* the zero position of the galvanometer when no current from the heart is flowing through it. It is the reference level from which all deflections except the QRS complex and ST junction are determined.

i. point. The pH at which the net electric charge on a particle or surface is zero.

i″so·feb″ri·fu′gine. An alkaloid, possessing some antimalarial activity, isolated from *Dichroa febrifuga,* which is the probable source of the Chinese antimalarial drug ch'ang shan. Isofebrifugine may be identical with α-dichroine.

i″so·flu′ro·phate. U.S.P. name for *diisopropyl fluorophosphate.*

i″so·gam′ete (eye″so·gam′eet) [*isos;* G. *gamos,* marriage]. A reproductive cell, similar in form and size to the cell with which it unites; found in certain protozoans and thallophytes.

i·sog′a·mous (eye·sog′uh·mus) [*isos; gamos*]. Characterized by the conjugation of gametes similar in size and shape. —**isogamy,** *n.*

i″so·gen′e·sis [*isos;* G. *genesis,* production]. Identity of origin of development. —**isog′enous,** *adj.*

i″so·ger′mi·dine. An ester alkaloid isolated from veratrum viride; on hydrolysis it yields germine.

i″so·ger′mine. An isomeric form of germine, obtained from the latter under certain conditions of chemical treatment. See also *pseudogermine.*

i·sog′na·thous (eye·sog′nuth·us, eye″so·nath us) [*isos;* G. *gnathos,* jaw]. Having jaws of equal size.

i′so·graft. Homograft.

isohalant. A proprietary containing ephedrine sulfate, chlorobutanol, and dextrose.

i″so·he″mag·glu′ti·nin (eye″so·hee″muh·glōō′ti-nin, eye″so·hem″uh·) [*isos;* G. *haima,* blood; L. *agglutinare,* to glue]. Isoagglutinin.

i″so·he·mol′y·sin (eye″so·hee·mol′i·sin, ·hem·ol′i-sin, ·hee″mo·lye′sin, ·hem″o·lye′sin) [*isos; haima;* G. *lysis,* a loosing]. A hemolysin produced by injecting red blood cells into an animal of the same species. An isohemolysin will destroy the red blood cells of any animal of the same species except the immunized individual. Syn., *isolysin.* —**isohemolyt′ic,** *adj.*

i″so·he·mol′y·sis [*isos; haima; lysis*]. The hemolytic action of an isohemolysin.

i″so·hy′dric shift. An increase in the base-binding capacity of hemoglobin which occurs upon oxygenation. It is due to the fact that HbO_2 (oxygenated hemoglobin) is a stronger acid than Hb (reduced hemoglobin) and thus binds more base.

i″so·i·co′ni·a (eye″so·eye·ko′nee·uh) [*isos;* G. *eikon,* image]. A condition in which the images are of equal size in the two eyes. —**isoicon′ic,** *adj.*

i″so·i·ko′ni·a. Isoiconia.

i″so·im″mu·ni·za′tion [*isos;* L. *immunis,* free from public service]. Immunization of a species of animal with antigens of the same species; for example, the development of anti-Rh serum may be produced by transfusing Rh-positive blood into an Rh-negative individual or by an Rh-negative woman being pregnant with an Rh-positive fetus.

i″so·i·on′ic point. The pH at which the number of protons dissociated from proton donors in a system equals the number of protons combined with proton acceptors. In solutions in which a protein is the only ionic species present, the isoionic point is identical with the isoelectric point.

i″so·lac′tose. A disaccharide synthesized by the action of a lactase on a solution of glucose and galactose.

i″so·la′tion [It. *isolare*, to isolate, from L. *insula*, island]. 1. *In medicine*, the separation of a patient from the rest of the community or from other patients because of a contagious disease (as in an isolation ward) or for reasons of therapy. 2. *In psychoanalysis*, the dissociation of an idea or memory from its emotional content or the feelings attached to it, or from other facts related to it, so as to render it a matter of indifference; a common defense mechanism against anxiety. 3. In a social sense, the separation of a person or group from others in the community; an inadequacy of personal contacts. —**i′solate,** *v.*

i″so·lec′i·thal (eye″so·less′i·thul) [G. *isos*, equal; *lekithos*, yolk]. Having yolk evenly distributed in the ovum, usually in small amount.

i″so·leu′cine (eye″so·lew′seen, ·sin). α-Amino-β-methyl-valeric acid, $C_2H_5.CH(CH_3).CH(NH_2).$-COOH. An essential amino acid.

i″so·leu′cyl. The univalent radical, CH_3CH_2CH-$(CH_3)CH(NH_2)CO$—, of the amino acid isoleucine.

i′so·log, i′so·logue (eye′so·log). One of a series of compounds of similar structure, but having different atoms of the same valency and usually of the same periodic group.

i″so·ly·ser′gic ac′id. $C_{16}H_{16}N_2O_2$; a parent constituent, along with lysergic acid, of certain ergot alkaloids; it may be obtained from such alkaloids by hydrolysis.

i″so·ly′sin (eye″so·lye′sin, eye·sol′i·sin). See *isohemolysin.*

i″so·mal′tose. An isomer of maltose claimed to be produced by the action of certain enzymes upon maltose; it may be identical with cellobiose.

i′so·mer [*isos;* G. *meros*, part]. One of two or more compounds having the same percentage composition but differing in the relative positions of the atoms within the molecule. See *isomerism.*

i·so′mer·ase [*isos; meros*]. Enzyme involved in establishing equilibrium between glucose-6-phosphate and fructose-6-phosphate and possibly other biochemical reactions.

i″so·mer′ic [*isos; meros*]. Pertaining to isomerism. Existing as an isomer of another substance.

i·som′er·ide (eye·som′ur·ide, ·id). See *isomer.*

i·som′er·ism (eye·som′ur·iz·um) [*isos; meros*]. The relationship between two isomers. The phenomenon wherein two or more compounds possess the same percentage composition but differ in the relative position of the atoms within the molecule and have different properties.

geometric i. That evidenced when substances have the same constitutional formula but differ in the special arrangement of the atoms and, consequently, in all of their physical properties and in most of their chemical properties. See stereo-*i.*

optical i. That indicated by substances having similar structural formulas and general properties but differing in their action on polarized light. See stereo-*i.*

stereo-i. That involving compounds of the same constitution but different configurations. Two types are recognized: *geometric isomerism* and *optical isomerism.*

structural i. That involving compounds with the same molecular formulas but distinctly different structures, as butane, $CH_3.CH_2.CH_2.CH_3$, and isobutane, $(CH_3)_3CH$; propylamine, CH_3.-$CH_2.CH_2.NH_2$, and trimethylamine, $(CH_3)_3N$.

i″so·meth′a·done. $(C_6H_5)_2C.CO.C_2H_5$
|
$CH_3.CH.CH_2.N(CH_3)_2$.
1,6-Dimethylamino-4,4-diphenyl-5-methyl-3-hexanone; an oily liquid. The hydrochloride of the levorotatory isomer has been employed as an analgesic and narcotic, though it is not as active as methadone.

i″so·met′ric [*isos;* G. *metron*, a measure]. Of the same dimensions.

i″so·me·tro′pi·a [*isos; metron;* G. *ōps*, eye]. Equality of kind and degree in the refraction of the two eyes.

i′so·morph. 1. *In chemistry*, one of two or more substances of different composition which have the same crystalline form. 2. *In chemistry*, one of a group of elements whose compounds with the same other atoms or radicals have the same crystalline form. 3. *In biology*, an animal or plant having superficial similarity to another which is phylogenetically different.

i″so·mor′phic [*isos;* G. *morphē*, form]. 1. *In genetics*, descriptive of genotypes of polysomic or polyploid organisms which, although containing the same number of linked genes in different combinations on homologous chromosomes, yet are similar in the series of gametes which they can produce. 2. *In chemistry*, pertaining to similar crystalline forms. —**isomor′phism,** *n.*; **isomor′phous,** *adj.*

i″so·mor′phous ir″ri·ta′tion ef·fect. See isomorphous provocative *reaction.*

isomyn. A trade name for amphetamine.

i″so·ni′a·zid. Generic name for the antituberculosis drug isonicotinic acid hydrazide. See *cotinazin, dinacrin, ditubin, nydrazid, pyricidin, rimifon.*

i″so·nic″o·tin′ic ac′id hy′dra·zide. $C_5H_4N.CO.$-$NH.NH_2$; isonicotinylhydrazide, forming nearly colorless crystals, soluble in water. It is employed as a therapeutic agent in treating human tuberculosis, being administered orally or intramuscularly, commonly along with either streptomycin or para-aminosalicylic acid or with both. Syn., *isoniazid, N-isonicotinylhydrazine.* See *cotinazin, dinacrin, ditubin, nydrazid, pyricidin, rimifon.*

N-i″so·nic″o·tin″yl·hy′dra·zine. Isonicotinic acid hydrazide.

1-i″so·nic″o·tin′yl-2-i″so·pro′pyl·hy′dra·zide. $C_5H_4N.CO.NH.NH.CH(CH_3)_2$; the isopropyl derivative of isonicotinic acid hydrazide, used similarly; but it is so much more toxic that it is available only for investigative purposes. Syn., *iproniazid.* See *marsilid.*

i″so·nip′e·caine. Meperidine hydrochloride.

i″so·ni′trile. An isocyanide.

isonorin sulfate. A trade-marked name for the sympathomimetic amine salt *isopropylarterenol sulfate.*

i″so·os·mot′ic. Referring or pertaining to a solution which has the same osmotic pressure as that of any reference physiological fluid, particularly that enclosed in red blood cells. An isoosmotic solution is also isotonic only when the tissue concerned, by virtue of its lack of permeability to the solutes present or to any interaction with them, maintains its normal state or tone. Syn., *isosmotic.*

i·sop′a·thy (eye·sop′uth·ee) [*isos;* G. *pathos*, disease]. The treatment of a disease by the administration of the causative agent or of its products, as the treatment of smallpox by the administration of variolous matter.

i″so·pel″le·tier′ine (eye″so·pel″i·teer′een, ·in, ·pel″et·yair′een, ·in, ·pi·let′i·reen, ·rin, ·pel″i·tee″-eh·reen′). One of the alkaloids of pomegranate bark. See *pelletierine.*

i″so·pen′ta·quine. $C_{18}H_{27}N_3O$; 8-(4-isopropylamino-1-methylbutylamino)-6-methoxyquinoline; a compound related to pamaquine and having a similar antimalarial activity: also referred to as *SN 13,274.*

i′so·phane ra′tio. See under *ratio.*

i″so·phen′ic [*isos;* G. *phainein,* to show]. Pertaining to different genes which produce similar phenotypic effects.

i″so·pho′ri·a [*isos;* G. *phoros,* bearing]. A condition in which the eyes lie in the same horizontal plane, the tension of the vertical muscles being equal in both eyes, and the visual lines lying in the same plane.

i·so′pi·a (eye·so′pee·uh) [*isos;* G. *ōps,* eye]. Equal acuteness of vision in the two eyes.

i″so·pi″lo·car′pine (·pye″lo·kahr′peen, ·pin). An alkaloid from jaborandi; stereo-isomeric with pilocarpine, and similar to it in physiologic effect.

i″so·plas′tic [*isos;* G. *plassein,* to form]. Transplanted from one individual to another of the same species, said of a graft. See *isograft* under *graft.*

i″so·pre·cip′i·tin [*isos;* L. *praecipitare,* to hurl against]. A precipitin which is active only against the serum of animals of the same species as that from which it is derived.

i″so·pren′a·line sul′phate. British Pharmacopoeia name for *isopropylarterenol sulfate.*

i′so·prene. CH_2:CH.C(CH_3):CH_2. Methyl butadiene, a hydrocarbon formed in the dry distillation of rubber.

i″so·pro′pa·nol. Isopropyl alcohol.

i″so·pro′pyl. The univalent hydrocarbon radical $(CH_3)_2CH$—.

i. vinyl ether. $(CH_3)_2$CH.O.CH:CH_2; a volatile, colorless, mobile liquid; boils at 56° C. and has a specific gravity of approximately 0.75 at 26° C. It is an inhalation anesthetic, with a potency approximately twice that of ethyl ether.

i″so·pro″pyl·a·ce′tic ac′id. Isovaleric acid.

i″so·pro′pyl al′co·hol. $(CH_3)_2$CHOH. Dimethyl carbinol. A homolog of ethyl alcohol; used similarly to it externally, but more poisonous if taken internally. Syn., *isopropanol.*

i″so·pro″pyl·ar·ter′e·nol. $(OH)_2C_6H_3$.CHOH.-NH.CH$(CH_3)_2$; α-(isopropylaminomethyl)protocatechuyl alcohol; a sympathomimetic amine closely related in its action to epinephrine and arterenol (norepinephrine), but whose action on the smooth muscle of blood vessels is much less pronounced than that of epinephrine or arterenol. The principal effects of isopropylarterenol occur in the bronchi; when administered sublingually or by oral inhalation isopropylarterenol salts are effective in treatment of asthma.

i. hydrochloride. $C_{11}H_{17}NO_3$.HCl, occurring as crystals, soluble in water. Syn., *isoproterenol hydrochloride.* See *aludrine hydrochloride, isuprel hydrochloride.*

i. sulfate. $(C_{11}H_{17}NO_3)_2.H_2SO_4$, occurring as crystals, soluble in water. Syn., *isoprenaline sulphate.* See *isonorin sulfate, norisodrine sulfate.*

i″so·pro·ter′e·nol hy″dro·chlo′ride. The United States Pharmacopeia name for *isopropylarterenol hydrochloride.*

i″so·pro″to·ver′ine. An isomeric form of protoverine, obtained from the latter under certain conditions of chemical treatment.

i·sop′ters (eye·sop′turz) [*isos;* G. *optēr,* observer]. The curves of relative visual acuity of the retina, at different distances from the macula, for form and for color.

i″so·quas′sin. $C_{22}H_{28}O_6$; a bitter principle of quassia, forming with neoquassin the molecular complex called *quassin.* Isoquassin is the ketone of neoquassin and is identical with picrasmin isolated from quassia by earlier investigators.

i″so·quin′o·line (eye″so·kwin′o·leen, ·lin). C_9H_7N. White, hygroscopic crystals. Numerous natural and synthetic alkaloids are derivatives of this substance. Also called *2-benzazine, leucoline.*

i″so·rau·wol′fine. An alkaloid, sometimes called *serpentinine,* from *Rauwolfia serpentina.*

i″so·ri″bo·fla′vin. 5,6-Dimethyl-9-(D-1′-ribityl)-isoalloxazine; an isomer of riboflavin, which is 6,7-dimethyl-9-(D-1′-ribityl)-isoalloxazine. Isoriboflavin is an effective metabolite antagonist for riboflavin in the rat, but not in certain bacterial systems.

i′so·scope [*isos;* G. *skopein,* to examine]. An instrument consisting of two sets of parallel vertical wires, one of which can be superimposed on the other; it is designed to show that the vertical lines of separation of the retina do not correspond exactly to the vertical meridians.

i″so·ser′ine. CH_2NH_2.CHOH.COOH; α-hydroxy-β-aminopropionic acid, isomeric with serine; it is an analog of β-alanine and inhibits the growth-promoting action of the latter.

i″sos·mot′ic. Isoosmotic.

I·sos′po·ra (eye·sos′po·ruh) [*isos;* G. *spora,* spore]. A genus of coccidia.

I. hominis. A species parasitic in the small intestine of man, but of doubtful pathogenicity.

i″so·spor·o′sis [*isos; spora;* G. *-osis,* condition]. Human infection by members of the genus *Isospora,* a coccidium. Only *I. belli* has been known to cause pathological symptoms.

i′so·stere. Generally, any of two or more compounds having essentially identical molecular configurations, including molecular volumes, and similar electrical fields. Criteria for deciding whether two dissimilar compounds are isosteres vary. —**isoster′ic,** *adj.*

i·sos′ter·ism. The relationship between two or more compounds which are isosteres. *In pharmacology,* the concept of isosterism involves the possibility that compounds having such a relationship may have the same or quite similar pharmacologic actions.

i″so·sthe·nu′ri·a (eye″so·sthi·new′ree·uh, eye″-sos·thi·) [*isos;* G. *sthenos,* strength; *ouron,* urine]. Inability of the kidneys to produce either a concentrated or dilute urine.

i′so·tel [G. *isotelēs,* bearing equal burdens]. A food factor capable of replacing another in a given diet for a specified species; thus, for the human species, carotene is isotelic with vitamin A; for the cat, it is not, since the cat is incapable of converting carotene into vitamin A. —**isotel′ic,** *adj.*

i′so·therm. 1. A graph or curve representing the dependence of one quantity upon another at constant temperature, e.g., the dependence of gas pressure upon volume. 2. Specifically, **Freundlich's** or **Langmuir's adsorption isotherm** is a graph representing the dependence of the quantity of dissolved substance by a solid upon the concentration of the dissolved substance: term encountered in discussions on the mechanism of drug action. —**i′sotherm,** *adj.*

i″so·ther′mal, i″so·ther′mic [G. *isos,* equal; *thermē,* heat]. Of equal or uniform temperature; without change in temperature.

i″so·thi″o·cy′a·nate. Any organic compound of

the formula RNCS, isomeric with but differing from RCNS, which is a thiocyanate.

i″so·tone. One of two or more species of atoms which contain the same number of neutrons.

i″so·ton′ic [*isos;* G. *tonos,* tension]. 1. Referring or pertaining to a solution in which a tissue, especially red blood cells, maintains the normal state or tone. See also *isoosmotic.* 2. *In physiology,* having uniform tension under pressure or stimuli.

i′so·tope [*isos;* G. *topos,* place]. An element which has the same atomic number as another but a different atomic weight. Many of the common elements have been shown to consist of several isotopes, the apparent atomic weight of the element actually representing an average of the atomic weights of the isotopes. —**isotop′ic,** *adj.*

i. dilution analysis, isotopic dilution analysis. A method of analysis for a component of a mixture in which a known amount of the same component, commonly labeled with a radioactive isotope of predetermined activity, is added to the mixture. A pure sample of the compound is then isolated, and from the decrease in activity of the tracer substance, the original concentration of the component may be calculated.

i. effect. The effect of difference of mass between isotopes of the same element on the rate of reaction, position of equilibrium, or both, of chemical reactions involving the isotopes; the effect may be particularly prominent in the case of an element of low atomic weight.

i. exchange reaction. A chemical reaction in which interchange of the atoms of a given element between two or more chemical forms of the element occurs, the atoms in one form being isotopically labeled so as to distinguish them from atoms in the other form. Thus study of the course of the reaction is made possible.

radioactive i. One exhibiting the property of spontaneous decomposition, usually referring to an element rendered radioactive by artificial means. Radioactive isotopes of C, N, P, Na, K, Cl, I, and some other elements, incorporated in the molecules of compounds which are fed or injected, can be traced readily because the radiations of such tagged atoms may be detected by sensitive apparatus such as the Geiger-Müller counter. Compounds isolated from the tissues can be shown, if radioactive, to be intermediary metabolic products of the material administered.

i″so·top′ic a·bun′dance. The relative number of atoms of a particular isotope in a particular sample of an element.

i″so·trop′ic (eye″so·trop′ick, ·tro′pick) [*isos;* G. *trepein,* to turn]. 1. Having the same shape and appearance, from whatever point observed. 2. Being singly and uniformly refractive.

i″so·va·ler′ic ac′id (eye″so·va·lerr′ick, ·va·leer′-ick). $(CH_3)_2.CH.CH_2.COOH$; the valeric acid of commerce, obtained from valerian root; it has been used medicinally in the form of the ammonium salt. See *valeric acid.* Syn., *isopropylacetic acid.*

i″so·va·ler′ic al′de·hyde. $(CH_3)_2CH.CH_2.CHO$. A pungent, oily liquid with an odor of apples; obtained from oxidation of amyl alcohol.

is′pa·ghul″ (iss′puh·gull″). The seeds of *Plantago ispaghula,* used as a purgative in India; they contain mucilage and are used for recurring bacillary dysentery.

Israel, James Adolf [*German surgeon,* 1848–1926]. Made substantial contributions to renal surgery, especially in tuberculosis. Was first to describe the ray fungus in human lesions (1878).

is′sue [OF. from L. *exire,* to go out]. 1. Offspring. 2. A bloody or purulent discharge from a wound or cavity.

isth·mec′to·my (iss·meck′to·mee, isth·) [G. *isthmos,* isthmus, neck; *ektomē,* excision]. Excision of an isthmus; specifically, excision of the isthmus of the thyroid gland in goiter.

isth′mus (iss′mus, isth′mus) [*isthmos*]. 1. The neck or constricted part of an organ. 2. The part of the brain which, situated axially, unites the forebrain, the cerebellum, and the spinal cord. —**isthmic,** *adj.*

aortic i. A constriction of the fetal aorta between the left subclavian and the ductus arteriosus.

gyral i. A narrow gyrus connecting two adjoining gyri; an annectant convolution.

i. hippocampi. See *i.* of gyrus fornicatus.

i. of fauces. The passage between the oral cavity and the oral pharynx.

i. of gyrus fornicatus. A narrow convolution connecting the hippocampal and callosal gyri.

i. of limbic lobe. See *i.* of gyrus fornicatus.

i. of thyroid gland. The narrow transverse part connecting the lobes of the thyroid gland. See Plate 45.

i. of uterine tube. That part of the uterine tube nearest the uterus.

i. rhombencephali. The constriction between the third primary brain vesicle and the midbrain.

Krönig's i. See Georg *Krönig.*

uterine i. The transverse constriction of the uterus, dividing it into two portions, the body and the cervix.

istizin. Trade-mark for the laxative and cathartic substance 1,8-dihydroxyanthraquinone, or *danthron.*

isuprel hydrochloride. A trade-marked name for the sympathomimetic amine salt *isopropylarterenol hydrochloride.*

i·su′ri·a (eye·sue′ree·uh, i·sue′ree·uh) [G. *isos,* equal; *ouron,* urine]. Excretion of equal amounts of urine in equal periods of time.

Itard, Jean Marie Gaspard [*French otologist,* 1775–1838]. Contributed to the knowledge of diseases of the ear. Invented a type of Eustachian catheter, called *Itard's catheter.*

itch [AS. *gicce*]. 1. An irritating sensation in the skin. 2. Any of various skin diseases accompanied by itching, particularly scabies.

barber's i. See *tinea* barbae.

Bedouin's i. Miliaria.

Caripito i. (car″ry·pee′to). Itch caused by hairs from the wings and abdomen of moths of the genus *Hylesia* (family Saturniidae), common among seamen from the port of Caripito, Venezuela.

collector's i. Schistosome dermatitis.

coolie i. A dermatosis associated with ancylostomiasis: also called *water i.*

copra i. An epizoonosis caused by the copra mite, *Tryoglyphus longior.*

cowlot i. See schistosome *dermatitis.*

Cuban i. A disease resembling a mild form of smallpox.

dhobie mark i. Dermatitis caused by a laundry-marking ink made from the anacardium or cashew nut.

frost-i. See *pruritus* hiemalis.

grain i. An eruption due to *Pediculoides ventricosus,* acquired by contact with grain or straw, which harbors the parasite. See *acarodermatitis urticarioides, prairie i.*

grocer's i. The urticovesicular eruption of the skin caused by bites of the mite *Glyciphagus domesticus.*

ground i. Local irritation of the skin resulting from the entrance of the larvae of any variety of *Ancylostoma* into the skin.

jockey i. Tinea cruris.

mad i. Infectious bulbar paralysis.

Malabar i. See *tinea* imbricata.

Mazzamarra i. An itch caused by ancylostomiasis.

Norwegian i. A variety of scabies, usually severe in type; has been seen in many countries, including the United States.

Philippine i. Alastrim.

pineapple i. A dermatitis following contact with pineapples, possibly caused by an acarus.

prairie i. See grain *i.*

sandhog's i. The patchy mottling of the skin with itching, found in decompression sickness (caisson disease).

Sawah i. Schistosome dermatitis of the Malay countries.

swamp i. Schistosome dermatitis.

swimmer's i. Schistosome dermatitis.

washerwoman's i. Dermatitis of the hands, a general term for various eruptions, usually a fungus infection or contact dermatitis; seen in those who have their hands frequently in water.

water i. Schistosome dermatitis.

itch'ing [*gicce*]. A sensation of tickling and irritation in the skin, producing the desire to scratch. Syn., *pruritus.*

itch mite. See *Sarcoptes scabiei.*

-ite [G. *-itēs*]. 1. *In mineralogy,* a suffix denoting *a mineral* or *rock.* 2. *In zoology,* a suffix denoting *a division of the body* or *of a part.*

-ite [L. *-atum*]. *In chemistry,* a suffix denoting *the salt* or *ester* from an acid with the termination *-ous.*

i'ter (eye'tur, it'ur) [L., journey]. A passageway.

i. ad infundibulum. The passage between the third ventricle of the brain and the infundibulum, 2.

i. chordae anterius. The aperture through which the chorda tympani nerve leaves the tympanum: also called *Huguier's canal.*

i. chordae posterius. The aperture through which the chorda tympani nerve enters the tympanum.

i. dentium. An opening in the alveolar process lingual to or between the roots of a deciduous tooth, occupied by an extension of the dental sac of the permanent (succedaneous) tooth.

-i'tis (-eye'tis, -ee'tis) [G., inflammation]. *In medicine,* a suffix denoting *a disease;* specifically, *an inflammatory disease of a* (specified) *part.*

Ito-Reenstierna test. See under *test.*

I.U. Immunizing unit; international unit.

I.V., i.v. Abbreviation for intravenous.

i'vo·ry [OF]. *ivoire,* from L. *ebur,* ivory]. The dentin, particularly of commerce, such as that obtained from the tusks of the elephant, walrus, or hippopotamus.

i'vo·ry black. Animal charcoal.

Ivy, Andrew Conway [*American physiologist,* 1893–]. Known for his researches concerning cancer, gastric ulcer, aviation medicine, and geriatrics. Contributed greatly to the knowledge of the hormones of the digestive tract.

ivy oak. Trade-mark for a solution in peanut oil of equal parts of the toxic principles derived from *Toxicodendron radicans* (common poison ivy) and *T. diversilobum* (Pacific poison oak). Used for prophylaxis and treating dermatitis produced by poison ivy and poison oak.

ivyol. Trade-mark for a solution in olive oil of the extracts of *Toxicodendron radicans* (common poison ivy); also the trade-mark for a similar solution of the extracts of *T. diversilobum* (Pacific poison oak). Used for prophylaxis and treatment in poison-ivy and poison-oak dermatitis, respectively.

Ix·o'des (ick·so'deez) [G. *ixōdēs,* like birdlime]. A genus of parasitic ticks, some species of which cause tick paralysis and are important vectors of diseases of cattle, sheep, and dogs, as well as transmitters of encephalomyelitis and tularemia to man.

ix"o·di'a·sis [*ixōdēs;* NL. *-iasis,* condition]. Lesions or disease caused by infestation with ticks.

ix·od'ic [*ixōdēs*]. Caused by or relating to ticks.

Ix·od'i·dae (ick·sod'i·dee) [*ixōdēs*]. A family of hard-bodied ticks, which includes the genera *Boöphilus, Amblyomma, Dermacentor, Haemaphysalis, Hyalomma, Ixodes,* and *Rhipicephalus,* all of some pathologic significance to man.

ix"y·o·my"e·li'tis [G. *ixys,* waist; *myelos,* marrow; *-itis,* inflammation]. Inflammation of the lumbar portion of the spinal cord. *Rare.*

JKL

J

J Symbol for Joule's equivalent, joule.

j Used as a Roman numeral (in prescriptions) as the equivalent of i for one, or at the end of a number as j, ij, iij, vj, vij, etc.

ja'ag·siek"te. A contagious disease of sheep, sometimes of goats and guinea pigs, resembling the more benign and diffuse forms of bronchiolar carcinoma in man.

jab"o·ran'di. See *Pilocarpus.*

jab'o·rine. A mixture of alkaloids, formerly believed to be a single alkaloid, from *Pilocarpus jaborandi.*

Jaboulay, Mathieu [*French surgeon,* 1860–1913]. Performed the first gastroduodenostomy (1892). Introduced sympathectomy to relieve vascular tension (1900). Introduced an operation for hydrocele in which he incised the sac and everted it about the spermatic cord. Invented a device, consisting of two cylinders which fit together, for use in lateral intestinal anastomosis; called *Jaboulay's button.*

Jaccoud, Sigismond [*French physician,* 1830–1913]. Known for his special investigations of the causes of albuminuria. Described a type of fever in tuberculous meningitis, with irregular, slow pulse; called *Jaccoud's dissociated fever.* Described prominence of the aorta in the region of the suprasternal notch as diagnostic of aortic dilatation; called *Jaccoud's sign.*

jack bean. 1. The seed of *Canavalia* from which urease is prepared for use in the estimation of urea. 2. A plant of the genus *Canavalia*

jack'et [F. *jaquette,* dim. from *jaque*]. 1. A short coat. 2. *In medicine,* a supporting, therapeutic, or restraining apparatus covering the upper part of the body.

celluloid j. One made principally of celluloid, fashioned over a plaster mold of the patient's body.

j. crown. An artificial crown of a tooth consisting of a covering of metal, porcelain, or acrylic.

leather j. One made of leather, sometimes equipped with apparatus, made over a body mold;

used principally in tuberculosis of the vertebrae and in flaccid paralysis.

plaster of Paris j. A casing applied by winding plaster of Paris bandages over padding, so as to encase the body in a hard mold from armpits to groin; used to immobilize the spine.

pneumonia j. A padded cotton or wool coat which may contain poultices and which encases the upper part of the body; sometimes employed in the care of patients with pneumonia.

strait-j. A restraining apparatus, not always conforming to the jacket type, used to prevent violently insane or irresponsible persons from injuring themselves or others.

jack'screw" [OF. *Jaques*, LL. *Jacobus*, ultimately from the Hebrew; *escroue*, from L. *scrofa*, sow]. *In orthodontia*, an appliance used for forcing apart the fragments of certain types of fractures and retaining them in a separated condition.

Jackson, Chevalier (1865–). American bronchoesophagologist and laryngologist who devised instruments and techniques for peroral endoscopy, contributed to laying the foundation for bronchoesophagology as a branch of medical science, and, with W. W. Babcock, introduced the Jackson-Babcock operation for radical removal of an esophageal diverticulum.

Jackson, Jabez North [*American surgeon*, 1868–1935]. Described a thin membrane extending from the parietal peritoneum on the right, across the anterior surface of the ascending colon to the inner side, from the cecum to the hepatic flexure. *Jackson's membrane* or *veil* sometimes gives rise to obstructive symptoms. Devised his incision for removal of the breast in carcinoma, in which he made a circular incision about the breast, prolonging the incision vertically to the axilla.

Jackson, John Hughlings (1835–1911). English neurologist who described seizures due to focal lesions of the cerebral cortex (1863); see Jacksonian *epilepsy*. He made a classic study of aphasia, and with J. A. L. Clarke, gave the first full description of syringomyelia (1867). He also described paralysis of half the palate, pharynx, and larynx, and flaccid paralysis of the homolateral sternocleidomastoid and part of trapezius (1872), called *Jackson's syndrome, or vagoaccessory-hypoglossal paralysis*. See also *reevolution*.

Jackson's sign. See under *sign*.

Jacob, Arthur [*Irish ophthalmic surgeon*, 1790–1874]. Described a rodent ulcer involving face and eyelid; called *Jacob's ulcer*. Described the layer of rods and cones in the retina; called *Jacob's membrane*.

Jacobaeus, Hans Christian [*Swedish surgeon*, 1879–1937]. Known for his ingenuity in adapting the cystoscope to other cavities of the body (1910), leading to the invention of the thoracoscope. Devised an operation of pneumonolysis in which he divided pleural adhesions with a galvanocautery (1916); called *Jacobaeus' operation*.

Jacobi, Abraham (1830–1919). American pediatrician who invented a laryngoscope, wrote numerous treatises on children's diseases, established the first free clinic for children, and, with Emil Noeggerath, founded the *American Journal of Obstetrics* (1862).

jac'o·bine. $C_{18}H_{25}NO_6$; an alkaloid obtained from *Senecio jacoboea* and certain other species of *Senecio*.

Jacobsohn's reflex. See under *reflex*.

Jacobson, Ludwig Levin [*Danish anatomist*, 1783–1843]. Described the vomeronasal organ, called *organ of Jacobson*, and the tympanic nerve and plexus, called *Jacobson's nerve*, *Jacobson's plexus*.

jac'o·dine. $C_{18}H_{25}NO_5$; an alkaloid obtained from *Senecio jacoboea* and certain other species of *Senecio*.

jac'o·nine. $C_{18}H_{25}NO_8$; an alkaloid obtained from *Senecio jacoboea*.

Jacquemier, Jean Marie [*French obstetrician*, 1806–79]. Described a bluish discoloration of the vaginal mucosa, appearing from about the sixth to the twelfth week of pregnancy; called *Jacquemier's sign, Chadwick's sign, Kluge's sign*.

Jacquet's erythema. See *erythema* gluteale.

jac"ti·ta'tion [L. *jactitare*, to bring forward in public, from *jactare*, to toss about]. A tossing about, great restlessness; a condition at times present in grave diseases.

jac"u·lif'er·ous [L. *jaculum*, dart; *ferre*, to bear]. Prickly, bearing spines.

Jadassohn, Josef [*German dermatologist*, 1863–1936]. Described maculopapular erythroderma (1892), called *Jadassohn's disease*. Described and named granulosis rubra nasi (1901). See *nevus*.

Jaeger, Eduard [*Austrian ophthalmologist*, 1818–84]. Introduced a method of testing acuteness of vision by means of lines of type of different sizes printed on cards. Called *Jaeger's test types*.

Jaeger test. See Naegeli *test*.

Jaesche, Georg Emanuel [*German surgeon*, 1815–76]. Known for his contributions to the development of plastic surgery. Devised operations for entropion and trichiasis. Devised an operation for distichia in which he transplanted the glands of Zeis away from the edge of the lid by excising a crescent-shaped piece of skin; called *Arlt-Jaesche technic*.

Jaffé, Max [*German biochemist*, 1841–1911]. Discovered urobilin in urine (1868). Isolated indican from urine (1877). In *Jaffé's test* a red color develops when picric acid is added to creatinine in alkaline solution.

Jakob, Alfons Maria (1884–1931). German psychiatrist who described a form of pseudosclerosis, called *Jakob's disease*.

Jaksch, Rudolf von [*Austrian physician in Czechoslovakia*, 1855–1947]. Described infantile pseudoleukemic anemia (1889), called *von Jaksch's anemia* or *disease*. See also von Jaksch-Pollak's *test*.

jal'ap [Sp. *jalapa*, from a town in Mexico] (*jalapa*). The tuberous root of *Exogonium purga*, a plant of the Convolvulaceae. Its active principle is a resin which contains a glycoside, convolvulin. Jalap is an active hydragogue cathartic, and is used to remove dropsical effusions by way of the intestine. Dose, 0.65–2.0 Gm. (10–30 gr.).

compound colocynth and j. pills (*pilulae colocynthidis et jalapae*). The vegetable cathartic pills; contain compound colocynth extract, hyoscyamus extract, jalap resin, leptandra extract, and podophyllum resin. The compound cathartic pills (*pilulae hydrargyri chloridi mitis compositae*) contain compound colocynth extract, mild mercurous chloride, jalap resin, and gamboge.

compound j. powder (*pulvis jalapae compositus*). Powdered jalap 35, potassium bitartrate 65. The salt increases the degree of subdivision of the jalap and enhances its hydragogue action. Dose, 2–4 Gm. (30–60 gr.).

j. resin (*resina jalapae*). An alcoholic jalap extract precipitated with water. Dose, 0.13–0.32 Gm. (2–5 gr.).

jal'a·pin [*jalapa*]. A name sometimes applied to the resin from jalap.

jal"a·pi·no'lic ac'id. $C_{15}H_{30}(OH)COOH$. An acid occurring as a constituent of glycosides of ipomoea.

Ja·mai'ca dog'wood. See *piscidia*.

jam'bul. *Eugenia jambolana*, the bark and seeds of which have been variously used in medicine.

James's powder. See *antimony* powder.

James'town weed. Old term for Jimson weed. See *stramonium.*

Janet, Pierre Marie Félix [*French psychiatrist,* 1859–1947]. Described psychasthenia (1903), also called *Janet's disease.*

Janeway, Edward Gamaliel [*American physician,* 1841–1911]. Described small hemorrhagic lesions occurring usually on the palms and soles in bacterial endocarditis; called *Janeway's nodes.*

Janeway, Theodore Caldwell [*American physician,* 1872–1917]. Invented a sphygmomanometer, called *Janeway's sphygmomanometer.*

jan'i·ceps [L. *Janus,* an Italian deity represented with two opposite faces; *caput,* head]. Conjoined twins in which there is a single head exhibiting two equal, opposite faces. Also called *cephalothoracopagus disymmetros.*

j. asymmetros. A janiceps with the two faces unequally developed; iniops.

Jansen, Albert [*German otolaryngologist,* 1859–1933]. Described an operation for disease of the frontal sinus in which he curetted the frontal sinus after removing the lower wall and the inferior portion of the anterior wall; called *Jansen's operation.*

Jansen, Barend Coenraad Petrus [*Dutch physiological chemist,* 1884–]. With Donath, isolated vitamin B_1 (1926). Devised a test for thiamine hydrochloride by means of potassium ferricyanide. Vitamin B_1 in aqueous solution is oxidized to thiochrome, which is extracted with isobutanol and its fluorescence determined.

Janský, Jan [*Czechoslovakian physician,* d. 1921]. Classified human blood in four groups (1907); see *blood groups.* Late infantile amaurotic familial idiocy is called *Bielschowsky-Janský disease.*

Janssen, Zacharias [*Dutch spectacle maker,* fl. 1600]. Credited with the construction of the first compound microscope (ca. 1590).

ja'nus. See *janiceps.*

j. asymmetros. See *iniops.*

Ja'nus green B (C.C.). A basic aniline dye, diethyl safranin. Used especially in the vital staining of mitochondria; has been used in the vital staining of fungi and protozoa. Also called *diazin green S.*

jap"a·con'i·tine (jap"uh·kon'i·teen, ·tin). The most poisonous of aconite alkaloids; obtained from *Aconitum japonicum.* On saponification, it hydrolyzes to benzoic acid and japaconine.

Ja·pan' tal'low. Japan wax.

Ja·pan' wax. A fat from the mesocarp of the fruit of *Rhus succedanea* of Japan and China; a pale-yellow solid: used as an ingredient of ointments. Syn., *Japan tallow, sumach wax, vegetable wax.*

ja"ra·ra'ca (zhah"ruh·rah'kuh, jah"ruh·rack'uh). A poisonous snake, a member of the genus *Bothrops,* found in Brazil.

Jarcho, Julius [*American gynecologist and obstetrician,* 1882–]. Invented a manometer for testing the patency of the uterine tubes; called *Jarcho's pressometer.* It is used also for the introduction of opaque mediums for hysterosalpingography and pyelography.

jar'gon [OF.]. Confused, unintelligible talk, gibberish, babble. Also see *agrammatism, aphasia.*

jar'gon·ize [*jargon*]. To utter unintelligible sounds; to speak in, or turn something into, jargon.

Jarisch-Herxheimer reaction. See under *reaction.*

Jarjavay, Jean François [*French physician,* 1815–69]. Described a depressor urethrae muscle, a slip of the sphincter urethrae membranaceae which joins the sphincter vaginae; called *Jarjavay's muscle.*

Jarvis, William Chapman [*American laryngologist,* 1855–95]. Inventor of a snare used for removing polypoid growths in the nose and throat; called *Jarvis' snare.*

Jat'ro·pha [G. *iatros,* physician; *trophē,* nourishment]. A genus of plants of the Euphorbiaceae. Also called *Jatropa.*

J. curcas. The source of purging nuts.

J. gossypifolia. The tua-tua plant, indigenous to South America, West Indies, and Africa; has been used as a purgative and as a cure for leprosy.

jaun'dice (jawn'dis, jahn'dis) [OF. *jaunisse,* from L. *galbus,* yellow]. Yellowness of the skin, mucous membranes, and secretions; due to bile pigments in the blood. Also see *icterus.*

acholuric j. That without demonstrable bile pigment in the urine. See hereditary *spherocytosis.*

arsenical j. That due to arsenical hepatitis.

black j. An extreme degree of jaundice.

catarrhal j. See infectious *hepatitis.*

chronic familial j. See hereditary *spherocytosis.*

clinical j. Icterus with yellowing of the skin and scleras; the icterus index is above 15.

congenital j. That appearing at, or shortly after, birth; due to defective development of the biliary passages.

constitutional j. Physiologic hyperbilirubinemia.

dissociated j. Selective retention of either bile pigment or bile salts; most frequently acholuric.

epidemic j. See infectious *hepatitis.*

familial acholuric j. See hereditary *spherocytosis.*

familial j. (a) Hemolytic jaundice. (b) Physiologic hyperbilirubinemia.

familial nonhemolytic j. See physiologic *hyperbilirubinemia.*

gravis neonatorum j. A severe degree of icterus neonatorum.

green j. That in which the discoloration of the skin is green or olive-colored.

hemolytic j. A chronic, microcytic anemia, characterized by increased erythrocyte fragility, reticulocytosis, spherocytosis, acholuric jaundice, and splenomegaly. There is a familial form now classified as hereditary spherocytosis in which splenectomy can be of great value; in the acquired form, splenectomy is of questionable value.

hepatocanalicular j. A rare form of chronic hepatic jaundice which may follow infectious hepatitis or the therapeutic use of arsenicals, sulfonamides, or thiouracil. Biliary cirrhosis is this type of jaundice. Bile pigments and bile salts are present in the urine; undamaged parenchymal cells and periportal infiltration, with no evidence of retention of bile, are indicated by biopsy.

hepatocellular j. That due to impairment of function of the liver cells.

hepatogenous j. That due to hepatic disease. It may be obstructive or hepatocellular.

hereditary nonhemolytic j. See physiologic *hyperbilirubinemia.*

homologous serum j. Homologous serum hepatitis.

hyperhemolytic j. That due to inability of the liver to excrete the quantity of pigment presented to it as the result of excessive hemolysis.

infectious j. See infectious *hepatitis.*

inoculation j. See homologous serum *hepatitis.*

intralobular j. Hepatocellular jaundice.

j. of the new born. See *icterus* neonatorum.

late arsphenamine j. See homologous serum *hepatitis.*

latent j. Increase in bile pigment in the blood, insufficient to show jaundice clinically but determinable by the icterus index (from 6 to 15).

malignant j. Icterus gravis.

mechanical j. See obstructive *j.*

Minkowski-Chauffard hemolytic j. See hereditary *spherocytosis.*

nuclear j. See *kernicterus.*

obstructive j. That due to interference with the outflow of bile by mechanical obstruction of the biliary passages, as by gallstones or tumor.

parenchymatous j. Hepatocellular jaundice.

posthepatic j. Obstructive *j.*: occasional usage.

postvaccinal j. See homologous serum *hepatitis.*

prehepatic j. Jaundice in which there is no apparent liver lesion, as hemolytic *j.* and physiologic hyperbilirubinemia.

regurgitation j. That due to secretion of bile pigment into the hepatic lymph channels and thence into the blood. It may be hepatocellular or obstructive. Also called *resorptive j.*

retention j. That due to the inability of the liver to excrete the bile pigment presented to it.

spirochetal j. A disease in man caused by the spirochete, *Leptospira icterohaemorrhagiae;* characterized by fever, nausea, headache, muscular pain, and jaundice. Also called *Weil's disease, spirochaetosis icterohaemorrhagica.*

syringe j. See homologous serum *hepatitis.*

toxic j. That associated with toxic hepatitis.

transfusion j. See homologous serum *hepatitis.*

Jauregg. See Julius *Wagner* von Jauregg.

Javal, Louis Emile [*French ophthalmologist,* 1839–1907]. Inventor of the astigmometer (1867). With Schiötz, invented an ophthalmometer (1881).

ja·van'i·cin. $C_{15}H_{14}O_6$; a red antibiotic substance derived from cultures of *Fusarium javanicum,* active against many bacteria but only slightly antifungal. **Oxyjavanicin** is produced simultaneously.

ja'va·nine. An alkaloid from the bark of various species of *Cinchona.*

jaw [perhaps from E. *chaw, chew,* with influence from F. *joue,* cheek]. Either of two bones, the upper jaw or maxilla, and the lower jaw or mandible, which form the skeleton of the mouth.

lumpy j. See *actinomycosis.*

phossy j. Phosphorus necrosis of the jaw.

snapping j. A condition characterized by an audible and palpable snap on opening and closing the mouth, usually caused by displacement of the meniscus in the mandibular joint.

wolf jaw. Bilateral cleft of the lip, jaw, and palate.

Jaworski, Valery [*Polish physician,* 1849–1925]. Described spiral bodies of mucus, *Jaworski's corpuscles,* found in the gastric secretion in cases of pronounced hyperchlorhydria.

jaw-wink'ing. See Marcus Gunn *phenomenon.*

Jeanselme, Antoine Edouard [*French dermatologist,* 1858–1935]. Known especially for his studies of syphilis. Described juxta-articular nodules, also called *Jeanselme's nodules.*

je"co·le'ic ac'id (jee"ko-lee'ick, jeck"o-). An acid occurring in the glycerides of cod liver oil.

Jeculin. A proprietary hematinic used in primary and secondary anemias.

Jed'dah ul'cer (yed'uh, jed'uh). See *oriental sore.*

jej"u·nec'to·my (jedg"oo·neck'to·mee) [L. *jejunus,* empty; G. *ektomē,* excision]. Excision of part or all of the jejunum.

jej"u·ni'tis (jedj"oo·nigh'tis) [*jejunus;* G. *-itis,* inflammation]. Inflammation of the jejunum.

jej'u·no- (jedj'oo·no-, ji·jew'no-), **jejun-** [*jejunus*]. *In medicine,* a combining form denoting *the jejunum.*

jej"u·no·ce·cos'to·my [*jejunus;* L. *caecus,* blind; G. *stoma,* mouth]. Formation of an anastomosis between the jejunum and the cecum by surgery.

jej"u·no·co·los'to·my [*jejunus;* G. *kolon,* colon; *stoma*]. The formation of an anastomosis between the jejunum and the colon by surgery.

jej"u·no·gas'tric. See *gastrojejunal.*

jej"u·no·il"e·i'tis [*jejunus;* G. *eilein,* to roll; *-itis,* inflammation]. Inflammation of the jejunum and the ileum.

jej"u·no·il"e·os'to·my [*jejunus; eilein;* G. *stoma,* mouth]. The formation of an anastomosis between the jejunum and the ileum by surgery.

jej"u·no·il'e·um [*jejunus; eilein*]. That part of the small intestine extending from the duodenum to the cecum.

jej"u·no·jej"u·nos'to·my (·jedj"oo·nos'to·mee) [*jejunus; jejunus;* G. *stoma,* mouth]. Surgical formation of an anastomosis between two parts of the jejunum.

jej"u·nor'rha·phy (jedj"oo·nor'uh·fee) [*jejunus;* G. *rhaphē,* a suture]. Suture of the jejunum.

jej"u·nos'to·my (jedj"oo·nos'to·mee) [*jejunus;* G. *stoma,* mouth]. The making of an artificial opening (jejunal fistula) through the abdominal wall into the jejunum.

jej"u·not'o·my (jedj"oo·not'o·mee) [*jejunus;* G. *tomē,* a cutting]. Incision into the jejunum.

je·ju'num [*jejunus*]. The second division of the small intestine extending between the duodenum and the ileum, and measuring about 8 feet (2.2 meters) in length. See Plate 13. —**jejunal,** *adj.*

Jellinek-Tillais' sign. See under *sign.*

jel'ly [L. *gelare,* to congeal]. A semisolid colloidal system of a liquid suspended in a solid, as water in gelatin.

contraceptive j. Any one of a number of viscous substances introduced into the vagina to prevent conception; designed to act both as an occlusive and as a vehicle for contraceptive chemicals.

electrode j. A jelly for improving the contact between skin and electrode in electrocardiography and electroencephalography.

glycerin j. A mixture of glycerin, gelatin, and other substances, e.g. zinc oxide.

K-Y j. Trade-mark for a lubricating jelly containing boric acid, glycerin, chondrus, and tragacanth.

Lieberkühn j. The alkali metaprotein having the consistency of a jelly, formed by the action of dilute sodium hydroxide solution on albumin.

mineral j. Petrolatum. Also called *petroleum j.*

petroleum j. Petrolatum.

vaginal j. Any one of a group of substances introduced into the vagina for the treatment of disease, or, more commonly, for contraceptive purposes.

Wharton's j. The mucoid connective tissue that constitutes the matrix of the umbilical cord.

jel'ly boot. See *Unna's paste boot.*

jel'ly of Whar'ton. See Wharton's *jelly.*

Jenner, Edward [*English physician,* 1749–1823]. Introduced inoculation with matter containing the virus of vaccinia, to produce immunity to smallpox. See smallpox *vaccine,* also called *Jennerian vaccine.*

Jenner, William [*English physician,* 1815–98]. Differentiated typhus from typhoid fever (1849).

Jenner's stain. See under *stain.*

Jensen, Carl Oluf [*Danish veterinary surgeon and pathologist,* 1864–1934]. Established the fact that cancer can be transmitted by inoculation. See Jensen's *sarcoma.*

Jensen, Edmund Zeuthen [*Danish ophthalmologist,* 1861–1950]. Described retinochoroiditis juxtapapillaris (1908), called *Jensen's disease.* It is characterized by the juxtapapillary location of the exudate, with retinal involvement and a sector defect in the visual field.

Jensen's method. See Hagedorn and Jensen's *method.*

Jephcott method. See under *method.*

je·quir'i·ty [Pg. *jequiriti*]. The seed of *Abrus precatorius.* An infusion containing abrin has been prepared from it and used in treating trachoma.

jerk [possibly imitative in origin]. A sudden, spasmodic movement; a term often applied to certain reflexes, as the jaw-jerk reflex, patellar reflex.

jer'vine (jur'veen, ·vin). The predominant alkaloidal constituent, an alkanolamine, of veratrum viride and veratrum album, practically inert physiologically.

jes"a·con'i·tine. $C_{35}H_{49}NO_{12}$; an alkaloid from the root of certain species of *Aconitum.*

Jesu Haly ('Alī ibn 'Īsā) [*Arabian ophthalmologist,* eleventh century]. His book on diseases of the eye was considered the standard throughout Europe and the East, and is said still to be in use among Arabian physicians.

Jes'u·its' bal'sam (bawl'sum). Compound benzoin tincture.

Jes'u·its' bark. Old term for Peruvian bark; the bark of several species of *Cinchona.* See *cinchona.*

Jes'u·its' drops. Compound benzoin tincture.

jet dust coun'ter. An instrument for determining the number of dust particles in the air. A measured sample of air is humidified and propelled at high velocity through a narrow aperture against a perpendicular plate to which the dust particles adhere. They are then counted under a microscope. Other instruments used for the same purpose are the konimeter, impinger, and precipitator. Also see *dust count.*

jet in·jec'tion. See *hypospray.*

Jewett, Hugh Judge [*American urologist,* 1903–]. Known for his operation of ureterointestinal anastomosis, in which a junction is made in two stages between ureter and sigmoid colon.

Jezler-Takata test. See Takata-Ara *test.*

jig'ger. See *Tunga penetrans.*

Jim'son weed. See *stramonium.*

jiu·jit'su. See *jujitsu.*

Jobert de Lamballe, Antoine Joseph [*French surgeon,* 1799–1867]. Known for his contributions to plastic surgery and to surgery of the intestinal tract. Described a potential hollow in the upper part of the popliteal space, called *Jobert's fossa.*

Jobling, James Wesley [*American physician,* 1876–]. Described an experimentally transmissible carcinoma of the rat, called *Flexner-Jobling tumor.* He also developed an antimeningitis serum.

jock'ey strap. The popular name given to a scrotal supporter; a suspensory.

Joffroy, Alix [*French physician,* 1844–1908]. With Charcot, demonstrated atrophy of the anterior horns of the spinal cord in poliomyelitis, and described the lesions of the spinal cord in muscular atrophy (1869). See also Joffroy's *reflex, sign.*

John of Arderne [*English physician,* 1306–90]. Made important contributions to the development of surgery. Described an operative method for the treatment of anal fistula.

Johne, Heinrich Albert [*German veterinarian,* 1839–1910]. Described a chronic type of enteritis of cattle, in which emaciation and recurrent diarrhea persist for months; called *Johne's disease.* On post-mortem examination, typical thickening and corrugation of the intestinal mucosa are found. The etiologic agent, *Mycobacterium paratuberculosis,* is called *Johne's bacillus.* See johnin *reaction.*

joh'nin (yo'nin). A vaccine prepared from cultures of *Mycobacterium paratuberculosis.* Also called *paratuberculin.*

Johnson, Clayton Richardson [*American radiologist,* 1896–]. Known for his methods and improvements in radiographic pelvimetry. Invented a stereoroentgenometer. The *Johnson method* is a procedure for interpreting a roentgenogram, based on cross-thread localization.

joint. Articulation. For joints listed by name, see Table of Joints in the Appendix. See Plate 2.

ball-and-socket j. See *enarthrosis.*

biaxial j. One in which movement is around two transverse axes at right angles to each other. The two varieties are the condyloid and the saddle joint.

Charcot's j. A neuropathic arthropathy in which articular cartilage and subjacent bone degenerate while hypertrophic changes occur at the joint edges and present an irregular deformity with instability of the joint. Most common in tabes dorsalis.

false j. A pseudarthrosis.

flail j. A condition of excessive mobility often following resection of a joint.

gliding j. One which allows only gliding movements; formed by the apposition of plane surfaces, or one slightly convex, the other slightly concave.

hinge j. A joint with only one axis of rotation. Syn., *ginglymus.*

incudostapedial j. The diarthrodial articulation between the lenticular process of the incus and the head of the stapes.

pastern j. The articulation between the proximal and second phalanges (great and small pastern bones) of any leg of a horse.

pivot j. One in which movement is limited to rotation; the movement is uniaxial, and in the longitudinal axis of the bones. Also called *trochoid joint.*

rotation j. A lateral ginglymus.

saddle j. One in which the opposing surfaces are reciprocally concavo-convex.

joint body. See *joint mouse.*

joint fu'sion. See *arthrodesis.*

joint-ill. A pyosepticemia of newborn animals resulting from an infection of the navel, characteristically accompanied by a suppurative arthritis.

joint mouse. A small loose body within a joint, frequently calcified, derived from synovial membrane, organized fibrin fragments of articular cartilage, or arthritic osteophytes: also called *joint body.*

Jolly, Friedrich (1844–1904). German neurologist who described a reaction, said to occur in certain amyotrophias, in which the contractility of a muscle which has been exhausted by faradism can still be excited by the influence of the will; inversely, when voluntary movements are impossible, the muscle can contract on faradization; called *Jolly's reaction.*

Jolly, Justin Marie Jules [*French histologist,* 1870–]. Described nuclear bodies, probably detritus from the nuclei, found in erythrocytes. Called *Jolly bodies, Howell-Jolly bodies.*

Jones, Robert [*English orthopedic surgeon,* 1858–1933]. Pioneer in tendon transplanting and bone grafting. Devised many orthopedic appliances, among them a modification of the Thomas splint, designed for fractures of the humerus; called *Jones splint.* See also Jones's *position.*

Jones, Thomas Wharton [*Scottish ophthalmologist,* 1808–91]. Remembered for his operation for the relief of ectropion, in which he made a V incision, closing it in the shape of a Y.

Jones test. See Boerner, Jones, and Lukens *test.*

Jonnescu. See *Ionescu.*

Jorissenne, Gustave [*Belgian physician,* b. 1846]. Described a sign of early pregnancy: the pulse rate is not increased when the patient changes from the horizontal to the erect position. Called *Jorissenne's sign.*

Joseph, Jacques [*German surgeon*, 1865–1934]. Made important contributions to the development of plastic surgery. Introduced an operation for complete reconstruction of the ear by implanting an ivory ear covered by a skin flap.

Joslin, Elliott Proctor [*American physician*, 1869–]. Known for his investigations into the cause and treatment of diabetes mellitus.

joule (jowl, jōōl) [after James Prescott *Joule*, English physicist, 1818–89]. A unit of energy, equivalent to the energy supplied by a power of 1 watt operating for 1 second. Symbol, J.

judg'ment [L. *judex*, judge]. The capacity to judge; the ability to draw correct conclusions from the material acquired by experience.

ju'do. See *jujitsu*.

ju'gal [L. *jugum*, yoke]. 1. Connecting or uniting, as by a yoke. 2. Pertaining to the zygoma, as the jugal point.

j. point. The craniometric point which is situated at the angle that the posterior border of the frontosphenoidal process of the zygoma makes with the superior border of its temporal process.

ju'glans (jew'glanz) [L., walnut]. The dried inner bark from the roots of *Juglans cinera*. The fluidextract is used as a cathartic and antiperiodic. Also called *butternut bark*.

ju'glone. $C_{10}H_6O_3$; 3-hydroxy-1,4-naphthoquinone, obtained from various species of *Juglans* (the walnut trees); a yellow, crystalline substance, slightly soluble in hot water; antifungal activity is claimed for it.

jug'u·lar (jug'yoo·lur, jōōg'yoo·lur) [L. *jugulum*, collarbone]. Pertaining to the neck above the clavicle, as the jugular vein.

jug'u·lar. The internal jugular vein. See Table of Veins in the Appendix.

juice [L. *jus*, broth]. 1. The liquid contained in vegetable or animal tissues. 2. Any of the secretions of the body.

gastric j. The secretion of the glands of the stomach; a clear, colorless liquid, having an acid reaction, and a specific gravity of about 1.006, and containing about 0.5% of solid matter. It contains hydrochloric acid, pepsin, rennin, and mucin.

intestinal j. The secretion of the intestinal glands, a pale yellow fluid, alkaline in reaction, having a specific gravity of 1.001, and possessing diastasic and proteolytic properties. It also, to a certain extent, emulsifies and decomposes fats.

pancreatic j. The secretion of the pancreas; a thick, transparent, colorless, odorless fluid, of a salty taste, and strongly alkaline, containing proteolytic, lipolytic, and amylolytic enzymes.

ju·jit'su, jiu·jit'su [Jap.]. A Japanese method of physical training used also as a system of self-defense without weapons. The opponent's own weight is used to overthrow him. Syn., *judo*.

ju'jube [F., from G. *zizyphon*, jujube]. The fruit of the jujube tree, *Zizyphus jujuba;* used for throat irrigation in the form of a lozenge or syrup.

j. paste. A paste containing the pulp of jujubes and used as a demulcent sialagogue. It is now made of gum arabic or of gelatin, variously flavored.

Jukes. A fictitious name given to the descendants of certain sisters in a study of the occurrence among them of crime, immorality, pauperism, and disease in relation to heredity.

Jukes unit. See Bourquin-Sherman *unit*.

ju·men'tous [L. *jumentum*, beast of burden]. Similar to that of a horse; applied to the odor of urine.

junc'tion [L. *junctio*, from *jungere*, to join]. The point or line of union of two parts; juncture; interface.

cementoenamel j. That between the enamel and the cementum of a tooth.

dentinocemental j. The interface between the dentin and the cementum in the root of a tooth.

dentinoenamel j. The interface between the enamel and dentin in the crown of a tooth.

dermoepidermal j. The site of a thin wavy membrane separating the basal cells of the epidermis from the underlying collagen fibrils of the dermis: demonstrated by the periodic acid Schiff stain and electron microscopy.

mucocutaneous j. The transition from skin to mucous membrane at the body orifices.

mucogingival j. The scalloped line between the gingiva and the alveolar mucosa.

myoneural j. The point of junction of a motor nerve with the muscle which it innervates: also called *neuromuscular j.*

sclerocorneal j. The boundary between the white, opaque sclera and the transparent cornea in the eye.

ureteropelvic j. The point at which the renal pelvis becomes the ureter proper; the upper isthmus of Schwalbe.

junc·tu'ra [L.]. 1. An articulation; a suture of bones. 2. A junction, as of tendons.

June cold. That type of hay fever caused by sensitivity to grass pollen. Syn., *hay fever*.

Jung, Carl Gustav (1875–). Swiss psychologist and psychiatrist; a pioneer in analytic psychology. He regarded the libido not as an expression of the sex instinct but as the will to live; he classified individuals as either extroverts or introverts, and made comparative and historical researches concerning the nature of the unconscious mind. See feeling-type, intuitional-type, sensational-type, thinking-type *personality*.

jun'gle ra'tion (rash'un, ray'shun). See under *ration*.

jung'le rot. Any cutaneous disturbance caused or induced by a tropic-like climate; most often cutaneous bacterial and mycotic infections: lay term.

ju'ni·per [L. *juniperus*] (*juniperus*). 1. The fruit of *Juniperus communis*, containing a volatile oil, resin, and fixed oil. 2. Any evergreen shrub or tree of the genus *Juniperus*.

j. oil (*oleum juniperi*). The volatile oil from the fruit of *J. communis*. A stimulant in chronic genitourinary disorders. Has been used as a diuretic.

j. tar. See cade *oil*.

junk [perhaps from L. *juncus*, bulrush]. A quilted cushion forming a sling in which to suspend a fractured limb. *Obs.*

Junod, Victor Théodore [*French physician*, 1809–81]. Invented a device, now obsolete, for producing passive congestion. *Junod's boot* consisted of a boot-shaped case enclosing the leg so that air could be removed from around the part.

ju"ris·pru'dence [L. *jurisprudentia*, from *jus*, law, *prudentia*, skill]. The science of law, its interpretation and application.

medical j. Legal medicine.

ju'ry [L. *jurare*, to swear]. A body of adult persons chosen according to law to attend a judicial tribunal and to determine the true verdict upon a matter being tried or inquired into.

coroner's j. That jury which attends a coroner's inquest, to determine the cause of a death.

j. of inquest. A coroner's jury.

jury mast. An iron rod fixed in a plaster jacket; used to support the head in disease or fracture of the cervical spine.

Juster's reflex. See under *reflex.*

jus′to ma′jor [L.]. Greater than normal, larger in all dimensions than normal; applied to a pelvis.

jus′to mi′nor [L.]. Abnormally small in all dimensions; said of a pelvis.

jute [Bengali *jūt*, from Skr. *jūta*, matted hair]. The bast fiber of several species of the genus *Corchorus*, grown chiefly in India and Ceylon: used in absorbent dressings.

ju′ve·nile (jew′vi·nil, ·nyle) [L. *juvenilis*, young]. Young; pertaining to youth or childhood. —**ju′venile,** *n.*

jux′ta- [L.]. A combining form denoting *nearness, situated near.*

jux″ta-ar·tic′u·lar. Near a joint.

jux″ta·glo·mer′u·lar [*juxta;* dim. from L. *glomus*, ball]. 1. Next to the glomerulus. 2. Referring to epithelioid cells near the glomerulus of the kidney.

jux″ta·po·si′tion [*juxta;* L. *positio*, from *ponere*, to place]. 1. Situation adjacent to another; close relationship; apposition. 2. The act of placing near.

jux″ta·py·lor′ic (juck″stuh·pye·lor′ick, ·pi·lor′ick) [*juxta;* G. *pylōros*, gatekeeper]. Near the pylorus.

K

K The chemical symbol for potassium (*kalium*).

K_a Symbol for the dissociation constant of an acid.

K_b Symbol for the dissociation constant of a base.

Kader, Bronislaw [*Polish surgeon*, 1863–1937]. Originated an operation for gastrostomy, in which a pleat is formed in the anterior gastric wall through which a catheter passes, the pleat being infolded by several rows of interrupted Lembert sutures.

Kaes, Theodor [*German neurologist*, 1852–1913]. Described a layer of fibers parallel to the tangential fibers in the cerebral cortex; called *Kaes's layer, Bekhterev's fibers.*

Kaf′fir pox. A mild form of smallpox. Syn., *alastrim.*

Kahler, Otto [*Austrian physician*, 1849–93]. Described multiple myeloma (1889). *Kahler's law* states that the ascending branches of the posterior spinal nerve roots, after entering the cord, pass successively from the root zone toward the mesial plane.

Kahn, Reuben Leon [*American bacteriologist*, 1887–]. Introduced a flocculation test for the diagnosis of syphilis (1923). The *Kahn test* requires an ether-purified alcohol extract of beef-heart muscle and cholesterol which, when correctly mixed with physiological NaCl solution, results in a suspension of unstable aggregates. When this is added in proper ratio to inactivated serum and shaken, the aggregates disperse, remaining so in the case of a negative serum. When positive serum is used, new stable aggregates or flocculi are formed.

Kahn's method. See Leiboff and Kahn's *method.*

kai″no·pho′bi·a (kigh″no·fo′bee·uh) [G. *kainos*, new; *phobos*, fear]. A morbid fear of anything new. —**kai′nophobe,** *n.*

Kaiserling's method. See under *method.*

kak″er·ga′si·a. See *merergasia.*

kak′ke. See *beriberi.*

kak′o-. See *caco-.*

kak′o·dyl. See *cacodyl.*

kak″or·rhaph″i·o·pho′bi·a [G. *kakorraphia*, contrivance of ill; *phobos*, fear]. Morbid fear of failure.

ka′la-a·zar′ (kah′lah-ah·zahr′, -ah′zahr, kal″uh-ay′zur, -az′ur). Visceral leishmaniasis; there are two types: the Indian type which affects older children and adults in India, Indo-China, and Sudan, and the Mediterranean type which attacks infants in countries bordering the Mediterranean. *Leishmania donovani* is the etiologic agent of both types. The chief lesion is marked by hyperplasia of the cells of the reticuloendothelial system, particularly of the spleen and liver, continued irregular fever, emaciation, anemia, and leukopenia.

ka·le′mi·a, kal″i·e′mi·a. See *potassemia.*

ka·lim′e·ter. See *alkalimeter.* —**kalimetry,** *n.*

ka′li·um. Potassium.

Kal′li·kak. A fictitious name given to the descendants of a Revolutionary War soldier in a study of the occurrence among them of feeblemindedness and immorality and the bearing of these on heredity.

kal″li·kre′in. A principle obtained from the pancreas, having peripheral vasodilating action: used for treatment of peripheral vascular disorders, angina pectoris, hypertension, etc.

ka·ma′la (kuh·may′luh, kam′uh·luh), **ka·me′la** (kuh·mee′luh) [Skr.]. Rottlera. The glands and hairs from the capsules of *Mallotus philippinensis* (kamala tree), found in Asia, Africa, and Australia. Purgative and anthelmintic; used for the expulsion of ascarid worms and tapeworms.

Kammerer, Frederic [*American surgeon*, 1856–1928]. Introduced, coincidently with Battle, a vertical abdominal incision in which the rectus sheath is opened, and medial retraction made, followed by vertical incision of the posterior rectus sheath and peritoneum for exposure of the abdominal cavity. The *Kammerer-Battle incision* is useful when exploration is desired.

Kanavel, Allen Buckner [*American surgeon*, 1874–1938]. Contributed to the knowledge of infections of the hand and to the development of surgery of the hand. Devised a technic for draining the thenar space by incision of the dorsal surface of the thumb-index web. Advocated full-thickness grafts, with all fat removed, for the relief of Dupuytren's contracture, called *Kanavel's method.* See also Kanavel's *sign.*

Kan′da·har sore. See *oriental sore.*

kan″ga·roo′ ten′don. A tendon obtained from the tail of the kangaroo; used for surgical ligatures and sutures.

kan′gri burn. A squamous epithelioma frequent on the skin of the abdomen and thighs of the natives of Kashmir, and attributed to the irritation caused by charcoal heaters worn beneath the clothing in cold weather. Also called *kangri cancer.*

ka′o·lin [F., from the Chinese, high hill]. A native, hydrated aluminum silicate, powdered and freed from gritty particles by elutriation; occurs as a soft, white or yellowish white powder, or as lumps; it is insoluble in water, cold dilute acids, and solutions of the alkali hydroxides. Externally, it is used for its protective influence and for its power of absorbing moisture. As a dusting powder, it is sometimes applied to freely discharging ulcers and similar affections. Internally, it acts as an adsorptive in the treatment of various forms of enteritis. Dose, 15–60 Gm. (½–2 oz.).

k. cataplasm (*cataplasma kaolini*). Contains kaolin 565 Gm., boric acid 45 Gm., thymol 0.5 Gm., methyl salicylate 2 cc., peppermint oil 0.5 cc., glycerin 387 Gm. Used as a carrier of heat in treating various local inflammations.

ka″o·li·no′sis [*kaolin;* G. *-ōsis*, condition]. Chronic inflammation of the lungs, occurring in workers in kaolin; a form of benign pneumonoconiosis.

kaomagma. A proprietary preparation containing aluminum hydroxide gel and kaolin. Used in intestinal disorders.

kaomin. A proprietary preparation containing bismuth subcarbonate, kaolin, magnesium hydroxide, sucrose, and vegetable mucilage. Used in intestinal disorders.

kaopectate. A proprietary preparation containing kaolin and pectin in an aromatic and carminative vehicle. Used in intestinal disorders.

Kaposi, Moritz [*Hungarian dermatologist*, 1837–1902]. Described multiple idiopathic hemorrhagic sarcoma (1872), called *Kaposi's sarcoma*, and xeroderma pigmentosum (1882), called *Kaposi's disease*. Described lymphodermia perniciosa (1885) and impetigo herpetiformis (1887).

kap′pa fac′tor. See under *factor*.

kappaxin. Trade-mark for a brand of menadione.

Kappeler, Otto [*German surgeon*, 1841–1909]. Described his operation for cholecystenterostomy performed in one stage. In *Kappeler's operation*, the gallbladder is emptied by puncture with a trocar, the margins of the opening being united, after enlargement, by a double row of sutures to the highest portion of the jejunum.

Kappers, Cornelius Ubbo Ariens (1877–1946). Dutch neuroanatomist, who made important contributions, with Edinger, to the concepts of the neo-, archi-, and paleo-subdivisions of the parts of the brain. His first paper on neurobiotaxis (1907) stated a theory which drew attention to certain general principles in comparative neuroanatomy.

ka·ra′ya gum (ka·rah′yuh, kar′ay·uh). An exudate from trees of the *Sterculia* or *Cochlospermum* species; with water, it swells to form a bulky mass. This hydrophilic property is utilized in industry and in pharmaceutical manufacturing. *In medicine*, karaya gum is sometimes employed as a mechanical laxative. Dose, a heaping teaspoonful. Also called *sterculia gum*.

Karell diet. See under *diet*.

Karrer, Paul (1889–). Swiss chemist noted for studies on the constitution of carotenoids, flavins, and vitamins A and B. Nobel laureate in chemistry (1938).

Karr's method. See under *method*.

ka″ry·en′chy·ma (care″ree·eng′ki·muh, ·en′ki·) [G. *karyon*, kernel; *egchyma*, instillation]. The clear ground substance occupying the meshes of the nuclear reticulum. Also called *karyolymph; nuclear sap*.

ka′ry·o-, ka′ry- [*karyon*]. A combining form meaning *nut* or *kernel;* used especially in biology to denote *relation to the karyon* or *nucleus of a cell*.

ka′ry·o·blast″ [*karyon;* G. *blastos*, germ]. The most immature cell of the erythrocyte series. Also called *megaloblast, proerythroblast*.

ka′ry·o·chrome″ [*karyon;* G. *chrōma*, color]. 1. A nerve cell which has a high nucleocytoplasmic ratio. 2. A nerve cell in which the nucleus stains intensely.

ka″ry·oc′la·sis. Old term for *karyorrhexis*.

ka′ry·o·cyte″. See *normoblast*.

ka″ry·og′a·my [*karyon;* G. *gamos*, marriage]. A conjugation of cells characterized by a fusion of the nuclei. —**karyogam′ic,** *adj.*

ka″ry·o·ki·ne′sis (care″ee·o·ki·nee′sis, ·kigh·nee′sis) [*karyon;* G. *kinēsis*, motion]. Mitosis or indirect cell division; especially the nuclear transformations, as opposed to *cytokinesis*. Also called *karyomitosis*. —**karyokinet′ic,** *adj.*

ka″ry·o·lo′bic [*karyon;* G. *lobos*, lobe]. Concerning a lobated nucleus. *O.T.*

ka′ry·o·lymph″. See *karyenchyma*.

ka″ry·ol′y·sis [*karyon;* G. *lysis*, a loosing]. The dissolution of the nucleus of the cell. —**karyolyt′ic,** *adj.*

ka′ry·o·mere [*karyon;* G. *meros*, a part]. A segment of a chromosome. See *chromomere*.

ka″ry·o·mi″cro·so′ma (·migh″kro·so′muh, ·mick″ro·so′muh) [*karyon;* G. *mikros*, small; *sōma*, body]. Old term for the chromatin particles of the nucleus.

ka″ry·o·mi′tome [*karyon;* G. *mitos*, thread]. Old term for the mitome threads of the nucleus. See *mitome*.

ka″ry·o·mi·to′sis (care″ee·o·mi·to′sis, ·migh·to′sis) [*karyon; mitos;* G. *-ōsis*, condition]. Karyokinesis.

ka′ry·on [G.]. Old term for the nucleus of a cell.

ka′ry·o·phage″ [*karyon;* G. *phagein*, to eat]. An intercellular parasite which destroys the nucleus of the infested cell.

ka′ry·o·plasm [*karyon;* G. *plasma*, anything formed]. Old term for nucleoplasm.

ka″ry·or·rhex′is [*karyon;* G. *rhēxis*, a breaking]. Fragmentation or splitting up of a nucleus into a number of pieces which become scattered in the cytoplasm.

ka′ry·o·some″, kar″y·o·so′ma [*karyon;* G. *sōma*, body]. 1. A chromatin nucleolus or false nucleolus, by differentiation from a true nucleolus or plasmosome. 2. A large, deeply staining body in the nucleus of many Protista, associated with the chromosomes or other structures.

ka″ry·os′ta·sis [*karyon;* G. *stasis*, a standing]. The stage of the nucleus between mitotic divisions. Also called *interkinesis, interphase, resting nucleus*.

kar″y·o·the′ca. Nuclear membrane.

kar″y·o·type′. The total of characteristics, including number, form, and size, of chromosomes and their grouping in a cell nucleus; it is characteristic of an individual, race, species, genus, or larger grouping.

Ka·sai′. A syndrome seen in the Belgian Congo, characterized by depigmentation of the skin, anemia, edema, and digestive disturbances, and attributed to iron deficiency: also called *Belgian Congo anemia*.

Kasanin-Vigotsky test. See under *test*.

Kashida's sign. See under *sign*.

kata-. See *cata-*.

kat″a·did′y·mus [G. *kata*, down; *didymos*, twin]. Duplication of the superior pole, as in diprosopia or dicephalism. Has been incorrectly used for inferior duplicity. Also called *superior duplicity*.

kat″a·pla′si·a. See *cataplasia*.

kat″a·ther·mom′e·ter [*kata;* G. *thermē*, heat; *metron*, a measure]. A double-bulbed, alcohol thermometer, graduated from 100°–90° F., which records how quickly air is cooling, thus permitting an estimate of evaporation of moisture from the body.

kat″a·to′ni·a. See *catatonia*.

Kat″a·ya′ma (cat″uh·yah′muh, kah″tuh·) [Jap.]. A genus of amphibious snails.

K. formosana. A species found in Formosa; one of the intermediate hosts of *Schistosoma japonicum*.

K. nosophora. A species found in Japan and along the coast of China; an intermediate host of *Schistosoma japonicum*.

ka·thep′sin. See *cathepsin*.

kath″i·so·pho′bi·a [G. *kathisis*, a sitting; *phobos*, fear]. Morbid fear of sitting down.

kath′ode. See *cathode.*

kat′i″on. See *cation.*

Katzman and Doisy method. See under *method.*

kau′ri (kou′ree) [Maori]. The fossilized resinous exudate from the Kauri pine; used largely in the arts. A solution in alcohol has been used as a substitute for collodion in treating wounds.

ka′va (kah′vah, kav′uh), **ka″va-ka′va** [Maori *kawa*, bitter]. 1. An intoxicating beverage prepared in the Hawaiian Islands from the root of *Piper methysticum.* 2. The root of *Piper methysticum*, containing a resin, kawine, and other constituents. The resin is a motor depressant.

ka′wine (kah′ween, ·win) [*kawa*]. A resin occurring in kava.

kayquinone. Trade-mark for a brand of menadione.

Kayser, Bernhard [*German ophthalmologist*, 1869–]. Described a sign of hepatolenticular degeneration. See Kayser-Fleischer *ring.*

kcal. Kilo calorie: occasional usage.

Keefer, Chester Scott [*American physician*, 1897–]. Known for his work on chemotherapy, especially in connection with the production and distribution of penicillin and streptomycin during World War II.

Keegan, Denis Francis [*Irish surgeon*, 1840–1920]. Remembered for his operation, a rhinoplasty according to the Indian method, the flap being derived from the side of the forehead.

Keeler, Leonarde [*American psychologist and criminologist*, 1903–1949]. Invented the lie detector, called *Keeler's lie detector*, *Keeler's polygraph.*

Keeley, Leslie E. [*American physician*, 1832–1900]. Introduced a method for treating alcoholics by means of a secret remedy said to contain strychnine and gold chloride. Called *Keeley* or *gold cure.*

Keen, William Williams [*American surgeon*, 1837–1932]. Contributed to the development of neurosurgery. With Silas Weir Mitchell and George Read Morehouse, made an important study of injuries of the peripheral nerves. Removed a meningioma (1888), and successfully tapped the ventricles of the brain (1889). Devised an operation of linear craniotomy, called *Keen's operation.* Called attention to the surgical complications of typhoid fever (1898).

keep′er [AS. *cēpan*]. The armature of a horseshoe magnet.

kef′ir. A beverage prepared, especially in certain European countries, from the milk of cows, sheep, or goats through fermentation by kefir grains, these containing unidentified species of yeast or bacterial organisms.

Kehr, Hans [*German surgeon*, 1862–1916]. Introduced an operation for the establishment of a direct connection between the smaller hepatic ducts and the alimentary tract. A segment of liver is resected so that several moderate-sized bile ducts are opened; this area is then sutured, preferably to the duodenum. Called *Kehr's operation.* See also Kehr's *sign.*

Kehrer, Ferdinand Adalbert (1883–). German neurologist who discovered the pain reflex in increased intracranial pressure called *auriculopalpebral reflex*, and first described pupillotonic pseudotabes, called *Adie's syndrome* or *pupil.*

Kehrer, Ferdinand Adolph [*German gynecologist and obstetrician*, 1837–1914]. Improved the classic technic of Cesarean section by opening the uterus at the level of the internal os by a transverse incision; called *Kehrer's operation.* Introduced an operation for depressed nipple in which a crescent of skin is excised on either side of the nipple to permit cicatricial contraction.

Keith, Sir Arthur (1866–1955). Scottish anthropologist and anatomist who, with Flack, discovered the sinoatrial node, called *node of Keith and Flack.*

Keith, Norman Macdonnell [*American physician*, 1885–]. With Rowntree and Geraghty, introduced a method of estimating the blood and plasma volume (1915); the method includes the intravenous injection of a dye.

kelene. A trade-mark for a brand of ethyl chloride.

ke′lis. 1. Localized scleroderma. 2. See *keloid.*

Keller's micromethod. See under *micromethod.*

Keller-Blake splint. See under *splint.*

Kelley, William Joseph [*American pediatrician*, 1908–]. Described a sign of pleural effusion in children, which consists of a preference for lying upon the back or propped up high in bed and avoidance of bending toward, or pressing upon, the affected side.

kel′lin. Khellin.

Kelling's test. See under *test.*

Kelly, Howard Atwood [*American surgeon*, 1858–1943]. Pioneer in the surgical treatment of uterine displacement. Catheterized the ureters in the male (1898). Devised an operation for ureteroureteral anastomosis in which a catheter served temporarily as a splint. Designed rectal and vesical specula, called *Kelly's specula*, and a special artery forceps, called *Kelly's forceps.* Introduced wax-tipped bougies for locating stones in the urinary tract (1901).

ke′loid [G. *kēlis*, spot; *eidos*, form]. A fibrous hyperplasia usually at the site of a scar, elevated, rounded, white, sometimes pink, firm and with ill-defined borders. There is predilection for the upper trunk and face, and the condition is observed especially in young adults, females, and Negroes. Composed of parallel bundles of hyalinized connective tissue covered by thin epidermis with atrophic interpapillary epithelium.

kelp [ME. *culp*]. 1. A common name for a group of large brown algae growing in the cool ocean waters. 2. Burnt seaweed from which potassium salts and iodine formerly were prepared.

Kelso, Richard Edward [*American pathologist*, 1910–]. Introduced a test for pregnancy. The *Kelso test* is a modification of the Aschheim-Zondek test.

kel′vin [after William Thomson, Lord *Kelvin*, British physicist, 1824–1907]. A commercial unit of electricity; 1000 watt-hours.

Kel′vin scale. An absolute scale of temperature which has its zero at $-273°$ C.

kemithal. Trade-mark (British) for 5-allyl-5(Δ^2-cyclohexenyl)-2-thiobarbituric acid, the sodium salt of which is used intravenously as an anesthetic.

Kendall, Edward Calvin [*American physiologist and chemist*, 1886–]. Isolated thyroxin (1914) and adrenal cortical hormones (1936); prepared Compound A by partial synthesis (1944); collaborated in the preparation of cortisone (Compound E) (1948). With Hench, Slocumb, and Polley first showed the influence of cortisone in rheumatic and related diseases (1948). Nobel laureate with Philip S. Hench and Tadeus Reichstein (1950).

ke″nes·the′si·a. See *cenesthesia.*

Kennedy, Foster [*American neurologist*, 1884–]. Described a syndrome of unilateral optic atrophy and contralateral choking of the optic nerve with anosmia. *Kennedy's syndrome* is due usually to a tumor underlying the frontal lobe of the cerebrum.

Kennedy's method. See Elvehjem and Kennedy's *method.*

Kenny, Elizabeth [*Australian nurse in the United States*, 1886–1952]. Introduced the *Kenny treatment* for anterior poliomyelitis. In the acute stage the affected muscles are treated with hot, moist packs. Passive exercise is started very early, and is followed as soon as possible by active exercise.

ken′o-, ken- [G. *kenos*, empty]. A combining form meaning *empty*.

ken″o·pho′bi·a [*kenos;* G. *phobos*, fear]. A morbid fear of large, empty spaces.

ken″o·tox′in [*kenos;* G. *toxikon*, poison]. A hypothetical poisonous substance developed in the tissues during their activity which has been said to be responsible for their fatigue and for sleep.

Kent, bundle of. See under *bundle.*

Kent mental test. See under *test.*

keph′a·lin [G. *kephalē*, head]. Cephalin.

keph′ir, keph′yr. See *kefir.*

kephrine hydrochloride. Trade-mark for methylamino-aceto-catechol hydrochloride. The substance is a white powder used as a local hemostat.

ker″a·phyl′lo·cele [G. *keras*, horn; *phyllon*, leaf; *kēlē*, tumor]. A horny tumor on the inner side of the wall of a horse's hoof.

ker″a·phyl′lous, ke·raph′yl·lous [*keras; phyllon*]. *In veterinary medicine*, composed of horny layers.

ker′a·sin. A cerebroside separated from the brain; contains sphingosine, galactose, and fatty acid.

ker″a·tal′gi·a [*keras;* G. *algos*, pain]. Pain in the cornea.

ker″a·tec·ta′si·a (kerr″uh·teck·tay′zhuh) [*keras;* G. *ektasis*, extension]. A protrusion of the cornea.

ker″a·tec′to·my [*keras;* G. *ektomē*, excision]. Surgical excision of a part of the cornea.

ke·rat′ic [*keras*]. Horny.

ker′a·tin [*keras*]. Any of a group of albuminoids or scleroproteins characteristic of horny tissues, hair, nails, feathers, etc., insoluble in protein solvents, and having a high content of sulfur. Two main groups are distinguished: eukeratins, which are not digested by common proteolytic enzymes, and pseudokeratins, which are partly digested. Both contain varied amino acids; cystine and arginine generally predominate.

ker″a·tin·i·za′tion [*keras*]. 1. Development of a horny quality in a tissue. 2. Process whereby keratin is formed. 3. Coating of pills with keratin.

ke·rat′i·nous [*keras*]. 1. Relating to keratin. 2. Horny.

kér′a·tite en ban″de·lette′. See band-shaped *keratitis.*

ker″a·ti′tis [*keras;* G. *-itis*, inflammation]. Inflammation of the cornea.

annular k. An inflammation around the periphery of the cornea. Also called *marginal k.*

band-shaped k. An inflammation occurring in the form of an opaque transverse band across the cornea opposite the palpebral fissure; sometimes seen in patients with rheumatoid arthritis, it may result from prolonged uveitis. Syn. *kératite en bandelette.*

dendritic k. A superficial form attributed to the virus of herpes simplex; characterized by a line of infiltration of the corneal tissue near the surface, developing later into an arborescent ulcer. Also called *furrow k., herpetic k., k. arborescens, mycotic k.*

exposure k. Inflammation of the cornea due to trauma from excessive drying or from foreign particles.

fascicular k. A form of phlyctenular keratitis marked by the formation of a fascicle of blood vessels.

gonococcic k. That caused by the gonococcus.

interstitial k. A form of keratitis in which the entire cornea is invested with a diffuse haziness, almost completely hiding the iris. The surface of the cornea has a ground-glass appearance. Later, blood vessels form in the superficial layers of the cornea from ciliary injection, and produce a dull-red color or the so-called salmon patch. Seen most frequently in children between 5 and 15, resulting from congenital syphilis. Syn., *syphilitic k.*

k. bullosa. The formation of large or small blebs upon the cornea in cases of iridocyclitis, glaucoma, interstitial keratitis, or senile guttate keratitis.

k. disciformis. A localized subacute nonsuppurative inflammation of the parenchyma characterized by a discoid opacity, due to infection by an agent of low virulence and usually following trauma or a virus infection.

k. hypopyon. That accompanied by the formation of pus. Also called *serpiginous k.*

k. neuroparalytica. Keratitis following lesion of the ophthalmic nerve, caused by mechanical irritation and drying of the cornea. Syn., *trophic k.*

k. parenchymatosa anaphylactica. An interstitial keratitis on an allergic basis.

k. punctata. The presence of white blood cells on the back of Descemet's membrane. Not a primary inflammation of Descemet's membrane, since the cells derive from the ciliary body as a result of its inflammation. Includes two varieties, **keratitis punctata leprosa** (that caused by leprosy), and **keratitis punctata profunda** (that of syphilitic origin). Syn., *descemetitis.*

k. purulenta. Old term for keratitis hypopyon.

k. pustuliformis profunda. That accompanied by the formation of deep pustules; due to acquired syphilis. Syn., *k. punctata profunda.*

k. rosacea. The occurrence of small, sterile infiltrates at the periphery of the cornea, which are approached but not invaded by small blood vessels. They are most frequently seen unaccompanied by acne rosacea, but are most severe in this connection.

lagophthalmic k. That due to the failure of the eyelids to close completely; a form of exposure keratitis.

lattice k. See familial corneal *dystrophy.*

oyster-shucker's k. A form due to corneal traumatism from pieces of embedded oyster shell.

parenchymatous k. Interstitial *k.*

phlyctenular k. See phlyctenular *conjunctivitis.*

reaper's k. That due to irritation from grain awns.

sclerosing k. An interstitial form associated with scleritis.

scrofulous k. See phlyctenular *k.*

superficial k. That affecting primarily the epithelium, Bowman's membrane, and superficial lamellae of the substantia propria.

syphilitic k. See interstitial *k.*

trachomatous k. See *pannus.*

traumatic k. That consequent upon wounds or injury of the cornea.

trophic k. See *k.* neuroparalytica.

tuberculous k. That associated with tuberculous infection.

xerotic k. See *keratomalacia.*

ker′a·to-, kerat- [*keras*]. 1. A combining form meaning *horn* or denoting *horny tissue.* 2. *In anatomy, medicine,* and *surgery,* a combining form denoting *the cornea.*

ker″a·to·ac″an·tho′ma. Usually a single epidermal nodule of 2 cm or less in diameter, located on exposed skin, characterized by acanthosis and increased keratin formation. It occurs in the upper age groups and in oil and tar workers. Syn., *molluscum sebaceum.*

ker″a·to·an″gi·o′ma (kerr″uh·to·an″jee·o′muh). See *angiokeratoma.*

ker′a·to·cele [*keras;* G. *kēlē*, hernia]. A hernia of Descemet's membrane through the cornea; descemetocele.

ker″a·to·cen·te′sis [*keras;* G. *kentēsis,* a pricking]. Corneal puncture.

ker″a·to·chro″ma·to′sis [*keras;* G. *chrōma,* color; *-ōsis,* increase]. Discoloration of the cornea.

ker″a·to·con·junc″ti·vi′tis [*keras;* LL. *conjunctivus,* connective; G. *-itis,* inflammation]. Simultaneous inflammation of the cornea and the conjunctiva.

epidemic k. A virus infection, usually affecting adults; is epidemic and self-limited.

k. sicca. That due to dryness or excess secretion of a tenacious mucoid discharge.

phlyctenular k. See phlyctenular *keratitis.*

ker″a·to·co′nus [*keras;* G. *kōnos,* cone]. A conic protrusion of the cornea.

ker″a·to·der′ma [*keras;* G. *derma,* skin]. A horny condition of the skin, especially of the palms and soles.

k. blennorrhagicum. See *keratosis* blennorrhagica.

k. climactericum. A circumscribed hyperkeratosis of the palms and soles occurring in women during the menopause, and accompanied chiefly by obesity and hypertension: also called *Haxthausen's disease.*

k. punctatum. See *keratosis* punctata.

ker″a·to·der·mat′o·cele. See *keratocele.*

ker″a·to·der′mi·a. See *keratoderma.*

ker″a·to·gen′e·sis [*keras;* G. *genesis,* production]. Development of horny growths.

ker″a·to·glo′bus [*keras;* L. *globus,* ball]. A globular protrusion of the cornea.

ker″a·to·hel·co′sis [*keras;* G. *helkōsis,* ulcerations]. Ulceration of the cornea.

ker″a·to·hy′a·lin (kerr″uh·to·high′uh·lin) [*keras;* G. *hyalos,* glass]. The substance of the granules in the stratum granulosum of keratinized stratified squamous epithelium; an early phase in the formation of keratin. **—keratohy′aline,** *adj.*

ker′a·toid [*keras;* G. *eidos,* form]. Hornlike.

ker″a·to·ir′i·do·scope (·irr′i·do·scope, ·eye′ri·do·, ·i·rid′o·) [*keras;* G. *iris,* iris; *skopein,* to examine]. An apparatus for examining the cornea and iris.

ker″a·to·i·ri′tis (kerr″uh·to·eye·rye′tis, ·i·rye′tis) [*keras; iris;* G. *-itis,* inflammation]. Combined inflammation of the cornea and the iris.

ker″a·to·leu·ko′ma (kerr″uh·to·lew·ko′muh) [*keras;* G. *leukōma,* white spot]. A leukoma or whitish opacity of the cornea.

ker″a·tol′y·sis [*keras;* G. *lysis,* a loosing]. 1. Exfoliation of the epidermis. 2. A congenital anomaly in which the skin is shed periodically. **—keratolyt′ic,** *adj.*

k. neonatorum. See *dermatitis exfoliativa neonatorum.*

ker″a·to·lyt′ic [*keras; lysis*]. An agent which causes exfoliation of the epidermis to a greater degree than that which occurs normally.

ker″a·to′ma. See *callositas.*

k. sulcatum plantarum. A pitted thickening of the soles seen in barefooted native adults in the tropics. Causative factors are obscure.

ker″a·to·ma·la′ci·a (kerr″uh·to·ma·lay′shee·uh, ·see·uh) [*keras;* G. *malakia,* softness]. A softening of the cornea. Syn., *xerotic keratitis.*

ker′a·tome [*keras;* G. *tomos,* cutting]. A knife with a trowel-like blade, for incising the cornea in the operation of iridectomy.

ker″a·tom′e·ter [*keras;* G. *metron,* a measure]. An instrument for measuring the curves of the cornea. **—keratometry,** *n.*

ker″a·to·my·co′sis (kerr″uh·to·migh·ko′sis) [*keras;* G. *mykēs,* fungus; *-ōsis,* condition]. 1. A fungoid growth in or on the cornea. 2. Tinea nigra: occasional usage. Syn., *k. nigricans palmaris.*

ker″a·to·nyx′is [*keras;* G. *nyxis,* a pricking]. Puncture of the cornea; especially, the needling of a soft cataract by puncture of the cornea.

ker′a·to·plas″ty [*keras;* G. *plassein,* to form]. Plastic operation upon the cornea, especially the transplantation of a portion of cornea. **—keratoplas′tic,** *adj.*

lamellar k. That in which the more superficial lamellae are replaced.

penetrating k. That in which the entire thickness of a portion of the cornea is replaced.

tectonic k. Corneal transplantation for repairing a fistulating or ectatic corneal cicatrix, with or without incarceration of the iris.

ker″a·tor·rhex′is [*keras;* G. *rhēxis,* a breaking]. Rupture of the cornea, due to ulceration or traumatism.

ker″a·to·scle·ri′tis [*keras;* G. *sklēros,* hard; *-itis,* inflammation]. Inflammation of the cornea and the sclera.

ker′a·to·scope [*keras;* G. *skopein,* to examine]. An instrument for examining the cornea and testing the symmetry of its meridians of curvature. Also called *Plácido's disk.*

ker″a·tos′co·py [*keras; skopein*]. Examination of the cornea with the keratoscope.

ker′a·tose [*keras*]. Horny.

ker″a·to′sis [*keras;* G. *-ōsis,* increase]. Any disease of the skin characterized by an overgrowth of the cornified epithelium.

arsenical k. A patchy keratosis occurring after long-continued ingestion of arsenic.

gonorrheal k. See *k.* blennorrhagica.

k. blennorrhagica. A disease characterized by horny growths, chiefly of the hands and feet, and occurring during the course of an attack of gonorrhea. Syn., *keratoderma blenorrhagica, gonorrheal k.*

k. follicularis. A disease characterized by horny, prominent projections occurring about the hair follicles; they are firmly adherent and produce a roughness. Also called *Darier's disease, psorospermosis.*

k. nigricans. See *acanthosis* nigricans.

k. palmaris et plantaris. A marked, congenital thickening of the volar surfaces of the hands and feet. This condition may be complicated with painful fissures. Sometimes called *congenital palmoplantar k.*

k. pharyngeus. A rare affection in which there is a hornlike outgrowth (composed of horny desquamated epithelium) from the crypts of the tonsils.

k. pilaris. A chronic affection of the skin marked by hard, conical elevations in the pilosebaceous orifices on the arms and thighs.

k. punctata. Keratosis of the palms and soles, characterized by numerous minute, crateriform pits set in patches of thickening of the stratum corneum. Syn., *keratoderma punctatum.*

k. seborrheica. Nummular and flat lesions covered with greasy scales; occurs in older people. The lesions are superficial and seldom become malignant.

k. senilis. A patchy keratosis of the skin of old people; found chiefly on the face and dorsal surfaces of the hands and feet, or those surfaces exposed to wind and sun. Some lesions may develop into epitheliomas.

k. universalis congenita. See *ichthyosis* congenita.

ker′a·to·tome″ (kerr′uh·to·tohm″, keh·rat′o·tohm). See *keratome.*

ker·a·tot′o·my [*keras;* G. *tomē,* a cutting]. Incision of the cornea.

delimiting k. Incision into the cornea at points outside the area of a serpiginous ulcer (Gifford's operation).

ke·rau″no·pho′bi·a [G. *keraunos*, thunderbolt; *phobos*, fear]. Morbid fear of lightning; a common symptom in psychoneurotic patients.

Kerckring, Theodor [*German physician and anatomist in Holland*, 1640–93]. Described the circular folds of the small intestine; called *Kerckring's folds* or *valves*. Described an independent ossification center in the occipital bone at the posterior margin of the foramen magnum; called *Kerckring's ossicle*.

ke·rec′to·my. See *keratectomy*.

ke′ri·on cel′si. A type of dermatophytosis of the scalp or beard, with deep, boggy infiltration. Also called *tinea kerion*.

ker′mes (kur′meez) [Ar. *qirmiz*]. The dried bodies of an insect found on *Quercus coccifera;* contains a purplish red coloring matter said to be the oldest dyestuff known; has been used in medicine.

ker·nic′ter·us (kair·nick′tair·ōōs, kur·nick′tuh-rus. *See* Notes § 35) [Ger., from *kern*, kernel; G. *ikteros*, jaundice]. Biliary pigmentation of gray matter of central nervous system, especially basal ganglions, accompanied by degeneration of nerve cells; occurring as a rare, usually fatal complication of icterus neonatorum commonly associated with erythroblastosis fetalis: also called *nuclear jaundice, nuclear icterus*.

Kernig's sign. See under *sign*.

Kernohan, James Watson (1897–   ). American pathologist who, with H. W. Woltman, described the crus syndrome.

ker′o·cele [G. *keras*, horn; *kēlē*, tumor]. *In veterinary medicine*, a horny tumor on the inner surface of the wall of a horse's hoof.

ker′o·sene″ oil. A liquid mixture of hydrocarbons distilled from petroleum: sometimes called *coal oil*.

Kerr's sign. See under *sign*.

ke′tene. $H_2C{:}CO$. A colorless gas of penetrating odor, forming acetic acid upon hydrolysis. It may be employed to effect acetylization of free amino and hydroxyl groups.

ke′to-, ket- [Ger. *keton*]. *In chemistry*, a combining form denoting *the presence of the ketone group*.

ke′to ac′id. Any compound containing both a ketone (—CO—) and a carboxyl (—COOH) group.

ke″to·a·dip′ic ac′id. $COOH.CO.CH_2.CH_2.CH_2.COOH$; α-ketoadipic acid; an intermediate compound in the biochemical conversion of lysine to glutaric acid.

ke″to·bem′i·done. $C_{15}H_{21}NO_2$; 4-(*m*-hydroxyphenyl)-1-methyl-4-piperidyl ethyl ketone; a narcotic related to morphine and causing true addiction: used experimentally as an analgesic.

ketochol. Trade-mark for a combination of the keto forms of the biliary acids in approximately the same proportions as found in normal human bile. The preparation is used in gallbladder disorders.

ke″to·cho·lan′ic ac′id (kee″to·ko·lan′ick). Cholic acid in which one or more of the secondary alcohol groups have been oxidized to ketone groups.

ke″to·gen′e·sis [*keton;* G. *genesis*, production]. The production of ketone, or acetone, bodies.

ke″to·glu·tar′ic ac′id (kee″to·glue·tarr′ick, ·tahr′-ick). $COOH(CH_2)_2CO.COOH$. A dibasic keto acid, an intermediate product in the metabolism of carbohydrates and proteins.

ke″to·hep′tose. A general term for monosaccharides consisting of a seven-carbon chain and containing a ketone group.

ke″to·hex′ose. A general term for monosaccharides consisting of a six-carbon chain and containing a ketone group.

ke″to·hy·drox″y·oes′trin (kee″to·high·drock″see-es′trin, ·ees′trin). See *estrone*.

ke′tol. Any compound containing both a ketone (—CO—) group and an alcohol (—OH) group.

ke′tole. Indole.

ke·tol′y·sis [*keton;* G. *lysis*, a loosing]. The dissolution of ketone bodies. —**ketolyt′ic,** *adj*.

ke′tone. An organic compound derived by oxidation from a secondary alcohol; it contains the characterizing group =CO.

ke″to·ne′mi·a [*keton;* G. *haima*, blood]. The presence of ketone bodies in the blood.

ke″to·nu′ri·a [*keton;* G. *ouron*, urine]. The presence of ketone bodies in the urine.

ke″to·pro″pi·on′ic ac′id. α-Ketopropionic acid; pyruvic acid.

ke″to·re·duc′tase (kee″to·ri·duck′tace, ·taze). An enzyme occurring in muscle, liver, and kidney, which converts diacetic acid into beta-oxybutyric acid.

ke′tose. A carbohydrate containing the ketone group =CO.

ke′to·side. Any glycoside that yields, on hydrolysis, a ketose.

ke·to′sis [*keton;* G. *-ōsis*, condition]. 1. A condition in which ketones are present in the body in excessive number. 2. The acidosis of diabetes.

k. threshold. The critical ratio at which ketone substances can be oxidized by the tissues as they are put forth by the liver. Ketosis occurs when the ketosis threshold has been passed and the liver is spilling out ketone substances faster than they can be oxidized by the tissues.

ke″to·ster′oid (kee″to·sterr′oyd, ·steer′oyd, ki-tos′ti·royd) [*keton;* G. *stereos*, solid; *eidos*, form]. One of a group of neutral steroids possessing ketone substitution, which produces a characteristic red color with *m*-dinitrobenzene in alkaline solution. The ketosteroids are principally metabolites of adrenal cortical and gonadal steroids; also called *17-ketosteroids*.

ke·tox′ime. An oxime resulting from action of hydroxylamine upon a ketone, having the general formula R(R′)C:NOH.

Key, Charles Aston [*English surgeon*, 1793–1849]. Ligated the external iliac artery for femoral aneurysm (1822), and the subclavian for axillary aneurysm in the following year.

Key, Ernst Axel Henrik [*Swedish physician and anatomist*, 1832–1901]. With M. G. Retzius, described the lateral apertures of the fourth ventricle; called *foramens of Key and Retzius, foramens of Luschka*. See under *aperture*. Key and Retzius described sensory nerve endings resembling Herbst's corpuscles, found in the skin of the beaks of certain birds; called *corpuscles of Key and Retzius*.

Keynes, Geoffrey Langdon [*English surgeon*, 1887–   ]. Contributed to the development of the treatment of mammary cancer by means of radium, also to the development of the use of blood transfusion and of thyroid surgery.

kg, kg. Kilogram.

khel′lin. $C_{14}H_{12}O_5$; 2-methyl-5,8-dimethoxyfuranochromone, reputed to be the therapeutically important constituent of the umbelliferous plant *Ammi visnaga*, the fruits of which have been used in Egypt as an antispasmodic in renal colic and ureteral spasm. A coronary vasodilator, it is claimed to be also a bronchodilator. Also called *kellin, chellin, visammin*.

khel′li·nin. $C_{19}H_{20}O_{10}$; 2-hydroxymethyl-5-methoxyfuranochrome glucoside; a minor constituent of *Ammi visnaga*. It has been claimed and denied to have coronary vasodilator action. Syn., *khellol-glucoside*.

khel′lol-glu′co·side. Khellinin.

kid′ney [ME. *kydney*]. One of the paired glandular organs situated retroperitoneally lateral to the spine, caudal to the spleen on the left and the liver on the right side. The kidney has a characteristic bean shape; convex laterally and concave on the medial border. The hilum at the medial border expands into a central cavity, the renal sinus, which contains the renal calyxes. The calyxes are cup-shaped tubes embracing the renal papillae and unite to form a funnel-shaped sac, the renal pelvis. In the adult each kidney weighs about 150 Gm. and measures about 11.5 × 6 × 3.5 cm. It is covered by a fairly dense fibrous capsule and embedded in perirenal fat. The kidney consists of a medulla and cortex. The medulla consists of eight to eighteen conical masses, the renal pyramids; the apexes of the pyramids converge toward the renal sinus and project into the lumens of the minor calyxes. The cortex lies immediately beneath the capsule, and dips in between adjacent pyramids; the parts between the pyramids are called renal columns of Bertin. The kidney helps to regulate the normal concentrations of blood constituents by the excretion of water and various substances usually considered as waste products; it probably also furnishes products which have to do with control of systemic blood pressure. The filtering, excreting, and reabsorbing functions of the kidney take place in the nephrons, each composed of a renal corpuscle and tubule. The renal corpuscle consists of a tuft of capillary loops, the glomerulus, and a glomerular (Bowman's) capsule. The latter consists of a simple squamous epithelium seated on a basement membrane. It has a visceral layer fitting closely over the loops of the glomerulus and a parietal layer which is continuous with the epithelium of the renal tubule. The part of the tubule near the glomerulus is the proximal convoluted tubule, continuous with the medullary loop or loop of Henle which consists of a descending and ascending limb, the latter communicating with the distal convoluted tubule and thence with the collecting tubule. The renal artery (or arteries) enters at the hilum and divides dichotomously to provide branches for the medulla, the so-called arcuate arteries at the junction of pyramid and medulla, and the interlobar arteries of the cortex; the veins are distributed in parallel. See Plates 7, 8, 9, 14, 45.

aglomerular k. (a) *In clinical medicine*, a kidney having a greatly diminished number of functioning glomeruli, found in chronic glomerulosclerosis and in other conditions in which scarring of the renal cortex is prominent. (b) A type found in some fishes in which glomeruli are entirely lacking: used in the study of renal physiology.

amyloid k. One which is the seat of amyloidosis.

cake k., caked k. Congenital fusion of both kidneys into a solid, irregularly lobate mass usually found over the sacrum. Syn., *clump k., lump k.*

cement k. A calcified kidney.

clump k. See cake *k.*

confluent k. Congenital fusion of two kidneys.

contracted k. The last stage of chronic glomerulonephritis, arteriolar nephrosclerosis, or chronic pyelonephritis.

cyanotic k. A chronically congested kidney, with resultant dilated veins, pigmentation, and some fibrosis.

cystic k. A kidney containing one to several cysts, usually unilateral.

definitive k. The metanephros.

disk, disc k. A congenital defect in which both kidneys are fused into one mass, usually on one side of the midline; one kidney is superimposed upon the other.

double k. A developmental condition in which one of the kidneys is subdivided into two.

ectopic k. A common congenital anomaly in which the kidney is held in abnormal position on its own or on the opposite side, where fusion with the other kidney may occur.

embryonic k. The mesonephros.

end-stage k. A chronic stage of renal disorder, with accompanying extensive scarring of the renal tissue.

fatty k. Fatty degeneration of the renal epithelium.

floating k. One which is displaced from its bed, becoming more freely movable, sometimes causing symptoms, as by kinking the ureter: also called *wandering k., ren mobilis.*

fused k. See horseshoe *k.*, sigmoid *k.*

head k. The pronephros.

horseshoe k. Greater or lesser degree of congenital fusion of the two kidneys, usually at lower poles.

intrathoracic k. One situated within the thoracic cavity as in some cases of diaphragmatic hernia.

k. stone. A concretion of the kidney. Syn., *renal calculus.*

large white k. Enlargement and pallor of kidney such as may be due to amyloidosis, marked nephrosis, chronic lipoid nephrosis, or chronic parenchymatous nephritis.

L-shaped k. See sigmoid *k.*

lump k. See cake *k.*

middle k. The mesonephros or Wolffian body.

monopyramidal k. See unilobar *k.*

movable k. See floating *k.*

multilobar k. One with more than one renal pyramid. Syn., *polypyramidal k.*

pelvic k. One abnormally located in the pelvis.

pigback k. The kidney of marked chronic passive hyperemia, with a longitudinal ridge over the vertex.

polycystic k. One containing a large number of cysts, usually of the congenital variety and most frequently bilateral.

polypyramidal k. See multilobar *k.*

primitive k. The pronephros.

sacculated k. Advance stage of hydronephrosis.

sigmoid k. A congenital anomaly resulting from the fusion of the lower pole of one kidney to the upper pole of the other: also called *L-shaped k., unilateral fused k.*

small white k. One of the forms of chronic glomerulonephritis.

surgical k. Suppurative inflammation or tuberculosis of kidney.

triple k. A developmental condition in which one of the kidneys is subdivided into three.

unilateral fused k. See sigmoid *k.*

unilobar k. One consisting of a single lobe, as in rats, dogs, and many other animals but not in man. Syn., *monopyramidal k.*

wandering k. See floating *k.*

waxy k. A kidney which is the seat of amyloidosis.

Kielland, Christian Caspar Gabriel [*Norwegian obstetrician*, 1871–1941]. Invented obstetric forceps with blades articulated to allow them to move over each other. The cephalic curves of the blades are like those of other obstetric forceps, but the pelvic curves are very slight. Called *Kielland's forceps.*

Kienböck, Robert (1871–). Austrian radiologist who described acute atrophy of bone, occurring with different conditions of the extremities, called *Kienböck's atrophy;* he also described aseptic necrosis of the lunate bone, called *Kienböck's disease.* **Kienböck's photometric unit** of x-ray dosage equals one-tenth of the erythema dose.

Kiernan, Francis (1800–1874). Irish surgeon and anatomist in England who described the portal canals in the liver, called *Kiernan's spaces.*

kie′sel·guhr″ (kee′zul·goor″). See purified siliceous *earth.*

Kiesselbach, Wilhelm [*German laryngologist,* 1839–1902]. Remembered for his description of a thin area of the nasal septum, frequently the site of epistaxis and likely to be the seat of perforation, called *Kiesselbach's area* or *triangle;* also called *Little's area.*

Kilian, Hermann Friedrich [*German gynecologist and obstetrician,* 1800–63]. Described pelvis spinosa and spondylolisthetic pelvis; each is known as *Kilian's pelvis.* The transverse line formed by the promontory of the sacrum is called *Kilian's line.*

Kiliani, Heinrich [*German chemist,* 1855–1945]. Made an important study of digitalis. Described the synthesis of a higher homolog of a compound, brought about by the formation of a nitrile, followed by hydrolysis; called *Kiliani's reaction.*

Killian, Gustav [*German laryngologist and rhinologist,* 1860–1921]. Introduced direct bronchoscopy (1898) and suspension laryngoscopy (1912). Devised an operation in which he excised the anterior wall of the frontal sinus and formed a permanent opening into the nose (1903); called *Killian's operation.*

kil′o- [G. *chilioi,* thousand]. A prefix meaning *thousand.*

kil′o·cal″o·rie, kil′o·cal″o·ry [*chilioi;* L. *calor,* heat]. A large calorie; the amount of heat required to raise 1 kg of water from 15° to 16° C.; used in the study of metabolism.

kil′o·gram [*chilioi;* G. *gramma,* a small weight]. One thousand grams, or about 2.2 pounds avoirdupois. Abbreviated, kg, kg.

kil′o·gram-me′ter, kil′o·gram-me′tre [*chilioi; gramma;* G. *metron,* a measure]. A unit of energy; the amount of energy required to raise one kilogram one meter; approximately 7.233 foot-pounds.

kil′o·joule″ (kill′o·jōōl″) [*chilioi;* after James P. *Joule,* English physicist]. A unit of heat, equivalent to 239.1 small calories.

kil′o·li″ter, kil′o·li″tre (kill′o·lee″tur) [*chilioi;* G. *litra,* a silver coin, pound]. One thousand liters, or 35.31 cubic feet. Abbreviated, kl, kl.

kil′o·me″ter, kil′o·me″tre (kill′o·mee″tur, ki-lom′i·tur) [*chilioi;* G. *metron,* a measure]. One thousand meters, or 1093.6 yards. Abbreviated, km, km.

kil′o·nem [*chilioi;* G. *nemein,* to feed on]. A unit of nutriment, equivalent to 667 calories.

kil′o·volt. Unit of electric power equal to 1000 volts. Abbreviated, kv, kv.

kil′o·watt″ (kill′o·wot″) [*chilioi;* after James *Watt,* Scottish mechanical engineer]. A unit of electric power; one thousand watts. Abbreviated, kw, kw.

kil′o·watt″ hour. A unit of energy equivalent to the energy supplied by a power of 1000 watts operating for 1 hour.

kil′u·rane [*chilioi;* G. *ouranos,* heaven]. A unit of radioactivity; one thousand uranium units.

Kimmelstiel-Wilson syndrome. See *intercapillary glomerulosclerosis.*

ki′nase (kigh′nace, kin′ace, kin′aze). A substance which acts on a zymogen to form an enzyme. See *activator.*

kin″e·ma·di·ag′ra·phy (kin″i·muh·dye·ag′ruh·fee) [G. *kinēma,* movement; *dia,* through; *graphein,* to write]. Cineroentgenography.

kin″e·mat′ics [*kinēma*]. The science of motion.

kin″e·mat′o·graph [*kinēma;* G. *graphein,* to write]. A device for making and demonstrating a continuous record of a moving body.

kin′e·plas″ty [G. *kinein,* to move; *plassein,* to form]. A method of amputation designed to provide direct transmission of voluntary motion from muscles in the stump to the artificial part. Now rarely used.

kin″e·ra″di·o·ther′a·py [*kinein;* L. *radius,* ray; G. *therapeia,* treatment]. X-ray therapy whereby the tube is moved in relation to the patient, or the patient in relation to the stationary tube. The object is the attainment of larger depth doses without overloading the skin.

kin′e·scope [*kinein;* G. *skopein,* to examine]. An instrument for testing the refraction of the eye; consists of a moving disk with a slit of variable width, through which the patient observes a fixed object.

ki·ne′si- (ki·nee′see-, kigh·nee′see-) [G. *kinēsis,* motion]. A combining form meaning *movement, motion.*

ki·ne′si·a (ki·nee′shuh, ·see·uh, ·zhuh, ·zee·uh, kigh·nee′·) [*kinēsis*]. 1. Any form of motion sickness, such as seasickness. 2. A suffix implying motion or movement, as hyperkinesia.

ki·ne″si·at′rics [*kinēsis;* G. *iatrikos,* skilled in the medical art]. The treatment of disease by systematic active or passive movements. Syn., *kinesitherapy, kinetotherapy.*

ki·ne′sic. See *kinetic.*

ki·ne″si·es·the″si·om′e·ter [*kinēsis;* G. *aisthēsis,* perception; *metron,* a measure]. An instrument for testing the muscular sense.

kin″e·sim′e·ter, ki·ne″si·om′e·ter [*kinēsis; metron*]. An instrument for determining quantitatively the motion of a part.

ki·ne″si·ol′o·gy [*kinēsis;* G. *logos,* word]. The science of the anatomy, physiology, and mechanics of purposeful muscle movement in man.

ki·ne″si·om′e·ter. See *kinesimeter.*

ki·ne′sis (ki·nee′sis, kigh·nee′sis) [G.]. The general term for transformation of physical forms of energy.

ki·ne′sis par′a·dox′a. The sudden and violent overexertion in walking and running observed in patients with paralysis agitans who, because of generalized muscular rigidity, are ordinarily inactive or sluggish. Also called *Souques' sign.*

ki·ne″si·ther′a·py. See *kinesiatrics.*

ki·ne″so·pho′bi·a [*kinēsis;* G. *phobos,* fear]. Morbid fear of motion.

kin″es·the′si·a (kin″ess·thee′zhuh, ·zee·uh), **kin″es·the′sis** [*kinēsis;* G. *aisthēsis,* sensation]. The muscle sense; the sense of perception of movement, weight, resistance, and position. Syn., *kinesthetic memory.* —**kinesthet′ic,** *adj.*

kin″es·the″si·om′e·ter [*kinēsis; aisthēsis;* G. *metron,* a measure]. Instrument for measuring the degree of muscle sense.

ki·net′ic (ki·net′ick, kigh·net′ick), **ki·ne′sic** [G. *kinētikos,* of motion]. Pertaining to motion; producing motion.

ki·net′ics [*kinētikos*]. The science of force as producing motion.

ki·ne′tism. The ability to initiate or perform independent movement.

ki·ne′to·chore (ki·nee′to·kor, ki·net′o·, kigh·) [G. *kinētos,* moving; *chōra,* space]. The constriction in the chromosome where the spindle fiber is attached.

ki·ne′to·plast. The blepharoplast and parabasal body in hemoflagellates.

ki·ne″to·ther′a·py (ki·nee″to·therr′uh·pee, ki-net″o·, kigh·). See *kinesiatrics.*

Kingsbury, Francis Bullard [*American biochem-*

ist, 1886–]. With C. P. Clark, devised permanent albumin standards used in the life-insurance method of determining protein in urine. The *Kingsbury-Clark albumin standards* consist of tubes of gelatin containing a small amount of formaldehyde, and graduated quantities of formazin in suspension. See also Kingsbury's *test.*

king's e'vil. Scrofula. So called because of a belief that it could be cured by the touch of the king. Obsolete term since the time of the Stuart monarchs.

Kingsley, Norman William [*American dentist,* 1829–1913]. Sometimes called the founder of modern orthodontics. Devised a splint for fractures of the maxilla. *Kingsley's splint* consists of a curved metal bar passing around the face with its lower edge at the level of the mandible, and a headpiece fixed in a plaster cast. A rubber band suspended from the headpiece may be stretched around the curved bar to exert downward traction.

King's operation. Arytenoidopexy.

King's stain. See *carbol-thionine* (*King*) under *stain.*

king's yel'low. See *arsenic* trisulfide.

kink. See *angulation.*

Kinnersley, Henry Wulf [*English biochemist,* 1877–1944]. With C. W. Carter and R. A. Peters, discovered vitamin B_5 (1930). With Peters, devised a thiamine test in which diazo-benzene-sulfuric acid in carbonate containing sodium hydroxide solution gives a red color with thiamine and formaldehyde; called *Peters-Kinnersley test.*

Kinney's law. See under *law.*

Kinnier Wilson. See S. A. K. *Wilson.*

ki'no (kee'no, kigh'no) [Mandingo *keno*] (*kino*). The dried juice obtained from the trunk of *Pterocarpus marsupium.* Powerful astringent; used chiefly in the treatment of diarrhea. Dose, 0.5–2.0 Gm. (8–30 gr.).

k. tincture (*tinctura kino*). Glycerin and 20% kino in alcohol. Dose, 2–4 cc. (30–60 min.).

ki"no·cen'trum (kigh"no·sen'trum, kin"o·) [G. *kinein,* to move; *kentron,* center]. The centrosome.

kin'o·plasm (kin'o·plaz·um, kigh'no·). See *archoplasm.*

ki"no·tan'nic ac'id (kee"no·tan'ick). The tannic acid found in kino.

ki·no'vin, kin'o·vin. Quinovin.

Kinyoun stain. See Ponder-Kinyoun *stain.*

ki'o·tome [G. *kiōn,* uvula; *tomos,* cutting]. An instrument for amputating the uvula.

ki·ot'o·my (kigh·ot'o·mee) [*kiōn;* G. *tomē,* a cutting]. Surgical removal of the uvula.

Kircher, Athanasius [*German scholar,* 1602–80]. Pioneer microscopist. Described microscopic "worms" in putrescent material and in blood taken from cases of plague (1658).

Kirchner, Wilhelm [*German otologist,* 1849–1935]. Described a diverticulum of the auditory tube; called *Kirchner's diverticulum.*

Kirkes, William Senhouse [*English physician,* 1823–64]. Gave a classic description of embolism due to intracardiac blood clots (1852).

Kirmisson, Edouard [*French surgeon,* 1848–1927]. Introduced an operation involving transplantation of the Achilles tendon, for talipes varus; called *Kirmisson's operation.*

Kirschner, Martin [*German surgeon,* 1879–1942]. Said to have been the first to operate successfully for the relief of pulmonary embolism (1942). Introduced a method of treating fractures by means of wires, called *Kirschner's wires,* passed through drill holes in the bone; called *Kirschner's traction.*

Kisch's reflex. See auriculopalpebral *reflex.*

Kitasato, Shibasáburo [*Japanese bacteriologist,* 1852–1931]. With von Behring, produced antitoxins for tetanus and diphtheria (1890). This discovery of passive immunization was the starting point of modern serotherapy. Independently of Yersin, he discovered the plague bacillus (1894), now called *Pasteurella pestis,* and also *Kitasato's bacillus.*

ki'tol [G. *kētos,* whale]. A precursor of vitamin A in whale-liver oil, which yields vitamin A on heating under low pressures.

Kjeldahl method. See under *method.*

Kjelland. See *Kielland.*

kl, kl. Kiloliter.

Klebs, Theodor Albrecht Edwin [*German bacteriologist,* 1834–1913]. Described glomerulonephritis (1870), called *Klebs's disease.* Made an experimental study in which syphilis was transmitted to apes. Discovered the diphtheria bacillus, called *Klebs-Loeffler bacillus,* now called *Corynebacterium diphtheriae.*

Kleb·si·el'la [after *Klebs*]. A genus of bacteria of the family Enterobacteriaceae; frequently associated with infections of the respiratory tract and pathologic conditions of other parts of the body.

K. granulomatis. See *Donovania granulomatis.*

K. pneumoniae. A species of short, plump, heavily capsulated, nonmotile, and Gram-negative bacteria, responsible for severe pneumonitis in man: formerly called *Bacillus mucosus capsulatum, Friedländer's bacillus, pneumobacillus.*

K. rhinoscleromatis. Encapsulated Gram-negative rod recovered from nasal granulomas of patients with rhinoscleroma: formerly called *Frisch's bacillus.*

klein"re'gel (kline"ray'gl) [Ger. *klein,* small; *Regel,* menstruation]. Scant uterine bleeding at the mid-interval of the menstrual cycle. It may be associated with midpains or mittelschmerz.

Kleitman, Nathaniel (1895–). American physiologist who has contributed to the knowledge of the physiology of sleep; exponent of the evolutionary theory that primitive alternation of sleep and wakefulness is subcortical, whereas diurnal sleep-wakefulness rhythm is cortical in origin.

Klemperer's tuberculin. See *P. T. O.*

klep"to·lag'ni·a [G. *kleptein,* to steal; *lagneia,* coition]. Sexual gratification induced by theft.

klep"to·ma'ni·a [*kleptein;* G. *mania,* madness]. A morbid desire to steal; obsessive stealing; a mental disorder in which the objects stolen are usually of symbolic value only, being petty and useless items.

klep"to·pho'bi·a [*kleptein;* G. *phobos,* fear]. 1. A morbid dread of thieves. 2. A morbid dread of becoming a kleptomaniac, observed in psychasthenia.

klim. Trade-mark for a powdered, dry, whole milk.

Kline test. A microscopic flocculation test for syphilis.

kli'no-. For words beginning with *klino-,* see words beginning *clino-.*

Klippel, Maurice [*French neurologist,* 1858–1942]. First to describe arthritic general pseudoparalysis (1892), called *Klippel's disease.* With Feil, described congenital fusion of the cervical vertebrae (1912). See Klippel-Feil *syndrome.*

klis"e·om'e·ter. See *cliseometer.*

klop"e·ma'ni·a. Old term for kleptomania.

klotogen. Trade-mark for a solution in oil of a vitamin-K concentrate.

Kluge, Karl Alexander Ferdinand [*German obstetrician,* 1782–1844]. Introduced his method for induction of premature labor by dilatation of the cervix with sponges. Described bluish discoloration of the vaginal mucosa as indicative of pregnancy; called *Kluge's sign, Jacquemier's sign, Chadwick's sign.*

Klumpke. See *Dejerine-Klumpke.*

km, km. Kilometer.

Knapp, Arnold Herman [*American ophthalmic surgeon,* 1869–]. Devised an operation for cataract in which a wide iridectomy is made and, after subluxation with special forceps, the lens is removed in the capsule by external pressure on the cornea.

Knapp, Herman Jakob [*American ophthalmologist,* 1832–1911]. Made important studies of the curvature of the cornea and of intraocular tumors.

knead′ing. Pétrissage.

knee [AS. *cnēo*]. The articulation between the femur and the tibia. Also see *genu.* See Table of Joints and Ligaments in the Appendix. See Plate 2.

snapping k. A condition in which the tibia on sudden extension of the knee rotates outward or glides forward on the femur with an audible snapping sound, occasionally caused by slipping of the biceps tendon or by displacement of one of the menisci.

knee′cap″ [*cnēo;* AS. *caeppe*]. The patella.

knee′-jerk″. See patellar *reflex.*

knee′-sprung″. *In veterinary medicine,* an alteration in the direction and articulation of the bones which form the carpus in the horse, so that, instead of the leg appearing as a vertical line, the knee (wrist) is more or less bent forward.

knife [AS. *cnīf*]. A cutting instrument of varying shape, size, and design, used in surgery and in dissecting; a scalpel. Also see *bistoury.*

amputating k. A long, pointed, single- or double-edged instrument, used for amputations.

cautery k. A knife to produce cautery, usually with an insulated handle and heated by electricity or in a flame.

electrosurgical k. See radio *k.*

radio k. One operating on a high-frequency current, which divides tissues by means of an electric spark; used in electrosurgery.

tenotomy k. See *tenotome.*

knit′ting [AS. *cnyttan*]. A lay term to indicate the process of union in a fractured bone.

knob [ME. *knobbe*]. 1. A rounded prominence or protuberance. 2. End-foot. See *end-feet.*

embryonic k. In many mammals, that part of the inner cell mass consisting of primary ectoderm and entoderm after the migration of the endodermal cells forming the yolk sac.

synaptic k. See *end-feet.*

trophoblastic k. In rodents, the mass of trophoblast cells apposite to, and resembling, the embryonic knob from which the placenta develops.

knock′-knee″. See *genu valgum.*

knock-out drops. Chloral hydrate: so-called because of the rapid action of small doses of the compound, sometimes given to a victim in food or drink to render him helpless.

Knopf, Sigard Adolphus [*American physician,* 1857–1940]. Advocated the training of tuberculous patients in the diaphragmatic type of respiration, in the hope of putting the lung apexes at rest; called *Knopf's treatment.*

knot [AS. *cnotta*]. 1. *In surgery,* the interlacing of the ends of a ligature, suture, bandage, sling, or cord, so placed that they remain fixed without slipping or detachment. 2. A small mass of cells or tissue.

clove-hitch k. One formed of two contiguous loops, placed around an object, such as a limb, the ends of the cord parallel and extending in opposite directions. This knot remains firm only so long as traction is applied.

double k. One in which the ends of the cord or suture are twisted twice around each other before tying; friction knot; surgeon's knot. It does not slip and can be adjusted.

enamel k. Cells in the enamel pulp in early stages of the enamel organ which have not yet differentiated into stellate reticulum. Also called *enamel node.*

false k. (a) See granny *k.* (b) External knotlike bulges of the umbilical cord caused by loops in the umbilical blood vessels.

granny k. A double knot in which, unlike the square knot, in the second loop the end of one cord is over, and the other under, its fellow; the loops, not being in the same plane, tend to slip. A false knot.

Hensen's k. See Hensen's *node.*

primitive k. Synonym for Hensen's node.

reef k. See square *k.* Also called *sailor's k.*

square k. A double knot in which the free ends of the second knot lie in the same plane as the ends of the first. The knot which is in most general use in surgery.

syncytial k. Protuberant masses of syncytiotrophoblast characteristic of placental villi.

true k. A knot of the umbilical cord formed by the fetus slipping through a loop in the cord.

Knott tech·nique′. See under *method.*

knuck′le [ME. *knokel*]. 1. An articulation of the phalanges with the metacarpal bones or with each other. 2. The distal convex ends of the metacarpals.

knuck′ling [*knokel*]. A condition in which the hoof of a horse is turned under; due to excessive flexion of the fetlock joint.

koagamin. Trade-mark for a hemostatic preparation representing an extract of the plant, shepherdspurse, and containing oxalic acid and related dicarboxylic acids.

koaxin. Trade-mark for a brand of menadione.

Kobert, Eduard Rudolf [*German biochemist,* 1854–1918]. Introduced *Kobert's test* for hemoglobin: The addition of zinc to the solution to be tested precipitates zinc hemoglobin, which turns red when an alkali is added.

Koch, Robert [*German bacteriologist,* 1843–1910]. Considered one of the founders of modern bacteriology. See *law of specificity of bacteria,* called *Koch's law* or *postulate.* Made an important study of the anthrax bacillus (1877). Demonstrated the bacterial character of traumatic infections (1878). Introduced improved methods of cultivating and staining bacteria. Discovered the tubercle bacillus (1882), formerly called *Koch's bacillus.* One of two bacilli which Koch discovered in two types of contagious conjunctivitis (1883) was later found by Weeks to be the causal agent of pinkeye; the *Koch-Weeks* bacillus is thought to be similar to *Hemophilus influenzae.* Influenzal conjunctivitis is called *Koch-Weeks conjunctivitis.* Koch discovered *Vibrio comma* and demonstrated its transmission by food, drinking water, clothing, etc. (1884). He introduced tuberculin (1890), which, though disappointing in the treatment of tuberculosis, proved useful in diagnosis. When tuberculin is injected into the skin of an animal or human being previously exposed to the tubercle bacillus, a local inflammatory reaction indicates continued hypersensitivity; called *Koch's phenomenon.* Nobel laureate (1905).

Koch-McMeekin's method. See under *method.*

Kocher, Emil Theodor [*Swiss surgeon,* 1841–1917]. Made important studies of the pathology and surgery of the thyroid gland. Nobel laureate (1909). Devised operations for excision of the tongue, the hip joint, the rectum, and the ankle joint, and for hernia repair. Devised a technic for radical amputation of the breast. Introduced a method of reducing dislocation of the shoulder by means of outward rotation of the humerus, flexion, and adduction with inward rotation; the gaping of the rent in the joint capsule permits reduction.

Called *Kocher's maneuver* or *method. Kocher's forceps* are serrated forceps. See also Kocher's *reflex.*

Kocks, Joseph [*German surgeon,* 1846–1916]. Remembered for his operation for relief of uterine displacements by shortening the broad ligaments through a vaginal approach.

Koeberlé, Eugène [*French surgeon,* 1828–1915]. Contributed to the development of gynecologic surgery. Introduced a type of hemostatic forceps, called *Koeberlé's forceps.*

Koebner, Heinrich [*German dermatologist,* 1838–1904]. Described epidermolysis bullosa (1886), called *Koebner's disease,* and the isomorphous provocative reaction, called *Koebner's phenomenon* (1878).

Koelliker, Rudolph Albert von. See *Kölliker.*

ko′ha. A Japanese drug, a cyanine dye derivative, given intravenously; claimed to stimulate the formation of leukocytes and new tissue and thus hasten wound healing. Also called *rainbow wave drug.*

Köhler, Alban [*German physician,* 1874–1947]. Improved the technic of radiography of the heart. Described osteochondrosis of the tarsal navicular bone, probably a form of aseptic necrosis, found in children; called *Köhler's disease, Köhler's tarsal scaphoiditis.*

Köhler's method of illumination. See under *method.*

Kohlrausch's law of migration of ions. See under *law.*

koidin. Trade-mark for a brand of menadione.

koi″lo·nych′i·a (koy″lo·nick′ee·uh) [G. *koilos,* hollow; *onyx,* nail]. An atrophic deformity of the nails in which the outer surface is concave, occurring in varied unrelated diseases, e.g., lichen planus and acanthosis nigricans, and also found as a familial defect: also called *spoon nail.*

koi·not′ro·py [G. *koinos,* common; *trepein,* to turn]. *In psychobiology,* the state of being socialized; the condition of being identified with the common interests of the people. —**koinotrop′ic,** *adj.*

Kojewnikoff's epilepsy. See continuous *epilepsy.*

ko′jic ac′id. $C_6H_6O_4$. 3-Hydroxy-5-hydroxymethyl-γ-pyrone, formed from glucose by the action of certain molds; it possesses antibiotic activity against various bacterial species.

ko′la [Temne *k'ola,* cola tree]. The dried cotyledon of *Cola nitida* or of other species of *Cola* (cola nut); the chief constituent is caffeine, with traces of theobromine also present. The therapeutic effect of kola is the same as that of other sources of caffeine, such as coffee and tea.

Kolle, Wilhelm [*German bacteriologist,* 1868–1935]. Developed a bacteriolytic serum used for the treatment of cerebrospinal meningitis. Introduced a vaccine of killed cholera bacilli, for use as a prophylactic; called *Kolle's cholera vaccine.*

kollidon. See *polyvinylpyrrolidone.*

Kölliker, Rudolph Albert von (1817–1905). Swiss histologist, anatomist, and zoologist, known for his pioneer work in histology and embryology. He proved that spermatozoa originate as cells in the testes, and described their function in fertilization. He isolated smooth muscle cells, described the relation of myelinated fibers to nerve cells, and described groups of myofibrils surrounded by sarcoplasm, called *Kölliker's columns,* and described granules seen in sarcoplasm, called *Kölliker's granules.*

Kolmer's test. See under *test.*

kolp-. For words beginning with *kolp-* not found here, see words beginning *colp-.*

kol′po-. See *colpo-.*

ko″ly·phre′ni·a [G. *kōlyein,* to hinder; *phrēn,* mind]. A condition in which there is abnormal inhibition of lower brain centers by the cortex.

Kondoléon, Emmanuel [*Greek surgeon,* 1879–1939]. Introduced an operation for the relief of elephantiasis in which strips of skin, subcutaneous tissue, and scarred fascia are removed; called *Kondoléon's operation.*

König, Franz (1832–1910). German surgeon who wrote on general and special surgery and tuberculosis of the bones and joints, and was the first to describe osteochondritis dissecans. The earliest type of autogenous graft in cranioplasty was the Mueller-König method of flap transposition, involving an interchange of scalp and dermato-periosteo-osteal flaps. He perfected the technique of osseous resection.

ko′ni·me″ter (ko′ni·mee″tur, ko·nim′i·tur), **ko′no·me″ter** (ko′no·mee″tur, ko·nom′i·tur) [G. *konis,* dust; *metron,* a measure]. An instrument for determining the number of dust particles in the air. A measured air sample is propelled against a perpendicular surface coated with an adhesive to which dust adheres. The particles are counted under a microscope. Also see *dust count.*

ko″ni·o·cor′tex [*konis;* L. *cortex,* bark, rind]. Granular cortex characteristic of sensory areas.

ko″ni·o′sis. See *coniosis.*

ko′no·me″ter. See *konimeter.*

konseal. Trade name for a form of cachet.

konsyl. A proprietary laxative prepared from *Plantago ovata.*

ko·phe′mi·a. See word *deafness.*

Koplik's sign. See under *sign.*

Koplik's spots. See Koplik's *sign.*

kop″o·pho′bi·a [G. *kopos,* exertion; *phobos,* fear]. Morbid fear of fatigue or exhaustion.

Kopp, Johann Heinrich [*German physician,* 1777–1858]. Described laryngismus stridulus which he ascribed to an enlarged thymus; called *Kopp's thymic asthma.*

kop″ro·ste′a·rin. See *coprosterol.*

Korff's fibers. See dentinogenic *fibers,* osteogenic *fibers.*

Kornhauser's quadruple stain. See under *stain.*

ko·ros′co·py. See *retinoscopy.*

Korotkov, Nikolai Sergeevich [*Russian physician,* 1874–]. Introduced the auscultatory method of determining blood pressure, applying a stethoscope to the brachial artery below the pressure cuff of a sphygmomanometer (1905); called *Korotkov's method.* The sounds heard in a normal individual as the cuff deflates are known as *Korotkov's sounds.* In *Korotkov's test* for collateral circulation in aneurysm, an artery is compressed above the aneurysm; if the blood pressure in the peripheral circulation is moderately high, the collateral circulation is considered good.

korotrin. Trade-mark for a brand of chorionic gonadotropin.

Korsakov, Sergei Sergeevich [*Russian neurologist,* 1853–1900]. Described polyneuritis with loss of memory, a retrograde amnesia associated with tendency to confabulation, caused by alcohol and severe deficiency of food intake (1887), called *Korsakov's syndrome* or *psychosis.*

ko″so·tox′in [Abyssinian *kussu;* G. *toxikon,* poison]. The chief active constituent of brayera.

Kossel, Albrecht [*German physiological chemist,* 1853–1927]. Made important studies of the chemistry of the cell and its nucleus. Nobel laureate (1910). Discovered histidine (1889) and thymine (1900). See also Kossel's *test* for hypoxanthine.

Kossel and Siegfried's protamine nucleus hypothesis. See under *hypothesis.*

kous′sin (kōōs′in) [Abyssinian *kussu*]. A resinous substance from brayera.

kous'so (kōōs'o). See *brayera.*

Kowarsky's plate. See under *plate.*

Kozhevnikov, Aleksei Yakovlevich (1836–1902). Russian neurologist, best known for his description of continuous epilepsy.

Kr Chemical symbol for krypton.

Krabbe, Knud H. [*Danish neurologist,* 1885–]. Described familial infantile diffuse cerebral sclerosis, called *Krabbe's disease.*

Kraepelin, Emil [*German psychiatrist,* 1856–1926]. Established the modern classification of mental disorders, introducing the clinical concepts of dementia precox (also known as *Morel-Kraepelin disease*) and manic depressive psychosis.

Krafft-Ebing, Richard von [*German psychiatrist,* 1840–1902]. Made a classic study of sexual psychopathology.

krait. See *Bungarus.*

Krajian's Congo stain. See under *stain.*

Krajian's rapid staining. See under *stain.*

Kramer-Tisdall method. See under *method.*

kra·me'ri·a [NL., after John George Henry *Kramer,* Austrian physician and botanist, eighteenth century]. The dried root of *Krameria triandra,* known in commerce as Peruvian rhatany, or of *Krameria argentea,* known in commerce as Para or Brazilian rhatany. An active astringent. Dose, 1–2 Gm. (15–30 gr.).

Kraske, Paul [*German surgeon,* 1851–1930]. Devised an operation for rectal carcinoma in which the coccyx and part of the sacrum are removed; called *Kraske's operation.*

K ra'tion [rash'un, ray'shun). See under *ration.*

kra·tom'e·ter [G. *kratos,* power; *metron,* a measure]. A device consisting of prisms. It is used for correcting nystagmus, or in orthoptic exercises.

krau·ro'sis [G. *krauros,* brittle; *-ōsis,* condition]. A progressive, sclerosing, shriveling process of the skin; due to glandular atrophy.

k. of penis. Balanitis xerotica obliterans.

k. of vulva. A disease of elderly women, characterized by pruritus, atrophy, and dryness of the genitalia. Stenosis of the vaginal orifice and epithelioma may develop.

Krause, Carl Friedrich Theodor [*German anatomist,* 1797–1868]. Described the accessory lacrimal glands of the upper eyelid; called *Krause's glands.*

Krause, Fedor Victor [*German surgeon,* 1857–1937]. Independently of Hartley, devised an operation of excision of the ganglion of the fifth cranial nerve for facial neuralgia, approaching through the temporal bone (1893); called *Hartley-Krause operation.* The full-thickness skin graft is known as the *Wolfe-Krause graft.* See under J. R. *Wolfe.*

Krause, Wilhelm [*German anatomist,* 1833–1910]. Described the intermediate disk, called *Krause's membrane.* See also Krause's *corpuscle.*

kre'a·tin. See *creatine.*

kre·at'i·nine. See *creatinine.*

Krebs, Hans Adolf [*English biochemist,* 1900–]. Formulated a theory of aerobic carbohydrate oxidation. Described a breakdown of carbohydrates through stages involving citric acid; this he called the citric acid cycle. See Krebs *cycle.* With Kurt Henseleit, postulated a theory of urea production by the liver, involving the breakdown of arginine to urea and ornithine; called *ornithine cycle, Krebs-Henseleit cycle.* Nobel Prize winner, with Fritz A. Lippmann, in medicine and physiology (1953).

kre"o·tox'in [G. *kreas,* flesh; *toxikon,* poison]. A meat poison or ptomaine that is formed by bacteria.

kre"o·tox'ism [*kreas; toxikon*]. Poisoning by infected meat.

Kretschmer, Ernst [*German psychiatrist,* 1888–]. Described various psycho-physical types, including the pyknic, leptosome, and athletic.

Kreysig, Friedrich Ludwig [*German physician,* 1770–1839]. Remembered for his description of a sign observed in adherent pericardium, in which retraction of the intercostal spaces occurs with the cardiac systole; called *Kreysig's sign, Heim-Kreysig sign.*

Krimer, Johann Franz Wenzel [*German surgeon,* 1795–1834]. Described his operation for cleft palate in which he made wide mucoperiosteal flaps dissected upward and united in the midline.

Krogh, August (1874–1949). Danish physiologist, known for outstanding investigations on the physiology of respiration and blood circulation, and particularly his studies of the anatomy and physiology of the capillaries. He discovered the regulation of the vasomotor mechanism of small vessels by studying how the circulation carries oxygen to the tissues. Nobel laureate in medicine and physiology (1920).

kro-kro. See *craw-craw.*

Kromayer, Ernst Ludwig Franz [*German dermatologist,* 1862–1933]. Known as the inventor of a small, water-cooled, mercury-vapor lamp with a quartz window which permits the emission of ultraviolet rays. *Kromayer's lamp* is for therapeutic use.

Krompecher, Edmund [*Hungarian pathologist,* 1870–1926]. Described basal-cell carcinoma or rodent ulcer (1900); called *Krompecher's tumor.*

Kronecker, Karl Hugo [*Swiss physiologist,* 1839–1914]. Studied the physiology of the heart. Described a point in the interventricular septum, puncture of which is said to cause fibrillary contractions of the ventricles; called *Kronecker's inhibitory center.* Introduced a solution of sodium chloride and sodium carbonate, known as *Kronecker's solution,* for use in the microscopical examination of fresh tissue.

Krönig, Georg [*German physician,* 1856–1911]. Described anterior and posterior areas of resonance over the apex of the lung; called *Krönig's areas* or *fields.* A narrow area of resonance connecting Krönig's fields over the shoulder is called *Krönig's isthmus.*

Krönlein, Rudolf Ulrich [*Swiss surgeon,* 1847–1910]. Described his operation for removal of orbital tumors without enucleating the eye.

Krüger and Schmid's method. See under *method.*

Krukenberg, Friedrich Ernst (1871–1946). German pathologist who described a bilaterally located carcinoma of the ovary, called *Krukenberg tumor* (1896). See also Krukenberg's *spindle.*

Kruse, Walther [*German bacteriologist,* 1864–1943]. Known for his research on bacillary dysentery. The *Shigella dysenteriae* is also called *Shiga-Kruse bacillus, Shiga bacillus.*

kry"mo·ther'a·py. See *crymotherapy.*

kryp'to-. See *crypto-.*

kryptok. Trade name of a bifocal lens.

kryp'ton [G. *kryptos,* hidden]. Kr = 83.80; a colorless, inert gaseous element which occurs in the atmosphere.

ku"bis·a·ga'ri (kōō"bis·uh·gah'ree), **ku"bis·ga'ri** (kōō"bis·gah'ree) [Jap.]. A paralytic vertigo, endemic in Japan.

Kühne, Willie [*German physiologist and histologist,* 1837–1900]. Pioneer investigator of enzymes. Made important contributions to the knowledge of the chemistry of digestion and of the physiology of muscles and nerves. Demonstrated that muscle proteins are coagulable (1859). Isolated trypsin

(1874). Extracted visual purple from the retina (1877).

Kuhnt, Hermann [*German ophthalmologist*, 1850–1925]. His name is associated with a number of operations: a canthoplasty, in which a flap of skin is cut from the lid to be turned into the wound at the canthus; for ectropion, in which a wedge-shaped portion of the conjunctiva and tarsus is excised; for symblepharon, in which skin grafts are used to prevent adhesions; for the radical cure of frontal sinus disease, in which the anterior wall of the sinus is removed with curetting of the mucous membrane.

Kull's method. See *Champy-Kull's method* under *stain.*

Kultschitzky's hematoxylin. See under *stain.*

Kultschitzky's myelin stain. See under *stain.*

Kümmell, Hermann [*German surgeon*, 1852–1937]. Remembered for his description of a form of traumatic spondylitis (1891) or compression fracture of vertebrae, which is known as *Kümmell's disease.*

Kumon method for indican. See under *method.*

Kundrat, Hans [*Austrian physician*, 1845–93]. Distinguished a type of lymphoid tumor called *Kundrat's lymphosarcoma.*

Kupffer cells. See under *cell.*

kur'chi (koor'chee) [Skr. *kūrcin*, long-bearded]. An extract of kurchi bark used in amebic dysentery: also called *Holarrhena antidysenterica.*

Kurlov, Mikhail Georgievich [*Russian physician*, 1859–]. Described inclusion bodies of unknown significance found in the lymphocytes and monocytes of the guinea pig; called *Kurlov bodies.* A cell containing one or more Kurlov bodies is known as a *Kurlov cell, Foà-Kurlov cell.*

Küss, Georges [*French physician*, 1867–1936]. Made important studies of tuberculosis in children. The primary lesion or Ghon tubercle, plus the satellite lymph node involvement, is known as the *primary complex, Küss-Ghon focus, Ghon complex.* Küss demonstrated that the children of tuberculous parents are not born with the disease, although they are likely to acquire it.

Kussmaul, Adolf [*German physician*, 1822–1902]. Made a study of the color phenomena of the fundus oculi (1845). With Maier, described periarteritis nodosa (1866), called *Kussmaul's disease, Kussmaul-Maier disease.* Gave a classic description of the labored breathing associated with diabetic coma (1874); called *air hunger, Kussmaul's respiration* or *sign.* Described voluntary mutism, sometimes observed in psychotic cases (1877); called *Kussmaul's aphasia.*

kus'so (kōōs'oh, kuss'oh). See *brayera.*

Küster, Ernst Georg Ferdinand von [*German surgeon*, 1839–1930]. Pioneer in performing thoracotomy for the relief of empyema (1889). Improved the technic of radical mastoidectomy. Devised an operation in which he resected the ureter for the relief of hydronephrosis (1892); called *Küster's operation.*

Küstner, Heinz (1897–). German gynecologist, who with Giles (Prausnitz) described local passive sensitization to a specific allergen. See Prausnitz-Küstner *test.*

Küstner, Otto Ernst [*German gynecologist*, 1849–1931]. Described a sign of ovarian dermoid cyst: the presence of a cystic tumor in the median line anterior to the uterus, disclosed by palpation; called *Küstner's sign.*

kv, kv. Kilovolt.

kw, kw. Kilowatt.

kwash·i·or'kor [Gold Coast, Africa, literally, red boy]. A deficiency disease, probably of animal protein or some associated factor, characterized by fatty infiltration of the liver, pigmentary changes of the skin, edema, and pancreatic dysfunction. In varying forms it is probably seen throughout the tropics and subtropics.

Kwilecki's method. See under *method.*

ky"a·nop'si·a. See *cyanopia.*

ky·es'te·in (kigh·ess'tee·in) [G. *kyein*, to be pregnant]. A filmy deposit upon decomposing urine, once thought to be diagnostic of pregnancy.

K-Y jelly. Trade-mark for a lubricating jelly containing boric acid, glycerin, chondrus, and tragacanth.

ky'mo·gram [G. *kyma*, wave; *gramma*, letter]. The record made on a kymograph.

ky'mo·graph [*kyma;* G. *graphein*, to write]. An instrument for recording physiologic cycles or actions in a patient or an experimental animal; consists of a clock- or motor-driven cylinder, covered with paper on which the record is made. Time intervals can be recorded simultaneously with the phenomena. —**kymograph'ic,** *adj.*

ky·mog'ra·phy (kigh·mog'ruh·fee) [*kyma; graphein*]. Use of the kymograph.

roentgen k. See *radiokymography.*

ky"no·pho'bi·a. See *cynophobia.*

kyn"u·re'nic ac'id (kin"yoo·ree'nick, ·ren'ick, kigh"new·). $C_{10}H_7NO_3$. γ-Hydroxy-β-quinoline carboxylic acid, a product of the metabolism of tryptophan occurring in the urine of some animals, but not of man.

ky·nur'e·nine (kigh·new'ri·neen, ·nin, kin"yoo-ree'neen, ·nin). An intermediate product, $C_{10}H_{12}N_2O_3$, of tryptophan metabolism isolated from the urine of certain animals, but not man.

ky"pho·ra·chi'tis (kigh"fo·ra·kigh'tis) [G. *kyphos*, hunchbacked; *rhachis*, spine]. Rachitic deformity of the thorax and spine, resulting in an anteroposterior hump. The pelvis is sometimes involved. —**kyphorachit'ic,** *adj.*

ky"pho·sco"li·o·ra·chi'tis [*kyphos;* G. *skolios*, curved; *rhachis;* G. *-itis*, inflammation]. A combined kyphosis and scoliosis due to rickets. The pelvis and thorax may be involved in the deformity. —**kyphoscoliorachit'ic,** *adj.*

ky"pho·sco"li·o'sis [*kyphos;* G. *skoliōsis*, obliquity]. Lateral curvature of the spine with vertebral rotation, associated with an anteroposterior hump in the spinal column. —**kyphoscoliot'ic,** *adj.*

ky·pho'sis (kigh·fo'sis) [G., a being hunchbacked]. Angular curvature of the spine, the convexity of the curve being posterior, usually situated in the thoracic region, and involving few or many vertebrae; the result of such diseases as tuberculosis, osteoarthritis, or rheumatoid arthritis of the spine, or an improper posture habit. Syn., *humpback, hunchback.* Also see *round shoulders.* —**kyphot'ic,** *adj.*

thoracic k. A posterior angular deformity of the spine in the thoracic area.

ky'rine (kigh'reen, ·rin). A tripeptide obtained by slow hydrolysis of certain proteins. *Obs.*

kyr·tom'e·ter. See *cyrtometer.*

ky'to-. See *cyto-.*

L

L. Latin.

L_+ Symbol for limes death.

L_0 Symbol for limes zero.

L- *In chemistry*, a prefix, written as a small capital letter: used to indicate the structural configuration of a particular asymmetric carbon atom, with reference to the standard substance L-glyceraldehyde, as distinguished from D-glyceraldehyde. For the basis of assigning this prefix, and of the significance of the usage of **L(+)-**, **L(−)**, **L_g**, and **L_s** see definition of **D-**.

l, l. Liter.

l. Left, left eye, libra, lethal.

***l*-** 1. *In chemistry*, abbreviation for *levorotatory*, referring to the direction in which the plane of polarized light is rotated by a substance; this usage may be confused with the following. 2. *In chemistry*, a prefix formerly used to indicate the structural configuration of a particular asymmetric carbon atom in a compound, in the manner that the small capital letter L- is now used.

La Chemical symbol for lanthanum.

lab, lab-fer′ment. Rennin. *Obs.*

Labarraque's solution. See chlorinated soda *solution.*

Labbé, Leon [*French surgeon*, 1832–1916]. *Labbé's triangle* is that area bounded by a horizontal line along the lower border of the cartilage of the ninth rib, by the left costal arch, and by the lower edge of the liver.

lab′da·cism. See *lambdacism.*

lab′da·num. See *ladanum.*

la′bi·a. Plural of labium.

la′bi·al·ism [L. *labium*, lip]. The tendency to pronounce any articulate sounds as if they were labial consonants, as *b*, *p*, or *m;* the addition of a labial or labiodental quality to an articulate sound.

La″bi·a′tae (lay″bee·ay′tee). Lamiaceae.

la′bile (lay′bil, lab′il) [L. *labilis*, apt to slip]. Unstable; readily changing; moving from place to place.

la·bil′i·ty. 1. *In psychiatry*, very rapid fluctuations in intensity and modality of emotions, usually without adequate external cause and with inadequate control of their expression, seen most dramatically in the affective reaction or in certain organic brain disorders. 2. *In chemistry*, readily susceptible to change, such as a spontaneous atomic rearrangement of an organic molecule.

la′bi·o- [L. *labium*, lip]. A combining form denoting *the lips, labial.*

la″bi·o·al·ve′o·lar [*labium;* L. *alveolus*, small hollow]. Pertaining to the lip and to the alveolar process of maxilla or mandible.

la″bi·o·cer′vi·cal [*labium;* L. *cervix*, neck]. Pertaining to a lip and a neck; pertaining to the labial surface of the neck of a tooth.

la″bi·o·den′tal [*labium;* L. *dens*, tooth]. Pertaining to the lips and the teeth.

la″bi·o·gin′gi·val (lay″bee·o·jin′ji·vul, ·jin·jy′vul) [*labium;* L. *gingiva*, gum]. Pertaining to the lips and gums.

la″bi·o·glos″so·la·ryn′ge·al [*labium;* G. *glōssa*, tongue; *larygx*, larynx]. Pertaining conjointly to lips, tongue, and larynx, as in labioglossolaryngeal paralysis, a form of bulbar paralysis.

la″bi·o·gres′sion. Location of the anterior teeth in front of their normal position.

la″bi·o·men′tal [*labium;* L. *mentum*, chin]. Relating to the lip and chin.

la″bi·o·pal′a·tine (lay″bee·o·pal′uh·tyne, ·tin) [*labium;* L. *palatum*, palate]. Relating to the lip and palate.

la′bi·o·plas″ty [*labium;* G. *plassein*, to form]. Cheiloplasty.

la′bi·um (pl. *labia*) [L.]. 1. A lip. 2. *In invertebrate zoology*, the lower lip as opposed to the labrum, the upper lip. See also *lip.* —**labial,** *adj.*

l. leporinum. OT for *harelip.*

l. majus. One of two folds (labia majora) of the female external genital organs, arising just below the mons pubis, and surrounding the vulval entrance. Also called *l. majus pudendi, major lip.* See Plate 41.

l. minus. One of the two folds (labia minora) at the inner surfaces of the labia majora. Also called *l. minus pudendi, minor lip.* See Plate 41.

la′bor [L., labor, toil]. Childbirth.

artificial l. That effected or aided by means other than the forces of the maternal organism.

dry l. That in which there is a deficiency of the liquor amnii, or in which there has been a premature rupture of the amniotic sac.

false l. Painful uterine contractions of the same intensity, occurring usually at irregular intervals, frequently several days before normal labor. It is not associated with progressive dilation or effacement of the cervix or descent of the presenting part.

induced l. Labor brought on by artificial means.

instrumental l. One requiring instrumental means to extract the child.

l. pains. The pains associated with childbirth.

mechanism of l. The mechanism by which a fetus and its appendages traverse the birth canal. See Plate 42.

mimetic l. False labor.

missed l. Retention of the dead fetus in the uterus beyond the period of normal gestation.

obstructed l. That which is mechanically blocked, as from a contracted pelvis or pelvic tumor. Its severity is relative to the size of the fetus and the maternal structures.

postponed l. Delayed beyond nine months.

precipitate l. The sudden expulsion of the fetus and its appendages.

premature l. Labor taking place before the normal period of gestation, but when the fetus is viable.

protracted l. Labor prolonged beyond the usual limit (10–20 hours in primiparas, 2–6 hours in multiparas).

rotation stage of l. That period in the mechanism of childbirth in which the presenting part turns about its vertical axis to accommodate itself to the birth canal. This turning may be internal, occurring before the birth of the presenting part, or external, occurring afterward.

spontaneous l. That requiring no artificial aid.

stages of l. Arbitrary divisions of the period of labor; the first begins with dilatation of the os and ends with complete dilatation; the second ends with the expulsion of the child; the third (placental) consists in the expulsion of the placenta.

lab′o·ra·to″ry [*labor*]. A place for experimental work in any branch of science.

general medical l. A large fully equipped U. S. Army laboratory in a theater of operations, with certain facilities comparable to those of the Army Medical Service Graduate School and Armed Forces Institute of Pathology.

l. unit. See medical *l.*

medical l. *In military medicine*, a medical establishment, generally a mobile unit, with personnel and equipment for medical tests and field research. Its main function is to prevent disease. There are two types: **general,** assigned to a theater of operations; **medical,** assigned on the basis of one to an army and one to each section of the communications zone.

Laborde's method. See under *artificial respiration.*

lab′ro·cyte [G. *labros*, boisterous; *kytos*, cell]. Mast cell. *Obs.*

la′brum, lab′rum [L., lip]. 1. A liplike structure. 2. *In invertebrate zoology*, the upper lip, as opposed to the labium, the lower lip.

l. glenoidale. The fibrocartilaginous ring that surrounds a socket in which the head of a large bone is received, such as the acetabulum or the glenoid cavity; glenoid lip.

lab′y·rinth [G. *labyrinthos*, labyrinth]. 1. An intricate system of connecting passageways; maze. 2. The system of intercommunicating canals and cavities that makes up the inner ear. —**labyrin′thine,** *adj.*

bony l. That part of the inner ear consisting of canals containing perilymph and the membranous labyrinth.

ethmoid l. That formed by the air cells in the lateral portions of the ethmoid bone.

membranous l. Those membranous canals corresponding to the shape of the bony labyrinth, suspended in the perilymph, and containing endolymph.

nasal l. The irregular cavity formed by the turbinate bones in the nasal passages.

osseous l. See bony *l.*

lab″y·rin·thec′to·my [*labyrinthos;* G. *ektomē*, excision]. The complete removal of the semicircular canals of the ear. Also see *hemilabyrinthectomy.*

lab″y·rin·thi′tis [*labyrinthos;* G. *-itis*, inflammation]. Inflammation of the labyrinth of the inner ear. Syn., *otitis interna.*

serous l. That due to bacterial infection, toxins, or trauma, marked by increased perilymphatic pressure without suppuration.

suppurative l. That due to bacterial invasion, characterized by all of the diagnostic evidence of infection, including production of pus cells.

toxic l. Inflammation of the labyrinth due to drugs which cause nausea and vertigo.

traumatic l. Inflammation of the labyrinth due to trauma, as a fractured skull or such functional labyrinthine surgery as a fenestration operation.

lab″y·rin·thot′o·my [*labyrinthos;* G. *tomē*, a cutting]. Incision into the labyrinth, specifically, into that of the inner ear.

lac [L.]. 1. Milk. 2. A term applied to various natural resins used in preparing shellac.

l. sulfuris. Sulfur milk or precipitated sulfur.

lac bismo. Trade-mark for bismuth magma.

lac′case. 1. An oxidizing enzyme present in many plants. 2. A class of oxidases which act on phenols.

lac′er·at″ed (lass′uh·ray″tid) [L. *lacerare*, to tear]. Torn.

lac″er·a′tion [L. *laceratio*, from *lacerare*]. 1. A tear. 2. The act of tearing or lacerating.

l. of perineum. A tearing of the wall separating the lower portion of the vagina and anal canal occurring occasionally during childbirth.

la·cer′tus [L., muscular part of the arm]. A small bundle of fibers.

l. fibrosus. An aponeurotic band from the biceps tendon to the fascia of the forearm.

Lach′e·sis (lack′i·sis) [G., one of the three Fates]. A genus of venomous pit vipers, the Crotalidae.

L. mutus. A species found in South America and in the extreme lower portion of Central America. Commonly known as the bushmaster, it attains a length of 11 or 12 feet and produces a powerful hemotoxic venom.

lach′ry·mal. See *lacrimal.*

la·cin′i·ate [L. *lacinia*, fringe]. Jagged, fringed; cut into narrow flaps, as laciniate ligament.

lac′moid. $[C_6H_2(OH)_3]_2:H.C_6H_3(OH)_2$; an acid-base indicator, prepared by interaction of resorcinol and sodium nitrite; it occurs as dark-violet scales or granules, slightly soluble in water. Syn., *resorcinol blue.*

lac′ri·mal [L. *lacrima*, a tear]. 1. Pertaining to the tears, or to the organs secreting and conveying the tears. 2. The lacrimal bone. See Table of Bones in the Appendix.

lac″ri·ma′le (lack″ri·mah′lee, ·may′lee) [*lacrima*]. The point where the posterior lacrimal crest meets the frontolacrimal suture. This point may occasionally be coincident with the dacryon, and cannot be located in skulls from which the lacrimal bones have been lost.

lac″ri·ma′tion [L. *lacrimare*, to shed tears]. Normal secretion of tears; also, excessive secretion, as in weeping.

lac′ri·ma″tor [*lacrimare*]. Any substance, as a gas, which irritates the conjunctiva and causes secretion of the tears; a tear gas.

lac′ri·mo·tome [L. *lacrima*, a tear; G. *tomos*, cutting]. A cutting instrument used in operating on the nasolacrimal duct or lacrimal sac.

lac″ri·mot′o·my [L. *lacrima*, a tear; G. *tomē*, a cutting]. Incision of the nasolacrimal duct.

lac·tac″i·de′mi·a (lack·tass″i·dee′mee·uh) [L. *lac*, milk; *acidus*, sour; G. *haima*, blood]. Presence of lactic acid in the blood.

lac″ta·cid′o·gen. Name originally given by Embden and Zimmerman to a hexose-diphosphoric acid isolated from tissue. *Obs.*

lac·tac″i·du′ri·a (lack·tass″i·dew′ree·uh) [*lac; acidus;* G. *ouron*, urine]. Lactic acid in the urine.

lac′ta·gogue. See *galactagogue.*

lac″tal·bu′min [*lac;* L. *albus*, white]. A simple protein contained in milk which resembles serum albumin and is of high nutritional quality.

lactalumina. Trade-mark for an aqueous suspension of aluminum hydroxide.

lac′tam. An organic compound, containing a —NH—CO— group in ring form, produced by the elimination of a molecule of water from certain amino acids. It is the keto form of its isomer, lactim.

lac·tam′ic ac′id. Alanine.

lac·tam′ide (lack·tam′id, ·ide, lack′tuh·mide, ·mid). $CH_3.CHOH.CONH_2$. The amide of lactic acid.

lac′tant [L. *lactare*, to suckle]. Suckling.

lac′tase. A soluble enzyme found in the animal body which hydrolyzes lactose to dextrose and galactose.

lac·tar″o·vi·o′lin. An antibiotic pigment, $C_{15}H_{14}O$, from *Lactarius deliciosus.*

lac′tate. A salt of lactic acid.

lac·ta′tion [*lactare*]. 1. Suckling; the period during which the child is nourished from the breast. 2. The formation or secretion of milk. —**lactational,** *adj.*

lac′te·al [L. *lac*, milk]. Pertaining to milk.

lac′te·al. Any of the lymphatics of the small intestine that take up the chyle.

lac·tes′cence [L. *lactescere*, to turn to milk]. Milkiness; often applied to the chyle.

lac′tic [L. *lac*, milk]. Pertaining to milk or its derivatives.

lac′tic ac′id. 2-Hydroxypropanoic acid or α-hydroxypropionic acid, existing in three forms: (a) D(−)-lactic acid, $CH_3.HCOH.COOH$, levorotatory, biochemically produced from methylglyoxal under certain conditions; (b) L(+)-lactic acid, $CH_3.HOCH.COOH$, dextrorotatory, the product of anaerobic glycolysis in muscle, hence called *sarcolactic acid;* (c) DL-lactic acid, a racemic mixture of (a) and (b), produced by the action of bacteria on sour milk and other foods, and prepared synthetically by fermentation of sugar or corn starch. The last form, medicinally important, occurs as a colorless, syrupy liquid, miscible with water; part of the acid exists as anhydride. It is used as an ingredient of infant-feeding formulas, and has been administered intraarticularly in treatment of arthritis; externally it is used in spermatocidal compositions, and sometimes as a caustic antiseptic.

l. a. dehydrogenase. An enzyme, in animal tissues, which catalyzes dehydrogenation of L(+)-lactic acid to pyruvic acid; an anaerobic dehydrogenase which functions in the presence of coenzyme I.

lac′tide. 1. The ring compound produced by interaction of two molecules of an α-hydroxyacid in such a way that the carboxyl group of one molecule is esterified with the hydroxyl group of the other and vice versa. 2. The ring compound formed, according to the preceding definition, from two molecules of lactic acid; it is

```
          O.CO
        /      \
  CH3CH          CHCH3.
        \      /
          CO.O
```

lac·tif′er·ous [*lac;* L. *ferre*, to carry]. Conveying or secreting milk. Syn., *lactigerous.*

lac′ti·fuge [*lac;* L. *fugare*, to put to flight]. Lessening the secretion of milk.

lac′ti·fuge. A drug or agent that lessens the secretion of milk.

lactigen. Trade-mark for a lipoprotein antigen prepared from sterilized milk. Used in nonspecific protein therapy.

lac·tig′e·nous (lack·tidj′i·nus) [*lac;* G. *genesthai*, from *gignesthai*, to be produced]. Producing milk.

lac·tig′er·ous (lack·tidj′i·rus). See *lactiferous.*

lac′tim. An organic compound, containing a —N:COH— group in ring form, produced by the elimination of a molecule of water from certain amino acids. It is the enol form of its isomer, lactam.

lac′tin. See *lactose.*

lac″ti·su′gi·um (lack″ti·sue′jee·um) [*lac;* L. *sugere*, to suck]. Breast pump.

lac·tiv′o·rous [*lac;* L. *vorare*, to devour]. Subsisting on milk.

lac′to-, lact- [*lac*]. A combining form meaning *milk.*

lac″to·ba·cil′lic ac′id. $C_{19}H_{36}O_2$; a fatty acid, probably a methyleneoctadecanoic acid, containing a cyclopropane ring, elaborated by *Lactobacillus arabinosus*, and apparently essential for the growth of the organism.

Lac″to·ba·cil′lus [*lac;* L. *bacillus*, small staff]. A genus of bacteria composed of microorganisms which are capable of producing lactic acid from carbohydrates and carbohydratelike compounds, and which are able to withstand a degree of acidity usually destructive to nonsporulating bacteria.

L. acidophilus. Gram-positive rod found in milk, feces, saliva, and carious teeth, nonpathogenic and unusually resistant to acid: also called *Bacillus acidophilus, L. gastrophilus*, and probably identical with *L. of Boas-Oppler* and *Bacillus vaginalis* (*Döderlein's bacillus*).

L. bifidus. A nonmotile, anaerobic, Gram-positive rod; the predominant organism in the intestine and feces of breast-fed infants.

L. bulgaricus. A species isolated from Bulgarian fermented milk.

L. casei factor. See *folic acid.*

L. gastrophilus. See *L. acidophilus.*

L. lactis Dorner. A microorganism used in the study of B_{12} since it requires this vitamin for growth.

L. of Boas-Oppler. Gram-positive rod originally found in the gastric juice of patients with carcinoma of the stomach, but bearing no known causative relationship to this; probably *L. acidophilus.*

lac′to·cele (lack′to·seel). Galactocele.

lac′to·crit [*lac;* G. *kritēs*, judge]. An apparatus for testing the quantity of fat in milk.

lac″to·fla′vin (lack″to·flay′vin, ·flav′in). Riboflavin.

lac′to·gen [*lac;* G. *genesthai*, from *gignesthai*, to be produced]. Any agent or substance which stimulates the secretion of milk.

lac″to·gen′ic [*lac; genesthai*]. Activating or stimulating the mammary glands.

lac″to·glob′u·lin [*lac;* L. *globulus*, small ball]. One of the proteins of milk.

lac·tom′e·ter [*lac;* G. *metron*, a measure]. An instrument for determining the specific gravity of milk.

lac′tone. An anhydro-ring compound produced by elimination of water from a molecule of an oxyacid.

lac·ton′ic ac′id. Galactonic acid.

lactopeptine. Trade-mark for a mixture of pepsin, diastase, and pancreatin with lactic acid and hydrochloric acid.

lac″to·per·ox′i·dase. A peroxidase present in milk: it has been isolated in crystalline form.

lac″to·phos′phate. A salt composed of a base united to lactic and phosphoric acids.

lac″to·pro′te·in [*lac;* G. *prōteios*, of first rank]. A protein in milk.

lac″tor·rhe′a. Galactorrhea.

lac·to′sa·zone. Characteristic osazone of lactose. See phenylhydrazine *test.*

lac′tose. $C_{12}H_{22}O_{11}$; 4-(β-D-galactopyranosido)-D-glucopyranose or 4-D-glucopyranosyl-β-D-galactopyranoside; a disaccharide representing D-glucose and D-galactose joined by a 1,4-glycosidic bond; on hydrolysis it is converted to these sugars. Two forms are known, *alpha-lactose* and *beta-lactose;* milk of mammals contains an equilibrium mixture of the two. Lactose of the U.S.P. is the alpha form; crystallization of this sugar at higher temperatures yields the beta form, which is more soluble in water. Both are used as nutrients and occasionally as diuretic agents; in pharmacy both are widely used as diluents and tablet excipients. Syn., *lactin, milk sugar.*

lac″to·su′ri·a [*lac;* G. *ouron*, urine]. The presence of lactose in the urine.

lac″to·ther′a·py. See *galactotherapy.*

lac″to·tox′in [*lac;* G. *toxikon*, poison]. A poisonous substance found in milk.

lac″to·veg″e·tar′i·an [*lac;* L. *vegetus*, lively]. One who lives on a diet of milk, eggs, and vegetables. —**lactovegetar′ian,** *adj.*

lac″tu·car′i·um (lack″too·kair′ee·um) [L. *lactuca*,

lettuce]. The concrete milky juice of *Lactuca virosa.* Contains a considerable amount of lactucerin, a mixture of acetyl esters of alpha-lactucerol and beta-lactucerol. Lactucarium is alleged to be sedative and anodyne; has been used in cough and nervous irritability.

lac·tu'cer·in. A mixture of acetyl esters of alpha-lactucerol and beta-lactucerol from lactucarium.

lac·tu'cer·ol. $C_{18}H_{30}O$. A crystalline substance from lactucerin; occurs in two isomeric forms, **alpha-lactucerol** and **beta-lactucerol.**

lac'tyl. The monovalent radical $CH_3.CHOH.CO$— derived from lactic acid.

la·cu'na [L., hole, opening]. 1. A little depression or space. 2. The space in the matrix occupied by a cartilage cell or by the body of a bone cell. —**lacunar,** *adj.*

blood l. Any one of the cavities containing maternal blood in the early syncytiotrophoblast before the development of the true villi; they become the intervillous spaces of the placenta.

Howship's lacunas. See John *Howship.*

lacunae urethrales. The openings of the urethral glands.

l. magna. An inconstant pouch extending upward from the dorsal wall of the navicular fossa of the penis.

l. musculorum. The space beneath the inguinal ligament which contains the iliopsoas muscle and femoral nerve.

l. vasorum. The space beneath the inguinal ligament which contains the femoral artery and vein.

l. venosa durae matris. Any small venous cleft between the layers of the dura mater, connecting the emissary and diploic veins with the venous sinuses.

urethral l. An orifice of one of the larger urethral glands (of Littré).

la·cu'nu·la [dim. from L. *lacuna,* hole]. A small or minute lacuna; an air space, as seen in a gray hair when magnified.

la·cu'nule. See *lacunula.*

la'cus. Lake.

lad'a·num [G. *lēdanon,* gum-ladanum, from the Persian]. The resin of various species of *Cistus,* growing in the Mediterranean region. Also called *labdanum.* **Ladanum oil** distilled from the resin is used in perfumery.

Ladd-Franklin, Christine [*American psychologist and logician,* 1847–1930]. Advanced a theory of color vision developed upon a basis of evolution (1892). From a primitive black-white substance operative in rod vision in retinas without cones, the first stage in the development of color vision is said to have produced yellow and blue substances and cones; in the final stage, red and green substances were produced from the yellow, finishing the series of substances for white, yellow, red, and green vision. Called *Ladd-Franklin theory of vision.*

la'dre·rie". A chronic cutaneous helminthiasis characterized by multiple painless nodules containing parts of Taenia (*Cysticercus cellulosae*).

Lady Webster dinner pills. Aloe and mastic pills.

Laehr-Henneberg hard palate reflex. In pseudobulbar paralysis, contraction of the orbicularis oris and lowering of the upper lip when the hard palate is tickled.

Laennec, René Théophile Hyacinthe [*French physician,* 1781–1826]. Invented the stethoscope, and made a basic study of auscultation. Gave classic descriptions of tuberculosis, lobar pneumonia, pleurisy, bronchiectasis, pneumothorax, emphysema, and hydatid cysts of the lung. See also Laennec's *cirrhosis,* Laennec's *thrombus.*

lae've (lee'vuh) [L. *lēvis,* smooth]. Smooth; nonvillous, as chorion laeve.

lae'vo- (lee'vo-), **laev-.** See *levo-.*

Lafayette mixture. Copaiba mixture.

lag [perhaps Middle Danish *lakka,* to go slowly]. 1. The space of time between the application of a stimulus and the resulting response. 2. See lag *phase.*

lag'am bal'sam (bawl'sum). A thick yellow liquid resembling Copaiba balsam.

la·ge'na (la·jee'nuh) [G. *lagynos,* flask]. The curved, flasklike organ of hearing in lower vertebrates corresponding to the cochlea of higher forms.

la·ge'ni·form (la·jee'ni·form, la·jen'i·) [*lagynos;* L. *forma,* form]. Flask-shaped.

lag·nei'a (lag·nigh'uh) [G., coition]. Satyriasis or nymphomania; erotomania.

lag"neu·o·ma'ni·a [G. *lagneuein,* to have sexual intercourse; *mania,* madness]. A mental disorder characterized by lustful, sadistic, lewd, and lecherous actions.

lag"oph·thal'mos [G. *lagōs,* hare; *ophthalmos,* eye]. A condition in which the eyes cannot be entirely closed: also called *lagophthmia.* —**lagophthalmic,** *adj.*

Lagrange, Pierre Félix [*French ophthalmologist,* 1857–1928]. Devised an operation combining iridectomy and sclerectomy, for the relief of glaucoma; called *Lagrange's operation.*

la grippe (lah grip). Old term for influenza.

la'i·ty [G. *laos,* people]. Nonprofessional people as opposed to any professional group.

lake [L. *lacus,* lake]. 1. A small, fluid-filled hollow or cavity; lacus. 2. A pigment prepared by precipitating a vegetable or animal coloring matter with a metallic compound.

blood l. See *hematoma.*

lacrimal l. The space at the inner canthus of the eye, near the puncta lacrimalis, in which the tears collect.

lake. To hemolyze.

la'ky [F. *laque*]. Lake-colored; of a purplish red; said of blood serum which has a transparent red color after hemolysis.

lal"i·o·pho'bi·a [G. *lalia,* talk; *phobos,* fear]. Morbid fear of talking or of stuttering. Also called *lalophobia.*

lal·la'tion [L. *lallare,* to sing lalla or lullaby]. 1. Any unintelligible stammering of speech, as word-salad or the prattling of a baby. 2. Pronunciation of the letter *r* so that it sounds like *l.*

lall'ing [*lallare*]. Speech marked by lallation.

lal"og·no'sis. Recognition of words.

la·lop'a·thy [G. *lalein,* to prattle; *pathos,* disease]. Any disorder of speech or disturbance of the function of language.

lal"o·pho'bi·a. See *laliophobia.*

lal"o·pho·mi'a·trist. A specialist dealing with defects in voice production, and especially with speech defects.

lal"o·ple'gi·a [*lalein;* G. *plēgē,* stroke]. Inability to speak, due to paralysis of the muscles concerned in speech, except those of the tongue.

lal"or·rhe'a. See *logorrhea.*

Lalouette, Pierre [*French physician,* 1711–92]. Described the pyramidal lobe of the thyroid gland. This is an inconstant and variable third lobe, rising usually from the isthmus or from the adjacent part of the left lobe. It may extend as far as the hyoid bone. Called *Lalouette's pyramid.*

Lamarck, Jean Baptiste Pierre Antoine de Monet de (1744–1820) French naturalist, comparative anatomist, and biologist, who classified animals as vertebrates and invertebrates. He antedated Darwin in postulating some elements of Darwin's theory of evolution.

La·marck′ism [after *Lamarck*]. The theory that organic evolution takes place through the inheritance of modifications caused by the environment, and by the effects of use and disuse of organs.

Lamballe. See *Jobert de Lamballe.*

lamb′da [G.]. 1. The eleventh letter of the Greek alphabet (Λ, λ). 2. Wavelength of light or other radiation. 3. The point where the sagittal suture meets the lambdoid suture.

lamb′da·cism [*lambda*]. 1. Difficulty in uttering the sound of the letter *l*. 2. Too frequent use of the *l* sound, or its substitution for the *r* sound.

lamb′doid [*lambda;* G. *eidos,* form]. Resembling the Greek letter lambda (Λ, λ), as lambdoid suture.

lam′bert [after Johann Heinrich *Lambert,* German physicist, 1728–77]. A photometric unit for describing the brightness of light reflected from a surface. One lambert is the equivalent of one lumen per sq. cm.

Lambert's law. See *law* of Lambert.

Lambl's excrescences. See under *excrescence.*

Lam′bli·a [from Wilhelm Dusan *Lambl,* Bohemian physician, 1824–95]. Synonym for *Giardia.*

lam·bli′a·sis. See *giardiasis.*

la·mel′la (pl. *lamellas*) [L., thin plate of metal]. 1. A thin scale or plate. 2. *In ophthalmology,* a medicated gelatin disk intended to be inserted under the eyelid.

circumferential l. A thin layer of bone deposited under the periosteum or endosteum.

concentric l. One of the plates of bone making up the Haversian systems in compact bone.

cornoid l. A horn plug penetrating the epidermis and having a central column of parakeratotic cells, microscopically diagnostic of porokeratosis.

enamel l. A thin organic sheet extending from the surface of the enamel toward and sometimes into the dentine of a tooth. It may be due to local developmental disturbance or a crack filled with organic matter.

ground l. See interstitial *l.*

Haversian l. One of the thin concentric layers of bone surrounding a Haversian canal.

interstitial l. One of the layers of bone of the regions between Haversian systems.

l. of bone. A thin layer of bone deposited during one period of osteogenic activity.

la·mel′lar, lam′el·lar [*lamella*]. Resembling a thin plate; composed of lamellas or thin plates, as lamellar cataract.

lame′ness [AS. *lama*]. Limping; weakness or partial loss of function of a leg, so that the gait is abnormal, whether due to acute disease, shortening, atrophy of muscle, pain, or to any other disturbance of the member. —**lame,** *adj., v.*

elbow l. Lameness in the horse, due to disease of the elbow joint.

intermittent l. See intermittent *claudication.*

lames foliacées [F.]. Fibrous tissue in a concentric arrangement, resembling Meissner tactile bodies, found in the intradermal type of nevus pigmentosus.

La″mi·a′ce·ae (lay″mee·ay′see·ee) [L. *lamium,* dead nettle]. A family of herbs, mostly aromatic. Syn., *Labiatae, Menthaceae.*

lam′i·na [L.]. A thin plate or layer. —**laminar, laminated,** *adj.*

alar l. See alar *plate.*

anterior elastic l. The condensed, outer layer of the substantia propria of the cornea. Also called *l. elastica anterior, Bowman's membrane.*

basal l. 1. A homogeneous membrane covering the inner surface of the choroid. Also called *Bruch's membrane.* 2. See basal *plate.*

buccogingival l. See vestibular *l.*

choriocapillary l. The inner layer of the choroid, consisting of a capillary plexus.

cribriform l. See cribriform *plate.*

dental l. The epithelial ingrowth into the jaw which gives rise to the enamel organs of the developing teeth.

external elastic l. See external elastic *membrane.*

external medullary l. Fibers lying along the outer border of the thalamus and separating it from the internal capsule.

internal medullary l. A delicate band of fibers which divides the thalamus into lateral and medial parts.

labial l. See labiogingival *l.*

labiodental l. The epithelial ingrowth which forms the labiogingival lamina and the dental lamina.

labiogingival l. The portion of the vestibular lamina opposite the lips: also called *labial l.*

l. affixa. The line of union of a cerebral hemisphere with the thalamus.

l. cribrosa. (a) That portion of the sclera which is perforated for the passage of the optic nerve. (b) The fascia covering the saphenous opening. (c) The anterior or posterior perforated space of the brain. (d) The perforated plates of bone through which pass branches of the cochlear or auditory nerve.

l. dura. 1. See *dura mater.* 2. The bone lining a dental alveolus: so called because of its apparent density in roentgenograms.

l. elastica. The layer of interlacing elastic fibers in the mucous membrane of the pharynx, larynx, and respiratory tree.

l. fornicis. The fornix. See Plate 18.

l. modioli. The upper part of the osseous spiral lamina.

l. muscularis mucosae. The layer or layers of smooth muscle at the deep face of the mucous membrane of the digestive tube.

l. papyracea. A thin, smooth, oblong plate of bone which closes in the ethmoidal cells and forms a large part of the medial wall of the orbit. Also called *os planum.*

l. perpendicularis. Perpendicular plate.

l. propria. (a) The middle or fibrous layer of the tympanic membrane. (b) See *l.* propria mucosae.

l. propria mucosae. The connective tissue of a mucous membrane. Syn., *tunica propria mucosae.*

l. quadrigemina. The alar plate of the midbrain from which the corpora quadrigemina are developed.

l. suprachorioidea. The delicate connective-tissue membrane uniting the choroid and sclerotic coats of the eye.

l. terminalis. The connecting layer of gray matter between the optic chiasma and the anterior commissure where it becomes continuous with the rostral lamina.

l. vasculosa chorioideae. The outer, pigmented layer of the choroid, composed of small arteries and veins.

l. vasculosa testis. The vascular connective tissue deep to the tunica albuginea testis.

lateral pterygoid l. The lateral pterygoid plate.

medial pterygoid l. The medial pterygoid plate.

neural l. The lateral portion of the neural arch of a vertebra.

osseous spiral l. The thin shelf of bone projecting from the modiolus and partially subdividing the cochlea; the basilar membrane completes the division.

periclaustral l. The layer of white matter between the claustrum and the cortex of the insula.

posterior elastic l. An elastic, transparent, homogeneous membrane covering the posterior surface of the substantia propria of the cornea. Also called *Descemet's membrane.*

reticular l. The hyaline membrane of the inner ear, extending between the heads of the outer rods of Corti and the external row of the outer hair cells.

rostral l. The thin continuation of the rostrum of the corpus callosum into the lamina terminalis. See Plate 18.

secondary spiral l. A short partition projecting from the outer wall of the cochlea in the lower part only.

spiral l. A thin plate in the ear, osseous in the inner part and membranous in the outer, which divides the spiral tube of the cochlea into the scala tympani and scala vestibuli. See osseous spiral *l.* and basilar *membrane.*

vestibular l. The vertical sheet of oral ectoderm which splits to form the vestibule of the mouth: also called *lip furrow band.*

lam'i·na·gram. See *tomogram.*

lam"i·nag'ra·phy. See sectional *radiography.*

lam"i·na'tion [*lamina*]. 1. Arrangement in plates or layers. 2. An operation in embryotomy consisting in cutting the skull in slices.

la'mine. A hemostatic alkaloid occurring in the flowers of *Lamium album.*

lam"i·nec'to·my [*lamina;* G. *ektomē,* excision]. Surgical removal of one or more neural laminas of the vertebrae, often including the spinous processes of the vertebrae.

lam"i·ni'tis [*lamina;* G. *-itis,* inflammation]. Inflammation of the laminas of a horse's hoof. It is often an accompanying symptom to founder.

lam"i·nog'ra·phy. See sectional *radiography.*

lam"i·not'o·my [*lamina;* G. *tomē,* a cutting]. Division of a neural lamina of a vertebra.

La'mi·um [L., dead nettle]. A genus of plants of the Labiatae. **L. album** is a species furnishing the alkaloid lamine.

lamp [G. *lampas,* torch]. An apparatus for furnishing artificial light or heat.

annealing l. An alcohol lamp used by dentists for annealing gold leaf.

carbon arc l. A source of therapeutic light, produced by an electric arc between carbon electrodes. Such light contains a mixture of wavelengths from 2200 to 40,000 angstroms. The intensity of various wavelengths between these limits may be altered by impregnation of the carbon electrodes with different salts.

carbon filament l. A luminous heater with maximum emission between 10,000 and 20,000 angstroms. About 30% of the energy is in the range with greatest penetrability.

cold quartz mercury vapor l. A mercury vapor lamp emitting radiations which are practically devoid of heat.

infrared l. A source of heat rays, which emanate from a surface heated to a temperature of 300° to 800° C. The spectral emission ranges through infrared from 8000 to 150,000 angstroms. Such rays have poor penetrability for skin.

mercury vapor l. A hollow fused quartz lamp filled with mercury vapor, producing radiations a large proportion of which are at the radiation emission line of 2540 angstroms, having high germicidal action. This is probably the most suitable source of ultraviolet radiations for routine therapeutic use.

slit l. An instrument designed for examination of the anterior segment of the eye. It produces a bright beam of parallel light and has a microscope which can be focused on any opaque structure of the cornea, iris, or lens.

sunlight l. One which at a measured distance produces rays which imitate in range and intensity the wave lengths of sunshine.

tungsten filament l. A lamp with filament made of tungsten.

Wood's l. See Robert Williams *Wood.*

lam'pas [F., cf. *lamper,* to guzzle]. *In veterinary medicine,* a congestion of the mucous membrane of the hard palate just posterior to the incisor teeth in horses.

lamp'black" [G. *lampas,* torch; AS. *blaec*]. A fine black substance, almost pure carbon, made by burning oils, tars, fats, or resins in an atmosphere deficient in oxygen. The similar product (sometimes called lampblack), obtained by allowing a gas flame to impinge on a cold surface, is more properly designated *gas black* or *carbon black.*

lam·proph'o·ny, lam"pro·pho'ni·a [G. *lampros,* clear, brilliant; *phōnē,* voice]. Clearness of voice. —**lamprophon'ic,** *adj.*

La'mus me·gis'tus. Synonym for *Panstrongylus megistus.*

lam'ziek·te (lahm'zeek·tuh) [S. Afr. D., lame-sickness]. A bone disease of cattle in South Africa, resulting from the eating of contaminated carrion. The disease is due to *Clostridium botulinum D.*

la'na (lay'nuh, lan'uh) [L.]. Wool. See *wool fat.*

lan'a·to·side. A natural glycoside from the leaves of *Digitalis lanata;* three such glycosides have been isolated and are designated **lanatoside A, lanatoside B,** and **lanatoside C,** formerly called digilanid A, digilanid B, and digilanid C, respectively. The aglycones are, respectively, digitoxigenin, gitoxigenin, and digoxigenin. All three lanatosides yield, on hydrolysis with acid, one molecule of D-glucose, three molecules of digitoxose, and one molecule of acetic acid. They are cardioactive.

Lancaster's advancement. See under *advancement,* 2.

lance [L. *lancea,* spear]. Cut or open, as with a lancet or bistoury.

Lancefield groups. See under *Streptococcus.*

Lancereaux, Étienne [*French physician,* 1829–1910]. Made important observations on syphilis. Described diabetes mellitus with extreme emaciation, often seen in association with pancreatic disease; called *Lancereaux's diabetes.* See also Lancereaux's *law* of thrombosis.

lan'cet [F. *lancette*]. A short, double-edged puncturing knife, once in common use for bleeding patients and for lancing the gums of teething children.

spring l. One in which the blade is thrust out by means of a small spring operating on a trigger; often used to obtain small quantities of blood for laboratory examinations.

lan'ci·na"ting [L. *lancinare,* to tear to pieces]. Tearing; shooting, sharply cutting, as lancinating pains. —**lancinate,** *v.*

Lancisi, Giovanni Maria [*Italian physician,* 1654–1720]. Made important contributions to epidemiology. Gave a classic description of aneurysm. See also *stria* longitudinalis, also called *stria of Lancisi.*

land'marks" [AS. *land; mearc*]. Superficial marks, as eminences, lines, and depressions, that serve as guides to, or indications of, deeper parts.

Landolt, Edmond [*French ophthalmologist,* 1846–1926]. Made important contributions to the knowledge of physiologic optics. Described small, elongated bodies lying between the rods and cones on the outer nuclear layer of the retina; called *Landolt's bodies.* The *Landolt ring* is an incomplete ring used as a test object for visual acuity.

Landouzy, Louis Théophile Joseph [*French physician,* 1845–1917]. Described spirochetal jaundice (1883), called *Landouzy's disease, Fiedler's disease,*

Weil's disease. Independently and with Dejerine, described facioscapulohumeral atrophy, called *Landouzy-Dejerine atrophy* or *type.* Neuralgia of the sciatic nerve with atrophy of part or all of the affected leg is known as *Landouzy's sciatica.* A form of purpura with serious systemic symptoms is called *Landouzy's purpura.* The *Landouzy-Grasset law,* named for Landouzy and Joseph Grasset, states that in disease of a single cerebral hemisphere, if there are spastic symptoms, the patient's head inclines toward the side of the affected muscles; if paralysis occurs, the head is turned toward the side of the cerebral lesion.

Landry de Thézillat, Jean Baptiste Octave (1826–1865). French physician who described acute ascending paralysis, also called *Landry's paralysis.*

Landsteiner, Karl (1868–1943). American pathologist who established the basis of blood grouping, discovered isoagglutinins in human blood serum and isoagglutinogens in blood cells (1900) and discovered three of the four main blood groups. The classification adopted by the Permanent Commission on Biology Standards, which designates the four groups as O, A, B, and AB, is also known as the *Landsteiner classification.* He was the first to transmit poliomyelitis from man to monkeys by injection of an emulsion of spinal cord from a fatal case (1909). Landsteiner and Alexander S. Wiener discovered the Rh factor (1940). Nobel laureate (1930).

Lane, William Arbuthnot [*Scottish surgeon in England,* 1856–1943]. Devised steel plates of various shapes, with holes for screws, for fixing fragments in position in cases of fracture; called *Lane's plates.* Described intestinal bends or twists, called *Lane's kinks; Lane's kink* usually refers to an obstructive twist of the ileum. Devised an operation of ileosigmoidostomy for the relief of chronic constipation; called *Lane's operation.* Intestinal stasis is known as *Lane's disease.*

la·nette' wax. An emulsifier, introduced in England as an ingredient of washable ointment bases; it is said to be approximated in composition by a mixture of 9 parts of cetyl alcohol and 1 part of sodium lauryl sulfate.

Lange's test. See under *test.*

Langenbeck, Bernhard Rudolph Konrad von [*German surgeon,* 1810–87]. Made numerous contributions to the development of orthopedic and plastic surgery. Modified the Indian method of rhinoplasty. Devised an operation for cleft palate in which closure was effected by means of periosteal flaps obtained from either side and sutured in the midline.

Langer, Carl von [*Austrian anatomist,* 1819–87]. Plotted lines indicating the direction of skin tension; called *Langer's lines.* These cleavage lines lie in the direction in which skin stretches least and perpendicular to the direction of greatest stretch. Thus, linear scars following the direction of skin tension usually spread little, whereas scars crossing the tension lines have an opposite tendency. Langer described an inconstantly present musculotendinous slip of the latissimus dorsi extending across the axilla anterior to the vessels; it inserts in the region of the pectoralis major, called *Langer's axillary arch.*

Langerhans, Paul [*German physician and anatomist,* 1847–88]. Described the islets of the pancreas (1869), called *islets* or *islands of Langerhans;* see *islet of pancreas.* Described two types of cells called *Langerhans' cells:* star-shaped cells in the stratum germinativum, and spindle-shaped cells in the lumens of the acini of the pancreas. See also stellate *corpuscle,* called *Langerhans' corpuscle.*

Langhans, Theodor [*German anatomist and pathologist in Switzerland,* 1839–1915]. Described the cytotrophoblast, called *layer* or *stria of Langhans.* The cells forming the cytotrophoblast are known as *Langhans' cells.* See also Langhans' giant *cell.*

Langley, John Newport (1852–1925). English physiologist who observed the action of pilocarpine on the heart (1875) and demonstrated that large amounts of nicotine painted on sympathetic ganglia blocked the passage of impulses across them (1889). He contributed greatly to the knowledge of the autonomic nervous system, coined the terms *preganglionic* and *postganglionic,* and described the parasympathetic system (1905), separating it from the sympathetic outflow by differences in response to adrenalin, pilocarpine, and other drugs.

lan'guor (lang'gur) [L.]. A condition of mind and/or body caused by exhaustion; lassitude.

Lannelongue, Odilon Marc [*French surgeon,* 1840–1911]. Transplanted the thyroid gland of an animal to a human being for the relief of thyroid deficiency (1890). Devised a number of operations, including one of craniectomy in which a narrow strip of parietal bone near the sagittal suture was resected, for decompression as in microcephaly. Called *Lannelongue's operation.*

lan"o·ce'ric ac'id (lan"o·seer'ick, lay"no·). A dibasic fatty acid occurring in wool fat.

lanolac. Trade-mark for a sodium-free milk.

lan'o·lin. See hydrous *wool fat.*

lan"o·palm'ic ac'id (lan"o·pal'mick, ·pahl'mick, lay"no·). A fatty acid present in wool fat.

lan·os'ter·ol, lan"o·ster'ol. $C_{30}H_{49}OH$; $\Delta^{8,24}$-lanostadiene-3β-ol; an unsaturated sterol from wool fat which differs from ordinary sterols in having three additional methyl groups attached to the ring system.

Lantermann's incisure. See *incisure* of Schmidt-Lantermann.

lan'tha·nide. Any chemical element of a series beginning with lanthanum, and including cerium, praseodymium, neodymium, promethium, samarium, europium, gadolinium, terbium, dysprosium, holmium, erbium, thulium, ytterbium, and lutetium, the group constituting the lanthanide series of elements, formerly called the *rare-earth elements.*

lan'tha·non. Any element belonging to the lanthanide series of elements.

lan'tha·num [G. *lanthanein,* to escape notice]. La = 138.92. A rare metallic element.

lan·thi'o·nine. $COOH.CHNH_2.CH_2.S.CH_2.CHNH_2.COOH$; β,β'-thiodialanine or bis (2-amino-2-carboxyethyl) sulfide; an amino acid obtained from wool, hair, feathers, and lactalbumin previously treated with mild alkali.

lan'tho·pine. $C_{23}H_{25}NO_4$; a minor alkaloid from opium.

la·nu'go [L., down]. 1. The downlike hair that covers the fetus about the fifth month of gestation. 2. The fine, downy hair that appears on all parts of the body except palms of hands and soles of feet, and those parts, such as the scalp, where other varieties of hair are found. —**lanuginous,** *adj.*

lan'u·lous [L. *lanula,* a small lock of wool]. Covered with short, fine hair.

lanum. Trade name for hydrous wool fat.

lap'a·chol. $C_{15}H_{14}O_3$; 2-hydroxy-3-(3-methyl-2-butenyl)-1,4-naphthoquinone; a yellow pigment in the grain of various woods.

la·pac'tic [G. *lapassein,* to empty]. 1. An evacuant. 2. Any purgative substance.

lap'a·ro-, lapar- [G. *lapara,* soft part of the body between the ribs and the hip]. *In medicine and* *surgery*, a combining form denoting *the flank* or, more loosely, *the abdomen*.

lap″a·ror′rha·phy [*lapara;* G. *rhaphē*, a suture]. Suture of the abdominal wall.

lap″a·rot′o·mist [*lapara;* G. *tomos*, cutting]. A surgeon who performs laparotomies. *Obs.*

lap″a·rot′o·my [*lapara;* G. *tomē*, a cutting]. 1. An incision through the abdominal wall; celiotomy. 2. The operation of cutting into the abdominal cavity through the loin or flank.

lap″a·ro·tra″che·lot′o·my (·tray″ki·lot′o·mee, ·track″i·lot′o·mee) [*lapara;* G. *trachēlos*, neck; *tomē*]. Low Cesarean section. The peritoneal cavity is not opened, the approach being through the cervix of the uterus.

Lapham, Maxwell E. (1899–). American obstetrician known for his research in breech presentation and on the effect of amytal on the uterus in obstetrics. He developed a simple, rapid procedure for laboratory diagnosis of early pregnancy, called the *Friedman-Lapham test*.

la′pis (lay′pis, lap′is) [L.]. A stone; an alchemic term applied to any nonvolatile substance.

l. calaminaris. Calamine.

l. imperialis. Silver nitrate. Also called *l. infernalis*.

l. mitigatus. Diluted silver nitrate.

l. pumicis. Pumice.

Laplace, Pierre Simon de [*French astronomer and physicist*, 1749–1827]. With Lavoisier, demonstrated by means of an ice calorimeter that respiration is a form of combustion.

lap′pa [L., bur]. The root of the common burdock, *Arctium lappa*, or of *Arctium minus*. Contains a bitter principle, a resin, and tannin. It has been used as an aperient, diuretic, and alterative.

lap″pa·con′i·tine. $C_{32}H_{44}N_2O_8$ or $C_{32}H_{42}N_2O_9$; an alkaloid from *Aconitum septentrionale*.

lap′sus [L., from *labi*, to fall]. A fall or slip; ptosis.

l. calami. Slip of the pen; from the psychoanalytic point of view, it reveals an unconscious desire.

l. linguae. Slip of the tongue, considered by psychoanalysts to reveal an unconscious desire.

l. palpebrae superioris. Ptosis of the eyelid.

l. pilorum. Alopecia.

l. unguium. Falling of the nails.

Laqueur, Ludwig [*German ophthalmologist*, 1839–1909]. Introduced the use of physostigmine as a miotic in the treatment of glaucoma (1876).

lar′bish. A form of larva migrans that is seen in Senegal.

lard [L. *laridum*, lard] (*adeps*). The purified internal fat of the abdomen of the domestic hog. Used in pharmacy chiefly as an ingredient of ointment and cerate bases.

benzoinated l. (*adeps benzoinatus*). Lard with 1% of benzoin; used as a mild antiseptic and ointment base.

lar·da′ceous [*laridum*]. 1. Resembling lard. 2. Containing diffuse amyloid infiltration.

largactil. Trade-mark for the antinauseant drug chlorpromazine hydrochloride.

lark′spur [AS. *lāwerce; spura*] (*delphinium*). The dried ripe seed of *Delphinium ajacis;* it contains the alkaloids ajacine and ajaconine.

l. tincture (*tinctura delphinii*). Larkspur 10% w/v in alcohol; used as a pediculicide.

larocaine hydrochloride. Trade-mark for *p*-aminobenzoyl-2, 2-dimethyl-3-diethylaminopropanol hydrochloride, an anesthetic of the procaine type used in surface and infiltration anesthesia in concentrations of 0.25–10.0%.

larodon. Trade-mark for phenyl-dimethyl-isopropyl-pyrazolon; the substance is a white, crystalline powder used as an analgesic and antipyretic.

larosan. Trade-mark for a compound of casein and calcium oxide.

larostidin. Trade-mark for a 4% solution of *l*-histidine hydrochloride used in gastroduodenal-ulcer therapy.

Laroyenne, Lucien [*French surgeon*, 1832–1902]. Known for his operation for draining a pelvic abscess by incising the rectouterine pouch, called *Laroyenne's operation*.

Larrey, Dominique Jean [*French army surgeon*, 1766–1842]. Devised numerous operations, including methods of amputation at the shoulder and hip joints. Improved the methods of treating war wounded, using advanced first-aid stations and fast ambulances.

Larrey's sign. See under *sign*.

Larson method. See under *method*.

lar′va (pl. *larvae*) [L. *larva*, ghost]. An immature, free-living stage in the life cycle of various animals which reach the adult form by undergoing a metamorphosis.

l. migrans. Infestation of the dermis by various larvae, characterized by bizarre red irregular lines which are broad at one end and fade at the other, produced by burrowing larvae, most commonly in the United States by those of *Ancylostoma braziliense*. Syn., *dermamyiasis linearis migrans oestrosa*.

lar′val [*larva*]. 1. Pertaining to or in the condition of a larva. 2. Pertaining to an abortive form of a disease, the full clinical syndrome not developing; as larval pneumonia, larval scarlet fever.

lar′vate [L. *larvatus*, masked]. Concealed; masked; applied to diseases and conditions that are hidden by more obvious conditions, or by some peculiarity of their symptoms.

lar′vi·cide [L. *larva*, ghost; *caedere*, to kill]. Any agent destroying insect larvae.

lar″yn·gal′gi·a [G. *larygx*, larynx; *algos*, pain]. Pain or neuralgia of the larynx.

la·ryn′ge·al cri′sis (la·rin′jul, ·jee·ul, lar″in·jee′ul). An acute laryngeal spasm, sometimes occurring in tabes dorsalis.

lar″yn·gec′to·my (lar″in·jeck′to·mee) [*larygx;* G. *ektomē*, excision]. Extirpation or partial excision of the larynx.

lar″yn·gem·phrax′is [*larygx;* G. *emphraxis*, stoppage]. Closure or obstruction of the larynx.

lar″yn·gis′mus (lar″in·jiz′mus, ·jis′mus) [*larygx*]. A spasm of the larynx. —**laryngismal,** *adj.*

l. stridulus. A spasmodic affection of the larynx, seen most commonly in rachitic infants and young children; characterized by a sudden crowing inspiration followed by an arrest of respiration of several seconds' duration, with increasing cyanosis, and ending with long, loud, whistling inspirations: also called *false croup, spasmodic croup*.

lar″yn·gi′tis [*larygx;* G. *-itis*, inflammation]. Inflammation of the larynx. It may be acute or chronic, catarrhal, suppurative, croupous (diphtheritic), tuberculous, or syphilitic. —**laryngit′ic,** *adj.*

chronic catarrhal l. The most common form of laryngitis; consists of a hypertrophic and an atrophic stage. Symptoms are hoarseness, pain, dryness of the throat, dysphagia, and cough.

diphtheritic l. Inflammation of the larynx occurring with diphtheria. A false membrane, difficult to remove, forms on the mucosa.

dry l. A form characterized by sensations of heat and by fatigue in the throat, persistent cough, and sometimes aphonia. Also called *l. sicca, Türck's trachoma*.

granulomatous l. That associated with multiple

small ulcers of the larynx, as found in tuberculosis of the larynx.

spasmodic l. See *laryngismus* stridulus.

tuberculous l. A type usually secondary to active tuberculosis of the lung. It usually attacks the vocal folds and arytenoid region and later extends as a markedly destructive lesion.

la·ryn′go- (la·ring′go-), **laryng-** [*larygx*]. A combining form signifying *the larynx.*

la·ryn′go·cele [*larygx;* G. *kēlē*, hernia]. A saccular dilatation of the mucosa of the larynx occurring at some site between the hyoid bone and the cricoid cartilage.

ventricular congenital l. An abnormally deep pocket between the true and false vocal folds.

la·ryn″go·cen·te′sis [*larygx;* G. *kentēsis*, a pricking]. Puncture of the larynx.

la·ryn″go·fis′sure [*larygx;* L. *fissura*, fissure]. 1. Division of the larynx for the removal of tumors or foreign bodies. 2. The aperture made in the operation of laryngofissure.

la·ryn′go·graph [*larygx;* G. *graphein*, to write]. An instrument for recording laryngeal movements. —**laryngog′raphy,** *n.*

lar″yn·gol′o·gist [*larygx;* G. *logos*, word]. One who specializes in laryngology.

lar″yn·gol′o·gy [*larygx; logos*]. The science of the anatomy, physiology, and diseases of the larynx. —**laryngolog′ic,** *adj.*

lar″yn·gom′e·try [*larygx;* G. *metron*, a measure]. The systematic measurement of the larynx.

la·ryn″go·pa·ral′y·sis [*larygx;* G. *paralysis*, paralysis]. Paralysis of the laryngeal muscles.

lar″yn·gop′a·thy [*larygx;* G. *pathos*, disease]. Any disease of the larynx.

la·ryn″go·phan′tom [*larygx;* G. *phantasma*, phantom]. An artificial larynx designed for illustrative purposes.

la·ryn″go·pha·ryn′ge·al (la·ring″go·fa·rin′jul, ·jee·ul, ·far″in·jee′ul) [*larygx;* G. *pharygx*, pharynx]. Pertaining conjointly to the larynx and pharynx.

la·ryn″go·phar″yn·gec′to·my (·far″in·jeck′to-mee) [*larygx; pharygx;* G. *ektomē*, excision]. Surgical removal of the larynx and a portion of the pharynx.

la·ryn″go·pha·ryn′ge·us [*larygx; pharygx*]. Old term for the inferior constrictor of the pharynx.

la·ryn″go·phar″yn·gi′tis [*larygx; pharygx;* G. *-itis*, inflammation]. 1. Inflammation of the laryngopharynx. 2. Inflammation of the larynx and the pharynx.

la·ryn″go·phar′ynx [*larygx; pharygx*]. The inferior portion of the pharynx. It extends from the level of the greater cornua of the hyoid bone to that of the inferior border of the cricoid cartilage: also called *hypopharynx, laryngeal pharynx.*

lar″yn·goph′o·ny [*larygx;* G. *phōnē*, voice]. The sound of the voice observed in auscultation of the larynx.

la·ryn′go·plas″ty [*larygx;* G. *plassein*, to form]. Plastic operation upon the larynx.

la·ryn″go·ple′gi·a [*larygx;* G. *plēgē*, stroke]. Paralysis of one or more muscles of the larynx.

la·ryn″go·pto′sis (la·ring″go·to′sis) [*larygx;* G. *ptōsis*, a falling]. Mobility and falling of the larynx; sometimes occurs in old age.

la·ryn″go·rhi·nol′o·gy (la·ring″go·rye·nol′o·jee) [*larygx;* G. *rhis*, nose; *logos*, word]. The branch of medicine which treats of diseases of the larynx and the nose.

la·ryn″gor·rha′gi·a [*larygx;* G. *rhēgnynai*, to burst]. Hemorrhage from the larynx.

lar″yn·gor′rha·phy [*larygx;* G. *rhaphē*, a suture]. Suture of the larynx.

la·ryn″gor·rhe′a, la·ryn″gor·rhoe′a (la·ring″go-ree′uh) [*larygx;* G. *rhoia*, flow]. Excessive secretion of mucus from the larynx, especially when it is used in phonation.

la·ryn″go·scle·ro′ma [*larygx;* G. *sklērōma*, induration]. Induration affecting the larynx. *Rare.*

la·ryn′go·scope [*larygx;* G. *skopein*, to examine]. A tubular instrument, combining a light system and a telescopic system, used in the visualization of the interior larynx and adaptable for diagnostic, therapeutic, and surgical procedures. —**laryngoscop′ic,** *adj.*

lar″yn·gos′co·pist [*larygx; skopein*]. An expert in laryngoscopy.

lar″yn·gos′co·py [*larygx; skopein*]. Examination of the interior of the larynx with the laryngoscope.

direct l. Examination of the interior of the larynx by direct vision with the aid of a laryngoscope.

indirect l. Examination of the interior of the larynx by means of a laryngeal mirror.

suspension l. A method of laryngoscopy devised by Killian, in which the head is suspended on a combined mouth gag and tongue spatula which are supported by a bar connected with a moving overhead crane. The advantages of the method are that it leaves both hands of the examiner free and gives excellent exposure of the larynx, as in examining laryngeal tumors.

la·ryn′go·spasm [*larygx;* G. *spasmos*, spasm]. Spasmodic closure of the glottis; laryngismus stridulus.

lar″yn·gos′ta·sis. Croup.

la·ryn″go·ste·no′sis [*larygx;* G. *stenōsis*, a being straitened]. Contraction or stricture of the larynx.

lar″yn·gos′to·my [*larygx;* G. *stoma*, mouth]. The establishing of a permanent opening into the larynx through the neck.

la·ryn″go·stro′bo·scope (·stro′bo·scope, ·strob′o-scope) [*larygx;* G. *strobos*, a whirling round; *skopein*, to examine]. A laryngoscope combined with an adjustable intermittent source of illumination, used in the observation of the vocal folds. —**laryngostrobos′copy,** *n.*

la·ryn″go·syr′inx (la·ring″go·sirr′inks) (pl. *laryngosyringes*) [*larygx;* G. *syrigx*, pipe]. A laryngeal tube.

la·ryn′go·tome [*larygx;* G. *tomos*, cutting]. A cutting instrument used in laryngotomy.

lar″yn·got′o·my [*larygx;* G. *tomē*, a cutting]. The operation of incising the larynx.

complete l. Incision of the larynx through its whole length.

inferior l. Incision of the larynx through the cricothyroid membrane.

median l. Incision of the larynx through the thyroid cartilage.

superior l. Incision of the larynx through the thyrohyoid membrane. Also called *subhyoid l., thyrohyoid l.*

la·ryn″go·tra′che·al (la·ring″go·tray′kee·ul) [*larygx;* G. *trachys*, rough]. Pertaining conjointly to the larynx and the trachea.

la·ryn″go·tra″che·i′tis (·tray″kee·eye′tis) [*larygx; trachys;* G. *-itis*, inflammation]. Inflammation of the larynx and the trachea.

la·ryn″go·tra″che·o·bron·chi′tis (·tray″kee·o-brong·kigh′tis) [*larygx; trachys;* G. *brogchos*, windpipe; *-itis*]. Acute inflammation of the mucosa of the larynx, trachea, and bronchi.

la·ryn″go·tra″che·os′co·py. Tracheoscopy.

la·ryn″go·tra″che·ot′o·my [*larygx; trachys;* G. *tomē*, a cutting]. Tracheotomy in which the cricoid cartilage and one or more of the upper rings of the trachea are divided.

la·ryn″go·xe·ro′sis (la·ring″go·zi·ro′sis) [*larygx;* G. *xēros*, dry; *-ōsis*, condition]. Dryness of the larynx.

lar'ynx [*larygx*]. The organ of the voice, situated between the trachea and the base of the tongue. It consists of a series of cartilages: the thyroid, the cricoid, and the epiglottis, and three pairs of cartilages: the arytenoid, corniculate, and cuneiform, all of which are lined by mucous membrane and are moved by the muscles of the larynx. The mucous membrane is, on each side, thrown into two transverse folds that constitute the vocal bands or folds, the upper being the false, the lower the true, vocal folds. By the approximation or separation of the vocal folds, the changes in the pitch of the voice are produced. The space between the vocal folds is termed the *glottis* and the margins the *rima glottidis*. See Plate 12. —**laryn'geal** (la·rin'jul, ·jee·ul, lar"in·jee'ul), *adj.*

las·civ'i·a [L. *lascivus*, wanton]. Satyriasis, nymphomania.

las·civ'i·ous [*lascivus*]. Libidinous; wanton; having an unlawful desire; lustful.

Lasègue, Ernest Charles [*French physician*, 1816–83]. Described a sign of sciatic nerve disease: elevation of the extended lower extremity produces pain in the nerve trunk. Called *Lasègue's sign. Lasègue's law* states that superficial lesions or simple functional ailments of an organ increase, whereas organic disease decreases the reflexes.

lash [ME. *lasche*]. 1. An eyelash. 2. A flagellum. *Obs.*

Lashmet and Newburgh's test. See under *test*.

Lassar's paste. See under *paste*.

las'si·tude [L. *lassitudo*, weariness, heaviness]. A state of exhaustion or weakness; debility.

la'tent [L. *latens*, lying hid]. Concealed; not manifest; potential. —**latency,** *n.*

lat'er·ad [L. *latus*, side; *ad*, toward]. Toward the lateral aspect.

lat'er·al [L. *lateralis*, from *latus*, side]. 1. At, belonging to, or pertaining to the side; situated on either side of the median vertical plane. 2. External, as opposed to medial (internal), away from the midline of the body.

lat"er·it'i·in I. An antibiotic substance isolated from cultures of *Fusarium latericium*, perhaps identical with enniatine A.

lat"er·it'i·in II. An antibiotic substance isolated from cultures of a species of *Fusarium*, possibly a strain of *F. latericium.*

lat"er·i'tious, lat"er·i'ceous (lat"ur·ish'us) [L. *latericius*, from *later*, brick]. Resembling brick dust, as the lateritious sediment of the urine.

lat"er·i·ver'sion. See *lateroversion*.

lat'er·o- [L. *latus*, side]. A combining form denoting *laterally, to one side.*

lat"er·o·ab·dom'i·nal [*latus;* L. *abdomen*, belly]. Pertaining to either lateral portion of the abdomen.

lat"er·o·duc'tion [*latus;* L. *ducere*, to lead]. Lateral movement, as of the eye.

lat"er·o·flex'ion (lat"ur·o·fleck'shun) [*latus;* L. *flectere*, to bend]. Bending or curving to one side; the alteration in position of the uterus in which the uterine axis is bent upon itself to one side.

lat"er·o·mar'gin·al [*latus;* L. *margo*, edge]. Placed on the lateral edge.

lat"er·o·pul'sion [*latus;* L. *pulsio*, a beating]. A tendency to move to one side in forward locomotion.

lat"er·o·spor'in. A multiple antibiotic, consisting of laterosporin A and laterosporin B, isolated from cultures of *Bacillus laterosporus*, active in vitro against a number of bacteria.

lat"er·o·tor'sion [*latus;* L. *torquere*, to twist]. A twisting to one side.

lat"er·o·ver'sion [*latus;* L. *vertere*, to turn]. The alteration in position of the uterus in which the entire uterine axis is displaced to one side.

la'tex (pl. *latices*) [L., liquid]. The milky juice of certain plants and trees. Rubber and gutta-percha are commercial products of latex.

l. cells. Cells giving rise to latex or milky juice.

lath'y·rism (lath'i·riz·um) [G. *lathyros*, a kind of pulse]. An affection produced by the use of meal from varieties of vetches, chiefly *Lathyrus sativus* and *L. cicera.* It is a form of spastic paraplegia with tremor, involving chiefly the legs. Syn., *lupinosis.*

la·tis"si·mo·con"dy·lar'is. The dorsoepitrochlearis muscle.

la·tis'si·mus [L., superlative of *latus*, wide]. Widest, as latissimus dorsi muscle. See Table of Muscles in the Appendix.

l. thoracis. BR name for the latissimus dorsi muscle.

la·trine' [L. *latrina*]. A water closet or privy, especially any of a number of types used in military installations, permanent or temporary.

Lat"ro·dec'tus [NL.]. A genus of small black spiders of the family Theridiidae which possesses potent venom and frequently causes serious symptoms in man. *L. basselti* of Australia and *L. luqubria* of Russia are toxic.

L. mactans. The species most dangerous in the Americas; the black widow or hourglass spider. The female of the species alone is dangerous.

lat'tah. A form of imitative neurosis in Malaya.

la'tus, -a, -um [L., wide]. Broad, as ligamentum latum, the broad ligament of the uterus.

Latzko, Wilhelm [*Austrian obstetrician*, 1863–1945]. Devised an operation of low Cesarean section in which the approach is extraperitoneal, with lateral displacement of the urinary bladder and peritoneal reflection. Called *Latzko's low Cesarean, Latzko's operation.*

laud'a·ble [L. *laudare*, to praise]. Healthy; formerly said of a copious pus thought to indicate an improved condition of the wound.

lau·dan'i·dine. $C_{20}H_{25}NO_4$; an alkaloid from opium.

lau'da·nine (law'duh·neen, ·nin). $C_{20}H_{25}NO_4$. One of the alkaloids of opium.

lau·dan'o·sine (law·dan'o·seen, ·sin, law'dun·o·). $C_{21}H_{27}NO_4$. A crystallizable alkaloid of opium.

lau'da·num [NL.]. Opium tincture.

laugh [AS. *hlehhan*]. Normally, an audible expression of mirth. —**laugh,** *v.*

canine l. Risus sardonicus.

sardonic l. Risus sardonicus.

Laughlen test. A flocculation test for syphilis.

laugh'ter [AS. *hleahtor*]. A succession of rhythmic, spasmodic expirations with open glottis and vibration of the vocal folds, expressing mirth.

compulsive l. That seen in schizophrenics; it is without cause and mirthless; the patient usually does not know he is laughing. Also called *obsessive l.*

Laumonier, Jean Baptiste Phillippe Nicolas René [*French anatomist and surgeon*, 1749–1818]. Described the carotid ganglion, also called *Laumonier's ganglion.*

Launois, Pierre Emile [*French physician*, 1856–1914]. With M. Cléret, described hypophyseal gigantism (1910), called *Launois' syndrome, Launois-Cléret syndrome.*

Laurence, John Zachariah [*English ophthalmic surgeon*, ca. 1829–1870]. With Moon, described familial retinitis pigmentosa associated with general defective development (1866). See Laurence-Moon-Biedl *syndrome.*

Laurentjew's phenomenon. See multiplication *phenomenon* of Laurentjew.

lau'ric ac'id. $CH_3(CH_2)_{10}COOH$. A fatty acid derived from cherry laurel and spermaceti.

lau'ro-, laur- [L. *laurus*, laurel]. *In chemistry*, a combining form denoting *lauric acid*.

lauron. Trade-mark for aurothioglycanide, a gold compound used for treatment of rheumatoid arthritis.

lau"ro·tet'a·nine (law"ro·tet'uh·neen, ·nin). $C_{19}H_{21}NO_4$. An alkaloid from the bark of *Litsea citrata*. A powerful poison, acting like strychnine on the spinal cord.

lau'rus [L.]. The leaves of *Laurus nobilis* (bay laurel) containing cineol, *l*-linalool, geraniol, eugenol, etc. Used as a spice.

Lauth, Ernest Alexandre [*Alsatian anatomist and physiologist*, 1803–37]. Described the venous sinus of the sclera (1829); called *Lauth's canal, Schlemm's canal*. See venous *sinus* of the sclera.

Lauth's violet. See *thionine* under *stain*.

la·vage' (lah·vahzh', lav'idj) [F.]. The irrigation or washing out of an organ, such as the stomach, bowel, urinary bladder, or paranasal sinus.

la·va'tion [L. *lavatio*, from *lavare*, to wash]. Lavage; ablution.

lav'en·der [ML. *lavendula*]. The flowers of *Lavandula officinalis*. The active principle is a volatile oil.

compound l. tincture (*tinctura lavandulae composita*). Contains lavender oil, rosemary oil, cinnamon, clove, myristica, and red saunders in a hydroalcoholic menstruum. A popular remedy for nausea and flatulence. Dose, 2–4 cc. (30–60 min.).

l. oil (*oleum lavandulae*). The volatile oil distilled with steam from the fresh flowering tops of *Lavandula officinalis;* contains not less than 30% of esters calculated as linalyl acetate. Used chiefly as a perfume; sometimes as a carminative.

l. spirit (*spiritus lavandulae*). Stimulant and carminative; 5% of oil in alcohol. Dose, 0.6–2.0 cc. (10–30 min.).

la·ven'du·lin. An antibiotic substance, containing sulfur, isolated from a variant of *Actinomyces lavendulae*, active in vitro against a variety of bacteria.

Laveran, Charles Louis Alphonse [*French army physician and bacteriologist*, 1845–1922]. Discovered malarial parasites in blood cells (1880). Nobel laureate (1907).

Lavoisier, Antoine Laurent [*French chemist*, 1743–94]. Called the founder of modern chemistry. Named oxygen, previously isolated by Priestley and Scheele, and discovered its function in combustion; is sometimes called the discoverer of oxygen. With Laplace, demonstrated by means of an ice calorimeter that respiration is a form of combustion.

law [AS. *lagu*]. 1. Statement of a relation or sequence of phenomena invariable under the same conditions. 2. A rule of conduct prescribed by authority.

Adrian-Bronk l. The intensity of excitation of a nerve is directly related to the frequency of discharge of the individual neuron and to the number of neurons.

all-or-nothing l. The response of a single fiber of cardiac muscle, skeletal muscle, or nerve to an adequate stimulus is always maximal. The strength of response depends upon the number of fibers stimulated.

average localization l. Visceral pain is most accurately localized in the least mobile viscera.

Bastian-Bruns l. See Henry C. *Bastian*.

Beer's l. The transmittance of light through a stable solution is an exponential function of the product of the concentration of solute and the length of path in the solution.

biogenetic l. See recapitulation *theory*.

Boyle's l. The osmotic pressure is proportional to the concentration of the solute if the temperature remains invariable.

Cannon's l. of denervation. When in a series of efferent neurons a unit is destroyed, an increased irritability to chemical agents develops in the isolated structure or structures, the effects being maximal in the part directly denervated.

Courvoisier's l. In jaundice due to impaction of a stone in the common duct, the gallbladder will usually be contracted; that due to extrinsic pressure on the common duct (e.g., carcinoma of head of the pancreas) the gallbladder will be distended.

Dalton's laws. See John *Dalton*.

Donder's l. *In ophthalmology*, when the position of the line of fixation is given with respect to the head, there is correspondingly a definite angle of torsion, independent of the observer's volition and the manner in which the line of fixation arrived in the position in question.

Driesch's l. (*of constant volume*). The differences in the total mass of the organ are due to the number and not to the volume of the cells, e.g., the renal or hepatic cells of a bull, man, or mouse have approximately equal size.

Einthoven's l. *In electrocardiography*, the algebraic sum of the potentials of lead I plus those of lead III is equal to the potentials of lead II.

eugenic sterilization l. One providing for the sterilization of persons with certain inheritable mental disorders and deficiencies, who have been committed to mental institutions, and of certain criminals.

Fechner's l. The intensity of a sensation produced by a stimulus varies directly as the logarithm of the numerical value of that stimulus.

Fick's l. of diffusion. The rate at which a dissolved substance diffuses through a medium (solvent) will depend upon the concentration of the substance diffusing.

Fuerbringer's l. The embryological origin of a muscle can be traced by its innervation.

Grotthus' l. Light must be absorbed in order to produce an effect. Frequently known as *Draper's l.*

isodynamic l. In metabolism, different foods are interchangeable in accordance with their caloric values.

Jadassohn-Lewandowsky l. Tubercles or tuberculoid structures tend to appear wherever microorganisms or their products are neutralized or overcome by the local immunological reactions. Thus chronic infections other than tuberculosis can produce the tuberculoid structure.

Kinney's l. A law of speech and hearing—a person with normal speech and hearing who subsequently loses all of his hearing, begins to show speech changes in a length of time that is directly proportional to the length of time that he had speech.

Kohlrausch's l. of migration of ions. Molecular conductivity of a binary electrolyte (one that dissociates into two univalent ions) is u plus v, where the symbol u is given to the part contributed by the cation and v to that contributed by the anion. These are constant values for the same ions, whatever salts they may form.

Lancereaux's l. of thrombosis. Marantic thromboses always occur at the points where there is the greatest tendency to stasis; that is, where the influence of the cardiac propulsion and of thoracic aspiration is least.

l. of Avogadro. Equal volumes of gases at the same pressure contain equal numbers of molecules.

l. of Blagden. The lowering of the freezing point is proportional to the concentration of the solution.

l. of Bunsen-Roscoe. The time required for a reaction to light is inversely proportional to the intensity of the light.

l. of definite proportions. Any chemical compound is formed always by the same elements in the same proportion by weight.

l. of Dulong and Petit. The specific heat of an element varies inversely as its atomic weight.

l. of filial regression. According to Galton, children whose parents deviate from the average of the population likewise deviate from the average in the same direction as the parents, but regress by about one-third of the parental deviation toward the mean. For example, children whose parents are 3 inches above the average stature are themselves on the average about 2 inches above the mean stature of the population.

l. of Howland and Kramer. A maxim concerned with the production and healing of rickets, based on the fact that the solubility product of total serum inorganic phosphorus times total serum inorganic calcium remains approximately constant (40–55 mg per 100 cc in growing children); it states that rickets will occur in children if the product is below 35, and will heal if it rises above 40. The law, with proper modifications, is applicable in cases of osteomalacia in adults (normal value for the product of the ions, 30–40 mg per 100 cc).

l. of independent assortment. The members of different gene-pairs segregate at miosis independently of one another, provided they are located on different pairs of homologous chromosomes.

l. of inverse squares. For point sources of radiant energy the intensity of the radiation at any point varies inversely as the square of the distance from the point source.

l. of Lambert. A mathematical expression of the amount of light absorbed when passed through a liquid or solid medium.

l. of Le Chatelier. A more general form of van't Hoff's principle of mobile equilibrium. See van't Hoff's *principle* of mobile equilibrium.

l. of mass action. The speed of a chemical reaction is proportional to the active masses of the reacting substances. Also called *Guldberg-Waage l.*

l. of Maxwell. The dielectric constant of a substance is identical with the square of its refractive index, as calculated for light of very long wave length or for electric waves.

l. of Müller. However excited, each nerve of special sense gives rise to its own peculiar sensation. Syn., *l. of specific energy.*

l. of multiple proportions. If more than one compound is formed by two elements, the weight of one of the elements remains constant, that of the other element varies as a multiple of the lowest amount of that element in the series of compounds.

l. of parsimony. Economy in the use of a specific means to an end.

l. of progress (Gaskell). The nervous system has been the dominant factor in evolution.

l. of reciprocal proportions. Two elements, which unite with each other, will unite singly with a third element in proportions which are the same as, or multiples of, the proportions in which they unite with each other.

l. of refraction. A ray of light passing from a rarer to a denser medium is turned toward a perpendicular to the surface and in passing from a denser to a rarer medium it is turned away from that perpendicular.

l. of refreshment. The rate of recovery of muscle from fatigue is proportional to its blood supply.

l. of segregation. The two members of any given pair of genes separate at miosis so that a mature germ cell receives one or the other member of each pair of genes.

l. of similars. The Hahnemann rule of homeopathy that like cures like.

L. of Small Numbers. See *Poisson distribution.*

l. of specific energy of nerve. A theory, first formulated by Johannes Müller, that each nerve of special sense gives rise to its own specific sensation, no matter how it is excited.

l. of specific irritability. Every sensory nerve reacts to one form of stimulus and gives rise to one form of sensation. If under abnormal circumstances it is stimulated by other forms of excitation, the sensation produced is the same.

l. of specificity of bacteria. As elucidated by Robert Koch, the microorganism must be present in every case of the disease; it must be capable of cultivation in pure culture; it must, when inoculated in pure culture, produce the disease in susceptible animals. To this has been added a fourth condition: that the organism must be recovered and again grown in pure culture. Also called *Koch's l., Koch's postulate.*

l. of the heart. The force or amplitude of contraction of the heart is proportional within physiologic limits to its diastolic length. Syn., *Starling's law.*

l. of the intestines. A stimulus applied to a given point in the intestinal wall initiates a band of constriction on the proximal side and relaxation on the distal side of the stimulated point.

l. of velocities. Any process, which is on the way to an equilibrium, becomes slower and slower as the final state is approached. Sometimes known as *Newton's l. of cooling.*

linkage l. Different gene-pairs tend to segregate together if they are located on the same pair of homologous chromosomes. Linked genes may be separated with a frequency which varies from 0 to 50%, depending chiefly upon the relative linear distances between them.

Mendel's laws. The laws of heredity. They refer to the way in which the hereditary units, the genes, pass from one generation to the next by way of the germ cells. In neo-Mendelian terms the principles may be stated as follows: Genes segregate at the time of maturation, with the result that a mature germ cell gets either the maternal or the paternal gene of any pair. Genes of different pairs segregate independently of one another, provided they are located on different pairs of chromosomes. If they are located on the same pair of chromosomes, they are linked and consequently segregate in larger or smaller blocks depending mainly on their relative distances apart on the chromosome, i.e., on the percentage of crossing over.

Newton's l. of cooling. The rate of cooling depends on the difference of temperature between the hot body and its surroundings, so that it steadily diminishes as the temperature difference becomes less. Generally known as the *l.* of *velocities.*

periodic l. If the elements are arranged in the sequence of their atomic weights, elements having similar characteristics recur regularly in the series, that is, most of the physical and chemical properties of the elements are periodic functions of their atomic weights. Also called *Mendeléev's l.*

Perrin's l. Particles constituting the internal phase of a colloidal system, if of sufficiently low concentration, must arrange themselves as a result of the influence of gravity, as do the molecules of gases under comparable conditions.

Pflüger's laws. Laws pertaining to the alteration of excitability and conduction of nerves during and after the application of direct electric current.

psychophysical l. See Fechner's *l.*

Rosenbach's l. See under Ottomar *Rosenbach.*
Rubner's laws. See under Max *Rubner.*
Spallanzani's l. See Lazaro *Spallanzani.*
Starling's l. See *l.* of the heart; also see Ernest Henry *Starling.*
Stokes's l. The relationship between velocity of fall of a spherical body as influenced by gravity and the radius of the particle, or the particle size.
van't Hoff's l. See Jacobus Henricus van't *Hoff.*
Weber's l. To excite a series of sensations differing by equal increments, the stimuli must increase in geometric proportion.
Weigert-Meyer l. A urological maxim which states that in cases of reduplication of the upper urinary tract, the lower ureteral orifice belongs to the upper pelvis (Weigert), or in cases where the two orifices are located side by side, the medial orifice belongs to the upper pelvis (Meyer).
Wolff's l. Every change in the use or static relations of a bone leads not only to a change in its internal structure and architecture but also to a change in its external form and function.

Läwen, George Arthur [*German surgeon,* 1876–]. Credited with introducing paravertebral injections in the treatment of angina pectoris (1922). Described a pathologic fracture of the cartilage of the patella (1925); called *Büdinger-Ludloff-Läwen disease.*

Lawson Tait. See *Tait.*

lax'a·tive [L. *laxare,* to lighten, relieve]. Aperient; mildly cathartic.

lax'a·tive. An agent that relieves constipation; a mild purgative.

lax'i·ty [L. *laxitas,* roominess]. 1. Lack or loss of tone, tension, or firmness. 2. Lack of strictness or precision. —**lax,** *adj.*

lay'er [AS. *lecgan*]. A deposited material of uniform, or nearly uniform, thickness, spread over a comparatively considerable area; cover; stratum.
basal-cell l. The deepest layer of cells in the germinative layer of a stratified epithelium.
basal l. The nondeciduate stratum basalis of the endometrium, containing the blind ends of the uterine glands. Syn., *stratum basalis.*
choriocapillary l. See choriocapillary *lamina.*
compact l. The superficial layer of the endometrium during the secretory phase of the menstrual cycle; it is characterized by the presence of many decidual cells in pregnancy. Syn., *stratum compactum.*
dermic l. The middle layer of the tympanic membrane.
ependymal l. A layer of elongated nuclei near the central canal of the neural tube. Syn., *nuclear l.*
external granular l. of the cerebellum. A granular layer in fetal and neonatal cerebellar cortex: also called *Obsteiner's l.*
external granular l. of the cerebrum. The second layer of the cerebral cortex, containing a large number of small pyramidal and granule cells. Also called *layer of small pyramidal cells.*
external pyramidal l. See *l.* of pyramidal cells.
ganglionic l. (a) The inner cell layer of the retina. (b) The deep layer of large pyramidal cells in the cerebral cortex: in the motor area it contains the giant pyramidal cells: also called *internal pyramidal l.*
germinative l. The deeper, proliferative layers of cells of the epidermis, including the basal-cell layer and the prickle-cell layer. Syn., *stratum germinativum, malpighian l.*
germ l. One of the epithelial layers of the blastula or blastocyst from which the various organs of the embryo are derived. See *ectoderm, entoderm, mesoderm.*
granular l. The layer deep to the molecular layer of the cerebellar cortex, containing a large number of granule cells.
granular l. of Tomes. A thin zone of imperfectly calcified dentin immediately under the cementum in the roots of teeth.
half-value l. *In roentgenology,* that thickness of a suitable absorber which reduces the intensity of a given x-ray beam to half of its initial value.
horny l. The stratum corneum of the epidermis.
infragranular l. The ganglionic layer and the layer of fusiform cells of the cerebral cortex collectively.
inner nuclear l. The layer of the retina made up chiefly of the cell bodies of the bipolar neurons.
internal granular l. The fourth layer of the cerebral cortex containing many small multipolar cells with short axons, and scattered small pyramidal cells.
internal pyramidal l. See ganglionic *l.* (b).
l. of fusiform cells. The deepest layer of the cerebral cortex, with irregular fusiform and angular cells, whose axons enter the subjacent white matter. Syn., *multiform l.*
l. of Henle. The outermost layer of the internal root sheath of hair.
l. of Huxley. The middle layer of the internal root sheath of hair.
l. of Langhans. The inner, cellular layer of the ectoderm of the chorion. Syn., *cytotrophoblast.*
l. of pyramidal cells. The third layer of the cerebral cortex, having a superficial stratum containing chiefly medium-sized pyramidal cells and a deeper stratum containing large pyramidal cells: also called *external pyramidal l.*
l. of rods and cones. Outer layer of the retina.
malpighian, Malpighian l. See germinative *l.*
mantle l. A layer of neuroblasts between the ependymal and marginal layers of the (developing) neural tube.
marginal l. A narrow nonnuclear zone in the external part of the neural tube.
molecular l. (a) The outermost layer of the cerebral or of the cerebellar cortex, made up of neuroglia, a few small ganglion cells, and a reticulum of myelinated and unmyelinated nerve fibers. (b) One of the two layers, inner and outer of the retina, made up of interlacing dendrites. Also called *plexiform layer.*
multiform l. See *l.* of fusiform cells.
nuclear l. See ependymal *l.*
Obersteiner's l. See external granular *l.* of the cerebellum.
osteogenic l. The deeper layer of periosteum, connected with the formation of bone.
outer nuclear l. The layer of the retina which contains the rod and cone granules, or cell bodies.
papillary l. The surface layer of the derma, extending into the papillae formed by the uneven line of union of the dermis and epidermis.
pigment l. The external layer of the embryonic optic cup or retina.
plexiform l. See molecular *l.*
prickle-cell l. The germinative layer of the epidermis exclusive of the basal cells.
reticular l. The deeper layer of the derma, composed of a dense network of collagenous and elastic fibers.
somatic l. The external layer of the lateral mesoderm after the formation of the coelom, forming a part of the somatopleure.
splanchnic l. The internal layer of the lateral mesoderm after the formation of the coelom, forming a part of the splanchnopleure.
spongy l. The middle zone of the endometrium during the secretory phase of the menstrual cycle,

characterized by the dilated portion of the glands and edematous connective tissue. Syn., *stratum spongiosum.*

subendocardial l. A layer of loose connective tissue binding the endocardium and myocardium together.

subendothelial l. The middle layer of the tunica intima of veins and of medium and larger arteries. It consists of collagenous and elastic fibers and a few fibroblasts.

suprachoroid l. See *lamina* suprachorioidea.

supragranular l. The external granular layer and layer of pyramidal cells of the cerebral cortex collectively.

tympanic covering l. The connective-tissue layer covering the lower surface of the basilar membrane of the cochlea.

vestibular covering l. The connective-tissue layer covering the upper surface of the basilar membrane of the cochlea.

lay·ette′ [F.]. A full outfit of garments, bedding, etc., for a newborn child.

lay′man [G. *laos*, people; AS. *mann*]. A member of the laity; a person not a member of a given professional group, as distinguished from a member of the group.

la′zar, laz′ar [G. *Lazaros*, from the Hebrew]. An old name for a leper, or for any person having a repulsive disease.

laz″a·ret′to [It.]. 1. A public hospital for the care of persons suffering from contagious diseases, especially lepers; a pesthouse. 2. A building or vessel used for quarantine.

Lazear, Jesse William [*American physician*, 1866–1900]. Member with Reed, Carroll, and Agramonte y Simoni of the United States Army Yellow Fever Commission which proved that yellow fever is transmitted to man by mosquitoes (1900).

lb. *Libra;* pound (usually avoirdupois).

℔. *Libra;* pound (usually apothecaries').

LCT 50 See median lethal gas *exposure.*

LD Lethal dose; the smallest dose that kills the test animal: also written L. D.

LD 50 dose. Median lethal dose: also written LD_{50}.

LD 100 dose. Total lethal dose: also written LD_{100}.

L. D. Perception of light difference; also, lethal dose.

L. D. A. Left dorsoanterior position of the fetus.

L. D. P. Left dorsoposterior position of the fetus.

L.D.S. Licentiate in Dental Surgery.

LE Lupus erythematosus.

L. E. 1. Left eye. 2. Lupus erythematosus.

leach′ing [AS. *leccan*]. The process of washing or extracting the soluble constituents from insoluble material.

lead (led) [AS. *lēad*] (*plumbum*). Pb = 207.21. A soft, bluish-gray, malleable metal, occurring in nature chiefly as the sulfide, PbS, known as *galena.* Its soluble salts are violent irritant poisons, formerly used as local astringents. Insoluble lead salts at one time were used as protectives, but due to the danger of absorption, the therapeutic use of lead compounds has been practically discontinued.

basic l. chromate. $PbO.PbCrO_4$. A red pigment. Syn., *chrome red.*

colloidal l. A dispersion of lead or one of its compounds; has been administered intravenously, with some good results, in treating cancer.

diluted l. subacetate solution. Lead subacetate solution diluted with approximately 30 volumes of water; applied externally. Syn., *l. water.*

l. acetate (*plumbi acetas*). $(CH_3COO)_2Pb.3H_2O$. Occurs as white crystals; a local astringent in 1–2% solution. Syn., *sugar of lead.*

l. and opium lotion (*lotio plumbi et opii*). Prepared from lead acetate, opium tincture, and water. An embrocation of doubtful value for sprains and bruises. Also called *l. and opium wash.*

l. arsenate. Approximately $PbHAsO_4$; a dense, white powder, insoluble in water, used as a constituent of insecticides.

l. arsenite. Approximately $Pb(AsO_2)_2$; a white powder, insoluble in water, used as a constituent of insecticides.

l. borosilicate. A mixture of the borate and silicate of lead; a constituent of certain optical glasses.

l. carbonate. Approximately $(PbCO_3)_2.Pb(OH)_2$; basic lead carbonate or lead subcarbonate; a white powder, insoluble in water: used chiefly as a pigment.

l. chloride. $PbCl_2$; a white, crystalline powder, sparingly soluble in water.

l. chromate. $PbCrO_4$. A yellow powder; used as a pigment. Syn., *chrome yellow.*

l. dioxide. PbO_2; a dark-brown powder, insoluble in water, used in preparation of electrodes, also as an oxidizing agent, and for industrial purposes. Syn., *lead peroxide.*

l. monoxide (*plumbi monoxidum*). PbO. A yellowish or reddish powder, almost insoluble in water. An ingredient of lead plaster; occasionally used as an ingredient of external applications for relieving inflammation. Also called *litharge, yellow l. oxide.*

l. nitrate. $Pb(NO_3)_2$; occasionally employed in solution as an astringent.

l. oleate. An unctuous material of varying composition; active ingredient of lead oleate plaster.

l. oleate ointment. See under *ointment.*

l. oleate plaster (*emplastrum oleatis*). Made by the interaction of lead monoxide, olive oil, and lard; formerly used as a protective for skin inflammations. Syn., *l. plaster.* Also called *diachylon plaster.*

l. orthoplumbate. Pb_2PbO_4 (or Pb_3O_4). An orange-red powder, almost insoluble in water; formerly used externally as a protective. Also called *minium, red l., red l. oxide.*

l. oxide. See *l.* monoxide and *l.* orthoplumbate.

l. peroxide. Lead dioxide.

l. plaster. See *l.* oleate plaster.

l. subacetate solution (*liquor plumbi subacetatis*). A solution of approximately $Pb_2O(CH_3COO)_2$; an externally applied astringent and sedative. Also called *Goulard's extract.* Also see diluted *l.* subacetate solution; *l.* water and laudanum.

l. tetraethyl. $Pb(C_2H_5)_4$. A colorless, inflammable liquid; used as an anti-knock ingredient in motor fuels. Acute or chronic poisoning may result from its inhalation.

l. water. See diluted *l.* subacetate solution.

l. water and laudanum. A mixture of lead subacetate solution with an equal volume of opium tincture; used as an external application to sprains and bruises.

sugar of l. See *l.* acetate.

white l. Lead carbonate; used in paints. Formerly used as an external astringent and protective.

lead (leed) [AS. *laēdan*]. A pair of terminals or electrodes situated within or upon the body, each connected either directly or through resistors to a recording instrument for the purpose of measuring the difference in electrical potential between them.

augmented unipolar limb l. A form of unipolar limb lead whose amplitude is increased 50 per cent. Two limb leads connected to a central terminal constitute one electrode, and a connection with the other limb constitutes the other lead.

bipolar limb l. See standard limb *l.*

CF l. Precordial lead paired with the left leg (so-called indifferent electrode) and connected to the galvanometer so that an upright deflection in the finished record represents positivity.

chest l. An electrocardiograph lead derived by placement of electrodes on the chest.

CL l. Precordial lead paired with the left arm (so-called indifferent electrode) and connected to the galvanometer so that an upright deflection in the finished record represents positivity.

CR l. Precordial lead paired with the right arm (so-called indifferent electrode) and connected to the galvanometer so that an upright deflection in the finished record represents positivity.

CV l. Precordial lead pairing with the precordial electrode and joining electrodes from the three extremities (central terminal). Connections are made with the galvanometer in such a way that the finished record presents upward deflections of positive value.

electrocardiogram l. A pair of terminals placed on the body surface which records electric potential differences due to cardiac action.

electroencephalographic l. A pair of terminals which measures the potential differences resulting from cerebral activity between two points on the skull.

esophageal l. An electrode placed in the esophagus adjacent to the heart and paired with an indifferent electrode; used to study atrial waves or posterior myocardial infarction.

extremity l. A standard limb *l.*

indirect l. An electrical connection in which all of the electrodes are distant from the current source, e.g., heart, brain, muscle, or spinal cord.

l. axis. See electric *axis.*

l. IV (R, L, F). Precordial electrode placed just external to the apex of the heart, paired with the right arm, left arm, and left leg, respectively.

precordial l. One taken from the precordium, one electrode being placed over the precordium and the other at some distant or indifferent region; precordial leads are CF, CL, CR, and CV.

semidirect l. An electrical connection in which the exploring electrode is placed in close proximity to the source of current (heart, brain, etc.), while the indifferent electrode or combination of electrodes is far removed.

standard limb l. An electrocardiographic connection between electrodes placed on two limbs: lead I, a combination of right and left arms; lead II, of right arm and left leg; lead III, of left arm and left leg. Syn., *bipolar limb l.*

unipolar l. An electrocardiogram taken with one electrode on a region with potential variations of considerable magnitude and another on a region with minimal potential changes.

unipolar limb l. *In electrocardiography,* one in which the exploring electrode is paired with an electrode that is relatively indifferent (central terminal).

voltage l. One taken by means of a precordial electrode paired with a central terminal (joining electrodes placed on the right arm, left arm, and left leg); V_1 right margin of sternum in fourth interspace, V_2 left margin of sternum in fourth interspace, V_3 midway between the left sternal margin and midclavicular line, V_4 midclavicular line, V_5 left anterior axillary line, V_6 midaxillary line, the latter three on a line to the apex and then horizontal from the apex. Also called *V lead.*

Leadbetter, Guy Whitman [*American orthopedic surgeon,* 1893–1945]. Devised a method of reduction in fracture of the femoral neck. The patient lies supine on a table, the anterior superior spines of the ilium being held firmly. The operator, facing the patient's feet, places his shoulder under the patient's calf to provide a fulcrum, and with both hands over the front of the leg above the ankle, exerts downward pressure on the long axis of the femur. Called *Leadbetter's procedure.*

lead′er (lee′dur) [AS. *lǣdan*]. A sinew or tendon. *Obs.*

lead′ing (led′ing) [AS. *lēad*]. Vernacular for chronic lead poisoning.

lead poi′son·ing. A form of poisoning due to the introduction of lead into the system. **Acute lead poisoning** is characterized by an immediate metallic taste and a burning sensation in the throat. Severe abdominal pain occurs, and, later, local paralysis and collapse. **Chronic lead poisoning** (saturnism or plumbism) occurs in persons long exposed to repeated absorption of small amounts of the element. There is anorexia, general lassitude, various dyspeptic symptoms, and obstinate constipation associated with violent pain. A blue line on the gums may appear, as may basophilic degeneration of the red blood cells. Various nervous symptoms may develop, such as the characteristic wrist drop.

leaf [AS. *lēaf*]. A term occasionally employed in anatomic descriptions of certain parts of the body, as the right or left leaf of the diaphragm.

Leake and Guy's method. See under *method.*

Le·ã′o's (lay·ow′o) **spread′ing de·pres′sion.** See under *depression.*

learn′ing dis·tur′bance or **de·fect′.** Any specific defect in the ability of a child to learn one of the basic academic disciplines, as strephosymbolia, or a general defect in learning to read or write, or in learning mathematics. It may be due to specific organic disorder, and is often complicated by habit disturbances.

Leber, Theodor [*German ophthalmologist,* 1840–1917]. Described a rare hereditary form of axial neuritis of the optic nerve (1871); called *Leber's optic atrophy.*

le Boë. See Franciscus *Sylvius.*

lec″a·nop′a·gus [*lekanē; pagos*]. Conjoined twins with union of the pelves and lower parts, and separate heads, necks, and upper thoraxes. Also called *dicephalus.*

lec″a·nor′in A. An antibiotic substance isolated from the lichen *Lecanora esculenta.*

lec″a·no·so″ma·top′a·gus [G. *lekanē,* basin; *sōma,* body; *pagos,* that which is fixed]. Equal twins conjoined by the pelves and thoraxes, or by the vertebral columns; a form of dicephalism.

Lecat, Claud Nicolas (1700–1768). French surgeon and anatomist. Dilatation of the bulbous portion of the urethra is known as *Lecat's gulf.*

Le Chatelier's law. See *law* of Le Chatelier.

le′che de hi·gue·ron′ (lay′chay day ee·gay·rohn′. *See* Notes § 35) [Sp.]. The crude sap of a bastard fig tree, *Ficus glabrata* or *F. doliara;* used in Central and South America as an anthelmintic, especially in trichuriasis.

lech″o·py′ra (leck″o·pye′ruh, leck·op′i·ruh) [G. *lechō,* woman in childbed; *pyr,* fire]. Puerperal fever.

lec′i·thal (less′i·thul) [G. *lekithos,* yolk]. Having a yolk; used especially in combination, as alecithal and telolecithal.

lec″ith·al′bu·min (less″ith·alb′yoo·min, ·alb·yoo′-min) [*lekithos;* L. *albus,* white]. A more or less stable compound of albumin and lecithin, found in various organs.

lec′i·thin (less′i·thin) [*lekithos*]. Any of a group of phospholipids of the general composition $CH_2OR_1.CHOR_2.CH_2OPO_2OHR_3$ in which R_1 and R_2 are fatty acids and R_3 is choline; a colorless to yellow-brown, waxy solid widely distributed in the body. —**lec′ithoid,** *adj.*

lec'i·thi·nase. An enzyme which catalyzes the breakdown of a lecithin to its constituents.

l. A. An enzyme catalyzing the removal of only one fatty acid from lecithin and yielding lysolecithin.

l. B. An enzyme catalyzing the removal of the fatty acid from lecithin or lysolecithin and yielding choline phosphate.

lec'i·tho·blast" (less'ith·o·blast", leh·sith'o·blast) [*lekithos;* G. *blastos,* germ]. The entoblast or primitive entoderm of the bilaminar blastodisk.

lec"i·tho·pro'te·in [*lekithos;* G. *prōteios,* of first rank]. A compound of lecithin with a protein molecule. See American Classification of Proteins in the Appendix.

lec"i·tho·vi·tel'lin. The lecithin-phosphoprotein complex as found in egg yolk.

lec'tin. A general term for blood-group specific agglutinins, occurring in seeds and other parts of certain plants; some lectins are also specific precipitins.

ledercillin. Trade-mark for a brand of penicillin G preparations for oral or topical use.

Lederer, Max [*American pathologist,* 1885–1952]. Known for his description of an acute hemolytic anemia of unknown cause associated with jaundice, fever, and severe systemic symptoms, but responding to blood transfusions (1925); called *Lederer's anemia.*

Leduc, Stéphane Armand Nicolas [*French physicist,* 1853–1939]. Remembered for his introduction of an interrupted, direct electric current used in the production of electric narcosis; called *Leduc's current.*

Lee, Robert (1793–1877). Scottish gynecologist and obstetrician in England who described the cervical ganglion found in the uterine nerve plexus, called *Lee's ganglion.*

Lee's test. See under *test.*

Lee-White method. See under *method.*

leech [AS. *lǣce*]. Any parasitic annelid of the class Hirudinea; some leeches have been detrimental, and some have aided medically. Infestation by leeches (hirudiniasis) may be either internal or external.

medicinal l. See *Hirudo medicinalis.*

leech'es [*lǣce*]. A mycotic disease of horses and mules characterized by localized lesions on the skin.

lees (leez) [OF. *lie*]. Dregs of vinous liquors.

Leeuwenhoek, Antonj van [*Dutch naturalist,* 1632–1723]. Pioneer microscopist, credited with the discovery of bacteria and protozoa, the first description of spermatozoa, which had been pointed out to him by a student, and the first reasonably accurate description of red blood cells. Described the crystalline lens and the rods of the retina.

Le Fort, Léon Clément (1829–1893). French surgeon who introduced an operation for uterine prolapse in which a rectangular area of vaginal mucosa is removed from the anterior and posterior walls of the vagina. These areas are then approximated by sutures, closing the vagina except for a small channel on either side. This is called *partial colpocleisis* or *Le Fort's operation.*

left [ME.]. Sinistral; opposite of right.

left. The left-hand side. Abbreviated, l.

left'-hand"ed. Having the left hand stronger or more expert than the right, or using the left hand in preference to the right.

leg [ON. *leggr*]. The lower extremity, especially that part from the knee to the ankle.

bowleg. Genu varum. See *bowleg.*

milk l. Phlegmasia alba dolens.

restless legs. A disease of unknown mechanism characterized by paresthesia of the muscles and bones, pain, and weakness, especially in the legs. Relief generally is afforded by moving the legs and walking. Also called *Wittmaack-Ekbom syndrome.*

rider's l. Strain of the adductor muscles of the thigh.

Legal, Emmo [*German physician,* 1859–1922]. Described paroxysmal pains and tenderness of the scalp in the region supplied by the auriculotemporal nerve, associated with pharyngotympanic inflammation; called *Legal's disease.* Devised a test for acetone. See Legal's *test.*

Legallois, Julien Jean César [*French physician,* 1770–1814]. Investigated the relation of the vagus nerve to respiration; reported bronchopneumonia following the bilateral section of the vagus. Credited with locating the respiratory center in the medulla (1812).

Legg, Arthur Thornton [*American orthopedic surgeon,* 1874–1939]. Described osteochondritis deformans juvenilis, called *Legg-Calvé-Perthes disease.*

le·git'i·ma·cy [L. *legitimus,* legitimate]. The state of being born within wedlock.

le·gu'me·lin, leg"u·me'lin. An albumin found in most leguminous seeds.

le·gu'min, leg'u·min. A globulin found in the seeds of many plants belonging to the Leguminosae. —**legu'minous,** *adj.*

Leiboff and Kahn's method. See under *method.*

Leichtenstern's phenomenon. See under *phenomenon.*

Leiner's disease. See *erythroderma* desquamativa.

lei'o- (lye'o-), **li'o-** [G. *leios,* smooth]. A combining form signifying *smooth.*

lei"o·der'ma·tous [*leios;* G. *derma,* skin]. Smooth-skinned.

lei"o·der'mi·a, li"o·der'mi·a [*leios; derma*]. A condition of abnormal smoothness and glossiness of the skin.

lei"o·my"o·fi·bro'ma (lye"o·my"o·figh·bro'muh) [*leios;* G. *mys,* muscle; L. *fibra,* fiber; G. *-ōma,* tumor]. A benign tumor composed of cells of smooth muscle and fibrous connective tissue.

lei"o·my·o'ma (lye"o·migh·o'muh) [*leios; mys; -ōma*]. A benign tumor consisting largely of smooth muscle cells; may be found in any position where there is preexisting smooth muscle. In the uterus, these tumors are usually multiple, and may reach a weight of several kilograms; in skin, they are usually small, though multiple and arranged in groups, and are at times painful. Also called *Huguier's disease, fibromyoma of uterus, myofibroma of uterus.*

malignant l., metastasizing l. Leiomyosarcoma.

lei"o·my"o·sar·co'ma [*leios; mys;* G. *sarkōma,* fleshy excrescence]. A malignant tumor composed in large part of smooth muscle cells, many of which are poorly differentiated or of embryonal form; multinucleated neoplastic cells are frequent. Also called *malignant* or *metastasizing l.*

lei·ot'ri·chous (lye·ot'ri·kus) [*leios;* G. *thrix,* hair]. Having smooth or straight hair.

lei"po·me'ri·a (lye"po·meer'ee·uh) [G. *leipein,* to leave; *meros,* part]. Congenital absence of one or more limbs.

Leishman's stain. See under *stain.*

Leishman-Donovan bodies. See under *body.*

Leish·ma'ni·a (leesh·may'nee·uh, ·man'ee·uh, lyshe·) [after William Boog *Leishman,* 1865–1926]. A genus of protozoan flagellates whose species are morphologically similar but differ in serologic reactions; transmitted to man by the bite of a species of *Phlebotomus.*

L. brasiliensis. That species confined largely to Central and South America. This parasite shows a predilection for the mucocutaneous borders of the nose and mouth and produces leishmaniasis americana. Syn., *L. peruviana, L. tropica* var. *americana.*

L. donovani. A species which is the etiologic agent of kala-azar, the visceral form of leishmaniasis.

L. infantum. A parasite, observed in the Mediterranean area, believed generally to belong to the species *L. donovani;* the causative agent of infantile leishmaniasis.

L. peruviana. *L. brasiliensis.*

L. tropica. This species affects primarily the skin and produces oriental sore.

L. tropica var. americana. *L. brasiliensis.*

leish″man·i′a·sis (leesh″mun·eye′uh·sis, lyshe″-mun·) [*Leishman;* NL. *-iasis,* condition]. A variety of visceral and superficial infections caused by protozoan parasites of the genus *Leishmania.* Several species of biting flies belonging to the genus *Phlebotomus* are chiefly responsible for transmission. In India, man constitutes the chief reservoir, but in the Mediterranean region infected dogs are considered to be the reservoirs for the infantile form of the disease.

cutaneous l. An Old World skin infection caused by *Leishmania tropica,* and a New World skin infection caused by *Leishmania brasiliensis.* See *oriental sore, leishmaniasis americana.*

infantile l. A form of kala-azar, observed primarily in small children in the Mediterranean area, clinically identical with that of adults. It is acquired from dogs who act as reservoirs for the parasite *Leishmania infantum.*

l. americana. A form of leishmaniasis caused by the *Leishmania brasiliensis,* differing primarily from oriental sore by the fact that in 10–20% of the cases the mucous membranes are involved, leading to extensive necrosis of the nose, mouth, and pharynx: also called *Bahia ulcer, Bauru ulcer, chiclero ulcer, bosch yaws, forest yaws, uta.* Syn., *American l., South American l., espundia.*

South American l. See *l.* americana. Syn., *L. tropica* var. *americana; L. peruviana.*

visceral l. See *kala-azar.*

Leloir, Henri Camille Chrysostome [*French dermatologist,* 1855–96]. Described an erythmoid variety of lupus vulgaris; called *Leloir's disease.*

le′ma [G. *lēmē,* a humor in the corner of the eye, rheum]. A collection of dried secretion of the tarsal glands at the inner canthus of the eye.

Lembert, Antoine [*French surgeon,* 1802–51]. Widely known and remembered for his introduction of an interrupted approximation suture adapted to uniting divided serous layers of intestine. This is regarded as having brought about a new concept of intestinal surgery, and is considered the basis for present-day gastric and intestinal surgery. Called *Lembert's suture.*

Le Mesurier, Arthur Baker [*Canadian surgeon,* 1889–]. With Gallie, devised an operation for the radical cure of inguinal hernia. See under *Gallie.*

-lem′ma [G. *lemma,* sheath, husk]. A combining form denoting *a sheath* or *envelope.*

lem′mo·cyte, lem′no·cyte [*lemma;* G. *kytos,* cell]. A formative cell for the neurilemma.

lem·nis′cus (pl. *lemnisci*) [G. *lēmniskos,* fillet]. A secondary sensory pathway of the central nervous system, which usually decussates and terminates in the thalamus.

lateral l. The secondary auditory pathway arising in the cochlear nuclei and terminating in the inferior colliculus and medial geniculate body; it crosses in the trapezoid body: formerly called *lateral fillet.*

medial l. That arising in the nucleus gracilis and nucleus cuneatus, crossing immediately as internal arcuate fibers, and terminating in the posterolateral ventral nucleus of the thalamus: formerly called *medial fillet.*

spinal l. The lateral and ventral spinothalamic tracts combined as they ascend in the brain stem.

trigeminal l. The secondary fibers from the main sensory nucleus of the trigeminal nerve and spinal nucleus of the trigeminal nerve, terminating in the posteromedial ventral nucleus of the thalamus: also called *trigeminothalamic tract.*

lem′no·blast [G. *lemma,* sheath, husk; *blastos,* germ]. A primitive neurilemma cell.

lem′no·cyte. See *lemmocyte.*

lem′on [F. *limon,* from Ar. *laymūn*]. The fruit of *Citrus limon.*

l. oil (*oleum limonis*). The volatile oil obtained by expression, without the aid of heat, from the fresh peel of the fruit of *C. limon;* its characteristic odor is due chiefly to citral, an aldehyde.

l. peel (*limonis cortex*). The outer yellow rind of the fresh ripe fruit of *C. limon;* it contains a volatile oil and the glycoside hesperidin.

l. tincture (*tinctura limonis*). An aromatic; prepared by macerating lemon peel with alcohol.

le″mo·pa·ral′y·sis [G. *laimos,* gullet; *paralysis,* paralysis]. Paralysis of the esophagus.

le″mo·ste·no′sis [*laimos;* G. *stenōsis,* a being straitened]. Constriction of the pharynx or esophagus.

Lempert, Julius [*American otologist,* 1891–]. Devised a one-stage fenestration operation for the improvement of hearing in otosclerosis; a permanently mobile window is formed in the lateral semicircular canal. Called *Lempert's operation.*

Lenard rays. See under *ray.*

Lenhartz diet. See under *diet.*

Lenhossék, Mihály [*Hungarian anatomist,* 1863–1937]. Contributed to the knowledge of the histology of the central nervous system. Described the ascending roots of the vagus and glossopharyngeal nerves; called *bundle of Lenhossék.*

len′i·ceps [L. *lenis,* mild, gentle; *caput,* head]. Obstetric forceps with short handles.

lenigallol. Trade-mark for a brand of pyrogallol triacetate.

len′i·tive [*lenis*]. Soothing, emollient, demulcent.

len′i·tive. An emollient remedy or application.

Lennander, Karl Gustaf (1857–1908). Swedish surgeon who described a laparotomy, in which he incised the anterior rectus sheath through a paramedian incision, retracted the rectus abdominis muscle laterally, and made a second incision through the posterior rectus sheath and peritoneum.

lens [L., lentil]. 1. A piece of glass or crystal for the refraction of rays of light. 2. The crystalline lens of the eye. See Plate 19.

absorption l. One used in spectacles, designed to prevent certain wavelengths from reaching the retina; may be a yellow or amber lens, which absorbs the upper range beyond violet (the actinic rays) which have been said to be harmful, or may be one designed to absorb a determined amount of the entire spectrum, as in antiglare glasses or sunglasses, which, while altering the apparent color, diminish visual acuity only when illumination is reduced to threshold.

achromatic l. A double lens, each part made of such optical glass that the one neutralizes the dispersive effects of the other, without affecting the refraction.

aplanatic l. A lens corrected for spherical aberration: also called *rectilinear l.*

apochromatic l. A compound lens corrected for spherical and chromatic aberration.

biconcave l. A negative or minus, thick-edged lens, having concave spherical surfaces upon its opposite sides; used in spectacles in the correction of myopia.

biconvex l. A positive or plus, thin-edged lens, having two convex surfaces; used in the correction of hyperopia.

bifocal l. See *bifocal.*

contact l. A lens for the correction of refractive errors, consisting of a plastic shell, the concavity of which is in contact with the globe of the eye; a layer of liquid is interposed between the lens and the cornea.

converging l. A double convex or planoconvex lens that focuses rays of light.

convexoconcave l. A lens having a convex and a concave surface, which would not meet if continued. Its properties are those of a convex lens of the same focal distance.

crystalline l. The lens of the eye, a refractive organ of accommodation; a biconvex, transparent, elastic body lying in its capsule immediately behind the pupil of the eye, suspended from the ciliary body by the ciliary zonule.

cylindrical l. A minus or plus lens, with a plane surface in one axis and a concave or convex surface in the axis at right angles to the first. Abbreviated, C., Cyl.

decentered l. One with the optic center not opposite to the pupil of the eye.

dispersing l. A concave lens.

eye l. That lens of a microscope which is nearest to the eye; the eyepiece.

im·mer′sion l. A lens, usually of high power, the lower end of which is immersed in a drop of some liquid, such as oil, that has nearly the same refractive index as glass, and is placed on the cover glass of the object under examination.

iseikonic l. A temporary lens, known as a fit-over; may be of two kinds, over-all or meridional.

negative l. A lens with a negative focal length, the edge of the lens being thicker than the center. The three negative lenses are, according to their figure: planoconcave, double concave or biconcave, and diverging concavoconvex.

optical center of l. That which lies on the lens axis; a ray of light passing through a lens so that its angular magnification is unity will pass through the optical center of the lens.

orthoscopic l. One which gives a flat, undistorted field of vision.

overcorrection of l. An aberration of a lens causing the light rays passing the central zones to focus at a point nearer to the lens than rays passing the outer zones.

periscopic l. One with concavoconvex or convexoconcave surfaces, the opposite sides being of different curvatures; known as a meniscus lens.

planoconcave l. A lens having one plane and one concave surface.

planoconvex l. A lens having one plane and one convex surface.

positive l. Any lens with a positive focal length; it is thicker in the center than around the circumference. There are three types of positive lenses: double convex or biconvex, planoconvex, and converging concavoconvex.

punktal l. One which is corrected for astigmatism in all powers throughout the entire field.

rectilinear l. See aplanatic *l.*

spherical l. One in which the curved surface, either concave or convex, is a segment of a sphere. Abbreviated, S, sph.

toric l. A lens wherein the curvatures in two meridians at right angles are different.

undercorrection of l. The spherical aberration which normally exists in a simple lens. Rays from the outer zones of the source are brought to a focus closer to the lens than the rays from the central portion.

lens·om′e·ter (len·zom′i·tur) [*lens;* G. *metron,* a measure]. An instrument for determining the refractive power of a lens.

len″ti·co′nus [*lens;* G. *kōnos,* cone]. A rare, usually congenital, anomaly of the lens; marked by a conical prominence upon its anterior or, more rarely, upon its posterior surface.

len·tic′u·lar [L. *lenticula,* lentil, dim. of *lens*]. 1. Pertaining to or resembling a lens. 2. Pertaining to the crystalline lens. 3. Pertaining to the lenticular nucleus of the brain.

len·tic′u·lar pro·gres′sive de″gen·er·a′tion. See hepatolenticular *degeneration.*

len·tic′u·late [*lenticula*]. Lens-shaped.

len·tic″u·lo·stri′ate [*lenticula;* L. *stria,* channel, furrow]. Pertaining to the lenticular nucleus of the corpus striatum, as lenticulostriate artery.

len·tic″u·lo·tha·lam′ic (len·tick″yoo·lo·tha·lam′-ick, ·thal′uh·mick) [*lenticula;* G. *thalamos,* chamber]. Extending from the lenticular nucleus to the thalamus, as the lenticulothalamic tract.

len′ti·form [L. *lens,* lentil; *forma,* form]. Lens-shaped or lentil-shaped.

len″ti·glo′bus [*lens;* L. *globus,* sphere]. A spherical bulging of the lens of the eye.

len·ti′go, len′ti·go (pl. *lentigines*) [L., a freckly eruption]. A dark-brown mark of small size, present on both exposed and covered areas of the skin, and, in distinction to freckles, not influenced by the sun. There is an increase in melanocytes in the basal layer and the rete pegs are elongated. —**lentig′inous** (len·tidj′i·nus), *adj.*

lentigines leprosae. The pigmented spots of macular leprosy.

l. maligna. Xeroderma pigmentosum.

len·ti′tis. See *phacitis.*

leocillin. Trade-mark for benzylpenicillin β-diethylaminoethyl ester hydriodide, reported to have specific action on lung tissue, and thus to be useful in treatment of pulmonary diseases.

Leonicenus, Nicolaus (Leoniceno) [*Italian physician,* 1428–1524]. Gave a classic description of syphilis (1497). He recognized the fact that the disease produces visceral as well as cutaneous lesions.

le″on·ti′a·sis [G. *lēon,* lion; NL. *-iasis,* condition]. A lionlike appearance of the face, seen in lepromatous leprosy.

l. ossea. An overgrowth of the bones of the face, through which the features acquire a lionlike appearance. Also called *megalocephaly.*

Leopold, Christian Gerhard [*German physician,* 1846–1911]. Formulated a law in obstetrics stating that insertion of the placenta into the posterior uterine wall pushes the uterine tubes forward, while insertion into the anterior wall causes them to turn backward and parallel to the longitudinal axis of the recumbent woman.

Lepehne-Pickworth method (for demonstration of cerebral capillary distribution). See benzidine and nitroprussic oxidase *method* for hemoglobin.

lep′er [G. *lepros,* scaly]. One affected with leprosy.

lep′i·do-, lepid- [G. *lepis,* scale]. A combining form meaning *a scale* or *scaly.*

lep″i·do′ma [*lepis;* G. *-ōma,* tumor]. A term proposed by Adami for a tumor arising from a lining membrane. *Obs.*

Lep″i·dop′ter·a [*lepis;* G. *pteron,* wing]. An order

of insects distinguished by featherlike scales and spirally coiled suctorial apparatus. The order includes butterflies, moths, and skippers. Their larvae may cause caterpillar dermatitis.

lep'o·thrix [G. *lepos*, scale; *thrix*, hair]. A skin condition in which masses of reddish, black, and yellow fungous material are found in nodular or diffuse distribution about the axillary or genital hair; usually seen in those who sweat freely. Also called *trichomycosis axillaris, trichomycosis rubra, trichomycosis flava nigra.*

lep'ra. Old term for leprosy.

l. mixta. Lepromatous leprosy accompanied by neural symptoms. *Obs.*

l. reaction. A febrile, acute hypersensitivity response of a patient having one of the major forms of leprosy as a result of aggressive treatment or overpotent lepromin test.

lep'rid [G. *lepra*, leprosy, from *lepros*, scaly]. See tuberculoid *leprosy.*

lep'ro·lin. A vaccine prepared from an acid-fast bacillus; used unsatisfactorily in the treatment of leprosy. The term is often used erroneously as a synonym for lepromin.

lep·rol'o·gist [*lepros;* G. *logos*, word]. One who makes a special study of leprosy.

lep·rol'o·gy [*lepros; logos*]. The special study of leprosy. —**leprolog'ic,** *adj.*

lep·ro'ma [*lepros;* G. *-ōma*, tumor]. The cutaneous nodular lesion of leprosy. —**leprom'atous,** *adj.*

lep'ro·min [*lepros*]. An emulsion prepared from ground and sterilized tissue containing the leprosy bacillus (*Mycobacterium leprae);* used for intradermal skin tests in leprosy but of little or no diagnostic utility.

lep"ro·pho'bi·a [*lepros;* G. *phobos*, fear]. Morbid dread of leprosy.

lep"ro·sar'i·um (lep"ro·sair'ee·um) [*lepros*]. An institution for the treatment of persons affected with leprosy.

lep'ro·ser"y, le·pro'ser·y. See *leprosarium.*

lep'ro·sin. A neutral, acid-fast, waxlike substance isolated from *Mycobacterium leprae*, consisting of a complex mixture of solid glycerides and waxes. Fatty acids liberated on saponification are myristic, palmitic, stearic, tetracosanic, and a new hydroxy acid, leprosinic acid. Glycerin is the only water-soluble component detected. Ether-soluble matter includes two higher, secondary, optically active alcohols.

lep"ro·sin'ic ac'id. A hydroxy acid occurring in the fatty acids of leprosin.

lep'ro·sy [*lepros*]. A chronic infectious disease occurring almost exclusively in tropical and subtropical countries; caused by *Mycobacterium leprae.* On the basis of clinical, bacteriologic, and immunologic features, the Havana (Pan-American) classification defined a lepromatous, a tuberculoid, and an indeterminate form. Syn., *Hansen's disease.*

anesthetic l. See tuberculoid *l.*

bacillary positive tuberculoid l. Major tuberculoid *l.*

corneal l. Infection of the cornea by the causative agent of leprosy, sometimes causing corneal tumors.

cutaneous l. Lepromatous *l.*

indeterminate l. A nonspecific form with clinical manifestations chiefly of the skin and peripheral nerves, differentiated from the two major types, lepromatous or tuberculoid, by the absence of lepra cells and tuberculoid structures, the scarcity of bacilli which, when found, are not bunched, and the tendency to arrest or spontaneous recovery. Lepromin test gives variable results. Some cases may transform into a major type.

intermediate l. Formerly, indeterminate *l.*

lazarine l. See Lucio *l.*

lepromatous l. The contagious form of leprosy, with lesions histologically characterized by lepra cells containing "cigar-bunches" or globi of bacilli and by lymphocytic infiltration. Clinically the skin may be first involved, showing lepromas insensible to heat, cold, and pain. The face is frequently a favorite site (*facies leontina*), especially the mucous membranes of the eyes and upper respiratory tract. All organs may be involved, but involvement of peripheral nerves, when present, develops slowly, and mutilations generally occur as a result of osteonecrosis. Lepromin test is negative, while body excretions and secretions of affected organs contain the organism. Also called *cutaneous l., nodular l.*

Lucio l. A form of lepromatous leprosy exhibiting diffuse, generalized eruptions of lepromatous infiltrations with necrotizing lesions. Lepromin test may produce a brief intense positive response. It is synonymous with **lazarine leprosy,** but some reserve this term for the ulcerative forms. Also called *spotted l., manchada, lepromatous erythema necroticans.*

maculoanesthetic l. See tuberculoid *l.*

major tuberculoid l. A form in which large numbers of *Mycobacterium leprae* are found, but not in bunches or globi.

malignant l. Lepromatous *l.*

neural l. See tuberculoid *l.*

nodular l. Lepromatous *l.*

ocular l. Complications in the eye resulting from leprosy or from secondary invasions due to its presence.

spotted l. See Lucio *l.*

tuberculoid l. The noncontagious form of leprosy, with lesions histologically characterized by a tuberculoid granulomatous structure and the absence of lepra cells; bacilli are absent or few, and, when present, are never bunched. Grossly, it is marked by peripheral nerve involvement, and mutilations result from septic processes which are associated with the neurological and trophic changes. Bacillary cutaneous involvement is minimal. The viscera are not affected. Lepromin test is positive in a high percentage of cases. This form is considered benign, as under hygienic conditions it is often nonprogressive, and shows a tendency toward spontaneous cure. During a hypersensitivity reaction, it may be transformed into lepromatous leprosy. Also called *neural l., anesthetic l., maculoanesthetic l., Hansenid, leprid, neuroleprid.*

white l. Vitiligo.

lep'ro·tene. A naturally occurring provitamin A.

lep'rous, lep·rot'ic [*lepros*]. Applied to lesions caused by *Mycobacterium leprae*, and to persons affected with leprosy.

lep·tan'dra [G. *leptos*, thin; *anēr*, man]. The dried rhizome and roots of *Veronicastrum virginicum.* Its active principle is unknown. Leptandra is cathartic. Dose, 1–4 Gm. (15–60 gr.).

l. extract (*extractum leptandrae*). One gram represents four grams of leptandra. Dose, 0.25 Gm. (4 gr.).

leptazol. The British Pharmacopoeia name for pentylenetetrazol. See *metrazol.*

lep'to-, lept- [*leptos*]. A combining form signifying *thin, small, weak, fine.*

lep"to·ce·pha'li·a, lep"to·ceph'a·ly [*leptos;* G. *kephalē*, head]. Abnormal smallness of the skull.

leptocephal'ic, *adj.*

lep"to·ceph'a·lus [*leptos; kephalē*]. An individual with an abnormally small head from premature union of the frontal and sphenoid bones.

lep″to·chro·mat′ic [*leptos;* G. *chrōma*, color]. Characterized by a finely differentiated chromatin reticulum.

lep′to·cyte. A thin erythrocyte of decreased volume in relation to its diameter, often characterized also by abnormal shape.

lep″to·cy′tic. 1. Of or pertaining to leptocytes. 2. Pertaining to a blood picture in which leptocytosis is evident microscopically, and in which the hypochromic microcytic anemia present is not amenable to iron therapy.

lep″to·cy·to′sis. A preponderance of leptocytes in the blood. See *thalassemia.*

hereditary l. Thalassemia.

lep″to·dac′ty·lous [*leptos;* G. *daktylos*, finger]. Characterized by slenderness of the fingers or toes, or both.

lep″to·don′tous [*leptos;* G. *odous*, tooth]. Having thin or slender teeth.

lep″to·me·nin′ges (lep″to·mi·nin′jeez) [*leptos;* G. *mēnigx*, membrane]. The arachnoid and the pia mater considered together.

lep″to·me·nin″gi·o′ma [*leptos; mēnigx;* G. *-ōma*, tumor]. A tumor of the pia mater or arachnoid.

lep″to·men″in·gi′tis [*leptos; mēnigx;* G. *-itis*, inflammation]. Inflammation of the pia mater and arachnoid of the brain or the spinal cord.

lep″to·men″in·gop′a·thy [*leptos; mēnigx;* G. *pathos*, disease]. Disease of the leptomeninges, or pia mater and arachnoid.

lep″to·me′ninx [*leptos; mēnigx*]. The pia mater or the arachnoid.

lep″to·mi″cro·gnath′i·a (·migh″kro·nath′ee·uh, ·nayth′ee·uh, ·migh″krog·nath′ee·uh, ·nayth′ee·uh) [*leptos;* G. *mikros*, small; *gnathos*, jaw]. A mild degree of micrognathia.

Lep″to·mi·cru′rus (lep″to·migh·kroor′us). A genus of coral snakes found in the Americas, with neurotoxic venom.

Lep″to·mo′nas, Lep·tom′o·nas [*leptos;* G. *monas*, unit]. A genus of the Trypanosomidae whose members are hemoflagellates of invertebrates.

lep′ton. An elementary particle of small mass, as the electron, positron, neutrino, or antineutrino.

lep″to·pel′lic [*leptos;* G. *pellis*, wooden bowl]. Having a very narrow pelvis.

lep″to·pho′ni·a [*leptos;* G. *phōnē*, voice]. Delicacy, gentleness, or weakness of the voice. —**leptophon′ic,** *adj.*

lep″to·pro·so′pi·a [*leptos;* G. *prosōpon*, face]. Narrowness of the face. —**leptoprosop′ic,** *adj.*

lep′tor·rhine″ (lep′to·ryne″, ·rin) [*leptos;* G. *rhis*, nose]. 1. *In craniometry*, designating an apertura piriformis that is relatively long and narrow; having a nasal index of 46.9 or less. 2. *In somatometry*, designating a nose that is long and narrow; having a height-breadth index of 55.0 to 69.9.

lep′to·scope. An optical device for measuring the thickness and composition of the plasma membrane of a cell.

Lep″to·spi′ra [*leptos;* G. *speira*, coil]. A genus of spirochetes able to survive in water; characterized by sharply twisted filaments with one or both extremities hooked or recurved. These organisms are not predominantly blood parasites, but are also found in other tissues.

L. autumnalis. The causative agent of a leptospirosis called *pretibial fever* in the United States and *autumnal fever* in the Far East.

L. canicola. The etiological agent of Stuttgart disease in dogs and of canicola fever in man.

L. grippotyphosa. The etiological agent of marsh fever.

L. hebdomadis. That species which is the causative agent of seven-day fever in the Far East.

L. icterohaemorrhagiae. A species which produces spirochetal jaundice in man.

lep″to·spi·rol′y·sin (lep″to·spy·rol′i·sin, ·spy″ro·lye′sin) [*leptos; speira;* G. *lysis*, a loosing]. A lysin operating on leptospiras.

lep″to·spi·ro′sis (lep″to·spy·ro′sis) [*leptos; speira;* G. *-ōsis*, condition]. Infection with *Leptospira.*

canine l. See Stuttgart *disease.*

lep′to·tene [*leptos;* G. *tainia*, ribbon]. *In cytology,* a stage in the prophase of mitosis in which the chromosomes have a slender, threadlike appearance.

Lep′to·thrix [*leptos;* G. *thrix*, hair]. A genus of unbranched filamentous organisms of the Chlamydobacteriaceae.

L. buccalis. A species which is a common inhabitant of the oral cavity. Pathogenic properties have been claimed for it, but its invasive power is probably slight.

lep″to·tri·cho′sis (lep″to·tri·ko′sis, ·try·ko′sis) [*leptos; thrix*]. Any disease caused by a species of *Leptothrix.*

l. of the conjunctiva. A conjunctivitis caused by members of the genus *Leptothrix;* usually associated with swelling of the lacrimal gland and preauricular lymph nodes. Also called *Parinaud's conjunctivitis.*

lep′tus. See *chigger.*

le·re′sis [G. *lērēsis*, silly talk]. Garrulousness; senile loquacity.

Leri, André [*French physician,* 1875–1930]. Described a phenomenon observed in spastic hemiplegia. If the fingers of a normal person are passively folded into the hollow of the hand and the wrist is then forcibly flexed, the arm flexes at the elbow. In spastic hemiplegia, this reflex is absent.

Leriche, René (1870–). French surgeon known for his operation of periarterial sympathectomy for the relief of vasomotor disturbances (1917), called *Leriche's operation.* He was the originator of arteriectomy (1917), of surgery of the sympathetic nervous system, and of ganglionic blocking by procaine, especially in surgery in the field of childbirth.

Les′bi·an·ism (lez′bee·un·iz·um, less′·) [G. *Lesbos*, Lesbos]. An abnormal affection between women; homosexuality between women. Syn., *Lesbian love, sapphism, tribadism.*

le′sion [L. *laesio*, a hurting]. The alteration, structural or functional, due to injury: commonly limited to morphological alterations.

discharging l. A brain lesion which may be accompanied by irregular discharge of motor impulses, as Jacksonian epilepsy.

focal l. One in a focus; usually applied to a circumscribed focus in the brain with such symptoms and signs as may lead to a diagnosis of its situation.

functional l. An alteration of function or functional capacity without demonstrable morphologic substrate.

initial l. See primary *l.*

lower motor neuron l. An injury to the cell body or axon of a lower motor neuron, characterized by flaccid paralysis of the muscle(s), innervated, diminished, or absent reflexes, muscle atrophy, reaction of degeneration (about two weeks after injury), and absence of pathological reflexes.

Luys body l. See *hemiballismus,* subthalamic *nucleus.*

peripheral l. One in the periphery of the body, especially in the peripheral nerves.

primary l. (a) In syphilis, the chancre. (b) In tuberculosis, the focus of the first infection, as the tuberculous, caseous mass near the hilum or periphery in the lung.

secondary l. One which follows, and is due to, a primary lesion, as the secondary, cutaneous lesions of syphilis; the involvement of mediastinal lymph nodes following pulmonary tuberculosis.

structural l. One in which there is demonstrable morphologic change.

systemic l. One which affects members of a system, such as the nervous system or hematopoietic system.

upper motor neuron l. An injury to the cell body or axon of an upper motor neuron, resulting in spastic paralysis of the muscle involved, hyperactive deep reflexes but diminished or absent superficial reflexes, little or no muscle atrophy, absence of reaction of degeneration, and the presence of pathological reflexes and signs.

vascular l. One which affects blood vessels.

Lesser's triangle. See under *triangle.*

le'thal [L. *letalis,* deadly, from *letum,* death]. Deadly; pertaining to or producing death. Abbreviated, l.

leth'ar·gy [G. *lēthargia,* drowsiness]. A morbid condition of drowsiness or stupor. —**lethar'gic,** *adj.*

le'the (leeth'ee) [G., forgetfulness]. Total loss of memory; amnesia. *Obs.*

letheon. An old trade name for ethyl ether used as an anesthetic.

Letonoff and Reinhold's method. See under *method.*

Letterer, Erich (1895–). German pathologist who described a form of nonlipid reticuloendotheliosis (1924), later described by the pediatrician Siwe from the clinical viewpoint. See Letterer-Siwe *disease.*

leu·cae'thi·op (lew·seeth'ee·op) [G. *leukos,* white; *Aithiops,* Ethiopian]. A Negro albino. —**leucaethiop'ic,** *adj.*

leu·ce'mi·a. See *leukemia.*

leu'cine (lew'seen, ·sin). $CH_3CH(CH_3)CH_2CH(NH_2)COOH$. The α-aminoisocaproic acid, an amino acid obtainable by the hydrolysis of milk and other protein-containing substances, and found in various tissues of the human body. It is essential to the growth of man. —**leucic,** *adj.*

leu"ci·no'sis [*leukos;* G. *-ōsis,* increase]. Excessive proportion or production of leucine, as in the liver.

leu"ci·nu'ri·a [*leukos;* G. *ouron,* urine]. The occurrence of leucine in the urine.

leu'co-, leuc-. See *leuko-.*

leu"co·fla'vin (lew"ko·flay'vin, ·flav'in). See *leucoriboflavin.*

leu"co·lac"to·fla'vin (lew"ko·lack"to·flay'vin, ·flav'in). See *leucoriboflavin.*

leu·co'ma. See *leukoma.*

leu·co'ma·ine (lew·ko'may·een, ·in, ·muh·een, ·in, lew'ko·myne). The name applied to any one of the nitrogenous bases normally developed by the metabolic activity of living organisms, as distinguished from the bases developed by putrefactive processes, and called ptomaines. —**leucomain'ic,** *adj.*

leu"co·ma·i·ne'mi·a (lew"ko·may·i·nee'mee·uh, ·migh·nee'mee·uh) [*leukos;* pto*maine;* G. *haima,* blood]. An excess of leucomaines in the blood.

Leu"co·nos'toc [*leukos;* NL. *Nostoc,* coined by Paracelsus]. A genus of saprophytic bacteria of the family Lactobacteriaceae. Species of this genus are found in milk, fermenting vegetables, and slimy sugar solutions.

leu·cop'sin. See *leukopsin.*

leu"co·ri"bo·fla'vin (lew"ko·rye"bo·flay'vin, ·flav'in, ·rib"o·). The dihydro compound resulting from reduction of riboflavin. It is colorless and shows no fluorescence: also called *leucoflavin.*

leu'co·sin [*leukos*]. A simple protein of the albumin type found in wheat and other cereals.

leu"co·tax'in. A substance which appears to be liberated by injured tissues and toward which phagocytes are positively chemotactic.

leu'co·tome. See *leukotome.*

leucovorin. A trade-mark for folinic acid (2) or 5-formyl-5,6,7,8-tetrahydrofolic acid.

leu'cyl. The univalent radical $(CH_3)_2CHCH_2CH(NH_2)CO$—, of the amino acid leucine.

leu"ka·ne'mi·a [*leukos;* G. *anaimia,* want of blood]. A blood disease having characteristics of leukemia and pernicious anemia: also called *erythroleukosis.*

leu·kas'mus (lew·kaz'mus, ·kas'mus). See *leukoderma, albinism.*

leu·ke'mi·a [*leukos;* G. *haima,* blood]. Any disease of the reticuloendothelial system characterized by uncontrolled proliferation of the leukocytes. Immature leukocytes usually are present in the blood, often in large numbers, and characteristically infiltrate various organs. Leukemias are classified on the basis of rapidity of course (acute, subacute, or chronic), the cell count, and the cell type. Also called *leukosis, leukocythemia.* —**leuke'mic,** *adj.*

acute l. A form with rapid onset and progress, characterized by severe anemia, hemorrhagic manifestations, and susceptibility to infection; the predominant cells in the bone marrow and peripheral blood are blast forms. Also called *lymphoblastic l., blast-cell l.*

aleukemic l. A form of leukemia in which the total leukocyte count is normal or low, despite leukemic changes in the tissues and qualitative changes in the blood. Syn., *leukopenic l., subleukemic l.*

basophilic l. A granulocytic leukemia in which the predominating cells belong to the basophilic series: also called *basophilocytic l., mast-cell l.*

blast-cell l. See stem-cell *l.*, acute *l.*

chloro-l. See *chloroma.*

chronic l. A form in which the expected duration of life is 1 to 20 years or more. The cell types are the less immature forms of the specific blood series (granulocytic, lymphocytic, or monocytic).

embryonal l. See stem-cell *l.*

eosinophilic l. A rare form in which the predominant cell type belongs to the eosinophilic series. Although the cells are relatively mature, the course is acute. Also called *eosinophilocytic l.*

giant-cell l. See megakaryocytic *l.*

granulocytic l. Leukemia in which the predominant cell types belong to the granulocytic series. Usually, cells of the neutrophilic series are most numerous. Syn., *myelocytic l., myelogenous l.* Also called *myeloid l., myelemia, myelocythemia, myelosis.*

hemoblastic l. See stem-cell *l.*

hemocytoblastic l. See stem-cell *l.*

histiocytic l. The Schilling type of monocytic leukemia.

l. of the skin. A state of the skin characterized by leukemic infiltration.

leukemic l. Leukemia in which the leukocyte count in peripheral blood is above 15,000 per cu. mm., and the cell types are in accord with the diagnosis of leukemia.

leukopenic l. See aleukemic *l.*

lymphatic l. See lymphocytic *l.*

lymphoblastic l. An acute lymphocytic leukemia.

lymphocytic l. A form of leukemia, acute or chronic, in which the predominating cell type belongs to the lymphocytic series. Syn., *lymphoid l., lymphogenous l.*

lymphogenous l. See lymphocytic *l.*

lymphoid l. See lymphocytic *l.*

lymphosarcoma-cell l. See *leukosarcoma.*

mast-cell l. See basophilic *l.*

megakaryocytic l. A rare form in which a large number of fragmented megakaryocytes are seen; probably a variant of granulocytic leukemia or a manifestation of Hodgkin's *disease.* Also called *giant-cell l., piastrenemia.*

monocytic l. A form in which the predominant cell type belongs to the monocytic series. Two types are differentiated on the basis of the predominant cell present in the peripheral blood: **Naegeli (myelomonocytic) type,** in which atypical monocytes in some ways resemble immature granulocytes; **Schilling type,** in which the predominant cells are very large, bizarre-shaped monocytes having a lacy chromatin structure. The Naegeli type is probably a variant of granulocytic leukemia; the Schilling type is a true monocytic leukemia, probably derived from the reticuloendothelium.

myeloblastic l. An acute granulocytic leukemia.

myelocytic l. See granulocytic *l.*

myelogenous l. Granulocytic leukemia.

myeloid l. See granulocytic *l.*

myelomonocytic l. See monocytic *l.*

Naegeli type l. See monocytic *l.*

neutrophilic l. A granulocytic leukemia in which the cells belong almost exclusively to the neutrophilic series: sometimes called *granulocytic leukemia.*

plasmacytic, plasmocytic l. A rare form in which plasmacytes appear in large numbers or are the predominant cell type: probably a variant of multiple myeloma.

Schilling type l. See monocytic *l.*

stem-cell l. An acute leukemia in which the type of cell is so primitive and undifferentiated that it is difficult or impossible to identify its series: also called *blast-cell l., hemoblastic l., hemocytoblastic l., embryonal l., undifferentiated-cell l.*

subacute l. A form with many features of acute leukemia, but of longer duration.

subleukemic l. Aleukemic leukemia: a term proposed as less self-contradictory.

undifferentiated-cell l. See stem-cell *l.*

leu·kem′id [*leukos; haima*]. A cutaneous lesion which accompanies leukemia.

leu·ke′moid [*leukos; haima;* G. *eidos,* form]. Similar to leukemia, but due to other conditions; usually refers to the presence of immature cells in the blood in conditions other than leukemia.

leu′kin. A substance, derived from leukocytes of certain animals, which is bactericidal or bacteriostatic against certain organisms, including typhoid and anthrax bacilli, and micrococci.

leu′ko-, leuk- [*leukos*]. 1. A combining form meaning *white, colorless.* 2. *In chemistry,* a combining form denoting a *colorless* or *weakly colored* compound. 3. *In medicine,* a combining form denoting a *whitish decolorization.*

leu′ko·blast [*leukos;* G. *blastos,* germ]. A general term for the parent cell of the leukocytes.

leu″ko·blas·to′sis [*leukos; blastos;* G. *-ōsis,* increase]. Excessive proliferation of immature leukocytes.

leu·ko′ci·din (lew·ko′si·din, ·koss′i·din, lew″ko-sid′in, ·sigh′din) [*leukos;* L. *caedere,* to kill]. A toxic substance capable of killing and destroying neutrophil leukocytes.

leu′ko·cyte [*leukos;* G. *kytos,* cell]. One of the colorless, more or less ameboid cells of the blood, having a nucleus and cytoplasm. Those found in normal blood are usually divided according to their staining reaction into **granular leukocytes,** consisting of neutrophils, eosinophils, and basophils, and **nongranular leukocytes,** consisting of lymphocytes and monocytes. Those found in abnormal blood consist of myeloblasts, promyelocytes, neutrophilic myelocytes, eosinophilic myelocytes, basophilic myelocytes, lymphoblasts, plasma cells, and Türk's irritation cells. Syn., *white blood cell, white corpuscle.* For methods of classifying leukocytes, see under *method.* See Plate 27.

acidophil l. See eosinophil *l.*

basophil l. One containing granules which stain deep purple (basic dye) with Wright's stain, and having a nucleus without distinct lobulation.

endothelial l. A histiocyte.

eosinophil l. One containing coarse round granules which stain pink to bright red (acid dye) with Wright's stain and usually having a bilobed nucleus.

granular l. One of those containing granules in their cytoplasm. Syn., *granulocyte.*

heterophil l. See neutrophil *l.*

lymphoid l. A nongranular leukocyte including lymphocytes and monocytes.

neutrophil l. A highly motile and phagocytic leukocyte having numerous fine granules which do not stain definitely either blue (basic dye) or red (acid dye). Its polymorphous nucleus may be ribbonlike, bandlike, or segmented, having two to seven lobules.

nongranular l. One with clear homogeneous cytoplasm, such as a lymphocyte or monocyte.

oxyphil l. Old term for eosinophil leukocyte.

polymorphonuclear l. The neutrophil leukocyte so-called because of its irregular-shaped and lobulated nucleus. Syn., *granulocyte.*

transitional l. Old term for monocyte.

leu″ko·cy·the′mi·a (lew″ko·sigh·theem′ee·uh). See *leukemia.*

leu″ko·cy′to·blast [*leukos; kytos;* G. *blastos,* germ]. The precursor of a leukocyte.

leu″ko·cy″to·gen′e·sis [*leukos; kytos;* G. *genesis,* generation]. The formation of leukocytes.

leu″ko·cy″to·ly′sin (lew″ko·sigh″to·lye′sin, ·sigh-tol′i·sin) [*leukos; kytos;* G. *lysis,* a loosing]. A lysin which disintegrates leukocytes.

leu″ko·cy·tol′y·sis (·sigh·tol′i·sis) [*leukos; kytos; lysis*]. The destruction of leukocytes. —**leukocytolyt′ic,** *adj.*

leu″ko·cy·to′ma (·sigh·to′muh) [*leukos; kytos;* G. *-ōma,* tumor]. A tumorlike mass composed of leukocytes.

leu″ko·cy·tom′e·ter (·sigh·tom′i·tur) [*leukos; kytos;* G. *metron,* a measure]. A graduated capillary tube used for counting leukocytes.

leu″ko·cy″to·pe′ni·a. See *leukopenia.*

leu″ko·cy″to·poi·e′sis [*leukos; kytos;* G. *poiēsis,* production]. The formation of leukocytes. —**leukocytopoiet′ic,** *adj.*

leu″ko·cy·to′sis (lew″ko·sigh·to′sis) [*leukos; kytos;* G. *-ōsis,* increase]. An increase in the leukocyte count above the upper limits of normal. It is physiologic during pregnancy and pathologic in many infections and toxemias. —**leukocytot′ic,** *adj.*

leu″ko·der′ma [*leukos;* G. *derma,* skin]. A condition of defective pigmentation of the skin, especially a congenital absence of pigment in patches or bands. —**leukodermic,** *adj.*

l. acquisitum centrifugum. A vitiligo manifested by small round areas of depigmentation, each with a brown mole in the center: also called Sutton's *disease, circumnevic* or *perinevoid vitiligo.*

l. colli. A condition coincident with the appearance of the macular eruption of cutaneous syphilis; characterized by mottled skin on the neck, chin, or rarely on other parts.

l. psoriaticum. An affection of the skin characterized by areas of hypopigmentation following psoriatic inflammation.

l. punctatum. An affection of the skin characterized by minute areas of hypopigmentation scattered through the melanosis following prolonged intake of arsenic.

l. syphiliticum. See *vitiligoid*, 2.

leu″ko·en·ceph″a·li′tis. See *staggers*.

leu″koe·ryth″ro·blas·to′sis. See myelophthisic *anemia*.

leu″ko·ker″a·to′sis. See *leukoplakia*.

leu′kol, leu′ko·lin. Quinoline.

leu″ko·lym″pho·sar·co′ma. Leukosarcoma.

leu·kol′y·sis. Leukocytolysis.

venom l. Destruction of leukocytes by the action of venom.

leu·ko′ma [G., white spot in the eye]. 1. An opacity of the cornea as a result of an ulcer, wound, or inflammation, which presents an appearance of ground glass. 2. Leukoplakia buccalis. 3. Leukosarcoma. Syn., *albugo*. —**leukom′atous, leukom′atoid,** *adj*.

leu·ko′ma·ine (lew·ko′may·een, ·in, ·muh·een, ·in, lew′ko·myne). See *leucomaine*.

leu″ko·mel″a·no·der′ma. See *vitiligoid*, 2.

leu″ko·my·o′ma (lew″ko·migh·o′muh). See *lipomyoma*.

leu″ko·nych′i·a (lew″ko·nick′ee·uh) [G. *leukos*, white; *onyx*, nail]. A whitish discoloration of the nails; due to the presence of air beneath them.

leu·kop′a·thy [*leukos;* G. *pathos*, disease]. Any deficiency of coloring matter. Albinism.

leu″ko·pe·de′sis [*leukos;* G. *pēdēsis*, a leaping]. Diapedesis of leukocytes through the walls of blood vessels.

l. gastrica. Leukocytes, particularly in increased numbers, in the gastric secretion.

leu″ko·pe′ni·a [*leukos;* G. *penia*, want]. A decrease below the normal number of leukocytes in the peripheral blood. For **idiopathic, malignant,** or **pernicious l.,** see *agranulocytosis*. —**leukopenic,** *adj*.

leu″ko·phleg·ma′si·a (·fleg·may′zhuh, ·zee·uh, ·shuh, ·see·uh) [*leukos;* G. *phlegmasia*, inflammation]. 1. A condition marked by dropsy, a pale flabby skin, and general edema. 2. Phlegmasia alba dolens.

leu″koph·thal′mous [*leukos;* G. *ophthalmos*, eye]. Having unusually white eyes.

leu″ko·pla′ki·a [*leukos;* G. *plax*, anything flat and broad]. A disease characterized by a whitish thickening of the epithelium of a mucous membrane. —**leukoplakial,** *adj*.

l. buccalis. One characterized by pearly-white or bluish white patches on the surface of the tongue or the mucous membrane of the cheeks, due to a hyperplasia of the epithelium.

l. oris. See *l.* buccalis.

l. vulvae. Occurrence of irregular white patches on the mucosa of the vulva. There is thickening of the epithelium and the papillae may be hypertrophied. Also see *kraurosis* of the vulva.

leu″ko·pla′si·a (lew″ko·play′zhuh, ·zee·uh). See *leukoplakia*.

leu″ko·pro′te·ase (·pro′tee·ace, ·aze). An enzyme in leukocytes which splits protein. In inflammation it causes liquefaction of necrotic tissue.

leu·kop′sin [*leukos;* G. *opsis*, vision]. Visual white, produced by reaction of light on rhodopsin (visual purple) derived from vitamin A: also spelled *leucopsin*.

leu″kor·rha′gi·a [*leukos;* G. *rhēgnynai*, to burst forth]. An excessive leukorrheal flow.

leu″kor·rhe′a [*leukos;* G. *rhoia*, flow]. A whitish, mucopurulent discharge from the female genital canal. —**leukorrheal,** *adj*.

leu″ko·sar·co′ma [*leukos;* G. *sarkōma*, fleshy excrescence]. 1. Lymphosarcoma which has invaded the blood stream and in which lymphosarcoma cells (malignant lymphoblasts and lymphocytes) are circulating: also called *leukolymphosarcoma, sarcoleukemia*. 2. Lymphocytic leukemia.

leu″ko·sar·co″ma·to′sis [*leukos; sarkōma;* G. *-osis*, condition]. A condition characterized by multiple sarcomatous tumors associated with a leukemic blood picture. Also see *leukosarcoma*.

leu′ko·scope [*leukos;* G. *skopein*, to examine]. An instrument formerly used for testing for color blindness.

leu·ko′sis. See *leukemia*.

leu″ko·tax′ine (lew″ko·tack′seen, ·sin) [*leukos;* G. *taxis*, arrangement]. A crystalline, nitrogenous substance present in inflammatory exudates, which exerts positive chemotaxis and appears to increase capillary permeability. It is probably produced by injured cells.

leu′ko·tome. An instrument for dividing nerve fibers of the white matter of the brain in leukotomy or lobotomy: also spelled *leucotome*.

leu·kot′o·my. See *lobotomy*.

leu″ko·tox′ic [*leukos;* G. *toxikon*, poison]. Destructive to leukocytes.

leu″ko·tox′in [*leukos; toxikon*]. A cytotoxin obtained from lymph nodes.

leu″ko·trich′i·a (lew″ko·trick′ee·uh) [*leukos;* G. *thrix*, hair]. Whiteness of the hair; canities. —**leukot′richous,** *adj*.

leu″ko·u″ro·bil′in (·yoor″o·bil′in, ·buy′lin) [*leukos;* G. *ouron*, urine; L. *bilis*, bile]. A colorless decomposition product of bilirubin.

leu′kous [*leukos*]. White.

Levaditi's method. See under *stain*.

lev′an. A fructosan polysaccharide, composed of furanose-type D-fructose (D-fructofuranose) units linked by 2,6-β-glycosidic bonds, elaborated from sucrose by certain microorganisms, as *Bacillus subtilis* and *Bacillus mesentericus*.

l. sucrase. An enzyme that catalyzes formation of levan from sucrose.

Le·vant′ nut. Old term for cocculus, dried fruit of *Anamirta cocculus*.

Le·vant′ worm′seed. See *santonica*.

lev″ar·ter′en·ol bi·tar′trate. The United States Pharmacopeia name for the levorotatory form of *norepinephrine bitartrate*.

le·va′tor [L., from *levare*, to lift up]. 1. That which raises or elevates, as levator palpebrae superioris, the muscle which widens the palpebral fissure or opens the eye. See Table of Muscles in the Appendix. 2. An instrument used for raising a depressed portion of the skull.

l. anguli oris. The caninus muscle.

l. anguli scapulae. The levator scapulae muscle: old term.

l. ani. The chief muscle of the pelvic diaphragm.

l. claviculae. An occasional muscle arising from the transverse process of the first or second cervical vertebra and extending to the lateral end of the clavicle.

levatores costarum. Small muscles which aid in raising the ribs.

levatores costarum longi. Certain lower levatores costarum muscles.

l. epiglottidis. A variant part of the genioglossus muscle inserted into the epiglottis.

l. glandulae thyroideae. An occasional slip of muscle extending from the body of the hyoid to the isthmus of the thyroid gland.

l. labii superioris. A portion of the quadratus labii superioris muscle.

l. labii superioris alaeque nasi. The quadratus labii superioris muscle.

l. menti. The mentalis muscle: old term.

l. palati. The levator veli palatini muscle.

l. palpebrae superioris. The muscle which raises the upper eyelid.

l. prostatae. A few medial fibers of the pubococcygeus part of the levator ani muscle.

l. scapulae. The muscle which raises the shoulder and rotates the inferior angle of the scapula medially.

l. veli palatini. The muscle which raises the soft palate.

le′ver (lee′vur, lev′ur) [*levare*]. A vectis or one-armed tractor, used in obstetrics.

le·vid′u·lin·ose. A trisaccharide occurring in manna; on hydrolysis it yields 1 molecule of glucose and 2 of mannose.

lev″i·ga′tion [L. *levigare*, to make smooth]. The reduction of a substance to a powder by grinding in water, followed by fractional sedimentation, in order to separate the coarser from the finer particles. Also see *porphyrization*. —**lev′igate,** *v.*

Levin, Abraham Louis [*American physician*, 1880–1940]. Devised a nasal gastroduodenal catheter, called a *Levin tube*, for use in connection with gastric and intestinal operations (1921).

Levinson test. See under *test*.

lev″i·ta′tion [L. *levitas*, lightness]. 1. The illusion of the suspension of a body in air; performed by modern magicians. 2. The subjective sense of rising into the air or being aloft without support, as in dreams or certain mental disorders.

le′vo-, lae′vo- (lee′vo-, lev′o-) [L. *laevus*, left]. 1. A combining form meaning *left, on the left side*. 2. *In chemistry*, a combining form signifying *levorotatory*.

le″vo·car′di·o·gram [*laevus;* G. *kardia*, heart; *gramma*, letter]. An electrocardiogram in which the initial ventricular deflections are associated only with left ventricular activity; produced by blocking the right atrioventricular bundle.

le″vo·con′dyl·ism. Deviation of the mandibular condyles toward the left.

levo-dromoran tartrate. Trade-marked name for the morphinelike synthetic analgesic substance levorphan tartrate.

le″vo·duc′tion [*laevus;* L. *ducere*, to lead]. Movement to the left, said especially of an eye.

le′vo·gram. See *levocardiogram*.

le″vo·gy′rate. See *levorotatory*.

le″vo·gy′rous [*laevus;* G. *gyros*, circle]. Rotating to the left, as the rotation of rays of polarized light.

levophed. A trade-mark for *l*-norepinephrine, a primary pressor amine, supplied in the form of the bitartrate salt.

le″vo·pho′bi·a [*laevus;* G. *phobos*, fear]. Morbid fear of objects on the left side of the body.

le″vo·pho′ri·a [*laevus;* G. *phoros*, bearing]. A tending of the visual lines to the left.

le″vo·ro·ta′tion [*laevus;* L. *rotare*, to turn round]. Rotation toward the left, especially of the plane of polarization of light.

le″vo·ro′ta·to″ry [*laevus; rotare*]. Rotating the plane of polarized light from right to left (counterclockwise).

lev·or′phan tar′trate. Generic name for levorotatory 3-hydroxy-N-methylmorphinan tartrate, a potent synthetic analgesic related chemically and pharmacologically to morphine. See *levo-dromoran tartrate, racemorphan hydrobromide*.

le″vo·tar·tar′ic ac′id (lee″vo·tahr·tar′ick, ·tahr-tahr′ick). The optical isomer of tartaric acid which rotates polarized light to the left.

Levret, André [*French obstetrician*, 1703–80]. Made numerous contributions to the development of obstetrics. Devised improved forceps with cephalic and pelvic curves; called *Levret's forceps*. *Levret's law* states that in placenta previa the insertion of the umbilical cord is marginal.

lev′u·lin [L. *laevus*, left]. A substance resembling starch occurring in some tubers; easily converted into levulose; synanthrose.

lev″u·lin′ic ac′id. $CH_3COCH_2CH_2COOH$. An acid obtained by boiling dextrose, sucrose, starch, or similar derivatives with dilute hydrochloric acid.

lev″u·lo′san (lev″yoo·lo′san, lev′yoo·lo·san, lev″-yoo·lo·san′) [*laevus*]. A sugar anhydride which yields levulose on hydrolysis; fructosan.

lev′u·lose [*laevus*]. $CH_2OH.CO.HOCH.HCOH.$-$HCOH.CH_2OH$; a monosaccharide occurring as such in many fruits and obtainable also by hydrolysis of sucrose and inulin; a white, crystalline powder, freely soluble in water, at least as sweet as sucrose: used for parenteral alimentation. It may have special utility for diabetic patients requiring parenteral carbohydrate, as insulin is not required for activation of its phosphorylating enzyme. Syn., *fructose,* D*-fructose, fruit sugar*.

lev″u·lo·se′mi·a [*laevus;* G. *haima*, blood]. Presence of levulose in the blood.

lev″u·lo·su′ri·a [*laevus;* G. *ouron*, urine]. Presence of levulose in the urine.

lev′u·rid. See *moniliid*.

Levy test. See Babcock-Levy *test*.

Lévy-Roussy syndrome. See under *syndrome*.

Lewandowsky, Felix [*German dermatologist*, 1879–1921]. Described rosacealike tuberculid, called *Lewandowsky's disease*.

Lewis, Thomas [*English cardiologist*, 1881–1945]. Pioneer in electrocardiography, by which he contributed to the analysis of cardiac arrhythmia. Studied atrial fibrillation. Described effort syndrome, a manifestation of neurocirculatory asthenia, in soldiers (1917).

lew′is·ite. $ClCH:CHAsCl_2$. Chlorovinyldichloroarsine; an oily substance having vesicant, lacrimatory, and lung irritant effects; it was developed for use as a chemical warfare agent.

lexo. Trade-mark for wafers containing soybean lecithin with thiamine hydrochloride and vitamins A and D.

Leyden, Ernst Viktor von [*German neurologist*, 1832–1910]. Described a type of hemiplegia resembling that noted by Gubler; called *Leyden's paralysis*. Described an atrophic type of progressive muscular dystrophy seen in children, and usually beginning in the pelvic girdle and thighs; called *Leyden-Möbius dystrophy*. Described fatty infiltration of the heart. Acute ataxia is known as *Leyden's ataxia* or *Leyden-Westphal ataxia*. See also *Charcot-Leyden crystals* under *crystal*.

Ley′den jar (lye′dun). A glass jar coated within and without, for its lower two-thirds, with metal foil, surmounted by a knobbed conductor in connection with the inner coating. It is designed for the temporary accumulation of electricity. A series of Leyden jars connected in parallel is known as a *Leyden battery*.

Leydig, Franz von [*German histologist*, 1821–1908]. Described the interstitial cells of the testis, thought to be the source of the male sex hormone; called *Leydig cells, Gley's cells*.

ley·dig·ar′che (lye·dig·ar′kee) [*Leydig;* G. *archē*, beginning]. The time at which production of androgen by the interstitial cells of the testis begins.

Ley′dig pause. The hypothetical time of physiological cessation of the function of the interstitial cells of the testis; the male climacteric.

Lf. Limit of flocculation.

L. F. A. Left frontoanterior position of the fetus.

L. F. P. Left frontoposterior position of the fetus.

L. G. V. Lymphogranuloma venereum. See venereal *lymphogranuloma*.

LH Luteinizing hormone.

Lhermitte's sign. See under *sign.*

Li Chemical symbol for lithium.

lib″er·a′tion [L. *liberatio*, from *liberare*, to set free]. The act of freeing.

l. of the arms. In breech presentations, a lowering of the arms of the fetus when they have become extended along the sides of the child's head.

li·bi′do (li·buy′do, li·bee′do) [L., longing]. 1. Sexual desire. 2. *In psychoanalysis*, the sum total of all instinctual forces; psychic energy. —**libid′-inous,** *adj.*

Libman, Emanuel [*American physician*, 1872–1946]. With Sacks, described a form of valvular and mural endocarditis. See atypical verrucous *endocarditis*. Lupus erythematosus disseminatus is known as *Osler-Libman-Sacks syndrome.*

li′bra [L., a balance]. A pound. A weight of twelve troy ounces. Abbreviated, l. Symbol, ℔.

lice. Plural of louse.

li′cense [L. *licentia*, license]. An official permit or authority conferring on the recipient the right and privilege of exercising his profession.

li·cen′ti·ate (lye·sen′shee·ate) [*licentia*]. One who practices a profession by the authority of a license.

li′chen (lye′kin, ·kun) [G. *leichēn*, lichen]. A generic term used to describe certain lesions of the skin which consist of solid papules with exaggerated skin markings. —**lichenoid,** *adj.*

l. chronicus simplex. The chronic stage of neurodermatitis characterized by lichenification of lesions in various regions. Also called *neurodermatitis circumscripta.*

l. corneus hypertrophicus. Thickening and induration of the skin, found in lichen chronicus simplex and the plaque type of lichen planus: also called *lichenificatio gigantea.*

l. nitidus. A chronic, inflammatory skin disease characterized by groups of tiny papules which are asymptomatic; found frequently in the genital region and the flexor region of a joint.

l. obtusus corneus. See *prurigo* nodularis.

l. pilaris. See *keratosis* pilaris.

l. planus. A common, inflammatory skin disease with an eruption of papules, broad and angular at the base, flat and glazed at the summit; slightly umbilicated, and of a dull purplish red color. The papules may be discrete or may coalesce, and itching may be slight or severe. The disease may be either acute and widespread or chronic and localized.

l. ruber acuminatus. See *pityriasis* rubra pilaris.

l. ruber moniliformis. A disease of unknown cause, with linear lesions of flat papules which resemble those of lichen planus; but it is probably a separate disease.

l. sclerosus et atrophicans. A chronic, atrophic disease of the skin in which the lesions evolve into white spots.

l. scrofulosus. See *tuberculosis* lichenoides.

l. spinulosus. A skin disease of children, probably due to a vitamin-A deficiency; characterized by spines protruding from hair follicles or follicular papules.

l. striatus. A rare, sudden, self-limited disorder of the skin, occurring mostly in children, appearing as long strips of small lichenoid papules, usually on the extremities.

l. tropicus. See *miliaria.*

l. urticatus. See *urticaria* papulosa.

li″chen·i·fi·cat′i·o gi·gan′te·a. See *lichen* corneus hypertrophicus.

li″chen·if·i·ca′tion (lye″kun·if·i·kay′shun, lye-ken″if·i·) [*leichēn*; L. *facere*, to make]. The process whereby the skin becomes leathery and hardened; often the result of chronic pruritus and the irritation produced by scratching or rubbing skin eruptions.

li″chen·i·for′min. An antibiotic substance isolated from cultures of *Bacillus licheniformis*, active in vitro against a variety of bacteria.

li′chen·in (lye′kun·in). $C_6H_{10}O_5$. Moss starch; a carbohydrate obtained from Iceland moss. Does not give the starch reaction with iodine. Insoluble in cold water; forms a jelly with hot water. See *Cetraria.*

li″chen·i·za′tion (lye″kun·i·zay′shun, ·eye·zay′-shun) [*leichēn*]. The development of lesions having the characteristics of lichen.

Lichtheim, Ludwig [*German physician*, 1845–1928]. Described subcortical aphasia, called *Lichtheim's disease.* Noted that in this disease the patient, although able to indicate by signs the number of syllables in a word, cannot articulate the word; called *Lichtheim's sign.* Drew attention to dorsolateral spinal degeneration associated with pernicious anemia; called *Lichtheim's syndrome.*

lic′o·rice, liq′uo·rice [G. *glykyrriza*, sweet-root]. Glycyrrhiza.

lid. Eyelid.

granulated lids. Trachoma.

l. lag. See von Graefe's *sign.*

li′do·caine hy″dro·chlo′ride. $(CH_3)_2.C_6H_3.NH.CO.CH_2N(C_2H_5)_2.HCl$; α-diethylamino-2,6-acetoxylidide or ω-diethylamino-2,6-dimethylacetanilid; a white, crystalline powder, soluble in water; a potent local anesthetic agent useful for infiltration and block anesthesia and also effective topically. Syn., *lignocaine hydrochloride.* See *xylocaine hydrochloride.*

Lieben's test. See under *test.*

Lieberkühn, Johann Nathanael [*German anatomist*, 1711–56]. Described the simple straight tubular glands of the intestinal mucous membrane (1745); called *crypts of Lieberkühn, Lieberkühn's glands, Galeati's glands, intestinal glands.*

Liebermann reaction. See under *reaction.*

Liebermann-Burchard test. See under *test.*

Liebermann-Burchardt cholesterol reaction. See *Schultz's sterol reaction method for cholesterol* under *stain.*

Liebig, Justus von [*German chemist*, 1803–73]. Pioneer investigator of metabolism. Credited with discovering chloral and hippuric acid. Was among the first to prepare chloroform. Devised a method of estimating urea. See also Liebig's *test* for cystine, Liebig's *test* for cyanide.

lie de·tec′tor. A polygraph used to reveal a repressed sense of guilt or a fear of detection in a subject who is confronted by questions pertaining to a misdemeanor or crime; it records sudden changes in pulse rate, respiration, and blood pressure.

Liefson's method. See under *stain.*

li′en [L.]. The spleen. —**lienal** (lye′i·nul, lye·ee′nul), *adj.*

l. accessorius. Accessory spleen.

li·en′cu·lus. See *lienunculus.*

li″e·ni′tis [*lien*; G. *-itis*, inflammation]. Splenitis.

li·e′no- (lye·ee′no-, lye·en′o-, lye′i·no-), **lien-** [*lien*]. A combining form denoting *the spleen; splenic.*

li·e′no·cele [*lien*; G. *kēlē*, hernia]. Hernia of the spleen.

li″en·og′ra·phy [*lien*; G. *graphein*, to write]. Radiography of the spleen.

li·e″no·ma·la′ci·a (·ma·lay′shuh, ·see·uh) [*lien*; G. *malakia*, softness]. Morbid softening of the spleen.

li·e″no·my″e·lo·ma·la′ci·a [*lien*; G. *myelos*, marrow; *malakia*]. Abnormal softening of the spleen and bone marrow.

li″e·nop′a·thy [*lien;* G. *pathos*, disease]. Disease of the spleen.

li·e″no·re′nal [*lien;* L. *renes*, kidneys]. Relating to the spleen and the kidney, as the lienorenal ligament, a fold of peritoneum between spleen and kidney.

li·e″no·tox′in [*lien;* G. *toxikon*, poison]. A cytotoxin with specific action on spleen cells.

li′en·ter″y [G. *leienteria*, passing one's food undigested]. A form of diarrhea in which undigested food is discharged. —**lienter′ic,** *adj.*

li″en·un′cu·lus [L., dim. from *lien*, spleen]. A detached part of the spleen; accessory spleen.

Liepmann, Hugo Carl (1863–1925). German neurologist who showed, in a study of alcoholic delirium, that hallucinations could be artificially produced, wrote on apraxia and differentiated the various forms, discovered the dominance of the left cortical hemisphere in right-handed individuals, and showed that isolated apraxia of the left side of the body is due to involvement of the corpus callosum.

Liesegang's phenomenon. See under *phenomenon.*

Lieutaud, Joseph [*French physician*, 1703–80]. Described the vesical trigone, formerly called *trigone of Lieutaud.*

life [AS. *līf*]. The sum of properties by which an organism grows, reproduces, and adapts itself to its environment; the quality by which an organism differs from inorganic or dead organic bodies.

average l. *In radiobiology*, the average amount of time an atom in a radioactive substance remains unchanged, equal to 1.443 of the radioactive half-life. Syn., *mean life.*

change of l. See *menopause.*

embryonic l. The life of the embryo.

expectation of l. See *expectation of life.*

mean l. Average *l.*

life ex·pec′tan·cy. See *expectation of life.*

lig′a·ment [L. *ligamentum*, band, tie]. 1. A band of flexible, tough, dense white fibrous connective tissue connecting the articular ends of the bones, and sometimes enveloping them in a capsule. 2. Certain folds and processes of the peritoneum. For ligaments listed by name, see Table of Joints and Ligaments in the Appendix. See Plate 2. —**ligamen′tous,** *adj.*

alar l. Lateral synovial folds of the capsule of the knee joint.

alar odontoid l. Either of the broad, strong ligaments arising on each side of the apex of the odontoid process and connecting the axis with the skull. Also called *check l., odontoid l.*

annular l. of the stapedial base. A ring of elastic fibers encircling the base of the stapes and binding it to the rim of the vestibular window.

anococcygeal l. That which connects the tip of the coccyx with the external sphincter of the anus.

apical dental l. A fibrous cord extending from the summit of the dens of the epistropheus to the occipital bone near the anterior margin of the foramen magnum. Also called *apical odontoid l., suspensory l.*

Arantius' l. See *ligamentum* venosum.

arcuate l. of diaphragm. One of the arched ligaments extending from the body of the diaphragm to the last rib and to the transverse process of the first lumbar vertebra.

arcuate l. of knee. That which extends from the back of the head of the fibula, arching medially over the popliteal tendon to join the capsule of the knee joint.

arcuate l. of pubis. The arched inferior portion of the capsule of the articulation between the two pubic bones: also called *subpubic l.*

auricular l. One of two extrinsic ligaments fixing the cartilage of the auricle to the temporal bone.

broad l. of uterus. A fold of peritoneum which extends laterally from the uterus to the pelvic wall and in which run the uterine blood vessels.

capsular l. A heavy fibrous structure surrounding a diarthrosis, and lined by synovial membrane. See Plate 2.

cardinal l. The lower portion of the broad ligament which is firmly united to the supravaginal portion of the cervix: also called *Mackenrodt's l.*

check l. A thickening of the orbital fascia running from the insertion of the medial rectus muscle to the medial orbital wall (**medial check ligament**) or from the insertion of the lateral rectus muscle to the lateral orbital wall (**lateral check ligament**).

circular l. Various fibers in the gingiva: old term.

Colles' l. The reflected *l.*

conoid l. A dense conical band of fibers attached by its apex to the base of the coracoid process medial to the trapezoid ligament and by its base to the coracoid tuberosity on the under surface of the clavicle.

coracoacromial l. A triangular ligament joining the coracoid process to the acromion.

coronary l. A reflection of the peritoneum between the liver and the diaphragm. Its right and left margins are called the **right triangular ligament** and the **left triangular ligament** of the liver.

coronary l. of knee. A thick inner portion of the capsular ligament of the knee joint which attaches the medial and lateral meniscus to the tibia.

costocoracoid l. See costocoracoid *membrane.*

cruciate l. of the ankle. A band of deep fascia on the dorsum of the foot.

cruciate l. of atlas. That formed by the transverse ligament of the atlas and two vertical bands of fibers, the superior and inferior limbs, passing from the transverse ligament to the occipital bone and to the body of the axis respectively.

cruciate ligaments of knee. Two ligaments crossing in the middle of the knee joint, designated as anterior and posterior by their attachment to the tibia.

deltoid l. The medial collateral ligament of the ankle joint.

dentate l. A narrow fibrous band separating the dorsal and ventral roots of the spinal cord throughout its entire length. Along its lateral border, triangular toothlike processes are fixed at intervals to the dura mater. Also called *denticulate l.*

diaphragmatic l. The bandlike part of the urogenital fold formed by the degeneration of the cranial mesonephric tubules. It extends from the diaphragm to the persisting part of the mesonephros and forms a portion of the suspensory ligament of the ovary.

dorsal carpal l. The extensor retinaculum.

falciform l. of liver. The ventral mesentery of the liver extending from the diaphragm to the umbilicus and containing the round ligament of the liver. See Plate 13.

fundiform l. of penis. That arising from the front of the sheath of the rectus abdominis muscle and the linea alba, splitting into two bands to encircle the root of the penis.

gastrocolic l. The mesentery or portion of the omentum between stomach and transverse colon produced by fusion of the embryonic mesocolon with part of the great omentum.

gastrohepatic l. The portion of the lesser omentum extending between the liver and the stomach.

gastrosplenic l. The fold of peritoneum passing

from the stomach to the spleen: also called *gastrosplenic omentum.*

Gruber's l. Petrosphenoid *l.*: old term.

hammock l. An arrangement of the periodontal membrane related to the growing end of the root of a tooth.

Henle's l. The lateral expansion of the tendinous insertion of the rectus abdominis muscle situated posterior to the conjoined tendon.

hepatocolic l. A prolongation of the hepatoduodenal ligament downward to the transverse colon.

hepatoduodenal l. The portion of the lesser omentum extending between the liver and the duodenum.

hepatorenal l. A fold of peritoneum extending from the inferior surface of the liver to the right kidney.

hyaloideocapsular l. The circular fibers at the area of contact of the vitreous humor and the posterior surface of the lens of the eye.

hyothyroid l. See thyrohyoid *l.*

iliofemoral l. A strong ligament extending from the anterior inferior iliac spine to the lesser trochanter and the intertrochanteric line. Also called *Y l.* See Plate 2.

iliolumbar l. A fibrous band radiating laterally from the transverse processes of the fourth and fifth lumbar vertebrae to attach to the pelvis by two main bands. The lower part blends with the anterior sacroiliac ligament and the upper is attached to the ilium and is continuous above with the lumbodorsal fascia. See Plate 2.

infundibulopelvic l. See suspensory *l.* of ovary.

inguinal l. The lower portion of the aponeurosis of the external oblique muscle extending from the anterior superior spine of the ilium to the tubercle of the pubis and the pectineal line. Also called *Poupart's l.* See Plate 2.

interfoveolar l. Tendinous bands of the transversalis fascia curving downward medial to the abdominal inguinal ring: formerly called *Hesselbach's l.*

interspinal l. Thin membranous bands connecting adjacent spinous processes of the vertebrae.

labial l. A ligamentous cord developing in the labial swellings that forms the distal end of the round ligament of the uterus.

laciniate l. A strong fibrous band extending from the medial malleolus to the calcaneus.

lacunar l. The part of the aponeurosis of the external oblique muscle which is reflected backward and laterally to be attached to the pectineal line. Its base is thin and sharp and forms the medial boundary of the femoral ring.

lateral umbilical l. One of two cordlike folds extending from the urinary bladder to the umbilicus representing the degenerated distal parts of the umbilical arteries.

lienorenal l. A short fold of peritoneum extending from the front of the left kidney to the hilum on the visceral surface of the spleen.

l. of Cooper. 1. Any of the fibrous bands which pass through the breast from the overlying skin to the underlying pectoral fascia. 2. A band of fibrous connective tissue overlying the pectineal line of the pubis.

Mackenrodt's l. The cardinal *l.*

median umbilical l. A fold of the peritoneum extending from the umbilicus to the urinary bladder containing vestiges of the urachus and its connective tissue. Also called *vesicoumbilical l.*

nuchal l. An elastic ligament extending from the external occipital protuberance and middle nuchal line to the spinous process of the seventh cervical vertebra.

odontoid l. See alar odontoid *l.*, apical dental *l.*

ovarian l. A band of connective tissue running from the uterine pole of the ovary to the side of the uterus.

palpebral l. The fibrous band running from the extremities of the tarsal plates to the wall of the orbit. There is a medial and a lateral one for each eye. Also called *tarsal l.*

pancreaticosplenic l. A fold of peritoneum uniting the tail of the pancreas with the lower part of the medial surface of the spleen.

patellar l. The ligament attaching the patella to the tuberosity of the tibia.

pectinate l. Trabecular tissue from the posterior elastic lamina which extends into the substance of the iris.

petrosphenoid l. A thickened portion of the dura mater joining the petrous apex with the posterior clinoid process: also called *Gruber's l.*

phrenicocolic l. A fold of peritoneum extending from the left colic flexure to the diaphragm serving to support the spleen.

proper l. of ovary. The terminal portion of the genital ridge uniting the caudal end of the embryonic ovary with the uterus.

pterygospinous l. A band of fibrous tissue extending from the lateral pterygoid plate to the spine of the sphenoid.

puboprostatic l. A thickening of the pelvic fascia running from the capsule of the prostate gland to the pubic bone; medial and lateral ones on each side are described: in the female called *pubovesical ligaments.*

pubovesical l. A thickening of the pelvic fascia running from the urinary bladder to the pubic bone; medial and lateral ones on each side are described: in the male called *puboprostatic ligaments.*

pulmonary l. A fold of pleura extending between the lower part of the mediastinal surface of the lung and the pericardium.

quadrate l. A thickened band extending from the neck of the radius to the inferior border of the annular ligament below the radial notch.

radiate l. A fibrous band connecting the anterior part of the head of each rib with the sides of two vertebrae and corresponding intervertebral disk.

reflected l. An occasional band of fibers of the superior crus of one inguinal ligament which crosses the midline to an attachment on the tubercle of the other pubic bone: also called *triangular fascia;* formerly *Colles' l.*

rhomboid l. One joining the cartilage of the first rib and the tuberosity of the clavicle.

round l. of femur. A flattened band extending from the fovea on the head of the femur to attach on either side of the acetabular notch between which it blends with the transverse ligament. Also called *ligamentum teres femoris.* See Plate 2.

round l. of liver. A fibrous cord running from the umbilicus to the notch in the anterior border of the liver. It represents the remains of the obliterated umbilical vein. Also called *ligamentum teres hepatis.*

round l. of uterus. A ligament running from the anterior surface of the lateral border of the uterus through the inguinal canal to the labium majus. Also called *ligamentum teres uteri.* See Plate 41.

sacrospinous l. A thin triangular band running from the spine of the ischium medially to the lateral margin of the sacrum and coccyx. See Plate 2.

sacrotuberous l. A ligament extending from the sacrum, coccyx, and posterior iliac spines to the tuberosity of the ischium. See Plate 2.

sphenomandibular l. A fibrous band extending from the angular spine of the sphenoid to the lingula of the mandibular foramen. It is derived from the embryonic Meckel's cartilage.

sphenomaxillary l. Old term for sphenomandibular ligament.

spiral l. The greatly thickened periosteum of the outer wall of the cochlear duct. See Plate 20.

stellate l. Radiate ligament.

stylohyoid l. A fibrous cord attached to the tip of the styloid process of the temporal bone and the lesser horn of the hyoid bone, derived from Reichert's cartilage.

subpubic l. The arcuate ligament of the pubis.

suspensory l. of lens. See ciliary *zonule.*

suspensory l. of ovary. A small peritoneal fold passing upward from the tubal end of the ovary to the peritoneum over the iliac vessels and psoas muscle. Also called *infundibulopelvic l.*

suspensory l. of penis. Fibers from the linea alba and symphysis pubis forming a strong fibrous band which extends to the upper surface of the root to blend with the fascial sheath of the penis.

sutural l. A thin layer of fibrous membrane separating bones forming an immovable articulation, as the bones of the skull.

tarsal l. See palpebral *l.*

thyrohyoid l. Thyrohyoid membrane.

transverse carpal l. See flexor *retinaculum* of the wrist.

transverse crural l. See superior extensor *retinaculum.*

transverse perineal l. The fibrous anterior margin of the urogenital diaphragm: formerly called *transverse pelvic l.*

trapezoid l. A broad quadrilateral ligament extending from the upper surface of the coracoid process to the oblique ridge on the under surface of the clavicle.

triangular l. Urogenital diaphragm.

triangular ligaments of liver. The right and left margins of the coronary ligament connecting the right and left lobes of the liver respectively with the diaphragm.

true lateral l. of bladder. A thickening of the pelvic fascia extending laterally on either side from the lower part of the urinary bladder or prostate gland.

uterosacral l. A concentric fold of peritoneum containing much fibrous tissue which passes backward from the cervix of the uterus on either side of the rectum to the posterior wall of the pelvis.

ventricular l. Ventricular fold.

vocal l. Vocal fold.

volar carpal l. A band of deep fascia of the wrist overlying the ulnar artery and nerve.

xiphocostal l. A ligament extending from the xiphoid cartilage to the cartilage of the eighth rib.

Y l. The iliofemoral *l.*

lig"a·men'to·pex"y [*ligamentum;* G. *pēxis,* a fixing]. Suspension of the uterus by shortening or fixation of the round ligaments.

lig"a·men'tum (pl. *ligamenta*) [L.]. Ligament.

ligamenta auricularia. Fibrous bands which aid in fixing the auricle against the head.

l. arteriosum. The remains of the fetal ductus arteriosus, extending from the pulmonary trunk to the arch of the aorta.

l. caudale. An embryonic ligament formed by the degeneration and fusion of the last two or three somites; it is attached to the dermis under the coccygeal glabella and is closely related to the caudal medullary vestige.

l. flavum. Yellow elastic tissue which connects the laminas of contiguous vertebrae.

l. nuchae. The nuchal ligament.

l. pulmonis. The pulmonary ligament.

l. reflexum. The reflected ligament.

l. teres femoris. See round *ligament* of the femur.

l. teres hepatis. See round *ligament* of the liver.

l. teres uteri. See round *ligament* of the uterus.

l. testis. A short embryonic ligament developing in the caudal genital ridge forming the upper part of the gubernaculum testis.

l. venosum. A ligament of the liver representing the remains of the embryonic ductus venosus.

li·ga'tion (lye·gay'shun) [L. *ligatio,* from *ligare,* to bind]. The operation of tying, especially arteries, veins, or ducts, with some form of knotted ligature. —**li'gate,** *v.*

lig'a·ture [L. *ligatura,* a band]. 1. A cord or thread for tying vessels. 2. The act of tying or binding; ligation.

absorbable l. One composed of animal tissue, such as catgut, which can be absorbed by the tissues.

chain l. One used by tying broad pedicles in sections, the whole mass being constricted in sections by a chain of interlocking ligatures.

double l. The ligation of a vessel at two points, the vessel being divided distal to both.

elastic l. One of live rubber, used for strangulation of tissue and the gradual cutting through of certain areas by constant pressure.

interlocking l. Chain ligature.

l. carrier. A specially designed forceps for passing or drawing ligatures through tissues.

nonabsorbable l. One which cannot be absorbed by the tissues, such as silkworm gut.

occluding l. One completely obstructing a vessel or channel.

light [AS. *lēoht*]. Electromagnetic radiations that give rise to the sensation of vision when the rays impinge upon the retina.

axial l. Light rays that are parallel to each other and to the optic axis.

black l. See Robert Williams *Wood.*

central l. See axial *l.*

diffused l. That reflected simultaneously from an infinite number of surfaces, or that which has been scattered by means of a concave mirror or lens.

Finsen l. Light from which the heat rays and most visible rays are absorbed by filters, leaving only blue, violet, and notably ultraviolet rays; used in phototherapy.

monochromatic l. See *monochromatic.*

oblique l. Light falling obliquely on a surface.

polarized l. Light which has undergone polarization.

quartz l. A lamp fitted with a quartz lens, used in radiant light therapy.

reflected l. Light thrown back from an illuminated object.

refracted l. Light rays that have passed from one medium into another and have been bent from their original course.

refrigerated l. See Finsen *l.*

transmitted l. The light passing through an object.

ultraviolet l. Invisible radiant energy having a wavelength of approximately 20 to 400.

Wood's l. See Robert Williams *Wood.*

light dif'fer·ence. 1. The difference between the two eyes in respect to their sensitiveness to light. 2. The smallest difference in illumination which can be distinguished by the eyes. Abbreviated, L. D.

light'en·ing [AS. *līgt*]. The sinking of the fetal head into the pelvic inlet with an accompanying descent of the uterus.

light'er·man's bot'tom. Inflammation of the bursa over the tuberosity of the ischium; due to prolonged sitting. Also called *weavers' bottom.*

light green S.F. yel′low·ish (C.C.). A dye derivative of brilliant green which fades rapidly; a valuable plasma stain. It has been used to stain bacteria, yeasts, algae, and plant cells.

light′ning pains. The lancinating pains of spinal root disease, coming on and disappearing with lightninglike rapidity, as in tabes dorsalis.

light sense test′er. Any instrument used to test the sensitivity of the eye to light.

perimetric l. s. t. An attachment for a perimeter which may be used for determining the light threshold of the eye at any desired position or positions in the visual field.

lig′ne·ous [L. *ligneus*, wooden]. Woody, or having a woody texture.

lig″ni·fi·ca′tion [L. *lignum*, wood; *facere*, to make]. The process by which the cell wall of a plant acquires greater rigidity by deposition of lignin.

lig′nin. $C_{20}H_{20}O_6$. A modification of cellulose, constituting the greater part of the weight of most dry wood. A substance deposited in the cell walls of plants.

lig′no·caine hy″dro·chlo′ride. British generic name for the local anesthetic agent lidocaine hydrochloride.

lig″no·cer′ic ac′id (lig″no·serr′ick, ·seer′ick). $C_{23}H_{47}COOH$. A fatty acid derived from kerasin.

lig′num [L.]. Wood.

l. benedictum. Guaiac wood.

l. cedrum. Cedar wood.

l. vitae. The tree, *Guajacum officinale*. See *guaiac.*

lig′ro·in. A liquid fraction obtained from petroleum; used as a solvent.

li·gus′ti·cum (li·gus′ti·kum, lye·). See *lovage.*

lik′mi·sis [G. *likmao* or *likmizo*, to winnow]. Chromatography: term suggested as being a more rational designation.

Lilienthal, Howard [*American surgeon*, 1861–1946]. Well known for his many contributions to the knowledge of thoracic surgery. He described low posterior mediastinotomy by resection of the ninth rib, with transillumination of the esophagus for ease of access. Described esophagogastrostomy through the posterior approach, implanting the lower end of the esophagus into the stomach wall by intussusception, using traction sutures through a secondary stomach incision; called *Lilienthal's operation.* Inventor of a guillotine type of costotome for use in removing the first rib; called *Lilienthal's costotome.*

Lillie's stains. See under *stain.*

lily of the val′ley. See *convallaria.*

limb [AS. *lim*]. 1. One of the extremities attached to the trunk and used for prehension or locomotion. 2. An elongated limblike structure, as one of the limbs of the internal capsule.

anterior l. of the internal capsule. That portion which lies between the caudate and lentiform nuclei.

artificial l. See *prosthesis*, 2.

ascending l. The portion of a renal tubule which extends from the bend in Henle's loop to the distal convoluted portion.

descending l. The portion of a renal tubule which extends from the proximal convoluted portion to the bend in Henle's loop.

pelvic l. A lower extremity.

posterior l. of the internal capsule. That portion which lies between the lentiform nucleus and the thalamus.

thoracic l. An upper extremity.

lim′ber·neck. An avian type of botulism; a disease caused by *Clostridium botulinum Cα* and characterized by muscular incoordination, weakness, and death.

lim′bus (pl. *limbi*) [L., border]. A border; the circumferential edge of any flat organ or part. —**limbic,** *adj.*

corneoscleral l. The circumference of the cornea at its junction with the sclera.

l. alveolaris. The alveolar crest.

l. corneae. See corneoscleral *l.*

l. fossae ovalis. The thick margin of the fossa ovalis of the heart, representing the margin of the foramen ovale in the embryonic septum secundum. Syn., *annulus ovalis.*

l. of the spiral lamina. A thickening of the periosteum at the border of the osseous spiral lamina of the cochlea; to it is attached the tectorial membrane.

l. palpebralis anterior. The rounded anterior edge of the margin of the eyelid from which the eyelashes grow.

l. palpebralis posterior. The sharp posterior edge of the margin of the eyelid that is applied to the eyeball; it is the point of transition of skin to the conjunctival mucous membrane.

l. sphenoidalis. The sharp anterior edge of the groove on the sphenoid bone for the optic commissure.

l. spiralis. See *l.* of the spiral lamina.

lime [AS. *lim*]. CaO, calcium oxide. See under *calcium.*

chlorinated l. (*calx chlorinata*). The product of the chlorination of lime; consists chiefly of calcium hypochlorite and calcium chloride. Employed as a disinfectant.

l. liniment. See carron *oil.*

l. milk. A milky fluid consisting of calcium hydroxide suspended in water.

l. water (*liquor calcii hydroxidi*). An aqueous solution containing 0.14% $Ca(OH)_2$ at 25° C. Used as an antacid. Dose, 30–120 cc. (1–4 fluidounces).

slaked l. Lime which has been acted on by water; it consists chiefly of calcium hydroxide.

lime [F.]. The fruit of *Citrus aurantifolia;* its juice is antiscorbutic and refrigerant.

li′men (pl. *limina*) [L., threshold]. 1. A boundary line. 2. See *threshold.*

l. insulae. The imaginary line separating the anterior perforated substance from the insula.

l. nasi. The boundary line between the osseous and the cartilaginous portions of the nasal cavity.

li′mes (pl. *limites*). [L.] Limit, boundary.

li′mes death (lye′meez). The least amount of toxin which, when mixed with one unit of antitoxin and injected into a guinea pig weighing 250 Gm., kills within five days. Symbol, L_+.

li′mes ze′ro. The greatest amount of toxin which causes no local edema when mixed with one unit of antitoxin and injected into a guinea pig weighing 250 Gm. Symbol, L_0.

lim′i·na. Plural of limen.

lim′i·nal [*limen*]. Pertaining to the limen or threshold, especially pertaining to the lowest limit of perception.

lim′it of floc″cu·la′tion. The dose of toxin per unit of a certain antitoxin in the mixture which flocculates more rapidly, under the same conditions, than all other mixtures, which contain other amounts of the same toxin per unit of the same antitoxin. Abbreviated, Lf.

lim′i·troph′ic. Controlling nutrition.

Lim·na′tis. A genus of aquatic leeches.

L. nilotica. A widely distributed species which produces internal hirudiniasis in man.

lim·nol′o·gy [G. *limnē*, marsh; *logos*, word]. The study of inland waters; particularly the study of biologic, chemical, and physical conditions in ponds, lakes, and streams.

lim'o·nene. $C_{10}H_{16}$; a monocyclic terpene hydrocarbon, existing in optically active and racemic forms, occurring in many volatile oils.

li'mo·nite (lye'mo·night, lim'o·). Ferric oxide, of the approximate formula $2Fe_2O_3.3H_2O$; a yellow powder. See *iron* oxide.

li·moph'thi·sis (li·mof'thi·sis, lye·) [G. *limos*, hunger; *phthisis*, a wasting away]. Wasting of the body, due to starvation.

limp [cf. AS. *lemphealt*, lame]. A halting gait. See *claudication*.

lin·al'o·ol (lin·al'o·ole, ·ol, ·awl, lin"uh·lool'). $C_{10}H_{17}OH$. An alcohol occurring in coriander, lavender, and bergamot oils. It exists in both dextrorotatory and levorotatory forms, designated *d*-linalool and *l*-linalool, respectively. *d*-Linalool, also called *coriandrol*, is the chief constituent of coriander oil.

lin'a·lyl ac'e·tate (ass'i·tayt). $C_{10}H_{17}OCOCH_3$. A constituent of lavender and other oils.

lin"a·ma'rin, lin·am'a·rin. The toxic glycoside of flaxseed.

Lind, James [*Scottish physician*, 1716–94]. Made important observations on tropical diseases. Gave a classic description of scurvy (1753). Is considered largely responsible for the fact that the British navy adopted lemon juice as a preventive of scurvy.

lin'dane. Generic name for the gamma isomer of 1,2,3,4,5,6-hexachlorocyclohexane ($C_6H_6Cl_6$), known also as benzene hexachloride, of a purity of not less than 99 per cent; a powerful insecticide.

Lindau, Arvid [*Swedish pathologist*, 1892–]. Studied angiomatosis of the central nervous system. Demonstrated that some cystic tumors of the cerebellum are due to angiomas, and that these vascular lesions can be found in other parts of the body, including the retina and abdominal organs. The cerebellar tumor is known as *Lindau's tumor*, and the retinal lesion as *von Hippel's disease*. The syndrome is called *von Hippel-Lindau's disease*.

Lindbergh, Charles Augustus [*American aviator*, 1902–]. With Carrel, devised a perfusion apparatus with which organs can be kept alive outside the body; called *Carrel-Lindbergh pump*. He also devised a flask with two chambers, one above the other, for cultivating a large number of tissue fragments in a thin layer of well oxygenated and constantly circulating medium, called *Lindbergh flask*.

line [L. *linea*, line]. 1. Extension of dimension having length, but neither breadth nor thickness. 2. *In anatomy*, anything resembling a mathematical line in having length without breadth or thickness; a boundary or guide-mark. 3. The 1/12 part of an inch. *Obs*. 4. *In genetics*, lineage; the succession of progenitors and progeny.

abdominal lines. Transverse lines of the abdominal wall: also called *striae albicantes gravidarum*.

alveolobasilar l. A line joining the basion and the alveolar point.

alveolonasal l. A line joining the nasal and alveolar points.

anocutaneous l. The junction between skin and mucous membrane at the anus.

anorectal l. The junction between the intestinal portion and the anal portion of the rectum.

anterior axillary l. A vertical line extending downward from the anterior fold of the axilla on the side of the trunk.

anterior gluteal l. A line beginning at the anterior extremity of the iliac crest and curving downward and backward to the upper part of the greater sciatic notch.

arcuate l. (a) The iliac portion of the iliopectineal line. (b) An arched thickening of the obturator fascia from which the levator ani muscle arises. Also called *arcus tendineus*.

auriculobregmatic l. One passing from the auricular point to the bregma, dividing the preauricular from the postauricular part of cranium.

base l. A line running backward from the infraorbital ridge through the middle of the external auditory meatus, and prolonged to the middle line of the head posteriorly.

basiobregmatic l. The line joining the basion and the bregma.

biauricular l. The line separating the anterior from the posterior portion of the skull; it extends from one external auditory meatus over the vertex to the other.

blue l. See lead *l.*

cement l. The optically demonstrable interface between older bone matrix and more recently formed matrix.

cervical l. The line about the neck of a tooth at the junction of enamel and cementum.

cleavage lines. See Carl von *Langer*.

costoarticular l. A line drawn between the sternoclavicular articulation and the tip of the eleventh rib.

costoclavicular l. See parasternal *l.*

epiphyseal l. 1. The scar left at the site of the epiphyseal plate after fusion of an epiphysis with the diaphysis of a long bone. 2. *In radiology*, an epiphyseal cartilage.

equipotential l. Isopotential *l.*

facial l. A straight line tangential to the glabella and some point at the lower portion of the face. Also called *Camper's l.*

genal l. A line running downward from the region of the zygomatic bone to join the nasal line; it is seen in the faces of children in certain diseases.

gingival l. A line about the crown of a tooth that conforms to the free margin of the gingiva.

iliopectineal l. The bony ridge marking the brim of the true pelvis, situated partly on the ilium and partly on the pubis.

imbrication l. One of the grooves in the surface of the dental enamel where lines of Retzius outcrop.

incremental l. One of the lines in sections of dentin (lines of Owen) and dental enamel (lines of Retzius) which mark zones of imperfect calcification at successive stages in the development of a tooth.

inferior gluteal l. A line extending from the anterior inferior spine of the ilium to the middle of the greater sciatic notch. Formerly called *inferior curved line of the ilium*.

inferior nuchal l. A transverse ridge extending from the median nuchal line across the outer surface of the occipital bone, a short distance below the superior nuchal line. Formerly called *inferior curved line of the occipital bone*.

inferior temporal l. A line arching across the side of the cranium, marking the upper limit of the temporal fossa and of the attachment of the temporalis muscle.

intercondyloid l. A ridge on the posterior surface of the lower end of the femur, forming the upper limit of the intercondyloid fossa.

intermediate l. A ridge on the iliac crest between the inner and outer lips.

intertrochanteric l. A line upon the anterior surface of the femur, between the neck and shaft, and extending from the tubercle of the greater trochanter to a point below the lesser trochanter.

intertubercular l. An imaginary transverse line drawn across the abdomen at the level of the tubercles on the iliac crests.

isoelectric l. Isopotential line.

isopotential l. The portion of an electrogram during which there is no potential difference between the two leading electrodes, and therefore no deflection from the base line.
Langer's lines. See Carl von *Langer*.
lead l. The blue line at the dental margin of the gums in chronic lead poisoning.
l. of demarcation. A line of division between healthy and gangrenous tissue.
l. of duty. 1. Authorized duty in service. 2. *In U. S. military medicine*, a classification of all sickness, injury, or death suffered by personnel in active military service, unless caused by individual fault or neglect and unless the disease, injury, or condition existed prior to, and was not aggravated by, service.
l. of fixation. An imaginary line drawn from the object viewed through the center of rotation of the eye.
l. of Gennari. See under *Gennari*.
l. of occlusion. Line joining the areas of contact of teeth in occlusion.
l. of regard. *In optics*, the line connecting the center of rotation of the eye with the point of fixation or of regard.
l. of sight. An imaginary line drawn from the object viewed to the center of the pupil.
lines of Owen. Incremental lines of dentin.
lines of Retzius. Incremental lines of enamel.
lines of Schreger. Radial dark and light bands in the dental enamel or similar bands concentric with the surface of the dentin, produced by differential refraction and reflection of light used in microscopical examination of sections.
longitudinal l. A longitudinal ridge on a nail produced by unequal growth.
mammary l. See milk *l.*
mammillary l. A vertical line passing through the center of the nipple.
median nuchal l. A ridge or crest on the occipital bone, extending from the external occipital protuberance to the foramen magnum. Syn., *external occipital crest.*
midaxillary l. A perpendicular line drawn from the apex of the axilla.
midclavicular l. A vertical line parallel to, and midway between, the midsternal line and a vertical line drawn downward through the outer end of the clavicle.
midsternal l. A vertical line through the middle of the sternum.
milk l. A ridge of thickened ectoderm, extending longitudinally between the bases of the limb buds, from which the mammary glands develop.
mylohyoid l. A ridge on the internal surface of the mandible, extending upward and backward from the sublingual fossa to the ramus. Also called *mylohyoid ridge.*
nasal l. A line from the upper margin of the ala nasi curving around the angle of the mouth, ending at the edge of the orbicularis oris; it is seen in diseases of the gastrointestinal tract.
nasobasilar l. A line drawn through the basion and the nasal point.
neonatal l. A prominent incremental line formed in the neonatal period in the enamel and dentine of a deciduous tooth.
nipple l. See mammillary *l.*
oblique l. of the fibula. The posteromedial border, beginning at the medial side of the head and continuing downward into the interosseous crest.
oblique l. of the mandible. Continuation of the anterior border of the ramus downward and forward onto the lateral surface of the mandible.
oblique l. of the radius. A ridge of bone extending laterally and downward from the radial tuberosity; it gives origin to the flexor digitorum sublimis and flexor pollicis longus muscles.
oblique l. of the thyroid cartilage. A line running downward and forward on the lateral side of each lamina.
obturator l. A sign seen roentgenologically in early inflammatory disease of the hip in children.
parasternal l. An imaginary vertical line midway between the lateral margin of the sternum and the mammillary line.
Pastia's lines. Red streaks in the lateral folds of the skin in the antecubital, axillary, and inguinal regions and the neck in severe scarlet fever: also called *Pastia's sign.*
pectineal l. That on the posterior surface of the femur, running downward from the lesser trochanter and giving attachment to the pectineus muscle.
popliteal l. An oblique ridge on the posterior surface of the tibia, extending from the fibular facet to the middle of the medial border.
posterior axillary l. A vertical line extending downward from the posterior fold of the axilla on the side of the trunk.
posterior gluteal l. A line beginning near the end of the posterior extremity of the crest of the ilium and curving downward to the posterior part of the greater sciatic notch. Formerly called *superior curved l. of the ilium.*
primitive l. See primitive *streak.*
pure l. See *pure line.*
quadrate l. A slight ridge extending downward from the middle of the intertrochanteric crest and giving attachment to the quadratus femoris muscle.
respiratory l. The line connecting the bases of the upward strokes in a tracing of the pulse.
scapular l. A vertical line drawn on the back through the inferior angle of the scapula.
semicircular l. The curved lower edge of the internal layer of the aponeurosis of the internal oblique muscle, where it ceases to cover the posterior surface of the rectus muscle. Also called *linea semicircularis of Douglas.*
semilunar l. A line, convex laterally, marking the transition of the internal oblique and transverse muscles of the abdomen to aponeuroses. Also called *linea semilunaris of Spigelius.*
sternal l. The median line of the sternum.
sternomastoid l. A line drawn from a point between the two heads of the sternocleidomastoid muscle to the mastoid process.
subcostal l. An imaginary transverse line drawn across the abdomen at the level of the lower border of the tenth costal cartilage.
superior nuchal l. A semicircular line passing outward and forward from the external occipital protuberance. Formerly called *superior curved line of the occipital bone.*
superior temporal l. A line arching across the side of the cranium and giving attachment to the temporal fascia.
supraorbital l. A line extending horizontally across the forehead immediately above the zygomatic process of the frontal bone.
temporal l. The ridge of bone curving upward and backward from the zygomatic process of the frontal bone; it divides into the superior and inferior temporal lines.
tension lines. See Carl von *Langer*.
terminal l. See iliopectineal *l.*
test l. A line for detecting shortening of the neck of the femur.
transpyloric l. A horizontal line drawn through a point midway between the jugular notch and the symphysis pubis.

transverse l. One of the lines of nails in the form of sulci limited proximally by slightly elevated ridges which appear at the lunula and progress forward with the growth of the nail until they disappear at the free edge. Also called *Beau's lines.*

trapezoid l. The line of attachment of the trapezoid ligament on the inferior surface of the outer portion of the clavicle.

visual l. An imaginary line drawn from a point looked at, through the nodal point of the eye, to the macula lutea.

white l. The linea alba.

Z l. See Z *disk.*

lin′e·a (pl. *lineae*) [L.]. Line.

l. alba. A tendinous raphe extending in the median line of the abdomen from the pubes to the xiphoid process; it is formed by the blending of the aponeuroses of the oblique and transverse muscles. See Plate 4.

l. aspera. A rough longitudinal ridge on the posterior surface of the middle third of the femur serving as attachment for muscles.

lineae albicantes. Glistening white lines seen in the skin, especially that of the abdomen, after reduction of extreme distention, as in pregnancy (*l.* gravidarum, striae gravidarum), excessive adiposity, tumors: produced by rupture of the elastic tissue fibers.

lineae gravidarum. Lineae albicantes.

l. nigra. A dark pigmented line often present in pregnant women and extending from the pubes upward in the median line.

l. sinuosa analis. The junction between the columnar and intermediate zones of the anal canal. Also called *anorectal junction.*

l. splendens. A longitudinal fibrous band of pia mater along the median line of the anterior surface of the spinal cord.

lin′e·ar cor″re·la′tion. A correlation between two variables in which the regression equation is represented by a straight line; a relationship that can be described graphically by a straight line.

lin′gua [L.]. The tongue. —**lingual,** *adj.*

l. nigra. See black hairy *tongue.*

l. plicata. Fissured tongue.

lin′gual (ling′gwal). The inferior and superior intrinsic longitudinal muscles of the tongue: old term.

Lin·guat′u·la (ling·gwach′oo·luh) [dim. from *lingua*]. A genus of the class Pentastomida, degenerate arthropods, endoparasites of vertebrates; commonly known as tongue worms.

L. serrata. A species found in the nose or paranasal sinuses of dogs and other carnivores; rarely infests man.

linguet. Trade-mark for a tablet designed to permit absorption of active ingredient through the buccal mucosa into the venous system.

lin′gu·la [dim. from *lingua*] 1. A small lobule between the anterior medullary velum and the central lobule of the cerebellum. 2. A tonguelike structure. —**lingular,** *adj.*

l. of the ear. The cartilaginous projection toward or into the upper portion of the lobe of the ear.

l. of the mandible. The prominent, thin process of bone partly surrounding the mandibular foramen.

l. of the sphenoid. A small, tonguelike process extending backward in the angle formed by the body of the sphenoid and one of its greater wings.

lin″guo·dis′tal [*lingua;* L. *distare,* to be distant]. Distally and toward the tongue, as the inclination of a tooth.

lin″guo·gin′gi·val (ling″gwo·jin′ji·vul, ·jin·jy′vul) [*lingua;* L. *gingiva,* gum]. Relating to the tongue and the gingiva.

lin′i·ment [L. *linire,* to smear]. A liquid intended for application to the skin by gentle friction.

li′nin. 1. A strongly purgative principle obtainable from *Linum catharticum,* or purging flax. 2. *In biology,* the substance of the achromatic network of the nucleus of a cell.

li·ni′tis (li·nigh′tis, lye·nigh′tis). Old term for gastritis.

l. plastica. Infiltrating scirrhous carcinoma of the stomach.

link′age [ME. *linke*]. 1. *In chemistry,* the lines used in structural formulas to represent valency connections between the atoms: a single line represents a valency of one, a double line a valency of two, etc. 2. *In genetics,* the association of genes located in the same chromosome.

Linnaeus, Carolus (von Linné) [*Swedish physician and naturalist,* 1707–78]. Known for his work in classifying minerals, plants, and animals. Classified diseases (1763). Said to have given the first description of aphasia (1745).

lin″o·le′ic ac′id (lin″o·lee′ick, li·no′lee·ick). $C_{17}H_{31}$-COOH; an unsaturated acid, 9,12-octadecadienoic acid, containing two double bonds, occurring in the glycerides of linseed and other oils. Syn., *linolic acid.*

li·no′le·in. The glyceride of linoleic acid found in all drying oils.

lin″o·le′nic ac′id (lin″o·lee′nick, ·len′ick). $C_{17}H_{29}$-COOH; an unsaturated acid, 9,12-15-octadecatrienoic acid, containing three double bonds, occurring in the glycerides of linseed and other oils: essential for normal nutrition.

li·no′lic ac′id. See *linoleic acid.*

lin″o·no·pho′bi·a [G. *linon,* anything made of flax; *phobos,* fear]. Morbid fear of string.

lin′seed [AS. *līnsǣd*] (*linum*). The dried ripe seed of *Linum usitatissimum;* it contains 30–40% of a fixed oil, together with wax, resin, tannin, gum, and protein. Linseed is demulcent and emollient; infusions of the whole seed have been used in respiratory infections, and the whole seed is sometimes employed as a laxative. Syn., *flaxseed.*

l. oil (*oleum lini*). The fixed oil obtained from linseed (oil that has been boiled or treated with a drier must not be used medicinally); used mostly in liniments and cerates, occasionally given for its laxative effect. Dose, 30–60 cc. (1–2 fluidounces).

lint [ME. *lynt*]. A loosely woven or partly felted mass of broken linen fibers, made by scraping or picking linen cloth. It was once much used as a dressing for wounds.

lin′tin [*lynt*]. Absorbent cotton rolled or compressed into sheets; used for dressing wounds.

Linzenmeier's blood sedimentation tube. See under *tube.*

li′o-. See *leio-.*

lip [AS. *lippa*]. 1. One of the two fleshy folds surrounding the orifice of the mouth. 2. One of the labia majora or labia minora. See *labium.* 3. A projecting margin; rim.

cleft l. Harelip.

glenoid l. See *labrum* glenoidale.

l. of the cervix of the uterus. One of two surrounding the external os.

rhombic l. The lateral ridge produced by the union of the tela chorioidea of the fourth ventricle with the alar plate of the rhombencephalon.

tympanic l. The upper margin of the internal spiral sulcus in the cochlea.

vestibular l. The lower margin of the internal spiral sulcus in the cochlea.

li′pa [G., oil]. Fat.

lip″a·ro·trich′i·a (lip″uh·ro·trick′ee·uh) [G. *liparos,* oily; *thrix,* hair]. Abnormal oiliness of the hair.

lip′a·rous [*liparos*]. Fat; obese.

li′pase (lye′pace, lip′ace). A fat-splitting enzyme contained in the pancreatic juice, in blood plasma, and in many plants. See Table of Normal Values of Blood Constituents in the Appendix.

pancreatic l. A fat-splitting enzyme secreted by the pancreas. Syn., *steapsin.*

lip″a·su′ri·a, li″pa·su′ri·a [G. *lipos,* fat; *ouron,* urine]. The presence of lipase in the urine.

lip·ec′to·my [*lipos;* G. *ektomē,* excision]. Excision of fatty tissue.

li·pe′mi·a, li·pae′mi·a (li·pee′mee·uh) [*lipos;* G. *haima,* blood]. The presence of a fine emulsion of fatty substances in the blood: also called *lipidemia, lipoidemia.* —**lipem′ic,** *adj.*

alimentary l. Lipemia due to the ingestion of a high-fat diet.

lip·fan′o·gen. Any lipid substance present in blood serum (e.g., long-chain soaps, monoglycerides) which can be taken up by animal cells in tissue culture and converted to visible fat granules: thought to play a role in atherogenesis.

lip′id (lip′id, lye′pid), **lip′ide** (lip′yde, ·id, lye′-pyde, ·pid) [*lipos*]. Any one of a group of fats and fatlike substances having in common the property of insolubility in water and solubility in the fat solvents. Included are fats, fatty acids, fatty oils, waxes, sterols, and esters of fatty acids containing other groups such as phosphoric acid (phospholipids), carbohydrates (glycolipids), etc. Also called *lipin.* See Table of Normal Values of Blood Constituents in the Appendix.

lip″i·de′mi·a. See *lipemia.*

lip″i·do′sis. See *lipoidosis.*

li′pin (lye′pin, lip′in). See *lipid.*

lipiodol. The trade-mark for an iodized poppy seed oil containing 10% or 40% iodine used as a substitute for inorganic iodides, or as a contrast medium for roentgenologic work.

Lipmann, Fritz A. (1899–). American biochemist, born in Germany; Nobel prize winner with Hans A. Krebs in medicine and physiology (1953). He discovered, isolated, and identified coenzyme A, and developed the concept of the generation and utilization of phosphate-bond energy in biochemical reactions.

lip′o-, lip- [*lipos*]. 1. *In medicine and physiology,* a combining form denoting *fat, fatty.* 2. *In chemistry,* a combining form denoting *a lipid.*

lipo-bismol. Trade-mark for an antisyphilitic preparation containing bismuth octyl oxyacetate: used in bismuth therapy in syphilis.

lip′o·blast [*lipos;* G. *blastos,* germ]. A formative fat cell, small or moderate in size, polyhedral, and having numerous tiny droplets of fat in its cytoplasm.

lip″o·blas·to′ma. See *liposarcoma.*

lip″o·blas·to′sis. Multiple lipomas in subcutaneous and visceral fat deposits: rare. Syn., *systemic multiple l.*

lip″o·ca′ic. A substance, probably a hormone, found in the pancreas which prevents deposition of lipids in the liver.

lip″o·cal″ci·no·gran″u·lo·ma·to′sis. Lipoidosis characterized by painless symmetric tumors in the bursae mucosae and musculature; microscopic examination reveals deposits of cholesterol and calcium, degeneration and necrosis of surrounding tissues, and replacement granulation tissue.

lip′o·cere. See *adipocere.*

lip″o·chon″dro·dys′tro·phy (lip″o·kon″dro·dis′-tro·fee) [*lipos;* G. *chondros,* cartilage; *dys-,* bad; *trophē,* nourishment]. Gargoylism.

lip″o·chon·dro′ma (lip″o·kon·dro′muh) [*lipos; chondros;* G. *-ōma,* tumor]. Chondroma containing fat cells.

lip′o·chrome [*lipos;* G. *chrōma,* color]. Any one of a group of fatlike substances containing a pigment or coloring matter, and occurring in natural fats, such as egg yolk. Also called *chromolipoid.*

lip′o·cyte [*lipos;* G. *kytos,* cell]. A fat cell.

lip″o·di·er′e·sis (lip″o·dye·err′i·sis). See *lipolysis.*

lip″o·dys′tro·phy [*lipos;* G. *dys-,* bad; *trophē,* nourishment]. A disturbance of fat metabolism in which the subcutaneous fat disappears over large areas of the body, but is unaffected in others.

cephalothoracic l. See progressive *l.*

intestinal l. A rare disease of unknown cause, described by George H. Whipple (1907), occurring almost exclusively in males over 30 years old, in which the intestinal mucosa and later the intestinal lymphatics become filled with fat, clinically very similar to sprue, and often associated with polyarthritis.

progressive l. Progressive loss of fat from face, neck, arms, thorax, and abdomen: also called *cephalothoracic l.*

lip″o·fi·bro′ma (lip″o·figh·bro′muh). See *fibrolipoma.*

lip″o·fi″bro·myx·o′ma [*lipos;* L. *fibra,* fiber; G. *myxa,* mucus; *-ōma,* tumor]. A mesodermal mixed tumor, containing fatty tissue, fibrous tissue, and mucoid or myxomatous tissue.

lip″o·fi″bro·sar·co′ma. A fibrosarcoma with lipomatous component.

lip″o·fus′cin [*lipos;* L. *fuscus,* dark]. Lipid-containing granules, possibly waste products, which stain black with silver in the presence of a reducing substance such as ascorbic acid; one of the wear-and-tear pigments.

lip″o·gen′e·sis [*lipos;* G. *genesis,* production]. The formation or deposit of fat. —**lipogenic,** *adj.*

li·pog′e·nous (li·podj′i·nus) [*lipos;* G. *genesthai,* from *gignesthai,* to be produced]. Fat-producing.

lip″o·gran″u·lo′ma [*lipos;* L. *granulum,* small grain; G. *-ōma,* tumor]. A nodule of fatty tissue, consisting of a center of degenerated and necrotic fat enclosed by granulation tissue. Due usually to trauma; may possibly be caused by faulty fat metabolism.

lip″o·gran·u·lo″ma·to′sis [*lipos; granulum; -ōma;* G. *-ōsis,* condition]. A condition marked by the presence of one or more lipogranulomas.

lip″o·he″mar·thro′sis. The extravasation of blood and lipids into the synovial sac following trauma.

lip·o′ic ac′id. $CH_2.CH_2.CH(CH_2)_4COOH$. α-Lipoic acid or 6,8-dithio-*n*-octanoic acid, occurring in yeast and liver, which replaces a growth factor necessary for oxidative decarboxylation of pyruvic acid by resting cells of *Streptococcus fecalis* and certain other organisms. Syn., *6-thioctic acid, protogen A.*

lip′oid (lip′oyd, lye′poyd) [*lipos;* G. *eidos,* form]. 1. Resembling fat or oil. 2. Having the character of a lipid; lipoidic.

lip′oid. Old term for *lipid,* particularly one of the intracellular lipids which contain nitrogen. The chemists have officially adopted the term *lipid,* but many histologists still use the old term *lipoid.*

lip″oi·de′mi·a. See *lipemia.*

lip″oi·do′sis [*lipos; eidos;* G. *-ōsis,* condition]. A general term for various conditions in which lipoproteins or lipids are deposited in different organs, particularly in the spleen or liver. Syn., *lipoid histiocytosis.* See *xanthomatosis,* Niemann-Pick *disease,* Hand-Schüller-Christian *disease.*

cerebroside l. See Gaucher's *disease.*

epidermal l. A term used by Sutton to define the reaction to fats in the epidermis and its appendages, especially the hair follicle, in acne.

l. corneae. Fatty deposits in the cornea.

l. cutis et mucosae. See lipid *proteinosis.*

lipoiodine. Trade-mark for ethyl diiodobrassidate, $C_{21}H_{39}I_2COOC_2H_5$, used where iodide therapy is indicated and as a contrast medium in roentgenray examinations.

lipo-lutin. Trade-mark for an oil solution of progesterone.

li·pol′y·sis [*lipos;* G. *lysis,* a loosing]. The decomposition of fat. —**lipolyt′ic,** *adj.*

li·po′ma [*lipos;* G. *-ōma,* tumor]. A tumor, which in the gross is obviously fatty; microscopically composed of fat cells usually of mature form but occasionally in part or wholly of embryonal type. —**lipom′atous, lipom′atoid,** *adj.*

embryonal-cell l. See *liposarcoma.*

fetal fat-cell l. See *liposarcoma.*

infiltrating l. See *liposarcoma.*

lipoblastic l. See *liposarcoma.*

primitive-cell l. See *liposarcoma.*

li·po″ma·to′sis [*lipos; -ōma;* G. *-ōsis,* condition]. Multiple lipomas. A general deposition of fat; obesity.

embryonal l. See *liposarcoma.*

lip″o·me′ri·a (lip″o·meer′ee·uh, lye″po·). See *leipomeria.*

lip″o·me·tab′o·lism [*lipos;* G. *metabolē,* change]. The absorption and metabolism of fat.

li·pom′pha·lus [*lipos;* G. *omphalos,* navel]. A fatty umbilical hernia.

lip″o·my·o·hem·an″gi·o′ma. A mesenchymoma.

lip″o·my·o′ma (lip″o·migh·o′muh) [*lipos;* G. *mys,* muscle; *-ōma,* tumor]. A mesenchymoma.

lip″o·my·o·sar·co′ma. A malignant mesenchymoma.

lip″o·myx·o′ma [*lipos;* G. *myxa,* mucus; *-ōma*]. See *liposarcoma.*

lip″o·myx″o·sar·co′ma. See *liposarcoma.*

Lip″o·nys′sus [*lipos;* G. *nyssein,* to prick]. A genus of small parasitic mites.

L. bacoti. The common rat mite; this species will attack man, producing an uncomfortable dermatitis, and is thought to be a vector of endemic typhus.

lip″o·pe′ni·a [*lipos;* G. *penia,* want]. Abnormal diminution of fat in tissues.

lip″o·pep′tide. Aminolipid. A poorly defined group of fatlike substances containing amino acids.

lip″o·pha′gic [*lipos;* G. *phagein,* to eat]. Absorbing or destroying fat; as lipophagic granuloma, in which there is subcutaneous fat necrosis with indurated areas of various sizes. —**lipopha′gia,** *n.*

lip′o·phil [*lipos;* G. *philein,* to love]. Having affinity for fatty tissue; lipotropic.

lip″o·phil′i·a. Affinity for fat.

lip″o·phre′ni·a (lip″o·free′nee·uh, lye″po·) [G. *leipein,* to be wanting; *phrēn,* mind]. Failure of mental capacity.

lip″o·pro′te·in [G. *lipos,* fat; *prōteios,* of first rank]. One of a group of conjugated proteins consisting of a simple protein combined with a lipid. See *protein.* See American Classification of Proteins in the Appendix.

lip″o·rho′din [*lipos;* G. *rhodon,* rose]. A red-colored lipochrome.

lip″o·sar·co′ma [*lipos;* G. *sarkōma,* fleshy excrescence]. A sarcoma arising in adipose tissue, usually of the thigh, groin, and buttock, and rarely in bone. Its microscopic structure varies from fully developed fat cells to completely anaplastic cellular sarcoma, and often includes areas resembling myxosarcoma or immature mesenchymal tissue. Immature and giant lipoblasts showing all stages of vacuolization are common. Also called *lipoblastoma, embryonal-cell lipoma, fetal fat-cell lipoma, infiltrating lipoma, lipoblastic lipoma, primitive-cell lipoma, embryonal lipomatosis, lipomyxoma, lipomyxosarcoma, myxolipoma, myxoliposarcoma, myxoma lipomatodes, primitive fat-cell tumor.*

li·po′sis [*lipos;* G. *-ōsis,* condition]. Lipomatosis.

li·po′si·tol. A name proposed by Folch and Woolley for inositol phospholipids.

lip″o·sol′u·ble [*lipos;* L. *solutum,* from *solvere,* to loosen]. Soluble in fats.

li·pos′to·my (li·pos′to·mee, lye·) [G. *leipein,* to be wanting; *stoma,* mouth]. The congenital absence of a mouth.

lip″o·thi·am′ide py″ro·phos′phate. A factor, representing α-lipoic acid joined to thiamine pyrophosphate by an amide bond, which, when added to enzyme preparations from *Escherichia coli,* effects oxidative decarboxylation of pyruvic acid to acetyl or succinyl coenzyme A.

lip″o·tro′pic (lip″o·tro′pick, ·trop′ick) [G. *lipos,* fat; *trepein,* to turn]. 1. Having an affinity for lipids, particularly fats and oils. 2. Having a preventive or curative effect on the development of fatty livers.

lip″o·vac′cine (lip″o·vack′seen, ·sin) [*lipos;* L. *vaccinus,* from *vacca,* cow]. A vaccine with a fatty or oily menstruum.

lip″o·vi·tel′lin. A lipoprotein occurring in egg yolk; a conjugated protein containing approximately 18 per cent of phospholipid.

lip″o·xan′thin (lip″o·zan′thin) [*lipos;* G. *xanthos,* yellow]. A yellow lipochrome.

li·pox′e·nous (li·pock′si·nus, lye·) [G. *leipein,* to leave; *xenos,* host]. Term applied to a parasite which leaves its host after completing its development. —**lipoxeny,** *n.*

li·pox′i·dase. An enzyme catalyzing oxidation of long-chain unsaturated fatty acids to short-chain fatty acids.

lip′pa. Lippitudo.

lip′ping [AS. *lippa*]. The perichondral growth of osteophytes which projects beyond the margin of the joint in degenerative joint disease.

lip″pi·tu′do, lip′pi·tude [L. *lippitudo,* blearedness, inflammation of the eyes]. A condition of the eyes marked by ulcerative marginal blepharitis; a state of being blear-eyed.

lip read′ing. The ability to understand what a person is saying by observing the movements of his lips and other facial muscles, without hearing him speak; important in instruction of the deaf.

Lipschütz, Benjamin [*Austrian dermatologist,* 1878–1931]. Described acute vulvar ulcer, nonvenereal in origin, possibly caused by *Bacillus crassis;* called *Lipschütz ulcer, disease.* The centrocyte is also known as the *Lipschütz cell.*

li·pu′ri·a [G. *lipos,* fat; *ouron,* urine]. The presence of fat in the urine.

liquaemin. Trade-mark for a sterile solution of the sodium salt of heparin.

liq″ue·fac′tion (lick″wi·fack′shun) [L. *liquefacere,* to make liquid]. The change to a liquid form, usually of a solid tissue to a fluid or semifluid state, due principally to occlusion of blood supply, or to bacterial or chemical corrosive action. Used in chemistry to indicate condensation of gases to liquid.

l. necrosis. See liquefactive *necrosis.*

liq′uid [L. *liquidus,* fluid]. A fluid or substance that flows readily. A state of matter intermediate between a solid and a gas, shapeless and fluid, taking the shape of the container and seeking the lowest level.

liq′uo·gel. A gel which, when melted, yields a sol of low viscosity.

liq′uor [L., liquid]. 1. Any of certain medicinal solutions, usually including aqueous solutions of nonvolatile substances, except those solutions which belong to the class of syrups, infusions, or decoctions. 2. An English designation for any liquid, as dye liquor, mother liquor, etc. 3. An alcoholic drink.

l. amnii. The liquid contained in the amniotic sac.

l. amnii spurius. The oxidation products formed by the mesonephros contained as a fluid in the sac of the allantois. Syn., *allantoic fluid.*

l. folliculi. Follicular fluid.

l. sanguinis. Old term for the blood plasma.

l. seminis. Old term for semen.

liq′uo·rice. See *licorice.*

Lisfranc de Saint Martin, Jacques [*French surgeon,* 1790–1847]. Described the scalene tubercle on the upper surface of the first rib for the insertion of the scalenus anterior muscle; called *Lisfranc's tubercle.* Partial amputation of the foot by disarticulation of the metatarsal bones from the tarsus is known as *Lisfranc's amputation.*

lisp [AS. *wlispian*]. Speak indistinctly; pronounce imperfectly the sibilant letters *s* and *z*, as by giving them the sound of *th*, and by giving the letter *l* the sound of *w*. See *sigmatism.*

Lissauer, Heinrich [*German neurologist,* 1861–91]. Described a type of dementia paralytica in which focal symptoms are predominant. The disease is characterized by convulsions, aphasia, monoplegia, etc. Called *Lissauer's paralysis.* The dorsolateral tract is also called *Lissauer's tract.*

lis″sen·ce·pha′li·a [G. *lissos,* smooth; *egkephalos,* brain]. Agenesia of the cerebral gyri, resulting in a smooth brain.

lis″sen·ceph′a·lous [*lissos; egkephalos*]. Having a brain with few or no convolutions.

lissephen. Trade-marked name for *mephenesin.*

Lister, Joseph [*English surgeon,* 1827–1912]. Considered the founder of antiseptic surgery; established the use of antiseptics in the operating room.

Lister, Joseph Jackson [*English optician and wine merchant,* 1786–1869]. Made important improvements in microscope lenses. Discovered the law of aplanatic foci.

Lis″ter·el′la. Synonym for *Listeria.*

Lis·te′ri·a [after Joseph *Lister*]. A genus of bacteria of the family Corynebacteriaceae. Its members are small, non-spore-forming, Gram-positive rods, motile by means of a single terminal flagellum.

L. monocytogenes. One cause of sporadic cases of purulent meningitis in man and the probable cause of an infectious mononucleosislike syndrome.

listerine. A proprietary antiseptic preparation containing, as active ingredients, thymol, eucalyptol, methyl salicylate, menthol, benzoic and boric acids.

Lis′ter·ism [*Lister*]. A general name for the antiseptic and aseptic treatment of wounds according to the principles of Joseph Lister.

Listing, Johann Benedict [*German physicist and physiologist,* 1808–82]. Devised a method of simplifying optical problems; in *Listing's reduced schematic eye* the two nodal points are represented by one point and the two principal points by one point. *Listing's law* states that when the eyeball moves from the position of rest, its angle of rotation is the same as if it rotated on an axis perpendicular to both the line of vision in its new position and the line of vision in its former position.

Liston, Robert [*Scottish surgeon in England,* 1794–1847]. Credited with introducing ether anesthesia in Europe (1846). Devised long-bladed knives, called *Liston's knives,* for use in amputations, and bone-cutting forceps, called *Liston's forceps.* Devised a straight splint for the side of the leg, or the body; called *Liston's splint.*

li′ter (lee′tur) [G. *litra,* pound]. The metric unit of volume. One liter is the volume occupied by 1 kg. of pure water at 4° C. and 760 mm. pressure. It is equal to 1.056 United States quarts. Abbreviated, l, l.

lith′a·gogue (lith′uh·gog) [G. *lithos,* stone; *agōgos,* leading]. Any agent which is supposed to expel calculi from the urinary bladder.

lith′arge (lith′ardj, li·thardj′). Lead monoxide.

lith·ec′to·my [*lithos;* G. *ektomē,* excision]. Old term for lithotomy.

li·the′mi·a, li·thae′mi·a (li·theem′ee·uh) [*lithos;* G. *haima,* blood]. A condition in which, owing to defective metabolism of the nitrogenous elements, the blood becomes charged with uric acid.

lith′i·a. Li_2O. Lithium oxide. **Lithia tablets** contain lithium citrate. **Lithia water** is a mineral water containing lithium salts in solution.

li·thi′a·sis [*lithos;* NL. *-iasis,* condition]. The formation of calculi in the body. —**lithiasic,** *adj.*

lith′ic [*lithos*]. 1. Pertaining to calculi. 2. Pertaining to lithium.

lith′ic ac′id. Uric acid.

lith″i·co′sis [G. *lithikos,* of stone; *-ōsis,* condition]. Silicosis occurring in stone cutters.

lith′i·um [G. *lithos,* stone]. Li = 6.940. A soft, silver-white metal belonging to the alkali group. It is the lightest solid element, having a specific gravity of 0.534. Salts of lithium have been used like salts of other alkali metals; the belief that the former have special value in gouty conditions is unfounded. Under certain conditions lithium salts are toxic.

l. benzoate (*lithii benzoas*). C_6H_5COOLi. One Gm. dissolves in 3 cc. of water; it has been used for the therapeutic effect of benzoates.

l. bromide (*lithii bromidum*). LiBr. One Gm. dissolves in 0.6 cc. of water; used for its bromide effect. Dose, 0.65–1.3 Gm. (10–20 gr.).

l. carbonate (*lithii carbonas*). Li_2CO_3. One Gm. dissolves in 78 cc. of water; its effect is probably similar to that of other carbonates.

l. citrate (*lithii citras*). $C_3H_4.OH.(COOLi)_3$. One Gm. dissolves in 1.4 cc. of water. An ingredient of lithia tablets.

l. iodide. $LiI.3H_2O$. Used like potassium iodide.

l. salicylate (*lithii salicylas*). $C_6H_4.OH.COOLi$. Very soluble in water. It has been used for the effect of salicylate ion.

lith′o-, lith- [*lithos*]. A combining form meaning *stone, calculus.*

lith′o·chol′ic ac′id (lith″o·kol′ick). $C_{24}H_{40}O_3$; 3(α)-hydroxycholanic acid, found in human and animal bile, also in gallstones from certain animals.

lith″o·di·al′y·sis (lith″o·dye·al′i·sis) [*lithos;* G. *dialysis,* dissolution]. 1. The solution of calculi in the urinary bladder. 2. The breaking of a vesical calculus previous to its removal.

lith″o·fel′lic ac′id. $C_{20}H_{36}O_4$. An acid occurring in the intestinal concretions of ruminants.

lith″o·gen′e·sis, li·thog′e·ny (li·thodj′i·nee) [*lithos;* G. *genesis,* production]. The formation of calculi or stones. —**lithogenet′ic, lithog′enous** (li·thodj′i·nus), *adj.*

lith′oid, li·thoi′dal [*lithos;* G. *eidos,* form]. Resembling a stone.

lith″o·kel″y·pho·pe′di·on [*lithos;* G. *kelyphos,* sheath; *paidion,* child]. A calcified fetus (lithopedion) enclosed in calcified fetal membranes.

lith″o·kel′y·phos. See *lithopedion.*

lith′o·labe [*lithos;* G. *labein,* from *lambanein,* to take]. An instrument for grasping and holding a vesical calculus during an operation for its removal. *Obs.*

li·thol′a·pax″y (li·thol′uh·pack″see, lith′o·luh·)

[*lithos;* G. *lapaxis,* evacuation]. The operation of crushing a urinary calculus in the bladder by means of the lithotrite, and then removing the fragments by irrigation, a procedure now performed by a transurethral approach: also called *lithotrity.*

lith″o·ne·phri′tis [*lithos;* G. *nephros,* kidney; *-itis,* inflammation]. Inflammation of the kidney, associated with the presence of renal calculi.

lith″o·ne·phrot′o·my [*lithos; nephros;* G. *tomē,* a cutting]. Lithotomy performed by means of an incision into the kidney parenchyma or the renal pelvis; renal lithotomy. *Rare.*

lith″o·pe′di·on [*lithos;* G. *paidion,* child]. A retained fetus that has become calcified.

lith′o·phone [*lithos;* G. *phōnē,* sound]. An instrument for detecting by sound the presence of calculi in the urinary bladder. *Obs.*

lith′o·scope [*lithos;* G. *skopein,* to examine]. An instrument for the visual detection and examination of vesical calculi; a cystoscope.

li·tho′sis [*lithos;* G. *-ōsis,* condition]. Pneumonoconiosis. *Obs.*

li·thot′o·mist [*lithos;* G. *tomos,* cutting]. 1. A surgeon who performs lithotomy. 2. A term applied in former times to an individual who cut for stone in the urinary bladder.

li·thot′o·my [*lithos;* G. *tomē,* a cutting]. The removal of a calculus, usually vesical, through an operative incision.

perineal l. A type in which the incision is made through the membranous urethra in the middle of the perineum. The calculus is then removed by means of a lithotrite or suitable forceps.

suprapubic l. A type in which the incision into the urinary bladder is made through the abdominal wall just above the symphysis, the stone being removed by forceps.

vaginal l. One in which the incision is made through the anterior vaginal wall.

lith′o·trip″sy, li·thot′rip·sy [*lithos;* G. *tripsis,* a rubbing]. The operation of crushing calculi in the urinary bladder.

lith″o·trip′to·scope. See cystoscopic *lithotrite.*

lith′o·trite [*lithos;* L. *tritum,* from *terere,* to rub]. An instrument for crushing a vesical calculus. —**lith-otrit′ic,** *adj.*

cystoscopic l. A lithotrite which operates under visual control by means of a cystoscopic attachment.

li·thot′ri·ty. See *litholapaxy.*

lith′ous [*lithos*]. Having the nature of a calculus. *Obs.*

li·thox″y·du′ri·a [*lithos;* G. *oxys,* sharp; *ouron,* urine]. Presence of xanthic oxide in the urine.

lith″u·re′sis [*lithos;* G. *ourēsis,* a making water]. Voiding of small calculi with the urine.

li·thu′ri·a [*lithos;* G. *ouron,* urine]. A condition marked by excess of lithic acid or its salts in the urine.

lit″mo·ci′din. An antibiotic substance elaborated by *Proactinomyces cyaneus* var. *antibioticus,* active in vitro against a variety of bacteria.

lit′mus [ON. *litmose,* a lichen used for dyeing]. A blue pigment obtained from *Roccella tinctoria,* a lichen. Employed for determining the presence of acids and alkalies.

blue l. paper. Unsized paper steeped in a solution of litmus; turns red on contact with acid solutions.

red l. paper. Unsized paper steeped in a solution of litmus colored red with acid; turns blue on contact with alkaline solutions.

li′tre (lee′tur). See *liter.*

Litten's sign. See diaphragmatic *sign.*

lit′ter [OF. *litiere,* from L. *lectus,* bed]. A stretcher or bed for carrying the sick or injured. It consists of parallel bars of wood or metal, the ends serving as handles, over which is stretched canvas for supporting the body. It may be made in the form of an open metal basket for greater safety, especially for transfer of persons from shore to ship or vice versa.

lit′ter re′lay point. *In military medicine,* the point where a new litter team takes over further movement of a casualty, and the first team returns for another casualty. The object is to provide short litter hauls for the bearers.

Little, William John [*English surgeon,* 1810–94]. Pioneer orthopedist. Described cerebral spastic paralysis of infants; called *Little's disease.*

Little's tube. See under *tube.*

Littré, Alexis [*French surgeon and anatomist,* 1658–1726]. Described the small mucous glands of the male urethra (1700); called *Littré's glands.* Described a hernia of Meckel's diverticulum; called *Littré's hernia.* In *Littré's operation* of inguinal colostomy a sigmoid loop is brought out on the left side through a small incision parallel to the inguinal ligament. See *spaces of Littré* under *space.*

lit·tri′tis. See *urethritis.*

Litzmann, Carl Conrad Theodor [*German gynecologist and obstetrician,* 1815–90]. Described the coxalgic, scoliotic, and kyphoscoliotic types of the female pelvis. Classified female pelves. See also posterior *asynclitism.*

live blood. Twitching of the eyelids.

li·ve′do re·tic″u·lar′is (li·vee′do reh·tick″yoo·lair′-iss). See *cutis* marmorata.

liv′er [AS. *lifer*]. The largest gland or organ in the body, weighing approximately 1750 Gm. in the adult. It lies in the right upper part of the abdomen immediately under the diaphragm and is attached to it by the falciform and other ligaments. There are two principal lobes: the larger right and the smaller left; in addition there are smaller divisions of the right lobe: the quadrate lobe and caudate lobe. The inferior surface has a depression, the cystic fossa, in which lies the gallbladder. The organ is covered by a capsule, from which extensions penetrate throughout the organ, dividing it into lobules. These extensions, which only incompletely surround the lobules, contain divisions of bile duct, hepatic artery and portal vein, the portal triad, the whole being called the portal canal. The lobules are composed of polyhedral cells arranged in cords which radiate from the central vein toward the portal canal. Between the cords are the sinusoids, lined by endothelium and special reticuloendothelial cells, the Kupffer cells. Coursing in the cords and surrounded by hepatic cells are the biliary intralobular canals, which originate in bile canaliculi between the hepatic cells and drain into the bile ducts in the portal canal. Functions of the liver are multiple, including secretion of bile, protein breakdown, storage of glycogen and fat, maintenance of composition of blood, and detoxification. See Plates 8, 10, 13, 14.

amyloid l. Amyloidosis of the liver.

beavertail l. A liver with a large flat left lobe, suggesting resemblance to the tail of a beaver.

cardiac l. One in which there is severe passive hyperemia with enlargement, often tenderness, and sometimes pulsation.

cirrhotic l. One which is the seat of cirrhosis.

corset l. One in which a vertical or oblique groove, with fibrosis, appears on the anterior surface at about the line of the costal margin, due to compression from tight stays (now rare).

fatty l. One which is the seat of fatty change, as fat infiltration, fatty degeneration, or both.

foamy l. One containing many gas-filled spaces which give the organ a spongy appearance and consistency; due to growth of gas-producing anaerobic bacteria, especially *Clostridium perfringens.*

gin-drinker's l. See Laennec's *cirrhosis.*

hobnail l. See Laennec's *cirrhosis.*

icing l. Chronic perihepatitis resulting in the formation of a hyalinized, thickened capsule resembling the icing on a cake; hyalocapsulitis.

infantile l. Biliary cirrhosis.

lardaceous l. See amyloid *l.*

l. breath. A sweetness in the breath which often occurs in patients with Laennec's cirrhosis.

l. extract (*extractum hepatis*). A dry, brownish, somewhat hygroscopic powder containing that soluble thermostable fraction of mammalian livers which increases the number of red blood cells in the blood of persons affected with pernicious anemia. The approximate antianemia potency in pernicious anemia is expressed in U.S.P. units (oral).

l. fluke. A trematode which lodges in the intrahepatic biliary passages, most frequently *Clonorchis sinensis,* rarely *Fasciola hepatica.*

l. injection (*injectio hepatis*). A sterile solution in water for injection of that soluble thermostable fraction of mammalian livers which increases the number of red blood cells in the blood of persons affected with pernicious anemia. The potency is expressed in terms oi the equivalent of cyanocobalamin.

l. solution (*liquor hepatis*). A brownish liquid containing that soluble thermostable fraction of mammalian livers which increases the number of red blood cells in the blood of persons affected with pernicious anemia. The approximate antianemia potency in pernicious anemia is expressed in U.S.P. units (oral).

l. spot. Chloasma.

nutmeg l. A liver the cross section of which shows a fine mottling of yellow and brown or dark red, somewhat suggestive of the cross section of a nutmeg. In marked passive hyperemia the enlarged red central zones of adjacent lobules fuse to form a network in the meshes of which are the peripheral zones, yellow because of fatty degeneration.

packet l. See syphilitic *l.*, syphilitic *cirrhosis* (b).

syphilitic l. Rarely, fine bands of connective tissue interlace to divide off small segments of hepatic tissue about a centimeter or two in transverse dimension, the so-called packet liver. See *hepar* lobatum.

waxy l. See amyloid *l.*

liv'er·wort" (liv'ur·wurt"). See *Hepatica.*

liv'e·tin. A protein occurring in the yolk of egg.

liv'id [L. *lividus,* of a leaden, bluish color]. Of a pale lead color; black and blue; discolored, as flesh from contusion or from hyperemia. —**livid'ity,** *n.*

li·vid'i·ty [*lividus*]. The state of having a black and blue discoloration.

cadaveric l. The reddish or bluish discoloration in the dependent parts of a corpse, due to the gravitation of laked blood. Syn., *livcr mortis.*

Livierato's sign. See abdominocardiac *sign,* orthocardiac *sign.*

li'vor [L., leaden color]. 1. Lividity. 2. Livid spots on a cadaver.

l. mortis. See cadaveric *lividity.*

lix·iv"i·a'tion. The extraction and separation of a soluble substance from a mixture with insoluble matter; as leaching of salts from ashes.

Lizars, John [*Scottish surgeon,* ca. 1787–1860]. Devised an operation for excision of the upper jaw, the incision running from the corner of the mouth to the zygoma; called *Lizars' operation.*

Ljubinsky's stain. See under *stain.*

Lloyd test. See Sawyer and Lloyd serum protection *test.*

L. M. A. Left mentoanterior position of the fetus.

L. M. P. Left mentoposterior position of the fetus; last menstrual period.

L. O. A. Left occipitoanterior position of the fetus.

Lo'a [Kongo dial. *lowa*]. A genus of filarial worms.

L. loa. Species which invades the subcutaneous tissues of man; the eye worm.

lo"a·i'a·sis. A filariasis of tropical Africa, caused by the filaria *Loa,* and characterized by diurnal periodicity of microfilariae in the blood and transient cutaneous swelling.

lobe [G. *lobos,* lobe]. A more or less rounded part or projection of an organ, separated from neighboring parts by fissures and constrictions. —**lo'bar, lo'bate,** *adj.*

accessory l. A small, separate part of the parotid gland, usually found immediately above the duct. Syn., *socia parotidis.*

anterior cerebellar l. A median unpaired structure including all that part of the cerebellum which lies on the rostral side of the primary fissure.

anterior l. of hypophysis. (a) The anterior part of the adenohypophysis. (b) In the lobar classifications of the pituitary gland, the anterior part separated from the posterior lobe by a thin cleft and the pars intermedia. Syn., *pars anterior, pars distalis.*

azygos l. A variable, partially separate portion of the upper medial part of the superior lobe of the right lung. When present, it is isolated from the main part of the lobe by a deep groove occupied by the azygos vein.

caudate l. The tailed lobe of the liver that separates the right extremity of the transverse fissure from the commencement of the fissure for the inferior vena cava. See Plate 13.

developmental l. One of the portions of a tooth germ which initiate enamel and dentin formation.

flocculonodular l. That part of the cerebellum consisting of the nodule of the vermis and the paired lateral flocculi.

frontal l. That part of the cerebral hemisphere in front of the central sulcus and above the lateral cerebral fissure. See Plates 16, 17.

Home's l. The subtrigonal gland.

intermediate l. of hypophysis. (a) The intermediate part of the adenohypophysis. (b) In the lobar classifications of the pituitary gland, the part separated by a thin cleft from the anterior lobe and in front of the posterior lobe: sometimes erroneously classified with the posterior lobe.

limbic l. Gyrus fornicatus.

occipital l. One of the lobes of the cerebrum, a triangular area at the occipital extremity.

olfactory l. See *rhinencephalon.*

optic lobes. Superior colliculi of lower vertebrates. Also called *corpora bigemina.*

orbital l. That part of the frontal lobe which rests on the orbital plate of the frontal bone.

parietal l. The cerebral lobe above the lateral cerebral fissure and behind the central sulcus.

posterior cerebellar l. That part of the cerebellum which lies on the posterior side of the primary fissure.

posterior l. of hypophysis. (a) The pars nervosa of the neurohypophysis. (b) In the lobar classification of the pituitary gland, the posterior part separated from the anterior lobe by a thin cleft and the pars intermedia: sometimes erroneously used to include the intermediate lobe (pars intermedia).

pulmonary l. One of the five lobes of the lung.

pyramidal l. An inconstant portion of the thyroid gland extending upward from the isthmus; it arises from the persisting caudal end of the thyroglossal duct. See Plate 45.

pyriform l. See pyriform *area.*

quadrate l. An oblong lobe on the inferior surface of the liver. See Plate 13.

renal l. One of the subdivisions of the kidney corresponding to a renal pyramid with its associated cortex; externally visible in the fetus and infant, or throughout life in some mammals.

semilunar l. A lobe on the upper surface of the cerebellum.

Spigelian l. See caudate *l.*

temporal l. That part of the cerebral hemisphere below the lateral cerebral fissure, continuous posteriorly with the occipital lobe. See Plates 16, 18.

lo·bec'to·my [*lobos;* G. *ektomē,* excision]. Excision of a lobe of an organ or gland; specifically, the excision of a lobe of the lung.

lo"be·lan'i·dine. $C_{22}H_{29}NO_2$; an alkaloid from lobelia.

lo"be·lan'ine. $C_{22}H_{25}NO_2$; an alkaloid from lobelia.

lo·be'li·a [after Matthias de *Lobel,* Flemish botanist, 1538–1616]. The leaves and tops of *Lobelia inflata;* contains several alkaloids including lobeline. Lobelia is a respiratory stimulant, but unreliable. Produces slowing of heart, vomiting, and even convulsion when given in large doses. Formerly employed as an expectorant, especially in the form of the fluidextract or tincture.

lobelin. Trade-mark for an injectable solution of the hydrochloride of alpha-lobeline used as a respiratory stimulant.

lo'be·line (lo'bi·leen, ·lin, lob'i·, lo·bee'·). 1. A mixture of alkaloids obtained from lobelia; these have been separated into alpha-, beta-, and gamma-forms. 2. Alpha-lobeline, $C_{22}H_{27}NO_2$, an alkaloid from lobelia having emetic, respiratory, and vasomotor actions similar to those of nicotine. The drug is potent, uncertain, and dangerous.

l. sulfate. The sulfate of lobeline 1, or 2.

lo'bi. Plural of lobus.

lo'bo·cyte. See segmented *cell.*

lo"bo·po'di·um [*lobos;* G. *pous,* foot]. A broad and thick pseudopodium.

lo·bot'o·my [*lobos;* G. *tomē,* a cutting]. Section of brain tissue. Also called *leukotomy.*

frontal l. Prefrontal *l.*

prefrontal l. Operative section of the white matter of the frontal lobes of the brain, as used in the treatment of certain mental disorders and intractable pain.

transorbital l. A lobotomy performed through the roof of the orbit.

Lobstein, Johann Georg Christian Friedrich Martin [*Alsatian pathologist,* 1777–1835]. Described osteogenesis imperfecta, called *Lobstein's disease.* Described ossification of the arteries. Introduced the term arteriosclerosis.

lob'ster-claw". See *bidactyly.*

lob'ule [dim. from G. *lobos,* lobe]. A small lobe or a subdivision of a lobe. —**lobular, lobulated,** *adj.*

anatomic l. of the liver. A polygonal prism with the central vein running through the center of its long axis, with branches of the portal vein, the interlobular bile ducts, branches of the hepatic artery and lymph vessels running in the periphery.

ansiform l. A lobule of the posterior lobe of the cerebellum, extending from the superior surface of the hemisphere around the posterior border to the inferior surface; the inferior and superior semilunar lobules and the biventral lobule collectively.

biventral l. The anterior, inferior part of the ansiform lobule of the cerebellum.

central l. A lobule of the superior vermis of the cerebellum.

cuneate l. See *cuneus.*

floccular l. One of the paired, small, irregular lobules on the inferior surface of the cerebellar hemisphere forming part of the flocculonodular lobe.

l. of the epididymis. One of the series of cones forming the head of the epididymis, composed of the coiled efferent ductules. Also called *vascular cone.*

l. of the testis. One of the conoid compartments of the testis, the cavity of which contains the terminal portions of one to three seminiferous tubules.

paracentral l. The quadrilateral convolution on the medial surface of the cerebral hemisphere, surrounding the upper end of the central sulcus.

paramedian l. A rounded lobule on the inferior surface of the cerebellum, medial to the ansiform lobule.

parietal lobules. Subdivisions of the parietal lobe of the cerebrum. The **inferior parietal lobule** is that containing the supramarginal gyrus and the angular gyrus; the **superior parietal lobule,** that separated from the inferior by the interparietal sulcus.

physiologic l. of the liver. That portion of the liver tissue which surrounds and is drained by an interlobular bile duct.

pulmonary l. A respiratory bronchiole and its branches, the alveolar ducts and alveolar sacs, all with pulmonary alveoli in their walls, constituting a physiologic unit of the lung.

quadrangular l. The greater portion of the superior surface of the cerebellar hemispheres.

quadrate l. See *precuneus.*

semilunar lobules. Portions of the ansiform lobule. The **inferior semilunar lobule** is that on the inferior surface of the cerebellum; the **superior semilunar lobule,** that on the superior surface.

lob'u·lus (pl. *lobuli*) [L.]. Lobule.

l. medius medianus. A small lobule of the middle lobe of the cerebellum comprising the folium and tuber of the vermis.

l. simplex. The most rostral part of the posterior lobe of the cerebellum, forming a broad crescentic band across the superior surface.

lo'bus (pl. *lobi*) [L., from G. *lobos,* lobe]. A lobe.

lo'cal [L. *localis,* from *locus,* place]. Limited to a part or place; not general.

lo"cal·i·za'tion [*localis*]. 1. The determination of the site of a lesion. 2. The limitation of a process to a circumscribed area.

cerebral l. (a) Determination of the position of the centers in the brain that preside over certain physiologic acts. (b) Determination of the seat of pathologic conditions interfering with the normal function of these centers.

experimental l. Localization of brain centers through experiments on animals.

lo'cal·ized [*localis*]. Confined to a particular situation or place.

lo'cal·i"zer [*localis*]. An instrument used in radiographic examination of the eye for localizing opaque foreign bodies.

lo'chi·a (lo'kee·uh, lock'ee·uh) [G., discharge after childbirth]. The discharge from the uterus and vagina during the first few weeks after labor. —**lochial,** *adj.*

l. alba. The whitish or yellowish white flow that takes place after the seventh day after labor.

l. cruenta. The sanguineous flow of the first few days after labor. Also called *lochia rubra.*

l. serosa. The serous discharge taking place about the fifth day after labor.

lo"chi·o·col'pos (lo"kee·o·kol'poss, lock"ee·o·) [*lo-*

chia; G. *kolpos,* vagina]. Distention of the vagina by retained lochia.

lo′chi·o·cyte [*lochia;* G. *kytos,* cell]. A decidual cell found in the lochia.

lo″chi·o·me′tra [*lochia;* G. *mētra,* uterus]. A collection of lochia in the uterus.

lo″chi·o·me·tri′tis [*lochia; mētra;* G. *-itis,* inflammation]. Puerperal metritis.

lo″chi·or·rha′gi·a [*lochia;* G. *rhēgnynai,* to burst forth]. Lochiorrhea.

lo″chi·or·rhe′a, lo″chi·or·rhoe′a (lo″kee·o-ree′uh, lock″ee·o·) [*lochia;* G. *rhoia,* flow]. An abnormal flow of the lochia.

lo″chi·os′che·sis (lo″kee·os′ki·sis, lock″ee·) [*lochia;* G. *schesis,* a checking]. Suppression or retention of the lochia.

lo″cho·me·tri′tis (lo″ko·mi·try′tis, lock″o·) [G. *lochos,* childbirth; *mētra,* uterus; *-itis,* inflammation]. Puerperal metritis.

lo″cho·per″i·to·ni′tis [*lochos;* G. *peritonaion,* membrane which contains the lower viscera; *-itis*]. Inflammation of the peritoneum following childbirth.

lo′ci (lo′sigh). Plural of locus.

Locke-Ringer's solution. See under *solution.*

lock′jaw″. See *tetanus.*

Lockwood, Charles Barrett (1856–1914). English surgeon who described a thickening of the orbital fascia extending below the eyeball from the cheek ligaments: called *suspensory ligament of Lockwood.* See also Lockwood's *sign* of chronic appendicitis.

lo′co dis·ease′. A poisoning produced in livestock by eating plants which take up selenium from the soil; the symptoms of the disease are loss of flesh, disordered vision, delirium, convulsive movements, and stupor, often terminating fatally.

lo″co·mo′tion [L. *locus,* place; *motio,* from *movere,* to move]. The act or power of moving from place to place. **—locomotive, locomotor,** *adj.*

lo′co weed. Those species of *Astragalus* which contain selenium.

loc″u·la′tion [L. *loculus,* little place]. The formation of loculi in tissue.

loc′u·lus (pl. *loculi*) [L.]. A small space or compartment. **—loc′ulated,** *adj.*

lo′cum te′nens (lo′kum ten′enz) [L.]. A physician who temporarily acts as a substitute for another physician.

lo′cus (pl. *loci*) [L.]. 1. A place, spot, or organ. 2. *In genetics,* the point on a chromosome occupied by a gene.

l. caeruleus. A bluish-tinted eminence on the floor of the fourth ventricle of the brain, subjacent to which is an aggregation of pigmented cells. It receives fibers from the intertrigeminal nucleus and most of its axons form the fasciculus of Probst. Also called *nucleus pigmentosus pontis.*

l. minoris resistentiae. A spot of diminished resistance.

l. perforatus. A name formerly given to the anterior and the posterior perforated substance at the base of the brain through which the blood vessels pass.

Loeb, Jacques [*American biologist,* 1859–1924]. Advanced the theory of tropisms (1890) and the mechanistic theory of life. Made important studies of parthenogenesis; raised fatherless frogs to maturity.

Loeb, Leo (1869–). American pathologist, first to culture cells artificially (1898). He analyzed factors governing successful transplantation and growth of normal tissues in vitro, made important studies of the transplantation of tumors, showed that the incidence of mammary cancer in mice could be reduced in a quantitative way by oophorectomy, in accordance with the time of life at which oophorectomy was performed, and described the formation of decidual tissue (deciduomata) in the uterus as a result of mechanical stimulation, called *Loeb's decidual reaction.*

Loeffler, Charles William (1887–). Swiss physician who first described a syndrome of transient eosinophilic infiltration of the lungs and eosinophilia, called *Loeffler's syndrome.*

Loeffler, Friedrich August Johannes [*German bacteriologist,* 1852–1915]. Discovered the glanders bacillus. Gave the first full description of the diphtheria bacillus (1884), called *Klebs-Loeffler bacillus.* With Frosch, was first to discover a filtrable virus to be the cause of a disease of animals (foot and mouth disease, 1897). See also Loeffler's *stain* for flagella; *Loeffler's alkaline methylene blue* under *stain.*

Loef″fler·el′la mal′le·i (lef″lur·el′uh). *Malleomyces mallei,* the causative agent of glanders.

Loewenberg, Benjamin Benno [*German surgeon,* b. 1836]. Devised special forceps for removing adenoid growths from the posterior nasopharynx, called *Loewenberg's forceps.*

Loewenthal, Wilhelm [*German physician,* 1850–94]. Described the tectospinal tract called *Loewenthal's tract.*

Loewi, Otto (1873–). American pharmacologist who demonstrated that stimulation of both the vagus and the accelerator nerve produces its effect on the heart by liberation of chemical substances identical with acetylcholine or epinephrine.

log″a·dec′to·my (log″uh·deck′to·mee, lo″guh·) [G. *logades,* whites of the eyes; *ektomē,* excision]. Excision of a piece of the conjunctiva.

log″a·di′tis (log″uh·dye′tis, lo″guh·) [*logades;* G. *-itis,* inflammation]. Old term for scleritis.

log″a·do·blen″nor·rhe′a [*logades;* G. *blenna,* mucus; *rhoia,* flow]. Inclusion blennorrhea.

log″ag·no′si·a (log″ag·no′see·uh, ·zee·uh, lo″gag·), **log″ag·no′sis** [G. *logos,* word; *agnōsia,* ignorance]. Aphasia; word blindness.

log″a·graph′i·a (log″uh·graf′ee·uh, ·gray′fee·uh, lo″guh·). Agraphia.

log″am·ne′si·a (log″am·nee′zhuh, ·zee·uh, lo″gam·) [*logos;* G. *amnēsia,* forgetfulness]. Word deafness; word blindness; sensory aphasia.

log′a·nin. $C_{25}H_{34}O_{14}$. A glycoside extracted from the seeds and pulp of the fruit of *Strychnos nux-vomica.*

log″a·pha′si·a (log″uh·fay′zhuh, ze·e·uh, lo″guh·) [*logos;* G. *aphasia,* speechlessness]. Motor aphasia.

log″o·clo′nia. See *logospasm.*

log″o·ko·pho′sis [*logos;* G. *kōphōsis,* deafness]. Word deafness; incapacity to understand spoken language.

log″o·ma′ni·a [*logos;* G. *mania,* madness]. A form of mental disorder characterized by talkativeness.

log″o·neu·ro′sis [*logos;* G. *neuron,* nerve; *-ōsis,* condition]. A neurosis associated with a speech defect. *Obs.*

log·op′a·thy [*logos;* G. *pathos,* disease]. Any disorder of the speech.

log″o·pe′dics, log″o·pe′di·a [*logos;* G. *pais,* child]. The study, knowledge, and treatment of defective speech.

log″o·pha′si·a (log″o·fay′zhuh, ·zee·uh) [*logos;* G. *phasis,* utterance]. A speech disturbance characterized by loss of the ability to articulate correctly. Syn., *dysarthria.*

log″o·ple′gi·a [*logos;* G. *plēgē,* stroke]. Loss of the power of uttering articulate speech.

log″or·rhe′a [*logos;* G. *rhoia,* flow]. Excessive loquacity; may be incoherent. Syn., *lalorrhea. tachylogia.*

log′o·spasm [*logos;* G. *spasmos,* spasm]. Explosive or spasmodic enunciation of words.

log″o·ther′a·py. The therapeutic influence of the spoken word.

log′wood″. See *hematoxylon.*

Lohmann reaction. See under *reaction.*

Lohmann's reagent. See under *reagent.*

lo·i′a·sis [Kongo dial. *lowa;* NL. *-iasis,* condition]. Filariasis caused by *Loa loa.* The infestation is acquired from bites by *Chrysops dimidiata* and *C. silacea* and involves the subcutaneous tissues, particularly those of the eye.

loin [OF. *loigne,* from L. *lumbus,* loin]. The lateral and posterior region of the body between the so-called false ribs and the iliac crest.

lol′ism (lol′iz·um, lo′liz·um) [L. *lolium,* darnel]. Poisoning by the seeds of *Lolium temulentum* (darnel ryegrass).

Lombroso, Cesare [*Italian physician and criminologist,* 1836–1909]. Advanced the theory that criminals constitute a definite physical and mental type.

Londe, Paul Fréderic Léon [*French neurologist,* 1864–1944]. Described progressive bulbar paralysis in early life; called *Fazio-Londe's atrophy.*

Long, Crawford Williamson [*American physician,* 1815–78]. Believed to have been the first to use ether as an anesthetic in a surgical operation (1842).

Long, John Harper [*American biochemist,* 1856–1918]. Introduced a method of determining the number of grams of solids in a liter of urine: the last two figures of the specific gravity of the specimen, determined at 25° C., are multiplied by the figure 2.6, which is called *Long's coefficient.*

lon·gev′i·ty [L. *longaevitas,* longevity]. Long life; length of life.

lon″gi·lin′e·al [L. *longus,* long; *linea,* line]. Referring to a long, lean type of body build. Syn., *asthenic, dolichomorphic, longitypical.*

lon″gi·ma′nous (lon″ji·may′nus, ·man′us) [*longus;* L. *manus,* hand]. Long-handed.

long′ing [AS. *langian*]. The earnest desire for anything; a condition often present to an abnormal degree during pregnancy.

lon″gi·ped′ate (lon″ji·ped′ate, ·pee′date) [L. *longus,* long; *pes,* foot]. Long-footed.

lon·gis′si·mus [superl. of *longus*]. The longest; applied to muscles, as longissimus dorsi. See Table of Muscles in the Appendix.

lon″gi·tu′di·nal [L. *longitudo,* length]. Lengthwise; in the direction of the long axis of a body.

lon″gi·tu″di·na′lis. The longitudinal intrinsic muscles of the tongue.

lon″gi·typ′i·cal [L. *longus,* long; G. *typikos,* conforming to type]. Referring to a long body type; dolichomorphic; longilineal.

lon′gus (long′gus) [L.]. A long muscle, as longus colli, a muscle attached to the anterior surfaces of the bodies of the cervical vertebrae. See Table of Muscles in the Appendix.

l. capitis. The rectus capitis anterior major muscle.

l. cervicis. The longus colli muscle.

l. colli. A deep muscle of the anterior neck region.

Looney and Dyer method for potassium in blood. See under *method.*

loop [ME. *loupe*]. 1. A bend in a cord or cordlike structure. 2. A platinum wire, in a glass handle, with its extremity bent in a circular form; used to transfer bacterial cultures.

Axenfeld's intrascleral nerve l. An anomalous loop of the ciliary nerve in the scleral layer of the eyeball.

bulboventricular l. The U-shaped or S-shaped loop of the embryonic heart involving chiefly the bulbus and ventricle.

lenticular l. Ansa lenticularis.

l. of Henle. The U-shaped section of a uriniferous tubule which is formed by a descending and an ascending limb.

Meyer's l. See Adolf *Meyer.*

Stoerk's l. See under Oscar *Stoerk.*

loose [ON. *lauss*]. Lax; without restraint.

loose′ness [*lauss*]. 1. The state of being free, loose, or unrestrained. 2. Colloquial term for diarrhea.

l. of the teeth. A condition of the teeth due to disease of the gums and the gradual destruction of the alveolar processes. See *periodontosis.*

Looss, Arthur [*German parasitologist,* 1861–1923]. In experiments on dogs, discovered the route of migration of the hookworm from the skin through the lung to the intestine.

L. O. P. Left occipitoposterior position of the fetus in utero.

lo′pho·dont (lo′fo·dont, lof′o·) [G. *lophos,* ridge; *odous,* tooth]. Having the crowns of the molar teeth formed in crests or ridges; opposed to *bunodont.*

lo·phoph′o·rine (lo·fof′o·reen, ·rin). $C_{13}H_{17}O_3N$. The most active of the alkaloids from mescal buttons. Has been used experimentally as a hypnotic.

lo·phot′ri·chous (lo·fot′ri·kus) [*lophos;* G. *thrix,* hair]. Pertaining to microorganisms characterized by a tuft of cilia or flagella at each pole.

lo·quac′i·ty (lo·kwass′i·tee) [L. *loquax,* talkative]. Volubility of speech; talkativeness; a condition that is frequently excessive in various forms of mental disorders.

Lorain, Paul Joseph [*French physician,* 1827–75]. Made a study of dwarfism and sexual infantilism; called *Lorain syndrome.* See *infantilism,* 1.

Lóránd, Sándor (Löwi) [*Hungarian gynecologist,* contemporary]. Devised a tocograph for recording the uterine contractions, measured through the medium of the anterior abdominal wall; called *Lóránd tocograph.*

lor·do′sis [G., a curvature of the spine]. Forward curvature of the lumbar spine. —**lordot′ic,** *adj.*

Lorente de Nó, Rafael (1902–). American neurophysiologist known for his contributions to the anatomy and physiology of the cerebral cortex.

Lorenz, Adolf [*Austrian surgeon,* 1854–1946]. Devised a so-called bloodless method of reducing congenital dislocation of the hip. The adductor muscles of the thigh were forcibly stretched and kneaded with the hand, the femur being brought into extreme abduction. The quadriceps femoris and hamstring muscles then were similarly treated, until all the muscles were sufficiently stretched to allow the femoral head to be slipped into the shallow acetabular cavity. The femoral head was held in place by extreme abduction and inward or outward rotation of the femur. A heavy plaster cast was then applied and kept intact for several months. Called *Lorenz method* or *technic.*

Loreta, Pietro [*Italian surgeon,* 1831–89]. Known for his operation of gastrotomy and digital dilatation for the relief of pyloric stenosis. *Loreta's operation* is now obsolete.

L or′gan·isms. See under *organism.*

lo·ri′ca [L., leather cuirass]. A protective external covering or case.

Lorrain Smith's stain. See *Nile blue A* under *stain.*

Lossen, Hermann Friedrich [*German surgeon,* 1842–1909]. Devised an operation of section of the second division of the fifth cranial nerve, without division of the masseter muscle; called *Lossen's operation.*

Lotheissen, Georg [*Swiss surgeon in Austria,* 1860–

]. Devised an improved operation, using the inguinal approach, for the radical cure of femoral hernia (1898); called *Lotheissen's operation.*

lo'ti·o (lo'shee·o, lo'tee·o) [L., from *lavare*, to wash]. A lotion.

lo'tion [*lotio*]. An aqueous solution or suspension for local application; a wash.

lo"to·fla'vine (lo"to·flay'veen, ·vin, ·flav'een, ·in) [G. *lōtos*, lotus; L. *flavus*, yellow]. A yellow pigment produced by the hydrolysis of lotusin.

Lo'tus [*lōtos*]. A genus of the Leguminosae. **L. arabicus** yields a toxic glycoside, lotusin, and a pigment, lotoflavine.

lo'tus·in. A toxic glycoside in *Lotus arabicus;* on hydrolysis yields HCN and the coloring matter lotoflavine.

Louis, Antoine [*French surgeon*, 1723–92]. Described the angle formed at the junction of the manubrium and the body of the sternum; called *angle of Louis.*

Louis, Pierre Charles Alexandre [*French physician*, 1787–1872]. Credited with introducing the statistical method in the study of disease (1825). Made important studies of tuberculosis and typhoid fever. Described the characteristic lenticular rose spots of typhoid fever (1829).

loupe (loop) [F.]. A magnifying lens.

binocular l. A binocular magnifier, consisting of a combination of lenses in an optical frame, worn like spectacles.

loup'ing ill (lou'ping, lo'ping). An enzootic and sometimes epizootic disease of sheep; a form of encephalomyelitis caused by a virus and transmitted by the tick *Ixodes ricinus.* The virus is infectious also for monkeys, mice, horses, and cattle. Infected animals display ataxia. Syn.. *ovine encephalomyelitis, trembling-ill.*

louse (pl. *lice*) [AS. *lūs*]. A small, wingless, dorsoventrally flattened insect which lacks true metamorphosis. An ectoparasite of birds and mammals, it is medically important as a vector of disease and as a producer of irritating dermatitis.

bird l. See *Mallophaga.*

body l. *Pediculus humanus* var. *corporis.*

crab l. *Phthirius pubis.*

head l. *Pediculus humanus* var. *capitis.*

rat l. *Polyplax spinulosa.* It carries the organism of murine typhus, *Rickettsia mooseri*, and transmits it to its rat host, but not to man.

lous'y [*lūs*]. Infested with lice. See *pediculosis, phthiriasis.* —**lousiness,** *n.*

lov'age (luv'idj) [OF. *luvesche*, from L. *Ligusticus*, Ligurian]. The root of *Levisticum officinale.* Formerly used as a stimulant, aromatic, carminative, and emmenagogue.

Lovén's reflex. See under *reflex.*

Lovibond unit. See under *unit.*

Löwenstein, Ernst [*Austrian pathologist*, 1878–]. *Löwenstein's medium* for the culture of tubercle bacilli is an egg-potato meal type.

Lower, Richard [*English physician*, 1631–91]. Made important contributions to the knowledge of the anatomy and physiology of the heart. Described the intervenous tubercle, also called *Lower's tubercle.* Experimented with blood transfusion.

Lowry substance. See *Brönsted and Lowry substance* under *acid.*

Lowsley, Oswald Swinney (1884–). American urologist who made an important study of the prostate, developed an operation for calculus in the renal pelvis, and an original method of repairing renal wounds. He also devised a three-stage operation for the repair of hypospadias, called *Lowsley's operation.*

lox'a bark. Pale cinchona; the bark of *Cinchona officinalis.*

lox'i·a. See *torticollis.*

lox'ic. See *loxotic.*

lox·ot'ic [G. *loxos*, slanting]. Slanting; twisted.

loz'enge [OF. *losenge*]. A medicated tablet; usually intended for throat medication; usually sweetened.

L. R. C. S. Licentiate of the Royal College of Surgeons.

L. R. C. S. E. Licentiate of the Royal College of Surgeons of Edinburgh.

L. R. C. S. I. Licentiate of the Royal College of Surgeons of Ireland.

L. R. F. P. S. Licentiate of the Royal Faculty of Physicians and Surgeons.

L. S. A. Licentiate of the Society of Apothecaries; left sacroanterior position of the fetus.

L. S. P. Left sacroposterior position of the fetus.

Lu Chemical symbol for lutetium.

Lubarsch, Otto [*German pathologist*, 1860–1933]. Described minute crystals found in the epithelial cells of the testis; called *Lubarsch's crystals.*

Luc, Henri [*French laryngologist*, 1855–1925]. Devised an operation for the relief of severe disease of the maxillary sinus (1889). In addition to the usual nasomaxillary opening, an opening is made in the anterior wall through a supradental fossa. Called *Caldwell-Luc operation.*

lu·can'thone hy"dro·chlo'ride. $C_{20}H_{24}N_2OS$.-HCl; 1-(2-diethylaminoethylamino)-4-methylthiaxanthone hydrochloride, a bright yellow crystalline powder, sparingly soluble in water, effective in the treatment of certain types of human schistosomiasis. Syn., *miracil D.* See *nilontin.*

Lucas, Richard Clement [*English surgeon*, 1846–1915]. Described distention of the abdomen early in rickets; called *Lucas' sign.*

Lucas and Beveridge method for cysteine. See under *method.*

Lucas-Championnière, Just Marie Marcellin [*French surgeon*, 1843–1913]. Credited with introducing antisepsis in France. Chronic pseudomembranous bronchitis is known as *Lucas-Championnière's disease.*

Luciani, Luigi (1840–1919). Italian physiologist who described three phases of cardiac activity preceding heart failure: attack, periodic rhythm, and crisis: known as *Luciani's phenomenon.* He studied the physiology of starvation in man; his studies of the physiology and pathology of the cerebellum in decerebellated dogs led to the theory of the function of the cerebellum as the center for tonic, sthenic, and static functions.

lu·cid'i·ty [L. *lucidus*, clear]. Clearness; the state of being of a clear mind. —**lu'cid,** *adj.*

lu'ci·dum. See *septum* lucidum, *stratum* lucidum.

lu·çif'er·ase. An oxidative enzyme which catalyzes the reaction between oxygen and luciferin to produce luminescence.

lu·cif'er·in [L. *lux*, light; *ferre*, to bring]. An organic substrate found in luminescent organisms which when oxidized in the presence of the enzyme, luciferase, emits light, as in fireflies and glowworms.

lu·cif'u·gal [*lux;* L. *fugere*, to flee]. Fleeing from, or avoiding, light.

Lu·cil'i·a [NL.]. A genus of blowflies whose species, **L. caesar, L. sericata,** may cause myiasis in man. Species of this genus have also been found feeding on human wounds and occasionally attacking the adjacent healthy tissue.

lu'cite. See *acrylics.*

Lücke reaction for hippuric acid. See under *reaction.*

lu'dic [L. *ludere*, to play]. Referring to the element of play in automatic action.

Ludloff, Karl [*German surgeon*, 1864–1947]. Described a pathologic fracture of the patellar cartilage (1910); called *Büdinger-Ludloff-Läwen disease.*

ludozan. Trade-mark for a synthetic aluminum sodium silicate used as antacid.

Ludwig, Karl Friedrich Wilhelm [*German physiologist*, 1816–95]. Invented the kymograph (1846). Contributed to the knowledge of endosmosis. Developed the theory that the kidney glomeruli filter a protein-free dilute urine which in passing through the tubules becomes concentrated because of the resorption of water; called *Ludwig's filtration theory.* Described the innervation of the submaxillary glands (1851). Investigated perfusion, using excised organs. With Élie de Cyon, is credited with discovering the vasomotor reflexes (1866).

Ludwig, Wilhelm Friedrich von [*German surgeon*, 1790–1865]. Described cellulitis of the floor of the mouth (1836); see Ludwig's *angina, muscle* of Ludwig.

Luer [*German instrument maker in France*, d. 1883]. Invented a glass syringe with a glass piston, for use in intravenous and hypodermic injections. Called *Luer syringe.*

lu'es (lew'eez) [L., pestilence]. A euphemism for syphilis. Also called *l. venerea.* —**luet'ic,** *adj.*

lu'e·tin [*lues*]. An extract of the killed cultures of several strains of the *Treponema pallidum;* used in skin tests for syphilis.

Lugol's solution. See under *stain.* See also strong *iodine* solution.

Lukens test. See Boerner, Jones, and Lukens *test*, Boerner-Lukens *test.*

luke'warm" [AS. *hlēow; wearm*]. Tepid; about the temperature of the body.

lumalgin. Trade-mark for a combination of luminal and acetylsalicylic acid in tablet form.

lum·ba'go [L., from *lumbus*, loin]. A general term for backache in the lumbar or lumbosacral region.

lum'bar [*lumbus*]. Pertaining to the loins.

lum"bar·i·za'tion. See *sacralization.*

lum'bo-, lumb- [*lumbus*]. A combining form denoting *the loin, lumbar.*

lum"bo·co·los'to·my [*lumbus;* G. *kolon*, colon; *stoma*, mouth]. Colostomy in the left lumbar region.

lum"bo·co·lot'o·my [*lumbus; kolon;* G. *tomē*, a cutting]. Incision of the colon through the lumbar region.

lum"bo·cos'tal [*lumbus;* L. *costa*, rib]. Pertaining to the loins and ribs, as lumbocostal arch.

lum"bo·dor'sal [*lumbus;* L. *dorsum*, back]. Pertaining to the lumbar and dorsal regions, as lumbodorsal fascia.

lum"bo·in'gui·nal (lum"bo·ing'gwi·nul) [*lumbus;* L. *inguen*, groin]. Pertaining to the lumbar and inguinal regions, as the lumboinguinal nerve, a branch of the genitofemoral, distributed to the skin on the front of the thigh.

lum"bo·is'chi·al (lum"bo·iss'kee·ul) [*lumbus;* G. *ischion*, hip-joint]. Pertaining to the ischium and lumbar part of the vertebral column.

lum"bo·sa'cral [*lumbus;* L. *os sacrum*, lowest bone of the spine]. Pertaining to the lumbar vertebrae and to the sacrum, as the lumbosacral plexus, the plexus made up of the lower lumbar and upper sacral nerves.

lum'bri·cal [L. *lumbricus*, earthworm]. Relating to, or resembling, an earthworm or *Lumbricus.*

lum'bri·cal. One of four small muscles in the hand or foot (L., *lumbricalis*, pl. *lumbricales*). See Table of Muscles in the Appendix.

Lum'bri·cus [L.]. A genus of earthworms, formerly erroneously regarded as an intestinal worm. See *Ascaris.*

lu'men (pl. *lumens, lumina*) [L., light]. 1. The space inside of a tube, as the lumen of a thermometer, blood vessel, duct. 2. The unit of flux of light; the flux in a unit of solid angle from a source of which the intensity is 1 candle.

residual l. The persisting lumen, or a portion thereof, of Rathke's pouch; found in the hypophysis between pars distalis and pars intermedia.

lu'mi·chrome. $C_{12}H_{10}N_4O_2$. 7,8-Dimethyl-alloxazine. An oxidation product of riboflavin.

lu"mi·fla'vin (lew"mi·flay'vin, ·flav'in) [*lumen;* L. *flavus*, yellow]. A derivative of riboflavin; produced by irradiation of riboflavin in alkaline solution.

luminal. Trade-mark for a brand of phenobarbital.

luminal sodium. Trade-mark for a brand of phenobarbital sodium.

lu'mi·nance. The amount of light emitted from a source and projected on a measuring surface, also called *brightness*, although, technically, brightness is a subjective quality of light as measured by the eye.

lu"mi·nes'cence [*lumen*]. An emission of light without a production of heat sufficient to cause incandescence. It is encountered in certain animals, as some protozoa and fireflies.

lu"mi·nif'er·ous [*lumen;* L. *ferre*, to bear]. Conveying or bearing light.

lu'mi·nol. 3-Aminophthalhydrazide. A substance which becomes strongly luminescent as it undergoes oxidation. See *chemiluminescence.*

lu"mi·nos'i·ty [*lumen*]. The property of emitting light.

lu·mis'ter·ol [*lumen;* G. *stereos*, solid]. The first product obtained in the irradiation of ergosterol with ultraviolet light; further irradiation produces calciferol (vitamin D_2).

lump [cf. D. *lompe*, mass]. 1. A small mass; a protuberant part. 2. Any localized swelling or tumor.

lump'y jaw. See *actinomycosis.*

lu'na·cy [L. *luna*, moon]. 1. *In legal medicine*, mental disorder in which the individual is not legally responsible; insanity. 2. Insanity: so-called because formerly believed to be caused by the moon. *Obs.* —**lu'natic,** *adj.*

lu'nar [*luna*]. Pertaining to the moon or to silver (*luna* of the alchemists).

l. caustic. Toughened silver nitrate.

lu'nate [L. *lunatus*, crescent-shaped]. Semilunar bone, one of the carpal bones. See Table of Bones in the Appendix.

lu'na·tic [L. *luna*, moon]. A psychotic person.

lu·nel'la. See *hypopyon.*

lung [AS. *lungen*]. The organ of respiration, in which the venous blood is oxidized by the air drawn through the trachea and bronchi into the alveoli. There are two lungs, a right and a left, the former consisting of three, the latter of two, lobes. The lungs are situated in the thoracic cavity, and are enveloped by the pleura. See Plates 5, 12, 13, 14.

cardiac l. See brown *induration.*

honeycomb l. An emphysematous lung, or occasionally a lung containing numerous small pus-filled cavities: nonspecific term.

iron l. A mechanical respirator; Drinker respirator; used in respiratory paralysis. Also called *artificial l.*

turtle l. See *bronchiectasis.*

lung'mo"tor [*lungen;* L. *motor*, from *movere*, to move]. An apparatus for pumping air or air and oxygen into the lungs.

lung'wort" (lung'wurt"). See *Verbascum.*

lunosol. Trade-mark for a preparation of colloidal silver chloride in liquid and ointment form. The preparations are used as an antiseptic and germicide on mucous membranes.

lu′nu·la, lun′u·la [L., little moon]. 1. The white, semilunar area of a nail near the root. 2. The thin, crescentic area of a semilunar valve of the heart, on either side of the nodule.

lu′pa·nine. $C_{15}H_{24}N_2O$; an alkaloid from various species of *Lupinus*.

lu′pe·ose. Stachyose.

lu′pine (lew′pin, ·peen) [L. *lupinus*, lupine]. A plant of the genus *Lupinus*. One or more poisonous alkaloids have been found in various species of the genus. The bruised seeds of *L. albus* have been used as an external application to ulcers.

lu·pin′i·dine (lew·pin′i·deen, ·din). An alkaloid obtained from various species of *Lupinus*.

lu′pin·ine (lew′pin·een, ·in) [*lupinus*]. An alkaloid from various species of *Lupinus*.

lu″pi·no′sis. See *lathyrism*.

lu·po′ma [L. *lupus*, wolf; G. *-ōma*, tumor]. The primary nodule of lupus.

α-lu·pu′lic ac′id. Humulon.

β-lu·pu′lic ac′id. Lupulon.

lu′pu·lin [NL. *lupulus*, dim. from *lupus*, hop] (*lupulinum*). The glandular trichomes separated from the strobiles of *Humulus lupulus*. It is reputedly antispasmodic and sedative.

lu′pu·lon, lu′pu·lone. $C_{26}H_{38}O_4$; an antibiotic constituent of humulus or hops. Syn. *β-lupulic acid*.

lu′pu·lus. See *humulus*.

lu′pus [L., wolf]. A chronic tuberculous disease of the skin and mucous membranes, characterized by the formation of nodules of granulation tissue. Syn., *lupus exedens, lupus vulgaris.* —**lupoid, lupiform,** *adj*.

chilblain l. A form of lupus erythematosus that is aggravated in the cold seasons.

discoid l. erythematosus. Usually a chronic, but occasionally acute, disease of the skin characterized by red, scaly patches of various sizes and configurations which induce atrophy and superficial scar formation. It is a capricious disease, the acute form of which is often fatal. The chronic form causes follicular plugging, and occurs in the exposed areas, as the face, scalp, and hands. It is not caused by the tubercle bacillus. It is divided into the following forms: chronic discoid, subacute, and acute varieties. The latter may be a different disease. Syn., *l. sebaceus, l. superficialis, ulerythema centrifugum.* Also called *l. erythematodes*.

disseminated follicular l. A variety of lupus confined to the face, especially in the situations usually occupied by acne. The papules vary from a large pinhead to a pea in size, conical and deep red. Syn., *acnitis*.

disseminated l. erythematosus. A highly fatal disease of unknown cause, characterized clinically by fever, muscle and joint pains, anemia, leukopenia, and frequently by a skin eruption similar to discoid lupus erythematosus. Pathologically it is characterized by alteration in the connective tissue, especially of the arterioles, and the presence of hematoxylin-staining bodies in areas of fibrinoid degeneration of involved tissues. Primarily involved are the kidney, spleen, and endocardium.

exanthematous l. erythematosus. Disseminated lupus erythematosus.

l. crustosus. A crusted form of lupus vulgaris.

l. endemicus. Oriental sore.

l. erythematosus cell. A mature polymorphonuclear neutrophil with a vacuole containing lyzed nuclear material which has been phagocytized, found in bone marrow and peripheral blood preparations from patients with systemic lupus erythematosus. Abbreviated LE or L.E. cell or body.

l. erythematosus (LE) test. A test for disseminated lupus erythematosus made by incubating serum from patients with normal bone marrow, normal leukocytes, or the patient's leukocytes. A positive test consists of the presence of LE cells, homogeneous basophilic masses in the polymorphonuclear leukocytes, and rosettes of leukocytes about a basophilic amorphous substance.

l. erythematosus unguium mutilans. A type of lupus erythematosus affecting the dorsum of both hands in which the nails become reduced to irregular, discolored, "worm-eaten" strips adherent to the ungual bed, with deformities of the ends of the fingers.

l. exedens. The ulcerating type of lupus vulgaris.

l. hypertrophicus. That variety of lupus in which new connective-tissue formation predominates over the destructive process, and markedly raised, thick patches result.

l. keloid. A scar tissue overgrowth in an area of lupus vulgaris.

l. of larynx. A condition caused by *Mycobacterium tuberculosis* which usually follows lupus of the nasopharynx or face: rarer and less destructive than tuberculous laryngitis. The nodules occur on the epiglottis or the arytenoepiglottic folds.

l. lymphaticus. See *lymphangioma* circumscriptum congenitale.

l. maculosus. A variety of lupus characterized by the eruption of very soft, smooth, brownish red, semitranslucent miliary nodules that develop in the connective tissue of otherwise healthy skin without subjective sensations.

l. miliaris disseminatus. A more acute form usually occurring in children and at times following measles. Many small lesions appear rapidly. May be fatal.

l. miliaris disseminatus faciei. A form of tuberculosis of the skin characterized by tiny nodules usually over the face and especially the eyelids. Occur in crops and may involute. More often seen in Negroes.

l. pernio. A tuberculous affection that is usually classified as a sarcoid of the Boeck type. This term has also been used for chilblain lupus.

l. sebaceus. See discoid *l.* erythematosus.

l. serpiginosus. Spreads peripherally while cicatrizing centrally.

l. superficialis. See discoid *l.* erythematosus.

l. tumidus. A form with edematous infiltration.

l. vegetans. The formation in the lupus process of a warty-looking patch liable to become inflamed.

l. verrucosus. See *l.* vegetans.

l. vulgaris. True tuberculosis of the skin. A diverse and variable disease. Nodules of the apple jelly type are usually seen. It is a slow-developing, scarring, and deforming disease, often asymptomatic, and often involving the face. Syn., *tuberculosis luposa*. See Plate 31.

lu″pus·car″ci·no′ma [*lupus*; G. *karkinos*, crab; *-ōma*, tumor]. A carcinoma developing on the site of a lupus.

Luschka, Hubert von [*German anatomist*, 1820–75]. Described the pharyngeal bursa, called *Luschka's bursa*. Noted an inconstant, small, cartilaginous nodule in the anterior portion of the vocal fold, called *Luschka's cartilage*. Described the lateral apertures of the fourth ventricle; called *foramens of Luschka, foramens of Key and Retzius*. See also *Luschka's glands* under *gland*.

Lusk, Graham [*American physiologist*, 1866–1932]. Contributed much to the knowledge of the physiology of metabolism, and made important studies of nutrition.

Lusk, William Thompson (1838–1897). American

obstetrician who described the retraction ring observed during labor, which, when pathologic, is also called *Lusk's contraction ring.*

Lust's reflex. See under *reflex.*

lu'sus na·tu'rae (na·tew'ree) [L.]. A freak of nature, a monstrosity.

lute [L. *lutum,* mud]. A pasty substance which hardens when dry; used to make joints waterproof in pharmaceutical apparatus.

lu'te·al [L. *luteus,* yellow]. Of or pertaining to the corpus luteum or to its principle, as the luteal hormone.

lu·te'ci·um. See *lutetium.*

lu'te·in [L. *luteus,* yellow]. 1. $C_{40}H_{56}O_2$; a yellow dihydroxy-α-carotene first isolated from egg yolk, but widely distributed in nature; it has been called *xanthophyll.* 2. A dried, powdered preparation of corpus luteum.

Lutembacher, René [*French cardiologist,* 1884–]. Described mitral stenosis associated with defect of the interatrial septum (1916); called *Lutembacher's complex, disease, syndrome.*

lu"te·no'ma, lu"te·in·o'ma. See *luteoma.*

lu'te·o- [L. *luteus,* yellow]. 1. A combining form signifying *orange yellow* or *brownish yellow.* 2. *In botany,* a combining form denoting *yellowish.* 3. *In chemistry,* a combining form used in naming a series of yellow ammoniacal cobaltic salts.

lu"te·o·blas·to'ma. See *luteoma.*

lu"te·o'lin. $C_{15}H_{10}O_6$; 3′,4,′5,7-tetrahydroxyflavone, occurring in many plants in glycosidic combination.

lu"te·o'ma [*luteus;* G. *-ōma,* tumor]. An ovarian tumor made up of cells resembling those seen in the corpus luteum: also called *carcinoma of corpus luteum, granulosa-cell carcinoma, lutenoma, luteinoma, luteoblastoma, struma ovarii luteinocellulare, lipid-cell tumor of ovary.*

lu"te·o·tro'phin. Trade-mark for a brand of prolactin.

lutesterone. Trade-mark for progesterone.

lu·te'ti·um. Lu = 174.99. A rare earth metal: formerly spelled *lutecium.*

lu'ti·din. Any dimethylpyridine, C_7H_9N, of which the commonest is the 2,6-isomer, obtained by distillation of tar and bone oils.

lutocylin. Trade-mark for progesterone.

lutocylol. Trade-mark for anhydrohydroxyprogesterone.

lux·a'tion. 1. A dislocation. 2. *In dentistry,* the partial or complete separation of a tooth from its socket as a result of trauma.

lux·u'ri·ant [L. *luxuriare,* to abound to excess]. Growing to excess, exuberant; specifically referring to the abnormal growth of certain body cells, as in granulation tissue.

lux'us [L.]. Excess.

heart l. Cardiac dilatation with hypertrophy of the left ventricle.

l. breathing. Excessively deep and forcible inspiration.

l. consumption. The metabolism of certain surplus protein material, which, though inside the body, does not form a component part of any of its tissues, but constitutes a kind of reservoir of force upon which the organism may draw. *Obs.*

Luys, Jules Bernard [*French neurologist,* 1828–97]. Described the degenerative process in the anterior horns of the spinal cord in progressive muscular atrophy (1860). Described a nucleus in the hypothalamus (1865), formerly called *corpus Luysii,* the destruction of which results in hemiballismus. He also contributed to the knowledge of thalamic functions.

ly"ca·con'i·tine. $C_{36}H_{46}N_2O_{10}$; an alkaloid from *Aconitum lycoctonum.*

ly·can'thro·py (lye·can'thro·pee) [G. *lykos,* wolf; *anthrōpos,* man]. A belief that one is a wolf or some other wild beast, common among schizophrenic patients. Syn., *lycomania.* **—lycan·throp'ic,** *adj.;* **ly'canthrope,** *n.*

ly'cine (lye'seen, ·sin). See *betaine.*

ly"co·ma'ni·a. See *lycanthropy.*

ly'co·pene. $C_{40}H_{56}$; a red carotenoid pigment occurring in ripe fruit, especially tomatoes.

ly"co·per'si·cin. The antibiotic substance, now known as *tomatine,* obtained from *Lycopersicon pimpinellifolium,* the red-currant tomato plant.

ly"co·po'di·um [*lykos;* G. *pous,* foot]. The spores of *Lycopodium clavatum,* occurring in the form of a light, fine, yellowish powder. Used as a desiccant and absorbent on moist and excoriated surfaces, and as an inert powder in which to embed pills to prevent their adhering to one another. Can also act as an allergen. Also called *club moss, witch meal, wolf's claw.*

ly'co·pus [*lykos; pous*]. Bugle weed, *Lycopus virginicus;* formerly used as an astringent and hemostatic.

ly"co·rex'i·a [*lykos;* G. *orexis,* longing]. A wolfish or canine appetite.

lye [AS. *lēah*]. 1. An alkaline solution obtained by leaching wood ashes. 2. A solution of sodium or potassium hydroxide.

ly"go·phil'i·a [G. *lygē,* twilight; *philein,* to love]. Morbid love of dark places.

lygranum. Trade-mark for antigens employed in the complement-fixation test and the Frei test for venereal lymphogranuloma. They are prepared by growing the virus on the chick embryo.

ly"ing-in'. 1. Confinement. 2. The puerperium.

Lyle-Curtman-Marshall method. See under *method.*

lymph [L. *lympha,* water]. 1. The fluid in the lymph vessels, collected from the interstitial fluid. 2. Old term for exudate. **—lymph'oid,** *adj.*

l. channel. Old term for tissue space or lymphatic.

l. follicle. Old term for lymph nodule.

l. nodes. Masses of lymphatic tissue 1–25 mm. long, often bean-shaped, intercalated in the course of lymph vessels, more or less well organized by a connective-tissue capsule and trabeculae into cortical nodules and medullary cords which form lymphocytes, and into lymph sinuses through which lymph filters, permitting phagocytic activity of reticular cells and macrophages. Syn., *lymph glands* (BNA). See Plate 11.

vaccine l. The virus of vaccine.

lym·phad"e·nec'to·my [*lympha;* G. *adēn,* gland; *ektomē,* excision]. Excision of a lymph node.

lym·phad"e·ni'tis [*lympha; adēn;* G. *-itis,* inflammation]. Inflammation of a lymph node.

aleukemic l. See lymphocytic *leukemia.*

dermatopathic l. See lipomelanotic *reticulosis.*

infectious l. Lymphadenitis associated with infectious diseases, e.g., scarlet fever, mumps, and diphtheria.

mesenteric l. Inflammation of the mesenteric lymph nodes, commonly tuberculous. The tuberculous form was formerly called *tabes mesenterica.*

purulent l. (of the lung). An invasion of the peribronchial lymph nodes by streptococci, causing the lymphatics to become occluded, thereby spreading the infection toward the surface of the lung. A small area of focal pleurisy ensues, swiftly followed by the exudation of a serofibrinous fluid, at first clear, but becoming full of streptococci and leukocytes.

scrofulous l. The small-celled caseous or suppurative hyperplasia of the lymph nodes. *Obs.*

tuberculous l. Tuberculous infection of the lymph nodes.

lym·phad"e·no'ma [*lympha; adēn;* G. *-ōma,* tumor]. A tumorlike enlargement of a lymph node, in which the architectural pattern is obliterated by proliferation of lymphocytes; it probably exists in two forms, the neoplastic and the hyperplastic.

malignant l. See *lymphoma.*

multiple l. See *lymphoma.*

lym·phad"e·no·ma·to'sis. Old term for Hodgkin's disease.

lym·phad"e·nop'a·thy [*lympha; adēn;* G. *pathos,* disease]. Disease of the lymph nodes.

dermatopathic l. A type of chronic hyperplastic lymphadenitis, the result of chronic exfoliative dermatitis and other dermatoses. The pathologic changes are called *lipomelanotic reticulosis.*

lym·phad"e·no'sis. Lymphocytic leukemia.

l. benigna cutis. See *lymphocytoma* cutis.

lym·phad"e·not'o·my [*lympha; adēn;* G. *tomē,* a cutting]. Incision of a lymph node.

lym'pha·gogue (lim'fuh·gog) [*lympha;* G. *agōgos,* leading]. An agent that stimulates the flow of lymph. —**lym'phagogue,** *adj.*

lym·phan"gi·ec'ta·sis (lim·fan"jee·eck'tuh·sis), **lym·phan"gi·ec·ta'si·a** (·eck·tay'zhuh, ·zee·uh, ·shuh, ·see·uh) [*lympha;* G. *aggeion,* vessel; *ektasis,* extension]. Dilatation of the lymphatic vessels. It may cause elephantiasis. —**lymphangiectat'ic,** *adj.*

lym·phan"gi·ec·to'des. See *lymphangioma* circumscriptum congenitale.

lym·phan"gi·ec'to·my [*lympha; aggeion;* G. *ektomē,* excision]. Excision of a pathologic lymphatic channel, as in surgery for cancer.

lym·phan"gi·o·en"do·the"li·o'ma [*lympha; aggeion;* G. *endon,* within; *thēlē,* nipple; *-ōma,* tumor]. A tumor composed of a congeries of lymphatic vessels, between which are many large mononuclear cells presumed to be endothelial cells.

lym·phan"gi·o'ma [*lympha; aggeion; -ōma*]. A dilated or varicose condition or tumor of the lymphatics: also called *simple l.* See also *hygroma.*

cavernous l. See *hygroma.*

cystic l. See *hygroma.*

l. circumscriptum congenitale. Lymphangiectodes; lupus lymphaticus; a very rare skin disease occurring in early life. Marked by the formation of straw-yellow vesicles, deeply situated in the skin, with thick and tense walls, and connected with the lymphatics. Of unknown cause.

l. tuberosum multiplex. A very rare skin disease; probably congenital; characterized by the formation of large, brownish-red papules or tubercles, the size of lentils, not arranged in groups or clusters, but scattered indiscriminately over the trunk. See *hygroma.*

lym·phan'gi·o·plas"ty (lim·fan'jee·o·plas"tee, lim·fan"jee·o·plas'tee) [*lympha; aggeion;* G. *plassein,* to form]. Replacement of lymphatics by artificial channels.

lym·phan"gi·o·sar·co'ma [*lympha; aggeion;* G. *sarkōma,* fleshy excrescence]. Lymphangioma or lymphangioendothelioma, invasive and containing poorly differentiated or undifferentiated cells.

postmastectomy l. A rare malignant neoplasm, histologically resembling lymphangiosarcoma, which occurs in women following radical removal of a breast and involving the arm on the same side: sometimes called *Stewart-Treves syndrome.*

lym·phan"gi·ot'o·my [*lympha; aggeion;* G. *tomē,* a cutting]. Cutting or dissection of lymphatic channels.

lym"phan·gi'tis [*lympha; aggeion;* G. *-itis,* inflammation]. Inflammation of a lymphatic vessel; it may be acute or chronic.

streptococcal l. (respiratory). Streptococcal infection of the lymphatics of the lower respiratory tract.

lym·phat'ic [L. *lymphaticus,* from *lympha*]. Pertaining to lymph.

lym·phat'ic. A vessel conveying lymph.

afferent l. A vessel conveying lymph to a lymph node.

efferent l. A vessel conveying lymph away from a lymph node.

lym·phat'ic block·ade'. The bits of fibrinous exudate that pass into the local lymphatics and the fibrinous network thrown about a wounded part, blocking the passage of foreign bodies, notably microorganisms, to other body parts.

lym·phat"i·cos'to·my [*lymphaticus;* G. *stoma,* mouth]. Formation of an opening into a lymphatic trunk, as the thoracic duct.

lym'pha·tism [L. *lympha,* water]. See *status lymphaticus.*

lym"phe·de'ma. See under *edema.*

lym'pho-, lymph- [*lympha*]. A combining form denoting *connection with,* or *relation to, lymph* or *the lymphatics.*

lym'pho·blast [*lympha;* G. *blastos,* germ]. A blast cell, considered a precursor or early form of lymphocyte. As in other blast cells, the nucleus has a chromatin structure finer than that of the lymphocyte but coarser than that of the myeloblast, and has a large single nucleolus. A clear perinuclear area is frequently seen in the cytoplasm.

lym"pho·blas·to'ma [*lympha; blastos;* G. *-ōma,* tumor]. A lymphosarcoma in which the predominant cell type has some of the features of lymphoblasts. The cells are larger and more pleomorphic, with fairly large, centrally placed vesicular nuclei; mitotic figures and multinucleation are numerous. See follicular *lymphoma.*

giant follicular l. See follicular *lymphoma.*

l. leucaemicum. The acute form of lymphocytic leukemia.

l. malignum. Hodgkin's disease.

scirrhous l. See Hodgkin's *disease.*

lym"pho·chlor·o'ma. See *chloroma.*

lym'pho·cyte [*lympha;* G. *kytos,* cell]. A cell formed primarily in lymphoid tissue in many parts of the body, as lymph nodes, spleen, and tonsils, morphologically identical with a class of agranular leukocytes in the peripheral blood, and usually classified according to size. The **small lymphocyte** is the smallest leukocyte (7–10μ), with markedly clumped chromatin in the nucleus, and scant cytoplasm forming a rim around the nucleus. The **large lymphocyte** varies in diameter 10–20μ; the nucleus is often irregularly shaped, shows moderately clumped chromatin, and has a much larger proportion of clear light-blue cytoplasm than the small lymphocyte. See Plate 26. —**lymphocyt'ic,** *adj.*

atypical lymphocytes. Abnormal mononuclear cells seen in infectious mononucleosis, sometimes divided into three types (*Downey cell* I, II, III) correlating with the degree of immaturity. Also see *viruscytes.*

plasmacytoid l. See *plasmacyte.*

young l. See *prolymphocyte.*

lym"pho·cy·the'mi·a (lim"fo·sigh·theem'ee·uh). See lymphocytic *leukemia.*

lym"pho·cy'tic se'ries. Lymphocytes (small, large, young), prolymphocytes, and lymphoblasts.

lym"pho·cy·to'ma (lim"fo·sigh·to'muh) [*lympha; kytos* G. *-ōma,* tumor]. A lymphosarcoma in which the predominant cell type closely resembles mature lymphocytes. In contrast to *lymphoblastoma,* cells show fewer mitotic figures and no multinucleation.

l. cutis. A dense infiltrate of mature lymphocytes and some reticulum cells in the dermis. In the localized type there is either a single lesion or a group of nodules; in the disseminated type a varying number of nodules, plaques, and tumors, from bluish-red to skin-color occur anywhere in the skin and may involve any organ of the body. Also called *Spiegler-Fendt sarcoid, lymphadenosis benigna cutis.*

lym"pho·cy"to·pe'ni·a [*lympha; kytos;* G. *penia,* want]. Decrease of the normal number of lymphocytes in the peripheral blood.

lym"pho·cy"to·poi·e'sis [*lympha; kytos;* G. *poiēsis,* production]. The genesis of lymphocytes.

lym"pho·cy·to'sis (lim"fo·sigh·to'sis). The condition of having an abnormally large number of lymphocytes in peripheral blood, seen with, or during convalescence from, certain acute infections, as pertussis, in chronic infections, as tuberculosis, infectious mononucleosis, or infectious hepatitis, and as an increase of abnormal lymphocytes in lymphocytic leukemia.

relative l. Percentage increase of lymphocytes in the differential leukocyte count, observed in most conditions associated with neutropenia.

lym"pho·der'mi·a [*lympha;* G. *derma,* skin]. Affection of the lymphatics of the skin.

l. perniciosa. Leukemic enlargement of the lymph nodes.

lym"pho·ep"i·the"li·o'ma [*lympha;* G. *epi,* on; *thēlē,* nipple; *-ōma,* tumor]. A rapidly growing tumor, regarded by many as a variant of an epidermoid carcinoma, found usually in the posterior nares, about the orifice of the auditory tube, in the vault of the pharynx in the tonsils, often with metastases to cervical lymph nodes. Microscopically there is an association of cells resembling lymphocytes and larger, indistinctly outlined, mononuclear cells of epithelial character. Responds readily to irradiation but often recurs. A more distinctly alveolated type sometimes occurs in which the epithelial cells are arranged as trabeculae.

lym·phog'en·ous (lim·fodj'in·us) [*lympha;* G. *genesthai,* from *gignesthai,* to be produced]. Producing lymph.

lym"pho·glan'du·la [*lympha;* L. *glandula,* dim. from *glans,* acorn]. BNA term for a lymph node.

lym"pho·go'ni·a [*lympha;* G. *gonos,* offspring]. Large lymphocytes having a relatively large nucleus deficient in chromatin, and a faintly basophil nongranular cytoplasm, observed in lymphocytic leukemia.

lym"pho·gran"u·lo'ma [*lympha;* L. *granulum,* little grain; G. *-ōma,* tumor]. Old term for Hodgkin's disease.

l. inguinale. See venereal *l.*

l. venereum. Venereal lymphogranuloma. Abbreviated, L. G. V.

venereal l. A virus disease characterized by an initial lesion, usually on the genitalia, followed by regional lymph-node enlargement and, at times, systemic involvement. The Frei test is a specific skin test for this condition. A venereal disease. Also called *fourth venereal disease, l. inguinale, l. venereum, lymphopathia venereum, Nicolas-Favre disease, Durand-Nicolas-Favre disease, Frei's disease.* Syn., *venereal adenitis.*

lym"pho·gran"u·lo·ma·to'sis. See Hodgkin's *disease.*

benign l. See *sarcoidosis.*

l. cu'tis. A specific autonomous venereal disease which typically involves the inguinal lymph nodes in a subacute inflammation.

venereal l. See venereal *lymphogranuloma.*

lym·phoi'do·cyte. See *hemocytoblast.*

lym"pho·ken'tric ac'id. A hydroxy acid, insoluble in water, in the urine of patients with lymphoid leukemia as a water-soluble conjugate. It causes proliferation of cells of the leukopoietic system and produces Hodgkin's-type lesions. It may be oxidized to myelokentric acid.

lym·pho'ma [*lympha; -ōma*]. Loosely, a group of malignant or premalignant conditions of lymphoid tissue in which splenomegaly and lymphadenopathy usually are present. These conditions, which may represent variations of each other, have similar clinical and pathological pictures, and generally include *Hodgkin's disease, lymphosarcoma, leukolymphosarcoma, reticulum-cell sarcoma, follicular lymphoma,* and *lymphocytic leukemia.* Also called *malignant* or *multiple lymphadenoma, lymphomatosis.* —**lymphomatoid,** *adj.*

benign l. See follicular *l.*

clasmatocytic l. See reticulum-cell *sarcoma.*

follicular l. A slowly progressive premalignant form of lymphoma, in which the lymph nodes show markedly enlarged follicles composed predominantly of closely packed, large reticuloendothelial cells; it usually mutates to one of the malignant forms of lymphoma. Syn., *Brill-Symmers disease, giant follicular l.* Also called *giant follicular lymphoblastoma, benign lymphoma, nodular lymphoma, lymphoreticulosis.*

granulomatous l. See Hodgkin's *disease.*

l. of orbit. A neoplastic disease of lymphoid cells occurring in the orbit and varying greatly in malignancy. Clinically and histologically it is difficult to distinguish the localized disease of low-grade malignancy from a focal manifestation of a generalized neoplasm of lymphoid cells, as lymphosarcoma and lymphocytic leukemia. Also called *ocular l., lymphomatosis of orbit.*

malignant l. Old term for Hodgkin's disease, or for lymphosarcoma.

nodular l. See follicular *l.*

ocular l. *L.* of orbit.

lym"pho·ma·to'sis. See *lymphoma.*

l. of orbit. See *lymphoma* of orbit.

lym"pho·path'i·a ve·ne're·um. Old term for venereal lymphogranuloma.

lym"pho·pe'ni·a. Decreased number of lymphocytes in the blood.

lym"pho·poi·e'sis [*lympha;* G. *poiēsis,* production]. Formation of lymphocytes. —**lymphopoiet'ic,** *adj.*

lym"pho·pro'te·ase. An enzyme, capable of catalyzing hydrolysis of proteins, occurring in lymphocytes.

lym"pho·re·tic"u·lo'ma (Hodgkin's). See Hodgkin's *disease.*

lym"pho·re·tic"u·lo'sis. Follicular lymphoma.

benign l. See cat-scratch *fever.*

lym'phor·rhage, lym"phor·ra'gi·a. 1. A flow of lymph from a ruptured lymphatic vessel. 2. Aggregation of lymphocytes. Usually those aggregates seen in muscle and rarely in other organs in myasthenia gravis or spirochetal jaundice (Weil's disease).

lym"phor·rhe'a [*lympha;* G. *rhoia,* flow]. A discharge of lymph from a wound, internally or externally.

lym"pho·sar·co'ma [*lympha;* G. *sarkōma,* fleshy excrescence]. A malignant tumor of lymphatic tissue, distinguished from lymphocytic leukemia only by the absence of malignant cells from the peripheral blood, in which the lymph nodes show diffuse masses of uniform rounded cells highly resembling lymphocytes (*lymphocytoma*) or lymphoblasts (*lymphoblastoma*), according to the degree of differentiation. Syn., *lymphocytic sarcoma.* Also see reticulum-cell *sarcoma.*

pleomorphic l. Hodgkin's sarcoma. See Hodgkin's *disease.*

reticulum-cell, reticular l. See reticulum-cell *sarcoma.*

lym"pho·sar"co·ma·to'sis [*lympha; sarkōma;* G.

-*ōsis*, condition]. A condition or diathesis marked by the development of lymphosarcoma.

lymph scro′tum. Elephantiasis of the scrotum.

lym·phu′ri·a [*lympha;* G. *ouron,* urine]. The presence of lymph in the urine.

lynoral. Trade-mark for ethynyl estradiol.

ly′o-, ly- [G. *lyein,* to loose]. A combining form signifying to *dissolve, loose.*

ly′o·chrome. See *flavin.*

ly″o·en′zyme. See extracellular *enzyme.*

ly′o·gel. A gel rich in liquid.

ly″o·gly′co·gen. That portion of glycogen in tissue readily extractable with water.

Lyon's tube. See under *tube.*

ly′o·phile (lye′o·file, ·fil), **ly″o·phil′ic.** Referring to the dispersed phase of a colloidal system when there is strong affinity between the dispersion medium and the dispersed phase. Also see *lyophobe.*

l. complement. Complement prepared by freezing guinea-pig serum and dehydrating it rapidly under high vacuum.

l. process. A desiccation procedure involving rapid freezing of the material to be dried followed by evaporation of the moisture at low temperature under vacuum. Also called *l. method.* See *cryochem, desivac.*

ly″o·phil·i·za′tion [*lyein;* G. *philein,* to love]. The process of rapidly freezing a substance (pollen, blood plasma, antitoxin, serum, etc.) at an unusually low temperature, and then quickly dehydrating the frozen mass in a high vacuum. —**lyophilized,** *adj.*

ly′o·phobe, ly″o·pho′bic. Referring to the dispersed phase of a colloidal system when there is lack of strong affinity between the dispersed phase and the dispersion medium. Also see *lyophile.*

ly′o·sol. A disperse system wherein a liquid is the dispersing medium for suspended liquid or solid particles.

ly″o·sorp′tion [*lyein;* L. *sorbere,* to suck in]. The preferential adsorption of the solvent constituent of a solution or of the dispersing medium of a colloidal system.

ly′o·trope. 1. One of a group of ions which, when arranged in a series, influence in the same order different phenomena which involve forces existing between the solvent and one or more other components of a solution. 2. A readily soluble substance. —**lyotrop′ic,** *adj.*

ly″pe·ma′ni·a (lye″pi·may′nee·uh, lip″i·) [G. *lypē,* grief; *mania,* madness]. Old term for melancholia.

ly″po·thy′mi·a (lye″po·thigh′mee·uh, lip″o·) [*lypē;* G. *thymos,* mind]. Old term for melancholia.

lyse. To cause or undergo lysis, 3: also spelled *lyze.*

ly·ser′gic ac′id. $C_{16}H_{16}N_2O_2$. A component of ergot alkaloids.

ly′si- (lye′si-, lis′i-), **lys-** [G. *lysis,* a loosing]. A combining form signifying *loosening.*

ly·sim′e·ter (lye·sim′i·tur) [*lysis;* G. *metron,* a measure]. An apparatus for determining the solubility of a substance.

ly′sin [*lysis*]. A cell-dissolving substance.

beta l. Certain thermostable bactericidal serum constituents; similar to leukins and obtained from granulocytes and perhaps from blood platelets. The relation of these factors to immunity is not clear.

ly′sine (lye′seen, ·sin). $NH_2CH_2(CH_2)_3CH(NH_2)$-COOH. The α-amino-ϵ-caproic acid, an amino acid obtainable by the hydrolysis of casein and other proteins. It is essential to the growth of man.

ly′sis [G.]. 1. Gradual decline in the manifestations of a disease, especially an infectious disease. Syn., *defervescence.* 2. Gradual fall of fever. 3. The solution of a cell or tissue by the action of a lysin, as the solution of erythrocytes by chemical substances, by alteration of environment, or by action of a specific immune hemolysin and complement. —**ly′tic,** *adj.*

osmotic l. Destruction of cells, e.g., erythrocytes, by hypotonic solutions.

-lysis [G.]. 1. A combining form signifying *dissolving, dissolution.* 2. *In biochemistry,* a combining form signifying *dissolution.* 3. *In chemistry,* a combining form signifying *decomposition.* 4. *In medicine,* a combining form denoting *relief* or *reduction, detachment,* or *paralysis.*

lysivane hydrochloride. A trade-marked name for 10-(2-diethylamino-1-propyl)phenothiazine hydrochloride, official in the International Pharmacopoeia as *profenamine hydrochloride:* used to treat parkinsonism.

ly″so·ceph′a·lin. A substance derived from cephalin by the removal of one of the fatty acid components of the molecule, by the action of an enzyme contained in cobra venom. It possesses powerful hemolytic properties.

ly″so·gen′e·sis. The production of lysins or lysis. —**lysogen′ic,** *adj.*

lysol. Trade-mark for a disinfectant containing orthophenylphenol as the principal germicidal ingredient.

ly″so·lec′i·thin (lye″so·less′i·thin) [*lysis;* G. *lekithos,* yolk of an egg]. A substance having strong hemolytic properties produced from lecithin by the action of snake venom, which removes unsaturated fatty acids from the lecithin molecule.

ly′so·zyme [*lysis;* G. *en,* in; *zymē,* leaven]. An enzyme found in tears, leukocytes, mucous secretions, egg albumin, and many plants. It exerts a strong antiseptic action, due to lysis of bacteria.

ly″so·zy·mu′ri·a. Lysozyme in the urine, found in patients demonstrating the nephrotic syndrome and in some normal children.

lys′sa. See *rabies.*

lys′sic [G. *lyssa,* rage]. Pertaining to rabies; due to rabies.

lys″so·dex′is [*lyssa;* G. *dēxis,* a bite]. The bite of a rabid dog.

lys′soid [*lyssa;* G. *eidos,* form]. Resembling rabies.

lys″so·pho′bi·a [*lyssa;* G. *phobos,* fear]. 1. Morbid fear of hydrophobia; hydrophobophobia. 2. Morbid fear of becoming insane.

Lyster, William John L. [*American Army physician,* 1869–1947]. Invented an apparatus for the rapid sterilization of water in camps. The water is placed in a large rubber-lined canvas bag, called a *Lyster bag,* which is fitted with faucets and with straps for suspension. Sterilization is accomplished by means of calcium hypochlorite contained in glass tubes, called *Lyster tubes,* which are broken and emptied into the bag.

ly′syl. The univalent radical, $H_2NCH_2CH_2CH_2$-$CH_2CH(NH_2)CO$—, of the amino acid lysine.

ly·te′ri·an (lye·teer′ee·un) [G. *lysis,* a loosing]. Indicative of a lysis, or of a favorable crisis terminating an attack of disease.

-lyt′ic [*lysis*]. A suffix signifying *lysis* or *a lysin.*

Lyt′ta ves″i·ca·to′ri·a. The Spanish fly; a species of Meloidae of the order Coleoptera. Characterized by the formation of cantharidin, a toxin which may produce blisters of the skin.

ly″xo·fla′vin. $C_{17}H_{20}N_4O_6$; the L-lyxose analog of riboflavin, first isolated from human cardiac muscle. It has no riboflavin activity but possesses growth-promoting activity in rats. Also spelled *lyxoflavine.*

lyx′ose (licks′ose). A synthetic pentose sugar that is isomeric with arabinose, ribose, and xylose.

lyze. See *lyse.*

Index of Illustrative Plates

PLATE 1

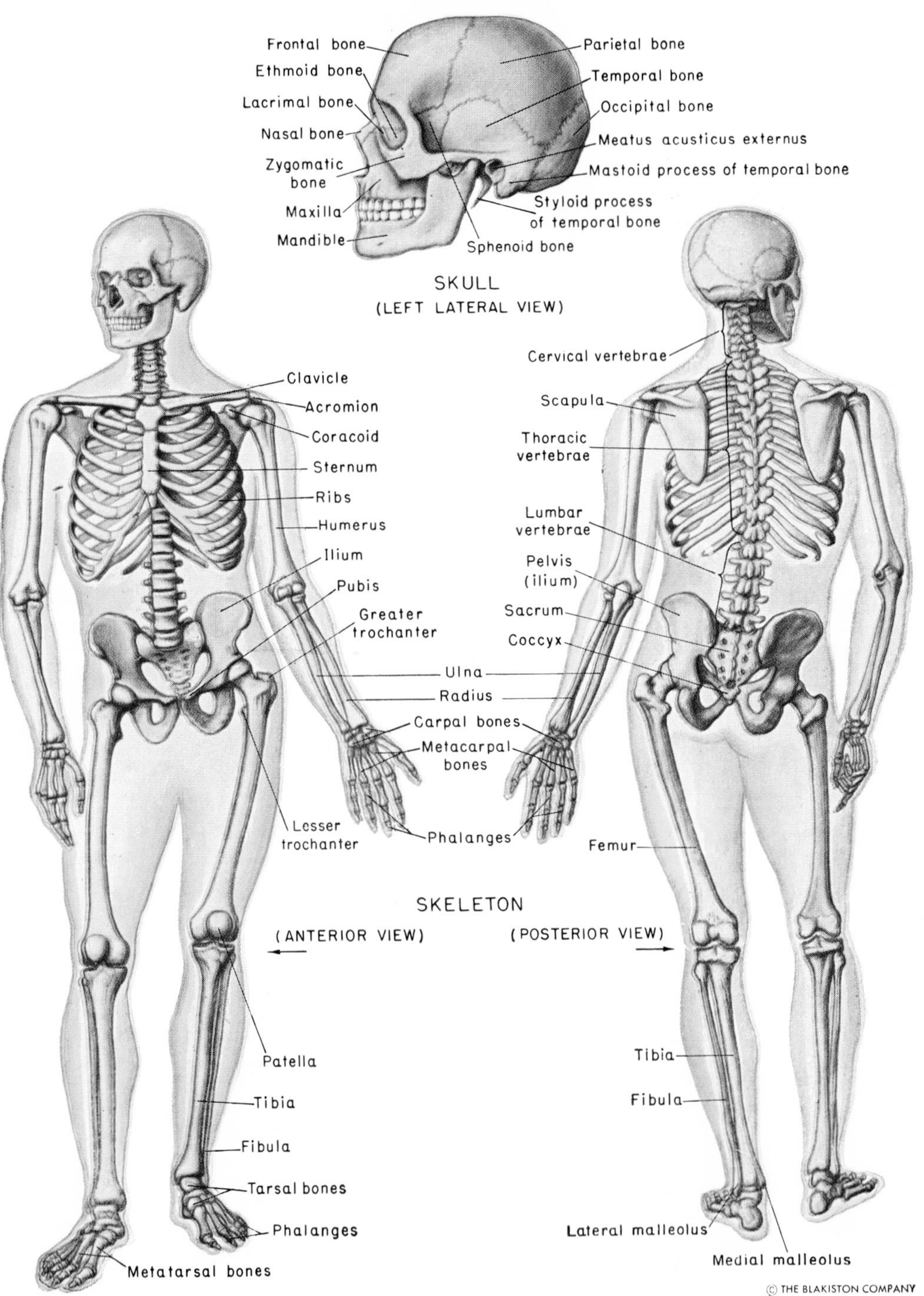
Frontal bone
Ethmoid bone
Lacrimal bone
Nasal bone
Zygomatic bone
Maxilla
Mandible
Parietal bone
Temporal bone
Occipital bone
Meatus acusticus externus
Mastoid process of temporal bone
Styloid process of temporal bone
Sphenoid bone
SKULL
(LEFT LATERAL VIEW)
Clavicle
Acromion
Coracoid
Sternum
Ribs
Humerus
Ilium
Pubis
Greater trochanter
Cervical vertebrae
Scapula
Thoracic vertebrae
Lumbar vertebrae
Pelvis (ilium)
Sacrum
Coccyx
Ulna
Radius
Carpal bones
Metacarpal bones
Phalanges
Lesser trochanter
Femur
SKELETON
(ANTERIOR VIEW)
(POSTERIOR VIEW)
Patella
Tibia
Fibula
Tarsal bones
Phalanges
Metatarsal bones
Tibia
Fibula
Lateral malleolus
Medial malleolus

SKELETON

PLATE 2

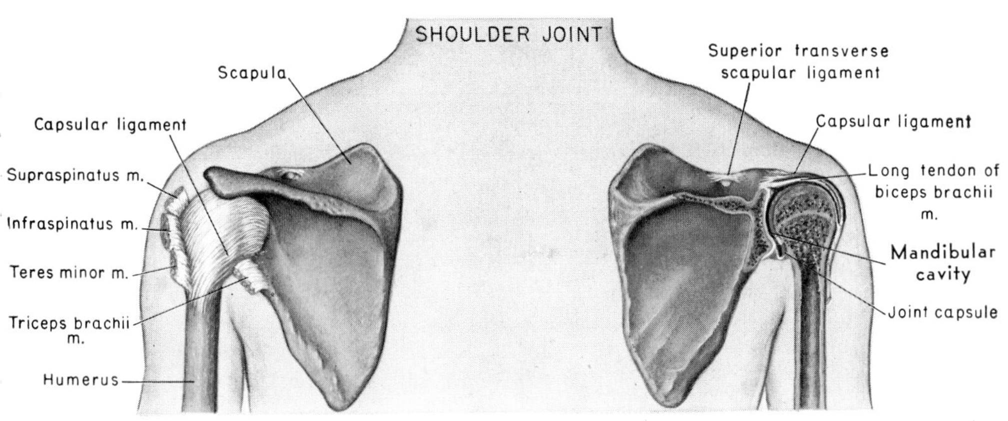
SHOULDER JOINT
Scapula
Capsular ligament
Supraspinatus m.
Infraspinatus m.
Teres minor m.
Triceps brachii m.
Humerus
Superior transverse scapular ligament
Capsular ligament
Long tendon of biceps brachii m.
Mandibular cavity
Joint capsule

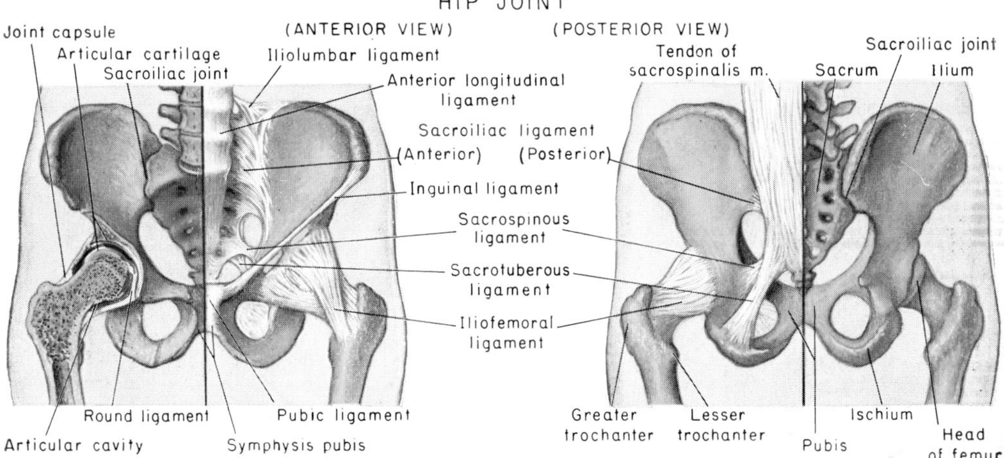
HIP JOINT
(ANTERIOR VIEW)
(POSTERIOR VIEW)
Joint capsule
Articular cartilage
Sacroiliac joint
Iliolumbar ligament
Anterior longitudinal ligament
Sacroiliac ligament
(Anterior)
(Posterior)
Inguinal ligament
Sacrospinous ligament
Sacrotuberous ligament
Iliofemoral ligament
Round ligament
Pubic ligament
Articular cavity
Symphysis pubis
Tendon of sacrospinalis m.
Sacroiliac joint
Sacrum
Ilium
Greater trochanter
Lesser trochanter
Pubis
Ischium
Head of femur

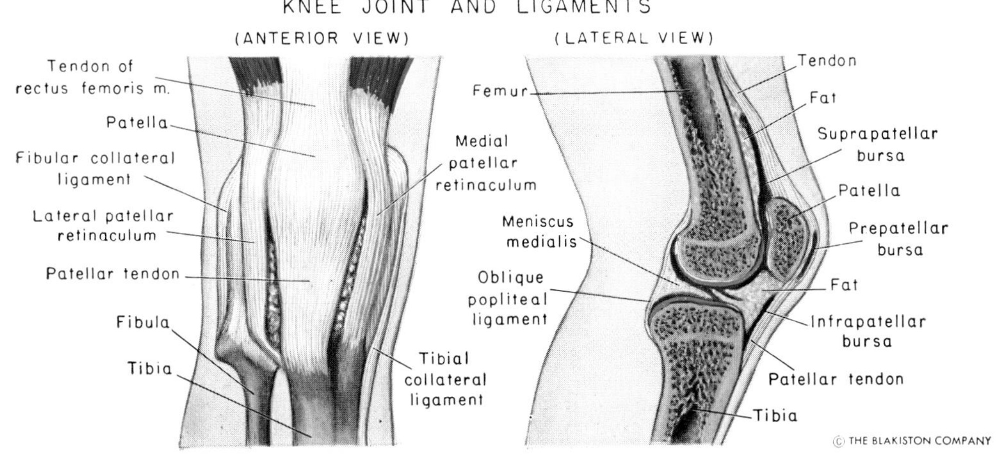
KNEE JOINT AND LIGAMENTS
(ANTERIOR VIEW)
(LATERAL VIEW)
Tendon of rectus femoris m.
Patella
Fibular collateral ligament
Lateral patellar retinaculum
Patellar tendon
Fibula
Tibia
Medial patellar retinaculum
Tibial collateral ligament
Femur
Meniscus medialis
Oblique popliteal ligament
Tendon
Fat
Suprapatellar bursa
Patella
Prepatellar bursa
Fat
Infrapatellar bursa
Patellar tendon
Tibia

JOINTS

PLATE 3

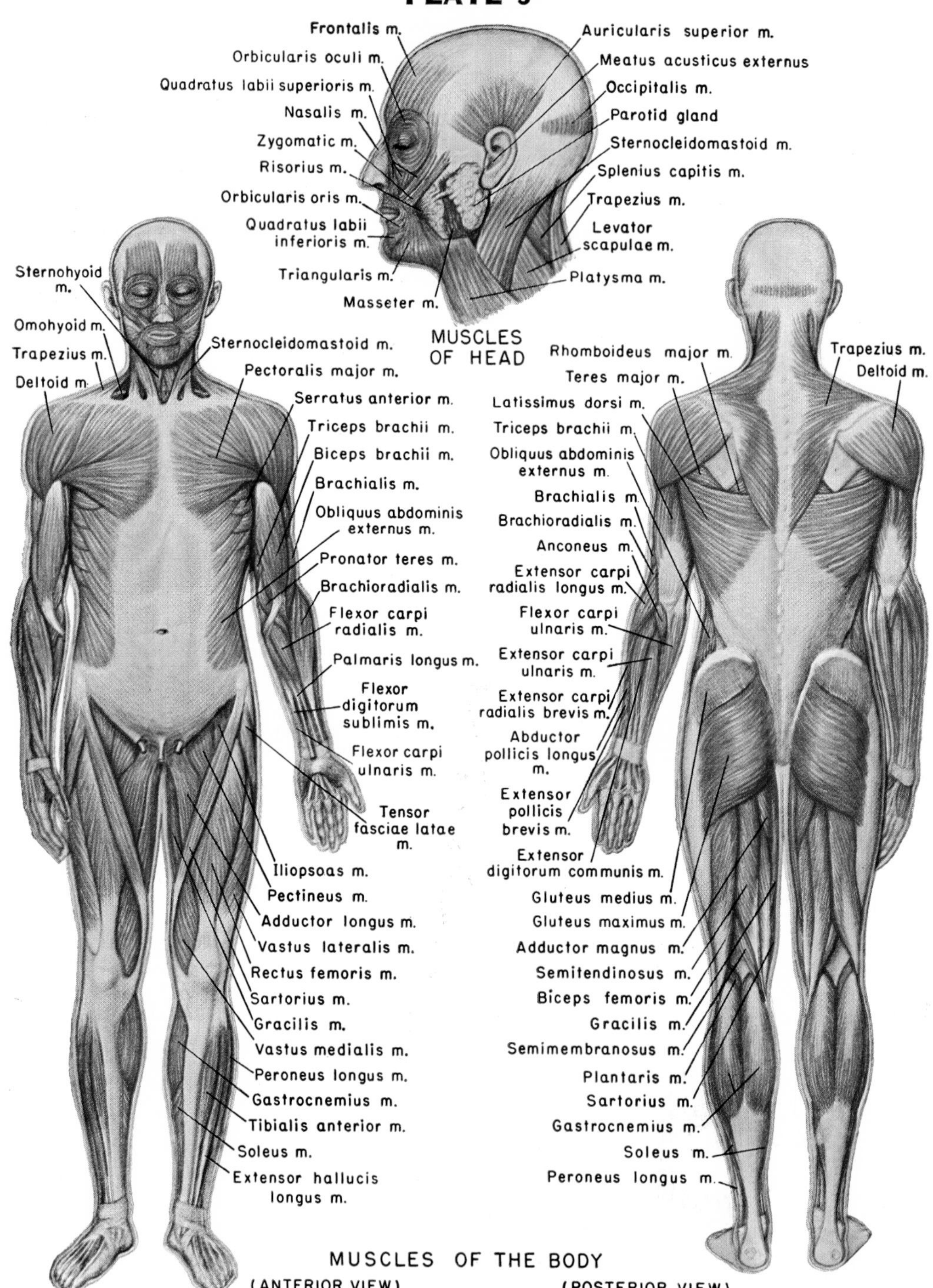
Frontalis m.
Orbicularis oculi m.
Quadratus labii superioris m.
Nasalis m.
Zygomatic m.
Risorius m.
Orbicularis oris m.
Quadratus labii inferioris m.
Triangularis m.
Masseter m.
Auricularis superior m.
Meatus acusticus externus
Occipitalis m.
Parotid gland
Sternocleidomastoid m.
Splenius capitis m.
Trapezius m.
Levator scapulae m.
Platysma m.
MUSCLES OF HEAD
Sternohyoid m.
Omohyoid m.
Trapezius m.
Deltoid m.
Sternocleidomastoid m.
Pectoralis major m.
Serratus anterior m.
Triceps brachii m.
Biceps brachii m.
Brachialis m.
Obliquus abdominis externus m.
Pronator teres m.
Brachioradialis m.
Flexor carpi radialis m.
Palmaris longus m.
Flexor digitorum sublimis m.
Flexor carpi ulnaris m.
Tensor fasciae latae m.
Iliopsoas m.
Pectineus m.
Adductor longus m.
Vastus lateralis m.
Rectus femoris m.
Sartorius m.
Gracilis m.
Vastus medialis m.
Peroneus longus m.
Gastrocnemius m.
Tibialis anterior m.
Soleus m.
Extensor hallucis longus m.
Rhomboideus major m.
Teres major m.
Latissimus dorsi m.
Triceps brachii m.
Obliquus abdominis externus m.
Brachialis m.
Brachioradialis m.
Anconeus m.
Extensor carpi radialis longus m.
Flexor carpi ulnaris m.
Extensor carpi ulnaris m.
Extensor carpi radialis brevis m.
Abductor pollicis longus m.
Extensor pollicis brevis m.
Extensor digitorum communis m.
Gluteus medius m.
Gluteus maximus m.
Adductor magnus m.
Semitendinosus m.
Biceps femoris m.
Gracilis m.
Semimembranosus m.
Plantaris m.
Sartorius m.
Gastrocnemius m.
Soleus m.
Peroneus longus m.
Trapezius m.
Deltoid m.

MUSCLES OF THE BODY

(ANTERIOR VIEW) (POSTERIOR VIEW)

MUSCLES

PLATE 4

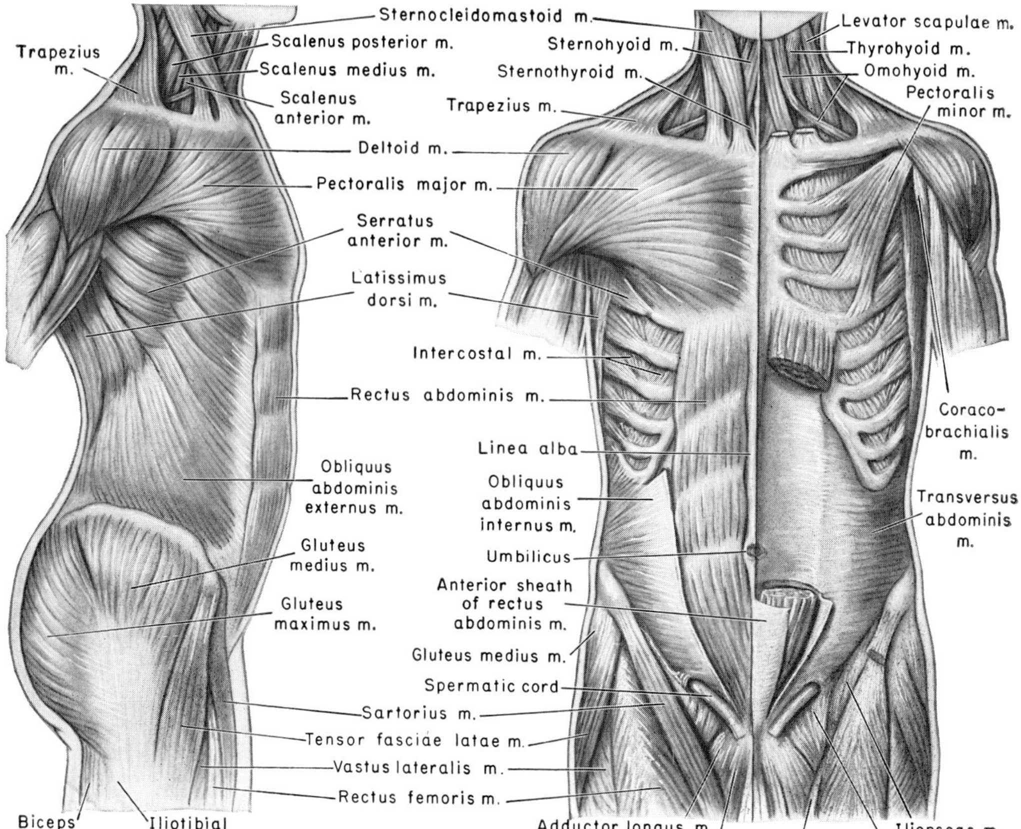

Trapezius m.
Sternocleidomastoid m.
Scalenus posterior m.
Scalenus medius m.
Scalenus anterior m.
Deltoid m.
Pectoralis major m.
Serratus anterior m.
Latissimus dorsi m.
Rectus abdominis m.
Obliquus abdominis externus m.
Gluteus medius m.
Gluteus maximus m.
Sartorius m.
Tensor fasciae latae m.
Vastus lateralis m.
Rectus femoris m.
Biceps femoris m.
Iliotibial band
Levator scapulae m.
Sternohyoid m.
Thyrohyoid m.
Sternothyroid m.
Omohyoid m.
Trapezius m.
Pectoralis minor m.
Intercostal m.
Coraco-brachialis m.
Linea alba
Obliquus abdominis internus m.
Transversus abdominis m.
Umbilicus
Anterior sheath of rectus abdominis m.
Gluteus medius m.
Spermatic cord
Adductor longus m.
Gracilis m.
Vastus medialis m.
Iliopsoas m.
Pectineus m.

MUSCLES OF SHOULDER, TRUNK, AND HIP

(RIGHT LATERAL VIEW) (ANTERIOR VIEW)

Abdominal inguinal ring
Subcutaneous inguinal ring
Femoral v.
Spermatic cord
Inguinal hernia
Femoral hernia

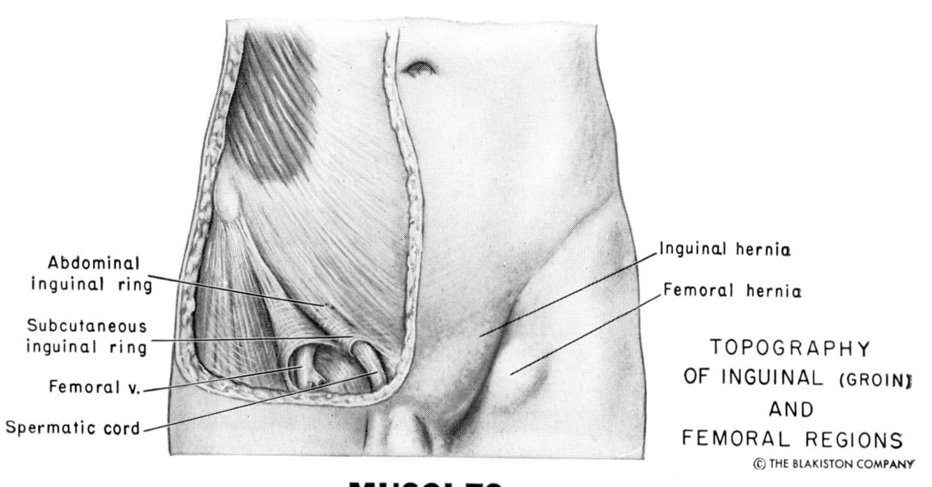

TOPOGRAPHY OF INGUINAL (GROIN) AND FEMORAL REGIONS

MUSCLES

PLATE 5

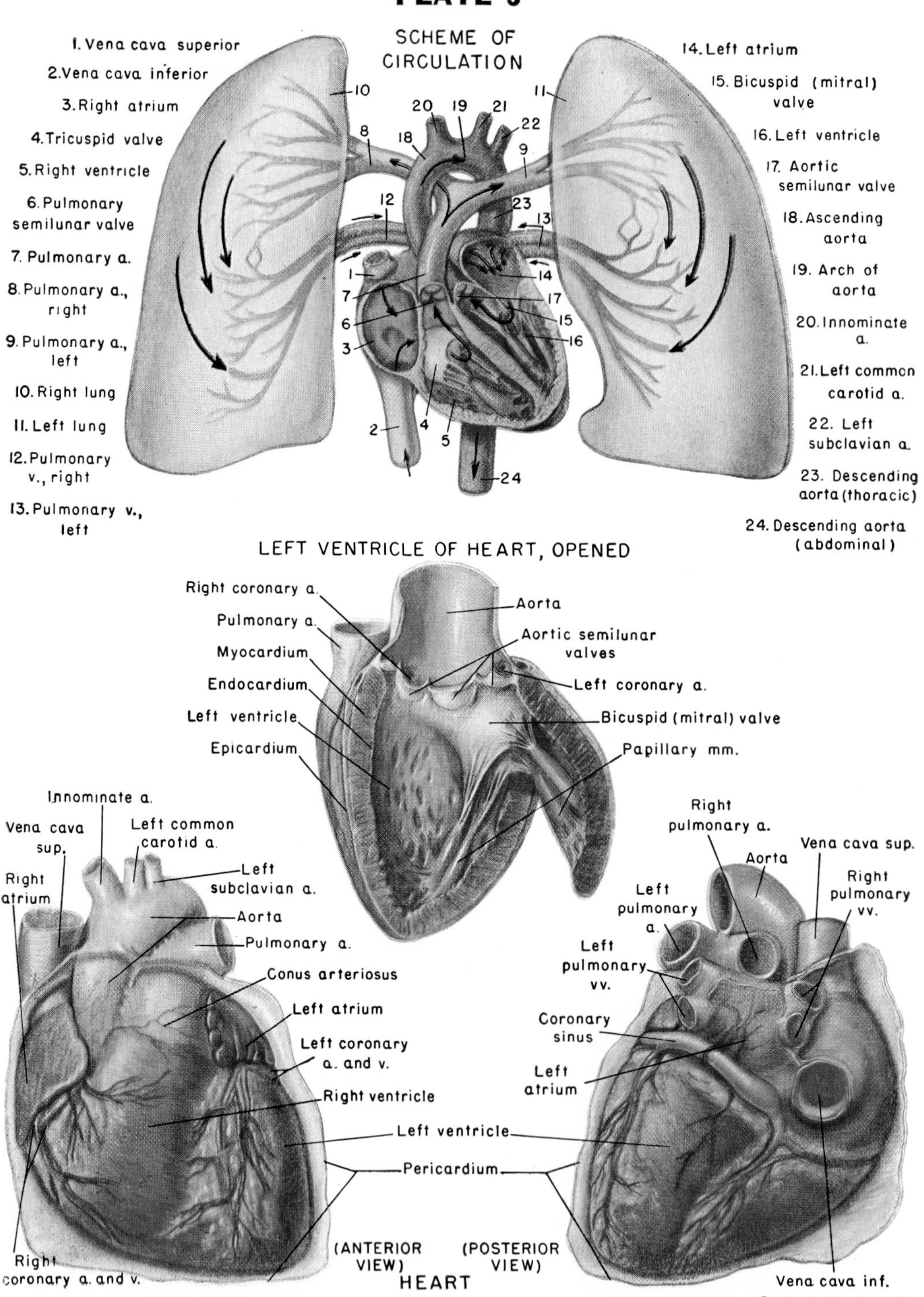

SCHEME OF CIRCULATION
1. Vena cava superior
2. Vena cava inferior
3. Right atrium
4. Tricuspid valve
5. Right ventricle
6. Pulmonary semilunar valve
7. Pulmonary a.
8. Pulmonary a., right
9. Pulmonary a., left
10. Right lung
11. Left lung
12. Pulmonary v., right
13. Pulmonary v., left
14. Left atrium
15. Bicuspid (mitral) valve
16. Left ventricle
17. Aortic semilunar valve
18. Ascending aorta
19. Arch of aorta
20. Innominate a.
21. Left common carotid a.
22. Left subclavian a.
23. Descending aorta (thoracic)
24. Descending aorta (abdominal)
LEFT VENTRICLE OF HEART, OPENED
Right coronary a.
Pulmonary a.
Myocardium
Endocardium
Left ventricle
Epicardium
Aorta
Aortic semilunar valves
Left coronary a.
Bicuspid (mitral) valve
Papillary mm.
Innominate a.
Vena cava sup.
Left common carotid a.
Right atrium
Left subclavian a.
Aorta
Pulmonary a.
Conus arteriosus
Left atrium
Left coronary a. and v.
Right ventricle
Left ventricle
Pericardium
Right coronary a. and v.
(ANTERIOR VIEW)
(POSTERIOR VIEW)
HEART
Right pulmonary a.
Aorta
Vena cava sup.
Right pulmonary vv.
Left pulmonary a.
Left pulmonary vv.
Coronary sinus
Left atrium
Vena cava inf.

BLOOD CIRCULATION

PLATE 6

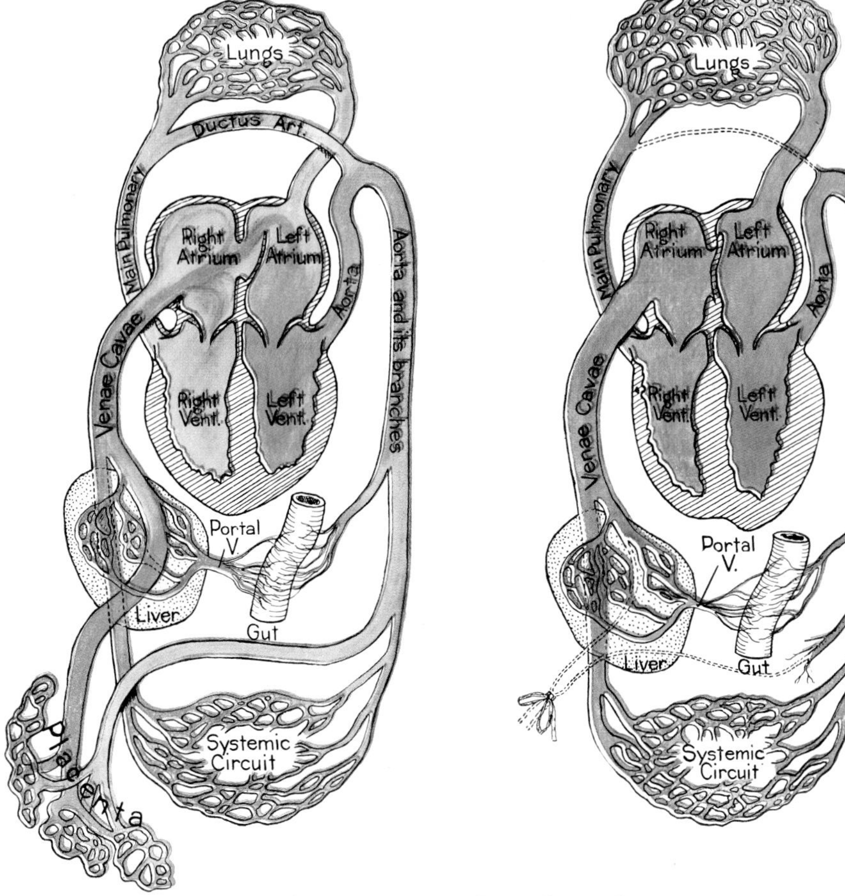

Lungs
Ductus Art.
Main Pulmonary
Right Atrium
Left Atrium
Aorta
Aorta and its branches
Venae Cavae
Right Vent.
Left Vent.
Portal V.
Liver
Gut
Placenta
Systemic Circuit
Lungs
Main Pulmonary
Right Atrium
Left Atrium
Aorta
Aorta and its branches
Venae Cavae
Right Vent.
Left Vent.
Portal V.
Liver
Gut
Systemic Circuit

(Left) Prenatal (fetal) circulation. (Right) Postnatal circulation.

(From Patten: "Human Embryology." Copyright, The Blakiston Company.)

Intima
Endothelium
Internal elastic membrane
Media
Muscle fibers
Connective tissue
Externa (adventitia)
External elastic membrane
Connective tissue
Vasa vasorum
Fat cells
For orientation
This portion is shown enlarged on the left

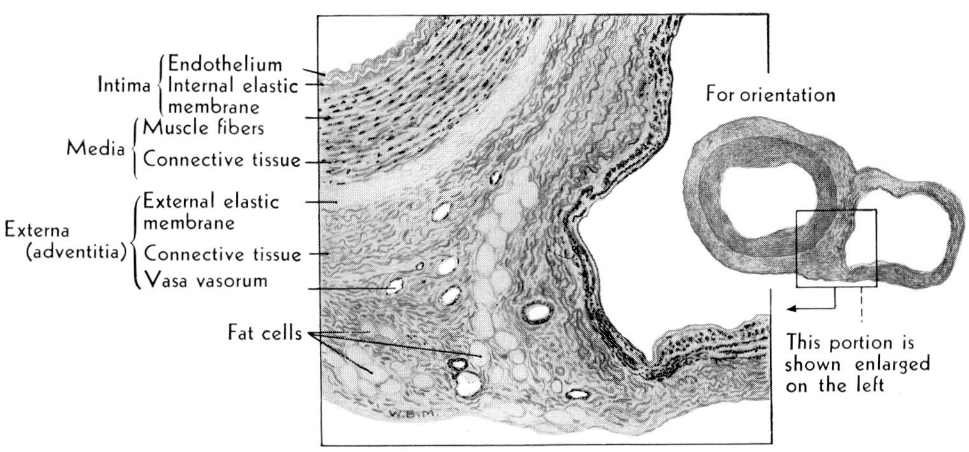

Section through human ulnar artery and vein, showing (left) wall of artery and (right) wall of vein.

(From Bremer-Weatherford: "Textbook of Histology." Copyright, The Blakiston Company.)

PRE- AND POSTNATAL BLOOD CIRCULATORY SYSTEMS

PLATE 7

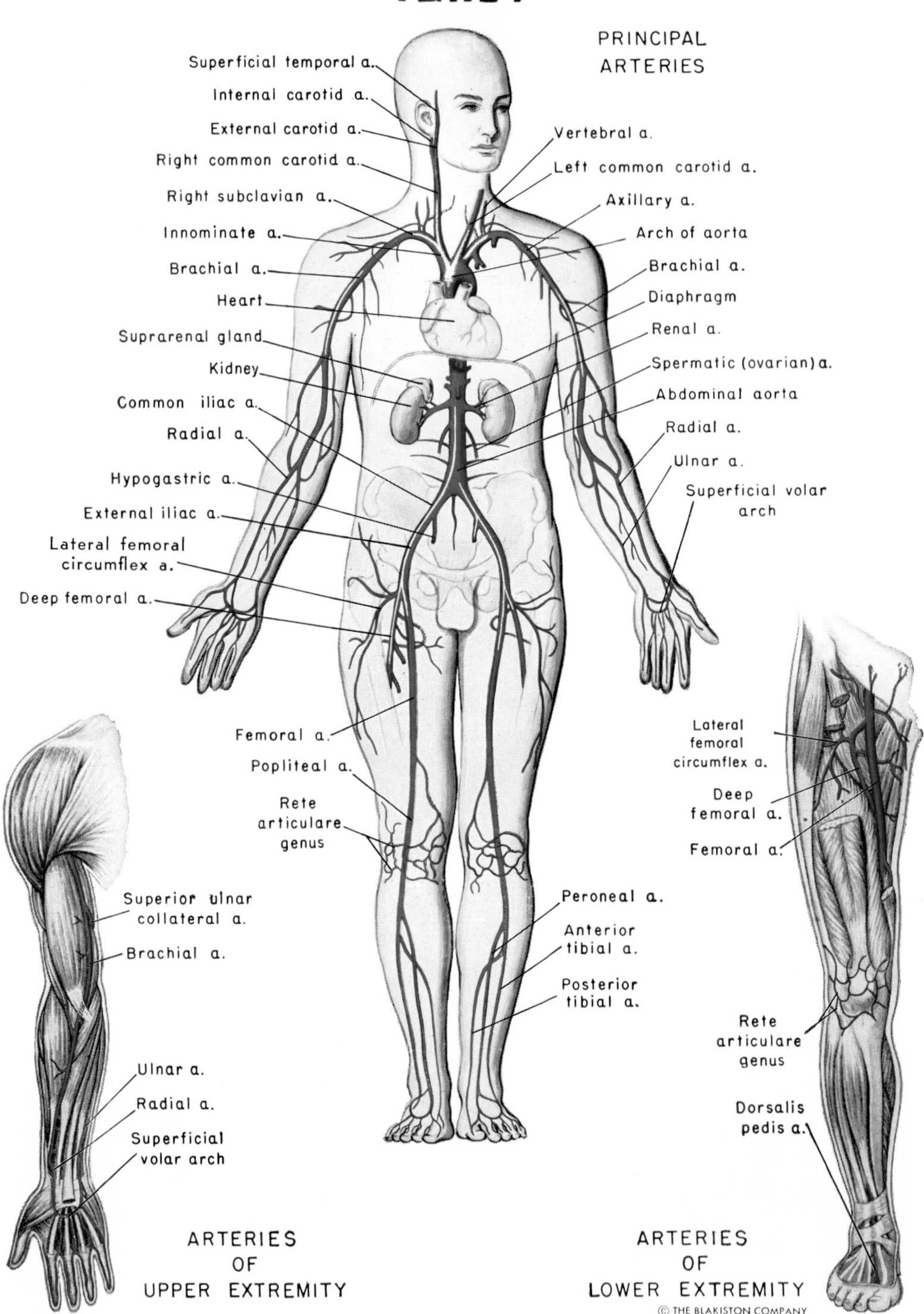
PRINCIPAL
ARTERIES
Superficial temporal a.
Internal carotid a.
External carotid a.
Right common carotid a.
Right subclavian a.
Innominate a.
Brachial a.
Heart
Suprarenal gland
Kidney
Common iliac a.
Radial a.
Hypogastric a.
External iliac a.
Lateral femoral
circumflex a.
Deep femoral a.
Vertebral a.
Left common carotid a.
Axillary a.
Arch of aorta
Brachial a.
Diaphragm
Renal a.
Spermatic (ovarian) a.
Abdominal aorta
Radial a.
Ulnar a.
Superficial volar
arch
Femoral a.
Popliteal a.
Rete
articulare
genus
Peroneal a.
Anterior
tibial a.
Posterior
tibial a.
Superior ulnar
collateral a.
Brachial a.
Ulnar a.
Radial a.
Superficial
volar arch
ARTERIES
OF
UPPER EXTREMITY
Lateral
femoral
circumflex a.
Deep
femoral a.
Femoral a.
Rete
articulare
genus
Dorsalis
pedis a.
ARTERIES
OF
LOWER EXTREMITY

ARTERIES

PLATE 8

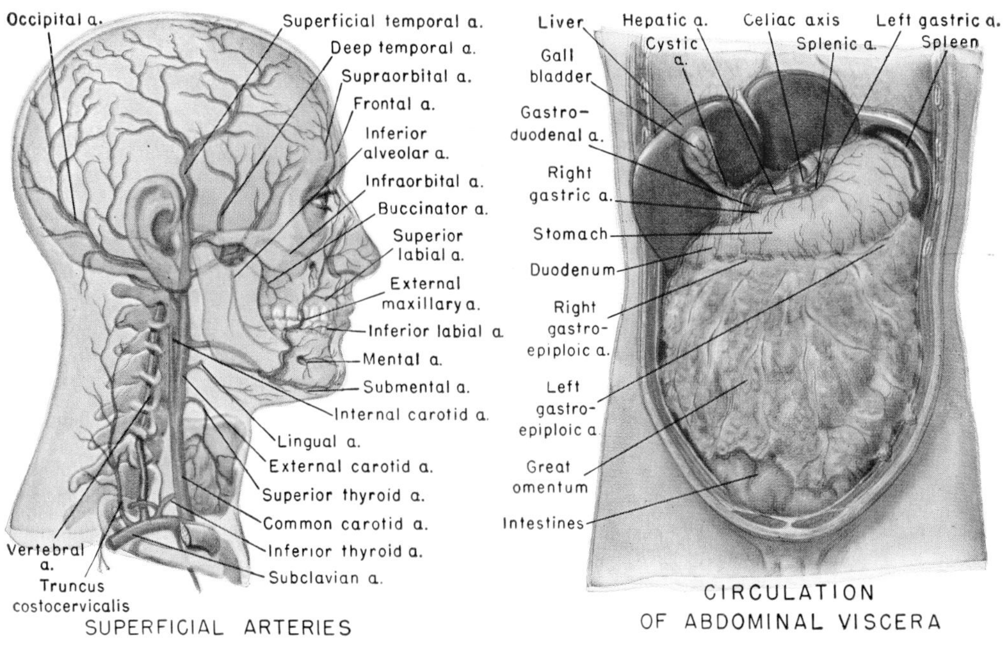

SUPERFICIAL ARTERIES OF HEAD AND NECK

CIRCULATION OF ABDOMINAL VISCERA

CIRCULATION OF DIGESTIVE TRACT

DEEP CIRCULATION OF ABDOMEN

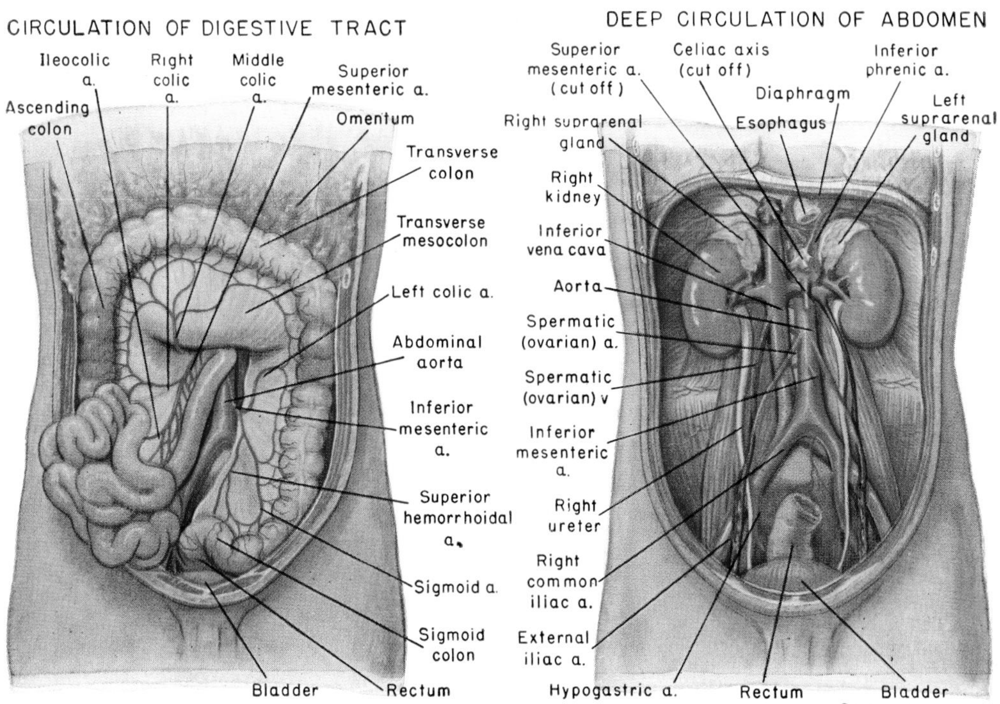

ARTERIES

PLATE 9

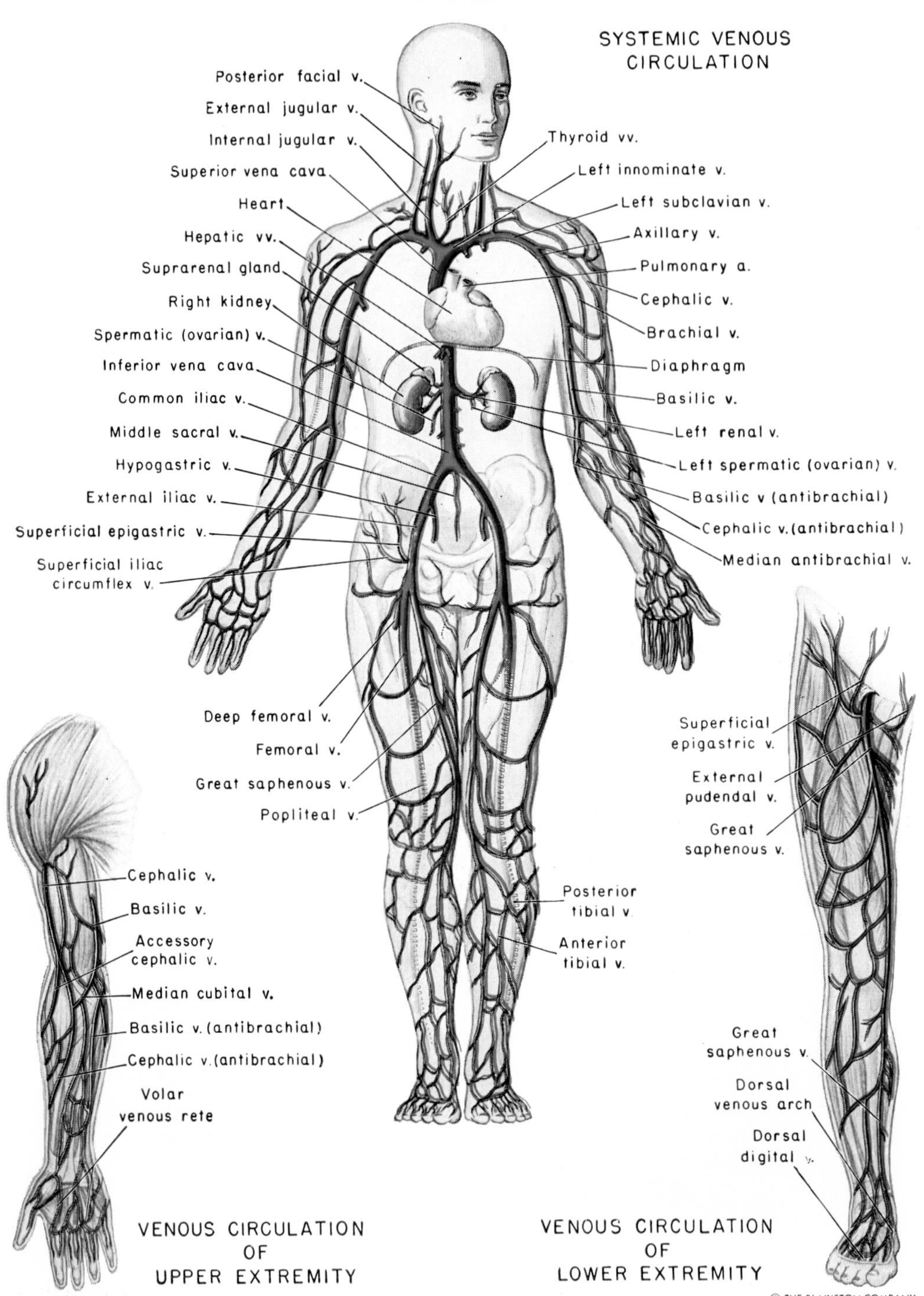
SYSTEMIC VENOUS CIRCULATION
Posterior facial v.
External jugular v.
Internal jugular v.
Superior vena cava
Heart
Hepatic vv.
Suprarenal gland
Right kidney
Spermatic (ovarian) v.
Inferior vena cava
Common iliac v.
Middle sacral v.
Hypogastric v.
External iliac v.
Superficial epigastric v.
Superficial iliac circumflex v.
Thyroid vv.
Left innominate v.
Left subclavian v.
Axillary v.
Pulmonary a.
Cephalic v.
Brachial v.
Diaphragm
Basilic v.
Left renal v.
Left spermatic (ovarian) v.
Basilic v (antibrachial)
Cephalic v.(antibrachial)
Median antibrachial v.
Deep femoral v.
Femoral v.
Great saphenous v.
Popliteal v.
Posterior tibial v.
Anterior tibial v.
Cephalic v.
Basilic v.
Accessory cephalic v.
Median cubital v.
Basilic v. (antibrachial)
Cephalic v. (antibrachial)
Volar venous rete
VENOUS CIRCULATION OF UPPER EXTREMITY
Superficial epigastric v.
External pudendal v.
Great saphenous v.
Great saphenous v.
Dorsal venous arch
Dorsal digital v.
VENOUS CIRCULATION OF LOWER EXTREMITY

VEINS

PLATE 10

PRINCIPAL VEINS OF HEAD AND NECK

Inferior sagittal sinus
Cavernous sinus
Frontal v.
Supraorbital v.
Pterygoid plexus
Inferior ophthalmic v.
Nasal vv.
Superior labial v.
Anterior facial v.
Posterior facial v.
Lingual v.
Superior thyroid v.
Middle thyroid v.
Inferior thyroid v.
Innominate v.
Superior sagittal sinus
Lateral ventricle
Straight sinus
Transverse sinus
Occipital sinus
Occipital v.
Deep cervical v.
External jugular v.
Internal jugular v.
Vertebral v.
Subclavian v.

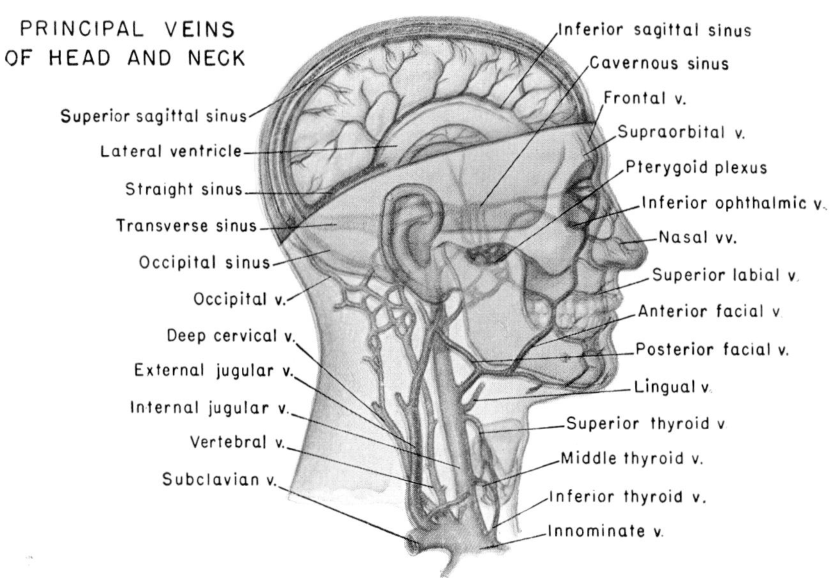

PORTAL VEIN AND PRINCIPAL TRIBUTARIES

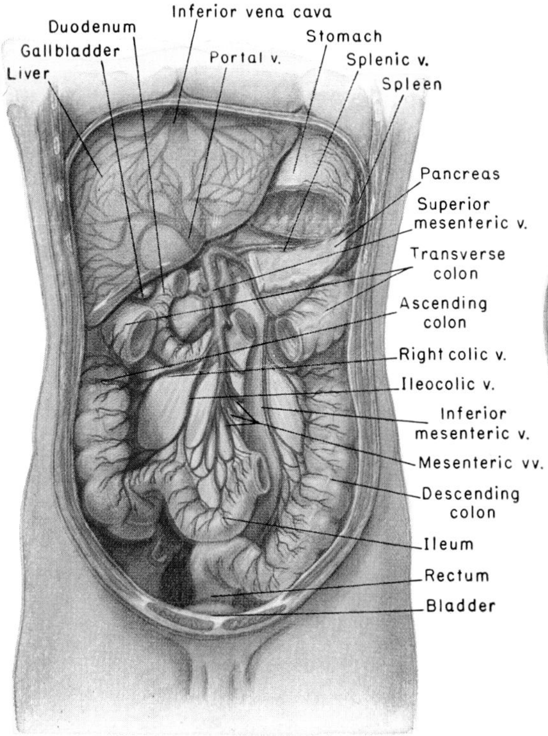

Inferior vena cava
Duodenum
Gallbladder
Liver
Portal v.
Stomach
Splenic v.
Spleen
Pancreas
Superior mesenteric v.
Transverse colon
Ascending colon
Right colic v.
Ileocolic v.
Inferior mesenteric v.
Mesenteric vv.
Descending colon
Ileum
Rectum
Bladder

PORTAL VEIN AND TRIBUTARIES

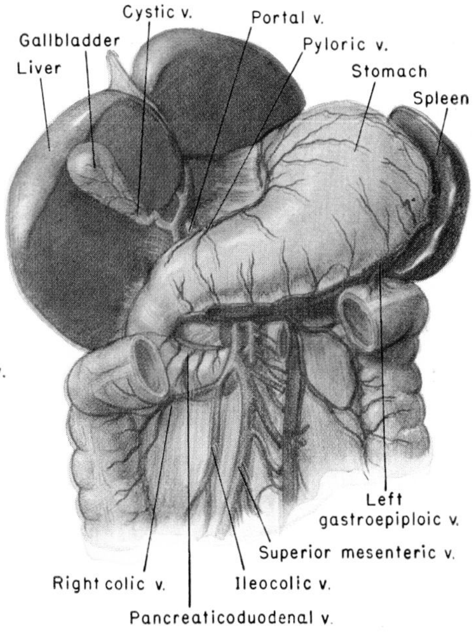

Cystic v.
Portal v.
Pyloric v.
Gallbladder
Liver
Stomach
Spleen
Left gastroepiploic v.
Superior mesenteric v.
Right colic v.
Ileocolic v.
Pancreaticoduodenal v.

VEINS

PLATE 11

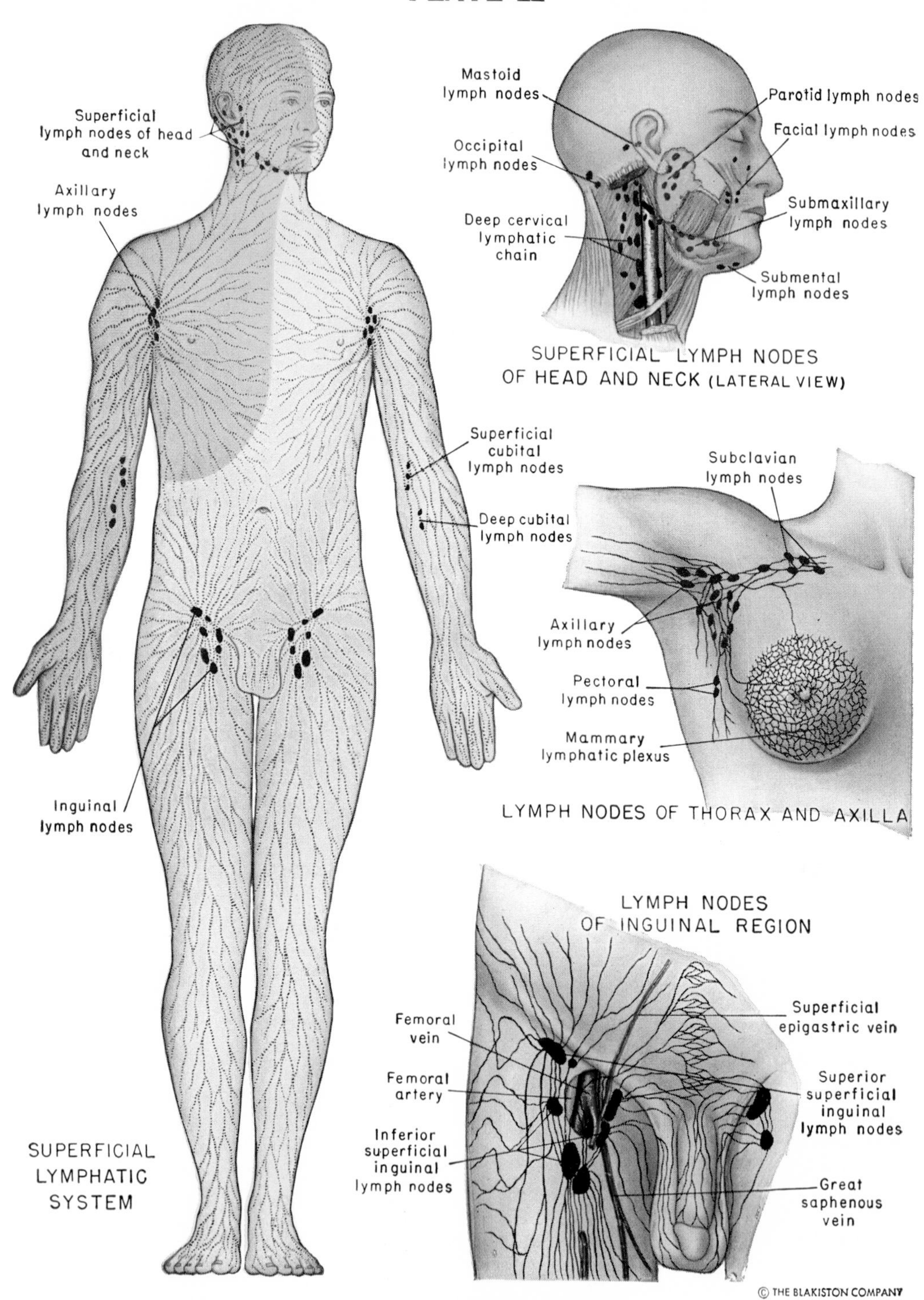

Superficial lymph nodes of head and neck
Axillary lymph nodes
Superficial cubital lymph nodes
Deep cubital lymph nodes
Inguinal lymph nodes
SUPERFICIAL LYMPHATIC SYSTEM
Mastoid lymph nodes
Parotid lymph nodes
Facial lymph nodes
Occipital lymph nodes
Deep cervical lymphatic chain
Submaxillary lymph nodes
Submental lymph nodes
SUPERFICIAL LYMPH NODES OF HEAD AND NECK (LATERAL VIEW)
Subclavian lymph nodes
Axillary lymph nodes
Pectoral lymph nodes
Mammary lymphatic plexus
LYMPH NODES OF THORAX AND AXILLA
LYMPH NODES OF INGUINAL REGION
Femoral vein
Femoral artery
Inferior superficial inguinal lymph nodes
Superficial epigastric vein
Superior superficial inguinal lymph nodes
Great saphenous vein

LYMPHATIC SYSTEM

PLATE 12

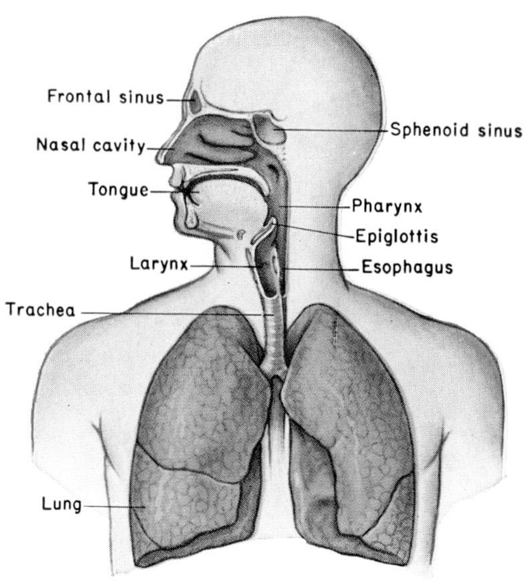

RESPIRATORY TRACT
(SCHEMATIC)

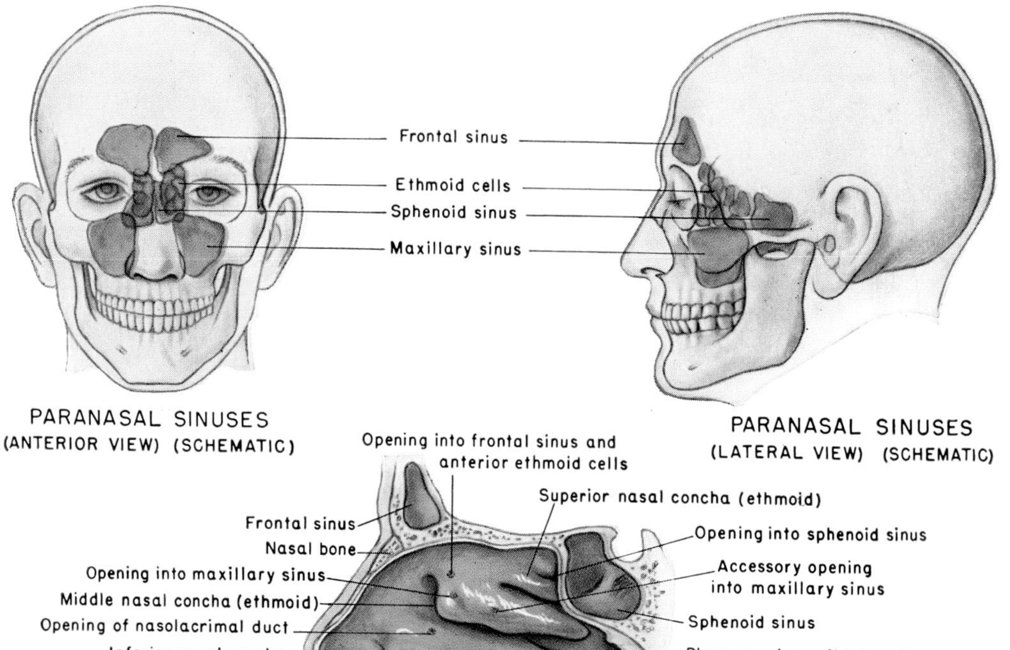

PARANASAL SINUSES
(ANTERIOR VIEW) (SCHEMATIC)

PARANASAL SINUSES
(LATERAL VIEW) (SCHEMATIC)

SAGITTAL SECTION THROUGH NOSE
(LATERAL VIEW)

RESPIRATORY TRACT

PLATE 13

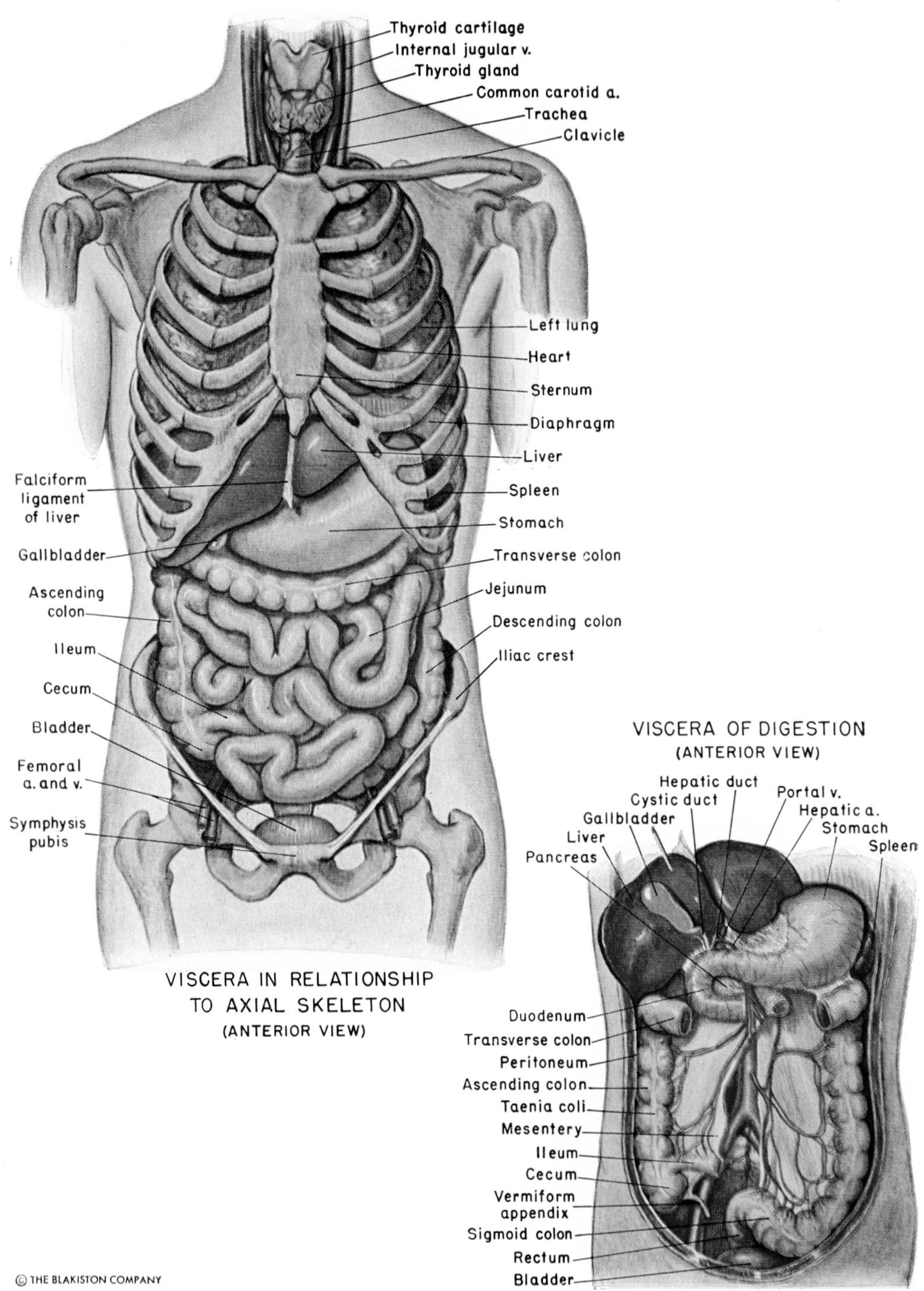

VISCERA IN RELATIONSHIP TO AXIAL SKELETON
(ANTERIOR VIEW)

VISCERA

PLATE 14

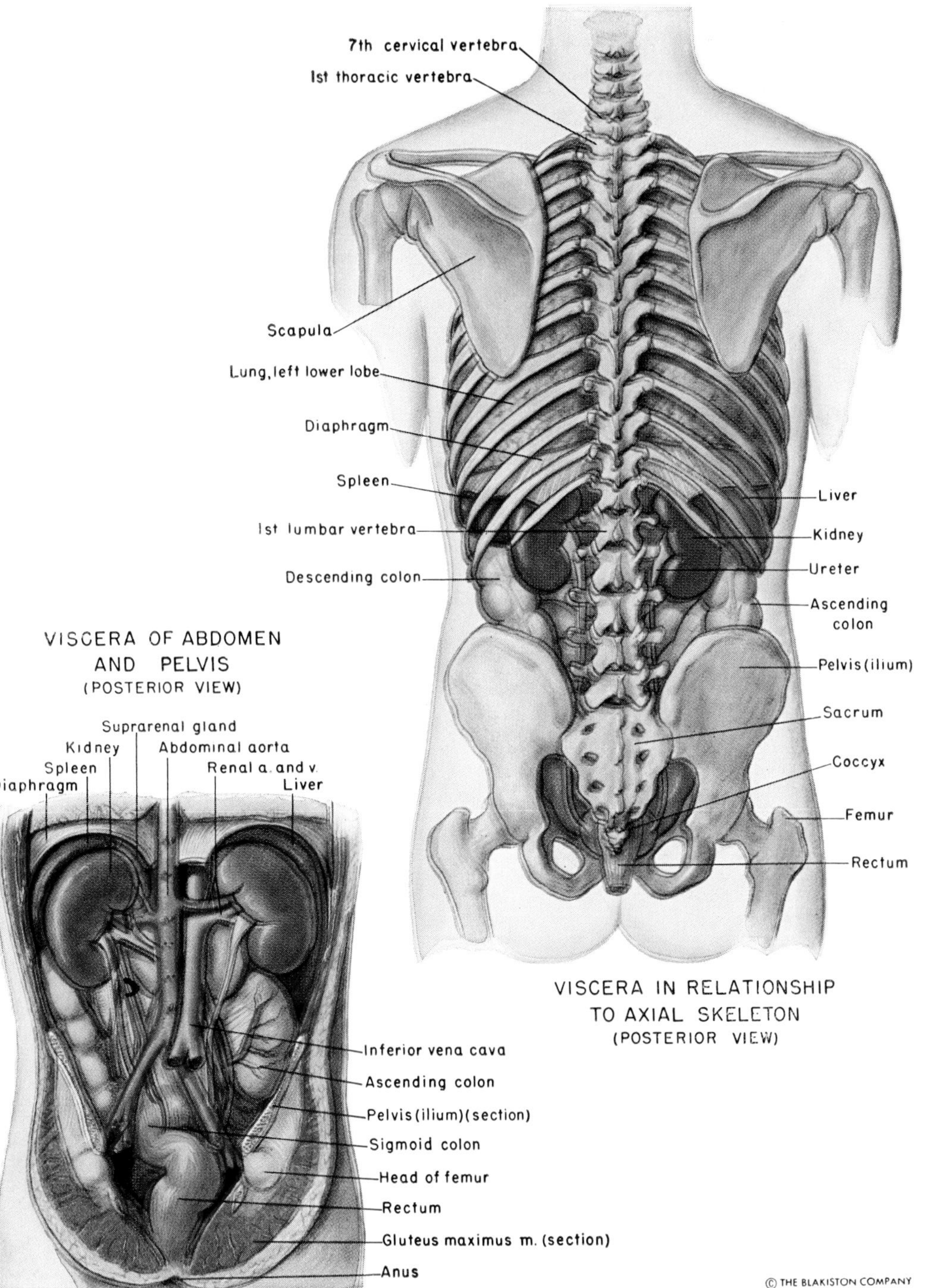

VISCERA OF ABDOMEN AND PELVIS
(POSTERIOR VIEW)

VISCERA IN RELATIONSHIP TO AXIAL SKELETON
(POSTERIOR VIEW)

VISCERA

PLATE 15

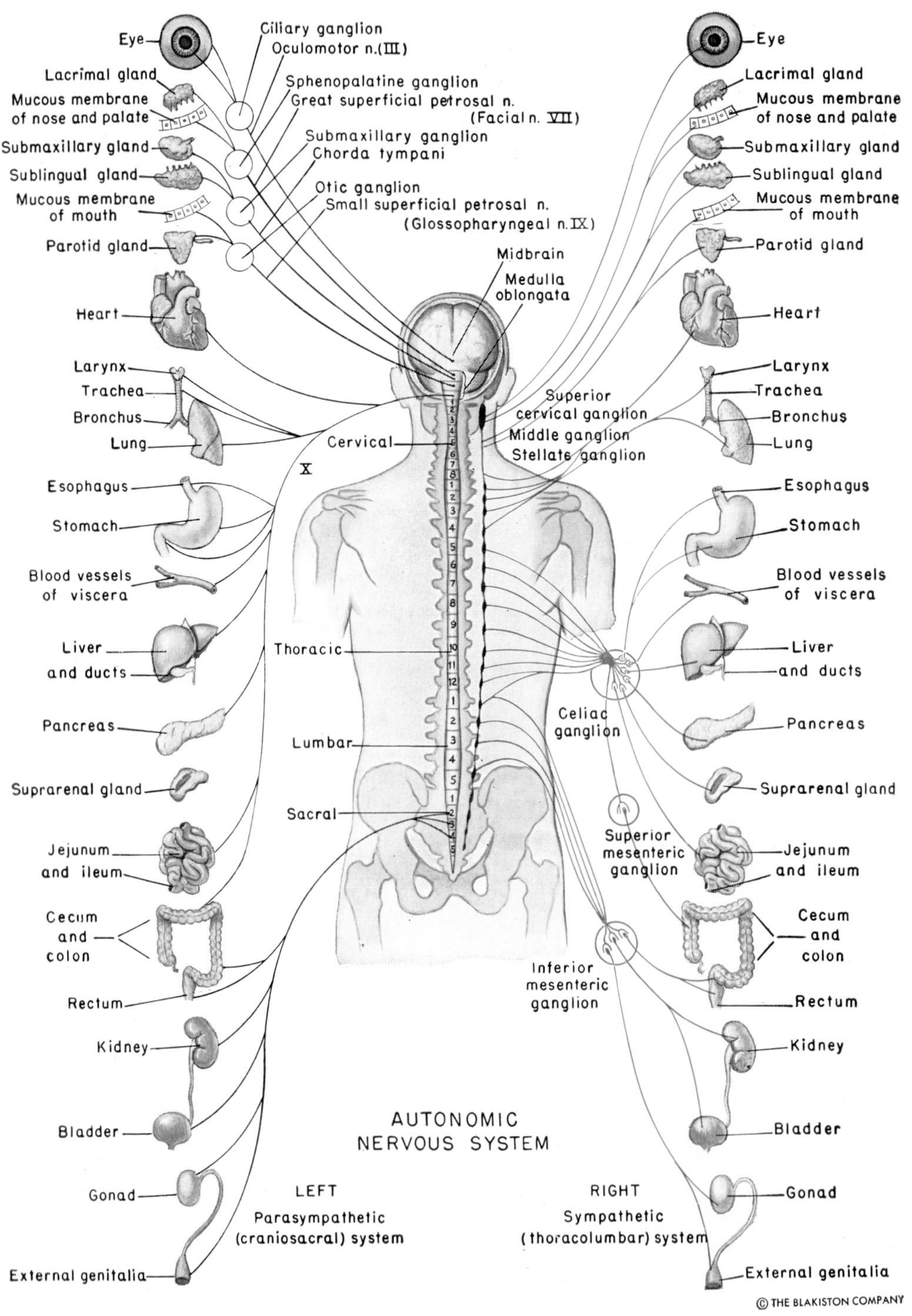
Eye
Ciliary ganglion
Oculomotor n.(III)
Lacrimal gland
Sphenopalatine ganglion
Great superficial petrosal n.
(Facial n. VII)
Mucous membrane of nose and palate
Submaxillary gland
Submaxillary ganglion
Chorda tympani
Sublingual gland
Otic ganglion
Small superficial petrosal n.
(Glossopharyngeal n. IX)
Mucous membrane of mouth
Parotid gland
Midbrain
Medulla oblongata
Heart
Larynx
Trachea
Bronchus
Lung
Superior cervical ganglion
Middle ganglion
Stellate ganglion
Cervical
X
Esophagus
Stomach
Blood vessels of viscera
Liver and ducts
Thoracic
Pancreas
Celiac ganglion
Lumbar
Suprarenal gland
Sacral
Superior mesenteric ganglion
Jejunum and ileum
Cecum and colon
Inferior mesenteric ganglion
Rectum
Kidney
AUTONOMIC NERVOUS SYSTEM
Bladder
Gonad
LEFT
Parasympathetic (craniosacral) system
RIGHT
Sympathetic (thoracolumbar) system
External genitalia

AUTONOMIC NERVOUS SYSTEM

PLATE 16

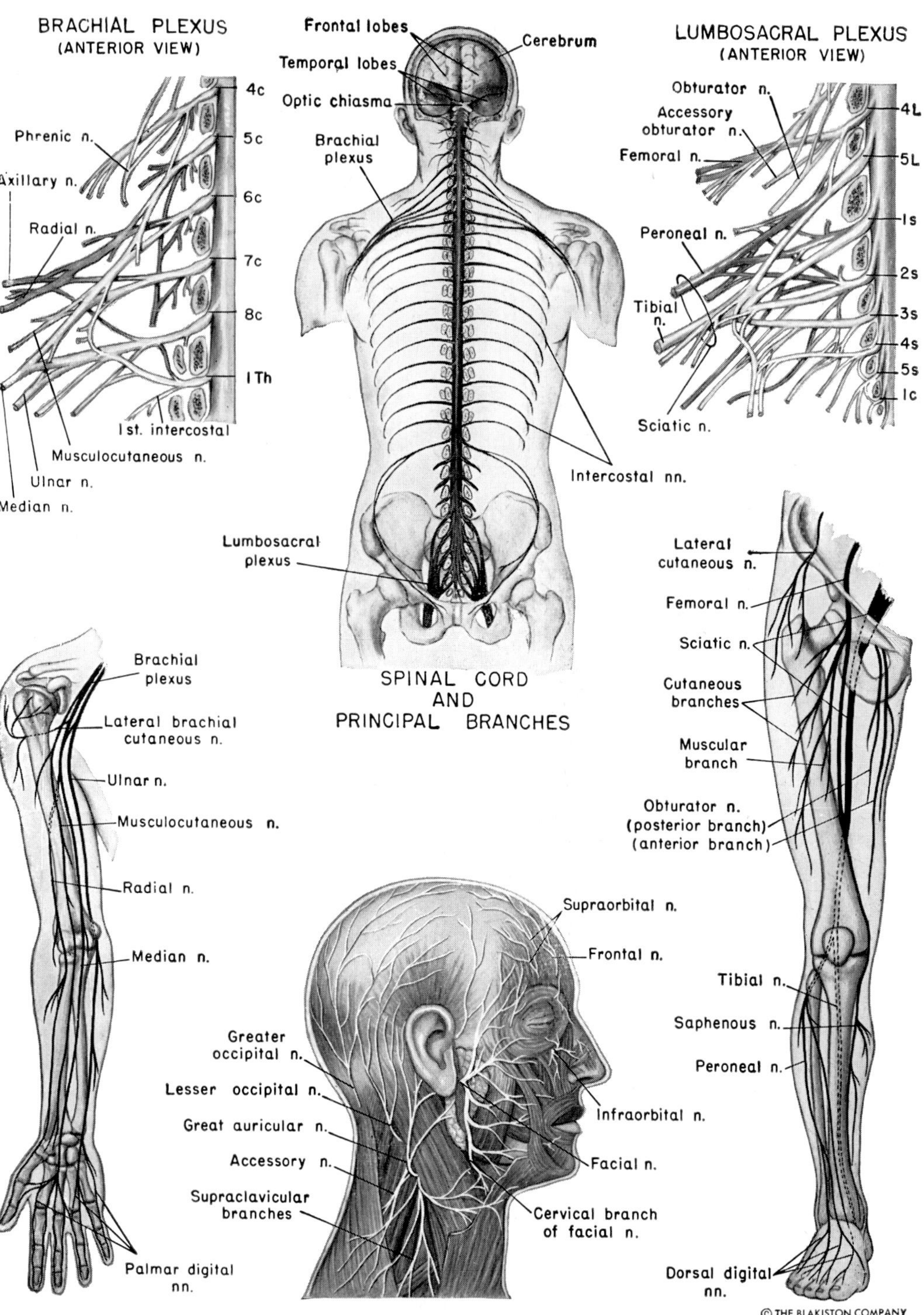

BRACHIAL PLEXUS
(ANTERIOR VIEW)
4c
Phrenic n.
5c
Axillary n.
6c
Radial n.
7c
8c
1Th
1st. intercostal
Musculocutaneous n.
Ulnar n.
Median n.
Frontal lobes
Cerebrum
Temporal lobes
Optic chiasma
Brachial plexus
Intercostal nn.
Lumbosacral plexus
LUMBOSACRAL PLEXUS
(ANTERIOR VIEW)
Obturator n.
4L
Accessory obturator n.
Femoral n.
5L
1s
Peroneal n.
2s
Tibial n.
3s
4s
5s
1c
Sciatic n.
Brachial plexus
Lateral brachial cutaneous n.
Ulnar n.
Musculocutaneous n.
Radial n.
Median n.
Palmar digital nn.
SPINAL CORD AND PRINCIPAL BRANCHES
Lateral cutaneous n.
Femoral n.
Sciatic n.
Cutaneous branches
Muscular branch
Obturator n.
(posterior branch)
(anterior branch)
Tibial n.
Saphenous n.
Peroneal n.
Dorsal digital nn.
Supraorbital n.
Frontal n.
Greater occipital n.
Lesser occipital n.
Great auricular n.
Accessory n.
Supraclavicular branches
Infraorbital n.
Facial n.
Cervical branch of facial n.

NERVOUS SYSTEM

PLATE 17

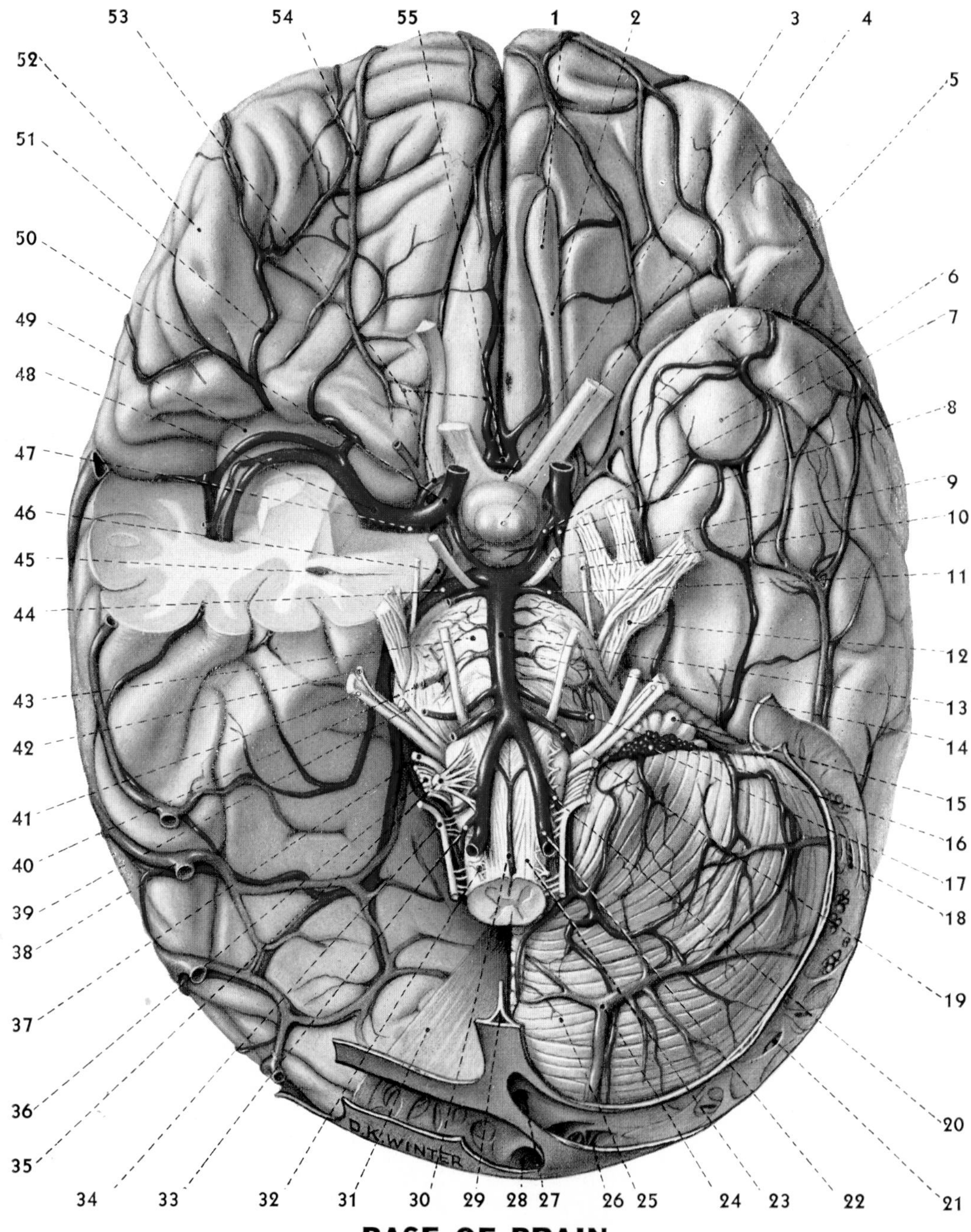

BASE OF BRAIN

Accessory n. (spinal accessory) (XI), **34.** Acoustic (auditory) n. (VIII), **41.** Anterior cerebral a., **53.** Anterior communicating a., **55.** Anterior inferior cerebellar a., **19.** Anterior spinal a., **30.** Basilar a., **13.** Brain stem, **23.** Cerebellar v., **24.** Cerebellar v.—opening of into sinus, **26.** Cerebellum, **25.** Choroid a., **8.** Choroid plexus of 4th ventricle, **17.** Confluens sinuum—opening of straight sinus into, **27.** Facial n. (VII), **39.** Flocculus, **15.** Frontal lobe, **52.** Ganglionic branches, **47.** Glossopharyngeal n. (IX), **37.** Hypoglossal n. (XII), **35.** Inferior frontal v., **54.** Inferior occipital v. to lateral sinus, **38.** Insula (island of Reil), **49.** Intermediary n. (Wrisberg), **42.** Internal auditory a. (a. auditiva interna), **16.** Internal carotid a., **50.** Lateral sinus—junction of with sigmoid sinus, **18.** Lateral sinus—opening of vein into, **21.** Lateral ventricle—inferior cornu, **45.** Middle cerebral a., **48.** Middle cerebral a.—cortical branch of, **51.** Occipital sinus, **29.** Oculomotor n. (III), **9.** Olfactory bulb, **1.** Olfactory tract, **2.** Optic chiasma, **3.** Pituitary (hypophysis cerebri), **4.** Pons, **43.** Pontile branch, **14.** Posterior cerebral a., **44.** Posterior cerebral v., **46.** Posterior communicating a., **7.** Posterior inferior cerebellar a., **33.** Posterior spinal a., **20.** Roots of 1st spinal n., **32.** Semilunar ganglion, **12.** Sigmoid sinus—junction of with lateral sinus, **18.** Sinus—opening of cerebellar v. into, **26.** Straight sinus—opening of into confluens sinuum, **27.** Superior cerebellar a., **11.** Superior sagittal sinus—opening of into confluens sinuum, **28.** Sylvian v., **5.** Temporal pole, **6.** Tentorium, **31.** Trigeminal n. (V)—motor root, **40.** Trochlear n. (IV), **10.** Vagus n. (X), **36.** Vertebral a., **22.**

PLATE 18

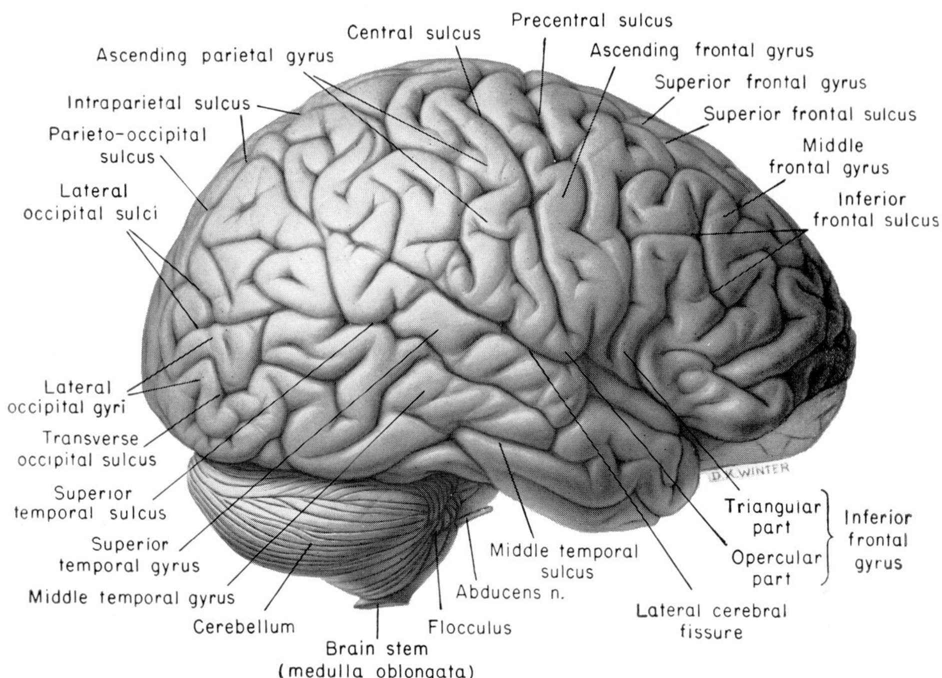
Central sulcus
Precentral sulcus
Ascending parietal gyrus
Ascending frontal gyrus
Superior frontal gyrus
Intraparietal sulcus
Superior frontal sulcus
Parieto-occipital sulcus
Middle frontal gyrus
Lateral occipital sulci
Inferior frontal sulcus
Lateral occipital gyri
Transverse occipital sulcus
Superior temporal sulcus
Superior temporal gyrus
Middle temporal gyrus
Cerebellum
Brain stem (medulla oblongata)
Flocculus
Abducens n.
Middle temporal sulcus
Lateral cerebral fissure
Triangular part
Opercular part
Inferior frontal gyrus
D.K. WINTER

Lateral View

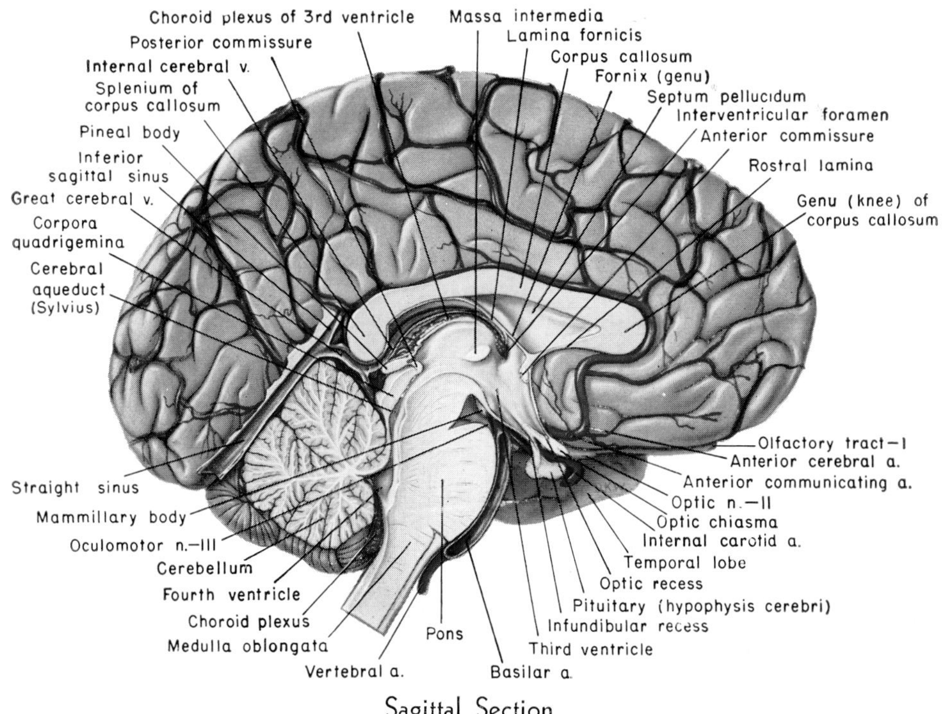
Choroid plexus of 3rd ventricle
Massa intermedia
Lamina fornicis
Posterior commissure
Corpus callosum
Internal cerebral v.
Fornix (genu)
Splenium of corpus callosum
Septum pellucidum
Interventricular foramen
Pineal body
Anterior commissure
Inferior sagittal sinus
Rostral lamina
Great cerebral v.
Genu (knee) of corpus callosum
Corpora quadrigemina
Cerebral aqueduct (Sylvius)
Olfactory tract—I
Anterior cerebral a.
Straight sinus
Anterior communicating a.
Optic n.—II
Mammillary body
Optic chiasma
Oculomotor n.—III
Internal carotid a.
Cerebellum
Temporal lobe
Fourth ventricle
Optic recess
Choroid plexus
Pituitary (hypophysis cerebri)
Infundibular recess
Pons
Medulla oblongata
Third ventricle
Vertebral a.
Basilar a.

Sagittal Section

BRAIN

PLATE 19

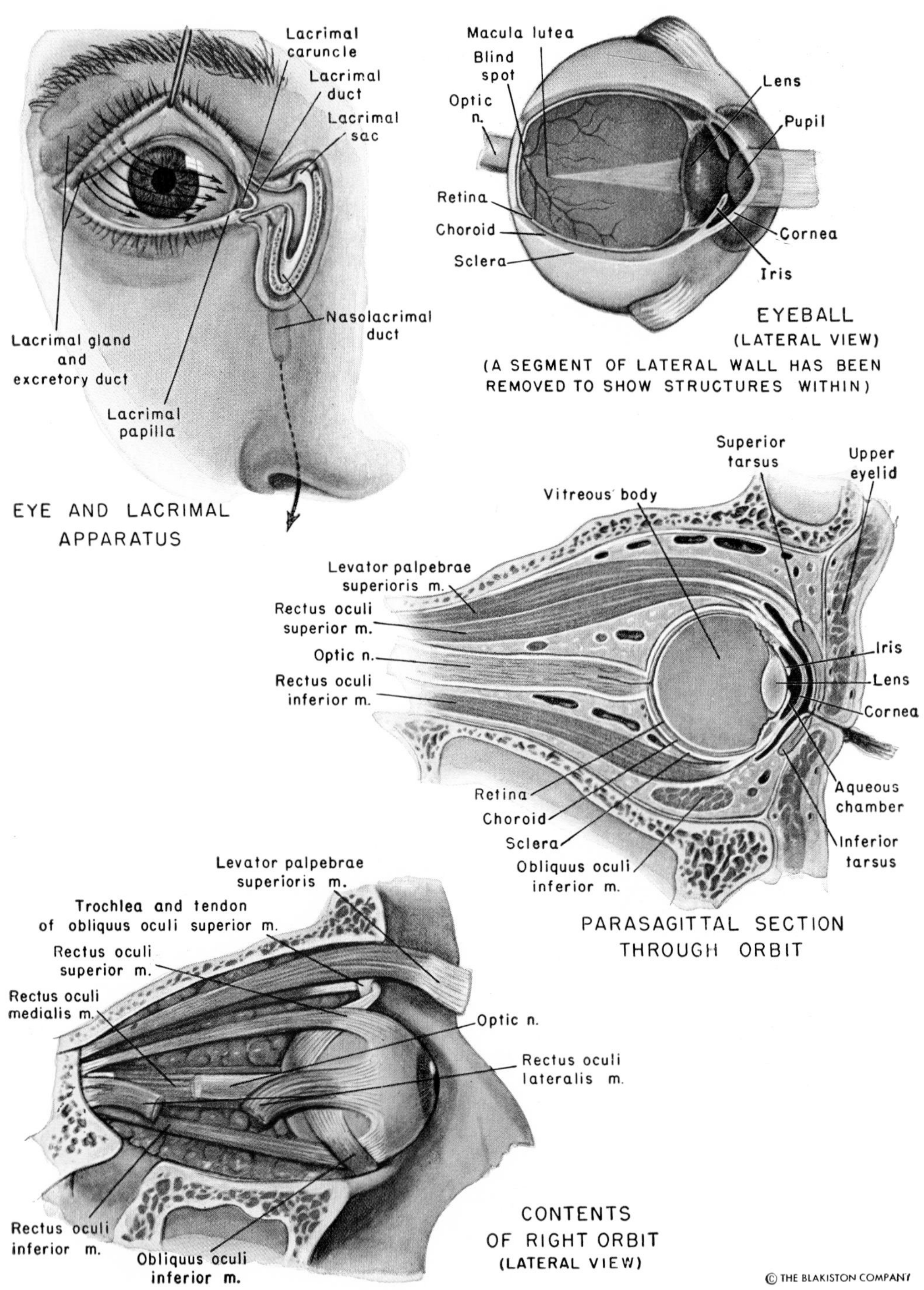

Lacrimal caruncle
Lacrimal duct
Lacrimal sac
Nasolacrimal duct
Lacrimal gland and excretory duct
Lacrimal papilla
EYE AND LACRIMAL APPARATUS
Macula lutea
Blind spot
Optic n.
Lens
Pupil
Retina
Choroid
Sclera
Cornea
Iris
EYEBALL (LATERAL VIEW)
(A SEGMENT OF LATERAL WALL HAS BEEN REMOVED TO SHOW STRUCTURES WITHIN)
Superior tarsus
Upper eyelid
Vitreous body
Levator palpebrae superioris m.
Rectus oculi superior m.
Optic n.
Rectus oculi inferior m.
Iris
Lens
Cornea
Aqueous chamber
Inferior tarsus
Retina
Choroid
Sclera
Obliquus oculi inferior m.
PARASAGITTAL SECTION THROUGH ORBIT
Levator palpebrae superioris m.
Trochlea and tendon of obliquus oculi superior m.
Rectus oculi superior m.
Rectus oculi medialis m.
Optic n.
Rectus oculi lateralis m.
Rectus oculi inferior m.
Obliquus oculi inferior m.
CONTENTS OF RIGHT ORBIT (LATERAL VIEW)

EYE

PLATE 20

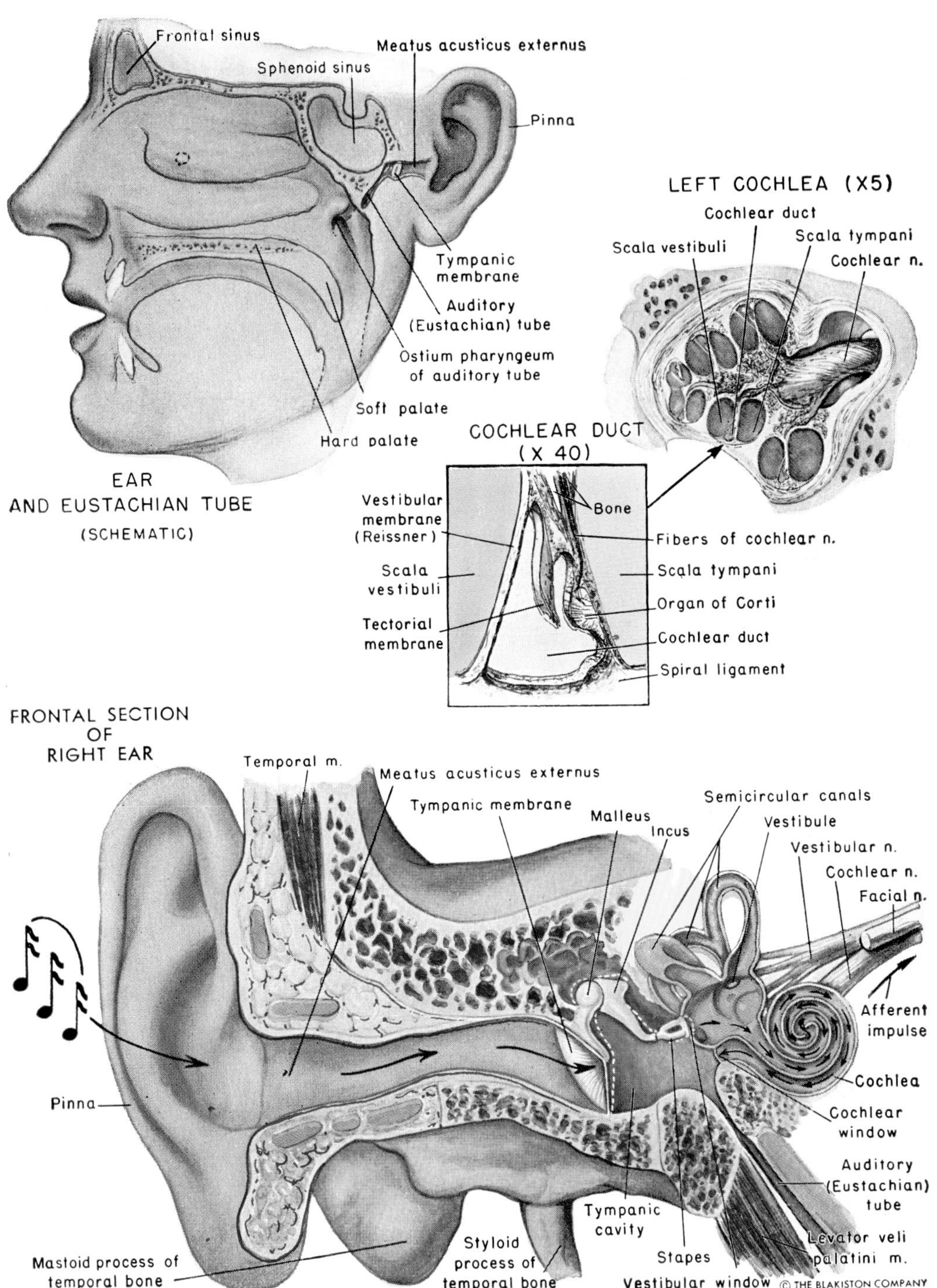

Frontal sinus
Sphenoid sinus
Meatus acusticus externus
Pinna
Tympanic membrane
Auditory (Eustachian) tube
Ostium pharyngeum of auditory tube
Soft palate
Hard palate
EAR AND EUSTACHIAN TUBE (SCHEMATIC)
LEFT COCHLEA (X5)
Cochlear duct
Scala vestibuli
Scala tympani
Cochlear n.
COCHLEAR DUCT (X 40)
Vestibular membrane (Reissner)
Bone
Fibers of cochlear n.
Scala vestibuli
Scala tympani
Organ of Corti
Tectorial membrane
Cochlear duct
Spiral ligament
FRONTAL SECTION OF RIGHT EAR
Temporal m.
Meatus acusticus externus
Tympanic membrane
Malleus
Incus
Semicircular canals
Vestibule
Vestibular n.
Cochlear n.
Facial n.
Afferent impulse
Cochlea
Cochlear window
Auditory (Eustachian) tube
Levator veli palatini m.
Pinna
Tympanic cavity
Stapes
Vestibular window
Mastoid process of temporal bone
Styloid process of temporal bone

EAR

PLATE 21

DECIDUOUS DENTITION

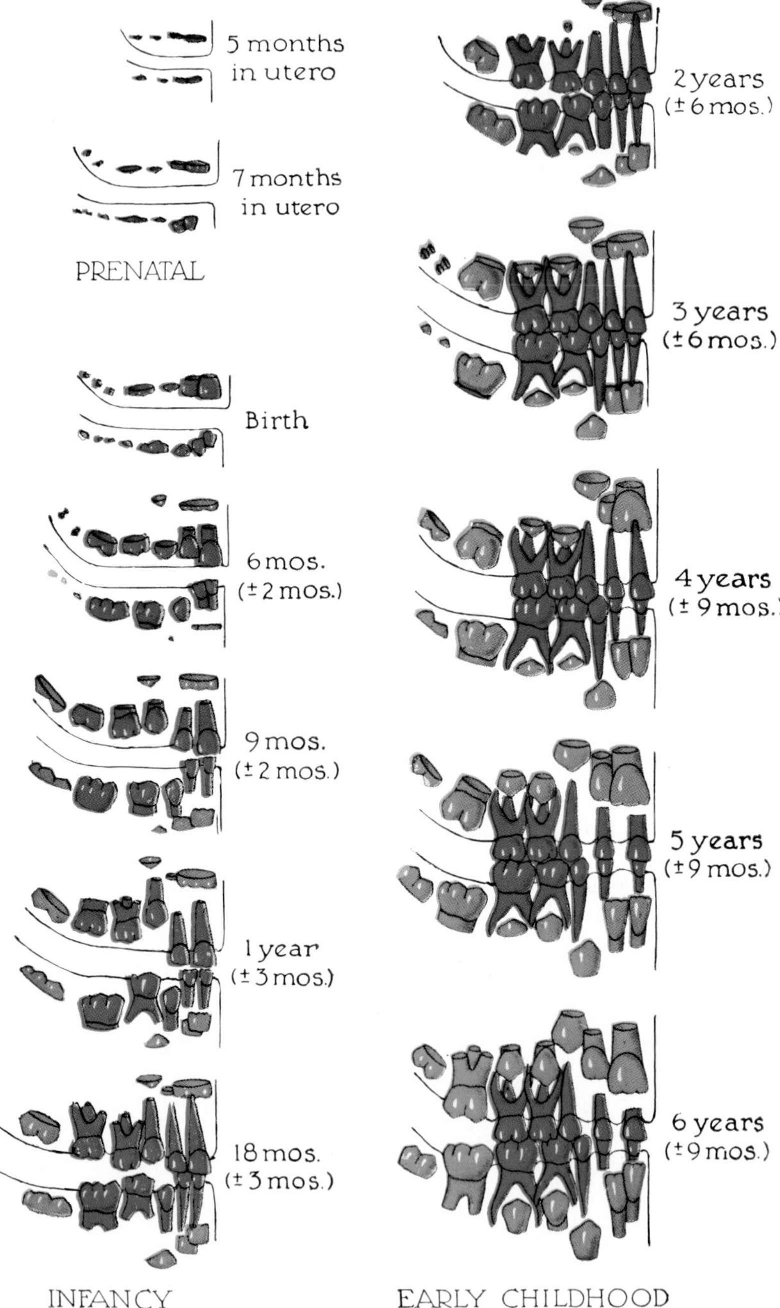

DEVELOPMENT OF HUMAN DENTITION

(Courtesy, Schour and Massler, American Dental Association.)

PLATE 22

MIXED DENTITION

PERMANENT DENTITION

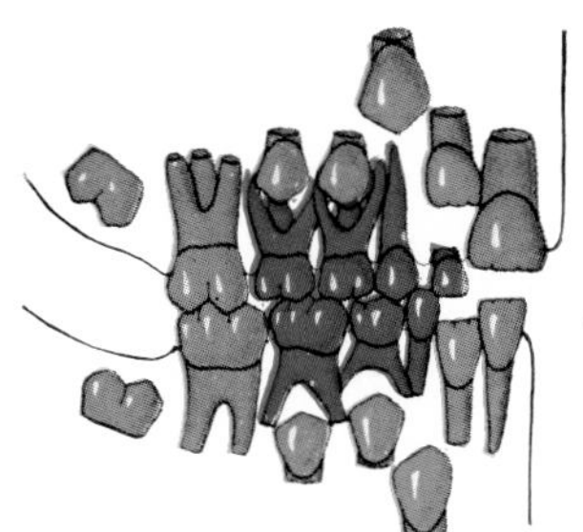

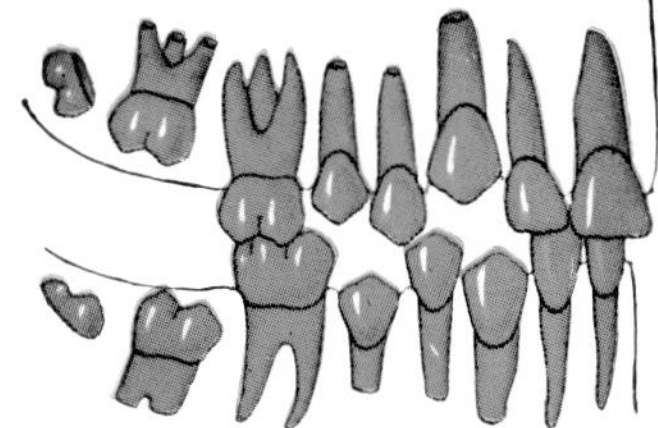

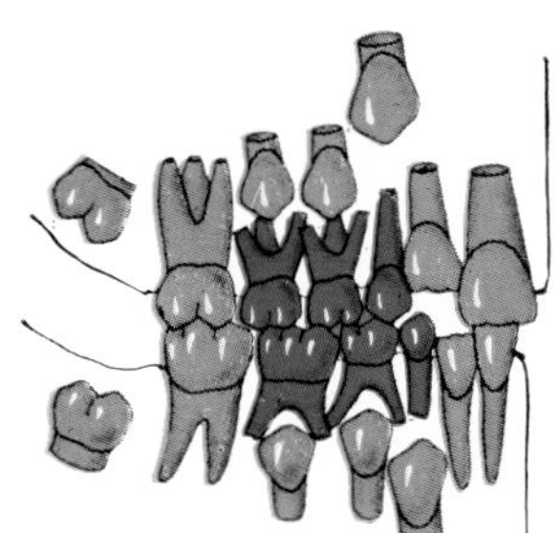

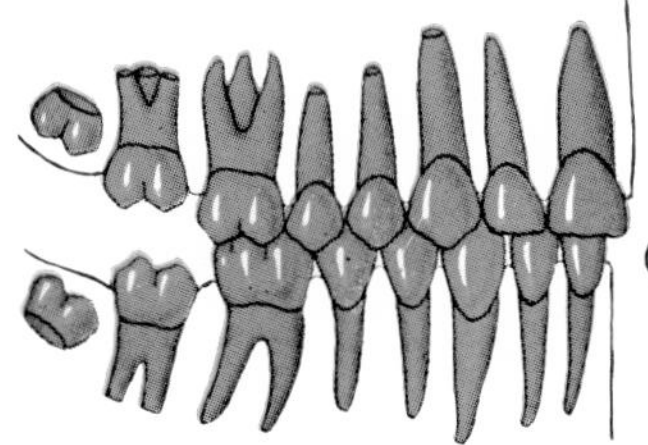

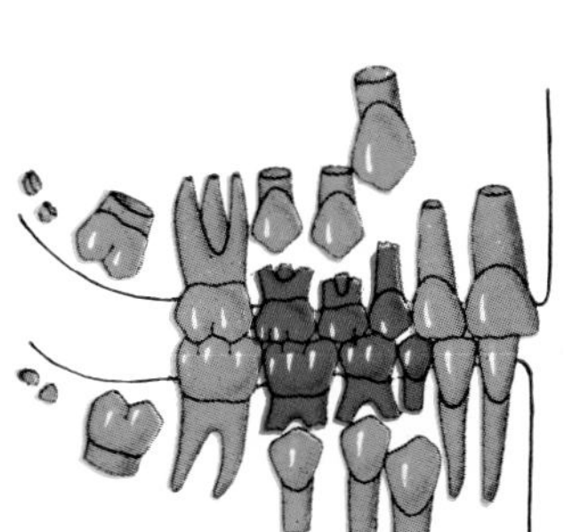

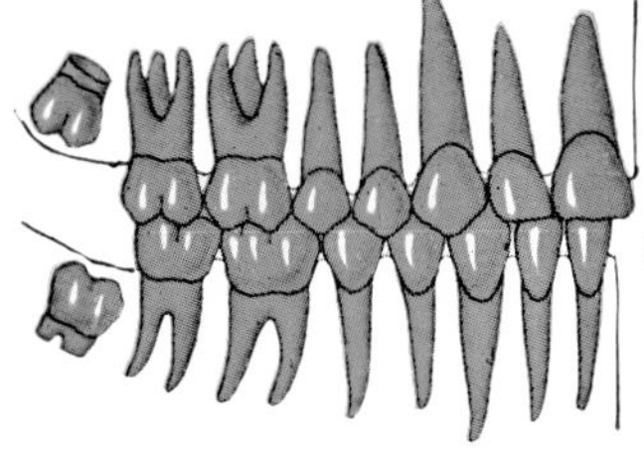

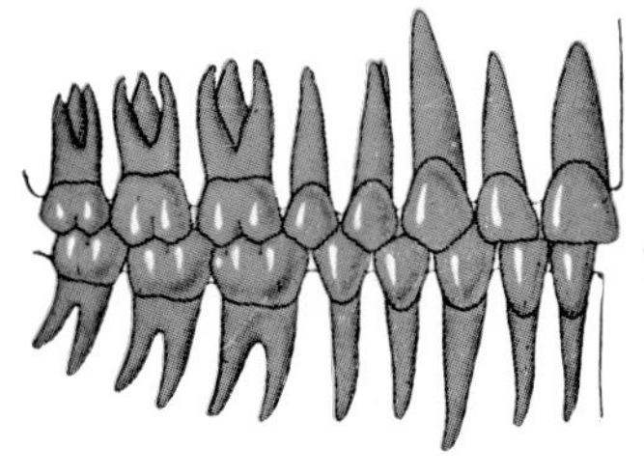

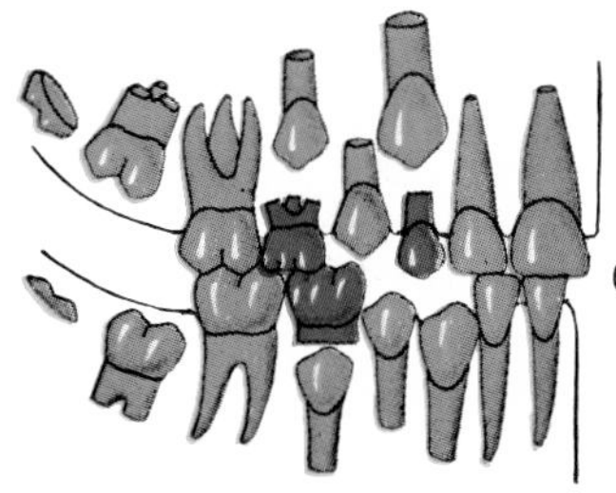

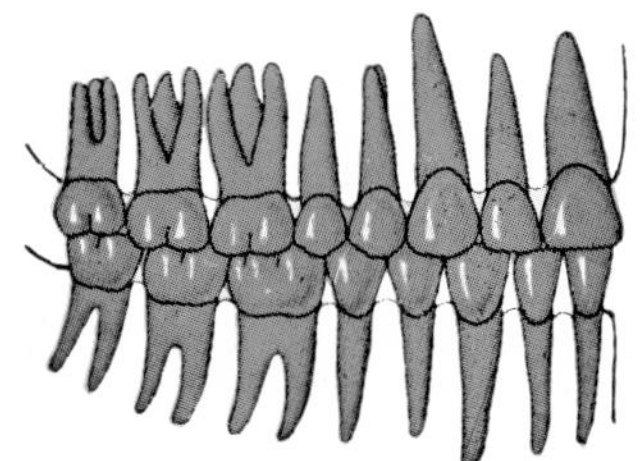

LATE CHILDHOOD
(SCHOOL AGE)

ADOLESCENCE
and ADULTHOOD

DEVELOPMENT OF HUMAN DENTITION

(Courtesy, Schour and Massler, American Dental Association.)

PLATE 23

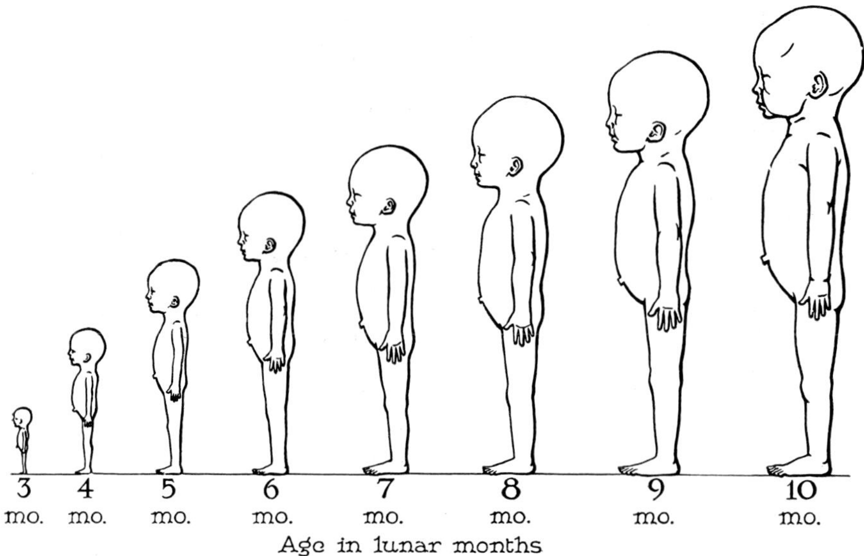

Prenatal growth. Eight fetal stages (based on the empirical formula of Calkins and Scammon: Proc. Soc. Exper. Biol. and Med., vol. 22, 1925).

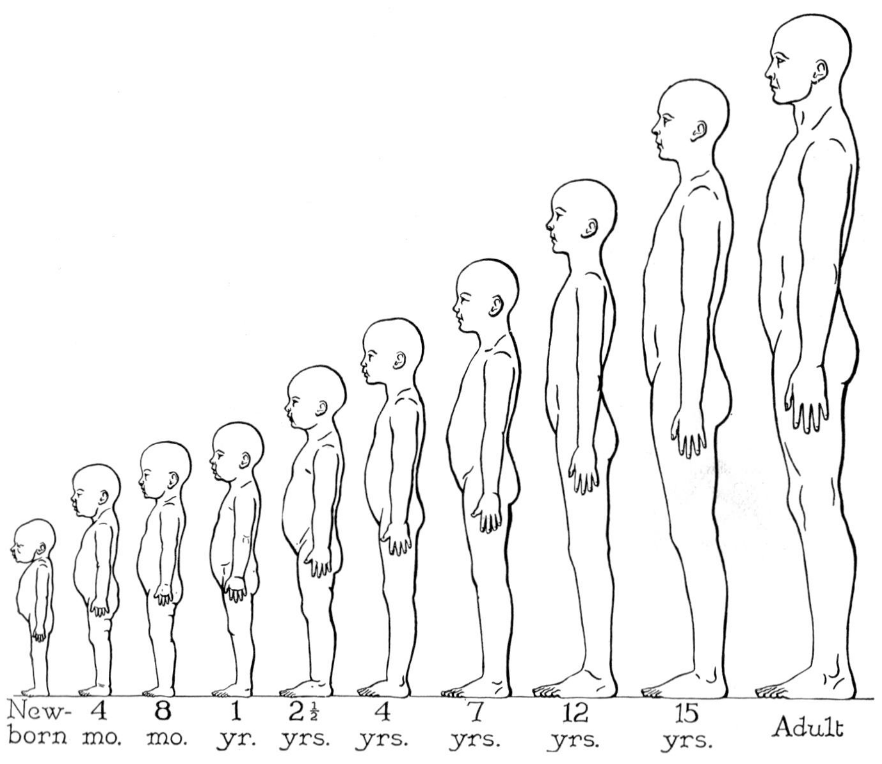

Postnatal growth. Ten postnatal stages.

GROWTH AND DEVELOPMENT OF FORM OF THE BODY (LEFT LATERAL VIEWS)

PLATE 24

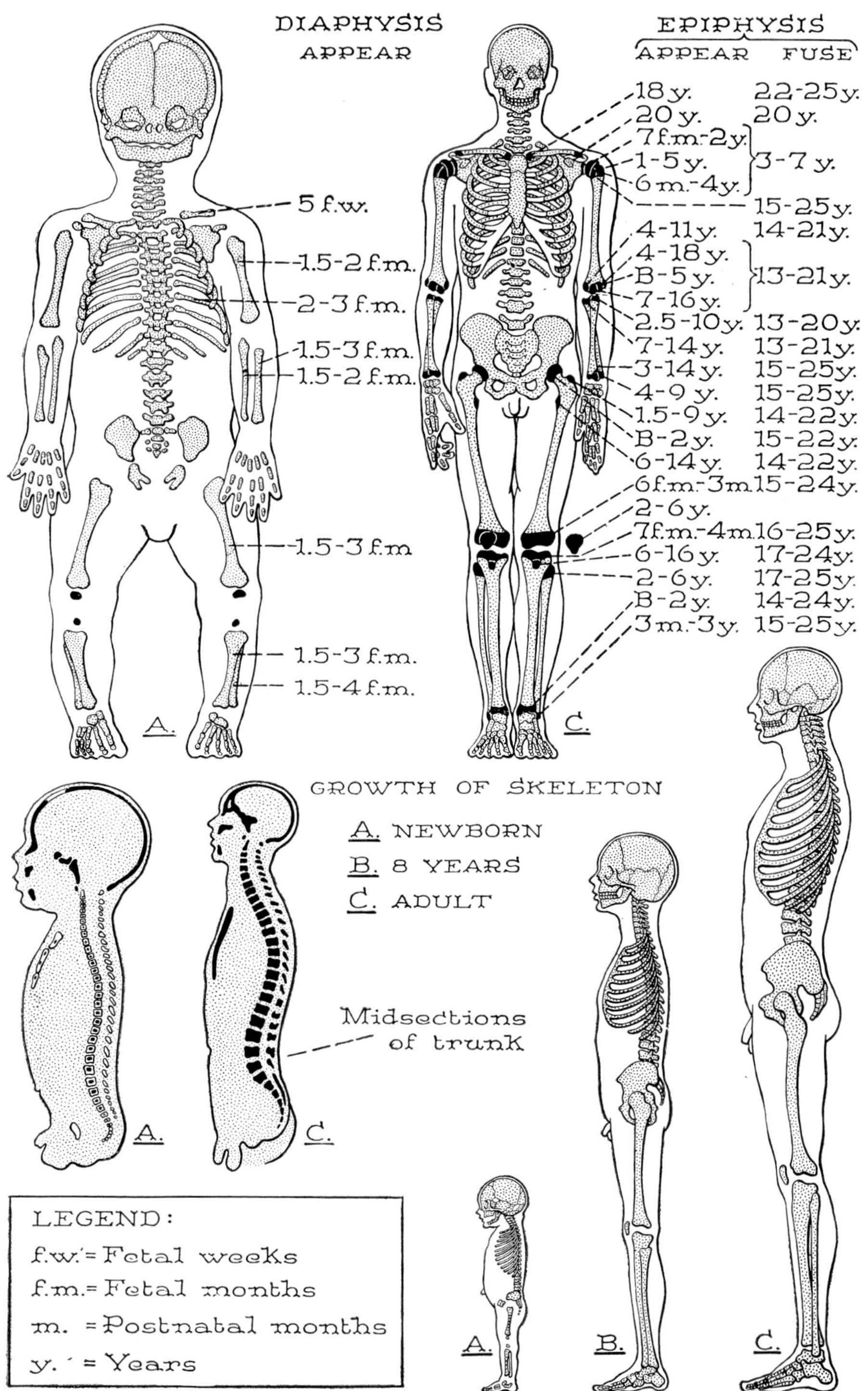

SKELETAL DEVELOPMENT

(From Morris: "Human Anatomy." Copyright, The Blakiston Company.)

PLATE 25

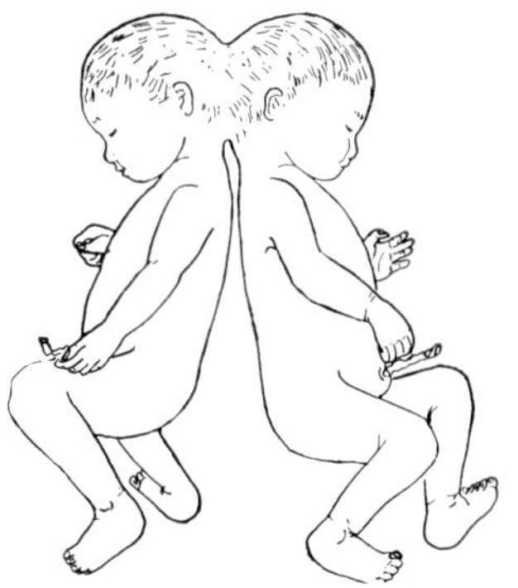
Craniopagus occipitalis

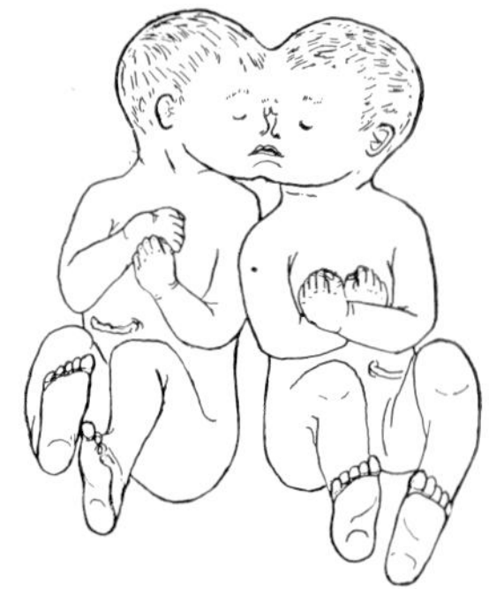
Craniopagus frontalis (Metopagus)

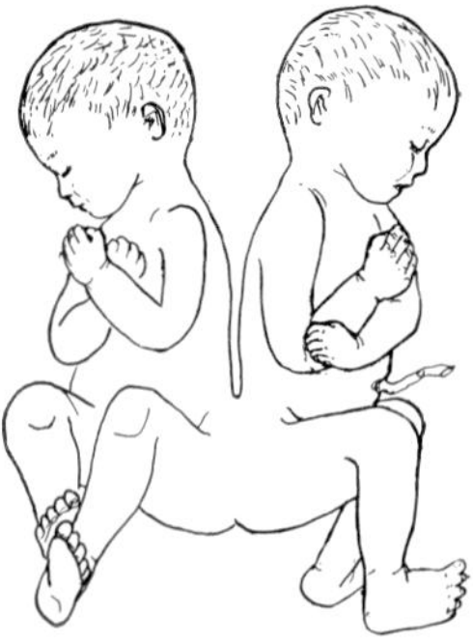
Pygopagus

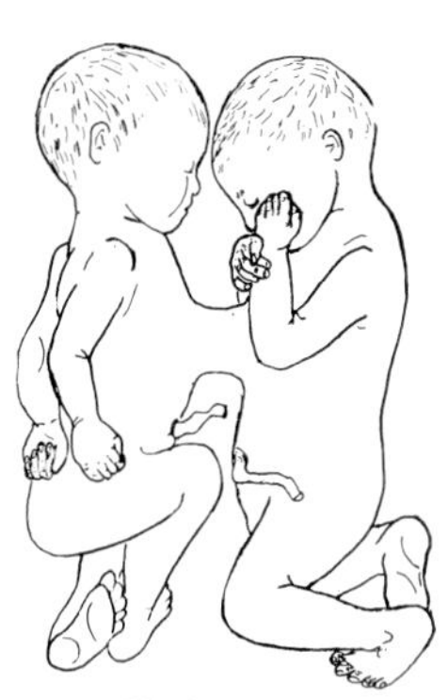
Xiphopagus

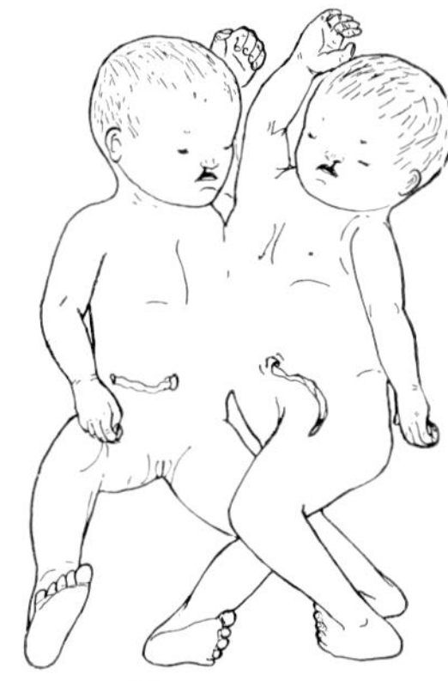
Thoracopagus

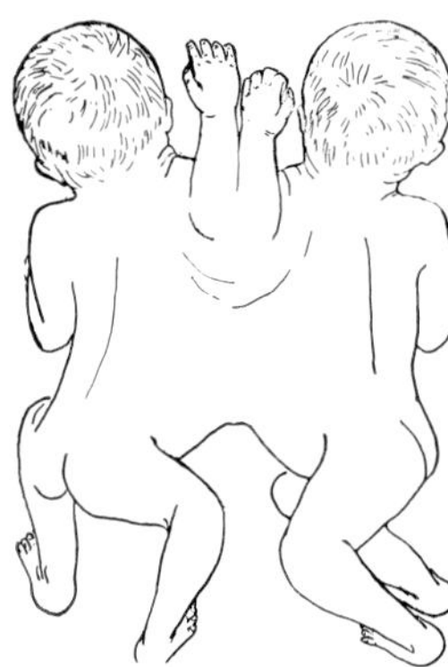
Thoracopagus

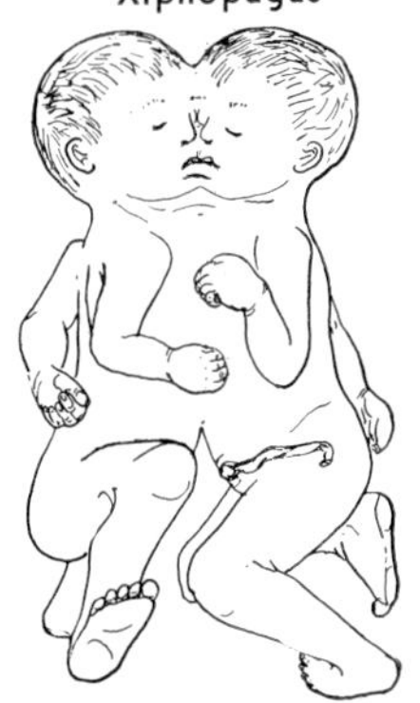
Prosopothoracopagus

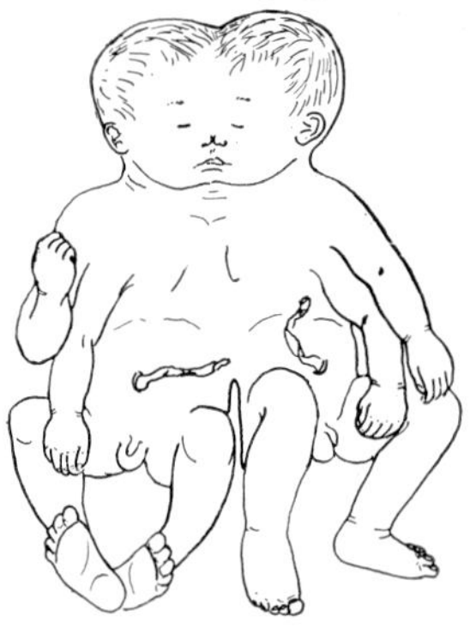
Cephalothoracopagus

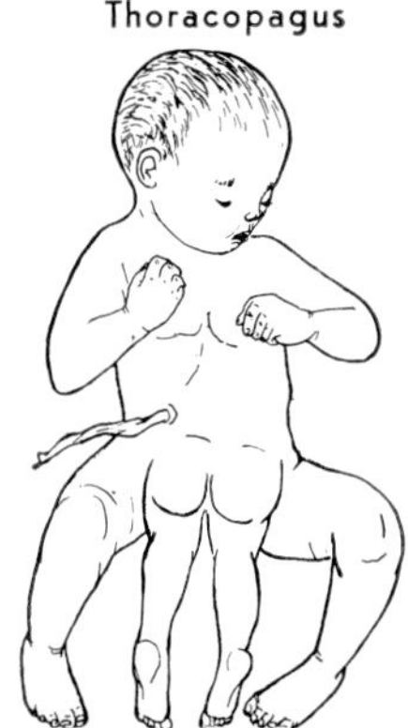
Dipygus parasiticus

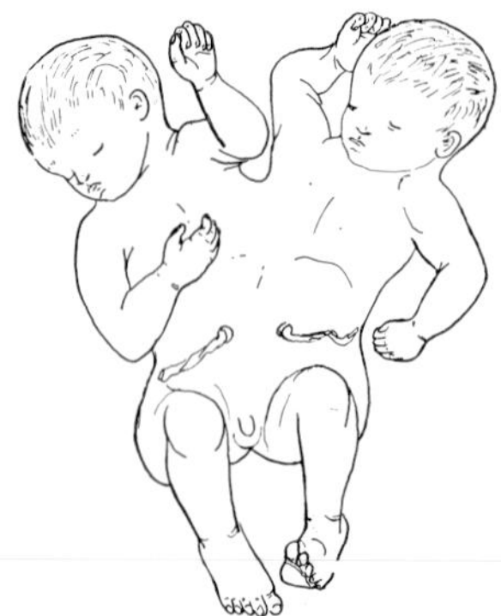
Dicephalus tetrabrachius

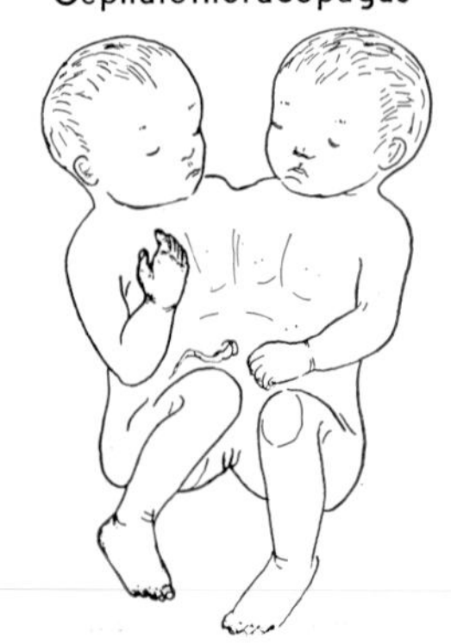
Dicephalus dibrachius

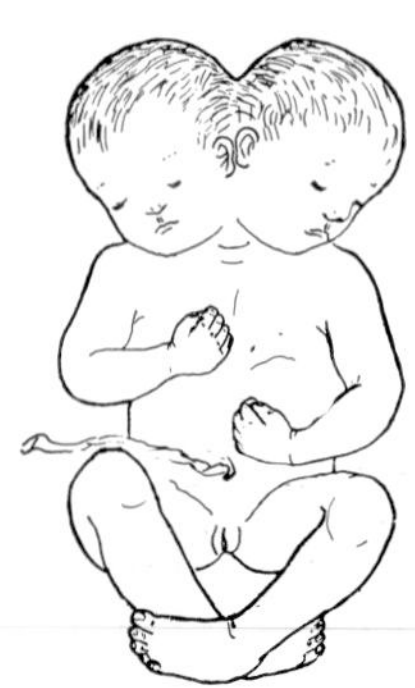
Diprosopus tetrotus

MONSTERS

PLATE 26

CELLS FROM SMEAR PREPARATION OF NORMAL HUMAN BLOOD, WRIGHT'S STAIN

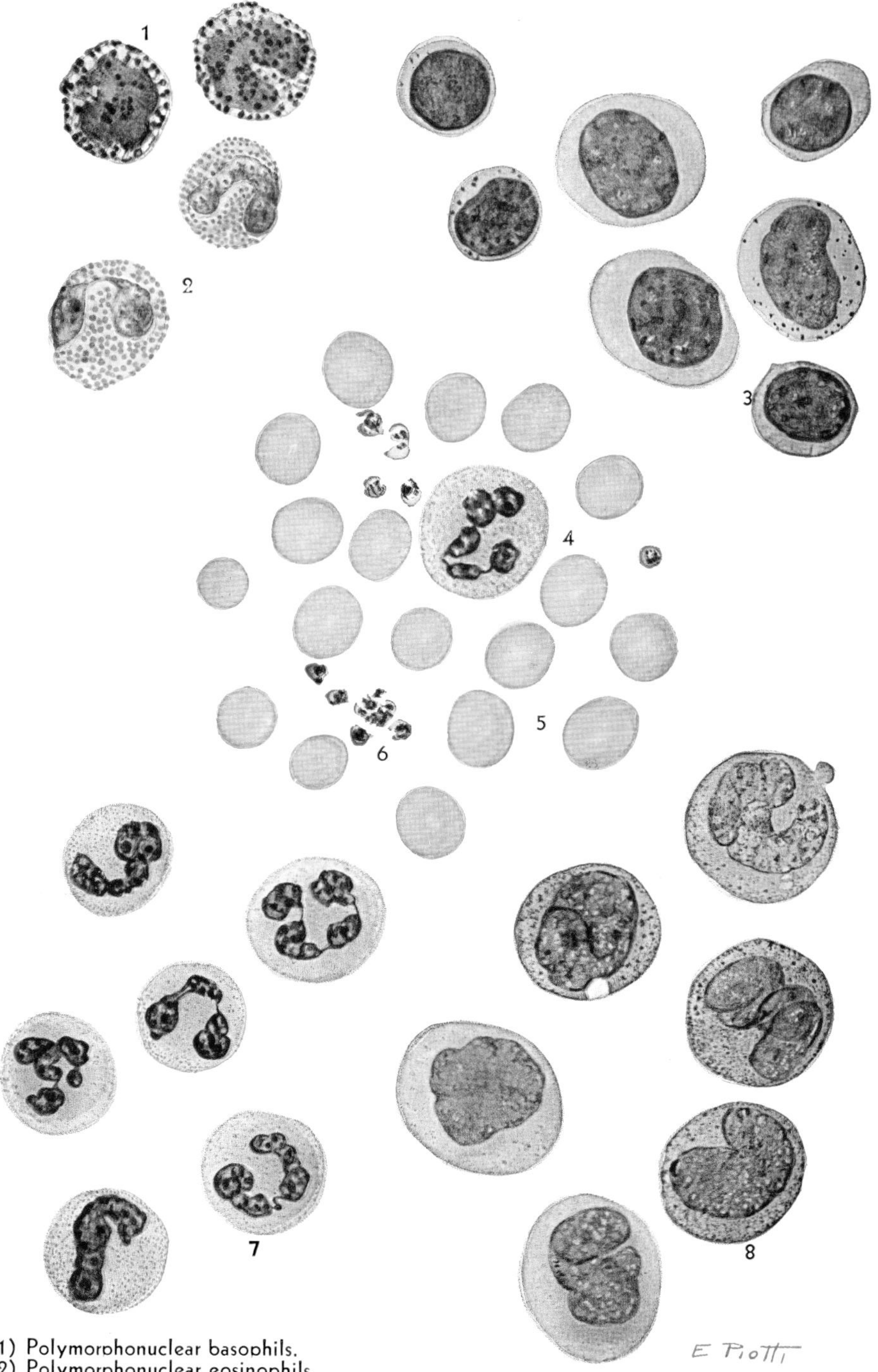

(1) Polymorphonuclear basophils.
(2) Polymorphonuclear eosinophils.
(3) Lymphocytes, some containing granules in the cytoplasm.
(4) Polymorphonuclear neutrophil.
(5) Erythrocytes.
(6) Blood platelets.
(7) Polymorphonuclear neutrophils.
(8) Monocytes; some containing more protoplasmic granules than others. (In the younger cells the nuclei tend to be rounded; in the adult cells they are horseshoe-shaped, indented, or lobed.)

NORMAL BLOOD CELLS

Plate 27. Malaria Parasites

A. Thick Films

A1. *Plasmodium vivax.* Characteristic for the species in thick films is the presence of the parasite in various stages of development together with the distinctive ameboid form. The heavily pigmented parasite in the right portion of the field is a gametocyte. The large purplish objects are leukocytes showing the usual distortion seen in thick films.

A2. *Plasmodium malariae.* Various developmental stages are present as in *P. vivax* but the parasites are smaller, more compact, lack the ameboid shape, and are heavily pigmented.

A3. *Plasmodium falciparum.* Only ring forms of the trophozoites are seen. These, together with the characteristically shaped gametocytes (crescents), make identification possible.

B. Internal Organs

B. "Cerebral" malaria. Smears taken post mortem from a fatal case of malignant tertian malaria. (From a case of Lt. J. J. Sapero, Medical Corps, U. S. Navy.)

B1. Smear from spleen. Almost one-third of the red cells are parasitized with *P. falciparum.* Note the mature schizont in the upper portion of the field and three monocytes containing pigment.

B2. Smear from brain. A capillary of the brain distended and "blocked" with red cells scarcely one of which has escaped being parasitized. A mature schizont is in the upper left part of the field.

B3. Smear from bone marrow. The parasites, though less numerous than in the smears from other organs, are present in considerable numbers. In the upper part of the field is a melaniferous leukocyte.

PLATE 27

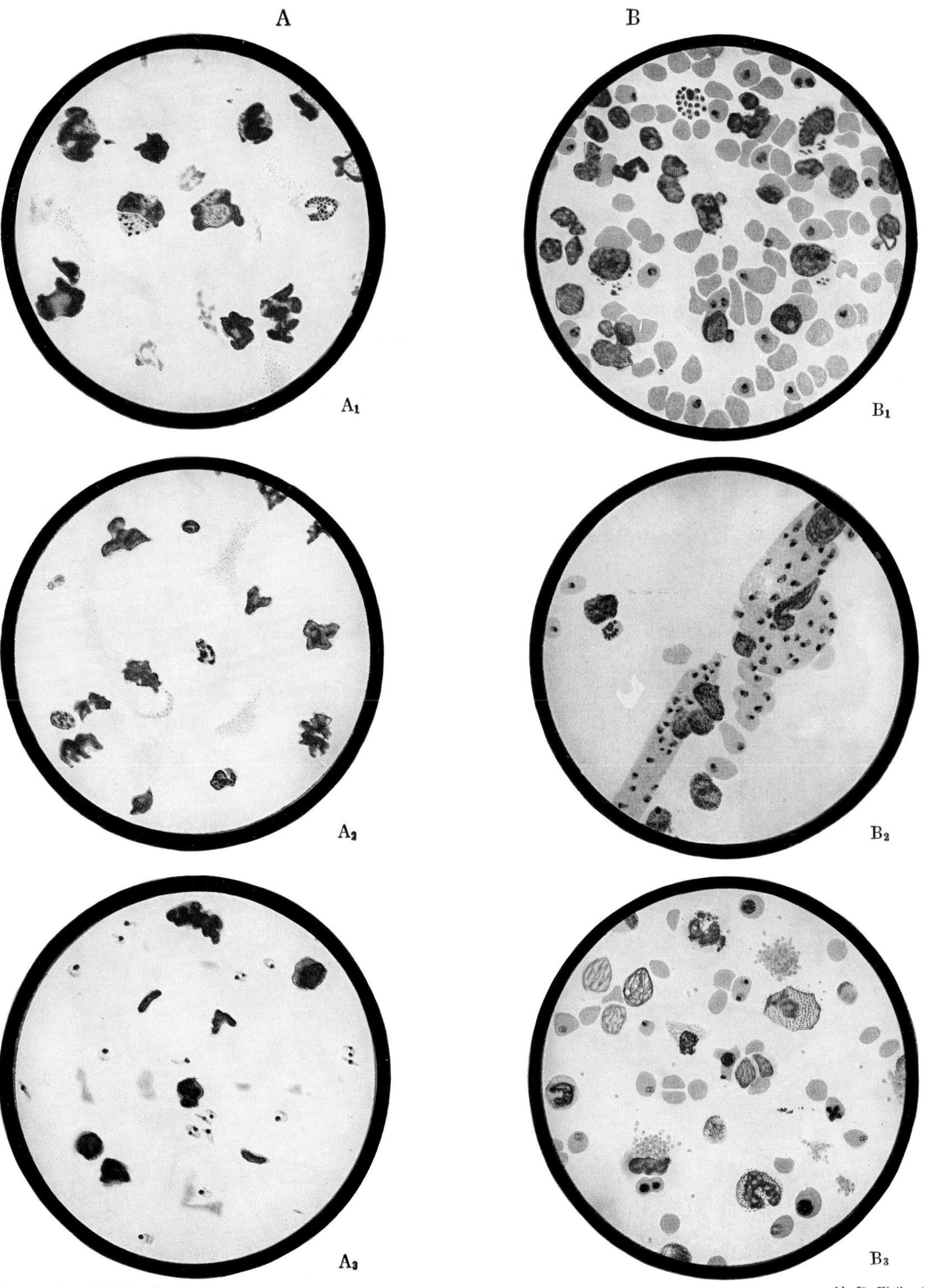

(U.S. Naval Medical School) (A. D. Wallace)

MALARIA PARASITES

(From Strong: "Stitt's Diagnosis, Prevention and Treatment of Tropical Diseases." Copyright, The Blakiston Company.)

Plate 28. Malaria Parasites

Benign Tertian Parasites

1. Normal red cell for comparison of size.
2. Trophozoite, young ring form.
3. Trophozoite, full grown. Red cell is enlarged and Schüffner's dots are present.
4. Schizont, young form, undergoing second nuclear division.
5. Schizont, quarter grown. Nuclei composed of fine chromatin granules in irregular clumps. Yellowish brown pigment is present.
6. Schizont, mature form. Nuclear division complete. Cytoplasm dividing preparatory to liberation of merozoites.
7. Macrogametocyte (female gametocyte). Cytoplasm is blue, chromatin eccentric, compact, deep red, and surrounded by a halo.
8. Microgametocyte (male gametocyte). Cytoplasm is greenish blue, chromatin central, diffuse, and light red.

Quartan Parasites

1. Trophozoite, young ring form. Fine black pigment granules are present.
2. Trophozoite, young band or equatorial form.
3. Trophozoite, a more mature oval form, showing beginning nuclear division.
4. Schizont, young, binucleate form, heavily pigmented.
5. Schizont, older band form. Pigment is more abundant about periphery.
6. Schizont, mature. Chromatin clumps form eight nuclear masses arranged around a central mass of pigment.
7. Macrogametocyte (female gametocyte). Chromatin is compact and deep red. Pigment abundant.
8. Microgametocyte (male gametocyte). Chromatin is diffuse and pale. Pigment abundant.

Malignant Tertian Parasites

1. Trophozoite, young, hairlike ring form.
2. Trophozoites, young ring forms. Characteristic multiple infection of a red cell showing also peripherally placed forms.
3. Trophozoite, full grown. Rarely seen in peripheral blood except in very heavy infections.

4, 5, 6. Schizonts in successive stages of maturity. Rarely seen in peripheral blood. Specimens from red cells in a brain capillary of a fatal case of cerebral malaria.

7. Macrogametocyte (female gametocyte). Shows characteristic crescent shape. Nucleus is compact, deeply stained. Pigment is clumped in center.
8. Microgametocyte (male gametocyte). Chromatin is pale staining and diffuse. Pigment is dispersed.

PLATE 28

BENIGN TERTIAN PARASITES (*Plasmodium vivax*)

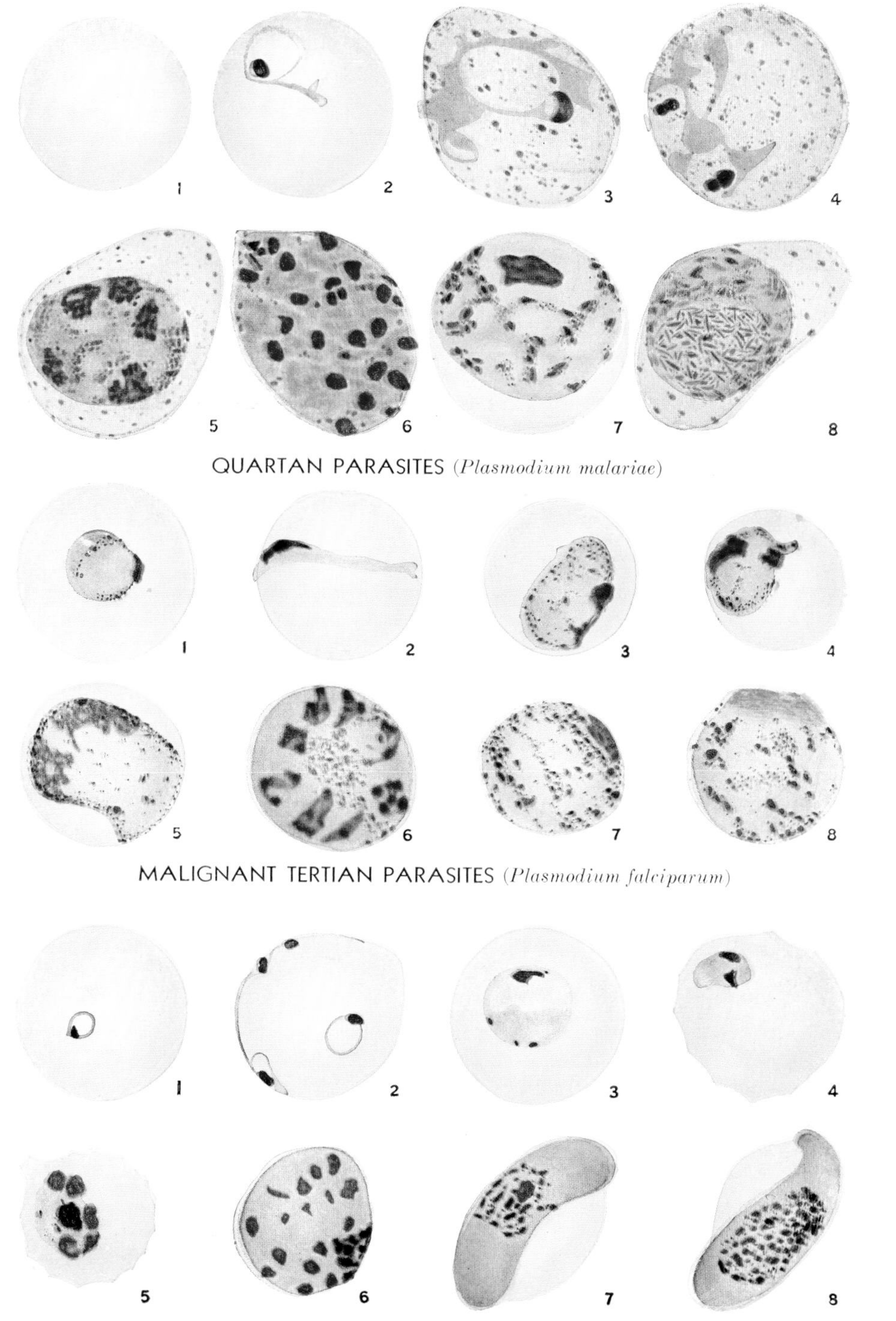

(U.S. Naval Medical School) (A. D. Wallace)

MALARIA PARASITES

PLATE 29

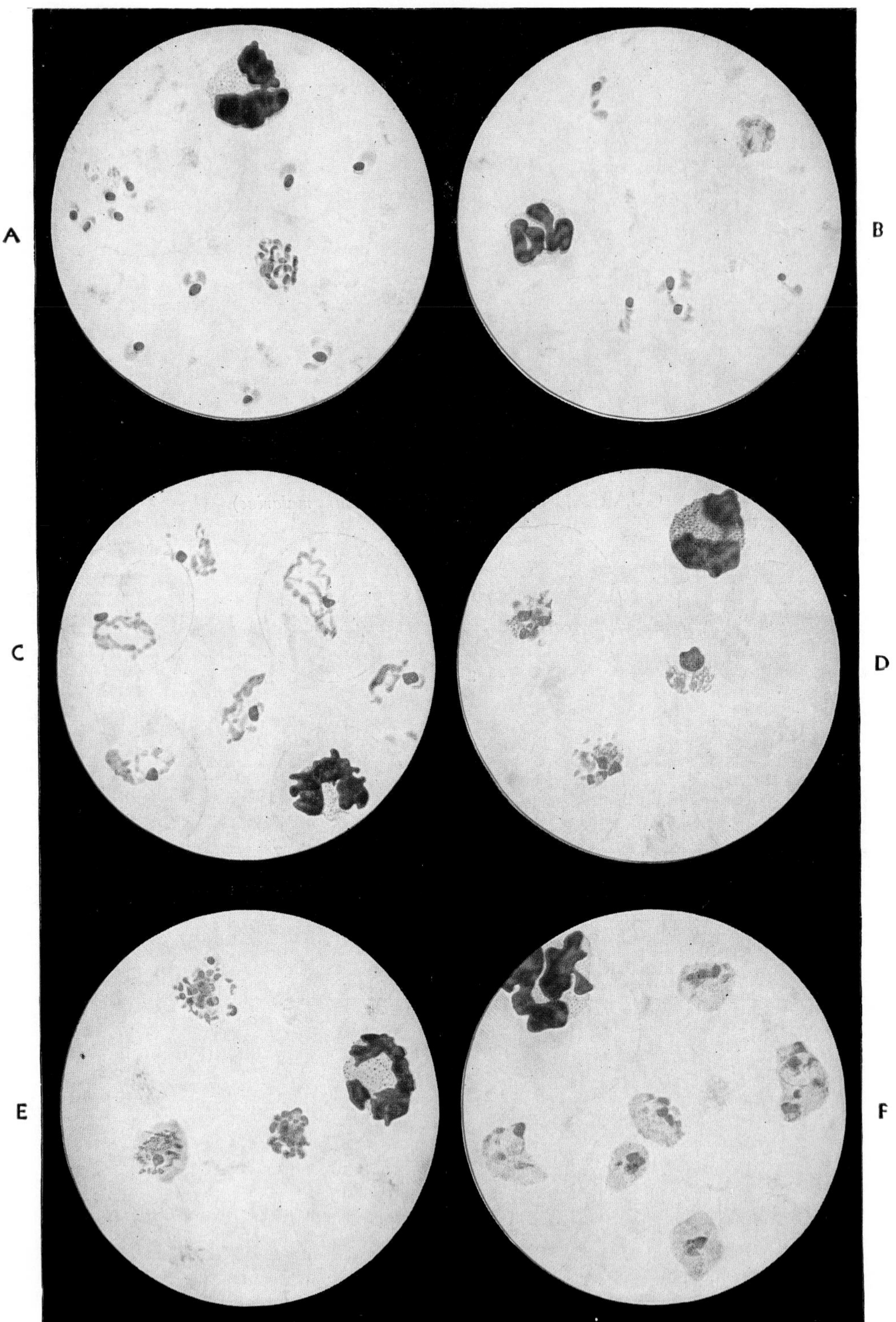

PLASMODIUM VIVAX IN THICK SMEARS, GIEMSA'S STAIN, USING BUFFER OF pH 6.8

MALARIA PARASITES

(From Stitt, Clough, and Branham: "Practical Bacteriology, Hematology, and Parasitology." Copyright, The Blakiston Company.)

PLATE 30

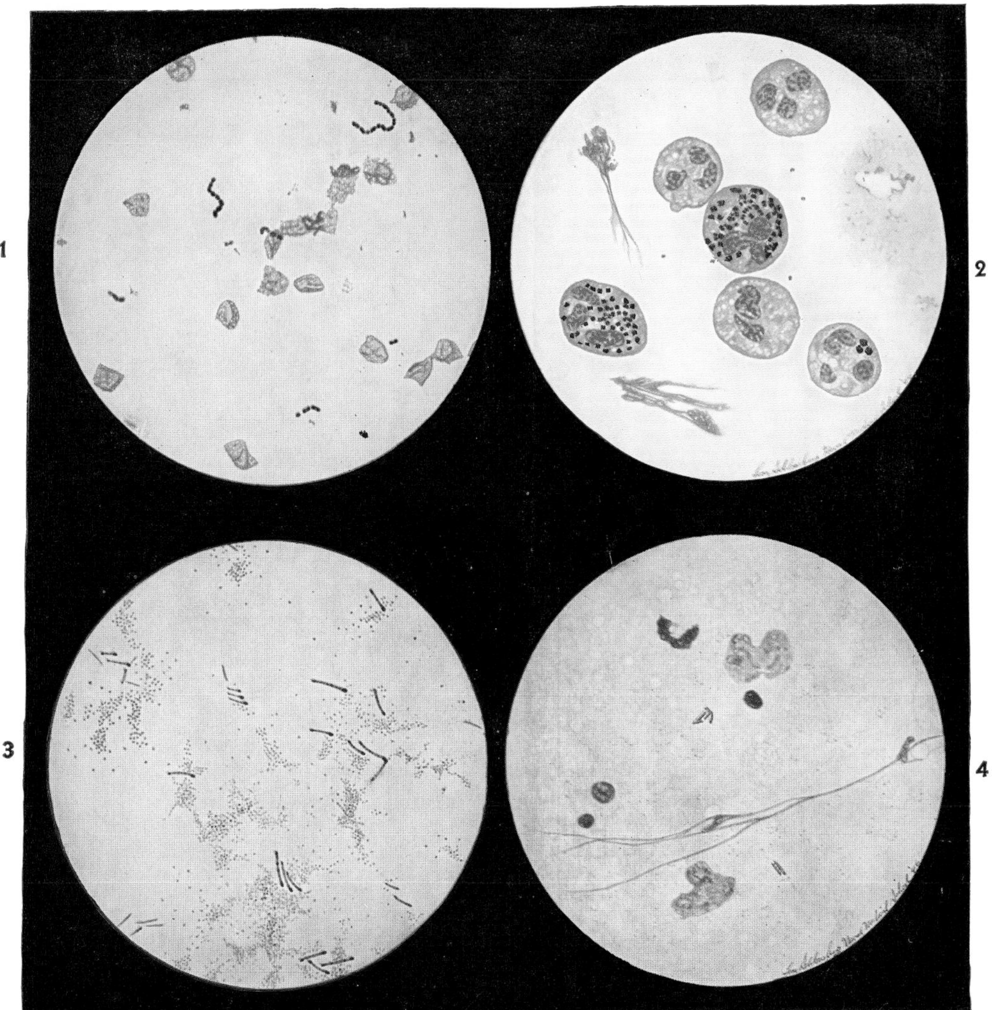

(1) Streptococcus pyogenes (Gram's stain).
(2) Neisseria gonorrhoeae (Gram's stain).
(3) Corynebacterium diphtheriae (Neisser's stain).
(4) Mycobacterium tuberculosis (Ziehl-Neelsen's stain).

BACTERIA

(From Stitt, Clough, and Branham: "Practical Bacteriology, Hematology, and Parasitology." Copyright, The Blakiston Company.)

CAPTION FOR PLATE 29

(A) Height of paroxysm: mature schizont with 14 merozoites; ruptured schizont; young trophozoites; segmented neutrophil.

(B) 6–8 hrs. after paroxysm: young trophozoites with diagnostic ameboid cytoplasm; gametocyte (female); segmented neutrophil.

(C) 20–30 hrs. after paroxysm: characteristic ameboid trophozoites; segmented neutrophil.

(D) 40 hrs. after paroxysm: two young schizonts; gametocyte (male); eosinophil.

(E) Before paroxysm: two nearly mature schizonts; gametocyte (female); segmented neutrophil.

(F) 30 hrs. after paroxysm: characteristic absence of lysis in parasitized cells; segmented neutrophil.

PLATE 31

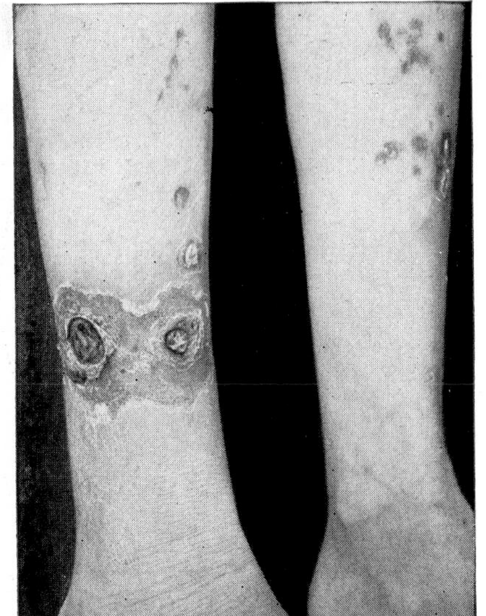

Ecthyma.

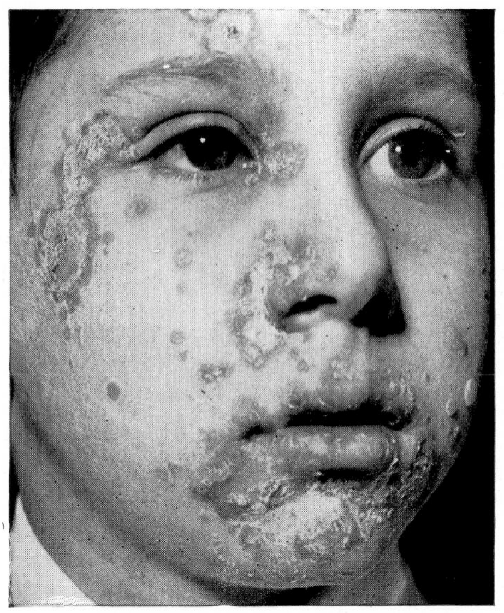

Impetigo contagiosa.

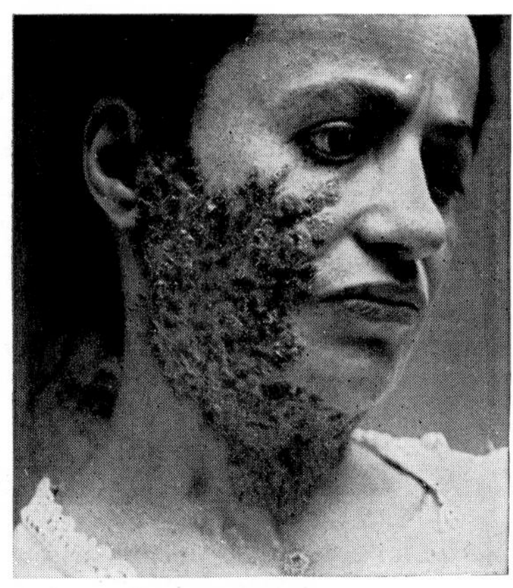

Lupus vulgaris.

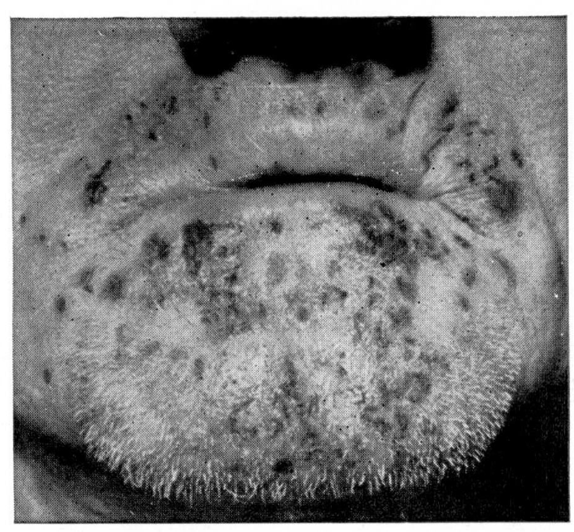

Sycosis coccygenica.

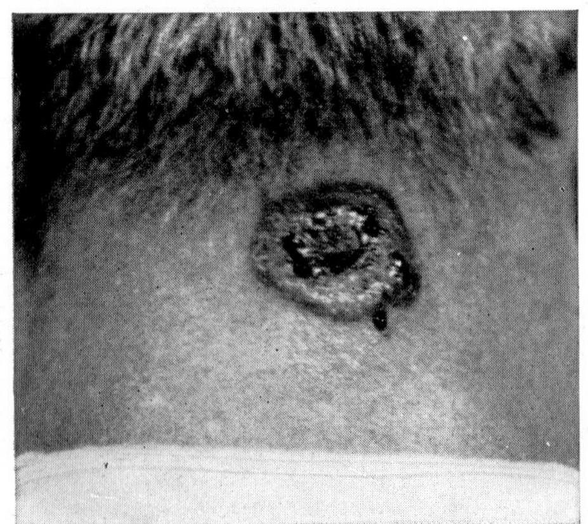

Anthrax pustule (Pennsylvania Hospital).

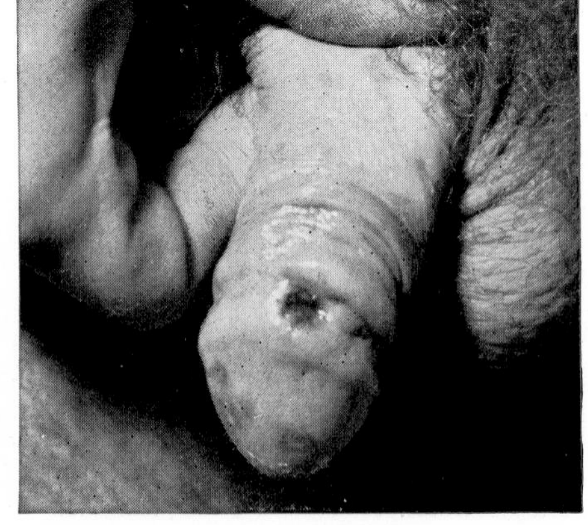

Syphilis (primary).

SKIN LESIONS

PLATE 32

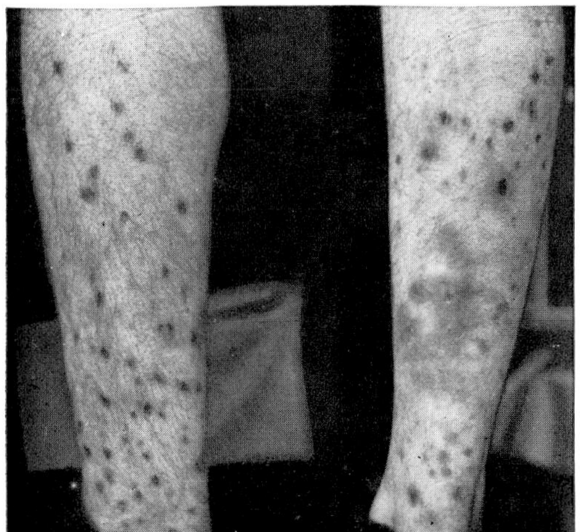
Erythema induratum.

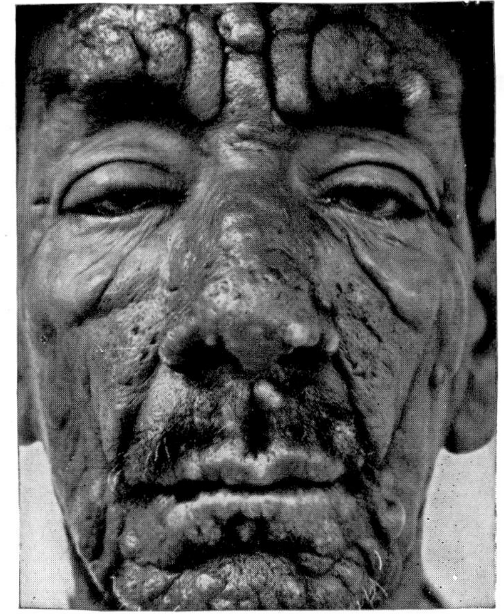
Leprosy.

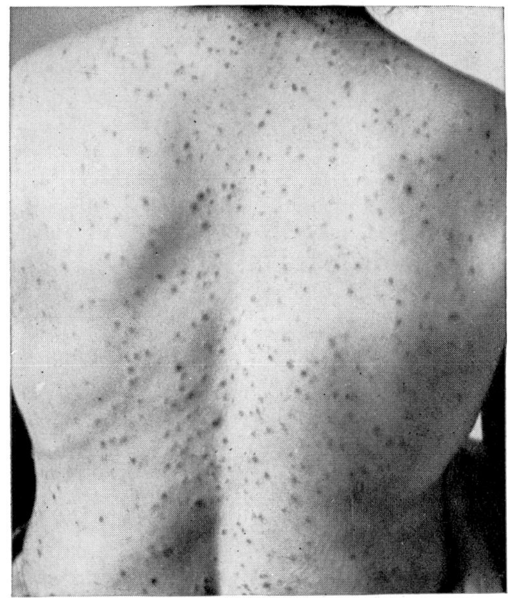
Syphilis (secondary).

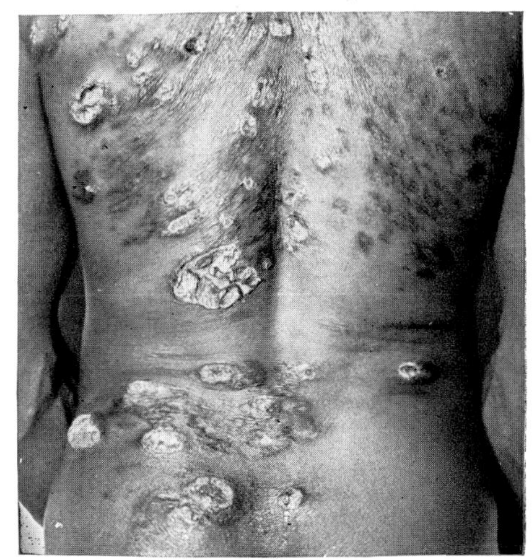
Syphilis (tertiary).

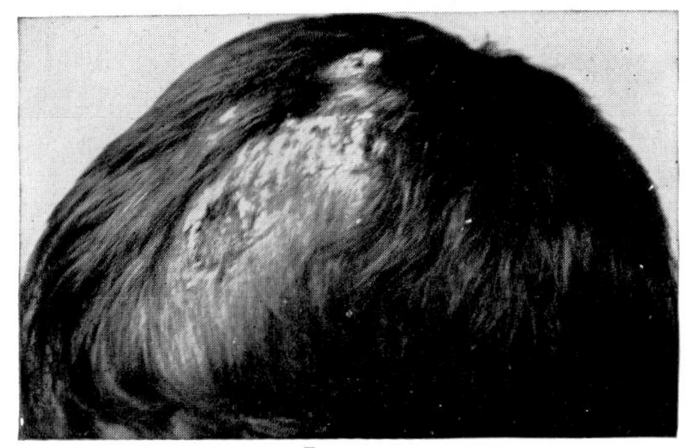
Favus.

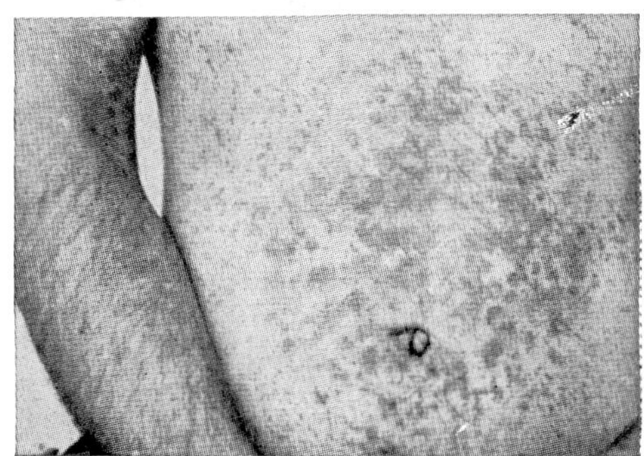
Tinea versicolor.

SKIN LESIONS

PLATE 33

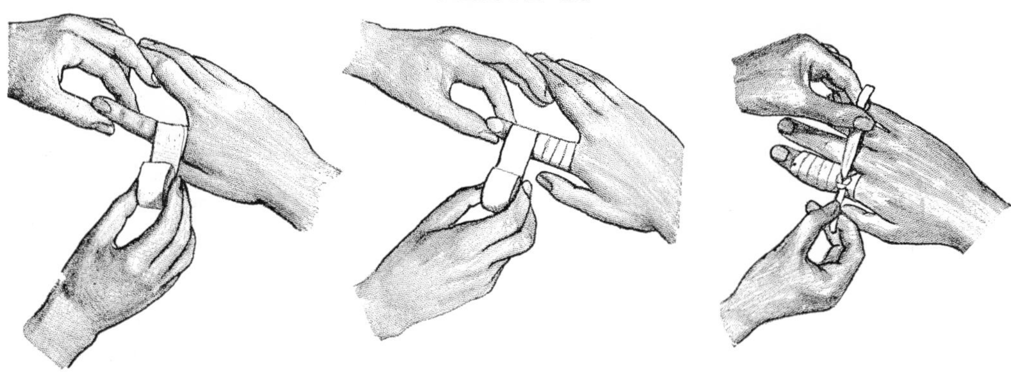

Spiral bandage for finger (or toe).

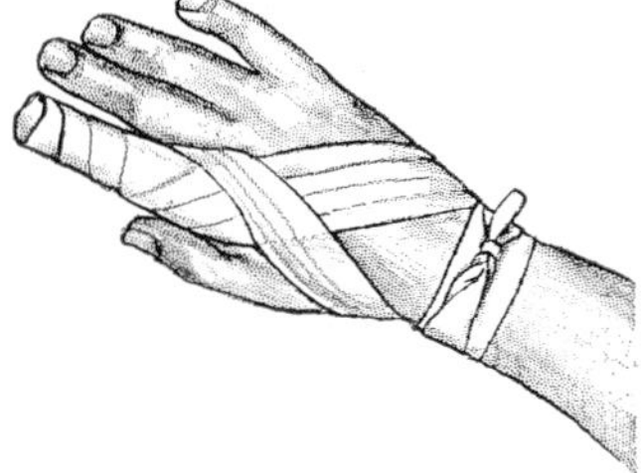

Spiral bandage to cover end of finger.

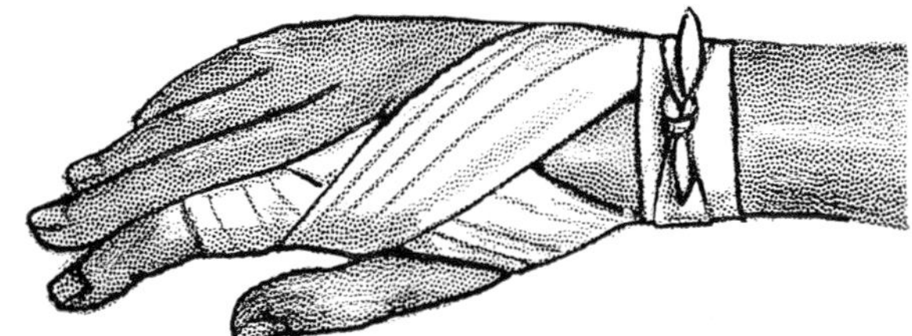

Spiral bandage for base of finger.

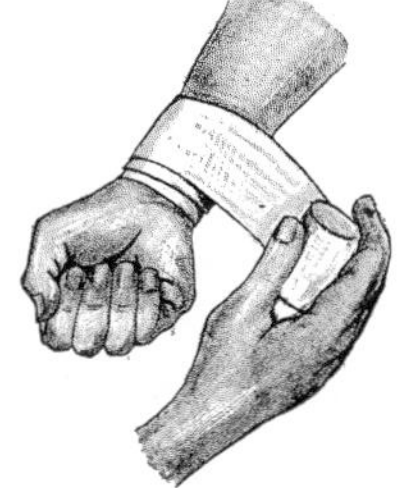

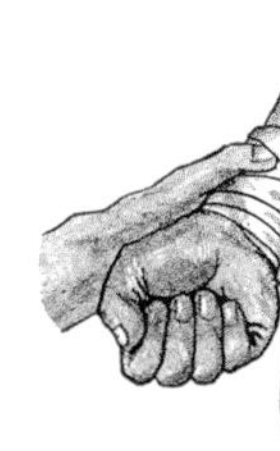

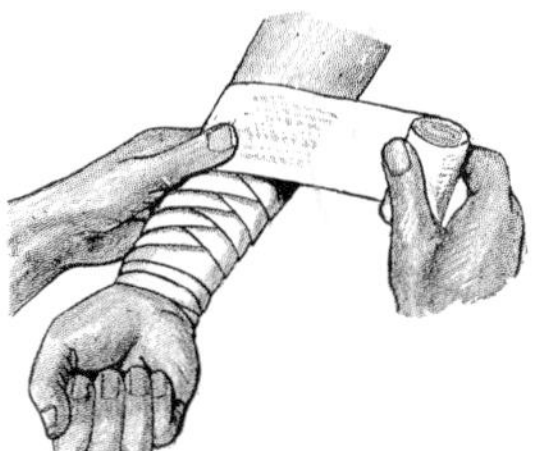

Spiral reverse bandage for limbs.

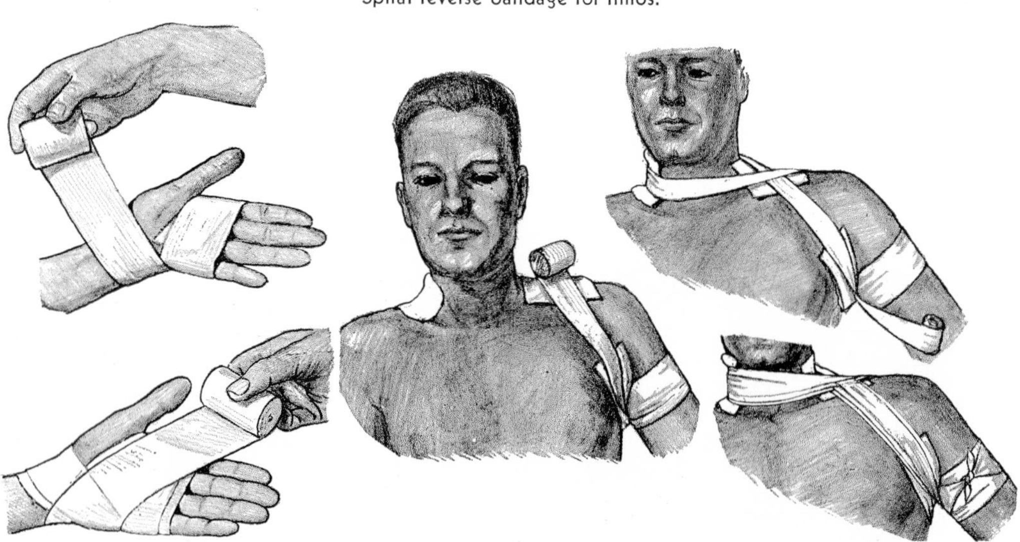

Figure-of-eight bandage of hand and wrist.

Figure-of-eight bandage of neck and axilla.

BANDAGES

PLATE 34

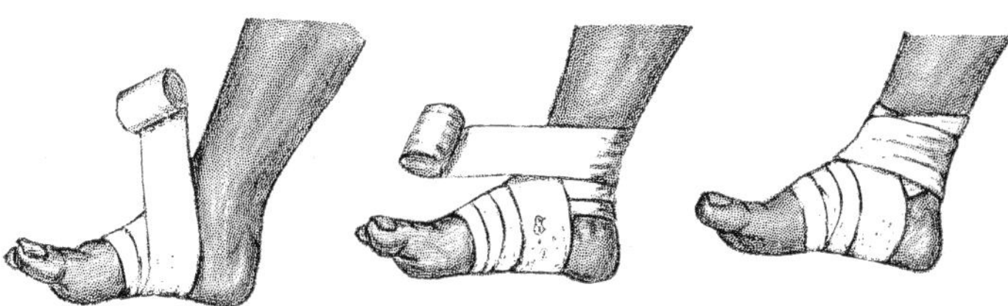

Figure-of-eight bandage of ankle.

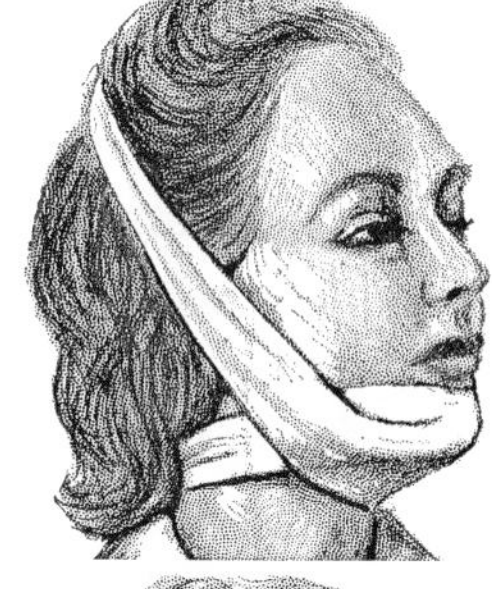

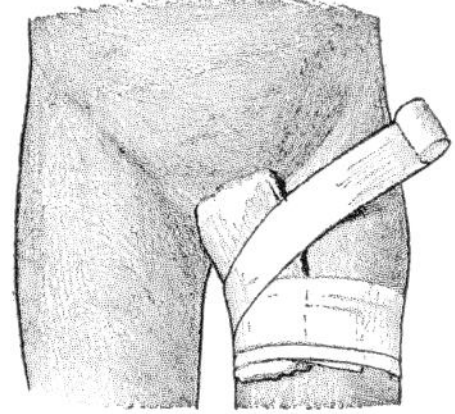

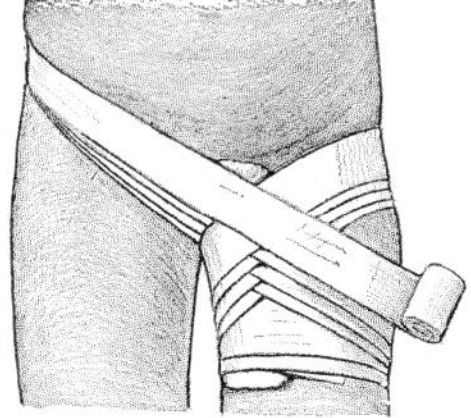

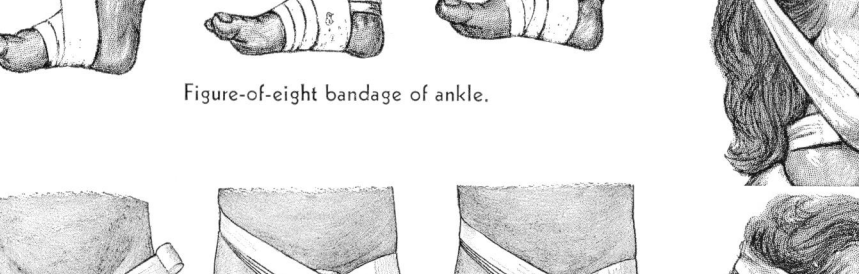

Spica bandage of groin.

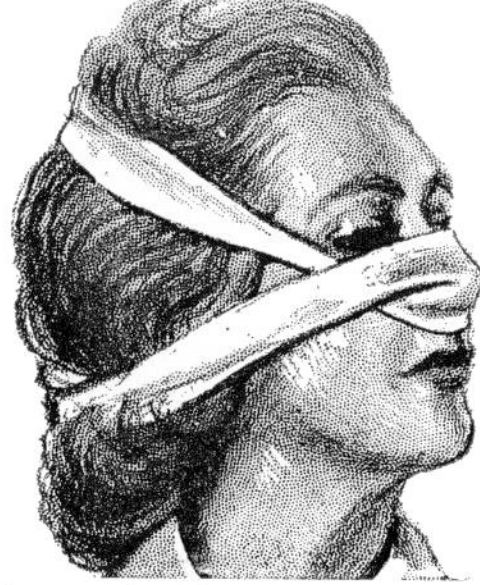

Four-tailed bandage (above) for chin, (below) for nose.

(From American Red Cross: "First Aid Textbook." Copyright, The American National Red Cross.)

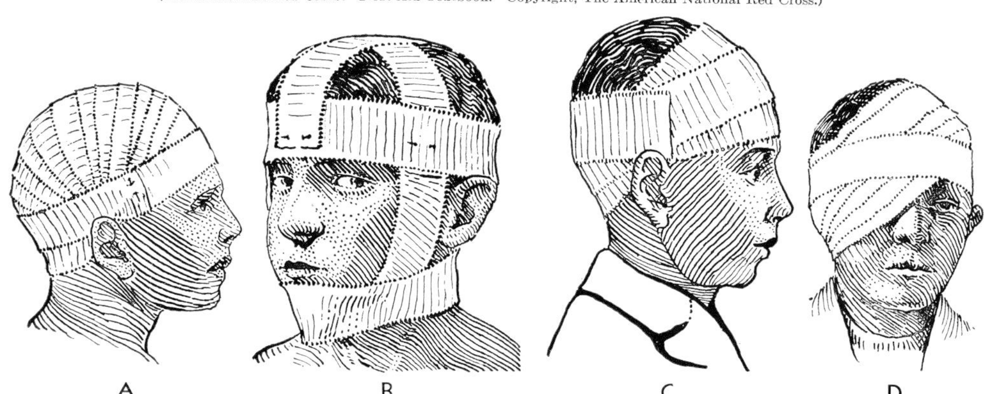

Bandages for head injuries: (A) Recurrent, for cranial injury, (B) Gibson's, (C) capeline, (D) recurrent, for eye injury.

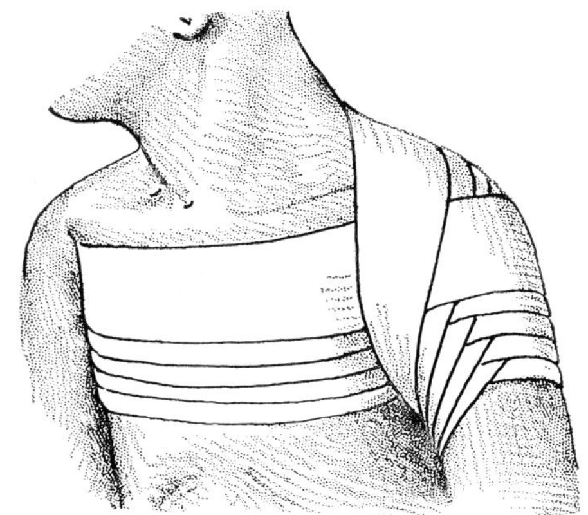

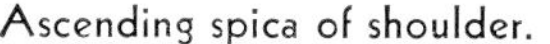

Ascending spica of shoulder.

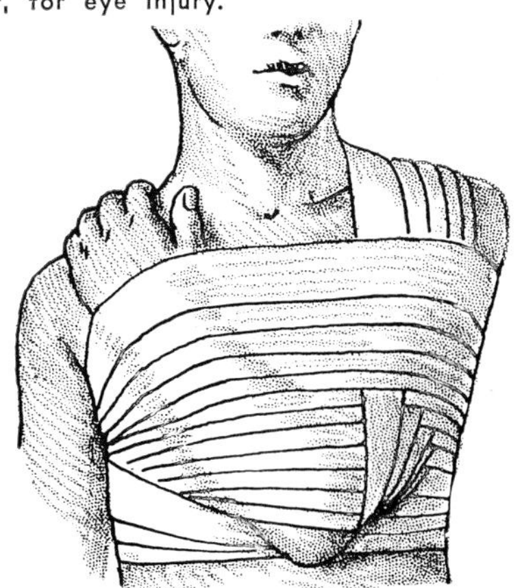

Velpeau's bandage for fractured clavicle.

(From Stewart-Lee: "Manual of Surgery." Copyright, The Blakiston Company.)

BANDAGES

PLATE 35

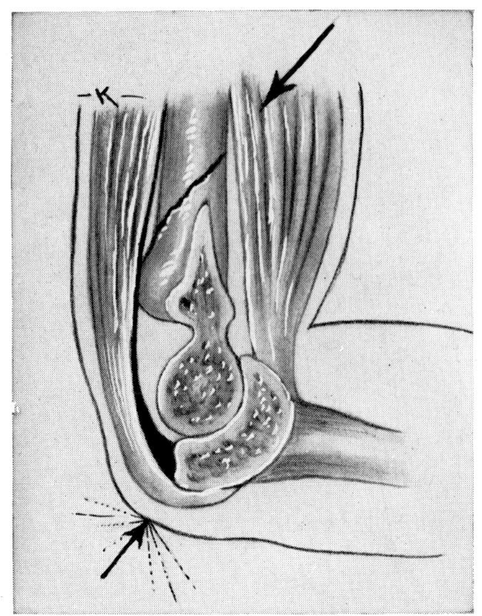

Forces.

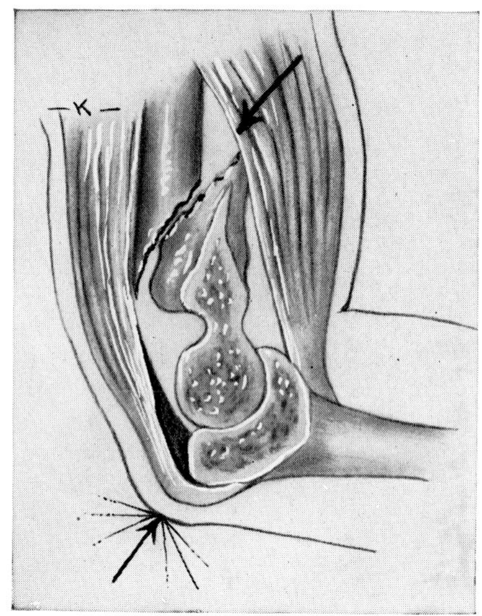

Resulting displacement.

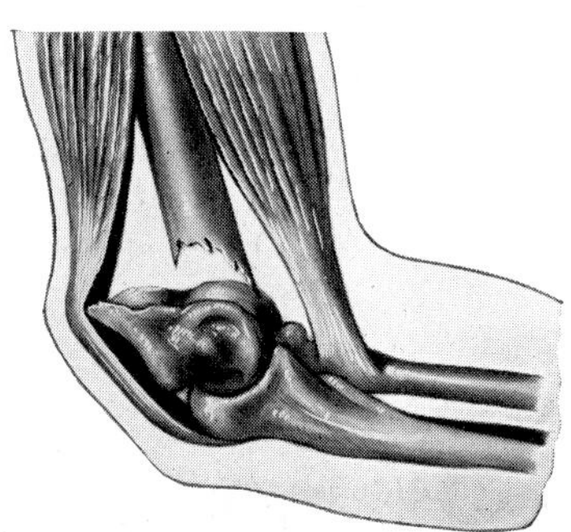

Supracondylar fracture of humerus with backward displacement of distal fragment.

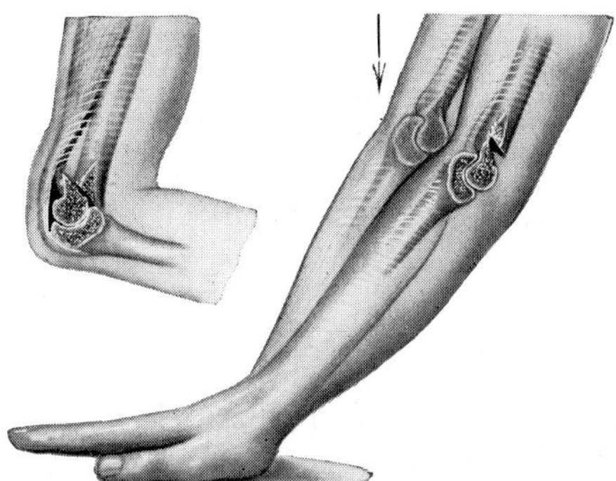

Forces resulting in this type of fracture.

PRODUCTION OF SUPRACONDYLAR FRACTURE OF HUMERUS

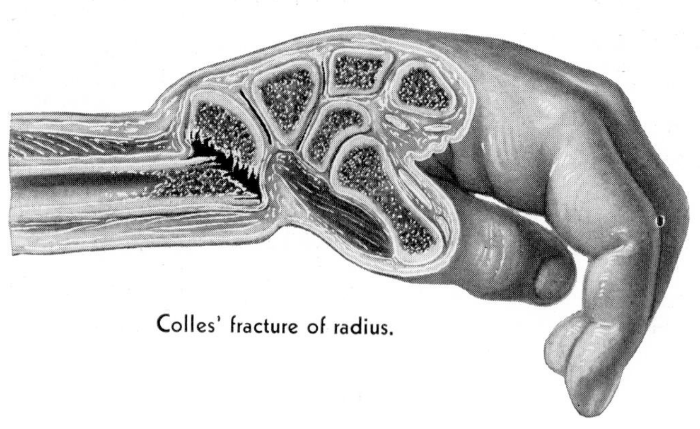

Colles' fracture of radius.

FRACTURES

PLATE 36

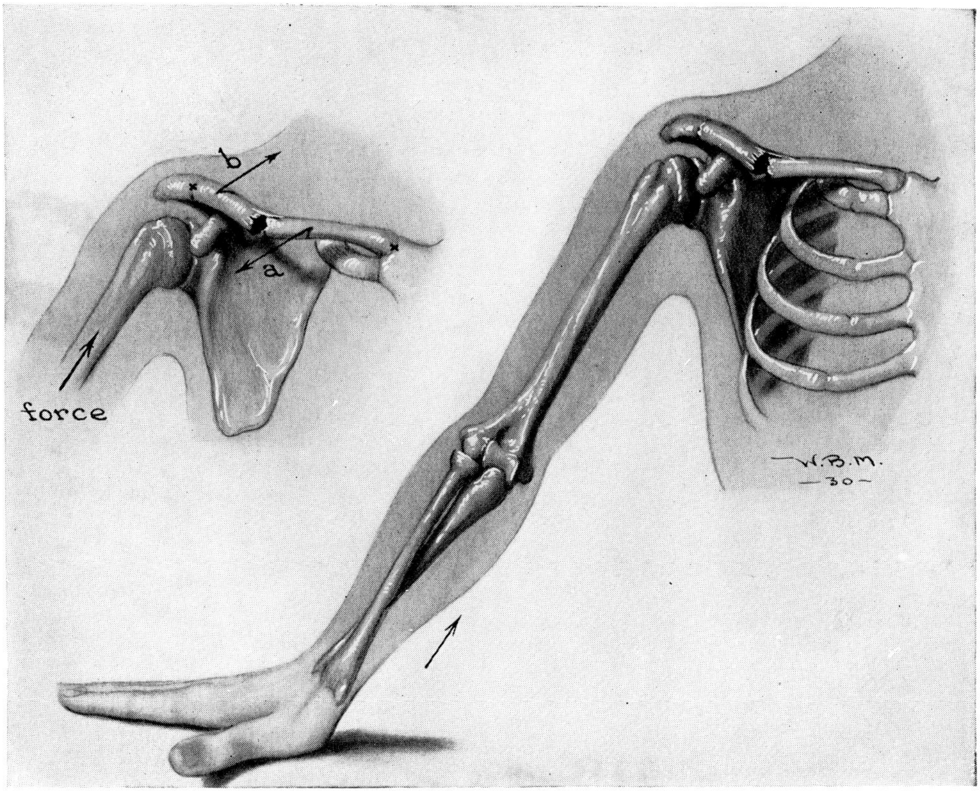

Mechanism producing fracture and upward displacement of clavicle.

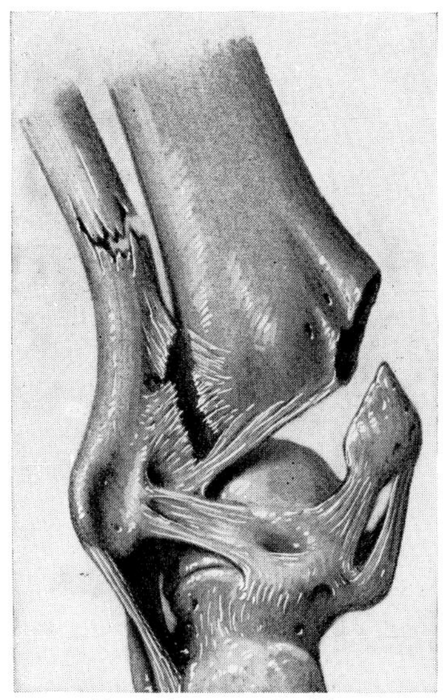

Pott's fracture of ankle.

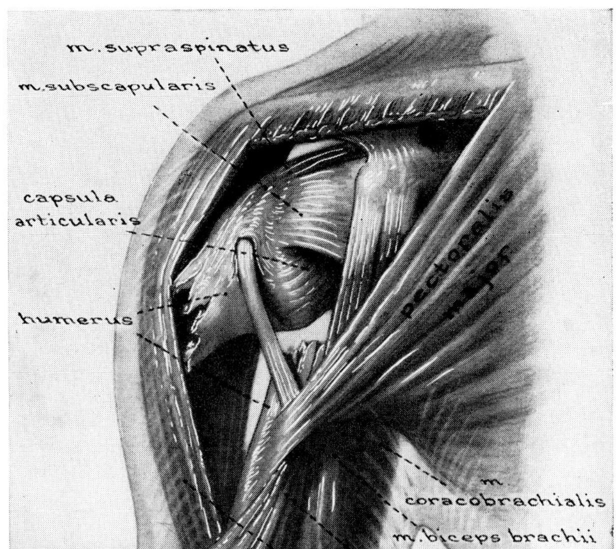

Fracture of surgical neck of humerus.

FRACTURES

PLATE 37

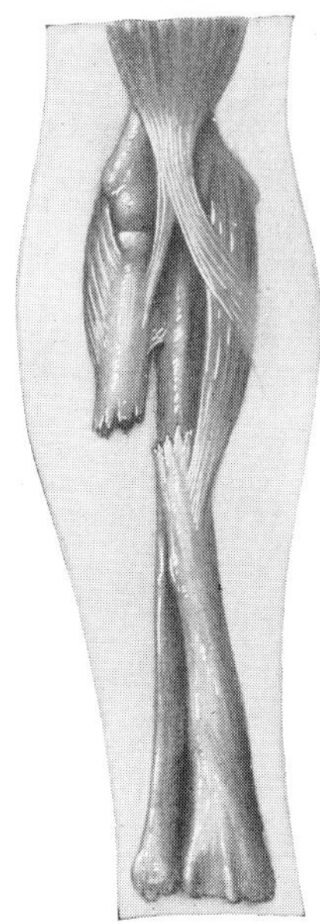

Displacement of fractured radius by contraction of pronator teres.

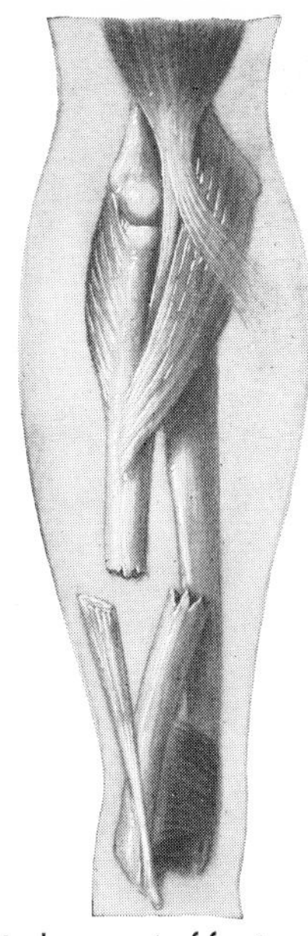

Displacement of fractured radius by contraction of pronator quadratus.

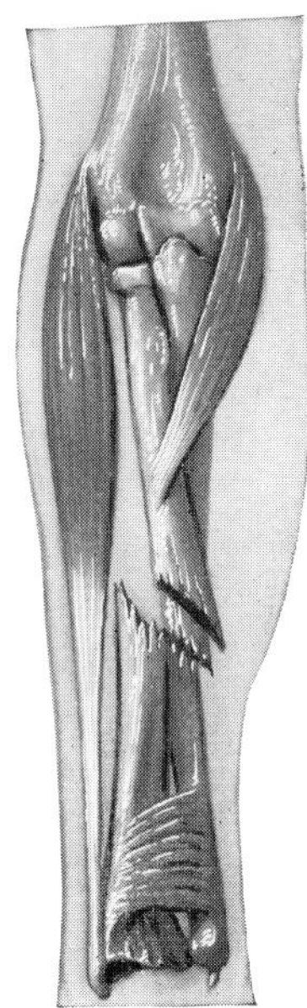

Fracture of both bones of forearm.

FRACTURES

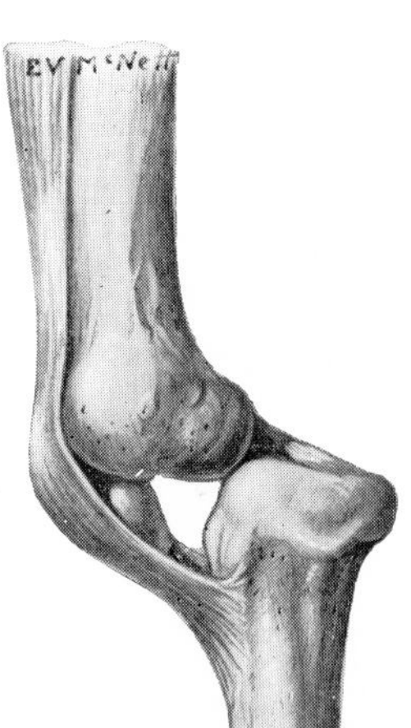

Posterior dislocation of leg.

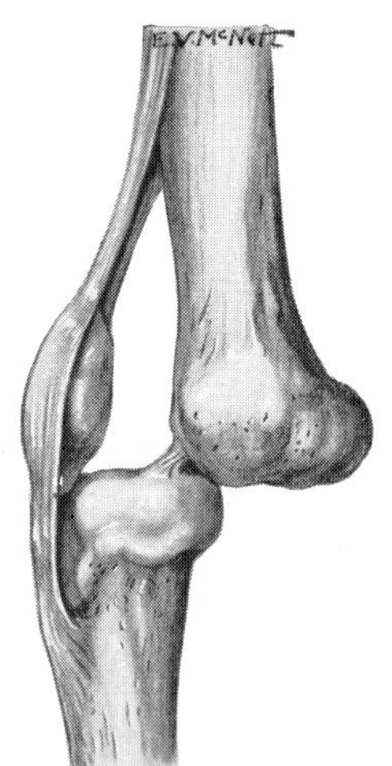

Anterior dislocation of leg.

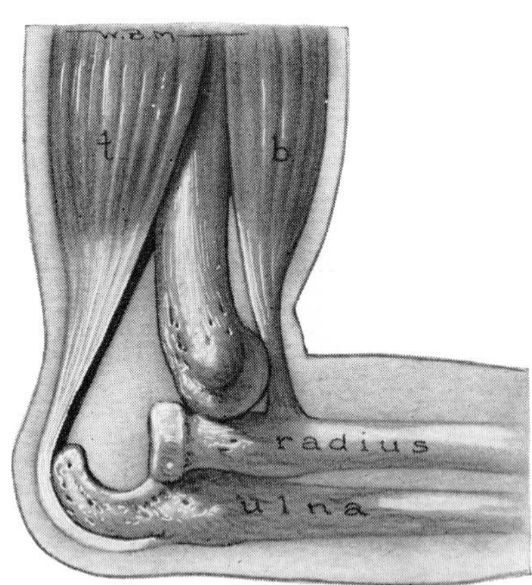

Posterior dislocation of elbow.

DISLOCATIONS

FRACTURES AND DISLOCATIONS

PLATE 38

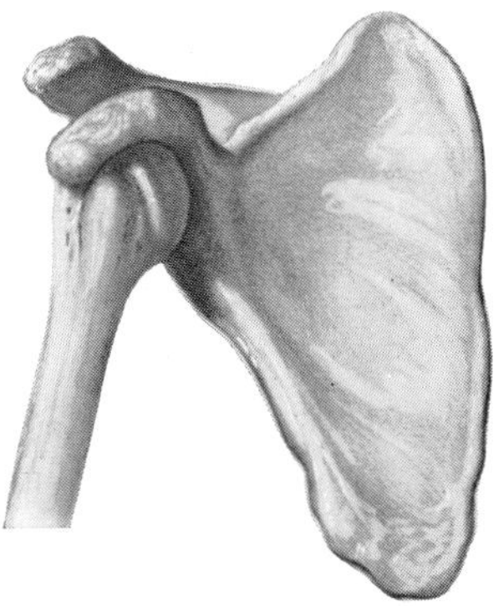

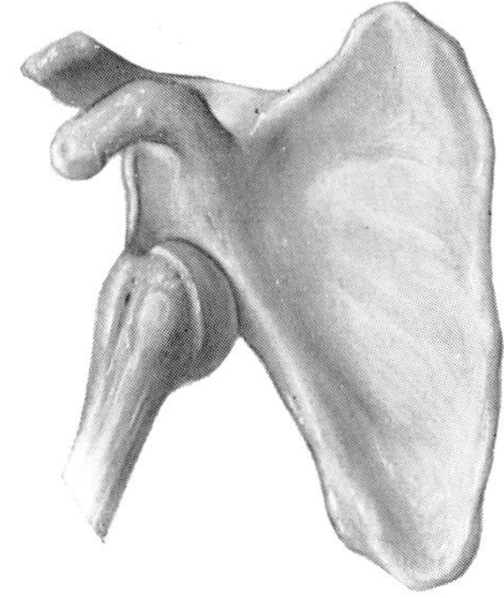

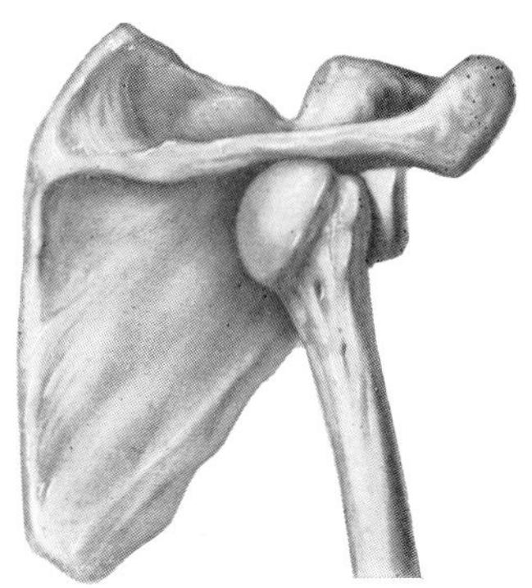

Dislocation of humerus. (Left) Subcoracoid. (Center) Subglenoid. (Right) Subspinous.

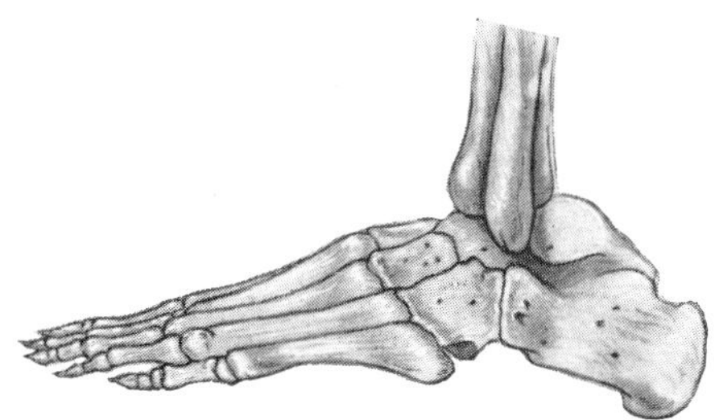

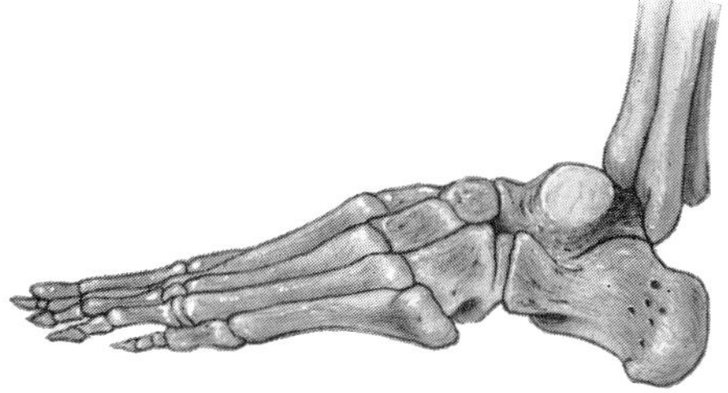

Dislocation of foot. (Left) Backward. (Right) Forward.

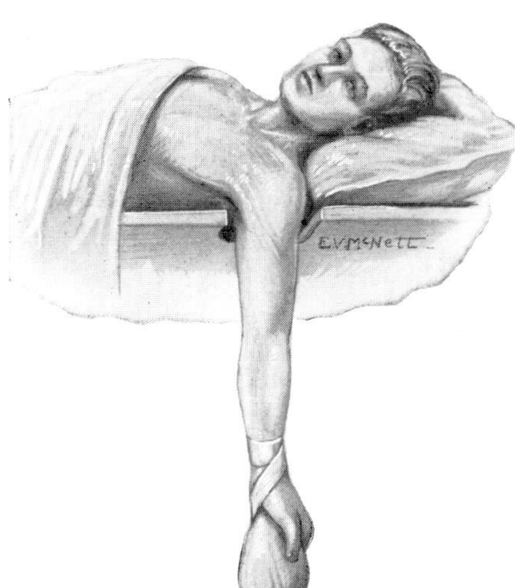

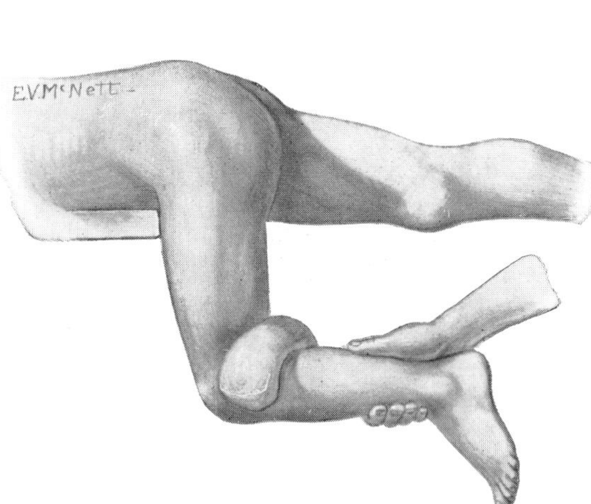

Stimson's method of passive reduction of dislocation. (Left) Humerus. (Right) Hip.

DISLOCATIONS

PLATE 39

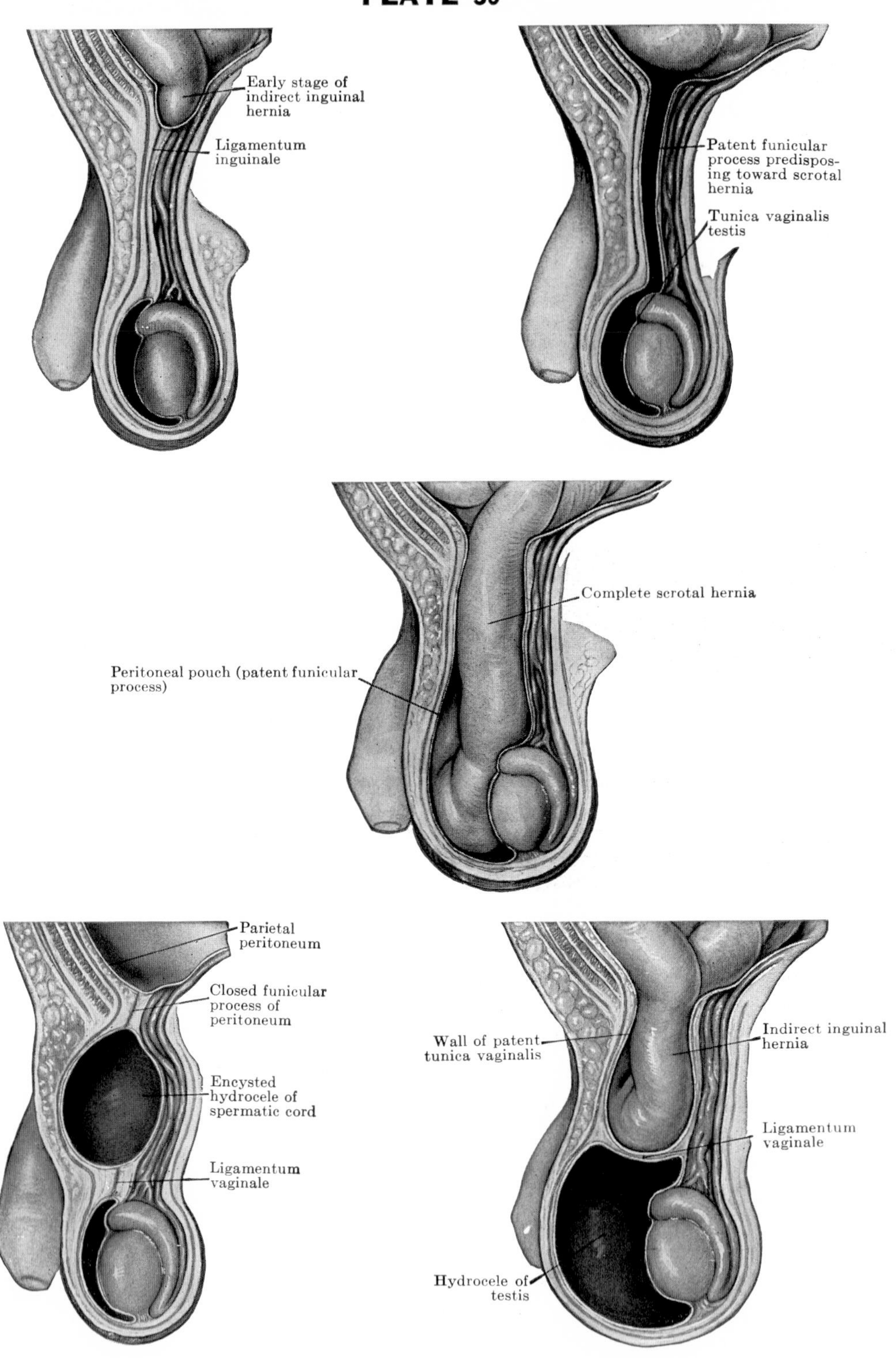

HERNIA

PLATE 40

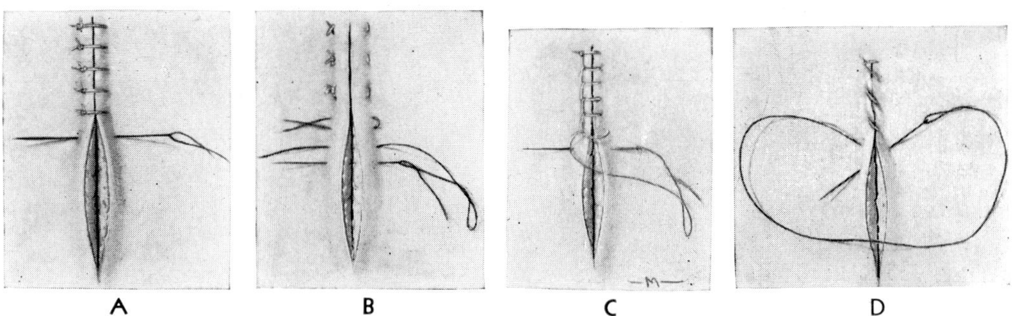

(A) Interrupted suture. (B) Mattress suture. (C) Blanket suture. (D) Continuous (glover's) suture.

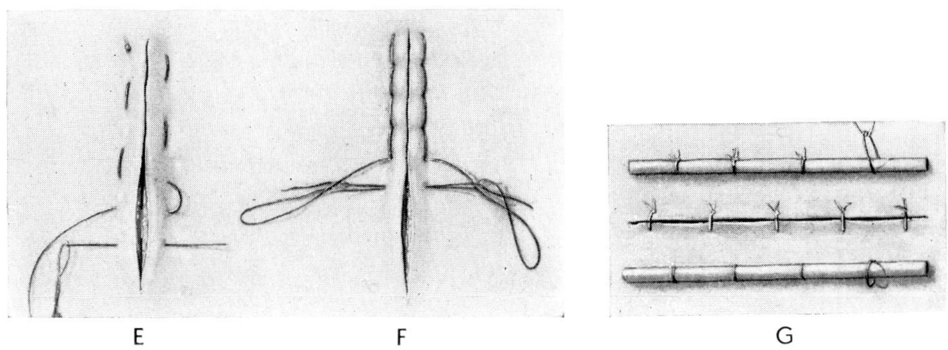

(E) Continuous mattress suture. (F) Cobbler's stitch. (G) Relaxation sutures over dental rolls.

SUTURES

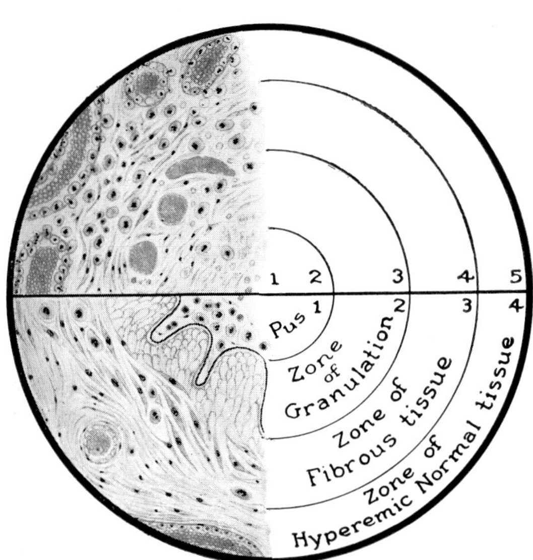

Diagram of spreading ulcer (above) and healing ulcer (below).

ULCER

SUTURES; ULCER

(From Stewart-Lee: "Manual of Surgery." Copyright, The Blakiston Company.)

PLATE 41

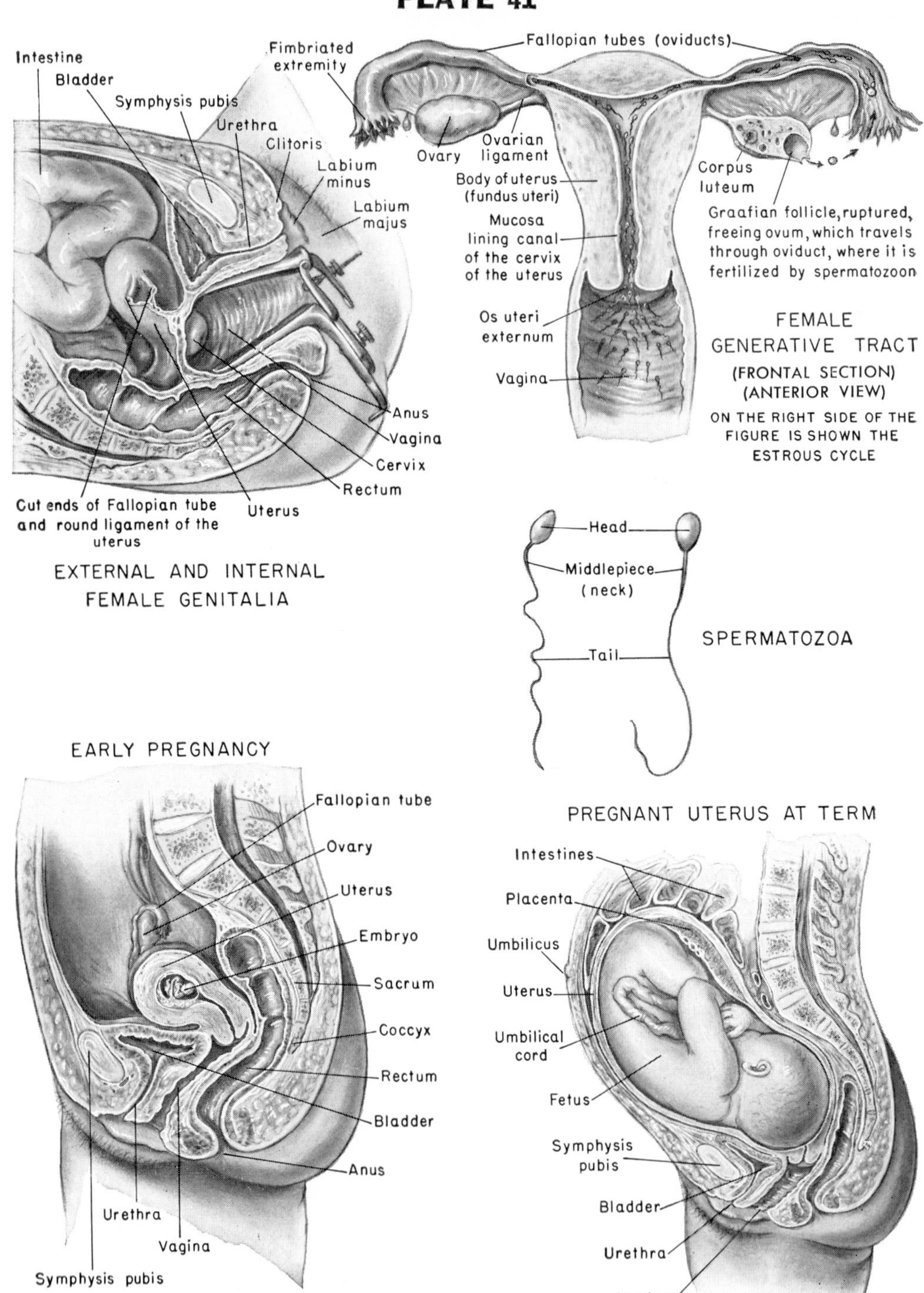
Intestine
Bladder
Symphysis pubis
Urethra
Clitoris
Labium minus
Labium majus
Fimbriated extremity
Anus
Vagina
Cervix
Rectum
Uterus
Cut ends of Fallopian tube and round ligament of the uterus
EXTERNAL AND INTERNAL FEMALE GENITALIA
Fallopian tubes (oviducts)
Ovary
Ovarian ligament
Body of uterus (fundus uteri)
Mucosa lining canal of the cervix of the uterus
Os uteri externum
Vagina
Corpus luteum
Graafian follicle, ruptured, freeing ovum, which travels through oviduct, where it is fertilized by spermatozoon
FEMALE GENERATIVE TRACT
(FRONTAL SECTION)
(ANTERIOR VIEW)
ON THE RIGHT SIDE OF THE FIGURE IS SHOWN THE ESTROUS CYCLE
Head
Middlepiece (neck)
Tail
SPERMATOZOA
EARLY PREGNANCY
Fallopian tube
Ovary
Uterus
Embryo
Sacrum
Coccyx
Rectum
Bladder
Anus
Urethra
Vagina
Symphysis pubis
PREGNANT UTERUS AT TERM
Intestines
Placenta
Umbilicus
Uterus
Umbilical cord
Fetus
Symphysis pubis
Bladder
Urethra
Vagina

GENITALIA—FEMALE

PLATE 42

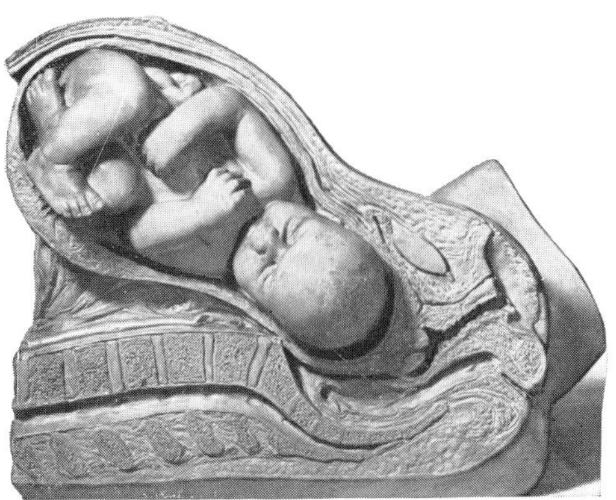

Uterus and fetus at term—head "floating"—cervix not yet dilated.

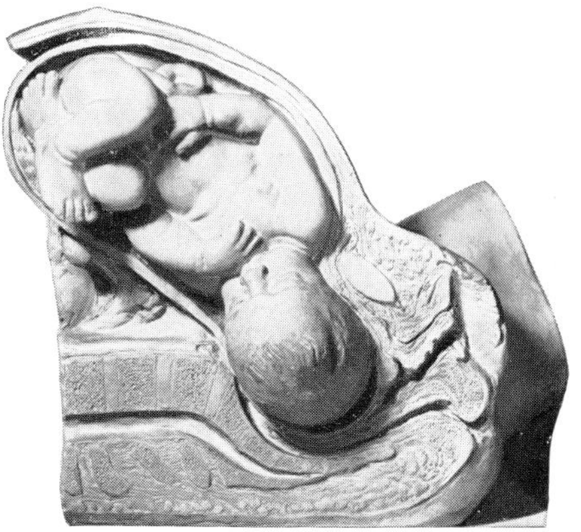

Uterus contracting—head "engaged" —cervix dilating.

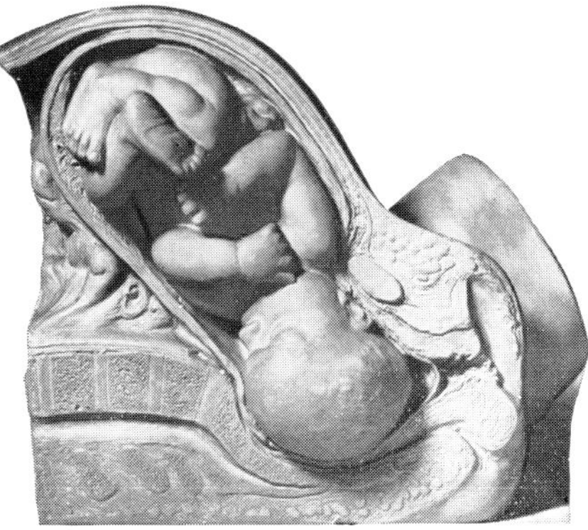

Progression of head to pelvic floor—cervix fully dilated—unruptured amnion preceding head and dilating birth canal.

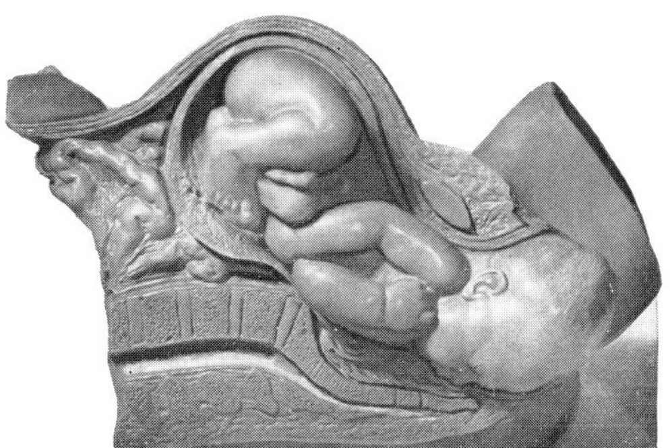

Emergence and rotation of head—caput succedaneum visible over right parietal bone.

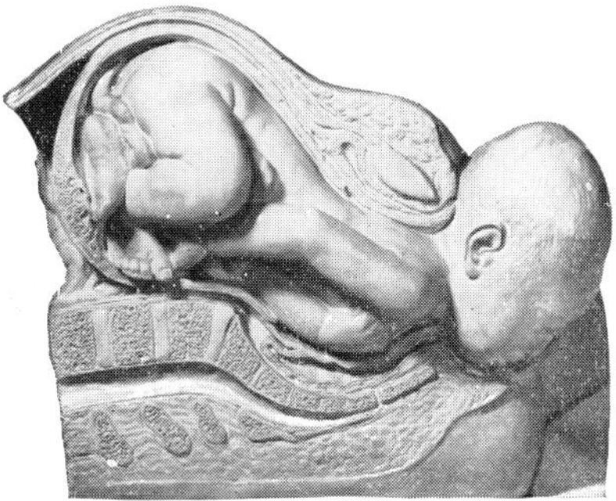

Extension of head after passing symphysis pubis. "Molding" of head is quite marked.

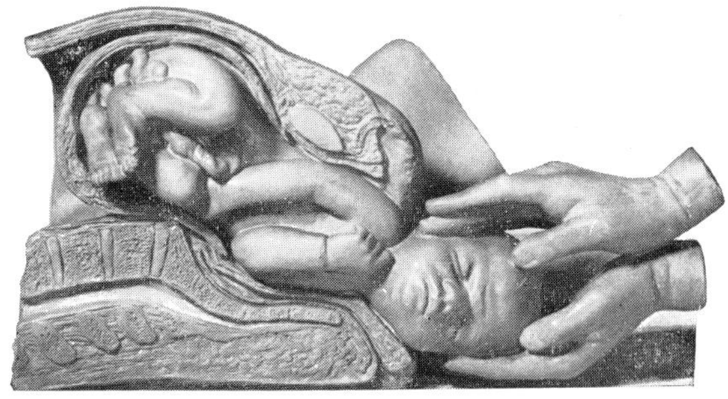

"Restitution" or return of head to original position—birth of anterior shoulder has begun.

CHILDBIRTH

(Courtesy of the Cleveland Health Museum.)

PLATE 43

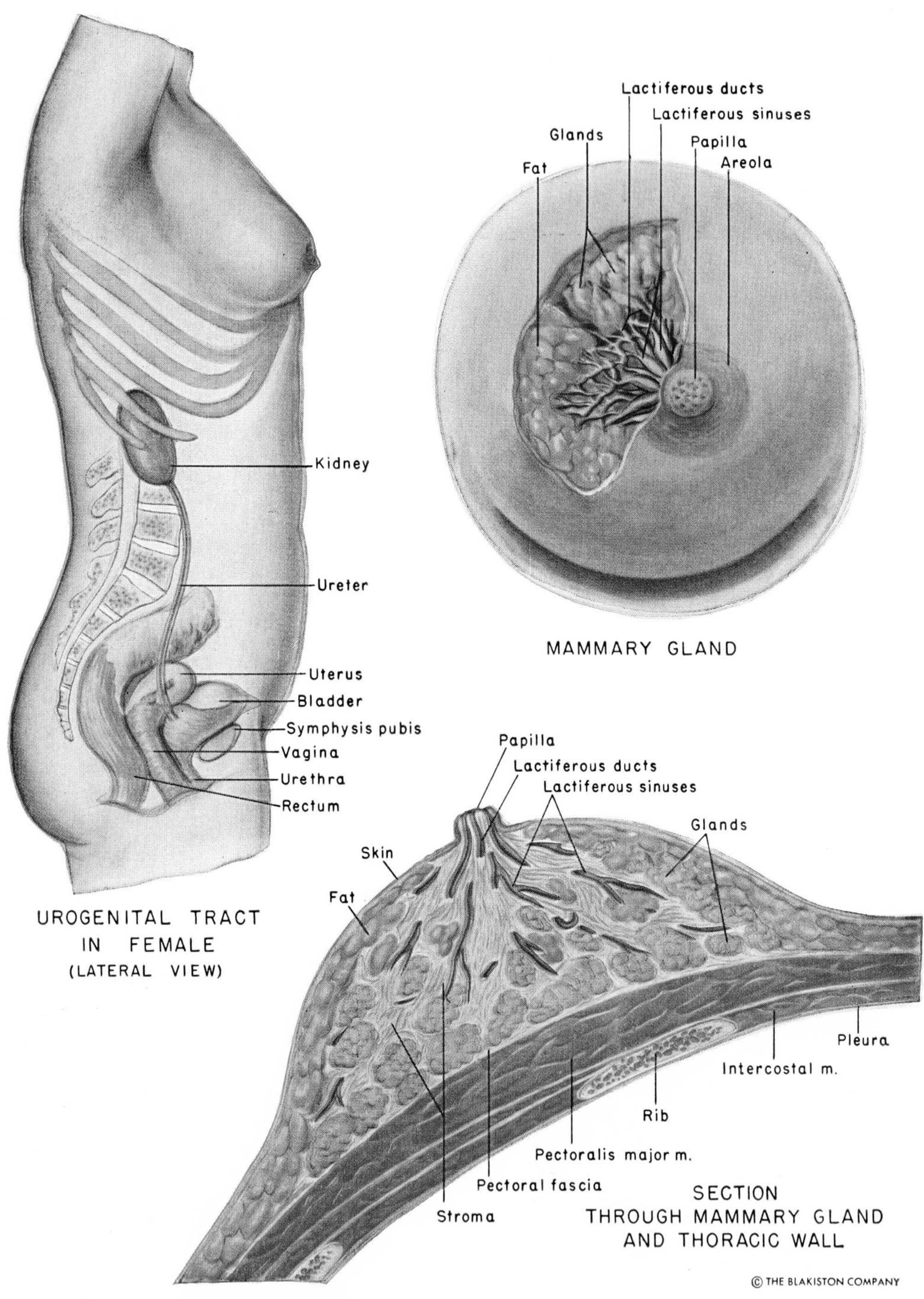

UROGENITAL TRACT—FEMALE; MAMMARY GLAND

PLATE 44

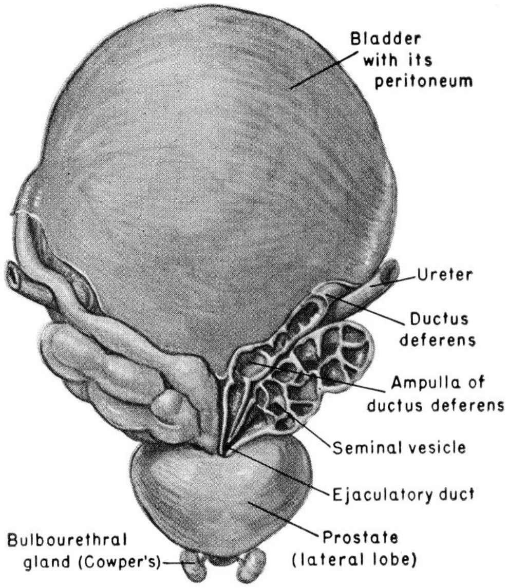

Bladder with its peritoneum
Ureter
Ductus deferens
Ampulla of ductus deferens
Seminal vesicle
Ejaculatory duct
Prostate (lateral lobe)
Bulbourethral gland (Cowper's)

MALE BLADDER, PROSTATE, AND SEMINAL VESICLES
(POSTERIOR VIEW)

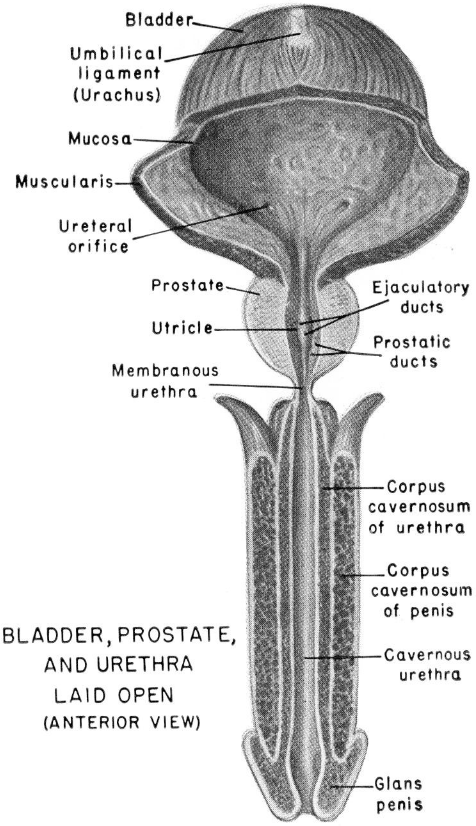

Bladder
Umbilical ligament (Urachus)
Mucosa
Muscularis
Ureteral orifice
Prostate
Utricle
Membranous urethra
Ejaculatory ducts
Prostatic ducts
Corpus cavernosum of urethra
Corpus cavernosum of penis
Cavernous urethra
Glans penis

BLADDER, PROSTATE, AND URETHRA LAID OPEN
(ANTERIOR VIEW)

VISCERA OF MALE PELVIS
(LATERAL VIEW)

Ductus deferens
Spermatic vv.
Bladder
Ureter
Seminal vesicles
Rectum
Prostate
Anus
Epididymis
Testis
Tunica vaginalis
Scrotum

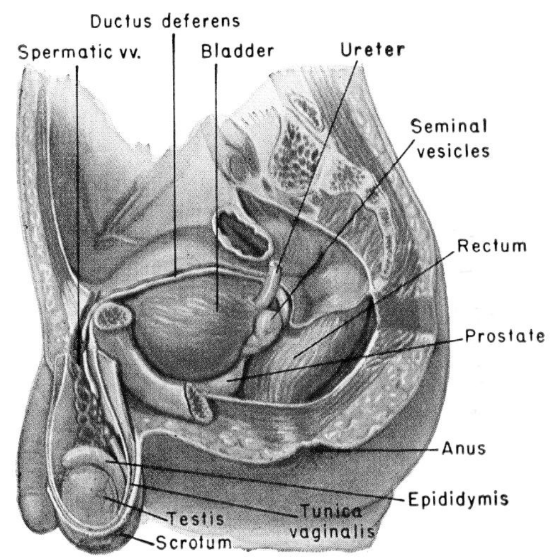

MALE PELVIS
(SAGITTAL SECTION)

Seminal vesicle
Ejaculatory duct
Bladder
Symphysis pubis
Urethra
Penis
Testis
Prostate

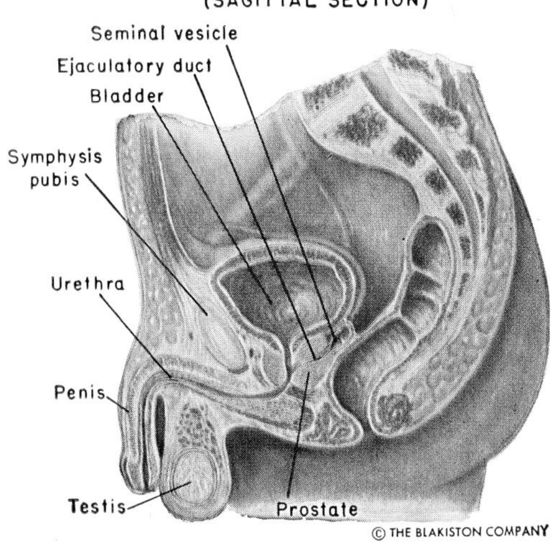

UROGENITAL TRACT—MALE

PLATE 45

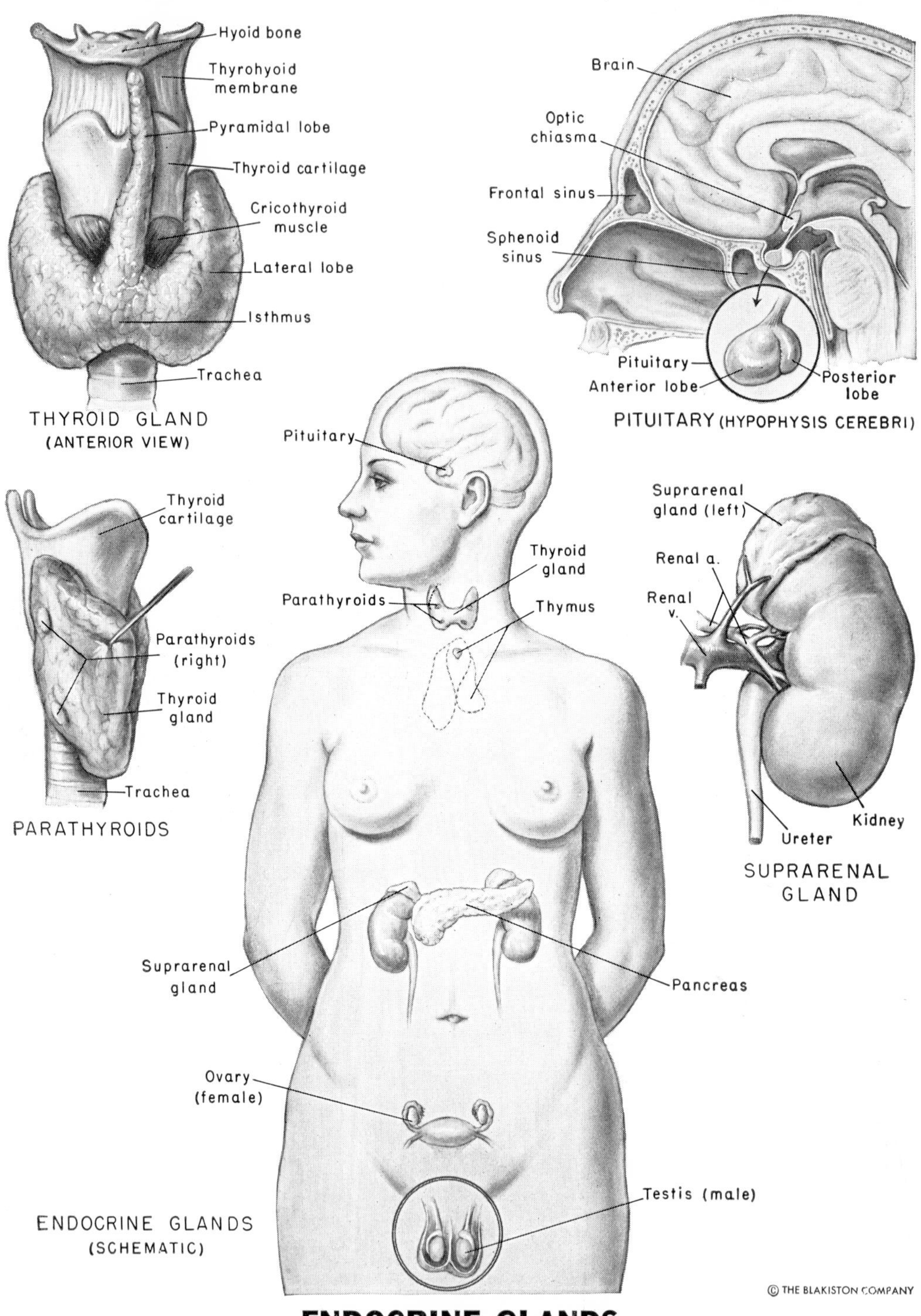

Hyoid bone
Thyrohyoid membrane
Pyramidal lobe
Thyroid cartilage
Cricothyroid muscle
Lateral lobe
Isthmus
Trachea
THYROID GLAND (ANTERIOR VIEW)
Brain
Optic chiasma
Frontal sinus
Sphenoid sinus
Pituitary
Anterior lobe
Posterior lobe
PITUITARY (HYPOPHYSIS CEREBRI)
Thyroid cartilage
Parathyroids (right)
Thyroid gland
Trachea
PARATHYROIDS
Pituitary
Thyroid gland
Parathyroids
Thymus
Suprarenal gland
Pancreas
Ovary (female)
Testis (male)
ENDOCRINE GLANDS (SCHEMATIC)
Suprarenal gland (left)
Renal a.
Renal v.
Kidney
Ureter
SUPRARENAL GLAND

ENDOCRINE GLANDS

M

M Roman numeral for one thousand.

M. An abbreviation for mass, molar, molecular weight; *misce*, mix.

M. *Misce*, mix.

m, m. Meter.

m- *In chemistry*, meta-.

mμ Millimicron or micromillimeter; the one-thousandth part of a micron.

MA Mental age.

M. A. Master of Arts; mental age.

Ma Chemical symbol for masurium.

ma Milliampere.

McBurney, Charles [*American surgeon*, 1845–1913]. Introduced an incision, for use in appendectomy, in which the muscle fibers are separated rather than cut. The external oblique muscle is divided for three or four inches parallel to the inguinal ligament. At right angles to the first incision, the internal oblique and the transversus muscles are split by blunt dissection down to the peritoneum, to give access to the right iliac fossa. Called *McBurney's incision*. See also McBurney's *point, sign*.

MacCallum, William George [*American pathologist*, 1874–1944]. His investigations with Voegtlin proved that calcium metabolism is controlled by the parathyroid glands (1909). Studied the mode of fertilization of malarial parasites (1897). See also MacCallum's *stain*.

McCarthy, Joseph Francis [*American urologist*, 1874–]. Introduced a modification of the cystoscope, for use in transurethral surgery; called *McCarthy's electrotome* or *resectoscope*.

McCarthy's reflex. See under *reflex*.

Macchiavello's stain. See *basic fuchsin* under *stain*.

McClintock, Alfred Henry [*Irish physician*, 1822–81]. Described a pulse rate of more than 100 a minute, an hour or more after parturition, as indicative of postpartum hemorrhage; called *McClintock's sign*.

McCormac's reflex. See under *reflex*.

McCoy, George Walter (1876–). American public health administrator who first recorded tularemia in rodents (1911) and with Charles W. Chapin isolated *Pasteurella tularensis* (1912).

McCrudden method (*for calcium and magnesium*). See under *method*.

McCullagh's method. See under *method*.

McDonald, Ellice (1876–). American surgeon who introduced a solution of sodium orthophenylphenate, sodium oleate, acetone, and alcohol for hand sterilization, called *McDonald's solution*.

McDowell, Ephraim [*American surgeon*, 1771–1830]. Performed ovariectomy by abdominal section (1809); called *McDowell's operation*.

mace [ME., cf. L. *macis*, a fictitious spice]. A spice derived from the dried covering of the seed of the nutmeg.

McEllroy test. See Folin-McEllroy *test*.

ma'cene (may'seen). $C_{10}H_{16}$. A hydrocarbon resulting from the distillation of nutmeg flowers.

mac'er·ate (mass'ur·ate) [L. *macerare*, to make soft]. Soften a solid or a tissue by steeping. —**macera'tion,** *n.*

mac'er·a"ter [*macerare*]. A vessel used for macerating a substance.

Macewen, William [*Scottish surgeon*, 1848–1924]. Made important contributions to the development of surgery of the brain. Described the suprameatal triangle, also known as *Macewen's triangle*. Devised an operation for inguinal hernia in which the ligated sac is used as a plug to close the internal inguinal ring; called *Macewen's operation*. Designed osteotomes in three sizes; called *Macewen's osteotomes*. Devised an operation of subcutaneous supracondylar cuneiform osteotomy for the relief of knock-knee; called *Macewen's osteotomy*. See also Macewen's *sign*.

McFarlane's method. See under *method*.

McGill, Arthur Fergusson [*English surgeon*, 1846–90]. Remembered for his prostatectomy by the suprapubic method; called *McGill's operation*.

Machado-Guerreiro reaction. See under *reaction*.

McHardy, George Gordon [*American physician*, 1910–]. With D. C. Browne, invented an esophageal dilator (1939), called *Browne-McHardy dilator*.

Mache, Heinrich [*Austrian physicist*, 1876–]. Introduced a unit of radioactive emanation. A *Mache unit* is the quantity of emanation which produces a saturation current of one one-thousandth of an electrostatic unit.

McIntosh test. Möller, McIntosh, and Van Slyke's test. See urea clearance *test*.

ma'cis. See *mace*.

Mackenrodt, Alwin Karl [*German gynecologist*, 1859–1925]. Remembered for his description of an operation for the relief of uterine retrodisplacement by vaginal fixation of the round ligaments; called *Mackenrodt's method, operation*. Devised an operation for plastic reconstruction of the vagina (1896). *Mackenrodt's ligament* is also called *cardinal ligament*.

Mackenzie, James [*Scottish cardiologist in England*, 1853–1925]. Made important contributions to the knowledge of atrial fibrillation. Gave the name x-disease to a syndrome of pathologic symptoms, including irregular respiration and pulse, sensitivity to cold, and dyspepsia, of unknown origin; also called *Mackenzie's disease*.

Mackenzie, Richard James [*Scottish surgeon*, 1821–54]. Devised a technic of amputation at the ankle joint. See Mackenzie's *amputation*.

Mackenzie, Stephen [*English physician*, 1844–1909]. Described paralysis of the tongue, soft palate, and vocal fold on the same side; called *Mackenzie's syndrome*.

Mackenzie, William (1791–1868). Scottish ophthalmologist who drew attention to increased intraocular tension in glaucoma. He also gave a classic description of sympathetic ophthalmia (1830).

McLean, Franklin Chambers [*American physiologist*, 1888–]. Contributed to the knowledge of the physiology of bone. Devised an index of urea secretion; called *McLean's formula, index*. D = Gm. of urea excreted in 24 hours; C = Gm. of urea per liter of urine; Wt. = body weight of the individual in kilograms; Ur = Gm. of urea per liter of blood.

$$\text{Index} = \frac{D\sqrt{C} \times 8.96}{\text{Wt.} \times \text{Ur}^2}$$

See also McLean and Van Slyke's *method.*

MacLean's test. See under *test.*

Macleod, John James Rickard (1876–1935). Scottish physiologist in America who made important studies of diabetes and was associated with Banting and Best in the discovery of insulin (1922). Nobel laureate with Banting (1923).

mac'ley·ine, mac·ley'ine. See *fumarine.*

ma·clu'rin. $C_{13}H_{10}O_6.H_2O$; pentahydroxybenzophenone; morintannic or moritannic acid; a light yellow, microcrystalline powder from the wood of *Chlorophora tinctoria* (*Morus tinctoria, Maclura tinctoria*): used in dyeing fabrics.

McMeekin's method. See Koch-McMeekin's *method.*

McMillan, Edwin M. (1907–). American physicist; Nobel prize winner in chemistry (1951) with Glenn T. Seaborg for the creation and discovery of the transuranium elements.

MacNeal, Ward J. [*American pathologist,* 1881–1946]. With Novy, devised a nutrient blood agar used especially for the cultivation of trypanosomes; called *Novy-MacNeal agar* or *medium.* Nicolle's modification of this for the cultivation of *Leishmania* is known as the *NNN medium.* See also MacNeal's tetrachrome *stain.*

McNeil test. See Schwartz-McNeil *test.*

Mac"ra·can"tho·rhyn'chus (mack"ruh·can"thoring'kus) [G. *makros,* long, large; *akantha,* spine; *rhygchos,* snout]. A genus of acanthocephalan worms.

M. hirudinaceus. A species attacking swine and formerly man in the Russian Volga valley.

mac"ra·cu'si·a (mack"ra·cue'zhuh, ·zee·uh, mack"ra·kōō'·) [*makros;* G. *akousis,* hearing]. A cerebral disorder simulating epilepsy, in which sounds are exaggerated.

mac"ren·ce·phal'ic, mac"ren·ceph'a·lous [*makros;* G. *egkephalos,* brain]. Having an abnormally large brain.

mac"ren·ceph'a·ly [*makros; egkephalos*]. The condition of having an abnormally large brain.

McReynolds, John Oliver [*American ophthalmologist,* 1865–1942]. Described a transplanting operation for the relief of pterygium; called *McReynold's transplant.*

mac'ro-, macr- [G. *makros,* long, large]. 1. *In anatomy* and *medicine,* a combining form denoting *an enlargement.* 2. *In botany* and *zoology,* a combining form signifying *having an unusually large* or *elongated part.*

mac"ro·bac·te'ri·um [*makros;* G. *baktērion,* little staff]. A large bacterium.

mac"ro·blast'. See *proerythroblast.*

mac"ro·ble·phar'i·a (mack"ro·bli·farr'ee·uh, ·fair'ee·uh) [*makros;* G. *blepharon,* eyelid]. Abnormal largeness of the eyelid.

mac"ro·bra'chi·a (mack"ro·bray'kee·uh) [*makros;* G. *brachiōn,* arm]. Excessive development of the arms.

mac"ro·car'di·us [*makros;* G. *kardia,* heart]. A fetus with a greatly enlarged heart.

mac"ro·ce·pha'li·a, mac"ro·ceph'a·ly [*makros;* G. *kephalē,* head]. Abnormal largeness of the head. —**macroceph'alous,** *adj.*

mac"ro·ceph'a·lus [*makros; kephalē*]. A fetus with excessive development of the head.

mac"ro·chei'li·a (mack"ro·kigh'lee·uh) [*makros;* G. *cheilos,* lip]. Excessive development of the lips; characteristic of certain Negro tribes and of cretins; in the latter due to lymphangioma of the lips and cheeks.

mac"ro·chei'ri·a (mack"ro·kigh'ree·uh) [*makros* G. *cheir,* hand]. Enlargement of the hands.

mac"ro·co·nid'i·um (pl. *macroconidia*) [*makros;* G. *konis,* dust]. *In botany,* a large and usually multicelled conidium.

mac'ro·cyte [*makros;* G. *kytos,* cell]. An erythrocyte having either a diameter or a mean corpuscular volume (MCV), or both, exceeding by more than two standard deviations that of the mean normal, as determined by the same method on the bloods of healthy persons of the patient's age and sex group: also called *macronormocyte.* See also macrocytic *anemia.* —**macrocyt'ic,** *adj.*

mac"ro·cy·to'sis (mack"ro·sigh·to'sis) [*makros; kytos;* G. *-ōsis,* condition]. The presence of macrocytes, or abnormally large erythrocytes, in the blood as determined microscopically or by measurement of cell volume.

mac"ro·dac·tyl'i·a, mac"ro·dac'ty·ly, mac"ro·dac'tyl·ism [*makros;* G. *daktylos,* finger]. Abnormally large fingers or toes.

mac"ro·don'ti·a [*makros;* G. *odous,* tooth]. The condition of having abnormally large teeth: also called *macrodentism.* Syn., *megalodontia.* —**mac'rodont,** *adj.*

mac"ro·gam'ete (mack"ro·gam'eet) [*makros;* G. *gamos,* marriage]. A relatively large, nonmotile reproductive cell of certain protozoans and thallophytes, comparable to an ovum of the metazoans.

mac"ro·ga·me'to·cyte (·ga·mee'to·sight, ·met'o·sight, ·gam'i·to·) [*makros; gamos;* G. *kytos,* cell]. The enlarged merozoite before maturation into the female cell, in propagative reproduction in sporozoa. See Plate 28.

ma·crog'a·my [*makros; gamos*]. Conjugation of two adult protozoan cells.

ma·crog'li·a. See *astrocytes.*

mac"ro·glob"u·lin·e'mi·a. A disorder of the blood, clinically manifested by a variable combination of generalized lymphadenopathy, hepatosplenomegaly, and increased lymphocytes in blood and bone marrow, together with normochromic anemia and hemorrhagic diathesis not associated with a disturbance of clotting time, bleeding time, prothrombin time, or platelet count. Diagnosis rests on the finding by ultracentrifugation of the macroglobulin, and perhaps also upon immunological characteristics. Also called *m. of Waldenström.*

mac"ro·glos'si·a [*makros;* G. *glōssa,* tongue]. Enlargement of the tongue.

mac"ro·gnath'ic (mack"ro·nath'ick, ·nay'thick, mack"rog·) [*makros;* G. *gnathos,* jaw]. Having long jaws; prognathous. —**macrog'nathism,** *n.*

mac"ro·gy'ri·a [*makros;* G. *gyros,* circle]. A congenital condition of excessively large convolutions of the brain.

mac"ro·lymph'o·cyte [*makros;* L. *lympha,* water; G. *kytos,* cell]. A large lymphocyte.

mac"ro·mas'ti·a [*makros;* G. *mastos,* breast]. Abnormal enlargement of the breast. Also called *macromazia.*

mac"ro·me'li·a [*makros;* G. *melos,* limb]. Abnormally large size of arms or legs.

ma·crom'e·lus [*makros; melos*]. An individual having excessively large limbs.

ma·crom'e·ly. See *macromelia.*

mac"ro·mer"o·zo'ite (mack"ro·merr"o·zo'ite, ·meer"o·zo'ite) [*makros;* G. *meros,* part; *zōion,* living being]. A large merozoite.

mac"ro·mo·lec'u·lar [*makros;* F. *molécule,* from L. *moles,* mass]. Having large molecules.

mac"ro·mon'o·cyte [*makros;* G. *monos,* alone; *kytos,* cell]. An abnormally large monocyte.

mac"ro·my'e·lo·blast [*makros;* G. *myelos,* marrow; *blastos,* germ]. An excessively large myeloblast.

mac″ro·nor′mo·blast [*makros;* L. *norma,* rule; G. *blastos,* germ]. A large normoblast or definitive erythroblast. See *proerythroblast.*

mac″ro·nor′mo·cyte. See *macrocyte.*

mac″ro·nu′cle·us [*makros;* L. *nucleus,* nut]. The vegetative or trophic nucleus of protozoa as contrasted with the micronucleus which is reproductive in function.

mac″ro·nych′i·a (mack″ro·nick′ee·uh) [*makros;* G. *onyx,* nail]. Excessive size of the nails.

mac′ro·phage [*makros;* G. *phagein,* to eat]. A phagocytic cell, not a leukocyte, belonging to the reticuloendothelial system. It has the capacity for storing certain aniline dyes, as trypan blue or lithium carmine, in its cytoplasm in the form of granules.

fixed m. A nonmotile macrophage, as that found in loose connective tissue (histiocyte), or lining the sinuses in the liver (Kupffer cell), the spleen, bone marrow, or lymph nodes.

free m. An actively ameboid macrophage found in an area of inflammation. Also called *inflammatory m.*

mac″ro·po′di·a, ma·crop′o·dy [*makros;* G. *pous,* foot]. Abnormal size of the foot or feet. Syn., *pes gigas, sciapody.*

mac″ro·pol′y·cytes [*makros;* G. *polys,* many, much; *kytos,* cell]. Unusually large, neutrophilic leukocytes with six or more lobes in the nucleus. Sometimes called *P.A. polys,* because they are commonly found in the peripheral blood of patients with pernicious anemia.

mac″ro·pro·so′pi·a [*makros;* G. *prosōpon,* face]. Abnormal enlargement of the face.

mac″ro·pro′so·pus (mack″ro·pro′so·pus, ·pro·so′-pus) [*makros; prosōpon*]. An individual with an abnormally large face: also spelled *macroprosopy.*

ma·crop′si·a, ma·crop′sy [*makros;* G. *opsis,* vision]. A disturbance of vision in which objects seem larger than they are. Syn., *megalopia.*

mac″ro·scop′ic [*makros;* G. *skopein,* to examine]. Large enough to be seen by the naked eye; gross; not microscopic.

mac″ros·mat′ic [*makros;* G. *osmē,* smell]. Possessing a highly developed sense of smell.

mac″ro·so′mi·a [*makros;* G. *sōma,* body]. Gigantism.

mac′ro·spore [*makros;* G. *spora,* seed]. 1. A spore of relatively large size. 2. One of the larger spores arising in the reproduction of certain protozoans, as Radiolaria. —**macrospor′ic,** *adj.*

mac″ro·sto′mi·a [*makros;* G. *stoma,* mouth]. Abnormally large mouth; a mild form of transverse facial cleft.

ma·cro′ti·a (ma·kro′shee·uh) [*makros;* G. *ous,* ear]. Abnormal largeness of the external ear.

mac′u·la (pl. *maculas, maculae*) [L., spot]. 1. A spot, usually upon the skin, not elevated above the surrounding level and distinguished by a discoloration. Syn., *macule.* 2. The area of most distinct vision of the retina. —**macular,** *adj.*

false m. The point on the retina of a squinting eye which receives the same impression as the macula of the fixing eye.

m. communis. The thickening in the medial wall of the otic vesicle, which divides to form the maculas, cristae, and organ of Corti of the internal ear.

m. corneae. A permanent corneal opacity from an ulcer or keratitis.

m. cribrosa. A small area of the wall of the vestibule perforated for the passage of the filaments of the vestibular nerve.

m. cribrosa inferior. A small area in the ampulla of the osseous superior semicircular canal perforated by nerve filaments to the corresponding ampulla of the membranous posterior semicircular canal.

m. cribrosa media. A small circular depression in the spherical recess of the vestibule perforated by filaments of the vestibular nerve to the saccule.

m. cribrosa superior. A small oval depression in the elliptical recess of the vestibule perforated by filaments of the vestibular nerve to the utricle and the superior and lateral semicircular canals.

m. densa. A thickening of the epithelium of the ascending limb of the loop of Henle, at the level of attachment to the vascular pole of the renal corpuscle.

maculae acusticae. The *m.* sacculi and *m.* utriculi.

m. germinativa. The nucleolus of the ovum.

m. lutea. The yellow spot of the retina; the point of clearest vision. See Plate 19.

m. sacculi. An oval thickened area in the anterior portion of the saccule where the saccular nerve filaments attach: also called *macula acustica sacculi.*

m. utriculi. An oval thickened area in the floor and anterior portion of the utricle where the utricular nerve filaments attach: also called *macula acustica utriculi.*

mac′ule. See *macula,* 1.

mac″u·lo·pap′u·lar [*macula;* L. *papula,* pustule]. Having the characteristics of a macule and a papule.

mad [AS. *gemǣed*]. 1. Colloquial term for insane. 2. Affected with rabies; rabid.

mad″a·ro′sis [G. *madaros,* bald; *-ōsis,* condition]. Loss of the eyelashes or eyebrows. —**madarot′ic, mad′arous,** *adj.*

mad′der. 1. The Eurasian herb *Rubia tinctorum* L. and other species. 2. The root of *Rubia tinctorum* L. and other species, used for dyeing and from which alizarin and purpurin may be obtained: formerly used medicinally. See also *ruberythric acid.*

Maddox, Ernest Edmund [*English ophthalmologist,* 1860–1933]. Devised a test for heterophoria by means of a glass rod or several parallel glass rods set in an opaque disk. When held before one eye, the *Maddox rod* converts the image of a candle flame into a line of light. The relative positions of the images seen by the two eyes indicate the degree of heterophoria.

mad″e·fac′tion [L. *madefactum,* from *madefacere,* to moisten]. The act of moistening. *Rare.*

Madelung, Otto Wilhelm (1846–1926). German surgeon who described a deformity of the wrist, called Madelung's *deformity.*

mad′i·dans (mad′i·danz, ·dance) [L. *madidare,* to moisten]. Weeping, oozing.

mad′ness [AS. *gemǣed*]. Colloquial term for mental disorder.

ma·du′ra foot (mad·oor′uh, mad·yoor′uh, mad′-yoo·ruh). See *mycetoma.*

Mad″u·rel′la [dim. from *Madura,* a city in southern India]. A genus of fungi of the Fungi imperfecti; species of this genus are often isolated in cases of mycetoma.

mad″u·ro·my·co′sis. See *mycetoma.*

Magath, Thomas Byrd [*American pathologist,* 1895–]. With A. H. Sanford devised a graduated tube for use in the hematocrit; called *Sanford and Magath's centrifuge tube.*

ma′gen·bla·se (mah′gen·blah·seh) [Ger. stomach bubble]. *In radiology,* the bubble of gas in the stomach normally located under the left side of the diaphragm after eating.

Magendie, François [*French physiologist,* 1783–1855]. Made important studies of the function of the cerebellum; of cardiac function; of the mechanics of deglutition, vomiting, and the venous flow; of vascular absorption; of the chemistry of blood and lymph; of the localized action of various drugs. With Pelletier, isolated emetine (1817). Gave the earliest clear description of the cerebrospinal fluid (1825). Described the medial foramen in the membranous roof of the fourth ventricle of the brain (1825); called *foramen of Magendie*. *Magendie's law* states that anterior spinal roots are motor; posterior roots are sensory.

mag'en·stras"se (mah'gun·shtrah"suh. *See* NOTES § 35) [Ger.]. A longitudinal groove in the mucous membrane of the stomach, along the lesser curvature from the cardiac end to the pyloric end. It is associated with the direct passage of food through the stomach, and is one of the most frequent sites of gastric ulcer.

ma·gen'ta [from *Magenta*, Italy]. Basic fuchsin.

acid m. Acid fuchsin.

mag'got [ME. *mathek*]. The larval form of an insect, especially of the order Diptera. Maggots have been used in the healing of suppurating wounds. Also see maggot *therapy*.

Congo floor m. See *Auchmeromyia luteola*.

mag'is·ter"y (madj'i·sterr"ee) [L. *magister*, master]. Formerly, a preparation considered to have especial virtue as a remedy.

bismuth m. Bismuth subnitrate.

tin m. Precipitated stannous oxide, SnO.

mag'is·tral (madj'i·strul). Pertaining to medicines prepared on prescription. *Obs.*

mag'ma [G. *magma*, thick unguent]. 1. Any pulpy mass; a paste. 2. *In pharmacy*, a more or less permanent suspension of a precipitate in water.

m. reticulare. The jellylike strands of extraembryonic mesoderm bridging the extraembryonic coelom of the young human embryo.

mag·na'li·um. An alloy of aluminum and magnesium.

magnamycin. Trade-mark for the antibiotic substance carbomycin.

Magnan, Valentin Jacques Joseph [*French psychiatrist*, 1835–1916]. Described an illusory sensation of a foreign body under the skin. The illusion is noted in cases of cocaine addiction. Called *Magnan's sign*.

mag·ne'sia (mag·nee'shuh, ·zhuh). Magnesium oxide; MgO.

calcined m. Magnesium oxide prepared by ignition of the carbonate.

heavy m. Magnesium oxide prepared by ignition of heavy magnesium carbonate.

light m. Magnesium oxide prepared by ignition of light magnesium carbonate.

m. magma. Milk of magnesia.

mag'ne·site. Native magnesium carbonate; used as a substitute for plaster of Paris.

mag·ne'si·um (mag·nee'zee·um, ·zhum, ·shee·um, ·shum) [G. *Magnēsie lithos*, Magnesian stone]. Mg = 24.32. A bluish white metal of the group to which calcium and barium belong. Abundantly distributed throughout inorganic and organic nature and essential to life; its salts are used in medicine. See Table of Normal Values of Blood Constituents in the Appendix. —**magnesic,** *adj.*

m. ammonium phosphate. $MgNH_4PO_4.6H_2O$; a white, crystalline salt, very slightly soluble in water; its formation provides the qualitative and quantitative basis of analyzing for magnesium or phosphate ion.

m. benzoate. $Mg(C_7H_5O_2)_2$; has been used in gout.

m. borate. $Mg(BO_2)_2.2Mg(OH)_2.7H_2O$. Used as a preservative.

m. bromide. $MgBr_2.6H_2O$; has been used as a sedative.

m. carbonate (*magnesii carbonas*). Basic or normal hydrated magnesium carbonate. Exists in two forms: light and heavy magnesium carbonate. Antacid and laxative. Dose, as antacid, 0.3–1.3 Gm. (5–20 gr.); as laxative, 2–8 Gm. (30–120 gr.).

m. chloride. $MgCl_2.6H_2O$; has been used as an aperient and cathartic.

m. citrate solution (*liquor magnesii citratis*). Used as a cathartic. Dose, 180–350 cc. (6–12 fluidounces).

m. hydroxide. $Mg(OH)_2$. Antacid and cathartic. Dose, 4–8 Gm. (60–120 gr.). Also called *m. hydrate*.

m. lactate. $Mg(C_3H_5O_3)_2.3H_2O$; has been used as a laxative.

m. mandelate. $(C_6H_5CHOHCOO)_2Mg$. A urinary antiseptic. Dose, 0.5–1.0 Gm. (8–15 gr.).

m. oxide. MgO. Obtained by calcining magnesium carbonate. Exists in two forms: light magnesia (*magnesii oxidum*) and heavy magnesia (*magnesii oxidum ponderosum*). Used as an antacid and laxative and as a dusting powder. Dose, as an antacid, 0.25–0.6 Gm. (4–10 gr.); as a laxative, 2–4 Gm. (30–60 gr.).

m. perborate. Approximately $Mg(BO_3)_2.7H_2O$. Yields 8–9% oxygen; used in dentifrices.

m. perchlorate. $Mg(ClO_4)_2$, and several hydrates thereof. The anhydrous salt is a white, very hygroscopic, granular or flaky powder, soluble in water, used in various chemical procedures for absorption of water. See *anhydrone, dehydrite*.

m. salicylate. $Mg(C_7H_5O_3).4H_2O$; has been used as an intestinal antiseptic and antirheumatic.

m. sulfate (*magnesii sulfas*). $MgSO_4.7H_2O$. Epsom salt, an active cathartic, especially useful in inflammatory affections. Dose, 4–30 Gm. (1–8 dr.).

m. trisilicate (*magnesii trisilicas*). Approximately $2MgO.3SiO_2$ with varying amounts of water. Almost insoluble in water; reacts slowly with acid; used as an antacid and adsorbent. Dose, 0.3–2.0 Gm. (5–30 gr.).

tribasic m. phosphate (*magnesii phosphas tribasicus*). $Mg_3(PO_4)_2$. A gastric antacid; almost insoluble in water. Dose, 0.6–2.0 Gm. (10–30 gr.).

mag'net [G. *Magnētis lithos*, magnet]. 1. Loadstone, iron that attracts iron. 2. Any body having the power to attract iron. See also *electromagnet*. —**magnet'ic,** *adj.*

giant m. A large, powerful, stationary magnet for extracting particles of steel from the eye.

horseshoe m. An iron magnet having the shape of a horseshoe.

m. operation. The operation of removing foreign bodies of steel from the eye by means of a magnet.

Mellinger m. A type of giant magnet, with a magnetized core held in the surgeon's hand, the coil being over the patient's eye, and devised for extracting steel particles from the eyeball.

permanent m. One whose magnetic properties are permanent.

temporary m. One which derives its magnetism from another magnet or from a galvanic current.

mag'net·ism [*Magnētis lithos*]. 1. The power possessed by a magnet to attract or repel other masses. 2. The force formerly supposed to be transmitted from man to man, an important factor in hypnotism or mesmerism. Also called *animal m.*

mag'net·ite. A naturally occurring oxide of iron of the composition Fe_3O_4.

mag"net·i·za'tion [*Magnētis lithos*]. The process of rendering a substance magnetic.

mag·ne"to·e·lec"tric'i·ty (mag·nee"to·, mag"-ni·to·, mag·net"o·) [*Magnētis lithos;* G. *ēlektron*, amber]. Electricity produced by moving an electric conductor through a magnetic field.

mag·ne′to·graph [*Magnētis lithos;* G. *graphein,* to write]. An instrument for determining the strength of a magnetic field.

mag·ne″to·in·duc′tion [*Magnētis lithos;* L. *inductio,* from *inductum,* to lead into]. The induction of an electric current by placing a permanent or temporary magnet within a coil of wire.

mag″ne·tom′e·ter [*Magnētis lithos;* G. *metron,* a measure]. A series of magnets suspended to record graphically variations in direction and intensity of magnetic force.

mag·ne″to-op′tic (mag·nee″to-op′tick, mag″nito-, mag·net″o-) [*Magnētis lithos;* G. *optikos,* of sight]. Pertaining to optic phenomena influenced by magnetic fields.

mag·ne″to·stric′tion. Magnetic phenomenon involving the change in length of a rod or tube of ferromagnetic material when it is exposed to a magnetic field parallel to its length.

mag·ne″to·ther′a·py [*Magnētis lithos;* G. *therapeia,* treatment]. The treatment of diseases by magnets.

mag′ne·tron. Microwave generator; a thermionic tube with a magnetic field acting transversely to the cathode-anode path.

mag″ni·fi·ca′tion [L. *magnificare,* from *magnus,* large; *facere,* to make]. Apparent enlargement, especially the enlargement of an object by means of lenses. —**mag′nify,** *v.*

mag′num [*magnus*]. Large, as in foramen magnum.

mag′num. An old term for capitate bone (os magnum). See Table of Bones in the Appendix.

Magnus, Rudolf (1873–1927). German physiologist in Holland, best known for his monograph on postural mechanisms, *Körperstellung* (1924). He demonstrated the functions of the otoliths as compared to those of the semicircular canals (1926). The postural reflexes, especially the righting and supporting reflexes, and the tonic neck and tonic labyrinthine reflexes are called *Magnus-de Kleijn reflexes* after him and his chief collaborator. He is also known for his technique of isolating a loop of small intestine and research on the physiology of the surviving intestine.

Magnus-Levy, Adolf [*German clinical physiologist in the United States,* 1865–1955]. Demonstrated that thyroid deficiency is associated with reduced metabolism, and is correctible by the administration of desiccated thyroid (1895). Made important studies of diabetic coma and of metabolism in multiple myeloma and introduced dehydration by the use of potassium salts.

Magnuson splint. See under *splint.*

ma·ha·ma′ri (mah·hah·mah′ree). See *plague.*

maid′en·head″ [AS. *maegden; hād*]. The hymen, the allusion being to the intact organ of the maid or virgin.

Maier, Rudolf [*German physician,* 1824–88]. Described a small, infundibular depression in the wall of the lacrimal sac; called *Maier's sinus.* With Kussmaul, described polyarteritis nodosa (1866), called *Kussmaul-Maier disease.*

ma·ieu″si·o·ma′ni·a (may·yōō″see·o·may′nee-uh·) [G. *maieusis,* delivery of a woman in childbirth; *mania,* madness]. Puerperal psychosis. *Obs.*

ma·ieu″si·o·pho′bi·a [*maieusis;* G. *phobos,* fear]. Morbid fear of childbirth.

ma·ieu′tic (may·yōō′tick, migh·yōō′tick) [G. *maieutikos,* skilled in midwifery]. A rubber bag used for dilating the cervix uteri.

ma·ieu′tics [*maieutikos*]. Obstetrics. —**maieu′tic,** *adj.*

maim [ME. *maymen*]. Deprive a person or animal of any part of the body; disable or cripple.

main en griffe′ (man ong grif′. *See* Notes § 35). See *clawhand.*

main en lorgnette (man ong lor·nyet′). See opera-glass *hand.*

Maisonneuve, Jacques Gilles Thomas [*French surgeon,* 1809–97]. Devised a urethrotome with a concealed knife which is retracted until the instrument reaches the stricture; called *Maisonneuve's urethrotome, maisonneuve.*

Maissiat, Jacques Henri [*French anatomist,* 1805–78]. Described the iliotibial tract, formerly called *Maissiat's band.*

Maitland, Hugh Bethune [*Canadian bacteriologist in England,* 1895–]. With Mary Cowan Maitland, developed a medium containing chicken kidney and serum, for the cultivation of vaccinia virus without tissue culture.

maize [Sp. *maíz,* from Taino *mahiz*]. Indian corn. A cereal grain; the seed of *Zea mays.* One of the principal foodstuffs. Deficient in niacin (nicotinic acid) and other vitamins. Consequently, pellagra is frequent among maize eaters.

Majocchi, Domenico [*Italian dermatologist,* 1849–1929]. Described purpura annularis telangiectodes, called *Majocchi's disease.*

ma′jor med′i·cal as·sem′bly. *In military medicine,* an aggregation of medical supplies and equipment identified by a consignee combination.

make [AS. *macian*]. *In electricity,* the establishing of the flow of an electric current.

mak′ro-. See *macro-.*

mal [F.]. Disease.

grand m. See grand mal *epilepsy.*

haut m. See grand mal *epilepsy.*

m. de caderas. A disease of South American countries, affecting domestic animals; characterized by fever, emaciation, and paralysis of the hind legs; probably due to a trypanosome.

m. de Cayenne. Elephantiasis.

m. de coit. See *dourine.*

m. del pinto. Pinta.

m. de mer. Seasickness.

m. de Morada. The cutaneous form of onchocerciasis.

m. de rosa. See *pellagra.*

m. des bassines. A dermatitis affecting those in the silkworm industry; due to handling cocoons.

m. de sole. See *pellagra.*

m. perforant. Tabetic, perforating ulcer of the foot.

petit m. See petit mal *epilepsy.*

mal- [L. *malus,* bad]. A combining form denoting *ill, bad.*

mal′a·chite green (mal′uh·kite) (C.C.). Tetramethyl-di-*p*-aminotriphenylcarbinol, a triphenylmethane dye. Violet-green crystals or powder with bronze luster; soluble in water or alcohol; used as a bacteriologic stain. Has been used as a wound antiseptic and also in the treatment of trypanosomiasis.

ma·la′ci·a (ma·lay′shee·uh, ·see·uh) [G. *malakia,* softness]. Softening of part of an organ or structure, the result of necrosis. Also see *encephalomalacia, osteomalacia.*

m. cordis. Softening of parts of the myocardium in infarction.

mal″a·co·pla′ki·a [G. *malakos,* soft; *plakion,* small slab]. Soft, pale plaques in the mucosa, especially of the urinary system, which are slightly elevated, well defined, and surrounded by a zone of hyperemia.

mal″a·die′ de Ro′ger (mal″a·dee′ duh ro′jay). See *ventricular septal defect.*

mal″ad·just′ment [L. *malus,* bad; F. *ajustement,* from *a,* to, *juste,* L. *justus,* right]. A state of faulty or inadequate conformity to one's environment, due to the inability to adjust one's desires, attitudes, or feelings to social requirements.

mal'a·dy [F. *malade*, sick]. Disease or illness.

ma·laise' (ma·layz'. *See* NOTES § 35) [F.]. A general feeling of illness, sometimes accompanied by restlessness, lack of appetite, and decreased energy.

mal''a·ko·pla'ki·a. See *malacoplakia*.

mal'an·ders [L. *malandria*, blisters]. A disease of the horse characterized by a furfuraceous eruption at the bend of the knee and on the inside of the hock. It is called malanders when affecting the foreleg and sallenders when affecting the hindleg.

ma'lar [L. *mala*, cheek]. Pertaining to the cheek or to the zygoma.

ma'lar. Old name for zygoma. See Table of Bones in the Appendix.

ma·lar'i·a (ma·lair'ee·uh) [It., from *mala aria*, bad air]. An infectious febrile disease, caused by four species of the protozoan genus *Plasmodium* (*P. falciparum, P. vivax, P. malariae, P. ovale*), characterized by intermittent fever, splenomegaly, debility, and anemia, and tending to run a chronic course. The acute, clinical attacks or paroxysms are characterized by chills, high fever, and profuse sweating; these usually alternate with periods of comparative well-being; they occur in regular cycles, e.g., every day, every other day, or every fourth day. The disease is transmitted naturally only by the *anopheles* mosquito. Older classifications of malaria were based on the organ system involved, as cerebral *m.*, gastrointestinal *m.*, thoracic *m.*, or on the most prominent symptom, as algid *m.* or bilious *m.* Syn., *Basra fever*. See Plates 27, 28, 29. —**malar'ial, malar'ious,** *adj.*

avian m. Malaria of birds and poultry due to numerous species of the genus *Plasmodium*.

benign tertian m. See vivax *m.*

equine m. Infectious anemia of horses.

falciparum m. A severe form caused by *Plasmodium falciparum*, characterized by paroxysms occurring at irregular intervals and often by the localization of the organism in a specific organ of the body, as the brain, lungs, intestinal mucosa, spleen, and kidney: also called *estivo-autumnal m.*, *malignant m.*, *malignant tertian m.*

ovale m. A form similar to vivax *m.*, caused by *Plasmodium ovale*.

quartan m. That caused by *Plasmodium malariae*, characterized by short paroxysms occurring every third day.

quotidian m. A form in which the paroxysms occur every day, usually caused by two concomitant infections by *Plasmodium vivax*.

subtertian m. Falciparum *m.*

tertian m. See vivax *m.*

vivax m. That caused by *Plasmodium vivax*, characterized by typical paroxysms occurring every two or three days, typically every second day: also called *benign tertian m.*, *tertian m.*

ma·lar''i·ol'o·gist [*malaria;* G. *logos*, word]. An expert in the diagnosis, treatment, and control of malaria.

ma·lar''i·ol'o·gy [*malaria; logos*]. The study of malaria.

ma·lar''i·o·ther'a·py [*malaria;* G. *therapeia*, treatment]. Treatment of neurosyphilis by infecting the patient with malaria.

Mal''as·se'zi·a [after Louis Charles *Malassez*, French physiologist, 1842–1909]. A genus of fungi.

M. furfur. That species which is the causative agent of pityriasis versicolor.

mal''as·sim''i·la'tion [L. *malus*, bad; *assimilare*, to make like]. Defective assimilation.

mal'ate. Any salt or ester of malic acid.

mal''di·ges'tion [*malus;* L. *digestio*, from *digerere*, to digest]. Disordered or imperfect digestion.

male [L. *masculus*, male]. 1. An individual of the male sex. The designative symbol is □, ♂ (that of the female is ○, ♀). 2. Of a double-bladed instrument, the blade which is received into a hollow of the other (female) blade. 3. *In botany*, a plant having stamens only. —**male,** *adj.*

ma·le'ate. Any salt or ester of maleic acid.

male fern. See *aspidium*.

ma·le'ic ac'id (ma·lee'ick, ma·lay'ick). COOH.-CH:CH.COOH. Cis-ethylene carboxylic acid. A dibasic acid, the cis-isomer of fumaric acid. Does not occur in nature.

ma·le'ic an·hy'dride. $C_4H_2O_3$; 2,5-furandione, occurring as white crystals, soluble in water to form maleic acid, used commercially in synthesis of resins, dye intermediates, and other substances. It causes burns when in contact with the skin.

Malfatti formol titration method. See under *method*.

mal''for·ma'tion [L. *malus*, bad; *formatio*, from *formare*, to form]. An abnormal development or formation of a part of the body; deformity.

Malgaigne, Joseph François [*French surgeon*, 1806–65]. Devised an operation of subastragalar disarticulation of the foot, called *Malgaigne's amputation*. He also described vertical fracture of the pelvis, called *Malgaigne's fracture*.

mal'ic ac'id (mal'ick, may'lick). $COOH.CH_2$.-CHOH.COOH. A dibasic hydroxy acid found in apples and many other fruits. Exists in two optically active isomers and a racemic form. The iron salt has been used medicinally for the effect of the metal.

ma·lig'nant [L. *malignus*, wicked, malignant]. Virulent; threatening life, as malignant tumors. —**malignancy,** *n.*

ma·lin'ger·er (ma·ling'gur·ur) [F. *malingre*, sickly]. One who feigns illness or inability, usually to escape military duty or to secure benefit from an alleged injury. —**malingering,** *n.*

mal''in''ter·dig·i·ta'tion (mal''in''tur·didj·i·tay'-shun) [L. *malus*, bad; *inter*, between; *digitus*, finger]. Abnormal occlusion of the teeth.

Mall, Franklin Paine [*American embryologist*, 1862–1917]. Developed a formula for estimating the age of human embryos with a vertex-breech length of 100 mm. or less. VB represents vertex-breech length in millimeters.

$$\text{Age in days} = \sqrt{VB \times 100}$$

When *Mall's formula* was introduced, the Peters embryo was thought to be three or four days old. Since the Peters embryo is now known to be about 14 days old, it is necessary to correct the formula as follows:

$$\text{Age in days} = \sqrt{VB \times 100} + 10$$

Founder of the laboratory of embryology of the Carnegie Institution.

mal'le·a·ble [L. *malleus*, hammer]. Capable of being beaten or rolled into thin sheets. —**malleabil'ity,** *n.*

mal''le·a'tion [*malleus*]. A spasmodic action of the hands, consisting in continuously striking any near object.

mal'le·in [*malleus*]. A fluid obtained from cultures of *Malleomyces mallei* (glanders bacillus). When injected into the circulation of an animal having glanders, it causes an elevation of temperature. Mallein has been recommended for use in the early diagnosis of glanders.

mal''le·o·in'cu·dal (mal''ee·o·ing'cue·dul, ·in'cue-dul) [*malleus;* L. *incus*, anvil]. Relating to the malleus and the incus.

mal·le'o·lus (pl. *malleoli*) [L., small hammer]. A part or process of bone having a hammerhead shape. —**malleolar,** *adj.*

lateral m. The lower extremity of the fibula. Also called *external m.* See Plate 1.

medial m. A process on the internal surface of the lower extremity of the tibia. Also called *internal m.* See Plate 1.

Mal″le·o·my′ces (mal″ee·o·migh′seez) [*malleus;* G. *mykēs*, fungus]. A genus of the family Parvobacteriaceae; composed of small, slender, Gram-negative, nonmotile, nonsporulating, rodlike bacteria sometimes developing into branched filaments.

M. mallei. That species which is the causative agent of glanders. Formerly called *Bacillus mallei.*

M. pseudomallei. That species which causes melioidosis in rodents and in man. Formerly called *Bacillus whitmori.*

mal″le·ot′o·my [*malleus;* G. *tomē*, a cutting]. 1. Incision or division of the malleus. 2. Division of the ligaments attached to the malleoli.

mal′let fin′ger. See under *finger.*

mal′le·us [L.]. 1. One of the ossicles of the internal ear, having the shape of a hammer. See Plate 20. See Table of Bones in the Appendix. 2. *In veterinary medicine*, glanders. —**mal′leal,** *adj.*

Mal·loph′a·ga [Gr. *mallos*, wool]. An order of small, wingless, flat insects which feed on hair, feathers, and epidermal scales, parasitic on birds and occasionally man; the bird lice.

Mallory, Frank Burr [*American pathologist*, 1862–1941]. Introduced a number of stains. See under *stain.*

Mal·lo′tus [G. *mallōtos*, fleecy]. A genus of trees and shrubs of the Euphorbiaceae. **M. philippinensis,** a species of India, yields the taeniafuge and dyestuff, kamala.

mal′low [L. *malva*, mallows]. Any plant of the genus *Malva.*

Malloy-Evelyn method for bilirubin in blood. See under *method.*

Malmsten, Per Henrik [*Swedish physician*, 1811–83]. Discovered *Balantidium coli* (1857).

mal″nu·tri′tion [L. *malus*, bad; *nutrire*, to nourish]. Imperfect nutrition. —**malnour′ish,** *v.*

mal″oc·clu′sion (mal″oc·clue′zhun) [*malus;* L. *occludere*, to close]. Any deviation from normal occlusion of the teeth; usually associated with abnormal developmental growth of the jaws.

Angle's classification of m. is based on the mesiodistal (anteroposterior) relations of the teeth, dental arches, and jaws which depend primarily upon the positions mesiodistally assumed by the first permanent molars on their erupting and locking.

Class I. Arches in normal mesiodistal relations.

Class II. Lower arch distal to normal in relation to the upper arch.

Division 1. Bilaterally distal, protruding upper incisors. Primarily, at least, associated with mouth-breathing.

Subdivision. Unilaterally distal, protruding upper incisors. Primarily, at least, associated with mouth-breathing.

Division 2. Bilaterally distal, retruding upper incisors. Normal breathers.

Subdivision. Unilaterally distal, retruding upper incisors. Normal breathers.

Class III. Lower arch mesial to normal in relation to upper arch.

Division. Bilaterally mesial.

Subdivision. Unilaterally mesial.

mal′o·nate. Any salt or ester of malonic acid.

ma·lo′nic ac′id (ma·lo′nick, ·lon′ick). COOH.-CH_2.COOH. A dibasic acid found in many plants and obtainable from malic acid by oxidation.

mal′o·nyl (mal′o·nyl, ·neel). $H_2C<\begin{matrix}CO—\\CO—\end{matrix}$. The bivalent radical of malonic acid.

mal″o·nyl·u·re′a. Barbituric acid.

Malpighi, Marcello [*Italian anatomist*, 1628–94]. Pioneer histologist. Discovered the capillary circulation (1661). Made important studies of the structure of the lungs (1661) and of the kidneys (1666). Described the metamorphosis of the silkworm (1669), and the development of the chick embryo as observed through the microscope (1673). Both the splenic corpuscles, or lymph nodules of the spleen, and the renal corpuscles, were called *Malpighian* (or *malpighian*) *bodies* or *corpuscles.* See also Malpighian (or malpighian) *pyramid.* The germinative layer of the epidermis was called the *Malpighian* (or *malpighian*) *layer.*

mal″po·si′tion [L. *malus*, bad; *positio*, from *ponere*, to place]. An abnormal position of any part or organ, as of the fetus.

mal·pos′ture [*malus;* L. *positura*, from *ponere*, to place]. Faulty posture.

mal″prac′tice [*malus;* G. *praktikos*, fit for doing]. Improper medical or surgical treatment, through carelessness, ignorance, or intent.

mal″pres″en·ta′tion (mal″prez″un·tay′shun, ·pree″zen·tay′shun) [*malus;* L. *praesentare*, to present]. Abnormal position of the child at birth, making delivery difficult or impossible.

mal″re·duc′tion [*malus;* L. *reductio*, from *reducere*, to bring back]. Faulty or incomplete reduction of a fracture.

malt (mawlt) [AS. *mealt*]. Grain, commonly of one or more varieties of barley, which has been soaked, made to germinate, and dried. The germinated grains contain diastase, dextrin, and maltose, as well as proteins. Malt is used as a nutrient in wasting diseases.

m. extract (*extractum malti*). A viscous, light-brown, aqueous extract. Dose, 4–15 cc. (1–4 fluidrachms).

Mal′ta fe′ver (mawl′tuh). See *brucellosis.*

malt′ase (mawl′tace, ·taze). An enzyme found in the saliva and pancreatic juice which converts maltose into dextrose.

Malthus, Thomas Robert [*English political economist*, 1766–1834]. Evolved the theory that population, in the absence of such checks on its growth as epidemics and war, tends to increase more rapidly than the food supply. Advocated sexual continence as a means of limiting the birth rate. Acceptance of Malthus' doctrines is called *Malthusianism.* The term is incorrectly applied to advocacy of restriction of the birth rate by means of birth control.

mal″to·bi′ose (mawl″to·buy′oce). Maltose.

mal″to·dex′trin. A form of dextrin convertible into maltose.

malt′ose (mawl′toce). $C_{12}H_{22}O_{11}.H_2O$; 4-(α-D-glucopyranosido)-D-glucopyranose, a reducing disaccharide representing two molecules of D-glucose joined by α-glycosidic linkage, and yielding two molecules of D-glucose on hydrolysis. It does not appear to exist free in nature, being a product of enzymatic hydrolysis of starch by diastase, as in malt. It exists in two forms, α-maltose and β-maltose. Syn., *maltobiose, malt sugar.*

mal″to·su′ri·a [AS. *mealt;* G. *ouron*, urine]. The presence of maltose in the urine.

mal·turned′ [L. *malus*, bad; AS. *turnian*]. Turned abnormally; applied to a tooth so turned on its long axis as to stand in malposition.

ma′lum [L.]. Disease.

m. Aegyptiacum. Diphtheria.

m. coxae senilis. Hypertrophic arthritis of the hip joint in the aged.

m. perforans pedis. Perforating ulcer of the foot.

m. pilare. Trichinosis.

m. venereum. Syphilis.

mal·un'ion [L. *malus,* bad; *unire,* to unite]. Incomplete or faulty union of the fragments of a fractured bone.

Mal'va [L., mallows]. The mallow; a genus of the Malvaceae. The leaves of **M. neglecta** and **M. sylvestris** are used as demulcents.

ma·man·pi·an' (mah·mahn·pee·ahn'. *See* NOTES § 35). See mother *yaws.*

mam'ba (mahm'bah) [Kaffir, snake]. Any snake of *Dendraspis,* a genus of venomous snakes of southern Africa, allied to cobras except that they have no hood. The common black mamba is *D. angusticeps.*

mam'e·lon [F. nipple]. One of the three elevations on the incisal edge of a recently erupted or little-worn incisor tooth.

mam'ma (pl. *mammae*) [L. *mamma,* breast]. The breast; the milk-secreting gland.

m. aberrans. Supernumerary breast. Also called *m. erratica.*

m. virilis. The male breast.

mam'mal [*mamma*]. An individual of the class Mammalia.

mam·mal'gi·a [*mamma;* G. *algos,* pain]. Pain in the mamma.

Mam·ma'li·a [*mamma*]. The highest class of vertebrates, including all animals that have hair and suckle their young. —**mamma'lian,** *adj.*

mam'ma·plas"ty [*mamma;* G. *plassein,* to form]. Plastic surgery of the breast.

mam'ma·ry [*mamma*]. Pertaining to the mammae.

mam·mec'to·my [*mamma;* G. *ektomē,* excision]. Excision or amputation of the breast.

mam'mi·form [*mamma;* L. *forma,* shape]. Shaped like a breast or nipple.

mam·mil'la (pl. *mammillae*) [L., nipple]. A small prominence or papilla; nipple.

mam'mil·lar"y (mam'i·lerr"ee, ·lair"ee) [*mammilla*]. Nipple-shaped; pertaining to a nipple; shaped like a breast.

mam'mil·la"ted [*mammilla*]. Covered with nipple-like protuberances.

mam"mil·la'tion [*mammilla*]. A granulation, especially on some mucous surface.

mam·mil'li·form [*mammilla;* L. *forma,* shape]. Nipple-shaped.

mam·mil'li·plas"ty [*mammill;* G. *aplassein,* to form]. Plastic surgery of the nipple. Syn., *thelyplasty.*

mam"mil·li'tis [*mammilla;* G. *-itis,* inflammation]. Inflammation of the mammilla, or nipple. Syn., *thelitis.*

mam"mil·lo·tha·lam'ic [*mammilla;* G. *thalamos,* chamber]. Connecting the mammillary body with the thalamus, as the mammillothalamic tract.

mam·mi'tis. See *mastitis.*

mam'mo·gen [L. *mamma,* breast; G. *genesthai,* from *gignesthai,* to be produced]. Old term for prolactin: also called *mammogenic hormone.* —**mammogen'ic,** *adj.*

mam·mog'ra·phy [*mamma;* G. *graphein,* to write]. Radiographic examination of the breast; performed after injecting the ducts of the mammary gland with an opaque contrast medium.

mam'mose (mam'ohss, ma·mohss') [*mamma*]. Having full or abnormally large breasts.

mam·mot'o·my [*mamma;* G. *tomē,* a cutting]. Mastotomy.

mam"mo·tro'pin [*mamma;* G. *tropos,* turning]. Prolactin: formerly spelled *mammotrophin.*

mam"mo·tro'phin. See *mammotropin.*

mam·pir'ra. A tiny ceratopogon midge of the tropics which causes urticaria and subjective symptoms of burning pruritus. Syn. *merutu.*

man. 1. *Homo sapiens;* the human race, mankind. 2. A male human being.

man'a·ca [Brazilian]. The dried root of *Brunfelsia hopeana.* Has been used as an antisyphilitic, diuretic, and cathartic.

man·cha'da. See Lucio *leprosy.*

Manchester operation. See under W. E. *Fothergill.*

Mancke's test. See insulin-glucose-water tolerance *test,* also called *Althausen-Mancke's test.*

man·da'mon. See *ammonium* mandelate.

M & B 693. A manufacturer's designation for sulfapyridine.

Mandelbaum, Maier (1881–1947). German physician who described filamentation of bacteria which is also called *Mandelbaum's reaction.*

man·del'ic ac'id (man·del'ick, ·dee'lick) (*acidum mandelicum*). $C_6H_5CH(OH)COOH$. Alpha-hydroxyphenylacetic acid, occurring as white crystals or powder; 1 Gm. dissolves in about 6.5 cc. of water. Employed, chiefly in the form of one of its salts, as a urinary antiseptic; for maximum efficiency the pH of the urine should be below 5.5. Dose, 2–4 Gm. (30–60 gr.). Also called *amygdalic acid, inactive mandelic acid, racemic mandelic acid.*

man·del"o·ni'trile. $C_6H_5.CH(CN).OH$; mandelic acid nitrile or benzaldehyde cyanhydrin, capable of existing in optically active and racemic forms. Hydrolysis of the racemic substance yields mandelic acid.

m. glucoside. $C_6H_5CH(CN).O.C_6H_{11}O_5$; a glucoside, existing in various plants in three isomeric forms, designated *d*-mandelonitrile glucoside (sambunigrin), *l*-mandelonitrile glucoside (prunasin), and *dl*-mandelonitrile glucoside (prulaurasin). On hydrolysis all three give D-glucose as the sugar, and *d*-mandelonitrile, *l*-mandelonitrile, and *dl*-mandelonitrile, respectively, as the aglycone.

man'di·ble, man·dib'u·la [L. *mandibula,* jaw]. The lower jawbone. See Plate 1. See Table of Bones in the Appendix. —**mandib'ular,** *adj.*

man·dib"u·lo·glos'sus. A variant portion of the genioglossus muscle extending from the posterior border of the mandible to the side of the tongue.

man·dib"u·lo·mar"gin·al'is. A variant part of the platysma muscle extending from the mastoid process forward over the angle of the mandible.

man"di·o'ca. See *manioc.*

Mandl, Felix (1892–). Austrian surgeon who, with F. Brunn, introduced the method of treating angina pectoris by the injection of alcohol into the sympathetic trunk (1924). He relieved osteitis fibrosa generalisata by extirpation of a parathyroid tumor (1925), and introduced infiltration of the frontal lobes instead of operation for intractable pain (1950).

Mandler fil'ter. See under *filter.*

Man·drag'o·ra [G. *mandragoras,* mandrake]. The mandrake. A genus of solanaceous plants. **M. officinarum** has been used as a narcotic and hypnotic; contains an alkaloid, mandragorine.

man·drag'o·rine (man·drag'o·reen, ·rin). A poisonous alkaloid from *Mandragora* resembling atropine in action.

man'drake [ME., from *mandragoras*]. Common name for *Mandragora.*

man'drin [F.]. A guide or stylet.

man"du·ca'tion [L. *manducatio,* from *manducare,* to chew]. The chewing or mastication of food. —**man'ducatory,** *adj.*

ma·neu'ver [F. *manoeuvre,* from L. *manu operari,* to work by hand]. Skillful procedure or manual method.

Jendrassik's m. A method used in neurological examination to facilitate testing of a peripheral reflex, wherein the patient is asked to interlink his hands and pull them apart at time of testing.

Prague m. Delivery of the after-coming head by

grasping the shoulders from below with two fingers of one hand, while the other hand draws the feet up over the abdomen of the mother.

ma·neu′ver. To manipulate.

manexin. Trade-mark for *mannitol hexanitrate.*

man′ga·nese (mang′guh·niece, ·neez, man′guh·) [It., from ML. *magnesia*]. Mn = 54.94. A brittle, hard, grayish-white metal resembling iron in its properties. Manganese salts are extensively used in medicine, but proof of their value is lacking.

m. butyrate. $Mn(C_4H_7O_2)_2$. A red, water-soluble powder; aqueous solutions have been administered intramuscularly in the treatment of furunculosis.

m. dioxide. MnO_2. A black powder, insoluble in water; has been used in treatment of amenorrhea, syphilis, and various skin diseases.

m. glycerophosphate (*mangani glycerophosphas*). $MnC_3H_5(OH)_2PO_4$. A white or pinkish-white powder, slightly soluble in water; has been used in neurasthenia.

m. hypophosphite (*mangani hypophosphis*). $Mn(PH_2O_2)_2.H_2O$. A pink, crystalline powder, soluble in water; has been used as a hematinic.

m. iodide. $MnI_2.4H_2O$. A yellowish-brown powder, soluble in water; has been given in the anemias of tuberculosis and syphilis. Dose, 0.12–0.25 Gm. (2–4 gr.).

m. peptonate. A brown powder, soluble in water, representing about 3% manganese; used in the treatment of anemias.

m. sulfate. $MnSO_4.4H_2O$; pale pink crystal, soluble in water; has been used as a cholagogue and in treating anemias.

soluble m. citrate (*mangani citras solubilis*). Manganese citrate. $[C_3H_4.OH.(COO)_3]Mn_3$; rendered soluble by the presence of sodium citrate; has been used as a tonic.

man·gan′ic (man·gan′ick, mang·gan′ick). Referring to manganese when it has a valence of four.

man′ga·nous (mang′guh·nus, man′guh·nus). Referring to manganese when it has a valence of two.

mange (mayndj) [ME. *manjewe;* cf. F. *manger*, to eat]. Infestation of the skin of mammals by mange mites which burrow into the epidermal layer of the skin; characterized by multiple lesions in the skin with vesiculation and papule formation accompanied by intense itching.

follicular m. That form produced by the *Demodex folliculorum* which parasitizes the hair follicles or sebaceous glands of man and domestic animals.

sarcoptic m. The form most common to man, caused by the *Sarcoptes scabiei.* See *scabies.*

man′go (mang′go) [Pg. *manga*, from Tamil *mānkāy*]. The fruit of *Mangifera indica;* the seeds have been used as an anthelmintic; and the bark has been used as an astringent and tonic to the mucous membranes.

man′go·steen (mang′go·steen). 1. Fruit of *Garcinia mangostana.* 2. $C_{10}H_{22}O_5$. A crystalline, bitter principle found in the pericarp of *Garcinia mangostana.*

ma′ni·a [G., madness]. 1. Excessive enthusiasm or excitement; a violent desire or passion. 2. A psychotic disorder. See manic depressive *reaction.* —**man′ic, ma′nic,** *adj.;* **maniac,** *n.*

Bell's m. Acute manic excitement.

brooding m. A morbid mental state characterized by an impulse to prolonged and anxious meditation.

histrionic m. Mania in which the patient assumes a dramatic manner, playing the role of an actor. *Obs.*

m. à potu. See pathologic *intoxication.*

periodic m. A succession of manic attacks. Also called *recurrent m.*

puerperal m. See puerperal *psychosis.*

transitory m. A form characterized by sudden onset and short duration (one hour to a few days).

man′ic-depres′sive re·ac′tion. See under *reaction.*

Man′i·hot [F., of Tupian origin]. A genus of the Euphorbiaceae; yields cassava.

man′i·kin [D. *manneken*, dim. from *man*, man]. 1. A model of the body; made of plaster, papier-mâché, or other material, and showing, by means of movable parts, the relations of the organs. 2. A model of a term fetus; used for the teaching of obstetrics. 3. A little man with normal proportion of parts; a dwarf; a homunculus.

man′i·oc, ma′ni·oc [F., of Tupian origin]. The cassava plant or its product, tapioca. See *Manihot.*

man′i·ple [L. *manipulus*, handful]. A handful. *Obs.*

ma·nip″u·la′tion [*manipulus*]. The use of the hands in a skillful manner, as reducing a dislocation, returning a hernia into its cavity, or changing the position of a fetus.

conjoined m. The use of both hands in obstetric or gynecologic procedure, one being in the vagina and the other on the abdomen.

Mann, Frank Charles (1887–). American physiologist and surgeon who, with Carl S. Williamson, produced an experimental peptic ulcer in dogs, called Mann-Williamson *ulcer.* With Jesse L. Bollman, he introduced an intestinal fistula in animal experimentation, called Mann-Bollman *fistula.*

Mann, John Dixon [*English physician*, 1840–1912]. Described disturbance of the normal muscle balance in the two orbits, so that one eye appears to be on a lower level than the other, in exophthalmic goiter. Called *Mann's sign.*

Mann, Ludwig [*German neurologist*, 1866–1936]. Described spastic hemiplegia of the extremities; in the *Wernicke-Mann type* of paralysis some groups of muscles are relatively less affected than others.

Mann's eosin-methyl blue stain. See under *stain.*

man′na [G., from the Hebrew]. The concrete, saccharine exudation of the flowering ash, *Fraxinus ornus.* A mild laxative; contains a sweet principle, mannite or mannitol, sugar, mucilage, and resin. Some specimens also contain a glycoside (fraxin).

m. sugar. Mannitol.

man′nan. See *mannosan.*

man″ni·no·tri′ose. A trisaccharide occurring in manna; on hydrolysis it yields one molecule of glucose and two of galactose.

man′ni·tan. $C_6H_{12}O_6$. A sweet, syrupy substance, the anhydride of mannitol.

man′nite. See *mannitol.*

man′ni·tol. $CH_2OH.HOCH.HOCH.HCOH.HCOH.CH_2OH$; D-mannitol; a hexahydric alcohol from manna and other plant sources, occurring as colorless crystals, freely soluble in water: sometimes used to measure the rate of glomerular filtration, and as an irrigating fluid in transurethral resection of the prostate; in pharmacy used as a diluent and excipient. Syn., *manna sugar, mannite.*

m. hexanitrate. $C_6H_8(O.NO_2)_6$; an ester formed by nitration of mannitol, occurring as explosive, colorless crystals, insoluble in water. It is supplied only in admixture with carbohydrates to render it nonexplosive. It exerts the vasodilator action of nitrite ion, acting within 15 to 30 minutes and remaining effective for 4 to 6 hours. Syn., *nitromannite, nitromannitol.* See *manexin, maxitate, nitranitol.*

man′ni·tose. See *mannose.*

man″no·car′o·lose. A polysaccharide of unique structure, synthesized by the mold *Penicillium charlesii*, consisting only of mannose residues.

man″no·ke″to·hep′tose. $CH_2HO.CO.(CHOH)_4.$-CH_2OH. A polysaccharide obtained from the avocado pear, *Persea gratissima.*

man·non′ic ac′id (ma·non′ick, ma·no′nick). CH_2-$OH(CHOH)_4COOH$. An acid derived by the oxidation of mannitol.

man″no·sac·char′ic ac′id. COOH.HOCH.-HOCH.HCOH.HCOH.COOH; the saccharic acid produced when both the aldehyde and primary alcohol groups of mannose are oxidized.

man′no·san. A polysaccharide, occurring in plants, which upon hydrolysis yields mannose. Sometimes called *mannan.*

man′nose. $C_6H_{12}O_6$. A fermentable monosaccharide obtained from manna. Occurs in two optically active forms.

man″no·tet′rose. Stachyose.

man″no·tri′ose. A trisaccharide having two molecules of galactose and one of glucose as the constituent monosaccharides, formed by partial hydrolysis of mannotetrose.

man″nu·ron′ic ac′id. CHO.HOCH.HOCH.-HCOH.HCOH.COOH; D-mannuronic acid; the uronic acid resulting when the primary alcohol group of mannose is oxidized to carboxyl.

ma·nom′e·ter [G. *manos,* rare; *metron,* a measure]. An instrument for measuring the pressure of liquids and gases. —**manomet′ric,** *adj.*

Hamilton m. A very accurate optical manometer which measures arterial pressure.

optical m. Device for the accurate registration of the details of pressure pulses, in which pressure changes are led through a rigid, fluid-filled system to a tense rubber or metallic membrane on which is mounted a small mirror. The deflections of a beam of light reflected from this mirror are recorded on moving photographic paper.

man″o·met′ric flames. Flames of different heights and characters seen in a rotating mirror and due to the reflection of a pulsating gas flame, when the supplying gas is set in motion by sound waves.

man·om′e·try. Use of manometers.

Cartesian diver m. That using a micromanometric technique for the gasometric determination of isolated enzymes and the metabolic activity of minute quantities of tissue.

man′o·scope [*manos;* G. *skopein,* to examine]. An instrument for measuring the density of gases.

Manson, Patrick [*Scottish physician and parasitologist,* 1844–1922]. Sometimes called the father of tropical medicine. Demonstrated that the mosquito *Culex fatigans* serves as intermediate host to the parasite which causes elephantiasis (1879); this is said to be the first report of an invertebrate vector in a disease of man. Studied intestinal schistosomiasis, also called *Manson's disease.* The blood fluke causing the disease is called *Schistosoma mansoni.*

Man″so·nel′la [NL., after *Manson*]. A genus of filarial worms transmitted to man by mosquitoes of the genus *Culicoides.*

M. ozzardi. A species which infests man but produces little tissue reaction.

Man·so′ni·a. A genus of mosquitoes which are important as vectors of human disease. Species of *Mansonia* subgenus *Mansonioides* are the principal carriers of *Wuchereria malayi,* and also are carriers of *Wuchereria bancrofti.*

man′tle [L. *mantellum,* mantle]. 1. Old term for that portion of the brain substance including the convolutions, corpus callosum, and fornix. 2. A mantle layer. See under *layer.*

Mantoux, Charles [*French physician,* 1877–1947]. Introduced intradermal injections of tuberculin as a test for hypersensitivity (1908). The method was introduced independently in the same year by Felix Mendel. Called *Mantoux test, Mendel's test.* Originally dilutions of old tuberculin were used, but today the term *Mantoux test* refers also to the intradermal injection of PPD (purified protein derivative) of the *Mycobacterium tuberculosis.*

ma·nu′bri·um [L., that which is grasped in the hand]. 1. A handle. 2. The first or upper piece of the sternum. —**manubrial,** *adj.*

m. of malleus. The handle-shaped process of the malleus of the ear.

man″u·duc′tion [L. *manus,* hand; *ducere,* to lead]. Operation performed by the hands in surgical and obstetric practice.

man″u·dy″na·mom′e·ter [*manus;* G. *dynamis,* power; *metron,* a measure]. An instrument which measures the force exerted by the thrust of an instrument.

ma′nus [L.]. The hand.

m. cava. Excessive concavity of the palm of the hand.

m. curta. Clubhand.

m. extensa. Clubhand with a backward deviation.

m. flexa. Clubhand with a forward deviation.

m. valga. Clubhand with ulnar deviation.

m. vara. Clubhand with radial deviation.

man″u·stu·pra′tion. Masturbation.

man′y·plies (men′ee·plize) [E. *many;* plural of *-ply,* fold]. The third compartment in the stomach of ruminants. See *omasum, psalterium.*

Manz, Wilhelm [*German ophthalmologist,* 1833–1911]. Described glandlike depressions in the ocular conjunctiva near the margin of the cornea. *Manz's utricular glands* are now thought to be simple epithelial invaginations.

mapharsen. Trade-mark for oxophenarsine hydrochloride crystallized with half a molecule of alcohol.

Maragliano, Edoardo [*Italian physician,* 1849–1940]. Introduced *Maragliano's serum* for the treatment of tuberculosis. Described areas of degeneration seen in red blood cells after exposure to air; called *Maragliano's degeneration.*

Ma·ran′ta. See *arrowroot.*

ma·ran′tic [G. *marantikos,* wasting away]. 1. Pertaining to marasmus. 2. Pertaining to slowed circulation.

ma·ras′mic ac′id. An antibiotic substance elaborated by the Basidiomycetes fungus *Marasmius conigenus,* active in vitro against a variety of organisms.

ma·ras′mus (ma·raz′mus) [G., a withering]. A gradual wasting of the tissues of the body from insufficient, imperfect food supply, or from poor absorption of a good food supply. —**marasmic, marasmoid,** *adj.*

mar′ble bones. See *osteopetrosis.*

mar″ble·i·za′tion [G. *marmaros,* marble]. The condition of being marked or veined like marble.

Marburg, Otto (1874–1948). Austrian neuroanatomist, known for his work on multiple sclerosis, malformations, diseases and injuries of the nervous system, and the neurology of the ear.

marc (mark, mar) [F., from *marcher,* to trample]. The residue remaining after the extraction of the active principles from a vegetable drug, or after the extraction of the juice or oil from fruits.

Marchand, Felix Jacob [*German pathologist,* 1846–1928]. Described the accessory adrenal bodies found in the broad ligament; called *Marchand's adrenals.*

march col·lec′ting post. *In military medicine,* a location on the route of march at which casualties who cannot continue to march are given medical treatment and moved to medical stations in the rear.

marche′-à-pet·it-pas, (marsh′ah·pet·i·pah′) [F.

a walk with little steps]. A shuffling gait, with no swing of the arms and rigid movement of the whole body, often seen in arteriosclerotic parkinsonism.

march foot. See march *fracture.*

Marchi, Vittorio (1851–1908). Italian neurohistologist who contributed greatly to neurohistology and the study of secondary degeneration of nerves by showing that products formed in degenerating myelin sheaths could be stained specifically by osmic acid after mordanting with a chromic salt. See *Marchi's method* under *stain.*

Marchiafava, Ettore (1847–1935). Italian pathologist who established the life cycle of *Plasmodium falciparum,* first described syphilitic cerebral arteritis (1877), and was first to observe primary degeneration of the corpus callosum in alcoholic patients (*Marchiafava's disease*). Nocturnal hemoglobinuria is known as *Marchiafava-Micheli syndrome.*

Marckwald, Max [*German surgeon,* 1844–1923]. Devised an operation in which he removed two wedge-shaped sections of the vaginal portion of the cervix uteri, for the relief of stenosis of the external uterine os; called *Marckwald's operation.*

mar'cor. Marasmus.

Maresch stain. See *Bielschowsky-Maresch diammine silver solution* under *stain.*

Marey, Étienne Jules [*French physiologist,* 1830–1904]. Inventor of the sphygmograph. Contributed to the knowledge of the circulation. *Marey's law* states that the heart rate is inversely related to pressure in the aortic arch and carotid sinus; increase in pressure produces cardiac slowing; decrease in pressure, acceleration: also called *Marey's reflex.*

Marfan, Antonin Bernard Jean [*French pediatrician,* 1858–1942]. Described progressive spastic paraplegia in children with hereditary syphilis; called *Marfan's disease.* Described arachnodactyly, unusual flexibility of the joints, and subluxation of the crystalline lens, often associated with spina bifida occulta; called *Marfan's syndrome.*

mar'fa·nil. 4-Amino-2-methylbenzenesulfonamide, or α-amino-*p*-toluenesulfonamide, or benzylaminesulfonamide, effective against organisms made resistant to other sulfonamides but more toxic than the latter. It is not antagonized by *p*-aminobenzoic acid. In the form of the hydrochloride it appears to be superior to other sulfonamides for local chemotherapy. Also called *homosulfanilamide* and *mesudin.* See *sulfamylon.*

mar'ga·rate. A salt or ester of margaric acid.

mar·gar'ic ac'id. $CH_3(CH_2)_{15}COOH$; a synthetic fatty acid. Mixtures of stearic and palmitic acids have erroneously been called by the same name.

mar'ga·rin. The glyceryl ester of margaric acid, $C_3H_5(C_{17}H_{33}O_2)_3$.

m.-needles. Fatty crystals found in putrid bronchitis and pulmonary gangrene.

mar''ga·ri·to'ma [G. *margaron,* pearl; *-ōma,* tumor]. A true primary cholesteatoma formation in the auditory canal. *Obs.*

Mar·gar'o·pus an''nu·la'tus. Synonym for *Boophilus annulatus.*

mar'gin [L. *margo,* edge]. The boundary or edge of a surface. **—marginal,** *adj.*

falciform m. The sharp, crescentic, lateral boundary of the fossa ovalis of the femoral triangle.

gingival m. The more or less rounded crest of the gingiva at the neck of a tooth. Syn., *gum margin.*

mar''gi·na'tion [*margo*]. Adhesion of leukocytes to the walls of capillaries in the early stage of inflammation.

mar'gi·no·plas''ty [*margo;* G. *plassein,* to form]. Plastic surgery of the marginal portion of the eyelid.

mar'go (pl. *margines*). Margin.

Marie, Pierre [*French neurologist,* 1853–1940]. Described acromegaly (1886), also called *Marie's syndrome.* With Charcot, described the peroneal form of progressive neuropathic muscular atrophy (1886), called *Charcot-Marie-Tooth disease* or *type.* Described hypertrophic pulmonary osteoarthropathy (1890), called *Marie-Bamberger disease,* and hereditary cerebellar sclerosis (1893) called *Marie's ataxia.* Ankylosing spondylitis (1898) is known as *Marie-Strümpell arthritis* or *Strümpell-Marie disease.* Hysterical glossolabial hemispasm is called *Brissaud-Marie syndrome.*

ma''ri·hua'na (mah''ri·hwah'nuh). See *cannabis.*

Marinesco, Georges (1864–1938). Rumanian pathologist who first used x-rays in the study of bone changes in acromegaly, studied degeneration of nerve cells and coined the term *chromatolysis* (1909). First to destroy the pituitary of dogs by cautery (1892), he was able to maintain his hypophysectomized animals alive for over two weeks. He also made many contributions to the knowledge of hereditary and familial diseases affecting the central nervous system. The name is also spelled *Marinescu.*

Mariotte, Edme [*French scientist,* 1620–84]. Made many contributions to the knowledge of physics and of the anatomy of the eye. Is credited with discovering the macula lutea. See also blind *spot* of Mariotte. Boyle's law is also known as *Mariotte's law;* see under Robert *Boyle.*

Marjolin's ulcer. See under *ulcer.*

mar'jo·ram [ME. *majoran*]. **Sweet marjoram,** *Majorana hortensis* of the Lamiaceae, is widely cultivated as a seasoning herb. Its chief constituent is a volatile oil containing camphor and borneol. **Wild marjoram** or origanum consists of the dried leaves and flowering top of *Origanum vulgare.* Possesses a volatile oil containing carvacrol and thymol. Several other species are used to produce oils that have been used in veterinary liniments and in microscopical technic.

mark [AS. *mearc,* cf. L. *margo,* edge]. Birthmark, a nevus.

port-wine m. See port-wine *nevus.*

Markee, Joseph Eldridge [*American anatomist,* 1904–]. Known for his studies of menstruation and uterine circulation as observed by means of intraocular transplants of endometrium. Described rhythmic, hormonally controlled phases of circulation in the endometrium; called the blush-and-blanch phenomenon.

Marriott method (for alkali reserve: alveolar carbon dioxide tension). See under *method.*

mar'row [ME. *marowe,* from AS. *mearg*]. The soft tissues contained in the medullary canals of long bones and in the interstices of cancellous bone.

hematopoietic m. See red *m.*

primary m. The embryonic marrow, before it becomes hematopoietic.

red m. Marrow of all bones in early life and of restricted locations in adulthood in which active formation of blood cells (hematopoiesis) is taking place. Syn., *myeloid tissue.*

spinal m. Old term for the spinal cord.

yellow m. Marrow which has lost its hematopoietic function and become largely replaced by fat cells.

mar·ru'bi·in (ma·rōō'bee·in) [L. *marrubium,* horehound]. The crystalline, neutral, bitter substance found in horehound.

mar·ru'bi·um (ma·rōō'bee·um) [L.]. Horehound. The dried leaves and tops of *Marrubium vulgare* of the Lamiaceae. Contains a volatile oil, a bitter principle (marrubiin), tannin, resin, and lignin. Used mainly in the form of candy or syrup for relieving sore throat.

Marsh's test. See under *test.*

Marshall, Eli Kennerly, Jr. [*American pharmacologist,* 1889–]. With A. C. Bratton, J. T. Litchfield, and H. J. White, introduced sulfaguanidine in the treatment of intestinal infections. With Bratton, L. B. Edwards, and E. Walker, introduced this treatment for acute bacillary dysentery in children (1941). See also Bratton and Marshall's *method* for determining concentrations of sulfonamides in blood and urine.

Marshall, John [*English surgeon and anatomist,* 1818–91]. Described a fold of the pericardium, between the left pulmonary artery and the left superior pulmonary vein, enclosing the fibrous remnant of part of the left common cardinal vein; called *ligament of the left vena cava, vestigial fold of Marshall.* This joins the oblique vein of the left atrium; see oblique *vein* of Marshall.

Marshall method. See Lyle-Curtman-Marshall *method.*

Marshall and Welker method. See under *method.*

marsh gas. The gaseous products, chiefly methane, formed from decaying, moist organic matter in marshes and mines.

marsh'mal"low. See *althea.*

marsilid. Trade-mark for iproniazid, an antituberculosis drug having the composition of 1-isonicotinyl-2-isopropyl hydrazine.

Marston, William Moulton [*American psychologist,* 1893–1947]. Introduced a systolic blood pressure test called *lie detector test, Marston deception test.*

mar·su"pi·al·i·za'tion [G. *marsippion,* little bag]. An operation for retention, degeneration, and parasitic cysts (such as hydatid, pancreatic, etc.) when extirpation of the cyst walls and complete closure are not possible. The cyst is evacuated and the walls sutured to the edges of the wound, leaving the packed cavity to close by granulation. The procedure has been used also in cases of extrauterine pregnancy when the placenta cannot be removed.

Martin, August Eduard [*German gynecologist,* 1847–1933]. Devised an operation of hysterectomy by the vaginal route; called *Martin's operation.*

Martin, Henry Newell [*American physiologist,* 1848–96]. Isolated the mammalian heart in a perfusion chamber (1881). With Edward Mussey Hartwell, demonstrated the function of the intercostal muscles in respiration.

Martinotti, Giovanni [*Italian pathologist,* 1857–1928]. Described nerve cells in the cerebral cortex with axons running toward the surface and ramifying horizontally; called *Martinotti's cells.*

Mar'ti·us yel'low (mahr'shus, ·shee·us) (C.C.). An acid nitro dye used as a stain and in preparing certain light filters for photomicrography. Also called *Manchester yellow, naphthol yellow.*

Marwedel, Georg [*German surgeon,* contemporary]. Devised a method of gastrostomy similar to Witzel's; called *Marwedel's operation.*

M + As. Symbol for compound myopic astigmatism.

mas'cu·line [L. *masculus,* male]. Having the qualities of a male. —**masculin'ity,** *n.*

mas"cu·lin·i·za'tion [*masculus*]. The induction of male secondary sex characteristics in a female or sexually immature animal.

mas"cu·lin·o'ma. See adrenocorticoid *adenoma* of ovary.

mas"cu·lin·o"vo·blas·to'ma. See adrenocorticoid *adenoma* of ovary.

mask [F. *masque,* from Ar. *maskharah,* buffoon]. 1. A bandage applied to the face. 2. The characteristic expressionless facies seen in certain pathologic conditions, notably paralysis agitans. 3. A gauze shield, fitted with tapes, to enclose the mouth and nose during surgical operations. 4. An apparatus for covering the nose and mouth in giving anesthetics.

Boothby-Lovelace m. A mask used in the administration of oxygen.

death m. A plaster of Paris mold of a dead person's face, taken soon after death.

ecchymotic m. The cyanotic facies of traumatic asphyxia.

m. of pregnancy. Irregularly shaped, yellowish patches of varying size which frequently appear on the face and neck during pregnancy.

parkinsonian m. See James *Parkinson,* and *parkinsonism.*

mask'ing [*maskharah*]. The interference of a given tone with the perception of other tones.

mas'o·chism" (maz'o·kiz"um, mass'o·) [after Leopold von Sacher-*Masoch,* Austrian novelist, 1836–95]. A sexual perversion in which pleasure is obtained in receiving cruel treatment, pain, and humiliation. —**masochist,** *n.*

Mason, James Tate [*American surgeon,* 1882–1936]. Introduced an incision permitting adequate exposure of any part of the upper abdomen, while protecting the nerve supply of the rectus muscles. *Mason's incision* begins below and to the left of the xiphoid process and extends downward along the left rectus to a point about one inch above the umbilicus, then across the midline to the right rectus, then downward along that muscle for one and one-half to two inches. Incisions in the muscle sheaths are connected transversely in a pattern following that of the skin incision. The muscles are then rolled outward, and the peritoneum is opened under the left rectus and transversely just above the umbilicus.

masque bil·i·are'. A condition, found more often in women, involving development of excess pigment in the eyelids: also called *periocular hyperpigmentation.*

mass [L. *massa,* from G. *maza,* barley-cake]. 1. An aggregation of particles of matter characterized by inertia. Abbreviated, M. 2. A cohesive substance that may be formed into pills.

atomic m. Mass of an element measured on an arbitrary scale and expressed relatively to mass 16 for oxygen. Also called *atomic weight.*

cell m. See *cell mass.*

epithelial m. The internal mass of cells derived from and covered by the germinal epithelium of the indifferent gonad.

ferrous carbonate m. (*massa ferri carbonatis*). Contains 36–41% $FeCO_3$; used in treating simple anemia and chlorosis. Dose, 0.3–1.0 Gm. (5–15 gr.). Also called *Vallet's m.*

interfilar m. Hyaloplasm.

m. defect. The difference between the mass number of an atom and the mass determined by a mass spectrograph; energy equivalent to the mass defect is considered to be the binding energy of the atom.

m. number. The whole number nearest the atomic weight of a given atomic species; the total number of nucleons (protons and neutrons) in the nucleus of the atom described.

mercury m. (*massa hydrargyri*). Contains 31–35% of mercury; used as an alterative and laxative. Dose, as an alterative, 0.06–0.2 Gm. (1–3 gr.); as a laxative, 0.3–1.0 Gm. (5–15 gr.). Also called *blue m., blue pill.*

Massa, Nicolo [*Italian physician,* d. 1569]. Described the neurologic effects of syphilis (1532).

mas·sage′ [F., from L. *massa*, mass]. The act of rubbing, kneading, or stroking the superficial parts of the body with the hand or with an instrument, for the purpose of modifying nutrition, restoring power of movement, breaking up adhesions, etc.

buttonhole method of cardiac m. A means of resuscitation after the heart has stopped beating. A buttonhole incision is made just below the xiphoid process, between the attachments of the two sides of the diaphragm; and the thumb of the right hand is thrust through the opening. The heart can then be compressed between the thumb, within the pericardium, and the fingers, beneath the diaphragm.

cardiac m. Manual massage of the heart in cases of cardiac standstill or ventricular fibrillation.

electrovibratory m. That performed by means of an electric vibrator.

vibratory m. Light, rapid percussion either by hand or by an electric apparatus.

mas′sa in″ter·me′di·a [BNA]. A mass of gray matter which joins the surfaces of the adjacent thalami across the third ventricle. It has no functional significance and is absent in over half of brains examined. See Plate 18.

mas·se′ter [G. *masētēr*, chewer]. A muscle of mastication, arising from the zygomatic arch, and inserted into the mandible. See Table of Muscles in the Appendix. —**masseter′ic,** *adj.*

mas·seur′ (mas·sur′. *See* NOTES § 35) [F.]. 1. A man who practices massage. 2. An instrument used for mechanical massage.

mas·seuse′ (mas·suz′. *See* NOTES § 35) [F.]. A woman who practices massage.

mas′si·cot. PbO. Lead oxide; litharge.

Massol, Léon [*Swiss bacteriologist*, 1837–1909]. *Lactobacillus bulgaricus* is known as *Massol's bacillus*.

Masson's trichrome stain. See under *stain*.

mas″so·ther′a·py [L. *massa*, mass; G. *therapeia*, treatment]. Treatment by massage.

mast″ad·e·ni′tis [G. *mastos*, breast; *adēn*, gland; *-itis*, inflammation]. Mastitis.

mast″ad·e·no′ma [*mastos;* G. *adēn*, gland; *-ōma*, tumor]. A glandular tumor of the breast.

mas·tal′gi·a [*mastos;* G. *algos*, pain]. Pain in the breast.

mast″a·tro′phi·a, mast·at′ro·phy [*mastos;* G. *atrophia*, want of food]. Atrophy of the breast.

mas·taux′y (mas·tawk′see) [*mastos;* G. *auxē*, growth]. Increase in size, or excessive size, of the breast.

mas·tec″chy·mo′sis (mas·teck″i·mo′sis) [*mastos;* G. *ek*, out of; *chymos*, juice; *-ōsis*, condition]. Ecchymosis of the breast.

mas·tec′to·my [*mastos;* G. *ektomē*, excision]. Excision, or amputation, of the breast.

radical m. Surgical removal of the entire breast and also of adjacent tissue, including the pectoralis minor muscle, part or all of the pectoralis major muscle, and all the lymphatic tissue of chest wall and axilla.

simple m. Surgical removal of the breast only.

mast″hel·co′sis [*mastos;* G. *helkosis*, ulceration]. Ulceration of the breast.

mas′tic [G. *mastichē*, mastic]. The resin flowing from the incised bark of the *Pistacia lentiscus*. Formerly used as a styptic, as a filling for teeth, and as a varnish in microscopy.

mas″ti·ca′tion [L. *masticare*, to chew]. The act of chewing. —**mas′ticatory,** *adj.*

mas″ti·ca′tor. The motor portion of the fifth cranial nerve.

mas′ti·ca·to″ry [*masticare*]. A remedy to be chewed, but not swallowed; used for its local action in the mouth.

m. surface. The occlusal or biting surface of a tooth.

mas′ti·che (mass′ti·kee) [G. *mastichē*, mastic]. Old term for mastic.

Mas″ti·goph′o·ra [G. *mastix*, whip; *phoros*, bearing]. A class of flagellated protozoa which includes both free-living and parasitic species.

mastisol. Trade name of a mastic varnish; used in the treatment of wounds.

mas·ti′tis [G. *mastos*, breast; *-itis*, inflammation]. Inflammation of the breast.

carcinomatous m. See inflammatory *carcinoma*.

chronic cystic m. Any of various noninflammatory conditions of the breast, more properly called *mammary dysplasias*. See *adenosis, cystic disease, mastodynia*.

interstitial m. Inflammation of the connective tissue of the breast.

lactation m. Puerperal *m.*

parenchymatous m. Inflammation of the proper glandular substance of the breast.

puerperal m. A complication of the early puerperium, in which part or all of the breast becomes indurated from retention of milk and engorgement of the tissues. Syn., *lactation m.*

suppurative m. Inflammation of the breast with the formation of pus.

mas′to-, mast- [*mastos*]. 1. A combining form denoting *the breast*. 2. A combining form denoting *mastoid*.

mas″to·car″ci·no′ma [*mastos;* G. *karkinōma*, from *karkinos*, crab; *-ōma*, tumor]. Mammary carcinoma.

mas″to·de·al′gi·a [G. *mastoeidēs*, like a breast; *algos*, pain]. Pain in, or over, the mastoid process.

mas″to·dyn′i·a [G. *mastos*, breast; *odynē*, pain]. A condition affecting females, usually of low fertility between the ages of 25 to 40, clinically characterized by pain in one or both breasts which is more marked during the premenstrual period. Pain may be referred to an area that is tender, firmer, and more granular than the surrounding mammary tissue. There is imperfect lobular development and increase in periductal and intralobular stroma of the breast due to endocrine imbalance. Also called *mazoplasia, mastoplasia*.

mas′toid [G. *mastoeidēs*, like a breast]. Breast-shaped, as the mastoid process of the temporal bone.

mas′toid. The mastoid process of the temporal bone which is classified by surgeons into four types: **pneumatic m.,** one completely honeycombed with air spaces; **diploic m.,** one possessing marrow within the bony substance; **sclerotic m.,** one composed of almost solid bone; **mixed m.,** one in which solid bone, air sinuses and cells, and marrow are all found.

mas″toid·ec′to·my [*mastoeidēs;* G. *ektomē*, excision]. Exenteration of the mastoid air cells.

modified radical m. An operation for the removal of as many potentially infected cells as is possible without disturbing hearing; a simple mastoidectomy is performed, the epitympanic air cells are exenterated without disturbing the ossicular chain, the posterior wall is partially taken down, and the perilabyrinthine cells are cleaned out.

radical m. The complete exenteration of mastoid, epitympanic, perilabyrinthine, and tubal air cells. The tympanic membrane, ossicular chain, middle ear mucous membrane, stapedius muscle, and tensor tympani muscle are also removed.

simple m. Exenteration of the air cells in the

mastoid process alone, without disturbing those air cells in the epitympanic space, the external auditory canal, or the perilabyrinthine area.

mas″toid·i′tis [*mastoeidēs;* G. *-itis,* inflammation]. Inflammation of the mastoid air cells: formerly called *mastoid abscess.*

mas″toid·ot′o·my [*mastoeidēs;* G. *tomē,* a cutting]. Incision into mastoid air cells or the mastoid antrum.

mas·ton′cus [G. *mastos,* breast; *onkos,* tumor]. Any tumor of the mammary gland or nipple.

mas·top′a·thy [*mastos;* G. *pathos,* disease]. Any disease or pain of the mammary gland.

mas′to·pex″y [*mastos;* G. *pēxis,* a fixing]. Surgical fixation of a pendulous breast.

mas″to·pla′si·a (mas″to·play′zhuh, ·zee·uh, ·shuh, ·see·uh) [*mastos;* G. *plassein,* to form]. Hyperplasia of breast tissue. Also see *mastodynia.*

mas′to·plas″ty [*mastos; plassein*]. Plastic surgery on the breast.

mas″tor·rha′gi·a [*mastos;* G. *rhēgnynai,* to burst forth]. Hemorrhage from the breast.

mas″to·scir′rhus (mas″to·skirr′us, ·sirr′us) [*mastos;* G. *skiros,* hard]. Hardening, or scirrhus, of the breast; usually cancer.

mas·to′sis [*mastos;* G. *-ōsis,* increase]. Hypertrophy of the breast.

mas·tos′to·my [*mastos;* G. *stoma,* mouth]. Incision into the breast.

mas·tot′o·my [*mastos;* G. *tomē,* a cutting]. Incision of the breast.

mas′tous [*mastos*]. Having large breasts.

mas″tur·ba′tion [L. *masturbari,* to defile oneself]. Production of an orgasm by self-manipulation of the genitalia. Also called *self-abuse, chiromania.*

ma·su′ri·um (ma·sue′ree·um, ma·zue′·) [from *Masuria,* a region in East Prussia]. Ma, atomic number 43; an element reported in 1925, but its existence not established. Subsequently it was prepared artificially and in 1947 it was named *technetium.*

Matas, Rudolph [*American surgeon,* 1860–]. Devised a technic of endoaneurysmorrhaphy (1888), called *Matas' operation.*

ma·te′ri·a al′ba [L.]. A soft, cheeselike, white deposit on the necks of teeth and adjacent gums, made up of epithelial cells, leukocytes, bacteria, and molds.

ma·te′ri·a med′i·ca [L.]. The science that treats of the sources and preparations of the substances used in medicine.

ma·te′ri·es mor′bi (ma·teer′ee·eez mor′buy, mor′-bee) [L.]. The material that is the cause of a disease. *Obs.*

ma·ter′nal [L. *maternus,* of a mother]. Pertaining to the mother.

ma·ter′ni·ty [*maternus*]. 1. Motherhood. 2. A lying-in-hospital. *Colloquial.*

Mathews method. See under *method.*

ma·ti′co (ma·tee′ko) [Sp., dim. from *Mateo,* Matthew]. The leaves of *Piper angustifolium,* of the Piperaceae. Aromatic and stimulant; has been used as a local and general hemostatic and as an alterative stimulant to mucous membranes.

ma′ting [MLG. *māt,* companion]. The meeting of individuals for sexual reproduction.

random m. A system of breeding in which individuals mate in accordance with the frequency with which they occur in the population; as a first approximation, mating in any human population is of this type.

mat″la·za·hua′tl (mat″lah·zuh·what′ul. *See* NOTES § 35). A form of typhus fever found in Mexico; tabardillo.

mat″ri·ca′ri·a [L. *matrix,* womb]. German camomile; the flower tops of *Matricaria chamomilla,* of the order Compositae. Contains a volatile oil and a bitter principle; has been used as an aromatic bitter.

ma′trine. $C_{15}H_{24}N_2O$; an alkaloid, existing in several forms, occurring in several *Sophora* species, and isomeric with lupanine.

ma′trix, mat′rix [L.]. 1. A mold; the cavity in which anything is formed. 2. That part of tissue into which any organ or process is set, as the matrix of a nail. 3. The intercellular substance of a tissue, as of cartilage.

interterritorial m. The lighter-stained area which separates the areas of territorial matrix from each other in hyalin cartilage. See territorial *m.*

territorial m. Matrix in hyalin cartilage differentiated into regions of high basophilia surrounding smaller or larger groups of cells.

mat′ter [L. *materia,* matter, wood]. 1. Any material or substance, described as having three states of aggregation, solid, liquid, or gaseous. 2. Pus.

central gray m. See *substantia grisea centralis.*

gray m. The gray substance of the central nervous system. Also called *substantia grisea.*

suspended m. Solid particles, oils, etc., which are either insoluble or not dissolved in a liquid.

white m. The white substance of the central nervous system. Also called *substantia alba.*

Mattioli, Pier Andrea [*Italian physician,* ca. 1500–77]. Author of an encyclopedia of pharmacology which was standard during the Renaissance.

mat′u·rate [L. *maturare,* to make ripe]. Bring to maturity; to ripen, especially to bring a boil to a head; to suppurate.

mat″u·ra′tion [*maturare*]. 1. The process of coming to full development. 2. The final series of changes in the growth and formation of the germ cells. It includes two divisions of the cell body but only one division of the chromosomes, with the result that the number of chromosomes in the mature germ cell is reduced to one-half the original number. The term also includes the cytoplasmic changes which occur in the preparation of the germ cell for fertilization.

ma·ture′ [L. *maturus,* ripe]. To become ripe.

ma·ture′. Full-grown, ripe.

ma·tu′ri·ty [L. *maturitas,* maturity]. The state or quality of being mature; full growth and development.

ma·tu′ti·nal [L. *matutinalis,* of the morning]. Occurring in the morning, as matutinal nausea.

Mauchart, Burkhard David [*German anatomist,* 1696–1751]. Remembered for his description of the lateral or alar odontoid ligaments; also called *Mauchart's ligaments.*

Maunoir, Jean Pierre [*Swiss surgeon,* 1768–1861]. Devised an operation for the construction of an artificial pupil. Described a congenital lymphatic cyst of the neck; called *Maunoir's hydrocele.*

Mau′rer's dots (mow′rerz). See under *dot.*

Mauriceau, François [*French surgeon,* 1637–1709]. Made numerous contributions to the development of obstetrics. Refuted the theory that the pelvic bones separate in normal labor. Described brow presentation, strangulation by the umbilical cord, and tubal pregnancy.

Mauthner, Ludwig (1840–94). Bohemian ophthalmologist in Austria who described the axolemma, called *axolemma of Mauthner, Mauthner's sheath.*

max·il′la (pl. *maxillae, maxillas*) [L., jaw]. The bone of the upper jaw. See Plate 1. See Table of Bones in the Appendix. —**max′illary,** *adj.*

max·il″lo·fa′cial [*maxilla;* L. *facies,* face]. Pertaining to the lower half of the face. *In plastic surgery,* pertaining to a subdivision called maxillofacial surgery.

max·il"lo-fron·ta'le (-fron·tah'lee, -fron·tay'lee) [*maxilla;* L. *frons*, forehead]. The point where the anterior lacrimal crest or its prolongation meets the frontomaxillary suture.

max·il"lo·tur'bi·nal. See inferior nasal *concha* in Table of Bones in the Appendix.

max'i·mal [L. *maximus*, greatest]. Pertaining to the maximum; highest; greatest.

Maximow, Alexander A. (1874–1928). Russian-American histologist renowned for important investigations of inflammation and hematopoiesis, and of the normal and pathological histogenesis of connective tissues. For Maximow's method, see under *stain*.

max'i·mum (pl. *maxima*) [*maximus*]. The greatest possible degree or amount of anything; the highest point attained or attainable by anything.

maxitate. Trade-mark for *mannitol hexanitrate*.

Maxwell's law. See *law* of Maxwell.

May ap'ple. See *podophyllum*.

May-Grünwald stain. See under *stain*.

Maydl, Karel [*Bohemian surgeon*, 1853–1903]. Devised an operation in which the ureters are transplanted into the rectum, for exstrophy of the bladder, and one of colostomy, in which the unopened colon is held in place by means of a glass rod until adhesions have formed. Each technic is called *Maydl's operation*.

Mayer, Karl [*Austrian neurologist*, 1862–1932]. Described a reflex occurring in normal individuals but not in those with hemiplegia. When the extended middle finger is flexed against resistance, the thumb goes into a position of extension and opposition. Called *Mayer's reflex*.

Mayer, Paul [*German histologist*, 1848–1923]. Introduced a number of histological techniques. See Mayer's albumen *fixative*, *Mayer's acid carmine*, *Mayer's hemalum*, etc., under *stain*.

may'hem [ME. *maymen*]. *In legal medicine*, the offense of depriving a person, by violence, of any limb, member, or organ, or causing any mutilation of the body.

Mayo, Charles Horace [*American surgeon*, 1865–1939]. Cofounder, with W. J. Mayo, of the Mayo Clinic in Rochester, Minnesota. Devised an operation for hallux valgus in which the head of the first metatarsal is excised and the flap containing the bursa is turned inward and sutured in place. Introduced an operation for varicose veins in which the varicosities are stripped out by means of a special dissector. Each is known as *Mayo's operation*.

Mayo, William James [*American surgeon*, 1861–1939]. Cofounder, with C. H. Mayo, of the Mayo Clinic in Rochester, Minnesota. Devised an operation for umbilical hernia in which the aponeuroses of the abdominal muscles are overlapped, after excision of the sac. Devised technics of choledochoduodenostomy, of posterior gastrojejunostomy, and of excision of the rectum for carcinoma. Each of these is known as *Mayo's operation*.

Mayo-Robson, Arthur William [*English surgeon*, 1853–1933]. Described a point of extreme tenderness, above and to the right of the umbilicus, in gallbladder disease; called *Mayo-Robson's point*. Introduced a position of the patient to facilitate operations on the gallbladder and bile ducts; in *Mayo-Robson's* (or *Robson's*) *position*, the lumbar and lower costal regions are raised by means of a sandbag or a mechanical device. *Mayo-Robson's* (or *Robson's*) *incision* in operations on the biliary tract is made vertically over the middle of the right rectus muscle, and if necessary is extended upward parallel to the costal margin, between the costal margin and the xiphoid process.

ma·zal'gi·a (may·zal'juh, ·jee·uh) [G. *mazos*, breast; *algos*, pain]. Mastalgia, or mastodynia.

maze [ME.]. A network of paths, blind alleys, and compartments; used in intelligence tests and in experimental psychology for developing learning curves.

ma'zic [G. *maza*, barley cake]. Pertaining to the placenta. *Obs.*

ma"zo·ca·coth'e·sis [*maza;* G. *kakos*, bad; *thesis*, a placing]. Faulty implantation of the placenta.

ma"zo·dyn'i·a. See *mastodynia*.

ma"zo·i'tis. See *mastitis*.

ma·zol'y·sis (may·zol'i·sis) [*maza;* G. *lysis*, a loosing]. Separation of the placenta.

maz"o·mor'ro. A dermatosis associated with ancylostomiasis.

ma·zop'a·thy (may·zop'uth·ee) [*maza;* G. *pathos*, disease]. Any disease of the placenta.

ma·zop'a·thy (may·zop'uth·ee) [G. *mazos*, breast; *pathos*]. Mastopathy.

ma'zo·pex"y [*mazos;* G. *pēxis*, a fixing]. Surgical fixation of a pendulous breast; mastopexy.

ma"zo·pla'si·a (may"zo·play'zhuh). See *mastodynia*.

Mazzini, Louis Yolando [*American serologist*, 1894–   ]. Introduced a microscopic flocculation test for syphilis. In the *Mazzini test* the usual heart-muscle antigen is supplemented with powdered egg yolk, which supplies additional lecithin and thus renders the antigen more reactive with syphilitic serums.

Mazzoni, Vittorio. A contemporary Italian physician who described a sensory nerve-ending similar to Krause's corpuscle (1891), called *Mazzoni's corpuscle, Golgi-Mazzoni's corpuscle*.

M. B. *Medicinae Baccalaureus*, Bachelor of Medicine.

MBC Abbreviation for maximum breathing capacity.

M. C., M. Ch. *Magister Chirurgiae*, Master of Surgery.

mc Abbreviation for millicurie.

μc Abbreviation for microcurie.

mcg, mcg. United States Pharmacopeia abbreviation for microgram: also written μg.

MCH Mean corpuscular hemoglobin: an expression, in absolute terms, of the average content of hemoglobin of the individual erythrocyte, calculated from the equation

$$\text{MCH} = \frac{\text{hemoglobin [(gm/100 ml)} \times 10]}{\text{erythrocyte count } (10^6/\text{mm}^3)}$$

and stated in micromicrograms (10^{-12} gm) per cell. Normal values are 28–32 μμg.

MCHC Mean corpuscular hemoglobin concentration: an expression, in absolute terms, of the average hemoglobin concentration per unit volume (per 100 ml) of packed red cells, calculated from the equation

$$\text{MCHC} = \frac{\text{hemoglobin [(gm/100 ml)} \times 100]}{\text{hematocrit}}$$

and stated in grams per 100 ml of packed red cells. Normal values for adults are 32–36 gm/100 ml.

MCV Mean corpuscular volume: an expression, in absolute terms, of the average volume of the individual erythrocyte, calculated from the equation

$$\text{MCV} = \frac{\text{hematocrit (per cent)} \times 10}{\text{erythrocyte count } (10^6/\text{mm}^3)}$$

and stated in cubic microns per cell. Normal values are 82–92μ^3.

M. D. *Medicinae Doctor*, Doctor of Medicine.

M. D. S. Master of Dental Surgery.

mead'ow saf'fron. See *colchicum*.

mean. See *arithmetic mean; geometric mean*.

mean af'ter·life'time". See *expectation of life.*

mean cor·pus'cu·lar he"mo·glo'bin. See *MCH.*

mean cor·pus'cu·lar he"mo·glo'bin con"cen·tra'tion. See *MCHC.*

mean cor·pus'cu·lar vol'ume. See *MCV.*

mea'sles [ME. *masel*]. 1. An acute, infectious disease, characterized by a morbilliform eruption and by catarrhal inflammation of the conjunctiva and of the air passages. After a period of incubation of nearly two weeks, the disease begins with coryza, cough, conjunctivitis, and the appearance of Koplik spots on the oral mucous membranes; on the third or fourth day chills and fever and dusky rose-red, maculopapular eruption appear, arranged in the form of crescentic groups, at times becoming confluent, usually appearing first on the face or behind the ears. In three or four days, the eruption gradually fades, and is followed by a branny desquamation. The symptoms are worse at the height of the eruption. The disease affects principally the young, is exceedingly contagious, and one attack usually confers immunity. It is caused by a virus. 2. *In veterinary medicine*, a disease of hogs, cattle, and sheep, due to the presence in the body of the larval form of the *Taenia solium* and larvae of other tapeworms. 3. Cysticerci.

black m. A grave variety of measles in which the eruption is hemorrhagic and the constitutional symptoms are profound.

German m. See *rubella.*

hemorrhagic m. See black *m.*

m. vaccine. The measles virus is grown on fertile eggs of the hen, thus attenuating the infective agent; injected under the skin or placed in the nose, it causes a very mild form of measles in some individuals but causes no symptoms at all in others.

meas'ly. 1. Infected with measles; having or spotted with measles. 2. Containing encysted Trichinella: said of meat.

meas'ure [L. *mensura*, measure]. For units of measure, see Tables of Weights and Measures in the Appendix.

me"a·ti'tis [L. *meatus*, a passing; G. *-itis*, inflammation]. Inflammation of the wall of a meatus.

me·a'to- [L. *meatus*, a passing]. *In surgery*, a combining form signifying *meatus* or *opening.*

me"a·tot'o·my [*meatus;* G. *tomē*, a cutting]. Incision into and enlargement of a meatus.

me·a'tus [L.]. An opening or passage. —**meatal,** *adj.*

auditory m. See *m.* acusticus externus and *m.* acusticus internus.

m. acusticus externus. The external auditory canal extending from the concha to the tympanic membrane. See Plates 1, 3, 20.

m. acusticus internus. The internal auditory canal.

m. nasopharyngeus. The communication between the nasopharynx and the nasal cavity.

m. urethrae. The orifice of the urethra.

urinary m. See *m.* urethrae.

mebaral. A trade-mark for *mephobarbital.*

Mec'ca bal'sam. See Gilead *balsam.*

mech'a·nism [G. *mēchanikos*, from *mēchanē*, machine]. 1. An aggregation of parts arranged in a mechanical way to perform a specific function. 2. The manner in which a mechanical act is performed, as the mechanism of labor. See Plate 42.

trigger m. A region of anoxia in the heart muscle which sets off ventricular extrasystoles or ventricular fibrillation.

mech"a·no·ther'a·py (meck"uh·no·therr'uh·pee) [*mēchanē;* G. *therapeia*, treatment]. Treatment of injury or disease by mechanical means. —**mechanotherapist,** *n.*

me"chlor·eth'a·mine hy"dro·chlo'ride. National Formulary designation for the nitrogen mustard methyl bis(β-chloroethyl)amine hydrochloride or 2,2-dichloro-N-methyldiethylamine hydrochloride, a white, crystalline powder supplied as a trituration with 9 parts of sodium chloride (*sterile mechlorethamine hydrochloride trituration*). Syn., *mustine hydrochloride.* See *mustargen hydrochloride.*

mecholin. See *mecholyl chloride.*

mecholyl bromide. Trade-mark for acetyl-beta-methylcholine bromide.

mecholyl chloride. Trade-mark for acetyl-beta-methylcholine chloride. The substance is a white, hygroscopic, crystalline powder. Used in certain conditions in which the effects of parasympathetic stimulation are desirable. See *methacholine chloride.*

me'cism [G. *mēkos*, length]. A condition marked by abnormal prolongation of one or more parts of the body.

Meckel, Johann Friedrich (The Elder) [*German anatomist*, ca. 1724–74]. Described the sphenopalatine ganglion, also called *Meckel's ganglion.* See also Meckel's *cavity.*

Meckel, Johann Friedrich (The Younger) [*German anatomist*, 1781–1833]. Described the cartilage bar of the mandibular arch; called *Meckel's cartilage.* Described the diverticulum ilei, the persistent proximal end of the yolk stalk; called *Meckel's diverticulum.* The yolk stalk is also known as *Meckel's stalk. Diverticulitis* of diverticulum ilei is also called *Meckel's diverticulitis.*

me'cli·zine hy"dro·chlo'ride. Generic name for the dihydrochloride of *p*-chlorobenzylhydryl-4-*m*-methylbenzylpiperazine, a compound effective in preventing motion sickness. See *bonamine, postafene.*

me·com'e·ter [G. *mēkos*, length; *metron*, a measure]. An instrument used in measuring newborn infants.

me"co·nal'gi·a [G. *mēkōn*, poppy; *algos*, pain]. Pain or neuralgia when the use of opium is discontinued.

mec'on·ate (meck'o·nate, mee'ko·nate). A salt of meconic acid.

mec"o·neu"ro·path'i·a (meck"o·new"ro·path'-ee·uh) [*mēkōn;* G. *neuron*, nerve; *pathos*, disease]. Nervous disorder due to the abuse of opium or its narcotic derivatives.

me·con'ic ac'id (mi·kon'ick, ·ko'nick). $C_7H_4O_7$. A dibasic acid found in opium. Nearly devoid of physiologic activity.

me·con'i·dine (mi·kon'i·deen, ·din). $C_{21}H_{23}NO_4$. An amorphous alkaloid of opium.

mec'o·nin, me'co·nin. $C_{10}H_{10}O_4$. A principle occurring in opium and hydrastis; has been used as a hypnotic.

mec"o·ni·or·rhe'a [G. *mēkōnion*, discharge from the bowels of newborn children; *rhoia*, flow]. An excessive discharge of meconium.

me·co'ni·um [*mēkōnion*]. The pasty, greenish mass, consisting of mucus, desquamated epithelial cells, bile, lanugo hairs, and vernix caseosa, that collects in the intestine of the fetus. It forms the first fecal discharge of the newborn and is not wholly voided until the third or fourth day after birth.

mec'o·no- [G. *mēkōn*, poppy]. A combining form signifying *opium.*

me·cys'ta·sis. A process in which a muscle increases in length but maintains its original degree of tension. Also called *mecystatic relaxation.*

me'di·a [L. *medius*, middle]. 1. The middle coat of a vein, artery, or lymph vessel; tunica media. See Plate 6. 2. Plural of medium.

transparent m. of the eye. The cornea, aqueous humor, lens, and vitreous humor.

me′di·ad [*medius;* L. *ad,* toward]. Toward the median plane or line.

me′di·al [*medius*]. Internal, as opposed to lateral (external); toward the midline of the body.

me″di·a·lec′i·thal (mee″dee·a·less′i·thul). See *mesolecithal.*

me′di·an [L. *medianus,* middle]. Situated or placed in the middle of the body or in the middle of a part of the body, as the arm.

me′di·an. That value on the numerical scale of classification in a frequency distribution below which and above which half the observations fall.

me″di·as″ti·ni′tis [ML. *mediastinus,* from *medius,* middle; G. *-itis,* inflammation]. Inflammation of the tissues of the mediastinum.

me″di·as·ti″no·per″i·car·di′tis (mee″dee·ass·tigh″no·, ·ass″ti·no·, ·ass″tigh·no·) [*mediastinus;* G. *perikardios,* about the heart; *-itis*]. Combined inflammation of the mediastinum and the pericardium. Also see *pericarditis.*

me″di·as″ti·not′o·my [*mediastinus;* G. *tomē,* a cutting]. Incision into the mediastinum.

me″di·as·ti′num [*mediastinus*]. 1. A partition separating adjacent parts. 2. The space left in the middle of the chest between the two pleurae, divided into the anterior, middle, posterior, and superior mediastinum. The anterior mediastinum contains the internal mammary vessels of the left side, loose areolar tissue, lymphatic vessels, and a few lymph nodes. The middle mediastinum contains the heart and pericardium, the ascending aorta, the superior vena cava, the bifurcation of the trachea, the pulmonary arteries and veins, and the phrenic nerves. The posterior mediastinum contains a part of the aorta, the greater and lesser azygos veins, the vagus and splanchnic nerves, the esophagus, the thoracic duct, and some lymph nodes. The superior mediastinum, that part lying above the pericardium, contains the origins of the sternohyoid and sternothyroid muscles, and part of the longus colli muscles, the transverse portion of the aortic arch, the innominate, left carotid, and subclavian arteries, the superior vena cava and the innominate veins, the left superior intercostal vein, the vagus, cardiac, phrenic, and left recurrent laryngeal nerves, the trachea, esophagus, and thoracic duct, the remains of the thymus and lymphatics. —**mediastinal,** *adj.*

m. testis. A septum in the posterior portion of the testis, formed by a projection inward of the tunica albuginea. Formerly called *body of Highmore.*

me′di·ate [L. *mediare,* to halve]. Indirect; performed through something interposed, as mediate percussion, percussion on a pleximeter.

med′i·ca·ble [L. *medicare,* to heal]. Amenable to cure.

med′i·cal [L. *medicus,* medical]. Pertaining to medicine, as medical ethics, medical books, medical school.

med′i·cal cen′ter. 1. A medical clinic usually serving a discrete geographical area. 2. A group of medical facilities, incorporating all the medical specialties, and possessing the capacity for medical education, and the diagnosis, care, and treatment of patients.

Med′i·cal Corps. In the U.S. Army and Navy Departments and the Air Force, the medical officers of the Regular Army, Navy, and Air Force, the National Guard, and the Reserve Corps, together with medical officers appointed from civil life during war.

Med′i·cal De·part′ment. In the U.S. Army and Navy Departments and the Air Force, a subdivision consisting of commissioned officers, nurses, and enlisted and civilian personnel, with a surgeon general as directing head.

med′i·cal de·tach′ment. *In military medicine,* (a) a unit, consisting of medical personnel, organic to regiments and separate battalions of arms and services other than medical: so named because its personnel are not of the same branch as the parent organization in the usual administrative sense; (b) an integral part of certain hospitals (base, general, field, evacuation, and station) composed of enlisted personnel performing both administrative and professional services.

med′i·cal eth′ics. The principles of conduct which physicians follow.

med′i·cal ex·am′in·er. 1. A medical officer appointed to an office of a municipality or state, whose duty it is to determine facts concerning causes of death and to testify thereto in courts of law. The medical examiner in many states and counties replaces the former coroner or coroner's jury. 2. An officer of a corporation or bureau, whose duty it is to determine facts relating to injuries and deaths alleged to have occurred, to place responsibility on the part of the corporation or other agency, and to make recommendations as to compensation. In certain cases, as in life insurance applications, etc., the examiner is charged with passing upon the state of health of the applicant.

med′i·cal group. In the U.S. Army, a command embracing clearing companies, collecting companies, ambulance companies, and those elements required for emergency treatment and evacuation of combat casualties.

med′i·cal reg′u·la″tor. An officer of the U.S. Medical Service of one of the armed services who regulates and controls the movement of patients between various medical treatment facilities.

med′i·cal ser′vice. The professional service of a U. S. military medical unit whose sections handle patients diagnosed in the various fields of medicine.

med′i·cal treat′ment fa·cil′i·ty. A U.S. Armed Forces installation through which medical service is furnished to individuals of the U.S. Armed Forces regardless of service affiliation.

med′i·cal troops. The enlisted personnel of the U.S. Army Medical Service, especially those who serve in a medical element assigned or attached to, or in support of a combat unit.

me·dic′a·ment, med′i·ca·ment [L. *medicamentum,* remedy]. A medicinal substance.

med″i·ca·men·to′sus [L., medicinal]. Pertaining to a drug or a drug eruption.

med″i·ca·men′tum [L.]. See *medicament.*

m. arcanum. A proprietary or secret remedy. *Obs.*

med′i·ca″ted [L. *medicare,* to heal]. Impregnated with a medicinal substance.

med″i·ca′tion [L. *medicatio,* from *medicare*]. 1. Impregnation with a medicine. 2. Treatment by medicines; the administration of medicines.

endermic m. See *cataphoresis.*

hypodermic m. Treatment by the introduction of medicines beneath the skin, usually by means of a hypodermic syringe.

preanesthetic m. Administration of drugs, such as sedatives and anticholinergic agents, before the patient is anesthetized to facilitate induction by thus allaying apprehension, by reduction of basal metabolic rate, and drying of oral and nasal secretions, thus reducing anesthetic requirements.

med′i·ca″tor [L., from *medicare*]. 1. A person who gives medicines for the relief of disease. *Obs.* 2. An applicator.

me·dic′i·nal [L. *medicinalis*, pertaining to medicine]. Pertaining to, due to, or having the nature of, a medicine, as medicinal rashes, eruptions on the skin following the internal administration of certain drugs.

med′i·cine [L. *medicina*, medicine]. 1. Any substance used for treating disease. 2. The science of treating disease; the healing art. In a restricted sense, that branch of the healing art dealing with internal diseases, which can be treated by a physician rather than by a surgeon.

anatomic m. That system which deals with the anatomic changes in diseased organs and their connection with symptoms manifested during life.

aviation m. That field which integrates and applies the fundamentals of medicine and the basic sciences to aviation; it deals with biological problems peculiar to aviation, including selection, maintenance and treatment of the flier, assistance in designing aircraft and related equipment to meet human requirements, adaptation of men to the conditions of flight, and the problems involved in evacuation of the sick and wounded by air: also called *aeromedicine*.

clinical m. The study of disease by the bedside of the patient.

constitutional m. That branch of medicine which deals with the relation between a patient's constitution and his susceptibility to disease. See *constitution*, 2.

domestic m. The treatment of disease or injuries, at home, by a layman.

experimental m. That based upon experiments on animals by the observation of pathologic changes in diseases induced in them and the effect of drugs administered.

forensic m. See legal *m.*

group m. (a) The practice of medicine by a number of physicians working in systematic association, with joint use of equipment and technical personnel, and with centralized administrative and financial organization. Its objectives are increased professional efficiency, improved medical care of the patient, and increased economic efficiency. (b) The practice of medicine carried on under a legal agreement in a community, by a body of registered physicians and surgeons, for the purpose of caring for a group of persons who have subscribed to such service by the payment of a definite sum for a specified time, which entitles each subscriber to medical care and hospitalization under definite rules and regulations.

internal m. That branch of medicine which treats of diseases that are nonsurgical.

legal m. That branch of medicine, involving any and all of its disciplines, employed by the legal authorities for the solution of legal problems. Syn., *forensic m.*

military m. That part of general medicine dealing with the character, epidemiology, prevention, and treatment of diseases and injuries which are brought about by the special conditions incident to military life. Syn., *war m.*

osteopathic m. The principles and practice of medicine as employed by osteopaths.

patent m. (a) Medicine, the manufacture of which is protected by a patent. (b) Term commonly applied to an advertised nostrum of secret composition.

physical m. A consultative, diagnostic, and therapeutic service coordinating and integrating the employment of physical and occupational therapy, and physical reconditioning on the professional management of the diseased and injured.

practice of m. The practical application of the principles taught by the theory of medicine.

preventive m. Any activity which seeks to prevent disease, prolong life, and promote physical and mental health and efficiency; especially, the science of the etiology and epidemiology of disease processes, dealing with the predisposing factors which increase an individual's vulnerability, the provoking factors which initiate or precipitate a disease process, and the perpetuating factors which in noninfective or degenerative diseases tend to cause their progression.

proprietary m. One, the manufacture of which is limited or controlled by an owner, because of a patent, copyright, or secrecy as regards its constitution or method of manufacture.

psychosomatic m. That branch of medicine dealing with psychic and physical components as a unit, and the interrelationship between them.

quack m. A medicine falsely advertised to the laity as being able to cure certain diseases.

regular school of m. A term formerly used to designate the great mass of the profession as contrasted with the homeopathic and eclectic schools.

socialized m. The control, direction, and financing of the medical care of a population by its government: assumption of legal, administrative, and financial responsibility for the practice of medicine by professional services and for the total care of the patients, as in the National Health Service of Great Britain.

social m. In its widest sense, an approach to the maintenance and advancement of health and to the prevention, amelioration, and cure of disease, which has its foundation in an inclusive and dynamic sociology and biology, i.e., in the study of man and the environment in which he is an integral component. Social medicine seeks to integrate clinical and social pathology and the workers in these fields, the methods of biostatistics, and the data thus obtained, and to be constantly guided by the concepts of normal variability of human beings, and their capacity for adaptability. Not to be confused with *socialized m.*

space m. A branch of aviation medicine concerned with the human factor encountered in flights under the space equivalent conditions in the upper atmosphere and under the conditions found in free interplanetary space.

state m. (a) Legal medicine. (b) Socialized medicine as exercised by a state or federal government.

tropical m. That branch of medical science concerned chiefly with diseases found commonly or exclusively in the tropical or subtropical regions.

veterinary m. That branch of medical practice which treats of the diseases and injuries of animals.

war m. See military *m.*

med″i·co·chi·rur′gi·cal (med″i·ko·kigh·rur′ji·kul) [L. *medicus*, medical; G. *cheirourgos*, working by hand, surgeon]. Pertaining conjointly to medicine and surgery.

med″i·co·le′gal [*medicus;* L. *legalis*, legal]. Relating both to medicine and law.

med″i·co·psy·chol′o·gy [*medicus;* G. *psychē*, soul; *logos*, word]. The study of mental diseases in relation to medicine.

med″i·co·sta·tis′tic [*medicus;* ML. *statisticus*]. Relating to medicine as connected with statistics.

Medin, Karl Oskar [*Swedish physician*, 1847–1927]. Drew attention to the epidemic character of acute anterior poliomyelitis, sometimes called *Heine-Medin disease.*

medinal. Trade-mark for a brand of barbital sodium.

Me·di′na worm. See *Dracunculus medinensis.*

me′di·o-, me′di- [L. *medius*, middle]. A combining

form meaning *middle;* used to denote *medially, relating to the middle* or *median plane,* or *intermediate.*

me″di·o·car′pal [*medius;* G. *karpos,* wrist]. Pertaining to the articulation between the two rows of carpal bones.

me″di·o·dor′sal [*medius;* L. *dorsum,* back]. Both median and dorsal; on the median line of the back.

me″di·o·fron′tal [*medius;* L. *frons,* forehead]. Pertaining to the middle of the forehead.

me″di·o·ne·cro′sis. Necrosis occurring in the tunica media of an artery, commonly associated with in a dissecting aneurysm.

m. aortae idiopathica cystica. Degeneration of the muscle and elastic fibers of the aorta. Syn., *medial necrosis of aorta.*

me″di·o·tar′sal [*medius;* G. *tarsos,* flat of the foot]. Pertaining to the middle articulations of the tarsal bones.

Med″i·ter·ra′ne·an dis·ease′. See familial erythroblastic *anemia.*

Med″i·ter·ra′ne·an fe′ver. See *brucellosis.*

me′di·um [L.]. 1. That in which anything moves or through which it acts. 2. *In bacteriology,* a substance used for the cultivation of bacteria; may be modified for certain purposes. Also see *culture.*

bismuth sulfite agar m. A highly selective medium for the isolation of *Salmonella typhosa* from feces, urine, sewage, and other infectious materials, especially valuable in detecting typhoid (and paratyphoid) carriers. The organisms reduce bismuth sulfite to the black sulfide. Also called *Wilson-Blair bismuth sulfite m.*

Bordet-Gengou m. See Jules Jean Baptiste Vincent *Bordet.*

Dorset's egg m. A medium of fresh egg yolk used with or without diluent, for culture of *Mycobacterium tuberculosis* and other microorganisms.

Hiss's serum water m. A medium used for determining fermentative capacities of bacteria, containing water, serum, glucose, and phenol red.

Kauffmann's tetrathionate broth m. See tetrathionate broth base *m.*

Kligler's triple sugar m. See triple sugar iron agar *m.*

Littman ox-gall m. A selective medium containing bile salts, crystal violet, and streptomycin, used in the primary isolation of fungi from specimens having a mixed bacterial and fungal flora.

Löwenstein-Jensen m. An egg-potato-glycerin medium used for culture of *Mycobacterium tuberculosis.*

mounting m. See *mountant.*

NNN m. A medium for culturing *Leishmania donovani* which consists of 1000 cc. of water, 50 Gm. of beef extract, 20 Gm. of agar, 20 Gm. of neopeptone, 5 Gm. of sodium chloride, and 10 per cent defibrinated rabbit's blood. Also called *Senekjie's m.*

rice-grain m. A medium of autoclaved rice grains in water, used for the confirmation and identification of the various species of *Microsporum* when microscopy is inconclusive.

selenite F m. A culture medium for the isolation of an organism causing an enteric infection.

Senekjie's m. See NNN *m.*

tellurite m. A medium containing sodium tellurite, used for the isolation and identification of *Corynebacterium diphtheriae* and of certain fungi; it inhibits many species of bacteria.

tetrathionate m. A nutrient broth for isolation of organisms in enteric infections.

tetrathionate broth base m. A selective liquid enrichment medium used to isolate *Salmonella typhosa* and other members of the Salmonella group in laboratory diagnosis of enteric infections: also called *Kauffmann's tetrathionate broth m.*

triple sugar iron agar m. A differential identification medium used to identify the Gram-negative enteric pathogens in routine stool examination. It indicates the ability of the organism to ferment lactose, saccharose, and dextrose to acid or gas or both and its ability to produce hydrogen sulfide.

trypsin digest agar m. A bacteriologic culture medium in which the products of meat digested with trypsin are substituted for meat extract.

Tween albumin m. of Dubos. A medium especially for the culture of *Mycobacterium tuberculosis.* To a culture medium of defined composition are added the wetting agent Tween 80 (trademark for polysorbate 80) and albumin, to lower the toxicity of the Tween 80 to some strains of the *Mycobacteria.*

urea m. A nutrient agar containing potassium biphosphate, glucose, urea, and phenol red. Urease activity is denoted by reduction of the pH. Such organisms as *Proteus* and *Aerobacter* are urease-positive; *Escherichia, Salmonella,* and *Shigella* are urease-negative.

Wilson-Blair bismuth sulfite m. See bismuth sulfite agar *m.*

me′di·us [L.]. 1. The middle. 2. The middle finger.

me·dul′la [L.]. 1. The marrow. 2. The medulla oblongata. 3. Anything resembling marrow in its structure or in its relation to other parts, as a fatty substance or marrow occupying certain cavities; the central parts of certain organs as distinguished from the cortex. —**med′ullary,** *adj.*

m. oblongata. The lowest part of the brain extending from the pons to the spinal cord. See Plates 15, 18.

m. ossium. Bone marrow.

m. ossium rubra. Red bone marrow.

m. spinalis. Old term for the spinal cord.

med′ul·la″ted (med′uh·lay″tid, mi·dull′ay·tid) [*medulla*]. Provided with a myelin sheath. Syn., *myelinated.*

med″ul·la′tion [*medulla*]. The process of acquiring a myelin sheath, as in the case of many nerve fibers in the course of their development.

med″ul·li·za′tion [*medulla*]. Conversion into marrow, as the replacement of bone tissue in the course of osteitis.

med′ul·lo·blast (med′uh·lo·blast, mi·dull′o·) [*medulla;* G. *blastos,* germ]. A primitive brain cell of the neural tube.

med″ul·lo·blas·to′ma (med″uh·lo·blas·to′muh, mi·dull″o·) [*medulla; blastos;* G. *-ōma,* tumor]. A malignant brain tumor with a tendency to spread in the meninges; most common in the cerebellum of children. The cells are small, with scanty cytoplasm, dense spheroid or oval nuclei, many mitoses, and a tendency to form pseudo rosettes. Also called *glioblastoma isomorphe, glioma sarcomatoides, embryonal neurogliocytoma, neurospongioma.*

med″ul·lo·ep″i·the·li·o′ma (med″uh·lo·ep″ith-ee·lee·o′muh, mi·dull″o·) [*medulla;* G. *epi,* on; *thēlē,* nipple; *-ōma*]. Old term for neuroepithelioma, ependymoma, or, loosely, for glioma.

Meduna's method. See under *method.*

meg′a-, meg- [G. *megas,* large]. A combining form used to signify *great, extended, enlarged.*

meg″a·car′di·a [*megas;* G. *kardia,* heart]. A large heart. Hypertrophy of the heart.

meg″a·ce′cum. Cecum with a markedly distended lumen.

meg″a·coc′cus [*megas;* G. *kokkos,* berry]. A large coccus.

meg″a·co′lon [*megas;* G. *kolon,* colon]. Hypertrophy and dilatation of the colon, usually first seen in childhood, associated with prolonged constipation and consequent abdominal distention. It appears in two primary forms: (1) **Hirschsprung's m.** (achalasic or congenital), characterized roentgenographically by narrowing and atony of the distal sigmoid and rectum, neuropathologically by absence in these structures of the myenteric plexuses, and therapeutically by the success of rectosigmoidectomy. (2) **idiopathic m.,** characterized roentgenographically by dilatation of the colon, including sigmoid and rectum, clinically by slower development and lower morbidity and mortality than in Hirschsprung's *m.* Its causes are unknown, but are presumed to result from faulty bowel habits, anal sphincter spasm, imbalance of the autonomic nervous system with overactivity of the thoracicolumbar portion. Megacolon may also be secondary to an obstructive lesion.

meg'a·dont [*megas;* G. *odous,* tooth]. Having abnormally large teeth; macrodont.

meg″a·du″o·de'num (meg″uh·dew″o·dee'num, ·dew·od'i·num) [*megas;* L. *duodeni,* twelve each]. Idiopathic dilatation of the duodenum.

meg'a·dyne [*megas;* G. *dynamis,* power]. A million dynes.

meg″a·e·soph'a·gus [*megas;* G. *oisophagos,* gullet]. A markedly enlarged esophagus.

meg″a·far'ad [*megas; Faraday*]. A million farads.

meg″a·ga·mete' (meg″uh·ga·meet', ·gam'eet) [*megas;* G. *gamos,* marriage]. Macrogamete.

meg″a·gna'thus (meg″uh·nayth'us) [*megas;* G. *gnathos,* jaw]. Large-jawed.

meg″a·kar'y·o·blast (meg″uh·kar'ee·o·blast) [*megas;* G. *karyon,* kernel; *blastos,* germ]. An immature, developing megakaryocyte. It is a large cell with nongranular, deeply basophilic cytoplasm, and a nucleus showing a fine chromatin structure and numerous nucleoli.

meg″a·kar″y·o·blas·to'ma [*megas; karyon; blastos;* G. *-oma,* tumor]. Old term for Hodgkin's disease.

meg″a·kar'y·o·cyte [*megas; karyon;* G. *kytos,* cell]. A giant cell of the bone marrow, 30–70μ, containing a large, irregularly lobulated nucleus; the progenitor of blood platelets. The cytoplasm contains fine azurophil granules.

lymphoid m. See *promegakaryocyte.*

meg″a·kar″y·oph'thi·sis (meg″uh·kar″ee·off'thisis, ·kar″ee·o·thigh'sis) [*megas; karyon;* G. *phthisis,* a wasting away]. A scarcity of megakaryocytes in the bone marrow in thrombocytopenia.

meg″a·lec'i·thal (meg″uh·less'i·thul) [*megas;* G. *lekithos,* yolk]. Large-yolked.

meg″a·ler·y·the'ma. See *erythema* infectiosum.

me·gal'gi·a [*megas;* G. *algos,* pain]. Excessively severe pain. *Obs.*

meg'a·lo-, megal- [*megas*]. A combining form meaning *large, great;* used especially to denote *abnormal enlargement.*

meg'a·lo·blast″ [*megas;* G. *blastos,* germ]. A large erythroblast with a characteristic nuclear pattern formed in marrow in liver principle deficiency anemias during relapse. The basophilic, polychromatophilic, and acidophilic (orthochromatic) forms mature to become nonnucleated megalocytes. Megaloblasts may appear in the peripheral blood. They resemble erythroblasts from embryos and fishes. Megaloblast is not synonymous with macronormoblast, but is the same as the proerythroblast of some authors.

meg″a·lo·car'di·a [*megas;* G. *kardia,* heart]. Auxesis; hypertrophy of the heart.

meg″a·lo·ce·phal'ic [*megas;* G. *kephalē,* head]. Large-headed; applied to a skull the capacity of which exceeds 1450 cc.

meg″a·lo·ceph'a·ly [*megas; kephalē*]. 1. The condition of having a very large head. 2. A disease characterized by progressive enlargement of the head, face, and neck, involving both the bony and the soft tissues. Also called *leontiasis ossea.*

meg″a·loc'er·us (meg″uh·los'ur·us) [*megas;* G. *keras,* horn]. A monstrosity with hornlike projections on the forehead.

meg″a·lo·chei'rous (meg″uh·lo·kigh'rus) [*megas;* G. *cheir,* hand]. Large-handed.

meg″a·lo·cor'ne·a [*megas;* L. *cornu,* horn]. An enlarged cornea.

meg'a·lo·cyte [*megas;* G. *kytos,* cell]. A large, nonnucleated, red blood corpuscle, usually oval, derived from a megaloblast. —**megalocyt'ic,** *adj.*

meg″a·lo·cy·to'sis (meg″uh·lo·sigh·to'sis) [*megas; kytos;* G. *-ōsis,* condition]. The occurrence of megalocytes and megaloblasts in the peripheral blood.

meg″a·lo·dac'ty·ly. See *macrodactylia.*

meg″a·lo·don'ti·a. Macrodontia. —**meg'alodont,** *adj.*

meg″a·lo·en'ter·on [*megas;* G. *enteron,* intestine]. An excessively large intestine.

meg″a·lo·gas'tri·a [*megas;* G. *gastēr,* belly]. Abnormal enlargement of the stomach.

meg″a·lo·glos'si·a. See *macroglossia.*

meg″a·lo·he·pat'i·a [*megas;* G. *hēpar,* liver]. Enlargement of the liver. *Obs.*

meg″a·lo·kar'y·o·blast. Megakaryoblast.

meg″a·lo·kar'y·o·cyte. See *megakaryocyte.*

meg″a·lo·ma'ni·a [*megas;* G. *mania,* madness]. The delusion of personal greatness, a symptom common in schizophrenic and other psychotic reactions. The patient expresses and acts out ideas of exalted attainment. —**megalomanic,** *adj;* **megalomaniac,** *n.*

meg″a·lo·me'li·a [*megas;* G. *melos,* limb]. Gigantism of one or more limbs.

meg″a·lo·ny·cho'sis (meg″uh·lo·ni·ko'sis) [*megas;* G. *onyx,* nail; *-ōsis,* condition]. Universal, noninflammatory hypertrophy of the nails.

meg″a·lo·pe'nis. Abnormally large penis.

meg″a·loph·thal'mus [*megas;* G. *ophthalmos,* eye]. Excessive largeness of the eyes.

meg″a·lo'pi·a, meg″a·lop'si·a. See *macropsia.*

meg″a·lo·po'di·a [*megas;* G. *pous,* foot]. The condition of having large feet.

meg″a·lo·splanch'nic [*megas;* G. *splagchnon,* inward parts]. Possessing large viscera, especially a large liver.

meg″a·lo·sple'ni·a. Old term for splenomegaly.

meg'a·lo·spore″ [*megas;* G. *spora,* seed]. A large spore; macrospore.

meg″a·lo·u·re'ter. A greatly enlarged ureter.

meg″a·mer″o·zo'ite (meg″uh·merr″o·zo'ite, ·meer″o·zo'ite) [*megas;* G. *meros,* part; *zōion,* living being]. A large merozoite. *Obs.*

meg″a·nu'cle·us [*megas;* L. *nucleus,* nut]. Formerly used for macronucleus.

meg'a·phone [*megas;* G. *phōnē,* sound]. An instrument used for assisting the hearing of the deaf, by means of large reflectors of the sound waves.

meg″a·pros'o·pous [*megas;* G. *prosōpon,* face]. Having an unusually large face.

meg″a·rec'tum [*megas;* L. *rectus,* straight]. A greatly enlarged rectum.

meg″a·sig'moid [*megas;* G. *sigmoeidēs,* of the shape of a sigma]. A greatly enlarged sigmoid colon.

meg'a·spore″. See *macrospore.*

meg'a·volt″ [*megas;* Alessandro *Volta*]. A unit equal to 1,000,000 volts.

Méglin, Jean Antoine [*French physician,* 1756–1824]. Described the point at which the anterior palatine nerve emerges from the greater palatine foramen; called *Méglin's point.*

meg′ohm″ [G. *megas*, large; G. S. *Ohm*]. An electric unit equal to 1,000,000 ohms.

meg″oph·thal′mus. See *megalophthalmus.*

me′grim. Old term for migraine.

Meibom, Heinrich [*German physician and anatomist*, 1638–1700]. Described the tarsal glands, also called *Meibom's glands, Meibomian glands.* Chalazion is also called *Meibomian cyst.*

Meier-Porges test. See under Otto *Porges.*

Meige, Henri [*French physician*, 1866–1940]. Described hereditary trophedema of the legs (1899); called *Meige's disease, Milroy's disease.*

Meigs, Arthur Vincent [*American physician*, 1850–1912]. Described the capillary vessels between the muscle fibers of the heart; called *Meigs's capillaries.*

Meigs, Joe Vincent [*American gynecologist*, 1892–]. Described fibroma of the ovary with ascites and hydrothorax; called *Meigs's syndrome.*

Meiklejohn-Cohen indican method. See *method.*

Meinicke's test. A flocculation test for syphilis.

mei′o- (migh′o-). See *mio-.*

mei″o·lec′i·thal, mi″o·lec′i·thal (migh″o·less′i-thul). Alecithal.

mei·o′sis (migh·o′sis) [G. *meiōsis*, diminution]. The nuclear changes which take place in the last two cell divisions in the formation of the germ cells. The chromosomes divide once but the cell body divides twice with the result that the nucleus of the mature egg or sperm contains the reduced (haploid) number of chromosomes. Also spelled *miosis.* Syn., *reduction division.* —**meiotic,** *adj.*

Meissner, Georg [*German anatomist and physiologist*, 1829–1905]. With Rudolph Wagner, described tactile nerve endings (1852) called *Meissner's* or *Wagner's corpuscles;* see Meissner's *corpuscle.* See also submucous *plexus,* also called *Meissner's plexus.*

mel. [L.] Honey.

mel- [G. *melos*, limb]. *In medicine,* a combining form signifying *limb.*

mel-, mel′o- [G. *mēla*, cheeks]. *In medicine,* a combining form meaning *cheek.*

me·lae′na (mi·lee′nuh). See *melena.*

me·la′gra, me·lag′ra [G. *melos*, limb; *agra*, a seizure]. Muscular pains in the extremities.

me·lal′gi·a [*melos;* G. *algos*, pain]. Pain or neuralgia in the extremities.

nutritional m. A syndrome of painful burning feet and, in severe cases, hands, revealing neurovascular symptoms with the predominant pathology in the blood vessels; it may be a pantothenic acid deficiency.

mel″an·cho′li·a, mel′an·chol″y [G. *melagcholia*, melancholy]. A form of mental disorder characterized by extreme depression, fear, brooding, and painful delusions. All activity is usually inhibited, but a melancholic patient may show psychomotor overactivity (agitated depression) or he may have many depressive ideas that shift rapidly (depressive mania). When mild, a melancholic state is called retardation. When average, it is called acute depression. When severe, it may become stuporous depression. —**melanchol′ic,** *adj.;* **melancho′-liac,** *n.*

climacteric m. That occurring at the menopause.

involutional m. A form of melancholia, arising during the involutional period; characterized by agitation, anxiety, and brooding in conjunction with narrow mental horizons and lack of adaptability. See involutional psychotic *reaction.*

m. agitata. (a) Old term for catatonia. (b) Agitated melancholia. A form associated with excessive motor excitement; usually implies association with manic-depressive psychosis or with involutional melancholia.

m. attonita. The morbid state characterized by muscular rigidity. Common in catatonia.

m. simplex. Simple depression. A mild form without delusions.

paranoid m. The depressive phase of manic-depressive psychosis when it assumes a paranoid appearance. Syn., *melancholic insanity.*

mel″a·ne′mi·a [G. *melas*, black; *haima*, blood]. The presence of melanin in the blood.

Me·la′ni·a [*melas*]. A genus of fresh-water snails whose species serve as important intermediate hosts of the trematodes *Paragonimus westermani* and *Metagonimus yokogawai.*

mel″an·id·ro′sis. A form of chromhidrosis in which the sweat is dark-colored or black.

mel″a·nif′er·ous [*melas;* L. *ferre*, to bear]. Containing melanin.

mel′a·nin [*melas*]. A group of black or dark brown pigments; produced by metabolic activity of certain specialized cells and containing carbon, nitrogen, hydrogen, oxygen, and probably sulfur; iron is probably an accidental impurity. Occurs naturally in the choroid coat of the eye, the skin, hair, cardiac muscle, and pia mater. Some evidence indicates that melanin is 5,6-dihydroxyindole-α-carboxylic acid, and results from the action of the enzyme tyrosinase on tyrosine.

mel′a·nism [*melas*]. Abnormal deposition of dark pigment (melanin) in tissues, in organs, or in the skin.

mel′a·no-, melan- [*melas*]. A combining form signifying *dark-colored,* or *relating to melanin.*

mel″a·no·am″e·lo·blas·to′ma. Ameloblastoma in which melanin is found.

mel′a·no·blast″ [*melas;* G. *blastos*, germ]. 1. An immature melanin-forming cell. 2. Old term for (a) *in biology,* an immature pigment cell, of neural crest origin in certain vertebrates; (b) *in medicine,* the mature melanin-elaborating cell.

mel″a·no·blas·to′ma. See *melanoma.*

mel″a·no·car″ci·no′ma. See *melanoma.*

mel′a·no·cyte″ [*melas;* G. *kytos*, cell]. A mature melanin-forming cell in the dermoepidermal junction; it may be dopa or tyrosinase positive. In hematoxylin- and eosin-stained section, it appears as a clear cell, in sections impregnated with silver, as a dendritic cell.

mel″a·no·der′ma, mel″a·no·der′mi·a [*melas;* G. *derma*, skin]. Black pigmentation of the skin. —**melanodermic,** *adj.*

mel″a·no·der″ma·ti′tis tox′i·ca. A contact dermatitis, clinically and histologically identical with Riehl's melanosis, due to tars, oils, or greases.

mel″a·no·der″ma·to′sis. An inflammatory condition of skin characterized by increased pigmentation.

mel″a·no·ep″i·the″li·o′ma. See *melanoma.*

me·lan′o·gen [*melas;* G. *genesthai*, from *gignesthai*, to be produced]. The colorless precursor which is transformed into melanin on oxidation. Patients, especially those with widespread melanomas, may excrete urine containing melanogen; on standing or oxidation, the urine becomes dark brown or black.

mel″a·no·gen′e·sis [*melas;* G. *genesis*, production]. The formation of melanin.

mel″a·no·glos′si·a [*melas;* G. *glōssa*, tongue]. Blacktongue.

mel′a·noid [*melas;* G. *eidos*, form]. Dark-colored; resembling melanosis.

mel″a·no′ma [*melas;* G. *-ōma*, tumor]. A malignant tumor derived from melanophores of skin, of the choroid, of the anus, of meninges, and perhaps of adrenals. The cells of the tumor are of immature type. Depending upon the content of melanins within the cells, the tumor varies from white (amelanotic *m.*) to black or blue-black. Also called *malignant m., melanoblastoma, melanocarcinoma, melanoepithelioma, melanosarcoma, melanotic whitlow, nevocarcinoma, nevomelanoma.*

amelanotic m. See *melanoma.*

juvenile m. A junction nevus which pathologically resembles malignant melanoma but which is clinically benign.

mel″a·no·ma·to′sis [*melas; -ōma;* G. *-ōsis,* increase]. 1. Widespread distribution of melanoma. 2. Diffuse melanotic pigmentation of the meninges.

mel″a·no·nych′i·a (mel″uh·no·nick′ee·uh) [*melas;* G. *onyx,* nail]. A condition in which the fingernails or toenails turn black.

mel′a·no·phage″. A cell containing phagocytized melanin.

mel′a·no·phore″, me·lan′o·phore [*melas;* G. *phoros,* bearing]. 1. A dendritic cell containing melanin in its cytoplasm and having contractile properties. Melanophores are partly responsible for color changes in many animals, when, in response to certain stimuli, the pigment granules disperse into the dendrites or are concentrated in the perikaryon. 2. *In medicine,* formerly, a melanophage.

mel″a·no·pla′ki·a [*melas;* G. *plax,* plate]. Pigmentation of the mucous membrane of the mouth, usually in patches and occasionally with leukoplakia superimposed.

mel″a·no·pro′te·in. A conjugated protein in which melanin is the associated chromogen.

mel″a·nor·rha′gi·a [*melas;* G. *rhēgnynai,* to burst forth]. Old term for melena.

mel″a·nor·rhe′a. Melena.

mel″a·no·sar·co′ma. See *melanoma.*

mel″a·no′sis [*melas;* G. *-ōsis,* condition]. Dark brown or brownish black pigmentation of surfaces by melanins or, in some instances, by hematogenous pigments. In the skin, melanosis is observed in such conditions as sunburn, Addison's disease, various dermatoses, and about the nipples and elsewhere in pregnancy. —**melanot′ic,** *adj.*

m. coli. Pigmentation of mucosa of the colon in innumerable, approximated, minute foci (shaven-beard appearance) due to hematogenous pigments; a similar appearance may be due to deposits of bismuth in bismuth poisoning.

m. iridis. The invasion of the iris by melanoblasts; a form of melanosis of the eye.

Riehl's m. Formerly, melanodermatosis involving the face, neck, axillary folds, breasts, umbilical and inguinal areas described by G. Riehl. Etiology was probably nutritional. Now, any brown pigmentary dermatosis of the exposed skin of face and neck and of various causations, e.g., hormonal disturbances and occupational irritants.

mel″a·no·trich′i·a lin′guae (mel″uh·no·trick′ee·uh ling′gwee). See black, hairy *tongue.*

mel″a·not′ri·chous (mel″uh·not′ri·kus) [*melas;* G. *thrix,* hair]. Black-haired.

mel″a·nu′ri·a [*melas;* G. *ouron,* urine]. The presence of black pigment in the urine, the result of oxidation of melanogens. —**melanuric,** *adj.*

mel·ar′sen. The disodium salt of N-(4,6-diamino-2-*s*-triazinyl)arsanilic acid; disodium *p*-melaminyl phenylarsonate, a pentavalent arsenical which has been used as a trypanocidal agent.

m. oxide. N-(4,6-Diamino-2-*s*-triazinyl)-*p*-aminophenyl arsine oxide, a trivalent arsenical differing from melarsen in having the —AsO group replace —AsO(ONa)$_2$; it possesses trypanocidal activity.

me·las′ma (mi·laz′muh). Melanoderma.

me·le′na, me·lae′na [*melas*]. The discharge of stools colored black by altered blood.

m. neonatorum. An extravasation of blood into the stomach and intestines of the newborn infant. occurring most often in the first few hours of life,

mel′e·tin. Quercetin.

me·lez′i·tose. Trisaccharide obtained from an exudate of the Douglas fir and the larch. Yields D-fructose on hydrolysis. Also called *melicitose.*

mel′i- [G.]. A combining form meaning *honey.*

Me′li·a [G., ash tree]. A genus of the Meliaceae. **M. azedarach** is indigenous to Asia, but naturalized in southern Europe and America. The bark and fruit have been used as an anthelmintic and antiperiodic. Also has been used as an emetic and cathartic, and, in large doses, as a narcotic. Usually given as a decoction.

mel″i·bi′ase. An enzyme from certain brewer's yeasts catalyzing the hydrolysis of melibiose to dextrose and galactose.

mel″i·bi′ose. $C_{12}H_{22}O_{11}$; a disaccharide resulting from hydrolysis of raffinose and also occurring naturally; it may be hydrolyzed to glucose and galactose.

mel″i·lot′ic ac′id. $OH.C_6H_4(CH_2)_2.COOH$. An acid found in *Melilotus* species and also obtainable from coumarin.

mel″i·lot′in. $COOH.CH{:}CH.C_6H_4.O.C_6H_{11}O_5$; a glucoside occurring in flowers of *Melilotus altissima* and *M. arvensis;* on hydrolysis it yields *o*-coumaric acid and D-glucose. Syn., *melilotoside.*

mel″i·lot′o·side. Melilotin.

Mel″i·lo′tus [G. *melilōton,* a kind of clover]. A genus of the Leguminosae.

M. officinalis. Yellow sweet clover; contains coumarin, melilotic acid, and a volatile oil. Has been used as a local anodyne.

melin. See *rutin.*

me″li·oi·do′sis [G. *mēlis,* glanders; *eidos,* form; *-ōsis,* condition]. An infectious granuloma similar to glanders; it is primarily a disease of rodents but is occasionally communicable to man. This disease has been observed in Rangoon and the surrounding area and is caused by the *Malleomyces pseudomallei.*

Me·lis′sa [G., bee]. A genus of plants of the Labiatae.

M. officinalis. Common balm; a species growing in southern Europe. Contains a volatile oil; has been used as a carminative, a diaphoretic, and a flavoring agent.

me·lis′sic ac′id. $CH_3(CH_2)_{28}COOH$. An acid occurring in beeswax.

me·lis″so·pho′bi·a [G. *melissa,* bee; *phobos,* fear]. A morbid fear of bees.

me·lis′syl. Myricyl.

m. al′co·hol. Myricyl alcohol.

mel′i·tin, mel′i·tine. A filtrate of a 20-day culture of *Brucella melitensis,* used for diagnosis of undulant fever.

me·li′tis [G. *mēla,* cheeks; *-itis,* inflammation]. Inflammation of the cheek.

mel″i·to·coc·co′sis. See *brucellosis.*

mel′i·tose. See *raffinose.*

mel″i·tox′in. Dicoumarin.

mel″i·tri′ose. Raffinose.

mel″i·tu′ri·a [G. *mēli,* honey; *ouron,* urine]. General term indicating the presence of any sugar in urine.

Mellinger magnet. See under *magnet.*

mel·lit′ic ac′id. $C_6(COOH)_6$; benzenehexacarboxylic acid; a crystalline substance occurring in certain coal and wood products and synthesized by oxidation of carbon with nitric acid.

mel·li′tum [L. *mellitus,* of honey]. *In pharmacy,* a honey; a preparation in which honey is the menstruum.

Mellon, Ralph R. (1883–). American bacteriologist, one of the earliest experimenters with sulfa drugs in America; he pioneered in the application of sulfathiazole in pneumonia.

Melnick method. See Hochberg-Melnick-Oser *method* for ascorbic acid.

mel′o-. See *mel-*, *melo-*.

mel″o·di·dy′mi·a [G. *melos*, limb; *didymos*, twin]. The presence of an accessory limb or limbs. *Obs.*

mel″o·did′y·mus [*melos; didymos*]. An individual with an accessory limb or limbs. *Obs.*

mel″o·ma′ni·a [G. *melos*, song; *mania*, madness]. A psychosis marked by an inordinate devotion to music. *Obs.* —**melomaniac,** *n.*

me·lom′e·lus [G. *melos*, limb; *melos*]. An individual with one or more rudimentary accessory limbs attached to a limb.

Me·loph′a·gus [*melos;* G. *phagein*, to eat]. A genus of ticks ectoparasitic on mammals and birds.

M. ovinus. That species known as the sheep tick which transmits *Rickettsia melophagi* and the trypanosomiasis of sheep.

mel″o·rhe″os·to′sis [*melos;* G. *rhein*, to flow; *osteon*, bone; *-ōsis*, condition]. A very rare condition of unknown cause in which certain bones, or parts of bones, undergo asymmetrical or local enlargement and sclerotic changes, typically confined to the bones of one extremity, with distortion of affected bone, limitation of movement in the joints between the bones, and marked pain: also called *Léri type of osteopetrosis, osteosi eburnizzante monomelica.*

me·los′chi·sis (mi·los′ki·sis) [G. *mēla*, cheeks; *schisis*, cleavage]. A congenital cleft of the cheek.

mel″o·trid′y·mus. See *dipygustripus.*

me·lo′tus [G. *mēla*, cheeks; *ous*, ear]. An individual showing congenital displacement of the ear, which lies on the cheek.

melt′ing point. The degree of temperature at which fusible solids begin to melt. Abbreviated, m.p.

Meltzer, Samuel James [*American physiologist*, 1851–1920]. With John Auer, developed a method of anesthesia by intratracheal insufflation (1909); called *Meltzer's method.*

mem′ber [L. *membrum*, limb]. A part of the body, especially a projecting part, as the leg or the arm.

mem′brane [L. *membrana*, membrane]. A thin layer of tissue surrounding a part, separating adjacent cavities, lining a cavity, or connecting adjacent structures. —**mem′branous,** *adj.*

anal m. The dorsal part of the cloacal membrane caudal to the urorectal septum.

animal m. A membrane made from animal tissues, used in dialyzing.

anterior atlanto-occipital m. A dense membrane extending from the ventral surface and cranial margin of the anterior arch of the atlas to the anterior border of the foramen magnum and inferior surface of the basilar part of the occipital bone.

arachnoid m. The arachnoid.

atlantoaxial m. One bridging the gap between the posterior arch of the atlas and the arch of the axis.

atlanto-occipital m. See anterior and posterior atlanto-occipital *m.*

basal m. of Bruch. That which forms the outer of the four layers of the choroid coat of the eye.

basement m. The delicate, noncellular membrane on which an epithelium is seated.

basilar m. The membranous portion of the spiral lamina separating the scala vestibuli from the scala tympani, extending from the base to the apex of the cochlea and supporting the organ of Corti: also called *cochlear zone.*

birth membranes. The two fetal membranes, inner amnion and outer chorion, which enclose the amniotic fluid. A portion of the chorion contributes to the placenta.

blastodermic m. See *blastoderm.*

Bowman's m. A thin membrane which separates the corneal epithelium from the substantia propria of the cornea.

brood m. The internal germinative layer of the hydatid cyst of *Echinococcus granulosus*, which on proliferation gives rise to scolices, brood capsules, or daughter cysts.

Bruch's m. See basal *m.* of Bruch.

bucconasal m. A thin epithelial membrane formed at the site of a primary choana by the apposition of stomodeal and olfactory epithelia. It ruptures during the seventh week.

buccopharyngeal m. The membrane separating stomodeum and pharynx, composed of ectoderm and endoderm. It ruptures in embryos of 2.5 mm. Syn., *oral m., pharyngeal m.*

cell m. See plasma *m.*

chorio-allantoic m. In Sauropsida, a vascular extraembryonic membrane formed by fusion of the allantois and chorion.

choroid m. That part of the vascular tunic, or uvea, of the eye which extends anteriorly as far as the ora serrata.

cloacal m. A delicate membrane of ectoderm and endoderm separating the embryonic hindgut from the external or ectodermal cloaca.

costocoracoid m. A dense layer of fascia extending between the subclavius muscle and the pectoralis minor, and forming the anterior portion of the sheath of the axillary vessels.

cricothyroid m. A ligamentous membrane between the cricoid and thyroid cartilages. Also called *cricovocal m., conus elasticus.*

croupous m. The yellowish white membrane forming in the larynx in laryngotracheobronchitis.

decidual m. One of the membranes formed by the superficial part of the endometrium during pregnancy. See *decidua basalis, decidua capsularis, decidua parietalis.*

Descemet's m. The posterior elastic lamina of the cornea which covers the posterior surface of the substantia propria.

diphtheritic m. A fibrinous layer formed on a mucous membrane or cutaneous surface and extending downward for a variable depth. It is the result of coagulation necrosis, generally brought about by the bacillus of diphtheria.

drum m. The tympanic membrane.

egg m. Any one of several membranes surrounding an ovum: The primary egg membrane is one formed by the ovum itself, such as the vitelline membrane; the secondary egg membrane is formed by the follicular cells of the ovary, as the zona pellucida; the tertiary egg membrane is one formed by secretions of the oviduct or uterus, as in sauropsids and monotremes.

elastic m. One composed of elastic fibrous tissue.

elastic m. of the larynx. The quadrangular membrane and the conus elasticus, or elastic cone.

Elford m. Graded collodion membrane filters employed for the determination of the relative size of different filtrable viruses.

exocoelomic m. A delicate, mesothelium-like membrane bounding the exocoelom of the blastocyst; continuous with the extraembryonic mesoderm and with the primary endoderm. It may be derived from either or both.

external elastic m. That of the wall of some arteries forming the boundary between the tunica media and tunica adventitia. See Plate 6.

external limiting m. (a) In the eye, the thin layer between the outer nuclear layer of the retina and that of the rods and cones. (b) *In embryology*, the membrane investing the outer surface of the neural tube.

extraembryonic m. Any of the membranes surrounding the embryo or fetus, shed at birth. See *amnion, chorion, yolk sac, allantois.*
false m. See diphtheritic *m.*
fenestrated m. One of the layers of elastic tissue in the tunica media and tunica intima of large arteries.
fetal membranes. The chorion, amnion, or allantois.
fibroserous m. Thin, transparent, glistening structures forming closed sacs that contain certain organs. They are the peritoneum, the two pleurae, the pericardium, the tunica vaginalis testis, the arachnoid, and synovial membranes.
germinal m. See *blastoderm.*
germ m. See *blastoderm.*
glassy m. Basement membrane of a clear, highly refractive nature, as in the maturing ovarian follicle or in a hair follicle.
granulosa m. The layer of small polyhedral cells within the theca of the Graafian follicle.
Henle's fenestrated m. See fenestrated *m.*
Heuser's m. The exocoelomic membrane.
hyalin m. (a) Basement membrane. (b) The membrane between the inner fibrous layer of a hair follicle and its outer root sheath. (c) The basement membrane of a Graafian follicle.
hyaloid m. The limiting membrane surrounding the vitreous body, and forming the suspensory ligament and zonule.
hyoglossal m. The membrane at the posterior portion of the tongue: unites the tongue to the hyoid bone and gives attachment to the posterior fibers of the genioglossus muscle.
hyothyroid m. See thyrohyoid *m.*
intercostal m. Either of the membranes between the ribs, which replaces the internal or external muscles.
internal elastic m. Forms the boundary between the tunica intima and the tunica media, being prominent in arteries of medium and small caliber. See Plate 6.
internal limiting m. (a) In the eye, the inner layer of the retina. (b) *In embryology,* the membrane which lines the lumen of the neural tube.
interosseous m. (a) Of the forearm, the strong fibrous membrane between the interosseous borders of the radius and ulna. (b) Of the leg, the strong fibrous sheet between the interosseous crests of the tibia and fibula.
intrachoroidal m. An ependymal membrane below the choroidal fissure in the embryo.
limiting m. The membrane surrounding the vitreous body. See hyaloid *m.*
meconic m. A layer within the rectum of the fetus, supposed to invest the meconium.
medullary m. Endosteum.
m. bone. Any bone that originates, not in cartilage, but in membrane, as some of the cranial bones.
mucous m. The membrane lining those cavities and canals communicating with the air. It is kept moist by the secretions of various types of glands.
Nasmyth's m. See enamel *cuticle* (a).
nictitating m. The winking membrane of the lower animals, represented in the human eye by the plica semilunaris.
Nitabuch's m. See *stria* of Nitabuch.
nuclear m. The layer of condensed protoplasm at the periphery of the nucleus.
obturator m. (a) That of the pelvis, the fibrous membrane closing the obturator foramen. (b) That of the stapes, the thin membrane between the crura and footplate.
oral m. See buccopharyngeal *m.*
oronasal m. A double layer of epithelium separating the nasal pits from the stomodeum of the embryo. Also called *bucconasal m.*
otolithic m. The gelatinous membrane covering the free surface of the sensory epithelium of the acoustic macula that bears the otoliths.
peridental m. See periodontal *m.*
perineal m. Fibrous membrane stretching across the pubic arch and dividing the urogenital triangle into a superficial and a deep portion: also called *inferior fascia of the urogenital diaphragm.*
periodontal m. The connective tissue between the root of a tooth and the bone of the alveolar process, or extending from the root into the gingiva. Syn., *pericementum.* Formerly called *peridental m.*
permeable m. One which permits the passage of water and certain dissolved substances.
persistent pupillary m. An anomaly of the eye, the result of the failure of the pupillary membrane of the fetus to disappear.
pharyngeal m. See buccopharyngeal *m.*
pituitary m. The Schneiderian membrane. *Obs.*
placental m. The tissues of the placenta separating the maternal and fetal blood streams. Syn., *placental barrier.*
plasma m. That surrounding the cytoplasm of every living cell, consisting of a fine flat network of elongated protein molecules to which lipid molecules are tightly bound. It maintains the life and integrity of the cellular interior.
pleuropericardial m. The embryonic membrane, derived from the septum transversum, that separates the pericardial coelom from the pleural canal.
pleuroperitoneal m. The embryonic membrane, derived in large measure from the septum transversum, that separates the pleural canal from the peritoneal part of the coelom. It forms a part of the diaphragm.
posterior atlanto-occipital m. A broad membrane extending from the posterior surface and cranial border of the posterior arch of the atlas to the posterior margin of the foramen magnum.
pseudoserous m. One presenting the moist, glistening surface of a serous membrane, but differing from it in structure, as the endothelium of the blood vessels.
pupillary m. A membrane formed by the mesoderm on the anterior surface of the lens epithelium in the embryo. It combines peripherally with pars iridica retinae to form the iris; centrally it disappears to form the pupil of the eye.
pyogenic m. The lining of an abscess cavity or a fistulous tract. The term should be restricted to the lining of an abscess that is spreading and in which the membrane produces pus.
quadrangular m. The membrane of the larynx which extends from the aryepiglottic folds above to the level of the ventricular folds below.
Reichert's m. The delicate basement membrane of the trophoblast cells in the nonplacental area of the rodent blastoderm. It persists for some time after the trophoblast cells migrate into the decidua.
Reissner's m. See vestibular *m.*
reticular m. The membrane covering the space of the outer hair cells of the cochlea.
round-window m. See secondary tympanic *m.*
Schneiderian m. The mucosa lining the nasal cavities and paranasal sinuses.
secondary tympanic m. The membrane closing the fenestra rotunda: also called *round-window m.*
semipermeable m. One which permits water to pass but which holds back salts and their ions.
serous m. A delicate membrane covered with flat, mesothelial cells lining closed cavities of the body.

Shrapnell's m. The pars flaccida of the tympanic membrane, that is the part filling the notch of Rivinus.

sternal m. The fibrous layer ensheathing the sternum in front and behind.

submucous m. See *tela* submucosa.

suprapleural m. The extrapleural fascia attached to the inner margin of the first rib and covering the dome of the pleura. Also called *Sibson's fascia.*

sutural m. Fibrous tissue between the sutures of the cranium.

synaptic m. The single membrane at the synapse, demonstrated by special staining as separating the cytoplasm of the terminal enlargement of an axon from the cytoplasm of the nerve cell. Syn., *synaptolemma.*

synovial m. The lining of an articular capsule, concerned with secretion of synovial fluid into the articular cavity; it is lacking over articular surfaces.

tectorial m. A jellylike membrane covering the organ of Corti in the internal ear. See Plate 20.

thyrohyoid m. The membrane joining the thyroid cartilage and hyoid bone. See Plate 45.

tympanic m. The drum membrane; the membrane separating the external from the middle ear. It consists of three layers: an outer or skin layer, a fibrous layer, and an inner mucous layer. See Plate 20.

undulating m. A membrane projecting laterally from certain protozoa, especially seen in trypanosomes.

urethral m. See urogenital *m.*

urogenital m. That part of the cloacal membrane cranial or ventral to the urorectal septum; it forms the floor of the urethral groove of the phallus.

vestibular m. A thin membrane within the semicircular ducts of the ear, stretching from the upper surface of the osseous spiral lamina to the outer wall of the cochlea, separating the cochlear duct from the scala vestibuli: also called *Reissner's m.* See Plate 20.

vitelline m. A structureless cytoplasmic membrane on the surface of the ovum.

vitreous m. The inner membrane of the choroid.

mem′brane po·ten′tial. Potential difference across the membrane of a living cell.

mem″bra·no·cra′ni·um [*membrana;* G. *kranion,* skull]. The membranous skull of the fetus, prior to ossification. Syn., *desmocranium.*

mem′brum [L.]. Member.

m. muliebre. The clitoris.

m. virile. The penis.

mem′o·ry [L. *memoria,* memory]. That faculty of the mind by which ideas and sensations are recalled.

anterograde m. Memory for events in the remote past; forgetfulness for recent occurrences, or retrograde amnesia, is implied.

cutaneous m. See *mnemodermia.*

kinesthetic m. See *kinesthesia.*

retrograde m. Memory for events in the recent past, as contrasted with retrograde amnesia, the loss of memory for recent events.

me·nac′me [G. *mēn,* month; *akmē,* prime]. The period of a woman's life during which menstruation persists.

men″a·di′ol. $C_{11}H_{10}O_2$; 2-methyl-1,4-naphthohydroquinone of 2-methyl-1,4-naphthalenediol, the alcohol obtained by reduction of the =CO groups of menadione.

m. diacetate. Acetomenaphthone.

m. sodium diphosphate. $C_{11}H_8Na_4O_8P_2.6H_2O$; the hexahydrate of the tetrasodium salt of 2-methyl-1,4-naphthalenediol diphosphate; a white to pink powder, hygroscopic, very soluble in water. It has the actions and uses of menadione. Syn., *sodium menadiol diphosphate.* See *synkavite.*

men·ad′i·one (men·ad′ee·ohn, men″uh·dye′ohn) (*menadionum*). $C_{11}H_8O_2$. The 2-methyl-1,4-naphthoquinone, occurring as a bright-yellow, crystalline powder; practically insoluble in water. Possesses vitamin-K activity in hemorrhagic diatheses due to prothrombin deficiency in the blood; in cases of biliary obstruction bile salts must be administered simultaneously. Dose, 1–2 mg. (1/60–1/30 gr.). Syn., *menaphthone, synthetic vitamin K, vitamin K_3.* See *kayquinone, koaxin, koidin, proklot, thyloquinone.*

m. sodium bisulfite (*menadioni sodii bisulfis*). $C_{11}H_8O_2.NaHSO_3.3H_2O$. A water-soluble compound containing 50% menadione; suited for parenteral administration. Dose, 2–3 mg. (1/30–1/20 gr.).

men′a·gogue″ (men′uh·gog″). Emmenagogue.

men·aph′thone. The British Pharmacopoeia name for menadione.

me·nar′che (mi·nar′kee) [*mēn;* G. *archē,* beginning]. The time when menstruation starts.

delayed m. Late onset of menstruation.

Mendel, Gregor Johann [*Austrian botanist,* 1822–84]. Discovered a principle, called *Mendel's law* or *Mendelian law,* governing the inheritance of certain characteristics: in a specific character the individual offspring is not intermediate between the parents, but is like one parent or the other, and a specific character may be dominant or recessive. For example, in crossing red and white flowers, Mendel found that the first generation of hybrids were all red, and when self-fertilized produced red- and white-flowering plants in the ratio of 3:1. See Mendelian *ratio.* In this case the red was dominant, the white recessive. When the second generation of hybrids was self-fertilized, the white bred true, as did one of each three reds; the remaining two reds produced both colors, again in the ratio of three dominant to one recessive. The term *Mendelism* applies to the body of knowledge growing out of Mendel's discovery; it refers to all inheritance through the chromosomes, in contradistinction to non-Mendelian inheritance depending on autonomous bodies in the cytoplasm. See also *Mendel's laws* under *law.*

Mendel, Kurt [*German neurologist,* 1874–1946]. Described dorsal flexion of the second to fifth toes in normal individuals when the dorsum of the foot is tapped; called *dorsocuboidal* or *cuboidodigital reflex, Mendel's dorsal reflex of the foot, Bekhterev-Mendel reflex.* Plantar flexion occurs in disease of the pyramidal tract.

Mendel's reaction test. See Mantoux *test.*

Mendeléev, Dimitri Ivanovich [*Russian chemist,* 1834–1907]. A discoverer of the periodic law, also called *Mendeléev's law.*

Men′del·ism. See under Gregor Johann *Mendel.*

men″el·lip′sis. Incorrect term for menolipsis.

me·ner′ik. A Siberian mental disease; a psychosis in which the patient is incoherent, disoriented, and perhaps violent.

menformon. Trade name for a purified estrogen.

men″hi·dro′sis (men″hi·dro′sis, ·high·dro′sis), **men″i·dro′sis** [G. *mēn,* month; *hidrōsis,* a sweating]. Replacement of the menstrual flow by bloody sweat.

Ménière, Prosper [*French otologist,* 1799–1862]. Described auditory vertigo, also called *Ménière's syndrome.* See under *syndrome.*

me·nin′ge·al [G. *mēnigx,* membrane]. Pertaining to the meninges.

me·nin″ge·or′rha·phy [*mēnigx;* G. *rhaphē,* suture]. 1. Suture of membranes. 2. Suture of the meninges of the brain or spinal cord.

me·nin′ges (mi·nin′jeez). Plural of meninx.

me·nin″gi·o·blas·to′ma, me·nin″gi·o·fi″bro·blas·to′ma. See *meningioma.*

me·nin″gi·o′ma [*mēnigx;* G. *-ōma,* tumor]. A tumor situated usually in the meninges, but occasionally in other parts of the central nervous system, probably derived from cells of the meningeal primordium. Grows by expansion but rarely it may be invasive. Also called *mesenchymal m., durosarcoma, dural endothelioma, endothelioma of meninges, endotheliosis of meninges, meningeal fibroblastoma, meningioblastoma, meningiofibroblastoma, meningiomatosis, meningiosarcoma, meningiothelioma, mesothelioma of meninges, psammoma of meninges, meningeal sarcoma.*

parasagittal m. A common form of benign brain tumor. It is slow-growing and nonfiltrable, developing along the course of the superior longitudinal sinus.

suprasellar m. One situated above the sella turcica.

me·nin″gi·o″ma·to′sis. Multiple meningiomas.

me·nin″gi·o·sar·co′ma. Meningioma.

me·nin″gi·o·the″li·o′ma. Meningioma.

me·nin′gism, men′in·gism [*mēnigx*]. 1. An acute, infectious state of meningeal irritation, usually associated with the specific fevers and pneumonias in childhood. 2. A hysterical state simulating meningitis.

men″in·gis′mus (men″in·jiss′mus, ·jiz′mus). See *meningism.*

men″in·git′i·des. Plural of meningitis.

men″in·gi′tis [*mēnigx; -itis*]. Inflammation of the membranes of the brain or cord; that of the dura is termed *pachymeningitis;* that of the piarachnoid, *leptomeningitis,* or simply meningitis. According to etiology, meningitis can be classified as *actinomycotic, oidiomycotic, sporotrichotic,* etc. —**meningit′ic,** *adj.*

acute aseptic m. See lymphocytic *choriomeningitis.*

acute benign lymphocytic m. See lymphocytic *choriomeningitis.*

acute pyogenic m. Acute inflammation of the meninges due to the streptococcus, pneumococcus, micrococcus, and pyogenic organisms other than the meningococcus.

aseptic m. See lymphocytic *choriomeningitis.*

bacteroides m. Meningitis due to anaerobic, Gram-negative, non-spore-bearing bacilli (*Bacteroides*).

basilar m. Inflammation of the meninges at the base of the brain.

cancerous m. Metastatic neoplasm of the meninges with mild inflammatory reaction. Polyradiculoneuritis sometimes results from the infiltration of nerve roots in contact with the diseased meninges.

cerebrospinal m. Inflammation of the meninges of the brain and spinal cord.

chronic aseptic m. Chronic nonbacterial meningitis of unknown cause.

encephalitic m. See *meningo-encephalitis.*

epidemic cerebrospinal m. An acute purulent inflammation of the meninges of endemic and epidemic incidence caused by the *Neisseria meningitidis* (meningococcus).

fulminating adrenal m. See Waterhouse-Friderichsen *syndrome.*

gonococcal m. Meningitis caused by the gonococcus organism.

gummatous m. A granulomatous infection of the meninges occurring in the third stage of syphilis.

influenzal m. Inflammation of the meninges due to infection with *Hemophilus influenzae,* most commonly occurring in infants.

leptospiral m. A form caused by a member of the genus *Leptospira,* sometimes accompanied by jaundice.

m. circumscripta spinalis. Arachnoiditis of the spinal cord only.

m. serosa circumscripta. Inflammation of the meninges with formation of cystic accumulations of fluid which cause symptoms of tumors.

m. serosa spinalis. Arachnoiditis of the spinal cord.

meningococcus m. See epidemic cerebrospinal *m.*

plasmodial m. Meningitis caused by some form of *Plasmodium.*

pseudotyphoid m. A nonfatal louse-borne variety affecting swineherds, characterized by fever, headache, muscular pain, digestive disturbance, and foul diarrhea with occasional rectal hemorrhages.

rickettsial m. Meningitis caused by some member of the Rickettsiae.

serous m. Meningitis associated with a cranial focus of infection, for example mastoiditis, without the passage of organisms into the cerebrospinal fluid.

spinal m. Inflammation of the meninges of the spinal cord, usually secondary to osteitis of the vertebrae.

sterile m. Meningitis without infection, usually resulting from subarachnoid injection of foreign materials such as gases, serums, or chemical compounds.

streptococcal m. A form usually caused by streptococci of group A, often following otitis media, mastoiditis, or petrositis.

syphilitic m. Inflammation of the meninges caused by syphilis.

torular m. See yeast *m.*

traumatic m. Meningitis resulting from the invasion of organisms after injuries to the head or spine.

tuberculous m. Inflammation of the meninges due to the tubercle bacillus which reaches the brain from a distant focus via the blood stream; the disease occurs most commonly in children.

virus m. Meningitis caused by a virus.

yeast m. Meningitis caused by a form of yeast such as *Torula.*

men″in·git″o·pho′bi·a (men″in·jit″o·fo′bee·uh) [*mēnigx;* G. *phobos,* fear]. 1. A morbid fear of meningitis. 2. A pseudomeningitis due to fear of that disease.

me·nin′go- (mi·ning′go-, mi·nin′go-, meh·ning′go-, meh·nin′go-), **mening-** [*mēnigx*]. A combining form meaning *membrane* or denoting *the meninges.*

me·nin″go·ar″te·ri′tis [*mēnigx;* G. *artēria,* artery; *-itis,* inflammation]. Meningeal arteritis.

me·nin′go·cele [*mēnigx;* G. *kēlē,* hernia]. A protrusion of the cerebral or spinal meninges through a defect in the skull or vertebral column. It forms a cyst filled with cerebrospinal fluid.

me·nin″go·ceph″a·li′tis. See *meningoencephalitis.*

me·nin″go·cer″e·bri′tis. See *meningoencephalitis.*

me·nin″go·coc·ce′mi·a (·cock·see′mee·uh) [*mēnigx;* G. *kokkos,* berry; *haima,* blood]. The presence of meningococci in the blood.

me·nin″go·coc′cus [*mēnigx; kokkos*]. Common name for the coccus *Neisseria meningitidis.* —**meningococcal, meningococcic** (·cock′sick), *adj.*

me·nin″go·cor′ti·cal [*mēnigx;* L. *cortex,* bark]. Pertaining to the meninges and the cortex.

me·nin′go·cyte [*mēnigx;* G. *kytos,* cell]. A flattened epithelioid cell lining a subarachnoid space, which may become phagocytic.

me·nin"go-en·ceph"a·li'tis. Inflammation of the brain and its membranes. —**menin'go-encephalit'ic,** *adj.*

brucellar m. Involvement of meninges during or after recovery from brucellosis.

me·nin"go-en·ceph'a·lo·cele. Hernia of the brain and its meninges through a defect in the skull.

me·nin"go-en·ceph"a·lo·my"e·li'tis. Combined inflammation of the meninges, brain, and spinal cord.

me·nin"go-en·ceph"a·lop'a·thy. Disease of the brain and meninges.

me·nin"go·my"e·li'tis [*mēnigx;* G. *myelos,* marrow; *-itis,* inflammation]. Inflammation of the spinal cord and its meninges.

me·nin"go·my'e·lo·cele [*mēnigx; myelos;* G. *kēlē,* hernia]. A protrusion of a portion of the spinal cord and membranes through a defect in the vertebral column.

men"in·gop'a·thy [*mēnigx;* G. *pathos,* disease]. Any disease of the cerebrospinal meninges.

me·nin"go·ra·dic'u·lar [*mēnigx;* L. *radicula,* small root]. Pertaining to the meninges and nerve roots (cranial or spinal).

me·nin"go·rha·chid'i·an (·ra·kid'ee·un) [*mēnigx;* G. *rhachis,* spine]. Pertaining to the spinal cord and its membranes.

me·nin"gor·rha'gi·a [*mēnigx;* G. *rhēgnynai,* to burst forth]. Hemorrhage from the meninges.

men"in·go'sis [*mēnigx;* G. *-ōsis,* condition]. The union of bones by membranes.

me·nin"go·vas'cu·lar [*mēnigx;* L. *vasculum,* small vessel]. Involving both the meninges and the cerebral blood vessels, as meningovascular syphilis. See *syphilis.*

men"in·gu'ri·a [*mēnigx;* G. *ouron,* urine]. The passage, or presence, of membranous shreds in the urine.

me'ninx (pl. *meninges*) [*mēnigx*]. A membrane, especially one of the brain or spinal cord; the meninges covering the brain and spinal cord consist of the dura, pia, and arachnoid.

m. primitiva. The layer of mesoderm surrounding the neural tube that forms the neurocranium and meninges.

men"is·cec'to·my (men"i·seck'to·mee) [G. *mēniskos,* any crescent-shaped body; *ektomē,* excision]. The surgical excision of a meniscus or semilunar cartilage.

men"is·ci'tis (men"i·sigh'tis, ·sky'tis) [*mēniskos;* G. *-itis,* inflammation]. An inflammation of any interarticular cartilage; specifically, of the semilunar cartilages of the knee joint.

me·nis'co·cyte [*mēniskos;* G. *kytos,* cell]. A sickle-shaped erythrocyte.

me·nis"co·cy·to'sis (mi·nis"ko·sigh·to'sis) [*mēniskos; kytos;* G. *-ōsis,* condition]. Sickle-cell anemia.

men"is·cot'o·my. Incorrect term for meniscectomy.

me·nis'cus (pl. *meniscuses, menisci*) [*mēniskos*]. 1. A crescent or crescentic body, especially an interarticular fibrocartilage. 2. A concavoconvex lens (positive meniscus) or a convexoconcave lens (negative meniscus). 3. The curved surface of a column of liquid.

m. lateralis. The external, semilunar fibrocartilage of the knee joint.

m. medialis. The internal, semilunar fibrocartilage of the knee joint. See Plate 2.

tactile m. See tactile *disk.*

men"i·sper'mine. $C_{18}H_{24}N_2O_2$; a crystalline alkaloid obtained from the seed coat of *Anamirta paniculata,* pharmacologically inactive.

men"i·sper'mum. The rhizome and roots of *Menispermum canadense.* It contains the alkaloid *menispine* and has been used as a substitute for sarsaparilla. Syn., *Canada moonseed, yellow parilla.*

men'o- [G. *mēn,* month]. A combining form meaning *month;* denotes *relation to the menses.*

men"o·ce'lis [*mēn;* G. *kēlis,* spot]. Dark, erythematous or hemorrhagic spots occurring upon the skin in failure of menstruation.

men"o·lip'sis [*mēn;* G. *leipsis,* omission]. The retention or absence of the menses.

men'o·pause (men'o·pawz) [*mēn;* G. *pausis,* a stopping]. The physiologic cessation of menstruation, usually between the forty-fifth and fiftieth years. Also called *climacteric.* —**menopausic, menopaus'al,** *adj.*

artificial m. Permanent cessation of menses and normal ovarian function from other than normal physiological cause, e.g., by surgical removal of the ovaries or by irradiation. Surgical removal of the uterus alone produces permanent cessation of menstruation, but not necessarily an artificial menopause if the ovaries continue to function cyclicly.

men"o·pha'ni·a [*mēn;* G. *phainein,* to appear]. The first appearance of the menses.

men"o·pla'ni·a [*mēn;* G. *planē,* a wandering]. A discharge of blood occurring at the menstrual period, but derived from some part of the body other than the uterus; vicarious menstruation.

men"or·rha'gi·a [*mēn;* G. *rhēgnynai,* to burst forth]. An excessive menstrual flow. Syn., *hypermenorrhea.*

functional m. Excessive menstruation due to no demonstrable anatomic or pathologic lesion; usually assumed to be due to endocrine dysfunction. Also called *primary m.*

men"or·rhal'gi·a [*mēn;* G. *rhoia,* flow; *algos,* pain]. Pelvic pain at menstrual periods other than characteristic midline cramp; characteristic of endometriosis.

men"or·rhe'a, men"or·rhoe'a [*mēn; rhoia*]. 1. The normal flow of the menses. 2. Excessive menstruation.

me·nos'che·sis (mi·nos'ki·sis, men"o·skee'sis) [*mēn;* G. *schesis,* a checking]. Retention of the menses.

men"o·sta'si·a (men"o·stay'zhuh, ·zee·uh), **me·nos'ta·sis** [*mēn;* G. *stasis,* a standing]. A suppression of the menstrual flow.

men"o·stax'is [*mēn;* G. *staxis,* a dripping]. Prolonged menstruation.

men"o·xe'ni·a (men"ock·see'nee·uh, men"o·zee'-nee·uh) [*mēn;* G. *xenos,* strange]. Irregularity of menstruation; vicarious menstruation. *Obs.*

mens [L.]. Mind. *Compos mentis,* of sound mind. *Non compos mentis,* of unsound mind. *Mens sana in corpore sano,* a sound mind in a sound body.

men'sa [L., table]. The chewing surface of the molars. *Obs.*

men'ses (men'seez) [L., months]. The recurrent monthly discharge of blood from the genital canal of a woman during sexual maturity.

men'stru·ant [L. *menstruus,* monthly]. Subject to, or capable of, menstruating.

men'stru·ant. One who menstruates.

men'stru·ate [L. *menstruare,* to menstruate]. Discharge the menses.

men"stru·a'tion [*menstruare*]. A periodic discharge of a sanguineous fluid from the uterus, occurring during the period of a woman's sexual maturity from puberty to the menopause. —**men'strual,** *adj.*

anovulatory m. That not preceded by the release of an ovum.

delayed m. Menstruation occurring later than expected from previous cyclic timing.

regurgitant m. A backflow through the uterine tubes.

supplementary m. Vicarious menstruation.

suppressed m. Nonappearance of the menstrual flow in patients who formerly menstruated. Syn., *menostasia*.

vicarious m. The discharge of blood at the time of menstruation from some place other than the vagina.

men'stru·um [L.]. A solvent.

Pitkin m. A medium developed to retard the release of water-soluble drugs injected subcutaneously or intramuscularly, composed of gelatin, dextrose, and glacial acetic acid: used in the administration of heparin in thromboembolic disease.

men'su·al (men'shoo·ul, men'sue·ul) [L. *mensualis*, monthly]. Monthly.

men"su·ra'tion (men"shoo·ray'shun, men"sue·) [L. *mensurare*, to measure]. The act of measuring; one of the methods of physical diagnosis.

men·tag'ra. See *sycosis*.

men'tal [L. *mentalis*, mental]. Pertaining to the mind.

men'tal [L. *mentum*, chin]. Pertaining to the chin. Syn., *genial*.

men'tal age. A score, derived from intelligence tests, expressed in terms of the age at which an average individual attains that score. Abbreviation, MA.

men'tal de·fi'cien·cy. 1. *In psychiatry*, a defect of intelligence existing since birth; it may be *primary* (hereditary or familial), that is, without demonstrated organic brain lesion or known prenatal cause, or *secondary*, that is, associated with a chronic organic brain disorder due to brain tissue anomalies, mongolism, prenatal maternal infectious diseases, or birth trauma. The degree of the defect may be indicated by the intelligence quotient for the specific test employed. 2. *In civil law*, the condition as defined by statute is frequently divided into three grades: idiocy, the lowest; imbecility, the intermediate; and moronity, the highest.

mild m. d. That in which there is primarily impairment of vocational capacities; the intelligence quotient is approximately 70 to 85.

moderate m. d. That in which there is impairment requiring special training and guidance; the intelligence quotient is generally about 50 to 70.

severe m. d. That in which there is impairment requiring custodial or complete protective care; the intelligence quotient is expected to be below 50.

men'tal dis·or'ders. *In psychiatry*, groups of related psychiatric conditions, called *reactions*, and divided into two major groups: 1. Those in which there is primary impairment of brain function, generally associated with an organic brain syndrome upon which diagnosis is based. The psychiatric picture is characterized by impairment of intellectual functions, including memory, orientation, and judgment, and by shallowness and lability of affect. Additional disturbances, described as *psychotic, neurotic*, or *behavioral reactions*, may be associated with these disorders, but are secondary to the diagnosis. When the syndrome is chronic, congenital, or produced in infancy or early childhood, with a primary defect in learning ability and intellectual development, the term *mental deficiency* is applied. 2. Those which are more directly the result of the individual's difficulty to adapt to his environment, and in which any associated disturbance of brain function is secondary to the psychiatric reaction.

men·ta'lis [*mentum*]. A muscle of the lower lip. See Table of Muscles in the Appendix.

men·tal'i·ty [L. *mentalis*, mental]. Mental endowment, capacity, or power; intellect.

men·ta'tion. The mechanism of thought; mental activity.

Menten, Maud Lenore [*American pathologist*, 1879–]. With L. Michaelis, evolved a theory of enzymatic behavior. In the *Michaelis-Menten theory* it is assumed that an enzymatic reaction proceeds by way of an intermediate compound of the enzyme and its substrate.

Men'tha [L., mint]. A genus of plants of the Lamiaceae; the mints.

M. piperita. Peppermint; the dried leaves and flowering tops have been used as an aromatic stimulant. Also has been used to relieve nausea, flatulence, and spasmodic pain in the stomach and bowel.

M. pulegium. European pennyroyal, the leaves and tops of which are used as a carminative. See also *hedeoma*.

M. viridis. Spearmint. The dried leaves and flowering tops of *M. spicata*. The properties and uses of *M. viridis* are similar to those of *M. piperita*.

Men·tha·ce·ae (men·thay'see·ee). Synonym for Lamiaceae.

men'thene. $C_{10}H_{18}$; a colorless, liquid hydrocarbon derived from menthol or from peppermint oil.

men'tho-, menth- [*mentha*]. A combining form denoting *menthol*.

men'thol (*menthol*). $C_{10}H_{19}OH$. An alcohol obtained from peppermint oil or other mint oils, or prepared synthetically; may be levorotatory (*l*-menthol) or racemic (*dl*-menthol), the latter being solely of synthetic origin. Occurs in colorless crystals, in fused masses, or as a crystalline powder; very slightly soluble in water but very soluble in alcohol. Used principally externally for its anesthetic, counterirritant, or antiseptic effects. Dose, 0.06–0.13 Gm. (1–2 gr.).

camphorated m. (*menthol camphoratum*). A liquid mixture of equal parts of menthol and camphor; used externally as a counterirritant and anodyne.

men'thone. $C_{10}H_{18}O$. The ketone of menthol; obtained from peppermint oil.

men'thyl. The monovalent radical $C_{10}H_{19}$.

men'to- [L. *mentum*, chin]. *In anatomy*, a combining form signifying *pertaining to the chin*.

men"to·hy'oid. A variant of the digastric muscle extending from the hyoid to the chin.

men'ton. See *gnathion*.

men"tu·lo·ma'ni·a. Masturbation.

men'tum [L.]. Chin.

men"y·an'thes (men"ee·an'theez) [perhaps from G. *mēn*, month; *anthos*, flower]. The dried leaves of *Menyanthes trifoliata;* contains a bitter principle, menyanthin; has been used as a simple bitter and a febrifuge. Also called *buckbean*.

men"y·an'thin. $C_{33}H_{50}O_{14}$. A bitter glycoside found in menyanthes.

meonine. Trade-mark for *methionine*.

mep'a·crine hy"dro·chlo'ride (mep'uh·krene, ·krin, mi·pack'reen, ·rin). British Pharmacopoeia name for quinacrine hydrochloride.

mep'a·crine meth"ane·sul'fo·nate. The name given by the British Pharmacopoeia to the salt quinacrine methanesulfonate. Used like quinacrine hydrochloride, but preferred over the latter for parenteral administration because of its greater solubility in water. Dose, intramuscularly, 0.05–0.1 Gm. (¾–1½ gr.).

me·per'i·dine hy"dro·chlo'ride (meh·perr'i·deen, ·din, mep'ur·i·deen", ·din"). $C_2H_5OOC.C(C_6H_5)$-$CH_2.CH_2.N(CH_3)CH_2.CH_2$.HCl. The hydrochloride of ethyl 1-methyl-4-phenylpiperidine-4-carboxylate. A colorless, crystalline powder, soluble in water. It exerts both the analgesic and sedative action of morphine and the antispasmodic action of atropine. Used to relieve pain, particularly that associated with smooth muscle spasm in the gastrointestinal, biliary, and genitourinary tracts. Effective for preanesthetic medication and for control of postoperative pain. May be used instead of opiates. Dose, 0.025–0.1 Gm. (3/8–1½ gr.), orally or intramuscularly. See *demerol hydrochloride, dolantin, isonipecaine, pethidine.*

me·phen′e·sin, meph″e·ne′sin. $CH_3.C_6H_4.OCH_2CHOHCH_2OH$; 3-*o*-toloxy-1,2-propanediol or 1,2-dihydroxy-3-(2-methylphenoxy) propane, colorless crystals, sparingly soluble in water; a skeletal muscle relaxant and sedative. See *avosyl, dioloxol, lissephen, myanesin, myoxane, oranixon, sinan, tolserol.*

me·phen′ter·mine. $C_6H_5CH_2C(CH_3)_2NHCH_3$; N-methyl-N-phenyl-*tertiary*-butylamine; a volatile, sympathomimetic amine used as a nasal decongestant. See *wyamine.*

m. sulfate. $(C_{11}H_{17}N)_2.H_2SO_4.2H_2O$; a white, crystalline powder, soluble in water: used parenterally in treatment of hypotensive states. See *wyamine sulfate.*

me·phit′ic [L. *mephitis*, noxious exhalation from the ground]. Foul or noxious; stifling, as mephitic gangrene, necrosis of bone associated with the evolution of offensive odors. *Obs.*

meph″o·bar′bi·tal. $C_{13}H_{14}N_2O_3$; 5-ethyl-1-methyl-5-phenylbarbituric acid; a white, crystalline powder, slightly soluble in water; a barbiturate characterized by slight hypnotic effect and marked anticonvulsant action, useful in the treatment of epilepsy. Syn., *methylphenobarbital, methylphenobarbitone, phemitone.* See *mebaral, prominal.*

mephyton. Trade-mark for 2-methyl-3-phytyl-1,4-naphthoquinone, identical with natural vitamin K_1 or phytonadione. The substance is employed intravenously, in the form of an aqueous emulsion stabilized with lecithin, as an antidote to anticoagulant-induced hypoprothrombinemia.

me·pip″er·phen′i·dol bro′mide. Generic name for the visceral anticholinergic agent supplied under the trade-marked name darstine bromide.

meprane dipropionate. Trade-mark for promethestrol dipropionate, a synthetic estrogen.

me″pro·bam′ate. Generic name for 2-methyl-2-*n*-propyl-1,3-propanediol dicarbamate, a substance having tranquilizing action. See *equanil, miltown.*

mep′y·ra·mine″ ma·le′ate. British Pharmacopoeia name for the antihistaminic salt pyrilamine maleate.

mEq, mEq. Milliequivalent.

me·ral′gi·a [G. *mēros*, thigh; *algos*, pain]. Neuralgic pain in the thigh.

m. paresthetica. Bernhardt's term for a paresthesia of the skin of the lower and outer aspect of the thigh in the region supplied by the lateral cutaneous nerve of the thigh: also called *Roth-Bernhardt disease, Roth's disease.*

me·ral′lu·ride (meh·ral′yoo·ride, ·rid). A combination of methoxyhydroxymercuripropylsuccinylurea and theophylline in approximately molecular proportions; a mercurial diuretic, the sodium derivative of which is administered parenterally. See *mercuhydrin.*

me·ra·lo′pi·a. Blurring of vision, with halos seen around objects viewed in a bright light: often associated with the administration of oxazolidine derivatives for the control of petit-mal seizures.

mer″a·mau·ro′sis [G. *meros*, part; *amaurōsis*, a darkening]. Partial amaurosis.

merbak. Trade-mark for the organomercurial topical antiseptic acetomeroctol.

mer′ba·phen. The double salt of sodium mercurichlorophenyl oxyacetate and diethylbarbituric acid, occurring as a white, crystalline powder; soluble in water: used as a diuretic. See *novasurol.*

mer·bro′min (*merbrominum*). The disodium salt of 2,7-dibromo-4-hydroxymercurifluorescein, occurring as iridescent, green scales or granules but forming a red solution with yellow-green fluorescence; freely soluble in water. Merbromin, introduced as mercurochrome, is a surgical disinfectant.

m. solution (*liquor merbromini*). A 2% (w/v) aqueous solution of merbromin.

mer·cap′tal, mer″cap·tal′. A product of the union of a mercaptan and an aldehyde.

mer·cap′tan, mer″cap·tan′. 1. An organic compound of the general formula R.SH, representing an alcohol R.OH, in which oxygen is replaced by sulfur. Syn., *thioalcohol, thiol.* 2. Ethyl mercaptan, C_2H_5SH.

mer·cap′tide, mer″cap·tide′. Any metallic derivative of a mercaptan in which the hydrogen of the SH group of the latter is replaced by metal.

mer·cap′tol. A compound resulting from the interaction of a ketone and a mercaptan, of the general formula $R'R''C(SR)_2$.

mer·cap″to·mer′in so′di·um. $C_{16}H_{25}HgNNa_2O_6S$; disodium N-[3-(carboxymethylmercaptomercuri)-2-methoxypropyl]-α-camphoramate; a hygroscopic, white solid, freely soluble in water; a mercurial diuretic, less irritating on injection and less toxic to the heart than other mercurial diuretics. See *thiomerin sodium.*

mer·cap″to·pu′rine. $C_5H_4N_4S$; 6-mercaptopurine, the mercapto analog of 6-aminopurine or adenine; a potent inhibitor of a strain of mouse sarcoma, possibly through its ability to block a metabolic step in conversion of adenine to guanine. It is under investigation as a possible chemotherapeutic agent in human neoplastic diseases.

mer″cap·tu′ric ac′id. Any detoxication product in which acetylated cysteine is conjugated with the foreign body undergoing the process of detoxication.

mercarbolide. Trade-mark for orthohydroxyphenylmercuric chloride, an externally applied antiseptic, germicide, and fungicide.

Mercier, Louis Auguste [*French urologist*, 1811–82]. Described the transverse ridge joining the openings of the ureters on the inner surface of the bladder and forming the posterior boundary of the triangle of the bladder; called *Mercier's bar.* Devised an operation of transurethral prostatectomy; called *Mercier's operation.*

mer″co·cre′sols. Generic name for the preparation marketed under the trade-marked name *mercresin.*

mercresin. Trade-mark for an acetone-alcohol solution containing secondary amyltricresols and mercarbolide. The solution is used as an antiseptic and germicide. See *mercocresols.*

mercuhydrin. Trade-mark for the mercurial diuretic meralluride.

mer·cu″ma·til′in, mer″cu·mat′i·lin. Generic name for a mercurial diuretic preparation containing 8-(2′-methoxy-3′-hydroxymercuripropyl) coumarin-3-carboxylic acid (known as *mercumallylic acid*) and theophylline, the combination being supplied under the trade-mark *cumertilin.*

m. sodium. Generic name for a preparation containing the sodium salt of the mercuri compound described in the preceding and theophylline, the combination being supplied under the trade-marked name *cumertilin sodium.*

mercurettes. Trade-mark for a preparation of metallic mercury in cacao butter, applied by inunction in syphilis.

mer′cu·ri- [L. *Mercurius*, god and planet]. A combining form signifying *mercury;* used in chemistry to denote *mercuric.*

mer·cu′ri·al [*Mercurius*]. Pertaining to or caused by mercury.

mer·cu′ri·al. Any preparation of mercury or its salts.

mer·cu″ri·a′lis [*Mercurius*]. An herbaceous European plant, *Mercurialis annua;* formerly used as a diuretic, emmenagogue, and vermifuge. Also called *mercury herb, French mercury.*

mer·cu′ri·al·ism [*Mercurius*]. Poisoning due to absorption of mercury.

mer·cu″ri·al·i·za′tion [*Mercurius*]. The act of bringing under the influence of mercury. —**mercu′rialize,** *v.*

mer·cu′ric [*Mercurius*]. Pertaining to mercury as a bivalent element.

m. benzoate. $Hg(C_6H_5COO)_2.H_2O$. A white, crystalline powder, slightly soluble in water; has been used for intramuscular injections in syphilis and locally in the treatment of gonorrhea.

m. cyanide. $Hg(CN)_2$. Colorless or white crystals, soluble in 13 parts of water; has been used hypodermically in treating syphilis, also as a local germicide. Dose, 0.004–0.008 Gm. (1/16–1/8 gr.).

m. lactate. $(C_3H_5O_3)_2Hg$. A white powder, soluble in water; has been used in the treatment of syphilis.

m. nitrate. $Hg(NO_3)_2$. A white or slightly yellow deliquescent salt, soluble in water. Applied locally, usually in ointment form, for its stimulating and antiseptic effects.

m. oxycyanide. Approximately $Hg(CN)_2.HgO$. A white powder, soluble in about 80 parts of water; used locally as an antiseptic, also intravenously in the treatment of syphilis.

m. salicylate (*hydrargyri salicylas*). A white powder of variable composition containing 54–59% Hg, practically insoluble in water; used locally as an antiseptic and, by intramuscular injection, in treating syphilis. Dose, by injection, 0.06 Gm. (1 gr.) 2 or 3 times a week.

m. succinimide (*hydrargyri succinimidum*). $C_8H_8N_2O_4Hg$. A white powder, soluble in 20 parts of water; used in the treatment of syphilis, generally hypodermically. Dose, 0.01–0.02 Gm. (1/6–1/3 gr.) daily.

m. sulfide. HgS. A scarlet powder, turning black on heating; insoluble in water; a stabilized colloidal solution of the chemical is used intramuscularly in the treatment of syphilis.

red m. iodide (*hydrargyri iodidum rubrum*). HgI_2. A scarlet-red amorphous powder, insoluble in water, but soluble in solutions of iodides; used locally as an antiseptic, occasionally also internally in syphilis. Dose, 0.003–0.005 Gm. (1/20–1/12 gr.).

red m. oxide (*hydrargyri oxidum rubrum*). HgO. An orange-red, crystalline powder, almost insoluble in water; used locally as antiseptic application to chancres, to ulcers, and to fungoid infections.

yellow m. oxide (*hydrargyri oxidum flavum*). HgO. A yellow powder, differing from the red variety in being more finely subdivided. Employed in the same manner as the red oxide but more effective because of the greater surface area of its particles.

mercurochrome. Trade-mark for the disodium salt of 2,7-dibromo-4-hydroxymercurifluorescein. See *merbromin.*

mercurophen. Trade-mark for sodium hydroxymercuri-*o*-nitrophenolate, used as a germicide.

mer″cu·ro·phyl′line in·jec′tion (mur″cue·ro·fill′-een, ·in) (*injectio mercurophyllinae*). A sterile aqueous solution of the sodium salt of β-methoxy-γ-hydroxymercuripropylamide of trimethylcyclopentanedicarboxylic acid ($C_{14}H_{24}NO_5HgNa$), called the mercuri compound, and of theophylline in approximately molecular proportions. The commercial product represents 10% of the mercuri compound and approximately 4% of theophylline. Employed intravenously as a diuretic. Dose, 1–2 cc. (15–30 min.). See *mercuzanthin.*

mer·cu′rous, mer′cu·rous [*Mercurius*]. Pertaining to compounds containing mercury as a univalent radical.

m. acetate. $Hg_2(C_2H_3O_2)_2$. White crystals, soluble in about 100 parts of water; has been used as a local application to syphilitic sores.

m. sozoiodolate. $HgC_6H_2I_2OSO_3$. A yellow powder, sparingly soluble in water; has been used locally in the treatment of syphilitic ulcerations, ozena, lupus, etc.

m. tannate. A variable substance containing 50% Hg; has been used as an antisyphilitic.

mild m. chloride (*hydrargyri chloridum mite*). HgCl. A white powder, insoluble in water; used as an antisyphilitic, cathartic, diuretic, and antiseptic. Dose, as alterative, 0.01–0.02 Gm. (1/6–1/3 gr.); as cathartic, 0.12–0.3 Gm. (2–5 gr.). Syn., *calomel.*

yellow m. iodide (*hydrargyri iodidum flavum*). HgI. A yellow, amorphous powder, practically insoluble in water; has been used as an antisyphilitic.

mer′cu·ry (*hydrargyrum*). Hg = 200.61. A shining, silver-white, liquid, volatile metal, having a specific gravity of 13.55. Insoluble in the ordinary solvents, in hydrochloric acid, and in sulfuric acid in the cold; dissolves in the last when boiled with it; readily soluble in nitric acid. Boils at 356.9° C., and solidifies at −38.9° C. Is found pure, but is obtained chiefly as the native sulfide, or cinnabar. Forms two classes of compounds: (a) the mercurous, those in which two atoms of the metal are combined with a bivalent radical, and (b) the mercuric, those in which one atom of the metal is combined with a bivalent radical. The mercuric salts are more soluble and more poisonous than the mercurous. Mercury in the form of its salts was formerly used as a purgative and cholagogue (calomel, blue mass, mercury with chalk), as an alterative in chronic inflammations, as an antisyphilitic, an antiphlogistic, an intestinal antiseptic, a disinfectant, a parasiticide, a caustic, and an astringent. The absorption of mercury in sufficient quantity causes poisoning, characterized by a coppery taste in the mouth, ptyalism, loosening of the teeth, sponginess of the gums; in severer cases, ulceration of the cheeks, necrosis of the jaws, marked emaciation; at times neuritis develops, and a peculiar tremor. The soluble salts when taken in excess act as intense gastrointestinal irritants.

ammoniated m. (*hydrargyrum ammoniatum*). NH_3HgCl. White precipitate; mercuric ammonium chloride; used chiefly locally to treat various skin conditions.

m. bichloride (*hydrargyri bichloridum*). $HgCl_2$. Corrosive sublimate; employed for the systemic effects of mercury as well as for its germicidal property. Dose, 0.0015–0.008 Gm. (1/40–1/8 gr.).

m. gallate. Approximately $Hg[C_6H_2(OH)_3COO]_2$. A greenish black powder containing about 37% of mercury; has been used as an alterative and antisyphilitic.

m. mass (*massa hydrargyri*). Blue mass; blue pill. Dose, as an alterative, 0.06–0.2 Gm. (1–3 gr.); as a laxative, 0.3-1.0 Gm. (5–15 gr.).

m. oleate (*oleatum hydrargyri*). Prepared by reaction of yellow mercuric oxide and oleic acid; has been used locally. Also see mercurial *ointment*.

m. with chalk (*hydrargyrum cum creta*). Gray powder; used as a laxative and antisyphilitic. Dose, as cathartic, 0.25–0.6 Gm. (4–10 gr.); as antisyphilitic, 0.03–0.06 Gm. (½–1 gr.).

mercuzanthin. Trade-mark for mercurophylline injection.

mer″er·ga′si·a (merr″ur·gay′zhuh, ·zee·uh, ·shuh, ·see·uh) [G. *meros*, part; *ergasia*, work]. *In psychobiology*, Meyer's term for a partial disturbance of the personality, as a neurotic or psychoneurotic reaction. Syn., *kakergasia*.

me·rid′i·an [L. *meridianus*, of midday]. A great circle surrounding a sphere and intersecting the poles.

m. of the eye. A line drawn around the globe of the eye and passing through the poles of the vertical axis (vertical meridian), or through the poles of the transverse axis (horizontal meridian). —**merid′ional,** *adj.*

Mering, Joseph von [*German physician*, 1849–1908]. Said to have produced glycosuria experimentally by the administration of phlorhizin (1886). With O. Minkowski, studied the diabetic syndrome following experimental pancreatectomy (1889). With E. Fischer, introduced the use of barbital.

mer″in·tho·pho′bi·a (merr″in·tho·fo′bee·uh, mi-rin″tho·) [G. *mērinthos*, cord; *phobos*, fear]. A morbid fear of being bound.

mer′i·spore [G. *meros*, part; *spora*, seed]. A segment or spore of a multicellular spore body.

me·ris′tic [G. *meristikos*, fit for dividing]. Pertaining to, or divided into, segments.

Merkel, Friedrich Siegmund [*German anatomist*, 1845–1919]. Described tactile nerve endings, called *Merkel's corpuscles, disks, tactile disks*. See tactile *disk*.

mer′o-, mer- [G. *meros*, part]. A combining form meaning *part*.

mer″o·a·cra′ni·a [*meros;* G. *a-*, not; *kranion*, skull]. Congenital absence of a part of the cranium.

mer″o·blas′tic [*meros;* G. *blastos*, germ]. Dividing only in part, referring to an egg in which the cleavage divisions are confined to the animal pole, owing to the presence of a large amount of yolk.

mer′o·crine (merr′o·kryne, ·krin) [*meros;* G. *krinein*, to separate]. Pertaining to glands in which the act of secretion leaves the cell intact. See *holocrine, apocrine*.

mer″o·gen′e·sis [*meros;* G. *genesis*, production]. Reproduction by segmentation; somite formation. *Rare.*

mer″o·mi″cro·so′mi·a [*meros;* G. *mikros*, small; *sōma*, body]. Abnormal smallness of some part of the body.

me·ro′pi·a [*meros;* G. *ōps*, eye]. Partial blindness; obscuration of vision.

mer″o·ra·chis′chi·sis (merr″o·ra·kiss′ki·sis) [*meros;* G. *rhachis*, spine; *schisis*, cleavage]. Partial spina bifida.

me·ros′mi·a (mi·ros′mee·uh, mi·roz′·, meh·) [*meros;* G. *osmē*, smell]. Partial loss of the sense of smell in that certain odors are not perceived.

mer″o·som′a·tous [*meros;* G. *sōma*, body]. Characterizing a monstrosity in which only part of the body is involved.

mer′o·some [*meros; sōma*]. A somite or metamere.

me·rot′o·my [*meros;* G. *tomē*, a cutting]. The section of a living cell for the study of the ulterior transformation of its segments; by extension it is also applied to experimental division of unicellular organisms, as amebas, etc.

mer″o·zo′ite, me″ro·zo′ite [*meros;* G. *zōion*, living being]. Any one of the segments resulting from the splitting up of the schizont in the asexual form of reproduction of sporozoa. See Plates 28, 29.

merphenyl. Trade-mark for certain phenylmercuric salt antiseptic preparations.

mer′sa·lyl (mur′suh·lil, ·leel) (*mersalyl*). NaOOC.-$CH_2O.C_6H_4.CO.NH.CH_2.CH(OCH_3).CH_2.HgOH$. The sodium salt of salicyl-(γ-hydroxymercuri-β-methoxypropyl)-amide-O-acetic acid, a white powder; 1 Gm. dissolves in about 1 cc. of water. Mersalyl was introduced as an antisyphilitic, but is now employed mainly as a diuretic; generally administered parenterally, in combination with theophylline. See *salyrgan*.

m. and theophylline injection (*injectio mersalylis et theophyllinae*). A sterile aqueous solution of approximately 10% of mersalyl and 5% of theophylline. The addition of theophylline reduces the toxicity and irritation of the mersalyl. Dose, 0.5–2.0 cc. (8–30 min.).

merthiolate. Trade-mark for thimerosal or sodium ethylmercurithiosalicylate, a bacteriostatic and fungistatic agent.

Me·ru′li·us [L. *merula*, blackbird]. A genus of fungi of the class Basidiomycetes. The mycelium of **M. lacrymans** causes dry rot in timber, and diseases (sometimes fatal) of the respiratory passages are attributed to the inhaled spores.

me·ru·tu′. See *mampirra*.

Méry, Jean [*French surgeon*, 1645–1722]. Described the bulbourethral glands (1684), called *Méry's glands, Cowper's glands*.

mer′y·cism [G. *mēryx*, a ruminating animal]. The voluntary regurgitation of food, remastication, and swallowing a second time; occurs in certain idiots and some psychiatric patients.

Merzbacher, Ludwig [*German physician in Argentina*, 1875–]. Described aplasia axialis extracorticalis congenita, also called *Merzbacher-Pelizaeus disease*. See under *aplasia*.

mes″a·con′i·tine. $C_{33}H_{45}NO_{11}$; a crystalline alkaloid occurring in several species of *Aconitum*.

mes″a·me′boid [G. *mesos*, middle; *amoibē*, change]. Minot's term for a primitive ameboid wandering cell of the mesoderm functioning as a hemocytoblast in the embryo and perhaps in the adult.

mes·an′to·in. Trade-mark for *methoin*.

mes″a·or·ti′tis [*mesos;* G. *aortē*, aorta; *-itis*, inflammation]. Inflammation of the middle coat of the aorta.

giant-cell m. A rare histologic lesion of the aorta consisting of patchy destruction of the elastic lamellae involving the middle third of the media with secondary inflammatory changes.

mes·ar″te·ri′tis [*mesos;* G. *artēria*, artery; *-itis*]. Inflammation of the middle coat of an artery.

mes·at″i·ceph′a·lus (mess″uh·ti·sef′uh·lus, mi-sat″i·) [G. *mesatos*, midmost; *kephalē*, head]. *In craniometry*, a person whose skull has a cephalic index of between 75 and 79. —**mesaticephal′ic,** *adj.*

mes″a·ti·pel′lic, mes″a·ti·pel′vic (mess″uh·ti-pel′vick, mi·sat″i·) [*mesatos;* L. *pelvis*, basin]. *In osteometry*, designating a pelvis in which the transverse diameter of the pelvic inlet is nearly equal to the conjugata vera; having a pelvic-inlet index of 90.0 to 94.9.

mes·cal′ [Sp. *mezcal*]. An intoxicant spirit distilled from Mexican pulque, a fermented beverage.

m. buttons. The dried tops from a species of cactus, *Lophophora williamsii;* capable of producing inebriation and hallucinations.

mes′ca·line. $C_{11}H_{17}NO_3$; 3,4,5-trimethoxyphenethylamine; a crystalline alkaloid from the flowering heads of *Anhalonium* or *Lophophora* cactus (*L. williamsii*): also spelled *mezcaline.*

mes·ec′to·derm [G. *mesos*, middle; *ektos*, outside; *derma*, skin]. That part of the mesenchyme derived from ectoderm, especially from the neural crest in the head region anterior to the somites. It is said to contribute to the formation of meninges; and, in some animals, the pigment cells or melanophores are derived from it.

mes·em′brin, mes·em′brine. $C_{17}H_{23}NO_3$; a tropane ester alkaloid, said to have cocainelike action, occurring in several *Mesembryanthemum* plants.

Mes·em″bry·an′the·mum. A large genus of largely South African herbs or subshrubs, including *M. acinaciforme* (more properly *Carpobrotus edulis*) which contains tannin and has been used in treating dysentery, *M. crystallinum* used as a diuretic, and *M. anatomicum* and *M. tortuosum*, both narcotic drugs containing the tropane ester alkaloid mesembrin.

mes″en·ceph″al·i′tis. Inflammation of the midbrain.

mes″en·ceph′a·lon [*mesos;* G. *egkephalos*, brain]. The midbrain; that part of the brain developed from the middle cerebral vesicle and consisting of the corpora quadrigemina and cerebral peduncles, and traversed by the cerebral aqueduct. —**mesencephal′ic,** *adj.*

mes″en·ceph·a·lot′o·my. Surgical incision of the spinothalamic tract in the midbrain, formerly used to control intractable pain, now in disuse because of resulting dysesthesia.

mes′en·chyme (mess′eng·kim, ·kyme, mess′un·), **me·sen′chy·ma** (mi·seng′ki·muh, ·sen′ki·muh, ·seng′kigh·muh, ·sen′kigh·muh) [*mesos;* G. *egchyma*, instillation]. The portion of the mesoderm that produces all the connective tissues of the body, the blood vessels, and the blood, the entire lymphatic system proper, and the heart; the nonepithelial portions of the mesoderm. —**mesen′chymal,** *adj.*

mes″en·chy″mo·blas·to′ma. A gonadal tumor. See *dysgerminoma, seminoma.*

mes″en·chy·mo′ma. A tumor of the soft tissues, of mesenchymal origin, composed of two or more mesenchymal elements other than fibrous tissue. Mesenchymomas are of particular interest because, showing various combination of adipose, cartilaginous, muscular, osteoid, vascular, and other tissues, they demonstrate the great variability of the pluripotential mesenchymal cell. The term *malignant* is reserved for those composed of tumor cells differentiating into two or more unrelated malignant forms other than differentiated fibrosarcomas. Syn., *mixed mesenchymal* or *mesodermal tumor.*

me·sen′na [Tigriña *mussenna*]. The bark of the Abyssinian tree *Albizzia anthelmintica;* used as a taeniafuge. Also called *musenna.*

mes″en·ter·ec′to·my [G. *mesos*, middle; *enteron*, intestine; *ektomē*, excision]. Excision of the mesentery or a part of it.

mes″en·ter″i·co·mes″o·col′ic [*mesos; enteron; mesos;* G. *kolon*, colon]. Relating to the mesentery and the mesocolon.

mes″en·ter″i·o′lum (mess″un·terr″ee·o′lum, ·tur-eye′o·lum) [*mesos; enteron*]. A little mesentery; especially the fold of peritoneum that sometimes connects the vermiform process with the mesentery. *O.T.*

mes″en·ter′i·o·pex″y. See *mesopexy.*

mes″en·ter″i·or′rha·phy [*mesos; enteron;* G. *rhaphē*, suture]. Surgical repair of a mesentery.

mes″en·ter″i·pli·ca′tion [*mesos; enteron;* L. *plicare*, to fold]. Mesenteriorrhaphy; reduction of folds of redundant mesentery by overlapping and suture.

mes″en·te′ri·um. A mesentery.

mes·en′ter·on [*mesos; enteron*]. Old term for midgut.

mes′en·ter″y [*mesos; enteron*]. A fold of the peritoneum that connects the intestine with the posterior abdominal wall; that of the small intestine is termed mesentery proper; that of the colon, cecum, and rectum, mesocolon, mesocecum, mesorectum, respectively. See Plate 13. —**mesenter′ic,** *adj.*

caval m. An embryonic mesentery, separated from the primitive mesentery of the stomach by the mesenteric recess, in which develops a part of the inferior vena cava and the caudate lobe of the liver.

dorsal m. The mesentery of the digestive tube attached to the dorsal abdominal wall.

ventral m. See lesser *omentum*, gastrohepatic *ligament*, hepatoduodenal *ligament*, ventral *mesogastrium.*

me·sen′to·derm [*mesos;* G. *entos*, within; *derma*, skin]. 1. The entodermal division of the mesoderm. 2. The indifferent tissue from which both entoderm and mesoderm are developed. 3. The portion of the mesoderm from which certain digestive-tract structures are derived.

mes″en·tor′rha·phy [*mesos; entos;* G. *rhaphē*, a suture]. Suture of the mesentery.

me′si·al (mee′zhul, ·zee·ul, mess′ee·ul, mee′see·ul). 1. Old term sometimes used for medial. 2. *In dentistry*, toward the midline following the curve of a dental arch.

me′si·o- (mee′zee·o-, mee′see·o-) [*mesos*]. *In dentistry*, a combining form which denotes the aspect of a tooth *facing the midline, following the dental arch.*

me″si·o·buc′cal [*mesos;* L. *bucca*, cheek]. Pertaining to surfaces between the mesial and buccal aspects of the teeth.

me″si·o·buc″co·oc·clu′sal (·o·clue′sul) [*mesos; bucca;* L. *occludere*, to close]. Pertaining to the mesial, buccal, and occlusal surfaces of a tooth.

me″si·o·clu′sion, me″si·o·oc·clu′sion (·o·clue′zhun) [*mesos; occludere*]. Occlusion of the teeth in which the mandibular teeth are in an anterior relationship to the maxillary teeth.

me″si·o·dis′tal [*mesos;* L. *distare*, to be distant]. Pertaining to a line or plane between the mesial and distal surfaces of a tooth.

me″si·o·gres′sion. The location of teeth anterior to their normal position.

me″si·o·in·ci′sal (·in·sigh′zul) [*mesos;* L. *incidere*, to cut into]. Pertaining to the mesial and incisal surfaces of a tooth or cavity.

me″si·o·la′bi·al [*mesos;* L. *labium*, lip]. Pertaining to the mesial and labial surfaces of a tooth.

me″si·o·lin′gual [*mesos;* L. *lingua*, tongue]. Relating to the junction of the mesial and lingual aspects of a tooth.

me″si·o·lin″guo·oc·clu′sal (·o·clue′sul) [*mesos; lingua;* L. *occludere*, to close]. Pertaining to the mesial, lingual, and occlusal surfaces of a tooth.

me″si·o·oc·clu′sal [*mesos; occludere*]. Pertaining to the mesial and occlusal surfaces of a tooth.

me″si·o·oc·clu′sion (·o·clue′zhun). See *mesioclusion.*

me·sit′y·lene. $C_6H_3(CH_3)_3$; 1,3,5-trimethylbenzene; a liquid hydrocarbon obtained from coal tar and crude petroleum, and also prepared synthetically, insoluble in water but miscible with alcohol, ether, and benzene.

Mesmer, Franz Anton [*German physician*, 1734–1815]. Introduced the concept of animal magnetism (1779). Hypnotism is also called *Mesmerism.*

mes′o- (mess′o-, mee′so-), **mes-** [G. *mesos*, middle]. 1. A combining form signifying *middle.* 2. *In anatomy*, a combining form denoting *an intermediate connective part, mesentery.* 3. *In medicine*, a combining form which denotes *partial* or *secondary.*

mes″o·ap·pen′dix [*mesos;* L. *appendix*, that which hangs to anything]. The mesentery of the vermiform appendix.

me″so·bi′lane. One of the products resulting from the reduction of bilirubin in the tissues by an enzyme manufactured in the reticuloendothelial system. See also *mesobilirubin.*

mes″o·bil″i·fus′cin. Either of two isomeric substances, each containing two pyrrole rings but not of definitely known structure, obtained as products of hydrolytic cleavage of mesobilirubinogen when the latter is prepared by reduction of bilirubin. They contribute significantly to the color of normal feces and may represent the prosthetic group of myobilin.

mes″o·bil″i·leu′kan. A colorless precursor of mesobilifuscin, apparently identical with promesobilifuscin.

mes″o·bil″i·rho′din. A product of dehydrogenation of the urobilin obtained from mesobilirubinogen. Mesobilirhodin is isomeric with mesobiliviolin, these substances differing only in the position of a side methyne bridge.

mes″o·bil″i·ru′bin. $C_{33}H_{40}N_4O_6$; a yellow, crystalline substance formed by reduction of bilirubin, probably by conversion of two vinyl groups to ethyl groups; it occurs in the small intestine and some claim to have found it in bile.

mes″o·bil″i·ru·bin′o·gen. $C_{33}H_{44}N_4O_6$; a colorless, crystalline substance formed by reduction of bilirubin through conversion of two vinyl groups to ethyl groups and two methyne bridges to methene bridges. By various oxidative processes it may be converted to urobilin, stercobilinogen, or stercobilin.

mes″o·bil″i·vi·o′lin. A product of dehydrogenation of the urobilin obtained from mesobilirubinogen. Mesobiliviolin is isomeric with mesobilirhodin, these substances differing only in the position of a side methyne bridge.

mes′o·blast [*mesos;* G. *blastos*, germ]. Synonym (*O.T.*) for mesoderm. —**mesoblas′tic,** *adj.*

mes″o·blas·te′ma [*mesos;* G. *blastēma*, offshoot]. The mesoderm as a whole.

mes″o·blas·tem′ic [*mesos; blastēma*]. Derived from the mesoblastema.

mes″o·car′di·um [*mesos;* G. *kardia*, heart]. One of the embryonic mesenteries of the heart.

dorsal m. The dorsal mesentery of the heart; its disappearance creates the transverse sinus of the pericardium.

ventral m. A ventral mesentery of the heart; not formed in human development.

mes′o·carp [*mesos;* G. *karpos*, fruit]. The middle layer of the pericarp.

mes″o·ce′cum [*mesos;* L. *caecus*, blind]. The mesentery that in some cases connects the cecum with the right iliac fossa.

mes″o·ce·phal′ic [*mesos;* G. *kephalē*, head]. *In somatometry*, designating a head having a relatively moderate relationship between its greatest length and breadth; having a cephalic index of 76.0 to 80.9.

mes″oc·ne′mic [*mesos;* G. *knēmē*, the tibia]. *In osteometry*, designating a tibia with a moderate mediolateral flattening of the proximal portion of the diaphysis; having a cnemic index of 65.0 to 69.9.

mes″o·co′lon [*mesos;* G. *kolon*, colon]. The mesentery connecting the colon with the posterior abdominal wall. It may be divided into ascending, descending, and transverse portions. See Plate 8. —**mesocol′ic,** *adj.*

sigmoid m. See *mesosigmoid.*

mes′o·conch [*mesos;* G. *kogchē*, mussel]. *In craniometry*, designating an orbit of medium height; having an orbital index of 76.0 to 84.9.

mes′o·derm [*mesos;* G. *derma*, skin]. The third germ layer, lying between the ectoderm and entoderm. It gives rise to the connective tissues, muscles, urogenital system, vascular system, and the epithelial lining of the coelom. —**mesoderm′al,** *adj.*

amniotic m. The extraembryonic mesoderm forming the external layer of the amnion, derived from trophoblast.

axial m. See paraxial *m.*

extraembryonic m. The earliest mesoderm of the embryo derived from the trophoblast that forms a part of the amnion, chorion and yolk sac, and the body stalk.

intermediate m. The unsegmented mass of mesoderm uniting the somite and the lateral mesoderm and from which the nephrogenic tissue of the embryonic and definitive kidneys is derived. Syn., *nephrotome.*

intraembryonic m. The mesoderm of the embryo formed largely from the primitive streak.

lateral m. The mesoderm lateral to the intermediate mesoderm. After formation of the coelom it is separated into the somatic and the splanchnic mesoderm.

paraxial m. The medial part of the mesoderm forming a platelike mass that eventually segments to form the somites.

protocardiac m. The mesoderm anterior to the buccopharyngeal membrane from which the heart and pericardial coelom develop.

somatic m. The external layer of the lateral mesoderm associated with ectoderm after formation of the coelom.

splanchnic m. The internal layer of the lateral mesoderm associated with entoderm after formation of the coelom.

mes″o·du″o·de′num (mess″o·dew″o·dee′num, ·dew·od′i·num, mee″so·) [*mesos;* L. *duodeni*, twelve each]. That part of the mesentery that sometimes connects the duodenum with the posterior wall of the abdominal cavity. Normally, the true duodenum has no mesentery in its fully developed state.

mes″o·e·soph′a·gus [*mesos;* G. *oisophagos*, gullet]. The dorsal mesentery of the lower end of the embryonic esophagus.

mes″o·gas′ter, mes″o·gas′tri·um [*mesos;* G. *gastēr*, belly]. The mesentery of the stomach.

dorsal m. The dorsal mesentery of the stomach. The great omentum is derived from it.

ventral m. The ventral mesentery of the stomach. See lesser *omentum*, gastrohepatic *ligament.*

mes″o·gle′a, mes″o·gloe′a (mess″o·glee′uh, mee″so·) [*mesos;* G. *gloios*, a glutinous substance]. The amorphous, gelatinous substance interposed between the entoderm and ectoderm in coelenterates, considered to be more or less homologous to the third germ layer of tripoblastic animals. Not to be confused with mesoglia.

me·sog′li·a [*mesos;* G. *glia*, glue]. A type of ameboid phagocyte found in the neuroglia, probably of mesodermal origin.

mes″o·gnath′ic, mes″o·gnath′ous [*mesos; gnathos*]. *In craniometry*, designating a condition of the upper jaw in which it has a mild degree of anterior projection with respect to the profile of the facial skeleton, when the skull is oriented on the Frankfort horizontal plane; having a gnathic index of 98.0 to 102.9.

mes″o·gna′thi·on (mess″o·nayth′ee·on, ·nath′-ee·on, mee″so·) [*mesos;* G. *gnathos,* jaw]. The hypothetical lateral portion of the premaxilla, considered separate from the mesial portion, the endognathion.

mes″o·in·o′si·tol. Inositol. See also *myoinositol.*

mes″o·lec′i·thal (mess″o·less′i·thul, mee″so·) [*mesos;* G. *lekithos,* yolk]. Having a moderate amount of yolk. Syn., *medialecithal.*

mes′o·mere [*mesos;* G. *meros,* part]. The middle portion of the mesothelial lining of the coelom of primitive chordates, forming nephrogenous tissue.

mes″o·me′tri·um. That portion of the broad ligament directly attached to the uterus.

mes′o·morph. *In the somatotype,* an individual exhibiting relative predominance of mesomorphy.

mes′o·mor″phy [*mesos;* G. *morphē,* form]. Component II of the somatotype, representing relative predominance of somatic structures or the bony and muscular framework of the body, derived from mesoderm. Mesomorphs tend toward massive strength and heavy muscular development. The counterpart on the behavioral evel is *somatotonia.* —**mesomorph′ic,** *adj.*

mes′on [*mesos*]. *In nuclear physics,* any of several different elementary particles, having a rest mass between that of a proton and an electron, the exchange of which between nucleons is believed to constitute the force which holds nucleons together in the nucleus of an atom. The various mesons are distinguished as mu, pi (two kinds), tau, V_1^0, V_2^0, $V\pm$, chi, and kappa; all are unstable See *mesotron, muon.*

mes″o·ne·phro′ma [*mesos;* G. *nephros,* kidney; *-ōma,* tumor]. A term used to cover a variety of benign or malignant tumors supposed to be, but not proved to be, derived from mesonephros (Wolffian body), and occurring in the genital tract. Included are extrauterine adenomyomas, cystic or solid tumors of the ovary situated near the hilus, and tumors resembling the adenomyosarcoma of the kidney. Also called *teratoid adenocystoma.*

m. ovarii. A cystic malignant tumor of the ovary which microscopically contains structures resembling primitive mesonephros. Its origin from the mesonephros is disputed. Also called *papilloendothelioma ovarii.*

mes″o·neph′ros [*mesos; nephros*]. The middle kidney of higher vertebrates; functional in the embryo, it is replaced by the metanephros. Syn., *Wolffian body.* —**mesoneph′ric,** *adj.*

caudal m. (a) The caudal part of the mesonephros, associated with the gonad, that does not undergo complete degeneration. (b) That part of the mesonephros caudal to the genital mesonephros, the tubules of which form the paradidymis or paroöphoron. Syn., *paragenitalis.*

cranial m. That part of the mesonephros, anterior to the gonad, that degenerates during development.

genital m. That part of the mesonephros opposite to the gonad, the tubules of which become the ductuli efferentes.

mes′o·pex″y [*mesos;* G. *pēxis,* a fixing]. The surgical fixation of a mesentery.

mes″o·phle·bi′tis. Inflammation of the middle coat of a vein.

mes″o·phrag′ma. See M *disk.*

mes·o′pic [*mesos;* G. *ōps,* face]. 1. *In craniometry,* designating a facial skeleton that is moderately wide and flat; having an orbitonasal index of 107.5 to 110.0. 2. *In somatometry,* designating a face that is moderately wide and flat; having an orbitonasal index of 110.0 to 112.9.

mesopin. A trade-mark for homatropine methylbromide.

me″so·por′phyr·in. $C_{32}H_{36}N_4(COOH)_2$; any of the 15 isomers obtained by addition of hydrogen to the double bond of each vinyl group (thereby forming an ethyl group) in the 15 isomers of protoporphyrin. Mesoporphyrin 9 is the reduced form of the protoporphyrin occurring in hemoglobin.

mes″o·pul′mo·num [*mesos;* L. *pulmo,* lung]. The embryonic mesentery of the lung attached to the mesoesophagus.

me·sor′chi·um (mi·sor′kee·um, meh·sor′·) [*mesos;* G. *orchis,* testis]. The mesentery of the fetal testis by which it is attached to the mesonephros; represented in the adult by a fold between testis and epididymis.

mes″o·rec′tum [*mesos;* L. *rectus,* straight]. The narrow fold of the peritoneum connecting the upper part of the rectum with the sacrum.

mes″o·rop′ter [*mesos;* G. *oros,* boundary; *optēr,* spy]. The normal position of the eyes when their muscles rest.

muscular m. The angle formed by the visual axes of the eyes when the lateral ocular muscles are at rest.

mes·or′rha·phy [*mesos;* G. *rhaphē,* a suture]. Suture of a mesentery.

mes′or·rhine [*mesos;* G. *rhis,* nose]. 1. *In craniometry,* designating an apertura piriformis approximately twice as long as it is wide; having a nasal index of 47.0 to 50.9. 2. *In somatometry,* designating a nose that is moderately long and wide; having a height-breadth index of 70.0 to 84.9.

mes″o·sal′pinx [*mesos;* G. *salpigx,* trumpet]. The upper part of the broad ligament which surrounds the uterine tube.

mes″o·sig′moid [*mesos;* G. *sigmoeidēs,* in the shape of a sigma]. The mesentery of the sigmoid flexure of the colon.

mesotan. Trade-mark for methoxymethyl salicylate, an ester of salicylic acid, analogous to methyl salicylate and used as a counterirritant.

mes″o·tar·tar′ic ac′id (mess″o·tahr·tar′ick, ·tahr-tahr′ick, mez″o·). Tartaric acid which is optically inactive by reason of internal compensation.

mes″o·ten′don [*mesos;* L. *tendere,* to stretch]. The fold of synovial membrane extending to a tendon from its synovial tendon-sheath.

mes″o·the″li·o′ma [*mesos;* G. *thēlē,* nipple; *-ōma,* tumor]. A primary tumor, either benign or malignant, of the cells forming the lining of the peritoneum, pericardium, or pleura. These cells may resemble mesothelial or endothelial cells, but their appearance may vary markedly from tumor to tumor, or within the same tumor. Also called *celioma, celothelioma, sarcoendothelioma, mesothelial sarcoma.*

m. of the genital tract. A small firm tumor arising from peritoneal cells and composed of multiple tubes lined by swollen and vacuolated cells which secrete a mucoid material, found in the uterus, ovarian tubes, canal of Nuck, epididymis, and spermatic cord.

mes″o·the′li·um [*mesos; thēlē*]. 1. The lining of the wall of the primitive body cavity situated between the somatopleure and splanchnopleure. 2. The simple squamous-cell epithelium lining the pleural, pericardial, peritoneal, and scrotal cavities. —**mesothe′lial,** *adj.*

mes″o·tho′ri·um. Either of the radioactive disintegration products, **mesothorium-1** ($MsTh_1$) and **mesothorium-2** ($MsTh_2$), formed from thorium and ultimately converted to radiothorium.

me·sot′o·my. The separation of an optically inactive mixture of isomers into its optically active components. Syn., *resolution.*

mes′o·tron. A meson, particularly the kind now known as the *mu meson. Obs.*

mes″o·var′i·um (mess″o·vair′ee·um, mee″so·) [*mesos;* NL. *ovarium,* from *ovum,* egg]. A peritoneal fold connecting the ovary and the broad ligament; in the embryo with the Wolffian body.

mes′quite (mess′keet, mess·keet′) [Sp. *mezquite*]. The tree or shrub, *Prosopis chilensis,* of the southwestern U. S., Mexico, and Hawaii. It yields a gum resembling acacia.

me·stil′bol. Generic name for the estrogen supplied under the trade-mark *monomestrol.*

mesudin. Marfanil.

met″a-, met- [G.]. 1. A prefix signifying *over, after, beyond, among, between, change,* or *transformation.* 2. *In chemistry,* a prefix denoting the 1,3 position of benzene derivatives. Symbol, *m-*. 3. *In chemistry,* denoting an acid or base containing one less molecule of water than the parent substance, commonly referred to as the ortho compound; as meta-phosphoric acid, HPO_3, from ortho-phosphoric acid, H_3PO_4. 4. *In medicine,* a prefix denoting *post-*. 5. *In anatomy,* a prefix denoting *dorso-*. 6. *In zoology,* a prefix denoting *a later* or *more highly developed form of* some *type,* as Metazoa.

met″a·bi·o′sis (met″uh·buy·o′sis) [G. *meta,* with; *biōsis,* way of life]. A form of symbiosis, in which only one of the organisms is benefited; the other may remain uninfluenced or injured.

met″a·bol′ic e″qui·lib′ri·um. See nutritive *equilibrium.*

met″a·bol′ic fail′ure. Advanced, progressive debility, characterized by rapid failure of mental and physical functions, terminating in death.

met″a·bo·lim′e·ter (met″uh·bo·lim′i·tur, mi-tab″o·, meh·tab″o·) [G. *metabolē,* change; *metron,* a measure]. An apparatus for estimating the rate of basal metabolism.

me·tab′o·lism [*metabolē*]. The phenomena of synthesizing foodstuffs into complex tissue elements (assimilation, anabolism) and complex substances into simple ones in the production of energy (disassimilation, catabolism). —**metabol′ic,** *adj.*

acid-base m. Those physiologic activities which pertain to the relative concentrations of hydrogen and hydroxyl ions.

aerobic m. Metabolism utilizing O_2.

anaerobic m. Metabolism carried on in the absence of O_2.

basal m. The minimum amount of energy expenditure necessary to maintain cellular activity when the body is at complete rest in a warm atmosphere 12–18 hours after the intake of food. Also see *basal metabolic rate.*

energy m. Physiologic activities concerned with the intake, interchange, and output of energy.

intermediary m. The intermediate chemical steps in the intracellular transformation of foodstuffs within the body.

protoporphyrin m. In liver diseases, such as cirrhosis and epidemic jaundice, the protoporphyrin level of the blood is raised.

me·tab′o·lite [*metabolē*]. A product of metabolic change.

essential m. A substance necessary for proper metabolism, such as vitamins.

me·tab′o·lize [*metabolē*]. Transform by means of metabolism.

met″a·bol′o·gy [*metabolē;* G. *logos,* word]. Study of the metabolic processes.

met″a·car′pal [G. *metakarpion,* bones forming the palm of the hand]. Pertaining to the metacarpus, or to a bone of it.

met″a·car·pec′to·my [*metakarpion;* G. *ektomē,* excision]. Excision of a metacarpal bone.

met″a·car″po·pha·lan′ge·al [*metakarpion;* G. *phalagx,* bone between two joints of the fingers]. Belonging to the metacarpus and the phalanges, as metacarpophalangeal ligaments. See Table of Joints and Ligaments.

met″a·car′pus [*metakarpion*]. That part of the hand between the carpus and the phalanges, consisting of five bones. See Table of Bones.

met″a·chlo′ral. A tasteless, polymeric form of chloral, said to have properties not unlike those of chloral hydrate.

metachloridine. Trade-mark for the synthetic antimalarial agent N^1-(5-chloro-2-pyrimidyl)metanilamide; $C_{10}H_9ClN_4O_2S$.

met″a·chro·ma′si·a (met″uh·kro·may′zhuh, ·zee·uh, ·see·uh, ·shuh) [G. *meta,* denoting change; *chrōma,* color]. The assumption of different colors or shades by different substances when stained by the same dye. —**metachromat′ic,** *adj.;* **metachro′matism,** *n.*

met″a·chro′sis [*meta;* G. *chrōsis,* coloring]. *In biology,* the change or play of colors seen in the squid, chameleon, and other animals.

met′a·coele (met′uh·seel) [G. *meta,* beyond; *koilia,* hollow]. The coelom proper, developing in the lateral plate of mesoderm.

met′a·cone [G. *meta,* behind; *kōnis,* cone]. The outer posterior (distobuccal) cusp of an upper molar tooth.

met″a·con′id, met″a·co′nid. The inner anterior (mesiolingual) cusp of a lower molar tooth.

met″a·con′ule, met″a·co′nule [*meta;* L. *conula,* from *conus,* cone]. A small intermediate cusp between the metacone and the protocone on the upper molar teeth of animals.

met″a·cor·tan′dra·cin. An early generic name for *prednisone.*

met″a·cor·tan′dra·lone. An early generic name for *prednisolone.*

met″a·cre′sol. $C_6H_4(CH_3)OH$. The meta form of cresol; a colorless liquid obtained from coal tar. It is a more powerful germicide than phenol, but is less toxic.

met″a·cres″yl·ac′e·tate. *m*-Cresylacetate.

met″a·cy·e′sis (met″a·sigh·ee′sis) [G. *meta,* beyond; *kyēsis,* pregnancy]. Extrauterine gestation.

met″a·di″i·o″do·an′l·lin. See *diiodoaniline.*

met″a·dra′sis [*meta;* G. *drasis,* strength]. Overwork of body or mind.

met″a·fil·tra′tion. Filtration through superimposed metallic strips with beveled edges, the system depending on the formation of a filter bed in the interstices between the strips.

met″a·gen′e·sis. Alternation of generations.

Met″a·gon′i·mus [G. *meta,* behind; *gonimos,* productive]. A genus of digenetic trematodes.

M. yokogawai. That species found most commonly in the Far East which infests the small intestine of man, producing a mild diarrhea.

met″a·gran′u·lo·cyte. See *metamyelocyte.*

met″a·kar′y·o·cyte [G. *meta; karyon,* kernel; *kytos,* cell]. A normoblast or micronormoblast. Also called *orthochromatic erythroblast.*

met″a·ken′trin. See luteinizing *hormone.*

met′al [G. *metallon,* mine]. An elementary substance usually characterized by hardness, malleability, ductility, fusibility, luster, its conduction of heat and electricity, and the basic character of its oxides. Symbol, M.

alkali m. Any of the metals lithium, sodium, potassium, rubidium, or cesium, belonging to group I in the periodic classification of chemical elements.

cheoplastic m. Any low fusing metal or alloy

which may be employed in cheoplasty. An alloy composed of tin, silver, and bismuth, with a small trace of antimony, is often used.

m. fume fever. See brass founder's *ague*.

met·al′de·hyde. $(C_2H_4O)_3$. A white, solid polymer of acetaldehyde.

me·tal″les·the′si·a (mi·tal″ess·thee′zhuh, ·zee·uh, meh·tal″·) [*metallon;* G. *aisthēsis*, perception]. The ability to distinguish between various metals by the sense of touch, presumed to occur in hysterical or hypnotized subjects.

me·tal′lic [*metallon*]. 1. Resembling metal. 2. *In physical diagnosis*, referring to a sound similar to that produced by metal. It is high-pitched, short in duration, and possesses overtones. A form of tympany.

m. tinkle. A faint, clear, bell-like sound, heard after a cough or deep breath in some cases of hydropneumothorax.

met′al·loid [*metallon;* G. *eidos*, form]. An element which has metallic properties in the free state but which behaves chemically as an amphoteric or nonmetallic element. **—met′aloid,** *adj.*

met″al·lo·pho′bi·a [*metallon;* G. *phobos*, fear]. A morbid fear of metals or metallic objects.

met″al·lo·por′phy·rin [*metallon;* G. *porphyra*, purple]. A compound formed by the combination of a porphyrin with a metal such as iron, copper, cobalt, nickel, silver, tin, zinc, manganese, or magnesium. Heme is a metalloporphyrin in which a porphyrin is combined with iron.

me·tal″lo·pro′te·in. A protein enzyme containing metal as an inherent portion of its molecule.

met·al′o·phil. Any of the reticular cells which stain with metallic salts, as silver carbonate. It may be a fixed or ameboid cell or a monocyte of peripheral blood.

met′a·mer. One of two or more compounds having the same number and kind of atoms but with a different distribution of the component radicals.

met′a·mere [G. *meta*, beyond; *meros*, part]. One of the linear series of more or less similar segments of the body of many animals.

met″a·mer′ic [*meta; meros*]. Pertaining to a metamere or metamerism.

me·tam′er·ism [*meta; meros*]. 1. The repetition of more or less similar parts or segments in the body of many animals, as exhibited especially by the Annelida, Arthropoda, and Vertebrata. See *pseudometamerism*. 2. The relationship existing between two or more metamers.

met″a·mor′phic [G. *metamorphōsis*, transformation]. Pertaining to metamorphosis.

met″a·mor·phop′si·a [*metamorphōsis;* G. *opsis*, vision]. A defect of vision in which objects appear distorted; due to disease of the retina or imperfection of the media.

met″a·mor′pho·sis (met″uh·mor′fo·sis, ·mor·fo′-sis) [G.]. A structural change or transformation. *In pathology*, a retrogressive change.

fatty m. Fatty degeneration, fat infiltration, or both.

sexual m. A variety of sexual perversion in which the individual has the tastes and feelings of, and assumes dress and habits of, the opposite sex.

met″a·mor′phous [*metamorphōsis*]. Amorphous, but with a tendency to crystallize.

metamucil. Trade-mark for a mixture of the powdered mucilaginous portion of blond psyllium seed and powdered anhydrous dextrose, about 50% of each: used as a laxative.

met″a·my′e·lo·cyte [G. *meta*, between; *myelos*, marrow; *kytos*, cell]. A cell of the granulocytic series intermediate between myelocyte and granular leukocyte, having a full complement of specific granules and an indented, bean-shaped (juvenile) nucleus: also called *metagranulocyte, juvenile cell*.

metandren. Trade-mark for methyltestosterone, a crystalline androgen.

met″a·neph″ro·gen′ic [G. *meta*, after; *nephros*, kidney; *genesthai*, from *gignesthai*, to be produced]. Capable of forming, or giving rise to, the metanephros.

met″a·neph′ros (pl. *metanephroi*) [*meta; nephros*]. The definitive or permanent kidney of reptiles, birds, and mammals. It develops from the caudal part of the nephrogenic cord in association with the ureteric bud from the mesonephric duct. **—metanephric,** *adj.*

met·an′il yel′low. Sodium salt of *m*-sulfanilic acid-azodiphenylamine. $NaSO_3.C_6H_4.N{:}N.C_6H_4.NH.C_6H_5$. Brownish yellow powder used as an indicator. Red at pH 1.2; yellow at pH 2.3. Also called *tropaeolin G, victoria yellow*.

met′a·phase (met′uh·faze) [*meta;* G. *phasis*, phase]. The middle stage of mitosis when the chromosomes lie nearly in a single plane at the equator of the spindle, forming the equatorial plate. It follows the prophase and precedes the anaphase.

metaphedrin. Trade-mark for an aqueous solution of ephedrine containing metaphen.

metaphen. Trade-mark for the anhydride of 4-nitro-3-hydroxy-mercuri-ortho-cresol, designated as nitromersol by the National Formulary.

met″a·phos·phor′ic ac′id. HPO_3. A clear, viscous liquid; the commercial product, occurring in sticks, contains about 17% Na_2O. Used as a reagent.

metaphyllin. Trade-mark for *aminophylline*.

me·taph′y·sis [G. *meta*, between; *physis*, growth]. 1. The region of growth between the epiphysis and diaphysis of a bone. Also called *epiphyseal plate*. 2. The growing end of the diaphysis.

met″a·phys·i′tis. Inflammation of a metaphysis.

met″a·pla′si·a (met″uh·play′zee·uh, ·see·uh, ·shuh, ·zhuh) [G. *meta*, denoting change; *plasis*, molding]. Transformation of one form of adult tissue to another, such as replacement of respiratory epithelium by stratified squamous epithelium. **—metaplas′tic,** *adj.*

agnogenic myeloid m. Marked myeloid metaplasia of the spleen, apparently the result of a compensatory reaction to failure of the hematopoietic function of bone marrow; presumably not a disease entity since the bone-marrow picture, hematological picture, and jaundice are variable.

myeloid m. The occurrence of hematopoietic tissue in areas of the body where it is not normally found.

prosoplastic m. Transformation in the direction of higher orders of differentiation.

regressive m. Transformation in the direction of lower orders of differentiation: also called *retrogressive atrophy*.

me·tap′la·sis [*meta; plasis*]. Fulfilled growth and development seen in the stage between anaplasis and cataplasis.

met′a·plasm (met′uh·plaz·um) [G. *metaplasma*, metaplasm]. The lifeless inclusions in protoplasm collectively.

met″a·pneu·mon′ic (met″uh·new·mon′ic) [G. *meta*, after; *pneumōn*, lung]. Secondary to, or consequent upon, pneumonia.

met″a·poph′y·sis. Old term for a mammillary process, as seen upon the lumbar vertebrae.

met″a·pro′te·in [*meta;* G. *prōteios*, of first rank]. A product of acid or alkaline hydrolysis of a protein. Soluble in weak acids and alkalis, insoluble in water. See *protein*. See American Classification of Proteins in the Appendix.

met″ar·te′ri·ole [G. *meta*, between; *artēria*, artery]. A blood vessel, intermediate in position and structural characteristics, between an arteriole and a true capillary. Also called *arteriolar capillary, precapillary, junctional capillary.*

met″a·ru′bri·cyte. See *normoblast*, 1.

met′a·sta·ble. Of intermediate stability; changing readily either to a more or a less stable state.

me·tas′ta·sis [G., removal]. The transfer of disease from a primary focus to a distant one by the conveyance of causal agents or cells through the blood vessels or lymph channels. —**metastat′ic,** *adj.*

cannon-ball m. Large spherical lesions of the lung which result from metastatic carcinoma, sometimes characteristic of metastasis from primary renal carcinoma: descriptive term from x-ray findings. Also called cotton-ball m.

me·tas′ta·size [*metastasis*]. Transfer disease into a distant part by metastasis.

Met″a·stron′gy·lus (met″uh·stron′ji·lus) [G. *meta*, beyond; *stroggylos*, round]. A genus of nematode parasites.

M. apri. Synonym for *M. elongatus.*

M. elongatus. A species common to hogs, occasionally to sheep and cattle, which infests the respiratory tract and produces a pneumonitis and bronchitis often fatal in young animals. A few cases of human infestation have been reported.

met″a·tar·sal′gi·a [G. *meta*, between; *tarsos*, flat of the foot; *algos*, pain]. Pain and tenderness in the metatarsal region.

Morton's m. A specific clinical type of metatarsalgia, described by T. G. Morton (1876), characterized by severe pain between the heads of the third and fourth metatarsal bones and due to a neurofibroma at the point of union of the digital branches from the medial and lateral plantar nerves: also called *Morton's foot* or *toe.*

met″a·tar·sec′to·my [*meta; tarsos;* G. *ektomē*, excision]. Excision of a metatarsal bone.

met″a·tar″so·pha·lan′ge·al [*meta; tarsos;* G. *phalagx*, bone between two joints of the fingers or toes]. Pertaining to the metatarsus and the phalanges, as the ligaments between these bones. See Table of Joints and Ligaments in the Appendix.

met″a·tar′sus [*meta; tarsos*]. The portion of the foot between the tarsus and the phalanges, containing five bones of the foot. See Table of Bones in the Appendix. —**metatarsal,** *adj.*

m. adductovarus. A congenital deformity of the foot; a deviation of the fore part of the foot toward the midline, associated with an elevation of its inner border, the heel remaining in a neutral or slightly valgus position. It is caused by soft tissue contracture with bony deformity, occurs only in older cases and is due to secondary adaptation. Syn., *skewfoot.*

m. adductus. A congenital deformity of the foot; deviation of the fore part of the foot toward the midline, the heel remaining in a neutral or slightly valgus position. At birth there is no bone deformity, the deviation of the metatarsals being produced by soft tissue contracture. In older cases bone deformity may develop due to secondary adaptation.

m. primus varus. An abnormality in the developmental process involving adduction of the first metatarsal.

m. varus. A congenital deformity of the foot; an elevation of the inner border of the fore part of the foot (varus), the heel remaining in a neutral or slightly valgus position.

met″a·thal′a·mus [*meta;* G. *thalamos*, chamber]. The lateral and medial geniculate bodies.

me·tath′e·sis [G., transposition]. A chemical reaction in which there is an exchange of radicals or elements of the type: $\overset{+-}{AB} + \overset{+-}{CD} = \overset{+-}{AD} + \overset{+-}{CB}$ with no change in valence. —**metathet′ic,** *adj.*

met″a·troph′ic [G. *meta*, beyond; *trophē*, nourishment]. Deriving sustenance from organic matter, said of bacteria.

Met″a·zo′a [*meta;* G. *zōion*, living being]. A subdivision of the animal kingdom, which includes all the multicellular forms, and so stands in contrast to the Protozoa.

Metchnikoff, Elie [*Russian biologist in France*, 1845–1916]. Developed the theory of phagocytosis. With P. P. E. Roux, introduced calomel ointment as a prophylactic against syphilis. For his researches on immunity, shared the Nobel prize with Paul Ehrlich (1908).

me·te′ci·ous, me·toe′ci·ous. See *heterecious.*

met″el·oi′dine. An alkaloid from certain *Datura* species.

met″em·pir′ic [G. *meta*, beyond; *empeirikos*, experienced]. Not derived from experience, but implied or presupposed by it.

met″en·ceph′a·lon [G. *meta*, behind; *egkephalos*, brain]. The cephalic part of the rhombencephalon, giving rise to the cerebellum and pons.

me″te·or′ic [G. *meteōros*, raised from the ground]. Pertaining to meteorism; also, pertaining to meteors or to atmospheric phenomena.

me′te·or·ism [*meteōros*]. Gaseous distention of the abdomen or intestine; tympanites.

me′te·or·o·graph″ (mee′tee·or·o·graf″, mee″tee·orr′o·graf) [*meteōros;* G. *graphein*, to write]. An apparatus for securing a continuous record of the pressure, temperature, humidity, and velocity of the wind.

me″te·or·ol′o·gy [*meteōros;* G. *logos*, word]. The science which treats primarily of atmospheric phenomena.

me″te·or·o·path″o·log′ic [*meteōros;* G. *pathos*, disease; *logos*]. Pertaining to the influence of weather on incidence, development, and course of disease.

me′ter [G. *metron*, a measure]. 1. The basic unit of linear measure of the metric system, 39.37 inches. Abbreviated, m, m. 2. An instrument for measuring and recording quantities, as a roentgen meter, which measures roentgen-ray quantities in roentgens by ionization. —**met′ric,** *adj.*

dose-rate m. *In radiology*, any instrument for measuring the radiation dose rate.

integrating dose m. *In radiology*, an ionization chamber and measuring system designed to determine the total radiation administered during a single exposure, usually designed to be placed on the patient's skin.

respiratory ventilation m. One which gives a relatively accurate measurement of inspiratory volume.

viscosity-effusion m. An instrument for determining the concentration of anesthetic gases during surgical anesthesia.

me·tes′trus [G. *meta*, after; *oistros*, gadfly]. The period that follows the estrus when there is marked invasion of the vaginal walls by leukocytes.

meth″a·cho′line chlo′ride (meth″uh·ko′leen, ·lin) (*methacholinae chloridum*). The pharmacopeial name for acetyl-β-methylcholine chloride. See *mecholyl chloride.*

meth′a·don. Methadone hydrochloride.

meth′a·done hy″dro·chlo′ride. $CH_3CH_2CO.C(C_6H_5)_2CH_2CH(CH_3)N(CH_3)_2.HCl$; *d,l*-6-dimethylamino-4,4,diphenyl-3-heptanone hydrochloride; a white, crystalline powder, soluble in water. Its actions are similar to those of morphine and it is used similarly. The *l* isomer is about 5 times as potent as the *d* isomer. Syn., *amidone* *hydrochloride, methadon.* See *adanon hydrochloride, dolophine hydrochloride.*

meth″am·phet′a·mine hy″dro·chlo′ride. [$C_6H_5CH_2CH(CH_3)N^+H_2CH_3]Cl^-$; *d*-1-phenyl-2-methylaminopropane hydrochloride; a methyl derivative of amphetamine or a desoxy derivative of ephedrine; it occurs as a white, crystalline powder, freely soluble in water. It is a central stimulant and vasoconstrictor. Syn., *desoxyephedrine hydrochloride, methylamphetamine hydrochloride.* See *desoxyn hydrochloride, dexoval hydrochloride, doxyfed hydrochloride, efroxine hydrochloride, methedrine, norodrin hydrochloride, semoxydrine hydrochloride, syndrox hydrochloride.*

meth′an·al. Formaldehyde.

meth′ane. CH_4. Marsh gas. The first member of the homologous series of paraffins having the general formula C_nH_{2n+2}. A colorless, odorless, inflammable gas.

meth″ane·ar·son′ic ac′id. Methylarsonic acid.

meth″a·no′ic ac′id. Formic acid.

meth′a·nol. Methyl alcohol.

meth·an′thel·ine bro′mide. $C_{21}H_{26}BrNO_3$; β-diethylaminoethyl-9-xanthenecarboxylate methobromide; a white or nearly white powder, very soluble in water; a parasympatholytic agent, producing the peripheral action of anticholinergic drugs, such as atropine, and the ganglionic blocking action of drugs such as tetraethylammonium chloride: useful whenever anticholinergic spasmolytic action is desired. See *banthine bromide.*

meth″a·phen′i·lene hy″dro·chlo′ride. Generic name for the antihistaminic substance N,N-dimethyl-N′-phenyl-N′-(2-thenyl)ethylenediamine hydrochloride; $C_{15}H_{20}N_2S.HCl$; marketed under the trade-marked name *diatrin hydrochloride.*

meth″a·pyr′i·lene hy″dro·chlo′ride. $C_{14}H_{19}N_3S.HCl$; 2-[(2-dimethylaminoethyl)-2-thenylamino]pyridine hydrochloride; a white, crystalline powder, very soluble in water; a histamine-antagonizing agent with low incidence of sedation. Syn., *thenylpyramine hydrochloride.* See *histadyl, semikon hydrochloride, thenylene hydrochloride.*

meth·ar′bi·tal. $C_9H_{14}N_2O_3$; 5,5-diethyl-1-methylbarbituric acid; a white, crystalline powder, slightly soluble in water; a barbiturate, less sedative than phenobarbital, useful in the treatment of various forms of epilepsy. See *gemonil.*

meth-di′a-mer-sul·fon′a·mides. A generic name for a mixture containing equal weights of sulfadiazine, sulfamerazine, and sulfamethazine.

methedrine. Trade-mark for *methamphetamine hydrochloride.*

met″he·mal′bu·min. A product of the combination of hematin and serum albumin, comparable to methemoglobin. Syn., *pseudomethemoglobin.*

met″he·mal″bu·mi·ne′mi·a. Methemalbumin in the blood of a patient in whom intravascular hemolysis is taking place.

met′heme. Hematin.

met·he″mo·glo′bin. The oxidized form of hemoglobin, in which the iron atom is trivalent, and which is not able to combine reversibly with oxygen. Found in the blood after poisoning by chlorates, nitrites, ferricyanides, quinones, peroxides, acetanilid, acetophenetidin, etc.; it is dark brown in color. Syn., *ferrihemoglobin.*

met·he″mo·glo″bi·ne′mi·a, met·hae″mo·glo″bi·ne′mi·a [G. *meta*, with; *haima*, blood; L. *globus*, ball; *haima*]. The presence of methemoglobin in the blood, causing cyanosis, dizziness, headache, diarrhea, and anemia.

met·he″mo·glo″bi·nu′ri·a, met·hae″mo·glo″bi·nu′ri·a [*meta; haima; globus;* G. *ouron*, urine]. The presence of methemoglobin in the urine.

me·the′na·mine (meth·ee′nuh·meen, ·min, meth″in·uh·meen′, meth″i·nam′in) (*methenamina*). $(CH_2)_6N_4$. Hexamethylenetetramine, occurring in colorless crystals or as a white, crystalline powder; 1 Gm. dissolves in 1.5 cc. of water. Used mainly as a urinary antiseptic; its effectiveness is dependent on hydrolyzing it, in acid urine, to formaldehyde. Dose, 0.3–1.3 Gm. (5–20 gr.). Syn., *hexamine.* See *formin, urotropin.*

m. tetraiodide. See *siomine.*

meth′ene. 1. The first member of the ethylene (alkene) series of unsaturated hydrocarbons, having the formula CH_2. It has never been isolated. 2. The hydrocarbon radical $CH_2=$. Syn., *methylene.*

meth′e·nyl. The trivalent radical, $\equiv CH$. Syn., *methine, methyne.*

m. tribromide. Bromoform.

m. trichloride. Chloroform.

m. triiodide. Iodoform.

methergine. Trade-mark for N-(α-hydroxy-methylpropyl)-*d*-lysergamide, an oxytocic useful for shortening the third stage of labor and for reducing blood loss. The compound is said to cause more prolonged contraction of the uterus than ergonovine.

me·thim′a·zole, me·thi′ma·zole. The generic namefor 1-methyl-2-mercaptoimidazole; $C_4H_6N_2S$; a white to buff powder, soluble in water, used as an antithyroid drug. See *tapazole.*

meth′ine, meth′yne. Methenyl.

meth·i′o·dal so′di·um. CH_2INaO_3S; sodium monoiodomethanesulfonate; a white, crystalline powder, soluble in water: used as a radiopaque medium, especially for visualization of the urinary tract. See *skiodan sodium.*

meth·i′o·nine (meth·eye′o·neen, ·nin). $CH_3.S.(CH_2)_2.CHNH_2.COOH$. α-Amino-γ-methylthiol-*n*-butyric acid. A naturally occurring amino acid, essential for normal growth and as a source of methyl groups for the synthesis of choline, creatine, etc., in vivo. May be useful in prevention and treatment of certain types of liver damage.

me·thi′o·nyl. The univalent radical, $CH_3SCH_2CH_2CH(NH_2)CO—$, of the amino acid methionine.

methocel. Trade-mark for methyl cellulose.

meth′od [G. *methodos*, following after, pursuit]. The manner of performance of any act or operation. The term embraces open and closed operations, reduction of fractures and dislocations, maneuvers and tests performed in a definite way and according to a described and practiced plan. For methods of treatment, see *treatment;* for methods of staining, see *stain;* for methods of making qualitative tests, see *test*, See also under *reaction* and under the designating name.

acetylene m. A method for estimating cardiac output by determining the arteriovenous difference in oxygen absorption or carbon dioxide elimination in a given period of time. The patient breathes into a bag filled with air and acetylene.

Achard-Castaigne m. See methylene blue *test.*

Achucárro's silver tannin m. (*for astrocytes*). See under *stain.*

acid hematin m. (*for hemoglobin*). Blood is diluted with tenth normal HCl, and the color is compared with glass standards or with a standard hematin solution. Modifications of this are the Haden-Hausser method, the Wintrobe method the Sahli method, and the Sanford, Sheard, and Osterberg method.

Addis' m. A method for counting the sediment (casts and cells) in a 24-hour urine.

alkaline hematin m. (*for hemoglobin*). Determination of hemoglobin in blood by photoelectric colorimetry of alkaline hematin.

Allen-Bourne m. (*for zymohexase*). A histochemical method based on the formation of triose phosphate, when the enzyme acts on hexose diphosphate, liberation of phosphate at room temperature in alkaline solution, and visualization of phosphate by the Gomori method.

alternate case m. A method of investigating the effects of different treatments by using alternate types of treatment on alternate patients who suffer from the same disease.

alternate paired case m. A method of investigating the effects of different treatments by pairing cases as to extent and similarity of disease, using one type of treatment on one pair and another type on the second pair.

Altmann-Gersh m. (*for tissue fixation*). Tissue is frozen quickly at liquid air temperatures, dehydrated at −30° C. in a low vacuum, and then prepared for examination.

Anfinsen m. (*for diphosphopyridine nucleotide*). A Cartesian-diver method based on conversion of hexose diphosphate to phosphoglyceric acid and phosphoglycerol in a bicarbonate buffer, where the amount of diphosphopyridine nucleotide (DPN) is the limiting factor. The phosphoglyceric acid produced causes liberation of CO_2 from the buffer; the amount of CO_2 is a measure of the diphosphopyridine nucleotide concentration.

Armitage m. A method for determining the presence of peroxidase in smears of blood or bone marrow. If yellow granules appear, the test is positive.

Arneth's m. A method of classifying neutrophils according to the shape of the nucleus, and the number of nuclear lobes. See also Joseph *Arneth.*

Arnold and Gunning's m. A modification of the Kjeldahl method used in determining total nitrogen.

Askenstedt's m. (Parker's modification) (*for indican*). Urine is precipitated with mercuric chloride. Indican is converted to indigo with Obermayer's reagent and extracted with chloroform which is diluted with alcohol. The blue color is compared with a standard solution of indigo.

Austin and Van Slyke's m. (*for blood chlorides*). Blood is laked with distilled water and the proteins are precipitated with picric acid. Procedure is completed as in McLean and Van Slyke's method.

Barber's m. A method for the isolation of a single microorganism by the use of a mechanically operated pipet under a microscopic field.

Barker's m. (*for thiocyanates*). Ferric nitrate acts upon the thiocyanate of a blood filtrate to produce a color which is compared with a standard.

Barrett m. A modification of the urease method for the determination of blood urea nitrogen, which includes the addition of a few drops of 10% sodium hypochlorite solution to the Nessler's reagent. This prevents any organic substance from clouding the final colored solution. The method can also be adapted for urine urea determinations.

Bauer-Feulgen m. (*for glycogen*). See *Bauer's method* under *stain.*

Bell's m. (*for calcium*). The diffusible fraction of blood calcium is crystallized by the addition of oxalic acid. After dilution, the crystals are counted in a Thoma chamber and compared with a standard solution.

Benedict and Franke's m. (*for uric acid in urine*). Diluted urine is treated with arsenophosphotungstic acid reagent and sodium cyanide and the blue color compared with a standard uric acid solution.

Benedict and Newton's m. (*for protein-free blood filtrate*). Blood is hemolyzed, and the proteins are precipitated with tungstomolybdic acid.

Benedict and Theis's m. (*for inorganic phosphate*). A trichloroacetic acid filtrate of serum is treated with molybdic acid and reduced with hydroquinone sulfite reagent.

Benedict's m. (a) (*for glucose*). Glucose in the urine is estimated by titrating the urine with Benedict's quantitative sugar reagent. (b) (*for total sulfur*). Sulfur in the urine is estimated by adding urine to Benedict's sulfur reagent and evaporating to dryness. Precipitation with $BaCl_2$ is followed by filtering, drying, and weighing. (c) (*for uric acid*). A tungstic acid blood filtrate is mixed with acid lithium chloride and silver nitrate. After centrifuging, the supernatant fluid is mixed with sodium cyanide and arsenotungstic color reagent and compared with a standard uric acid solution in a colorimeter.

Benedict's picrate m. (*for glucose in urine*). Color produced by picric acid reduction is compared with permanent inorganic standards which represent definite concentrations of sugar. Also called *life insurance m.*

Bensley-Hoerr m. (*for isolation of mitochondria*). A method of isolation of mitochondria based on differential centrifugation. The cells of a tissue are broken up by various methods of incomplete homogenization, and the mitochondria freed from other cell constituents and tissue fragments by repeated centrifugation at speeds determined by the size and density of the particular mitochondria. Now important in the study of the oxidative enzymes.

Bensley's m. (*for glycogen*). See under *stain.*

benzidine and nitroprusside oxidase m. (*for hemoglobin*). Place sections for 30 minutes at 37° C. in fresh benzidine and nitroprusside reagent; agitate frequently; wash in distilled water; place in 0.04 to 0.05 per cent hydrogen peroxide at 37° C. for 30 minutes, shaking frequently; wash in distilled water; dehydrate and mount. Blood cells are colored black while other structures remain gray.

Bessey-Lowry-Brock-Lopez m. (*for vitamin A and carotene*). A method based on destruction of vitamin A by ultraviolet light and absorption measurements by a spectrophotometer.

Bessey-Lowry-Brock m. (*for phosphatase*). A colorimetric method based on the splitting of *p*-nitrophenyl phosphate by the enzyme to give the yellow salt of *p*-nitrophenol.

Bethe m. (*for chitin*). A method based on treatment of tissue with aniline hydrochloride, hydrochloric acid, and potassium dichromate to give a green color.

Bier's m. (a) A method of producing anesthesia in a limb by intravenous injections of ½% cocaine after the part has been rendered bloodless by elevation and constriction. (b) Anesthesia of the lower part of the body produced by the injection of an anesthetic agent into the spinal membranes.

biopsy m. for sex determination. A method, devised by Murray L. Barr, of determining the sex-chromosome constitution of an individual of doubtful sex by microscopic examination of sections of excised skin.

blind-test, cross-over m. A clinical test in which the subjects are divided into two or more statistically comparable groups. Under identical conditions, one group is given a medication and the other a placebo; after a period, the groups are reversed; thus each group serves as control both for itself and the other group.

Bloch m. (*for dopa oxidase*). A histochemical method based on conversion of dihydroxyphenylalanine to melanin on exposure to tissue containing dopa oxidase. Leukocytes and melanoblasts turn black due to their dopa-oxidase content. See dopa *reaction*.

Bodansky's m. (*for serum phosphatase*). The difference between inorganic phosphate before and after incubation with sodium glycerophosphate substrate is a measure of phosphatase activity.

Boettiger m. (*for glycogen*). A colorimetric method based on the color development through the action of diphenylamine on glycogen.

Borchardt m. (*for gold*). A histochemical method using silver nitrate followed by nitric acid to localize gold.

Bordley-Hendrix-Richards m. (*for creatinine*). An adaptation of Folin's method to capillary-tube colorimetry.

Bordley-Richards m. (*for uric acid*). An adaptation of Folin's method to capillary-tube colorimetry.

Borsook m. (*for allantoin*). A colorimetric method based on the enzymatic conversion of allantoin to allantoic acid, acid hydrolysis of the acid to urea and glyoxylic acid, and the measurement of the latter.

Bott m. (*for sodium*). A capillary-tube colorimetric method based on the precipitation of uranyl zinc sodium acetate and the reaction of the latter with diphenylthiocarbazone to give a red color.

Bourne m. (a) (*for alkaline phosphatase*). A histochemical method based on the action of the enzyme on glycerophosphate and calcium chloride to produce calcium phosphate and the staining of the latter with alizarin sulfonate. (b) (*for ascorbic acid*). A histochemical method based on reduction of silver nitrate by ascorbic acid. (c) (*for sulfhydryl groups*). A histochemical method using acetic acid, nitroprusside, ammonium sulfate, and ammonium hydroxide to obtain a purplish-blue color.

Bratton and Marshall's m. (*for sulfonamides in blood and urine*). A colorimetric method based upon the amount of purplish red azo dye formed by the coupling of diazotized sulfanilamide with N-(1-naphthyl) ethylene diamine dihydrochloride. This method may be used for any sulfonamide derivative in which the amino group is free or can be made free.

breath alcohol m. A method for rapidly measuring the concentration of alcohol in the expired air of an individual to determine whether or not he is intoxicated. Trade names for instruments used are *alcometer*, *drunkometer*, *intoximeter*.

Breh and Gaebler's m. (*for potassium*). Potassium is precipitated from a chloride-free blood filtrate as potassium silver cobaltinitrite which is estimated colorimetrically.

Broda m. (*for magnesium*). A histochemical method using quinalizarin to give a blue color, titian yellow to give a red color, and azo blue to give a violet color.

brucine m. (*for determination of nitrates*). The development of a yellow color by brucine in the presence of nitrates and concentrated sulfuric acid. It will detect 5 micrograms of nitrate and may be used for quantitative estimation.

Buist's m. See under *artificial respiration*.

Butler and Tuthill's m. (*for sodium*) (Weinbach's modification). Sodium is precipitated from a blood filtrate as uranyl zinc sodium acetate which is titrated with sodium hydroxide.

Cajal's gold-sublimate m. See under *stain*.

carbon tetrachloride m. (*for pollen*). Partially dried staminate flowers are soaked in carbon tetrachloride and gently beaten with a pestle to loosen the pollen from the anthers. This is strained through muslin which passes only the carbon tetrachloride and pollen. The desired pollen is then obtained by passing the suspension through a Buchner filter.

Carere-Comes Siena orange m. (*for potassium*). A histochemical method based on the development of an orange color with Siena orange solution (sodium dipicrylamine).

Castañeda's rat-lung m. A method for the production of vaccine in which high concentrations of Rickettsiae are obtained.

Castel m. (a) (*for arsenic*). A histochemical method using copper acetate to obtain a green salt of arsenic. (b) (*for bismuth*). A histochemical method based on treating tissue with a solution of brucine sulfate, sulfuric acid, and potassium iodide to obtain red granules.

cat m. A method of assay for digitalis.

cerimetric m. A titrimetric method using ceric salt. See Lindner-Kirk cerimetric *m.* and Heck-Brown-Kirk cerimetric *m.*

Chèvremont-Combaire m. (*for riboflavin*). A histochemical method based on reduction of riboflavin to leucoriboflavin and reoxidation to red granules of rhodoflavin.

Christeller m. (*for gold*). A histochemical method using stannous chloride to localize gold.

Christopher's m. of spleen index. This consists of two measurements: the umbilicus-nipple and the umbilicus-apex (of spleen). A correction is obtained from a table.

chromate m. (*for lead*). A histochemical method based on precipitation of yellow lead chromate.

Claude m. (a) (*for isolation of mitochondria*). A method based on differential centrifugation for the separation of mitochondria from neoplastic cells developed after injection of leukemic cells into rats. The advantages of this source of material are the scant blood supply, uniformity of cell type, and abundance of mitochondria. (b) (*for isolation of microsomes*). A differential centrifugation method for isolation of microsomes.

Claude-Potter m. (*for isolation of chromatin*). A method based on differential centrifugation of the nuclei of spleen and liver cells.

Conway-Byrne diffusion m. (*for ammonia and nitrogen*). A microcolorimetric method based on diffusion of ammonia from an alkalinized solution to a standard acid solution followed by titration.

Conway m. (*for chloride*). A method based on the oxidation of chloride to chlorine by acid permanganate, absorption of chlorine by iodide, and estimation of iodine liberated by titration or colorimetry.

Cooke-Ponder m. (*for classifying leukocytes*). A method of making a differential neutrophil count in which five different types of cells are classified according to the number of nuclear lobes.

Copenhagen m. See under *artificial respiration*.

copper sulfate m. (*for specific gravity and hemoglobin*). Drops of plasma or whole blood are put into a graded series of copper sulfate solutions of known specific gravity. Line charts are used for the conversion of plasma or whole blood gravities into hemoglobin or protein concentrations.

Corper and Cohn m. (*for tubercle bacilli in sputum*). Five to 20 cc. of homogenized sputum are mixed with 2 cc. of oxalic acid and put in a 50-cc. centrifuge tube and then 40 cc. of sterile saline are added. After centrifuging for 25–30 minutes, the supernatant fluid is cultured for tubercle bacilli.

Cox's yolk-sac m. A method for the production of vaccine in which high concentrations of Rickettsiae are obtained.

Crämer m. (*for nitrate*). A histochemical method based on the interaction of a nitrate with nitron to give a birefringent insoluble salt.

Crétin m. (*for minerals*). A histochemical method using gallic acid to obtain blue color for calcium, bright green for barium, blue-green for strontium and cadmium, yellowish rose for magnesium, violet-brown for iron, dull yellow for zinc and lead, and pure yellow for silicon.

Crêtin-Pouyanne m. (*for nickel*). A histochemical method based on the precipitation of nickel as lilac or blue nickel ammonium phosphate.

Cunningham-Kirk-Brooks m. (*for chloride*). An electrotitrimetric method using silver-silver amalgam electrodes and determining the titration end point by plotting the volume of silver nitrate added against the resulting electromotive force values.

cyanmethemoglobin m. (*for hemoglobin*). Photoelectric colorimetry of hemoglobin in blood after reduction to the cyanmethemoglobin form.

da Fano's cobalt nitrate m. for Golgi apparatus. See under *stain.*

Dalldorf m. See suction *test.*

Danzer and Hooker's m. (*for capillary blood pressure*). The observer measures the external pressure necessary to obliterate the flow of blood through capillaries while they are being observed microscopically.

Denis' m. (*for serum magnesium*). Calcium is removed as oxalate and magnesium is precipitated as magnesium ammonium phosphate which is estimated colorimetrically.

diaphanol m. (*for chitin*). A method for softening chitin, using diaphanol.

Diethelm's m. (*for bromide in blood*). The bromide in a blood filtrate reacts with gold chloride to produce a color which is measured colorimetrically.

diffraction m. See halo *m.*

dilatometric m. Measurement of the volume changes accompanying a chemical reaction, as indicated by the displacement of a drop of the reaction mixture in a vertical column of a nonaqueous medium.

displacement m. See Arthur Walter *Proetz.*

Dounce-Lan m. (*for isolation of nuclei*). A method for isolation of nuclei of avian erythrocytes, based on hemolysis of cells by saponin and isolation of nuclei by differential centrifugation.

Dounce m. (*for isolation of nuclei*). A method based on rupture of cells at pH of 6.5 and separation of nuclei by differential centrifugation.

Drinker's m. See under *artificial respiration.*

Dubos-Brachet m. (*for ribonucleic acid*). A histochemical method using ribonuclease to break down ribonucleic acid and remove its basophilic staining properties.

Dunn m. (*for hemoglobin*). A method for detection of hemoglobin in tissues and erythrocytes, based on staining with aniline and counterstaining with safranin. Hemoglobin stains dark blue to bluish gray.

Edwards-Scholander-Roughton m. (*for total nitrogen*). A syringe capillary method based on the extraction of all the nitrogen and part of the oxygen with carbon dioxide, absorption of the oxygen and carbon dioxide with alkaline hydrosulfite, and the measurement of the nitrogen which remains.

Einarson's gallocyanin chrome alum m. (*for Nissl bodies*). See under *stain.*

electrophoresis m. The introduction of antigens into the skin by means of an induced current. This produces less trauma than a scratch or intradermal test.

Elftman-Elftman m. (*for gold*). A histochemical method using hydrogen peroxide to obtain rose to blue colloidal gold.

Elvehjem and Kennedy's m. (*for iron*). The urine is ashed, the ash dissolved, and the iron present determined colorimetrically as thiocyanate.

epidermic m. A method of administering medicinal substances by applying them to the skin.

Esbach's m. (*for albumin in urine*). Picric acid is added to urine to precipitate protein which settles to the bottom of a graduated tube.

ester wax m. A method of embedding tissues which are unusually tough or of varied consistency.

Evans blue m. A dye-dilution method using Evans blue (T-1824) for the determination of blood volume, cardiac output, and residual blood volume in the heart.

Eve's m. See under *artificial respiration.*

Exton's m. (*for specific gravity*). A method for determining the specific gravity of small amounts of fluid by suspending it in an immiscible medium of the same specific gravity as the specimen.

falling-drop m. A method of determining the specific gravity of a solution by determining the time taken for a drop of known size to fall a given distance in a nonmiscible fluid of known density.

Farley, St. Clair, and Reisinger's m. A method of classifying neutrophils into filament and nonfilament types according to the shape of the nucleus.

Farmer and Abt's m. (*for ascorbic acid in blood*). Plasma is deproteinized, centrifuged, and titrated with 2,6-dichlorobenzenoneindophenol.

Faust's zinc sulfate centrifugal flotation m. A method of concentrating cysts of protozoa in the stool by using centrifugal flotation with zinc sulfate of specific gravity 1.180.

Fell-O'Dwyer m. See under *artificial respiration.*

fermentation m. (*for glucose*). The CO_2 evolved when urine undergoes fermentation with yeast is measured.

Fishberg and Dolin's m. (*for serum proteins*). Serum is diluted and acidified. The color of the added indicator is an index of protein concentration.

flash m. A method of pasteurizing milk by heating it to 178° F. and then chilling it promptly.

flotation m. A technic employed for separating ova and larvae from stool specimens. The stool is put into a salt solution where it sinks while the ova and larvae, due to their smaller specific gravity, rise to the surface.

Folin and Denis' m. (a) (*for phenols*). Phenols with a solution of phosphotungstic-phosphomolybdic acid and alkali yield a blue color proportional to their concentration. (b) (*for Bence-Jones protein*). The urine is heated to 60° C. and centrifuged. The precipitated protein is washed with alcohol, dried, and weighed.

Folin and Svedberg's m. (*for urea*). Urease is added to a blood filtrate to produce ammonium carbonate after which the ammonia is distilled off and determined colorimetrically after nesslerization.

Folin and Wu's m. (a) (*for protein-free blood filtrate*). Blood is laked and the proteins removed by precipitation with tungstic acid. (b) (*for nonprotein nitrogen*). The nitrogen in the blood filtrate is estimated by the Kjeldahl method; the ammonia formed is determined colorimetrically after direct nesslerization. (c) (*for glucose in blood*). The blood filtrate is heated with a copper solution and phosphomolybdic acid is added to form a blue color which is compared with a standard. (d) (*for total acidity*). Twenty-five cc. of a mixed 24-hour urine are titrated with tenth normal sodium hydroxide using phenolphthalein for an indicator.

Folin and Youngburg's m. (*for urea*). Ammonia is removed from urine by an ion-exchange zeolite. The urea is decomposed with urease and the filtrate is nesslerized.

Folin, Cannon, and Denis' m. (*for epinephrine*). Epinephrine is extracted from the suprarenals with acid. The amount is then determined by its reducing power on the uric acid reagent of Folin and Denis.

Folin-Farmer m. (*for total nitrogen*). A micromethod using the Kjeldahl procedure except that the ammonia solution is nesslerized and compared colorimetrically.

Folin-Shaffer m. (*for uric acid*). Phosphates and organic matter are removed with uranium acetate. Uric acid is precipitated as ammonium urate which is titrated with potassium permanganate.

Folin's m. (a) (*for uric acid*). A tungstic acid filtrate is mixed with a phosphotungstic acid reagent which produces a blue color that is compared with a standard. (b) (*for amino-acid nitrogen*) (Danielson's modification). The color developed by amino acids with β-naphthoquinonesulfonic acid is compared with a standard. (c) (*for ammonia*). Alkali is used to set free the ammonia of the urine. The ammonia is collected in a measured amount of acid which is then titrated. (d) (*for creatinine*). Creatinine in urine yields a red color with picric acid in alkaline solution which may be compared with a standard. (e) (*for protein*). Protein precipitated by heat and acetic acid is centrifuged, washed, dried, and weighed.

Forsgren m. (*for bile acids*). A histochemical method treating the tissue with barium chloride, acid fuchsin, phosphomolybdic acid, and aniline blue-orange G stain to obtain reddish-blue granules.

Frame, Russell, and Wilhelmi's m. (*for amino-acid nitrogen*). The amino nitrogen groups in a protein-free blood filtrate combine with β-naphthoquinone sulfonate to form highly colored compounds which may be compared colorimetrically with a standard.

Friedemann and Graeser's m. (*for lactic acid*). Glucose of the blood is removed and the lactic acid converted to acetaldehyde which is combined with sodium bisulfite. The bound sulfite is then determined iodometrically.

Gersh-Macallum m. (*for potassium*). A histochemical method employing the freezing-drying process; potassium is precipitated as yellow sodium potassium cobaltinitrite.

Glick acidimetric m. (*for esterase, lipase, and cholinesterase*). Titrimetric methods based on the neutralization of the acid liberated with an alkaline buffer medium and measurement of the loss in alkalinity of the buffer with acid. Butyrate, tributyrin, and acetylcholine are used as subtrates for esterase, lipase, and cholinesterase, respectively.

Glick-Linderstrøm-Lang-Holter m. (*for inorganic phosphate*). A microtitrimetric method based on precipitating the phosphate as magnesium ammonium phosphate, dissolving the latter in hydrochloric acid, and titrating the excess acid with ammonium acetate.

Glick m. (*for ascorbic acid*). A titrimetric method based on extraction of ascorbic acid with metaphosphoric acid, the conversion of dehydroascorbic acid, if present, to ascorbic acid with hydrogen sulfide, and titration with 2,6-dichlorophenolindophenol.

Goldblatt m. The production of experimental persistent hypertension by the permanent constriction of the main renal arteries with a special clamp devised for the purpose.

Gomori m. (*for glycogen and mucin*). A histochemical method using chromic acid and silver nitrate-methanamine to obtain grayish to black granules of glycogen and mucin. Melanin and insoluble calcium salts also stain black with this method.

Gomori's acid phosphatase m. See under *stain*.

Gomori's alkaline phosphatase m. See under *stain*.

Gomori's lipase m. See under *stain*.

Gouilliart m. (*for hemoglobin*). A method for detection of hemoglobin in tissues and erythrocytes, using potassium iodide in glacial acetic acid to obtain birefringent crystals of protoiodoheme.

Graff m. (*for cytochrome oxidase*). A histochemical method based on conversion of Nadi reagent to indophenol to obtain a blue color.

Graham alphanaphthol pyronin m. (*for oxidase granules*). See under *stain*.

Greenberg's m. (*for serum proteins*). Proteins are separated with sodium sulfate and determined colorimetrically after treatment with a phenol reagent.

Griffith's m. (*for hippuric acid*). Hippuric acid is extracted with ether. The residue from the ether distillation is treated with bromine and sodium hypobromite. Hippuric acid nitrogen is then determined by the Kjeldahl method.

Hackmann m. (*for sulfonamides*). A method by which colorless sulfonamides can be demonstrated by diazotizing with nitrous acid and coupling with alpha-naphthylamine. In frozen dried tissues, colored sulfonamides can be seen directly.

Haden-Hausser m. (*for hemoglobin*). An acid hematin method, in which the color is compared with a glass standard scale through a microscope in a special hemoglobinometer having a wedge-shaped dilution channel.

Haden m. A simplification of the Folin-Wu method for making protein-free filtrates in which the acid and tungstate solutions are combined before adding to the blood instead of adding separately.

Hagedorn and Jensen's m. (*for blood sugar*). Blood is precipitated with zinc hydroxide, filtered, and used to reduce potassium ferricyanide which is then titrated with sodium thiosulfate.

Hale m. (*for hyaluronic acid*). A histochemical method based on the combination of hyaluronic acid with iron and the development of a blue color by ferrocyanide.

halo m. A method for determining the mean diameter of a group of erythrocytes. A beam of white light is passed through an unstained blood film, the resulting spectrum is projected on a screen; the diameter of the halo on the screen varies inversely with the mean diameter of the erythrocytes. Also called *diffraction m.*

Hammerschlag m. (*for specific gravity of blood*). See under Albert *Hammerschlag*.

Hammett-Chapman m. (*for bile acids*). A histochemical method of treating tissue with ammonium hydroxide, nitroprusside, and ammonium sulfate.

Hand-Edwards-Caley m. (*for mercury*). A histochemical method based on the reduction of the mercuric form by stannous chloride and the mercurous form by thioglycollic acid to obtain black spheres of metallic mercury.

Hanus m. (*for iodine number*). See under *iodine*.

Heatley m. (*for glycogen*). A microtitrimetric

method based on the isolation of glycogen from tissue, hydrolysis with hydrochloric acid, and estimation of glucose produced by Linderstrøm-Lang-Holter method.

Heck-Brown-Kirk cerimetric m. (*for reducing sugars*). A titrimetric method using ceric sulfate for titration.

Hellige m. (*for hemoglobin*). A colorimetric method for determination of hemoglobin by comparing acid hematin (prepared by diluting blood 1 to 100 with hydrochloric acid) with a revolving disk of 18 known glass standards.

Henriques-Sørensen m. for amino-acid nitrogen. If formaldehyde is added to a solution of amino acids, a reaction takes place with the formation of derivatives which are strongly acid in reaction due to the destruction of the basic properties of the amino groups. The carboxyl groups may then be titrated using phenolphthalein as an indicator. The acidity as shown by the titration is a measure of the amino-acid nitrogen present.

Herter-Foster m. (*for indole*). To 10 ml. of unknown, 2 drops of 2% solution of beta-naphthoquinone sodium monosulfonate and 2 ml. of 10% NaOH are added; the mixture is allowed to stand for 15 minutes, then shaken with 2 ml. of chloroform. A red color indicates the presence of indole.

Hildebrand m. for hydrogen-ion concentration. An electrometric method for the determination of hydrogen-ion concentration.

Hittorf m. for ionic mobilities. The determination of the mass of the particles passing from one electrode chamber to the other in a given time under the influence of an applied electric field.

Hochberg-Melnick-Oser m. for ascorbic acid. Ascorbic acid is determined in the presence of other reducing substances by photometric measurement of the rate of decolorization of the dye, 2,6-dichlorophenol indophenol.

Höjer m. for vitamin C. A quantitative technic based on the histologic examination of the incisors of guinea pigs after a test period of 14 days.

Holter-Doyle m. (*for catalase*). A titrimetric method based on the oxidation of iodide to iodine, by oxygen liberated from hydrogen peroxide, and titration of iodine with thiosulfate.

Horowitz-Beadle m. for choline. Measurement of choline by the growth stimulation of a mutant strain of *Neurospora crassa,* produced artificially by exposure to ultraviolet radiation. Methionine, which can replace choline for the microorganism, is removed by absorption of the extract on an ion-exchange silicate followed by elution with sodium chloride solution.

Hortega's silver m. (*for oligodendrocytes*). See under *stain.*

Hotchkiss m. (*for polysaccharides*). A histochemical method based on oxidation of hydroxyl groups in the polysaccharide to aldehydes and the coloring of the aldehydes with Feulgen reaction.

Howard's m. See under *artificial respiration.*

Howell's m. (*for coagulation time*). Venous blood is put into a test tube of 21 mm. diameter, coagulation time being complete when the clot is firm enough to permit inversion of the tube.

Hulett and Bonner m. A method for the preparation of standard HCl from a constant boiling solution.

Humphrey m. (*for iron*). A histochemical method using dinitroresorcinol to obtain a bright dark-green color against a reddish or brown background.

Hunter and Givens' modification of the Krüger-Schmid m. The Krüger-Schmid process is combined with the microchemical colorimetric method for uric acid. The modification is recommended where the amount of uric acid present is minute.

hypobromite m. A method of estimating the quantity of urea in body fluids, based upon the fact that when urea is acted upon by sodium hypobromite it is decomposed into nitrogen, carbon dioxide, and water. From the volume of nitrogen evolved the quantity of urea can be determined.

India ink m. A method of isolating and observing a single bacterium.

investing m. The process of enveloping or covering wholly or in part an object such as a denture, tooth, wax form, crown, orthodontic band, etc., with some heat-resisting investment compound before vulcanizing, soldering, or casting.

iodometric permanganate m. See Siwe *m.*

isotope-dilution m. A procedure in which a known quantity of an elemental isotope is introduced into a system containing an unknown amount of that element; after equilibration the concentration or specific activity of the isotope in the system is used to calculate the amount of element originally present. When the isotope is part of a chemical compound, then the amount of that compound can be determined.

Jackson m. (*for lipid*). A histochemical method, using acetic-carbol-Sudan III to stain those lipids (red) which are refractory to ordinary Sudan-staining methods.

Jephcott m. A method for the preparation of insulin from finely minced pancreas.

Kaiserling's m. A method of preparing museum specimens to preserve their color. There are three steps: (a) Fix organs for one to 14 days in: formalin 40 cc., water 2000 cc., potassium nitrate 30 Gm., and potassium acetate 60 Gm. (b) Restore optimum color by immersing in 80% ethyl alcohol for 10 to 60 minutes. (c) Keep permanently in: glycerin 500 cc., 1% aqueous arsenious acid 200 cc., water 2300 cc., potassium acetate 250 Gm., thymol 2.5 Gm.

Karr's m. (*for urea*). Similar to Folin and Svedberg's method except that the ammonium carbonate is nesslerized directly in the presence of gum ghatti as a protective colloid.

Katzman and Doisy m. A method for the preparation of chorionic gonadotrophin from human pregnancy urine.

Kirk-Bentley m. (*for iron*). A microtitrimetri- method based on the reduction of iron by cadc mium amalgam, the addition of excess ceric sulfate, and the titration of the excess with ferrous ammonium sulfate.

Kjeldahl m. (*for total nitrogen*). A method to determine the amount of nitrogen in an organic compound. Concentrated sulfuric acid reacts with the material to produce ammonia which is distilled into an acid solution. The excess of acid is determined by titration with standard alkali solution.

Knott m. Ultraviolet irradiation of blood.

Koch-McMeekin's m. (*for nonprotein nitrogen*). The organic matter is digested with sulfuric acid and hydrogen peroxide and the resulting solution is nesslerized. May also be used for total nitrogen of urine.

Köhler's m. of illumination. A method of microscopical illumination in which an image of the source is focused in the lower focal plane of the microscope condenser, and the condenser, in turn, focuses an image of the lamp lens in the object field.

Kramer-Tisdall m. (*for serum calcium*) (Clark-

Collip modification). Calcium is precipitated from serum as oxalate and titrated with potassium permanganate.

Kretchmer-Holman-Burr m. (*for iodine number*). See under *iodine.*

Krüger and Schmid's m. (*for determination of uric acid and purine bases*). The principle involved is the precipitation of both uric acid and the purine bases in combination with copper oxide and the subsequent decomposition of this precipitate by means of sodium sulfide. The uric acid is then precipitated by HCl and the purine bases are separated from the filtrate in the form of their copper or silver compounds. The nitrogen content of the precipitates is determined by the Kjeldahl method and the corresponding values for uric acid and purine bases calculated. See also Hunter and Givens' modification of the Krüger-Schmid *m.*

Kumon m. for indican. A specific procedure based upon the color reaction between indican and ninhydrin.

Kwilecki's m. (*for albumin*). A solution of ferric chloride is added to urine before proceeding with Esbach's method.

Laborde's m. See under *artificial respiration.*

Laidlow m. (*for dopa oxidase*). An adaptation of Bloch's *method.*

Larson m. for allantoin in urine. Urine is treated with phosphotungstic acid to remove interfering substances. Basic lead acetate is then added to remove excess phosphotungstic acid and residual interfering substances. Excess lead is removed by sulfuric acid and excess acid neutralized by sodium hydroxide. The solution is then boiled with Folin ammoniacal reagent and acid molybdate reagent added to the cool solution. A colorimetric comparison is made against a 1.0 mg. allantoin standard.

Laskowski m. (*for isolation of nuclei*). A method for isolation of nuclei of avian erythrocytes, based on hemolysis of cells by lysolecithin and isolation of nuclei by differential centrifugation.

Lazarow m. A method for isolation of lipoprotein and glycogen particles from liver cells, based on differential centrifugation. The resulting red precipitate, containing lipoprotein and glycogen, is treated with diastase to obtain pure lipoprotein.

Leake and Guy's m. (*for platelets*). Consists of diluting the blood in order to count the platelets in a solution composed of formalin 6 cc., sodium oxalate 1.6 Gm., crystal violet 0.01 Gm., and water 94 cc.

Lee-White m. A modification of Howell's method of measuring coagulation time of blood.

Leiboff and Kahn's m. (*for urea*). Urea in a blood filtrate is converted to ammonia by acid hydrolysis under pressure and directly nesslerized.

Lepehne-Pickworth m. (*for demonstration of cerebral capillary distribution*). See benzidine and nitroprusside oxidase *m.* (for hemoglobin).

Leschke m. (*for urea*). A histochemical method based on treatment with mercuric nitrate followed by hydrogen sulfide to obtain black mercuric sulfide precipitate at the site of urea in the tissue.

Letonoff and Reinhold's m. (*for inorganic sulfate in serum*). After deproteinization with uranium acetate, the sulfate is precipitated, dissolved, and determined colorimetrically.

Levy m. (*for total nitrogen*). A microcolorimetric method based on the nesslerization of an acid-digested sample.

Levy-Palmer m. (*for total nitrogen*). A colorimetric method based on the reaction of ammonia with excess hypobromite and measurement of the excess iodometrically.

life insurance m. (*for protein*). Clarified urine is treated with sulfosalicylic acid and the turbidity is compared with artificial standards.

Lillie's azure-eosin m. See *Lillie's azure eosinates in buffered solutions* under *stain.*

Linderstrøm-Lang-Duspiva m. (*for protease*). A microtitrimetric method based on exposure of peptides to protease and titration of the carboxyl groups of the proteolytic products with tetraethylammonium hydroxide.

Linderstrøm-Lang-Engel m. (*for amylose*). A titrimetric method based on the measurement of an increase in reducing sugar after the action of the enzyme on starch.

Linderstrøm-Lang-Glick m. (*for cholinesterase*). A Cartesian-diver method based upon the fact that when a choline ester is broken down in a bicarbonate buffer, the acid produced causes equivalent liberation of carbon dioxide which is measured by the Warburg apparatus.

Linderstrøm-Lang-Holter m. (a) (*for protease*). A titrimetric method based upon the addition of acetone indicator to the products and the titration of their amino groups with hydrochloric acid. (b) (*for reducing sugars*). A microtitrimetric method based on reduction of iodide to iodine and titration of the latter with thiosulfate.

Linderstrøm-Lang-Lanz m. (*for peptidase*). A dilatometric method using DL-alanylglycine as the substrate for peptidase.

Linderstrøm-Lang m. (*for combined potassium and sodium*). A microtitrimetric method based on the conversion of potassium and sodium to chlorides by an ashing reagent, removal of other chlorides, and electrometric titration of the residual chloride with silver nitrate.

Linderstrøm-Lang-Palmer-Holter m. (*for chloride*). A method using the same principle as Cunningham-Kirk-Brooks *m.*

Linderstrøm-Lang-Weil-Holter m. (*for arginase*). (a) *Urease m.* A titrimetric method based on the action of the enzyme on arginine to liberate urea, the action of urease on urea to release ammonia, and the measurement of ammonia. (b) *Acetone-alcohol m.* A method based on titration of ornithine and urea, formed on the breakdown of arginine by acetone-alcohol mixture.

Lindner-Kirk cerimetric m. (*for calcium*). A titrimetric method based on the precipitation of calcium as oxalate, treatment with excess ceric sulfate, and titration of the excess with ferrous ammonium sulfate.

Loele m. (*for alphanaphthol oxidase*). A histochemical method based on the effect of the enzyme on alphanaphthol dissolved in potassium hydroxide to give violet or black granules.

Looney and Dyer m. for potassium in blood. Potassium is precipitated from the protein-free, chloride-free serum filtrate as the insoluble potassium silver cobaltinitrite. The washed precipitate is decomposed by alkali to liberate the nitrite, which is then determined colorimetrically.

Lowry-Lopez-Bessey m. (*for ascorbic acid*). A colorimetric method based on the conversion of ascorbic acid to dehydroascorbic acid which is treated with 2,4-dinitrophenylhydrazine to give an osazone; the osazone is treated with sulfuric acid to give a colored dehydration product.

Lowry-Lopez m. (*for inorganic phosphate*). A method using the same principle as the Siwe *m.*, using ascorbic acid for reduction.

Lucas and Beveridge m. for cysteine. A procedure for preparing cysteine from human hair by means of cuprous oxide.

Lundsteen-Vermehren m. (*for inorganic phosphate and phosphatase*). A microcolorimetric method based on the same principle as the Siwe *m.*, using amidol for reduction.

Lyle-Curtman-Marshall m. A modification of the benzidine test for blood in which the benzidine reagent is prepared by a different procedure.

Macallum m. (a) A method for changing organic iron to free ferric form, using nitric or sulfuric acid in alcohol. (b) (*for potassium*). See Gersh-Macallum *m.*

McCrudden m. (*for calcium and magnesium*). Calcium is precipitated as calcium oxalate and is either ignited and weighed as CaO or determined volumetrically by titration with potassium permanganate. Magnesium ammonium phosphate is precipitated, ignited, and then weighed as pyrophosphate.

McCullagh's m. (*for iodine*). Iodine is converted to iodide, then oxidized to iodate which liberates iodine from an excess of added iodide. The iodine is then titrated with sodium thiosulfate.

McFarlane's m. (*for copper*). Sodium diethyldithiocarbamate is added to an extracted ashed blood and the blue color which develops is extracted with amyl alcohol and compared with a standard.

McGunkin m. (*for catalase*). A histochemical method based on the oxidation of benzidine by the oxygen liberated from hydrogen peroxide, to give a blue color which changes to brown.

MacKee-Herrmann-Baker-Sulzberger m. (*for sulfonamides*). A histochemical method based on the formation of a yellow to orange precipitate of *p*-dimethylaminobenzylidene derivative when sulfonamides react with *p*-dimethylaminobenzaldehyde.

McLean and Van Slyke's m. (*for chlorides*). The excess of silver nitrate which has been used to precipitate chlorides from oxalated plasma is titrated with potassium iodide and starch.

Malfatti formol titration m. A method based on the reaction that takes place when formalin solution is added to a solution containing ammonium salts. An acid reaction is produced in the mixture which is then titrated with standard alkali using phenolphthalein as an indicator. Amino acids give the same reaction so that the result of titration represents ammonia plus amino-acid nitrogen.

Mallory-Parker m. (*for lead and copper*). (a) *Hematoxylin m.* A method by which lead appears grayish blue and copper intense blue. (b) *Methylene blue m.* A method by which lead appears intense blue and copper, pale blue.

Malloy-Evelyn m. for bilirubin in blood. Blood is treated with Ehrlich's reagent and the bilirubin reacts to form a colored compound, azorubin or azobilirubin. The quantity of azorubin formed is determined photometrically.

Marriott m. (*for alkali reserve: alveolar carbon dioxide tension*). By rebreathing air under certain definite conditions, a sample is obtained whose carbon dioxide tension is virtually that of venous blood. The collected alveolar air is allowed to pass rapidly through a standard sodium bicarbonate solution to which an indicator has been added. The reaction of the saturated solution will depend on the relative amounts of the alkaline bicarbonate and the acid carbon dioxide present. This in turn will depend on the tension of carbon dioxide in the air with which the mixture has been saturated. High tensions of CO_2 change the reaction of the solution toward the acid side. Low tensions have the reverse effect; hence the reaction of such a solution is a measure of the tension of CO_2 in the air with which it has been saturated.

Marshall and Welker m. A procedure for the preparation of hemoglobin.

Marshall Hall's m. See under *artificial respiration.*

Mathews m. A procedure for distinguishing fermentable sugar (glucose) from nonfermentable reducing substances (lactose, etc.) by the use of yeast.

Maximow's hematoxylin-azure II-eosin m. (*for blood-forming organs*). See under *stain.*

Meduna's m. Convulsion therapy in dementia precox.

Meiklejohn-Cohen indican m. A photometric modification which is based upon calibration of the photometer with standard indican solutions.

Mendel-Bradley m. (*for zinc*). A histochemical method based on precipitation of zinc by nitroprusside and the treatment of the precipitate with sulfide to obtain a deep-purple color.

Menke m. (*for isolation of chloroplasts*). A method based on grinding leaves, suspending them in phosphate, and precipitating the chloroplasts by ammonium sulfate.

Menten-Junge-Green m. (*for alkaline phosphatase*). A histochemical method based on the liberation of betanaphthol from calcium betanaphthol phosphate and the reaction of betanaphthol with diazotized alphanaphthylamine to obtain a reddish-purple precipitate.

metatrophic m. A therapeutic method of modifying the nutrition by changes in the food, with a view of administering some drug, as suppression of sodium chloride in food of epileptics in order to reinforce the action of bromides.

m. for alkali reserve. See Van Slyke and Cullen's *m.*

m. for ascorbic acid. See Farmer and Abt's *m.*

m. for Bence-Jones protein. See Folin and Denis' *m.* (b).

m. for bromide in blood. See Diethelm's *m.*

m. for capillary blood pressure. See Danzer and Hooker's *m.*

m. for carbon dioxide combining power. See Van Slyke and Cullen's *m.* for alkali reserve. Also called *carbon dioxide capacity.*

m. for cholesterol. See Schoenheimer and Sperry's *m.*

m. for copper. See McFarlane's *m.*

m. for creatinine. See Folin's *m.* (d).

m. for digitalis. See cat *m.*

m. for epinephrine. See Folin, Cannon, and Denis' *m.*

m. for hemoglobin. See acid hematin *m.*

m. for hippuric acid. See Griffith's *m.*

m. for icterus index. See Meulengracht's *m.*

m. for indican. See Askenstedt's *m.*

m. for iodine. See McCullagh's *m.*

m. for lactic acid. See Friedemann and Graeser's *m.*

m. for magnesium. See Denis' *m.*

m. for phosphatase. See Bodansky's *m.*

m. for phosphate. See Benedict and Theis's *m.*

m. for pollen. See carbon tetrachloride *m.*

m. for potassium. See Breh and Gaebler's *m.*

m. for prothrombin activity. See one-stage *m.* and two-stage *m.*

m. for serum amylase. See Somogyi's *m.*

m. for sodium. See Butler and Tuthill's *m.*

m. for sulfonamides. See Bratton and Marshall's *m.*

m. for sulfur. See Letonoff and Reinhold's *m.* and Benedict's *m.* (b).

m. for thiocyanates. See Barker's *m.*

m. for total acidity of urine. See Folin and Wu's *m.* (d).

m. for urobilinogen. See Wallace and Diamond's *m.*

m. of least squares. The method of finding a statistical constant or the equation of a straight line or curve in such a manner that the sum of the squares of the deviations about the mean, line, or curve is a minimum.

methods for amino-acid nitrogen. See Folin's *m.* (b), and Frame, Russel, and Wilhelmi's *m.*

methods for ammonia. See Folin's *m.* (c), and permutit *m.*

methods for bile pigment. See Meulengracht's *m.* and van den Bergh's *m.*

methods for calcium. See Bell's *m.* and Kramer-Tisdall *m.*

methods for chlorides. See Whitehorn's *m.*, Van Slyke's *m.*, Austin and Van Slyke's *m.*, and McLean and Van Slyke's *m.*

methods for classifying leukocytes. See Arneth's *m.*, Schilling's *m.*, Cooke-Ponder *m.*, and Farley, St. Clair, and Reisinger's *m.*

methods for glucose. See Benedict's *m.* (a), Folin and Wu's *m.* (c), Hagedorn and Jensen's *m.*, Benedict's picrate *m.*, and fermentation *m.*

methods for iron. See Wong's *m.*, and Elvehjem and Kennedy's *m.*

methods for nonprotein nitrogen. See Folin and Wu's *m.* (b) and Koch-McMeekin's *m.*

methods for phenols. See Theis and Benedict's *m.*, and Folin and Denis' *m.* (a).

methods for protein-free blood filtrate. See Folin and Wu's *m.* (a), Benedict and Newton's *m.*

methods for proteins in urine. See Folin's *m.*, (e), and life insurance *m.*

methods for serum proteins. See Greenberg's *m.*, and Fishberg and Dolin's *m.*

methods for specific gravity. See falling-drop *m.* and copper sulfate *m.*

methods for total nitrogen. See Kjeldahl *m.*, Folin-Farmer *m.*, and Koch-McMeekin's *m.*

methods for urea. See Folin and Svedberg's *m.*, Karr's *m.*, Myers' *m.*, Leiboff and Kahn's *m.*, Folin and Youngburg's *m.*, and hypobromite *m.*

methods for uric acid. See Folin's *m.* (a), Benedict's *m.* (c), Benedict and Franke's *m.*, and Folin-Shaffer *m.*

methylene blue m. See Mallory-Parker *m.* (b).

Mett m. (*for determination of peptic activity*). Small glass tubes, filled with coagulated egg albumin, are introduced into the solution to be tested and kept for a definite length of time in the incubator. The protein column is digested at both ends of the tube to an extent depending on the amount of pepsin present.

Meulengracht's m. (*for bile pigment*). The yellow color of serum is compared with a standard potassium dichromate solution. Also called the icteric index.

Michaelis indicator m. A method for a colorimetric determination of hydrogen-ion concentration without the use of buffer solutions. The procedure is most simply carried out by using a single-color indicator.

Milovidov m. (*for starch*). A staining method using toluidine blue, gentian violet, or methyl green, which give blue, violet, and green colors, respectively.

Mirsky-Pollister m. A procedure for the preparation of chromonucleoprotein from liver.

Monaldi m. Drainage and continuous aspiration. See under Vincenzo *Monaldi.*

Montgomery m. (*for hydrogen ion*). A capillary tube colorimetric method for determination of hydrogen ion concentration.

Morris's wet-film m. A technique for staining tissue removed from the brain either by craniotomy or with a brain needle. Films of tissue are spread on a slide and fixed while still wet.

moving-boundary m. See moving-boundary *electrophoresis.*

Myers and Wardell m. (*for cholesterol*). The serum or plasma is dried on plaster of Paris and extracted with chloroform. The total cholesterol of the extract is determined colorimetrically by the Liebermann-Burchard reaction with acetic anhydride and sulfuric acid.

Myers' m. (*for urea*). Urea is converted to ammonium carbonate with urease. The ammonia is aerated off and determined by nesslerization.

Najjar riboflavin m. The riboflavin is extracted with acetic acid-pyridine-butanol mixture after interfering urinary pigments are oxidized with permanganate. The concentration of riboflavin in the extract is measured fluorometrically.

Neish m. (*for isolation of chloroplasts*). A method for isolation of chloroplasts from leaves, based on grinding and differential centrifugation.

Neumann m. for total phosphorus. The organic matter is destroyed by digestion with a mixture of sulfuric and nitric acids or some other oxidizing agent. The phosphorus is then precipitated as the phosphomolybdate and determined gravimetrically or volumetrically.

Newcomer m. for hemoglobin. Hemoglobin is converted to acid hematin with hydrochloric acid and then compared with a yellow groundglass filter, which approaches the spectroscopic properties of acid hematin, in a balancing type of colorimeter.

Newton m. for uric acid determination. Interfering material in the blood filtrate is removed by the acid silver chloride precipitation method. The uric acid remaining is determined colorimetrically by reaction at room temperature in the presence of cyanide with a special arsenotungstate reagent.

Nielsen's m. See under *artificial respiration.*

Norberg titrimetric m. (*for potassium*). A microtitrimetric method based on the precipitation of potassium as chloroplatinate, the conversion of chloroplatinate to iodoplatinate, and the titration of the latter with thiosulfate.

Ochoa-Peters m. (*for thiamine*). A gasometric method based on the stimulating effect of thiamine on decarboxylation of pyruvic acid by yeast and the measurement of carbon dioxide liberated by the Warburg apparatus.

Ogata and Ogata's silver m. (*for chromaffin cells*). See under *stain.*

Okamoto m. (*for metals*). A histochemical method based on development of a reddish-violet precipitate by most metals upon their reaction with *p*-dimethylaminobenzydilene rhodanine.

Okkels m. (*for gold*). A histochemical method using ultraviolet light to obtain black gold granules.

one-stage m. (*for prothrombic activity*). A method for determination of plasma prothrombic activity by the addition of thromboplastin and calcium to decalcified plasma. The clotting time or prothrombin time is then used as an index of prothrombin concentration.

Ormsby's m. (*for urea*). A blood filtrate is heated with biacetyl monoxime in acid solution and a yellow color develops. The color is deepened by oxidation with potassium persulfate and compared colorimetrically with a standard urea solution similarly treated.

Orr-Trueta m. Treatment of severe open wounds, especially in compound fractures, by packing with petroleum gauze after careful debridement and reduction, and applying a plaster cast, which is left on for 6 to 8 weeks: used most frequently in military surgery.

Oster-Mulinos m. A method for differentiation of aldehydes from nonaldehydes giving the Feulgen reaction; the purple color developed by Feulgen reaction can be eliminated by sodium hydroxide in both and can be restored by hydrochloric acid in aldehydes but not in nonaldehydes.

Oster-Schlossman m. (*for amine oxidase*). A histochemical method based on Feulgen reaction of the aldehyde formed as the product of action of the enzyme on tyramine.

Palmer m. for hemoglobin. The diluted blood is treated with carbon monoxide gas before the photometric reading is taken. This method is more accurate than the direct photometric method, since it is free from any error due to the presence of carbon monoxide hemoglobin in the blood as drawn.

Pap m. (*for reticulum*). A special staining method for reticulum fibers, using ammoniacal silver nitrate.

Parker's m. for indican. See Askenstedt's *m.*

Penfield's m. for glia. See *Penfield's method* under *stain.*

permutit m. (*for ammonia*). Urine is shaken with a permutit ion-exchanger to remove the ammonia which is set free with alkali, followed by nesslerization and comparison with a standard.

Peters m. A procedure for determining urinary creatine under conditions whereby the diluted sample is treated by methods similar to those used for blood filtrates, thus permitting the determination of both blood and urine creatine in essentially the same manner.

Pohl m. (*for ultraviolet intensity*). A photochemical method in which the index is the time required for the ultraviolet energy to produce a blue color in a solution containing potassium iodide, sodium thiosulfate, and starch.

polar m. A method of applying electricity; the pole, the distinctive effect of which is wanted, is placed over some part to be treated, and the other pole over some indifferent part.

Pollack m. (*for calcium*). A histochemical method using sodium alizarin sulfonate to give a red precipitate.

Popper m. (*for lipids*). A histochemical method using phosphine 3R which gives neutral fats a silver-white fluorescence on a brown background.

Post-Laudermilk m. (*for cellulose*). A staining method for cellulose by applying iodine and lithium chloride to the fibers to obtain blue, yellow, or green color.

Prague m. (*for delivery of the aftercoming head*). See under *maneuver.*

Price-Jones m. See Cecil *Price-Jones.*

Prochownick's m. See under *artificial respiration.*

prone pressure m. See *Schafer* (*prone pressure*) *m.* under *artificial respiration.*

Pryce slide-culture m. A method of preparing sputum, body fluid, or tissue for examination for *Mycobacterium tuberculosis.* A smear is made, air-dried, incubated, and stained for acid-fast bacilli.

pulp traction m. A means of finger extension limited to compound fracture of the phalanges, where the corresponding flexor surfaces of the fingers are wounded. A stainless steel wire is passed through the pulp in the distal phalanx, and then is attached to a banjo hand splint, using rubber bands for traction.

quartz-rod m. (*for illuminating living organs*). The use of a fused quartz rod to conduct light from an intense source to a living internal organ, to permit direct microscopic study in situ while maintaining experimental conditions which disturb as little as possible the structures and processes to be observed. The normal temperature of the illuminated living structures is maintained with a slowly flowing isotonic and isothermal wash solution.

Quick and Csonka m. (*for conjugated glucuronic acids*). The compound is extracted with ether, hydrolyzed with dilute acid, and finally determination of the liberated glucuronic acid is made by a copper reduction method.

Quick m. See one-stage *m.*

Ralph m. (*for hemoglobin*). A method for the detection of hemoglobin in tissues and erythrocytes by using benzidine and hydrogen peroxide to obtain a black color.

Ramón y Cajal's gold-sublimate m. See *Cajal's gold-sublimate m.* under *stain.*

Ramsay m. (*for iron*). A microtitrimetric method using titanous sulfate for titration.

Rapkine m. (*for sulfhydryl groups*). A histochemical method of treating tissue with zinc acetate, nitroprusside, ammonium sulfate, and ammonium hydroxide to obtain a red color.

Rasorian m. In phlebotomy, repeated bleeding.

Rehfuss m. (*for fractional gastric analysis*). See under M. E. *Rehfuss.*

Reinhold and Shiels m. (*for blood cholesterol*). The serum or plasma is dried on anhydrous sodium sulfate and extracted with chloroform. The total cholesterol of the extract is determined colorimetrically by the Liebermann-Burchard reaction with acetic anhydride and sulfuric acid. A modification of the Myers and Wardell method.

Riggs and Stadie m. (*for peptic activity*). Enzyme activity is measured photometrically as the decrease in turbidity of a standardized homogenized suspension of coagulated egg white under specified conditions.

rocking m. See *Eve's m.* under *artificial respiration.*

Roe-Kahn m. (*for blood calcium*). Calcium is precipitated from the protein-free serum filtrate as tricalcium phosphate, which is then determined colorimetrically.

Roese-Gottlieb m. (*for analysis of milk fat*). The milk is made alkaline and extracted repeatedly with petroleum benzine and the filtered extract evaporated to dryness in a flask.

Rosenfield-Tuft m. A variation of the one-stage *m.* of Quick.

Roth's m. A method for the intravenous injection into a mouse using a tin mailing tube to hold the body while the tail protrudes from one end.

Roughton-Scholander m. Micromethod for determination of gases in capillary blood, using a glass syringe fused to a graduated capillary tube which has a cuplike expansion at its free end. With appropriate procedure and reagents, separate determinations can be made for O_2, CO_2, CO, and N_2. Also called *syringe-capillary m.*

rowing m. See under *artificial respiration.*

Russel m. (*for ammonia*). A colorimetric method based on the reaction of phenol and hypochlorite with ammonia in alkaline solution to give an intense blue product.

Sahli m. (*for hemoglobin*). An acid hematin method, in which the acid hematin solution is diluted in a special graduated tube by dropwise addition of water until it matches a glass standard.

Sahyun m. (*for amino acids*). A method based on the color developed by the reaction between amino acids and β-naphthoquinone-4-sulfonic acid in alkaline solution. Heating develops the color.

Sanford, Sheard, and Osterberg m. (*for hemoglobin*). Blood is diluted with 0.1 per cent sodium carbonate, and the resulting oxyhemoglobin is read in a special photoelectric colorimeter with a green glass filter.
Satterthwaite's m. See under *artificial respiration.*
Schafer (prone pressure) m. See under *artificial respiration.*
Schales and Schales m. (*for blood chlorides*). The sample is titrated with standard mercuric nitrate solution at the proper acidity in the presence of diphenylcarbazone as indicator. Chlorides present react with the added mercuric ions to form soluble, but undissociated, mercuric chloride. When an excess of mercuric ion has been added, the indicator turns purple.
Schilling's m. A method of classifying neutrophils. See Victor *Schilling.*
Schmidt-Nielsen m. (a) (*for lipids*). A microtitrimetric method based on saponification of lipids by alcoholic alkali in the presence of toluol, liberation of free fatty acids by excess mineral acid, solution of the fatty acids in the toluol phase, and titration of the toluol phase. (b) (*for iodine number*). See under *iodine.*
Schmorl's alizarin SX m. for calcium. See under *stain.*
Schneider m. (*for uranium*). A histochemical method based on the precipitation of dark-brown uranium ferrocyanide.
Schoenheimer and Sperry's m. (*for cholesterol*). The cholesterol is precipitated from an acetone alcohol extract with digitonin. The digitonide undergoes the Liebermann-Burchard reaction and the color is compared with a standard.
Schroeder's m. See under *artificial respiration.*
Schulze m. (*for chitin*). A staining method which consists of subjecting half of the specimen to the Zander method and the other half to iodine followed by sulfuric acid. The latter test gives a brown color with chitin and a blue color with cellulose.
Schultze's m. See under *artificial respiration.*
Schultz's sterol reaction m. for cholesterol. See under *stain.*
sedimentation m. A method of concentrating helminth eggs by washing stools one or more times and discarding the supernatant fluid. Water or fluids of greater density may be used so long as the specific gravity of the wash is less than that of the eggs.
Semenoff m. (*for succinic dehydrogenase*). A histochemical method based on the reduction of methylene blue by the enzyme.
Sendroy m. (a) (*for chloride*). A colorimetric method based on the conversion of chloride in acid solution to silver salt by silver iodate and reaction of the liberated iodate with potassium iodide to give free iodine which is titrated by thiosulfate. (b) (*for calcium*). A colorimetric method based on the precipitation of calcium as oxalate, treatment with excess ceric sulfate, and reaction of the excess with potassium iodide to liberate yellow-free iodine.
Sen m. (*for urease*). A histochemical method based on decomposition of urea on exposure to urease with formation of carbonic acid which is converted to cobalt carbonate and the latter to a brown or black precipitate of cobalt sulfide.
Serra m. (*for arginine and arginine-containing proteins*). A method using the same principle as Thomas *m.*
Serra-Queiroz Lopes m. (*for inorganic phosphate*). A histochemical method based on the same principle as the Siwe *m.*, using benzidine for reduction.
Shinowara, Jones, and Reinhart m. A procedure for phosphorus determination, using stannous chloride as reducing agent, which requires as little as 0.06 ml. of serum.
Shock and Hastings m. A procedure for determining the hydrogen-ion concentration of blood by use of a special pipet which not only permits the determination of cell volume as well as plasma pH, but also makes possible the transfer of the diluted plasma to the manometric apparatus for CO_2 determination.
Shohl and King m. A procedure for the colorimetric determination of hydrogen-ion concentration of gastric contents.
Sicka m. A hemoglobinometric method using reduced hemoglobin as pigment and requiring a special comparator.
silver impregnation methods. See under *stain.*
Silvester's m. See under *artificial respiration.*
Siwe m. (a) (*for calcium*). Titrimetric methods based on the precipitation of calcium by oxalate: **iodometric permanganate m.** Calcium oxalate precipitate is dissolved in acid, an excess of permanganate is added followed by iodide, and the iodine liberated by excess permanganate is titrated with thiosulfate. **Acidimetric m.** Calcium oxalate is converted to calcium carbonate by heating, and an excess of hydrochloric is added and titrated with sodium hydroxide. (b) (*for inorganic phosphate*). A colorimetric method based on conversion of phosphate to phosphomolybdic acid and the reduction of the latter by aminonaphtholsulfonic acid.
Snell-Strong m. (*for riboflavin*). Riboflavin is determined by measurement of the growth stimulation of *Lactobacillus casei.* The acid produced by the microorganism is determined by titration with sodium hydroxide.
Sobel-Kaye m. (*for calcium*). A method using the same principle as the Siwe *m.* (a), determining the excess acid iodometrically.
Somogyi's m. (*for serum amylase*). *First method:* Amylase of serum acts upon starch to form a reducing sugar which is determined by Somogyi's copper-iodometric procedure. *Second method* (rapid, clinical method): The amyloclastic effect of amylase is measured by means of color reaction with iodine.
stasis tadpole m. A method used for assay of the thyroid-stimulating hormone.
Stehle gasometric m. (*for urea*). A determination based on the liberation of nitrogen by treatment with hypobromite.
Steiger m. (*for vitamin A and carotene*). A histochemical method using sulfuric acid to produce a dark-blue color.
Stimson's m. A method for reducing a dislocated shoulder or hip joint by continuous traction with a 10-pound weight. The patient is placed on a canvas sling, and the dislocated extremity passed through a hole in the sling, hanging free of the floor for about 5 to 6 minutes, after which reduction occurs without pain. See Plate 38.
Stockholm and Koch m. (*for total sulfur*). A procedure for complete oxidation of biological material in which strong hydrogen peroxide and nitric acid are used.
Stoddard and Drury m. (*for fatty acids in blood*). The blood is extracted with alcohol-ether, the extract saponified, the fatty acids separated, filtered, washed, dissolved in alcohol, and titrated with phenol blue as indicator.
Stoll's m. A technic for estimating the number of ova in stool specimens in which the solid feces are disintegrated with N/10 sodium hydroxide.
Summerson-Barker m. (*for lactic acid in blood*).

The glucose and other interfering material of the protein-free blood filtrate are removed by treatment with copper sulfate and calcium hydroxide. An aliquot of the resulting solution is heated with concentrated sulfuric acid to convert lactic acid to aldehyde, which is then determined colorimetrically by reaction with *p*-hydroxydiphenyl in the presence of copper ions.

Sumner m. (*for glucose in urine*). Urine is heated with a dinitrosalicylic acid reagent which is reduced by the sugar, and the resultant color is compared with standards.

Sumner-Somers m. A modification of a method for the preparation of glucose-1-phosphate.

Sunderman m. A method for calculating the approximate concentration of total base in the serum by measuring the specific conductance and the specific gravity or protein of the serum.

surface fixation m. (*for brucellosis*). A loopful of a mixture of antigen, stained black with hematoxylin, and serum is placed on a filter paper; the edge of the paper is dipped in isotonic NaCl solution, or droplets of the solution may be placed over the antigen. When the serum contains antibodies, the antigen is fixed to the paper and not washed away by the NaCl.

syringe-capillary m. Roughton-Scholander *m.*

Tallquist m. (*for hemoglobin*). A crude, semiquantitative method for the determination of hemoglobin content in which the color of a spot of blood is matched to lithographed standards.

Terry's m. A method for the rapid preparation of tissue sections by using a slice 0.5 to 1 mm. thick and covering the exposed surface with a modified polychrome methylene blue stain.

Theis and Benedict's m. (*for blood phenols*). Diazotized *p*-nitroaniline reacts with phenols to produce an orange color which is compared with a standard.

thick film m. A method of making a blood smear in order to increase the chances of finding parasites in the blood.

thin film m. A method of making blood smears for microscopical examination.

Thomas-Lavollay m. (*for iron*). A histochemical method using hydroxyquinoline and ammonium hydroxide. Iron appears as a greenish-black precipitate.

Thomas m. (*for arginine and arginine-containing proteins*). A histochemical method based on development of an orange-red color when arginine reacts with alphanaphthol and hypobromite or hypochlorite in alkaline medium.

Thunberg and Ahlgren m. (*for study of tissue oxidations*). Finely divided tissue is suspended in a solution containing methylene blue, phosphate solution to regulate the acidity, and the substance whose action it is desired to determine. After subjection to partial vacuum, the tube is placed in a water bath, and the time required for the methylene blue to be decolorized is determined. This is a measure of the rate of oxidation in the mixture.

Tirmann-Schmelzer m. for ionic iron. See under *stain.*

transparent-chamber m. Insertion of a chamber with a transparent top and bottom into a suitable part of an animal, e.g., a rat's back or rabbit's ear, to permit microscopic study of enclosed cells or tissues.

transtympanic m. A surgical approach, working backward on the outer wall of the attic, using the external acoustic meatus, to the regions of the middle ear and mastoid process: useful in performing fenestration and radical mastoidectomy. It eliminates blind groping for landmarks through a sclerotic mastoid cortex.

turbidity m. for standardizing vaccines. A method of estimating the number of bacteria in a suspension by diluting them to correspond with the density of a standard nephelometer tube.

Turchine-Castel-Kien m. A method for the differentiation of ribonucleic from desoxyribonucleic acid based on hydrolysis by hydrochloric acid and staining by a phenyl- (or methyl-) trihydroxyfluorene. Ribonucleic acid gives a yellow-pink, and desoxyribonucleic acid gives a blue-violet color.

two-stage m. (*for prothrombin activity*). A method of determination of plasma prothrombic activity by the addition of thromboplastin and calcium to decalcified and defibrinated plasma (*first stage*) and the estimation of the thrombin which evolves by the addition of fibrinogen (*second stage*).

van den Bergh's m. (*for bile pigment*) (Gibson and Goodrich modification). Plasma or serum is diazotized with Ehrlich's reagent and the red color developed is compared with a standard.

Van Slyke and Cullen's m. (*for alkali reserve*). Fresh oxalated plasma is brought into equilibrium with expired air so that it combines with as much carbon dioxide as it is able to hold under normal tension. The plasma is then acidified and the carbon dioxide given off is measured.

Van Slyke and Kirk m. A nitrous acid procedure for determining the α-amino acid nitrogen content of urine.

Van Slyke and Neill m. A manometric method of analysis of gases in blood and other solutions.

Van Slyke and Palmer m. (*for organic acids in urine*). Carbonates and phosphates are precipitated and the filtrate titrated with acid from pH 8 to pH 2.7. In diabetes this titration approximates closely the amount of β-hydroxybutyric and acetoacetic acids in the urine.

Van Slyke, MacFadyen, and Hamilton ninhydrin m. (*for amino-acid nitrogen*). The urine sample, previously freed from urea by treatment with urease, is heated at 100° in a closed reaction vessel with ninhydrin. Amino acids present yield carbon dioxide quantitatively under these conditions.

Van Slyke's m. (*for acetone bodies in urine*). The method is based on a combination of Shaffer's oxidation of β-hydroxybutyric acid to acetone and Denigè's precipitation of acetone as a basic mercuric sulfate compound. Glucose and certain other interfering substances are removed by precipitation with copper sulfate and calcium hydroxide. Preservatives other than toluene or copper sulfate should not be used.

Van Slyke's m. (*for chlorides*). Proteins are oxidized and chlorides precipitated with silver nitrate. Excess silver is titrated with thiocyanate.

Van Slyke titration m. (*for plasma bicarbonate*). Plasma is treated with an excess of standard acid which is titrated back with standard alkali to the original pH of the plasma as drawn.

Van Wagtendonk-Simonson-Hackett m. (*for glycogen*). A colorimetric method using Lugol's solution.

Volhard and Löhlein m. (*for peptic activity*). The pepsin is added to casein solution. The unaltered casein is salted out. The filtrate from this contains the digestion products of casein which can be estimated by titration.

Volhard-Arnold m. (*for chlorides in urine*). The urine is acidified with nitric acid and the chlorides are precipitated with a measured excess of standard silver nitrate solution. The silver chloride formed is filtered off and in the filtrate the excess silver nitrate is titrated back with standard ammonium thiocyanate solution. Ferric ammonium sulfate is used as an indicator. A red color due to the formation of ferric thiocyanate indicates that an excess of thiocyanate is present and that the end-point has been reached.

Volhard-Harvey m. (*for chlorides in urine*). Differs from the Volhard-Arnold method in that the excess of silver nitrate is titrated directly without filtering and hence in the presence of the silver chloride. The procedure is thus more rapid but the end-point is more difficult to determine.

Volterra m. (*for phenols in urine*). The urine is distilled from slightly alkaline solution to obtain the free volatile phenols in the distillate. After acidification, a second distillate is obtained; this represents the conjugated volatile phenols present. Ether extraction of the remaining fluid separates the aromatic hydroxy-acids from "residual phenols." Each fraction, after proper preparation, is treated with the phosphotungstic-phosphomolybdic acid color reagent of Folin and Ciocalteu and the resulting color compared with that obtained from a standard phenol solution.

Von Kóssa's $AgNO_3$ m. (*for demonstration of calcification*). See under *stain.*

Wachstein-Zak m. (*for bismuth*). A histochemical method based on the oxidation of bismuth sulfide, the form occurring in tissues, to sulfate by hydrogen peroxide and conversion of the sulfate to orange-red brucine iodide salt.

Walker m. (*for inorganic phosphate*). A capillary colorimetric-tube method based on the same principle as the Siwe method, using stannous chloride for reduction.

Walker-Reisinger m. A capillary tube microcolorimetric adaptation of the Summer dinitrosalicylic acid method of determining the amount of reducing substances in blood or urine.

Wallace and Diamond's m. (*for urobilinogen*). A series of dilutions of urine is carried to the point where the red color resulting from the reaction between urobilinogen and Ehrlich's aldehyde reagent is just discernible.

Waterhouse m. (*for copper*). A microhistochemical method using sodium diethyl dithiocarbamate to obtain a yellow product with copper.

Watson m. A method for the determination of urobilin and urobilinogen in urine and feces.

Webster, Hill, and Eidinow m. (*for ultraviolet radiation*). The fading of the blue color in an acetone-methylene blue solution is measured by comparison with known standards.

Weigl's m. A method for the production of vaccine against human typhus made from triturated intestine of lice infected by rectal injection of rickettsia.

Weil m. (*for trypsin*). A titrimetric method based on the employment of casein as the substrate and enterokinase as the activator, the addition of formol, and titration with tetramethylammonium hydroxide.

Weil-Russel m. (*for phosphatase*). A capillary colorimetric method using the same reactions as the Siwe method.

Weinbach m. (*for sodium in blood*). After deproteinization, the sodium in the filtrate is precipitated in alcoholic medium as the triple salt, uranyl zinc sodium acetate, which is washed, dissolved in water, and titrated with standard sodium hydroxide.

Welker and Tracy m. Aluminum hydroxide cream, when added to urine, will remove albumin so that a nitrogen partition can be made.

Westerbrink m. (*for thiamine*). An adaptation of the Ochoa-Peters method to the Cartesian diver.

Westergren m. A method to determine the blood sedimentation rate in which normal for men is 0 to 15 and for women is 0 to 20 mm. in one hour.

Westfall-Findley-Richardson m. (*for chloride*). A capillary colorimetric method based on the reaction of chloride with silver chromate to liberate the yellow chromate ion. Addition of diphenylcarbazide gives an intense purple-red color.

Whitehorn's m. (*for blood chlorides*). Chlorides from a blood filtrate are precipitated with silver nitrate and the excess silver is titrated with a standard thiocyanate solution.

Wiggers and Dean m. A method for the optical registration of heart sounds using a stethoscope bell attached by a rubber tube to a sound recorder consisting of a capsule protected from outside vibrations by a housing having a conical vent to equalize pressures.

Wigglesworth m. (*for chloride*). A microtitrimetric method for chloride, based on the addition of excess silver nitrate and back-titration with thiocyanate.

Wijs m. (*for iodine number*). See *Hanus m.* under *iodine number* under *iodine.*

Wilbur and Addis m. A spectroscopic procedure for the determination of urobilinogen.

Willis salt flotation m. A method for concentration of helminth eggs in which feces and concentrated sodium chloride solution are mixed, allowing the eggs to gravitate to the top of the solution where they are collected and examined.

Willstätter, Waldschmidt-Leitz, and Hesse m. (*for amylolytic activity*). The reducing sugar formed is determined by hypoiodite titration.

Wintrobe-Landsberg m. See under M. M. *Wintrobe.*

Wintrobe m. (*for hemoglobin*). An acid hematin method, using a special hemometer with a yellow glass standard.

Wohlgemuth m. A method for the quantitative determination of amylase in feces.

Wolff m. A procedure for the protein concentration of the gastric contents.

Wong's m. (*for iron*). Blood is treated with sulfuric acid and potassium persulfate. The proteins are removed with tungstic acid and the iron in the filtrate is determined colorimetrically.

xanthydrol m. (*for urea*). A histochemical method based on fixation of tissue in xanthydrol in acetic acid to precipitate dixanthylurea which is birefringent under the polarizing microscope.

Yasuda m. (*for iodine number*). See *Kretchmer-Holman-Burr m.* under *iodine number* under *iodine.*

Youngburg and Folin m. (*for urea*). The diluted urine is treated with an alcoholic urease solution to convert urea into ammonia, and the ammonia present is then determined by direct nesslerization.

Zander m. (*for chitin*). A method based on the treatment of tissue with fresh iodine in potassium iodide followed by zinc chloride to give a violet color.

Ziehl-Neelsen m. (*for Mycobacterium tuberculosis*). See *carbolfuchsin solution* under *stain.*

Zinsser's agar slant tissue culture m. A method for the production of vaccine in which high concentrations of Rickettsiae are obtained.

meth′o·in. 3-Methyl-5-phenyl-5-ethylhydantoin; an antiepileptic substance especially useful in grand mal seizures. See *mesantoin.*

meth″o·ma′ni·a. See *methylepsia.*

me·tho′ni·um. A generic name for a homologous series of compounds containing the ion $(CH_3)_3$-$N^+(CH_2)_nN^+(CH_3)_3$. The compounds in which n is 5 (pentamethonium), 6 (hexamethonium), or

10 (decamethonium) possess therapeutically useful actions.

meth·or′phi·nan hy″dro·bro′mide. A former generic name for the substance now designated *racemorphan hydrobromide*.

meth·ox′a·mine hy″dro·chlo′ride. $(CH_3O)_2.C_6H_3.CHOH.CH(CH_3)NH_2.HCl$; β-hydroxy-β-(2,5-dimethoxyphenyl)isopropylamine hydrochloride, occurring as colorless or white crystals or a white crystalline powder, freely soluble in water. It possesses prompt, potent pressor action useful in maintaining blood pressure during anesthesia, treating circulatory collapse (hypotension) caused by myocardial infarction, and counteracting hypotensive effect of hexamethonium compounds. See *vasoxyl hydrochloider*.

meth·ox′y·chlor. Bis-(*p*-methoxyphenyl)trichloroethane, an effective insecticide of low toxicity for human beings and animals.

meth·ox″y·phen′a·mine hy″dro·chlo′ride. $CH_3O.C_6H_4.CH_2.CH(CH_3).NH.CH_3.HCl$; β-(*o*-methoxyphenyl)isopropylmethylamine hydrochloride; a crystalline, white powder, freely soluble in water; a sympathomimetic compound whose predominant actions are bronchodilatation and inhibition of smooth muscle; its pressor activity is minimal. See *orthoxine hydrochloride*.

meth′yl. The univalent radical CH_3. —**methyl′ic,** *adj*.

meth″yl·a·cet′y·lene. Allylene.

meth″yl·al′, meth′yl·al. $CH_2(OCH_3)_2$. Dimethoxymethane; a water-soluble liquid; formerly used as a hypnotic and antispasmodic.

meth′yl al′co·hol. CH_3OH. A colorless, narcotic liquid, obtained in the destructive distillation of wood and by synthesis. Syn., *carbinol, methanol, wood alcohol, wood spirit*.

meth′yl al′de·hyde. Formaldehyde.

meth″yl·am′ine (meth″il·am′een, ·in, ·a·meen′). CH_3NH_2. A colorless gas formed during putrefaction of fish and in cultures of the *Vibrio comma* (comma bacillus).

meth″yl·am·phet′a·mine hy″dro·chlo′ride. Methamphetamine hydrochloride.

meth′yl an·thran′i·late. $NH_2.C_6H_4.COOCH_3$; methyl 2-aminobenzoate; the odoriferous constituent of a number of essential oils.

meth″yl·ar·son′ic ac′id. $CH_3AsO(OH)_2$; a crystalline substance, freely soluble in water, the disodium salt of which has been employed therapeutically in the same manner as sodium cacodylate: sometimes misspelled *methylarsinic acid*. Syn., *methanearsonic acid*.

meth′yl·ate. A compound formed from methyl alcohol by the substitution of the hydrogen of the hydroxyl by a base. —**methylated,** *adj*.

meth″yl·a′tion. The process of substituting a methyl group for a hydrogen atom.

meth″yl·at′ro·pine bro′mide (meth″il·at′ro·peen, ·pin). See *atropine* methylbromide.

meth″yl·at′ro·pine ni′trate. See *atropine* methylnitrate.

meth″yl·ben′zene. Toluene.

meth″yl·benz″e·tho′ni·um chlo′ride. $C_{28}H_{44}ClNO_2.H_2O$; benzyldimethyl{2-[2-(*p*-1,1,3,3-tetramethylbutylcresoxy)ethoxy]ethyl}ammonium chloride, forming colorless crystals, readily soluble in water; a quaternary ammonium salt with surface-active and disinfectant properties: used especially for bacteriostasis of urea-splitting organisms in diaper dermatitis. See *diaparene chloride*.

meth″yl·ben″zo·yl·ec′go·nine. Cocaine.

meth′yl blue. Sodium triphenyl-pararosaniline trisulfonate; an antiseptic used as a local application in diphtheria. Not to be confused with methylene blue.

meth′yl bro′mide. CH_3Br; bromomethane; a colorless gas at ordinary temperature, liquefying to a colorless liquid, slightly soluble in water, freely soluble in alcohol. A high concentration in air causes local irritation and lung injury. It is used in organic synthesis, also as a refrigerant, and fire-extinguishing agent.

meth′yl bu′tyr·ate. $CH_3(CH_2)_2COO.CH_3$; a colorless liquid, sparingly soluble in water, miscible with alcohol: used in the formulation of fruit essences.

meth″yl·car′bi·nol. Alcohol, 2.

methyl cellosolve. Trade-marked name for ethylene glycol monomethyl ether; $CH_3.O.CH_2.CH_2OH$; a colorless liquid, soluble in water: used as an industrial solvent.

meth″yl·cel′lu·lose. A methyl ether of cellulose, occurring as a grayish-white fibrous powder, swelling in water to produce a clear to opalescent, viscous, colloidal solution: used in the treatment of chronic constipation because it imparts bulk and blandness to the stool; *in pharmacy*, used to produce stable dispersions.

meth′yl chlo′ride. CH_3Cl. A liquid local anesthetic; when applied as a spray it volatilizes rapidly and produces a localized freezing.

meth′yl chlo′ro·form. CH_3CCl_3. A volatile liquid, obtained by chlorinating ethyl chloride. It is anesthetic.

meth″yl·cho·lan′threne (meth″il·ko·lan′threen). $C_{21}H_{16}$; 3-methylcholanthrene or 20-methylcholanthrene; a pentacyclic hydrocarbon obtained by degradation of desoxycholic acid and certain cholesterol derivatives; a potent carcinogen when applied locally.

meth′yl cy′a·nide. Acetonitrile.

meth′yl·ene [G. *methy*, wine; *hylē*, wood, material]. The bivalent hydrocarbon radical, $=CH_2$.

meth′yl·ene blue (*coeruleum methylenum*). $C_{16}H_{18}ClN_3S.3H_2O$. An aniline dye belonging to the class of thiazines; it occurs as dark green crystals or as a crystalline powder having a bronzelike luster. Solutions have a deep blue color. The medicinal grade of the dye is employed, by intravenous injection, in the treatment of hydrocyanic acid or carbon monoxide poisoning; it has also been used in a variety of systemic infections. It is an ingredient of many biologic staining solutions. Syn., *methylthionine chloride*.

meth′yl·ene chlo′ride. CH_2Cl_2; a colorless, volatile liquid; its vapor is not flammable. It has been used as an anesthetic for minor operations, but principally used as a solvent. Also called *dichloromethane, methylene bichloride*.

meth′yl·ene ci″tryl·sal″i·cyl′ic ac′id. See *novaspirin*.

meth′yl·ene vi′o·let (C.C.). A weakly basic thiazine dye; an oxidation product of methylene blue; used as a blood stain.

meth″yl·en′o·phil (meth″il·en′o·fill, ·ee′no·fill). Capable of being stained with methylene blue. methylenophilous.

meth″yl·ep′si·a [*methy; lēpsis*, a seizing]. Morbid desire for intoxicating drink. Syn., *methomania, methylmania*.

meth′yl e′ther. $(CH_3)_2O$. Dimethyl oxide; a gas having anesthetic properties.

meth″yl·eth″yl·a·ce′tic ac′id. See under *valeric acid*.

meth′yl for′mate. $HCOOCH_3$; a colorless, flammable liquid, soluble in water, used as a fumigant and larvicide for fruit, cereals, and tobacco.

meth″yl·gly·ox′al. CH_3COCHO. The aldehyde of pyruvic acid, capable of transformation into glycogen by the liver.

meth'yl green (C.C.). An aniline dye; used in staining tissues.

meth"yl·hex"ane·a'mine. $CH_3.CH_2.CH(CH_3).$-$CH_2.CH(CH_3).NH_2$; 1,3-dimethylamylamine; a colorless to pale-yellow liquid, very slightly soluble in water; a volatile sympathomimetic amine used as an inhalant for its local vasoconstrictor action on nasal mucosa. See *forthane.*

1-meth"yl·hex'yl·a·mine. The sympathomimetic agent known by the generic name *tuaminoheptane* and the trade-marked name *tuamine.* Syn., 2-*aminoheptane.*

meth'yl hy'drate. Methyl alcohol.

meth'yl hy'dride. CH_4. Methane or marsh gas.

meth"yl·hy·drox"y·ben·zo'ic ac'id (meth"il-high·drock"see·ben·zo'ick). Cresotic acid.

meth'yl i'o·dide. CH_3I. A colorless liquid, insoluble in water. Has been used as a vesicant. Syn., *iodomethane.*

meth'yl lac'tate. $CH_3.CH(OH).COOCH_3$; a colorless, transparent liquid, decomposed by water, miscible with most organic liquids: used as a solvent for cellulose derivatives.

meth"yl·ma'ni·a. See *methylepsia.*

meth"yl·mer·cap'tan. CH_3SH. Methyl hydrosulfide gas, found normally in the intestines through protein decomposition. It has a highly disagreeable odor.

meth'yl meth·ac'ryl·ate. See *acrylics.*

meth"yl·meth'ane. See *ethane.*

meth"yl·mor'phine (meth"il·mor'feen, ·fin, ·morfeen'). See *codeine.*

2-meth"yl-1,4,-naph"tho·qui·none'. Menadione.

meth"yl·nic"o·tin·am'ide. [$CH_3.C_5H_5N^+$.-$CONH_2$]OH^-; N^1-methylnicotinamide; the principal excretory product of nicotinamide, eliminated in the urine.

meth'yl or'ange (C.C.). Dimethylaminoazobenzene sodium sulfonate, an indicator used in volumetric analysis.

meth"yl·par'a·ben (*methylparabenum*). $C_6H_4.OH.$-$COOCH_3$. Methyl parahydroxybenzoate, a white powder, soluble in 400 parts of water; an antiseptic used to preserve medicinal preparations. See *nipagin M, solbrol.*

meth"yl·par"a·fy'nol. 3-Methyl-1-pentyn-3-ol; a hypnotic supplied under the trade-mark *dormison.*

meth'yl par"a·hy·drox"y·ben'zo·ate (par"uh-high·drock"see·ben'zo·ate). Methylparaben.

meth"yl·phe"no·bar'bi·tal. Mephobarbital.

meth"yl·phe"no·bar'bi·tone. British Pharmacopoeia name for *mephobarbital.*

meth"yl·phe'nol. Cresol.

meth"yl·psy'cho·trine. $C_{29}H_{38}N_2O_4$; O-methylpsychotrine; an alkaloid occurring in ipecac.

meth"yl·pu'rine (meth"il·pure'een, ·in). Any compound in which one or more methyl radicals have been introduced into the purine nucleus. Among the more important compounds of this type are caffeine, theobromine, and theophylline.

meth'yl red. Dimethylaminoazobenzene-*o*-carboxylic acid; an indicator used in volumetric analysis.

meth"yl·ros·an'i·line chlo'ride (meth"il·ro·zan'-i·leen, ·lin) (*methylrosanilinae chloridum*). Hexamethylpararosaniline chloride, usually containing also pentamethylpararosaniline chloride and tetramethylpararosaniline chloride. A dark green powder or glistening pieces with a metallic luster; soluble in 30 to 40 parts of water to form a purple solution. Used as an anthelmintic and bactericide, being active against Gram-positive organisms. Also used in the treatment of burns, and as a biologic stain. Also called *gentian violet, methyl violet, crystal violet.*

meth'yl sal'i·cyl"ate (sal'i·sil"ate, sa·liss'i·late, sal"i·sil'ate) (*methylis salicylas*). $C_6H_4(OH)$-$COOCH_3$. Synthetic wintergreen oil; an oily liquid of a peculiar odor, identical with the essential constituent of wintergreen oil; used internally in rheumatism and externally as a counterirritant. Dose, 0.3–1.2 cc. (5–20 min.).

meth"yl·ste·ar'ic ac'id. 10-Methylstearic acid, more commonly known as *tuberculostearic acid.*

meth"yl·sul'fo·nal. See *sulfonethylmethane.*

meth"yl·tes·tos'ter·one. 17-Methyl testosterone. $C_{20}H_{30}O_2$. An orally effective male sex hormone. See *metandren, neo-hombreol-M, oreton-M.*

meth'yl the"o·bro'mine. Caffeine.

meth"yl·thi'o·nine chlo'ride (meth"il·thigh'o-neen, ·nin). Methylene blue.

meth"yl·thi"o·u'ra·cil. $C_5H_6N_2OS$; 6-methyl-2-thiouracil or 4-hydroxy-2-mercapto-6-methylpyrimidine; a white crystalline powder, slightly soluble in water, having the action and uses of propylthiouracil, and useful with patients unable to tolerate or refractory to other antithyroid drugs.

meth'yl vi'o·let. Methylrosaniline chloride.

meth'yl vi'o·let 2B (C.C.). A mixture consisting mainly of pentamethylpararosaniline chloride with some hexamethylpararosaniline chloride and tetramethylpararosaniline chloride; it is germicidal. See *gentian* violet, *methylrosaniline chloride.*

meth'yl yel'low. See *dimethyl aminoazobenzene.*

meth'yne. Methenyl.

meth'y·sis [G. *methysis*, drunkenness]. Intoxication.

meticortelone. Trade-mark for *prednisolone.*

meticorten. Trade-mark for *prednisone.*

met"my·o·glo'bin. The oxidized form of myoglobin, analogous to methemoglobin.

met"o·don·ti'a·sis [G. *meta*, after; *odontiasis*, teething]. 1. The second dentition. 2. Loosely, any abnormality of teething.

me·toe'ci·ous (mi·tee'shus, ·see·us). See *heterecious.*

metol. Trade-mark for *methyl-para-aminophenol.*

me·top'a·gus [G. *metōpon*, forehead; *pagos*, that which is fixed]. Twins united at the foreheads. Syn., *craniopagus frontalis.*

met"o·pan·tral'gi·a [*metōpon*; G. *antron*, cave; *algos*, pain]. Pain or neuralgia of the frontal sinus. *Obs.*

me·top'ic, me·to'pic [*metōpon*]. 1. Relating to the forehead; frontal. 2. Pertaining to or describing a cranium having a mediofrontal suture.

me·to'pi·on [G., forehead]. The craniometric point where the line that connects the highest points of the frontal eminences crosses the sagittal plane.

me·to'pi·um [*metōpion*]. Metopon.

me·to'pi·um. Expressed almond oil.

me·to'pon, met'o·pon [G., forehead]. *In anatomy,* old term for forehead.

met'o·pon hy"dro·chlo'ride. $C_{18}H_{21}NO_3.HCl$. Methyl dihydromorphinone hydrochloride. A derivative of morphine having at least double its analgesic effectiveness and about the same duration of action. It is nearly devoid of emetic action. Tolerance appears to develop more slowly and to disappear more quickly, and physical dependence builds up more slowly than with morphine. Therapeutic analgesic doses produce little or no respiratory depression and much less mental dullness than does morphine, and it is relatively highly effective by oral administration. It is employed in treating the chronic suffering of cancer. Dose, 6–9 mg. ($\frac{1}{10}$–$\frac{3}{20}$ gr.).

met'o·pryl. $CH_3CH_2CH_2.O.CH_3$. *n*-Propyl methyl ether, a colorless liquid, isomeric with, but less volatile than, ethyl ether. It is under investigation to determine its usefulness as a general anesthetic.

met·ox′e·nous. See *heterecious.*

me·tral′gi·a. Metrodynia.

met″ra·pec′tic (met″ruh·peck′tick, mee″truh·) [G. *mētra*, womb; *apechein*, to keep away from]. Referring to a disease which is transmitted through the mother, but which she herself escapes (such as hemophilia).

met″ra·to′ni·a (met″ruh·to′nee·uh, mee″truh·) [*mētra;* G. *atonia*, slackness]. Atony of the uterus.

met″ra·tro′phi·a [*mētra;* G. *atrophia*, want of food]. Atrophy of the uterus.

me·traux′e (meh·trawk′see) [*mētra;* G. *auxē*, increase]. Hypertrophy or enlargement of the uterus.

metrazol. A trade-mark for pentamethylenetetrazol (pentylenetetrazol), $CH_2.(CH_2)_4.C{:}N.N{:}N$, a white, crystalline powder, soluble in water. In doses of 0.1 Gm. ($1\frac{1}{2}$ gr.) the compound is a circulatory and respiratory stimulant; in doses of 0.4–0.5 Gm. (6–$7\frac{1}{2}$ gr.) given intravenously it produces convulsions and has been used in the shock treatment of mental depressions and in the catatonic form of schizophrenia. See *cardiazol, leptazol.*

me′tre. See *meter.*

me′trec (mee′treck). *In optics*, a unit of curvature; the curvature of a surface whose radius of curvature is one meter: contraction of meter-curvature.

met″rec·ta′si·a (met″reck·tay′zhuh, ·zee·uh, mee″treck·) [*mētra;* G. *ektasis*, extension]. Enlargement of the nonpregnant uterus.

met″rec·to′pi·a (met″reck·to′pee·uh, mee″treck·), **me·trec′to·py** [*mētra;* G. *ektopos*, away from a place]. Displacement of the uterus.

me·tre′mi·a [*mētra;* G. *haima*, blood]. Congestion of the uterus.

met″reu·ryn′ter (met″roo·rin′tur, mee″troo·) [*mētra;* G. *eurynein*, to make broad]. An inflatable bag for dilating the cervical canal of the uterus.

met·reu′ry·sis (met·roor′i·sis) [*mētra;* G. *eurys*, broad]. Dilatation of the uterine cervix with the metreurynter.

me′tri·a [*mētra*]. 1. Any uterine affection. 2. Any inflammatory condition during the puerperium.

met′ric sys′tem. The most widely used system of weights and measures in the world today, originated in France about 1790, now the officially adopted system in most countries, and nearly universally employed for scientific purposes. It is a decimal system based primarily on the meter as the fundamental *unit of length.* The meter is approximately one ten-millionth of the distance from the equator to the North Pole. It is defined as the distance between two scratches on a platinum-iridium bar, designated as the international prototype meter, deposited at the International Bureau of Weights and Measures at Sèvres, near Paris. It is equivalent to exactly 39.37 U.S. inches, the inch being so defined by statute. The basic *unit of mass*, and *of weight*, is the gram, defined as 1/1000 of the international prototype kilogram, also deposited at the International Bureau of Weights and Measures. The main *unit of capacity* is the liter, which is the volume of a kilogram of water at the temperature of maximum density under normal atmospheric pressure, and which very closely approximates 1000 cubic centimeters, 1/1000 of a cubic meter. Multiples of the principal units are designated by the prefixes deca- meaning 10, hecto- meaning 100, and kilo- meaning 1000. For fractional units the corresponding prefixes are deci-, 1/10; centi-, 1/100; and milli-, 1/1000. The following equivalents of U.S. units in metric units are close enough for most purposes:

1 inch = 2.54 centimeters
1 ounce (avoirdupois) = 28.35 grams
1 pound (avoirdupois) = 453.6 grams
1 fluidounce = 29.57 milliliters (or cubic centimeters)
1 quart = 0.9463 liter
1 minim = 0.0617 milliliter (or cubic centimeter)

Also see Tables of Weights and Measures in the Appendix.

met″ri·o·ce·phal′ic [G. *metrios*, moderate; *kephalē*, head]. Applied to a skull in which the arch of the vertex is moderate in height, neither acrocephalic (pointed) nor platycephalic.

me·tri′tis [G. *mētra*, womb; *-itis*, inflammation]. Inflammation of the uterus, involving the endometrium and myometrium.

puerperal m. Inflammation of the uterus following childbirth.

me′tro- (mee′tro-, met′ro-), **metr-** [*mētra*]. A combining form denoting *relation to the uterus.*

me′tro·cele [*mētra;* G. *kēlē*, hernia]. Hernia of the uterus.

me′tro·clyst [*mētra;* G. *klyzein*, to wash]. An instrument for giving uterine douches.

me″tro·col′po·cele (mee″tro·kol′po·seel, met″ro·) [*mētra;* G. *kolpos*, vagina; *kēlē*, hernia]. Protrusion or prolapse of the uterus into the vagina, with prolapse of the anterior vaginal wall.

me″tro·cys·to′sis (mee″tro·sis·to′sis, met″ro·) [*mētra;* G. *kystis*, bladder; *-ōsis*, condition]. 1. The formation of uterine cysts. 2. The condition giving rise to uterine cysts.

me′tro·cyte [*mētra;* G. *kytos*, cell]. A large, uninuclear spheroidal cell whose protoplasm contains hemoglobin, and which is supposed to be the source of the red cells of the blood. *Rare.* Syn., *megaloblast, polychromatic erythroblast.*

me″tro·dy″na·mom′e·ter [*mētra;* G. *dynamis*, power; *metron*, a measure]. An instrument for measuring uterine contractions.

me″tro·dyn′i·a [*mētra;* G. *odynē*, pain]. Pain in the uterus; metralgia.

me″tro·ec·ta′si·a (mee″tro·eck·tay′zhuh, ·zee·uh, met″ro·). Metrectasia.

me″tro·en″do·me·tri′tis [*mētra;* G. *endon*, within; *mētra; -itis*, inflammation]. Combined inflammation of the uterus and endometrium. *Rare.*

met·rog′ra·phy [*mētra;* G. *graphein*, to write]. Roentgenography of the uterus through the injection of contrast mediums into the uterine cavity; uterography.

me·trol′o·gy [G. *metron*, a measure; *logos*, word]. The science that deals with methods of measurement and units of measure.

me″tro·lym″phan·gi′tis (mee″tro·lim″fan·jy′tis, met″ro·) [G. *mētra*, womb; L. *lympha*, water; G. *aggeion*, vessel; *-itis*, inflammation]. Inflammation of the lymphatic vessels of the uterus; uterine lymphangitis.

me″tro·ma·la′ci·a (mee″tro·ma·lay′shee·uh, ·see·uh, met″ro·) [*mētra;* G. *malakia*, softness]. Softening of the tissues of the uterus.

met′ro·nome. An instrument for indicating exact time intervals, usually by means of a pendulum and an audible clicking device.

me″tro·pa·ral′y·sis [*mētra;* G. *paralysis*, paralysis]. Uterine paralysis, usually that which may occur immediately following childbirth.

me″tro·path′i·a hem″or·rha′gi·ca. Abnormal uterine bleeding, now generally considered to be of endocrine origin.

me·trop′a·thy [*mētra;* G. *pathos*, disease]. Any uterine disease. —**metropath′ic,** *adj.*

me″tro·per″i·to·ni′tis [*mētra;* G. *peritonaion*, membrane which contains the lower viscera; *-itis*, inflammation]. 1. Combined inflammation of uterus and peritoneum. 2. Peritonitis secondary to inflammation of the uterus. 3. Inflammation of the peritoneum about the uterus.

me″tro·pex′i·a, me′tro·pex″y. See *hysteropexy.*

me″tro·phle·bi′tis [*mētra;* G. *phleps,* blood vessel; *-itis*]. Inflammation of the veins of the uterus.

me″trop·to′sis [*mētra;* G. *ptōsis,* a falling]. Uterine prolapse.

me″tror·rha′gi·a (mee″tro·ray′juh, ·jee·uh, met″-ro·) [*mētra;* G. *rhēgnynai,* to burst forth]. Uterine hemorrhage independent of the menstrual period: also called *intermenstrual flow, polymenorrhea.*

me″tror·rhe′a, me″tror·rhoe′a [*mētra;* G. *rhoia,* flow]. Any pathologic discharge from the uterus.

me″tror·rhex′is [*mētra;* G. *rhēxis,* a breaking]. Rupture of the uterus.

me″tro·sal″pin·gi′tis [*mētra;* G. *salpigx,* tube; *-itis,* inflammation]. Inflammation of the uterus and oviducts.

me″tro·sal″pin·gog′ra·phy (mee″tro·sal″ping-gog′ruh·fee, met″ro·) [*mētra; salpigx;* G. *graphein,* to write]. Radiography of uterus and oviducts after injecting an iodized oil contrast medium into the cervical canal under pressure. Same as hysterosalpingography and uterosalpingography.

me′tro·scope [*mētra;* G. *skopein,* to examine]. An instrument for examining the uterus.

me″tro·stax′is [*mētra;* G. *staxis,* a dripping]. Slight but persistent uterine hemorrhage.

me″tro·ste·no′sis [*mētra;* G. *stenōsis,* a being straitened]. Abnormal contraction of the cavity of the uterus.

me′tro·tome (mee′tro·tohm, met′ro·tohm) [*mētra;* G. *tomos,* cutting]. An instrument for incising the uterine neck.

me·trot′o·my. See *hysterotomy.*

me·try″per·ci·ne′sis (mi·try″pur·si·nee′sis, mee″-try·) [*mētra;* G. *hyper,* over; *kinēsis,* motion]. Excessive uterine contraction.

me·try″per·e′mi·a. See *metremia.*

me·try″per·es·the′si·a (mi·try″pur·ess·thee′zhuh, ·zee·uh, mee″try·) [*mētra; hyper;* G. *aisthēsis,* perception]. Hyperesthesia of the uterus.

me·try″per·tro′phi·a [*mētra; hyper;* G. *trophē,* nourishment]. Hypertrophy of the uterus.

Mett method for determination of peptic activity. See under *method.*

metubine iodide. Trade-marked name for *dimethyltubocurarine iodide.*

metycaine hydrochloride. Trade-marked name for the local anesthetic substance piperocaine hydrochloride.

Meulengracht diet. See under *diet.*

Meulengracht's method. See under *method.*

mev Abbreviation for 1 million electron volts.

Mex′i·can scam′mo·ny. See *ipomea.*

Meyer, Adolf (1866–1950). American psychiatrist and neurologist who developed the concept of *psychobiology,* and introduced the term in the United States (1915). This approach to psychiatry as a biological and social science has left a deep imprint upon American psychiatry. He also described that portion of the optic radiation which curves around the inferior horn of the lateral ventricle subjacent to the temporal cortex and ends in the calcarine fissure, called *Meyer's loop.*

Meyer, Georg Hermann von [*German anatomist,* 1815–92]. Described an aggregation of glands opening on the surface of the posterior part of the tongue; called *Meyer's glands* or *organ.* A line extended from the axis of the big toe, passing through the center of the heel in the normal foot, is known as *Meyer's line.*

Meyer-Overton theory. See under *theory.*

Meyerhof, Otto (1884–1951). German biochemist who studied the relationship between chemical reactions and energetic transformations in living tissues, mainly in muscle. With A. V. Hill, he was named Nobel laureate in medicine and physiology (1922). See Meyerhof *cycle.*

Meyerhof scheme. See Meyerhof *cycle.*

Meynert, Theodor Hermann [*German neurologist and psychiatrist in Austria,* 1833–92]. Described the fasciculus retroflexus, also called *Meynert's bundle* or *fasciculus.* See also Meynert's *commissure,* solitary *cells* of Meynert.

Meynet, Paul Claude Hyacinthe [*French physician,* 1831–92]. Described nodular growths sometimes found attached to tendon sheaths and joint capsules in rheumatic conditions; called *Meynet's nodosities.*

mez·cal′ (mess·kahl′, mez·kahl′). See *mescal.*

mez·cal′ine. See *mescaline.*

me·ze′re·on. See *mezereum.*

me·ze′re·um [NL., from Ar. *māzariyūn*]. The dried bark of *Daphne mezereum* and other species of *Daphne,* of the Thymeleaceae. It contains a glycoside, daphnin, and an acrid resin. Locally applied, mezereum is an irritant and vesicant, and has been used to stimulate indolent ulcers. Internally, it has been employed in syphilis, scrofula, chronic rheumatism, and various skin diseases.

mez·quite′ (mess·keet′, mess·kee′tay). See *mesquite.*

Mg Chemical symbol for magnesium.

mg, mg. Milligram, milligrams.

mg %, mg. %. Milligrams per cent.

mgh, mgh. Milligram-hour; the radium dosage obtained by the application of one milligram of radium element for one hour.

mho, mho. The unit of electric conductance; the reciprocal of the ohm.

mi′a·neh. See *relapsing fever.*

Mibelli, Vittorio [*Italian dermatologist,* 1860–1910]. Described angiokeratoma and porokeratosis, each of which is also called *Mibelli's disease.*

mi′ca [L.]. 1. A crumb. 2. A silicate mineral occurring in the form of thin, shining, transparent scales.

mi·ca′ce·ous (migh·kay′shus, ·shee·us) [*mica*]. Resembling mica; composed of crumbs; friable.

mi·celle′ (mi·sell′), **mi·cel′la** (mi·sell′uh, migh-sell′uh) [dim. from *mica*]. 1. One of the fundamental submicroscopic structural units of protoplasm. 2. Originally, a highly hydrated and charged colloidal aggregate, now extended to include also any unit of structure composed of an aggregate or oriented arrangement of molecules, as in cellulose and rubber.

Michaëlis, Gustav Adolf [*German obstetrician,* 1798–1848]. Made an important study of pelvic deformities. A diamond-shaped area formed over the sacrum by the sacrospinalis and gluteus maximus muscles is known as *Michaëlis' rhomboid.*

Michaelis, Leonor [*American physical and physiological chemist,* 1875–1949]. With Menten, evolved a theory of enzymatic behavior. In the *Michaelis-Menten theory* it is assumed that an enzymatic reaction proceeds by way of an intermediate compound of the enzyme and its substrate.

Michaelis indicator method. See under *method.*

Michailow's test. See under *test.*

Michel clip. See skin *clip.*

Micheli syndrome. Nocturnal hemoglobinuria. Also called *Marchiafava-Micheli syndrome.*

mi″cra·cous′tic (migh″kruh·kōō′tick) [G. *mikros,* small; *akoustikos,* of hearing]. Pertaining to or adapted to the hearing of very faint sounds.

mi″cra·cous′tic. An instrument adapted to the audition of very faint sounds.

mi″cren·ceph′a·lon [*mikros;* G. *egkephalos,* brain]. 1. An abnormally small brain. 2. Obsolete term for the cerebellum.

mi″cren·ceph′a·lous [*mikros; epkephalos*]. Having an abnormally small brain.

mi″cren·ceph′a·ly [*mikros; egkephalos*]. The condition of having an abnormally small brain.

mi′cro-, micr- [*mikros*]. 1. A combining form meaning *small* or *petty*, or *one-millionth*. 2. A combining form denoting *microscopic*. 3. *In botany*, a combining form signifying *very small in a specified feature*. 4. *In chemistry*, a combining form signifying *of* or *pertaining to very small amounts of material*. 5. *In medicine*, a combining form signifying *abnormally small*.

mi″cro·ab′scess. An abscess which is seen only microscopically.

Munro's m. One frequently occurring in, or directly below, the stratum corneum of the epidermis and containing chiefly degenerating polymorphonuclear leukocytes and epithelial cells, found in seborrheic dermatitis, psoriasis, and other skin lesions.

Pautrier's m. One occurring in the epidermis, primarily containing lymphocytic and histiocytic cells; it is pathognomonic of mycosis fungoides. Syn., *Darier's abscess*.

mi″cro·a″er·o·phil′ic. A term applied to microorganisms which require free oxygen for their growth, but which thrive best when the oxygen is less in amount than that in the atmosphere.

mi″cro·a·nal′y·sis. See microchemical *analysis*.

mi″cro·a·nat′o·mist. See *histologist*. *Obs.*

mi″cro·au′di·phone [*mikros;* L. *audire*, to hear; G. *phōnē*, sound]. An instrument for rendering very slight sounds audible.

Mi″cro·bac·te′ri·um [*mikros;* G. *baktērion*, dim. of *baktron*, staff]. A genus of small non-spore-forming bacteria commonly found in milk. It is not killed readily during pasteurization of milk. It is harmless and has no relation to the *Microbacterium multiforme psittacosis* of Levinthal.

Mi″cro·bac·te′ri·um mul′ti·forme″ psit″ta·co′sis. A term formerly proposed for the pleomorphic elementary bodies of psittacosis virus considered as the causative organism of psittacosis.

mi′crobe [*mikros;* G. *bios*, life]. A living organism of very small size; microorganism: applied to bacteria, especially those of a pathogenic nature. Also see *dissociation*, 4. —**micro′bial, micro′bian, micro′bic,** *adj.*

blue-pus m. *Pseudomonas aeruginosa.*

mi·cro′bi·cide (migh·kro′bi·side) [*mikros; bios;* L. *caedere*, to kill]. Destructive to microbes.

mi·cro′bi·cide. An agent that destroys microbes. Syn., *germicide*. —**microbici′dal,** *adj.*

mi″cro·bin·ert′ness. Failure to support microbial growth because of absence of necessary nutrients. *Obs.* —**microbinert,** *adj.*

mi″cro·bi·ol′o·gist (migh″kro·buy·ol′o·jist) [*mikros; bios;* G. *logos*, word]. An expert in microbiology.

mi″cro·bi·ol′o·gy [*mikros; bios; logos*]. The science of the nature, life, and actions of microorganisms. —**microbiolog′ic,** *adj.*

mi″cro·bi″o·pho′bi·a (migh″kro·buy″o·fo′bee·uh, migh″kro·bee″o·, migh·kro″bee·o·). See *microphobia*.

mi″cro·bi·ot′ic (migh″kro·buy·ot′ick) [*mikros;* G. *biōtikos*, of life]. Any antibacterial substance produced by molds, bacteria, or other organisms; an antibiotic or antibacterial.

mi′cro·bism. Infection with microbes.

latent m. The presence in the body of inactive organisms awaiting favorable conditions to become active.

mi′cro·blast [*mikros;* G. *blastos*, germ]. 1. An immature blood cell. 2. A small, nucleated, red blood cell.

mi″cro·bleph′a·ron, mi″cro·ble·pha′ri·a (migh″kro·bli·fay′ree·uh), **mi″cro·bleph′a·rism** [*mikros;* G. *blepharon*, eyelid]. Abnormal smallness of the eyelids.

mi″cro·bra′chi·a (migh″kro·bray′kee·uh) [*mikros;* L. *brachium*, arm]. Abnormally (congenital) small arms.

mi″cro·brach″y·ce·pha′li·a (·brack″i·si·fay′lee·uh, ·bray″ki·) [*mikros;* G. *brachys*, short; *kephalē*, head]. Brachycephalia combined with microcephaly.

mi″cro·bu·ret′ [*mikros;* F. *burette*, cruet]. An apparatus for delivering or measuring small quantities of liquids or gases.

mi″cro·cal′o·rie, mi″cro·cal′o·ry [*mikros;* L. *calor*, heat]. A small calorie; the quantity of heat necessary to raise the temperature of 1 Gm. of water from 15° to 16° C. Also see *calorie*.

mi″cro·car′di·a [*mikros;* G. *kardia*, heart]. Congenital smallness of the heart.

mi″cro·car′di·us [*mikros; kardia*]. An individual with an abnormally small heart.

mi″cro·cen′trum [*mikros;* G. *kentron*, point]. The centrosome or central apparatus constituting a lesser center of cell activity in contrast to the nucleus.

mi″cro·ceph′a·lus [*mikros;* G. *kephalē*, head]. An individual with an unusually small head.

mi″cro·ceph′a·ly [*mikros; kephalē*]. A congenital hypoplasia of the cerebrum with a thick skull and early closure of the fontanels, resulting in a small head. —**microcephal′ic, microceph′alous,** *adj.*

mi″cro·chei′li·a (migh″kro·kigh′lee·uh) [*mikros;* G. *cheilos*, lip]. Abnormal smallness of the lips.

mi″cro·chem′is·try [*mikros;* G. *chymos*, juice]. 1. The study of chemical reactions, using small quantities of materials, frequently less than 1 mg., and often requiring special small apparatus and microscopical observation. 2. The chemistry of individual cells and minute organisms. —**microchemical,** *adj.*

mi″cro·chi′ri·a (migh″kro·kigh′ree·uh) [*mikros;* G. *cheir*, hand]. Smallness of the hand to an unnatural degree.

microcidin. A brand of betanaphthol sodium.

Mi″cro·coc·ca′ce·ae (migh″kro·cock·ay′see·ee) [*mikros;* G. *kokkos*, berry]. A family of bacteria containing the genera *Micrococcus*, *Gaffkya*, *Sarcina*, and *Staphylococcus*.

mi″cro·coc′cin. An antibiotic substance derived from a species of *Micrococcus* resembling *Micrococcus varians*, active in vitro against a variety of bacteria.

Mi″cro·coc′cus [*mikros; kokkos*]. A genus of bacteria of the family Micrococcaceae.

M. albus. *M. pyogenes* var. *albus*.

M. ascoformans. The causative organism of botryomycosis in horses.

M. aureus. *M. pyogenes* var. *aureus*.

M. catarrhalis. Bacteria found in the secretions of patients afflicted with the common cold, but not supposed to be the causative agent.

M. citreus. A common laboratory contaminant; formerly called *Staphylococcus citreus*.

M. gazogenes. Synonym for *Veillonella gazogenes*.

M. gonorrheae. Synonym for *Neisseria gonorrhoeae*.

M. intracellularis meningitidis. Synonym for *Neisseria meningitidis*.

M. lanceolatus. Synonym for *Diplococcus pneumoniae*.

M. melitensis. Synonym for *Brucella melitensis*.

M. meningitidis. Synonym for *Neisseria meningitidis*.

M. parvulus. Synonym for *Veillonella parvula*.

M. pneumoniae. Synonym for *Diplococcus pneumoniae.*

M. pyogenes. Pathogenic Gram-positive cocci, having a tendency to form grapelike clusters, often the cause of boils, abscesses, and other pathogenic lesions. *M. pyogenes* var. *albus* (formerly called *Staphylococcus albus*) is an organism whose colony is white on nutrient agar, usually considered of low pathogenicity. *M. pyogenes* var. *aureus* (formerly called *Staphylococcus aureus*) is an organism whose colony is golden or orange-yellow on nutrient agar; this species has the highest pathogenicity.

M. tetragenus. A species of parasitic cocci frequently found on the mucous membranes of the upper respiratory tract. They occur typically in tetrads or groups of four and are of low grade virulence. Syn., *Gaffkya tetragena.* See Table of the Most Common Microorganisms Pathogenic to Man in the Appendix.

mi″cro·co′lon [*mikros;* G. *kolon,* colon]. An abnormally small colon.

mi″cro·co·nid′i·um (pl. *microconidia*) [*mikros;* G. *konis,* dust]. *In botany,* a small and single-celled conidium.

mi″cro·co′ri·a. Miosis.

mi″cro·cor′ne·a [*mikros;* L. *corneus,* horny]. Abnormal smallness of the cornea.

mi″cro·cos′mic salt. Sodium ammonium phosphate.

mi″cro·cou′lomb (migh″kro·kōō′lom, ·kōō·lom′). The one-millionth part of a coulomb.

mi″cro·cous′tic (migh″kro·kōōs′tick). Synonym of *micracoustic.*

mi″cro·crys′tal·line [*mikros;* G. *krystallos,* rock-crystal]. Composed of crystals of microscopic size.

mi″cro·cu′rie [*mikros; Curie*]. The amount of a radioactive substance which undergoes 3.7×10^4 disintegrations per second: equivalent to one-millionth of a curie. Abbreviated, *μc.*

mi′cro·cyst [*mikros;* G. *kystis,* bladder]. A cyst of small size, visible only microscopically.

mi″cro·cy′tase. An enzyme in leukocytes capable of digesting microorganisms.

mi′cro·cyte [*mikros;* G. *kytos,* cell]. An erythrocyte having either a diameter or a mean corpuscular volume (MCV) or both more than two standard deviations below the mean normal, determined by the same method on the bloods of healthy persons of the patient's age and sex group. —**microcyt′ic,** *adj.*

mi″cro·cy·the′mi·a. A blood condition characterized by abnormally small erythrocytes.

mi″cro·cy·to′sis (migh″kro·sigh·to′sis) [*mikros; kytos;* G. *-ōsis,* condition]. A condition of the blood, characterized by a preponderance of microcytes, as observed microscopically or determined by measurement of cell volume.

mi″cro·dac·tyl′i·a, mi″cro·dac′ty·ly [*mikros;* G. *daktylos,* finger]. Abnormal smallness of one or more fingers or toes. —**microdac′tylous,** *adj.*

mi″cro·dent′ism. See *microdontia.*

mi″cro·de·ter″mi·na′tion [*mikros;* L. *determinare,* to enclose within boundaries]. The identification of minute amounts of a substance.

mi″cro·dis·sec′tion [*mikros;* L. *dissecare,* to cut in pieces]. Dissection with the aid of a microscope.

mi′cro·dont [*mikros;* G. *odous,* tooth]. Having abnormally small teeth.

mi″cro·don′ti·a [*mikros; odous*]. The condition of having one or more abnormally small teeth: also called *microdentism.* Syn., *microdontism.*

mi″cro·dont·ism [*mikros; odous*]. Microdontia.

mi″cro·drep′a·no·cyt·ic dis·ease′. A rare, hereditary anemia resulting from the presence of both thalassemia and sickle-cell traits, characterized by marked hypochromia, microcythemia, sicklemia, target cells, and marked anisocytosis and poikilocytosis. The clinical signs and symptoms, when present, are those of sickle-cell anemia. The sickled, hypochromic microcytes are called *microdrepanocytes.* Also called *sickle-cell-thalassemia disease.*

mi″cro·e·lec″tro·pho·ret′ic [*mikros;* G. *ēlektron,* amber; *phorēsis,* from *pherein,* to bear]. Pertaining to electrophoresis of minute quantities of solutions.

mi″cro·e·lec″tro·pho·ret′ic cells. Both flat and cylindrical cells, the flat cell containing a layer of colloidal sol 0.6 mm. in depth, and the cylindrical cell consisting of a capillary tube through which colloidal particles pass under the influence of an electric field.

mi″cro·e·ryth′ro·cyte (·eh·rith′ro·sight, ·err′ithro·). See *microcyte.*

mi″cro·far′ad. The one-millionth part of a farad.

mi″cro·fi·lar′i·a (migh″kro·fi·lay′ree·uh) (pl. *microfilariae*) [*mikros;* L. *filum,* thread]. The embryonic or prelarval forms of filarial worms; slender motile forms, 150–300 μ in length, found in the blood stream and tissues. On ingestion by the proper blood-sucking insects the microfilariae pass through developmental stages in the body of the host and become infestive larvae.

sheathed microfilariae. Microfilariae encased in a delicate membrane which usually protrudes beyond the ends of the parasite. The membrane is thought to be the remains of the egg shell. When the membrane or shell breaks, an unsheathed microfilaria results.

mi″cro·flu″o·ro·met′ric scan′ner. A device for the differential detection of cancer cells based on the principle that cancer cells absorb more basic fluorescent dye than normal cells. Cancer cells fluoresce more under long-wave ultraviolet light, and the amount of light emitted can be measured by a microphotometer.

mi″cro·frac′ture [*mikros;* L. *fractura,* fracture, from *frangere,* to break]. One of several minute multiple fractures in bone.

mi″cro·gam′ete (migh″kro·gam′eet, ·ga·meet′) [*mikros;* G. *gamos,* marriage]. A male reproductive cell in certain Protozoa, corresponding to the sperm cell in Metazoa.

mi″cro·ga·me′to·cyte [*mikros; gamos;* G. *kytos,* cell]. The cell which produces the microgametes in Protozoa. See Plate 28.

mi·crog′a·my (migh·krog′uh·mee) [*mikros; gamos*]. Fusion of male and female reproductive cells in certain Protozoa and Algae.

mi″cro·gas′tri·a. Abnormal smallness of the stomach.

mi″cro·gen′e·sis [*mikros;* G. *genesis,* production]. Abnormally small development of a part.

mi″cro·ge′ni·a [*mikros;* G. *geneion,* chin]. Abnormal smallness of the chin.

mi″cro·gen′i·tal·ism [*mikros;* L *genitalis,* genital]. Having extremely undersized genital organs. See *hypogenitalism.*

mi·crog′li·a (migh·krog′lee·uh) [*mikros;* G. *glia,* glue]. Small neuroglia cells of the central nervous system, having long processes and exhibiting ameboid and phagocytic activity under pathologic conditions. Probably mesodermal in origin.

mi″cro·glos′si·a [*mikros;* G. *glōssa,* tongue]. Abnormal smallness of the tongue.

mi″cro·gna′thi·a (migh″kro·nay′thee·uh, ·nath′ee·uh, migh″krog·) [*mikros;* G. *gnathos,* jaw]. Abnormal smallness of the jaws, especially of the lower jaw. —**microg′nathous, micrognath′ic,** *adj.*

mi″cro·go′ni·o·scope [*mikros;* G. *gōnia,* angle;

skopein, to examine]. An apparatus for measuring extremely small angles, as in ophthalmology.

mi′cro·gram [*mikros;* G. *gramma*, scruple]. One one-thousandth of a milligram. Symbol, μg. Sometimes called *gamma*, a designation which should be abandoned.

mi′cro·graph [*mikros;* G. *graphein*, to write]. 1. A pantographic device for enabling one to draw sketches on a very small scale. 2. An instrument that magnifies the vibrations of a diaphragm and records them on a moving photographic film.

mi·crog′ra·phy (migh·krog′ruh·fee) [*mikros; graphein*]. 1. A description of bodies studied under the microscope. 2. Very minute writing.

mi″cro·gy′ri·a (migh″kro·jy′ree·uh, ·jirr′ee·uh) [*mikros;* G. *gyros*, circle]. Abnormal smallness of the convolutions of the brain.

mi′crohm [*mikros;* after G. S. *Ohm*]. One one-millionth of an ohm.

mi″cro·in·cin″er·a′tion [*mikros;* L. *in*, in; *cinis*, ashes]. Reduction of microscopic sections to ash on a quartz slide, for microscopic study of the amounts and distribution of inorganic components of tissues and cells.

mi″cro·in·jec′tion [*mikros;* L. *injectio*, from *inicere*, to throw into]. The injection of solutions into cells by means of a micropipet.

mi″cro·len′ti·a [*mikros;* L. *lens*, lentil]. Having an abnormally small crystalline lens.

mi″cro·leu′ko·blast (migh″kro·lew′ko·blast) [*mikros;* G. *leukos*, white; *blastos*, germ]. A small leukoblast.

mi′cro·li″ter. A millionth of a liter, or a thousandth of a milliliter.

mi′cro·lith [*mikros;* G. *lithos*, stone]. A microscopic calculus.

mi″cro·li·thi′a·sis [*mikros; lithos;* NL. *iasis*, condition]. The formation of very minute calculi.

m. alveolaris pulmonum. A rare form of pulmonary calcification of uncertain cause in which, at autopsy, a great many minute, spherical, concentrically calcified bodies (calcospherites or microliths) together usually with osseous nodules of larger size are found: first described by Ludwig Puhr (1933).

mi″cro·ma′ni·a [*mikros;* G. *mania*, madness]. A delusional state in which the patient believes himself diminutive in size and mentally inferior.

mi″cro·ma·nip′u·la″tive tech·nique′. 1. A procedure or technique designed to investigate living or preserved biological material on the microscopic level by means of microdissection, microinjection, and other manual maneuvers. 2. Any technique demanding small, careful, and delicate manipulation, usually under a microscope.

mi″cro·ma·nip′u·la″tor [*mikros;* L. *manipulus*, handful]. A device for moving exceedingly fine instruments, under the magnification of a microscope, for dissection of cells or for other operations involving minute objects.

mi″cro·mas′ti·a [*mikros;* G. *mastos*, breast]. Abnormal smallness of the breasts. Syn., *micromazia.*

mi″cro·ma′zi·a [*mikros;* G. *mazos*, breast]. Abnormal smallness of the breasts.

mi″cro·me′li·a, mi·crom′e·ly (migh·krom′i·lee) [*mikros;* G. *melos*, limb]. Abnormal smallness of the limbs.

mi·crom′e·lus (migh·krom′i·lus) [*mikros; melos*]. An individual characterized by the presence of abnormally small limbs.

mi·crom′e·ter (migh·krom′i·tur) [*mikros;* G. *metron*, a measure]. 1. An instrument designed for measuring minute distances, or apparent diameters; used with a microscope or telescope. 2. (migh′kro·mee″tur, migh·krom′i·tur). The millionth part of a meter; a micron, generally represented by the Greek letter μ. —**micrometry,** *n.*

eyepiece m. A micrometer to be used with the eyepiece of a microscope. Also called *ocular m.*, *filar ocular m.*

screw m. A fine screw with a scale attached showing the distance passed at each fraction of a revolution.

stage m. A micrometer placed on the stage of a microscope and used with the objective lenses.

mi·crom′e·ter disk. A glass disk engraved with a suitable scale, used at the diaphragm of a micrometer ocular. The scale can be focused by the eye lens and seen in the field of view.

mi″cro·meth′od [*mikros;* G. *methodos*, a following after]. A method of laboratory examination in which very small quantities of the substances to be examined are used.

Keller's m. (*for urea*). The solution resulting from incubation of a protein-free blood filtrate with urease and buffer is nesslerized and compared colorimetrically with a similarly treated standard urea solution.

mi″cro·mi′cron [*mikros; mikros*]. The millionth part of a micron, generally denoted by μμ.

mi′cro·mil [*mikros;* L. *mille*, thousand]. A micromillimeter.

mi″cro·mil′li·me″ter [*mikros; mille;* G. *metron*, a measure]. The one-millionth part of a millimeter or the one-thousandth part of a micron. Incorrectly used to denote the one-thousandth part of a millimeter or the one-millionth part of a meter. Symbol, mμ. Also called *millimicron.*

mi″cro·mon″o·spo′rin [*mikros;* G. *monos*, alone; *spora*, seed]. An antibiotic substance produced by species of the genus *Micromonospora* of the family Streptomycetaceae.

mi″cro·mo′to·scope [*mikros;* L. *motum*, from *movere*, to move; G. *skopein*, to examine]. An apparatus for photographing and exhibiting motile microorganisms.

mi″cro·my·e′li·a (migh″kro·migh·ee′lee·uh) [*mikros;* G. *myelos*, marrow]. Abnormal smallness of the spinal cord.

mi″cro·my′e·lo·blast [*mikros; myelos;* G. *blastos*, germ]. An extremely small myeloblast.

mi″cro·my″e·lo·lym′pho·cyte [*mikros; myelos;* L. *lympha*, water; G. *kytos*, cell]. A small lymphocyte of myeloid tissue, regarded as a hemocytoblast.

mi′cron [*mikros*]. The one-thousandth part of a millimeter, or the one-millionth part of a meter. Generally represented by the Greek letter μ.

mi′cro·nee″dles [*mikros;* AS. *nǣdl*]. Exceedingly fine glass needles for use in microdissection with a micromanipulator.

mi·cron′e·mous (migh·kron′i·mus) [*mikros;* G. *nēma*, thread]. Furnished with short filaments.

mi″cro·nu′cle·us [*mikros;* L. *nucleus*, nut]. 1. A small or minute nucleus. 2. *In biology*, the paranucleus, or the nucleolus. 3. The reproductive nucleus of protozoa as contrasted with the macronucleus.

mi″cro·nu′tri·ents [*mikros;* L. *nutrire*, to nourish]. The vitamins and minerals occurring in traces essential for growth, development, and health. The essential minerals are also called trace minerals.

mi″cro·nych′i·a (migh″kro·nick′ee·uh) [*mikros;* G. *onyx*, nail]. The presence of one or more small nails which in every other respect seem normal.

mi″cro·or′chism. Congenital hypoplasia of the testes; when severe, it may be associated with the eunuchoid state.

mi″cro·or′gan·ism [*mikros;* G. *organon*, instrument for making or doing a thing]. A microscopic organism, either animal or plant, especially a bacterium or protozoan. For a list of the microorganisms pathogenic to man, see Table in the Appendix. —**microorgan'ic,** *adj.*

pyogenic m. A microorganism producing pus; usually staphylococci and streptococcin but may other organisms may produce pus.

mi"cro·par'a·site [*mikros;* G. *parasitos,* parasite]. A parasitic microorganism.

mi"cro·pe'nis [*mikros;* L. *penis,* penis]. Abnormal smallness of the penis. Syn., *microphallus.*

mi'cro·phage [*mikros;* G. *phagein,* to eat]. 1. A neutrophil granulocyte in tissues. 2. Formerly a small phagocyte.

mi"cro·pha'ki·a [*mikros;* G. *phakos,* lentil]. A congenital or developmental anomaly in which there is an abnormally small crystalline lens.

mi"cro·phal'lus [*mikros;* G. *phallos,* phallus]. Abnormal smallness of the penis. Syn., *micropenis.*

mi"cro·pho'bi·a [*mikros;* G. *phobos,* fear]. 1. Morbid fear of microbes. 2. Morbid fear of small objects.

mi'cro·phone [*mikros;* G. *phōnē,* sound]. An instrument in which feeble sounds modulate an electric current which can be amplified so that the sounds become audible.

mi"cro·pho'ni·a, mi·croph'o·ny (migh·krof'o-nee) [*mikros; phōnē*]. Weakness of voice.

mi"cro·pho'no·graph [*mikros; phōnē;* G. *graphein,* to write]. A combination of microphone and phonograph used for the recording of sounds.

mi"cro·pho'no·scope [*mikros; phōnē;* G. *skopein,* to examine]. A binaural stethoscope with a membrane in the chestpiece to accentuate the sound.

mi"cro·pho'to·graph [*mikros;* G. *phōs,* light; *graphein,* to write]. 1. A photograph of microscopic size. 2. Photomicrograph.

mi"cro·pho·tom'e·ter [*mikros; phōs;* G. *metron,* a measure]. A photometric device, made to fit onto the microscope tube, which measures the intensity of light reflected or transmitted from the specimen.

mi"croph·thal'mi·a [*mikros;* G. *ophthalmos,* eye]. Synonym for microphthalmus.

mi"croph·thal'mus [*mikros; ophthalmos*]. 1. A condition in which the eyeball is abnormally small. Also called *microphthalmia, nanophthalmus, nanophthalmos, nanophthalmia.* 2. A person manifesting such a condition.

mi"cro·phys'ics [*mikros;* G. *physikos,* natural]. That branch of science which deals with electrons, atoms, and molecules.

mi'cro·phyte [*mikros;* G. *phyton,* plant]. Any microscopic plant, especially one that is parasitic.

mi·cro'pi·a (migh·kro'pee·uh). See *micropsia.*

mi"cro·pi·pet' [*mikros;* F., dim. of *pipe,* tube]. An exceedingly fine pipet used in microinjection.

mi"cro·pla'nar [*mikros;* L. *planus,* flat]. Anastigmatic objective of perfect correction, designed especially for use in photographing small objects, like embryos, and for microprojection.

mi"cro·ple·thys·mog'ra·phy. The recording of small volume changes. —**microplethys'mogram,** *n.*; **microplethys'mograph,** *n.*

mi"cro·po'di·a [*mikros;* G. *pous,* foot]. Unnatural smallness of the feet.

mi·crop'o·dy. See *micropodia.*

mi"cro·po·lar'i·scope (migh"kro·po·lar'i·scope) [*mikros;* L. *polus,* pole; G. *skopein,* to examine]. A polariscope used in connection with a microscope.

mi"cro·pro·jec'tion [*mikros;* L. *projectio,* from *proicere,* to throw before]. The projection of the image of microscopic objects on a screen.

mi"cro·pro·so'pi·a [*mikros;* G. *prosōpon,* face]. Congenital abnormal smallness of the face. —**micropros'opy,** *n.*

mi"cro·pro'so·pus (migh"kro·pro'so·pus, ·pro·so'-pus) [*mikros; prosōpon*]. An individual with a small and imperfectly developed face.

mi·crop'si·a (migh·crop'see·uh) [*mikros;* G. *opsis,* vision]. Disturbance of visual perception in which objects appear smaller than their true size.

mi"cro·psy'chi·a (migh"kro·sigh'kee·uh) [*mikros;* G. *psychē,* soul]. Feeblemindedness. *Obs.*

mi'cro·pus (migh'kro·pus, migh·kro'pus, mick'ro-pus) [*mikros;* G. *pous,* foot]. Abnormal smallness of the feet; a congenital defect.

mi"cro·pyk"nom'e·ter. An instrument for determining the specific gravity of minute amounts of liquids or solutions.

mi'cro·pyle [*mikros;* G. *pylē,* gate]. A minute opening in the investing membrane of many ova, permitting entrance of the sperm.

mi"cro·ra"di·og'ra·phy. Radiography using a photographic emulsion so fine that enlargement (of the order of 100 times) does not reveal silver grains of the emulsion, thereby permitting great magnification of the original image of a very small object.

mi"cro·res'pi·ra"tor. An instrument used to measure metabolic activity of minute amounts of tissue.

mi"cro·rrhi'ni·a [*mikros;* G. *rhis,* nose]. Congenital atrophy or smallness of the nose.

mi"cro·ruth'er·ford [*mikros;* after Ernest *Rutherford,* English physicist, 1871–1937]. A unit equivalent to $1/_{1,000,000}$ of a rutherford or 1 disintegration per second. See *rutherford.* Abbreviated, μrd.

mi"cro·scel'ous (migh"kro·skell'us, migh·kros'kil-us) [*mikros;* G. *skelos,* leg]. Short-legged.

mi'cro·scope [*mikros;* G. *skopein,* to examine]. An apparatus through which minute objects are rendered visible. It consists of a lens, or group of lenses, by which a magnified image of the object is produced.

binocular m. A microscope having two oculars, one for each eye, so that the object is seen with both eyes.

centrifuge m. A high-speed centrifuge provided with windows which permit microscopic observation of the material being sedimented.

compound m. One that consists of two or more lenses or lens systems, of which one, the objective, placed near the object, gives a large and inverted real image; the other, the ocular, acting like a simple microscope, gives an enlarged virtual image of the real image.

corneal m. A microscope used to examine the cornea in the living patient.

electron m. A device for directing streams of electrons by means of electric and magnetic fields, in a manner similar to the direction of visible light rays by means of glass lenses in an ordinary microscope. Since electrons carry waves of much smaller wave lengths than light waves, correspondingly greater magnifications are obtainable. The electron microscope will resolve detail fifty to one hundred times finer than the optical microscope. Images can be studied on a fluorescent screen or recorded photographically.

fluorescence m. A microscope with quartz lenses, which transmit ultraviolet wavelengths, or any microscope used in fluorescence studies.

Greenough binocular m. A binocular microscope equipped with erecting prisms; it has an objective for each tube and so is truly stereoscopic.

phase m. A compound microscope with an annular diaphragm at the front focal plane of the condenser and a diffraction plate at the back focal plane of the objective of the bright-field compound microscope. By suitable choice of diffraction plate the image contrast may be varied to give increased visibility.

proton m. A microscope, similar to the electron microscope, utilizing protons rather than electrons and having a magnifying power of 600,000 diameters.

reflecting m. One using mirror pairs in the objective, thus extending the range of achromatism throughout the optical spectrum.

simple m. One of one or more lenses or lens systems acting as a single lens. The rays of light that enter the observer's eye after refraction through these lenses proceed directly from the object itself.

slit-lamp m. An apparatus which, in combination with the corneal microscope, enables the physician to observe the endothelium on the posterior surface of the cornea. See *ultramicroscope.*

television m. A television camera fitted to a microscope; large audiences may simultaneously view microscopic phenomena.

mi″cro·scop′ic, mi″cro·scop′i·cal [*mikros; skopein*]. 1. Pertaining to the microscope. 2. Visible only with the aid of a microscope. 3. Colloquial term for "of extremely small size."

mi·cros′co·pist (migh·kros′ko·pist) [*mikros; skopein*]. One who is skilled in the use of the microscope.

mi·cros′co·py, mi′cro·sco″py [*mikros; skopein*]. The use of the microscope; examination with the microscope.

bright-field m. Microscopy utilizing transillumination of the specimen with light rays in the optical axis of the microscope.

fluorescence m. Study by means of the microscope of the emission of radiant energy which is the result of the absorption of radiation of different wavelength.

phase m. A method for controlling the contrast in the image by means of absorption and optical path difference within the microscope. Transparent materials with small optical path differences or of low absorption contrast may be examined with phase microscopy when bright-field microscopy fails to reveal detail. Also called *phase difference m., phase contrast m.*

mi″cros·mat′ic. Having a poorly developed sense of smell. Man is classified as a microsmatic animal.

mi′cro·some [*mikros;* G. *sōma*, body]. A noncommittal term for any granule found in a cell.

mi″cro·so′mi·a [*mikros; sōma*]. Abnormal smallness of the whole body. Syn., *dwarfism, nanosomia.*

mi″cro·spec·trog′ra·phy [*mikros;* L. *spectrum*, image; G. *graphein*, to write]. Spectrographic methods applied to the study of the composition of protoplasm.

mi″cro·spec″tro·pho·tom′e·try. Measurement at different wavelengths of light absorbed, reflected, or emitted by objects in a microscopic field.

mi″cro·spec′tro·scope [*mikros; spectrum;* G. *skopein*, to examine]. A spectroscope used in connection with the ocular of a microscope, and by means of which the spectrums of microscopic objects can be examined.

mi″cro·spher′o·cyte. A characteristically small, spheroidal erythrocyte observed in congenital hemolytic icterus.

mi″cro·sphyg′my [*mikros;* G. *sphygmos*, pulse]. Diminished amplitude of the pulse with small oscillometric index.

mi″cro·sphyx′i·a [*mikros;* G. *sphyxis*, pulse]. Weakness or smallness of the pulse.

mi″cro·splanch′nic [*mikros;* G. *splagkna*, inward parts]. Synonym for hypovegetative.

Mi″cro·spo·rid′i·a [*mikros;* G. *sporos*, seed]. An order of Sporozoa which infest chiefly invertebrates, insects in particular.

mi″cro·spo′rin [*mikros; sporos*]. Extract prepared from a culture of a species of *Microsporum;* used intracutaneously or as patch test to determine sensitivity to the fungus.

Mi″cro·spo′ron [*mikros; sporos*]. Former name for a genus of fungi.

M. audouini. Synonym for *Microsporum audouini.*

M. furfur. Synonym for *Malassezia furfur.*

M. minutissimus. Synonym for *Nocardia minutissima.*

mi″cro·spo·ro′sis [*mikros; sporos;* G. *-ōsis*, condition]. Dermatophytosis caused by a species of *Microsporum.*

Mi″cro·spo′rum, Mi·cros′po·rum (migh·kros′po·rum) [*mikros; sporos*]. A genus of dermatophytes which attack only the hair and the skin.

M. audouini. That species which is sometimes the causative agent of tinea capitis maculosus. This species produces low-grade scaling lesions.

M. canis. That species which causes the kerion type of tinea capitis, an inflammatory form.

M. gypseum. That species which is found mainly in South America and is one cause of dog favus. This, too, is an inflammatory form. Syn., *Achorion gypseum.*

M. lanosum. *M. canis.*

mi″cro·steth′o·phone [*mikros;* G. *stēthos*, breast; *phōnē*, voice]. A stethoscope which amplifies the sounds heard.

mi″cro·steth′o·scope [*mikros; stēthos;* G. *skopein*, to examine]. A stethoscope which amplifies the sounds heard.

mi″cro·sto′mi·a [*mikros;* G. *stoma*, mouth]. Abnormal smallness of the mouth.

mi″cro·sur′ger·y [*mikros;* G. *cheirourgia*, a working by hand]. Surgery practiced on single cells or ova, using a microscope and special minute cutting instruments.

mi″cro·syr′inge. See *syrette.*

mi″cro·the′li·a [*mikros;* G. *thēlē*, nipple]. Congenital hypoplasia of the nipple of the breast.

mi′cro·therm [*mikros;* G. *thermē*, heat]. An organism in which the life processes are carried on at a low temperature.

mi·cro′ti·a (migh·kro′shee·uh) [*mikros;* G. *ous*, ear]. Abnormal smallness of the external ear(s).

mi′cro·tome [*mikros;* G. *tomos*, cutting]. An instrument for making thin sections of tissues for microscopical examination, the tissues usually being embedded in paraffin or celloidin.

freezing m. One in which the tissue is frozen, in order to secure the hardness required for properly cutting sections of tissue that is fixed but not embedded in a hardening medium.

mi·crot′o·my (migh·krot′o·mee) [*mikros;* G. *tomē*, a cutting]. Section cutting.

mi″cro·trau′ma. Injury resulting from repeated mechanical stimuli which individually are not recognizably injurious.

Mi·cro′tus (migh·kro′tus) [*mikros;* G. *ous*, ear]. A genus of field voles of the Orient that may transmit leptospirosis, rat-bite fever, and tsutsugamushi disease.

mi″cro·u′nit [*mikros;* L. *unitas*, unity]. A unit of minute measurements; the one-millionth part of an ordinary unit.

mi′cro·volt [*mikros;* Alessandro *Volta*, Italian physicist, 1745–1827]. One one-millionth of a volt.

mi′cro·wave. The region of the electromagnetic spectrum extending from a few tenths of a millimeter to a few meters, the limits varying to some degree according to the investigator.

mi·crox′y·cyte (migh·crock′si·sight) [*mikros;* G. *oxys,* sharp; *kytos,* cell]. A cell containing fine oxyphil granules and a more or less pigmented nucleus, occurring in the peritoneal fluid of infected subjects. *Rare.*

mi·crox′y·phil [*mikros; oxys;* G. *philein,* to love]. An oxyphil leukocyte.

mi″cro·zo′on [*mikros;* G. *zōion,* a living being]. A microscopic animal.

mi″cro·zo·o·sper′mi·a. Abnormally small living sperms in the semen.

mi′crur·gy. The art and science of manipulation, under the magnification of a microscope, including microdissection, microinjection, and various techniques using the micromanipulator.

Mi″cru·roi′des (migh″kroo·roy′deez) [*mikros;* G. *oura,* tail; *eidos,* form]. A genus of coral snakes with neurotoxic venom; found in the Americas.

Mi·cru′rus (migh·kroor′us) [*mikros; oura*]. A genus of elapine snakes commonly known as coral snakes, found in the Americas. Their venom is neurotoxic.

mic′tion. See *micturition.*

mic′tu·rate [L. *mictus,* a making water]. Urinate.

mic″tu·ri′tion (mick″choo·rish′un) [L. *micturire,* to make water]. The act of passing urine. Syn., *miction.*

mid- [AS. *midd*]. A combining form denoting *the middle.*

mid″ax·il′la [*midd;* L. *axilla,* armpit]. The center of the axilla. —**midax′illary,** *adj.*

mid′bod″y [*midd;* AS. *bodig*]. A mass of granules formed in the equator of the spindle during the anaphase and early telophase of mitosis.

mid′brain″ [*midd;* AS. *bragen*]. The mesencephalon. See Plate 15.

mid″fron′tal. Pertaining to the middle of the forehead.

midge [AS. *mycge*]. An insect of those Diptera which comprise the family Chironomidae; small, delicate forms usually smaller than mosquitoes. The genus *Culicoides* is the most important medically.

midg′et [dim. from *mycge*]. An adult who has never reached full growth. Such persons are usually fully formed, but are low in the scale of reproductivity, especially if mated to another midget.

mid′gut″ [AS. *midd; guttas*]. The middle portion of the embryonic digestive tube, opening ventrally into the yolk sac.

mid′pain″ [*midd;* L. *poena,* penalty]. Intermenstrual pain. See *mittelschmerz.*

mid′riff [AS. *midhrif*]. The diaphragm. Loosely used for the upper part of the abdomen.

mid′wife″ [AS. *midd; wīf*]. A woman, trained or experienced, who attends other women in labor.

mid′wife″ry [*midd; wīf*]. Obstetrics.

mi′graf. A portable microscope and camera combined; designed for the observation of microscopic objects and for making a quick and permanent record of them.

mi′graine (migh′grain, mi·grain′, mee′grain) [F., from G. *hēmi-,* half, *kranion,* skull]. A paroxysmal intense pain in the head, preceded or accompanied by characteristic sensory or motor disturbances or both, with vasomotor or psychic phenomena. The attack is probably the result of functional, vasomotor disturbances in the intracranial branches of the carotid artery. The etiology is unknown. Also called *sick headache.* —**migrain′ous,** *adj.*

abdominal m. Recurrent attacks of abdominal pain associated with migraine.

facioplegic m. Paralysis of facial muscles sometimes accompanying migraine.

ocular m. An attack of migraine accompanied by amblyopia or other visual disturbances.

ophthalmic m. See ocular *m.*

ophthalmoplegic m. A rare form of migrainous headache, perhaps not a true migraine, which is accompanied by temporary paralysis of muscles innervated by the third cranial nerve.

mi′grate [L. *migrare,* to migrate]. Move from one place to another.

mi·gra′tion [L. *migratio,* from *migrare*]. A wandering.

external m. The passage of the ovum from an ovary to the oviduct.

internal m. of the ovum. The passage of the ovum through the oviduct into the uterus.

m. of leukocytes. One of the phenomena of inflammation, consisting in the passage of leukocytes through the vessel wall into the connective tissues.

m. of ovum. The passage of an ovum from the ovary to the oviduct and uterus.

transperitoneal m. The passage of an ovum from one ovary to the oviduct of the opposite side.

mi′kro-. See *micro-.*

mi′kron. Micron.

Mikulicz-Radecki, Johann von (1850–1905). Rumanian surgeon in Austria and Germany who devised a technique of plastic reconstruction of the esophagus after resection for cancer, and an operation for disease of the maxiliary sinus, the antrum being perforated from the nasal cavity. He developed an operation of colonic resection performed in stages, for carcinoma, called *Mikulicz operation.* The loop of bowel is externalized, then removed; the resulting artificial anus is made into a fecal fistula, which later is closed. A technique of pylorotomy, now rarely used, is called the *Heineke-Mikulicz operation.* Chronic hypertrophic enlargement of the lacrimal and salivary glands is known as *Mikulicz's disease.* See also Mikulicz *cell, drain.*

mil·am′me″ter. Milliammeter.

mil′dew [AS. *meledēaw*]. A common name for minute fungi parasitic on plants, and also found on dead vegetable substances such as textiles, clothes, etc.

Miles, William Ernest [*English surgeon,* 1869–1947]. Known for his one-stage abdominoperineal resection of the rectum for carcinoma; called *Miles's operation.*

Milian, Gaston [*French dermatologist,* 1871–1945]. Described erythema following the administration of arsphenamine; called *Milian's erythema.* See also Milian's ear *sign.*

mil″i·a′ri·a [L. *miliarius,* of millet]. An acute inflammatory skin disease, the lesions consisting of vesicles and papules, which may be accompanied by a pricking or tingling sensation. It occurs especially in summer and in the tropics, often in the folds of the skin. Syn., *prickly heat, heat rash, strophulus, lichen tropicus, wildfire rash.* Also called *miliaria rubra, Bedouin's itch.*

m. crystallina. A skin condition in which the sweat accumulates under the superficial horny layers of the epidermis to form small, clear, transparent vesicles. Syn., *sudamen.*

m. profunda. The skin reaction seen in the sweat-retention syndrome. The skin is uniformly studded with many discrete normal skin-colored papules located around a sweat pore. There are no subjective symptoms.

m. pustulosa. A sweat-retention pustular dermatosis which is secondary to the skin damage caused by another dermatitis. The pustules are usually sterile or may contain nonpathogenic cocci.

mil′i·ar″y (mil′ee·err″ee, ·air″ee, mil′yuh·ree) [*miliarius*]. 1. Of the size of a millet seed, 0.5 to 1.0 mm., as miliary aneurysm, miliary tubercle. 2. Characterized by the formation of numerous lesions the size of a millet seed distributed rather uniformly throughout one or more organs, especially as in miliary tuberculosis.

milibis. Trade-mark for bismuth glycolylarsanilate or glycobiarsol, a compound of pentavalent arsenic and bismuth, used in intestinal amebiasis.

mi·lieu′ ex·té′rieur′ (mee′lyuh′ ex·tay′ryur′. *See* NOTES §35) [F.]. Literally, the external environment.

mi′lieu′ in·té′rieur′ (mee′lyuh′ ahn·tay′ryur′. *See* NOTES §35) [F.]. Literally, the internal environment. Claude Bernard's concept of the *milieu intérieur*, now fundamental for modern physiology, postulates that the living organism exists not so much in its gaseous or aqueous external environment (*milieu extérieur*) as within its aqueous internal environment. Formed by circulating liquid, the blood plasma and interstitial fluid including lymph, this *milieu intérieur* bathes all tissue elements, and is the medium in which all elementary exchanges of nutrient and waste materials take place. Its stability is the primary condition for independent existence of the organism, and the mechanisms by which stability is achieved ensure maintenance of all conditions necessary to the life of tissue elements.

mil′i·um [L., millet]. A disease of the skin characterized by the formation of small, pearly, noninflammatory elevations or globoid masses situated mainly on the face or genitalia. They often become quite hard and may last for years.

colloid m. A rare skin disease characterized by the presence, especially on the face, of minute, shining, flat, or slightly raised lesions of a pale lemon or bright lemon color. It is a form of colloid degeneration of the skin, affecting persons of middle or advanced age.

milk [AS. *meoluc*]. 1. The whitish fluid secreted by the mammary gland for the nourishment of the young. It is composed of carbohydrates, proteins, fats, mineral salts, vitamins, antibodies. 2. Any whitish fluid resembling milk, as cocoanut milk. 3. A suspension of certain metallic oxides, as milk of magnesia, iron, bismuth, etc.

AVERAGE COMPOSITION OF MILKS OF VARIOUS MAMMALS

(From "Allen's Commercial Organic Analysis," Vol. IX, The Blakiston Company)

Species	*Water* %	*Casein* %	*Albumin* %	*Fat* %	*Lactose* %	*Ash* %
Human	87.41	0.91	1.23	3.76	6.29	0.31
Cow	87.27	2.95	0.52	3.66	4.91	0.69
Goat	84.14	3.04	0.99	6.00	5.02	0.81
Sheep	81.90	4.57	1.26	6.52	4.82	0.93
Buffalo	82.14	4.29	0.49	7.44	4.81	0.83
Camel	87.04	3.49	0.40	2.76	5.57	0.74
Horse	90.68	1.27	0.75	1.17	5.77	0.36
Ass	89.88	0.73	1.31	1.50	6.09	0.49
Reindeer	68.2	8.4	2.0	17.1	2.08	1.5

acidophilus m. Milk inoculated with cultures of *Lactobacillus acidophilus;* used in various enteric disorders to provide a change of bacterial flora.

adapted m. Milk that is modified to suit the digestive capacity of the child.

after-milk. The stripping, or the last milk obtained at each milking.

albumin m. Milk high in casein and fat, but poor in lactose and salts, a preparation devised by Finkelstein.

bacillary m. Proprietary milk containing *Lactobacillus bulgaricus.*

blue m. Milk which develops a bluish tint due to contamination with *Pseudomonas cyanogenes.*

buddeized m. Sterilization of milk by adding hydrogen peroxide (H_2O_2) and heating; the heat causes decomposition of the hydrogen peroxide, liberating oxygen.

buttermilk. That which remains after churning butter.

casein m. See albumin *m.*

centrifugalized m. Milk from which the cream has been separated by whirling it in a centrifuge.

certified m. Milk, the purity of which is certified by a special commission of physicians, bacteriologists, or sanitarians.

citric acid m. A special preparation in which 4 Gm. of dehydrated citric acid is added to one quart of milk.

condensed m. Milk that is partially evaporated and enriched by the addition of sugar.

diabetic m. One that contains only a small amount of lactose.

dialyzed m. Milk with the sugar removed by dialysis through a parchment membrane.

evaporated m. Milk treated with heat to lose about half of its water content. It is then canned and sterilized, and usually fortified by ultraviolet radiation. Popular in making infants' formulas.

fore-milk. (a) That first withdrawn at each milking. (b) Colostrum.

fortified m. That which is enriched by the addition of albumin, cream, or vitamins.

homogenized m. Milk especially processed so that the fat globules are very minute and emulsification is so complete that the cream does not separate from the rest of the milk.

hydrochloric acid m. Acidified milk, prepared by adding 5 cc. of one-tenth normal hydrochloric acid to 100 cc. of milk.

lemon juice m. An acid milk made by adding 22 cc. of lemon juice to one quart of milk.

litmus m. One which contains litmus; used as an indicator in bacteriology.

metalized m. That containing minute traces of iron, copper, and magnesium; used in treating anemia.

m. crust. Seborrhea of the scalp in nursing infants; a form of eczema.

m. cure. Treatment of disease by a diet of milk or milk products.

modified m. One altered so that its composition approximates mother's milk.

pasteurized m. One treated by pasteurization.

peptonized m. Milk partially digested by the use of pepsin or pancreatic extract.

perhydrase m. See buddeized *m.*

protein m. One containing a high percentage of protein, and a low percentage of sugar and fat.

red m. One with a red tint due to contamination by blood or certain microorganisms, or to the ingestion of madder root.

ropy m. Milk that becomes viscid so that it may be drawn out into a stringy mass; caused by a growth of bacteria, *Alcaligenes viscosus.*

skim m. Milk after the cream is removed.

soft curd m. Milk that is treated by boiling or by the addition of cream or sodium citrate, to produce a soft, flocculent curd.

sour m. Milk containing lactic acid produced by the lactic acid bacteria normally present.

uterine m. A whitish fluid found between the placental villi of the pregnant uterus.

uviol m. Milk sterilized by exposure to ultraviolet rays.

vegetable m. Synthetic milk expressed from various vegetables, as the soybean: used to replace natural milk for those with milk allergy.

vinegar m. An acid milk made by adding one ounce of vinegar to 15 ounces of cow's milk.

vitamin-D m. Cow's milk fortified by the direct addition of vitamin D, by exposure to ultraviolet rays, or by feeding irradiated yeast to the animals.

witch's m. Milk sometimes secreted from the breasts of the newborn.

milk a'gent. A filtrable substance found in the milk and organs of certain inbred strains of mice, which is essential for the production of mammary carcinoma in the offspring of these mice.

milk-drinker's syndrome. Milk poisoning. See pathologic *calcification* (c).

milk fe'ver. See under *fever.*

milk'ing [*meoluc*]. 1. The process of expressing milk from the mammary gland, manually or mechanically. 2. Pressing a finger along a compressible tube or duct in order to squeeze out the contents.

Milkman, Louis Arthur (1895–). American radiologist known for his description of a clinical and roentgenological syndrome associated with a certain degree of bone decalcification. See Milkman's *syndrome.*

Millar, John [*Scottish physician in England,* 1733–1805]. Described laryngismus stridulus, called *Millar's asthma.*

Millard, Auguste Louis Jules [*French physician,* 1830–1915]. Described a syndrome, due to a lesion in the pons, of paralysis of the lateral rectus muscle and often of the peripheral facial muscles on the side of the lesion, with paralysis of the limbs on the other side. Called *Millard-Gubler syndrome.* Alternate hemiplegia of various types is known as *Millard-Gubler syndrome, Gubler's paralysis, Weber-Gubler syndrome.* See also Hermann David *Weber.*

mil'le·pedes (mil'i·peedz). See *millipedes.*

Miller, Thomas Grier [*American physician,* 1886–]. With W. O. Abbott, developed an intestinal drainage tube. See Miller-Abbott *tube.*

Mil'ler oc'u·lar disk. See Miller *disk.*

mil'let seed. The edible seed of a grass; frequently used to designate the approximate size of small lesions or tumors, being about 2 mm. in diameter.

mil'li- [L. *mille,* thousand]. A combining form denoting *a thousand* or *a thousandth.*

mil"li·am'me"ter [*mille;* A. M. *Am*père; G. *metron,* a measure]. An ammeter which records electric current in milliamperes. Used in measuring currents passing through a roentgen-ray tube.

mil"li·am'pere [*mille; Ampère*]. One one-thousandth of an ampere. Abbreviated, ma.

mil"li·am'pere·me"ter. Obsolete term for milliammeter.

mil'li·bar [*mille;* G. *baros,* weight]. Unit of atmospheric pressure, the one-thousandth part of a bar.

mil'li·cu"rie [*mille; Curie*]. The amount of a radioactive substance which undergoes 3.7×10^7 disintegrations per second, equivalent to one-thousandth of a curie. Abbreviated, mc.

mil'li·cu"rie-hour'. A dosage unit of radon; the amount of radiation emitted by a millicurie of radon multiplied by time of treatment in hours.

mil"li·e·quiv'a·lent [*mille;* L. *aequus,* equal; *valere,* to be strong]. The weight of a substance contained in, represented by, or equivalent to 1 cc. of a solution of specified normality, usually one-normal. Abbreviated, mEq.

mil'li·gram [*mille;* G. *gramma,* scruple]. One one-thousandth of a gram. Abbreviated, mg, mg.

mil'li·gram"age. See *milligram-hour.*

mil'li·gram-hour'. A dosage unit of radium; the amount of radiation emitted by a milligram of radium multiplied by the time of treatment in hours. Abbreviated, mgh, mgh.

mil'li·grams per cent. *In biochemistry,* indicating milligrams of a substance per 100 cc. of blood. Symbol, mg %, mg. %.

Millikan rays. See under *ray.*

mil'li·li"ter (mil'i·lee"tur) [*mille;* G. *litra,* pound]. The one one-thousandth part of a liter, for all practical purposes equivalent to a cubic centimeter. Abbreviated, ml, ml.

mil'li·me"ter [*mille;* G. *metron,* a measure]. One one-thousandth of a meter. Abbreviated, mm, mm.

mil"li·mi'cron [*mille;* G. *mikros,* small]. One one-thousandth of a micron. Also called *micromillimeter.* Symbol, mμ.

mil'li·mol [*mille;* L. *moles,* mass]. One one-thousandth of a gram molecule. —**millimol'ar,** *adj.*

mil"li·nor'mal [*mille;* L. *normalis,* made according to the square]. Containing a thousandth part of the quantity designated as normal.

mil"li·os'mol. The concentration of an ion in a solution expressed as milligrams per liter divided by atomic weight. In univalent ions, milliosmolar and milliequivalent values are identical; in divalent ions, 1 milliosmol equals 2 milliequivalents. —**millios'molar,** *adj.*

mil'li·pedes, mil'le·pedes (mil'i·peedz) [*mille;* L. *pes,* foot]. Wingless, vermiform arthropods with two pairs of legs on each body segment. Some species are incriminated as hosts of *Hymenolepis diminuta.*

mil"li·ruth'er·ford [*mille;* after Ernest *Rutherford,* English physicist, 1871–1937]. A unit of radioactivity representing 10^3 disintegrations per second. Abbreviated, mrd.

mil'li·volt. One one-thousandth of a volt.

mil'li·volt sec'ond. A measurement of an electric current, equal to one one-thousandth of a volt per second.

Millon's reagent. See under *reagent.*

Mills, Charles Karsner [*American neurologist,* 1845–1931]. Described unilateral progressive ascending paralysis (1900), called *Mills's disease.* Described unilateral descending paralysis (1906).

milontin. Trade-mark for N-methyl-α-phenylsuccinimide; $CH_2.CO.N(CH_3).CO.CH(C_6H_5)$; an anticonvulsant drug effective in petit mal.

mil·pho'sis [G. *milphōsis,* falling off of the eyelashes]. Baldness of the eyebrows.

Milroy, William Forsyth [*American physician,* 1855–1942]. Described hereditary edema of the legs (1892); called *Milroy's* or *Meige's disease.*

miltown. A trade-mark for *meprobamate.*

milz'brand" (milts'bront". *See* Notes § 35) [Ger.]. Anthrax.

mi·me'sis (mi·mee'sis, migh·mee'sis) [G., imitation]. 1. Mimicry, as of an organic disease. 2. The assumption of the symptoms of one disease by another disease. Also called *mimosis.* —**mimet'ic, mim'ic,** *adj.*

mim·ma'tion [Ar. *mīm,* the letter m.] The unduly frequent use of the sound of the letter M in speech.

min. Minim.

mind [AS. *gemynd*]. 1. The understanding; the reasoning and intellectual faculties considered as a whole. 2. *In psychiatry,* the psyche.

mind cure. The alleged cure of disease through mental influence; mental healing.

Min"der·e'rus spir'it. See *ammonium* acetate solution.

min'er·al [NL. *minera*, ore]. An inorganic chemical compound found in nature, especially one that is solid.

m. glycerin. Petroleum.

m. oil. Petroleum; also the liquid petrolatum used medicinally.

m. pitch. Bitumen.

m. water. Water naturally or artificially impregnated with sufficient inorganic salts to give it special properties.

min"er·al·o·cor'ti·coid. An adrenal cortical steroid hormone that primarily regulates mineral metabolism and, indirectly, fluid balance.

min'er·al spring. A spring reputed to be of value in restoring health, especially to persons with arthritic disease, through the action of the minerals in its waters.

Mingazzini, Giovanni (1859–1929). Italian pathologist who contributed to knowledge of the lenticular nucleus and the disorders resulting from lesions in it and to knowledge of the corpus callosum.

min'im [L. *minimus*, least]. A unit of volume in the apothecaries' system; it equals 1/60 fluidrachm or about 1 drop (of water). Symbol, ♏. Abbreviated, min.

min'i·mal [*minimus*]. Least; lowest. Of doses, the smallest quantity that is effective.

min'i·mum (pl. *minima*) [*minimus*]. The least; the lowest; the lowest intensity or level; threshold.

m. cognoscibile. *In physiologic optics*, the lowest limit at which recognition of complicated detail of form occurs.

m. discernibile. The smallest discernible light difference, i.e., the differential threshold of light sense.

m. legibile. *In physiologic optics*, the lowest limit at which recognition of letters or numbers occurs.

m. separabile. *In physiologic optics*, visual acuity for more than one detail. Originally, the minimum angular distance by which two stars must be separated to be perceived as two. See minimum separable *acuity*.

m. visibile. The smallest amount of light (expressed in watts of light energy) just perceptible, i.e., the absolute threshold of light sense.

Minkowski, Oskar [*Lithuanian pathologist in Germany*, 1858–1931]. Noted the relation of enlargement of the pituitary gland to acromegaly (1887). With von Mering, studied the diabetic syndrome following experimental pancreatectomy (1889). Described congenital familial cholemia, which is also called *Chauffard-Minkowski syndrome.*

mi·nom'e·ter. An instrument for measuring the total amount of radiation which passes through the dosimeter from the time it is charged until the remaining charge is measured.

Minor, Lazar Salomovich [*Russian neurologist*, 1855–]. Described central hematomyelia, also called *Minor's disease*, and essential tremor, also called *Minor's tremor.*

mi'nor [L., less]. Less; lesser; smaller.

mi'nor. An individual under legal age; one under the authority of parents or guardians.

mi'nor med'i·cal as·sem'bly. *In military medicine*, an aggregation of medical supplies and/or equipment, not assigned consignee combinations, such as kits and chests.

Minot, George Richards [*American physician*, 1885–1950]. With William Parry Murphy, introduced the *Minot-Murphy diet*, consisting chiefly of liver, in the treatment of pernicious anemia (1926). This led to the present-day therapeutic use of liver extracts. Nobel laureate with W. P. Murphy and G. H. Whipple (1934).

mint. See *Mentha.*

mi'o- [G. *meiōn*, smaller, less]. 1. A combining form denoting *smaller, less.* 2. *In medicine*, a combining form denoting *decrease* or *contraction.*

mi"o·car'di·a [*meiōn;* G. *kardia*, heart]. The systolic diminution of the volume of the heart

mi"o·did'y·mus, mi·od'y·mus [*meiōn;* G. *didymos*, twin]. A dicephalic monster with a small head fused occipitally with a large head.

mi"o·lec'i·thal. See *meiolecithal.*

mi·o'pus (migh·o'pus, migh'o·pus) [*meiōn;* G. *ōps*, face]. A type of diprosopus in which one face is rudimentary.

mi·o'sis (migh·o'sis) [G. *meiōsis*, diminution]. 1. Constriction of the pupil of the eye. 2. See *meiosis.*

senile m. Miosis associated with increase in the connective tissue and hyalinization of the septa of the sphincter pupillae muscle, seen usually in the aged.

mi·ot'ic [G. *meiōtikos*, diminishing]. 1. Pertaining to, or characterized by, miosis. 2. Causing contraction of the pupil.

mi·ot'ic. An agent which constricts the pupil.

mi"ra·cid'i·um [G. *meirakidion*, youthful person]. The first larval form of the digenetic trematodes which develops from the fertilized ovum and which emerges from the egg as a ciliated, free-swimming, pear-shaped organism. On penetration into the tissue of an appropriate species of snail the miracidium undergoes metamorphosis into a sporocyst.

miracil D. Lucanthone hydrochloride; a drug useful in the treatment of certain types of human schistosomiasis. See *nilodin.*

Mirault, Germanicus [*French surgeon*, 1796–1879]. Devised an operation in which the lingual arteries were tied as a preliminary to excision of the tongue, and one for the plastic repair of unilateral harelip by means of a flap turned down on one side and attached to the opposite side. Each is known as *Mirault's operation.*

mir'bane oil. Nitrobenzene.

mire (meer) [L. *mirare*, to wonder]. Figures used upon the perimeter bar of the ophthalmometer; by noting the variations of their images, as reflected by different meridians of the cornea, the measurement of corneal astigmatism is effected.

mir'ror [*mirare*]. A polished surface for reflecting light or forming images of objects placed in front of it; used in rhinoscopy, ophthalmoscopy, laryngoscopy, dentistry, etc.

concave m. One with a concave reflecting surface.

convex m. A mirror with a convex reflecting surface.

frontal m. A head mirror.

head m. A circular mirror with a central perforation, strapped to the head by a band, and used to throw light on parts to be examined.

laryngeal m. A small circular mirror affixed to a long handle, used in laryngoscopy; a similar instrument is used by dentists, in the examination of the teeth.

plane m. A mirror with a flat reflecting surface.

mir'ror writ'ing. A peculiar kind of writing in which the letters appear backward, as if seen in a mirror.

Mirsky-Pollister method. See under *method.*

mis·an'thro·py (mi·san'thro·pee, mi·zan'·) [G. *misanthrōpos*, hating mankind]. An aversion to society; hatred of mankind. —**mis'anthrope,** *n.*

mis·car'riage [AS. *mis-;* ONF. *cariage*]. 1. Expulsion of the fetus before it is viable. 2. Abortion.

mis·car'ry [*mis-;* ONF. *carier*]. Give birth to a nonviable fetus.

mis′ce (miss′ee) [L., imperative of *miscere*, to mingle]. Mix, a direction placed under the ingredients of compound prescriptions, and usually abbreviated M.

mis″ce·ge·na′tion [*miscere;* L. *genus*, race]. Intermarriage or interbreeding of different races of man.

mis′ci·ble [*miscere*]. Capable of mixing or dissolving in all proportions.

mis′o- (miss′o-, migh′so-), **mis-** [G. *misein*, to hate]. A combining form denoting *hatred, hating.*

mi·sog′a·my (mi·sog′uh·mee, migh·sog′·) [*misein;* G. *gamos*, marriage]. Aversion to marriage. —**misogamist,** *n.*

mi·sog′y·ny (mi·sodj′i·nee, migh·sodj′·) [*misein;* G. *gynē*, woman]. Hatred of women. —**misogynist,** *n.*

mi·sol′o·gy (mi·sol′o·jee, migh·sol′·), **mis″o·lo′gi·a** [*misein;* G. *logos*, word]. Unreasoning aversion to intellectual or literary matters, or to argument or speaking.

mis″o·ne′ism [*misein;* G. *neos*, new]. Hatred or horror of novelty or change. —**misoneist,** *n.*

mis″o·pe′di·a [*misein;* G. *pais*, child]. Morbid hatred of all children, but especially of one's own.

mis″o·psy′chi·a (miss″o·sigh′kee·uh, miss″op·, my″so·, my″sop·) [*misein;* G. *psychē*, life]. Morbid disgust with life; hatred of living. *Obs.*

mist. *Mistura;* mixture.

mis′tle·toe [AS. *misteltān*]. The woody parasites *Viscum album* (European mistletoe) and *V. flavescens* (American mistletoe). Preparations of the former may be useful in hypertension.

Mitchell, Silas Weir [*American physician, physiologist, and author*, 1829–1914]. Made important studies of the physiologic effects of various poisons, especially snake venoms, and of the physiology of the cerebellum. With George Read Morehouse and William Williams Keen, studied injuries of the peripheral nerves. Gave a classic description of erythromelalgia (1872), called *Mitchell's disease.* Advocated rest in bed in the treatment of functional nervous disease; called *Weir Mitchell treatment.*

mite [AS. *mīte*]. Any representative of a large group of small arachnids, which together with the larger ticks constitute the order Acarina.

chicken m. *Dermanyssus gallinae.*

follicular m. *Demodex folliculorum.*

grain itch m. *Pediculoides ventricosus.*

harvest m. *Trombicula irritans.*

itch m. *Sarcoptes scabei.*

mange m. Any species of the Sarcoptoidea.

rat m. *Liponyssus bacoti.*

red m. Any member of the genus *Trombicula.*

sarcoptic m. See itch *m.*

mith′ri·date [G. *Mithridates*, king of Pontus, ca. 132–63 B.C.]. An old confection believed to contain an antidote to every known poison.

mi′ti·cide. A substance destructive to mites. —**mitici′dal,** *adj.*

mit′i·gate [L. *mitigare*, to soften]. Allay, make milder; moderate.

mi′tis [L.]. Mild.

mit″o·chon′dri·a (mit″o·kon′dree·uh, my″to·) [G. *mitos*, thread; *chondrion*, granule]. Cytoplasmic organelles in the form of granules, short rods, or filaments, present in all cells. —**mitochon′drial,** *adj.*

mit″o·chon′dri·on. Singular of mitochondria.

mit″o·gen′e·sis (mit″o·jen′i·sis, my″to·) [*mitos;* G. *genesis*, production]. Formation as a result of mitosis. —**mitogenic, mitogenet′ic,** *adj.*

mi′tome [*mitos*]. The threads of the reticulum of the cytoplasm of a cell (cytomitome) or of the nucleoplasm (karyomitome).

mit′o·plasm. See *chromatin.*

mi·to′sis (mi·to′sis, my·to′sis) [*mitos;* G. *-ōsis*, condition]. 1. Indirect nuclear division; usually divided into a series of stages: prophase, metaphase, anaphase, and telophase. Syn., *karyokinesis.* 2. The indirect division of the cytoplasm and nucleus. —**mitot′ic,** *adj.*

abortive m. See pathologic *m.*

anastral m. Mitosis occurring without the formation of asters.

heterotypic m. Applied to the first miotic division in the maturation of the germ cells; the reduction division.

homeotypic m. Applied to the second miotic division in the maturation of the germ cells; an equational division.

pathologic m. Irregular, atypical, asymmetric and multipolar mitosis, an indication of malignancy: also called *abortive m.*

mit′o·some (mit′o·sohm, my′to·) [*mitos;* G. *sōma*, body]. A cytoplasmic body derived from the spindle fibers of the preceding mitosis. Also called *spindle remnant.*

mi′tral [G. *mitra*, girdle, headband]. 1. Resembling a bishop's miter. 2. Pertaining to the atrioventricular valve of the left side of the heart. See also mitral *cell.*

fish-mouth m. Advanced degree of constriction of the mitral orifice of the heart.

mi′troid [*mitra;* G. *eidos*, form]. Shaped like a miter cap.

Mitsuda's test. See lepromin *test.*

mit′tel·schmerz [Ger., middle pain]. Pain or discomfort in the lower abdomen of women occurring midway in the intermenstrual interval, thought to be secondary to the irritation of the pelvic peritoneum by fluid or blood escaping from the point of ovulation in the ovary.

mixed chan′cre (shang′kur). A lesion, the result of infection with both *Treponema pallidum* and *Hemophilus ducreyi* (Ducrey's bacillus).

mix″o·sco′pi·a [G. *mixis*, intercourse; *skopein*, to examine]. A form of sexual perversion in which the orgasm is excited by the sight of coitus. —**mixoscop′ic,** *adj.*

mix′ture [L. *mixtura*, from *miscere*, to mingle]. *In pharmacy*, a preparation made by incorporating insoluble ingredients in a liquid vehicle, preferably with the aid of a suitable suspending agent so that the insoluble substances do not readily settle out. Occasionally the term is applied to aqueous solutions, containing two or more solutes. For mixtures not found here, see under the names of the most active ingredients. Also see *emulsion.*

Basham's m. See *iron* and *ammonium acetate solution.*

brown m. Compound opium and glycyrrhiza mixture.

carminative m. (*mistura carminativa*). Composed of opium tincture, 25 cc.; magnesium carbonate, 65 Gm.; potassium carbonate, 3 Gm.; volatile oils, syrup, and water sufficient to make 1000 cc. Dose for an infant, 0.3–0.6 cc. (5–10 min.). Also called *Dalby's carminative.*

copaiba m. An aqueous emulsion containing 12.5 per cent copaiba; formerly used as a diuretic. Syn., *Lafayette m.*

expectorant m. (*mistura pectoralis*). A nauseating expectorant prepared from fluidextracts of senega and squill, camphorated opium tincture, ammonium carbonate, and tolu balsam syrup. Dose, 4 cc. (1 fluidrachm). Also called *Stoke's expectorant.*

freezing m. A mixture of salt and snow or ice, which absorbs heat in undergoing solution.

Lafayette m. Copaiba mixture.

Mi·ya·ga″wa·nel′la (for Yoneji *Miyagawa*, Japanese bacteriologist [1885–]). Proposed name for a genus of large viruses, family Chlamydozoaceae, which includes the causative agents of venereal lymphogranuloma (*M. lymphogranulomatosis*), of a type of viral pneumonia (*M. pneumoniae*), of psittacosis (*M. psittacii*), ornithosis (*M. ornithosis*), and several other animal diseases.

ml, ml. Milliliter.

MLD Minimal lethal dose.

mm, mm. Millimeter.

Mn Chemical symbol for manganese.

mne″mas·the′ni·a (nee″mass·thee′nee·uh) [G. *mnēmē*, memory; *astheneia*, weakness]. Weakness of memory not due to organic disease.

mne′mic hy·poth′e·sis (nee′mick, nem′ick). A hypothesis that a stimulus or irritant, when continuous, tends to produce a habit which may persist even when the stimulus ceases; these stimuli are supposed to leave impressions on the cells affected, such impressions being called engrams.

mne″mo·der′mi·a. Pruritus and discomfort of the skin hours and days after the cause of the symptoms has been removed and recovery well established, usually stimulated by scratching or rubbing, sometimes by heat and other stimuli. Syn., *cutaneous memory.*

mne·mon′ics (nee·mon′icks) [G. *mnēmonikos*, of memory]. The science of cultivation of the memory by systematic methods.

mne′mo·tech″ny, mne′mo·tech″nics (nee′mo-teck″·). Mnemonics.

Mo Chemical symbol for molybdenum.

moan [ME. *mone*]. To utter a low, dull sound expressive of suffering. —**moan,** *n.*

mobenate. Trade-mark for sodium benzylsuccinate.

mo′bile med′i·cal serv′ice u′nit. A mobile unit of the U.S. Army Medical Service composed of a number of professional teams and necessary service elements.

mo′bile op′ti·cal u′nit. A U.S. Army Medical Department installation, equipped to make or repair spectacles in the field; no refraction or eye examination is done.

mo·bil′i·ty [L. *mobilitas*, mobility]. The condition of being movable.

mo″bi·li·za′tion [L. *mobilis*, movable]. 1. The act of rendering an ankylosed part movable. 2. Freeing an organ during surgical operation to make it accessible. 3. The liberation of a substance stored in the body, as the mobilization of glycogen stored in the liver. —**mo′bilize,** *v.t.*

Möbius, Paul Julius [*German neurologist*, 1853–1907]. Described periodic ophthalmoplegic migraine, called *Möbius' disease.* An atrophic type of progressive muscular dystrophy, seen in children, is known as *Leyden-Möbius dystrophy;* this usually begins in the pelvic girdle and thighs. See also Möbius' *sign.*

mo·dal′i·ty. A form of sensation, such as touch, pressure, vision, or audition.

mode [L. *modus*, a measure]. That value in a series of observations which occurs most frequently.

mod′el [L. *modulus*, small measure]. 1. The form or material pattern of anything to be made, or already existing. 2. A reproduction in plaster or metal of any object, as a tooth or the dental arch; made by pouring the material into an impression taken from that object. Also see *cast.*

compound m. *In dentistry*, one constructed of plaster, stone, or investment material prepared from dental impressions; used in jaw fractures to fashion wax models for the construction of dental splints.

investment compound m. See compound *m.*

Rutherford-Bohr atom m. A concept of atomic structure: the positive charge is located in a centrally located nucleus, negatively charged electrons, in elliptical orbits around the nucleus.

mod′er·a·tor. A substance (e.g., graphite, water, heavy water, beryllium, paraffin) used to slow down the motion of nuclear particles, especially to slow down neutrons to a thermal equilibrium state and thus to promote a chain reaction.

mo·di′o·lus [L., the nave of a wheel]. The central pillar or axis of the cochlea, around which the spiral canal makes two and one-half turns.

mod′u·la″tor. A receptive sensory end organ in light-adapted eyes, of relatively infrequent type, occurring in narrow spectral sensitivity curves or absorption bands in three preferential regions of the spectrum, 5800–6000 angstroms, 5200–5400 angstroms, and 4500–4700 angstroms, thought to be related to color sensation and discrimination.

mod′u·lus [L., small measure]. 1. The measure of a force, of properties of mass, or their effects. 2. A constant which converts a proportionality into an equality.

mo′dus [L.]. A mode or method.

m. operandi. The method of doing something.

Moeller, Julius Otto Ludwig [*German physician*, 1819–87]. Described infantile scurvy (1859), also called *Moeller-Barlow disease.*

Moeller's glossitis. See chronic superficial *glossitis.*

Moeller's method. See under *stain.*

Mo·ën′a an·om′a·ly. See PTC deficiency *disease.*

Moens, Adriann Isebree [*Dutch physiologist*, 1847–91]. Introduced a formula for determining the velocity of the pulse wave; called *Moens' equation* or *formula.*

mog″i·graph′i·a (modj″i·graf′ee·uh, ·gray′fee·uh) [G. *mogis*, with difficulty; *graphein*, to write]. Writer's cramp.

mog″i·la′li·a [*mogis;* G. *lalia*, talk]. Difficult or painful speech, as stammering or stuttering. Syn., *molilalia.*

mog″i·pho′ni·a [*mogis;* G. *phōnē*, sound]. Difficulty in speaking, excited by an effort to sing or speak loudly.

Mohr's salt. Ferrous ammonium sulfate.

Mohrenheim, Joseph Jacob von [*Austrian surgeon*, d. 1799]. Described the infraclavicular fossa, called *Mohrenheim's fossa.*

moi′e·ty. A part or portion, especially of a molecule, generally complex, having a characteristic chemical or pharmacological property.

moist [L. *mucidus*, moldy]. Damp; slightly wet; characterized by the presence of fluid.

mol. See *gram molecule.*

mo′lal [L. *moles*, mass]. Pertaining to moles of a solute per 1000 Gm. of solvent. Also see *molar*, 2.

mo′lar [L. *molaris*, from *mola*, mill]. A grinding tooth; a grinder. Abbreviated, M. —**molar′i·form,** *adj.*

dome-shaped molars. Small first molars with cusps abnormally close together; their imperfect development is due to congenital syphilis. Also called *Fournier's molars, Moon's molars, mulberry molars.*

peg m. A molar, usually the third, of diminutive size.

six-year molars. The first of the permanent molar teeth.

twelve-year molars. The second permanent molars.

mo′lar [L. *moles*, mass]. 1. Pertaining to masses, in contradistinction to molecular. 2. Pertaining to moles of solute in a definite volume of solution, usually 1 liter. Also incorrectly called *molal.*

mo·las′ses [L. *mel*, honey]. The syrupy liquid

obtained in the refining of sugar. It contains a considerable quantity of uncrystallizable sugar, and coloring matter. Combined with sulfur it is employed as a domestic remedy for constipation.

mold [L. *modulus,* small measure]. A cavity or form in which a thing is shaped.

acrylic m. *In dental surgery,* a plastic stent used in the edentulous mouth, when all or part of the mandible has been lost, to secure immobilization for an intraoral skin graft for restoring the contour of the face.

mold. To make conform to a given shape, as the fetal head.

mold [ME. *moul*]. Any one of those saprophytic fungi which form slimy or cottony growths on foodstuffs, leather, etc.

mold'ing [L. *modulus,* small measure]. The act of shaping or modeling, as changing the shape of a child's head in vertex presentations, resulting from pressure during labor.

mole [L. *moles,* mass]. 1. A mass formed in the uterus by fetal membranes or a fetus, the growth of which has become arrested or which has undergone degeneration. 2. See *nevus.*

blood m. A mass of coagulated blood and retained fetal membranes and placenta, sometimes found in the uterus after an abortion.

blue-black m. See *melanoma.*

Bren's m. See tuberous *m.*

carneous m. See fleshy *m.*

common m. See *nevus.*

cystic m. See *hydatidiform m.*

destructive m. See *chorioadenoma.*

false m. One not containing any tissues derived from a fetus or fetal membranes.

fleshy m. 1. A blood mole which has become more solid and has assumed a fleshy appearance. 2. The more or less amorphous remains of a dead fetus in the uterine cavity.

hairy m. See hairy *nevus.*

hematoma m. See tuberous *m.*

hydatidiform m. One formed by a proliferation and cystic degeneration of the chorionic villi. It may be partial or complete, involving the entire placenta. When trophoblastic proliferation is extensive, invasion of the blood vessels of the uterine wall may occur, but metastases rarely occur. Also called *hydatid m.*

invasive m. See *chorioadenoma.*

malignant m. of placenta. See *chorioadenoma.*

pigmented m. See pigmented *nevus.*

true m. One which is the remains of a fetus or fetal membranes.

tubal m. Remains of a fetus or fetal membranes in incomplete tubal abortion which have become infiltrated with blood.

tuberous m. A blood mole of highly nodular appearance, due to multiple localized hematomas of varying size under the amnion and chorionic membrane: also called *Bren's m., tuberous subchorial hematoma, ovum tuberculosum.*

vesicular m. See hydatidiform *m.*

mole, mol [*moles*]. A gram molecule, or formula weight expressed in grams. —**mo'lar,** *adj.*

mo·lec'u·lar dis"til·la'tion. Distillation performed under a very high vacuum and a short path between the distilland and the condenser so that on the average a molecule of distilland will reach the condenser surface without colliding with another molecule: more properly called *short-path, high-vacuum distillation.* See Hickman molecular distillation *process.*

mol'e·cule [dim. from *moles*]. 1. A minute mass of matter. 2. The smallest quantity into which a substance can be divided and retain its characteritics properties; or the smallest quantity that can exist in a free state. —**molec'ular,** *adj.*

mol"i·la'li·a. See *mogilalia.*

mo·li'men, mo'li·men (pl. *molimina*) [L., endeavor]. 1. Effort. 2. *In physiology,* laborious functioning. 3. *In gynecology,* nervous or circulatory symptoms accompanying menstruation.

Molisch's test. See under *test.*

Moll, Jacob Antonius [*Dutch ophthalmologist,* 1832–1914]. Described the ciliary glands, also called *Moll's glands.*

Möller, McIntosh, and Van Slyke's test. See urea clearance *test.*

Moller test. See Fabricus-Moller urine *test.*

Mollier's quadruple stain. See under *stain.*

mol·li'ti·es (mo·lish'ee·eez) [L.]. Softness.

m. ossium. See *osteomalacia.*

mol·lus'cum [L. *molluscus,* soft]. 1. A term applied to certain diseases of the skin. 2. A chronic skin disease with pulpy nodules. —**molluscous,** *adj.*

m. contagiosum. A chronic disease of the skin, characterized by the formation of pinhead-sized to pea-sized, rounded, sessile or pedunculated, waxlike elevations of a yellowish white or pinkish color, usually with central umbilication. The lesions on microscopical examination are found to contain peculiar ovoid, sharply defined bodies—molluscum bodies—which generally are considered to be forms of epithelial degeneration (the older idea that they are parasitic inclusion bodies has been abandoned). Syn., *m. epitheliale.*

m. epitheliale. See *m.* contagiosum.

m. fibrosum. Neurofibromatosis.

m. sebaceum. See *keratoacanthoma*

Moloney test. See under *test.*

Moloy, Howard Carman [*American gynecologist,* 1903–1953]. With W. E. Caldwell, classified varieties of the female pelvis according to measurement and form (1933). Called *Caldwell-Moloy classification.*

molt, moult (mohlt) [ME. *mouten,* from L. *mutare,* to change]. To shed skin, feathers, or hair.

mo·lyb'date. Any salt of molybdic acid.

mo·lyb'de·nous. See *molybdic.*

mo·lyb'de·num (mo·lib'di·num, mol"ib·dee'num) [G. *molybdaina,* piece of lead]. Mo = 95.95. A heavy metallic element. Its principal oxide, molybdite, MoO_3, forms molybdic acid.

mo·lyb'dic [*molybdaina*]. Containing trivalent or hexavalent molybdenum.

mo·lyb'dic ac'id. H_2MoO_4. Molybdic hydroxide. Colorless needles; soluble in alkalis. Used as a reagent.

mo·lyb'do-, molybd- [G. *molybdos,* lead]. 1. A combining form meaning *lead.* 2. *In chemistry,* a combining form denoting *molybdous.* 3. *In medicine,* a combining form denoting *lead poisoning.*

mo·lyb'dous. Containing divalent molybdenum.

mo·lys"mo·pho'bi·a (mo·liz"mo·fo'bee·uh, mo-lis"mo·) [G. *molysmos,* pollution; *phobos,* fear]. Morbid dread of infection or contamination.

mo'ment [L. *momentum,* moment]. The arithmetic mean of the deviations of the observations in a frequency distribution from any selected value, each raised to the same power. First power for first moment, second power for second moment, etc.

mo·men'tum [L., from *movere,* to move]. The mass of a body multiplied by its linear velocity.

mon-. See *mono-.*

mon'ad, mo'nad [G. *monas,* unit]. 1. A univalent element or radical. 2. Any of the small flagellate protozoa. 3. In miosis, one of the elements of the tetrad produced by the pairing and splitting of homologous chromosomes. Each monad is separated into a different daughter cell as the result of the two miotic divisions.

Monakow, Constantin von [*Russian neurologist in Switzerland,* 1853–1930]. Reported contralateral hemiplegia due to occlusion of the anterior choroid artery; called *Monakow's syndrome.* The rubrospinal tract is also called *Monakow's bundle, fibers, tract.*

Monaldi, Vincenzo [*Italian physician,* 1899–]. Introduced a method of draining pulmonary cavities in advanced tuberculosis, with the object of facilitating eventual closure by natural processes. Negative pressure is maintained within a cavity by means of a rubber catheter passing through the chest wall. Called *Monaldi drainage* or *method.*

mon″al·kyl′a·mine. See *alkylamine.*

mon·am′ide. An amide formed by the replacement of a hydrogen in one molecule of ammonia by an acid radical.

mon·am′ine (mon·am′een, ·in). An amine formed by the replacement of a hydrogen in one molecule of ammonia by an alkyl radical.

mon″a·my′cin. An antibiotic extracted from the green actinomycete found about the roots of the banana plant, highly active against Gram-positive bacteria.

Mo·nar′da [after *Nicolas Monardes,* Spanish physician and botanist, 1493–1588]. A genus of labiate plants, comprising **M. didyma,** the Oswego beebalm, **M. fistulosa,** the wild bergamot, and **M. punctata,** the horsemint. The last is diaphoretic, carminative, and stimulant. It is also a source of thymol.

mon·ar′thric [G. *monos,* alone; *arthron,* joint]. Pertaining to one joint.

mon″ar·thri′tis [*monos;* G. *arthritis,* arthritis]. Arthritis affecting only a single joint.

mon″ar·tic′u·lar [*monos;* L. *articulus,* joint]. Pertaining to one joint.

mon·as′ter [*monos;* G. *astēr,* star]. 1. The chromosomes in the equatorial plate at the end of the prophase of mitosis; the "mother-star." 2. The single aster formed in an aberrant type of mitosis, in which the chromosomes are doubled but the cell body does not divide.

mon″a·the·to′sis [*monos;* G. *athētos,* not fixed; *-ōsis,* condition]. Athetosis affecting one limb or side.

mon″a·tom′ic [*monos;* G. *atomos,* uncut]. 1. Having but one atom of replaceable hydrogen, as a monatomic acid. 2. Having only one atom, as a monatomic molecule. 3. Having the combining power of one atom of hydrogen, as a monatomic radical. 4. Formed by the replacement of one hydrogen atom in a compound by a radical, as a monatomic alcohol.

Mönckeberg, Johann Georg [*German pathologist,* 1877–1925]. Described medial arteriosclerosis (1903), also called *Mönckeberg's arteriosclerosis* or *disease.*

Mondeville, Henri de [*French surgeon,* ca. 1260–ca. 1320]. Pioneer advocate of cleanliness in surgery. Among the first to regard suppuration as a harmful development, not a natural stage of healing.

Mondino de' Luzzi (Mondinus, Mundinus) [*Italian anatomist,* ca. 1270–ca. 1326]. Author of a textbook of anatomy (1316) regarded as standard for more than two centuries.

mo·ne′sia (mo·nee′shuh, ·zhuh, ·see·uh, ·zee·uh) [of unknown origin]. An extract from the Brazilian tree *Pradosia lactescens.* Has been used as a stomachic, alterative, and astringent.

mo·nes′trus [G. *monos,* alone; *oistros,* gadfly]. Having only one estrus period in each sexual season, said of animals.

Monge, Carlos (1884–). Peruvian physician who described discrete forms of chronic mountain sickness affecting natives and men acclimatized at high altitudes, and relieved by descent to sea level, called *Monge's disease.* See chronic mountain *sickness.*

mon′go·lism [Mongolian *Mongol*]. A type of idiocy having some similarities to myxedema and cretinism; characterized by a broad face, flat or stubby nose, obliquely set eyes, open mouth, fat and soft skin, and flaccid muscles. Also called *mongolian idiocy.*

mon′go·loid. Having physical characteristics resembling those of mongolism.

mo·nil′e·thrix, mon″i·leth′rix [L. *monile,* necklace; G. *thrix,* hair]. A congenital and hereditary disease of the hair; characterized by dryness and fragility of the scalp hair with nodes regularly or irregularly along the hair shaft, giving it a beaded appearance. Also called *moniliform hair, beaded hair.*

Mo·nil′i·a. Synonym for *Candida.*

mo″ni·li′a·sis (mo″ni·lye′uh·sis, mon″i·) [*monile;* NL. *-iasis,* condition]. A condition produced by infection with a fungus of the genus *Candida,* usually *C. albicans.* Various parts of the body may be involved: skin, mucous membrane, nails, bronchi, lungs, vagina, and gastrointestinal tract. Rarely, a septicemia may occur. Also see *thrush, intertrigo, onychomycosis, paronychomycosis, perlèche, erosio interdigitalis blastomycetica.*

oral m. An infection in the mouth by *Candida albicans,* precancerous when chronic, occurring alone or in association with beta hemolytic streptococcus or diphtheria organism.

pharyngeal m. (a) An infection of the throat by *Candida albicans.* (b) A condition of the throat caused by debilitating systemic disease, diabetes, or unhygienic conditions.

mon′i·lid. See *candidid.*

mo·nil′i·form [*monile;* L. *forma,* form]. Constricted or jointed at intervals, as antennae; resembling a string of beads.

Mo·nil″i·for′mis [*monile; forma*]. A genus of acanthocephalan worms.

M. moniliformis. A species of worms which infests some mammals and accidentally man.

mo·nil′i·id [*monile*]. A secondary eruption characterized by sterile, grouped, vesicular lesions. It is a result of hypersensitivity and hematogenous spread from the primary focus which is caused by *Candida.* Also called *levurid.*

mon′i·tor·ing. *In nuclear science,* the periodic or continuous determination of the amount of ionizing radiation or radioactive contamination in an occupied region, or in or on personnel, as a safety measure for health protection.

Moniz. See *Egas Moniz.*

monks′hood. Aconite.

Monneret, Jules Edouard Auguste [*French physician,* 1810–68]. Drew attention to the soft, slow, full pulse associated with jaundice; called *Monneret's pulse.*

mon′o-, mon- [G. *monos,* alone]. 1. A combining form meaning *single, one,* or *alone.* 2. (mon′o-, mo′no-). *In chemistry,* a combining form denoting the presence of *one atom* or *group* of that to the name of which it is attached.

mon″o·ac′id (mon″o·ass′id, mo″no·), **mon″o·a·cid′ic** (mon″o·a·sid′ick, mo″no·). 1. Having one replaceable hydroxyl group (OH), as a monoacid base. 2. Capable of uniting directly with a molecule of a monobasic acid, with half a molecule of a dibasic acid, etc.

mon″o·ar·tic′u·lar. Monarticular.

mon″o·bas′ic (mon″o·bay′sick, mo″no·). Having one hydrogen which can be replaced by a metal or positive radical, as a monobasic acid.

mon′o·blast [*monos;* G. *blastos,* germ]. The undifferentiated progenitor of the monocytes. The nucleus has a finely granular to lacy chromatin structure, nucleoli are present, the cytoplasm shows more gray-blue than other blast cells, and may have pseudopods. Auer bodies are often present.

mon″o·blep′si·a, mon″o·blep′sis [*monos;* G. *blepsis,* act of sight]. 1. A condition in which either eye has a better visual power than both together. 2. The form of color blindness in which but one color can be perceived.

mon″o·bra′chi·us (mon″o·bray′kee·us) [*monos;* G. *brachiōn,* arm]. An individual lacking one arm congenitally.

mon″o·bra′chi·us. Characterizing a one-armed condition, congenital or acquired.

mon″o·bro′ma·ted (mon″o·bro′may·tid, mo″no·). Containing one atom of bromine in the molecule.

monocaine. Trade-mark for 2-isobutylaminoethyl-*p*-aminobenzoate, a local anesthetic. See *butethamine.*

mon″o·car′di·an [*monos;* G. *kardia,* heart]. Having a heart with a single atrium and ventricle.

mon″o·car′di·o·gram. Vectorcardiogram.

mon″o·cel′lu·lar [*monos;* L. *cellula,* small storeroom]. Unicellular.

mon″o·ceph′a·lus [*monos;* G. *kephalē,* head]. A monster consisting of a single head, with two bodies more or less completely fused. Syn., *cephalothoracopagus.*

mon″o·chlo″ro·a·ce′tic ac′id. $CH_2Cl.COOH$; colorless or white, deliquescent crystals, very soluble in water: used in manufacturing dyes and organic chemicals.

mon″o·chlo″ro·ac′e·tone (mon″o·klor″o·ass′i·tone, mo″no·) 1-Chloro-2-propanone. $CH_2Cl.-CO.CH_3$. Used in organic syntheses. In mice it inhibits cell glycolysis and stimulates tumor formation by chemical agents. Also called *chloroacetone.*

mon″o·chlor″o·meth′ane. Methyl chloride.

mon″o·chlo″ro·phe′nol. See *chlorophenol.*

mon′o·chord [G. *monochordos,* with but one string]. Old instrument for testing hearing, particularly for the higher tones of speech.

mon″o·cho·re′a (mon″o·ko·ree′uh) [G. *monos,* alone; *choreia,* dance]. Chorea confined to a single part of the body.

mon″o·chor·i·on′ic (mon″o·kor·ee·on′ick) [*monos;* G. *chorion,* chorion]. Having a common chorion, as monochorionic twins.

mon″o·chro′ic [*monos;* G. *chroia,* color]. See *monochromatic.*

mon″o·chro′ma·sy, mon″o·chro·ma′si·a (mon″o·kro·may′zhuh, ·zee·uh, ·shuh, ·see·uh) [*monos;* G. *chrōma,* color]. See total *colorblindness.*

mon″o·chro′mat, mon″o·chro′mate [*monos; chrōma*]. A person in whom all the variations of the world of color are reduced to a system of one color.

mon″o·chro·mat′ic. 1. Referring to or possessing one color or substantially one wavelength of light. 2. *In color optics,* having no variation in hue and saturation, and varying only in brightness.

mon″o·chro′ma·tism. See total *colorblindness.*

mon″o·chro·mat′o·phil [*monos; chrōma;* G. *philein,* to love]. Exhibiting a strong affinity for a single stain.

mon″o·chro′ma·tor [*monos; chrōma*]. A light-dispersing instrument used to obtain light of substantially one wave length, or at least of a very narrow band of the spectrum.

mon″o·chro′mic. See *monochroic.*

mon″o·clin′ic [*monos;* G. *klinein,* to incline]. Applied to crystals in which the vertical axis is inclined to one, but is at a right angle to the other, or lateral axis.

mon″o·coc′cus [*monos;* G. *kokkos,* berry]. A coccus occurring singly, not united in chains, pairs, or groups.

mon″o·cra′ni·us [*monos;* G. *kranion,* skull]. A double monster having a single cranium: also called *monocephalus, cephalothoracopagus.*

mon″o·cro′ta·line (mon″o·kro′tuh·leen, ·lin, mo″no·). A toxic alkaloid, $C_{16}H_{23}NO_6$, from *Crotalaria spectabilis* and *C. retusa.* Many species of this genus are used as soil-enriching legumes.

mon″o·crot′ic [*monos;* G. *krotos,* a beating]. Having but a single beat (as the normal pulse) for each cardiac systole; not dicrotic.

mon·oc′u·lar [*monos;* L. *oculus,* eye]. 1. Pertaining to or affecting only one eye, as monocular diplopia; performed with one eye only, as monocular vision. 2. Having a single ocular or eyepiece, as a monocular microscope.

mon·oc′u·lus [*monos; oculus*]. 1. A monster with but one eye; cyclops. 2. *In surgery,* a bandage for covering one eye.

mon″o·cy·e′sis (mon″o·sigh·ee′sis) [*monos;* G. *kyēsis,* pregnancy]. Pregnancy with but one fetus.

mon″o·cys′tic [*monos;* G. *kystis,* bladder]. Composed of, or containing, but one cyst.

mon′o·cyte [*monos;* G. *kytos,* cell]. A large, mononuclear leukocyte with a more or less deeply indented nucleus, slate-gray cytoplasm, and fine, usually azurophilic granulation: synonymous with, or related to, the large mononuclear cell, transitional cell, resting wandering cell, clasmatocyte, endothelial leukocyte, or histiocyte of other classification. See Plates 26, 27. —**monocyt′ic,** *adj.*

mon″o·cy·te′mic (mon″o·sigh·tee′mick) [*monos; kytos;* G. *haima,* blood]. Producing, or having the ability to produce, monocytes.

mon″o·cyt′ic se′ries. The cells concerned in the development of the adult monocyte. See *monoblast, promonocyte.*

mon″o·cy·to′ma. A rare tumor which may be derived from a stem cell of the reticular system.

mon″o·cy″to·pe′ni·a [*monos; kytos;* G. *penia,* poverty]. Diminution in the number of large mononuclear leukocytes in the peripheral circulation.

mon″o·cy·to′sis (mon″o·sigh·to′sis) [*monos; kytos;* G. *-ōsis,* increase]. Increase in the number of large mononuclear leukocytes in the peripheral circulation.

mon″o·dac′ty·lism [*monos;* G. *daktylos,* finger]. The presence of only one toe or finger on the foot or hand.

mon″o·der′mo·ma. See *teratoma.*

mon″o·di·plo′pi·a [*monos;* G. *diploos,* double; *ōps,* eye]. Double vision with a single eye.

mon″o·dro′mi·a [*monos;* G. *dromos,* course]. Unidirectional conduction in muscle or nerve.

mo·nog′a·my [*monos;* G. *gamos,* marriage]. Marriage with only one person at a time.

mon″o·gas′tric [*monos;* G. *gastēr,* belly]. Having one digestive cavity.

mon″o·ger′mi·nal [*monos;* L. *germen,* sprout]. Having or developing from a single ovum, as twins with but one chorionic sac.

mo·nog′o·ny [*monos;* G. *gonē,* offspring]. Asexual reproduction. Syn., *agamogony, agamocytogony.* —**monogonous,** *adj.*

mon″o·hy′brid [*monos;* G. *hybris,* outrage]. An individual or type heterozygous in respect to a particular pair of genes.

mon″o·hy′drate. A crystal containing one molecule of water of crystallization. —**monohydrated,** *adj.*

mon″o·hy′dric. Containing one replaceable hydrogen atom, as a monohydric alcohol or a monohydric acid.

mon″o·hy′drol. Hydrol.

mon″o-i·de′ism (mon″o-eye·dee′iz·um) [*monos;* G. *idea,* idea]. A mental condition marked by the domination of a single idea; induced by suggestion or hypnosis, wherein an elementary idea or image is left isolated and is not synthesized or associated with other ideas or impressions. Persistent and complete preoccupation with one idea.

mon″o·i·o″do·a·ce′tic ac′id. $CH_2I.COOH$; colorless or white crystals, soluble in water. Salts of the acid markedly inhibit absorption of glucose through interference with the enzyme system involved in phosphorylation of glucose; the sodium salt is used in studies of carbohydrate metabolism. Also called *iodoacetic acid.*

mon″o·ke′tone. A ketone containing one CO group.

mon″o·loc′u·lar. See *unilocular.*

mon″o·ma′ni·a [*monos;* G. *mania,* madness]. A form of mental disorder in which the patient's thoughts and actions are dominated by one subject or one idea, as in paranoia. —**monomaniac,** *adj., n.*

mon″o·mel′ic [*monos;* G. *melos,* limb]. Pertaining to one limb, as monomelic hyperostosis.

m. hyperostosis. See *melorheostosis.*

mon′o·mer. The simplest molecular form of a substance, as distinguished from a *dimer* or from a *polymer.*

mon″o·mer′ic [*monos;* G. *meros,* part]. Consisting of a single piece or segment.

monomestrol. Trade-mark for the monomethyl ether of diethylstilbestrol, a white, crystalline powder, practically insoluble in water but soluble in oil; it is employed as an estrogen. See *mestilbol.*

mon″o·mo′ri·a. Melancholia. *Obs.*

mon″o·mor′phic [*monos;* G. *morphē,* form]. Having or existing in only one form.

mon″o·mor′phous [*monos; morphē*]. Having a single form or the same appearance; not polymorphous.

mo·nom′pha·lus [*monos;* G. *omphalos,* navel]. Conjoined twins with a common umbilical cord.

mon″o·neph′rous [*monos;* G. *nephros,* kidney]. Limited to one kidney.

mon″o·neu′ral [*monos;* G. *neuron,* nerve]. 1. Pertaining to a single nerve. 2. Receiving branches from but one nerve; said of muscles.

mon″o·neu·ri′tis [*monos; neuron;* G. *-itis,* inflammation]. Neuritis affecting a single nerve.

m. multiplex. Neuritis affecting simultaneously single nerves remote from each other.

mon″o·nu′cle·ar. Possessing only one nucleus.

mon″o·nu′cle·ar cell. A monocyte or a histiocyte: occasional usage.

mon″o·nu″cle·o′sis [*monos;* L. *nucleus,* nut; G. *-ōsis,* condition]. A condition of the blood or tissues in which there is an increase in the number of large mononuclear leukocytes or monocytes above the normal.

infectious m. A communicable disease of unknown etiology, with fever, sore throat, generalized swollen lymph nodes, especially those of the posterior cervical area, and an increase in abnormal mononuclear cells. There may be a rubelliform eruption and enlargement of the spleen. Also called *Pfeiffer's disease, glandular fever, lymphocytic angina, monocytic angina.* Syn., *acute benign lymphoblastosis.*

mon″o·nu′cle·o·tide. A product obtained by hydrolytic decomposition of nucleic acid; it is a compound of phosphoric acid, a hexose or pentose, and a purine or pyrimidine base such as guanine, adenine, cytosine, or uracil.

mon″o·pa·re′sis (mon″o·pa·ree′sis, ·par′i·sis) [*monos;* G. *paresis,* paralysis]. Paresis of a single part of the body, as of one limb.

mon″o·pha′gi·a [*monos;* G. *phagein,* to eat]. 1. Desire for a single article of food. 2. The eating of a single daily meal.

mo·noph′a·gism [*monos; phagein*]. Habitual eating of a single article of food.

mon″o·pha′si·a (mon″o·fay′zhuh, ·zee·uh) [*monos;* G. *phasis,* utterance]. A form of aphasia in which speech is limited to a single syllable, word, or phrase.

mon″o·pha′sic (mon″o·fay′zick) [*monos; phasis*]. Having a single phase.

mon″o·pho′bi·a [*monos;* G. *phobos,* fear]. Morbid dread of being alone.

mon″o·phos′phate. A phosphate with but one atom of phosphorus in the molecule.

mon″oph·thal′mi·a [*monos;* G. *ophthalmos,* eye]. Congenital absence of one eye. Also called *unilateral anophthalmia.*

mon″o·phy·let′ic (mon″o·figh·let′ick) [*monos;* G. *phyletikos,* of a tribe]. Pertaining to, or derived from, a single original ancestral type; opposed to *polyphyletic.*

mon″o·phy′o·dont [*monos;* G. *phyein,* to grow; *odous,* tooth]. Having but a single set of teeth, the permanent ones.

mon″o·ple′gi·a [*monos;* G. *plēgē,* a stroke]. Paralysis of a single limb or of a single muscle or group of muscles. It is designated as brachial, crural, or facial, when affecting the arm, the leg, or the face, respectively, and as central or peripheral, according to the seat of the causal lesion.

mon″o·po′di·a [*mono;* G. *pous,* foot]. The condition of having but one lower limb.

sirenoid m. Congenital absence of a lower limb in gastroschisis.

mon′ops. See *cyclops.*

mo·nop′si·a. See *monophthalmia.*

mon″o·psy·cho′sis (mon″o·sigh·ko′sis) [*monos;* G. *psychōsis,* a giving soul or life to]. Old term for monomania.

mon″o·pty′chi·al (mon″o·tye′kee·ul) [*monos;* G. *ptychē,* fold]. Arranged in a single layer, as the epithelial cells of some glands.

mon′o·pus [*monos;* G. *pous,* foot]. An individual with congenital absence of one foot or leg.

mon″o·ra·dic′u·lar [*monos;* L. *radicula,* small root]. Having only one root, said of teeth.

mon·or′chid (mon·or′kid) [*monos;* G. *orchis,* testis]. A person who has but one testis, or in whom only one testis has descended into the scrotum.

mon·or′chid·ism, mon·or′chism [*monos; orchis*]. Congenital absence of one testis. —**monorchid,** *adj.*

mon″o·rrhi′nous [*monos;* G. *rhis,* nose]. Having a single median nasal cavity.

mon″o·sac′cha·ride (mon″o·sack′uh·ride, ·rid, mo″no·). A carbohydrate which cannot be hydrolyzed to a simpler carbohydrate, hence called a *simple sugar;* chemically, a polyhydric alcohol having reducing properties associated with an actual or potential aldehyde or ketone group. It may contain 3–10 carbon atoms, and on this basis be classified as a triose, tetrose, pentose, hexose, heptose, octose, nonose, or decose. A diose, glycolaldehyde, is by some classed as a monosaccharide, but does not exhibit the characteristic properties of the class.

mon″o·scel′ous [*monos;* G. *skelos,* leg]. One-legged. *Rare.*

mon′ose. See *monosaccharide.*

mon″o·so′di·um glu′ta·mate. $HOOC.CH(NH_2)$-CH_2CH_2COONa. White or nearly white powder, very soluble in water; possesses a meatlike taste.

Employed to impart meat flavor to foods and to enhance other natural food flavors. Syn., *sodium glutamate, MSG.*

mon″o·som′a·tous (mon″o·som′uh·tus, ·so′muh-tus) [*monos;* G. *sōma,* body]. Pertaining to a monstrosity involving a single individual.

mon′o·some [*monos; sōma*]. Accessory chromosome.

mon″o·so′mus [*monos; sōma*]. A double monster with a fused trunk and two heads.

Mon″o·spo′ri·um [*monos;* G. *sporos,* seed]. A genus of the Fungi imperfecti. The species **M. apio-spermum** and **M. scleriotiale** have been isolated in cases of white-grained mycetoma.

mo″no·ste′a·rin. Glyceryl monostearate.

mon″o·stot′ic. Involving only one bone.

mon″o·stra′tal [*monos;* L. *stratum,* covering]. Arranged in a single layer or stratum.

mon″o·symp″to·mat′ic [*monos;* G. *symptōmati-kos,* accidental]. Having but one dominant symptom.

mon″o·ter′pene. A terpene having a composition represented by $C_{10}H_{16}$.

mon″o·ther′mi·a [*monos;* G. *thermē,* heat]. Evenness of body temperature.

mon·o′tic, mon·ot′ic [*monos;* G. *ous,* ear]. Pertaining to or affecting but one of the ears.

mo·not′o·cous [*monos;* G. *tokos,* childbirth]. Producing one young at a birth.

mo·not′ri·chous (mo·not′ri·kus), **mon″o·trich′ic** (mon″o·trick′ick) [*monos;* G. *thrix,* hair]. Characterizing a unicellular organism in which there is but one flagellum.

mon″o·trop′ic. Describing a substance occurring in one crystalline form only.

mon″o·va′lent, mo·nov′a·lent. See *univalent.*

mo·nox′e·nous [*monos;* G. *xenos,* host]. *In parasitology,* confined to a single species of host.

mon·ox′ide. 1. An oxide containing a single oxygen atom. 2. A popular name for carbon monoxide.

mon″o·zy·got′ic (mon″o·zye·got′ick, ·go′tick) [*monos; zygōtos,* yoked]. Developed from a single fertilized egg or zygote, as identical twins.

Monro, Alexander (Primus) [*Scottish anatomist,* 1697–1767]. Described an intratendinous bursa of the olecranon (1726); called *Monro's bursa.* Is sometimes credited with describing the structures named for his son.

Monro, Alexander (Secundus) [*Scottish anatomist,* 1733–1817]. Made a study of the nervous system. Described the interventricular foramen, also called *foramen of Monro,* and the hypothalamic sulcus, also called *sulcus of Monro.*

mons (pl. *montes*) [L., mountain]. *In anatomy,* an eminence.

m. pubis. The eminence in front of the body and superior ramus of the os pubis.

m. veneris. The mons pubis of the female.

Monsel's salt. Ferric subsulfate.

Monsel's solution. Ferric subsulfate solution.

mon′ster [L. *monstrum,* evil omen]. A fetus (rarely an adult) which, through congenital faulty development, is incapable of properly performing the vital functions, or which, owing to an excess or deficiency of parts, differs markedly from the normal type of the species; a teratism. For a simplified classification of monsters, see Table in the Appendix. See Plate 25.

mon′stri·cide [*monstrum;* L. *caedere,* to kill]. The killing of a monster.

mon·strip′a·ra [*monstrum;* L. *parere,* to bring forth]. A woman who has given birth to one or more monsters.

mon·stros′i·ty [*monstrum*]. 1. The condition of being a monster. 2. A monster. See Plate 25.

mon′tan wax. A hard wax obtained by extraction of lignite; a dark-brown substance which becomes white on bleaching, insoluble in water, soluble in chloroform and carbon tetrachloride: a substitute for carnauba and beeswax.

Monteggia, Giovanni Battista [*Italian surgeon,* 1762–1815]. Dislocation of the hip toward the anterior superior iliac spine is known as *Monteggia's dislocation.* A fracture of the upper shaft of the ulna, associated with a dislocation of the head of the radius, is known as *Monteggia's fracture-dislocation.*

Montenegro's test. See under *test.*

Montgomery, William Fetherston [*Irish obstetrician,* 1797–1859]. Described epithelial depressions in the uterine mucosa; called *Montgomery's cups.* See also *areolar glands,* under *gland;* also called *Montgomery's tubercles* or *glands.*

mon·tic′u·lus [L., small mountain]. A small elevation.

m. cerebelli. The prominent central portion of the superior vermiform process of the cerebellum.

mont″mo·ril′lo·nite. $Al_2Si_4O_{10}(OH)_2.nH_2O$; the principal mineral constituent of bentonite and fuller's earth, occurring as a white or grayish to rose-blue claylike substance with a smooth, greasy texture.

mood [AS. *mōd,* mind]. *In psychology,* a sustained emotional or feeling tone, such as in mania or melancholia.

moogrol. Trade-mark for *ethyl chaulmoograte.*

Moon, Robert Charles [*American ophthalmologist,* 1844–1914]. With Laurence, described familial retinitis pigmentosa associated with general defective development (1866). See Laurence-Moon-Biedl *syndrome.*

Moon's molars. See *dome-shaped molars,* under *molar.*

Moore, Austin Talley [*American orthopedic surgeon,* 1899–]. Known for his device for maintaining position in intracapsular fractures. It consists of a large metal pin with threaded ends for holding a nut, the metal rod being passed through the cortical bone of the femur into the femoral head. Several pins are used, all joined by wire to prevent extrusion; called *Austin Moore's pins.*

Moore, Charles Hewitt [*English surgeon,* 1821–70]. With Charles Murchison, introduced an operation for aneurysm in which a fine wire is introduced into the aneurysmal sac (1864). Formulated certain principles on which the modern surgical treatment of cancer is based (1867).

Moore, Robert Foster [*English ophthalmologist,* 1878–]. Introduced the treatment of neoplasms of the choroid by means of intraocular radon seeds (1930); called *Foster Moore's technic.*

Moore, Thomas [*English biochemist,* 1900–]. Introduced a unit of vitamin A equal to 60 international units; called *blue unit of Moore.*

Moore's test. See under *test.*

Mooren, Albert [*German ophthalmologist,* 1828–99]. Rodent ulcer of the cornea is known as *Mooren's ulcer.*

Mooser test. See Neill-Mooser *test.*

mor·ad′e·ine (mor·ad′ee·een, ·in). An alkaloid from the bark of *Pogonopus tubulosus,* of South America.

mor″a·men′ti·a (mor″uh·men′shuh). The state of being entirely without moral sense. *Obs.*

moranyl. A trade-mark for *suramin.*

Morax, Victor [*French ophthalmologist,* 1866–1935]. In the same year as Axenfeld, isolated *Hemophilus duplex,* also called *Moraxella lacunata, Morax-Axenfeld bacillus* (1896). Chronic conjunctivitis caused by this diplobacillus is known as *Morax-Axenfeld conjunctivitis.*

Mor″ax·el′la [after Victor *Morax*]. A genus of bacteria, family Parvobacteriaceae.

M. lacunata. The type species of the genus. It is a nonmotile, Gram-negative, short rod, occurring singly, in pairs, or in short chains. Also called *Morax-Axenfeld bacillus.*

mor'bi (mor'buy) [L. *morbus*, disease]. Of a disease, as materies morbi, the agent producing a disease.

mor'bid [L. *morbidus*, diseased]. Pertaining to disease or diseased parts, as morbid anatomy, an old term for pathologic anatomy.

mor·bid'i·ty [*morbidus*]. 1. The quality of disease or of being diseased. 2. The conditions inducing disease. 3. The ratio of the number of sick individuals to the total population of a community.

mor·bid'i·ty rate. The number of cases of a specific disease in a calendar year in a given place per 100,000 actual or estimated population at the middle of the year.

mor·bif'ic [L. *morbus*, disease; *facere*, to make]. Old term for producing disease; pathogenic.

mor·bil'li (mor·bil'eye) [ML.]. Old term for measles. —**morbilliform,** *adj.*

mor'bus [L.]. Obsolete term for disease.

cholera m. See *cholera* morbus.

m. anglicus. Rickets.

m. arcuatus. Icterus.

m. caducus. Epilepsy.

m. caeruleus. Congenital cyanosis due to venoarterial shunt: also called *maladie bleu.*

m. cardiacus. See *m.* cordis.

m. castrensis. Classic epidemic typhus.

m. coeliacus. See celiac *disease.*

m. cordis. Chronic cardiac disease.

m. coxae. Hip disease; tuberculous coxitis.

m. cucullaris. Pertussis; whooping cough.

m. divinus. Epilepsy.

m. gallicus. Syphilis.

m. hungaricus. Classic epidemic typhus.

m. maculosis Werlhofi. See idiopathic thrombocytopenic *purpura.*

m. maculosus neonatorum. A fatal disease occurring during the first few days of life and consisting of hemorrhages in various parts of the body.

m. magnus. Epilepsy.

m. major. Epilepsy.

m. medicorum. The mania of those who seek the advice of physicians for imaginary diseases.

m. miseriae. Any disease due to poverty.

m. Pageti papillae. See Paget's *disease* (b).

m. phlyctenoides. Pemphigus.

m. pulicaris. Classic epidemic typhus.

m. regius. Jaundice.

m. sacer. Epilepsy.

m. saltatorius. Chorea.

m. vesicularis. Pemphigus.

m. virgineus. Chlorosis.

m. vulpis. Alopecia.

mor"cel·la'tion [F. *morceller*, to divide into pieces]. The act of reducing to fragments, as the fetus in embryotomy; the removal of a tumor or fetus piecemeal. *Obs.*

mor·da'cious [L. *mordax*, biting]. Biting, pungent.

mor'dant [L. *mordere*, to bite]. A substance, such as alum, phenol, aniline oil, that fixes the dyes used in coloring textiles or in staining tissues and bacteria.

Morel, Ferdinand [*French psychiatrist*, 1888–]. Described as a stigma of degeneracy a large, prominent ear in which the ridges and grooves appear to have been obliterated; called *Morel ear.* Metabolic craniopathy is known as *Morel's syndrome, Morgagni's syndrome, Stewart-Morel syndrome* (for Morel and R. M Stewart). Dementia precox is also called *Morel-Kraepelin disease.*

Morgagni, Giovanni Battista [*Italian anatomist and pathologist,* 1682–1771]. Considered the founder of the science of pathologic anatomy. Described aortic insufficiency, mitral stenosis, and angina pectoris (1761). Gave a classic description of heart block (1761), called *Morgagni's disease, Stokes-Adams syndrome.* Metabolic craniopathy is known as *Morgagni's syndrome.* Small mucous glands in the male urethra are known as the *glands of Morgagni* or *Littré's glands,* and their orifices are called the *lacunas of Morgagni.* The middle lobe of the prostate is called *Morgagni's caruncle.* The *columns of Morgagni* are the vertical folds of the rectum. The spaces between them just above the anal canal are known as the *sinuses of Morgagni;* here the columns join to form the *valves of Morgagni.* The term *sinus of Morgagni* also refers to the space between the upper border of the levator veli palatini and the base of the skull; this is closed by the pharyngeal aponeurosis. The laryngeal ventricle is known as the *ventricle of Morgagni.* The superior nasal concha is called *Morgagni's concha.* See also Morgagnian *cataract, hydatid* of Morgagni, *foramen* of Morgagni.

Morgan, Thomas Hunt (1866–1945). American geneticist who discovered the function of chromosomes in heredity; his studies of Drosophilae provided evidence that the chromosome actually bears the genes. Nobel laureate in medicine and physiology (1933).

Morgan's bacillus. See *Proteus morganii.*

morgue [F.]. 1. A place where unknown dead are exposed for identification. 2. A place where dead bodies are stored pending disposition.

mo'ri·a [G. *mōria*, folly]. 1. A dementia characterized by talkativeness and silliness. 2. A morbid desire to joke.

mor'i·bund [L. *moribundus*, dying]. In a dying condition.

Morison, James Rutherford [*English surgeon,* 1853–1939]. With David Drummond, devised an operation of omentopexy to relieve ascites in cirrhosis of the liver by establishing collateral circulation (1896). A similar technic was introduced independently by Talma (1898). The operation is known as the *Morison-Talma* or *Talma-Morison operation.* Also see *hepatorenal pouch.*

Mörner's reagent. See under *reagent.*

morn'ing sick'ness. Nausea and vomiting occurring on arising, an early symptom of pregnancy.

Moro reflex. See under *reflex.*

Moro test. See under *test.*

mo'ron [G. *mōros*, dull, stupid]. One afflicted with moronity.

mo·ron'i·ty [*mōros*]. The highest grade of mental deficiency in which the subject's mental age is from 7 to 12 years and his I.Q. between 50 and 74. Syn., *morosis.*

mo·ro'sis. See *moronity.*

mor·phe'a [G. *morphē*, form]. Localized scleroderma.

mor'phi·a. See *morphine.*

mor'phine (mor'feen, ·fin, mor·feen') (*morphina*). $C_{17}H_{19}NO_3.H_2O$. Discovered by Sertürner in 1806. A colorless or white crystalline alkaloid obtained from opium, to which the chief effects of the latter are due. Differs from opium in being less constipating, and less likely to produce disagreeable aftereffects. Frequently acts as an allergen. Because of its insolubility in water morphine is used principally in the form of its salts. Dose, of morphine salts, 0.005–0.032 Gm. ($\frac{1}{12}$–$\frac{1}{2}$ gr.).

m. acetate. $C_{17}H_{19}NO_3.C_2H_4O_2.3H_2O$. Once popular but now rarely used because of its instability.

m. hydrochloride (*morphinae hydrochloridum*). $C_{17}H_{19}NO_3.HCl.3H_2O$; a morphine salt much used in Great Britain but not in the United States.

m. stearate. $C_{17}H_{19}NO_3.C_{17}H_{35}COOH$, contains 50% of morphine; used in oil or fat vehicles.

m. sulfate (*morphinae sulfas*). $(C_{17}H_{19}NO_3)_2.H_2SO_4.5H_2O$; in this country the most frequently prescribed morphine salt.

m. tartrate. $(C_{17}H_{19}NO_3)_2.C_4H_6O_6.3H_2O$, formerly official in the British Pharmacopoeia; recommended for hypodermic use because it is slightly more soluble in water than either the hydrochloride or the sulfate.

mor′phin·ism [G. *Morpheus*, god of dreams]. 1. The condition caused by the habitual use of morphine. 2. The morphine habit.

mor″phi·no·ma′ni·a, mor″phi·o·ma′ni·a [*Morpheus;* G. *mania*, madness]. A morbid craving for morphine.

mor″pho·bi·om′e·try. The statistics of the shape, size, and structure of living things or parts thereof. **—morphobiomet′ric,** *adj.*

mor″pho·gen′e·sis [G. *morphē*, form; *genesis*, production]. The morphologic transformations including growth, alterations of germinal layers, and differentiation of cells and tissues during development. Also called *topogenesis.* **—morphogenet′ic,** *adj.*

mor·phog′e·ny. See *morphogenesis.*

mor′pho·line. C_4H_9NO; tetrahydro-1,4,*2H*-oxazine; a colorless, hygroscopic, oily base with an ammonialike odor, possessing caustic, alkaline properties, soluble in water and miscible with organic solvents: used as a solvent for resins, waxes, shellac, and dyestuffs.

mor·phol′o·gy [*morphē;* G. *logos*, word]. The branch of biology which deals with structure and form. It includes the anatomy, histology, and cytology of the organism at any stage of its life history. **—morpholog′ic, morpholog′ical,** *adj.;* **morphol′ogist,** *n.*

mor·phom′e·try [*morphē;* G. *metron*, a measure]. The measurement of the forms of organisms.

Morquio, Luis (1867–1935). Uruguayan physician known for his description (1929) of chondro-osteodystrophy, also called *Morquio-Brailsford disease.*

mors [L.]. Death.

m. putativa. Apparent death.

m. subita. Sudden death.

mor′sal [L. *morsus*, a biting]. Relating to the cutting or grinding portion of a tooth; occlusal.

Morson's napelline. See British *aconitine.*

mor′sus [L.]. A bite.

m. stomachi. See *cardialgia.*

m. ventriculi. See *cardialgia.*

mor′tal [L. *mortalis*, mortal]. Liable to death or dissolution; terminating in death; causing death; deadly.

mor·tal′i·ty [L. *mortalitas*, mortality]. 1. The quality of being mortal. 2. The death rate.

mor′tar [L. *mortarium*, large basin or trough in which mortar is made]. An urn-shaped vessel of porcelain, iron, or glass; used for pulverizing substances by means of a pestle.

mor″ti·fi·ca′tion. Old term for gangrene.

mor″ti·na·tal′i·ty [L. *mors*, death; *natalis*, natal]. The stillbirth rate.

Morton, Dudley J. (1894–). American orthopedist who described Morton's *syndrome.*

Morton, Thomas George (1835–1903). American surgeon who described a specific type of metatarsalgia.

Morton, William Thomas Green [*American dentist*, 1819–68]. Independently of Crawford W. Long, discovered the anesthetic properties of sulfuric ether, and demonstrated its value first in tooth extraction and later in a surgical operation performed by John Collins Warren (1846). Sometimes called the discoverer of ether anesthesia, although probably the credit should go to Long.

mor′tu·ar″y (mor′choo·err″ee) [L. *mortuarius*, of the dead]. A morgue.

mor′tu·ar″y. Relating to death or burial.

mor′u·la (mor′yoo·luh, mor′oo·luh) [dim. from L. *morum*, mulberry]. A type of solid blastula, without a blastocoele but having central cells not reaching the free surface. Frequently used, incorrectly, for the late cleavage stage of the mammalian ovum.

Mo′rus. See *mulberry.*

Morvan, Augustin Marie [*French physician*, 1819–97]. Described a form of syringomyelia characterized by atrophy and analgesic paralysis of the forearms and hands and by paronychia; called *analgesic panaris, Morvan's disease.*

mor′vin. See *mallein.*

moryl. Trade-mark for carbachol.

mo·sa′ic [ML. *musaicus*, from G. *Museios*, belonging to the Muses]. 1. A pattern made on a surface by the assembly and arrangement of many small pieces. 2. *In genetics*, an individual with adjacent tissues of different genetic constitution, as a result of mutation, somatic crossing over, or chromosome elimination. 3. *In embryology*, an egg in which the cells of the early cleavage stages have already a type of cytoplasm which determines its later fate. See *regulative.* 4. *In plant pathology*, a plant infected with a virus which produces a characteristic spotting, as in tobacco mosaic disease.

mo·sa′ic bone. Microscopically, bone appearing as though formed of small pieces fitted together, due to cement lines indicating regional alternating periods of osteogenesis and osteoclasis; characteristic of Paget's disease.

mo·sa′ic fun′gus. See under *fungus.*

Moschcowitz, Alexis Victor [*American surgeon*, 1865–1933]. Introduced improvements in the technic of the operation for femoral hernia by the inguinal approach. Devised an operation for rectal prolapse in which an abdominal approach is made and the rectum is sutured to the pelvic fascia to obliterate the cul-de-sac. Each operation is called *Moschcowitz's operation.*

Moschcowitz, Eli [*American physician*, 1879–]. Contributed to the knowledge of sclerosis of arteries and veins. Made important studies of the natural history of diseases.

Mosenthal test. See under *test.*

Mosetig-Moorhof, Albert von [*Austrian surgeon*, 1838–1907]. Introduced iodoform dressings in surgery (1882). Introduced a bone wax consisting of iodoform, spermaceti, and sesame oil; called *Mosetig-Moorhof's bone wax.*

mos·qui′to [Sp., from L. *musca*, fly]. An insect of the family Culicidae.

Moss, William Lorenzo [*American hematologist*, 1876–]. Independently of Janský, demonstrated that human blood can be classified in four groups (1910); see *blood groups.*

moss [ME. *mos*]. Low green bryophytic plants of the class Musci.

Ceylon m. See *agar*, 1.

club m. See *lycopodium.*

Iceland m. See *Cetraria.*

Irish m. See *Chondrus.*

reindeer m. *Cladonia rangiferina.*

Mossman fever. A fever noted among agricultural workers in the Mossman District of Australia. It is transmitted by a mite of the genus *Trombicula*, and is characterized by swelling of the inguinal lymph nodes.

Mosso, Angelo [*Italian physiologist*, 1846–1910]. Made many contributions to the knowledge of physiology. Introduced an ergograph for the study of voluntary contraction of muscle (1890).

Made important studies in fatigue (1891). Engaged in researches on the action of respiration at high altitudes (1897). Inventor of a sphygmomanometer (1895).

mos'sy foot. See *chromoblastomycosis.*

Moszkowicz, Ludwig [*Austrian surgeon,* 1873–]. Devised a test to determine the proper site for amputation of a limb, as in gangrene. The limb is elevated until pallor is observed. An elastic bandage or a tourniquet is then applied as high as possible on the limb, to obstruct the artery, and is left in place for a few minutes. When the bandage or tourniquet is removed a hyperemic blush spreads rapidly over the well-vascularized areas, but pallor persists where the blood supply is inadequate. Amputation should not be performed within the paler areas. Called *Moszkowicz's test, hyperemia test of Moszkowicz.*

Motais, Ernst [*French ophthalmologist,* 1845–1913]. Devised an operation for ptosis in which the middle portion of the tendon of the superior rectus muscle of the eyelid is transplanted into the eyelid; called *Motais' operation.*

moth'er [AS. *mōdor*]. 1. A female parent. 2. The source of anything.

moth'er [MD. *modder,* filth]. A slimy film formed on the surface of fermenting liquid, as on vinegar.

moth patch'es. Chloasma. *Obs.*

mo'tile (mo'til) [L. *motum,* from *movere,* to move]. Able to move; capable of spontaneous motion, as a motile flagellum.

mo·til'i·ty [*motum*]. Ability to move spontaneously.

gastric m. The movements of the stomach walls, including those caused by gastric secretions and peristalsis.

mo'tion [L. *motio,* from *movere*]. 1. The act of changing place; movement 2. An evacuation of the bowels; the matter evacuated.

passive m. The movement produced by external agency and not by the person himself.

vermicular m. Peristalsis.

mo'tion sick'ness. A syndrome characterized by nausea, vertigo, and vomiting; occurs as the result of the motion of a ship, airplane, train, or automobile. See *airsickness, seasickness.*

mo"to·neu'ron. See motor *neuron.*

mo"to·neu"ro·ni'tis. See Guillain-Barré *syndrome.*

mo'tor [L., from *movere*]. That which causes motion.

club m. See plastic *m.*

knob m. See plastic *m.*

loop m. See plastic *m.*

m. end-plate. Myoneural junction. An area of specialized structure beneath the sarcolemma where a motor nerve fiber makes functional contact with a muscle fiber.

m. meal. See under *test meal.*

m. oculi. The third cranial or oculomotor nerve supplying all the extrinsic muscles of the eye except the superior oblique and lateral rectus. *Obs.*

m. points. The points on the surface of the body where the various branches of the motor nerves supplying the muscles may be excited by electric stimuli.

plastic m. A tissue motor fashioned from muscle or tendon covered with skin, in the form of a knob, loop, or tunnel to which is attached a loop or ring; devised in certain kineplastic amputations and used in connection with a prosthesis, notably in amputations of the upper extremity. Where the point of attachment is a knob, it is known as a club motor; where the attachment is formed by joining opposing tendons and muscles, it is called a loop motor; where it is in the form of a tunnel through the muscle, it is referred to as a tunnel motor.

tunnel m. See plastic *m.*

mo'tor. Pertaining to or involving motion, as a motor cell, motor center, motor nerve.

Mott, Frederick Walter (1853–1926). English neurologist who demonstrated the thalamic connections of the medial lemniscus, and showed that the projection of impulses from each ear was bilateral.

Mott, Valentine [*American surgeon,* 1785–1865]. Known for his vascular and bone surgery. Ligated the innominate artery (1818). Ligated the carotid artery for tumor of the jaw (1822). Ligated the common iliac artery (1827) and the subclavian (1831). Amputated successfully at the hip joint (1824).

mot'tled en·am'el. A dappled condition of the teeth caused by hypocalcification or hypoplasia with or without later extraneous staining; chronic dental fluorosis.

mot'tling [L. *mustela,* weasel]. A spotted condition.

mouches vo·lantes'. See *muscae volitantes.*

mou"lage' (mōō"lahzh') [F.]. A mold or cast made directly from any portion of the body, used especially to show a surface lesion or defect.

mould. See *mold.*

mound [D. *mond,* protection]. An elevation.

anal m. *In embryology,* a mound produced by the anterior median union of the anal tubercles.

mound'ing [*mond*]. The rising in a lump of muscle fibers when struck by a slight, firm blow. It is observed in the thin and feeble, and in certain diseases, as pulmonary tuberculosis and advanced locomotor ataxia. See *myoedema.*

moun'tain balm. *Eriodictyon californicum.*

moun'tain sick'ness. See *chronic mountain sickness* under *sickness.*

moun'tant [F. *montant,* from *monter,* to rise]. Any medium such as balsam or glycerin in which histological sections or specimens are embedded on slides for microscopic study. Syn., *mounting medium.*

mouse'pox'. A contagious disease of mice characterized by a puffy appearance about the face and inflammation of the foot pads. At autopsy the liver is pale and mottled; the proximal portion of the small intestine is hemorrhagic; and there is pulmonary congestion and consolidation. The disease is highly contagious, and is usually fatal.

mouth [AS. *mūth*]. 1. The commencement of the alimentary canal; the cavity in which mastication takes place. In a restricted sense, the aperture between the lips. 2. The entrance to any cavity or canal.

primitive m. See *blastopore.*

trench m. Vincent's stomatitis.

mouve·ment' de ma·nège' (moov·mahn' duh ma·nezh'. *See* NOTES §35) [F.]. The movement of the trunk to the same side as that on which a unilateral lesion has been produced experimentally in the frontal lobe, in front of the areas controlling the arm, face, and jaw.

move'ment [L. *movere,* to move]. The act of moving.

accessory m. See *synkinesia.*

active m. Movement effected without any outside help.

ameboid m. A movement produced in certain cells, as the white blood cells, by the protrusion of processes of the cytoplasm into which the whole cell then seems to flow; so called from the resemblance of the movement to that of the ameba.

angular m. The movement between two bones that may take place forward or backward, inward or outward.

associated automatic m. See *synkinesia.*

associated movements. Synergic, coincident, or consensual movements of muscles other than the leading one, which are involuntarily connected with its action; as in reading both eyeballs move alike although one eye may be blind.

bowel m. Lay term for: (a) the evacuation of feces; an act of defecation; (b) the feces evacuated by defecation; a stool.

Brownian m. A physical phenomenon, a form of communicated motion observed in aggregations of minute particles, and consisting of a rapid oscillating movement without change of the relative position of the moving particles. Also called *pedesis.*

ciliary m. A lashing movement produced by delicate hairlike processes termed cilia, as on the epithelium of the respiratory tract and in certain microorganisms.

circus m. Rapid, circular movements or somersaults, produced by injury on one side to some part of the posture-controlling mechanisms of the nervous system, as the vestibular apparatus or the cerebral peduncles.

dead beat m. A movement of the string of the electrocardiograph which shows no preliminary overshooting of its proper mark.

eccentric m. Any movement of the mandible away from centric occlusion.

fetal m. The movement of the fetus in the uterus.

forced m. Movement of the body from injury of the motor centers or the conducting paths.

gliding m. The simplest movement that can take place in a joint, one surface gliding or moving over another, without any angular or rotatory movement.

ideomotor m. Unconscious movement when the attention is otherwise absorbed.

index m. Movement of the cephalic part of the body about the fixed caudal part.

molecular m. See Brownian *m.*

passive m. Movement effected by the aid of some outside agency.

percussion movements. *In massage,* a series of blows delivered to the surface of a region in rapid succession: called beating, clapping, hacking, slapping, and tapping. Syn., *tapotement.*

rolling m. The rolling of an animal on its long axis.

segmenting m. of the small intestine. Spaced constrictions of the intestinal lumen at successive points along the intestine, acting to expose repeatedly new surfaces of the intestinal contents to the action of digestive juices.

Swedish m. Kinetotherapy. See *kinesiatrics.*

synkinetic m. See *synkinesia.*

vermicular m. Peristalsis.

nox'a [Jap. *moe kusa,* burning herb]. A combustible material which is applied to the skin and ignited for the purpose of producing an eschar or counterirritant. It is made with the down of dried leaves of several species of *Artemisia.* **Artificial moxa** is made from cotton saturated with niter.

electric m. A faradic brush used as an active electrode upon dry skin.

Moynihan, Berkeley George Andrew [*English surgeon,* 1865–1936]. Introduced several procedures in gastrointestinal surgery. Devised a clamp called *Moynihan's clamp.* Hunger pain three or more hours after eating, indicative of duodenal ulcer, is known as *Moynihan's symptom complex.*

Mo"zam·bique' ul'cer. See tropical *ulcer.*

m.p. Melting point.

MPI. Multiphasic personality inventory. See *Minnesota multiphasic personality inventory* under *test.*

M. R. C. Medical Reserve Corps.

M. R. C. P. Member of the Royal College of Physicians.

M. R. C. P. E. Member of the Royal College of Physicians of Edinburgh.

M. R. C. P. I. Member of the Royal College of Physicians of Ireland.

M. R. C. S. Member of the Royal College of Surgeons.

M. R. C. S. E. Member of the Royal College of Surgeons of Edinburgh.

M. R. C. S. I. Member of the Royal College of Surgeons of Ireland.

M. R. C. V. S. Member of the Royal College of Veterinary Surgeons.

mrd Millirutherford.

M. S. Master of Surgery, Master of Science.

M. Sc. Master of Science.

MSG Monosodium glutamate.

MSH Melanocyte-stimulating hormone.

$MsTh_1$ Mesothorium-1.

$MsTh_2$ Mesothorium-2.

M. U., M. u. Mache unit.

m. u. Mouse unit.

Much, Hans Christian R. (1880–1932). German physician who described Gram-positive, nonacid-fast granules, seen in sputum, which he believed to be modified tubercle bacilli, called *Much's bacilli, granules.* With Holzmann, he claimed that the serum of a dementia precox patient inhibited hemolysis by cobra venom; this is called the *Much-Holzmann reaction.*

mu'cic acid. COOH.HCOH.HOCH.HOCH.-HCOH.COOH; the dibasic acid resulting from oxidation of D-galactose or from carbohydrates yielding this sugar. Syn., D-*galactosaccharic acid.*

mu·cif'er·ous [L. *mucus,* mucus; *ferre,* to bear]. Producing or secreting mucus.

mu'ci·gen [*mucus;* G. *genesthai,* from *gignesthai,* to be produced]. A substance producing mucin; it is contained in epithelial cells that form mucus. —**mucig'enous,** *adj.*

mu'ci·lage (mew'si·lidj) [*mucus*]. *In pharmacy,* a solution of a gum in water. Mucilages (mucilagines) are employed as applications to irritated surfaces, particularly mucous membranes, as excipients for pills, and to suspend insoluble substances. The most important are **acacia mucilage** and **tragacanth mucilage.** —**mucilag'inous,** *adj.*

mu"ci·la'go. See *mucilage.*

mu'cin [*mucus*]. A mixture of glycoproteins that forms the basis of mucus. It is soluble in water and precipitated by alcohol or acids. —**mucinous,** *adj.*

gastric m. Trade name for a product made from hog stomach linings and intended for use in the treatment of peptic ulcers as a demulcent and adsorbent.

mu'cin·o·blast", mu·cin'o·blast [*mucus;* G. *blastos,* germ]. The cell which forms a mucous cell.

mu·cin'o·gen [*mucus;* G. *genesthai,* from *gignesthai,* to be produced]. The antecedent principle from which mucin is derived.

mu'cin·oid [*mucus;* G. *eidos,* form]. 1. Resembling mucin. 2. Mucoid.

mu·cip'a·rous [*mucus;* L. *parere,* to bring forth]. Secreting or producing mucus.

mu'co-, muc- [*mucus*]. A combining form denoting *relation to mucus* or *mucous membrane.*

mu"co·al·bu'mi·nous. See *mucoserous.*

mu'co·cele [*mucus;* G. *kēlē,* tumor]. 1. A mucous tumor. 2. An enlarged lacrimal sac.

mu"co·co·li'tis. See mucous *colitis.*

mu"co·col'pos [*mucus;* G. *kolpos,* vagina]. A collection of mucus in the vagina.

mu"co·cu·ta'ne·ous [*mucus;* L. *cutis,* skin]. Pertaining to a mucous membrane and the skin, and to the line where these join.

mu′co·derm [*mucus;* G. *derma,* skin]. The nituca propria of a mucous membrane. *Obs.*

mu″co·en″ter·i′tis [*mucus;* G. *enteron,* intestine; *-itis,* inflammation]. Inflammation of the mucous membrane of the intestine.

mu″co·hem″or·rhag′ic (mew″ko·hem″o·radj′ick) [*mucus;* G. *haimorrhagikos,* liable to bleeding]. Related to, or accompanied by, mucus and blood.

mu′coid [*mucus;* G. *eidos,* form]. Resembling mucus.

mu′coids [*mucus; eidos*]. A group of glycoproteins, differing from true mucins in their solubilities and precipitation properties. They are found in cartilage, in the cornea and crystalline lens, in white of egg, and in certain cysts and ascitic fluids.

mu·co′i·tin-sul·fu′ric ac′id. A component of the mucin of saliva; on hydrolysis, yields sulfuric acid, glucuronic acid, glucosamine, and acetic acid.

mu·con′ic ac′id. HOOC.CH: CH.CH: CH.COOH. An oxidation product of benzene resulting from detoxication of the latter in the animal body.

mu″co·per″i·os′te·um [*mucus;* G. *periosteos,* around the bones]. Periosteum with a closely associated mucous membrane.

mu″co·pol″y·sac′cha·ride. A polysaccharide containing an amino sugar as well as uronic acid units.

mu″co·pro′te·in. A glycoprotein, particularly one in which the sugar component is chondroitinsulfuric or mucoitinsulfuric acid.

mu″co·pu′ru·lent [*mucus;* L. *purulentus,* purulent]. Containing mucus mingled with pus.

mu′co·pus″ [*mucus;* L. *pus,* pus]. A mixture of mucus and pus.

Mu′cor [L., moldiness]. A genus of the class Phycomycetes, including fungi, which produce a nonseptate mycelium. The genus includes some of the black bread molds; species are secondary invaders but rarely primary invaders and are also common allergens. Also called *Absidia.*

mu″co·rif′er·ous [*mucor;* L. *ferre,* to bear]. Covered with a moldlike substance.

mu′cor·in [*mucor*]. An albuminoid substance from many species of the mucorinous molds.

mu″cor·my·co′sis (mew″kor·migh·ko′sis) [*mucor;* G. *mykēs,* fungus; *-ōsis,* condition]. An infection with certain species of the fungus *Mucor.* Species of this genus have been reported in cases of paronychia, otomycosis, and pulmonary lesions. These organisms are common secondary contaminants and seldom produce disease.

mu·co′sa [L. *mucosus,* mucous]. A mucous membrane; tunica mucosa. —**muco′sal,** *adj.*

alveolar m. The vestibular mucous membrane between the attached gingiva and the fornix of the vestibule of the mouth.

mu″co·san·guin′e·ous (mew″ko·sang·gwin′ee·us) [L. *mucus,* mucus; *sanguen,* blood]. Consisting of mucus and blood.

mu″co·se′rous [*mucus;* L. *serum,* whey]. Mucous and serous; containing mucus and serum.

mu′co·sin [*mucus*]. A term suggested for mucin from nasal, uterine, and bronchial mucous membranes, because of their special viscous properties, as contrasted with mucins from other regions.

mu″co·si′tis. Inflammation of mucous membranes.

mu·cos′i·ty [L. *mucosus,* mucous]. Sliminess.

mu″co·stat′ics. *In dentistry,* a method of obtaining an impression with minimum displacement or distortion of the oral mucosa.

mucotin. A trade-mark for an antacid composition known by the generic name *almagucin.*

mu′cous [L. *mucus,* mucus]. Relating to mucus; secreting mucus, as mucous gland; depending on the presence of mucus, as mucous rales.

mu″co·vis·ci·do′sis. See pancreatic *fibrosis.*

mu′cro·nate [L. *mucronatus,* pointed]. Tipped with a sharp point.

mu′cu·lent [L. *muculentus,* sniveling]. Rich in mucus. *Rare.*

Mu·cu′na [Tupi *mucunā*]. A genus of leguminous herbs. The hairs of the pods of *Stizolobium pruritum* (cowage) were formerly used as a vermifuge and counterirritant.

mu′cus [L.]. The viscid liquid secreted by mucous glands. It consists of water, mucin, inorganic salts, epithelial cells, leukocytes, etc., held in suspension.

Mueller, Paul [*Swiss research chemist,* 1899–]. In 1939, he discovered the insecticidal action of DDT, for which work he was awarded the Nobel prize in physiology and medicine in 1948.

Mueller's snake. See *Pseudelaps muelleri.*

mu″guet′ (mew″gay′. *See* Notes § 35) [F.]. Thrush.

mu·i′ra pu·a′ma (mōō·eer′uh pōō·ah′muh, ·am′uh). The dried root of *Liriosma ovata.* Used by the Brazilian aborigines in dysentery and as an aphrodisiac.

mu·laire′. A subcutaneous lesion occurring in verruga peruana which presses against the skin, finally eroding it. This lesion looks very much like that produced by the same disease in mules.

mul′ber·ry [ME. *mulberie,* from G. *moron,* mulberry]. A tree of the genus *Morus. M. nigra* is the source of a juice or a syrup used as a drink in fevers and added to gargles in pharyngitis. The leaves of *M. alba* are used as food for silkworms.

m. calculus. See mulberry *calculus.*

m. mark. Nevus.

m. mass. See *morula.*

Mulder's test. See xanthoproteic *test.*

mu″li·e′bri·a (mew″lee·ee′bree·uh, ·eb′ree·uh) [L. *muliebris,* of a woman]. The female genitals.

mu″li·eb′ri·ty [L. *muliebritas,* from *muliebris*]. 1. Womanliness. 2. Puberty in the female. 3. Assumption of female qualities by the male.

mul′lein (mul′in). See *Verbascum.*

Müller, Carl (1886–). Norwegian physician known for describing Müller's *syndrome.*

Müller, Heinrich [*German anatomist,* 1820–64]. Discovered visual purple (1851). Demonstrated electric current in contraction of frog's heart (1856). See also Müller's *fibers.*

Muller, Hermann Joseph [*American geneticist,* 1890–]. Known for his research on the artificial transmutation of genes by means of roentgen rays. Nobel laureate (1946).

Müller, Johannes [*German anatomist and physiologist,* 1801–58]. A pair of embryonic ducts on the external surface of the mesonephric ducts are called *Müllerian ducts.* In the female they become the oviducts and vagina, the lower extremity becoming the hymen. In the male they leave vestiges, the prostatic utricle and the appendices testis. See also *utricle.* Discovered chondrin and glutin (1837). See also Müller's *tubercle.* See *law* of Müller, *law* of specific energies of nerve.

Müller, Leopold [*Czechoslovakian ophthalmologist,* 1862–1936]. Remembered for his description of an operation for retinal detachment, in which he resected the sclera; called *Müller's operation.* See *muscle* of Müller.

Müller, Otto Friedrich [*Danish microscopist,* 1730–84]. Made a systematic classification of bacteria. Said to have coined the terms bacillus and spirillum.

Müller, Rudolf [*Austrian dermatologist,* 1877–1934]. Introduced a complement-fixation reaction, with Maurice Oppenheim, used in the diagnosis of gonorrhea; called *Müller-Oppenheim reaction.*

Müller's fixing fluid. See under *fixing fluid.*

Müller's test. See under *test.*

mul·tan′gu·lum [L. *multus,* many; *angulus,* angle]. A bone with many angles. Also called *multangular.*

m. majus. The trapezium, lateral carpal bone of the distal row. Also called *greater multangular*. See Table of Bones in the Appendix.

m. minus. The trapezoid bone, second carpal bone of the distal row. Also called *lesser multangular*. See Table of Bones in the Appendix.

mul′ti- [*multus*]. 1. A combining form meaning *many, much*. 2. *In medicine*, a combining form signifying *affecting many parts*.

mul″ti·cap′su·lar [*multus;* L. *capsula*, little box]. *In biology*, composed of many capsules.

mul″ti·cel′lu·lar [*multus;* L. *cellula*, small storeroom]. Having many cells.

Mul′ti·ceps [*multus;* L. *caput*, head]. A genus of tapeworms.

M. multiceps. A species which in its larval form causes gid in sheep and also infests other herbivorous animals. Human infestation is rare.

M. serialis. A species which in its adult form infests the intestinal tract of the dog. Human infestation is rare.

mul″ti·cos′tate [*multus;* L. *costa*, rib]. Having many ribs.

mul″ti·cus′pid [*multus;* L. *cuspis*, point]. Having several cusps, as the molar teeth. Also called *multicuspidate*.

mul″ti·den′tate [*multus;* L. *dentatus*, toothed]. Having many teeth or toothlike processes.

mul″ti·dig′i·tate (mul″ti·didj′i·tate) [*multus;* L. *digitatus*, having fingers or toes]. Having many digits or digitate processes.

mul″ti·fa·mil′i·al [*multus;* L. *familia*, family]. Attacking several successive generations of a family, as certain diseases.

mul″ti·fe·ta′tion. See *superfetation*.

mul′ti·fid [L. *multifidus*, divided into many parts]. Divided into many parts.

mul·tif′i·dus. A deep muscle of the back. See Table of Muscles in the Appendix.

m. spinae. Multifidus muscle: old term.

mul″ti·flag′el·late (mul″ti·fladj′i·late) [L. *multus*, many; *flagellare*, to whip]. Having many flagella.

mul′ti·form [*multus;* L. *forma*, form]. Polymorphic.

mul″ti·gan′gli·on·ate [*multus;* G. *gagglion*]. Having many ganglions.

mul″ti·glan′du·lar [*multus;* L. *glandulae*, glands of the throat]. Pertaining to several glands, as multiglandular secretions, a mixture of secretions from two or more glands.

mul″ti·grav′i·da [*multus;* L. *gravidus*, pregnant]. A pregnant woman who has had two or more previous pregnancies.

mul″ti·in·fec′tion [*multus;* L. *infectio*, from *inficere*, to infect]. A mixed infection.

mul″ti·lo′bar, mul″ti·lo′bate, mul″ti·lob′ed [*multus;* G. *lobos*, lobe]. Composed of many lobes.

mul″ti·lob′u·lar [*multus; lobos*]. Having many lobules.

mul″ti·loc′u·lar [*multus;* L. *loculus*, little place]. Many-celled; polycystic.

mul″ti·mam′mae (mul″ti·mam′ee) [*multus;* L. *mamma*, breast]. Polymastia; the presence of more than two breasts in a human being. *Obs.*

mul″ti·nod′u·lar [*multus;* L. *nodulus*, little knot]. Having many nodules.

mul″ti·nu′cle·ar, mul″ti·nu′cle·a″ted [*multus;* L. *nucleus*, nut]. Having two or more nuclei.

mul·tip′a·ra [*multus;* L. *parere*, to bring forth]. A pregnant woman who has already borne one or more children.

mul″ti·par′i·ty (mul″ti·par′i·tee) [*multus; parere*]. The condition of having borne several children. —**multip′arous,** *adj.*

mul′ti·ple [L. *multiplex*, that has many folds]. Manifold; affecting many parts at the same time, as multiple sclerosis.

mul″ti·po′lar [L. *multus*, many; *polus*, pole]. Having more than one pole, as multipolar nerve cells, those having more than one process.

mul″ti·va′lent, mul·tiv′a·lent [*multus;* L. *valere*, to be strong]. Capable of combining with more than one atom of a univalent element.

mum″mi·fi·ca′tion [Ar. *mūmiya*, mummy, from Per. *mūm*, wax; L. *facere*, to make]. The change of a part into a hard, dry mass; dry gangrene.

mum′mi·fied [*mūmiya; facere*]. Dried, as mummified pulp, the condition of the dental pulp when it is affected by dry gangrene.

mumps [E. dial., *mump*, lump or bump]. An acute infectious disease caused by a virus; characterized by swelling of the parotid and at times of the other salivary glands as well as the pancreas, ovaries, and testes. After a period of incubation of from two to three weeks, the disease begins with fever, pain below the ear, and swelling of the parotid gland. In the course of a week, the swelling subsides without suppuration. One attack usually confers immunity. Syn., *epidemic parotitis*.

metastatic m. Complication involving organs other than the salivary glands, such as the testis or ovary.

Münchmeyer [*German physician*, nineteenth century]. Described progressive ossifying myositis (1869); also called *Münchmeyer's disease*.

mun·dif′i·cant [L. *mundificare*, to make clean]. Having the power to cleanse, purge, or heal. —**mundif′icant,** *n.*

Mundinus. See *Mondino de' Luzzi*.

Munsell, Hazel E. (1891–). American chemist who, with H. C. Sherman, introduced the rat-growth unit, called the *Sherman-Munsell unit*.

Munson-Walker values. Standard values for the quantitative measurement of sugar concentration.

mu′on. The mu meson.

mu′ral [L. *murus*, wall]. Pertaining to a wall, as a mural fibroid, mural abscess, or mural pregnancy.

mu·rex′ide. $C_8H_4O_6N_5NH_4.H_2O$. Ammonium purpurate; a purple coloring matter resulting from uric acid by treatment with nitric acid and then neutralizing with ammonia. Formerly used as a dye.

mu′ri·ate. An old term for a chloride. —**muriated,** *adj.*

mu″ri·at′ic [L. *muriaticus*, from *muria*, brine]. Pertaining to brine.

mu″ri·at′ic ac′id. An old term for hydrochloric acid.

mur′mur [L., humming, roaring]. A blowing or rasping sound heard on auscultation.

accidental m. A murmur due to an accidental circumstance such as compression of an artery by the stethoscope.

anemic m. A hemic murmur.

aneurysmal m. The murmur or bruit heard over an aneurysm.

aortic m. One produced at the aortic orifice.

apex m. One heard best in the area directly over the apex of the heart. Also called *apical m.*

arterial m. The sound made by the arterial current.

attrition m. A pericardial murmur.

Austin Flint m. See Flint's *m.*

blood m. See hemic *m.*

Bright's m. A creaking sound heard over the heart in pericarditis or pleurisy.

cardiac m. Any adventitious sound heard over the region of the heart. In relation to their seat of generation, cardiac murmurs are designated as mitral, aortic, tricuspid, and pulmonary; according to the period of the heart's cycle at which they occur they are divided into systolic, those occurring during systole; diastolic, those occurring in diastole; and presystolic, those occurring just before systole.

cardiopulmonary m. One produced by the impact of the heart against the lung.

continuous m. One lasting throughout systole and diastole, as in patent ductus arteriosus, arteriovenous aneurysm, and venous hum at the base of the neck.

diastolic m. A cardiac murmur occurring during diastole.

direct m. A murmur produced by obstruction to the blood as it is passing in its normal direction.

Duroziez's m. The double murmur heard over the femoral artery in aortic regurgitation.

endocardial m. A murmur produced within the cavities of the heart.

exocardial m. A murmur connected with the heart, but which is produced outside of its cavities.

Flint's m. An apical diastolic murmur sometimes heard in aortic regurgitation. It is probably due to the fact that because of the extreme ventricular dilatation the valves cannot be forced back against the walls and produce a relative narrowing of the atrioventricular orifice.

Fraentzel m. One heard in patients with mitral stenosis, loudest at the beginning and end of diastole.

friction m. A sound produced by the rubbing of two inflamed serous surfaces upon each other.

functional m. See innocent *m.*

Graham Steell m. A murmur of pulmonary valve incompetence: it may occur in cases of severe mitral stenosis and cardiac insufficiency.

heart m. A cardiac murmur.

hemic m. A murmur heard over the heart or jugular bulb in severe anemia, due to decreased viscosity of the blood and increased rapidity of the blood stream. Syn., *bruit de diable.*

humming-top m. See venous *hum.*

indirect m. One produced by the blood flowing in a direction contrary to the normal current.

innocent m. One occurring in the absence of structural changes in the heart, usually faint, of blowing quality, and systolic in time. Syn., *functional m.*

inorganic m. A murmur not due to valvular lesions. A hemic or functional murmur.

lapping m. One which occurs following rupture of the aorta.

machinery m. A loud, continuous, rough cardiac murmur heard in cases of patent ductus arteriosus.

mitral m. One produced at the mitral orifice.

muscular m. (a) The sound heard on auscultation of a contracting muscle. (b) The first sound of the heart.

musical m. A cardiac murmur having a musical quality.

organic m. A murmur due to structural changes in the heart.

paradox m. A systolic murmur prolonged so as to appear to be followed by a diastolic murmur.

pericardial m. A murmur produced in the pericardium.

placental m. A sound attributed to the circulation of the blood in the placenta. Formerly called *placental bruit.*

presystolic m. A cardiac murmur occurring just before systole.

pulmonary m. One produced at the pulmonary orifice.

regurgitant m. One due to regurgitation.

respiratory m. The sound produced by the air entering and escaping from the lungs during respiration.

Roger m. A long loud systolic murmur heard best to the left of the sternum in the third or fourth intercostal space in cases of uncomplicated congenital interventricular septal defect.

steam-tug m. One which accompanies aortic obstruction and insufficiency.

systolic m. A cardiac murmur occurring during systole.

to-and-fro m. A pericardial murmur heard during both systole and diastole.

tricuspid m. One produced at the tricuspid orifice.

venous m. One occurring in a vein.

vesicular m. A fine inspiratory breath sound heard over the chest during normal breathing.

whiffing m. A humming rushing sound heard in the veins in anemia.

whistling m. See whiffing *m.*

Murphy, John Benjamin [*American surgeon,* 1857–1916]. Internationally known as surgeon, educator, and inventor. He exercised a great influence in many surgical fields, including orthopedic surgery. Contributed to the knowledge of ankylosed joints and their treatment. Invented the metal button used in rapid, end-to-end anastomosis of divided intestine (1892), called *Murphy button.* Introduced a method of approach to the hip joint especially adapted to arthroplasty; called *Murphy's operation.* Described punch tenderness at the costovertebral angle in perinephritic abscess; called *Murphy sign, punch.* Described sign of cholecystitis. See Murphy's *sign.*

Murphy, William Parry [*American physician,* 1892–]. With George Richards Minot, introduced the *Minot-Murphy diet,* consisting chiefly of liver, in the treatment of pernicious anemia (1926). This led to the present-day therapeutic use of liver extracts. Nobel laureate with G. R. Minot and G. H. Whipple (1934).

mur·ri′na (muh·rye′nuh, moo·ree′nuh) [Sp. *morriña*]. A form of trypanosomiasis caused by *Trypanosoma hippicum,* seen in horses and mules, with cattle acting as reservoir hosts; characterized by weakness, emaciation, edema, anemia, enlarged spleen, and paralysis.

Mus [L., mouse]. A genus of small rodents including the common house mouse (**Mus musculus**) and other small species. Some members of the genus are medically important as intermediate hosts and reservoir hosts of diseases transmissible to man.

mu·sar′in. An antibiotic substance elaborated by Meredith's actinomycete, named for the banana plant, *Musa sapientum,* host to the parasitic *Fusarium oxysporum* var. *cubense,* against which it is active.

Mus′ca [L., fly]. A genus of flies of the family Muscidae.

M. domestica. The most important species, the common housefly; it carries and frequently transmits the causal agents of a number of diseases, including typhoid fever, infantile diarrhea, bacillary and amebic dysentery, cholera, trachoma, and tuberculosis.

M. vetustissima. The Australian housefly.

M. vicina. The common housefly of the Orient.

mus′cae vol″i·tan′tes (mus′ee vol″i·tan′teez, mus′kee) [L.]. Floating specks in the field of vision, due to opacities in the media of the eye. Also called *mouches volantes.*

mus′ca·rine (mus′kuh·reen, ·rin, mus·kay′·) [L. *muscarius,* pertaining to flies]. A poisonous alkaloid obtained from certain mushrooms, as *Agaricus muscarius.* Stimulates the parasympathetic nerves and so slows the heart; increases the secretions of the salivary and lacrimal glands and of the intestine; produces contraction of the pupil.

mus″ca·rin′ic ac′tion. Peripheral drug effects similar to those produced by muscarine, resulting in parasympathetic stimulation at the receptor levels.

mus′ca·rin·ism [*muscarius*]. Mushroom poisoning.

mus′ci·cide (mus′i·side) [L. *musca*, fly; *caedere*, to kill]. An agent which is poisonous or destructive to flies.

Mus′ci·dae (mus′i·dee) [*musca*]. A family of the Diptera, which includes the common houseflies.

mus′cle [L. *musculus*, muscle]. 1. Muscle tissue composed of individual muscle fibers or muscle cells. Classified by microscopical appearance as nonstriated (smooth) or striated; by volitional control as voluntary or involuntary; by location in the body as skeletal, cardiac, or visceral. 2. A contractile organ composed of muscle tissue, effecting the movements of the organs and parts of the body; particularly, that composed of a belly of skeletal muscle tissue attached by tendons to bone on either side of a joint effecting movements at the joint by contraction of the belly drawing the more movable attachment, the insertion, toward the more fixed attachment, the origin. For muscles listed by name, see Table of Muscles in the Appendix. See Plates 3, 4. —**muscular,** *adj.*

accessory m. A muscle slip additional to a muscle, as scalenus minimus, a muscle inserted on the first rib in addition to the scalenus anterior.

antagonistic m. One acting in opposition to another, as the triceps, which extends the elbow, in opposition to the biceps, which flexes the elbow.

antigravity muscles. Muscles, chiefly extensors, the contraction of which support the body against gravity, as in standing.

appendicular m. A muscle inserted on the upper or lower extremity.

articular m. A muscle inserted in part into the fibrous capsule of a joint, holding the capsule taut in sudden movements of the joint.

axial m. One attached to the vertebral column.

bicipital m. One having two heads or attachments of origin.

bipennate m. A muscle whose fibers are inserted on two sides of a central tendon.

Brücke's m. The meridional portion of the ciliary muscle.

cardiac m. The muscle of the heart.

ciliary m. The smooth muscle of the ciliary body. See Table of Muscles in the Appendix.

circumpennate m. A muscle whose fibers are inserted on all sides of a central tendon.

conjoined m. The combined insertion of internal oblique abdominal and transverse abdominal muscles into the pubis in cases where muscle fibers are present in the insertion.

cutaneous m. One having an insertion into the skin or both origin and insertion in the skin.

dermal m. See cutaneous *m.*

digastric m. One having two muscular bellies joined by a central tendon.

extrinsic m. One which has its origin outside, its insertion into an organ, as a rectus muscle of the eye. See intrinsic *m.*

fibulocalcaneus m. An occasional muscle arising from the lower third of the fibula and inserted into the tendon of the quadratus plantae or of the flexor digitorum longus, found as an anterior or a medial variant.

fibulotibialis m. An occasional small muscle arising from the medial side of the head of the fibula and inserted into the posterior surface of the tibia beneath the popliteus.

fixation m. One which holds a part from moving to allow more accurate control of a distal part, as a muscle which holds the wrist steady to allow more precise control of finger movement.

fusiform m. A spindle-shaped muscle.

intercostal muscles. Muscles lying between adjacent ribs, divided into external and internal, and sometimes a third group, the intermediate, as a subdivision of the internal. See Table of Muscles in the Appendix.

intra-aural m. One in the ear, particularly inside the tympanic cavity; includes the tensor tympani and the stapedius muscles.

intrinsic m. One which has both its origin and its insertion within an organ, as the transverse muscle of the tongue. See extrinsic *m.*

involuntary m. One not under the control of the will; usually consists of smooth muscle tissue and lies within a viscus, or is associated with skin.

mimetic m. One of the muscles of facial expression.

multicipital m. One having more than two heads or attachments of origin.

multipennate m. See circumpennate *m.*

m. of Bell. A band of smooth muscle of the urinary bladder, running from the orifice of the ureter toward the median lobe of the prostate gland in the male and toward the neck of the bladder in the female.

m. of Ganser. (a) The accessorius ad flexorem carpi radialis muscle. (b) The accessorius ad flexorem profundum digitorum muscle. (c) The accessorius ad pollicem muscle.

m. of Gegenbaur. The auriculofrontalis muscle.

m. of Gruber. The peroneocalcaneus externus muscle.

m. of Henle. The epicraniotemporalis muscle.

m. of Holl. The ischiobulbosus muscle.

m. of Horner. Lacrimal part of orbicularis oculi muscle.

m. of Houston. The compressor venae dorsalis muscle.

m. of Jung. The procerus muscle.

m. of Klein. The compressor labii muscle.

m. of Landström. Smooth muscle fibers in the fascia about the eyeball; the smooth muscle associated with the levator palpebrae superioris muscle is a portion of it.

m. of Ludwig. The aryvocalis muscle.

m. of Macallister. The fibulocalcaneus medialis muscle.

m. of Müller. (a) The orbital muscle. (b) The tarsal muscles. (c) The innermost, circular portion of the ciliary muscle.

m. of Raux. The rectourethralis muscle.

m. of Riolan. Ciliary portion of the orbicularis oculi muscle.

m. of Santorini. (a) The risorius muscle. (b) The incisurae helicis muscle.

m. of Sappey. The temporalis superficialis muscle.

m. of Treitz. (a) Muscle tissue sometimes associated with the suspensory ligament of the duodenum; it arises from the right crus of the diaphragm and inserts on the duodenum at the jejunal junction: also called *suspensory m. of the duodenum.* (b) The rectococcygeus muscle.

m. of Wood. The extensor carpi radialis intermedius muscle.

nonstriated m. See smooth *m.*

papillary m. The muscular eminences in the ventricles of the heart from which the chordae tendineae arise. See Plate 5.

pectinate m. One of the small muscular columns traversing the inner surface of the auricles of the heart.

pennate m. One whose fibers are inserted on a central tendon.

postaxial m. One on the posterior aspect of an extremity.

postural m. See antigravity *m.*

preaxial m. One on the anterior aspect of an extremity.

red m. A muscle which appears red in the fresh state; in the fibers of red muscles, the longitudinal striation is more prominent and the transverse striation is somewhat irregular. The red color probably is due to muscle hemoglobin and cytochrome.

skeletal m. One attached to a bone or bones of the skeleton and concerned in body movements.

smooth m. One consisting of spindle-shaped, unstriped muscle cells and found in the walls of viscera and blood vessels; involuntary muscle: also called *nonstriated m.*, *unstriated m.*

striated m. Muscle consisting of cross-straited muscle fibers.

striped m. See striated *m.*

supernumerary m. See accessory *m.*

suspensory m. of duodenum. The *m.* of Treitz.

synergistic m. One which, though not directly concerned as a prime mover in a particular act, helps some other muscle to perform the movement more efficiently.

tensor m. of the choroid. The outer portion of the ciliary muscle.

tricipital m. One having three heads.

two-joint m. A muscle which crosses two joints and effects the movements at each joint.

unipennate m. One whose fibers are inserted obliquely into one side of a tendon.

unstriated m. See smooth *m.*

unstriped m. See smooth *m.*

vestigial m. One that is rudimentary in man but well developed in lower animals.

visceral m. (a) Muscle of a viscus. (b) Muscle associated with the visceral skeleton.

voluntary m. One directly under the control of the will. Also called skeletal *m.*

white m. Skeletal muscle which appears paler in the fresh state than red muscle, and is associated with slow movements.

mus′cle plate. See *myotome*, 2.

mus′cle sense. See *proprioception.*

mus′cle splint′ing, guard′ing. The involuntary limitation of motion of an extremity, or the rigidity of trunk muscles, by muscle spasm.

mus″cu·lar′is mu·co′sae (mus″cue·lar′is mew-ko′see). The single or double thin layer of smooth muscle in the deep portion of some mucous membranes, as in most of the digestive tube.

mus″cu·lar′i·ty [*musculus*]. The quality of being muscular.

mus′cu·la·ture [*musculus*]. The muscular system of the body, or a part of it.

mus′cu·lo-, muscul- [*musculus*]. A combining form denoting *relating to the muscles.*

mus″cu·lo·ap″o·neu·rot′ic [*musculus;* G. *apo*, from; *neuron*, nerve]. Composed of muscle and of fibrous connective tissue in the form of a membrane.

mus″cu·lo·cu·ta′ne·ous [*musculus;* L. *cutis*, skin]. Pertaining to or supplying the muscles and skin, as the musculocutaneous nerve of the arm. See Table of Nerves in the Appendix.

mus″cu·lo·fas′ci·al (mus″cue·lo·fash′ee·ul) [*musculus;* L. *fascia*, band]. Consisting of both muscular and fascial elements, as in an amputation flap.

mus″cu·lo·fi′brous. Pertaining to a tissue which is partly muscular and partly fibrous connective tissue.

mus″cu·lo·phren′ic [*musculus;* G. *phrēn*, midriff]. Pertaining to or supplying the muscles of the diaphragm, as the musculophrenic artery. See Table of Arteries in the Appendix.

mus″cu·lo·spi′ral [*musculus;* G. *speira*, coil]. 1. Old term for radial, as the musculospiral or radial nerve. 2. Referring to the radial groove on the posterior surface of the humerus.

mus″cu·lo·ten′di·nous [*musculus;* L. *tendere*, to stretch]. Pertaining to both muscle and tendon.

mus′cu·lus. See *muscle.*

mush′room [ME. *muscheron*]. A fleshy fungus of the Basidiomycetes. See fly *agaric.*

mu″si·co·ma′ni·a (mew″zi·ko·may′nee·uh) [G. *mousikos*, musical; *mania*, madness]. Monomania for, or insane devotion to, music. *Obs.*

mu″si·co·ther′a·py [*mousikos;* G. *therapeia*, treatment]. The use of music in the treatment of mental and nervous diseases.

musk [G. *moschos*, from the Sanskrit]. The dried secretions from the preputial glands of musk deer. Occurs in grains or lumps, possessing a peculiar, penetrating odor. Was formerly employed for the treatment of low fevers and nerve exhaustion but today is employed only in the manufacture of perfumery.

artificial m. One of several musk substitutes, as xylene musk, ketone musk, and musk ambrette, each having a characteristic composition. Used in perfumery; also has had some usage in medicine based on reported antispasmodic action.

Musken's tonometer. See under *tonometer.*

musk root. Sumbul.

mus′sa·nine (mus′uh·neen, ·nin). An alkaloid resembling saponin, from the bark of *Acacia anthelmintica.* Also called *musenine.*

mus″si·ta′tion [L. *mussitare*, to mutter]. Speechless movement of the lips.

Mussy, François de. See *Guéneau de Mussy.*

mus′tard [L. *mustum*, must]. 1. A plant of the genus *Brassica.* 2. The dried ripe seed of *Brassica alba* or *B. nigra.*

black m. The finely ground seeds of *Brassica nigra.* Contains a fixed oil; a pungent, irritant, essential oil; an enzyme (myrosin); and a glycoside (sinigrin).

m. flour. Black and white mustard seeds mixed and pulverized.

m. paper. Charta sinapis. See m. *paper.*

nitrogen m. See under *nitrogen.*

red m. Black mustard.

volatile oil of m. Allyl isothiocyanate.

white m. The finely ground seeds of *Brassica hirta;* contains the same constituents as black mustard except for a different glycoside (sinalbin). Used as a condiment or as a counterirritant and stimulant.

mustargen hydrochloride. A trade-marked name for mechlorethamine hydrochloride, a cytotoxic agent acting mainly on proliferating cells.

mus′tine hy″dro·chlo′ride. Mechlorethamine hydrochloride.

mu′ta·cism. See *mytacism.*

mu′ta·gen. Any substance or agent causing a genetic mutation.

mu′tant [L. *mutare*, to change]. An individual with characteristics different from those of the parental type, or the stock established from such individuals; due to a genetic constitution that includes a mutation.

mu″ta·ro·ta′tion [*mutare;* L. *rotatio*, rotation]. A change in optical rotation of solutions of certain sugars occurring while standing and continuing until equilibrium between the isomeric forms present in the solution is attained.

mu′tase [*mutare*]. An enzyme which simultaneously catalyzes the oxidation of one molecule and reduction of another molecule of the substrate. See Table of Enzymes in the Appendix.

aldehyde m. An enzyme, occurring in liver and yeast, which catalyzes conversion of two molecules of acetaldehyde to one each of acetic acid and ethyl alcohol.

mu·ta'tion [L. *mutatio*, from *mutare*]. 1. A change of small or moderate extent, which represents a definite stage in the gradual evolution of an organism, such as may be recognized in a series of fossils from successive geologic strata (Waage, 1868). 2. A change in the characteristics of an organism produced by an alteration of the hereditary material. The alteration in the germ plasm may involve an addition of one or more complete sets of chromosomes, the addition or loss of a whole chromosome, or some change within a chromosome, ranging from a gross rearrangement, loss or addition of a larger or smaller section, down through minute rearrangements to a change at a single locus. The latter are gene mutations, or simply mutation in the restricted use of the term.

induced m. That produced by experimental treatment, as by x-rays.

lethal m. One causing death of the organism during any stage of its development.

natural m. Mutation in nature which forms the basic materials for evolution.

somatic m. A mutation during the course of development in a somatic cell, resulting in a mosaic condition.

spontaneous m. Natural mutation.

mute [L. *mutus*, silent]. Unable to articulate.

mu″ti·la'tion [L. *mutilatio*, from *mutilare*, to mutilate]. The act of maiming or disfiguring; depriving of a limb, member, part, or organ.

mu'tism [L. *mutus*, silent]. The condition or state of being speechless.

deaf-m. The condition of being both deaf and mute.

hysterical m. That of psychic or hysterical origin, seen in stupors and in schizophrenic patients; there is an obstinate and voluntary silence, although the vocal organs are uninjured and there is no visible lesion of the cerebral speech centers.

mu'tu·al·ism [L. *mutuus*, borrowed]. The living together of two organisms of different species, for the advantage that each derives from the other. Syn., *symbiosis*.

muz'zle [ML. *musellum*]. The projecting jaws and nose of an animal; a snout.

my. Symbol for myopia.

Mya, Giuseppe [*Italian pediatrician*, 1857–1911]. Described congenital megacolon, called *Mya's disease, Hirschsprung's disease*.

my·al'gi·a (migh·al'juh, ·jee·uh) [G. *mys*, muscle; *algos*, pain]. Pain in the muscles; muscular rheumatism. —**myalgic,** *adj.*

nuchal m. An allergic reaction to certain specific substances in which the patient suffers from pulling, drawing, tightness, and aching in the cervical muscles.

spastic m. See muscle-contraction *headache*.

myanesin. A trade-mark for *mephenesin*.

my″as·the'ni·a (migh″ass·thee'nee·uh, ·ass·thi-nigh'uh) [*mys*; G. *astheneia*, weakness]. Muscular debility. —**myasthe'nic,** *adj.*

congenital m. Myasthenia present at birth, involving the muscles symmetrically.

m. gravis pseudoparalytica. A disease characterized by an abnormal exhaustibility of the voluntary muscles, manifesting itself in a rapid diminution of contractility, both when the muscle is activated by the will and when stimulated by electric current. It may be associated with overactivity of the lymphatic tissues of the thymus. —**myasthen'ic,** *adj.*

neonatal m. Myasthenia occurring in children of myasthenic mothers.

my″a·to'ni·a [*mys*; G. *a-*, not; *tonos*, tone]. Absence of muscular tone. Syn., *amyotonia*.

m. congenita. See *amyotonia* congenita.

my·ce″li·an·am'ide. An antibiotic substance derived from *Penicillium griseofulvum*, having no activity against Gram-negative bacteria but active against other bacteria.

my·ce'li·oid (migh·see'lee·oyd) [G. *mykēs*, fungus; *hēlos*, nail; *eidos*, form]. Moldlike, as colonies of bacteria having the appearance of mold colonies.

my·ce'li·um [*mykēs*; *hēlos*]. The vegetative filaments of fungi, usually forming interwoven masses. —**mycelial,** *adj.*

racquet m. Hyphal configuration in which the distal end of hyphal cells in many fungi (including *Microsporum audouini*) is swollen.

my·ce'tes (migh·see'teez) [*mykēs*]. The fungi.

my·ce'tin. An antibiotic substance derived from *Streptomyces violaceus*, active against Gram-positive but not against Gram-negative bacteria.

my·ce″to·gen'ic (migh·see″to·jen'ick, migh-set″o·), **my″ce·tog'e·nous** (migh″si·todj'i·nus) [*mykēs*; G. *genesthai*, from *gignesthai*, to be produced]. Produced or caused by fungi.

my·ce'toid, my'ce·toid [*mykēs*; G. *eidos*, form]. Resembling a fungus.

my″ce·to'ma [*mykēs*; G. *-ōma*, tumor]. 1. A chronic infection affecting usually the foot but may be found in other parts. Nodules of variable size appear in skin and subcutaneous tissues, which break down with discharge of oily serosanguineous pus in which are small granules, the color of which varies from case to case, black, white, red, or intermediate shades. Microscopically, masses of fungi simulating actinomyces granules lie in abscesses, which are surrounded by granulation tissue and fibrosis. Occurs most frequently in tropical and subtropical regions. Due to a wide variety of fungi of the classes Schizomycetes, Ascomycetes, and Fungi imperfecti. Syn., *madura foot, maduromycosis*. 2. Any tumor mass occurring in tissues which is largely composed of fungous elements.

mycifradin sulfate. Trade-marked name for the sulfate of the antibiotic *neomycin*.

my'co-, myc- [*mykēs*]. 1. A combining form meaning *fungus*. 2. A combining form signifying *mucus* or *mucous membrane*.

my″co·an″gi·o·neu·ro'sis (migh″ko·an″jee·o-new·ro'sis) [L. *mucus*, mucus; G. *aggeion*, vessel; *neuron*, nerve; *-ōsis*, condition]. A neurosis accompanied by a hypersecretion of mucus, producing mucous colitis.

My″co·bac·ter″i·a'ce·ae (migh″ko·back·teer″ee-ay'see·ee) [G. *mykēs*, fungus; *baktērion*, small staff]. A family of the order Actinomycetales; contains one genus, *Mycobacterium*.

My″co·bac·te'ri·um [*mykēs*; *baktērion*]. A genus of rod-shaped, aerobic bacteria of the family Mycobacteriaceae. Species of this genus are rarely filamentous and occasionally branch but produce no conidia. They are Gram-positive, and stain with difficulty, but are acid-fast.

M. leprae. That species which is the causative organism of leprosy: formerly called *Bacillus leprae*.

M. paratuberculosis. The causative agent of a chronic enteritis of cattle, sheep, and deer, non-pathogenic for man. See Johne's *disease*.

M. tuberculosis. A species of bacilli which produces tuberculosis in mammals; is subdivided into the **Mycobacterium tuberculosis** var. **hominis** var. **bovis,** and var. **muris.** Also called *Bacillus tuberculosis*. See Plate 30.

M. ulcerans. The causative agent of a chronic or subacute ulceration of the skin and subcutaneous tissue on the upper or lower extremity: also called *Barnsdale bacillus*.

my″co·ci′din. An antibiotic substance extracted from a mold of the Aspergillaceae family. It is active, in vitro, against *Mycobacterium tuberculosis*.

my′coid [*mykēs;* G. *eidos*, form]. Resembling, or appearing like, a fungus; fungoid.

my′co·in. An antibiotic believed to be identical with *Escherichia coli* factor, corylophilline, notatin, penatin, and penicillin-B.

α-my·col′ic ac′id. A fatty acid, of high molecular weight, isolated from a human test strain of *Mycobacterium tuberculosis*.

my·col′o·gy [*mykēs;* G. *logos*, word]. The science of fungi.

my″co·myr″in·gi′tis (·mirr″in·jigh′tis, migh″rin·). See *myringomycosis*.

my″co·phe·nol′ic ac′id. An antibiotic derived from *Penicillium brevi-compactum* and *P. stoloniferum*, in vitro active against a variety of microorganisms.

my″coph·thal′mi·a [*mykēs;* G. *ophthalmia*, ophthalmia]. Ophthalmia due to a fungus.

my′cose. Trehalose.

my·co′sis (pl. *mycoses*) (migh·ko′sis; *pl.* migh·ko′-seez) [*mykēs;* G. *-ōsis*, condition]. An infection caused by a fungus. It may be a **superficial mycosis** as in tinea capitis, tinea barbae, when the fungus first invades the stratum corneum, later the hair follicle, and eventually the deeper portions of the hair; or it may be a **deep mycosis** where the infection is essentially or potentially systemic, as in actinomycosis, mycetoma, and coccidioidomycosis. —**mycot′ic,** *adj*.

m. fungoides. A form of lymphoma, with special cutaneous manifestations, characterized by eczematoid areas, infiltrations, nodules, tumors, and ulcerations; possibly a cutaneous form of Hodgkin's *disease:* also called *fibroma fungoides*. Syn., *granuloma fungoides*.

m. fungoides d'emblée. The presence of mycosis fungoides without previous erythema or plaques.

secondary m. See *mycotization*.

my·cos′ter·ol. Any sterol occurring in yeast or fungi.

my″co·sub·til′in. An antibiotic derived from a strain of *Bacillus subtilis*, active in vitro against a variety of yeasts and fungi.

my·cot″i·za′tion. Superimposition of a mycotic infection on a nonfungous lesion; secondary mycosis.

mycozol. Trade-mark for a fungicidal ointment containing chloretone, salicylic acid, and mercury salicylate.

myc″ter·o·pho′ni·a [G. *myktēr*, nostril; *phōnē*, sound]. A nasal quality of the voice.

my·de′sis (migh·dee′sis) [G. *mydēsis*, dampness]. 1. Putrefaction. 2. A discharge of pus from the eyelids.

mydriasine. Trade-mark for atropine methylbromide.

my·dri′a·sis (mi·dry′uh·sis, migh·dry′·) [G., dilatation of the pupil]. Dilatation of the pupil of the eye. —**mydriat′ic,** *adj., n.*

alternating m. Mydriasis which, by normal light and convergence reaction, attacks first one eye and then the other; due to disorder of the central nervous system. Also called *leaping m., springing m.*

paralytic m. That due to the paralysis of the oculomotor nerve.

spasmodic m. That caused by overaction of the sympathetic or dilator nerve of the iris. Also called *spastic m.*

spinal m. That produced by irritation of the ciliospinal center of the spinal cord.

my·ec′to·my (migh·eck′to·mee) [G. *mys*, muscle; *ektomē*, excision]. Excision of a portion of muscle.

my·ec′to·py [*mys;* G. *ektopos*, away from a place]. The abnormal placement of a muscle.

my″e·lap′o·plex″y. Hemorrhage into the spinal cord. *Obs.*

my″e·lat′ro·phy [G. *myelos*, marrow; *atrophia*, want of nourishment]. Atrophy of the spinal cord.

my″el·e′mi·a. See granulocytic *leukemia*.

my″e·len·ceph′a·lon [*myelos;* G. *egkephalos*, brain]. The lower part of the embryonic hindbrain, from which the medulla oblongata develops. —**myelencephal′ic,** *adj.*

my·el′ic (migh·el′ick) [*myelos*]. Pertaining to the spinal cord.

my′e·lin [*myelos*]. 1. The white, fatty substance forming a sheath of some nerves, also called *white substance of Schwann*. 2. A complex mixture of lipins extracted from nervous tissue; it is doubly refractile and contains phosphatides and cholesterol.

my″e·li·nat′ed. Provided with a myelin sheath; medullated.

my″e·li·na′tion [*myelos*]. Myelinization.

my″e·lin′ic [*myelos*]. 1. Relating to myelin. 2. Medullated. *Rare.*

my″e·li·ni·za′tion [*myelos*]. The process of supplying or accumulating myelin during the development, or repair, of nerves.

my″e·lin·o·cla′sis. Demyelination; destruction of the myelin.

acute perivascular m. Postinfection encephalitis.

my″e·li·no·gen′e·sis. Myelinization.

my″e·li·nop′a·thy [*myelos;* G. *pathos*, disease]. Any disease of the myelin.

my″e·li·no′sis [*myelos;* G. *-ōsis*, condition]. Decomposition of fat with the formation of myelin.

my″e·li′tis [*myelos;* G. *-itis*, inflammation]. 1. Inflammation of the spinal cord. 2. Inflammation of the bone marrow. See *osteomyelitis*. —**myelit′ic,** *adj.*

acute ascending m. An ascending form of inflammation of the spinal cord, usually occurring as a manifestation of anterior poliomyelitis or of postvaccinal or postexanthematous myelitis. It may be simulated by a progressive diphtheritic polyneuritis or by the toxic effect of tick bites. Also called *Landry's paralysis*.

acute m. Acute inflammation of the spinal cord.

amyotrophic syphilitic m. See syphilitic *amyotrophia*.

apoplectiform m. Paralysis of sudden onset, due to inflammation of the spinal cord.

disseminated m. Diffuse, irregular, patchy inflammatory lesions of the spinal cord.

funicular m. See subacute combined *degeneration* of spinal cord.

neurooptic m. See *neuroencephalomyelopathy*.

postvaccinal m. Inflammation of the spinal cord which sometimes follows vaccination. Also see acute ascending *m.*

pressure m. Myelitis from pressure on the cord.

syphilitic m. Inflammation of the spinal cord due to syphilis.

transverse m. Inflammation extending across the spinal cord at a specific level.

my′e·lo-, myel- [*myelos*]. A combining form denoting *myelin, the spinal cord,* or *the bone marrow*.

my′e·lo·blast″ [*myelos;* G. *blastos*, germ]. The youngest of the precursor cells of the granulocytic series, having a nucleus with a finely granular or homogeneous chromatin structure and nucleoli and intensely basophilic cytoplasm: also called *granuloblast.*

my″e·lo·blas·te′mi·a [*myelos; blastos;* G. *haima,* blood]. Presence of myeloblasts in the circulating blood.

my″e·lo·blas′tic [*myelos; blastos*]. Originating from, or characterized by, the presence of myeloblasts.

my″e·lo·blas·to′ma [*myelos; blastos;* G. *-ōma,* tumor]. A malignant tumor composed of undifferentiated myeloid cells.

my″e·lo·blas·to′sis [*myelos; blastos;* G. *-ōsis,* condition]. A manifestation of myeloblastic leukemia characterized by the presence of myeloblasts in the circulating blood and a proliferation of myeloblasts in hematopoietic and other tissues and other viscera.

my′e·lo·cele″ [*myelos;* G. *kēlē,* hernia]. Spina bifida, with protrusion of the spinal cord.

my″e·lo·chlo·ro′ma. See *chloroma.*

my″e·lo·cys′to·cele [*myelos;* G. *kystis,* bladder; *kēlē*]. A hernial protrusion, in spina bifida, in which there is accumulation of fluid in the central canal of the spinal cord.

my′e·lo·cyte″ [*myelos;* G. *kytos,* cell]. 1. Any cell concerned in development of granular leukocytes. See *granulocytic series.* 2. A granular leukocyte, precursor in the stage of development intermediate between the myeloblast and metamyelocyte, characterized by granularity of the cytoplasm. The early cells of this stage (*promyelocytes* or *progranulocytes*) include *myelocyte A* and *B.* **Myelocyte A** has fewer than ten usually nonspecifically staining granules, which cover the nucleus and are present in greatest number in the myelocyte B stage; in **myelocyte B,** the nonspecifically staining granules decline, so that few or none are present, while specific (basophilic, eosinophilic, neutrophilic) granules appear. The specific ones are fully developed, and attain greatest number in the *late* or *differentiated myelocyte,* **myelocyte C;** these granules, unlike nonspecific ones of this series, do not cover the nucleus. In myelocyte A and B the nucleus is round and usually centrally placed; in myelocyte C, the nucleus may be eccentrically placed. —**myelocyt′ic,** *adj.*

my″el·o·cy·the′mi·a. See granulocytic *leukemia.*

my″e·lo·cy·to′ma. See *myeloma.*

my″e·lo·cy·to′sis (·sigh·to′sis) [*myelos; kytos;* G. *-ōsis,* increase]. An excess of myelocytes in the blood.

my″e·lo·dys·pla′si·a (migh″i·lo·dis·play′zhuh, ·zee·uh, ·shuh, ·see·uh) [*myelos;* G. *dys-,* bad; *plassein,* to form]. Defective development of the spinal cord, especially in its lumbosacral portion.

my″e·lo·en·ceph″a·li′tis [*myelos;* G. *egkephalos,* brain; *-itis,* inflammation]. Inflammation of both spinal cord and brain.

my″e·lo·fi·bro′sis (migh″i·lo·figh·bro′sis) [*myelos;* L. *fibra,* fiber; G. *-ōsis,* condition]. Fibrosis of the bone marrow.

my″el·o·gen′e·sis. The development of the myelin sheath of a nerve fiber.

my″e·lo·gen′ic, my″e·log′e·nous (migh″i·lodj′i-nus) [*myelos;* G. *genesthai,* from *gignesthai,* to be produced]. Produced in, or by, bone marrow, as in myelogenic leukemia, leukemia due to disease of the bone marrow. Also see *granulocytic series.*

my′e·lo·gone″ [*myelos;* G. *gonē,* offspring]. A primitive blood cell of the bone marrow from which the myeloblast develops.

my′e·lo·gram [*myelos;* G. *gramma,* letter]. Radiograph of the spinal cord, made after the injection of a contrast medium into the subarachnoid space.

my″e·log′ra·phy [*myelos;* G. *graphein,* to write]. Roentgenographic demonstration of the spinal subarachnoid space, after the introduction of contrast mediums such as lipiodol, air, or pantopaque.

my′e·loid [*myelos;* G. *eidos,* form]. Pertaining to bone marrow. Also see *granulocytic series.*

m. reaction. A proliferation of the cells of the granulocytic series with appearance in the blood stream of immature granulocytes and an increased number of granulocytes, seen in association with many infectious diseases, as rubella, scarlet fever, etc.; not a leukemic process.

my″e·lo·ken′tric ac′id. A keto acid, insoluble in water, in the urine of patients with myeloid leukemia as a water-soluble conjugate. It causes proliferation of cells of the leukopoietic system, and produces Hodgkin's-type lesions. It may be reduced to lymphokentric acid.

my″e·lo·lym·phan″gi·o′ma. See *elephantiasis.*

my″e·lo·lym′pho·cyte [*myelos;* L. *lympha,* water; G. *kytos,* cell]. A small lymphocyte formed in the bone marrow.

my″e·lo′ma [*myelos;* G. *-ōma,* tumor]. A primary malignant tumor of bone marrow, generally composed of tumor cells which are uniform, small, and superficially resemble plasmacytes, or dominated by variegated, large cells. Mixtures appear, and the cytologic variations are considered to represent stages in maturation of the tumor cells. It appears most commonly as **multiple m.** or Kahler's disease, characterized by diffuse osteoporosis or areas of bone destruction often resulting in pathologic fractures and bone pain, by anemia, hyperglobulinemia, the finding of Bence-Jones protein, hypercalcemia, and increased number of cells resembling immature plasmacytes in bone marrow. Infrequently it appears as a **solitary m.,** identified by microscopical examination, exclusion of multiple myeloma, and examination of bone marrow. Rarely, a primary **extramedullary m.** occurs, almost exclusively in the upper respiratory and digestive tracts. In older classifications also called, according to predominant cytologic appearance, *erythroid m., hemic m., lymphocytic* or *lymphoid m., myeloid m., plasma cell m., plasmacytic* or *plasmocytic m., plasmacytoma, plasmocytoma, plasmona, plasmacytic* or *plasmocytic sarcoma, myelocytic sarcoma,* or *myeloid tumor.*

endothelial m. See Ewing's *sarcoma.*

my″e·lo·ma·la′ci·a (migh″i·lo·ma·lay′shee·uh, ·see·uh) [*myelos;* G. *malakia,* softness]. Softening of the spinal cord.

my″e·lo·ma·to′sis [*myelos;* G. *-ōma,* tumor; *-ōsis,* increase]. Multiple myeloma.

my″e·lo·men″in·gi′tis [*myelos;* G. *mēnigx,* membrane; *-itis,* inflammation]. Inflammation of the spinal cord and its meninges.

my″e·lo·me·nin′go·cele″ [*myelos; mēnigx;* G. *kēlē,* hernia]. Spina bifida with protrusion of a meningeal sac containing elements of the spinal cord or cauda equina.

my′e·lo·mere″ [*myelos;* G. *meros,* part]. A segment of the spinal cord; a neuromere.

my″e·lo·mon′o·cyte″ [*myelos;* G. *monos,* alone; *kytos,* cell]. A monocyte developing in the bone marrow.

my′el·on. The spinal cord.

my″e·lo·neu·ri′tis (migh″i·lo·new·rye′tis) [*myelos;* G. *neuron,* nerve; *-itis,* inflammation]. Multiple neuritis combined with myelitis.

my″e·lo·pa·ral′y·sis [*myelos;* G. *paralysis,* paralysis]. Spinal paralysis.

my″e·lo·path′ic [*myelos;* G. *pathos,* disease]. Relating to disease of the spinal cord.

my″e·lop′a·thy [*myelos; pathos*]. Any disease of the spinal cord, or of myeloid tissues.

toxic m. Any disease of the spinal cord caused by toxic substances.

transverse m. Disease of the spinal cord localized to a definite cross-sectional level of the cord.

my″e·lop′e·tal [*myelos;* L. *petere,* to seek]. Moving toward the spinal cord.

my″e·loph′thi·sis [*myelos;* G. *phthisis,* a wasting away]. 1. Synonym for tabes dorsalis. 2. Aplastic anemia.

my′e·lo·plaque. See *myeloplax.*

my′e·lo·plast″ [*myelos;* G. *plassein,* to form]. A leukocyte of the bone marrow.

my′e·lo·plax″ (migh′i·lo·placks″) [*myelos;* G. *plax,* anything flat and broad]. A giant cell of the marrow; a myeloplaque; an osteoclast. *Obs.*

my″e·lo·ple′gi·a [*myelos;* G. *plēgē,* a stroke]. Paralysis of spinal origin.

my″e·lo·poi·e′sis [*myelos;* G. *poiēsis,* production]. The process of formation and development of the blood cells in the bone marrow.

ectopic m. The formation in the adult of erythrocytes and granulocytes in regions other than bone marrow. Also called *extramedullary m., extramedullary hematopoiesis.*

my′e·lo·pore″ [*myelos;* G. *poros,* passage]. An opening in the spinal cord.

my″e·lo·pro·lif′er·a·tive dis·or′ders, syn′-drome. Those hematological conditions in which there is diffuse or irregular abnormal proliferative activity of all the hematopoietic bone marrow cells: a concept which postulates that such disorders as chronic granulocytic leukemia, megakaryocytic leukemia, polycythemia vera, agnogenic myeloid metaplasia, and acute erythremia are closely related. Syn., *panmyelosis, panmyelopathy.*

my″e·lo·ra·dic″u·li′tis [*myelos;* L. *radicula,* small root; G. *-itis,* inflammation]. Inflammation of the spinal cord and roots of the spinal nerves.

my″e·lo·ra·dic″u·lo·dys·pla′si·a (·dis·play′zhuh, ·zee·uh, ·shuh, ·see·uh) [*myelos; radicula;* G. *dys-,* prefix meaning bad; *plassein,* to form]. Congenital abnormality of the spinal cord and roots of the spinal nerves.

my″e·lo·ra·dic″u·lop′a·thy [*myelos; radicula;* G. *pathos,* disease]. Disease of the spinal cord and roots of the spinal nerves.

my″e·lo·rrha′gi·a [*myelos;* G. *rhēgnynai,* to burst forth]. Hemorrhage into the spinal cord.

my″e·lo·sar·co′ma. Myeloma.

my″e·los′chi·sis [*myelos;* G. *schisis,* cleavage]. Complete or partial failure of the neural plate to form a neural tube, resulting in a cleft spinal cord.

my″e·lo·scin·to′gram. A myelogram using human serum albumin labeled with radioactive iodine as the localizing substance.

my″e·lo·scin·tog′ra·phy. A technique of introducing iodinated human serum albumin, containing radioactive iodine-131 as a tracer substance, into the spinal subarachnoid space and then of determining the distribution of the radioactive iodine-131 and a profile of the tissue by means of a scintiscanner.

my″e·lo·scle·ro′sis [*myelos;* G. *sclērōsis,* a hardening]. 1. Sclerosis of the spinal cord. 2. A rare, slowly progressing disease of the skeletal system of unknown cause, characterized by an irregular increase of fibrous or bony tissue or both in the bone marrow; a form of agnogenic myeloid metaplasia. Splenomegaly with extramedullary hematopoiesis is the most prominent symptom.

my″e·lo′sis [*myelos;* G. *-ōsis,* condition]. 1. Myelocytosis. 2. The formation of myeloid tumors. 3. Granulocytic leukemia.

acute erythremic m. Acute erythremia.

funicular m. See subacute combined *degeneration* of spinal cord.

leukopenic m. See aleukemic *leukemia.*

my″e·lo·spon′gi·um (migh″i·lo·spon′jee·um, ·spun′jee·um) [*myelos;* G. *spoggion,* dim. of *spoggos,* sponge]. A network in the wall of the neural tube of the embryo, composed of protoplasmic fibers of the spongioblasts.

my″e·lo·syr·in′go·cele. See *syringomyelocele.*

my·en′ta·sis (migh·en′tuh·sis) [G. *mys,* muscle; *entasis,* a straining]. The extension or stretching of a muscle.

my″en·ter′ic [*mys;* G. *enteron,* intestine]. Relating to the muscular coat of the intestine.

my·en′ter·on [*mys; enteron*]. The muscular coat of the intestine.

Myers' method. See under *method.*

Myers and Wardell method for cholesterol. See under *method.*

my″es·the′si·a (migh″ess·thee′zhuh, ·zee·uh) [*mys;* G. *aisthēsis,* perception]. Muscle sense; the perception of a muscular contraction.

my′ia·sis (migh′yuh·sis, migh·eye′uh·sis) [G. *myia,* fly; NL. *-iasis,* condition]. Invasion by the larvae of flies. The type of disease produced depends upon the area or cavity invaded; may be aural, nasal, intestinal, ophthalmic, cutaneous, etc.

my″io·de·op′si·a, my″io·des·op′si·a (migh″yo·, migh″eye·o·) [G. *myioeidēs,* like a fly; *opsis,* vision]. The condition in which muscae volitantes appear.

my·io′sis (migh·yo′sis, migh″eye·o′sis). See *myiasis.*

my″la·ceph′a·lus [G. *mylē,* mill; *a-,* not; *kephalē,* head]. A placental parasitic twin (omphalosite) which has but vestiges of a head and limbs, hence is only a degree above an amorphic fetus.

my′ler·an. $CH_3.SO_2.O(CH_2)_4O.SO_2.CH_3$; 1,4-dimethanesulfonyloxybutane; a drug used experimentally, with some degree of success, in the treatment of myelogenous leukemia.

my′lo-, myl- [*mylē*]. A combining form denoting *molar.*

my·lo′dus (pl. *mylodontes*) [*mylē;* G. *odous,* tooth]. A molar tooth. *Obs.*

my″lo·glos′sus [*mylē;* G. *glōssa,* tongue]. 1. That portion of the superior constrictor of the pharynx which arises from the mylohyoid ridge of the lower jaw. 2. An anomalous slip joining the styloglossus.

my″lo·hy′oid [*mylē;* G. *hyoeidēs,* shaped like the letter upsilon]. Pertaining to the region of the lower molar teeth and the hyoid bone, as mylohyoid muscle. Also called *mylohyoidean.* See Table of Muscles in the Appendix.

my″lo·phar·yn′ge·al. A portion of the superior constrictor muscle of the pharynx.

my′o-, my- [G. *mys,* muscle]. *In medicine,* a combining form denoting *a muscle.*

my″o·arch″i·tec·ton′ic (migh″o·ark″i·teck·ton′-ick) [*mys;* G. *architektonikos,* of a master-builder]. Pertaining to the structure and arrangement of muscle fibers.

my″o·bil′in. A brown pigment excreted in feces in conditions associated with rapid atrophy or destruction of muscle tissue. It appears to consist of a protein component and a prosthetic group, mesobilifuscin.

my′o·blast [*mys;* G. *blastos,* germ]. A cell which develops into a muscle fiber. —**myoblas′tic,** *adj.*

my″o·blas·to′ma [*mys; blastos;* G. *-ēma,* tumor]. See granular-cell *m.*

embryonal m. A mesenchymoma.

granular-cell m. A tumor of controversial origin, considered by many to be made up of myoblasts, widely distributed but most frequently found in the extremities, trunk, and tongue. It is composed of large polygonal cells with deeply staining nuclei and cytoplasm containing many fine acidophilic granules. It is usually benign, but may form one of two types of malignant granular-cell myoblastomas. Also called *granular myoblastoma, myoblastic myoma, myoblastoma, epulis of newborn, granular-cell neurofibroma, embryonal rhabdomyoblastoma, Abrikosov's tumor.*

granular-cell m. of ear canal. See glomus jugulare *tumor.*

malignant granular-cell m. A malignant tumor showing two different forms. The less common one morphologically resembles the benign type. The more common type is organoid in appearance with larger cells growing in masses outlined by fibrous septa. The cytoplasm of the cells, while granular, may be vacuolated; some contain lipid material. These tumors are usually found in the striated muscles of the extremities and often metastasize. Also called *malignant myoblastoma, polymorphous sarcoma, alveolar soft-part sarcoma.*

my″o·car′di·al in″suf·fi′cien·cy. See *cardiac failure.*

my″o·car·di′tis [*mys;* G. *kardia,* heart; *-itis,* inflammation]. Inflammation of the myocardium.

acute bacterial m. Myocarditis caused by bacterial infection.

acute isolated m. See Fiedler's *m.*

Fiedler's m. An inflammation of the myocardium unrelated to known forms of infection and commonly causing myocardial failure: also called *acute isolated m., idiopathic m., interstitial m.*

idiopathic m. See Fiedler's *m.*

interstitial fibroid m. Inflammation of the stroma of an already diseased, fibrotic heart, seen in recurring rheumatic fever.

interstitial m. See Fiedler's *m.*

rheumatic m. A myocarditis of unknown etiology characterized by the formation of Aschoff nodules in the myocardium.

suppurative m. Inflammation of the myocardium characterized by a purulent exudate, either localized or diffuse.

my″o·car′di·um [*mys; kardia*]. The muscular tissue of the heart. See Plate 5. —**myocardial,** *adj.*

myocardone. Trade-mark for a purified and concentrated heart-muscle extract, used therapeutically in various heart diseases.

my″o·car·do′sis [*mys; kardia;* G. *-ōsis,* condition]. Any noninflammatory disease of the myocardium.

myochrysine. Trade-mark for an ampuled solution of gold sodium thiomalate, $C_4H_3O_4SAuNa_2$, used by intramuscular injection in rheumatoid arthritis, pulmonary tuberculosis, and lupus erythematosus.

my″o·clo′ni·a [*mys;* G. *klonos,* confused motion]. Any disorder characterized by myoclonus.

infectious m. Chorea.

my″o·clo′nus (migh″o·klo′nus, migh·ock′lo·nus) [*mys; klonos*]. Clonic spasm of a muscle or of various muscles. —**myoclonic,** *adj.*

palatal m. Rhythmic contractions of the palate seen in patients with lesions in the brain stem when these lesions involve the olives or their connections with the tegmentum. Also called *palatal nystagmus.*

Unverricht's familial m. A hereditary form of myoclonic epilepsy most frequently affecting the tongue, pharynx, and diaphragm; occurs mainly in girls about 10 years of age.

my′o·coele. The cavity of a myotome, 2.

my′o·cyte [*mys;* G. *kytos,* cell]. A muscle cell.

Anitschkow m. See Anitschkow *cell.*

my″o·dys·to′ni·a [*mys;* G. *dys-,* bad; *tonos,* tone]. A condition in parkinsonism marked by the rapid response of the muscles to faradic stimulation, contrasted with the prolonged and interrupted contraction time.

my″o·dys′tro·phy [*mys; dys-;* G. *trophē,* nourishment]. Degeneration of muscles.

my″o·e·de′ma [*mys;* G. *oidēma,* swelling]. Edema of a muscle.

my″o·e·las′tic [*mys;* G. *elaunein,* to drive]. Pertaining to the layer of intimately interrelated smooth muscle cells and elastic fibers in bronchi and bronchioles.

my″o·ep″i·the′li·al [*mys;* G. *epi,* on; *thēlē,* nipple]. Referring to contractile cells of ectodermal origin.

my″o·ep″i·the″li·o′ma. A slow-growing sweat-gland tumor appearing as a solitary or rarely multiple, firm, well circumscribed intracutaneous nodule usually less than 2 cm in diameter. The two types of cells found are the secretory and the myoepithelial cells. Also called *myoepithelial tumor, myoepithelial sweat-gland tumor, nodular hidradenoma.*

my″o·fas′ci·al (migh″o·fash′ee·ul) [*mys;* L. *fascia,* band]. Pertaining to the fasciae of muscles, as myofascial inflammation.

my″o·fas·ci′tis (migh″o·fa·sigh′tis) [*mys; fascia;* G. *-itis,* inflammation]. A term, both anatomic and descriptive, indicating low back pain of obscure pathology, with symptoms severe enough to indicate probable inflammatory origin.

my″o·fi′bril [*mys;* L. *fibra,* fiber]. A fibril found in the cytoplasm of muscle.

my″o·fi·bro′ma (migh″o·figh·bro′muh). See *leiomyoma.*

my″o·fi″bro·sar·co′ma. A leiomyosarcoma with rich fibromatous component: occasional term.

my″o·ge·lo′sis [*mys;* L. *gelare,* to freeze; G. *-ōsis,* condition]. A hardened region in a muscle; specifically, hard nodules localized at the head of a muscle.

my′o·gen. Collectively, the water-soluble proteins of muscle, largely located in the sarcoplasm and consisting of various enzymes.

my″o·gen′ic [*mys;* G. *genesthai,* from *gignesthai,* to be produced]. Of muscular origin, used in myogenic contraction of muscle, as opposed to neurogenic contraction.

my″o·glo′bin [*mys;* L. *globus,* ball]. Myohemoglobin, muscle hemoglobin; the form of hemoglobin occurring in the muscle fibers. It differs somewhat from blood hemoglobin in showing a displacement of the spectral absorption bands toward the red, a higher oxygen affinity, and a hyperbolic dissociation curve, a smaller Bohr effect, a lower affinity for carbon monoxide, and a lower molecular weight. It serves as a short-time oxygen store, carrying the muscle from one contraction to the next.

my″o·glo″bin·u′ri·a. The presence of free myoglobin in the urine, seen in Haff disease, trauma, aschemia, and other primary lesions of striated muscle which result in muscle necrosis.

paroxysmal paralytic m. A rare disease of unknown cause characterized by sudden painful muscle spasms, probably corresponding to the onset of focal necrosis in the affected muscles, and excretion of a brownish urine, found to contain myoglobin. It may be a sporadic varient of Haff disease.

traumatic m. That following severe physical damage to striated muscle as the result of crushing injuries, high-voltage currents, or even extreme physical punishment.

my″o·gnath′us [*mys;* G. *gnathos,* jaw]. A form of double monster in which a rudimentary head is joined to the jaw of the autosite by means of muscle and integument only.

my′o·gram [*mys;* G. *gramma,* letter]. The tracing made by the myograph.

my′o·graph [*mys;* G. *graphein,* to write]. An instrument for recording the phases of a muscular contraction. —**myograph'ic,** *adj.*

my″o·he'ma·tin (migh″o·hee'muh·tin, ·hem'uh·tin). A respiratory enzyme; an iron porphyrin compound allied to hematin; important in animal and plant tissue oxidation.

my″o·he″mo·glo'bin (·hee″mo·glo'bin, ·hem″o·) [*mys;* G. *haima,* blood; L. *globus,* ball]. Myoglobin.

my″o·he″mo·glo″bin·u'ri·a. Myoglobinuria.

my·oi'des (migh·oy'deez) [*mys;* G. *eidos,* form]. See *platysoma.*

my″o·in·o'si·tol. New name proposed for the common inositol, sometimes called *mesoinositol,* to distinguish it from the eight other possible stereoisomers.

my″o·ki'nase, my·ok'i·nase. An enzyme present in muscle tissue which enables myosin to bring about the reaction by which two moles of adenosinediphosphate yield one mole of adenylic acid and one mole of adenosinetriphosphate. It also facilitates the action of hexokinase in catalyzing the reaction between glucose or fructose and adenosinetriphosphate by which glucose-6-phosphate or fructose-6-phosphate and adenosinediphosphate are formed.

my″o·ki·ne'si·o·gram″ [*mys;* G. *kinēsis,* motion; *gramma,* letter]. The curve obtained in myokinesiography.

my″o·kin″es·i·og'ra·phy. 1. A method of recording graphically the movement of muscle either in vivo or in vitro. 2. Specifically, a method for studying muscle action during walking; it reveals disturbances in motor activity and coordination.

my″o·ky'mi·a (migh″o·kigh'mee·uh, ·kim'ee·uh) [*mys;* G. *kyma,* wave]. Constant quivering of a muscle. See *myoclonus.*

my″o·li·po'ma. A mesenchymoma.

my·ol'o·gy (migh·ol'o·jee) [*mys;* G. *logos,* word]. The science of the nature, structure, functions, and diseases of muscles.

my·o'ma (migh·o'muh) [*mys;* G. *-ōma,* tumor]. A tumor derived from muscle. When it is derived from smooth muscle, it is called a **leiomyoma;** when derived from striated muscle, it is called a **rhabdomyoma.** —**myom'atous,** *adj.*

myoblastic m. See granular-cell *myoblastoma.*

m. striocellulare. Rhabdomyoma.

m. telangiectoides. A myoma with many blood vascular spaces, often cavernous. Also called *angiomyoma.*

my″o·ma·la'ci·a (migh″o·ma·lay'shee·uh, ·see·uh) [*mys;* G. *malakia,* softness]. Degeneration, with softening, of muscle tissue.

m. cordis. Softening of a portion of the heart muscle, usually resulting from thrombosis or embolism.

my″o·mec'to·my [*mys;* G. *-ōma,* tumor; *ektomē,* excision]. Excision of a uterine or other myoma.

my·ome' dar·to·ïque' (migh·ome' dar·to·eek') [F.]. A solitary leiomyoma occurring usually in the external genitalia or rarely in the nipples.

my'o·mere. Old term for myotome, 2.

my″o·me·tri'tis [*mys;* G. *mētra,* womb; *-itis,* inflammation]. Inflammation of the uterine muscular tissue.

my″o·me'tri·um [*mys; mētra*]. The uterine muscular structure.

my'o·neme [*mys;* G. *nēma,* thread]. One of the long contractile fibrillae in protozoa.

my″o·neu'ral [*mys;* G. *neuron,* nerve]. 1. Pertaining to both muscle and nerve. 2. Relating to the nerve endings in muscle tissue.

my″o·pal'mus [*mys;* G. *palmos,* quivering motion]. Twitching of the muscles.

my″o·pa·ral'y·sis [*mys;* G. *paralysis,* paralysis]. Paralysis of a muscle or muscles.

my″o·pa·re'sis (migh″o·pa·ree'sis, ·par'i·sis) [*mys;* G. *paresis,* paralysis]. Slight paralysis of muscle.

my″o·path'i·a ra·chit'i·ca (ra·kit'i·kuh). The muscular atonia of rachitic infants.

my″o·path'ic [*mys;* G. *pathos,* disease]. Depending upon or relating to disease of the muscles.

my·op'a·thy, my″o·path'i·a [*mys; pathos*]. Any disease of the muscles.

my'ope [G. *myōps,* closing or contracting the eyes]. A person affected with myopia.

my″o·per″i·car·di'tis [G. *mys,* muscle; *perikardios,* around the heart]. A combination of pericarditis with myocarditis.

my·o'pi·a (migh·o'pee·uh) [G. *myōps,* closing or contracting the eyes]. Nearsightedness; an optical defect, usually due to too great length of the anteroposterior diameter of the globe, whereby the focal image is formed in front of the retina. Symbol, my. —**myop'ic,** *adj.*

high m. A degree of myopia greater than 6.5 diopters.

low m. One less than 2 diopters.

malignant m. Rapidly progressing myopia.

progressive m. of children. Continuous increase of myopia, due to increasing growth of the eyeball.

twilight m. A phenomenon of normal eyes in which they become myopic in dim light, a factor of great importance in night flying.

my'o·plasm [G. *mys,* muscle; *plasma,* anything formed]. The cytoplasm of a muscle cell or fiber.

my'o·plas″ty [*mys;* G. *plassein,* to form]. Plastic surgery on a muscle or group of muscles.

my″o·por·tho'sis [G. *myōps,* closing or contracting the eyes; *orthōsis,* a making straight]. The correction of myopia.

my″o·psy·chop'a·thy (migh″o·sigh·kop'uth·ee) [G. *mys,* muscle; *psychē,* soul; *pathos,* disease]. A disease of the muscles associated with feebleness or defect of mind. Syn., *myopsychosis.*

my″o·psy·cho'sis (migh″o·sigh·ko'sis). Myopsychopathy.

myorgal. Trade-mark for a preparation of nucleosides free of choline, histamine, and epinephrine. The preparation is used as a vasodilator.

my·or'rha·phy (migh·orr'uh·fee) [G. *mys,* muscle; *rhaphē,* suture]. Suture of a muscle.

my'o·san [*mys*]. A protein derivative of the class of proteans which is formed by the action of dilute acid or water on myosin.

my″o·sar·co'ma [*mys;* G. *sarkōma,* fleshy excrescence]. A sarcoma derived from muscle.

granular-cell m. See malignant granular-cell *myoblastoma,* 1.

my″o·schwan·no'ma. See *neurilemmoma.*

my″o·scle·ro'sis [*mys;* G. *sklērōsis,* hardening]. Fibrous myositis.

my'o·sin [*mys*]. One of the principal proteins occurring in muscle, comprising up to one-half of the total muscle protein. It combines with actin to form actomyosin, and as such is believed to be responsible for the birefringent, contractile, and elastic properties of muscle. It is closely associated with the enzyme adenosine triphosphatase (ATPase). Its coagulation after death is the cause of rigor mortis.

my″o·si'tis [*mys;* G. *-itis,* inflammation]. Inflammation of muscle, usually referring to voluntary muscle. —**myosit'ic,** *adj.*

fibrous m. Chronic myositis with formation of fibrous tissue.

gas-gangrene m. Inflammation of a muscle followed by or concomitant with a necrotizing infection by anaerobic gas-producing bacteria.

interstitial m. Inflammation of the stroma of muscle.

ischemic m. Inflammatory reaction in muscle due to marked reduction of blood supply, as by prolonged tight bandaging of a fracture.

m. ossificans. Myositis with formation of bone. It includes a circumscribed form, with bone formation in a scar; a traumatic form with bone formation in the injured part of the muscle; and a multiple progressive form, characterized by bone formation in many foci in muscles, tendons, ligaments, etc., beginning in early life and progressively increasing.

parenchymatous m. Inflammation affecting the muscle fibers.

rheumatoid m. That characterized by focal inflammation, lesions occurring in muscles during the course of rheumatoid arthritis.

trichinous m. That due to *Trichinella spiralis* in the muscle.

my″o·stat′ic [*mys;* G. *statikos,* causing to stand]. Referring to a muscle of fixed length in relaxation, as in myostatic contracture.

my″o·su′ture [*mys;* L. *sutura,* a sewing together]. Suture of a muscle; myorrhaphy.

my″o·syn″o·vi′tis. Inflammation of synovial membranes and surrounding musculature.

my″o·tac′tic [*mys; tactum,* from L. *tangere,* to touch]. Relating to muscular sense.

my·ot′a·sis (migh·ot′uh·sis) [*mys;* G. *tasis,* a stretching]. Stretching of a muscle. —**myotat′ic,** *adj*

my″o·ten″o·si′tis [*mys;* G. *tenōn,* tendon; *-itis,* inflammation]. Inflammation of a muscle and its tendon.

my″o·te·not′o·my [*mys; tenōn;* G. *tomē,* a cutting]. Surgical division of muscles and tendons.

my′o·tome [*mys;* G. *tomos,* cutting]. 1. An instrument for performing myotomy. 2. That part of a somite that differentiates into skeletal muscle. Syn., *muscle plate.* 3. The muscle group innervated by a single spinal nerve.

head m. One of the specialized head somites present in many vertebrate embryos that give rise to the eye muscles.

my·ot′o·my (migh·ot′o·mee) [*mys;* G. *tomē,* a cutting]. Division of a muscle, particularly through its belly.

my″o·to′ni·a [*mys;* G. *tonos,* tone]. Tonic muscular spasm.

m. acquisita. A disease of unknown cause characterized by tonic muscular spasm.

m. atrophica. See muscular *dystrophy.*

m. congenita. A congenital and usually hereditary disease characterized by tonic spasms in the voluntarily moved muscles. Also called *Thomsen's disease.*

m. congenita intermittens. See *paramyotonia congenita.*

m. dystrophica. See muscular *dystrophy.*

my″ot′ro·phy. Nutrition of muscle

myoxane. Trade-mark for *mephenesin.*

myr′cene. $C_{10}H_{16}$; 7-methyl-3-methylene-1,6-octadiene; a terpene hydrocarbon occurring in myrcia oil and other volatile oils.

myr·i·a′chit (meer·yah′chit. *See* Notes § 35). See *palmus,* 1.

myr′i·a·gram [G. *myrioi,* ten thousand; *gramma,* scruple]. Ten thousand grams.

myr″i·a·li′ter (mirr″ee·uh·lee′tur) [*myrioi;* G. *litra,* pound]. Ten thousand liters.

myr″i·a·me′ter [*myrioi;* G. *metron,* a measure]. Ten thousand meters.

myr′i·a·pods. Millipedes and centipedes.

my·ri′ca [G. *myrikē,* tamarisk]. The dried bark of the root of *Myrica cerifera* and *M. pennsylvanica;* formerly used as an astringent and tonic. Also employed in diarrhea. Also called *bayberry bark.*

myr′i·cin. Myricyl palmitate, $C_{30}H_{61}O_2C_{16}H_{31}$, a constituent of beeswax.

myr′i·cyl. The univalent hydrocarbon radical $CH_3(CH_2)_{29}$—. Syn., *melissyl.*

m. alcohol. $CH_3(CH_2)_{28}CH_2OH$; an alcohol present in beeswax as a palmitate ester, known as *myricin.* Syn., *melissyl alcohol.*

my·rin′ga [ML., from G. *mēnigx,* membrane]. The tympanic membrane.

myr″in·gec′to·my (mirr″in·jeck′to·mee). See *myringodectomy.*

myr″in·gi′tis (mirr″in·jy′tis, my″rin·) [*mēnigx;* G. *-itis,* inflammation]. Inflammation of the tympanic membrane.

m. bullosa. Myringitis with bullous lesions on the tympanic membrane. These may contain serum or blood.

my·rin″go·dec′to·my [*mēnigx;* G. *ektomē,* excision]. Excision of a part or of the whole of the tympanic membrane.

my·rin″go·my·co′sis (mi·ring″go·migh·ko′sis) [*mēnigx;* G. *mykēs,* fungus; *-ōsis,* condition]. An infection of the eardrum due to fungi, usually as the result of spread from the external auditory canal; an otomycosis.

my·rin′go·plas″ty [*mēnigx;* G. *plassein,* to form]. A plastic operation on the tympanic membrane. —**myringoplast′ic,** *adj.*

my·rin′go·tome [*mēnigx;* G. *tomos,* cutting]. Instrument used in incising tympanic membrane.

myr″in·got′o·my [*mēnigx;* G. *tomē,* a cutting]. Incision of the tympanic membrane.

my′rinx. See *myringa.*

my·ris′ti·ca (mi·ris′ti·kuh, migh·ris′·). Nutmeg.

my·ris′tic ac′id (mi·ris′tick, migh·ris′tick). $CH_3(CH_2)_{12}COOH$. A fatty acid occurring in the glycerides of many fats.

my·ris′ti·cin. $C_{11}H_{12}O_3$. A liquid constituent of myristica (nutmeg) oil.

my·ris′ti·col. $C_{10}H_{16}O$. An oily substance extracted from nutmeg oil.

my·ris′tin. $(C_{14}H_{27}O_2)_3C_3H_5$. Glyceryl trimyristate, a component of spermaceti, nutmeg butter, and other fats.

my′ro·nate. A salt of myronic acid.

my·ron′ic ac′id (migh·ron′ick, mi·ron′ick). $C_{10}H_{19}NS_2O_{10}$. The acid component of the glycoside, sinigrin, found in black mustard, which on hydrolysis yields allyl isothiocyanate.

myr′o·sin (mirr′o·sin, migh′ro·sin). An albuminous ferment found in mustard seed; liberates the mustard oil from potassium myronate.

myrrh (mur) [G. *myrra*]. A gum resin obtained from *Commiphora molmol, C. abyssinica,* or other species of *Commiphora.* Contains a volatile oil, a resin myrrhin, and a gum; used as an aromatic stimulant mouthwash. Has been used as a local application in various forms of stomatitis.

myrticolorin. See *rutin.*

myr′til·lin (mur′ti·lin) [L. *myrtus,* myrtle]. An extract from the berries of *Vaccinium myrtillus,* one of the Ericaceae with insulinlike properties. Has been used to reduce glycosuria in diabetes.

myr′tle [*myrtus*]. The dried leaves of *Myrtus communis;* its volatile oil yields myrtol.

myr′tol (mur′tole, ·tol, ·tawl) [*myrtus*]. A constituent of the essential oil of myrtle; formerly used in bronchial and pulmonary affections as antiseptic.

mysoline. Trade-mark for 5-phenyl-5-ethylhexahydropyrimidine-4:6-dione; $C_6H_5.C_2H_5.C-(CONH)_2CH_2$; a white crystalline substance, sparingly soluble in water: effective in initial clinical trials on patients subject to attacks of epilepsy.

my″so·pho′bi·a [G. *mysos,* defilement; *phobos,* fear]. Abnormal dread of contamination or of dirt.

my′ta·cism [G. *mytakismos,* fondness for the letter

mu]. Excessive or faulty use of the letter *m*, and its substitution for other sounds. Syn., *mutacism.*

myth″o·ma′ni·a [G. *mythos*, story; *mania*, madness]. A morbid tendency to lie or to exaggerate; a condition seen in certain psychiatric patients.

myth″o·pho′bi·a [*mythos;* G. *phobos*, fear]. A morbid dread of stating what is not absolutely correct.

myt″i·lo·tox′in. A poisonous principle found in mussels.

myt″i·lo·tox′ism [G. *mytilos*, mussel; *toxikon*, poison]. Mussel poisoning, with paralysis of the central and peripheral nervous system.

mytolon chloride. Trade-marked name for 2,5-*bis*(3-diethylaminopropylamino)-benzoquinone-*bis*-benzyl chloride; $C_{34}H_{50}Cl_2N_4O_2$: a curariform compound used as a skeletal muscle relaxant in surgical anesthesia.

my·u′rous (migh·yoor′us) [G. *mys*, mouse; *oura*, tail]. Tapering like the tail of the mouse; said of the pulse when it is progressively growing feeble. *Obs.*

myvizone. Trade-mark for *amithiozone.*

myx·ad″e·ni′tis [G. *myxa*, mucus; *adēn*, gland; *-itis*, inflammation]. Inflammation of a mucous gland.

m. labialis. Inflammation of the mucous membrane of the lips; characterized by painless papules. See also *cheilitis glandularis.*

myx·ad″e·no′ma. See *myxoadenoma.*

myx″as·the′ni·a (mix″ass·thee′nee·uh, mix·ass″-thi·nigh′uh) [*myxa;* G. *astheneia*, weakness]. Overdryness of the mucosa or impairment of the power to secrete mucus. *Rare.*

myx″e·de′ma [*myxa;* G. *oidēma*, swelling]. A constitutional disorder, occurring usually in adults or older children; due to decrease or absence of thyroid hormone resulting from atrophy, removal, lack of normal stimulation, inhibition of hormone formation, or prevention of hormone utilization, as with drugs. It is characterized by a sallow, puffy appearance, especially of the face and hands, low basal metabolic rate (−25 to −40%), increased sensitivity to cold, dryness of skin and absence of sweating, dryness and sparseness of the hair, brittleness of the nails, paresthesia, apathy, lethargy, delayed cerebration, retarded reflexes, slow, thick, coarse speech, anemia, increased glucose tolerance, change in plasma protein levels, hypercholesterolemia, cardiac dilatation, bradycardia, and low-voltage electrocardiogram. It is completely controlled by the continued administration of a sufficient dose of desiccated thyroid orally or thyroxin intravenously. Also called *Gull's disease, athyrea, athyreosis.* —**myxedem′atous,** *adj.*

childhood m. That occurring before puberty.

circumscribed m. A rare condition arising in patients who have had hyperthyroidism; characterized by the appearance of small or large, raised, solid, reddish or reddish brown, sharply circumscribed areas over the shins; heavily infiltrated with a mucinous material. It does not respond to thyroid feeding. Also called *localized m, m. circumscriptum thyrotoxicum, trophedema of Basedow.*

m. circumscriptum thyrotoxicum. See circumscribed *m.*

operative m. That arising as a result of removal of a large part of the thyroid gland. Syn., *cachexia strumipriva.*

pituitary m. A rare type of myxedema developing in association with, and probably resulting from, pituitary deficiency, as in pituitary adenoma.

myx·id′i·o·cy [*myxa;* G. *idiōteia*, want of education]. Cretinism.

myx″i·o′sis [*myxa;* G. *-ōsis*, condition]. A mucous discharge. *Obs.*

myx′o-, myx- [*myxa*]. A prefix meaning *relating to mucus* or *mucoid.* A combining form meaning *mucus;* denotes a *mucous gland* or *mucous tissue.*

myx″o·ad″e·no′ma [*myxa;* G. *adēn*, gland; *-ōma*, tumor]. Adenoma with a myxomatous component; an adenoma of a mucous gland.

myx″o·chon″dro·fi″bro·sar·co′ma (mick″so-kon″dro·) [*myxa;* G. *chondros*, cartilage; L. *fibra*, fiber; G. *sarkōma*, fleshy excrescence]. A malignant tumor composed of a mixture of myxomatous, chondromatous, and fibromatous elements.

myx″o·chon·dro′ma. See *chondromyxoma.*

myx″o·chon″dro·sar·co′ma [*myxa; chondros;* G. *sarkōma*, fleshy excrescence]. A chondrosarcoma showing extensive myxomatous degeneration: also called *chondrosarcoma myxomatodes.* Syn. *chondromyxosarcoma.*

myx′o·cyte [*myxa;* G. *kytos*, cell]. A large cell polyhedral or stellate, found in mucous tissue.

myx″o·fi·bro′ma (mick″so·figh·bro′muh) [*myxa;* L. *fibra*, fiber; G. *-ōma*, tumor]. A fibroma with a myxomatous component.

m. of breast. See *cystosarcoma phylloides.*

m. of nerve sheath. See *neurofibroma.*

myx″o·fi″bro·sar·co′ma [*myxa; fibra;* G. *sarkōma*, fleshy excrescence]. A malignant tumor composed of myxomatous and fibrosarcomatous elements. Often mucoid degeneration in a fibrosarcoma, that is, fibrosarcoma myxomatodes.

m. of breast. See *cystosarcoma phylloides.*

myx″o·gli·o′ma (mick″so·glye·o′muh) [*myxa;* G. *glia*, glue; *-ōma*, tumor]. A gelatinous form of glioma.

myx′oid [*myxa;* G. *eidos*, form]. Like mucus.

myx″o·li·po′ma [*myxa;* G. *lipos*, fat; *-ōma*]. See *liposarcoma.*

myx″o·li·po″sar·co′ma. See *liposarcoma.*

myx·o′ma [*myxa; -ōma*]. A connective-tissue tumor, composed of cells of stellate and spindle form with processes separated by mucoid material. Tissue of similar type is frequently seen in foci in other connective-tissue tumors. Also called *m. simplex, m. gelatinosum, m. medullare.* —**myx-om′atous,** *adj.*

cystic m. One with an accumulation of mucoid so as to resemble cysts. Also called *cystoid m.*

giant mammary m. See *cystosarcoma phylloides.*

intracanalicular m. See intracanalicular *fibroadenoma.*

intracanalicular m. (of breast). See *cystosarcoma phylloides.*

malignant m. One displaying infiltrative growth, usually a myxoma of the heart.

m. cavernosum. A cystic *m.*

m. fibrosum. See *fibromyxoma.*

m. lipomatodes. See *liposarcoma.*

odontogenic m. One of the jaws, considered to be of dental origin, and usually seen in young individuals.

telangiectatic m. One with a rich vascular component. Also called *m. telangiectodes, vascular m.*

myx″o·ma·to′sis [*myxa; -ōma;* G. *-ōsis*, condition]. The presence of numerous myxomas.

infectious m. An infectious disease in rabbits, transmitted by a virus, with widespread lesions resembling myxomas.

Myx″o·my·ce′tes (mick″so·migh·see′teez) [*myxa;* G. *mykēs*, fungus]. A class of fungi, known as the slime molds, none of which is pathogenic to man; resemble protozoa in some respects.

myx″o·neu·ro′ma [*myxa;* G. *neuron*, nerve; *-ōma*, tumor]. 1. A neuroma, or more often a neurofibroma, with a myxomatous component, occurring in peripheral nerves. 2. Mucoid form of meningioma. 3. A gelatinous form of glioma.

myx″or·rhe′a [*myxa;* G. *rhoia,* flow]. A copious mucous discharge.

myx″o·sar·co′ma [*myxa;* G. *sarkōma,* fleshy excrescence]. A sarcoma with a myxomatous component.

m. of breast. See *cystosarcoma phylloides.*

myx′o·spore [*myxa;* G. *sporē,* seed]. A spore produced in the midst of a gelatinous mass without a distinct ascus or basidium.

My″zo·my′ia [G. *myzein,* to suck; *myia,* fly]. A subgenus of the genus *Anopheles,* the mosquito which transmits the malarial parasite.

N

N 1. Chemical symbol for nitrogen. 2. Abbreviation for normal.

N- *In chemistry,* symbol prefixed to a radical which is attached to the nitrogen atom.

n 1. A unit of neutron dosage corresponding to the roentgen. 2. Symbol for refractive index.

n. Abbreviation for nasal.

n- *In chemistry,* normal.

N. A. Numerical aperture.

Na Chemical symbol for sodium (*natrium*).

Naboth, Martin [*German anatomist,* 1675–1721]. Known eponymically for his description of the mucous follicles of the cervix uteri about the external os; called *Naboth's follicles* or *glands.* He also described the small retention cysts formed by the Nabothian follicles which are called *Nabothian cysts* or *ovules.* The discharge of thin mucus from the pregnant uterus, which accumulates as the result of excessive secretion of the uterine glands, is known as *Nabothian menorrhagia.*

na′cre·ous (nay′kree·us, nack′ree·us) [Ar. *naqqārah,* drum]. Resembling mother-of-pearl.

N. A. D. No appreciable disease.

Naegele, Franz Karl [*German obstetrician,* 1778–1851]. Once named the Euclid of obstetrics for his geometric description of biparietal obliquity (*Naegele's obliquity*), the lateral inclination of the fetal head at the superior pelvic strait (1819); described the obliquely contracted pelvis, with ankylosis of one sacroiliac synchondrosis, and imperfect development of the sacrum (1839) (*Naegele pelvis*). Invented an obstetric extraction instrument equipped with cephalic and pelvic curves and attached axis-traction bar; called *Naegele's forceps.*

Naegeli, Otto [*Swiss physician,* 1871–1938]. Devised a maneuver for relief of epistaxis, in which upward traction of the patient's head is made with one hand of the physician under the patient's occiput and the other under the jaw; called *Naegeli's maneuver.*

Naegeli test. See under *test.*

nae′paine hy″dro·chlo′ride. $NH_2.C_6H_4.COOCH_2.CH_2.NH.CH_2(CH_2)_3CH_3.HCl$; 2-amylaminoethyl-*p*-aminobenzoate hydrochloride; a white powder, soluble in water; its actions resemble those of cocaine hydrochloride, but the solution does not cause mydriasis: used to produce corneal anesthesia. See *amylsine hydrochloride.*

nae′vus (nee′vus). See *nevus.*

Naffziger, Howard Christian [*American surgeon,* 1884–]. Distinguished neurosurgeon. Described the scalenus syndrome, called *Naffziger's syndrome.* Described excision of the superior and lateral walls of the orbit for the relief of progressive exophthalmos; called *Naffziger's operation.* See also Naffziger's *test.*

na·ga′na (na·gah′nuh) [Zulu]. An infectious disease of domestic animals, especially equine animals in East Africa, caused by the *Trypanosoma brucei.* It is transmitted by the bite of the tsetse fly.

naganol. Trade name for *suramin.*

Na′ga sore (nah′guh). See tropical *ulcer.*

Nagel's test. See under *test.*

Nageotte, Jean [*French pathologist,* 1866–1948]. Known for his association with Babinski in the study of the syndrome of contralateral hemiplegia. See under *Babinski.*

Nagler's reaction. See under *reaction.*

nail [AS. *naegel*]. 1. The horny structure covering the dorsal aspect of the terminal phalanx of each finger and toe. It consists of intimately united, horny epithelial cells probably representing the stratum corneum of the epidermis. 2. A metallic (usually stainless steel or vitallium) elongated rod with one sharp and one blunt end, used in surgery to anchor bone fragments. Syn., *pin.*

clover-leaf n. An intramedullary nail which in cross section is shaped like a clover leaf: used particularly for internal fixation of fractures of the femur.

eggshell n. A nail which assumes a semitransparent, bluish white hue resembling the color of the shell of an egg. The nail plate is thinned and shows a tendency to curve upward at the free border. Hyperhidrosis may be an associated condition.

Hippocratic n. See clubbed *finger.*

ingrowing n. An overlapping of the nail by the adjacent tissues, often attended by painful ulceration and exuberant granulations. It is most common in the great toe.

intramedullary n. One inserted through the medullary canal of a tubular bone to provide internal immobilization of fractures. It is long enough to pass across the fracture site to obtain fixation in both fragments of the bone.

Jewett angle n. A nail, 2, for internal fixation of intertrochanteric fractures; a single piece of metal with a three-flanged nail to be driven into the head and neck of the femur and an attached flat plate to conform to the side of the femur shaft.

Küntscher n. A stainless steel rod used for intramedullary fixation of fractures of long bones, especially the femur, tibia, humerus, radius, and ulna: also called *Küntscher intramedullary n.*

n. bed. A vascular tissue, corresponding to the corium and the germinative layer of the skin, on which a nail rests.

n. culture. *In bacteriology,* a stab-culture showing a growth along the needle track, and on the surface a buttonlike projection, giving the appearance of a nail driven into the gelatin.

n. en raquette. A dystrophy of the nail in which the nail, usually that of the thumb, appears wider than normal, its transverse curvature diminished so that the nail seems flat. The effect is that of a miniature tennis racket.

n. fold. The fold of skin bounding the sides and proximal portion of a nail.

n. groove. The sulcus between the nail fold and the nail bed.

n. root. The part of the body of the nail covered by the proximal nail fold.

n. wall. See *n.* fold.

Neufeld n. *In orthopedics*, a V-shaped device for internal fixation of intertrochanteric fractures; a nail inserted into the neck of the femur merges with a rounded plate which is fastened to the side of the femur with screws.

parrot-beak n. A nail curved like a parrot's beak.

Smith-Petersen n. A three-flanged nail used to fix fractures of the neck of the femur. It is inserted from laterally on the shaft just below the greater trochanter, through the neck, and into the head of the femur.

spoon n. See *koilonychia.*

Steinmann's n. See Fritz *Steinmann.*

Thornton n. A nail, 2, for internal fixation of intertrochanteric fractures; a metallic plate is screwed on to the end of a Smith-Petersen nail and secured to the shaft of the femur with screws.

turtle-back n. A nail curved in all directions; a condition seen in certain trophic disturbances.

nail bit′ing. Onychophagia; a nervous affliction or neurotic reaction in adolescents and children, manifested by the habit of biting the fingernails down to the quick. The habit is difficult to break and frequently persists into middle age.

Naiman's test. See under *test.*

Na′ja (nah′juh) [Skr. *nāga*, snake]. A genus of venomous snakes of the family Elapidae; commonly known as cobras.

N. haje. The Egyptian cobra which has a markedly hemolytic venom.

N. hannah. The king cobra; an aggressive and large species of snakes. It possesses a powerful neurotoxic venom.

N. naja. The well-known Indian or Asiatic cobra which is smaller and commoner than the king cobra. The species possesses a neurotoxic venom.

Najjar riboflavin method. See under *method.*

na′ked [AS. *nacod*]. Unclothed; nude.

nalline hydrochloride. Trade-marked name for *nalorphine hydrochloride.*

nal·or′phine hy″dro·chlo′ride. $C_{19}H_{21}NO_3.HCl$; N-allylnormorphine hydrochloride; a derivative of morphine, occurring as a white, crystalline powder, soluble in water. It exerts little or no analgesic effect and antagonizes such narcotic analgesics as morphine, meperidine, and methadone; it is useful as an antidote in treating accidental overdosage or to combat alarming symptoms of extreme narcosis produced by morphine and other narcotic analgesics. See *nalline hydrochloride.*

nam′bi u′vu. A disease of dogs in Brazil; marked by icterus and bleeding from the ear; caused by a blood parasite. Syn., *canine yellow fever.* Also called *bleeding ear, blood plague.*

nan′di·nine. $C_{19}H_{19}NO_4$; an alkaloid from the root bark of *Nandina domestica*, a shrub of the Berberidaceae family.

na′nism (nay′niz·um, nan′iz·um) [G. *nanos*, dwarf]. Abnormal smallness from arrested development; dwarfism.

na″no·ceph′a·lus (nay″no·sef′uh·lus, nan″o·) [*nanos;* G. *kephalē*, head]. A fetus with a dwarfed head.

na″no·cor′mi·a [*nanos;* G. *kormos*, trunk]. See *nanosoma.*

na″no·cor′mus [*nanos; kormos*]. See *nanosomus.*

na′noid (nay′noyd, nan′oyd) [*nanos;* G. *eidos*, form]. Dwarflike.

na·nom′e·lus [*nanos;* G. *melos*, limb]. An individual characterized by undersized limbs.

nan″oph·thal′mi·a, nan·oph·thal′mos, nan″oph·thal′mus [*nanos;* G. *ophthalmos*, eye]. A type of microphthalmus in which eyeball, orbit, and palpebral fissure are all abnormally small.

na″no·so′ma, na″no·so′mi·a [*nanos;* G. *sōma*, body]. Dwarfism.

nanosomia pituitaria. Pituitary dwarfism.

na″no·so′mus [*nanos; sōma*]. An individual with a dwarfed body.

na′nus (nay′nus, nan′us) [L., from *nanos*]. A dwarf. —**nanous, nanus,** *adj.*

na′palm. An aluminum soap, prepared from naphthenic acids and the fatty acids of coconut oil, used for producing gels of gasoline for incendiary munitions.

nape [ME.]. The back of the neck; the nucha.

na·pel′line (na·pel′een, ·in, nap′ul·een, ·in). $C_{22}H_{33}O_3N$. An alkaloid of *Aconitum napellus:* employed as an anodyne and antineuralgic.

na′pex. That portion of the scalp just below the occipital protuberance.

naph·az′o·line hy″dro·chlo′ride (naf·az′o·leen, ·lin). $C_{14}H_{14}N_2.HCl$; 2-(1-naphthylmethyl)-2-imidazoline hydrochloride; a white, crystalline powder, freely soluble in water; a vasoconstrictor which, when applied to nasal and ocular mucous membranes, causes prolonged reduction of local swelling and congestion. See *privine hydrochloride.*

naph′tha (naf′thuh) [G., naphtha]. 1. Formerly, any strong-smelling, inflammable, volatile liquid. 2. A mixture of low-boiling hydrocarbons distilled from petroleum and bituminous shale.

coal tar n. A fraction distilled from coal tar; contains benzene, toluene, xylene, and similar hydrocarbons.

petroleum n. The more volatile part of petroleum collected during distillation and known as crude naphtha, or again separated by distillation into gasoline, benzene, and refined naphtha.

shale n. Naphtha distilled from bituminous shale.

wood n. Mainly methyl alcohol and acetone obtained by the distillation of wood.

naphthalan. Trade-mark for a substance obtained from the distillation of a variety of naphtha and used as a protective dressing.

naph′tha·lene [*naphtha*]. $C_{10}H_8$. A hydrocarbon crystallizing in large, silvery, rhombic plates, insoluble in cold water, but slightly soluble in hot water, readily soluble in methyl and ethyl alcohols, chloroform, ether, and benzene. It is antiseptic, and has been used in intestinal putrefaction and in typhoid fever, and locally, in scabies and pruritus. It is the most commonly used moth repellent. See naphthalene *poisoning.*

naph″tha·lene·a·ce′tic ac′id. $C_{10}H_7CH_2.COOH$. A substance found to have plant-growth-regulating properties.

naph″tha·lene·sul·fon′ic ac′id. 1. Any of the sulfonic acid derivatives of naphthalene. 2. Either of the two crystalline acids having the composition $C_{10}H_7.SO_3H$, distinguished by the prefixes α- and β-; both are employed in various syntheses.

naph′tha·lol. See *betol.*

naph′tha·mine (naf′thuh·meen, ·min). Methenamine.

naph′thene. 1. Any cyclic hydrocarbon of the general formula C_nH_{2n}: sometimes called *cycloparaffin.* 2. The naphthalene ring system.

naph·the′nic ac′id. 1. $C_6H_{11}.COOH$; hexahydrobenzoic acid or cyclohexanecarboxylic acid, occurring in crystals, slightly soluble in water, employed in insecticide formulations and for various industrial uses. 2. Any of a group of carboxylic acids derived from naphthenes, occurring in certain petroleums.

naph″thi·on′ic ac′id. $NH_2.C_{10}H_6SO_2OH$. A compound which has been used as an antidote for nitrite poisoning; also used in the treatment of iodism.

naph′tho-, naphth- [*naphtha*]. A combining form denoting *relationship to naphthalene* or *its ring structure.*

naph′thol. $C_{10}H_7OH$. A substance found in coal tar existing in two isomeric forms, **alphanaphthol** and **betanaphthol. Alphanaphthol** occurs in colorless prisms and is sparingly soluble in water; occasionally used as an intestinal antiseptic. **Betanaphthol** occurs as a crystalline powder, soluble in 100 parts of water; it has been used in dyspepsia and as an intestinal antiseptic in diarrhea and typhoid fever. Locally, it is used in eczema, prurigo, herpes, and favus.

naph′thol·ate. A naphthol compound in which a base replaces the hydrogen atom in the hydroxyl.

α-naph″thol·benz′e·in. $(HO.C_{10}H_6)_2{:}C(C_6H_5)$-OH; a reddish-brown powder, insoluble in water, soluble in alcohol: used as an indicator for acids and bases.

naph′thol yel′low S $C_{10}H_4N_2O_8SK_2.3H_2O$; the potassium (or sodium) salt of 2,4-dinitro-1-naphthol-7-sulfonic acid; a light-yellow or orange-yellow powder, soluble in water. A pure grade, when certified, is used for coloring foods, drugs, and cosmetics, and called F. D. & C. Yellow No. 2.

naph″tho·qui·none′. $C_{10}H_6O_2$; either of two compounds derived from naphthalene: 1,4-naphthoquinone (α-naphthoquinone), derivatives of which have vitamin-K activity, or 1,2-naphthoquinone (β-naphthoquinone), used as a reagent.

naph′thyl. $C_{10}H_7$. The radical of naphthalene.

naph″thyl·a′mine. $C_{10}H_9N$; either of two compounds, α-naphthylamine or β-naphthylamine, the former being 1-aminonaphthalene, the latter 2-aminonaphthalene. Both occur as white to reddish crystals, slightly soluble in water; inhalation of their dust or vapor may result in urinary-bladder tumors.

α-naph″thyl·thi″o·u·re′a. See *ANTU.*

naphuride sodium. Trade-mark for suramin sodium.

Napier's aldehyde test. See under *test.*

na′pi·form (nay′pi·form, nap′i·) [L. *napus,* a kind of turnip; *forma,* shape]. Turnip-shaped.

Narath, Albert [*Austrian surgeon,* 1864–1924]. Introduced an operation of omentopexy to relieve ascites in cirrhosis of the liver by establishing collateral circulation (1905). The omentum is brought forward into a subcutaneous pocket and loosely sutured in place. Called *Narath's operation.*

nar′ce·ine (nahr′see·een, ·in). $C_{23}H_{27}O_8N.3H_2O$. An alkaloid contained in opium. It is sparingly soluble in water and alcohol, and forms fine, silky, inodorous, bitter crystals. It has been used as a substitute for morphine.

nar′cism. See *narcissism.*

nar·cis′sine (nahr·sis′een, ·in). An alkaloid obtained from the daffodil *Narcissus pseudonarcissus.*

nar·cis′sism [G. *Narkissos,* a beautiful youth who fell in love with his own reflection]. 1. Self-love, frequently without genitality as an object. 2. *In psychoanalysis,* fixation of the libido upon one's own body. Syn., *ego erotism, narcism.* —**narcissis′tic,** *adj.;* **narcissist,** *n.*

nar′co- [G. *narkoun,* to benumb]. A combining form signifying *narcosis, numbness,* or *stupor.*

nar″co·an·al′y·sis. The chemical induction of a quickly reversible sleep during which a trained interrogator elicits memories and feelings not expressed in the patient's wakeful state because of either willful or unconscious resistance: used in the treatment of psychoneurotic and psychosomatic reactions (*narcotherapy, narcosynthesis*), and occasionally in the investigation of suspected criminals. Intravenous solutions of sodium amytal or thiopental (often called *truth serums*) are the commonest narcotics used.

nar″co·hyp′ni·a [*narkoun;* G. *hypnos,* sleep]. Waking numbness; a peculiar state in which the patient feels numb on awaking.

nar″co·hyp·no′sis [*narkoun; hypnos;* G. *-ōsis,* condition]. A state of deep sleep induced by hypnosis. Also called *hypnonarcosis.*

nar′co·lep″sy [*narkoun;* G. *lēpsis,* a seizing]. An uncontrollable tendency to attacks of deep sleep of short duration. Has been observed in epilepsy, encephalitis, and in tumors of the third ventricle and hypothalamus. Also called *Gélineau's disease, Gélineau-Redlich syndrome.* —**narcolep′tic,** *n.*

nar·co′ma [*narkoun*]. Stupor from the use of a narcotic. —**narcom′atous,** *adj.*

nar″co·ma′ni·a [*narkoun;* G. *mania,* madness]. A morbid craving for narcotics (medicinal or psychologic) in order to escape painful stimuli. —**narcomaniac,** *n.*

narconumal. Trade-mark for N-methyl alurate, a hypnotic recommended as a surgical anesthetic and general nerve sedative.

nar″co·pep′si·a [*narkoun;* G. *pepsis,* digestion]. Old term for slow or torpid digestion.

nar·co′sis [G., a benumbing]. A state of profound stupor, unconsciousness, or arrested activity.

nar′co·spasm [G. *narkoun,* to benumb; *spasmos,* spasm]. Spasm accompanied by stupor.

nar″co·syn′the·sis. See *narcoanalysis.*

nar″co·ther′a·py. See *narcoanalysis.*

nar·cot′ic [G. *narkōtikos,* narcotic]. 1. A drug that produces stupor, complete insensibility, or sleep, as opium, chloral, and cannabis. There are three main groups: the opium group which produces sleep, the belladonna group which produces illusions and delirium, and the alcohol group which produces exhilaration and sleep. 2. An individual addicted to the use of narcotics. —**narcot′ic,** *adj.*

nar·cot′i·co- [*narkōtikos*]. A combining form meaning *narcotic.*

nar·cot′i·co-ac′rid. Both narcotic and irritant. Also called *narcotico-irritant.* See *acronarcotic.*

nar′co·tine (nahr′ko·teen, ·tin). $C_{22}H_{23}NO_7$. An alkaloid occurring in opium, second in abundance to morphine. Sudorific and antipyretic, but not narcotic. Dose, 0.06–0.2 Gm. (1–3 gr.).

nar′co·tism [G. *narkoun,* to benumb]. The condition resulting from the use of a narcotic.

nar′co·tize [*narkoun*]. Put under the influence of a narcotic; render unconscious by means of a narcotic.

nar″e·ga′mi·a [L.]. Goanese ipecacuanha; the bark of *Naregamia alata,* having properties due to an alkaloid, naregamine; used as an emetic.

na·reg′a·mine (na·reg′uh·meen, ·min). An alkaloid contained in *Naregamia alata.*

na·rin′gin. The bitter glycoside of grapefruit rind.

na′ris (pl. *nares*) [L.]. A nostril. One of a pair of openings at the anterior part (anterior nares) or at the posterior part (posterior nares) of the nasal cavities.

na′sal (nay′zul) [L. *nasus,* nose]. Pertaining to the nose. Abbreviated, n.

na′sal. The nasal bone. See Table of Bones in the Appendix.

na·sa′lis. A muscle of facial expression. See Table of Muscles in the Appendix.

na′sal step. See *Roenne's nasal step.*

nas′cent (nass′unt, nay′sunt) [L. *nasci,* to be born]. Pertaining to gaseous substances at the moment of their liberation from chemical combination.

na″si·o·al·ve′o·lar (nay″zee·o·, nay″see·o·). [L.

nasus, nose; *alveolus*, small hollow]. Relating to, or connecting, the nasion and the alveolar point.

na′si·on (nay′zee·on, nay′see·on) [*nasus*]. The craniometric point where the sagittal plane intersects the nasofrontal suture.

na·si′tis (nay·sigh′tis, ·zigh′tis). See *rhinitis. Obs.*

Nasmyth, Alexander [*Scottish anatomist and dentist*, d. 1848]. Described the primary enamel cuticle, called *Nasmyth's membrane.*

na′so- (nay′zo-) [L. *nasus*, nose]. *In anatomy*, a combining form denoting *connection with*, or *relation to, the nose.*

na″so·cil′i·ar″y (nay″zo·sil′ee·err″ee) [*nasus;* L. *cilium*, eyelid]. Applied to a nerve distributed to the nose, the ethmoid sinuses, and the eyeball. See Table of Nerves in the Appendix.

na″so·fron′tal [*nasus;* L. *frons*, forehead]. Pertaining to the nasal and the frontal bones.

na″so·gen′i·tal [*nasus;* L. *genitalis*, genital]. Pertaining to a correlation that exists between functional changes in the reproductive organs and changes in the nasal mucosa.

na″so·la′bi·al [*nasus;* L. *labium*, lip]. Pertaining to the nose and lip.

na″so·la·bi·a′lis. A portion of the orbicularis oris muscle.

na″so·lac′ri·mal [*nasus;* L. *lacrima*, tear]. Pertaining to the nose and the lacrimal apparatus, as the nasolacrimal duct.

na″so·max′il·lar·y. Pertaining to the nasal and maxillary bones.

na″so·pal′a·tine (nay″zo·pal′uh·tyne, ·tin) [*nasus;* L. *palatum*, palate]. Pertaining to both the nose and the palate, as the nasopalatine nerve. See Table of Nerves in the Appendix.

na″so·phar·yn·gi′tis. Inflammation of the nasal passages and pharynx.

na″so·pha·ryn′go·scope [*nasus;* G. *pharygx*, pharynx; *skopein*, to examine]. An electrically lighted instrument for inspecting the nasopharynx.

na″so·phar′ynx [*nasus; pharygx*]. The space behind the posterior nares and above a horizontal plane through the lower margin of the palate: also called *epipharynx.* —**nasopharyn′geal,** *adj.*

na″so-spi·na′le (nay″zo-spy·nah′lee). A craniometric point located in the sagittal plane where it meets a line joining the lowest points on the nasal margins. If this falls within the substance of the anterior nasal spine, a point on the left side wall of the nasal spine is used for taking measurements.

na″so·tur′bi·nal [*nasus;* L. *turbinatus*, cone-shaped]. The ridgelike elevation midway between the anterior extremity of the middle nasal concha and the roof of the nose in most lower mammals. In man its rudimentary homolog is the agger nasi.

Nasse, Christian Friedrich [*German physician*, 1778–1851]. Noted that hemophilia occurs only in males but may be transmitted by females. The phenomenon previously had been described by Otto (1803), but is known as *Nasse's law.*

na′sus [L.]. The nose.

n. aduncus. Hook nose.

n. cartilagineus. Cartilaginous part of the nose.

n. externus. The external nose.

n. incurvus. Saddle nose.

n. osseus. The bony part of the nose.

n. simus. Pug nose.

na′tal [L. *natalis*, natal]. Native; connected with one's birth.

na·tal′i·ty (nay·tal′i·tee) [*natalis*]. *In medical statistics*, the birth rate.

na·tal′o·in. The aloin derived from Natal aloes.

Na·tal′ sore. See *oriental sore.*

na′tant [L. *natare*, to swim]. Swimming or floating on the surface of a liquid.

na′tes (nay′teez) [L. *natis*, rump]. Old term for buttocks. —**na′tal,** *adj.*

Na′tion·al For′mu·lar″y (for′mew·lerr″ee). A formulary published by the American Pharmaceutical Association; it is officially recognized by the Federal Food, Drug, and Cosmetic Act. Abbreviated, N. F.

Na′tion·al Health Serv′ice. *In Great Britain*, a government agency under the Ministry of Health, operative since 1948, charged with providing health services for the entire population. Its purpose is to supply hospitalization, preventive medicine, family medical, dental, and nursing services, medicines, appliances, and other requirements for complete, comprehensive medical services; it is financed by the national government. Free choice of a physician by a patient and the acceptance of him by the doctor have been preserved. The legal charge to the patient for services is nothing or minimal. Remuneration, also governed by law, is on a salary or capitation basis; for dentists, on a fee-for-service basis.

Na′tion·al In′sti·tutes of Health. A division of the U.S. Public Health Service that is devoted to research in public health and the diseases of man. It controls the manufacture and sale of biologic products by licensure.

na′tive [L. *nativus*, innate]. Of indigenous origin or growth; occurring in its natural state; not artificial, as native albumins, a class of proteins occurring ready-formed in the tissues.

nat·re′mi·a. 1. Sodium in the blood. 2. Hypernatremia: erroneous usage.

na′tri·um. See *sodium.*

na″tri·u·ret′ic. A medicinal agent which inhibits reabsorption of cations, particularly sodium, from urine. —**natriuret′ic,** *adj.*

na′tron. Native sodium carbonate, $Na_2CO_3.10H_2O$.

na′trum. Sodium.

nat′u·ar″y (nach′oo·err″ee, nay′choo·) [L. *natus*, from *nasci*, to be born]. A lying-in ward or hospital. *Obs.*

nat′u·ral [L. *naturalis*, natural]. Not abnormal or artificial.

nat′u·ral se·lec′tion. Darwin's theory of evolution, according to which organisms tend to produce progeny far above the means of subsistence; a struggle for existence ensues which results in the survival of those with favorable variations. Since the favorable variations accumulate as the generations pass, the descendants tend to diverge markedly from their ancestors, and to remain adapted to the conditions under which they live.

naturin. Trade name for thin membranous eluting disks made from animal skin.

na′tur·o·path″. One who professes to heal the sick exclusively by the use of natural remedies, such as light, heat, cold, water, fruits, etc. —**naturop′athy,** *n.*

Naunyn, Bernard [*German physician*, 1839–1925]. Wrote especially on the gallbladder and pancreas, and studied metabolism in diabetes. Credited with introducing the term *acidosis.*

nau·pa′thi·a (naw·payth′ee·uh, ·path′ee·uh, naw″puh·thee′uh) [G. *naus*, ship; *pathos*, disease]. Seasickness. *Obs.*

nau′se·a [L., from G. *nautia*, seasickness]. A feeling of discomfort in the region of the stomach, with aversion to food and a tendency to vomit. —**nauseous,** *adj.*

creatic n. Morbid aversion to meat.

nau′se·ant [L. *nauseare*, to be seasick]. Any agent that produces nausea. —**nau′seant,** *adj.*

Na′val Med′i·cal Cen′ter. An installation of the United States Navy similar in character and purpose to the Army Medical Center.

na′vel [AS. *nafela*]. The umbilicus.

enamel n. See under *enamel*.

na·vic′u·lar [L. *navicula*, small boat]. Boatshaped.

na·vic′u·lar. A carpal or tarsal bone; the scaphoid bone of the hand or the foot. See Table of Bones in the Appendix.

navicular fossa. 1. A depression between the vaginal aperture and the fourchette. 2. The dilated distal portion of the urethra in the glans penis.

na·vic″u·lar·thri′tis [*navicula;* G. *arthritis*, arthritis]. Inflammation of the distal sesamoid bone in the horse; causes chronic lameness due to incomplete extension of the joint. Also called *navicular disease*.

na·vic″u·lo·cu′boid [*navicula;* G. *kyboeidēs*, like a cube]. Relating to the navicular and the cuboid bones, as naviculocuboid ligament.

na·vic″u·lo·cu·ne′i·form [*navicula;* L. *cuneus*, wedge; *forma*, shape]. Relating to the navicular and cuneiform bones.

navigan. Trade-mark for the hydrochloride of N-hydroxy-ethyl-piperidine-acetyl-tropic acid, a remedy for seasickness.

Nb Chemical symbol for niobium, formerly known as columbium.

N. C. A. Neurocirculatory asthenia.

Nd Chemical symbol for neodymium.

NDGA Abbreviation for nordihydroguaiaretic acid.

Ne Chemical symbol for neon.

near point. The punctum proximum; the point nearest the eye at which an object can be seen distinctly.

absolute n. p. That near point for either eye alone at which no effort at accommodation is made.

convergence n. p. See relative *n. p.*

relative n. p. That near point for both eyes at which accommodation is brought into play.

near-sight. See *myopia*.

ne″ar·thro′sis [G. *neos*, new; *arthrōsis*, articulation]. A new and abnormally produced articulation in the sequence of a fracture, dislocation, or disease of the bone.

ne′ben·kern″ (nay′bun·kairn″). See *paranucleus. Obs.*

neb′u·la [L., mist, fog]. 1. A faint, grayish opacity of the cornea. 2. A spray, a liquid intended for use in an atomizer.

neb″u·lar′in, neb″u·lar′ine. An antibiotic substance derived from the fungus *Agaricus* (*Clitocybe*) *nebularis*.

ne·bu′li·um [*nebula*]. A hypothetical element formerly believed to exist in nebulas; evidence for its existence is now attributed to formation of ionized oxygen and nitrogen.

neb″u·li·za′tion. Atomization.

neb′u·lize [*nebula*]. Convert into a spray or vapor.

neb′u·li″zer. Atomizer.

Ne·ca′tor [L., slayer]. A genus of nematode hookworms.

N. americanus. That species widely distributed in the tropical regions of the Western Hemisphere and throughout southern United States; produces the infestation necatoriasis.

nec″a·to·ri′a·sis [*necator;* NL. *-iasis*, condition]. Infestation of man with the American hookworm, *Necator americanus*, whose infestive larvae enter the skin usually at the interdigital regions and may produce a ground itch and vesicular lesions. The adult parasite is found in the small intestine and during the larval migration to the intestine damage to the lungs is commonly incurred.

neck [AS. *hnecca*]. 1. The constricted portion of the body connecting the head with the trunk. 2. The narrow portion of any structure serving to join its parts. 3. The line of junction of the crown and root of a tooth.

anatomic n. The constricted portion of the humerus, just below the articular surface, serving for the attachment of the capsular ligament.

bison n. Excess adiposity of the neck, seen in Cushing's syndrome.

n. of the bladder. That portion of the urinary bladder immediately surrounding the internal urethral orifice.

n. of the gallbladder. The constricted S-shaped portion of the gallbladder between the fundus and the cystic duct.

surgical n. The constricted part of the humerus just below the tuberosities.

wryneck. See *torticollis*.

nec″ro·bac″il·lo′sis (neck″ro·bas″i·lo′sis) [G. *nekros*, corpse; L. *bacillum*, small staff; G. *-ōsis*, condition]. A disease of animals caused by *Actinomyces necrophorus*.

Nec″ro·ba·cil′lus [*nekros; bacillum*]. A highly pleomorphic, non-spore-forming, Gram-negative anaerobe found in feces, in abscesses of various organs, and in chronic ulcerative colitis. Also called *Bacterium necrophorum, Actinomyces necrophorus*.

nec″ro·bi·o′sis (neck″ro·buy·o′sis) [*nekros;* G. *biōsis*, way of life]. Physiologic death of a cell or group of cells, in contrast to necrosis or pathologic death of cells, and to somatic death or death of the entire organism. —**necrobiot′ic,** *adj.*

n. lipoidica. A cutaneous disease, characterized by multiple yellow to red plaques generally on the extremities, occurring mostly in female diabetics. There is connective-tissue necrosis with an accumulation of macrophages containing lipids. Also called *Oppenheim-Urbach disease, n. lipoidica diabeticorum.*

nec″ro·cy·to′sis (neck″ro·sigh·to′sis) [*nekros;* G. *kytos*, cell; *-ōsis*, condition]. Death of cells.

nec″ro·cy″to·tox′in [*nekros; kytos;* G. *toxikon*, poison]. A toxin produced by the death of cells.

nec″ro·gen′ic, ne·crog′e·nous (neh·krodj′i·nus) [*nekros;* G. *genesthai*, from *gignesthai*, to be produced]. Originating from dead substances.

nec″ro·ma′ni·a [*nekros;* G. *mania*, madness]. 1. A morbid desire for death or attraction to dead bodies. 2. See *necrophilism*.

nec″ro·mi·me′sis [*nekros;* G. *mimēsis*, imitation]. 1. A delusional state in which the patient believes himself to be dead. 2. Simulation of death by a deluded person.

ne·croph′a·gous, ne·croph′a·gic [*nekros;* G. *phagein*, to eat]. Pertaining to the eating of carrion, or putrid meat.

nec″ro·phil′i·a, ne·croph′il·y [*nekros;* G. *philein*, to love]. 1. Necrophilism 2. A longing for death.

ne·croph′il·ism [*nekros; philein*]. Sexual perversion in which dead bodies are violated; insane sexual desire for a corpse. —**nec′rophile,** *n.*

ne·croph′i·lous [*nekros; philein*]. Subsisting on dead matter; used in qualifying certain bacteria.

ne·croph′il·y. See *necrophilia*, 2; *necrophilism*.

nec″ro·pho′bi·a [*nekros;* G. *phobos*, fear]. 1. Insane dread of dead bodies. 2. Thanatophobia; extreme dread of death.

nec′rop·sy [*nekros;* G. *opsis*, sight]. The examination of a dead body; autopsy; post-mortem examination.

ne·crose′ (neh·krohss′, ·krohz′, neck′rohss) [*nekros*]. To undergo necrosis or tissue death.

nec′ro·sin [*nekros*]. A substance isolated from inflamed areas; said to be capable of injuring body cells.

ne·cro′sis [G., mortification]. The pathologic death of a cell or group of cells in contact with living cells. —**necrot′ic,** *adj.;* **nec′rotize,** *v.*

anemic n. See aseptic *n.*

aseptic n. Necrosis without infection and inflammation: also called *anemic n., avascular n., bland n., quiet n., simple n., spontaneous n.*

avascular n. See aseptic *n.*

bland n. See aseptic *n.*

caseation n. That occurring typically in tuberculosis, with formation of a cheesy substance.

central n. Necrosis of the liver around the central vein of the lobule.

coagulation n. A variety characterized by cell death in situ with preservation of cell form and arrangement; most frequent in infarction.

colliquative n. See liquefactive *n.*

diphtheritic n. Necrosis of the mucous membrane; characterized by the formation of a tough, leathery membrane composed of coagulated cells and fibrin.

embolic n. Coagulation necrosis in an anemic infarct following embolism.

fat n. Necrosis in adipose tissue, commonly accompanied by the production of soaps from the hydrolyzed fat, and seen most frequently in association with pancreatitis and less often in injuries to adipose tissue (traumatic fat n.).

ischemic n. Death of tissue due to occlusion of an artery supplying the region.

liquefactive n. A type resulting in liquefaction of the involved tissue.

mammary-fat n. Destruction of fatty tissue of the breast as a result of certain conditions, such as stagnation of duct contents and accumulation within the ducts of irritant substances, tumors, or trauma. It is followed by a regenerative process in which phagocytes, plasma cells, and foreign-body giant cells are prominent.

medial (muscle) n. The death of cells located in the muscular coat of the walls of arteries.

phosphorus n. A necrosis of bone, especially of the lower jaw, occurring in those exposed to the fumes of phosphorus.

postpartum pituitary n. See Sheehan's *syndrome.*

quiet n. See aseptic *n.*

radium n. Necrosis due to an overdose of radium in the treatment of carcinoma.

simple n. See aseptic *n.*

spontaneous n. See aseptic *n.*

subcutaneous n. of the newborn. Adiponecrosis neonatorum.

traumatic fat n. A type resulting from trauma, found most often in the breast and subcutaneous region, and involving inflammation with hemorrhage and leukocytic invasion. See mammary-fat *n.*

Zenker's hyaline n. Coagulation necrosis of striated muscle, especially rectus abdominis, occurring in typhoid fever and other infectious diseases. The muscle fibers are swollen, fragmented, homogeneous, and acidophilic; nuclei are usually absent. Also called *Zenker's hyalin* or *hyaline degeneration, waxy degeneration.*

nec″ro·sper′mi·a [G. *nekros*, corpse; *sperma*, seed]. Impotence due to loss of motility of the spermatozoa.

nec″ro·zo·o·sper′mi·a [*nekros;* G. *zōion*, living being; *sperma*, seed]. A condition in which spermatozoa are present but are immobile and without evidence of life.

Nec·tan′dra. See *Ocotea.*

nec·tar′e·ous (neck·tair′ee·us) [G. *nektar*, nectar]. Agreeable to the taste. *Rare.*

nec′ta·ry [*nektar*]. *In biology*, that part of a flower which secretes nectar.

N.E.D. Abbreviation for normal equivalent deviation.

Nedden, Max Wilhelm zur [*German ophthalmologist*, 1870–   ]. Described a bacillus sometimes found in ulcer of the cornea, called *zur Nedden's bacillus.*

nee′dle [AS. *nǣdl*]. A sharp-pointed steel instrument, used for puncturing or for sewing tissue; of various shapes, sizes, and edges, the sewing needle having an eye for carrying suture material through the parts.

aneurysm n. One fixed on a handle, half curved and at a right angle to the handle, with an eye at the point; used for passing a ligature about a vessel.

aspirating n. A hollow needle for withdrawing fluid from a cavity.

brain n. A biopsy needle used in neurosurgery.

cataract n. One used for operating upon a cataract or its capsule.

curved n. One with a curve of any degree up to a full semicircle.

cutting n. One with a sharp edge, either curved or straight.

discission n. One used for inserting into the capsule of the lens for breaking up a cataract.

electrosurgical n. See *acusector.*

exploring n. A hollow needle or a trocar with a grooved side, which allows the passage of fluid along it after it is plunged into a part where fluid is suspected.

hypodermic n. A hollow needle, used with a hypodermic syringe.

malleable n. An especially annealed stainless-steel or German-silver pliable, nonbreakable needle which assumes, through ligamental and bony pressure, the proper curves within the vertebral canal for continued or serial injections without stress: used for continuous spinal, caudal, or peridural anesthesia.

radium needles. Steel or platinum-iridium-walled, needle-shaped containers filled with radium salt and used in radium therapy.

round n. Any needle which is circular in cross section without a cutting edge; may be either curved or straight.

spinal n. A hollow needle equipped with obturator, used for spinal or sacral anesthesia or lumbar puncture.

surgical n. Any sewing needle used in surgical operations.

Tuohy n. A needle with a directional bevel for accurately inserting and positioning a small catheter into the subarachnoid or peridural spaces.

Turkel and Bethell n. An instrument consisting of an outer guiding or splitting needle and an inner trephine needle and stylet for bone-marrow biopsy or for infusion of solutions into the marrow.

nee′dle car′ri·er. See *needle holder.*

nee′dle for′ceps. See *needle holder.*

nee′dle hold′er. A handle, usually in the form of a self-locking forceps, for clasping a surgical needle.

nee′dling [*nǣdl*]. The discission with a needle, as of a cataract, to afford entrance to the aqueous humor and cause absorption of the lens.

n. in aneurysm. Formerly, the passage of needles into the sac of an aneurysm.

n. of the heart. The aspiration of an overdistended right atrium; cardiocentesis.

n. of the kidney. Puncture of the kidney substance for locating a stone.

Neelsen stain. See *carbolfuchsin solution* under *stain*, Ziehl-Neelsen *method.*

ne″en·ceph′a·lon [*neos;* G. *egkephalos*, brain]. The neopallium and the phylogenetically new acquisitions of the cerebellum and thalamus collectively: also spelled *neoencephalon.*

ne′frens (nee′frenz) (pl. *nefrendes*) [L., that cannot bite]. Without teeth; edentate, whether nurslings or aged persons. *Rare.*

Neftel's disease. See *atremia.*

neg′a·tive [L. *negativus*, negative]. 1. Denying; contradicting; opposing. 2. Of quantities, less than nothing. 3. *In physics*, opposed to a quality termed positive. Symbol, −.

neg′a·tiv·ism. Markedly reduced activity in which the subject ignores inner stimuli or is indifferent, and even resistant, to suggestions and commands: a symptom of mental illness, usually schizophrenia.

active n. That in which the individual does the opposite of what he is asked to do.

passive n. That in which the individual does not do what he is expected to do.

neg′a·tron [L. *negare*, to deny; G. ēlek*tron*, amber]. A term suggested for replacing electron; counterpart to positron.

neg′li·gence. *In medical jurisprudence*, an act of commission or omission which, without regard to circumstances, violates a statute or is obviously opposed to the dictates of accepted medical practices.

contributory n. Failure to exercise ordinary care or performance of a voluntary act, by a patient, which contributes to a resultant injury.

Negri, Adelchi [*Italian physician and pathologist*, 1876–1912]. Remembered for his discovery of the inclusion bodies noted in the Purkinje cells and cells of the hippocampus which are diagnostic of rabies; called *Negri bodies*.

Negro's sign. See cogwheel *rigidity*.

Neil Robertson stretcher. See under *stretcher*.

Neill method. See Van Slyke and Neill *method*.

Neill-Mooser test. See under *test*.

Neisser, Albert Ludwig Siegmund [*German physician*, 1855–1916]. Celebrated discoverer of the gonococcus (1879). Introduced, with August von Wassermann and Carl Bruck, the specific blood test used in the detection of syphilis (1906).

Neisser, Max [*German bacteriologist*, 1869–1938]. With R. Lubowski, noted the phenomenon of complement deviation (1901), which was described independently in the same year by Friedrich Wechsberg. When excessive amounts of antibody are introduced, the excess may combine with complement and thereby prevent part or all of the complement from reacting with the antigen-antibody complex. Called *Neisser-Wechsberg phenomenon*. See also Neisser's *stain*.

Neis·se′ri·a (nigh·seer′ee·uh, nigh·serr′ee·uh, nigh′-seh·ree″uh) [Albert *Neisser*]. A genus of Gram-negative, anaerobic cocci of the family Neisseriaceae.

N. catarrhalis. A species found in the respiratory tract; appears to excite catarrhal inflammation and sometimes pneumonia in man.

N. discoides. An anaerobic species of unknown pathogenicity found in the intestinal and genitourinary tracts.

N. flavescens. A species found in the spinal fluid in certain cases of clinical meningitis.

N. gonorrhoeae. The type species of this genus; the causative agent of gonorrhea. See Plate 30.

N. intracellularis. Synonym for *N. meningitidis*.

N. meningitidis. Species which causes epidemic cerebrospinal meningitis: also called *Diplococcus intracellularis meningitides, Neisseria intracellularis*.

N. orbiculata. An anaerobic species found in the respiratory tract; of unknown pathogenicity.

N. reniformis. An anaerobic species found in the respiratory tract; of unknown pathogenicity.

N. sicca. A species which apparently is the causative agent of kidney infection; found in the blood stream in cases of clinical endocarditis.

Nélaton, Auguste [*French surgeon*, 1807–73]. Introduced a soft rubber catheter called *Nélaton's catheter*, and a probe tipped with rough porcelain for locating bullets, called *Nélaton's probe*. Described pelvic hematocele. A variable muscle band in the rectum three to four inches above the anus is called *Nélaton's fibers* or *sphincter*. Subastragalar disarticulation, usually with wedging between tibia and fibula, is called *Nélaton's disarticulation*. Operations for stones, ankylosed wrist, rhinoplasty, arthroplasty of elbow or hip, excision of shoulder by transverse incision, have been called *Nélaton's operations*. A line drawn from the anterior superior iliac spine to the tuberosity of the ischium is called *Nélaton's line*. In dislocated hip the tip of the greater trochanter of the femur is above this line.

n electron. See under *electron*.

nem″a·thel′minth (nem″uh·thel′minth, nee″-muh·) [G. *nēma*, thread; *helmins*, worm]. Any roundworm of the phylum Nemathelminthes.

Nem″a·thel·min′thes (nem″uh·thel·min′theez, nee″muh·) [*nēma; helmins*]. The phylum of the roundworms, which includes the true roundworms or nematodes, the hair snakes, and acanthocephalan worms.

Nem″a·to′da (nem″uh·to′duh, nee″muh·) [*nēma;* G. *eidos*, form]. A class of the phylum Nemathelminthes; the true roundworms. Members of the class are bilaterally symmetrical, unisexual, without a proboscis, and have a body cavity not lined with epithelium.

nem′a·tode (nem′uh·toad, nee′muh·) [*nēma; eidos*]. Any worm of the class Nematoda.

nem″a·tol′o·gy (nem″uh·tol′o·jee, nee″muh·) [*nēma;* G. *logos*, word]. That portion of the science of parasitology concerned with the study of nematode worms.

nem″a·to·sper′mi·a (nem″uh·to·spur′mee·uh, nee″muh·to·) [*nēma;* G. *sperma*, seed]. Spermatozoa with long, threadlike tails, as those found in human semen. *Rare*.

nembutal. Trade-mark for *pentobarbital sodium*.

nemural. Trade-mark for *drocarbil*, a veterinary anthelmintic.

Nencki, Marcellus von [*Polish physician*, 1847–1901]. Remembered for his introduction of a test for indole. *Nencki's test for indole* uses nitrous and nitric acids, which produce a red coloration in the solution tested.

ne′o-, ne- [G. *neos*, new]. 1. A combining form meaning *new* or *recent*. 2. *In biology*, a combining form signifying *an immature form, a recently formed part*, or *an abnormal new formation*. 3. *In chemistry*, a combining form denoting *a new compound*.

ne″o·aj′ma·line. An alkaloid from *Rauwolfia serpentina*.

neo-antergan maleate. Trade-marked name for the antihistaminic substance, pyrilamine maleate.

neoantimosan. See *fuadin*.

ne″o·ars″phen·a·mine′ (nee″o·ars″fen·uh·meen′, ·fen·am′een, ·in) (*neoarsphenamina*). Chiefly sodium 3:3′-diamino-4:4′-dihydroxyarsenobenzene-N-methylenesulfoxylate, $(NH_2)(OH)C_6H_3As{:}As{-}C_6H_3(OH)(NH.CH_2.O.SONa)$. An antisyphilitic. A yellow powder, very soluble in water to form a neutral solution; has the advantage over arsphenamine in not requiring neutralization before injection. Dosage requires caution. See *neosalvarsan, neodiarsenol*, and *neokharsivan*. Also called *novarsenobenzol, arsphenamine-S*.

ne″o·ar·thro′sis [G. *neos*, new; *arthrōsis*, articulation]. A false joint.

ne″o·blas′tic [*neos;* G. *blastos*, germ]. Pertaining to, or of the nature of, new tissue.

neocaine. Trade-mark for procaine hydrochloride.

ne″o·cal′a·mine (nee″o·kal′uh·meen, ·min) (*neocalamina praeparata*). A mixture of red ferric oxide, 3; yellow ferric oxide, 4; zinc oxide, 93. It is used for the same purposes as calamine but has a standardized, reproducible color which more nearly matches that of the average skin.

n. liniment (*linimentum neocalaminae*). Neocalamine, 15; olive oil, 50; calcium hydroxide solution, to 100.

n. lotion (*lotio neocalaminae*). Neocalamine, 15; bentonite magma, 40; water, to 100.

n. ointment (*unguentum neocalaminae*). Neocalamine, 15; wool fat, 12.5; petrolatum, 37.5; liquid petrolatum, 10; water, 25.

phenolated n. lotion (*lotio neocalaminae phenolata*). Neocalamine lotion, 99; liquefied phenol, 1.

ne″o·cer″e·bel′lum [G. *neos*, new; L. *cerebellum*, small brain.] Phylogenetically the most recent part of the cerebellum: the simple lobule, the folium and tuber vermis, and the lateral paired ansiform and paramedian lobules. It receives cerebral cortex impulses via the corticopontocerebellar tract.

neocid. Trade-mark for *chlorophenothane*.

ne″o·cin′cho·phen (nee″o·sing′ko·fen) (*neocinchophenum*). $C_{19}H_{17}O_2N$. The ethyl ester of 6-methyl-2-phenylquinoline-4-carboxylic acid; it is a white to pale-yellow powder, nearly insoluble in water. Its actions and uses are the same as those of cinchophen, but it appears to be less toxic. Dose, 0.3 Gm. (5 gr.). See *tolysin*.

ne″o·cor′tex. That part of the cerebral cortex which is phylogenetically the most recent in development; it includes all of the cortex except the olfactory portions, the hippocampal regions, and the piriform areas. Syn., *isocortex*.

ne″o·cys·tos′to·my [G. *neos*, new; *kystis*, bladder; *stoma*, mouth]. A surgical procedure whereby a new opening is made into the urinary bladder.

ureteroileal n. A surgical procedure in which an isolated segment of the ileum is used for a portion of a ureter.

ne″o·den·ta′tum. The phylogenetically new ventrolateral part of the dentate nucleus.

neodiarsenol. Trade-mark for a brand of neoarsphenamine.

ne″o·di′a·ther″my. See short-wave *diathermy*.

ne″o·dym′i·um [G. *neos*, new; *didymos*, twin]. Nd = 144.27. A rare earth metal occurring in cerium and lanthanum minerals.

ne″o·en·ceph′a·lon. See *neencephalon*.

ne″o-en′do·thrix. A type division of the genus *Trichophyton*.

ne·og′a·la. Colostrum. *Obs.*

ne″o·gen′e·sis [*neos;* G. *genesis*, production]. Regeneration of tissues. —**neogenet′ic,** *adj.*

ne″o·ger′mi·trine. A triester alkaloid, hypotensively active, isolated from veratrum viride; on hydrolysis it yields germine, two moles of acetic acid, and one mole of 2-methylbutyric acid.

neohetramine hydrochloride. A trade-marked name for the antihistaminic substance thonzylamine hydrochloride.

neo-hombreol. A trade-mark for testosterone propionate, a male sex hormone derivative.

neo-hombreol-M. A trade-mark for methyltestosterone.

neohydrin. Trade-mark for the orally effective mercurial diuretic known by the generic name *chlormerodrin*.

neo-iopax. A trade-mark for sodium iodomethamate, a radiopaque medium. See *iodoxyl*.

ne″o·i″so·co′de·ine. Pseudocodeine.

neokharsivan. A trade-mark for neoarsphenamine.

neolin. A trade-mark for N,N′-dibenzylethylenediamine dipenicillin G. See *benzathine penicillin G*.

ne·ol′o·gism [*neos;* G. *logos*, word]. *In psychiatry*, meaningless, or newly coined, words uttered by the insane.

ne″o·mem′brane [*neos;* L. *membrana*, membrane]. A new or false membrane.

ne″o·mor′phism [*neos;* G. *morphē*, form]. *In biology*, the development of a new form.

ne″o·my′cin [*neos;* G. *mykēs*, fungus]. An antibiotic substance isolated from cultures of *Streptomyces fradiae;* a polybasic compound. It exhibits activity against a variety of Gram-positive and Gram-negative bacteria. The sulfate, administered orally, is used as an intestinal antiseptic in surgery of the large bowel and anus; the salt is used for topical application in treatment or prevention of susceptible infections of the skin and the eye. See *mycifradin sulfate*.

ne′on [*neos*]. Ne = 20.183. A chemically inert, gaseous element occurring, in small amounts, in air.

neonal. Trade-mark for 5-*n*-butyl-5-ethylbarbituric acid, a drug employed as a hypnotic and sedative. See *butethal*.

ne″o·na′tal. Newborn.

ne″o·na′tal mor·tal′i·ty rate. The number of deaths reported among infants under one month of age in a calendar year per 1,000 live births reported in the same year and place.

ne′o·nate. See *neonatus*.

ne″o·na·to′rum [*neos;* L. *natus*, born]. Pertaining to the newborn.

ne″o·na′tus, ne′o·nate [*neos; natus*]. A newly born infant. —**neona′tal,** *adj.*

neo-oestranol I. Trade-mark for a brand of diethylstilbestrol.

ne″o-ol′ive. The olive with the exception of its small medial portion which is part of thepaleoolive.

ne″o·pal′li·um [*neos;* L. *pallium*, cover]. The cerebral hemisphere with the exception of the rhinencephalon. —**neopallial,** *adj.*

neo-penil. Trade-mark for penicillin G diethylaminoethylester hydroiodide, known also by the generic name *penethamate hydroiodide;* a salt of benzyl penicillin of low solubility and prolonged action.

ne″o·pen′tane. $(CH_3)_4C$; 2,2-dimethylpropane or tetramethylmethane; a hydrocarbon, gaseous at room temperature, occurring in petroleum naphtha, and also prepared by synthesis.

ne·oph′il·ism [*neos;* G. *philein*, to love]. Morbid or undue desire for novelty.

ne″o·pho′bi·a [*neos;* G. *phobos*, fear]. Dread of new scenes or of novelties.

ne″o·phren′i·a (nee″o·fren′ee·uh, ·free′nee·uh) [*neos;* G. *phrēn*, mind]. Mental deterioration in early youth.

ne′o·pine (nee′o·peen, ·pin, ·pyne). $C_{18}H_{21}NO_3$; an alkaloid, isomeric with codeine, occurring in opium: sometimes called *β-codeine*.

ne″o·pla′si·a (nee″o·play′zhuh, ·zee·uh, ·shuh, ·see·uh) [*neos;* G. *plassein*, to form]. 1. Formation of new tissue. 2. Formation of tumors or neoplasms.

ne′o·plasm [*neos;* G. *plasma*, anything formed]. Any new growth; usually applied to a tumor, an aberrant new growth. —**neoplast′ic,** *adj.*

metastatic n. A metastatic tumor.

ne′o·prene. Generic name for synthetic rubber made by polymerization of 2-chloro-1,3-butadiene. Neoprene vulcanizates are markedly resistant to oils, greases, chemicals, sunlight, ozone, and heat.

neoprontosil. A trade-mark for disodium 4′-sulfamidophenyl-2-azo-7-acetylamino-1-hydroxynaphthalene-3,6-disulfonate, $(NaSO_3)_2.NHCOCH_3.$-$OH.C_{10}H_3.N{:}N.C_6H_4.SO_2.NH_2$, the red dye, moderately soluble in water, first used by Domagk in his epochal chemotherapeutic studies. The substance is still occasionally employed for the same purposes as sulfanilamide. Dose, 3–4 Gm. (45–60 gr.) initially, then 1 Gm. (15 gr.) every 4 hours.

Prontosil soluble, prontosil red, streptozon-S, streptocid rubrum, and *azosulfamide* are other trade-marks for the same drug.

ne″o·pyr″i·thi′a·mine. A structural analog of thiamine in which the thiazole ring is replaced by pyridine, being, specifically, 1-[(4-amino-2-methyl)-5-pyrimidylmethyl]-2-methyl-3-(β-hydroxyethyl)pyridinium bromide hydrobromide; a powerful antagonist of thiamine. Originally what was believed to be this compound was called *pyrithiamine,* which proved to be a mixture of compounds. To avoid confusion the pure substance was designated *neopyrithiamine.*

ne″o·quas′sin. $C_{22}H_{30}O_6$; a bitter principle of quassia, forming with isoquassin the molecular complex called *quassin.*

ne″o·sal′var·san. A name given by Ehrlich to the substance now officially designated neoarsphenamine.

ne″o-sen″si·bil′i·ty. See gnostic *sensibility.*

neo-silvol. Trade-mark for a compound of silver iodide with a soluble gelatin base containing 18–22% silver iodide in colloidal form, a drug employed as an antiseptic on mucous membranes.

neostam stibamine glucoside. A brand of stibamine glucoside, a pentavalent organic antimony compound employed in the treatment of kala-azar.

neostibosan. Trade-mark for the pentavalent antimonial preparation ethylstibamine.

ne″o·stig′mine (nee″o·stig′meen, ·min). The dimethylcarbamic ester of 3-hydroxyphenyl-dimethylamine, available only in the form of its salts. The neostigmine component has some of the properties of the related compound physostigmine; the former is used to prevent atony of the intestinal and urinary-bladder musculature, and for symptomatic control of myasthenia gravis.

n. bromide (*neostigminae bromidum*), $Br.N(CH_3)_3.C_6H_4.OOC.N(CH_3)_2$, a salt which, because of its lesser hygroscopicity, is suited for use in tablets. Dose, 15–30 mg. (¼–½ gr.), three times daily. See *prostigmine bromide.*

n. methylsulfate (*neostigminae methylsulfas*). The salt used for hypodermic injection. Dose, 0.5–1.0 mg. (1/120–1/60 gr.). See *prostigmine methylsulfate.*

ne″o·stri·a′tum (nee″o·stry·ay′tum) [G. *neos,* new; L. *striare,* to furnish with channels]. The caudate nucleus and putamen combined; the phylogenetically new part of the corpus striatum.

neo-synephrine hydrochloride. Trade-mark for the hydrochloride of the levo isomer of a synthetically prepared derivative of phenylethylamine, widely used as a pressor substance. See *phenylephrine hydrochloride.*

ne·ot′e·ny [*neos;* G. *teinein,* to stretch]. *In zoology,* sexual maturity in the larval stage; pedogenesis.

ne″o·vi′ta·min A. $C_{20}H_{30}O$; 5-*cis*-vitamin A; an isomer of vitamin A occurring to approximately 35 per cent of the total vitamin-A content of various liver oils and in about the same proportion in synthetic vitamin-A concentrates. Certain of its physical properties differ from those of vitamin A, but it appears to have the same biological potency.

neph′a·lism [G. *nēphalismos,* soberness]. Total abstinence from alcoholic liquors.

neph″e·lom′e·ter [G. *nephelē,* cloud; *metron,* a measure]. An apparatus for ascertaining the number of bacteria in a suspension, or the turbidity of a fluid.

Zeis's n. The Pulfrich photometer mounted in a horizontal position and equipped with a turbidity gage.

neph″e·lom′e·try [*nephelē; metron*]. The determination of the degree of turbidity of a fluid.

nephr-. See *nephro-.*

ne·phral′gi·a [G. *nephros,* kidney; *algos,* pain]. Pain in a kidney.

ne″phrec·ta′si·a (nee″freck·tay′zhuh, ·zee·uh, ·shuh, ·see·uh, nef″reck·) [*nephros;* G. *ektasis,* extension]. Dilatation of a kidney.

ne·phrec′to·mize [*nephros;* G. *ektomē,* excision]. To remove a kidney.

ne·phrec′to·my [*nephros; ektomē*]. Excision of a kidney.

abdominal n. Nephrectomy performed through an abdominal incision.

lumbar n. Nephrectomy through an incision in the loin.

transthoracic n. Nephrectomy performed through a thoracic approach and an incision through the diaphragm.

neph′ric [*nephros*]. Pertaining to the kidney; renal.

ne·phrid′i·um (pl. *nephridia*) [*nephros*]. One of the segmentally arranged, paired, coiled, excretory tubules of many invertebrates, notably the annelid worms.

ne·phrit′i·des. Plural of nephritis: general term for the varieties thereof.

ne·phri′tis [G.]. Inflammation of the kidney. If the inflammation is primarily of the glomeruli, the disease is called glomerulonephritis. Nephritis caused by an infection ascending from the ureter is called pyelonephritis. —**nephrit′ic,** *adj.*

acute diffuse interstitial n. Nephritic complication of bacterial, rickettsial, and virus infections; the symptoms usually occur earlier than when glomerulonephritis follows a streptococcal infection.

chronic parenchymatous n. Chronic glomerulonephritis with marked changes in the renal tubules, as fibrosis, atrophy, cloudy swelling, hydropic or fatty degeneration, and dilatation with formation of cystic spaces.

embolic n. A rare form of acute nephritis in which the focal lesions develop in only part of the glomerulus. It usually occurs in subacute bacterial endocarditis, but sometimes in acute bacterial and acute rheumatic endocarditis, and in septicemias with no endocarditis. Hematuria with or without proteinuria is common, but renal insufficiency is not usually present. Also called *thrombotic n.*

glomerular n. See *glomerulonephritis.*

interstitial n. An essentially exudative inflammation of the interstitial tissue; inflammatory cells may be present diffusely or focally.

nephrotoxic n. A type produced experimentally in animals by the injection of serum containing antibodies to the animals' kidney proteins, thus simulating glomerulonephritis.

scarlatinal n. The acute catarrhal nephritis arising in the course of, or during the convalescence from, scarlet fever.

syphilitic n. A rare type which may occur in the later stages of syphilis, and perhaps in prenatal syphilis.

thrombotic n. See embolic *n.*

trench n. A type of acute glomerulonephritis which occurred in epidemic form in the front lines during World War I.

tubular n. (a) Inflammation of renal tubules. (b) Renal disorders in which the lesions are primarily in the tubules. See *nephrosis,* 1.

neph′ro-, nephr- [G. *nephros,* kidney]. A combining form meaning *kidney.*

neph″ro·ab·dom′i·nal [*nephros;* L. *abdomen,* abdomen]. Pertaining to the kidneys and abdomen.

neph″ro·cal″ci·no′sis [*nephros;* L. *calx,* lime; G. *-ōsis,* condition]. Renal calcinosis, marked by the precipitation of deposits of calcium phosphate in the kidney tubules.

neph″ro·cap·sec′to·my, neph″ro·cap″su·lec′-to·my [*nephros;* L. *capsula,* little box; G. *ektomē,* excision]. Excision of the capsule of a kidney.

neph″ro·cap″su·lot′o·my [*nephros; capsula;* G. *tomē,* a cutting]. Incision of the renal capsule.

neph″ro·car′di·ac [*nephros;* G. *kardia,* heart]. Pertaining to the kidney and the heart.

neph′ro·coele (nef′ro·seel) [*nephros;* G. *koilia,* cavity]. The embryonic cavity in a nephrotome.

neph″ro·col′o·pex″y [*nephros;* G. *kolon,* colon; *pēxis,* a fixing]. The surgical anchoring of a kidney and the colon by means of the nephrocolic ligament.

neph″ro·co″lop·to′sis [*nephros; kolon;* G. *ptōsis,* a falling]. Downward displacement of a kidney and the colon.

neph″ro·cys″tan·as″to·mo′sis [*nephros;* G. *kystis,* bladder; *anastomōsis,* outlet]. The surgical formation of an opening between the renal pelvis and the urinary bladder.

neph″ro·cys·ti′tis [*nephros; kystis;* G. *-itis,* inflammation]. Inflammation of both the urinary bladder and kidney.

neph″ro·dys′tro·phy. See *nephrosis,* 1.

neph″ro·gen′ic [*nephros;* G. *genesthai,* from *gignesthai,* to be produced]. 1. Having the ability to produce kidney tissue. 2. Of renal origin.

ne·phrog′e·nous (ni·frodj′i·nus) [*nephros; genesthai*]. Of renal origin.

neph′roid [*nephros;* G. *eidos,* form]. Kidney-shaped; reniform; resembling a kidney.

neph′ro·lith [*nephros;* G. *lithos,* stone]. A calculus of the kidney.

neph″ro·li·thi′a·sis [*nephros; lithos;* NL. *-iasis,* condition]. The formation of renal calculi, or the diseased state that leads to their formation.

neph″ro·lith′ic [*nephros; lithos*]. Pertaining to, or affected with, a nephrolith.

neph″ro·li·thot′o·my [*nephros; lithos;* G. *tomē,* a cutting]. An incision of the kidney for the removal of a calculus.

ne·phrol′y·sin, neph″ro·ly′sin [*nephros;* G. *lysis,* a loosing]. A toxic substance capable of disintegrating kidney cells.

ne·phrol′y·sis [*nephros; lysis*]. 1. The disintegration of the kidney by the action of a nephrolysin. 2 The operation of loosening a kidney from surrounding adhesions. —**nephrolyt′ic,** *adj.*

neph·ro′ma [*nephros;* G. *-ōma,* tumor]. The clear-cell carcinoma of the renal parenchyma.

mesoblastic n. See Wilm's *tumor.*

neph′ro·mere. See *nephrotome.*

neph′ron (pl. *nephrons, nephroi*) [*nephros*]. The renal unit, consisting of the glomerular capsule, its glomerulus, and the attached uriniferous tubule.

neph″ro·path′ic. Of or pertaining to any disease of the kidney.

ne·phrop′a·thy. See *nephrosis,* 1.

neph′ro·pex″y [*nephros;* G. *pēxis,* a fixing]. Surgical fixation of a floating kidney.

neph″ro·poi′e·tin (nef″ro·poy′i·tin, ·poy·ee′tin) [*nephros;* G. *poiein,* to produce]. A substance supposed to stimulate growth of renal tissue.

neph″rop·to′sis, neph″rop·to′si·a (nef″rop·to′-shuh, ·see·uh, ·zhuh, ·zee·uh) [*nephros;* G. *ptōsis,* a falling]. Prolapse of the kidney.

neph″ro·py″e·li′tis [*nephros;* G. *pyelos,* trough; *-itis,* inflammation]. Inflammation of the pelvis of the kidney; pyelonephritis.

neph″ro·py′e·lo·plas″ty [*nephros; pyelos;* G. *plassein,* to form]. A plastic operation on the pelvis of the kidney.

neph·ror′rha·phy [*nephros;* G. *rhaphē,* a suture]. 1. The stitching of a floating kidney to the posterior wall of the abdomen or to the loin. 2. Suturing a wound in a kidney.

neph′ros [G.]. The kidney.

neph″ro·scle·ro′sis [*nephros;* G. *sclerōsis,* a hardening]. Involvement of the kidney in hypertensive vascular disease. Gives rise to disturbances in renal function and a clinical picture identical with that of chronic glomerulonephritis.

arterial n. Arteriosclerosis of the kidney, causing a reduction in blood supply and atrophy of the parenchyma, with resulting fibrosis of the kidney. Often accompanies arteriosclerosis in the aged. Also called *senile arteriosclerctic n.*

arteriolar n. Diffuse fibrosis of the kidney due to arteriolar disease.

malignant n. Nephrosclerosis characterized by rapidly progressive renal disease and marked interference with renal function; associated with malignant hypertension. There is sclerosis or hyaline necrosis of renal arterioles or sometimes acute exudative arteriolitis.

ne·phro′sis [*nephros;* G. *-ōsis,* condition]. 1. *In pathology,* degenerative or retrogressive renal lesions, as distinct from inflammation (*nephritis*) or vascular involvement (*nephrosclerosis*), especially as applied to tubular lesions (*tubular nephritis*): also called *nephropathy, nephrodystrophy.* 2. Clinically, and loosely, nephrotic syndrome.

acute n. Renal tubular degeneration occurring in either the proximal or distal segments of the nephron, including the mild degeneration associated with infectious diseases as well as the chemical nephroses and other intoxications.

amyloid n. A form of chronic nephrosis due to excessive deposition of amyloid in the kidney, especially in the glomeruli, and sometimes resulting in the nephrotic syndrome.

chemical n. An acute, severe renal-tubule nephrosis caused by exogenous chemical poisons, such as mercury bichloride, ethylene glycol, bismuth, carbon tetrachloride, uranium nitrate, and others. Pathologically, the kidneys are swollen and grayish-white; clinically, the patient develops oliguria, then anuria, often dying of uremia.

cholemic n. That accompanying severe jaundice, characterized by yellowish pigment casts in the collecting tubules and mild degeneration of the convoluted tubules.

chronic n. A slowly progressing degeneration associated with metabolic diseases, such as gout or diabetes.

fat n. A clinically silent, reversible, purely tubular, histologic entity characterized by lipid deposition in the epithelial cells of the proximal convoluted tubules, occurring in severe diabetes and in poisonings due to phosphorus, carbon tetrachloride, chloroform, and other halogenated organic compounds.

hemoglobinuric n. See lower nephron *n.*

ischemic n. See lower nephron *n.*

lipemic n. See lipoid *n.*

lipoid n. A relatively rare chronic disease of young children, characterized clinically by severe proteinuria, edema, hypoproteinemia, albumin-globulin ratio reversal, and hypercholesterolemia. When hematuria is absent, the condition is called **pure lipoid n.,** when present, **mixed lipoid n.** The proteinuria is due to a glomerular lesion which is morphologically not evident; the tubules are the seat of degeneration and lipid deposition. The cause is unknown, although some believe it to be a stage of glomerulonephritis. Treatment is symptomatic; about 50 per cent of patients recover. Also called *lipemic n., membranous glomerulonephritis.*

lower nephron n. A patchy nephrosis involving mainly the distal segments of the nephrons; pathologically, there is cloudy swelling, a segmental necrosis, and casts in the distal and collection tubules. Initially there is renal insufficiency, often oliguria progressing to anuria and uremia. This condition occurs following crushing injuries (*crush syndrome*), in severe transfusion reaction and burns, black-water fever, toxemias of pregnancy, favism, and in sulfonamide, mushroom, and carbon tetrachloride poisoning. It is thought to be caused by partial ischemia in conjunction with injurious substances such as myoglobin, hemoglobin (*hemoglobinuric n.*), or exogenous poisons. Also called *ischemuric tubulorrhexis.*

mercurial n. Nephrosis due to mercury bichloride poisoning.

toxic n. Tubular lesions including cloudy swelling, fatty and hyaline degeneration, and necrosis caused by toxins and other injurious agents released into the blood stream during acute infectious or metabolic disturbances.

neph′ro·stome, neph″ro·sto′ma [*nephros;* G. *stoma*, mouth]. The opening of a nephron or of a nephridium into the coelom in lower vertebrates and many invertebrates. —**nephrosto′mal,** *adj.*

ne·phros′to·my [*nephros; stoma*]. The formation of a fistula leading to the pelvis of a kidney.

neph′ro·tome [*nephros;* G. *tomos*, cutting]. The narrow mass of mesoderm connecting somites and lateral mesoderm, from which the pronephros, mesonephros, metanephros, and their ducts develop. Also called *intermediate cell mass, mesomere, nephromere.*

ne·phrot′o·my [*nephros;* G. *tomē*, a cutting]. Incision of the kidney.

abdominal n. One through an abdominal incision.

lumbar n. One through an incision in the loin.

neph″ro·tox′ic [*nephros;* G. *toxikon*, poison]. 1. Pertaining to nephrotoxin. 2. Destructive to the kidney cells; nephrolytic.

neph″ro·tox′in [*nephros; toxikon*]. A cytotoxin which has a supposedly specific action on the cells of the kidney.

neph″ro·tro′pic. Referring to a medicinal agent which affects predominantly a function of the kidney. —**nephrotro′pic,** *n.*

neph″ro·tu·ber″cu·lo′sis [*nephros;* L. *tuberculum*, small swelling; G. *-ōsis*, condition]. Disease of the kidney due to the tubercle bacillus.

neph″ro·u″re·ter·ec′to·my [*nephros;* G. *ourētēr*, ureter; *ektomē*, excision]. The excision of a kidney and whole ureter at one operation.

nep″i·ol′o·gy (nep″ee·ol′o·jee, nee″pee·) [G. *nēpios*, infant; *logos*, word]. That branch of pediatrics which treats of young infants. *Rare.*

nep·tu′ni·um [L. *Neptunius*, of Neptune]. Np = 237 ca. An element, atomic number 93, obtained by bombarding ordinary uranium with neutrons. Undergoes transformation into plutonium.

ne″re·an′tin. See *nerianthin.*

Neri's sign. A sign of sciatica. See under *sign.*

ne″ri·an′thin, ne″re·an′tin. A crystalline glycoside obtained from the leaves of *Nerium oleander.*

ne′ri·in. A glycoside from the bark and leaves of *Nerium oleander*. It belongs to the digitalis group.

ne″ri·o·do′re·in. A glycoside from *Nerium oleander*. See *nerium.*

ne′ri·um [G. *nērion*, oleander]. The leaves and bark of *Nerium oleander*. The extractive principles, in small doses, act as a cardiac tonic, resembling digitalis.

Nernst, Walther Hermann [*German physicist,* 1864–1941]. Known for his invention of an incandescent electric lamp with metallic oxide filaments, called *Nernst lamp.* Nobel laureate (1920).

ner′ol. $C_{10}H_{17}OH$; 2,6-dimethyl-2,6-octadien-8-ol; an unsaturated alcohol found in many essential oils; the *trans* isomer of geraniol.

ner′o·li oil (nerr′o·lee, neer′o·lee) [It., supposedly after an Italian princess]. Orange flower oil.

nerve [L. *nervus*, nerve]. A bundle of nerve fibers, usually outside the brain or spinal cord; the nerve fibers are held together by connective tissue called endoneurium inside the nerve bundle and perineurium, the enclosing sheath. A collected bundle of nerve fibers within the brain and spinal cord is usually called a nerve tract. For nerves listed by name, see Table of Nerves; for those not given here, see alphabetical entry. See Plate 16.

accelerator n. The cardiac sympathetic nerve, stimulation of which causes acceleration of the heart's action.

accessory (eleventh cranial) n. A nerve with motor and parasympathetic components, having both a bulbar origin along the lateral aspect of the medulla oblongata and a spinal origin from the upper 5 or 6 cervical segments. The bulbar part (*internal ramus*) runs with the vagus, sending motor fibers via the recurrent laryngeal nerve to the striate muscles of larynx and pharynx, and parasympathetic fibers to thoracic and abdominal viscera. The spinal portion (*external ramus*) innervates via the cervical plexus (C-2, 3, 4) parts of the trapezius and sternocleidomastoid muscles.

adrenergic nerves. Postganglionic sympathetic fibers which, upon stimulation, release an adrenergic substance at their terminations.

afferent n. One that transmits impulses from the periphery to the central nervous system; a sensory nerve.

autonomic n. A nerve of the autonomic nervous system.

cerebrospinal n. Any nerve taking origin from the brain or spinal cord.

cholinergic nerves. See *cholinergic.*

cochlear n. A sensory nerve, attached on the brain stem at the lower border of the pons, which innervates the spiral organ (of Corti) of the cochlea.

cranial nerves. Nerves arising directly from the brain stem and making their exit to the periphery via openings in the skull: **I. olfactory, II. optic, III. oculomotor, IV. trochlear, V. trigeminal, VI. abducens, VII. facial** (including *nervus intermedius*), **VIII. acoustic** (*cochlear* and *vestibular*), **IX. glossopharyngeal, X. vagus, XI. accessory, XII. hypoglossal.** Usually described and numbered as 12 pairs, the first two are not true nerves but nerve-fiber tracts of the brain; the caudal 10 pairs originate from nuclei in the brain stem, except for that part of XI which has a spinal root.

depressor n. One which, upon stimulation, lowers the blood pressure either in a local part or throughout the body.

effector n. See efferent *n.*

efferent n. One conducting impulses from the central nervous system to the periphery, as to a muscle.

excitoreflex n. A visceral nerve, excitation of which brings about a reflex action.

extrinsic n. One which conveys nervous impulses to an organ from the central nervous system or from the ganglionated chain of the sympathetic nervous system. It may synapse with a secondary neuron which lies within the organ. See intrinsic *n.*

facial (seventh cranial) n. A motor nerve, attached to the brain stem at the inferior border

of the pons, which innervates the stapedius, stylohyoid, posterior belly of the digastric, and the muscles of facial expression. It also has parasympathetic and sensory components, running by way of the nervus intermedius.
femoral n. A motor and somatic sensory nerve which is attached at the second, third, and fourth lumbar segments of the cord (lumbar plexus). The motor portion innervates the pectineus, the quadriceps femoris, and the articularis genus muscles; the sensory portion innervates the skin of the anterior aspect of the thigh, the medial aspect of the leg, and the skin of the hip and knee joints.
frontal n. A somatic sensory nerve, attached to the ophthalmic, which innervates the skin of the upper eyelid, the forehead, and the scalp.
glossopharyngeal n. The ninth cranial nerve with motor, sensory (special and visceral), and parasympathetic components. Motor fibers pass from the nucleus ambiguus to the stylopharyngeus and muscles of soft palate and pharynx; sensory fibers supply the posterior third of the tongue and taste buds there, the pharynx, middle-ear and mastoid air cells; parasympathetic fibers pass from the inferior salivary nucleus via the otic ganglion to the parotid gland.
hypoglossal (twelfth cranial) n. A motor nerve, attached to the medulla oblongata, which innervates the intrinsic and extrinsic muscles of the tongue.
inhibitory n. Any nerve which, upon stimulation, lowers the activity of a center or organ.
intrinsic n. One which innervates the muscles, glands, or mucous membrane of an organ. It may be the nerve fiber either of a sensory neuron or of a postganglionic neuron of the sympathetic system.
mandibular n. A motor (masticator nerve) and somatic sensory nerve, attached to the trigeminus, which innervates the tensor tympani, tensor veli palatini, mylohyoid, anterior belly of the digastric, and muscles of mastication, the lower teeth, the mucosa of the anterior two-thirds of the tongue, the floor of the mouth, the cheek and the skin of the lower portion of the face, and the meninges.
maxillary n. A somatic sensory nerve, attached to the trigeminus, which innervates the meninges, the skin of the upper portion of the face, the upper teeth, and the mucosa of the nose, palate, and cheeks.
mixed n. A nerve composed of both afferent and efferent fibers.
motor n. Any nerve composed chiefly or wholly of motor fibers.
n. avulsion. Operation of tearing a nerve from its central origin by traction.
n. block. The interruption of the passage of impulses through a nerve, as by chemical, mechanical, or electric means.
n. ending. The termination of a nerve at the periphery or in the nerve centers.
n. gases. See under *gas.*
n. grafting. The transplantation of a portion of a nerve to reestablish the continuity of a severed nerve.
n. of Arnold. The auricular branch of the vagus.
n. of Bell. The long thoracic nerve.
n. of Cotunnius. The nasopalatine nerve.
n. of Cruveilhier. An occasional lingual branch of the seventh cranial nerve.
n. of Cyon. In the rabbit, a separate branch of the vagus which carries sensory fibers concerned in cardiac depressor action.
n. of Eisler. The greater coccygeal perforating nerve, only occasionally present, arising from the fourth and fifth sacral nerves.
n. of Jacobson. The tympanic branch of the ninth cranial nerve.
n. of Lancisi. The medial longitudinal striae.
n. of Scarpa. The nasopalatine nerve.
n. of Vidius. The nerve of the pterygoid canal.
n. of Vieussens. The ansa subclavia.
n. of Wrisberg. 1. The intermedius branch of the ninth cranial nerve. 2. The medial cutaneous nerve of the arm.
n. tract. A bundle of nerve fibers having the same general origin and destination within the nervous system; as a rule, all fibers of a nerve tract serve the same or a very similar function. See *tract.*
oculomotor n. The third cranial nerve whose motor fibers arise from nuclei in the central gray matter at the level of the superior colliculus and supply the levator palpebrae superioris and all extrinsic eye muscles except the lateral rectus and superior oblique, and whose parasympathetic component arises from the Edinger-Westphal nucleus and goes to the ciliary ganglion, from which short fibers pass to the ciliary and sphincter pupillae muscles.
olfactory (first cranial) n. A sensory nerve, attached to the olfactory bulb, which innervates the olfactory mucosa.
ophthalmic n. A somatic sensory nerve, attached to the trigeminal, which innervates the skin of the forehead, the upper eyelids, the anterior portion of the scalp, the orbit, the eyeball, the meninges, the nasal mucosa, the frontal, ethmoidal, and sphenoidal air sinuses.
optic (second cranial) n. A sensory nerve, attached at the optic tracts, which innervates the retina.
parasympathetic n. A nerve of the parasympathetic nervous system.
pelvic splanchnic n. See *nervus* erigens.
peripheral n. (a) Specifically, one whose distribution is to the skin or to superficial structures of the body. (b) Often used to denote any nerve which is a branch of the central nervous system.
phrenic n. A motor nerve, arising from the third, fourth, and fifth cervical (cervical plexus) segments of the cord. It innervates the diaphragm.
pilomotor n. A nerve causing contraction of one of the arrectores pilorum muscles.
pneumogastric n. Old name for vagus nerve.
pressor n. An afferent nerve, stimulation of which excites the vasomotor center.
respiratory n. One of two nerves supplying important muscles of respiration: the external is the long thoracic, the internal is the phrenic, nerve.
sacral n. Any of the motor, somatic sensory, parasympathetic, and visceral sensory nerves (there are five pairs) attached at the sacral segments of the cord, which innervate the posterior divisions to the muscles and skin of the lower back and sacral region, the anterior divisions to the sacral plexus supplying the muscles and skin of the lower extremity and perineum, and branches to the hypogastric and pelvic plexuses supplying the pelvic viscera and the genitalia.
secretory n. An efferent nerve, stimulation of which causes increased activity of the gland to which it is distributed.
segmental n. A nerve that supplies the structures derived from one of the original body somites, as an intercostal nerve.
sensory n. A nerve which conducts afferent impulses from the periphery to the central nervous system, as those mediating sensations of pain, touch, and temperature.
somatic n. One of the nerves supplying somatic

structures, as voluntary muscles, skin, tendons, joints, and parietal serous membranes.

sphenopalatine n. A somatic sensory nerve, attached to the maxillary, which innervates the nose and palate via the sphenopalatine ganglion and the palatine nerves.

spinal n. A nerve arising from the spinal cord and making its exit through an intervertebral foramen. There are 31 pairs of spinal nerves: 8 cervical, 12 thoracic, 5 lumbar, 5 sacral, and 1 coccygeal.

splanchnic n. A nerve carrying nerve fibers from the lower thoracic paravertebral ganglions to the collateral ganglions. The **greater splanchnic nerve** arises from the fifth to ninth or tenth thoracic ganglions and goes to visceral nerve plexuses in the thorax and to the celiac plexus. The **lesser splanchnic nerve** arises from the ninth and tenth thoracic ganglions and goes to the celiac plexus. The **lowest** or **least splanchnic nerve** arises from the lowest thoracic ganglion and goes to the renal plexus.

sudomotor nerves. The nerves which excite the sweat glands to activity.

sympathetic n. A nerve of the sympathetic nervous system.

vasoconstrictor n. See vasomotor *nerves*.

vasodilator n. See *vasomotor nerves* under *nerve*.

vasomotor nerves. Those concerned with controlling the caliber of blood vessels. They are of two types: those which cause constriction of the blood vessel or **vasoconstrictor nerves,** and those which cause dilation of the blood vessel or **vasodilator nerves.** Ordinarily vasomotor is synonymous with vasoconstrictor.

visceral n. Any nerve supplying a visceral structure.

nerve sup·ply′. The nerves of an organ or structure; distinguished as **extrinsic n. s.,** that which connects the organ or structure with the central nervous system, and as **intrinsic n. s.,** that portion of the nerve supply entirely contained within the structure or organ, as the myenteric and submucous plexuses of the intestine.

nerve trac′ing. A method used by chiropractors for locating nerves and studying their pathology. It depends on the patient's reports about areas of tenderness or pain when adjoining areas are pressed upon by the operator.

ner′vi (nurv′eye). Plural of nervus.

nerv′ine. Allaying nervous excitement.

nerv′ine. A medicament for treating nervous disorders; nerve tonic.

ner′vone. A cerebroside occurring in brain tissue; its characteristic fatty acid is nervonic acid.

ner·von′ic ac′id. $C_{23}H_{45}COOH$. An unsaturated acid, related to lignoceric acid, believed to exist in nervone.

ner′vo·sism [L. *nervus*, nerve]. 1. Neurasthenia or nervousness. 2. An obsolete doctrine that all morbid phenomena are caused by alterations of nerve force.

ner·vos′i·ty [L. *nervositas*, strength, thickness]. Excessive nervousness.

ner″vo·ta′bes (nur″vo·tay′beez) [*nervus;* L. *tabes*, a wasting]. A disturbance resembling tabes clinically, but due to parenchymatous neuritis and not to spinal-cord changes.

nerv′ous ex·haus′tion. A state of fatigue and discomfort due to emotional causes. See *neurasthenia*.

nerv′ous·ness [*nervus*]. A popular term denoting excessive excitability of the nervous system; characterized by shaken mental poise, muscle tremors or weakness, and an uncomfortable awareness of self.

nerv′ous sys′tem. 1. The entire nervous apparatus of the body, including the brain, brain stem, spinal cord, cranial and peripheral nerves, and ganglions. 2. A functional or anatomic part of the nervous apparatus of the body.

autonomic n. s. The nervous system supplying, and exerting a regulatory influence over, involuntary muscle, glands, viscera, etc.; divided into sympathetic and parasympathetic nervous systems. See Plate 15.

central n. s. The brain and spinal cord.

cerebrospinal n. s. The brain, spinal cord, and cranial and spinal nerves.

craniosacral autonomic n. s. The parasympathetic system composed of those nerves whose preganglionic fibers exit from the central nervous system by way of the third, seventh, ninth, and tenth cranial nerves, and the second, third, and fourth sacral nerves.

involuntary n. s. Old term for autonomic *n. s.*

parasympathetic n. s. The craniosacral division of the autonomic nervous system, consisting of preganglionic nerve fibers carried in cranial and sacral nerves, outlying ganglions, postganglionic fibers, and associated afferent nerve fibers; in general, innervating the same structures and having a regulatory function opposite to that of the sympathetic nervous system.

peripheral n. s. The autonomic nervous system and the cerebrospinal nerves; the peripheral portions of the nervous system conducting impulses to and from the central nervous system.

somatic n. s. That part of the nervous system exercising control over skeletal muscle and relating the organism to its environment.

sympathetic n. s. (a) The entire autonomic nervous system. (b) The thoracolumbar division of the autonomic nervous system; the ganglionated sympathetic trunk, sympathetic plexuses, and the associated preganglionic, postganglionic, and afferent nerve fibers.

thoracolumbar autonomic n. s. The sympathetic nervous system composed of those nerves whose preganglionic fibers exit from the spinal cord by way of the thoracic and upper lumbar spinal nerves.

vegetative n. s. See autonomic *n. s.*

visceral n. s. See autonomic *n. s.*

ner′vus (pl. *nervi*) [L.]. Nerve.

nervi nervorum. Nerve filaments going to the nerve sheaths.

nervi vasorum. Small nerves which innervate the walls of the blood vessels.

n. erigens. Sacral parasympathetic fibers which pass through the pelvic plexus to terminal ganglions in the pelvic viscera and are concerned with the emptying mechanisms of the urinary bladder, rectum, and uterus, and with erection of the genital organs. Syn., *pelvic splanchnic nerve.*

n. furcalis. The fourth lumbar nerve which forks to send fibers to both the lumbar and sacral plexus.

n. intermedius. The intermedius branch of the seventh cranial or facial nerve: formerly called *glossopalatine nerve, Wrisberg's n., Wrisberg's pars intermedius.*

n. ischiadicus. The sciatic nerve.

n. pelvicus. The nervus erigens.

Nesbit, Reed Miller [*American urologist*, 1898–]. Known for his introduction of an operation for relief of advanced bladder and urethral tuberculosis; he performed a double-barrel type of sigmoid colostomy, after which the lower bowel was made sufficiently aseptic to eliminate the hazard of infection in subsequent ureteral transplantation according to the technic of Robert C. Coffey.

ne′sis. Suture. *Obs.*

ness′ler·i″zing [after A. *Nessler*, German chemist, 1827–1905]. The process of using Nessler's reagent.

Nessler's reagent. See under *reagent.*

nest [AS.]. A group, as of ova or insects.

cell n. (a) An isolated mass of epithelial cells surrounded by connective tissue, as in carcinoma. (b) A large number of chondrocytes surrounded by a single primary capsule.

nes·tei′a (neh·sty′uh) [G., fast]. 1. Fasting. 2. The jejunum. *Rare.*

nes″ti·at′ri·a (nes″tee·at′ree·uh, ·ay′tree·uh, neh-sty″uh·try′uh) [*nēsteia;* G. *iatreia,* treatment]. Treatment by fasting; the hunger-cure.

nes″ti·os′to·my [G. *nēstis,* jejunum; *stoma,* mouth]. Jejunostomy. *Rare.*

nes′tis [G.]. 1. Fasting. 2. The jejunum.

nes″ti·ther′a·py. Old term for nestiatria.

nethamine. A trade-mark for *l*-N-ethylephedrine.

net·ran′eu·rysm (net·ran′yoo·riz·um) [G. *nētron,* spindle; *aneurysma,* aneurysm]. A fusiform aneurysm. *Rare.*

ne·trop′sin. $C_{32}H_{48}N_{18}O_4$; an antibiotic substance produced by the actinomycete *Streptomyces netropsis.*

net′tle. See *urtica.*

net′tle rash. See *urticaria.*

Nettleship, Edward [*English ophthalmologist,* 1845–1913]. Described urticaria pigmentosa (1869), also called *Nettleship's disease.*

net′work″ [AS. *net; worc*]. The arrangement of fibers or vessels in a reticulum. See *rete.*

Neubauer, Johann Ernst [*German anatomist,* 1742–77]. Described the deep thyroid artery, an occasional branch of the innominate, called arteria thyreoidea ima or *Neubauer's artery.* Described the large ganglion formed by the union of the lower cervical and first thoracic ganglions, called *Neubauer's ganglion.*

Neubauer, Otto [*German physician,* 1874–]. Introduced an improvement on the platform of the blood counting chamber by means of a system of engraved lines which divide the chamber into nine primary squares, each divided into many smaller squares. Called *Neubauer's ruling for counting chamber.*

Neuber, Gustav Adolf [*German surgeon,* 1850–1932]. Introduced decalcified bone drainage tubes called *Neuber's tubes.*

Neufeld, Fred [*German bacteriologist,* 1869–1904]. With Willi Rimpau, described bacteriotropins (1904). With Ludwig Haendel published work on pneumococcic serum (1910). See also Neufeld quellung *test,* also called *Neufeld reaction.*

Neumann, Ernst [*German pathologist,* 1834–1918]. Remembered for his description of changes occurring in bone marrow in leukemia (1870). The first to use the term myelogenous leukemia. Described nucleated red corpuscles in the bone marrow developing into erythrocytes, called *Neumann's corpuscles.* The lining of some dentinal tubules is also called *Neumann's sheath.*

Neumann, Heinrich (1873–1939). Austrian otolaryngologist, best known for his introduction of a method of opening the labyrinth, called *Neumann's operation.*

Neumann, Isidor (1832–1906). Austrian dermatologist who described porokeratosis under the name of dermatitis circumscripta herpetiformis (1875), also called *Mibelli's disease,* and pemphigus vegetans (1886), which is also called *Neumann's disease.*

Neumann method for total phosphorus. See under *method.*

neu′ral [G. *neuron,* nerve]. Pertaining to nerves or nervous tissue.

neu·ral′gi·a [*neuron;* G. *algos,* pain]. Severe paroxysmal pain along the course of a nerve; not associated with demonstrable structural changes in the nerve. According to their anatomic situation, the following forms of neuralgia are described: trigeminal neuralgia, tic douloureux, or prosopalgia; supraorbital neuralgia; cervico-occipital neuralgia; cervicobrachial and brachial neuralgia; intercostal neuralgia, sciatica, or ischialgia; coccygodynia; visceral neuralgia (as hepatic, gastric, intestinal, uterine, ovarian neuralgia). The pain of neuralgia is sharp, stabbing, and paroxysmal, lasting usually but a short time; tenderness is often present at the points of exit of the nerve (points douloureux), and the paroxysm can be produced by contact with specific areas (trigger zones). Intercostal neuralgia is at times associated with herpes zoster. —**neuralgic,** *adj.*

articular n. Neuralgia of a joint.

atypical n. Facial pain, due to various causes, differing from facial neuralgia by being continuous, deep-seated, and beyond the distribution of the trigeminal nerve.

brachial plexus n. Neuralgia of the brachial plexus, manifested in the neck and shoulder and extending into the arm and hand.

ciliary n. Neuralgic pain of the eye, brow, or temple.

coccygeal n. See *coccygodynia.*

crural n. See lumbosacral *n.*

dental n. Toothache.

facial n. Neuralgia over the region of facial distribution of the trigeminal nerve. Also called *trifacial n., trigeminal n.*

geniculate n. One involving the geniculate ganglion of the facial nerve, causing pain in the middle ear and auditory canal.

glossopharyngeal n. Neuralgic pain of the throat and base of the tongue, relieved by cutting the affected parts of the glossopharyngeal nerve.

lumbosacral n. Pain along the branches of the lumbosacral plexus.

obturator n. See lumbosacral *n.*

occipital n. Neuralgia over the region of distribution of the greater occipital nerve.

phrenic n. Pain referred to the shoulder or arm from diseased viscera, e.g., pericarditis or adrenal tumor.

pudendal plexus n. Neuralgia of the lower two or three sacral nerves, manifested in the perineum, scrotum, penis, and testes.

Seeligmueller's n. Bilateral neuralgia of the auriculotemporal nerves with pain extending over the vertex, characteristic of neurosyphilis.

sphenopalatine n. Sluder's neuralgia. Neuralgia caused by infection of the nasal sinuses, which is referred to the root of the nose, the upper teeth, the eyes, and even to the ears, the mastoid regions and the occiput.

trifacial n. Old term for trigeminal neuralgia.

trigeminal n. See facial *n.*

tympanic n. Neuralgia of the tympanic branch of the glossopharyngeal nerve, manifested in the ear and neck.

neu·ral′gi·form [*neuron; algos;* L. *forma,* form]. Resembling neuralgia.

neu·ram″e·bim′e·ter [*neuron;* G. *amoibē,* requital; *metron,* a measure]. The nerve-reply measurer; an instrument devised and used in psychophysics to obtain the reaction time of nervous impressions.

neur″a·min′ic ac′id. $C_{11}H_{23}NO_9$; an acid, of unknown structure, isolated from the ganglioside fraction of brain lipid and from the mammary gland of certain experimental animals.

neur″a·min-lac′tose. A carbohydrate derivative isolated from the mammary gland of rats; on hydrolysis it yields neuraminic acid and lactose.

neu″ra·poph′y·sis [*neuron;* G. *apophysis*, process]. Either one of the two apophyses on each vertebra which blend and form the neural arch, or the dorsal wall of the spinal foramen.

neu″ra·prax′i·a [*neuron;* G. *apraxia*, nonaction]. Injury to a nerve in which the nerve fiber itself undergoes no degeneration, although there may be localized degeneration of the myelin sheath. Recovery is spontaneous, complete, and rapid.

neu″ras·the′ni·a [*neuron;* G. *astheneia*, weakness]. A group of symptoms formerly ascribed to debility or exhaustion of the nerve centers. The symptoms include fatigability, lack of energy, various aches and pains, and disinclination to activity. Some individuals have many symptoms, in others the symptoms center upon some particular organ or region. It is now classified, according to specific features, as *conversion reaction, psychophysiologic nervous-system reaction, psychophysiologic autonomic and visceral disorder.*

abdominal n. That in which gastrointestinal symptoms predominate.

professional n. That manifested in the individual's total or partial inability to use the organ or organs commonly employed in his occupation, as the inability of a writer to write due to a spasm or a painful feeling of fatigue in his arm.

neu·rax′is [*neuron;* L. *axis*, axis]. 1. The cerebrospinal axis; the neural tube. 2. An axis cylinder. *Obs.*

neu″rax·i′tis [*neuron; axis;* G. *-itis*, inflammation]. 1. Inflammation of an axon. 2. Encephalitis.

neu·rax′on [*neuron;* G. *axōn*, axis]. Axon of a nerve cell. *Obs.*

neu″rec·ta′si·a (new″reck·tay′zhuh, ·zee·uh, ·shuh, ·see·uh), **neu·rec′ta·sis** [*neuron;* G. *ektasis*, extension]. Nerve stretching.

neu·rec′to·my [*neuron;* G. *ektomē*, excision]. Excision of a part of a nerve.

neu″rec·to′pi·a, neu·rec′to·py [*neuron;* G. *ektopos*, away from a place]. Displacement, or other abnormality, of the distribution of a nerve.

neu″ren·ter′ic [*neuron;* G. *enteron*, intestine]. Pertaining to the embryonic neural canal and the intestinal tube.

neu·rep″i·the′li·um [*neuron;* G. *epi*, on; *thēlē*, nipple]. See *neuroepithelium.*

neu·rer′gic (new·rur′jick) [*neuron;* G. *ergon*, work]. Pertaining to the activity of a nerve. *Rare.*

neur″ex·e·re′sis (new″reck·si·ree′sis, ·serr′i·sis), **neur″ex·ai′re·sis** (new″reck·sigh′ri·sis, ·sigh·ree′-sis) [*neuron;* G. *exairesis*, a taking out]. The surgical extraction, or avulsion, of a nerve.

neu′ri- [*neuron*]. A combining form denoting a nerve.

neu·ri′a·sis [*neuron;* NL. *-iasis*, condition]. Hysterical hypochondriasis.

neu·ri′a·try [*neuron;* G. *iatreia*, treatment]. The study and treatment of nervous diseases.

neu′ri·dine (new′ri·deen, ·din). A basic substance said to be present in brain tissue, identical with spermine.

neu″ri·lem′ma [*neuron;* G. *lemma*, sheath]. The thin cellular sheath of peripheral nerve fibers, covering the axon directly or covering the myelin sheath when this is present: also called *neurolemma, sheath of Schwann.*

neu″ri·lem·mi′tis [*neuron; lemma; -itis*, inflammation]. Inflammation of the neurilemma.

neu″ri·lem·mo′ma [*neuron; lemma;* G. *-ōma*, tumor]. A solitary encapsulated benign tumor occurring in the peripheral, cranial, and sympathetic nerves, which arises from the sheath of Schwann: also called *myoschwannoma, peripheral glioma, perineural fibroblastoma, perineural glioma, schwannoglioma, schwannoma*, specific *nerve-sheath tumor.*

malignant n. See malignant *schwannoma.*

neu″ri·lem″mo·sar·co′ma. See malignant *schwannoma.*

neu′rine (new′reen, ·rin). $(CH_3)_3N(OH)CH{=}CH_2$. A product of bacterial decomposition of lecithin.

neu″ri·no′ma [*neuron;* G. *-ōma*, tumor]. See acoustic-nerve *tumor.*

acoustic n. An intracranial neoplasm involving the acoustic-nerve sheath. There is an associated tinnitus in one ear and deafness in the late stages.

malignant n. See malignant *schwannoma.*

neu″ri·no·ma·to′sis. See *neurofibromatosis.*

neu′rit, neu′rite [*neuron*]. Old term for axon.

neu·ri′tis [*neuron;* G. *-itis*, inflammation]. Lesions of a nerve or nerves; either degenerative or inflammatory, with pain, hypersensitivity, anesthesia or paresthesia, paralysis, muscular atrophy, and lost reflexes in the part supplied. There are numerous forms, according to cause, pathology, location, and number of nerves involved, such as acute, chronic, or syphilitic. —**neurit′ic,** *adj.*

adventitial n. That affecting the nerve sheath.

alcoholic n. Neuritis of chronic alcoholism, presumably due to thiamine deficiency as a result of deficient food intake.

ascending n. That extending from the periphery of a nerve to the brain or cord.

axial n. A form affecting the central part of the nerve.

degenerative n. That involving the nerve fibers; usually multiple neuritis.

descending n. Neuritis extending from the brain or cord to the periphery of the nerve.

diabetic n. See diabetic *polyneuritis.*

diphtheritic n. Neuritis of the cranial or spinal nerves, as a sequel of diphtheria.

disseminated n. Segmental neuritis.

endemic n. Beriberi.

infectious n. An acute multiple neuritis, probably due to a virus disease.

interstitial n. See Guillan-Barré *syndrome.*

ischemic n. A type produced by ischemia of the nerves, seen in Buerger's disease, arteriosclerosis, and polyarteritis nodosa.

mononeuritis. Involvement of a single nerve.

multiple n. Simultaneous involvement of several nerves, usually symmetrical; due to poisons such as alcohol, arsenic, lead, or mercury, or to diseases such as diphtheria, typhoid, or syphilis. Also called *polyneuritis.*

nutritional n. Neuritis caused by vitamin-B deficiency; pellagra neuritis.

optic n. See *papillitis.*

paralytic brachial n. Pain and paralysis in the arm and shoulder during recovery from an infection or disease, differentiated from poliomyelitis by objective sensory changes and the absence of marked pleocytosis.

parenchymatous n. Degenerative neuritis.

pellagra n. A nutritional neuritis.

retrobulbar n. Inflammation of the optic nerve posterior to the eyeball.

sciatic n. Due to involvement of the sciatic nerve; sciatica.

segmental, segmentary n. Neuritis affecting a segmental nerve.

serum n. Neuritis following injection of serum, presumably caused by perineural urticaria and edema, usually involving the middle roots of the brachial plexus.

thenar n. Atrophy of the thenar eminence with no associated pain.

toxic n. That due to some poisonous substance. See multiple *n.*

traumatic n. Neuritis due to trauma.

neu'ro-, neur- [*neuron*]. A combining form denoting *a nerve, nervous tissue,* or *the nervous system.*

neu"ro·ab"i·ot'ro·phy. Idiopathic degeneration of nerve cells.

neu"ro·a·nas"to·mo'sis [*neuron;* G. *anastomōsis,* an opening]. Surgical anastomosis of nerves.

neu"ro·a·nat'o·my [*neuron;* G. *anatomē,* dissection]. The anatomy of the nervous system.

neu"ro·ar'thri·tism [*neuron;* G. *arthritis,* arthritis]. A combined nervous and gouty diathesis.

neu"ro·ar·throp'a·thy [*neuron;* G. *arthron,* joint; *pathos,* disease]. Manifestations of disease in both joints and the nervous system.

neu"ro·as·the'ni·a. See *neurasthenia.*

neu"ro·as"tro·cy·to'ma. A rare tumor found usually on the floor of the third ventricle and in the temporal lobes, histologically exhibiting neuronal elements within predominant astrocytic elements: also called *cerebroma, gangliocytoma, ganglioglioma, ganglioneuroblastoma, ganglioneuroma, glioneuroblastoma, glioneuroma, spongioneuroblastoma.*

neu"ro·bi·ol'o·gy [*neuron;* G. *bios,* life; *logos,* word]. Biology of the nervous system.

neu"ro·bi"o·tax'is [*neuron; bios;* G. *taxis,* arrangement]. The tendency of nerve cells, during development, to be drawn toward the source of their nutrition and activity.

neu'ro·blast [*neuron;* G. *blastos,* germ]. A formative cell of a neuron, derived from ectoderm of the neural plate.

apolar n. A neuroblast without protoplasmic processes.

neu"ro·blas·to'ma [*neuron; blastos;* G. *-ōma,* tumor]. See *sympathicoblastoma.*

neu"ro·blas·to·ma·to'sis. See *neurofibromatosis.*

neu"ro·cal"o·rim'e·ter [*neuron;* L. *calor,* heat; G. *metron,* a measure]. An instrument for measuring the heat of a nerve.

neu"ro·ca·nal' [*neuron;* L. *canalis,* channel]. The central canal of the spinal cord. *O.T.*

neu'ro·cele [*neuron;* G. *koilia,* cavity]. The system of cavities and ventricles in the central nervous system. *O.T.*

neu"ro·cen'trum [*neuron;* G. *kentron,* center of a circle]. Old term for the body of a vertebra. —**neurocentral,** *adj.*

neu"ro·chem'is·try [*neuron;* G. *chymos,* juice]. The chemistry of nervous tissue.

neu"ro·cho"ri·o·ret"i·ni'tis (·kor"ee·o·ret"i·nigh'tis) [*neuron;* G. *chorion,* skin; L. *rete,* net; G. *-itis,* inflammation]. Chorioretinitis combined with optic neuritis.

neu"ro·cho"roid·i'tis (new"ro·kor"oy·dye'tis) [*neuron;* G. *choroeidēs,* choroid; *-itis*]. Combined inflammation of the choroid body and optic nerve.

neu"ro·cir'cu·la·to"ry [*neuron;* L. *circulare,* to encircle]. Concerned with both the nervous and the vascular systems, as neurocirculatory asthenia.

n. syndrome. See neurocirculatory *asthenia.*

neu·roc'la·dism [*neuron;* G. *klados,* branch]. A theoretical, neurotropic phenomenon in which regeneration of injured neuraxons is considered to occur by the production of collateral or terminal branches, in response to the attraction of external, mechanical, or chemical stimuli.

neu"ro·cra'ni·um [*neuron;* G. *kranion,* skull]. The brain case, or cranial portion of the skull.

neu"ro·cu·ta'ne·ous [*neuron;* L. *cutis,* skin]. Pertaining to the innervation of the skin.

neu'ro·cyte" [*neuron;* G. *kytos,* cell]. A nerve cell; a neuron; the essential element of nervous structures. Neurons are cells specialized as conductors of impulses.

neu"ro·cy·to'ma. See *sympathicoblastoma.*

neu"ro·de·al'gi·a [G. *neuroeidēs,* like sinews; *algos,* pain]. Retinal pain.

neu"ro·de"a·tro'phi·a [*neuroeidēs;* G. *atrophia,* want of nourishment]. Atrophy of the retina. *Obs.*

neu"ro·den'drite [G. *neuron,* nerve; *dendritēs,* of a tree]. A dendrite of a neuron.

neu"ro·den'dron. See *dendrite.*

neu"ro·der"ma·ti'tis [*neuron;* G. *derma,* skin; *-itis,* inflammation]. A skin disorder characterized by localized, often symmetrical, patches of pruritic dermatitis with lichenification. It appears characteristically on the neck, antecubital and popliteal spaces in women of nervous temperament. **N. circumscripta** is also called *lichen chronicus simplex.*

n. disseminata. (a) An eczematous dermatitis precipitated by psychogenic factors. (b) Atopic dermatitis with psychogenic factors predominating.

neu"ro·der"ma·to·my"o·si'tis [*neuron; derma;* G. *mys,* muscle; *-itis*]. A disease of inflammatory or infectious nature, manifested by neuritic pain, with induration of the skin, subcutaneous tissue, and underlying muscles.

neu"ro·der"ma·to'sis [*neuron; derma;* G. *-ōsis,* condition]. A neurotic skin affection.

neu"ro·der"ma·tro'phi·a [*neuron; derma;* G. *atrophia,* want of nourishment]. Atrophy of the skin from nervous disturbance.

neu"ro·di·as'ta·sis (new"ro·dye·ass'tuh·sis) [*neuron;* G. *diastasis,* separation]. Stretching of nerves; neurectasia.

neu"ro·dy·nam'i·a (new"ro·dye·nam'ee·uh) [*neuron;* G. *dynamis,* strength]. Nervous strength or energy. —**neurodynamic,** *adj.*

neu"ro·dyn'i·a (new"ro·din'ee·uh, ·dye'nee·uh). See *neuralgia.*

neu"ro·e·lec"tro·ther"a·peu'tics [*neuron;* G. *ēlektron,* amber; G. *therapeutikos,* therapeutic]. The treatment of nervous affections by means of electricity.

neu"ro·en·ceph"a·lo·my"e·lop'a·thy. See *neuromyelitis optica.*

neu"ro·en'do·crine (new"ro·en'do·kryne, ·krin) [*neuron;* G. *endon,* within; *krinein,* to separate]. Pertaining to the nervous and endocrine systems in anatomic or functional relationship; as the hypothalamic nuclei and the pituitary gland constitute a neuroendocrine apparatus.

neu"ro·ep"i·der'mal [*neuron;* G. *epidermis,* outer skin]. Relating to the nerves and the skin.

neu"ro·ep"i·the·li·o'ma [*neuron;* G. *epi,* on; *thēlē,* nipple; *-ōma,* tumor]. A tumor derived from primitive neuroepithelium, containing cells of small cuboidal or columnar form with a tendency to form true rosettes, occurring in the retina, central nervous system, and occasionally in peripheral nerves: also called *diktyoma, esthesioneuroblastoma, esthesioneuroepithelioma.* N. of retina is also called *glioblastoma of retina, glioma of retina, neuroblastoma of retina, retinoblastoma, retinocytoma.*

olfactory n. A rare neuroepithelioma occurring in the nasal cavity of adults, which may infiltrate the paranasal sinuses: also called *olfactory esthesioneuroepithelioma.*

neu"ro·ep"i·the'li·um [*neuron; epi; thēlē*]. The highly specialized epithelial structures constituting the terminations of the nerves of special sense, as the rod and cone cells of the retina, the olfactory cells of the nose, the hair cells of the internal ear, the gustatory cells of the taste buds. —**neuroepithelial,** *adj.*

neu"ro·fi'bril [*neuron;* L. *fibra,* fiber]. A fibril of a nerve cell, usually extending from the processes and traversing the cell body.

neu″ro·fi·bro′ma (new″ro·figh·bro′muh) [*neuron; fibra;* G. *-ōma,* tumor]. A tumor characterized by diffuse proliferation of peripheral nerve elements; it may occur as a solitary and localized phenomenon but more commonly as part of the condition known as *neurofibromatosis.* Also called *perineural fibroblastoma, endoneural fibroma, fibroma of nerve sheath, perineural fibroma, fibromyxoma of nerve sheath, myxofibroma of nerve sheath, neurofibromyxoma.*

granular-cell n. See granular-cell *myoblastoma.*

malignant n. See malignant *schwannoma.*

multiple n. See *neurofibromatosis.*

n. gangliocellulare. See *ganglioneuroma.*

plexiform n. See plexiform *neuroma.*

neu″ro·fi·bro″ma·to′sis (·figh·bro″muh·to′sis) [*neuron; fibra; -ōma;* G. *-ōsis,* condition]. A condition characterized by the presence in the skin, or along the course of peripheral nerves, of neurofibromas. Usually the tumors are multiple, from a few to hundreds, gradually increasing in both number and size, and are painless. There is a hereditary tendency and, occasionally, malignancy supervenes. Also called *von Recklinghausen's disease, Smith-Recklinghausen's disease, multiple n., neurinomatosis, neuroblastomatosis, multiple neurofibroma* or *neuroma, fibroma molluscum.*

neu″ro·fi·bro·myx·o′ma. See *neurofibroma.*

neu″ro·fi″bro·sar·co′ma. See malignant *schwannoma.*

neu″ro·fi″bro·si′tis [*neuron; fibra;* G. *-itis,* inflammation]. A fibrositis which involves fibers of a nerve and also of muscle.

neu″ro·gan·gli·i′tis [*neuron;* G. *gagglion,* encysted tumor on a tendon; *-itis*]. Inflammation of a ganglion. *Obs.*

neu″ro·gas′tric [*neuron;* G. *gastēr,* belly]. Relating to the nerves and the stomach.

neu″ro·gen′e·sis [*neuron;* G. *genesis,* production]. The formation of nerves.

neu″ro·gen′ic [*neuron;* G. *genesthai,* from *gignesthai,* to be formed]. 1. Of nervous origin, as neurogenic tumors. 2. Stimulated by the nervous system, as neurogenic muscular contractions.

neu·rog′e·nous (new·rodj′i·nus) [*neuron; genesthai*]. Originating in the nervous system.

neu·rog′e·ny (new·rodj′i·nee). See *neurogenesis.*

neu·rog′li·a [*neuron;* G. *glia,* glue]. 1. A general term for the fibrous and cellular, nonnervous, supporting elements of the nervous system, chiefly derived from ectoderm. Includes the ependyma, the epithelial lining of the choroid plexuses, neuroglia proper, microglia; also, in the peripheral nervous system, the neurilemma sheath cells of nerves and the satellite cells of ganglions. 2. Specifically neuroglia proper, comprising the astrocytes and the oligodendroglia cells of the central nervous system. —**neurog′lial,** *adj.*

neu·rog′li·a·cyte″ [*neuron; glia;* G. *kytos,* cell]. A neuroglia cell.

neu·rog″li·o′ma [*neuron; glia;* G. *-ōma,* tumor]. A tumor composed of neuroglial tissue; a glioma.

ganglionar n. A glioma containing ganglion cells.

neu·rog″li·o′sis [*neuron; glia;* G. *-ōsis,* condition]. A condition of multiple neurogliomas developing diffusely throughout the nervous system.

neu′ro·gram [*neuron;* G. *gramma,* letter]. *In psychiatry,* Morton Prince's term for the record of theoretic changes imprinted on the brain by life's experiences.

neu″ro·his·tol′o·gy [*neuron;* G. *histos,* web; *logos,* word]. The histology of the nervous system.

neu″ro·hu′mor [*neuron;* L. *humor,* moisture]. The chemical excitor in a neuron which, supposedly, activates a neighboring neuron or a muscle. Chemical substances are liberated at the visceral endings of stimulated nerves, thus sympathin is produced by stimulation of postganglionic sympathetic fibers, whereas acetylcholine is produced at the endings of stimulated parasympathetic nerves.

neu″ro·hu′mor·al [*neuron; humor*]. Pertaining to certain qualities in substances which serve as agents to transmit nervous influence across synapses and myoneural junctions.

neu″ro·hyp·nol′o·gy [*neuron;* G. *hypnos,* sleep; *logos,* word]. The study of hypnotism. *Obs.*

neu″ro·hy·poph′y·sis (new″ro·high·pof′i·sis) [*neuron;* G. *hypophysis,* attachment underneath]. The neural portion of the pituitary gland, developing as a downward evagination of neural ectoderm from the floor of the diencephalon. It has three subdivisions: inferiorly the *pars nervosa (infundibular process, pars neuralis, pars posterior, posterior lobe of the hypophysis);* the *stalk (infundibulum, infundibular stem);* and uppermost the *median eminence of the tuber cinereum.*

neu′roid [*neuron;* G. *eidos,* form]. Resembling a nerve or nerve substance.

neu′roid tube. Nevus cells arranged in thin columns in an intradermal nevus. The columns have the appearance of neural sheaths.

neu″ro·in·duc′tion [*neuron;* L. *inductio,* a leading into]. Suggestion.

neu″ro·in′su·lar com′plex [*neuron;* L. *insula,* island; *complexus,* an encircling]. Small intimate aggregates of islet cells and ganglion cells in the pancreas.

neu″ro·ker′a·tin [*neuron;* G. *keras,* horn]. The insoluble protein substance found in the myelin sheath, particularly after fixation in alcohol. It is usually in the form of a network.

neu″ro·lem′ma. See *neurilemma.*

neu″ro·lep′rid. See tuberculoid *leprosy.*

neu·rol′o·gist [*neuron;* G. *logos,* word]. One versed in neurology, usually a physician who specializes in the diagnosis and treatment of disorders of the nervous system.

neu·rol′o·gy [*neuron; logos*]. The study of the anatomy, physiology, and pathology of the nervous system. —**neurolog′ic,** *adj.*

neu″ro·lu′es (new″ro·lew′eez). Neurosyphilis.

neu′ro·lymph [*neuron;* L. *lympha,* water]. The cerebrospinal fluid. *Obs.*

neu·rol′y·sin, neu″ro·ly′sin [*neuron;* G. *lysis,* a loosing]. A cytolysin having specific action upon nerve cells.

neu·rol′y·sis [*neuron; lysis*]. 1. Exhaustion of a nerve by overstimulation. 2. Nerve stretching to relieve excessive tension. 3. The loosening of adhesions binding a nerve. 4. The disintegration of nerve tissue. —**neurolyt′ic,** *adj.*

neu·ro′ma [*neuron;* G. *-ōma,* tumor]. Any tumor of the nervous system, as originally described by Virchow. These tumors have since been classified into special groups on a basis of histology. See also *pseudoneuroma.* —**neurom′atous,** *adj.*

acoustic n. See acoustic nerve *tumor.*

amputation n. See *pseudoneuroma.*

amyelinic n. One composed of unmyelinated fibers.

appendiceal n. A tumorlike growth of nerve fibers, and often of ganglion cells, in chronic fibrotic lesions of the vermiform process.

fibrillary n. See plexiform *n.*

ganglion-celled n. See *astroblastoma.*

ganglionic n. See *ganglioneuroma.*

multiple n. See *neurofibromatosis.*

myelinic n. One composed of myelinated fibers.

n. cutis. A cutaneous neurofibroma.

n. gangliocellulare. See *ganglioneuroma.*

n. telangiectodes. One with a rich content of blood vessels, often cavernous in type.

n. verum. See *ganglioneuroma.*

plexiform n. A tumor or tumorlike mass of whorls of myelinated and unmyelinated nerve fibers and of connective tissue. Occurs in early life and probably is congenital. There is doubt as to whether it is neoplasm, anomaly, or hamartoma.

neu″ro·ma·la′ci·a (new″ro·ma·lay′shee·uh, ·see·uh) [*neuron;* G. *malakia,* softness]. A softening of nerve tissue. *Obs.*

neu″ro·ma·to′sis [*neuron;* G. *-ōma,* tumor; *-ōsis,* condition]. A tendency to form multiple neuromas. See *neurofibromatosis.*

neu″ro·mech′a·nism [*neuron;* G. *mēchanē,* machine]. The correlated structure and function of the nervous system in relation to a bodily activity.

neu′ro·mere [*neuron;* G. *meros,* part]. An embryonic segment of the brain or spinal cord.

neu·rom′er·y [*neuron; meros*]. The segmentation of the central nervous system.

neu″ro·mi·me′sis (new″ro·mi·mee′sis, ·migh·mee′-sis) [*neuron;* G. *mimēsis,* imitation]. A group of hysterical phenomena resembling true organic disease. —**neuromimet′ic,** *adj.*

neu″ro·mus′cu·lar [*neuron;* L. *musculus,* muscle]. Pertaining jointly to nerves and muscles, as neuromuscular junction.

neu″ro·my′al, neu″ro·my′ic. Neuromuscular.

neu″ro·my″e·li′tis [*neuron;* G. *myelos,* marrow; *-itis,* inflammation]. Inflammation of the spinal cord and of nerves.

n. optica. A morbid process, probably due to a virus or an infectious toxic agent, involving the optic nerve and the white and gray matter of the cord. It is closely allied to other demyelinating diseases, such as multiple sclerosis and encephalomyelitis disseminata. Also called *optic neuroencephalomyelopathy, neuropticomyelitis, Devic's disease* or *syndrome.*

neu″ro·my′on. A functional unit composed of a muscle fiber and its nerve supply. See motor *unit.* —**neuromy′ic,** *adj.*

neu″ro·my″o·path′ic [*neuron;* G. *mys,* muscle; *pathos,* disease]. Relating to disease of both muscles and nerves.

neu″ro·my″o·si′tis [*neuron; mys;* G. *-itis,* inflammation]. Myositis associated with neuritis.

neu′ron, neu′rone [*neuron*]. The complete nerve cell, including the cell body or perikaryon, axon, and dendrites; specialized as a conductor of impulses. —**neuron′al,** *adj.*

adjustor n. See internuncial *n.*

afferent n. One which conducts impulses to a nerve center; in the peripheral nervous system, that neuron which conducts impulses to nuclei in the central nervous system.

autonomic n. One which is a component of the autonomic nervous system.

efferent n. One conducting impulses away from a nerve center; in the peripheral nervous system, a neuron conducting impulses away from the central nervous system.

exciter n. A postganglionic *n.*

intercalated n. One interposed between the sensory and motor neurons of a reflex pathway.

internuncial n. One interposed between the initial and terminal neurons of a nervous pathway: also called *adjustor neuron.*

motor n. An efferent neuron. The **lower motor neuron** or final common pathway has its cell body located in the anterior gray column of the spinal cord or in brain stem nuclei, and its axon passes by way of a peripheral nerve to skeletal muscle. The **upper motor neuron** may be any descending efferent neuron synapsing with a lower motor neuron, or more specifically, an efferent neuron having its cell body in the motor cortex and essential to fine voluntary muscular activity. See also under *lesion.*

n. pathway. The successive neurons over which a given impulse is thought to be transmitted.

n. pattern. The theoretic pathways which determine an instinct, reflex, sensation, or other nervous response.

postganglionic n. A neuron of the autonomic nervous system having its cell body in a ganglion, the axon extending to an organ or tissue.

preganglionic n. One of the autonomic nervous system which has its cell body in the brain or spinal cord, its axon terminating in a ganglion.

sensory n. One which conducts impulses arising in a sense organ or at sensory endings.

sympathetic n. One belonging to the thoracolumbar autonomic nervous system.

neu′ron doc′trine. The doctrine (based on the work of van Gehuchten, His, Forel, and Ramón y Cajal) that the basic unit of the central nervous system is a nerve cell with its processes which, having no direct anatomic continuity with other functionally related cells, acts upon another nerve cell solely through a discontinuous interphase, the synapse: opposed to the theory that nerve cells in the central nervous system are united in a syncytium.

neu″ro·ne′vus. See blue *nevus.*

neu″ro·ni′tis [*neuron; -itis*]. Inflammation of a neuron or nerve cell.

infective n. See Guillain-Barré *syndrome.*

neu″ro·nog′ra·phy. The study of neuron connections.

physiological n. The mapping of functional neuron connections by action current recording, after local stimulation of the cortical area by strychnine.

neu·ro″no·pha′gi·a [*neuron;* G. *phagein,* to eat]. The destruction of neurons by phagocytes.

neu′ro·path [*neuron;* G. *pathos,* disease]. One who is predisposed to disorders of the nervous system.

neu″ro·path′ic [*neuron; pathos*]. 1. Characterized by a diseased or imperfect nervous system. 2. Depending upon, or pertaining to, nervous disease.

neu″ro·path′ic es′char (es′kahr). Bedsore; decubitus ulcer.

neu·rop′a·thist [*neuron; pathos*]. Neurologist.

neu″ro·path″o·gen′e·sis [*neuron; pathos;* G. *genesis,* production]. The development of a disease of the nervous system.

neu″ro·pa·thol′o·gy [*neuron; pathos;* G. *logos,* word]. Pathology of diseases of the nervous system.

neu·rop′a·thy [*neuron; pathos*]. Any nervous disease.

hereditary sensory radicular n. A heredofamilial disease characterized by perforating ulcers of the feet, shooting pains, and deafness. There is primary degeneration of dorsal root ganglia with amyloid deposits in some.

progressive hypertrophic interstitial n. See J. J. *Dejerine.*

neu″ro·phleg′mon [*neuron;* G. *phlegmonē,* inflammation]. Neuritis. *Obs.*

neu″ro·pho′ni·a [*neuron;* G. *phōnē,* voice]. A rare choreic disease of the larynx and muscles of expiration, characterized by the utterance of sharp, spasmodic cries.

neu″ro·phys″i·ol′o·gy [*neuron;* G. *physis,* nature; *logos,* word]. The physiology of the nervous system.

neu′ro·pil [*neuron;* G. *pilos,* felt]. Nervous tissue consisting of a feltwork of nonmyelinated nerve fibers; gray matter with few nerve-cell bodies; usually a region of synapses between axons and dentrites.

neu′ro·plasm [*neuron;* G. *plasma,* anything formed]. The protoplasm filling the interstices of the fibrils of nerve cells.

neu′ro·plas″ty [*neuron;* G. *plassein,* to form]. A plastic operation on the nerves.

neu″ro·po′di·um [*neuron;* G. *podion,* small foot]. A bulblike expansion of the terminal of an axon in one type of synapse. *Rare.* Also called *end-foot, end-bulb.*

neu′ro·pore [*neuron;* G. *poros,* passage]. The anterior or posterior terminal aperture of the embryonic neural tube before complete closure occurs (about the 20–25 somite stage).

anterior n. One at the cephalic end of the neural tube.

posterior n. One at the caudal end of the neural tube.

neu″ro·psy·chi′a·try [*neuron;* G. *psychē,* soul; *iatreia,* treatment]. The branch of medical science dealing with both nervous and mental diseases.

neu″ro·psy·chol′o·gy [*neuron; psychē;* G. *logos,* word]. A system of psychology based on neurology.

neu″ro·psy·chop′a·thy (new″ro·sigh·kop′uth·ee) [*neuron; psychē;* G. *pathos,* disease]. A mental disease based upon, or manifesting itself in, nervous disorders or symptoms. —**neuropsychopath′ic,** *adj.*

neu″ro·psy·cho′sis (new″ro·sigh·ko′sis). Old term for psychosis. Also see *psychotic disorders.*

neu·rop″ti·co·my″e·li′tis. See *neuromyelitis optica.*

neu″ro·rec′i·dive (new″ro·ress′i·deev, ·div, ·ray-see·deev′). See *neurorelapse.*

neu″ro·re·cur′rence. See *neurorelapse.*

neu″ro·re·lapse′ [*neuron;* L. *relapsum,* from *relabi,* to slip back]. Acute syphilitic meningitis, occurring usually during the treatment of early syphilis. Syn., *neurorecidive, neurorecurrence.*

neu″ro·ret″i·ni′tis [*neuron;* L. *rete,* net; G. *-itis,* inflammation]. Inflammation of both the optic nerve and the retina.

neu·ror′rha·phy [*neuron;* G. *rhaphē,* a suture]. The operation of suturing a divided nerve.

neu″ror·rhex′is [*neuron;* G. *rhēxis,* a breaking]. Avulsion of a nerve, as in the treatment of persistent neuralgia; neurexeresis.

neu″ror·rhyc′tes hy″dro·pho′bi·ae (new″ro-rick′teez high″dro·fo′bee·ee). A Negri body; that is, an inclusion body occasionally seen in the cytoplasm or processes of cerebral or cerebellar nerve cells in rabies.

neu″ro·sar·co′ma [*neuron;* G. *sarkōma,* fleshy excrescence]. A sarcoma of the general order of a neuroma.

neu″ro·scle·ro′sis [*neuron;* G. *sklērōsis,* a hardening]. Sclerosis of nervous tissue.

neu″ro·se·cre′tion [*neuron;* L. *secretio,* a dividing]. The process of elaboration and discharge of colloidlike granules and masses by nerve cells which, during phases of such activity, assume the appearance of gland cells.

neurosine. Trade-mark for a liquid preparation of bromides, with hyoscyamus, belladonna, cascara sagrada, and humulus.

neu·ro′sis (pl. *neuroses*) [*neuron;* G. *-ōsis,* condition]. A disorder of the psyche or psychic functions. See *psychoneurotic disorder.* —**neurosal.** *adj.*

anxiety n. *In psychoanalysis,* a psychoneurosis characterized by emotional instability, irritability, apprehension, and a sense of utter fatigue; caused by incomplete repression of emotional problems. It is associated with visceral phenomena such as tachycardia, palpitation, nausea, a sense of suffocation, diarrhea, tremors, and perspiration. Now, depending upon specific manifestations, it is more properly classified as (a) *anxiety reaction;* (b) one of the *psychophysiologic autonomic and visceral disorders.*

blast n. (a) A nervous disorder developing after rapid and extreme changes in atmospheric pressure without producing any external evidence of injury. (b) A disorder caused by detonation of explosives; often terminated by sudden death, necropsy findings showing multiple brain hemorrhages.

combat neuroses. War neuroses.

compensation n. A neurotic reaction, motivated by the uncontrollable desire to receive a monetary award for damages or injuries, a common complication in traumatic neurosis: also called *indemnity n., pension n.*

compulsion n. See obsessive compulsive *reaction.*

fright n. An intense terror reaction to an external frightful situation, as an earthquake or a dangerous fire. *Rare.*

occupational n. (a) One in which the occupation of the individual appears to be the precipitating cause. (b) A disorder affecting groups of muscles used in the performance of special movements. Syn., *copodyskinesia,* professional *neurasthenia.*

sensory n. Abnormalities of sensation, neurotic in origin, e.g., neurotic pruritis.

traumatic n. One in which an injury is the precipitating cause.

vasomotor n. See *angioneurosis.*

war neuroses. Mental disorders following exhaustion or emotional stress in warfare; include hysterias, neurasthenias, and psychasthenias.

neu′ro·sism. Neurasthenia.

neu″ro·skel′e·tal. Pertaining to nervous and skeletal muscular tissues.

neu′ro·somes [*neuron;* G. *sōma,* body]. Old term for minute granules of variable size seen in nerve cells. Some are undoubtedly mitochondria.

neu′ro·spasm [*neuron;* G. *spasmos,* spasm]. Nervous spasm or twitching of a muscle.

neu″ro·spon·gi·o′ma. See *medulloblastoma.*

neu″ro·spon′gi·um (new″ro·spun′jee·um, ·spon′-jee·um) [*neuron;* G. *spoggion,* dim. from *spoggos,* sponge]. The inner, reticular layer of the retina.

Neu·ros′po·ra [*neuron;* G. *spora,* seed]. A generic name for one of the fungi, more commonly known as the bread mold, which is used as a bioassay organism in enzyme studies.

neu″ro·ste·ar′ic [*neuron;* G. *stear,* fat]. Pertaining to nervous tissue and fat.

neu″ro·sur′geon [*neuron;* G. *cheirourgos,* working by hand]. One who specializes in surgery of the brain and the nervous system.

neu″ro·sur′ger·y [*neuron; cheirourgos*]. Surgery of the nervous system.

neu″ro·su′ture [*neuron;* L. *sutura,* a sewing together]. The suture of a nerve.

neu″ro·syph′i·lis [*neuron;* NL. *syphilis*]. Syphilitic infection of the nervous system.

asymptomatic n. Neurosyphilis diagnosed only on the basis of pathological findings in the cerebrospinal fluid. In the early form, within two years after primary infection, serological tests give varied results. Late forms (*latent neurosyphilis, preparetic neurosyphilis, paresis sine paresi*), detected after more than two years, show a positive serological test and often a Lange test of the luetic type.

latent n. Late asymptomatic *n.*

preparetic n. Late asymptomatic *n.*

neu″ro·the·ci′tis [*neuron;* G. *thēkē,* case; *-itis,* inflammation]. Inflammation of a nerve sheath.

neu″ro·ther′a·py [*neuron;* G. *therapeia,* treatment]. The treatment of nervous diseases. Also called *neurotherapeutics.*

neu·rot′ic [*neuron*]. 1. Pertaining to or affected with a neurosis. 2. Pertaining to the nerves.

neu·rot′ic. An emotionally unstable individual.

neu·rot′i·ca [*neuron*]. Functional nervous disorders.

neu·rot′i·cism [*neuron*]. A neurotic condition, character, or trait.

neu·rot″i·za′tion [*neuron*]. 1. The regeneration of a divided nerve. 2. Surgical implantation of a nerve into a paralyzed muscle. 3. Providing an anatomic structure with a nerve supply.

neu″rot·me′sis [*neuron;* G. *tmēsis*, a cutting]. Condition in which the connective-tissue structures and nerve constituents have been interrupted. In the regeneration of new nerve fibers, the new axons grow in misdirected confusion and spontaneous regeneration of the complete nerve trunk rarely occurs.

neu″ro·tol′o·gy [*neuron;* G. *ous*, ear; *logos*, word]. That branch of medical science dealing with the structure and functions of the internal ear, its nervous connections with the brain, and its central pathways within the brain.

neu′ro·tome [*neuron;* G. *tomos*, cutting]. 1. An instrument for the division or dissection of a nerve. 2. One of the segments of the embryonic neural tube. Also called *neuromere.*

neu·rot′o·my [*neuron;* G. *tomē*, a cutting]. The surgical division or dissection of some or all of the fibers of a nerve.

opticociliary n. The surgical division of the optic nerve and the cutting of all ciliary nerves passing through the sclera in the region of the optic nerve.

neu″ro·ton′ic [*neuron;* G. *tonos*, tension]. Having a tonic effect upon the nerves.

neu″ro·tox′in [*neuron;* G. *toxikon*, poison]. A toxin capable of destroying nerve tissue. —**neurotoxic,** *adj.*

neu″ro·trau′ma (new″ro·traw′muh, ·trou′muh) [*neuron;* G. *trauma*, wound]. Injury to a nerve.

neu″ro·trip′sy [*neuron;* G. *tripsis*, a rubbing]. The crushing of a nerve.

neu″ro·troph′ic, neu″ro·tro′phic [*neuron;* G. *trophē*, nourishment]. Relating to the influence of nerves upon the nutrition and maintenance of normal condition in tissues.

neu″ro·trop′ic [*neuron;* G. *trepein*, to turn]. That which turns toward, or has an affinity for, nervous tissue.

neu·rot′ro·pism [*neuron; trepein*]. The attraction said to be exercised upon regenerating nerve fibers by substances in the peripheral portion of the severed nerve. The theory has been somewhat discredited by recent observations.

neu″ro·var″i·co′sis [*neuron;* L. *varicosus*, full of dilated veins]. A varicosity on a nerve fiber, or the formation of one.

neu″ro·vas′cu·lar [*neuron;* L. *vasculum*, small vessel]. Pertaining to both the nervous and vascular structures.

neu′ru·la. *In embryology*, the stage following the gastrula stage in Amphibia. It is characterized by the development of the neural plate and axial embryonic structures and corresponds to the somite stage in human development.

Neusser, Edmund von [*Austrian physician*, 1852–1912]. Described basophilic granules about the nucleus of a leukocyte; called *Neusser's granules.*

neu′tral [L. *neutralis*, neuter]. 1. Inert; on neither one side nor the other. 2. Neither alkaline nor acid; bland and soothing, inactive. —**neutral′ity,** *n.*

n. acriflavine. See *acriflavine.*

n. mixture. An 8% potassium citrate solution prepared extemporaneously by reaction of potassium bicarbonate and citric acid.

neu″tra·li·za′tion [*neutralis*]. 1. That process or operation that counterbalances or cancels the action of an agent. 2. *In medicine*, the process of checking the operation of any agent that produces a morbid effect. 3. *In chemistry*, a change of reaction to that which is neither alkaline nor acid.

neu′tral·ize [*neutralis*]. Render neutral; render inert; counterbalance an action or influence.

neu′tral red (C.C.). Dimethyl-diaminotoluphenazine hydrochloride, a dye used as an indicator and as a vital stain, suggested for use as a test of gastric function: also called *toluylene red.*

neu·tri′no (new·tree′no) [L. *neuter*, neither]. A hypothetical atomic particle having the mass of the electron but without an electric charge.

neut′ro·clu″sion, neut′ro·oc·clu″sion. Occlusion in which the mesiobuccal cusp of the upper first molar interdigitates with the buccal groove of the lower first molar.

neu′tro·cyte [*neuter;* G. *kytos*, cell]. A neutrophil granulocyte.

neu′tron [*neuter*]. An atomic nuclear particle with mass = 1 and charge = 0. A constituent of all atomic nuclei except ${}_1H^1$. (Isotopes differ from one another solely by the number of neutrons in their nuclei.) Free neutrons with various kinetic energies are produced by nuclear reactions, including fission. Conversely neutrons because of their lack of charge produce nuclear reactions, including fission, most easily. These two facts are the basis of the fission chain reaction. The biologic effects of neutron irradiation are higher than those predicted on the basis of ionization alone. This may be the effect of transmutation added to ionization.

neu′tron ther′apy. See under *therapy.*

neu″tro·pe′ni·a [*neuter;* G. *penia*, poverty]. A decrease below the normal standard in the number of neutrophils in the peripheral blood.

malignant n. See *agranulocytosis.*

neu′tro·phil [*neuter;* G. *philein*, to love]. Stained readily by neutral dyes.

neu′tro·phil. 1. Any histologic element readily stainable with neutral dyes. 2. The polymorphonuclear leukocyte of the blood, which contains neutrophil granules in its cytoplasm. See Plate 26.

neu″tro·phil′i·a [*neuter; philein*]. 1. An affinity for neutral dyes. 2. Great increase of neutrophil leukocytes in the blood or tissues.

ne′vose [L. *naevus*, mole]. Spotted, having nevi.

ne″vo·xan″tho·en″do·the″li·o′ma. A group or groups of yellowish-brown nodules, found usually on the extremities in early childhood, histologically characterized by the presence of many histiocytes, foam cells, and foreign-body giant cells: considered as a juvenile form of histiocytoma or xanthogranuloma.

ne′vus (pl. *nevi*) [*naevus*]. 1. Any lesion containing nevus cells. 2. *In dermatology*, a cutaneous hamartoma; a birthmark. —**ne′void,** *adj.*

bathing-trunk n. A pigmented nevus, localized chiefly to the lumbar and central portions of the body, often of the hairy type, called *nevus pellinus.*

blue n. A nevus composed of a great mass of spindle-shaped pigmented melanocytes in the middle and lower two-thirds of the derma. Malignant degeneration rarely occurs.

cobblestone n. See *n.* elasticus.

compound n. A pigmented nevus composed of the features of both the junction and intradermal nevus.

dermal epidermal n. See junction *n.*

epithelial n. A nevoid proliferation, either present at birth or developing later in life, in which hyperplasia of epithelial cells occurs without the presence of nevus cells.

generalized keratotic n. See systematized *n.*
hairy n. A pigmented nevus covered with downy or stiff hairs: also called *hairy mole, n. pilosus.*
intradermal n. A pigmented nevus consisting of nevus cells located chiefly or entirely in the derma, with little or no dermoepidermal junctional proliferation. The deeply placed nevus cells tend to be more fibrillar in type. This nevus is more common in adult life.
Jadassohn's n. See *n.* sebaceus.
Jadassohn-Tièche n. See blue *spot.*
junction n. A pigmented nevus exhibiting marked proliferation of nevus cells in the epidermis or at the dermoepidermal junction, usually in nests, with relatively few located in the derma. Such nevi are found most commonly in childhood on the trunk, thighs, and arms. Decreasing in frequency with age, they are occasionally seen in adults, notably on the hands and feet, and are suspected of being predisposed to development of malignant melanomas.
linear n. A cutaneous nevus which occurs in bunches or streaks, and clinically is most often of warty appearance.
n. acneiformis unilateralis. See *n.* comedonicus.
n. arachnoideus. See spider *n.*
n. araneus. See spider *n.*
n. comedonicus. A unilateral verrucous nevus with hard follicular accretions simulating comedones of acne: also called *n. acneiformis unilateralis, n. follicularis.*
n. elasticus. A dermal nevus of connective tissue which histologically simulates scleroderma: also called *cobblestone n., paving-stone n., zosteriforme n.*
n. epitheliomato-cylindromatosus. See *cylindroma.*
n. flammeus. Port-wine nevus.
n. lipomatodes. An elevated pigmented nevus with connective tissue and fat hypertrophy. Rare.
n. lipomatosus. See *lipoma.*
n. papillaris, n. papillomatosus. A papillomatous pigmented nevus.
n. pellinus. A markedly hairy nevus which has the appearance of pelt or fur.
n. pigmentosus. See pigmented *n.*
n. pilosus. See hairy *n.*
n. sebaceus. A single lesion formed by an aggregate of sebaceous glands, usually as a linear streak, most often present since birth on the scalp and face: also called *Jadassohn's n.*
n. spilus. A smooth, flat, pigmented nevus devoid of hair.
n. spongiosus albus. A rare genodermatosis of the oral and anogenital mucosa, characterized by a white tint and a spongy appearance with numerous small clear follicular openings: also called *congenital leukokeratosis mucosa oris, white-sponge n. of mucosa.*
n. unilateralis, unius lateralis. A linear warty growth (*verrucous n.*) in lines or bands limited to one side of the body.
n. vasculosus. A strawberry mark.
nonpigmented n. A common nevus composed of clear cells containing little or no pigment.
paving-stone n. See *n.* elasticus.
pigmented n. A pigmented mole, varying in color from light fawn to blackish, sometimes hairy, frequently papillary and hyperkeratotic, characterized by clear cells (celles claires), nevus cells, and intermediate forms. Pigmented nevi have a variable appearance, influenced by age and anatomic location, and, for practical purposes, are divided into *intradermal* (*resting*), *junction* (*active*), and *compound* (*intermediary*) nevi.
port-wine n. A congenital hemangioma characterized by one or several red to purplish flat or slightly elevated patches, most often on the face. Variations in color from red to blue depend principally upon the degree of oxygenation of the blood. Syn., *n. flammeus, port-wine mark.*
spider n. A type of telangiectasis characterized by a central, elevated, tiny red dot, pinhead in size, from which blood vessels radiate like spokes of a wheel. Syn., *n. araneus, n. arachnoideus, stellar n.*
systematized n. A linear epithelial nevus which contains no nevus cells, but shows hyperkeratosis, vacuolation, and degenerative changes in the granular layer: also called *generalized keratotic n.*
verrucous n. A warty brownish growth which often shows linear distribution. Histologically there is hyperkeratosis, acanthosis, and papillomatosis. Also called *hard n., epidermal n., keratotic n., acanthotic n.*
white-sponge n. of mucosa. See *n.* spongiosus albus.
zosteriforme n. See *n.* elasticus.

new'born'. A term applied to infants up to two or three days of age. Syn., *neonatal.*

Newburgh's test. See Lashmet and Newburgh's *test.*

Newcastle disease. See under *disease.*

Newcomer, Harry Sidney (1887–). American physician who invented a small colorimeter with colored glass standards, called the *Newcomer hemoglobinometer.*

Newcomer method for hemoglobin. See acid hematin *method.*

new growth. A circumscribed, new formation of tissue, characterized by abnormality of structure or location. Syn., *neoplasm.*

Newman, David [*Scottish surgeon,* 1854–1924]. Remembered for his operation of nephropexy in which he split the renal capsule and sutured the kidney to the overlying lumbar muscles.

Newton, Isaac [*English natural philosopher and physicist,* 1642–1727]. Celebrated for his studies in gravitation and his laws applied to pure physics. Described chromatic aberration, also called *Newtonian aberration.* See also *Newtonian constant* under *G.*, 1; Newton's *law* of cooling.

Newton's method. See Benedict and Newton's *method.*

Newton method for uric acid determination. See under *method.*

nex'us [L., a binding together]. A tying or binding together, as the grouping of several causes which bring about an infectious disease; interlacing.

N. F. National Formulary.

Ni Chemical symbol for nickel.

ni'a·cin. Nicotinic acid.

ni"a·cin·am'ide. Nicotinamide.

nib'ble [cf. LG. *nibbelen*]. To eat in small bits.

nicamide. Trade-mark for *nikethamide.*

nic'co·lum [NL. *niccolum*]. Nickel.

niche (nitch) [F., from L. *nidus*, nest]. A recess.
enamel n. A depression between the lateral dental lamina, the dental lamina itself, and the enamel organ. Syn., *enamel crypt.*

nick'el [Ger.]. Ni = 58.69. A metal of silver-white luster, resembling iron in physical properties.
n. bromide. $NiBr_2.3H_2O$. Has been used in epilepsy. Dose, 0.3–0.5 Gm. (5–8 gr.).
n. carbonyl. $Ni(CO)_4$; nickel tetracarbonyl; a yellow, volatile liquid. It may explode when heated; vapors are poisonous and may cause irritation, congestion, and edema of lungs.
n. chloride. $NiCl_2.6H_2O$. Has been used as a tonic in anemia. Dose, 0.13 Gm. (2 gr.).
n. methylkinase. A soluble enzyme system,

obtained from the liver of animals, which catalyzes aerobic or anaerobic transfer of methyl groups from L-methionine to nicotinamide in the presence of magnesium ion and adenosinetriphosphate.

n. sulfate. $NiSO_4.6H_2O$. Has been used as a tonic. Dose, 0.032–0.065 Gm. (½–1 gr.).

nick'ing [of uncertain origin]. 1. Notching. 2. Incising of the ventral muscles of the base of a horse's tail, causing the tail to be carried higher.

A-V n. The nicking of a retinal vein by pressure from the artery.

Nicklès, François Joseph Jérôme [*French chemist*, 1821–69]. Demonstrated the method of distinguishing glucose from cane sugar by heating the sugar at 100° C. with carbon tetrachloride. Cane sugar is turned black in the process while glucose is not. Called *Nicklès' test.*

Nicol, William [*Scottish physicist*, 1768–1851]. Devised a polished prism of Iceland-spar cut diagonally across the principal axis, the sections being joined by means of Canada balsam. *Nicol's prism* reflects the ordinary rays of light out of the field while polarized rays are transmitted.

Nicola, Toufick [*American orthopedic surgeon*, 1894–]. Known for his operation for the relief of habitual dislocation of the shoulder, by transplant of the long head of the biceps. Called *Nicola's operation, procedure.*

Nicolaier, Arthur [*German physician*, 1862–]. Credited with the discovery of the bacillus of tetanus (1884), called *Nicolaier's bacillus.* He failed to demonstrate the organism in pure culture.

Nicolas, Joseph [*French physician*, 1868–]. Known for his contributions to the knowledge of venereal lymphogranuloma (1913), called *Nicolas-Favre* and *Durand-Nicolas-Favre disease.*

Nicolle, Charles Jules Henri [*French bacteriologist*, 1866–1936]. Made important studies of kala-azar and typhus. With C. Comte and E. Conseil, demonstrated that typhus is transmitted by the body louse (1909). Nobel laureate (1928). See also *NNN medium* under *Novy.*

Nicolle's carbol-crystal violet. See under *stain.*

Nicolle's carbol-thionine. See under *stain.*

Ni·co"ti·a'na (ni·ko"shee·ay'nuh, ·ah'nuh) [after Jean *Nicot*, French diplomat, 1530–1600]. See *tobacco.*

nic"o·tin·am'ide (nick"o·tin·am'ide, ·id, nick"o·tin'uh·mide, ·mid) (*nicotinamidum*). $C_5H_4N.CONH_2$. Nicotinic acid amide, occurring as a white, crystalline powder; 1 Gm. dissolves in about 1 cc. of water. It is a specific for pellagra, like nicotinic acid, but avoids the unpleasant flushing of the skin so often produced by the latter. Dose, same as for nicotinic acid. Syn., *niacinamide.*

nic'o·tine (nick'o·teen, ·tin) [*Nicot*]. A liquid, poisonous alkaloid found in the leaves of the tobacco plant, and responsible for the effects of tobacco.

nic"o·tin'ic ac'id (*acidum nicotinicum*). $C_5H_4N.COOH$. Beta- or 3-pyridinecarboxylic acid; occurs as a white, crystalline powder; 1 Gm. dissolves in 60 cc. of water. A specific for the treatment of pellagra. Dose, dependent on the needs of the patient; the maximum is 0.5 Gm. (8 gr.) per day (in 10 doses of 50 mg. each). Also called *niacin, P.P. factor.* See Table of Vitamins in the Appendix.

nic"o·tin'ic ac'tion. Peripheral drug effects similar to those produced by nicotine; small doses result in stimulation of autonomic ganglia and many myoneural junctions, including skeletal muscle; all turn to depression with large doses.

nic·ta'tion. See *nictitation.*

nic'ti·ta"ting [L. *nictare*, to wink]. Winking, as nictitating membrane, a vestigial fold in the human eye.

nic"ti·ta'ti·o (nick"ti·tay'shee·o) [*nictare*]. A clonic form of eyelid spasm.

nic"ti·ta'tion [*nictare*]. Abnormal frequency of winking.

ni·da'tion (nigh·day'shun, ni·) [L. *nidus*, nest]. The implantation of the fertilized ovum in the endometrium (decidua) of the pregnant uterus.

ni'dus (pl. *nidi*) [L.]. 1. A focus of infection. 2. Old term for a nucleus in the central nervous system. —**nidal,** *adj.*

Nielsen, Holger (contemporary). Danish Army officer, who devised the Holger Nielsen resuscitation technique (1932). See under *artificial respiration.*

Niemann, Albert [*German pediatrician*, 1880–1921]. First described the disease which is now known as *Niemann-Pick disease.* See under *disease.*

Niewenglowski's rays. See under *ray.*

night blind'ness. The condition of reduced dark adaptation, resulting temporarily from vitamin-A deficiency or permanently from retinitis pigmentosa or other peripheral retinal diseases. Syn., *nyctalopia.*

night'-bloom"ing ce're·us. See *Cactus grandiflorus.*

night cry. A shrill cry uttered by a child during sleep; sometimes symptomatic of physical disorders, as in the early stages of hip disease; sometimes of psychic origin.

Nightingale, Florence [*English nurse*, 1820–1910]. Immortalized as the founder of modern nursing service and famous throughout the world for her devotion to the English soldiers in the Crimean War. She created a woman's nursing service at Scutari and Balaklava (1860). From funds donated, she organized a school of nursing bearing her name. She was known far and wide as The Lady with the Lamp.

Nightingale test. See Anderson-Nightingale dilution *test.*

night'mare" [AS. *neaht; mara*]. A terrifying dream which usually awakens the sleeper; characterized by great distress and a sense of oppression or suffocation.

night pain. Pain, usually in the hip or knee, occurring during muscular relaxation of the limb in sleep; often a symptom of disease of the joints.

night pal'sy (pawl'zee). Numbness of the extremities occurring during the night, or on waking in the morning, affecting women about the period of the menopause.

night'shade [AS. *nihtscada*]. A name applied to plants of the family Solanaceae.

deadly n. A poisonous plant, *Atropa belladonna.* See *belladonna.*

night sweat. Profuse nocturnal sweating. A frequent accompaniment of any diurnal fever and, by tradition, associated especially with pulmonary tuberculosis.

night ter'rors. See *night cry.*

night vi'sion. The ability to see at night. Nocturnal visual efficiency is determined by the ability to perform visual tasks at light intensities below the cone threshold, that is, at scotopic levels of illumination.

n. v. tester. A self-recording group testing device for determining the ability to discriminate the break in a Landolt ring at eight different levels of illumination. The testing distance is 20 feet.

portable n. v. tester. An instrument used by the School of Aviation Medicine for measuring the threshold of the dark-adapted eye at a distance of 15 inches from the eyes. The test object is a Landolt ring subtending a visual angle of two degrees. The background is a disk of self-luminous paint, the brightness of which can be varied by a series of neutral density filters.

ni·gran′i·line (nigh·gran′i·leen, ·lin). Aniline black, a black dye obtained by the oxidation of aniline, used as a histological stain. Also called *nigrosine.*

nig′ri·cans (nig′ri·kanz, nigh′gri·) [L. *nigricare,* to be blackish]. Black or blackish.

ni·gri′ti·es (nigh·grish′ee·eez) [L., blackness]. Black, hairy tongue.

ni′gro·sine (nigh′gro·seen, ·sin). Any one of several black or dark blue aniline dyes; variously used in bacteriologic and histologic technics.

NIH National Institutes of Health.

ni′hil·ism (nigh′hi·liz·um, nigh′i·) [L. *nihil,* nothing]. 1. Pessimism in regard to the efficacy of drugs. 2. *In psychiatry,* the content of delusions encountered in depressed or melancholic states. The patient insists that his inner organs no longer exist, and that his relatives have passed away.

ni·keth′a·mide. $C_5H_4N.CON(C_2H_5)_2$. The diethylamide of nicotinic acid, occurring either as a colorless to yellow oily liquid or as a crystalline solid, soluble in water. Stimulates medullary centers; used as an analeptic, and for its respiratory stimulant effects. A 25% aqueous solution, for oral or parenteral use, is the principal dosage form. Dose, 1–4 cc. (15–60 min.). See *anacardone, coromine, corvotone, nicamide.*

Nile blue A (C.C.). A basic oxazine dye, of value as a fat stain. See under *stain.*

nilodin. Trade-mark for lucanthone hydrochloride, a drug useful in treating certain types of human schistosomiasis. See *miracil D.*

ninhydrin. Trade name of triketohydrindene hydrate. A water-soluble substance which gives a color reaction with proteins and amino acids. Also used in Abderhalden's test for pregnancy.

ni·o′bi·um (nigh·o′bee·um) Nb = 92.91; chemical element No. 41; a steel-gray, lustrous metal, formerly called *columbium.*

ni·o′po (nigh·o′po). A snuff made from the seeds of *Piptadenia peregrina,* said to produce an intoxication approaching frenzy.

nipagin A. Trade-mark for ethyl parahydroxybenzoate; used as a preservative.

nipagin M. Trade-mark for methyl parahydroxybenzoate. See *methylparaben.*

niph″a·blep′si·a [G. *nipha,* snow; *ablepsia,* blindness]. Snow blindness.

niph″o·typh·lo′sis [*nipha;* G. *typhlōsis,* a blinding]. Snow blindness.

nip″i·ol′o·gy. See *nepiology.*

nip′pers [ME. *nippen*]. An instrument for seizing small bodies.

bone n. An instrument for grasping small bits of bone; a small bone-trimming forceps.

nip′ple [perhaps dim. from AS. *nebb,* beak]. The conical projection in the center of the mamma, containing the outlets of the milk ducts. Also called *papilla.* See Plate 43.

cracked n. One in which the epidermis is broken.

crater n. See retracted *n.*

n. line. A vertical line drawn on the surface of the chest through the nipple.

n. protector. A device worn by nursing women to protect the nipple. Also called *nipple shield.*

retracted n. One below the surrounding level.

nir′va·nol (nur′vuh·nole, ·nol, ·nawl, nur·vah′·). $C_{11}H_{12}O_2N_2$. Phenylethylhydantoin, a sedative and soporific. Formerly used in the treatment of chorea, producing "nirvanol sickness," characterized by morbilliform rash and fever.

Nisbet, William [*British physician,* 1759–1822]. Described inflammatory nodules, sometimes ulcerative, in the penis, following acute lymphangitis secondary to chancroid.

nisentil hydrochloride. Trade-marked name for the synthetic analgesic *dl*-alpha-1,3-dimethyl-4-phenyl-4-propionoxypiperidine hydrochloride, known by the generic names *alphaprodine hydrochloride* and *prisilidene hydrochloride.*

nis′in. An antibiotic substance derived from *Streptococcus lactis,* active, in vitro, against a number of bacterial species; it protects mice against certain experimental infections.

Nissl, Franz [*German neurologist,* 1860–1919]. Remembered for his description of degeneration of ganglion cells (1892), called *Nissl's degeneration.* Described a stain, *Nissl's methylene blue* and chromophilic bodies of various sizes and shapes in nerve cells, called *Nissl bodies, substance.*

nisulfadine. Trade-mark for 2-(*p*-nitrophenylsulfonamido)-pyridine, a drug for the treatment of ulcerative colitis.

nisulfazole. Trade-mark for para-nitrosulfathiazole, a drug for the treatment of ulcerative colitis.

ni′sus [L., effort]. 1. Any strong effort or struggle. 2. The periodic desire for procreation manifested in the spring season by certain species of animals; called **nisus formativus.** 3. The contraction of the diaphragm and abdominal muscles for the expulsion of feces, urine, or a fetus.

nit [AS. *hnitu*]. The egg or larva of a louse.

Nitabuch, stria of. See under *stria.*

ni′ter [G. *nitron,* sodium carbonate]. Potassium nitrate or saltpeter. Also spelled *nitre.*

Chile n. Sodium nitrate.

cubic n. Sodium nitrate.

rough n. Magnesium chloride.

sweet spirit of n. (*spiritus aethylis nitritis*). Ethyl nitrite spirit. An alcoholic solution of ethyl nitrite. A popular diaphoretic in mild fevers. Dose, 2–4 cc. (30–60 min.).

ni′ton. Radon. Symbol, Nt.

ni′tra·gin. A nitrifying, bacterial ferment obtained from the root tubercles of leguminous plants.

ni′tra·mine (nigh′truh·meen, ·min, nigh·tram′in, nigh″truh·meen′). See *tetryl,* 2.

nitranitol. Trade-mark for *mannitol hexanitrate.*

ni′trate. A salt of nitric acid.

ni·tra′tion. The process of combining or reacting with nitric acid.

nitrazine. Trade-mark used for a dye, sodium dinitrophenylazo-naphthol disulfonate, used as an indicator. Strips of paper treated with this dye are used for the determination of the pH of urine.

ni′tre. Niter.

ni′tric ac′id (*acidum nitricum*). A liquid containing 67–71% HNO_3, the remainder being water; possesses a characteristic, highly irritating odor and is very caustic and corrosive. Occasionally employed internally, well diluted with water, for the same purpose as hydrochloric acid and also as a hepatic stimulant; externally, employed as an escharotic, particularly for venereal and phagedenic ulcers. Dose, 0.2–0.5 cc. (3–8 min.), well diluted with water.

fuming n. a. Nitric acid containing more or less nitrogen tetroxide, a gas which gives it a reddish color and causes it to fume.

ni″tri·fi·ca′tion [G. *nitron,* sodium carbonate; L. *facere,* to make]. The conversion of the nitrogen of ammonia and organic compounds into nitrites and nitrates, a process constantly going on in nature under the influence of certain bacteria and other agencies.

ni′tri·fi″er [*nitron; facere*]. A microorganism that participates in the process of nitrification; bacteria of the genus *Nitrosomonas* oxidize ammonium to nitrite; bacteria of the genus *Nitrobacter* oxidize nitrite to nitrate.

ni′trile (nigh′trile, ·tril). An organic compound containing the monovalent CN group.

ni′trite [*nitron*]. A salt of nitrous acid. See *amyl* nitrite, *ethyl* nitrite, *potassium* nitrite, *sodium* nitrite. The nitrites produce dilatation of the blood vessels, diminution of the blood pressure, increased rapidity of the pulse, and depression of the motor centers in the spinal cord. They are used as antispasmodics in asthma and angina pectoris, in spasmodic dysmenorrhea, tetanus, epileptic and hysterical convulsions, and in cases of arteriosclerosis with high arterial tension. Full doses in man give rise to flushing of the face, throbbing, and headache.

ni′tri·toid [*nitron;* G. *eidos,* form]. Like a nitrite.

ni″tri·tu′ri·a [*nitron;* G. *ouron,* urine]. The presence of nitrates or nitrites, or both, in the urine when voided.

nitro-, nitr- [*nitron*]. 1. A combining form denoting *the presence of the monovalent radical NO_2.* 2. A combining form denoting *combination with nitrogen.*

ni″tro·ben′zene. $C_6H_5NO_2$. An oily, sweetish liquid made by the action of strong nitric acid on benzene; it is employed as a flavoring agent under the name of artificial oil of bitter almonds or oil of mirbane. It is a powerful poison, resembling hydrocyanic acid in action.

ni″tro·ben′zol. Nitrobenzene.

ni″tro·cel′lu·lose. See *pyroxylin.*

ni″tro·chlo′ro·form. See *chloropicrin.*

ni″tro·er′y·throl. $C_4H_6(NO_3)_4$. Erythrityl tetranitrate, prepared by nitration of the alcohol erythrol (tetrahydroxybutane); it explodes on percussion. It is used in the same manner as nitroglycerin. Dose, 0.015–0.06 Gm. (¼–1 gr.).

ni″tro·fur·an′toin. $C_8H_6N_4O_5$; N-(5-nitro-2-furfurylidene)-1-aminohydantoin; a yellow powder, practically insoluble in water. It exhibits a wide spectrum of antibacterial activity against both Gram-positive and Gram-negative organisms, and is useful in treating bacterial infections of the urinary tract. See *furadantin.*

ni″tro·fur′a·zone. $C_6H_6N_4O_4$. 5-Nitro-2-furaldehyde semicarbazone, a derivative of furfural possessing bacteriostatic and bactericidal properties. It is a lemon yellow, crystalline powder, very slightly soluble in water. See *furacin.*

ni′tro·gen [*nitron;* G. *genesthai,* from *gignesthai,* to be produced]. N = 14.008. A nonmetallic element existing free in the atmosphere, of which it constitutes about 77% by weight. A colorless, odorless gas, incapable of sustaining life. Chemically it is relatively inert, and combines directly with but few elements. An important constituent of all animal and vegetable tissues. See Table of Normal Values of Blood Constituents in the Appendix.

blood urea n. Nitrogen in the form of urea found in whole blood or serum; normal range is 8–20 mg. per 100 ml.

n. balance. The difference between the nitrogen intake (as protein) of an individual and his total nitrogen excretion. If the nitrogen intake equals the nitrogen excretion, a subject is in nitrogen equilibrium. If the nitrogen intake exceeds the nitrogen excretion, the nitrogen balance is positive. If the nitrogen excretion is greater than the nitrogen intake, the nitrogen balance is negative.

n. cycle. The fixation of atmospheric nitrogen and the nitrification of inorganic nitrogen compounds by bacteria, the synthesis of these into protein by plants and consumption by animals, with ultimate degradation to inorganic nitrogen compounds and molecular nitrogen.

n. dioxide. N_2O_2. A toxic gas resulting from the decomposition of nitric acid.

n. fixation. Conversion of free nitrogen in the air into compounds, such as ammonia and nitric acid and salts or derivatives of the same, accomplished naturally through electrical discharges in the atmosphere, through the agency of certain soil organisms, also by various industrial synthesis methods.

n. fixers. Certain bacteria, as *Azotobacter,* capable of transforming atmospheric nitrogen into nitrogenous compounds in the cell.

n.-lag. The time elapsing between the ingestion of a protein and the appearance in the urine of an amount of nitrogen equal to that taken in.

n. monoxide. Nitrous oxide.

n. mustard. Any of a series of nitrogen analogs of dichlorodiethylsulfide of which *tris* (β-chloroethyl)amine, $N(CH_2CH_2Cl)_3$, and methyl-*bis* (β-chloroethyl)amine, $CH_3N(CH_2CH_2Cl)_2$, in the form of water-soluble hydrochloride salts, intravenously administered, have been found useful in the treatment of Hodgkin's disease, lymphosarcoma, and chronic leukemia. Methyl *bis* (β-chloroethyl)amine hydrochloride is officially recognized as *mechlorethamine hydrochloride* (*sterile*). The nitrogen mustards possess vesicant properties and are of interest as potential chemical warfare agents.

n. pentoxide. The solid substance N_2O_5; reacts with water to form nitric oxide.

n. tetroxide. N_2O_4. A toxic gas resulting from oxidation of nitrogen dioxide. Also called *n. peroxide.*

nonprotein n. The fraction of nitrogen in the blood, tissues, urine, and excreta, not precipitated by the usual protein precipitants such as sodium tungstate. Symbol, N. P. N.

ni·trog′e·nous (nigh·trodj′i·nus) [*nitron; genesthai*]. Containing nitrogen.

ni″tro·glyc′er·in (nigh″tro·gliss′ur·in). $C_3H_5(NO_3)_3$. Glonoin, glyceryl trinitrate; a colorless, oily liquid produced by the action of sulfuric and nitric acids upon glycerin. A powerful explosive; physiologically, has the actions of the nitrites, but is more persistent than amyl nitrite, which it most resembles. Dose, 0.3–1.2 mg. (1/200–1/50 gr.).

n. spirit (*spiritus glycerylis trinitratis*). A 1% alcoholic solution. Dose, 0.06–0.12 cc. (1–2 min.).

n. tablets (*tabellae glycerylis trinitratis*). Glyceryl trinitrate tablets; commonly available in potencies of 0.3, 0.4, 0.6, and 1.2 mg. (1/200, 1/150, 1/100, and 1/50 gr.).

ni″tro·hy″dro·chlo′ric ac′id (*acidum nitrohydrochloricum*). Prepared by mixing 1 volume of nitric acid and 4 volumes of hydrochloric acid; contains the component acids together with nitrosyl chloride and chlorine. Increases the flow of bile and is used in cholecystitis. Dose, 0.2–0.3 cc. (3–5 min.), well diluted. Syn., *nitromuriatic acid.*

diluted n. a. (*acidum nitrohydrochloricum dilutum*). A solution of 22 cc. of nitrohydrochloric acid diluted with water to 100 cc. Dose, 0.6–1.3 cc. (10–20 min.), well diluted.

ni″tro·man′nite. Mannitol hexanitrate.

ni″tro·man′ni·tol. Mannitol hexanitrate.

ni″tro·mer′sol (*nitromersol*). $C_7H_5O_3NHg$. The anhydride of 4-nitro-3-hydroxy-mercuri-orthocresol, containing about 57% of mercury; it is a brownish yellow to yellow powder, or occurs in granules. It is insoluble in water, but dissolves in solutions of alkalies. It is employed as a germicide. See *metaphen.*

n. solution (*liquor nitromersolis*). Nitromersol 0.2 Gm., sodium hydroxide 0.04 Gm., monohydrated sodium carbonate 0.425 Gm., in water to 100 cc.

n. tincture (*tinctura nitromersolis*). Nitromersol

0.5 Gm., sodium hydroxide 0.1 Gm., acetone 10 cc., alcohol 50 cc., water to 100 cc.

ni·trom′e·ter (nigh·trom′i·tur) [*nitron;* G. *metron,* a measure]. An apparatus for collecting and measuring nitrogen evolved during a chemical reaction.

ni″tro·mu″ri·at′ic ac′id. See *nitrohydrochloric acid.*

ni′tron. 4,5-Dihydro-1,4-diphenyl-3,5-phenylamino-1,2,4-triazole: used in Crämer's nitrate method.

ni″tro·prus′side. Any salt containing the anion $[Fe(CN)_5NO]^{=}$.

ni·tro′so- (nigh·tro′so-) [*nitron*]. A combining form signifying *combination with nitrosyl,* the univalent NO.

ni·tro″so·ni′tric ac′id. Fuming nitric acid containing nitrous acid gas.

ni·tro′syl (nigh·tro′sil, nigh″tro·seel′, nigh′tro·sil). The univalent radical NO.

ni′trous [*nitron*]. 1. Containing nitrogen as a trivalent positive element. 2. Pertaining to or derived from nitrous acid.

n. ether. $C_2H_5NO_2$. Ethyl nitrite, a very volatile liquid having properties similar to those of amyl nitrite.

n. oxide. N_2O. A colorless gas; used as a general anesthetic in dentistry and in surgery. Also called *hyponitrous oxide, laughing gas, nitrogen monoxide.*

ni′trous ac′id. HNO_2. An unstable solution prepared by passing N_2O_3 into water.

Nitze, Max [*German urologist,* 1848–1906]. Introduced an electrically lighted cystoscope (1877). Author of an important monograph on the science of cystoscopy (1889).

nizin. Trade-mark for a brand of zinc sulfanilate.

NK *Nomenklatur Kommission;* the committee appointed to revise the BNA. The recommendations of this committee, published in 1935, have not been widely adopted.

N.L.N.E. National League of Nursing Education.

N. N. R. New and Nonofficial Remedies; a book describing substances that have been approved by the Council on Pharmacy and Chemistry of the American Medical Association.

No. *Numero,* number, to the number of.

no″as·the′ni·a [G. *nous,* mind; *astheneia,* weakness]. Mental feebleness.

Nobel, Alfred Bernard [*Swedish manufacturer of munitions,* 1833–96]. The inventor of dynamite, he provided (1895) for a yearly distribution of prizes for noteworthy advances in literature, chemistry, physics, and medicine, as well as in the cause of international peace. The recipient is known as *Nobel laureate* or *prizeman.*

Noble, Charles Percy [*American gynecologist,* 1863–1935]. Introduced a posture assumed for examination of the kidney. The patient stands with torso flexed and supported by the extended arms; known as *Noble's posture.*

no′ble gas′es. The inert gases, helium, neon, argon, krypton, xenon, and radon, so called because they will not enter into chemical combination with any other element.

Nocard, Edmond Isidore Etienne [*French veterinarian,* 1850–1903]. With Pierre Paul Roux published an early study on filtrable viruses (1898). Discovered the virus of psittacosis. Described a diphtheroid bacillus producing pseudotuberculosis in cattle, sheep, and horses; called *Preisz-Nocard bacillus.*

No·car′di·a [*Nocard*]. A genus of aerobic fungi of the family Actinomycetaceae.

N. asteroides. A species which is an aerobic and acid-fast actinomycete; causes pulmonary, brain, and subcutaneous lesions, usually without granules.

N. madurae. A species which is one of the causes of white-grained mycetoma.

N. minutissima. A species which causes the chronic infection of the stratum corneum known as erythrasma.

N. somaliensis. A species which is one of the causes of white-grained mycetoma.

N. tenuis. A species which is the causative agent of trichomycosis axillaris.

no·car′din. An antibiotic substance elaborated by the fungus *Nocardia coeliaca,* active, in vitro and to some extent in vivo, against some strains of *Mycobacterium tuberculosis.*

no″car·di·o′sis [*Nocard;* G. *-ōsis,* condition]. Actinomycosis caused by certain species of the aerobic actinomycetes, *Nocardia.* The disease is indistinguishable from that caused by *Actinomyces bovis.*

granulomatous n. A granulomatous reaction to infection with the fungus *Nocardia.*

Nocht-Romanovsky stain. See under *stain.*

no″ci·cep′tive [L. *nocere,* to hurt; *capere,* to take]. Referring to sensory nerves which mediate impulses stimulated by trauma; pain receptors.

no″ci·fen′sor [*nocere;* L. *defendere,* to protect]. A term introduced by Lewis to denote efferent fibers which release chemical substances at their terminals, which stimulate the pain endings.

no″ci·per·cep′tion [*nocere;* L. *perceptio,* from *percipere*]. Perception of pain by the central nervous system.

no″ci·per·cep′tor [*nocere;* L. *percipere,* to perceive]. One of the peripheral nerves concerned in the reception of pain stimuli.

noc″tal·bu″mi·nu′ri·a [L. *nox,* night; *albus,* white; G. *ouron,* urine]. Excretion of albumin in night urine only.

noc·tam″bu·la′tion [*nox;* L. *ambulare,* to walk]. Sleep walking.

noc″ti·pho′bi·a [*nox;* G. *phobos,* fear]. Morbid fear of night.

Noc·tu′i·dae (nock·tew′i·dee) [L. *noctua,* night owl]. A family of the Lepidoptera; owlet moths. Caterpillars of this family have irritating hairs which cause caterpillar dermatitis in man.

noc·tu′ri·a [L. *nox,* night; G. *ouron,* urine]. 1. Nocturnal enuresis. 2. Frequency of urination at night. Syn., *nycturia.*

noc·tur′nal [L. *nocturnalis,* nocturnal]. Pertaining to night, as nocturnal emission, discharge of semen without coitus during sleep.

noc″u·fen′sor. A term suggested by Thomas Lewis to replace nocifensor.

noc′u·ous [L. *nocuus,* hurtful]. Noxious; hurtful; venomous.

node [L. *nodus,* knot]. 1. A knob, or protuberance. 2. A point of constriction. 3. A small, rounded organ. **—nod′al,** *adj.*

atrioventricular n. A small mass of interwoven Purkinje fibers of the conduction system in the central fibrous body of the heart. Syn., *Tawara n.*

auriculoventricular n. See atrioventricular *n.*

Bouchard's nodes. Enlargement of the proximal interphalangeal joints, seen in gout.

Cloquet's n. The highest deep inguinal lymph node situated in the femoral ring: also called *Rosenmueller's n.*

Ewald's n. See signal *n.*

Heberden's n. Nodose deformity of the fingers in multiple degenerative joint disease.

hemal n. A node of lymphatic tissue, situated in the course of blood vessels, and containing large numbers of erythrocytes. Hemal nodes are frequent in ruminants, but probably do not occur in man, although even normal lymph nodes may contain erythrocytes in the parenchyma.

hemolymph n. See hemal *n.*
Hensen's n. In the embryo, an accumulation of cells at the anterior end of the primitive streak, through which the neurenteric canal passes from the outside into the blastodermic vesicle. Also called *primitive n., primitive knot.*
Janeway n. See Edward Gamaliel *Janeway.*
juxta-articular n. See under *nodule.*
lymph n. See under *lymph.*
n. of Keith and Flack. See sinoatrial *n.*
n. of Ranvier. The region, in a myelinated nerve, of a local constriction in the myelin sheath. The axis cylinder (or axon) is also slightly constricted at the node.
Osler's n. See William *Osler.*
preacher's n. See singer's *n.*
Rosenmueller's n. See Cloquet's *n.*
signal n. Metastatic tumor in supraclavicular lymph node, usually on the left side, and most frequently secondary to primary carcinoma in abdomen or thorax: also called *Ewald's n., sentinel n., Virchow's n., Virchow's signal n.*
singer's n. An inflammatory or fibrous nodule on the free margin of the vocal cords, seen in those who use their voices professionally: also called *preacher's n., singer's* or *vocal nodule, chorditis nodosa, chorditis tuberosa.*
sinoatrial n. A dense network of Purkinje fibers of the conduction system at the junction of the superior vena cava and the atrium. Syn., *n. of Keith and Flack.*
supraclavicular signal n. See signal *n.*
syphilitic n. Localized swelling on bones due to syphilitic periostitis.
Tawara n. See atrioventricular *n.*
Virchow's n. See signal *n.*
vocal nodes. See singers' *n.*

no'dose [L. *nodosus,* knotty]. Characterized by nodes; jointed or swollen at intervals.

no·dos'i·ty [*nodosus*]. 1. State of being nodose. 2. A node.

nod'u·lar sub·ep·i·der'mal fi·bro'sis. See *dermatofibroma.*

nod'ule [L. *nodulus,* little knot]. 1. A small node. 2. A small aggregation of cells. 3. Specifically, *in dermatology,* one of the primary skin lesions, a circumscribed solid elevation of varying size. Syn., *tubercula.* —**nod'ular,** *adj.*
aggregate nodules. Groups of lymph nodules massed together in the wall of an organ, as the Peyer's patches of the small intestine.
agminated nodules. See *aggregate nodules* under *nodule.*
Aschoff n. The specific lesion of rheumatic fever; a small area of necrosis surrounded by Aschoff cells and a few lymphocytes, located perivascularly in the myocardium and occasionally found elsewhere. Syn., *Aschoff body.*
Bizzozero nodules. Small nodular thickenings of the intercellular bridges of the epidermis.
Gamna nodules. See *siderotic nodules* under *nodule.*
Gandy-Gamna nodules. See *siderotic nodules* under *nodule.*
juxta-articular nodules. Subcutaneous tumors of poorly vascularized connective tissue, without elastic fibers, which may contain necrotic areas, found in patients with late syphilis or yaws. The tumors are hard in consistency and are found about the joints of the upper extremity, especially the elbow, and on the legs. Nodes have been reported in patients without syphilis or yaws.
Koeppe's nodules. Nonspecific gray lumps found on the pupillary margin in a variety of inflammatory diseases of the uvea.
lymph n. A small mass of dense lymphatic tissue in which new lymphocytes are formed.
milker's nodules. Small, raised, bluish-red, firm, rarely purulent nodules found on the hands and arms of slaughterhouse workers and dairy farmers: probably vaccinia.
n. of cerebellum. The nodulus.
nodules of Arantius. Those of the semilunar valves, formerly called the bodies of Arantius, corpora Arantii.
Osler's nodules. Painful or tender cutaneous nodules, observed commonly at the tips of fingers or toes, and due to embolic phenomena, as in subacute bacterial endocarditis.
rheumatic nodules. Subcutaneous nodules occurring in both rheumatic fever and rheumatoid arthritis about the elbows, knees, ankles, and other points of pressure along tendon sheaths. The skin over the lesion may be normal in color or slightly erythematous. The nodules result from granulomatous inflammation, and are characterized by necrosis of connective tissue with peripheral fibrosis.
Schmorl's nodules. Herniation of the nucleus pulposus of the intervertebral disk into a softened spongy substance of a vertebra. When extensive, the result is kyphosis with wedge-shaped vertebrae.
siderotic nodules. Small yellow to brown foci seen in some spleens, and less often in other organs. They consist of necrotic, fibrillar, and cellular material encrusted with salts of iron and calcium, and may be the result of focal hemorrhage.
singer's n. See singer's *node.*
solitary lymphatic n. An independent lymph nodule, as in some mucous membranes.
subcutaneous n. Usually a rheumatic nodule.
triticeous n. Corpus triticeum; a small, cartilaginous nodule in the thyrohyoid ligament.
typhus n. A focal collection of lymphocytes, plasmacytes, and large mononuclear cells around or near small blood vessels: a common feature of rickettsial diseases.
vocal n. See singer's *node.*

nod'u·lus [L.]. 1. Nodule. 2. The nodule of the cerebellum; one of the anterior subdivisions of the vermis of the cerebellum.

no'dus. See *node.*

no"e·gen'e·sis [G. *noēma,* thought; *genesis,* production]. *In psychology,* a term that denotes the utmost degree of creativeness attainable by the mind. *Rare.*

Noeggerath, Emil [*American gynecologist and obstetrician,* 1827–95]. Introduced the operation of epicystotomy (1858). Pioneer in pointing out the effects of latent gonorrhea in the production of sterility in women (1872).

no"e·mat"a·chym'e·ter (no"i·mat"uh·kim'i·tur) [G. *noēma,* thought; *tachys,* swift; *metron,* a measure]. An apparatus for estimating the time taken in recording a simple perception.

no"e·mat'ic [*noēma*]. Pertaining to thought or to any mental process.

Noguchi, Hideyo [*Japanese bacteriologist in America,* 1876–1928]. With S. Flexner, made important study of snake venom. Cultivated *Treponema pallidum* (1911). Obtained pure culture of *Treponema pallidum* from a case of paralytic dementia (1913), thus establishing its connection with syphilis. Isolated *Bacillus granulosis* from trachoma (1927). Modified the Wassermann test for syphilis. See also Noguchi's *test.*

no'ma [G. *nomē,* a feeding]. A stomatitis, often fatal, starting in debilitated children during convalescence from disease, usually one of the exanthemas. It begins in the mucous membrane, becomes gangrenous, and ulcerates through the cheek. Also called *cancrum oris, gangraena oris, gangrenous stomatitis, European noma.*

n. of penis. An extremely rare gangrenous ulceration of the penis, seen in young boys.

n. pudendi. An ulceration similar to noma of penis, occurring about the genital region of female children. Also called *n. vulvae.*

no·mad'ic [G. *nomas*, roaming]. Spreading; said of ulcers.

no'men·cla·ture. A systematic arrangement of the distinctive names employed in any science. See *BNA, BR.*

nom'o·gram. See *nomograph.*

nom'o·graph [G. *nomos*, law; *graphein*, to write]. A graph on which appear graduated lines for all variables in a formula, arranged in such a manner that the value of one variable can be read on the appropriate line from a knowledge of the values of the other variables; as the DuBois nomograph for estimation of surface area.

nom"o·top'ic [*nomos;* G. *topos*, place]. Occurring at the usual site. *Rare.*

non- [L., not]. A prefix meaning *not.*

no'na. See lethargic *encephalitis.*

non·ac'cess [*non;* L. *accessus*, from *accedere*, to approach]. *In legal medicine*, the absence of opportunity for sexual intercourse.

non"ad·he'rent [*non;* L. *adhaerere*, to stick to]. Not connected to an adjacent organ or part.

non"al·ler'gic [*non;* G. *allos*, other; *ergon*, work]. Unrelated to allergy.

no'nan [L. *nonus*, ninth]. Having an exacerbation every ninth day.

no"nane·di·o'ic ac'id. Azelaic acid.

non·a'que·ous (non·ay'kwee·us, ·ack'wee·us) [L. *non*, not; *aqua*, water]. Not consisting of, or pertaining to, water; said of organic solvents.

non com'pos men'tis [L.]. Of unsound mind.

non"con·duc'tor [*non;* L. *conductor*, from *conducere*, to conduct]. Any substance not transmitting electricity or heat.

non"dis·junc'tion [*non;* L. *disjunctio*, a separation]. The failure of homologous material and paternal chromosomes to separate at meiosis; also applied to the failure of sister chromosomes to separate in an ordinary mitosis.

non"e·lec'tro·lyte. A substance which in solution does not dissociate into ions and is therefore unable to conduct an electric current.

non'fixed med'i·cal treat'ment fa·cil'i·ty. *In U.S. Army medicine*, a medical treatment facility capable of being moved from place to place and designed to operate tactically in that manner. It includes evacuation hospitals, mobile army surgical hospitals, unit dispensaries (aid stations), collecting stations, clearing stations, holding stations, NP treatment stations, and convalescent centers.

Nonidez chloral hydrate method. See under *stain.*

no"ni·grav'i·da (no"ni·grav'i·duh, non"i·) [L. *nonus*, ninth; *gravidus*, pregnant]. A woman pregnant for the ninth time.

no·nip'a·ra [*nonus;* L. *parere*, to bring forth]. A woman who has been in labor nine times.

non"lu·et'ic [L. *non*, not; *lues*, pestilence]. Not due to syphilitic infection.

non"ma·lig'nant [*non;* L. *malignus*, wicked]. Lacking any features of malignant disease, usually referring to tumors. Syn., *benign.*

non·med'ul·la"ted. Having no myelin sheath; amyelinated; unmyelinated.

non·mo'tile (non·mo'til) [*non;* L. *motum*, from *movere*, to move]. Not having the power of spontaneous motion.

non·my·el'i·na"ted. Amyelinated.

Nonne, Max (1861–). German neurologist credited with the first description of hereditary edema, now called *Milroy's disease.* He described a group of symptoms resulting from hereditary cerebellar disease. See hereditary cerebellar *ataxia*, Nonne-Apelt's *test.*

non·nu'cle·a·ted. Without a nucleus, as a mature erythrocyte.

non'ose. A monosaccharide which contains nine carbon atoms in the molecule.

non·par'ous. Nulliparous.

non·pro'te·in [L. *non*, not; G. *prōteios*, of first rank]. Not derived from protein, as nonprotein nitrogen; not containing protein, as nonprotein fraction of an extract.

non·pro'te·in ni'tro·gen (of the blood). The total N of the blood less that of the proteins.

non"py·o·gen'ic (non"pye·o·jen'ick) [*non;* G. *pyon*, pus; *genesthai*, from *gignesthai*, to be produced]. Not inducing the formation of pus.

non·re"a·gin'ic [*non;* L. *re-*, back; *agere*, to act]. Referring to conditions in which reagins are not demonstrable, as nonreaginic allergy.

non"re·frac'tive [*non;* L. *refractum*, from *refringere*, to break up]. Not possessing properties permitting the refraction of light rays.

non"re·straint' [*non;* L. *restringere*, to bind back]. The treatment of insanity without any forcible means of compulsion.

non·sex'u·al. Asexual.

non"spe·cif'ic [*non;* L. *species*, a particular sort]. Referring to relations that are not specific, but general.

non"spe·cif'ic pro'te·in ther'a·py. Treatment which recognizes that stock and autogenous vaccines may owe a part of their value in disease therapy to nonspecific effects; for example peptone, milk, normal serum, etc., have been employed to replace bacterial products.

non·sup'pu·ra"tive [*non;* L. *suppurare*, to form pus]. Uninfected; surgically clean; not forming pus.

non·sur'gi·cal [*non;* G. *cheirourgos*, working by hand]. Not surgical; nonoperative.

non·vi'a·ble [*non;* L. *vita*, life]. Incapable of living.

non'yl. The univalent hydrocarbon radical $CH_3(CH_2)_8$—.

non·yl'ic ac'id. Pelargonic acid.

no"o·klo'pi·a (no"o·klo'pee·a). See *castrophrenia.*

no'o·psy"che (no'o·sigh"kee) [G. *nous*, mind; *psychē*, soul]. Mental or reasoning processes.

Noorden, Carl Harko von [*German physician*, 1858–1944]. Known for his important investigations of diabetes (1895). Contributed to the knowledge of metabolism (1900–10). Introduced special oatmeal diet in diabetes and other conditions, called *von Noorden treatment.*

N.O.P.H.N. National Organization for Public Health Nursing.

nor- [L. *norma*, rule]. A prefix indicating the *parent compound* from which another is derived.

nor"a·dren'a·lin, nor"a·dren'a·line. Norepinephrine.

nor'bi·o·tin. A homolog of biotin containing one less CH_2 group in the side chain; it is an antagonist of biotin toward some bacteria but is capable of replacing biotin in certain of its functions toward other oganisms.

Nordau, Max Simon [*German physician and author*, 1849–1923]. Author of *Degeneration* (1892–93), in which he tried to correlate genius and insanity. Degeneracy has since been known as *Nordauism.*

Nordhausen sulfuric acid. Fuming sulfuric acid; sulfuric acid containing sulfur trioxide.

nor"di·hy"dro·guai"a·ret'ic ac'id. $(OH)_2C_6H_3$-

$CH_2.CH(CH_3).CH(CH_3).CH_2.C_6H_3(OH)_2$; 4,4′-(2,3-dimethyltetramethylene)dipyrocatechol; a substance in resinous exudates of many plants and also prepared synthetically; it occurs in crystals, slightly soluble in hot water but soluble in organic liquids. It is used as an antioxidant in fats and oils. Abbreviated NDGA.

nor″e·phed′rine (nor″eh·fed′rin, nor·ef′i·dreen, ·drin). The 1-phenyl-2-aminopropanol, representing ephedrine in which the methyl radical of the amino group is replaced by hydrogen. See *propadrine hydrochloride.*

nor·ep″i·neph′rine. $(OH)_2C_6H_3.CHOH.CH_2.NH_2$; 3,4-dihydroxyphenylaminoethanol; a demethylated epinephrine. The levorotatory isomer is formed at sympathetic nerve endings as a mediator of functional activity; it is probably the postulated *sympathin E.* Therapeutically it is useful for maintenance of blood pressure in acute hypotensive states caused by surgical and nonsurgical trauma, central vasomotor depression, and hemorrhage; the bitartrate salt is commonly employed. Syn., *arterenol, noradrenalin.* See *levophed.*

norisodrine sulfate. A trade-marked name for the sympathomimetic amine salt isopropylarterenol sulfate.

nor′ite fac′tor. See under *factor.*

nor·leu′cine (nor·lew′seen, ·sin). $CH_3(CH_2)_3CH(NH_2)COOH$. Alpha-amino-caproic acid, a component of many proteins.

nor·leu′cyl. The univalent radical, $CH_3CH_2CH_2CH_2CH(NH_2)CO$—, of the amino acid norleucine.

norm [L. *norma*, rule]. A standard.

nor′ma (pl. *normae*) [L.]. *In anatomy*, a view or aspect, essentially of the skull.

n. anterior. Norma facialis.

n. basilaris. That directed toward the inferior aspect of the skull.

n. facialis. That directed toward the face.

n. inferior. Norma ventralis.

n. lateralis. A profile view.

n. occipitalis. That directed toward the back of the skull.

n. sagittalis. The skull seen in a sagittal section.

n. superior. Norma verticalis.

n. ventralis. The inferior aspect of the skull.

n. verticalis. The aspect viewed from above, or that directed toward the top of the skull.

nor′mal [L. *normalis*, from *norma*]. 1. Conforming to some ideal norm or standard; pertaining to the central values of some homogeneous group, as that which is typical of or acceptable to a majority or dominant group; average, common, mean, median, standard, typical, usual, ideal, modal. 2. *In medicine* and *psychology*, "healthy," i.e., lacking observable or detectable clinical abnormalities, deficiencies, or diseases; also, pertaining to or describing a value or measurement obtained in an ideal group by a particular method, such as may be found in the Table of Normal Values of Blood Constituents in the Appendix; i.e., a value which in itself is not significant of disease; pertaining to the **normal variability** of an individual's anatomical, physiological, and psychological pattern within the parameters of age, sex, social and physical anthropological factors, population or segment thereof to which the individual belongs, and variability in time, activity, etc. **Normal variability** frequently is used to cover the values falling within some range, usually the 95 per cent range of some factor or factors (mental, physical, emotional, social) measured in a random or selected sample of population or even an individual by standardized methods and recording systems during many observations. 3. *In chemistry*, referring to solutions containing the equivalent weight of a substance, in grams, in a liter. Abbreviated, N. 4. *In mathematics*, pertaining to a right angle, i.e., to a perpendicular line or plane. —**normalcy, normality,** *n.*

nor′mal bed ca·pac′ity. *In military medicine*, space for patients' beds measured in terms of the number of beds that can be set up in wards or rooms designed for patients' beds, spacing beds 8 feet between centers (approximately 100 square feet per bed); capacity for normal peacetime use.

nor′mal de′vi·ate. *In biological assay*, conversion of a percentage response, e.g., cases which responded to a certain dose, into the deviation on the normal frequency curve to which the percentage is equivalent, and used to obtain a linear relation between log dose and percentage response: also called *normal equivalent deviate.* See *probit.*

nor′mal dis″tri·bu′tion. *In statistics*, a frequency distribution, specified by its mathematical form and two constants: the mean and the standard deviation. This distribution is continuous and bell-shaped; 95% of the area covered by the distribution curve lies within two standard deviations below and two above the mean. This distribution describes adequately some individual biological measurements and many random sample measurements.

nor′mal prob″a·bil′i·ty curve. The curve represented by the equation $y = \frac{1}{\sigma\sqrt{2\pi}} \cdot e^{-\frac{x^2}{2\sigma^2}}$ in which the ordinate y shows the relative frequency of differences or deviations from the mean represented by the corresponding abscissa x in a large group of observations; σ represents the standard deviation of the distribution; π equals 3.1416 . . . ; e equals 2.7182 . . .

norm·er′gy [L. *norma*, rule; G. *ergon*, work]. *In allergy*, a normal degree of capacity to react. —**normer′gic,** *adj.*

nor′mo·blast [*norma;* G. *blastos*, germ]. 1. *In hematology*, the smallest of the nucleated precursors of the erythrocyte, and of slightly larger size than the adult erythrocyte. It has almost a full complement of hemoglobin, and shows a small, centrally placed chromatic and pyknotic nucleus. It is usually considered that a single normoblast gives rise to a single erythrocyte. Also called *acidophilic, eosinophilic,* or *orthochromatic erythroblast, karyocyte, metarubricyte, meta nitricyte.* 2. In some terminologies, any nucleated cell of the erythrocytic series.

acidophilic n. See *normoblast*, 1.

basophilic n. An early erythroblast.

early n. An early erythroblast.

intermediate n. See polychromatic *n.*

orthochromatic n. The last of the nucleated erythrocyte precursors with totally acidophilic cytoplasm.

polychromatic n. A normoblast in which cytoplasmic polychromatophilia is well established, indicating progression of hemoglobin synthesis: also called *intermediate n.*

pyknotic n. See *normoblast*, 1.

nor″mo·chro·mat′ic. Pertaining to the microscopic appearance of cells of the erythrocytic series which show normal staining characteristics, and are considered to have their full complement of hemoglobin and no residual basophilic material in their cytoplasm. —**normochroma′sia,** *n.*

nor″mo·chro′mi·a [*norma;* G. *chrōma*, color]. Blood with the normal hemoglobin content.

nor″mo·chro′mic. Pertaining to a blood picture

in which the erythrocytes have a mean corpuscular hemoglobin (MCH) or color index and a mean corpuscular hemoglobin concentration (MCHC) or saturation index within (plus or minus) two standard deviations of the mean normal as determined by the same method on the bloods of healthy persons of the same age and sex group. See normochromic normocytic *anemia*.

nor′mo·cyte [*norma;* G. *kytos,* cell]. An erythrocyte having both a diameter and a mean corpuscular volume (MCV) within (plus or minus) two standard deviations of the mean normal determined by the same method on the bloods of healthy persons of the same age and sex group. —**normocyt′ic,** *adj.*

nor″mo·cy·to′sis (nor″mo·sigh·to′sis) [*norma; kytos;* G. *-ōsis,* condition]. A normal state of the cells of the blood.

nor″mo·gly·ce′mi·a. Normal concentration of glucose in the blood.

nor″mo·ten′sive. Referring to normal blood pressure.

nor″mo·ther′mi·a. A state of normal temperature.

nor″mo·ton′ic [*norma;* G. *tonos,* tension]. Relating to normal muscular tonus.

nor″mo·to′pi·a. Normal location.

nor″mo·vo·le′mi·a [*norma;* L. *volumen,* volume; G. *haima,* blood]. The blood volume found in normal healthy individuals.

nor·nic′o·tine (nor·nick′o·teen, ·tin). A minor alkaloid occurring in tobacco. It is chemically related to nicotine and has similar action, but is less toxic.

Norris, Charles [*American physician,* 1867–1935]. With Alwin M. Pappenheimer and Thomas Flournoy, reported discovery of a spirochete in an American case of relapsing fever (1906).

North, Elisha [*American physician,* 1771–1843]. Remembered for being the first to describe spotted fever, or epidemic cerebrospinal meningitis, in his published work (1811).

Northrop, John Howard [*American scientist,* 1891–]. Known for his achievements in isolating crystallized enzymes and virus proteins in pure form. Nobel laureate with W. M. Stanley (1946).

nor·val′ine. $CH_3(CH_2)_2CH(NH_2)COOH$. α-Amino-n-valeric acid. An amino-acid component of casein, globin, and the protein of horns.

nose [AS. *nosu*]. The prominent organ in the center of the face; the upper part (regio olfactoria) constitutes the organ of smell, the lower part (regio respiratoria) the beginning of the respiratory tract, in which the inspired air is warmed, moistened, and deprived of impurities. See Plate 12.

bridge of n. The prominence formed by the junction of the nasal bones.

hammer n. Rhinophyma.

saddle n. One with a depression in the bridge due to the loss of the septum.

telescope n. Depression below the root of the nose as a result of necrosis of the septum and vomer, seen in leprosy.

nose′bleed″ [*nosu;* AS. *blēdan*]. A hemorrhage from the nose. Syn., *epistaxis.*

nose clip. A rubberized, spring-steel device worn by swimmers and divers to prevent the passage of water into the nose.

nose drops. A preparation containing medicaments, which is administered by placing drops in the nose.

nose′piece″ [*nosu;* OF. *pece*]. A mechanical device screwed into the object end of the tube of the microscope, for holding an objective.

revolving n. A device to be screwed on to the end of the microscope tube to permit the mounting of two to four objectives, any of which may be swung into place, ready for use, by turning the nosepiece into the desired position.

nos·er″es·the′si·a (noss·err″ess·thee′zhuh, ·zee·uh) [G. *noseros,* unhealthy; *aisthēsis,* perception]. Perverted sensibility.

nos′o-, nos- [G. *nosos,* disease]. A combining form signifying *disease.*

nos″o·chor″o·lo′gi·a (noss″o·kor″o·lo′jee·uh). See *nosochthonography.*

nos″och·tho·nog′ra·phy (noss″ock·tho·nog′ruh-fee) [*nosos;* G. *chthōn,* earth; *graphein,* to write]. Geography of endemic diseases; medical geography.

nos″o·co′mi·al [*nosos;* G. *komein,* to attend to]. 1. Pertaining to a hospital. *Obs.* 2. Applied to disease caused or aggravated by hospital life. *Obs.*

nos″o·co′mi·um [*nosos; komein*]. A hospital. *Obs.*

no·sog′e·ny (no·sodj′i·nee) [*nosos;* G. *genesthai,* from *gignesthai,* to be produced]. The development of diseases. —**nosogenet′ic,** *adj.*

nos″o·ge·og′ra·phy. See *nosochthonography.* —**nosogeograph′ic,** *adj.*

no·sol′o·gy [*nosos;* G. *logos,* word]. The science of the classification of diseases. —**nosolog′ic,** *adj.*

nos″o·ma′ni·a [*nosos;* G. *mania,* madness]. 1. A morbid dread of disease. 2. A delusion that one is suffering from disease.

no·som′e·try. See *morbidity rate.*

nos″o·par′a·sites [*nosos;* G. *parasitos,* parasite]. Microorganisms found in conjunction with a disease process which, while capable of modifying the course of the disease, are not its cause. *Obs.*

nosophen. Trade-mark for iodophthalein.

nos″o·pho′bi·a [*nosos;* G. *phobos,* fear]. The exaggerated fear of disease; pathophobia.

nos′o·phyte [*nosos;* G. *phyton,* plant]. Any pathogenic vegetable microorganism.

No″sop·syl′lus [*nosos;* G. *psylla,* flea]. A genus of fleas.

N. fasciatus. A species of rat fleas which may transmit plague.

nos″o·tax′y. Classification of diseases.

nostal. Trade-mark for 5-isopropyl-5-β-bromallyl barbituric acid, used as a hypnotic. See *propallylonal.*

nos·tal′gi·a [G. *nostos,* return home; *algos,* pain]. Homesickness. —**nostalgic,** *adj.*

nos·tal′gy [*nostos; algos*]. Nostalgia.

nos″to·ma′ni·a [*nostos;* G. *mania,* madness]. Nostalgia amounting to monomania.

nos·top′a·thy. Pathogenic homecoming, as observed in veterans discharged from military service or others who have spent a considerable length of time in institutions such as hospitals or prisons. The situational factor of returning home represents a major psychological stress which precipitates illness. The stress may be a fear of assuming adult responsibilities, a reaction against a dependency situation, guilt feelings, or difficulties in controlling instinctual rivalry.

nos″to·pho′bi·a. A fear of returning home.

nos′tras [L., of our country]. Denoting a disease belonging to the country in which it is described, in contradistinction to a similar disease originating elsewhere, as cholera nostras as distinguished from Asiatic cholera.

nos′trate [*nostras*]. Endemic.

nos′tril [AS. *nosthyrl*]. One of the external orifices of the nose. Syn., *naris.*

nos′trum [neut. sing. of L. *noster,* our]. A quack medicine; a secret medicine.

no·tal′gi·a [G. *nōton,* back; *algos,* pain]. Any pain in the back. *Obs.*

n. paresthetica. A sensory disturbance of the region supplied by the posterior branches of the lumbar nerves; occurs occasionally in vertebral lesions.

no″tan·ce·pha′li·a [*nōton;* G. *a-*, not; *kephalē*, head]. Congenital absence of the occipital part of the cranium.

no″tan·en″ce·pha′li·a [*nōton;* G. *anegkephalos*, without brain]. Congenital absence of the cerebellum.

no·ta′tin. An antibiotic from *Penicillium notatum;* soluble in water, insoluble in organic solvents. It acts in the presence of glucose on Gram-positive and Gram-negative bacteria. Also called *corylophilline*, *Escherichia coli factor*, *mycoin*, *penatin*, *penicillin-B*.

no·ta′tion. A system of symbols to indicate in brief form more extensive ideas or data.

dental n. One to indicate the type and location of a tooth in the dentition. Commonly a vertical line separates right and left sides, and a horizontal line the upper from the lower teeth. Palmer's numerical notation for the permanent human dentition is:

	87654321	12345678	
right			left
	87654321	12345678	

For the deciduous dentition:

	V IV III II I	I II III IV V	
right			left
	V IV III II I	I II III IV V	

For example, 2| means lower right lateral permanent incisor; |III is upper left deciduous canine.

Another system uses I_1 I_2 C P_1 (or pm_1) P_2 M_1 M_2 M_3 for the permanent teeth and i_1 i_2 c m_1 m_2 for the deciduous set (I for incisor, C for canine, P for premolar, M for molar).

notch [perhaps from OF. *osche*, from *oschier*, to notch]. A deep indentation. —**notched,** *adj*.

acetabular n. A notch in the lower border of the acetabulum.

angular n. A notch in the lesser curvature of the stomach formed at the junction of its body and the pyloric portion. Also called *angular incisure.*

anterior cerebellar n. A broad, flat depression on the anterior margin of the upper surface of the cerebellum, between the two hemispheres.

cardiac n. A notch in the anterior border of the left lung, occupied by the heart within the pericardium.

clavicular n. A depression on each superior lateral aspect of the upper end of the sternum articulating with the clavicles.

costal n. One of the facets on the lateral border of the sternum for articulation with the costal cartilages.

ethmoidal n. The gap between the two orbital plates of the frontal bone, filled in the articulated skull by the cribriform plate of the ethmoid.

frontal n. A notch in the superior orbital margin, medial to the supraorbital notch, which transmits the frontal artery and nerve.

gastric n. See angular *n.*

greater sciatic n. A notch between the spine of the ischium and the posterior inferior iliac spine; it is converted into a foramen by the sacrospinous and sacrotuberous ligaments.

infrasternal n. The depression in the anterior abdominal wall, superficial to the xiphoid cartilage.

interlobar n. A fissure separating the superior and inferior lobes of the left lung.

interspinous n. The notch between the posterior superior and posterior inferior iliac spines.

intertragic n. The notch between the tragus and the antitragus of the external ear.

jugular n. of the occipital bone. A concavity in the inferior border, posterior to the jugular process, which, in the articulated skull, forms the posterior part of the jugular foramen.

jugular n. of the sternum. The depression on the upper surface of the manubrium between the two clavicles.

jugular n. of the temporal bone. A small notch in the petrous portion which corresponds to the jugular notch of the occipital bone, with which it forms the jugular foramen.

lacrimal n. A notch on the inner margin of the orbital surface of the maxilla which receives the lacrimal bone.

lesser sciatic n. The notch below the spine of the ischium which is converted to a foramen by the sacrotuberous and sacrospinous ligaments; it transmits the tendon of the obturator internus and the internal pudendal vessels and pudendal nerve.

mandibular n. The deep concavity between the condyloid and coronoid processes of the mandible.

mastoid n. See digastric *groove.*

median prostatic n. A notch in the posterior border of the base of the prostate.

nasal n. (a) The concave medial margin of the anterior surface of the maxilla; the lateral margin of the apertura piriformis. (b) An uneven interval between the internal angular processes of the frontal bone which articulates with the nasal and maxillary bones.

n. of Rivinus. Tympanic *n.*: old term.

pancreatic n. A groove in the pancreas for the superior mesenteric artery and vein, separating the uncinate process from the rest of the head of the pancreas.

parietal n. The angle formed by the squamous and mastoid portions of the temporal bone.

postcondylar n. A notch in the lower surface of the occipital bone between the condyle and the foramen magnum.

posterior cerebellar n. A narrow notch separating the cerebellar hemispheres posteriorly.

radial n. A depression on the lateral surface of the coronoid process of the ulna for articulation with the head of the radius.

sacrococcygeal n. The lateral notch at the point of union of the coccyx and sacrum.

scapular n. The notch in the upper border of the scapula at the base of the coracoid process for the passage of the suprascapular nerve.

semilunar n. The concavity on the proximal end of the ulna for articulation with the trochlea of the humerus.

sphenopalatine n. A deep notch separating the orbital and sphenoid processes of the palatine bone.

supraorbital n. Supraorbital foramen.

suprasternal n. The jugular notch of the sternum.

tentorial n. See *incisure* of the tentorium.

thyroid n. A deep notch in the upper margin of the thyroid cartilage between the two laminas.

trochlear n. The semilunar notch.

tympanic n. The gap in the tympanic sulcus occupied by the flaccid, highest portion of the tympanic membrane. Also called *incisure of Rivinus.*

ulnar n. A depression on the medial surface of the lower end of the radius for articulation with the head of the ulna.

umbilical n. A deep notch in the anterior border of the liver, marking the attachment of the falciform ligament.

vertebral n. One of the concavities above and below the pedicles of the vertebrae; in the articulated vertebral column, the notches of contiguous pairs of bones form the intervertebral foramens.

note [L. *nota*, mark]. A sound.

amphoric n. A low-pitched, hollow sound, obtained over a large cavity of the chest, or over pneumothorax.

bell n. A clear, ringing note brought out by percussing with coins over pneumothorax.

cracked-pot n. A note with a peculiar clinking quality, heard on percussion over a superficial pulmonary cavity.

percussion n. The sound elicited on percussion, usually described as flat, dull, resonant, or tympanitic.

note′-blind″ness. See *amusia.*

No·te′chis (no·tee′kiss). A genus of poisonous terrestrial snakes belonging to the family Elapidae.

N. scutatus. That species found in Australia which possesses a very powerful neurotoxic venom; known as the tiger snake.

no″ten·ceph′a·lo·cele [G. *nōton*, back; *egkephalos*, brain; *kēlē*, hernia]. An occipital hydrencephalocele.

no″ten·ceph′a·lus [*nōton; egkephalos*]. An individual with occipital encephalocele, or more usually hydrencephalocele.

Nothnagel, Carl Wilhelm Hermann (1841–1905). One of the leading clinicians of his time, especially eminent for his knowledge of gastrointestinal and chronic diseases. He described a general vasoconstricting storm, producing paroxysmal hypertension, with or without angina pectoris, sometimes called *Nothnagel's disease* or *syndrome* (also see *acroparesthesia*), and also described unilateral oculomotor paralysis with ipsilateral cerebellar ataxia, due to a lesion involving the third cranial nerve or nucleus and the brachium conjunctivum.

no′ti·fi″a·ble [L. *notificare*, to make known]. Pertaining to a disease which must be made known to health authorities.

no′to·chord (no′to·kord) [G. *nōton*, back; *chordē*, string]. An elongated cord of cells enclosed in a structureless sheath, which is the primitive axial skeleton of the embryo. It serves as a focal axis about which the vertebral bodies develop and persists as the nuclei pulposi of the intervertebral disks. Also called *chorda dorsalis.* —**notochord′al,** *adj.*

No″to·ed′res (no″to·ed′reez). A genus of mange mites whose species infest cats and rats, producing serious lesions.

no″to·gen′e·sis [*nōton;* G. *genesis*, production]. The development of the notochord.

no·tom′e·lus [*nōton;* G. *melos*, limb]. A monster in which supernumerary limbs are attached to the back.

novaldin. Trade-mark for sodium phenyldimethylpyrazolon-methylaminomethane sulfonate, an antipyretic and analgesic substance.

novarsan. A trade-mark for neoarsphenamine.

novarsenobenzol. Neoarsphenamine.

novaspirin. Trade-mark for a brand of salicitrin; methylene citrylsalicylic acid. The substance is used as an analgesic.

novasurol. Trade-mark for *merbaphen.*

novatophan. Trade-mark for methyl cinchophen.

novatrin. A trade-mark for homatropine methylbromide.

novatropine. Trade-mark for the methylbromide of the alkaloid homatropine. The substance is used in the treatment of gastrointestinal spasm and hyperchlorhydria.

novocain. Trade-mark for a brand of procaine hydrochloride.

Novy, Frederick George [*American bacteriologist,* 1864–]. With MacNeal, devised a nutrient blood agar used especially for the cultivation of trypanosomes; called *Novy-MacNeal agar* or *medium.* Nicolle's modification of this for the cultivation of *Leishmania* is known as the *NNN medium.*

nox′ious (nock′shus) [L. *noxius*, harmful]. Harmful; poisonous or deleterious.

Noyes, Henry Drury [*American ophthalmologist,* 1832–1900]. Described and introduced a number of operations in ophthalmic surgery, such as those for the relief of cataract, entropion, and staphyloma. His operation for strabismus consists of advancement of the elongated tendon.

NP *In U. S. Army medicine,* neuropsychiatric.

Np Chemical symbol for neptunium.

NPH An insulin of intermediate duration of action, the *N* referring to neutral, the *P* to protamine, and the *H* to Hagedorn, in whose laboratory the product was originally developed.

N. P. N. Nonprotein nitrogen.

n-rays. A nonluminous radiation of lower wave length than visible light. Emitted by an x-ray tube, the sun, or a Welsbach burner; passes through thin metals, and increases the luminosity of phosphorescent bodies. Discovered by Blondlot.

Nt Chemical symbol for niton.

nu′bile (new′bil) [L. *nubilis*, marriageable]. Marriageable; of an age for childbearing. —**nubil′ity,** *n.*

nu·cel′lus [L. *nucella*, little nut]. *In botany,* the central part or nucleus of an ovule.

nu′ces (new′seez). Plural of nux.

nu′cha (new′kuh) [Ar. *nukhā*, spinal marrow]. The nape of the neck. —**nuchal,** *adj.*

Nuck, Anton [*Dutch anatomist,* 1650–92]. Described a diverticulum, a shallow, peritoneal invagination in the female homologous to the processus vaginalis in the male; called *Nuck's diverticulum, canal of Nuck.* The hydrocele sometimes seen in this canal is called *Nuck's hydrocele.*

nu′cla·den. See *myorgal.*

nu′cle·ar [L. *nucleus*, nut]. Pertaining to, or resembling, a nucleus.

nu′cle·ar dis″in·te·gra′tion. Any transformation or change involving atomic nuclei.

nu′cle·ar fis′sion. *In chemistry* and *in physics,* the splitting of certain heavy nuclei into two large fragments, accompanied by the emission of neutrons and the release of large amounts of energy.

nu′cle·ar re·ac′tion. See under *reaction.*

nu′cle·ar re·ac′tor. An apparatus in which nuclear fission may be sustained in a self-supporting chain reaction. It includes fissionable material such as uranium or plutonium (referred to as *fuel*), and generally a moderating material such as carbon or beryllium or heavy water; also, a reflector to conserve escaping neutrons, and provision for heat removal. Syn., *pile, reactor.*

nu′cle·ase (new′klee·ace, ·aze). An enzyme capable of splitting nucleic acids to nucleotides, nucleosides, or the components of the latter. Nucleases are found in animal organs, as liver, pancreas, and thymus, and in germinating seeds. See Table of Enzymes in the Appendix.

nu′cle·a″ted [L. *nucleatus*, having a kernel]. Possessing a nucleus.

nu″cle·a′tion. The starting of chemical or physical changes at discrete points in a system, as the formation of nuclei for condensation of vapors or for formation of crystals in a liquid.

nu′cle·i (new′klee·eye). Plural of nucleus.

nu·cle′ic ac′id. One of a group of compounds found in nuclei and cytoplasm. See *desoxyribonucleic acid, ribonucleic acid.*

nu′cle·ide. A compound of nuclein with some metal, as iron, copper, silver, mercury, etc.

nu′cle·i·form″, nu·cle′i·form″ [L. *nucleus*, nut; *forma*, form]. Resembling a nucleus.

nu′cle·in. Any one of a group of ill-defined complexes of protein and nucleic acid occurring in the nuclei of cells. On hydrolysis, they yield simple proteins and nucleic acid.

n. therapy. The employment of nuclein from different glands and blood serum in the treatment of disease.

nu′cle·in·ase (new′klee·in·ace, ·aze). An enzyme which resolves nucleic acid into nucleotides.

nu″cle·in′ic ac′id. See *nucleic acid.*

nu′cle·o-, nucle- [*nucleus*]. A combining form signifying *relating to a nucleus.*

nu″cle·o·al·bu′min [*nucleus;* L. *albus*, white]. A compound of nucleic acid and albumin.

nu″cle·o·chy·le′ma (·kigh·lee′muh) [*nucleus;* G. *chylos*, juice]. Old term for nuclear sap or juice. See *nucleohyaloplasm.*

nu′cle·o·chyme (new′klee·o·kime) [*nucleus;* G. *chymos*, juice]. Nucleochylema.

nu″cle·o·cy″to·plas′mic (·sigh″to·plaz′mick) [*nucleus;* G. *kytos*, cell; *plasma*, anything formed]. Referring to both the nucleus and cytoplasm of a cell, as nucleocytoplasmic ratio.

nu″cle·of′u·gal (new″klee·off′yoo·gul, new″klee·o-few′gul) [*nucleus;* L. *fugere*, to flee]. Moving away from a nucleus.

nu″cle·o·his′tone [*nucleus;* G. *histos*, web]. A basic protein from cell nuclei.

nu″cle·o·hy′a·lo·plasm (·high′uh·lo·plaz·um, ·high·al′o·plaz·um) [*nucleus;* G. *hyalos*, glass; *plasma*, anything formed]. Old term for the viscous fluid material occupying space in the nucleus not taken by the nucleolus, linin, or chromatin. Now called *nuclear sap, nuclear juice.*

nu′cle·oid [*nucleus;* G. *eidos*, form]. Shaped like a nucleus.

nu′cle·oid. A finely granular or fibrillar substance in certain erythrocytes, which resembles a nucleus.

nu′cle·ol. See *nuclein.*

nu′cle·ole. See *nucleolus.*

nu·cle′o·li·form [*nucleolus*, dim. from *nucleus;* L. *forma*, form]. Resembling a nucleolus.

nu·cle′o·lin [*nucleolus*]. The substance of which the nucleolus is composed.

nu·cle′o·loid [*nucleolus;* G. *eidos*, form]. Resembling a nucleolus.

nu·cle′o·lus [L.]. A small spherical body within the cell nucleus. Syn., *plasmosome.* **—nucleolar,**

false n. See *karyosome.*

true n. See *plasmosome.*

nu″cle·o·mi″cro·so′ma [L. *nucleus*, nut; G. *mikros*, small; *sōma*, body]. Any one of the many minute bodies that make up each fiber of the nuclear framework.

nu′cle·on. Protons and neutrons: collective term.

nu″cle·on′ics. The study of atomic nuclei, including the application of nuclear science in all fields of specialization; nuclear technology.

nu″cle·op′e·tal (new″klee·op′i·tul, new″klee·o-pet′ul) [*nucleus;* L. *petere*, to seek]. Seeking the nucleus; said of the movement of the male pronucleus toward the female pronucleus.

Nu″cle·oph′a·ga [*nucleus;* G. *phagein*, to eat]. A parasite which destroys the nuclei of amebas.

nu′cle·o·plasm [*nucleus;* G. *plasma*, anything formed]. The protoplasm of the nucleus. Syn., *karyoplasm.*

nu″cle·o·pro′te·id. See *nucleoprotein.*

nu″cle·o·pro′te·in [*nucleus;* G. *prōteios*, of first rank]. A protein constituent of cell nuclei, consisting of nucleic acid and a basic protein. On hydrolysis, nucleoproteins yield purine bases, pyrimidine bases, phosphoric acid, and a carbohydrate. *adj.* See American Classification of Proteins in the Appendix.

nu″cle·o·re·tic′u·lum [*nucleus;* L. *reticulum*, little net]. Any network contained within a nucleus.

nu″cle·o·si′dase. An enzyme that catalyzes the hydrolysis of a nucleoside into its component pentose and purine or pyrimidine base.

nu′cle·o·side. A glycoside resulting from the removal of phosphate from a nucleotide. It is a combination of a sugar (pentose) with a purine or pyrimidine base.

nu″cle·o·spin′dle [*nucleus;* AS. *spinel*]. A mitotic spindle formed from the nuclear substance, as in some forms of anastral mitosis.

nu″cle·o·ti′dase (new″klee·o·tye′dace, ·daze, new″klee·ot′i·). One of a group of nucleophosphatases which split phosphoric acid from nucleotides, leaving nucleosides.

nu′cle·o·tide. The combination of a purine or pyrimidine base with a sugar and phosphoric acid. The basic structural unit of nucleic acid.

phosphopyridine nucleotides. See *phosphopyridine nucleotides.*

nu″cle·o·tox′in [*nucleus;* G. *toxikon*, poison]. A toxin derived from cell nuclei; any toxin affecting the nuclei of cells.

nu′cle·us (pl. *nuclei*) [L.]. 1. The differentiated central protoplasm of a cell; its trophic center. 2. A collection of nerve cells in the central nervous system concerned with a particular function. 3. A stable and characteristic complex of atoms to which other atoms may be attached. 4. The center around which the mass of a crystal aggregates. 5. The center of an atom consisting of protons, neutrons, and alpha particles.

abducens n. A nucleus lying under the floor of the fourth ventricle at the junction of the pons and medulla which gives origin to the abducens nerve.

accessory n. of the facial nerve. A small group of motor cells, dorsomedial to and functionally a part of the facial nucleus.

ambiguous n. A column of cells lying in the lateral half of the reticular formation whose cells give origin to efferent fibers of the glossopharyngeal and vagus nerves. Also called *n. ambiguus.*

amygdaloid n. Gray matter which is continuous with the cortex of the hippocampal gyrus lying in the amygdaloid tubercle at the tip of the inferior horn of the lateral ventricle; part of olfactory pathways.

angular n. See superior vestibular *n.*

anterior hypothalamic n. See *hypothalamus, anterior region.*

anterior median n. Vertical plate of small cells, in front of and ventral to the Edinger-Westphal nucleus, which perhaps represents the rostral continuation of the latter.

anterior nuclei of the thalamus. The nuclei which occupy the anterior part of the thalamus and are separated from the rest of it by the limbs of the internal medullary lamina. They receive fibers from the mammillothalamic tract and send fibers to the gyrus cinguli.

anterior ventral n. of the thalamus. One of the nuclei of the ventral division of the lateral nuclei of the thalamus which receives fibers from the globus pallidus and sends fibers to the corpus striatum: also called *n. ventralis anterior.*

arcuate n. (a) An irregular small flattened cellular mass located in the medulla ventral to the pyramids. (b) The posteromedial ventral nucleus of the thalamus, which receives fibers from the secondary trigeminal tract.

association nuclei of the thalamus. Nuclei which receive fibers from other thalamic nuclei or

from sensory collaterals and send their efferent fibers to the association areas of the cortex.
atomic n. See *nucleus*, 5.
basal magnocellular n. See dorsal *n.* of Clarke.
basal olfactory nuclei. A collective name applied to the gray substance of the olfactory tract, olfactory trigone, olfactory area, gyrus subcallosus, and parolfactory area.
branchiomotor n. of the facial nerve. See facial *n.*
caudate n. An elongated arched gray mass which projects into and forms part of the lateral wall of the lateral ventricle; part of the corpus striatum.
central magnocellular n. See *n.* proprius of dorsal horn.
central n. of the thalamus. See centromedian *n.* of the thalamus.
centrodorsal n. See *n.* proprius of dorsal horn.
centromedian n. of the thalamus. One of the medial nuclei of the thalamus, partly embedded in the internal medullary lamina: also called *central n. of the thalamus, n. centrum medianum.*
cleavage n. The nucleus of the ovum which controls or initiates cleavage. It may be syngamic, parthenogenetic, or androgenic.
cochlear nuclei. Nuclear masses in which the fibers of the cochlear nerve terminate. These are the ventral cochlear nucleus and the dorsal cochlear nucleus located, respectively, ventrad and dorsad to the restiform body.
commissural n. The collection of nerve cells in the medulla oblongata formed by the junction of the nuclei of the solitary tract at the posterior end of the fourth ventricle.
conjugation n. The segmentation nucleus.
cornucommissural nuclei. Two cell columns extending the length of the spinal cord and occupying the medial margin of the dorsal and ventral horn. These nuclei probably relay impulses across the midline.
cuneate n. The collection of nerve cells lying in the dorsal aspect of the medulla oblongata in which the fibers of the fasciculus cuneatus terminate and which give origin to part of the fibers of the medial lemniscus. Formerly called *nucleus of Burdach.*
Deiters' n. The lateral vestibular nucleus.
dentate n. A large, irregular, ovoid, flattened mass located in the medullary center of the cerebellum whose cells give rise to fibers that form the brachium conjunctivum.
descending vestibular n. See spinal vestibular *n.*
disseminate n. See *n.* proprius of ventral horn.
dorsal accessory olivary n. See accessory *olive.*
dorsal lateral n. This and the posterior lateral nuclei are in the dorsal division of the lateral nuclei of thalamus. They are continuous with the pulvinar, receive fibers from other thalamic nuclei, and connect with the cortex of the parietal lobe.
dorsal motor n. of the vagus. The column of cells in the medulla oblongata at the floor of the fourth ventricle which gives origin to preganglionic parasympathetic fibers of the vagus nerve.
dorsal n. of Clarke. A nucleus at the base of the dorsal gray horn of the spinal cord; contains the cells of origin of the dorsal spinocerebellar tract. Also called *Clarke's column, n. dorsalis, basal magnocellular n., spinocerebellar n.*
dorsal paramedian n. A band of small cells in the dorsal aspect of the reticular formation of the medulla oblongata on either side of the midline just beneath the ependyma extending the entire length of the fourth ventricle.
dorsal sensory n. of the vagus. A column of nerve cells in the medulla oblongata lateral to the dorsal motor nucleus of the vagus in which part of the fibers of the solitary tract terminate.
dorsomedial hypothalamic n. See *hypothalamus, middle region.*
dorsomedial n. of the thalamus. One of the medial nuclei of the thalamus, located between the internal medullary lamina and the wall of the third ventricle, consisting of a medial part which receives fibers from the midline nuclei and sends fibers to the hypothalamus, and a lateral part which receives fibers from the thalamic nuclei and sends fibers to the frontal lobe: also called *n. medialis dorsalis.*
Edinger-Westphal n. A nucleus in the midbrain dorsomedial to the oculomotor nucleus which gives origin to preganglionic parasympathetic fibers for the constrictor pupillae and ciliary muscle of the ciliary body: also called the *pupilloconstrictor center.*
emboliform n. A nucleus in the medullary portion of the cerebellum located mediad to the upper part of the dentate nucleus. It receives afferent fibers from the paleocerebellum and sends efferent fibers into the brachium conjunctivum.
entopeduncular n. Cells located along the fibers of the ansa lenticularis, which apparently receive fibers from the putamen and caudate nucleus and contribute fibers to the ansa lenticularis. Syn., *n. of the ansa lenticularis.*
external cuneate n. A group of cells lateral to the cuneate nucleus whose axons form the dorsal external arcuate fibers: also called *magnocellular n. of dorsal column, n. of Monakow.* Syn., *lateral cuneate nucleus.*
facial n. An ovoid collection of nerve cells in the lateral portion of the reticular formation of the pons, giving origin to motor fibers of the facial nerve.
fastigial n. A nucleus in the cerebellum situated dorsad to the upper end of the fourth ventricle which receives fibers from the vestibular nerve and superior vestibular nucleus and sends efferent fibers into the brain stem.
germinal n. Synonym for pronucleus.
globose n. A nucleus of the cerebellum located between the fastigial and emboliform nuclei. Receives fibers from the paleocerebellum and sends efferent fibers to the red nucleus.
glossopharyngeal nuclei. See *n. ambiguus, inferior salivatory n., n. of tractus solitarius.*
gracilis n. A nucleus in the dorsal aspect of the medulla oblongata in which fibers of the fasciculus gracilis terminate and which gives origin to part of the fibers of the medial lemniscus. Formerly called *nucleus of Goll.*
gustatory n. A nucleus in the medulla oblongata medial to the nucleus of the solitary tract in which terminate the gustatory fibers of the chorda tympani, glossopharyngeal and vagus nerves.
habenular n. The nucleus of the habenula which serves as an olfactory correlation center.
hypoglossal n. A long and cylindrical nucleus located lateral to the midline extending throughout most of the length of the medulla oblongata whose cells give origin to the motor fibers of the hypoglossal nerve.
inferior central n. The nucleus of the raphe.
inferior olivary n. A conspicuous convoluted gray band opening medially, dorsal to the pyramids, occupying the entire upper two-thirds of the medulla oblongata, the cells of which give rise to most of the fibers of the olivocerebellar tract: also called *oliva, olive, inferior olive, olivary body.*
inferior salivatory n. An ill-defined nucleus anterior to the ambiguous nucleus which sends

preganglionic autonomic fibers to the otic ganglion via the glossopharyngeal nerve. Concerned in the regulation of secretion of the parotid gland.

intercalated mammillary n. One in the mammillary body, lateral to the medial mammillary nucleus.

intercalated n. A nucleus of the medulla oblongata in the central gray matter of the ventricular floor located between the hypoglossal nucleus and the dorsal motor nucleus of the vagus.

intermediomedial n. Diffusely organized cell group in the intermediate gray column of the spinal cord, most prominent in the upper cervical segments, which sends their axons to the lateral white funiculus of the same side.

interpeduncular n. A nucleus of the brain stem located between the cerebral peduncles, in which terminate the fibers of the habenulopeduncular tract.

interstitial n. of Cajal. A small nucleus in the dorsomedial part of the tegmentum just anterior to the oculomotor nucleus. It receives fibers from the vestibular nuclei, globus pallidus, superior colliculi, and substantia nigra. It contributes fibers to the medial longitudinal fasciculus.

intertrigeminal n. A small group of cells located near the motor nucleus of the trigeminal nerve. This nucleus receives collaterals from the mesencephalic nucleus; and its axons send collaterals to the motor nucleus of the trigeminal nerve, and go to the locus caeruleus.

intralaminar nuclei of the thalamus. Diffusely organized thalamic nuclei located in the internal medullary lamina. The lateral central nucleus, paracentral nucleus, parafascicular nucleus, and submedial nucleus, belong to this group.

lacrimatory n. One located near the superior salivatory nucleus at the junction of the pons and medulla. Its axons go to the sphenopalatine ganglion.

lateral central n. of the thalamus. One of the intralaminar nuclei of the thalamus, located dorsally in the internal medullary lamina.

lateral cuneate n. See external cuneate *n.*

lateral hypothalamic n. See *hypothalamus, middle region.*

lateral mammillary n. A nucleus in the mammillary body, ventrolateral to the intercalated mammillary nucleus.

lateral nuclei of the thalamus. The nuclei lying between the internal medullary lamina and the internal capsule. The anterior ventral, dorsal lateral, lateral ventral, posterior lateral, posterolateral ventral, posteromedial ventral nuclei, and the reticular nucleus of the thalamus belong to this group.

lateral reticular n. A nucleus, in the lateral part of the reticular formation, which receives spinoreticular fibers from the dorsal gray columns of the spinal cord and perhaps also collaterals from the ventral spinocerebellar tract. Its axons contribute to the ventral external arcuate fibers.

lateral sympathetic n. Cells of the intermediolateral cell column of the spinal cord, extending from the eighth cervical to the second lumbar segment.

lateral ventral n. of the thalamus. One of the nuclei of the ventral division of the lateral nuclei of the thalamus which receives fibers from the superior cerebellar peduncle and sends fibers to the motor cortex and premotor cortex of the frontal lobe.

lateral vestibular n. A group of scattered large cells at the caudal border of the pons between the restiform body and the spinal tract of the trigeminal nerve. Also called *Deiters' n.*

lenticular n. The globus pallidus and putamen considered together.

lentiform n. Old term for lenticular nucleus.

magnocellular n. of the dorsal column. See external cuneate *n.*

main sensory n. of the trigeminal nerve. A large gray mass in the tegmentum dorsolateral to the entering fibers of the fifth nerve in which most of the afferent fibers terminate. Probably concerned with touch and pressure.

mammilloinfundibular n. The posterior and lateral hypothalamic nuclei collectively, which together furnish the efferent fibers to the lower levels of the brain stem.

marginal n. See posteromarginal *n.*

masticator n. The motor nucleus of the trigeminal nerve.

medial accessory olivary n. See accessory *olive.*

medial mammillary n. The main nucleus of the mammillary body located on its medial aspect.

medial nuclei of the thalamus. The nuclei located between the midline nuclei of the thalamus and the internal medullary lamina, including the centromedian and dorsomedial nuclei.

medial sympathetic n. A column of cells extending from the third lumbar segment to the conus terminalis, lying along the medial border of the ventral horn in the lumbar and upper sacral segments and mingled with the inferior portion of the intermediolateral column in the lower sacral segments. Its axons go to the pelvic ganglia. Also called *n. myoleioticus.*

medial vestibular n. A nucleus of the floor of the fourth ventricle medial to the vestibular root and lateral to the ala cinerea. Also called *principal vestibular n.*, *triangular n.*, and *n. of Schwalbe.*

mesencephalic n. of the trigeminal nerve. A flat column of large round cells ventrolateral to the aqueduct of the midbrain whose cells give origin to the mesencephalic root of the trigeminal nerve.

midline nuclei of the thalamus. Diffusely organized thalamic nuclei, located near the wall of the third ventricle and in the massa intermedia, which are connected to the hypothalamic and intralaminar nuclei.

motor n. A nucleus giving origin to a motor nerve.

motor n. of the spinal cord. A group of somatic motor cells located in the ventral horn, whose axons go to striated voluntary muscles.

motor n. of the trigeminal nerve. An ovoid column of cells in the reticular formation dorsal to the superior olivary nucleus which gives origin to motor fibers of the trigeminal nerve.

motor reticular n. Diffuse cell groups in the reticular formation. Their axons, mostly uncrossed, bifurcate into ascending and descending branches and form the reticulobulbar, reticulospinal, reticulo-olivary, and reticuloreticular tracts. They receive fibers from secondary afferent neurons, the red nucleus, tectum of the midbrain, and corpus striatum.

n. of the ansa lenticularis. See entopeduncular *n.*

n. of Bekhterev. See superior vestibular *n.*

n. centrum medianum. See centromedian *n.* of thalamus.

n. conterminalis. Retropyramidal nucleus.

n. of Darkshevich. A nucleus located at the edge of the central gray matter dorsomediad to the red nucleus in the upper midbrain. It sends crossed and uncrossed fibers to the medial longitudinal fasciculus. Also called *n. of the posterior commissure.*

n. dorsalis. See dorsal *n.* of Clarke.

n. eminentiae teretis. The lateral extension of the dorsal paramedian nucleus.

nuclei of the hypothalamus. See *hypothalamus.*
n. of the inferior colliculus. An ovoid mass of cells in the body of the inferior colliculus.
n. intercalatus. See intercalated *n.*
n. of the lateral lemniscus. A group of nerve cells of the upper pons in the course of the lateral lemniscus. It receives fibers from the lateral lemniscus and sends its axons medially to cross the midline.
n. magnocellularis pericornaulis. See posteromarginal *n.*
nuclei of the mammillary body. See *hypothalamus, caudal region.*
n. medialis dorsalis. See dorsomedial *n.* of thalamus.
n. of Monakow. See external cuneate *n.*
n. myoleioticus. See medial sympathetic *n.*
n. of origin. A collection of nerve cells in the central nervous system giving rise to the fibers of a nerve or a nerve tract.
n. of Perlia. A medially placed cell group of the oculomotor nuclei which has been regarded as the mesencephalic center for convergence of the eyes.
n. pigmentosus pontis. See *locus caeruleus.*
n. of the posterior commissure. See *n.* of Darkshevich.
n. prepositus. A group of large cells, extending from the oral limits of the hypoglossal nucleus to the caudal limit of the abducens nucleus, which receives fibers from the periependymal tract and medial vestibular nucleus and which sends fibers to the reticular formation and probably also to the hypoglossal, dorsal motor vagus, and secretory nuclei.
n. proprius of the dorsal horn. A poorly defined cell column in the head and cervix of the dorsal horn, which gives origin to the long crossed spinothalamic and spinotectal fibers: also called *central magnocellular n., centrodorsal n., spinothalamic n.*
n. proprius of the ventral horn. Small cells, scattered between the somatic motor cells in the ventral horn, which may serve for intranuclear connections: also called *disseminate n.*
n. pulposus. The pulpy body at the center of an intervertebral disk; a remnant of the notochord.
n. of the raphe. A collection of nerve cells in the midportion of the reticular formation of the medulla oblongata.
n. reuniens. One of the midline nuclei of the thalamus, located in the massa intermedia and adjacent ventricular wall.
n. of Roller. A group of cells lying ventrad to the hypoglossal nucleus: also called *sublingual nucleus.*
n. ruber. See red *n.*
n. of Schwalbe. The medial or principal vestibular nucleus.
n. of the spinal tract of the trigeminal nerve. The column of cells lying medial to the entire length of the spinal tract of the trigeminal nerve in which the fibers of the tract terminate.
n. sympathicus lateralis. The lateral sympathetic nucleus.
n. of the tegmental field. Cells scattered among the fibers of the tegmental field, considered a continuation of the mesencephalic reticular formation.
n. of termination. A collection of nerve cells in which the axons of a nerve tract or a nerve root terminate.
n. of the tractus solitarius. A column of cells in the medulla oblongata surrounding the solitary tract and in which part of the fibers of the solitary tract terminate.
n. of the trapezoid body. A group of cells scattered among the fibers of the trapezoid body.
n. ventralis anterior. See anterior ventral *n.* of thalamus.
n. ventralis lateralis. See lateral ventral *n.* of thalamus.
oculomotor n. A wedge-shaped nucleus lying just rostrally to the trochlear nucleus a little below the aqueduct near the median line. It gives origin to motor fibers for the extrinsic muscles of the eye supplied by the oculomotor nerve.
oocyte n. The nucleus of the primordial female gamete.
parabducens n. Group of cells in the reticular formation, near the motor cells of the abducens nucleus, which send fibers to the oculomotor nucleus by way of the medial longitudinal fasciculus.
parabigeminal n. A group of cells, ventrolateral to the inferior colliculus and lateral to the lateral lemniscus, which apparently send fibers to the lateral nuclei of the pons.
paracentral n. of the thalamus. One of the intralaminar nuclei of the thalamus, ventrolateral to the dorsomedial nucleus.
parafascicular n. of the thalamus. One of the intralaminar nuclei of the thalamus, ventral to the caudal portion of the dorsomedial nucleus.
parataenial n. of the thalamus. One of the midline nuclei of the thalamus, located near the stria medullaris thalami.
paraventricular n. of the hypothalamus. A thin flat plate of large cells in the anterior hypothalamus whose axons combine with those of the supraoptic nucleus to form the supraopticohypophyseal tract.
paraventricular n. of the thalamus. One of the midline nuclei of the thalamus, located in the dorsal ventricular wall.
perifornical n. Mantle of hypothalamic cells surrounding the anterior columns of the fornix.
peripeduncular n. The layer of cells covering the dorsal surface of the crus cerebri, lateral to the substantia nigra.
pontine (pontile) n. Scattered collections of nerve cells located throughout the pons.
pontobulbar n. A group of cells, which caudally are dorsolateral to, and rostrally ventral to, the inferior cerebellar peduncle.
posterior hypothalamic n. See *hypothalamus, middle region.*
posterior lateral n. See dorsal lateral *n.*
posterior nuclei of the thalamus. The pulvinar, medial, and lateral geniculate bodies, and the suprageniculate nucleus.
posterolateral ventral n. of the thalamus. A column of cells, lying lateral to the posteromedial ventral nucleus, which receives the fibers of the ventral and lateral spinothalamic tracts and medial lemniscus.
posteromarginal n. A thin layer of cells in the zona spongiosa, most prominent in the lumbosacral segments, whose axons go to the lateral white column and bifurcate into ascending and descending fibers, probably forming intersegmental tracts: also called *n. magnocellularis pericornualis, marginal n.*
posteromedial ventral n. of the thalamus. A sharply defined column of cells ventral to the central nucleus of the thalamus which receives sensory fibers from the nucleus of the spinal tract of the trigeminal nerve and from the main sensory nucleus of the trigeminal nerve: also called *semilunar nucleus.*
premammillary n. A small group of cells on the anterosuperior aspect of the medial mammillary nucleus.
preolivary nuclei. Two nuclei, the **internal** and

external preolivary nuclei, ventral to the superior olive and intercalated in the secondary auditory pathways.
principal vestibular n. See medial vestibular *n.*
protamine n. See Kossel and Siegfried's protamine nucleus *hypothesis.*
red n. A large oval nucleus, situated in the midbrain and thalamus ventrad to the cerebral aqueduct, which in the fresh brain has a pink color. It receives fibers from the brachium conjunctivum and gives fibers to the rubrospinal tract.
reticular n. of the subthalamus. A nucleus consisting of the nucleus of the tegmental field and cells scattered along the thalamic and lenticular fasciculi.
reticular n. of the thalamus. One of the lateral nuclei of the thalamus which is located between the external medullary lamina and internal capsule, and is continuous ventrally with the zona incerta.
retropyramidal n. The lateral extension of the nucleus of the raphe. Also called *nucleus conterminalis.*
salivatory, salivary nuclei. See superior and inferior salivatory *n.*
segmentation n. The nucleus that appears shortly after the fusion of the male and female pronuclei; the last step in the process of fertilization; it is so called because within it cleavage is first established.
sensibilis proprius n. A group of cells of varied size, lying ventromedial to the substantia gelatinosa Rolandi.
semilunar n. The posteromedial ventral nucleus of the thalamus.
spinal accessory n. A small and discontinuous strand of cells having considerable length in the caudal extreme of the medulla oblongata and the first five segments of the cervical spinal cord, lying in the rostral end of the motor horn of the cord, lateral to the motor cells of the upper cervical roots.
spinal vestibular n. A nucleus dorsolateral to the tractus solitarius which is the terminal nucleus for the spinal vestibular tract. Also called *descending vestibular n.*
spinocerebellar n. See dorsal *n.* of Clarke.
spinothalamic n. See *n.* proprius of the dorsal horn.
sublingual n. See *n.* of Roller.
submedial n. of the thalamus. One of the intralaminar nuclei of the thalamus, ventral to the dorsomedial nucleus: also called *ventromedial n.*
subthalamic n. A biconvex nucleus between the internal capsule and the cerebral peduncle, receiving fibers from the globus pallidus. Formerly called *corpus Luysii.*
superior central n. A group of cells in the reticular formation in the upper pontile levels.
superior olivary n. See superior *olive.*
superior salivatory n. An ill-defined nucleus in the reticular formation caudal to the facial nucleus which sends preganglionic fibers to the submaxillary ganglion via the nervus intermedius, facial, and chorda tympani nerves and to the sphenopalatine ganglion via the greater superficial petrosal nerve. It is concerned in the regulation of secretion of the submaxillary, sublingual, and lacrimal glands.
superior vestibular n. A nucleus dorsal to the lateral vestibular nucleus at the lateral limit of the fourth ventricle. Also called *angular n., n. of Bekhterev.*
suprageniculate n. One of the posterior nuclei of the thalamus, ventral to the pulvinar and dorsomedial to the medial geniculate body.
supramammillary n. A layer of large cells on the dorsal aspect of the medial mammillary nucleus, which is continuous with the interpeduncular nucleus.
supraoptic n. of the hypothalamus. A well-defined crescent-shaped nucleus which straddles the optic tract lateral to the chiasma. Its efferent fibers combine with those of the paraventricular nucleus to form the supraopticohypophyseal tract.
supraspinal n. Somatic motor cells of the first cervical nerve, which are located in the ventral gray column of the spinal cord and extend into the medulla for a short distance.
supratrigeminal n. A nucleus near the motor nucleus of the trigeminal nerve and functionally similar to the intertrigeminal nucleus.
tectal nuclei. The fastigial, globose, and emboliform nuclei of the cerebellum.
tegmental nuclei. Groups of nerve cells located in the tegmentum of the midbrain.
thalamic nuclei. See all of the anterior, lateral, medial, midline, and posterior *nuclei,* and intralaminar *nuclei* of the thalamus.
triangular n. See medial vestibular *n.*
trigeminal n. See motor *n.* of the trigeminal nerve.
trochlear n. A nucleus in the midbrain ventral to the central canal and dorsal to the medial longitudinal fasciculus giving rise to motor fibers of the trochlear nerve.
tuberal n. Circular cell groups, in the lateral part of the tuber cinereum, which often produce small eminences on the basal surface of the hypothalamus.
vagal nuclei. See dorsal motor *n.* of the vagus, dorsal sensory *n.* of the vagus, *n.* ambiguus, *n.* of the tractus solitarius.
ventral n. of the thalamus. A nucleus of the thalamus which may be subdivided into other groups of nuclei. It serves as a somesthetic relay system receiving fibers from the medial lemniscus, spinothalamic tracts, and secondary trigeminal tract.
ventromedial hypothalamic n. See *hypothalamus, middle region.*
ventromedial n. of the thalamus. See submedial *n.* of thalamus.

nu'clide. A species of atom characterized by the constitution of its nucleus, in particular by the number of protons and neutrons in the nucleus.

nu'dic ac'id. Either of two antibiotic substances, nudic acid A and nudic acid B, produced by the basidiomycete *Tricholoma nudum.*

nud'ism [L. *nudus,* naked]. 1. *In psychiatry,* a more or less complete intolerance of clothing; a morbid tendency to remove the clothing. 2. The practice of a cult, nudists, who profess to believe in the benefits of a society in which clothes are discarded.

Nuel, Jean Pierre (1847–1920). Belgian ophthalmologist who described the triangular space between the outer hair cells and the outer pillars of the organ of Corti, called *Nuel's space.* He also introduced an operation for relief of corneoscleral rupture, the conjunctiva being drawn over the opening by means of a special suture.

Nuhn, Anton [*German anatomist,* 1814–89]. Remembered for his description of the anterior lingual gland, called *Nuhn's gland, Blandin's gland.*

nui'sance [OF., from L. *nocere,* to harm]. *In legal medicine,* that which is noxious, offensive, or troublesome; applied to persons or things.

nujol. A trade-mark for liquid petrolatum.

nul·lip'a·ra [L. *nullus,* none; *parere,* to bring forth]. A woman who has never borne a child. —**nulliparous,** *adj.;* **nullipar'ity,** *n.*

Numa Pompilius [*second legendary king of Rome,* 715–673 B. C.]. Known medically for his law ordering the operation of abdominal incision for women dying in late pregnancy or childbirth, in order to save the child; called *lex regia.* Under the Caesars the lex regia became known as *lex caesaria.*

numb [ME. *nume,* taken]. Having impaired cutaneous sensibility.

num'ber [L. *numerus,* number]. 1. The total count of units. 2. A numeral, designating place in a series. Abbreviated, No. Symbol, #.

acetyl n. See under *acetyl.*

acid n. See *acid number.*

atomic n. The total number of protons in an atom or the number of orbital electrons in the neutral atom. Each element has a characteristic atomic number.

iodine n. See under *iodine.*

mass n. See under *mass.*

Reichert-Meissl n. A measure of the soluble, volatile fatty-acid content of a fat or oil; the number of cubic centimeters of 0.1 N KOH (one-tenth normal potassium hydroxide) required to neutralize the soluble, volatile fatty acids obtained from 5.0 Gm. of fat or oil. The Reichert-Meissl number is important in identifying certain fats and oils and in detecting their adulteration.

saponification n. The number of milligrams of potassium hydroxide required to neutralize the free acids and saponify the esters contained in 1 Gm. of oil, fat, wax, or other substance of similar composition. Also called *saponification value.*

turnover n. The number of molecules with which an enzyme can react in a certain period of time, usually one minute.

volatile fatty-acid n. See Reichert-Meissl *n.*

numb'ness [ME. *nume,* taken]. Partial, or local, anesthesia with torpor; deficiency of sensation. Obdormition.

nu·mer'i·cal ap'er·ture. The product of the sine of half the angular aperture of a lens, and the index of the medium through which the light passes. A mathematical relationship discovered by Abbe between the resolving power of an objective and its aperture. Microscope objectives and condensers are largely designated by the numerical aperture (generally abbreviated N. A.) value.

num'mi·form [L. *nummus,* coin; *forma,* form]. Having the form of a coin.

num'mu·lar [L. *nummularius,* of money]. Resembling a coin in form, as nummular sputum; resembling rouleaux or rolls of coin.

num"mu·la'tion [L. *nummulus,* dim. of *nummus,* coin]. The aggregation of blood cells into coinlike rolls or rouleaux.

Nuñez Andrade dis·ease'. A trombidiosis seen in Mexico, caused by *Neoschoengastia nunezi,* characterized by hemorrhages, pustules, and scarring umbilicated papules.

nun·na'tion [*nūn,* the Arabic letter n]. The frequent, or abnormal, use of the *n* sound.

nupercaine hydrochloride. Trade-marked name for the local anesthetic substance dibucaine hydrochloride or cinchocaine hydrochloride.

nurse [L. *nutrix,* nurse]. 1. To suckle an infant. 2. To care for a sick person.

nurse. 1. One who cares for an infant or young child, also called a nursemaid. 2. One who cares for a sick person, often under the supervision of a physician.

Army n. A commissioned officer of the U. S. Army Nurse Corps, who provides nursing care of personnel treated or hospitalized in Army medical treatment facilities.

attending n. One who visits patients in their homes.

community n. One employed by a subdivision of the government to assist in the medical care and supervise the health in a definite locality.

district n. See community *n.*

dry n. One who cares for but does not suckle the baby.

general duty n. One assigned to a ward or division of a hospital and performing many different duties for all the patients.

graduate n. One who has been graduated from a recognized school of nursing.

head n. One who is in charge of a ward or division of a hospital.

hospital n. One who works for a hospital rather than for one special patient or physician.

practical n. One skilled in the care of the sick but who has not been graduated from a regular nursing school or passed an examination to qualify as a graduate nurse.

private duty n. See private *n.*

private n. One who works exclusively for one patient at a time and is employed by him whether in a hospital or a home.

probationer n. One who has recently entered nurses' training and is still under probation. This usually lasts three months, at the successful conclusion of which the girl becomes a student nurse.

public health n. A graduate nurse working for a public health official, or a public health agency to assist in safeguarding the health of the people in her district. She gives instruction and actual care to the people in their homes and helps in the prevention of disease.

registered n. A graduate nurse who has passed the state board examination and is thus qualified to be a nurse, and is legally entitled to add R.N. to the name.

school n. A graduate nurse who visits the children in one or more schools, assisting the school physician in his duties.

scrub n. One who is part of an operating team, being scrubbed, gowned, and surgically clean to assist the operating surgeon.

special n. (a) A private nurse taking special care of one patient. (b) One well trained in a particular specialty.

student n. One in nurses' training school.

trained n. One who has trained in, and been graduated from, a nurses' training school.

visiting n. See community *n.*

wet n. A woman who furnishes breast feeding to an infant not her own.

nurse corps. The women nurses in the Army and Navy, who have ranks, titles, and status as officers, corresponding to the officer component of the Armed Services.

nurs'ing [L. *nutrix,* nurse]. 1. Obtaining milk from a breast by an infant. 2. Giving milk to an infant from a breast. 3. Caring for the sick.

foster n. Suckling of the young by an animal not the mother. Used in cancer research for suckling of young mice of one strain by females of a different strain.

n. bottle. A bottle fitted with a rubber tip or nipple for feeding infants not nursed from the breast.

nurs'ling [*nutrix*]. An infant that is nursed.

Nussbaum, Johann Nepomuk von [*German surgeon,* 1829–90]. Prolific writer who contributed more than 80 monographs on various subjects connected with surgery and surgical pathology. Inventor of an apparatus to assist the hand in writing where muscular power or coordination is lacking; called *Nussbaum's bracelet.* Introduced a prolonged chloroform anesthesia, using a preliminary dose of morphine, a procedure which was adopted extensively in surgical practice; called *Nussbaum's narcosis*.

Nussbaum, Moritz [*German histologist*, 1850–1915]. Described small cells in the pyloric glands, called *Nussbaum's cells*.

nu·ta′tion [L. *nutare*, to nod]. Nodding or oscillation, as nutation of the sacrum, a partial rotation of the sacrum on its transverse axis, whereby the distance between the upper extremity or the lower extremity and the anterior pelvic wall is increased.

nut′gall″ (nut′gawl″) [AS. *hnutu;* L. *galla*, gall-nut] (*galla*). The excrescence on young twigs of *Quercus infectoria*, caused by the deposition of eggs of the insect *Cynips tinctoria*, and the subsequent response of the plant to the stimulating action of a secretion of the insect larva. Nutgall contains about 70% of gallotannic acid, an astringent.

nut′meg [ME. *notemuge*]. 1. Any plant of the genus *Myristica*. 2. The dried ripe seed of *Myristica fragrans* deprived of its covering (mace). A spice; used as a condiment, a corrective, and a mild flavoring agent; also has slight narcotic properties.

nut′meg liv′er. Cirrhotic liver.

nu′tri·ent [L. *nutrire*, to nourish]. Affording nutrition. **—nu′tri·ent,** *n.*

nu′tri·lite [*nutrire*]. A substance which, in small amounts, functions in the nutrition of microorganisms.

nu′tri·ment [L. *nutrimentum*, nourishment]. Anything that nourishes.

nu·tri′tion [*nutrire*]. 1. The sum of the processes concerned in the growth, maintenance, and repair of the living body as a whole, or of its constituent parts. 2. Nourishment; food. **—nutritional,** *adj.*

nu·tri′tious [*nutrire*]. Nutritive.

nu′tri·tive [*nutrire*]. Affording nutrition.

nu′tri·to″ry [*nutrire*]. Pertaining to the processes of nutrition.

nu′tri·ture. Nutritional status.

nu′trix [L., nurse]. A wet nurse. *Obs.*

Nuttall, George Henry Falkiner [*American biologist*, 1862–1937]. Well remembered for his description, with William H. Welch, of gas bacillus infection by *Bacillus aerogenes capsulatus* (1892), now called *Clostridium perfringens*. He had previously demonstrated the bactericidal qualities of defibrinated blood (1904).

nux (pl. *nuces*) [L., nut]. Musky nut. The nutmeg; myristica.

n. vomica (*nux vomica*). The seed of *Strychnos nux-vomica*, an Indian tree of the Loganiaceae. Contains several alkaloids, the most important being strychnine and brucine. The official drug is required to contain not less than 1.15% strychnine. Has been used in small doses as a bitter tonic, but its action is principally that of strychnine. Dose, 0.06–0.25 Gm. (1–4 gr.).

n. vomica extract (*extractum nucis vomicae*). Contains 7.0–7.75% strychnine. Dose, 15–30 mg. (¼–½ gr.).

n. vomica fluidextract (*fluidextractum nucis vomicae*). Contains 1.05–1.25% (w/v) strychnine. Dose, 0.06–0.2 cc. (1–3 min.).

n. vomica tincture (*tinctura nucis vomicae*). Contains 0.105–0.125% (w/v) strychnine. Dose, 0.6–2.0 cc. (10–30 min.).

nyctal. Trade-mark for carbromal.

nyc·tal′gi·a [G. *nyx*, night; *algos*, pain]. Pain, which occurs chiefly during the night.

nyc′ta·lope [*nyx;* G. *alaos*, blind; *ōps*, eye]. One who cannot see at night. See *night blindness*.

nyc″ta·lo′pi·a. See *night blindness*.

nyc′ter·ine (nick′tur·yne, ·een, ·in) [G. *nykterinos*, nightly]. 1. Occurring in the night. 2. Obscure.

nyc″to·phil′i·a [G. *nyx*, night; *philein*, to love]. Preference for night or darkness.

nyc″to·pho′bi·a [*nyx;* G. *phobos*, fear]. A morbid fear of night and of darkness.

nyc″to·pho′ni·a [*nyx;* G. *phōnē*, voice]. The hysterical loss of the voice during the day, in one who is capable of speaking during the night.

nyc″to·typh·lo′sis. Night blindness.

nyc·tu′ri·a. See *nocturia*.

nydrazid. Trade-mark for a brand of isoniazid; an antituberculosis drug having the composition of isonicotinic acid hydrazide.

nyg′ma [G., prick]. A punctured wound. *Obs.*

Nylander reagent. See under *reagent*.

Nylander's test. See under *test*.

ny′lic stand′ard. A standard of weight in accordance with height and age, as adopted by the New York Life Insurance Company.

nymph [G. *nymphe*, maiden]. The immature stage of an insect, during which the wing pads first appear and the reproductive organs have not developed to the functional stage.

nym′pha (pl. *nymphae*) [G.]. A minor lip of the vulva.

nym·phec′to·my [*nympha;* G. *ektomē*, excision]. Surgical removal of one or both minor lips.

nym·phi′tis [*nympha;* G. *-itis*, inflammation]. Inflammation of the minor lips.

nym′pho·lep″sy [*nympha;* G. *lēpsis*, a seizing]. Ecstasy of an erotic type.

nym″pho·ma′ni·a [*nympha;* G. *mania*, madness]. Excessive sexual desire on the part of a woman. **—nymphomaniac,** *adj., n.*

nym·phon′cus [*nympha;* G. *ogkos*, mass]. Tumor or swelling of the minor lip. *Rare.*

nym·phot′o·my [*nympha;* G. *tomē*, a cutting]. Incision of one or both minor lips.

nys·tag′mic [G. *nystagmos*, drowsiness, from *nystazein*, to doze, to hang the head]. Pertaining to, or suffering from, nystagmus.

nys·tag′mi·form [*nystagmos;* L. *forma*, form]. Resembling nystagmus.

nys·tag′mo·graph [*nystagmos;* G. *graphein*, to write]. An apparatus for recording the movements of the eyeball in nystagmus.

nys″tag·mog′ra·phy [*nystagmos; graphein*]. The study and recording of the movements of the eyeballs in nystagmus.

nys·tag′moid [*nystagmos;* G. *eidos*, form]. Resembling true nystagmus in certain particulars.

nys·tag′mus [*nystagmos*]. An oscillatory movement of the eyeballs. It may be congenital or dependent on intracranial disease, as meningitis or multiple sclerosis. **—nystagmic,** *adj.*

labyrinthine n. That occurring when the labyrinths are irritated or diseased. Syn., *vestibular n.*

lateral n. Oscillation of the eyes in the horizontal meridian.

miner's n. Nystagmus caused by darkness.

optokinetic n. That which occurs in normal individuals when a succession of moving objects traverses the field of vision, or when the individual moves past a succession of stationary objects.

oscillatory n. That which occurs when vision in both eyes has long been extremely poor, as an occupational disorder such as miners' nystagmus, and as a congenital defect. Also called *pendulous n.*

palatal n. Rhythmic contractions of the palate possibly due to lesions of the brain stem involving the inferior olivary nuclei or their connections with the tegmentum.

positional n. That which occurs only when the patient's head is placed in an abnormal plane.

pseudonystagmus. That due to visual defect,

usually of the macula, as choroidal degeneration, or bilateral congenital toxoplasmosis.

rhythmic n. That form in which the eyes slowly wander a few degrees in one direction and then are jerked back. Observed normally in passengers in a moving vehicle who watch the landscape, and pathologically usually in lesions of the vestibular apparatus or its connections.

rotatory n. An oscillatory, partial rolling of the eyeball around the visual axis.

spontaneous ocular n. Nystagmus as a result of complete blindness or defective central vision.

vertical n. Oscillatory movement in the vertical meridian.

vestibular n. See labyrinthine *n.*

Nysten, Pierre Hubert [*French pediatrician,* 1774–1817]. Editor and compiler of Littré and Robin's *Dictionary of Medicine* (1865). Proposed a law of rigor mortis; *Nysten's law* states that it is first observed in the muscles of mastication, later extends to the facial and cervical muscles, and finally involves the lower extremities.

nyx′is [G., a pricking]. Surgical puncture or paracentesis. *Obs.*

O

O Chemical symbol for oxygen.

O. Abbreviation for *oculus* eye; *octarius,* a pint; opening of an electric circuit; occiput.

o- *In chemistry,* ortho-.

oak [AS. *āc*]. A genus of trees, *Quercus,* of the Fagaceae. The dried inner bark of *Quercus alba,* white oak, contains a characteristic tannic acid known as quercitannic acid. It is employed in the tanning industry and has been used medicinally as an astringent.

oa′kum (o′kum) [AS. *ācumba*]. The loose fiber made by picking old hemp rope to pieces. Oakum was formerly used as a dressing for wounds, and (in the form of pads) to absorb the lochial discharges.

o″a·ri·al′gi·a [G. *ōiarion,* small egg; *algos,* pain]. Ovarian neuralgia; ovarialgia. *Rare.*

o·ar′i·o- (o·air′ee·o-). For words beginning with *oario-,* see *ovario-* or *oophor-.*

o·a′sis [G. *oasis,* name of fertile areas in the Libyan desert]. *In surgery,* an isolated spot of normal tissue situated in a pathologic area.

ob- [L.]. A prefix signifying *on, against, in front of,* or *toward.*

ob″ce·ca′tion (ob″si·kay′shun) [L. *occaecatio,* a hiding]. Partial blindness.

ob″dor·mi′tion (ob″dor·mish′un) [L. *obdormire,* to fall asleep]. Numbness of a part due to interference with nervous function; the state of a part when it is said to be asleep.

ob·duc′tion [L. *obductio,* a covering]. A post-mortem examination; an autopsy; a necropsy. *Obs.*

o·be′li·on [dim. from G. *obelos,* spit]. The point where the line which joins the parietal foramens crosses the sagittal suture.

Ober, Frank Roberts [*American orthopedic surgeon,* 1881–   ]. Devised a number of operative procedures in orthopedic surgery which bear his name. Described a test for contraction of the fascia lata in sciatica or low back pain, called *Ober's sign.* Introduced an operation for relief of paralysis of the gastrocnemius muscle, in which he isolated and divided the tendons of the peroneus longus and tibialis posterior, exposed the tendo achillis and drilled a hole in the calcaneus. The freed tendons were drawn behind the tendo achillis and passed through the hole described, their ends being sutured to the tendo achillis. Introduced an operation in paralysis of the quadriceps femoris muscle, in which he transplanted the tendons of the tensor of the fascia lata and the sartorius muscles into the patellar tendon by means of tunneling. Each operation is called *Ober's operation.*

Obermayer's reagent. See under *reagent.*

Obermayer's test. See under *test.*

Obermeier, Otto Hugo Franz [*German physician,* 1843–73]. Discovered *Borrelia recurrentis,* the cause of European relapsing fever (1868); also called *Spirochaeta obermeieri.*

Oberst, Max [*German surgeon,* 1849–1925]. Introduced a form of block anesthesia using a dilute solution of cocaine over the course of a nerve trunk (1889).

o·bese′ [L. *obesus,* from *obedere,* to eat oneself fat]. Extremely fat; corpulent. —**obesely,** *adv.;* **obeseness,** *n.*

o·be′si·ty (o·bee′si·tee, o·bess′i·tee) [L. *obesitas,* fatness]. Generalized weight excess, due to accumulation of fat, beyond 10 to 20 per cent of the normal range for the particular age, sex, and height. It is generally due to excess food intake, often because of psychogenic factors, rarely to endocrine disturbances and heredofamilial factors.

buffalo o. The type of obesity usually seen in Cushing's syndrome, confined chiefly to the trunk, face, and neck: also called *adrenocortical o.*

endocrine o. That due to dysfunction of the endocrine glands.

hypothalamic o. That resulting from a disturbance of function of the appetite-regulating centers of the hypothalamus.

o′bex [L., bolt, barrier]. Thin triangular lamina formed by the meeting of the taeniae choroideae of the fourth ventricle over the caudal limit of the cavity.

ob″fus·ca′tion [L. *offuscatio,* a darkening]. Mental confusion.

ob·jec′tive [L. *objectum,* from *obicere,* to cast before]. 1. Pertaining to an object or to that which is contemplated or perceived, as distinguished from that which contemplates or perceives. 2. Pertaining to those relations and conditions of the body perceived by another, as objective signs of disease.

ob·jec′tive. The lens of a microscope nearest the object.

fluorite o. The optical properties of fluorite make possible the attainment of a high order of correction. All apochromats contain at least one fluorite element, and the high powers may contain three such elements. Lenses which are classed as fluorite objective are achromatic objectives of high power. Also called *semiapochromatic o.*

monochromatic o. An objective corrected for use with monochromatic light, as, for example, the quartz objective corrected for the 2750 A. line.

oil-immersion o. *In microscopy,* an objective designed for use when oil with a refractive index close to that of glass replaces air between the objective and the object.

semiapochromatic o. An objective containing fluorite, intermediate in quality between an achromat and an apochromat. Also called *fluorite o., semiapochromat o.*

ob′li·gate [L. *obligatus*, from *obligare*, to bind around]. Constrained; bound; not facultative, as an obligate anaerobe, one that can live only as an anaerobe.

ob·lique′ (o·bleek′, o·blike′) [L. *obliquus*, sidelong]. 1. Not direct; aslant; slanting. 2. *In botany*, unequal-sided.

ob·lique′. *In anatomy*, an oblique muscle, as the external or internal oblique of the abdomen, or the superior or inferior oblique of the eye.

ob·liq′ui·ty [L. *obliquitas*, a sidelong direction]. The state of being oblique. Particularly, *in obstetrics*, a term used for a theory of the mechanism of labor.

biparietal o. Anterior asynclitism.

Litzmann's o. See posterior *asynclitism*.

Naegele's o. See anterior *asynclitism*.

ob·li′quus (ob·lye′kwus, ·lick′wus) [L.]. Designation of various muscles, as obliquus abdominis externus. See Table of Muscles in the Appendix.

ob·lit″er·a′tion [L. *obliteratio*, from *obliterare*, to blot out]. 1. The complete removal of a part by disease or surgical operation; extirpation. 2. Complete closure of a lumen. 3. The complete loss of memory or consciousness of certain events.

ob″mu·tes′cence [L. *obmutescere*, to lose one's speech]. Aphonia; loss of voice. *Rare.*

ob·nu″bi·la′tion [L. *obnubilare*, to cover with clouds]. A form of mental haze preceding loss of consciousness.

ob·ses′sion [L. *obsessio*, a besieging]. An idea or emotion that persists in an individual's mind in spite of any conscious attempts to remove it; an imperative idea, as in psychoneurosis. —**obsessive,** *adj.*

ob·ses′sive com·pul′sive re·ac′tion. See under *reaction.*

ob·ses′sive ru′mi·na″tive state. A form of psychoneurotic disorder (perhaps part of a depressive reaction) very similar to obsessive compulsive reaction, characterized by continuous morbid preoccupation with certain ideas, usually trivial or inconsequential, to the exclusion of other interests, but without compulsive acts.

ob″so·les′cence [L. *obsolescere*, to grow old]. The state of becoming old or obsolete.

ob″ste·tri′cian (ob″steh·trish′un) [L. *obstetrix*, midwife]. One who practices obstetrics.

ob·stet′rics [*obstetrix*]. The branch of medicine that cares for women during pregnancy, labor, and the puerperium. —**obstetric, obstetrical,** *adj.*

ob″sti·pa′tion [L. *obstipatio*, close pressure]. Intractable constipation. *Obs.*

ob·struc′tion [L. *obstructio*, a building before]. 1. The state of being occluded or stenosed, applied especially to hollow viscera, ducts, and vessels. 2. The act of occluding or blocking. 3. An obstacle. —**obstructive,** *adj.*

intestinal o. Any hindrance to the passage of the fecal stream.

mitral o. See mitral *stenosis.*

partial o. Incomplete obstruction.

pyloric o. A spasm or failure to relax of the pyloric sphincter.

ureteral o. Any hindrance to the flow of urine through the ureter to the bladder.

urinary o. Any hindrance to the passage of urine through the urinary system, specifically to the evacuation of urine from the bladder.

ob·struc′tive at″e·lec′ta·sis. See under *atelectasis.*

ob′stru·ent [L. *obstruere*, to build before]. Obstructive; tending to obstruct. —**ob′struent,** *n.*

ob·tund′ [L. *obtundere*, to strike against, to dull]. Blunt or dull; lessen, as to obtund sensibility.

ob·tund′ent [*obtundere*]. Soothing, quieting; a remedy that relieves or overcomes irritation or pain. *Obs.*

ob″tu·ra′tion [L. *obturare*, to stop up]. 1. The closing of an opening or passage. 2. A form of intestinal obstruction in which the lumen of the intestine is occupied by its normal contents or by foreign bodies. *Rare.*

ob′tu·ra″tor [*obturare*]. 1. Closing an opening. 2. Pertaining to the obturator membrane, muscles, etc. See Tables of Muscles, Nerves, and Arteries in the Appendix.

ob′tu·ra″tor. 1. Any obturator muscle. 2. A solid wire or rod contained within a hollow needle or cannula. Obturators may be bayonet-pointed for piercing tissues, or obliquely faced at the end for fitting, exactly, large aspirating needles. The term includes the metal carriers within urethroscopes and cystoscopes, etc. 3. An appliance which closes a cleft or fissure of the palate.

o. externus. The outer obturator muscle.

o. internus. The inner obturator muscle.

ob·tuse′ [L. *obtusus*, from *obtundere*, to strike against, to dull]. 1. Blunt. 2. *Of angles*, greater than 90°.

ob·tu′sin. An antibiotic derived from a species of Basidiomycetes, active principally against Gram-positive bacteria.

ob·tu′sion (ob·tew′zhun) [L. *obtusio*, from *obtundere*]. The blunting or weakening of normal sensation, a symptom of certain diseases.

oc·cip′i·tal (ock·sip′i·tul) [L. *occiput*, back part of the head]. Pertaining to, or in relation with, the occiput.

oc·cip′i·tal. The occipital bone. See Table of Bones in the Appendix.

oc·cip″i·ta′lis (ock·sip″i·tah′lis, ·tay′lis) [*occiput*]. The posterior sheet of the epicranius muscle.

o. minor. A variant of the posterior sheet of the epicranius muscle.

oc·cip′i·tal·ize [*occiput*]. Incorporate with the occipital bone; fuse the atlas with the occipital bone.

oc·cip′i·to- (ock·sip′i·to-) [*occiput*]. *In anatomy*, a combining form denoting *occipital.*

oc·cip″i·to·an·te′ri·or [*occiput;* L. *anterior*, foremost]. Having the occiput directed toward the front, as the occipitoanterior position of the fetus in the uterus.

oc·cip″i·to·ax′i·al [*occiput;* L. *axis*, axis]. Pertaining to the occipital bone and the axis.

oc·cip″i·to·fron′tal [*occiput;* L. *frons*, forehead]. Pertaining to the occiput and forehead, or to the occipitofrontal muscle (epicranius).

oc·cip″i·to·fron·ta′lis (ock·sip″i·to·fron·tah′lis, ·tay′lis). The epicranius muscle.

oc·cip″i·to·pos·te′ri·or [*occiput;* L. *posterior*, posterior]. Having the occiput directed backward, as the occipitoposterior position of the fetus in the uterus.

oc·cip″ito·scap″u·lar′is. A variant of the rhomboideus major muscle extending to the occipital bone.

oc′ci·put (ock′si·put) [L.]. The back part of the head.

oc·clu′si·o [L. *occlusus*, from *occludere*, to close up]. Closure.

o. pupillae. Obliteration of the pupil.

o. pupillae lymphatica. Obliteration of the pupil by a false membrane.

oc·clu′sion (o·clue′zhun) [*occludere*]. 1. A closing or shutting up. 2. The state of being closed or shut. 3. The absorption, by a metal, of gas in large quantities, as of hydrogen by platinum. 4. The full meeting or contact in a position of rest of the masticating surfaces of the upper and lower teeth; erroneously called articulation of teeth. 5. *In neurophysiology,* the deficit in muscular tension when two afferent nerves which share certain motoneurons in the central nervous system are stimulated simultaneously, as compared to the sum of tensions when the two nerves are stimulated separately. **—occlude′,** *v.*

afunctional o. Congenital nonocclusion.

balanced o. *In prosthetic dentistry,* one designed to assure stability of artificial dentures during excursive movements of the jaw. *In periodontics,* one in which the forces of occlusion are conducive to maximum periodontal health.

buccal o. Occlusion, 4, occurring when a premolar or a molar tooth is situated lateral to the line of occlusion.

centric o. The relation of the incisal edges and the inclined planes of the teeth when the jaws are closed in the position of rest.

coronary o. Occlusion of a branch of the arterial system that supplies blood to the heart muscle.

distal o. Occlusion, 4, occurring when a tooth is situated posterior to its normal position.

eccentric o. The relation of the inclined planes of the teeth when the jaws are closed in any of the excursive movements of the mandible.

labial o. Occlusion, 4, occurring when an incisor or canine tooth is situated external to the line of occlusion.

lingual o. Occlusion, 4, occuring when a tooth is situated internal to the line of occlusion.

mesial o. That occurring when a tooth is more anterior than normal (especially the cheek teeth). Opposite of distal occlusion.

puerperal tubal o. The agglutination of mucosal folds of the uterine tube occurring about one week after labor, presumably from a mild gonococcus infection and producing one-child sterility.

traumatic o. An abnormal occlusal stress leading to injury of the periodontium.

tubal o. Loss of patency of the oviduct.

oc·clu′sive [*occludere*]. Closing or shutting up, as an occlusive surgical dressing.

oc″clu·som′e·ter. Gnathodynamometer.

oc·cult′, oc′cult [L. *occultus,* from *occulere,* to cover]. Hidden; concealed; not evident, as occult blood, the blood in excrement or secretion not clearly evident to the naked eye, or occult disease, any disease the nature of which is not readily determined.

oc″cu·pa′tion·al dis·ease′. One caused by the occupation of the patient. It may be organic, as lead poisoning, or functional. See occupational *neurosis.*

oc″cu·pa′tion·al ther′a·py. The teaching of trades and arts as a means for the rehabilitation of patients handicapped physically or mentally.

oc′cu·pied beds. *In military medicine,* a number of operating beds in a medical treatment facility currently assigned to patients, excluding beds for patients on leave or absent without leave.

o·cel′lus [L., little eye]. 1. One of the simple eyes or pigmented spots of invertebrate animals. 2. One of the colored eyelike spots on feathers, flowers, etc.

ocenol. Trade-mark for *oleyl alcohol.*

och′e·us (ock′ee·us) [G.]. The scrotum. *Obs.*

och·le′sis (ock·lee′sis) [G. *ochlos,* crowd]. A morbid condition produced by crowding many people together in a small space with a lack of ventilation.

och″lo·pho′bi·a (ock″lo·fo′bee·uh) [*ochlos;* G. *phobos,* fear]. Morbid fear of crowds.

o·chrom′e·ter [G. *ōchros,* paleness; *metron,* a measure]. An instrument for measuring the capillary blood pressure.

o″chro·no′sis, o·chron′o·sis [*ōchros;* G. *-ōsis,* condition]. A blue or brownish blue pigmentation of cartilage and connective tissue, especially around joints, by a melanotic pigment. The condition is frequently accompanied by alkaptonuria and occurs in those who have had phenol, in large quantities, applied to skin or mucous membrane for a long time. A disturbed metabolism of aromatic compounds is associated with this condition. **—ochronot′ic,** *adj.*

Ochsner, Albert John [*American surgeon,* 1858–1925]. Renowned surgeon, diagnostician, and educator. Author of an important paper on the cause and prevention of diffuse peritonitis complicating appendicitis (1901).

Ochsner, Alton (1896–). American surgeon, known for his studies on the thoracic sympathetic nervous system and the peripheral vascular system. With Karl Nather he introduced an operation for subphrenic abscess, and with Michael E. DeBakey, a special technique of esophagogastrostomy.

oc′i·mene. $C_{10}H_{16}$; 2,6-dimethyl-1,5,7-octatriene; a terpene constituent of many plants.

O″co·te′a (o″ko·tee′uh, o·ko′tee·uh, o·cot′ee·uh) [NL., from the Indian]. A large genus of tropical trees of the family Lauraceae.

O. rodioei. A tropical South American tree; greenheart ocotea. Its bark contains tannic acid, resin, sugar, albumin, various salts, and two alkaloids, bebeerine and sepeerine. It is reputedly tonic, astringent, and has been used in malarial fevers.

oc′ta-, oct- [L. *octo,* eight]. A combining form meaning *eight.*

oc′ta·caine. β-Octyl-2-amino-β,β-dimethylethyl *p*-aminobenzoate hydrochloride. A local anesthetic.

oc′tad [*octo*]. An octavalent element or radical.

oc′tad. Having a valence of eight.

oc″ta·dec·a·di″e·no′ic ac′id. 9,12-Octadecadienoic acid or linoleic acid.

oc″ta·dec·a·tri″e·no′ic ac′id. 9,12,15-Octadecatrienoic acid or linolenic acid.

oc″ta·meth′yl py″ro·phos″phor·am′ide. $[(CH_3)_2N]_2(O)P.O.P(O)[N(CH_3)_2]_2$; bis[bisdimethylaminophosphonous] anhydride; a colorless, viscous liquid, soluble in water; a systemic insecticide and also a potent anticholinesterase agent, with selective action on peripheral cholinesterase: employed in treating myasthenia gravis. Abbreviated OMPA.

oc′tan [*octo*]. Returning every eighth day, as an octan fever.

oc′tane. C_8H_{18}. The eighth member of the paraffin or marsh gas series.

oc″ta·no′ic ac′id. Caprylic acid.

oc·ta′ri·us [*octo*]. An eighth part of a gallon; a pint. Abbreviated, O.

oc″ta·va′lent, oc·tav′a·lent [*octo;* L. *valere,* to be strong]. Having a valence of eight.

oc′tene. See *octylene.*

oc″ti·grav′i·da [*octo;* L. *gravidus,* pregnant]. A woman pregnant for the eighth time.

octin. Trade-mark for 6-methylamino-2-methylheptene, $C_8H_{15}.NH.CH_3$, a colorless, oily liquid which causes relaxation of smooth muscle. The substance is available commercially in preparations containing the hydrochloride or mucate salt.

oc·tip′a·ra [*octo;* L. *parere,* to bring forth]. A woman who has been in labor eight times.

oc′to-, oct- [*octo*]. A combining form meaning *eight.*

octofollin. Trade-mark for a brand of benzestrol.

oc′to·pine. A compound, found in the muscles of scallops and other marine invertebrates, representing a molecule of arginine and one of alanine joined in such a way as to share a nitrogen atom.

oc″to·roon′ [*octo;* quad*roon,* from Sp. *cuarterón*]. The offspring of a white person and a quadroon; a person who has one-eighth part of Negro blood.

oc′to·ses. A group of the monosaccharides with the formula $C_8H_{16}O_8$.

octrite. Trade-mark for octyl nitrite, used by inhalation as a vasodilator.

oc′tyl. The radical C_8H_{17}—.

o. ni′trite. $C_8H_{17}NO_2$; a liquid used like amyl nitrite, by inhalation, as a vasodilator; it is less likely to cause methemoglobinemia than is amyl nitrite. See *octrite.*

oc′tyl·ene. One of a group of liquid unsaturated hydrocarbons of the formula C_8H_{16}.

oc′u·lar [L. *ocularis*, of the eyes]. Pertaining to or in relation with the eye.

oc′u·lar. The lens assembly of a microscope, telescope, or other optical instrument that is nearest the eye; an eyepiece.

compensating o. A lens that compensates for axial aberration of the objective.

Huygenian o. A lens consisting of two planoconvex lenses, the convexities being directed toward the objective; the lower lens is the field lens, the upper, the eye lens.

Ramsden o. A positive ocular with two planoconvex lenses, the convex sides facing each other; used in micrometry.

telaugic oculars. Oculars with an extremely high exit pupil, so that spectacles can be worn with comfort.

wide-field oculars. Oculars with a wide field of view, now used especially in biobjective dissecting microscopes.

oc″u·len′tum [L. *oculus*, eye]. An ointment for use in the eye.

oc′u·list. See *ophthalmologist.*

oc′u·lo-, ocul- [*oculus*]. A combining form denoting *the eye* or *ocular.*

oc″u·lo·gy·ra′tion (ock″yoo·lo·jye·ray′shun) [*oculus;* L. *gyrare*, to turn around in a circle]. Movement of the eyeballs.

oc″u·lo·gy′ric [*oculus;* G. *gyros*, circle]. Referring to movements of the eyes.

oc″u·lo·mo′tor [*oculus;* L. *motor*, from *movere*, to move]. Pertaining to the movement of the eye, or to the oculomotor nerve.

oc″u·lo·my·co′sis (ock″yoo·lo·migh·ko′sis) [*oculus;* G. *mykēs*, fungus; *-ōsis*, condition]. Any disease of the eye or its appendages, due to the presence of a fungus.

oc″u·lo·phren″i·co·re·cur′rent [*oculus;* G. *phrēn*, mind; L. *recurrere*, to run back]. Referring to the recurrent laryngeal and phrenic nerves associated with Horner's syndrome, as in oculophrenicorecurrent paralysis.

oc″u·lo·zy″go·mat′ic [*oculus;* G. *zygōma*, bolt, bar]. Pertaining to the eye and the zygoma.

oc′u·lus (pl. *oculi*) [L.]. An eye. Abbreviated, O.

oculi marmarygodes. See *metamorphopsia.*

o. caesius. Glaucoma.

o. dexter. The right eye. Abbreviated, O. D.

o. duplex. A bandage covering both eyes.

o. lacrimans. Epiphora.

o. leporinus. Lagophthalmos.

o. purulentus. Hypopyon.

o. simplex. See *monoculus.*

o. sinister. The left eye. Abbreviated, O. S.

o. uterque. Each eye. Abbreviated, O. U. Also called *o. unitas.*

o″cy·o·din′ic (o″see·o·din′ick, o″sigh·o·) [G. *ōkys*, swift; *ōdis*, pangs of childbirth]. Oxytocic; hastening the delivery of the fetus.

O. D. *Oculus dexter*, right eye.

od (od, ode) [G. *hodos*, way]. The force supposed to produce the phenomena of mesmerism. *Obs.* —**od′ic,** *adj.*

o″dax·es′mus (o″dacks·ez′mus) [G. *odaxēsmos*, biting]. The biting of the tongue, lip, or cheek, during an epileptic seizure.

Oddi, Ruggero [*Italian physician*, nineteenth century]. Described the opening of the common bile duct at the ampulla of Vater. See *sphincter* of Oddi.

o″don·tag′ra, o″don·ta′gra [G., from *odous*, tooth; *agra*, a seizing]. Toothache. *Obs.*

o″don·tal′gi·a [G., toothache]. Toothache. —**odontal′gic,** *adj.*

phantom o. Pain felt in the space from which a tooth has been removed.

o″don·tal′gic [*odontalgia*]. A remedy for toothache.

o″don·tec′to·my [G. *odous*, tooth; *ektomē*, excision]. Surgical removal of a tooth.

o·don′ter·ism [*odous*]. Chattering of the teeth. *Obs.*

o″don·tex·e′sis. [*odous;* G. *exēsis*, removal]. Removal of deposits such as salivary calculus from the teeth.

o″don·thar′pa·ga. See *dentagra*, 1.

o·dont″he·mo′di·a (o·dont″hi·mo′dee·uh, o·don″-thi·) [*odous;* G. *haimōdia*, sensation of having the teeth set on edge]. Hemodia; excessive sensibility of the teeth. *Obs.*

o″don·thy′a·lus (o″don·thigh′uh·lus, o″dont-high′). Enamel. *Obs.*

o·don′ti·a [*odous*]. Any abnormality of the teeth.

o. deformis. Deformity of the teeth, arising either from error of shape or position, or from malformation of the jaws or alveolar border.

o. incrustans. Calculus of the teeth.

o″don·ti′a·sis [G., teething]. Dentition; the cutting of teeth.

o″don·ti′a·try, o·don″ti·at′ri·a (o·don″tee·at′-ree·uh, o·don″tee·uh·tree′uh) [*odous;* G. *iatreia*, medicine]. Dentistry. *Obs.* —**odontiatrist,** *n.*

o·don′tic [*odous*]. Relating to teeth.

o·don′tin·oid [*odous;* G. *eidos*, form]. Resembling, or having the nature of, teeth.

o″don·ti′tis [*odous;* G. *-itis*, inflammation]. Inflammation of the teeth.

o·don′to-, odont- [*odous*]. A combining form meaning *tooth.*

o·don″to·a·mel″o·sar·co′ma. See *ameloblastosarcoma.*

o·don″to·at·lan′tal [*odous;* G. *atlas*, axis]. Old term for atlantoaxial.

o·don′to·blast [*odous;* G. *blastos*, germ]. One of the cells covering the dental papilla or dental pulp, concerned with the formation of the dentin.

o·don″to·blas·to′ma [*odous; blastos;* G. *-ōma*, tumor]. A tumor developing from the mesenchymal portion of the tooth germ.

o·don″to·bo·thri′tis [*odous;* G. *bothrion*, small trench; *-itis*, inflammation]. Inflammation of a tooth socket. *Obs.*

o·don″to·both′ri·um [*odous; bothrion*]. The alveolus of a tooth. *Obs.*

o·don′to·cele [*odous;* G. *kēlē*, tumor]. A dentoalveolar cyst.

o·don″to·ce·ram′ic [*odous;* G. *keramos*, potter's clay]. Pertaining to porcelain teeth.

o″don·to·cha′lix (o″don·tock′uh·licks) [*odous;* G. *chalix*, gravel, rubble]. Dental cement. *Obs.*

o·don″to·chi·rur′gi·cal (·kigh·rur′ji·kul) [*odous;* G. *cheirourgos*, working with the hands]. Pertaining to dental surgery.

o″donto·cla′sis [*odous;* G. *klasis*, a breaking]. The process of resorption of the dentin of a tooth.

o·don′to·clast [*odous;* G. *klastos*, broken in pieces]. A multinuclear cell, morphologically identical to an osteoclast, which is associated with resorption of tooth roots.

o·don″toc·ne′sis [*odous;* G. *knēsis*, itching]. A painful itching sensation in the gums, as that preceding cutting of the teeth. *Obs.*

o·don″to·dyn′i·a (o·don″to·din′ee·uh, ·dye′nee·uh) [*odous;* G. *odynē*, pain]. Toothache. *Obs.*

o·don″to·gen′e·sis [*odous;* G. *genesthai*, to become]. 1. Development of a tooth. 2. Dentinogenesis.

o″don·tog′e·ny (o″don·todj′i·nee) [*odous; genesthai*]. The origin and development of teeth. —**odontogen′ic,** *adj.*

o·don′to·glyph [*odous;* G. to *glyphein.* carve]. An instrument for scraping teeth.

o·don′to·gram [*odous;* G. *gramma*, letter]. A record made by an odontograph.

o·don′to·graph [*odous;* G. *graphein*, to write]. An instrument for recording the inequalities of the surface of teeth and the thickness of the enamel.

o″don·tog′ra·phy [*odous; graphein*]. The descriptive anatomy of the teeth. —**odontograph′ic,** *adj.*

o·don″to·hy″per·es·the′si·a (·high″pur·ess·thee′-zhuh, ·zee·uh) [*odous;* G. *hyper*, beyond; *aisthēsis*, perception]. Hypersensitiveness of dentin or nerves of the teeth.

o·don′toid [*odous;* G. *eidos*, form]. Resembling a tooth; toothlike, or pertaining to the dens of the axis, as odontoid ligament.

o·don′to·lith. Dental calculus.

o″don·tol′o·gist [*odous;* G. *logos*, word]. A dental surgeon.

o″don·tol′o·gy [*odous; logos*]. The branch of science dealing with the anatomy and diseases of the teeth.

o·don″to·lox′i·a, o″don·tol′ox·y (o″don·tol′uck-see, o·don′to·lock″see) [*odous;* G. *loxos*, slanting]. Irregularity or obliquity of the teeth.

o″don·tol′y·sis [*odous;* G. *lysis*, dissolution]. The loss of calcified tooth substance by dissolution.

o″don·to′ma [*odous;* G. *-ōma*, tumor]. A tumor or tumorlike hyperplasia which develops from one or more parts of a tooth germ. Resulting tissue may be soft, calcified, or a mixture of both.

composite o. A tumor composed of various histologic elements of the tooth germ.

simple o. A tumor composed of only one histologic element of the tooth germ.

o·don′tome. See *odontoma.*

o·don″to·ne·cro′sis [*odous;* G. *nekrōsis*, mortification]. Necrosis or decay of the tissues of the teeth; dental caries.

o·don″to·neu·ral′gi·a [*odous;* G. *neuron*, nerve; *algos*, pain]. Neuralgia due to diseased teeth.

o·don″to·par″al·lax′is [*odous;* G. *parallaxis*, alternation]. Irregularity of the teeth; deviation of one or more of the teeth from the natural position.

o″don·top′a·thy [*odous;* G. *pathos*, disease]. Any disease of the teeth.

o·don″to·per″i·os′te·um. See *periodontium.*

o·don″to·pho′bi·a [*odous;* G. *phobos*, fear]. Morbid fear of teeth (usually animals' teeth).

o·don′to·plast. Odontoblast.

o·don″to·ple·ro′sis [*odous;* G. *plērōsis*, filling]. The filling of teeth. *Obs.*

o·don″to·pri′sis (o·don″to·pry′sis, o″don·top′ri-sis) [*odous;* G. *prisis*, a sawing]. Grinding of the teeth.

o·don″top·to′si·a (o·don″top·to′shuh, ·see·uh), [*odous;* G. *ptōsis*, a falling]. Falling out of teeth. *Obs.*

o·don″to·ra′di·o·graph [*odous;* L. *radius*, ray; G. *graphein*, to write]. A radiograph of the teeth.

o·don″tor·rha′gi·a [*odous;* G. *rhēgnynai*, to burst forth]. Hemorrhage from the socket of a tooth.

o″don·tos′chi·sis (o″don·tos′ki·sis) [*odous;* G. *schisis*, cleavage]. Splitting of a tooth.

o·don′to·schism (o·don′to·skiz·um, ·siz·um) [*odous;* G. *schismē*, cleft]. A fissure in a tooth.

o·don′to·scope [*odous;* G. *skopein.* to examine]. 1. A dental mirror used for inspecting the teeth. 2. A magnifying device for inspection of tooth surfaces.

o″don·tos′co·py [*odous; skopein*]. The recording of the occlusion or bite of the teeth for purposes of identification.

o·don″to·sei′sis (o·don″to·sigh′sis) [*odous;* G. *seisis*, a shaking]. Looseness of the teeth from partial or total destruction of the alveolar processes; caused most frequently by gum disease. *Obs.*

o″don·to′sis, od″on·to′sis [*odous;* G. *-ōsis*, condition]. The formation and development of the teeth.

o·don″to·ste·re′sis [*odous;* G. *sterēsis*, deprivation]. Loss of the teeth. *Obs.*

o·don″to·syn″er·is′mus (o·don″to·sin″ur·iz′mus) [*odous;* G. *synerizein*, to contend together]. Chattering of the teeth. *Obs.*

o·don″to·the′ca [*odous;* G. *thēkē*, case]. The follicle of a tooth; the dental sac. *Obs.*

o·don″to·ther′a·py [*odous;* G. *therapeia*, treatment]. The treatment of diseases of the teeth. *Obs.*

o″don·tot′o·my [*odous;* G. *tomē*, a cutting]. Cutting into a tooth.

prophylactic o. Opening and filling structural imperfections of the enamel to prevent dental caries.

o·don″to·trip′sis [*odous;* G. *tripsis*, a rubbing]. The natural abrasion or wearing away of the teeth.

o″don·tot′ry·py [*odous;* G. *trypa*, hole]. Perforation of a tooth to remove pus.

o′dor [L.]. A scent, smell, or perfume; a fragrance.

o″dor·if′er·ous [*odor;* L. *ferre*, to bear]. Emitting an odor.

o″do·rim′e·try [*odor;* G. *metron*, a measure]. The measuring of the effect of odors upon the nasal sensory organs.

O'Dwyer, Joseph P. [*American otolaryngologist*, 1841–98]. Introduced the first satisfactory method of laryngeal intubation for diphtheria, and was the inventor of the metal tube and intubator (1884) known as *O'Dwyer's tube.* These tubes are made in several sizes and, after introduction, are left in the larynx for several days before removal or replacement. Devised a method for artificial respiration; see *Fell-O'Dwyer method* under *artificial respiration.*

od′yl, od′yle (od′il, o′dil). See *od.*

o·dyn″a·cou′sis (o·din″uh·kōō′sis), **o·dyn″a·cu′-sis** (o·din″uh·cue′sis, ·kōō′sis, o″din·uh·, od″in-uh·) [G. *odynē*, pain; *akousis*, a hearing]. Pain caused by noises.

-o·dyn′i·a, -o·dy′ni·a [*odynē*]. A combining form meaning *state of pain.*

o·dyn″o·pha′gi·a (o·din″o·fay′juh, ·jee·uh, o″din·o·, od″in·o·). Old term for dysphagia.

o·dyn″o·pho′bi·a [*odynē;* G. *phobos*, fear]. Morbid dread of pain; algophobia.

o″dy·nu′ri·a [*odynē;* G. *ouron*, urine]. The painful passage of urine. *Obs.*

oe-. For words beginning with *oe-* not found here, see words beginning *e-.*

oe·de′ma (i·dee′muh). See *edema.*

oed′i·pal. Pertaining to the Oedipus complex: also spelled *edipal.*

oed′i·pism. See *edipism.*

Oed′i·pus com′plex. See under *complex.*

Oehl, Eusebio [*Italian anatomist*, 1827–1903]. Author of a monograph on the histology of the skin (1857). Described the stratum lucidum of the epidermis, which is also called *Oehl's layer.*

o e·lec′tron. See under *electron.*

oe·nan″tho·tox′in (i·nanth″o·tock′sin, ee″-nanth·o·) [G. *oinanthē*, vine; *toxikon*, poison]. A toxic resinous principle from *Oenanthe crocata*, a poisonous plant (water hemlock) of Europe.

oenethyl. Trade-mark for 2-methylaminoheptane,

$C_8H_{19}N$, used intramuscularly or intravenously as a vasopressor in spinal anesthesia.

Oertel, Max Joseph [*German physician*, 1835–97]. Remembered for his description of circulatory disturbance due to cardiac disease. For these and for obesity he advised diet, reduction of body fluids by low intake of fluid, muscular exercises, including systematic mountain climbing and gymnastics; called *Oertel's method* or *treatment*.

oe·soph′a·go- (i·sof′uh·go-). See *esophago-*.

oe·soph″a·go·sto·mi′a·sis [G. *oisophagos*, gullet; *stoma*, mouth; NL. *-iasis*, condition]. A condition due to the presence of a parasitic worm of the genus *Oesophagostomum*.

Oe″soph·a·gos′to·mum (ee″sof·uh·gos′to·mum, i·sof″uh·) [*oisophagos; stoma*]. A genus of nematodes parasitic in the intestines, particularly the cecum, of gorillas, monkeys, and apes; rarely infests man.

oe·soph′a·gus (i·sof′uh·gus). See *esophagus*.

oes·tra′di·ol (es·tray′dee·ole, ·ol, ·awl, es·trad′ee·, es″truh·dye′·). Estradiol.

oes·tri′a·sis, es·tri′a·sis [G. *oistros*, gadfly; NL. *-iasis*, condition]. Myiasis due to the larva of the *Oestrus*.

Oes′tri·dae (es′tri·dee) [*oistros*]. A family of botflies (warble flies), some species of which produce larvae which live under the skin of cattle, causing a characteristic swelling called the warble. Also see *warbles*.

oes′trin (es′trin) [*oistros*]. Estrin.

oes′tri·ol (es′tree·ole, ·ol, ·awl) [*oistros*]. Estriol.

oes″tro·gen′ic (es″tro·jen′ick) [*oistros;* G. *genesthai*, from *gignesthai*, to be produced]. Estrogenic.

oes′trone (es′trone) [*oistros*]. Estrone.

oes′trum (es′trum) [*oistros*]. Estrus.

Oes′trus (es′trus) [*oistros*]. A genus of botflies.

O. ovis. Species which infests the nose of sheep and sometimes attacks the conjunctiva, the outer nares, and buccal regions of man.

oes′trus [*oistros*]. Estrus.

of′fal [E. *off, fall*]. Refuse of any kind.

of·fi′cial [L. *officialis*, of duty]. Referring to medicines recognized by, and conforming to the standards of, the United States Pharmacopeia or the National Formulary.

of·fic′i·nal [L. *officina*, a workshop]. On sale without prescription.

Ogata and Ogata's method. See under *stain*.

Ogston, Alexander [*Scottish surgeon*, 1844–1929]. Described operations for flatfoot and knock-knee. Also described an operation for opening the frontal sinus by trephining; called *Ogston's operation, Ogston-Luc operation*.

Oguchi, Chuta [*Japanese ophthalmologist*, 1875–1945]. Described congenital night blindness in Japan, called *Oguchi's disease*.

Ohara, Hachiro [*Japanese physician*, contemporary]. Described a disease similar to, or identical with, tularemia (yato byo) in Japan (1930); also called *Ohara's disease*.

Ohlmacher's fixing fluid. See under *fixing fluid*.

Ohm, Georg Simon [*German physicist*, 1787–1854]. Postulated a law stating that the strength of an electric current varies directly as the electromotive force, and inversely as the resistance; called *Ohm's law*.

ohm [*Ohm*]. The unit of electric resistance, equal to one thousand million units of resistance of the centimeter-gram-second system of electromagnetic units. The **international ohm,** adopted 1893, is the resistance of a column of mercury 106.3 centimeters long and weighing 14.4521 grams at 0°C. Its cross section is 1 $mm.^2$

ohm′-am′me″ter. A combined ohmmeter and ammeter.

ohm′me″ter [*Ohm;* G. *metron*, a measure]. Apparatus for measuring electric resistance in ohms.

-oid [G. *eidos*, form]. A suffix signifying *like* or *resembling*.

o·id″i·o·my′cin [G. *ōion*, egg; *mykēs*, fungus]. A vaccine prepared from the fungus *Candida albicans*.

o·id″i·o·my·co′sis (·migh·ko′sis). See *moniliasis*.

O·id′i·um [dim. of *ōion*]. A genus of fungi with characteristics intermediate between those of the yeasts and those of the molds.

O. albicans. Synonym for *Candida albicans*.

O. dermatitidis. Synonym for *Blastomyces dermatitidis*.

oi·kol′o·gy [G. *oikos*, home; *logos*, word]. 1. The science of the home. 2. Old term for ecology.

oi″ko·ma′ni·a, oi″ki·o·ma′ni·a. See *ecomania*.

oi″ko·pho′bi·a [*oikos;* G. *phobos*, fear]. Morbid fear of home, or of a house.

oi′ko·site [*oikos;* G. *sitos*, old term for food]. Parasite fixed to its host; an ectoparasite.

oil [L. *oleum*, from G. *elaion*]. A liquid, immiscible with water.

ajowan o. That from the fruit of *Trachyspermum ammi;* contains up to 50% of thymol. Syn., *ptychotis o.*

allspice o. See pimenta *o.*

almond o. (*oleum amygdalae expressum*). The fixed oil from the kernels of varieties of *Prunus amygdalus* (*Amygdalus communis*). Used as an emollient. Syn., *sweet almond o.*

amber o. (*oleum succini*). A product of the dry distillation of amber, formerly used as rubefacient and, internally, in amenorrhea, hysteria, and whooping cough.

aniseed o. See anise *o.*

anise o. (*oleum anisi*). The volatile oil containing 80–90% of anethol obtained from the fruit of *Pimpinella anisum* or *Illicium verum.* Syn., *aniseed o.*

arachis o. Peanut oil.

arbor vitae o. See cedar leaf *o.*

balm o. See melissa *o.*

banana o. Amyl acetate.

basil o. That from the Indian plant, *Ocimum basilicum;* consists principally of *l*-linalool and methyl cinnamate.

bay o. The volatile oil from leaves of *Pimenta racemosa.* It yields from 50–65% of phenols. A perfume oil. Syn., *myrcia o.*

behen o. A fixed oil from seeds of *Moringa apatera* and *M. oleifera.* A flavoring oil. Also called *ben o.*

benne o. Sesame oil.

bergamot o. (*oleum bergamottae*). A volatile oil obtained by expression from the rind of the fresh fruit of *Citrus aurantium* var. *bergamia*, yielding not less than 36% of esters calculated as linalyl acetate. A perfume oil.

betel o. The volatile oil from betel leaves; used as a local stimulant.

betula o. The volatile oil from *Betula lenta;* methyl salicylate.

bitter almond o. (*oleum amygdalae amarae*). The volatile oil from the dried ripe kernels of *Amygdalus communis.* It contains over 80% of benzaldehyde and from 2–4% of hydrogen cyanide. Dose, 0.016–0.06 cc. (¼–1 min.). The British Pharmacopoeia recognizes under the title *purified volatile oil of bitter almond* an oil obtained by distillation from the seeds of bitter almonds, peach kernels, or apricot kernels from which the fixed oil has been previously expressed. Contains not less than 95% of benzaldehyde and no hydrogen cyanide. Used as a flavor.

bitter orange o. (*oleum aurantii amari*). A

volatile oil from the fresh peel of the fruit of *Citrus aurantium.* A flavor.

bone o. An oil obtained by destructive distillation of bone or deer's horn: formerly used as an antispasmodic. Syn. *Dippel's o.*

bouchi o. Oil of bouchi (*Psoralea corylifolia*) used in leukoderma or vitiligo and the skin lesions of pinta. It may accelerate repigmentation.

cade o. The empyreumatic volatile oil from the wood of *Juniperus oxycedrus;* used in skin diseases. It contains cadinene, guaiacol, and cresol. Also called *juniper tar.*

cajeput o. (*oleum cajuputi*). Obtained by distillation from leaves and twigs of species of *Melaleuca.* Contains 50–65% of cineol. A stimulating expectorant, anthelmintic, and, externally, rubefacient and antiparasitic.

camphorated o. Camphor liniment (*linimentum camphorae*). A solution of camphor (20 Gm.) in cottonseed oil (80 Gm.); a popular liniment.

camphor o. A volatile oil obtained from the camphor tree, *Cinnamomum camphora;* used as a solvent, occasionally as a rubefacient.

caraway o. (*oleum cari*). A volatile oil distilled from the fruit of *Carum carvi,* yielding 50–60% of carvone, $C_{10}H_{14}O$. A flavor.

carbolized o. Phenolated oil.

cardamom o. (*oleum cardamomi*). A volatile oil distilled from the seeds of *Elettaria cardamomum.* A flavor.

carron o. Lime liniment, a mixture consisting of equal parts of linseed oil and lime water. Used in the treatment of burns.

cassia o. See cinnamon *o.*

castor o. (*oleum ricini*). The fixed oil obtained from the seed of *Ricinus communis;* the oil contains glycerides of ricinoleic acid which confer on it its cathartic property.

cedar leaf o. (*oleum cedri folii*). A volatile oil from the leaves of *Thuja occidentalis,* containing not less than 60% of ketones, chiefly thujone and fenchone. Formerly used in menstrual disorders, occasionally as a counterirritant. Syn., *arbor vitae o., thuja o.*

chamomile o. A volatile oil from chamomile flowers which has been used as an aromatic bitter.

champaca o. A volatile perfume oil from the flowers of *Michelia champaca.*

chaulmoogra o. (*oleum chaulmoograe*). The fixed oil expressed from the seed of various species of *Hydnocarpus,* containing principally glycerides of chaulmoogric and hydnocarpic acids. Long used in treatment of leprosy. Dose, 0.3–0.6 cc. (5–10 min.) increased gradually to 4 cc. (1 fluidrachm). Used externally in local treatment and as a counterirritant. Syn., *hydnocarpus o.*

chenopodium o. (*oleum chenopodii*). A volatile oil from the overground portion of the flowering and fruiting plant of *Chenopodium ambrosioides* var. *anthelminticum.* Contains over 65% of ascaridol, $C_{10}H_{16}O_2$. An anthelmintic. Dose, 0.2–0.3 cc. (3–5 min.) for well-nourished adults.

cinnamon o. (*oleum cinnamomi*). The volatile oil distilled with steam from leaves and twigs of *Cinnamomum cassia* and rectified by distillation. Contains 80–90% of cinnamic aldehyde. A carminative and local stimulant. Also germicidal and fungicidal. Dose, 0.06–0.2 cc. (1–3 min.). Syn., *cassia o.*

citronella o. A volatile oil from *Cymbopogon nardus.* Contains up to 93% of geraniol and citronellal. Its value as an insect repellent is said to be due to methyl heptenone.

clove o. (*oleum caryophylli*). The volatile oil distilled with steam from the dried flower buds of *Syzygium aromaticum.* Contains over 82% of eugenol. A local anesthetic, especially for toothache; a carminative. Dose, 0.12–0.4 cc. (2–6 min.).

coconut o. That present in the fruit of the coconut palm, *Cocos nucifera,* to the extent of 30–40%. Liquefies at about 23° C. Used chiefly in soap manufacture for its high lathering quality.

cod-liver o. See *cod-liver oil.*

colza o. See *rape oil.*

copaiba o. A volatile oil consisting chiefly of caryophyllene.

coriander o. (*oleum coriandri*). The volatile oil from the fruit of *Coriandrum sativum.* Contains 45–65% of coriandrol, $C_{10}H_{18}O$. A flavoring oil.

corn o. (*oleum maydis*). The fixed oil from the seed of *Zea mays.* A food and a solvent for injectable medicaments, especially hormones.

cottonseed o. (*oleum gossypii seminis*). The fixed oil from the seed of cultivated species of *Gossypium.*

croton o. (*oleum tiglii*). A fixed oil from the seed of *Croton tiglium.* A drastic purgative. Dose, 0.03–0.12 cc. (½–2 min.). Causes pustular eruptions when applied to the skin. Well diluted with a suitable vehicle, it is rubefacient.

cypress o. A volatile oil from the leaves and twigs of *Cupressus sempervirens.* Its vapors were once used in whooping cough.

dill o. (*oleum anethi*). The volatile oil from *Anethum graveolens.* Contains 40–65% of carvone, $C_{10}H_{14}O$. A carminative. Dose, 0.06–0.2 cc. (1–3 min.).

dwarf pine needle o. (*oleum pini pumilionis*). The volatile oil steam-distilled from the leaves of *Pinus mugo.* It contains bornyl acetate, levopinene, sylvestrene, and other principles. An inhalant in bronchitis; it has been used as an expectorant and antirheumatic. Syn., *pine needle o.*

erigeron o. A volatile oil consisting chiefly of α-limonene with some terpineol obtained from species of *Erigeron;* it has been used in diarrhea and internal hemorrhage.

essential o. Volatile oil.

ethereal o. (*oleum aethereum*). A volatile liquid consisting of equal volumes of ether and a so-called heavy oil of wine made up of ethyl esters of sulfuric acid.

eucalyptus o. (*oleum eucalypti*). The volatile oil from the leaves of *Eucalyptus globulus* or other species. It contains over 70% of eucalyptol. A local antiseptic and stimulating expectorant. Dose, 0.2–0.6 cc. (3–10 min.).

expressed nutmeg o. Mace oil or nutmeg butter; a solid oil obtained by hot expression of bruised nutmegs.

fennel o. (*oleum foeniculi*). The volatile oil steam-distilled from the fruit of *Foeniculum vulgare.* Contains about 60% of anethol. A carminative and flavoring oil. Dose, 0.2–0.3 cc. (3–5 min.).

fern o. Aspidium oleoresin; a vermifuge.

fir o. See Siberian fir *o.*

fixed o. Oil obtained from a vegetable or animal source, consisting chiefly of glyceryl esters of various fatty acids, and containing a higher proportion of esters of unsaturated acids than do fats.

flaxseed o. Linseed oil.

fusel o. A by-product, formed from protein materials, in the production of ethyl alcohol by fermentation; it consists chiefly of isoamyl alcohol with varying quantities of other alcohols. Syn., *commercial amyl alcohol.*

garlic o. The volatile oil present in garlic to the extent of about 0.1%. Chiefly allyl disulfide and allyl-propyl disulfide.

gaultheria o. (a) Methyl salicylate. (b) Volatile

oil consisting principally of methyl salicylate from *Gaultheria procumbens*.
gray o. Mercurial liquid used in syphilis.
gurjun o. See gurjun *balsam*.
haarlem o. A proprietary mixture of turpentine oil and sulfur balsam.
halibut-liver o. See *halibut-liver oil.*
haliver o. A refined halibut-liver oil, rich in vitamins A and D.
hydnocarpus o. Chaulmoogra oil.
iodized o. (*oleum iodatum*). An iodine addition product of vegetable oils, containing 38–42% of organically combined iodine. Used for the therapeutic effect of iodine and as an x-ray contrast medium.
jasmine o. A volatile oil from the flowers of *Jasminum odoratissimum, J. sambac, J. officinale* var. *grandiflorum*. A perfume oil.
juniper o. See cade *o*.
lavender o. (*oleum lavandulae*). The volatile oil steam-distilled from the fresh flowering tops of *Lavandula officinalis*, containing not less than 30% of esters calculated as linalyl acetate ($C_{10}H_{17}.C_2H_3O_2$). A perfume oil; carminative. Dose, 0.06–0.3 cc. (1–5 min.).
lemon o. (*oleum limonis*). The volatile oil expressed from the fresh peel of the fruit of *Citrus limon*. Contains chiefly *d*-limonene and phellandrene with 7–8% of citral and some citronellal.
linaloe o. A volatile oil obtained from species of *Bursera;* used in perfumery as a source of linalyl acetate.
linseed o. (*oleum lini*). A fixed oil obtained from the dried ripe seeds of *Linum usitatissimum.*
mace o. Expressed nutmeg oil.
maize o. Corn oil.
melissa o. A volatile oil from the leaves and tops of *Melissa officinalis;* has been used as a diaphoretic. Syn., *balm o.*
mineral o. Any mixture of liquid hydrocarbons obtained from liquid petrolatum. When refined to meet U.S.P. standards for liquid petrolatum, it is sometimes known as *white mineral oil.*
mirbane o. Nitrobenzene.
mustard o. A volatile oil, essentially allyl isothiocyanate, obtained from the dried ripe seed of *Brassica nigra* or *B. juncea*. A powerful rubefacient and blister.
myrcia o. Bay oil.
myristica o. (*oleum myristicae*). The volatile oil distilled with steam from the dried kernels of the ripe seed of *Myristica fragrans*. It contains chiefly *d*-pinene, *d*-camphene, and dipentene, and some myristicin. Syn., *nutmeg o.*
neroli o. Orange flower oil.
nutmeg o. Myristica oil.
o. of vitriol. Sulfuric acid.
olive o. (*oleum olivae*). The fixed oil from the ripe fruit of *Olea europaea;* composed chiefly of glyceryl esters of oleic and palmitic acids. It is used as a nutrient, laxative, emollient, and an ingredient of liniments, ointments, and plasters.
orange flower o. (*oleum aurantii floris*). A complex volatile oil distilled from the fresh flowers of *Citrus aurantium* and used for its odor. Syn., *neroli o.*
orange o. (*oleum aurantii*). A volatile oil obtained by expression from the fresh peel of *Citrus sinensis*. It consists chiefly of *d*-limonene. A flavor.
origanum o. The volatile oil distilled from the leaves of species of *Origanum* or marjoram.
palm o. Fixed oil from the fruit and seed of *Elaeis guineensis*. It contains chiefly palmitin, also some stearin and linolein: used mainly in the manufacture of soap and candles.
parsley seed o. The oleoresin of parsley seed containing apiol, apiolin, and myristicin. Also called *apiol, liquid apiol.*
patchouli o. An oil distilled from the leaves of *Pogostemon cablin* and *P. heyneanus*. Used as a fixative in perfumery.
peanut o. (*oleum arachidis*). Refined fixed oil obtained from seed kernels of one or more cultivated varieties of *Arachis hypogaea*, containing a large proportion of glycerides of oleic acid and smaller amounts of glycerides of linoleic, hypogeic, arachidic, and lignoceric acids: used as a vehicle for injections. Syn., *arachis oil.*
peppermint o. (*oleum menthae piperitae*). The volatile oil steam-distilled from the overground parts of the flowering plant of *Mentha piperita*, containing not less than 5% of esters calculated as menthyl acetate, and not less than 50% of total menthol, free and combined. Colorless liquid of strong, characteristic odor. Carminative and flavor. Dose, 0.1 cc. (1½ min.).
persic o. (*oleum persicae*). The oil expressed from the kernels of varieties of *Prunus armeniaca* (apricot kernel oil), or from the kernels of varieties of *Prunus persica* (peach kernel oil); occurs as a clear, pale straw-colored or colorless oily liquid and is composed chiefly of the glycerides of the higher fatty acids. Possesses the emollient properties of other fixed oils and has been used as a substitute for expressed almond oil.
phenolated o. (*oleum phenolatum*). Consists of 5% of phenol in olive oil. An emollient, mild antiseptic, and anesthetic.
pimenta o. (*oleum pimentae*). A volatile oil distilled from the fruit of *Pimenta officinalis;* yields not less than 65% of phenols, chiefly eugenol. Carminative and flavor. Syn., *allspice o.*
pine needle o. Dwarf pine needle oil.
pine o. Siberian fir oil.
pine tar o. See rectified *tar* oil.
poppyseed o. The fixed oil expressed from the seeds of *Papaver somniferum*. It contains none of the alkaloids of opium. British Pharmacopoeia requires that it be used in preparing the official iodized oil, obtained by treating the oil with hydriodic acid.
ptychotis o. See ajowan *o*.
rectified birch tar o. (*oleum betulae empyreumaticum rectificatum*). The pyroligneous oil obtained by dry distillation of the wood and bark of *Betula pendula* and related species.
rectified turpentine o. (*oleum terebinthinae rectificatum*). May be prepared by redistilling turpentine oil after mixing with a solution of sodium hydroxide. A carminative in flatulent colic, a stimulant expectorant, and a rubefacient. As an enema with soapy water, it is used as a strong cathartic. Dose, 0.3–0.6 cc. (5–10 min.).
rock o. Petroleum.
rose geranium o. An odorous volatile oil from *Pelargonium graveolens, P. odoratissimum,* and other species.
rosemary o. The volatile oil distilled with steam from the fresh flowering tops of rosemary. Contains at least 1.5% of esters calculated as bornyl acetate and 10% of total borneol, free and as esters. Used as a carminative and in rubefacient liniments. Dose, 0.2–0.4 cc. (3-6 min.).
rose o. (*oleum rosae*). The volatile oil distilled with steam from the fresh flowers of *Rosa gallica, R. damascena, R. alba,* and *R. centifolia,* and varieties of these species; a perfume and flavoring agent: also called *otto of rose, attar of rose.*
Russian o. A liquid petrolatum obtained originally from Russia and consisting chiefly of naphthenes of the general formula C_nH_{2n}. These derivatives of cyclopentane and cyclohexane are said

to emulsify more readily and thus cause less leakage than a product composed of members of the paraffin series. Certain American wells yield a similar product.

sandalwood o. (*oleum santalis*). The volatile oil from the heart wood of *Santalum album*. Contains chiefly santalol and santalyl acetate. Used in gonorrheal urethritis as a mild antiseptic. **Australian sandalwood oil** is obtained from *Eucarya spicata* (*Santalum spicatum*). Syn., *santal o.*

sapucainha o. A fixed oil derived from *Carpotroche brasiliensis*, containing hydnocarpic, chaulmoogric, gorlic (dehydro-chaulmoogric), palmitic, and oleic acids. It is used in leprosy.

sassafras o. (*oleum sassafras*). The volatile oil from the roots of *Sassafras albidum*. Contains about 80% of safrol. A carminative and antiseptic. Toxic in overdose. Dose, 0.12–0.4 cc. (2–6 min.).

savin o. A strongly irritant volatile oil from *Juniperus sabina* which has been used as an emmenagogue. Its action is said to arise from a systemic poisoning and not from a specific effect.

sesame o. (*oleum sesami*). A fixed oil obtained from the seed of one or more cultivated varieties of *Sesamum indicum;* occurs as a pale yellow, oily liquid. It is a semidrying oil. Contains about 75% of olein with smaller amounts of the glycerides of linoleic, palmitic, stearic, and myristic acids. Used for pharmaceutical purposes, especially as a solvent for certain hormones. Syn., *teel o.*, *benne o.*

Siberian fir o. (*oleum abietis*). A volatile oil from the leaves of *Abies sibirica*, containing about 40% of bornyl acetate. An expectorant in chronic bronchitis.

soy o. The fixed oil obtained from the soybean; a pale-yellow to brownish-yellow liquid consisting of glycerides of oleic, linoleic, linolenic, palmitic, and stearic acids: used in the manufacture of paints and soaps, also as a food. Also written *soya o.*, *soybean o.*

spearmint o. (*oleum menthae viridis*). The volatile oil from the overground parts of the flowering plant of *Mentha spicata*, yielding at least 50% of carvone. A flavor.

spike o. The volatile oil from the European lavender, *Lavandula latifolia*. Also called *spike lavender o.*

spruce o. A volatile oil from the hemlock spruce, *Tsuga canadensis*. Has been used in veterinary liniments.

star anise o. The volatile oil from *Illicium verum*. See anise *o.*

stone o. Petroleum.

sweet birch o. The volatile oil from the bark of *Betula lenta*, consisting principally of methyl salicylate.

sweet o. Olive oil.

tar o. See rectified *tar* oil.

teaberry o. The volatile oil from the leaves of *Gaultheria procumbens*, consisting essentially of methyl salicylate. Syn., *wintergreen o.*

teel o. Sesame oil.

theobroma o. (*oleum theobromatis*). A yellowish white solid consisting chiefly of the glycerides of stearic, palmitic, oleic, and lauric acids, obtained from the roasted seeds of *Theobroma cacao*. It melts between 30° and 35° C. and is used in the preparation of suppositories, in ointments, and as an emollient. Also called *cocoa butter*.

thuja o. Cedar leaf oil.

thyme o. A volatile oil from the flowering plant of *Thymus vulgaris;* it yields not less than 20% of phenols, chiefly thymol.

tung o. The fixed oil obtained from seeds of *Aleurites cordata;* a pale yellow liquid used in paints and varnishes and for other industrial uses.

turpentine o. (*oleum terebinthinae*). The volatile oil distilled from the oleoresin obtained from *Pinus palustris* and other species of *Pinus* which yield exclusively terpene oils. Also called *turpentine spirits*.

volatile o. Oil characterized by volatility, variously obtained from tissues of certain plants, particularly odoriferous ones. The oil may exist as such in the plant or may be formed during the process of obtaining it, as by hydrolytic or pyrolytic action. Volatile oils may contain a variety of chemical compounds, e.g., hydrocarbons, alcohols, ethers, aldehydes, ketones, acids, phenols, esters, and sulfur and nitrogen compounds. Syn., *essential oil*.

wheat germ o. An oil obtained from the embryo of choice *Triticum vulgare*. A group of chemically related substances have been separated from this oil, to which were given the name tocopherols; they possess the activity of vitamin E. One of these, α-tocopherol, is especially active biologically. It is suggested that wheat germ oil has a field of application in habitual and in threatened abortion.

white mineral o. Liquid petrolatum.

wintergreen o. Teaberry oil.

wood o. Dipterocarpus oleoresin; gurjun balsam.

ylang ylang o. A volatile perfume oil obtained from the flowers of the southern Asiatic tree, *Cananga odorata*.

oil red O. An acid monoazo dye; a fat stain; it stains more intensely and more quickly than Sudan III.

oil sug'ars (*oleosacchara*). Preparations made by triturating 100 Gm. of sucrose with 2 cc. of the prescribed oil.

oi·no·ma'ni·a [G. *oinos*, wine; *mania*, madness]. 1. A form of mental disorder characterized by an irresistible craving for, and consequent indulgence in, drink. 2. Delirium tremens.

oint'ment [L. *unguentum*, ointment]. A semisolid preparation used for a protective and emollient effect or as a vehicle for the local or endermic administration of medicaments. Ointment bases are composed of various mixtures of fats, waxes, animal and vegetable oils, and solid and liquid hydrocarbons, or, in the so-called washable or water-soluble bases, there may be from 50 to 75% of water incorporated into an emulsified product. For ointments not listed here, see under qualifying word or most important ingredient.

ammoniated mercury o. Contains 5% ammoniated mercury in a base of liquid petrolatum and white ointment. Syn., *white precipitate o.*

basilicon o. Rosin cerate.

benzoic and salicylic acid o. (*unguentum acidi benzoici et salicylici*). The U.S.P. XV preparation contains 6% of benzoic acid and 3% of salicylic acid. An antiparasitic. Syn., *Whitfield's o.*, *compound benzoic acid o.*

calomel o. Mild mercurous chloride ointment.

citrine o. Mercuric nitrate ointment.

compound benzoic acid o. See benzoic and salicylic acid *o.*

diachylon o. Lead oleate ointment.

Hebra's itch o. Compound sulfur ointment.

hydrophilic o. An official oil-in-water type of ointment base, containing stearyl alcohol, white petrolatum, propylene glycol, polyoxyethylene stearate, and water, preserved with methylparaben and propylparaben.

lead oleate o. Contains 50% lead oleate plaster, 49% white petrolatum, 1% lavender oil. Syn., *diachylon o.*

mercurial o. Two forms are official: **mild m. o.** contains 10% mercury and is applied in pediculosis pubi; **strong m. o.** contains 50% mercury and has been used as an antisyphilitic inunction.

mercuric nitrate o. Represents approximately 11% of mercuric nitrate in a lard base. Syn., *citrine o.*

mild mercurous chloride o. Contains 30% mild mercurous chloride in a base of hydrous wool fat and white petrolatum; used as an antiseptic. Syn., *calomel o.*

protective o. *In military medicine,* a substance used by a service personnel for protection against blister-gas burns and for limited decontamination of the person and, in emergency, of equipment.

simple o. White ointment.

stainless iodized o. (*unguentum iodatum denigrescens*). Prepared from iodine, oleic acid, paraffin, and petrolatum. No free iodine is present. Its value for any purpose is questionable. Also called *stainless iodine ointment.*

white o. (*unguentum album*). An official ointment base containing 5% of white wax and 95% of white petrolatum: also called *simple o.*

white precipitate o. Ammoniated mercury ointment.

Whitfield's o. Benzoic and salicylic acid ointment.

Wilkinson's o. Compound sulfur ointment.

yellow o. (*unguentum flavum*). An official ointment base containing 5% of yellow wax and 95% of petrolatum.

zinc o. Zinc oxide ointment.

Oken, Lorenz [*German naturalist and physiologist,* 1779–1851]. Remembered for his description of the Wolffian body; also called *Oken's body.*

-ol. *In organic chemistry,* a suffix denoting an alcohol or a phenol, both characterized by the presence of the —OH group.

O. L. A. *Occipitolaevoanterior;* left occipitoanterior position of the head of a fetus in labor.

o′le·a. Plural of oleum.

o″le·ag′i·nous (o″lee·adj′i·nus) [L. *oleagineus,* of the olive-tree]. Oily.

o″le·an′der. See *nerium.*

o″le·an′drin. See *folinerin.*

o″le·an·o′lic ac′id. $C_{30}H_{48}O_3$; a pentacyclic carboxylic acid occurring both free and as esters or glycosides in many plants: identical with caryophyllin.

o′le·ate [L. *olea,* olive-tree]. 1. A salt of oleic acid. 2. A pharmaceutical preparation made by a solution of medicinal ingredients in oleic acid.

o″le·cra″nar·thri′tis (o″li·kray″nahr·thry′tis, o·leck″ran·ahr·thry′tis) [*ōlekranon;* G. *arthritis,* arthritis]. Inflammation of the elbow joint.

o″le·cra″nar·throc′a·ce (o″li·kray″nahr·throck′uh·see, o·leck″ran·ahr·) [*ōlekranon;* G. *arthron,* joint; *kakē,* badness]. Inflammation of the elbow joint.

o″le·cra″nar·throp′a·thy (o″li·kray″nahr·throp′uth·ee, o·leck″ran·ahr·) [*ōlekranon; arthron;* G. *pathos,* disease]. A disease of the elbow joint.

o·lec′ra·noid [*ōlekranon;* G. *eidos,* form]. Resembling or pertaining to the olecranon, as the olecranoid fossa, the fossa at the dorsal side of the distal end of the humerus for the reception of the olecranon.

o·lec′ra·non, o″le·cra′non [*ōlekranon*]. The large process at the upper extremity of the ulna. —**olec′ranal,** *adj.*

o·lef′i·ant gas (o·lef′ee·unt, o·lee′fee·unt, o″li·figh′unt). Old term for ethylene.

o′le·fine (o′li·feen), **ol′e·fin** (ol′i·fin). Any member of the ethylene series of hydrocarbons; unsaturated compounds of the general formula C_nH_{2n}.

o·le′ic ac′id (o·lee′ick, o′lee·ick) (*acidum oleicum*). An unsaturated acid, $CH_3(CH_2)_7CH{:}CH(CH_2)_7COOH$, obtained from fats and fixed oils. Brownish yellow, oily liquid insoluble in water, miscible with alcohol. Used in the preparation of oleates and ointments.

o. a. series. Unsaturated fatty acids having one double bond and corresponding to the general formula, $C_nH_{2n-1}COOH$.

o′le·in. Glyceryl oleate, $(C_{17}H_{33}COO)_3C_3H_5$, the chief constituent of olive oil and occurring in varying amounts in most other fixed oils. A colorless or yellowish, tasteless, and odorless oil; insoluble in water. Solidifies at −4° to −5° C. Syn., *triolein.*

o′le·o- [L. *oleum,* oil]. 1. A combining form meaning *oil.* 2. *In chemistry,* a combining form signifying *olein, oleic.*

oleo-bi. Trade-mark for a suspension of bismuth oleate in olive oil representing 5% of Bi. The substance is used as an antiluetic.

o″le·o·mar′ga·rine [*oleum;* F., from G. *margaron,* pearl]. A butter substitute made by hydrogenation of a mixture of vegetable oils.

o″le·om′e·ter. 1. A hydrometer used to determine the specific gravity of oils, or calibrated in the range of specific gravity of oils. 2. An apparatus for determining the content of oil in a material.

o″le·op′tene. See *eleoptene.*

o″le·o·res′in (o″lee·o·rez′in) [*oleum;* L. *resina,* resin]. A substance consisting chiefly of a mixture of an oil, either fixed or volatile, and a resin, sometimes with other active constituents, extracted from plants by means of a volatile solvent.

o″le·o·sac′cha·ra (o″lee·o·sack′uh·ruh) [*oleum;* G. *sakchar,* sugar]. Oil sugars. Prepared by triturating 100 Gm. of sugar with 2 cc. of the prescribed oil.

o″le·o·ther′a·py [*oleum;* G. *therapeia,* treatment]. The treatment of disease by the administration of oils. Also called *eleotherapy.*

o″le·o·tho′rax [*oleum;* G. *thōrax,* thorax]. A condition in which the lung is compressed in tuberculosis by using injections of sterile oil.

o″le·o·vi′ta·min [*oleum;* vitamin]. A solution of a vitamin in oil.

o. A (*oleovitamina A*). Fish-liver oil or an oil solution containing not less than 50,000 U.S.P. units (15 milligrams) of vitamin A and not more than 500 U.S.P. units (12.5 micrograms) of vitamin D per gram.

o. A and D (*oleovitamina A et D*). A fish-liver oil or edible vegetable-oil solution of vitamins A and D.

synthetic o. D (*oleovitamina D synthetica*). A solution of activated ergosterol (vitamin D_2, calciferol, viosterol) or activated 7-dehydrocholesterol (vitamin D_3), in an edible vegetable oil. It contains not less than 10,000 U.S.P. units (250 micrograms) of vitamin D per gram.

o′le·um (pl. *olea*) [L.]. 1. Oil. 2. Fuming sulfuric acid; a solution of sulfur trioxide in concentrated sulfuric acid.

o′le·yl al′co·hol. $CH_3(CH_2)_7CH{:}CH(CH_2)_7CH_2OH$. The commercial product is a mixture of aliphatic alcohols consisting chiefly of oleyl alcohol, *cis*-9-octadecen-1-ol, an oily liquid, insoluble in water but soluble in various organic liquids. It is used as an emulsifying aid in formulation of dermatologic and cosmetic preparations. See *ocenol.*

ol·fac′tion [L. *olfacere,* to smell]. The function of smelling. —**olfactory,** *adj.*

ol″fac·tom′e·ter [*olfacere;* G. *metron,* a measure]. An instrument for determining the power of smell.

ol·fac′to·ry es·the″si·o·neu″ro·ep·i·the″li·o′ma. See olfactory *neurepithelioma.*

ol·fac′to·ry nerve. See under *nerve.*

o·lib′a·num [Ar. *al-lubān*]. A gum resin produced by various species of *Boswellia*. Has been used as a substitute for Peruvian and tolu balsams, as an inhalation in laryngeal and bronchial inflammations, for fumigation, and in plasters. Syn., *frankincense.*

ol″i·ge′mi·a (ol″i·ghee′mee·uh) [G. *oligos*, little; *haima*, blood]. A state in which the total quantity of the blood is diminished. See *hydremia.*

ol″i·ger·ga′si·a (ol″i·ghur·gay′zhuh, ·zee·uh, ·shuh, ·see·uh) [*oligos*; G. *ergasia*, work]. *In psychiatry,* Adolf Meyer's term for all types of feeblemindedness and mental deficiency.

ol″ig·hid′ri·a (ol″ig·hid′ree·uh, ·high′dree·uh, ol″i-ghid′ree·uh), **ol″i·gid′ri·a** (ol″i·ghid′ree·uh, ·jid′-ree·uh) [*oligos*; G. *hidrōs*, perspiration]. Deficiency of perspiration.

ol″ig·hy′dri·a (ol″ig·high′dree·uh, ·hid′ree·uh, ol″i-ghid′ree·uh) [*oligos*; G. *hydōr*, water]. Deficiency of the fluids of the body.

ol′i·go-, olig- [*oligos*]. A combining form meaning *few, scant;* used in medicine to denote *deficiency.*

ol″i·go·am′ni·os. Oligohydramnios.

ol″i·go·blen′ni·a [*oligos*; G. *blenna*, mucus]. A deficient secretion of mucus.

ol″i·go·cho′li·a (ol″i·go·ko′lee·uh) [*oligos*; G. *cholē*, bile]. A deficiency of bile.

ol″i·go·chro·ma′si·a (·kro·may′zhuh, ·zee·uh, ·shuh, ·see·uh) [*oligos*; G. *chrōma*, color]. A decreased amount of hemoglobin in the red cells, which present a pale appearance.

ol″i·go·chro·me′mi·a [*oligos*; *chrōma*; G. *haima*, blood]. Deficiency of hemoglobin in the blood.

ol″i·go·chy′li·a (ol″i·go·kigh′lee·uh) [*oligos*; G. *chylos*, juice]. Deficiency of chyle.

ol″i·go·cy·the′mi·a (ol″i·go·sigh·thee′mee·uh) [*oligos*; G. *kytos*, cell; *haima*, blood]. A reduction in the total quantity of erythrocytes in the body.

ol″i·go·cy·the′mic nor″mo·vo·le′mi·a (ol″i·go-sigh·thee′mick, ·themm′ick). A normal blood volume with a decrease in red cells.

ol″i·go·dac′ry·a [*oligos*; G. *dakryon*, tear]. Deficiency of the tears.

ol″i·go·dac·tyl′i·a [*oligos*; G. *daktylos*, finger]. A condition characterized by a deficiency of fingers or toes.

ol″i·go·den″dro·blas·to′ma [*oligos*; G. *dendron*, tree; *blastos*, germ; *-ōma*, tumor]. A glial tumor similar to the oligodendroglioma, but composed of somewhat larger cells showing more cytoplasm, larger nuclei with less dense chromatin, and mitotic figures.

ol″i·go·den′dro·cyte [*oligos*; *dendron*; G. *kytos*, cell]. See *oligodendroglia.*

ol″i·go·den·drog′li·a [*oligos*; *dendron*; G. *-glia*, glue]. Small supporting cells of the nervous system, located about the nerve cells, between nerve fibers (perineural satellites) and along blood vessels (perivascular satellites) and characterized by spheroidal or ovoid nuclei and fine cytoplasmic processes with secondary divisions. Syn., *oligodendrocyte, oligoglia.*

ol″i·go·den″dro·gli·o′ma (ol″i·go·den″dro·glye·o′-muh, ·den″drog·lee·o′muh) [*oligos*; *dendron*; *glia*; G. *-ōma*, tumor]. A slowly growing glioma of cerebrum, rarely of septum lucidum, fairly large and well defined, with a tendency to focal calcification. Microscopically, most of the cells are small, with richly chromatic nuclei and scanty, poorly staining cytoplasm without processes or neuroglia. Astrocytes in various stages of differentiation are often present. Also called *oligodendrocytoma, oligodendroma.*

ol″i·go·den″dro·gli·o″ma·to′sis [*oligos*; *dendron*; *glia*; *-ōma*; G. *-ōsis*, condition]. Diffuse dissemination of oligodendroglioma tumor tissue through the leptomeninges and, sometimes, also into the ependymal lining of the cerebral ventricles.

ol″i·go·den·dro′ma. See *oligodendroglioma.*

ol″i·go·don′ti·a [*oligos*; G. *odous*, tooth]. The condition of having few teeth.

ol″i·go·dy·nam′ic (ol″i·go·dye·nam′ick, ·di·nam′-ick) [*oligos*; G. *dynamis*, power]. 1. Active in small quantities. 2. Pertaining to toxic effects produced by direct contact of cells with minimal quantities of metals.

ol″i·go·el′e·ment. An element which, though present in low concentration, possesses a relatively high degree of activity.

ol″i·go·ga·lac′ti·a (ol″i·go·ga·lack′tee·uh, ·shee·uh) [*oligos*; G. *gala*, milk]. Deficiency in the secretion of milk.

ol″i·go·gen′ic [*oligos*; G. *genesthai*, from *gignesthai*, to be produced]. Referring to hereditary characters which are determined by one or a few genes.

ol″i·go·gen′ics [*oligos*; *genesthai*]. Old term for birth control.

ol″i·gog′li·a. See *oligodendrocyte.*

ol″i·go·hy·dram′ni·os (ol″i·go·high·dram′nee·os) [*oligos*; G. *hydōr*, water; *amnion*, membrane around the fetus]. Deficiency of the amniotic fluid.

ol″i·go·hy′dri·a (ol″i·go·high′dree·uh, ·hid′ree·uh). See *olighydria.*

ol″i·go·hy·dru′ri·a (ol″i·go·high·droor′ee·uh) [*oligos*; *hydōr*; G. *ouron*, urine]. Urine with a relative diminution of water; highly concentrated urine.

ol″i·go·lec′i·thal (ol″i·go·less′i·thul) [*oligos*; G. *lekithos*, yolk]. Having little yolk. Syn., *meiolecithal.*

ol″i·go·ma′ni·a [*oligos*; G. *mania*, madness]. Mental disorder on only a few subjects. *Obs.*

ol″i·go·me′lus [*oligos*; G. *melos*, limb]. Excessive congenital thinness of the limbs, or a deficiency in their number.

ol″i·go·men″or·rhe′a [*oligos*; G. *mēn*, month; *rhoia*, flow]. Abnormally infrequent menstruation: distinguished from *hypomenorrhea.*

ol″i·go·nu′cle·o·tide. A depolymerization product of a nucleic acid, characterized by a lower degree of aggregation of nucleotide units.

ol″i·go·phos″pha·tu′ri·a [*oligos*; G. *phōsphoros*, lightbringer; *ouron*, urine]. A decrease in the amount of phosphates in the urine.

ol″i·go·phre′ni·a [*oligos*; G. *phrēn*, mind]. Feeblemindedness; mental deficiency. —**oligophren′ic,** *adj.*

phenylpyruvic o. A mental deficiency associated with a metabolic disturbance wherein phenylalanine is not completely oxidized and phenylpyruvic acid accumulates. Syn., *phenylpyruvic amentia.* Also called *imbecillitas phenylpyruvica.*

ol″i·gop·noe′a (ol″i·gop·nee′uh, oli·gop′nee·uh) [*oligos*; G. *pnoē*, breath]. Respiration diminished in depth or frequency.

ol″i·go·psy′chi·a (ol″i·go·sigh′kee·uh, ol″i·gop·) [*oligos*; G. *psychē*, soul]. Mental deficiency. *Obs.*

ol″i·gop·ty′a·lism (ol″i·gop·ty′uh·liz·um, ol″i·go·) [*oligos*; G. *ptyalon*, saliva]. Deficient secretion of saliva.

ol″i·go·py′rene [*oligos*; G. *pyrēn*, stone of a fruit]. A term descriptive of abnormal sperm cells which contain only a part of the full complement of chromosomes. See *apyrene, eupyrene.*

ol″i·go′ri·a [G., an esteeming lightly]. An abnormal apathy or indifference to persons or to environment, as in melancholia.

ol″i·go·sac′cha·ride. Any carbohydrate of a class comprising disaccharides, trisaccharides, tetrasaccharides, and, according to some authorities, pentasaccharides: so named because they yield on hydrolysis a small number of monosaccharides.

ol″i·go·si·a′li·a (ol″i·go·sigh·ay′lee·uh, ·al′ee·uh, ·see·ay′lee·uh, ·al′ee·uh) [G. *oligos*, little; *sialon*, saliva]. Deficiency of saliva.

ol″i·go·sper′mi·a [*oligos;* G. *sperma*, seed]. Scarcity of spermatozoa in the semen.

ol″i·go·trich′i·a (ol″i·go·trick′ee·uh) [*oligos;* G. *thrix*, hair]. Scantiness or thinness of hair.

ol″i·go·zo″o·sper′mi·a [*oligos;* G. *zōon*, animal; *sperma*, seed]. Deficiency of the spermatozoa in the spermatic fluid.

ol″i·gu·re′sis. See *oliguria.*

ol″i·gu′ri·a [*oligos;* G. *ouron*, urine]. A diminution in the quantity of urine excreted.

ol″i·gyd′ri·a. See *olighydria.*

o·lis″ther·o·chro′ma·tin. The material found in the constricted portion of a chromosome.

o·lis″ther·o·zone′ [*olistheros;* G. *zōnē*, belt]. An area of constriction of a chromosome, important in identification of chromosomes.

ol′ive [L. *oliva*, from G. *elaia*]. 1. The oil tree, *Olea europaea*, of the Oleaceae. The value of the olive lies chiefly in its fruit, from which a fixed oil (**olive oil**) is expressed. Olive oil consists chiefly of olein and palmitin, and is used as a nutritive food; in medicine as a laxative; as an emollient external application to wounds or burns, and as an ingredient of liniments, ointments, and plasters. Formerly used in the treatment of gallstones and as an anthelmintic. 2. The inferior olivary nucleus. 3. An oval eminence on the anterior, ventrolateral surface of the medulla oblongata; it marks the location of the inferior olivary nucleus, which lies just beneath the surface. —**olivary,** *adj.*

accessory o. One of two small masses of gray matter: (a) the medial accessory olivary nucleus, lying medial to the inferior olive, and (b) the dorsal accessory olivary nucleus, lying dorsal to the inferior olive.

inferior o. See inferior olivary *nucleus.*

superior o. A small mass of gray matter situated on the dorsal surface of the lateral part of the trapezoid body of the pons immediately above the inferior olive.

Oliver, George [*English physician*, 1841–1915]. Discovered, with Sharpey-Schafer, the existence of an adrenal pressor substance (1894), later named epinephrine by Abel. Devised a test for albumin in urine; called *Oliver's test.*

Oliver, William Silver [*English physician*, 1836–1908]. Described a pulsation of the larynx elicited by grasping it between the thumb and index finger while the patient is erect; it is indicative of aneurysm of the aortic arch or certain mediastinal tumors; called *Oliver's sign, Oliver-Cardarelli's symptom.*

ol″i·vif′u·gal [L. *oliva*, from G. *elaia; fugere*, to flee]. In a direction away from the inferior olivary nucleus.

ol″i·vip′e·tal [*oliva;* L. *petere*, to seek]. Toward the inferior olivary nucleus.

ol″i·vo·pon″to·cer·e·bel′lar. Pertaining to the inferior olivary nucleus, pons, and cerebellum.

Ollier, Léopold Louis Xavier Edouard [*French surgeon*, 1830–1900]. Described dyschondroplasia (1889); also called *Ollier's disease.* Introduced intermediate-thickness skin grafts (1872), called *Ollier's grafts, method.* Later, the method was modified by Carl Thiersch and called *Ollier-Thiersch method.* The method of skin grafting perfected by Ollier and Thiersch consisted of sheets of epidermis only, or of all skin elements removed from the donor area with razor, knife, or in later years by a mechanically operated contrivance or dermatome, and held or sutured in place upon the skin defect. Ollier devised operations for excision of the elbow, for excision of the knee, for excision of the scapula, and for excision of the shoulder, each of which was once called *Ollier's operation.*

-ol′o·gy [G. *logos*, word]. A combining form signifying *a science*, or *a special line of study.*

ol″o·pho′ni·a [G. *oloos*, destructive; *phōnē*, voice]. Abnormal speech due to malformation of the vocal organs.

O. L. P. Abbreviation for *occipitolaevoposterior*, the left occipitoposterior position of the head of the fetus in labor.

Olshausen, Robert von [*German gynecologist*, 1835–1915]. Said to have been the first to perform the operation of suturing the round ligaments and a portion of the broad ligaments to the abdominal wall for the relief of retrodisplacement of the uterus (1886); called *Olshausen's operation.* Described operation of vaginectomy or extirpation of the vagina (1895).

o·lym′pi·an fore′head. The abnormally high and vaulted forehead seen in children with congenital syphilis.

-o′ma [G., tumor]. A suffix signifying *a morbid affection*, usually a tumorlike nodule or swelling.

o″ma·ceph′a·lus [G. *ōmos*, shoulder; *a-*, not; *kephalē*, head]. A placental parasitic twin in which there is imperfect development of the head and absence of upper extremities.

o·ma′gra (o·may′gruh, o·mag′ruh, o′mag·ruh) [*ōmos;* G. *agra*, a seizing]. Gout in the shoulder.

o″mar·thral′gi·a [*ōmos;* G. *arthron*, joint; *algos*, pain]. Pain in the shoulder joint.

o″mar·thri′tis [*ōmos;* G. *arthritis*, arthritis]. Inflammation of the shoulder joint.

o″mar·throc′a·ce (o″mahr·throck′uh·see) [*ōmos;* G. *arthron*, joint; *kakē*, badness]. Disease of the shoulder joint. *Obs.*

o·ma′sum [L., bullock's tripe]. The third compartment of the stomach of a ruminant. Also called *manyplies, psalterium.*

om″bro·pho′bi·a [G. *ombros*, rain; *phobos*, fear]. A morbid fear of rain.

o″men·tec′to·my [L. *omentum*, membrane which encloses the bowels; G. *ektomē*, excision]. Excision of a portion of the omentum; omentumectomy.

o·men″to·fix·a′tion. See *omentopexy.*

o·men′to·pex·y [*omentum;* G. *pēxis*, a fixing]. The surgical operation of suspending the great omentum, by suturing it to the abdominal wall.

o″men·tor′rha·phy [*omentum;* G. *rhaphē*, a suture]. Suture of an omentum.

o·men′tum [L.]. Apron; a fold of the peritoneum connecting the abdominal viscera with the stomach. —**omental,** *adj.*

gastrocolic o. See great *o.*

gastrohepatic o. See lesser *o.*

gastrosplenic o. The gastrosplenic ligament.

great o. A fold of peritoneum attached to the greater curvature of the stomach above and, after dipping down over the intestine, returning to fuse with the transverse mesocolon. Between the ascending and descending folds is the cavity of the great omentum. Also called *gastrocolic o.* See Plate 8.

lesser o. A fold of peritoneum passing from the lesser curvature of the stomach to the transverse fissure of the liver. On the right its edge is free and encloses all the structures issuing from or entering the transverse fissure of the liver: portal vein, hepatic artery, bile duct, nerves and lymphatics. Behind the free edge is the epiploic foramen. Also called *gastrohepatic o.*

o·men″tum·ec′to·my (o·men″tuh·meck′to·mee) [*omentum; ektomē*]. The surgical excision of any portion of the great omentum; omentectomy.

o·mi′tis [G. *ōmos*, shoulder; *-itis*, inflammation]. Inflammation of the shoulder. *Obs.*

om"ma·tid'i·um (pl. *ommatidia*) [L., from G. *ommatidion*, dim. of *omma*, eye]. One of the functional prismatic units of a compound eye, as in most arthropods.

omnadin. Trade-mark for a brand of prolipin, a sterile solution of protein obtained from nonpathogenic bacteria, various animal fats, and lipoids derived from bile. The substance is used for nonspecific lipoprotein therapy.

omni-beta. Trade-mark for a vitamin-B complex preparation in elixir and capsule form.

om·niv'o·rous [L. *omnivorus*, all-devouring]. Subsisting on all kinds of food.

o'mo-, om- [G. *ōmos*, shoulder]. A combining form meaning *the shoulder*.

o"mo·cer"vi·ca'lis. The levator claviculae muscle.

o"mo·hy'oid [*ōmos;* G. *hyoeidēs*, shaped like the letter upsilon]. Pertaining conjointly to the scapula and the hyoid bone, as the omohyoid muscle, which is attached to these bones. See Table of Muscles in the Appendix.

o"mo·ver'te·bral. Pertaining to the scapula and vertebrae.

OMPA Abbreviation for octamethyl pyrophosphoramide.

om"pha·lec'to·my [G. *omphalos*, navel; *ektomē*, excision]. Excision of the navel.

om·phal'ic [*omphalos*]. Pertaining to the umbilicus, as the omphalomesenteric duct or vitelline duct: that which connects the yolk sac with the fetal intestine during the first three months of intrauterine life.

om"pha·li'tis [*omphalos;* G. *-itis*, inflammation]. Inflammation of the navel.

om'pha·lo-, omphal- [*omphalos*]. A combining form meaning *the navel, umbilicus*.

om"pha·lo·an"gi·op'a·gus [*omphalos;* G. *aggeion*, vessel; *pagos*, that which is fixed]. See *omphalosite*. —**omphaloangiopagous,** *adj.*

om·phal'o·cele (om·fal'o·seel, om'fuh·lo·). See under umbilical *hernia*.

om"pha·lo·cho'ri·on (om"fuh·lo·kor'ee·on) [*omphalos;* G. *chorion*, chorion]. A chorion, or that part of one supplied by the omphalomesenteric blood vessels of the yolk sac. Also called *chorion omphaloideum, yolk sac placenta*.

om"pha·lo·cra"ni·o·did'y·mus [*omphalos;* G. *kranion*, skull; *didymos*, twin]. A double monster in which the parasite is attached to the cranium of the autosite by an umbilical cord.

om"pha·lo·did'y·mus. Gastrodidymus.

om"pha·lo·gen'e·sis [*omphalos;* G. *genesis*, production]. The development of the yolk sac.

om"pha·lo·mes"en·ter'ic [*omphalos;* G. *mesenterion*, membrane to which the intestines are attached]. Pertaining conjointly to the umbilicus and mesentery, as the omphalomesenteric artery.

om"pha·lo·mon"o·did'y·mus [*omphalos;* G. *monos*, alone; *didymos*, twin]. A twin monster in which the fetuses are joined at the umbilicus.

om"pha·lop'a·gus [*omphalos;* G. *pagos*, that which is fixed]. A double monster united at the umbilicus. Syn., *gastrodidymus*.

om"pha·lo·prop·to'sis [*omphalos;* G. *proptōsis*, a fall forward]. Abnormal protrusion of the navel.

om'pha·los [G.]. The umbilicus.

om·phal'o·site, om'pha·lo·site [*omphalos;* G. *sitos*, food]. The parasitic member of asymmetric uniovular twins. The parasite has no heart, or only a vestigial one, deriving its blood supply from the placenta of the more or less normal twin (autosite). Syn., *placental parasite, acardius, omphaloangiopagus, chorioangiopagus, allantoidoangiopagous twin, adelphosite*.

om"pha·lo·so'tor [*omphalos;* G. *sōtēr*, preserver]. An instrument for replacing a prolapsed umbilical cord.

om"pha·lo·tax'is [*omphalos;* G. *taxis*, arrangement]. Reposition of the prolapsed umbilical cord.

om·phal'o·tome [*omphalos;* G. *tomos*, cutting]. An instrument for dividing the umbilical cord.

om"pha·lot'o·my [*omphalos;* G. *tomē*, a cutting]. The cutting of the umbilical cord.

om'pha·lo·trip"sy [*omphalos;* G. *tripsis*, a rubbing]. Separation of the umbilical cord by a crushing instrument.

o'nan·ism [*Onan*, son of Judah]. 1. Incomplete coitus; coitus interruptus. 2. Masturbation. —**o'nan·ist,** *n.*

Onanoff's reflex. See under *reflex*.

on'cho- (ong'ko-). See *onco-*.

On"cho·cer'ca [G. *ogkos*, mass; *kerkos*, tail]. A genus of filarial worms.

O. caecutiens. Synonym for *O. volvulus*.

O. volvulus. A species which infests man, forming fibrous nodular tumors with encapsulation of the adult worms in the subcutaneous connective tissue, and often causing severe ocular disease when microfilariae invade the tissues of the eye.

on"cho·cer·ci'a·sis (ong"ko·sur·sigh'uh·sis, ·kigh'-uh·sis) [*ogkos; kerkos;* NL. *-iasis*, condition]. Infestation with the filarial worm *Onchocerca volvulus;* produces tumors of the skin, papular dermatitis, and ocular complications in man. Syn., *blinding filaria*.

on"cho·cer·co'ma. The fibrous nodular lesion of onchocerciasis which contains the adult worms (*Onchocerca*), usually located at a site at which a bone is close to the surface.

on"cho·cer·co'sis. Onchocerciasis.

on"cho·der·ma·ti'tis. Onchocerciasis; specifically, the cutaneous manifestations of it.

on'co-, oncho- [*ogkos*]. A combining form meaning *bulk;* used in medicine to denote *a tumor*.

on'co·cyte [*ogkos;* G. *kytos*, cell]. Columnar-shaped cells with granular eosinophilic cytoplasm, found in salivary and certain endocrine glands, nasal mucosa, and other locations; they represent dedifferentiation of parenchymal cells and may occur singly or in aggregates (oncocytomas).

on"co·cy·to'ma, on·ko·cy·to·ma. Rare tumor occurring primarily in the parotid gland but also in the submaxillary, hypophysis, thyroid, and other locations, composed of oncocytes, which may be in a lymphoid stroma.

on"co·gen'e·sis [*ogkos;* G. *genesthai*, from *gignesthai*, to be produced]. The process of tumor formation. —**oncogenic,** *adj.*

on'co·graph [*ogkos;* G. *graphein*, to write]. An instrument that records the changes of volume of an organ in an oncometer.

on·cog'ra·phy [*ogkos; graphein*]. The recording of measurements by an oncometer.

on·col'o·gy [*ogkos;* G. *logos*, word]. The study or science of neoplastic growth.

On"co·me·la'ni·a. A genus of amphibious snails.

O. hupensis. A species found in the Yangtze basin; one of the intermediate hosts of *Schistosoma japonicum*.

O. hydrobiopsis. A species found in Leyte and other of the Philippine Islands; an intermediate host of *Schistosoma japonicum*.

on·com'e·ter [*ogkos;* G. *metron*, a measure]. An instrument for measuring variations in the volume of an organ, as of the kidney or spleen, or of an extremity.

on·com'e·try [*ogkos; metron*]. Measurement by means of an oncometer. —**oncomet'ric,** *adj.*

on·co'sis. Any condition marked by the development of tumors. —**oncot'ic,** *adj.*

on′co·sphere [*ogkos;* G. *sphaira*, sphere]. The hexacanth embryo of tapeworms.

-one [G. *-ōnē*, indicating female descendant]. A suffix in organic chemistry meaning a *ketone.*

o·nei′rism (o·nigh′riz·um) [G. *oneiros*, dream]. A cerebral automatism analogous to the dream state, as a dream prolonged to the waking period. —**onei′ric,** *adj.*

o·nei″ro·dyn′i·a (o·nigh″ro·din′ee·uh) [*oneiros;* G. *odynē*, pain]. Disquietude of the mind during sleep; painful dreaming; nightmare. *Obs.*

o″nei·rog′mus (o″nigh·rog′mus) [G., effusion during sleep]. Seminal emission during sleep. *Obs.*

o″nei·rol′o·gy [G. *oneiros*, dream; *logos*, word]. The science, or scientific view, of dreams.

o″nei·ron′o·sus [*oneiros;* G. *nosos*, disease]. Disorder manifesting itself in dreams; morbid dreaming.

o″nei·ros′co·py [*oneiros;* G. *skopein*, to examine]. Diagnosis of mental conditions by the analysis of dreams.

one-min′ute de·na″tur·a′tion val′ue. The percentage of fetal type of hemoglobin present in total hemoglobin of blood, obtained by the following method: 0.1 cc of an approximately 10% stroma-free hemoglobin solution is exposed to 1.6 cc of 0.12 *N* NaOH solution for exactly 1 minute, after which 3.4 cc of a reagent to precipitate the chromogens and to stop the denaturation process is added. This reagent consists of 1 cc 10 *N* HCl added to 400 cc of half-saturated $(NH_4)_2SO_4$ solution. After filtration the undenatured hemoglobin (type F) is determined by photoelectric colorimetry at 540 mμ, and its concentration is expressed as the percentage of the initial amount of hemoglobin.

o″ni·o·ma′ni·a [G. *ōnios*, to be bought; *mania*, madness]. A mania for buying.

on′ion [L. *unio*, a kind of single onion]. The *Allium cepa* and its bulb. The latter contains a volatile oil resembling garlic oil and consisting principally of allyl sulfide, $(C_3H_5)_2S$. The onion has been used as a diuretic and expectorant; locally it has been applied as a rubefacient poultice.

on′ion·peel″ der′ma·tomes. The arrangement of the zones or segments of pain and thermal sensibility on the face; the zones have a concentric arrangement centering about the mouth and nose and represent the primitive lamination of the spinal nucleus of the trigeminal nerve.

on·kin′o·cele [G. *ogkos*, mass; *is*, fiber; *kēlē*, tumor]. Inflammation of the tendon sheaths, attended by swelling. *Rare.*

on″ko·cy·to′ma. See *oncocytoma.*

on″o·mat″o·ma′ni·a [G. *onoma*, name; *mania*, madness]. An irresistible impulse to repeat certain words.

on″o·mat″o·pho′bi·a [*onoma;* G. *phobos*, fear]. Morbid fear of hearing a certain name.

on″o·mat″o·poi·e′sis [*onoma;* G. *poiēsis*, production]. 1. The formation of words in imitation of a sound. 2. *In psychiatry*, the extemporaneous formation of words on the basis of sound association; frequently a symptom of schizophrenia.

O·no′nis [G.]. A genus of leguminous plants. The diuretic root of **O. spinosa,** restharrow, a shrub of Europe, is used in dropsy and gout. It contains saponinlike principles.

on·tog′e·ny, on″to·gen′e·sis (on·todj′i.nee) [G. *ōn*, pres. part. of *einai*, to be; *genesthai*, from *gignesthai*, to be produced]. The origin and development of the individual organism from fertilized egg to adult, as distinguished from phylogenesis, the evolutionary history of the race or group to which the individual belongs. —**ontogenet′ic,** *adj.*

on″y·al′ai (on″ee·al′ay, o″nee·al′ay·ee). An African disease of obscure origin. Characterized by distended vesicles of mucous membranes of the cheeks and hard palate. The tongue is often swollen. The skin and mucous membranes show hemorrhages; there is anemia and thrombocytopenia with prolonged bleeding but not prolonged clotting time; hematuria may occur. Syn., *tropical thrombocytopenia.*

on″y·chal′gi·a ner·vo′sa (on″i·kal′juh, ·jee·uh, o″ni·). Extreme sensitivity of apparently normal nails. Also called *hyperesthesia unguium.*

on″y·cha·tro′phi·a (on″i·kuh·tro′fee·uh, o″ni·kuh·), **on″y·chat′ro·phy** [G. *onyx*, nail; *atrophia*, want of nourishment]. 1. Atrophy of nails. 2. Failure of development of the nail.

on″y·chaux′is (on″i·kawk′sis, o″ni·) [*onyx;* G. *auxein*, to increase]. Hypertrophy of the nail.

on″y·chec′to·my (on″i·keck′to·mee, o″ni·) [*onyx;* G. *ektomē*, excision]. Excision of a fingernail or toenail.

on″y·chex″al·lax′is (on″i·keck″suh·lack′sis) [*onyx;* G. *exallaxis*, alteration]. Degeneration of nails.

o·nych′i·a (o·nick′ee·uh) [*onyx*]. Inflammation of the nail matrix.

o. craquelé. Fragility and fracture of the nail.

o. maligna. A form occurring in debilitated persons; characterized by an ulcer in the matrix of the nail, which becomes discolored and is thrown off.

o. punctata. A nail characterized by numerous small, punctiform depressions.

o. simplex. Onychia without much ulceration, with loss of the nail and its replacement by a new one.

o. superficialis ondulata. A rare type seen in secondary syphilis, characterized by superficial waves and ripples across the nail.

on′y·chin (on′i·kin) [*onyx*]. A hard substance found in nails; probably a type of keratin.

on′y·cho- (on′i·ko-), **onych-** [*onyx*]. A combining form meaning *a nail* or *claw.*

on″y·choc′la·sis (on″i·cock′luh·sis) [*onyx;* G. *klasis*, a breaking]. Breaking of a nail.

on″y·cho·cryp·to′sis [*onyx;* G. *kryptos*, hidden; *-ōsis*, condition]. Ingrowing of a nail. Syn., *unguis incarnatus.*

on″y·cho·dys′tro·phy [*onyx;* G. *dys-*, bad; *trophē*, nourishment]. Any distortion of a nail; a symptom seen in several diseases.

on″y·cho·gen′ic [*onyx;* G. *genesthai*, from *gignesthai*, to be produced]. Relating to the formation of the nails.

on″y·cho·gry·pho′sis (on″i·ko·grye·fo′sis, ·rgi·fo′-sis). Incorrect term for onychogryposis.

on″y·cho·gry·po′sis (on″i·ko·grye·po′sis, ·gri·po′-sis) [*onyx;* G. *grypōsis*, a crooking]. A thickened, ridged, and curved condition of a nail.

on″y·cho·hel·co′sis [*onyx;* G. *helkōsis*, ulceration]. Ulceration of the nail.

on″y·cho·het″er·o·to′pi·a [*onyx;* G. *heteros*, other; *topos*, place]. An anomaly consisting of the presence of abnormally situated nails, as on the lateral aspect of the terminal phalanges. Most often occurs on the little finger.

on′y·choid (on′i·koyd) [*onyx;* G. *eidos*, form]. Resembling a fingernail in form or texture.

on″y·chol′y·sis (on″i·kol′i·sis) [*onyx;* G. *lysis*, a loosing]. A slow process of loosening of a nail from its bed, beginning at the free edge and progressing gradually toward the root.

on″y·cho′ma (on″i·ko′muh) [*onyx;* G. *-ōma*, tumor]. A tumor of the nail bed.

on″y·cho·ma·de′sis [*onyx;* G. *madēsis*, loss of hair]. Spontaneous separation of a nail from its bed beginning at the proximal end and progressing rapidly toward the free edge until the nail plate falls off. Syn., *defluvium unguium*.

on″y·cho·ma·la′ci·a (on″i·ko·ma·lay′shee·uh, ·see·uh) [*onyx;* G. *malakia,* softness]. Abnormally soft nails.

on″y·cho·my·co′sis (on″i·ko·migh·ko′sis) [*onyx;* G. *mykēs,* fungus; *-ōsis,* condition]. A disease of the nails due to fungi.

on″y·cho·pac′i·ty (on″i·ko·pas′i·tee) [*onyx;* L. *opacus,* shaded]. White spots within the nail. Syn. *leukonychia.*

on″y·chop′a·thy (on″i·cop′uth·ee) [*onyx;* G. *pathos,* disease]. Any disease of the nails. —**onychopath′ic,** *adj.*

on″y·cho·pha′gi·a [*onyx;* G. *phagein,* to eat]. The habit of biting the nails at the free edge.

on″y·choph′a·gist (on″i·kof′uh·jist) [*onyx; phagein*]. One addicted to biting the fingernails.

on″y·cho·phy′ma [*onyx;* G. *phyma,* growth]. Disease of the nails.

on″y·chop·to′sis (on″i·cop·to′sis) [*onyx;* G. *ptōsis,* a falling]. Downward displacement of the nails.

on″y·chor·rhex′is (on″i·ko·reck′sis) [*onyx;* G. *rhēxis,* a bursting]. Longitudinal striation of the nail plate, with or without the formation of fissures.

on″y·chor·rhi′za [*onyx;* G. *rhiza,* root]. The root of the nail.

on″y·cho·schiz′i·a (on″i·ko·skiz′ee·uh, ·shiz′ee·uh) [*onyx;* G. *schizein,* to split]. An ungual dystrophy consisting of lamination of the nail in two or more superimposed layers.

on″y·cho·stro′ma [*onyx;* G. *strōma,* mattress]. The matrix or bed of the nail.

on″y·chot″il·lo·ma′ni·a (on″i·cot″i·lo·may′-nee·uh) [*onyx;* G. *tillein,* to pluck; *mania,* madness]. The neurotic picking at a nail until it is permanently altered.

on″y·chot′o·my (on″i·cot′o·mee) [*onyx;* G. *tomē,* a cutting]. Surgical incision into a fingernail or toenail.

on′yx (on′icks, o′nicks) [G.]. 1. A nail of the fingers or toes. 2. A collection of pus between the corneal lamellas at the most dependent part.

o″nyx·i′tis, on″yx·i′tis [*onyx;* G. *-itis,* inflammation]. Onychia.

o′o- (o′o-) [G. *ōion,* egg]. A combining form meaning *an egg.*

o″o·ceph′a·lus (o″o·sef′uh·lus). See *trigonocephalus.*

o′o·cyst [*ōion;* G. *kystis,* bladder]. The encysted zygote in the life history of some sporozoa. See *ookinete.*

o′o·cyte [*ōion;* G. *kytos,* cell]. An egg cell before the completion of the maturation process. Its full history includes its origin from an oogonium, a growth period, and the final meiotic divisions.

primary o. One in the growth phase preceding the first maturation division.

secondary o. One preceding the second maturation division.

o″o·gen′e·sis [*ōion;* G. *genesis,* production]. The process of the origin, growth, and formation of the ovum in its preparation for fertilization. —**oogenet′ic,** *adj.*

o″o·go′ni·um (pl. *oogonia*) [*ōion;* G. *gonos,* offspring]. 1. A cell which, by continued division, gives rise to oocytes. 2. An ovum in a primary follicle immediately before the beginning of maturation.

o″o·ki·ne′sis (o″o·ki·nee′sis, ·kigh·nee′sis) [*ōion;* G. *kinēsis,* movement]. The mitotic phenomena in the egg cell during maturation and fertilization.

o″o·ki·nete′ (o″o·ki·neet′, ·kigh·neet′, ·kin′eet, o′o-kin·eet) [*ōion;* G. *kinēteos,* to be moved]. The elongated, motile zygote in the life history of some sporozoan parasites; as that of the malaria parasite as it bores through the epithelial lining of the mosquito's intestine, in the wall of which it becomes an oocyst. —**ookinet′ic,** *adj.*

o″o·lem′ma. See *zona pellucida.*

o″o·pho·rec′to·my (o″o·fo·reck′to·mee, o·off″o·) [G. *ōiophoros,* bearing eggs; *ektomē,* excision]. Excision of an ovary.

bilateral partial o. Any partial removal of ovarian tissue from both ovaries.

o″o·pho·ri′tis [*ōiophoros;* G. *-itis,* inflammation]. Inflammation of an ovary.

o·oph′o·ro-, oophor- [*ōiophoros*]. A combining form denoting *an ovary* or *ovarian.*

o·oph″o·ro·cys·tec′to·my [*ōiophoros;* G. *kystis,* bladder; *ektomē,* excision]. Removal of an ovarian cyst.

o·oph″o·ro·cys·to′sis [*ōiophoros; kystis;* G. *-ōsis,* condition]. The formation of ovarian cysts.

o·oph″o·ro·hys″ter·ec′to·my [*ōiophoros;* G. *hystera,* womb; *ektomē,* excision]. Removal of the uterus and ovaries.

o·oph″o·ro′ma fol·lic″u·la′re. See Brenner *tumor.*

o·oph″o·ro·ma·la′ci·a (o·off″o·ro·ma·lay′shee·uh, ·see·uh) [*ōiophoros;* G. *malakia,* softness]. Softening of the ovary. *Rare.*

o·oph″o·ro·ma′ni·a [*ōiophoros;* G. *mania,* madness]. Insanity due to ovarian disorder. *Obs.*

o·oph′o·ron [*ōiophoros*]. The ovary.

o·oph″o·ro·path′i·a [*ōiophoros;* G. *pathos,* disease]. Any disease of the ovary.

o·oph′o·ro·pex″y [*ōiophoros;* G. *pēxis,* a fixing]. Surgical fixation of an ovary.

o·oph′o·ro·plas″ty [*ōiophoros;* G. *plassein,* to form]. Plastic surgery on the ovary.

o·oph″o·ro·sal″pin·gec′to·my [*ōiophoros;* G. *salpigx,* tube; *ektomē,* excision]. Excision of an ovary and oviduct.

o·oph″o·ro·sal″pin·gi′tis [*ōiophoros; salpigx;* G. *-itis,* inflammation]. Inflammation of an ovary and oviduct.

o″o·pho·ros′to·my [*ōiophoros;* G. *stoma,* mouth]. The establishment of an opening into an ovarian cyst for drainage. Also called *oophorocystostomy.*

o″o·phor′rha·phy [*ōiophoros;* G. *rhaphē,* suture]. Operation of suturing an ovary to the pelvic wall.

o′o·plasm [G. *ōion,* egg; *plasma,* anything formed]. The cytoplasm of the egg; it includes the yolk or deutoplasm, as well as the more active cytoplasm.

o″o·por′phy·rin [*ōion;* G. *porphyra,* purple]. A porphyrin occurring in the pigment from the eggshells of certain birds.

o′o·sperm [*ōion;* G. *sperma,* seed]. A fertilized egg; a zygote.

O·os′po·ra [*ōion;* G. *spora,* seed]. A genus of fungi which reproduce by mycelial fragmentation.

O. madurae. Synonym for *Nocardia madurae.*

O. minutissima. Synonym for *Nocardia minutissima.*

o″o·the′co-. For words beginning with *ootheco-*, see words beginning *ovario-* or *oophor-*.

o′o·tid [*ōion*]. The ovum after the completion of the maturation divisions, by which one ootid and three polar bodies are found.

o′o·type [*ōion;* G. *typos,* impression]. A muscular dilatation of the oviduct of certain trematode worms, in which secretory cells furnish shell substance to the ova.

o·pac″i·fi·ca′tion (o·pas″i·fi·kay′shun) [L. *opacus,* shaded; *facere,* to make]. 1. The process of becoming opaque. 2. The formation of an opacity.

o·pac′i·ty (o·pas′i·tee) [*opacus*]. 1. The condition of being impervious to light. 2. An opaque spot, as opacity of the cornea or lens.

o″pal·es′cent [G. *opallios,* opal]. Showing a play of colors; reflecting light; iridescent.

o″pa·les′cin, o·pal′i·sin [*opallios*]. A protein found in milk; it forms opalescent solutions.

o·paque′ [L. *opacus*, shaded]. Dark; obscure; not transparent; impervious to light.

o·pei′do·scope (o·pye′do·scope) [G. *ops*, voice; *eidos*, form; *skopein*, to examine]. An instrument for studying the vibrations of the voice.

o′pen [AS.]. 1. Exposed to the air, as an open wound. 2. Interrupted, as an open circuit, one through which an electric current cannot pass.

o′pen·ing [*open*]. An orifice; a hole or gap.

primary anal o. The orifice of the endodermal anal canal of the embryo.

saphenous o. An opening in the fascia lata at the upper part of the thigh through which passes the great saphenous vein: also called *fossa ovalis.*

secondary anal o. The definitive anal orifice formed by the growth of the external or ectodermal anal part of the cloaca.

op″er·a·bil′i·ty [L. *operari*, to work]. The qualities or state which permit surgical operation without the expectation of a fatal result.

op′er·a·ble [*operari*]. Admitting of an operation; referring to a condition where operation is not contraindicated.

op″e·ra′tion [L. *operatio*, a working, from *operari*]. 1. Anything done or performed, especially with instruments; a surgical procedure by a surgeon in which the method follows a definite routine. 2. The mode of action of anything; the specific action of a drug. For operations not listed below, see under the qualifying word.

ablative o. One in which a part is removed.

anastomotic o. One where two hollow organs, vessels, or ducts are joined by suture so that their contents may flow from one to the other.

Blalock-Taussig o. See Alfred *Blalock.*

bloodless o. One performed with little or no loss of blood.

Brock o. Valvulotomy of a stenosed pulmonary valve.

capital o. One which may threaten life; a grave or serious operation.

compensating o. *In ophthalmology*, tenotomy of the associated antagonist in cases of diplopia from paresis of one of the ocular muscles.

cosmetic o. A surgical operation to improve the appearance of a defective or unsightly part.

crescent o. For lacerated perineum, involving the vaginal entrance only; a crescent-shaped denudation is made from the vulvovaginal entrance, the angles of which extend into the vulvovaginal sulci.

elective o. One in which the time for operation may be set in advance, as a tonsillectomy.

emergency o. One which must be done at once to save the patient from an extension of the disease or from death.

endaural o. A fenestration operation, called *Lempert's o.* See Julius *Lempert.*

exploratory o. One performed for the purpose of diagnosis, often an abdominal operation.

fenestration o. *In otology*, the establishment of a window in the horizontal semicircular canal, for the treatment of otosclerosis.

finger fracture o. of the mitral valve. One for the relief of mitral stenosis in which the finger of the operator is used to increase the size of the stenosed opening.

high o. The application of forceps to the fetal head at the superior strait.

interposition o. An operation occasionally performed in aged women for relief of cystocele and prolapse of the uterus, performed through vaginal incision. The body of the uterus is fastened below the urinary bladder, and the pelvic floor is repaired.

interval o. One done between acute attacks of a disease, as an interval appendectomy.

Judet's o. Replacement of the head of the femur by an acrylic prosthesis to relieve arthritis deformans, congenital dislocation in the adult, pseudoarthrosis of the femoral neck.

Keller o. Arthroplasty of the first metatarsophalangeal joint to correct hallux valgus or hallux rigidus.

major o. A capital operation.

minor o. An operation which does not threaten life; one in which there is little or no danger.

palliative o. One designed to make the patient more comfortable when the condition cannot be cured.

plastic o. A reconstructive operation.

Pott's o. Side-to-side anastomosis of pulmonary artery and aorta in cases of tetralogy of Fallot.

prophylactic forceps o. The routine delivery by forceps in head presentations as soon as the head has come to rest on the pelvic floor.

radical o. One which seeks to extirpate or remove the causative factor of the disease or condition.

reconstructive o. One done to repair a defect, either congenital or acquired.

Semiramidian o. Castration. *Historical.*

shelf o. An arthroplastic procedure in the open reduction of a congenitally displaced hip, in which a bony shelf is inserted, by bone grafting, into the upper portion of the acetabulum so as to hold the femoral head and prevent its slipping out of the shallow joint cup.

Taarnhoj o. Surgical decompression of the semilunar ganglion and preganglionic roots for relief of trigeminal neuralgia.

Z-plastic relaxing o. An operation for the relaxation of scar contractures, effected by a Z incision, with transposition of the flaps. Syn., *Z-plasty.*

op′er·a″tor [L., a worker, from *operari*]. 1. A surgeon. 2. One who gives treatments, especially those involving mechanotherapy. 3. An expert technician, as in roentgenology.

o·per′cu·lum [L., lid]. 1. A lid or cover, as operculum ilei, the ileocecal valve. 2. The convolutions covering the insula. —**opercular,** *adj.*

frontoparietal o. The portion of the cerebral gyri overlying the upper part of the insula: also called *o. proper, parietal o.*

o. proper. The frontoparietal operculum.

orbital o. The portion of the orbital gyri of the cerebrum overlying the insula.

parietal o. The frontoparietal operculum.

temporal o. The portion of the temporal lobe overlying the insula.

trophoblastic o. The operculum, formed from the trophoblast, closing the wound in the endometrium made by the implanting ovum.

o·phi′a·sis [G., bald place on the head]. Alopecia areata in which the baldness progresses in a serpentine form about the hair margin. Usually seen in children.

o·phid″i·o·pho′bi·a [G. *ophis*, serpent; *phobos*, fear]. Morbid fear of snakes.

o′phid·ism [*ophis*]. Poisoning from snake venom.

oph′i·o·phobe″, o′phi·o·phobe″ [*ophis; phobos*]. A person who has an unusual dread of snakes.

oph″i·o′sis [*ophis;* G. *-ōsis*, condition]. Circumscribed baldness with scaliness.

oph″ry·i′tis [G. *ophrys*, brow; *-itis*, inflammation]. Inflammation of the eyebrow.

oph′ry·on (off′ree·on, o′free·on) [*ophrys*]. *In craniometry*, the point where the sagittal plane intersects an arc drawn horizontally from the frontotemporalia across the frontal bone.

oph″ry·o′sis [*ophrys;* G. *-ōsis*, condition]. Spasm of the muscles of the eyebrow.

oph″ryph·thei·ri′a·sis (off″rif·thigh·rye′uh·sis) [*ophrys;* G. *phtheiriasis,* morbus pedicularis]. Pediculosis of the eyebrows and eyelashes.

oph′rys [*ophrys*]. The eyebrow. —**ophryt′ic,** *adj.*

oph·thal″ma·cro′sis [G. *ophthalmos,* eye; *makros,* large; *-ōsis,* condition]. Enlargement of the eyeball.

oph″thal·ma′gra (off″thal·may′gruh, ·mag′ruh) [*ophthalmos;* G. *agra,* a seizing]. Painful ophthalmic symptoms attributable to an attack of gout.

oph″thal·mal′gi·a [*ophthalmos;* G. *algos,* pain]. Neuralgia of the eye.

oph″thal·mec″chy·mo′sis (off″thal·meck″i·mo′-sis) [*ophthalmos;* G. *ekchymōsis,* ecchymosis]. An effusion of blood into the conjunctiva.

oph″thal·mec′to·my [*ophthalmos;* G. *ektomē,* excision]. Excision, or enucleation, of the eye.

oph″thal·men·ceph′a·lon [*ophthalmos;* G. *egkephalos,* brain]. The visual nervous mechanism; the retina, optic nerves, optic chiasm, optic tract, and visual centers.

oph·thal′mi·a [G.]. Inflammation of the eye, especially one in which the conjunctiva is involved.

catarrhal o. Simple conjunctivitis; a hyperemia of the conjunctiva with a mucopurulent secretion.

caterpillar hair o. Inflammation of the conjunctiva or of the cornea, the result of penetration of the tissues by caterpillar hairs. Syn., *o. nodosa.*

Egyptian o. Obsolete term for trachoma.

gonorrheal o. An acute and severe form of purulent conjunctivitis, caused by infection by the *Neisseria gonorrhoeae.* Syn., *gonorrheal conjunctivitis.*

granular o. See *trachoma.*

jequirity o. That due to poisoning by jequirity.

neuroparalytic o. Disease of the eye from lesion of the semilunar ganglion or branches of the fifth nerve supplying the eyeball.

o. electrica. Conjunctivitis due to intense electric light.

o. neonatorum. A gonorrheal or purulent ophthalmia of the newborn. Also called *acute infectious conjunctivitis.*

o. nivalis. Snow blindness.

o. nodosa. See caterpillar hair *o.*

phlyctenular o. See phlyctenular *conjunctivitis.*

purulent o. Conjunctivitis with a purulent discharge.

scrofulous o. See phlyctenular *conjunctivitis.*

spring o. A form common in the spring, usually an allergy to tree pollen.

strumous o. Old term for phlyctenular *conjunctivitis.*

sympathetic o. A severe destructive inflammation, a form of iridocyclitis secondary to injury or disease of the fellow eye.

varicose o. That associated with a varicose state of the veins of the conjunctiva.

oph·thal′mi·a″ter (off·thal′mee·ay″tur, off·thal″-mee·ay′tur) [G. *ophthalmos,* eye; *iatros,* physician]. An oculist or ophthalmologist.

oph·thal″mi·at′rics [*ophthalmos;* G. *iatrikos,* skilled in the medical art]. The treatment of eye diseases. *Obs.*

oph·thal′mic [*ophthalmos*]. Pertaining to the eye.

oph·thal′mic nerve. See under *nerve.*

oph″thal·mi′tis [*ophthalmos;* G. *-itis,* inflammation]. Inflammation of the eye. —**ophthalmit′ic,** *adj.*

sympathetic o. That following injury of the fellow eye.

oph·thal′mo-, ophthalm- [*ophthalmos*]. A combining form meaning *eye.*

oph·thal″mo·blen″nor·rhe′a [*ophthalmos;* G. *blenna,* mucus; *rhoia,* flow]. Blennorrhea of the conjunctiva.

oph″thal·moc′a·ce (off″thal·mock′uh·see) [*ophthalmos;* G. *kakē,* badness]. Disease of the eye. *Obs.*

oph·thal′mo·cele. See *exophthalmos.*

oph·thal″mo·cen·te′sis [*ophthalmos;* G. *kentēsis,* a pricking]. Surgical puncture of the eye.

oph·thal″mo·co′pi·a [*ophthalmos;* G. *kopos,* fatigue]. Fatigue of visual power; asthenopia.

oph·thal″mo·di″ag·no′sis [*ophthalmos;* G. *diagnōsis,* a deciding]. Diagnosis by means of the ophthalmo-reaction.

oph·thal″mo·di″a·phan′o·scope [*ophthalmos;* G. *diaphainein,* to show through; *skopein,* to examine]. An instrument for examining the fundus of the eye by transillumination through the mouth.

oph·thal″mo·di″a·stim′e·ter [*ophthalmos;* G. *diastasis,* separation; *metron,* a measure]. An instrument used for determining the proper adjustment of lenses to the axes of the eyes.

oph·thal″mo·do·ne′sis [*ophthalmos;* G. *donein,* to shake]. A tremulous or oscillatory movement of the eye.

oph·thal″mo·dy″na·mom′e·ter (off·thal″mo-dye″nuh·mom′i·tur, ·din″uh·mom′i·tur) [*ophthalmos;* G. *dynamis,* power; *metron,* a measure]. 1. An instrument for measuring the power of convergence of the eyes. 2. An instrument which measures the pressure necessary to collapse the retinal blood vessels.

oph·thal″mo·dyn′i·a (off·thal″mo·din′ee·uh, ·dye′nee·uh) [*ophthalmos;* G. *odynē,* pain]. Neuralgic pain referred to the eye.

oph·thal″mo·fun′do·scope [*ophthalmos;* L. *fundus,* bottom; G. *skopein,* to examine]. An apparatus for examining the fundus of the eye.

oph″thal·mog′ra·phy [*ophthalmos;* G. *graphein,* to write]. Descriptive anatomy of the eye.

oph·thal″mo·gy′ric [*ophthalmos;* G. *gyros,* circle]. Pertaining to, or causing, movements of the eye.

oph·thal″mo·i″co·nom′e·ter [*ophthalmos;* G. *eikōn,* image; *metron,* a measure]. An apparatus for measuring the retinal image.

oph·thal″mo·ko′pi·a. See *ophthalmocopia.*

oph·thal″mo·leu′ko·scope [*ophthalmos;* G. *leukos,* white; *skopein,* to examine]. An instrument for testing color sense by means of polarized light.

oph·thal′mo·lith″ [*ophthalmos;* G. *lithos,* stone]. A calculus of the eye or lacrimal duct.

oph″thal·mol′o·gist [*ophthalmos;* G. *logos,* word]. One skilled or specializing in ophthalmology.

oph″thal·mol′o·gy [*ophthalmos; logos*]. The science of the anatomy, physiology, and diseases of the eye. —**ophthalmolog′ic,** *adj.*

oph·thal″mo·ly′ma [*ophthalmos;* G. *lymē,* maltreatment]. Destruction of the eye.

oph·thal″mo·ma·cro′sis [*ophthalmos;* G. *makros,* large; *-ōsis,* condition]. Enlargement of the eye.

oph·thal″mo·ma·la′ci·a (off·thal″mo·ma·lay′-shee·uh, ·see·uh) [*ophthalmos;* G. *malakia,* softness]. Abnormal softness or subnormal tension of the eye.

oph·thal″mo·mel″a·no′ma [*ophthalmos;* G. *melas,* black; *-ōma,* tumor]. A melanotic tumor, usually sarcoma, of the eye.

oph·thal″mo·mel″a·no′sis [*ophthalmos; melas;* G. *-ōsis,* condition]. 1. The formation of an ophthalmomelanoma. 2. The growth itself.

oph″thal·mom′e·ter [*ophthalmos;* G. *metron,* a measure]. 1. An instrument for measuring refractive errors, especially astigmatism. 2. An instrument for measuring the capacity of the chambers of the eye. 3. An instrument for measuring the eye as a whole.

oph″thal·mom′e·try [*ophthalmos; metron*]. Most commonly, the determination of refractive errors of the eye, mainly by measuring the astigmatism of the cornea.

oph·thal″mo·my·co′sis (off·thal″mo·migh·ko′sis) [*ophthalmos;* G. *mykēs,* fungus; *-ōsis,* condition]. Any disease of the eye or its appendages due to the presence of a fungus.

oph·thal″mo·my′ia·sis (·migh′yuh·sis, ·migh-eye′uh·sis) [*ophthalmos;* G. *myia,* fly; NL. *-iasis,* condition]. Infestation of wounds about the eye by eggs of flies from which larvae develop.

habronemic o. A granulomatous disease of the eyelids of the horse, caused by any of three species of the nematode *Habronema.* It has been suggested that the "blue eye" or "bung eye" of Australian bushmen may be due to this parasite.

oph·thal″mo·my·i′tis (·migh·eye′tis) [*ophthalmos;* G. *mys,* muscle; *-itis,* inflammation]. Inflammation of the ocular muscles.

oph·thal″mo·my″o·si′tis. See *ophthalmomyitis.*

oph·thal″mo·my·ot′o·my (off·thal″mo·migh·ot′-o·mee) [*ophthalmos; mys;* G. *tomē,* a cutting]. Division of a muscle or muscles of the eye.

oph·thal″mo·neu·ri′tis [*ophthalmos;* G. *neuron,* nerve; *-itis,* inflammation]. Inflammation of the ophthalmic nerve.

oph″thal·mop′a·thy [*ophthalmos;* G. *pathos,* disease]. Any disease of the eye.

external o. An affection of the eyelids, cornea, conjunctiva, or muscles of the eye.

internal o. Any disease affecting the eyeball.

oph·thal″mo·pha·com′e·ter, oph·thal″mo-pha·kom′e·ter [*ophthalmos;* G. *phakos,* lentil; *metron,* a measure]. An instrument for measuring the radius of curvature of the crystalline lens.

oph·thal″mo·phan′tom [*ophthalmos;* G. *phantasma,* apparition]. A model or mask for practicing operations on the eye.

oph·thal″mo·phas″ma·tos′co·py (off·thal″mo-faz″muh·tos′ko·pee) [*ophthalmos;* G. *phasma,* apparition; *skopein,* to examine]. Ophthalmoscopic and spectroscopic examination of the interior of an eye.

oph·thal″mo·pho′bi·a [*ophthalmos;* G. *phobos,* fear]. Morbid dislike of being stared at.

oph″thal·moph′thi·sis (off″thal·mof′thi·sis, off-thal″mo·tye′sis, off·thal″mof·thigh′sis) [*ophthalmos;* G. *phthisis,* a wasting away]. Phthisis bulbi; shrinking of the eyeball.

oph·thal″mo·phy′ma [*ophthalmos;* G. *phyma,* growth]. Swelling of the eyeball.

oph·thal′mo·plas″ty [*ophthalmos;* G. *plassein,* to form]. Plastic surgery of the eye or accessory parts. —**ophthalmoplas′tic,** *adj.*

oph·thal″mo·ple′gi·a [*ophthalmos;* G. *plēgē,* a stroke]. Paralysis of the ocular muscles. —**ophthalmopleg′ic,** *adj.*

nuclear o. A form due to a lesion of the nuclei of origin of the motor nerves of the eyeball.

o. externa. Paralysis of the extrinsic ocular muscles.

o. interna. Paralysis of the intrinsic muscles of the eye—those of the iris and ciliary body.

partial o. A form in which only some of the muscles are paralyzed.

progressive o. A form in which all of the muscles of both eyes gradually become paralyzed.

total o. That form involving the intrinsic muscles, as well as the extrinsic muscles, of the eyeball.

oph·thal″mop·to′sis [*ophthalmos;* G. *ptōsis,* a falling]. Protrusion of the eyeball; exophthalmos.

oph·thal′mo-re·ac′tion. A temporary inflammation of the conjunctiva due to the instillation of one drop of a 1% solution of tuberculin into the eye of a tuberculous subject.

oph·thal″mor·rha′gi·a [*ophthalmos;* G. *rhēgnynai,* to burst forth]. Hemorrhage from the eye.

oph·thal″mor·rhe′a [*ophthalmos;* G. *rhoia,* flow]. A watery or sanguineous discharge from the eye.

oph·thal″mor·rhex′is [*ophthalmos;* G. *rhēxis,* a breaking]. Rupture of the eyeball.

oph·thal′mos [G.]. The eye.

oph·thal′mo·scope [*ophthalmos;* G. *skopein,* to examine]. An instrument for examining the interior of the eye. It consists essentially of a mirror with a hole in it, through which the observer looks, the concavity of the eye being illuminated by light reflected from the mirror into the eye and seen by means of the rays reflected from the eye ground back through the hole in the mirror. The ophthalmoscope is fitted with lenses of different powers that may be revolved in front of the observing eye, and these neutralize the ametropia of either the patient's or the observer's eye, thus rendering clear the details of the fundus oculi. Many opthalmoscopes now in use are of the portable type and are fitted with a battery in the handle so that bedside examinations may be made. —**ophthalmoscop′ic,** *adj.*

stereo o. An ophthalmoscope with two eyepieces.

oph″thal·mos′co·pist [*ophthalmos; skopein*]. One versed in ophthalmoscopy.

oph″thal·mos′co·py [*ophthalmos; skopein*]. The examination of the interior of the eye by means of an ophthalmoscope.

direct o. The method of the erect or upright image, the observer's eye and the ophthalmoscope being brought close to the eye of the patient.

indirect o. The method of the inverted image; the observer's eye is placed about 16 inches from that of the patient, and a 20 D. biconvex lens is held about two inches in front of the observed eye, thereby forming an aerial inverted image of the fundus.

medical o. Ophthalmoscopy as an aid to internal medicine in the diagnosis of such diseases as manifest themselves in changes in the fundus of the eye.

metric o. That for measuring refraction.

oph·thal′mo·spasm [*ophthalmos;* G. *spasmos,* spasm]. Ocular spasm.

oph·thal″mo·spin′ther·ism [*ophthalmos;* G. *spinthēr,* spark]. A condition of the eye in which there is a visual impression of luminous sparks.

oph″thal·mos′ta·sis [*ophthalmos;* G. *stasis,* a standing]. Fixation of the eye during an operation upon it.

oph·thal′mo·stat [*ophthalmos;* G. *statos,* standing]. An instrument used in fixing the eye in any position during an ophthalmic operation.

oph·thal″mo·sta·tom′e·ter [*ophthalmos; statos;* G. *metron,* a measure]. An instrument for determining the position of the eyes.

oph·thal″mo·sta·tom′e·try [*ophthalmos; statos; metron*]. The measurement of the position of the eyes.

oph·thal″mo·ste·re′sis [*ophthalmos;* G. *sterēsis,* deprivation]. Loss or absence of one or both eyes.

oph·thal″mo·syn′chy·sis (off·thal″mo·sin′ki·sis) [*ophthalmos;* G. *sygchysis,* mixture]. Effusion into the interior chambers of the eye.

oph·thal″mo·ther·mom′e·ter [*ophthalmos;* G. *thermē,* heat; *metron,* a measure]. A device for recording local temperature in eye diseases.

oph″thal·mot′o·my [*ophthalmos;* G. *tomē,* a cutting]. The dissection or incision of the eye.

oph·thal″mo·to·nom′e·ter [*ophthalmos;* G. *tonos,* tension; *metron,* a measure]. An instrument for measuring intraocular tension.

oph·thal″mo·to·nom′e·try [*ophthalmos; tonos; metron*]. Measurement of intraocular tension.

oph·thal′mo·trope [*ophthalmos;* G. *trepein,* to turn]. An instrument used for the demonstration of the direction and the position that the eye takes under the influence of each of its muscles, and the position of the false image in the case of paralysis of a given muscle.

oph·thal″mo·tro·pom′e·ter [*ophthalmos; trepein;* G. *metron,* a measure]. An instrument for measuring the movement of the eyeballs.

oph·thal″mo·tro·pom′e·try [*ophthalmos; trepein; metron*]. The measurement of the movement of the eyeballs.

oph·thal″mo·vas′cu·lar [*ophthalmos;* L. *vasculum,* small vessel]. Pertaining to the blood vessels of the eye.

oph·thal″mo·xe·ro′sis (off·thal″mo·zi·ro′sis). See *xerophthalmia.*

oph·thal″mo·xy′sis (off·thal″mo·zye′sis, ·mocks-eye′sis) [*ophthalmos;* G. *xysis,* a scraping]. Treatment by scraping or scarification of the conjunctiva. *Rare.*

oph·thal″mox·ys′ter (off·thal″mock·siss′tur, ·mo-ziss′tur), **oph·thal″mox·ys′trum** [*ophthalmos;* G. *xystēr,* scraper]. An instrument for scraping or scarifying the conjunctiva.

oph·thal′mu·la [*ophthalmos*]. A scar of the eye.

oph·thal′mus [*ophthalmos*]. The eye.

-o′pi·a, -o′py [G. *ōps,* eye]. A combining form denoting a *defect of the eye.*

o″pi·an′ic ac′id. An acid, $C_{10}H_{10}O_5$, obtained from narcotine.

o″pi·an′ine. Old term for narcotine.

o′pi·ate [G. *opion,* poppy juice]. A preparation of opium; a substance that brings on rest or inaction; that which quiets uneasiness or dulls the feelings.

Opie, Eugene Lindsay [*American pathologist,* 1873–]. Known for his researches in the histology and pathology of the pancreas and its relation to diabetes mellitus.

o′pin. Porphyroxine.

o″pi·o·ma′ni·a [G. *opion,* poppy juice; *mania,* madness]. A morbid desire for opium; opium habit. —**opiomaniac,** *n.*

o″pi·o·pha′gi·a, o″pi·oph′a·gism, o″pi·oph′a·gy [*opion;* G. *phagein,* to eat]. The eating of opium.

o′pi·o·phile [*opion;* G. *philein,* to love]. An addict of opium; an opium smoker or eater.

o·pis′then [G., behind]. *In biology,* the hind part of the body of an animal.

o·pis′the·nar [*opisthen;* G. *thenar,* palm of the hand]. The back of the hand. Also see *thenar.*

o·pis′thi·on [G. *opisthios,* hinder]. *In craniometry,* the point where the sagittal plane cuts the posterior margin of the foramen magnum.

o·pis′tho-, o·pisth′- [G. *opisthen,* behind]. Combining form meaning *behind* or *backward.*

o·pis″tho·cra′ni·on [G. *opisthen,* behind; *kranion,* skull]. Not a set craniometric point, but that point, wherever it may lie in the sagittal plane on the occipital bone, which marks the posterior extremity of the longest diameter of the skull, measured from the glabella. Also called *maximum occipital point.*

op″is·thog′na·thism (op″iss·thog′nuh·thiz·um, ·thohn′uh·thiz·um, o″pis·) [*opisthen;* G. *gnathos,* jaw]. Recession of the lower jaw.

o·pis″tho·neph′ros [*opisthen;* G. *nephros,* kidney]. The mesonephros of certain Anamniota, in which the functional kidney arises from all nephrotomes caudal to the pronephros: proposed term.

o·pis″tho·po·rei′a (o·pisth″o·po·rye′uh) [*opisthen;* G. *poreia,* mode of walking]. Involuntary walking backward in an attempt to go forward; occurs in parkinsonism.

o·pis″thor·chi′a·sis (o·pis″thor·kigh′uh·sis, op″-iss·) [*opisthen;* G. *orchis,* testis; NL. *-iasis,* condition]. Infestation of the liver with the fluke *Opisthorchis felineus.*

Op″is·thor′chis (op″iss·thor′kis, o″pis·) [*opisthen; orchis*]. A genus of trematodes or flukes.

O. felineus. A species naturally parasitic to cats, dogs, foxes, and hogs, and accidentally to man. Produces hepatic lesions and extensive hyperplasia of the biliary ducts.

O. noverca. A species parasitic to dogs and occasionally found in man.

O. viverrini. A natural parasite of civet cat and an important human infestation in the Laos country of northern Siam.

op″is·thot′o·nos, op″is·thot′o·nus (op″iss·thot′o-nos, o″pis·) [*opisthen;* G. *tonos,* tension]. A condition in which, from a tetanic spasm of the muscles of the back, the head and lower limbs are bent backward and the trunk is arched forward. —**opisthoton′ic, opisthotonoid,** *adj.*

o′pi·um [G. *opion,* poppy juice]. The air-dried juice from unripe capsules of *Papaver somniferum,* or its variety *album.* It contains a number of alkaloids, of which morphine is the most important, since it represents the chief properties of the drug. Crude opium contains 5–15% morphine, 2–8% narcotine, 0.1–2.5% codeine, 0.5–2.0% papaverine, 0.15–0.5% thebaine, 0.1–0.4% narceine, and lesser amounts of cryptopine, laudanine, and other alkaloids. These bases occur in opium combined with meconic and lactic acids. Opium acts as a narcotic, dulls pain and discomfort, and produces deep sleep, which may be preceded by a stage of mental excitement and exhilaration; on awakening there may be headache, nausea, or vomiting. Small doses do not depress the respiration, but large doses do so in a marked degree. It causes gastric spasm and constipation, and lessens all secretions except that of the skin; it produces contraction of the pupil. When taken in poisonous doses it causes unconquerable drowsiness, passing into deep sleep, with slow, full respiration, slow pulse, and contracted pupils; later cyanosis develops, the respiration becomes exceedingly slow, and the pulse rapid and feeble; death takes place from failure of the respiration. The habitual use of opium or morphine leads to stubborn addiction. The drug is used for the relief of pain of all forms except that due to cerebral inflammation; in inflammation of serous membranes; in spasmodic conditions; in acute colds; for cough, vomiting, diarrhea, and certain forms of dyspnea, particularly that from heart disease.

camphorated o. tincture (*tinctura opii camphorata*). Contains opium, anise oil, benzoic acid, and camphor. It is used as an anodyne and in diarrheas. Dose, for an infant, 0.3–1.3 cc. (5–20 min.); for an adult, 4–15 cc. (1–4 fluidrachms). Syn., *paregoric.*

compound o. and glycyrrhiza mixture (*mistura opii et glycyrrhizae composita*). Contains camphorated opium tincture, glycyrrhiza fluidextract, antimony potassium tartrate, ethyl nitrite spirit, glycerin, and water. A nauseating expectorant. Dose, 4–15 cc. (1–4 fluidrachms). Also called *brown mixture, compound glycyrrhiza mixture.*

denarcotized o. Opium freed of certain nauseating constituents by extraction with petroleum benzin. Also called *deodorized o.*

granulated o. (*opium granulatum*). A coarse powder containing from 10–10.5% of anhydrous morphine. Dose, 0.03–0.2 Gm. (½–3 gr.).

ipecac and o. powder (*pulvis ipecacuanhae et opii*). Contains 10% each of ipecac and opium. A diaphoretic and sedative. Dose, 0.2–0.6 Gm. (3–10 gr.). Syn., *Dover's powder.*

o. extract (*extractum opii*). Prepared by maceration or percolation with hot water, contains 20% of anhydrous morphine. Dose, 0.01–0.06 Gm. (⅙–1 gr.).

o. tincture (*tinctura opii*). Contains 1% of anhydrous morphine. Dose, 0.3–0.6 cc. (5–10 min.). Also called *laudanum, deodorized opium tincture.*

powdered o. (*opium pulveratum*). Contains 10–10.5% of anhydrous morphine. Dose, 0.03–0.2 Gm. (½–3 gr.).

op′o- [G. *opos*, juice]. *In pharmacology*, a combining form meaning *juice.*

op″o·bal′sam (op″o·bawl′sum), **op″o·bal′sa·mum** (op″o·bal′suh·mum, ·bawl·sam′um). See Gilead *balsam.*

op″o·ceph′a·lus [G. *ōps*, eye; *kephalē*, head]. A monster characterized by fusion of the ears, one orbit, and absence of mouth and nose.

op″o·del′doc. A soap liniment.

liquid o. Camphor and soap liniment.

solid o. Solid soap liniment. Also called *camphorated soap liniment.*

op″o·did′y·mus, o·pod′y·mus [*ōps;* G. *didymos*, twin]. A monster with a single body and skull but with two distinct faces. Syn., *diprosopus.*

Oppenheim, Hermann [*German neurologist*, 1858–1919]. Known for his description of amyotonia congenita (1900); also called *Oppenheim's disease.* Described torsion spasm or dystonia musculorum deformans, which is also called *Ziehen-Oppenheim's disease* (1911). See also Oppenheim *reflex.*

Oppenheim, Maurice (1876–1949). American dermatologist who described necrobiosis lipoidica, which is also called *Oppenheim-Urbach disease, Oppenheim disease.* See also *Müller-Oppenheim reaction* under Rudolf *Müller.*

op″pi·la′tion [L. *oppilatio*, an obstructing]. 1. Obstruction; a closing of the pores. 2. A constipating agent or remedy. *Obs.* —**op′pilative,** *adj., n.*

op·po′nens (o·po′nenz) [L. *opponere*, to oppose]. Opposing; applied to certain muscles that bring one part opposite another, as opponens pollicis, a muscle placing the thumb opposite the little finger. See Table of Muscles in the Appendix.

o. digiti minimi. BR term for the opponens digiti quinti muscle.

op·por·tu′nist. *In bacteriology*, an organism incapable of inducing disease in a healthy host, but producing severe to fatal infections in a less resistant or injured host; e.g., certain types of *Escherichia coli* and the fusospirochetal group of synergistic organisms.

-ops [G. *ōps*, eye]. *In botany and zoology*, a combining form meaning *-eyed.*

-op′si·a, -op′sy [G. *opsis*, vision]. A combining form denoting a *condition of vision.*

op·sig′e·nes (op·sidj′i·neez) [G. *opse*, late; *genesthai*, from *gignesthai*, to be produced]. Born late, referring to certain body tissues which come into use long after birth, as the wisdom teeth.

op·sin′o·gen, op′so·gen [G. *opsōnein*, to buy victuals; *genesthai*]. A substance producing an opsonin.

op″si·nog′e·nous (op″si·nodj′i·nus) [*opsōnein; genesthai*]. Capable of producing an opsonin.

op″si·om′e·ter. See *optometer.*

op″si·o·no′sis (op″see·o·no′sis, op″see·on′o·sis) [G. *opsis*, vision; *-ōsis*, condition]. A disease of the eye, or of vision.

op″si·u′ri·a [G. *opse*, late; *ouron*, urine]. Condition in which more urine is excreted during fasting than after a meal. *Obs.*

op′so·gen. Opsinogen.

op″so·ma′ni·a [G. *opson*, cooked food; *mania*, madness]. Intense craving for dainties or some special food. —**opsomaniac,** *n.*

op′so·nin, op·so′nin [*opsōnein*]. A substance occurring in blood serum which is necessary to prepare bacteria for phagocytosis. It occurs normally and may be increased by immunization. —**op·son′ic,** *adj.*

immune o. An opsonin in the serum resulting from infection or inoculation with dead bacteria of the same species, and active only against the microorganism that created it. See *bacteriotropin.*

op·son″i·za′tion [*opsōnein*]. The process by which bacteria are rendered susceptible to phagocytosis.

op′so·nize [*opsōnein*]. Prepare microorganisms for phagocytosis.

op″so·no·cy″to·pha′gic (op″so·no·sigh″to·fay′·jick, ·sigh·tof′uh·jick) [*opsōnein;* G. *kytos*, cell; *phagein*, to eat]. Pertaining to the phagocytic activity of blood containing serum opsonins and homologous leukocytes.

op″so·nom′e·try [*opsōnein;* G. *metron*, a measure]. The estimation of the opsonic index.

op·son″o·ther′a·py [*opsōnein;* G. *therapeia*, treatment]. The treatment of disease by increasing the opsonic power of the blood.

optalidon. A proprietary tablet containing isobutylallylbarbituric acid, aminopyrine, and caffeine.

op″tes·the′si·a (op″tess·thee′zhuh, ·zee·uh) [G. *optikos*, of sight; *aisthēsis*, perception]. Visual sensibility.

op′tic [*optikos*]. Pertaining to the eye.

op′ti·cal [*optikos*]. 1. A synonym for optic. 2. Pertaining to light and the science of optics.

op′ti·cal an′ti·pode. See *enantiomorph.*

op′ti·cal den′si·ty. See *absorbance.*

op′ti·cal flat. A glass or quartz plate or disk, ground flat until any remaining unevenness can be measured only by interferometric methods, the maximum departure from flatness usually being less than 1/10 of a wavelength of sodium light.

op′ti·cal glass. An especially fine glass made under the most carefully controlled conditions. There are many kinds, some with low index and high dispersion values and some with high index and low dispersion.

op′ti·cal path dif′fer·ence. The product of the thickness of a specimen times its index of refraction.

op·ti′cian [*optikos*]. A maker of optical instruments or lenses.

dispensing o. One who retails spectacles and ophthalmic lenses.

op·ti′cian·ry. The application of the art and science of optics to the compounding, filling, and adapting of ophthalmic prescriptions.

op′tic nerve. See under *nerve.*

op″ti·co·chi″as·mat′ic (op″ti·ko·kigh″az·mat′ick), **op″ti·co·chi·as′mic** (·kigh·az′mick) [*optikos;* G. *chiasma*, a placing crosswise]. Pertaining to the optic nerve and optic chiasma.

op″ti·co·cil′i·ar″y [*optikos;* L. *cilium*, eyelid]. Pertaining to the optic and ciliary nerves.

op′ti·coele (op′ti·seel). The cavity of the optic vesicle.

op″ti·co·pu′pil·lar″y [*optikos;* L. *pupilla*, pupil]. Pertaining to the optic nerve and the pupil.

op′tics [*optikos*]. That branch of physics treating of the laws of light, its refraction and reflection, and of its relation to vision.

electron o. Science of the emission and propagation of electrons and of the factors controlling and modifying their flow, especially when applied to electron microscopy.

physiological o. That branch of optics dealing with the eye.

op·tim′e·ter [*optikos;* G. *metron*, a measure]. Optometer.

op′ti·mum [L. *optimus*, best]. The temperature or other condition at which vital processes are carried on with the greatest activity. Between the minimum and maximum temperatures or other conditions. —**optimal,** *adj.*

op′to- [G. *optikos*, of sight]. A combining form denoting *vision* or *optic*.

optochin. Trade-mark for ethylhydrocupreine, a potent pneumococcide employed as the base and also in the form of the hydrochloride.

op′to·gram [*optikos;* G. *gramma*, letter]. An image made on the retina by the sensitiveness to light of pigment in the eye.

op·tom′e·ter [*optikos;* G. *metron*, a measure]. An instrument for determining the strength of vision, especially the degree of refractive error that is to be corrected.

prism o. An instrument for prismatic testing of the refraction of the eye.

skiascope o. One designed for the determination of the refraction of the eye by retinoscopy.

op·tom′e·trist [*optikos; metron*]. One who measures the degrees of visual powers, without the aid of a cycloplegic or mydriatic; a refractionist.

op·tom′e·try [*optikos; metron*]. Measurement of the visual powers.

op″to·my·om′e·ter (op″to·migh·om′i·tur) [*optikos;* G. *mys*, muscle; *metron*]. An instrument for measuring the strength of the extrinsic muscles of the eye.

op′to·type [*optikos;* G. *typos*, impression]. A test type used in testing the acuity of vision.

O·pun′ti·a (o·pun′shee·uh, ·tee·uh) [G. *Opous*, city in Locris]. Prickly pear; a genus of the Cactaceae, represented by numerous species, many of which, as **O. reticulata** and **O. tuna,** have slight medicinal properties.

o′ra [L., edge, margin]. Margin.

o. serrata. The serrated margin of the sensory portion of the retina, behind the ciliary body.

o′ra. Plural of os (meaning "mouth").

o′rad [L. *os*, mouth; *ad*, toward]. Toward the mouth, or the oral region.

oradiol. Trade-mark for *ethynyl estradiol*.

o′ral [*os*]. Pertaining to the mouth.

o′ral char′ac·ter. A Freudian term applied to persons who, during the developmental period, have undergone an unusual degree of oral stimulation through poor feeding habits and otherwise and who thereby have laid the basis for a particular type of character, usually characterized by a general attitude of carefree indifference and by dependence on a mother or mother substitute to provide for their needs throughout life with little or no effort of their own.

o·ra′le (o·rah′lee, o·ray′lee) [*os*]. *In craniometry*, the point on the anterior portion of the hard palate where the line, drawn tangent to the lingual margins of the alveoli of the medial incisor teeth, and projected upon the hard palate, crosses the sagittal plane.

or′ange G (C.C.). An acid monoazo dye; used as a counterstain with nuclear stains.

or′ange I (C.C.). $NaSO_3.C_6H_4.N{:}N.C_{10}H_6.OH$; sodium azo-α-naphtholsulfanilate; a reddish-brown powder, soluble in water. When certified, a pure form, used to color foods, drugs, and cosmetics, is known as F. D. & C. Orange No. 1. Syn., *tropaeolin 000*.

or′ange II (C.C.). An acid monoazo dye; used in histologic staining.

oranixon. Trade-mark for *mephenesin*.

oravax. Trade-mark for a polyvalent catarrhal vaccine in enteric coated tablets containing killed bacteria of species common to the upper respiratory tract. The tablets are used for prophylaxis against the common cold.

Orbeli, Leon Abgarovich [*Russian scientist*, 1882–]. Noted that fatigue in a muscle stimulated by its motor nerve is reduced by concurrent stimulation of its sympathetic nerve supply; called *Orbeli effect*.

or·bic′u·lar [L. *orbicularis*, circular]. Circular; applied to circular muscles, as the orbicular muscle of the eye (orbicularis oculi) or of the mouth (orbicularis oris).

or·bic″u·la′re (or·bick″yoo·lah′ree) [*orbicularis*]. The orbicular bone, a tubercle at the end of the long process of the incus; it is separate in early fetal life.

or·bic″u·lar′is [L.]. The ring muscle of the eye (orbicularis oculi) or mouth (orbicularis oris). See Table of Muscles in the Appendix.

o. palpebrarum. Orbicularis oculi muscle: old term.

or′bit [L. *orbita*, track, course]. The bony cavity containing the eye, which is formed by the frontal, sphenoid, ethmoid, nasal, lacrimal, maxillary, and palatal bones. See Plate 19. —**orbital,** *adj.*

or′bi·tal. Any of certain fibers of smooth muscle bridging the inferior orbital fissure. —**or′bital,** *adj.*

or″bi·ta′le (or″bi·tah′lee, ·tay′lee) [*orbita*]. *In craniometry*, the lowest point on the inferior margin of the orbit. It is not a measuring point; it is used in conjunction with the poria to orient the skull on the Frankfort horizontal plane.

or′bi·tal height. *In craniometry*, the greatest vertical width of the external opening of the orbit.

or″bi·ta′li·a. Plural of orbitale.

or″bi·to·na′sal (or″bi·to·nay′zul) [*orbita;* L. *nasus*, nose]. Relating to the orbit of the skull and the nasal cavity.

or″bi·to·nom′e·ter. A device used to measure the repressibility of the eye into the orbit in cases of exophthalmic goiter.

or″bi·to·nom′e·try. The measurement of the resistance of the globe of the eye to retrodisplacement.

or″bi·to·sphe′noid bone. The orbital portion of the sphenoid bone, separate in certain lower vertebrates and in embryos, represented by the small wing of the sphenoid bone in mammals.

or″bi·tot′o·my [*orbita;* G. *tomē*, a cutting]. Incision into the orbit.

or′ce·in, or·ce′in (C.C.). $C_{28}H_{24}N_2O_7$. Brownish red, crystalline powder synthesized from orcin; insoluble in water, soluble in alcohol. Used in microscopy as a stain.

or″che·i′tis (or″kee·eye′tis). See *orchitis*.

or·ches″tro·ma′ni·a (or·kes″tro·may′nee·uh) [G. *orchēstra*, space in the Greek theater in which the chorus danced; *mania*, madness]. Dancing mania; chorea, or St. Vitus' dance.

or′chi- (or′ki-). See *orchio-*.

or′chic (or′kick) [G. *orchis*, testis]. Pertaining to the testis.

or″chi·dec′to·my. See *orchiectomy*.

or″chi·di′tis. See *orchitis*.

or″chi·dop′a·thy [*orchis;* G. *pathos*, disease]. Disease of a testis.

or·chid′o·pex″y. See *orchiopexy*.

or·chid′o·plas″ty [*orchis;* G. *plassein*, to form]. Orchioplasty; plastic surgery of a testis.

or″chi·dor′rha·phy. See *orchiopexy*.

or″chi·dot′o·my [*orchis;* G. *tomē*, a cutting]. Incision into the testis.

or″chi·ec′to·my [*orchis;* G. *ektomē*, excision]. Surgical removal of one or both testes; castration.

or″chi·en·ceph″a·lo′ma [*orchis;* G. *egkephalos*, brain; *-ōma*, tumor]. An encephaloid carcinoma of the testis.

or″chi·ep″i·did″y·mi′tis [*orchis;* G. *epididymis*, epididymis; *-itis*, inflammation]. Inflammation of both testis and epididymis.

or′chi·o- (or′kee·o-), **or′chi-** [*orchis*]. A combining form meaning *testis*.

or″chi·o·ca·tab′a·sis [*orchis;* G. *katabasis*, descent]. The normal descent of the testis into the scrotum.

or′chi·o·cele [*orchis;* G. *kēlē*, hernia]. *In surgery*, a complete scrotal hernia.

or″chi·op′a·thy [*orchis;* G. *pathos*, disease]. Any disease of the testis.

or′chi·o·pex″y (or′kee·o·peck″see, or″kee·o·peck′-see) [*orchis;* G. *pēxis*, a fixing]. Surgical fixation of a testis, as in a plastic operation for relief of an undescended testis.

or′chi·o·plas″ty [*orchis;* G. *plassein*, to form]. Any plastic operation on the testis.

or″chi·ot′o·my. See *orchidotomy.*

or′chis (or′kiss) [G.]. Testis.

or·chi′tis (or·kigh′tis) [*orchis;* G. *-itis*, inflammation]. Inflammation of the testis. —**orchit′ic,** *adj.*

mumps o. Orchitis due to the mumps virus. It may occur without the usual parotitis associated with mumps.

or·chit′o·my (or·kit′o·mee). See *orchidotomy.*

or·chot′o·my (or·kot′o·mee). See *orchidotomy.*

or′cin (or′sin), **or′cin·ol** [L. *Orcus*]. 3,5-Dihydroxytoluene. $C_6H_3(CH_3)(OH)_2.H_2O$. White crystals, reddened by exposure to air, freely soluble in water, ether, or alcohol. Prepared from many species of lichens. A reagent for pentoses and certain other substances.

or′der [L. *ordo*, order]. 1. Systematic arrangement. 2. *In biology*, the taxonomic group below a class and above a family.

or′der·ly [*ordo*]. A male hospital attendant.

or′di·nate [L. *ordinare*, to regulate]. The vertical line of the two coordinates used in plotting the interrelationship of two sets of data. The horizontal one is called the abscissa.

or″e·go·nen′sin. An antibiotic substance produced by *Ganoderma oregonense.*

orestralyn. Trade-mark for *ethynyl estradiol.*

oreton. Trade-mark for a brand of testosterone propionate in ampuls for intramuscular injection.

oreton F. Trade-mark for testosterone in pellets for subcutaneous implantation.

oreton M. Trade-mark for methyl testosterone in tablets for oral use.

o·rex′is, o·rex′i·a [G. *orexis*, longing for]. Appetite.

orf [AS]. A virus disease of sheep and goats transmitted to man (in whom it is called *contagious pustular dermatitis*), characterized by red papules with depressed centers containing a clear or sometimes purulent serum. Syn., *sheep pox, sheep thrush.*

or′gan [G. *organon*, instrument, tool]. A differentiated part of an organism adapted for a definite function.

accessory organs of the eye. The fasciae, ocular muscles, eyebrows, eyelids, conjunctiva, and lacrimal apparatus.

adipose organs. The fat lobules; regarded as distinct organs rather than simple tissue. Also called *fat organs.*

enamel o. The epithelial ingrowth from the dental lamina which covers the dental papilla, furnishes a mold for the shape of a developing tooth, and forms the dental enamel.

gustatory o. A taste bud.

o. of Corti. The end organ of hearing; the sensory part of the cochlear duct: also called *papilla of Huschke.* See Plate 20.

o. of Golgi. A sensory nerve end organ resembling a neuromuscular spindle at the surface of a muscle next to its tendon. Also called *neurotendinal spindle, Golgi's corpuscle, tendon organ of Golgi.*

o. of Jacobson. See vomeronasal *o.*

organs of generation. Those that are functional in reproduction.

organs of Zuckerkandl. Paraganglions.

sense o. A receptor.

sex organs. Those pertaining entirely to the sex of the individual; in the male, the external generative organs, the penis and testes, and the internal, the prostate, deferential ducts, and seminal vesicles; in the female, the external generative organs, the vulva, vagina, and clitoris, and the internal, the uterus, uterine tubes, and ovaries. In woman the breasts are considered as secondary sex organs.

shock o. The organ or tissue which exhibits the most marked response to the antigen-antibody interaction in hypersensitivity, as the lungs in allergic asthma, or the skin in atopic or contact dermatitis.

tendon o. of Golgi. See *o.* of Golgi.

vomeronasal o. A slender tubule ending in a blind sac; situated in the anteroinferior part of the nasal septum; vestigial in man.

or″gan·elle′, or′gan·elle [dim. from *organon*]. A specialized structure or part of a cell having a definite function to perform, as the contractile vacuole of many Protozoa.

or·gan′ic [*organon*]. 1. Having, pertaining to, or characterized by organs; pertaining to living substances; affecting the structure of organs. 2. *In chemistry*, of or pertaining to compounds of carbon.

or·gan′ic brain dis·or′der. *In psychiatry*, a basic mental condition characteristic of diffuse impairment of brain-tissue function from any cause, characterized by impairment of orientation, judgment, memory, the intellectual functions, e.g., calculation, learning, and knowledge, and by lability and shallowness of affect. The degree of severity is generally commensurate with the severity of the precipitating basic organic lesion upon which the diagnosis is based, but may be associated with psychotic, neurotic, or behavioral reactions.

acute o. b. d. One resulting from temporary, reversible, diffuse impairment of brain-tissue function, with a basic disturbance of the sensorium. It may be due to acute intracranial or systemic infections, drug, poison, or alcohol intoxication, trauma, circulatory or metabolic disturbances, convulsive disorders, or diseases of obscure etiology.

chronic o. b. d. One resulting from relatively permanent and irreversible, diffuse impairment of brain-tissue function, or the sequel of a pathological process involving the brain which has responded to specific therapy, often ushered in by the acute form. It may be associated with syphilis of the central nervous system, various forms of intoxication or poisoning, brain trauma, cerebral arteriosclerosis and other cerebral circulatory disturbances, convulsive disorders, senile brain disease, disturbances of metabolism, growth, or nutrition, intracranial neoplasms, or diseases whose causes are obscure. Included in this classification are also those mental disorders, formerly called *secondary mental deficiency*, associated with congenital brain-tissue anomalies, mongolism, prenatal maternal infectious diseases, or birth trauma, and characterized primarily by defective ability to learn. See also *mental deficiency.*

or·gan′i·cism. See *holism.*

organidin. Trade-mark for a preparation of an iodine compound with an organic base.

or′gan·ism [*organon*]. Any living thing, plant or animal, having regard especially to the fact that it consists of differentiated parts with specialized functions, so related to one another as to form a unified whole. For a list of organisms pathogenic to man, see Table in the Appendix.

coprozoic organisms. Organisms living in feces and other excreta.

L organisms. Abbreviation for pleuropneumonialike organisms.

pleuropneumonialike organisms. See *pleuropneumonialike organisms.*

pus o. See pyogenic *microorganism.*

or″gan·i·za′tion [*organon*]. 1. The systematic interrelationships of the structurally and functionally differentiated parts to form an integrated whole. 2. A part of the repair process occurring in an injury that has destroyed tissue; the ingrowth of capillaries and fibroblasts into thrombi or blood clots.

or′gan·i″zer [*organon*]. Spemann's term for the region of the dorsal lip of the blastopore, comprising chordamesoderm, that is self-differentiating and capable of inducing the formation of medullary plate in the adjacent ectoderm; the primary organizer. A second-grade (or higher) organizer, coming into play after the laying down of the main axis of the body induced by the primary organizer is completed, is any part of the embryo which exerts a morphogenetic stimulus on an adjacent part or parts, as in the induction of the lens by the optic vesicle. Also called *organizator, organization center.*

or′ga·no- [*organon*]. 1. A combining form meaning *organ.* 2. *In chemistry,* a combining form signifying *organic.*

or·gan′o·gel. A hydrogel in which the dispersion medium is an organic liquid instead of water.

or″ga·no·gen′e·sis [*organon;* G. *genesis,* production]. The formation of the various organs of the plant or animal body. —**organogenet′ic,** *adj.*

or″ga·nog′e·ny. Organogenesis.

or′gan·oid [*organon;* G. *eidos,* form]. Resembling an organ.

or″ga·nol′o·gy [*organon;* G. *logos,* word]. The science that treats of the organs of plants and animals.

or″ga·no·me·tal′lic. Pertaining to compounds having a carbon to metal linkage.

or″ga·nos′co·py [*organon;* G. *skopein,* to examine]. The examination of an organ with a special lens system, such as a cystoscope, esophagoscope, or laryngoscope.

or·gan′o·sol. A colloidal solution in which the continuous phase or dispersion medium is an organic liquid, as alcohol, benzene, ether, etc.

or″ga·no·ther′a·py [*organon;* G. *therapeia,* treatment]. The treatment of diseases by means of animal organs or their extracts.

or″ga·no·troph′ic (or″guh·no·trof′ick, ·tro′fick) [*organon;* G. *trophē,* nourishment]. Relating to the nutrition of living organs.

or″ga·no·trop′ic [*organon;* G. *trepein,* to turn]. 1. Pertaining to substances which act on the organs of the body. 2. Having affinity for the tissues. —**organot′ropism, organot′ropy,** *n.*

or″gan·ot′ro·pism [*organon; trepein*]. Ehrlich's theory that certain poisons manifest a definite chemical affinity for certain components of cells.

or′ga·num. See *organ.*

or′gasm (or′gaz·um) [G. *orgasmos,* orgasm]. Intense excitement, especially that occurring during sexual intercourse; the culmination or climax of the sexual act, followed by ejaculation of the seminal fluid or, in the female, by relaxation and detumescence. —**orgas′tic,** *adj.*

or·gas′mo·lep″sy (or·gaz′mo·lep″see) [*orgasmos;* G. *lēpsis,* a seizing]. A sudden loss of muscle tone during sexual orgasm, accompanied by a transitory loss of consciousness.

or′i·dine. $C_5H_{11}NO_2$; a substance, isomeric with betaine, obtained from rice hulls, occurring as white crystals, soluble in water.

oridine. Trade-mark for the calcium salt of the iodized fatty acids of cottonseed oil, used in iodine therapy.

o″ri·en′tal sore. A form of cutaneous leishmaniasis caused by infection with *Leishmania tropica* and transmitted by some species of *Phlebotomus.* It is characterized by ulcerated granulomatous lesions of the skin which lead to hypertrophy of the stratum corneum and hypertrophy and proliferation of the papillæ. Necrosis and ulceration occur as well as secondary infections with bacteria. Syn., *Delhi boil, Aleppo boil, tropical sore, Biskra button, Bagdad boil, Kandahar sore, Delhi sore, Delasoa sore, oriental button, Tashkend ulcer.*

o″ri·en·ta′tion [L. *oriens,* from *oriri,* to rise]. 1. The act of determining one's relation to time (**temporal orientation**) or to space (**spatial orientation**) or to other individuals (**personal orientation**). 2. The relative position of the substitution elements or radicals in the benzene ring.

or′i·fice [L. *orificium,* opening]. An opening, an entrance to a cavity or tube. —**orifi′cial,** *adj.*

or″i·fi′ci·um (or″i·fish′ee·um) [L.]. Orifice.

o·rig′a·num. See *marjoram.*

or′i·gin [L. *origo,* origin]. The beginning or starting point of anything.

o. of a muscle. The end of attachment of a muscle which remains relatively fixed during contraction of the muscle.

Or′i·za′ba jal′ap. See *ipomea.*

o·riz′a·bin. See *jalapin.*

ormicet. Trade-mark for aluminum formate.

or′mo·sine (or′mo·seen, ·sin). A crystalline alkaloid from the seeds of *Ormosia dasycarpa,* of South America. Has been used as a narcotic.

Ormsby's method. See under *method.*

or′ni·thine (or′ni·theen, ·thin). $NH_2.(CH_2)_3.CHNH_2.COOH$. α,δ-Diamino-valeric acid. An amino acid derived from the excrement of birds, but not found in native proteins. It is postulated as an intermediate in a cyclic process of urea formation in the body (Krebs-Henseleit cycle).

Or″ni·thod′o·rus (or″ni·thod′o·rus, or″nith·o·dor′us) [G. *ornis,* bird; *doros,* leathern bag]. A genus of soft ticks of the family Argasidae containing many species parasitic to man, some of which produce painful bites and inflammatory lesions. Several species are vectors of relapsing fever spirochetes, e.g., **O. moubata** in Africa, **O. talaje** in tropical America, **O. rudis** in subtropical regions of the United States.

or″ni·tho′sis [*ornis;* G. *-ōsis,* condition]. A psittacosislike disease found in birds other than parrots and parakeets, particularly pigeons and domestic fowl. The virus causing ornithosis differs from that of psittacosis; similar strains have been isolated in cases of atypical pneumonia in man.

or′ni·thyl. The univalent radical, $H_2NCH_2CH_2CH_2CH(NH_2)CO$—, of the amino acid ornithine.

or′o-. See *orrho-.*

o′ro- [L. *os,* mouth]. A combining form meaning *mouth* or *oral.*

o·ron′o·sus. See *mountain sickness.*

o″ro·phar′ynx [L. *os,* mouth; G. *pharygx,* pharynx]. The oral pharynx, situated below the level of the lower border of the soft palate and above the larynx, as distinguished from the nasopharynx and laryngeal pharynx. —**oropharyn′geal,** *adj.*

or′o·sin [G. *oros,* serum]. Old term for the total coagulable protein of serums.

or′o·sin hy·poth′e·sis. A concept of the interconnection of certain soluble proteins with each other and the nonprotein constituents of the tissue; used to denote an interrelationship among various proteins found in plasma or serum by physical and chemical means.

or·ot′ic ac′id. $C_5H_4N_2O_4$; 1,2,3,6-tetrahydro-2,6-dioxo-4-pyrimidinecarboxylic acid or uracil-4-carboxylic acid; a pyrimidine precursor in animal tissues.

O·ro′ya fe′ver (o·ro′yuh, o·roy′uh). See under *fever*.

or′phol. Bismuth betanaphthol.

or′pi·ment. Native arsenic trisulfide.

Orr, Hiram Winnett (1877–). American surgeon celebrated for his method (1923) of treating severe wounds complicated by infections and compound fractures. See Orr-Trueta *method*.

or·rhag′o·gus. See *hydragogue*.

or′rho-, or′o- [G. *orros*, whey]. A combining form meaning *serum*.

or″rho·men″in·gi′tis [G. *orros*, whey; *mēnigx*, membrane; *-itis*, inflammation]. Inflammation of a serous membrane. *Obs.*

or′rhos [*orros*]. Serum; whey.

or′ris [perhaps from G. *iris*, iris]. The peeled and dried rhizome of *Iris germanica florentina* or *Iris pallida*. Valued chiefly for its pleasant odor.

o. root. A powder from certain varieties of iris; used in various cosmetics, toothpastes, etc. It is a common sensitizer, both by contact or by inhalation.

orsanine. Trade-mark for sodium-4-acetyl-amino-2-hydroxyphenylarsonate, a drug related to acetarsone. Has been used in the treatment of trypanosomiasis.

ortal sodium. Trade-marked name for hexethal sodium, a barbiturate having short duration of action.

or″thi·auch′e·nus (orth″ee·awk′i·nus) [G. *orthios*, steep; *auchēn*, neck]. A skull in which the angle formed between the radius fixus and the line joining the basion and the inion is between 38° and 49°.

or″thi·o·chor′dus (orth″ee·o·kor′dus) [*orthios;* G. *chordē*, chord]. A skull in which the angle formed between the radius fixus and the line joining the hormion and the basion is between 33.2° and 52°.

or″thi·o·cor′y·phus [*orthios;* G. *koryphē*, head]. A skull in which the angle formed between the radius fixus and the line joining the bregma and the lambda is between 29° and 41°.

or″thi·o·don′tus [*orthios;* G. *odous*, tooth]. A skull in which the angle between the radius fixus and the line joining the alveolar and subnasal points is between 88° and 121°.

or″thi·o·me·to′pus [*orthios;* G. *metōpon*, forehead]. A skull in which the angle between the radius fixus and the line joining the bregma and the nasal point is between 47° and 60°.

or″thi·o·pis′thi·us [*orthios;* G. *opisthen*, behind]. A skull in which the angle between the radius fixus and the line joining the lambda and the inion is between 84° and 95°.

or″thi·o·pis·tho·cra′ni·us [*orthios; opisthen;* G. *kranion*, skull]. A skull in which the angle formed between the radius fixus and the line joining the lambda and the opisthion is 107°–119°.

or″thi·o·pro·so′pus [*orthios;* G. *prosōpon*, face]. A skull in which the angle formed between the radius fixus and the line joining the nasion and the alveolar point is between 89.4° and 100°.

or″thi·op′y·lus [*orthios;* G. *pylē*, gate]. A skull in which the angle formed between the radius fixus and the line joining the middle point of the anterior margin of the foramen magnum and the middle point of the posterior margin of the foramen magnum is between 15.5° and 24°.

or″thi·or·rhi′nus [*orthios;* G. *rhis*, nose]. A skull in which the angle formed between the radius fixus and the line joining the nasion and the subnasal point is between 87.5° and 98°.

or″thi·u·ra·nis′cus [*orthios;* G. *ouraniskos*, vaulted ceiling roof of the mouth]. A skull in which the angle formed between the radius fixus and a line joining the posterior border of the incisive fossa and the alveolar point is between 40° and 60°.

or′tho-, orth- [G. *orthos*, straight]. 1. A combining form denoting *straight, normal*, or *true*. 2. *In chemistry*, a prefix indicating the neighboring or 1,2 positions on the benzene ring. Symbol, *o-*.

or″tho·bo′ric ac′id. Boric acid.

or′tho·caine (*orthocaina*). British Pharmacopoeia title for the methyl ester of *m*-amino-*p*-hydroxybenzoic acid, $HO.C_6H_3(NH_2)COOCH_3$, a local anesthetic used in ointment form, as a dusting powder, or in alcoholic solution. It has been used as a gastric anesthetic. See *orthoform*.

or″tho·ceph′a·ly [*orthos;* G. *kephalē*, head]. The condition of having a skull with a vertical index of from 70.1° to 75°.

or″tho·chlo″ro·phe′nol. $C_6H_4Cl.OH$. A compound of high germicidal activity and high toxicity.

or″tho·cho·re′a (orth″o·ko·ree′uh) [*orthos;* G. *choreia*, dance]. Choreic movements in the erect posture.

or″tho·chro·mat′ic [*orthos;* G. *chrōma*, color]. A term originally used in photography to denote correctness in the rendering of colors; orthochromatic emulsions are not sensitive to red, and may be developed under a red safe light.

or″tho·cra′si·a (orth″o·kray′see·uh, ·zee·uh) [*orthos;* G. *krasis*, mixing]. A condition in which there is no idiosyncrasy. *Rare.*

ortho-creme. Trade-mark for a contraceptive vaginal cream.

or″tho·cre′sol. $CH_3.C_6H_4.OH$. One of the isomers of cresol. It has the weakest germicidal activity of the three isomers.

or″tho·dac′ty·lous [*orthos;* G. *daktylos*, finger]. Having straight digits.

or″tho·den′tin. The mammalian type of dentin; it contains processes, but not cell bodies, of odontoblasts.

or″tho·di′a·gram [*orthos;* G. *diagramma*, figure marked out by lines]. A tracing of the outer contours and exact size of an organ, usually the heart; made by illuminating the edge of the organ with parallel x-rays through a small, movable aperture and marking the outer edge of the shadow cast upon a fluoroscopic screen.

or″tho·di′a·graph [*orthos;* G. *diagraphein*, to mark out by lines]. A fluoroscopic apparatus for making orthodiagrams.

or″tho·di·ag′ra·phy [*orthos; diagraphein*]. Determining by the aid of roentgen rays the exact dimensions of an internal organ, especially the heart, by the shadow which it throws upon the fluorescent screen.

or″tho·dol″i·cho·ceph′a·lous (orth″o·dol″i·ko·sef′uh·lus, ·do″li·ko·sef′uh·lus) [*orthos;* G. *dolichos*, long; *kephalē*, head]. Having a long and straight head; having a vertical index between 70.1° and 75°, and a transverso-vertical index between 70° and 74.9°.

or″tho·don′ti·a. Old term for orthodontics.

or″tho·don′tics [*orthos;* G. *odous*, tooth]. The branch of dentistry concerned with the treatment of malocclusion.

or″tho·dont′ist [*orthos; odous*]. A practitioner of orthodontics.

orthoform. A trade-mark for methyl *m*-amino-*p*-hydroxybenzoic acid. See *orthocaine*.

or″tho·gen′e·sis [*orthos;* G. *genesis*, production]. The doctrine that phylogenetic evolution takes place according to system in certain well-defined and limited directions, and not by accident in many directions. —**orthogenet'ic, orthogenic,** *adj.*

or"thog·nath'ic [*orthos;* G. *gnathos*, jaw]. *In craniometry,* designating a condition of the upper jaw in which it is in an approximately vertical relationship to the profile of the facial skeleton, when the skull is oriented on the Frankfort horizontal plane; having a gnathic index of 97.9 or less.

or'tho·grade [*orthos;* L. *gradus*, step]. Walking or standing in the upright position.

ortho-gynol. Trade-mark for a contraceptive vaginal jelly.

or"tho·hy·drox"y·ben·zo'ic ac'id (orth"o·high-drock"see·). Salicylic acid.

or"tho·ki·net'ic. See Brownian *movement.*

or"tho·mes"o·ceph'a·lous (orth"o·mez"o·sef'uh-lus) [G. *orthos*, straight; *mesos*, middle; *kephalē*, head]. *In craniometry,* designating a skull with a transverso-vertical index between 75.1° and 79.9°, and a vertical index between 70.1° and 75°.

or·thom'e·ter [*orthos;* G. *metron*, a measure]. An instrument for measuring the relative degree of protrusion of the eyes. Also called *exophthalmometer.*

or"tho·pe'dic [*orthos;* G. *pais*, child]. Pertaining to orthopedics, as orthopedic surgery.

or"tho·pe'dics [*orthos; pais*]. That branch of surgery concerned with corrective treatment of deformities, diseases, and ailments of the locomotor apparatus, especially those affecting limbs, bones, muscles, joints, and fasciae, whether by apparatus, manipulation, or open operation; formerly, devoted to the correction and treatment of deformities in children.

or"tho·pe'dist [*orthos; pais*]. One who practices orthopedic surgery; a specialist in orthopedics.

or"tho·per·cus'sion [*orthos;* L. *percussio*, from *percutere*, to strike]. Percussion in which the distal phalanx of the percussing finger is held at right angles to the surface.

or"tho·phe·nan'thro·line (·fi·nan'thro·leen, ·lin). $C_{12}H_8N_2.H_2O$. A white, crystalline powder which forms a complex with ferrous ions and is used as an indicator in oxidation reduction systems in volumetric analysis.

or"tho·pho'ri·a [*orthos;* G. *phoros*, bearing]. 1. A tending of the visual lines to parallelism. 2. Normal balance of eye muscles.

or"tho·phos·phor'ic ac'id. Phosphoric acid.

or"thop·ne'a [*orthos;* G. *pnoē*, breath]. A condition in which there is need to sit up to breathe more easily, usually associated with cardiac asthma. —**orthopneic,** *adj.*

or"tho·prax'is [*orthos;* G. *praxis*, a doing]. Correction of the deformities of the body.

or"tho·psy·chi'a·try (orth"o·sigh·kigh'uh·tree) [*orthos;* G. *psychē*, soul; *iatreia*, treatment]. A subdivision of psychiatry primarily concerned with the prevention and treatment of behavior disorders. Mental hygiene and preventive methods are the main interests of orthopsychiatry.

Or·thop'ter·a [*orthos;* G. *pteron*, wing]. An order of insects including the grasshoppers, crickets, cockroaches, etc.

or·thop'tic [*orthos;* G. *optikos*, optic]. Pertaining to normal binocular vision.

or·thop'tics [*orthos; optikos*]. The science of rendering visual reactions and responses right and efficient, usually by some form of exercise or training. These measures include the treatment of amblyopia, the education of stereopsis, and the treatment of muscle imbalances and strabismus.

or·thop'to·scope [*orthos; optikos;* G. *skopein*, to examine]. An instrument used in orthoptic training.

or"tho·roent"gen·og'ra·phy (orth"o·rent"ghin-og'ruh·fee) [*orthos; Röntgen;* G. *graphein*, to write]. Orthodiagraphy.

or'tho·scope [*orthos;* G. *skopein*, to examine]. 1. An instrument for examination of the eye through a layer of water, whereby the curvature, and hence the refraction, of the cornea is neutralized, and the cornea acts as a plane medium. 2. An instrument for use in drawing the projections of skulls.

or"tho·scop'ic [*orthos; skopein*]. 1. Pertaining to an orthoscope or to orthoscopy. 2. Pertaining to lenses cut from near the periphery of a large lens. 3. Having normal vision.

or·thos'co·py [*orthos; skopein*]. The examination of the eye with the orthoscope.

or·tho'sis [G. *orthōsis*, a making straight]. The straightening of a deformity. —**orthot'ic,** *adj.*

or"tho·stat'ic [G. *orthos*, straight; *statikos*, causing to stand]. Pertaining to, or caused by, standing upright, as orthostatic albuminuria, which occurs when the patient stands on his feet or exercises for long periods of time, but which disappears after a period of rest in bed.

orthosympathetic system. See thoracicolumbar *system.*

or'tho·tast [*orthos;* G. *tassein*, to arrange]. A device for straightening curvatures of long bones. It has also been used as a tourniquet.

or"tho·ter'i·on (orth"o·teer'ee·on) [*orthos*]. An apparatus for straightening curved limbs.

or·thot'o·nus [*orthos;* G. *tonos*, tension]. Tetanic cramp in which the body lies rigid and straight. —**orthoton'ic,** *adj.*

or·thot'ro·pism [*orthos;* G. *trepein*, to turn]. Vertical, upward, or downward growth. —**orthotrop'ic,** *adj.*

orthoxine. Trade-mark for beta-(*ortho*-methoxyphenyl)isopropylmethylamine, a sympathomimetic amine available as the hydrochloride salt. See *methoxyphenamine.*

o. hydrochloride. Trade-marked name for the sympathomimetic compound, methoxyphenamine hydrochloride.

Orth's fix'ing flu'id. See under *fixing fluid.*

o·ryz'a·min. Thiamine hydrochloride.

or"y·zen'in. A glutelin from rice.

O. S. *Oculus sinister*, left eye.

Os Chemical symbol for osmium.

os (pl. *ora*) [L.]. The mouth.

o. uteri externum. The external opening of the cervix of the uterus: also called *o. uteri.* See Plate 41.

o. uteri internum. The opening of the junction of the cervix and body of the uterus.

pinhole o. An extreme degree of atresia of the os uteri, seen in young and undeveloped women.

os (pl. *ossa*) [L.]. A bone.

o. acetabuli. An ossific center in the triradiate cartilage: also called *cotyloid bone.* There is an anterior one between the iliac and pubic portions of the acetabulum and a posterior one between the iliac and ischial portions.

o. acromiale. The acromion when not united to the scapula.

o. articulare. See *articular.*

o. basioticum. A separate center of ossification between the basal part of the occipital bone and the sphenoid; the os prebasioccipitale.

o. bregmaticum. An occasional sutural bone, caused by the presence of a separate center of ossification in the anterior fontanel.

o. breve. A short bone.

o. calcis. Old term for calcaneus, the bone of the heel.

o. centrale. An occasional ossicle found on the dorsal aspect of the carpus between any pair of the navicular, capitate, and lesser multangular bones, in many mammals.

o. clitoridis. A bone in the septum of the clitoris, in some mammals.

o. cordis. A bone in the fibrous triangle of the heart, between the atrioventricular and aortic orifices, in some mammals.

o. coxae. Hipbone.

o. entomion. A supernumerary bone situated at the entomion.

o. epiptericum. A supernumerary bone situated near the pterion.

o. falciforme. A sickle-shaped ossicle at the lower end of the radius in moles.

o. ilium. The ilium.

o. incisivum. The incisive bone; premaxilla.

ossa intercalaria. Wormian bones: old term.

o. interfrontale. An occasional accessory ossicle in the anterior part of the metopic suture.

o. intermetatarseum. An occasional wedge-shaped bone on the dorsal aspect of the foot between the medial cuneiform and first and second metatarsal bones.

o. interparietale. A supernumerary bone in the sagittal suture.

o. ischii. The ischium.

o. japonicum. The divided zygomatic bone, a racial characteristic of the Japanese.

o. lenticulare. The lenticular process: incorrect usage.

o. magnum. Old term for the capitate, the third bone of the second row of the carpus.

o. novum. Bone prepared for grafting by implanting os purum in another site until soft tissues have become associated with it.

o. odontoideum. The dens of the epistropheus when it persists as a separate ossicle.

o. orbiculare. The lenticular process of the incus.

o. orbitale. The upper of two portions into which the zygomatic bone is sometimes divided by a horizontal suture.

o. pedis. The distal phalanx of a horse's foot. Syn., *coffin bone.*

o. penis. A bone in the septum of the penis in some mammals, as the dog: seen rarely, as a pathological condition, in man.

o. prebasioccipitale. The os basioticum.

o. pubis. The pubic bone.

o. purum. Bone for grafting, processed to remove soft tissue and proteins. It is kept dry and boiled before use.

o. styloideum. The styloid process of the third metacarpal when it occurs as a separate ossicle.

o. suprasternale. A suprasternal bone.

o. trigonum. An ossicle due to the separation of the lateral tubercle of the posterior surface of the talus and ossification from a distinct center.

o. Vesalii. 1. An occasional accessory ossicle between the hamate and fifth metacarpal. 2. An occasional accessory ossicle at the base of the fifth metatarsal.

o. zygomaticum. The cheekbone.

o'sa·zone. Compound formed by reaction of a sugar with phenylhydrazine in the presence of acetic acid: used in the identification of sugars.

os'che·a (oss'kee·uh). Scrotum. —**oscheal,** *adj.*

os'che·o- (oss'kee·o-), **os'che-** [G. *oscheon*]. A combining form meaning *the scrotum.*

Os"cil·la'ri·a ma·la'ri·ae (oss"i·lay'ree·uh ma·lay'ree·ee). Old term for the malarial plasmodia, *Plasmodium falciparum, P. malariae,* and *P. vivax.*

os"cil·la'tion [L. *oscillatio*, from *oscillare*, to swing]. A swinging or vibration; also any tremulous motion.

os'cil·la"tor [*oscillare*]. An apparatus used in mechanical therapeutics.

os'cil·lo·graph" [L. *oscillum*, swing; *graphein*, to write]. An apparatus for recording oscillations. —**oscillograph'ic,** *adj.*

cathode-ray o. An instrument in which a pencil of electrons, striking a fluorescent screen, will trace a graph of any two variables that have been converted into electric equivalents. Its virtue is absence of mechanical inertia, and hence the ability to record changes of extreme rapidity with absolute accuracy.

os"cil·lom'e·ter [*oscillum;* G. *metron*, a measure]. An instrument for measuring oscillations, as those seen in taking blood pressures. —**oscillomet'ric,** *adj.*

os"cil·lom'e·try [*oscillum; metron*]. Measurement or detection of oscillations of any type, especially circulatory, usually by means of a string galvanometer.

os"cil·lop'si·a [*oscillum;* G. *opsis*, vision]. Oscillating nystagmus of disseminated sclerosis, usually occurring only during walking.

os·cil'lo·scope [*oscillum;* G. *skopein*, to examine]. A cathode-ray vacuum tube so constructed as to portray visually the deflections or oscillations of electromotive forces as a function of time: also called *cathode-ray o.* See cathode-ray *oscillograph.*

os'cine. Scopoline.

Os·cin'i·dae (oss·in'i·dee) [L. *oscen*, singing bird]. A family of the Diptera, which contains many species of small active flies known as eye gnats; contains the medically important genera *Hippelates, Siphunculina,* and *Oscinis.* Syn., *Chloropidae.*

Os'ci·nis [*oscen*]. A genus of flies of the family Oscinidae.

O. pallipes. A species which feeds on conjunctival exudates.

os'ci·tan·cy [L. *oscitare*, to yawn]. The disposition to yawn; drowsiness. *Obs.*

os"ci·ta'tion [L. *oscitatio*, from *oscitare*]. Yawning.

os"cu·la'tion [L. *osculatio*, from *osculari*, to kiss]. 1. Anastomosis of vessels. 2. Kissing.

os'cu·lum [L., little mouth]. A small aperture.

-ose [F. gluc*ose*]. 1. A suffix denoting *carbohydrate.* 2. A suffix denoting a *substance derived by hydrolysis of a protein.*

Oser method. See Hochberg-Melnick-Oser *method* for ascorbic acid.

Oseretsky test. See under *test.*

Osgood, Robert Bayley [*American orthopedic surgeon,* 1873–]. Known for his description of tibial tuberosity lesions occurring in adolescents (1903); called *osteochondrosis of tuberosity of tibia, Osgood-Schlatter disease.* Introduced his operation for the relief of so-called tennis elbow, in which he incised from the epicondyle downward, and exposed and excised the involved bursa.

Osgood-Haskins test. See under *test.*

O'Shaughnessy's operation. See *cardiomentopexy.*

-o'sis [G.]. Suffix signifying: 1. State, process, or condition, as psych*osis*, neur*osis*, osm*osis*. 2. *In pathology,* a diseased condition, as nephr*osis;* specifically, a disease caused by a fungus; a mycosis. 3. Increase or formation, as leucocyt*osis.*

Osler, William [*English physician of Canadian birth,* 1849–1919]. For years his *Principles and Practice of Medicine* has been a standard textbook. He described (1901) hereditary hemorrhagic telangiectasis, called *Osler-Rendu-Parkes-Weber disease.* Independently of Vaquez, described primary polycythemia, called *Osler's disease, Osler-Vaquez disease.* Described acute bacterial endocarditis. Small, painful swellings on hands and feet, especially on the tips of toes and fingers, associated with this disease, are called *Osler's nodes.* Compiled a bibliography of his own library of 7500 titles, now at McGill University. See Osler-Libman-Sacks *syndrome*.

os′mate (oz′mate, os′mate). A salt of osmic acid.

os·mat′ic (os·mat′ick, oz·mat′ick) [G. *osmē*, smell]. Characterized by a sense of smell.

os·me′sis (os·mee′sis, oz·mee′sis) [G., a smell]. The act of smelling. *Obs.*

os″mes·the′si·a (oz″mess·thee′zhuh, ·zee·uh, os″-mess·) [G. *osmē*, smell; *aisthēsis*, perception]. Olfactory sensibility.

os′mic ac′id (oz′mick, os′mick). OsO_4. A crystalline substance employed as a histologic stain and reagent; has been used internally, in the form of the potassium salt, in rheumatic affections and in epilepsy.

os′mics (oz′micks) [*osmē*]. The science of smell.

os″mi·dro′sis (oz″mi·dro′sis, os″mi·) [*osmē*; G. *hidrōsis*, sweat]. The secretion of a malodorous perspiration; bromhidrosis.

os′mi·um (oz′mee·um, os′) [*osmē*]. Os = 190.2. A heavy metallic element belonging to the platinum group. —**os′mic,** *adj.*

os′mo- [*osmē*]. A combining form meaning *smell, odor.*

os′mo- (os′mo-, oz′mo-) [G. *ōsmos*, impulse]. A combining form denoting *osmosis.*

os″mo·dys·pho′ri·a [G. *osmē*, smell; *dys-*, bad; *phoros*, bearing]. Intolerance of certain odors.

os′mol. One thousand milliosmols.

os″mo·lar′i·ty. The osmotic effectiveness of an ion present in a biological fluid. In plasma, sodium makes up about 92% of the osmotically effective bases. Also see *milliosmol.*

os·mol′o·gy (os·mol′o·jee, oz·) [*osmē*; G. *logos*, word]. The science of odors and the sense of smell.

os·mol′o·gy [G. *ōsmos*, impulse; *logos*]. That part of physical science treating of osmosis.

os·mom′e·ter (os·mom′i·tur, oz·) [G. *osmē*, smell; *metron*, a measure]. An instrument for testing the sense of smell; an olfactometer.

os·mom′e·ter [G. *ōsmos*, impulse; *metron*]. An apparatus for measuring osmosis.

os″mo·pho′bi·a [G. *osmē*, smell; *phobos*, fear]. A morbid fear of odors.

os′mo·phor. A group or radical that imparts odor to a compound.

os″mo·re·cep′tors. The (postulated) nerve endings in the hypothalamus which respond to changes in osmotic pressure of the blood by regulating the secretion of the neurohypophyseal antidiuretic hormone (ADH).

os″mo·reg″u·lar′i·ty [G. *ōsmos*, impulse; L. *regula*, rule]. Affecting or regulating the extent and rate of osmosis.

os·mo′sis (os·mo′sis, oz·) [*ōsmos*]. The passage of a solvent through a membrane from a dilute solution into a more concentrated one.

os·mot′ic (os·mot′ick, oz·) [*ōsmos*]. Pertaining to osmosis, particularly to osmotic pressure.

os·phre″si·ol′o·gy (os·free″zee·ol′o·jee) [G. *osphrēsis*, sense of smell; *logos*, word]. The science of the sense of smell and its organs, and of odors. *Obs.*

os·phre″si·om′e·ter (os·free″zee·om′i·tur). Osmometer; olfactometer.

os·phre′sis [G.]. The sense of smell; olfaction. *Obs.*

os″phy·al′gi·a [G. *osphys*, loins; *algos*, pain]. Any pain in the hip or loins; sciatica. *Obs.*

os″phy·i′tis [*osphys*; G. *-itis*, inflammation]. Lumbar inflammation; coxitis. *Obs.*

os″phy·o·my″e·li′tis [*osphys*; G. *myelos*, marrow; *-itis*]. Myelitis of the lumbar portion of the spinal cord. *Obs.*

os′sa. Plural of os (meaning "bone").

os′se·in, os′se·ine (oss′ee·in) [L. *osseus*, of bone]. 1. Collagen. 2. The organic framework of osseous tissue.

os′se·let [dim. from L. *os*, bone]. A hard nodule on the inner aspect of the horse's knee.

os″se·o·al·bu′mi·noid. A tough, elastic, and fibrous protein in bone, believed to be a constituent of the lining of the Haversian canals.

os″se·o·car″ti·lag′i·nous (oss″ee·o·kahr″ti·ladj′i-nus) [L. *osseus*, of bone; *cartilago*, cartilage]. Pertaining to or composed of both bone and cartilage.

os″se·o·fi′brous. Pertaining to or composed of both bone and fibrous tissue.

os″se·o·mu′coid [*osseus*; L. *mucus*, mucus; G. *eidos*, form]. A mucin or glycoprotein obtained from bone.

os′se·ous [*osseus*]. Bony; composed of or resembling bone.

os′si·cle [L. *ossiculum*, dim. of *os*, bone]. A small bone; particularly, one of three small bones in the tympanic cavity: the malleus, incus, and stapes.

Kerckring's o. See Theodor *Kerckring.*

o. of Bertin. See *concha* sphenoidalis.

os″si·cu·lec′to·my [*ossiculum*; G. *ektomē*, excision]. The removal of one or more of the ossicles of the middle ear.

os″si·cu·lot′o·my [*ossiculum*; G. *tomē*, a cutting]. Surgical incision involving the tissues about the ossicles of the ear.

os·sif′er·ous [L. *os*, bone; *ferre*, to bear]. Containing or producing bone tissue.

os·sif′ic [*os*; L. *facere*, to make]. Producing bone.

os″si·fi·ca′tion [*os*; *facere*]. The formation of bone; the conversion of tissue into bone. See Plate 24.

pathologic o. Bone development in unusual sites or abnormal bone formation. Metaplastic or heteroplastic bone may be observed in soft tissues.

os·sif′lu·ence [*os*; L. *fluere*, to flow]. Osteolysis.

os·sif′lu·ent [*os*; *fluere*]. Breaking down and softening bony tissue, as an ossifluent abscess.

os′si·form [*os*; L. *forma*, form]. Bonelike.

os′si·fy (oss′i·figh) [*os*; L. *facere*, to make]. To turn into bone.

os·tal′gi·a [G. *osteon*, bone; *algos*, pain]. Pain in a bone: also spelled *ostealgia.* —**ostalgic,** *adj.*

os″tal·gi′tis [*osteon*; *algos*; G. *-itis*, inflammation]. Inflammation of a bone attended by pain.

os′te·al [*osteon*]. Osseous, bony; pertaining to bone.

os″te·al″le·o′sis [*osteon*; G. *alloiōsis*, alteration]. A metamorphosis of the substance of bone, as exemplified in osteosarcoma.

os″te·an″a·gen′e·sis [*osteon*; G. *anagennēsis*, regeneration]. Regeneration of bone.

os″te·a·naph′y·sis [*osteon*; G. *anaphysis*, a growing again]. The reproduction of bone tissue. Syn., *osteanagenesis.*

os″te·ar·throt′o·my. See *osteoarthrotomy.*

os·tec′to·my, os″te·ec′to·my [*osteon*; G. *ektomē*, excision]. Excision of a bone or a portion of a bone.

os·tec′to·py [*osteon*; G. *ektopos*, away from a place]. Displacement of bone: also spelled *osteectopia.*

os′te·in, os′te·ine (os′tee·in, os·tee′in). See *ossine.*

os″te·i′tis [*osteon*; G. *-itis*, inflammation]. Inflammation of bone. —**osteit′ic,** *adj.*

condensing o. A form usually involving both marrow and periosteum and resulting in the filling of the medullary cavity with a dense bony mass; new bone usually forms on the surface, so that the bone becomes heavier and denser than normal.

dentoalveolar o. See alveolar *pyorrhea.*

gummatous o. A chronic form due to syphilis and characterized by the formation of gummas in the cancellous tissue of the epiphysis, in the shaft of a bone, or in the periosteum.

o. carnosa. Inflammation of bone with an excess of fungous granulations.

o. condensans ilii. A condition in which the normal bony structure of the portion of the ilium along the sacroiliac joint is altered, probably as a result of mechanical strain on the joint.

o. cystica of Jüngling. Osseous lesions of sarcoidosis. The phalanges of fingers and toes appear on roentgenograms to have cysts. They represent replacement of bone and marrow by sarcoid nodules. Syn., *osteitis tuberculosa multiplex cystoides.*

o. deformans. See Paget's *disease* (a).

o. fibrosa cystica. Hyperparathyroidism: a disease due to hyperplasia or adenoma of the parathyroid gland resulting in an abnormal calcium and phosphorus metabolism. It is characterized clinically by thinning of the bony skeleton, often in the form of cysts. Also called *von Recklinghausen's* or *Engel-Recklinghausen's disease.* Syn., *osteitis fibrosa generalisata.*

o. fibrosa disseminata. See fibrous *dysplasia.*

o. fibrosa generalisata. See *o.* fibrosa cystica.

o. fungosa. A simple, inflammatory hyperplasia of the medulla and of the compact substance of bone; characterized by fungoid granulations and leading to new ossification or destructive chronic inflammation.

o. interna. Osteomyelitis of the alveolar process resulting from infection of a tooth.

o. pubis. Inflammation of the periosteum over the pubic symphysis and sometimes of the ischii, as a complication of surgical operation on the urinary bladder or prostate: more frequent in males.

o. tuberculosa multiplex cystoides. See *o.* cystica of Jüngling.

rarefying o. See *osteoporosis.*

renal o. A disorder of calcium metabolism, with secondary hyperparathyroidism, resulting from phosphorus retention, caused by tubular or glomerular disease of the kidney which produces acidosis and renal insufficiency. The disease is not affected by the administration of the parathyroid hormone, but only by a cure for the acidosis. Therapy includes an alkaline salt, vitamin D, and a calcium salt. Also called *renal rickets.*

sclerotic o. See *osteopetrosis.*

os·tem'bry·on [*osteon;* G. *embryon,* embryo]. An ossified fetus.

os"tem·py·e'sis (os"tem·pye·ee'sis, ·pee·ee'sis) [*osteon;* G. *empyēsis,* suppuration]. Suppuration of bone.

os'te·o-, os'te- [*osteon*]. A combining form meaning *bone.*

os"te·o·an"a·gen'e·sis [*osteon;* G. *anagennēsis,* regeneration]. Osteanagenesis.

os"te·o·an'eu·rysm. Aneurysm of the blood vessels of a bone; a pulsating tumor of a bone. See also osteogenic *sarcoma.*

os"te·o·ar·threc'to·my. Surgical excision or partial excision of the bony portion of a joint.

os"te·o·ar·thri'tis. Degenerative joint disease.

ochronotic o. A rare degenerative arthropathy associated with the diseased cartilage of ochronosis, usually accompanied by alkaptonuria: also called *alkaptonuric o.*

os"te·o·ar·throp'a·thy [*osteon;* G. *arthron,* joint; *pathos,* disease]. Any disease of bony articulations.

hypertrophic pulmonary o. Clubbing of the fingers and toes associated with enlargement of the ends of the long bones, encountered in chronic pulmonary disease: also called *osteopulmonary arthropathy.*

os"te·o·ar·thro'sis [*osteon;* G. *arthrōsis,* articulation]. Old term for degenerative joint disease.

os"te·o·ar·throt'o·my [*osteon;* G. *arthron,* joint; *tomē,* a cutting]. Surgical excision or partial excision of the bony portion of a joint.

os'te·o·blast" [*osteon;* G. *blastos,* germ]. Any one of the cells of mesenchymal origin concerned in the formation of bony tissue. —**osteoblast'ic,** *adj.*

os"te·o·blas·to'ma [*osteon; blastos;* G. *-ōma,* tumor]. See osteogenic *sarcoma.*

os"te·o·camp'si·a [*osteon;* G. *kampsis,* a bending]. Curvature of a bone without fracture, as in osteomalacia. *Obs.*

os"te·o·car"ci·no'ma [*osteon; karkinōma*]. An ossifying carcinoma; carcinoma of a bone.

os"te·o·car"ti·lag'i·nous (os"tee·o·kahr"ti·ladj'i·nus) [*osteon;* L. *cartilago,* cartilage]. Pertaining to or composed of both bone and cartilage.

os"te·o·chon'dral, os"te·o·chon'drous. Composed of both bone and cartilage.

os"te·o·chon·dri'tis (·kon·dry'tis) [*osteon;* G. *chondros,* cartilage; *-itis,* inflammation]. Inflammation of both bone and cartilage. The term is sometimes used for *osteochondrosis.*

o. deformans juvenilis. Formerly, osteochondrosis of the head of the femur, seen especially in children: also called *arthritis deformans juvenilis, caput deformatum, coxa plana, osteochondritis deformans coxae juvenilis,* and associated with the names of J. Calvé, A. J. Legg, G. C. Perthes, and J. H. Waldenström. Syn., *osteochondrosis deformans juvenilis.*

o. dissecans. A joint affection, first described by F. König, characterized by partial or complete detachment of a fragment of articular cartilage and underlying bone: also called *osteochondrosis dissecans.*

syphilitic o. Syphilitic involvement of the epiphyseal cartilage during infancy, characterized by irregular calcification of the epiphyses and thickening of the distal ends of long bones. The extremities are usually symmetrically involved.

vertebral o. See *osteochondrosis.*

os"te·o·chon"dro·dys·pla'si·a [*osteon; chondros;* G. *dys-,* prefix meaning hard, bad, unlucky; *plassein,* to form]. Abnormal development of bony and cartilaginous structures.

os"te·o·chon"dro·dys·tro'phi·a de·for'mans (os"tee·o·kon"dro·dis·tro'fee·uh di·for'manz). Chondro-osteodystrophy.

os"te·o·chon·dro'ma (·kon·dro'muh) [*osteon; chondros;* G. *-ōma,* tumor]. 1. A tumor originating in bone or cartilage, occasionally from other structure, which histologically contains both bone and cartilage. It is not malignant but is marked by a predilection for local recurrence after surgery. 2. The solitary form of exostosis.

os"te·o·chon"dro·ma·to'sis [*osteon; chondros; -ōma;* G. *-ōsis,* condition]. 1. The presence of several osteochondromas. 2. Chondromatosis in which some ossification is present.

os"te·o·chon"dro·myx·o'ma. An osteochondroma with a myxoid component.

os"te·o·chon"dro·myx"o·sar·co'ma. An osteosarcoma.

os"te·o·chon"dro·sar·co'ma [*osteon; chondros;* G. *sarkōma,* fleshy excrescence]. An osteosarcoma.

os"te·o·chon·dro'sis. A process involving ossification centers chiefly during periods of rapid growth, characterized by avascular necrosis followed by slow regeneration. Osteochondrosis of the lunate bone was described by A. Kienböck; of the tarsal navicular bone by A. Köhler; of the primary and secondary growth centers of vertebral bodies by J. Calvé and H. W. Scheuermann, respectively; of a metatarsal head, usually the second, by A. H. Freiberg and A. Köhler; of the tibial tuberosity by R. B. Osgood and C. Schlatter; of an accessory center of ossification in the patella by Johansson and Sinding-Larsen. It is seen most frequently in the head of the femur, where it has been called *osteochondritis deformans juvenilis:* formerly often called *osteochondritis.*

o. deformans juvenilis. See *osteochondritis* deformans juvenilis.

o. deformans tibiae. Nonrachitic bowing of the legs seen in very young, and less frequently in older children, which usually improves spontaneously: also called *Blount-Barber syndrome.*

o. dissecans. See *osteochondritis* dissecans.

os″te·o·chon′drous. Osteochondral.

os″te·oc′la·sis [*osteon;* G. *klasis,* a breaking]. 1. The fracture of a long bone without resort to open operation, for the purpose of correcting deformity. 2. The destruction of bony tissue; the resorption of bone.

os′te·o·clast″ [*osteon;* G. *klastos,* broken in pieces]. 1. A powerful surgical apparatus or instrument through which leverage can be brought to bear at the point desired to effect osteoclasis or the forcible fracture of a long bone. 2. One of the large multinuclear cells found in association with the resorption of bone. —**osteoclas′tic,** *adj.*

os″te·o·clas·to′ma [*osteon; klastos;* G. *-ōma,* tumor]. Giant-cell tumor, 1, of bone.

os′te·o·cope″. See osteocopic *pain.*

os″te·o·cra′ni·um [*osteon;* G. *kranion,* skull]. The ossified cranium as distinguished from the chondrocranium.

os″te·o·cys·to′ma [*osteon;* G. *kystis,* bladder; *-ōma,* tumor]. A cystic bone tumor.

os′te·o·cyte″ [*osteon;* G. *kytos,* cell]. A bone cell.

os″te·o·den′tin (os″tee·o·den′teen, ·tin) [*osteon;* L. *dens,* tooth]. A tissue intermediate in structure between bone and dentin.

os″te·o·der″ma·to·plas′tic [*osteon;* G. *derma,* skin; *plassein,* to form]. Pertaining to the formation of osseous tissue in dermal structures.

os″te·o·der′mi·a [*osteon; derma*]. Bony formations in the skin.

os″te·o·di·as′ta·sis (·dye·ass′tuh·sis) [*osteon;* G. *diastasis,* separation]. Separation of bone (as an epiphysis) without true fracture. *Obs.*

os″te·o·dyn′i·a [*osteon;* G. *odynē,* pain]. A pain in a bone.

os″te·o·dys·tro′phi·a. Osteodystrophy.

o. deformans. See Paget's *disease.*

o. fibrosa. See fibrous *dysplasia.*

os″te·o·dys′tro·phy. Any defective bone formation such as the bone defects seen in rickets, dwarfism, etc.; also spelled *osteodystrophia.* See also *dystrophy.*

renal o. See renal *rickets.*

os″te·o·e·piph′y·sis. Old term for epiphysis.

os″te·o·fi″bro·chon·dro′ma. An osteochondroma.

os″te·o·fi″bro·li·po′ma [*osteon;* L. *fibra,* fiber; G. *lipos,* fat; *-ōma,* tumor]. A tumor of bony, fibrous, and fatty components.

os″te·o·fi·bro′ma (os″tee·o·figh·bro′muh) [*osteon; fibra; -ōma*]. An osteoma with a rich fibrous component; a fibroma with osseous metaplasia.

os″te·o·fi″bro·sar·co′ma. An osteosarcoma.

os″te·o·fi·bro′sis (·figh·bro′sis) [*osteon; fibra;* G. *-ōsis,* condition]. Fibrosis of bone; a change involving mainly the red bone marrow.

os′te·o·gen [*osteon;* G. *genesthai,* from *gignesthai,* to be produced]. The substance from which osteogenic fibers are formed.

os″te·o·gen′e·sis [*osteon;* G. *genesis,* production]. The development of bony tissue; ossification; the histogenesis of bone.

o. imperfecta. A defect of bone formation and calcification, of unknown cause but often hereditary or familial, characterized by bone fragility and blue sclerae. The first of many fractures may occur at or before birth (prenatal type), in infancy (postnatal type), or later in childhood (**o. imperfecta tarda**). Many severe cases are dwarfed. In the survivors, otosclerosis and deafness may develop (Van der Hoeve's syndrome) and hyperplastic callus formation may accompany the disease. On the basis of the radiographic appearance, the disease is divided into a thick-bone type, usually severe prenatal cases; a thin-bone type, a few prenatal and all postnatal cases; and **o. imperfecta cystica,** the rare type in which cystic changes of bone are also seen. Also called *fragilitas ossium, osteopsathyrosis, periosteal dysplasia, Lobstein's disease, Eddowes' disease.*

os″te·o·gen′ic, os″te·o·ge·net′ic [*osteon;* G. *genesthai,* from *gignesthai,* to be produced]. Pertaining to osteogenesis, as osteogenic layer, the deep layer of periosteum from which bone is formed.

os″te·og′e·nous (os″tee·odj′i·nus). Osteogenic.

os″te·og′e·ny (os″tee·odj′i·nee). See *osteogenesis.*

os″te·o·ha·lis″ter·e′sis [*osteon;* G. *hals,* salt; *sterēsis,* deprivation]. A loss of the mineral constituents of bone frequently resulting in softening and deformity of the bone. *Obs.*

os″te·o·hy″per·troph′ic [*osteon;* G. *hyper,* beyond; *trophē,* nourishment]. Pertaining to overgrowth of bone.

os′te·oid [*osteon;* G. *eidos,* form]. The young hyaline matrix of true bone in which the calcium salts are deposited.

os′te·oid. Resembling bone.

os″te·o·lip″o·chon·dro′ma (os″tee·o·lip″o·kon·dro′muh, ·lye″po·kon·dro′muh) [*osteon;* G. *lipos,* fat; *chondros,* cartilage; *-ōma,* tumor]. A chondroma with osseous and fatty elements.

os′te·o·lith [*osteon;* G. *lithos,* stone]. A petrified or fossil bone.

os″te·ol′o·gy [*osteon;* G. *logos,* word]. The science of anatomy and structure of bones.

os″te·ol′y·sis [*osteon;* G. *lysis,* a loosing]. 1. Resorption of bone. 2. Degeneration of bone.

os″te·o′ma [*osteon;* G. *-ōma,* tumor]. 1. A benign bony tumor seen particularly in the membrane bones of the skull and exhibiting a tendency to extend into the orbit or paranasal sinuses. Histologically, it is composed of osteoblasts, forming osteoid and osseous tissue, and may become compact. Classified according to location, it may be central, endosteal, cortical, or periosteal. 2. Loosely, a nonneoplastic or neoplastic lesion, such as a hyperostosis, a fibrous dysplasia, or an exostosis (osteochondroma). —**osteo′matoid,** *adj.*

cavalryman's o. An exostosis at the attachment of the adductor longus or adductor magnus muscle.

fibrous o. Ossifying fibroma.

osteoid o. A small benign tumor of bone, composed of a nidus of well-vascularized connective tissue and osteoid matrix surrounded by atypical trabeculae of dense new bone, occurring almost exclusively in younger age groups and characteristically accompanied by severe pain.

o. cutis. Bony deposits in the skin and subcutaneous tissue, usually secondary to some other skin lesion: also called *osteosis cutis.*

o. durum. Hard, dense osteoma with little marrow. Also called *o. eburneum.*

o. eburneum. An ivorylike osteoma.

o. medullare. An osteoma with conspicuous marrow spaces.

o. spongiosum. One which is spongy because of coarse bands of cancellous bone.

os″te·o·ma·la′ci·a. [*osteon;* G. *malakia,* softness]. A disorder of bone characterized by failure of calcium salts to be deposited in newly formed osteoid, leading to weakened bones. The product of total serum inorganic calcium and total serum inorganic phosphorus is below the normal adult level (see *law of Howland and Kramer*). Its causes include lack of vitamin D or resistance to it, failure to absorb it, as in steatorrhea, renal acidosis, hypercalciuria and others. Syn., *adult rickets*. —**osteomala'cial, osteomala'cic,** *adj.*

juvenile o. Rickets.

os"te·om'e·try [*osteon;* G. *metron*, a measure]. The study of the proportions and measurements of the skeleton. —**osteomet'ric,** *adj.*

os"te·o·mu'coid. See *osseomucoid.*

os"te·o·my"e·li'tis [*osteon;* G. *myelos*, marrow; *-itis*, inflammation]. Inflammation of the marrow of bone. —**osteomyelit'ic,** *adj.*

chronic hemorrhagic o. See giant-cell *tumor*, 1.

chronic sclerosing o. A low-grade chronic osteomyelitis, described by Carl Garré, which stimulates bone-marrow formation, characterized by marked increase in bone density, without pus. The marrow may be replaced by granulation or fibrous tissue. Also called *sclerotic nonsuppurative o.*

hematogenous o. An infection of the bone, transmitted through the blood stream and localized on the diaphyseal side of the epiphysis, usually caused by *Micrococcus pyogenes.*

suppurative o. A complication or late sequel of enteric fevers, e.g., typhoid or *Salmonella* infections.

os"te·o·my"e·log'ra·phy [*osteon; myelos;* G. *graphein*, to write]. Roentgenography of bone marrow and marrow spaces.

os"te·o·myx"o·chon·dro'ma. An osteochondroma with a myxoid component.

os'te·on, os·te·one'. A concentric lamellar (Haversian) system in compact bone.

os"te·o·ne·cro'sis [*osteon;* G. *nekrōsis*, mortification]. Necrosis of bone in mass.

os"te·o·neph·rop'a·thy. Any of a variety of syndromes, involving bone changes, accompanying renal disease, e.g., renal rickets, nephrocalcinosis, amino-diabetes, and idiopathic hypercalciuria.

os"te·o·neu·ral'gia [*osteon;* G. *neuron*, nerve; *algos*, pain]. Neuralgia of bone. *Obs.*

os"te·o·pae'di·on (os"tee·o·pee'dee·un). See *lithopedion.*

os'te·o·path, os"te·op'a·thist [*osteon;* G. *pathos*, disease]. One who practices osteopathy.

os"te·o·path'i·a. Any bone disease or defect.

o. condensans disseminata. Osteopoikilosis.

o. hyperostotica (scleroticans) multiplex infantilis. See Engelmann's *disease.*

o. striata. An unusual congenital osseous defect characterized by the roentgenographic finding of striation of the skeleton and particularly of the metaphyses of long bones. It may be related to dyschondroplasia and osteopoikilosis.

os"te·op'a·thy [*osteon; pathos*]. A school of healing which teaches that the body is a vital mechanical organism whose structural and functional integrity are coordinate and interdependent, the perversion of either constituting disease. Its major effort in treatment is in manipulation, but surgery and the specialties are also included. —**osteopath'ic,** *adj.*

os"te·o·pe·cil'i·a. See *osteopoikilosis.*

os"te·o·pe'di·on [*osteon;* G. *paidion*, little child. A calcified fetus. Syn., *lithopedion.*

os"te·o·per"i·os·ti'tis [*osteon;* G. *periosteos*, around the bones; *-itis*, inflammation]. Combined inflammation of bone and its periosteum.

os"te·o·pe·tro'sis [*osteon;* G. *petros*, stone; *-ōsis*, condition]. A rare developmental error of unknown cause but of familial tendency, characterized chiefly by excessive radiographic density of most or all of the bones. Clinically there may be a tendency toward bone fracture, anemia, and optic atrophy. The extent to which the bones are involved varies. Pathologically, bones show sclerotic changes with fibrosis of the marrow. Also called *o. generalisata, Albers-Schönberg disease, ivory bones, marble bones, osteosclerosis (fragilis generalisata), rheostosis.*

Léri type of o. See *melorheostosis.*

os'te·o·phage [*osteon;* G. *phagein*, to eat]. An osteoclast, 2.

os"te·oph'o·ny [*osteon;* G. *phōnē*, sound]. The transmission of sound through bone.

os"te·oph'thi·sis [*osteon;* G. *phthisis*, a wasting away]. Wasting of the bones. *Obs.*

os'te·o·phyte" [*osteon;* G. *phyton*, plant]. A bony outgrowth.

os'te·o·plaque" (os'tee·o·plack") [*osteon;* G. *plax*, anything flat and broad]. A layer of bone; a flat osteoma.

os'te·o·plast". See *osteoblast.*

os"te·o·plas'tic [*osteon;* G. *plassein*, to form]. 1. Pertaining to the formation of bone tissue. 2. Pertaining to reparative operations upon bone.

os'te·o·plas"ty [*osteon; plassein*]. Plastic operations on bone.

os"te·o·poi"ki·lo'sis [*osteon;* G. *poikillein*, to work in various colors; *-ōsis*, condition]. A bone affection of unknown cause, giving rise to no symptoms and discovered by chance on roentgenographic examination when ellipsoidal dense foci are seen in all bones: also called *osteopathia condensa disseminata.*

os"te·o·po·ro'sis [*osteon;* G. *poros*, passage; *-ōsis*]. Enlargement of the marrow and Haversian spaces of the bone at the expense of the solid parts. Trabeculae become fewer and thinner; compact bone tends to resemble cancellous, with resulting fragility. —**osteoporot'ic,** *adj.*

disuse o. Demineralization with loss of matrix, involving the bones of all or a part of an extremity in which function has been impaired, or the entire skeleton when total physical activity is limited. Senility, menopause, and systemic disease are predisposing conditions.

malnutrition o. That resulting from negative mineral and nitrogen balances and deficiencies of vitamins essential for maintenance of proper calcium and phosphorus distribution in the body and for ossification.

postmenopausal o. A diffuse osteoporosis, often severe, chiefly involving the spine and pelvis, which may follow artificial or physiological menopause, and is caused by the hormonal deficiency and concomitant inadequate bone formation.

senile o. Osteoporosis in the aged, due to deficient osteoid formation. Blood calcium, phosphorus, and phosphatase levels are all normal or low.

os"te·op·sath"y·ro'sis (os"tee·op·sath"i·ro'sis, os"-tee·o·sath"i·) [*osteon;* G. *psathyros*, crumbling; *-ōsis*]. Old term for osteogenesis imperfecta.

os"te·o·ra"di·o·ne·cro'sis [*osteon;* L. *radius*, ray; G. *nekrōsis*, mortification]. Bone necrosis due to irradiation by roentgen or radium rays.

os"te·or·rha'gi·a [*osteon;* G. *rhēgnynai*, to burst forth]. Hemorrhage from a bone. *Rare.*

os"te·or'rha·phy [*osteon;* G. *rhaphē*, a suture]. The suturing or joining of bones.

os"te·o·sar·co'ma. Osteogenic sarcoma. —**osteosarco'matous,** *adj.*

os"te·o·scle·ro'sis. See *osteopetrosis.*

os"te·o'sis [*osteon;* G. *-ōsis*, condition]. Bone formation.

ivory o. Osteoma eburneum.

o. cutis. See *osteoma* cutis.

os"te·o·spon"gi·o'ma (os"tee·o·spon"jee·o'muh. ·spun"jee·o'muh) [*osteon;* G. *spoggia*, sponge;

-ōma, tumor]. A tumor consisting of cancellous bone.

os″te·o·stix′is [*osteon;* G. *stixis*, a pricking]. Surgical puncturing of a bone.

os″te·o·su′ture [*osteon;* L. *sutura*, suture]. Suture of bone.

os″te·o·syn″o·vi′tis (os″tee·o·sin″o·vy′tis, ·sigh″-no·vy′tis) [*osteon;* G. *syn*, with; *ōion*, egg; *-itis*, inflammation]. Synovitis complicated with osteitis of adjacent bones.

os″te·o·syn′the·sis [*osteon;* G. *synthesis*, a putting together]. Fastening the ends of a fractured bone together by mechanical means, such as a plate.

os″te·o·ta′bes (os″tee·o·tay′beez) [*osteon;* L. *tabes*, a wasting away]. Bone degeneration beginning with the destruction of the cells of the bone marrow, which disappears in parts and is replaced by soft gelatinous tissue; later the spongy bone diminishes, and lastly the compact bone.

os″te·o·throm·bo′sis [*osteon;* G. *thrombōsis*, a blocked vein]. Thrombosis of the veins of a bone.

os′te·o·tome″ [*osteon;* G. *tomos*, cutting]. An instrument for cutting bone. Specifically, an instrument somewhat similar to a chisel but without the beveled edge, used for cutting long bones, generally with the aid of a surgical mallet.

os″te·o·to″mo·cla′si·a (os″tee·o·to″mo·clay′zhuh, ·zee·uh, ·shuh, ·see·uh, os·tee·ot″o·mo·), **os″te·o·to·moc′la·sis** (os″tee·o·to·mock′luh·sis, os·tee·ot″o·) [*osteon; tomos;* G. *klaein*, to break]. The correction of a pathologically curved bone by forcible bending following partial division by a osteotome.

os″te·ot′o·my [*osteon;* G. *tomē*, a cutting]. 1. The division of a bone. 2. Making a section of a bone for the purpose of correcting a deformity.

cuneiform o. An ostectomy in which a wedge of bone is removed.

linear o. A simple division of a bone.

subcutaneous o. Osteotomy, usually by Macewen's technic, in which a small incision is made in the skin over the bony area to be divided, the bone itself being unexposed, and the operation completed by the sense of touch.

os′te·o·tribe [*osteon;* G. *tribein*, to rub]. A bone rasp. Formerly called *osteotrite.*

os″te·ot′ro·phy [*osteon;* G. *trophē*, nourishment]. Nutrition of bony tissue.

Osterberg method. See Sanford, Sheard, and Osterberg *method.*

os·ti′tis. See *osteitis.*

os′ti·um (pl. *ostiums, ostia*) [L., door, mouth, entrance]. A mouth or aperture. **—ostial,** *adj.*

o. abdominale. The orifice of the oviduct communicating with the peritoneal cavity.

o. atrioventriculare. Either the right or left atrioventricular opening.

o. internum. The uterine opening of the oviduct.

o. maxillare. The opening of the maxillary air sinus.

o. pharyngeum. The pharyngeal opening of the auditory tube. See Plate 12.

o. tympanicum. The tympanic opening of the auditory tube.

o. vaginae. The external orifice of the vagina.

os·to′sis. Osteosis.

os″tre·o·tox·is′mus (os″tree·o·tock·siz′mus) [G. *ostreon*, oyster; *toxikon*, poison]. Poisoning due to eating diseased or deteriorated oysters.

Ostwald-Folin pipet. See under *pipet.*

o·syr′i·tin. See *rutin.*

OT, O.T. 1. *In anatomy*, old term, in opposition to BNA term. 2. Original, or old, tuberculin. Also abbreviated T.O.

o·tal′gi·a [G. *ous*, ear; *algos*, pain]. Earache. **—otalgic,** *adj.*

o″tan·tri′tis [*ous;* L. *antrum*, cave; G. *-itis*, inflammation]. Inflammation of the mastoid antrum.

o″thel·co′sis (o″thel·ko′sis, oat″hel·ko′sis) [*ous;* G. *helkōsis*, ulceration]. Ulceration of the ear. *Obs.*

o·the″ma·to′ma [*ous;* G. *haima*, blood; *-ōma*, tumor]. Hematoma of the external ear, usually the pinna.

ot″hem·or·rha′gi·a (oath″em·o·ray′juh, ·jee·uh, ·radj′uh, ·radj′ee·uh, oat″hem·o·) [*ous; haima;* G. *rhēgnynai*, to burst]. Hemorrhage from the ear.

ot″hem·or·rhe′a (oat″hem·o·ree′uh, oath″em·o·) [*ous; haima;* G. *rhoia*, flow]. A sanguineous discharge from the ear.

o′tic [G. *ōtikos*, of the ear]. Pertaining to the ear.

o″ti·co·din′i·a [*ōtikos;* G. *dinē*, whirling]. Vertigo from ear disease.

Otis, Fessenden Nott [*American urologist*, 1825–1900]. Used local anesthesia in urology (1884). Introduced his operation for internal urethrotomy, in which he divided the stricture from within, using a specially constructed urethrotome.

o·ti′tis [G. *ous*, ear; *-itis*, inflammation]. Inflammation of the ear. **—otit′ic,** *adj.*

acute suppurative o. Acute inflammation of the middle ear, with formation of pus, caused by such organisms as hemolytic streptococci, pneumococci, and/or nonhemolytic streptococci.

furuncular o. The formation of furuncles in the external auditory meatus.

mycotic o. externa. Infection of the external auditory canal due to fungi; an otomycosis.

o. externa. Inflammation of the external ear.

o. interna. Inflammation of the internal ear.

o. labyrinthica. Inflammation of the labyrinth.

o. mastoidea. Inflammation confined to the mastoid cells; mastoid disease.

o. media. Inflammation of the middle ear. A tuberculous type is associated with active pulmonary tuberculosis, but runs an independent course.

o. parasitica. Inflammation caused by a parasite.

o. sclerotica. Inflammation of the inner ear with hardening of the tissues. See *otosclerosis.*

o′to-, ot- [*ous*]. A combining form meaning *the ear.*

o″to·blen″or·rhe′a [*ous;* G. *blenna*, mucus; *rhoia*, flow]. Any discharge of mucus from the ear.

o″to·ca·tarrh′ [*ous;* G. *katarroos*, running down]. Catarrh of the ear. *Rare.*

o″to·ceph′a·lus [*ous;* G. *kephalē*, head]. A monster characterized by a union or close approach of the ears, by absence of the lower jaw, and an ill-developed mouth. See *synotus, agnathus.*

o″to·clei′sis (o″to·kly′sis) [*ous;* G. *kleisis*, a closing]. Occlusion of the ear.

o″to·co′ni·um (pl. *otoconia*) [*ous;* G. *konis*, dust]. Otolith; a soft substance over the two maculae acusticae containing many crystals of calcium carbonate 1–15μ long (large ear stones of fishes are called otoliths). **—otoconial,** *adj.*

o′to·cyst [*ous;* G. *kystis*, bladder]. 1. In invertebrates, an auditory vesicle, otocell, or otidium. 2. In vertebrates, the embryonic auditory vesicle.

o″to·dyn′i·a [*ous;* G. *odynē*, pain]. Pain in the ear.

o″to·gen′ic, o·tog′e·nous (o·todj′i·nus) [*ous;* G. *genesthai*, from *gignesthai*, to be produced]. Originating or arising within the ear.

o″to·hem′i·neur″as·the′ni·a [*ous;* G. *hēmi-*, half; *neuron*, nerve; *astheneia*, weakness]. A condition in which hearing is limited exclusively to one ear, without the evidence of any material lesion of the auditory apparatus.

o″to·lar″yn·gol′o·gist [*ous;* G. *larygx*, larynx; *logos*, word]. One skilled in the practice of otology, rhinology, and laryngology.

o″to·lar″yn·gol′o·gy [*ous; larygx; logos*]. A medical

specialty including otology, rhinology, laryngology, and, usually, peroral endoscopy.

o·to·lith [*ous;* G. *lithos*, stone]. One of the calcareous concretions within the membranous labyrinth of the ear, especially the large ear stones of fishes.

o·tol′o·gist [*ous;* G. *logos*, word]. One versed in otology.

o·tol′o·gy [*ous; logos*]. The science of the ear, its anatomy, functions, and diseases. —**otolog′ic, otolog′ical,** *adj.*

otomide. A proprietary solution of sulfanilamide, urea, and chlorobutanol in glycerin; intended for the treatment of infections of the middle and external ear.

o″to·my″as·the′ni·a [*ous;* G. *mys*, muscle; *astheneia*, weakness]. 1. Weakness of the muscles of the ear. 2. Defective hearing due to a paretic condition of the tensor tympani or stapedius muscle.

O″to·my′ces (o″to·migh′seez, o·tom′i·seez) [*ous;* G. *mykēs*, fungus]. Fungous growth within the ear.

O. Hageni. A fungus with green conidia, sometimes found in the external canal of the ear.

O. purpureus. A dark red fungous growth in the ear.

o″to·my·co′sis (o″to·migh·ko′sis) [*ous; mykēs;* G. *-ōsis*, condition]. The growth of fungi within the ear, or the diseased condition caused thereby.

o″to·neu·ral′gi·a. See *otalgia.*

o″to·neur″as·the′ni·a [*ous;* G. *neuron*, nerve; *astheneia*, weakness]. A condition of deficient sensitivity of the auditory apparatus.

o″to·pha·ryn′ge·al (o″to·fa·rin′jul, ·jee·ul, ·far″in-jee′ul) [*ous;* G. *pharygx*, pharynx]. Pertaining to the ear and the pharynx.

o′to·plas″ty [*ous;* G. *plassein*, to form]. Plastic surgery of the external ear.

o″to·pol′y·pus [*ous;* G. *polypous*, many-footed]. A polyp occurring in the ear.

o″to·py″or·rhe′a [*ous;* G. *pyorroia*, discharge of matter]. A purulent discharge from the ear.

o″to·py·o′sis (o″to·pye·o′sis) [*ous;* G. *pyōsis*, suppuration]. Suppuration within the ear.

o″to·rhi·nol′o·gy (o″to·rye·nol′o·jee) [*ous;* G. *rhis*, nose; *logos*, word]. Literally, the study of diseases of the ears and the nose only. The terms most frequently employed for the study of the diseases of the ear, nose, and throat are *otolaryngology* and *otorhinolaryngology.*

o″tor·rha′gi·a [*ous;* G. *rhēgnynai*, to burst forth]. A discharge of blood from the external auditory meatus.

o″tor·rhe′a [*ous;* G. *rhoia*, flow]. A discharge from the external auditory meatus.

cerebrospinal o. Drainage of cerebrospinal fluid from the ear, usually the result of a posterior fossa basilar skull fracture, rarely from erosion of the petrous portion of the temporal bone caused by tumor.

o″to·sal′pinx [*ous;* G. *salpigx*, trumpet]. Old term for the auditory tube.

o″to·scle·rec′to·my. See *ossiculectomy.*

o″to·scle·ro′sis [*ous;* G. *sklērōsis*, hardening]. A clinical entity, the symptom being progressive impairment of hearing. The end result of the pathologic process is the laying down of new bone around the oval window, the cochlea, or both. Erroneously thought to be new bone growth around any of the ossicles. —**otosclerot′ic,** *adj.*

o′to·scope [*ous;* G. *skopein*, to examine]. An apparatus designed for examination of the ear and for rendering the tympanic membrane visible.

o·tos′co·py [*ous; skopein*]. Visualization of the auditory canal and tympanic membrane by means of the otoscope. —**otoscop′ic,** *adj.*

otosmosan. Trade-mark for a solution of sulfathiazole and urea in glycerin used in infections of the middle and external ear.

o·tot′o·my [*ous;* G. *tomē*, a cutting]. Dissection of the ear; incision of any of the tissues of the external auditory meatus or the ear proper.

ot′ri·vin. 2-Anilinomethyl-2-imidazoline; a drug which inhibits cholinesterase destruction, thus intensifying and prolonging the action of acetylcholine and leading to increased activity of the parasympathetic system: used as vasoconstrictor.

Otto, Adolph Wilhelm [*German surgeon,* 1786–1845]. Described osteoarthritic protrusion of the acetabulum into the pelvis; called *Otto's disease.* The resulting pelvic deformity is called *Otto's pelvis.*

Otto, John Conrad [*American physician,* 1774–1844]. The first to describe hemophilia fully, and to note that it does not occur in women but may be transmitted by them (1803). This phenomenon was also noted by Nasse (1820), and is known as *Nasse's law.*

O. U. *Oculus uterque*, each eye.

oua″ba·gen′in (wah″buh·jenn′in). $C_{23}H_{34}O_8$; the aglycone of ouabain; a steroid, slightly soluble in water.

oua·ba′in (wah·bah′in, ·bay′in, wah′bah·in, ·bay·in). $C_{29}H_{44}O_{12}.8H_2O$; a crystalline glycoside obtained from the seeds of *Strophanthus gratus* and the wood of *Acokanthera schimperi*, sparingly soluble in water. On hydrolysis it yields a molecule each of ouabagenin and rhamnose. It has digitalislike action.

Oudin current. See under *current.*

ou′la (oo′luh) [G. *oulon*, gum]. Ula; the gingiva. *Obs.*

ou′loid (ōō′loyd) [G. *oulē*, scar; *eidos*, form]. Resembling a scar.

ou″lor·rha′gi·a (ōō″lo·ray′juh, ·jee·uh) [G. *oulon*, gum; *rhēgnynai*, to burst forth]. Hemorrhage from the gums.

ounce [L. *uncia*, twelfth part of a pound]. A unit of measure or weight. See Tables of Weights and Measures in the Appendix. See also *fluidounce.*

avoirdupois o. The sixteenth part of the avoirdupois pound, or 437.5 gr. (28.35 Gm.). Abbreviated, oz.

troy o. The twelfth part of the troy pound, or 480 gr. (31.10 Gm.). Symbol, ℥.

ou·ra′ri (oo·rah′ree). See *curare.*

ou′ro- (oor′o-). See *uro-.*

-ous (-us) [L. *-osus*]. 1. A suffix meaning *full of* or *having.* 2. *In chemistry*, a suffix denoting the *lower* of two valences assumed by an element.

out′flow [ME. *out;* AS. *flōwan*]. *In neurology*, the transmission of efferent impulses, particularly of the autonomic nervous system; these are divided into thoracolumbar and craniosacral outflows.

out′let [*out;* ME. *leten*]. The lower aperture of the pelvic canal.

out′pa″tient [*out;* L. *patiens*, from *pati*, to suffer]. A hospital patient who does not occupy a bed in the institution.

o. service. Medical and dental care furnished at a medical-treatment facility when hospitalization is not required.

out·spo′ken [Ger. *ausgesprochen*, pronounced]. *Of symptoms*, pronounced, strongly marked.

o′va [L.]. Plural of ovum, an egg.

o′val [L. *ovum*, egg]. 1. Egg-shaped. 2. Pertaining to an ovum.

o″val·bu′min [*ovum;* L. *albus*, white]. The albumin of egg white.

o·val′o·cyte [*ovum;* G. *kytos*, cell]. An elliptical erythrocyte: incorrectly spelled *ovalcyte.*

o″va·lo·cy·to′sis (o″vuh·lo·sigh·to′sis, o·val″o·). Elliptocytosis: incorrectly spelled *ovalcytosis.*

o·va′ri·a. Plural of ovarium.

o·va″ri·al′gi·a [NL. *ovarium*, from *ovum;* G. *algos*, pain]. Neuralgic pain in the ovary: also spelled *oarialgia*.

o·va′ri·an [*ovarium*]. Pertaining to the ovaries.

o·va′ri·an pseu″do·myx·o′ma. See pseudomucinous *cystadenoma*.

o·va″ri·ec′to·my [*ovarium;* G. *ektomē*, excision]. Excision of an ovary; oophorectomy.

o·va′ri·o-, ovari- [*ovarium*]. A combining form denoting *an ovary* or *ovarian*.

o·va′ri·o·cele″ [*ovarium;* G. *kēlē*, tumor]. Tumor of the ovary; hernia of an ovary.

vaginal o. Invasion of the vaginal wall by one or both ovaries.

o·va″ri·o·cen·te′sis [*ovarium;* G. *kentēsis*, a pricking]. Puncture of an ovary or of an ovarian cyst.

o·va″ri·o·cy·e′sis (o·vair″ee·o·sigh·ee′sis) [*ovarium;* G. *kyēsis*, pregnancy]. Ovarian pregnancy.

o·va″ri·o·dys·neu′ri·a [*ovarium;* G. *dys-*, bad; *neuron*, nerve]. Ovarian neuralgia.

o·va″ri·o·gen′ic [*ovarium;* G. *genesthai*, from *gignesthai*, to be produced]. Arising in the ovary.

o·va″ri·o·hys″ter·ec′to·my [*ovarium;* G. *hystera*, womb; *ektomē*, excision]. Surgical removal of one or both ovaries and the uterus.

o·va″ri·o·lyt′ic [*ovarium;* G. *lyein*, to loose]. Producing disorganization of ovarian tissue.

o·va″ri·on′cus [*ovarium;* G. *ogkos*, mass]. An ovarian tumor. *Rare.*

o·va″ri·or·rhex′is [*ovarium;* G. *rhēxis*, a breaking]. Rupture of an ovary.

o·va″ri·o·sal″pin·gec′to·my. See *oophorosalpingectomy*.

o·va″ri·o·ste·re′sis [*ovarium;* G. *sterēsis*, deprivation]. Extirpation of an ovary. *Rare.*

o·va″ri·os′to·my. See *oophorostomy*.

o·va″ri·ot′o·my [*ovarium;* G. *tomē*, a cutting]. Literally, incision of an ovary. As generally used, removal of an ovary; oophorectomy.

o·va″ri·o·tu′bal [*ovarium;* L. *tubus*, tube]. Pertaining to an ovary and oviduct.

o″va·ri′tis. See *oophoritis*.

o·va′ri·um (pl. *ovaria*) [NL.]. An ovary or oophoron.

o′va·ry [*ovarium*]. 1. One of a pair of glandular organs giving rise to ova. It consists of a fibrous framework or stroma, in which are embedded the ovarian follicles, and is surrounded by a serous covering derived from the peritoneum. See Plates 41, 45. 2. The dried, undefatted, and powdered ovary of cattle, sheep, or swine; one part represents approximately six parts by weight of fresh glands. Has been used as a therapeutic agent but probably is devoid of physiologic action. Syn., *desiccated ovarian substance*.

bilateral polycystic ovaries. Multiple cysts of both ovaries, generally associated with enlargement of these organs, and often with amenorrhea and/or abnormal uterine bleeding, infertility, and frequently hirsutism. See Stein-Leventhal *syndrome*.

undescended ovaries. A rare congenital anomaly in which the ovaries fail to descend to normal position, accompanied by amenorrhea, poorly developed secondary sexual characters, and limitation of growth. The other genitalia may be developed normally and the body configuration is female.

o″va·tes′tis. Ovotestis.

o′ver·bite″. The extent to which the upper anterior teeth overlap the lower when the dentition is in the position of rest.

o″ver·cor·rec′tion. *In optics*, an aberration of a lens causing the light rays passing the central zones to focus at a point nearer to the lens than rays passing the outer zones.

o′ver·de·pen′den·cy. See *passive-dependent personality* under passive-aggressive *personality*.

o′ver·de·ter″mi·na′tion [AS. *ofer;* L. *determinare*, to limit, determine]. *In psychoanalysis*, the state of having more than one etiologic factor.

o″ver·ex·ten′sion [*ofer;* L. *extensio*, from *extendere*, to stretch out]. Excessive extension; extension beyond the normal point or line.

o′ver·flow″ [*ofer;* AS. *flōwan*]. The escape of liquid from a filled vessel or viscus when more liquid is added.

o′ver·growth″ [*ofer;* AS. *grōwan*]. Hypertrophy or hyperplasia.

o′ver·jet″. The extent to which the upper incisors project in front of the lower incisors when the dentition is in the position of rest.

o″ver·ly′ing [*ofer;* AS. *licgan*]. A cause of death in infants sleeping with adults; suffocation occurs when one of the adults lies upon the child.

o″ver·max′i·mal [*ofer;* L. *maximus*, greatest]. Beyond the normal maximum, as the overmaximal contraction of a muscle.

o″ver·pro·duc′tion the′o·ry. Loss of elements or parts may be followed by overproduction of such parts during repair. Formerly called *Weigert's law*.

o″ver·reach′ [*ofer;* AS. *rǣcan*]. Strike the toe of the hindfoot against the heel or shoe of the forefoot; said of a horse.

o″ver·rid′ing [*ofer;* AS. *rīdan*]. The slipping of an end of a fragment of a fractured bone over the other fragment. Said also of toes which overlap.

o′ver·strain″ [*ofer;* OF. *estraindre*, from L. *stringere*, to draw tight]. To strain to excess.

o′ver·strain″. A condition resulting from exhausting effort.

Overton theory. See Meyer-Overton *theory*.

o′ver·tone″ [*ofer;* G. *tonos*, tone]. A harmonic tone heard above the fundamental tone.

psychic o. An associated impression contributing to a mental image.

o′ver·weight″ [*ofer;* AS. *wiht*]. Exceeding normal weight, usually meaning an excess of more than 10%.

o′vi- [L. *ovum*, egg]. A combining form meaning *egg;* used to denote *ovum*.

o″vi·cap′sule [*ovum;* L. *capsula*, small box]. Old term for an egg case, or for an ovarian follicle.

o′vi·duct [*ovum;* L. *ductus*, from *ducere*, to conduct]. The duct serving to transport the ovum from the ovary to the exterior, or to an organ such as the uterus. In mammals, the oviduct is also called the uterine or fallopian tube. See Plate 41. —**ovidu′cal, oviduc′tal,** *adj.*

o·vif′er·ous [*ovum;* L. *ferre*, to bear]. Producing or bearing ova.

o″vi·fi·ca′tion [*ovum;* L. *facere*, to make]. The production of ova.

o′vi·form [*ovum;* L. *forma*, form]. Egg-shaped; oval.

o″vi·gen′e·sis [*ovum;* G. *genesis*, production]. Oogenesis.

o″vi·ge·net′ic. See *ovigenous*.

o·vig′e·nous (o·vidj′i·nus) [*ovum;* G. *genesthai*, from *gignesthai*, to be produced]. Producing ova, as the ovigenous layer, the outer layer of the ovary, in which the follicles containing the ova are situated.

o′vi·germ [*ovum;* L. *germen*, sprout]. A cell producing or developing into an ovum.

o·vig′er·ous (o·vidj′ur·us) [*ovum;* L. *gerere*, to bear]. Producing or carrying ova.

o′vine [LL. *ovinus*, from *ovis*, sheep]. 1. Relating to or derived from sheep. 2. Sheeplike.

o·vip′a·rous [*ovum;* L. *parere*, to bring forth]. Laying eggs; bringing forth young in the egg stage of development. —**ovipara,** *n.*

o″vi·po·si′tion (o″vi·po·zish′un) [*ovum;* L. *positio*, a placing]. The act of laying or depositing eggs by the females of oviparous animals. —**ovipos′it,** *v.*

o″vi·pos′i·tor (o″vi·poz′i·tur) [*ovum;* L. *positor,* from *ponere,* to place]. An organ, common among insects, composed of several modified rings of somites, forming the end of the abdomen, and employed in depositing the eggs.

o′vi·sac [*ovum;* L. *saccus,* sack]. Old term for an ovarian follicle.

o′vi vi·tel′lus (o′vye vye·tel′us, o′vee). Yolk of egg; the substance is sometimes used in pharmacy as an emulsifying agent.

o′vo-. See *ovi-.*

o′vo·cen″ter, o″vo·cen′ter [*ovum;* G. *kentron,* center]. The centrosome of the ovum during fertilization.

ovocylin. Trade-mark for a brand of estradiol.

ovocylin dipropionate. Trade-marked name for estradiol dipropionate: formerly called *di-ovocylin.*

o′vo·cyte. See *oocyte.*

o″vo·fla′vin (o″vo·flay′vin, ·flav′in) [*ovum;* L. *flavus,* yellow]. A flavin separated from eggs; it is identical with riboflavin.

o″vo·gen′e·sis. See *oogenesis.*

o″vo·glob′u·lin [*ovum;* L. *globulus,* little ball]. The globulin of white of egg.

o″vo·go′ni·um. See *oogonium.*

o′void [*ovum;* G. *eidos,* form]. Egg-shaped.

o″vo·mu′cin. A glycoprotein from egg white.

o″vo·mu′coid [*ovum;* L. *mucus,* mucus; *eidos*]. A glycoprotein obtained from white of egg.

o′vo·plasm [*ovum;* G. *plasma,* anything formed]. The cytoplasm of the unimpregnated ovum.

o″vo·tes′tis, o″va·tes′tis [*ovum;* L. *testis,* testis]. A rare form of hermaphroditism in which an ovary and a testis are combined.

o′vo·tid. See *oocyte.*

o″vo·vi·tel′lin (o″vo·vye·tel′in, ·vi·tel′in) [*ovum;* L. *vitellus,* yolk of an egg]. A protein contained in egg yolk; a white, granular substance, soluble in dilute acids and in alkalies.

o″vo·vi·vip′a·rous (o″vo·vye·vip′uh·rus) [*ovum;* L. *viviparus,* that brings forth its young alive]. Reproducing by means of eggs hatched within the body. —**ovoviviparism,** *n.*

ov′u·lar [*ovum*]. Relating to an ovule or ovum.

ov″u·la′tion [*ovum*]. The maturation and escape of the ovum.

ov′ule [*ovum*]. 1. A small egg; one in an early stage of development. 2. The egg before its escape from the ovarian follicle.

ov″u·log′e·nous (o″view·lodj′i·nus) [*ovum;* G. *genesthai,* from *gignesthai,* to be produced]. Producing ovules.

o′vum (pl. *ova*) [L.]. 1. A female germ cell; an egg cell; a cell which is capable of developing into a new member of the same species, in animals usually only after maturation and fertilization. The human ovum (see Plate 41) is a large, spheroidal cell containing a large mass of cytoplasm and a large nucleus (germinal vesicle), within which is a nucleolus (germinal spot). 2. The early human embryo from the time of fertilization until the bilaminar blastodisk is formed.

alecithal o. One having little or no yolk.

centrolecithal o. One having a central yolk surrounded by cytoplasm, as in insects.

dropsical o. One in which the embryo has entirely disappeared or is represented by only a nodule of degenerated tissue. The amniotic vesicle is distended by an amount of fluid far out of proportion to the duration of pregnancy.

holoblastic o. One having total or complete cleavage.

isolecithal o. One having little yolk evenly distributed in the cytoplasm.

meroblastic o. One having partial cleavage, limited to the cytoplasmic region.

o. tuberculosum. See tuberous *mole.*

primordial o. An ovum present in the germinal epithelium of the embryonic ovary, frequently considered to serve as a parent cell for the oogonia.

telolecithal o. One having the yolk concentrated at one pole or in one hemisphere.

Owen, Richard [*English anatomist,* 1804–92]. Celebrated paleontologist. Described *Trichinella spiralis* (1835). Described incremental lines of the dentin; called *Owen's lines, Salter's lines.*

ox- *In chemistry:* 1. Short for *oxal-.* 2. Combining form denoting *presence of oxygen.*

ox′a- *In chemistry,* a combining form denoting the *presence of oxygen* in place of carbon.

ox′al-, ox′al·o-. *In chemistry,* a combining form denoting *oxalic.*

ox″al·a·ce′tic ac′id. Oxaloacetic acid.

ox′a·late. Any salt or ester of oxalic acid.

ox″a·le′mi·a [*oxalis;* G. *haima,* blood]. Excess of oxalates in the blood.

ox·al′ic [*oxalis*]. *In chemistry,* pertaining to an oxalic acid.

ox·al′ic ac′id. $HOOC.COOH.2H_2O$. A poisonous dibasic or dicarboxylic acid occurring in many plants. Used as a reagent and in many industries and the arts, chiefly for its bleaching properties.

ox′a·lism [*oxalis*]. Poisoning by oxalic acid or potassium binoxalate. It is characterized by gastroenteritis with nephritis, collapse, cyanosis, mydriasis, labored breathing, and dyspnea.

ox″al·o·a·ce′tic ac′id. $HOOC.CH_2.CO.COOH$. A metabolic product in carbohydrate metabolism; it may be produced by oxidation of malic acid or by addition of a molecule of carbon dioxide to one of pyruvic acid. Also called *oxalacetic acid.*

ox″al·o′sis. A condition in which there is widespread deposition of calcium oxalate crystals in tissues, especially the kidneys and bone marrow, associated with recurrent calcium oxalate urinary calculi and renal insufficiency: possibly due to an inborn error of metabolism.

ox·al″o·suc·cin′ic ac′id. $COOH.CO.HC(COOH).CH_2.COOH$; an intermediate substance in the Krebs or tricarboxylic acid oxidation cycle, formed by addition of carbon dioxide to α-ketoglutaric acid or by dehydrogenation of isocitric acid.

ox″a·lu′ri·a [*oxalis;* G. *ouron,* urine]. The presence of oxalic acid or oxalates in the urine.

ox″a·lu′ric ac′id. $NH_2.CO.NH.CO.COOH$. An acid occasionally found in traces in normal human urine.

ox·am′i·dine (ocks·am′i·deen, ·din). See *amidoxim.*

oxamycin. A name assigned to *cycloserine.*

ox′a·tyl. Carboxyl.

ox′a·zine. One of 13 isomeric heterocyclic compounds of the general formula C_4H_5NO, each containing four carbon atoms, one oxygen atom, and one nitrogen atom in the ring; two double bonds are present in each ring.

ox″a·zol′i·dine. The heterocyclic compound $O.CH_2.NH.CH_2.CH_2$, from which medicinal derivatives have been prepared. See *trimethadione.*

ox bile (*fel bovis*). The fresh bile of the ox, *Bos taurus.* See *bile.*

o. b. extract (*extractum fellis bovis*). Contains sodium salts of ox bile acids standardized to be equivalent to not less than 45% of cholic acid. Used in deficiencies of bile secretion.

ox gall (gawl). Ox bile.

ox′i·dant [G. *oxys,* sharp; L. *acidus,* sour]. An oxidizing agent.

ox′i·dase (ock′si·dace, ·daze). Any enzyme which promotes an oxidation reaction. See Table of Enzymes in the Appendix.

amino acid o. An enzyme capable of causing the oxidation of amino acids; **D-amino acid oxidase** occurs in most animal tissues and is specific for the oxidation of D-amino acids to keto acids; **L-amino acid oxidase** occurs in animal tissues in much lower concentrations than the D-enzyme and is specific for the oxidative deamination of the naturally occurring L-amino acids.

choline o. An enzyme causing the oxidation of choline.

indophenol o. A heme-containing enzyme in living cells which, in the presence of oxygen and cytochrome C, oxidizes *p*-aminodimethylaniline so that it will form indophenol blue with α-naphthol. The enzyme is probably identical with Warburg's respiratory enzyme and with cytochrome oxidase.

monophenol o. A copper-containing protein enzyme which catalyzes the oxidation of monophenols, including tyrosine. It is probably identical with tyrosinase and perhaps also with polyphenol oxidase.

phenol o. A group of enzymes that catalyze the oxidation of phenolic compounds. They contain copper and utilize molecular oxygen directly.

polyphenol o. A copper-containing protein enzyme which catalyzes the oxidation of polyphenols. It is probably identical with tyrosinase and perhaps also with monophenol oxidase.

xanthine o. A flavoprotein enzyme catalyzing the oxidation of certain purines.

ox″i·da′tion [*oxys*; *acidus*]. 1. An increase in positive valence of an element (or a decrease in negative valence) occurring as a result of the loss of electrons. Each electron so lost is taken on by some other element, thus accomplishing a reduction of that element. 2. Originally, the process of combining with oxygen.

anodic o. An electrochemical process by which certain articles are given a thin coating of oxide, usually for the purpose of retarding corrosion, by immersing them as the anodes in an oxidizing electrolyte bath.

beta o. Oxidation of the carbon atom which is in the beta position with reference to a functional group in the molecule. The theory of beta oxidation as a mechanism of fatty acid catabolism has been extensively investigated and was at one time widely accepted. It involves an oxidation of the beta carbon atom followed by the loss of two carbon atoms.

multiple alternate o. A theory of fatty acid oxidation proposed by Jowett and Quastel, according to which a simultaneous oxidation to the ketone stage occurs on every alternate C atom of a fatty acid, followed by scission at each fourth carbon to give acetoacetic acid. The theory is no longer tenable.

omega o. The oxidation of a fatty acid at the end of the chain opposite to that where the carboxyl group occurs, thereby forming a dicarboxylic acid, which may then undergo beta oxidation from both ends of the chain.

ox′ide [*oxys*; *acidus*]. A binary compound of oxygen and another element or radical.

acid o. An oxide of a nonmetal which produces an acid when combined with water; an anhydride.

basic o. An oxide of a metal which produces a base when combined with water.

ox′i·dize [*oxys*; *acidus*]. To produce an oxidation or increase in positive valence (or decrease in negative valence) through the loss of electrons. The oxidizing agent is itself reduced in the reaction; that is, it takes on the electrons which have been liberated by the element being oxidized.

ox″i·do-re·duc′tase. An enzyme catalyzing a reaction in which two molecules of a compound interact so that one molecule is oxidized and the other reduced, with a molecule of water entering the reaction.

ox′ime. Any compound resulting from the action of hydroxylamine upon an aldehyde or ketone; the former yields an oxime having the general formula RCH:NOH, called *aldoxime;* the latter yields an oxime of the general formula R(R′)C:NOH, called *ketoxime.*

ox·im′e·ter [*oxys*; G. *metron*, a measure]. An instrument measuring the per cent of blood hemoglobin saturated with oxygen. In common medical practice it is attached to the earlobe; in experimental techniques it may be employed elsewhere. The amount of light traversing the earlobe is measured by a galvanometer activated by the photoelectric cell. The oxygen saturation is then determined according to previous calibrations. **—oxim′etry,** *n.*

oxine. Trade name for *hydroxyquinoline.*

oxo-ate "B". Trade-mark for calcium orthoiodoxybenzoate, $(C_6H_4(IO_2)COO)_2Ca.8H_2O$, used as an antiarthritic.

ox″o·eth″a·no′ic ac′id. Glyoxylic acid.

ox″o·i·som′er·ase. An enzyme which catalyzes the interconversion of glucose-6-phosphate and fructofuranose-6-monophosphate.

oxone. Trade name of a preparation of fused sodium peroxide, used for the manufacture of oxygen.

ox″o·phen·ar′sine hy″dro·chlo′ride (ock″so·fen-ahr′seen, ·sin) (*oxophenarsinae hydrochloridum*). 3-Amino-4-hydroxyphenylarsinoxide hydrochloride, $(NH_2)(OH)C_6H_3AsO.HCl$, employed as an antisyphilitic. Mapharsen is a trade-mark for the hemialcoholate of this product.

ox′y- [*oxys*]. 1. A combining form meaning *sharp, acid, acute, shrill, quick.* 2. *In botany*, a combining form signifying *pointed* or *smooth.* 3. *In medicine*, a combining form denoting *acuteness of perception, swift, sharp in pitch*, or *acute.*

ox′y- [*oxys*]. 1. A prefix meaning *oxygen;* used to denote *one oxygen atom united to two different atoms.* 2. A prefix denoting *the presence of the hydroxyl group.*

ox″y·a·can′thine (ock″see·a·can′theen, ·thin). $C_{37}H_{40}N_2O_6$. An alkaloid of berberis, occurring in small quantities.

ox″y·ac′e·tone (ock″see·ass′i·tone). Acetol; acetyl carbinol. A reducing agent used in organic syntheses.

ox′y·ac″id [*oxys;* L. *acidus*, sour]. Any acid containing oxygen.

ox″y·a·co′a. See *oxyakoia.*

ox″y·aes·the′si·a. See *oxyesthesia.*

ox″y·a·koi′a, ox″y·a·co′a [*oxys;* G. *akoē*, hearing]. Increased acuteness of hearing, or sensitiveness to noises. *Rare.*

ox″y·a′phi·a (ock″see·ay′fee·uh, ·af′ee·uh) [*oxys;* G. *haphē*, touch]. Abnormal acuteness of the sense of touch.

ox″y·a″si·at′i·co·side″. A derivative of the antibiotic substance asiaticoside which is active against experimental infections with *Mycobacterium tuberculosis.*

ox″y·bi′o·tin. An analog of biotin in which oxygen replaces the sulfur atom of biotin.

ox″y·blep′si·a [*oxys;* G. *blepsis*, sight]. Acuteness of vision.

ox″y·cam′phor. $C_{10}H_{16}O_2$. An oxidation product of camphor; it has been used in cardiac and pulmonic dyspnea.

oxycel. Trade-mark for an absorbable oxidized cellulose material used in surgical hemostasis.

ox″y·ceph′a·ly [*oxys;* G. *kephalē*, head]. A condition in which the head is roughly conical in shape.

Caused by premature closure of the coronal or lambdoid sutures, or both, which induces compensatory development in the region of the bregma. It is also caused by artificial pressure on the frontal and occipital regions of the heads of infants to alter the shape. Commonly known as *sugar-loaf head, steeple head, tower head,* or *tower skull.* Syn., *acrocephaly.*

ox″y·chlo′ride. Any compound containing both —OH and —Cl attached to the same element; a compound containing the —OCl radical.

ox″y·chro′ma·tin [*oxys;* G. *chrōma,* color]. That part of the chromatin having an affinity for acid dyes.

ox″y·ci·ne′sis [*oxys;* G. *kinēsis,* motion]. Excessive movements, particularly of the limbs, observed in the manic phase of manic-depressive psychosis. *Obs.*

ox″y·cor″ti·co·ster′oid. An oxysteroid originating in the adrenal cortex.

ox′y·dase. See *oxidase.*

ox″y·den′dron [*oxys;* G. *dendron,* tree]. The leaves of the sorrel tree, *Oxydendrum arboreum;* has been used as a diuretic in dropsy.

ox″y·es·the′si·a (ock″see·ess·thee′zhuh, ·zee·uh) [*oxys;* G. *aisthēsis,* perception]. A condition of increased acuity of sensation.

ox′y·gen [*oxys;* G. *genesthai,* from *gignesthai,* to be produced] (*oxygenium*). O = 16. A colorless, tasteless, odorless gas, constituting one-fifth of the atmosphere, eight-ninths of water, and about one-half the crust of the globe; it supports combustion, and is essential to life of animals. It combines with most elements, and is carried by the blood from the lungs to the tissues.

o. acid. An acid which contains oxygen.

o. capacity. The maximum amount of oxygen absorbed by a given amount of blood when it is equilibrated with an excess of oxygen expressed in volume per cent (cc. per 100 cc.). See Table of Normal Values of Blood Constituents in the Appendix.

o. content. Oxygen in volume per cent present in blood at a given moment. See Table of Normal Values of Blood Constituents in the Appendix.

o. debt. The amount of O_2 needed to metabolize the lactic acid and other accumulated products of anaerobic metabolism of muscle during severe exercise; the volume of O_2 required after the completion of exercise in excess of O_2 consumption in the resting state for an equivalent length of time. Syn., *oxygen deficit, recovery oxygen.*

o. deficit. Oxygen debt.

o. saturation. Oxygen content divided by oxygen capacity expressed in volume per cent.

o. tent. An airtight chamber enclosing the patient's head and shoulders in which the oxygen content of the atmosphere can be maintained at a higher than normal level.

recovery o. Oxygen debt.

ox′y·gen·ase″. An enzyme that makes it possible for atmospheric oxygen to be utilized by the organism or in the system in which it occurs.

ox″y·ge·na′tion. The saturation of a substance with oxygen, either by chemical combination or by mixture. —**ox′ygenated,** *adj.*

ox″y·geu′si·a (ock″si·gew′see·uh, ·jew′see·uh) [*oxys;* G. *geusis,* taste]. Marked acuteness of the sense of taste.

ox″y·hem′a·tin (ock″si·hem′uh·tin, ·hee′muh·tin). $C_{34}H_{32}N_4O_7Fe$. The coloring matter of oxyhemoglobin; on oxidation, it yields hematinic acid; on reduction, hematoporphyrin.

ox″y·hem″a·to·por′phy·rin. A pigment sometimes found in urine; it is related to hematoporphyrin.

ox″y·he″mo·glo′bin (ock″si·hee″mo·glo′bin, ·hem″o·glo′bin) [*oxys;* G. *haima,* blood; L. *globus,* ball]. Oxidized hemoglobin. See *hemoglobin.*

ox″y·ja·van′i·cin. An antibiotic substance produced, along with javanicin, by *Fusarium javanicum.*

ox″y·la′li·a (ock″si·lay′lee·uh, ·lal′ee·uh) [*oxys;* G. *lalia,* talk]. Rapid speech.

oxyl-iodide. Trade-mark for cinchophen hydriodide, $C_{16}H_{11}O_2N.HI$, an analgesic and antirheumatic.

ox′y·mel [*oxys;* G. *meli,* honey]. 1. A mixture of honey, water, and vinegar or dilute acetic acid. 2. Any preparation containing honey and vinegar (or acetic acid) as a vehicle.

ox″y·nar′co·tine (ock″si·nahr′ko·teen, ·tin). An alkaloid, $C_{22}H_{23}NO_8$, related to narcotine and separable from crude narceine.

ox″y·ner′vone, ox″y·ner′von. A galactolipin, isolated from nerve tissue, reported to contain oxynervonic acid.

ox″y·ner·von′ic ac′id. $C_{23}H_{44}.OH.COOH$. An unsaturated acid, the hydroxy derivative of nervonic acid, reported to exist in oxynervone.

ox″y·neu′rine (ock″si·new′reen, ·rin). See *betaine.*

ox·yn′tic [G. *oxynein,* to make acid]. Secreting acid, formerly applied to the parietal cells of the stomach.

ox″y·o′pi·a [G. *oxys,* sharp; *ōps,* eye]. Increased acuity of vision.

ox″y·op′ter [*oxys;* G. *optēr,* spy]. The unit of acuity of vision; it is the reciprocal of the visual angle expressed in degrees.

ox″y·o′sis. Acidosis. *Obs.*

ox″y·os·phre′si·a (ock″see·os·free′zhuh, ·zee·uh, ·shuh, ·see·uh) [*oxys;* G. *osphrēsis,* sense of smell]. Marked or abnormal acuteness of sense of smell.

ox·yp′a·thy [*oxys;* G. *pathos,* disease]. A constitutional condition due to faulty elimination of unoxidized acids, which unite with fixed alkalies of the body. *Obs.*

α-ox″y·phen′a·zine. See *pyo compounds.*

ox″y·phe·non′i·um bro′mide. Generic name for diethyl(2-hydroxyethyl)methyl-ammonium bromide α-phenylcyclohexaneglycolate, available under the trade-marked name antrenyl bromide; the substance is an anticholinergic agent used in treating peptic ulcer and gastrointestinal spasm.

ox′y·phil, ox′y·phile [*oxys;* G. *philein,* to love]. 1. Attracting acid dyes. 2. Pertaining to histologic elements that attract acid dyes. Syn., *acidophil, eosinophil.*

ox″y·phil′i·a. See *eosinophilia.*

ox″y·pho′ni·a [*oxys;* G. *phōnē,* voice]. Shrillness of voice.

ox″y·pol″y·gel′a·tin [*oxys;* G. *polys,* many; L. *gelare,* to freeze]. An oxidized, polymerized gelatin used experimentally as a blood plasma substitute.

ox″y·pro′line. Hydroxyproline.

ox″y·quin′o·line (ock″si·kwin′o·leen, ·lin). Hydroxyquinoline.

ox′y·rhine (ock′si·ryne, ·rin) [*oxys;* G. *rhis,* nose]. 1. Possessing a sharp-pointed nose or snout. 2. Having an acute olfactory sense.

ox″y·ster′oid. A steroid having an oxygen atom, thereby forming an alcohol or a ketone group, at some specified position: e.g., an 11-oxysteroid has the oxygen atom present at the number 11 carbon atom of the steroid nucleus.

ox″y·tet″ra·cy′cline. Generic name for an antibiotic substance produced by the growth of the soil fungus *Streptomyces rimosus,* or by any other means; $C_{22}H_{24}N_2O_9$, marketed as the hydrochloride under the trade-marked name *terramycin hydrochloride;* a white, crystalline powder, soluble in water. It represents tetracycline in which a hydrogen atom is replaced by a hydroxyl group, and is active against a number of Gram-positive and Gram-negative bacteria, rickettsias, and several viruses. See also *chlortetracycline.*

ox″y·thi′a·mine. A compound differing from thiamine in having an OH group in place of the NH_2 group of thiamine; a powerful antagonist of thiamine.

ox″y·to′ci·a (ock″si·to′shee·uh, ·see·uh) [*oxys;* G. *tokos,* childbirth]. Rapid childbirth.

ox″y·to′cic [*oxys; tokos*]. A drug that hastens parturition. —**oxyto′cic,** *adj.*

ox″y·to′cin. The hormone extracted from the neurohypophysis which increases contraction of the uterine muscles in late pregnancy or during parturition; it has been isolated in pure form and synthesized. Syn., *alpha-hypophamine.* See *pitocin.*

ox″y·u·ri′a·sis. See *enterobiasis.*

ox″y·u′rid [*oxys;* G. *oura,* tail]. The human pinworm or seatworm. See *Enterobius vermicularis.*

Ox″y·u′ris ver·mic″u·la′ris. Synonym for *Enterobius vermicularis.*

-o′yl. Suffix indicating a radical formed from an organic acid when OH is removed from the latter, as the radical RCO— from RCOOH.

oz. Ounce (avoirdupois).

o·ze′na [G. *ozē,* bad smell]. A chronic disease of the nose accompanied by a fetid discharge. It is due to atrophic rhinitis, syphilitic ulceration, or caries. Also called *rhinitis sicca.*

o·zo′ce·rite, o·zo′ke·rite. Ceresin.

o″zo·chro′ti·a (o″zo·kro′shuh, ·see·uh) [G. *ozein,* to smell; *chrōs,* skin]. An offensive odor of the skin. —**ozoch′rotous,** *adj.*

o·zo′ke·rite. Ceresin.

o′zone [*ozein*]. O_3. An allotropic form of oxygen, the molecule of which consists of three atoms; a common constituent of the atmosphere. It is a powerful oxidizing agent and is used as a disinfectant for swimming pools, etc.

o′zo·nide. A compound of ozone with certain unsaturated organic substances. Such derivatives of fixed oils have been applied locally to infected areas for the bactericidal effect of the nascent oxygen released by the oils.

o″zos·to′mi·a [*ozein;* G. *stoma,* mouth]. A foul odor of the breath of oral origin.

P

P Chemical symbol for phosphorus; premolar.

P. Pharmacopeia; position; *pugillus,* handful; *punctum proximum,* near point.

p- *In chemistry,* para-.

Pa Chemical symbol for protactinium.

PABA Para-aminobenzoic acid.

pab′u·lum [L.]. Food; any nutrient.

Pacchioni, Antonio [*Italian anatomist,* 1665–1726]. Well-known pupil of Malpighi. Described arachnoidal granulations, called *Pacchionian bodies.* Noted for studies of the cerebrum and dura.

pace′mak″er [L. *passus,* step; ME. *maken*]. That portion of the right atrium of the heart, normally the sinoatrial node, where the stimulus for the heart beat originates.

ectopic p. A source of impulse initiation outside of the sinoatrial node.

idioventricular p. A focus of impulse initiation in the ventricle.

wandering p. A phenomenon in which the pacemaker shifts away from the sinoatrial node but remains within the atrium or atrioventricular node; recognized only by the electrocardiogram.

pach′y- (pack′ee-) [G. *pachys,* thick]. A combining form meaning *thick.*

pach″y·ac′ri·a [*pachys;* G. *akra,* extremity]. A condition marked by clubbing of the fingers and toes, and thickening of the skin of the extremities. Formerly called *acropachyderma, pseudoacromegaly.* See hypertrophic pulmonary *osteoarthropathy.*

pach″y·bleph′a·ron [*pachys;* G. *blepharon,* eyelid]. Thickening of the eyelids.

pach″y·bleph″a·ro′sis [*pachys; blepharon;* G. *-ōsis,* condition]. Chronic thickening and induration of the eyelids.

pach″y·ceph′a·ly, pach″y·ce·pha′li·a [*pachys;* G. *kephalē,* head]. Unusual thickness of the walls of the skull. —**pachycephal′ic, pachyceph′alous,** *adj.*

pach″y·chi′li·a, pach″y·chei′li·a (pack″i·kigh′lee·uh, ·kil′ee·uh) [*pachys;* G. *cheilos,* lip]. Increased thickness of one or both lips.

pach″y·chro·mat′ic [*pachys;* G. *chrōma,* color]. Having a coarse chromatin network.

pach″y·dac·tyl′i·a, pach″y·dac′ty·ly [*pachys;* G. *daktylos,* finger]. A condition characterized by great thickness of the fingers.

pach″y·der′ma·tous [*pachys;* G. *derma,* skin]. Abnormally thick-skinned.

pach″y·der′mi·a, pach″y·der′ma [*pachys; derma*]. 1. Abnormal thickening of the skin. 2. Elephantiasis. —**pachydermial,** *adj.*

occipital p. A rare disease of the scalp characterized by thickened skin thrown into folds; limited to the occipital region of the scalp.

p. laryngis. Extensive thickening of the mucous membrane of the larynx.

p. lymphangiectatica. A diffuse form of lymphangioma. Consists of lymph-filled sacs and at times produces extreme deformities.

pach″y·glos′si·a [*pachys;* G. *glōssa,* tongue]. Abnormal thickness of the tongue.

pach″y·gy′ri·a [*pachys;* G. *gyros,* circle]. Flattening and broadening of the gyri of the cerebrum.

pach″y·hem′a·tous [*pachys;* G. *haima,* blood]. Referring to thickening of the blood.

pach″y·hy·men′ic (pack″i·high·men′ick). See *pachydermatous.*

pach″y·lep″to·men″in·gi′tis [*pachys;* G. *leptos,* thin; *mēnigx,* membrane; *-itis,* inflammation]. Combined inflammation of the pia and dura.

pach″y·lo′sis [G. *pachylos,* thickish; *-ōsis,* condition]. A thick, dry, harsh, and scaly skin, especially of the legs.

pach″y·men″in·gi′tis (pack″i·men″in·jy′tis) [G. *pachys,* thick; *mēnigx,* membrane; *-itis,* inflammation]. Inflammation of the dura. —**pachymeningit′ic,** *adj.*

epidural p. Inflammation of the epidural space and the external aspect of the dura, usually resulting from tuberculosis of the spine.

hemorrhagic p. See chronic subdural *hematoma.*

hypertrophic cervical p. Most common form of hypertrophic spinal pachymeningitis.

hypertrophic spinal p. A localized or diffuse hypertrophy of the dura mater, resulting from syphilis or unknown causes, giving rise to symptoms of irritation of spinal roots and compression of the spinal cord. It attacks any level of the spinal cord or brain but most often the lower cervical region.

p. cervicalis hypertrophica. See hypertrophic cervical *p.*

p. externa. See epidural *abscess.*

p. interna hemorrhagica. See chronic subdural *hematoma.*

pyogenic p. Infection of the dura with pyogenic organisms, usually secondary to cranial osteitis.

spinal p. Inflammation of the spinal dura.

syphilitic p. Inflammation of the dura due to syphilis.

pach″y·men″in·gop′a·thy [*pachys; mēnigx;* G. *pathos*, disease]. Disease of the dura mater, or pachymeninx.

pach″y·me′ninx [*pachys; mēnigx*]. The dura mater.

pa·chyn′sis (pa·kin′sis) [G., a thickening]. A thickening, as of a membrane. —**pachyntic,** *adj.*

pach″y·o·nych′i·a (pack″ee·o·nick′ee·uh) [G. *pachys*, thick; *onyx*, nail]. Thickening of the nails.

p. congenita. A rare congenital anomaly characterized by dystrophic changes of the nails, palmar and plantar hyperkeratosis, anomalies of the hair, follicular keratosis of the knees and elbows, and dyskeratosis of the cornea. Probably a type of ectodermal defect.

pach″y·o′ti·a (pack″ee·o′shuh, ·shee·uh) [*pachys;* G. *ous*, ear]. Abnormal thickness of the ears.

pach″y·pel″vi·per″i·to·ni′tis [*pachys;* L. *pelvis*, basin; G. *peritonaion*, membrane which contains the lower viscera; *-itis*, inflammation]. Pelvic peritonitis with a fibrous deposit over the uterus.

pach″y·per″i·os·to′sis [*pachys;* G. *periosteos*, around the bones; *-ōsis*, condition]. Pathologic alteration of the long bones in which the periosteum is greatly thickened.

pach″y·per″i·to·ni′tis [*pachys;* G. *peritonaion*, membrane which contains the lower viscera; *-itis*, inflammation]. Thickening of the peritoneum by inflammation.

pa·chyp′o·dous (pa·kip′o·dus) [*pachys;* G. *pous*, foot]. Having thick feet.

pach″y·rhi′nic, pach′y·rhine (pack″i·rye′nick) [*pachys;* G. *rhis*, nose]. Having a thick or unusually broad and flat nose.

pach″y·sal·pin′go-o″o·the·ci′tis. See *pachysalpingo-ovaritis.*

pach″y·sal·pin′go-o″va·ri′tis. Inflammation of the ovary and oviduct with thickening of the parts.

pach′y·tene [G. *pachytēs*, thickness]. Applied to a stage in miosis or mitosis, following synapsis, in which the homologous chromosome threads shorten and thicken and coil about each other.

pach′y·tes (pack′i·teez). Pachyblepharon.

pa·chyt′ic (pa·kit′ick) [G. *pachys*, thick]. Thick.

pach″y·vag″i·ni′tis (pack″i·vadj″i·nigh′tis) [*pachys;* L. *vagina*, sheath; G. *-itis*, inflammation]. Vaginitis accompanied by thickening of the vaginal walls.

pac′i·fi″er [L. *pacificare*, to pacify]. Any article, such as a rubber nipple, placed in the mouths of irritable or teething children to quiet or pacify them.

Pacini, Filippo [*Italian anatomist*, 1812–83]. Described the lamellar corpuscle (1835); called *Pacini's corpuscle, Pacinian corpuscle, corpuscle of Vater-Pacini.* See Pacinian *corpuscle.*

pack [M.E. *pakke*]. A dressing or blanket, either dry or soaked, hot or cold, that is laid upon or wrapped about the body or part.

cold p. A blanket wrung out of cold water and wrapped about the body.

hot p. A blanket wrung out of hot water and wrapped about the body.

mud p. A dressing soaked in hot muds or moors.

periodontal p. A dressing placed between and about the teeth in treatment of periodontal disease.

surgical p. A pack used in an operative wound to secure hemostasis.

wet p. A blanket wrung out of warm or cold water.

Packard, Francis Randolph (1870–1950). American otolaryngologist and medical historian; author of *History of Medicine in the United States*, the standard textbook of American medical history.

pack′er [ME. *pakke*]. A tapered surgical instrument equipped with a point ending in a shoulder, for inserting gauze or other dressings into a cavity; used generally in conjunction with an aural, vaginal, or other speculum.

pack′ing frac′tion. The difference between the actual mass of an isotope and the nearest whole number divided by this whole number, usually expressed as parts in 10,000; it is related to the loss of energy and therefore loss of mass involved in the formation of atomic nuclei from protons and neutrons.

Pacquelin. See *Paquelin.*

pad [of uncertain origin]. 1. A small cushion stuffed with cotton, hair, etc., for supporting any part of the body. 2. Compress.

dinner p. A removable pad of felt, cotton, or other material placed over the abdomen prior to the application of a plaster jacket, to allow for normal distention after eating.

fat p. *In anatomy*, any mass of fatty tissue.

foot p. Cushionlike mass of connective tissue covered by a heavily keratinized hairless epidermis, found on the flexor surface of the carpus and digits of certain animals.

hard p. A disease of dogs, paradistemper, characterized by an encephalitis and paralysis as well as a hardening of the foot pads.

incisive p. See incisive *papilla.*

p. of corpus callosum. The splenium of the callosum.

sucking p. A fatty mass situated between the masseter and the buccinator muscles, well developed in infancy; the buccal fat pad: also called *corpus adiposum buccae.*

Padgett, Earl Calvin [*American surgeon*, 1893–1946]. Made many contributions to plastic surgery. Devised an operation for reconstruction of the lip using transplanted tubular grafts from the scalp and neck; called *Padgett's operation.* Especially known for his invention of an instrument for cutting even thickness of skin of any given calibration, for grafting, called *Padgett's dermatome.*

pae-. For words beginning with *pae-*, see words beginning *pe-*.

Pagenstecher, Alexander [*German ophthalmologist*, 1828–79]. Introduced an ophthalmic ointment of yellow oxide of mercury and petrolatum, called *Pagenstecher's ointment.* Inventor of a special type of suture made of flax or linen thread coated with celluloid; called *Pagenstecher's suture.* Assisted by his brother, Hermann, devised several operations. An operation for cataract in which the lens is removed in a closed capsule using pressure on the cornea is called *Pagenstecher's operation.*

Paget, James (1814–1899). English surgeon who described osteitis deformans and a mammary carcinoma. See Paget's *disease.*

pagitane hydrochloride. Trade-marked name for 1-phenyl-1-cyclopentyl-3-piperidino-1-propanol hydrochloride, a drug used in the symptomatic treatment of Parkinson's disease. See *cycrimine hydrochloride.*

pa″go·plex′i·a [G. *pagos*, frost; *plēxis*, stroke]. Numbness from cold; frostbite.

-pa·gus [G. *pagos*, that which is fixed]. A suffix used by I. Geoffroy Saint-Hilaire to express superior and inferior duplicity in conjoined twins.

PAH, PAHA Para-aminohippuric acid.

pai·dol′o·gy (pay·dol′o·jee, pye·dol′·). Pedology.

pain [L. *poena*, penalty]. 1. A disturbed sensation causing suffering or distress. 2. A rhythmic contraction of the uterus during labor; labor pain. —**pain′ful, pain′less,** *adj.*

bearing-down p. A feeling of distress with a sensation of dragging of the pelvic organs; occurs in labor and in pelvic inflammatory disease.

boring p. A severe feeling of distress simulating the action of a drill or other piercing instrument.

dilating p. That accompanying the stretching of the cervix in the first stage of labor.

excentric p. Radiating pain symptomatic of spinal disease, due to irritation of the posterior nerve roots; it is felt to be in peripheral areas, thus accounting for the name.

expulsive p. A bearing-down sensation accompanying the last two stages of labor.

false p. Mild, recurring lower abdominal cramps, occurring late in pregnancy, but not followed by labor.

fulgurant p. The intense darting pain affecting principally the limbs of patients suffering from locomotor ataxia. Also called *lancinating p.*, *lightning p.*, *shooting p.*

girdle p. A painful sensation as of a cord tied about the waist; it is a symptom of organic disease of the spinal cord.

growing pains. Soreness of variable degree, duration, and kind in muscles and occasionally in joints in children and adolescents, sometimes during systemic infections, and often as a minor manifestation of rheumatic fever.

heterotopic p. See referred *p.*

homotropic p. Soreness felt at the site of trauma.

intermenstrual p. Lower abdominal pain occurring between menstrual periods, apparently associated with ovulation. Also called *Mittelschmerz.*

labor p. The pains of childbirth associated with the first stage of labor.

lancinating p. See fulgurant *p.*

osteocopic p. The boneache that characterizes syphilis.

p. joy. Hysterical enjoyment of suffering.

phantom limb p. Pain which seems to the individual to be located in an amputated limb.

referred p. Pain whose origin is not in the area in which it is felt; for example, pain felt under the right scapula due to gallbladder disease.

starting p. Pain caused by a spasmodic contraction of the muscles just before the onset of sleep. It occurs in inflammatory joint diseases.

terebrating p. See boring *p.*

paint′er's col′ic. Lead colic. See under *colic*, 2.

pair pro·duc′tion. The formation of a positron and a negatron when an x-ray loses its energy in passing close to the nucleus of an atom, occurring only when x-rays have energy of 1 million electronvolts or above.

Pajot, Charles [*French obstetrician*, 1816–96]. Described a hook which he introduced for decapitation of the fetal head in difficult labor; called *Pajot's hook. Pajot's maneuver* or *method* in labor was a strong, downward pull with one hand over the lock of the obstetric forceps, while the other was used for horizontal traction. Said to have been used by other obstetricians many years earlier. Also called *Saxtorph's maneuver.*

pal′a·dang″. A pintalike condition seen in Guam.

pa′lae·o-. See *paleo-.*

pal′a·ta. Plural of palatum.

pal′ate [L. *palatum*, palate]. The roof of the mouth. It is composed of the **hard palate,** formed by the palatal process of the maxillary bones and the palatine bones with their covering mucous membranes, and the **soft palate,** or velum palati, consisting of an aggregation of muscles, the tensor palati, levator veli palatini, azygos uvulae, palatoglossus, and palatopharyngeus, and their covering mucous membrane. See Plates 12, 20. —**palatine** (pal′uh·tyne, ·tin), **palatal,** *adj.*

artificial p. A plate of hard material used as an obturator to close a fissure in the palate.

cleft p. A congenital deformity characterized by incomplete closure of the lateral halves of the palate. The soft palate and the uvula, the hard palate, or all together, may be involved. It may or may not be associated with cleft lip or cleft alveolar process.

gothic p. An enormously high palatal arch.

premaxillary p. See primary *p.*

primary p. The embryonic palate corresponding approximately to the premaxillary region.

primitive p. *In embryology*, that part of the median nasal process that forms the median part of the upper lip and the primary palate.

secondary p. The embryonic palate formed by the union of the palatine processes of the maxillary processes; the definitive palate.

pal′ate-hook″. A surgical instrument for retracting the uvula.

pal′ate-my′o·graph. An instrument for taking a tracing of the movements of the soft palate.

pa·lat′ic [*palatum*]. Palatal, palatine. *Rare.*

pa·lat′i·form [*palatum*; L. *forma*, form]. Resembling the palate.

pal′a·tine [*palatum*]. The palatine bone. See Table of Bones in the Appendix.

pal″a·ti′tis [*palatum*; G. *-itis*, inflammation]. Inflammation of the palate.

pal′a·to- [*palatum*]. A combining form denoting *the palate.*

pal″a·to·glos′sal [*palatum*; G. *glōssa*, tongue]. Pertaining to the palate and the tongue, as the palatoglossal muscle.

pal″a·to·glos′sus [*palatum*; *glōssa*]. The muscle within the anterior pillar of the fauces; it connects the soft palate with the tongue; the glossopalatinus. See Table of Muscles in the Appendix.

pal′a·to·graph″ [*palatum*; G. *graphein*, to write]. An instrument for the recording of palatal movements.

pal″a·to·max′il·lar″y (·mack′si·lerr″ee) [*palatum*; L. *maxilla*, jaw]. Pertaining to the palate and the maxilla.

pal″a·to·my′o·graph. See *palate-myograph.*

pal″a·to·na′sal (pal″uh·to·nay′zul) [*palatum*; L. *nasus*, nose]. Pertaining to the palate and the nose.

pal″a·top′a·gus par″a·sit′i·cus. See *epipalatum.*

pal″a·to·pha·ryn′ge·al (·fa·rin′jul, ·jee·ul, ·far″·in·jee′ul) [*palatum*; G. *pharygx*, pharynx]. Pertaining conjointly to the palate and the pharynx, as the pharyngopalatine muscle or arch.

pal″a·to·pha·ryn′ge·us (pal″uh·to·fa·rin′jee·us, ·far″in·jee′us) [*palatum*; *pharygx*]. The muscle in the posterior pillar of the fauces, connecting the soft palate with the lateral wall of the pharynx below, the pharyngopalatinus. See Table of Muscles in the Appendix.

pal′a·to·plas″ty [*palatum*; G. *plassein*, to form]. Plastic surgery of the palate.

pal″a·to·ple′gi·a [*palatum*; G. *plēgē*, stroke]. Paralysis of the soft palate.

pal″a·to·pter′y·goid (pal″uh·to·terr′i·goyd) [*palatum;* G. *pterygoeidēs*, like a wing]. Relating to the palate bone and pterygoid processes of the sphenoid bone; pterygopalatine.

pal″a·tor′rha·phy [*palatum;* G. *rhaphē*, suture]. Suture of a cleft palate.

pal″a·to·sal·pin′ge·us [*palatum;* G. *salpigx*, trumpet]. A portion of the levator veli palatini.

pal″a·tos′chi·sis (pal″uh·tos′ki·sis) [*palatum;* G. *schisis*, cleavage]. Cleft palate.

pal′a·tum (pl. *palata*) [L.]. The palate.

p. durum. Hard palate.

p. fissum. Cleft palate.

p. mobile. The soft palate. Also called *p. molle.*

pa″le·en·ceph′a·lon. The brain with the exception of the neencephalon; the phylogenetically old part of the brain: also spelled *paleoencephalon.*

pa′le·o-, pa′lae·o- [G. *palaios*, old, ancient]. A combining form meaning *old, ancient;* used to denote *early, primitive, long ago.*

pa″le·o·cer″e·bel′lum [*palaios;* L. *cerebellum*, small brain]. Phylogenetically old parts of the cerebellum: the anterior lobe, composed of lingula, central lobule, and culmen, and the posterior part of the posterior lobe, composed of pyramis, uvula, and paraflocculus; may include the flocculonodular lobe.

pa″le·o·en·ceph′a·lon. See *paleencephalon.*

pa″le·o·gen′e·sis. See *palingenesis.*

pa″le·o·ki·net′ic (pay″lee·o·ki·net′ick, ·kigh·net′·ick) [*palaios;* G. *kinētikos*, of motion]. Referring to motor nervous mechanisms of submammals, represented in mammals by the extrapyramidal systems, which are the pathways concerned with postural and automatic associated movements.

pa″le·on·tol′o·gy [*palaios;* G. *ōn*, pres. part. of *einai*, to be; *logos*, word]. The science and study of fossil remains.

pa″le·o-ol′ive. The accessory nuclei and the most medial portion of the main nucleus which form, phylogenetically, the oldest part of the olive.

pa″le·o·pal′li·um [*palaios;* L. *pallium*, mantle]. The lateral olfactory lobe, or pyriform lobe of lower forms; in the higher mammals, especially in man, it forms the uncus and adjacent anterior part of the hippocampal gyrus.

pa″le·o·pa·thol′o·gy [*palaios;* G. *pathos*, disease; *logos*, word]. A branch of pathology dealing with diseases of ancient times demonstrated in human and animal remains.

pa″le·o·stri·a′tum (pay″lee·o·strye·ay′tum) [*palaios;* L. *striare*, to furnish with channels]. The globus pallidus; the phylogenetically old part of the corpus striatum.

pa″le·o·thal′a·mus [*palaios;* G. *thalamos*, chamber]. The nuclei of the midline of the thalamus, which are nucleus parataenialis, nucleus paraventricularis anterior, nucleus paraventricularis posterior, nucleus centralis medialis, and nucleus grisea centralis; definite function unknown.

pal″i·ki·ne′si·a (pal″i·ki·nee′shuh, ·see·uh, ·zhuh, ·zee·uh, pal″i·kigh·), **pal″i·ki·ne′sis** (pal″i·ki·nee′sis, ·kigh·nee′sis) [G. *palin*, backward, again; *kinēsis*, motion]. Constant and involuntary repetition of movements. Also spelled *palicinesia.*

pal″i·la′li·a [*palin;* G. *lalia*, talk]. Pathologic repetition of words or phrases.

pal″in·dro′mi·a [*palin;* G. *dromos*, course]. Recurrence or growing worse of a disease; a relapse. —**palindrom′ic,** *adj.*

pal″in·gen′e·sis [*palin;* G. *genesis*, production]. The development of characteristics during ontogeny which are regarded as inherited from ancestral species; opposed to *cenogenesis.* See recapitulation *theory.*

pal″i·op′si·a [*palin;* G. *opsis*, vision]. Visual perseveration in time; recurrence of a visual impression after the stimulus has ceased.

pal″i·phra′si·a (pal″i·fray′zhuh, ·zee·uh) [*palin;* G. *phrasis*, speech]. Pathologic repetition of words or phrases.

pal″ir·rhe′a, pal″ir·rhoe′a [*palin;* G. *rhoia*, flow]. 1. The recurrence of a mucous discharge. 2. Regurgitation.

pal·la′di·um [G. *Pallas*, epithet of Athena] (*palladium*). Pd = 106.7. Silver-white, fairly ductile, hard metal, somewhat softer than platinum, belonging to the platinum group of metals; also available as a black powder and as spongy masses; soluble in nitric acid, hot sulfuric acid, and aqua regia. It has many uses in gold, silver, and copper alloys and as a catalyst in many manufacturing processes.

p. chloride. $PdCl_2.2H_2O$; red or brown-red crystals; soluble in water and alcohol. Has been suggested as a local antiseptic and internally in tuberculosis.

pal″lan·es·the′si·a (pal″an·ess·thee′zhuh, ·zee·uh) [G. *pallein*, to shake; *anaisthēsia*, lack of sensation]. Absence of pallesthesia.

pal″les·the′si·a (pal″ess·thee′zhuh, ·zee·uh) [*pallein;* G. *aisthēsis*, perception]. Sensation similar to that felt when a vibrating tuning fork is touched; the sense of vibration.

pal″li·a′tion [L. *palliatus*, cloaked]. Alleviation; the act of soothing or moderating, without really curing. —**pal′liate,** *v.;* **pal′liative,** *adj.*

pal′li·a″tive [*palliatus*]. A drug relieving or soothing the symptoms of a disease without curing it.

pal″lid·oid·o′sis. See *Treponema cuniculi.*

pal′li·dum [L. *pallidus*, pale]. The globus pallidus, medial pale portion of the lenticular nucleus of the brain. —**pallidal,** *adj.*

pal′li·um [L., cloak]. Old term for the cerebral cortex and superficial white matter of a cerebral hemisphere.

pal′lor [L., paleness]. Paleness, especially of the skin and mucous membranes.

palm [L. *palma*, palm]. 1. The inner or flexor surface of the hand; the hollow of the hand. 2. A palm tree. —**pal′mar,** *adj.*

p. oil. See under *oil.*

pal·ma′ris [L.]. One of two muscles, palmaris longus and palmaris brevis, inserted into the fascia of the palm. See Table of Muscles in the Appendix.

pal′ma·tine. $C_{21}H_{23}NO_5$; an alkaloid first isolated from calumba (*Jateorrhiza palmata*) but widely distributed in species of *Berberis.*

pal′ma·ture [L. *palma*, palm]. Union of the fingers; may be congenital or due to burns, wounds, or other trauma.

pal·mel′lin [NL. *palmella*, from G. *palmos*, vibration]. A red coloring-principle of a fresh-water alga, the *Palmella cruenta*, resembling hemoglobin.

Palmer method. See Van Slyke and Palmer *method.*

Palmer method for hemoglobin. See under *method.*

pal′min. Palmitin.

pal′mi·ped [L. *palma*, palm; *pes*, foot]. Having webbed feet.

pal′mi·tate. A salt or ester of palmitic acid.

pal·mit′ic [*palma*]. 1. Relating to or derived from palm oil. 2. Relating to palmitin.

pal·mit′ic ac′id. $CH_3(CH_2)_{14}COOH$. A saturated acid occurring in the glycerides of many fats and oils. Syn., *cetic acid, hexadecanoic acid.*

pal′mi·tin. $C_3H_5(C_{16}H_{31}O_2)_3$; glyceryl tripalmitate or glyceryl palmitate; an ester of glycerin with palmitic acid; a crystallizable and saponifiable solid found in vegetable and animal fats and oils;

insoluble in water, sparingly soluble in alcohol, and freely soluble in the organic solvents.

pal′mi·tyl. The univalent hydrocarbon radical $CH_3(CH_2)_{15}$—. Syn., *cetyl, hexadecyl.*

pal·mod′ic [G. *palmōdēs,* palpitating]. Pertaining to, resembling, or affected with, palmus.

pal″mo·plan′tar [L. *palma,* palm; *planta,* sole of the foot]. Pertaining to both the palms of the hands and the soles of the feet.

pal′mus [G. *palmos,* palpitation]. 1. A convulsive tic, with echolalia and abulia; frequently a manifestation of hysteria or schizophrenia. 2. Palpitation, throbbing, pulsation, twitching, jerkiness. 3. The heartbeat.

pal′pa·ble [L. *palpare,* to touch softly]. 1. Capable of being touched or palpated. 2. Evident.

pal·pa′tion [L. *palpatio,* a stroking, from *palpare*]. *In physical diagnosis,* the laying of the hand on a part of the body or the manipulation of a part for the purpose of ascertaining its condition or that of underlying organs. —**pal′pate,** *v.*

bimanual p. The use of the two hands in examining an organ.

pal″pa·to·per·cus′sion [*palpare;* L. *percussio,* a striking]. Combined palpation and percussion.

pal′pe·bra (pal′pi·bruh, ·brah, pal·pee′bruh) (pl. *palpebrae*) [L., eyelid]. The eyelid. —**palpebral,** *adj.*

p. inferior. The lower eyelid.

p. superior. The upper eyelid.

pal′pe·brate [L. *palpebrare,* to wink frequently]. Furnished with eyelids.

pal′pe·brate. To wink.

pal″pe·bra′tion [L. *palpebratio,* a blinking]. The act of winking; nictitation.

pal″pe·bri′tis. See *blepharitis.*

pal′pi·tate [L. *palpitare,* to palpitate]. Flutter, tremble, or beat abnormally fast; applied especially to the heart.

pal″pi·ta′tion [L. *palpitatio,* from *palpitare*]. A fluttering or throbbing, especially of the heart; any heart action of which the patient is conscious.

Pal's myelin stain. See under *stain.*

pal′sy (pawl′zee) [G. *paralysis,* paralysis]. A synonym for paralysis, used to designate special types. For terms not found here, see under *paralysis.*

Bell's p. Peripheral paralysis of the facial nerve.

birth p. A paralysis due to injury sustained during parturition; the common form is the Erb-Duchenne syndrome, or obstetric paralysis with deltoid involvement from injury to the brachial plexus. Also used as a synonym for spastic diplegia.

brachial birth p. Paralysis of the arm due to injury of the brachial plexus during birth. It may involve the entire arm, the upper arm (Erb-Duchenne type), or the forearm (Klumpke type).

bulbar p. Progressive degeneration of motor conduction pathways in the bulbar region of the brain. See progressive bulbar *paralysis.*

cerebral p. Paralysis due to a lesion of the brain. Also used as a synonym for spastic diplegia.

congenital cerebral p. Spastic diplegia.

cranial nerve p. Paralysis of those areas of the body controlled by the cranial nerves, usually caused by, and accompanying, some other disorder.

crutch p. Paralysis of the arm due to pressure of the crutch in the axilla.

diver's p. Caisson disease.

drummer's p. Paralysis of the extensor of the distal phalanx of the thumb occurring in drummers.

Erb's p. See Erb-Duchenne *paralysis.*

hod-carrier's p. Paralysis of the long thoracic nerve, from continuous muscular effort with the arms above the shoulder or from carrying heavy objects on the shoulder, characterized by unilateral "winging" of the scapula.

infantile cerebral p. Cerebral spastic infantile paralysis. See spastic *diplegia.*

Klumpke's p. Weakness of the hand and forearm due to injury of the lower roots of the brachial plexus.

lead p. Weakness of the hand grasp and paralysis of the extensors of the wrist and fingers resulting from degenerative changes in the posterior interosseous branch of the radial nerve produced by lead poisoning.

painter's p. Lead palsy.

pressure p. Paralysis due to pressure on a nerve.

printer's p. A rare form of paralysis due to polyneuritis in chronic antimony poisoning occurring in printers.

progressive bulbar p. See progressive bulbar *paralysis.*

pseudobulbar p. See pseudobulbar *paralysis.*

scriveners' p. Writers' cramp.

shaking p. See idiopathic *parkinsonism.*

wasting p. Progressive muscular atrophy.

Paltauf, Arnold [*Austrian physician,* 1860–93]. Described a form of dwarfism associated with lymphatism; called *Paltauf's nanism.*

Paltauf, Richard [*Austrian pathologist,* 1858–1924]. Described lymphogranulomatosis (1897), also called *Hodgkin's disease, Paltauf-Sternberg's disease.*

pal′u·dal (pal′yoo·dul, pa·lew′dul) [L. *palus,* swamp]. Malarial. *Obs.*

pal′u·dide [*palus*]. A cutaneous eruption supposed to be due to malaria. *Obs.*

pal′u·dism. See *malaria.*

paludrine hydrochloride. A trade-mark for chloroguanide hydrochloride.

pa·lus′tral [L. *paluster,* swampy]. Malarial. *Obs.*

Pal-Weigert method. See *Weigert's method* under *stain.*

pal″y·ster′ol. $C_{29}H_{50}O$; a sterol containing one double bond in the 5,6-position, occurring in certain marine invertebrates of the phylum Coelenterata.

pam′a·quine naph′tho·ate (pam′uh·kween, ·kwin) (*pamaquinae naphthoas*). $C_{42}H_{45}N_3O_7$. The methylene-bis-β-hydroxynaphthoate of 6-methoxy-8-(1-methyl-4-diethylamino)butylaminoquinoline; a yellow to orange-yellow, odorless powder; insoluble in water, but soluble in alcohol. Used as an antimalarial. Rapidly destroys gametocytes of all forms of malaria, including estivo-autumnal. Also as a gametocide for prophylaxis. Also called *aminoquin naphthoate.* See *plasmochin.* Dose, 0.01–0.02 Gm. (1/6–1/3 gr.); total daily dose, 0.06 Gm. (1 gr.).

pam·pin′i·form [L. *pampinus,* tendril; *forma,* form]. Having the form of a tendril, used particularly for the pampiniform plexus of veins in the spermatic cord.

pan [AS. *panne*]. A low, flat-bottomed vessel.

bed p. A large, flat, oval pan, usually of agate or enameled ware or stainless steel, serving as a receptacle for the fecal discharges and urine of patients confined to bed.

brain p. The skull.

pan- [G. *pas,* the whole, all]. A combining form meaning *all, every;* used in medicine to signify *general* or *affecting all or many parts.*

pan″a·ce′a [G. *panakeia,* universal remedy]. A cure-all; a quack remedy.

pan″ag·glu′ti·nin. An agglutinin lacking specificity, which agglutinates erythrocytes of various types.

Pan″a·ma′ bark. Quillaja bark.

Pan A·mer′i·can San′i·tar″y Bu′reau. A technical international organization of the Americas responsible to the member states through technical representatives of these states whose concerns include prevention of epidemics, the collection and dissemination of epidemiological data, consultation services, improvement of health administration in the member states, and promotion of liaison between them; a regional office of the World Health Organization since 1949.

pan′a·ris, pa·na′ris. See *paronychia.*

analgesic p. Painless lesions of the phalanges in syringomyelia.

pan″a·ri′ti·um. See *paronychia.*

pan″ar·te·ri′tis [G. *pas,* whole, all; *artēria,* artery; *-itis,* inflammation]. 1. Inflammation of all the coats of an artery. 2. Inflammation of several arteries at the same time.

pan″ar·thri′tis [*pas;* G. *arthritis,* arthritis]. Inflammation of many joints.

Panas, Photinos [*Greek ophthalmologist,* 1832–1903]. Noted clinician in Paris and author of a well-known textbook (1894). Introduced an operation for relief of ptosis, in which he raised the tarsal portion of the lid by sutures which allowed the occipitofrontalis muscle to assume the function of the levator palpebrae superioris; called *Panas' operation.*

pan·at′ro·phy [G. *pas,* whole, all; *atrophia,* want of food]. 1. Atrophy affecting every part of a structure. 2. General atrophy.

Pa′nax [G., universal remedy]. A genus of plants of the Araliaceae. See *ginseng.*

pan″car·di′tis [G. *pas,* whole, all; *kardia,* heart; *-itis,* inflammation]. General inflammation of the heart.

pan·cav″er·no·si′tis. See *cavernitis.*

Pancoast, Henry Khunrath [*American roentgenologist,* 1875–1939]. Known for his description of an apical pulmonary tumor accompanied by Horner's syndrome, pain, bone destruction, and atrophy of hand muscles; called *Pancoast syndrome.*

Pancoast, Joseph [*American surgeon,* 1805–82]. Operated successfully for exstrophy of the urinary bladder with epispadias (1859). Introduced an operation for the relief of facial neuralgia in which he divided the mandibular branch of the trigeminal nerve as it emerged from the foramen ovale; called *Pancoast's operation.*

pan″co·lec′to·my [*pas;* G. *kolon,* colon; *ektomē,* excision]. Surgical removal of the entire colon.

pan·col″po·hys″ter·ec′to·my. See *panhysterocolpectomy.*

pan′cre·as (pan′kree·us, pang′kree·us) (pl. *pancreata, pancreases*) [G. *pagkreas*]. A compound racemose gland, from six to eight inches in length, lying transversely across the posterior wall of the abdomen. Its right extremity, the head, lies in contact with the duodenum; its left extremity, the tail, is in close proximity to the spleen. It secretes a limpid, colorless fluid that digests proteins, fats, and carbohydrates. The secretion is conveyed to the duodenum by the pancreatic duct. It furnishes an important internal secretion, insulin, from the islets of Langerhans. See Plates 10, 13, 45. —**pancreat′ic,** *adj.*

accessory p. A small mass of glandular structure similar to the pancreas and adjacent to it.

annular p. An anomalous form of the pancreas encircling the duodenum.

dorsal p. The embryonic pancreas arising as a diverticulum of the dorsal duodenal wall; it forms most of the adult organ.

lesser p. A small, partially detached portion of the gland, lying posteriorly to its head, and occasionally having a separate duct that opens into the pancreatic duct proper.

p. extract. See *insulin, lipocaic, pancreatin.*

p. of Aselli. Lymph nodes near the pancreas.

tail of p. The splenic end of the pancreas.

ventral p. The embryonic pancreas arising as a diverticulum of the common bile duct; it forms a part of the adult organ.

pan″cre·a′ta. A plural of pancreas.

pan″cre·a·tec′to·my [*pagkreas;* G. *ektomē,* excision]. Excision of the pancreas.

pan″cre·at″i·co·du″o·de′nal (pan″kree·at″i·ko·dew″o·dee′nul, ·dew·od′i·nul, pang″kree·) [*pagkreas;* L. *duodeni,* twelve]. Pertaining to the pancreas and the duodenum, as the pancreaticoduodenal arteries. See Table of Arteries in the Appendix.

pan″cre·at″i·co·du″o·de·nos′to·my. See *pancreatoduodenostomy.*

pan″cre·at″i·co·en″ter·os′to·my [*pagkreas;* G. *enteron,* intestine; *stoma,* mouth]. The surgical anastomosis of the pancreatic duct or a pancreatic fistulous tract with the small intestine.

pan″cre·at″i·co·gas·tros′to·my [*pagkreas;* G. *gastēr,* belly; *stoma*]. The surgical anastomosis of a pancreatic fistulous tract with the pyloric portion of the stomach.

pan″cre·at″i·co·je″ju·nos′to·my (·jee″jew·nos′-to·mee, ·jedj″oo·nos′to·mee) [*pagkreas;* L. *jejunus,* empty; *stoma*]. Anastomosing the pancreatic duct with the jejunum.

pan″cre·at″i·co·li·thot′o·my [*pagkreas;* G. *lithos,* stone; *tomē,* a cutting]. The surgical removal of a stone in the pancreatic duct.

pan″cre·at″i·co·splen′ic (·splen′ick, ·splee′nick) [*pagkreas;* G. *splēnikos,* of the spleen]. Pertaining to the pancreas and the spleen.

pan′cre·a·tin (*pancreatinum*). A substance containing enzymes, principally pancreatic amylase (amylopsin), trypsin, and pancreatic lipase (steapsin), obtained from the fresh pancreas of the hog, *Sus scrofa* var. *domesticus,* or of the ox, *Bos taurus;* it is a cream-colored amorphous powder with a faint odor. Used for its enzymatic action in various forms of digestive failure but of doubtful activity.

pan″cre·a·ti′tis [*pagkreas;* G. *-itis,* inflammation]. Inflammation of the pancreas. The acute form may be hemorrhagic, suppurative, or gangrenous. The onset of acute pancreatitis is usually sudden, with severe abdominal pain, vomiting, tympanites, and tenderness of the abdomen. Chronic pancreatitis may be interlobular, with an increase of interlobular connective tissue, or interacinar, in which the interacinar spaces are invaded and the islets of Langerhans involved. —**pancreatit′ic,** *adj.*

pan″cre·a·to·du″o·de·nec′to·my (·dew″o·di-neck′to·mee, ·dew·od″i·neck′to·mee). See *duodenopancreatectomy.*

pan″cre·a·to·du″o·de·nos′to·my [*pagkreas;* L. *duodeni,* twelve; G. *stoma,* mouth]. The anastomosis of a portion of the pancreas, especially a fistulous tract into the duodenum.

pan″cre·a·to·en″ter·os′to·my [*pagkreas;* G. *enteron,* intestine; *stoma*]. Anastomosing the pancreatic duct with some part of the small intestine.

pan″cre·a·tog′e·nous. Arising in the pancreas.

pan″cre·a·to·li′pase. Lipase found in the pancreatic juice.

pan″cre·at′o·lith [*pagkreas;* G. *lithos,* stone]. A calculus of the pancreas. Syn., *pancreolith.*

pan″cre·a·to·li·thec′to·my [*pagkreas; lithos;* G. *ektomē,* excision]. Surgical removal of a pancreatic calculus.

pan″cre·a·to·li·thot′o·my [*pagkreas; lithos;* G. *tomē,* a cutting]. Operative removal of calculus from the pancreas. Also called *pancreolithotomy.*

pan″cre·a·tol′y·sis, pan″cre·ol′y·sis [*pagkreas;* G. *lysis*, a loosing]. Destruction of the pancreas. —**pancreatolyt′ic,** *adj.*
pan″cre·a·tot′o·my [*pagkreas;* G. *tomē*, a cutting]. Incision of the pancreas.
pan″cre·ec′to·my. See *pancreatectomy.*
pan′cre·o·lith. See *pancreatolith.*
pan″cre·o·li·thot′o·my. See *pancreatolithotomy.*
pan″cre·ol′y·sis. See *pancreatolysis.*
pan″cre·op′a·thy, pan″cre·o·path′i·a [*pagkreas;* G. *pathos*, disease]. Disease of the pancreas.
pan′cre·o·zyme″ [*pagkreas;* G. *zymē*, leaven]. A ferment similar to but not identical with secretin.
pan″cre·o·zy′min. A crude extract of the intestinal mucosa which stimulates the secretion of pancreatic enzymes.
pancrobilin. Trade-mark for a preparation containing desiccated pancreas and extract of ox bile.
pan″cy·to·pe′ni·a. Reduction of all three formed elements of the blood: erythrocytes, leukocytes, and platelets; panhematopenia.
pan·de′mi·a, pan′de·my [G. *pandēmia*, the whole people]. An epidemic that attacks all persons.
pan·dem′ic [*pandēmia*]. Epidemic over a wide geographic area.
Pander, Heinrich Christian von [*German embryologist*, 1794–1865]. With Karl E. Baer, described the splanchnopleural layer of the mesoderm. Described embryonic cellular masses from which blood vessels develop, called *Pander's islands.* A lenticular mass of gray matter below the thalamus is called *Pander's nucleus.*
pan·dic″u·la′tion [L. *pandiculari*, to stretch one's self]. The act of stretching the limbs, especially on waking from sleep, accompanied by yawning.
Pandy's reagent. See under *reagent.*
Pandy's test. See under *test.*
pan″e·lec′tro·scope [G. *pas*, whole, all; *ēlektron*, amber; *skopein*, to examine]. An inspection apparatus for use in proctoscopy, esophagoscopy, urethroscopy, etc. It throws concentrated light through the whole tube, thus illuminating the spot that is to be inspected.
pan·en′do·scope. A modification of the cystoscope, utilizing a foroblique lens system, permitting adequate visualization of both the urinary bladder and the urethra.
pan″es·the′si·a (pan″ess·thee′zhuh, ·zee·uh) [G. *panaisthēsia*, full vigor of the senses]. General or total sensation; cenesthesia. —**panesthet′ic,** *adj.*
Paneth, Josef [*German physician*, 1857–90]. Described the coarsely granular cells found in the crypts of Lieberkühn in the small intestine; called *cells of Paneth.*
pang [ME. *prange*]. A momentary, sharp pain.
breast p. Angina pectoris.
brow p. See *migraine, hemicrania*, 2.
Pangborn test. A flocculation test for syphilis.
pan′gene, pan′gen. See hypothetical *units.*
pan·gen′e·sis [G. *pas*, whole, all; *genesis*, production]. Darwin's comprehensive theory of heredity and development, according to which all parts of the body give off gemmules which aggregate in the germ cells. During development they are sorted out from one another and give rise to parts similar to those of their origin.
pan·glos′si·a [G. *pagglōssia*, garrulity]. Excessive or psychotic garrulity.
pan·hem″at·o·pe′ni·a. See *pancytopenia.*
pan″hi·dro′sis [G. *pas*, whole, all; *hidrōsis*, a sweating]. Generalized perspiration.
pan·hy′grous [G. *panygros*, quite damp]. Damp as to the entire surface.
pan·hy″po·pi·tu′i·ta·rism. See *hypopituitarism.*
pan″hys·ter·ec′to·my [G. *pas*, whole, all; *hystera*, womb; *ektomē*, excision]. Total extirpation of the uterus.
pan·hys″ter·o·col·pec′to·my [*pas; hystera;* G. *kolpos*, vagina; *ektomē*]. Complete removal of the uterus and vagina.
pan·hys″ter·o-o″o·pho·rec′to·my. Excision of the entire uterus and one or both ovaries.
pan·hys″ter·o·sal″pin·gec′to·my (·sal″pin·jeck′-to·mee) [*pas; hystera;* G. *salpigx*, trumpet; *ektomē*]. Excision of the entire uterus and the oviducts.
pan·hys″ter·o·sal·pin″go-o″o·pho·rec′to·my. Excision of the uterus, oviducts, and ovaries.
pan′ic [G. *panikos*, from *Pan*, Pan]. An extreme anxiety attack in which the anxious person becomes incapacitated temporarily.
pa·nic″u·la′tine. $C_{29}H_{35}NO_7$; an alkaloid from *Aconitum paniculatum.*
pan″im·mu′ni·ty [*pas;* G. *immunitas*, freedom from public services]. General immunity to disease.
pa·niv′o·rous [L. *panis*, bread; *vorare*, to devour]. Subsisting on bread; bread-eating.
Panizza, Bartolomeo [*Italian anatomist*, 1785–1867]. Remembered for having located the visual function in the posterior portion of the occipital lobes of the brain (1855), reported also a year later by Joseph Swann. Described two lymphatic plexuses in the lateral fossae of the preputial frenum, called *Panizza's plexuses.*
pan″me·tri′tis. Widespread inflammation of the entire uterus, often accompanied by cellulitis of the broad ligaments.
pan·mne′si·a (pan·nee′zhuh, ·zee·uh) [G. *pas*, whole, all; *mnēsios*, of memory]. A potential remembrance of all impressions.
panmycin. Trade-mark for the antibiotic substance tetracycline, commonly supplied as the hydrochloride.
pan″my·e·loph′thi·sis (pan″migh·i·lof′thi·sis, pan·migh″i·lof·thigh′sis) [*pas;* G. *myelos*, marrow; *phthisis*, a wasting away]. A general wasting of the bone marrow. *O.T.*
pan″my·e·lo′sis (pan″migh·i·lo′sis) [*pas; myelos;* G. *-ōsis*, increase]. See *myeloproliferative disorders.*
pan·my″e·lo·tox″i·co′sis [*pas; myelos;* G. *toxikon*, poison; *-ōsis*, condition]. A condition in which all elements of the bone marrow are affected.
pan·nic″u·li′tis [L. *panniculus*, small piece of cloth; G. *-itis*, inflammation]. Inflammation of the abdominal panniculus adiposus.
nodular nonsuppurative p. That form characterized by the formation of painful nodules in the subcutis; relapses occur frequently. Also called *Christian-Weber disease.*
pan·nic′u·lus [L.]. A membrane or layer.
p. adiposus. The layer of subcutaneous fat.
p. carnosus. The layer of muscles contained in the superficial fascia. It is well developed in some lower animals, but in man is represented mainly by the platysma.
pan′nus [L., cloth]. 1. Vascularization and connective-tissue deposition beneath the epithelium of the cornea. 2. Chloasma. 3. Connective tissue overgrowing the articular surface of a diarthrodial joint.
allergic eczematous p. That associated with phlyctenular keratitis.
p. carateus. Pinta.
p. carnosus. One that has acquired a considerable thickness. Also called *p. crassus.*
p. degenerativus. That occurring in blind degenerated eyes following diseases such as cyclitis, glaucoma, or retinal detachment.
p. hepaticus. Chloasma.
p. siccus. An old pannus composed of connective tissue and poor in vessels. Also called *p. degenerativus.*

p. tenuis. Slight pannus.

p. trachomatosus. That occurring with trachoma.

pan″oph·thal·mi′tis [G. *pas*, whole, all; *ophthalmos*, eye; *-itis*, inflammation]. Inflammation of all the tissues of the eyeball. Also called *panophthalmia.*

p. purulenta. A severe form, with great protrusion of the eyeball and formation of pus, usually resulting in blindness.

pan″os·te·i′tis [*pas;* G. *osteon*, bone; *-itis*]. An inflammation of all parts of a bone.

pan″o·ti′tis [*pas;* G. *ous*, ear; *-itis*]. A diffuse inflammation of all parts of the ear, usually beginning in the internal ear.

panparnit. Trade-mark for the β-diethylaminoethyl ester of 1-phenylcyclopentanecarboxylic acid, a muscle relaxant.

pan·phar′ma·con [*pas;* G. *pharmakon*, drug]. A panacea. *Obs.*

pan″phle·bi′tis. Inflammation of all the coats of a vein.

pan·pho′bi·a. See *pantophobia.*

panrone. Trade-mark for *amithiozone.*

Pansch, Adolf [*German anatomist*, 1841–87]. Described a cerebral fissure extending from the lower end of the central fissure to the occipital lobe; called *Pansch's fissure.*

pan″scle·ro′sis [G. *pas*, whole, all; *sklērōsis*, a hardening]. Complete hardening of a part.

pan·si″nus·i′tis (pan·sigh″nuh·sigh′tis, ·sin″yoo-sigh′tis, ·sigh″new·sigh′tis) [*pas;* L. *sinus*, a bent surface; G. *-itis*, inflammation]. Inflammation of all the paranasal sinuses.

Pan·stron′gy·lus (pan·stron′ji·lus) [*pas;* G. *stroggylos*, round]. A genus of bugs of the family Reduviidae, the assassin or cone-nosed bugs.

P. megistus. A species which transmits *Trypanosoma cruzi* in South America.

pant [OF. *pantaisier*, to be breathless]. Breathe hard or quickly.

pan″ta·mor′phi·a [G. *pas*, whole, all; *amorphia*, formlessness]. General deformity. —**pantamorphic,** *adj.*

pan″tan·en·ce·pha′li·a [*pas;* G. *anegkephalos*, without brain]. Total congenital absence of the brain. —**pantanencephal′ic,** *adj.*

pan″tan·en·ceph′a·lus [*pas; anegkephalos*]. A monster showing complete absence of the brain.

pan·tan″ky·lo·bleph′a·ron (pan·tang″ki·lo·blef′-uh·ron) [*pas;* G. *agkylos*, crooked, bent; *blepharon*, eyelid]. Complete ankyloblepharon.

pan″ta·pho′bi·a [*pas;* G. *a-*, not; *phobos*, fear]. Total absence of fear.

pan″ta·som′a·tous (pan″tuh·som′uh·tus, ·so′muh-tus) [*pas;* G. *sōma*, body]. Involving the entire body.

pan″ta·tro′phi·a, pan·tat′ro·phy [*pas;* G. *atrophia*, want of nourishment]. Complete or general atrophy.

pan″te·the′ine. The β-aminoethanethiol ester of pantothenic acid, occurring naturally; a growth factor for *Lactobacillus bulgaricus.*

pan′te·thine. The disulfide of pantetheine, occurring naturally. Some lactic acid bacteria show preference for pantethine over pantothenic acid as a growth factor.

panthenol. Trade-mark for *pantothenyl alcohol.*

pan·ther′a·pist [*pas;* G. *therapeia*, treatment]. One who treats upon the basis of any available remedial agent.

panthesine. Trade-mark for the N-diethylleucinol ester of para-aminobenzoic acid. The substance is used for both infiltration anesthesia in 0.2% solution and for surface anesthesia in strengths of from 5–10% in solution or in ointment form.

pan′to-. See *pan-.*

pan′to·caine. A term occasionally applied to tetracaine hydrochloride.

pan′to·graph″ [*pas;* G. *graphein*, to write]. An instrument for the mechanical copying of diagrams, etc., upon the same scale, or upon an enlarged or a reduced scale.

pan·to′ic ac′id. $CH_2OH.C(CH_3)_2.CHOH.COOH$; the fragment of pantothenic acid remaining after cleavage of β-alanine; it replaces pantothenic acid as a growth factor for certain organisms.

pantopaque. A proprietary compound, ethyl iodophenylundecylate, used in roentgenographic visualization of the spinal subarachnoid space.

pan″to·pho′bi·a [*pas;* G. *phobos*, fear]. Morbid fear of everything; a symptom present in some cases of psychasthenia.

pantopon. Trade-mark for a preparation containing all the alkaloids of opium in the form of hydrochlorides, and in the relative proportion in which they occur in the whole gum. Used in place of opium and morphine.

pan″top·to′sis [*pas;* G. *ptōsis*, a falling]. A condition in which several viscera are prolapsed.

pan″to·scop′ic. See *bifocal.*

pan″to·som′a·tous (pan″to·som′uh·tus, ·so′muh-tus) [*pas;* G. *sōma*, body]. Characterizing a monstrosity in which the whole or nearly the whole body is affected.

pan″to·then′ate. Any salt or ester of pantothenic acid.

pan″to·then′ic ac′id. $CH_2OH.C(CH_3)_2CHOH.-CONH.CH_2.CH_2COOH$. α,γ-Dihydroxy-β,β-dimethylbutyryl-β -alanide; a substance widely distributed in nature and believed to be present in animal tissues essentially as a component of coenzyme A. Absence of this factor of the vitamin-B complex gives rise to dermatitis in chicks; it also appears to be essential for nutrition of rats, but its importance in human nutrition has not been established. It is employed chiefly in the form of calcium pantothenate. See Table of Vitamins in the Appendix. Syn., *chick antidermatitis factor, filtrate factor, pantoyl-β-alanine.*

pan″to·then′yl al′co·hol. $CH_2OH.C(CH_3)_2-CHOH.CONH.CH_2.CH_2.CH_2OH$; α,γ-dihydroxy-N-(3-hydroxypropyl)-β, β-dimethylbutyramide; a viscous liquid, freely soluble in water. In the body it is converted to pantothenic acid, and because of the greater stability of the alcohol, is sometimes used in place of the acid. See *panthenol.*

pan″to·yl-β-al′a·nine. Pantothenic acid.

pan″to·yl·tau′rine. $HOCH_2.C(CH_3)_2.CHOH.CO.-NH.CH_2.CH_2.SO_3H$. A substance antagonistic to pantothenic acid for a variety of microorganisms but not to those which can synthesize pantothenic acid. Also called *thiopanic acid.*

pan·trop′ic [*pas;* G. *trepein*, to turn]. Polytropic; having affinity for or affecting many tissues; applied to viruses.

Panum, Peter Ludvig [*Danish physiologist*, 1820–85]. Made important contributions to knowledge of putrefactive processes (1856). Described embolism (1864). In his early years made an important study and report of an epidemic of measles in the Faroe Islands (1846) which has become famous in the history of epidemiology. His serum globulin was once known as *Panum's casein.*

pa′nus [L., swelling]. 1. An inflamed, nonsuppurating lymph node. 2. Venereal lymphogranuloma: old term.

p. faucium. An inflamed lymph node in the throat.

p. inguinalis. A bubo.

pan″zo·ot′ic [G. *pas*, whole, all; *zōion*, living being].

In veterinary medicine, affecting many species of animals.

pap [perhaps from L. *papa*, the word with which infants call for food]. A soft, semiliquid food.

pa·pa′in (pa·pay′in, pay′puh·in). An enzyme obtained from the juice of the fruit and leaves of *Carica papaya;* occurs as a white, or grayish-white, slightly hygroscopic powder; incompletely soluble in water and glycerin; contains enzymes similar to pepsin, but acting in acid, neutral, or alkaline medium. Used to aid digestion in chronic dyspepsia and gastric fermentation; externally as a solvent of false membranes and on warts, etc.; also used to treat erythrocytes in testing for Rh antibodies. Dose, 0.1–0.3 Gm. (2–5 gr.). Also called *papayotin.*

Papanicolau, George Nicholas (1883–). American anatomist who popularized the study of exfoliated cells, primarily as a means for detection of cancer. See *cytological cancer techniques.*

Pa·pa′ver [L.]. A genus of herbs of the Papaveraceae; the poppy. See *opium.*

pa·pav″er·al′dine. $C_{20}H_{19}NO_5$; 6,7-dimethyl-1-veratroylisoquinoline; an alkaloid occurring in, or formed during extraction of, opium.

pa·pav′er·a″mine. $C_{21}H_{25}NO_6$; an alkaloid from opium.

pa·pav′er·ine (pa·pav′ur·een, ·in, pa·pay′vur·). $C_{20}H_{21}O_4N$. An alkaloid obtained from opium, belonging to the benzyl isoquinoline group (it is not a morphine derivative); occurs as a white, crystalline powder.

p. hydrochloride (*papaverinae hydrochloridum*). $C_{20}H_{21}O_4N.HCl$, the hydrochloride of an alkaloid obtained from opium; occurs as white crystals, or as a white, crystalline powder; 1 Gm. is soluble in about 40 cc. of water; it is soluble in alcohol and chloroform. Papaverine relaxes smooth muscle in general, although different organs are affected in a varying degree. It is also a rather feeble central analgesic and a local anesthetic. It is used in all kinds of gastric and intestinal spasms, in biliary colic, and in bronchial spasm. Dose, 0.06–0.2 Gm. (1–3 gr.).

pa·paw′ [Sp. *papayo*, papaw tree]. 1. The seed of *Asimina triloba;* has been used as an emetic. 2. See *papaya.*

pa·pa′ya (pa·pah′yuh, pa·pay′uh) [Sp., fruit of the papaw]. Melon tree; papaw; *Carica papaya*, a tree of the Passifloraceae. The unripe fruit yields a milky juice containing papain.

pap″a·yo′tin (pap″uh·yo′tin, pa·pah′yo·tin, pa·pay′o·tin). See *papain.*

pa′per [G. *papyros*, papyrus]. A processed material pressed into thin sheets; made from wood pulp, cloth, or other substances.

articulating p. See *articulating paper.*

blistering p. Paper saturated with cantharides; used for producing vesication.

filter p. An unglazed paper used for filtration.

indicator p. Strong white filter paper, saturated with the proper strength indicator solution or other particular substance, and dried. These papers are used for testing acidity or alkalinity, pH, or for the presence or absence of a particular substance. Also called *test p.*

mustard p. A mixture of powdered black mustard and an adhesive spread on paper or a thin cloth. When applied to the skin, it acts as a rubefacient. Syn., *charta sinapis.*

pa·pes′cent. Having the consistence of pap.

pa·pil′la (pl. *papillae*) [L., nipple]. 1. A small, nipplelike eminence. 2. A pimple or pustule. —**pap′illary,** *adj.*

alpine p. A narrow and elongated papilla of the corium; seen in several skin diseases.

anal p. Any of the small elevations occasionally present on the free margins of the anal valves or at the bases of the rectal columns: also called *papilla of Morgagni.*

basilar p. The organ of Corti.

bile p. See duodenal *p.*

circumvallate p. See vallate *p.*

conical p. A variant form of filiform *p.*

dental p. The mass of connective tissue over which fits the enamel organ of a developing tooth. It forms the dentin and dental pulp.

dermal p. An elevation of the corium into a corresponding depression in the overlying epidermis.

duodenal p. The eminence on the duodenal mucosa at the opening of the common bile duct. Also called *papilla of Vater.*

engorged p. Choked disk. See *papillitis.*

filiform p. Any one of the papillae occurring on the dorsum and margins of the oral part of the tongue, consisting of an elevation of connective tissue covered by a layer of epithelium. Variously divided to appear shredded.

foliate p. One of the papillae, similar in structure to the vallate papillae, found on the posterolateral margin of the tongue of many mammals, but vestigial or absent in man.

fungiform p. One of the low, broad papillae scattered over the dorsum and margins of the tongue.

genital p. The primitive penis or clitoris.

gustatory p. A papilla of the tongue which is furnished with taste buds.

Huschke's p. Formerly, the organ of Corti.

incisive p. The oval or pear-shaped thickening of the palatine mucous membrane overlying the incisive fossa (a) and containing vestiges of the nasopalatine ducts: also called *palatine p., incisive pad.*

interdental p. That portion of the gingiva between two contiguous teeth: also called *interproximal gingiva.*

lacrimal p. A small, conical eminence on the eyelid at the inner canthus pierced by the lacrimal punctum. See Plate 19.

lenticular p. One of the irregularly distributed, low folds of mucous membrane in the anterior part of the dorsum of the base of the tongue.

lingual p. Any one of the papillae on the tongue.

mammary p. The nipple of the breast. See Plate 43.

optic p. See optic *disk.*

palatine p. See incisive *p.*

renal p. The summit of any one of the renal pyramids projecting into the renal pelvis.

tactile p. A little eminence of the corium containing a tactile corpuscle.

vallate p. One of the large, flat papillae, each surrounded by a trench, in a group anterior to the sulcus terminalis of the tongue. Sny., *circumvallate p.*

vascular p. A dermal papilla containing capillary loops.

pap′il·late [L. *papillatus*, shaped like a bud]. Having small papillary or nipplelike projections.

pap″il·lec′to·my [L. *papilla*, nipple; G. *ektomē*, excision]. Surgical removal of a papilla or papillae.

pa·pil″le·de′ma [*papilla;* G. *oidēma*, swelling]. Edema of the optic nerve. If severe, it may result in choked disk or papillitis.

pap″il·lif′er·ous [*papilla;* L. *ferre*, to bear]. Bearing or containing papillae, as a papilliferous cyst.

pa·pil′li·form [*papilla;* L. *forma*, form]. Shaped like a papilla.

pap″il·li′tis [*papilla;* G. *-itis*, inflammation]. 1. Inflammation of a papilla. 2. Inflammation of the optic disk: also called *optic neuritis.*

necrotizing p. Necrosis and inflammation of renal papillae, probably resulting from ischemia, and usually associated with acute pyelonephritis, especially in patients with diabetes mellitus.

pap″il·lo″cys·to′ma. See serous *cystadenoma.*

pap″il·lo′ma [*papilla;* G. *-ōma,* tumor]. A neoplastic growth of surface epithelium, supported on cores or papillae of vascularized connective tissue. May arise from skin, mucous membranes, or glandular ducts, such as those of mammary glands, glandular acini, and acinar spaces of adenomas and adenocarcinomas. Similar growths may arise from serous surfaces and are covered with mesothelial cells. The epithelial papillomas are benign, but tend to recur unless completely eradicated. They may be caused by a virus, as those of the skin. Others, as those of the urinary bladder, may be due to chemical factors such as the products of anilines. —**papillom′atous,** *adj.*

cylindrical-cell p. One covered by simple or stratified columnar epithelium. Also called *soft p.*

ductal p. A tumor of the breast limited to the mammary duct system, characterized by atypical papillary structures: also called *intraductal p.*

p. choroideum. That derived from choroid plexus and covered with ependymal cells.

psammomatous p. See serous *cystadenoma.*

pseudomucinous p. See pseudomucinous *cystadenoma.*

squamous-cell p. A papilloma covered by stratified squamous epithelium. Also called *hard p.*

pap″il·lo″ma·to′sis [*papilla; -ōma;* G. *-ōsis,* condition]. The widespread formation of papillomas; also the state of being affected with multiple papillomas.

infectious oral p. of dogs. A viral disease of young dogs, characterized by the formation of multiple pedunculated growths on the oral mucosa. The growths disappear spontaneously and leave the animal with a high degree of immunity.

infectious p. of cattle. A viral disease of cattle, characterized by the formation of warts on various parts of the body.

papular p. See juvenile *acanthosis.*

verrucose p. of mouth. Warty vegetations in the mouth that are very difficult to cure. Growths appear similar to the condyloma acuminatum seen on the genitalia.

pa·pil″lo·ret″i·ni′tis [*papilla;* L. *rete,* net; G. *-itis,* inflammation]. Inflammation of the optic disk and retina.

Papin, Denis [*French physicist,* 1647–1714]. Introduced an apparatus for boiling organic material under pressure in a closed vessel; called *Papin's digester.*

papoid. Trade name for a papain preparation.

pa·poose′ root. *Caulophyllum thalictroides,* the blue cohosh.

Pappenheim, Artur [*German pathologist,* 1870–1916]. Leading hematologist. Devised numerous stains and laboratory methods. See Pappenheim-Saathoff methyl green-pyronin *stain,* also *Pappenheim's method* and *Pappenheim's solution,* under *stain.*

Pappenheimer, Alwin Max [*American pathologist,* 1877–]. With Charles Norris and Thomas Flournoy reported discovery of a spirochete in an American case of relapsing fever (1906).

pap′pose [G. *pappos,* down]. Covered with fine downy hair.

pap′pus [*pappos*]. The fine downy hair first appearing on the cheeks and chin.

pa·pri′ka (pa·pree′kuh, pap′ri·kuh) [Hung. *paprika,* Turkish pepper]. The dried pulverized capsules of *Capsicum annuum.* Contains vitamin C. Also called *Spanish pepper, Turkish pepper.*

pap″u·la′tion [L. *papula,* pimple]. The stage, in certain eruptions, marked by papule formation.

pap′ule, pap′u·la [*papula*]. A small, circumscribed, solid elevation of the skin, varying in size from that of a pin point to that of a split pea. —**papular,** *adj.*

moist p. The syphilitic condyloma.

pap″u·lif′er·ous [*papula;* L. *ferre,* to bear]. Covered with papules.

pap″u·lo·er″y·them′a·tous (pap″yoo·lo·err″ith-em′uh·tus, ·eem′uh·tus) [*papula;* G. *erythēma,* redness]. Having a papular eruption superimposed on a generalized erythema.

pap″u·lo·pus′tu·lar [*papula;* L. *pustula,* blister]. Characterized by both papules and pustules.

pap″u·lo·squa′mous [*papula;* L. *squama,* scale]. Characterized by both papules and scales.

pap″u·lo·squa′mous re·ac′tion. See under *reaction.*

pap″u·lo·ve·sic′u·lar [*papula;* L. *vesicula,* little blister]. Characterized by both papules and vesicles.

pap″y·ra′ce·ous (pap″i·ray′shus, ·see·us) [G. *papyros,* papyrus]. Resembling paper, as the papyraceous plate of the ethmoid bone.

p. fetus. See *fetus* papyraceus.

Paquelin, Claude André [*French surgeon,* 1836–1905]. Introduced a thermocautery, a hollow platinum point kept at a uniform temperature by a current of hot vapor (1877); called *Paquelin cautery.*

par′a-, par- [G. *para,* beside, near, beyond]. 1. A prefix signifying *beyond, beside, near.* 2. *In chemistry,* a prefix (to a derivative of the benzene ring) indicating the substitution of two atoms of hydrogen situated opposite each other, in the 1,4-position. Symbol, *p-*. 3. *In medicine,* a prefix denoting *a faulty* or *abnormal condition, associated in an accessory capacity, remotely* or *indirectly related to,* or *almost, closely resembling.*

par″a-ac″et·phe·net′i·din (par″uh-ass″et·fi·net′-i·din, par″uh-a·set″·). See *acetophenetidin.*

par″a-am″e·bi′a·sis. Amebid.

par″a-a·mi″no·ben″zene·ar·son′ic ac′id. Arsanilic acid.

par″a-a·mi″no·ben·zo′ic ac′id (par″uh-a·mee″-no·ben·zo′ick, par″uh-am″i·no·). $C_6H_4NH_2COOH$. A yellowish-red, crystalline subtance considered a member of the B complex group of vitamins. Under some experimental conditions it corrects premature graying of hair. It inhibits the action of sulfonamides,and is essential for the metabolism of certain bacteria; it is used in the biosynthesis of folic acid and related substances. It is of clinical value in the treatment of rickettsial diseases. Syn., *PABA.* Also called *vitamin H′, vitamin* B_x, *vitamin V.* See Table of Vitamins in the Appendix.

par″a-a·mi″no·hip·pu′ric ac′id. $NH_2.C_6H_4.CONH.CH_2.COOH$; *p*-aminobenzoylaminoacetic acid: used to test renal function by its excretion in the urine after intravenous injection; also to test liver function by measuring the extent of its synthesis from orally administered para-aminobenzoic acid as determined from para-aminohippuric acid blood levels. Abbreviated, PAH, PAHA.

par″a-a·mi″no·sal″i·cyl′ic ac′id. $C_6H_3(NH_2)(OH)(COOH)$. 4-Aminosalicylic acid or 4-amino-2-hydroxybenzoic acid, a white, crystalline substance, soluble in water. It is bacteriostatic against tubercle bacilli and is used clinically in the treatment of tuberculosis. Also called *aminosalicylic acid* and abbreviated PAS, PASA.

par″a-am″y·loi·do′sis. See primary *amyloidosis.*

par″a-an″al·ge′si·a (par″uh-an″al·jee′zee·uh, ·see·uh). Analgesia limited to the lower half of the body.

par″a-an″es·the′si·a (-an″ess·thee′zhuh, ·zee·uh). Anesthesia of the body below the waist.

par″a-ap·pen″di·ci′tis. Inflammation of the connective tissue adjacent to that part of the appendix not covered with peritoneum.

par″a·bi·o′sis (par″uh·buy·o′sis) [G. *para*, beside; *biōsis*, a way of life]. The experimental fusing together of two individuals or embryos so that the effects of one partner upon the other may be studied. —**parabiot′ic,** *adj.*

par″a·blep′sis [G., a looking askance]. False or perverted vision.

par·a′bo·loid dark′-field con·den′ser. A lens of paraboloid shape, the vertex end being ground back so that its focus can be brought into coincidence with the specimen on the slide. A central stop is provided to block the central rays. It is used chiefly for medium-power work.

par″a·bu′li·a [G. *para*, beyond; *boulē*, will]. Abnormality of volitional action.

par″a·bux′ine. $C_{24}H_{48}NO$; an alkaloid from *Buxus sempervirens*, the common box shrub.

par·ac″an·tho′ma [G. *para*, near; *akantha*, prickle; *-ōma*, tumor]. A new growth affecting the prickle-cell layer of the skin.

par·ac″an·tho′sis [*para; akantha;* G. *-ōsis*, condition]. A process characterized by some anomaly of the prickle-cell layer of the epidermis.

par″a·ca·ri′nal [*para;* L. *carina*, keel]. Beside a carina, especially the urethral carina.

par″a·car′mine (par″uh·kahr′min, ·myne). A staining solution containing calcium chloride and carminic acid in 75% alcohol.

par″a·ca′se·in. A digestion product of casein, formed through the action of rennin.

par′a·cele [G. *para*, beside; *koilia*, cavity]. Old term for the lateral ventricle of the brain.

Paracelsus (Aureolus Philippus Theophrastus) (Bombastus ab Hohenheim) [*Swiss physician, chemist, and reformer*, 1493–1541]. Regarded by many as the pioneer of modern chemists. Suggested the hereditary transmission of syphilis (1529). Recommended mercury in the treatment of syphilis, or, as he called it, French gonorrhea. Noted association of cretinism and exophthalmic goiter. The use of chemical agents alone in treating disease is known as the *Paracelsian method.*

par″a·cen·te′sis [G. *parakentēsis*, a tapping]. Puncture; especially the puncture or tapping of the wall of a cavity by means of a hollow needle or trochar, to draw off the contained fluid.

abdominal p. Puncture of the abdominal wall with an abdominal trochar and cannula, usually for the relief of ascites.

p. bulbi. Surgical puncture of the eye.

p. oculi. Surgical puncture of the eye.

p. of the bladder. The puncture of the urinary bladder wall with a vesical trochar for the relief of obstruction or to provide constant drainage.

p. of the chest. The insertion of a needle or trochar into the pleural cavity for the relief of pleural effusion.

p. of the pericardium. The insertion of a hollow needle into the pericardium in pericarditis with effusion.

p. of the tympanum. The insertion of a paracentesis needle or knife through the tympanic membrane, for the relief of otitis media.

par″a·cen′tral [G. *para*, near; *kentron*, center of a circle]. Situated near the center, as paracentral lobule.

par″a·ceph′a·lus [G. *para*, beside; *kephalē*, head]. A placental parasitic twin (omphalosite) characterized by a rudimentary, misshapen head and defective trunk and limbs.

par″a·cer″a·to′sis. Parakeratosis.

par″a·cet·al′de·hyde. See *paraldehyde.*

par″a·chlor·phe′nol. $C_6H_4(Cl)OH$. A substitution product of phenol. It is antiseptic, disinfectant, and is employed in a 2% to 3% ointment in erysipelas. Also spelled *parachlorophenol.*

p. paste. A paste of equal parts of lanolin, petrolatum, starch, and parachlorphenol; it is used in lupus.

par″a·chol′er·a (par″uh·kol′ur·uh) [G. *para*, near; *cholera*, cholera]. A disease resembling Asiatic cholera but caused by a different organism.

par″a·cho′li·a (par″uh·ko′lee·uh) [G. *para*, beyond; *cholē*, bile]. 1. Any abnormality in the secretion of bile. 2. The prodrome of disturbed liver-cell activity, in consequence of which bile is present in the blood and lymph.

par″a·chor′dal (par″uh·kor′dul) [G. *para*, beside; *chordē*, string]. 1. Adjoining the cephalochord; situated at the side of the cranial part of the notochord of the embryo. 2. Pertaining to the cartilaginous basis of the cranium in the embryo.

par″a·chor′dal. One of two bars of cartilage extending alongside the cephalic notochord in the human fetus. Also called *parachordalia.*

par″a·chro′ma [G. *para*, beyond; *chrōma*, color]. Change in color, as of the skin.

par″a·chro′ma·tism [*para; chrōma*]. False, or incorrect, perception of color, not true colorblindness, which it may approach more or less completely.

par″a·chro″ma·to·blep′si·a. See *parachromatism.*

par″a·chro″ma·top′si·a [*para; chrōma;* G. *opsis*, vision]. Colorblindness.

par″a·chro″ma·to′sis. See *parachroma.*

par″a·chro′mo·phore [*para; chrōma;* G. *phoros*, bearing]. Pigment excreted or retained either within cells or in the capsule surrounding the cell. It is not an integral part of the cytoplasm of the cell. The term is applied to bacteria and fungi. —**parachromophor′ic, parachromophor′ous,** *adj.*

par·ac′me (par·ack′mee) [*para;* G. *akmē*, highest point]. 1. The degeneration or decadence of a group of organisms after they have reached their acme of development. 2. The period of decline of a disease.

Par″a·coc·cid″i·oi′des (par″uh·cock·sid″ee·oy′deez) [G. *para*, near; *kokkos*, berry; *eidos*, form]. See *Blastomyces.*

P. brasiliensis. See *Blastomyces brasiliensis.*

par″a·coc·cid″i·oi″do·my·co′sis (par″uh·cock·sid″ee·oy″do·migh·ko′sis) [*para; kokkos; eidos;* G. *mykēs*, fungus; *-ōsis*, condition]. South American blastomycosis.

par′a·coele (par′uh·seel). See *paracele.*

par″a·co·li′tis [G. *para*, beside; *kolon*, colon; *-itis*, inflammation]. Inflammation of the tissue adjacent to the colon, not covered by peritoneum.

par″a·co′lon [*para; kolon*]. A group of bacteria intermediate between the *Escherichia-Aerobacter* genera and the *Salmonella-Shigella* group. Culturally, these organisms may be confused with the nonlactose-fermenting pathogenic bacteria found in the intestinal tract. Some of the paracolon bacilli probably produce disease.

par″a·col·pi′tis [*para;* G. *kolpos*, vagina; *-itis*, inflammation]. Inflammation of the connective tissue about the vagina.

par″a·col′pi·um [*para; kolpos*]. The connective tissue about the vagina.

par″a·con′dy·lar [*para;* G. *kondylos*, knuckle]. Situated alongside a condyle or a condylar region.

par'a·cone [*para;* G. *kōnos,* cone]. The mesiobuccal cusp of an upper molar tooth.

par"a·con'id, par"a·co'nid [*para; kōnos*]. The mesiolingual cusp of a lower molar tooth.

par"a·co'to [*para;* Pg. *cotó-cotó*]. A South American tree, *Ocotea pseudocoto* of the Lauraceae, the bark of which contains a neutral substance, paracotoin.

par"a·co'to·in (par"uh·ko'to·in, ·ko·to'in). $C_{12}H_8O_4$. A crystalline substance obtained from paracoto bark; closely resembles cotoin in physiologic action.

par"a·cre'sol. C_7H_8O. One of the three isomeric forms of cresol.

par"a·cu'si·a (par"a cue'zhuh, ·see·uh), **par"a·cu'sis** (par"a cue'sis) [G. *parakousis,* defect of hearing]. Any perversion of the sense of hearing.

p. acris. Excessively acute hearing, rendering the person intolerant of sounds.

p. duplicata. A condition in which all or only certain sounds are heard double.

p. imaginaria. Tinnitus.

p. localis. Difficulty in estimating the direction of sounds, met with in unilateral deafness, or when the two ears hear unequally.

p. obtusa. Difficulty in hearing.

p. Willisii. A condition of deafness in which the hearing is better in a noisy place, as in a train or factory.

par"a·cy·e'sis (par"uh·sigh·ee'sis) [G. *para,* beyond; *kyēsis,* pregnancy]. Extrauterine pregnancy.

par"a·cys'tic [G. *para,* beside; *kystis,* bladder]. Situated near, or alongside, the urinary bladder.

par"a·cys·ti'tis [*para; kystis;* G. *-itis,* inflammation]. Inflammation of the connective tissue surrounding the urinary bladder.

par"a·cy'tic (par"uh·sigh'tick) [*para;* G. *kytos,* cell]. Lying among cells.

par"a·de·ni'tis [*para;* G. *adēn,* gland; *-itis,* inflammation]. Inflammation of the areolar tissue about a gland.

par"a·den'tal [*para;* L. *dens,* tooth]. Near, or beside, a tooth.

par"a·den·to'sis. See *periodontosis.*

par"a·di"ag·no'sis [G. *para,* near; *diagnōsis,* a distinguishing]. A diagnosis that is almost correct.

par"a-di·chlo"ro·ben'zene. $C_6H_4Cl_2$; colorless or white crystals, insoluble in water, soluble in various organic liquids: used to kill moths and their larvae, also certain other insects.

par"a·did'y·mis [*para;* G. *didymos,* testis]. The atrophic remains of the paragenital tubules of the mesonephros, which separate from the mesonephric duct and lie near the convolutions of the epididymal duct. Also called *organ of Giraldès.*

paradione. Trade-marked name for *paramethadione.*

par"a·diph·the'ri·al, par"a·diph"the·rit'ic [*para;* G. *diphthera,* leather]. Remotely or indirectly related to diphtheria.

par"a·dis·tem'per. See hard *pad.*

par"a·dox'i·a sex"u·al'is. Sexual excitement occurring independently of the period of the physiologic processes in the generative organs; the abnormal exhibition of sexual instincts in childhood, prior to puberty, or in the senile years.

par"a·du"o·de'nal (par"uh·dew"o·dee'nul, ·dew·od'i·nul) [G. *para,* beside; L. *duodeni,* twelve]. On either side of the duodenum, as the paraduodenal mesenteric recess.

par"a·dys'en·ter"y [G. *para,* near; *dysenteria,* dysentery]. A mild form of dysentery.

par"a·ep'i·lep"sy [*para;* G. *epilēpsis,* epileptic fit]. An abortive epileptic attack, consisting only of the aura.

par"a-e·ryth'ro·blast. An erythroblast with indented rather than spheroidal nuclei.

par'af·fin. 1. Any saturated hydrocarbon having the formula C_nH_{2n+2}. These compounds constitute the **paraffin series.** Also called *alkane.* 2. (*paraffinum*). A purified mixture of solid hydrocarbons obtained from petroleum; occurs as a white, more or less translucent, mass, showing a crystalline structure; it is insoluble in water and alcohol, but freely soluble in ether. *In pharmacy,* it is used chiefly to give stiffness to ointments.

chlorinated p. (*paraffinum chlorinatum*). A liquid paraffin which has been treated with chlorine; occurs as a light yellow to light amber, clear, thick, oily liquid; immiscible with water, slightly miscible with alcohol. It is used solely as a solvent for dichloramine-T. Solutions up to 8% may be prepared. The chlorine contained in the preparation is therapeutically without action. See *chlorcosane.* Also see *parresine.*

light liquid p. See light liquid *petrolatum.*

liquid p. See liquid *petrolatum.*

par"af·fi·no'ma [L. *parum,* too little; *affinis,* akin; G. *-ōma,* tumor]. A nodular mass of inflammatory, granulation, or scar tissue, due to injection of paraffin into the tissues.

par"a·floc'cu·lus [G. *para,* beside; dim. from L. *floccus,* flock of wool]. A small lobule of the cerebellum found in mammals other than man.

par'a·form. See *paraformaldehyde.*

par"a·form·al'de·hyde. $(CH_2O)_n$. A polymer of formaldehyde, or, more properly, a mixture of polyoxymethylenes, as there are many formaldehyde groups involved in the polymerization. It is formed when solutions of formaldehyde are allowed to evaporate; occurs as a white, friable mass or a white powder with a slight odor of formaldehyde, slowly soluble in cold water, insoluble in alcohol. It is employed as a convenient form for generating small quantities of formaldehyde gas for disinfecting purposes. Also called *paraform, trioxymethylene.*

Par"a·fos·sar'u·lus. A genus of snails, species of which are known to transmit the trematode parasite *Clonorchis sinensis.*

par"a·fuch'sin (par"uh·fo͝ok'sin, ·fo͝ok'sin). See *pararosaniline.*

par"a·gam'ma·cism, par"a·gam"ma·cis'mus [G. *para,* beyond; *gamma,* third letter of the Greek alphabet]. Inability to pronounce the hard *g* and *k,* other consonants being substituted.

par"a·gan"gli·o'ma [G. *para,* beside; *gagglion,* encysted tumor on a tendon; *-ōma,* tumor]. A nonfunctioning tumor derived from the paraganglionic cells of the sympathetic and parasympathetic nervous systems, having the same structure as pheochromocytoma, but composed of cells of less bizarre appearance and without chromaffin granules in the cytoplasm. The tumors are encapsulated and highly vascular. They may be located in the adrenal medulla, retroperitoneal and mediastinal ganglia, in the carotid body, in connection with the glossopharyngeal nerve and its branches in the middle ear, ganglion nodosum in the vagus nerve, tumors of the ciliary ganglion, and, doubtfully, in Zuckerkandl's bodies. Also see *pheochromocytoma.*

functioning p. See *pheochromocytoma.*

nonchromaffin p. See carotid body *tumor.*

nonchromaffin p. of the middle ear. See glomus jugulare *tumor.*

par"a·gan'gli·on ca·rot'i·cum. See carotid body *tumor.*

par"a·gan"gli·o·neu·ro'ma. See *paraganglioma.*

par"a·gan'gli·ons [*para; gagglion*]. Groups of paraganglionic or chromaffin cells scattered along the ventral surface of the aorta, especially in the fetus. Also called *abdominal paraganglions of Zuckerkandl.*

par″a·gan′gli·on tym·pan′i·cum. See glomus jugulare *tumor*.

par″a·gen″i·tal′is [*para;* L. *genitalis*, genital]. The functional part of the mesonephros caudal to the genital part in lower vertebrates, or in the embryo of higher vertebrates. In higher forms, it persists as the vestigial paradidymis or paroophoron.

par″a·geu′si·a (par″ug·yōō′see·uh, par″uh·jew′-see·uh), **par″a·geu′sis** (par″ug·yōō′sis, par″uh-jew′sis) [G. *para*, beyond; G. *geusis*, sense of taste]. Perversion of the sense of taste. —**parageusic,** *adj.*

par″ag·glu″ti·na′tion [G. *para*, beside; L. *agglutinare*, to glue]. Agglutination of colon bacilli and cocci with the serum of patients infected with or recovering from infection with dysentery bacilli. The property of paragglutination disappears when the bacteria are subcultured.

par″a·glos′sa [*para;* G. *glōssa*, tongue]. Swelling of the tongue; a hypertrophy of the tongue, usually congenital.

par″a·glos′si·a [*para; glōssa*]. Inflammation of the muscles and connective tissues under the tongue.

par″a·gnath′ous [*para;* G. *gnathos*, jaw]. 1. Having upper and lower jaws of equal length, their tips falling together, as in certain birds. 2. Pertaining to paragnathus.

par″a·gnath′us [*para; gnathos*]. 1. An individual having a supernumerary jaw. 2. A parasitic fetus or part attached to the jaw laterally. See *epignathus*.

par″a·gom·pho′sis [*para;* G. *gomphōsis*, a bolting together]. Impaction of the fetal head in the pelvic canal.

par″a·go″ni·mi′a·sis [*para;* G. *gonimos*, generative; NL. *-iasis*, condition]. The condition of being infested by species of the genus *Paragonimus*, especially *P. westermani*.

Par″a·gon′i·mus [*para; gonimos*]. A genus of trematode worms.

P. westermani. Species of lung flukes which in the adult stage cause tissue destruction, inflammation, and hemorrhage.

par″a·gram′ma·tism [G. *paragrammizein*, to alter by changing a letter]. Aphasia marked by inability to speak grammatically, or by the use of improper words.

par″a·gran″u·lo′ma. A term used only as *Hodgkin's paragranuloma*. See Hodgkin's *disease*.

par″a·graph′i·a (par″uh·graf′ee·uh, ·gray′fee·uh) [G. *para*, beyond; *graphein*, to write]. 1. Perverted writing; a form of aphasia in which letters or words are misplaced or improperly used. 2. A loss of ability to express ideas in writing, usually the result of a brain lesion. —**paragraphic,** *adj.*

par″a·he″mo·phil′i·a. A hemorrhagic disorder characterized by a deficiency of proaccelerin. Syn., *Owren's disease*.

par″a·he·pat′ic [G. *para*, near; *hēpar*, liver]. About or near the liver.

par″a·hep″a·ti′tis [*para; hēpar;* G. *-itis*, inflammation]. Inflammation of structures about or near the liver.

par″a·hex′yl. Synhexyl.

par″a·hor′mone [*para;* G. *hormaein*, to excite]. A waste product which exerts a secondary stimulating action.

par″a·hy·drox″y·ben·zo′ic ac′id (par″uh·high-drock″see·). $C_6H_4.OH.COOH$. An isomer of salicylic acid; its esters are powerful antiseptics used to preserve various medicinal products.

par″a·hyp·no′sis [G. *para*, beyond; *hypnos*, sleep; *-ōsis*, condition]. Abnormal sleep, as that of hypnotism or of narcosis.

par″a·in″flu·en′za [G. *para*, near; It. *influenza*, influence]. 1. Similar to influenza; conditions due to influenza. 2. *In bacteriology*, organisms having all but a few of the growth characteristics of *Hemophilus influenzae*. —**parainfluenzal,** *adj.*

par″a·ker″a·to′sis [*para;* G. *keras*, horn; *-ōsis*]. The retention of nuclei in the stratum corneum of the epidermis. Usually associated with some inflammation in the prickle-cell layer, resulting in a disturbance in the process of keratinization. Occurs normally in the stratified squamous epithelium of true mucous membranes.

p. gonorrheica. See *keratosis* blennorrhagica.

p. scutularis. A condition believed to be a very rare and unusual form of psoriasis.

p. variegata. A retiform type of parapsoriasis that is an intermediate between lichen planus and psoriasis; a chronic disease with hyperemia in a patchy network.

par″a·lac′tic ac′id. Sarcolactic acid.

par″a·la′li·a [G. *para*, beyond; *lalia*, talk]. Disturbance of the faculty of speech, characterized by distortion of sounds.

par″al·bu′min [*para;* L. *albus*, white]. A protein substance found in ovarian cysts.

par·al′de·hyde (*paraldehydum*). $(CH_3COH)_3$. A polymer of acetaldehyde, occurring as a colorless, transparent liquid, with a strong characteristic odor and a disagreeable taste; 1 cc. dissolves in 8 cc. of water; miscible with alcohol, ether, and chloroform. Used as a somnifacient where rapid action is desired. A disadvantage is the unpleasant odor it imparts to the breath. Dose, 2–6 cc. (30–60 minims). Syn., *paracetaldehyde*.

par″a·lep·ro′sis [G. *para*, near; *leprōsis*, leprosy]. Attenuated or modified form of leprosy.

par′a·lep″sy [*para;* G. *lēpsis*, a seizing]. Psycholepsy.

par″a·le·re′ma [*para;* G. *lērēma*, silly talk]. Mild delirium or delirious utterance.

par″a·le·re′sis [G., delirium]. Mild delirium, or moderate mental disturbance.

par″a·lex′i·a [G. *para*, beyond; G. *lexis*, speech]. Disturbance in reading, marked by the substitution or transposition of words or syllables. —**paralexic,** *adj.*

par″al·ge′si·a (par″al·jee′zee·uh, ·see·uh) [*para;* G. *algos*, pain]. An abnormal, painful sensation; painful paresthesia. —**paralgesic,** *adj.*

par·al′gi·a [*para; algos*]. Any perverted and disagreeable cutaneous sensation, as of formication, cold, or burning.

par′al·lax [G., in turn]. The apparent displacement of an object, caused by a change in the position of the observer, or by looking at the object alternately first with one eye and then with the other. —**parallac′tic,** *adj.*

binocular p. The angle of convergence of the visual axes.

crossed p. That in which the object moves away from the uncovered eye. Also called *heteronymous p.*

homonymous p. That in which the object moves toward the uncovered eye.

mental p. A slight personal equation in observation, due to one's standpoint.

stereoscopic p. See binocular *p.*

vertical p. That in which the object moves upward or downward.

par′al·lel·ism [G. *para*, beside; *allēlōn*, of one another]. 1. The state or condition of being parallel; the quality of being similar or of corresponding. 2. See *isopathy*.

p. of disease. The tendency of some diseases to simulate others.

par″al·lel·om′e·ter [*para; allēlōn;* G. *metron*, a measure]. *In dentistry*, an instrument used for paralleling attachments and abutments for bridges.

pa·ral′ler·gy [*para;* G. *allos,* other; *ergon,* work]. Sensitivity to nonspecific proteins, induced by specific sensitization.

par″a·lo′gi·a [G., false form]. Difficulty in thinking logically.

thematic p. A condition in which the thought is unduly concentrated on one subject.

pa·ral′o·gism [G. *para,* beyond; *logos,* word]. *In logic,* the error of considering effects or unrelated phenomena as the cause of a condition. —**paralo·gis′tic,** *adj.*

par″a·lu′te·in cells. The epithelioid cells of the corpus luteum, derived from the theca interna of the ovarian follicle. Also called *theca lutein cells.*

par′a·ly″sant (par′uh·lye″zunt). See *paralyzant.*

pa·ral′y·sis [G.]. Loss of muscle function or of sensation, caused by injury to nerves or by destruction of neurons. A slight loss of function is called *palsy.* Paralyses may be classified according to etiology, as *alcoholic* or *lead;* according to part involved, as *facial* or *hypoglossal;* according to function, as *flaccid* or *spastic;* or according to some characteristic, as *ascending* or *crossed.*

abducens p. Paralysis of the abducens nerve.

abductor p. Paralysis of the posterior cricoarytenoid muscle. Also called *posticus p.*

accommodation p. Paralysis of the ciliary muscles of the eye.

acute ascending p. A syndrome of varied etiology, characterized by flaccid paralysis beginning in the muscles of the legs and spreading upward to involve the muscles of the arms and other parts of the body. It may occur in anterior poliomyelitis, postvaccinal or postexanthematous myelitis. Also called *Landry's p.*

alcoholic p. That due to alcoholic neuropathy.

alternating p. Paralysis due to injury of various cranial nerves or their nuclei on one side, with a contralateral hemiplegia.

ambiguospinothalamic p. A unilateral paralysis of the soft palate and larynx with contralateral loss of deep sensibility and of pain and temperature sense: also called *Avellis' syndrome.*

amyotrophic p. That seen in muscular atrophy.

anapeiratic p. A neurosis in which the subject believes he is paralyzed from excessive use of his limbs.

anterior spinal p. Anterior poliomyelitis.

arsenical p. Paresthesia and peripheral neuritis developing in the later stages of arsenic poisoning.

ascending p. Paralysis progressing upward, due to involvement of spinal nerves or the spinal cord.

associated p. A common paralysis or spasm of associated muscles.

axillary p. Paralysis of the axillary nerve resulting in the loss of function of the deltoid muscle; usually due to fracture or dislocation of the humerus, or to pressure from a crutch.

basal ganglionic p. One due to destruction of cells in the basal ganglions.

Bell's p. Peripheral paralysis of the facial nerve.

birth p. Paralysis caused by injury of the brain or brachial plexus during birth.

brachial p. Paralysis of an arm.

brachiofacial p. Paralysis involving the face and arm.

Brown-Séquard's p. Ipsilateral motor paralysis and contralateral loss of sensation for pain and temperature, due to a unilateral lesion of the spinal cord such as compression by a tumor or traumatic hemisection.

bulbar p. See progressive bulbar *p.*

capsular p. That due to an injury of the internal capsule.

central p. Paralysis due to a lesion of the brain or spinal cord.

cerebral p. That due to a lesion of the brain.

cerebral spastic infantile p. See spastic *diplegia.*

cervical sympathetic p. See Horner's *syndrome.*

circumflex p. See axillary *p.*

compression p. That caused by pressure on a nerve.

conjugate p. Lack of coordinate movements of the eyes, such as inability of both eyes to track concomitantly a moving object across the field of vision.

crossed p. Paralysis of the arm and leg of one side, associated with contralateral paralysis of the face or oculomotor nerve.

cruciate p. Crossed *p.*

crural p. Paralysis involving chiefly the thigh.

crutch p. Paralysis of the muscles of the upper extremity, due to traumatic neuritis of the brachial plexus and especially of the radial nerve from pressure of the crutch head.

diphtheritic p. That due to the effect of diphtheria toxin upon some part of the nervous system, usually the motor components of the cranial nerves or the motor nerves to the extremities.

diver's p. See caisson *disease.*

epidural ascending spinal p. A low-grade inflammation of the dura associated with thrombophlebitis of the meningorachidian veins; characterized by pain in the back, chest, or legs, followed by paralysis, loss of sensibility, and incontinence. Also called *Spiller's syndrome.*

Erb-Duchenne p. Paralysis of the fifth and sixth cervical nerve roots, involving chiefly the functions of the biceps, deltoid, brachialis, and brachioradialis muscles.

Erb's syphilitic p. See Wilhelm Heinrich *Erb.*

essential p. Paralysis without characteristic anatomic lesions.

extraocular p. That involving the extrinsic muscles of the eye.

facial p. Paralysis of the muscles of expression of the face. There are two types, the central or supranuclear type, and the peripheral or infranuclear type.

familial periodic p. A hereditary disease of unknown etiology; characterized by periodic attacks of flaccid muscular paralysis, which develop abruptly and last from a few hours to several days.

flaccid p. A condition in which a muscle manifests loss of muscular tone, diminished or absent tendon reflexes, and, eventually, atrophy and the electric reaction of degeneration.

functional motor p. See hysterical *p.*

functional p. See hysterical *p.*

general p. See general *paresis.*

general p. of the insane. See general *paresis.*

ginger p. A polyneuritis or acroneuropathy caused by the adulteration of liquor with triorthocresylphosphate. The neural involvement is almost purely motor in distribution, involving the distal portions of the legs and arms.

glossolabial p. Paralysis of the tongue and lips in bulbar paralysis.

glossolabiopharyngeal p. One involving the tongue, lips, and pharynx, occurring in bulbar palsy. Also called *labioglossopharyngeal p.*

hysterical p. Muscle weakness or paralysis without loss of reflex activity, in which no organic nerve lesion can be demonstrated.

infantile p. Poliomyelitis; especially, acute anterior poliomyelitis.

infantile spastic p. See spastic *diplegia.*

infectious bulbar p. An acute virus disease of cattle characterized by a short incubation period, intense itching, paralysis of the larnyx and eyes, and a rapid course. It may also occur in suckling pigs. dogs, cats, horses, and rats. Syn., *pseudorabies, Aujeszky's disease, mad itch.*

infranuclear p. Paralysis of the motor function of a cranial nerve, due to a lesion of the nerve peripheral to its nucleus.

ischemic p. That of a part due to stoppage of the circulation, as in certain cases of embolism or thrombosis, or in Volkmann's paralysis.

jake p. Paralysis due to peripheral neuritis, caused by the ingestion of Jamaica ginger.

Jamaica ginger p. See jake *p.*

juvenile p. General paralysis in young persons.

Landry's p. See acute ascending *p.*

lead p. One due to peripheral neuritis from lead poisoning.

mimetic p. Paralysis of the facial muscles.

mixed p. Associated motor and sensory paralysis.

motor p. The loss of voluntary control of skeletal muscle, due to functional or organic interruption at any point in the motor pathway from the cerebral cortex to, and including, the muscle fiber.

myopathic p. That in which the interruption of voluntary control is in the muscle.

nuclear p. Paralysis from lesions of the nuclei of origin of the nerves.

obstetric p. One due to injury of some part of the nervous system at birth.

occupational p. Muscular weakness and atrophy due to nerve compression or overexertion in certain occupations.

ocular p. Paralysis of the extraocular muscles, of the optic nerve, or of the ciliary muscle.

oculomotor p. Paralysis of the oculomotor nerve, due to lesions.

oculophrenicorecurrent p. That of the recurrent laryngeal and phrenic nerves with associated Horner's syndrome, such as may occur in cancer of the lung with mediastinal extension.

p. agitans. See idiopathic *parkinsonism.*

periodic p. A recurrent paralysis. Also see familial periodic *p.*

peripheral p. Paralysis due to any disease of peripheral nerves.

phonetic p. Paralysis of the vocal folds.

postdiphtheritic p. Paralysis which may occur when the other symptoms of diphtheria are diminishing, usually during the two months following the acute phase of the disease. It may affect the ciliary muscles, the palate, the respiratory muscles, or the extremities. Respiratory failure is the most serious consequence.

postdormital p. Transient paralysis at the end of sleep, with spontaneous recovery, often associated with narcolepsy.

predormital p. Transient paralysis at the beginning of sleep, with spontaneous recovery, often associated with narcolepsy.

pressure p. That due to pressure on a nerve trunk.

progressive bulbar p. Progressive and symmetrical paralysis of the muscles of the tongue, throat, face, and sometimes of the larynx, due to degenerative changes in the motor nuclei of the medulla oblongata.

pseudobulbar p. Symmetrical disease of both cerebral hemispheres, involving the centers or paths of the tracts to cranial nerves in the brain stem; resembles disease of the medulla oblongata and causes voluntary paralysis of swallowing, articulation, and chewing movements, with retention of bulbar reflexes.

pseudohypertrophic muscular p. Loss or diminution of the power of motion, accompanied by enlarged, and apparently hypertrophied, muscles. The most important type is progressive muscular dystrophy, also called *Landouzy-Dejerine p.*

Saturday night p. Paralysis due to compression of the radial nerve against the humerus during sleep, or when the arm is hung over the edge of a chair or bench during alcoholic stupor.

sensory p. Loss of sensation due to disease of sensory nerves, pathways, or centers in the nervous system.

spastic p. A condition in which a group of muscles manifest increased tone, exaggerated tendon reflexes, depressed or absent superficial reflexes, and sometimes clonus.

spinal p. A central paralysis caused by injury to the spinal cord.

supranuclear p. That of the motor function of a nerve, due to a lesion in pathways or centers above its nucleus or cells of origin.

tegmental mesencephalic p. See Benedikt *syndrome.*

tick-bite p. A flaccid type of paralysis occurring in animals, and occasionally in man, during the attachment of a tick. The paralysis will disappear a few hours after removal of the tick. The cause is unknown, but it is thought to be a toxin generated in the tick. Syn., *tick p.*

Todd's p. A temporary paralysis which sometimes follows a focal Jacksonian convulsive seizure.

tourniquet p. Pressure paralysis caused by too long application of a tourniquet to a limb while checking hemorrhage. It is most common in the nerves of the arm.

vagoaccessory-hypoglossal p. See under John H. *Jackson.*

vasomotor p. Paralysis of the vasomotor mechanism with resultant atony and dilatation of the blood vessels.

vestibular p. Loss of vestibular function, often caused by streptomycin therapy, manifested by vertigo, aural noises, headache, nausea, and vomiting, followed by disturbances of gait, posture, and vision.

Volkmann's p. Paralysis of a hand due to constriction of the blood supply when tight splints or casts are applied to the forearm. See ischemic *p.*

Weber's crossed p. See Hermann David *Weber.*

writer's p. Writer's cramp, a form of occupational neurosis.

par″a·lyt′ic [G. *paralytikos*, paralytic]. Pertaining to, or affected with, paralysis.

par″a·lyt′ic. A person affected with paralysis.

par′a·ly″zant, par′a·ly″sant (par′uh·lye″zunt) [G. *paralysis*, paralysis]. Causing paralysis. —**par′alyzant, par′alysant,** *n.*

par′a·ly″zer [*paralysis*]. 1. Anything that will produce paralysis. 2. Any agent which will inhibit a chemical reaction.

par″a·mag·net′ic [G. *para*, beyond; *Magnētis lithos*, magnet]. Having a magnetic permeability greater than unity. —**paramag′netism,** *n.*

paramammary route of Gerota. See Dumitru *Gerota.*

par″a·mas·ti′tis [G. *para*, beside; *mastos*, breast; *-itis*, inflammation]. Inflammation of the connective tissue about the mammary gland.

par″a·mas″toid·i′tis [*para*; G. *mastoeidēs*, like a breast; *-itis*]. Inflammation of the squamous portion of the temporal bone, from extension following mastoiditis.

Par″a·me′ci·um (par″uh·mee′shee·um, ·see·um) [G. *paramēkēs*, oblong]. A genus of ciliate Protozoa, various species of which are used as test and experimental unicellular animals, because of their large size and ease of culture. Commonly called the "slipper animalcule."

par″a·me′di·an [G. *para*, near; L. *medianus*, middle]. Situated near the median line, as paramedian sulcus, old term for a fissure present in the cervical portion of the spinal cord, not far from the posterior median fissure, and separating the fasciculus gracilis from the fasciculus cuneatus.

par″a·me′ni·a [G. *para*, beyond; *mēn*, month]. Difficult or disordered menstruation.

pa·ram′e·ter [G. *para*, beside; *metron*, a measure]. An arbitrary constant which characterizes a mathematical expression by its values.

par″a·meth″a·di′one. Generic name for 3,5-dimethyl-5-ethyloxazolidine-2,4-dione; $C_7H_{11}NO_3$; a colorless liquid sparingly soluble in water, used in the treatment of petit mal epilepsy. See *paradione*.

par″a·met′ric (par″uh·met′rick, ·mee′trick) [*para;* G. *mētra*, womb]. Pertaining to the tissues about the uterus.

par″a·met′rism [*para; mētra*]. Painful spasm of the smooth muscular fibers of the broad ligaments.

par″a·me·tri′tis [*para; mētra;* G. *-itis*, inflammation]. Inflammation of the connective tissue about the uterus; pelvic cellulitis. —**parametrit′ic,** *adj.*

p. anterior. That in which the inflammation is limited to the loose, vesicouterine connective tissue, or to that between the symphysis and the bladder. The swelling is anterior, and the pus generally tracks into the bladder, vagina, or inguinal region.

p. chronica atrophicans. Inflammatory hypertrophy of the connective tissue of the pelvis, progressing to cicatricial atrophy.

p. chronica posterior. Chronic, inflammatory processes in the rectouterine ligaments, causing fixation of the uterus at the level of the internal os, anteflexion by shortening of the folds, and torsion of the uterus when only one fold is shortened.

remote p. Parametritis marked by formation of abscesses in places more or less remote from the focus of the disease.

par″a·me′tri·um [*para; mētra*]. The connective tissue surrounding the uterus. —**parametrial,** *adj.*

par″a·me·trop′a·thy [*para; mētra;* G. *pathos*, disease]. Disease of the parametrium.

par″a·mim′i·a [G. *paramimeisthai*, to imitate]. A form of aphasia characterized by the faulty use of gestures.

par″a·mi′tome [G. *para*, beside; *mitos*, thread]. The fluid portion of the cell substance contained in the meshes of the mitome.

par″am·ne′si·a (par″am·nee′zhuh, ·zee·uh) [G. *para*, beyond; *amnēsia*, forgetfulness]. Perversion of memory, in which experiences and phantasies are confused.

par″a·mo′lar [*para;* L. *molaris*, from *mola*, mill]. A usually peg-shaped, occasionally molariform, supernumerary tooth occurring next to the mesiobuccal aspect of a second or third molar.

p. tubercle. An accessory lobe or cusp on the mesiobuccal side of a second or third molar tooth, believed to represent a rudimentary paramolar.

par″a·mon″o·chlor·phe′nol. See *parachlorphenol.*

par″a·mor′phine (par″uh·mor′feen, ·fin, par″uh-mor·feen′). See *thebaine.*

par″a·mor′phism. *In chemistry*, a change of molecular structure without alteration of chemical constitution, as when a mineral changes from one modification to another. —**paramorphic,** *adj.*

par″a·mu′cin. A colloid isolated from ovarian cysts; it differs from mucin and pseudomucin by reducing Fehling's solution before boiling with acid.

par″a·mu′si·a (par″uh·mew′zhuh, ·zee·uh) [G. *paramousos*, discordant with]. A form of aphasia in which there is perversion of the musical sense, resulting in the production of improper notes and intervals.

par″a·my′e·lo·blast″. A myeloblast with an indented rather than spheroidal nucleus, present in some acute leukemias.

par·am′y·loid. Atypical amyloid.

par″a·my·oc′lo·nus mul′ti·plex (par″uh·migh-ock′lo·nus, ·migh″o·klo′nus). A rare degenerative disease occurring in adult life manifested by irregular rapid muscular twitching (myoclonic shocks). The seat of the disease is in the basal ganglions.

par″a·my″o·sin′o·gen [G. *para*, near; *mys*, muscle; *genesthai*, from *gignesthai*, to be produced]. One of the proteins of muscle plasma, coagulating at 47° C.

par″a·my″o·to′ni·a con·gen′i·ta. A rare, heredofamilial condition characterized by persistent contraction of the muscles of the neck, face, and extremities when the body is exposed to cold. Also called *Eulenburg's disease.*

par″a·na′sal (par″uh·nay′zul) [*para;* L. *nasus*, nose]. Located next to, or near, the nasal cavities.

par″a·ne·phri′tis [G. *para*, beside; *nephros*, kidney; *-itis*, inflammation]. 1. Inflammation of the adrenal gland. 2. Inflammation of the connective tissue adjacent to the kidney.

par″a·neph′ros [*para; nephros*]. Old term for adrenal gland.

par″a·neu′ral [*para;* G. *neuron*, nerve]. Beside or near a nerve, as paraneural analgesia, analgesia resulting from injection of an analgesic solution into the immediate vicinity of a nerve trunk.

pa·ran′gi (pa·ran′jee, pa·rang′ghee). See *yaws.*

par″a-ni″tro·sul″fa·thi′a·zole. $C_9H_7N_3O_4S_2$; a yellow powder, very slightly soluble in water: used intrarectally as an antibacterial agent in treatment of ulcerative colitis. See *nisulfazole.*

par″a·noi′a [G., derangement]. A rare form of paranoid reaction characterized by the slow development of a complex paranoid system, often built upon a delusion, and particularly isolated from much of the normal stream of consciousness, the remaining personality being intact despite a chronic course. The patient generally considers himself superior and possessing unique or even divine gifts. Compare paranoid type of *schizophrenic reaction.* —**paranoid,** *adj.;* **paranoiac,** *adj., n.*

litigious p. That in which the main symptom is a desire to initiate lawsuits which have no rational basis.

par′a·noid·ism [*paranoia*]. The condition of a person affected with paranoia.

par′a·noid per″son·al′i·ty. See under *personality.*

par″a·noid re·ac′tions. See under *reaction.*

par′a·noid state. A form of paranoid reaction characterized by delusions of persecution and sometimes of grandeur, but without the systematization and manifestations of bizarre fragmentation and deterioration of the schizophrenic reaction. Its duration is variable, though usually short.

par″a·no′mi·a. See *aphasia.*

par·an′tral [*para;* L. *antrum*]. Situated near an air sinus, as an accessory air cell of a paranasal or mastoid sinus.

par″a·nu′cle·in. A compound of nucleic acid and protein, derived either by partial degradation of nucleoproteins or by direct combination. Syn., *nucleoalbumin, paranucleoprotein, pseudonuclein.*

par″a·nu″cle·o·pro′te·in. See *paranuclein.*

par″a·nu′cle·us [G. *para*, beside; L. *nucleus*, kernel]. 1. A small spherical body lying in the cytoplasm of a cell near the nucleus, and perhaps extruded by the latter. 2. A mitochondrial aggregation of a spermatid, which becomes drawn out to form the envelope of the axial filament. Also called *nebenkern.* —**paranuclear, paranucleate,** *adj.*

par″a·ox″y·eth·yl·ac″e·tan′i·lid (·ass″i·tan′i·lid). See *acetophenetidin.*

par″a·pan″cre·at′ic (par″uh·pan″kree·at′ick, ·pang″kree·at′ick) [*para;* G. *pagkreas,* pancreas]. Situated beside or near the pancreas, as parapancreatic abscess.

par″a·pa·re′sis (par″uh·pa·ree′sis, ·par′i·sis) [*para;* G. *paresis,* paralysis]. Partial paralysis of the lower extremities. *Obs.* —**paraparet′ic,** *adj.*

par″a·path′i·a. See *psychoneurosis.*

par″a·pep′tone. See *peptone.*

par″a·per·tus′sis. An acute infection of the respiratory tract resembling pertussis, but caused by such bacteria as *Brucella bronchiseptica, B. abortus,* or *Hemophilus influenzae:* distinguished from pertussis only by bacteriological examination.

par″a·pha′si·a (par″uh·fay′zhuh, ·zee·uh) [*para;* G. *aphasia,* speechlessness]. A form of aphasia in which words are spoken freely but are inappropriate in translating ideas. Syn., *agrammatism, jargon aphasia.* —**paraphasic,** *adj.*

par″a·phe′mi·a [G. *para,* beyond; *phēmē,* speech]. Aphasia marked by employment of wrong words. *Rare.*

par″a·phe″ne·tol·car·bam′ide (·kahr·bam′ide, ·id, ·kahr′buh·mide, ·mid). See *dulcin.*

par″a·phen″yl·ene″di·am′ine. $C_6H_4(NH_2)_2$. A crystalline substance used in the manufacture of certain hair dyes, and giving rise to eczema of the scalp and eyelids, or to poisoning marked by vomiting and diarrhea.

pa·ra′phi·a (pa·ray′fee·uh, pa·raf′ee·uh) [*para;* G. *haphē,* touch]. Abnormality of the sense of touch. *Rare.*

par″a·phil′i·a. Sexual perversion. —**paraphil′iac,** *adj., n.*

par″a·phi·mo′sis (par″uh·figh·mo′sis, ·fi·mo′sis) [G. *para,* beside; *phimōsis,* stopping up of an orifice]. Retraction and constriction, especially of the prepuce behind the glans penis: also called *Spanish collar.*

p. oculi. Retraction of the eyelid behind the eyeball.

par″a·pho′bi·a [G. *para,* near; *phobos,* fear]. A slight degree of phobia; phobia which the person can control by effort.

par″a·pho′ni·a [G. *para,* beyond; *phōnē,* voice]. Any abnormal condition of the voice.

p. puberum. The harsh, deep, irregular voice noticed in boys at puberty.

pa·raph′o·ra [G. *paraphora,* a going aside]. 1. Slight mental derangement or distraction. 2. Unsteadiness due to intoxication.

par″a·phra′si·a (par″uh·fray′zhuh, ·zee·uh) [G. *paraphrasis,* paraphrase]. A form of aphasia characterized by incoherence of speech.

p. vesana. Jumbling of words and ideas.

par″a·phre·ne′sis [G. *para,* beyond; *phrēn,* mind]. Amentia; delirium. *Obs.*

par″a·phre′ni·a [*para; phrēn*]. 1. Old term for paranoia. 2. Dementia precox or schizophrenia.

par″a·phre·ni′tis [*para; phrēn;* G. *-itis,* inflammation]. Inflammation of the tissues adjacent to the diaphragm.

pa·raph′y·sis [G., attachment]. 1. *In biology,* one of sterile filaments among reproductive bodies of various kinds in certain cryptogams. 2. A median outgrowth from the roof of the brain in front of the epiphysis in certain lower vertebrates.

par″a·pla′si·a. See *paraplasm,* 2.

par′a·plasm [G. *paraplasma,* from *para,* beyond; *plasma,* anything formed]. 1. Hyaloplasm. 2. Malformed substance.

par″a·plas′tic [G. *paraplassein,* to transform]. 1. Of the nature of paraplasm. 2. Having morbid formative powers. 3. Misshapen.

par″a·plas′tin [*paraplassein*]. A lininlike substance in the nucleus.

par″a·plec′tic [G. *paraplēktikos,* suffering with hemiplegia]. Pertaining to, or afflicted with, paraplegia.

par″a·ple′gi·a [G. *paraplēgiē,* hemiplegia]. Paralysis of the lower limbs. —**paraplec′tic, parapleg′ic, paraplegiform,** *adj.*

alcoholic p. Paralysis of the legs resulting from alcoholic neuritis.

ataxic p. A slowly progressive degeneration of the posterior and lateral columns of the spinal cord; characterized clinically by spasticity, weakness, and incoordination of the legs.

cerebral p. Paralysis of both legs due to a bilateral cerebral lesion, as in meningioma of the falx, thrombosis of the superior sagittal sinus, or congenital cerebral lesions.

congenital spastic p. Spastic paralysis of the legs in infants, due to a congenital lesion of the brain: also called *infantile spastic p., cerebral diplegia, Little's disease.*

flaccid p. Paralysis of both legs with muscular hypotonia and diminished, or absent, tendon reflexes.

hysterical p. A psychogenic form, due to an emotional upset.

infantile spasmodic p. See double *athetosis.*

p. in extension. Paraplegia with extension of the legs; seen following incomplete transection of the spinal cord.

p. in flexion. Paraplegia with flexion of the legs; seen following complete transection of the spinal cord.

peripheral p. That due to disease of the peripheral nerves.

progressive spastic p. A progressive heredofamilial condition characterized by spastic paralysis of the legs and weakness; due to spinal-cord lesions of the crossed pyramidal tracts.

senile p. Spastic paralysis of the legs due to arteriosclerosis of the arteries supplying the spinal cord.

spastic p. Paralysis of the legs with increased muscular tone and hyperactive tendon reflexes; commonly seen in multiple sclerosis and other diseases involving the pyramidal tracts of the spinal cord, and after birth injury.

par″a·pneu·mo′ni·a [G. *para,* near; *pneumonia*]. A disease presenting the symptoms of lobar pneumonia, but not due to the pneumococcus.

pa·rap′o·plex″y [*para;* G. *apoplēxia,* madness]. A masked or slight form of apoplexy.

par″a·prax′i·a [*para;* G. *praxis,* a doing]. A condition in which certain intentional acts are imperfectly accomplished, as a slip of the tongue.

par″a·proc·ti′tis [G. *para,* beside; *prōktos,* anus; *-itis,* inflammation]. Inflammation of the connective tissue about the rectum.

par″a·proc′ti·um (par″uh·prock′shee·um, ·prock′tee·um) [*para; prōktos*]. The connective tissue that surrounds the rectum.

par″a·pros″ta·ti′tis [*para;* G. *prostatēs,* one who stands before; *-itis,* inflammation]. Inflammation of tissues surrounding the prostate gland.

par″a·pso·ri′a·sis (par″uh·so·rye′uh·sis) [G. *para,* near; *psōriasis,* itch]. A group of rare skin diseases characterized by red, scaly lesions resembling lichen planus or psoriasis. All types are resistant to treatment and usually present no subjective symptoms.

par″a·psy·chol′o·gy [G. *para,* beyond; *psychē,* soul; *logos,* word]. The study of psi phenomena (extrasensory perception and psychokinesis), i.e., of phenomena of personality that do not submit to physical explanation.

par″a·pyk″no·mor′phous [G. *para*, near; *pyknos*, close-packed; *morphē*, form]. Nissl's term for nerve cells in which the arrangement of the stainable portion of the cell body is intermediate between that of pyknomorphous and apyknomorphous cells. *Obs.*

par″a·rec′tal [G. *para*, beside; L. *rectus*, straight]. Beside, or near, the rectum.

par″a·rho′ta·cism. See *rhotacism.*

par″a·ros·an′i·line (par″uh·ros·an′i·leen, ·lin). A basic dyestuff of the triphenylmethane group.

par″a·sa′cral [*para;* L. *os sacrum*, lowest bone of the spine]. Beside, or near, the sacrum.

par″a·sag′it·tal (par″uh·sadj′i·tul) [*para;* L. *sagitta*, arrow]. Referring to any plane parallel and lateral to the sagittal plane.

par″a·sal″pin·gi′tis [*para;* G. *salpigx*, trumpet; *-itis*, inflammation]. Inflammation of the tissues around an oviduct.

par″a·se·cre′tion [G. *para*, beyond; L. *secretio*, from *secernere*, to separate]. Any abnormality of secretion; any substance abnormally secreted.

par″a·sex·u·al′i·ty. Any sexual perversion.

par′a·site [G. *parasitos*, parasite]. 1. An organism that lives on or in another organism known as the host, from which it obtains nourishment during all or part of its existence. 2. *In teratology*, a fetus or fetal parts attached to or included in another fetus. —**parasit′ic,** *adj.*

ectoparasite. See *ectoparasite.*

endoparasite. See *endoparasite.*

facultative p. One capable of being free-living as well as parasitic.

incidental p. One that establishes itself in a host in which it does not ordinarily live.

obligate p. One incapable of living without a host.

occasional p. One which seeks its host periodically to obtain nourishment. Also called *periodic p.*

permanent p. One which remains in or on the body of the host until maturity and sometimes for its entire life.

placental p. See *omphalosite.*

specific p. One which always lives on its present host.

temporary p. One which is free-living during part of its life.

par″a·sit′ic cap′ture. *In nuclear physics*, any absorption of a neutron which does not result either in fission or formation of another element.

par″a·sit′i·cide [*parasitos;* L. *caedere*, to kill]. Destructive to parasites.

par″a·sit′i·cide. An agent capable of destroying parasites, especially the parasites living upon or in the skin.

par″a·sit′i·cin. See *flavicin.*

par′a·sit·ism (par′uh·sigh·tiz·um) [*parasitos*]. Relation a parasite bears to its host; state of being infested or infected with parasites.

par′a·si·tize (par′uh·sigh·tize, par′uh·si·tize) [*parasitos*]. Infest; invade as a parasite.

par″a·si′to- [*parasitos*]. A combining form signifying *parasite.*

par″a·si″to·gen′ic (par″uh·sigh″to·jen′ick) [*parasitos;* G. *genesthai*, from *gignesthai*, to be produced]. 1. Produced by parasites. 2. Favoring parasitism.

par″a·si·tol′o·gy (par″uh·sigh·tol′o·jee) [*parasitos; logos*]. The science and study of organisms that obtain nourishment at the expense of the hosts on or in which they live. —**parasitol′ogist,** *n.*

par″a·si″to·pho′bi·a [*parasitos;* G. *phobos*, fear]. Morbid dread of parasites.

par″a·si·to′sis (par″uh·sigh·to′sis, ·si·to′sis) [*parasitos;* G. *-ōsis*, condition]. Any disease dependent upon the presence of parasites.

par″a·si″to·trop′ic [*parasitos;* G. *trepein*, to turn]. Having a special affinity for parasites.

par″a·si″to·trop′ic. A substance, such as a drug or a chemical agent, with an affinity for parasites. —**parasi′totrope,** *adj., n.;* **parasitot′ropy,** *n.;* **parasitot′ropism,** *n.*

par″a·small′pox [G. *para*, near; AS. *smael; pocc*]. A mild form of smallpox.

par′a·some, par″a·so′ma [*para;* G. *sōma*, body]. An irregular body found in the cytoplasm near the nucleus. See *paranucleus*, 1.

par″a·spa′di·as [G. *paraspaein*, to draw aside]. An acquired condition in which the urethra opens on one side of the penis.

par′a·spasm [G. *paraspasmos*, a drawing sideways]. Spasm involving the lower extremities, as in spastic paraplegia.

par″a-sprue′. A dietary disease characterized by chronic watery diarrhea, weight loss, a sore red tongue, and macrocytic anemia. It differs from true sprue in that it shows less emaciation, no swollen lower abdomen, no dry skin, no dysphagia, and in having pale, frothy stools with the fat content above 40 per cent.

par″a·ste″a·to′sis [G. *para*, beyond; *stear*, fat; *-ōsis*, condition]. An altered condition of the sebaceous secretion.

par″a·ster′nal [G. *para*, beside; *sternon*, chest]. Beside or near the sternum, as parasternal line.

par″a·sym″pa·thet′ic [*para;* G. *sympathēs*, sympathetic]. Pertaining to the craniosacral portion of the autonomic nervous system.

par″a·sym″pa·thet′ic sys′tem. See craniosacral *system.*

par″a·sym·path″i·co·to′ni·a. See *vagotonia.*

par″a·sym″pa·tho·lyt′ic [*para; sympathēs;* G. *lyein*, to loose]. Blocking the action of parasympathetic nerve fibers.

par″a·sym″pa·tho·mi·met′ic [*para; sympathēs;* G. *mimesis*, imitation]. Referring to drugs having an effect similar to that produced when the parasympathetic nerves are stimulated.

par″a·syn·ap′sis [*para;* G. *synapsis*, contact]. The side-by-side union of homologous chromosomes in preparation for the reduction division of meiosis.

par″a·syph′i·lis [*para;* NL. *syphilis*]. A series of morbid manifestations not having the anatomicopathologic characteristics of syphilis, but apparently of syphilitic origin; e.g., tabes, general paresis. *Obs.*

par″a·sys′to·le (par″uh·sis′to·lee). See parasystolic *rhythm.*

par″a·te·re″si·o·ma′ni·a [G. *paratērēsis*, observation; *mania*, madness]. A mania for observing, or seeing new sights; peeping mania.

par″a·ter′mi·nal [G. *para*, near; L. *terminus*, end]. Near a terminal.

par″a·the·li·o′ma. See stromal *endometriosis.*

parathesin. A brand of ethyl aminobenzoate.

parathion. Trade name for *O,O*-diethyl-*O*-*p*-nitrophenyl thiophosphate, a liquid insecticide having pronounced cholinesterase-inhibiting action.

par″a·thor′mone. A hormone from the parathyroids. See *parathyrin.*

par″a·thy′mi·a [G. *para*, beyond; *thymos*, mind]. Perversion of mood in which the emotions are out of harmony with the real situation.

par″a·thy′rin. A hormone produced in the parathyroid glands, which regulates phosphorus and calcium metabolism. Also called *parathormone, parathyroid hormone.*

par″a·thy′roid. [G *para*, near; *thyreoeidēs*, shield-shaped]. One of several (usually four) small endocrine glands which lie posterior to the capsule of the thyroid gland, or imbedded in the gland, and near the superior and inferior thyroid arteries. Their hormone has a powerful effect on the rate of renal phosphorus excretion and the level of blood calcium. Their complete removal causes tetany and death. See Plate 45. —**parathy'roid,** *adj.*

p. in·jec'tion. A sterile solution in water of the water-soluble principle or principles of the parathyroid glands, which have the property of relieving the symptoms of parathyroid tetany and of increasing the calcium content of the blood serum in man and other animals. It is obtained from the fresh parathyroid glands of healthy, domesticated animals which are used for food by man. The continuation and regulation of the dose must be controlled by determinations of the serum calcium. Also called *solution of parathyroid, parathyroid extract.*

par"a·thy"roid·ec'to·my [*para; thyreoeidēs;* G. *ektomē,* excision]. Excision of a parathyroid gland.

par"a·thy"ro·pri'val [*para; thyreoeidēs;* L. *privus,* deprived of]. Pertaining to the condition due to loss of function, or removal, of the parathyroid glands.

par"a·thy"ro·tro'pic hor'mone, principle. The hypothetical adenohypophyseal hormone regulating the activity of the parathyroid glands.

par"a·thy"ro·tro'pin. See *parathyrotropic hormone.*

par"a·ton'sil·lar [*para;* L. *tonsillae,* tonsils]. Near, or around, the tonsil, as paratonsillar abscess.

par"a·tra·cho'ma. See inclusion *conjunctivitis.*

par"a·tri·cho'sis (par"uh·tri·ko'sis, ·try·ko'sis) [G. *para,* beyond; *trichōsis,* hairy growth]. A condition in which the hair is either imperfect in growth or develops in abnormal places.

par"a·trip'sis [G., friction]. 1. A rubbing or chafing. 2. A retardation of catabolic processes.

par"a·troph'ic [G. *paratrophos,* reared in the same house]. Parasitic; obtaining nourishment from living organic matter.

pa·rat'ro·phy [G. *para,* beyond; *trophē,* nourishment]. Perverted or abnormal nutrition.

par"a·tu·ber'cu·lin. See *johnin.*

par"a·typh·li'tis [G. *para,* near; *typhlos,* cecum; *-itis,* inflammation]. Inflammation of the connective tissue near the cecum.

par"a·ty'phoid [*para;* G. *typhōdēs,* delirious]. An acute generalized disease of man caused by the paratyphoid bacteria, *Salmonella schottmuelleri* and *S. choleraesuis.* The disease resembles typhoid fever both clinically and pathologically but tends to be less severe.

par"a·u·re'thral [G. *para,* beside; *ourēthra,* urethra]. Beside the urethra.

par"a·u'ter·ine. Beside or adjacent to the uterus.

par"a·vac·cin'i·a (par"uh·vack·sin'ee·uh) [G. *para,* near; L. *vaccinus,* of cows]. An eruption consisting of small vesicles outside the vaccinated area, which are not vaccinial.

par"a·vag'i·nal. Beside the vagina.

par"a·vag"i·ni'tis (par"uh·vadj"i·nigh'tis) [*para; vagina;* G. *-itis,* inflammation]. Inflammation of the connective tissue surrounding the vagina.

par"a·ver'te·bral [*para;* L. *vertebra,* joint]. Occurring or situated near the spinal column, as paravertebral analgesia.

par"a·ves'i·cal [*para;* L. *vesica,* bladder]. Situated near the urinary bladder.

par"a·vi"ta·min·o'sis. A disease associated indirectly with a vitamin deficiency.

par"a·xan'thine (par"uh·zan'theen, ·thin). $C_7H_8N_4O_2$. 1,7-Dimethylxanthine. A crystalline substance found in normal urine and isomeric with theobromine, which it resembles in its action upon the organism, causing muscular rigidity, dyspnea, and less reflex excitability.

par·ax'i·al [G. *para,* near; L. *axis,* axis]. 1. Lying near the axis of the body. 2. Referring to the space or rays closely surrounding the principal axis of a lens system.

par·ax'on [G. *para,* beside; *axōn,* axle]. Old term for a collateral of an axon.

par"a·zo'on [*para;* G. *zōion,* living being]. An animal parasite.

parch'ment crack'ling. The peculiar sound elicited by pressure on the cranial bones in rachitic and syphilitic children. It is due to a localized thinning of the bones.

parch'ment skin. An atrophic type of epidermis seen in xeroderma pigmentosum, senile skin, and in some skins exposed to the wind and sun.

Pardee, Harold Ensign Bennett [*American cardiologist,* 1886–]. The first to describe the constant changes in electrocardiograms in coronary disease (1920). Described the slight elevation of R-T or S-T waves in a curve with a sharply negative T observed in the electrocardiogram of a subject with a healing or a healed myocardial infarction; called *Pardee's sign.* The coronary T wave is also called the *Pardee T wave.*

Paré, Ambroise [*French surgeon,* 1510–90]. Probably the greatest surgeon of his age. Author of a treatise on gunshot wounds (1545). Advocated the mild treatment of wounds in contrast to the popular methods of cauterization by fire and boiling oil. Introduced the ligature in vascular surgery in place of cautery. His *Works of Ambroise Paré* (1575) was a leading authority of the times.

par·ec'ta·sis, par"ec·ta'si·a (par"eck·tay'zhuh, ·zee·uh, ·shuh, ·see·uh) [G. *parektasis,* a stretching out]. Excessive stretching or dilatation.

paredrine. $OH.C_6H_4.CH_2.CHNH_2.CH_3$. Trade-mark for a substance related to benzedrine but differing from it in the presence of a hydroxyl group in the benzene ring: used as the hydrobromide, as a mydriatic. The dilation of the pupil is not accompanied by loss of accommodation or increase of intraocular pressure.

par"e·gor'ic (par"i·gorr'ick, ·gor'ick). See camphorated *opium* tincture.

pa·rei'ra (pa·ray'ruh, pa·rair'uh) [Pg. *parreira brava,* wild vine]. The root of *Chondodendron tomentosum,* formerly called pareira brava. Contains the alkaloid bebeerine (pelosine). It was formerly employed as a bitter tonic and in chronic inflammations of the urinary passages. The plant has been identified as the source of tube curare, which contains the paralyzant alkaloids *d*-tubocurarine and curine.

par"e·le'i·din. See *keratin.*

parenamine. Trade-mark for certain preparations of protein hydrolysate prepared from casein.

pa·ren'chy·ma (pa·reng'ki·muh) [G. *paregchyma,* anything poured in beside]. The essential or specialized part of an organ as distinguished from the supporting connective tissue. —**parenchymal, parenchym'atous,** *adj.*

par"en·chym"a·ti'tis (par"eng·kim"uh·tye'tis, par"en·) [*paregchyma;* G. *-itis,* inflammation]. Inflammation of parenchyma.

par'e·nol (par'i·nole, ·nol, ·nawl). A stable, bland, absorbable ointment base composed of 65% white or yellow petrolatum, 15% wool fat, and 20% distilled water.

par'ent [L. *parens,* parent]. 1. A father or mother. 2. *In radiochemistry,* a radioactive nuclide the disintegration of which gives rise either to a radioactive or a stable nuclide, called the *daughter.*

p. image. Primordial parent.

primordial p. *In psychoanalysis,* the primitive or original parent; the source of all life; the stage prior to the differentiation of mother and father: also called *parent image.*

par·en'ter·al [G. *para,* beside; *enteron,* intestine]. Outside of the intestine; not via the alimentary tract.

par·en'ter·al. A subcutaneous, intravenous, intramuscular, or intrasternal injection.

par″ep·i·thym'i·a (par″ep·i·thim'ee·uh, ·thigh'-mee·uh) [G. *para,* beyond; *epithymia,* yearning]. A morbid desire or craving.

par″e·reth'i·sis [*para;* G *erethizein,* to excite]. Abnormal or perverted excitement. *Obs.*

par″er·ga'si·a (par″ur·gay'zhuh, ·zee·uh, ·shuh, ·see·uh) [*para;* G. *ergasia,* a working]. *In psychiatry,* Meyer's term for psychoses manifesting withdrawal, deep regression, delusions, and hallucinations, as schizophrenia and paranoia.

pa·re'sis, par'e·sis [G., a letting go, paralysis]. A slight paralysis; incomplete loss of muscular power; weakness of a limb. —**paret'ic,** *adj.*

agitated p. A type of general paresis characterized by sudden violent and destructive excitement.

general p. A late form of neurosyphilis involving chiefly the cortex of the frontal and temporal lobes, characterized clinically by mental changes, tremors, disturbances of speech, apoplectiform and epileptiform seizures, and pupillary changes: also called *dementia paralytica, general paralysis* (of the insane).

p. sine paresi. Late asymptomatic neurosyphilis.

parturient p. A disease of cows, occurring shortly after calving, characterized by motor and sensory nervous paralysis, not accompanied by fever, but always by hypocalcemia. Syn., *milk fever.*

par″es·the'si·a (par″ess·thee'zhuh, ·zee·uh) [*para;* G. *aisthēsis,* perception]. A perverted sensation of tingling, crawling, or burning of the skin, which occurs in peripheral neuritis and spinal-cord lesions. —**paresthet'ic,** *adj.*

Bernhardt's p. Abnormal sensations, especially of numbness, with hyperesthesia and pain on exertion, in the region supplied by the lateral cutaneous nerve of the thigh. Also called *Bernhardt's disease.*

pa·reu'ni·a (pa·rōō'nee·uh) [G. *pareunos,* lying beside]. Coitus.

par·fo'cal [L. *par,* equal; *focus,* hearth]. Pertaining to microscopical oculars and objectives which are so constructed or so mounted that, in changing from one to another, the image remains in focus.

Parham, Frederick William [*American surgeon,* 1856–1927]. With E. D. Martin, introduced a metal band of aluminum or steel which was placed about the ends of fractured long bones for immobilization until union had taken place; called *Parham-Martin band.*

par″hi·dro'sis (par″hi·dro'sis, ·high·dro'sis), **par″-i·dro'sis** [G. *para,* beyond; *hidrōsis,* a sweating]. Any abnormal secretion of sweat.

par'i·cine (par'i·seen, ·sin). An amorphous alkaloid obtained from the bark of *Cinchona succirubra.*

pa'ri·es (pair'ee·eez) (pl. *parietes*) [L.]. An enveloping or investing structure or wall.

p. anterior. Anterior wall.

p. caroticus tympani. Carotid or anterior wall of the tympanic cavity.

p. inferior. Inferior wall.

p. jugularis tympani. The jugular wall or floor of the tympanic cavity.

p. labyrinthicus tympani. Labyrinthic or inner wall of the tympanic cavity.

p. lateralis. Lateral wall.

p. mastoideus tympani. The mastoid or posterior wall of the tympanic cavity.

p. medialis. The medial wall.

p. membranaceus tracheae. The posterior wall of the trachea into which the tracheal cartilages do not extend.

p. membranaceus tympani. The membranous or outer wall of the tympanic cavity.

p. posterior. Posterior wall.

p. superior. Superior wall.

p. tegmentalis tympani. The tegmental wall of the tympanic cavity.

pa·ri'e·tal [*paries*]. 1. Forming or situated on a wall, as the parietal layer of the peritoneum. 2. Pertaining to, or in relation with, the parietal bone of the skull, as the parietal foramen.

pa·ri'e·tal. The parietal bone. See Table of Bones in the Appendix.

pa·ri'e·to- [*paries*]. *In anatomy,* a combining form signifying *parietal.*

pa·ri″e·to·fron'tal [*paries;* L. *frons,* forehead]. Pertaining to both the parietal and frontal bones or lobes; frontoparietal.

pa·ri″e·to·mas'toid [*paries;* G. *mastoeidēs,* like a breast]. Pertaining to the parietal bone and the mastoid portion of the temporal bone; mastoparietal.

pa·ri″e·to-oc·cip'i·tal (pa·rye″i·to-ock·sip'i·tul) [*paries;* L. *occiput,* back part of the head]. Pertaining to the parietal and occipital bones or lobes.

pa·ri″e·to·squa·mo'sal [*paries;* L. *squamosus,* scaly]. Pertaining to the parietal bone and the squamous portion of the temporal bone.

pa·rig'e·nin (pa·ridg'i·nin, par″i·jee'nin). $C_{27}H_{44}O_3$; the steroidal aglycone of parillin, a glycoside of sarsaparilla; identical with *sarsasapogenin.*

pa·ril'lin. A glycoside from sarsaparilla; on hydrolysis, it yields the aglycone parigenin.

Parinaud, Henri [*French ophthalmologist,* 1844–1905]. Known for his description with Galezowski of an infectious conjunctivitis which is transferred from animals to man (1889); called *Parinaud's conjunctivitis, leptotrichosis of the conjunctiva.* Described a syndrome characterized by a paralysis of upward gaze. *Parinaud's syndrome* is indicative of a lesion in the midbrain.

Par'is green. $Cu(C_2H_3O_2)_2.3Cu(AsO_2)_2$. Copper acetoarsenite; occurs as an emerald green powder; insoluble in water. It is used extensively for dusting on potato vines to destroy the so-called potato bug or Colorado beetle. Also used as a pigment. Care must be taken in its use, as it is extremely poisonous. Also called *imperial, Schweinfurth, Vienna,* or *parrot green.*

par·isth'mi·on (pa·riss'mee·on, pa·risth'·, pa·rist'·) [G., tonsil]. A tonsil. *Obs.*

par'i·ty [L. *parere,* to bring forth]. Condition of a woman with regard to the number of children she has borne.

par'i·ty [L. *paritas,* equality]. Similarity approaching equality; equivalence.

Park, Henry [*English surgeon,* 1744–1831]. Described arteriovenous aneurysm in which the dilatation communicates with two vessels, also called *Park's aneurysm.*

Park, William Hallock [*American bacteriologist,* 1863–1939]. Widely known as head of the New York City Health Department. With Jacobi and Anna Williams, was responsible for the rapid acceptance of diphtheria antitoxin by American physicians. Described, with Anna Williams, a strain of diphtheria bacillus from which antitoxin was made; called *Park-Williams bacillus.*

Parker, George Howard [*American zoologist,* 1864–]. Known for his important studies of the nervous system of lower animals and vertebrates

(1919). Introduced a hardening and preserving fluid consisting of a 1% formaldehyde solution in 70% alcohol, called *Parker's fluid.*

Parker, Ralph Robinson (1888–1949). American entomologist who developed, with R. R. Spencer, Rocky Mountain spotted-fever vaccine.

Parker, Willard (1800–1884). American surgeon, first in America to operate by abdominal incision for appendicitis (1864). In this he was preceded in England by Henry Hancock (1848). An incision for appendectomy made over the area of dullness is called *Parker's incision.* He performed cystotomy for inflammation or rupture of the urinary bladder (1851).

Parker's method. See Askenstedt's *method.*

Parkinson, James (1755–1824). English physician remembered for his classical treatise (1817) on a widespread neurological symptom complex which he described as: "Involuntary tremulous motion with lessened muscular power, with a propensity to bend the trunk forward and to pass from a walking to a running pace, the senses and intellects being uninjured." The affliction is now best known as *parkinsonism,* classified as idiopathic or symptomatic of a variety of associated conditions.

par′kin·son·ism, Par′kin·son·ism [after James *Parkinson*]. A neurological symptom complex, occurring in association with several distinct factors and idiopathically characterized by four major symptoms: rigidity, tremor, akinesia, and loss of spontaneous and automatic movement. As a consequence of rigidity, there may be a fixed facial expression, abnormal posture, poor balance, festinating and propulsive gait, weakness and fatigue, and difficulties in speaking, chewing, and swallowing. There is a marked relationship between the intensity of the symptoms to emotional stress and their disappearance in sleep. Syn., *Parkinson's disease* or *syndrome.*

arteriosclerotic p. That appearing in individuals with cerebral arteriosclerosis, clinically differentiated by commencing most frequently in or after the sixth decade, and in an evanescent manner. Involvement is always bilateral, with rigidity the chief feature, tremor usually delayed, less marked, and not characteristic, and rapid progression of existing symptoms. Pathologically the changes are bilateral, most often in the globus pallidus, and commonly include capillary occlusion and foci of softening.

hemi-parkinsonism. Disease of the extrapyramidal system of the brain, manifested by tremor and rigidity of the extremities on one side.

idiopathic p. The classical form, coming on in the fifth and sixth decade of life, more often in males, and showing a distinct hereditary tendency. It is clinically characterized by sudden onset in a previously well individual, with tremor in one extremity, slight rigidity of arm and leg, and some asymmetry of the face of the same side. Tremor and rigidity are progressive and spread to the other side. The pathogenesis is most often ascribed to degenerative changes in, or centering about, the globus pallidus, putamen, caudate nucleus, and substantia nigra. There is a prominent accumulation of lipid material in the nerve cells of the globus pallidus and other scattered areas of the extrapyramidal system, suggesting metabolic defect, an aging process, or combination of these. Syn., *paralysis agitans, shaking palsy.*

intoxication p. That developing within months or a few years in survivors of acute poisoning from carbon monoxide, less commonly from nitrous oxide, manganese, carbon disulfide, or phosphorus. In carbon monoxide intoxication, characteristic bilateral necrosis of the anterior portion of the globus pallidus has been established.

postencephalitic p. That occurring as a sequel to lethargic encephalitis (epidemic e., von Economo's disease) within a variable period, from days to many years, after the acute process. Clinically distinct, it is characterized by commencing almost exclusively before the age of forty, by a history of varying degrees of lethargy, and very slow but steady evolution of the classical symptom complex. Patients frequently exhibit oculogyric and other ocular disorders. Pathologically, changes in the substantia nigra are most often demonstrable, but the essential process is unknown.

symptomatic p. That associated with known factors, as lethargic encephalitis, arteriosclerosis, trauma, syphilis, and intoxications.

syphilitic p. That associated, usually at autopsy, with neurosyphilis but most likely coincidental.

traumatic p. That following trauma to a limb or the brain, occurring very rarely, and most likely due to the emotional stress of the trauma which unmasks the previously controlled or latent symptoms.

parlodion. Trade-mark for a shredded form of pure concentrated collodion (cellulose nitrate): used for imbedding microscope specimens and preparing membranes.

Parnum's test. See under *test.*

par″o·don·ti′tis [G. *para,* beside; *odous,* tooth; *-itis,* inflammation]. Inflammation of the tissues near, or surrounding, a tooth.

par″o·don′ti·um (par″o·don′shee·um) [*para; odous*]. The alveolar process, periodontal membrane, and gingival tissue in the region of a tooth socket.

par″o·dyn′i·a [L. *parere,* to bring forth; G. *odynē,* pain]. Difficult parturition. *Obs.*

paroidin. Trade-mark for a brand of parathyroid injection.

paroleine. Trade-mark for a brand of liquid petrolatum.

par·ol′i·var″y (par·ol′i·verr″ee) [G. *para,* near; L. *olivarius,* of olives]. Situated near the olivary body.

par″o·ni′ri·a (par″o·nigh′ree·uh, ·nirr′ee·uh) [G. *para,* beyond; *oneiros,* dream]. Morbid dreaming.

p. ambulans. Sleepwalking. *Obs.*

par″o·nych′i·a (par″o·nick′ee·uh) [G. *para,* beside; *onyx,* nail]. A suppurative inflammation about the margin of a nail. —**paronychial,** *adj.*

mycotic p. An inflammatory process at the base of the nails usually associated with *Candida albicans* infection.

p. diphtheritica. That due to *Corynebacterium diphtheriae.*

p. tendinosa. Old term for tenosynovitis with involvement of the flexor tendons in the hand.

par″o·nych″o·my·co′sis (par″o·nick″o·migh·ko′-sis) [*para; onyx;* G. *mykēs,* fungus; *-ōsis,* condition]. A fungous infection around the nails.

par″o·ny·cho′sis (par″o·ni·ko′sis) [*para; onyx; -ōsis*]. 1. A diseased condition of the structures about the nails. 2. Growth of a nail in unusual places.

par″o·oph″o·ri′tis [*para;* G. *ōiophoros,* bearing eggs; G. *-itis,* inflammation]. 1. Inflammation of the parovarium. 2. Inflammation of the tissues about the ovary.

par″o·oph′o·ron [*para; ōiophoros*]. A vestigial, caudal group of mesonephric tubules located in or about the broad ligament of the uterus, homologous with the male paradidymis. They usually disappear in the adult.

par″oph·thal′mi·a [*para;* G. *ophthalmos,* eye]. Inflammation about the eye.

par″oph·thal·mon′cus [*para; ophthalmos;* G. *ogkos*, mass]. A tumor near the eye.

pa·ro′pi·a [*para;* G. *ōps*, eye]. The angle of the eyelid toward the temple.

pa·ro′pi·on [*para; ōps*]. An eye screen.

par·op′si·a, par·op′sis [*para;* G. *opsis*, vision]. Disordered or false vision.

par·op′tic [*para;* G. *optikos*, of sight]. Pertaining to colors produced by the diffraction of light rays.

par″o·ra′sis [G. *para*, beyond; *horasis*, a seeing]. Any perversion of vision or of color perception; a hallucination.

par″o·rex′i·a [*para;* G. *orexis*, yearning]. A perverted appetite.

par·os′mi·a (par·oz′mee·uh, par·os′·) [*para;* G. *osmē*, smell]. A perversion of the sense of smell. May be present in organic brain disease, in schizophrenia (olfactory hallucinations), or in psychoneurotic conditions. See also *cacosmia*.

par″os·phre′sis. See *parosmia*.

par″os·ti′tis [G. *para*, beside; *osteon*, bone; *-itis*, inflammation]. Inflammation of the tissue adjacent to the periosteum: also spelled *parosteitis*.

par″os·to′sis [*para; osteon;* G. *-ōsis*, condition]. The abnormal formation of bone outside of the periosteum, or in the connective tissue surrounding the periosteum: also spelled *parosteosis*.

pa·ro′tic (pa·ro′tick, ·rot′ick) [*para;* G. *ous*, ear]. Situated near, or about, the ear.

pa·rot′id [G. *parōtis*, from *para*, *ous*]. 1. Situated near the ear, as the parotid gland. 2. Pertaining to, or affecting, the parotid gland.

pa·rot″id·ec′to·my [*para; ous;* G. *ektomē*, excision]. Excision of a parotid gland.

pa·rot″id·i′tis. See *parotitis*.

pa·rot″i·do·scle·ro′sis [*para; ous;* G. *sklērōsis*, a hardening]. Fibrous induration of the parotid gland.

par″o·ti′tis [*para; ous;* G. *-itis*, inflammation]. Inflammation of the parotid gland, as in mumps; inflammation of the lymph node overlying the parotid (parotid bubo). —**parotit′ic.** *adj.*

epidemic p. Mumps.

infectious p. Any infection of the parotid gland, including the mumps virus and bacterial agents complicating systemic disease, as well as an infection complicating obstruction of the parotid duct.

metastatic p. That secondary to disease elsewhere; it occurs in infectious fevers, as typhoid fever, and usually goes on to suppuration.

phlegmonous p. One which is the seat of pus formation. Also called *suppurative p.*

par′ous [L. *parere*, to bring forth]. Having borne one or more children.

par″o·va′ri·an (par″o·vair′ee·un) [G. *para*, beside; L. *ovarius*, egg-keeper]. 1. Situated near the ovary. 2. Pertaining to the parovarium.

par″o·va″ri·ot′o·my [*para; ovarius;* G. *tomē*, a cutting]. Excision of a parovarian cyst.

par″o·va·ri′tis [*para; ovarius;* G. *-itis*, inflammation]. Inflammation of the parovarium.

par″o·va′ri·um (par″o·vair′ee·um) [*para; ovarius*]. The remnant of the Wolffian body of the female; the homolog of the caput epididymidis in the male. Also called *epoophoron, organ of Rosenmueller*.

par′ox·ysm [G. *paroxysmos*, irritation]. 1. The periodic increase or crisis in the progress of a disease; a sudden attack, a sudden reappearance of symptoms, or a sudden increase in the intensity of existing symptoms. 2. A spasm or fit; a convulsion.

parpanit. See *panparnit*.

Parr turbidimeter. A turbidimeter designed for the determination of sulfur by observation of the light dispersed by a suspension of barium sulfate, into which the sulfur has been converted. The source of light is a filament lamp in the base of the instrument.

parresine. Trade-mark for a protective dressing composed of paraffin, gum elemi, japan wax, asphalt, and eucalyptol.

Parrot, Joseph [*French physician*, 1829–83]. With Pasteur, gave what was probably the first description of the pneumococcus. Primary infantile atrophy or marasmus is called *Parrot's atrophy of the newborn*. Syphilitic pseudoparalysis due to epiphyseal separation is known as *Parrot's disease*. Nodes on the frontal and parietal bones found in hereditary syphilis are called *Parrot's nodes*.

par′rot fe′ver. See *psittacosis*.

Parry, Caleb Hillier [*English physician*, 1755–1822]. Confirmed work of Heberden on angina pectoris (1799), and considered it due to coronary arterial disease. He reported a series of toxic goiter cases with careful description (1825), usually called *Graves's disease*, also called *Parry's disease*. He also described facial hemiatrophy (1825).

pars (pl. *partes*) [L.]. A part.

p. alveolaris. The alveolar process of maxilla or mandible.

p. anterior. (a) The anterior part of the adenohypophysis. See *p.* distalis. (b) The anterior lobe of hypophysis (b).

p. basilaris. Basilar process of the occipital bone.

p. buccalis. Term formerly used for *adenohypophysis*.

p. cavernosa urethrae. The cavernous or spongy portion of the male urethra.

p. ciliaris retinae. The part of the retina in front of the ora serrata.

p. convoluta. The convoluted part or labyrinth of the kidney.

p. distalis. (a) The anterior part of the adenohypophysis, consisting of clumps and cords of cells (acidophil, basophil, chromophobe primarily) and a diffuse vascular bed. (b) The anterior lobe of the hypophysis (b).

p. flaccida. Shrapnell's membrane.

p. glandularis. Term formerly used for *adenohypophysis*.

p. horizontalis ossis palatini. The horizontal plate of the palatine bone.

p. intercartilaginea. The portion of the rima glottidis between the arytenoid cartilages.

p. intermedia. (a) The intermediate part of the adenohypophysis, consisting chiefly of an irregular row of follicles of pale cells and containing pale-staining colloidal material, and some rows of basophilic cells extending into the neurohypophysis. Its function in man is not known. In some species, it produces the hormone intermedin, causing the pigment-containing cells of the animal to expand. (b) The intermediate lobe of the hypophysis (b). (c) Term formerly used for *nervus intermedius*.

p. intermembranacea. The portion of the rima glottidis between the vocal folds.

p. iridica retinae. The uveal tract.

p. laryngea pharyngis. The laryngopharynx.

p. mastoidea. The mastoid portion of the temporal bone.

p. membranacea septi. The membranaceous part of the interventricular septum situated near the root of the aorta.

p. membranacea urethrae. The membranous portion of the male urethra.

p. nasalis pharyngis. The nasopharynx.

p. nervosa. (a) The inferior part of the neurohypophysis, exhibiting neurosecretory granules and Herring bodies when properly stained. Syn., *infundibular process*. (b) The posterior lobe of the hypophysis (b): also called *p. neuralis*.

p. neuralis. See *p. nervosa*, (b).

p. olfactoria. See olfactory *region*.

p. oralis pharyngis. The oropharynx.

p. perpendicularis ossis palatini. The vertical plate of the palatine bone.

p. petrosa ossis temporalis. The petrous portion of the temporal bone.

p. posterior. (a) The pars nervosa of the neurohypophysis. (b) The posterior lobe of the hypophysis (b).

p. prostatica urethrae. The prostatic portion of the male urethra.

p. pylorica. The pyloric portion of the stomach.

p. spongiosa urethrae. See *p.* cavernosa.

p. tensa. All of the tympanic membrane except the pars flaccida or Shrapnell's membrane.

p. tuberalis. The upward extension of the anterior part of the adenohypophysis, containing predominantly agranular chromophobic cells. Its function is as yet unknown.

p. tympanica ossis temporalis. The tympanic portion of the temporal bone.

parsidol hydrochloride. A trade-marked name for 10-(2-diethylamino-1-propyl)phenothiazine hydrochloride, official in the International Pharmacopoeia as *profenamine hydrochloride:* used in the treatment of parkinsonism.

pars'ley [ME. *persely*, G. *petroselinon*, rock parsley]. *Petroselinum crispum*, a plant of the Umbelliferae, containing a volatile oil. From the seed an oily liquid, termed *apiol*, is obtained. The root has been used as a diuretic in renal diseases and dropsy; the juice of the fresh herbs and the fruit were formerly employed as antiperiodics; apiol has been used as an emmenagogue.

p. camphor. Apiol.

p. oleoresin. Liquid apiol.

par'the·nine (pahr'thi·neen, ·nin). An alkaloid from *Parthenium hysterophorus;* has been used as an antipyretic and antineuralgic.

Par·the'ni·um [G. *parthenion*, from *parthenos*, virgin]. A genus of herbs of the Compositae. **P. hysterophorus** contains several alkaloids, one of which (parthenine) seems to be the active principle.

par"the·no·gen'e·sis [*parthenos;* G. *genesis*, production]. A modification of sexual reproduction, in which the organism develops from an unfertilized egg. It occurs chiefly in certain insects, crustacea, and worms. —**parthenogenet'ic,** *adj.*

par'tial [L. *pars*, part]. Incomplete; finished in part only.

par·tic"i·pa'tion. See *law* of participation.

par'ti·cle [L. *particula*, a little bit]. A small portion or piece of a substance.

alpha p. A particle, carrying two positive charges, ejected from the nucleus of a radioactive atom. When ejected in a stream, these particles are known as alpha rays. Each alpha particle is equivalent to the nucleus of a helium atom.

beta p. One of the radiations emitted by certain radioactive materials, identical with the electrons found in the outer structure of all atoms. It has a unit negative charge equal and opposite to the positive charge of the proton and is nearly weightless, having less than $1/1800$ the mass of a proton.

colloid p. One, smaller than particles visible under the optical microscope, which forms colloid solutions.

p. accelerator. Any device for accelerating atomic particles.

par·tic'u·late [*particula*]. Composed of particles.

par·ti'tion [L. *partitio*, a dividing]. The distribution of a substance or ions between two immiscible liquids, or between a liquid and a gas.

p. of urinary nitrogen and sulfur. The percentage of the total nitrogen and total sulfur of the urine which appears in the form of any particular nitrogen constituent or in any particular form of sulfur is regulated directly by the extent of the total nitrogen and sulfur elimination.

par'tridge·ber"ry [ME. *partriche;* AS. *berie*]. A trailing plant, *Mitchella repens*, which has been used as a diuretic, tonic, and emmenagogue.

par·tu'ri·en·cy [L. *parturire*, to bring forth]. The state of being in labor.

par·tu'ri·ent [*parturire*]. 1. Being in labor; giving birth. 2. Traversed during birth, as the parturient canal.

par·tu"ri·fa'cient (pahr·tew"ri·fay'shunt) [*parturire;* L. *facere*, to make]. Promoting labor.

par·tu"ri·fa'cient. An agent that induces labor.

par·tu"ri·om'e·ter [*parturire;* G. *metron*, a measure]. An instrument to determine the progress of labor by measuring the expulsive force of the uterus.

par"tu·ri'tion (pahr"tew·rish'un, pahr"chew·) [L. *parturitio*, from *parturire*]. The act of giving birth to young. See Plate 42.

par'tus [L., a bringing forth]. The bringing forth of offspring; labor.

p. agrippinus. Labor with breech presentation.

p. caesareus. Cesarean section.

p. difficilis. Dystocia.

p. immaturus. Premature labor.

p. maturus. Labor at term.

p. precipitatus. Precipitate labor.

p. serotinus. Labor unduly prolonged.

p. siccus. Dry labor.

pa·ru'lis [G. *paroulis*, gumboil]. 1. Abscess of the gum. 2. Incorrectly, a gumboil.

par"um·bil'i·cal [G. *para*, beside; L. *umbilicus*, navel]. In the region of the navel.

par"um·bil'i·cal. The parumbilical vein. See Table of Veins in the Appendix.

par'vi- [L. *parvus*, small, little]. A combining form meaning *small, little;* sometimes used instead of the more common *micro-*.

par"vi·cel'lu·lar [L. *parvus*, small; *cellula*, small storeroom]. Pertaining to, or composed of, small cells.

par"vi·loc'u·lar. Pertaining to small loculi.

par'vule [L. *parvulus*, very small]. A small pill or pellet; a granule.

PAS, PASA Para-aminosalicylic acid.

Pascal, Blaise [*French scientist and philosopher*, 1623–62]. Proponent of a law of physics that pressure exerted anywhere on a mass of fluid is transmitted equally in all directions; called *Pascal's law*.

pas"cha·chur'da (pas"kuh·koor'duh). See *oriental sore*.

Paschen, Enrique [*German bacteriologist*, 1860–1936]. Described elementary bodies found in the inclusion (Guarnieri) bodies of smallpox and vaccinia. They are thought to represent virus particles. Called *Paschen bodies*.

Paschutin, Victor Vasilyevich [*Russian physician*, 1845–1901]. Remembered for his investigations in diabetes mellitus (1871); described degeneration peculiar to the disease, called *Paschutin's degeneration*.

pas'sage [*passus*]. 1. A channel or lumen. 2. The act of passing from one place to another. 3. The introduction of an instrument into a cavity or channel. 4. An evacuation of the bowels.

air passages. The nares, nasal cavities, pharynx, mouth, larynx, trachea, and bronchial tubes.

cloacal p. See cloacal *duct*.

false p. A false channel, especially one made by the unskillful introduction of an instrument into the urethra.

Passavant's bar, cushion. See under *cushion*.

pas″si·flo′ra [L. *passio*, passion, suffering; *flos*, flower]. The rhizome of *Passiflora incarnata* (passionflower); has been used as a sedative and anodyne. Dose of the fluidextract, 0.2–0.6 cc. (3–10 min.).

pas′sion [*passio*]. 1. Pain; suffering. *Obs.* 2. An intense emotion of the mind; fervid desire, overpowering emotion. 3. A specific intense excitement, as rage or ardent affection. —**passional,** *adj.*

ileac p. A disorder marked by severe pain, fecal vomiting, and spasm of the abdominal muscles. *Obs.*

sexual p. See *erotic.*

pas′sive [L. *passivus*, passive]. Not active; not performed or produced by active efforts, but by causes coming from without.

pas′siv·ism [*passivus*]. A form of sexual perversion in which one person submits to the will of another in unnatural erotic acts. —**passivist,** *n.*

pas′ta [L., paste, from G. *pasta*, barley porridge]. A paste.

paste [*pasta*]. An ointmentlike preparation of one or more medicinal substances, such as zinc oxide, coal tar, starch, or sulfur, in a hydrogel or fatty base. They are generally intended for dermatologic use and are less greasy and more absorptive than ointments.

paste boot. See *Unna's paste boot.*

pas′tern [L. *pastorius*, pertaining to shepherds]. That part of a horse's leg between the fetlock joint and the coronet of the hoof.

Pasteur, Louis [*French scientist and bacteriologist*, 1822–95]. Generally regarded as the founder of modern bacteriology. His study of wine fermentations disclosed causative organisms, and disposed finally of the theory of spontaneous generation. With Joubert, discovered *vibrion septique*, the first pathogenic anaerobe to be identified. This led to Pasteur's distinction between aerobic and anaerobic bacteria. Experimented with attenuated virus in chicken cholera. Confirmed Koch's work on anthrax, and, with Chamberland and Roux, developed the first attenuated bacterial culture to be used therapeutically. With the same workers discovered the rabies virus in the blood (1884), and first used attenuated vaccine as a prophylactic (1885). See also *rabies.* With Parrot, made probably the first observation of a pneumococcus. Cultivated the streptococcus of puerperal sepsis. The Pasteur Institute in Paris was established for his investigations.

Pasteur-Chamberland filter. See under *filter.*

Pasteur effect. The inhibition of fermentation when anaerobic conditions are replaced by abundant O_2 supply.

Pas″teur·el′la (pas″tur·el′uh) [*Pasteur*]. A genus of bacteria of the tribe Pasteurelleae and of the family Parvobacteriaceae. Species are small, Gram-negative, bipolar staining, often ovoid, and are parasites of man, birds, and other higher animals.

Past. avicida. A species pathogenic for birds and mammals known as the fowl cholera bacillus; it is the type species of this genus.

Past. aviseptica. Synonym for *Past. avicida.*

Past. bollingeri. Synonym for *Past. boviseptica.*

Past. boviseptica. A species which produces hemorrhagic septicemia of cattle, known as shipping fever.

Past. pestis. Species known as the plague bacillus; is pathogenic to man and produces bubonic or glandular plague and plague pneumonia.

Past. pseudotuberculosis. A species which is similar to *Past. pestis;* causes an infection of rodents and occasionally of man.

Past. suilla. Synonym for *Past. suiseptica.*

Past. suiseptica. Species which is the etiologic agent of swine plague.

Past. tularensis. The causative organism of tularemia, a disease of rodents, and of rabbits in particular, which is transmitted to man: also called *Brucella tularensis.*

pas″teur·i·za′tion (pas″tur·i·zay′shun, ·eye·zay′-shun, pas″choor·) [*Pasteur*]. Arresting the process of fermentation in milk, wine, and other organic fluids by heating them at 60° or 70° C. for about 40 minutes. Destroys the common pathogens found in milk.

pas′teur·i″zer [*Pasteur*]. An instrument employed in pasteurization.

pas′til (pas′til), **pas·tille′** (pas·teel′, ·til′) [L. *pastillus*, little roll]. 1. A small mass composed of aromatic substances and employed in fumigation. 2. A troche. 3. A paper disk, chemically coated, which changes color on exposure to x-rays; used to determine the dosage.

past point′ing. A test in which the patient is asked to point at a fixed object alternately with the eyes open and closed. A constant error with the eyes closed indicates a cerebellar lesion. Also called *Bárány's pointing test.*

pa·ta′gi·um. See *pterygium*, 3.

patch [ME. *pacche*]. An irregular spot or area.

butterfly p. A patch of lupus erythematosus on the cheeks and nose. A similar patch is often the site of erysipelas.

MacCallum's p. Roughened, tawny area of inflammation of the left atrium, on the posterior wall above the mitral valve ring, rheumatic in origin, and often associated with mitral stenosis.

moth p. Chloasma.

mucous p. A characteristic lesion of secondary syphilis, occurring as a whitish papule or superficial ulcer on mucous membranes and at mucocutaneous junctions. Syn., *condyloma latum, moist papule.*

Peyer's patches. See Johann Conrad *Peyer.*

soldier's patches. Opaque white spots on the epicardium, of unknown origin, probably due to friction. Also called *soldier's plaques.*

patch′ou·li, patch′ou·ly (patch′oo·lee, pa·chōō′-lee) [Tamil *paccilai*, green leaf]. The herb, *Pogostemon heyneanus*, or other species of *Pogostemon*, the source of **patchouli oil;** used as a fixative in perfumes.

pate [ME.]. The crown or top of the head.

pa·tel′la [L., small dish]. A sesamoid bone in front of the knee, developed in the tendon of the quadriceps femoris muscle; the kneecap. See Table of Bones in the Appendix. See Plates 1, 2. —**patellar,** *adj.*

p. biparta. A developmental variation of the patella, in which a portion (usually the upper lateral part) develops from a distinct center of ossification and remains as a separate ossicle in the adult.

p. cubiti. An anomalous sesamoid bone lying proximal to the olecranon within the tendon of the triceps brachii muscle.

pa·tel′la·pex″y [*patella;* G. *pēxis*, a fixing]. The operation of fixing the patella to the lower end of the femur to stiffen or stabilize the knee joint in flail joint cases of infantile paralysis, by the production of a partial arthrodesis. *Obs.*

pat″el·lec′to·my [*patella;* G. *ektomē*, excision]. The surgical removal or excision of a patella.

pa′ten·cy [L. *patere*, to be open]. The state of being open.

pa′tent, pat′ent [*patere*]. Open; exposed.

Paterson, Robert [*Scottish physician*, 1814–89]. Described round or oval microscopic bodies found in molluscum contagiosum; called *Paterson's bodies* or *corpuscles*.

Paterson's syndrome. See Plummer-Vinson *syndrome*.

path, path'way". *In neurology*, a neuron pathway.

final common p. The anterior horn cell (motoneuron): Sherrington's term.

pa·the'ma [G., suffering]. Any disease or morbid condition. *Obs.*

path"er·ga'si·a (path"ur·gay'zhuh, ·zee·uh, ·shuh, ·see·uh) [G. *pathos*, disease; *ergasia*, a working]. *In psychiatry*, a term applied by Adolf Meyer to personality maladjustments associated with organic or structural changes in the body or with gross functional disturbances.

path'er·gy, path·er'gi·a [*pathos;* G. *ergon*, work]. 1. An unusually intense response to an allergen, in which the individual becomes sensitive not only to the specific substance but to others; hyperergy. 2. A subnormal response to an allergen; hypoergy.

pa·thet'ic [G. *pathētos*, subject to suffering]. 1. Pertaining to or causing feelings. 2. Denoting the fourth cranial nerve: old term.

path'e·tism [G. *pathētos*, subject to suffering]. Hypnotism, mesmerism, animal magnetism. *Obs.*

path'e·tist [*pathētos*]. A mesmerizer, a hypnotist. *Obs.*

path'o-, path- [G. *pathos*, disease]. A combining form denoting *disease, pathologic.*

path"o·don'ti·a [*pathos;* G. *odous*, tooth]. The branch of dental science which treats of the diseases of the teeth.

path'o·gen [*pathos;* G. *genesthai*, from *gignesthai*, to be produced]. Any agent which is capable of producing disease. The term is usually restricted to living agents.

path"o·gen'e·sis [*pathos;* G. *genesis*, production]. The course of development of disease, including the sequence of processes or events from inception to the characteristic lesion or disease.

path"o·gen'ic [*pathos; genesthai*]. Pertaining to the capacity to produce disease, as a pathogenic microorganism.

path"o·ge·nic'i·ty (path"o·ji·nis'i·tee) [*pathos; genesthai*]. The capacity to produce disease.

pa·thog"no·mon'ic [*pathos;* G. *gnōmonikos*, skilled in a thing]. Characteristic of a disease, distinguishing it from other diseases.

path"og·nos'tic. See *pathognomonic.*

path"o·le'si·a (path"o·lee'zhuh, ·zee·uh) [*pathos;* G. *lēsis*, a willing]. Any impairment or weakness of the will. *Rare.*

path"o·log'ic men·dac'i·ty. Pathologic lying; persistent habitual lying without external need or actual advantage, involving both falsifications of real events and development of phantasies. The individual may have complete insight, or the condition may be part of a psychoneurotic or psychotic reaction.

pa·thol'o·gist [*pathos;* G. *logos*, word]. A person trained and experienced in the study and practice of pathology.

pa·thol'o·gy [*pathos; logos*]. That branch of biological science which deals with the nature of disease, through study of its causes, its process, and its effects, together with the associated alterations of structure and function. —**patholog'ic, patholog'ical,** *adj.*

cellular p. The study of changes in cells as the basis of disease.

chemical p. The study of diseased structures and processes by the application of chemical methods.

comparative p. That which compares disease in various animals, including man, to arrive at resemblances and differences which may clarify disease as a phenomenon of nature.

dermal p. The pathology of diseases of the skin.

experimental p. That which utilizes experimental methods for the study of disease in animals and in man.

general p. A study of disturbances which are common to various tissues and organs of the body, as degenerations, hypertrophy, atrophy, neoplasms, etc.

geographic p. A study of the distribution of diseases and their manifestations in various parts of the world.

gynecologic p. The pathology of the female sexual organs and associated structures.

humoral p. Historical, but invalid, theory that disease is caused by alterations in constitution of the blood and various secretions. The term is now occasionally applied to effects of immune bodies in blood, tissue fluids, exudates, and secretions.

medical p. The study of diseases not of surgical importance.

ophthalmic p. The pathology of the eye and associated structures.

physiologic p. Utilization of physiology in the study of disease.

special p. Application of the laws of general pathology to individual organs or systems.

surgical p. The study of diseases in the realm of surgery.

veterinary p. Pathology of animals, principally domestic.

path"o·ma'ni·a [*pathos;* G. *mania*, madness]. Moral insanity. *Obs.*

pa·thom'e·try [*pathos;* G. *metron*, a measure]. Estimation of the number of people suffering from a disease and the conditions which increase or decrease this number. —**pathomet'ric,** *adj.*

path"o·mi·me'sis (path"o·mi·mee'sis, ·migh·mee'-sis) [*pathos;* G. *mimēsis*, imitation]. Imitation of the symptoms and signs of a disease; occurs in hysteria and in malingering. Syn., *pathomimicry.*

path"o·mim'ic·ry [*pathos;* G. *mimikos*, of a mime]. Pathomimesis.

path"o·pho'bi·a [*pathos;* G. *phobos*, fear]. Exaggerated dread of disease. *Obs.*

path"o·phor'ic [*pathos;* G. *phorein*, to bear]. Carrying or transmitting disease, said of certain insects.

path·oph'o·rous. See *pathophoric.*

path"o·psy·chol'o·gy [*pathos;* G. *psychē*, soul; *logos*, word]. That branch of science dealing with the mental processes during disease, from the viewpoint of general, rather than medical, psychology. See *psychopathology.*

pa·tho'sis [*pathos;* G. *-ōsis*, condition]. A diseased condition, abnormality, or pathologic finding.

pa'tient [L. *pati*, to suffer]. A person under the care of a physician; a sick person.

ambulant p. An ambulatory patient.

bed p. A patient who is confined to bed or who, by nature of his disability, must take exercises in bed.

convalescent p. One in the stage of recovery from disease or injury.

litter p. *In military medicine*, a patient unable to walk and requiring medical care.

mental p. (a) In common usage, any patient who requires psychiatric care and treatment. (b) *In military medicine*, when used in connection with the evacuation of patients, those psychiatric cases requiring security accommodations aboard a ship, train, or other vehicle.

nontransportable p. *In military medicine*, a casualty whose physical condition is so poor that extended evacuation without proper medical treatment would seriously endanger life or limb.

troop-class p. *In military medicine*, an ambulant

patient who requires little medical care while en route during evacuation.

Patrick, Hugh Talbot [*American neurologist*, 1860–1938]. Described dolorogenic areas of the skin, mucous membrane of the cheeks, sides of the tongue, upper and lower lips, within the area of distribution of the fifth cranial nerve, stimulation of which initiates a paroxysmal attack of trigeminal neuralgia; called *Patrick's trigger areas.*

pat″ri·lin′e·al [L. *pater*, father; *linea*, line]. Pertaining to descent through the male line.

pat′ten [OF. *patten*]. A metal support serving as a high sole and attached to the shoe on the sound leg, to prevent weight bearing in hip disease and to permit the employment of traction apparatus on the affected leg.

pat′tern [ME. *patron*]. Example, model, design.

action p. Crile's term for the brain impulses which induce certain actions peculiar to the individual. Such impulses may be wholly or partly congenital, or acquired.

juvenile T p. Persistence of inverted or diphasic T waves (ST-T complexes), found in precordial electrocardiograms of normal children.

mixed QT p. of electrocardiogram. That showing the initial ventricular deflections of one of the previous groups and the final ventricular deflections of the other, as Q_1T_3, or Q_3T_1.

Q_1T_1 p. of electrocardiogram (atypical). A pattern similar to that of the typical form, but with a high amplitude of the QRS group in lead I and a Q wave which is not prominent or is missing.

Q_1T_1 p. of electrocardiogram (typical). A pattern in recent, healing, and healed anterior infarction, low amplitude of QRS in lead I, prominent Q wave in lead I, deep S wave in leads II and III, progressive changes in the final ventricular deflections. At first, the latter consist of elevation of the S-T segment and fusion with the T wave in lead I and depression and fusion of this segment with the T wave in lead III. After a variable period of time, the displacement of S-T disappears, and T becomes sharply inverted in lead I, and sharply upright in lead III.

Q_3T_3 p. of electrocardiogram (atypical). A pattern similar to that of the typical form, but which does not show all of the details described for it.

Q_3T_3 p. of electrocardiogram (typical). A pattern in recent, healing, and healed posterior infarction, low amplitude of QRS in lead II, prominent Q wave in leads II and III, no Q wave in lead I, progressive changes in the final ventricular deflection. At first the latter consists of elevation of the S-T segment and fusion with T in leads II and III and depression and fusion of the segment with T in lead I. After a variable period of time, the displacement of the S-T segment disappears, and the T wave becomes sharply upright in lead I and sharply inverted in leads II and III.

pat′u·lin. An antibacterial substance originally prepared from *Penicillium patulum.* See *clavacin.*

pat′u·lous [L. *patulus*, standing open]. Expanded; open.

pau′cine. $C_{27}H_{39}N_5O_5$; an alkaloid from the seed of the owala tree, *Pentaclethra macrophylla.*

Paul, Constantin Charles Théodore [*French physician*, 1833–96]. Widely known as a cardiologist. Described a feeble apex beat with forcible impulse over the rest of the heart as indicative of adherent pericardium; called *Paul's sign.*

Paul, Frank Thomas [*English surgeon*, 1851–1941]. Introduced, coincidently with Samuel J. Mixter, a glass drainage tube with flanged edges for temporary use in intestinal operations; called *Paul's tube, Paul-Mixter's tube.* This was later modified and, in its present form, is regarded as a right-angled glass drainage tube with a flange to allow the placing of a purse string bowel suture about it. Paul devised an operation for obstructed colon similar to the Mikulicz operation; called *Paul-Mikulicz operation, enterectomy in stages.*

Paul of Aegina (Paulus). Greek physician of the late 7th century, famous in Alexandria; author of an early compilation on medicine and surgery. He wrote the first recorded description of lead poisoning.

Paul's test. See under *test.*

Paul-Bunnell test. See under *test.*

Pauling, Linus Carl (1901–). American chemist who received the Nobel prize in chemistry (1954) for research in the structure of proteins and immunochemistry, widely known for his determinations of the structure of crystals and molecules and of the nature of chemical bonds.

Paul·lin′i·a [after Christian Franz *Paullini*, German botanist, 1643–1712]. A genus of woody vines. The seeds of **P. cupana** are the source of guarana.

pau″lo·car′di·a [G. *paula*, pause; *kardia*, heart]. A subjective sensation of intermission or momentary stoppage of the heartbeat.

paunch [L. *pantex*, paunch]. 1. Colloquial term for the abdominal cavity and its contents. 2. *In veterinary medicine*, the rumen.

pause [G. *pausis*, a stopping]. A temporary stop or rest.

compensatory p. Any pause which, immediately succeeding a premature beat, compensates by its length for the prematurity of the beat. Also called *returning cycle.*

pau″si·me′ni·a (paw″si·mee′nee·uh, paw″zi·). See *menopause.*

Pauzat, Jean Eugène [*French physician*, contemporary]. Described osteoplastic periostitis of the metatarsal bones, called *Pauzat's disease.*

pa′vaex (pay′vex). See *pavex.*

pavatrine. Trade-mark for β-diethylaminoethyl fluorene-9-carboxylate hydrochloride; $C_{13}H_9$.-$COOC_2H_4N(C_2H_5)_2$.HCl. The substance is an antispasmodic, inducing muscular relaxation through its effects upon the autonomic nervous system, as well as upon involuntary muscle. Used in the alleviation of dysmenorrhea and in the management of gastrointestinal disturbances.

pave′ment-ep″i·the′li·um. Epithelium consisting of flattened, scalelike cells fitted together by their edges like the tiles of a pavement. *Obs.*

pave′ment·ing [L. *pavimentum*, pavement]. A stage in the process of tissue inflammation in which the blood stream in the capillaries becomes slowed, the leukocytes gravitating out of the central current to become adherent to the vessel walls.

paveril. Trade-mark for *dioxyline.* The drug is supplied as a phosphate salt.

paveril phosphate. Trade-marked name for the antispasmodic and peripheral vasodilator substance dioxyline phosphate.

pa′vex, pa′vaex [*pa*ssive *va*scular *ex*ercise]. A positive-negative pressure apparatus for passive vascular exercise in the treatment of thromboangiitis obliterans.

Pavlov, Ivan Petrovich (1849–1936). Russian physiologist known for his contributions to our knowledge of cardiac and digestive physiology, of the central nervous system, and psychophysiology. He discovered, independently of W. H. Gaskell, the special innervation of the heart, and also the secretory innervation of the pancreas (1888); developed an experimental technique of "sham feeding," and by establishing salivary, pancreatic, and biliary fistulas in dogs, studied the secretion of the digestive glands (1889–1904). He investigated gastric secretion by means of a small portion of stomach completely separated from the main stomach but retaining its vagal nerve branches, which communicated with the exterior (*Pavlov's pouch*). Applying these procedures to the long-term study of secretion in healthy animals, he discovered the conditioned reflex (first English publication, 1928), and then concentrated on the activity of higher nervous centers as determined by the conditioned reflex. Nobel laureate in physiology and medicine (1904).

pa'vor [L.]. Fright; fear.

p. nocturnus. Night cry; nightmare.

Pavy, Frederick William [*English physician*, 1829–1911]. Known for his studies in metabolism. Made important investigations in diabetes mellitus (1862). Described recurrent or cyclic albuminuria (1885), called *Pavy's disease*. Described a type of arthritis seen in some cases of typhoid fever, which is known as *Pavy's joint*. Introduced a modification of Fehling's solution; *Pavy's solution* is used in testing for sugar.

Pawlik, Karel J. [*Czechoslovakian surgeon*, 1849–1914]. Described the triangle on the anterior wall of the vagina which corresponds to the trigonum vesicae and is called *Pawlik's triangle*. Described the anterior columns of the vagina which form the lateral boundaries of Pawlik's triangle and serve as landmarks in locating the opening of the ureters; known as *Pawlik's folds*.

paw'paw [Sp. *papayo*, papaw tree]. Papaw. See *papaya*.

Payr, Erwin [*German surgeon*, 1871–1947]. Introduced an operation for draining hydrocephaly by means of transplanted blood vessels lying in the ventricles. Developed a crushing forceps used before cutting, in gastrointestinal resection; called *Payr's clamp*. Described colonic stasis due to kinking at the splenic or hepatic flexures; called *Payr's disease*.

paytine. $C_{21}H_{24}N_2O.H_2O$; an alkaloid from white cinchona bark, *Payta alba*.

P. B. *Pharmacopoeia Britannica*, British Pharmacopoeia.

Pb Chemical symbol for lead (*plumbum*).

P. B. E. A tuberculin prepared from bovine tubercle bacilli; similar to Koch's new tuberculin.

PBI Protein-bound iodine in the blood.

P. D. Doctor of Pharmacy.

Pd Chemical symbol for palladium.

Peacock, Thomas Bevill (1812–1882). English physician who noted the congenital anomaly of the heart, later called the *tetralogy of Fallot*.

Péan, Jules Emile [*French surgeon*, 1830–98]. Resected the pylorus and extirpated fibroids through the vaginal approach. Devised a position used for operating, with the patient lying on a low table and the surgeon seated on a high chair placed between the patient's legs; called *Péan's position*. Inventor of the simple hemostat called *Péan's forceps*.

Pearl, Raymond [*American biologist and statistician*, 1879–1940]. Widely known as a vital statistician. Contributed studies in genetics (1915) and the growth of population in the United States since 1790 (completed in 1920).

pearl [ML. *perla*]. A rounded aggregation of squamous epithelial cells, concentrically arranged, seen in certain carcinomas and also in sites of epithelial union of embryonically open hiatuses, e.g., palatine raphe: also called *epithelial p.*

Pearson, George [*English physician*, 1751–1828]. Introduced an aqueous solution of sodium arsenate, one-tenth the strength of the liquor sodii arsenatis; called *Pearson's solution*.

peat [ME. *pete*]. The product of the spontaneous decomposition of plants, especially swamp plants, in many cases mixed with sand, loam, clay, lime, iron pyrites, or ocher.

Pecquet, Jean [*French anatomist*, 1622–74]. Discovered the thoracic duct, in dogs, the most important channel through which lymph and chyle are carried to the blood; called *Pecquet's duct*. The dilated abdominal portion in which it begins is called the *receptaculum chyli*, *Pecquet's cistern* or *reservoir*.

pec'tase. An enzyme, found associated with pentose in fruits, which converts the pectose into pectin.

pec'ten [L., comb]. 1. Old term for os pubis. 2. The middle third of the anal canal.

p. ossis pubis. The pectineal line of the pubis, a continuation of the ileopectineal line.

pec"te·no'sis [L. *pecten*, comb; G. *-ōsis*, condition]. Induration of the pecten, or middle third of the anal canal.

pec'tic ac'id. A complex acid, partially demethylated, obtained from the pectin of fruits.

pec'tin [G. *pēktos*, congealed] (*pectinum*). Pectin is a purified carbohydrate product obtained from the dilute acid extract of the inner portion of the rind of citrus fruits, or from apple pomace. It consists chiefly of partially methoxylated polygalacturonic acids; a coarse or fine powder, yellowish white in color, almost odorless, and with a mucilaginous taste; it is almost completely soluble in 20 parts of water, forming a viscous, opalescent colloidal solution which flows readily and is acid to litmus paper; it is insoluble in alcohol.

p. insulin. A slowly absorbed preparation of insulin in a viscous medium containing 4 to 5 per cent pectin and adjusted to pH 4.0 to 4.4. See *decurvon*.

p. paste (*pasta pectini*). Contains 7.5% of pectin in a vehicle of glycerin and isotonic solution of three chlorides. Used as an application for the treatment of bed sores and ulcers.

thin p. paste (*pasta pectini tenuis*). Contains 3.5% of pectin. Because of its lesser viscosity it is preferred in extensive excoriations and ulcerated conditions of the skin.

pec'tin·ase. The enzyme capable of transforming pectin into sugars and galacturonic acid.

pec'ti·nate [L. *pecten*, comb]. Arranged like the teeth of a comb.

pec·tin'e·al [*pecten*]. 1. Comb-shaped. 2. Pertaining to the pecten or os pubis.

pec·tin'e·us, pec"ti·ne'us [*pecten*]. A muscle arising from the pubis and inserted on the femur. See Table of Muscles in the Appendix.

pec'tin·ose. See *arabinose*.

pec"ti·za'tion. *In colloid chemistry*, the transformation of sols into gels. *Obs.* See *coagulation*, *flocculation*.

pec'to·ral [L. *pectoralis*, of the breast]. Pertaining to the chest, as the pectoral muscles, which connect the arm and the chest.

pec"to·ra'lis (peck"to·rah'lis, ·ray'lis) [L.]. One of two muscles, major and minor, on the anterior aspect of the chest. See Table of Muscles in the Appendix.

p. major. The larger muscle of the anterior thoracic wall.

p. minimus. A variant of the pectoralis minor muscle, extending from the cartilage of the first rib to the coracoid process.

p. minor. The smaller and deeper muscle of the anterior thoracic wall.

pec"to·ril'o·quy [L. *pectus*, breast; *loqui*, to speak]. Exaggerated bronchophony, in which there is distinct transmission of articulate speech in addition to increased intensity of the voice sounds. Heard over consolidations which are either large in extent or located in proximity to a major air passage.

whispered p. The transmission of whispered voice sounds having the same characteristics and the same significance as above.

pec′tose [G. *pēktos*, congealed]. The water-insoluble pectin substance occurring in various unripe fruits. It is converted into the water-soluble pectin by the combined action of weak acid and heat, or, in the fruit, by the enzyme pectase, as the fruit ripens. Also called *pectinogen, protopectin.*

pec′tous [*pēktos*]. Relating to pectin or pectose.

pec′tus [L.]. The chest or breast.

p. carinatum. See pigeon *breast.*

p. excavatum. See funnel *breast.*

pe″dar·throc′a·ce (pee″dahr·throck′uh·see, ped″-ahr·) [G. *pais*, child; *arthron*, joint; *kakē*, evil]. A necrotic ulceration or caries of the joints of children.

pe·dat′ro·phy, pe″da·tro′phi·a [*pais;* G. *atrophia*, a want of food]. 1. Any wasting disease of childhood. 2. Tabes mesenterica.

ped′er·as″ty [G. *paiderastia*, love of boys]. Sexual intercourse through the anus; practiced on boys. See also *sodomy.* —**pederast,** *n.*

pe·de′sis [G. *pēdēsis*, a leaping]. The dancing, oscillating motion of the particles of any substance sufficiently powdered and suspended in a suitable liquid.

ped″i·al′gi·a (ped″ee·al′juh, ·jee·uh, pee″dee·) [L. *pes*, foot; G. *algos*, pain]. Pain in the foot.

pe″di·at′rics (pee″dee·at′ricks, ped″ee·) [G. *pais*, child; *iatrikos*, of a physician]. The branch of medicine dealing with children's diseases. —**pediatric,** *adj.*

pe″di·at′rist, pe″di·a·tri′cian. A specialist in children's diseases.

ped′i·at″ry (ped′ee·at″ree, pi·dye′uh·tree) [*pais;* G. *iatreia*, medical treatment]. Pediatrics.

ped′i·cel·late [L. *pediculus*, little foot]. Pedunculated.

ped′i·cle [*pediculus*]. A slender process acting as a foot or stem, as the pedicle of a tumor.

vertebral p. The portion of bone projecting backward from each side of the body of a vertebra, and connecting the lamina with the body.

pe·dic′te·rus [G. *pais*, child; *ikteros*, jaundice]. Jaundice of the newborn; icterus neonatorum.

pe·dic′u·lar [L. *pediculus*, louse]. Lousy; pertaining to lice.

pe·dic″u·la′tion [L. *pediculus*, little foot]. The process of developing a pedicle.

pe·dic″u·la′tion [L. *pediculus*, louse]. The state of one suffering from pediculosis.

pe·dic′u·li·cide [*pediculus;* L. *caedere*, to kill]. An agent which destroys lice.

Pe·dic″u·loi′des (pi·dick″yoo·loy′deez) [*pediculus;* G. *eidos*, form]. A genus of mites.

P. ventricosus. A microscopically small mite which infests straw, stored grain, and cotton. Among laborers handling cereals and cotton it causes outbreaks of a dermatitis (*acarodermatitis urticarioides*) which may be marked in severe cases by fever and nausea.

pe·dic″u·lo·pho′bi·a [*pediculus;* G. *phobos*, fear]. Morbid dread of infestation with lice.

pe·dic″u·lo′sis [*pediculus;* G. *-ōsis*, condition]. A skin disease due to infestation by lice, characterized by intense pruritus and cutaneous lesions.

p. capitis. Infestation of the scalp with the species *Pediculus humanus* var. *capitis* occurring chiefly in women and girls with long hair.

p. corporis. Infestation of the skin of the body with the species *Pediculus humanus* var. *corporis.* In cases of long standing the chronic scratching gives rise to pigmentation and lichenification of the skin, the so-called *vagabond's disease.*

p. palpebrarum. That of the eyebrows and the eyelashes. See also *p.* pubis.

p. pubis. An infestation of the pubic hair with the *Phthirius pubis*, the crab louse; may spread over the body and involve the axillas, eyebrows, and eyelashes.

pe·dic′u·lous [*pediculus*]. Infested with lice.

Pe·dic′u·lus [L., louse]. A genus of small parasitic insects known as lice, whose species produce dermatitis and transmit diseases, such as typhus fever, trench fever, and relapsing fever.

P. humanus var. capitis. The head louse; important as a vector of disease and produces pediculosis capitis.

P. humanus var. corporis. The body louse; important as a vector of disease and causes pediculosis corporis.

ped′i·cure [L. *pes*, foot; *cura*, care]. Care of the feet.

ped′i·palp [NL. *pedi*, from G. *pedion*, sole, instep; NL. *palpus*, a feeler]. One of the pincer appendages of *Arachnida* for attaching the animal to its host while sucking.

pe·di′tis [*pes;* G. *-itis*, inflammation]. An inflammation of the pedal bone of a horse.

Pedley's method. See Shohl and Pedley's *method.*

pe″do·bar″o·ma·crom′e·ter (pee″do·, ped″o·) [G. *pais*, child; *baros*, weight; *makros*, large; *metron*, a measure]. An instrument for weighing and measuring infants. *Obs.*

pe″do·ba·rom′e·ter [*pais; baros; metron*]. An instrument for weighing a child. *Obs.*

pe″do·don′tics [*pais; odous*]. The branch of dentistry which treats abnormal oral and dental conditions occurring in childhood: also called *pedodontia, pedodontology.*

pe″do·don′tist [*pais odous*]. One who specializes in pedodontics.

pe″do·don·tol′o·gy. See *pedodontics.*

ped″o·dy″na·mom′e·ter [L. *pes*, foot; G. *dynamis*, power; *metron*, a measure]. An instrument for measuring the muscular strength of the leg.

pe″do·gen′e·sis. See *neoteny.*

pe·dol′o·gist [G. *pais*, child; *logos*, word]. A specialist in pediatrics.

pe·dol′o·gy [*pais; logos*]. The science, or sum of knowledge, regarding childhood, its diseases, hygiene, etc.

pe·dom′e·ter [*pais;* G. *metron*, a measure]. An instrument for weighing and measuring a newborn child. —**pedometry,** *n.*

pe·dom′e·ter [L. *pes*, foot; *metron*]. An instrument which registers the number of footsteps in walking. —**pedometry,** *n.*

pe″do·no·sol′o·gy. See *pedology.*

pe·dop′a·thy [*pes;* G. *pathos*, disease]. Disease of the foot.

pe″do·phil′i·a [G. *pais*, child; *philein*, to love]. Fondness for children; usually, love of children by adults for sexual purposes.

pe″do·pho′bi·a [*pais;* G. *phobos*, fear]. Morbid dislike or fear of children.

pe·dun′cle (pi·dung′kul, ped′ung·kul, pee′dung·kul) [L. *pedunculus*, little foot]. A narrow part acting as a support. —**peduncular, pedunculate, pedunculated,** *adj.*

cerebral p. One of two large bands of white matter containing descending axons of upper motor neurons which emerge from the underside of the cerebral hemispheres to approach each other as they enter the rostral border of the pons. Between the peduncles, which form the ventral part of the mesencephalon, lies the interpeduncular fossa. Syn., *crus of the cerebrum.*

inferior cerebellar p. A large bundle of nerve fibers running from the medulla oblongata to the cerebellum. It contains the dorsal spinocerebellar tract from the nucleus dorsalis of the spinal cord, olivocerebellar fibers from the inferior olivary nuclei, dorsal external arcuate fibers from the lateral cuneate nucleus, and ventral external arcuate fibers from the arcuate and lateral reticular nuclei. Syn., *restiform body.*

middle cerebellar p. One of the bands of white matter joining the pons and the cerebellum: also called *pontocerebellar tract.* Syn., *brachium pontis.*

p. of the pineal body. A delicate white band passing forward from each side of the pineal body along the edge of the third ventricle.

superior cerebellar p. A large band of nerve fibers which arise in the dentate and emboliform nuclei of the cerebellum, form the dorsolateral part of the rostral portion of the fourth ventricle, decussate in the region of the inferior colliculi, and end in the red nucleus and thalamus. Syn., *brachium conjunctivum.*

peel′ing [ME. *pelen* from L. *pilare,* to deprive of the hair]. A term applied to the process of desquamation, as after any inflammation of the skin. It is a result of disturbed keratinization of epidermis.

Peet, Max Minor [*American surgeon,* 1885–1949]. Known for his operation for the relief of hypertension, in which he removed subdiaphragmatically the greater and lesser splanchnic nerves and the ninth, tenth, eleventh, and twelfth thoracic ganglions.

peg [ME. *pegge*]. 1. A pointed pin of wood, metal, or other material. 2. A wooden leg.

bone p. A peg or screw fashioned of beef bone, used in bone operations to secure immobility.

peg′a·nine (peg′uh·neen, ·nin). *l*-Peganine. An alkaloid, $C_{11}H_{12}N_2O$, from the leaves of *Adhatoda vasica* and *Peganum harmala.* A bronchial dilator. Syn., *vasicine.*

pei″no·ther′a·py (pye″no·therr′uh·pee) [G. *peina,* hunger; *therapeia,* treatment]. The cure of disease by deprivation of food. *Rare.*

Pekelharing, Cornelis Adrianus [*Dutch physiologist,* 1848–1922]. Known for his theory of blood coagulation. According to *Pekelharing's theory,* thrombin supplies calcium which unites with fibrinogen to form fibrin.

Pel, Pieter Klazes [*Dutch physician,* 1852–1919]. Described the ocular crises in tabes (1898), called *Pel's crises.* Described pseudoleukemia or lymphadenoma with periodic pyrexia (1885), which was investigated by Wilhelm Ebstein at about the same time. Called *Pel-Ebstein's disease.* See also Pel-Ebstein *fever.*

Pel, von. See Alexander von *Poehl.*

pe·la′da, pe·lade′ (pi·lahd′, pi·lad′) [F.]. Alopecia areata of the scalp.

pel′age [F., from L. *pilus,* hair]. The hairy covering of the body.

pel″ar·gon′ic ac′id. The fatty acid, $CH_3.(CH_2)_7.$-COOH; formed artificially by oxidation of oleic acid; occurs naturally in the glycerides of certain oils.

pel″ar·go′nin. $C_{27}H_{30}O_{15}$; a glycoside in flowers of certain pelargonium species and of several other plants.

p electron. See under *electron.*

Pelger, Karel [*Dutch physician,* 1885–1931]. Described an anomalous appearance of the nuclei of leukocytes consisting of coarse nuclear structure, division of neutrophils into not more than two segments, and a pear-shaped nuclear outline of segmented cells; observed in constitutional disease of bone marrow; called *Pelger's nuclear anomaly.*

pel″i·com′e·ter. Pelvimeter.

pel″i·di′si (pel″i·dee′see, ·dee′zee) [L. *p*ondus *d*ecies *li*neare *di*visio *s*edent*i*s altitudo]. According to Pirquet, the cube of the sitting height of a person expressed in centimeters is approximately the weight in grams of a normal person. The ratio, as expressed in the following formulas, is called the pelidisi.

$$\frac{\text{10 times the weight}}{\text{sitting height}^3} = 100\%$$

or

$$\frac{\sqrt[3]{\text{10 times the weight}}}{\text{sitting height}} = 100\%$$

pel″i·o′sis (pel″ee·o′sis, pee″lee·) [G., extravasation of the blood]. Purpura.

p. rheumatica. See Schönlein's *purpura.*

Pelizaeus, Friedrich [*German neurologist,* b. 1850]. Described aplasia axialis extracorticalis congenita, also called *Merzbacher-Pelizaeus disease.* See under *aplasia.*

pel·lag′ra (pi·lag′ruh, pi·lay′gruh) [It., from L. *pellis,* skin; G. *agra,* a seizing]. A syndrome resulting from nicotinic acid deficiency, characterized by dermatitis of sun-exposed surfaces, glossitis and stomatitis, diarrhea, and in severe cases by disturbances of the central nervous system. It may be due to faulty diet, or it may occur secondarily to various diseases, especially of the digestive system. Other vitamin deficiencies often coexist. —**pellag′rous,** *adj.*

p. sine pellagra. Pellagra without the erythematous rash.

pel·la′grin [*pellagra*]. One afflicted with pellagra.

Pellegrini, Augusto [*Italian surgeon, contemporary*]. Described posttraumatic calcification of the medial collateral ligament of the knee; called *Pellegrini-Stieda disease.*

pel′let [L. *pila,* ball]. A small pill.

Pelletier, Pierre Joseph [*French chemist,* 1788–1842]. Made important discoveries of active principles of drugs. Isolated emetine (1817), strychnine (1819), and quinine (1820).

pel″le·tier′ine (pel″i·teer′een, ·in, pel″et·yair′·, pi-let′i·reen, ·rin, pel″i·tee″eh·reen′) [*Pelletier*]. A liquid alkaloid obtained together with an isomeric body, isopelletierine, also a liquid alkaloid, from pomegranate bark. These are also called *punicine* and *isopunicine.* It is used as a taeniafuge, chiefly in the form of the tannate.

p. tannate (*pelletierinae tannas*). A mixture in varying proportions of the tannates of several alkaloids obtained from pomegranate, *Punica granatum* Linné. A light yellow, amorphous powder; 1 Gm. dissolves in about 250 cc. of water. Insoluble in chloroform. Most important of the several alkaloids present are pelletierine (punicine) and isopelletierine. Used as an anthelmintic and taeniafuge. The tannate is the least dangerous form of the drug since its slight solubility prevents rapid absorption. Dose, 0.1–0.3 Gm. (2–5 gr.) followed by an active cathartic.

pel′li·cle [L. *pellicula,* small skin]. 1. A thin membrane, or cuticle. 2. A film on the surface of a liquid. —**pellic′ular, pellic′ulous, pellic′ulate,** *adj.*

pel·lic′u·la [L.]. Epidermis.

pel′li·to″ry. See *pyrethrum.*

pel′lo·tine (pel′o·teen, ·tin). $C_{13}H_{19}NO_3$. An alkaloid from the Mexican cactus, *Lophophora williamsii.* Produces central nervous system depression.

pel·lu′cid [L. *pellucere,* to shine through]. Transparent; translucent; not opaque.

pel′o- [G. *pēlos,* mud]. A combining form meaning *mud.*

pe'loid. Generic term for muds and moors used in physical therapy; they may be purely mineral as fango, a volcanic residue, mainly mineral, as sea mud or liman, or mainly vegetable, as moors or peats.

pel·ol'o·gy (pel·ol'o·jee). The study of mud and similar substances.

pe·lop'si·a [G. *pelas*, near; *opsis*, vision]. A defect of vision characterized by illusions of abnormal nearness of objects.

pel'o·sine (pel'o·seen, pi·lo'seen). An alkaloid derived from *Cissampelos pareira*. Syn., *bebeerine*.

pel"o·ther'a·py. Treatment with mud.

pel·ta'tin. Either of two related constituents identified as α-peltatin and β-peltatin, obtained from the rhizome and roots of *Podophyllum peltatum*. β-Peltatin contains a methoxyl (OCH_3) group in place of a hydroxyl (OH) group in α-peltatin; both are related to podophyllotoxin. Both are active, when applied topically, against certain wartlike neoplasms.

pel'vic ham'mock. A canvas sling, generally attached to an overhead bed frame, used to suspend the lower part of the trunk and pelvis in pelvic fractures.

pel"vi·en·ceph"a·lom'e·try [L. *pelvis*, basin; G. *egkephalos*, brain; *metron*, a measure]. Measurement of the maternal pelvis and fetal skull by means of radiographic examination.

pel·vim'e·ter [*pelvis; metron*]. An instrument for measuring the pelvic dimensions.

pel·vim'e·try [*pelvis; metron*]. The measurement of the dimensions of the pelvis.

AVERAGE MEASUREMENTS OF THE ADULT FEMALE PELVIS COVERED BY THE SOFT PARTS

Between iliac spines	26	cm.
Between iliac crests	29	"
External conjugate diameter	20¼	"
Internal conjugate diagonal	12¾	"
True conjugate, estimated	11	"
Right diagonal	22	"
Left diagonal	22	"
Between trochanters	31	"
Circumference of pelvis	90	"

combined p. A combination of external and internal pelvimetry.

digital p. Measurement of the pelvis by means of the hand.

external p. Measurement of external diameters of the pelvis, to estimate the dimensions of the internal parts.

internal p. Measurement of the internal dimensions of the pelvis by hand or by pelvimeter.

manual p. See digital *p*.

pel"vi·o·li·thot'o·my [*pelvis;* G. *lithos*, stone; *tomē*, a cutting]. Removal of a kidney stone from the renal pelvis.

pel"vi·o·ne"o·cys·tos'to·my. A surgical procedure in which the renal pelvis is anastomosed to the urinary bladder in cases of hydronephrotic ectopic kidneys: rarely used.

pel"vi·o·ra"di·og'ra·phy. Measurement of the pelvis and fetal head by radiography. A number of methods are utilized, all of which are concerned with correcting the distortion that occurs in roentgenograms.

pel"vi·ot'o·my [*pelvis; tomē*]. 1. Incision of the renal pelvis. 2. Pelvisection.

pel'vis (pl. *pelves*) [L.]. 1. A basin or basin-shaped cavity, as the pelvis of the kidney. 2. The bony ring formed by the two innominate bones and the sacrum and coccyx. 3. The cavity bounded by the bony pelvis. The cavity consists of two parts: the true pelvis and the false pelvis, which are separated by the iliopectineal line. The entrance of the true pelvis, corresponding to this line, is known as the inlet or superior strait; the outlet or inferior strait is bounded by the symphysis pubis, the tip of the coccyx, and the two ischia. See Plates 1, 14, 44. —**pelvic,** *adj.*

android p. A female pelvis with a deeper cavity and more conical shape, similar to the normal male pelvis.

anthropoid p. The type of female pelvis resembling that of the great apes, a long, narrow, oval pelvis with the anteroposterior diameter greater than the transverse.

assimilation p. An anomaly of the pelvis, in which the transverse processes of the last lumbar vertebra may be transformed and fused with the sacral vertebrae.

asymmetrical p. One in which the two lateral halves are markedly dissimilar in contour.

beaked p. One in which the pubic bones are compressed laterally so as to approach each other, and are pushed forward; a condition seen in osteomalacia.

bifid p. A congenital anomaly of the renal pelvis in which there are two major calyces.

brachypellic p. Oval type of pelvis having a transverse diameter more than one and less than three centimeters greater than the anteroposterior diameter.

brim of the p. The pelvic inlet.

contracted p. One having one or more major diameters reduced in size, interfering with parturition.

cordate p. One with a heart-shaped inlet.

coxalgic p. An obliquely contracted pelvis, due to unequal pressure of the femora in unilateral disease of the hip in early life.

coxarthrolisthetic p. A unilateral or bilateral transversely contracted pelvis, resulting from softening about the acetabulum with projection of the head of the femur into the pelvic cavity.

dolichopellic p. See anthropoid *p*.

dwarf p. Deformity of the pelvis seen in true hypoplastic, chondrodystrophic, cretin, and rachitic dwarfs.

false p. That part above the iliopectineal line.

fetal p. See infantile *p*.

flat p. Deformity of the pelvis in which all anteroposterior diameters are shortened but the transverse diameters are practically normal.

funnel p. A deformity in which the usual external measurements are normal while the outlet is contracted, the transverse diameter of the latter being eight centimeters or less.

generally contracted p. One having all diameters symmetrically shortened; a small normally shaped pelvis.

generally enlarged p. One having all diameters symmetrically enlarged; a large normally shaped pelvis.

greater p. The false pelvis.

gynecoid p. A female pelvis in which the inlet is round instead of oval or blunt heart-shaped.

infantile p. An adult pelvis retaining the infantile shape.

justamajor p. A generally enlarged pelvis.

justaminor p. A generally contracted pelvis.

kyphorachitic p. A deformity of the pelvis associated with rickets in which changes are slight because the effect of kyphosis tends to counterbalance that of rickets.

kyphoscoliorachitic p. A deformity of the pelvis resembling the kyphorachitic type because the kyphotic and rachitic effects counterbalance each other. However, a considerable degree of oblique deformity of the superior strait is usually present.

kyphoscoliotic p. A deformity of the pelvis varying in character with the predominance of the kyphosis or scoliosis of the vertebral column.

kyphotic p. One characterized by increase of the conjugata vera, but decrease of the transverse diameter of the outlet, through approximation of the ischial spines and tuberosities. Associated with kyphosis of the vertebral column.

lesser p. The true pelvis.

masculine p. A female pelvis resembling the normal male pelvis; an android pelvis.

mesatipellic p. See gynecoid *p.*

Naegele p. An obliquely contracted pelvis with ankylosis of one sacroiliac synchondrosis, underdevelopment of the associated sacral ala, and other distorting defects producing an obliquely directed conjugata vera.

obliquely contracted p. A deformed pelvis with unequal oblique diameters.

osteomalacic p. A distorted pelvis characterized by a lessening of the transverse and oblique diameters, with great increase of the anteroposterior diameter.

p. aequabiliter justo major. A generally enlarged pelvis.

p. aequabiliter justo minor. A generally contracted pelvis.

p. fissa. Congenital cleft of the pubic symphysis. Syn., *split p.*

p. major. The false pelvis.

p. minor. The true pelvis.

p. nana. A generally contracted pelvis tending toward the infantile type, with persistence of cartilage at all the epiphyses; dwarf pelvis.

p. spinosa. One deformed by sharp bony outgrowths which may injure maternal soft parts, but rarely present an obstacle to labor.

platypelloid p. Flat pelvis. Also spelled *platypellic p.*

pseudospider p. A congenitally small, long, thin renal pelvis which resembles the pyelogram of certain renal tumors.

rachitic p. One characterized by a sinking in and forward of the sacrovertebral angle, with a flaring outward of the iliac crests and increased separation of the iliac spines.

renal p. The expansion of the proximal end of the ureter which receives the major and minor calyxes within the renal sinus.

Robert p. A transversely contracted pelvis having a rudimentary sacrum, undeveloped sacral alae, and much narrowed oblique and transverse diameters.

scoliotic p. A pelvis with slight asymmetry depending upon the situation and degree of scoliosis of the vertebral column.

simple flat p. One in which the only deformity consists in a shortening of the anteroposterior diameter.

split p. A form in which there is congenital separation of the pubic bones at the symphysis, often associated with exstrophy of the urinary bladder; pelvis fissa.

spondylolisthetic p. A deformity resulting from a forward displacement of the centrum of the last lumbar vertebra.

transversely contracted p. One having a reduced transverse diameter.

true p. That part of the pelvic cavity situated below the iliopectineal line.

pel'vi·scope. An endoscope for examination of the pelvic organs of the female.

pel"vi·sec'tion [*pelvis;* L. *sectio*, a cutting]. A cutting through of one or more of the bones of the pelvis. *Obs.*

pem'mi·can [Cree *pemikkân*]. A concentrated food consisting of powdered dried buffalo meat or venison mixed with melted fat; also a similar preparation, as of dried beef, suet, raisins, and sugar; used by explorers, etc.

pem'phi·goid [G. *pemphix*, pustule]. A bullous disease like pemphigus vulgaris but more benign and self-limited, perhaps a bullous variant of dermatitis herpetiformis. Oral involvement may be absent and is usually mild. Upon rupture of the bullae, the eroded areas do not increase much in size and tend to heal.

pem'phi·gus (pem'fi·gus) [G. *pemphix*, pustule]. An acute or chronic disease of the skin characterized by the appearance of bullae which develop in crops or continuous succession. —**pemphigoid,** *adj.*

familial benign p. A vesicular and bullous dermatitis localized to the sides of the neck, the axillary spaces, and other flexor surfaces. It is distinctly familial, and is possibly a variant of keratosis follicularis. Also called *Hailey-Hailey disease.*

p. acutus. A type once thought to be associated with septic wounds and vaccination, and now considered to be an acute micrococcal infection with septicemia.

p. chronicus. See *p. vulgaris.*

p. erythematosus. A relatively benign form of chronic pemphigus combining features of lupus erythematosus, characterized by small bullae on the forehead, sternal skin, and upper back: also called *Senear-Usher syndrome.*

p. foliaceus. A rare type characterized by crops of flaccid blebs which recur and rupture, producing a marked scaliness and generalized exfoliation.

p. neonatorum. An acute form of micrococcal or streptococcal infection of the skin occurring in infants, probably more properly called *impetigo contagiosa.* It may be a form of bullous impetigo.

p. tropicus. A pyoderma in tropical climates.

p. vegetans. A form characterized by oral lesions followed by skin eruptions which rupture, leaving a raw surface on which vegetative or papillary growths develop.

p. vulgaris. A form that is usually chronic, characterized by successive crops of blebs which leave pigmented spots when they are healed.

pen"al·ge'si·a (pen"al·jee'zee·uh, ·see·uh) [G. *penia*, poverty; *algēsis*, sense of pain]. Reduction in the number of pain and touch spots in trigeminal neuralgia.

pen'a·tin. An antibiotic from *Penicillium notatum;* it is identical with corylophilline, *Escherichia coli* factor, mycoin, notatin, and penicillin-B.

pen'du·lous [L. *pendere*, to hang]. Hanging down loosely.

pen"e·tham'ate hy"dro·i'o·dide. Generic name for penicillin G diethylaminoethylester hydroiodide; a salt of benzyl penicillin characterized by low solubility and prolonged action, no longer available because of its toxicity. See *neopenil.*

pen'e·trance [L. *penetrare*, to penetrate]. The percentage of organisms having a given genetic constitution which show the corresponding hereditary character. Also see *expressivity.*

pen'e·tra"ting [*penetrare*]. Entering beyond the surface, as a penetrating wound, one that pierces the wall of a cavity or enters an organ.

pen"e·tra'tion [L. *penetratio*, from *penetrare*]. 1. The act of penetrating or piercing into. 2. Of a microscope, the focal depth. 3. The entrance of the penis into the vagina.

pen"e·trom'e·ter [*penetrare;* G. *metron*, a measure]. An instrument for estimating the penetrating power or hardness of a roentgen-ray beam.

Penfield, Wilder Graves (1891–). Canadian neurosurgeon who, with Foerster, described an operation for the relief of traumatic epilepsy in which he excised the cortical scar; called *Foerster-Penfield operation.* See also *Penfield's method* under *stain.*

pe·nic′i·din (peh·nis′i·din, pen″i·sigh′din). An antibiotic from species of *Penicillium;* soluble in ether, alcohol, and chloroform; insoluble in petroleum ether. It is active against Gram-negative and Gram-positive bacteria.

pen″i·cil′la·mine. $(CH_3)_2C(SH)CH(NH_2)COOH$. An amino acid obtained from all penicillins upon treatment with hot dilute mineral acid.

pen″i·cil′lase. See *penicillinase.*

pen″i·cil′late [L. *penicillum,* a painter's brush]. Ending in a tuft of hairs.

pen″i·cil′lic ac′id. An antibiotic from species of *Penicillium,* particularly *P. puberulum;* soluble in water. It is a rather weak antibiotic, active largely against Gram-positive bacteria, but is more active against Gram-negative bacteria than is penicillin.

pen″i·cil′li·form [*penicillum;* L. *forma,* form]. Penicillate; ending in a tuft of hairs.

pen″i·cil′lin [*penicillum*]. An antibacterial produced from strains of *Penicillium notatum.* Several penicillins are known, having the formula $C_9H_{11}O_4SN_2R$. In penicillin F (known in the United Kingdom as penicillin I), R is the Δ^2-pentenyl ($—CH_2CH:CHCH_2CH_3$) group; in penicillin G (penicillin II), R is benzyl ($C_6H_5CH_2—$); in penicillin X (penicillin III), R is *p*-hydroxybenzyl ($C_6H_4OHCH_2—$); in penicillin K, R is *n*-heptyl ($CH_3CH_2CH_2CH_2CH_2CH_2CH_2—$); in penicillin O, a biosynthetic derivative useful in patients sensitive to penicillin G, R is allylmercaptomethyl ($CH_2:CHCHSCH_2—$). Crystalline sodium or potassium salts, especially of penicillin G, are most commonly employed; other derivatives are described below. Aqueous solutions are most stable at a pH between 5 and 7; any deviation inactivates the drug, the rate depending on the temperature and pH. The action of penicillin upon bacteria is chiefly bacteriostatic and not bactericidal. It is a potent inhibitor of the growth of nearly all Gram-positive bacteria, certain Gram-negative cocci, and spirochetes; it has a high degree of specificity. Its bacterial activity is not interfered with by bacterial extracts, *p*-amino-benzoic acid, peptones, pus, blood, or body fluids, and it may be used either locally or systemically. Penicillin is not believed to cause organic injury; but it has considerable power of sensitization, and may produce serious toxic reactions. Sensitivity reactions vary from mild erythema to severe serum sickness and even death from anaphylactic shock. Penicillin is rapidly excreted by the kidneys; effective blood levels are maintained by administering poorly soluble salts which release the antibiotic slowly or by giving simultaneously a substance, like probenecid, which decreases the rate of excretion of penicillin.

benzathine p. G. Generic name for N,N′-dibenzylethylenediamine dipenicillin G, an oral dosage form which yields higher blood levels of penicillin than are obtainable with equivalent amounts of other dosage forms of the antibiotic. See *benzethacil, bicillin, neolin.*

chloroprocaine p. O. A crystalline salt of 2-chloroprocaine and penicillin O, similar to procaine penicillin G, especially useful for patients who are allergic to penicillin G. See *depo-cer-o-cillin.*

L-ephenamine p. G. A salt of penicillin G with L-ephenamine (N-methyl-1,2-diphenyl-2-hydroxyethylamine), a base which has antiallergic activity; the salt has low solubility in aqueous or oily dispersion media and thus has long duration of action. See *compenamine.*

p. B. An antibiotic identical with corylophilline, *Escherichia coli* factor, mycoin, notatin, and penatin.

p. G diethylaminoethylester hydroiodide. A salt of benzyl penicillin characterized by low solubility and prolonged action; it produces relatively high concentrations of penicillin in lung tissue, sputum, and cerebrospinal fluid. Because of severe anaphylactoid and fatal reactions it has been withdrawn from the market. Syn., *penethamate hydroiodide.* See *neo-penil.*

p. G procaine. The procaine salt of benzyl penicillin, a sparingly soluble salt of the penicillin which releases the antibiotic slowly to give prolonged effective blood levels. The procaine component minimizes pain of injection. Penicillin G procaine is commonly administered in suspension in aqueous or oily medium. Also written *procaine penicillin G.*

p. V. Phenoxymethyl penicillin, a biosynthetic form poorly soluble in acid media and resistant to destruction by gastric juice.

pen″i·cil′lin·ase. Any enzyme, found in many bacteria, which antagonizes the antibacterial action of penicillin.

pen″i·cil″li·o′sis. Lesions of ear, skin, and occasionally lungs, caused by certain species of *Penicillium.*

Pen″i·cil′li·um [*penicillum*]. A genus of fungi of the Ascomycetes in which the fruiting organs have a brushlike form. The species **Penicillium chrysogenum, P. citrinum, P. claviforme, P. notatum, P. patulum, P. puberulum, P. spinulosum** are used in the production of antibiotics. Species are also common allergens.

pen″i·cil·lo′ic ac′id. Any one of the dicarboxylic acids formed when the lactam ring in a penicillin is opened by the action of alkalies or penicillinase.

pen″i·cil′lus (pl. *penicilli*) [L., painter's brush]. One of the tufts of fine twigs into which the arteries of the spleen subdivide. —**penicil′lar,** *adj.*

pe·nil′lic ac′id. Any one of the dicarboxylic acids resulting when a penicillin is subjected to a mild acid treatment; the penillic acids are isomeric with the corresponding penicillins.

pe′nis [L.]. The male organ of copulation. Its essential parts consist of the corpus cavernosum urethrae enclosing the urethra and forming the glans, and the two corpora cavernosa, all covered by fascia and skin. See Plate 44. —**pe′nile,** *adj.*

chordeic p. See *chordee.*

concealed p. A congenital anomaly in which the penis, in this condition usually only rudimentary, is hidden within the scrotum or perineal skin.

p. captivus. One held in the vagina during copulation by spasm of the perineal muscles of the female.

p. clamp. A clamp which is fitted upon the shaft of the penis to retain anesthetic or antiseptic solutions in the urethra, for control of incontinence, or training an enuretic.

p. envy. *In psychoanalysis,* the envy of the young female child for the penis which she does not possess, or which she thinks she has lost (thus forming a part of the castration complex). The wish for the penis is replaced normally by the wish for a child, or by denial of its absence and the compulsion to behave like a man.

webbed p. A marked chordee associated with penoscrotal hypospadias, in which the penis is integral with the scrotum.

pen′nate [L. *penna,* feather]. Like a feather.

pen′ni·form [*penna;* L. *forma,* form]. Shaped like a feather; said of certain muscles.

pen″ny·roy′al. *Mentha pulegium.* See *hedeoma.*

pen′ny·weight″ [AS. *penig; wiht*]. A weight of 24 grains. Abbreviated, dwt, dwt.

pe·nol′o·gist [G. *poinē*, penalty; *logos*, word]. One who makes a study of crime, its cause and prevention.

pe·nol′o·gy [*poinē; logos*]. The science treating of crime, its punishment and prevention; the study of the management of prisons. —**penolog′ic,** *adj.*

pe″no·scro′tal [L. *penis*, penis; *scrotum*, scrotum]. Pertaining to the penis and the scrotum.

Penrose drain. A latex nasogastric tube. See cigarette *drain.*

pen′ta-, pent- [G. *pente*, five]. A combining form meaning *five.*

pen″ta·ba′sic [*pente;* G. *basis*, base]. Having five replaceable hydrogen atoms.

pen″ta·chlo″ro·phe′nol. C_6Cl_5OH; needlelike crystals, almost insoluble in water but forming a water-soluble sodium salt: used as a preservative of wood, glue, and other substances and for control of slime and algae.

pen′tad [*pente*]. An element or radical having a valence of five.

pen″ta·dac′tyl [*pente;* G. *daktylos*, finger]. Having five fingers or toes upon each hand or foot.

3-pen″ta·dec″yl·cat′e·chol. $C_{21}H_{36}O_2$; a constituent of the irritant oil of *Rhus toxicodendron* and other species of *Rhus:* used as a standard allergen in patch tests to determine sensitivity to poison ivy.

pen″ta·e·ryth′ri·tol tet″ra·ni′trate. Pentaerythrityl tetranitrate.

pen″ta·e·ryth′ri·tyl tet″ra·ni′trate. $(CH_2NO_3)_4C$; a vasodilator similar to erythrityl tetranitrate, claimed by some to be superior to the latter: useful in preventing attacks of angina pectoris in some cases and in treating intermittent claudication. Syn., *pentaerythritol tetranitrate.* See *peritrate tetranitrate.*

pen″ta·gen′ic [*pente;* G. *genesthai*, from *gignesthai*, to be produced]. Referring to genotypes of polysomic or polyploid organisms which contain five different alleles for any given locus.

pen″ta·hy·drox″y·hex·o′ic ac′id. Galactonic acid.

pen′tal. C_5H_{10}. See *amylene hydrate.*

pentalogy of the Cuban School. Congenital heart lesion consisting of tetralogy of Fallot associated with an interatrial septal defect.

pen″ta·me′tho′ni·um. One of a homologous series of polymethylene bis(trimethylammonium) ions, of the general formula $(CH_3)_3N^+(CH_2)_nN^+(CH_3)_3$, in which n is 5. It possesses ganglion-blocking action, effecting reduction in blood pressure. It is used clinically in the form of one of its salts, commonly the bromide or iodide. Also designated *C5.*

pen″ta·meth″yl·ene·tet′ra·zol. See *metrazol.*

pen″ta·meth″yl·ros·an′i·line. See *methylrosaniline chloride.*

pen·tam′i·dine (pen·tam′i·deen, ·din). A diamidine, 4:4′-diamidino-1:5 diphenoxypentane or 4,4′-[pentamethylenedioxy]dibenzamidine, useful in treatment of African trypanosomiasis and kala-azar. It has also been shown to inhibit strongly the growth of bacteria in wounds and to be of value in the treatment of multiple myeloma.

pen′tane. Chemical name for one of the three isomeric hydrocarbons of the paraffin series, having the formula C_5H_{12}. All are liquids.

pen″tane·di·o′ic ac′id. Glutaric acid.

pen′ta·quine (pen′tuh·kween, ·kwin). 6-Methoxy-8-(5′-isopropylaminopentylamino)-quinoline, an effective remedial agent in malaria, especially when given with quinine. It appears to be too toxic for prophylactic use. Introduced as SN 13,276. The phosphate is the usual dosage form.

Pen·tas′to·ma, Pen″ta·sto′ma [G. *pente*, five; *stoma*, mouth]. A genus of blood-sucking arthropods which are endoparasites of vertebrates. One species, **P. najae,** has been reported to infest the upper respiratory tract of man.

pen′tas·tomes [*pente; stoma*]. A group of endoparasites known as tongue worms which infest man; includes the genera *Linguatula, Armillifer,* and *Pentastoma.*

pen″ta·tom′ic [*pente;* G. *atomos*, uncut]. 1. Containing five atoms. 2. Having five replaceable hydrogen atoms in the molecule.

Pen″ta·trich″o·mo′nas [*pente;* G. *thrix*, hair; *monas*, unit]. A generic name improperly applied to the five-flagellated variety of *Trichomonas hominis.*

pen″ta·vac′cine [*pente;* L. *vaccinus*, of cows]. A vaccine composed of five different kinds of organisms.

pen″ta·va′lent, pen·tav′a·lent [*pente;* L. *valere*, to be strong]. Having a valence of five.

pent·dy′o·pent. The red pigment, containing two pyrrole rings, obtained when a propentdyopent is reduced with sodium dithionite.

pen′tene. 1. Chemical name for one of the isomeric hydrocarbons of the olefin series, having the formula C_5H_{10}, of which five are possible. 2. See *amylene hydrate.*

pen·te″no·lac′tone. A cyclic group,

$$\overline{\text{—C:CH.CO.O.CH}_2}$$

commonly found in the structure of cardioactive steroidal aglycones, being attached to the number 17 carbon atom.

pen·tet′ra·zol. International Pharmacopoeia name for pentylenetetrazol, more exactly designated pentamethylenetetrazol.

pentnucleotide. Trade-mark for the sodium salts of the pentose nucleotides from the ribonucleic acid of yeast. The preparation is used in infectious conditions accompanied by leukopenia or neutropenia.

pen″to·bar′bi·tal so′di·um (pen″to·bahr′bi·tawl, ·tal, ·tol) (*pentobarbitalum sodicum*). $C_{11}H_{17}O_3N_2Na$. Sodium ethyl-(1-methyl-butyl) barbiturate. A white, odorless, slightly bitter, crystalline powder. Freely soluble in water and alcohol. One of the more rapidly acting hypnotics, extensively used as a preanesthetic sedative. Also used as an anticonvulsant in strychnine or cocaine poisoning by slow intravenous injection. Dose, as a hypnotic, 0.1 Gm. (1½ gr.); as a preanesthetic sedative, 0.2 Gm. (3 gr.); as an anticonvulsant, 0.3–0.5 Gm. (5–8 gr.). Also called *soluble pentobarbital.* See *nembutal.*

pen″to·lin′i·um bi·tar′trate. Generic name for pentamethylene-1:5-bis(1′-methylpyrrolidinium bitartrate); $C_{15}H_{32}N_2^{++}.2C_4H_5O_6^-$; a ganglionic blocking agent used in the management of hypertension. See *ansolysen.*

pen′to·san. A complex carbohydrate capable of forming a pentose by hydrolysis.

pen·to′sa·zone (pen·to′suh·zone, pen″to·say′zone). A reaction product of pentose and phenylhydrazine, used to identify and distinguish pentoses from other monosaccharides.

pen′tose. Any one of a class of carbohydrates containing five atoms of carbon. The pentoses are not fermentable, and, on boiling with dilute hydrochloric acid, yield furfural.

p. nucleic acid. Ribose nucleic acid.

p. nucleotide. See *pentnucleotide.*

pen′to·side (pen′to·side, ·sid). A glycoside in which the sugar component is a pentose; nucleosides are pentosides.

pentostam. Trade-mark for a preparation of sodium stibogluconate.

pen″to·su′ri·a [G. *pente*, five; *ouron*, urine]. The presence of pentose in the urine.

pentothal sodium. Trade-mark for the monosodium salt of 5-ethyl-5-(1-methylbutyl) thiobarbituric acid, known also as *thiopental sodium* and *thiopentone soluble*. The solution is used as a general anesthetic by intravenous injection.

pent·ox′ide. An oxide containing five atoms of oxygen.

pen′tyl. Chemical name for the univalent radical of five carbon atoms. The name amyl is used interchangeably.

pen″tyl·ene·tet′ra·zol. See *metrazol*.

Penzoldt, Franz [*German physician*, 1849–1927]. Introduced a solution for testing for the presence of acetone, and another for the presence of glucose in the urine. Each method is called *Penzoldt's method*.

pe″o·til″lo·ma′ni·a [G. *peos*, penis; *tillein*, to pluck; *mania*, madness]. The nervous habit of constantly pulling the penis; not masturbating.

pe′po [G. *pepōn*, ripe]. Seed of the pumpkin, *Cucurbita pepo;* it is a taeniafuge.

Pepper, William (Senior) [*American physician and clinician*, 1843–98]. Celebrated figure in American medicine. Recorded bone marrow changes in progressive pernicious anemia (1875).

Pepper, William (Junior) [*American physician*, 1874–1947]. Widely known clinician and educator. Described congenital sarcoma of the liver and adrenals; called *Pepper type of adrenal mediastinal tumor* (1901). Described a syndrome connected with tumor of the right adrenal, in which he noted that metastasis is limited largely to the liver substance; called *Pepper's syndrome*.

pep′per [G. *peperi*, pepper]. The dried, unripe fruit of various species of *Piper*. Due to the widespread cultivation of pepper a large number of varieties exist. The important constituents of pepper are chavicine, piperine, piperidine, volatile oil, and resin. A small quantity of a volatile alkaloid has also been found. Pepper is used as a condiment and in medicine. Its chief use in medicine is to excite the languid stomach and correct flatulence. Also see *capsicum*.

pep′per·mint [*peperi;* G. *mintha*, mint]. Consists of the dried leaf and flowering top of *Mentha piperita*. Peppermint contains about 1.0%–1.25% of a volatile oil together with tannin, resin, and gum. Used as an aromatic stimulant to allay nausea, relieve spasmodic pains of the stomach and bowels, expel flatus, or cover the taste or qualify the nauseating or griping effects of other medicines. Also see peppermint *oil*.

p. spirit (*spiritus menthae piperitae*). Peppermint essence; a 10% solution of the oil in alcohol, rendered green by maceration of the coarsely ground leaves in the alcohol.

pep′si·gogue [G. *pepsis*, digestion; *agōgos*, leading]. Referring to the secretagogue effect of substances which stimulate the discharge of pepsin in the gastric secretion; contrasted with the effect of histamine, which stimulates the secretion of hydrochloric acid but not of pepsin.

pep′sin (*pepsinum*). A substance containing a proteolytic enzyme obtained from the glandular layer of the fresh stomach of the hog, *Sus scrofa* var. *domesticus;* occurs as transparent or translucent scales, granular or spongy masses, yellow to light brown in color; freely soluble in water; nearly insoluble in alcohol. Pepsin is useful to secure the digestion of protein food in the stomach. It is seldom indicated, because the gastric juice usually contains sufficient pepsin to perform gastric digestion. May be given with hydrochloric acid in those cases in which there is an absence of free hydrochloric acid in the stomach contents. Dose, 0.6–4.0 Gm. (10–60 gr.). Pepsin is contained in the following preparations: **compound pepsin elixir** (*elixir pepsini compositum*), also called lactated pepsin elixir and compound digestive elixir, dose, 8 cc. (2 fluidrachms); **pepsin and rennin elixir** (*elixir pepsini et rennini*), also called pepsin essence, dose, 8 cc. (2 fluidrachms); **pepsin elixir** (*elixir pepsini*), dose, 8 cc. (2 fluidrachms); **saccharated pepsin** (*pepsinum saccharatum*), dose, 4–8 Gm. (1–2 dr.).

pep·sin′o·gen [G. *pepsis*, a cooking; *genesthai*, from *gignesthai*, to be produced]. The antecedent substance or zymogen of pepsin, present in the cells of the gastric glands, which during digestion is converted into pepsin.

pep″si·no·ther′a·py [*pepsis;* G. *therapeia*, treatment]. The employment of pepsin as a digestant in the treatment of dyspepsia.

pep′tic [G. *peptikos*, promoting digestion]. 1. Pertaining to pepsin. 2. Pertaining to digestion, as peptic ulcer. See peptic *ulcer*.

pep′ti·dase. An enzyme which splits peptides to amino acids. See Table of Enzymes in the Appendix.

pep′tide. A compound of two or more amino acids containing one or more peptide groups, —CO.-NH—. An intermediate between the amino acids and peptones in the synthesis of proteins. See American Classification of Proteins in the Appendix.

pep″ti·do·lyt′ic [G. *peptos*, cooked; *lysis*, a loosing]. Causing the digestion or splitting up of peptides into amino acids.

pep″ti·za′tion. 1. The liquefaction of a gel to a sol. 2. The bringing of a solid material into colloidal suspension.

pep″to·gen′ic, pep·tog′e·nous (pep·todj′i·nus) [*peptos;* G. *genesthai*, from *gignesthai*, to be produced]. Producing pepsin or peptones.

pep·tol′y·sis. See *peptonolysis*.

pep′tone. A derived protein produced by the hydrolysis of natural protein either by an enzyme or by an acid. Complete hydrolysis of protein yields amino acids. Peptones, as well as proteoses, which are similar to peptones, are intermediate compounds between proteins and amino acids. Dried peptone occurs as a reddish yellow to brown powder, with characteristic odor; it is soluble in water but insoluble in alcohol; peptone is not coagulated by heat or precipitated on the addition of ammonium or zinc sulfate. It is used for the preparation of culture mediums in certain bacteriologic tests, and is occasionally given as a nutrient. Also called *meat peptone, beef peptone*, See American Classification of Proteins in the Appendix. —**pepton′ic,** *adj.*

venom p. A peptone found in the venom of certain serpents.

pep″to·ne′mi·a [*peptos;* G. *haima*, blood]. The presence of peptone in the blood.

pep′to·nize [*peptos*]. 1. Convert into peptones; predigest. 2. Digest with pepsin.

pep″to·nol′y·sis [*peptos;* G. *lysis*, a loosing]. The hydrolysis or digestion of peptones; peptolysis.

pep″to·nu′ri·a [*peptos;* G. *ouron*, urine]. The presence of peptones in the urine.

enterogenous p. Peptonuria due to disease of the intestine.

hepatogenous p. That accompanying certain liver affections.

nephrogenous p. Peptonuria of renal origin.
puerperal p. That of the puerperal state.
pyogenic p. That produced by suppuration in the body.

per- [L., through, very]. 1. A prefix signifying *throughout, completely, thoroughly, over,* or *very, extremely.* 2. *In chemistry,* a prefix denoting the highest valence of a series.

per″a·ceph′a·lus (pur″a·sef′uh·lus, perr″a·) [L. *per,* through; G. *akephalos,* headless]. A placental parasitic twin which lacks head and arms and has a defective or absent thorax, the body being reduced to little more than the pelvis and legs.

per″ac′id. That acid, of a series of acids formed by a particular element, which contains the highest proportion of oxygen.

per″a·cid′i·ty (pur″a·sid′i·tee) [L. *per-,* very; *acidus,* sour]. Excessive acidity.

per″a·cute′ (pur″a·cute′) [*per-;* L. *acutus,* sharp]. Very acute; unusually sharp: said of pain.

perandren. Trade-mark for the propionic acid ester of synthetic testosterone in oil.

per a′num [L.]. By the anus, said of the administration of certain drugs or nutrient substances.

per″a·to·dyn′i·a [*G. peras,* boundary; *odynē,* pain]. Pain at the cardiac extremity of the stomach.

perazil hydrochloride. A trade-marked name for chlorcyclizine hydrochloride, an antihistaminic compound.

per″ben·zo′ic ac′id. $C_6H_5COO_2H$; peroxybenzoic acid, occurring as crystalline leaflets of very acrid odor, very volatile, almost soluble in water, and freely soluble in most organic liquids: used in chemical synthesis and analysis.

per·bo′rate (pur·bor′ate). A salt of perboric acid.

per·bo′ric ac′id. The hypothetical acid, HBO_3, from which perborates are derived.

per·ca′ine (pur·kay′een, ·in, pur′kay·een, ·in). See *nupercaine hydrochloride.*

per cent [L. *per centum,* by the hundred]. Indicating milligrams of a substance per 100 cc. of a fluid; more properly *milligrams per cent.*

per·cen′tile (pur·sen′tile, ·til) [*per centum*]. Any of the values of a variable which separate the entire distribution into 100 groups of equal frequency.

per·cep′tion [L. *perceptio,* from *percipere,* to perceive]. Recognition in response to sensory stimuli; the act or process by which the memory of certain qualities of an object is associated with other qualities impressing the senses, thereby making possible recognition of the object. —**perceptive,** *adj.*
depth p. The ability to estimate depth or distance between points in the field of vision.
extrasensory p. (**ESP**). Direct awareness without the use of the senses; telepathy, clairvoyance, or precognition. See psi *phenomena.*
space p. Knowledge, through the senses, of the area, dimensions, or position occupied, of any space.
stereognostic p. The recognition of objects by touch.

per″cep·tiv′i·ty [*percipere*]. The faculty or capability of receiving impressions.

per″cep·to′ri·um. See *sensorium.*

per·chlo′rate. A salt of perchloric acid.

per″chlor·hy′dri·a. See *hyperchlorhydria.*

per·chlo′ric ac′id. $HClO_4$ A powerful oxidizing acid used in chemical analysis.

per·chlo″ro·eth′yl·ene. Tetrachloroethylene.

per·clu′sion [L. *percludere,* for *praecludere,* to close]. Inability to execute any movement.

per″co·la′tion [L. *percolatio,* from *percolare*]. The process of extracting the soluble constituents of a substance by allowing a suitable solvent to pass through a column of the powdered substance placed in a long, conical vessel, the percolator. —**per′colate,** *v., n.*

per′co·la″tor [*percolare*]. A long, conical vessel with a delivery tube at the lower extremity; used for extracting the soluble constituents of a substance, packed in the percolator, by means of a suitable solvent passing through it.

per′co·morph [L. *perca,* perch; G. *morphē,* form]. A fish of the order Acanthopteri (Percomorphi), which includes the genera *Thunnus, Xiphias, Stereolepis, Scomber,* and others.
p.-liver oil. A mixture containing the fixed oils from the fresh livers of the percomorph fishes and not more than 50% of other fish-liver oil. It has a potency of not less than 60,000 U.S.P. units of vitamin A and not less than 8500 U.S.P. units of vitamin D per gram. It is marketed under the trade-mark oleum percomorphum.

percorten. A trade-mark for desoxycorticosterone acetate.

per·cus′sion [L. *percussio,* a striking]. The act of firmly tapping the surface of the body with a finger or a small hammer to elicit sounds, or vibratory sensations, of diagnostic value.
auditory p. That in which attention is concentrated upon the character of the sounds produced.
auscultatory p. That in which the sound is received through a stethoscope, the bell of which is placed on the skin, while the examiner either scratches the skin surface or percusses lightly in the near vicinity.
definitive p. Percussion whose purpose is to outline the borders of a viscus.
direct p. Striking the skin directly with the pads of one or two fingers without the interposition of a pleximeter. Also called *immediate p.*
indirect p. That effected by placing a pleximeter against the skin surface to receive the tap. Also called *mediate p.*
orthopercussion. The use of a cylindrical pleximeter, placed with its long axis perpendicular to the surface of the body, for the purpose of sharply demarcating the border of an internal organ, especially the heart. The two distal phalanges of a finger flexed at a right angle, or a glass rod or other mechanical object, may be used as pleximeter.
palpatory p. Direct percussion, in which attention is concentrated upon the sensation of resistance detected by the one or two fingers used as a plexor.
qualitative p. That used to determine the physical state of the underlying tissues.
threshold p. The determination of the border of a viscus by the transition from no sound to the least audible sound, when percussion strokes of minimum force are used.

per·cus′sor [L., from *percutere,* to strike]. A person who performs percussion.

per″cu·ta′ne·ous [L. *per,* through; *cutis,* skin]. Performed through the skin.

Perdrau's method. See under *stain.*

pe·rei′rine (peh·ray′reen, ·rin, peh·rye′·). $C_{19}H_{24}ON_2$(?). An amorphous alkaloid found in the bark of *Geissospermum laeve.* Formerly used as an antiperiodic.

Perez, Fernand [*Argentinian bacteriologist,* 1863–1935]. Isolated and named *Coccobacillus foetidus ozaenae,* the supposed cause of ozena (1899); also called *Perez' bacillus,* now called *Salmonella foetida.*

per′for·ans (pur′fur·anz) [L. *perforare,* to pierce through]. Penetrating or perforating; a term applied to a muscle, artery, or nerve perforating a part.

per′for·ate [*perforare*]. *In biology*, pierced with small holes.

per″fo·ra″ted [*perforare*]. Pierced through.

per″fo·ra′tion [*perforare*]. 1. The act or occurrence of piercing or boring into a part, especially into the wall of a hollow organ or viscus. 2. A hole made through a part or wall of a cavity, produced by a variety of means.

per′fo·ra″tor [*perforare*]. An instrument for perforating, especially one for performing craniotomy on the fetus.

per″fo·ra·to′ri·um [*perforare*]. The pointed tip differentiated from the acrosome in the spermatozoa of some animals.

per″fri·ca′tion [L. *perfricare*, to rub all over]. Inunction.

per·fu′sion [L. *perfusio*, from *perfundere*, to pour over]. 1. A pouring of fluid. 2. The passage of a fluid through spaces. 3. The introduction of fluids into tissues by their injection into arteries.

perhydrol. Trade-mark for a 30 per cent solution of hydrogen peroxide.

per″i- [G., about, around]. A prefix signifying *about, beyond, around, near;* especially, *enclosing a part* or *affecting the tissues around a part.*

per″i·ad″e·ni′tis [*peri;* G. *adēn*, gland; *-itis*, inflammation]. Inflammation of the tissues that surround a gland or lymph node.

p. mucosa necrotica recurrens. A disorder characterized by recurring necrotic or ulcerative lesions occurring on the buccal and pharyngeal mucosa. Begins as a small, smooth, hard nodule that sloughs, leaving a deep crateriform depression. May occur on the tongue or genitalia as well. Described by R. L. Sutton, Sr. (1911).

per″i·a″lien·i′tis (perr″ee·ayl″yen·eye′tis, ·ay″lee-en·eye′tis) [*peri;* L. *alienus*, foreign; *-itis*]. Noninfectious inflammation due to a foreign body. Also called *foreign-body reaction, perixenitis.*

per″i·a′nal [*peri;* L. *anus*, anus]. Situated or occurring around the anus.

per″i·an″gi·i′tis [*peri;* G. *aggeion*, vessel; *-itis*, inflammation]. Inflammation of the outer coat of, or the tissues surrounding, an artery, vein, or lymphatic vessel.

per″i·an″gi·o·cho·li′tis (perr″ee·an″jee·o·ko·lye′-tis) [*peri; aggeion;* G. *cholē*, bile; *-itis*]. Inflammation of the tissues surrounding the biliary ducts.

per″i·a″or·ti′tis [*peri;* G. *aortē*, aorta; *-itis*]. Inflammation of the tissues surrounding the aorta.

per″i·ap′i·cal. Around an apex.

per″i·ap·pen″di·ci′tis [*peri;* L. *appendix*, appendage; G. *-itis*, inflammation]. Inflammation of the tissue around the vermiform process, or of the serosal region of the appendix.

per″i·ap″pen·dic′u·lar [*peri; appendix*]. Surrounding the vermiform, or any other, appendix.

per″i·ar·te′ri·al [*peri;* G. *artēria*, artery]. Surrounding an artery.

per″i·ar″te·ri′tis [*peri; artēria;* G. *-itis*, inflammation]. Inflammation of the adventitia of an artery and the periarterial tissues.

disseminated necrotizing p. See *polyarteritis* nodosa.

p. nodosa. See *polyarteritis* nodosa.

per″i·ar·thri′tis [*peri;* G. *arthron*, joint; *-itis*]. Inflammation of the tissues about a joint.

p. calcarea. Calcification of the musculotendinous cuff of the shoulder joint.

p. of the shoulder. See frozen *shoulder.*

scapulohumeral p. See frozen *shoulder.*

per″i·ar·tic′u·lar [*peri;* L. *articulus*, joint]. About a joint.

per″i·a′tri·al [*peri;* L. *atrium*, atrium]. Situated around the atria of the heart.

per″i·au·ric′u·lar [*peri;* L. *auricula*, external ear]. Around the external ear.

per″i·ax′i·al [*peri;* L. *axis*, axis]. Surrounding an axis.

per″i·blep′sis [G. *periblepsis*, a gazing around]. The wild look of a patient in delirium. Also called *periblepsia.*

per″i·bron′chi·al (perr″i·brong′kee·ul) [G. *peri*, about, around; *brogchos*, windpipe]. Surrounding or occurring about a bronchus.

per″i·bron″chi·o′lar (perr″i·brong″kee·o′lur, ·brong·kigh′o·lur) [*peri;* G. *brogchia*, bronchial tubes]. Surrounding the bronchioles.

per″i·bron″chi·o·li′tis (·brong″kee·o·lye′tis) [*peri; brogchia;* G. *-itis*, inflammation]. Inflammation of the tissues around the bronchioles.

per″i·bron·chi′·tis [*peri;* G. *brogchos*, windpipe; *-itis*]. Inflammation of the tissues around bronchi.

per″i·bro′sis [G., ulceration]. Ulceration at the canthus of the eyelid.

per″i·cap′il·lar″y (perr″i·cap′i·lerr″ee) [G. *peri*, about, around; L. *capillus*, hair]. Surrounding a capillary.

per″i·car″di·ec′to·my [G. *perikardios*, around the heart; *ektomē*, excision]. Excision of a part of the pericardium.

per″i·car″di·o·cen·te′sis [*perikardios;* G. *kentēsis*, a pricking]. Puncture of the pericardium.

per″i·car″di·ol′y·sis [*perikardios;* G. *lysis*, a loosing]. Cardiolysis.

per″i·car″di·o·pleu′ral (perr″i·kahr″dee·o-ploor′ul) [*perikardios;* G. *pleura*, rib]. Relating to the pericardium and to the pleura.

per″i·car″di·or′rha·phy [*perikardios;* G. *rhaphē*, a suture]. The suturing of a wound in the pericardium.

per″i·car″di·os′to·my [*perikardios;* G. *stoma*, mouth]. The establishing by surgical means of an opening into the pericardium, for repair of wounds of the heart or for drainage of the pericardial sac.

per″i·car″di·ot′o·my [*perikardios;* G. *tomē*, a cutting]. Incision of the pericardium.

per″i·car·di′tis [*perikardios;* G. *-itis*, inflammation]. Inflammation of the pericardium. The symptoms are slight fever, precordial pain and tenderness, cough, dyspnea, and rapid pulse. In the early stage, there is a distinct friction sound on auscultation, and sometimes a fremitus on palpation. In the stage of effusion, there are bulging of the precordia and a triangular area of dullness, the base of which is downward; the heart sounds are muffled. In chronic pericarditis with adhesions, there is often systolic retraction of the precordia. The causes of pericarditis are rheumatic fever, tuberculosis, septicemia (as in pneumonia), nephritis, or extension of infection from neighboring parts. —**pericardit′ic,** *adj.*

acute p. An acute inflammation of the pericardium, characterized by serous, fibrinous, purulent, or hemorrhagic exudate.

adhesive p. That in which the two layers of pericardium tend to adhere by means of fibrous adhesions, usually the result of the organization of acute exudate: also called *concretio cordis.*

carcinomatous p. That due to metastatic carcinoma of the pericardium.

constrictive p. A chronic pericarditis in which dense scar tissue in the pericardium interferes either with venous return to the atria or diastolic filling of the ventricles, with consequent reduction in cardiac output: also called *Pick's disease* (for Friedel *Pick*), *chronic cardiac compression.* See *Beck's triads* under Claude S. *Beck.*

dry p. A form without effusion.

external p. That affecting the outer layer of the parietal pericardium.

fibrinous p. A form in which the pericardium is covered with a fibrinous exudate, first soft and buttery in consistence, but later organizing.

fibropurulent p. A form in which there is an exudate containing an abundance of neutrophil granulocytes as well as fibrin.

hemorrhagic p. A form in which the fluid contains blood, found most often in tuberculous pericarditis.

localized p. A form giving rise to white areas, the so-called milk spots.

moist p. That attended by an effusion.

p. obliterans. A form leading to obliteration of the cavity by the adhesions of the layers.

purulent p. A variety in which the effused fluid becomes purulent. Syn., *suppurative p.*

rheumatic p. An inflammation of the pericardium due to rheumatic fever.

serofibrinous p. A form in which there is but little fibrin, but a considerable quantity of serous fluid.

suppurative p. See purulent *p.*

tuberculous p. Acute or chronic pericarditis, usually secondary to tuberculosis of the lungs, pleura, mediastinum, or peribronchial lymph nodes.

uremic p. A fibrinous form occurring in uremia, and probably of chemical origin.

per″i·car′di·um [*perikardios*]. The closed membranous sac enveloping the heart. Its base is attached to the central tendon of the diaphragm; its apex surrounds, for a short distance, the great vessels arising from the base of the heart. It consists of an outer fibrous coat, derived from the cervical fascia, and an inner serous coat. The sac normally contains from 5–20 Gm. of clear, serous liquid. The part in contact with the heart (visceral pericardium) is termed the epicardium; the other is the parietal pericardium. See Plate 5. —**pericardiac, pericardial,** *adj.*

bread-and-butter p. A peculiar appearance produced in fibrinous pericarditis by the rubbing of the two surfaces of the membrane over each other.

shaggy p. A pericardium upon which, as the result of fibrinous pericarditis, thick, loose, shaggy layers of fibrin are deposited.

per′i·carp [G. *perikarpion*, case of fruit]. *In botany*, the mature ovary wall.

per″i·ce′cal [G. *peri*, around; L. *caecum*, cecum]. Surrounding the cecum.

per″i·ce·ci′tis [*peri; caecum;* G. *-itis*, inflammation]. Inflammation of the serosa of the cecum. Syn., *perityphlitis.*

per″i·cel′lu·lar [*peri;* L. *cellula*, small storeroom]. Surrounding a cell.

per″i·ce″men·ti′tis (perr″i·see″men·tye′tis, ·sem″-en·tye′tis) [*peri;* L. *caementum*, quarrystone; G. *-itis*, inflammation]. Inflammation of the periodontal membrane; periodontitis.

per″i·ce·men″to·cla′si·a (·si·men″to·clay′zhuh, ·zee·uh, ·shuh, ·see·uh) [*peri; caementum;* G. *klasis*, a breaking]. Breaking down of the periodontium with absorption of the alveolar bone.

per″i·ce·men′tum [*peri; caementum*]. Periodontal membrane. —**pericemen′tal,** *adj.*

per″i·cha·rei′a (perr″i·kah·rye′uh) [G., excessive joy]. Sudden vehement or abnormal rejoicing; a symptom in certain psychoses, such as mania or general paresis.

per″i·chol″an·gi′tis (perr″i·kol″an·jy′tis, ·ko″lan-jy′tis) [G. *peri*, about, around; *cholē*, bile; *aggeion*, vessel; *-itis*, inflammation]. Inflammation in the tissues around the bile ducts. Syn., *periangiocholitis.*

per″i·chol″e·cys′tic (·kol″i·sis′tick, ·ko″li·) [*peri; cholē;* G. *kystis*, bladder]. Around the gallbladder.

per″i·chol″e·cys·ti′tis (·kol″i·sis·tye′tis, ·ko″li·) [*peri; cholē; kystis;* G. *-itis*, inflammation]. Inflammation of the serosa or tissues around the gallbladder.

per″i·chon·dri′tis (perr″i·kon·dry′tis) [*peri;* G. *chondros*, cartilage; *-itis*]. Inflammation of perichondrium. —**perichondrit′ic,** *adj.*

per″i·chon′dri·um (perr″i·kon′dree·um) [*peri; chondros*]. The fibrous connective tissue covering cartilage, except articular surfaces. —**perichondral,** *adj.*

per″i·chon·dro′ma [*peri; chondros;* G. *-ōma*, tumor]. A tumor of the perichondrium.

per′i·chord [*peri;* G. *chordē*, string]. The sheath of the notochord. —**perichor′dal,** *adj.*

per″i·cho′roid (perr″i·kor′oyd), **per″i·cho·roi′dal** (perr″i·ko·roy′dul) [*peri;* G. *chorioeidēs*, choroid]. Surrounding the choroid.

per″i·cla′si·a (perr″i·clay′zhuh, ·zee·uh, ·shuh, ·see·uh). See *periodontoclasia.*

per″i·col′ic [*peri;* G. *kolon*, colon]. Surrounding or about the colon.

per″i·co·li′tis [*peri; kolon;* G. *-itis*, inflammation]. Inflammation of the peritoneum or tissues around the colon. Also called *pericolonitis.*

per″i·col·pi′tis. See *paracolpitis.*

per″i·con′chal (perr″i·kong′kul) [*peri;* G. *kogchē*, mussel]. Surrounding the concha of the ear.

per″i·con·chi′tis (perr″i·kong·kigh′tis) [*peri; kogchē;* G. *-itis*, inflammation]. Inflammation of the periosteum or lining membrane of the orbit. *Obs.*

per″i·cor′ne·al [*peri;* L. *corneus*, horny]. Surrounding the cornea.

per″i·cor″o·ni′tis [*peri;* L. *corona*, crown; G. *-itis*, inflammation]. Inflammation of the tissue surrounding the coronal portion of the tooth, usually a partially erupted third molar.

per″i·cow″per·i′tis [*peri;* after William *Cowper*, English surgeon; *-itis*]. Inflammation of the tissues about Cowper's glands. *Obs.*

per″i·cra′ni·um [G. *perikranios*, around the skull]. The periosteum on the outer surface of the cranial bones. —**pericranial,** *adj.*

per″i·cys′tic [G. *peri*, about, around; *kystis*, bladder]. 1. Surrounding a cyst. 2. Surrounding a bladder, either the gallbladder or the urinary bladder.

per″i·cys·ti′tis [*peri; kystis;* G. *-itis*, inflammation]. 1. Inflammation surrounding a cyst. 2. Inflammation of the peritoneum or other tissue surrounding the urinary blader.

per″i·cys′ti·um [*peri; kystis*]. 1. The vascular wall of a cyst. 2. The tissues surrounding a bladder.

per′i·cyte. 1. A histiocyte occurring outside the wall of a vessel. 2. A special cell, according to some authorities, sometimes seen around a capillary or capillary arteriole, with dendritic processes about the vessel and exhibiting contractile properties, and thus similar to Rouget cells: also called *p. of Zimmerman.*

per″i·cy′ti·al (perr″i·sish′ee·ul, ·sish′ul, ·sit′ee·ul) [*peri;* G. *kytos*, cell]. Surrounding a cell.

per″i·dec′to·my. See *perimitry.*

per″i·den·drit′ic [*peri;* G. *dendritēs*, of a tree]. Surrounding a dendrite.

per″i·den′tal [*peri;* L. *dens*, tooth]. Surrounding a tooth or its root; periodontal.

per″i·den·ti′tis [*peri; dens;* G. *-itis*, inflammation]. Inflammation around a tooth; periodontitis.

per′i·derm [*peri;* G. *derma*, skin]. The superficial transient layer of epithelial cells of the embryonic epidermis. Syn., *epitrichium.*

per″i·di″ver·tic″u·li′tis [*peri;* L. *diverticulum*, bypath; G. *-itis*, inflammation]. Inflammation of the structures surrounding a diverticulum.

per″i·du″o·de·ni′tis [*peri;* L. *duodeni,* twelve; *-itis*]. Inflammation, acute, chronic, or with fibrous adhesions, in the tissues surrounding the duodenum.

per″i·du′ral. Situated about the dura mater, especially outside that of the spinal cord.

per″i·en·ceph″a·li′tis [*peri;* G. *egkephalos,* brain; *-itis*]. Inflammation of the pia mater and the cortex of the brain.

per″i·en·ceph″a·lo·men″in·gi′tis [*peri; egkephalos;* G. *mēnigx,* membrane; *-itis*]. See *periencephalitis.*

per″i·en·ter′ic [*peri;* G. *enteron,* intestine]. Situated around the enteron; perivisceral.

per″i·en″ter·i′tis [*peri; enteron;* G. *-itis,* inflammation]. Inflammation of the intestinal peritoneum.

per″i·ep·en′dy·mal [*peri;* G. *ependyma,* upper garment]. Surrounding the ependyma.

per″i·e″so·phag′e·al (perr″ee·ee″so·fadj′ee·ul, ·fadj′ul) [*peri;* G. *oisophagos,* esophagus]. Situated, or occurring just outside of, or around, the esophagus.

per″i·e·soph″a·gi′tis [*peri; oisophagos;* G. *-itis,* inflammation]. Inflammation of the tissues that surround the esophagus.

per″i·fis′tu·lar [*peri;* L. *fistula,* tube]. Around or about a fistula.

per″i·fol·lic′u·lar. Surrounding a follicle.

per″i·fol·lic″u·li′tis [*peri;* L. *folliculus,* small bag; G. *-itis,* inflammation]. Inflammation around the hair follicles.

p. capitis abscedens et suffodiens. A rare form of suppurating and cicatrizing disease of the scalp. Nodules and abscesses occur that terminate with scars. A chronic recurring disease that is resistant to treatment.

superficial pustular p. Impetigo follicularis.

per″i·gan″gli·i′tis [*peri;* G. *gagglion,* encysted tumor on a tendon; *-itis*]. Inflammation of the tissues surrounding a ganglion.

per″i·gan″gli·on′ic [*peri; gagglion*]. Situated, or occurring, around a ganglion.

per″i·gas′tric [*peri;* G. *gastēr,* belly]. Surrounding, or in the neighborhood of, the stomach.

per″i·gas·tri′tis [*peri; gastēr;* G. *-itis,* inflammation]. Inflammation of the serosa of the stomach.

per″i·glan′du·lar [*peri;* L. *glandulae,* glands of the throat]. Pertaining to the tissue surrounding a gland.

per″i·glot′tic [*peri;* G. *glōttis,* glottis]. Situated around the base of the tongue and the epiglottis.

per″i·glot′tis [G., covering of the tongue]. The mucous membrane of the tongue. *O.T.*

per″i·gnath′ic (perr″i·nath′ick, ·nay′thick) [G. *peri,* about, around; *gnathos,* jaw]. Situated about the jaws.

per″i·he·pat′ic [*peri;* G. *hēpar,* liver]. Surrounding, or occurring around, the liver.

per″i·hep″a·ti′tis [*peri; hēpar;* G. *-itis,* inflammation]. Inflammation of the peritoneum surrounding the liver.

chronic hyperplastic p. See *polyserositis.*

per″i·her′ni·al [*peri;* L. *hernia,* hernia]. Around or surrounding a hernia.

per″i·hi′lar. Around a hilus.

per″i·hys·ter′ic [*peri;* G. *hystera,* womb]. Around the uterus; periuterine.

per″i·je″ju·ni′tis (perr″i·jee″jew·nigh′tis, ·jedj″oo-nigh′tis) [*peri;* L. *jejunus,* empty; G. *-itis,* inflammation]. Inflammation of the peritoneal coat or tissues around the jejunum.

per″i·kar′y·on [*peri;* G. *karyon,* nut]. 1. The cell body of a neuron, containing the nucleus and a well-defined nucleolus. 2. A circumnuclear cytoplasmic mass.

per″i·ker·at′ic [*peri;* G. *keras,* horn]. Surrounding the cornea.

per″i·lab″y·rin·thi′tis [*peri;* G. *labyrinthos,* labyrinth; *-itis,* inflammation]. Inflammation in the osseous labyrinth of the internal ear.

per″i·la·ryn′ge·al (perr″i·la·rin′jul, ·jee·ul, ·lar″in-jee′ul) [*peri;* G. *larygx,* larynx]. Situated, or occurring, around the larynx.

per″i·lar″yn·gi′tis [*peri; larygx;* G. *-itis,* inflammation]. Inflammation of the areolar tissue surrounding the larynx.

per′i·lymph [*peri;* L. *lympha,* water]. The fluid separating the membranous from the osseous labyrinth of the internal ear.

per″i·lym·phan′ge·al, per″i·lym·phan′gi·al [*peri; lympha;* G. *aggeion,* vessel]. Situated, or occurring, around a lymphatic vessel.

per″i·lym″phan·gi′tis [*peri; lympha; aggeion;* G. *-itis,* inflammation]. Inflammation of the tissues surrounding a lymphatic vessel.

per″i·lym·phat′ic [*peri;* L. *lymphaticus,* from *lympha*]. 1. Pertaining to the perilymph. 2. Situated or occurring about a lymphatic vessel.

per″i·mas·ti′tis [*peri;* G. *mastos,* breast; *-itis,* inflammation]. Inflammation of the fibroadipose tissues around the mammary gland.

per″i·men″in·gi′tis. See *pachymeningitis.*

per·im′e·ter [G. *perimetron,* circumference]. 1. Circumference or border. 2. An instrument for measuring the extent of the field of vision. It consists ordinarily of a flat, narrow, metal plate bent in a semicircle, graduated in degrees, and fixed to an upright at its center by a pivot, on which it is movable. Variously colored disks are moved along the metal plate, and the point noted at which the person, looking directly in front of him, distinguishes the color.

per″i·met′ric [G. *peri,* about, around; *mētra,* womb]. Situated around the uterus.

per″i·met′ric [G. *perimetron,* circumference]. Pertaining to perimetry.

per″i·me·tri′tis [G. *peri,* about, around; *mētra,* womb; *-itis,* inflammation]. Inflammation of the tissues about the uterus. —**perimetrit′ic,** *adj.*

per″i·me′tri·um [*peri; mētra*]. The serous covering of the uterus.

per″i·met″ro·sal″pin·gi′tis [*peri; mētra;* G. *salpigx,* tube; *-itis,* inflammation]. A collective name for periuterine inflammations.

per·im′e·try [G. *perimetron,* perimeter]. The measuring of the field of vision.

per·im′i·trist. One who performs perimitry.

per·im′i·try. 1. The removal of a strip of conjunctival and subconjunctival tissue from about the cornea for the relief of pannus. 2. The cutting of the conjunctiva at the limbus prior to enucleation. Formerly called *peridectomy, peritomy.*

per″i·my″e·li′tis [G. *peri,* around, about; *myelos,* marrow; *-itis,* inflammation]. 1. Inflammation of the pia mater of the spinal cord. 2. Inflammation of the endosteum.

per″i·my″o·si′tis [*peri;* G. *mys,* muscle; *-itis*]. Inflammation of the connective tissues around muscle.

per″i·mys′i·um (perr″i·mizh′ee·um, ·miz′ee·um, ·miss′ee·um) [*peri; mys*]. The connective tissue enveloping bundles of muscle fibers. —**perimysial,** *adj.*

p. externum. The epimysium.

p. internum. The endomysium.

per″i·ne′o- [G. *perineos,* space between the anus and the scrotum]. A combining form denoting *relating to the perineum.*

per″i·ne′o·cele [*perineos;* G. *kēlē,* hernia]. Perineal hernia.

per″i·ne″o·col″po·rec″to·my″o·mec′to·my

[*perineos;* G. *kolpos*, vagina; L. *rectus*, straight; G. *mys*, muscle; *ektomē*, excision]. Excision of a myoma by incision of the perineum, vagina, and rectum. *Obs.*

per″i·ne·om′e·ter. Instrument used to measure the strength of voluntary muscle contractions about the vagina and urethra.

per″i·ne′o·plas″ty [*perineos;* G. *plassein*, to form]. Plastic operation upon the perineum.

per″i·ne·or′rha·phy [*perineos;* G. *rhaphē*, suture]. Suture of the perineum, usually for the repair of a laceration occurring during labor.

per″i·ne″o·scro′tal [*perineos;* L. *scrotum*, scrotum]. Relating to the perineum and scrotum.

per″i·ne″o·syn′the·sis [*perineos;* G. *synthesis*, a putting together]. A plastic operation upon the perineum in which a graft of vaginal mucosa is made to cover the wound; a variety of perineorrhaphy. *Obs.*

per″i·ne·ot′o·my [*perineos;* G. *tomē*, a cutting]. Incision through the perineum; in gynecologic surgery, an incision into and repair of the perineum for the purpose of enlarging the introitus.

per″i·ne″o·vag′i·nal (perr″i·nee″o·vadj′i·nul, ·va-jy′nul) [*perineos;* L. *vagina*, vagina]. Relating to the perineum and vagina.

per″i·ne″o·va·gi″no·rec′tal [*perineos; vagina;* L. *rectus*, straight]. Relating to the perineum, vagina, and rectum.

per″i·neph′ric [G. *peri*, around; *nephros*, kidney]. Situated or occurring around a kidney, as perinephric abscess.

per″i·ne·phri′tis [*peri;* G. *nephros*, kidney; *-itis*, inflammation]. Inflammation of the tissues surrounding a kidney. —**perinephrit′ic,** *adj.*

per″i·neph′ri·um [*peri; nephros*]. The connective and adipose tissue surrounding a kidney. —**perinephrial,** *adj.*

per″i·neph′ros. See *perinephrium.*

per″i·ne′um [G. *perineos*, space between the anus and scrotum]. 1. That portion of the body included in the outlet of the pelvis, bounded in front by the pubic arch, behind by the coccyx and sacrotuberous ligaments, and at the sides by the tuberosities of the ischium. In the male it is occupied by the anal canal, membranous urethra, and root of the penis; in the female by the anal canal, urethra, root of the clitoris, and vaginal orifice; in both sexes by the muscles, fasciae, vessels, and nerves of these structures. 2. The region between the anus and the scrotum in the male; between the anus and the posterior commissure of the vulva in the female. —**perineal,** *adj.*

primary p. A temporary perineum, present in the embryo after rupture of the cloacal membrane, formed by the caudal end of the urorectal septum with its endodermal covering. Also called *primitive perineal body.*

per″i·neu′ral an″al·ge′si·a (an″al·jee′zee·uh, ·see·uh). Analgesia resulting from injection of an analgesic solution into the immediate vicinity of a nerve trunk to the area.

per″i·neu′ri·al fi″bro·blas·to′ma. See neurogenic *sarcoma.*

per″i·neu·ri′tis [G. *peri*, around; *neuron*, nerve; *-itis*, inflammation]. Inflammation of the perineurium.

retrobulbar p. Inflammation of the sheath of the orbital part of the optic nerve.

per″i·neu′ri·um [*peri; neuron*]. The connective-tissue sheath investing a fasciculus or primary bundle of nerve fibers. —**perineurial,** *adj.*

per″i·nu′cle·ar [*peri;* L. *nucleus*, kernel]. Surrounding a nucleus.

per″i·oc′u·lar [*peri;* L. *oculus*, eye]. Surrounding the eye, as the periocular space, the space between the globe of the eye and the orbital walls.

pe′ri·od [G. *periodos*, a going around, cycle]. Duration; measure of time. The space of time during which anything is in progress or an event occurs.

childbearing p. The time of life, from puberty to the menopause, during which a woman is capable of reproduction.

gestation p. The period of pregnancy. The average length of human gestation is taken as ten lunar months (280 days) from the onset of the last menstrual period with a variation between 250 and 310 days. See Table of the Duration of Pregnancy in the Appendix.

incubation p. The time required for an infective agent to produce symptoms.

isoelectric p. A period of the heart's cycle in which the galvanometric string stands at zero.

lag p. A period of delayed growth observed following the transfer of an old bacterial culture to a new medium.

last menstrual p. Abbreviated, L.M.P. See gestation *p.*, menstrual *p.*

latent p. (a) Incubation period. (b) *In physiology*, the time intervening between the application of a stimulus and the appearance of the resulting phenomenon. (c) *In radiology*, the elapsed time between the exposure to radiation and the appearance of morphologic or physiologic effects.

menstrual p. The menses. Also called *monthly p.*

patent p. The time in parasitic disease during which parasites are demonstrable in the body.

postsphygmic p. Period of isometric relaxation of the heart muscle at the beginning of diastole.

presphygmic p. Period of isometric contraction of the heart muscle at the beginning of ventricular systole.

reaction p. The time required for the body to respond to some form of stimulation or injury.

refractory p. The period following adequate stimulation of an irritable tissue, divided into: the brief **absolute refractory p.** in which no stimulus, however strong, can excite a response; and the **relative refractory p.** of decreased excitability. It occurs only in tissues subject to the all-or-nothing law (e.g., nerve, striated muscle, heart).

respiratory p. The interval between two successive inspirations.

safe p. The nonovulatory phase of the menstrual cycle, when conception cannot occur. Since the time of ovulation is variable in different women, the safe period is also variable.

per·i′o·date (pur·eye′o·date). A salt of periodic acid.

pe″ri·od′ic [G. *periodikos*, periodical]. Recurring at more or less regular intervals.

per″i·od′ic ac′id (pur″eye·od′ick). $HIO_4.2H_2O$. A colorless, crystalline acid used as an oxidizing agent.

pe″ri·o·dic′i·ty [*periodikos*]. Recurrence at regular intervals.

pe″ri·od′ic ta′ble. A table of chemical elements arranged according to the law that chemical and physical properties of elements are periodic functions of their atomic numbers.

per″i·o·don′tal, per″i·o·don′tic [G. *peri*, around; *odous*, tooth]. 1. Surrounding a tooth, as the periodontal membrane, which covers the cement of a tooth. 2. Pertaining to the periodontium or to periodontia.

per″i·o·don′tics, per″i·o·don′ti·a [*peri; odous*]. That branch of dentistry dealing with the science and treatment of periodontal disease.

per″i·o·don′tist [*peri; odous*]. One who is versed in and practices periodontia.

per″i·o·don·ti′tis [*peri; odous;* G. *-itis*, inflammation]. Inflammation of the periodontal membrane: also called *periodontitis simplex*.

chronic periapical p. Localized nodule of organizing and cicatrizing inflammation at or near the apex of a tooth; a dental granuloma.

complex p. Periodontitis secondary to periodontosis: sometimes used as a synonym for *periodontosis*.

periapical p. Inflammation at the apex of a tooth.

Vincent's p. See necrotizing ulcerative *gingivitis*.

per″i·o·don′ti·um (perr″ee·o·don′shee·um) [*peri; odous*]. The investing and supporting tissues surrounding a tooth; namely, the periodontal membrane, the gingiva, and the alveolar bone.

per″i·o·don″to·cla′si·a (perr″ee·o·don″to·clay′-zhuh, ·zee·uh, ·shuh, ·see·uh) [*peri; odous;* G. *klasis*, a breaking]. General term for periodontal diseases that result in the destruction of the periodontium.

per″i·o·don·tol′o·gy. The science and study of the periodontium and periodontal diseases.

per″i·o·don·to′sis [*peri; odous;* G. *-ōsis*, condition]. A degenerative disturbance of the periodontium, characterized by degeneration of connective-tissue elements of the periodontal membrane and by bone resorption: also called *cementopathia, dentoalveolitis*.

pe″ri·od′o·scope [G. *periodos*, cycle; *skopein*, to examine]. A calendar in the form of a movable dial, used in determining the probable date of confinement.

per″i·o·dyn′i·a [*periodos;* G. *odynē*, pain]. Severe general pain throughout the body.

per″i·om·phal′ic [G. *peri*, around; *omphalos*, navel]. Around, or near, the umbilicus.

per″i·o·nych′i·a (perr″ee·o·nick′ee·uh) [*peri;* G. *onyx*, nail]. Inflammation around the nails.

per″i·o·nych′i·um (perr″ee·o·nick′ee·um) [*peri; onyx*]. The border of epidermis surrounding an entire nail.

per″i·o″o·pho·ri′tis [*peri;* G. *ōiophoros*, bearing eggs; *-itis*, inflammation]. Inflammation of the peritoneum, ovary, and the adjacent connective tissues.

per″i·o·oph″or·o·sal″pin·gi′tis [*peri; ōiophoros;* G. *salpigx*, trumpet; *-itis*]. Inflammation of the tissues surrounding an ovary and oviduct.

per″i·o″o·the·ci′tis. Perioophoritis. *Obs.*

per″i·o″o·the″co·sal″pin·gi′tis. Old term for perioophorosalpingitis.

per′i·o″ple [*peri;* G. *oplē*, hoof]. The outer layer of horny tissue of the hoof secreted by the perioplic ring. It extends downward over the wall of the hoof, acting as an impervious protective covering.

per″i·op·tom′e·try [*peri;* G. *optos*, visible; *metron*, a measure]. The measurement of the limits of the visual field.

per″i·or′al [*peri;* L. *os*, mouth]. Surrounding the mouth; circumoral.

per″i·or′bit, per″i·or′bi·ta [*peri;* L. *orbita*, path]. The periosteum within the orbit. —**periorbital,** *adj.*

per″i·or″bi·ti′tis [*peri; orbita;* G. *-itis*, inflammation]. Inflammation of the periorbit.

per″i·os″te·i′tis. See *periostitis*.

per″i·os′te·o·phyte″ [G. *periosteos*, around the bones; *phyton*, plant]. A morbid osseous formation upon or proceeding from the periosteum.

per″i·os″te·ot′o·my [*periosteos;* G. *tomē*, a cutting]. An incision into periosteum.

per″i·os′te·um [*periosteos*]. A fibrous membrane investing the surfaces of bones, except at the points of tendinous and ligamentous attachment and on the articular surfaces, where cartilage is substituted. —**periosteal,** *adj.*

per″i·os·ti′tis [*periosteos;* G. *-itis*, inflammation]. Inflammation of periosteum. It may be acute or chronic, the latter being the more frequent form. It is caused by trauma or infection. The exudative forms show a serous, fibrinous, leukocytic, or purulent exudate. The proliferative forms are characterized by local or diffuse formation of collagenous fibrous tissue or bone. —**periostit′ic,** *adj.*

per″i·os·to′ma [*periosteos;* G. *-ōma*, tumor]. Any morbid osseous growth occurring on or surrounding a bone.

per″i·os·to′sis [*periosteos;* G. *-ōsis*, condition]. An osseous formation on the exterior of a bone.

per″i·o′tic (perr″ee·o′tick, ·ot′ick) [G. *peri*, around; *ous*, ear]. 1. Situated about the ear. 2. Of or pertaining to the parts immediately about the internal ear.

per″i·o″va·ri′tis. See *perioophoritis*.

per″i·o′vu·lar [*peri;* L. *ovum*, egg]. Surrounding the ovum.

per″i·pach″y·men″in·gi′tis (perr″i·pack″i·men″-in·jy′tis) [*peri;* G. *pachys*, thick; *mēnigx*, membrane; *-itis*, inflammation]. Inflammation of the connective tissue outside the dura mater.

per″i·pan″cre·a·ti′tis [*peri;* G. *pagkreas*, pancreas; *-itis*]. Inflammation of the tissues around the pancreas.

per″i·pap′il·lar″y (perr″i·pap′i·lerr″ee) [*peri;* L. *papilla*, nipple]. Occurring or situated around the circumference of a papilla, and especially of the optic disk.

per″i·phak′us (perr″i·fack′us, ·fay′kus) [*peri;* G. *phakos*, lens]. The capsule surrounding the crystalline lens.

per″i·pha·ryn′ge·al (perr″i·fa·rin′jul, ·jee·ul, ·far″-in·jee′ul) [*peri;* G. *pharygx*, pharynx]. Surrounding the pharynx.

pe·riph′er·al ref′er·ence. That condition in which, from 10 to 14 weeks following section of a peripheral sensory nerve, tactile and painful stimuli and stimuli of cold, applied within the originally anesthetic area, elicit mixed sensations at the edge of the area of sensory change. This gradually disappears as the true stimulated point becomes perceptible.

pe·riph′er·a·phose″ (peh·rif′ur·a·fohz″, perr″i-ferr′uh·fohz) [G. *periphereia*, circumference; *a-*, not; *phōs*, light]. An aphose originating in the peripheral organs of vision (the optic nerve or the eyeball).

pe·riph′er·o·phose″ (peh·rif′ur·o·fohz″) [*periphereia; phōs*]. A phose originating in the peripheral organs of vision (the optic nerve or the eyeball).

pe·riph′er·y [*periphereia*]. Circumference; the external surface. —**peripheral,** *adj.*

per″i·phle·bi′tis [G. *peri*, around; *phleps*, vein; *-itis*, inflammation]. Inflammation of the tissues about a vein. —**periphlebit′ic,** *adj.*

Per″i·pla·ne′ta (perr″i·pla·nee′tuh) [*peri;* G. *planētēs*, wanderer]. A genus of cockroaches; the species **P. americana** and **P. orientalis** have served as obligatory hosts for the tapeworm *Hymenolepis diminuta* and may transmit pyogenic bacteria, helminthic ova, and protozoan cysts mechanically.

per″i·pleu·ri′tis (perr″i·ploor·eye′tis) [*peri;* G. *pleura*, rib; *-itis*, inflammation]. Inflammation of the tissues outside the parietal pleura.

pe·rip″lo·bi′ose. $C_{13}H_{24}O_9$; the disaccharide obtained on hydrolysis of periplocin. Hydrolysis of periplobiose yields the monosaccharides cymarose ($C_7H_{14}O_4$) and D-glucose.

pe·rip′lo·cin, per″i·plo′cin. $C_{36}H_{56}O_{13}$; a cardioactive steroidal glycoside from *Periploca graeca;* acid hydrolysis yields periplogenin and the sugar periplobiose. Syn., *glucoperiplocymarin, periplocoside.*

pe·rip″lo·cy·mar′in. $C_{30}H_{46}O_8$; a cardioactive steroidal glycoside from *Periploca graeca;* acid hydrolysis yields periplogenin and the sugar cymarose ($C_7H_{14}O_4$).

pe·rip″lo·gen′in. $C_{23}H_{34}O_5$; the steroidal aglycone of periplocin and periplocymarin; a desoxostrophanthidin.

per″i·por·i′tis. Miliaria pustulosa.

per″i·por′tal [*peri;* L. *porta,* gate]. Surrounding the portal vein and its branches.

per″i·proc′tal, per″i·proc′tic [*peri;* G. *prōktos,* anus]. Surrounding the anus or rectum.

per″i·proc·ti′tis [*peri; prōktos;* G. *-itis,* inflammation]. Inflammation of the connective tissue about the rectum or anus.

per″i·pro·stat′ic [*peri;* G. *prostatēs,* one who stands before]. Situated or occurring around the prostate.

per″i·pros″ta·ti′tis [*peri; prostatēs;* G. *-itis,* inflammation]. Inflammation of the tissue situated around the prostate.

per″i·py″e·li′tis. Inflammation about the renal pelvis.

per″i·py·e′ma (perr″i·pye·ee′muh) [G., suppuration around, about]. Suppuration about an organ or tissue. *Rare.*

per″i·py″le·phle·bi′tis [G. *peri,* around; *pylē,* gate; *phleps,* vein; *-itis,* inflammation]. Inflammation of the tissues surrounding the portal vein.

per″i·py·lor′ic (perr″i·pye·lor′ick, ·pi·lor′ick) [*peri;* G. *pylōros,* gate-keeper]. Surrounding the pylorus.

per″i·rec′tal [*peri;* L. *rectus,* straight]. About the rectum.

per″i·rec·ti′tis. See *periproctitis.*

per″i·re′nal [*peri;* L. *renes,* kidneys]. Around a kidney.

per″i·rhi′nal [*peri;* G. *rhis,* nose]. Situated about the nose or nasal cavities.

per″i·sal″pin·gi′tis [*peri;* G. *salpigx,* trumpet; *-itis,* inflammation]. Inflammation of the peritoneal covering of a uterine tube.

per″i·sal·pin″go-o″va·ri′tis. See *perioophorosalpingitis.*

per″i·sal′pinx [*peri; salpigx*]. The peritoneum covering the upper border of a uterine tube.

per″i·sig″moid·i′tis [*peri;* G. *sigmoeidēs,* in the shape of sigma, semicircular; *-itis,* inflammation]. Inflammation of the tissues, especially the peritoneum, covering the sigmoid flexure of the colon.

per″i·sin′u·ous (perr″i·sin′yo͞o·us) [*peri;* L. *sinus,* hollow]. Surrounding a sinus.

per″i·si″nus·i′tis (·sigh″nuh·sigh′tis, ·sin″yoo·, ·sigh″new·) [*peri; sinus;* G. *-itis,* inflammation]. Inflammation of the tissues around a sinus, especially a sinus of the dura mater.

per″i·sper″ma·ti′tis [*peri;* G. *sperma,* seed; *-itis*]. Inflammation around the spermatic cord, with an effusion of fluid; a funicular hydrocele.

per″i·splen′ic, per″i·sple′nic [*peri;* G. *splēn,* spleen]. Situated near the spleen.

per″i·sple·ni′tis [*peri; splēn;* G. *-itis,* inflammation]. Inflammation of the peritoneum covering the spleen.

p. cartilaginea. Hard, inflammatory overgrowth of the capsule of the spleen. Also called *hyalin capsulitis.*

per″i·spon·dyl′ic [*peri;* G. *spondylos,* for *sphondylos,* vertebra]. Around a vertebra.

per″i·spon″dy·li′tis [*peri; spondylos;* G. *-itis,* inflammation]. Inflammation of the tissues around the vertebrae.

per″i·stal′sis [G. *peristaltikos,* clasping and compressing]. A progressive wave of contraction seen in tubes provided with longitudinal and transverse muscular fibers. It consists in a narrowing and shortening of a portion of the tube, which then relaxes, while a distal portion becomes shortened and narrowed. By means of this movement the contents of this tube are forced toward the opening. —**peristal′tic,** *adj.*

reversed p. Peristaltic movement opposite to the normal direction.

per″i·stal′tic rush. An exaggerated peristaltic wave that sweeps extensively over the intestine.

per″i·staph′y·line (perr″i·staf′i·lyne, ·lin, ·leen) [G. *peri,* around; *staphylē,* uvula]. Situated near the uvula.

per″i·staph″y·li′tis [*peri; staphylē;* G. *-itis,* inflammation]. Inflammation of the tissues surrounding the uvula.

per″i·sta′sis [G., a standing round]. According to Ricker's hypothesis, the early stage of the vascular changes in inflammation. The inactivity of vasoconstrictors leads to hyperemia in arterioles, venules, and capillaries. Subsequently, vasoconstriction in the distal segments of the arterioles leads to increased slowing of the blood current, the stage of prestasis. As more proximal segments of arterioles become constricted, the current is further slowed or stopped, the stage of rubrostasis. As arteriolar constriction is subsequently reduced, circulation is resumed, the stage of poststasis or postrubrostasis. This theory supposes a neurogenic basis for these vascular changes. Syn., *peristatic hyperemia.*

pe·ris′to·le. Peristalsis.

per″i·sto′ma, pe·ris′to·ma. See *peristome.*

per′i·stome [G. *peri,* around; *stoma,* mouth]. 1. *In biology,* the parietal region surrounding the mouth, as the oral disk of a polyp. 2. A fringe of hygroscopic teeth, which lines the opening of the capsule in mosses.

per′is·ton. A preparation of polyvinylpyrrolidone, employed as a substitute for whole blood or plasma.

per″i·syn·o′vi·al [G. *peri,* around; NL. *synovia*]. Situated or occurring around a synovial membrane.

per″i·tec′to·my [*peri;* G. *ektomē,* excision]. Excision of a ring of conjunctiva around, and near to, the cornea.

per″i·ten·din′e·um [*peri;* L. *tendere,* to stretch]. The white, fibrous sheath covering the fiber bundles of tendons.

per″i·ten″di·ni′tis [*peri; tendere;* G. *-itis,* inflammation]. Inflammation of the sheath and tissues around a tendon. Syn., *peritenonitis.*

p. calcarea. Calcific deposits in tendons and regional tissues which cause pain and limit motion of the parts.

per″i·ten′on [*peri;* G. *tenōn,* tendon]. Sheath of a tendon.

per″i·ten″o·ni′tis. See *peritendinitis.*

per″i·the″li·o′ma [*peri;* G. *thēlē,* nipple; *-ōma,* tumor]. See *hemangiopericytoma.*

per″i·the′li·um [*peri; thēlē*]. The connective tissue accompanying the capillaries and smaller vessels. —**perithelial,** *adj.*

per″i·thy″roid·i′tis [*peri;* G. *thyreoeidēs,* shield-shaped; *-itis,* inflammation]. Inflammation of the capsule of the thyroid gland.

pe·rit′o·my [*peri;* G. *tomē,* a cutting]. 1. Excision of a strip of conjunctiva around the cornea, for the treatment of pannus. 2. Obsolete term for circumcision.

per″i·to·ne′a·tome. The areas of the peritoneum supplied with sensory fibers from a single spinal nerve.

per″i·to·ne″o·cen·te′sis [G. *peritonaion,* membrane which contains the lower viscera; *kentēsis,* a pricking]. Puncture of the peritoneal cavity, as for the removal of ascitic fluid.

per″i·to·ne·op′a·thy [*peritonaion;* G. *pathos*, disease]. Any disease or abnormality of the peritoneum.

per″i·to·ne″o·per″i·car′di·al [*peritonaion;* G. *perikardios*, around the heart]. Pertaining to the peritoneum and the pericardium.

per″i·to·ne′o·pex″y [*peritonaion;* G. *pēxis*, a fixing]. Fixation of the uterus by the vaginal route in the treatment of retroflexion of this organ.

per″i·to·ne′o·scope [*peritonaion;* G. *skopein*, to examine]. A long, slender telescope, equipped with sheath, obturator, biopsy forceps, sphygmomanometer bulb and tubing, scissors, syringe, for the visualization of the gas-inflated peritoneal cavity. It is introduced into the peritoneal cavity through a small incision in the abdominal wall and permits diagnosis of abdominal and pelvic tumors, biliary disease, and other intraabdominal diseases. —**peritoneos′copy,** *n.*

per″i·to·ne·ot′o·my [*peritonaion;* G. *tomē*, a cutting]. Incision into the peritoneum.

per″i·to·ne′um [*peritonaion*]. The serous membrane lining the interior of the abdominal cavity and surrounding the contained viscera. See Plate 13. —**peritoneal,** *adj.*

per″i·to·ni′tis [*peritonaion;* G. *-itis*, inflammation]. Inflammation of the peritoneum.

acute p. That with an abrupt onset and rapid course, characterized by abdominal pain, tenderness, vomiting, constipation, and fever. May be due to irritation or bacterial infection, the latter being the more serious.

adhesive p. That characterized by the formation of fibrous bands between peritoneal surfaces.

aseptic p. A type due to irritation of the peritoneum by chemicals, either occurring naturally, as from bile, or introduced from without, as by antiseptic solutions, by x-ray or radium, or by mechanical means, as during the course of an operation.

chronic p. That due to infection of the peritoneum by tuberculosis or actinomycosis, or occurring as a residual peritonitis from an acute attack.

diffuse p. A type in which the inflammation is widespread over all, or almost all, of the peritoneum. Also called *generalized p.*

gelatinous p. See *pseudomyxoma* peritonei.

localized p. That in which only a part of the peritoneum is involved, as a local area of inflammation associated with appendicitis.

pelvic p. That which involves only the pelvic peritoneum, frequently associated with infection of the uterine tubes in women.

pneumococcal p. That caused by pneumococci.

primary p. One in which the infection is carried to the peritoneum by the blood or lymph stream.

puerperal p. One following childbirth; associated with infection of the uterus and adnexa.

purulent p. That characterized by the formation of pus.

secondary p. The most usual type of peritonitis, due to extension of infection from neighboring parts, the rupture of a viscus or an abscess, trauma, or as a result of irritation.

streptococcal p. That caused by streptococci.

tuberculous p. Invasion of the peritoneal cavity by *Mycobacterium tuberculosis*, occurring most often in adolescents and young adults, and characterized by abdominal distention, anemia, anorexia, weakness, and loss of weight.

per′i·to·nize [*peritonaion*]. Cover with peritoneum by operative procedures.

per″i·ton′sil·lar [G. *peri*, around; L. *tonsilla*, tonsil]. About a tonsil.

per″i·ton″sil·li′tis [*peri; tonsilla;* G. *-itis*, inflammation]. Inflammation of the tissues surrounding a tonsil.

per″i·tra′che·al (perr″i·tray′kee·ul, ·tra·kee′ul) [*peri;* G. *trachys*, jagged]. Surrounding the trachea.

per″i·tra″che·i′tis (·tray″kee·eye′tis) [*peri; trachys;* G. *-itis*, inflammation]. Inflammation of the connective tissue about the trachea.

peritrate tetranitrate. A trade-marked name for the vasodilator substance pentaerythrityl tetranitrate.

per″i·trich′i·al (perr″i·trick′ee·ul) [*peri;* G. *thrix*, hair]. Surrounding a hair follicle.

pe·rit′ri·chous (peh·rit′ri·kus), **pe·rit′ri·chal** (peh·rit′ri·kul) [*peri; thrix*]. Pertaining to flagella projecting from the whole body of a bacterial cell.

per″i·trun′cal [*peri;* L. *truncus*, trunk]. Perivascular and peribronchial conjointly, as peritruncal carcinoma of the lung.

per″i·typh′lic [*peri;* G. *typhlon*, cecum]. Surrounding the cecum.

per″i·typh·li′tis [*peri; typhlon;* G. *-itis*, inflammation]. Inflammation of the peritoneum surrounding the cecum and vermiform process. —**peri-typhlit′ic,** *adj.*

per″i·um·bil′i·cal [*peri;* L. *umbilicus*, navel]. Surrounding the umbilicus.

per″i·un′gual [*peri;* L. *unguis*, nail]. Around a nail.

per″i·u″re·ter′ic [*peri;* G. *ourētēr*, ureter]. Surrounding one or both ureters.

per″i·u·re″ter·i′tis [*peri; ourētēr;* G. *-itis*, inflammation]. Inflammation of the tissues around a ureter.

per″i·u·re′thral [*peri;* G. *ourēthra*, urethra]. Surrounding the urethra.

per″i·u″re·thri′tis [*peri; ourēthra;* G. *-itis*, inflammation]. Inflammation of the connective tissue about the urethra.

per″i·u′ter·ine (perr″i·yōō′tur·in, ·yōō′tuh·ryne) [*peri;* L. *uterus*, womb]. About the uterus.

per″i·u′vu·lar [*peri;* ML. *uvula*, uvula]. Situated near the uvula.

per″i·vag′i·nal (perr″i·vadj′i·nul, ·va·jy′nul) [*peri;* L. *vagina*, vagina]. About the vagina.

per″i·vag″i·ni′tis (·vadj″i·nigh′tis). See *paracolpitis.*

per″i·vas′cu·lar [*peri;* L. *vasculum*, vessel]. About a vessel.

per″i·vas″cu·li′tis [*peri; vasculum* G. *-itis*, inflammation]. Inflammation of the perivascular sheaths, including the adventitia.

per″i·ve′nous [*peri;* L. *vena*, vein]. Investing a vein; occurring around a vein.

per″i·ves′i·cal [*peri;* L. *vesica*, bladder]. Situated about, or surrounding, the urinary bladder.

per″i·ve·sic″u·li′tis [*peri; vesica;* G. *-itis*, inflammation]. Inflammation around a seminal vesicle.

per″i·vis′cer·al (perr″i·vis′ur·ul) [*peri;* L. *viscera*, inner parts]. Surrounding a viscus or viscera.

per″i·vis″cer·i′tis [*peri; viscera;* G. *-itis*, inflammation]. Inflammation around a viscus or viscera.

per″i·vi·tel′line (perr″i·vi·tel′yne, ·in, perr″i·vit′i·lin, ·vy′ti·lyne) [*peri;* L. *vitellus*, yolk]. Surrounding the vitellus or yolk, as perivitelline space, the space between the zona pellucida and vitellus.

per″i·xe·ni′tis (perr″i·zi·nigh′tis) [*peri;* G. *xenos*, stranger; *-itis*, inflammation]. Inflammation around a foreign body embedded in the tissues.

Perkins, Elisha [*American physician*, 1741–99]. Inventor of the famous metallic tractors. By drawing them across the skin he proposed to draw out from the part affected any inflammation or painful disorder. He was exposed as a charlatan and the method soon fell into disuse. The rods were called *Perkins' tractors*, the belief in their efficacy being known as *Perkinism.*

perle (purl) [F.]. A capsule for administration of medicine.

per·lèche′ (pur·lesh′, perr·lesh′. *See* NOTES § 35) [F.]. A superficial, inflammatory condition occurring at the angles of the mouth with resultant fissuring. It is more prevalent in children, but is also seen in adults. Although it has been regarded as an infection, it is often a symptom of riboflavin deficiency.

Perlia's nucleus. See *nucleus* of Perlia.

per′ma·nent [L. *permanere*, to stay to the end]. Lasting; fixed; enduring, as permanent teeth, the teeth of the second dentition.

per′ma·nent par′tial dis″a·bil′i·ty. *In military medicine*, a complete loss of any part of the body or permanent impairment of any bodily function, other than that producing permanent total disability, which results from injury (occupational or other).

per·man′ga·nate. A salt of permanganic acid.

per″man·gan′ic ac′id. $HMnO_4$. A monobasic acid known chiefly in the form of its salts.

permapen. Trade-mark for *benzathine penicillin G.*

per″me·a·bil′i·ty [L. *permeabilis*, that can be passed through]. *In physiology*, the property of membranes which permits transit of molecules and ions by solution in, or adsorption to, membranes, and by mechanical passage through fine pores.

capillary p. The permeability of the capillary wall to proteins of high molecular weight.

per′me·a·ble [*permeabilis*]. Affording passage; pervious.

per″me·a′tion [L. *permeare*, to pass through]. The act of passing through; specifically, the extension of a malignant tumor, especially carcinoma, by continuous growth through lymphatics.

permutit. Trade-mark for certain synthetic solid substances used for the purpose of exchanging a component ion, such as sodium, for other ions, such as calcium and magnesium, present in water or an aqueous solution in contact with the solid. An important use of such substances is for softening water. The trade-mark is also applied to equipment used with the ion-exchanging substances.

per·ni′cious [L. *perniciosus*, destructive]. Highly destructive; of intense severity; fatal.

per′ni·o. See *chilblain.*

per″ni·o′sis [L. *pernio*, chilblain; G. *-ōsis*, condition]. Any dermatitis resulting from chilblain.

per″noc·ta′tion [L. *pernoctare*, to pass the night]. Wakefulness; insomnia. *Obs.*

pernoston. Trade-mark for 5-*sec.*-butyl-5-β-bromallyl barbituric acid. The substance is used as a hypnotic and sedative. See *butallylonal.*

p. sodium. The sodium salt of pernoston. Used as a hypnotic by intravenous or intramuscular injection.

pe″ro·bra′chi·us (peer″o·bray′kee·us) [G. *pēros*, maimed; *brachiōn*, arm]. A developmental defect in which the forearms and hands are malformed or wanting.

pe″ro·ceph′a·lus [*pēros;* G. *kephalē*, head]. An animal with anomalies of the head and face.

pe″ro·chi′rus, pe″ro·chei′rus (peer″o·kigh′rus) [*pēros;* G. *cheir*, hand]. Congenital absence or stunted growth of the hand.

pe″ro·cor′mus [*pēros;* G. *kormos*, trunk]. Congenital defect of the trunk.

pe″ro·dac·tyl′i·a [*pēros;* G. *daktylos*, finger]. Defective development of the fingers or toes.

pe″ro·dac′ty·lus [*pēros; daktylos*]. An individual having congenitally defective and partially absent fingers and/or toes.

pe″ro·me′li·a [*pēros;* G. *melos*, limb]. Teratic malformation of the limbs.

pe·rom′e·lus [*pēros; melos*]. An individual with congenitally deficient, stunted, or misshapen limbs.

pe·rom′e·ly [*pēros; melos*]. Congenital deficiency or malformation of the limbs.

per″o·ne′al [G. *peronē*, fibula]. Pertaining to the fibular side of the leg, as peroneal nerve. See Table of Nerves in the Appendix.

per″o·ne′o- (perr″o·nee′o-) [*peronē*]. A combining form denoting *connection with* or *relation to the fibula.*

per″o·ne″o·cal·ca′ne·us. An occasional extra slip of the tibialis posterior muscle.

p. externus. A variable slip of insertion of the peroneus brevis muscle into the calcaneus.

p. internus. The fibulocalcaneus medialis muscle.

per″o·ne″o·cu·boi′de·us. An occasional slip of insertion of the peroneus brevis muscle into the cuboid.

per″o·ne″o·tib″ia′lis. The fibulotibialis muscle.

per″o·ne′us ac″ces·so′ri·us. An occasional extra slip of the peroneus longus or brevis muscle.

p. a. digiti quinti. A variant of the peroneus brevis muscle.

p. a. quartus. The peroneocalcaneus externus muscle.

p. a. tertius. The third peroneal muscle.

per″o·ne′us bre′vis. The shorter of the peroneal muscles.

per″o·ne′us lon′gus. The longer peroneal muscle.

pe·ro′ni·a [G. *pēroun*, to maim]. Mutilation; malformation.

pe″ro·pla′si·a (peer″o·play′zhuh, ·zee·uh, ·shuh, ·see·uh) [G. *pēros*, maimed; *plassein*, to form]. A malformation due to abnormal development.

pe′ro·pus [*pēros;* G. *pous*, foot]. An individual with congenitally malformed feet.

per·o′ral (pur·or′ul) [L. *per*, through; *os*, mouth]. Passed or performed through the mouth.

per os [L.]. By way of, or through, the mouth, as in the administration of medicines.

per-os-cillin. Trade-mark for a penicillin calcium tablet.

pe·ro′sis [G. *pērōsis*, maiming]. The condition of abnormal or defective formation.

pe″ro·so′mus [G. *pēros*, maimed; *sōma*, body]. A monster presenting malformation of the body.

pe″ro·splanch′ni·ca (peer″o·splangk′ni·kuh) [*pēros;* G. *splagchnon*, inner parts]. Malformation of the viscera.

per·os′se·ous [L. *per*, through; *os*, bone]. Through bone.

per·ox′i·dase (per·ock′si·dace, ·daze). A conjugated, nonporphyrin enzyme, found largely in plant tissues and to a lesser extent in animal tissues, which catalyzes reactions in which hydrogen peroxide is an electron acceptor, i.e., of the type: $AH_2 + H_2O_2 \rightarrow A + 2H_2O$.

per·ox′ide. That oxide of any base which contains the most oxygen.

per·ox′i·dize. Oxidize completely.

per″pen·dic′u·lar [L. *perpendicularis*, from *perpendiculum*, plumb line]. At right angles to any given line or plane; at right angles to the horizontal.

per pri′mam [L.]. By first intention, said of normal wound healing.

per rec′tum [L.]. By way of the rectum.

Perrin, Maurice [*French surgeon*, 1826–89]. Described snapping hip, called *Perrin-Ferraton's disease.* Sometimes confused with dislocation, it is due to movement of a band of the fascia lata over the greater trochanter of the femur.

Perrin's law. See under *law.*

per′salt″. A salt which contains the maximum amount of the acid radical.

per·seu′lose. A ketoheptose obtained from the juice of the avocado following oxidation by *Bacterium xylinum.*

per·sev″er·a′tion [L. *perseverare,* to persist]. Persistent repetition of words or some activity.

per·sim′mon [Algonquian in origin]. The tree, *Diospyros virginiana.* Its fruit, edible when fully ripe but otherwise highly astringent, and its bark have been used in diarrhea.

per′son·al [L. *personalis,* of a person]. Pertaining to a person, as personal equation, the peculiar difference of individuals in their relation to various orders of stimuli.

per″son·al′i·ty [*personalis*]. 1. The totality of traits and the habitual modes of behavior of the individual as they impress others; the physical and mental qualities peculiar to the individual, and which have social connotations. Regarded by psychoanalysts as the resultant of the interaction of the instincts and the environment. 2. *In psychiatry,* an individual with a certain basic personality pattern which resists efforts at change by either the person himself or others.

aggressive p. See passive-aggressive *p.*

alternating p. One which allows the individual to live alternatingly as two different persons.

Bernreuter p. inventory. See under *test.*

Brown p. inventory. See under *test.*

compulsive p. *In psychiatry,* one characterized by chronic, excessive, or obsessive concern with adherence to standards of conscience or of conformity resulting in inhibited, rigid, overly conscientious behavior.

cycloid p. One which is characterized by recurring states of increased mental and motor activity, alternating with periods of reduced animation bordering on depression.

dissociated p. See split *p.*

dual p. See alternating *p.*

emotionally unstable p. *In psychiatry,* one characterized by undependable judgment and behavior under minor stress.

extroverted p. One in which instinctual energy or libido is directed from the individual and toward the environment.

feeling-type p. One in which the total attitude or reaction is dictated by feeling or emotional tone; one of Jung's functional types of personality.

inadequate p. One showing no obvious mental or physical defect, but characterized by inappropriate or inadequate response to intellectual, social, emotional, and physical demands. The behavioral pattern shows inadaptability, ineptitude, poor judgment, lack of physical and emotional stamina, and social incompatibility.

introverted p. One in which instinctual energy is weak and such inadequate libido is directed inwardly upon the individual himself.

intuitional-type p. One directed by unconscious indications or by vaguely conscious stimuli; one of Jung's functional types of personality.

Minnesota multiphasic p. inventory. See under *test.*

multiple p. One which is capable of dissociation into several or many other personalities at the same time, whereby the delusion is entertained that the one person is many separate persons; a symptom in schizophrenic patients.

neurotic p. One which exhibits symptoms or manifestations intermediate between normal character traits and true neurotic features.

paranoid p. One characterized by the tendency to project hostile feelings so that he always is or easily becomes suspicious of others and is quick to feel persecuted and jealous. Often there are related features of schizoid personality.

passive-aggressive p. A general term for one exhibiting one of three types of behavior: (1) *passive-dependent,* characterized by helplessness, indecisiveness, and a tendency to cling to and seek support from others; (2) *passive-aggressive,* in which aggressiveness and hostility are expressed quietly by such reactions as stubbornness, pouting, procrastination, inefficiency, "doing nothing," or passive obstructionism; (3) *aggressive,* in which irritability, temper tantrums, and destructive behavior are the dominant manifestations of frustration.

p. disorders. *In psychiatry,* a group of disorders characterized by pathological trends in personality structure, with minimal subjective anxiety, manifested, in most instances, by a lifelong pattern of abnormal action or behavior, rather than mental or emotional symptoms. These disorders comprise three main groups: *personality pattern disturbances, personality trait disturbances,* and *sociopathic personality disturbances.*

p. formation. *In psychoanalysis,* the arrangement of the basic constituents of personality.

p. pattern disturbance. *In psychiatry,* a term for an abnormal personality development which can rarely if ever be altered therapeutically in its inherent structure: said of more or less cardinal or arch personality types.

p. trait disturbance. *In psychiatry,* an inability to maintain emotional equilibrium and independence under more or less severely stressful situations because of the disturbances in emotional development. Psychoneurotic features are relatively insignificant. Sometimes individuals exhibiting these disturbances are called immature, but physical immaturity need not be present.

psychopathic p. One characterized by emotional immaturity with marked defects of judgment, prone to impulsive behavior without consideration of others and without evidence of learning by experience.

schizoid p. One given to seclusiveness, emotional rigidity, introversion, and unsocial behavior. See schizophrenic *reaction.*

sensational-type p. One in which sensation, rather than reflective thinking or feeling, dictates action or attitude; Jung's fourth functional type of personality.

sociopathic p. disturbance. *In psychiatry,* a personality disorder characterized primarily in terms of the pathologic relationship between the individual and the society and the moral and cultural environment in which he lives, as well as personal discomfort and poor relationships with others. Sociopathic reactions may be symptomatic of severe personality disorders, psychoneurotic or psychotic reactions, or organic brain injury or disease, the recognition of which then forms the basic diagnosis. See antisocial *reaction,* dyssocial *reaction, sexual deviation.*

split p. One in which there is a separation of various components of the normal personality unit, and each segregation functions as an entity apart from the remaining personality structure; observed in hysteria and the schizophrenic reactions.

syntonic p. One in which there is harmony and appropriateness of thinking, feeling, and action; one which is in harmony with the environment.

thinking-type p. One in which actions and attitudes are ruled predominantly by deliberation and reflective thought rather than by feeling, intuition, or sensation; the first of the four functional types of personality according to Jung.

per″spi·ra′tion [L. *perspirare,* to breathe everywhere]. 1. The secretion of sweat. 2. The sweat.

fetid p. See *bromhidrosis, bromohyperhidrosis.*
insensible p. That which takes place constantly, the fluid being evaporated as fast as excreted.
sensible p. Visible drops or beads of sweat.

per·spire′ [*perspirare*]. To sweat.

per·sul′fate. A salt of persulfuric acid, $H_2S_2O_8$, an acid obtained by electrolytic oxidation of sulfuric acid. It represents the highest valence of sulfur.

per·sul′fide. A sulfide that contains more atoms of sulfur than are required by the normal valence of sulfur, as, for example, in Na_2S_2.

Perthes, Georg Clemens [*German surgeon,* 1869–1927]. Described osteochondritis deformans juvenilis, called *Legg-Calvé-Perthes disease.* Introduced a test for the patency of the deep veins of the leg, called *Perthes' test.*

Pertik, Ottó [*Hungarian pathologist,* 1852–1913]. Described a diverticulum of the nasopharyngeal space amounting to an abnormally deep lateral pharyngeal fossa, called *Pertik's diverticulum.*

per″tur·ba′tion [L. *perturbatio,* disturbance]. Restlessness or disquietude; great uneasiness.

per·tus′sal [L. *per-,* very; *tussis,* cough]. Like whooping cough. Also called *pertussoid.*

per·tus′sis. See *whooping cough.*

Pe·ru′vi·an bark. Old term for cinchona.

per·vap″o·ra′tion [*per-;* L. *vaporatio,* a steaming]. A method of concentration of colloidal and crystalloidal solutions by means of a dialytic membrane either without raising the temperature or by heating without boiling.

per·ver′sion (pur·vur′zhun, ·shun) [L. *perversio,* from *pervertere,* to turn about]. 1. The state of being turned away from the normal or correct. 2. *In psychopathology,* deviation from the normal or average in sexual practices, as homogenitality or fellatio. —**per′vert,** *n.*

per″vi·gil′i·um (pur″vi·jill′ee·um) [L., a watching all night]. 1. Insomnia; wakefulness. *Obs.* 2. See *coma* vigil.

pervitin hydrochloride. Trade-mark for methamphetamine.

per′y·lene. $C_{20}H_{12}$; *peri*-dinaphthalene; a pentacyclic hydrocarbon found in coal tar, occurring as crystals, insoluble in water, and sparingly to freely soluble in various organic liquids.

pes (pl. *pedes*) (payz, pace, *pl.* pee′deez) [L.]. A foot or footlike structure. For other terms concerning pes, see under *talipes.*
p. anserinus. (a) The radiate branching of the facial nerve after its exit from the facial canal. (b) The junction of the tendons of the sartorius, gracilis, and semitendinosus muscles. *O.T.*
p. cavus. Permanently elevated heel associated with an exaggerated curve of the foot resulting from contracture of the plantar fascia.
p. contortus. Clubfoot; talipes.
p. gigas. Macropodia. An abnormally large foot.
p. pedunculi. See *basis* pedunculi.
p. planovalgus. See *flatfoot.*
p. planus. Flatfoot.

pes′sa·ry [L. *pessarium,* pessary]. 1. An appliance of varied form placed in the vagina. 2. Any suppository or other form of medication placed in the vagina for therapeutic purposes. *Obs.*
cradle p. A cradle-shaped pessary once commonly used in the correction of uterine displacements.
cup p. A type of pessary for uterine prolapse in which the cervix rests in a cup held in by a belt and straps.
diaphragm p. The occlusive diaphragm for contraception.
doughnut p. A ring pessary for uterine prolapse.
prolapse p. Any of several types of rings or cups inserted into the vagina for the purpose of holding up the uterus.
retroversion p. Any type of pessary, such as the Smith-Hodge, used to correct a retroverted uterus.
ring p. A round or ring-shaped pessary.
stem p. A device for insertion into the cervical canal, to prevent conception or to stimulate an infantile uterus.

pes′su·lus, pes′sum [L. *pessulus,* bolt; *pessum,* pessary]. A pessary.

pest [L. *pestis,* pest]. 1. An annoying, destructive, or infectious organism; often, large numbers of such organisms, as a cockroach or rat pest. 2. A plague; pestilence; in the old medical literature, any major epidemic. 3. Bubonic plague.

pes′te lo′ca. See Venezuelan equine *encephalitis.*

pest′house″ [*pestis;* AS. *hūs*]. A hospital for persons sick with pestilential diseases.

pes′ti·cide. A substance destructive to pests, especially to insects.

pes′tis [L.]. Pest or plague.
p. ambulans. Plague with first-degree cutaneous manifestations in which the patient is ambulatory.
p. minor. Plague with few systemic manifestations.

pes′tle (pess′ul) [L. *pistillum,* pestle]. The device for rubbing substances in a mortar.

pe·te′chi·a (pi·tee′kee·uh, pi·teck′ee·uh) (pl. *petechiae*) [It. *petecchia*]. A minute, rounded spot of hemorrhage on a surface such as skin, mucous membrane, serous membrane, or on a cross-sectional surface of an organ. —**petechial,** *adj.*

pe·te·chi·om′e·ter. An instrument for the detection of increased capillary fragility by the application of suction to the skin.

Peters, Rudolph Albert [*English biochemist,* 1889–]. With C. W. Carter and H. W. Kinnersley, discovered vitamin B_5 (1930). With Kinnersley, devised a thiamine test in which diazo-benzene-sulfuric acid in carbonate containing sodium hydroxide solution gives a red color with thiamine and formaldehyde; called *Peters-Kinnersley test.*

Peters embryo. An early human embryo discovered by H. Peters and described by him in 1899.

Peters method. See under *method.*

Peters reaction. See Wilkinson and Peters benzidine peroxidase *reaction.*

Petersen, Ferdinand [*German surgeon,* 1845–1908]. Introduced a type of suprapubic lithotomy called *Petersen's operation.* Designed a rubber bag to be inserted into the rectum and inflated for the purpose of pushing the bladder forward so that it could be opened more easily in cystotomy; called *Petersen's bag.*

peth′i·dine (peth′i·deen, ·din). Meperidine hydrochloride.

pe·ti′o·lus [L. *petiolus,* little leg]. A stem, stalk, or petiole; as the petiolus of the epiglottis.

Petit, François Pourfoir du [*French physician and physiologist,* 1664–1741]. Discovered the vasomotor nerves (1727). Described spaces in the ciliary zonule of the eye; called *canals of Petit, zonular spaces.*

Petit, Jean Louis [*French surgeon,* 1674–1750]. One of the founders of the French school of surgery. Described bone softening (1723). Developed several variations on the tourniquet. Adapted the technic of trephining to opening the mastoid bone in cases of mastoiditis, which became standard procedure. Best known for his description of the lumbar triangle, the space bounded by the posterior border of the external oblique muscle in front, the anterior border of the latissimus dorsi posteriorly, its base being formed by the crest of the ilium; called *Petit's triangle.*

pe·tit′ mal′ (puh·tee′ mal′). See petit mal *epilepsy.*

PETN Pentaerythrityl tetranitrate.

Petragnani, Giovanni (1893–). Italian bacteriologist who introduced a culture medium containing malachite green, for isolation of *Mycobacterium tuberculosis*, called *Petragnani's medium*.

Petri, Julius [*German bacteriologist*, 1852–1921]. Known for his introduction of the shallow, cylindrical, covered glass vessels for bacterial cultures in which colonies may be observed without removing the cover; the *Petri dish* is in use the world over. Described a test for proteins called *Petri's test*.

pet″ri·fac′tion [G. *petra*, rock; L. *facere*, to make]. The process of changing to stone, as petrifaction of the fetus. See *lithopedion*.

pé″tris·sage′ (pay″tri·sahzh′) [F.]. Kneading massage; the muscles are picked up or lifted from the bones and rolled, squeezed, or wrung.

pet″ro·bas′i·lar (pet″ro·bas′i·lur, ·ba·zil′ur) [G. *petros*, stone; *basis*, base]. Pertaining to the petrous part of the temporal bone and the basilar part of the occipital bone.

pet′ro·chem″i·cal. A chemical obtained from petroleum.

Petroff, Strashimis Alburtus [*American bacteriologist*, 1882–]. Introduced an egg and gentian violet culture medium (1915). *Petroff's egg medium* is used for cultivation of *Mycobacterium tuberculosis*.

petrogalar. Trade-mark for an emulsion of liquid petrolatum; also with other supporting agents—magnesia magma, nonbitter fluidextract cascara sagrada, and phenolphthalein.

pet″ro·la′tum (*petrolatum*). A purified, semisolid mixture of hydrocarbons obtained from petroleum. Occurs as an unctuous mass, varying in color from yellowish to light amber; insoluble in water, freely soluble in benzene and chloroform. Used as a bland, protective dressing and as a base for ointments. Also called *petroleum jelly, yellow petrolatum*.

hydrophilic p. An ointment base, capable of absorbing aqueous solutions, containing 3% cholesterol, 3% stearyl alcohol, 8% white wax, and 86% petrolatum.

light liquid p. (*petrolatum liquidum leve*). A mixture of liquid hydrocarbons obtained from petroleum: used in sprays for the nose and throat though with risk of injury to lungs. Also called *light liquid paraffin, light white mineral oil*.

liquid p. (*petrolatum liquidum*). A mixture of liquid hydrocarbons obtained from petroleum; a colorless, transparent, oily liquid, insoluble in water and alcohol. Miscible with fixed oils but not with castor oil. Used as a vehicle for medicinal agents to be applied externally or to the mucous membranes of the nose and throat. Also used internally for its mechanical action in constipation. Also called *liquid paraffin, white mineral oil*.

liquid p. emulsion (*emulsum petrolati liquidi*). Contains 50% of liquid petrolatum. Used in constipation. Dose, 30 cc. (1 fluidounce). Also called *mineral oil emulsion*.

liquid p. emulsion with phenolphthalein. Contains 50% (v/v) of liquid petrolatum and 0.4% (w/v) of phenolphthalein.

p. gauze. Absorbent gauze saturated with white petrolatum to the extent of not less than 4 times the weight of the gauze: used as an emollient dressing, packing, or drain.

white p. (*petrolatum album*). Petrolatum wholly or nearly decolorized. Used the same as petrolatum.

pe·tro′le·um [G. *petros*, stone; L. *oleum*, oil]. A complex mixture of hydrocarbons consisting chiefly of the paraffins and cycloparaffins or of cyclic aromatic hydrocarbons, with small amounts of benzene hydrocarbons, sulfur, and oxygenated compounds. Occurs as a dark-yellow to brown or greenish-gray, oily liquid; insoluble in water and only partially soluble in alcohol. It has been used as an expectorant and vermifuge, and externally in skin diseases. Industrially, it is a source of a great number of compounds.

p. benzin. See *benzin*.

p. ether. See *benzin*.

p. jelly. See *petrolatum*.

p. naphtha. See *benzin*.

pet″ro·mas′toid [*petros;* G. *mastoeidēs*, shaped like a breast]. Pertaining to the petrous and mastoid portions of the temporal bone.

pet″ro-oc·cip′i·tal (pet″ro-ock·sip′i·tul). Pertaining to the petrous portion of the temporal bone and to the occipital bone.

pet″ro·pha·ryn′ge·us (pet″ro·fa·rin′jee·us, ·far″-in·jee′us) [*petros;* G. *pharygx*, pharynx]. A small muscle arising from the lower surface of the petrous portion of the temporal bone, and blending with the constrictors of the pharynx; a part of the salpingopharyngeus.

pe·tro′sa [L. *petrosus*, rocky]. The petrous portion of the temporal bone: also called *petrous pyramid*. —**petrosal,** *adj*.

pe·tro′sal nerve. Any of several small nerves passing through the petrous part of the temporal bone and usually attached to the geniculate ganglion. See Table of Nerves in the Appendix.

pet″ro·si′tis [*petrosus;* G. *-itis*, inflammation]. Inflammation of the petrous portion of the temporal bone, usually from extension of a mastoiditis or from middle-ear disease.

pet″ro·sphe′noid [G. *petros*, stone; *sphēnoeidēs*, wedge-shaped]. Pertaining to the petrous portion of the temporal bone and the sphenoid bone.

pet″ro·squa′mous [*petros;* L. *squama*, scale]. Pertaining to the petrous and squamous portions of the temporal bone.

pet′rous (pet′rus, pee′trus) [*petros*]. Stony; of the hardness of stone.

pet′rox (pet′rocks, pee′trocks). See *petroxolin*.

pe·trox′o·lin. A liquid or solid preparation made with a vehicle or base composed of light liquid petrolatum with soft ammonia soap and alcohol and containing medicinal substances. Petroxolins were used by external application.

solid p. (*petroxolinum spissum*). Solid petrox, a yellowish-brown solid preparation containing yellow wax, light liquid petrolatum, oleic acid, strong solution of ammonia, lavender oil, and alcohol: formerly used as a base for the application of various medicinal substances, especially Peruvian balsam.

Pettenkofer, Max Josef von [*German chemist and hygienist*, 1818–1901]. Studied the etiology of cholera, including conditions necessary for its spread. Founded the first laboratory of experimental hygiene (1862). His system of sewage disposal in Munich resulted in the elimination of typhoid fever from the city, a landmark in the history of sanitation. Made important investigations in respiration. With Voit, studied the metabolism of proteins, carbohydrates, and fats. Introduced a test for bile. See Pettenkofer's *test*.

Petzval theory. See under *theory*.

Peu′mus (pew′mus) [Sp. *peumo*]. A genus of evergreen shrubs native to Chile, having one species, **P. boldus,** the boldutree, source of boldo.

pex′is [G. *pēxis*, a fixing]. Fixation. *Obs.*

-pex′y, -pex′i·a [*pēxis*]. *In surgery*, a combining form denoting *fixation*.

Peyer, Johann Conrad [*Swiss naturalist and anatomist*, 1653–1712]. Known for his description of the aggregations of lymph nodules in the mucous membrane of the ileum opposite the mesenteric attachment (1677), called *aggregate* or *agminated* *nodules; Peyer's patches, nodules, nodes, glands; aggregate follicles.*

Peyronie, François de la (1678–1747). French surgeon who described a penile disease, called *Peyronie's disease.*

Peyrot, Jean Joseph [*French surgeon,* 1843–1918]. Described the obliquely oval thorax seen in large pleural effusions; called *Peyrot's thorax.*

Pfannenstiel, Hermann Johann (1862–1909). German gynecologist who described an incision for entering the abdominal cavity; he employed a long, horizontally placed incision curving over the mons pubis so that the pubic hair rendered the scar practically unnoticeable (1900), called *Pfannenstiel's incision.*

Pfaundler, Meinhard von [*German physician,* 1872–1939]. Described filamentation, also called *Pfaundler's reaction.*

Pfeiffer, Emil [*German physician,* 1846–1921]. Described infectious mononucleosis (1889), also called *Pfeiffer's disease.* This had been described by Nil F. Filatov (1885) under the name of idiopathic adenitis.

Pfeiffer's bacillus. *Hemophilus influenzae.*

Pfeif″fer·el′la (pfigh″fur·el′uh, figh″fur·) [after Richard F. J. *Pfeiffer,* German bacteriologist, 1858–1945]. Old term for a genus of bacteria now called *Malleomyces.*

P. whitmori. A motile, Gram-negative rod which is the causative organism of melioidosis. Syn., *Malleomyces pseudomallei.*

Pflüger, Eduard Friedrich Wilhelm [*German physiologist,* 1829–1910]. Formulated laws of polar excitation and muscle contraction, called *Pflüger's laws.* See also Pflüger's *tube.*

P. G. *Pharmacopoeia Germanica,* German Pharmacopoeia.

pH Symbol introduced by Sørensen; used in expressing hydrogen-ion concentration. It signifies the logarithm, on the base ten, of the reciprocal of the hydrogen-ion concentration. A pH above seven represents alkalinity in an aqueous medium; below seven, acidity.

pha·cen′to·cele [G. *phakos,* lentil, lens; *entos,* within; *kēlē,* hernia]. Displacement of the crystalline lens into the anterior chamber of the eye.

pha·ci′tis (fa·sigh′tis) [*phakos;* G. *-itis,* inflammation]. Inflammation of the lens of the eye.

phac′o- (fack′o-, fay′ko-), **phac-** [*phakos*]. A combining form denoting *a lens* or *the lens of the eye.*

phac″o-an″a·phy·lax′is. Anaphylaxis to the crystalline lens. If extracapsular cataract extraction has been performed on one eye, the patient may become sensitized to the lens protein, so that breakage of the other lens capsule, with release of lens protein, allows anaphylactic reaction, due to the previous sensitization.

phac′o·cele. See *phacentocele.*

phac′o·cyst [*phakos;* G. *kystis,* bladder]. The capsule of the crystalline lens.

phac″o·cys·tec′to·my [*phakos; kystis;* G. *ektomē,* excision]. Excision of a part of the capsule of the crystalline lens.

phac″o·er′i·sis [*phakos;* G. *erysis,* a drawing]. An operation for cataract employing suction.

phac″o·hy″men·i′tis [*phakos;* G. *hymēn,* membrane; *-itis,* inflammation]. Inflammation of the capsule of the crystalline lens.

pha′coid (fay′koyd, fack′oyd) [*phakos;* G. *eidos,* form]. Lens-shaped.

pha·col′y·sis [*phakos;* G. *lysis,* a loosing]. 1. Dissolution or disintegration of the crystalline lens. 2. An operation for the relief of high myopia, consisting in discission of the crystalline lens followed by extraction. —**phacolyt′ic,** *adj.*

phac″o·ma·to′sis [*phakos;* G. *-ōma,* tumor; *-ōsis,* condition]. One of a group of diseases, hereditary and developmental in origin, which produce a host of symptoms but which are all characterized by the presence of spots, tumefactions, and cysts joined to other congenital malformations in various parts of the body, especially in the central nervous system. Three distinct syndromes can be recognized: Tuberous sclerosis (phacomatosis of Bourneville), von Hippel-Lindau's disease (angiophacomatosis retinae et cerebelli), and von Recklinghausen's disease (neurofibromatosis, neurofibrophacomatosis).

phac″o·met″a·cho·re′sis (fack″o·met″uh·kor·ee′sis, fay″ko·) [*phakos;* G. *metachōrēsis,* withdrawal]. Dislocation of the crystalline lens.

phac″o·met″e·ce′sis [*phakos;* G. *metoikēsis,* migration]. Displacement of the crystalline lens into the anterior chamber of the eye.

pha·com′e·ter [*phakos;* G. *metron,* a measure]. An instrument for determining the refractive power of lenses. Usually called *lensometer.*

phac″o·pla·ne′sis [*phakos;* G. *planēsis,* a making to wander]. Displacement of the crystalline lens of the eye from the posterior to the anterior chamber and back again.

phac″o·scle·ro′sis [*phakos;* G. *sklērōsis,* a hardening]. Hardening of the crystalline lens.

phac′o·scope [*phakos;* G. *skopein,* to examine]. An instrument for observing the accommodative changes of the lens. —**phacos′copy,** *n.*

phac″o·sco·tas′mus [*phakos;* G. *skotasmos,* a becoming dark]. Clouding of the crystalline lens.

phae′o·chrome (fay′o·krome). Chromaffin. *Obs.*

Phae″o·phy′ce·ae. A class of brown algae.

phae″o·ret′in (fee″o·ret′in). $C_{14}H_8O_7$; a resinous extract from rhubarb root, various species of the genus *Rheum,* occurring as a yellowish-brown powder soluble in alcohol and alkalies.

phage (faydj). See *bacteriophage.*

-phage (-faydj), **-phag** [G. *phagein,* to eat]. A combining form denoting *an eater;* used especially to denote *a phagocyte.* See also *bacteriophage.*

phag″e·de′na, phag″e·dae′na (fadj″i·dee′nuh) [G. *phagedaina,* cancerous sore]. A rapidly spreading destructive ulceration of soft parts. —**phageden′ic,** *adj.*

p. geometrica. Pyoderma gangrenosum with chronic burrowing ulcers.

p. tropica. Tropical ulcer.

sloughing p. Gangrene.

phag″o·car″y·o′sis. Phagokaryosis.

phag′o·cyte [G. *phagein,* to eat; *kytos,* cell]. A cell having the property of engulfing and digesting foreign or other particles or cells harmful to the body. **Fixed phagocytes** include the cells of the reticuloendothelial system and fixed macrophages (histiocytes). **Free phagocytes** include the leukocytes and free macrophages. —**phagocy′tal, phagocyt′ic,** *adj.*

phag″o·cy′to·blast [*phagein; kytos;* G. *blastos,* germ]. A cell giving rise to phagocytes. *Obs.*

phag″o·cy·tol′y·sis (fag″o·sigh·tol′i·sis) [*phagein; kytos;* G. *lysis,* a loosing]. Destruction or dissolution of phagocytes. —**phagocytolyt′ic,** *adj.*

phag″o·cy·to′sis (fag″o·sigh·to′sis) [*phagein; kytos;* G. *-ōsis,* condition]. Ingestion of foreign or other particles, principally bacteria, by certain cells. —**phagocy′tize, phagocy′tose,** *v.*

phag″o·dy″na·mom′e·ter [*phagein;* G. *dynamis,* power; *metron,* measure]. An apparatus for estimating the force exerted in chewing.

phag″o·kar″y·o′sis (fag″o·kar″ee·o′sis) [*phagein;* G. *karyon,* kernel; *-ōsis,* condition]. Supposed phagocytic action by the cell nucleus.

pha·gol′y·sis [*phagein;* G. *lysis,* a loosing]. Destruction or dissolution of phagocytes; phagocytolysis.

phag″o·ma′ni·a [*phagein;* G. *mania,* madness]. An insatiable craving for food.

phag″o·ther′a·py [*phagein;* G. *therapeia,* treatment]. Treatment by superalimentation; overfeeding.

phak′o-. See *phaco.*

phal″a·cro′sis [G. *phalakrōsis,* baldness]. Baldness; alopecia. *Rare.* —**phalacrot′ic, phalac′rous,** *adj.*

phal″a·my′cin. An antibiotic substance produced by a variant of *Streptomyces noursei.* It inhibits a variety of Gram-positive bacteria.

phal″an·gec′to·my (fal″an·jeck′to·mee) [G. *phalagx,* bone between two joints of the fingers or toes; *ektomē,* excision]. Surgical excision of a phalanx of a finger or toe.

pha·lan′ges (fay·lan′jeez, fa·lan′jeez). Plural of phalanx.

phal″an·gi′tis [*phalagx;* G. *-itis,* inflammation]. Inflammation of a phalanx.

p. syphilitica. See *dactylitis* syphilitica.

pha·lan″gi·za′tion [*phalagx*]. A plastic operation in which a metacarpal bone is separated from its fellows and surrounded with skin, thus forming a substitute for a finger or thumb.

pha·lan″go·pha·lan′ge·al (fa·lang″go·fa·lan′jul, ·jee·ul) [*phalagx; phalagx*]. Pertaining to the successive phalanges of the digits, as in phalangophalangeal amputation, removal of a finger or toe at the first or second phalangeal joints.

pha′lanx (fay′langks, fal′angks) (pl. *phalanges*) [*phalagx*]. 1. One of the bones of the fingers or toes. See Table of Bones in the Appendix. See Plate 1. 2. One of the delicate processes of the headplate of the outer rod of Corti projecting beyond the inner rod. —**phalan′geal,** *adj.*

ungual p. The terminal phalanx.

phal′lic [G. *phallos,* phallus]. Pertaining to the penis. See *phallus.*

phal′li·cism [*phallos*]. Phallic worship.

phal′lin. A toxalbumin obtained from the death cup fungus, *Amanita phalloides.*

phal·loi′dine. A peptide from the poisonous mushroom *Amanita phalloides;* on hydrolysis it yields cystine, alanine, and allohydroxy-L-proline.

phal′lo·plas·ty. Plastic construction or repair of the penis.

phal′lus [*phallos*]. 1. The penis. 2. The indifferent embryonic structure derived from the genital tubercle that, in the male, differentiates into the penis, and, in the female, into the clitoris. —**phallic, phalliform, phalloid,** *adj.*

phan′er·o·gam″ [G. *phaneros,* manifest; *gamos,* marriage]. A plant which bears seeds. —**phanerogam′ic,** *adj.*

phan″er·o·gen′ic [*phaneros;* G. *genesthai,* from *gignesthai,* to be produced]. Having a known cause; the opposite of *cryptogenic.*

phan″er·o·ma′ni·a [*phaneros;* G. *mania,* madness]. A neurotic condition in which a person pays undue attention to or cannot resist the impulse to touch some external part or growth, such as a pimple, a hair, or a hangnail; a compulsion reaction.

phan″er·o′sis [*phaneros;* G. *-ōsis,* condition]. The act of passing from a transparent to a visible state.

phanodorn. Trade-mark for a rapidly eliminated hypnotic and sedative, cyclohexenylethylbarbituric acid or cyclobarbital.

phan′tasm [G. *phantasma,* apparition]. An illusive perception of an object that does not exist; an illusion or hallucination. —**phantas′mic,** *adj.*

phan·tas″ma·to·mo′ri·a (fan·taz″muh·to·mor′ee·uh) [*phantasma;* G. *mōria,* folly]. Childishness, or dementia, with absurd fancies or delusions.

phan·tas″mo·sco′pi·a [*phantasma;* G. *skopein,* to examine]. The seeing of phantasms; hallucinations involving ghosts.

phan′ta·sy [G. *phantasia,* appearance]. 1. Visionary imagination; the faculty of reproducing unreal, phantasmic notions or sensuous impressions. 2. An image. 3. Fantasy.

phan′tom. *In radiology,* an object, made of beeswax or pressed-wood composition and sometimes consisting of water, which simulates a tissue in its behavior toward radiation and permits determination of the dose of radiation delivered to the surface of and within the simulated tissue through measurements with ionization chambers placed within the phantom material.

phan′tom limb. A psychological phenomenon frequently occurring in amputees: the patient feels sensations, and sometimes pain, in the missing limb.

phar′ci·dous [G. *pharkis,* wrinkle]. Wrinkled; rugose; full of wrinkles. *Obs.*

Phar. D. *Pharmaciae Doctor,* Doctor of Pharmacy.

phar′ma·cal [G. *pharmakon,* drug]. Pertaining to pharmacy.

phar″ma·ceu′tic (fahr″muh·sue′tick), **phar″ma·ceu′ti·cal** [G. *pharmakeutikos,* of drugs]. Pertaining to pharmacy.

phar″ma·ceu′tist. See *pharmacist.*

phar′ma·cist [G. *pharmakon,* drug]. An apothecary, a druggist.

phar′ma·co- [*pharmakon*]. A combining form denoting *drug.*

phar″ma·co·dy·nam′ics (fahr″muh·ko·dye·nam′icks, ·di·nam′icks) [*pharmakon;* G. *dynamis,* power]. The science of the action of drugs. —**pharmacodynamic,** *adj.*

phar″ma·cog′no·sist [*pharmakon;* G. *gnōsis,* knowledge]. One versed in pharmacognosy.

phar″ma·cog′no·sy [*pharmakon; gnōsis*]. The science of crude drugs.

phar″ma·cog′ra·phy. See *pharmacognosy.*

phar″ma·col′o·gist [*pharmakon;* G. *logos,* word]. A specialist in pharmacology.

phar″ma·col′o·gy [*pharmakon; logos*]. The science of the nature and properties of drugs, particularly their actions. —**pharmacolog′ic, pharmacolog′ical,** *adj.*

phar″ma·co·ma′ni·a [*pharmakon;* G. *mania,* madness]. A morbid craving for medicines, or for self-medication.

phar″ma·co·pe′dics. The scientific study of drugs and medicinal substances.

phar″ma·co·pe′ia, phar″ma·co·poe′ia (fahr″muh·ko·pee′uh) [G. *pharmakopoiia,* preparation of drugs]. A collection of formulas and methods for the preparation of drugs, especially a book of such formulas recognized as a standard, as the United States Pharmacopeia, the British Pharmacopoeia. The former is issued every five years under the supervision of a national committee. Abbreviated, P. —**pharmacope′al,** *adj.*

phar″ma·co·pho′bi·a [*pharmakon;* G. *phobos,* fear]. Morbid dislike or fear of medicine.

phar′ma·co·phore. A particular grouping of atoms within a molecule which is considered to confer pharmacological activity to a substance.

phar″ma·co·psy·cho′sis (fahr″muh·ko·sigh·ko′sis) [G. *pharmakon,* drug; *psychōsis,* from *psychē,* soul, *-ōsis,* condition]. Psychosis associated with drugs or alcohol.

phar″ma·co·ther′a·py [*pharmakon;* G. *therapeia,* treatment]. The treatment of disease by means of drugs.

phar′ma·cy [*pharmakon*]. 1. The art of preparing, compounding, and dispensing medicines. 2. A drug store.

pharmagel. Trade-mark for a brand of gelatin particularly designed for the preparation of emulsions and available in two types based upon the method of manufacture.

p. A. A gelatin prepared from acid-treated precursors, used without other emulsifying agents at a pH of about 3.2.

p. B. A gelatin prepared from alkali-treated precursors, used at a pH of about 8.0. Pharmagel B may be used alone or in combination with other emulsifying agents.

phar″yn·gal′gi·a [G. *pharygx*, pharynx; *algos*, pain]. Pain in the pharynx.

phar″yn·gec′to·my (far″in·jeck′to·mee) [*pharygx;* G. *ektomē*, excision]. Excision of a part of the pharynx.

phar″yn·gem·phrax′is (far″in·jem·frack′sis) [*pharygx;* G. *emphraxis*, stoppage]. Obstruction of the pharynx.

phar″yn·gis′mus [*pharygx*]. Spasm of the pharynx.

phar″yn·gi′tis [*pharygx;* G. *-itis*, inflammation]. Inflammation of the pharynx. —**pharyngit′ic,** *adj.*

acute p. A form due to exposure to cold, to the action of irritant substances, or to certain infectious causes, and characterized by pain on swallowing, by dryness, later by moisture, and by congestion of the mucous membrane. Also called *catarrhal p.*

atrophic p. A form attended by atrophy of the mucous membrane.

beta-hemolytic streptococcal p. A type caused by beta-hemolytic streptococci of Lancefield group A.

chronic p. A form that is generally the result of repeated acute attacks, and is associated either with hypertrophy of the mucous membrane (**hypertrophic pharyngitis**) or with atrophy (**atrophic pharyngitis**).

diphtheritic p. That characterized by the presence of a false membrane, the product of the action of the *Corynebacterium diphtheriae:* also called *croupous p.*

follicular p. See granular *p.*

granular p. A form of chronic pharyngitis in which the mucous membrane has a granular appearance. Also called *clergyman's sore throat.*

nonstreptococcal exudative p. A disease of unknown etiology, suspected of being viral, which closely resembles streptococcal pharyngitis, but in which group A streptococci are not found.

p. sicca. The atrophic form characterized by a very dry state of the mucous membrane.

pha·ryn′go- (fa·ring′go-), **pharyng-** [*pharygx*]. A combining form meaning *pharynx.*

pha·ryn′go·cele [*pharygx;* G. *kēlē*, hernia]. A hernia or pouch of the pharyngeal mucosa projecting through the pharyngeal wall.

pha·ryn″go·dyn′i·a [*pharygx;* G. *odynē*, pain]. Pain referred to the pharynx.

pha·ryn″go·ep″i·glot′tic [*pharygx;* G. *epiglōttis*, epiglottis]. Pertaining to the pharynx and the epiglottis.

pha·ryn″go·ep″i·glot′ti·cus [*pharygx; epiglōttis*]. Muscular fibers derived from the stylopharyngeus and inserted into the side of the epiglottis and the pharyngoepiglottic ligament.

pha·ryn″go·e″so·phag′e·al (fa·ring″go·ee″so-fadj′ul, ·fadj′·ee·ul, ·ee″so·fuh·jee′ul) [*pharygx;* G. *oisophagos*, gullet]. Pertaining to the pharynx and esophagus.

pha·ryn″go·e·soph′a·gus [*pharygx; oisophagos*]. The pharynx and esophagus considered as one organ.

pha·ryn″go·glos′sal [*pharygx;* G. *glōssa*, tongue]. Pertaining conjointly to the pharynx and the tongue.

pha·ryn″go·glos′sus [*pharygx; glōssa*]. Muscular fibers extending from the superior constrictor of the pharynx to the base of the tongue.

pha·ryn″go·ker″a·to′sis [*pharygx;* G. *keras*, horn; *-ōsis*, condition]. Thickening of the mucous lining of the pharynx with formation of a tough and adherent exudate.

pha·ryn″go·la·ryn′ge·al (fa·ring·go·la·rin′jul,″ ·jee·ul, ·lar″in·jee′ul) [*pharygx;* G. *larygx*, larynx]. Pertaining both to the pharynx and to the larynx.

pha·ryn″go·lar″yn·gi′tis [*pharygx; larygx;* G. *-itis*, inflammation]. Simultaneous inflammation of the pharynx and larynx.

pha·ryn′go·lith [*pharygx;* G. *lithos*, stone]. A calcareous concretion in the walls of the pharynx.

phar″yn·gol′o·gy [*pharygx;* G. *logos*, word]. The science of the pharyngeal mechanism, functions, and diseases.

phar″yn·gol′y·sis [*pharygx;* G. *lysis*, a loosing]. Paralysis of the pharyngeal muscles.

pha·ryn″go·max′il·lar″y (·mack′si·lerr″ee) [*pharygx;* L. *maxilla*, jaw]. Relating to the pharynx and the maxilla.

pha·ryn″go·my·co′sis (fa·ring″go·migh·ko′sis) [*pharygx;* G. *mykēs*, fungus; *-ōsis*, condition]. Disease of the pharynx due to the action of fungi.

pha·ryn″go·na′sal [*pharygx;* L. *nasus*, nose]. Pertaining to the pharynx and the nose, as pharyngonasal cavity.

pha·ryn″go·pal′a·tine (fa·ring″go·pal′uh·tyne, ·tin) [*pharygx;* L. *palatum*, palate]. Relating to the pharynx and the palate.

pha·ryn″go·pal″a·ti′nus. See *palatopharyngeus.*

pha·ryn″go·pa·ral′y·sis. See *pharyngoplegia.*

phar″yn·gop′a·thy [*pharynx;* G. *pathos*, disease]. Any disease of the pharynx.

pha·ryn″go·pe·ris′to·le (·peh·ris′to·lee). See *pharyngostenia.*

pha·ryn′go·plas″ty [*pharygx;* G. *plassein*, to form]. Plastic surgery of the pharynx.

pha·ryn″go·ple′gi·a (fa·ring″go·plee′juh, ·jee·uh, far″ing·go·) [*pharygx;* G. *plēgē*, stroke]. Paralysis of the muscles of the pharynx.

pha·ryn″go·rhi·ni′tis (fa·ring″go·rye·nigh′tis) [*pharygx;* G. *rhis*, nose; *-itis*, inflammation]. Pharyngitis with rhinitis; inflammation of the pharyngeal and nasal mucosa.

pha·ryn″go·rhi·nos′co·py (·rye·nos′ko·pee). See *posterior rhinoscopy* under *rhinoscopy.*

pha·ryn″gor·rha′gi·a (fa·ring″go·ray′juh, ·jee·uh, far″ing·go·) [*pharygx;* G. *rhēgnynai*, to burst forth]. Hemorrhage from the pharynx.

pha·ryn″gor·rhe′a [*pharygx;* G. *rhoia*, flow]. A mucous discharge from the pharynx.

pha·ryn″go·scle·ro′ma [*pharygx;* G. *sklērōma*, induration]. Pharyngeal scleroma.

pha·ryn′go·scope [*pharygx;* G. *skopein*, to examine]. An instrument for use in examining the pharynx. —**pharyngos′copy,** *n.*

pha·ryn′go·spasm [*pharygx;* G. *spasmos*, spasm]. Spasmodic contraction of the pharynx. —**pharyngospasmod′ic,** *adj.*

pha·ryn″go·ste′ni·a [*pharygx;* G. *stenos*, narrow]. Narrowing or stricture of the pharynx. —**pharyngos′tenous,** *adj.*

pha·ryn″go·ther′a·py [*pharygx;* G. *therapeia*, treatment]. The treatment of diseases of the pharynx by direct applications or irrigations.

pha·ryn′go·tome [*pharygx;* G. *tomos*, cutting]. An instrument for incising the pharynx.

phar″yn·got′o·my [*pharygx;* G. *tomē*, a cutting]. Incision into the pharynx.

anterior p. An approach to the oral pharynx by an incision above the hyoid bone and a separation of the suprahyoid structures.

lateral p. Incision into one side of the pharynx.

pha·ryn″go·ton″sil·li′tis [*pharygx;* L. *tonsilla*, tonsil; G. *-itis*, inflammation]. Inflammation of the pharynx and the tonsils.

pha·ryn″go·xe·ro′sis (fa·ring″go·zi·ro′sis) [*pharygx;* G. *xēros*, dry; *-ōsis*, condition]. Dryness of the pharynx.

phar′ynx [*pharygx*]. The musculomembranous tube situated back of the nose, mouth, and larynx, and extending from the base of the skull to a point opposite the sixth cervical vertebra, where it becomes continuous with the esophagus. It is lined by mucous membrane, covered in its upper part with pseudostratified ciliated epithelium, in its lower part with stratified squamous epithelium. On the outside of this is a layer of fibrous tissue, the **pharyngeal aponeurosis.** This in turn is surrounded by the muscular coat. The upper portion of the pharynx, communicating with the nose through the posterior nares, is known as the **nasopharynx,** and functionally belongs to the respiratory tract; the lower portion, divided into the **oropharynx** and **laryngopharynx,** is common to the respiratory and digestive tracts. The pharynx communicates with the middle ear by means of the auditory tube. See Plate 12. —**pharyn′geal,** *adj.*

primitive p. The embryonic pharynx with its characteristic visceral arches, grooves, and pouches.

phase (faze) [G. *phasis*, appearance]. 1. The condition or stage of a disease or of biologic, chemical, and physiologic functions at a given time. 2. A solid, liquid, or gas which is homogeneous throughout and physically separated from another phase by a distinct boundary.

ejection p. The phase of ventricular systole during which blood is pumped into the aorta.

group p. *In immunology*, that characterized by antigens shared by only a few other species or types.

lag p. The early period of slow growth of bacteria when first inoculated in a culture medium.

maximal ejection p. The period of early systole during which the largest volume of blood per unit time is discharged by the ventricles.

meiotic p. The stage of the reduction division in meiosis.

negative p. The temporary lessening of the amount of antibody in the serum immediately following a second inoculation of antigen. See opsonic *index*.

p. variation. See bacterial *variation.*

positive p. The increase in opsonic index which follows the negative phase.

reduced ejection p. The period of late systole during which diminishing volumes of blood per unit of time are discharged by the ventricles.

specific p. *In immunology*, that characterized by the presence of specific flagellar antigens.

pha·se′o·lin (fa·see′o·lin). A simple protein of the globulin type which occurs in kidney beans.

pha′sic ir·reg″u·lar′i·ty (fay′zick). A disorder consisting of a periodic slowing of the heart for a few seconds, unrelated to the respiratory cycle; occurs in convalescence from acute fevers, and sometimes during the administration of digitalis. It is a vagal effect, as it is abolished by atropine, but the manner of its production is unknown.

pha′sin. A poisonous agglutinin, said to be an alkaloid, obtained from soybean and other beans, occurring as a white, amorphous powder, and inactivated by boiling. A 1 per cent solution agglutinates red cells of all animals.

phat′ne (fat′nee). See *alveolus*, 1.

phat″nor·rha′gi·a [G. *phatnē*, socket; *rhēgnynai*, to burst forth]. Hemorrhage occurring from a tooth socket.

pheas′ant's eye. Adonis; an extract from *Adonis vernalis.*

phel·lan′drene. $C_{10}H_{16}$; either of two isomeric substances: *α-phellandrene*, 5-isopropyl-2-methyl-1,3-cyclohexadiene, or *β-phellandrene*, 3-isopropyl-6-methylene-1-cyclohexane; both occur in dextrorotatory and levorotatory forms in various volatile oils.

Phelps, Abel Mix [*American surgeon,* 1851–1902]. Introduced his operation for the relief of clubfoot, in which he divided all soft parts on the inner side of the foot; called *Phelps's operation.*

phemerol chloride. Trade-mark for *p-tert*-octylphenoxyethoxyethyldimethylbenzylammonium chloride, a quaternary ammonium compound, sometimes referred to as a cationic detergent. The substance occurs as colorless crystals, very soluble in water; used as an antiseptic and fungicide. The combination of detergent and antiseptic properties suggests its use for cleansing wounds. See *benzethonium chloride.*

phem′i·tone. Former British Pharmacopoeia title for *methylphenobarbitone* or *mephobarbital.*

phen-, phe′no- (fee′no-, fen′o-) [G. *phainein*, to bring to light]. A combining form denoting *derivation from benzene.*

-phen [*phainein*]. A combining form for *phene.*

phen′a·caine hy″dro·chlo′ride (fen′uh·cane, fee′-nuh·cane) (*phenacainae hydrochloridum*). CH_3CN-$(NC_6H_4OC_2H_5).(NH.C_6H_4OC_2H_5).HCl.H_2O$. Ethenyl-*p*-diethoxydiphenylamidine hydrochloride; white, odorless crystals or crystalline powder; 1 Gm. dissolves in 50 cc. of water; freely soluble in alcohol. Used as a local anesthetic, especially for anesthesia in the eye. See *holocaine hydrochloride.*

phe·nac′e·mide. Generic name for the synthetic anticonvulsant drug phenylacetylurea.

phe·nac′e·tin (fi·nass′i·tin). Acetophenetidin.

phe·nac″e·tu′ric ac′id. $C_6H_5CH_2CO.NH.CH_2$-COOH. Glycine conjugate of phenylacetic acid, one form in which the latter is excreted following ingestion by animals.

phen″a·dox′one. British generic name for the analgesic substance 6-morpholino-4:4-diphenylheptan-3-one, supplied under the names *heptalgin* and *heptazone.*

phe″na·kis′to·scope, phae″na·kis′to·scope (fee″nuh·kis′to·scope, fen″uh·) [G. *phenakistēs*, imposter; *skopein*, to examine]. That form of stroboscope in which the figures and slits revolve in the same direction. Also called *direct stroboscope.*

phe·nam′i·dine (fi·nam′i·deen, ·din). A diamidine, 4:4′-diamidinodiphenyl ether, reported to have therapeutic merit against pathogenic trypanosomes. It also inhibits growth of bacteria in wounds.

phe·nan′threne. $C_{14}H_{10}$. A hydrocarbon isomeric with anthracene, and found with it in coal tar.

phenarsen. A trade-mark for dichlorophenarsine hydrochloride.

phenarsenamine. A Canadian brand of arsphenamine.

phe·nar′sone sulf·ox′y·late. $NaO.OH.O.AsC_6H_3$.-$OH.NH.CH_2OSONa$. Sodium 3-amino-4-hydroxyphenylarsonate-N-methanal sulfoxylate. A pentavalent arsenical which may be used in the treatment of *Trichomonas vaginalis* vaginitis and central nervous system syphilis. The drug must be used with caution. See *aldarsone.*

phe′nate, phen′ate. A compound of phenol and a base; a carbolate.

phen′a·zone. Antipyrine.

phene (feen) [G. *phainein*, to bring to light]. *In chemistry*, benzene.

phenergan hydrochloride. Trade-marked name for *promethazine hydrochloride.*

phen·eth′yl. The monovalent radical $C_6H_5CH_2$-CH_2.

phen·eth′yl al′co·hol. $C_6H_5CH_2CH_2OH$; 2-phenylethanol or β-phenylethyl alcohol; a liquid with a floral odor, occurring in some essential oils and also prepared by synthesis: used in perfume and flavor formulations, and recommended as an antibacterial agent for ophthalmic preparations. Also called *phenylethyl alcohol*.

phe·net'i·din. $NH_2.C_6H_4.OC_2H_5$. Aminoethyoxybenzene, of which three isomers exist. The para-isomer frequently appears in the urine following administration of acetophenetidin.

phe·net″i·di·nu'ri·a. The presence of phenetidin in the urine.

phe·net'sal, phen'et·sal. $C_6H_4OH.CO.O.C_6H_4$-$(NHCH_3CO)$. Acetyl-*p*-aminophenyl salicylate. White, odorless crystals. The actions of phenetsal resemble those of phenyl salicylate. Used as an antirheumatic, antipyretic, and analgesic. Externally it has been applied in psoriasis and itching skin diseases. Dose, 0.3–1 Gm. (5–15 gr.). Externally in 10% ointment. See *salophen*.

phen″go·pho'bi·a [G. *pheggos*, light; *phobos*, fear]. A morbid fear of daylight.

phe'nic ac'id (fee'nick, fen'ick). See *phenol*.

phe'nic al'co·hol. Phenol.

phen'i·cin. An antibiotic substance derived from *Penicillium phoeniceum* and *P. rubrum*, active against several bacteria: also written *phoenicin*.

phe·nin'da·mine (fi·nin'duh·meen, ·min). $C_{19}H_{19}N$. 2-Methyl-9-phenyl-2,3,4,9-tetrahydro-1-pyridindene, an antihistaminic substance. See *thephorin*.

phen″in·di'one. Generic name for 2-phenylindane-1,3-dione, an anticoagulant effective when administered orally.

phen·ir'a·mine. A shorter generic name for *prophenpyridamine*.

phen·meth'y·lol. Benzyl alcohol.

phe″no·bar'bi·tal (fee″no·bahr'bi·tawl, ·tal, ·tol, fen″o·) (*phenobarbitalum*). $C_{12}H_{12}O_3N_2$. Phenylethylbarbituric acid; white, glistening, small crystals; slightly soluble in water, soluble in alcohol. Used as a hypnotic in nervous insomnia and conditions of excitement of the nervous system. Due to the slowness and persistence of its action it is used as a sedative and antispasmodic in epilepsy. Dose, 0.015–0.12 Gm. (¼–2 gr.). Syn., *phenylethylmalonylurea, phenobarbitone*. See *luminal*.

elixir p. (*elixir phenobarbitali*). Contains 4 Gm. of phenobarbital per liter. Dose, 4 cc. (1 fluidrachm).

p. sodium (*phenobarbitalum sodicum*). The sodium derivative of phenobarbital; very soluble in water and soluble in alcohol. The effects of phenobarbital sodium are similar to phenobarbital except that it is more rapidly absorbed. Dose, 0.015–0.12 Gm. (¼–2 gr.). Also called *soluble phenobarbitone, soluble phenobarbital*. See *luminal sodium*.

phe″no·bar'bi·tone. See *phenobarbital*.

phe'no·coll. $C_2H_5O.C_6H_4.NHCOCH_2NH_2$; aminoacetophenetidin; a crystalline base, salts of which have been used as antipyretics and analgesics.

phen'o·cop″y, phe'no·cop″y. An experimentally produced effect on the body which copies the appearance of genetic effects; *e.g.*, tanning produced by ultraviolet light which duplicates hereditary pigmentation.

phe'no·din. Hematin.

phe'nol (fee'nole, ·nol, ·nawl, fi·nole'). 1. (*phenol*). C_6H_5OH. Hydroxybenzene; obtained from coal tar or prepared synthetically; colorless to light pink, needle-shaped crystals; 1 Gm. dissolves in 15 cc. of water, soluble in alcohol and glycerin; undiluted it whitens and cauterizes the skin and mucous membranes; used as an antiseptic, germicide, disinfectant, escharotic, and local anesthetic. Phenol has also been used for the treatment of tetanus by hypodermic injection. Also called *carbolic acid, phenyl alcohol, phenyl hydrate*. 2. Any hydroxy derivative of aromatic hydrocarbons which has the OH group directly attached to the ring.

camphorated p. (*phenol camphoratum*), (*camphor-phenol*). Contains 30% of phenol and 60% of camphor in liquid petrolatum.

liquefied p. (*phenol liquefactum*), (*liquefied carbolic acid*). Phenol maintained in the liquid condition by the presence of 10% of water.

p. coefficient. A figure representing the relative strength of an antiseptic, as compared with phenol acting on the same organism and for the same length of time.

p. glycerite (*glyceritum phenolis*), (*glycerite of carbolic acid*). Contains 20% of liquefied phenol in an aqueous-glycerin vehicle.

p. ointment (*unguentum phenolis*), (*ointment of carbolic acid*). Contains 2% of phenol in yellow ointment.

p. red. See *phenolsulfonphthalein*.

phe'no·lase. An enzyme which catalyzes oxidation of phenolic substances.

phe'no·late. A compound of a phenol in which the hydrogen of the hydroxyl group is replaced by a univalent metal.

phe″nol·phthal'ein (fee″nole·thal'een, ·thal'ee·in, ·fthal'ee·in, fee″nol·, fee″nawl·) (*phenolphthaleinum*). $(C_6H_4OH)_2CO.C_6H_4CO$; a white or faintly yellowish powder; almost insoluble in water, soluble in alcohol. Used as a laxative in the treatment of simple constipation, increasing both peristalsis and secretion throughout the whole intestinal tract. A frequent allergen. Dose, 0.03–0.2 Gm. (½–3 gr.).

yellow p. An impure form of phenolphthalein, having a canary yellow color; is two or three times as active as the white form.

phe″nol·phthal'in. 4′,4″-Dihydroxytriphenylmethane-2-carboxylic acid, prepared from phenolphthalein with zinc and sodium hydroxide. Used as a reagent for detecting the presence of blood.

phe″nol·sul'fo·nate. A salt or ester of phenolsulfonic acid.

phe″nol·sul″fone·phthal'ein. Phenolsulfonphthalein.

phe″nol·sul·fon'ic ac'id. $C_6H_4.OH.SO_3H$. Of the three isomers, ortho-, meta-, and para-, the last is used, in the form of salts, as an intestinal antiseptic. Syn., *sulfocarbolic acid*.

phe″nol·sul″fon·phthal'ein (*phenolsulfonphthaleinum*). $C_{19}H_{14}O_5S$; bright-red to dark-red, crystalline powder; 1 Gm. dissolves in about 1300 cc. of water and about 350 cc. of alcohol. Used for determining the functional activity of the kidneys. 1 cc. of a sterile solution containing 6 mg. (¹⁄₁₀ gr.) as the monosodium salt is injected intramuscularly or intravenously. The degree of renal defect is estimated by adding solution of sodium hydroxide to the voided urine, and comparing with a standard. Phenolsulfonphthalein is also used as an indicator; yellow, pH 6.8, red, pH 8.4. Also spelled *phenolsulfonephthalein*. Syn., *phenol red*.

p. injection (*injectio phenolsulfonphthaleini*). Phenolsulfonphthalein ampuls; a sterile solution of phenolsulfonphthalein in isotonic solution of sodium chloride made with water for injection and rendered soluble with sodium bicarbonate or sodium hydroxide.

phe″nol·tet″ra·chlo″ro·phthal'ein. A dye used intravenously in the form of the sodium salt for the determination of the functional activity of the liver.

phe″nol·tet″ra·i·o″do·phthal′ein so′di·um (fee″nole·tet″ruh·eye·o″do·thal′een). See *phentetiothalein sodium.*

phe″no·lu′ri·a [G. *phainein,* to bring to light; *ouron,* urine]. The presence of phenols in the urine.

phe·nom′e·non (pl. *phenomena*) [G. *phainomenon,* neut. pres. part. from *phainesthai,* to appear]. An event or manifestation, generally of an unusual character.

adhesion p. Thrombocytobarin reaction; a phenomenon in which clumping of platelets or bacteria and spirochetes occurs in the presence of their specific immune serums. It has been used to distinguish between closely allied species or between varieties of the same species.

Argyll Robertson p. See under *pupil.*

Arthus p. See Nicolas Maurice *Arthus.*

autokinetic p. A nocturnal visual illusion manifested through the oculovestibular apparatus and characterized by apparent movement of a fixed point of light following staring at the light.

bulldog p. Closure of the jaws in response to a tap on the lower jaw, seen in experimental animals following ablation of both suppressor bands (8s and 24s) in the cerebral cortex.

clasp-knife p. See clasp-knife *rigidity.*

conglutination p. Normal bovine serum increases the agglutination of erythrocytes in the presence of antibodies and complement, suggested as a method for detecting antibodies too weak to cause agglutination.

diaphragm p. See diaphragmatic *sign.*

Donath-Landsteiner p. See Donath-Landsteiner *test.*

double pain p. The phenomenon of feeling two successive sensations of pain following a single pain stimulus, e.g., a pinprick. A brief sensationless interval, whose duration is directly proportional to the distance between the site of stimulus and site of interpretation (cerebral cortex), separates the two sensations, which are thus considered to be due to the presence of two sets of nerve fibers (delta and C fibers) with different conduction rates.

Dupuys-Dutemps' p. A paradoxical lid retraction present in peripheral facial paralysis.

entoptic p. One of the visual sensations generated within the eye.

face p. See Chvostek's *sign.*

Fuchs' p. A paradoxical lid retraction associated with eye movements during the healing stage of oculomotor paresis, characterized by spasmodic raising of the lid which had suffered from ptosis.

Gowers' p. Pain produced along the entire course of the sciatic nerve by passive dorsal flexion of the foot in sciatica.

great toe p. See Babinski *reflex.*

Hoffmann's p. Increased galvanic irritability of the sensory nerves in tetany.

Houssay p. The rare occurrence of pituitary hypofunction in a true diabetic, causing amelioration of the diabetes. See also Bernardo Alberto *Houssay.*

immune-adherence p. An immunologically specific in vitro reaction involving normal human erythrocytes, microorganisms sensitized with antibody, phagocytic cells, and complement resulting in enhanced phagocytosis. It forms the basis of the *Treponema pallidum* immobilization test.

interference p. *In microbiology,* a condition in which an infectious agent may so alter the host that for a time the host is less susceptible to a second infectious agent.

jaw-winking p. Winking of the eye sometimes seen with movements of the jaw, as in individuals who have recovered from herpes zoster.

knee p. See patellar *reflex.*

Koch p. See Robert *Koch.*

Koebner's p. See isomorphous provocative *reaction.*

Leichtenstern's p. The violent jerk of a patient with cries of pain when any part of the skeleton is tapped; seen in meningitis.

Liesegang's p. A precipitation of colloids in the form of concentric rings, which occurs in stone formation.

Lucio's p. See Lucio *leprosy.*

Marcus Gunn p. A congenital syndrome of unknown cause in which opening the mouth causes the apparently paretic upper lid to rise suddenly, usually unilateral. Syn., *jaw-winking p.*

Marin Amat p. Closure of the eye when the mouth is open or in the process of mastication, found during the recovery period of peripheral facial palsy. Syn., *inverse Marcus Gunn p.*

Meirowsky p. The increase in epidermal pigment in excised skin, from living or post-mortem donors, after incubation at 37° C. or higher or on exposure to ultraviolet light.

multiplication p. of Laurentiev. The concept that each vagus fiber to the gastrointestinal tract branches terminally to innervate a large number of enteric ganglion cells.

p. of local skin reactivity. See Shwartzman *p.*

Piltz-Westphal p. Contraction of the pupils on firm closure of the lids or their attempted closure against resistance, demonstrable in 35 per cent of normal individuals.

platysma p. In hemiplegia, when the patient opens the mouth widely, there occurs an exaggerated contraction of the platysma on the opposite or unaffected side.

pronation p. Immediate return to pronation position of the hand on the affected side of the hemiplegic patient when both hands are passively supinated and suddenly released.

psi phenomena. *In parapsychology,* personal experiences or events defying physical explanation, e.g., clairvoyance, precognition, and telepathy.

puppet-head p. Sudden dropping forward of the head which causes the eyeballs to look upward; the reverse occurs when the head is elevated; a sequela of encephalitis.

quellung p. See Neufeld quellung *test.*

Quinquaud's p. A sideward oscillating movement in all the fingers, probably due to intermittent contraction of the interosseous muscles; in almost any disease with tremors.

Raynaud's p. The color changes of digits seen in Raynaud's syndrome, particularly when occurring secondarily to known arteriolar disease.

rebound p. Sudden withdrawal of strong resistance to a movement causes marked rebound; ipsilateral to cerebellar lesion.

release p. Hyperreflexia induced by a lesion of the brain stem and release of the effect of the cerebral cortex.

Rust's p. Use of the hands to support the head during change of position; in tuberculous caries of the upper cervical vertebrae.

satellite p. The characteristic arrangement of the colonies of *Hemophilus influenzae* in association with *Micrococcus aureus.* The bacilli form satellites at a distance from the coccal colonies.

Schiff-Sherrington p. Hyperreflexia of the forelimbs after the spinal cord is severed below the cervical enlargement.

setting-sun p. A sign associated with hydrocephaly where, because of tightness of the scalp, the upper eyelids are pulled up and expose the sclera above the iris.

Shwartzman p. A phenomenon of local tissue reactivity in the skin and various organs to bacterial filtrates. Active principles responsible for the phenomenon were identified as antigenic soluble exotoxins. The phenomenon is produced by a preparatory (intradermal, intraparenchymal, or intravenous) injection of the active substance, followed by an intravenous injection of the active substance 24 hours later. The lesion produced at the site of preparation is severe hemorrhagic necrosis. The phenomenon was first observed, but incorrectly interpreted by Giuseppe Sanarelli.

simile p. The basis of homeopathy: like is cured by like.

staircase p. The increases in height of muscle contractions early in a series of responses to stimuli of constant intensity. Contractions are increased by residual effects of previous contractions, probably metabolic products.

Staub-Traugott p. See under Hans *Staub*.

stress p. See general adaptation *syndrome*.

tibialis p. A marked dorsiflexion at the ankle occurring in attempts to draw the leg toward the body in pyramidal tract injury.

toe p. A movement of flexion and abduction of the toe caused by a sudden blow on the toe-ends; seen in upper motor neuron damage.

Tyndall p. See *Tyndallization*.

von Stockert p. Quick induction of sleep, caused by certain visual stimuli; after acute stages of encephalitis lethargica.

Vulpian-Heidenhain-Sherrington p. Stimulation of intact sensory nerve fibers in atrophic muscles may produce enough antidromic impulses generating sufficient acetylcholine to cause a slow, small, maintained contraction.

Wenckebach p. A recurring pulse pause in partial heart block.

phen″o·pro′pa·zine hy″dro·chlo′ride. Profenamine hydrochloride.

phe″no·sul′fa·zole. Generic name for N-(2-thiazolyl)-1-phenol-4-sulfonamide; $OH.C_6H_4.$-$SO_2NH.C_3H_2NS$, employed experimentally in treating poliomyelitis but found ineffective. See *darvisul*.

phe″no·thi′a·zine (fee″no·thigh′uh·zeen, ·zin). $C_{12}H_9NS$. Thiodiphenylamine; occurs as a weak yellow-green to weak olive-green powder; insoluble in water, soluble in alcohol. It is used at present chiefly by veterinarians for its vermifuge action. Dose varies, depending on animal's size.

phe′no·type [G. *phainein*, to show; *typos*, impression]. 1. The sum total of visible traits which characterize the members of a group. 2. A group of individuals who look alike, but differ in their genetic make-up. —**phenotyp′ic,** *adj.*

phe·nox′y. The univalent radical C_6H_5O.

phe·nox″y·a·ce′tic ac′id. $C_6H_5O.CH_2COOH$; phenoxyethanoic acid or O-phenylglycolic acid, occurring in needlelike crystals, sparingly soluble in water, freely soluble in alcohol; a fungicide.

phe·nox″y·benz′a·mine hy″dro·chlo′ride. Generic name for N-phenoxyisopropyl-N-benzyl-β-chloroethylamine, an adrenergic blocking agent. See *dibenzyline*.

phe·noz′y·gous [*phainein;* G. *zygon*, yoke]. Pertaining to an anomaly of development in which the cranium is considerably narrower than the broadest part of the face.

phen·tet″i·o·thal′e·in so′di·um (fen·tet″eye·o·thal′ee·in, ·thal′een, ·thay′lee·in). $NaO.O:C.$-$C_6I_4.C:C_6H_4OC_6H_4ONa$. The disodium salt of a dye, phenoltetraiodophthalein. Bronze-purple, odorless granules; soluble in water and alcohol. Used for the roentgenologic examination of the gallbladder and simultaneous test of hepatic function. Dose, 0.04 Gm. per kg. of body weight, total dose need not exceed 2.5 Gm. Syn., *phenoltetraiodophthalein sodium*.

phen·tol′a·mine. Generic name for 2-[(*m*-hydroxy-N-*p*-tolylanilino)-methyl]-2-imidazoline, supplied under the trade-marked name *regitine:* intended for use in diagnosis between essential hypertension and that resulting from pheochromocytoma.

phenurone. Trade-mark for *phenacemide*.

phen′yl, phe′nyl. The univalent radical, C_6H_5—. —**phenyl′ic,** *adj.*

phen″yl·ac″et·al′de·hyde. $C_6H_5.CH_2CHO$; a colorless liquid with a strong hyacinthlike odor, polymerizing and becoming viscous on standing, slightly soluble in water: used as attractant in insect control and in perfumery.

phen″yl·ac″et·am′ide. See *acetanilid*.

phen″yl·a·ce′tic ac′id. $C_6H_5.CH_2.COOH$; crystals, soluble in water; a product of apparently faulty metabolism of phenylalanine, also of normal metabolism of phenyl derivatives of fatty acids having an even number of carbon atoms.

phen″yl·a·ce″tyl·glu′ta·mine. $H_2N.CO(CH_2)_2$-$(CHNHOCCH_2C_6H_5)COOH$. A conjugated form of phenylacetic acid excreted in man and the chimpanzee.

phen′yl a·ce″tyl·sal″i·cyl′ate. $C_6H_4(OCH_3CO)$-$COOC_6H_5$. A white, tasteless powder, insoluble in water; hydrolyzed in the intestines. An analgesic, antipyretic and mild intestinal antiseptic. Dose, 0.5–1 Gm. (7½–15 gr.). See *spiroform*.

phen″yl·ac″e·tyl·u·re′a. $C_6H_5.CH_2.CONH.CO$-NH_2; a white, crystalline substance, very slightly soluble in water, prepared by synthesis; an anticonvulsant with minor sedative action, useful in treating epilepsies. Syn., *phenacemide*. See *phenurone*.

α-phen″yl·a·cryl′ic ac′id. Atropic acid.

phen″yl·al′a·nine (fen″il·al′uh·neen, ·nin, fee″-nil·). $C_6H_5CH_2CH(NH_2)COOH$. α-Amino-β-phenylpropionic acid, an amino acid essential in human nutrition.

phen′yl al′co·hol. See *phenol*.

phen″yl·am′ine. See *aniline*.

phen″yl·benz·am′ide (·ben·zam′id, ·ben′zuh-myde, ·mid). Benzanilide.

phen″yl·bu′ta·zone. Generic name for 3,5-dioxo-1,2-diphenyl-4-*n*-butylpyrazolidine, supplied under the trade-marked name *butazolidin* for use in treatment of arthritis and allied disorders.

phen″yl·car′bi·nol. Benzyl alcohol.

phen″yl·car·byl′a·mine chlo′ride. $C_6H_5NCCl_2$; a lacrimatory agent having potential utility in chemical warfare.

phen″yl·cin″cho·nin′ic ac′id. Cinchophen.

phen′yl cy′a·nide. Benzonitrile.

phen″yl·di·bro″mo·ar′sine. $C_6H_5AsBr_2$; a lung irritant having potential utility in chemical warfare.

phen″yl·di·chlo″ro·ar′sine. $C_6H_5AsCl_2$; a lung irritant having potential utility in chemical warfare.

phen′yl·ene (fen′i·leen, fee′ni·leen). The bivalent radical, C_6H_4.

phen″yl·ene·di′a·mine. Any of three isomeric crystalline substances of the formula $C_6H_4(NH_2)_2$, distinguished by the prefixes *ortho-*, *meta-*, and *para-*. All are used in manufacturing dyes, and the *para*-compound has been used as a hair dye, causing toxic reactions.

phen″yl·eph′rine hy″dro·chlo′ride. Generic name for the sympathomimetic substance available under the trade-marked name *neo-synephrine hydrochloride*.

phen″yl·eth″yl·a·mine′. $C_6H_5CH_2CH_2NH_2$; 1e amino-2-phenylethane; a liquid, slightly solublin water, produced by enzymatic decarboxylation of phenylalanine: also called *β-phenylethylamine.* Syn., *phenethylamine.*

phen″yl·eth″yl·bar″bi·tu′ric ac′id. See *phenobarbital.*

phen″yl·eth″yl·mal″o·ny·lu′re·a. See *phenobarbital.*

phen″yl·glu·co′sa·zone. $C_{18}H_{22}N_4O_4$. A yellow, crystalline compound produced in the phenylhydrazine test for glucose.

phen′yl hy′drate. See *phenol.*

phen″yl·hy′dra·zine (fen″il·high′druh·zeen, ·zin, fee″nil·). $C_6H_5.NH.NH_2$. A colorless to pale-yellow to red-brown liquid, sparingly soluble in water and miscible with alcohol. It is used as a reagent for sugars, aldehydes, and ketones, and in other chemical reactions. Phenylhydrazine base must not be used medicinally.

p. hydrochloride. $C_6H_5.NH.NH_2.HCl$, occurs as white, silky leaflets; soluble in water and alcohol; discolors in light and air. It is used in the treatment of polycythemia. It must be used with caution as excessive doses cause fatty degeneration of the liver. Dose, 0.1–0.2 Gm. (1½–3 gr.) two or three times a week.

phen″yl·hy′dra·zone. The product resulting from the interaction of phenylhydrazine with an aldehyde or ketone.

phe·nyl′ic ac′id. Phenol.

2-phen″yl·in″dane-1,3-di′one.

```
          CO
         /  \
   C6H4      CH.C6H5
         \  /
          CO
```

A white powder, insoluble in water, soluble in alcohol. It is an orally effective anticoagulant. Syn., *phenindione.*

phen″yl·ke″to·nu′ri·a. The presence of a phenylketone in the urine.

phen″yl·mer·cu′ric ac′e·tate (ass′i·tayt). $C_6H_5.Hg.C_2H_3O_2$; occurs as small, white, lustrous prisms; soluble in about 600 parts of water but more soluble in alcohol. Used as an antiseptic, germicide, and fungicide.

phen″yl·mer·cu′ric bor′ate. See *merphenyl borate.*

phen″yl·mer·cu′ric chlo′ride. C_6H_5HgCl; occurs as white, leafy crystals, practically insoluble in water. Used as an antiseptic, germicide, and fungicide.

phen″yl·mer·cu′ric ni′trate. $C_6H_5Hg.OH.C_6H_5.HgNO_3$, basic phenylmercuric nitrate; occurs as a white or grayish white powder; soluble in about 1250 parts of water; slightly soluble in alcohol. Used as an antiseptic, germicide, and fungicide.

phen″yl·mer·cu′ric pic′rate. See *merphenyl picrate.*

phen′yl meth′yl al′co·hol. Benzyl alcohol.

phen′y·lon. Antipyrine.

o-phen″yl·phe′nol. $C_6H_5.C_6H_4.OH$; 2-hydroxydiphenyl, occurring as white, flaky crystals, insoluble in water, soluble in alkali solutions and most organic solvents: used in various formulations as a germicide and fungicide.

phen″yl·pro″pa·nol′a·mine hy″dro·chlo′ride. $C_6H_4.CHOH.CH(CH_3).NH_2.HCl$; *dl*-norephedrine hydrochloride; a white, crystalline powder, freely soluble in water, chemically and pharmacologically analogous to ephedrine, its action being more prolonged: used as a bronchial dilator and nasal vasoconstrictor. See *propadrine hydrochloride.*

phen″yl·pro″pyl·meth′yl·a·mine. $C_6H_5.CH(CH_3).CH_2.NH.CH_3$; *dl*-N,β-dimethylphenethylamine; a volatile liquid, slightly soluble in water, employed as a nasal vasoconstrictor by inhalation. The hydrochloride is applied topically for the same purpose. See *vonedrine.*

phen″yl·py·ru′vic ac′id (fen″il·pye·roo′vick, ·pi-roo′vick, fee″nil·). $C_6H_5CH_2.CO.COOH$. A metabolic product of phenylalanine; the state of mental deficiency known as phenylpyruvic oligophrenia is characterized by excretion of the acid.

phen″yl·py·ru′vic a·men′ti·a (a·men′shee·uh, ·shuh). See phenylpyruvic *oligophrenia.*

phen″yl·quin″o·line-car″box·yl′ic ac′id (fen″il-kwin″o·leen-, ·lin-, fee″nil·). Cinchophen.

phen′yl sal′i·cyl″ate (*phenylis salicylas*). $OH.C_6H_4.COO.C_6H_5$. A white, crystalline powder; very slightly soluble in water, freely soluble in alcohol. Phenyl salicylate is hydrolyzed in the small intestine by the pancreatic juice, yielding phenol and salicylic acid. For this reason it is used as an internal antiseptic in the treatment of enteritis and intestinal fermentation. Dose, 0.3–1.0 Gm. (5–15 gr.). Syn., *salol.*

phen″yl·sul′fate. A salt of phenylsulfuric acid.

phen″yl·sul·fur′ic ac′id. $C_6H_5OSO_3H$. A phenol ester of sulfuric acid.

phen″yl·thi″o·u·re′a. $C_6H_5.NH.CS.NH_2$; needle-like crystals, slightly soluble in water, of interest as a substance which tastes bitter to most persons, but is tasteless to others: also called *phenylthiocarbamide.*

phen′y·toin so′di·um. Diphenylhydantoin sodium.

phe′o·chrome (fee′o·krome). Chromaffin. *Obs.*

phe″o·chro″mo·blas·to′ma [G. *phaios*, gray; *chrōma*, color; *blastos*, germ; *-ōma*, tumor]. A tumor of the same order as pheochromocytoma, but made up of less well differentiated cells, the pheochromoblasts, and considered more malignant as evidenced by invasion of the capsule, direct extension, and metastases. Syn., *chromaffinoblastoma, malignant chromaffinoma, malignant pheochromocytoma.*

phe″o·chro′mo·cyte [*phaios; chrōma;* G. *kytos*, cell]. Obsolete term for chromaffin cell.

phe″o·chro″mo·cy·to′ma (fee″o·kro″mo·sigh·to′-muh) [*phaios; chrōma; kytos;* G. *-ōma*, tumor]. A tumor of the sympathetic nervous system, found most often in the adrenal medulla but occasionally in other sites such as Zuckerkandl's bodies and in the thorax. It is made up largely of pheochromocytes, or chromaffin cells, derivatives of the primitive neurocytes, with a strong affinity for taking up chrome salts. May be accompanied by the adrenal-sympathetic syndrome of spasmodic or persistent hypertension. Also called *chromaffinoma, chromaffin* or *chromophile tumor.*

malignant p. See *pheochromoblastoma.*

phe″o·phor′bide. The product resulting when magnesium and the alcohol phytol are removed from chlorophyll by treatment with strong acid.

phe″o·phy′tin. The product formed by replacement of magnesium in chlorophyll by hydrogen. The corresponding copper and iron derivatives of chlorophyll, which may be considered **magnesium pheophytin,** are called **copper pheophytin** and **iron pheophytin.** They are sometimes referred to simply as chlorophylls.

phe·then′y·late. The generic name for 5-phenyl-5-(2-thienyl)hydantoin, $C_{13}H_{10}N_2O_2S$, a synthetic anticonvulsant. See *thiantoin.*

Ph. G. Graduate in Pharmacy; German Pharmacopoeia.

phi′al. See *vial.*

Phi″a·loph′o·ra [G. *phialē*, a bowl; *phoros*, bearing]. A genus of fungi.

P. verrucosa. A species which is one of the causative agents of chromoblastomycosis.

-phil′i·a [G. *philein*, to love]. A combining form meaning *love of;* used to denote *a tendency toward* or *a craving for*. Also see *-phobia*.

phi·li′a·ter, phil″i·a′ter [*philein;* G. *iatēr*, physician]. 1. A student of medicine. *Obs.* 2. A dabbler in medicine. *Obs.*

Philipson's reflex. See under *reflex*.

phil′ly·rin. $C_{27}H_{34}O_{11}$. A crystalline glucoside found in the bark and leaves of various species of *Phillyrea;* has been used as an antipyretic.

phil″o·cy′tase [*philein;* G. *kytos*, cell]. Metchnikoff's name for the intermediate body of Ehrlich; an amboceptor. *Obs.*

phil″o·ne′ism [*philein;* G. *neos*, new]. Abnormal love of novelty; the reverse of misoneism.

phil″o·pa·trid″o·ma′ni·a [*philein;* G. *patris*, fatherland; *mania*, madness]. Uncontrollable desire to return home; excessive nostalgia, or homesickness. *Obs.*

phil′ter, phil′tre [G. *philtron*, love charm]. A love potion; a preparation supposed to be efficacious in exciting sexual passion.

phil′trum [*philtron*]. The depression on the surface of the upper lip immediately below the septum of the nose.

phi·mo′sis (figh·mo′sis, fi·mo′sis) [G., a stopping up]. Elongation of the prepuce and constriction of the orifice, so that the foreskin cannot be retracted to uncover the glans penis. —**phimot′ic,** *adj*.

phleb-. See *phlebo-*.

phleb·an″gi·o′ma [G. *phleps*, vein; *aggeion*, vessel; *-ōma*, tumor]. A venous aneurysm.

phleb″ar·te″ri·ec·ta′si·a [*phleps;* G. *artēria*, artery; *ektasis*, extension]. Varicose aneurysm.

phleb″ar·te″ri·o·di·al′y·sis (fleb″ahr·teer″ee·o·dye·al′i·sis) [*phleps; artēria;* G. *dialysis*, separation]. Arteriovenous aneurysm.

phleb″ec·ta′si·a, phle·bec′ta·sis [*phleps;* G. *ektasis*, extension]. Dilatation of a vein; varicosity.

phle·bec′to·my [*phleps;* G. *ektomē*, excision]. Excision of a vein or a portion of a vein.

phleb″ec·to′pi·a [*phleps;* G. *ektopos*, away from a place]. The displacement, or abnormal position, of a vein.

phleb″em·phrax′is [*phleps;* G. *emphraxis*, stoppage]. Plugging of a vein.

phleb″ep·a·ti′tis [*phleps;* G. *hēpar*, liver; *-itis*, inflammation]. Inflammation of veins within the liver.

phleb″eu·rys′ma (fleb″yoo·riz′muh). See *varix*.

phleb″ex·ai·re′sis (fleb″ecks·eye·ree′sis) [*phleps;* G. *exairesis*, a taking out]. Excision of a vein.

phle·bis′mus (fli·biz′mus) [*phleps*]. Undue prominence or swelling of a vein.

phle·bi′tis [*phleps;* G. *-itis*, inflammation]. Inflammation of a vein; is generally suppurative (**suppurative phlebitis**), and is the result of the extension of suppuration from adjacent tissues. It leads to the formation of a thrombus within the vein (**thrombophlebitis**), which may break down and cause the distribution of septic emboli to various parts of the body. When not due to a suppurative process (**plastic, adhesive,** or **proliferative phlebitis**), it may give rise to obliteration of the vein. Symptoms are pain and edema of the affected part, redness along the course of the vein, the latter appearing as a hard, tender cord. —**phlebit′ic,** *adj*.

blue p. See *phlegmasia* cerulea dolens.

infectious p. That due to infection.

pelvic p. Inflammation of the veins in the pelvis.

sclerosing p. A type in which the veins become permanently occluded by scar formation.

sinus p. Phlebitis of the sinuses of the dura mater.

phleb′o-, phleb- [*phleps*]. A combining form meaning *vein*.

phleb″o·car″ci·no′ma [*phleps;* G. *karkinōma*, cancer]. Extension of carcinoma to the walls of a vein.

phle·boc′ly·sis (fli·bock′li·sis, fleb″o·kly′sis) [*phleps;* G. *klysis*, a drenching]. The injection of a saline solution into a vein.

phleb′o·gram [*phleps;* G. *gramma*, letter]. 1. A roentgenogram of a vein after injection of the artery, whose capillary bed it drains, with a roentgenopaque material, such as diodrast. 2. A tracing of the venous pulse by the sphygmograph.

phleb′o·graph [*phleps;* G. *graphein*, to write]. An instrument for recording a venous pulse.

phle·bog′ra·phy [*phleps; graphein*]. The anatomy and physiology of the veins.

phleb′oid [*phleps;* G. *eidos*, form]. 1. Pertaining to a vein; venous. 2. Resembling a vein.

phleb′o·lith [*phleps;* G. *lithos*, stone]. A hard concretion sometimes found in veins, produced by calcareous infiltration of a thrombus. —**phlebolith′ic,** *adj*.

phleb″o·li·thi′a·sis [*phleps; lithos;* NL. *-iasis*, condition]. The formation of phleboliths.

phleb″o·ma·nom′e·ter [*phleps;* G. *manos*, thin; *metron*, a measure]. An apparatus for the direct measurement of venous pressure.

phleb″o·phle·bos′to·my [*phleps; phleps;* G. *stoma*, mouth]. An operation in which an anastomosis is made between veins.

phleb″o·phlo·go′sis. See *phlebitis*.

phleb′o·plas″ty [*phleps;* G. *plassein*, to form]. Plastic operation for the repair of veins.

phleb″o·ple·ro′sis [*phleps;* G. *plērōsis*, a filling up]. Distention of the veins.

phleb″or·rha′gi·a [*phleps;* G. *rhēgnynai*, to burst forth]. Venous hemorrhage.

phle·bor′rha·phy [*phleps;* G. *rhaphē*, suture]. Suture of a vein.

phleb″or·rhex′is [*phleps;* G. *rhēxis*, a breaking]. Rupture of a vein.

phleb″o·scle·ro′sis [*phleps;* G. *sklērōsis*, a hardening]. 1. Sclerosis of a vein. 2. Chronic phlebitis.

phle·bos′ta·sis [*phleps;* G. *stasis*, a standing]. The temporary removal of some of the blood from the general circulation by means of compression of the veins in the extremities. Syn., *bloodless phlebotomy*.

phleb″o·ste·no′sis [*phleps;* G. *stenōsis*, a being straitened]. Constriction of a vein.

phleb″o·strep′sis [*phleps;* G. *strepsis*, a turning round]. Torsion, or twisting, of a vein.

phleb″o·throm·bo′sis [*phleps;* G. *thrombōsis*, a becoming curdled]. Formation of a thrombus in a vein.

phleb′o·tome [*phleps;* G. *tomos*, cutting]. A cutting instrument used in phlebotomy.

Phle·bot′o·mus [*phleps; tomos*]. A genus of small blood-sucking sandflies of the family Psychodidae. The species **P. argentipes** transmits the flagellates of kala-azar in India, **P. chinensis** in China; **P. papatasii** is the vector of pappataci fever, sandfly fever of the Balkans. **P. verrucarum** is the vector for *Bartonella bacilliformis*, the causative agent of bartonellosis or Carrión's disease (Oroya fever and verruca peruviana).

phle·bot′o·my [*phleps;* G. *tomē*, a cutting]. The opening of a vein for the purpose of bloodletting. —**phlebot′omist,** *n*.

bloodless p. See *phlebostasis*.

phlegm (flem) [G. *phlegma*, phlegm]. 1. A viscid, stringy mucus, secreted by the mucosa of the air passages. 2. One of the four humors of the old writers.

phleg·ma′si·a [G., turgescence]. Inflammation.

p. adenosa. See *adenitis.*

p. alba dolens. Milk leg, a painful swelling of the leg beginning either at the ankle and ascending, or at the groin and extending down the thigh, its usual cause being infection after labor.

p. cellularis. Cellulitis.

p. cerulea dolens. Acute, fulminating, deep venous thrombosis, characterized by pain, edema, and cyanosis of the extremities: also called *blue phlebitis.*

p. dolens. See *p.* alba dolens.

p. lactea. See *p.* alba dolens.

p. malabarica. See *elephantiasis* arabum.

p. membranae mucosae gastropulmonalis. See *aphthae tropicae* under *aphtha.*

p. myoica. Myositis.

phleg·mat′ic [G. *phlegmatikos,* abounding in phlegm]. 1. Of the nature of phlegm. 2. Characterized by an apathetic, sluggish temperament.

phleg′mon [G. *phlegmonē,* inflammation]. Suppurative inflammation of a part, especially the connective tissues. —**phlegmonous,** *adj.*

phlo′em [G. *phloos,* bark]. *In botany,* that portion of a fibrovascular bundle lying beneath the epidermis which consists of sieve tubes, companion cells, and associated fibers or parenchyma; leptome. Also see *xylem.*

phlo·gis′ton. The name, introduced by Stahl in the 17th century, of the hypothetical component of combustible substances. Such substances were thought to be compounds of phlogiston with another component; on combustion the phlogiston escaped, leaving the other component. The theory was abandoned following the discovery of oxygen and of its role in combustion.

phlog″o·gen′ic, phlo·gog′e·nous [G. *phlox,* flame; *genesthai,* from *gignesthai,* to be produced]. Producing inflammation.

phlo·go′sin. A crystalline substance found in cultures of pyogenic cocci, which can produce inflammation.

phlo·go′sis. Old term for inflammation.

phlog″o·zel′o·tism [*phlox;* G. *zēlōtēs,* zealot]. An old craze for ascribing to every disease an inflammatory origin.

phlor′e·tin, phlo·re′tin. $C_{15}H_{14}O_5$. A product of the hydrolysis of phlorhizin. Its administration in suitable doses, like that of phlorhizin, is followed by glycosuria.

phlo·rhi′zin (flo·rye′zin, flor′i·zin). $C_{21}H_{24}O_{10}.2H_2O$. A glycoside derived from the bark and root of apple, cherry, pear, and other trees; occurs as light, white, silky needles; slightly soluble in water, and soluble in alcohol. Phlorhizin causes the appearance of a considerable amount of glucose in the urine. The drug has been suggested as a test for kidney function. It has also been used as an antiperiodic. Also called *phlorizin, phloridzin, phlorrhizin.*

phlor″o·glu′cine (flor″o·glōō′seen, ·sin). See *phloroglucinol.*

phlor″o·glu′ci·nol. $C_6H_6O_3.2H_2O$. Used as a reagent for hydrochloric acid in gastric juice, for lignin, pentosans, pentoses, etc.

phlox′ine (flock′seen, ·sin) (C.C.). A red acid dye of the xanthine series; used as a counterstain with blue nuclear dyes.

phlyc·te′na [G. *phlyktaina,* blister]. A vesicle· —**phlyctenar, phlyctenous,** *adj.*

phlyc·ten′ule (flick·ten′yōōl, flick′ten·yōōl″), **phlyc·ten′u·la** [dim. from *phlyktaina*]. A minute phlyctena; a little vesicle or blister. —**phlyctenular,** *adj.*

phlyc·ten″u·lo′sis [*phlyktaina;* G. *-ōsis,* condition]. The presence of phlyctenules.

-phobe [G. *phobos,* fear]. A combining form denoting *one having a phobia.*

pho′bi·a [*phobos*]. A specific neurotic fear, symbolic of a neurotic conflict and its resulting anxiety. See Table of Phobias in the Appendix. Also see phobic *reaction.* —**pho′bic,** *adj.*

-pho′bi·a [*phobos*]. A combining form denoting *fear* or *dread.* Also see *-philia.*

pho″bo·dip′si·a [*phobos;* G. *dipsa,* thirst]. Hydrophobia. *Obs.*

pho″bo·pho′bi·a [*phobos; phobos*]. A morbid dread of being afraid.

Phocas, B. Gerasimo [*French physician,* 1861–1937]. Described a form of chronic mastitis, characterized by the presence of multiple fibrous nodules; called *Phocas' disease.*

pho″co·me′li·a, pho·com′e·ly [G. *phōkē,* seal; *melos,* limb]. Absence or markedly imperfect development of arms and forearms, thighs and legs, but with hands and feet present.

pho·com′e·lus [*phōkē; melos*]. An individual with phocomelia.

phoen′i·cin. Phenicin.

Pho′ma [G. *phōis,* blister]. A genus of fungi whose species may act as common allergens and as laboratory contaminants.

pho′nal, phon′ic (fon′ick, fo′nick) [G. *phōnē,* voice]. Pertaining to the voice or to sound.

pho″nas·the′ni·a [*phōnē;* G. *astheneia,* want of strength]. Weakness of voice, especially that resulting from bodily exhaustion.

pho·na′tion [*phōnē*]. The production of vocal sound or articulate speech.

subenergetic p. Hypophonia.

superenergetic p. Hyperphonia.

pho′na·to″ry [*phōnē*]. Pertaining to phonation, as the phonatory cord, the vocal fold.

phon·au′to·gram (fone·aw′to·gram) [*phōnē;* G. *autos,* self; *gramma,* letter]. The diagram of a phonautograph.

phon·au′to·graph (fone·aw′to·graf) [*phōnē; autos;* G. *graphein,* to write]. An apparatus for recording automatically the vibrations of the air produced by the voice.

phone [*phōnē*]. A vocal sound.

pho′neme [G. *phōnēma,* sound]. An auditory hallucination of hearing words.

pho·nen′do·scope [G. *phōnē,* voice; *endon,* within; *skopein,* to examine]. A variety of stethoscope which intensifies the auscultatory sounds by the use of two diaphragms. *Obs.*

pho·net′ic [G. *phonētikos,* vocal]. 1. Pertaining to sounds. 2. Pertaining to the voice.

pho·net′ics [*phōnētikos*]. The science dealing with the mode of production of sounds.

pho″ni·at′rics, pho·ni′a·try (fo·nigh′uh·tree, fo″-nee·at′ree) [G. *phōnē,* voice; *iatros,* physician]. The study and treatment of the voice.

phon′ic. See *phonal.*

pho′ni·ca [*phōnē*]. Diseases affecting the vocal organs. *Obs.*

phon′ics. The science of teaching pronunciation and oral reading by the sounds for which the letters stand: distinguished from *phonetics.*

pho′nism [*phōnē*]. A sensation, of sound or hearing, due to the effect of sight, touch, taste, or smell, or even to the thought of some object, person, or general conception.

pho′no-, phon- [*phōnē*]. A combining form meaning *sound* or *voice.*

pho″no·car′di·o·gram″ [*phōnē;* G. *kardia,* heart; *gramma,* letter]. A graphic record of heart sounds.

pho″no·car′di·o·graph″ [*phōnē; kardia;* G. *graphein,* to write]. An instrument for registering the sounds of the heart. —**phonocardiograph′ic,** *adj.*

pho″no·car″di·og′ra·phy [*phōnē; kardia; graphein*]. The graphic recording of heart sounds and murmurs by electric reproduction, using microphone, amplifier, and galvanometer, or by transmission of the vibrations to a delicate membrane, the oscillations of which are optically recorded, as in the Wiggers and Dean method. Syn., *stethography.*

pho″no·chor′da (fo″no·kor′duh) [*phōnē;* G. *chordē,* string]. A vocal fold. *Obs.*

pho′no·gram [*phōnē;* G. *gramma,* letter]. A written record of a sound.

pho′no·graph [*phōnē;* G. *graphein,* to write]. An instrument for recording and reproducing vocal and other sounds.

pho·nol′o·gy [*phōnē;* G. *logos,* word]. The science and study of vocal sound. Phonetics.

pho″no·ma′ni·a [G. *phonos,* slaughter; *mania,* madness]. Homicidal mania.

pho″no·mas·sage′ [G. *phōnē,* sound; F. *massage,* massage]. Stimulation and exercise of tympanic membrane and ossicular chain, by alternating pressure and suction in the external auditory meatus.

pho·nom′e·ter [*phōnē;* G. *metron,* a measure]. An instrument for measuring the pitch and intensity of vocal sounds. —**phonometry,** *n.*

pho″no·my·oc′lo·nus (fo″no·migh·ock′lo·nus, ·migh″o·klo′nus) [*phōnē;* G. *mys,* muscle; *klonos,* turmoil]. A condition in which a sound is heard on auscultation over a muscle, denoting fibrillary contractions, which may be so fine as to be invisible.

pho″no·my·og′ra·phy (·migh·og′ruh·fee) [*phōnē; mys;* G. *graphein,* to write]. Recording of sounds made by the contraction of a muscle.

pho·nop′a·thy [*phōnē;* G. *pathos,* disease]. Any disorder or disease of the voice. *Rare.*

pho″no·pho′bi·a [*phōnē;* G. *phobos,* fear]. 1. A fear of speaking; fear of one's own voice. 2. Morbid dread of any sound or noise.

pho″no·pho·tog′ra·phy [*phōnē;* G. *phōs,* light; *graphein,* to write]. Photography of sound waves produced in phonation.

pho·nop′si·a [*phōnē;* G. *opsis,* vision]. The perception of color sensations by auditory sensations.

phor′bin. The metal-free ring system characteristic of chlorophylls, composed of four pyrrole rings on one of which is fused a cyclopentane ring. It closely resembles the porphyrin ring system of heme.

-pho′ri·a [G. *phorein,* to bear]. *In ophthalmology,* a combining form meaning *bearing;* used to denote *turning of the visual axis,* as in exophoria.

Phor′mi·a. A genus of blowflies.

P. regina. This species normally deposits its eggs or larvae in the decaying flesh of dead animals, but may be a secondary invader of neglected wounds and sores. The maggots may attack living tissue when dead tissue is not available.

phor′o·blast [G. *phoros,* bearing; *blastos,* germ]. Fibroblast. *Obs.*

phor′o·cyte [*phoros;* G. *kytos,* cell]. A connective-tissue cell. *Obs.*

pho·rol′o·gy [*phoros;* G. *logos,* word]. The science pertaining to disease carriers. *Obs.*

pho·rom′e·ter [*phoros;* G. *metron,* a measure]. An instrument for measuring the relative strength of the ocular muscles.

phor″o-op·tom′e·ter. An apparatus for optical testing of muscular defects.

phor·op′ter [*phoros;* G. *optēr,* one who looks]. A sight-testing device containing 36 lenses; by manipulating the dials, over 61 billion combinations are possible. It adds automatically and rapidly the magnifications of its combinations, thus obviating the tedious shifting of refracting lenses into trial frames by hand.

phor′o·scope [*phoros;* G. *skopein,* to examine]. An apparatus for testing vision, consisting of a trial frame for lenses, fixed to a bench or table.

phor′o·tone [*phoros;* G. *tonos,* tension]. An apparatus for exercising the eye muscles.

phose (fohz) [G. *phōs,* light]. The subjective sensation of light or color, as scotoma scintillans of migraine. Also see *aphose, centraphose, centrophose, chromophose, cyanophose, erythrophose, peripheraphose, peripherophose.*

phos′gene. $COCl_2$. Carbonyl chloride; a colorless gas used in chemical warfare and in chemical syntheses.

phos·gen′ic. See *photogenic.*

phos′pha·gen. Phosphocreatine.

phosphaljel. Trade-mark for an aluminum phosphate gel containing 4% of aluminum phosphate. The product has antacid and astringent properties analogous to those of aluminum hydroxide gel, but does not interfere with phosphate absorption. Used in the treatment of peptic ulcer.

phos′pha·tase (fos′fuh·tace, ·taze). A type of enzyme that catalyzes the hydrolysis of esters of phosphoric acid. Numerous phosphatases are known to exist, and they play an important role in carbohydrate metabolism, in nucleotide metabolism, in phospholipid metabolism, and in bone formation. See Table of Normal Values of Blood Constituents in the Appendix.

phos′phate. A salt of phosphoric acid.

acid p. One in which only one or two of the hydrogen atoms of phosphoric acid have been replaced by metals.

normal p. One in which the three hydrogen atoms of phosphoric acid are substituted by metals.

p. cycle. A cycle of continuous phosphorylation and dephosphorylation reactions which provides for conversion of energy derived from certain metabolic processes to useful cellular work.

phos″pha·te′mi·a [G. *phōsphoros,* light-bringer; *haima,* blood]. The presence of phosphates in the circulating blood; especially, hyperphosphatemia.

phos′pha·tide. See *phospholipid.*

phos″pha·tid′ic ac′id. Any ester of glycerin in which two of its alcohol groups are esterified with long-chain fatty acids, and the other alcohol group is esterified with phosphoric acid, with two acidic groups of the phosphoric acid being unsubstituted. Salts of phosphatidic acids have been isolated from plant tissues and beef heart.

phos″pha·tu′ri·a [*phōsphoros;* G. *ouron,* urine]. A condition in which an excess of phosphates is passed in the urine; more properly called *hyperphosphaturia.*

phos′phene [G. *phōs,* light; *phainein,* to show]. A subjective, luminous sensation caused by pressure upon the eyeball. Also called *pressure p.*

p. of accommodation. A phosphene produced by the effort of accommodation.

phos′phide. A compound containing phosphorus in its lowest valence state (−3).

phos′phine (fos′feen, ·fin). 1. Hydrogen phosphide, PH_3, a poisonous gas of alliaceous odor. 2. A substitution compound of PH_3, bearing the same relation to it that an amine does to ammonia.

phos′phite. A salt of phosphorous acid.

phos′pho-, phosph- [G. *phōsphoros,* light bringer]. A combining form denoting *phosphorous* or *phosphoric.*

phos″pho·a·mi″no·lip′id (fos″fo·a·mee″no·lip′id, ·lye′pid, fos″fo·am″i·no·). A compound lipid that contains phosphorus and an amino group.

phos″pho·ar′gi·nine (fos″fo·ahr′ji·neen, ·nin). Arginine phosphate. A phosphoric acid derivative of arginine which contains an energy-rich phosphate bond. Phosphoarginine is believed to play a role in invertebrate muscle metabolism similar to that of phosphocreatine in the muscle of vertebrates.

phos″pho·cre′a·tine (fos″fo·kree′uh·teen, ·tin). $C_4H_{10}O_5N_3P$. Phosphagen. Creatine phosphate. Creatinephosphoric acid. A phosphoric acid derivative of creatine which contains an energy-rich phosphate bond. Phosphocreatine is present in muscle and other tissues, and during the anaerobic phase of muscular contraction it breaks down to yield creatine and phosphate and makes energy available for the contractile process.

phos″pho·di·es′ter·ase. An enzyme catalyzing hydrolysis of one ester linkage in phosphoric acid esters containing two ester linkages.

phos″pho·e·nol″py·ru′vic ac′id. 2-Phosphoenolpyruvic acid; $CH_2{:}CO \sim P(O)(OH)_2.COOH$; a high-energy phosphate formed by dehydration of 2-phosphoglyceric acid; it reacts with adenosinediphosphate to form adenosinetriphosphate and enolpyruvic acid.

phos″pho·fruc″to·mu′tase. The enzyme which catalyzes the conversion of fructose-1-phosphate to fructose-6-phosphate.

phos″pho·ga·lac″to·i·so′mer·ase. An enzyme which catalyzes conversion of galactose-1-phosphate to glucose-1-phosphate.

phos″pho·glu″co·mu′tase. The enzyme which catalyzes the conversion of glucose-1-phosphate to glucose-6-phosphate.

phos″pho·glu·con′ic ac′id. $COOH(CHOH)_4CH_2$-OPO_3H_2; 6-phospho-D-gluconic acid, a product of the oxidation of glucose-6-phosphate by triphosphopyridine nucleotide in the presence of glucose-6-phosphate dehydrogenase.

phos″pho·glyc″er·al′de·hyde. $CHO.CHOH.CH_2$-OPO_3H_2. An intermediate product in carbohydrate metabolism; it may give rise to glycerin utilized in fat synthesis.

2-phos″pho·gly·cer′ic ac′id. $COOH.HCOPO_3H_2$.-CH_2OH; an intermediate compound in carbohydrate metabolism, specifically between 3-phosphoglyceric acid and phosphoenolpyruvic acid.

3-phos″pho·gly·cer′ic ac′id. $COOH.HCOH.CH_2$-OPO_3H_2; an intermediate product in carbohydrate metabolism, specifically between 1,3-diphosphoglyceric acid and 2-phosphoglyceric acid.

phos″pho·glyc″er·o·mu′tase. An enzyme which catalyzes conversion of 3-phosphoglyceric acid to 2-phosphoglyceric acid.

phos″pho·gly″co·pro′te·in. See *nucleoprotein, nucleoalbumin.*

phos″pho·hex″o·i·som′er·ase (·eye·som′ur·ace). The enzyme which catalyzes the conversion of glucose-6-phosphate to fructose-6-phosphate.

phos″pho·hex″o·ki′nase. The enzyme which catalyzes the formation of fructose-1,6-diphosphate through transfer of phosphate from adenosinetriphosphate to fructose-6-phosphate.

phos″pho·lip′id (fos″fo·lip′id, ·lye′pid). A type of lipid compound which is an ester of phosphoric acid and contains, in addition, one or two molecules of fatty acid, an alcohol, and a nitrogenous base. They are widely distributed in nature and include such substances as lecithin, cephalin, and sphingomyelin. See Table of Normal Values of Blood Constituents in the Appendix. Syn., *phosphatide, phospholipin.*

phos″pho·lip′in. See *phospholipid.*

phos″pho·mo·lyb′dic ac′id. $H_3PO_4.12MoO_3$.-$12H_2O$. A yellow solid used as a reagent.

phos″pho·mon″o·es′ter·ase (fos″fo·mon″o·ess′-tur·ace, ·aze, fos″fo·mo″no·). An enzyme catalyzing hydrolysis of phosphoric acid esters containing one ester linkage.

phos″pho·ne·cro′sis, phos″phor·ne·cro′sis. See phosphorus *necrosis.*

phos·pho′ni·um. The hypothetical univalent radical PH_4; it is analogous to ammonium, NH_4.

phos″pho·nu′cle·ase (fos″fo·new′klee·ace, ·aze). An enzyme which splits nucleotides into nucleosides and phosphoric acid. Also called *nucleotidase.*

phos″pho·pro′te·in. A conjugated protein consisting of a compound of protein with a phosphorus-containing substance other than nucleic acid or lecithin. See American Classification of Proteins in the Appendix.

phos″pho·pyr′i·dine nu′cle·o·tides (fos″fo·pirr′-i·deen, ·din). Complex compounds containing nicotinic acid amide, a pentose, adenine, and phosphoric acid.

diphosphopyridine nucleotide. Coenzyme I; cozymase.

triphosphopyridine nucleotide. Coenzyme II.

phos″pho·py·ru′vic ac′id. $CH_2{:}CO(PO_3H_2)$-$COOH$. An intermediate substance obtained in the breakdown of glycogen to lactic acid and the resynthesis of glycogen from lactic acid.

phos′phor. A substance which phosphoresces.

phos′pho·ra″ted [G. *phōsphoros*, light bringer]. Containing phosphorus, as phosphorated oil, a 1% solution of phosphorus in expressed almond oil.

phos″pho·res′cence [*phōsphoros*]. 1. The continuous emission of light from a substance without any apparent rise in temperature, produced after exposure to heat, light, or electric discharges. 2. The faint green glow of white phosphorus exposed to air, due to its slow oxidation. 3. *In radiology*, the emission of radiation by a substance as a result of previous absorption of radiation of shorter wavelength. —**phosphores′cent,** *adj.;* **phosphoresce,** *v.i.*

phos″phor·hi·dro′sis (fos″for·hi·dro′sis, ·high-dro′sis), **phos″phor·i·dro′sis** [*phōsphoros;* G. *hidrōsis*, sweating]. The secretion of phosphorescent sweat; a very rare condition.

phos″pho·ri″bo·mu′tase. An enzyme which catalyzes interconversion of ribose-5-phosphate and ribose-1-phosphate.

phos·phor′ic ac′id (*acidum phosphoricum*). H_3PO_4. Orthophosphoric acid; occurs as a colorless, odorless liquid of a syrupy consistence and contains 85% of H_3PO_4; miscible with water and alcohol.

diluted p. a. (*acidum phosphoricum dilutum*). An aqueous solution containing 10 Gm. of H_3PO_4 per 100 cc.

phos′pho·rism [*phōsphoros*]. Chronic phosphorus poisoning.

phos″phor·ne·cro′sis. See phosphorus *necrosis.*

phos″phor·ol′y·sis. A chemical reaction by which the elements of phosphoric acid are incorporated into the molecule of a compound.

phos·pho′rous ac′id (fos·for′us, fos′for·us). H_3PO_3. A yellow, crystalline acid used as a reducing agent and as a reagent.

phos′pho·rus [*phōsphoros*] (*phosphorus*). P = 30.975. A nonmetallic element occurring in two allotropic forms, white or yellow phosphorus and amorphous or red phosphorus. The red form occurs as a reddish-brown powder having a specific gravity of 2.19; it is nonpoisonous and is not inflammable in air; insoluble in the solvents in which the yellow form is soluble. The yellow form when recently made is an almost colorless or yellowish, semitransparent mass having a specific gravity of 1.82; with age it becomes darker and waxy in appearance; has a disagreeable odor, and when exposed to air emits poisonous fumes which have an odor resembling garlic; on longer exposure it may ignite spontaneously; 1 Gm. is soluble in about 400 cc. of dehydrated alcohol, in about 40 cc. of chloroform, in about 102 cc. of dehydrated ether, in about 31.5 cc. of benzene, or in about 0.9 cc. of carbon disulfide; practically insoluble in water. The yellow form should be kept under water and should not be handled with bare hands as it may cause burns when in contact with the skin. Little is known of the effects of elemental phosphorus when administered in therapeutic dose. See Table of Normal Values of Blood Constituents in the Appendix.

p. pentachloride. PCl_5; white to pale-yellow, fuming, deliquescent, crystalline masses, soluble in water with decomposition and release of considerable heat: used as a catalyst.

p. pentoxide. P_2O_5; a white, amorphous, bulky powder, rapidly absorbing moisture from air, slowly soluble in water with evolution of heat: used as a dehydrating agent.

p. trioxide. P_2O_3; colorless crystals, soluble in water, ether, or carbon disulfide.

phos′pho·ryl. The trivalent radical PO.

phos·phor′yl·ase. An enzyme widely distributed in animals, plants, and microorganisms. It is specific for the formation of glucose-1-phosphate (Cori ester) from glycogen and inorganic phosphate.

phos″pho·ryl·a′tion. The term used for the esterification of compounds with phosphoric acid.

phos″pho·ryl·cho′line (fos″fo·ril·ko′leen, ·lin, ·kol′een, ·in). An ester of choline and phosphoric acid which constitutes a portion of the lecithin molecule.

phos″pho·ser′ine. $(HO)_2OPO.CH_2.CH(NH_2)$-COOH; a phosphoric acid ester of serine; the chief, possibly the only, phosphate containing component of phosphoproteins.

phos″pho·trans·a·cet′y·lase. The enzyme which catalyzes the reversible transfer of an acetyl group from acetyl coenzyme A to a phosphate, with formation of acetyl phosphate.

phos″pho·tri′ose i·som′er·ase. Triose isomerase, an enzyme in the Embden-Meyerhof scheme, catalyzing the interconversion of 3-phosphoglyceraldehyde and phosphodihydroxyacetone.

phos″pho·tung′stic ac′id. Approximately P_2O_5.-$24WO_3.25H_2O$. A white or yellowish-green crystalline acid used as a reagent.

phos′sy jaw. Phosphorous necrosis of the jaw.

phos·vi′tin. A phosphoprotein isolated from the vitellin fraction of egg yolk.

pho·tal′gi·a [G. *phōs*, light; *algos*, pain]. Pain arising from too great intensity of light.

pho·tau″gi·o·pho′bi·a (fo·taw″jee·o·fo′bee·uh) [*phōs;* G. *augein*, to glitter; *phobos*, fear]. A shrinking from the glare of light.

phote [*phōs*]. A unit of intensity of illumination.

pho′tech″y (fo′teck″ee) [*phōs;* G. *echein*, to have]. Radioactive power exhibited by a substance which has been exposed to radiation.

photelometer. A trade-marked device combining a point source of light, a photoelectric cell, and spectral filters for the rapid and fairly accurate quantitation of unknown substances.

pho″tes·the′si·a, pho″taes·the′si·a (fo″tess-thee′zhuh, ·zee·uh) [*phōs;* G. *aisthēsis*, sensation]. 1. Sensitiveness to light. 2. Photophobia.

pho′tic [*phōs*]. Relating to light.

pho′tism [G. *phōtismos*, illumination]. A visual sensation, as of color or light, produced by hearing, taste, smell, touch, or temperature, or even by the thought of some object, person, or general conception. Also see *phonism*.

pho′to- [G. *phōs*, light]. A combining form meaning *light*.

pho″to·ac·tin′ic [*phōs;* G. *aktis*, ray]. Emitting both luminous and actinic rays.

pho″to·bac·te′ri·um [*phōs;* G. *baktērion*, small staff]. A bacterial organism which is light-producing or phosphorescent.

pho″to·bi·ot′ic (fo″to·buy·ot′ick) [*phōs;* G. *biōtikos*, of life]. Living in the light exclusively.

pho″to·ca·tal′y·sis. Catalysis of a chemical reaction effected by exposure to light, either in the visible or ultraviolet region.

pho″to·chem′i·cal [*phōs;* G. *chymos*, juice]. Pertaining to chemical action produced directly or indirectly by means of radiation.

pho″to·chem′is·try [*phōs; chymos*]. The study of chemical reactions produced directly or indirectly by means of radiation.

pho′to·chrome [*phōs;* G. *chrōma*, color]. Pertaining to colored light.

pho″to·col″or·im′e·ter [*phōs;* L. *color*, color; G. *metron*, a measure]. A colorimeter consisting of one or more photoelectric cells as indicators and various colored filters for examining certain parts of the spectrum.

pho″to·con″duc·tiv′i·ty. The increase in electrical conductivity of a substance when illuminated.

pho″to·con·junc″ti·vi′tis. See actinic *conjunctivitis*.

pho″to·der″ma·to′sis. A dermatitis of exposed skin caused by the sun's rays or artificial rays; most often caused by ultraviolet rays.

pho″to·dis·in″te·gra′tion. Nuclear disintegration initiated by an incoming high-energy photon.

pho·tod′ro·my (fo·tod′ro·mee) [*phōs;* G. *dromos*, course]. The movement of particles suspended in a fluid toward the light (positive) or away from it (negative).

pho″to·dy·nam′ic (fo″to·dye·nam′ick, ·di·nam′-ick) [*phōs;* G. *dynamis*, power]. Pertaining to the energy of light.

pho″to·dyn′i·a [*phōs;* G. *odynē*, pain]. Pain arising from too great intensity of light; extreme photophobia.

pho″to·dys·pho′ri·a [*phōs;* G. *dysphoria*, discomfort]. Intolerance of light; photophobia.

pho″to·e·lec′tric col″or·im′e·ter. A colorimeter for determining the concentration of the colored component of a solution, consisting of one or more combinations of calibrated filters and photoelectric cells for measurement of the color.

pho″to·e·lec″tric′i·ty [*phōs; ēlektron*]. Electricity produced under the influence of light or other radiations, such as ultraviolet and x-rays. When irradiated by such radiations, certain metals give off photoelectrons. —**photoelec′tric,** *adj.*

pho″to·e·lec′tron [*phōs; ēlektron*]. An electron set into swift motion by the impact of a photon, and to which the primary photon transmits all of its energy.

pho″to·flu″or·os′co·py [*phōs;* L. *fluere*, to flow; G. *skopein*, to examine]. Fluoroscopy permitting recording of fluoroscopic images on photographic film. Also called *fluororoentgenography, photofluorography*.

pho′to·gene [*phōs;* G. *genesthai*, from *gignesthai*, to be produced]. 1. A retinal impression; an afterimage. 2. A liquid derived from bituminous shale.

pho″to·gen′e·sis [*phōs;* G. *genesis*, production]. The production of light or of phosphorescence.

pho″to·gen′ic, pho·tog′e·nous [*phos;* G. *genesthai*, from *gignesthai*, to be produced]. Producing light.

pho′to·gram [*phōs;* G. *gramma*, letter]. A photographic record, as an enlargement obtained by the microscope. Preferably called *photomicrograph*.

pho″to·ki·net′ic (fo″to·ki·net′ick, ·kigh·net′ick)

[*phōs;* G. *kinētikos,* of motion]. Causing movement by means of the energy of light.

pho″to·ky′mo·graph [*phōs;* G. *kyma,* wave; *graphein,* to write]. An instrument for the optical recording of physiologic cycles or actions; a photographic camera having a cylindrical lens, moving photographic paper, and a device for the recording of time intervals simultaneously with the physiologic phenomena.

pho·tol′y·sis [*phōs;* G. *lysis,* a loosing]. Decomposition by the action of light.

pho′to·lyte [*phōs; lysis*]. A substance that is decomposed by the action of light.

pho″to·mag′net·ism [*phōs;* G. *Magnētis lithos,* magnet]. Magnetism produced in certain substances by the action of light.

pho″to·ma′ni·a [*phōs;* G. *mania,* madness]. 1. The increase of maniacal symptoms under the influence of light. 2. A morbid desire for light.

pho″to·mes′on. A meson ejected from a nucleus by an impinging photon.

pho·tom′e·ter [*phōs;* G. *metron,* a measure]. 1. An instrument for measuring the intensity of light. 2. An instrument for testing the sensitiveness of the eye to light, by determining the minimum illumination in which the object is visible.

flame p. One used especially for the quantitative determination of sodium and potassium in biological fluids. A sample when sprayed into a flame emits light which is resolved into its spectrum; a photoelectric cell measures the intensity of light of the wavelength corresponding to the particular element under analysis.

pho·tom′e·try [*phōs; metron*]. The measurement of the intensity of light.

flame p. The measurement of the intensity of the emission spectra of any element which is introduced into a gas flame as an atomized solution.

internal standard flame p. Flame photometry in which the intensity of the unknown element is simultaneously compared with a fixed or known concentration of another element, usually lithium.

pho″to·mi′cro·graph [*phōs;* G. *mikros,* small; *graphein,* to write]. A photograph of a minute or microscopic object, usually made with the aid of a microscope, and of sufficient size for observation with the naked eye. —**photomicrog′raphy,** *n.*

pho″to·mo′tor [*phōs;* L. *motor,* from *movere,* to move]. Pertaining to a muscular response to light stimuli, as the constriction of the pupil.

pho′ton [*phōs*]. A quantum of energy of visible light or any other electromagnetic radiation.

pho″to·neu′tron. A neutron released from a nucleus in a photonuclear reaction.

pho·ton′o·sus [*phōs;* G. *nosos,* disease]. A diseased condition arising from continued exposure to intense or glaring light, as snowblindness.

pho″to·nu′cle·ar re·ac′tion. See under *reaction.*

pho″to·par″es·the′si·a (·par″ess·thee′zhuh, ·zee·uh) [*phōs;* G. *para,* beyond; *aisthēsis,* perception]. Defective, or perverted, retinal sensibility.

pho″to·path″o·log′ic [*phōs;* G. *pathos,* disease; *logos,* word]. Pertaining to an abnormality related to light.

pho·top′a·thy. See *photonosus.*

pho″to·per·cep′tive [*phōs;* L. *perceptio,* from *percipere,* to perceive]. Capable of receiving and perceiving rays of light.

pho″to·phil′ic [*phōs;* G. *philein,* to love]. Seeking or loving light.

pho″to·pho′bi·a [*phōs;* G. *phobos,* fear]. Intolerance or morbid fear of light. See *phengophobia.* —**photophobic,** *adj.*

pho′to·phone [*phōs;* G. *phōnē,* sound]. An apparatus for the graphic recording of sound by means of light waves.

pho′to·phore [*phōs;* G. *phoros,* bearing]. An electric light for endoscopes.

pho″toph·thal′mi·a [*phōs;* G. *ophthalmia,* ophthalmia]. Inflammation of the eyes due to excessively strong light, as a welder's arc light or sunlight on snow.

industrial p. That resulting from occupations using insufficiently screened sources of light rich in the shorter wavelengths: also called *flash-eye.*

solar p. See *snowblindness.*

pho″to·po·lym″er·i·za′tion. The polymerization of a substance when exposed to light.

pho″to·pro′ton. A proton released from a nucleus in a photonuclear reaction.

pho·top′si·a [*phōs;* G. *opsis,* vision]. Subjective sensations of sparks or flashes of light occurring in certain pathologic conditions of the optic nerve, the retina, or the brain. —**photoptic,** *adj.*

pho·top′sin. The protein moiety of iodopsin.

pho″top·tom′e·ter [*phōs;* G. *optikos,* of sight; *metron,* a measure]. An instrument for determining visual acuity.

pho″top·tom′e·try [*phōs; optikos; metron*]. The measurement of the perception of light.

pho″to·ra″di·om′e·ter [*phōs;* L. *radius,* ray; *metron*]. An instrument for the measurement of the quantity of x-rays passing through a given surface. *Obs.*

pho″to·re·cep′tive [*phōs;* L. *receptum,* from *recipere,* to receive]. Capable of receiving and perceiving rays of light.

pho″to·ret″i·ni′tis. See sun *blindness.*

pho″to·roent″gen·og′ra·phy (fo″to·rent″ghin·og′ruh·fee). See *fluorography.*

pho·tos′co·py. See *skiascopy.*

pho″to·sen″si·tiv′i·ty [*phōs;* L. *sentire,* to feel]. 1. The capacity of an organ or organism to be stimulated to activity by light. 2. The absorption of a certain portion of the spectrum by a chemical system. —**photosen′sitive,** *adj.*

pho″to·sen″si·ti·za′tion [*phōs; sentire*]. Abnormal condition of the skin, making it hyperreactive to exposure to ultraviolet radiation or natural sunlight. It may be produced by the ingestion of fluorescent dyes, endocrine products, or heavy metals.

pho″to·shock′. A type of shock treatment in psychotherapy in which an intermittently flashing light is used after administration of a sensitizing drug.

pho″to·syn′the·sis [*phōs;* G. *synthesis,* a putting together]. The process by which simple carbohydrates are synthesized from carbon dioxide and water by the chloroplasts of living plant cells in the presence of light.

pho″to·tax′is [*phōs;* G. *taxis,* arrangement]. Response to a stimulus of light.

pho″to·ther′a·py [*phōs;* G. *therapeia,* treatment]. Treatment with light rays, including the invisible infrared and ultraviolet radiations.

pho′to·ti″mer [*phōs;* AS. *tima*]. A clocklike device used to provide a proper interval of time for photographic plate or film exposures.

pho·tot′o·nus [*phōs;* G. *tonos,* tension]. State of sensitiveness to light. —**phototon′ic,** *adj.*

pho″to·to′pi·a [*phōs;* G. *ōps,* eye]. A subjective sensation of light.

pho″to·troph′. An autotrophic bacterium able to utilize light energy for metabolism: also called *photosynthetic autotroph.* —**phototroph′ic,** *adj.*

pho·tot′ro·pism [*phōs;* G. *trepein,* to turn]. The tendency shown by most plants to turn or bend toward the greater light.

pho′to·tube [*phōs;* L. *tubus,* tube]. A radio tube which furnishes a current of about 2×10^{-8} amp. which, through a resistance of 1 megohm, provides an input to the amplifier of 2×10^{-2} volts in the operation of a photoelectric plethysmograph.

pho·tu′ri·a [*phōs;* G. *ouron,* urine]. The passage of phosphorescent urine.

phrag′mo·plast [G. *phragmos,* an enclosure; *plassein,* to form]. The spindle during cytokinesis in plant cells possessing rigid cell membranes.

phre·nal′gi·a [G. *phrēn,* midriff, heart, mind; *algos,* pain]. Melancholia. *Obs.*

phren″as·the′ni·a [*phrēn;* G. *astheneia,* weakness]. Mental defect; feeblemindedness. —**phrenasthen′ic,** *adj., n.*

phren″a·tro′phi·a [*phrēn;* G. *atrophia,* want of food]. Atrophy of the brain; idiocy. *Obs.*

phren″em·phrax′is [*phrēn;* G. *emphraxis,* stoppage]. Crushing of a phrenic nerve with a hemostat to produce temporary paralysis of the diaphragm: a form of collapse therapy used in the treatment of pulmonary tuberculosis.

phre·ne′si·a (fri·nee′zhuh, ·zee·uh) [*phrēn*]. Encephalitis. *Obs.* —**phrenesiac** (fri·nee′zee·ack), *n.*

phre·ne′sis [*phrēn*]. Frenzy; delirium; insanity. *Obs.* —**phrenet′ic,** *adj.*

-phre′ni·a [*phrēn*]. A combining form denoting *mental disorder.*

phren′ic [*phrēn*]. 1. Pertaining to the diaphragm. 2. Pertaining to the mind. See also Table of Arteries and Table of Nerves in the Appendix.

phren″i·cec′to·my (fren″i·seck′to·mee) [*phrēn;* G. *ektomē,* excision]. Resection of a section of a phrenic nerve or removal of an entire phrenic nerve.

phren″i·co·col′ic. See *phrenocolic.*

phren″i·co·ex·er′e·sis [*phrēn;* G. *exairesis,* removal]. Avulsion of a phrenic nerve.

phren″i·co·gas′tric. See *phrenogastric.*

phren″i·co·splen′ic (fren″i·ko·splen′ick, ·splee′nick). See *phrenosplenic.*

phren″i·cot′o·my [*phrēn;* G. *tomē,* a cutting]. Surgical division of a phrenic nerve in the neck for the purpose of causing a one-sided paralysis of the diaphragm, with consequent immobilization and compression of a diseased lung.

phren″i·co·trip′sy [*phrēn;* G. *tripsis,* a rubbing]. Crushing of a phrenic nerve.

phre·ni′tis [*phrēn;* G. *-itis,* inflammation]. 1. Inflammation of the brain. 2. Inflammation of the diaphragm. 3. Acute delirium. —**phren′ic, phrenit′ic,** *adj.*

phren′o-, phren- [*phrēn*]. A combining form denoting *relation to the diaphragm.*

phren″o·bla′bi·a [*phrēn;* G. *blabē,* harm]. Any disorder of the mind. *Obs.*

phren″o·car′di·a [*phrēn;* G. *kardia,* heart]. A neurasthenic condition associated with dyspnea and pain in the region of the heart. A symptom-complex in anxiety neurosis.

phren″o·col′ic [*phrēn;* G. *kolon,* colon]. Pertaining to the diaphragm and the colon.

phren″o·gas′tric [*phrēn;* G. *gastēr,* belly]. Pertaining conjointly to the stomach and the diaphragm.

phren″o·glot′tic [*phrēn;* G. *glōttis,* glottis]. Pertaining to the diaphragm and the glottis.

phren″o·glot·tis′mus [*phrēn; glōttis*]. Spasm of the glottis ascribed to disease of the diaphragm.

phren″o·he·pat′ic [*phrēn;* G. *hēpar,* liver]. Pertaining to the diaphragm and liver.

phren″o·lep′si·a [*phrēn;* G. *lēpsis,* a seizing]. Insanity. *Obs.*

phre·nol′o·gy [*phrēn;* G. *logos,* word]. An old science based on the theory that the various faculties of the mind occupy distinct and separate areas in the brain cortex, and that the predominance of certain faculties can be ascertained from modifications of the parts of the skull overlying the areas where these faculties are located. *Obs.*

phren″o·pa·ral′y·sis. See *phrenoplegia.*

phren′o·path [*phrēn;* G. *pathos,* disease]. An alienist. *Obs.* —**phrenop′athy,** *n.*

phren″o·ple′gi·a [*phrēn;* G. *plēgē,* stroke]. Paralysis of the diaphragm.

phren′o·sin. A complex lipid obtained chiefly from white matter and containing sphingosine, cerebronic acid, and a sugar, usually galactose: also called *cerebron.*

phren″o·sin′ic ac′id. $C_{24}H_{48}O_3$. Cerebronic acid. A hydroxy fatty acid which is a component of the glycolipid (cerebroside) phrenosin.

phren″o·spasm′. See *cardiospasm.*

phren″o·splen′ic (fren″o·splen′ick, ·splee′nick) [*phrēn;* G. *splēn,* spleen]. Pertaining to the diaphragm and the spleen.

phric″to·path′ic [G. *phriktos,* to be shuddered at; *pathos,* disease]. Pertaining to, or accompanied by, a shuddering sensation.

phron″e·mo·pho′bi·a [G. *phronēma,* thought; *phobos,* fear]. A morbid dread of thinking.

phro·ne′sis [G., practical wisdom]. Soundness of mind, or of judgment.

phryn″o·der′ma (frin″o·dur′muh, fry″no·) [G. *phrynos,* toad; *derma,* skin]. Dryness of the skin with follicular hyperkeratosis; due to vitamin-A deficiency.

phry·nol′y·sin (fri·nol′i·sin, fry″no·lye′sin, frin″o·) [*phrynos;* G. *lysis,* a loosing]. The lysin or toxin of the fire toad, *Bombinator igneus;* it is hemolytic for the blood of various animals.

phthal-. See *phthalo-.*

phthal′ate (thal′ate). Any salt of phthalic acid.

phthal′ic ac′id (thal′ick). $C_6H_4(COOH)_2$. A colorless crystalline acid used in organic syntheses.

phthal′ic an·hy′dride. $C_6H_4(CO)_2O$. The anhydride of phthalic acid. Can act as an allergen.

phthal′i·dyl (thal′i·dil, ·deel). 3-(α-Aminopropyl)-phthalide hydrochloride, a substance having analgesic properties.

phthal′o- (thal′o-), **phthal-** [na*phthal*ene]. *In chemistry,* a combining form for *phthalic.*

phthal″yl·sul″fa·thi′a·zole. $C_{17}H_{13}N_3O_5S_2$; 2-(N^4-phthalylsulfanilamido)thiazole; a white or faintly yellowish-white crystalline powder, practically insoluble in water. It is poorly absorbed from the gastrointestinal tract, by virtue of which a sufficiently high concentration develops in the lumen of the large bowel to suppress growth of bacteria and make the drug useful in treatment of disease and in surgery of the colon. See *sulfathalidine.*

phthei·ri′a·sis (thigh·rye′uh·sis). See *pediculosis.*

phthi′o·col (thigh′o·coal, ·kol, ·kawl). $C_{11}H_8O_3$; 2-hydroxy-3-methyl-1,4-naphthoquinone; an antibiotic substance, isomeric with plumbagin, derived from *Mycobacterium tuberculosis,* active, in vitro, against a number of bacteria, and having some vitamin-K activity.

phthi·o′ic ac′id (thigh·o′ick). A cyclic fatty acid produced by *Mycobacterium tuberculosis.* When applied to the body, it produces a local reaction characterized by the appearance of a cheesy nodule similar to that observed in tuberculosis.

phthi·ri′a·sis (thigh·rye′uh·sis, thi·rye′·) [G. *phtheiriasis,* morbus pedicularis]. Pediculosis pubis; infestation by the pubic louse *Phthirius pubis.*

phthir″i·o·pho′bi·a (thirr″ee·o·fo′bee·uh, thighi″ree·o·) [G. *phtheir,* louse; *phobos,* fear]. Morbd-dread of lice.

Phthir′i·us [*phtheir*]. A genus of true lice.

P. pubis. Species which infests the pubic region of man, and has been implicated in the transmission of louse-borne typhus fever, louse-borne relapsing fever, etc.; the crab louse.

phthis″i·ol′o·gy (tiz″ee·ol′o·jee, thiz″ee·ol′o·jee)

[G. *phthisis*, a wasting away; *logos*, word]. The study or science of tuberculosis. *Obs.*

phthis″i·o·pho′bi·a (tiz″ee·o·fo′bee·uh, thiz″ee·o·) [*phthisis;* G. *phobos*, fear]. Morbid fear of tuberculosis.

phthis″i·o·ther′a·py [*phthisis;* G. *therapeia*, treatment]. The treatment of tuberculosis. *Obs.*

phthi′sis (thigh′sis, tye′sis) [G.]. 1. Old term for tuberculosis, especially pulmonary tuberculosis. 2. Old term for any disease characterized by emaciation and loss of strength, especially diseases of the lungs. —**phthis′ic, phthis′ical,** *adj.*

abdominal p. Old term for tuberculous infection of the intestines, peritoneum, or both. In children, usually involves the mesenteric and retroperitoneal lymph nodes.

fibroid p. Chronic, slowly progressive, pulmonary tuberculosis with extensive fibrosis and mild symptoms.

flax-dresser's p. A fibroid pneumonia resulting from the inhalation of particles of flax.

florid p. Acute pneumonic pulmonary tuberculosis, with rapid progression and fatal termination, usually within one to four months.

miner's p. Fibrosis of the lungs occurring in miners. Also called *miner's asthma.* Also see *silicosis.*

p. bulbi. Shrinking of the eyeball.

p. corneae. Cicatrical shrinking of the cornea.

renal p. Tuberculosis of the kidney.

phy″co·bi′lin. A metal-free pigment, found in algae, in which an open-chain tetrapyrrole group, related to bile pigments, is linked to a globulinlike protein.

phy′co·chrome [G. *phykos*, seaweed; *chrōma*, color]. The complex blue-green pigment that masks the green of the chlorophyll in certain algae.

phy″co·col′loid. A class name for polysaccharides, derived from brown or red seaweeds, which form colloidal dispersions with water.

phy″co·cy′a·nin [*phykos;* G. *kyanos*, blue]. *In biology*, a blue pigment, characteristic of the Cyanophyceae, blue-green algae. Active in photosynthesis.

phy″co·e·ryth′rin. A red, protein-containing pigment found in the chloroplasts of most red algae.

Phy″co·my·ce′tes (figh″ko·migh·see′teez) [*phykos;* G. *mykēs*, fungus]. A class of fungi, with a generally nonseptate mycelium. This group includes the common black bread mold and water mold.

phyg″o·ga·lac′tic [G. *phygein*, to avoid; *gala*, milk]. Stopping the secretion of milk.

phyg″o·ga·lac′tic. An agent that checks the secretion of milk.

phy·lax′is (figh·lack′sis) [G., a watching]. The activity of the body in defending itself against infection.

phy·let′ic (figh·let′ick) [G. *phyletikos*, of a tribe]. Pertaining to a stock or to a race.

phyllicin. Trade-mark for a brand of theophylline calcium salicylate.

phyl″lo·e·ryth′rin. A porphyrin pigment resulting from degradation of chlorophyll, found in the bile of ruminants, in bovine gallstones, and in dog feces: claimed to be identical with cholehematin.

phyl″lo·por′phy·rin. See *porphyrin.*

phyl″lo·qui·none′. Phytonadione.

phy·log′e·ny, phy″lo·gen′e·sis (figh·lodg′i·nee) [G. *phylon*, tribe; *genesis*, production]. The evolution of a group or species of animals or plants from the simplest form; the evolution of the species, as distinguished from ontogenesis, the evolution of the individual. —**phylogenet′ic,** *adj.*

phy′lum (pl. *phyla*) [*phylon*]. A primary division of the animal or vegetable kingdom.

phy′ma [G., growth]. 1. A tumor or new growth of varying size, composed of any of the structures of the skin or subcutaneous tissue. 2. A localized plastic exudate larger than a tubercle; a circumscribed swelling of the skin. —**phymatoid,** *adj.*

phy″ma·tor·rhy′sin (figh″muh·to·rye′sin, ·riss′in, figh″muh·tor′i·sin) [*phyma;* G. *rhysis*, issue]. A pigment found in hair and melanotic new growths.

phy″ma·to′sis [*phyma;* G. *-ōsis*, condition]. Any disease characterized by the formation of phymas or nodules.

Phys″a·lop′te·ra [G. *physallis*, bubble; *pteron*, wing]. A genus of nematode worms of the family Strongylidae.

P. caucasica. The only species infesting man, commonly found in natives of tropical Africa.

phys·co′ni·a [G. *physkōn*, potbelly]. Any abdominal enlargement, especially from tympanites. *Obs.*

physeptone. Trade-mark for *methadone hydrochloride.*

phys″i·an′thro·py [G. *physis*, nature; *anthrōpos*, man]. The study of the constitution of man, his diseases, and their remedies.

phys″i·at′rics [*physis;* G. *iatrikos*, skilled in the medical art]. Physical medicine.

phys″i·at′rist. A physician specializing in physical medicine.

phys′ic [G. *physikos*, of nature]. 1. The science of medicine. 2. A medicine, especially a cathartic.

phys′ic. To administer medicines; to purge.

phys′i·cal [*physikos*]. 1. Pertaining to nature; pertaining to the body or material things. 2. Pertaining to physics.

phys′i·cal in·spec′tion. *In military medicine*, a physical check made by direct observation and, when indicated, a partial examination to ascertain the presence of any acute or chronic communicable disease, vermin infestation, or gross deterioration of physical status.

phys′i·cal med′i·cine. See under *medicine.*

phys′i·cal pro′file se′ri·al. *In military medicine*, an estimate of over-all ability of an individual to perform military duties by consideration of his physical and mental condition. Six factors, designated PULHES, are expressed numerically: *P*hysical capacity or stamina, *U*pper extremities, *L*ower extremities, *H*earing (including ear defects), *E*yes, and neuropsychiatric evaluation.

phys′i·cal re″con·di′tion·ing. 1. A treatment phase aimed at restoring and/or maintaining physical and psychological fitness of hospital patients through progressively graded activities during their hospitalization. 2. *In military medicine*, a section of physical medicine service.

phy·si′cian [G. *physis*, nature]. One who is authorized to practice medicine.

house p. A physician who lives in a hospital and is constantly available, as an intern.

resident p. A physician living in the hospital for further training after an internship. Also called *resident.*

phys′i·cist [G. *physikos*, of nature]. One skilled in physical science.

Physick, Philip Syng [*American surgeon*, 1768–1837]. Introduced the stomach tube in America (1805). Devised an operation for artificial anus (1826). Devised a method of iridectomy in which he removed a circular piece by means of a cutting forceps; called *Physick's operation.* Invented a tonsillotome (1828).

phys″i·co·chem′i·cal (fizz″i·ko·kem′i·kul) [G. *physikos*, of nature; *chymos*, juice]. Pertaining to the borderland area where physics and chemistry overlap.

phys″i·co·gen′ic [*physikos;* G. *genesthai*, from *gignesthai*, to be produced]. Produced by physical causes.

phys″i·co·py·rex′i·a (fizz″i·ko·pye·reck′see·uh) [*physikos;* G. *pyressein,* to be feverish]. Artificial fever produced by physical means for its therapeutic effect.

phys′ics [*physikos*]. The science of the phenomena and laws of nature, especially that treating of the properties of matter and of the forces governing it.

health p. The study of various methods of protecting personnel from ionizing radiation.

nuclear p. The branch of physics dealing with the structure and behavior of atomic nuclei.

phys″i·no′sis (fizz″i·no′sis) [G. *physis,* nature; *nosos,* disease]. Any disease due to physical agents. *Obs.*

phys″i·og′no·my (fizz″ee·og′no·mee) [G. *physiognōmonia,* physiognomy]. 1. The countenance. 2. The science of determining character by a study of the face.

phys″i·og·no′sis (fizz″ee·og·no′sis) [G. *physis,* nature; *gnōsis,* knowledge]. Determination of disease through facial characteristics and expression. *Obs.*

phys″i·o·log′ic (fizz″ee·o·lodj′ick), **phys″i·o·log′i·cal** [G. *physiologikos,* of inquiry into nature]. 1. Pertaining to physiology. 2. Pertaining to natural or normal processes, as opposed to those that are pathologic.

phys″i·o·log″i·co·an″a·tom′ic (fizz″ee·o·lodj″i-ko·an″uh·tom′ick) [*physiologikos;* G. *anatomikos,* relating to anatomy]. Pertaining to physiology and anatomy.

phys″i·ol′o·gist [G. *physiologos,* one who inquires into natural phenomena]. One versed in physiology.

phys″i·ol′o·gy (fizz″ee·ol′o·jee) [*physiologos*]. The science that treats of the functions of living organisms or their parts, as distinguished from morphology, etc.

animal p. The physiology of animals.

antenatal p. That which concerns the fetus in utero.

applied p. Physiologic knowledge used in interpretation of problems arising in medical practice, public health, or industry.

aviation p. The study of physiologic problems in flying.

cellular p. The physiology of cells.

comparative p. The comparative study of the physiology of different animals and plants.

experimental p. Experiments carried on in a physiologic laboratory with experimental animals or man.

pathologic p. The study of disordered functions or of functions modified by disease.

plant p. The physiology of plants.

special p. The physiology of special organs.

phys″i·o·med′i·cal·ism [G. *physis,* nature; L. *medicus,* medical]. The professed use of natural remedies only, poisons and minerals being rejected. *Obs.*

phys″i·o·pa·thol′o·gy. See physiologic *pathology.*

phys″i·o·ther′a·py. See physical *medicine.*

phy·sique′ [F.]. Physical structure or organization; body build.

phy″so·hem″a·to·me′tra (figh″so·hem″uh·to-mee′truh, ·hee″muh·to·mee′truh) [G. *physa,* breath; *haima,* blood; *mētra,* uterus]. An accumulation of gas, or air, and blood in the uterus, as in decomposition of retained menses, or placental tissue.

phy″so·hy″dro·me′tra [*physa;* G. *hydōr,* water; *mētra*]. An accumulation of gas and fluid in the uterus.

phy″so·me′tra [*physa; mētra*]. A distention of the uterus with gas.

phy″so·py″o·sal′pinx [*physa;* G. *pyon,* pus; *salpigx,* trumpet]. Pyosalpinx with formation of gas in the uterine tube.

phy″so·stig′ma [*physa;* G. *stigma,* mark]. The dried ripe seed of *Physostigma venenosum,* the calabar bean. Of several alkaloids reported present, physostigmine (eserine) is the most important.

phy″so·stig′mine (figh″so·stig′meen, ·min). $C_{15}H_{21}O_2N_3$. An alkaloid obtained from the seeds of *Physostigma venenosum;* slightly soluble in water, soluble in the organic solvents; occurs as white crystals, becoming red on exposure to air and light. Extremely poisonous. Syn., *eserine.*

p. salicylate (*physostigminae salicylas*). $C_{15}H_{21}O_2N_3.HC_7H_5O_3$. The salicylate of an alkaloid usually obtained from the dried ripe seed of *Physostigma venenosum;* white or slightly yellow, odorless crystals, becoming red on long exposure to light and air; 1 Gm. dissolves in 75 cc. of water and 16 cc. of alcohol. Used as a parasympathetic stimulant. It inactivates the cholinesterase and provides for a longer and more intense skeletal muscle tone. Through its parasympathetic activity, it is useful in postoperative intestinal atony and as a miotic in glaucoma and other diseases of the eye. As a depressant to the spinal cord, it has been used in tetanus and strychnine poisoning. Also used in the treatment of myasthenia gravis. Extremely poisonous. Dose, 0.001–0.0025 Gm. ($\frac{1}{60}$–$\frac{1}{24}$ gr.); for instillation in the eye, 0.25–1% solutions. Also called *eserine salicylate.*

p. sulfate $(C_{15}H_{21}O_2N_3)_2.H_2SO_4$. White or slightly yellowish, deliquescent powder. Reddens on exposure to light or air; very soluble in water and alcohol. Extremely poisonous. It is the preferred form in veterinary medicine. Also called *eserine sulfate.*

phy″so·ven′ine. $C_{14}H_{18}N_2O_3$; an alkaloid from the seed of *Physostigma venenosum.*

phy′tase. An enzyme occurring in plants, especially cereals, which catalyzes hydrolysis of phytic acid to inositol and phosphoric acid.

phy′tic ac′id. $C_6H_6O_6(H_2PO_3)_6$. Inositol-hexaphosphoric acid, a constituent of cereal grains. By forming an insoluble salt, it is said to prevent utilization of calcium in the cereal.

phy′tin. The calcium or magnesium salt of inositol-hexaphosphoric acid; a constituent of cereal grains. Also a trade-mark for same.

phy′to-, phyt- [G. *phyton,* plant]. A combining form meaning *plant;* used to denote *vegetation* or *a vegetable parasite.*

phy″to·be′zoar (figh″to·bee′zor, ·bez′or) [*phyton;* Per. *bād-zahr,* antidote]. A bezoar or ball of vegetable fiber sometimes found in the stomach.

phy″to·chem′is·try [*phyton;* G. *chymos,* juice]. Vegetable or plant chemistry.

phy″to·flu′ene. $C_{40}H_{64} \pm 2H$; a polyene hydrocarbon, occurring in the vegetable kingdom in chlorophyll-free tissues which contain considerable amounts of carotenoid pigments, as a pale-orange, viscous oil, insoluble in water and alcohol, soluble in ether and benzene.

phy″to·gen′e·sis, phy·tog′e·ny (figh·todj′i·nee) [*phyton;* G. *genesis,* production]. The science of the origin and development of plants. —**phytogenet′ic,** *adj.*

phy·tog′e·nous (figh·todj′i·nus) [*phyton;* G. *genesthai,* from *gignesthai,* to be produced]. Produced by plants.

phy″to·hor′mone. Any plant hormone.

phy′toid [*phyton;* G. *eidos,* form]. Plantlike; referring to certain animals and organs.

phy′tol. $C_{20}H_{39}OH$; an unsaturated aliphatic alcohol present in chlorophyll as an ester; a colorless liquid, insoluble in water but soluble in most organic solvents: used in synthesis of γ-tocopherol and vitamin K_1.

phy″to·lac′ca [*phyton;* NL. *lacca*, lac] (*phytolacca*). The dried root of *Phytolacca americana.* It yields a water-soluble material, containing a saponin, and an alcoholic extract containing a resinlike material which depresses the central nervous system. The saponin component is a local irritant and produces emesis. The therapeutic usefulness of phytolacca is obscure, but it has been used internally in chronic rheumatism and locally in the form of an ointment.

phy″to·lac′cin (figh″to·lack′sin) [*phyton; lacca*]. A resinoid, or the precipitate from a tincture of the root of *Phytolacca decandra.*

phy·tom′e·lin (figh·tom′i·lin). See *rutin.*

phy″to·mon′ic ac′id. $C_{20}H_{40}O_2$. A liquid saturated fatty acid isolated from the lipid fraction extracted from *Phytomonas tumefaciens.*

phy″to·na·di′one. $C_{31}H_{46}O_2$; the U.S.P. name for 2-methyl-3-phytyl-1,4-naphthoquinone, occurring in green plants but usually prepared by synthesis; a clear, yellow, very viscous, odorless or nearly odorless liquid, insoluble in water, soluble in alcohol: used therapeutically to promote prothrombin formation. Syn., *phylloquinone, 3-phytylmenadione, vitamin K_1.*

phy′ton·cide. An antibacterial and protozoacidal substance produced by various plants; certain of which, notably those produced by plants of the genus *Allium*, are volatile.

phy″to·par′a·site [*phyton;* G. *parasitos*, parasite]. A vegetable parasite.

phy″to·path″o·gen′ic [*phyton;* G. *pathos*, disease; *genesthai*, from *gignesthai*, to be produced]. Causing disease in plants.

phy″to·pa·thol′o·gy [*phyton; pathos;* G. *logos*, word]. 1. The science of diseases of plants. 2. The science of diseases due to vegetable organisms.

phy·toph′a·gous (figh·tof′uh·gus) [*phyton;* G. *phagein*, to eat]. 1. Plant-eating. 2. Vegetarian.

phy″to·phar″ma·col′o·gy [*phyton;* G. *pharmakon*, drug; *logos*, word]. That branch of pharmacology concerned with the effects of drugs on plant growth. —**phytopharmacolog′ical,** *adj.*

phy″to·pho″to·der″ma·to′sis. A dermatitis associated with contact with, or ingestion of, a plant and followed by exposure to the sun, as dermatitis bullosa striata praetensis.

phy″to·pneu″mo·no·co″ni·o′sis [*phyton;* G. *pneumōn*, lung; *konis*, dust; *-ōsis*, condition]. A condition marked by inflammatory nodules in the lungs, caused by the inhalation of vegetable particles.

phy″to·pre·cip′i·tin [*phyton;* L. *praecipitare*, to precipitate]. A precipitin produced by immunization with protein of vegetable origin.

phy·to′sis (figh·to′sis) [*phyton;* G. *-osis*, condition]. 1. Any disease due to the presence of vegetable parasites. 2. The production of disease by vegetable parasites. 3. The presence of vegetable parasites.

phy″to·ste′a·rin [*phyton;* G. *stear*, fat]. Old term for phytosterol.

phy·tos′ter·in (figh·tos′tur·in). Old term for phytosterol.

phy·tos′ter·ol (figh·tos′tur·ole, ·ol, ·awl, figh″to-steer′·). Any sterol occurring in a plant oil or fat.

phy·tos′ter·ol·in. A glycoside of phytosterol.

phy″to·throm″bo·kin′ase (·kin′ace, ·aze, ·kigh′-nace, ·naze). A thrombokinase prepared from yeast or plant sources.

phy″to·tox′ic. 1. Pertaining to a phytotoxin. 2. Pertaining to or describing a substance poisonous to plants.

phy″to·tox′in [*phyton;* G. *toxikon*, poison]. A toxin derived from a plant, such as abrin, ricin, and crotin.

phy″to·vi·tel′lin (figh″to·vi·tell′in, ·vye·tell′in) [*phyton;* L. *vitellus*, yolk]. A vegetable protein resembling vitellin.

3-phy″tyl·men″a·di′one. Phytonadione.

P.I. International Protocol (*Protocol Internationale*): the designation affixed in the U.S.P. to drugs on which international agreement as to composition has been reached.

pi′a, pi′a ma′ter. The vascular membrane enveloping the surface of the brain and spinal cord, and consisting of a plexus of blood vessels held in a fine areolar tissue. —**pial,** *adj.*

pi·an′ (pee·an′, pye′an, pee·ahn′, pyahn). Yaws.

pi·an′-bois″. See *leishmaniasis* americana.

pi″a·rach′noid (pee″uh·rack′noyd) [L. *pius*, tender; G. *arachnoeidēs*, like a cobweb]. The pia and arachnoid considered as one structure: also called *leptomeninx, leptomeninges;* also spelled *pia-arachnoid.*

pi″as·tre·ne′mi·a. See megakaryocytic *leukemia.*

pi·blok′to. A state of hysterical excitement exhibited by Eskimos, particularly women, in which the individual becomes irrational, often destructive.

Pic, Adrien [*French physician*, 1863–1943]. Described, with Louis Bard, typical symptoms of carcinoma of the head of the pancreas, including progressive icterus, cachexia, distended gallbladder, and loss of weight; called *Bard-Pic syndrome.*

pi′ca (pye′kuh) [L., magpie]. 1. A desire for strange foods; may occur in chlorosis and during pregnancy. 2. A craving to eat strange articles, as hair, dirt, or sand; the recurrence in later life of the infantile tendency of bringing everything to the mouth.

pi·ca′cic ac′id. An antibiotic produced by the fungus *Coprinus picaceus;* a pale-yellow oil, sparingly soluble in water, soluble in organic liquids. It forms soluble sodium and potassium salts.

Piccolomini, Archangelo [*Italian anatomist*, 1526–1605]. Striae acusticae are also known as *striae of Piccolomini.*

Pic′e·a (pis′ee·uh, pye′see·uh) [L., pitch pine]. A genus of coniferous trees.

P. abies. The Norway spruce.

P. glauca. The white spruce.

P. mariana. The black spruce.

pic′e·in (pis′ee·in, pye′see·in). $C_{14}H_{18}O_7$. A glycoside from the leaves of the Norway spruce, *Picea abies*, or from *Salix nigra*, a willow.

pi′cene. $C_{22}H_{14}$; a pentacyclic hydrocarbon, 1,2-7,8-dibenzphenanthrene, found in tar oils from soft coal and in petroleum residues from the cracking process. It occurs as crystals, difficultly soluble in most solvents.

pic′e·ous (pis′ee·us, pye′see·us) [*picea*]. Resembling pitch.

pi′chi (pee′chee) [Araucan, small thing]. The stems and leaves of *Fabiana imbricata*, growing in South America. It has been used as a terebinthinate diuretic in the treatment of cystitis.

Pick, Arnold [*Czechoslovakian physician*, 1851–1924]. Known for his study and description of circumscribed cerebral atrophy, accompanied by aphasia and progressive dementia (1892); also called *Pick's disease.* See also lobar *sclerosis.*

Pick, Friedel [*German physician*, 1867–1926]. Described pseudocirrhosis of the liver with pericarditis (1896); called *polyserositis, mediastinopericarditis, Pick's disease, Friedel Pick's disease.* Described a syndrome of liver enlargement with recurring ascites but without cardiac symptoms or icterus; called *Pick's syndrome.*

Pick, Ludwig [*German pediatrician,* 1868–1935]. Described a form of xanthomatosis. See Niemann-Pick *disease.*

Pickworth method. See benzidine and nitroprussic oxidase *method* for hemoglobin.

pic'o·line. C_6H_7N; either of two isomeric substances, *α-picoline,* 2-methyl-pyridine, or *β-picoline,* 3-methylpyridine, found in coal tar and bone oil. Both are colorless liquids, miscible with water and alcohol: used as solvents, intermediates, in dye and resins industries, and in insecticides.

pic"o·lin'ic ac'id. $C_5H_4N.COOH$; *o-* or 2-pyridine-carboxylic acid; an isomer of nicotinic acid, occurring as a white crystalline powder, sparingly soluble in cold water, and, as a metabolite analog of nicotinic acid, displacing it in certain bacteria.

pic"ra·con'i·tine. See *picroaconitine.*

pic"ra·don'i·din. A glucoside obtained from adonis. It has a digitalislike action.

Pic·rae'na (pick·ree'nuh). See *Picrasma.*

picragol. Trade-mark for *silver picrate.*

pic·ram'ic ac'id. $C_6H_2.OH.(NO_2)_2.NH_2$; 4,6-dinitro-2-aminophenol; a reduction product of picric acid, occurring as red crystals, slightly soluble in water, and appearing in urine following ingestion of picric acid: used as a reagent for albumin and in synthesis of dyes.

Pic·ras'ma (pick·raz'muh) [G. *pikrasmos,* bitterness]. A genus of the Simarubaceae. The wood of **P. excelsa** is the source of Jamaica quassia, containing α-picrasmin and β-picrasmin. It sometimes is employed in the form of an infusion as a bitter tonic and as a rectal injection for threadworms in children.

pic·ras'min. $C_{22}H_{28}O_6$; a bitter principle of quassia, identical with isoquassin isolated from quassia by later investigators.

pic'rate. A salt of picric acid.

pic'ric ac'id. Trinitrophenol.

pic"ro·a·con'i·tine (pick"ro·a·kon'i·teen, ·tin), **pic"ra·con'i·tine.** $C_{32}H_{45}O_{10}N$. Benzaconine; a bitter powder derived from aconite. Its action is similar to that of aconitine but less potent.

pic"ro·car'mine (pick"ro·kahr'min, ·meen, ·myne). One of a variety of mixtures of carmine, ammonia, and picric acid, used as a stain for tissues.

pic"ro·form'ol. A fixing agent consisting of a mixture of a saturated solution of picric acid 75 parts and formol 25 parts, to which 5 parts of acetic acid are added immediately before using. Also called *Bouin's fixing fluid.*

pic"ro·lon'ic ac'id. $C_{10}H_8N_4O_5$; 3-methyl-4-nitro-1-(*p*-nitrophenyl)-5-pyrazolone, occurring as yellow leaflets, sparingly soluble in water: used as a reagent for alkaloids and basic amino acids, also for calcium.

pic"ro·pod"o·phyl'lin (·pod"o·fill'in, ·po"do·fill'in, ·po·dof'i·lin). $C_{22}H_{22}O_8$; a nontoxic, crystalline substance isomeric with podophyllotoxin and formed by alkaline hydrolysis of it in alcoholic solution; it appears to be physiologically inert.

pic"ro·tox'in (*picrotoxinum*). $C_{30}H_{34}O_{13}$. A glycoside obtained from the seed of *Anamirta cocculus;* occurs as shining, prismatic crystals or a microcrystalline powder; stable in air but is affected by light. One gram dissolves in about 350 cc. of water and in about 5 cc. of boiling alcohol. Picrotoxin is a stimulant to apparently all the efferent centers of the cerebrospinal axis, affecting the cerebrum, the medulla, and the spinal cord. Used as one of the most reliable agents in poisoning by the barbiturates. Dose, 1.0–3.0 mg. ($\frac{1}{60}$–$\frac{1}{20}$ gr.) by intravenous injection, repeated at half-hour intervals as required. Also called *cocculin.*

p. injection (*injectio picrotoxini*). A sterile solution of picrotoxin in isotonic sodium chloride solution. Picrotoxin injection usually available contains 3.0 mg. ($\frac{1}{20}$ gr.) per 1 cc.

pie'dra (pee·ay'drah) [Sp., stone]. A nodular growth on the hair of the scalp, beard, or mustache. The type known as **black piedra** is found in tropical regions and is caused by the fungus *Piedraia hortai,* which infests only the hair shafts of the scalp. **White piedra,** a rarer form, occurs in temperate regions and is caused by the fungus *Trichosporon beigelii* which infests the hair of the beard and mustache. Also called *tinea nodosa, Beigel's disease, piedra nostros.*

pi"es·es·the'si·a (pye"ess·ess·theezh'uh, ·theez'-ee·uh, pye"ez·ess·) [G. *piesis,* compression; *aisthēsis,* perception]. Perception of the sense of pressure.

pi"e·sim'e·ter, pi"e·som'e·ter. See *piezometer.*

pi·e"zo·e·lec'tric ef·fect' (pye·ee"zo·i·leck'trick). The development of electric charges by certain crystals when subjected to strain. Conversely, if such crystals are located in an oscillating electric field, they will produce resonant vibrations. The latter effect is the principle of the recording part of some pen-writing (or stylus) recording electrocardiographs.

pi"e·zom'e·ter [G. *piezein,* to compress; *metron,* a measure]. 1. An apparatus for measuring the degree of compression of gases or fluids. 2. An apparatus for testing the sensitiveness of the skin to pressure. 3. A simple liquid manometer.

Piffard, Henry Granger [*American dermatologist,* 1842–1910]. Introduced a paste for testing urine for sugar. It contains sodium tartrate, sodium hydroxide, and copper sulfate. Called *Piffard's paste.*

pi'geon-toed. Walking with the feet turned in.

pig'ment [L. *pigmentum,* pigment]. 1. A dyestuff; a coloring matter. 2. Any organic coloring matter of the body. See Plate 28. 3. Any stain used in microscopical work. 4. Any medicinal agent applied externally to the skin, like paint. —**pigmented,** *adj.*

bile pigments. Pigments found in bile or derived from it. They include bilirubin, urobilinogen, urobilin, and biliverdin.

blood pigments. Pigments normally found in blood. See *hemoglobin, bilirubin.*

carboxyhemoglobin p. One used in hemoglobinometry. A solution of it is almost permanent when sealed in an atmosphere of carbon monoxide.

cholera-blue p. A color base obtained by dissolving cholera-red in concentrated sulfuric acid and then neutralizing with caustic soda.

cholera-red p. A color base found in cultures of cholera bacilli which, upon addition of mineral acids, gives a violet color. On rendering the solution alkaline and shaking it with benzol, the cholera-red is obtained in brownish red lamellas. Distillation of cholera-red with zinc dust gives indole.

hematogenous p. Any pigment derived from hemoglobin, including heme, hemosiderin, methemoglobin, and bile pigments.

hepatogenous p. See bile *pigments.*

iris p. The chemically pure pigment of the bovine eye; triturated with water, it is used for tattooing corneal opacities.

metabolic p. A pigment formed by the metabolic action of cells. Melanin is the type of metabolic pigments.

wear-and-tear pigments. Pigments, as hemofuscin, hemosiderin, and lipochrome, observed in increased amounts in tissues of older individuals.

pig'men·tar"y (pig'men·terr"ee) [L. *pigmentarius,*

of paints]. Pertaining to or containing pigment; characterized by the formation of pigment.

pig″men·ta′tion [L. *pigmentatus*, painted]. Deposition of or discoloration by pigment.

endogenous p. That, pathologic in character, due to increased amounts or abnormal distribution of natural body pigments or due to a new pigment elaborated in the body, as in Addison's disease or xanthomatosis.

exogenous p. That due to pigments introduced from without, as in pneumoconiosis or tattooing.

pathologic p. An abnormal amount, distribution, or composition of pigment in a tissue.

pig·men″to·gen′e·sis [L. *pigmentum*, pigment; G. *genesis*, production]. The origin of pigment.

pig·men′to·phage [*pigmentum;* G. *phagein*, to eat]. A phagocyte which destroys pigment, especially that of hairs.

pig·men′tum ni′grum [L.]. The dark coloring matter which lines the choroid coat of the eye.

pig′my. See *pygmy.*

Pignet, Maurice-Charles-Joseph [*French military surgeon*, 1871–]. Introduced a formula for the determination of standards of physical condition of recruits for the army, which he proposed as $F = H - (C + W)$. F is the empirical factor, H the height in centimeters, C the chest measurement in centimeters on deep inspiration, and W the weight in kilograms. If F is less than 10, the applicant is classed as exceptionally strong; if between 10 and 15, he is strong; if between 15 and 20, he is good; if between 20 and 25, he is fair; if above 30, he is very weak. A similar formula was published by J. A. Black using English weights and measures. Called *Black's formula; Pignet's factor* or *formula.*

pig′weed [ME. *pigge;* AS. *wēod*]. A plant of the genus *Chenopodium;* frequently causes allergy.

pi·i′tis (pye·eye′tis). Old term for leptomeningitis.

pil. *Pilula*, pill.

pi′lar, pi′la·ry (pye′luh·ree, pil′uh·ree) [L. *pilus*, hair]. Pertaining to the hair.

pi·las′tered [L. *pīla*, pillar]. Flanged so as to have a fluted appearance; arranged in pilasters or columns, as pilastered femur.

Pilcz's reflex. See under *reflex.*

pile [L. *pĭla*, ball]. A hemorrhoid.

blind p. One which does not bleed.

external p. A hemorrhoid which is located outside the anal sphincter.

internal p. A hemorrhoid which is located inside the anal sphincter.

sentinel p. The thickened wall of the anal pocket at the lower end of an anal fissure.

pile [L. *pīla*, pillar]. 1. A battery. 2. A nuclear reactor. The term *pile* arose from the construction of early reactors by piling graphite blocks and pieces of uranium and uranium oxide.

thermoelectric p. A number of bars or plates in which two kinds of metal are conjoined (thermocouples). When the junctions are heated, an electric current is generated by which temperature can be measured.

pile [L. *pilus*, hair]. The hair or hairs collectively of any part of the integument.

pi′le·ous [*pilus*]. Pertaining to hair; hairy.

piles. See *hemorrhoids.*

pi′li (pye′lye). Plural of pilus.

pi″li·a′tion, pil″i·a′tion [*pilus*]. The formation and production of hair.

Pi·lif′er·a. Animals with hair: term suggested for *mammals.* Syn., *Trichozoa.*

pil′i·form, pi′li·form [*pilus;* L. *forma*, form]. Having the appearance of hair; filiform.

pi′li·gan (pee′li·gahn) [G. *pilos*, felt; *genesthai*, from *gignesthai*, to be produced]. The plant *Lycopodium saururus*, found in South America and Africa. It contains the alkaloids saururine, $C_{10}H_{19}N$, sauroxine, $C_{17}H_{26}ON_2$, and piliganine, $C_{15}H_{24}ON_2$. It is also stated to contain a resin. It is used as an emetocathartic. Other species of *Lycopodium*, as *L. selago* and *L. polytrichoides*, have been used as cathartics.

pil′i·ga·nine (pill′i·guh·neen, ·nin, pye·lig′uh·). An alkaloid obtained from *Lycopodium saururus.* See *piligan.*

pi″li·mic′tion [*pilus;* L. *mictio*, from *mingere*, to make water]. The passing of urine containing hairlike filaments.

pill [L. *pĭla*, ball]. A small, solid body, of a globular, ovoid, or lenticular shape, containing one or more medicinal substances and used for internal administration.

pil′lar [L. *pīla*, pillar]. A columnar structure acting as a support.

anterior p. of the fornix. A band of white matter on each side passing from the anterior extremity of the fornix to the base of the brain.

p. of the fauces. One of the folds of mucous membrane on each side of the fauces.

posterior p. of the fornix. One of two bands passing from the posterior extremities of the fornix into the descending horn of the lateral ventricle.

pil′let [L. *pĭla*, ball]. A little pill, or pellet.

pil′le·us, pil′le·um [L., felt cap]. The caul or membrane which sometimes covers a child's head during birth.

pi′lo-, pil- [L. *pilus*, hair]. A combining form meaning *hair.*

pi″lo·car′pi·dine. $C_{10}H_{14}N_2O_2$; a liquid alkaloid from *Pilocarpus jaborandi.*

pi″lo·car′pine (pye″lo·kahr′peen, ·pin, pill″o·). $C_{11}H_{16}N_2O_2$. An alkaloid obtained from various species of *Pilocarpus (jaborandi);* occurs as a colorless to yellow, viscid liquid or crystals; freely soluble in water and alcohol.

p. hydrochloride (*pilocarpinae hydrochloridum*). $C_{11}H_{16}N_2O_2.HCl$, the hydrochloride of an alkaloid obtained from the dried leaflets of *Pilocarpus jaborandi* or of *Pilocarpus microphyllus;* colorless, translucent, faintly bitter, hygroscopic crystals; 1 Gm. is soluble in about 0.3 cc. of water and about 3 cc. of alcohol. For uses and dose, see *pilocarpine* nitrate. Also called *pilocarpine muriate.*

p. nitrate (*pilocarpinae nitras*). $C_{11}H_{16}N_2O_2.HNO_3$, the nitrate of an alkaloid obtained from the dried leaflets of *Pilocarpus jaborandi* or of *Pilocarpus microphyllus;* shining, white crystals; 1 Gm. is soluble in 4 cc. of water and 75 cc. of alcohol. Pilocarpine is the physiologic antagonist of atropine, exciting those nerve endings which are paralyzed by that alkaloid. It is used chiefly as a sudorific, in conjunction with some form of external heat, and in the treatment of postoperative urinary retention. It is widely employed by ophthalmologists as a miotic. Dose, 0.003–0.006 Gm. ($\frac{1}{20}$–$\frac{1}{10}$ gr.); as a miotic, 0.5–1% solution.

pi″lo·car′pus (pye″lo·kahr′pus, pill″o·) [G. *pilos*, felt; *karpos*, fruit]. The dried leaflets of *Pilocarpus jaborandi*, or of *Pilocarpus microphyllus* and other species of *Pilocarpus.* A number of alkaloids have been obtained from various species of pilocarpus, the principal one being pilocarpine. Syn., *jaborandi.*

pi″lo·cys′tic [L. *pilus*, hair; G. *kystis*, bladder]. Pertaining to encysted tumors containing hair and fat.

pi″lo·e·rec′tion. Erection of the hair.

pi″lo·mo′tor [*pilus;* L. *motor*, from *movere*, to move]. Causing movement of the hair, as the pilomotor muscles.

pi″lo·ni′dal [*pilus;* L. *nidus*, nest]. Pertaining to or containing an accumulation of hairs in a cyst.

pi'lose, pi'lous [L. *pilosus*, hairy]. Hairy.

pi"lo·se·ba'ceous [L. *pilus*, hair; *sebaceus*, tallow-candle]. Pertaining to the hair follicles and sebaceous glands, as the pilosebaceous apparatus, the hair follicle and its attached oil gland.

pi·lo'sis (pye·lo'sis) [*pilus;* G. *-ōsis*, increase]. The abnormal or excessive development of hair.

pi·los'i·ty (pye·los'i·tee, pi·los'i·tee) [L. *pilosus*, hairy]. The state of being pilose or hairy.

pil'u·la (pl. *pilulae*) [L. *pilula*, little ball]. A pill. Abbreviated, pil. —**pilular,** *adj.*

pil'ule [*pilula*]. A small pill.

pi'lus (pl. *pili*) [L.]. 1. A hair. 2. *In biology*, a fine, slender, hairlike body.

pili annulati. See *ringed hair.*

pili tactiles. Tactile hairs.

pili torti. A rare, congenital deformity of the hair, characterized by short, broken, twisted hairs presenting the appearance of stubble.

pi·mel'ic ac'id. $COOH(CH_2)_5COOH$; heptanedioic acid, occurring as crystals, soluble in water. Biotin may derive part of its molecule from pimelic acid which is interchangeable with biotin for some microorganisms.

pim"e·li'tis (pim"i·lye'tis, pye"mi·lye'tis) [G. *pimelē*, fat; *-itis*, inflammation]. Inflammation of any adipose tissue; also, inflammation of connective tissue in general.

pim"e·lo·pte·ryg'i·um (pim"i·lo·teh·ridj'ee·um, pye"mi·lo·) [*pimelē;* G. *pterygion*, small wing]. A fatty outgrowth on the conjunctiva.

pim"e·lor·rhe'a [*pimelē;* G. *rhoia*, flow]. 1. An excessive fatty discharge. 2. Diarrhea with excessive fat in the stools.

pim"e·lor·thop'ne·a (pim"i·lor·thop'nee·uh, ·lor"-thop·nee'uh, pye"mi·) [*pimelē;* G. *orthopnoia*, breathing only in an upright position]. Orthopnea due to obesity.

pim"e·lu'ri·a [*pimelē;* G. *ouron*, urine]. The excretion of fat in the urine; lipuria.

pi·men'ta [Sp. *pimienta*]. The nearly ripe fruit of *Pimenta officinalis*, an evergreen tree. The fruit yields from 1 to 4% of a volatile oil. It sometimes is used as an aromatic carminative in flatulence and as an adjuvant to tonics and purgatives. Syn., *allspice*. Sometimes spelled *pimento*.

pim"pi·nel'la [NL., from L. *piper*, pepper]. The dried rhizome and roots of *Pimpinella saxifraga* or other species. It contains pimpinellin, isopimpinellin, isobergaptene, volatile oil, and an acrid resin. It sometimes is used as a carminative, in certain types of diarrhea, and as a local stimulant in toothache. From the dried ripe fruit of *Pimpinella anisum* is obtained a volatile oil. See anise *oil*.

pim'ple [L. *papula*, pimple]. Lay term for a small pustule or papule.

pin. See *nail*, 2.

Austin Moore's pins. See Austin Talley *Moore*.

Steinmann's p. See Fritz *Steinmann*.

pin'a·coid [G. *pinax*, tablet; *eidos*, form]. Denoting polyhedral forms having only two parallel faces, as in some condensed systems of large molecules.

pin'a·col. 1. $(CH_3)_2C.OH.C.OH(CH_3)_2$; 2,3-dimethyl-2,3,-butanediol or tetramethylethyleneglycol; a crystalline substance, slightly soluble in cold water. 2. Any of a group of glycols of the type of $R_2C.OH.C.OH.R_2$, where R is a hydrocarbon radical.

pin"a·cy'a·nol. A basic xanthine dye of the cyanine group, used as a supravital stain for mitochondria, and for the staining of frozen sections.

Pinard, Adolphe [*French obstetrician*, 1844–1934]. Described a sign of breech presentation after the sixth month of pregnancy, in which a sharp pain is elicited upon pressure over the fundus uteri (1878), called *Pinard's sign.* He advocated a special technic in breech deliveries in which the knee of the fetus is pushed to one side and a foot brought down for traction purposes, called *Pinard's maneuver.*

pince"ment' (pans·mahng'. *See* Notes § 35) [F.]. In massage, a pinching or nipping of the tissues.

pin'cers [F. *pince*]. 1. Forceps. 2. The two median upper or lower incisor teeth of a horse.

Pinck'ney·a (pink'nee·uh) [after Charles Cotesworth *Pinckney*, American statesman, 1746–1825]. A genus of the Rubiaceae. **P. pubens** is a small tree of the southern United States. The bark is astringent and tonic and has been used in intermittent fevers.

pine [L. *pinus*, pine]. A general name for coniferous trees. Various varieties of this genus yield many substances used in medicine and in commerce, as turpentine, resin, tar, pitch, and many volatile oils.

compound white p. syrup (*syrupus pini albae compositus*). Used as a mild expectorant in subacute bronchitis. Dose, 4–8 cc. (1–2 fluidrachms).

p. camphor. Pinol, a terpene found in pine needles.

p. cone oil. A volatile oil from the cones of *Abies picea.*

p. leaf oil. A volatile oil distilled from pine needles.

p. needle oil. Oil of dwarf pine needles.

p. oil. A crude turpentine obtained by distillation of pine wood.

white p. (*pinus alba*). The dried inner bark of *Pinus strobus*. It contains a glycoside, coniferin, together with about 10% of tannin and some mucilage and oleoresin. White pine bark is used as an ingredient in cough syrups. Also called *white pine bark.*

pin'e·al [L. *pinea*, pine cone]. Referring to the pineal gland, or epiphysis cerebri.

pin"e·al·blas·to'ma. See *pinealoma.*

pin"e·al·cy·to'ma. See *pinealoma.*

pin"e·a·lec'to·my [*pinea;* G. *ektomē*, excision]. Surgical removal of the pineal gland.

pin'e·al·ism, pi·ne'al·ism [*pinea*]. Disturbances due to abnormality in the secretion of the pineal gland.

pin"e·a·lo'ma [*pinea;* G. *-ōma*, tumor]. An uncommon, usually small, frequently invasive tumor of the pineal gland composed of varying proportions of the large, round, parenchymal cells or the small, dense, stromal cells. Symptoms usually are due to hydrocephaly caused by obstruction of the cerebral aqueduct. Also called *pinealblastoma, pinealcytoma, pineal germinoma, pineal seminoma, pineal tumor, pineoblastoma.*

Pinel, Philippe [*French alienist*, 1745–1826]. Remembered for his advocacy of reforms in the treatment of the insane (1792). His *Mental Alienation* advocated abolition of forcible restraints (1801).

pi'nene. $C_{10}H_{16}$. 2.7.7-Trimethyl-Δ^2-bicyclo (1.1.3) heptene. A terpene or hydrocarbon found in many essential oils. It is the chief constituent in turpentine oil. Occurs as a colorless, aromatic liquid; slightly soluble in water, soluble in alcohol and ether.

pin"e·o·blas·to'ma. See *pinealoma.*

pine tar (*pix pini*). A product obtained by the destructive distillation of the wood of *Pinus palustris*, or other species of *Pinus;* a very viscid, blackish brown, noncrystalline liquid, with an empyreumatic, terebinthinate odor; it is slightly soluble in water and is miscible with alcohol. The composition is largely phenolic. The constituents include benzol, toluol, xylol, styrol, naphthalene, phenol, cresol, phlorol, etc. It sometimes is employed externally as a stimulating and antiseptic application in skin diseases. Internally it is used as a stimulating expectorant in subacute or chronic bronchitis. Dose, 0.3–0.6 Gm. (5–10 gr.). Also called *pix liquida.* See rectified *tar* oil.

p. t. ointment (*unguentum picis pini*), (*unguentum picis liquidae*). Contains 50% of pine tar in yellow ointment.

pin·guec′u·la [L. *pinguiculus,* somewhat fat]. A small, yellowish white patch situated on the conjunctiva, between the cornea and the canthus of the eye; it is composed of connective tissue.

pin′guid [L. *pinguis,* fat]. Fat; unctuous.

pi′ni·form, pin′i·form [L. *pinus,* pine; *forma,* form]. Shaped like a pine cone.

pink′eye″. 1. A contagious, mucopurulent conjunctivitis occurring especially in horses. 2. Acute contagious conjunctivitis in man. Also called *Koch-Weeks conjunctivitis.*

pink′root″. See *Spigelia.*

Pinkus, Felix (1868–1947). German dermatologist who described lichen nitidus (1901), called *Pinkus' disease.*

pin′na [L., feather]. The projecting part of the external ear; the auricle. See Plate 20. —**pinnal,** *adj.*

pi′no·cyte (py′no·sight, pin′o·) [G. *pinein,* to drink; *kytos,* cell]. A phagocytic cell exhibiting pinocytosis.

pi″no·cy·to′sis (pye″no·sigh·to′sis, pin″o·) [*pinein; kytos;* G. *-ōsis,* condition]. Drinking by cells, as opposed to phagocytosis, eating by cells.

pi″no·syl′vine. $(OH)_2C_6H_3.CH:CH.C_6H_5$; 3,5-dihydroxystilbene; a crystalline compound occurring in the heartwood of *Pinus sylvestris:* said to have many times the bactericidal activity of phenol.

Pins, Emil [*Austrian physician,* 1845–1913]. Described a sign in pericarditis in which the symptoms which simulate pleurisy disappear when the patient assumes the knee-chest position; called *Pins's sign.*

pint [OF. *pinte*]. The eighth part of a gallon; 16 fluidounces. Symbol, O. (*octarius*). Abbreviated, pt. An **imperial pint** contains 20 fluidounces.

pin′ta (pin′tuh, peen′tah) [Sp., spot]. A disease of the skin seen most frequently in tropical America, characterized by dyschromic changes and hyperkeratosis in patches of the skin; caused by the spirochete *Treponema carateum* which is morphologically identical with the spirochetes of syphilis and of yaws. Also called *carate, azul, spotted sickness, mal del pinto, piquite, Puru-puru, Quitiqua, Tinna.*

pin′worm″. See *Enterobius vermicularis.*

pi″o·ne′mi·a [G. *piōn,* fat; *haima,* blood]. The presence of an emulsion of fine oil globules in the blood, sometimes found in diabetes; a form of lipemia.

Pi·oph′i·la (pye·off′i·luh) [*piōn;* G. *philein,* to love]. A genus of small, black, dipterous insects containing the species **P. casei,** the cheese fly, which deposits its eggs preferably on cheese but also on ham, bacon, and other fatty foods. The larvae, commonly called cheese skippers, are a cause of intestinal myiasis.

Piorry, Pierre Adolphe [*French physician and clinician,* 1794–1879]. Reintroduced percussion using an intermediary element. Invented a pleximeter for this purpose (1866).

pi″or·thop·ne′a [G. *piōn,* fat; *orthopnoia,* breathing only in an upright position]. Orthopnea due to obesity.

pi′o·scope [*piōn;* G. *skopein,* to examine]. A variety of lactoscope, an instrument for measuring the butter-fat content of milk.

pip [L. *pituita,* slime]. A contagious disease of fowls characterized by a secretion of thick mucus in the throat and mouth.

Pi′per [L., pepper]. A genus of Piperaceae. See *pepper.*

pi·per′a·zine (pi·perr′uh·zeen, ·zin, pip′ur·uh·zeen, ·zin, pip″ur·ay′zin). $(CH_2)_4(NH)_2.6H_2O$. Diethylenediamine. The anhydrous base occurs as colorless, volatile crystals; freely soluble in water or glycerin, less soluble in alcohol. Has been used in the treatment of uric acid gravel and calculi and in gout. Dose, 0.3–0.6 Gm. (5–10 gr.).

pi·per′i·dine (pi·perr′i·deen, ·din, pye·perr′i·, pip′ur·i·deen, ·din, pye′pur·i·). $C_5H_{11}N$; hexahydropyridine; a volatile, liquid base found in small amounts in black pepper and also obtained by alkaline hydrolysis of piperine, soluble in water and alcohol: used as a reagent.

pip′er·ine (pip′ur·een, ·in, pye′pur·). $C_{17}H_{19}NO_3$; 1-piperoylpiperidine, an alkaloid from several varieties of pepper, occurring in crystals, almost insoluble in water, soluble in alcohol: used as an insecticide, antipyretic, and carminative.

pi·per′i·tone. $C_{10}H_{16}O$; 4-isopropyl-1-methyl-1-cyclohexen-3-one, occurring in dextrorotatory, levorotatory, or racemic forms in various volatile oils: used in perfumes, in dentifrices, etc., for its mintlike taste and odor.

pip′er·o·caine hy″dro·chlo′ride. $C_6H_5CO.O.CH_2.CH_2.CH_2.NC_5H_9.CH_3.HCl$; 3-benzoxy-1-(2-methylpiperidino)propane hydrochloride, occurring as white crystals or crystalline powder, freely soluble in water: used for topical, infiltrative, regional, spinal, and caudal anesthesia. See *metycaine hydrochloride.*

pip′er·o·nal (pip′ur·o·nal, pye·perr′o·nal). Dioxymethylene-protocatechuic aldehyde, $CH_2OO.C_6H_3.CHO$. Used in perfume. A pediculicide in 5% solution with castor oil and alcohol. Also called *heliotropin, piperonyl aldehyde.*

pip″er·o′va·tine (pip″ur·o′vuh·teen, ·tin, pye″pur·). $C_{16}H_{21}O_2N$. An alkaloid from the fruits of *Piper ovatum;* occurs as colorless crystals, soluble in alcohol, insoluble in water. It is said to act as a depressant of both motor and sensory nerves, and as a stimulant to the spinal cord.

pip″er·ox′an hy″dro·chlo′ride. Generic name for 2-(1-piperidylmethyl)-1,4-benzodioxan hydrochloride; $C_{14}H_{19}NO_2.HCl$; an adrenolytic agent used in differential diagnosis of hypertension. See *benodaine hydrochloride.*

pi·pet′, pi·pette′ (pi·pet′, pee·pet′) [F., dim. from *pipe,* tube]. A graduated open glass tube used for measuring or transferring definite quantities of liquids.

braking p. A micropipet in which a brake is inserted between the mouthpiece and the tip. The brake is a constriction which limits the flow of air and permits finer control of fluid movement.

Ostwald-Folin p. One which has less surface per unit volume than the ordinary pipet and no sharp shoulders to impede drainage. Favored in microanalysis.

syringe p. One having a small hypodermic syringe.

pip·sis′se·wa (pip·sis′i·wah, ·wuh) [Algonquian in origin]. Common name for the genus *Chimaphila.* See *chimaphila.*

pip′syl chlo′ride. $I.C_6H_4.SO_2Cl$; *p*-iodophenylsulfonyl chloride; a reagent which reacts nearly quantitatively with free amino groups of the amino acids in protein hydrolysates to give corresponding pipsylamino acids of the type of $I.C_6H_4.SO_2NHR$.

pip″to·nych′i·a (pip″to·nick′ee·uh) [G. *piptein,* to fall; *onyx,* nail]. Shedding of the nails.

pi·quite′. Pinta.

pi·qûre′ (pi·cure′. *See* NOTES § 35) [F.]. Puncture.

Piria, Raffaele [*Italian chemist*, 1815–65]. Known for his test for tyrosine in which he used sulfuric acid, barium carbonate, and ferric chloride, a violet color being considered a positive reaction. Isolated salicin (1839).

pir′i·form, pyr′i·form (pirr′i·form, pye′ri·form) [L. *pirum*, pear; *forma*, form]. The piriformis.

pir′i·form, pyr′i·form. Pear-shaped.

pir″i·for′mis [L. *pirum*, pear; *forma*, form]. A muscle arising from the front of the sacrum and inserted into the greater trochanter of the femur.

Pirogoff, Nickolai Ivanovich [*Russian surgeon*, 1810–81]. Author of a topographic anatomy (1852–59). One of the first to use ether in Europe. Introduced an osteoplastic operation for amputation of the foot resembling Syme's, in which part of the calcaneus was retained; see Pirogoff's *amputation*.

piromen, pyromen. Trade-mark for a complex polysaccharide derived from *Pseudomonas aeruginosa;* when intravenously injected in the form of a colloidal aqueous dispersion the product acts as a nonanaphylactogenic pyrogen and is useful for producing therapeutic fever and also for eliciting a euphoric effect in subpyrexial doses.

Pir″o·nel′la. A genus of operculated snails.

P. conica. That species which serves as the first intermediate host of the fluke *Heterophyes heterophyes* in Egypt.

Pi″ro·plas′ma (pye″ro·plaz′muh). Synonym for *Babesia*.

pi″ro·plas·mo′sis (pye″ro·plaz·mo′sis) [L. *pirum*, pear; G. *plasma*, anything formed; *-ōsis*, condition]. Infection of mammals other than man with sporozoa of the genera *Babesia* and *Theileria*. —**piroplasmot′ic,** *adj.*

bovine p. See Texas *fever*.

canine p. A type occurring in dogs characterized by hemoglobinuria, jaundice, weakness, and high temperature.

equine p. See equine biliary *fever*.

ovine p. A disease of sheep caused by the *Babesia ovis;* characterized by anemia, hemoglobinuria, fever, icterus, and weakness.

Pirquet von Cesenatico, Clemens Peter [*Austrian physician and pediatrician*, 1874–1929]. Introduced a type of tuberculin test in which the material is applied to a superficial abrasion of the skin (1907); called *von Pirquet test, reaction*. Described serum sickness, with Bela Schick (1905). Made important investigations in the etiology of cancer (1929). Introduced the term allergy (1907).

pis·cid′i·a [L. *piscis*, fish; *caedere*, to kill]. The dried bark of *Piscidia piscipula* (*P. erythrina*). Contains piscidic acid, $C_{11}H_{10}O_7$, a dibasic acid, and a neutral principle, piscidin, $C_{29}H_{24}O_8$. Piscidia possesses some anodyne power and has been used for the relief of neuralgia and in whooping cough. Syn., *Jamaica dogwood*.

pis′ci·din, pis·ci′din. See under *piscidia*.

pi″si·an·nu·la′ris. A variant of the abductor digiti quinti muscle inserted into the transverse carpal ligament.

pis′iform (pis′iform) [L. *pisum*, pea; *forma*, form]. A small bone on the inner and anterior aspect of the carpus. See Table of Bones in the Appendix.

pi′si·form. Pea-shaped.

pi″si·met″a·car′pus. A variant of the abductor digiti quinti muscle inserted into the fifth metacarpal.

pi″si·un″ci·na′tus. A variant of the abductor digiti quinti muscle inserted into the hamulus of the hamate.

Piso. See Guillaume le *Pois*.

pit [AS. *pytt*, from L. *puteus*, well]. A depression, as the pit of the stomach; the armpit.

anal p. The proctodeum.

auditory p. The embryonic invagination of the auditory placode that later becomes the otocyst or auditory vesicle: also called *otic p.*

basilar p. The depression upon the palatal surface of an upper incisor tooth, at the base of the cingulum.

ear p. See *fistula* auris congenita.

gastric p. One of the depressions in the gastric mucosa into which open the gastric glands.

olfactory p. One formed about the olfactory placode in the embryo by the growth of the median and lateral nasal processes; the anlage of part of the nasal cavity: also called *nasal p.*

otic p. See auditory *p.*

p. of the stomach. A name popularly given to that part of the abdomen just below the sternum and between the cartilages of the false ribs. Also called *scrobiculus cordis*.

primitive p. A minute pit at the anterior end of the primitive groove in the embryo just caudal to the primitive node; it may form the opening into the neuroenteric canal.

pitch [L. *pix*, pitch]. A heavy liquid or dark residue obtained by the distillation of tar; as, pine pitch, Burgundy pitch, coal tar pitch. It forms a lustrous brittle mass when cold, and a semisolid to syrupy mass according to the degree of heat to which it is subjected. It contains many organic compounds which differ according to its origin.

black p. The black residue obtained by distilling pine tar. It consists of rosin and empyreumatic products of rosin.

Burgundy p. The resinous exudation obtained from the stem of *Picea abies;* occurs as a reddish-brown or yellowish-brown solid, soluble in glacial acetic acid and boiling alcohol but partly soluble in cold alcohol. It is very fusible and softens and becomes adhesive at body temperature. It contains pimaric acid, which is a mixture of the dextro and levo forms, an amorphous resin acid, pinic acid, and a volatile oil. Has been used in chronic rheumatic pains and in chronic affections of the chest or abdomen.

Canada p. The resinous exudation from *Tsuga canadensis* (*Abies canadensis*). It is a hard, brittle, opaque, dark reddish brown substance. It softens and becomes adhesive at moderate temperatures. The constituents are a resin and a small quantity of volatile oil. Has been used as a mild rubefacient, analogous to Burgundy pitch in its properties.

pitch [ME. *picchen*]. That quality of sound which depends upon the rapidity of the vibrations that produce the sound.

pitch′blende [G. *pechblende*]. A massive form, having a pitchlike luster, of the mineral uraninite; a native uranium oxide, also containing radium.

Pitfield, Robert L. [*American physician*, 1870–1942]. Devised a method for staining flagella, known as *Smith-Pitfield method*.

pi·the′coid, pith′e·coid [G. *pithēkos*, ape; *eidos*, form]. Pertaining to the anthropoid apes.

pith′i·a·tism, pi·thi′a·tism [G. *peithein*, to persuade; *iatos*, curable]. 1. A condition caused by suggestion. See *hysteria*. 2. Treatment of disease by suggestion. —**pithiat′ic,** *adj.*

pith″i·at′ric [*peithein;* G. *iatrikos*, skilled in the medical art]. Capable of being relieved by suggestion or persuasion, as certain hysterical conditions.

Pitkin, George P. [*American surgeon*, 1885–1943]. Introduced a solution of procaine used in spinal anesthesia. See *spinocain*.

pitocin. Trade-mark for an aqueous solution containing the oxytocic principle of the neurohypophysis (oxytocin), with less than one-half unit of pressor activity per cc.

pi·tom′e·ter [after Henri *Pitot*, French physicist, 1695–1771; G. *metron*, a measure]. An instrument which records the rate of flow of fluids.

Pitres, Jean Albert [*French physician*, 1848–1928]. Known for his study of the cortical motor centers describing a series of sections through the brain used in post-mortem examinations, called *Pitres' sections*.

pitressin. Trade-mark for an aqueous solution containing the pressor and diuretic-antidiuretic principle of the neurohypophysis (vasopressin), with less than one unit of oxytocic activity per cc.

p. tannate in oil. A suspension in vegetable oil of a water-insoluble tannate of the pressor and diuretic-antidiuretic principle of the neurohypophysis: used where the prolonged action of pitressin is desired.

pit′ted [AS. *pytt*, from L. *puteus*, well]. Marked by indentations or pits, as from smallpox.

pit′ting [*puteus*]. 1. The formation of pits. 2. The quality of preserving, for a short time, indentations made by pressing with the finger.

pi·tu′i·cyte [L. *pituita*, phlegm; G. *kytos*, cell]. The characteristic cell of the neurohypophysis.

pi·tu′i·tar″y (pi·tew′i·terr″ee) [*pituita*]. 1. Secreting mucus or phlegm. 2. Pertaining to, or designating, the pituitary body.

pi·tu′i·tar″y. The pituitary body or gland; the hypophysis cerebri. The human pituitary is a small, rounded organ averaging about 0.5 Gm. in weight. It lies in the sella turcica of the sphenoid bone, and is attached by a stalk to the floor of the brain. A classification of the mammalian pituitary, based on embryogenesis, morphology, and functions, divides this gland into two: the *adenohypophysis*, derived from Rathke's pouch of buccal ectoderm, with subdivisions into the pars distalis, pars intermedia, and pars tuberalis; and the *neurohypophysis*, derived from the neural ectoderm from the floor of the diencephalon. Other classifications divide the hypophysis into anterior, intermediate, and posterior lobes, or only into anterior and posterior lobes. The name *pituitary* was given this organ because it was erroneously thought to secrete the mucus of the nose; it is now recognized as the master gland of internal secretion. The recognized adenohypophyseal hormones are adrenocorticotropin, thyrotropin, growth hormone, follicle-stimulating hormone, luteinizing hormone, and prolactin; those extracted from the neurohypophysis are antidiuretic hormone and oxytocin. See Plates 17, 18, 45, and Table of Hormones, B, in the Appendix.

desiccated anterior p. (*pituitarium anterius*). The dried, partially defatted, and powdered adenohypophysis of cattle, sheep, and swine, occurring as a gray or yellowish-gray amorphous powder, only partially soluble in water. Present evidence has not yet demonstrated that any of the six generally accepted hormones are absorbable from the alimentary canal; its use as a remedial agent is therefore in question. Also called *pituitary anterior lobe, desiccated pituitary anterior lobe, pituitary body anterior lobe*.

desiccated posterior p. (*pituitarium posterius*). The cleaned, dried, and powdered lobe obtained from the pituitary body of domesticated animals which are used for food by man; occurs as yellowish or grayish, amorphous powder and has a characteristic odor; only partially soluble in water. Also called *pituitary, hypophysis sicca*.

desiccated whole p. (*pituitarium totum*). The dried, partially defatted, and powdered pituitary gland of cattle, sheep, or swine; occurs as a gray or yellowish gray, amorphous powder. Any effects obtained by the oral administration of this drug probably are due to the stimulating action of the posterior lobe fractions. Also called *pituitary gland, desiccated pituitary substance, pituitary body*.

pituitrin. Trade-mark for a brand of posterior pituitary injection.

pituitrin-S. Trade-mark for a solution of posterior pituitary, double the strength of the official solution.

pit′u·rine. An alkaloid from a species of *Duboisia*, related to nicotine.

pit″y·ri′a·sis [G., branlike eruption on the skin]. A fine, branny desquamation of the skin.

p. capitis. Dermatitis seborrheica.

p. lichenoides et varioliformis acuta. A noncommunicable, acute or subacute skin eruption characterized by vesicles and pustules that form crusts and later scars; usually runs a course of one to three months: also called *Habermann's disease*.

p. linguae. Transitory benign plaques of the tongue.

p. nigra. See *tinea* nigra.

p. pilaris. See *keratosis* pilaris.

p. rosea. A self-limited skin disease of the trunk, usually acute; characterized by pale red patches with fawn-colored centers. The etiologic agent is unknown. Also called *p. circinata, herpes tonsurans maculosus*.

p. rubra. A chronic, inflammatory skin disease usually involving the whole body. The skin is deep red and covered by whitish scales. The disease varies in duration from months to years and is generally fatal. It was described by F. von Hebra (1857). Also called *Hebra's p.*

p. rubra pilaris. A chronic, mildly inflammatory skin disease in which firm, acuminate papules form at the mouths of the hair follicles with horny plugs in these follicles. By coalescence scaly patches are formed. Also called *lichen ruber acuminatus*.

p. simplex. Dermatitis seborrheica.

p. steatoides. Dermatitis seborrheica when large waxy scales are formed, usually associated with pruritus and alopecia.

p. versicolor. A chronic skin disease characterized by yellowish-brown desquamating macules, involving principally the trunk and caused by the fungus *Malassezia furfur*.

pit′y·roid [G. *pityron*, bran; *eidos*, form]. Branny.

Pit″y·ro·spor′um (pit″i·ro·spor′um, ·ros′por·um) [*pityron;* G. *spora*, seed]. A genus of fungi which is yeastlike in character.

P. ovale. A species found in the hair follicles and on the skin in seborrheic dermatitis; of unknown pathogenicity.

piv′ot. *In dentistry*, old term for dowel.

piv′ot clack. An old method for attaching a crown to a decayed tooth root.

piv′ot·ing [F. *pivot*]. The fixation of an artificial crown to a tooth by a dowel.

PK Psychokinesis.

pK The negative logarithm of the dissociation constant of an acid or a base; it is equivalent to the hydrogen-ion concentration (expressed in pH units) at which there is an equimolecular concentration of the acidic and basic components of any given buffer system.

Place, Edwin Hemphill [*American physician*, 1880–]. The first to report Haverhill fever, with Lee Sutton and Otto Willner (1926).

pla·ce′bo [L., I shall please]. A medicine having no pharmacologic effect, but given for the purpose of pleasing or humoring the patient.

pla·cen′ta [L., cake]. The organ on the wall of the

uterus to which the embryo is attached by means of the umbilical cord and through which it receives its nourishment. It is developed, about the third month of gestation, from the chorion of the embryo and the decidua basalis of the uterus. The villi of the chorion enlarge and are received into depressions of the decidua, and around them form blood sinuses into which, by diffusion, the waste materials brought from the fetus by the umbilical arteries pass, and from which the blood receives oxygen and food material being returned to the fetus by the umbilical vein. It also serves an endocrine function by producing hormones. At term the placenta weighs one pound, is one inch thick at its center, and seven inches in diameter. The lay term is *afterbirth.* See Plate 41. —**placental, placentoid,** *adj.*

abruption of p. Premature detachment of the placenta.

accessory p. See *p.* succenturiata.

adherent p. One that fails to separate from the uterine wall after childbirth.

annular p. One extending around the interior of the uterus in the form of a belt.

battledore p. One in which the insertion of the cord is at the margin of the placenta.

bilobed p. See duplex *p.*

bipartite p. A placenta with two divisions.

circumvallate p. A placenta with an irregular elevation on the fetal surface close to the circumference. Syn., *p. extrachoriala, p. neppiformis.*

discoid p. One shaped like a disk.

duplex p. A placenta with two or more parts separated by membranes, whose vessels do not communicate but unite just before entering the umbilical cord. Syn., *bilobed p.*

endotheliochorial p. A type in which syncytial chorionic epithelium is in direct contact with the endothelium of uterine blood vessels: found in carnivores.

epitheliochorial p. A type in which the endothelial, connective tissue, and epithelial layers are present in both the uterus and the chorion. The fetal circulation must pass through all of them. This type is found in the sow.

fundal p. One attached at the fundus.

hemochorial p. A type in which the chorionic ectoderm is in direct contact with maternal blood: found in rabbits, insectivores, bats, and anthropoids.

hemoendothelial p. A type in which the endothelium of vessels of chorionic villi is in direct contact with maternal blood: found in the rat and guinea pig.

horseshoe p. In twin pregnancy, a condition in which two placentas are joined.

incarcerated p. One retained by irregular contraction of the uterus.

maternal p. The external layer developed from the decidua basalis.

multipartite p. One with more than three lobes and vessels which may emerge to form the umbilical cord directly or may first communicate with one or more of the other lobes. Syn., *multilobed p., septuplex p.*

p. accreta. A placenta which has partially grown into the uterine myometrium (cleavage zone in basal decidua incompletely developed).

p. cirsoides. One in which the umbilical vessels have a varicose arrangement.

p. diffusa. See *p.* membranacea.

p. extrachoriala. See circumvallate *p.*

p. fenestrata. An irregular, four-sided variety of placenta with an opening near the center.

p. increta. One which has grown into the uterine myometrium at all contact areas (no cleavage zone).

p. membranacea. One in which the entire ovum is covered by functioning chorionic villi. Syn., *p. diffusa.*

p. neppiformis. See circumvallate *p.*

p. percreta. One which has grown into and through the entire uterine myometrium.

p. previa. A placenta superimposed upon and about the internal os, a condition producing serious hemorrhage during labor.

p. previa centralis. A condition in which the center of the placenta is directly above the internal os.

p. previa marginalis. A condition in which the edge of the placenta meets, but does not overlap, the internal os.

p. previa partialis. A condition in which the edge of the placenta overlies, but does not completely obstruct, the internal os.

p. reflexa. A condition in which a thickening occurs in the peripheral portion of the placenta, giving it a rolled-back appearance.

p. reniformis. A kidney-shaped placenta.

p. spuria. An adjacent, though separate, portion of placental tissue, apparently serving no role in fetal nourishment.

p. succenturiata. An anomalous formation in which one or more accessory lobules are developed in the membrane at a greater or lesser distance from the margin of the placenta, but connected with the latter by vascular channels. Syn., *accessory p.*

retained p. One not expelled by the uterus after labor.

Schultze's p. A mechanism in which the retroplacental hematoma forms in the center, causing this portion to present before the periphery.

septuplex p. See multipartite *p.*

syndesmochorial p. A type in which the chorionic ectoderm is in contact with uterine connective tissue: occurs in ruminants.

tripartite p. A three-lobed one connected by vessels, membranes, and a thinned portion of placenta.

velamentous p. A placenta with the umbilical cord springing from the outer border.

plac″en·ta′tion (plass″en·tay′shun) [*placenta*]. Formation and mode of attachment of the placenta.

pla·cen′tin [*placenta*]. Placental extract formerly used in the cutireaction for pregnancy.

plac″en·ti′tis (plass″en·ty′tis) [*placenta;* G. *-itis,* inflammation]. Inflammation of the placenta.

plac″en·tog′ra·phy [*placenta;* G. *graphein,* to write]. Roentgenography of the placenta after delivery, using a contrast medium.

plac″en·tol′y·sin (plass″en·tol′i·sin, pla·sen″to-lye′sin) [*placenta;* G. *lysis,* a loosing]. A cytolysin formed in the blood of an animal which has received injections of placental tissue emulsions from some other animal.

plac″en·to′ma [*placenta;* G. *-ōma,* tumor]. A neoplasm springing from a retained portion of the placenta.

plac″en·to′sis. See intervillous *thrombosis.*

pla·cen″to·ther′a·py [*placenta;* G. *therapeia,* treatment]. The remedial use of preparations of the placenta of animals.

Plácido da Costa, Antonio (1848–1916). Portuguese ophthalmologist who introduced the keratoscope in examinations of the eye (1882), called *Plácido's disk.*

plac′ode [G. *plax,* anything flat and broad; *eidos,* like]. A platelike epithelial thickening, frequently marking, in the embryo, the anlage of an organ or part.

auditory p. The dorsolateral ectodermal anlage of the internal ear: also called *otic p.*

dorsolateral p. One of a series of ectodermal placodes from which nerves and sense organs of the acoustic and lateral-line systems develop.

epibranchial p. One of a series at the dorsal ends of the visceral grooves that, in some vertebrates, contributes to the adjacent cranial ganglion.

lens p. The ectodermal anlage of the lens of the eye; its formation is induced by the presence of the underlying optic vesicle.

olfactory p. The ectodermal anlage of the olfactory region of the nasal cavity.

otic p. See auditory *p.*

plad″a·ro′ma [G., abundance of fluids]. A soft wart or tumor of the eyelid.

pla″gi·o·ce·phal′ic, pla″gi·o·ceph′a·lous [G. *plagios*, oblique; *kephalē*, head]. Designating a type of pronounced oblique deformation of the skull.

pla″gi·o·ceph′a·lism. See *plagiocephaly.*

pla″gi·o·ceph′a·ly [*plagios; kephalē*]. A type of strongly asymmetric cranial deformation, in which the anterior portion of one side and the posterior portion of the opposite side of the skull are developed more than their counterparts, so that the maximum length of the skull is not in the midline but on a diagonal. Due to a number of causes, such as prenatal, developmental (disordered sequence of suture closure), mechanical (intentional or unintentional). Syn., *wry-head.*

plague [L. *plaga*, plague]. 1. Any contagious, malignant, epidemic disease. 2. A contagious disease endemic in eastern Asia, and in former times occurring epidemically in Europe and Asia Minor. It is an acute febrile disease characterized by inflammation of the lymphatics, with the production of buboes, primary or secondary pneumonia, petechiae and diffuse hemorrhages, and a high mortality. Caused by *Pasteurella pestis.* Primarily a disease of rodents, transmitted to man by fleas.

black p. The plague which decimated the European nations in the 14th century, so called because of the high incidence of hemorrhages.

bubonic p. The usual form of plague, characterized by bubo formation, formerly prevalent in various parts of the world.

cattle p. See *rinderpest.*

fowl p. An acute septicemic disease of domesticated birds caused by *Pasteurella avicida*, characterized by fever, and manifested by weakness, prostration, and a profuse diarrhea.

hunger p. Relapsing fever.

levantine p. The plague of the eastern part of Europe.

lung p. Pleuropneumonia of cattle.

murine p. *Pasteurella pestis* infection of the rat, transmitted from rat to rat and from rat to man primarily by the flea.

p. sore. A sore resulting from the plague.

p. spot. The petechia characteristic of the plague.

p. vaccine. One used for the active immunization against plague; may be of either killed or attenuated living cultures of the organism.

pneumonic p. An extremely virulent type with lung involvement and a high mortality rate.

Siberian cattle p. See *anthrax.*

swine p. See *swine plague.*

sylvatic p. The type transmitted by rodents other than the rat, especially prevalent in wooded or rural areas.

plak·al′bu·min. A protein derived from egg albumin by the action of a proteinase elaborated by *Bacillus subtilis.*

pla′na. Plural of planum.

Planck, Max [*German physicist*, 1858–1947]. Known for his contributions which form the basis of the quantum theory. Nobel laureate (1918).

Planck's con′stant. See quantum *constant.*

plane [L. *planum*, level ground]. Any flat, smooth surface, especially any assumed or conventional surface, whether tangent to the body or dividing it. For subentries not found here, see under *planum.*

alveolocondylean p. The plane of Broca, tangent to the anteroinferior border of the maxillary alveolus and the inferior surfaces of the occipital condyles.

axiobuccolingual p. One parallel with the long axis of a tooth, passing through both the buccal and lingual surfaces.

axiolabiolingual p. One parallel with the long axis of an incisor tooth and passing through its labial and lingual surfaces.

base p. A theoretic horizontal plane upon which an artificial denture is set up.

bite p. An imaginary plane extending from the edge of the upper lip, at rest and relaxed, backward at right angles to the sagittal plane, and parallel with a line drawn from the anterior nasal spine to the lower border of the external auditory meatus. This is the plane to which the bite is constructed. Also called *occlusion plane* (Wilson).

Bolton nasion p. A line joining the Bolton point and nasion on the lateral roentgenogram. It marks the junction of the face and cranium.

cleavage p. 1. The area in a cell or developing ovum where cell division take place. Also see *cleavage.* 2. Any plane in the body along which organs or structures may be separated with minimal damage.

coronal p. A frontal plane, especially one in the head.

datum p. Any one of a number of horizontal planes, determined by certain craniometric points, used by craniometrists in the comparative study of skulls and the making of standardized comparable craniometric records.

fascial p. Any plane in the body which is oriented along a layer of fascia. It usually represents a cleavage plane, and is used for exposure in surgery; it may limit or direct the spread of infection.

focal p. The area perpendicular to the axis of a lens or lens system where an object forms its image.

Frankfort horizontal p. An anthropometric plane for orienting heads of the living as well as skulls in a definite position, so that measurements and contours of a series will be comparable. The F-H was proposed at the Craniometric Congress held in Munich in 1877, and was formally adopted by the International Congress of Anthropologists in Frankfurt-am-Main in 1884, whence its name. The plane was defined as being determined by *four* points, viz. the two *poria* and the two *orbitalia.* In anthropometric practice, only the two poria and left orbitale are the *three* points used to determine the plane, since only in perfectly symmetrical heads or skulls would four points fall in the plane. The plane was adopted because it can be determined easily on the living, making comparison between head and skull possible, and it approximates quite closely the position in which the head is carried during life.

frontal p. Any plane parallel with the long axis of the body and perpendicular to the median plane.

horizontal p. (a) Any transverse plane at right angles to the long axis of the body. (b) *In dentistry*, a plane at right angles with the long axis of a tooth.

inclined p. Any one of the inclined cuspal surfaces of a tooth.

infracostal p. See subcostal *p.*

intertubercular p. A horizontal plane passing

through the tubercles on the crests of the ilia. This plane usually lies at the level of the fifth lumbar vertebra.

lower horizontal p. See intertubercular *p.*

median p. One drawn vertically in the longitudinal axis of the body.

midepigastric p. See transpyloric *p.*

midsagittal p. The median plane.

nuchal p. See *planum* nuchale.

occipital p. See *planum* occipitale.

orbitale p. See *planum* orbitale.

parasagittal p. Any vertical plane parallel to the median plane.

p. of incidence. The plane containing a light ray incident to a surface.

p. of inlet of pelvis. A plane passing through the sacral promontory and the upper border of the symphysis pubis.

p. of outlet of pelvis. A plane passing through the lower border of the symphysis pubis and the tip of the coccyx.

popliteal p. The flat surface on the posterior aspect of the distal end of the femur between condyles.

principal p. A plane normal to the principal axis of a lens, passing through a principal point.

rotate p. *In biology*, wheel-shaped and flat.

sagittal p. A plane which bisects a bilaterally symmetrical body; the median plane.

standard horizontal p. See horizontal *p.*

sternal p. See *planum* sternale.

subcostal p. A horizontal plane passing through the lowest points of the costal arch or the lowest points of the tenth costal cartilages. This plane usually lies at the level of the third lumbar vertebra.

temporal p. See *planum* temporale.

transpyloric p. A horizontal plane through the body at the level of the second lumbar vertebra; the pylorus usually lies in this plane.

transverse p. One at right angles to the long axis of the body; horizontal plane.

umbilical p. A horizontal plane passing through the umbilicus; this plane usually lies at the level of the intervertebral disk between the third and fourth lumbar vertebrae.

upper horizontal p. See subcostal *p.*

visual p. One which passes through the axis of vision of both eyes.

pla′ni·ceps (play′ni·seps, plan′i·) [L. *planus*, flat; *caput*, head]. Flatheaded.

pla·nig′ra·phy. See sectional *radiography.*

pla·nim′e·ter [*planus;* G. *metron*, a measure]. An instrument which measures the area of a plane surface by tracing the periphery.

plan′ing. A method of plastic surgery whereby skin, hardened by freezing, is abraded by means of a burr, sandpaper, or rotating steel-wire brush, to remove permanently scars, pock marks, and superficial skin blemishes.

plank′ton [G. *plagkton*, from *plazesthai*, to wander]. General term for free-floating plants and animals in sea water.

plan′o-, plan- [G. *planos*, a wandering]. A combining form signifying *wandering.*

pla′no- [L. *planus*, flat]. A combining form signifying *flat* or *level.*

pla″no·cel′lu·lar [*planus;* L. *cellula*, small storeroom]. Flat-celled.

pla″no·con′cave [*planus;* L. *concavus*, hollow]. Concave on one surface and flat on the opposite side.

pla″no·con′ic [*planus;* G. *kōnos*, cone]. Having one side flat and the other conical.

pla″no·con′vex [*planus;* L. *convexus*, rounded]. Plane on one side and convex on the other.

plan′o·cyte [G. *planos*, a wandering; *kytos*, cell]. A wandering cell. *Obs.*

pla′no·gram. See *vectorcardiogram, monocardiogram.*

plan″o·ma′ni·a [*planos;* G. *mania*, madness]. A morbid desire for wandering; an impulse to throw off social restraints and live in the wilds.

Pla·nor′bis [L. *planus*, flat; *orbis*, circle]. A genus of fresh-water snails species of which act as intermediate hosts of the flukes causing schistosomiasis in man.

plan′ta [L.]. The sole of the foot.

Plan·ta′go [L.]. Plantain. A genus of weeds, some of which are used medicinally.

P. psyllium. A species, the seeds of which are used in chronic constipation.

plan·ta′go seed (*plantaginis semen*). The cleaned, dried, ripe seed of *Plantago psyllium* or of *P. indica*, known in commerce as Spanish or French psyllium seed; or of *P. ovata*, known in commerce as blonde psyllium or Indian plantago seed. It contains a mucilaginous principle called xylin together with protein, fixed oil, pentosans, and galactans. It is used almost exclusively in medicine in chronic constipation. The gum of the spermoderm, being largely indigestible, retains water and thereby gives bulk and softness to the fecal masses. Dose, 4–15 Gm. (1–4 drams). The seeds should be soaked in water before taking. Also called *psyllium seed, plantain seed.*

plan′tain (plan′tin). See *Plantago.*

plan′tar [L. *planta*, the sole of the foot]. Pertaining to the sole of the foot, as plantar fascia, the dense triangular aponeurosis occupying the sole of the foot beneath the integument.

plan·tar′is (plan·tar′is) [*planta*]. A small muscle of the calf of the leg. See Table of Muscles in the Appendix.

plan′tar wart. A type of verruca, usually multiple, occurring on the sole of the foot; may become quite painful, as the wart cannot grow out from the surface because of pressure. Also called *verruca plantaris.*

plan·ta′tion. A general term including *implantation, replantation,* and *transplantation.*

plan′ti·grade [*planta;* L. *gradi*, to walk]. Walking on the entire sole of the foot, as man and the bear.

plan′u·la [dim. from L. *planus*, flat]. *In embryology*, the embryo at the stage of the two primary germ layers of ectoderm and endoderm in coelenterates.

pla′num (pl. *plana*) [L.]. A plane, or level surface. For subentries not found here, see under *plane.*

p. nuchale. The rough, external surface of the squama occipitalis lying below the superior nuchal lines.

p. occipitale. The relatively smooth, triangular, external surface of the occipital squama lying above the superior nuchal lines.

p. orbitale. The smooth, triangular, superior surface of the maxilla which forms the floor of the orbit.

p. popliteum. A relatively smooth, triangular area on the posterior surface of the distal end of the femur, between the diverging lips of the linea aspera.

p. sternale. The ventral surface of the body of the sternum.

p. temporale. A relatively flat area lying below the linea temporalis inferior and composed of portions of the frontal and parietal bones, great wing of the sphenoid, and squama temporalis.

plaque (plack, plahk) [F.]. A patch.

agar p. See under *agar.*

bacterial plaques. See dental *plaques.*

blood plaques. See *blood* platelets.

dental plaques. Thin, transparent films on the surfaces of teeth made up of mucin and colloidal material secreted by the salivary glands. Depending on the predominant component, mucinous and bacterial plaques are recognized.

milk plaques. Pale-gray plaques in the epicardium without disruption of the continuity of the mesothelium, usually well-defined, roughly circular areas. Cause is unknown. Also called *soldier's spots.*

mucinous plaques. See dental *plaques.*

plasm (plaz′um) [G. *plasma,* anything formed]. 1. Plasma. 2. Old term for a part of the substance of a cell.

germ p. The material basis of inheritance; it is located in the chromosomes.

plas′ma (plaz′muh) [G.]. The fluid portion of blood or lymph, composed of a mixture of many proteins in a crystalloid solution and corresponding closely to the interstitial fluid of the body.

normal human p. The sterile plasma obtained by pooling approximately equal amounts of the liquid portion of citrated whole blood from eight or more healthy humans. The cell-free plasma is separated, sterility tests made, a preservative added, and the plasma distributed into final containers. The plasma so obtained may be stored in three ways: as liquid plasma at a temperature between 2° and 5° C.; by rapid freezing; or by desiccating the frozen plasma in a high vacuum at temperatures below freezing. Plasma is capable of serving all the purposes for which whole blood is employed, except restoration of the hemoglobin, and has the advantages that human plasmas are rarely incompatible with each other and that it can be stored for long periods of time. Also called *citrated normal human p.*

p. accelerator globulin. Proaccelerin.

p. cell. See *plasmacyte.*

p. hydrolysate. An artificial digest of protein derived from bovine blood plasma prepared by a method of hydrolysis sufficient to provide more than half of the total nitrogen present in the form of alpha amino nitrogen. It provides the approximate nutritive equivalent of the source protein in the form of its constituent amino acids. See *travamin.*

p. proteolytic enzyme. Collectively, the proteolytic enzyme (or enzymes) active at or near neutrality; plasmin or fibrinolysin.

p. thromboplastin antecedent (PTA). A clotting factor in normal blood, necessary for the normal elaboration of plasma thromboplastin activity, and distinct from plasma thromboplastinogen and plasma thromboplastin component (PTC). The deficiency of this is called *PTA deficiency.*

p. thromboplastin component (PTC). A clotting factor present in normal blood, necessary for the normal elaboration of plasma thromboplastin activity and distinct from plasma thromboplastinogen and plasma thromboplastin antecedent. The deficiency of this is called *PTC deficiency, hemophilia B,* or *Christmas disease.*

p. thromboplastinogen. See *thromboplastinogen.*

p. tryptase. A proteolytic enzyme, present in plasma in an inactive form, which may be identical with plasmin and fibrinolysin.

p. volume expander. Any synthetic or other blood substitute. See *dextran, periston.*

plas′ma·blast [*plasma;* G. *blastos,* germ]. The stem cell of the plasmacytes. The nucleus has the fine granular structure typical of other blasts, and nucleoli are present. Cytoplasm is characteristically gray-blue-green in color. Also called *lymphoblastic plasma cell.*

plas′ma·cules. See *hemoconia.*

plas′ma·cyte. A fairly large, deeply basophilic mononuclear cell with a lightly staining zone about the centrosome. The nucleus is eccentric with its chromatin arranged in irregular clumps or in a wheel-spoke pattern. They may be multinucleated, and are normally present in bone marrow and other body tissues. They are increased in chronically inflamed regions and multiple myeloma. They are considered by some to be an abnormal form of lymphocyte and by others to be an independent cell series. Also called *plasma cell, Unna's plasma cell, Marschalko's plasma cell, plasmacytoid lymphocyte, myeloma cell.* —**plasmacyt′ic,** *adj.*

plas″ma·cyt′ic se′ries. The cells concerned in the development of plasmacytes. See *plasmablast, proplasmacyte.*

plas″ma·cy′toid lym′pho·cyte. See *plasmacyte.*

plas″ma·cy·to′ma. See *myeloma.*

plas″ma·cy·to′sis. 1. An increase in number of plasmacytes in the spleen, lymph nodes, bone marrow, kidney, or liver. 2. An increase in number of plasmacytes in peripheral blood, occurring in certain infections, usually of virus origin, and occasionally in serum sickness and multiple myeloma.

plas′ma·gel (plaz′muh·jell) [*plasma;* L. *gelare,* to freeze]. That portion of the cytoplasm of a cell whose physical property is that of a gel.

plas′ma·gene [*plasma;* G. *genesthai,* from *gignesthai,* to be produced]. Any independently self-reproducing hereditary particle of the cytoplasm, which is part of the intimate cytoplasmic organization.

plas″ma·lem′ma. Plasma membrane; the cell membrane.

plas·mal′o·gen. One of a group of lipids in which a fatty acid aldehyde in acetal linkage replaces the two fatty acid groups of either α- or β-cephalin. Syn., *acetal-phosphatide.*

plas″ma·pher′e·sis (plaz″muh·ferr′i·sis, ·feer′i·sis) [*plasma;* G. *aphairesis,* a taking away]. The operation of venesection into sodium citrate solution, centrifugalization, washing the blood cells in physiological salt solution and returning them (without the plasma) into the donor's circulation.

plas′ma skim′ming. The phenomenon of plasma without erythrocytes flowing into a side branch of a blood vessel, the erythrocytes continuing along the main channel.

plas′ma·some [*plasma;* G. *sōma,* body]. A granule in cytoplasm.

plas″ma·ther′a·py [*plasma;* G. *therapeia,* treatment]. Treatment, as for shock, by the intravenous injection of blood plasma.

plas·mat′ic (plaz·mat′ick) [*plasma*]. Pertaining to plasma.

plas″ma·tog′a·my [*plasma;* G. *gamos,* marriage]. Cell union in which the nucleus of each remains.

plas″ma·tor·rhex′is. See *plasmorrhexis.*

plas″ma·to′sis [*plasma;* G. *-ōsis,* condition]. The liquefaction of cell substance.

plas′mic (plaz′mick) [*plasma*]. Of, or pertaining to, protoplasm or cytoplasm.

plas′min. A proteolytic enzyme, present in inactive form as plasminogen, occurring in plasma, and responsible for slow digestion and lysis of fibrin clots: sometimes called *plasma tryptase* and *fibrinolysin,* though it is not certain that all these substances are identical.

p. inhibitor. See *antiplasmin.*

plas·min′o·gen. The inactive form of plasmin; when blood is shed over injured tissues, it is converted to plasmin.

plas′mo- (plaz′mo-), **plasm-** [*plasma*]. A combining form meaning *plasma.*

plasmochin. Trade-mark for a brand of pamaquine naphthoate.

plas′mo·crin [*plasma;* G. *krinein,* to separate]. A term applied to crystalloid-filled vacuoles in the cytoplasm of secretory cells, representing a stage in the development of secretory granules.

plas′mo·cyte. See *plasmacyte.*

plas″mo·cy·to′ma (plaz″mo·sigh·to′muh) [*plasma; kytos;* G. *-ōma,* tumor]. Myeloma made up largely of plasma cells.

p. with leukemia. See plasmacytic *leukemia.*

plas·mo·des′m. See *intercellular bridges* under *bridge.*

plas·mo′di·blast. See *syncytiotrophoblast.*

Plas·mo′di·i·dae (plaz·mo′dee·i·dee) [*plasma;* G. *eidos,* form]. A family of the Haemosporidia; contains the genus *Plasmodium* which includes the malaria plasmodia of man, birds, and lower animals.

plas·mo″di·tro′pho·blast (plaz·mo″di·tro′fo-blast, ·trof′o·blast). See *syncytiotrophoblast.*

Plas·mo′di·um [*plasma; eidos*]. A genus of protozoa that causes malaria in birds, lower animals, and man. —**plasmodial,** *adj.*

P. falciparum. That species which is the cause of estivo-autumnal or malignant tertian malaria. See Plates 27, 28.

P. malariae. That species which is the etiologic agent of quartan malaria. See Plates 27, 28.

P. ovale. The species of protozoa which causes tertian or ovale malaria.

P. vivax. That species which causes vivax or benign tertian malaria. See Plates 27, 28, 29.

Plas″mo·dro′ma. A subphylum of protozoa in which the organisms move by means of flagella or pseudopodia. Includes the medically important classes Rhizopoda, Mastigophora, Cnidosporidia, and Sporozoa.

plas·mog′a·my [*plasma;* G. *gamos,* marriage]. Cell fusion.

plas′mo·gen [*plasma;* G. *genesthai,* from *gignesthai,* to be produced]. Formative protoplasm; germ plasm; bioplasm.

plas·mol′y·sis [*plasma;* G. *lysis,* a loosing]. Shrinkage of a cell or its contents, due to withdrawal of water by osmosis. —**plasmolyt′ic,** *adj.*

plas′mo·lyze [*plasma;* G. *lyein,* to loose]. Bring about dissolution or shrinkage of cell protoplasm.

plas·mo′ma. See *myeloma.*

plas′mon [*plasma*]. The hereditary properties of the egg cytoplasm; it stands in contrast to the genome.

plas″mo·nu·cle′ic ac′id. Ribonucleic acid.

plas·mop′ty·sis [*plasma;* G. *ptysis,* a spitting]. The escape of protoplasm from a cell, due to rupture of the cell wall.

plas′mo·quin. See *plasmochin.*

plas″mor·rhex′is [*plasma;* G. *rhēxis,* a breaking]. The rupture of a cell and the escape or loss of the protoplasm.

plasmosan. Trade-mark for *polyvinylpyrrolidone.*

plas·mos′chi·sis (plaz·mos′ki·sis) [*plasma;* G. *schisis,* cleavage]. Protoplasmic fragmentation or cleavage.

plas′mo·sin [*plasma*]. A nucleoprotein found in the cytoplasm of cells; one of the structure proteins.

plas′mo·some [*plasma;* G. *sōma,* body]. 1. The true nucleolus, distinguished from the karyosomes in the nucleus. 2. Old term for any cytoplasmic granule.

plas″mo·trop′ic [*plasma;* G. *trepein,* to turn]. Producing excessive hemolysis in the liver, spleen, and bone marrow.

plas·mot′ro·pism [*plasma; trepein*]. Destruction of red cells in the organs producing them, as the spleen and bone marrow. *Obs.*

plas′mo·zyme [*plasma;* G. *zymē,* leaven]. Prothrombin; thrombogen.

plas′te·in. A product of interaction between a protein digest and either pepsin or papain.

plas′ter [G. *emplastron,* plaster]. 1. Substance intended for external application, made of such materials and of such consistency as to adhere to the skin. 2. Calcined gypsum or calcium sulfate.

adhesive p. (*emplastrum adhaesivum*). A mixture having pressure-sensitive adhesive properties, spread evenly upon fabric, the back of which may be coated with a water-repellent film. The adhesive mixture usually consists of rubber, resins, waxes with one or more fillers of absorbent powder, such as zinc oxide, orris root, or starch. Types of adhesive plaster, differing in the kind of fabric used, intended for special uses, are extensively employed. Also called *adhesive tape.*

court p. A solution of isinglass made with alcohol, glycerin, and hot water spread on silk and allowed to dry. Used to hide blemishes or close small wounds.

mustard p. That made by mixing mustard and flour with water.

p. of Paris. See *calcium* sulfate.

plas′tic [G. *plastikos,* fit for molding]. 1. Formative; concerned with building up tissues, restoring lost parts, repairing or rectifying malformations or defects, etc., as plastic surgery, plastic operation, plastic repair. 2. Capable of being molded.

plas′tic. Material, such as celluloid, proteins, resins, etc., which can be molded during processing, by heat or pressure.

plas′tic force. The generative force of the body.

plas·tic′i·ty (plas·tiss′i·tee) [*plastikos*]. The quality of being plastic.

plas″ti·ciz′er. A substance incorporated in an organic formulation or substance to maintain it in a plastic condition, preventing or retarding cracking or development of brittleness.

plas′tic lymph. The inflammatory exudate that covers wounds or inflamed serous surfaces, and becomes organized by the development in it of blood vessels and connective tissues.

plas′tics [*plastikos*]. *In dentistry,* those filling materials, such as amalgam, gutta-percha, and various cements, which are soft at the time of insertion, and may then be shaped and molded.

plas′tid [G. *plassein,* to form]. 1. A hypothetical elementary organism; a cytode. 2. Any of certain small cytoplasmic bodies in plant cells, regarded as seats of the chemical activities of the cells.

plas′ti·dule [*plassein*]. See *biophore.*

plas′tin [*plassein*]. The substance forming the more solid portion of protoplasm, such as the linin or the cytospongioplasm.

plas″to·dy·na′mi·a (plas″to·dye·nay′mee·uh, ·nam′ee·uh [G. *plastos,* formed; *dynamis,* power]. Growth potential.

plas·tog′a·my [*plastos;* G. *gamos,* marriage]. Cytoplasmic fusion as contrasted with nuclear fusion.

plas′to·gene [*plastos;* G. *genesthai,* from *gignesthai,* to be produced]. The basic self-reproducing unit of the plastids of plants.

plas′to·some. See *mitochondria.*

-plas′ty [G. *plassein,* to form, mold]. Combining form denoting *plastic surgery.* See *plastic* (*adj.*), 1.

plate [OF.]. 1. A flattened part, especially a flattened process of bone. 2. A thin piece of metal or some other substance to which artificial teeth are attached. 3. *In microbiology,* a shallow, cylindrical, covered culture dish; also such a dish containing solid cultural medium suitable for the growth of microorganisms; a petri dish. 4. *In orthopedics,* a metallic device used with screws or bolts for internal fixation of bone.

agar-streak p. See under *agar.*

alar p. The lateral wall of the neural tube dorsal

to the sulcus limitans, associated with sensory nerves. Syn., *alar lamina*.

anal p. The anal membrane.

auditory p. The bony plate forming the roof of the external auditory meatus.

axial p. The primitive streak of the embryo.

basal p. of cranium. A cartilaginous plate of the embryonic cranium representing the fused parachordal plates of lower forms. It is the predecessor of the occipital bone.

basal p. of gravid uterus. That part of the decidua basalis incorporated into the placenta, including its covering of basal ectoderm from the trophoblast.

basal p. of neural tube. The lateral wall of the neural tube ventral to the sulcus limitans; motor in function. Syn., *basal lamina*.

base p. *In dentistry*, a rigid or semirigid substance adapted to a cast. It is part of a bite plate, and is sometimes incorporated in a completed denture.

bite p. *In dentistry*, a base plate and the plastic material attached to it, used to establish the proper relationship of the jaws to each other and to adjacent oral structures.

cardiogenic p. An area of splanchnic mesoderm at the cephalic margin of the embryonic area below the coelom that gives rise to the endothelial tubes of the embryonic heart.

cell p. The equatorial thickening of the spindle fibers from which the intercellular septum arises in the division of plant cells. It is vestigial in some animals. Syn., *midbody*.

chorionic p. The chorionic membrane of the placental region, formed externally by the trophoblast layer and internally by a fibrous lining layer of mesoderm.

cloacal p. The cloacal membrane.

closing p. Any epithelial membrane, usually bilaminar, closing a potential orifice; especially one separating a visceral groove and pouch.

cough plates. Those coated with boiled potato, glycerin, agar, and blood mixture, on which a pertussis patient coughs.

cribriform p. 1. The horizontal plate of the ethmoid bone, part of the floor of the anterior cranial fossa, perforated for the passage of the olfactory nerves. 2. The bone lining a dental alveolus: also called *alveolar bone proper, lamina dura*.

culture p. A culture of bacteria within a Petri dish.

cuticular p. An oar-shaped plate associated with the supporting cells of the organ of Corti.

cutis p. The dermatome.

dorsal p. One of the two longitudinal ridges on the dorsal surface of the embryo which subsequently join to form the neural canal.

end-p. See motor end-*p*.

epiphyseal p. (a) The broad, articular surface with slightly elevated rim on each end of the centrum of a vertebra. Syn., *epiphyseal disk.* (b) The thin cartilage mass between an epiphysis and the shaft of a bone; the site of growth in length. It is obliterated by epiphyseal union.

equatorial p. The compressed mass of chromosomes aggregated at the equator of the nuclear spindle during karyokinesis.

floor p. The ventral wall of the embryonic neural tube, ependymal in structure.

foot p. The flat part of the stapes.

frontal p. In the fetus, a cartilaginous plate interposed between the lateral parts of the ethmoid cartilage and the lesser wings and anterior portion of the sphenoid bone.

Kowarsky's p. A small plate composed of two layers of copper used in preparation of heat-fixed blood smears.

Lane p. See William Arbuthnot *Lane*.

lateral p. The thickened side walls of the neural tube.

lateral pterygoid p. A broad, thin plate whose lateral surface forms part of the medial wall of the infratemporal fossa and gives attachment to the external pterygoid muscle, and whose medial surface forms part of the pterygoid fossa and gives attachment to the internal pterygoid muscle.

meatal p. A solid mass of cells seen in a two-month embryo, formed by the ingrowth of ectoderm from the bottom of the branchial groove toward the tympanic cavity.

medial pterygoid p. A long, narrow plate whose lateral surface forms part of the pterygoid fossa and whose medial surface constitutes the lateral boundary of the choana. Its lower extremity forms a hook, the pterygoid hamulus, for the tendon of the tensor veli palatini.

medullary p. Neural plate, dorsal plate.

Moore blade p. See Austin Talley *Moore*.

motor end-p. A small mass of sarcoplasm formed beneath the sarcolemma at the junction of nerve and muscle fibers. It receives the terminal ramifications of the naked axis cylinder of a somatic motor nerve.

muscle p. A myotome.

nail p. The nail.

neural p. The thickened ectodermal plate overlying the head process that differentiates into the neural tube.

notochordal p. A plate of cells representing the root of the head process of the embryo after the latter becomes vesiculated. The plate becomes intercalated in the dorsal wall of the vesicle and later consolidates into the notochord.

nuclear p. (a) The metaphase chromosomes arranged along the equatorial plate. (b) The septum which sometimes divides the nucleus in amitotic division.

oral p. See stomodeal *p*.

orbital p. One of two thin, triangular plates of the frontal bone which form the vaults of the orbits.

paper-disk p. A filter-paper disk soaked with an antibiotic test solution and placed on the surface of seeded agar plates, to determine the zone of inhibition resulting from the diffusion of the antibiotic into the surrounding medium in the course of incubation.

parachordal p. See basal *p*. of cranium.

perpendicular p. A thin, flat, polygonal lamina of the ethmoid bone which assists in forming the septum of the nose.

petri, Petri p. See *plate*, 3: also called *petri dish*.

pour p. A bacterial culture in which the culture is incorporated into a medium, poured into a sterile petri dish, and allowed to solidify.

primitive joint p. The primary rudiment of a joint which is formed by a separate thickening of mesenchyme between the thickenings which are the forerunners of the bones to be joined.

primitive p. The floor of the primitive groove.

prochordal p. A region of thickened endoderm immediately anterior to the notochord and in direct contact with the ectoderm. It forms a part of the buccopharyngeal membrane.

pterygoid plates. Two plates into which the pterygoid process of the sphenoid bone divides.

roof p. The dorsal wall of the embryonic neural tube, ependymal in structure.

screening p. One using solid media for distinguishing the effect of some particular agent on bacteria, e.g., incorporation of antibiotics and notation of zones of inhibition, and susceptibility of *Salmonella typhi* to different bacteriophage types.

Sherman p. See Harry Mitchell *Sherman.*

sinus p. A median plate of epithelium within the glans penis of the embryo which later takes part in the formation of the external urethral orifice.

slotted p. *In orthopedics,* a steel plate with slots at either end in which screws are placed, allowing for compression of fractured bone fragments while being maintained in contact.

spiral p. Spiral lamina.

stomodeal p. A sheet of ectoderm and endoderm which separates the stomodeum from the originally blind end of the foregut. Also called *oral p., buccopharyngeal membrane.*

streak p. A bacterial culture within a Petri dish formed by streaking across the culture medium with a loopful of bacterial suspension.

sucking p. *In dentistry,* a plate constructed so as to be held in place largely by atmospheric pressure.

tarsal p. A thin, elongated plate of dense connective tissue which contributes to the form and support of an eyelid.

terminal p. The thin plate of bone of an epiphysis laid down on the metaphyseal surface preceding epiphyseal union.

Townsend and Gilfillan p. A plate used for treating, by open reduction, tibial shatter fractures; the plate is screwed to the tibial shaft, and extends upward to receive a bolt transfixing the condylar fragments.

tympanic p. The bony sides and floor of the external auditory meatus.

urethral p. A solid plate of endodermal cells, derived from the endoderm of the urogenital membrane, that temporarily obliterates the cavity of the phallic part of the urogenital sinus and later forms a large part of the penile urethra.

vacuum p. *In dentistry,* a plate on which artificial teeth are mounted, having an air chamber to assist in its retention in the mouth.

pla·teau′ [F.]. In operating Geiger counter tubes, the voltage range over which the number of impulses recorded is nearly constant.

plate cul′ture. A method of obtaining pure cultures of bacteria by the inoculation of a solid cultural medium in a petri dish with microorganisms. The inoculum may be distributed over the surface of the medium (streak plate) or incorporated within it (pour plate).

plate′let [dim. from OF. *plate,* plate]. See *blood* platelets, *thrombocyte.* See Plate 26.

pla′ting [*plate*]. *In microbiology,* the inoculation of solid cultural medium in a dish with microorganisms. The inoculum may be distributed over the surface of the medium or incorporated within it.

pla·tin′ic [Sp. *plata,* silver]. Referring to a compound containing platinum as a tetravalent element.

plat′i·nous [*plata*]. Referring to a compound containing platinum as a divalent element.

plat′i·num [*plata*]. Pt = 195.23. A silver-white metal occurring natively or alloyed with other metals. It is fusible only at very high temperatures, and is insoluble in all acids except nitrohydrochloric. On account of these properties, it is extensively used for chemical apparatus, crucibles, foils, wire; it is also employed as a reagent. Platinum occurs, aside from its ordinary metallic form, as a spongy mass (spongy platinum) and as a fine metallic powder (platinum black), which is capable of absorbing many times its volume of oxygen, and hence acts as a powerful oxidizing agent. Platinum forms two types of compounds: platinous, in which it is divalent, and platinic, in which it is tetravalent. It is no longer used medicinally.

Platner, Johann Zacharias [*German physician,* 1694–1747]. Remembered for his part in drawing attention to the tuberculous origin of kyphosis of the spine (1744). Described crystals of sodium glycocholate and taurocholate from urine containing an excess of bile; called *Platner's crystals.*

plat′ode, plat′oid [G. *platys,* broad; *eidos,* form]. *In biology,* broad or flat, as a worm.

plat″o·nych′i·a (plat″o·nick′ee·uh) [*platys;* G *onyx,* nail]. Rare dystrophy of the nail; consisting of a modification of its greatest curvature, which, instead of being transverse, as normally, is lengthwise.

p. acuta abrata. Psoriasiform eruption and lesions of fingernails, consisting of round, whitish, soft, thickened spots in the center of each nail except that of the middle finger.

platradon. Trade name for platinum radon seeds.

plat′y-, plat- [G. *platys,* broad]. A combining form meaning *broad, flat.*

plat″y·ba′si·a (plat″i·bay′see·uh) [*platys;* G. *basis,* base]. A developmental deformity of the occipital bone and upper cervical spine, in which the foramen magnum is small and misshapen, the atlas is occipitalized, and the odontoid process of the axis impinges on the brain stem. It is accompanied by neurologic symptoms and signs referable to changes in the medulla, cervical spinal cord, and lower cranial nerves.

plat″y·ce′li·an (plat″i·see′lee·un, ·sell′ee·un), **plat″y·ce′lous** (plat″i·see′lus, ·sell′us) [*platys;* G. *koilos,* hollow]. Concave in front and convex behind.

plat″y·ce·phal′ic [*platys;* G. *kephalē,* head]. Characterizing a person having a skull with a flat vertex. —**platyceph′aly,** *n.*

plat″yc·ne′mi·a (plat″ick·nee′mee·uh) [*platys;* G. *knēmē,* leg]. *In osteometry,* a pronounced mediolateral flattening of the diaphysis of the tibia, determined by a cnemic index of 64.9 or less: also called *platycnemism.*

plat″yc·ne′mic [*platys; knēmē*]. Designating a tibia with a marked mediolateral flattening.

plat″y·co′ri·a, plat″y·co·ri′a·sis [*platys;* G. *korē,* pupil]. Expansion of the pupil; mydriasis.

Plat″y·hel·min′thes (plat″i·hel·minth′eez) [*platys;* G. *helmins,* worm]. A phylum of flatworms characterized by bilaterally symmetrical, many-celled, leaf-shaped bodies lacking a body cavity and usually containing both sexual elements. Includes the medically important classes Trematoda and Cestoda.

plat″y·hi·er′ic (plat″i·high·err′ick) [*platys;* G. *hieron osteon,* os sacrum]. *In osteometry,* designating a sacrum that is greater in width than in length, with a hieric index of 106 or more.

plat″y·mer′ic (plat″i·merr′ick, ·meer′ick) [*platys;* G. *mēros,* thigh]. *In osteometry,* designating a femur with a moderate anteroposterior compression and an increased mediolateral diameter in the proximal portion of the diaphysis; having a platymeric index of 75.0 to 84.9.

plat″y·mor′phi·a [*platys;* G. *morphē,* form]. A flatness in the formation of the eye and shortening of the anteroposterior diameter, resulting in hyperopia.

plat″y·o′pi·a [*platys;* G. *ōps,* eye]. Relative flatness of the root of the nose with relation to the biorbital width, designated by craniometric methods by an orbitonasal index of 107.5 or less.

plat″y·o′pic [*platys; ōps*]. 1. *In craniometry,* designating a facial skeleton that is flat; having an orbitonasal index of 107.5 or less. 2. *In somatometry,* designating a face that is flat; having an orbitonasal index of 109.9 or less.

plat″y·pel′lic [*platys;* G. *pella,* basin]. *In osteometry,* designating a pelvis with a transverse diameter considerably greater than the conjugata vera, having a pelvic-inlet index of 89.9 or less.

plat″y·pel′loid. See *platypellic.*

plat′yr·rhine (plat′i·ryne, ·rin) [*platys;* G. *rhis,* nose]. 1. *In somatometry,* having a broad and flat nose with a height-breadth index of 85.0 or more. 2. *In craniometry,* having a very wide apertura piriformis with a nasal index of 51.0 or more. 3. *In taxonomy,* pertaining to the Platyrrhina or New World monkeys, so named because of their broad nasal septum and wide space between the nostrils. The term is practically replaced in its application to the human nose by *chamaerrhine.*

pla·tys′ma (pla·tiz′muh) [G., flat object]. A subcutaneous muscle in the neck, extending from the face to the clavicle. Formerly called *platysma myoides.* See Table of Muscles in the Appendix.

plat″ys·ten″ce·pha′li·a, plat″ys·ten·ceph′a·ly [G. *platys,* broad; *egkephalos,* brain]. The condition of a skull very wide at the occiput and with prominent jaws.

Plaut, Hugo Karl [*German physician,* 1858–1928]. Described a type of ulcerative membranous infection, chiefly of the tonsils; called *Plaut's angina, Vincent's angina, Plaut-Vincent's disease.*

plavolex. A trade-mark for *dextran.*

Playfair, William Smoult [*English physician,* 1836–1903]. Remembered as the advocate in England of the rest cure for neurasthenia, first proposed and used by Silas Weir Mitchell; called *Weir Mitchell treatment, Playfair's treatment.*

pledg′et [uncertain in origin]. A small, flattened compress of cotton, gauze, etc.

plei′o- (ply′o-), **pleo-** [G. *pleiōn,* more]. A combining form meaning *more.*

plei·ot′ro·pism (plye·ot′ro·piz·um) [*pleiōn;* G. *trepein,* to turn]. The occurrence of multiple effects produced by a given gene. —**pleiotrop′ic,** *adj.*

ple″o·chro′ic [*pleiōn;* G. *chroia,* color]. The capacity of a substance to show more than one color.

ple·och′ro·ism (plee·ock′ro·iz·um) [*pleiōn; chroia*]. The property possessed by some bodies, especially crystals, of presenting different colors when viewed in the direction of different axes. —**pleochroit′ic, pleochromat′ic,** *adj.*

ple″o·cy·to′sis (plee″o·sigh·to′sis) [*pleiōn; kytos;* G. *-ōsis,* condition]. Increase of cells in the cerebrospinal fluid.

ple″o·mas′ti·a, ple″o·ma′zi·a [*pleiōn;* G. *mastos,* breast]. See *polymastia.*

ple″o·mor′phism [*pleiōn;* G. *morphē,* form]. The occurrence of widely different forms of the same species; applied especially to bacteria and to malignant cells. —**pleomorphic, pleomorphous,** *adj.*

ple′o·nasm (plee′o·naz·um) [G. *pleonasma,* superfluity]. Any deformity marked by superabundance of certain organs or parts. —**pleonas′tic,** *adj.*

ple″o·nec′tic [G. *pleonektikos,* greedy]. 1. Pertaining to, or characterized by, pleonexia. 2. Pertaining to blood having more than the normal saturation of oxygen.

ple″o·nex′i·a [G., greediness]. 1. Excessive desire to have or to possess. 2. Increased body resistance.

ple″on·os″te·o′sis [G. *pleiōn,* more; *osteon,* bone; *-ōsis,* condition]. Excessive or premature ossification.

p. of Léri. A rare hereditary condition characterized by thickening and deformity of the digits, limited joint movements, short stature, and mongoloid facies.

ple″o·no′tus [*pleiōn;* G. *ous,* ear]. An earlike appendage located on the neck; cervical auricle.

ple″ro·cer′coid [G. *plērēs,* full; *kerkos,* tail; *eidos,* form]. The second larval stage in the second intermediate host of certain cestodes.

ple·ro′sis [G., a filling]. 1. The restoration of lost tissue. 2. Plethora.

ple″si·o·gnath′us [G. *plēsios,* near; *gnathos,* jaw]. An accessory mouth in the parotid region.

ple″si·o·mor′phism (plee″see·o·mor′fiz·um, pless″ee·o·) [*plēsios;* G. *morphē,* form]. Similarity in form.

ple″si·o′pi·a (plee″see·o′pee·uh, pless″ee·) [*plēsios;* G. *ōps,* eye]. Increased convexity of the crystalline lens, producing myopia.

pless″es·the′si·a (pless″ess·thee′zhuh, ·zee·uh) [G. *plēssein,* to strike; *aisthēsis,* perception]. Palpatory percussion performed by placing the left middle finger firmly against the body surface and percussing with the index finger of the right hand, allowing it to remain in contact with the left finger for a few seconds.

ples·sim′e·ter. See *pleximeter.*

ples′sor. See *plexor.*

pleth′o·ra, ple·tho′ra [G., fullness]. A state characterized by excess of blood in the body. —**plethor′ic,** *adj.*

p. apocoptica. A temporary increase in the volume of the blood in other parts of the body, caused by forcing blood from a part to be amputated.

ple·thys′mo·gram. A record made by a plethysmograph.

ple·thys′mo·graph (pli·thiz′mo·graf, ·thiss′mo·graf) [G. *plēthysmos,* a making multiple; *graphein,* to write]. A device for ascertaining the change in volume of an organ or part, through an increase in the quantity of the blood therein.

pleth″ys·mog′ra·phy (pleth″iz·mog′ruh·fee, pleth″iss·) [*plēthysmos; graphein*]. Measurement of volume changes of an extremity or of an organ.

pleu′ra (pl. *pleurae*) [G., rib]. The serous membrane enveloping the lung (**pulmonary** or **visceral pleura**), and lining the internal surface of the thoracic cavity (**parietal pleura**). —**pleural,** *adj.*

costal p. The portion of the parietal pleura which lines the bony wall of the thoracic cavity.

diaphragmatic p. The reflection of the parietal pleura upon the upper surface of the diaphragm.

mediastinal p. A continuation of the parietal pleura covering the side of the mediastinum.

pericardiac p. The portion of the parietal pleura contiguous to the pericardium.

pleu″ra·cen·te′sis. See *pleurocentesis.*

pleu″ra·cot′o·my [*pleura;* G. *tomē,* a cutting]. Incision of the thoracic wall and pleura, usually exploratory. Also called *thoracotomy.*

pleu·ral′gi·a [*pleura;* G. *algos,* pain]. Pain in the pleura or in the side; intercostal neuralgia. —**pleuralgic,** *adj.*

pleu·ram′ni·on [*pleura;* G. *amnion,* inner membrane around the fetus]. An amnion developing by folds, as in sauropsidans and some mammals. See *schizamnion.*

pleu″ra·poph′y·sis [*pleura;* G. *apophysis,* process]. One of the lateral processes of a vertebra, having the morphologic valence of a rib. —**pleurapophys′eal,** *adj.*

pleur′a·tome. The areas of the pleura supplied with sensory fibers from a single spinal nerve.

pleu·rec′to·my [*pleura;* G. *ektomē,* excision]. Excision of any portion of the pleura.

pleu′rin. An antibiotic derived from a species of Basidiomycetes.

pleu′ri·sy [G. *pleuritis,* pleurisy]. Inflammation of the pleura; pleuritis.

acute p. A type with a sudden onset in which the exudate may be fibrinous, fibrinoserous, purulent, putrid, or hemorrhagic. It may develop in the course of bacteremia, bacteria occasionally being recovered, or originate from infection of the underlying lung as a part of pneumonia, or from inflammatory processes in the mediastinum or other neighboring structures. Characterized by fever, pain with breathing, and crepitation or friction sounds on auscultation.

adhesive p. A form of fibrinous pleurisy in which fibrinous bands extend from the parietal to the visceral pleura.

chronic p. A slowly developing type, usually adhesive, as that seen in tuberculosis.

diaphragmatic p. Pleurisy of the upper surface of the diaphragm.

encapsulated p. Walled-off pocket of exudate in the pleural space.

fibrinous p. Pleurisy in which there is a fibrinous exudate; it may be the primary infection or a complication of another inflammatory condition of the lung or of infections such as pericarditis or periostitis of the ribs. Also called *dry p.*

hemorrhagic p. A type in which the exudate is serosanguineous, usually associated with tuberculosis or a malignant disease.

interlobar p. Localized inflammation of pleural surfaces between the lobes of the lung.

plastic p. A form of adhesive pleurisy in which a small amount of exudate causes extensive pleural changes resulting in a decrease of the hemithorax.

p. root. Asclepias.

purulent p. Empyema; pyothorax; suppurative inflammation of the pleura.

rheumatic p. A type which is fibrinous, later becoming fibrinoserous: a complication of rheumatic fever.

serous p. Pleurisy with effusion.

suppurative p. See *empyema.*

pleu·rit′ic [G. *pleuritikos*, suffering from pleurisy]. Pertaining to, affected with, or of the nature of, pleurisy.

pleu·ri′tis. See *pleurisy.*

pleu′ro-, pleur- [G. *pleura*, rib]. A combining form denoting *connection with the pleura* or *with a side* or *rib.*

pleu″ro·cen·te′sis [*pleura;* G. *kentēsis*, a pricking]. Puncture of the pleura. Also called *thoracentesis.*

pleu″ro·cen′trum (pl. *pleurocentra*) [*pleura;* G. *kentron*, center]. The lateral half of a vertebral body, as in a cleft centrum, or when only a lateral half is ossified. Also called *hemicentrum.* —**pleurocentral,** *adj.*

pleu″ro·chol″e·cys·ti′tis (·kol″i·sis·tye′tis, ·ko″li·) [*pleura;* G. *cholē*, bile; *kystis*, bladder; *-itis*, inflammation]. Inflammation of the gallbladder, with involvement of the pleura.

pleu″ro·cu·ta′ne·ous [*pleura;* L. *cutis*, skin]. In relation with the pleura and the skin, as pleurocutaneous fistula.

pleu′ro·dont [*pleura;* G. *odous*, tooth]. Having teeth affixed to the side of the bone which supports them, as certain lower vertebrates. See *acrodont, thecodont.*

pleu″ro·dy′ni·a [*pleura;* G. *odynē*, pain]. A syndrome of unknown cause, characterized by abrupt onset and severe pain, most commonly in the abdominal wall and intercostal spaces, and generally accompanied by mild fever.

epidemic p. That observed in epidemics and occurring usually in children and young adults. Syn., *Bornholm disease, devil's grip, epidemic myalgia.*

pleu″ro·gen′ic, pleu·rog′e·nous (ploo·rodj′i·nus) [*pleura;* G. *genesthai*, from *gignesthai*, to be produced]. Originating in the pleura.

pleu″ro·hep·a·ti′tis [*pleura;* G. *hēpar*, liver; *-itis*, inflammation]. Inflammation of the liver and diaphragmatic part of the pleura.

pleu′ro·lith [*pleura;* G. *lithos*, stone]. A calculus in the pleura or the pleural space.

pleu·rol′y·sis [*pleura;* G. *lysis*, a loosing]. Separation of the parietal pleura from the chest wall.

pleu·ro′ma. Mesothelioma of the pleura.

pleu″ro·me′lus [*pleura;* G. *melos*, limb]. An individual having a parasitic or accessory limb arising from the thorax laterally.

pleu″ro·mu·til′in. An antibiotic, $C_{22}H_{34}O_5$, isolated from culture liquids of the Basidiomycete *Pleurotus mutilus.*

pleu″ro·per″i·car′di·al [*pleura;* G. *perikardios*, around the heart]. Pertaining to both pleura and pericardium.

pleu″ro·per″i·car·di′tis [*pleura; perikardios;* G. *-itis*, inflammation]. Pleurisy associated with pericarditis.

pleu″ro·pneu·mo′ni·a. Combined pleurisy and pneumonia.

bovine p. A disease of cattle, characterized by extensive consolidation and subpleural effusion in one or both lungs, caused by a pleuropneumonialike organism (proposed name, *Bovimyces pleuropneumoniae*) numerous in the serous exudate. It spreads slowly in herds, and occurs throughout the world except in India, western Europe, and North America.

pleu″ro·pneu·mo′nia·like or′gan·isms. Highly pleomorphic, filterable microorganisms, usually stained by special methods, which can be cultured on infusion mediums enriched by high concentrations of serum or ascitic fluid. One form is the causative agent of bovine pleuropneumonia. Pathogenicity for man has not been established, but it is suggested that the organisms may contribute to, or cause inflammation of, the cervix, arthritis, Reiter's syndrome, and a venereal disease not yet named. Abbreviated, PPLO or L organisms.

pleu″ro·pneu″mo·ni′tis. Inflammation of the lungs and pleura.

radiation p. See radiation *pneumonitis.*

pleu″ro·pros″o·pos′chi·sis (ploor″o·pros″o·pos′ki·sis) [*pleura;* G. *prosōpon*, face; *schisis*, cleavage]. A general term for oblique and transverse facial clefts.

pleu″ro·pul′mo·nar″y (ploor″o·pul′mo·nerr″ee) [*pleura;* L. *pulmo*, lung]. Pertaining to the pleura and the lungs.

pleu·ros′co·py [*pleura;* G. *skopein*, to examine]. Examination of the pleural cavity. See *thoracoscopy.*

pleu″ro·so′ma [*pleura;* G. *sōma*, body]. Fissure of both abdomen and thorax with lateral eventration and atrophy or imperfect development of the arm on the side of the eventration.

pleu″ro·so″ma·tos′chi·sis (ploor″o·so″muh·tos′ki·sis) [*pleura; sōma;* G. *schisis*, a cleavage]. Lateral abdominal fissure.

pleu″ro·so′mus [*pleura; sōma*]. A monster exhibiting pleurosoma.

pleu′ro·spasm [*pleura;* G. *spasmos*, spasm]. Cramp, or spasm in the side, of pleural origin.

pleu″ros·thot′o·nos. See *pleurothotonos.*

pleu″ro·thot′o·nos [G. *pleurothen*, from the side; *tonos*, tension]. A form of tetanic spasm of the muscles in which the body is bent to one side.

pleu′ro·tin. An antibiotic substance derived from the fungus *Pleurotus griseus*, active, in vitro, against several species of bacteria.

pleu·rot′o·my [G. *pleura*, rib; *tomē*, a cutting]. Incision into the pleura.

pleu″ro·ty′phoid [*pleura;* G. *typhōdēs*, delirious]. Typhoid fever with involvement of the pleura.

pleu"ro·vis'cer·al [*pleura;* L. *viscera,* inner organs]. Pertaining to the pleura or side, and to the viscera.

plex'i·form [L. *plexus,* a twining; *forma,* form]. Resembling a network or plexus.

plexiglas. Trade-mark for a transparent plastic.

plex·im'e·ter [G. *plēxis,* stroke; *metron,* a measure]. 1. A finger, usually the left third finger, held firmly against the skin to receive the stroke in indirect percussion. 2. A small, thin, oblong plate of hard but flexible material, such as ivory or rubber, used for the same purpose. Also called *plessimeter.*

plex'or [*plēxis*]. 1. A finger, when used to tap the surface of the body in performing percussion. 2. A small hammer with rubber head used for the same purpose. Also called *percussion hammer.*

plex'us [L., a twining]. A network of interlacing nerves or anastomosing blood vessels or lymphatics. See Tables of Nerves and of Veins in the Appendix. —**plexal,** *adj.*

anococcygeal p. A nerve plexus formed from the anterior branches of the fifth sacral and coccygeal nerves and part of the anterior branch of the fourth sacral nerve.

anterior sacral p. A venous plexus which connects the sacral intervertebral veins with the lumbar and pelvic veins.

aortic p. A fine network of sympathetic nerves surrounding the aorta; continuous around both the thoracic and abdominal portions of the aorta through the aortic opening in the diaphragm.

atrial p. A nerve plexus found in the embryo surrounding the atrial region of the heart.

Auerbach's p. See myenteric *p.*

axillary p. A plexus of lymph nodes and lymphatic vessels in the axilla.

basilar p. A venous plexus over the basilar part of the occipital bone connecting the two inferior petrosal sinuses and the marginal and internal vertebral plexuses. See Table of Veins in the Appendix.

Batson's p. See vertebral venous *system.*

brachial p. A plexus of nerves located in the neck and axilla and composed of the anterior rami of the lower four cervical and first thoracic nerves. See Plate 16.

bulbar p. A nerve plexus found in the embryo surrounding the bulbus cordis.

cardiac p. A network of nerves situated at the base of the heart. The superficial part lies beneath the arch of the aorta just anterior to the right pulmonary artery. The deep part of the cardiac plexus lies anterior to the bifurcation of the trachea between it and the arch of the aorta. Each portion contains nerve fibers of both sympathetic and vagal origin.

carotid plexuses. Nerves of the sympathetic system surrounding the internal, external, and common carotid arteries, respectively.

cavernous p. 1. A nerve plexus associated with the corpus cavernosum of the penis or clitoris. 2. A sympathetic plexus in the cavernous sinus surrounding the internal carotid artery.

cavernous p. of nasal conchae. See *p.* cavernosi concharum.

celiac p. A large sympathetic plexus lying in front of the aorta around the origin of the celiac artery. It is formed by fibers from the splanchnic and vagus nerves and is distributed to the abdominal viscera.

cephalic ganglionated p. The four parasympathetic ganglions in close topographic relation to the branches of the fifth cranial nerve, known as the ciliary, sphenopalatine, otic, and submandibular ganglions, and connected by fine nerve filaments with the superior cervical ganglion of the sympathetic system.

cervical p. A plexus in the neck formed by the anterior branches of the upper four cervical nerves.

cervical posterior p. A nerve plexus derived from the posterior branches of the first, second, and third cervical nerves lying beneath the semispinalis muscle. Also called *posterior cervical p. of Cruveilhier.*

cervicothoracic p. The cervical and brachial plexuses considered together.

chorioid p. See choroid *p.*

choroid p. One of the longitudinal, lobulated, invaginated processes, consisting of a vascular plexus and a covering of ependyma, which project into the third, fourth, and lateral ventricles of the brain.

coccygeal p. One formed by the union of the anterior branches of the coccygeal nerve and the fifth sacral nerve with a communicating filament from the fourth sacral nerve.

corneal p. A nerve plexus of the cornea, derived from the ciliary nerves and divided into three parts: an **annular c. p.** about the periphery of the cornea; a **subepithelial c. p.** beneath the corneal epithelium; an **intraepithelial c. p.**

coronary p. A continuation of the cardiac plexus, arbitrarily divided into a larger posterior part which accompanies the left coronary artery and is distributed chiefly to the left atrium and ventricle and a smaller anterior part which follows the right coronary artery and is distributed to the right atrium and ventricle.

crural p. A nerve plexus surrounding the upper portion of the femoral artery. Syn., *femoral p.*

cystic p. A nerve plexus near the gallbladder.

deferential p. A nerve plexus surrounding the ductus deferens and seminal vesicle.

dental p. A plexus of nerve fibers in the alveolar canals of each jaw. That of the upper jaw is formed by branches of the infraorbital (maxillary) nerve and that of the lower jaw is derived from the inferior alveolar nerve.

diaphragmatic p. A nerve plexus near the inferior phrenic artery.

enteric p. The myenteric and submucosal plexuses considered together.

epigastric p. Celiac plexus.

esophageal p. A nerve plexus surrounding the esophagus.

extraspinal p. A large venous plexus extending the length of the vertebral column and lying between it and the multifidus muscle.

facial p. A nerve plexus enveloping part of the external maxillary artery.

femoral p. A nerve plexus surrounding the femoral artery. Syn., *crural p.*

gastric p. Any nerve plexus associated with the stomach. The **anterior g. p.** lies along the anterior surface of the lesser curvature of the stomach; its fibers are derived mainly from the left vagus, a few from the right vagus, and some sympathetic fibers. The **posterior g. p.** lies along the posterior surface of the lesser curvature; its fibers are derived mainly from the right vagus. The **inferior g. p.** accompanies the left gastroepiploic artery; its fibers are derived from the splenic plexus. The **superior g. p.** accompanies the left gastric artery, and receives fibers from the celiac plexus.

gastroduodenal p. A branch of the celiac plexus distributed to the stomach and duodenum.

hemorrhoidal p. (a) A venous plexus surrounding the lower part of the rectum. (b) Inferior and middle nerve plexuses derived from the pelvic plexus and located near the rectum.

hepatic p. A sympathetic nerve network accompanying the hepatic artery to the liver.
hypogastric p. A large sympathetic nerve plexus lying just in front of the promontory of the sacrum. Also called *presacral nerve.*
iliac p. A nerve plexus surrounding the common iliac artery.
infraorbital p. A nerve plexus under the levator labii superioris muscle.
intercellular p. A network of dendrites and axonic ramifications surrounding the cells in a sympathetic ganglion.
intermediate p. A nerve plexus found in the embryo between the bulbar and atrial plexuses.
intramural p. One located within the wall of an organ, as the submucous or myenteric plexus.
laryngeal venous p. A venous plexus draining blood from the larynx to the anterior and inferior laryngeal veins and communicating with the pharyngeal venous plexus.
lingual p. A nerve plexus surrounding the lingual artery.
lumbar p. One formed by the anterior divisions of the upper four lumbar spinal nerves in the posterior part of the psoas major muscle.
lumbosacral p. A network formed by the anterior branches of lumbar, sacral, and coccygeal nerves which for descriptive purposes are divided into the lumbar, sacral, and pudendal plexuses. See Plate 16.
mammary lymphatic p. One originating in the walls of the ducts and between the lobules of the mamma which also drains the overlying skin, areola, and nipple. The efferent vessels empty into the pectoral group of axillary nodes laterally, the sternal group medially, and occasionally the subclavian nodes superiorly. See Plate 11.
mammary venous p. A venous plexus draining blood from the mammary glands to the axillary vein.
maxillary plexuses. Nerve plexuses found around the external and internal maxillary arteries.
Meissner's p. See submucous *p.*
meningeal p. A nerve plexus found about the middle meningeal artery.
mesenteric p. A sympathetic nerve plexus surrounding the mesenteric arteries. That accompanying the superior mesenteric artery is derived from the celiac plexus and that surrounding the inferior mesenteric artery is derived from the aortic plexus.
myenteric p. A nerve plexus situated between the circular and longitudinal muscle layers of the digestive tube. Also called *Auerbach's p.*
nasopalatine p. A plexus uniting the nasopalatine nerves in the incisive foramen.
obturator p. See subsartorial *p.*
occipital p. A sympathetic network around the occipital artery.
ophthalmic p. A sympathetic plexus surrounding the ophthalmic artery.
ovarian p. (a) A network of veins in the broad ligament. (b) A nerve plexus distributed to the ovaries.
pampiniform p. A network of veins in the spermatic cord in the male, and in the broad ligament near the ovary in the female.
pancreaticoduodenal p. A sympathetic plexus whose nerve fibers are distributed to the duodenum and the pancreas.
parotid p. The branches of the facial nerve in close relation to the parotid gland.
patellar p. A nerve network situated in front of the patella.
pelvic p. A nerve plexus situated at the side of the rectum and urinary bladder and distributed to the pelvic viscera.
pericellular p. *In pathology,* newly formed nerve fibers which arise from the cell body or adjacent axon or cell and grow in circles around the cells in spinal ganglions, forming an interlocking network of fibers.
perivascular p. A network of nerve fibers which innervate the blood vessels. They may bring about vasoconstriction or vasodilation.
pharyngeal p. (a) A nerve plexus innervating the pharynx. (b) A plexus of veins situated at the side of the pharynx.
phrenic p. A nerve network which accompanies the inferior phrenic artery to the diaphragm.
p. cavernosi concharum. Venous plexuses found in the mucous membrane overlying the inferior nasal concha.
p. cavernosus. A nerve plexus distributed to the cavernous tissue of the penis or clitoris.
p. of Cruveilhier. See cervical posterior *p.*
p. venosus seminalis. A venous plexus about the seminal vesicles.
popliteal p. A nerve plexus surrounding the popliteal artery.
posterior cervical p. of Cruveilhier. See cervical posterior *p.*
prevertebral p. The collateral ganglions and nerve fibers of the sympathetic nervous system such as the cardiac, celiac, and hypogastric plexuses.
prostatic p. (a) A nerve plexus situated at the side of the prostate whose fibers are distributed to the urethra, prostate, and penis. (b) A venous plexus found in the areolar tissue around the prostate gland.
pterygoid p. A plexus of veins which accompanies the internal maxillary artery between the pterygoid muscles. See Table of Veins in the Appendix. See Plate 10.
pudendal p. (a) A plexus formed by the anterior branches of the second, third, and fourth sacral nerves. (b) A venous plexus lying around the urinary bladder and prostate. See Table of Veins in the Appendix.
pulmonary p. A nerve plexus composed chiefly of vagal fibers situated on the anterior and posterior aspects of the bronchi and accompanying them into the substance of the lung.
pyloric p. A nerve plexus which innervates the region of the pylorus.
renal p. A nerve plexus derived from the celiac and abdominal aortic plexuses; it accompanies the renal artery and is distributed to the kidney.
sacral p. (a) A nerve plexus formed by the anterior branch of the first, and contributions from the anterior branches of the second and third sacral nerves. (b) A venous plexus. See anterior sacral *p.*
sinocarotid p. Nerve fibers supplying the carotid sinus.
solar p. See celiac *p.*
spermatic p. A nerve plexus derived from the aortic and renal plexuses and running on each side with the internal spermatic artery to the testis.
sphenoid p. The upper part of the internal carotid plexus.
splenic p. A nerve plexus accompanying the splenic artery.
stroma p. A nerve plexus derived from the ciliary nerves found in the substantia propria of the cornea.
subclavian p. A nerve plexus found about the subclavian artery.
subepithelial p. A nerve plexus found beneath the epithelial cells of the cornea. It is a continuation of the stroma plexus.

submucous p. A nerve network lying in the submucosa of the digestive tube. Also called *Meissner's p.*

subpapillary p. A flat network of small, thin-walled vessels in the deeper part of the papillary layer and in the superficial part of the reticular layer of the dermis: also called *venous p.*

subperitoneal p. An arterial plexus, in the extraperitoneal fat of the lumbar region, formed by twigs from the lumbar, inferior phrenic, iliolumbar, hepatic, renal, and colic arteries.

subpleural p. An arterial plexus in the mediastinum, derived from small twigs of the pericardiacophrenic and intercostal arteries.

subsartorial p. A nerve network situated beneath the sartorius muscle. Syn., *obturator p.*

subtrapezial p. A nerve plexus lying beneath the trapezius muscle.

suprarenal p. A sympathetic nerve plexus surrounding the adrenal gland.

sympathetic p. A general term used to describe branches of sympathetic nerves surrounding organs or vessels. Each is named from the structure with which it is associated.

thyroid impar p. A venous plexus found in the substance of the thyroid gland and on its surface beneath the capsule; also called *p. thyreoideus impar.*

thyroid p. A sympathetic nerve plexus in the region of the thyroid gland. The superior part goes to the thyroid gland and the inferior part surrounds the external carotid and inferior thyroid arteries and is distributed to the larynx and pharynx as well as the thyroid gland.

tonsillar p. A nerve network whose fibers are distributed to the tonsils, fauces, and nearby region of the soft palate.

tympanic p. A nerve network formed by the tympanic branch of the glossopharyngeal, the lesser superficial petrosal and tympanopetrosal branches of the facial and sympathetic nerves derived from the internal carotid plexus.

uterine p. (a) A venous plexus on the walls of the uterus and extending into the broad ligament. (b) A nerve plexus supplying the cervix and lower part of the uterus.

uterovaginal p. (a) A nerve plexus on each side of the uterine cervix, composed of the pelvic part of the hypogastric plexus and the third and fourth sacral nerves. (b) A venous plexus at the cervix of the uterus, draining into the hypogastric vein.

vaginal p. (a) A nerve network supplying the walls of the vagina. (b) A plexus of veins near the entrance to the vagina.

venous p. See subpapillary *p.*

ventricular p. A nerve plexus found in the ependyma of the ventricles. It has been described in the cat and monkey.

vertebral p. (a) A sympathetic nerve plexus surrounding the vertebral and basilar arteries. (b) A plexus of large veins associated with the vertebral column throughout its length. They may be subdivided into the anterior and posterior external, and the anterior and posterior internal longitudinal plexus.

vesical p. (a) A sympathetic plexus surrounding the vesical arteries. (b) A venous plexus about the lower part of the urinary bladder and base of the prostate gland.

vesicopudendal p. The vesical and pudendal venous plexuses, collectively.

pli'ca (pl. *plicae*) [L. *plicare*, to fold]. A fold. For terms not listed here, see under *fold.* —**plicate,** *adj.;* **plica'tion** *n.*

alar p. One of the fringelike folds of the synovial membrane of the knee joint, on either side of the articular surface of the patella.

axillary p. A fold of skin and muscle which bounds the axilla anteriorly or posteriorly.

cecal p. A fold of peritoneum, the unfused portion of the ascending mesocolon, which forms the right boundary of the cecal fossa.

ciliary p. One of the small folds between the ciliary processes.

circular p. See *circular folds* under *fold.*

duodenojejunal p. An inconstant fold of peritoneum extending to the left from the duodenojejunal flexure to the posterior abdominal wall; it may contain the main stem of the inferior mesenteric vein.

duodenomesocolic p. An inconstant fold of peritoneum extending from the ascending part of the duodenum to the posterior abdominal wall.

gastropancreatic p. A fold of peritoneum on the posterior wall of the omental bursa, extending from the pancreas to the right side of the cardia of the stomach. It contains the left gastric artery.

genital p. Genital ridge.

longitudinal duodenal p. A fold in the medial wall of the descending portion of the duodenum extending upward from the papilla marking the opening of the common bile duct.

malleolar p. One of the two ligamentous bands, anterior and posterior, on the medial surface of the tympanic membrane, extending from either side of the tympanic notch to the lateral process of the malleus.

patellar synovial p. A fold of synovial membrane in the knee joint which extends from the infrapatellar fatty mass to the anterior part of the intercondyloid notch; its free margins form the alar plicae.

plicae iridis. Radiating folds on the posterior surface of the iris.

plicae palmatae cervicis. See *arbor vitae,* 2.

p. lacrimalis. See Hasner's *valve.*

p. of the ampulla. One of the longitudinal folds of the tunica mucosa of the ampulla of Vater.

p. polonica. A matted condition of the hair caused by filth and neglect. Syn., *Polish plait.*

rectouterine plicae. Two folds of peritoneum extending from the cervix of the uterus on either side of the rectum to the sacrum, and forming the lateral boundaries of the mouth of the rectouterine pouch. See uterosacral *ligament.*

rectovesical p. A peritoneal fold extending from the posterior part of the urinary bladder to the rectum and sacrum: also called *sacrogenital fold.*

semilunar p. The thin fold of mucous membrane across the supratonsillar fossa, between the palatine arches.

septal p. One of several folds occasionally in the fetus on the posteroinferior portion of the nasal septum.

sublingual p. Sublingual fold; the elevation of the mucous membrane of the floor of the mouth, on either side of the tongue, caused by the projection of the sublingual gland.

synovial p. A fold of the synovial membrane of a joint, extending toward or between the articular surfaces; it may contain fat or provide for the course of vessels.

transverse vesical p. A variable fold of peritoneum extending from the urinary bladder laterally to the pelvic wall; it is seen only when the viscus is empty.

tubal plicae. Folds of the tunica mucosa in the uterine tubes.

ureteric p. A transverse ridge on the internal surface of the urinary bladder formed by each ureter as it passes through the wall, marking the upper angle of the trigone on either side.

urorectal plicae. The lateral folds that fuse to form the urorectal septum of the embryo.

pli·cot'o·my (plye·cot'o·mee) [*plicare;* G. *tomē*, a cutting]. Division of the posterior fold of the tympanic membrane.

Plimmer, Henry George [*English protozoologist*, 1856–1918]. Remembered for his study of sodium antimony tartrate in the treatment of trypanosomiasis of rats; called *Plimmer's salt.*

Plinius, Gaius (Pliny) [*Roman naturalist*, 23–79]. Author of *Historia Naturalis* in many volumes, an encyclopedia of the natural sciences.

plo'cach (plo'cake). Cholera in sheep.

plomb (plum) [F. *plomber*, to stop a tooth]. Any plastic material, usually paraffin, used as an extrapleural tampon to close a tuberculous pulmonary cavity; a form of collapse therapy.

plom·bage' (plawm·bahzh'. *See* NOTES § 35) [*plomber*]. The extrapleural compression of a tuberculous pulmonary cavity by the use of a plastic material, usually paraffin. A form of collapse therapy. *Obs.*

plo·ra'tion [L. *ploratio*, from *plorare*, to cry aloud]. Lacrimation. *Obs.*

Plotz, Harry [*American physician and bacteriologist*, 1890–1947]. Described a type of bacillus found in typhus, called *Plotz bacillus.*

plug [MD. *plugge*]. Something that occludes a circular opening or channel, as a tooth filling.

cervical p. See mucous *p.*

epithelial p. A temporary mass of epithelial cells closing the embryonic external naris.

mucous p. The mass of inspissated mucus which occludes the cervix uteri during pregnancy and is discharged at the beginning of labor.

yolk p. The mass of yolk protruding into the blastopore of amphibian gastrulas as a result of epiboly.

plug'ger [*plugge*]. See *condenser*, 4.

foil p. One used for condensing gold foil in a prepared cavity of a tooth.

plug'ging. See *tampon.*

plum·ba'gin. $C_{11}H_8O_3$; 5-hydroxy-2-methyl-1,4-naphthoquinone; an antibiotic, isomeric with phthiocol, found in the root bark of *Plumbago europaea*, *P. zeylanica*, and *P. rosea*, and also prepared synthetically. It is active, in vitro, against several species of bacteria, and has been used therapeutically in *Staphylococcus* infections causing furuncles and acne.

plum·ba'go [L., a species of lead ore]. Native graphite. Black lead. Used in the manufacture of pencils, crucibles, and as a lubricant.

plum'bic [L. *plumbum*, lead]. Describing a compound of tetravalent lead.

plum'bism (plum'biz·um) [*plumbum*]. Lead poisoning.

plum'bite. A salt derived from lead hydroxide, $Pb(OH)_2$, of the types, $MHPbO_2$ or M_2PbO_2.

plum'bum. See *lead.*

Plummer, Andrew [*Scottish physician*, 1698–1756]. Introduced a compound pill of calomel and antimony, called *Plummer's pill.*

Plummer, Henry Stanley [*American physician*, 1874–1936]. Described a syndrome of dysphagia, glossitis, and hyperchromic anemia (1912), also described by D. R. Paterson (1919) and Porter P. Vinson (1922); called *Plummer-Vinson syndrome.* With W. M. Boothby, advocated treatment of exophthalmic goiter with iodine (1923); called *Plummer's treatment.* Described a method of palpating the thyroid gland, in which the right lobe is felt by the examiner's left hand with the fingers behind the sternomastoid muscle and the thumb in front. With the fingers of the other hand, the structures in the anterior part are pressed toward the palpating fingers. Known as *Plummer's method.*

plump'er [MD. *plomp*]. Formerly, one of a pair of pads worn in the cheeks to give them a rounded appearance; artificial dentures are now sometimes built up to produce the same effect.

plu"ri·glan'du·lar [L. *plus*, more; *glans*, acorn]. Referring to more than one gland or to the secretions of more than one gland, as in pluriglandular extract, a mixture of extracts from several glands.

plu"ri·grav'i·da [*plus;* L. *gravidus*, pregnant]. A woman during her third and subsequent pregnancies; multigravida.

plu"ri·loc'u·lar [*plus;* L. *loculus*, little place]. Having more than one compartment or loculus; multilocular.

plu·rip'a·ra [*plus;* L. *parere*, to bring forth]. A woman who has given birth to several children; a multipara.

plu"ri·par'i·ty [*plus; parere*]. The condition of having borne several children.

plu·rip'o·tent. Characterizing a cell or embryonic tissue capable of producing more than one type of cell or tissue.

plu"to·ma'ni·a [G. *ploutos*, wealth; *mania*, madness]. A false belief that one is the possessor of great wealth; greed for wealth.

plu'to·nism [L. *Plutonius*, Plutonian]. A disease caused by exposure to plutonium, manifested in experimental animals by graying of the hair, liver degeneration, and tumor formation. There is no record of its having attacked a human being.

plu·to'ni·um [*Plutonius*]. Pu = 242 *ca.* An element, atomic number 94, obtained from neptunium and capable of undergoing fission with the release of large amounts of energy.

Pm. 1. Symbol for promethium. 2. Premolar.

PMI Abbreviation, used clinically, for *p*oint of *m*aximal *i*mpulse.

PMS Pregnant mare's serum hormone.

PNA Ribonucleic acid.

pne"o·dy·nam'ics (nee"o·dye·nam'icks, ·di·nam'icks) [G. *pnein*, to breathe; *dynamikos*, powerful]. The dynamics of respiration.

pne'o·graph (nee'o·graf) [*pnein;* G. *graphein*, to write]. An instrument for recording the force and character of the current of air during respiration.

pne·om'e·ter (nee·om'i·tur). See *spirometer.*

pne'o·scope. See *pneumograph.*

pneu'ma- (new'muh-), **pneum-** [G. *pneuma*, breath]. A combining form meaning *wind* or *air.*

pneu"mar·thro'sis (new"mahr·thro'sis) [*pneuma;* G. *arthron*, joint; *ōsis*, condition]. Air or gas in a joint.

pneu·mat'ic (new·mat'ick) [G. *pneumatikos*, of the breath]. Pertaining to air or gas; may be compressed, rarefied, or under normal pressure.

pneu·mat'ics (new·mat'icks) [*pneumatikos*]. The branch of physics treating of the dynamic properties of air and gases.

pneu"ma·ti·za'tion. The progressive development of, or the state of having, air-filled cavities in bones, lined by a mucous membrane, as the accessory nasal sinuses or mastoid air cells. —**pneu'matize,** *v.*

pneu'ma·to- (new'muh·to-) [G. *pneuma*, air, breath]. 1. A combining form meaning *air;* used to denote *respiration.* 2. *In medicine*, a combining form denoting *the presence of air* or *gas in a part.*

pneu"ma·to·car'di·a [*pneuma;* G. *kardia*, heart]. The presence of air or gas in the chambers of the heart.

pneu'ma·to·cele", pneu·mat'o·cele" [*pneuma;* G. *kēlē*, tumor]. A sac or tumor containing gas; especially the scrotum filled with gas. Syn., *pneumonocele, pneumocele.*

pneu″ma·to·dysp·ne′a (new″muh·to·disp·nee′uh, ·disp′nee·uh, new·mat″o·) [*pneuma;* G. *dyspnoia,* difficulty of breathing]. Emphysematous dyspnea.

pneu′ma·to·gram″, pneu·mat′o·gram″ [*pneuma;* G. *gramma,* letter]. A tracing showing the frequency, duration, and depth of the respiratory movements.

pneu′ma·to·graph″, pneu·mat′o·graph″. See *pneumograph.*

pneu″ma·tol′o·gy [*pneuma;* G. *logos,* word]. 1. The science of respiration. 2. The science of gases; also their use as therapeutic agents.

pneu″ma·tom′e·ter [*pneuma;* G. *metron,* a measure]. An instrument for measuring the pressure of inspiration or expiration by the force exerted upon a column of mercury contained in a U-tube.

pneu″ma·tom′e·try [*pneuma; metron*]. 1. The measurement of the force in respiration. It is used as a means of diagnosis. 2. The treatment of pulmonary and circulatory diseases by means of a pneumatic apparatus.

pneu″ma·tor′ra·chis (new″muh·tor′uh·kis) [*pneuma;* G. *rhachis,* spine]. The presence of air in the spinal canal.

pneu″ma·to′sis [G., inflation]. Air or gas in abnormal situations in the body.

p. cystoides intestinalis. Cystlike dilatations of the lymph spaces of the intestinal wall due to gas-forming organisms or mechanical causes.

pneu″ma·tu′ri·a [G. *pneuma,* air, breath; *ouron,* urine]. Voiding urine containing free gas.

pneu′ma·type [*pneuma;* G. *typos,* impression]. Breath picture. The deposit formed upon a piece of glass by the moist air exhaled through the nostrils when the mouth is closed. It is employed in the diagnosis of nasal obstruction. Slate paper may be used, pulverized sulfur or boric acid being blown upon the moistened surface to make a permanent record.

pneu·mec′to·my. See *pneumonectomy.*

pneu″men·ceph″a·log′ra·phy. See *pneumoencephalography.*

pneu′mo- (new′mo-). A combining form meaning *air* or *lung.* See also *pneumato-, pneumono-.*

pneu″mo·an″gi·og′ra·phy. The outlining of the vessels of the lung, chiefly the pulmonary artery and its branches, by means of a radiopaque material. When done as an antemortem study, the roentgenographic technique is similar to that used in angiocardiography.

pneu″mo-ar·throg′ra·phy. Radiographic examination of joints into which air has been injected. —**pneumoar′throgram,** *n.*

pneu″mo·ba·cil′lus [G. *pneumōn,* lung; dim. from L. *bacillum,* stick]. *Klebsiella pneumoniae.*

pneu″mo·bul′bar [*pneumōn;* G. *bolbos,* bulb]. Pertaining to the lungs and to the respiratory center in the medulla.

pneu′mo·cele. See *pneumatocele.*

pneu″mo·cen·te′sis [*pneumōn;* G. *kentēsis,* a pricking]. Puncture of a lung with needle or trocar; usually done to obtain tissue or exudate for diagnostic study, or to establish communication with a cavity.

pneu″mo·ceph′a·lus [*pneumōn;* G. *kephalē,* head]. The presence of air or gas within the cranial cavity.

traumatic p. That following injuries, chiefly to the frontal part of the skull.

pneu″mo·chol″e·cys·ti′tis. Cholecystitis associated with gas in the gallbladder.

pneu″mo·coc′cal [*pneumōn* G. *kokkos,* berry]. Pertaining to or caused by pneumococci.

pneu″mo·coc·ce′mi·a (new″mo·cock·see′mee·uh) [*pneumōn; kokkos;* G. *haima,* blood]. The presence of pneumococci in the blood.

pneu″mo·coc′cide [*pneumōn; kokkos;* L. *caedere,* to kill]. A substance which destroys pneumococci. —**pneumococci′dal,** *adj.*

pneu″mo·coc″co·su′ri·a [*pneumōn; kokkos;* G. *ouron,* urine]. Presence of pneumococci in the urine.

pneu″mo·coc′cus (pl. *pneumococci*) [*pneumōn; kokkos*]. Old term for *Diplococcus pneumoniae.*

pneu″mo·co′lon [*pneumōn;* G. *kolon,* colon]. Distention of the colon, as a diagnostic measure.

pneu″mo·co″ni·o′sis. Chronic inflammation of the lungs caused by the inhalation of dust. All of the recognized forms are due to mineral dusts. The predominant reaction is fibrosis, which varies in type with the etiologic dust. Silicosis and asbestosis are the main forms of pneumoconiosis known to cause disability. Other forms, known as benign pneumoconioses, in which the reaction is limited to the stromal tissues, are anthracosis, due to carbon dust, siderosis, due to iron dust, calcicosis, due to marble dust, and baritosis, due to barium dust. Also see *berylliosis.*

benign p. Any of the numerous forms of pneumoconiosis which do not cause progressive disease or disability.

diatomaceous earth p. A distinctive type of pneumoconiosis occurring in workers engaged in the mining and processing of diatomaceous earth; disabling and nondisabling forms have been described.

Welsh coal-miner's p. A form of anthracosis in which areas of focal emphysema surround carbon deposits, and areas of conglomerate fibrosis may occur in the absence of either silica or the tubercle bacillus (*Mycobacterium tuberculosis*), seen occasionally in the United States.

pneu″mo·cra′ni·um [*pneumōn;* G. *kranion,* skull]. Presence of air or gas beneath the dura or within the ventricles of the brain.

pneu″mo·cys·tog′ra·phy [*pneumōn; kystis;* G. *graphein,* to write]. Radiography of the urinary bladder following its injection with air. —**pneumocyst′ogram,** *n.*

pneu″mo·der′ma [*pneumōn* G. *derma,* skin]. Air or gas collected under, or in, the skin.

pneu″mo·dy·nam′ics (new″mo·dye·nam′icks, ·di·nam′icks) [*pneumōn;* G. *dynamikos,* powerful]. Pneodynamics.

pneu″mo·en·ceph′a·lo·gram″ [*pneumōn;* G. *egkephalos,* brain; *gramma,* letter]. Roentgenographic picture of the brain after the replacement of cerebrospinal fluid with air or gas, which has been injected through a needle into the spinal subarachnoid space.

pneu″mo·en·ceph″a·log′ra·phy [*pneumōn; egkephalos;* G. *graphein,* to write]. A method of visualizing the ventricular system and subarachnoid pathways of the brain by roentgenography after removal of spinal fluid followed by the injection of air or oxygen into the lumbar subarachnoid space.

pneu″mo·en″ter·i′tis [*pneumōn;* G. *enteron,* intestine; *-itis,* inflammation]. Inflammation of the lungs and of the intestine.

pneu″mo·gas′tric. The tenth cranial nerve: old term.

pneu′mo·graph [*pneumōn;* G. *graphein,* to write]. Apparatus for recording respiratory excursion.

pneu·mog′ra·phy [*pneumōn; graphein*]. 1. Roentgenography of the lung. 2. The recording of the respiratory excursions.

pneu″mo·he″mo·per″i·car′di·um (·hee″mo·perr″i·kahr′dee·um, ·hem″o·) [*pneumōn;* G. *haima,* blood; *perikardios,* around the heart]. The presence of air and blood in the pericardial cavity.

pneu″mo·he″mo·tho′rax (·hee″mo·thor′acks, ·hem″o·). See *hemopneumothorax.*

pneu″mo·hy″dro·per″i·car′di·um [*pneumōn;* G. *hydōr*, water; *perikardios*]. An accumulation of air and fluid in the pericardial sac.

pneu″mo·hy″po·der′ma [*pneumōn;* G. *hypo*, under; *derma*, skin]. Subcutaneous emphysema.

pneu″mo·ko″ni·o′sis. See *pneumoconiosis.*

pneu′mo·lith [*pneumōn;* G. *lithos*, stone]. A calculus or concretion occurring in a lung.

pneu″mo·li·thi′a·sis [*pneumōn; lithos;* NL. *-iasis*, condition]. The occurrence of calculi or concretions in a lung. Also called *pneumonolithiasis.*

pneu·mol′y·sis [*pneumōn;* G. *lysis*, a loosing]. Old term for pneumonolysis.

pneu″mo·me″di·as·ti′num [*pneumōn;* L. *medius*, middle]. Air in the mediastinal tissues.

pneu·mom′e·try. Measurement of lung capacity in the living individual, including vital capacity, maximum breathing capacity, tidal volume, residual volume, etc.

pneu″mo·my·co′sis (new″mo·migh·ko′sis). See *pneumonomycosis.*

pneu′mon-. See *pneumono-.*

pneu″mo·nec′to·my [*pneumōn;* G. *ektomē*, excision]. Excision of an entire lung: also called *pneumectomy.*

cautery p. The removal of a lung by cautery.

pneu·mo′ni·a [G., from *pneumōn*]. A disease resulting from inflammation of the lungs; pneumonitis.

aspiration p. That resulting from the inhalation of a foreign body, usually fluids or food particles, from the pharynx into the air passages of the lungs, usually in the course of a general anesthesia.

bronchial p. See *bronchopneumonia.*

central p. Occasional term for a pneumonia with consolidated areas near the hilum, giving rise to relatively few signs.

chemical p. That caused by inhalation of a chemical irritant, particularly beryllium.

chronic p. Long-standing lung infection.

dermal p. *In bacteriology* and *immunology*, an experimental pathologic process produced by injecting virulent pneumococci into the skin of rabbits.

double p. Involvement of both lungs.

fibroid p. See organizing *p.*

Friedländer p. That due to infection with *Klebsiella pneumoniae* (Friedländer's bacillus).

hypostatic p. Infection of dependent parts of lungs which are hyperemic due to staying in one position for long periods of time, usually seen in elderly patients.

influenza p. That due to infection by *Hemophilus influenza.*

interstitial p. Infection particularly of the stroma of the lungs including the peribronchial tissues and the septa between alveoli. It may originate from the pleura or mediastinum.

lipid, lipoid p. That due to aspiration of oily substances, particularly from nose drops, mineral oil, or cod-liver oil. More common in children or in adults when the cough reflex is impaired. The inflammation is often chronic and is mostly in lower lobes.

lobar p. An acute febrile disease involving one or more lobes of the lung, due to infection by one of the pneumococci. Characterized by abrupt onset, fever, dyspnea, pain, cough, rusty sputum, and general toxic symptoms. Typically, the fever drops by crisis after about a week. The involved lung is consolidated, gradually returning to normal by resolution.

lobular p. Bronchopneumonia.

Löffler's p. See Loeffler's *syndrome.*

massive p. One which involves a large area of a lung, or an entire lung.

metastatic p. A type due to the presence in the lungs of infected emboli.

migratory p. Pneumonic infection which seems to shift from one part of the lungs to another.

organizing p. That in which the healing process is characterized by organization and cicatrization of the exudate rather than by resolution and resorption.

pneumococcal p. That due to infection by pneumococci. See lobar *p.*, *bronchopneumonia.*

p. alba. Diffuse interstitial fibrosis of the alveolar walls of the fetal lung due to prenatal syphilis; the lungs are white and often atelectatic at birth.

primary atypical p. Bronchopneumonia of unknown etiology, not secondary to any other acute infectious disease. Suspected of being caused by any one of several different strains of filtrable virus. Typically endemic, but may appear in mild epidemic form. Characterized clinically by failure to respond to sulfonamides and penicillin, absence of characteristic blood changes, tendency to protracted course and delayed resolution, and a generally good prognosis.

rheumatic p. Pneumonia in the acute stage of rheumatic fever.

staphylococcal p. A serious type caused by *Micrococcus pyogenes* var. *aureus.* Epidemics of this disease may follow influenza.

streptococcal p. A pneumonia, usually caused by the Lancefield group A streptococci, either primary or complicating an upper respiratory infection.

terminal p. That occurring in the course of other diseases and resulting in death.

tuberculous p. An exudative reaction in the lung caused by *Mycobacterium tuberculosis.* Usually it is an extensive lesion which clinically and roentgenologically simulates pneumonia caused by other organisms. It is often designated *tuberculous bronchopneumonia, bronchopneumonic tuberculosis, tuberculous lobar pneumonia,* or *lobar pneumonic tuberculosis*, depending on its distribution.

vagus p. Pneumonia following section of the vagi in the lower animals; due to aspiration of food into the air passages.

virus p. See primary atypical *p.*

pneu·mon′ic (new·mon′ick) [G. *pneumonikos*, of the lungs]. 1. Pertaining to pneumonia. *Obs.* 2. Pertaining to the exudative form of pulmonary tuberculosis, when sufficiently extensive to simulate either lobar pneumonia or bronchopneumonia.

pneu″mo·ni′tis (new″mo·nigh′tis) [G. *pneumōn*, lung; *-itis*, inflammation]. Inflammation of the lung.

eosinophilic p. See Loeffler's *syndrome.*

radiation p. That following large doses of radiation to the chest, characterized by edema, lymphectasia, injury to the epithelial elements, and formation of a well-defined hyaline membrane, and in the late stage, thickening of alveolar walls, patchy atelectasis, and endothelial swelling of capillaries. Respiratory function is usually significantly decreased; the only symptom may be a nonproductive cough.

pneu′mo·no- (new′mo·no-, new·mo′no-, new-mon′o-), **pneumon-** [*pneumōn*]. A combining form meaning *lung.*

pneu′mo·no·cele″. See *pneumatocele.*

pneu″mo·no·cen·te′sis. See *pneumocentesis.*

pneu″mo·no·coc′cic types (·cock′sick). Subdivisions of *Diplococcus pneumoniae*, based on their polysaccharide haptene or specific soluble substance (SSS). At present, over 30 such types have been distinguished.

pneu″mo·no·co″ni·o′sis. See *pneumoconiosis.*

pneu″mo·no·ko″ni·o′sis. See *pneumoconiosis.*

pneu″mo·nol′y·sis [*pneumōn;* G. *lysis,* a loosing]. The loosening of any portion of lung adherent to the chest wall; a form of collapse therapy used in the treatment of pulmonary tuberculosis.

extrapleural p. The separation of an area of parietal pleura from the chest wall. Also see *apicolysis.*

intrapleural p. The severance of adhesion bands between the visceral and parietal layers of pleura. May be closed when performed by the use of a thoracoscope, and open when an incision is made through the chest wall to permit direct vision.

pneu″mo·no·my·co′sis (·migh·ko′sis) [*pneumōn;* G. *mykēs,* fungus; *-ōsis,* condition]. Any disease of the lungs due to infestation by a fungus.

pneu″mo·nop′a·thy [*pneumōn;* G. *pathos,* disease]. Any abnormality of the lungs.

pneu·mo′no·pex″y (new·mo′no·peck″see, new-mon′o·, new·mo″no·peck′see) [*pneumōn;* G. *pēxis,* a fixing]. Fixation of lung tissue to the chest wall.

pneu″mo·nor′rha·phy [*pneumōn;* G. *rhaphē,* suture]. Suture of a lung.

pneu″mo·no′sis [*pneumōn;* G. *-ōsis,* condition]. Any noninfective degenerative disease of the lungs. *Obs.*

traumatic p. *In aviation medicine,* acute non-inflammatory pathologic changes produced in the lungs by large momentary deceleration. The principal changes are hemorrhage, emphysema, and laceration. These changes, in accordance with their location, type, and magnitude, may cause sudden death or variable clinical pulmonary signs and symptoms.

pneu″mo·not′o·my [*pneumōn;* G. *tomē,* a cutting]. Surgical incision of a lung.

pneu·mop′a·thy [*pneumōn;* G. *pathos,* disease]. Any abnormality of the lungs.

pneu″mo·per″i·car·di′tis [*pneumōn;* G. *perikardios,* around the heart; *-itis,* inflammation]. Pericarditis with the formation of gas in the pericardial sac.

pneu″mo·per″i·car′di·um [*pneumōn; perikardios*]. The presence of air in the pericardial sac. It is due to traumatism or to communication between the pericardium and the esophagus, stomach, or lungs, and is marked by tympany over the precordial region and peculiar, metallic heart sounds.

pneu″mo·per″i·to·ne′um [*pneumōn;* G. *peritonaion,* membrane which contains the lower viscera]. 1. The presence of gas in the peritoneal cavity. 2. Injection of a gas into the periotoneal cavity, as in special radiography of the abdomen.

transabdominal p. Injection of gas through the abdominal wall to outline pelvic organs and tumors in x-rays of the pelvic region.

pneu″mo·per″i·to·ni′tis [*pneumōn peritonaion;* G. *-itis,* inflammation]. Peritonitis with the presence of gas in the peritoneal cavity.

pneu′mo·pex″y. See *pneumonopexy.*

pneu″mo·py·el′o·gram″ [*pneumōn;* G. *pyelos,* trough; *gramma,* letter]. A pyelogram in which air or oxygen is used as the contrast medium instead of an opaque solution.

pneu″mo·py″o·per″i·car′di·um [*pneumōn;* G. *pyon,* pus; *perikardios,* around the heart]. Air or gas and pus in the pericardial sac.

pneu″mo·ra′chis (new″mo·ray′kis, new·mor′uh-kis) [*pneumōn;* G. *rhachis,* spine]. A collection of gas in the spinal canal, accidental or by injection of air for diagnostic purposes.

pneu″mo·ra″di·og′ra·phy [*pneumōn;* L. *radius,* ray; G. *graphein,* to write]. Radiography of a region, as of a joint or of the abdomen, following the injection of air into a cavity.

pneu″mo·roent″gen·og′ra·phy (new″mo·rent″-ghin·og′ruh·fee). See *pneumoradiography.*

pneu″mo·scle·ro′sis [*pneumōn;* G. *sklērōsis,* a hardening]. Fibrosis of the lungs.

pneu″mo·tax′ic cen′ter. See under *center.*

pneu″mo·tax′is. Pertaining to the control of respiration. —**pneumotax′ic,** *adj.*

pneu″mo·tho′rax [*pneumōn;* G. *thōrax,* thorax]. The presence of air or gas in a pleural cavity. May occur from perforating wounds of the chest, accidental or operative, by the rupture of an abscess or cavity of the lung, or the rupture of an air sac or bronchiole. Syn., *intrapleural pneumothorax.*

artificial p. The production of a pneumothorax by the introduction into a pleural cavity, through a needle, of air or other gas to produce collapse and immobility of a lung, with obliteration of cavities. Used in the treatment of pulmonary tuberculosis.

closed p. One having no opening through the chest wall. It may be artificial or spontaneous, due to a rupture of an air passage, air sac, or bronchiole.

extrapleural p. One in which the parietal pleura is stripped from the thoracic wall, and the air or gas introduced within the space so formed, as in apicolysis.

idiopathic p. See spontaneous *p.*

open p. One with a penetrating wound of the thoracic wall.

spontaneous p. The pneumothorax occurring from causes other than the introduction of air or gas into a pleural cavity from without. Extreme physical exertion appears as the major cause. Also called *idiopathic p.*

valvular p. A type of open pneumothorax known as a *sucking wound,* in which a margin of the wound acts as a valve. Air enters the pleural space with an inhalation, and is prevented by the valve from escaping during exhalation. Therefore, the air tension in the pleural space increases. Also called *tension p.*

pneu·mot′o·my. See *pneumonotomy.*

pneu″mo·tox′in [*pneumōn;* G. *toxikon,* poison]. A toxin of the pneumococcus; true exogenous toxins have not been found. The capsular polysaccharides may play a role in pathogenesis but cannot be considered as toxins. Parker described a necrotizing toxic factor; a capillary poison or spreading factor has also been reported to exist in these organisms by Julianelle and Reimann.

pneu″mo·ty′phoid. See *pneumotyphus.*

pneu″mo·ty′phus [*pneumōn;* G. *typhos,* delusion]. 1. Typhoid fever beginning with pneumonia dependent upon the typhoid bacillus. 2. Pneumonia occurring in the course of typhoid fever.

pneu″mo·ven′tri·cle. A form of pneumocephalus in which air enters the ventricles of the brain through the accessory sinuses of the skull: sometimes seen as a complication of skull fracture.

pneu″mo·ven·tric″u·log′ra·phy [*pneumōn;* L. *ventriculus,* ventricle; G. *graphein,* to write]. A method of depicting the ventricular system of the brain by roentgenography, after the fluid content has been removed and air has been injected. Also called *ventriculography.*

pneu′sis (new′sis) [G., a breathing]. Respiration.

pnig′ma (nig′muh) [G., a choking]. Strangulation. *Obs.*

pni″go·pho′bi·a (nigh″go·fo′bee·uh) [G. *pnigein,* to choke; *phobos,* fear]. The fear of choking that sometimes accompanies angina pectoris.

Po Chemical symbol for polonium.

pock [AS. *pocc*]. A pustule of an eruptive fever, especially of smallpox.

pocked [*pocc*]. Pitted; marked with pustules.

pock′et [AF. *pokete*]. *In anatomy,* a blind sac, or

sac-shaped cavity. A diverticulum communicating with a cavity.

gingival p. An abnormally deep gingival sulcus associated with gingivitis.

intraoral p. An artificially created pocket within the mouth, lined with grafted skin, used to hold a prosthetic appliance in the restoration of facial contours due to the loss of half or more of the mandible.

periodontal p. An abnormally deep gingival sulcus, associated with periodontosis, whose extension apically is at the expense of detached periodontal fibers and resorption of the alveolar crest: also called *intraosseus p.*

pyorrhea p. See gingival *p.*, periodontal *p.*

pock′-marked″. Pitted with the indentations of the smallpox pustule.

po·dag′ra, pod′a·gra [G., gout]. Gout, especially of the great toe or the joints of the foot.

po·dal′gi·a [G. *pous*, foot; *algos*, pain]. Pain in the foot.

po·dal′ic [*pous*]. Pertaining to the feet, as podalic version, the operation of changing the position of the fetus in the uterus to bring the feet to the outlet.

pod″ar·thri′tis [*pous;* G. *arthron*, joint; *-itis*, inflammation]. Inflammation of the joints of the feet.

pod″ar·throc′a·ce (pod″ahr·throck′uh·see) [*pous; arthron;* G. *kakos*, bad]. Caries of the articulations of the feet. *Obs.*

po·dar′thrum [*pous; arthron*]. *In biology*, the foot joint or metatarsophalangeal articulation. *Obs.*

pod″e·de′ma [*pous;* G. *oidēma*, swelling]. Edema of the feet.

pod″el·co′ma [*pous;* G. *helkōma*, ulcer]. Madura foot. See *mycetoma.*

pod″en·ceph′a·lus [*pous;* G. *egkephalos*, brain]. A monster with partial acrania in the parietal region, with protrusion of the cranial contents from the top of the head.

po·di′a·try [*pous;* G. *iatreia*, medical treatment]. Treatment of disorders of the feet; chiropody. Unofficial synonym for chiropody. —**podi′atrist, podiat′rist,** *n.*

pod″o·brom″hi·dro′sis (pod″o·brohm″hi·dro′sis, ·high·dro′sis, pod″o·brom″·) [*pous;* G. *brōmos*, stench; *hidrōs*, sweat; *-ōsis*, condition]. Offensive sweating of the feet.

pod′o·derm. The modified, highly vascular corium found under the horny layer of the hoof in ungulates; it furnishes nutrition to the hoof.

pod″o·dyn′i·a (pod″o·din′ee·uh, ·dye′nee·uh) [*pous;* G. *odynē*, pain]. Pain in the foot, especially a neuralgic pain in the heel unattended by swelling or redness.

po·dom′e·ter [*pous;* G. *metron*, a measure]. An instrument which registers the number of footsteps in walking; preferably called *pedometer.*

pod″o·phyl′lin, pod·oph′yl·lin. See *podophyllum* resin.

pod″o·phyl″lo·res′in (·rez′in). See *podophyllum.*

pod″o·phyl″lo·tox′in. $C_{22}H_{22}O_8$; a crystalline polycyclic substance obtained from the rhizome and roots of *Podophyllum peltatum*, insoluble in water but soluble in alcohol. It has cathartic properties, but is probably not the principal cathartic constituent of the drug; applied topically, it is active against certain wartlike neoplasms.

pod″o·phyl′lum [G. *pous*, foot; *phyllon*, leaf] (*podophyllum*). The dried rhizome and roots of *Podophyllum peltatum*, containing podophyllotoxin, α-peltatin, β-peltatin, and an amorphous resin called *podophylloresin;* a slow but active cathartic, rarely used in the crude state, podophyllum resin being the form most frequently used. Also called *mandrake, May apple.*

Indian p. The dried rhizome and roots of *Podophyllum emodi* (*P. hexandrum*), containing podophyllotoxin, demethylpodophyllotoxin, picropodophyllin glucoside, and resin; α-peltatin and β-peltatin have not been found in it. It is used like the podophyllum from *P. peltatum.*

p. resin (*resina podophylli*). A light brown to greenish yellow amorphous powder, obtained by pouring an alcoholic extract of podophyllum into acidified cold water. It is an active cathartic, often used in combination with milder laxatives in chronic constipation. Applied locally, it is active against many wartlike neoplasms.

poe-. For words beginning with *poe-*, see under *pe-*.

Poehl, Alexander Vasilyevich von (von Pel) [*Russian chemist*, 1850–98]. Remembered for his isolation of spermin from the testis (1891). Introduced his test for presence of cholera bacilli, using concentrated sulfuric acid.

po·go′ni·on [G. *pōgōnion*, little beard]. The most anterior point of the chin on the symphysis of the mandible.

Pohl method. See under *method.*

Pohl's test. See under *test.*

-poi·et′ic [G. *poiētikos*, productive]. A combining form denoting *making* or *producing.*

poi′ki·lo·blast″ [G. *poikilos*, diversified; *blastos*, germ]. A nucleated red blood cell of irregular shape and size.

poi′ki·lo·cyte″ [*poikilos;* G. *kytos*, cell]. A large, red blood cell of irregular shape.

poi″ki·lo·cy·the′mi·a (poy″ki·lo·sigh·thee′mee·uh) [*poikilos; kytos;* G. *haima*, blood]. The presence of poikilocytes in the blood.

poi″ki·lo·cy·to′sis (poy″ki·lo·sigh·to′sis) [*poikilos; kytos;* G. *-ōsis*, condition]. Abnormality in shape of circulating red corpuscles.

poi″ki·lo·der′ma [*poikilos;* G. *derma*, skin]. A skin syndrome characterized by pigmentation, telangiectasia, and, usually, atrophy.

p. of Civatte. See reticulated pigmented *p.*

p. vasculare atrophicans. A widespread cutaneous disease with atrophy, telangiectasia, pigmentation, and purpura. It may occur in association with, or as an end result of, other cutaneous diseases.

reticulated pigmented p. A variety of Riehl's melanosis, located on the neck as a symmetric, pigmented, teleangiectatic, and atrophic erythroderma with retiform arrangement: also called *p. reticulare of Civatte, p. of Civatte, Civatte's disease.*

poi″ki·lo·der″ma·to·my″o·si′tis [*poikilos; derma;* G. *mys*, muscle; *-itis*, inflammation]. Poikiloderma in association with muscular sclerosis.

poi″ki·lo·ther′mism, poi″ki·lo·ther′my (poy″ki·lo·thur′miz·um) [*poikilos; thermē*]. The condition of having a variable body temperature, usually slightly higher than that of the environment, as in all animals except birds and mammals. See *cold-blooded.* —**poikilother′mic, poikilother′mal, poikilother′mous,** *adj.*

poi″ki·lo·throm′bo·cyte [*poikilos;* G. *thrombos*, clot; *kytos*, cell]. A blood platelet of abnormal shape.

poi″ki·lo·zo·o·sper′mi·a. Variability in the shapes of spermatozoa.

point [OF. *point*, from L. *pungere*, to prick]. 1. The sharp end of an object, especially one used to pierce anything. 2. The limit at which anything occurs, as the melting point, freezing point. 3. A mark made by a sharp object; a minute spot.

alveolar p. The midpoint on the anterior surface of the superior alveolar arch, used in craniometry.

anterior focal p. One of the conjugate foci.

auricular p. Central point of the external auditory meatus.

boiling p. The temperature at which a liquid has a vapor pressure equal to the barometric pressure.
Bolton p. A point in the median line midway between the postcondylar notches on the occipital bone, the posterior termination of the Bolton plane. It is located as the most superior point in the profile of the postcondylar notches when viewed in the lateral roentgenogram.
Bolton registration p. The center of the Bolton cranial base, a point midway on a perpendicular from the Bolton plane to the center of sella turcica.
cardinal points. (a) *In obstetrics*, the four points of the pelvic inlet toward which the occiput of the fetus may be directed in a case of pregnancy with head presentation; the four points are the two sacroiliac articulations and the two ileopectineal eminences. (b) *In ophthalmology*, the six optical points that determine the direction of the rays entering or emerging from a series of refracting mediums.
condenser points. Instruments used for packing gold foil or amalgam into prepared cavities in teeth.
contact points. The points on the proximal surfaces of teeth which touch neighboring teeth.
craniometric p. Any one of the points on the skull used in craniometry. Among the more important are the following: acanthion, asterion, basion, bregma, dacryon, glabella, gnathion, gonion, inion, jugal point, lambda, metopion, nasion, obelion, ophryon, and opisthion. Also see *pterion*.
critical p. The temperature above which a gas cannot be liquefied by pressure.
deaf points. See deaf *field*.
dew p. The temperature at which the atmospheric moisture is deposited as dew.
disparate p. One of those points on the retina whence images are projected, not to the same, but to different points in space.
election p. *In surgery*, that point at which a certain operation is done by preference.
Erb's p. A point from 2 to 3 cm. above the clavicle and in front of the transverse process of the sixth cervical vertebra. Electric stimulation at this point produces contraction of the various muscles involved in Erb's paralysis.
far p. The remotest point of distinct vision.
fixiation p. The point of sharpest vision in the retina; the point where the visual axis meets the retina.
flash p. Lowest temperature at which vapor of a combustible liquid may be ignited.
focal p. See *focus*, 2.
freezing p. The temperature at which a pure liquid is in equilibrium with its solid form, or at which the solid form of the solvent is in equilibrium with a solution.
Gaussian points. Pair of axial points of a lens system, one corresponding to each side of the system and its appropriate focal point, locating object and image planes for which the image is the same size as the object and erect. Also called *nodal points*.
homologous points. *In roentgenology*, the same points on the two films of a stereogram.
hysterogenous p. See hysterogenic *zone*.
identical points. Corresponding points of the two retinas, upon which the rays from an object must be focused so that it may be seen as one.
infraorbital p. The lowest point on the anterior margin of the orbit.
isoelectric p. The pH at which the net electric charge on a particle or surface is zero.
lacrimal points. The lacrimal puncta.
McBurney's p. A point halfway between the umbilicus and the anterior superior iliac spine. A point of extreme tenderness in appendicitis.
malar p. The most prominent point on the outer surface of the zygomatic bone.
maximum occipital p. The point on the squama of the occipital bone which is farthest from the glabella.
melting p. The temperature at which a fusible solid begins to melt. Abbreviated, m.p.
mental p. See *gnathion*.
motor p. A point on the skin over a muscle at which electric stimulation will cause contraction of the muscle.
nasal p. See *nasion*.
near p. The nearest point at which the eyes can accommodate to see distinctly.
nodal p. See *Gaussian points* under *point*.
occipital p. The most posterior portion of the occiput in the sagittal plane.
painful p. Any point on the skin along the course of a nerve upon which pressure will cause pain; seen in neuritis.
p. of convergence. A conjugate focus upon which the light rays converge.
p. of divergence. A conjugate focus from which the light rays proceed.
p. of maximal impulse (PMI). The small area of the chest wall against which the left ventricle proximal to the apex is thrust during systole, normally found by palpation or inspection in or about the fifth left intercostal space inside the midclavicular line. Used in physical examination, the location, force, and quality of the point of maximal impulse may give important indications of cardiac and pulmonary abnormalities. Less properly called *apex beat* (*spitzenstoss*). See *herzstoss*.
points douloureux. See painful *p.*
posterior focal p. One of the conjugate foci. See under *focus*.
pressure points. Points of marked sensibility to pressure or weight, arranged like the temperature spots, and showing a specific end apparatus arranged in a punctate manner and connected with the pressure sense.
principal p. One of the two points in the optical axis of a lens that are so related that lines drawn from these points to the corresponding points in the object and its image are parallel.
reflection p. The point from which a ray of light is reflected.
refraction p. The point at which a ray of light is refracted.
spinous p. A sensitive point over a spinous process.
subnasal p. The middle point of the lower border of the nasal orifice.
supraclavicular p. That point stimulation of which causes contraction of the arm muscles.
triple p. The temperature and pressure at which the solid, liquid, and vapor phases of a substance may coexist.
vaccine p. A needle coated at one end with vaccine lymph.
vital p. A spot in the medulla oblongata corresponding to the seat of the respiratory center, puncture of which causes death.
Voillemier's p. A point on the linea alba 6–7 cm. below a line drawn between the two anterior superior spines of the ilium; suprapubic puncture of the urinary bladder is made at this point in fat or edematous subjects.

point'ing [*point*]. The coming to a point.
p. of an abscess. The process whereby pus forms or collects near the surface.

Poirier, Paul [*French surgeon*, 1853–1907]. Described the nasolambdoid line used in cranial topography. *Poirier's line* begins at the nasofrontal groove, extending around the base of the skull to a point just above the lambda; used as an aid in locating the lateral cerebral fissure and the left inferior frontal gyrus.

Pois, Guillaume le (**Piso**) [*Dutch naturalist*, 1611–78]. Remembered for his introduction of ipecacuanha into Europe (1648). Identified cases of yaws in Brazil.

poise [after Jean Léonard Marie *Poiseuille*, French physiologist, 1799–1869]. The unit of viscosity. The force in dynes necessary to be applied to an area of 1 sq. cm. between two parallel planes 1 sq. cm. in area and 1 cm. apart to produce a difference in streaming velocity between the liquid planes of 1 cm. per second.

Poiseuille, Jean Léonard Marie [*French physiologist*, 1799–1869]. Inventor of a hemodynamometer. Stated a law that the rapidity of current in capillary tubes is proportional to the square of their diameter; called *Poiseuille's law*. Noted the existence of a relatively slow-moving peripheral portion of the blood stream in minute vessels; called *Poiseuille's layer, space*.

poi'son [L. *potio*, a drink]. A substance that, being in solution in the blood or acting chemically on the blood, either destroys life or impairs seriously the functions of one or more of the organs of the body. Also see *poisoning*.

blood and nerve p. *In military medicine*, war gas which is absorbed into the body by breathing, by ingestion, or through the skin, and which affects the nervous and respiratory systems and various body functions.

capillary poisons. Substances such as peptones and foreign proteins which increase the flow of lymph, presumably by an injurious effect on the capillaries.

cellular poisons. Cytolysins.

irritant p. One that causes irritation at the point of entrance or at the point of elimination.

muscle p. A substance that impairs or destroys the proper functions of muscles.

narcotic p. One affecting the cerebral centers, producing stupor.

poi'son·ing [*potio*]. The condition caused by a poison. For poisonings not listed here, see the specific causative compound or agent.

acetanilid p. Symptoms: collapse, cyanosis. Treatment: evacuation, warmth, stimulants, artificial respiration.

acetophenetidin p. Similar to acetanilid poisoning.

acetylsalicylic acid p. See *p.* from salicylates.

aconite p. Symptoms: sudden collapse, slow, feeble, and irregular pulse and respirations, tingling in the mouth and extremities, giddiness, great muscular weakness, sometimes pain in the abdomen, marked anesthesia of skin, clear mind, convulsions at times. Treatment: tannic acid solution for washing out stomach, digitalis, stimulants, absolute quiet in recumbent position.

aconitum napellus p. See aconite *p.*

alcohol p. Symptoms: confusion of thought, giddiness, tottering gait, slight cyanosis, narcosis from which patient can be aroused, full pulse, deep, stertorous breathing, injection of eyes, low temperature; convulsions may occur. Treatment: stomach evacuation, coffee, stimulants.

alkali p. Ammonia, lye, washing soda, and quicklime poisoning fall into this category. Symptoms: intense gastroenteritis, often with bloody vomiting and purging, swollen lips and tongue covered with detached epithelium, violent dyspnea, characteristic odor. Treatment: dilution, vegetable acids (lemon juice or diluted vinegar), demulcents.

aniline p. A poisoning occurring commonly in industry. Symptoms: methemoglobin formation, headache, cyanosis, dyspnea, convulsions, and collapse. Treatment: warmth, stimulants, artificial respiration.

antimony p. Symptoms: metallic taste, violent vomiting which may become bloody, feeble pulse, pain and burning in the stomach, violent serous purging which becomes bloody, cramps in the extremities, thirst, great debility, sometimes prostration, collapse, unconsciousness, and convulsions without vomiting or purging. Treatment: tannic acid, demulcent drinks, opium, alcohol, external heat.

antipyrine p. Symptoms: headache, nausea, vomiting, a rash like that of measles, vertigo, drowsiness, deafness, confusion of ideas, cyanosis, collapse. Treatment: recumbent position, warmth, stimulants, oxygen, artificial respiration. Also called *phenazone p.*

apomorphine p. Symptoms: violent vomiting, paralysis of motor and sensory nerves, delirium, depression of respiration and of heart. Treatment: cardiac and respiratory stimulants.

arsenic p. Symptoms: violent, burning pain in the stomach, retching, thirst, purging of blood and mucus with flakes of epithelium, tenesmus, suppression of urine, sense of constriction in throat, small and frequent pulse. Treatment: gastric lavage, saline cathartics, colonic irrigation, enema, dimercaprol.

aspirin p. See *p.* from salicylates.

atropine p. Symptoms: heat and dryness of the mouth and throat, widely dilated pupils, scarlet rash, noisy delirium, quick pulse (at first corded, later feeble), rapid respirations (early strong, late shallow and feeble), retention of urine, sometimes convulsions, collapse, and paralysis. Treatment: tannic acid, stimulants, coffee, pilocarpine, artificial respiration, stomach and urinary bladder evacuation. Also called *homatropine p.*

barbiturate p. See *p.* from barbiturates.

barium sulfide p. That occurring from the use of certain depilatories. Symptoms: violent intestinal colic, cardiac irregularity. Treatment: gastric lavage, magnesium sulfate.

belladonna p. That caused by the deadly nightshade. See atropine *p.*

benzene p. If taken by mouth, symptoms: pyrexia, excitement followed by narcosis, paralysis, gastrointestinal irritation, aspiration pneumonia. Treatment: dilution with oil, evacuation. If from the toxic fumes, symptoms: the initial stage resembles alcoholic intoxication followed by narcosis, convulsions, and paralysis. Treatment: stimulants, artificial respiration.

borax p. See boric acid *p.*

boric acid p. Symptoms: profound depression, hepatitis. Treatment: evacuation, fluid, dextrose intravenously.

brucine p. See strychnine *p.*

caffeine p. Symptoms: burning pain in the throat, giddiness, faintness, nausea, numbness, abdominal pain, great thirst, dry tongue, tremor of extremities, diuresis, weak pulse, cold skin, collaspe. Treatment: emetics, stimulants, warmth.

calabar-bean p. See physostigma venenosum *p.*

camphor p. Symptoms: characteristic odor, giddiness, disturbance of vision, delirium, cyclic convulsions, clammy skin, smarting in the urinary organs, quick and weak pulse. Treatment: stomach evacuation.

cannabis indica p. Symptoms: pleasurable intoxication, heavy sleep. Treatment: stomach evacuation. Also called *Indian hemp p.*

cantharis vesicatoria p. See *p.* from cantharides.

carbolic acid p. See phenol *p.*
carbona p. See carbon tetrachloride *p.*
carbon disulfide p. Symptoms: vomiting, weakness, convulsions, coma. Treatment: evacuation, artificial respiration.
carbon monoxide p. Symptoms: headache, giddiness, loss of muscular power, unconsciousness, dilated pupils, labored breathing, coma, cherry-red skin color. Treatment: fresh air, artificial respiration, stimulants, oxygen, coffee, bleeding and replacement with healthy blood.
carbon tetrachloride p. Symptoms: unconsciousness, asphyxial convulsions, cardiac fibrillation, hepatitis. Treatment: evacuation, artificial respiration, dextrose intravenously.
chloral hydrate p. Symptoms: deep sleep, loss of muscular power, lividity, diminished reflexes, weak pulse, slowed respirations, contracted pupils during sleep, but dilated on waking, low temperature. Treatment: stomach evacuation, application of heat to the extremities, massage, coffee by rectum, strychnine, amyl nitrite, artificial respiration.
chlorinated lime p. That caused by the poisonous component of Labarraque's solution, Javelle water, or bleaching fluid. Symptoms: local irritation, gastrointestinal and pulmonary. Treatment: evacuation, sodium thiosulfate in water, milk and raw eggs.
chloroform p. Symptoms: excitement and intoxication followed by anesthesia and unconsciousness, later profound narcosis, progressively or suddenly failing pulse and respirations. Treatment: draw tongue forward, artificial respiration; if chloroform has been taken by mouth, evacuation of stomach.
chromic acid p. See chromium trioxide *p.*
chromium trioxide p. Symptoms: dark yellow stains, abdominal pain, vomiting and purging, collapse. Treatment: stomach evacuation, chalk, milk, or albumin, demulcent drinks.
coal gas p. See carbon monoxide *p.*
coal oil p. See benzene *p.*
coal tar p. See phenol *p.*
cocaine p. Symptoms: faintness, giddiness, nausea, small, rapid, and intermittent pulse, dilated pupils, severe prostration, slow and feeble respiration. Treatment: stimulants, amyl nitrite, artificial respiration.
codeine p. See opium *p.*
colchicum autumnale p. Symptoms: not unlike those of malignant cholera; griping pain in the stomach, vomiting and continuous purging of seromucous material, intense thirst, muscular cramps, great prostration, collapse, dilated pupils, pain in the extremities. Treatment: stomach evacuation, tannic acid, morphine.
conium maculatum p. Symptoms: weakness of the legs, gradual loss of all voluntary power, nausea, ptosis, dilatation of pupils, inability to speak or swallow. Treatment: stomach evacuation, tannic acid, stimulants, warmth, artificial respiration, atropine.
creosote p. See phenol *p.*
cresol p. See phenol *p.*
croton tiglium p. Symptoms: intense pain in abdomen, vomiting, purging, watery stools, pinched face, small and thready pulse, moist skin, collapse. Treatment: stomach evacuation, demulcent drinks, morphine, poultices to abdomen. Also called *croton oil p.*
cyanogen p. See hydrocyanic acid *p.*
Datura stramonium p. Symptoms and treatment similar to those of atropine poisoning.
depilatory p. See barium sulfide *p.*
digitalis p. Symptoms: purging, with severe pain, violent vomiting, vertigo, feeble pulse (although heart action is tumultuous), delirium, and asphyxial convulsions. Treatment: stomach evacuation, tannic acid, recumbent position.
food p. A type of poisoning due to food contaminated by bacterial toxins or by certain living bacteria, particularly those of the *Salmonella* group, and staphylococci. The term is also used to include symptoms due to foods naturally poisonous, such as fungi (see mushroom *p.*), botulism, mussel poisoning, and poisoning due to chemicals or allergens in food. Of the food poisonings, that due to bacterial contamination is the most frequent, but botulism is the most serious; two-thirds of the victims die. In food poisoning due to bacterial contamination of the food, the symptoms are: violent diarrhea, retching, prostration, dizziness, and cramps in the abdomen; symptoms generally appear from two to six hours after the food is eaten. Treatment: evacuation of stomach; fasting for at least 24 hours, then liquid diet for two days, bed rest.
foxglove p. See digitalis *p.*
gasoline p. See benzene *p.*
gelsemium sempervirens p. Symptoms: appear in about twenty minutes; great muscular weakness, diplopia, ptosis, squint, widely dilated pupils, dimness of vision, labored respiration, weak pulse. Treatment: evacuation of stomach, atropine, stimulants, artificial respiration.
green hellebore p. See veratrum *p.*
hellebore p. See veratrum *p.*
hemlock p. See conium maculatum *p.*
hydrochloric acid p. Symptoms: pain throughout digestive tract, vomiting, feeble pulse, clammy skin, collapse, eschars externally, yellow stains on clothing, but none on skin. Treatment: demulcent drinks, oil, stimulants (intravenous injection). Also called *muriatic acid p.*
hydrocyanic acid p. Symptoms: sudden unconsciousness, slow, labored respirations, slow pulse, staring eyes, purple face, general convulsions, then relaxation and collapse, odor of peach kernels; death may be almost instantaneous. Treatment: stomach tube if possible, alternate cold and warm effusions, artificial respiration.
hyoscyamus p. See atropine *p.*
Indian tobacco p. See lobelia inflata *p.*
iodine p. Symptoms: pain in throat and stomach, vomiting, purging, vomit yellow from iodine, or blue if starch is present in stomach, giddiness, faintness, convulsive movements. Treatment: stomach evacuation, starch, morphine.
iodoform p. Symptoms: slight delirium, drowsiness, high temperature, rapid pulse. Treatment: gastric lavage.
jaborandi p. See pilocarpine *p.*
Jamestown weed p. Symptoms and treatment similar to those of atropine poisoning.
kerosene p. See benzene *p.*
laudanum p. See opium *p.*
lead p. Symptoms: sweet metallic taste, vomiting of white matter, great thirst, pain in abdomen, usually rigid abdominal muscles, constipation or diarrhea with black stools, cramps in the legs, paralysis of the extremities, convulsions; in the chronic forms, a blue line at the margin of the gums, basophilic stippling of the red cells. Treatment: stomach evacuation, Epsom or Glauber's salts, milk, morphine.
lobelia inflata p. Symptoms: severe vomiting, with intense depression and prostration, giddiness, tremors, convulsions, collapse. Treatment: stomach evacuation, tannic acid, warmth, recumbent position.
manganese p. That which results from the inha-

lation of manganese dust or fumes. Symptoms: resemble paralysis agitans. Treatment: preventive.

meadow-saffron p. See colchicum autumnale *p.*

mercury bichloride p. Symptoms: acrid metallic taste, burning heat in throat and stomach, vomiting, diarrhea with bloody stools, white and shriveled lips and tongue, small and frequent pulse, nephrosis, and colitis, death in coma or convulsions. Secondary symptoms: hectic fever, coppery taste, fetid breath, gums swollen, salivation. Treatment: albumin in some form, raw white of egg or flour; immediate stomach evacuation; reducing agents, sodium formaldehyde sulfoxylate, calcium sulfide, sodium hypophosphide or thiosulfate.

mesothorium p. Biological damage to tissue as a result of exposure to radiations of mesothorium.

metal p. That due to inhalation of fumes of molten brass or zinc. Symptoms: chill, sweating, nausea, thirst, fever, leukocytosis. Treatment: emetics, laxatives, milk, and sodium bicarbonate.

methyl alcohol p. See wood alcohol *p.*

methyl salicylate p. See *p.* from salicylates.

monkshood p. See aconite *p.*

morphine p. See opium *p.*

mushroom p. Symptoms with most poisonous species: delayed gastroenteritis and hepatitis. Treatment: evacuation, dextrose injection.

naphthalene p. That caused by overdoses of naphthalene for therapeutic purposes or by eating or sucking naphthalene moth balls. Symptoms: listlessness and anorexia followed by emesis, fever, abdominal pain, hemoglobinuria, and blood changes caused by acute hemolytic anemia. Treatment: blood transfusion and alkali therapy.

narceine p. See opium *p.*

nicotine p. See tobacco *p.*

nitric acid p. Symptoms: yellow stains on skin; otherwise similar to sulfuric acid poisoning. Treatment: alkalies, soap, demulcents, stimulants.

nitrobenzene p. A type of poisoning important in industrial medicine with symptoms and treatment similar to aniline poisoning.

nitroglycerin p. Symptoms: throbbing headache, pulsation over entire body, dicrotic pulse, flushed face, mental confusion, anxiety, sudden collapse. Treatment: recumbent position.

nux vomica p. See strychnine *p.*

opium p. Symptoms: preliminary mental excitement, followed soon by weariness, sensation of weight in the limbs, sleepiness, diminished sensibility, pin-point pupils, slow and strong pulse and respiration; patient can be roused with difficulty; later, rousing becomes impossible; slow, irregular, and stertorous respiration, rapid and feeble pulse. Treatment: evacuate stomach with mustard or stomach tube, arouse patient to maintain respiration by exercise, with cold and hot ablutions alternately, or stimulate by atropine or coffee if pulse fails, and apply external heat.

oxalic acid p. Symptoms: hot, acrid taste, burning, vomiting, collapse, sometimes general paralysis, numbness, and stupor. Treatment: lime or chalk.

Paris green p. See arsenic *p.*

phenacetin p. Acetophenetidin poisoning; similar to acetanilid poisoning.

phenol p. Symptoms: immediate burning pain from mouth to stomach, giddiness, loss of consciousness, collapse, partial suppression of urine, which is smoky in color; characteristic odor; white, corrugated patches in mouth. Treatment: gastric lavage with dilute alcohol.

phosphorus p. Symptoms: vomiting and pain; vomit may be luminous in the dark; characteristic odor; after several days deep jaundice, coffee-colored vomit, hepatic tenderness, albuminuria, marked fall in temperature, coma, failure of pulse and respiration. Treatment: copper sulfate as an emetic, then as an antidote in small doses with opium; liquid paraffin.

physostigma venenosum p. Symptoms: giddiness, prostration, loss of power in the lower limbs, muscular twitching, contracted pupils, clear mind. Treatment: stomach evacuation, atropine.

pilocarpine p. Symptoms: copious sweating, dizziness, salivation, vomiting, diarrhea, myopia, pupils much contracted. Treatment: stomach evacuation, stimulants, atropine.

p. from antimony compounds. See antimony *p.*

p. from arsenic compounds. See arsenic *p.*

p. from barbiturates. Symptoms: narcosis, sometimes preceded by excitement; prolonged sleep, stupor or coma. Treatment: gastric lavage, picrotoxin or metrazol.

p. from bromides. Symptoms: vomiting, lethargy, hebetude, profound sleep, cramps, acne, mania. Treatment: sodium chloride.

p. from cantharides. Symptoms: burning in mouth and stomach, vomiting and purging, soon becoming bloody, tenesmus, salivation, aching pains in the back, strangury, priapism, unconsciousness only very late; convulsions at times. Treatment: stomach evacuation, demulcent drinks, morphine, hot bath for the strangury; anesthetics may be necessary for the pain.

p. from cyanogen compounds. See hydrocyanic acid *p.*

p. from hypnotics. See *p.* from barbiturates.

p. from iodine compounds. See iodine *p.*

p. from lead salts. See lead *p.*

p. from salicylates. Symptoms: nausea and vomiting, deafness, delirium, confusion, dyspnea, coma, collapse. These are complicated with local irritation for salicylic acid, acetylsalicylic acid, and methylsalicylate. The acids also produce acidosis. Treatment: evacuation, alkalies.

p. from sulfonamides. Symptoms: nausea and vomiting, fever, delirium, skin eruptions, hemolysis, nephritis, granulocytopenia, cyanosis. Treatment: fluids.

prussic acid p. See hydrocyanic acid *p.*

ptomaine p. Incorrect term for food poisoning.

radiation p. Any illness which results when a radioactive material gains access to the body where it acts as an internal poison producing localized or systemic effects or both.

roach poison p. See sodium fluoride *p.*

salicylic acid p. See *p.* from salicylates.

santonin p. Symptoms: disturbance of color vision; objects first assume a bluish tinge, then yellow; tinnitus, dizziness, pain in the abdomen, failure of respiration, convulsions, stupor. Treatment: evacuate stomach, mitigate convulsions with ether.

savin p. Symptoms: pain, vomiting, bloody stools and tenesmus, disordered respirations, coma, convulsions, and collapse. Treatment: evacuation of stomach, castor oil in large doses.

selenium p. A form of poisoning, seldom if ever acute in man, which is due to the ingestion of selenium in water and plant foods during a long period of years and characterized by general debility with degenerative changes in the liver and kidneys. Also called *alkali disease, loco disease.*

silver salts p. Symptoms: pain, vomiting, and purging; vomit white and cheesy, rapidly turning black in the sunlight; vertigo, coma, convulsions, paralysis, and marked disturbance of respiration. Treatment: salt and water, stomach evacuation, a large amount of milk.

sodium fluoride p. That due to a poison found

in roach powder. Symptoms: violent gastroenteritis. Treatment: gastric lavage, calcium salts.

Spanish fly p. See *p.* from cantharides.

stramonium p. See atropine *p.*

strophanthus p. See digitalis *p.*

strychnine p. Symptoms: tetanic convulsions in paroxysms at intervals varying from five minutes to half an hour; opisthotonos during paroxysm; prominent eyeballs; pupils dilated, impeded respiration, feeble and rapid pulse, anxiety. Treatment: evacuate stomach; tannic acid followed by an emetic; keep patient quiet; ether or barbiturates to control convulsions; artificial respiration if indicated.

sulfuric acid p. Symptoms: vomiting, often of tarry matter, black stains, pain throughout digestive tract, feeble pulse, clammy skin, profuse and bloody salivation. Treatment: chalk, magnesia, soap, demulcent drinks.

thorn-apple p. Symptoms and treatment similar to those of atropine poisoning.

tobacco p. Symptoms: nausea, vomiting, weakness, weak pulse, cold and clammy skin, collapse, contracted pupils, then dilated. Treatment: stomach evacuation, tannic acid, recumbent position, artificial respiration.

tung-nut p. That caused by the tung nut. Symptoms: gastroenteritis and fluid and electrolyte deficiencies; later cyanosis, paresthesia, mydriasis, irregular respirations, reflex changes; sometimes renal dysfunction may occur.

veratrum p. That caused by both the white (album) and the green (viride) varieties of veratrum, which have the same effect. Symptoms: pain and burning in the alimentary tract, vomiting and diarrhea, slow, weak pulse, labored respiration, sometimes convulsions. Treatment: stomach evacuation, opium, stimulants, coffee, warmth, recumbent position.

white hellebore p. See veratrum *p.*

wintergreen oil p. See *p.* from salicylates.

wood alcohol p. Symptoms: inebriation, gastroenteritis, prolonged coma, blindness. Treatment: gastric lavage, fluids, dextrose intravenously.

yellow jasmine p. See gelsemium sempervirens *p.*

poi'son i'vy. A climbing vine, *Toxicodendron radicans* (also called *Rhus toxicodendron* and *Rhus radicans);* contains an oleoresin (urushiol) which causes a form of dermatitis venenata.

poison-ivy extract. Trade name for a solution of a resin extracted from the fresh leaves of *Toxicodendron radicans:* used for the prevention or treatment of the symptoms of the dermatitis produced through contact with *Toxicodendron radicans.* See *ivyol.*

poi'son nut. Nux vomica.

poi'son oak. *Toxicodendron quercifolium* (also called *Rhus toxicodendron* Linné but not the *R. toxicodendron* of American authors, which is poison ivy); produces a contact dermatitis similar to that produced by poison ivy. **Western poison oak** is the *Toxicodendron diversilobum* (also known as *Rhus diversiloba*).

poison-oak extract. Trade name for a solution of a resin extracted from the fresh leaves of *Toxicodendron quercifolium:* used for the prevention or treatment of the symptoms of the dermatitis produced through contact with *Toxicodendron quercifolium.* See *ivyol.*

poi'son·ous. Having the properties of a poison.

poi'son su'mac. A smooth shrub, *Toxicodendron vernix* (also called *Rhus vernix* and *Rhus venenata);* contains an oil which makes the plant poisonous to the touch; produces eruptions resembling poison-ivy dermatitis.

poison-sumac extract. Trade name for a solution of a resin extracted from the fresh leaves of *Toxicodendron vernix:* used for the prevention or treatment of symptoms of dermatitis resulting from contact with *Toxicodendron vernix.*

Poisson distribution. *In statistics,* a discrete mathematical distribution, often called the Law of Small Numbers, that may be regarded as an approximation of the binomial distribution when *p* (probability) is small and *n* (number) large.

poke'ber"ry, poke'root. See *phytolacca.*

po'ker back. Complete stiffness of the spine, usually due to ankylosing spondylitis or rheumatoid arthritis of the spine.

po'lar. Of, pertaining to, or having a pole; *in chemistry,* used to describe any compound whose molecules are composed of atoms which share their common electron pairs unequally and thereby effect a separation of positive and negative centers of electricity to form a dipole.

po'lar bod'ies. The two minute cells given off successively by the ovum during the maturation divisions. They mark the animal pole. Also called *polar cells, polocytes, polar globules.*

po"lar·im'e·ter [L. *polus,* pole, from G. *polos;* G. *metron,* a measure]. An instrument for making quantitative studies on the rotation of polarized light by optically active substances.

po"lar·im'e·try. The use of the polarimeter.

po·lar'i·scope [*polus;* G. *skopein,* to examine]. An instrument for studying the polarization of light; a polarimeter.

po·lar"i·stro·bom'e·ter [*polus;* G. *strobos,* a whirling round; *metron,* a measure]. A form of polarimeter or saccharimeter that furnishes a delicate means of fixing the plane of polarization as rotated by the sugar solution under examination.

po·lar'i·ty [*polus*]. 1. The state or quality of having poles or points of intensity with mutually opposite qualities. 2. The electrically positive or negative condition of a battery or other electric terminals. 3. Demonstration of sedation of a nerve sensation at or near the positive electrode, and of irritation at or near the negative electrode; of anelectrotonus of muscular contraction near the positive electrode and of catelectrotonus near the negative.

po"lar·i·za'tion [*polus*]. 1. The act of polarizing or the state of being polarized. 2. A condition produced in a ray of light by absorption, reflection, or refraction, by means of which the vibrations are restricted and take place in one plane only (plane polarization) or in curves (circular or elliptic polarization). The plane of polarization is altered or rotated when the light is passed through a quartz crystal or solutions of certain substances (rotatory polarization). 3. The deposit of gas bubbles (hydrogen) on the electronegative plate of a galvanic battery, whereby the flow of the current is impeded. 4. Acquisition of electric charges of opposite sign, as across semipermeable membranes in polarization of cell membranes in living tissues.

p. of electrodes. Acquisition of charges on electrodes used to lead off from solutions or living tissues; due to migration of ions.

po'lar·ize [*polus*]. Endow with polarity; place in a state of polarization.

po'lar·i"zer [*polus*]. An object, such as a Nicol prism, by means of which light is polarized.

po·lar'o·gram. The current-voltage curve obtained in polarographic analysis.

po·lar'o·graph [*polus;* G. *graphein,* to write]. An instrument used in polarography.

po"lar·og'ra·phy [*polus; graphein*]. A method of chemical analysis based on the interpretation of the current-voltage curve characteristic of a solution of an electrooxidizable or electroreducible substance when it is electrolyzed with the dropping mercury electrode. —**polarograph'ic,** *adj*.

polaroid. Trade-mark for a specially prepared cellulose film containing oriented iodoquinine sulfate crystals, mounted between two glass plates. Used as a substitute for Nicol prisms, in polariscopes, and for microscopes, reading glasses, and windshields to avoid glare.

pole [*polus*]. 1. Either extremity of the axis of the body, as of the fetus, the crystalline lens, etc. 2. One of two points at which opposite physical qualities, for example, of electricity or of magnetism, are concentrated; specifically, the electrodes of a galvanic battery, or of other generators of electricity.

animal p. (a) The formative pole of an ovum distinguished by having more cytoplasm, pigment, etc. (b) In the mammalian blastocyst, the pole containing the inner cell mass. Also called *apical p., germinal p.*

frontal p. The tip of the frontal lobe of the cerebrum.

negative p. The active pole of a battery; the electropositive element. Also called *cathode*.

occipital p. The tip of the occipital lobe of the cerebrum.

p. changer. A switch or key for changing or reversing the direction of an electric current.

positive p. The inactive pole of a source of electricity, as a battery, consisting of an electronegative element. Also called *anode*.

temporal p. The tip of the temporal lobe of the cerebrum. See Plate 17.

vegetal p. The relatively inactive, yolk-laden pole of an ovum. Also called *vegetative p., antigerminal p.*

po'li·en·ceph"a·li'tis. See *polioencephalitis*.

pol"i·het"er·ox'e·nous [G. *polys*, many; *heteros*, different; *xenos*, host]. Pertaining to parasites having more than one intermediate host.

po'li·o (po'lee·o) [G. *polios*, gray]. Short for poliomyelitis.

po'li·o-, po'li- [*polios*]. A combining form meaning *gray;* used to denote *relation to the gray matter of the brain.*

po'li·o·en·ceph"a·li'tis [*polios;* G. *egkephalos*, brain; *-itis*, inflammation]. Inflammation of the gray matter of the brain.

anterior superior p. An inflammatory disease of the gray matter about the third ventricle, about the anterior portion of the fourth, and of that about the cerebral aqueduct, characterized by ophthalmoplegia, chiefly external, and a peculiar somnolent state.

inferior p. An inflammatory disease of the medulla oblongata.

p. acuta. An acute inflammation of the cerebral cortex; in children it gives rise to infantile cerebral palsy.

p. hemorrhagica. Inflammation of the gray matter with hemorrhage.

posterior p. Inflammation of the gray matter in the vicinity of the fourth ventricle.

superior hemorrhagic p. An inflammatory disease of the gray matter around the third ventricle.

po'li·o·en·ceph"a·lo·me·nin"go·my"e·li'tis [*polios; egkephalos;* G. *mēnigx*, membrane; *myelos*, marrow; *-itis*]. Inflammation of the gray matter of the brain and spinal cord and of their meninges.

po'li·o·en·ceph"a·lo·my"e·li'tis [*polios; egkephalos; myelos; -itis*]. Any inflammation of the gray matter of the brain and spinal cord, more specifically anterior poliomyelitis with encephalitis.

po'li·o·en·ceph"a·lop'a·thy [*polios; egkephalos;* G. *pathos*, disease]. Any disease of the gray matter of the brain.

po'li·o·my"e·len·ceph"a·li'tis [*polios;* G. *myelos*, marrow; *egkephalos; -itis*, inflammation]. Poliomyelitis and polioencephalitis existing together.

po'li·o·my"e·li'tis [*polios; myelos; -itis*]. 1. A common virus disease of man which usually runs a mild or abortive course, characterized by upper respiratory and gastrointestinal symptoms, but which may progress to involve the central nervous system and result in a nonparalytic or paralytic form of the disease, the latter being the classical form of acute anterior poliomyelitis. It is endemic with epidemic flare-ups. 2. Formerly, any inflammation of the gray matter of the spinal cord. —**poliomyelit'ic,** *adj*.

abortive p. An early form, diagnosed by inference during an epidemic, characterized clinically only by relatively mild symptoms of upper respiratory infection, headache, gastrointestinal disturbances, nausea, and vomiting, but which does not progress to involvement of the central nervous system. Definite diagnosis rests upon isolation of the virus and serological reactions.

acute anterior p. An acute inflammation of the anterior horns of the gray matter of the spinal cord. It is most common in children, producing a paralysis of certain muscle groups or of an entire limb. The onset is sudden, with fever, gastrointestinal complaints, and pain in the affected muscles, and the paralysis is usually most extensive in the beginning, a certain amount of improvement taking place subsequently. The affected muscles atrophy rapidly, the reflexes in them are lost, and reaction of degeneration develops. From contraction of antagonistic muscles, deformities occur later in life. Also called *infantile paralysis, epidemic paralysis, acute wasting paralysis, Heine-Medin's disease.*

anterior spinal p. Anterior poliomyelitis, acute or chronic.

ascending p. A type similar to Landry's paralysis. The paralysis starts in the toes, rapidly extends to the legs, thighs, trunk, and finally to the muscles of respiration.

bulbar p. A form in which lesions are concentrated in the medulla of the brain; motor cranial nuclei and respiratory and circulatory centers may be affected.

bulbospinal p. A form involving the medulla and spinal cord.

chronic anterior p. See progressive muscular *atrophy*.

encephalitic p. That in which, in addition to bulbar and spinal lesions, there is more diffuse involvement of the brain. Principal symptoms include anxiety, hyperexcitability, signs of upper motor neuron lesion, muscular tremors, delirium, coma, and occasionally convulsions.

metallic p. A form of toxic neuritis due to metal poisoning where the paralysis is so severe that it simulates poliomyelitis.

myelitic p. A type characterized by pain in the back, abdomen, and sometimes the lower limbs, flaccid paraplegia, sensory loss extending to the trunk, and retention of urine. The end result is spastic paraplegia and sphincter disturbances.

nonparalytic p. A form generally characterized by pain and stiffness in the muscles of the axial skeleton, especially of the neck and back, mild fever, and often increased amounts of proteins and number of leukocytes in the cerebrospinal fluid. This may be the clinical maximum of the disease. Definitive diagnosis rests upon isolation of the virus and serological reactions.

paralytic p. A form with a variable combination of signs of damage to the central nervous system, including flaccid paralysis, weakness, incoordination, muscle spasms, muscle tenderness, hyperesthesia, and disturbance of consciousness: subdivided, on the basis of anatomical structures involved, into acute anterior or spinal, bulbospinal, bulbar, and encephalitic types.

spinal p. See acute anterior *p.*

spinobulbar p. See bulbospinal *p.*

syphilitic p. See syphilitic *amyotrophia.*

po′li·o·my″e·lop′a·thy [*polios; myelos;* G. *pathos,* disease]. Disease of the gray matter of the spinal cord and medulla oblongata.

po′li·o·plasm″ (po′lee·o·plaz″um) [*polios;* G. *plasma,* anything formed]. Granular cytoplasm.

po′li·o′sis [*polios;* G. *-ōsis,* condition]. A condition characterized by the absence of pigment in the hair. Syn., *canities.*

po′li·o·thrix. See *canities.*

Po′lish plait. See *plica* polonica.

Politzer, Adam [*Austrian otologist,* 1835–1920]. Described otosclerosis (1895). Introduced a method of testing hearing. A tuning fork held in front of the nares will be heard only by an unaffected ear during swallowing; called *Politzer's test.* See also Politzer *bag.*

po·litz″er·i·za′tion (po·lit″sur·i·zay′shun, ·eye-zay′shun, po″lit·sur·, pol″it·sur·) [*Politzer*]. The production of sudden increased air pressure in the nasopharynx to inflate the middle ear, by means of compression by a Politzer bag.

poll (pole) [ME. *pol*]. *In veterinary medicine,* that part of a horse's neck lying just posterior to the occiput.

Pollak's test. See von Jaksch-Pollak's *test.*

pol″la·ki·u′ri·a (pol″uh·kee·yoor′ee·uh, ·kigh-yoor′ee·uh) [G. *pollakis,* often; *ouron,* urine]. Abnormally frequent micturition.

pol·lan′tin [L. *pollen,* fine flour; G. *anti,* against]. A hay-fever antitoxin obtained from the blood of horses inoculated with pollen extract. Also called *Dunbar's serum.*

pol′len [L.]. The fecundating element produced in the anthers of flowering plants.

pol″le·no′sis [*pollen;* G. *-ōsis,* condition]. Hay fever or asthma caused by contact with pollen to which the patient is specifically sensitive.

pol′lex [L.]. The thumb. —**pol′li·cis,** *adj.*

p. valgus. A thumb abnormally bent toward the ulnar side.

p. varus. A thumb abnormally bent toward the radial side.

Pollister method. See Mirsky-Pollister *method.*

pol·lu′tion [L. *pollutum,* from *polluere,* to defile]. 1. The act of defiling or rendering impure, as pollution of drinking water. 2. The discharge of semen without sexual intercourse, as in nocturnal emission.

nocturnal p. A nocturnal, involuntary seminal discharge. *Obs.*

self-p. Masturbation. *Obs.*

po′lo·cyte [L. *polus,* pole; G. *kytos,* cell]. One of the small cells or bodies formed during the maturation divisions of the ovum. Syn., *polar body.*

po·lo′ni·um [ML. *Polonia,* Poland]. Po = 210. The first radioactive element isolated by Pierre and Marie Curie from pitchblende (1898); a product of disintegration of radium. Syn., *radium-F.*

pol·toph′a·gy [G. *poltos,* porridge; *phagein,* to eat]. Complete chewing of the food before swallowing it.

po′lus [L.]. A pole.

pol′y- [G. *polys,* many]. 1. A combining form meaning *much* or *many.* 2. *In medicine,* a combining form denoting *excessive, affecting many parts,* or *of diverse origin.*

Pólya, Eugene [*Hungarian surgeon,* 1876–1944]. Distinguished for his important contributions to the technic of gastrointestinal surgery. His gastroenterostomy is accomplished by the use of small Payr clamps placed upon the duodenum after freeing it with the pyloric end of the stomach, the duodenum being divided, the stomach retracted, and the duodenum closed. The stomach is clamped at a point distal to the freed portion in which all vessels have been secured. A loop of jejunum is brought through an opening in the transverse mesocolon and united to the posterior wall of the stomach, forming a posterior gastroenterostomy. Called *Pólya's method, Pólya's operation.*

pol″y·ac′id (pol″ee·ass′id) [G. *polys,* many; L. *acidus,* sour]. Applied to a base or basic radical capable of yielding two or more hydroxyl groups, as $Ba(OH)_2$, $Fe(OH)_3$.

pol″y·aes·the′si·a (pol″ee·ess·thee′zhuh, ·zee·uh). See *polyesthesia.*

pol″y·am′ine (pol″ee·am′in, pol″ee·uh·meen′). Nonspecific term referring to compounds possessing two or more amine groups.

pol″y·am′ine-meth′yl·ene res′in. Generic name for a synthetic acid-binding resin obtained by the polymerization of an aromatic amine and formaldehyde or of a polyamine, a phenol, and formaldehyde. Such a resin is useful clinically as a gastric antacid and to prevent acidosis when carbacrylic resin is used for its sodium-depleting effect. Also called *polyamine-formaldehyde resin.* See also *carbacrylamine resins.*

pol′y·an″dry [*polys;* G. *anēr,* man]. A social state in which is recognized the marriage of one woman with more than one man at the same time.

polyansyn. Trade-mark for a sterile solution of the various anterior pituitary factors.

pol″y·ar″te·ri′tis [*polys;* G. *artēria,* artery; *-itis,* inflammation]. Inflammation of a number of arteries at the same time.

p. nodosa. An acute and sometimes recurrent disease of unknown cause, frequently fatal and occurring at any age. The characteristic lesion is an irregularly distributed segmental panarteritis resulting in nodules and hemorrhage along the involved arteries. Histologically necrosis, edema, and cellular exudate, frequently including eosinophils, make up the lesions. It has been regarded by some as a reaction of hypersensitivity, and is grouped as a collagen disease. Also called *periarteritis nodosa, disseminated necrotizing periarteritis.*

pol″y·ar′thric [*polys;* G. *arthron,* joint]. Pertaining to many joints.

pol″y·ar·thri′tis [*polys;* G. *arthritis,* arthritis]. Inflammation of many joints, sometimes used to mean acute rheumatic fever.

epidemic tropical acute p. A self-limited syndrome of unknown cause, first described among Australian soldiers (1942), characterized by acute polyarthritis, mild fever, lymphadenopathy, and transient rash: also called *fox-hole arthritis, Bougainville rheumatism.*

pol″y·ar·tic′u·lar [*polys;* L. *articulus,* joint]. Affecting many joints.

pol″y·a·tom′ic [*polys;* G. *atomos,* uncut]. 1. Containing several atoms. 2. Having several hydrogen atoms replaceable by bases.

pol″y·ba′sic [*polys;* G. *basis,* base]. Applied to an acid having several hydrogen atoms replaceable by bases.

pol″y·ba′sic ac′id. Any acid which contains several replaceable hydrogen atoms.

pol′y·blast [*polys;* G. *blastos,* germ]. A free macrophage of inflamed connective tissue.

pol″y·bleph′a·ron [*polys;* G. *blepharon,* eyelid]. A supernumerary eyelid. Also called *polyblepharia, polyblephary.*

pol″y·cel′lu·lar [*polys;* L. *cellula,* small storeroom]. Having many cells.

pol′y·cen′tric [*polys;* G. *kentron*, center]. Having many centers or nuclear points.

pol″y·chei′ri·a (·kigh′ree·uh) [*polys;* G. *cheir*, hand]. The state of having a supernumerary hand. —**pol″y·chei′rous,** *adj.*

pol″y·cho′li·a (·ko′lee·uh) [*polys;* G. *cholē*, bile]. Excessive secretion of bile.

pol″y·chro′ism [*polys;* G. *chroia*, color]. A property possessed by certain crystals, under polarized light, of exhibiting different absorption colors which vary as the polarizing instrument is rotated.

pol″y·chro·ma′si·a, pol″y·chro·ma′ti·a. See *polychromatophilia.*

pol″y·chro·mat′ic [G. *polys*, many; *chrōmatikos*, of color]. Many-colored.

pol″y·chro′ma·to·phil″. See polychromatophilic *erythrocyte.* See also *reticulocyte*, 1.

pol″y·chro″ma·to·phil′i·a [*polys; chrōma; philein*]. The presence in the blood of polychromatophilic cells. Also called *polychromasia, polychromophilia.*

pol″y·chro″ma·to·phil′ic [*polys; chrōma; philein*]. Susceptible to staining with more than one dye.

pol″y·chro′mi·a [*polys; chrōma*]. Increased or abnormal pigmentation.

pol″y·chro′mo·phil. See *polychromatophil.*

pol″y·chro″mo·phil′i·a. See *polychromatophilia.*

pol″y·chy′li·a (·kigh′lee·uh) [*polys;* G. *chylos*, juice]. Excessive formation of chyle. —**polychylic,** *adj.*

pol″y·clin′ic [*polys;* G. *klinikos*, of a bed]. A hospital in which many diseases are treated.

pol″y·clo′ni·a [*polys;* G. *klonos*, confused motion]. An affection said to be distinct from tic and chorea but marked by clonic spasms.

pol″y·co′ri·a [*polys;* G. *korē*, pupil]. The existence of more than one pupil in an iris.

pol″y·cy′clic (·sigh′click, ·sick′lick) [*polys;* G. *kyklos*, cycle]. 1. Describing a molecule which contains two or more groupings of atoms in the form of rings or closed chains. 2. *In dermatology*, pertaining to cutaneous lesions exhibiting many confluent rings or arcs.

polycycline. Trade-mark for tetracycline, commonly supplied as the hydrochloride.

pol″y·cy·e′sis (·sigh·ee′sis) [*polys;* G. *kyēsis*, pregnancy]. Multiple pregnancy.

pol″y·cys′tic [*polys;* G. *kystis*, bladder]. Containing many cysts.

pol″y·cys′tic o′va·ries. See Stein-Leventhal *syndrome.*

pol″y·cy·the′mi·a (·sigh·thee′mee·uh) [*polys;* G. *kytos*, cell; *haima*, blood]. A condition characterized by an increased number of erythrocytes.

myelopathic p. See primary *p.*

p. hypertonica. That associated with hypertension but without splenomegaly: described by F. Gaisböck.

p. vera. See primary *p.*

primary p. A rare disease in which the red blood cells are greatly increased in number, with an absolute increase in the total mass of red cells per kilogram of body weight. Characterized by a red cyanosis, disturbances of the central nervous system and gastrointestinal tract, epistaxis, and usually a marked splenomegaly. Also called *p. rubra, erythremia, Vaquez's disease, Osler's disease, erythrocytosis megalosplenica, myelopathic p.*

secondary p. That resulting from a physiologic response to oxygen unsaturation of arterial blood, as in the fetus, in certain forms of congenital and acquired heart disease, chronic pulmonary disease, etc. Syn., *anoxemic erythrocytosis.*

splenomegalic p. That associated with enlargement of the spleen. See primary *p.*

pol″y·dac′tyl·ism. See *polydactyly.*

pol″y·dac′ty·ly [G. *polys*, many; *daktylos*, finger]. The existence of supernumerary fingers or toes.

pol″y·de·fi′cien·cy [*polys;* L. *deficientia*, from *deficere*, to be wanting]. Deficiency of more than one vitamin or other food factor.

pol″y·dip′si·a [*polys;* G. *dipsa*, thirst]. Excessive thirst. Syn., *anadipsia.*

psychogenic p. Polydipsia due to psychological causes. It may be differentiated from organic polydipsia by the patient's ability to produce a concentrated urine.

pol″y·e·lec′tro·lyte [*polys;* G. *ēlektron*, amber; *lytos*, soluble]. Any substance of high molecular weight which behaves as an electrolyte, such as proteins, polysaccharides, and synthetic rubber.

pol″y·em′bry·o·ny [*polys;* G. *embryon*, embryo]. *In biology*, the instance of a zygote giving rise to more than one embryo.

pol″y·e′mi·a [*polys;* G. *haima*, blood]. An excess of blood over the normal amount in the body.

pol″y·ene′. A compound which contains three or more double bonds joining carbon atoms in the compound.

pol″y·es·the′si·a [*polys;* G. *aisthēsis*, perception]. An abnormality of sensation in which a single touch is felt in two or more places at the same time.

pol″y·es′trus. In animals, the existence of several estrus periods during each sexual season.

pol″y·eth′yl·ene. A long-chain plastic polymer containing 200 to 1000 or more ethylene units per molecule. In the form of flexible tubing and film a pure form of the plastic is useful in surgical procedures. See *polythene.*

Po·lyg′a·la [*polys;* G. *gala*, milk]. A genus of herbaceous or shrubby plants of some 260 species.

P. senega. A species of North America; therapeutically the most important. See *senega.*

pol″y·ga·lac′ti·a (·ga·lack′tee·uh, ·shee·uh) [*polys; gala*]. Excessive secretion of milk.

pol″y·gal′ic ac′id. An active glycosidal principle from senega.

po·lyg′a·lin. A glycosidal saponin derived from senega. Polygalic acid.

po·lyg′a·mous [*polys;* G. *gamos*, marriage]. 1. Pertaining to the social state of having more than one wife or husband at one time, more particularly the former. 2. Having both unisexual and hermaphrodite flowers on one plant. —**polygamy,** *n.*

pol″y·gas′tri·a [*polys;* G. *gastēr*, belly]. Excessive production of gastric juice.

pol″y·gas′tric. 1. Having several bellies, as certain muscles. 2. Having more than one stomach.

pol″y·gen′ic [*polys;* G. *genesthai*, from *gignesthai*, to be produced]. Referring to hereditary characters which are determined by many genes.

pol″y·glan′du·lar [*polys;* L. *glans*, acorn]. Pluriglandular; applied to a condition in which two or more unrelated endocrine disorders coexist in a patient.

pol″y·glo·bu′li·a, pol″y·glob′u·lism. See *polycythemia.*

pol″y·gnath′us [*polys;* G. *gnathos*, jaw]. A monster in which a parasitic twin or part is attached to the jaws of the host.

po·lyg′o·nal [G. *polygōnon*, polygon]. Having many angles.

pol″y·gon′in. $C_{21}H_{20}O_{10}$; a glucoside from the root of *Polygonum cuspidatum* (Japanese fleeceflower), a plant having purgative properties. Syn., *cuspidatin.*

pol′y·graph. An instrument for recording pulsations simultaneously, such as the radial and jugular pulses. There are photographic registration and inkwriting models.

pol″y·gyr′i·a (pol″i·jirr′ee·uh, ·jye′ree·uh) [*polys;* G. *gyros*, circle]. The existence of an excessive number of convolutions in the brain.

pol″y·he′dral [G. *polyedros*, with many seats]. Having many surfaces.

pol″y·he′mi·a (·hee′mee·uh, ·hem′ee·uh). See *polyemia.*

pol″y·hi·dro′sis, pol″y·i·dro′sis. See *hyperhidrosis.*

pol″y·hy′brid [G. *polys*, many; L. *hybrida*, offspring of a tame sow and a wild boar]. An individual heterozygous for many pairs of genes.

pol″y·hy·dram′ni·os (·high·dram′nee·os) [*polys;* G. *hydōr*, water; *amnion*, inner membrane around the fetus]. An excessive production of amniotic fluid.

pol″y·hy·dru′ri·a (·high·droor′ee·uh) [*polys; hydōr;* G. *ouron*, urine]. A large increase in fluid content of the urine.

pol″y·in·fec′tion [*polys;* L. *infectio*, from *inficere*, to infect]. Infection resulting from the presence of more than one type of organism.

pol″y·lec′i·thal (·less′i·thul) [*polys;* G. *lekithos*, yolk]. Having much yolk. Syn., *megalecithal, telolecithal.*

pol″y·lep′tic [*polys;* G. *lēptikos*, from *lambanein*, to seize]. Characterized by numerous remissions and exacerbations.

pol″y·mas′ti·a, pol″y·ma′zi·a [*polys;* G. *mastos*, breast]. The presence of more than two breasts.

pol″y·mas′ti·gate, pol″y·mas′ti·gous [*polys;* G. *mastix*, whip]. Having several flagella.

pol″y·me′li·a [*polys;* G. *melos*, limb]. The presence of more than the normal number of limbs.

pol″y·me′lus, pol″y·me′li·us [*polys; melos*]. Having more than the normal number of limbs.

pol″y·me′ni·a (·mee′nee·uh, ·men′ee·uh) [*polys;* G. *mēn*, month]. Menorrhagia.

pol″y·men″or·rhe′a. See *metrorrhagia.*

pol′y·mer [*polys;* G. *meros*, part]. The product resulting when two or more molecules of the same substance combine; the molecular weight of the product is a whole multiple of the molecular weight of the starting compound.

pol″y·me′ri·a [*polys; meros*]. The presence of extra or supernumerary parts of the body.

pol″y·mer′ic [*polys; meros*]. 1. Exhibiting polymerism. 2. Pertaining to muscles which are derived from two or more myotomes.

po·lym′er·ide [*polys; meros*]. One of a series of polymeric compounds. Syn., *polymer.*

po·lym′er·ism, pol′ym·er·ism [*polys; meros*]. 1. The existence of more than a normal number of parts. 2. A form of isomerism in which the molecular weights of certain substances, called polymers, are multiples of the molecular weights of simpler substances from which they are produced.

pol″y·mer·i·za′tion, po·lym″er·i·za′tion. General term for a reaction in which a complex molecule of relatively high molecular weight is formed by the union of a number of simpler molecules, which may or may not be alike; the reaction may or may not involve elimination of a by-product, e.g., water or ammonia.

addition p. A type which does not involve elimination of a by-product.

condensation p. A type which does involve elimination of a by-product.

simple p. A type of addition polymerization which involves only a single molecular species. See *copolymerization.*

pol′y·mer·ize, po·lym′er·ize [*polys; meros*]. Form a compound from several single molecules of the same substance, the molecular weight of the new compound being a multiple of the molecular weight of single molecules which have combined.

po·l″ymi·cro′bic (·migh·kro′bick, ·krob′ick) [*polys;* in. *mikros*, small; *bios*, life]. Containing many kinds of microorganisms.

pol′y·morph [*polys;* G. *morphē*, form]. A polymorphonuclear leukocyte.

pol″y·mor′phic, pol″y·mor′phous [*polys; morphē*]. 1. Having or occurring in several forms, as a substance crystallizing in several forms. 2. *In clinical medicine*, referring to the symptomatology of a disease process; polysymptomatic.

pol″y·mor′phism [*polys; morphē*]. The state of being polymorphic.

pol″y·mor″pho·cel′lu·lar [*polys; morphē;* L. *cellula*, small storeroom]. Having cells of many forms.

pol″y·mor′pho·cyte [*polys; morphē;* G. *kytos*, cell]. A cell having a polymorphic nucleus, especially a granular leukocyte.

pol″y·mor″pho·nu′cle·ar [*polys; morphē;* L. *nucleus*, kernel]. Having a nucleus which is lobated, the lobes being connected by more or less thin strands of nuclear substance; for example, the nucleus of a neutrophil leukocyte.

pol″y·my·oc′lo·nus (·migh·ock′lo·nus, ·migh″o-klo′nus). See *paramyoclonus multiplex.*

pol″y·my″o·si′tis [*polys;* G. *mys*, muscle; *-itis*, inflammation]. Simultaneous inflammation of many muscles.

pol″y·myx′in. A generic term for a group of related polypeptide antibiotic substances derived from cultures of various strains of the spore-forming soil bacterium *Bacillus polymyxa* (*B. aerosporus*); the individual substances are differentiated by affixing A, B, C, D and E to the name *polymyxin.* Polymyxin B, the least toxic of the group, is bactericidal against most Gram-negative microorganisms; it is used clinically, by intramuscular injection of the water-soluble sulfate salt, in treating pseudomonal (pyocyaneal) bacteremia, meningitis and urinary-tract infection, and meningitis caused by certain other Gram-negative bacilli. See *aerosporin.*

pol″y·ne′sic (·nee′sick, ·ness′ick) [*polys;* G. *nēsos*, island]. Occurring in several foci, as polynesic sclerosis.

pol″y·neu′ral, pol″y·neu′ric [*polys;* G. *neuron*, nerve]. Pertaining to, or supplied by, several nerves.

pol″y·neu·ral′gi·a [*polys; neuron;* G. *algos*, pain]. Neuralgia in which many nerves are involved.

pol″y·neu·ri′tis [*polys; neuron;* G. *-itis*, inflammation]. Multiple neuritis. —**polyneurit′ic,** *adj.*

diabetic p. A slowly progressive polyneuritis occurring in diabetes. It first affects the legs, then the arms, with paresthesias, muscular weakness, and loss of deep reflexes accompanied by dryness and scaling of the skin. It is believed to be due to a metabolic disorder.

hematoporphyrinuric p. That associated with hematoporphyrinuria, caused by poisoning with barbiturates or sometimes by the therapeutic use of hematoporphyrin.

infectious p. Guillain-Barré syndrome.

Jamaica ginger p. Inflammation of the nerves of the extremities due to toxic effects of triorthocresylphosphate through ingestion of quantities of Jamaica ginger.

pol″y·neu″ro·my″o·si′tis [*polys; neuron;* G. *mys*, muscle; *-itis*]. A disease in which there is concurrent inflammation in several peripheral nerves and muscles.

pol″y·neu·rop′a·thy [*polys; neuron;* G. *pathos*, disease]. An affection of several nerves, as in alcoholism and thiamin deficiency; polyneuritis. See multiple *neuritis.*

pol″y·nu′cle·ar, pol″y·nu′cle·ate. 1. See *multinuclear.* 2. Polymorphonuclear: erroneous usage.

pol″y·nu′cle·ate. See *multinuclear.*

pol″y·nu″cle·ot′i·dase. An enzyme which depolymerizes nucleic acid to form mononucleotides.

pol″y·nu′cle·o·tide [*polys;* L. *nucleus,* kernel]. A nucleic acid composed of four mononucleotides.

pol″y·o·don′ti·a [*polys;* G. *odous,* tooth]. The presence of supernumerary teeth.

pol″y·o·nych′i·a (·nick′ee·uh) [*polys;* G. *onyx,* nail]. The occurrence of supernumerary nails on fingers or toes.

pol″y·o′pi·a, pol″y·op′si·a [*polys;* G. *ōps,* eye]. A condition in which more than one image of an object is formed upon the retina.

p. monophthalmica. The phenomenon of multiple vision with a single eye.

pol″y·or′chid·ism, pol″y·or′chism [*polys;* G. *orchis,* testis]. The presence of more than two testes in one person.

pol″y·or′chis (·or′kis) [*polys; orchis*]. One who has more than two testes.

pol″y·o·rex′i·a [*polys;* G. *orexis,* longing]. Excessive hunger, or appetite; bulimia.

pol″y·or″ga·no·sil·ox′ane. Any synthetic polymer consisting of a chain of alternate links of silicon atoms and oxygen atoms, the two other bonds of the tetravalent silicon atom generally being attached to an organic group. They are represented by the general formula:

```
      R       R       R
      |       |       |
    —Si—O—Si—O—Si—
      |       |       |
      R       R       R
```

Commonly known as *silicones,* these substances may be limpid or viscous fluids or semisolid to solid substances. The fluids impart to glass surfaces a water-repellent film, resulting in complete drainage of aqueous solutions, and serve as antifoam and skin-protective agents. A puttylike form, *silicone bouncing putty,* has characteristics of deformability useful in ailments requiring therapeutic exercise of the fingers.

pol″y·or·rho″men″in·gi′tis. Polyorrhymenitis: erroneous usage. See *polyserositis.*

pol″y·or·rhy″men·i′tis. See *polyserositis.*

pol″y·o·stot′ic. Involving more than one bone.

pol″y·o′ti·a [*polys;* G. *ous,* ear]. A congenital defect in which there is more than one auricle on one or both sides of the head.

pol′yp [G. *polypous,* many-footed]. A pedunculated mass composed of neoplastic tissue or other structure, found especially on mucous membranes, as those of the nose, urinary bladder, stomach, large intestine, or uterus. —**polypous,** *adj.*

adenocarcinomatous p. One in which the nodule is an adenocarcinoma.

adenomatous p. One in which the nodule is an adenoma.

fibrinous p. One composed of fibrin or organized fibrin.

inflammatory polyps. See *pseudopolyposis.*

mucous p. A localized inflammatory proliferation of mucous membrane or of connective tissue, with mucoid degeneration.

nasal p. One in which pedunculated or sessile, edematous masses project from the nasal mucosa, with infiltration by cells of acute or chronic inflammation.

placental p. One composed of retained placental fragments, sometimes apparently proliferated.

pulp p. See hyperplastic *pulpitis.*

vascular p. A pedunculated angioma.

pol″y·pap″il·lo′ma. See *yaws.*

pol″y·pa·re′sis (·pa·ree′sis, ·par′i·sis) [G. *polys,* many; *paresis,* paralysis]. General progressive paralysis of the insane, or paralytic dementia.

pol″y·path′i·a [*polys;* G. *pathos,* disease]. The presence of several diseases at one time, or the frequent recurrence of disease.

pol″y·pep′ti·dase. One of the enzymes which hydrolyze proteins and molecular fragments of proteins.

pol″y·pep′tide [*polys;* G. *peptos,* cooked]. A compound containing two or more amino acids united through the peptide linkage —CO.NH—.

pol″y·pep″ti·de′mi·a [*polys; peptos; haima,* blood]. The presence of polypeptides in the blood.

pol″y·pep″ti·dor·rha′chi·a (·pep″tid·o·ray′kee·uh, ·rack′ee·uh) [*polys; peptos;* G. *rhachis,* spine]. 1. The presence of polypeptides in the cerebrospinal fluid. 2. Toxic meningitis caused by polypeptides in the cerebrospinal fluid.

pol″y·pep′tin. An antibiotic substance derived from a member of the *Bacillus circulans* group, *B. krzemieniewski:* originally known as *circulin,* a name now applied to another antibiotic. It is bactericidal as well as bacteriostatic against a number of species of bacteria.

pol″y·pha′gi·a [*polys;* G. *phagein,* to eat]. Excessive eating; increased intake of food; bulimia.

pol″y·pha·lan′gism [*polys;* G. *phalagx,* bone between two joints of the fingers and toes]. An extra phalanx in a finger or toe.

pol″y·phar′ma·cy [*polys;* G. *pharmakon,* drug]. The prescription of many drugs at one time; the excessive use of drugs.

pol″y·pho′bi·a [*polys;* G. *phobos,* fear]. Morbid fear of many things.

po·lyph′o·ny [*polys;* G. *phōnē,* voice]. The condition of multiple effects produced by a given gene. Syn., *pleiotropism.*

pol″y·phy·let′ic (·figh·let′ick) [*polys;* G. *phyletikos,* of a tribe]. Referring to origin from many lines of descent; opposed to *monophyletic.*

pol″y·phy′le·tism. See polyphyletic *theory* of hematopoiesis.

pol″y·phy′o·dont [G. *polyphyēs,* manifold; *odous,* tooth]. Having more than two successive sets of teeth at intervals throughout life.

pol″y·pif′er·ous [G. *polypous,* many-footed; L. *ferre,* to bear]. Bearing or originating polyps.

pol′y·plast [G. *polys,* many; *plassein,* to form]. 1. Formed of many different structures. 2. Having undergone many modifications during the process of development. *Rare.*

pol′y·ploid [*polys;* G. *-ploos,* -fold; *eidos,* form]. Denoting a condition in which the chromosome number is a multiple of the normal gametic number.

pol″yp·ne′a, pol″yp·noe′a [*polys;* G. *pnoia,* breath]. Very rapid respiration; panting.

pol″y·po′di·a [*polys;* G. *pous,* foot]. The condition of having supernumerary feet.

Pol″y·po′di·um [*polys; pous*]. A genus of ferns of several species said to have medicinal virtues.

P. vulgare. A species common in Europe and America. Contains in the rhizome a purgative fixed oil, an anthelmintic resin, and a glycoside samambain. Has also been used as an expectorant in chronic catarrh and asthma.

pol′yp·oid [G. *polypous,* many-footed; *eidos,* form]. Resembling a polyp.

pol″y·po′rin. An antibiotic substance derived from the polypore fungus *Polystictus sanguineus.* It is effective, by local application, against *Staphylococcus aureus, S. pyogenes,* and *S. viridans.*

po·lyp′o·rous [*polys;* G. *poros,* passage]. Having many small openings; cribriform.

pol″y·po′sis [G. *polypous,* many-footed; *-ōsis,* condition]. The condition of being affected with polyps.

acquired multiple p. Multiple pedunculated adenomas of the gastrointestinal tract, found most frequently in the rectum and sigmoid, which have a marked tendency to malignant degeneration. Syn., *polypoid adenomatosis*.

hereditary multiple p. A rare form transmitted as a Mendelian dominant by both sexes and manifesting itself early in life. The polyps may cover the entire small intestine and colon or be limited to either; melanin spots of oral mucosa, lips, and digits may be associated when the lesions occur in the small intestine. Malignant degeneration is common.

p. coli. Multiple polyps of the large intestine.

p. ventriculi. Multiple polyps of gastric mucosa. When associated with chronic atrophic gastritis may be called état mamelonné.

pol″y·pty′chi·al (pol″i·tye′kee·ul) [G. *polys*, many; *ptychē*, fold]. Arranged in more than one layer, as the epithelial cells of some glands.

pol′y·pus (pl. *polypi*). See *polyp*.

pol″y·ra·dic″u·li′tis [G. *polys*, many; L. *radicula*, small root; G. *-itis*, inflammation]. Inflammation or degeneration of spinal ganglions, nerve roots, or peripheral nerves. Also called *polyneuroradiculitis*.

pol″y·ra·dic″u·lo·neu·ri′tis. See Guillain-Barré *syndrome*.

pol″y·sac′cha·ride (·sack′uh·ride, ·rid) [*polys;* G. *sakchar*, sugar]. A carbohydrate which is formed by the condensation of two or more, usually many, monosaccharides. Examples are cellulose and starch. They do not go into true solution in water, and usually form hydrophilic colloids.

bacterial p. A substance of polysaccharide nature elaborated by bacteria. Such substances are of particular importance in immunologic phenomena, since they usually possess antigenic properties.

capsular p. A polysaccharide found in the capsule of bacteria, for example, of a pneumococcus, determining its type specificity. It may act as a hapten.

pol″y·sce′li·a (·see′lee·uh) [*polys;* G. *skelos*, leg]. Excess in the number of legs.

po·lys′ce·lus [*polys; skelos*]. A monster having supernumerary legs.

pol″y·se″ro·si′tis [*polys;* L. *serum*, whey; G. *-itis*, inflammation]. Widespread, chronic, fibrosing inflammation of serous membranes, especially in the upper abdomen. This may be associated with persistent ascites of chronic passive hyperemia. Also called *Pick's disease* (for Friedel Pick), *multiple serositis, Concato's disease, chronic hyperplastic perihepatitis, polyorrhymenitis*.

pol″y·si″nus·i′tis [*polys;* L. *sinus*, curve; *-itis*]. Simultaneous inflammation of several air sinuses.

pol″y·som′a·tous (·som′uh·tus, ·so′muh·tus) [*polys;* G. *sōma*, body]. Taruffi's descriptive term for monstrosities involving more than one body.

pol″y·so′mi·a [*polys; sōma*]. A polysomatous condition.

pol″y·so′mic [*polys; sōma*]. 1. Referring to organisms with more than two of any given chromosome, or having more than two sets of chromosomes, as tetraploids, hexaploids, etc. 2. See *polyploid*.

pol″y·so′mus [*polys; sōma*]. A general term embracing all grades of duplicity, triplicity, etc. It includes monochorionic twins, conjoined twins, equal or unequal, placental parasitic twins, and all grades of double monsters. See *polysomatous*.

pol″y·sor′bate 80. The United States Pharmacopeia name for a complex mixture of polyoxyethylene ethers of mixed partial oleic esters of sorbitol anhydride, available under the trademarked name *Tween 80*.

pol″y·sper′mi·a, pol″y·sper′mism [*polys;* G. *sperma*, seed]. The secretion and discharge of an excessive quantity of seminal fluid.

pol′y·sper″my, pol″y·sper′my [*polys; sperma*]. Impregnation of an ovum by more than one spermatozoon.

pol″y·sphyg′mo·graph [*polys;* G. *sphygmos*, pulse; *graphein*, to write]. An instrument by means of which tracings can be taken simultaneously of the cardiac movements, the arterial pulse, and the respiration.

pol″y·stich′i·a (·stick′ee·uh) [*polys;* G. *stichos*, row]. A condition in which the eyelashes are arranged in more than the normal number of rows.

pol″y·stic′tin. An antibiotic substance derived from the fungus *Polystictus versicolor;* it is weakly bacteriostatic.

pol″y·stom′a·tous (·stom′uh·tus, ·sto′muh·tus) [*polys;* G. *stoma*, mouth]. Having many mouths or apertures.

pol″y·sty′rene. A clear, lightweight plastic prepared by reaction and polymerization of ethylene and benzene and used particularly in the manufacture of containers and general laboratory ware such as beakers and funnels. Marketed as *styron, lustron, laolin, bakelite polystyrene*.

pol″y·sus·pen′soid. A colloid system in which there are several phases in different degrees of dispersion.

pol″y·symp″to·mat′ic. *In clinical medicine*, referring to a pathological process having manifold symptoms, which may not all occur simultaneously or in the same patient.

pol″y·ter′pene. See *terpene*.

pol″y·the′li·a, pol″y·the′lism (pol″i·theel′iz·um, pol′ith·i·liz·um) [G. *polys*, many; *thēlē*, nipple]. The presence of supernumerary nipples.

polythene. A trade-mark for polyethylene.

po·lyt′o·cous [*polys;* G. *tokos*, offspring]. Producing many young at a birth.

pol″y·trich′i·a (·trick′ee·uh), **pol″y·tri·cho′sis** (·tri·ko′sis) [*polys;* G. *thrix*, hair]. Excessive development of hair. Syn., *hypertrichosis*.

pol″y·tro′phi·a, po·lyt′ro·phy [*polys;* G. *trophē*, nourishment]. Abundant or excessive nutrition.

pol″y·trop′ic (·trop′ick, ·tro′pick) [*polys;* G. *trepein*, to turn]. Having affinity for or affecting more than one type of cell; applied to viruses. Syn., *pantropic*.

pol″y·un′gui·a [*polys;* L. *unguis*, nail]. Polyonychia.

pol″y·u′ri·a [*polys;* G. *ouron*, urine]. The passage of an excessive quantity of urine. —**polyuric,** *adj., n.*

pol″y·va′lent, po·lyv′a·lent [*polys;* L. *valere*, to be strong]. Multivalent; used especially in polyvalent serum, one obtained either by immunizing animals with different strains of the same bacterium, or by mixing serums derived from different animals immunized with various strains.

pol″y·vi′nyl al′co·hol (·vy′nil, ·vin′il). $(CH_2{:}CHOH)_n$; a cream-colored powder, soluble in water and insoluble in most organic solvents. It is used as an adhesive, emulsifier, and sizing agent for paper.

pol″y·vi″nyl·pyr·rol′i·done. A synthetic polymer of high molecular weight formed by interactions of formaldehyde, ammonia, hydrogen, and acetylene; a faintly yellow solid, resembling albumin, soluble in water with formation of a colloidal solution: used as a nonantigenic plasma expander and in preparing repository forms of certain drugs with which it combines loosely. Abbreviated, PVP. See *periston*.

po·made′ (po·mayd′, po·mahd′) [F. *pommade*, from L. *pomum*, apple]. A perfumed ointment for applying to the scalp.

pome′gran″ate (pom′gran″it, pum′·, pum·gran′it, pom·). See *pelletierine* tannate.

pom″pho·ly·he′mi·a. Bubbles in the blood.

pom′pho·lyx [G., bubble]. A skin disease characterized by vesicles and bullae on the palms of the hands and soles of the feet. Lesions recur in crops with a tendency to chronicity, and are usually deep-seated. The disease is not rare as formerly was taught; its cause is unknown. Also called *chiropompholyx, dyshidrosis.*

pom′phus. See *wheal.*

po′mum A·da′mi. Latin, apple of Adam: old term for the prominence in front of the neck caused by the projection of the thyroid cartilage. Syn., *Adam's apple.*

pon′ceau 3R. $C_{19}H_{16}N_2Na_2O_7S_2$; sodium cumeneazo-β-naphthol disulfonate; a dark-red powder, soluble in water. A pure grade of it, when certified, is used as a dye for foods, drugs, and cosmetics: designated F. D. & C. Red No. 1.

Poncet, Antonin [*French surgeon,* 1849–1913]. Described multiple tuberculous arthritis (1897); also called *Poncet's disease.* Introduced perineal urethrostomy and an operation for lengthening the Achilles tendon for the relief of talipes equinus; both are called *Poncet's operation.*

Pond's extract. A fluidextract of *Hamamelis virginiana.*

Ponder, Eric [*American physiologist,* 1898–]. Described a method of making a differential neutrophil count; see Cooke-Ponder *method.* Introduced a stain for diphtheria bacilli; see Ponder-Kinyoun *stain.* Author of numerous studies of the red blood cell.

pon′der·a·ble [L. *ponderabilis,* that can be weighed]. Having weight.

Ponfick, Emil [*German physician,* 1844–1913]. Known for his investigations in actinomycosis, especially of the role played by *Actinomyces* in its causation in human beings and animals (1880–82). Described achromacytes in the blood; called *Ponfick's shadows.* See also *achromacyte.*

pon′o·graph, po′no·graph [G. *ponos,* toil, pain; *graphein,* to write]. An apparatus for determining and registering sensitiveness to pain or fatigue.

pon″o·pal·mo′sis (pon″o·pal·mo′sis, po″no·) [*ponos;* G. *palmos,* throbbing; *-ōsis,* condition]. Condition in which slight exertion produces palpitation of the heart.

pon′os, po′nos [G.]. The Mediterranean form of kala-azar.

pons (ponz) (pl. *pontes*) [L., bridge]. 1. A process or bridge of tissue connecting two parts of an organ. 2. The pons, a convex white eminence situated at the base of the brain. It consists of fibers and nuclei which receive impulses from the cerebral cortex, and send fibers to the contralateral side of the cerebellum by way of the brachium pontis. Also called *pons varolii.* See Plates 17, 18. —**pon′tile, pon′tine** (pon′tyne), *adj.*

pon′tic [*pons*]. Portion of a prosthetic bridge which is between the abutments and serves as the artificial substitute for a lost tooth, or teeth. Syn., *dummy.*

pon″to·bul′bar [*pons;* L. *bulbus,* bulb]. Pertaining to the pons and to the medulla oblongata.

pontocaine hydrochloride. Trade-mark for a brand of tetracaine hydrochloride.

Pool-Schlesinger's sign. See under *sign.*

pop′lar bud (*populi gemma*). The air-dried, closed, winter leaf bud of *Populus candicans,* known in commerce as balm of Gilead buds, or of *Populus tacamahacca* (*Populus balsamifera*), known in commerce as balsam poplar buds. It contains, in addition to a small amount of the glycosides salicin and populin, an oleoresin allied in its composition to turpentine. The therapeutic action of poplar bud is analogous to that of the turpentines. It has been used externally as a mild counterirritant in muscular rheumatism and internally as a stimulating expectorant in subacute or chronic bronchitis.

pop″li·te′al, pop·lit′e·al [L. *poples,* ham of the knee]. Pertaining to or situated in the ham, as popliteal artery, popliteal nerve, popliteal space.

pop″li·te′us, pop·lit′e·us [*poples*]. 1. The ham or hinder part of the knee joint. 2. A muscle on the back of the knee joint. See Table of Muscles in the Appendix.

p. minor. A rare variant of the popliteus muscle arising from the femur medial to the plantaris and inserted into the posterior ligament of the knee joint.

Popper, Erwin [*German pathologist,* contemporary]. With Karl Landsteiner, transmitted poliomyelitis to the monkey (1909).

pop′py [AS. *popig*]. See *opium.*

pop′u·lin. $C_{20}H_{22}O_8.2H_2O$; a crystalline glycoside obtained from various species of *Populus* and also prepared by synthesis. Syn., *populoside, salicin benzoate.*

pop′u·lo·side. Populin.

Pop′u·lus. See *poplar bud.*

pore [G. *poros,* passage]. 1. A minute opening on a surface. 2. Opening of the duct of a sweat gland. Also see *porus.*

alveolar p. One of the minute openings in the walls of the pulmonary alveoli, affording communication between neighboring alveoli: also called *pore of Cohn.*

taste p. The minute opening through which project the gustatory bristles of a taste bud. Also called *gustatory p.*

po·ren″ce·pha′li·a, po″ren·ceph′a·ly [*poros;* G. *egkephalos,* brain]. Congenitally deficient development of the cerebral cortex and gray matter so that the lateral ventricles communicate with the brain surface and are lined by a continuation of the piarachnoid. —**porenceph′alous, porencephal′ic,** *adj.*

po″ren·ceph″a·li′tis [*poros; egkephalos;* G. *-itis,* inflammation]. Encephalitis with a tendency to form cavities.

po″ren·ceph′a·lus [*poros; egkephalos*]. An individual exhibiting porencephalia.

Porges, Otto (1879–). Austrian physician who, with K. Spiro, discovered gamma globulin (1903). He first described hypoglycemia in Addison's disease.

Porges-Pollatschek reaction. See under *reaction.*

po′ri (por′eye). Plural of porus.

po″ri·o·ma′ni·a [G. *poreia,* journey; *mania,* madness]. Uncontrollable impulse to wander away from home; fugue.

po′ri·on (pl. *poria*) [G. *poros,* passage]. The point on the upper margin of the porus acusticus externus. The two poria and the left orbitale define the Frankfort horizontal plane.

por·nog′ra·phy [G. *pornē,* prostitute; *graphein,* to write]. 1. A treatise on prostitution. 2. Obscene writing, painting, etc.

por″o·ceph″a·li′a·sis [G. *poros,* passage; *kephalē,* head; NL. *-iasis,* condition]. Infestation of the lungs, liver, trachea, and nasal cavities of man with any of the varieties of *Porocephalus.*

Por″o·ceph′a·lus [*poros; kephalē*]. A genus of wormlike arthropods parasitic in man.

por″o·ker″a·to′sis. A genodermatosis characterized by a collar of elevated hyperkeratosis about an irregular patch of depressed atrophic skin; microscopically, horn plugs or cornoid lamella in the dermis are diagnostic, but are not necessarily located in the openings of sweat glands as the name *porokeratosis* implies. Syn., *hyperkeratosis excentrica.*

po·ro′ma [G., hardened part]. A callosity.

por″o·plas′tic [G. *poros*, passage; *plassein*, to form]. Porous and plastic, as poroplastic felt, a porous, readily molded felt, used in the preparation of splints and jackets.

po·ro′sis [*poros;* G. *-ōsis*, condition]. Rarefaction; increased roentgen translucency; formation of vacuoles or pores; cavity formation.

po·ros′i·ty [*poros*]. The condition or quality of being porous.

po′rous [*poros*]. Having pores.

por′phin. A heterocyclic ring consisting of four pyrrole rings linked by methine (—CH═) bridges; the basic structure of chlorophyll, hemoglobin, the cytochromes, and certain other related substances.

por″pho·bi′lin. A product derived from hemoglobin which may be excreted in urine.

por″pho·bi·lin′o·gen (por″fo·buy·lin′o·jen). One of the derivatives of hemoglobin which makes the urine a Burgundy-red color.

por·phy′ri·a [G. *porphyra*, purple dye]. An inborn error of metabolism characterized by the presence of pathologic quantities of porphyrins in blood and other tissues, in feces and urine, and other clinical symptoms, including dark discoloration of urine.

acute intermittent p. The form appearing in young adults, usually not marked by cutaneous lesions but by such symptoms as abdominal colic, paresis, paralysis, and psychic disturbances.

congenital p. The form appearing in early childhood, characterized by vesicular and eczematoid dermatitis on skin directly exposed to the sun. These lesions may scar the skin. Teeth may be red at the gingival margin. Also called *erythropoietic p.*, *photosensitive p.*

p. cutanea tarda. The form appearing in late adulthood, characterized by photosensitivity, pigmentation of the skin, and hepatic dysfunction.

por′phy·rin. A heterocyclic ring derived from porphin by replacing the eight hydrogen atoms attached to the carbon atoms of the pyrrole rings of porphin by various organic groups. In the center of the ring a metal, e.g., iron (in heme) or magnesium (in chlorophyll), may or may not be present.

por″phy·ri·nu′ri·a (por″fi·ri·new′ree·uh, por″figh·ri·) [*porphyra;* G. *ouron*, urine]. The excretion of an abnormal amount of a porphyrin, commonly believed to be uroporphyrin I, in the urine: also called *porphyruria.*

por″phy·ri·za′tion [*porphyra*]. Pulverization; reduction to a fine powder, usually performed on a tablet of porphyry.

por″phy·rop′sin. A purple carotenoid protein that occurs in the rods of the retinas of certain fresh-water fish. It participates in a retinal cycle identical in arrangement with that of rhodopsin or visual purple.

por″phy·rox′ine. $C_{19}H_{23}NO_4$; carbonyl-dihydrocodeine; an alkaloid found in opium. Syn., *opin.*

por″phyr·u′ri·a. Porphyrinuria.

por′poise heart. A preponderance of the right ventricle, seen in underwater swimmers, not evidence of disease.

por·ri′go [L., dandruff]. An old term applied to several diseases of the scalp. —**porrig′inous,** *adj.*

p. decalvans. Alopecia areata.

p. favosa. Favus.

Porro, Edoardo [*Italian obstetrician*, 1842–1902]. Remembered for his early employment of Cesarean section. He combined the operation with hysterectomy (1876); called *Porro's operation.*

por′ta (pl. *portae*) [L., gate]. The hilus of an organ through which the vessels enter.

p. hepatis. The transverse fissure of the liver through which the portal vein enters the organ.

p. vestibuli. A narrow orifice between the sinus venosus and the atrium in the embryonic heart.

por·ta·ca′val, por·to·ca′val [*porta;* L. *cavus*, hollow]. Pertaining to the portal vein and the inferior vena cava.

por′tal [*porta*]. The porta or hilus of an organ. —**por′tal,** *adj.*

intestinal p. The opening of the foregut or of the hindgut into the midgut or yolk sac.

porte″pol′ish·er. *In dentistry*, an instrument used for holding a polishing point, stick or brush.

Porter, William Henry [*Irish physician*, 1790–1861]. Described the tracheal tug as a finding in aortic aneurysm; called *Porter's sign.*

Portes, Louis [*French obstetrician*, contemporary]. Described Cesarean section followed by temporary exteriorization of the uterus and secondary reintegration (1924); called *Portes operation.*

por′ti·o (por′shee·o, por′tee·o) (pl. *portiones*) [L.]. 1. Portion. 2. Portio vaginalis uteri, the vaginal portion of the uterus.

p. pylorica ventriculi. The pyloric extremity of the stomach.

port′-wine′ mark. See port-wine *nevus.*

po′rus (pl. *pori*) [G. *poros*, passage]. A pore, foramen.

p. acusticus externus. The opening of the external auditory canal.

p. acusticus internus. The opening of the internal auditory canal into the cranial cavity.

p. crotaphitico-buccinatorius. A foramen formed in about 10% of skulls by a bar of bone developing between the base of the lateral pterygoid lamina and the under surface of the great wing of the sphenoid bone. Syn., *pterygoalar foramen.*

p. opticus. The opening in the center of the lamina cribrosa transmitting the central artery of the retina.

p. sudoriferus. A sweat pore.

Posadas, A. [*Argentinian physician*, contemporary]. Remembered for his descriptions of coccidioidomycosis, also called *valley fever, Posadas' disease.*

po″si·o·ma′ni·a (po″see·o·may′nee·uh, pos″ee·o·) [G. *posis*, drinking; *mania*, madness]. Dipsomania.

po·si′tion [L. *positio*, a putting]. Place; location; attitude; posture. Abbreviated, P.

anatomic p. Attitude of a person standing erect with arms at the sides and palms forward.

apparent p. *In ophthalmology*, the position in space to which the mind projects a visual image.

bronchoscopic p. Posture of the patient in which he lies supine with head hyperextended to bring larynx and trachea in a straight line so as to permit introduction of the bronchoscope.

dorsal p. Attitude of a person lying on his back.

dorsosacral p. The posture of a patient lying on the back with the legs flexed on the thighs and the thighs flexed on the abdomen and abducted.

Edebohls' p. See Simon's *p.*

flipper p. One representing the figure of a seal, the body stiff, the arms extended and rotated inward with the wrists flexed, the legs rigid, with pronated feet. The attitude is indicative of hemorrhage into the midbrain or brain stem following fracture of the bones of the middle or posterior cranial fossa.

Fowler's p. The posture which the recumbent patient assumes when the head of the bed is raised 18 to 20 inches, or a similar position achieved by the use of a back rest.

high pelvic p. See Trendelenburg's *p.*

Jones's p. Hyperflexion of the forearm on the arm, in the treatment of elbow fractures involving the condyles.

knee-chest p. A position assumed by a patient resting on knees and chest as an exercise after childbirth, or for the purposes of examination and treatment.

knee-elbow p. Posture in which the patient lies upon the knees and elbows, the head resting upon the hands.

lateroabdominal p. See Sims' *p.*

lithotomy p. See dorsosacral *p.*

mentoanterior p. A presentation of the fetus *in utero* in which the head is sharply extended so that the occiput of the fetus is in contact with its back, and the face looks downward and anteriorly.

mentoposterior p. A face presentation of the fetus in which the head is sharply extended so that the occiput is in contact with the back, and the face looks downward and posteriorly.

physiologic rest p. *In dentistry,* the relaxed position of the mandible.

p. effect. *In genetics,* the view that the expression of a gene depends in part upon its relations to adjacent genes—*i.e.,* upon its position in the chromosome.

p. of function. An essential primary position of the hand, of importance during prolonged immobilization following injury to the hand or digits. The hand is hyperextended at the wrist at an angle of 45 degrees, the fingers being flexed at 45 degrees at their metacarpophalangeal and interphalangeal joints. The thumb is rotated and adducted so that its flexor surface is opposite the flexor surface of the index finger.

p. of the fetus. The relation of the presenting part of the fetus to the cardinal points. For the vertex, the face, and the breech there are four positions each: a right anterior, a right posterior, a left anterior, and a left posterior. For each of the shoulders there is an anterior and a posterior position. In order to shorten and memorize these positions, the initials of the chief words are made use of, as follows: for vertex presentations the word occiput is abbreviated O., and preceded by the letter R. or L. for right or left, and followed by A. or P. according to whether the presenting part is anterior or posterior. We thus have the initials L.O.A., left occipito-anterior, to indicate that the presenting occiput is upon the anterior left side. In the same way are derived the terms L.O.P., R.O.A., R.O.P. For facial presentations we have in the same way L.F.A., left frontoanterior, L.F.P., R.F.A., R.F.P. For breech or sacral presentations, L.S.A., L.S.P., R.S.A., R.S.P., and for shoulder or dorsal presentations, L.D.A., L.D.P., R.D.A., R.D.P.

protrusive p. *In dentistry,* that reached when the mandible is thrust forward bringing the upper and lower incisors into contact.

Simon's p. The dorsal posture with the legs and thighs flexed, the hips elevated, and the thighs abducted.

Sims's p. Posture of a patient lying on the left side with the right knee and thigh drawn up, the left arm placed along the back, and the chest inclined forward. Also called *semiprone p.*

Trendelenburg's p. The posture of a patient lying on a table which is tilted upward 45 degrees, with the legs and feet hanging over the upper end of it.

Walcher's p. Posture of a patient lying on the back with the thighs and legs hanging over the edge of the table. Used during a difficult delivery to lengthen the true conjugate.

pos'i·tive [L. *positivus*, positive]. *In mathematics* and *physiology,* denoting one of two quantities or conditions assumed as primary or fundamental; opposed to one assumed as negative; denoting a quantity greater than zero. Symbol, +.

pos'i·tron (poz'i·tron) [*positivus*; G. elek*tron*, amber]. An elementary particle having the mass of an electron but carrying a unit positive charge. It is evanescent, dissipating itself as radiation as soon as it encounters an electron, which is annihilated with it.

pos"i·tro'ni·um. A combination of a positron and an electron (negatron). The mean life of the combination is about 10^{-7} second, the particle being annihilated by conversion to one or more photons.

po·sol'o·gy [G. *posos*, how much; *logos*, word]. That branch of medical science dealing with the dosage of medicines.

post- [L.]. A prefix denoting *after, behind,* or *subsequent.*

post'a·fene. The dihydrochloride of *p*-chlorobenzylhydryl-4-*m*-methylbenzylpiperazine, a compound effective in preventing motion sickness. See *bonamine, meclizine hydrochloride.*

post·a'nal. Situated behind the anus.

post"an·es·thet'ic. Occurring after anesthesia.

post"ap·o·plec'tic [*post;* G. *apoplēktos*, stricken with paralysis]. Coming on, or occurring, after a stroke of apoplexy, as postapoplectic coma, the coma that often succeeds an apoplectic stroke.

post·au'di·to"ry [L. *post*, behind; *audire*, to hear]. Situated behind the auditory nerve, or ear.

post·ax'i·al [*post;* L. *axis*, axis]. Situated behind the axis: in the arm, behind the ulnar aspect; in the leg, behind the fibular aspect.

post·bra'chi·al (pohst·bray'kee·ul, ·brack'ee·ul) [*post;* L. *brachium*, arm]. Situated posterior to the arm.

post·cap'il·lar"y (pohst·cap'i·lerr"ee) [*post;* L. *capillaris*, from *capillus*, hair]. The terminal part of a capillary network which opens into a venule. Syn., *venous capillary.*

post·car'di·nal [*post;* L. *cardinalis*, principal]. Pertaining to the pair of cardinal veins draining the posterior part of the embryo.

post·ca'va [*post;* L. *cavus*, hollow]. The inferior or ascending vena cava. —**postcaval,** *adj.*

post·cen'tral [*post;* G. *kentron*, center]. 1. Situated behind a center. 2. Situated behind the fissure of Rolando, or central fissure of the brain, as the postcentral gyrus.

post·ci'bal [L. *post*, after; *cibus*, food]. Occurring after meals. *Obs.*

post"cla·vic'u·lar [L. *post*, behind; *clavicula*, small key]. Situated behind the clavicle.

post·co'i·tal [L. *post*, after; *coitus*, coition]. After sexual intercourse.

post"con·nu'bi·al [*post;* L. *connubium*, marriage]. Coming on, or occurring, after marriage.

post"con·vul'sive [*post;* L. *convulsio*, convulsion]. Coming on after a convulsion.

post·cor'di·al [L. *post*, behind; *cor*, heart]. Situated behind the heart.

post"di·crot'ic (·dye·krot'ick) [L. *post*, after; G. *dikrotos*, double beating]. Coming after the dicrotic wave of the pulse, as postdicrotic wave, a wave often following the dicrotic wave in the sphygmographic tracing.

post"di·ges'tive (·di·jes'tiv, ·dye·jes'tiv) [*post;* L. *digestio*, digestion]. Occurring after digestion.

post"diph·the·rit'ic [*post;* G. *diphthera*, leather; *-itis*, inflammation]. Occurring after an attack of diphtheria, as postdiphtheritic paralysis.

post"em·bry·on'ic [*post;* G. *embryon*, embryo]. Occurring after the embryonic stage; fetal.

post"en·ceph"a·lit'ic [*post;* G. *egkephalos*, brain; *-itis*]. Occurring after and presumably as a result of encephalitis.

post"ep·i·lep'tic [*post;* G. *epilēptikos*, epileptic]. Occurring after an epileptic attack.

pos·te′ri·ad [L. *posterior*, comp. from *posterus*, coming after; *ad*, to or toward]. Toward the posterior part of the body.

pos·te′ri·or [L.]. Situated behind or to the back of a part.

pos′ter·o- [L. *posterus*, coming after]. A combining form signifying *posterior*.

pos″ter·o·an·te′ri·or [*posterus;* L. *anterior*, foremost]. From the back to the front of the body, as in describing the direction of x-rays traversing the patient. Also see *dorsoventral*.

pos″ter·o·ex·ter′nal [*posterus;* L. *externus*, external]. Occupying the outer side of a back part, as the posteroexternal column of the spinal cord. —**posteroexternad,** *adv.*

pos″ter·o·in·ter′nal [*posterus;* L. *internus*, internal]. Occupying the inner side of a back part, as the posterointernal column of the spinal cord. —**posterointernad,** *adv.*

pos″ter·o·lat′er·al [*posterus;* L. *lateralis*, lateral]. Situated behind and at the side of a part. —**posterolaterad,** *adv.*

pos″ter·o·me′di·al [*posterus;* L. *medius*, middle]. Situated posteriorly and toward the midline. —**posteromediad,** *adv.*

pos″ter·o·me′di·an [*posterus; medius*]. Situated posteriorly and in the midline.

pos″ter·o·su·pe′ri·or [*posterus;* L. *superior*, higher]. Situated behind and above a part.

post″e·rup′tive [L. *post*, after; *eruptio*, a bursting forth]. Following eruption.

post″e·so·phag′e·al (·ee·so·fadj′ee·ul, ·fay′jee·ul) [L. *post*, behind; G. *oisophagos*, gullet]. Situated behind the esophagus.

post·fe′brile (·fee′bril, ·feb′ril, ·rile) [L. *post*, after; *febris*, fever]. Occurring after a fever.

post″gan·gli·on′ic (·gang·glee·on′ick, ·gang·lee·) [L. *post*, behind; G. *gagglion*, encysted tumor on a tendon]. Situated behind, or after, a ganglion.

post″gas·trec′to·my. After removal of part or all of the stomach, as postgastrectomy treatment.

post·gle′noid [*post;* G. *glēnoeidēs*, like a socket]. Situated behind the glenoid fossa of the temporal bone, as the postglenoid tubercle.

post″hem·i·pleg′ic (·hem·i·pledj′ick, ·plee′jick) [L. *post*, after; G. *hēmiplēgēs*, half-struck]. Occurring after or following an attack of hemiplegia.

post″hem·or·rhag′ic (·hem·o·radj′ick) [*post;* G. *haimorrhagia*, hemorrhage]. Occurring after a hemorrhage.

pos·thet′o·my [G. *posthē*, prepuce; *tomē*, a cutting]. Circumcision.

pos·thi′tis [*posthē;* G. *-itis*, inflammation]. Inflammation of the prepuce.

pos′tho·lith [*posthē;* G. *lithos*, stone]. A preputial calculus. *Obs.*

post′hu·mous (pos′tew·mus) [L. *postumus*, last]. 1. Occurring after death. 2. Born after the death of the father, or by Cesarean section after the death of the mother. 3. Published after the death of the writer.

post″hyp·not′ic [L. *post*, after; *hypnōtikos*, inclined to sleep]. Succeeding the hypnotic state; acting after the hypnotic state has passed off, as posthypnotic suggestion.

post·ic·ter′ic [*post;* G. *ikteros*, jaundice]. Of, relating to, or designating the period or condition following jaundice.

post′i·cus [L.]. Old term for posterior.

post″in·flu·en′zal. Occurring after influenza.

post″ma·lar′i·al (pohst″ma·lair′ee·ul) [*post;* It. *malaria*, from *mala aria*, bad air]. Occurring as a sequel of malaria.

post mortem. Latin, after death.

post″mor′tem, post″mor′tem. Occurring after death.

post″mor′tem, post″-mor′tem. An examination of the body after death; an autopsy. —**post-mortal,** *adj.*

post·na′ris [L. *post*, behind; *naris*, nostril]. The posterior naris; the choana.

post·na′sal [*post;* L. *nasus*, nose]. Situated behind the nose, or in the nasopharynx.

post·na′tal [L. *post*, after; *natalis*, natal]. Subsequent to birth, as a postnatal disease.

post″ne·crot′ic [*post;* G. *nekrōtikos*, causing mortification]. 1. Occurring after death. 2. Occurring after the death of a tissue or a part.

post″ne·crot′ic scar′ring. See postnecrotic *cirrhosis*.

post″neu·rit′ic [*post;* G. *neuron*, nerve; *-itis*, inflammation]. Occurring after neuritis.

post·nod′u·lar [L. *post*, behind; *nodulus*, little knot]. Situated behind the nodulus of the cerebellum.

post·oc′u·lar [*post;* L. *oculus*, eye]. Behind the eye.

post·op′er·a″tive [L. *post*, after; *operari*, to operate]. Occurring after an operation, as insanity, hernia; following closely upon an operation.

post·o′ral [L. *post*, behind; *os*, mouth]. Situated behind the mouth; posterior to the first visceral arch.

post·pal′a·tine (·pal′uh·tyne, ·tin) [*post;* L. *palatum*, palate]. Behind the uvula.

post″pa·lu′dal (·pa·lew′dul, ·pal′yoo·dul) [L. *post*, after; *palus*, swamp]. Postmalarial. *Obs.*

post″par·a·lyt′ic [*post;* G. *paralysis*, paralysis]. Following an attack of paralysis.

post-par′tum. Following childbirth, as post-partum hemorrhage.

post″pha·ryn′ge·al (·fa·rin′jul, ·jee·ul, ·far″in-jee′ul) [L. *post*, behind; G. *pharygx*, pharynx]. Situated behind the pharynx; old term for retropharyngeal.

post·pran′di·al [L. *post*, after; *prandium*, meal]. After a meal.

post″pu·bes′cent [*post;* L. *pubescere*, to reach the age of puberty]. Occurring subsequent to puberty.

post″pyc·not′ic [*post;* G. *pyknōsis*, condensation]. Occurring subsequent to pycnosis.

post″py·ram′i·dal [L. *post*, behind; G. *pyramis*, pyramid]. Situated behind the pyramidal tract.

post·ro′ta·to″ry [L. *post*, after; *rotare*, to revolve]. After rotation, as postrotatory ocular nystagmus.

post″scar·la·ti′nal (pohst″skahr·luh·tee′nul, ·ty′-nul) [*post;* OF. *escarlate*]. Occurring after scarlet fever.

post″ste·not′ic. Referring to area distal to (beyond) the stenosis of a valve or aorta.

post″syph·i·lit′ic [*post;* NL. *syphilis*, syphilis]. Following syphilis.

post″trau·mat′ic [*post;* G. *trauma*, wound]. Pertaining to any process, such as inflammation, following traumatic injury to a part.

post″trau·mat′ic per″son·al′i·ty dis·or′der. A psychosis resulting from direct injury to the head or brain. Symptoms include headache, emotional instability, fatigability, sometimes convulsions.

post·ty′phoid [*post;* G. *typhōdēs*, delirious]. Following typhoid.

pos′tu·late [L. *postulare*, to demand]. 1. A proposition assumed without proof. 2. A condition which must be fulfilled, as Koch's postulate.

Koch's p. See *law* of specificity of bacteria.

pos′tur·al [L. *positura*, from *ponere*, to place]. Pertaining to posture or position; performed by means of a special posture, as postural treatment.

pos′ture [*positura*]. Position or bearing, especially of the body.

jackknife p. One in which the patient reclines on his back with shoulders elevated, legs flexed on thighs, and thighs at right angles to abdomen;

the posture assumed when the upper and lower planes of the Gatch surgical bed are elevated.

post·vac′ci·nal (pohst·vack′si·nul) [L. *post*, after; *vaccinus*, of cows]. Following vaccination.

po′ta·ble [L. *potare*, to drink]. Drinkable; fit to drink.

Potain, Pierre Carl Edouard [*French physician*, 1825–1901]. Inventor of an air sphygmomanometer (1889). Described a syndrome of dyspepsia with cardiac dilatation and accentuation of the second pulmonic sounds in gastrectasis; called *Potain's syndrome*. Described pleuropulmonary congestion, also called *Potain's type of congestion*.

Pot′a·mon [G. *potamos*, river]. A genus of fresh-water crabs, species of which have been incriminated in the transmission of the fluke, *Paragonimus westermani*.

pot″a·mo·pho′bi·a [*potamos;* G. *phobos*, fear]. Morbid fear of sheets of water.

pot′ash″. Potassium carbonate.

caustic p. See *potassium* hydroxide.

p. lye. See *potassium* hydroxide.

sulfurated p. (*potassa sulfurata*). A mixture composed chiefly of potassium polysulfides and potassium thiosulfate; occurs in irregular pieces, liver-brown, when freshly made, changing to a greenish yellow, and has an odor of hydrogen sulfide; 1 Gm. is soluble in about 2 cc. of water; alcohol dissolves only the sulfides. Used as a parasiticide and to stimulate and soften the skin in chronic cutaneous diseases. It may be used either as a lotion or an ointment. Also called *liver of sulfur*.

po·tas′sa. Potassium carbonate.

pot·as·se′mi·a (pot·as see′mee·uh). 1. Potassium in the blood. 2. Hyperpotassemia.

po·tas′si·um [D. *potasch*] (*kalium*). K = 39.100. Light, malleable, ductile lumps, rods, or spheres. Reacts violently with water. A small amount of potassium in the blood is essential for proper function of the various organs of the body. In sufficient quantity the potassium ion is a universal depressant affecting especially the central nervous system and circulation. Salts of potassium are extensively used in medicine. See Table of Normal Values of Blood Constituents in the Appendix.

dibasic p. phosphate. K_2HPO_4. Occurs as white granules; very soluble in water. Also called *dipotassium phosphate, dipotassium hydrogen phosphate, p. phosphate*.

effervescent p. citrate (*potassii citras effervescens*). Contains about 20% potassium citrate, and is used similarly. Dose, 4–8 Gm. (1–2 dr.).

monobasic p. phosphate. KH_2PO_4. Occurs as colorless crystals or white granular powder; 1 Gm. dissolves in 4.5 cc. of water. Also called *p. biphosphate, p. acid phosphate, p. dihydrogen phosphate, monopotassium phosphate*.

p. acetate (*potassii acetas*). CH_3COOK. Occurs as colorless crystals or a white, crystalline powder; 1 Gm. dissolves in 0.5 cc. of water. Used as a saline diuretic, also as an expectorant and in rheumatism. Dose, 1–4 Gm. (15–60 gr.).

p. argenticyanide. Silver potassium cyanide.

p. arsenite solution (*liquor potassii arsenitis*). Represents 1% of arsenic trioxide. Used in malarial affections and chorea and for the general action of the arsenical preparations. Dose, 0.2–0.3 cc. (3–5 min.). Also called *Fowler's solution*.

p. bicarbonate (*potassii bicarbonas*). $KHCO_3$. Colorless crystals or white granular powder; 1 Gm. dissolves in 2.8 cc. of water. Rarely used, but efficient as a gastric antacid. Dose, 0.65–2.0 Gm. (10–30 gr.).

p. bichromate. See *p.* dichromate.

p. bifluoride. KHF_2; potassium acid fluoride, occurring as colorless crystals, soluble in water: used in etching glass and in metallurgy.

p. binoxalate. $KHC_2O_4.H_2O$. White crystals, soluble in water. Used to remove ink stains, to scour metals, to clean wood, and as a mordant in dyeing. Syn., *sal acetosella*.

p. bismuth tartrate. See *bismuth* and *p.* tartrate.

p. bitartrate (*potassii bitartras*). $KHC_4H_4O_6$. Occurs as slightly opaque crystals or a white, crystalline powder; 1 Gm. dissolves in 162 cc. of water. It is diuretic and aperient. When given in full dose it has a mild laxative action but is used mostly in conjunction with other laxatives. Dose, diuretic, 1–3 Gm. (15–45 gr.); cathartic. 8–23 Gm. (2–6 dr.). Also called *cream of tartar, acid p. tartrate*.

p. bromide (*potassii bromidum*). KBr. White cubical crystals or granular powder; 1 Gm. dissolves in 1.5 cc. of water. Used as a nerve sedative, in epilepsy, and to quiet nervous excitability in neurasthenia and hysteria. Dose, 0.6–2.0 Gm. (10–30 gr.).

p. car″ba·cryl′ate. The generic name for the potassium form of cross-linked polyacrylic polycarboxylic cation exchange resins. Such a resin, used in combination with carbacrylic resin, is useful clinically for removal of sodium from intestinal fluid with minimum disturbance of potassium ion equilibrium. See also *carbacrylamine resins*.

p. carbonate (*potassii carbonas*). $K_2CO_3.1\frac{1}{2}H_2O$. White granular powder; 1 Gm. dissolves in 1 cc. of water, insoluble in alcohol. Rarely used internally; used chiefly in pharmaceutical and chemical manipulations.

p. chlorate (*potassii chloras*). $KClO_3$. Colorless, odorless, lustrous crystals or a white, granular powder; 1 Gm. dissolves in 16.5 cc. of water; insoluble in alcohol. Potassium chlorate may explode on heating or when in contact with organic substances. Internal use has been discontinued. Used chiefly in mouth washes and gargles.

p. chloride (*potassii chloridum*). KCl. Colorless crystals or a white, granular powder; 1 Gm. dissolves in 2.8 cc. of water, insoluble in alcohol; used chiefly in correcting potassium deficiency states.

p. chloroplatinate. K_2PtCl_6; orange-yellow crystals or yellow powder, slightly soluble in cold water, insoluble in alcohol; a precipitation form for quantitative estimation of potassium: also called *platinic potassium chloride*.

p. citrate (*potassii citras*). $K_3C_6H_5O_7.H_2O$. Transparent crystals or a white, granular powder; 1 Gm. dissolves in 1 cc. of water. Used as a systemic alkali, a saline diuretic, and as an expectorant. Dose, 1.0–3.0 Gm. (15–45 gr.).

p. citrate solution (*liquor potassii citratis*). Contains 8 Gm. of potassium citrate per 100 cc. Dose, 15 cc. (4 fluidrachms).

p. cyanide. KCN. White, amorphous pieces or white, granular powder; 1 Gm. dissolves in 2 cc. of water. A violent poison. No longer used medicinally.

p. dichromate. $K_2Cr_2O_7$. Orange-red crystals, granules or powder; 1 Gm. dissolves in 6.3 cc. of water. Has many commercial and technical uses.

p. ferricyanide. $K_3Fe(CN)_6$; ruby-red crystals, slowly but freely soluble in water: used industrially and as a reagent. Syn., *red prussiate of potash*.

p. ferrocyanide. $K_4Fe(CN)_6.3H_2O$; yellow, slightly efflorescent crystals, freely soluble in water: used industrially and as a reagent. Syn., *yellow prussiate of potash*.

p. guaiacolsulfonate (*potassii guaiacolsulfonas*). $C_6H_3.OH.OCH_3.SO_3K$. White crystals or a crystalline powder; 1 Gm. dissolves in 7.5 cc. of water. Used as an expectorant. Dose, 0.3–1.3 Gm. (5–20 gr.).

p. guaiacolsulfonate syrup (*syrupus potassii guaiacolsulfonatis*). Contains 7.5 Gm. of potassium guaiacolsulfonate per 100 cc. Dose, 4–8 cc. (1–2 fluidrachms).

p. hydroxide (*potassii hydroxidum*). KOH; occurs as white or nearly white lumps, small pellets or rods; 1 Gm. dissolves in 1 cc. of water; very caustic to tissue. Used externally as an escharotic. Syn., *caustic potash.*

p. hydroxide solution (*liquor potassii hydroxidi*). Contains 5% of potassium hydroxide. Used for pharmaceutical purposes.

p. hypophosphite (*potassii hypophosphis*). KH_2PO_2; white, opaque plates or crystalline powder; 1 Gm. dissolves in 0.6 cc. of water. Formerly used as a nerve stimulant, but of doubtful value.

p. iodate. KIO_3; white crystals or crystalline powder, soluble in water: used as an oxidizing agent in analytical chemistry.

p. iodide (*potassii iodidum*). KI; transparent crystals or a white, granular powder; 1 Gm. dissolves in 0.7 cc. of water: variously used for the effect of iodide ion.

p. iodide ointment (*unguentum potassii iodidi*). Contains 10% of potassium iodide.

p. iodide solution (*liquor potassii iodidi*). Contains 100 Gm. of potassium iodide per 100 cc. Dose, 0.3–1.0 cc. (5–15 min.).

p. mercuric iodide. K_2HgI_4; occurs as yellow crystals, deliquescent in air; soluble in alcohol and in potassium iodide solution and yields a clear solution with one part of water. Used externally for skin disinfection, irrigations and disinfection of instruments and of excreta and discharges.

p. nitrate (*potassii nitras*). KNO_3; occurs as colorless prisms or a white, crystalline powder; 1 Gm. dissolves in 3 cc. of water. No longer used internally. Used in conjunction with stramonium leaves in asthmatic powders. Syn., *saltpeter.*

p. nitrite. KNO_2. A white or slightly yellow salt, soluble in water. Has been used for the same purposes, and in the same dose, as sodium nitrite.

p. percarbonate. $K_2C_2O_6.H_2O$; a white, granular mass, soluble in water with liberation of oxygen, used for detecting tubercle bacilli stained with fuchsin, in photography to decompose traces of sodium thiosulfate, and in chemical analysis. See *antihypo.*

p. permanganate (*potassii permanganas*). $KMnO_4$; occurs as dark purple crystals; 1 Gm. dissolves in 15 cc. of water. Used as a bactericide, oxidant, and astringent. For local use the strength of solution varies from 1 part in 4000 as a wash for mucous membranes, up to 3 or 4% in skin diseases.

p. quadroxalate. Potassium tetroxalate.

p. sodium tartrate (*potassii sodii tartras*). Occurs as colorless crystals or white crystalline powder; 1 Gm. dissolves in 1 cc. of water. Used as a saline cathartic. Dose, 4–15 Gm. (1–4 dr.). Syn., *Rochelle salt.*

p. sulfate (*potassii sulfas*). K_2SO_4. Occurs as white granules or powder; 1 Gm. dissolves in 10 cc. of water. Used as a mild purgative. Dose, 1–8 Gm. (15 gr.–2 dr.).

p. tartrate. $(K_2C_4H_4O_6)_2.H_2O$. White crystals, very soluble in water. Used as a diuretic and laxative, and as a refrigerant in fevers. Dose, 4–15 Gm. (1–4 drachms). Syn., *sal vegetabile.*

p. tetroxalate. $KHC_2O_4.H_2C_2O_4.2H_2O$; colorless or white crystals, sparingly soluble in water, used in analytical chemistry, in metal polishes, and for removing rust and ink stains: improperly called *essential salt of lemons, potassium quadroxalate.*

p. thiocyanate (*potassii thiocyanas*). KSCN. Occurs as colorless, transparent crystals; 1 Gm. dissolves in 9.5 cc. of water. Used in arterial hypertension. Dose, 0.12–0.3 Gm. (2–5 gr.). Also called *potassium sulfocyanate, potassium rhodanate.*

tribasic p. phosphate. K_3PO_4. Occurs as white granular powder; very soluble in water. Also called *tripotassium phosphate.*

po·ta'to nose. See *rhinophyma.*

po'ten·cy [L. *potentia*, power]. 1. Power of the male to perform the sexual act. 2. *In homeopathy,* the degree of dilution of a drug.

po·ten'tial [*potentia*]. Capable of acting or doing work, as potential energy.

po·ten'tial. *In electricity,* a state of tension or of difference in energy capable of doing work. If two bodies of different potential are brought into contact, a current is established between them that is capable of producing electric effects.

action p. Changes in electric potential at the surface of a nerve or muscle occurring at the moment of their excitation; consisting of a very brief period of negativity (spike potential) followed by secondary oscillations in potential (afterpotentials).

autonomous potentials. Continuous potentials arising spontaneously from neurons in the absence of stimulation.

bio-electric p. The difference of electric potential between the inside and the outside of a cell.

biological p. *In psychoanalysis,* any latent physical or psychological ability not currently available to the individual but capable of development by him.

biotic p. Soil yield in terms of living growth useful to man.

critical p. The point at which the electrokinetic or zeta potential between the immobile and mobile ionic layers is lowered by addition of electrolytes so that the double layers of colloidal particles collapse, and the particles aggregate and precipitate.

demarcation, demarkation p. See *injury potential.*

disease p. The sum of adverse health factors present in a community, which have a bearing upon the probable incidence of disease to be anticipated.

electrochemical p. The potential drop across all of the ionic layers from the surface of the particle to the solution. Also called *epsilon p.*

electrocortical p. Potential differences observed from leads applied to the surface of the cerebral cortex. Also called *cortical p.*

electrokinetic p. A potential at the interface between the semipermeable membrane and a solution on either side. See bio-electric *p.* Also called *zeta p.*

electrotonic p. (a) Potential led off by electrometers on either side of bipolar electrodes when a nerve is being stimulated by direct current. (b) Potential developed by cells as a result of metabolic activity and circuited through surrounding tissue.

evoked p. The electric response of any neuron to stimulation.

ground p. Electric potential of the earth, arbitrarily used as a standard reference point for all electric measurements.

injury p. See *injury potential.*

ionization p. The lowest potential that removes an electron from an atom.

membrane p. See *membrane potential.*

Nernst p. The total drop of potential (at a standard state) across the interface, dependent solely on the activity of the ions in the external medium.

oxidation-reduction p. The relative emf exerted by a nonreacting electrode in a solution at 25° C. as measured against that exerted by a normal hydrogen electrode.

$$E = E_0 + \frac{RT}{nF} \log_e \frac{[\text{oxidant}]}{[\text{reductant}]}$$

spike p. See action *p.*

Stern p. The potential between the immobile ion layer and the particle surface; it is equal to the electrochemical potential minus the electrokinetic potential.

streaming potentials. Potentials which result from the streaming of fluids, such as occurs in the flow of blood through the vessels.

po·ten″ti·a′tion. 1. The effect of a substance, when added to another, of making the latter more potent as a drug. 2. *In homeopathic medicine,* the process of making a drug more effective by physical manipulation, as by a high degree of subdivision of a solid by thorough and prolonged trituration.

po′tion [L. *potio,* drink]. A drink or draught.

po″to·cy·to′sis (po″to·sigh·to′sis) [L. *potare,* to drink; *kytos,* cell; *-ōsis,* condition]. Submicroscopic "sipping" or engulfing of fluid by the cytoplasm of cells, as opposed to *pinocytosis,* or microscopically visible imbibition of water by cells.

po″to·ma′ni·a [*potare;* G. *mania,* madness]. Delirium tremens. *Obs.* Also called *mania à potu.*

Pott, Percivall [*English surgeon,* 1714–88]. One of the most successful of the English surgeons of his time, his name is associated with a number of pathologic conditions. Described chimney sweep's cancer of the scrotum, an occupational disease (1775). Author of a treatise on rupture (1756) and one on hydrocele (1762). Best known for his description of the spinal curvature or kyphosis of the spine resulting from tuberculosis (1779); called *Pott's disease.* The eponym has persisted to this day, although Pott did not recognize the tuberculous nature of the disease. Described fracture of the fibula occurring three inches above the ankle, sometimes accompanied by a splitting of the medial malleolus (1765); called *Pott's fracture.* Described senile gangrene, also known as *Pott's gangrene.* See also Pott's puffy *tumor.*

pouch [OF. *pouche*]. A sac or pocket.

abdominovesical p. One formed by the reflection of the peritoneum from the anterior abdominal wall onto the distended urinary bladder; it contains the lateral and medial inguinal fossae.

branchial p. See pharyngeal *p.*

coelomic p. One of a series of evaginations from the wall of the archenteron of lower vertebrates that form the mesodermal somites of the embryo.

craniobuccal p. See Rathke's *p.*

guttural p. One of a pair of mucous sacs which are ventral diverticula of the auditory tube in Equidae, located between the base of the cranium and the atlas dorsally and the pharynx ventrally.

hepatorenal p. That portion of the peritoneal cavity situated behind the right lobe of the liver and in front of the right kidney and right portion of transverse mesocolon: also called *pouch of Morison.*

laryngeal p. A blind pouch of mucosa opening into the lateral part of the ventricle of the larynx.

Pavlov p. See Ivan Petrovich *Pavlov.*

pharyngeal p. One of a series of five paired lateral sacculations of the embryonic pharynx corresponding to the ectodermal grooves between the pharyngeal arches.

p. of Morison. Hepatorenal *p.*

Prussak's p. See *recess* of tympanic cavity (b). See also Alexander *Prussak.*

Rathke's p. A dorsal diverticulum of the stomodeum that develops into the oral or epithelial parts of the hypophysis: also called *craniobuccal p.*

rectouterine p. That part of the peritoneal cavity between the rectum and the posterior surface of the uterus. Also called *p. of Douglas.*

rectovesical p. That part of the peritoneal cavity between the urinary bladder and the rectum in the male. Also called *rectovesical excavation.*

vesicouterine p. That part of the peritoneal cavity between the anterior surface of the uterus and the urinary bladder: also called *uterovesical p.*

visceral p. See pharyngeal *p.*

Zenker's p. Diverticulum of the hypopharynx.

pou·drage′ (poo·drazh′) [F., powdering]. The therapeutic introduction of an irritating powder (talcum) on a serous surface to stimulate the formation of adhesions for the obliteration of the pleural space, as in **pleural p.** or for the development of corollary circulation, as in **epicardial p.**

Poulet, Alfred [*French physician,* 1848–88]. Described rheumatoid osteoperiostitis, also called *Poulet's disease.*

poul′tice (pole′tiss) [L. *puls,* porridge]. A soft, semiliquid mass made of some cohesive substance mixed with water, and used for application to the skin for the purpose of supplying heat and moisture or acting as a local stimulant.

mustard p. One containing a mixture of dry mustard and flour in water to form a paste and spread on a cloth.

Poulton, Edward Palmer [*English physiologist,* 1883–1939]. Remembered for his useful investigations of CO_2, particularly the partition of CO_2 between plasma and corpuscles in oxygenated and in reduced blood (with J. Joffa, 1920). Devised an oxygen tent, also called *Poulton's tent.*

poul′try chinch. *Hematosiphon inodora.*

pound [L. *pondo,* pound]. A unit of measure of weight. The **troy pound** contains 12 ounces, or 5760 grains, or 372.96 grams. Symbol, ℔. The **avoirdupois pound** contains 16 ounces, or 7000 grains, or 453.6 grams. Abbreviated, lb. See Table of Weights and Measures in the Appendix.

foot-pound. The force necessary to raise one pound through the height of one foot.

Poupart, François [*French surgeon,* 1616–1708]. Celebrated surgeon to the court of Louis XIV. Described the ligament extending from the anterior superior spine of the ilium to the spine of the pubis and pectineal line; called *inguinal ligament, Poupart's ligament.* Described a vertical line drawn from the center of the clavicle to Poupart's ligament; called *Poupart's line.*

Pourfoir. See François Pourfoir du *Petit.*

pow′der [L. *pulvis,* dust]. 1. A group of pharmaceutical preparations of definite formula, official in the United States Pharmacopeia or National Formulary, and consisting of intimate mixtures of finely divided medicinal substances. 2. *In pharmacy,* a single dose of medicine placed in powder paper; or may mean a dusting powder, douche powder, or other bulk powder to be administered by the teaspoonful or used externally, all being prepared extemporaneously.

absorbable dusting p. A biologically absorbable powder prepared from cornstarch by introducing certain ether linkages, and containing also 2% of magnesium oxide: used as a surgeon's glove lubricant. Also called *starch-derivative dusting powder.*

Dover's p. A powder prepared from ipecac 10%, opium 10%, and lactose 80%: used as a diaphoretic.

dusting p. Any fine powder used to dust on the skin to absorb or diminish its secretions or allay irritation.
gray p. See *mercury* with chalk.
impalpable p. A powder so fine that its separate particles cannot be felt.
insect p. A powder employed to destroy or ward off insects, formerly consisting usually of the powdered flowers of species of *Chrysanthemum*, known commonly as pyrethrum. Newer preparations may contain DDT or gammexane as active ingredients.
Sippy p. 1. A mixture of precipitated calcium carbonate 23%, sodium bicarbonate 77%: known as Sippy powder No. 1; also called *sodium bicarbonate* and *calcium carbonate powder*. 2. A mixture of magnesium oxide 50%, sodium bicarbonate 50%: known as Sippy powder No. 2; also called *sodium bicarbonate* and *magnesium oxide powder*.

pow′dered stom′ach (*stomachus pulveratus*). Powdered stomach is the dried and powdered, defatted wall of the stomach of the hog, *Sus scrofa* var. *domesticus;* occurs as a granular substance with a slight, not unpleasant, meaty odor, and is practically insoluble in water. It contains factors which cause an increase in the number of red blood cells in the blood of persons suffering from pernicious anemia. The activity is readily destroyed when the preparation is suspended in a hot liquid. It is used solely in the treatment of anemia, especially pernicious anemia. Dose, one U.S.P. unit daily, administered in a half glassful of water, milk, or fruit juice. Also called *dried stomach*. See *ventriculin*.

Powell, Cecil F. (1903–). British physicist known for his research on the discharge of electricity in gases and on the development of the photographic method in nuclear physics; Nobel laureate in physics (1950) for studies on the structure of the atom.

pow′er [F. *pouvoir*, from L. *posse*, to be able]. 1. Ability to produce an effect. 2. *In optics*, the magnification given by a lens or prism.
p. breeder. A nuclear reactor designed to produce both useful and powerful nuclear fuel.
p. reactor. A nuclear reactor capable of producing useful mechanical power, as by generating heat of sufficient intensity to permit its reasonably efficient conversion into work.
refractive p. The measure of influence which a transparent body exercises on the velocity of light which passes through it.

Power test. See Cutler-Power-Wilder *test*.

pox [ME. *pokkes*]. 1. Any vesicular or pustular disease. 2. Common term for syphilis. See *chickenpox, cowpox, horsepox, smallpox, whitepox*.
Ambonese p. The papules in yaws: old term.
fowl p. A disease of birds caused by a virus; characterized by wartlike nodules on the skin, particularly of the head.
kaffir p. Alastrim or mild variola.
milk p. A mild form of smallpox.
rickettsial p. Rickettsialpox.
sheep p. See *orf*.
Spanish p. Early syphilis: old term, English usage.
swine p. A frequent disease of hogs characterized by pox lesions on the body and inner surfaces of the legs. It is a benign infection and usually occurs in young pigs.

Pozzi, Samuel Jean [*French gynecologist*, 1846–1918]. Remembered for his description of backache and leukorrhea without enlargement of the uterus, found in some cases of endometritis; known as *Pozzi's syndrome*.

PP Pellagra preventive (factor).

P.p. *Punctum proximum*, near point.

P.P.D. Purified protein derivative; a form of tuberculin which is a dry powder, dry diluted with lactose, and is relatively constant in its activity.

P.P. factor. Goldberger's term for the pellagra preventive factor present in vitamin-B complex; identical with niacin (nicotinic acid).

PPLO Pleuropneumonialike organisms.

p.p.m. Parts per million.

ppt. Precipitate.

Pr Chemical symbol for praseodymium.

Pr. Abbreviation for presbyopia.

P.r. *Punctum remotum*, far point.

prac′tice [G. *praktikos*, fit for action]. The routine application of the principles of medicine to the diagnosis and treatment of disease.

prac′tice. To perform the duties of a physician.

prae-. See *pre-*.

prae·pu′ti·um (pree·pew′shee·um). See *prepuce*.

prag″mat·ag·no′si·a (prag″mat·ag·no′see·uh, ·zee·uh) [G. *pragma*, thing; *agnōsia*, lack of acquaintance]. Inability to recognize an object.
visual p. Object blindness.

prag″mat·am·ne′si·a (·am·nee′zhuh, ·zee·uh) [*pragma;* G. *amnēsia*, amnesia]. Loss of the ability to remember the appearance of an object.
visual p. A mental condition marked by a loss of ability to call up the visual image of an object.

Prague ma·neu′ver. See under *maneuver*.

pran′di·al (L. *prandium*, meal). Of or pertaining to a meal, especially a dinner.

pranone. Trade-mark for anhydrohydroxyprogesterone or ethisterone.

pranturon. Trade-mark for the gonadotropic substance obtained from pregnancy urine.

pra″se·o·dym′i·um (pray″zee·o·dim′ee·um, pray″see·o·, prass″ee·o·) [G. *prasios*, leek-green; *didymos*, twin]. Pr = 140.92. A rare earth metal. The principal valency is three. and its salts are generally green in color.

pra·tique′ (prah·teek′, prat′ick. *See* Notes § 35) [F.]. The bill of health given to vessels by a health officer.

Prausnitz, Carl Willy. See Carl Prausnitz *Giles*.

Pravaz, Charles Gabriel [*French physician*, 1791–1853]. Inventor of a hypodermic syringe fitted with a long slender cannula and trocar (1853); called *Pravaz's syringe*. Invented modern galvanocautery (1853).

-prax′i·a [G. *praxis*, a doing]. A combining form meaning *action, doing*.

prax·in′o·scope [*praxis;* G. *skopein*, to examine]. A modified stroboscope adapted to laryngologic instruction.

prax″i·ol′o·gy [*praxis;* G. *logos*, word]. The science of conduct.

pre- [L. *prae*, before]. A prefix signifying *before*.

pre·ag′o·nal [*prae;* G. *agōn*, struggle]. Immediately preceding the death agony.

pre″al·bu″mi·nu′ric [*prae;* L. *albus*, white; *ouron*, urine]. Occurring before the appearance of albuminuria.

pre·am′pul·lar·y. Before an ampulla, as the sphincter of Boyden proximal to the ampulla of Vater.

pre·a′nal [*prae;* L. *anus*, anus]. Situated in front of the anus.

pre″an·es·thet′ic [*prae;* G. *anaisthēsis*, lack of sensation]. Before anesthesia.

pre″an·ti·sep′tic [*prae;* G. *anti*, against; *sēpsis*, decay]. Pertaining to the time before the use of antisepsis in surgery.

pre″a·or′tic (pree″ay·or′tick) [*prae;* G. *aortē*, aorta]. Situated in front of the aorta.

pre″a·sep′tic [*prae;* G. *a-*, not; *sēpsis*]. Pertaining to the period before the introduction of aseptic surgery.

pre″a·tax′ic [*prae;* G. *ataxia,* confusion]. Occurring before ataxia.

pre″au·ric′u·lar [*prae;* L. *auricula,* external ear]. Situated in front of the auricle.

pre·ax′i·al [*prae;* L. *axis,* axis]. Situated in front of the axis of the body or of a limb.

pre·can′cer·ous (pree·can′sur·us). Pertaining to any pathological condition of a tissue which is likely to develop into cancer.

pre·cap′il·lar″y (pree·cap′i·lerr″ee) [*prae;* L. *capillaris,* from *capillus,* hair]. An arteriole with weakly developed media preceding capillaries. Syn., *arterial capillary, arteriocapillary, precapillary arteriole.*

pre·car′di·ac (pree·kahr′dee·ack) [*prae;* G. *kardia,* heart]. Anterior to the heart.

pre·car′di·nal (pree·kahr′di·nul) [*prae;* L. *cardinalis,* principal]. Pertaining to the pair of cardinal veins anterior to the common cardinal vein of the embryo, draining the head and neck.

pre·car′ti·lage (pree·kahr′ti·lidj) [*prae;* L. *cartilago,* cartilage]. Compact, cellular embryonic connective tissue just before it differentiates into cartilage.

pre·ca′va (pree·kay′vuh) [*prae;* L. *cavus,* hollow]. The superior, or descending, vena cava.

pre·cen′tral (pree·sen′trul) [*prae;* G. *kentron,* center]. Situated in front of the central fissure of the brain.

pre·chor′dal (pree·kor′dul) [*prae;* G. *chordē,* string]. Situated in front of the notochord.

pre·cip′i·tant [L. *praecipitare,* to precipitate]. Any reagent causing precipitation.

pre·cip′i·tate [*praecipitare*]. 1. An insoluble compound deposited in a solution of a substance on the addition of a reagent which produces a chemical reaction or otherwise decreases solubility. Abbreviated, ppt. 2. The product of the reaction between precipitinogen and precipitin.

red p. Red mercuric oxide.

white p. Ammoniated mercury.

yellow p. Yellow mercuric oxide.

pre·cip′i·tate. To throw down in an insoluble form.

pre·cip′i·tate. Headlong; hasty, as precipitate labor.

pre·cip′i·ta″ted chalk. See precipitated *calcium* carbonate.

pre·cip″i·ta′tion [L. *praecipitatio,* from *praecipitare*]. The process of making substances insoluble by the addition of a reagent, evaporation, freezing, or electrolysis.

co-precipitation. The simultaneous precipitation of more than one compound.

fractional p. The separation of substances by precipitating them in increasing order of solubility.

pre·cip′i·ta″tor [L., from *praecipitare*]. A type of instrument used for determining the number of dust particles in the air. In the **electric precipitator,** a high electric potential is created between two surfaces. When a measured sample of air is passed through this field, the dust particles adhere to one of the surfaces. In the **thermal precipitator,** a heated wire is suspended in a narrow slot between two cooled glass cover slips, and the dust particles from an air sample passed through the slot adhere to the cover slips. The collected particles are counted under a microscope. Other instruments used for the same purpose are the konimeter, impinger, and jet dust counter. Also see *dust count.*

pre·cip′i·tin [*praecipitare*]. An antibody to a soluble antigen. A precipitate is formed when the soluble antigen is layered over the antibody or mixed with it.

pre·cip″i·tin′o·gen [*praecipitare;* G. *genesthai,* from *gignesthai,* to be produced]. Any substance capable of causing the production of a precipitin.

pre·cip′i·tin·oid″ [*praecipitare;* G. *eidos,* form]. An inactive precipitin modified by heating to 60° C. The precipitinoid retains the capacity to combine with the precipitinogen, while not causing its precipitation.

pre·clin′i·cal (pree·klin′i·kul) [L. *prae,* before; G. *klinikos,* of a bed]. 1. Occurring prior to the period in which recognized symptoms or signs make diagnosis possible. 2. Referring to medical studies undertaken before the study of patients.

pre·co′cious [L. *praecox,* ripe before its time]. Developing at an age earlier than usual.

pre·coc′i·ty (pri·kos′i·tee) [*praecox*]. Early development or maturity; applied especially to great development of the mental faculties at an early age.

pre·cog·ni′tion. The foreknowledge, apart from rational forecasting or logical inference, of future events.

pre″col·lag′e·nous (pree″ko·ladj′i·nus) [L. *prae,* before; G. *kolla,* glue; *genesthai,* from *gignesthai,* to be produced]. Characterizing an incomplete stage in the formation of collagen.

pre·co′ma di″a·bet′i·cum (pree·ko′muh) [L.]. See *coma;* diabetic *acidosis.*

pre·con′scious (pree·kon′shus). See *foreconscious.*

pre″con·vul′sant [L. *prae,* before; *convulsio,* convulsion]. Relating to the stage of a disease preceding convulsions.

pre″con·vul′sive [*prae; convulsio*]. Referring to the period just prior to the occurrence of an epileptic seizure.

pre·cor′di·um, pre·cor′di·a [*prae;* L. *cor,* heart]. The area of the chest overlying the heart. —**precor′dial,** *adj.*

pre·cos′tal (pree·kos′tul) [*prae;* L. *costa,* rib]. Situated in front of the ribs.

pre·cu′ne·us [*prae;* L. *cuneus,* wedge]. A lobule of the parietal lobe, situated in front of the cuneus of the occipital lobe. —**precuneal,** *adj.*

pre·den′tin. Uncalcified dentinal matrix.

pre″di·crot′ic (pree″dye·krot′ick) [*prae;* G. *dikrotos,* double beating]. Preceding the dicrotic wave or elevation of the sphygmographic tracing.

pre″di·gest′ed (pree″di·jest′id, ·dye·jest′id) [*prae;* L. *digestum,* from *digerere,* to digest]. Partly digested by artificial means before being taken into the stomach.

pre″di·ges′tion (pree″di·jes′chun, ·dye·jes′chun) [*prae;* L. *digestio,* from *digerere*]. The partial digestion of food before it is eaten.

pre″dis·po′sing (pree″dis·po′zing) [*prae;* OF. *disposer*]. Rendering the body susceptible to a disease, as predisposing cause.

pre″dis·po·si′tion (pree″dis·po·zish′un) [*prae;* L. *dispositio,* arrangement]. The state of having special susceptibility to a disease or condition.

pred·nis′o·lone. Generic name for $\Delta^{1,4}$-pregnadiene-11β, 17α, 21-triol-3,20-dione; a synthetic steroid related to prednisone in the same way that hydrocortisone is related to cortisone, and having potent joint antiinflammatory activity. Syn., *metacortandralone.* See *meticortelone.*

pred′ni·sone. Generic name for $\Delta^{1,4}$-pregnadiene-17α, 21-diol-3, 11, 20-trione; a synthetic steroid containing one more double bond than cortisone. It is more potent than cortisone in suppressing inflammatory joint changes, without causing sodium and water retention. Syn., *metacortandracin.* See *deltra, meticorten.*

pre″dor·mi′tion (pree″dor·mish′un) [*prae;* L. *dormitio,* a sleeping]. Applied to the stage of unconsciousness immediately preceding actual sleep.

pre″ec·lamp′si·a [*prae;* G. *eklampsis,* a shining forth]. A disease, occurring in the latter half of pregnancy, characterized by an acute elevation of blood pressure and usually by edema and proteinuria, but without convulsions or coma. See *eclampsia*, 2.

pre·ep″i·glot′tic [*prae;* G. *epiglōttis*, epiglottis]. Anterior to the epiglottis.

pre″e·rup′tive [*prae;* L. *eruptio*, eruption]. Preceding eruption.

pre″for·ma′tion [*prae;* L. *formatio*, a shaping]. The theory which regards development as merely the unfolding or growth of the organism already fully formed in miniature, and contained in the germ cell (egg or sperm).

pre·fron′tal [*prae;* L. *frons*, forehead]. Situated in the anterior part of the frontal lobe of the brain.

pre·fron′tal leu·cot′o·my. See *prefrontal lobotomy*.

pre·fron′tal lo·bot′o·my. A method of treating mental disorders, particularly melancholia and psychasthenia, by severing the white fibers connecting the prefrontal and frontal lobes with the thalamus.

pre″gan·gli·on′ic (pree″gang·glee·on′ick, ·gang-lee·on′ick) [*prae;* G. *gagglion*, encysted tumor on a tendon]. Situated in front of, or preceding, a ganglion.

pre·glob′u·lin (pree·glob′yoo·lin) [*prae;* L. *globulus*, little ball]. A poorly defined protein found in cell protoplasm. *Obs.*

preg′nan·cy [L. *praegnans*, pregnant]. Being with child; the state of the woman from conception to childbirth. The duration of pregnancy in woman is approximately 280 days. To estimate the date of confinement, take the first day of the last menstrual period, count back three months, and add one year and seven days. See Ely's Table of the Duration of Pregnancy in the Appendix. See Plate 41.

abdominal p. Gestation with the fetus lying within the peritoneal cavity.

ampullar p. Gestation in the outer portion of the uterine tube.

bigeminal p. Twin pregnancy.

cervical p. A rare condition in which, from atrophy of the decidual membranes, the impregnated ovum is implanted in the cervical canal, where it develops until the uterus expels it.

cornual p. Gestation occurring in one horn of a two-horned uterus.

ectopic p. Extrauterine gestation.

extrauterine p. Gestation outside of the cavity of the uterus.

false p. See phantom *p.*

heterotopic p. Double gestation, with one fetus inside and the other outside the uterine cavity.

hydatid p. Gestation in which the chorionic sac degenerates into a hydatidiform mole.

interstitial p. Gestation in the uterine part of a uterine tube. Also called *intramural p.*

intraligamentary p. Gestation within the broad ligament.

membranous p. Gestation in which there has been a rupture of the amniotic sac and the fetus is in direct contact with the wall of the uterus.

mesenteric p. Tuboligamentary gestation.

molar p. Gestation in which the ovum has been converted into a fleshy tumor mass (mole).

multiple p. Gestation with two or more fetuses present within the uterus.

ovarian p. Gestation within the ovary.

parietal p. Interstitial gestation.

phantom p. Enlargement of the abdomen and often other symptoms simulating gestation, usually due to hysteria. Syn., *pseudocyesis*.

plural p. See multiple *p.*

p. test See under *test*.

sarcofetal p. Gestation with the presence of both a fetus and a mole.

sarcohysteric p. False pregnancy due to a mole.

signs of p. The three so-called absolute signs are ballottement, fetal movements, and fetal heart sounds.

tubal p. Gestation within an oviduct.

tuboabdominal p. Gestation which develops in the ampulla and extends into the peritoneal cavity.

tuboligamentary p. Gestation arising in an oviduct with extension into the broad ligament.

tubo-ovarian p. Gestation arising in an oviduct and extending into the ovary.

tubouterine p. See interstitial *p.*

twin p. Gestation with two fetuses.

uteroabdominal p. Gestation with one fetus in the uterus and another within the peritoneal cavity.

utero-ovarian p. Gestation with one fetus in the uterus and another in the ovary.

uterotubal p. Gestation with one fetus in the uterus and another in an oviduct.

preg′nan·cy rate. The number of pregnancies actually experienced in relation to the number of ova that theoretically might have been fertilized.

5-α-preg′nane. Allopregnane.

preg·nane′di·ol (preg·nan′dee·ole, ·dye·ole, ·ol, ·awl). $C_{21}H_{36}O_2$. A metabolite of progesterone, found in the urine during the progestational phase of the menstrual cycle and in pregnancy urine.

preg″nane·di′one. $C_{21}H_{32}O_2$; 3,20-pregnanedione; a steroid hormone occurring in pregnancy urine of mares; a dihydro derivative of progesterone.

preg′nant [L. *praegnans*, pregnant]. With child; gravid.

preg″nen·in′o·lone (preg″nen·in′o·loan, preg″-neen·). Anhydrohydroxyprogesterone or ethisterone.

preg·nen′o·lone. $C_{21}H_{32}O_2$; Δ^5-pregnen-3β-ol-20-one; a steroid oxidation product of cholesterol and stigmasterol, apparently effective in reducing fatigue and formerly believed of value as an antiarthritic agent.

pregnyl. Trade-mark for a preparation of the chorionic gonadotropin of human pregnancy urine.

pre·hal′lux (pree·hal′ucks) [L. *prae*, before; *hallex*, great toe]. A supernumerary digit attached to the great toe on its medial aspect.

pre″hem·i·pleg′ic (pree″hem·i·pledj′ick, ·plee′-jick) [*prae;* G. *hēmiplēgēs*, half-struck]. Occurring before an attack of hemiplegia, as prehemiplegic chorea.

pre·hen′sile (pri·hen′sil, ·sile) [L. *prehensum*, from *prehendere*, to seize]. Adapted for grasping, as the tail of certain species of monkeys.

pre·hen′sion [L. *prehensio*, from *prehendere*]. The act of grasping or seizing.

Preiser, Georg Karl Felix [*German orthopedic surgeon*, 1879–1913]. Described traumatic osteoporosis of the navicular bone of the wrist; called *Preiser's disease*.

Preisz, Hugo von [*Hungarian bacteriologist*, 1860–1940]. Described a diphtheroid bacillus, pathogenic for sheep and horses. It produces a form of pseudotuberculosis. Called *Preisz-Nocard bacillus*.

pre″lo·co·mo′tion [L. *prae*, before; *locus*, place; *motum*, from *movere*, to move]. The movements of a child who has not yet learned to walk, which indicate the intention of moving from one place to another.

pre′lum [L.]. A press.

p. abdominale. The squeezing of the abdominal viscera between the diaphragm and the rigid abdominal wall, as in the processes of defecation, micturition, and parturition.

pre″ma·lig′nant. See *precancerous.*

pre″ma·ni′a·cal [L. *prae,* before; G. *mania,* madness]. Previous to, or preceding, an attack of insanity.

premarin. Trade-mark for a preparation of conjugated estrogens, chiefly in the form of sodium estrone sulfate, administered orally.

pre″ma·ture′ [L. *praematurus,* too early]. Occurring before the proper time, as premature labor.

pre″ma·ture′ beat. *In cardiology,* a beat occurring before the next expected impulse and followed usually by a pause which may or may not be compensatory.

pre″max·il′la [L. *prae,* before; *maxilla,* jaw]. The intermaxillary bone. —**premaxillary,** *adj.*

pre″med·i·ca′tion [*prae·* L. *medicare,* to heal]. The administration of drugs before an operation, primarily to quiet the patient and to facilitate the administration of the anesthetic.

pre·men′stru·al (pree·men′stroo·ul) [*prae;* L. *menstrualis,* monthly]. Preceding menstruation.

pre·mo′lar (pree·mo′lur) [*prae;* L. *molaris,* from *mola,* mill]. In each quadrant of the human dentition, one of the two teeth between the canine and the first molar; a bicuspid. The term is often used incorrectly to signify a deciduous molar. The premolars replace the deciduous molars.

pre″mo·ni′tion [L. *praemonitio,* forewarning]. A warning of some future experience or event, usually tragic; a foreboding.

pre·mon′i·to″ry [L. *praemonitum,* from *praemonere,* to forewarn]. Giving previous warning or notice, as in premonitory symptoms, the nonspecific signs of impending illness before specific indications begin. Also called *prodromal.*

pre·mon′o·cyte. See *promonocyte.*

pre″mu·ni′tion (pree″mew·nish′un) [L. *praemunitio,* a fortifying beforehand]. An immunity which depends upon a persistent latent infection, such as an immunity in malaria due to long-continued quiescent infection.

pre·my′e·lo·blast″ (pree·migh′i·lo·blast″) [L. *prae,* before; G. *myelos,* marrow; *blastos,* germ]. A young form of myeloblast.

pre·my′e·lo·cyte″ (pree·migh′i·lo·sight″). See *promyelocyte.*

pre″nar·co′sis [*prae;* G. *narkōsis,* a benumbing]. Preliminary, light narcosis produced prior to general anesthesia.

pre·na′tal (pree·nay′tul) [*prae;* L. *natalis,* natal]. Existing or occurring before birth.

prenderol. Trade-mark for 2,2-diethyl-1,3-propanediol, a skeletal muscle relaxant.

pre″ne·o·plas′tic [*prae;* G. *neos,* new; *plassein,* to form]. Before the development of a definite tumor. See *precancerous.*

pre·nid′a·to″ry (pree·nid′uh·tor″ee, ·nigh′duh·tor″ee) [*prae;* L. *nidus,* nest]. Before nidation.

pre″oc·cip′i·tal (pree″ock·sip′i·tul) [*prae;* L. *occiput,* back part of the head]. Situated anterior to the occipital region, as the preoccipital notch, a notch indicating the division between the occipital and temporal lobes of the brain.

prep″a·ra′tion [L. *praeparatio,* from *praeparare,* to make ready beforehand]. 1. The act of making ready. 2. Anything made ready, especially, in anatomy, any part of the body prepared or preserved for illustrative or other uses. 3. *In pharmacy,* any compound or mixture made after a formula.

corrosion p. See under *corrosion.*

cover-glass p. One used in examining cells of blood or of any other fluid. A small drop of blood or other fluid is placed on a thin, square cover glass. A second cover glass is dropped on the first. As soon as the fluid has stopped spreading, the two cover glasses are pulled apart horizontally; after air drying, the material is stained with an appropriate stain and studied under the microscope.

hanging-drop p. A preparation using a special slide containing a circular concavity, or a regular slide with a petroleum jelly ring, in which a drop of solution to be examined microscopically can be suspended without spreading over the slide.

heart-lung p. A set-up for the study of the effects of mechanical or physical factors upon cardiac behavior, consisting of an apparatus for establishing a temporary, artificially controlled, circulatory system outside the body of the experimental animal while the lesser circulation remains undisturbed.

Klatsch p. A cover-glass preparation made by pressing the cover glass lightly on a bacterial colony in plate culture.

Langendorf p. An isolated mammalian heart preparation in which the coronary vessels are perfused in warm oxygenated Locke-Ringer or Tyrode solution.

Lawen-Trendelenburg p. A preparation used in perfusion of the hindleg of a toad.

pre″pa·tel′lar [L. *prae,* before; *patella,* kneepan]. Situated in front of the patella.

pre·pat′ent pe′ri·od (pree·pat′unt, ·pay′tunt). The period in parasitic disease between the introduction of the organism and its demonstration in the body.

prephysin. Trade-mark for a preparation of chorionic gonadotropin.

pre·pol′lex [*prae;* L. *pollex,* thumb]. A supernumerary digit attached to the thumb on its radial aspect.

pre·pon′der·ance [L. *praeponderare,* to be of greater weight]. 1. The state of being greater in weight or force. 2. A term used in electrocardiography as either (a) **left preponderance,** designating the effect of left ventricular hypertrophy due to a variation in the normal $\frac{\text{Right}}{\text{Left}}$ ventricular weight ratio (normal 1.4–2.0): abnormal left axis deviation, increased duration of QRS, and sometimes inversion of T_1 and T_2; or (b) **right preponderance,** designating the effect of right ventricular hypertrophy: abnormal right axis deviation, deep S_1, tall R_3, and $R_3 > R_2$, and sometimes increased duration of QRS.

ventricular p. Relative increase in the weight of the muscle of one ventricle as compared to that of the other, in hypertrophied hearts.

pre·po′ten·cy [L. *praepotentia,* superior power]. The ability of one parent to impress individual characteristics upon offspring to a marked degree. It has now been explained as Mendelian dominance. *Obs.*

pre·po′tent [L. *praepotens,* very powerful]. Having a marked tendency to transmit individual characters to offspring. *Obs.*

pre″psy·chot′ic (pree″sigh·cot′ick) [L. *prae,* before; G. *psychē,* soul]. Of or pertaining to the mental state that precedes or is potentially capable of preceding a psychosis.

pre·pu′ber·al (pree·pew′bur·ul) [*prae;* L. *puber,* adult]. Prior to puberty.

pre″pu·bes′cent [*prae;* L. *pubescere,* to reach the age of puberty]. Prepuberal.

pre′puce [L. *praeputium,* foreskin]. The foreskin of the penis, a fold of skin covering the glans penis; also, the similar fold over the glans clitoridis. —**prepu′tial,** *adj.*

pre″pu·cot′o·my [*praeputium;* G. *tomē,* a cutting]. An incision into the prepuce; an incomplete circumcision.

pre″py·lor′ic (pree″pye·lor′ick) [L. *prae*, before; G. *pylōros*, gatekeeper]. Placed in front of, or preceding, the pylorus.

pre″ra·chit′ic (pree″ra·kit′ick) [*prae;* G. *rhachis*, spine]. Pertaining to the interval previous to the time when rickets becomes obvious.

pre·rec′tal (pree·reck′tul) [*prae;* L. *rectus*, straight]. Situated in front of the rectum.

pre·re′nal (pree·ree′nul) [*prae;* L. *renes*, kidneys]. Situated in front of the kidney.

pre″re·pro·duc′tive [*prae;* L. *re-*, again; *producere*, to bring before]. Relating to the period of life preceding puberty.

pre·ret′i·nal (pree·ret′i·nul) [*prae;* L. *rete*, net]. Anterior to the internal limiting membrane of the retina, as preretinal hemorrhage.

pre·sa′cral. Lying in front of the sacrum, as a presacral nerve.

pres″by·a·cu′si·a (prez″bee·a·cue′shuh, ·a·kōō′shuh), **pres″by·a·cou′si·a** (prez″bee·a·koo′shuh). See *presbycusis.*

pres″by·at′rics (prez″bee·at′ricks, press″bee·) [G. *presbys*, old man; *iatrikos*, skilled in the medical art]. That branch of medicine which deals with the diseases of old age. Syn., *geriatrics.*

pres″by·cu′sis (prez″bi·cue′sis, ·kōō′sis, press″bi·), **pres″by·cou′sis** (prez″bi·kōō′sis, press″bi·) [*presbys;* G. *akousis*, hearing]. The lessening of the acuteness of hearing that occurs with advancing age.

pres″by·der′ma. Senile skin.

pres″by·o·phre′ni·a (prez″bee·o·free′nee·uh, ·fren′ee·uh, press″bee·o·) [*presbys;* G. *phrēn*, mind]. Failure of the sense of location and memory in the aged, frequently the normal condition of old age; the general concomitant of senility. —**presbyophren′ic,** *adj.*

pres″by·o′pi·a (prez″bee·o′pee·uh, press″bee·) [*presbys;* G. *ōps*, eye]. The condition of vision in the aged, due to diminished power of accommodation from impaired elasticity of the crystalline lens, whereby the near point of distinct vision is removed farther from the eye. Abbreviated, Pr. —**presbyop′ic,** *adj.;* **pres′byope,** *n.*

pres″by·o·sphac′e·lus (prez″bee·o·sfass′i·lus, press″bee·o·) [*presbys;* G. *sphakelos*, gangrene]. Senile gangrene.

pres·byt′i·a (prez·bish′uh, ·bit′ee·uh, press·). See *presbyopia.*

pres″by·ti·at′rics. See *presbyatrics.*

pres·byt′ic [G. *presbytēs*, old man]. Suffering from presbyopia.

pres′by·tism. See *presbyopia.*

pre″schiz·o·phren′ic (pree″skiz·o·fren′ick) [L. *prae*, before; G. *schizein*, to split; *phrēn*, mind]. Pertaining to symptoms and personality characteristics which usually precede a schizophrenic psychosis.

pre″scle·ro′sis [*prae;* G. *sklērōsis*, a hardening]. The vascular condition which precedes arteriosclerosis. —**presclerot′ic,** *adj.*

pre·scribe′ [L. *praescribere*, to write before]. Give instructions concerning the use of a remedy.

pre·scrip′tion [L. *praescriptio*, from *praescribere*]. Written instructions designating the preparation and use of substances to be administered. See Table of the More Common Latin or Greek Terms and Abbreviations Used in Prescription Writing in the Appendix.

shotgun p. Old term for a prescription containing many ingredients; written with the expectation that some one of the ingredients might prove helpful. Such prescriptions are now seldom used.

pre″se·nil′i·ty [L. *prae*, before; *senilis*, aged]. Premature old age. —**presen′ile,** *adj.*

pre·sent′ [L. *praesentare*, to place before]. Appear first at the os uteri, applied to a part of the fetus.

pres″en·ta′tion (prez″un·tay′shun, pree″zen·) [L. *praesentatio*, from *praesentare*]. That part of the fetus which is palpated through the cervix uteri at the beginning of labor. The relation of the part of the fetus to the birth canal determines the type of presentation.

breech p. The presentation of the buttocks and/or the feet first at the cervix; called double breech or complete breech if both buttocks and feet appear first; frank breech if the buttocks alone are the presenting part, the legs being bent so that the feet lie against the face.

brow p. That in which the brow of the child presents at the cervix.

cephalic p. That in which any part of the head is the presenting part.

compound p. Prolapse of an extremity of the fetus alongside the presenting part.

face p. The presentation of the face with the chin leading at the cervix during labor.

footling p. Presentation with the feet foremost.

p. of cord. Descent of the umbilical cord between the presenting part and the membranes at the beginning of labor.

transverse p. That in which the child is turned with its long axis across that of the birth canal; the presenting part may be the shoulder, back, or abdomen.

vertex p. The most usual type of presentation with the occiput the presenting part. See Plate 42.

pre·sent′ing com·plaints′. The symptoms of which the patient is aware and which bring him to the physician.

presidon. A trade-mark for pyrithyldione, a sedative and hypnotic no longer used because it may produce agranulocytosis.

pre·sphe′noid (pree·sfee′noyd) [L. *prae*, before; G. *sphēnoeidēs*, wedge-shaped]. The anterior portion of the body of the sphenoid, ossifying from a separate center.

pre·sphyg′mic (pree·sfig′mick) [*prae;* G. *sphygmos*, pulse]. Pertaining to the period preceding the pulse wave, the isometric phase of systole.

press·om′e·ter. A manometer for measuring pressure in the uterus and kidneys after injection of radiopaque media in doing pyelography and uterosalpingography (hysterosalpingography).

pres′sor [L. *pressor*, from *premere*, to press]. Producing a rise in blood pressure.

pres″so·re·cep′tor [*premere;* L. *receptor*, from *recipere*, to receive]. A nerve ending, located in the wall of the carotid sinus and aortic arch, sensitive to stretching induced by changes of blood pressure within the vessels or direct pressure from without. It sends afferent impulses to medullary centers to cause reflex vasodilatation and fall of blood pressure when stretched as by increase of systemic pressure and a reflex rise in systemic pressure when blood pressure within the carotid sinus and aortic arch is suddenly lessened. Syn., *baroceptor, baroreceptor.*

pres″so·sen′si·tive [*premere;* L. *sentire*, to feel]. Stimulated by changes in blood pressure, as nerve endings in the carotid sinus.

pres′sure [L. *pressura*, a pressing]. Force, weight, or tension.

abdominal p. Pressure upon the viscera, as when the diaphragm is contracted while the belly-wall muscles are contracted, as in urination and defecation. Also called *strain, squeeze, bearing down, prelum abdominale.*

afterpressure. The sense of pressure that remains for a brief period after the removal of an object from the surface of the body.

alveolar p. The combined pressures of oxygen,

carbon dioxide, nitrogen, and water vapor in the alveoli. At body temperature, water vapor exerts a pressure of about 48 mm. Hg.

ambient p. *In aviation medicine*, the pressure which surrounds a flier or his aircraft; the atmospheric pressure to which he is exposed.

arterial p. The tension of the arterial wall due to the pressure of the blood within the arteries.

atmospheric p. The pressure of the atmosphere; it equals about fifteen pounds to the square inch at sea level.

back p. effect. Pulmonary and venous engorgement; occurring when the ventricles are unable to pump blood from the venous to the arterial system as fast as it is received; damming back of the blood.

bipolar p. Pressure on the two ends of a bone. It is used in differentiating fractures from contusions, producing pain in the case of the former.

blood p. The pressure of the blood against the walls of the vessels or of the heart. It is measured by means of the manometer. Also see *blood pressure*.

colloid osmotic p. See oncotic *p.*

critical p. That pressure on a gas or vapor which will, at the critical temperature, convert it into a liquid.

endocardial p. The pressure of the blood within the heart.

hydrostatic p. A pressure created in a fluid system by the energy of muscular contraction not utilized in motion, as blood pressure created by the heart beat. A fluid system may also exert such pressure as a result of the effect of gravity.

imbibition p. Pressure due to the increase in volume of a gel as a result of the imbibition of liquid.

intraabdominal p. The pressure exerted upon the walls by the abdominal viscera. See abdominal *p.*

intracranial p. The pressure of the contents of the cranium upon its walls.

intraesophageal p. Air pressure within the esophagus, closely reflecting intrapleural pressure.

intraocular p. See intraocular *tension.*

intrapleural p. Normally, the negative pressure existing between the parietal and visceral pleura. In pneumothoraxes, this may be a negative, atmospheric, or positive pressure.

intrathoracic p. The pressure of the intrathoracic organs upon the walls of the chest.

negative p. The force of suction; also, absence of pressure.

oncotic p. The osmotic pressure exerted by colloids in a solution which varies owing to the variation of colloidal molecules or aggregations of micelles.

osmotic p. The pressure developed when a solution and its solvent component are separated by a membrane permeable to the solvent only, or when two solutions of different concentration of the same solute are similarly separated.

partial p. In a mixture of gases, the pressure exerted by one of the gases is said to be the partial pressure of that gas. In such a mixture the partial pressures of the gases are exerted independently of each other.

p. breathing. *In aviation medicine*, breathing by introduction of a suitable gas mixture into the lungs at a pressure above the ambient pressure exerted on the external surface of the chest.

pulse p. The difference between the systolic and diastolic blood pressure.

solution p. The tendency of the molecules or ions to leave the surface of a solute and pass into the solvent. Varies in different solute-solvent combinations.

vapor p. The pressure of a liquid, solid, or solution which is exerted by a vapor when a state of equilibrium has been reached between the liquid, solid, or solution and its vapor.

venous p. The tension of the blood within the veins.

pres′sure cone. The bulging of the brain stem and neighboring cerebellum into the foramen magnum as a result of a sharp pressure gradient between intracranial and intraspinal pressures, as in brain edema.

pre·sta′sis [L. *prae*, before; G. *stasis*, a standing]. A term used by the pathologist Ricker to designate a greater degree of dilatation of the precapillary arterioles, capillaries, and postcapillary venules than in peristasis. The blood flow is still more slowed but is not at a standstill. It is also characterized by the passage of red blood cells through the capillary walls (diapedesis), resulting in hemorrhages in the surrounding tissues. There is a constriction of the artery above. Syn., *prestatic hyperemia.*

pre·su·bic′u·lum. The area of transition between hippocampus proper and the subiculum.

pre·sup′pu·ra″tive [*prae;* L. *suppurare*, to gather matter]. Pertaining to an early stage of inflammation, prior to suppuration.

pre·syl′vi·an fis′sure. The anterior branch of the Sylvian fissure.

pre·sys′to·le (pree·sis′to·lee) [*prae;* G. *systolē*, contraction]. The period of the heart's pause preceding the systole.

pre″sys·tol′ic [*prae; systolē*]. Preceding the systole of the heart, as the presystolic murmur, presystolic thrill; usually refers to the time immediately preceding the first heart sound.

pre″thy·rog′e·nous (pree″thigh·rodj′i·nus) [*prae;* G. *thyreos*, shield; *genesthai*, from *gignesthai*, to be produced]. Pertaining to an atypical variety of thyroid disease.

pre″thy·roid′e·an (pree″thigh·roy′dee·un) [*prae;* G. *thyreoeidēs*, shield-shaped]. In front of the thyroid cartilage.

pre″trans·fer′ence. *In psychoanalysis*, the arousal of feelings in a patient when he perceives the therapist as a primordial parent or as a part of himself.

pre·u″re·thri′tis [*prae;* G. *ourēthra*, urethra; *-itis*, inflammation]. Inflammation of the vestibule of the vagina, around the urethral orifice.

prev′a·lence [L. *praevalere*, to prevail]. The number of cases of a disease existing in a population at any given time.

pre·ven′tive med′i·cine. See under *medicine.*

pre·ven′tive med′i·cine com′pa·ny. *In military medicine*, a unit designed to control rodents and insect vectors and to supervise hygiene and sanitation in armies, divisions, and installations as deemed necessary by the surgeon. It consists of survey, control, and sanitation platoons varying in number.

pre·ven′tive med′i·cine of′fi·cer. *In military medicine*, a medical officer attached to a command to supervise the sanitary arrangements of the command and the measures taken to prevent the spread of disease; an assistant to the surgeon of the command: formerly called *medical inspector.*

pre″ven·to′ri·um [L. *praevenire*, to come before]. A sanatorium devoted to the care of children who are thought to be predisposed to tuberculosis because of positive tuberculin tests and poor home environment.

pre″ven·tric″u·lo′sis [L. *prae*, before; *ventriculum*, ventricle; G. *-ōsis*, condition]. Cardiospasm. *Rare.*

pre″ver·tig′i·nous (pree″vur·tidj′i·nus) [*prae;* L. *vertigo*, a whirling around]. Dizzy, with a tendency to fall prone.

pre·ves'i·cal (pree·vess'i·kul) [*prae;* L. *vesica*, bladder]. Situated in front of the urinary bladder.

pre'vi·a [L. *praevius*, going before]. Coming before, or in front of, as placenta previa.

pre·vil'lous [L. *prae*, before; *villus*, shaggy hair]. Before the formation of villi; applied to the chorionic vesicle.

Prévost, Jean Louis [*French physician*, 1790–1850]. The first to observe segmentation in the frog's egg (1827), marking a great step in the knowledge of embryology. Known to have used defibrinated blood in animal transfusions (1821).

Preyer, Wilhelm Thierry [*German physiologist*, 1841–97]. Author of a history of hypnotism (1881). Described involuntary movement of the ears in auditory stimulation; called *Preyer's reflex*. Devised a test for carbon monoxide in the blood. See Preyer's *test*.

pre'zone. See *prozone*.

pre·zo'nu·lar, pre·zon'u·lar [L. *prae*, before; *zonula*, little zone]. Pertaining to the posterior chamber of the eye.

pre″zy·ga·poph'y·sis (pree″zye·guh·pof'i·sis, pree″zig·uh·) [*prae;* G. *zygon*, yoke; *apophysis*, process]. An anterior or superior zygapophysis; a superior articular process of a vertebra.

pri'a·pism [G. *Priapos*, Priapus]. Persistent erection of the penis, usually unaccompanied by sexual desire.

Price-Jones, Cecil [*English hematologist*, 1863–1943]. Described a method for direct measurement of red blood cells, the recording being in the form of a graph of the distribution of the diameters of the red cells in a stained blood specimen (1910); called *Price-Jones' method* or *curve*.

prick'ly heat. See *miliaria*.

Priessnitz, Vincenz [*German farmer*, 1799–1851]. Strong advocate of hydrotherapy. Author of a treatise on the cold-water cure (ca. 1835). His cold-water compress is called *Priessnitz's bandage*.

Priestley, Joseph [*English clergyman and chemist*, 1733–1804]. Isolated oxygen (1774), which he called dephlogisticated air. Is often credited with the discovery of oxygen. See also *Lavoisier* and *Scheele*.

pri'ma·quine phos'phate. $C_{15}H_{21}N_3O.2H_3PO_4$; 8-(4-amino-1-methylbutylamino)-6-methoxyquinoline diphosphate; an orange-red crystalline powder, soluble in water: used therapeutically for treatment of malaria, being effective in all races. Its action is on the exoerythrocytic stage of the parasite.

pri'ma·ry [L. *primarius*, of the first rank]. First, immediate, as primary union, healing by first intention.

Pri'mates (pry'mates) [L. *primas*, principal, from *primus*, first]. The highest order of the vertebrate class Mammalia; includes man, apes, monkeys, and lemurs.

pri″me·ve'rin. $C_{20}H_{28}O_{13}$; 2-hydroxy-4-methoxymethyl benzoate-2-primeveroside; a glycoside occurring in several species of primrose (*Primula*). On enzymatic hydrolysis, it yields one molecule each of 2-hydroxy-4-methoxymethyl benzoate and primeverose.

pri″me·ve'rose. $C_{11}H_{20}O_{10}$; 6-(β-D-xylosido)-D-glucose; a disaccharide produced by enzymatic hydrolysis of primeverin, gaultherin, and certain other glycosides. Hydrolysis of it yields one molecule each of D-glucose and D-xylose.

pri″mi·grav'i·da [L. *primus*, first; *gravidus*, pregnant]. A woman who is pregnant for the first time.

pri·mip'a·ra (pry·mip'uh·ruh) [*primus;* L. *parere*, to bear]. A woman bearing, or giving birth to, her first child. —**primiparous,** *adj.*

pri″mi·par'i·ty. Condition of being a primipara.

pri·mi'ti·ae (pry·mish'ee·ee) [L., first things of their kind]. The part of the amniotic fluid discharged before the extrusion of the fetus at birth.

prim'i·tive [L. *primitivus*, primitive]. First-formed; original, as primitive groove.

pri·mor'di·al (pry·mor'dee·ul) [L. *primordius*, original]. Existing in the beginning; first-formed; primitive; original; of the simplest character.

pri·mor'di·um (pry·mor'dee·um) [*primordius*]. The earliest discernible indication of an organ or part, as **acousticofacial primordium,** the mass of neural crest tissue that differentiates into the ganglions of the seventh and eighth cranial nerves. Syn., *anlage*.

prim'rose [L. *primus*, first]. A plant of the genus *Primula*, some species of which cause contact dermatitis.

prin'ceps [L., chief]. First; original; main, as the nucleus princeps, the main sensory nucleus of the trigeminal nerve.

prin'ci·ple [L. *principium*, beginning]. 1. A constituent of a compound representing its essential or characteristic properties. 2. A rule or basis of action.

anterior pituitarylike p. See anterior pituitarylike *substance*.

antianemia p. See antianemia *factor*.

Bernoulli's p. The lateral pressure of a fluid passing through a tube of varying diameter is least at the most constricted part where velocity is greatest, and is most at the widest part where velocity is least.

displacement p. One applying to the examination of certain accessory nasal sinuses, where failure of the testing solution to enter the sinus is pathognomonic of disease.

Fick p. See Adolf *Fick*.

Gillespie's bicolor p. Colorimetric determination of pH without the use of standard buffer solutions.

isopathic p. The apparently paradoxical rule that a feeling of guilt can be relieved by an exhibition of the cause of the guilt, namely, hate. Formerly called *homeopathic p.*

melanophore-dilating p. See melanocyte-stimulating *hormone*.

phylogenetic p. The rehearsal in childhood of reminiscences of the prehistory of mankind.

pleasure p. The instinctive endeavor to escape from unpleasant situations; the desire to obtain the greatest possible gratification with the smallest possible effort.

posterior pituitary p. See posterior pituitary *substance*.

p. of Carnot and Clausius. Free energy always tends to diminish. The second law of thermodynamics is one of the forms of this principle.

p. of inertia. See repetition-compulsion *p.*

proximate p. The active constituent of a drug, as an alkaloid, glycoside, etc.

reality p. The modification of the pleasure principle brought about by the demands of reality or parental and social demands.

repetition-compulsion p. The instinct to repeat earlier experiences, irrespective of any advantage to be obtained.

Stewart p. A principle applied to the determination of total flow of blood by injection of a dye into an artery. $F = \frac{R}{V - A}$, where F = total flow through organ, R = constant rate of dye injection (mg./min.), V = concentration of dye in venous blood from organ, and A = concentration of dye in arterial blood by virtue of recirculation.

van't Hoff's p. of mobile equilibrium. Any change of the temperature of a system in equilibrium is followed by a reverse thermal change within the system.

Pringle, John James [*English dermatologist*, 1855–1922]. Described sebaceous adenoma (1890); also called *Pringle's disease*, *Pringle's type of adenoma*.

prin'ter·s ac'e·tate. See basic *aluminum* acetate.

priodax. Trade-mark for *iodoalphionic acid.*

Pri"o·nu'rus [G. *priōn*, saw; *oura*, tail]. A genus of scorpions; species of this genus inflict stings which are painful and very poisonous.

P. australis. A well-known species of tropical scorpions found in North Africa. An antivenin has been prepared from members of this species which is effective against the stings of all North African scorpions.

Prior, J. [*German physician*, nineteenth century]. With Finkler, isolated *Vibrio proteus*, also called *Finkler-Prior spirillum* or *vibrio.*

priscoline. Trade-mark for a phenyl-substituted alkyl imidazoline, phenylmethyl imidazoline, or benzylimidazoline. The substance exerts a dilator effect on minute arteries and arterioles.

pri·sil'i·dene hy"dro·chlo'ride. Generic name for the synthetic analgesic *dl*-alpha-1,3-dimethyl-4-phenyl-4-propionoxypiperidine hydrochloride: also called *alphaprodine hydrochloride.* See *nisentil hydrochloride.*

prism [G. *prisma*, anything sawn]. 1. A solid whose bases or ends are similar plane figures and whose sides are parallelograms. 2. *In optics*, a transparent solid with triangular ends and two converging sides. It breaks up white light into its component colors, and bends the rays of light toward the side opposite the angle (the base of the prism), and is used to measure or correct imbalance of the ocular muscles.

enamel p. One of the prismatic columns of from four to six sides composing the enamel of the teeth, closely packed together and generally vertical to the surface of the underlying dentin. Syn., *enamel rod.*

Nicol p. One prepared from two obliquely bisected parts of a rhombohedron of calcite; used for production and analysis of polarized light.

Risley's p. A pair of prisms of equal strength with the faces apposing, so that by rotation of one, the power is gradually increased from zero to the total of their values.

pris·mat'ic (priz·mat'ick) [*prisma*]. Prism-shaped; produced by the action of a prism, as prismatic colors.

pris'moid [*prisma;* G. *eidos*, form]. Resembling a prism.

pris"mop·tom'e·ter (priz"mop·tom'i·tur) [*prisma;* G. *optikos*, of sight; *metron*, a measure]. An instrument for estimating refractive defects of the eye by means of two prisms placed base to base.

pris'mo·sphere [*prisma;* G. *sphaira*, ball]. A combination of a prism and a globular lens.

priv'i·leged com·mu"ni·ca'tion. *In medical jurisprudence*, information furnished by a patient to a physician to assist the physician in diagnosis or therapy. According to universal medical ethics, such information may not be disclosed without consent of the patient. Not all courts of law recognize this privilege.

privine hydrochloride. Trade-mark for the vasoconstrictor substance *naphazoline hydrochloride.*

p. r. n. *Pro re nata;* according as circumstances may require.

pro- [G. and L.]. A prefix signifying *for, before, in front of.*

pro·ac·cel'er·in. The precursor of accelerin. Syn., *factor V, plasma accelerator globulin.*

pro·ac"ti·no·my'cin [G. *pro*, before; *aktis*, ray; *mykēs*, fungus]. An antibiotic substance derived from *Nocardia* (*Proactinomyces*) *gardneri;* active, in vitro, against a number of bacteria. Proactinomycin A, B, and C have been described.

pro"ag·glu'ti·noid [L. *pro*, in favor of, *agglutinare*, to glue; *eidos*, form]. An agglutinoid having a stronger affinity for the agglutinogen than is possessed by the agglutinin.

pro'al [G. *pro*, in front of]. Having a forward direction or movement. *Rare.*

pro·am'ni·on [*pro;* G. *amnion*, inner membrane around the fetus]. That part of the embryonic area at the sides and in front of the head of the developing embryo, which remains without mesoderm for a considerable period.

pro·at'las [*pro;* G. *atlas*, first of the neck vertebrae]. An accessory vertebral element occasionally present between the atlas and the occipital bone.

prob'a·ble er'ror. A value which is 0.67449 times the standard error of any statistical constant.

pro·band'. See *propositus.*

pro'bang. A rod of whalebone or other flexible material, used for making local applications to the esophagus or larynx or for removing foreign bodies.

ball p. A probang having an ivory bulb attached to one end.

bristle p. One having on the end a sheath of bristles or horsehair that can be made to spread like an umbrella as the instrument is drawn out. Also called *horsehair p.*

sponge p. One with a small sponge at one end.

pro·bar'bi·tal cal'ci·um. Generic name for calcium 5-ethyl-5-isopropyl barbiturate. See *ipral calcium.*

pro·bar'bi·tal so'di·um. Generic name for sodium 5-ethyl-5-isopropyl barbiturate. See *ipral sodium.*

probe [L. *probare*, to test]. 1. A slender, flexible rod, for exploring or dilating a natural channel, as the lacrimal duct, or for following a sinus or the course of a wound. 2. A stiff rod, usually pointed at one end, used for separating tissues in dissection. 3. The act of using a probe. —**probe,** *v.*

pro·ben'e·cid. Generic name for *p*-(di-*n*-propylsulfamyl)-benzoic acid, $(CH_3CH_2CH_2)_2N.SO_2.C_6H_4.COOH$, an agent that selectively and reversibly inhibits the transport mechanism responsible for tubular secretion of penicillin, para-aminosalicylic acid, para-aminohippuric acid, and phenol red. Premedication with probenecid results in increased blood levels of penicillin and para-aminosalicylic acid when these drugs are subsequently administered. It is also of therapeutic value in gout, presumably by blocking reabsorption of urate. See *benemid.*

pro'bit. In biological assay, equal to the normal equivalent deviation increased by five: used to make all normal equivalent deviation values positive.

pro·bos'cis (pro·bos'iss) [G., means of providing food]. The cylindrical projection from the face, above or below the orbit, with or without a cavity, which represents the nose in various grades of cyclopia and ethmocephalus.

pro'caine (pro'cane, pro'kay·een, ·in, pro·cane') 1. The base *p*-aminobenzoyl-diethylaminoethanol, from which certain salts, such as the hydrochloride, are prepared. See *procaine hydrochloride.* 2. A synonym for procaine hydrochloride.

pro'caine am'ide hy"dro·chlo'ride. *p*-Amino-N-(2-diethylaminoethyl)benzamide hydrochloride; $NH_2C_6H_4CONHCH_2CH_2N(C_2H_5)_2.HCl$; white to tan crystals, very soluble in water: useful in the treatment of ventricular arrhythmias and extrasystoles. Unlike procaine hydrochloride, it is only slightly hydrolyzed by plasma enzymes, hence has prolonged action. See *pronestyl hydrochloride.*

pro′caine hy″dro·chlo′ride (*procainae hydrochloridum*). $H_2N.C_6H_4.CO.O.CH_2.CH_2.N(C_2H_5)_2.HCl$; *p*-aminobenzoyl-diethylaminoethanol hydrochloride; occurs as small, white crystals, or as a white, crystalline powder; 1 Gm. dissolves in 1 cc. of water and in 30 cc. of alcohol. It is employed as a local anesthetic in solutions from 1% to 4%. Procaine exhibits no local vasoconstriction as does cocaine, and the anesthesia is more localized and increased in duration by the addition of solution of epinephrine hydrochloride in the proportion of 1:1000. It is also employed as a spinal anesthetic for relaxation of short duration, but is relatively ineffective when applied to intact mucous membranes. There are also available the following salts of the procaine base: procaine benzoate (*aminocaine*), procaine borate, procaine butyrate, and procaine nitrate. These salts resemble procaine hydrochloride in their action and uses. Syn., *procaine.* Also see *novocain.*

pro·cal′lus [L. *pro*, before; *callus*, hardened skin]. The organized blood clot which forms in an early stage of repair of a fractured bone.

pro·ce′lous (pro·see′lus) [G. *pro*, in front of; *koilos*, hollow]. Concave in front and convex behind.

pro″ce·phal′ic [*pro;* G. *kephalē*, head]. *In biology,* pertaining to the front of the head.

pro·cer′coid (pro·sur′koyd) [*pro;* G. *kerkos*, tail; *eidos*, form]. The first larval stage in the first intermediate host of some cestodes.

pro·ce′rus. A muscle of facial expression. See Table of Muscles in the Appendix.

proc′ess, pro′cess [L. *processus*, process]. 1. A course of action; a group of phenomena, as an inflammatory process. 2. A prominence or outgrowth, as the spinous process of a vertebra, the axis cylinder process of a nerve. 3. *In chemistry,* a method of procedure; reaction; test.

accessory p. A small tubercle situated at the back part of the base of the transverse process of one of the lower thoracic and lumbar vertebrae.

acromion p. Acromion.

alar p. One of a pair of processes arising from the lower part of the anterior border of the cribriform plate of the ethmoid, articulating with the frontal bone and completing the cecal foramen of the frontal bone.

alveolar p. The border of the maxilla or mandible in which the alveoli, or bony sockets of the teeth, are embedded.

ameloblastic p. The cytoplasmic projection of an enamel-forming cell beyond the level of the terminal bar apparatus. Syn., *Tomes's p.*

anterior clinoid p. A prominent process that juts backward from the medial extremity of the lesser wing of the sphenoid bone behind the optic foramen.

anterior p. of the malleus. A long, delicate process that passes from the neck of the malleus forward to the petrotympanic fissure, to which it is connected by the anterior ligament of the malleus. Formerly called *long process, processus gracilis.*

articular p. See inferior articular *p.* and superior articular *p.*

auditory p. The lateral border of the tympanic part of the temporal bone; the area of attachment of the cartilage of the auricle.

axis cylinder p. Axon of a nerve cell.

basilar p. A strong, quadrilateral plate of bone forming the anterior portion of the occipital bone, in front of the foramen magnum.

birth p. The act of giving birth to young. See Plate 42.

caudate p. (a) The elevated portion of the liver extending from the caudate lobe to the under surface of the right lobe. (b) The lower end of one of the divisions of the antihelix of the external ear.

ciliary p. Circularly arranged choroid foldings continuous with the iris in front.

clinoid p. See anterior clinoid *p.*, posterior clinoid *p.*, and middle clinoid *p.*

cochleariform p. The curved terminal portion of the bony semicanal for the tensor tympani muscle forming a pulley over which the tendon of the muscle plays.

conchal p. See descending *p.*

condyloid p. The posterior process on the upper border of the ramus of the lower jaw.

conoid p. See conoid *tubercle.*

coracoid p. A beak-shaped process of the scapula.

coronoid p. (a) A thin, flattened process projecting from the anterior portion of the upper border of the ramus of the mandible and serving for the insertion of the temporal muscle. (b) A triangular projection from the upper end of the ulna, forming the lower part of the semilunar notch.

costal p. An embryonic rib primordium, the ventrolateral outgrowth of the caudal, denser half of a sclerotome.

deep p. A tonguelike extension of the submandibular gland which passes around the posterior border of the mylohyoid muscle and then extends forward along with the submandibular duct.

descending p. A downward prolongation of the inferior border of the lacrimal bone which articulates with the lacrimal process of the inferior nasal concha, and assists in forming the canal for the nasolacrimal duct.

ensiform p. Old term for xiphoid process, the cartilaginous tip at the lower end of the sternum.

ethmoid p. One of the projections from the superior border of the inferior nasal concha.

excitation p. The process underlying the action current.

facial p. of the parotid. A triangular portion of the parotid gland which extends forward, overlapping the masseter muscle.

falciform p. A thin extension of the sacrotuberous ligament to the ramus of the ischium.

freezing-drying p. Sudden cooling of tissue to very low temperatures and dehydration of the frozen material in a vacuum. The advantages of this method over use of fixing and dehydrating solutions are minimal chemical changes in tissue, a minimum of shifting of diffusible components, and a greater preservation of cytoplasmic inclusions.

frontal p. A prismatic extension from the body of the maxilla, forming part of the medial margin of the orbit and of the lateral side of the nasal cavity.

frontonasal p. The anterior region of the embryonic head that later develops into the frontal, median nasal, and lateral nasal processes. Also called *nasofrontal p.*

frontosphenoidal p. The thick, serrated, superior angle of the zygomatic bone which articulates with the zygomatic process of the frontal bone and with the great wing of the sphenoid.

funicular p. The portion of the tunica vaginalis that surrounds the spermatic cord. See Plate 39.

globular p. The inferior, bilateral bulbous expansions of the median nasal process that fuse in the midline to form the philtrum of the upper lip and adjacent premaxilla. It is erroneously used as synonymous with median nasal process.

glossohyal p. A small vestigial process from the anterior surface of the hyoid bone, prominent in some mammals.

hamate p. See uncinate *p.* of the ethmoid bone.
hamular p. (a) A hooklike process of bone on the lower extremity of the medial pterygoid plate, around which the tendon of the tensor palati muscle bends. (b) The hooklike termination of the lacrimal crest.
head p. The notochord or notochordal plate formed as an axial outgrowth of the primitive node.
Hickman molecular distillation p. A commercially important process for the concentration of vitamin A from fish-liver oils by distillation under high vacuum with a short path between the surface of the oil and the condenser.
inferior articular p. One of a pair of processes projecting downward from a vertebral arch and articulating with a superior articular process of the vertebra next below.
inferior tegmental tympanic p. A narrow plate of bone which proceeds from the anterior margin of the anterior pyramidal surface of the temporal bone and forms part of the petrotympanic fissure.
infraorbital p. The anterior angle of the zygomatic bone, sharp and pointed, which articulates with the maxilla and occasionally forms the superior boundary of the infraorbital foramen.
infundibular p. The pars nervosa of the neurohypophysis.
intrajugular p. A curved process found in some skulls which projects from the floor of the jugular notch and partially or completely divides the jugular foramen.
jugular p. A rough process external to the condyle of the occipital bone.
lacrimal p. A short process of the inferior nasal concha that articulates with the descending process of the lacrimal bone.
lateral nasal p. The embryonic process or fold bounding the lateral margin of the olfactory pit that forms a side and wing of the nose.
lateral palatine p. See palatal *p.*
lateral p. of the malleus. A slight projection from the root of the manubrium of the malleus, lying in contact with the tympanic membrane. Formerly called *short p.*
lateral p. of the talus. A process passing downward and laterally from the lateral surface of the talus bone.
lenticular p. The extremity of the long process of the incus, covered with cartilage and articulating with the stapes.
long p. of the incus. A slender process that descends vertically from the body of the incus and articulates with the head of the stapes.
long p. of the malleus. See anterior *p.* of the malleus.
lyophile p. A method for drying in vacuo plasma or serums from the frozen state.
mammillary p. One of the tubercles on the posterior part of the superior articular processes of the lumbar vertebrae.
mandibular p. The chief part of the embryonic mandibular arch that forms the lower jaw.
marginal p. A prominence situated on the lateral margin of the frontosphenoidal process of the zygoma.
mastoid p. The protruding part of the temporal bone felt behind the ear. See Plates 1, 20.
maxillary palatal p. See maxillary *p.* of the palatine bone.
maxillary p. of the embryo. An embryonic outgrowth from the dorsal part of the mandibular arch that forms the lateral part of the upper lip, the upper cheek region, and the upper jaw except the premaxilla.
maxillary p. of the inferior nasal concha. A thin plate of bone descending from the ethmoid process of the inferior nasal concha, and hooking over the lower edge of the orifice of the antrum.
maxillary p. of the palatine bone. A variable projecting lamina of the anterior border of the palate bone which is directed forward and closes in the lower and back part of the opening of the maxillary sinus. Syn., *maxillary palatal p.*
maxillary p. of the zygomatic bone. A rough, triangular process from the anterior surface of the zygomatic bone which articulates with the maxilla.
medial angular p. of the frontal bone. The medial end of the supraorbital margin.
median nasal p. The entire region between the olfactory sacs and below the frontonasal sulcus of the embryo. It forms the bridge, mobile septum, and anterior portion of the cartilaginous septum of the nose, the philtrum of the lip, and the premaxillary portion of the upper jaw.
middle clinoid p. Usually a small tubercle situated behind the lateral end of the tuberculum sellae. In some skulls it is not present and in others it is large and joins with the anterior clinoid process.
muscular p. A stout process from the lateral angle of the base of the arytenoid cartilage into which are inserted the cricoarytenoid muscles.
nasal p. of the frontal bone. The downward projection of the nasal part of the frontal bone which terminates as the nasal spine.
nasal p. of the maxilla. The frontal process of the maxilla.
nasofrontal p. See frontonasal *p.*
notochordal p. See head *p.*
odontoblastic p. The cytoplasmic process of an odontoblast which lies in a dentinal tubule. Syn., *Tomes's fiber.*
odontoid p. The toothlike process of the axis which ascends and articulates with the atlas.
olecranon p. A bony eminence on the upper and back part of the ulna. In extension of the forearm it fits into the olecranon fossa of the humerus.
opercular p. A caudal outgrowth of the hyoid arch that helps obliterate the cervical sinus.
orbital p. of the palatine bone. A process directed upward and outward from the upper portion of the palatine bone.
orbital p. of the zygomatic bone. A thick plate projecting backward and medially from the orbital margin.
palatal p. (a) A ventromedial outgrowth of the embryonic maxillary process that develops into the definitive palate. Also called *palatine p., lateral palatine p.* (b) A thick process projecting horizontally mediad from the medial aspect of the maxilla, forming part of the floor of the nasal cavity and part of the roof of the mouth. Also called *palatine p. of the maxilla.*
papillary p. A short, rounded process extending inferiorly from the caudate lobe of the liver behind the portal fissure. In the fetus it is large and is in contact with the pancreas.
paramastoid p. In some skulls, a downward projection from the lateral part of the jugular process which may articulate with the transverse process of the atlas: also called *paraoccipital p.*
paraoccipital p. See paramastoid *p.*
petrosal p. A sharp process of the sphenoid bone located below the notch for the passage of the abducens nerve, which articulates with the apex of the petrous portion of the temporal bone and forms the medial boundary of the foramen lacerum.
phalangeal p. An outward prolongation of one

of the outer rods of the spiral organ, or organ of Corti.

plantar p. of the navicular bone. The most prominent point on the plantar surface of the navicular bone of the foot.

postauditory p. A pointed extension of the squamous temporal which forms the lateral wall of the tympanic antrum and helps form the posterior wall of the external auditory meatus.

posterior clinoid p. One of the two short bony extensions from the superior angles of the dorsum sellae which give attachment to the tentorium cerebelli.

posterior p. of the talus. A prominent tubercle on the posterior surface of the talus to which the posterior talofibular ligament is attached.

postglenoid p. A process of the temporal bone situated immediately in front of the petrotympanic fissure, separating the mandibular fossa from the external auditory meatus.

progressive processes. Those which continue after the requirements of the organisms have been satisfied.

protoplasmic p. Any slender extension of cytoplasm from the body of a cell.

pterygoid p. of the sphenoid bone. One descending perpendicularly from the point of junction of the body with the greater wing of the sphenoid bone, and consisting of a lateral and a medial plate.

pterygospinous p. A spine from the posterior portion of the lateral pterygoid plate which gives attachment to the pterygospinous ligament.

pyramidal p. A tuberosity projecting backward and laterally from the junction of the horizontal and vertical parts of the palatine bone, fitting into a notch between the inferior extremities of the pterygoid plates and articulating anteriorly with the tuberosity of the maxilla. Syn., *tuberosity of the palatine bone.*

random p. See stochastic *p.*

retromandibular p. The medial, narrow portion of the parotid gland filling the fossa behind the mandible.

short p. of the incus. A conical process projecting almost horizontally backward from the body of the incus and attached by ligamentous fibers to the margin of the opening leading into the tympanic antrum.

short p. of the malleus. See lateral *p.* of the malleus.

sphenoidal p. A thin plate of bone directed upward and inward from the vertical plate of the palatine bone.

sphenoidal p. of the septal cartilage. The posterior extension, variable in size, of the septal cartilage between the vomer and perpendicular plate of the ethmoid.

sphenoidal turbinated p. A small, curved plate of bone which forms the anterior wall of each sphenoidal air sinus: also called *sphenoidal concha.*

sphenomaxillary p. An inconstant downward prolongation of the greater wing of the sphenoid.

spinous processes of the ilium. The spines of the ilium, anterior and posterior superior, and anterior and posterior inferior.

spinous p. of a vertebra. The prominent backward projection from the middle of the posterior portion of the arch of a vertebra.

stochastic p. *In statistics,* random process, covering practically all the theory of probability from coin-tossing to harmonic analysis: used mostly when a time parameter is introduced.

styloid p. of the fibula. See *apex* of the head of the fibula.

styloid p. of the radius. A projection from lateral border of lower extremity of the radius.

styloid p. of the temporal bone. A sharp spine about an inch in length, descending downward, forward, and inward from the inferior surface of the petrous portion of the temporal bone. See Plates 1, 20.

styloid p. of the third metacarpal. A projection from the lateral side of the base of the third metacarpal.

styloid p. of the ulna. A projection from the inner and posterior portion of the lower extremity of the ulna.

sulcate p. An inconstant process of the palatine bone connecting the orbital process with the sphenoidal process.

superior articular p. One of a pair of processes projecting upward from the side of the vertebral arch and articulating with an inferior articulating process of the vertebra above.

supracondylar p. A small projection, found in rare instances, about two inches above the medial epicondyle of the humerus, with which it connects by a fibrous band, and under which the median nerve and brachial vessels may pass.

temporal p. The posterior angle of the zygomatic bone by which it articulates with the zygomatic process of the temporal bone.

Tome's p. See ameloblastic *p.*, odontoblastic *p.*

transverse p. A process projecting outward from the side of a vertebra, at the junction of the pedicle and the lamina.

trochlear p. A variable process on the lateral surface of the calcaneus which separates the tendons of the peroneus longus and the peroneus brevis muscles.

tubal p. An occasional spur of bone projecting backward from the middle portion of the posterior border of the medial pterygoid plate.

unciform p. The hamulus of the hamate bone.

uncinate p. of the ethmoid bone. A hooklike projection from the inferior portion of either labyrinth; it articulates with the ethmoidal process of the inferior turbinate bone.

uncinate p. of the pancreas. An extension from the head of the pancreas to the left behind the superior mesenteric vessels.

vaginal p. of the peritoneum. A tube of peritoneum which evaginates through the inguinal canal into the scrotum (or labium majus) during embryonic life. In the male the distal portion persists as the tunica vaginalis testis. In the female a portion occasionally persists, forming the canal of Nuck.

vaginal p. of the sphenoid bone. A projection from the inferior surface of the body of the sphenoid bone, running horizontally inward from near the base of the medial pterygoid plate.

vaginal p. of the temporal bone. A sheathlike plate of bone extending backward from carotid canal to mastoid process; it separates behind into two laminas enclosing the styloid process.

vermiform p. A tubular diverticulum of the cecum. Also called *vermiform appendix.*

vertebral p. One of the processes projecting from a vertebra—e.g., transverse process, superior articular process, inferior articular process.

vocal p. The anterior process of the arytenoid cartilage.

xiphoid p. The elongated process projecting caudad from the lower end of the sternum between the cartilages of the seventh ribs. It usually becomes osseous after the age of 50.

zygomatic p. of the frontal bone. A strong, prominent lateral projection from the supraorbital margin of the frontal bone which articulates with the zygomatic bone.

zygomatic p. of the maxilla. A rough, triangular, serrated eminence which articulates with the maxillary process of the zygomatic bone.

zygomatic p. of the temporal bone. A long projection from the lower part of the squamous portion of the temporal bone, articulating with the zygomatic bone.

pro·ces″so·ma′ni·a [*processus;* G. *mania,* madness]. A mania for litigation.

pro·ces′sus [L.]. A process.

p. gracilis. See anterior *process* of the malleus.

pro·chei′li·a. A condition in which a lip is farther forward than is normal. Cf. *retrocheilia.*

pro·chei′lon (pro·kigh′lon) [G. *pro,* in front of; *cheilos,* lip]. The prominence in the middle of the upper lip.

procholon. Trade-mark for dehydrocholic acid, an oxidation product of cholic acid derived from natural bile acids.

pro·chon′dral (pro·kon′drul) [G. *pro,* before; *chondros,* cartilage]. Prior to the formation of cartilage.

pro·chor′dal (pro·kor′dul) [G. *pro,* in front of; *chordē,* string]. Situated in front of the notochord.

pro″cho·re′sis (pro″kor·ee′sis) [G., a going forth]. The propulsion of food through the gastrointestinal tract. *Obs.*

Prochownick's method. See under *artificial respiration.*

pro·chro′ma·tin [G. *pro,* before; *chrōma,* color]. Paranuclein, the substance composing the nucleolus of a cell.

proc″i·den′ti·a (pross″i·den′shuh, ·shee·uh, pro″-si·) [L., a falling forward]. The falling or sinking down of a part. Prolapse, prolapsus.

pro″con′dy·lism. Forward deviation of the mandibular condyles.

pro″con·ver′tin. A precursor in normal blood of convertin or SPCA.

pro″con·ver′tin-con·ver′tin. See *convertin.*

pro′cre·ate [L. *procreare,* to beget]. Beget.

pro″cre·a′tion [L. *procreatio,* from *procreare*]. The act of begetting offspring. —**pro′creative,** *adj.*

proc·ta′gra (prock·tay′gruh, prock′tuh·gruh, prock·tag′ruh) [G. *prōktos,* anus; *agra,* a hunting]. Sudden pain in the anal region.

proc·tal′gi·a [*prōktos;* G. *algos,* pain]. Neuralgic pain in the anus or rectum.

p. fugax. Acute severe pain of coccyx and anorectal regions.

proc″ta·tre′si·a (prock″ta·tree′zhuh, ·zee·uh, ·shuh, ·see·uh) [*prōktos;* G. *atrētos,* not perforated]. An imperforate condition of the anus or rectum.

proc″tec·ta′si·a (prock″teck·tay′zhuh, ·zee·uh, ·shuh, ·see·uh), **proc·tec′ta·sis** [*prōktos;* G. *ektasis,* extension]. Dilatation of the anus or rectum.

proc·tec′to·my [*prōktos;* G. *ektomē,* excision]. Excision of the anus and rectum, usually through the perineal route.

proc·ten′cli·sis (prock·teng′kli·sis, prock″ten·kly′-sis) [*prōktos;* G. *egklisis,* displacement]. Stricture of the rectum or anus.

proc″teu·ryn′ter (prock″tew·rin′tur) [*prōktos;* G. *eurynein,* to make wide]. An instrument for dilating the anus or rectum.

proc·ti′tis [*prōktos;* G. *-itis,* inflammation]. Inflammation of the anus or rectum.

circumscribed hypertrophic p. A well-demarkated annular lesion of the rectal mucosa confined to the region of the sphincteric ring, characteristically exhibiting thick folds and deep sulci and causing severe pain with bleeding on defecation.

gonorrheal p. A self-limited inflammatory disease of the rectum due to gonococcal infection, producing severe rectal burning and itching and usually subsiding within one month, regardless of treatment. It is seen in epidemics among infants with gonorrheal vaginitis, in adult females having venereal disease, and more rarely in male sexual perverts.

proc′to-, proct- [*prōktos*]. A combining form meaning *anus;* used to denote *the rectum.*

proc′to·cele [*prōktos;* G. *kēlē,* hernia]. The extroversion or prolapse of the mucous coat of the rectum.

vaginal p. A hernia of the rectum appearing in the vagina.

proc·toc′ly·sis [*prōktos;* G. *klysis,* a drenching]. The infusion of fluids by rectal tube.

proc″to·co·li′tis [*prōktos;* G. *kolon,* colon; *-itis,* inflammation]. Inflammation of the rectum and colon.

proc″to·co″lon·os′co·py [*prōktos; kolon;* G. *skopein,* to examine]. Inspection of the interior of the rectum and lower colon.

proc″to·col′po·plas″ty [*prōktos;* G. *kolpos,* vagina; *plassein,* to form]. Closure of a rectovaginal fistula.

proc″to·cys′to·plas″ty [*prōktos;* G. *kystis,* bladder; *plassein*]. A plastic operation on the rectum and the urinary bladder for repair of rectovesical fistula. *Obs.*

proc″to·de′um [*prōktos;* G. *hodaios,* on the way]. A pitlike, ectodermal depression formed by the growth of the anal hillocks surrounding the anal part of the cloacal membrane. Upon rupture of the latter, it forms part of the anal canal. Also called *anal pit, primitive anus.*

proc″to·dyn′i·a [*prōktos;* G. *odynē,* pain]. Pain about the anus or in the rectum.

proc·tol′o·gist [*prōktos;* G. *logos,* word]. One versed in diseases of the anus and rectum.

proc·tol′o·gy [*prōktos; logos*]. The science of the anatomy, functions, and diseases of the rectum and anus. —**proctolog′ic,** *adj.*

proc″to·pa·ral′y·sis [*prōktos;* G. *paralysis,* paralysis]. Paralysis of the external anal sphincter muscle.

proc′to·pex″y [*prōktos;* G. *pēxis,* a fixing]. The fixation of the rectum by anchoring it into the hollow of the sacrum by means of sutures passing externally across the sacrum. Also called *rectopexy.*

proc″to·pho′bi·a [*prōktos;* G. *phobos,* fear]. A morbid dread or apprehension of pain, common in persons with diseases of the rectum.

proc′to·plas″ty [*prōktos;* G. *plassein,* to form]. Plastic surgery of the anus.

proc″to·ple′gi·a. Proctoparalysis.

proc″top·to′si·a (prock″top·to′shuh, ·see·uh, ·zhuh, ·zee·uh) [*prōktos;* G. *ptōsis,* a falling]. Anal prolapse. *Obs.*

proc·tor′rha·phy [*prōktos;* G. *rhaphē,* suture]. The plaiting of the enlarged and prolapsed rectal walls by suture, to reduce the circumference.

proc″tor·rhe′a [*prōktos;* G. *rhoia,* flow]. Escape of mucus through the anus.

proc′to·scope [*prōktos;* G. *skopein,* to examine]. An instrument for inspecting the anal canal and rectum.

proc·tos′co·py [*prōktos; skopein*]. Ocular inspection of the anal canal and rectum with the aid of special instruments.

proc″to·sig″moid·ec′to·my [*prōktos;* G. *sigmoeidēs,* crescent-shaped; *ektomē,* excision]. The abdominoperineal excision of the anus and rectosigmoid, with the formation of an abdominal colostomy.

proc″to·sig″moid·i′tis. Inflammation of the rectum and sigmoid colon.

proc″to·sig″moid·os′co·py. See *sigmoidoscopy.*

proc′to·spasm [*prōktos;* G. *spasmos,* spasm]. Spasm or tenesmus of the rectum.

proc·tos′ta·sis [*prōktos;* G. *stasis,* a standing].

Constipation due to nonresponse of the rectum to the defecation stimulus.

proc″to·ste·no′sis. Stricture of the anus or rectum.

proc·tos′to·my [*prōktos;* G. *stoma*, mouth]. The establishment of a permanent artificial opening into the rectum.

proc·tot′o·my. Incision into the rectum or anus, especially for stricture or imperforate anus: described as external if the incision is below the external sphincter, and internal if above it.

pro·cum′bent [L. *procumbens*, leaning forward]. 1. Prone; lying face down. 2. *In dentistry*, said of a tooth whose long axis approaches horizontality. —**procum′bency,** *n.*

pro·cur′sive [L. *procurrere*, to rush forward]. Running forward, as procursive epilepsy, a form in which the patient runs during the epileptic attack.

pro″cur·va′tion [L. *procurvus*, curved forward]. Forward inclination of the body.

pro·cu′tin. A substance capable of specifically increasing the capacity of an excitant to produce a reaction in the sensitive skin, or of increasing the capacity of the skin to react to an excitant.

pro·dig′i·o′sin (pro·didj″ee·o′sin). $C_{20}H_{25}N_3O$; an antibiotic substance derived from *Serratia marcescens* (*Bacillus prodigiosus, Chromobacterium prodigiosum*), inactive against ten representative species of bacteria but bacteriostatic against *B. subtilis, C. diphtheriae*, and *S. aureus*.

prod′ro·mal, pro·dro′mal [G. *prodromos*, running before]. Relating to early manifestations or symptoms; premonitory.

pro′drome (pl. *prodromata*) [*prodromos*]. An early manifestation of impending disease, before the specific symptoms begin. —**prod′romal, prod′romous, prodrom′ic,** *adj.*

prod′uct [L. *productum*, from *producere*, to produce]. 1. Effect; result; that which is produced. 2. *In chemistry*, the compound formed by a reaction.

addition p. A compound resulting from the direct union of two substances.

solubility p. The product of the concentrations of the ions of a substance in a saturated solution of the substance, each concentration term being raised to the power equal to the number of ions represented in a molecule of the substance. Also called *precipitation value.*

split-product. A decomposition product, as of a hydrolytic reaction.

pro·duc′tive [*producere*]. Forming or capable of forming new tissue.

pro″en·ceph′a·lus [G. *pro*, in front of; *egkephalos*, brain]. Partial acrania in the frontal region with encephalocele or hydrencephalocele.

pro·en′zyme. The substance in a living cell from which an enzyme is formed.

pro″e·ryth′ro·blast [*pro;* G. *erythros*, red; *blastos*, germ]. A basophilic erythroblast, the youngest and largest cell of the erythrocyte precursors. Nucleoli are present. In normal bone marrow these cells are rare. In some classifications, the proerythroblast is synonymous with the megaloblast. Also called *lymphoid hemoblast, macroblast, macronormoblast, promegaloblast, pronormoblast, rubriblast.*

pro·e·ryth′ro·cyte. See *reticulocyte.*

Proescher's oil-red-pyridine. See under *stain.*

pro·es′tro·gen. A substance, in itself weakly estrogenic, which is converted to a more active estrogen in the body.

pro·es′trus [*pro;* G. *oistros*, gadfly]. A phase of the estrous cycle in mammals preceding heat; characterized by growth of the endometrium and follicular development in the ovary.

Proetz, Arthur Walter [*American otolaryngologist*, 1888–]. Known for his employment of a special method of treating infections of the paranasal sinuses by filling them with fluid using negative pressure; called *Proetz's treatment, displacement method.*

pro·fen′a·mine hy″dro·chlo′ride. International Pharmacopoeia name for 10-(2-diethylamino-1-propyl)phenothiazine hydrochloride or N(2-diethylamino-1′-propyl)dibenzoparathiazine; $C_{19}H_{24}N_2S.HCl$; a white, crystalline powder, slightly soluble in cold water: used in the treatment of parkinsonism. Syn., *ethopropazine hydrochloride, phenopropazine hydrochloride.* See *lysivane hydrochloride, parsidol hydrochloride.*

pro·fer′ment. See *proenzyme.*

pro·fes′sion·al [L. *professio*, profession]. 1. Pertaining to a profession; in keeping with ethics. 2. Produced by the practice of a profession, as professional neuritis (writers' cramp, etc.).

pro·fes′sion·al serv′ice u′nit. A mobile unit of the U.S. Army Medical Service composed of professional teams and necessary service elements.

Proficher, Georges Charles [*French physician*, 1873–]. Described a group of symptoms associated with deposits of subcutaneous calcareous nodules, especially in the periarticular tissues, associated with a tendency to atrophy, and atrophic and nervous symptoms; called *Proficher's disease* or *syndrome.*

pro·fla′vine (pro·flay′veen, ·vin). $C_{13}H_{11}N_3$. 2,8-Diaminoacridine. Its salts are used for their antiseptic effect in the treatment of wounds, urethritis, gingivitis, gonorrheal conjunctivitis, and other conditions requiring the use of a germicide.

p. dihydrochloride. $C_{13}H_{11}N_3.2HCl.2H_2O$. Orange-red to brown-red crystals. 1 Gm. dissolves in about 10 cc. of water.

p. sulfate. $C_{13}H_{11}N_3.H_2SO_4.H_2O$. A reddish brown, crystalline powder; 1 Gm. dissolves in about 300 cc. of water.

pro·flu′vi·um [L., a flowing forth]. A flux or discharge.

p. alvi. Diarrhea.

p. lactis. Excessive flow of milk.

pro·fun′da [fem. of L. *profundus*, deep]. Deep-seated; a term applied to certain arteries and veins.

pro·fun′dus [L., deep]. Deep-seated; applied to certain muscles and nerves.

pro·gas′ter. See *archenteron.*

pro·gen′er·ate [L. *pro*, before; de*generare*, to depart from its race or kind]. One endowed with superior faculties; a genius.

pro·gen′e·sis [G. *pro*, before; *genesis*, production]. The development and fate of the germ cells before fertilization or blastogenesis.

pro·gen′i·tor [L.]. An ancestor.

prog′e·ny (prodj′i·nee) [L. *progenies*, offspring]. Offspring; descendants.

pro·ge′ri·a [G. *progērōs*, prematurely old]. Premature senility; a morbid state showing symptoms both of infantilism and senility. Also called *Hutchinson-Gilford disease.*

p. of adults. A familial and hereditary multiple tissue nevus characterized by stunting of growth. It involves the skin, producing tautness and thinning, and premature baldness. Other involvements include bilateral juvenile cataracts, pluriendocrine dysfunction, osteoporosis, and calcification in muscles, ligaments, and arteries, especially of the lower extremities. Also called *Werner's syndrome.*

p. of children. A nonfamilial disorder, appearing several months after birth, characterized by cessation of growth, senilelike changes, large skull, birdlike features, atrophic skin, and usually severe mental defects.

pro″ges·ta′tion·al. Old term for progravid.

pro·ges′ter·one (pro·jes′tur·ohn). $C_{21}H_{30}O_2$. A diketone having the composition of pregnene-3-20-dione. Like other sex hormones, it is a steroid. It is the hormone found in the corpus luteum; occurs as a white, crystalline powder. The hormone occurs in two crystalline forms of identical physiologic potency; both forms are insoluble in water, but soluble in alcohol, most organic solvents, and vegetable oils. The value of progesterone as a remedial agent is not well established. It has been used in recurrent abortions and in threatened abortion. It is also used in various disturbances of menstruation. Progesterone is effective only after parenteral administration. It is available, in oil solution, under various trade-marked names, including *lutesterone, lutocylin, progestin, progestone,* and *proluton.* See Table of Hormones in the Appendix.

progestin. Trade-mark for a brand of progesterone.

progestone. Trade-mark for a brand of progesterone.

progestoral. Trade-mark for anhydrohydroxyprogesterone or ethisterone.

pro·glot′tid [G. *pro,* before; *glōtta,* tongue]. A segment of a tapeworm.

pro·glot′tis. Proglottid.

pro·gnath′ic [*pro;* G. *gnathos,* jaw]. *In craniometry,* designating a condition of the upper jaw in which it projects anteriorly with respect to the profile of the facial skeleton, when the skull is oriented on the Frankfort horizontal plane; having a gnathic index of 103.0 or more.

prog′na·thism [*pro; gnathos*]. The condition of having projecting jaws. **—prognath′ic, prog′nathous,** *adj.*

alveosubnasal p. The projection of the subnasal portion of the maxillary alveolus beyond the line of the facial profile.

prog·nose′ (prog·noce′, ·noze′) [G. *prognōsis,* foreknowledge]. Forecast the course and outcome of a particular case of a disease, illness, or injury. *Rare.*

prog·no′sis [G.]. A prediction of the duration, course, and termination of a disease, based on all information available in the individual case and knowledge of how the disease behaves generally. **—prognos′tic,** *adj.*

prog·nos′ti·cate [*prognōsis*]. Give a prognosis.

prog″nos·ti′cian (prog″nos·tish′un) [G. *prognōstikos,* foreknowing]. One who is versed in prognosis.

pro″gon·o′ma [G. *pro,* before; *gonos,* seed; *-ōma,* tumor]. A nodular or tumorlike mass due to embryonal displacement, resulting in structures resembling those of primitive forms of the species, as exemplified in hairy moles.

pro·gran′u·lo·cyte″. See *promyelocyte, myelocyte.*

pro·grav′id [*pro;* L. *gravidus,* pregnant]. Referring to the lutein phase or second growth phase of the endometrium; the glands become tortuous and irregularly sacculated, and the secretion contains glycogen. In pregnancy the progravid changes progress for six to eight weeks; in the nonpregnant uterus for about ten days. Syn., *progestational.*

pro·gres′sion [L. *progressio,* a going forward]. The act of advancing or moving forward.

backward p. A backward walking, a rare symptom of certain nervous lesions, such as Parkinsonism.

crosslegged p. Walking with the legs almost crossing, a condition sometimes observed in bilateral hip disease and in cerebral spastic palsy.

pro·gres′sive [*progressio*]. Gradually extending.

progynon B. Trade-mark for alpha-estradiol benzoate in oil for intramuscular injection.

progynon DH. Trade-mark for estradiol in tablets, solution, ointment, suppositories, and nasal spray.

progynon DP. Trade-mark for estradiol dipropionate in oil for intramuscular injection.

pro″in·va′sin I. An enzyme which accompanies and protects the hyaluronidase of pathogenic bacteria and snake venoms. It acts by destroying antinvasin I, an enzyme in blood plasma which is capable of destroying hyaluronidase, and thereby interferes with this defense mechanism of the host against the action of hyaluronidase.

pro″i·o·sys′to·le (pro″ee·o·sis′to·lee) [G. *prōïos,* early in the day; *systolē,* contraction]. Premature heart beat. *Rare.*

pro″i·o′ti·a (pro″ee·o′shee·uh), **pro″i·o′tes** (pro″ee·o′teez) [*prōïos*]. Sexual precocity.

pro·jec′tion [L. *projectio,* a throwing forward]. 1. The act of throwing forward. 2. A part extending beyond its surroundings. 3. The referring of impressions made on the organs of sense to the position of the object producing them. 4. *In psychopathology,* a mental dynamism whereby a person overcomes his feeling of inadequacy or guilt by transferring to other persons or to objects the responsibility for such inadequacy. The most prominent mental mechanism in paranoia.

pro·kar′y·o·cyte. See *erythroblast.*

pro·ki′nase (pro·kigh′nace, ·naze, pro·kin′ace, ·aze). A proteolytic enzyme found in extracts of the pancreas and demonstrated to pass into the pancreatic secretion.

proklot. Trade-mark for a brand of menadione.

pro·la′bi·um [L. *pro,* in front of; *labium,* lip]. 1. Exposed part of the lip. 2. Central prominence of the lip.

pro·lac′tin. The adenohypophyseal hormone which stimulates lactation in the mammalian breast: also called *galactin, mammary-stimulating hormone, mammogenic hormone, mammogen, mammotropin, luteotropin.* Syn., *lactogenic hormone.*

pro·lam′ine (pro·lam′een, ·in, pro′luh·meen, ·min). Gliadin. A vegetable protein, soluble in 80% alcohol, insoluble in water, absolute alcohol, or neutral solvents. See American Classification of Proteins in the Appendix.

pro′lan-A. A follicle-stimulating hormone: old term.

pro′lan-B. A luteinizing hormone which has been isolated from swine and sheep pituitaries.

pro·lapse′ [L. *prolapsus,* a falling]. The falling or sinking down of a part.

frank p. Complete displacement downward of the uterus and inversion of the vagina, with both structures hanging outside the vulva.

internal p. Intussusception of the upper portion of the rectum and the rectosigmoid into the lower rectum; a concealed prolapse of the rectum.

mucosal p. *In proctology,* protrusion of the mucous membrane of the rectum into the anal canal.

p. of the cord. Premature expulsion of the umbilical cord during parturition.

p. of the iris. Protrusion of the iris through a corneal wound.

p. of the uterus. Displacement of the uterus downward, sometimes outside the vulva. Syn., *descensus* or *prolapsus uteri.*

pro·lap′sus [L.]. Prolapse.

p. ani. Extrusion of the lower division of the intestinal tract through the external sphincter of the anus.

p. uteri. Prolapse of the uterus.

pro·lep′sis [G., anticipation]. In a periodic disease, the return of an attack or paroxysm before the expected time or at progressively shorter intervals. **—proleptic,** *adj.*

pro·leu′ko·cyte (pro·lew′ko·sight). Leukoblast.

pro·lif′er·ate [L. *proles,* offspring; *ferre,* to bear].

Multiply; generate by increase in number. —**proliferative, proliferous,** *adj.*

pro·lif″er·a′tion [*proles; ferre*]. Multiplying, as by cellular division.

pro·lif′ic [*proles*]. Fruitful.

pro·lig′er·ous (pro·lidj′ur·us) [*proles;* L. *gerere,* to bear]. Germinating; producing offspring.

pro′lin·ase. The enzyme which hydrolyzes proline peptides to proline and simpler peptides.

pro′line (pro′leen, ·lin). $C_5H_9O_2N$. Alpha- or 2-pyrrolidine carboxylic acid, an amino acid resulting from the hydrolysis of proteins.

pro·li′pase. Inactive form of steapsin found in pancreatic juice.

proluton. Trade-mark for a brand of progesterone.

pro′lyl. The univalent radical,

$$\overline{HN.CH_2.CH_2.CH_2.CHCO}—,$$

of the amino acid proline.

pro·lym′pho·cyte [G. *pro,* before; L. *lympha,* water; G. *kytos,* cell]. A cell of the lymphocyte series intermediate in maturity between the lymphoblast and the lymphocyte. A peroxidase negative cell of the size of a large lymphocyte but with a larger nucleus, whose chromatin structure is finer than that of the large lymphocyte but coarser than that of the lymphoblast. It is rarely seen in normal adult blood but frequently in the blood of children and in blood in various infectious states.

promacetin. Trade-mark for sodium 4,4′-diaminodiphenylsulfone-2-N-acetylsulfonamide; $C_{14}H_{14}N_3NaO_5S_2$: used in treatment of leprosy.

promanide. Trade-mark for disodium *p,p′*-sulfonyldianiline-N,N′-diglucoside disulfonate; $C_{22}H_{34}N_2Na_2O_{18}S_2$; a drug used in the treatment of leprosy and accessible surface tuberculous lesions. See *promin.*

pro·meg″a·kar′y·o·cyte″ [*pro;* G. *megas,* large; *karyon,* kernel; *kytos*]. The precursor of a megakaryocyte. It is smaller than the megakaryocyte; the nucleus becomes indented; cytoplasm is lightly basophilic, and contains fine granules. Also called *lymphoid megakaryocyte.*

pro·meg′a·lo·blast″. See *proerythroblast.* Also see *megaloblast.*

pro·meg″a·lo·kar′y·o·cyte″. See *promegakaryocyte.*

pro″mes·o·bil″i·fus′cin. A colorless precursor of mesobilifuscin, apparently identical with mesobilileukan.

pro·meth′a·zine hy″dro·chlo′ride. $C_{17}H_{20}N_2S.HCl$; N-(2′-dimethylamino-2′-methyl)ethylphenothiazine hydrochloride; a white to faint-yellow powder, very soluble in water; an antihistaminic substance. See *phenergan hydrochloride.*

pro″me·thes′trol di·pro′pi·o·nate. Generic name for 3,4-bis(*m*-methyl-*p*-propionoxyphenyl)hexane, or dimethylhexestrol dipropionate, a synthetic estrogen. See *meprane dipropionate.*

pro·me′thi·um. Pm. The name adopted for element 61, which has been called also *cyclonium, florentium,* and *illinium.*

promin. Trade-mark for disodium *p,p′*-sulfonyldianiline-N,N′-diglucoside disulfonate; $C_{22}H_{34}N_2Na_2O_{18}S_2$; a drug used in the treatment of leprosy and accessible surface tuberculous lesions. See *promanide.*

prominal. Trade-mark for *mephobarbital.*

prom′i·nence [L. *prominentia,* a jutting out]. 1. A projection, especially on a bone. 2. The state of projecting or standing out.

genital p. An accumulation of cells on the ventral aspect of the embryonic cloaca, from which the generative organs are developed.

laryngeal p. The tubercle of the thyroid cartilage: often called *Adam's apple.*

prom′i·zole. Trade-mark for 2,4′-diamino-5-thiazolylphenyl sulfone. This compound is a sulfone, as distinguished from other sulfanilamide congeners, which are sulfonamides: used in the treatment of tuberculosis and leprosy, in the latter disease proving especially promising.

prom·ne′si·a (prom·nee′zhuh). See *paramnesia.*

pro·mon′o·cyte, pre·mon′o·cyte [G. *pro,* L. *prae,* before; G. *monos,* single; *kytos,* cell]. 1. An immature monocyte derived from a monoblast. The nucleus is spheroidal or moderately indented, and a nucleolus may be visible. Also called *young monocyte, premonocyte.* 2. One of the transitional stages between the lymphocyte and monocyte.

prom′on·to·ry [L. *promontorium,* promontory]. A projecting prominence.

double p. An anomaly in which the body of the first sacral vertebra is displaced farther forward than those below it, so that its lower margin projects beyond the general surface.

false p. See double *p.*

p. of the middle ear. The outward protrusion on the inner wall of the middle ear formed by the basal turn of the cochlea.

p. of the sacrum. The prominence formed by the angle between the upper extremity of the sacrum and the last lumbar vertebra.

pro·my′e·lo·cyte [G. *pro,* before; *myelos,* marrow; *kytos,* cell]. The earliest myelocyte stage derived from the myeloblast; it contains a few granules, some of which may be nonspecific and azurophilic, while others may be characteristic of the type of granulocyte into which the myelocyte develops. In early forms the nucleus may be covered by the nonspecific granules and still contain small nucleoli. Also called *premyelocyte, progranulocyte A.* Syn., *myelocyte A* and *B, progranulocyte.*

pro′nate [L. *pronare,* to bend forward]. 1. Turn the forearm so that the palm of the hand is down or toward the back. 2. In the foot, to turn the sole outward with the lateral margin of the foot elevated; to evert: the preferable term.

pro·na′tion [*pronare*]. 1. The condition of being prone; the act of placing in the prone position. 2. The turning of the palm of the hand downward.

pro·na′tor [*pronare*]. That which pronates, as pronator teres and pronator quadratus, muscles of the forearm attached to the ulna and radius. See Table of Muscles in the Appendix.

p. radii teres. The pronator teres muscle: old term.

prone [L. *pronus,* leaning forward]. Lying with the face downward; the opposite of *supine.*

prone pres′sure meth′od. See Schafer method under *artificial respiration.*

pro·neph′ros (pl. *pronephroi*) [G. *pro,* before; *nephros,* kidney]. The primitive or head kidney, derived from the cranial part of the nephrogenic cord. Vestigial in mammalian embryos, its duct, the pronephric duct, is taken over by the mesonephros and called the mesonephric or Wolffian duct. —**pronephric,** *adj.*

pronestyl hydrochloride. A trade-marked name for *procaine amide hydrochloride.*

prong [ME. *prange*]. The root of a tooth.

pro′no·grade [L. *pronus,* leaning forward; *gradi,* to walk]. Walking or standing on all fours, as the quadrupeds.

pro·nor′mo·blast [G. *pro,* before; L. *norma,* rule; G. *blastos,* germ]. A young normoblast. Also see *proerythroblast.*

pro·nor′mo·cyte. See *reticulocyte.*

pron′to·sil. $(NH_2)_2.C_6H_3.N{:}N.C_6H_4.SO_2.NH_2$.2,4-Diaminoazobenzene-4′-sulfonamide. A reddish crystalline powder; soluble in water. This drug was the forerunner of the sulfanilamide group of drugs.

p. album. See *sulfanilamide.*

p. soluble. See *neoprontosil.*

prontylin. Trade-mark for a brand of sulfanilamide.

pro·nu'cle·us [G. *pro,* before; L. *nucleus,* kernel]. One of the two nuclear bodies of a newly fertilized ovum, the male pronucleus and the female pronucleus, the fusion of which results in the formation of the germinal (cleavage) nucleus.

proof gal'lon. A gallon of proof spirit.

proof spir'it. A mixture of ethyl alcohol and water containing 50% by volume of C_2H_5OH.

pro·o'tic (pro·o'tick, ·ot'ick) [G. *pro,* in front of; *ous,* ear]. In front of the ear.

pro"o·va'ri·um. See *epoophoron.*

pro"pa·di'ene. The gaseous hydrocarbon CH_2:C:CH_2. Syn., *allene.*

propadrine hydrochloride. Trade-mark for the sympathomimetic amine *phenylpropanolamine hydrochloride.*

pro"pae·deu'tics (pro"pi·dew'ticks) [G. *pro,* before; *paideutikos,* of teaching]. Preliminary instruction. —**propaedeutic,** *adj.*

prop'a·gate [L. *propagare,* to generate]. Produce offspring. —**propaga'tion,** *n.*

pro·pal'i·nal [G. *pro,* in front of; *palin,* backward]. *In biology,* pertaining to the forward and backward action of the jaws of some animals.

prop"al·lyl'o·nal. Generic title for 5-isopropyl-5-β-bromallyl barbituric acid. See *nostal.*

pro·pam'i·dine (pro·pam'i·deen, ·din). *p,p'*-(Trimethylenedioxy)dibenzamidine. NH:C(NH_2).C_6H_4.O.$(CH_2)_3$O.C_6H_4C(NH_2):NH. A diamidine derivative used as a surgical antiseptic.

p. isethionate. $C_{21}H_{32}N_4O_{10}S_2$; the isethionate salt of propamidine, occurring as hygroscopic crystals or granular powder, soluble in water: used in treatment of early stages of African trypanosomiasis and of leishmaniasis.

pro'pan·al. Propionaldehyde.

pro'pane. The gaseous hydrocarbon $CH_3CH_2CH_3$, occurring in natural gas and in solution in crude petroleum.

1,2-pro"pane·di'ol. Propylene glycol.

pro"pa·no'ic ac'id. Propionic acid.

pro'pa·none. Acetone.

pro'pene. Propylene.

pro"pent·dy'o·pent. Either of the two colorless compounds, each containing two pyrrole rings, obtained when heme, bilirubin, or any other pigment containing four pyrrole rings is oxidized with hydrogen peroxide in alkaline solution. On reduction with sodium dithionite, a propentdyopent is converted to a red pigment known by the generic name *pentdyopent.*

pro'pe·nyl, prop'e·nyl. 1. The monovalent radical CH_3.CH:CH—, derived from propylene. 2. The trivalent glyceryl radical —CH_2.CH.CH_2—.

p. ethyl ether. CH_3CH:CH.O.C_2H_5; an inhalation anesthetic which produces irritation of the upper respiratory tract.

pro·pep'sin. The zymogen of pepsin, found in the cells of the gastric glands.

pro·pep'tone. Hemialbumose. See *peptone.*

pro"pep·to·nu'ri·a [G. *pro,* before; *peptos,* cooked; *ouron,* urine]. The presence of propeptone in the urine.

pro·per'din [*pro;* L. *perdere,* to destroy; *-in,* protein]. A euglobulin of molecular weight greater than 1,000,000, found in the serum of higher animals, including man, which appears to be a nonspecific antibodylike substance, distinct from classical specific antibody. It destroys certain bacteria and viruses, lyses certain red blood cells, and requires magnesium ion and serum factors resembling complement for its action. Highly purified from human and bovine serum, it represents less than 0.03% of total serum protein.

pro"per·i·to·ne'al [G. *pro,* in front of; *peritonaion,* membrane which contains the lower viscera]. Situated in front of the peritoneum.

pro'phase (pro'fayz) [G. *pro,* before; *phasis,* phase]. The first stage of mitosis, in which the chromosomes are organized from nuclear materials as elongate spiremes.

pro"phen·pyr·id'a·mine, pro"phen·pyr"i·dam'ine. 1-Phenyl-1-(2-pyridyl)-3-dimethylaminopropane, an antihistaminic substance. Syn., *pheniramine.* See *trimeton.*

pro"phy·lac'tic [G. *prophylaktikos,* prophylactic]. Pertaining to prophylaxis.

pro"phy·lac'tic. A remedy or agent that prevents the development of disease.

p. kit. An individual tube or packet containing chemicals, for use in the prevention of venereal disease.

pro"phy·lax'is [G. *prophylax,* advanced guard]. 1. Prevention of disease; measures preventing the development or spread of disease. 2. *In military medicine,* measures taken to prevent or reduce the harmful effects of chemical agents.

Credé p. A 0.1% solution of silver nitrate for the prevention of ophthalmia neonatorum.

dental p. The prevention of dental and oral diseases by preventive measures, especially the mechanical cleansing of the teeth.

pro"pi·on·al'de·hyde. CH_3CH_2CHO; methylacetaldehyde; a liquid with a suffocating odor, soluble in water: used in synthesis of various compounds and as an attractant for the codling moth. Syn., *propanal, propyl aldehyde.*

pro'pi·o·nate. A salt of propionic acid.

Pro"pi·on"i·bac·te'ri·um (pro"pee·on"i·back·teer'ee·um, pro"pee·o"ni·) [G. *prōtos,* first; *piōn,* fat; *baktērion,* little staff]. A genus of bacteria of the family Lactobacteriaceae, which ferment hexases to predominantly propionic and acetic acids.

pro"pi·on'ic ac'id (pro"pee·on'ic, ·o'nick). CH_3.CH_2.COOH. A liquid acid of pungent odor; in the form of its calcium and sodium salts, it is used as a fungicide. Syn., *propanoic acid.*

pro"pi·on'o- (pro"pee·on'o-, ·o'no-), **propion-** [*prōtos; piōn*]. *In chemistry,* a combining form signifying *propionic.*

pro·plas'ma·cyte (pro·plaz'muh·sight) [G. *pro,* before; *plasma,* anything formed; *kytos,* cell]. 1. The precursor of the plasmacyte (plasma cell), usually larger than the adult cell, with a nucleus which has a finer chromatin structure and which is not necessarily eccentrically placed: frequently seen in multiple myeloma. Also called *lymphoblastic* or *myeloblastic plasma cell.* 2. Türk's irritation cell.

pro·pos'i·tus [L.]. The individual or index case, who is the starting point of a family pedigree or genealogical chart. Syn., *proband.*

proposote. Trade-mark for *creosote phenylpropionate.*

pro·pri'e·tar"y [L. *proprietarius,* owner]. Any chemical, drug, or similar preparation used in the treatment of diseases, if such an article is protected against free competition as to name, product, composition, or process of manufacture, by secrecy, patent, copyright, or any other means.

pro·pri'e·tar·y. Of or pertaining to a proprietary or a propriator; protected by copyright or patent; made, marketed, or operated by a person or persons having the exclusive right to do so, as a proprietary medicine, a proprietary school.

pro″pri·o·cep′tion [L. *proprius*, one's own; *perceptio*, perception]. Appreciation of position, balance, and changes in equilibrium on the part of the muscular system, especially during locomotion.

pro″pri·o·cep′tive im′pul·ses. Afferent nerve impulses originating in receptors in muscles, tendons, joints, and vestibular apparatus of internal ear. Their reflex functions are concerned with locomotion and maintenance of posture.

pro″pri·o·cep′tor [*proprius; perceptum*, from *percipere*, to perceive]. A receptor located in a muscle, tendon, joint, or vestibular apparatus, whose reflex function is locomotor or postural.

pro′pri·us [L.]. Individual; special, as extensor indicis proprius muscle, the special extensor of the index finger.

prop·tom′e·ter [G. *proptōsis*, a fall forward; *metron*, a measure]. An instrument for measuring the amount of exophthalmos.

prop·to′sis (prop·to′sis, pro·to′sis) [G., a fall forward]. 1. A falling downward. 2. Prolapse. 3. Exophthalmos.

pro·pul′sion [L. *propulsus*, a driving forth]. 1. Act of pushing or driving forward. 2. A falling forward in walking, as observed in paralysis agitans.

pro′pyl. The univalent radical $CH_3CH_2CH_2$, derived from propane.

pro′pyl ac′e·tate. $CH_3.COO.C_3H_7$; a colorless liquid, having an odor of pears, sparingly soluble in water, miscible with alcohol: used in formulation of perfumes and flavors and as a solvent.

pro″pyl·a·ce′tic ac′id. The normal valeric acid.

pro′pyl al′co·hol. $C_3H_7.OH$; *n*-propyl alcohol; a colorless liquid synthetically produced, miscible with water, alcohol, and ether. Syn., *ethyl carbinol, propylic alcohol.*

pro′pyl al′de·hyde. Propionaldehyde.

pro″pyl·a·mine′. $C_3H_7NH_2$; 1-aminopropane; a colorless, alkaline liquid with a strong odor of ammonia, miscible with water: used as an antispasmodic, antirheumatic, etc.

pro′pyl a·mi″no·ben′zo·ate. $H_2N.C_6H_4.CO.OC_3H_7$; a white, crystalline powder, slightly soluble in water, freely soluble in alcohol: used, like ethyl aminobenzoate, as a local anesthetic.

pro′pyl bu′ty·rate. $C_3H_7.CO_2.C_3H_7$; a colorless liquid, slightly soluble in water, miscible with alcohol and ether.

pro′pyl·ene, prop′yl·ene. 1. C_3H_6; the unsaturated hydrocarbon, $CH_3CH{:}CH_2$, a homolog of ethylene and isomer of cyclopropane; a colorless gas. 2. The monovalent radical, $CH_2CH{:}CH—$. 3. The bivalent radical, $—CH(CH_3)CH_2—$.

pro′pyl·ene di·chlo′ride. $CH_3.CHCl.CH_2Cl$; 1,2-dichloropropane; a flammable, mobile liquid with an odor of chloroform, slightly soluble in water, miscible with organic solvents: used as an oil and fat solvent and in dry cleaning.

pro′pyl·ene gly′col. $CH_3CHOHCH_2OH$; 1,2-dihydroxypropane; occurs as a colorless, practically odorless, viscous liquid; completely miscible with water and many organic solvents. Used as a solvent for many medicinals. Syn., *1,2-propanediol.*

pro″pyl·hex′e·drine. Generic name for the volatile sympathomimetic amine sold under the trademark *benzedrex.*

pro″pyl·par′a·ben (*propylparabenum*). $C_6H_4.OH.COOC_3H_7$. Propyl parahydroxybenzoate, a white powder, soluble in about 2000 parts of water; a bacteriostatic to preserve medicinal preparations.

pro′pyl pro′pi·o·nate. $CH_3.CH_2.COO.C_3H_7$; a colorless liquid, slightly soluble in water, miscible with most organic liquids: used as a solvent.

pro″pyl·thi″o·u′ra·cil. The 6-*n*-propyl derivative of thiouracil, used like the latter as an antithyroid drug, but more effective and less toxic in therapeutic doses.

pro′pyne. Allylene.

pro re na′ta [L.]. According to the circumstances of the case. Abbreviated, p. r. n.

pro·ren′nin. The zymogen of rennin or chymosin.

pro·ru′bri·cyte [G. *pro*, before; L. *ruber*, red; G. *kytos*, cell]. A cell in the formative stages of red blood cells, in which the chromatin is clumped and a nucleolus is present. See *erythroblast, proerythroblast.*

pro·se′cre·tin. The precursor of secretin; it is secreted by the epithelium of the small intestine.

pro·sect′ [L. *prosecare*, to cut away]. Dissect a subject or part for purposes of anatomic teaching or demonstration.

pro·sec′tor [L., from *prosecare*]. One who prepares subjects for anatomic dissection or to illustrate didactic lectures.

pros″en·ceph′a·lon [G. *pros*, toward; *egkephalos*, brain]. The forebrain or anterior brain vesicle of the embryo that subdivides into telencephalon and diencephalon. From it are derived the cerebral hemispheres, olfactory lobes, corpus striatum, and various parts of the thalamus, as well as the third and the lateral ventricles.

pro·sep′ta·zine (pro·sep′tuh·zeen, ·zin). $C_6H_5CH_2.NH.C_6H_4.SO_2.NH_2$. Benzyl sulfanilamide; occurs as a white powder, slightly soluble in water. Used in streptococcic and gonococcic infections. Also called *chemodyn, septazine.*

pro·se′ro·zyme. See *prothrombin.*

Proskauer, Bernhard [*German bacteriologist*, 1851–1915]. Described a qualitative test for the presence of acetylmethylcarbinol or, more correctly, for diacetyl. Used to differentiate the *Bacillus aerogenes* from the colon bacillus, the first forming acetylmethylcarbinol while the colon bacillus does not; called *Proskauer* or *Voges-Proskauer reaction.*

Proske and Watson's test. See under *test.*

pros′o·coele, pros′o·cele. The cavity of the prosencephalon.

pros″o·dem′ic [G. *prosō*, onward; *dēmos*, people]. Pertaining to disease spread by individual contact, as opposed to one spread by general means such as the water or milk supply.

pros′op-, pros′o·po- [G. *prosōpon*, face]. A combining form meaning *face.*

pros″op·ag·no′si·a (*of Wolpert*). Simultagnosia characterized by inability to recognize a human face though its separate details are perceived.

pro·sop′a·gus. See *prosopopagus.*

pros″o·pal′gi·a [G. *prosōpon*, face; *algos*, pain]. Neuralgic pain in the distribution of the trigeminal nerve. Also called *facial neuralgia, tic douloureux.* —**prosopalgic,** *adj.*

pro·sop′ic [*prosōpon*]. 1. *In craniometry*, designating a facial skeleton that is convex or projects anteriorly in the midline; having an orbitonasal index of 110.0 or more. 2. *In somatometry*, designating a face that is convex or projects anteriorly in the midline; having an orbitonasal index of 113.0 or more.

pros″o·po″a·nos′chi·sis (pross″o·po″a·noss′ki·sis) [*prosōpon;* G. *anō*, upward; *schisis*, cleavage]. Oblique facial cleft, or frontomaxillary fissure.

pros″o·po″di·ple′gi·a (pross″o·po″dye·plee′jee·uh, pross″o·pod″i·) [*prosōpon;* G. *dis*, twice; *plēgē*, stroke]. Bilateral facial paralysis.

pros″o·po·dyn′i·a [*prosōpon;* G. *odynē*, pain]. Facial pain, or neuralgia.

pros″o·po″neu·ral′gi·a. See *prosopalgia.*

pros″o·pop′a·gus [*prosōpon;* G. *pagos*, that which is fixed]. Unequal conjoined twins in which the parasitic twin, or parts of one, is attached to the face elsewhere than in the region of the jaws.

pros″o·po·ple′gi·a [*prosōpon;* G. *plēgē,* stroke]. Facial palsy; it may be unilateral (monoplegia facialis) or bilateral (diplegia facialis). —**prosopopleg′ic,** *adj.*

pros″o·pos′chi·sis (pross″o·poss′ki·sis) [*prosōpon;* G. *schisis,* cleavage]. Congenital facial cleft, from mouth to orbit (oblique facial cleft), or from the mouth to just in front of the auditory meatus (transverse facial cleft).

pros′o·po·spasm [*prosōpon;* G. *spasmos,* spasm]. Risus sardonicus.

pros″o·po·ster″no·did′y·mus. See *prosopothoracopagus.*

pros″o·po·ster″no·dym′i·a [*prosōpon;* G. *sternon,* chest; di*dymos,* twin]. The condition exhibited by a prosopothoracopagus.

pros″o·po·thor″a·cop′a·gus [*prosōpon;* G. *thōrax,* thorax; *pagos,* that which is fixed]. Conjoined twins united by the upper abdomen, chest, and face. Syn., *hemipagus.*

pros″o·po·to′ci·a [*prosōpon;* G. *tokos,* childbirth]. Face presentation in parturition. *Obs.*

pros′o·pus va′rus [L.]. Congenital hemiatrophy of the face and cranium, resulting in marked facial obliquity.

pros′tate [G. *prostatēs,* one who stands before]. The organ surrounding the neck of the urinary bladder and beginning of the urethra in the male (prostatic urethra). It consists of two lateral lobes and a middle lobe, and is composed of muscular and glandular tissue; a distinct capsule surrounds it. It often becomes enlarged in advanced life, and may then interfere with the emptying of the urinary bladder. See Plate 44. —**prostat′ic,** *adj.*

pros″ta·tec′to·my [*prostatēs;* G. *ektomē,* excision]. Excision of part or all of the prostate. It includes transurethral prostate resection of the median lobe or lateral lobes by electrocoagulation, by the use of various punches and resectoscopes (punch operation).

perineal p. The removal of the prostate by a U-shaped or V-shaped incision in the perineum, using a special prostatic retractor or a modification.

retropubic p. Removal of the prostate by an approach through the prevesical space.

suprapubic p. Removal of prostate by incision into urinary bladder through abdominal (suprapubic) route in a one- or two-stage operation.

transurethral p. Removal of the prostate by means of an operating cystoscope.

pros′ta·tism [*prostatēs*]. The condition caused by chronic disorders of the prostate, especially chronic, nonmalignant prostatic enlargement.

pros′ta·tism sans pros′tate. A term for the obstructive phenomena that occur without prostatic enlargement. They are due to fibrotic and degenerative processes of the median bar (bar of the bladder). *Rare.*

pros″ta·ti′tis [*prostatēs;* G. *-itis,* inflammation]. Inflammation of the prostate gland. —**prostatit′ic,** *adj.*

gonococcic p. That due to gonococcal infection.

pros″ta·to·cys·ti′tis [*prostatēs;* G. *kystis,* bladder; *-itis*]. Inflammation of the prostate and urinary bladder.

pros·tat′o·gram [*prostatēs;* G. *gramma,* letter]. A radiograph of the prostate gland, made after injecting a radiopaque substance into the orifices of the tubuloalveolar units through the urethral route.

pros″ta·tog′ra·phy [*prostatēs;* G. *graphein,* to write]. Radiography of the prostate gland after injecting a radiopaque substance into the orifices of the tubuloalveolar units through the urethral route.

pros·tat′o·lith [*prostatēs;* G. *lithos,* stone]. A prostatic calculus.

pros″ta·to·li·thot′o·my (pross″tuh·to·li·thot′o-mee, pro·stat″o·) [*prostatēs; lithos;* G. *tomē,* a cutting]. Removal of a stone or calculus from the prostate gland.

pros″ta·tor·rhe′a [*prostatēs;* G. *rhoia,* flow]. A thin urethral discharge coming from the prostate gland.

pros″ta·tot′o·my [*prostatēs;* G. *tomē,* a cutting]. Incision into the prostate gland.

pros″ta·to·ve·sic″u·li′tis [*prostatēs;* L. *vesicula,* vesicle; G. *-itis,* inflammation]. Inflammation of the seminal vesicles combined with prostatitis.

pro·ster′num. A cartilage bone ventral to the manubrium and attached to the clavicles of some amphibians and primitive mammals. In man, it is occasionally represented by an anomalous pair of suprasternal bones.

pros′the·sis (pl. *prostheses*) [G., addition]. 1. Replacement or substitution. 2. An artificial substitute for a missing part, as denture, hand, leg, eye. —**prosthet′ic,** *adj.*

dental p. An appliance to replace missing teeth, as a denture, crown, or bridgework.

maxillofacial p. A substitute for a jaw, nose, or cheek, when the loss is too extensive for surgical repair alone.

temporary p. An artificial limb used early following amputation and in preparation for the permanent apparatus.

pros·thet′ic group. 1. The group formed by a substance that is combined with a simple protein to form a complex protein, as the chromophoric group in chromoproteins. 2. The group formed by an organic radical not derived from an amino acid, that enters into the complex molecule of a conjugated protein. 3. The nonprotein component, or coenzyme, of certain enzyme systems.

pros·thet′ics [G. *prosthetikos,* adding]. The branch of surgery which deals with prostheses.

pros′the·tist [G. *prosthesis,* addition]. One who makes artificial limbs, artificial dentures, or external organs or parts.

pros′thi·on [G. *prosthios,* foremost]. That point on the alveolar border of the upper jaw which projects farthest anteriorly in the midsagittal plane, between the middle incisor teeth.

pros″tho·don′ti·a. That branch of dentistry which deals with the restoration of teeth by artificial means.

pros″tho·don′tics. See prosthetic *dentistry.*

pros″tho·don′tist [G. *prosthesis,* addition; *odous,* tooth]. A dentist who specializes in prosthetic dentistry.

prostigmine. Trade-mark for neostigmine, **prostigmine bromide** and **prostigmine methylsulfate** being available commercially.

pros″ti·tu′tion [L. *prostitutio,* from *prostituere,* to expose publicly]. The condition or act of using the body for sexual intercourse for a monetary consideration.

pros′trate [L. *prostratum,* from *prosternere,* to throw to the ground]. Lying at full length.

pros′trate. To reduce to exhaustion.

pros′trat·ed (pross′tray·tid) [*prostratum*]. Exhausted; stricken down.

pros·tra′tion [*prostratum*]. 1. The condition of being prostrate. 2. Extreme exhaustion.

heat p. Exhaustion due to exposure to excessive heat, as from the sun or from heated rooms.

nervous p. Old term for neurasthenia.

pro″tac·tin′i·um [G. *pro,* before; *aktis,* ray]. Pa = 231. A radioactive element occurring in pitchblende and yielding actinium on disintegration. Atomic number, 91.

pro·tal′bu·mose. See *albumose.*

pro′ta·mine (pro′tuh·meen, ·min, pro·tam′een, ·in). 1. One of a group of simple proteins occurring in the sex cells of fishes, as salmine, sturine. See American Classification of Proteins in the Appendix. 2. An amine isolated from spermatozoa and fish spawn; $C_{16}H_{32}O_2N_9$.

p. insulin. A combination of insulin hydrochloride and protamine from the trout, exerting a more prolonged action than insulin alone.

p. sulfate. A water-soluble salt of protamine which combines with heparin to counteract the anticoagulant effect of the latter but has anticoagulant action of its own; intravenously administered it is used in treatment of heparin overdosage.

pro·ta·nom′a·ly. See partial *protanopia.*

pro″tan·o′pi·a [G. *prōtos*, first; *a-*, not; *ōps*, eye]. Defective red vision; green-sightedness. See *dichromatism.* —**protanop′ic,** *adj.*

partial p. Decreased ability to perceive red. Syn., *protanomaly.*

pro·tar′gin (pro·tahr′jin). See mild *silver* protein and strong *silver* protein.

protargol. Trade-mark for a strong silver protein.

pro′te·an (pro′tee·un, pro·tee′un) [G. *Prōteus*, sea god who assumed different shapes when seized]. Taking on many shapes, as a protean disease, protean eruption.

pro′te·an. One of a group of derived proteins, insoluble products due to the action of water or enzymes. See American Classification of Proteins in the Appendix.

pro′te·ase (pro′tee·ace, ·aze). An enzyme which digests proteins.

pro·tec′tive [L. *protectum*, from *protegere*, to cover over]. Affording defense or immunity.

pro·tec′tive. 1. A covering or shield which protects. 2. A specific dressing, as oiled silk or rubber, used to prevent ingress of water.

pro·te′ic [G. *prōteios*, of first rank]. Relating to protein.

pro′te·id [*prōteios*]. Obsolete term for protein.

pro·te′i·form [G. *Prōteus;* L. *forma*, form]. Having various forms.

pro′te·in (pro′tee·in, pro′teen) [G. *prōteios*, of first rank]. One of a group of complex nitrogenous substances of high molecular weight which are found in various forms in animals and plants and are characteristic of living matter. On hydrolysis they yield amino acids. For proteins listed by name, see American Classification of Proteins in the Appendix. Also see Table of Normal Values of Blood Constitutents in the Appendix.

adequate proteins. Those proteins which furnish the body with all nitrogenous compounds necessary for maintenance and growth.

autologous p. A protein found normally in the human body.

bacterial p. A toxic protein formed by bacterial action.

bearer p. See *apoenzyme.*

Bence Jones p. A mixture of proteins in the urine, occurring most frequently in association with multiple myeloma, but occasionally with leukemia, lymphosarcoma, and Hodgkin's disease. Composed of a group of proteins which, when present in urine, have the characteristic property of being precipitated out of solution when warmed to 58° C., of redissolving at a much higher temperature, and reprecipitating on cooling.

coagulated proteins. A class of protein derivatives produced by heating solutions of various proteins. Coagulation of protein is believed to involve a preliminary denaturation which is followed by precipitation.

complete proteins. Adequate proteins.

conjugated p. A protein combined with a nonprotein group, other than a salt of a simple protein.

C-reactive p. An abnormal protein appearing in serum in the presence of any systemic inflammatory disease. Increases during active rheumatic fever are considered of value in establishing differential diagnosis.

defensive p. One of the proteins existing in the blood and rendering the system immune to infectious diseases.

denatured p. A protein whose structure and properties have been altered, mainly by the action of physical agents.

derived p. A synthetic protein, a polypeptide, or any product obtained from proteins by the action of acids, alkalies, enzymes, or heat.

foreign p. A protein which differs from the proteins of the animal or person into whom it is introduced.

globular p. One of the supposed closed cyclic molecules of certain types in which an imaginary polyhedron surface holds a definite number of hexagonal configurations.

Hektoen, Kretschmer, and Welker p. A nonblood protein occasionally excreted by the kidneys. It is distinct from other proteins in its precipitin reactions, its behavior with heat and in crystalline form.

immune p. An antitoxin.

iron-porphyrin p. One of a large group of proteins which contain iron and porphyrin; these include hemoglobin, the cytochromes, cytochrome oxidase, catalase, peroxidase, etc.

native p. A protein in its original state; a protein which has not been altered in composition or properties.

plasma proteins. The proteins present in blood plasma consisting of fibrinogen, albumins, and globulins.

p. hydrolysate. An artificial digest of protein derived by acid, enzymatic, or other hydrolysis of casein, lactalbumin, fibrin, or other suitable proteins that supply the approximate nutritive equivalent of the source protein in the form of its constituent amino acids. They are required to have more than half of the total nitrogen present in the form of alpha amino nitrogen. See *amigen, aminonat, aminosol, hyprotigen, parenamine, protolysate.*

serum proteins. The proteins present in the serum from clotted blood, differing from plasma proteins only in the absence of fibrinogen. See Table of Normal Values of Blood Constituents in the Appendix.

silver p. See *protein silver.*

simple p. One of a group of proteins which, upon hydrolysis, yield exclusively amino acids; included are globulins, glutelins, histones, prolamines, and protamines.

specific p. One possessing capabilities of acting as an allergen.

tissue p. That part of the body protein present in the solid tissues as distinguished from the circulating protein of the blood.

pro′te·in·ase (pro′tee·in·ace, ·aze). One of the subgroups of proteases or proteolytic enzymes which act directly on the native proteins in the first step of their conversion to simpler substances. See Table of Enzymes in the Appendix.

pro″te·in·e′mi·a (pro″tee·in·ee′mee·uh). 1. Protein in the blood. 2. Sometimes, hyperproteinemia.

pro″te·in″o·chro′mo·gen. Obsolete term for tryptophan.

pro″te·in·o′sis [*prōteios*]. The accumulation of protein in the tissues.

lipid p. A rare skin condition with a hereditary tendency which is the result of a disturbed fat metabolism. Yellow-colored plaques are seen about the joints and a fibrous sclerosing process occurs about face and mouth, and may involve the larynx. Also called *lipoidosis cutis et mucosae.*

pro′te·in sil′ver. Any combination of silver and protein. Also called *silver protein.* See mild *silver* protein, strong *silver* protein.

pro″te·in·u′ri·a [*prōteios;* G. *ouron*, urine]. The presence of protein in the urine.

proteolac. Trade-mark for a solution of peptones and proteoses obtained from defatted milk and used in nonspecific protein therapy.

pro″te·ol′y·sis [*prōteios;* G. *lysis*, a loosing]. The enzymatic or hydrolytic conversion of proteins into simpler substances. —**proteolyt′ic,** *adj.*

pro″te·o·me·tab′o·lism [*prōteios;* G. *metabolē*, change]. The processes of digestion, absorption, and utilization of proteins. —**proteometabol′ic,** *adj.*

pro″te·o·pep′tic [*prōteios;* G. *peptos*, cooked]. Pertaining to protein digestion.

pro′te·ose [*prōteios*]. One of a group of derived proteins intermediate between food proteins and peptones. Soluble in water, not coagulable by heat, but precipitated by saturation with ammonium or zinc sulfate. See American Classification of Proteins in the Appendix.

pro″te·o·su′ri·a [*prōteios;* G. *ouron*, urine]. The presence of proteoses in the urine.

Prot″er·og′ly·pha [G. *proteros*, earlier; *glyphein*, to carve]. One of the two principal groups of venomous snakes; includes the Elapidae (cobras and allies) and Hydrophiidae (sea snakes).

pro″te·u′ri·a. See *proteinuria.*

Pro′teus [G., sea god who assumed different shapes when seized]. A genus of the tribe Proteae belonging to the family Enterobacteriaceae. Species of this genus, **Pr. hydrophilus, Pr. mirabilis,** and **Pr. vulgaris,** have been associated with a variety of pathologic conditions, such as pleuritis, peritonitis, cystitis, and suppurative abscesses. *Pr. vulgaris* was formerly called *Bacillus proteus.* The species **Pr. morganii** has been isolated in cases of summer diarrhea of infants.

prothricin. Trade-mark for an isotonic buffered solution of tyrothricin and propadrine used in the symptomatic treatment of nasal congestion.

pro·throm′base. See *prothrombin.*

pro·throm′bin [G. *pro*, before; *thrombos*, clot]. The protein precursor in plasma of thrombin: also called *prothrombase, thrombinogen;* formerly called *proserozyme, serozyme, thrombogen.* See *thromboplastin.* —**prothrom′bic,** *adj.*

fraction A p. That portion of prothrombin which disappears when citrated or oxalated plasma or blood stands in contact with air.

fraction B p. That portion of prothrombin which disappears in the animal body where there is vitamin-K deficiency.

p. time. (a) Time which elapses from the addition of thromboplastin and calcium to decalcified plasma until the appearance of a clot. Widely used is the one-stage method devised by Armand J. Quick. Prothrombin time is influenced by many variables besides the concentration of prothrombin. (b) The clotting time of a mixture of calcium and decalcified plasma. *Obs.*

pro·throm″bi·ne′mi·a [*pro; thrombos;* G. *haima*, blood]. An excess of prothrombin in the blood plasma.

pro·throm″bi·no·pe′ni·a [*pro; thrombos;* G. *penia*, want]. Decrease in the prothrombin content of the blood. Syn., *hypoprothrombinemia.*

pro·throm″bo·ki′nase. The inactive precursor form of thrombokinase. Its activation may be autocatalytic, with calcium ions serving as an accessory factor.

pro·thy′mi·a [G. *prothymos*, eager]. Intellectual alertness.

pro′tides [G. *prōteios*, of first rank]. Old term for simple proteins.

pro·ti′o·dide. A salt containing the least amount of iodine of the iodides of the same base.

Pro·tis′ta [G. *prōtistos*, very first]. A group of organisms which includes the unicellular plants and animals.

pro″tis·tol′o·gist [*prōtistos;* G. *logos*, word]. A specialist in the study of the unicellular plants and animals.

pro″tis·tol′o·gy [*prōtistos; logos*]. The study of unicellular plants and animals.

pro′ti·um. The predominant constituent of ordinary hydrogen; the atom consists of one proton and one electron and therefore has an atomic weight of approximately one. Symbol, H^1. Sometimes called *light hydrogen.*

pro′to-, prot- [G. *prōtos*, first]. 1. A combining form meaning *first.* 2. *In chemistry,* a combining form meaning *the lowest of a series of compounds of the same elements.*

pro″to·al′bu·mose. See *albumose.*

pro″to·a·nem′o·nin. $C_5H_4O_2$; 5-methylene-2-oxodihydrofuran; an antibacterial substance derived from *Anemone pulsatilla;* a yellow, vesicant oil which polymerizes rapidly. In vitro it is active against a number of bacterial species.

pro″to·bi·ol′o·gy. See *bacteriophagology.*

Pro″to·bi′os bac·te″ri·oph′a·gus. D'Herelle's term for bacteriophage.

pro′to·blast [*prōtos;* G. *blastos*, germ]. A blastomere produced by mosaic cleavage which is destined to form a particular structure or organ in development. —**protoblas′tic,** *adj.*

pro″to·cat″e·chu′ic ac′id. $C_6H_3(OH)_2COOH$; 3,4-dihydroxybenzoic acid; a white to brownish crystalline powder, which discolors in air, sparingly soluble in water.

pro″to·chlo′ride. See *proto-*, 2.

pro′to·col [G. *prōtokollon*, first leaf of a papyrus roll]. 1. The original notes or records of an experiment, autopsy, or clinical examination. 2. The records from which a document is prepared.

pro′to·cone [G. *prōtos*, first; *kōnos*, cone]. 1. In the Cope-Osborn theory of origin of mammalian molar teeth, the primitive single cusp of a reptilian tooth. 2. The mesiolingual cusp on an upper molar.

pro″to·con′id, pro″to·co′nid [*prōtos; kōnos*]. The mesiobuccal cusp on a molar tooth of the lower jaw.

pro″to·cu·ra′rine (pro″to·cue·rah′reen, ·rin, ·cure′-uh·reen, ·rin). A poisonous alkaloid said to be derived from curare.

pro′to·derm. See *blastoderm*, 2.

pro″to·di″as·tol′ic [*prōtos;* G. *diastolē*, a drawing asunder]. The first diastolic action in an embryo.

pro″to·e·las′tose. A poorly defined product of the digestion of elastin.

pro″to·fi′bril. The fine filaments, seen under the electron microscope, of which fibrils are composed.

pro·tog′a·la. See *colostrum.*

pro″to·gas′ter [*prōtos;* G. *gastēr*, belly]. The primitive intestinal cavity of a gastrula. Also called *archenteron, progaster.*

pro′to·gen. A multiple factor in liver, which has been separated into protogen A and protogen B, essential for growth of certain protozoa. Protogen

A appears to be identical with α-lipoic acid, which is a dithiooctanoic acid; protogen B is a thiosulfinyloctanoic acid.

pro″to·glob′u·lose. A poorly defined product of the digestion of globulin.

pro″to·i′o·dide. See *protiodide.*

pro″to·leu′ko·cyte (pro″to·lew′ko·sight) [*prōtos;* G. *leukos,* white; *kytos,* cell]. One of the minute lymphoid cells found in the red bone marrow and also in the spleen.

protolysate. Trade-mark for a protein hydrolysate for oral administration; a casein hydrolysate prepared by digestion with fish ceca.

pro·tol′y·sis. Any reaction in which a proton (hydrogen ion) is transferred, as: $HCl + H_2O = H_3O^+ + Cl^-$.

pro·to·me′rite [*prōtos;* G. *meros,* part]. The anterior portion of a cephaline gregarine.

pro·tom′e·ter. See *proptometer.*

pro″to·met′ro·cyte [*prōtos;* G. *mētēr,* mother; *kytos,* cell]. Mother cell of both white and red blood cells. *Obs.*

Pro″to·mon″a·di′na [*prōtos;* G. *monas,* unit]. An order of the flagellate Protozoa; it contains many parasitic forms, notably the trypanosomes.

pro″to·my·o′sin·ose (pro″to·migh·o′sin·oce, ·migh·oss′in·oce, ·migh′o·sin·oce). A poorly defined product of the digestion of myosin.

pro′ton [*prōtos*]. A subatomic particle identical with the nucleus of the hydrogen atom. It has a positive electric charge numerically equal to the negative charge on the electron; its mass is equal to 6×10^{-23} Gm. The atomic number of an element is equivalent to, and defined by, the number of protons in its nucleus.

pro″to·neu′ron [*prōtos;* G. *neuron,* nerve]. A term proposed by G. H. Parker (1918) to characterize a hypothetical unit of the nerve net of the lowest metazoa. Such a unit transmits impulses indiscriminately in all directions, and has none of the polarization of the phylogenetically later synaptic system of neurons of animals in which there is a central nervous system.

pro″to·path′ic [*prōtos;* G. *pathos,* disease]. Designating primitive sensibility, as opposed to more discriminating, or epicritic, sensation.

pro″to·pep′si·a [*prōtos;* G. *pepsis,* digestion]. A primary process of digestion, as that of starches by the saliva. *Obs.*

pro″to·phile′. A substance which has an affinity for, and forms combinations with, protons (hydrogen ions).

pro′to·phyte [*prōtos;* G. *phyton,* plant]. Any plant of the lowest and most primitive type. The Schizomycetes, or bacteria, may be classed as protophytes, with other low vegetable forms. They have no visible reproductive organs.

pro′to·pine (·peen). See *fumarine.*

pro″to·pla′sis [*prōtos;* G. *plasis,* a molding]. The primary formation of tissue.

pro′to·plasm [*prōtos;* G. *plasma,* anything formed]. The viscid material constituting the essential substance of living cells, upon which all the vital functions of nutrition, secretion, growth, reproduction, irritability, and motility depend.

pro″to·plas′mic, pro″to·plas·mat′ic [*prōtos; plasma*]. Pertaining to, or composed of, protoplasm.

pro′to·plast [*prōtos;* G. *plassein,* to form]. 1. A cell. 2. Protoplasm.

pro″to·por·phy′ri·a [*prōtos;* G. *porphyra,* purple dye]. The presence of protoporphyrin in red blood cells.

pro″to·por′phy·rin. $C_{32}H_{32}N_4(COOH)_2$. Any of the 15 metal-free porphyrins having as substituents 4 methyl, 2 vinyl, and 2 propionic acid ($-CH_2CH_2COOH$) groups. The particular arrangement of these groups represented by *protoporphyrin 9* is the one occurring in hemoglobin.

pro″to·pro′te·ose [*prōtos;* G. *prōteios,* of first rank]. Primary proteose; further digestion changes it into deuteroproteose.

pro′to·spasm [*prōtos;* G. *spasmos,* spasm]. A spasm beginning in one part and extending to others.

pro″to·sul′fate. Of a series of sulfates, that one which contains relatively the smallest amount of sulfuric acid.

pro″to·tox′in [*prōtos;* G. *toxikon,* poison]. A dissociation product of toxins differing from deuterotoxins and tritotoxins in having a stronger affinity than either for the antitoxins.

pro″to·troph′ic (pro″to·trof′ick, ·tro′fick) [*prōtos;* G. *trophē,* nourishment]. Applied to organisms which do not require organic matter or have not the faculty of decomposing protein material.

pro″to·tro′py. The migration of a proton or hydrogen atom within a compound to form an isomer of the compound; a type of change included within the broad scope of tautomerism.

pro″to·ver′a·trine. An ester alkaloid isolated from both veratrum viride and veratrum album and subsequently found to consist of protoveratrine A and protoveratrine B. Protoveratrine A is a tetraester, and yields, on hydrolysis, protoverine, two moles of acetic acid, and one mole each of 2-methylbutyric acid and methylethylglycolic acid. Protoveratrine B is also a tetraester; on hydrolysis, it yields protoverine, two moles of acetic acid, and one mole each of 2-methylbutyric acid and 2,3-dihydroxy-2-methylbutyric acid. It appears to be identical with neoprotoveratrine and veratetrine. Both protoveratrines possess hypotensive activity.

pro″to·ver′ine. $C_{27}H_{43}NO_8$; a highly hydroxylated alkanolamine base, steroidal in character, various esters of which constitute certain of the alkaloids of veratrum viride and veratrum album. It is isomeric with germine and cevine, which are also parent bases of other alkaloids in the veratrums.

pro″to·ver′te·bra [*prōtos;* L. *vertebra,* vertebra]. 1. Originally, a somite. 2. More correctly, the condensed caudal half of a sclerotome, from which most of a vertebra is derived. Also called *primitive vertebra.* —**protovertebral,** *adj.*

Pro″to·zo′a [*prōtos;* G. *zōion,* living being]. The phylum of unicellular animals, subdivided into the subphylum Plasmodroma which contains the medically important classes Rhizopoda, Mastigophora, and Sporozoa, and into the subphylum Ciliophora which contains the class Ciliata. For a list of the protozoa pathogenic to man, see Table in the Appendix. —**protozo′an,** *adj.*

pro″to·zo′a·cide [*prōtos; zōion;* L. *caedere,* to kill]. An agent that will kill protozoa. —**protozo′-acide,** *adj.*

pro″to·zo′al [*prōtos; zōion*]. See *protozoan.*

pro″to·zo′an. A protozoon.

pro″to·zo·i′a·sis [*prōtos; zōion;* NL. *-iasis,* condition]. Infection by protozoa.

pro″to·zo·ol′o·gist [*prōtos; zōion;* G. *logos,* word]. One versed in protozoology.

pro″to·zo·ol′o·gy [*prōtos; zōion; logos*]. The study of protozoa.

pro″to·zo′on (pl. *protozoa*) [*prōtos; zōion*]. Any member of the phylum Protozoa.

pro″to·zo′o·phage, pro″to·zo′o·phag [*prōtos; zōion;* G. *phagein,* to eat]. Cell which is phagocytic to protozoa.

pro·tract′. 1. To extend in time; to prolong. 2. *In anatomy,* to extend or protrude a part of the body, as the tongue or mandible; to draw forward.

pro′trac·tor. 1. *In surgery,* an instrument formerly

used in debridement. 2. *In anatomy*, an extensor: old term.

pro·trude′ [L. *protrudere*, to thrust forward]. Project. Assume an abnormally prominent position, as a tooth which is thrust forward out of line.

pro·tru′sion [L. *protrusum*, from *protrudere*]. The condition of being thrust forward, as the protrusion of the incisor teeth —**protru′sive,** *adj.*

pro·tryp′sin. See *trypsinogen.*

pro·tu′ber·ance [L. *protuberare*, to swell out]. A knoblike projecting part.

external occipital p. The central prominence on the outer surface of the flat portion of the occipital bone.

frontal p. The prominence of the frontal bone.

internal occipital p. A slight central prominence on the inner surface of the tabular portion of the occipital bone.

laryngeal p. The subcutaneous bulging in the midline of the neck produced by the anterior margin of the thyroid cartilage.

mental p. The elevation of the body of the mandible.

parietal p. The eminence of the parietal bone, situated near the sagittal suture.

pro″ty·ros′in·ase (pro″tye·ross′in·ace, ro′sin·ace). An inactive precursor of the enzyme tyrosinase.

proud flesh. Exuberant granulation tissue.

Prout, William [*English physiologist*, 1785–1850]. Discovered that the gastric juice contains hydrochloric acid (1824), an important landmark in the history of physiological chemistry.

prove [L. *probare*, to try]. *In homeopathy*, test the action of a drug on a normal healthy person, and note the effects, both subjective and objective.

pro·ver′te·bra. See *scleromere.*

pro·vi′ta·min [L. *pro*, before; *vita*, life; *am*monia]. A precursor of a vitamin. That which assumes vitamin activity upon activation or chemical change within the body, as ergosterol, which upon ultraviolet irradiation is converted in part to calciferol (D_2); or β-carotene, which in the liver is hydrolyzed to vitamin A.

pro·voc′a·tive [L. *provocativus*, called forth]. Tending to excite or provoke; arousing signs, symptoms, or reactions, similar to those of a disease phenomenon.

Prowazek-Halberstaedter bodies. See under *body.*

prox′i·mal [L. *proximus*, nearest]. Nearest to the body or the median line of the body, or to some other point considered as the center of a system.

prox′i·mal. *In dentistry*, the proximal surface of a tooth is that next to the adjacent tooth. Syn., *approximal, interproximal.*

prox′i·mate (prock′si·mit) [L. *proximare*, to draw near]. Nearest; immediate, as proximate cause.

prox″i·mo·a·tax′i·a [L. *proximus*, nearest; G. *ataxia*, disorder]. Lack of coordination in the muscles of the proximal part of the limbs; in opposition to *acroataxia.*

prox″i·mo·buc′cal [*proximus;* L. *bucca*, cheek]. Pertaining to the proximal and buccal surfaces of a tooth.

prox″i·mo·la′bi·al [*proximus;* L. *labium*, lip]. Pertaining to the proximal and labial surfaces of a tooth.

prox″i·mo·lin′gual [*proximus;* L. *lingua*, tongue]. Relating to the proximal and lingual surfaces of a tooth.

prox. luc. [L.]. *Proxima luce;* the day before.

pro′zone [G. *pro*, before; *zōnē*, girdle, zone]. That portion of the low dilution range of bacteria in which the homologous serums fail to agglutinate the bacteria, the same serums agglutinating the bacteria in high dilution; more common and extensive with old or heated serums.

pro″zy·go′sis. See *syncephalus.*

pro·zy′mo·gen [*pro;* G. *zymē*, leaven; *genesthai*, from *gignesthai*, to be produced]. An intracellular substance which becomes zymogen.

P.R.U. $\frac{1 \text{ mm. Hg}}{1 \text{ ml./min.}}$. A unit of peripheral resistance which is comparable to the ohm in electricity.

pru′i·nate [L. *pruina*, hoarfrost]. Appearing as if covered with hoarfrost.

pru·ri′go [L., itching]. A chronic inflammatory disease of the skin characterized by small, pale papules and severe itching. The papules are deeply seated and are most prominent on the extensor surfaces of the limbs. The disease begins in early life. There are two forms of the disease: **prurigo mitis,** comparatively mild, and **prurigo ageia** or **ferox,** severe. —**prurig′inous,** *adj.*

p. aestivalis. Hydroa vacciniforme.

p. dermographia. A type seen at friction sites associated with dermographia. Psychogenic disturbances are usually present and accentuate the itching.

p. nodularis. A chronic skin disease which occurs chiefly in women and is characterized by pruritic, nodular, and verrucous lesions. It is regarded as an atypical nodular form of neurodermatitis circumscripta, unrelated to the prurigos. Syn., *lichen obtusus corneus.*

summer p. Hydroa vacciniforme.

pru·ri′tus [L., itching]. Itching, an uncomfortable sensation due to irritation of a peripheral sensory nerve; a symptom rather than a disease. —**prurit′ic,** *adj.*

bath p. A burning sensation varying from a slight pricking to an intense itching experienced by some persons after a bath.

p. ani. A common itching condition in and about the anus, especially in men; may be due to several causes.

p. hiemalis. A form affecting certain persons only in winter, especially in dry climates. Syn., *frost-itch, winter itch.*

p. senilis. The pruritus of the aged, probably caused by a lack of oil in the skin; accompanies the atrophy of the skin in old age.

p. vulvae. Intense or mild itching of the vulva and at times adjacent parts. May lead to atrophy, lichenification, and even malignancy. Etiology is varied.

psychogenic p. Severe itching of skin on a psychogenic basis.

punctate p. Patchy areas of itching with no cutaneous lesions; occurs especially over bony prominences.

Prussak, Alexander [*Russian otologist*, 1839–1907]. Described fibers in the tympanic membrane running from the ends of the tympanic notch to the lateral process of the malleus, bounding the lower lateral aspect of the pars flaccida of the tympanum (Shrapnell's membrane); called *Prussak's fibers.* A membranous pouch in the attic of the middle ear between the neck of the malleus and the pars flaccida is called *Prussak's space* or *pouch.*

Prus′sian blue. $Fe_4[Fe(CN)_6]_3$. Ferric ferrocyanide; occurs as dark blue powder or lumps; insoluble in water, alcohol, and dilute acids. It was formerly used as a tonic. Also called *Berlin blue.*

prus′si·ate (prush′ee·ate, pruss′·, prōō′·, prōōsh′·). Any salt of prussic or hydrocyanic acid; a cyanide; particularly a ferricyanide or ferrocyanide.

red p. of potash. Potassium ferricyanide.

yellow p. of potash. Potassium ferrocyanide.

prus′sic ac′id (pruss′ick, prōō′sick). Hydrocyanic acid.

diluted p. a. Diluted hydrocyanic acid.

psal·te′ri·um (sawl·teer′ee·um, sal·teer′·). 1. See *omasum.* 2. See hippocampal *commissure.*

psam′mism [G. *psammos,* sand]. The treatment of disease with sand baths. Syn., *ammism, ammotherapy.*

psam·mo′ma (sam·o′muh) [*psammos;* G. *-ōma,* tumor]. A firm, fibrous tumor found in the membranes of the brain, the choroid plexus, and in other parts; characterized by the presence of concentrically laminated calcareous nodules.

p. of meninges. See *meningioma.*

psam″mo·sar·co′ma [*psammos;* G. *sarkōma,* fleshy excrescence]. A psammoma with sarcomatous features, or a sarcoma containing psammoma bodies.

psam′mous [*psammos*]. Sandy or sabulous.

psel″a·phe′sis (sel″uh·fee′sis) [G., a touching]. The tactile sense. *Obs.*

psel′lism (sel′iz·um), **psel·lis′mus** [G. *psellismos,* a stammering]. 1. Stuttering or stammering. 2. Defective speech due to harelip or to cleft palate.

psellismus mercurialis. The unintelligible, hurried, jerking speech accompanying mercurial tremor.

pseud-. See *pseudo-.*

pseu″da·con′i·tine (sue″da·kon′i·teen, ·tin), **pseu″do·a·con′i·tine.** $C_{36}H_{49}NO_{12}$. An extremely poisonous alkaloid from *Aconitum ferox.*

pseu″da·cous′ma (sue″da·kōōs′muh, ·kōōz′muh, ·kouz′muh). See *pseudacusis.*

pseu·dac″ro·meg′a·ly [G. *pseudēs,* false; *akron,* extremity; *megas,* large]. Enlargement of the face and extremities without any involvement of the pituitary gland.

pseu″da·cu′sis (sue″da·cue′sis, ·kōō′sis) [*pseudēs;* G. *akousis,* hearing]. A disturbance of hearing in which the person's own voice sounds strange or peculiar, being altered in pitch and quality.

pseu″da·graph′i·a (sue″da·graf′ee·uh, ·gray′-fee·uh) [*pseudēs;* G. *agraphos,* unwritten]. 1. Incomplete agraphia, in which a person can copy correctly but is unable to write independently of an original. 2. The form of agraphia in which meaningless words are written.

pseu″dal·bu″mi·nu′ri·a [*pseudēs;* L. *albus,* white; G. *ouron,* urine]. False albuminuria. See *pseudoalbuminuria.*

pseu″dam·ne′si·a (sue″dam·nee′zhuh, ·zee·uh) [*pseudēs;* G. *amnēsia,* amnesia]. Spurious amnesia; a condition resembling amnesia, but of a transient character, usually associated with organic brain disease.

pseu·dan′gi·na. See *pseudoangina.*

pseu″dan·ky·lo′sis [*pseudēs;* G. *agkylōsis,* stiffening of the joints]. A false joint; a false or fibrous ankylosis.

pseu′da·phe (sue′duh·fee), **pseu·daph′i·a** (sue-daf′ee·uh, sue·day′fee·uh). Pseudesthesia.

pseu″dar·thro′sis [*pseudēs;* G. *arthrōsis,* jointing]. A false joint: also spelled *pseudoarthrosis.*

Pseu·dech′is (sue·deck′is, sue′dee·kis) [*pseudēs;* G. *echis,* viper]. A genus of snakes of the Elapidae.

P. porphyriacus. Species of poisonous terrestrial snakes found in Australia; known as the black snake; possesses a hemolytic venom.

P. scutellatus. A species of snakes known as the giant brown snake or taipan found in Australia and New Guinea; attains a length of nine feet.

Pseu′de·laps (sue′di·laps) [*pseudēs;* G. *elops,* serpent]. A genus of snakes of the Elapidae.

P. muelleri. Species of venomous snakes found in New Guinea, the Bismarck Islands, and other islands of the southwest Pacific. Also called *Mueller's snake.*

pseu·del′minth (sue·del′minth) [*pseudēs;* G. *helmins,* worm]. Any wormlike object mistaken for an endoparasitic worm.

pseu″den·ceph′a·lus [*pseudēs;* G. *egkephalos,* brain]. A type of anencephaly in which the cranial vault is completely, or nearly completely, absent; the upper cervical vertebrae are cleft, and the brain is represented by a mass of membranes, blood vessels, connective and possibly nervous tissue at the base of the skull.

pseu″des·the′si·a (sue″dess·thee′zhuh, ·zee·uh) [*pseudēs;* G. *aisthēsis,* sensation]. An imaginary sensation for which there is no corresponding object, as a sensation referred to parts of the body that have been removed by accident or surgical operation. Ghost or phantom sensations.

pseu″di·a′ter (sue″dee·ay′tur) [*pseudēs;* G. *iatēr,* physician]. A quack, or charlatan.

pseu′do- (sue′do-), **pseud-** [*pseudēs*]. 1. A combining form meaning *false, deceptive resemblance to a disease* or *condition.* 2. *In chemistry,* a combining form meaning *resemblance to* or *isomerism with a compound.*

pseu″do·a·ceph′a·lus [*pseudēs;* G. *akephalos,* headless]. A placental parasitic twin (omphalosite) which is apparently headless, but which has a rudimentary cranium and its contents buried in the superior part of the main mass.

pseu″do·a·con′i·tine. See *pseudaconitine.*

pseu″do·ag·glu″ti·na′tion. Rouleaux formation and clumping tendency of erythrocytes, occurring as a result of the increased concentration of plasma proteins, particularly fibrinogen.

pseu″do·a·graph′i·a. See *pseudagraphia.*

pseu″do·al·bu″mi·nu′ri·a [*pseudes;* L. *albus,* white; G. *ouron,* urine]. False albuminuria; the presence in the urine of protein derived from blood, pus, or special secretions and mixed with the urine during its transit through the urinary passages.

pseu″do·al·ve′o·lar [*pseudēs;* L. *alveolus,* small hollow]. Simulating an alveolus or alveolar structure.

pseu″do·an″a·phy·lac′tic [*pseudēs;* G. *anaphylassein,* to guard]. Resembling anaphylactic action.

pseu″do·an″a·phy·lax′is. See anaphylactoid *reaction.*

pseu″do·a·ne′mi·a [*pseudēs;* G. *anaimia,* want of blood]. Pallor and appearance of anemia without blood changes to support the diagnosis. Also called *apparent anemia.*

pseu″do·an·gi′na (sue″do·an·jy′nuh, ·an′ji·nuh) [*pseudēs;* L. *angina,* quinsy]. A mental disorder characterized by pain in the chest at the apex of the heart and at times radiating down the left arm, with no evidence of organic disease. A psychosomatic complex in a neurotic person with precordial anxiety.

pseu″do·an″gi·o′ma [*pseudēs;* G. *aggeion,* vessel; *-ōma,* tumor]. 1. Recanalized thrombus of the portal vein. 2. The formation of a temporary angioma, as is sometimes seen in healing stumps.

pseu″do·an″o·rex′i·a [*pseudēs;* G. *anorexia,* want of appetite]. Rejection of food because of gastric distress.

pseu″do·ap′o·plex″y [*pseudēs;* G. *apoplēxis,* apoplexy]. A condition resembling apoplexy, but unaccompanied by cerebral hemorrhage.

pseu″do·ap·pen″di·ci′tis [*pseudēs;* L. *appendix,* appendage; G. *-itis,* inflammation]. A condition simulating appendicitis, but with no lesion of the vermiform process.

pseu″do·a·tax′i·a. See *pseudotabes.*

pseu″do·ath″er·o′ma [*pseudēs;* G. *atherōma,* tumor full of gruellike matter]. Multiple sebaceous cysts; soft, painless tumors in or beneath the skin.

pseu″do·a·tro″pho·der′ma col′li. A rare skin disease characterized by depigmented areas surrounded by hyperpigmented skin. Often found about the neck but may occur elsewhere. Skin in center of lesion appears atrophic.

pseu″do·blep′si·a, pseu″do·blep′sis [*pseudēs;* G. *blepsis*, sight]. A visual hallucination; a distorted visual image.

pseu″do·bulb′ar [*pseudēs;* L. *bulbus*, bulb]. Not really bulbar, that is, not concerned with the medulla oblongata, as pseudobulbar paralysis.

pseu″do·car′ti·lage [*pseudēs;* L. *cartilago*, cartilage]. An embryonic type of cartilage in which but little matrix is formed, as that of the notochord. Also called *fibrohyaline tissue, vesicular supporting tissue, chondroid tissue, notochordal tissue.*

pseu′do·cast [*pseudēs;* ME. *casten*]. Structures such as mucous threads, epithelial cells, vegetable fibers, masses of bacteria, or debris which morphologically resemble tubular casts.

pseu′do·cele [*pseudēs;* G. *koilia*, cavity]. Old term for the cavity of the septum pellucidum of the brain. Formerly called *fifth ventricle, pseudoventricle.*

pseu″do·chan′cre (sue″do·shang′kur) [*pseudēs;* F. *chancre*]. An indurated sore simulating chancre.

pseu″do·chel″e·ryth′rine. Sanguinarine.

pseu″do·chol′es·tane. Coprostane.

pseu″do·cho·les″te·a·to′ma (·ko·les″tee·uh·to′muh) [*pseudēs;* G. *cholē*, bile; *stear*, fat; *-ōma*, tumor]. An aggregation of epithelial-cell debris resembling cholesteatoma.

pseu″do·cho″li·nes′ter·ase (·ko″li·nes′tur·ace, ·aze). An enzyme which catalyzes the hydrolysis of acetylcholine but which differs from cholinesterase in that it is nonspecific and hydrolyzes esters other than choline esters.

pseu″do·cho·re′a (sue″do·ko·ree′uh) [*pseudēs;* G. *choreia*, dance]. Spurious chorea, usually hysterical in origin.

pseu″do·chrom″es·the′si·a (sue″do·krohm″ess-thee′zhuh, ·zee·uh) [*pseudēs;* G. *chrōma*, color; *aisthēsis*, perception]. A condition in which each of the vowels of a word (whether seen, heard, or remembered) seems to have a distinct visual tint. See *photism, phonism.*

pseu″do·chrom″hi·dro′sis (sue″do·krohm″hi-dro′sis, ·high·dro′sis) [*pseudēs; chrōma;* G. *hidrōsis*, sweating]. A form of colored sweat in which the color changes occur after the sweat is excreted, possibly as a result of action by chromatogenous microorganisms.

pseu″do·chro′mi·a [*pseudēs; chrōma*]. A false or incorrect perception of color.

pseu″do·chro′mo·some [*pseudēs; chrōma;* G. *sōma*, body]. Old term for one of the filamentous types of mitochondria.

pseu″do·cir·rho′sis (sue″do·si·ro′sis) [*pseudēs;* G. *kirros*, orange-colored; *-ōsis*, condition]. A condition characterized by enlargement of the liver, due to obstruction of the hepatic vein, inferior vena cava, or adhesive pericarditis. Also called *Pick's syndrome.*

pseu″do·co·caine′. $C_{17}H_{21}NO_4$; a dextrorotatory stereoisomer of cocaine; a narcotic which causes true addiction. A tartrate salt, known as *psicaine*, has been used as a surface anesthetic. Syn., *d-cocaine, isococaine.*

pseu″do·co′de·ine. $C_{18}H_{21}NO_3$; an isomer of codeine produced synthetically, less effective as an analgesic agent than codeine. Syn., *neoisocodeine.*

pseu″do·col′loid [*pseudēs;* G. *kolla*, glue; *eidos*, form]. A mucoid material, found particularly in ovarian cysts.

p. of the lips. A condition of yellow-orange tumors in the lips and mucosa of the mouth.

pseu″do·col″o·bo′ma [*pseudēs;* G. *kolobōma*, mutilation]. A scarcely noticeable fissure of the iris, the remains of the embryonic ocular fissure, which has almost, but not perfectly, closed.

pseu″do·con·hy′drine. $C_8H_{17}NO$; 5-hydroxy-2-propylpiperidine; an alkaloid from conium.

pseu″do·cox·al′gi·a. See *osteochondritis* deformans juvenilis.

pseu″do·cri′sis [*pseudēs;* G. *krisis*, turning point]. A false crisis; a sudden fall of temperature resembling the crisis of a disease, but subsequently followed by a rise of temperature and a continuation of the fever. It is common in pneumonia.

pseu′do·croup″. False croup; laryngismus stridulus.

pseu″do·cy·e′sis (sue″do·sigh·ee′sis) [*pseudēs;* G. *kyēsis*, pregnancy]. Phantom pregnancy; the belief, on the part of a woman, in the existence of pregnancy when none exists, a condition due to a disorder of metabolism, growth, nutrition, or a psychic factor.

pseu″do·cyl′in·droid [*pseudēs;* G. *kylindros*, rolling stone; *eidos*, form]. A band of mucus or any substance in the urine simulating a renal cast.

pseu′do·cyst″ [*pseudēs;* G. *kystis*, bladder]. A saclike space containing liquid, semiliquid, or gas but without a definite lining membrane.

pseu″do·de·men′ti·a [*pseudēs;* L. *dementia*, madness]. A condition of apathy resembling dementia, but without the mental degenerative changes.

pseu″do·diph·the′ri·a. See *diphtheroid.*

pseu″do·di″ver·tic′u·lum. A pouch, formed by healing of a peptic ulcer, which may have the appearance of a diverticulum.

pseu″do·e·de′ma [*pseudēs;* G. *oidēma*, swelling]. A condition simulating edema.

pseu″do·en″do·me·tri′tis [*pseudēs;* G. *endon*, within; *mētra*, womb; *-itis*, inflammation]. A condition resembling endometritis marked by changes in the blood vessels, hyperplasia of the glands, and atrophy.

pseu″do·e″o·sin′o·phil. The polymorphonuclear leukocyte of avian blood which contains elongated red granules: also called *heterophil.*

pseu″do·e·phed′rine (sue″do·eh·fed′rin, ·ef′i-dreen, ·drin). $C_6H_5.HCOH.(CH_3NH)CH.CH_3$; *d*-$\psi$-ephedrine or *d*-isoephedrine; an alkaloid from the leaves of *Ephedra distachya;* a stereoisomer of ephedrine.

pseu″do·ep′i·lep″sy [*pseudēs;* G. *epilēpsis*, epileptic fit]. A disorder simulating epilepsy.

pseu″do·ep″i·the·li·om′a·tous hy″per·pla′si·a. An irregular, penetrating acanthosis accompanied by chronic inflammation in the dermis, found in chronic ulcers of the skin and chronic granulomatous infections. The reaction simulates squamous-cell carcinoma.

pseu″do·es·the′si·a (sue″do·ess·thee′zhuh, ·zee·uh). See *pseudesthesia.*

pseu″do·fluc″tu·a′tion [*pseudēs;* L. *fluctuatio*, a wavering motion]. A tremor simulating fluctuation, sometimes observed on tapping lipomas.

pseu″do·gan′gli·on. An enlargement on a nerve trunk which resembles a ganglion in form but which does not contain ganglion cells.

pseu″do·ger′mine. An isomeric form of germine, obtained from the latter under certain conditions of chemical treatment. See also *isogermine.*

pseu″do·geu″ses·the′si·a (sue″do·gew″sess·thee′-zhuh, ·zee·uh, sue″do·jew″·) [*pseudēs;* G. *geusis*, taste; *aisthēsis*, perception]. A condition in which color sensations accompany the sense of taste.

pseu″do·geu′si·a (sue″do·gew′see·uh, ·jew′see·uh) [*pseudēs; geusis*]. A false perception, or hallucination, of taste, which may often be an aura in some types of focal epilepsy.

pseu″do·gli·o′ma (sue″do·glye·o′muh) [*pseudēs;* G. *glia*, glue; *-ōma*, tumor]. A name given to inflammatory changes of the vitreous body, due to iridochoroiditis, and resembling glioma of the retina.

pseu″do·glob′u·lin [*pseudēs;* L. *globulus*, little ball]. A protein, one of the class of globulins; distinguished from the euglobulins by its solubility in distilled water, as well as in dilute salt solutions.

pseu″do·glu·co′sa·zone (sue″do·glōō·ko′suh·zone, ·koss′uh·zone, ·glōō″ko·say′zone). A crystalline substance sometimes in normal urine which gives the phenylhydrazine test for sugar.

pseu″do·gon″or·rhe′a [*pseudēs;* G. *gonorroia*, gonorrhea]. A simple nonspecific urethritis.

pseu″do·gyn″e·co·mas′ti·a. See under *gynecomastia.*

Pseu″do·ha′je (sue″do·hah′jee) [*pseudēs;* Ar. *hayyah*, snake]. A genus of arboreal cobras of the family Elapidae whose species possess a neurotoxic venom; found in the forests of central and west Africa.

pseu″do·hal·lu″ci·na′tion. A vivid perception without external stimulus (hallucination) recognized by the individual as an hallucinatory, hypnagogic, or hypnopompic experience.

pseu″do·hem″i·a·car′di·us [*pseudēs;* G. *hēmi-*, half; *a-*, not; *kardia*, heart]. A placental parasitic twin (omphalosite) which has no apparent thorax: also called *pseudothorax, acephalus athorus.*

pseu″do·he″mo·phil′i·a (sue″do·hee″mo·fill′ee·uh, ·hem″o·fill′ee·uh) [*pseudēs;* G. *haima*, blood; *philein*, to love]. A condition characterized by prolonged bleeding time but without the delayed coagulation time of true hemophilia. The platelets are normal in number but impaired in quality.

hereditary p. See hereditary hemorrhagic *diathesis.*

pseu″do·her·maph′ro·dite [*pseudēs;* G. *Hermaphroditos*, Hermaphrodite]. An individual with congenitally malformed external genitalia resembling one sex while the gonads are those of the opposite sex. —**pseudohermaphrodit′ic,** *adj.*

pseu″do·her·maph′ro·dit·ism. The condition of being a pseudohermaphrodite.

female p. Gynandry; a condition simulating hermaphroditism in which the external sexual characteristics are in part or wholly of male aspect, but internal female genitalia are present. Syn., *pseudohermaphroditismus femininus.*

male p. Androgyny; a condition simulating hermaphroditism in which the individual has external sexual characteristics of female aspect, but has testes (usually undescended). Syn., *pseudohermaphroditismus masculinus.*

pseu″do·hy″dro·ne·phro′sis [*pseudēs;* G. *hydōr*, water; *nephros*, kidney; *-ōsis*, condition]. The presence of a cyst near the kidney which resembles hydronephrosis.

pseu″do·hy″dro·pho′bi·a [*pseudēs; hydōr;* G. *phobos*, fear]. A dread of hydrophobia, often producing a condition resembling the disease. Syn., *cynophobia, lyssophobia.*

pseu″do·hy·per′tro·phy (sue″do·high·pur′tro·fee) [*pseudēs;* G. *hyper*, over; *trophē*, nourishment]. False hypertrophy; increase in the size of an organ on account of overgrowth of an important tissue. It is accompanied by diminution in function. —**pseudohypertroph′ic,** *adj.*

pseu″do·hy·po·par″a·thy′roid·ism. A condition exhibiting essentially the signs, symptomatology, and chemical findings of hypoparathyroidism, but due to an inability of the body to respond to parathyroid hormone, and not to a deficiency thereof. Administration of the hormone is not followed by a phosphate diuresis. Pathologically the parathyroid glands are normal or hyperplastic. Patients with the condition frequently exhibit round faces with short heavy-set figures, premature epiphyseal closure of the metacarpal and metatarsal joints resulting in shortening of digits, and subcutaneous foci of ectopic ossification. First described by F. Albright and coworkers (1942).

pseu″do·il′e·us [*pseudēs;* G. *eileos*, intestinal obstruction]. 1. An acute attack of severe abdominal pain with distention, resembling obstructive ileus but without apparent morphologic change. 2. Acute dilatation of the stomach.

pseu″do·i″so·chro·mat′ic [*pseudēs;* G. *isos*, equal; *chrōma*, color]. Pertaining to the different colors which appear alike to the colorblind. See color threshold *test*, Ishihara's *test.*

pseu″do·jaun′dice (sue″do·jawn′dis, ·jahn′dis) [*pseudēs;* OF. *jaunisse*, from L. *galbus*, yellow]. Yellow discoloration of the skin from causes other than hepatic disease.

pseu″do·jer′vine. An alkaloidal constituent, being an alkanolamine, of veratrum viride and veratrum album; it is practically inert physiologically.

pseu″do·ker′a·tin. A keratin that is partly digested by the common proteolytic enzymes, as distinguished from those keratins, classified as eukeratins, which are not digested.

pseu″do·leu·ke′mi·a. See leukemoid *reaction.*

infantile p. See infantile pseudoleukemic *anemia.*

pseu″do·li·thi′a·sis [*pseudēs;* G. *lithos*, stone; NL. *-iasis*, condition]. A condition in which the symptoms point to the existence of a calculus in the biliary or urinary passages but where no stone can be demonstrated.

pseu″do·lo′gi·a fan·tas′ti·ca. A syndrome marked by a single, elaborate phantasy, of which the patient gives full details. The phantasy includes real occurrences added to a fantastic basis.

pseu″do·lys′sa. Lyssophobia.

pseu″do·mal′a·dy [*pseudēs;* OF. *maladie*]. An imaginary or simulated illness.

pseu″do·ma·lar′i·a [*pseudēs;* It. *malaria*, malaria]. A toxemic disease simulating malaria. *Rare.*

pseu″do·mam′ma [*pseudēs;* G. *mammē*, breast]. A structure simulating a mammary gland sometimes occurring in dermoid cysts.

pseu″do·ma′ni·a [*pseudēs;* G. *mania*, madness]. 1. A mental disorder in which the patient accuses himself of crimes of which he is innocent. 2. A mania characterized by lying. 3. An excited mental state in hysteria which simulates true mania.

pseu″do·mel″a·no′sis [*pseudēs;* G. *melas*, black; *-ōsis*, condition]. The staining of tissues, usually after death, by dark brown or black pigments commonly derived from hemoglobin.

pseu″do·mem′brane [*pseudēs;* L. *membrana*, membrane]. A false membrane, as in diphtheria. —**pseudomembranous,** *adj.*

pseu″do·men″in·gi′tis [*pseudēs;* G. *mēnigx*, membrane; *-itis*, inflammation]. A group of symptoms resembling those produced by meningitis, but with absence of the lesions of meningeal inflammation; meningism.

pseu″do·me′ninx [*pseudēs; mēnigx*]. A false membrane.

pseu″do·men″stru·a′tion [*pseudēs;* L. *menstruare*, to menstruate]. Bloody vaginal discharge in newborn infants, ceasing after a few days.

pseu″do·me·tam′er·ism [*pseudēs;* G. *meta*, beyond; *meros*, part]. False metamerism, as seen especially in the linear series of segments of the Cestoda. Each segment, or proglottid, contains a complete set of both male and female reproductive organs.

pseu″do·met·he″mo·glo′bin (sue″do·met·hee″·mo·glo′bin, ·hem″o·glo′bin). See *methemalbumin.*

pseu″do·mi″cro·ceph′a·lus [*pseudēs;* G. *mikros*, small; *kephalē*, head]. Abnormally small brain due to partial atrophy of one cerebral hemisphere, or to changes in the cerebrum ascribable to fetal encephalitis or fetal hydrocephaly.

Pseu″do·mo′nas [*pseudēs;* G. *monas*, unit]. A genus of bacteria of the family Pseudomonadaceae; members are small, motile, aerobic, and Gram-negative.

Ps. aeruginosa. A species of bacteria pathogenic to man; it is the causative agent of various suppurative infections in man. In the multiplication of *Ps. aeruginosa*, pigments are liberated which give pus a blue-green color. Also called *Ps. pyocyanea, Bacillus pyocyaneus, blue-pus microbe.*

Ps. cyanogenes. Motile rods which form a blue pigment. Formerly called *Bacillus lactis cyanogenes.*

Ps. jaegeri. A species pathogenic to chickens.

Ps. pyocyanea. Synonym for *Ps. aeruginosa.*

pseu″do·mor′phine. $C_{34}H_{36}N_2O_6.3H_2O$; dehydromorphine; a dimolecular base formed by the oxidation of morphine in alkaline solution occurring as a crystalline powder, insoluble in cold water and in alcohol.

pseu″do·mu′cin [G. *pseudēs*, false; L. *mucus*, mucus]. A substance allied to mucin, found in proliferative cysts. —**pseudomucinous,** *adj.*

pseu″do·myx·o′ma [*pseudēs;* G. *myxa*, mucus; *-ōma*, tumor]. An epithelial tumor which contains much mucus, but so interspersed with tissue that grossly it suggests myxoma.

p. peritonei. A widespread implantation in the peritoneal cavity of nodules secondary to pseudomucinous tumors of the ovary or rupture of a mucocele of the appendix: also called *gelatinous ascites* or *peritonitis, Werth's tumor.*

pseu″do·nar′co·tism [*pseudēs;* G. *narkōtikos*, benumbing]. A hysterical simulation of narcotism.

pseu″do·ne′o·plasm [*pseudēs;* G. *neos*, new; *plasma*, anything formed]. 1. A phantom tumor. 2. A temporary swelling, generally of inflammatory origin. —**pseudoneoplas′tic,** *adj.*

pseu″do·neu·ri′tis [*pseudēs;* G. *neuron*, nerve; *-itis*, inflammation]. A disease simulating a neuritis.

pseu″do·neu·ro′ma [*pseudēs; neuron;* G. *-ōma*, tumor]. A massed proliferation of Schwann cells with mesodermal elements and neurites developing at the proximal end of an injured nerve, such as occurs in amputation stumps; not a neoplasm: also called *amputation* or *traumatic neuroma.*

pseu″do·nu′cle·in. See *paranuclein.*

pseu″do·nu·cle′o·lus [*pseudēs;* L. *nucleolus*, little nut]. A false nucleolus, or karyosome.

pseu″do·nys·tag′mus [*pseudēs;* G. *nystagmos*, drowsiness]. Symptoms resembling nystagmus but without the regular rhythmic movements of true nystagmus.

pseu″do·oph·thal″mo·ple′gi·a. A rare disorder in which the patient cannot move his eyes on command or fix his eyes on an object in the peripheral field of vision, but is able to follow slowly moving objects to some extent.

pseu″do·os″te·o·ma·la′ci·a (sue″do·os″tee·o·ma·lay′shee·uh, ·see·uh) [*pseudēs;* G. *osteon*, bone; *malakia*, softening]. Rachitis in which the pelvic basin is distorted so as to resemble in form that of osteomalacia.

pseu″do·pa·ral′y·sis [*pseudēs;* G. *paralysis*, paralysis]. An apparent motor paralysis which is caused by voluntary inhibition of motor impulses because of pain, incoordination, or other causes.

pseu″do·par″a·ple′gi·a [*pseudēs;* G. *paraplēgiē*, hemiplegia]. Spurious paraplegia.

pseu″do·par′a·site [*pseudēs;* G. *parasitos*, parasite]. 1. Any object resembling a parasite. 2. A commensal.

pseu″do·pa·re′sis (sue″do·pa·ree′sis, ·par′i·sis) [*pseudēs;* G. *paresis*, paralysis]. An affection resembling paresis, but regarded as distinct from the ordinary forms; a form of chronic alcoholic brain disease. *Obs.*

pseu″do·pe·lade′ (sue″do·pi·lahd′, ·pi·lad′). See *alopecia, cicatrisata.*

pseu″do·pep′tone. See *hemialbumose, propeptone.*

pseu″do·pho″tes·the′si·a (sue″do·fo″tess·thee′-zhuh, ·zee·uh) [*pseudēs;* G. *phōs*, light; *aisthēsis*, perception]. Ability to experience photisms.

Pseu″do·phyl·lid′e·a [*pseudēs;* G. *phyllon*, leaf]. Order of the class Cestoda or tapeworms.

pseu″do·ple′gi·a [*pseudēs;* G. *plēgē*, stroke]. Simulated or hysterical paralysis.

pseu″do·po′di·o·spore″ [*pseudēs;* G. *podion*, from *pous*, foot; *spora*, seed]. An ameboid swarm spore; an amebula.

pseu″do·po′di·um, pseu′do·pod [*pseudēs; pous*]. 1. A temporary protrusion of a portion of the cytoplasm of an ameboid cell, as an aid to locomotion or for engulfing particulate matter. 2. *In allergy*, an irregular projection of the margin of a wheal.

pseu″do·pol·y·po′sis. An acquired form of polyposis of the colon, secondary to ulcerative colitis or amebic dysentery, in which tufts of mucosa have a pedunculated appearance due to adjacent ulcers or scars. Malignant degeneration may be secondary to the associated chronic ulceration. Also called *inflammatory polyps.*

pseu″do·preg′nan·cy. See phantom *pregnancy.*

pseu″do·pseu″do·hy″po·par·a·thy′roid·ism. A rare condition, described by F. Albright (1952), similar to pseudohypoparathyroidism, but with normal serum phosphorus and calcium levels.

pseu·dop′si·a [*pseudēs;* G. *opsis*, vision]. Visual hallucination, or error of visual perception.

pseu″do·pte·ryg′i·um (sue″do·ti·ridj′ee·um, ·teh-ridj′ee·um) [*pseudēs;* G. *pterygion*, little wing]. False, or cicatricial, pterygium.

pseu″dop·to′sis, pseu″do·pto′sis [*pseudēs;* G. *ptōsis*, a falling]. A condition resembling ptosis, caused by a fold of skin and fat descending below the edge of the eyelid.

pseu′do·pus″ [*pseudēs;* L. *pus*, pus]. A liquid that resembles pus in appearance only.

pseu″do·pyr″i·dox′ine (·pirr″i·dock′seen, ·sin). A pyridoxine derivative believed to be widely distributed in natural products, which has a biologic activity for *Streptococcus lactis* much greater than pyridoxine. See *pyridoxine.*

pseu″do·ra′bies. 1. Hydrophobophobia. 2. Infectious bulbar paralysis. See Aladár *Aujeszky.*

pseu″do·re·ac′tion [*pseudēs;* cf. F. *réaction*]. A nonspecific reaction. A localized reaction following the intracutaneous inoculation of a test substance, due to impurities contained in the material. The reaction may be of an allergic nature and is frequently observed in the Schick test for immunity to diphtheria.

pseu″do·rick′ets. See renal *rickets.*

pseu″do·rhon′cus [*pseudēs;* G. *rhogchos*, wheezing]. A false or spurious rhonchus; a deceptive auscultatory sound.

pseu″do·sar·co′ma (*of breast*). See *cystosarcoma phylloides.*

pseu″do·scar″la·ti′na (sue″do·skahr″luh·tee′nuh) [*pseudēs;* ME. *scarlat*]. A febrile disease associated with a rash like that of scarlatina.

pseu″do·scle·ro′sis [*pseudēs;* G. *sklērōsis*, a hardening]. An affection similar in symptoms to multiple sclerosis of the nervous system. A familial degenerative disease, poorly defined but characterized by gradual development of tremors, rigidity, and mental deterioration. A greenish ring at the outer edge of the cornea is considered pathognomonic. Closely allied to progressive lenticular degeneration. Also called *Creutzfeldt-Jakob disease.*

pseu″do·sil″i·cot′i·cum. See talcum-powder *granuloma.*

pseu″do·small′pox. An epidemic disease of South America and Africa. It resembles smallpox and may be a mild form of variola. Also called *alastrim, amaas, Kaffir milk pox.*

pseu·dos′mi·a (sue·doz′mee·uh, sue·dos′·) [*pseudēs;* G. *osmē*, smell]. Perversion of the sense of smell; an olfactory hallucination. A disorder frequently observed in the uncinate type of epilepsy.

pseu″do·sto′ma [*pseudēs;* G. *stoma*, mouth]. An apparent aperture between endothelial cells that have been stained with silver nitrate.

pseu″do·strat′i·fied [*pseudēs;* L. *stratum*, covering; *facere*, to make]. Characterizing an epithelium in which the cells all reach the basement membrane, but are of different lengths, with their nuclei lying at different levels, thus producing the appearance of several layers of cells.

pseu″do·ta′bes (sue″do·tay′beez) [*pseudēs;* L. *tabes*, a wasting away]. 1. A disease simulating tabes dorsalis or tabes mesenterica. 2. The ataxic form of alcoholic multiple neuritis.

pupillotonic p. See Adie's *syndrome.*

pseu″do·tet′a·nus [*pseudēs;* G. *tetanos*, stretched]. Symptoms simulating tetanus without the presence of *Clostridium tetani.*

Pseu″do·thel·phu′sa [*pseudēs;* NL.]. A genus of crayfish, species of which may act as intermediate hosts of the fluke, *Paragonimus westermani.*

pseu″do·tho′rax [*pseudēs;* G. *thōrax*, thorax]. A placental parasitic twin (omphalosite) in which there is no apparent thorax.

pseu″do·tin·ni′tus. Objective tinnitus.

pseu″do·trich″i·no′sis. See *dermatomyositis.*

pseu″do·tro′pine (sue″do·tro′peen, ·pin). An optically inactive isomer of tropine.

pseu″do·trun′cus ar·ter″i·o′sus. A congenital malformation of the heart in which there is a high ventricular septal defect with over-riding aorta and absent or rudimentary pulmonary artery. Circulation to the lungs is by way of the bronchial arteries.

pseu″do·tu·ber″cu·lo′sis [*pseudēs;* L. *tuberculum*, small swelling; G. *-ōsis*, condition]. A general term for a pulmonary infection caused by a variety of fungi or bacteria other than the tubercle bacillus; found in man and lower animals.

pseu″do·tu′mor. A pseudoneoplasm.

inflammatory p. of the orbit. A self-limiting disease in which inflammation and degeneration of orbital fat and extraocular muscles result in proptosis.

p. cerebri. A condition characterized by increased intracranial pressure of unknown origin. In some cases it may be the result of occlusion of the large intracranial venous sinuses.

pseu″do·ty′phoid [*pseudēs;* G. *typhōdēs*, delirious]. Spurious typhoid, a disease simulating typhoid fever, but in which the true lesions of this disease as well as the typhoid bacilli are absent.

pseu″do·vac′u·oles [*pseudēs;* L. *vacuus*, empty]. Transparent bodies containing pigment, found by Laveran in blood of malarial patients.

pseu″do·ven′tri·cle [*pseudēs;* L. *ventriculus*, ventricle]. The so-called fifth ventricle of the brain; the cavity of the septum pellucidum. *O.T.*

pseu″do·vom′it·ing [*pseudēs;* L. *vomitus*, vomiting]. Passive regurgitation of material from the stomach, without expulsive effort.

pseu″do·xan·tho′ma e·las′ti·cum (·zan·tho′muh). A chronic disease of the skin, characterized by an eruption of yellowish plaques, slightly elevated, with an especial predilection for certain parts of the skin, as the lower abdomen, axilla, sides of neck, in which it differs from true xanthoma. Commonly associated with angioid streaks of the retina. At times it shows a familial tendency, but is apt to be recessive in character. It is histologically a degeneration of the elastic tissue of the skin. Also called *Groenblad-Strandberg syndrome.*

pseu·dy′drops [*pseudēs;* G. *hydrōps*, dropsy]. False dropsy.

psi′caine (sigh′kane, sigh′kay·een, ·in). $(COOH.COOH)_2NCH_3.C_7H_{10}(COOCH_3)O.COC_6H_5$. *d-ψ-*Cocaine bitartrate; occurs as white crystals; soluble in water. Used as a local anesthetic.

psi′cose. $CH_2OH.CO.HOCH.HOCH.HOCH.CH_2OH$; L-psicose; a ketose sugar.

psi·lo′sis (sigh·lo′sis) [G., a stripping bare]. 1. Old term for sprue. 2. Falling out of the hair. —**psilot′ic,** *adj.*

psi phe·nom′e·na. See under *phenomenon.*

psit″ta·co′sis (sit″uh·ko′sis) [G. *psittakos*, parrot; *-ōsis*, condition]. An acute febrile disease caused by a polytropic virus. Characterized in man by pneumonia and in parrots and related species by enteritis.

pso′as (so′us) [G. *psoa*, muscles of the loins]. One of two muscles, **psoas major** and **psoas minor.** Psoas major arises from the bodies and transverse processes of the lumbar vertebrae and is inserted into the lesser trochanter of the femur. Psoas minor has a similar origin and is inserted on the pubis. See Table of Muscles in the Appendix.

p. magnus. Old name for the psoas major.

p. parvus. Old name for the psoas minor muscle.

psod′y·mus (sod′i·mus) [*psoa;* G. *didymos*, twin]. A monster with two heads and chests and conjoined abdominal and pelvic cavities. Also called *dicephalus tetrabrachius, ilioxiphopagus.*

pso·i′tis (so·eye′tis) [*psoa;* G. *-itis*, inflammation]. Inflammation of the psoas major muscle.

pso″mo·pha′gi·a (so″mo·fay′juh, ·jee·uh), **pso·moph′a·gy** (so·mof′uh·jee) [G. *psōmos*, bit; *phagein*, to eat]. The swallowing of food without thorough chewing. —**psomophag′ic,** *adj.*

pso′ra. Psoriasis.

pso′ra·line (sor′uh·leen, ·lin). See *caffeine.*

pso″ri·as′i·form (sor″eye·ass′i·form) [G. *psōriasis*, itch; L. *forma*, form]. Like psoriasis.

pso·ri′a·sis (so·rye′uh·sis) [G.]. A chronic inflammatory skin disease characterized by the development of reddish patches covered with silvery-white imbricated scales. The disease affects especially the extensor surfaces of the body and the scalp.

arthropathic p. See psoriatic *arthropathy.*

p. buccalis. See *leukoplakia* buccalis.

p. circinata. Psoriasis in which the central part of the lesion disappears and leaves a ring-shaped patch. Also called *p. orbicularis.*

p. diffusa. A form in which there is coalescence of large contiguous lesions affecting large areas of the body.

p. discoidea. A form in which the patches are the size of small coins. Also called *p. nummularis.*

p. follicularis. A form in which scaly lesions are located at the openings of sweat and sebaceous glands.

p. guttata. See *p.* punctata.

p. gyrata. Psoriasis with a serpentine arrangement of the patches.

p. inveterata. One with persistent infiltrated lesions which often fissure and become covered with heavy scales.

p. palmaris. A form affecting the palms of the hands.

p. punctata. A form in which the lesions consist of minute red papules which rapidly become surmounted by pearly scales.

p. rupioides. A variety in which large conical crusts marked by concentric rings occur.

p. universalis. A form in which the lesions are all over the body.

pustular p. 1. An acute reaction in chronic psoriasis. The pustules are sterile and probably are macroscopic forms of Munro's microabscesses. 2. Pustulosis palmaris et plantaris; this latter may be a limited form of psoriasis or a bacterid.

pso″ri·at′ic (sor″ee·at′ick) [G. *psōriatikos*, of the itch]. Pertaining to or affected with psoriasis.

pso″roph·thal′mi·a (sor″off·thal′mee·uh) [G. *psōra*, itching; *ophthalmia*, ophthalmia]. Blepharitis ciliaris.

pso′ro·sperms. See *corps ronds.*

P. S. P. Phenolsulfonphthalein test.

psy′cha·go″gy, psy″cha·go′gi·a [G. *psychē*, soul; *agōgos*, leading]. A reeducational, psychotherapeutic procedure which stresses the proper socialization of the individual. —**psychagog′ic,** *adj.*

psy·chal′gi·a (sigh·kal′jee·uh) [*psychē;* G. *algos*, pain]. Pains in the head, ascribed by depressed patients to anxiety, or to some psychic rather than a physical cause: also spelled *psychalalgia.*

psy·cha′li·a (sigh·kay′lee·uh) [*psychē*]. A morbid state attended by auditory and visual hallucinations. *Obs.*

psy″chas·the′ni·a (sigh″kass·thee′nee·uh, ·thi-nigh′uh) [*psychē;* G. *astheneia*, want of strength]. A term coined by Janet which applies to all psychoneuroses containing compulsive, obsessive, and phobic tensions. A nervous state characterized by an urge to think, feel, or do something which at the same time is recognized by the patient as being senseless, silly, or irrational. *Rare.* —**psychasthen′ic,** *adj.*

psy″cha·tax′i·a [*psychē;* G. *ataxia*, confusion]. Impaired power of mental concentration; mental confusion or groping.

psych·au′di·to″ry (syke·aw′di·to″ree) [*psychē;* L. *auditorius*, of hearing]. Pertaining to the conscious or intellectual interpretation of sounds.

psy′che (sigh′kee) [G.]. The mind as a functional entity, serving to adjust the total organism to the needs or demands of the environment.

psy′che·ism (sigh′kee·iz·um) [*psychē*]. Mesmerism; animal magnetism.

psy″chen·to′ni·a (sigh″ken·to′nee·uh) [*psychē;* G. *entonia*, from *entonos*, intense]. Mental strain or overwork.

psy·chi′a·ter (sigh·kigh′uh·tur) [*psychē;* G. *iatēr*, physician]. An alienist; a psychiatrist.

psy″chi·at′ric (sigh″kee·at′rick, sick″ee·at′rick) [*psychē;* G. *iatrikos*, skilled in the medical art]. Pertaining to psychiatry.

psy″chi·at′rics [*psychē; iatrikos*]. The theory or practice of psychiatry.

psy·chi′a·trist [*psychē;* G. *iatros*, physician]. A specialist in psychiatry.

psy·chi′a·try (si·kigh′uh·tree) [*psychē;* G. *iatreia*, medical treatment]. The treatment of diseases of the mind.

psy′chic, psy′chi·cal [G. *psychikos*, of the soul]. 1. Pertaining to the mind or psyche. 2. Sensitive to nonphysical forces.

psy′chics [*psychikos*]. Psychology.

psy″chi·no′sis (sigh″ki·no′sis). Any disease of the mind. *Obs.*

psy·chlamp′si·a (sigh·clamp′see·uh) [G. *psychē*, soul; *lampsis*, a shining]. Mania, viewed as a discharging phenomenon of perverted cerebral activity. *Obs.*

psy′cho- (sigh′ko-), **psych-** [*psychē*]. A combining form denoting *mind, mental processes, psychologic methods.*

psy″cho·an″al·ge′si·a. The relief of pain by psychological means, principally by assurance of and explanations to the patient, suggestion, and therapeutic measures as music.

psy″cho·a·nal′y·sis (sigh″ko·an·al′i·sis) [*psychē;* G. *analysis*, a loosing]. 1. The method developed by Sigmund Freud for the exploration and synthesis of patterns in emotional thinking and development; a technic used in the treatment of a wide variety of emotional disorders, particularly the neuroses. Relies essentially upon the free associations of the patient to produce valuable information of which the patient was formerly unaware, by bringing to conscious manipulation ideas and experiences from the unconscious divisions of the psyche. 2. The body of data and theory based on the discoveries of this method; concerned chiefly with the conflict between infantile instinctual striving and parental or social demand, and the manner in which this conflict affects emotional growth, character development, and the formation of mental and emotional disorders.

psy″cho·an′a·lyst (sigh″ko·an′uh·list) [*psychē; analysis*]. One who practices psychoanalysis.

psy″cho·au′di·to″ry. See *psychauditory.*

psy″cho·bi·ol′o·gist (sigh″ko·buy·ol′o·jist) [*psychē;* G. *bios*, life; *logos*, word]. One who specializes in psychobiology.

psy″cho·bi·ol′o·gy [*psychē; bios; logos*]. An approach to the study of personality, introduced in the United States and emphasized by Adolf Meyer, in which the individual is considered as a whole within his whole situation, that is, not only as a physical organism but as the sum of and reacting to his environment. As a school of psychiatry, psychobiology stresses that mental disorders, like normal behavioral processes, are dynamic adaptive reactions of the individual to stress or conflict, and are the understandable results of the psychobiological development of the individual.—**psychobiolog′ic, psychobiolog′ical,** *adj.*

psy″cho·ci·ne′si·a (sigh″ko·si·nee′shuh, ·see·uh, ·zhuh, ·zee·uh). See *psychokinesia.*

psy″cho·co′ma [*psychē;* G. *kōma*, deep sleep]. Mental stupor. *Obs.*

psy″cho·cor′ti·cal [*psychē;* L. *cortex*, bark]. Pertaining to that part of the cerebral cortex concerned in the perception of sensations.

psy″cho·di″ag·nos′tics [*psychē;* G. *diagnōstikos*, able to distinguish]. The evaluation of the personality, as furnished by the Rorschach method.

Psy·chod′i·dae (sigh·cod′i·dee) [G. *psychē;* butterfly; *eidos*, form]. A family of the Diptera, which includes the moth flies, moth midges, and sand flies. The most important genus is *Phlebotomus.*

psy″cho·dom′e·ter [G. *psychē*, soul; *hodos*, way; *metron*, a measure]. An instrument for measuring the rapidity of psychic processes.

psy″cho·dom′e·try [*psychē; hodos; metron*]. The measurement of the rapidity of psychic processes.

psy″cho·dra′ma [*psychē;* G. *drama*, deed or act]. *In psychotherapy*, the reenactment of events from the patient's life, with the patient as either spectator or actor: a technique for obtaining cathartic relief.

psy″cho·dy·nam′ics (sigh″ko·dye·nam′icks, ·di-nam′icks) [*psychē;* G. *dynamikos*, powerful]. The study of psychology from the point of view of the causative factors in mental activity. —**psychodynam′ic,** *adj.*

psy″cho·ep′i·lep″sy. See idiopathic *epilepsy*.

psy″cho·gal″va·nom′e·ter [*psychē;* Luigi *Galvani;* G. *metron*, a measure]. A device for recording electrodermal responses to various mental stimuli which provoke emotional reactions. Its practical application is the lie detector, which indicates the emotional reactions of one who is suppressing the truth.

psy″cho·gen′ic o′ver·lay. Exaggeration of symptoms beyond what one would expect from the organic cause, and therefore presumed to be of functional origin.

psy″cho·gen′e·sis [*psychē;* G. *genesis*, production]. 1. The development of mental characteristics. 2. The process by which activities or ideas originate in the mind, or psyche. 3. The origin of psychic activity contributing to a psychosis. —**psychogen′ic, psychogenet′ic,** *adj.*

psy·chog′e·ny (sigh·kodj′i·nee) [*psychē;* G. *genesthai*, from *gignesthai*, to be produced]. 1. See *psychogenesis*. 2. The development of the mind. *Obs.*

psy″cho·geu′sic (sigh″ko·gew′sick, ·jew′sick) [*psychē;* G. *geusis*, taste]. Pertaining to perception of taste.

psy·chog′no·sis (sigh·cog′no·sis, sigh″cog·no′sis) [*psychē;* G. *gnōsis*, knowledge]. Diagnosis or recognition of mental and psychic conditions. *Rare.* —**psychognos′tic,** *adj.*

psy′cho·gram [*psychē;* G. *gramma*, letter]. A chart or table of personality traits.

psy″cho·graph′ic [*psychē;* G. *graphein*, to write]. 1. Relating to a chart of the personality traits of an individual. 2. *In psychiatry*, relating to the natural history of the mind.

psy″cho·ki·ne′si·a (sigh″ko·ki·nee′shuh, ·see·uh, ·zhuh, ·zee·uh, sigh″ko·kigh·), **psy″cho·ki·ne′sis** (sigh″ko·ki·nee′sis, ·kigh·nee′sis) [*psychē;* G. *kinēsis*, motion]. Explosive or impulsive maniacal action; a lack of inhibition of primitive instincts leading to violent and hasty actions.

psy″cho·ki·ne′sis. 1. See *psychokinesia*. 2. The direct action of mind on matter.

psy″cho·lag′ny [*psychē;* G. *lagneia*, coition]. Sexual excitement induced by mental concepts.

psy′cho·lep″sy [*psychē;* G. *lēpsis*, a seizure]. A sudden intense psychic depression, lasting for a short time. —**psycholep′tic,** *adj.*

psy″cho·log′ic screen′ing. The use of psychologic tests, usually for large groups, as a means of determining general fitness for any specific duty, such as army service.

psy·chol′o·gist [*psychē;* G. *logos*, word]. One who specializes in psychology.

psy·chol′o·gy [*psychē; logos*]. The science which studies the functions of the mind, such as sensation, perception, memory, thought, and, more broadly, the behavior of an organism in relation to its environment. —**psycholog′ic, psycholog′ical,** *adj.*

abnormal p. The study of the irregular and pathologic mental phenomena, such as hallucinations and delusions, which occur in mental illnesses.

analytic p. See *analytic psychology*.

animal p. That branch of psychology which investigates the behavior of animals.

applied p. That branch of psychology which emphasizes practical rather than theoretical objectives. It includes medical, industrial, educational, clinical, and similar branches of psychology. Refers also to the interpretation of data in history, literature, and such fields according to psychologic principles.

depth p. That relating to all unconscious mental activity.

dynamic p. 1. *In psychiatry*, specifically the Freudian concepts which ascribe to the energy of the libido a potent role in mental symptoms. 2. *In psychology*, an approach which emphasizes the cause-and-effect relations between conscious and unconscious phenomena and stresses the process nature of personality.

experimental p. The study of psychologic phenomena by experimental methods.

gestalt, Gestalt p. A system or theory of psychology which emphasizes the wholeness and organized structure of every experience. It maintains that psychologic processes and behavior cannot be described adequately by analyzing the elements of experience alone, and emphasizes sudden learning by insight rather than by trial and error or association.

individual p. A system developed by Alfred Adler. The individual is regarded as an indivisible unit of human society; his individual traits are compared, in terms of a striving for superiority which is assumed to exist in everyone, and then restated to provide a composite picture of a single tendency expressed in many ways.

industrial p. Psychology applied to problems in industry dealing chiefly with the selection and mental health of personnel.

physiologic p. That branch of psychology which investigates the structure and functions of the nervous system and bodily organs in their relationship to behavior.

psy·cho′ma (sigh·ko′muh) [*psychē;* G. *-ōma*, morbid affection]. Psychic forces based on a general sensation of substances. *Obs.*

psy″cho·math″e·mat′ics [*psychē;* G. *mathēmatikos*, fond of learning]. Mathematics associated with or applied to psychology; the application of mathematical formulas to designate variations in mental capacities.

psy·chom′e·try (sigh·kom′i·tree), **psy″cho·met′rics** [*psychē;* G. *metron*, a measure]. The measurement of the duration and intensity of psychic processes. Frequently applied to mean the measurement of intelligence. —**psychomet′ric,** *adj.*

psy″cho·mo′tor [*psychē;* L. *motor*, from *movere*, to move]. Pertaining to voluntary movement, as the psychomotor area, disposed chiefly along each side of the central fissure of the cerebral hemisphere.

psy″cho·neu″ro·log′ic (sigh″ko·new″ro·lodj′ick) [*psychē;* G. *neuron*, nerve; *logikos*, possessed of reason]. Pertaining to a condition characterized by both psychic and organic neural components.

psy″cho·neu·ro′sis [*psychē; neuron;* G. *-ōsis*, condition]. A group of reactions now classified as psychoneurotic disorders.

psy″cho·neu·rot′ic [*psychē; neuron*]. Relating to, or affected by, a psychoneurosis.

psy″cho·neu·rot′ic dis·or′ders. *In psychiatry*, a group of reactions characterized chiefly by anxiety, which may be directly felt and expressed or unconsciously controlled by means of a defense mechanism, the recognition of which becomes the basis for the specific diagnostic term applied. In contrast to psychotic disorders, there is no gross disorganization of personality in relation to external reality. Individuals suffering from psychoneurotic disorders usually present a history of unusual difficulties in development related to special stresses or deprivations in early life, which influence the form of the disorder in terms of symptoms and susceptibilities.

psy″cho·nom′ics [*psychē;* G. *nomikos*, relating to laws]. That science dealing with the laws of the mind; psychology. —**psychonomic,** *adj.*

psy·chon′o·my (sigh·kon′o·mee) [*psychē;* G. *nomos*, law]. Psychonomics.

psy″cho·no·se′ma [*psychē;* G. *nosēma*, disease]. Any mental disease. *Obs.*

psy″cho·pa·re′sis (sigh″ko·pa·ree′sis, ·par′i·sis) [*psychē;* G. *parēsis*, a slackening]. Enfeeblement of the mind. *Rare.*

psy′cho·path [*psychē;* G. *pathos*, disease]. A morally irresponsible person; one who continually comes in conflict with accepted behavior and the law. See sociopathic *personality* disturbance.

psy″cho·path′i·a [*psychē; pathos*]. Psychopathy.

p. chirurgicalis. A mania for being operated upon.

p. sexualis. See *sexual deviation.*

psy·chop′a·thist (sigh·cop′uth·ist) [*psychē; pathos*]. Old term for psychiatrist.

psy″cho·pa·thol′o·gist [*psychē; pathos;* G. *logos*, word]. One who specializes in the pathology of mental diseases.

psy″cho·pa·thol′o·gy [*psychē; pathos; logos*]. The pathology of mental diseases.

psy·chop′a·thy (sigh·cop′uth·ee) [*psychē; pathos*]. Any disease of the mind. —**psychopath′ic,** *adj.*

psy″cho·pho″nas·the′ni·a [*psychē;* G. *phōnē*, voice; *astheneia*, want of strength]. A speech difficulty of mental origin.

psy″cho·phys′ics [*psychē;* G. *physikos*, natural]. 1. The study of mental processes by physical methods. 2. The study of the relation of stimuli to the sensations which they produce, especially the determination of the differences of stimulus required to produce recognizable differences of sensation; experimental psychology. —**psychophysical,** *adj.*

psy″cho·phys″i·o·log′ic. Pertaining to the mind and its relation to the physiology of the body.

psy″cho·phys″i·o·log′ic au″to·nom′ic and vis′cer·al dis·or′ders. Symptoms arising from chronic and exaggerated forms of the normal physiologic organic components of emotion but with the subjective awareness of the emotion repressed. If long continued, may lead to structural changes in the affected organs, e.g., peptic ulcer. These disorders differ from conversion (hysterical) reactions in that they involve over- or underactivity of organs and viscera innervated by the autonomic nervous system, fail to alleviate anxiety, are physiologic rather than symbolic in origin. Diagnosis, based on the principal symptomatic manifestations of the organ system involved, is specified as *psychophysiologic skin reaction, musculoskeletal reaction* (to be differentiated from conversion reaction), *respiratory reaction, cardiovascular reaction* (cardiac neurosis), *hemic* and *lymphatic reaction, gastrointestinal reaction* (gastric neurosis), *genitourinary reaction, endocrine reaction, nervous system reaction* (including neurasthenia), and some *reactions of organs of special senses.* It covers the former diagnoses of organ neuroses and anxiety states

psy″cho·phys″i·ol′o·gy [*psychē;* G. *physis*, nature; *logos*, word]. Physiologic psychology; mental physiology.

psy″cho·ple′gi·a [*psychē;* G. *plēgē*, stroke]. Mental impairment of sudden onset. *Rare.* —**psychople′gic,** *adj.*

psy″cho·ple′gic [*psychē; plēgē*]. A drug which lessens excitability and suppresses receptivity.

psy″cho·rhyth′mi·a (sigh″ko·rith′mee·uh, ·rith′mee·uh) [*psychē;* G. *rhythmos*, any regular recurring motion]. A mental condition in which there is involuntary repetition of previous volitional behavior.

psy″chor·rha′gi·a (sigh″ko·ray′juh, ·jee·uh) [*psychē;* G. *rhēgnynai*, to burst forth]. The death agony. *Obs.*

psy″cho·sen·so′ri·al. Psychosensory.

psy″cho·sen′so·ry [*psychē;* L. *sensum*, from *sentire*, to feel]. Pertaining to perception of sensory impulses at conscious levels.

psy″cho·sex′u·al [*psychē;* L. *sexualis*, sexual]. Relating to the mental and emotional aspects of sexuality as contrasted to the strictly physical or endocrine manifestations.

psy·cho′sin (sigh·ko′sin). A cerebroside derivative obtained by boiling with barium hydroxide. Psychosin consists of a combination of sphingosine and galactose.

psy·cho′sis (sigh·ko′sis) [G., a giving soul to]. A mental disorder characterized by disintegration of the personality and its break with reality. See *psychotic disorder.* —**psychot′ic,** *n., adj.*

affective-reaction p. See manic-depressive *reaction,* affective *reaction.*

alcoholic p. Psychosis caused by alcoholism; chronic alcoholic delirium.

arteriosclerotic p. Psychic disturbance in which arteriosclerosis is the exciting cause.

climacteric p. A psychic reaction associated with menopause.

degenerative p. A psychosis in which puerilism is exhibited.

exhaustive p. Essentially the same as collapse delirium, but a more severe mental disorder.

famine p. See *p.* induced by starvation.

gestational p. One arising during pregnancy.

involutional p. See involutional psychotic *reaction.*

manic-depressive p. See manic-depressive *reaction.*

organic p. A psychosis associated with demonstrable organic disease. See *organic brain disorder.*

postinfectious p. Mental disturbance following acute disease, such as pneumonia or typhoid fever.

p. induced by starvation. A psychosis seen in war-torn countries when starvation is severe and widespread.

puerperal p. Any psychotic reaction in a woman during childbirth or the postpartum period.

reactive p. A psychosis which is supposed to be precipitated by an environmental condition. Also called *situational p.*

senile p. A psychosis occurring in old age.

therapeutic p. *In psychoanalysis,* a temporary regression during therapy accompanied by primitive means of dealing with drives which provide the basis for massive resynthesis of personality.

toxic p. Psychic disorders caused by toxins or toxic agents, such as opium or alcohol.

psy″cho·so·mat′ic [G. *psychē*, soul; *sōma*, body]. Of or pertaining to the mind and body, as in affections with an emotional background having both mental and bodily components. Especially relating to a system of medicine which emphasizes the interdependence of mental processes and physical or somatic functions. See *psychophysiologic autonomic and visceral disorders.*

psy″cho·sur′ger·y [*psychē;* G. *cheirourgia*, a working by hand]. Frontal lobotomy, or operative section of the frontothalamic fibers of the brain; used in the treatment of certain mental disorders.

psy″cho·tech′nics [*psychē;* G. *technikos*, skillful]. The application of psychologic principles to economics and social sciences.

psy″cho·ther″a·peu′tics. See *psychotherapy.*

psy″cho·ther′a·py [*psychē;* G. *therapeia*, treatment]. 1. The treatment of disease by suggestion. 2. The treatment of mental diseases.

psy·chot′ic de·pres′sive re·ac′tion. See under *reaction.*

psy·chot′ic dis·order. *In psychiatry,* the reaction of an individual to external or internal stress or injury, characterized generally by severe affective disturbance, profound introspection, and withdrawal from reality, with failure to test and evaluate external reality adequately, formation of delusions or hallucinations, and regression presenting the appearance of personality disintegration. In contrast to organic brain syndromes, there is no impairment of orientation, memory, or intellect, though these may be difficult to examine readily, but differentiation from the *psychoneurotic disorders* may require long and acute observations. Included in this grouping are the affective, paranoid, and schizophrenic reactions. A psychotic reaction may also accompany a symptomatic clinical picture, as in chronic brain syndromes associated with senile changes or alcohol intoxication. Formerly called *psychosis*.

psy′cho·trine. $(CH_3O)_3C_{25}H_{26}N_2.OH$; an alkaloid found in ipecac.

psy·chral′gi·a (sigh·kral′jee·uh), **psy″chro·al′gi·a** [G. *psychros*, cold; *algos*, pain]. A condition characterized by a painful subjective sense of cold.

psy′chro- [*psychros*]. A combining form meaning *cold*.

psy″chro·es·the′si·a (sigh″kro·ess·thee′zhuh, ·zee·uh) [*psychros;* G. *aisthēsis*, perception]. Subjective sensation of cold.

psy″chro·lu′si·a [*psychros;* G. *lousis*, a bathing]. Cold bathing.

psy·chrom′e·ter (sigh·krom′i·tur) [*psychros;* G. *metron*, a measure]. A hygrometer for determining the atmospheric moisture by observing the difference in the indication of two identical thermometers, the bulb of one being kept dry, and the other wet, with a water-soaked wick; both are swung through the air to facilitate evaporation from the wet bulb.

psy″chro·phil′ic [*psychros;* G. *philein*, to love]. Pertaining to cold-loving organisms; applied to microorganisms which develop best from 15°–20° C. Syn., *crymophilic*.

psy″chro·pho′bi·a [*psychros;* G. *phobos*, fear]. 1. Morbid fear of cold. 2. Morbid sensibility to cold.

psy′chro·phore [*psychros;* G. *phoros*, bearing]. An instrument for applying cold to deeply seated parts, as a double-current catheter for applying cold to the posterior part of the urethra.

psy″chro·ther′a·py [*psychros;* G. *therapeia*, treatment]. The treatment of disease by the use of cold.

psy′co·sin, psy·co′sin. The galactoside of sphingol.

psyl′li·um seed (sil′ee·um). See *plantago seed.*

Pt Chemical symbol for platinum.

pt. Pint.

PTA Plasma thromboplastin antecedent.

PTA de·fic′i·en·cy. Hemorrhagic disorder due to deficiency of plasma thromboplastin antecedent.

ptar′mic (tahr′mick) [G. *ptarmikos*, causing to sneeze]. Pertaining to the act of sneezing; sternutative.

ptar′mic. A substance that produces sneezing.

ptar′mus (tahr′mus) [G. *ptarmos*, sneezing]. Sneezing.

PTC Abbreviation for phenylthiocarbamide, plasma thromboplastin component.

PTC de·fic′i·en·cy. Deficiency of plasma thromboplastin component; Christmas disease.

ptel′e·or·rhine (tel′ee·o·ryne, ·rin) [G. *ptelea*, elm; *rhis*, nose]. Pertaining to a facial type in which the nostrils are asymmetric.

pter′i·dine. Any compound characterized by the presence of a ring system composed of fused pyrimidine and pyrazine rings. Folic acid, the pterins, and many other substances contain such a ring system.

pter′i·do·phyte″, pter·id′o·phyte [G. *pterido-*, from *pteris*, fern; *phytos*, grown]. One of a division of the plant kingdom, which includes the ferns and their allies.

pter′in (terr′in). Any pigment, containing a pteridine ring system, occurring in the wings of butterflies and, by extension, in mammalian tissues.

pter′i·on (terr′ee·on, teer′ee·on) [G. *pteron*, wing]. The region (not a point) surrounding the sphenoparietal suture where the frontal bone, parietal bone, squama temporalis, and greater wing of the sphenoid bone come together most closely.

pter′o- (terr′o-) [*pteron*]. A combining form meaning *feather, wing.*

pter·o′ic ac′id. $C_{14}H_{12}N_6O_3$; *p*-[(2-amino-4-hydroxy-6-pteridylmethyl)amino]benzoic acid, being folic acid (pteroylglutamic acid) without its glutamic acid component. The formyl derivative of pteroic acid (rhizopterin) appears to be a precursor of folic acid.

pter″o·yl·glu·tam′ic ac′id. Folic acid. See Table of Vitamins in the Appendix.

pte·ryg′i·um (teh·ridj′ee·um, ti·ridj′·) [G. *pterygion*, anything like a wing; disease of the eye when a membrane grows over it from the inner corner]. 1. A triangular patch of mucous membrane growing on the conjunctiva, usually on the nasal side of the eye. The apex of the patch points toward the pupil, the fan-shaped base toward the canthus. 2. See *eponychium*, 2. 3. Any fold of skin extending abnormally from one part of the body to another. —**pterygial,** *adj.*

pter′y·go- (terr′i·go-) [G. *pteryx*, wing]. A combining form denoting *connection with*, or *relation to, the pterygoid process.*

pter′y·goid (terr′i·goyd) [*pteryx;* G. *eidos*, form]. 1. Wing-shaped, as the pterygoid process of the sphenoid bone. 2. Pertaining to the pterygoid canal, pterygoid process, pterygoid plexus, etc.

pter″y·go·man·dib′u·lar [*pteryx;* L. *mandibula*, jaw]. Pertaining to the pterygoid process and the mandible.

pter″y·go·max′il·lar″y (terr″i·go·mack′si·lerr″ee) [*pteryx;* L. *maxilla*, jaw]. Pertaining to the pterygoid process and the maxilla.

pter″y·go·pal′a·tine (terr″i·go·pal′uh·tyne, ·tin) [*pteryx;* L. *palatum*, palate]. Situated between the pterygoid process of the sphenoid bone and the palatine bone, as the pterygopalatine canal.

pter″y·go·pha·ryn′ge·us [*pteryx;* G. *pharygx*, pharynx]. The part of the superior constrictor of the pharynx which arises from the medial pterygoid process.

pter″y·go·sper′min. An antibiotic substance derived from the root of *Moringa pterygosperma*, active, in vitro, against several bacterial species.

pter″y·go·spi′nous [*pteryx;* L. *spina*, thorn]. Pertaining to a pterygoid process and to the angular spine of the sphenoid bone.

pti·lo′sis (ti·lo′sis) [G., disease of the eyelids]. Falling out of the eyelashes.

P. T. O. Perlsucht tuberculin original; a tuberculin prepared from bovine tubercle bacilli, in the same manner as Koch's original tuberculin. Also called *Klemperer's tuberculin.*

pto′maine (to′mayn, to·mayn′, to′may·een, ·in) [G. *ptōma*, fallen body]. An amino compound which results from the decomposition of proteins or dead animal matter by microorganisms; should not be confused with those bacterial products which cause food poisoning.

pto·mat″i·nu′ri·a [*ptōma;* G. *ouron*, urine]. The presence of ptomaines in the urine.

pto′sis (to′sis) [G., a falling]. Prolapse, abnormal depression, or falling down of an organ; applied especially to drooping of the upper eyelid, due to paralysis or atrophy of the levator palpebrae superioris. —**ptosed, ptot′ic,** *adj.*

abdominal p. Enteroptosis.

congenital p. An anomaly of drooping upper eyelids due to absent or incomplete innervation of the levatores palpebrarum muscles.

p. iridis. Prolapse of the iris.

p. sympathetica. See Horner's *syndrome.*

-pto'sis [G.]. A combining form meaning *a lowered position of an organ.*

P. T. R. Perlsucht tuberculin rest; a tuberculin prepared from bovine tubercle bacilli.

pty·al'a·gogue (tye·al'uh·gog) [G. *ptyalon*, saliva; *agōgos*, leading]. A medicine producing a flow of saliva. Syn., *ptyalogogue.*

pty"a·lec'ta·sis (tye"uh·leck'tuh·sis) [*ptyalon;* G. *ektasis*, a stretching]. Dilatation of the duct of a salivary gland, either spontaneous or produced surgically.

pty'a·lin [*ptyalon*]. A diastatic enzyme found in saliva, having the property of hydrolyzing starch to dextrin, maltose, and glucose, and hydrolyzing sucrose to glucose and fructose. Also called *ptyalase, salivary diastase.*

pty"a·lin'o·gen [*ptyalon;* G. *genesthai*, from *gignesthai*, to be produced]. The zymogen of ptyalin.

pty'a·lism [*ptyalon*]. Salivation.

pty'a·lo·cele (tye'uh·lo·seel, tye·al'o·seel) [*ptyalon;* G. *kēlē*, tumor]. A cyst containing saliva; usually due to obstruction of the duct of a salivary gland.

sublingual p. Ranula.

pty"a·lo·gen'ic [*ptyalon;* G. *genesthai*, from *gignesthai*, to be produced]. Of salivary origin.

pty·al'o·gogue (tye·al'o·gog) [*ptyalon;* G. *agōgos*, leading]. A medicine causing a flow of saliva. Syn., *ptyalagogue.*

pty"a·log'ra·phy (tye"uh·log'ruh·fee) [*ptyalon;* G. *graphein*, to write]. Roentgenography of the salivary glands or their ducts.

pty'a·lo·lith [*ptyalon;* G. *lithos*, stone]. A salivary calculus: also spelled *ptyalith.*

pty"a·lo·li·thi'a·sis (tye"uh·lo·li·thigh'uh·sis) [*ptyalon; lithos;* NL. *-iasis*, condition]. The formation, or presence, of a salivary calculus.

pty"a·lor·rhe'a [*ptyalon;* G. *rhoia*, flow]. Excessive flow of saliva.

pty'a·lose (tye'uh·loce) [*ptyalon*]. A sugar found in saliva. Syn., *maltose.*

pty"a·lo'sis [*ptyalon;* G. *-ōsis*, condition]. Salivation. Also called *ptyalism.*

pty'o·crine (tye'o·kryne, ·krin, ·kreen). See *apocrine.*

pty·oc'ri·nous (tye·ock'ri·nus) [G. *ptyon*, fan; *krinein*, to separate]. Obsolete term for apocrine.

pty'sis (tye'sis) [G., spitting]. The act of spitting.

ptys'ma (tiz'muh) [G., sputum]. Saliva.

ptys'ma·gogue (tiz'muh·gog) [*ptysma;* G. *agōgos*, leading]. A drug that promotes the secretion of saliva.

P. U. Pregnancy urine, signifying the chorionic gonadotropic hormone found in such urine.

Pu Chemical symbol for plutonium.

pu'ber [L., adult]. One who has arrived at the age of puberty.

pu'ber·tas, pu·ber'tas [L.]. Puberty.

p. plena. Complete puberty.

p. precox. Puberty at a very early age.

pu'ber·ty [*pubertas*]. The period at which the generative organs become capable of exercising the function of reproduction; signalized in the boy by a change of voice and discharge of semen, in the girl by the appearance of the menses. —**puberal,** *adj.*

precocious p. That occurring before eight years of age.

premature p. That occurring between the ages of eight and ten.

pu·ber'u·lic ac'id. $C_8H_6O_6$. An antibiotic from *Penicillium puberulum;* occurs in almost colorless crystals. It is active largely against Gram-positive bacteria.

pu·ber"u·lon'ic ac'id. $C_8H_4O_6$. An antibiotic from *Penicillium puberulum;* occurs in bright yellow prisms. It is a weak antibiotic agent active largely against Gram-positive bacteria.

pu'bes (pew'beez) [L., pubic hair; the private parts]. 1. The hairy region covering the pubic bone. 2. The two pubic bones considered together; that portion of the hipbones forming the front of the pelvis.

pu·bes'cence [L. *pubescere*, to become pubescent]. 1. Hairiness; the presence of fine, soft hairs. 2. Puberty, or the coming on of puberty. —**pubescent,** *adj.*

pu"be·trot'o·my [L. *pubes*, the private parts; G. *ētron*, abdomen; *tomē*, a cutting]. Pelvic section through the pubes. *Obs.*

pu'bic [*pubes*]. Pertaining to the pubes.

pu"bi·ot'o·my [*pubes;* G. *tomē*, a cutting]. The operation of dividing the pubic bone to facilitate delivery in cases of pelvic malformation. *Obs.*

pu'bis [NL., from *pubes*]. Os pubis; the pubic bone, that portion of the hipbone forming the front of the pelvis. See Table of Bones in the Appendix. See Plates 1, 2.

pub'lic health. 1. The health of a population or community. 2. Specifically, the health of a community in terms of organized effort on the part of the community to carry out such preventive medicine measures which the individual cannot perform for himself: e.g., large-scale sanitation, control of communicable diseases, advancement of hygiene, medical and nursing services, and general development of such means and methods as will best maintain and promote the health and efficiency of the population. See social *medicine.*

Pub'lic Health Serv'ice. See *United States Public Health Service.*

pu'bo- [*pubes*]. *In anatomy,* a combining form denoting *relation to the pubes* or *pubis.*

pu"bo·cap'su·lar [*pubes;* L. *capsula*, little box]. Pertaining to the os pubis and the capsule of the hip joint. Used to denote a collateral ligament of the hip joint.

pu"bo·cav"er·no'sus. A variable part of the ischiocavernosus muscle.

pu"bo·coc·cyg'e·al (pew"bo·cock·sidj'ee·ul) [*pubes;* G. *kokkyx*, cuckoo]. 1. Pertaining to the pubic bone and the coccyx. 2. A muscle, part of the levator ani.

pu"bo·coc·cyg'e·us. A part of the levator ani muscle.

pu"bo·fem'o·ral [*pubes;* L. *femur*, upper part of the thigh]. Pertaining to the os pubis and the femur, as the pubofemoral ligament, a collateral ligament of the hip joint capsule.

pu"bo·per"i·to·ne·al'is. A variant of the transverse abdominal muscle.

pu"bo·pro·stat'ic [*pubes;* G. *prostatēs*, one who stands before]. Pertaining to the pubic bone and the prostate gland.

pu"bo·rec·tal'is. A part of the levator ani muscle.

pu"bo·trans·ver·sal'is. A variant of the transverse abdominal muscle.

pu"bo·ves'i·cal [*pubes;* L. *vesica*, bladder]. Pertaining to the pubic bone and the urinary bladder.

pu"bo·ves·i·cal'is. A portion of the levator ani muscle.

pu'chi·in. An antibiotic substance derived from the Chinese water chestnut *Eleocharis tuberosa*, active, in vitro, against several bacterial species.

pu"den·dag'ra (pew"den·dag'ruh, ·day'gruh) [L. *pudendus*, that of which one ought to be ashamed; G. *agra*, seizure]. Pain in the genital organs.

pu·den'dum (pl. *pudenda*) [*pudendus*]. The external genital organs, especially of the female. —**pudendal,** *adj.*

p. muliebre. The vulva.

pu'dic [L. *pudicus*, shameful, modest]. Old term for pudendal.

Puente's disease. Simple glandular cheilitis.

pu'er·i·cul"ture (pew'ur·i·kul"chur, pew·err'i·) [L. *puer*, boy; *cultura*, cultivation]. The specialty of child training.

pu'er·il·ism [L. *puerilis*, boyish]. Childishness. —**puerile,** *adj.*

pu"er·i'ti·a (pew"ur·ish'ee·uh) [L., boyhood]. Second childhood.

pu·er'per·a (pew·ur'pur·uh) [L. *puerperus*, bringing forth children]. A woman who is in labor or has recently been delivered.

pu·er'per·al (pew·ur'pur·ul) [*puerperus*]. Pertaining to, caused by, or following childbirth, as puerperal convulsions, puerperal eclampsia.

pu·er'per·al·ism [*puerperus*]. The state brought about by pathologic conditions of pregnancy.

pu·er'per·ant [*puerperus*]. A woman who has been recently delivered.

pu"er·pe'ri·um (pew"ur·peer'ee·um) [L., childbirth]. 1. The state of a woman in labor, or of one who has just been delivered. 2. The period from delivery to the time when the uterus has regained its normal size, which is about six weeks.

puff'ball" [ME. *puf; bal*]. Any of the fungi Lycoperdaceae which discharge their ripe spores like dust when struck. Many are edible when unripe.

Pugh's test. See under *test.*

pu·gil'lus. Handful. Abbreviated, P.

pu'le·gone. $C_{10}H_{16}O$; 1-methyl-4-isopropylidene-3-cyclohexanone; a liquid constituent of many volatile oils from plants of the Labiatae family.

Pu'lex [L., flea]. A genus of fleas.

P. irritans. The human flea; a species which is the intermediate host and transmitter of *Dipylidium caninum* and *Hymenolepis diminuta*, and may spread plague. It is parasitic on the skin of man and also infests hogs, dogs, and other mammals.

Pulfrich photometer. An instrument used to determine the concentration of a solution by matching its color to a solution of known concentration, observed at the same time.

pu"li·car'is (pew"li·kair'iss) [L. *pulicaris*, of fleas]. Marked with little spots like flea bites.

PULHES See *physical profile serial.*

pu"li·ca'ti·o (pew"li·kay'shee·o) [L. *pulicare*, to produce fleas]. The state of being infested with fleas.

Pu·lic'i·dae (pew·liss'i·dee) [L. *pulex*, flea]. A family of fleas or Siphonaptera of which the most important to man are the genera *Pulex*, *Xenopsylla*, and *Ctenocephalides*.

pu'li·cide [*pulex;* L. *caedere*, to kill]. An agent capable of killing fleas.

Pul·lu·lar'i·a. A genus of thick-walled black fungi with budding spores, common as laboratory contaminants. Syn., *Dematium.*

pul'lu·late [L. *pullulare*, to put forth]. Germinate, bud.

pul"lu·la'tion [*pullulare*]. The act of sprouting or budding, a mode of reproduction seen in the yeast plant.

pul'mo- [L., lung]. A combining form meaning *lung.*

pul'mo·nar"y (pul'mo·nerr"ee, pŏŏl'mo·) [L. *pulmonarius*, of the lungs]. Pertaining to, or affecting, the lungs or any anatomic component of the lungs. Syn., *pulmonic.*

pul"mo·nec'to·my. See *pneumonectomy.*

pul·mon'ic. See *pulmonary.*

pul"mo·ni'tis. See *pneumonia.*

pul'mo"tor (pul'mo"tur, pŏŏl'mo"tur) [L. *pulmo*, lung; *motor*, from *movere*, to move]. An apparatus for resuscitating persons who have been asphyxiated; it expels the gas from the lungs, introduces oxygen, and automatically establishes artificial respiration.

pulp [L. *pulpa*, solid flesh]. 1. The soft, fleshy part of fruit. 2. The soft part in the interior of an organ, as the pulp of the spleen, the pulp of a tooth. —**pulp'al, pulp'ar,** *adj.*

dental p. The soft vascular tissue which fills the pulp chamber and the root canals of a tooth and is responsible for its vitality. It consists of connective tissue, blood vessels, and nerves. A superficial layer of cells, the odontoblasts, supplies branching processes which occupy tubules in the dentin. Also called *tooth p.*

digital p. The sensitive, elastic, convex prominence on the palmar or plantar surface of the terminal phalanx of a finger or toe.

enamel p. The cells between the outer and inner enamel epithelium of the enamel organ. They include the stellate reticulum and the stratum intermedium.

p. of the finger. See digital *p.*

p. of the intervertebral disk. The soft substance in the center of the intervertebral disks, the remains of the notochord.

red p. See *spleen*, red pulp *cords.*

splenic p. The proper substance of the spleen.

white p. See *spleen.*

pul'pa. See *pulp. Obs.*

pul·pal'gi·a [*pulpa;* G. *algos*, pain]. Pain in the dental pulp.

pul·pa'tion [*pulpa*]. The act or process of reducing to a pulp.

pul'pec'to·my [*pulpa;* G. *ektomē*, excision]. Excision or extirpation of a dental pulp.

pulp"i·fac'tion [*pulpa;* L. *facere*, to make]. Conversion into a pulpy substance.

pulp'i·form [*pulpa;* L. *forma*, form]. Similar to, or resembling, pulp.

pulp'i·fy [*pulpa;* L. *facere*, to make]. Reduce to a pulpy condition.

pulp·i'tis [*pulpa;* G. *-itis*, inflammation]. An inflammation of the dental pulp.

hyperplastic p. A chronic inflammatory response characterized by protrusion of the pulp of a tooth through an opening in the pulp chamber, usually seen in young individuals with a deep carious lesion that exposes the pulp. Syn., *hypertrophic pulp, pulp polyp.*

pulp·ot'o·my [*pulpa;* G. *tomē*, a cutting]. The surgical removal of part of the pulp of a tooth.

pulp'stone". See *denticle*, 2.

pulp'y [*pulpa*]. Resembling pulp; characterized by the formation of a substance resembling pulp.

pulque. See *aguamiel.*

pul'sate [L. *pulsare*, to beat]. Beat or throb.

pul'sa·tile (pul'suh·til) [*pulsare*]. Pulsating; throbbing.

pul"sa·til'la (*pulsatilla*). The dried herb of *Anemone pulsatilla*, *A. pratensis*, or *A. patens.* The drug yields a volatile oil from which can be separated a crystallizable, intensely acrid substance known as pulsatilla camphor or anemonin. It is a powerful local irritant, and when taken in sufficient amount produces gastroenteritis with vomiting and purging, and often with evidence of kidney irritation. In large doses it is a powerful depressant to the central nervous system and to the heart. There is no evidence that it possesses any therapeutic virtues not ascribable to its local irritating effect. Also called *pasqueflower.*

pul·sa'tion [L. *pulsatio*, from *pulsare*]. A beating or throbbing.

suprasternal p. Pulsation at the suprasternal notch. It may be due to aneurysm, a dilated aortic arch, or the presence of an anomalous artery.

pul·sa'tor [L., from *pulsare*]. A mechanical device

which produces pulsations; used in physical therapy.

pulse [L. *pulsus*, a striking, from *pellere*, to strike]. The intermittent change in the shape of an artery due to an increase in the tension of its walls following the contraction of the heart. The pulse is usually counted at the wrist (radial pulse), but may be taken over any artery that is palpable, as the temporal, brachial, femoral, dorsalis pedis, etc.

alternating p. A variety in which there are alternations in amplitude of pulse waves, that is, large pulsations alternating with small ones in cycles of equal length. It occurs in normal hearts with excessive tachycardia, and may occur with a slow rate if the myocardium is impaired. Also called *pulsus alternans*.

anacrotic p. One with a notch in the ascending limb, palpable and seen on sphygmograms, especially in aortic stenosis.

anatricrotic p. A pulse wave with three breaks on the ascending curve.

angry p. Wiry pulse.

ardent p. One with a quick, full wave which seems to strike the finger at a single point.

bigeminal p. See *bigeminy*.

capillary p. An intermittent filling and emptying of the capillaries of the skin. It is common in aortic regurgitation, and is seen under the fingernail or on the forehead.

collapsing p. See water-hammer *p*.

contracted p. A small pulse with high tension.

Corrigan's p. See water-hammer *p*.

decurtate p. A progressively decreasing pulse.

dicrotic p. One in which the dicrotic wave or recoil wave is exaggerated. It is observed when the arterial tension is low, and gives to the finger the impression of two beats.

entoptic p. The subjective illumination of a dark visual field with each heart beat, a condition sometimes noted after violent exercise, and due to the mechanical irritation of the rods by the pulsating retinal arteries.

febrile p. That characteristic of fever: full, soft, and frequent, and exhibiting a well-marked dicrotism.

filiform p. A small, thready, almost imperceptible pulse.

formicant p. A small, feeble pulse likened to the movements of ants.

frequent p. One recurring at short intervals.

full p. One in which the artery is filled with a large volume of blood and conveys a feeling of being distended.

funic p. The arterial tide in the umbilical cord.

gaseous p. A full, compressible pulse.

goat-leap p. A pulse marked by a weak pulsation succeeding a strong one.

guttural p. One felt in the throat.

hard p. One characterized by high tension and rigidity.

high-tension p. One due to increase of the peripheral resistance, together with a corresponding increase in the force of the ventricular systole. It is gradual in its impulse, long in duration, slow in subsiding, with difficulty compressible, and the artery between the beats feels like a firm round cord.

hyperdicrotic p. A pulse in which the dicrotic wave is abnormally palpable.

incisura p. One showing a sharp fall in pulse pressure.

infrequent p. One which has a slower rate than normal.

intermittent p. One in which one or more beats are dropped.

intricate p. A pulse that is irregular, small, and infrequent.

irregular p. One in which the beats occur at irregular intervals, or in which the force, or both rhythm and force, varies.

jerky p. A pulse in which the artery is suddenly and markedly distended, as in aortic regurgitation.

jugular p. Pulsation of the jugular veins.

low-tension p. One sudden in its onset, short, and quickly declining. It is easily obliterated by pressure.

monocrotic p. One in which dicrotism is absent.

paradoxic p. One that is weaker during inspiration, a condition sometimes observed in acute and chronic cardiac compression. Syn., *pulsus paradoxus*.

pistol-shot p. The pulse produced by rapid distention and collapse of an artery, as occurs classically in aortic regurgitation. This produces an auscultatory phenomenon resembling a pistol shot.

plateau p. The prolonged pulse, usually with an anacrotic interruption, seen in aortic stenosis.

pressure p. The recorded pressure variations in a given heart chamber or blood vessel during the cardiac cycle; pressure curve.

quadrigeminal p. A pulse in which a pause occurs after every fourth beat.

quick p. One that strikes the finger rapidly, but also leaves it rapidly.

Quincke's p. A capillary pulse due to a high pulse pressure; seen classically in aortic regurgitation and elicited clinically by applying light pressure to a fingernail. See capillary *p*.

respiratory p. The modification in the pulse produced by respiration.

running p. A very weak, frequent pulse with low tension in the arteries, one pulse wave running into the next with no apparent interval; it is observed after hemorrhage.

soft p. A pulse that is readily compressed.

supradicrotic p. A pulse in which the preceding dicrotic wave falls on the ascending limb of the next pulse wave (in tachycardia).

thready p. One that is scarcely perceptible, feeling like a thread under the finger.

tricrotic p. A pulse in which the three waves normally present are abnormally distinct.

trigeminal p. A pulse in which a pause occurs every third beat.

ultrasonic p. A pulse of ultrasonic energy. See also *ultrasonoscope*.

unequal p. A pulse unequal in symmetrical arteries.

vagus p. A slow pulse due to the inhibitory action of the vagus on the heart.

venous p. A pulse observed in a vein.

vermicular p. A pulse imitating the movement of a worm.

vibrating p. A hard pulse with a wave arising quickly, giving the impression under the finger of the vibrations of a piece of tense catgut.

water-hammer p. The pulse observed in aortic regurgitation, characterized by a rapid rise and fall, combined with large amplitude.

wiry p. A small, rapid, tense pulse, which feels like a cord. Observed in acute peritonitis.

pulse breath. A peculiar, audible pulsation of the breath corresponding to the heart beats; observed in cases of dry cavities of the lungs, with thick walls not separated from the heart by permeable lung tissue.

pulse clock. A sphygmograph.

pulse curve. The tracing of the pulse, called a sphygmogram and made by the sphygmograph.

pulse cy'cle. The period between the beginning and end of a pulse wave.

pulse def'i·cit. The difference between the auscultatory heart rate and the rate of the peripheral pulse determined palpably.

pulse'less [L. *pulsus*, a striking, from *pellere*, to strike; AS. *-lēas*, free from]. Devoid of pulse or pulsation.

pulse pres'sure. See under *pressure*.

pulse wave. See under *wave*.

pul·sim'e·ter [*pulsus;* G. *metron*, a measure]. An instrument for determining the rate or force of the pulse.

pul'sion [L. *pulsio*, a striking]. The act of pushing forward.

p. diverticulum. That caused by pressure from within.

pul·som'e·ter. See *pulsimeter*.

pul'sus [L.]. The pulse.

p. bisferiens. A pulse wave surmounted by two peaks.

p. celer. A quick, short pulse.

p. celer et altus. A quick, full pulse, seen especially in aortic regurgitation.

p. debilis. A weak pulse.

p. duplex. A dicrotic pulse.

p. durus. A hard, incompressible pulse.

p. irregularis perpetuus. The pulse of atrial fibrillation which is perpetually irregular in rate and amplitude.

p. paradoxus. See paradoxic *pulse*.

p. parvus. A pulse small in amplitude.

p. parvus et tardus. The small, slowly rising pulse characteristic of aortic stenosis.

p. tardus. A pulse with a gradual ascent to the peak.

pul·ta'ceous [L. *puls*, porridge]. Having the consistence of pulp; mushy; soft.

pulv. *Pulvis;* powder.

pul'ver·ize [L. *pulvis*, dust, powder]. Reduce a substance to a powder. —**pulveriza'tion,** *n.*

pul·vi'nar [L., couch]. A nuclear mass forming the posterior tubercle of the thalamus.

pul'vis. Abbreviated, pulv. See *powder*.

pulvule. Trade-mark for a capsule containing a powdered drug.

pu'mex. See *pumice*.

pum'ice (pum'iss) [L. *pumex*, pumice stone]. A substance of volcanic origin, consisting chiefly of complex silicates of aluminum, potassium, and sodium; occurs as a very light, hard, rough, porous gray mass, or as a gritty, gray-colored powder. It is used in the arts as an abrasive, either in the original form, or in the powdered form as a basis for metal polish. *In pharmacy*, it is used to assist in distributing the particles of extracts, tar, and resins to facilitate solution.

pump [ME. *pumpe*, probably imitative in origin]. An apparatus which draws up a fluid into a hollow chamber, or, after sucking up the fluid, forcibly ejects it from one end.

air p. One used to exhaust the air from a chamber, or to force more air into a chamber already containing air.

blood p. A device capable of pumping blood rapidly into an artery or vein of a severely exsanguinated patient.

breast p. A pump for removing milk from the breast.

dental p. See saliva *ejector*.

stomach p. One for removing the contents of the stomach in cases of poisoning.

pump'kin seed. The dried, ripe seed of several varieties of *Cucurbita pepo*. The active constituents are resinous in character. It is used as an anthelmintic and taeniafuge. Dose, 30–60 Gm. (1–2 oz.), shelled and bruised, stirred in a thick syrup and flavored. It should be followed by a cathartic.

punch [ME. *ponchon*]. A surgical instrument for perforating or cutting out a disk or segment of resistant tissue, as cartilage, bone.

cervical p. See under *clamp*.

punch drunk. A postconcussional syndrome occurring in prize fighters.

punc'tate, punc'tat·ed (punk'tay·tid) [L. *punctum*, point]. Dotted; full of minute points.

punc·tic'u·lum [dim. from *punctum*]. A small point.

punc'ti·form [*punctum;* L. *forma*, form]. 1. Having the nature or qualities of a point; seeming to be located at a point, as a punctiform sensation. 2. *In bacteriology*, denoting very minute colonies.

punc'to·graph. [L. *punctum*, point; *graphein*, to write]. A radiographic instrument for the surgical localization of foreign bodies, as bullets embedded in the tissues.

punc'tum (pl. *puncta*) [L.]. Point.

puncta lacrimalia. The orifices of the lacrimal ducts in the eyelids near the inner canthus.

puncta vasculosa. Minute red spots studding the cut surface of the white central mass of the fresh brain. They are produced by the blood escaping from divided blood vessels.

puncta dolorosa. Tender or painful points at the exit or in the course of nerves; the seat of neuralgia.

p. proximum. Near point. Abbreviated, P., P.p.

p. remotum. Far point. Abbreviated, P.r.

punc'ture [L. *punctura*, puncture]. 1. A hole made by the piercing of a pointed instrument. 2. The procedure of making a puncture.

cisternal p. Puncture of the cisterna magna with a hollow needle, for diagnostic or therapeutic purposes: also called *cranial puncture*.

diabetic p. Puncture on the floor of the fourth ventricle, which produces glycosuria.

exploratory p. The puncture of a cyst or cavity for removal of a portion of the contents for examination.

lumbar p. Puncture of the spinal canal, usually between the third and fourth lumbar vertebrae, for the removal of fluid or the introduction of drugs or serums.

spinal p. See lumbar *p.*

splenic p. Needle biopsy of the spleen.

sternal p. Puncture of the manubrium with a hollow needle to obtain bone marrow specimens in disease of the hematopoietic system.

tibial p. A puncture method used in children to secure smears of marrow cells. A sternal puncture needle is used in the middle of the shaft of the tibia.

ventricular p. Puncture into one of the lateral ventricles of the brain to introduce air in ventriculography.

punc'tured [*punctura*]. Produced by a prick, or a piercing instrument, weapon, or missile, as a punctured wound.

pun'gent [L. *pungere*, to pierce into]. Acrid; penetrating; producing a painful sensation.

Pu'ni·ca [L. *Punicum malum*, pomegranate]. A genus of polypetalous plants.

P. granatum. See under *pelletierine* tannate.

pu'ni·cine (pew'ni·seen, ·sin). See *pelletierine*.

punk'to·graph. See *punctograph*.

pu·nu'dos (poo·nōō'dos, pew'new·dos). A disease resembling leprosy, found in Guatemala.

P. U. O. Pyrexia of unknown origin.

pu'pa [L., girl]. The stage, usually quiescent, in the life history of some insects, which follows the larval period and precedes the adult imago. —**pupal,** *adj.*

pu'pil [L. *pupilla*, pupil of the eye]. The aperture in the iris of the eye for the passage of light. See Plate 19. —**pupillary,** *adj.*

Adie's p. An anomaly of the pupil which includes abnormality in the size of the pupil (usually eccentrically dilated) and delay in, but not loss of, the reaction of the pupil either to light or in accommodation. Sometimes called *tonic pupil.* See Adie's *syndrome.*

Argyll Robertson p. One that constricts on accommodation, but not to light; it is seen in tabes dorsalis, and occasionally in other diseases. Also called *Argyll Robertson sign.*

artificial p. An aperture made by iridectomy when the normal pupil is occluded.

cat's-eye p. An elongated, slitlike pupil.

Hutchinson's p. A widely dilated, inactive pupil which demonstrates no reflex activity, seen in severe concussion injuries to the head, usually ipsilateral to the side of injury.

multiple p. The presence of bands dividing the pupil into several portions, due to persistence of portions of the fetal pupillary membrane.

pinhole p. Contraction of the iris until the pupil is scarcely larger than a pin's head. It is seen in opium poisoning, after the use of miotics, in certain cerebral diseases, and in locomotor ataxia. Also called *pinpoint p.*

pseudo Argyll Robertson p. One reacting neither directly nor consensually to ordinary light but which may constrict slightly to bright light; convergence-accommodation response is delayed, but there is a normal response to homatropine and eserine. The cause is unknown. Also called *Adie's pupil.*

tonic p. See Adie's *p.*

pu·pil'la [L.]. The pupil of the eye.

pu"pil·lom'e·ter [*pupilla;* G. *metron,* a measure]. An instrument for measuring the pupil of the eye.

pu"pil·lo·sta·tom'e·ter (pew"pi·lo·sta·tom'i·tur, pew·pill"o·) [*pupilla;* G. *statos,* standing; *metron,* a measure]. An instrument for measuring the exact distance between the centers of the two pupils.

pu"pil·lo·ton'ic pseu"do·ta'bes. Adie's syndrome.

Purcell, Edward Mills (1912–). American physicist, known for his extensive research in electron ballistics, cyclotron development, microwave radar, and nuclear magnetism. In 1952 he shared the Nobel prize with Felix Bloch for work in the exploration of the atomic nucleus.

Purdy, Charles Wesley [*American physician,* 1846–1901]. Known for his contributions to methods of urinalysis. Introduced a modification of Fehling's solution for quantitative estimation of glucose, called *Purdy's solution.* Introduced a test for albumin in the urine. See Purdy's *test.*

pure [L. *purus,* free from dirt]. 1. Free from mixture or contact with that which weakens or pollutes; containing no foreign or extraneous material. 2. Chaste.

pure line. All the progeny of a single completely homozygous individual, reproducing by self-fertilization. By extension, applied also to organisms with biparental reproduction where the condition of complete homozygosis is realized, and to the progeny of a single individual reproducing asexually. See *clone.*

pur'ga·tin. See *anthrapurpurin* acetate.

pur·ga'tion [L. *purgatio,* a cleansing]. 1. The evacuation of the bowels by means of purgatives. 2. Cleansing.

pur'ga·tive [L. *purgativus,* purgative]. Producing purgation.

pur'ga·tive. A purge.

pur'ga·tol. See *anthrapurpurin* acetate.

purge [L. *purgare,* to cleanse]. To cause free evacuation of the bowel.

purge. A drug that causes free evacuation of the bowel.

purg'ing [*purgare*]. A condition in which there is rapid and continuous evacuation of the bowels.

pu'ri·fied [L. *purificare,* to make clean]. Cleansed; freed from extraneous matter.

pu'ri·form [L. *pus,* pus; *forma,* form]. In the form of or resembling pus.

pu'rine (pure'een, ·in). The synthetic substance $C_5H_4N_4$, having the following structure:

```
N=CH
|   |
HC  C—NH
‖   ‖    \
‖   ‖     CH
‖   ‖    //
N—C—N
```

Various derivatives of this structure, generically called *purines* and including the xanthines and uric acid, are widely distributed in nature.

endogenous purines. Those originating from nuclein cleavage during metabolic processes.

exogenous purines. Those derived from the purine bodies of foodstuffs.

pu'ri·ty. *In optics,* the percentage contribution to luminous intensity by the dominant wavelength in a beam of light.

Purkinje, Johannes Evangelista von [*Bohemian physiologist,* 1787–1869]. One of the early users of the microtome. Pointed out the importance of fingerprints (1823). Studied ciliary epithelial motion (1835). First to use the term protoplasm (1839). Images on the retina from shadows of blood vessels are called *Purkinje's images.* Observed that fields of different color and equal brightness become unequally bright when illumination is decreased in brightness; called *Purkinje's phenomenon.* See also *Purkinje cells* under *cell, Purkinje fibers* under *fiber,* germinal *vesicle, Purkinje-Sanson images* under *image.*

Purmann, Matthaeus Gottfried [*German military surgeon,* 1648–1721]. One of the most famous of the army surgeons of his time. His methods of treatment were largely empirical. He is said to have extirpated the aneurysmal sac as a cure for aneurysm; called *Purmann's method* (1690).

purodigin. A trade-mark for digitoxin.

pu"ro·hep"a·ti'tis [L. *pus,* pus; G. *hēpar,* liver; *-itis,* inflammation]. Suppurative inflammation of the liver.

pu"ro·mu'cous [*pus;* L. *mucus,* mucus]. Consisting of mucus mixed with pus; mucopurulent.

pu"ro·thi'o·nin. An antibiotic substance derived from wheat flour, effective in inhibiting the growth, in vitro, of *Streptococcus viridans.*

pur'pu·ra [L., purple]. A condition in which hemorrhages occur in the skin, mucous membranes, serous membranes, and elsewhere. The two general types of lesion seen in the skin are petechiae and ecchymoses. —**purpu'ric,** *adj.*

allergic p. 1. Any purpura, thrombocytopenic or nonthrombocytopenic which results from an allergic reaction. 2. Henoch-Schönlein purpura. In this disorder, the cutaneous manifestations include erythematous and urticarial exanthema. Also called *anaphylactoid p.*

essential p. See idiopathic thrombocytopenic *p.*

hemorrhagic p. See idiopathic thrombocytopenic *p.*

Henoch's p. A nonthrombocytopenic purpura associated with gastrointestinal pain and bleeding and with erythematous or urticarial exanthema. The distinction between this disorder, Schönlein's *p.*, and allergic *p.* is not clear.

idiopathic thrombocytopenic p. Thrombocytopenic purpura of unknown cause. In some cases agglutinins of blood platelets have been demonstrated. Also called *essential p.*, *primary p.*, *thrombocytolytic p.*, *land scurvy*, *morbus maculosis Werlhofi*, *Werlhof's disease*.

mechanical p. That due to violent muscular contractions or application of a tourniquet, not associated with any other blood or vascular defects.

orthostatic p. Purpura, probably due to weakness of capillary walls, which sometimes develops in the lower extremities after long standing.

primary p. See idiopathic thrombocytopenic *p.*

p. annularis telangiectodes. An eruption of purpuric spots, grouped in ring form and accompanied by telangiectasis: described by D. Majocchi.

p. fulminans. A grave form, occurring principally in children with acute infectious disease, of short duration, and usually fatal.

p. hyperglobulinemia. Hemorrhagic diathesis attributed to elevation of the concentration of globulin in the serum.

p. necrotica. A condition characterized by enormous ecchymotic skin lesions which in later stages become necrotic and gangrenous.

p. rheumatica. See Schönlein's *p.*

p. senilis. One in which capillary resistance is low in old persons, thus creating a marked tendency to bruises.

p. simplex. A mild form not associated with well-defined defects of blood-clotting mechanisms or mucous-membrane bleeding: often familial and particularly prone to occur in females.

p. urticans. That associated with urticaria. See *urticaria* hemorrhagica.

quinidine p. Purpura following the use of quinidine, often associated with thrombocytopenia.

rheumatic p. See Schönlein's *p.*

Schönlein's p. A nonthrombocytopenic form marked by tenderness and pain of the joints or limbs, associated with periarticular effusions, and mild fever, and with erythematous or urticarial exanthema: also called *peliosis rheumatica* or *rheumatic purpura*. The distinction between this disorder, Henoch's *p.*, and allergic *p.* is not clear.

senile p. Purpura occurring in elderly persons of both sexes, clinically characterized by the large (1–4 cm), irregular but well-defined ecchymoses localized on the extensor surfaces of the forearm, the back of the hand but not fingers, and the face. The condition is not linked to any recognizable systemic disorder or dietary deficiency; histologically, it is constantly associated with extreme thinning and other degenerative changes of the exposed skin, and the lesions are thought to be due to minor trauma affecting inadequately supported superficial vessels.

symptomatic p. That which may accompany acute infectious diseases or chronic diseases such as malignant tumors, nephritis, and blood dyscrasias, and following administration of certain drugs. Also called *secondary p.*

thrombocytolytic p. See idiopathic thrombocytopenic *p.*

thrombocytopathic p. That associated with a normal number of qualitatively defective platelets.

thrombocytopenic p. That associated with thrombocytopenia.

thrombotic thrombocytopenic p. A rare, highly fatal disorder characterized by acute thrombocytopenic purpura and diffuse formation of thrombi in the capillaries. Hemolytic anemia and transitory focal neurological signs often accompany the clinical picture. The thrombi are thought by many to be the result of action of agglutinins of platelets. Also called *Moschkowitz's syndrome*.

toxic p. That caused by various poisons such as arsenic, phosphorus, phenolphthalein, heparin.

pur′pu·rin. $C_{14}H_8O_5$. 1. A dye present with alizarin in madder-root, but also prepared artificially. 2. Uroerythrin, a red pigment sometimes present in urinary deposits.

pur″pu·ri·nu′ri·a [*purpura;* G. *ouron*, urine]. The presence of purpurin in the urine; porphyruria.

pur″pu·ro·gal′lin. $C_{11}H_4(OH)_4O$; a dicyclic tropolone derivative, having a red color, formed by oxidation of pyrogallol, and also found in various galls in glycosidal combination.

purr [imitative in origin]. A low-pitched murmur.

pur′ring thrill. A fine, trembling vibration like the purring of a cat, perceived by palpation over the precordia. It may be due to aneurysm or to mitral stenosis.

Purtscher, Otmar [*German ophthalmologist*, 1852–1927]. Described traumatic angiopathy of the retina (1912); also called *liporrhagia retinalis*, *Purtscher's disease*.

pu′ru·lence (pure′yoo·luns) [L. *purulentia*, purulent mass]. The quality or state of containing pus. Also called *purulency*.

pu′ru·lent (pure′yoo·lunt) [L. *purulentus*, purulent]. Containing, consisting of, or forming pus.

pu′ru·loid [pure′yoo·loyd) [*purulentus;* G. *eidos*, form]. Resembling pus; puriform.

pu·ru″pu·ru′. Pinta.

pus [L.]. A semifluid, creamy, yellow or greenish yellow product of inflammation composed mainly of leukocytes and serum. The color varies with the causative organism.

blue p. Pus having a blue-green color because of the pigments liberated by the multiplication of *Pseudomonas aeruginosa*.

pus-tube. Lay term for pyosalpinx.

pus′tu·lant [L. *pustula*, blister]. 1. Causing the formation of pustules. 2. An irritant substance giving rise to the formation of pustules.

pus″tu·la′tion [*pustula*]. The formation of pustules.

pus′tule [*pustula*]. A small, circumscribed elevation of the skin containing pus. —**pustular, pustulose, pustulous,** *adj.*

malignant p. Anthrax. See Plate 31.

pus′tu·li·form″ [*pustula;* L. *forma*, form]. Resembling a pustule.

pus″tu·lo·der′ma [*pustula;* G. *derma*, skin]. Any skin disease characterized by the formation of pustules.

pus″tu·lo′sis pal·mar′is et plan·tar′is. Any chronic resistant noninfectious dermatitis chiefly of palms and soles. The pustules are sterile, deep-seated, and appear in continuous crops. It includes several entities: pustular bacterid, and what has been pustular psoriasis (Barber). Syn., *pustular acrodermatoses*.

pu·ta′men [L., that which falls off in pruning]. The outer darker part of the lenticular nucleus of the brain.

Putnam, James Jackson [*American neurologist*, 1846–1918]. Remembered for his contributions to the knowledge of pathologic anatomy and the physiology of the nervous system. Described pernicious anemia with dorsolateral sclerosis; called *Putnam's type of spinal sclerosis*, *Putnam-Dana syndrome*.

pu″tre·fac′tion [L. *putrefactio*, from *putrefacere*, to become rotten]. The decomposition of organic matter under the influence of microorganisms, accompanied by the development of disagreeable odors. The products include gases, as ammonia, hydrogen sulfide, methane, and others; acids, as acetic, lactic, butyric, and others; and toxic substances, as indole, skatole, phenol, and others.

Cadaverine and putrescine are toxic products known as ptomaines.

pu″tre·fac′tive [*putrefacere*]. Pertaining to or causing putrefaction.

pu′tre·fy [*putrefacere*]. Render putrid.

pu·tres′cent. Undergoing putrefaction. —**putres′cence,** *n.*

pu·tres′cine (pew·tress′een, ·in). $NH_2(CH_2)_4NH_2$; tetramethylenediamine; a product of decarboxylation of ornithine and also found in putrefying flesh: formerly believed to be responsible for food poisoning, and referred to as a ptomaine.

pu′trid [L. *putridus*, rotten]. Rotten; characterized by putrefaction.

pu′tro·maine. A ptomaine developed in putrefactive processes.

PVP Abbreviation for polyvinyl pyrrolidone.

py·ae′mi·a. See *pyemia*.

py″ar·thro′sis [G. *pyon*, pus; *arthron*, joint; *-ōsis*, condition]. Suppuration of a joint.

pyc″no·ep′i·lep″sy. See *pyknolepsy*.

pyc·nom′e·ter [G. *pyknos*, compact, thick; *metron*, a measure]. An instrument for the determination of the specific gravity of fluids.

pyc″no·mor′phous, pyk″no·mor′phous [*pyknos;* G. *morphē*, form]. Applied to nerve cells in which the chromophil substance of the cytoplasm is compactly arranged.

pyc″no·phra′si·a (pick″no·fray′zhuh, ·zee·uh) [*pyknos;* G. *phrasis*, speech]. Thickness of speech.

pyc·no′sis [G. *pyknōsis*, dense mass]. 1. Thickening; inspissation. 2. A degenerative change in cells whereby the nucleus is condensed and shrinks to a dense, structureless mass of chromatin. —**pycnot′ic,** *adj.*

py·ec′chy·sis (pye·eck′i·sis) [G. *pyon*, pus; *ekchysis*, outflow]. Effusion of pus.

py″e·lec·ta′si·a (pye″i·leck·tay′zhuh, ·zee·uh, ·shuh, ·see·uh) [G. *pyelos*, trough; *ektasis*, extension]. Dilatation of a renal pelvis.

py″e·li′tis. Inflammation of the pelvis of a kidney. —**pyelit′ic,** *adj.*

calculous p. That due to calculi.

p. cystica. A type of nonspecific chronic inflammatory reaction of the kidney pelvis, characterized by the pressure of numerous minute translucent cysts scattered over the surface of the pelvic mucosa. The cysts are apparently due to metaplasia of the epithelial cells resulting in the formation of glandular acini or cysts.

py′e·lo- [*pyelos*]. A combining form denoting *relation to the pelvis of the kidney.*

py″e·lo·cys·ti′tis [*pyelos;* G. *kystis*, bladder; *-itis*, inflammation]. Pyelitis with cystitis.

py′e·lo·gram″ [*pyelos;* G. *gramma*, letter]. A roentgenogram of the renal pelvis and ureter.

pseudospider p. See pseudospider *pelvis*.

py″e·log′ra·phy [*pyelos;* G. *graphein*, to write]. Roentgenography of a renal pelvis and ureter which have been filled with an opaque solution. Also see *urography*.

retrograde p. That following ureteral catheterization and the filling of the upper urinary tract with a contrast medium as part of a cystographic procedure. Syn., *retrograde urography*.

py″e·lo·li·thot′o·my [*pyelos;* G. *lithos*, stone; *tomē*, a cutting]. Removal of a renal calculus through an incision into the pelvis of a kidney.

py″e·lo·ne·phri′tis [*pyelos;* G. *nephros*, kidney; *-itis*, inflammation]. Interstitial inflammation of one or both kidneys, usually involving both parenchyma and pelvis, due to bacterial invasion from the middle and lower urinary tracts or the periureteral lymphatics (**ascending p.**) or from the blood stream (**descending p., hematogenous p.**). —**pyelonephrit′ic,** *adj.*

py′e·lo·plas″ty [*pyelos;* G. *plassein*, to form]. Plastic repair of the renal pelvis.

py″e·lo·pli·ca′tion (pye″i·lo·plye·kay′shun, ·pli·kay′shun) [*pyelos;* L. *plicare*, to fold]. Reducing an enlarged renal pelvis by plicating or suturing the infolded walls.

py″e·los′co·py [*pyelos;* G. *skopein*, to examine]. Fluoroscopic examination of the pelvis of a kidney.

py″e·los′to·my [*pyelos;* G. *stoma*, mouth]. Incision into the renal pelvis.

py″e·lot′o·my [*pyelos;* G. *tomē*, a cutting]. Incision of the renal pelvis.

py″e·lo·u·re″ter·og′ra·phy. See *pyelography*.

py″e·lo·ve′nous back′flow″. The phenomenon of drainage from the renal veins into the inferior vena cava, due to back pressure.

py·em′e·sis (pye·em′i·sis) [G. *pyon*, pus; *emesis*, vomiting]. Vomiting of pus.

py·e′mi·a (pye·ee′mee·uh) [*pyon;* G. *haima*, blood]. A disease due to the presence of pyogenic microorganisms in the blood and the formation, wherever these organisms lodge, of embolic or metastatic abscesses. —**pyemic,** *adj.*

arterial p. That produced by disorganization of a cardiac thrombus and the dissemination of emboli through the arterial circulation.

cryptogenic p. A condition in which the primary suppuration occurs in the deeper tissues of the body.

otogenous p. Pyemia originating in the ear.

py″en·ceph′a·lus [*pyon;* G. *egkephalos*, brain]. Suppuration within the brain.

py·gal′gi·a (pye·gal′juh, ·jee·uh) [G. *pygē*, rump; *algos*, pain]. Pain in the buttocks.

pyg·ma′li·on·ism [G. *Pygmaliōn*, sculptor who fell in love with a statue he carved]. The psychopathic condition in which an individual falls in love with a creation of his own.

pyg′my [G. *pygmaios*, dwarfish, from *pygmē*, a measure of length]. A small person or dwarf.

py″go·a·mor′phus [G. *pygē*, rump; *a-*, not; *morphē*, form]. A monster with a teratoma in the sacral region.

py″go·did′y·mus [*pygē;* G. *didymos*, twin]. Conjoined twins united by the buttocks. Syn., *pygopagus*.

py·gom′e·lus (pye·gom′i·lus) [*pygē;* G. *melos*, limb]. A monster with an accessory limb or limbs attached to the buttock.

py·gop′a·gus (pye·gop′uh·gus) [*pygē;* G. *pagos*, that which is fixed]. Conjoined twins united in the sacral region. See Plate 25.

py″go·par″a·si′tus [*pygē;* G. *parasitos*, parasite]. A monster consisting of unequal conjoined twins with the parasite attached to the nates of the autosite. Special monsters of this general type were called by Taruffi pygomelus, pygoamorphus, and pygoteratoides.

py″go·ter″a·toi′des (pye″go·terr″uh·toy′deez) [*pygē;* G. *teras*, monster; *eidos*, form]. A monster with teratoid tumors in the region of the sacrum.

py′ic [G. *pyon*, pus]. Purulent. *Obs.*

py′in [*pyon*]. An albuminous substance of complex constitution occurring in pus. It may be separated by adding sodium chloride and filtering.

pyk′nic [G. *pyknos*, thick, compact]. Referring to a constitutional body type marked by roundness of contour, amplitude of body cavities, and considerable subcutaneous fat.

pyk′no-. For words beginning *pykno-* not found here, see words beginning *pycno-*.

pyk′no·lep″sy [*pyknos;* G. *lēpsis*, a seizure]. A very mild form of epileptic variant, resembling petit mal. It appears as a fleeting mental blankness associated with a momentary stare. There are no tonic seizures, no falls, and no convulsions or true losses of consciousness. Electroencephalogram shows large, slow, delta waves.

Pylarino, James [*Italian physician,* 1659–1715]. One of the earliest immunologists to employ inoculation with smallpox virus (1701).

py″lem·phrax′is [G. *pylē,* gate; *emphraxis,* stoppage]. Obstruction of the portal circulation. *Rare.*

py″le·phle·bec′ta·sis, py″le·phleb″ec·ta′si·a (pye″li·fleb″eck·tay′zhuh, ·zee·uh, ·shuh, ·see·uh) [*pylē;* G. *phleps,* vein; *ektasis,* extension]. Dilatation of the portal vein, usually caused by some obstruction in the liver, but it may be due to relaxation of the vessel walls from some disturbance of innervation.

py″le·phle·bi′tis [*pylē; phleps;* G. *-itis,* inflammation]. Inflammation of the portal vein. The condition is usually secondary to disease of the intestine, is generally suppurative in character, and gives rise to the symptoms of pyemia.

py″le·throm″bo·phle·bi′tis [*pylē;* G. *thrombos,* clot; *phleps; -itis*]. Inflammation and thrombosis of the portal vein.

py″le·throm·bo′sis [*pylē; thrombos;* G. *-ōsis,* condition]. Thrombosis of the portal vein.

py″lo·ral′gi·a [G. *pylōros,* gate-keeper; *algos,* pain]. Pain in the region of the pylorus.

py″lo·rec′to·my [*pylōros;* G. *ektomē,* excision]. Excision of the pylorus; partial gastrectomy.

py·lor″i·ste·no′sis (pye·lor″i·sti·no′sis, pi·lor″i·) [*pylōros;* G. *stenōsis,* a being straitened]. Constriction of the pylorus.

py″lor·i′tis [*pylōros;* G. *-itis,* inflammation]. Inflammation of the pylorus.

py·lor′o- (pye·lor′o-, pi·lor′o-), **pylor-** [*pylōros*]. A combining form meaning *relating to the pylorus.*

py·lor″o·col′ic [*pylōros;* G. *kolon,* colon]. Pertaining to or connecting the pyloric end of the stomach with the transverse colon.

py·lor″o·di′la·tor (pye·lor″o·dye′lay·tur, ·dye·lay′-tur, ·di·lay′tur, pi·lor″o·) [*pylōros;* L. *dilator,* from *dilatare,* to dilate]. An appliance for dilating the pyloric orifice of the stomach.

py·lor″o·di·o′sis (pye·lor″o·dye·o′·sis, pi·lor″o·) [*pylōros;* G. *diōsis,* a pushing asunder]. Dilatation of the pylorus by the finger or an instrument, as a bougie. *Obs.*

py·lor″o·gas·trec′to·my [*pylōros;* G. *gastēr,* belly; *ektomē,* excision]. Resection of the pyloric end of the stomach; pylorectomy.

py·lor″o·my·ot′o·my (pye·lor″o·migh·ot′o·mee, pi·lor″o·) [*pylōros;* G. *mys,* muscle; *tomē,* a cutting]. The division, anteriorly, of the pyloric muscle, without incision through the mucosa, for congenital pyloric stenosis in infants: also called *Ramstedt's operation, Fredet-Ramstedt operation.*

py·lor′o·plas″ty [*pylōros;* G. *plassein,* to form]. An operation upon the pylorus, usually for stenosis due to ulcer, which may involve removal of a portion of the pylorus but which, in principle, divides the pylorus on the gastric and duodenal sides transversely, the wound being closed by sutures which convert it into a transverse incision. It provides a larger opening from stomach to duodenum. Also see *pylorotomy.*

py·lor″op·to′sis, py·lor″op·to′si·a [*pyloros;* G. *ptōsis,* a falling]. Downward displacement of the pylorus.

py·lor″o·sche′sis (pye·lor″o·skee′sis, pi·lor″o·, pye″lo·ros′ki·sis) [*pylōros;* G. *schesis,* a checking]. Obstruction of the pylorus.

py″lor·os′co·py [*pylōros;* G. *skopein,* to examine]. Inspection of the pylorus.

py·lor′o·spasm″ [*pylōros;* G. *spasmos,* spasm]. Spasm of the pylorus.

py·lor″o·ste·no′sis [*pylōros;* G. *stenōsis,* a being straitened]. Stenosis, or stricture, of the pylorus.

py″lor·os′to·my [*pylōros;* G. *stoma,* mouth]. Incision into the pylorus, as in the formation of a gastric fistula.

py″lor·ot′o·my [*pylōros;* G. *tomē,* a cutting]. An incision into or through the pylorus in the axis of the canal, converting it by sutures from a longitudinal to a transverse wound. Also called *pyloroplasty, Finney's operation, Heineke-Mikulicz operation, gastroduodenostomy.*

py·lo′rus (pye·lor′us, pi·lor′us) [*pylōros*]. 1. The circular opening of the stomach into the duodenum. 2. The fold of mucous membrane and muscular tissue surrounding the aperture between the stomach and the duodenum. 3. The final portion of the stomach, preceding the duodenum. —**pylor′ic,** *adj.*

py′o-, py- [G. *pyon,* pus]. A combining form meaning *suppuration, accumulation of pus* or *related to pus formation.*

py″o·ar·thro′sis. See *pyarthrosis.*

py′o·cele [*pyon;* G. *kēlē,* tumor]. Accumulation of pus in the tunica vaginalis testis.

py″o·ceph′a·lus [*pyon;* G. *kephalē,* head]. Pus within the cranium, especially in the cerebral ventricles.

py″o·che′zi·a (pye″o·kee′zee·uh) [*pyon;* G. *chezein,* to ease oneself]. Discharge of pus with or in the stool.

py″o·coc′cus [*pyon;* G. *kokkos,* berry]. Any pus-producing coccus.

py″o·col′po·cele [*pyon;* G. *kolpos,* womb; *koilia,* hollow]. A suppurating cyst of the vagina.

py″o·col′pos [*pyon; kolpos*]. An accumulation of pus within the vagina.

py′o com′pounds. A group of antibiotically active substances derived from *Pseudomonas aeruginosa.* They are designated as *pyocyanase, α-oxyphenazine* or *hemipyocyanin, pyocyanin* (*E*), *pyo I, pyo II, pyo III, pyo IV, pyo Ib* and *pyo Ic.* They are active, in vitro, against a number of bacterial species.

py″o·cy′a·nase (pye″o·sigh′uh·nace, ·naze). An antibiotic from *Pseudomonas aeruginosa;* soluble in ether and alcohol. Activity is due largely to unsaturated fatty acids. It has a lytic action on many Gram-positive and Gram-negative bacteria; it is active in vivo and has a low toxicity.

py″o·cy·an′ic (pye″o·sigh·an′ick) [*pyon;* G. *kyanos,* dark blue]. Pertaining to blue pus, or to pyocyanin.

py″o·cy′a·nin. An antibiotic from *Pseudomonas aeruginosa;* soluble in chloroform. It is active largely against Gram-positive bacteria; it has a limited toxicity.

py″o·cy″a·nol′y·sin (pye″o·sigh″uh·nol′i·sin, ·sigh·an″o·lye′sin) [*pyon; kyanos;* G. *lysis,* a loosing]. A hemolysin produced in broth cultures by *Pseudomonas aeruginosa.*

py′o·cyst″ [*pyon;* G. *kystis,* bladder]. A cyst containing pus.

py″o·der′ma [*pyon;* G. *derma,* skin]. Any pus-producing skin lesion or lesions, used in referring to groups of furuncles, pustules, or even carbuncles.

p. faciale. An intensely red or cyanotic erythema of the face with superficial and deep abscesses and cystic lesions.

p. gangrenosum. A pyogenic ulceration, usually of the trunk, often with large irregular ulcers; usually associated with ulcerative colitis.

py″o·der″ma·ti′tis [*pyon; derma;* G. *-itis,* inflammation]. A skin disease produced by infection with pyogenic organisms.

p. vegetans. See *dermatitis* vegetans.

py″o·der″ma·to′sis [*pyon; derma;* G. *-ōsis,* condition]. An inflammation of the skin in which pus formation occurs.

py·og′e·nes (pye·odj′i·neez) [*pyon;* G. *genesthai*, from *gignesthai*, to be produced]. Pus-producing.

py″o·gen′e·sis [*pyon;* G. *genesis*, production]. The formation of pus. —**pyogenic, pyogenet′ic, pyog′enous,** *adj.*

py″o·he″mo·tho′rax (pye″o·hee″mo·thor′acks, ·hem″o·thor′acks) [*pyon;* G. *haima*, blood; *thōrax*, thorax]. Pus and blood in the pleural cavity.

py′oid [G. *pyoeidēs*, like purulent matter]. Resembling pus.

pyoktanin. Trade-mark for methylrosaniline chloride.

py″ok·ta·ni′num au′re·um. Auramine O.

py″ok·tan′in yel′low. Auramine O.

py″o·lab″y·rin·thi′tis [G. *pyon*, pus; *labyrinthos*, labyrinth; *-itis*, inflammation]. Suppurative inflammation of the labyrinth of the ear.

py″o·lip′ic ac′id. An antibiotic substance derived from *Pseudomonas aeruginosa* (*pyocyanea*), active, in vitro, against *Mycobacterium tuberculosis*.

py″o·me′tra [*pyon;* G. *mētra*, uterus]. A collection of pus in the uterus.

py″o·my″o·si′tis [*pyon;* G. *mys*, muscle; *-itis*, inflammation]. Suppurative myositis.

py″o·ne·phri′tis [*pyon;* G. *nephros*, kidney; *-itis*]. Suppurative inflammation of a kidney.

py″o·neph″ro·li·thi′a·sis [*pyon; nephros;* G. *lithos*, stone; NL. *-iasis*, condition]. The presence of pus and calculi in a kidney.

py″o·ne·phro′sis [*pyon; nephros;* G. *-ōsis*, condition]. An accumulation of pus in the pelvis and calyces of a kidney. —**pyonephrot′ic,** *adj.*

py″o-o·va′ri·um. Ovarian abscess.

py″o·per″i·car·di′tis [*pyon;* G. *perikardios*, around the heart; *-itis*, inflammation]. Suppurative pericarditis.

py″o·per″i·car′di·um [*pyon; perikardios*]. The presence of pus in the pericardium.

py″o·per″i·to·ne′um [*pyon;* G. *peritonaion*, membrane which contains the lower viscera]. The presence of pus in the peritoneal cavity.

py″o·per″i·to·ni′tis [*pyon; peritonaion;* G. *-itis*, inflammation]. Suppurative inflammation of the peritoneum.

py″o·pha′gi·a [*pyon;* G. *phagein*, to eat]. The swallowing of pus.

py″oph·thal′mi·a [*pyon;* G. *ophthalmia*, ophthalmia]. Purulent ophthalmia.

py″o·phy·lac′tic [*pyon;* G. *phylaktikos*, preservative]. A defense against pus or pus formation.

py″o·phy″so·me′tra [*pyon;* G. *physa*, wind; *mētra*, uterus]. The presence of pus and gas in the uterus.

py″o·pneu″mo·per″i·car·di′tis (pye″o·new″mo·perr″i·car·dye′tis, pye″op·) [*pyon;* G. *pneuma*, breath; *perikardios*, around the heart; *-itis*, inflammation]. Pericarditis complicated by the presence of pus and gas in the pericardium.

py″o·pneu″mo·per″i·car′di·um [*pyon; pneuma; perikardios*]. Pus and air or gas in the pericardium.

py″o·pneu″mo·per″i·to·ne′um [*pyon; pneuma;* G. *peritonaion*, membrane which contains the lower viscera]. Pus and gas in the peritoneal cavity.

py″o·pneu″mo·per″i·to·ni′tis [*pyon; pneuma; peritonaion;* G. *-itis*, inflammation]. Suppurative inflammation of the peritoneum associated with gas in the abdominal cavity.

py″o·pneu″mo·tho′rax (pye″o·new″mo·thor′acks, pye″op·) [*pyon; pneuma;* G. *thōrax*, thorax]. An accumulation of air and pus in the pleural cavity.

py″o·poi·e′sis [*pyon;* G. *poiēsis*, production]. Pus formation. —**pyopoiet′ic,** *adj.*

py·op′ty·sis (pye·op′ti·sis) [*pyon;* G. *ptysis*, a spitting]. The expectoration of pus.

py″or·rhe′a, py″or·rhoe′a [G. *pyorroia*, discharge of matter]. A purulent discharge.

alveolar p. Periodontal disease in which a purulent exudate is a feature. *Obs.*

py″o·sal″pin·gi′tis [*pyon;* G. *salpigx*, trumpet; *-itis*, inflammation]. Purulent inflammation of the uterine or auditory tube.

py″o·sal·pin″go-o″o·pho·ri′tis. Combined suppurative inflammation of an ovary and oviduct.

py″o·sal′pinx [*pyon; salpigx*]. An accumulation of pus in an oviduct.

py·o′sis (pye·o′sis) [*pyon;* G. *-ōsis*, condition]. Suppuration; pus formation.

Castellani's p. See *jungle rot.*

Corlett's p. A bullous staphylodermatitis.

tropical p. Ecthyma.

py″o·sper′mi·a. Leukocytes in the seminal fluid.

py″o·stat′ic [*pyon;* G. *statikos*, causing to stand]. Preventing the formation of pus.

py″o·stat′ic. An agent arresting the formation of pus.

py″o·ther′a·py [*pyon;* G. *therapeia*, treatment]. The use of pus in the treatment of disease. *Obs.*

py″o·tho′rax [*pyon;* G. *thōrax*, thorax]. An accumulation of pus in the pleural cavity. Syn., *empyema.*

py″o·u′ra·chus (pye″o·yoo′ra·kus) [*pyon;* G. *ourachos*, urachus]. The presence of pus in or about the urachus.

py″o·u·re′ter (pye″o·yoor·ee′tur, ·yoor′i·tur) [*pyon;* G. *ourētēr*, ureter]. An accumulation of pus in a ureter.

py″o·xan′thin (pye″o·zan′thin), **py″o·xan′those** (pye″o·zan′thoce) [*pyon;* G. *xanthos*, yellow]. A yellow pigment sometimes found in pus, and resulting from the oxidation of pyocyanin.

pyr′a·cin. Either of two substances, α-pyracin (2-methyl-3-hydroxy-4-hydroxymethyl-5-carboxypyridine) and β-pyracin (2-methyl-3-hydroxy-4-carboxy-5-hydroxymethylpyridine); both are metabolite analogs of pyridoxine.

py″ra·hex′yl. Synhexyl.

pyr′a·mid [G. *pyramis*, pyramid]. Any conical eminence of an organ; especially a body of longitudinal nerve fibers on each side of the anterior median fissure of the medulla oblongata. —**pyram′idal,** *adj.*

malpighian, Malpighian p. See renal *p.*

petrous p. The petrous portion of the temporal bone. See *petrosa.*

p. of the stapedius muscle. See *p.* of the tympanum.

p. of the tympanum. A hollow conical process on posterior wall of the tympanum; the stapedius muscle passes through an aperture at its apex.

p. of the vermis. Pyramid of the cerebellum, a subdivision of the cerebellar vermis between the uvula and the tuber.

p. of the vestibule. The anterior end of the vestibular crest of the osseous labyrinth.

renal p. One of the conical masses composing the medullary substance of the kidney.

py·ram″i·da′lis (pi·ram″i·dah′lis, ·day′lis) [*pyramis*]. 1. A small muscle, enclosed in the sheath of the rectus abdominis, arising from the pubic crest, and inserted into the linea alba. See Table of Muscles in the Appendix. 2. Old name for triquetrum. See Table of Bones in the Appendix.

p. nasi. Old name for procerus muscle.

pyramidon. Trade-mark for a brand of aminopyrine.

pyr″a·mid·ot′o·my. Sectioning of the lateral corticospinal (pyramidal) tract.

spinal p. Pyramidotomy at the level of the second cervical vertebra, for alternating tremor.

pyr′a·min. 2-Methyl-4-amino-5-hydroxymethylpyrimidine; a hydrolytic cleavage product of thiamine excreted in the urine and also obtained in the presence of the enzyme thiaminase.

py′ran. The six-membered heterocyclic compound C_5H_6O, of which three isomers are possible. Certain natural compounds are often characterized as derivatives of a pyran and the pyranose form of certain sugars indicates structural relationship of the latter to a pyran.

py″ra·nis′a·mine. An earlier designation for the antihistaminic substance pyrilamine.

py′ra·nose. That isomeric form of certain sugars and glycosides having a structural analogy to a pyran. See also *furanose.*

pyr″a·zin·am′ide, pyr″a·zin′a·mide. Generic name for pyrazine-carboxylic acid amide; $C_4H_3N_2.CONH_2$; a drug under clinical investigation as a therapeutic agent in human tuberculosis. See *aldinamide.*

pyr′a·zine. 1. The 1,4-isomer of diazine, $C_4H_4N_2$, in which the nitrogen atoms are separated by two carbon atoms; a white, crystalline substance, freely soluble in water. 2. Any derivative of 1.

pyr′a·zole. CH:CH.NH.N:CH; a heterocyclic compound, isomeric with imidazole, being the ultimate parent compound of certain therapeutically useful analgesic drugs. See also *pyrazolone.*

py·raz′o·lone. $C_3H_6N_2O$; one of three isomeric derivatives of pyrazole, differentiated as 3-pyrazolone, 4-pyrazolone, and 5-pyrazolone. They differ from pyrazole in containing two additional hydrogen atoms and a keto group. Certain derivatives of 5-pyrazolone, notably aminopyrine and antipyrine, possess analgesic activity.

py·rec′tic (pye·reck′tick) [G. *pyretikos,* feverish]. Pyretic, feverish.

py′rene. $C_{16}H_{10}$; a tetracyclic hydrocarbon in coal tar, occurring in colorless crystals, insoluble in water.

py′re·nin (pye′ri·nin, pye·ree′nin) [G. *pyrēn,* stone of a fruit]. The substance of the plasmosome. Syn., *paranuclein.*

py·reth′rin I. $C_{21}H_{28}O_3$; the pyrethrolone ester of chrysanthemum-monocarboxylic acid, a viscous liquid, insoluble in water but soluble in alcohol. It is an insecticidal constituent of pyrethrum flowers and is itself used as an insecticide.

py·reth′rin II. $C_{22}H_{28}O_5$; the pyrethrolone ester of chrysanthemum-dicarboxylic acid monomethyl ester; a viscous liquid, insoluble in water but soluble in alcohol. It is an insecticidal constituent of pyrethrum flowers and is itself used as an insecticide.

py·re′thrum (pye·reeth′rum) [G. *pyrethron*]. Pellitory; the root of *Anacyclus pyrethrum:* formerly used as a sialagogue and masticatory in headache, toothache, and neuralgic affections of the face.

py·re′thrum flow′ers. The flower heads of *Chrysanthemum cinerariaefolium, C. coccineum* (*C. roseum*), and *C. Marschallii.* Should not be confused with pyrethrum, the root. Pyrethrum flowers are highly toxic to lower forms of life, especially insects and worms, and are used as insect powder under the names Dalmatian insect powder and Persian insect powder. The insecticidal power is probably due to two related compounds, pyrethrin I and pyrethrin II. While it is chiefly used as an insecticide, it has been used as a medicinal agent by protecting human beings from infection by disease-carrying insects, such as mosquitoes, fleas, and lice. It is also used as a local application in the treatment of pediculosis. An ointment containing an extract from powdered pyrethrum flowers (*C. cinerariaefolium*), **pyrethrum ointment,** is used in the treatment of scabies. The ointment is applied to the entire body following a thorough cleansing with soap and water.

py·ret′ic (pye·ret′ick) [G. *pyretikos,* feverish]. Pertaining to or affected with fever.

pyr′e·to- (pirr′i·to-, pye′ri·to-) [G. *pyretos,* burning heat]. A combining form meaning *fever.*

py·ret′o·gen (pye·ret′o·jin) [*pyretos;* G. *genesthai,* from *gignesthai,* to be produced]. Any agent which induces fever.

pyr″e·to·ge·ne′si·a (pirr″i·to·ji·nee′zee·uh, ·see·uh, pye″ri·to·), **pyr″e·to·gen′e·sis** [*pyretos;* G. *genesis,* production]. The origin and process of fever.

pyr″e·to·gen′ic, pyr″e·tog′e·nous (pirr″i·todj′i·nus, pye″ri·) [*pyretos;* G. *genesthai,* from *gignesthai,* to be produced]. Causing or producing fever.

pyr″e·tog′ra·phy [*pyretos;* G. *graphein,* to write]. A treatise on fevers.

pyr″e·tol′o·gist [*pyretos;* G. *logos,* word]. A specialist in fevers.

pyr″e·tol′o·gy (pirr″i·tol′o·jee, pyr″ri·) [*pyretos; logos*]. The science of the nature of fevers.

pyr″e·tol′y·sis [*pyretos;* G. *lysis,* a loosing]. Reduction of a fever.

pyr″e·to·ther′a·py [*pyretos;* G. *therapeia,* treatment]. Treatment of disease by the induction of fever in the patient.

pyr″e·to·ty·pho′sis (pirr″i·to·tye·fo′sis, pye″ri·to·) [*pyretos;* G. *typhos,* smoke; *-ōsis,* condition]. Old term for delirium in fever.

py·rex″e·o·pho′bi·a (pye·reck″see·o·fo′bee·uh) [G. *pyressein,* to be feverish; *phobos,* fear]. A morbid fear of fever; febriphobia.

py·rex′i·a (pye·reck′see·uh) [*pyressein*]. Elevation of temperature above the normal; fever. —**pyrexial,** *adj.*

pyr″go·ceph′a·ly. See *acrocephaly.* —**pyrgocephal′ic, pyrgocephalous,** *adj.*

pyr·he″li·om′e·ter (pyre·hee″lee·om′i·tur, pirr-hee″·) [G. *pyr,* fire; *hēlios,* sun; *metron,* a measure]. An instrument for measuring the total intensity of solar radiation.

pyribenzamine. Trade-mark for the antihistaminic substance N,N-dimethyl-N′-benzyl-N′-(alpha-pyridyl) ethylenediamine, available as the hydrochloride salt. See *tripelennamine hydrochloride.*

pyricidin. Trade-mark for a brand of *isoniazid.*

py·rid′a·zine. 1. The 1,2-isomer of diazine; $C_4H_4N_2$; a liquid in which the two nitrogen atoms are adjacent to each other. 2. Any derivative of 1.

pyr′i·dine (pirr′i·deen, ·din). C_5H_5N. A heterocyclic compound, first of a series of homologous bases, occurring as a colorless liquid with a persistent odor; miscible with water in all proportions; miscible with alcohol. Used as a solvent in industry; has been used as an antiseptic and germicide.

2-pyr″i·dine·car″box·yl′ic ac′id. Picolinic acid.

3-pyr″i·dine·car″box·yl′ic ac′id. Nicotinic acid.

pyr·i·din″o·pro′te·in en′zyme. A dehydrogenase-type enzyme which functions with diphosphopyridine nucleotide (coenzyme I) or triphosphopyridine nucleotide (coenzyme II) as the coenzyme.

pyridium. Trade-mark for phenylazo-α,α-diamino-pyridine monohydrochloride used in acute and chronic urogenital infections.

pyr″i·dox′al. The 4-aldehyde of pyridoxine, an essential component of enzymes concerned with amino-acid decarboxylation and with transamination, and therefore with amino-acid synthesis.

pyr″i·dox′a·mine. The amine of pyridoxine in which NH_2 replaces the OH group in position 4; obtained in transamination of pyridoxal.

pyr″i·dox′ic ac′id. 2-Methyl-3-hydroxy-4-carboxy-5-hydroxymethyl pyridine, a decomposition product occurring in urine following ingestion of pyridoxine by man.

pyr″i·dox′ine (pirr″i·dock′seen, ·sin). $C_8H_{11}O_3N$. 2-Methyl-3-hydroxy-4,5-di(hydroxymethyl)-pyridine; the term pyridoxine is synonymous with vitamin B_6; the hydrochloride occurs as a white, crystalline powder with a saline taste; 1 Gm. is soluble in 4.5 cc. of water and in about 91 cc. of alcohol; it is reasonably stable in solutions having a pH below 5. The importance of pyridoxine in human nutrition is not yet definitely established; in rats it is an antidermatitis factor. Convulsions and hypochromic anemia have been observed to develop in pyridoxine-deficient infants. **Pyridoxine hydrochloride,** intravenously administered, provides relief from the nausea and vomiting of pregnancy, but is not effective in all cases. It has value in treatment of irradiation sickness.

pyr′i·dyl. The monovalent radical C_5H_4N, from pyridine.

pyr′i·form. See *piriform.*

py·ril′a·mine, pyr·il′a·mine. Generic name for the antihistaminic base N-*p*-methoxybenzyl-N′,N′-dimethyl-N-α-pyridylethylenediamine; $C_{17}H_{23}N_3O$: originally called *pyranisamine.* It is most commonly used in the form of the maleate salt. Syn., *mepyramine.* See *neo-antergan.*

pyr″i·meth′a·mine. Generic name for 2,4-diamino-5-*p*-chlorophenyl-6-ethylpyrimidine, an antimalarial agent. See *daraprim.*

py·rim′i·dine (pye·rim′i·deen, ·din, pi·rim′·). 1. Any six-membered cyclic compound containing four carbon and two nitrogen atoms in the ring, the nitrogen atoms being separated by one carbon atom. To this group belong barbituric acid and its derivatives, the nucleic acid hydrolysis products thymine, uracil, and cytosine, and many other compounds of physiologic or therapeutic importance. 2. $C_4H_4N_2$. 1,3-Diazine, a solid melting between 20° and 22° C.; soluble in water.

pyr″i·thi′a·mine. A mixture of compounds, originally believed to be a single compound representing a structural analog of thiamine in which the thiazole ring is replaced by pyridine. The pure substance is now called *neopyrithiamine.*

pyr″i·thyl·di′one. Generic name for 3,3-diethyl-2,4-dioxotetrahydropyridine; a sedative and hypnotic substance no longer used because it may produce agranulocytosis. See *presidon.*

py′ro- (pye′ro-, pirr′o-), **pyr-** [G. *pyr*, fire]. 1. A combining form signifying *fire* or *heat.* 2. *In chemistry*, a combining form denoting *a substance derived by the action of heat.* 3. *In medicine*, a combining form denoting *fever.*

py″ro·bor′ic ac′id. $H_2B_4O_7$. An acid obtained from boric acid by heating. Also called *tetraboric acid.*

py″ro·cat′e·case. An enzyme catalizing oxidative breakdown of pyrocatechol.

py″ro·cat′e·chin. See *pyrocatechol.*

py″ro·cat′e·chin mon″o·ac′e·tate. Guaiacetin.

py″ro·cat″e·chin·u′ri·a (pye″ro·cat″i·ki·new′ree·uh, pirr″o·) [*pyr;* Malay *kāchū;* G. *ouron*, urine]. The presence of pyrocatechol in the urine.

py″ro·cat′e·chol (pye″ro·cat′i·chole, ·coal, ·kol, ·kawl, pirr″o·). $C_6H_4(OH)_2$. *o*-Dihydroxybenzene; occurs as colorless leaflets; soluble in water and alcohol. Used in solution or ointment as an antiseptic. It is also used in photography as a developer. Also called *pyrocatechin, catechol, oxyphenic acid.*

py″ro·cit′ric ac′id. Citraconic acid.

py′ro·din. $C_6H_5.(NH)_2COCH_3$. Acetylphenylhydrazine; occurs as white crystals, slightly soluble in cold water, but soluble in hot water and alcohol. It is a powerful antipyretic but has a destructive action on red blood cells. It has been employed in skin diseases. See *hydracetin.*

py″ro·gal′lic ac′id. Pyrogallol.

py″ro·gal′lol (pye″ro·gal′ole, ·ol, ·awl, ·ga·lole′, pirr″o·). $C_6H_3(OH)_3$. 1,2,3-Trihydroxybenzene; occurs as light, white, or nearly white odorless leaflets or fine needles; on exposure to air and light it acquires a grayish tint; 1 Gm. is soluble in 2 cc. of water and about 1.5 cc. of alcohol. Pyrogallol is an active irritant and in concentrated solution, caustic. It is somewhat germicidal, but inferior to phenol. Internally it is actively poisonous. Used solely as an application in various skin diseases, especially psoriasis; it is generally applied in the form of an ointment in strengths of from 2 to 10%. Also called *pyrogallic acid.*

p. monoacetate. $(OH)_2C_6H_3O.CO.CH_3$; available only in the form of a 67% solution in acetone, a reddish brown syrupy liquid. It is very vigorous in action and is to be used only in the most obstinate cases of psoriasis. Applied by painting once daily, followed in half an hour by zinc oxide powder or paste. See *eugallol.*

p. triacetate. $C_6H_3(COOCH_3)_3$; occurs as a white, crystalline powder; soluble in water and alcohol. It is used in psoriasis, lupus, acute and subacute eczema of children, and other skin diseases. It is applied in the form of a paste containing from 5 to 10% of the drug, usually with zinc oxide. Also called *triacetyl pyrogallol.* See *lenigallol.*

py″ro·gal″lol·phthal′ein. $C_{20}H_{12}O_7$. A brownish red powder obtained by the interaction of pyrogallol and phthalic acid. It is used as an indicator. Syn., *gallein.*

py′ro·gen [G. *pyr*, fire; *genesthai*, from *gignesthai*, to be produced]. The protein organic matter or complex polysaccharide of a fever-producing nature which is found frequently in sterile water. It is produced by a certain group of bacteria which enter and develop in the water during distillation and subsequent storage and are killed during sterilization, thus leaving their bodies and products of decomposition in the solution. They are said to be responsible for the majority of reactions following intravenous injections.

py″ro·gen′ic [*pyr; genesthai*]. Producing fever.

py″ro·glob′u·lin. A globulin, abnormally present in blood serum, which coagulates on heating.

py″ro·glob″u·li·ne′mi·a. The abnormal condition in which blood serum contains heat-coagulable globulin (pyroglobulin); a high correlation of this condition with multiple myeloma has been observed.

py″ro·glos′si·a [G. *pyr*, fire; *glōssa*, tongue]. A burning sensation of the tongue.

py″ro·guai′a·cin (pye″ro·gwye′uh·sin, pirr″o·) [*pyr;* Sp. *guayacán*]. A component of guaiac.

py″ro·lag′ni·a [*pyr;* G. *lagneia*, coition]. Sexual gratification attained by the sight of fires; sexual excitement accompanying pyromania.

py″ro·lig′ne·ous [*pyr;* L. *ligneus*, wooden]. Pertaining to the destructive distillation of wood.

py″ro·lig′ne·ous ac′id. The crude acid obtained by the destructive distillation of wood; it contains acetic acid.

py″ro·lu′site (pye″ro·lew′sight, pye·rol′yoo·sight). MnO_2. A native manganese dioxide.

py·rol′y·sis (pye·rol′i·sis) [*pyr;* G. *lysis*, a loosing]. The decomposition of organic substances by heat. —**pyrolyt′ic,** *adj.*

py″ro·ma′ni·a [*pyr;* G. *mania*, madness]. A monomania for incendiarism. —**pyromaniac,** *n.*

pyromen. See *piromen.*

py·rom′e·ter (pye·rom′i·tur) [*pyr;* G. *metron*, a measure]. An instrument for measuring temperatures too high to be estimated by the ordinary thermometer.

py″ro·mu′cic ac′id. Furoic acid.

py'rone. Any derivative of two of the three possible pyrans in which one or, less frequently, two oxygen atoms are attached to the same number of carbon atoms in the ring; also, certain derivatives of such pyrones, some of which are of medicinal importance.

py'ro·nin (C.C.). Tetraethyldiaminoxanthene; used as a histologic stain. Includes **pyronin B** and **pyronin G.**

py"ro·pho'bi·a [*pyr;* G. *phobos,* fear]. Morbid dread of fire.

py"ro·phos'pha·tase. An enzyme catalyzing hydrolysis of esters containing two or more molecules of phosphoric acid to form a simpler phosphate ester.

py"ro·phos'phate. A salt of pyrophosphoric acid.

py"ro·phos·phor'ic ac'id. $H_4P_2O_7$. A crystalline acid, certain salts of which, notably iron, have been used medicinally.

py·rop"to·thy'mi·a (pye·rop"to·thigh'mee·uh) [*pyr;* G. *ptoein,* to frighten; *thymos,* mind]. A form of mental disorder in which the person imagines himself enveloped in flame.

py'ro·punc"ture [*pyr;* L. *punctura,* puncture]. Puncturing with hot needles; ignipuncture.

py"ro·ra·ce'mic ac'id. Pyruvic acid.

py"ro·ra·ce'mic al'co·hol. See *acetyl* carbinol.

py'ro·scope [*pyr;* G. *skopein,* to examine]. Instrument used in determining high temperatures.

py·ro'sis (pye·ro'sis) [G. *pyrōsis,* firing]. An affection of the stomach characterized by a burning sensation, accompanied by eructations of an acrid, irritating fluid; heartburn.

py·rot'ic [G. *pyrōtikos,* heating]. 1. Pertaining to pyrosis. 2. Caustic.

py"ro·tox'in [G. *pyr,* fire; *toxikon,* poison]. A toxic agent generated in the course of the febrile process.

py·rox'y·lin (pye·rock'si·lin, pye"rock·sil'in) (*pyroxylinum*). A product obtained by the action of a mixture of nitric and sulfuric acids on cotton; consists chiefly of cellulose tetranitrate ($C_{12}H_{16}O_6$-$(NO_3)_4$); occurs as a yellowish white, matted mass of filaments, resembling raw cotton in appearance but harsh to the touch. It is exceedingly inflammable; dissolves slowly in 25 parts of a mixture of 3 volumes of ether and 1 volume of alcohol. It is used as a protective covering in the form of collodion. Also called *soluble guncotton.*

pyr·role' (pi·role', pirr'ole) [G. *pyrros,* fiery; L. *oleum,* oil]. NH.CH:CH.CH:CH. A colorless liquid occurring in bone oil and to a slight extent in coal tar. Many complex natural compounds, such as hemoglobin and chlorophyll, contain pyrrole components in their structure. See also *porphin ring, porphyrin.*

pyr·rol'i·dine. C_4H_9N; tetrahydropyrrole; an almost colorless, liquid base found in tobacco and carrot leaves.

pyr·rol"i·done·car"box·yl'ic ac'id. $C_5H_7NO_3$; 2-pyrrolidone-5-carboxylic acid; a urinary excretion form of unnatural D-glutamic acid, the latter losing a molecule of water and undergoing cyclization in the metabolic process.

pyr'ro·line. C_4H_7N; 2,5-dihydropyrrole; an almost colorless, liquid base prepared synthetically.

py·ru'vate. A salt or ester of pyruvic acid.

py·ru'vic ac'id (pye·roo'vick, pi·roo'vick). CH_3.-CO.COOH. An organic acid which is a normal intermediate in carbohydrate and protein metabolism. Excess quantities of pyruvic acid accumulate in blood and tissues in thiamine deficiency. Syn., *ketopropionic acid.*

py·u'ri·a (pye·yoor'ee·uh) [G. *pyon,* pus; *ouron,* urine]. The presence of pus in the urine. —**pyu'ric,** *adj.*

abacterial p., amicrobic p. Presence of a large number of leukocytes in the urine when no causative agent can be demonstrated, frequently associated with marked inflammation of the urinary bladder.

Q

Q$_{CO_2}$ The rate of evolution of carbon dioxide, in microliters given off in 1 hour by 1 mg. (dry weight) of tissue.

Q$_{O_2}$ The oxygen consumption in terms of the number of microliters consumed in 1 hour by 1 mg. (dry weight) of tissue; by convention, the consumption of oxygen is given a negative value.

Q$_{10}$ The increase in the rate of a chemical reaction for an increase in temperature of 10° C.

q electron. See under *electron.*

Q enzyme. See under *enzyme.*

Q fe'ver. See under *fever.*

q. h. *Quaque hora;* every hour.

q. 2 h. *Quaque secunda hora;* every second hour.

q. 3 h. *Quaque tertia hora;* every third hour.

q. i. d. *Quater in die;* 4 times a day.

q. l. *Quantum libet;* as much as is desired.

q. p. *Quantum placet;* as much as you please.

QRS See QRS *complex* of electrocardiography, QRS *interval.*

q. s. *Quantum sufficit;* as much as suffices.

qt. Quart.

quack [D. *kwakzalven,* to boast of one's salves]. A pretender to medical skill; a medical charlatan.

quack'er·y [*kwakzalven*]. The practice of medicine by a quack.

quack'sal·ver [D. *kwakzalver*]. A quack or mountebank; a peddler of his own medicines and salves.

quad·ran'gu·lar (kwod·rang'gew·lur) [L. *quadrangulum,* quadrangle]. Having four angles, as the quadrangular lobe, the square lobe of the cerebellum.

quad'rant (kwod'runt) [L. *quadrans,* a fourth part]. 1. The fourth part of a circle, subtending an angle of 90°. 2. One of the four regions into which the abdomen may be divided for purposes of physical diagnosis. 3. A sector of one-fourth of the field of vision of one or both eyes. —**quadran'tic,** *adj.*

quad"ran·ta·no'pi·a (kwod"ran·tuh·no'pee·uh), **quad"ran·ta·nop'si·a** [*quadrans;* G. *a-,* not; *ōps,* eye]. Loss of vision in about one-quarter of the visual field.

quad'rate [L. *quadratum,* from *quadrare,* to make square]. Square, four-sided, as quadrate cartilages, small, quadrangular, cartilaginous plates often found in the alae of the nose.

quad·ra'tus [*quadrare*]. A squared figure; a muscle having four sides, as the quadratus lumborum of the back, attached to the crest of the ilium and the twelfth rib. See Table of Muscles in the Appendix.

q. menti. The quadratus labii inferioris muscle.

quad′ri- [cf. L. *quattuor*, four]. A combining form meaning *four*.

quad′ri·ceps [*quattuor;* L. *caput*, head]. Four-headed, as a quadriceps muscle.

quad′ri·ceps. The large extensor muscle of the thigh. See Table of Muscles in the Appendix.

q. surae. The muscle mass comprising the gastrocnemius, soleus, and plantaris. *Obs.*

quad″ri·cus′pid. Having four cusps.

quad″ri·gem′i·na. The corpora quadrigemina.

quad″ri·gem′i·nal [*quattuor;* L. *geminus*, twin]. Fourfold; consisting of four parts, as the corpora quadrigemina.

quad·rip′a·ra [*quattuor;* L. *parere*, to bring forth]. A woman who is bearing, or has borne, her fourth child. —**quadriparous,** *adj.*

quad″ri·par′i·ty [*quattuor; parere*]. The state of having borne four children.

quad″ri·ple′gi·a [*quattuor;* G. *plēgē*, stroke]. Paralysis affecting the four extremities of the body.

quad″ri·tu·ber′cu·lar [*quattuor;* L. *tuberculum*, swelling]. Having four tubercles or cusps.

quad″ri·u′rate. A mixture of a urate with uric acid obtained from urine or blood, formerly believed to be a compound.

quad″ri·va′lent (kwod″ri·vay′lunt, kwod·riv′uh-lunt) [*quattuor;* L. *valere*, to be strong]. *In chemistry*, having a combining power equivalent to that of four hydrogen atoms. —**quadrivalence,** *n.*

quad·roon′ [Sp. *cuarterón*, from L. *quartus*, fourth]. The offspring of a white person and a mulatto.

quad′ru·ped [L. *quattuor*, four; *pes*, foot]. A four-footed animal. —**quadru′pedal,** *adj.*

quad′ru·plet (kwod′roo·plet, kwod·rōō′plet) [L. *quadruplus*, fourfold]. Any one of four children born at one birth.

Quain, Richard [*English physician*, 1816–98]. Described fatty degeneration of the heart; called *Quain's fatty degeneration.*

qua′ker but′tons. Nux vomica.

qua·lim′e·ter (kwol·im′i·tur) [L. *qualis*, of what kind; G. *metron*, a measure]. An instrument for measuring degree of penetration of roentgen rays.

qual′i·ta″tive [L. *qualitas*, quality]. Pertaining to quality.

qual′i·ty. *In radiobiology*, the approximate characterization of radiation with respect to its penetrating power.

quan′ta. Plural of quantum.

quan′tal sum·ma′tion (kwon′tul). Excitatory effects produced by the quantity or number of impulses reaching specific structures.

quan·tim′e·ter (kwon·tim′i·tur) [L. *quantus*, how much; G. *metron*, a measure]. An instrument for measuring the quantity of roentgen rays. Also see *dosimeter.*

quan′ti·ta″tive [L. *quantitas*, quantity]. Pertaining to quantity.

quan′tum [L., how much]. As much as.

q. libet. As much as is desired. Abbreviated, q.l.

q. placet. As much as you please. Abbreviated, q.p.

q. sufficit. As much as suffices. Abbreviated, q.s.

q. vis. As much as you wish. Abbreviated, q.v.

quan′tum (pl. *quanta*). 1. Quantity or amount. 2. A discrete portion of energy, of definite amount. See quantum *constant.*

quar′an·tine [It. *quarantina*, from L. *quadraginta*, forty]. 1. The limitation of freedom of movement of such susceptible persons or animals as have been exposed to communicable disease, for a period of time equal to the longest usual incubation period of the disease to which they have been exposed. 2. The place of detention of such persons. 3. The act of detaining vessels or travelers from suspected ports or places for purposes of inspection or disinfection.

absolute q. *In military medicine*, a quarantine in which normal duties are suspended and all contacts are avoided.

shotgun q. The extemporized and unauthorized establishment of a cordon against a place suspected of being the seat of an epidemic of a communicable disease.

working q. *In military medicine*, limitation of freedom of movement of such susceptible persons or animals as have been exposed to a communicable disease, for a period of time equal to the longest usual incubation periods of the disease to which they have been exposed. Regular duties are performed but measures are taken to prevent the spread of diseases.

quart [L. *quartus*, fourth]. In the U.S.A., the fourth part of a gallon; 0.9463 liter. Abbreviated, qt. An **imperial quart** contains about 20% more than the **U. S. quart.**

quar′tan (kwor′tun) [*quartus*]. Recurring on the fourth day.

quar′tan. A form of intermittent malarial fever in which the paroxysms occur approximately every 72 hours, that is, on the first, fourth, seventh days, etc.

double q. A form of intermittent malarial fever in which there are two concurrent cycles of quartan fever, not synchronous with each other, ordinarily resulting in fever on two successive days.

triple q. A form of intermittent malarial fever in which there are three concurrent cycles of quartan fever, not synchronous with each other, ordinarily resulting in fever every day.

quar′ter [L. *quartarius*, fourth part]. 1. *In veterinary anatomy*, that part of the horse's hoof between the heel and the toe. 2. The fourth part of a slaughtered animal.

quar′ter crack. *In veterinary medicine*, a fissuring of the inner or outer aspect of the wall of the hoof in the horse.

quar′ter e′vil. Obsolete term for blackleg.

quar·tip′a·ra (kwor·tip′uh·ruh) [L. *quartus*, fourth; *parere*, to bring forth]. A woman who has borne four children. —**quartiparous,** *adj.*

quartz. A crystalline silicon dioxide, SiO_2; when pure, in colorless hexagonal crystals. Used in chemical apparatus and for optical and electric instruments.

quartz rod. See quartz rod *method.*

quas′si·a (kwosh′ee·uh, kwosh′uh) [NL., from *Quassi*, a Surinam Negro who first used it about 1730]. The wood of *Picrasma excelsa*, known as **Jamaica quassia,** or of *Quassia amara*, known as **Surinam quassia.** A simple bitter, used in dyspepsia. An infusion is used as an enema against seatworms. Also called *bitter wood.*

quas′sin (kwoss′in, kwass′in) [*Quassi*]. A bitter substance from quassia; a molecular complex of isoquassin and neoquassin in approximately equal amounts. It has been used as a bitter tonic.

qua·ter′na·ry [L. *quarternarius*, consisting of four each]. 1. Consisting of four elements or substances, as quaternary solutions. 2. Fourth in order or stage, as quaternary syphilis. 3. Referring to compounds in which four similar atoms of a radical, as the hydrogen atoms in the ammonium radical, have been replaced by organic radicals. See *quaternary ammonium compounds* under *compound.*

Quatrefages de Bréau, Jean Louis Armand de [*French anthropologist*, 1810–92]. One of the most eminent in his field. Published important work on craniology and on pygmies and their descent (1887). Described the parietal angle; also called *angle of Quatrefages.*

quat'tu·or [L.]. Four.

que"bra·bun'da (kee"bruh·bun'duh, kay"brah-bo͞on'dah). A tropical disease of horses and swine simulating beriberi of humans.

que·brach'a·mine. $C_{19}H_{26}N_2$; an alkaloid of quebracho.

que·bra'chine (kay·brah'cheen ·chin, kee·brah'-cheen, ·chin, ·keen, ·kin). An alkaloid of quebracho found to be identical with yohimbine.

que·bra'cho (kay·brah'cho, kee·brah'cho, ·ko) [Sp.]. The name of several hard-wooded trees of South America. The **white quebracho** is *Aspidosperma quebracho-blanco*, of the family Apocynaceae. It contains aspidospermine, quebrachamine, quebrachine (yohimbine), and possibly other alkaloids.

Queckenstedt, Hans Heinrich Georg (1876–1918). German neurologist, known for his studies of cerebrospinal fluid. See Queckenstedt's *sign*.

Queckenstedt-Stookey test. See under *test*.

queen's'-de·light'. See *stillingia*.

queens'root". See *stillingia*.

quelicin chloride. Trade-marked name for *succinylcholine chloride*.

Quénu, Eduard André Victor Alfred [*French surgeon*, 1852–1933]. Developed a method of thoracoplasty involving division of the ribs to promote retraction, for the treatment of empyema; called *Quénu's operation, quenuthoracoplasty*.

quer'ce·tin (kwur'si·tin). $C_{15}H_{10}O_7$; 3,3',4',5,7-pentahydroxyflavone; the aglycone of quercitrin, rutin, and other glycosides, found especially in various rinds and barks, but widely distributed in the plant kingdom. It occurs as a yellow, crystalline powder, practically insoluble in water. It has been suggested to be the active component of rutin in decreasing capillary fragility and is used similarly. Syn., *flavin, meletin*. See *quertine*.

quer'ci- (kwur'si-) [L. *quercus*, oak]. A combining form meaning *an oak*.

quer'cin. A bitter, crystallizable carbohydrate, $C_6H_{12}O_6$, from acorns and oak bark.

quer"ci·tan'nic ac'id. The tannic acid from oak bark.

quer"ci·tan'nin. Quercitannic acid.

quer'cite. $C_6H_7(OH)_5$. Pentahydroxycyclohexane. White, sweet crystals; found in acorns. Also called *quercitol, acorn sugar*.

quer'ci·tol. See *quercite*.

quer'ci·trin. $C_{21}H_{20}O_{11}.2H_2O$. A glycoside found in the bark of *Quercus tinctoria* and in many other plants.

quer'cus [L.]. The dried inner bark of *Quercus alba*. See *oak*.

quertine. A trade-mark for *quercetin*.

Quervain, Fritz de [*Swiss surgeon*, 1868–1940]. Described tenosynovitis of the extensor and abductor muscles of the thumb, called *Quervain's disease, tendovaginitis stenosans*.

Query, Leon Camille [*French physician*, 1868–]. Introduced an antiserum obtained from monkeys who had been infected with *Treponema pallidum;* called *Quéry's serum*.

Quévenne's iron. See reduced *iron*.

Queyrat's erythroplasia. See *erythroplasia* of Queyrat.

quick [AS. *cwic*]. A vital, tender part, as the bed of a nail.

quick. Manifesting life and activity, as a fetus.

Quick and Csonka method. See under *method*.

quick'en·ing [*cwic*]. The first feeling on the part of the pregnant woman of fetal movements, occurring between the fourth and fifth months of pregnancy.

quick'lime" [*cwic;* AS. *līm*]. Calcium oxide; unslaked lime.

Quick's hippuric acid synthesis test. See hippuric acid *test*.

quick'sil"ver. Mercury.

Quick's test (*for prothrombin*). See one-stage *method*.

Quil·la'ja (kwi·lay'yuh, ·juh), **Quil·la'ia** [Sp. *quillái*]. A genus of trees of the family Rosaceae.

quil·la'ja [*quillái*]. The dried inner bark of *Quillaja saponaria*. It contains a saponin, quillain (quillaic acid), which is very toxic. Rarely used as a nauseating expectorant. Externally, it is a stimulant and detergent. Also called *soapbark, Panama bark*.

Quimby, Edith H. (1891–). American radiological physicist, known for her research in the standardization of x-rays and radium dosage and in the biological effects of radiation, in the application of x-rays, radium, and radioactive isotopes to medicine, and in the comparison of different types of radiations.

quin-, quin'o- [Sp. *quina*, from Quechua *quinquina*, cinchona bark]. A combining form denoting *quina* (cinchona bark) or *quinine*.

quin'a·crine hy"dro·chlo'ride (kwin'uh·kreen, ·krin) (*quinacrinae hydrochloridum*). $C_{23}H_{30}ClN_3O.2HCl.2H_2O$. A bright yellow, crystalline powder; odorless; of bitter taste; 1 Gm. dissolves in about 35 cc. of water. Aqueous solutions are yellow and show a greenish fluorescence. An acridine derivative, which destroys the asexual forms (trophozoites) of the malarial organism, completely suppressing the disease, but usually with recurrence when the administration is discontinued. It has the same scope and approximately the same effectiveness as quinine. Dosage for suppression, 0.1 Gm. daily; for treatment of attack, 0.2 Gm. every six hours for five doses, then 0.1 Gm. t.i.d. for six days. It may cause nausea and is best taken as tablets of 0.1 Gm. with meals. It is also used as an anthelmintic, in a single dose of 0.5 Gm. with 0.5 Gm. of sodium bicarbonate. It gives a yellow color to the urine and sometimes to the skin. Syn., *mepacrine hydrochloride*. See *atabrine dihydrochloride, chinacrin hydrochloride*.

quin'a·crine meth"ane·sul'fon·ate. A salt used like quinacrine hydrochloride but preferred over the latter for parenteral administration because of its greater solubility in water. See *mepacrine methanesulfonate*.

quin"al'bar'bi·tone so'di·um. British generic name for the barbiturate introduced under the trade-marked name seconal sodium. Syn., *secobarbital sodium*.

qui·nal'dine (kwi·nal'deen, ·din). $C_{10}H_9O$. Methylquinoline. An antipyretic similar to quinoline.

quin"al·din'ic ac'id. $C_{10}H_7NO_2.2H_2O$; quinoline-2-carboxylic acid; a crystalline powder, moderately soluble in water: used for quantitative estimation of copper, zinc, and uranium.

quin·al'gen. See *analgen*.

quin"a·liz'a·rin. $C_{14}H_8O_6$; an organic compound which turns blue in the presence of magnesium: used to detect magnesium in tissues.

qui·nam'i·dine (kwi·nam'i·deen, ·din). $C_{19}H_{24}N_2O_2$. An alkaloid from various species of *Cinchona*.

qui·nam'ine (kwi·nam'een, ·in, kwin'uh·meen, ·min). $C_{19}H_{24}N_2O_2$. An alkaloid of the cinchonas.

quince seed. See *cydonium*.

Quincke, Heinrich Irenaeus [*German physician*, 1842–1922]. Widely known for his description of angioneurotic edema (1882), previously described by John Laws Milton (1876); called *Quincke's disease*. He introduced the method of spinal puncture (1891), one of the chief clinical procedures in the diagnosis of disorders affecting the central nervous system. With Ernst Roos (1903), distinguished *Endamoeba histolytica* from *E. coli.* See also Quincke's *pulse.*

qui·ne′tum. Totaquine.

quin·hy′drone (kwin·high′drone, kwin′hi·drone). A substance representing equimolecular concentrations of quinone and hydroquinone; green prisms with pungent taste, soluble in hot water, alcohol, ether. Employed to prepare an electrode in pH determinations.

quin′ic ac′id. $C_7H_{12}O_6$. Hexahydrotetrahydroxybenzoic acid, found in cinchona bark and in several other plants.

quin′i·cine (kwin′i·seen, ·sin). A cinchona alkaloid, isomeric with quinine.

quin′i·dine (kwin′i·deen, ·din). $C_{20}H_{24}N_2O_2$. An alkaloid of cinchona bark isomeric with quinine. Like quinine, it is useful as an antimalarial although rarely employed. Used chiefly to restore normal rhythm in atrial fibrillation.

q. sulfate (*quinidinae sulfas*). $(C_{20}H_{24}N_2O_2)_2.H_2SO_4.2H_2O$. Fine, needlelike, white crystals which darken on exposure to light; odorless, of bitter taste. 1 Gm. dissolves in 100 cc. of water or in 10 cc. of alcohol. Used chiefly in atrial fibrillation. To determine possible hypersensitivity evidenced by headache, increased palpitation, nausea, vomiting, etc., a test dose of 0.2 Gm. (3 gr.) is given and repeated in 2 hours. In the absence of untoward symptoms, therapeutic dosage is begun. Dose, 0.2–0.4 Gm. (3–6 gr.) at intervals to provide a total dose of 1–2 Gm. (15–30 gr.) in 24 hours.

qui′nine (kwye′nyne, kwi·neen′, kwin′een) [Sp. *quina*, from Quechua *quinquina*, cinchona bark] (*quinina*). $C_{20}H_{24}N_2O_2.3H_2O$. An alkaloid obtained from cinchona. A white, odorless, microcrystalline powder of intensely bitter taste. It is somewhat efflorescent in dry air. Quinine kills the asexual forms (trophozoites) of the malarial organisms, and effectively arrests the malarial attacks, although there are usually recurrences which may again be suppressed by quinine. It is also analgesic and antipyretic and is used as such in colds and other fevers. Also employed as a bitter tonic in convalescence, and as a stimulant to the parturient uterus. The larger doses produce cinchonism. Quinine alkaloid is but slightly soluble, and usually administered as quinine sulfate in capsules, tablets, or pills, or suspended in chocolate syrup; also given as the hydrochloride or acid sulfate in solution, which, however, have a very bitter taste. The quinine hydrochloride or quinine and urea hydrochloride solution may be injected by vein in emergencies, but may produce sudden cardiac arrest. Intramuscular or hypodermic injection is inadvisable as it may produce gangrene. The oral dosage of quinine salts in malarial attacks is 1 Gm. (15 gr.) t.i.d. for two days, followed by 0.6 Gm. (10 gr.) t.i.d. for five days. It is best given before meals. Dose, in colds, 0.1–0.2 Gm. (1½–3 gr.) every two or three hours.

q. acetylsalicylate. Used as an antipyretic and analgesic. Dose, 0.06–0.3 Gm. (1–5 gr.).

q. acid sulfate. See *q.* bisulfate.

q. and urea hydrochloride (*quininae et ureae hydrochloridum*). A double salt. $C_{20}H_{24}N_2O_2.HCl.CO(NH_2)_2.HCl.5H_2O$. Contains 58–65% of anhydrous quinine. White, crystalline powder soluble in 1 part of water or 3 parts of alcohol. Used hypodermically in severe malaria. A sclerosing agent for varicose veins. Dose, 0.13–0.65 Gm. (2–10 gr.).

q. and urethan injection. A sterile solution in water for injection of approximately 2 parts of quinine hydrochloride and 1 part of urethan: used principally as a sclerosing agent in treatment of varicose veins.

q. bisalicylosalicylate. See *quinisal.*

q. bismuth iodide. Contains 18.0–20.1% of bismuth, 48.7–53.5% of iodine, and about 30% of anhydrous quinine. Used for the systemic effect of bismuth in the treatment of syphilis.

q. bisulfate (*quininae bisulfas*). $C_{20}H_{24}N_2O_2.H_2SO_4.7H_2O$. White, crystalline powder soluble in 10 parts of water. Dose, 0.13–1.0 Gm. (2–15 gr.). Syn., *q. acid sulfate.*

q. dihydrochloride (*quininae dihydrochloridum*). $C_{20}H_{24}N_2O_2.2HCl$. White, odorless powder; 1 Gm. dissolves in 0.6 cc. of water. Dose, 0.13–0.65 Gm. (2–10 gr.).

q. ethylcarbonate (*quininae aethylcarbonas*). $C_{23}H_{28}N_2O_4$. Fine, white, odorless needles; only slightly soluble in water; soluble in 3 parts of alcohol. Dose, 1–2 Gm. (15–30 gr.). Also called *euquinine.*

q. formate. $C_{20}H_{24}N_2O_2.HCOOH$. Dose, subcutaneous, 0.1–0.2 Gm. (1½–3 gr.). Syn., *quinoform.*

q. hydrobromide (*quininae hydrobromidum*). $C_{20}H_{24}N_2O_2.HBr.H_2O$. Small, white needles or scale-like crystals; odorless, efflorescent. Soluble in 40 parts of water or 1 part of alcohol. Used as antimalarial and in exophthalmic goiter. Dose, 0.13–0.65 Gm. (2–10 gr.).

q. hydrochloride (*quininae hydrochloridum*). $C_{20}H_{24}N_2O_2.HCl.2H_2O$. White, silky, glistening needles; odorless, efflorescent. Soluble in 16 parts of water or 1 part of alcohol. Dose, 0.13–0.65 Gm. (2–10 gr.).

q. lactate. $C_{20}H_{24}N_2O_2.CH_3.CHOH.COOH$. White, odorless, crystalline powder soluble in 3 parts of water. The aqueous solution is practically neutral and useful for subcutaneous administration of quinine. Dose, 0.06–0.3 Gm. (1–5 gr.).

q. phosphate (*quininae phosphas*). Approximately $(C_{20}H_{24}N_2O_2)_3.2H_3PO_4.5H_2O$. White, crystalline powder soluble in 600 parts of water. Dose, 0.13–0.65 Gm. (2–10 gr.).

q. salicylate (*quininae salicylas*). $C_{20}H_{24}N_2O_2.C_6H_4.OH.COOH.H_2O$. White needles or powder; odorless. Becomes pink on standing. Intended for use in rheumatism, myalgia, etc. Dose, 0.32–1.0 Gm. (5–15 gr.).

q. sulfate (*quininae sulfas*). $(C_{20}H_{24}N_2O_2)_2.H_2SO_4.2H_2O$. Fine, white needles; odorless; acquires a brown tint on exposure to light. One Gm. dissolves in 810 cc. of water or in 120 cc. of alcohol. The most popular salt of quinine. Dose, 0.13–0.65 Gm. (2–10 gr.).

q. tannate (*quininae tannas*). Contains 30–35% of anhydrous quinine. A pale yellow, amorphous powder. Dose, 0.2–1.0 Gm. (3–15 gr.).

qui′nin·ism (kwye′nyne·iz·um, kwi·neen′·, kwin′-een·), **qui′nism** [*quina*]. Cinchonism.

quin″in·o·der′ma. A drug dermatitis following the ingestion of quinine or its derivatives.

quinisal. Trade-mark for quinine bisalicylosalicylate, representing approximately 38% of anhydrous quinine. The substance is used as antirheumatic and febrifuge.

quin″i·zar′in. $C_{14}H_8O_4$; 1,4-dihydroxyanthraquinone; orange to red crystals, soluble in water. It has been used in experimental studies of vitamin-K antagonists.

quin′o·chromes. Blue, fluorescent products formed by the oxidation of vitamin B_1. Also see *thiochrome.*

quin′o·form. Quinine formate.

quin′oid. Referring to the molecular structure

```
          C=C
         /   \
      =C       C=
         \   /
          C=C
```

characteristic of quinones and believed to be responsible for the color of certain benzene derivatives.

qui·noi′dine (kwi·noy′deen, ·din). See *chinoidine.*

quin′ol. See *hydroquinone.*

quin′o·line (kwin′o·leen, ·lin). A tertiary amine, C_9H_7N, occurring in coal tar. The cinchona alkaloids may be considered as derivatives of this compound. A colorless liquid which becomes brown on exposure to air. It is antiseptic. Used chiefly as a solvent and in the synthesis of derivatives. Various salts have been used as antipyretics and antirheumatics.

q.-2-carboxylic acid. Quinaldinic acid.

qui·none′ (kwi·nohn′, kwin′ohn). 1. $C_6H_4O_2$; either of two isomeric derivatives of benzene, characterized by the presence of two oxygen atoms in place of two hydrogen atoms and containing one less double bond in the ring. *Ortho*-quinone, also called *o*-benzoquinone, contains the oxygen atoms in 1,2-position; *para*-quinone, also called *p*-benzoquinone, contains the oxygen atoms in 1,4-position. 2. Any derivative of either of the compounds defined in 1.

quin′o·rin. A glycoside from cinchona.

quin″o·tan′nic ac′id. See *cinchotannin.*

quin″o·tox′ine (kwin″o·tock′seen, ·sin). Quinicine.

qui·no′va·tine (kwi·no′vuh·teen, ·tin). An alkaloid, $C_{23}H_{26}N_2O_4$, occurring in the bark of *Cinchona cordifolia* var. *Pelletieriana.* Also called *aricine.*

qui·no′vic ac′id. $C_{30}H_{46}O_5$. A complex acid occurring in cinchona bark.

quin′o·vin, qui·no′vin [*quina*]. $C_{38}H_{62}O_{11}$. Kinovin, a bitter glycoside found in the bark of cinchona and other Rubiaceae.

quin·ox′a·line. $C_8H_6N_2$; the dicyclic compound 1,4-benzodiazine; a colorless, crystalline powder, slightly soluble in water: used in many syntheses, including those of medicinals.

quinoxyl. Trade-mark for a brand of chiniofon.

Quinquaud, Charles Eugène [*French physician,* 1841–94]. Described a method of measuring blood volume by means of CO (1882); called *Quinquaud-Gréhant's method.* Described folliculitis decalvans, an inflammation about the hair follicles attended with patchy baldness (1888); also called *Quinquaud's disease.* See also Quinquaud's *phenomenon.*

quin″que·tu·ber′cu·lar [L. *quinque,* five; *tuberculum,* swelling]. Having five tubercles or cusps.

quin′sy (kwin′zee) [G. *kynagchē,* dog-quinsy]. Acute inflammation of the tonsil and peritonsillar tissue, usually tending to suppuration. Also called *peritonsillar abscess.*

lingual q. Quinsy originating in the lingual tonsil and involving the tongue.

quin′tan [L. *quintus,* fifth]. Recurring on the fifth day.

quin′tan. An intermittent fever, the paroxysms of which recur every 96 hours; that is, on the fifth, ninth, thirteenth days, etc.

quin·tip′a·ra [*quintus;* L. *parere,* to bring forth]. A woman who has borne five children, or who is in labor for the fifth time.

quin′tu·plet, quin·tu′plet [L. *quintuplex,* fivefold]. One of five children who have been born at one birth.

qui·nu′cli·dine. $C_7H_{13}N$; 1-azabicyclo[2,2,2]octane or 1,4-ethylenepiperidine; a dicyclic, crystalline base, very soluble in water, representing one of the two principal structural units of quinine and other cinchona alkaloids, the other unit being quinoline.

Quitiqua. Pinta.

Quittenbaum, Carl Friedrich [*German surgeon,* 1793–1852]. Credited with being the first to establish extirpation of the spleen (1836).

quit′tor, quit′ter [ME. *quiture*]. *In veterinary medicine,* a disease of the lateral cartilages of the foot caused by injury and infection, resulting in the formation of a fistulous tract in the region of the coronet over the quarter.

quotane. Trade-mark for 1-(β-dimethylaminoethoxy)-3-*n*-butylisoquinoline hydrochloride; $C_{17}N_{25}N_2OCl$; a potent topical anesthetic useful in the treatment of dermatological diseases.

quo·tid′i·an [L. *quotidianus,* daily]. Recurring every day.

quo·tid′i·an. An intermittent fever, the paroxysms of which recur daily.

double q. A fever having two paroxysms a day, usually differing in character.

quo′tient [L. *quotiens,* how often]. The result of the process of division.

accomplishment q. *In psychology,* the ratio of achievement age to mental age. Also called *achievement q.* Abbreviated, AQ.

achievement q. Accomplishment *q.*

blood q. The result obtained by dividing the quantity of hemoglobin in the blood by the number of erythrocytes, expressed in each case as a percentage of the normal amount.

developmental q. The mathematical expression of the relation between developmental age and actual or chronologic age. To keep the related factors clear for easy reference, it is often expressed as a fraction,

$$\frac{\text{developmental age}}{\text{actual (chronologic) age}}$$

rather than worked out as a quotient. Developmental age may be determined by serial x-ray pictures leading to standards for epiphyseal development, body measurement (height, weight, etc.), mental and motor tests, or the grid method (Wetzel).

D/N q. The ratio of glucose to nitrogen in the urine.

economy q. The ratio of total gain of intake of water over total output of water at any one load. It measures the relative role of gain and of loss during attempts at recovery of water balance.

intelligence q. See *intelligence quotient.*

nonprotein respiratory quotients. The ratio of the volume of carbon dioxide given off to the volume of oxygen consumed after the subtraction from these gas volumes of the amounts utilized in protein metabolism.

protein q. The result of dividing the amount of globulin in the blood plasma by the amount of albumin in it.

respiratory q. Abbreviated, R. Q. (a) The ratio of the volume of carbon dioxide evolved by respiring cells or tissues to the volume of oxygen consumed in the same time. (b) The result obtained by dividing the carbon dioxide expired by the oxygen absorbed. This is normally

$$\frac{4.5}{5} = 0.9$$

velocity q. The volume of water restored or removed, relative to the increment to be restored or removed, per interval of time.

q.v. 1. *Quantum vis;* as much as you wish. 2. *Quod vide;* which see.

R

R Symbol for electrical resistance.
R. Réaumur, right.
® Symbol indicative of registered trade-mark status for a name.
r Symbol for roentgen.
R *Recipe,* take; used in prescription writing.
−R Rinne's test negative. See Rinne's *test.*
+R Rinne's test positive. See Rinne's *test.*
R_F *In chromatography,* the ratio of the distance traveled by a substance undergoing diffusion to the distance traveled by the solvent; the ratio is characteristic of the substance.
Ra Chemical symbol for radium.
rab′bit fe′ver. See *tularemia.*
rab″e·la′i·sin. A glycoside from *Lophopetalum toxicum;* its action is similar to that of digitalis.
rabellon. Trade-mark for a tablet containing belladonna alkaloids.
ra′bi·ate [L. *rabiatum,* from *rabiare,* to be mad]. Rabid.
rab′ic, ra′bic [L. *rabies,* madness]. Pertaining to rabies.
rab′id [L. *rabidus,* mad]. Affected with rabies; pertaining to rabies.
ra′bies (raybeez, ray′bee·eez) [L.]. An acute infectious disease of animals caused by a filtrable virus transmitted to other animals and man by the bite of infected animals. Many animals are subject to the disease, but it occurs most frequently in the wolf, the cat, and the dog, and is chiefly propagated by the last. The virus has a special affinity for the nervous system, and is found in secretions, particularly in the saliva. In man there are usually three stages of the disease; the first or preliminary, marked by restlessness, apprehension, and obvious ill health; the second or furious stage, in which the patient is hyperactive and has spasms of the muscles of swallowing and respiration; and the third or paralytic stage, which is marked in the beginning by drooling saliva, due to poor muscular control, and terminates fatally with a general paralysis ascending the spinal column. See also *pseudorabies.* —**rabiat′ic,** *adj.*

r. fixed virus. A term applied by Pasteur to virus that is so high in virulence for rabbits by successive intracerebral transfers that it will kill the animals in a period of six or seven days.

r. prophylaxis. The daily inoculation of an exposed person with emulsions of spinal cord from infected rabbits. The first injection is made with cord which has been dried for 14 days, successive inoculations being from progressively fresher cord. Other methods have been employed to inactivate the vaccine, such as chloroform and phenol. Also called *Pasteur treatment.*

r. vaccine. An emulsion made from the spinal cords of rabbits infected with rabies. Also see *r.* prophylaxis, Flury *strain.*

Rabinowitch, Israel Mordecai [*Canadian physician,* 1891–   ]. Known for his studies in the dietetic treatment of diabetes mellitus. Advocated diet of low caloric value with relatively low fat and high carbohydrate content.
race [F., from It. *razza*]. A poorly defined minor subdivision of a species. —**ra′cial,** *adj.*
ra·ce′mic (ra·see′mick, ·sem′ick) [L. *racemus,* a bunch of grapes]. Composed of equal parts of dextrorotatory and levorotatory forms of optical isomers and, therefore, optically inactive.
ra·ce′mic ac′id. An optically inactive mixture of dextrorotatory and levorotatory forms of tartaric acid.
rac″e·mi·za′tion. Conversion of the optically active form of a compound to its racemic form, commonly by heating.
rac″e·mor′phan hy″dro·bro′mide. Generic name for racemic 3-hydroxy-N-methylmorphinan hydrobromide; $C_{17}H_{22}NO.HBr$; formerly known as *methorphinan hydrobromide;* a potent synthetic analgesic related chemically and pharmacologically to morphine. The levorotatory component of the base, designated by the generic name *levorphan,* is approximately twice as potent as the mixture; levorphan tartrate is the available salt. See *dromoran hydrobromide, levo-dromoran tartrate.*
rac′e·mose (rass′i·mose) [L. *racemosus,* full of clusters]. Resembling a bunch of grapes.
racephedrine. Trade name for racemic ephedrine. The substance is readily soluble in water or alcohol and is used like ephedrine. Dose, 30–50 mg. (½–¾ gr.). Also called *d-l-ephedrine.*

r. hydrochloride. The corresponding hydrochloride, soluble in 4 parts of water or 25 parts of alcohol.

race su′i·cide. The gradual extinction of a human population through the voluntary widespread limitation of family size.
ra′chi-. See *rachio-.*
ra″chi·an″al·ge′si·a (ray″kee·an″al·jee′zee·uh, ·see·uh) [G. *rhachis,* spine; *analgēsia,* want of feeling]. Spinal anesthesia. *Obs.*
ra″chi·an″es·the′si·a (ray″kee·an″ess·thee′zhuh, ·zee·uh) [*rhachis;* G. *anaisthēsia,* lack of sensation]. Spinal anesthesia. *Obs.*
ra″chi·as′mus [*rhachis*]. Spasm of the muscles at the back of the neck, as seen in the early part of many epileptic attacks. *Rare.*
ra′chi·cele (ray′ki·seel) [*rhachis;* G. *kēlē,* hernia]. Hernial protrusion of the contents of the spinal canal in spina bifida. It includes spinal meningocele, myelomeningocele, and myelocystocele (syringomyelocele).
ra″chi·cen·te′sis [*rhachis;* G. *kentēsis,* a pricking]. Puncture into the subarachnoid space; lumbar puncture.
ra·chil′y·sis (ra·kil′i·sis) [*rhachis;* G. *lysis,* a loosing]. A method of treating lateral curvature of the spine by mechanical counteraction of the abnormal curves.
ra′chi·o- (ray′kee·o-), **ra′chi-** [*rhachis*]. A combining form meaning *the spine.*
ra″chi·o·camp′sis [*rhachis;* G. *kampsis,* a bending]. Curvature of the spine.
ra″chi·o·cen·te′sis. See lumbar *puncture.*
ra″chi·o·dyn′i·a (ray″kee·o·din′ee·uh, ·dye′nee·uh) [*rhachis;* G. *odynē,* pain]. Spasmodic pain in the spinal column.
ra″chi·om′e·ter [*rhachis;* G. *metron,* a measure]. An instrument used to measure the degree of spinal deformities.
ra″chi·op′a·thy [*rhachis;* G. *pathos,* disease]. Any disease of the spine. *Obs.*

ra″chi·o·ple′gi·a [*rhachis;* G. *plēgē*, stroke]. Spinal paralysis.

ra″chi·o·sco″li·o′sis (ray″kee·o·sko″lee·o′sis, ·skol″ee·o′sis) [*rhachis;* G. *skoliōsis*, obliquity]. Lateral curvature of the spine.

ra′chi·o·tome″ [*rhachis;* G. *tomos*, cutting]. A cutting instrument used in operations upon the vertebrae.

ra″chi·ot′o·my [*rhachis;* G. *tomē*, a cutting]. The operation of cutting into the vertebral column.

ra·chip′a·gus (ra·kip′uh·gus) [*rhachis;* G. *pagos*, that which is fixed]. Conjoined twins (diplopagi) united back to back by any portion of the vertebral column.

ra″chi·re·sis′tance. Resistance of the spinal nerves to a specific local anesthetic agent, related possibly to excessive myelinization of axons or thick perineural sheath or acid pH, seen in acidosis and infections.

ra′chis (ray′kis) [*rhachis*]. The vertebral column. —**rachid′ial, rachid′ian,** *adj.*

ra·chis′chi·sis (ra·kiss′ki·sis) [*rhachis;* G. *schisis*, cleavage]. Synonym for spina bifida.

ra·chit′a·min (ra·kit′uh·min). Vitamin D. *Obs.*

ra″chi·ter′a·ta [*rhachis;* G. *teras*, monster]. A collective term for all anomalies involving the spine.

ra·chit′ic [*rhachis;* G. *-itis*, inflammation]. Affected with, resembling, or produced by, rickets.

ra·chit′ic ro′sa·ry. The row of nodules appearing on the ribs at the junctions with their cartilages; often seen in rachitic children. Also called *beading of the ribs, rachitic beads.*

ra·chi′tis (ra·kye′tis). Rickets.

ra′chi·tism (ray′ki·tiz·um, rack′i·) [*rhachis; -itis*]. Tendency to rickets.

rach″i·to·gen′ic (rack″i·to·jen′ick) [*rhachis; -itis;* G. *genesthai*, from *gignesthai*, to be produced]. Producing rickets, as a vitamin-D deficient diet.

ra·clage′ (rah·klahzh′) [F.]. The destruction of a soft growth by rubbing, as with a brush or harsh sponge.

ra·cle·ment′ (rah·kluh·mahng′. *See* NOTES § 35). Raclage.

rad. *Radix*, root.

ra·dec′to·my [L. *radix*, root; G. *ektomē*, excision]. Resection of the root of a tooth, in whole or in part.

ra′di·al [L. *radius*, spoke, ray, exterior bone of the forearm]. 1. Radiating; diverging from a common center. 2. Pertaining to, or in relation to, the radius or bone of the forearm, as the radial artery. See Table of Arteries in the Appendix.

ra″di·a′lis (ray″dee·ah′lis, ·ay′lis) [*radius*]. Pertaining to the radius; a term applied to various arteries, nerves, and muscles, as flexor carpi radialis.

ra′di·an [*radius*]. An arc whose length is equal to the radius of the circle of which it is a part.

ra′di·ant [L. *radiare*, to furnish with beams]. Emitting rays, as radiant energy, energy traveling in the form of electromagnetic waves.

ra″di·a′tion [L. *radiatio*, a shining]. 1. The act of radiating or diverging from a central point, as radiation of light; divergence from a center, having the appearance of rays. 2. The emission and propagation of energy through space or through a material medium in a form having certain characteristics of waves, including the energy commonly described as electromagnetic and that of sound; usually, electromagnetic radiation, classified, according to frequency, as Hertzian, infrared, visible, ultraviolet, x-ray, and gamma ray; also, by extension, such corpuscular emissions as alpha and beta particles and cosmic rays. 3. *In neurology*, certain groups of fibers that diverge after leaving their place of origin. —**ra′di·ate,** *v., adj.*

acoustic r. Old term for auditory radiation.

annihilation r. The production of two photons when an electron and a positron unite and are annihilated.

auditory r. A large bundle of fibers in the posterior part of the internal capsule, running from the medial geniculate body to the superior and transverse temporal gyri. Also called *geniculotemporal r.* or *tract, acoustic r.*

corpus callosum r. A radiation of the corpus callosum fibers in the medullary center of each cerebral hemisphere.

corpuscular r. Subatomic particles such as electrons, protons, or neutrons, or combinations of these particles such as deuterons, alpha rays, traveling at high velocities.

corticostriate r. Fibers running between the corpus striatum and the equatorial zone of the cortex.

electromagnetic r. Radiation which is propagated through space or matter in the form of electromagnetic waves.

fluorescent r. Radiation that is emitted by fluorescent bodies.

fractionation r. Method of administration of roentgen rays or radium in fractions of the total dose spread over a period of days.

geniculotemporal r. See auditory *r.*

heterogeneous r. Radiation containing more than one wavelength.

homogeneous r. Radiation containing only one wavelength.

interstitial r. Radiation by inserting radium or radon directly into the tissue.

ionizing radiations. Radiations which directly or indirectly produce ionization.

irritative r. Ultraviolet radiation to the point of producing erythema.

mitogenetic r. A kind of radiation said to be produced in cells and tissues, which induces or is induced by the process of mitosis. Also called *Gurvich r.*

monochromatic r. Electromagnetic radiation which has either one wavelength or photons of the same energy level.

monoenergetic r. Radiation in which the particles or photons all have equal energy.

optic r. The geniculocalcarine tract, connecting the lateral geniculate body with the calcarine occipital area of the cortex: also called *optic r. of Gratiolet.*

photochemical r. Radiation which is part of the spectrum that produces chemical reactions.

protraction r. Decrease of the rate of application of a given dose of roentgen rays or radium rays.

r. injury. See under *injury.*

r. pneumonitis. See under *pneumonitis.*

r. poisoning. See under *poisoning.*

relative biological effectiveness of r. The inverse ratio of tissue doses of two different types of radiation that produces a particular biologic response under identical conditions.

secondary r. *In nuclear science*, particles or photons produced by the interaction with matter of a radiation that is regarded as primary.

sensory r. See thalamic *r.*

solar r. Radiation from the sun.

stem r. *In radiology*, roentgen rays emitted from areas of the roentgen-ray tube other than the target, especially from the target support.

striothalamic r. A system of fibers connecting the corpus striatum with the thalamus and the subthalamic region.

supervoltage r. *In radiology,* roentgen radiation produced by voltages of 500–2000 kilovolts.

thalamic radiations. Nerve fibers running from the thalamus to the cerebral cortex (*thalamocortical tract*) and from the cortex to the thalamus (*corticothalamic tract*).

ultraviolet r. Radiation comprising ultraviolet wavelengths.

ra″di·a′tion sick′ness. See under *sickness.*

ra″di·a′tion ther′a·py. See under *therapy.*

rad′i·cal [L. *radix,* root]. Belonging to a root; going to the root, or attacking the cause, of a disease; the opposite of conservative.

rad′i·cal. 1. A group of atoms that acts as a unit, but commonly does not exist in the free state, as NH_4, ammonium, or C_6H_5, phenyl. 2. The haptophore group of an antibody.

rad′i·cle [L. *radicula,* small root]. 1. A little root, as the radicle of a nerve, one of the ultimate fibrils of which a nerve is composed, or radicle of a vein, one of the minute vessels uniting to form a vein. 2. See *radical,* 1, 2.

rad″i·cot′o·my. See *rhizotomy.*

ra·dic′u·lar [*radicula*]. Pertaining to a root or to a radicle; specifically, pertaining to the roots of the spinal nerves or to those of teeth.

ra·dic″u·lec′to·my [*radicula;* G. *ektomē,* excision]. Excision or resection of a spinal nerve root.

ra·dic″u·li′tis [*radicula;* G. *-itis,* inflammation]. Inflammation of a nerve root.

acute brachial r. See shoulder girdle *syndrome.*

ra·dic″u·lo·my″e·lop′a·thy [*radicula;* G. *myelos,* marrow; *pathos,* disease]. Disease of the spinal cord and roots of the spinal nerves.

ra·dic″u·lo·neu·ri′tis [*radicula;* G. *neuron,* nerve; *-itis,* inflammation]. Inflammation of a spinal nerve root.

ra·dic″u·lo·neu·rop′a·thy [*radicula; neuron;* G. *pathos,* disease]. Disease of the peripheral spinal nerves and their roots.

ra·dic″u·lop′a·thy [*radicula; pathos*]. Disease of the roots of spinal nerves.

ra′di·o- [L. *radius,* ray]. 1. A combining form meaning *pertaining to radiant energy* or *to radium.* 2. A combining form meaning *relating to the radius.*

ra″di·o·ac·tin′i·um [*radius;* G. *aktis,* ray]. A radioactive product of actinium. It gives off alpha rays and disintegrates into actinium x.

ra″di·o·ac′tive [*radius;* L. *activus,* active]. Emitting radiant energy.

ra″di·o·ac·tiv′i·ty [*radius; activus*]. A property of certain substances of spontaneously emitting alpha particles, beta particles, or gamma rays from the nucleus of the atom. —**radioac′tive,** *adj.*

artificial r. That produced artificially by bombardment with high-velocity particles, as in a cyclotron or betatron or by other means. Also called *induced r.*

ra″di·o·au′to·graph [*radius;* G. *autos,* self; *graphein,* to write]. A direct photographic record of the distribution of a radioactive substance in an organism or tissue section: often used to detect a diseased tissue, such as a tumor or hyperactive endocrine gland. Also called *autoradiograph, autoradiogram, radioautogram.*

ra″di·o·au·tog′ra·phy. The process of making a radioautograph.

ra′di·obe [*radius*]. A peculiar, microscopic formation that is produced in sterilized bouillon by radium radiation, and that has the appearance of bacteria.

ra″di·o·bi·ol′o·gy [*radius;* G. *bios,* life; *logos,* word]. That branch of science devoted to the study of the results of radiation upon the body.

ra″di·o·car′pe·us. The flexor carpi radialis brevis muscle.

ra″di·o·chem′is·try [*radius;* G. *chymos,* juice]. That branch of chemistry which deals with radioactive phenomena.

ra″di·o·cir″cu·log′ra·phy. A technique for measuring and registering radioactivity of blood as it circulates through blood vessels.

ra″di·o·co′balt. Any radioactive isotope of cobalt, especially that having a mass number of 60 (Co^{60}), which has a half-life of 5.2 years and emits a negative beta particle and two gamma rays for each atom of cobalt that decays. In the form of metallic cobalt its radiation is used in the therapy of malignancies.

ra″di·o·col′loid. Any colloidal aggregate of radioactive substances.

ra″di·o·cur·a·bil′i·ty. The condition of being susceptible to cure or elimination by irradiation: said of cancer cells.

ra″di·o·cys·ti′tis [*radius;* G. *kystis,* bladder; *-itis,* inflammation]. Cystitis following x-ray or radium therapy.

ra′di·ode [*radius;* G. *hodos,* way]. An electric attachment for the application of radium.

ra″di·o·der″ma·ti′tis. See roentgen *dermatitis.*

ra″di·o·di″ag·no′sis [*radius;* G. *diagnōsis,* a distinguishing]. The diagnosis of disease by means of radiography or radioscopy.

ra″di·o·don′ti·a [*radius;* G. *odous,* tooth]. Radiography of the teeth and adjacent tissues.

ra″di·o·don′tist [*radius; odous*]. A specialist in radiography of the teeth and adjacent tissues.

ra″di·o·el′e·ment [*radius;* L. *elementum,* element]. An element with radioactive properties.

ra″di·o·gen′ic. Referring to a substance or state resulting from a radioactive transformation, as radiogenic lead resulting from disintegration of radium, or radiogenic heat produced within the earth by disintegration of radioactive substances.

ra″di·o·gold′. Any radioactive isotope of gold, especially that having a mass number of 198 (Au^{198}), which has a half-life of 2.69 days and emits a negative beta particle and a gamma ray for each atom of gold that decays. In the form of a colloidal dispersion of the metal it is used, by injection, in the therapy and palliation of neoplastic disease and in the treatment of neoplastic effusions, also as a tracer in various studies involving gold.

ra′di·o·graph″ [*radius;* G. *graphein,* to write]. To make a photograph on a sensitive film by projection of roentgen rays through a part of the body.

ra′di·o·graph″. A roentgen-ray photograph: also called *roentgenogram.*

ra″di·og′ra·pher [*radius; graphein*]. One skilled in radiography; an x-ray technician.

ra″di·og′ra·phy [*radius; graphein*]. The practice or act of making radiographs. —**radiograph′ic,** *adj.*

sectional r. The technic of making radiographs of plane sections of solid objects; its purpose is to show detail in a predetermined plane of the body, while blurring the images of structures in other planes. The methods used differ slightly and have been designated stratigraphy, tomography, planigraphy, x-ray focusing, vertigraphy, laminagraphy, and body-section roentgenography. In all, the radiographs are produced by movement of the film during exposure in a direction reciprocal and proportional to the simultaneous movement of the tube.

ra″di·o·hu′mer·al [L. *radius,* exterior bone of the forearm; *humerus,* upper part of the arm]. Pertaining to the radius and the humerus.

ra″di·o·i′o·dine (ray″dee·o·eye′o·dyne, ·deen, ·din) [L. *radius,* ray; G. *ioeidēs,* violetlike]. Any radioactive isotope of iodine, especially that having a mass number of 131 (I^{131}), which has a half-life of 8 days and emits two negative beta particles and several gamma rays for each atom of iodine that decays. In the form of sodium iodide it is used, by intravenous or oral administration, in the treatment of hyperthyroidism and cancer of the thyroid, also for various diagnostic purposes; in the form of diiodofluorescein, in the diagnosis and localization of brain tumors; in the form of iodinated serum albumin, for determination of plasma volume, peripheral vascular flow, circulation time, etc. It has many uses as a tracer in reactions involving iodine.

ra′di·o·i′ron [*radius;* AS. *iren*]. Any radioactive isotope of iron, especially that having a mass number of 59 (Fe^{59}), which has a half-life of 46 days and emits two negative beta particles and two gamma rays for each atom of iron that decays. In the form of ferric ammonium citrate it has been used in the study of iron metabolism, in determination of blood volume with red cells labeled with the radioisotope, and in various studies on blood transfusion.

ra″di·o·i′so·tope. A radioactive isotope, very commonly of an element which is stable. While certain isotopes of normally stable elements exist naturally in radioactive form, many are prepared only artificially, as by bombarding an element with neutrons, protons, deuterons, or alpha particles in a nuclear reactor or in an accelerating device such as the cyclotron or cosmotron; the bombarded element may form a radioactive isotope of the same element or of another element. By virtue of its radioactivity, a radioisotope is used either for the effect of its radiations, such use often being diagnostic or therapeutic, or as a tracer added to the stable form of a compound to follow the course of the latter in a particular sequence of reactions in living organisms or even in an inanimate system.

ra″di·o·ky·mog′ra·phy (ray″dee·o·kigh·mog′ruh-fee) [*radius;* G. *kyma*, wave; *graphein*, to write]. A method of obtaining a graphic record of movement of the silhouette of an organ or tissue on a single film.

Ra″di·o·la′ri·a [dim. from *radius*]. A subclass of Rhizopoda, which have a chitinous capsule between the endoplasm and the ectoplasm.

ra″di·ol′o·gist [*radius;* G. *logos*, word]. A physician specializing in radiology.

ra″di·ol′o·gy [*radius; logos*]. That branch of medicine which deals with radioactive substances, x-rays, and other ionizing radiations and with their utilization in the diagnosis and treatment of disease. —**radiolog′ic,** *adj.*

ra″di·o·lu′cent [*radius;* L. *lucere*, to shine]. Partly or wholly transparent to roentgen rays or other forms of radiation. —**radiolucency,** *n.*

ra″di·o·lu″mi·nes′cence [*radius;* L. *lumen*, light]. That luminescence brought about by radioactive rays striking an obstacle or screen treated with a suitable substance.

ra″di·o·mag·ne′si·um. Radioactive isotope of magnesium, produced artificially by bombardment with high energy positively charged atomic particles or with neutrons.

ra″di·o·man·om′e·try. The measurement of pressures due to the incidence of radiation on matter.

ra″di·om′e·ter [*radius;* G. *metron*, a measure]. 1. An instrument for measuring the intensity of thermal radiation. 2. An instrument for measuring the quality or penetration of x-rays.

ra″di·o·mi·crom′e·ter. A sensitive thermopile used for detection of very small changes of radiant energy.

ra″di·o·mi·met′ic. Capable of producing in tissue biological effects similar to those of ionizing radiation.

ra′di·on [*radius*]. A particle thrown off by a radioactive substance.

ra″di·o·ne·cro′sis [*radius;* G. *nekrōsis*, mortification]. Destruction or ulceration of tissues caused by radiation.

ra″di·o·neu·ri′tis [*radius;* G. *neuron*, nerve; *-itis*, inflammation]. A form of neuritis due to exposure to x-rays or radium rays.

ra″di·o·ni′tro·gen [*radius;* G. *nitron*, sodium carbonate; *genesthai*, from *gignesthai*, to be produced]. The radioactive isotope of nitrogen, having a mass number of 13 (N^{13}), which has a half-life of 10.1 minutes and emits a positive beta particle for each atom of nitrogen that decays.

ra″di·o·paque′ (ray″dee·o·payk′) [*radius;* L. *opacus*, shady]. Not transparent to the x-ray; not permitting the passage of radiant energy. —**radiopac′ity,** *n.*

ra″di·o·par′ent [*radius;* L. *parere*, to appear]. Transparent to the x-ray; permitting the passage of radiant energy. —**radioparency,** *n.*

ra″di·o·pa·thol′o·gy [*radius;* G. *pathos*, disease; *logos*, word]. Study of tissue changes brought about by radiation.

ra″di·o·pel·vim′e·try [*radius;* L. *pelvis*, basin; *metron*, a measure]. Radiographic procedure for making accurate measurements of the maternal pelvis and fetal skull. Also called *pelviencephalometry.*

ra″di·o·phos′pho·rus. The radioactive isotope of phosphorus, having a mass number of 32 (P^{32}), which has a half-life of 14.3 days and emits a negative beta particle for each atom of phosphorus that decays. In the form of disodium hydrogen phosphate it is used, by intravenous or oral administration, in the treatment of polycythemia vera and in various ways as a diagnostic agent, as in the determination of blood volume, and also as a tracer in various studies involving phosphorus.

ra″di·o·po·tas′si·um. Any radioactive isotope of potassium, especially that having a mass number of 42 (K^{42}), which has a half-life of 12.5 hours and emits two negative beta particles and a gamma ray for each atom of potassium that decays. In the form of various potassium salts, administered intravenously or orally, it has been used in studies of potassium metabolism, in localization of brain tumors, and in other tracer studies involving potassium.

ra″di·o·prax′is [*radius;* G. *praxis*, a doing]. The use of radiant energy either in therapy or for other purposes.

ra″di·o·re·sist′ance. Relative resistance of tissues or organisms to the injurious effects of radiation.

ra″di·os′co·py [*radius;* G. *skopein*, to examine]. The process of securing an image of an object upon a fluorescent screen by means of radiant energy.

ra″di·o·sen″si·tiv′i·ty [*radius;* L. *sentire*, to feel]. Sensitivity of tissues or organisms to various types of radiations, such as x-rays or rays from radioactive materials. —**radiosen′sitive,** *adj.*

ra″di·o·sil′i·con [*radius;* L. *silex*, flint]. Radioactive isotope of silicon, produced artificially by bombardment with high energy positively charged atomic particles or with neutrons.

ra″di·o·so′di·um. Any radioactive isotope of sodium, especially that having a mass number of 24 (Na^{24}), which has a half-life of 14.9 hours and emits a negative beta particle and two gamma rays for each atom of sodium that decays. In the form of sodium chloride it is used, by intravenous administration, in various diagnostic studies, as of peripheral vascular disease, circulation time, sodium metabolism, etc.

ra″di·o·ster″e·os′co·py [*radius;* G. *stereos*, solid; *skopein*, to examine]. The application of the principle of the stereoscope, obtaining a viewpoint for the left eye and one for the right by corresponding displacement of the x-ray tube along the plane of the film, and duplication of these geometric conditions in viewing the two radiographs in a properly constructed stereoscopic view box.

ra″di·o·stron′ti·um. Any radioactive isotope of strontium. That of mass number 89 (Sr^{89}), which has a half-life of 54 days and emits a negative beta particle for each atom of strontium that decays, has been used in treatment of bone tumors; that of mass number 90 (Sr^{90}), which has a half-life of 24 years and also emits a negative beta particle for each atom of strontium that decays, has been used for radiation therapy of benign conditions of the eye.

ra″di·o·sul′fur. Any radioactive isotope of sulfur, especially that having a mass number of 35 (S^{35}), which has a half-life of 87.1 days and emits a gamma ray for each atom of sulfur that decays. It has been incorporated in various compounds as a tracer element to study the metabolism of these and related compounds.

ra″di·o·sur′ger·y [*radius;* G. *cheirourgia*, a working by hand]. The use of radium in surgical therapy.

ra″di·o·tel·lu′ri·um [*radius;* L. *tellus*, earth]. Any of a group of radioactive isotopes of tellurium, ranging in mass number from 118 to 133 and with a range of half-life from about 25 minutes to about 143 days.

ra″di·o·ther″a·peu′tic. Of or pertaining to therapeutic use of radiant energy.

ra″di·o·ther″a·peu′tic (ray″dee·o·therr″uh·pew′-tick) [*radius;* G. *therapeutikos*, inclined to serve]. Referring to therapeutic use of radiant energy.

ra″di·o·ther″a·peu′tics. See *radiotherapy.*

ra″di·o·ther′a·py [*radius;* G. *therapeia*, treatment]. The treatment of disease by means of x-rays, radium rays, and other radioactive substances.

ra″di·o·ther′my [*radius;* G. *thermē*, heat]. 1. Treatment by radiant heat. 2. Short-wave diathermy.

ra″di·o·tho′ri·um. Any of a group of radioactive isotopes of thorium, ranging in mass number from 226 to 234 and with a range of half-life from about 31 minutes to about 10^{10} years.

ra″di·o·tox·e′mi·a [*radius;* G. *toxikon*, poison; *haima*, blood]. Toxemia induced from overexposure to any radioactive substance.

ra″di·o·trans·par′ent [*radius;* L. *trans*, across; *parere*, to appear]. Permitting the passage of radiations; used notably in connection with x-rays. The opposite of radiopaque.

ra″di·o·ul′nar [L. *radius*, exterior bone of the forearm; *ulna*, arm]. Pertaining to the radius and ulna.

ra′di·um [L. *radius*, ray]. Ra = 226.05. A highly radioactive metallic element. Discovered in 1898 by Pierre and Marie Curie, who separated it from pitchblende by a tedious process. The chloride or bromide of radium is usually used. Radium salts emit continuously heat, light, and three other distinct kinds of radiation (alpha particles, beta particles, and gamma rays).

ra′di·um can′non. *In radiology*, a tube resembling a gun barrel, allowing radiation only in a straight line; used in deep therapy.

ra′di·um-F Ra-F. Polonium.

ra″di·um·i·za′tion [*radius*]. Exposure to radium rays.

ra′di·us [L., exterior bone of the forearm]. The outer of the two bones of the forearm. See Table of Bones in the Appendix. See Plate 1.

r. fixus. A line drawn from the hormion to the inion.

ra′dix (pl. *radices*) [L., root]. A root. For special terms, see under *root*. Abbreviated, rad.

r. arcus vertebrae. A root or pedicle of the vertebral arch.

radolatum. Trade-mark for an ultraviolet-irradiated liquid petrolatum used as a bactericide.

ra′don [L. *radius*, ray]. Rn = 222. A decay product of radium; a colorless, gaseous, radioactive element. Also called *radium emanation.*

ra′don seed. A small capillary tube, of glass, containing radon, suitable for implantation in tissues; the tube may be placed inside a small gold or platinum tube.

raf′fin·ase. An enzyme which hydrolyzes raffinose with the splitting-off of fructose. Probably identical with saccharase.

raf′fin·ose. $C_{18}H_{32}O_{16}.5H_2O$. A trisaccharide found in sugar beets, cottonseed meal, and molasses. On hydrolysis, it yields glucose, fructose, and galactose.

ra′fle (ray′ful, rah′ful) [F.]. An eruptive pustular disease of cattle in northern France.

rag′pick″er′s dis·ease′. Anthrax occurring in ragpickers.

rag′weed″ [AS. *ragg; wēod*]. Any of several species of the genus *Ambrosia;* its pollen is the most important allergen in the central and eastern United States. Its pollinating period is from the middle of August to the time of frost.

Rail″li·e·ti′na (rye″lee·i·tye′nuh, ·tee′nuh). A genus of tapeworms.

R. celebensis. A species of tapeworms; infestations of man reported in Tokyo and in Formosa.

R. madagascariensis. A species which infests man.

R. quitensis. A species which infests man; reported from Ecuador.

rail′way″ fe′ver. See shipping *fever.*

rail′way″ sick′ness. Car sickness; a form of motion sickness occurring as a result of the movement of a train. See *airsickness.*

rail′way″ spine. See under *spine.*

rale (rahl) [F.]. An abnormal sound arising within the lungs or air passages and heard on auscultation over the chest. There is no agreement among authorities concerning a classification of these sounds. A very large number of descriptive terms have been used in the past, many of them based on fanciful considerations of the physical conditions held responsible for their production. The modern tendency is to discard most of the qualifying adjectives formerly used and to characterize rales by such simple and self-explanatory terms as coarse, medium (moderately coarse), and fine. The adjectives moist and dry are also widely used, but in a descriptive sense only. They are not intended to imply that the sound has originated in a moist or dry physical environment. Some authors hold that all rales originate in the presence of abnormal moisture. No type of rale is pathognomonic of a specific disease, such as pneumonia, tuberculosis, bronchiectasis, etc., or of a physical condition such as pulmonary cavity or consolidation. There is fairly general, though not complete, agreement regarding the significance of the following terms.

amphoric r. Coarse, tinkling sounds accompanying bronchiectasis and lung cavitation, caused by fluid splashing in a cavity which connects with a bronchus.

atelectatic r. See crepitant *r.*

cavernous r. A hollow, metallic sound accompanying far-advanced tuberculosis, caused by the expansion and contraction of a pulmonary cavity during respiration.

clicking r. A weak, sticky sound heard during

inspiration, accompanying the early stages of pulmonary tuberculosis, and caused by air passing through soft material in the smaller bronchi.

consonating r. A moderately coarse rale which sounds unusually loud and close to the ear, as though it were reinforced by transmission through the area of consolidated lung with which it is usually associated.

crepitant r. A fine, dry, crackling sound, simulated by the rubbing together of hairs, or by the sprinkling of salt on a hot stove; often heard as a transient phenomenon around the inferior margins of normal lungs during the first few forced inspirations.

Hirtz's r. A moist, metallic sound accompanying tuberculous softening.

latent r. See post-tussive *r.*

marginal r. See crepitant *r.*

mucous r. A sound similar to one heard when blowing through a pipe into soapy water, heard in patients with emphysema, and caused by viscid bubbles bursting in the bronchial tubes.

post-tussive r. That form not heard during either natural or forced breathing, but elicited only by the use of a short cough delivered at the end of a forced expiration.

rhonchus r. An extremely coarse type of rale which originates only in the larger air passages and sets up vibrations which usually can be palpated on the surface of the chest in addition to being heard with a stethoscope.

sibilant r. A dry, high-pitched, hissing or whistling sound heard most often in cases of bronchiolar spasm.

sonorous r. A dry, low-pitched, resonant, snoring sound heard most often in cases of bronchiolar spasm.

subcrepitant r. A crackling sound similar to crepitant rale, but coarser and lower pitched.

vesicular r. Crepitant rale.

R. A. M. C. Royal Army Medical Corps.

ram·e′a·lin. An antibiotic produced by the fungus *Stereum rameale;* a yellow viscous oil.

ra′mi (ray′migh). Plural of ramus.

ram″i·fi·ca′tion [L. *ramus,* branch; *facere,* to make]. 1. The act or state of branching. 2. A branch.

ram′i·fy (ram′i·figh) [*ramus; facere*]. Form branches; branch.

ram″i·sec′tion, ram′i·sec″tion [*ramus;* L. *sectio,* from *secare,* to cut]. Surgical division of the rami communicantes of the sympathetic nervous system.

ram″i·sec′to·my. See *ramisection.*

Ramon, Gaston [*French bacteriologist,* 1885–   ]. Known for his quantitative in vitro test for the determination of the potency in flocculation units of diphtheria toxins and antitoxins; called *Ramon's flocculation test.* He is the discoverer of toxoids (1923).

Ramón y Cajal, Santiago [*Spanish neurologist,* 1852–1934]. Generally considered the greatest Spanish medical scientist; he was the founder of the Spanish school of neurologists, and a Nobel laureate with Golgi in 1906. In 1909 he published "Histologie du système nerveux," which is still the great classic in this field. Celebrated for his many innovations in staining nervous tissue. See *Cajal's silver methods* and *Cajal's gold-sublimate method,* under *stain.* Astrocytes are also called *Cajal's cells.*

Ramon-Zoeller's reaction. See under C. *Zoeller.*

ra′mose [L. *ramosus,* full of branches]. Having many branches; branching.

ra′mous [L. *ramus,* branch]. Having many branches; branching.

Ramsden, Jesse [*English optician,* 1735–1800]. Inventor of the Ramsden ocular.

Ramstedt, Conrad [*German surgeon,* 1867–   ]. Widely known for his work in developing the operation for relief of congenital pyloric stenosis, called *Ramstedt's operation, Fredet-Ramstedt operation.* See *pyloromyotomy.*

ram′u·lus (pl. *ramuli*) [L., little branch]. A small branch, or ramus.

ra′mus (pl. *rami*) [L.]. 1. A branch, especially of a vein, artery, or nerve. 2. A slender process of bone projecting like a branch or twig from a large bone, as the ramus of the lower jaw, or the superior or inferior ramus of the pubis. —**ramal,** *adj.*

conjoined r. In the adult pelvis, the united inferior ramus of the pubis and ramus of the ischium.

gray r. communicans. A communicating branch of the sympathetic trunk connecting it with a peripheral nerve. Also called *postganglionic r.*

r. anastomoticus. A branch of a nerve which communicates with a neighboring nerve or with a plexus. Also, a communicating artery between two neighboring arteries.

r. cardiacus. A cardiac branch of the vagus nerve.

r. caroticus. A branch of the glossopharyngeal nerve to the carotid sinus.

r. communicans. An anastomotic branch of a nerve, applied especially to the white and gray rami communicantes.

r. descendens cervicis. A branch of the cervical plexus entering into the formation of the ansa hypoglossi.

r. descendens nervi hypoglossi. See *descendens hypoglossi.*

r. inferior ossis ischii. The bar of bone extending from the ischial tuberosity to the inferior ramus of the pubis: in some descriptions called *ramus of the ischium.*

r. inferior ossis pubis. The bar of bone extending from the symphyseal portion of the pubis to the ramus of the ischium.

r. mandibulae. The heavy flat sheet of bone extending upward from each extremity of the body of the mandible.

r. muscularis. Any unnamed branch of an artery to a muscle.

r. superior ossis ischii. The bar of bone extending upward from the ischial tuberosity toward the acetabulum: in some descriptions called *body of the ischium.*

r. superior ossis pubis. The bar of bone extending from the symphyseal portion of the pubis toward the acetabular portion.

white r. communicans. A communicating nerve connecting the sympathetic trunk with the dorsal and ventral roots of a spinal nerve. Also called *preganglionic r.*

ran′cid [L. *rancidus,* stinking]. Having the characteristic odor and taste of fat which has undergone oxidative and/or hydrolytic decomposition.

ran·cid′i·ty [*rancidus*]. The state of being rancid.

Ran′di·a [NL., after Isaac *Rand,* English botanist of the eighteenth century]. A genus of shrubs of the Rubiaceae.

R. aculeata. A species of West India; ink berry, indigo plant. The juice of the fruit has been used as a dye and astringent.

R. dumetorum. A species of India; the fruit has been used as a native fish poison. Has been used as an antispasmodic and emetic.

R. longiflora. A species of Bengal, of which the bark has been used in intermittent fever.

Randolph, Jacob [*American surgeon,* 1796–1848]. Said to have introduced litholapaxy in America (1831).

range [OF.]. The difference between the lowest and the highest values in a series of observations.

ra'nine (ray'nyne, ·nin) [L. *rana*, frog]. Pertaining to a ranula or to the region in which a ranula occurs.

Ranke, Hans Rudolph [*Dutch anatomist*, 1849–87]. Known for his description of an angle formed by a line drawn from the midline of the maxillary alveolar process to the midpoint of the frontonasal suture, and the horizontal plane of the skull; called *Ranke's angle.*

Ranke, Karl Ernst [*German physician*, 1870–1926]. Formulated a hypothesis stating that tuberculosis exhibits three stages: (1) a primary lesion, usually the pulmonary focus, established ordinarily in childhood; (2) subsequent generalization as a result of sensitization, commonly followed by healing, occasionally by death from miliary tuberculosis; and (3) localization or organ tuberculosis, the result of the development of chronic form. Called *Ranke's hypothesis.*

Rankin, Fred Wharton (1886–1954). American surgeon known for his contributions to abdominal surgery, especially his abdominoperineal resection of the rectum for carcinoma, called *Rankin's operation.*

Ransohoff, Joseph [*American surgeon*, 1853–1921]. A leader in surgery in his day. Described discission of the pulmonary pleura in treatment of chronic empyema; called *Ransohoff's operation.*

Ranson, Stephen Walter (1880–1942). American neuroanatomist, one of the foremost teachers of neurology in America, who studied amyelinated afferent fibers in peripheral nerves, pointed out their importance in the conduction of painful stimuli, and carried on important studies on the hypothalamus. See Ranson's pyridine silver *stain.*

ran'u·la [L., little frog]. A retention cyst of a salivary gland, situated beneath the tongue. —**ran'ular,** *adj.*

Ra·nun'cu·lus [L., crowfoot]. A genus of acrid herbs. Many species are both poisonous and irritating. —**ranuncula'ceous,** *adj.*

Ranvier, Louis Antoine [*French histologist and pathologist*, 1835–1922]. Described regular, local constrictions of myelinated nerve fibers of the peripheral nerves, called *nodes of Ranvier.* See also *Ranvier's gold chloride method* under *stain.*

Raoult, François Marie [*French physicist*, 1830–99]. Proposed a law relating the freezing point of a solution and the vapor pressure to molecular concentration; called *Raoult's law.*

rape [L. *rapere*, to seize]. 1. *In legal medicine*, intimate sexual contact by a male with a female, not his wife, without her consent, by compulsion through violence, threats, stealth, or deceit. Laws vary as to whether contact with or penetration of the female genitalia is required to constitute rape; in some laws "without consent" means psychologically or physically incapable of resisting the male. Also called *rape of the first degree.* 2. *In veterinary medicine*, the forcible sexual intercourse of the male while the female is not in heat.

statutory r. The violation of a female under the age of consent as fixed in the state or country in which the attack occurs: also called *rape of the second degree.*

rape oil. The semidrying oil from the seeds of *Brassica campestris, B. napus*, and other species. Used as a food and for industrial purposes. Syn., *colza oil.*

ra·pha'ni·a [G. *rhaphanos*, radish]. A disease characterized by spasms of the limbs. Has been attributed to a poisonous principle in the seeds of the wild radish, which become mixed with grain. *Obs.*

raph'a·nin. $C_{17}H_{26}N_3O_3S_5$ or $C_{17}H_{26}N_3O_4S_5$; a liquid antibiotic principle obtained from the seeds of the radish, *Raphanus sativus*, freely soluble in water, and active, in vitro, against several species of bacteria.

ra'phe (ray'fee) [G. *rhaphē*, seam]. A seam or ridge, especially one indicating the line of junction of two symmetrical halves.

amniotic r. The point of fusion of the amniotic folds over the embryo in sauropsidans and certain mammals.

buccal r. The scarlike vestige of the union of the parts of the cheek derived respectively from the maxillary and mandibular processes.

horizontal r. of the eye. That portion of the meridian of the eye at which the arcs of nerve fibers from the upper and lower temporal quadrants meet: functionally a sharp line in certain optic nerve fiber lesions. Also called *median r.*

palatine r. The narrow ridge of mucosa in the median line of the palate.

perineal r. The ridge of skin in the median line of the perineum.

r. exterior. The stria longitudinalis medialis.

r. inferior corporis callosi. The raphe on the inferior surface of the corpus callosum.

r. of the ampulla. The longitudinal ridge on the roof of the ampulla of the semicircular canal.

r. of the penis. A continuation of the raphe of the scrotum upon the penis.

r. of the pharynx. A fibrous band in the median line of the posterior wall of the pharynx.

r. of the pons. The intersection of the fibers at the midline as seen in transection.

r. of the scrotum. A median ridge dividing the scrotum into two lateral halves; it is continuous posteriorly with the raphe of the perineum, anteriorly with the raphe of the penis.

r. of the tongue. A median furrow on the dorsal surface of the tongue corresponding to the fibrous septum which divides it into symmetrical halves.

r. palati duri. See palatine *r.*

r. postoblongata. The posterior median fissure of the medulla oblongata.

r. superior corporis callosi. The longitudinal raphe in the middle of the superior surface of the corpus callosum.

Stilling's r. A narrow band connecting the pyramids of the medulla oblongata.

rap'tus [L., from *rapere*, to seize]. Any sudden attack or seizure; rape. *Obs.*

r. haemorrhagicus. A sudden hemorrhage. *Obs.*

r. maniacus. Transient frenzy. *Obs.*

r. melancholicus. Sudden and vehement melancholy. *Obs.*

r. nervorum. Cramp or spasm. *Obs.*

rar"e·fac'tion (rair"i·fack'shun, rar"i·fack'shun) [L. *rarefactum*, from *rarefacere*, to make thin]. The act of rarefying or of decreasing the density of a substance, especially the air.

r. of bone. The process of rendering bone more radiolucent by a decrease in the mineral content.

rar'e·fy (rair'i·figh, rar'i·figh) [*rarefacere*]. Make less dense or more porous.

rar'i·tas [L., rarity]. Rarity.

r. dentium. Fewness of teeth; less than the usual number of teeth, with or without interspaces between them.

ra·sce'ta (ra·see'tuh). Old term for the transverse lines or creases on the palmar surface of the wrist.

Rasch, Hermann [*German obstetrician*, 1873–]. Described a sign of early pregnancy in which fluctuation of the amniotic fluid is obtained as in ballottement; called *Rasch's sign.*

rash [OF. *rasche*, from L. *radere*, to scrape]. A lay term used for nearly any skin eruption but more commonly for acute inflammatory dermatoses.

brown-tail r. A common form of caterpillar dermatitis caused by the brown-tail moth, *Euproctis chrysorrhea.*

cable r. An eruption of acneform lesions caused by contact with chlorinated waxes used to coat electric cables. A type of chloracne.

canker r. Scarlet fever.

caterpillar r. See caterpillar *dermatitis.*

diaper r. See *erythema* gluteale.

drug r. See *dermatitis* medicamentosa.

heat r. Miliaria.

nettle r. Urticaria.

serum r. A dermatosis coincident with serum sickness; a result of injection of antitoxin.

vaccination r. A rash which sometimes follows vaccination; it is usually transitory but sometimes assumes an eczematous or erythematous form.

wandering r. Transitory benign plaques of the tongue.

wildfire r. See *miliaria.*

ra'sion [L. *rasio,* from *radere*]. The scraping of drugs with a file.

Rasmussen, Fritz Waldemar [*Danish physician,* 1834–77]. Remembered for his description of tuberculous aneurysm of the terminal pulmonary arteries; also called *Rasmussen's aneurysm.* This frequently results in rupture into a tuberculous cavity and serious hemorrhage.

Rasori, Giovanni [*Italian physician,* 1766–1837]. Known for his theory of counter stimuli, substances which diminish excitability by producing an opposite effect from that of the stimulant; called *Rasorianism, doctrine of Rasori.* Advocated repeated bleeding, known as *Rasori's method,* Rasorian *method.*

Ra·so'ri·an (ray·zor'ee·un) [*Rasori*]. Following the teachings of Rasori; contrastimulant.

ra'sor·ite. A native hydrate of borax, $Na_2B_4O_7$.-$4H_2O$; an important source of this chemical.

ras'pa·to''ry [ML. *raspatorium*]. A rasp or file for trimming rough surfaces or margins of bone or for removing the periosteum.

rasp'ber''ry. The fruit of *Rubus idaeus,* a plant of the Rosaceae. A syrup is used as a vehicle and as a drink in fevers.

rat [AS. *raet*]. A rodent which lives in close proximity to man, in homes, barns, wharves, ships, garbage dumps, etc. Rats are notorious disease carriers, harboring many varieties of intestinal parasites and being responsible especially for the transmission of bubonic plague, as well as a distinct septic disease, rat-bite fever.

rat'a·ny, ra·tan'hi·a. See *krameria.*

rat-bite fe'ver. See rat-bite *fever.*

rate [L. *ratum,* from *reri,* to calculate]. Measurement against a standard.

basal metabolic r. The amount of energy expended per unit of time under basal conditions, usually expressed as large calories per square meter of body surface (or kilograms of body weight) per hour.

case fatality r. The number of deaths from a specific disease per 100 persons suffering from the same disease.

cerebral metabolic r. The rate at which oxygen is consumed in the brain, calculated by multiplying the rate of cerebral blood flow by the difference in oxygen content between the arterial blood and the blood in the jugular vein.

decay r. *In radiobiology,* the rate of decay of a radioactive substance, usually expressed as disintegrations per gram per unit time.

disintegration r. See decay *r.*

dose r. *In radiology,* the amount of radiation administered per unit time. Syn., *dosage r.*

infant mortality r. The number of deaths reported among infants under one year of age in a calendar year per 1000 live births reported in the same year and place.

maternal mortality r. The number of deaths reported as due to puerperal causes in a calendar year per 1000 live births reported in the same year and place.

morbidity r. The number of cases of a disease per year for a certain number of the population.

pregnancy r. The number of pregnancies actually experienced in relation to the number of ova that theoretically might have been fertilized.

prevalence r. The number of cases of a disease occurring per unit of population at any given time.

pulse r. The number of pulsations of an artery per minute.

reproduction r. The number of total births to women of reproductive age (15 to 49 years) divided by the number of women of the same age in the population.

sedimentation r. The rate at which red cells settle out of citrated blood; the rate is somewhat more rapid in females than in males. Increases in sedimentation rate occur during menstruation, pregnancy, and in a number of pathologic states. ESR is the abbreviation for erythrocyte sedimentation rate.

Rathke, Martin Heinrich (1783–1860). German anatomist known for his early description of the pituitary gland. He described a persistent part of a paramesonephric duct opening into the prostatic utricle, called *Rathke's duct.* The cystic form of craniopharyngioma is called *Rathke's pouch.*

rat'in [AS. *raet*]. A preparation of bacteria of the genus *Salmonella,* used in food-poisoning outbreaks to destroy the rat population (which may act as vectors) by starting an epidemic disease in rats. However, the use of such preparations may be dangerous, for some of the rats may survive and become healthy carriers.

ra'tio [L.]. A proportion.

absorption r. A quantitative analysis by means of a colorimeter. The ratio between the amount of light-absorbing substance in a solution and the coefficient of light extinction (the amount of light of a specific wavelength absorbed by a 1% solution of a substance in a layer 1 cm. thick) in that solution.

albumin-globulin r. (A/G). The ratio of the albumin to the globulin concentration in blood serum. Normal value = 1.3–1.8. Values below 1.0 are said to be inverted and are associated with various pathologic processes.

birth-death r. The number of births per 100 deaths reported in the same population during the same calendar year.

body-weight r. Body weight in grams divided by height in centimeters.

cell-color r. The ratio between the percentage of erythrocytes in blood and the percentage of hemoglobin.

concentration r. The ratio of the concentration of a substance in the urine to its concentration in the blood or blood serum.

critical r. The ratio between an obtained difference and the standard error of that difference.

curative r. See therapeutic *r.*

differential absorption r. *In radiobiology,* the ratio of the concentration of a radioactive substance in a given organ or tissue to the concentration that would be obtained if the same amount of radioactive material were administered and uniformly distributed throughout the body.

D:N r. (dextrose-nitrogen r.). The ratio of the dextrose to the nitrogen in the urine. In the totally diabetic animal, the average value is 3.65, which is approached in severe human diabetes. It is considered as a measure of the conversion of protein to carbohydrate in the absence of carbohydrate intake.

G:N r. See D:N *r.*

human blood r. In malarial investigations, the percentage of freshly fed mosquitoes which contain human blood.

innervation r. The proportion of skeletal muscle fibers innervated by a nerve fiber in a motor unit.

i'so·phane r. The proportion in which insulin and protaine combine in preparations containing both. See isophane *insulin.*

karyoplasmic r. See nucleocytoplasmic *r.*

ketogenic-antiketogenic r. The ratio between those substances in the diet which give rise to ketone bodies and those which prevent or minimize this process. It may be calculated from the formula:

$$\text{Ratio} = \frac{2.4P + 3.43F}{3.2P + 0.75F + 5.56G}$$

where P, F, and G represent respectively the grams of protein, fat, and glucose metabolized. Ketonuria occurs when the ratio exceeds 1.0 and becomes severe when the ratio exceeds 2.0.

M:E r. Myeloid: erythroid ratio.

Mendelian r. The approximate numerical relation between various types of progeny in crosses involving sharply contrasted characters that conform to Mendel's law of heredity; the typical ratios for the F_2 generation are 3:1 for one pair of characters, 9:3:3:1 for two pairs.

monocyte-lymphocyte r. The ratio between monocytes and lymphocytes in the blood; has been used as a diagnostic criterion in the study of tuberculosis.

myeloid:erythroid r. The ratio of leukocytes of the granulocytic series to nucleated erythrocyte precursors in an aspirated sample of bone marrow. The limits of normal are 0.6:1 to 2.7:1. In most anemias the ratio is below unity; in severe infection or granulocytic leukemia the ratio may be markedly increased.

nucleocytoplasmic r. The ratio between the measured cross-sectional area or the estimated volume of the nucleus of a cell to its cytoplasm.

nucleoplasmic r. See nucleocytoplasmic *r.*

photosynthetic r. The ratio of oxygen evolved to the carbon dioxide assimilated during the process of photosynthesis.

sex r. The relative number of males and females in the population, usually stated as the number of males per 100 females.

therapeutic r. The ratio of the therapeutically effective dose to the lethal dose per kilogram of body weight as determined on experimental animals, usually expressed by dividing the effective dose by the lethal dose. The curative ratio is a corresponding fraction of the curative dose divided by the lethal dose. These ratios measure the margins of safety.

ra'tion (rash'un, ray'shun) [*ratio*]. A daily allowance of food or drink. In the armed services, the term usually means the complete subsistence for one man for one day.

A r. See field *r.*

B r. The overseas hospital ration.

C r. An emergency ration of canned goods.

D r. An emergency ration of chocolate bars. *Obs.*

emergency r. One of concentrated foods of little bulk which can be carried when troops are separated from field kitchens.

field r. A complete ration corresponding to the garrison ration, and served to troops in wartime.

Filipino r. That formerly prescribed for Philippine scouts.

five-in-one r. A ration for five men for one day or one for five days.

garrison r. The peacetime ration with a fixed monetary value based upon the cost of a specified list of food items.

jungle r. A ration for use in tropical warfare.

K r. A complete emergency ration for three meals put up in pocket size.

mountain r. A ration for use in mountain warfare. See five-in-one *r.*

travel r. A ration designed for troops separated from cooking facilities while traveling otherwise than by marching.

ra'tion·al (rash'un·ul) [L. *rationalis*, reasonable]. 1. Based upon reason; reasonable. 2. *In therapeutics*, opposed to empirical.

ra"tion·al·i·za'tion [*rationalis*]. A mode of adjustment to difficult and unpleasant situations; characterized by an attempt to justify or defend an unacceptable attitude or trait, its mode of expression, or its consequences or sequelae by withholding, misrepresenting, or falsifying essential facts, by blaming an incidental cause, or by comparing oneself with others in such manner as to excuse oneself.

rats'bane" [AS. *raet; bana*]. 1. Arsenic trioxide. 2. A name given to any rat poison containing arsenic.

rat'tle [ME. *ratelen*, probably imitative]. A rale.

rat'tle·snake" [*ratelen;* AS. *snaca*]. Any species of poisonous snake of the genera *Crotalus* and *Sistrurus.*

Rau, Johannes Jacobus [*Dutch anatomist*, 1668–1719]. Described the anterior process of the malleus; see under *process.* Also called *Folian process, Ravian process, process of Rau.*

Rauber, August Antinous [*German anatomist*, 1845–1917]. Remembered for his description of the most external of the three layers of cells which form the blastodisk of the embryo; called *Rauber's layer.* See also Rauber's *cell.*

rausch'brand (roush'brahnt). See *blackleg.*

Rau·wol'fi·a (raw·wol'fee·uh) [L., after Leonhard *Rauwolf*, German botanist, 16th century]. A genus of tropical trees and shrubs, mostly poisonous, of the Apocynaceae family. The dried root of *R. serpentina* has been used in India for centuries as a purgative, anthelmintic, and antidote for snake and insect bites; it has recently been advocated as a hypotensive agent and sedative. It contains the alkaloids ajmaline, ajmalinine, ajmalicine, reserpine, serpentine, and serpentinine; under certain climatic conditions it may also contain isoajmaline, neoajmaline, and other bases.

rau·wol'fine (raw·wol'feen, ·fin). An alkaloid, sometimes called *ajmaline*, from *Rauwolfia serpentina.*

rau·wols'cine. $C_{21}H_{26}N_2O_3$; an active principle of *Rauwolfia canescens.*

Ravaton, Hugues [*French military surgeon*, eighteenth century]. Described an external disarticulation of the hip through a racket incision; called *Ravaton's amputation* or *method.*

Rawlinson, Christopher [*English physician*, eighteenth century]. Wrote an early report on a probable case of perforating ulcer (1727).

Rawson, Arthur Joy [*American scientist*, 1896–]. With W. O. Abbott, developed a double-barreled gastroenterostomy tube.

Ray, Isaac [*American physician*, 1807–81]. Early student of the medicolegal implications of insanity. Pioneer in legal medicine. Described moral insanity; known as *Ray's mania.*

ray [L. *radius*, ray]. 1. A beam of light or other radiant energy. 2. A stream of discrete particles, such as alpha rays or beta rays. 3. Radial streak

of different color in an organ, as medullary rays of the kidney.
actinic rays. See *chemical rays* under *ray.*
alpha rays. Positively charged helium nuclei emitted from radioactive substances.
astral rays. See *aster.*
Becquerel rays. Rays emitted from uranium.
beta rays. Electrons with high velocities emitted from radioactive substances.
cathode r. The stream of electrons emanating from the cathode of a Crookes tube and passing in straight lines regardless of the anode. They are capable of deflection with a magnet, and produce fluorescence and heat wherever they impinge.
chemical rays. Solar rays that produce chemical change.
cortical rays. See *medullary rays* under *ray.*
cosmic r. A very penetrating radiation originating outside the earth's atmosphere, capable of producing ionization in passing through air or other matter. *Primary cosmic rays* probably consist of atomic nuclei, mainly protons, having energies up to 10^{15} electron volts; they are absorbed in the upper atmosphere. *Secondary cosmic rays* are produced when primary rays interact with nuclei and electrons in the earth's atmosphere; these consist mainly of mesons, protons, neutrons, electrons, and photons.
gamma r. Electromagnetic radiation emitted by the nucleus of an atom when it has excess energy: also called *photon.*
grenz rays. Electromagnetic radiations of about two angstrom units, useful in roentgen-ray therapy of the skin because of their limited power of penetration. They are on the borderline or limit of utilizable and chemically employable roentgen wavelengths.
hard rays. Roentgen rays from a tube operated on a high potential. They have short wavelengths and high penetrating powers. Also see *soft rays.*
Hertzian rays. Radiant energy having longer wavelengths than infrared; used for radio transmissions.
homocentric rays. Light rays that have a common focus or are parallel.
incident r. The ray of light which forms the angle of incidence.
infrared rays. Radiant heat with wavelengths between visible light and Hertzian waves.
infraroentgen rays. See *grenz rays* under *ray.*
Lenard rays. Cathode rays outside the vacuum tube, secured by means of an aluminum window.
medullary rays. Raylike extensions of medullary substance of the kidney projected from the base of the medullary pyramid into the cortex: also called *cortical r.*
Millikan rays. Cosmic rays, composed of high-energy photons and electrons.
monochromatic r. Radiation of a single sharply defined wavelength.
neutron r. A stream of neutrons obtained by bombardment in a cyclotron.
Niewenglowski's rays. Certain luminous rays emitted from phosphorescent substances which have been exposed to sunlight.
n-rays. Those named after the initial letter of the town Nancy; reportedly a form of ether waves discovered by Blondlot.
photographic rays. See *ultraviolet rays* under *ray.*
primary r. The roentgen ray as it emerges from the roentgen-ray tube.
rays of Sagnac. Secondary rays emanating from metals on which roentgen rays fall.
roentgen rays. The radiant energy of short wave lengths discovered by Röntgen, and named x-rays by him. A vacuum tube of glass (called a Geissler tube, a Hittorf, a Crookes, or a Coolidge tube) is used with two wires sealed through the glass. These wires are connected with the two poles of a high-voltage generator, and Röntgen found that the rays had peculiar penetrative powers through matter opaque to other ether rays, and that by means of these rays photographs (shadowgrams) may be taken of bones, metallic substances, etc., situated in the tissues; they readily traverse living tissues; they have no appreciable effect on the vitality of bacteria, but are effective in certain diseases.
scattered r. The roentgen ray which has been scattered by a reflecting collision from its original path.
secondary r. See secondary *electron.*
soft rays. Rays coming from a tube operated on a relatively low voltage; they are readily absorbed. Also see *hard rays* under *ray.*
ultraviolet rays. Light waves too short to affect the retina. They can be reflected, refracted, and polarized; they will not traverse many bodies that are pervious to the rays of the visible spectrum; they produce photographic and photochemical effects, and destroy rapidly the vitality of bacteria.
uranium rays. See *Becquerel rays* under *ray.*
x-rays. See *roentgen rays* under *ray.*

Raybin, Harry W. [*American chemist,* contemporary]. Described a reaction for vitamin B. When dibromoquinone-chloroimide is added to borax solution, an orange color results. The color can be extracted with chloroform and its intensity measured; called *Raybin's reaction.*

Rayer, Pierre François Olive [*French dermatologist,* 1793–1867]. Described pituitary obesity (1823). Described xanthoma (1828), also called *Rayer's disease.* Made observations on glanders (1837).

ray-formosil. Trade-mark for a buffered aqueous solution of formic and silicic acids used intramuscularly in the treatment of arthritis and rheumatism.

Raygat's test. See hydrostatic *test.*

Rayleigh, John William Strutt, Baron (1842–1919). English physicist who discovered, with William Ramsay, the element argon (1894). He was a pioneer in physical optics and acoustics and devised a test for red-green colorblindness, called *Rayleigh test.* Nobel laureate (1904).

Raymond, Fulgence [*French neurologist,* 1844–1910]. Widely known in his time as the successor to Charcot in his clinic. Made many contributions to the knowledge of spinal sclerosis, pseudotabes, and psychasthenia. Described a type of apoplexy, marked by premonitory hemiparesthesia, called *Raymond's type of paralysis.*

Raynaud, Maurice [*French physician,* 1834–81]. Famous for his description and observation (1862) of a syndrome of vascular spasm in digital arteries; see Raynaud's *phenomenon, syndrome.*

Rb Chemical symbol for rubidium.

RBC, Rbc Red blood cell.

RBE *In radiobiology,* relative biological effectiveness (of radiation).

R. C. P. Royal College of Physicians.

R. C. S. Royal College of Surgeons.

R. D. Reaction of degeneration.

rd Rutherford.

R. D. A. The right dorsoanterior position of the fetus.

R. D. P. The right dorsoposterior position of the fetus.

R. E. Right eye.

Re Chemical symbol for rhenium.

re-. A prefix signifying *back* or *again.*

re″ac·quired′ [L. *re-*, again; *acquirere*, to acquire]. Acquired a second time.

re·ac′tion [*re-;* L. *actio*, from *agere*, to do]. 1. A response to stimulus. 2. *In chemistry*, the interaction of two or more chemical substances; or, the result of a test of the hydrogen-ion concentration of a solution by means of an indicator, classified as neutral, acid, or alkaline. For reactions not listed here, see under *test*, *method*, *reflex*, or the qualifying adjective; see also under the proper name.

abortin r. See brucellergen *r.*

Adamkiewicz r. One given by a protein containing tryptophan, being a violet color produced at the junction of a glacial acetic acid solution of the protein superimposed on concentrated sulfuric acid. The reaction is attributed to the presence of glyoxylic acid in the acetic acid.

addition r. The direct union of two or more molecules to form a new molecule.

adjustment r. Transient situational personality disorder occurring in reaction to some significant person, immediate situation, or internal emotional conflict: in infancy, frequently manifested by undue apathy or excitement and by feeding and sleeping difficulties; in childhood, by such habit disturbances as nail-biting, enuresis, thumbsucking, or tantrums, by disturbance of social conduct as truancy or sexual offenses, or by neurotic traits, such as tics; in adolescence, frequently characterized by vacillations with reference to impulses and emotional tendencies. Adjustment reactions of middle or old age usually accentuate previous disturbances or precipitate latent disorders.

adult situational r. *In psychiatry*, a transient situational personality disorder characterized by superficial maladjustment to a new or difficult environmental situation, and manifested by temporary anxiety, alcoholism, poor efficiency, or unconventional behavior.

affective r. *In psychiatry*, a disorder characterized by primary and severe disturbance of mood, with resultant and consonant mental and behavioral disturbances.

agglutination r. The clumping of cellular antigens, as bacteria, upon mixture with immune serum.

alarm r. The sum of all nonspecific phenomena elicited by sudden exposure to stimuli, which affect large portions of the body and to which the organism is quantitatively or qualitatively not adapted; the first stage of the general adaptation syndrome: term introduced by Hans Selye.

allergic r. A reaction based on hypersensitivity to an antigen.

amphoteric r. The reaction of a compound as an acid or base depending upon the substrate.

anamnestic r. The prompt and efficient production of antibodies following the second injection of a specific antigen.

anaphylactic r. Antigen-antibody reaction in hypersensitive host. See *anaphylaxis.*

anaphylactoid r. A reaction similar to anaphylaxis elicited by introduction into the host of a substance which has not been used to produce a hypersensitive state. The reaction is not so severe nor so generalized as true anaphylaxis.

antigen-antibody r. A combination of an antigen with its specific antibody.

antisocial r. *In psychiatry*, a sociopathic personality disorder characteristic of chronically antisocial individuals who are always in trouble, profiting neither from experience nor punishment and maintaining no real loyalties to any person, group, or code. They are frequently callous, hedonistic, emotionally immature, and irresponsible, and exhibit a marked ability to rationalize their behavior so that it appears warranted and reasonable. This includes some individuals formerly classified as *psychopaths.*

anxiety r. *In psychiatry*, a psychoneurotic disorder characterized by diffuse anxious expectation not restricted to definite situations, persons, or objects, and frequently associated with somatic symptoms: formerly called *anxiety state.*

argentaffin r. Reduction of ammoniacal silver hydroxide by polyphenols, polyamines, and aminophenols.

arousal r. The electrical change from rhythms characteristic of the cerebral cortex of a sleeping or anesthetized animal to rhythms more nearly resembling those recorded during the waking condition, produced by stimulation of parts of the reticular activating system, and leading to signs of arousal in the animal.

Aschheim-Zondek r. Follicular growth and luteinization produced by substances in the urine of pregnant women, while the urine following oophorectomy and the menopause contains only the follicle growth-stimulating substance. Also see Aschheim-Zondek *test.*

axon r. See primary *degeneration.*

azo r. Conversion to an azo compound.

biuret r. One given by compounds which contain acid amide groups in close proximity, as by biuret (when formed from urea and certain of its derivatives), by certain proteins, etc. A red-violet to blue-violet color is produced on adding a cupric sulfate solution to an alkaline solution of the specimen.

Bloch's dopa r. See under *stain.*

brucellergen r. A skin reaction produced by the intradermal injection of *Brucella* antigen.

bufo r. A biologic pregnancy test: when urine, containing chorionic gonadotropic hormone from a pregnant woman is injected into a male toad, spermatozoa migrate from the testes to the urinary bladder and can be demonstrated in the toad's urine.

cadaveric r. Total loss of electrical response in the affected muscles, as in the acute stage of familial periodic paralysis.

Cannizzaro r. A reaction of certain aldehydes, when treated with a strong base, such that one molecule is oxidized to the corresponding acid while another is reduced to the corresponding alcohol.

carbylamine r. One for primary amines, in which a characteristic unpleasant odor of an isocyanide is evolved on heating the amine with chloroform and an alcohol solution of potassium hydroxide.

cholera red r. A nonspecific test for the cholera vibrio in which a pink color develops upon the addition of 8 drops of sulfuric acid to a 24-hour growth of the organism in 10 cc. of peptone broth.

complement-fixation r. An antigen-antibody combination with complement. Also see *fixation* of complement, complement-fixation *test.*

conjunctival r. See conjunctival *test.*

consensual r. (a) A reaction which is independent of the will. (b) A crossed reflex.

constitutional r. An immediate or delayed reaction following the administration of an allergen and occurring at sites other than that of its administration (local reaction) and other than that of the original symptoms (focal reaction). Usually associated with local or focal reactions or both.

conversion r. *In psychiatry*, a psychoneurotic disorder in which the impulse causing anxiety is converted into functional symptoms in organs or parts of the body, usually those under mainly voluntary nervous control and thus different from psychophysiologic autonomic and visceral disorders. The symptoms seem to lessen felt anxiety and ordinarily are symbolic of the underlying mental conflict. Conversion reactions may include anesthesia (anosmia, blindness, or deafness), paralysis (paresis, aphonia, monoplegia, or hemiplegia), or dyskinesia (tic, tremor, posturing, or catalepsy). Formerly classified as *conversion hysteria*.

cross r. A reaction between an antibody and an antigen which is closely related to, but not identical with, the specific antigen.

cutaneous r. (a) A specific allergic evanescent reaction of the skin resulting from the application of a specific antigen to the skin. If an irritative reaction can be eliminated, it demonstrates specific circulating antibodies. (b) When a bacterial antigen is used for a skin test, it will give a positive reaction in 24 to 48 hours (tuberculin type). Also called *dermal r.*

decidual r. The reaction of tissues, especially the endometrium, to pregnancy; marked by the development of characteristic decidual cells from fibroblasts.

dehydro*iso*androsterone color r. A test helpful in determining the presence of adrenal tumor.

delayed r. An inflammatory lesion of the skin or other phenomenon occurring hours or days after contact between allergen or atopen and hypersensitive tissue cells. Such a reaction may be either local at the site of contact or systemic or constitutional.

depressive r. *In psychiatry*, a psychoneurotic disorder in which the anxiety is partially relieved by depression and self-depreciation, frequently precipitated by an immediate and definite situation, such as the loss of a person or object, and associated with guilt feelings. Syn., *reactive depression*.

desmoplastic r. See *desmoplasia*.

diazo r. A color test using Ehrlich's diazo reagent. See van den Bergh's *test*.

Diels-Alder r. The condensation of 1,3-butadiene and similarly constituted dienes with a variety of unsaturated aldehydes, ketones, esters, and quinones to give six-membered rings: also called *diene reaction*.

dissociative r. *In psychiatry*, a neurotic disorder leading to gross disorganization of the personality, which may take the form of depersonalization, dissociation, stupor, fugue, amnesia, dream state, somnambulism, or of aimless running or freezing: formerly classified as a form of conversion hysteria.

distant r. A specific response to an allergen occurring at a site remote from that of its introduction or application.

dopa r. (*for melanoblasts*). A reaction involving 3,4-dihydroxyphenylalanine, which stains melanoblasts black when used under special conditions. See also Bloch *method*.

dyssocial r. *In psychiatry*, a sociopathic personality disorder characteristic of individuals who manifest disregard for the usual social codes and who often come in conflict with them as the result of having lived all their lives in an abnormal moral environment. Their deviations may be the result of adherence to the values and norms of their own predatory, criminal, or other social group, toward which they exhibit strong loyalties.

early r. A response becoming clinically manifest and reaching its maximum within several minutes after sensitive tissue is exposed to an excitant. It usually refers to wheal and flare reactions, to scratch or intracutaneous tests, or to an anaphylactic or anaphylactoid reaction. Syn., *immediate r.*

eczematoid r. See *eczematoid reaction*.

epiblastotropic r. One affecting the ectoderm. That reaction in yaws which produces lesions in the epidermis, as differentiated from *panblastotropic*, affecting three embryonic layers, which occurs in syphilis.

false-negative r. An erroneous or deceptive negative reaction.

false-positive r. An erroneous or deceptive positive reaction.

Feulgen r. A reaction specific for aldehydes based on formation of a purple-colored compound when aldehydes react with fuchsin-sulfuric acid. Desoxyribonucleic acid, but not ribonucleic acid, gives this reaction after the removal of its purine bases by acid hydrolysis.

first-order r. See unimolecular *r.*

focal r. A response (exacerbation or recurrence) at the site of an active, quiescent, or healed lesion distant from the place of introduction or the point of origin of the exciting agent.

galvanic skin r. (a) The psychogalvanic reflex. See under *reflex*. (b) A local galvanic skin reaction to moderately intense mechanical, thermal, electrical, or chemical stimuli, occurring in the area of stimulation as well as surrounding area, due to the development of a current within the tissues. It is independent of the psychogalvanic reflex, which may be superimposed.

Georgi-Sachs r. See Georgi-Sachs *test*.

gross stress r. *In psychiatry*, a transient personality disorder, in which, under conditions of great or unusual stress, a normal personality utilizes neurotic mechanisms to deal with overwhelming danger, differing from neurosis and psychosis with respect to clinical history, reversibility of reaction, and transient character. The stress, either physical or emotional, may occur in combat or civilian catastrophe.

Hanke and Koessler's p-diazobenzenesulfonic acid reactions. Reactions used for the detection and quantitative determination of histidine, histamine, and other imidazoles (giving a pink color), phenol, *o*- and *m*-cresol (yellow color), *p*-cresol, *p*-hydroxyphenylpropionic, *p*-hydroxy-phenylacetic, and *p*-hydroxyphenyllactic acids (red color), and tyrosine and tyramine (bluish red on adding hydroxylamine).

Hopkins-Cole r. See glyoxylic acid *test*.

id r. See *-id*.

immediate r. Early *r.*

immune r. A reaction which demonstrates the presence of an antibody.

indo r. A reaction based on formation of green or blue indamine when phenol or an aromatic monoamine acts on an aromatic paradiamine.

indophenin r. A reaction, shown by indole and other five-membered heterocyclic compounds, based on employment of isatin and sulfuric acid to give a reddish-violet color.

infusion r. An acute febrile response to the infusion of pyrogenic agents present as contaminants in parenteral fluids.

interplasmic reactions. Reactions taking place in interspaces between the protoplasmic micelles or molecules of cytoplasm.

inverse r. of drugs. *In homeopathy*, the effect of a *similimum*, i.e., of a drug which restores to normal in the ill the set of symptoms and signs it produces in healthy persons.

involutional psychotic r. A psychotic reaction occurring in the involutional period, usually in individuals of compulsive personality without previous disability due to manic-depressive reaction, characterized most commonly by depression and sometimes by paranoid ideas. It tends to be prolonged; there are excessive worry, intractable insomnia, guilt, anxiety, agitation, delusional ideas, and somatic concerns.

isomorphous provocative r. The appearance of cutaneous lesions at sites of trauma, originally observed in psoriasis, now applied equally to diseases such as lichen planus, atopic dermatitis, necrobiosis lipoidica: described by Heinrich Koebner. Syn., *isomorphous irritation effect, Koebner's phenomenon.*

isotope exchange r. See under *isotope.*

Ito-Reenstierna r. See under *test.*

Jaffé's r. See Jaffé's *test.*

Jarisch-Herxheimer r. An acute systemic reaction following initial dose of a therapeutic agent, characterized by fever, chill, and malaise, with exacerbations of the clinical signs of the infection being treated, most commonly seen in the treatment of syphilis: thought to be due to rapid release of large amounts of the antigen.

johnin r. A diagnostic skin test for paratuberculosis in cattle.

Kober r. The property of estrogenic steroids to develop a pink color with phenol in sulfuric acid, which permits their quantitative assay.

Lepra r. An acute inflammatory phase of leprosy, possibly a manifestation of hypersensitivity, sometimes ascribed to overtreatment.

lengthening r. Sudden inhibition of the stretch reflex when extensor muscles are subjected to an excessive degree of stretching by forceful flexion of a limb. Also see stretch *reflex.*

leukemoid r. See *leukemoid reaction.*

Liebermann r. Proteins containing tryptophane give a violet or bluish color in the presence of hydrochloric acid if the protein has been previously treated with alcohol and ether.

local r. The phenomena or lesions occurring at the site of application of an exciting agent.

local static r. A postural reflex in which only one part of the body, such as a limb, is involved.

Loeb's decidual r. See Leo *Loeb.*

Lohmann r. The transference of a phosphate radical from adenosinetriphosphate (ATP) to creatine, or to adenosinediphosphate (ADP) from creatine phosphate.

longitudinal r. Distal displacement of cutaneous points for electric stimulation of muscles due to degeneration of motor neurons.

Lücke r. for hippuric acid. Nitrobenzene is formed upon the addition of concentrated nitric acid to hippuric acid.

Machado-Guerreiro r. A complement-fixation test which employs antigen from cultures of *Trypanosoma cruzi* and usually is not positive before the thirtieth day for Chagas' disease and kala-azar.

magnet r. Reflex extension of the leg initiated by pressure of the foot against a surface.

Mandelbaum's r. See *filamentation.*

manic-depressive r. One of a group of psychotic reactions, fundamentally marked by severe mood swings and a tendency to remission and recurrence. Illusions, delusions, and hallucinations are often associated with the change of affect. The **manic type** of this reaction is characterized by elation or irritability, overtalkativeness, flight of ideas, and increased motor activity; the **depressive type** exhibits outstanding depression of mood, mental and motor retardation, and inhibition. Marked mixture of these phases is the **mixed type,** continuous alteration of phases is the **circular type.**

Mantoux r. See Mantoux *test.*

Mendel r. See Mantoux *test.*

Millon r. See Millon's *reagent.*

Mitsuda r. Lepromin test.

monomolecular r. See unimolecular *r.*

Moro's r. See Moro *reflex,* Moro *test.*

myasthenic r. That in which the normal tetanic contraction of a muscle under direct current stimulation becomes less intense and of shorter duration with every consecutive stimulus and finally ceases, the muscle being exhausted.

myeloid r. See *myeloid reaction.*

myotonic r. Increase in irritability seen in the myotonias.

Naegeli r. See Naegeli *test.*

Nagler's r. The opalescence produced in human serum when alpha toxin of *Clostridium welchii* is added, due to the splitting of free lecithin into phosphocholine and a diglyceride.

α-naphthol r. See Molisch's *test* (a).

nasal mucosa r. Chemical reactions in the nasal mucosa. Normally, the pH value of the nasal mucosa is on the acid side; in disease it may change toward the alkaline side.

neutralization r. The loss of poisonous properties of a toxin upon mixture with its corresponding antitoxin. Also see *neutralization.*

neutral r. That occurring at pH 7.

Nickerson-Kveim r. See under *test.*

ninhydrin r. A reaction given by all proteins and typical amino acids and by all compounds containing at least one free amino group and one free carboxyl group. A positive result is a blue color which develops on boiling. The color is intensified by the presence of pyridine. Proline and hydroxyproline do not give the test and histidine after some delay develops a red color. The reaction is highly sensitive.

Nissl r. See primary *degeneration.*

nitro r. A reaction which differentiates between indoles and pyrroles, based on treatment with equal parts of sulfuric and nitric acids. Benzene ring compounds including indoles give a yellow color; pyrroles remain colorless.

nitrosamine r. A reaction in which the imino groups of indoles and pyrroles are changed by nitrous acid to nitrosamine which, on addition of Liebermann reagent, results in a green color.

nuclear r. A process in which an atomic nucleus reacts with another nucleus, an elementary particle, or a photon to produce one or more other nuclei and possibly neutrons or photons.

obsessive compulsive r. A psychoneurotic disorder in which anxiety relates to unwanted thoughts and repetitive impulses to perform acts against which the individual usually fights and which he may consider abnormal, inappropriate, or absurd, but which he cannot control and by which he is dominated. The acts often become organized into rituals, and include such forms as touching, counting, hand-washing, and excessive neatness.

ophthalmic r. See conjunctival *test.*

oxidation-reduction r. A chemical reaction in which an ion loses electrons and another ion gains an equal number of electrons.

panblastotropic r. One which affects three embryonic layers, as in syphilis.

papulosquamous r. A skin reaction characterized clinically by discrete lesions, scaling, and, usually, erythema, and microscopically acanthosis and parakeratosis, seen most commonly in psoriasis, pityriasis rosea, early syphilis, and lichen planus, often called the *erythematosquamous diseases.*

paradoxical pupillary r. Dilatation of the pupil by epinephrine following removal of the superior cervical ganglion.

paranoid reactions. Psychotic reactions in which the patients exhibit persistent delusions, usually of persecution or grandeur, but ordinarily do not have hallucinations. Affective responses and behavior are consistent with the delusional thinking. It should be differentiated from the paranoid type of *schizophrenic reaction*.

peroxidase r. Any reaction indicating the presence of peroxidase in the cytoplasm of cells; usually the enzyme oxidizes the reagent to a deeply colored precipitate manifested as granulations.

Pfaundler's r. See thread *r.*

phloroglucinol-hydrochloric acid r. Bial's test for pentoses. See under *test.*

phobic r. A psychoneurotic disorder in which the patient's anxiety is fixed to some symbolic idea, object, or situation, so that the anxiety may be controlled by avoiding the feared object or situation. The subject may be unconscious of the origin of the anxiety. Formerly called *phobia*, inclusive of some forms of anxiety hysteria. Example: *syphilophobia* as a defense against the anxiety caused by sexual temptation.

photonuclear r. A nuclear reaction induced by a photon.

photosynthetic r. In general, the synthesis of chemical compounds effected by means of radiant energy, especially light; in particular, the synthesis of carbohydrate and related substances from carbon dioxide and water in tissues containing chlorophyll.

Porges-Pollatschek r. A test for pregnancy in which an intracutaneous injection of posterior pituitary secretion causes a red area to appear about the injection site if the woman is not pregnant; in a pregnant woman no reaction is observed.

Prausnitz-Küstner r. A reaction of local hypersensitivity produced by intradermal injection of blood serum from a hypersensitive person; a method of passive transfer of hypersensitivity. The reaction forms the basis of the passive transfer *test.*

precipitin r. The precipitation of a soluble antigen upon mixture with the specific immune serum.

prognostic moccasin venom r. An intradermal reaction employing moccasin venom as a test substance. A positive test indicates a purpurin state, usually associated with thrombocytopenia. Also used for prognosis; a positive which becomes negative is favorable.

pseudolepra r. A mild lepra reaction in which there are cutaneous hypersensitivity responses, but the patient's general condition is not affected. The skin lesions may resemble histologically both the tuberculoid and lepromatous forms of leprosy.

psychosomatic r. See *somatization.*

psychotic depressive r. An affective reaction in which the patient is severely depressed and manifests evidence of grossly misinterpreting reality, with occasional hallucinations and delusions. It differs from the depressive type of the manic-depressive reactions by absence of previous history of depressions or cyclothymia, and the frequent incidence of situational precipitating factors.

quellung r. Swelling of the capsule of a bacterium when in contact with its antigen.

r. of degeneration. The reaction of a degenerated muscle to a direct current in which the anodal closing contraction becomes first equal to the cathodal closing contraction and, later, greater than it. Abbreviated, R. D.

r. velocity. Velocity directly proportional to the active masses of reactants (raised to the power equal to the number of molecules of reactant) present at a time, *t.*

recurrent r. Reappearance or exacerbation of a local reaction.

Reinhold and Shiels r. See Reinhold and Shiels *method.*

Rh r. The result of Rh testing; namely, either Rh positive or Rh negative.

Romieu r. A test for tryptophan in proteins. Fixed tissue is treated with a drop of phosphoric acid to give a red or violet color.

Sakaguchi r. A reaction, shown by arginine, based on its action on alphanaphthol and hypobromite or hypochlorite, to give an orange-red color.

Schardinger r. The reaction demonstrates the presence of oxidase in milk by anaerobic oxidation in the presence of a hydrogen acceptor (methylene blue).

schizophrenic r. See *schizophrenic reaction.*

Schoenheimer and Sperry's r. See Schoenheimer and Sperry's *method.*

Schultz-Dale r. See Schultz-Dale *test.*

scratch r. See scratch *test.*

scrotal r. Inflammation of the scrotum and tunica vaginalis in male guinea pigs, due to infection with spotted fever rickettsiae. Necrosis of the skin frequently occurs.

semicarbazide r. A reaction used for detection of aldehydes and ketones based on conversion of semicarbazide to semicarbazone which is a yellow compound.

shortening r. Reflex contraction of extensor muscles when a flexed limb is extended by some external agent, acting to maintain the joints of the limb under a certain degree of tension.

Shwartzman r. See under *phenomenon.*

skin r. Exposure of the skin to an excitant. Typical examples are (a) the scratch test, (b) the intracutaneous test, and (c) the patch test.

Solera r. (*for thiocyanate in saliva*). This test depends upon the liberation of iodine through the action of thiocyanate upon iodic acid.

somatization reactions. See *psychophysiologic autonomic and visceral disorders.*

specific r. In allergy, phenomena produced by an agent which is identical with or immunologically related to one that previously produced alteration in capacity to react.

Straus r. Painful swelling of the testes of a rat two days after the intraperitoneal injection of *Pfeifferella whitmori*, the causative organism of melioidosis.

symptomatic r. A reaction following testing or therapeutic injection of an allergen or atopen and characterized by the occurrence or reproduction of the original symptoms under investigation or treatment.

systemic r. A reaction involving the entire body; usually a reaction against an injurious agent.

Takata r. A reaction to show the presence of neurosyphilis.

thalleioquin r. A characteristic green color is produced when quinine is treated with a solution of bromine or chlorine followed by ammonia. Addition of acid causes a blue, then red color.

therapeutic r. See therapeutic *test.*

thread r. The formation of long chains of bacillary forms of bacteria when grown in immune serum after agglutination. Syn., *filamentation, Mandelbaum's r., Pfaundler's r.*

thrombocytobarin r. See adhesion *phenomenon.*

toxin-antitoxin r. See neutralization *r.*

transfusion r. The complex of symptoms resulting from a transfusion of incompatible blood with consequent intravenous agglutination of red blood cells and hemolysis of the agglutinated cells.

tuberculin r. A localized inflammation of tissues when subjected to contact with tuberculin. It consists usually of hyperemia and induration. In severe reactions, known as the Koch phenomenon, necrosis and sloughing occur. A positive tuberculin reaction indicates that the body has been sensitized by the presence of tubercle bacilli.

tunica r. Enlargement of the scrotum of male guinea pigs, with reddening of the scrotal skin and adhesions between testes and tunica vaginalis, due to infection with epidemic or murine typhus.

unimolecular r. A reaction in which only one molecule is concerned, such as the decomposition of N_2O_5. Also called *monomolecular r.*, *first-order r.*

van den Bergh r. See van den Bergh's *test.*

vestibular r. The response of the labyrinth to sound vibrations.

Voges-Proskauer r. One used to detect the presence of acetylmethylcarbinol in bacterial cultures.

Voisenet-Rhode r. Tryptophan gives color reactions in the presence of aromatic aldehydes. With *p*-dimethylaminobenzaldehyde in sulfuric acid it gives a red-violet color.

von Pirquet r. See von Pirquet *test.*

Weidel r. (*for xanthine*). A small amount of the substance to be tested is brought into solution in bromine water. It is evaporated to dryness, and ammonia fumes are allowed to come into contact with the dry residue. The presence of xanthine is shown by development of a red color.

Weil-Felix r. The agglutination of certain strains of *Proteus vulgaris* (OX 19, OX 2, OX 1C) by the serums of patients with certain rickettsial infections, probably due to the presence of similar antigens in both *Proteus* and *Ricksettsia.*

Wernicke hemianopic pupillary r. See Wernicke's *sign.*

wheal r. The occurrence of a wheal at the site of a cutaneous test.

Wilkinson and Peters benzidine peroxidase r. To 10 ml. of the milk to be tested add 2 ml. of a 4% alcoholic solution of benzidine, sufficient acetic acid to coagulate the milk, and finally 2 ml. of a 3% solution of hydrogen peroxidase. Raw milk yields an immediate blue color.

xanthoprotein r. A test for proteins based on treatment with concentrated nitric acid. The yellow color which develops changes to deep orange on alkalization with ammonia.

Zimmermann r. A colorimetric procedure for the estimation of 17-ketosteroids. It involves treatment with *m*-dinitrobenzene and potassium hydroxide in an alcoholic solution.

re·ac′tion for·ma′tion. *In psychoanalysis,* the development of conscious, socially acceptable activity which is the antithesis of repressed or rejected unconscious desires.

re·ac′tion time. The interval between the application of a stimulus and the beginning of the response.

re·ac′ti·vate [*re-;* L. *activus,* active]. 1. To make active again, as by the addition of fresh normal serum containing complement to an immune serum which has lost its complement through age, heat, etc. 2. To restore complementary activity to a serum, deprived of one or several of its C′ components, by the addition of these components.

re″ac·ti·va′tion [*re-; activus*]. Rendering active again by the addition of complement or one or several of its components to a serum which has become inactive.

multiplicity r. The reactivation of bacteriophage inactivated by ultraviolet light, when such particles are adsorbed onto a single sensitive bacterial cell. It may also occur between two compatible pairs of viruses.

re·a′gent [*re-;* L. *agere,* to do]. 1. Any substance involved in a chemical reaction. 2. A substance used for the detection or determination of another substance by chemical or microscopical means.

acid molybdate r. A solution of 40 Gm. of sodium molybdate, 100 cc. of distilled water, 55 cc. of 85% phosphoric acid, 40 cc. of cool 25% sulfuric acid, and 20 cc. of 99% acetic acid used for the colorimetric estimation of cuprous oxide.

Almén's r. Dissolve 5 Gm. of tannic acid in 240 ml. of 50% alcohol and add 10 ml. of 25% acetic acid: used for detection in urine of nucleoprotein, with which it produces a precipitate.

antimony trichloride r. See Pincus *r.*

arsenophosphotungstic r. A solution of sodium tungstate 100 Gm., arsenic acid 50 Gm., 25 cc. of 85% phosphoric acid, and 20 cc. of concentrated hydrochloric acid in distilled water to make 1000 cc. Used in the determination of blood uric acid.

Barfoed's r. A solution of 4.5 Gm. of crystallized copper acetate and 1.2 cc. of 50% acetic acid in 100 cc. of water, used in the detection of monosaccharides.

Benedict's qualitative r. A solution containing 17.3 Gm. of crystallized copper sulfate, 173 Gm. of sodium or potassium citrate, 200 Gm. of crystallized sodium carbonate, and distilled water to make 1000 cc., used for qualitative urine sugar determination.

Benedict's quantitative r. A solution containing 18 Gm. of copper sulfate, 200 Gm. of crystallized sodium carbonate, 200 Gm. of sodium or potassium citrate, 125 Gm. of potassium sulfocyanate, 5 cc. of 5% potassium ferrocyanide, and distilled water to make 1000 cc., used for the quantitative determination of urine sugar.

Benedict's uric acid r. A solution of 100 Gm. of sodium tungstate, 50 Gm. of pure arsenic acid, 25 cc. of 85% phosphoric acid, 20 cc. of concentrated hydrochloric acid, and 600 cc. of distilled water, used in blood uric acid determination.

Benedict and Hitchcock's uric acid r. A solution of 9 Gm. of crystalline disodium hydrogen phosphate and 1 Gm. of sodium dihydrogen phosphate in 500 cc. of hot distilled water, used in blood uric acid determination.

benzidine and nitroprusside r. Dissolve 100 mg. of benzidine in 0.5 cc. of glacial acetic acid. Add 20 cc. of distilled water. Dissolve 100 mg. of sodium nitroprusside in 10 cc. of distilled water. Mix the two solutions and add 70 cc. of distilled water: used in testing for the presence of hemoglobin in urine.

benzidine r. A mixture of equal parts of a saturated solution of benzidine and 3% hydrogen peroxide used in testing for occult blood.

Bial's r. A solution of 500 cc. of 30% hydrochloric acid, 25 drops of 10% ferric chloride solution, and 1 Gm. of orcinol, used in the detection of pentose.

biuret r. $C_2H_3O_2N_3H_2O$. A condensation product of urea used as a reagent.

Boas' r. A solution of 5 Gm. of resublimed resorcinol and 3 Gm. of cane sugar in 100 cc. of alcohol, used in testing for free hydrochloric acid.

Castel r. A solution of 0.25 Gm. brucine sulfate, 2–3 drops concentrated sulfuric acid, 2 Gm. potassium iodide in 100 ml. of distilled water: used for localization of bismuth.

diazo r. See Ehrlich's diazo *r.*

Ehrlich's diazo r. Solution A contains 0.5 Gm. of sodium nitrite and 100 cc. of water. Solution B contains 1 Gm. of sulfanilic acid, 10 cc. of concentrated hydrochloric acid, and 200 cc. of water. For use, mix one part of A with 100 parts of B.

Urine containing certain aromatic compounds produces a pink color when added to the reagent.

Ehrlich's r. A solution containing 10 Gm. of para-dimethyl-amino-benzaldehyde, 75 cc. of concentrated hydrochloric acid, and 75 cc. of water, used in testing for urine urobilinogen, phenols, aryl amines, and heterocyclic compounds.

Esbach's r. A solution of 1 Gm. of picric acid, 2 Gm. of citric acid, and distilled water to make 100 cc., used in the quantitative determination of urine albumin.

Exton's quantitative r. A solution of 50 Gm. of sulfosalicylic acid, 10 Gm. of sodium sulfate, 25 cc. of 0.4% aqueous solution of bromphenol blue, and distilled water to make 100 cc., used in the quantitative determination of urine albumin.

Exton's r. A solution of 200 Gm. of sodium sulfate, 50 Gm. of sulfosalicylic acid, and distilled water to make 1000 cc., used to detect urine albumin.

Fehling's r. Two solutions, one containing 34.64 Gm. of crystalline copper sulfate in 500 cc. of water, the other containing 173 Gm. of Rochelle salt and 100 Gm. of potassium hydroxide in 500 cc. of water, used as a qualitative test for urine dextrose.

Florence's r. A solution of 2.54 Gm. of iodine, 1.65 Gm. of potassium iodide, and 30 cc. of distilled water, used to test for semen.

Folin's r. 1. A solution of 100 Gm. of sodium tungstate and 80 cc. of 85% orthophosphoric acid in 750 cc. of water, used in blood-sugar determinations. 2. A mixture of 5 volumes of saturated picric acid and 1 volume of 10% sodium hydroxide: used in creatinine determination.

Folin-Ciocalteu's r. A solution of 100 Gm. of sodium tungstate, 25 Gm. of sodium molybdate, 50 cc. of 85% phosphoric acid, and 100 cc. of concentrated hydrochloric acid in 700 cc. of water, used for blood alkaline phosphatase determination.

Fouchet's r. A solution of 25 Gm. trichloracetic acid in 100 ml. of distilled water, to which is added 10 ml. of an aqueous solution of ferric chloride (10 Gm./100 ml.): used in the Harrison spot test for bilirubin.

Frohde's r. A 0.1% solution of sodium molybdate in concentrated sulfuric acid; used for the detection of alkaloids.

group r. A reagent which identifies a group of substances of similar chemical nature.

Günzberg's r. Dissolve 2 Gm. of phloroglucinol and 1 Gm. of vanillin in 100 ml. of 95% alcohol.

Haines's r. A solution containing 2 Gm. of pure copper sulfate, 16 cc. of distilled water, 16 cc. of pure glycerin, and 156 cc. of 5% potassium hydroxide, used to test for urine sugar.

Kober r. A mixture of sulfuric acid and phenol (of betanaphthol) used for the colorimetric determination of estrogens.

Lieberman r. Concentrated sulfuric acid and 5% phenol used in nitrosamine reaction.

Lohmann's r. Add 25 ml. of concentrated nitric acid to 100 Gm. of mercuric nitrate octahydrate, followed by 25 ml. of water. Warm to dissolve.

Millon's r. A solution of mercuric nitrate and nitrite in a mixture of the corresponding acids prepared by dissolving metallic mercury in concentrated nitric acid. On heating, it gives a red color with proteins containing the tyrosine group and with substances, other than proteins, containing the hydroxy-phenyl group.

Mörner's r. A solution of 1 cc. of formalin, 55 cc. of concentrated sulfuric acid, and 45 cc. of distilled water, used to test for tyrosine.

Nadi (*na*phthol, *di*methyl) **r.** A mixture of β-naphthol with dimethyl-para-phenylene diamine, used as a test for indophenol oxidase.

Nessler's r. An aqueous solution of 5% potassium iodide, 2.5% mercuric chloride, and 16% potassium hydroxide, used in testing for ammonia.

Nylander r. Digest 2 Gm. of bismuth subnitrate and 4 Gm. of Rochelle salt in 100 ml. of a 10% solution of potassium hydroxide. Cool and filter.

Obermayer's r. A solution of 2 Gm. of ferric chloride in 1 liter of strong hydrochloric acid, used in testing for urine indican.

Pandy's r. A saturated solution of 10 Gm. of phenol crystals in 100 cc. of water, used in testing for spinal-fluid protein.

Pauly diazo r. One used in paper chromatography to demonstrate the presence of histidine and tyrosine.

Pincus r. A solution of antimony trichloride which gives a blue color with most 17-keto-steroids, but not with dehydro*iso*androsterone: useful in the determination of excessive amounts of this steroid.

pyrogallate r. (*alkaline*). Prepare a solution of potassium hydroxide by dissolving 160 Gm. in 130 ml. of water. In 200 ml. of this solution dissolve 10 Gm. of pyrogallic acid.

Roberts' r. A solution of one part of pure nitric acid to five parts of saturated solution of magnesium sulfate, used to test for urine albumin.

Schiff's r. A solution of 0.25 Gm. of acid fuchsin in 1000 cc. of water decolorized by sulfur dioxide: used in testing for aldehydes the presence of which causes a blue color.

Schweitzer r. To 10 parts of ammonium hydroxide (sp. gr. 0.9), add three parts of distilled water. To this mixture, add a slight excess of copper carbonate, shake vigorously, and allow to stand overnight. Siphon off the clear, supernatant liquid.

silver iodate r. Ammoniacal silver iodate added to plasma to precipitate the silver chloride: used in the determination of serum chlorides.

sodium cyanide-urea r. An aqueous solution of 1 part sodium cyanide and 4 parts urea used to determine blood uric acid, which, when added to a protein-free filtrate, produces a blue color in the presence of uric acid.

sodium cobaltinitrite r. A complex aqueous solution of cobaltous nitrate and sodium nitrite, used for the determination of potassium.

specific r. A reagent which identifies a single chemical substance.

Stokes's r. A reagent containing 2 Gm. of ferrous sulfate, 3 Gm. of tartaric acid, and 100 cc. of water, used in testing for blood.

Sulkowitch r. A solution containing 2.5 Gm. of oxalic acid, 2.5 Gm. of ammonium oxalate, 5 cc. of glacial acetic acid, and water to make 150 cc., used to test for urine calcium.

Tanret r. Dissolve 1.35 Gm. of mercuric chloride in 25 ml. of water, add to this solution 3.32 Gm. of potassium iodide dissolved in 25 ml. of water, then make the total solution up to 60 ml. with distilled water and add 20 ml. of glacial acetic acid to the mixture.

Töpfer's r. A 0.5% solution of dimethylamino-azobenzene in 95% alcohol, most commonly used as an indicator to detect free hydrochloric acid in the gastric contents.

Tsuchiya's r. A reagent containing 1.5 Gm. of phosphotungstic acid, 95 cc. of 96% alcohol, and 5 cc. of concentrated hydrochloric acid, used to test for urine albumin.

uric acid r. of Folin and Denis. An aqueous solution of sodium tungstate, phosphoric acid, and alcohol added to a solution of lithium carbonate and phosphoric acid, used in the determination of uric acid in the blood.

Winkler r. Cuprous chloride 40 Gm., ammonium chloride 50 Gm., distilled water to 150 ml. Mix the solution with ammonium hydroxide (sp. gr. 0.9) in the proportion of 3:1 for use.

zinc uranyl acetate r. An aqueous solution containing uranyl acetate and zinc acetate (in the proportion of 1 part of the former to 3 parts of the latter), also acetic acid: used in the determination of sodium. The sodium is precipitated as sodium zinc uranyl acetate.

re′a·gin [*re-; agere*]. 1. One of a group of antibodies in serum characterized in part by interacting with allergens or atopens (atopic reagin) and responsible for such manifestations of hypersensitivity in man as hay fever and asthma. 2. The antibodylike substance in serum and cerebrospinal fluid concerned with the flocculation of the alcohol-soluble lipids of normal tissue in the complement-fixation and flocculation reactions in syphilis.

re·al′gar. Arsenic disulfide, As_2S_2; a pigment.

ream′er [cf. ME. *remen*, to make room]. A surgical instrument used for gouging out holes or enlarging those already made, especially in bone operations.

re″am·i·na′tion. The introduction of an amino group into a compound from which an amino group had previously been removed.

re″am·pu·ta′tion [L. *re-*, again; *amputatio*, from *amputare*, to cut away]. An amputation upon a member on which the operation has already been performed.

re·an′i·mate [*re-;* L. *animare*, to animate]. Revive; resuscitate; restore to life, as a person apparently dead.

Réaumur, René Antoine Ferchault de [*French physiologist,* 1683–1757]. Renowned for his knowledge of natural history and his studies in gastric digestion. Made many contributions to knowledge of the insects. Best remembered for his thermometer (1731), called *Réaumur thermometer, Réaumur's scale.* Isolated gastric juice (1752).

re·bound′ [OF. *rebondir*, to spring back]. In reflex activity, a sudden contraction of a muscle following its relaxation; associated with a variety of forms of reflex activity. Seen most typically following the cessation of an inhibitory reflex.

re·cal″ci·fi·ca′tion (ree·kal″si·fi·kay′shun) [L. *re-*, again; *calx*, lime; *facere*, to make]. The supposed restoration of lime salts to bone matrix.

re·cal′ci·fied clot′ting time. The clotting time of decalcified blood or plasma upon the readdition of calcium ions: also called *recalcification time.*

Récamier, Joseph Claude Anthelm [*French gynecologist and obstetrician,* 1774–1852]. One of the first to study the spread of cancer, he coined the name metastasis (1829). Is said to have employed uterine curettage, called *Récamier's operation.* Developed a vaginal speculum (1842), called *Récamier's speculum.*

re″ca·pit″u·la′tion [L. *re-*, again; *capitulum*, chapter]. The summarizing of the main points of a subject; the repetition of the steps of a process, as recapitulation theory.

re·ceiv′er [L. *recipere*, to receive]. 1. The vessel receiving the products of distillation. 2. In an air pump, the jar in which the vacuum is produced.

rec″ep·tac′u·lum (ress″ep·tack′yoo·lum, ree″sep·) [L.]. A receptacle; a small container.

r. chyli. The saclike beginning of the thoracic duct opposite the last thoracic vertebra.

re·cep′tive [L. *receptum*, from *recipere*, to receive]. Having the quality of, or capacity for, receiving.

re·cep′tor [L., receiver, from *recipere*]. 1. A peripheral nerve ending in the skin and special sense organs. 2. A name given by Ehrlich to the atomic lateral chain or haptophorous group, which, existing in each cell in addition to its nucleus, combines with intermediary bodies such as toxins, food molecules, and foreign substances. Also see side-chain *theory.*

deflation r. Vagal nerve fibers which are stimulated by deflation of the lung and reflexly induce inspiration.

free r. An antibody, agglutinin, lysin, etc.

inflation r. See stretch *r.*

r. of the first order. One with a single anchoring or haptophore group.

r. of the second order. One containing a haptophore and a functional, fermentative, or zymophore group.

r. of the third order. One possessing two haptophore groups and a zymophore group.

stretch r. One responding to mechanical deformation brought about by the stretching of the tissue in which the receptor is embedded, e.g., the stretch receptors stimulated by inflation of the lung which, via ascending vagal nerve fibers, reflexly inhibit the respiratory center. See Hering-Breuer *reflex.*

re·cess′, re′cess [L. *recessus*, from *recedere*, to withdraw]. A fossa, ventricle, or ampulla; an anatomic depression.

chiasmal r. See optic *r.*

cochlear r. An elliptic pit below the oval window of the vestibule, forming part of the cochlea. It contains small foramens for the passage of nerves from the duct of the cochlea.

costodiaphragmatic r. A potential space formed by apposition of the costal and diaphragmatic layers of the parietal pleura.

costomediastinal r. A potential space formed by contact of the costal layer with the mediastinal layer of the parietal pleura.

duodenojejunal r. An occasional pouch of the mesentery on the right side of the jejunum and near its union with the duodenum: also called *duodenojejunal fossa.*

elliptical r. An oval depression in the roof and medial wall of the vestibule lodging the utricle. It contains small foramens for the passage of branches of the acoustic nerve to the utricle and to the ampulla of the superior and lateral semicircular ducts. Also called *utricular r.*

epitympanic r. The attic of the tympanic cavity.

hepatorenal r. That formed by the hepaticolic ligament.

ileocecal r. The ileocecal fossa.

incisive r. A depression on the nasal septum immediately above the incisive canal.

infundibular r. A recess in the anterior part of the floor of the third ventricle extending through the tuber cinereum into the infundibulum. See Plate 18.

intersigmoid r. The subsigmoid fossa.

labyrinthine r. A diverticulum of the otic vesicle which finally becomes the endolymphatic duct and sac.

laryngopharyngeal r. The lower pyramidal part of the pharynx from which open the esophagus and the larynx.

lateral r. The lateral extension of the fourth ventricle in the angle between the cerebellum and the medulla oblongata.

lienal r. An extension of the omental bursa behind the gastrosplenic ligament.

mesenteric r. A recess in the primitive gastric mesentery, formed by an invagination of the peritoneum on the right side, that separates the definitive gastric mesentery from the caval mesentery and gives rise to the omental bursa, its vestibule, and the infracardiac bursa.

nasopalatine r. A depression near the lower margin of the nasal septum above the incisive canal.

omental recesses. Portions of the omental bursa called respectively the superior recess behind the liver, the inferior recess, and the lienal recess in the region of the spleen.

optic r. A recess in front of the infundibular recess which extends downward and forward above the optic chiasma. See Plate 18.

paraduodenal r. An occasional small pouch of peritoneum situated to the left of the last part of the duodenum.

peritoneal recesses. Pockets behind or around organs in the peritoneal cavity, as paraduodenal recesses.

pharyngeal r. A lateral mucosal diverticulum of the pharynx situated behind the opening of the auditory tube. Also called *Rosenmueller's r.*

pineal r. A recess in the roof of the third ventricle extending posteriorly into the stalk of the pineal body.

piriform r. A small space lateral to the laryngeal orifice, bounded laterally by the thyroid cartilage and thyrohyoid membrane and medially by the aryepiglottic fold. Also spelled *pyriform r.* Syn., *piriform sinus.*

pneumoenteric r. In certain mammals, a peritoneal recess between the left lung bud and the esophagus; on the right side it is comparable to the infracardiac bursa.

preoptic r. See optic *r.*

pyriform r. See piriform *r.*

r. of pelvic mesocolon. A small peritoneal pouch found beneath the sigmoid mesocolon on the posterior abdominal wall. Also called *intersigmoid r.*

r. of tympanic cavity. (a) Anterior and posterior pouches of the mucous membrane covering the lateral wall of the tympanic cavity and found on either side of the manubrium of the malleus. Also called *r. of Tröltsch.* (b) A superior recess situated between the flaccid part of the tympanic membrane and the neck of the malleus. Also called *Prussak's space*, or *pouch.*

retrocecal r. An occasional pouch of peritoneum extending upward between the cecum and posterior abdominal wall.

retroduodenal r. An occasional small pouch of peritoneum situated behind the transverse portion of the duodenum extending upward from below.

sacciform r. of the wrist. An elongation of synovial membrane extending between the radius and ulna at their distal articulation.

sphenoethmoidal r. A small space between the sphenoid bone and the superior nasal concha.

spherical r. A depression in the medial wall of the vestibule which lodges the saccule. Small foramens in the recess transmit branches of the acoustic nerve to the saccule.

suprapineal r. A posterior recess of the third ventricle extending backward as a diverticulum from the ependyma of the roof.

tubotympanic r. The dorsal wing of the first pharyngeal pouch and possibly part of the second, which forms the tympanic cavity of the middle ear and the auditory tube.

umbilical r. A dilated portion of the left branch of the adult portal vein, marking the position of the left umbilical vein.

utricular r. See elliptical *r.*

re·ces′sion [L. *recessio*, from *recedere*]. The gradual withdrawal of a part from its normal position, as recession of the gums from the necks of teeth.

re·ces′sive [*recedere*]. *In biology*, a characteristic of one of the parents of a hybrid which is found in the minority of the offspring, in contrast to the dominant characteristic of the other parent. See recessive *character; dominant; Mendel's law* under Gregor Johann *Mendel.* —**reces′sive,** *adj.*

re·ces′sus. See *recess.*

re·cid″i·va′tion [L. *recidivatus*, from *recidivus*, falling back]. 1. The relapse of a patient recovering from a disease. 2. *In criminology*, a relapsing into crime.

re·cid′i·vism [*recidivus*]. The repetition of criminal or delinquent acts; bad behavior.

re·cid′i·vist [*recidivus*]. 1. A patient who returns to a hospital for treatment, especially an insane person who so returns. 2. *In criminology*, a confirmed, relapsed, or habitual criminal.

rec″i·div′i·ty (ress″i·div′i·tee) [*recidivus*]. Tendency to return or to relapse.

rec′i·pe (ress′i·pee) [L., imperative of *recipere*, to receive]. 1. The heading of a physician's prescription, signifying *take.* Symbol, ℞. 2. The prescription itself.

Recklinghausen, Friedrich Daniel von [*German pathologist*, 1833–1910]. Greatly distinguished in his field; described neurofibromatosis, also called *von Recklinghausen's disease.* Described hemochromatosis (1889). Generalized osteitis fibrosa cystica is called *von Recklinghausen's disease of bone;* see under *osteitis.* Described minute lymph channels present in connective tissue, called *von Recklinghausen's canals.*

rec″li·na′ti·o (reck″li·nay′shee·o). See *reclination.*

r. palpebrarum. Ectropion.

rec″li·na′tion [L. *reclinare*, to bend back]. An operation for cataract, in which the lens was pushed back into the vitreous chamber. *Obs.* Also called *couching.*

Reclus, Paul (1847–1914). French surgeon who described bilateral polycystic disease of the female breast (1883), also called *Reclus disease.* See cystic *disease* of breast.

re·com″bi·na′tion. *In radiobiology*, the coming together of two or more ionized or activated atoms, radicals, or molecules.

re″com·po·si′tion [L. *recompositum*, from *recomponere*, to put together again]. Reunion of parts or constituents after temporary dissolution.

re″com·pres′sion [L. *re-*, again; *compressio*, a pressing together]. Resubjection to increased atmospheric pressure; a procedure used in treating caisson workers or divers who develop symptoms of caisson disease on returning to normal pressures.

re″con·stit′u·ent [*re-;* L. *constituere*, to set up]. A medicine which promotes continuous repair of tissue waste or makes compensation for its loss.

re·con″sti·tu′tion (ree·kon″sti·tew′shun) [*re-;* L. *constitutio*, from *constituere*]. Continuous repair of progressive destruction of tissues.

re″con·struc′tion. 1. *In medical-history taking* and *psychoanalysis*, the integration into a significant whole of facts which are presented first without consciousness of their relationship. 2. Reproduction, usually with enlargement of the form, of an embryo, organ system, or part by assemblage of properly spaced and oriented outlines of serial sections. Common methods are **graphic reconstruction,** resulting in a two-dimensional drawing, and **Born wax-plate reconstruction,** by which a three-dimensional model is obtained.

re·cov′er·y [L. *recuperare*, to recover]. Restoration from illness.

rec′re·ment [L. *recrementum*, refuse]. A substance secreted from a part of the body, as a gland, and again absorbed by the body. —**recremen′tal, recrementi′tial, recrementi′tious,** *adj.*

re″cru·des′cence [L. *recrudescere*, to become raw

again]. An increase in the symptoms of a disease after a remission or a short intermission.

re·cruit′ment (ri·kroot′mint) [F. *recrutement*, from *recroître*, to grow again]. A serial discharge of the neurons which innervate groups of muscle fibers.

re·cruit′ment test. See under *test*.

rec·tal′gi·a [L. *rectus*, straight; G. *algos*, pain]. Pain in the rectum; proctalgia.

rec′tal shelf. See *Blumer's shelf*.

rec·tec′to·my. See *proctectomy*.

rec″ti·fi·ca′tion [L. *rectificatio*, from *rectus; facere*, to make]. 1. A straightening, as rectification of a crooked limb. 2. The redistillation or fractional distillation of liquids to obtain a product of higher purity or greater concentration of the desired constituent.

rec·ti′tis. See *proctitis*.

rec′to- [*rectus*]. A combining form denoting *the rectum* or *rectal*.

rec″to·ab·dom′i·nal [*rectus;* L. *abdomen*, belly]. Relating to the rectum and the abdomen.

rec′to·cele [*rectus;* G. *kēlē*, hernia]. Prolapse of the rectum into the vagina.

rec·toc′ly·sis [*rectus;* G. *klysis*, a drenching]. The slow instillation of a liquid into the rectum.

rec″to·coc·cyg′e·al (reck″to·cock·sidj′ee·ul) [*rectus;* G. *kokkyx*, cuckoo]. Pertaining to the rectum and the coccyx.

rec″to·coc·cyg′e·us. A band of mixed smooth and striate muscle fibers extending from front of coccyx to back of rectum.

rec″to·co·li′tis [*rectus;* G. *kolon*, colon; *-itis*, inflammation]. Inflammation of the mucosa of the rectum and colon combined.

rec″to·co·lon′ic [*rectus; kolon*]. Pertaining to the rectum and the colon.

rec″to·cys·tot′o·my [*rectus;* G. *kystis*, bladder; *tomē*, a cutting]. Incision of the urinary bladder through the rectum. *Obs.*

rec″to·fis′tu·la [*rectus;* L. *fistula*, tube]. Fistula of the rectum.

rec″to·gen′i·tal [*rectus;* L. *genitalis*, genital]. Pertaining to the rectum and the genital organs.

rec″to·la′bi·al [*rectus;* L. *labium*, lip]. Relating to the rectum and the labia pudendi.

rec′to·pex″y, rec″to·pex′y [*rectus;* G. *pēxis*, a fixing]. Fixation of the rectum to the pelvic wall by suturing.

rec″to·pho′bi·a. See *proctophobia*.

rec′to·plas″ty. See *proctoplasty*.

rec″to·rec·tos′to·my [*rectus; rectus;* G. *stoma*, mouth]. Surgical anastomosis between two parts of the rectum.

rec″to·ro·man′o·scope [*rectus;* L. *Romanus*, Roman; G. *skopein*, to examine]. A speculum used in examining the rectum and the sigmoid flexure.

rec′to·scope [*rectus; skopein*]. A rectal speculum. —**rectos′copy,** *n.*

rec″to·sig′moid [*rectus;* G. *sigmoeidēs*, crescent-shaped]. The rectum and sigmoid portion of the colon considered together.

rec″to·sig″moid·ec′to·my. Surgical excision of the rectum and sigmoid colon.

rec″to·sig″moid·os′co·py [*rectus; sigmoeidēs;* G. *skopein*, to examine]. Ocular inspection of the rectum and sigmoid flexure of the colon with the aid of special instruments.

rec″to·ste·no′sis [*rectus;* G. *stenōsis*, a being straitened]. Stenosis of the rectum.

rec·tos′to·my. See *proctostomy*.

rec·tot′o·my. See *proctotomy*.

rec″to·u·re′thral [*rectus;* G. *ourēthra*, urethra]. Pertaining to the rectum and the urethra.

rec″to·u·re·thra′lis. A small band of smooth muscle fibers running from the rectum to the membranous part of the urethra in the male.

rec″to·u′ter·ine [*rectus;* L. *uterus*, womb]. Pertaining to the rectum and uterus, as a small band of smooth muscle fibers running from front of the rectum to the uterus, corresponding to the rectovesicalis in the male.

rec″to·vag′i·nal (·vadj′i·nul, ·va·jye′nul) [*rectus;* L. *vagina*, sheath]. Pertaining to the rectum and the vagina.

rec″to·vag″i·no·ab·dom′i·nal (·vadj″i·no·ab·dom′i·nul) [*rectus; vagina;* L. *abdomen*, belly]. Pertaining to a method of combined examination in the female.

rec″to·ves′i·cal [*rectus;* L. *vesica*, bladder]. Pertaining to the rectum and the urinary bladder.

rec″to·ves·i·ca′lis. Smooth muscle fibers running between the rectum and the base of the urinary bladder.

rec′tum [*rectus*]. The lower part of the large intestine, extending from the sigmoid flexure to the anal canal. It begins opposite the third sacral vertebra and passes downward to terminate at the anal canal. See Plates 8, 10, 13, 14. —**rectal,** *adj.*

rec′tus [L.]. Straight; applied to anything having a straight course, as rectus abdominis muscle. See Table of Muscles in the Appendix.

r. accessorius. A rare variant of the vastus lateralis muscle in which a few fibers arise from the rim of the acetabulum.

re·cum′ben·cy [L. *recumbere*, to recline]. The reclining position.

re·cum′bent [*recumbere*]. Leaning back; reclining.

re·cu′per·ate [L. *recuperare*, to recover]. Regain strength or health.

re·cu″per·a′tion [L. *recuperatio*, from *recuperare*]. Convalescence; restoration to health.

re·cu′per·a″tive (ri·cue′pur·ay″tiv, ri·cue′pur·uh-tiv) [*recuperare*]. Pertaining to, or tending to, recovery of health or strength.

re·cur′rence [L. *recurrere*, to run back]. 1. The return of symptoms or a disease. 2. Reappearance of a neoplasm after apparently complete removal.

re·cur′rent [*recurrere*]. 1. Returning. 2. *In anatomy,* turning back in its course, as recurrent laryngeal nerve.

re″cur·va′tion [L. *recurvare*, to curve backward]. The act or process of bending backward.

red [AS. *rēad*]. The least refractive of the spectral colors. For other terms containing red, see under noun.

Chinese r. Mercuric sulfide.

Red Cross So·ci′e·ty. An international organization whose primary purpose is to care for the wounded, the sick, and prisoners in wartime. A more recent function is the relief of human suffering from catastrophe or any other cause.

Redi, Francesco [*Italian naturalist,* 1626–97]. Author of the first scientific treatise on poisoning by venomous snakes (1664), in which he showed that the poison must be injected to be effective. In his study of insects, dealt the first serious blow to the theory of spontaneous generation.

re′di·a (pl. *rediae*) [NL., after *Redi*]. *In parasitology,* the second larval stage of a trematode, which results from the development of a parthenogenetic egg of the first larval stage.

re″dif·fer·en″ti·a′tion [L. *re-*, again; *differentia*, difference]. The return to a position of greater specialization in actual and potential functions.

red. in pulv. *Redactus in pulverem;* reduced to powder.

red·in″te·gra′tion [L. *redintegratio*, from *redintegrare*, to make whole again]. 1. The complete restitution of a part that has been injured or destroyed. 2. See *reintegration*.

red′out [AS. *rēad; ūt*]. A condition met with by

flyers, in which acceleration is centripetal and the blood is driven toward the head. There is a bursting headache, and vision is blurred as by a red mist.

re′dox. A reduction-oxidation reaction, state, or system.

redoxon. A brand of ascorbic acid.

re′dox po·ten′tial. The electrical potential developed when a suitable inert electrode is in contact with a solution containing both the oxidized and the reduced forms of one or more substances. The potential is a function of the ratio of the activities (concentrations) of oxidant and reductant, and also provides a measure of the relative oxidizing (or reducing) power of the system.

re·dresse′ment [Fr.]. 1. A second dressing of a wound. 2. Correction of a deformity.

red′root″ [*rēad;* AS. *rōt*]. A perennial herb of the genus *Lachnanthes*, the root of which is sometimes used as a dye.

re·duce′ [L. *reducere*, to lead back]. 1. Restore a part to its normal relations, as to reduce a hernia or fracture. See Plate 38. 2. *In chemistry,* bring back to the metallic form; deprive of oxygen. 3. Lose weight by dietetic regimen.

re·duced′ [*reducere*]. 1. Restored to the proper place. 2. *In chemistry,* having undergone reduction, i.e., accepted electrons. 3. Diminished in size.

re·du′ci·ble [*reducere*]. Capable of being reduced.

re·duc′tant [*reducere*]. A reducing agent.

re·duc′tase (ri·duck′tace, ·taze). An enzyme causing reduction. *Obs.*

cytochrome C r. A flavoprotein enzyme system isolated from yeast; also, a similar one from liver; the oxidized form of flavoprotein is highly active in oxidizing reduced coenzyme II, while the reduced form of the flavoprotein readily reduces oxidized cytochrome C.

re·duc′tion. 1. *In chemistry,* (a) an increase in the negative valence of an element (or a decrease in positive valence) occurring as a result of the gain of electrons. Each electron so gained is taken from some other element, thus accomplishing an oxidation of that element; (b) originally, the process of separation from oxygen, or the combining with hydrogen. 2. *In medicine,* the restoration by surgical or manipulative procedures of a dislocated joint or a fractured bone to normal anatomic relationships.

closed r. That performed without making a surgical incision.

open r. That performed by making a surgical incision through the soft parts to the site of the fracture or dislocation.

re·duc′tion di·vi′sion. See *meiosis.*

re·duc′tone. A substance, probably HOCH:-C(OH)CHO, the enolic form of hydroxymalonic dialdehyde. It is a strong reducing agent.

re·du′pli·ca″ted [L. *reduplicatus*, redoubled]. Doubled, as reduplicated heart sounds.

re·du″pli·ca′tion [L. *reduplicatio*, repetition]. A doubling.

r. of the heart sounds. A doubling of either the first or the second sound of the heart. It occurs in hypertension, increased pulmonary pressure, and myocardial disease, but may also occur without clinical significance.

Red″u·vi′i·dae (red″yoo·vye′i·dee, ree″dew·) [L. *reduvia*, hangnail]. A family of the Heteroptera, commonly called assassin bugs and kissing bugs. They normally prey on other insects and only occasionally attack man. Their bite may be extremely painful and toxic. They are sometimes confused with the related bloodsucking Triatomidae.

Re·du′vi·us [*reduvia*]. A genus of bugs of the family Reduviidae.

R. personatus. The reduviid or kissing bug which is an avid bloodsucker and has a potent salivary toxin; attacks the face, particularly the lips, often causing pain.

Reed, Dorothy (Mendenhall) [*American pathologist,* 1874–]. Described the giant polynuclear cells which are the most constant feature of the lesions of Hodgkin's disease (1903), called *Dorothy Reed cells, Reed-Sternberg cells.*

Reed, Walter [*American Army surgeon,* 1851–1902]. Chairman of the celebrated United States Army Yellow Fever Board. His *Experimental Yellow Fever* (1901) published the proof that yellow fever is caused by a filtrable virus transmitted to man by a mosquito, *Aëdes aegypti.*

re″ed·u·ca′tion [L. *re-*, again; *educatio*, from *educare*, to rear]. The development of the processes of adjustment in an individual who has acquired these processes and then lost them.

reef′ing. See *plication.*

Reenstierna reaction. See Ito-Reenstierna *test.*

Reenstierna test. See Ito-Reenstierna *test.*

re″ev·o·lu′tion [L. *re-*, again; *evolutio*, from *evolvere*, to unroll]. Hughlings Jackson's term for a symptom following an epileptic attack, which consists of three stages: suspension of power to understand speech (word deafness); perception of words and echolalia without comprehension; return to conscious perception of speech with continued lack of comprehension.

re″ex·ci·ta′tion [*re-;* L. *excitatio*, from *excitare*, to rouse up]. Reentrance of the excitation wave into tissue that has recovered from a refractory state.

re·fec′tion [L. *refectio*, a restoring]. The phenomena of vitamin-B-complex synthesis by the bacterial flora of the intestine. With diets of certain composition, the amount of bacterial synthesis of vitamins is sufficiently increased that rats can grow and reproduce on a diet devoid of vitamin-B complex. Man's dietary requirement for certain vitamins and other nutrients may be controlled to a considerable extent by the nature and extent of refection.

re·fine′ [L. *re-*, again; *finire*, to finish]. Purify a substance, extract it from raw material, or remove impurities from it.

re·flect′ed [L. *reflectere*, to bend back]. 1. Cast or thrown back. 2. *In anatomy,* turned back upon itself, as visceral peritoneum from the surface of an organ to become parietal peritoneum.

re·flec′tion [*reflectere*]. 1. A bending or turning back; specifically, the turning back of a ray of light from a surface upon which it impinges without penetrating. 2. In membranes, as the peritoneum, the folds which are made in passing from the wall of the cavity over an organ and back again to the wall which bounds such cavity.

re·flec′tor [*reflectere*]. A device for reflecting light or sound.

re′flex [L. *reflexus*, from *reflectere*]. An involuntary, invariable, adaptive response to a stimulus.

abdominal r. Contraction of the abdominal muscles, induced by friction on the corresponding side of the abdominal wall.

acceleratory r. Any reflex originating in the vestibular organ in response to a change in the rate of movement. In linear acceleration, the response is a placing reflex independent of proprioceptive sensations; in angular acceleration, the response is the vestibulo-ocular reflex.

accommodation r. The occurrence of constriction of the pupils, convergence of the eyes, and increased convexity of the lens when the eyes adjust for near vision.

Achilles tendon r. Plantar flexion of the foot, produced by contraction of the calf muscles when the Achilles tendon receives a sharp blow.

acoustic r. See auditory *r.*
acquired r. Conditioned reflex.
acromial r. Flexion of the forearm induced by a sharp blow upon the acromion.
adductor r. Contraction of the adductors of the thigh, produced by tapping the medial condyle of the femur or any point along the inner side of the leg.
allied reflexes. Those elicited from different regions, producing common or reinforced protagonistic actions.
anal r. Contraction of the external anal sphincter in response to a scratch upon the skin in the perianal region.
ankle clonus r. Clonic contractions of the calf muscles in response to pressure against the sole of the foot.
antagonistic reflexes. Reflexes in response to different stimuli which elicit opposing effects, as the flexion and extension of a limb with resulting dominance of the stronger reflex. The nociceptive (pain) reflexes usually predominate.
anticus r. Dorsal flexion and inversion of the foot, induced by percussion of the tibialis anticus (tibialis anterior) muscle.
antigravity reflexes. Reflexes which, through contraction of the extensor muscles, support the body against the effect of gravity.
Argyll Robertson r. See Argyll Robertson *pupil.*
attitudinal reflexes. Reflex adjustments of the skeletal muscles to keep the trunk and limbs in a proper relationship to the position of the head.
audito-oculogyric r. Movement of the eyes toward the source of a sudden sound.
auditory r. Brief closure of the eyes, resulting from eighth nerve stimulation by the sudden production of a sound: also called *acoustic r., cochlear r.*
aural r. Any reflex which involves the auditory mechanism.
auriculopalpebral r. Closure of the eyelids in response to noxious stimuli when intracranial pressure is increased: also called *Kisch's r., Kehrer's r.*
auriculopressor r. A reflex rise in the heart rate due to rise of pressure in the right atrium. See Bainbridge *r.*
auropalpebral r. See cochleopalpebral *r.*
axon r. One occurring without involvement of a nerve cell body; results from a stimulus applied to a terminal branch of a sensory nerve, and gives rise to an impulse that ascends to a collateral branch down which it is conducted to an effector organ; believed to be important in the local regulation of blood vessels.
Babinski r. An abnormal reflex characterized by extension of the great toe upon stroking of the sole of the foot: also called *Babinski's sign.*
Bainbridge r. A reflex acceleration of the heart and rise of arterial pressure due to rise of pressure in the right atrium and roots of great veins. Also called *cardiovascular r., right heart r.*
behavior r. Conditioned reflex.
Bekhterev's r. (a) Facial contraction on the same side as irritation of the nasal mucosa. Syn., *nasal r.* (b) Dilatation of the pupil on exposure to light, occasionally seen in tabes and dementia paralytica. Syn., *paradoxic pupillary r.* (c) Dorsal flexion of the foot with flexion of the knee and hip on the same side upon release of a foot passively bent in a plantar direction; seen in pyramidal tract disease. (d) A normal response characterized by contraction of the lower abdominal muscles on stroking of the skin of the inner surface of the thigh. Syn., *hypogastric r.*
Bekhterev-Mendel r. Extension of the second to fifth toes induced by percussion of the dorsum of the foot in normal individuals; flexion occurs in the presence of pyramidal tract disease. Syn., *Mendel's dorsal r. of the foot, dorsocuboidal r., cuboidodigital r., tarsophalangeal r.*
Bezold r. A depressor and cardiac-decelerating reflex which has its afferent origin in receptors located in the heart, particularly the left ventricle, and lungs. The efferent pathway is from medullary centers over the vagus and sympathetic nervous systems. The reflex is activated by veratrum alkaloids and, possibly, by the changes of myocardial infarction.
biceps r. Contraction of the biceps brachii muscle induced by percussion of its tendon.
body-righting r. A righting reflex initiated by asymmetrical stimulation of pressure receptors on the surface of the body. It may be a body-righting reflex acting on the head, which tends to keep the head orientated in relation to the surface with which the body is in contact, or it may be acting on the body, which ensures orientation of the body in reaction to the surface with which it is in contact.
bone r. A reflex presumed to be elicited by stimulus applied to a bone, but really a muscle stretch reflex.
Brain's r. Extension of the paralyzed flexed arm when a patient with hemiplegia assumes the quadrupedal position. See quadrupedal extensor *r.*
Brissaud's r. Contraction of the tensor of the fascia lata on stimulation of the sole of the foot.
Brudzinski's r. See *Brudzinski's signs* under *sign.*
bulbocavernosus r. See penile *r.*
Capps's pleural r. Shock induced by mechanical irritation, as with a trocar, of an inflamed pleura.
cardiovascular r. See Bainbridge *r.*
carotid body r. One arising in the epithelioid of the carotid body and affecting respiration and blood pressure. See *chemoreceptor.*
carotid sinus r. That arising in the carotid sinus and affecting blood pressure, heart rate, and respiration. See *pressoreceptor.*
cerebral cortex r. Contraction of the pupil when, in a darkened room, the patient's attention is directed to a light that is visible to his peripheral retina. Also called *Haab's r.*
Chaddock's r. (a) Extension of the great toe on stimulation around the lateral malleolus, seen in pyramidal tract lesions. (b) Flexion of the wrist and extension and fanning of the fingers caused by irritation of the ulnar aspect of the lower forearm in hemiplegia.
chain r. A series of consecutive reflexes, each of which is initiated by the preceding one, resulting in an integrated action.
chemical r. One initiated by hormones or other chemical substances in the blood, as a carotid sinus reflex. Also called *humoral r.*
chin r. See jaw-jerk *r.*
Churchill-Cope r. Rapid, shallow respirations due to engorgement of the pulmonary vessels.
ciliary r. The normal constriction of the pupil in accommodation of the eye.
ciliospinal r. Dilatation of the ipsilateral pupil on pinching the skin on one side of the neck. Syn., *cutaneous pupillary r.*
cochlear r. See auditory *r.*
cochleo-orbicular r. See cochleopalpebral *r.*
cochleopalpebral r. Contraction of the orbicularis oculi muscle after hearing a sudden, unexpected sound. Syn., *Gault's r., cochleo-orbicular r., auropalpebral r.*
conditioned r. A reflex acquired as a result of repeated association and training, as opposed to a natural reflex.

conjunctival r. Closure of the eyelids induced by touching the conjunctiva. Syn., *lid r.*
consensual light r. See crossed *r.*
consensual r. See crossed *r.*
contact r. A reflex flexion and elevation of a limb resulting from gentle stimulation of the dorsum of the foot.
contralateral r. An overflow response on the opposite side when a reflex is elicited on one side of the body.
convulsive r. Incoordinated convulsive muscular contractions.
coordinated r. A coordinated reaction of several muscles in orderly progression.
corneal r. See conjunctival *r.*
corneomandibular r. Deflection of the lower jaw to the opposite side when the cornea of one eye is irritated, the mouth being open.
coronary r. See intercoronary *r.*
cough r. A cough caused by irritation of the laryngeal mucosa.
cranial r. Any reflex whose paths are connected directly with the brain by cranial nerves.
cremasteric r. Retraction of the testis on the same side induced by stimulation of the skin on the front and inner surface of one thigh.
crossed extension r. The extension of the limb opposite to that in which a flexor reflex is induced.
crossed r. A response on one side of the body induced by stimulation of the other side. Syn., *consensual r.*, *indirect r.*
cuboidodigital r. See Bekhterev-Mendel *r.*
cutaneous pupillary r. See ciliospinal *r.*
cutaneous r. Wrinkling or gooseflesh in response to irritation of the skin.
dartos muscle r. See scrotal *r.*
deep r. Any muscle stretch reflex, including the so-called tendon reflexes and periosteal reflexes.
deep r. of Bekhterev. See Bekhterev's *r.* (c).
defecation r. See rectum *r.*
defense r. Protective reflex.
deglutition r. See swallowing *r.*
delayed r. A reflex occurring an abnormally long while after the stimulus.
depressor r. A reflex fall in blood pressure or vasodilatation, which may be evoked by a variety of stimuli, as increased pressure in the carotid sinus.
determinate r. One referred back to the region of stimulation.
digital r. Sudden flexion of the terminal phalanx of the thumb and of the second and third phalanges of some other finger, elicited by snapping the terminal phalanx of the patient's middle or index finger. Also called *Hoffmann's sign.*
direct light r. Contraction of the sphincter pupillae induced by a ray of light thrown upon the retina. Also called *direct pupillary r.*
direct r. A reflex response on the same side as that of the stimulus.
dorsal r. See lumbar *r.*
dorsocuboidal r. See Bekhterev-Mendel *r.*
elbow r. See triceps *r.*
Erben's r. Slowing of the pulse, presumed to be due to vagus irritability, when the head and trunk are bent strongly forward.
erector spinae r. See lumbar *r.*
esophagosalivary r. Salivation induced by stimulation of the distal portion of the cut esophagus, the vagi being intact. See Rogers' *r.*
extensor thrust r. See extensor *thrust.*
external auditory meatus r. See auriculopalpebral *r.*
exteroceptive r. Any reflex elicited by stimulation of an exteroceptor. The reflex arc is a multineuron arc.
eyeball compression r. Slowing of the heart caused by pressure on the eyeball. Syn., *oculocardiac r.*
eye closure r. (a) Closure of the eyelids on tapping the supraorbital nerve. (b) Closure of the eyelids on stimulation of the external ear canal Syn., *Kisch's r.*
fascial r. A deep muscle stretch reflex elicited by a sudden tap over a fascia.
faucial r. Gagging or vomiting produced by irritation of the fauces.
femoral r. Extension of the knee and flexion of the toes induced by irritation of the skin over the upper anterior surface of the thigh.
finger-thumb r. Apposition and adduction of the thumb, associated with flexion at the metacarpophalangeal joint on firm passive flexion of the third to the fifth finger at the proximal joints.
fixation r. A reflex manifested by fixation of the eyes so that the image is kept on the fovea of both.
flexion r. Flexion or withdrawal of a limb in response to a noxious stimulus.
fontanel r. See Grünfelder's *r.*
foveolar r. The bright reflection of light seen with the ophthalmoscope when it is directed upon the fovea.
front-tap r. Contraction of the calf muscles induced by percussion over the stretched muscles of the extended leg.
gag r. See pharyngeal *r.*
gastrocolic r. Peristalsis of the colon induced by the entrance of food into the empty stomach.
gastroileac r. Physiologic relaxation of the ileocecal valve, resulting from food in the stomach.
gastrosalivary r. Salivation following the introduction of food into the stomach.
Gault's r. See cochleopalpebral *r.*
Geigel's r. See inguinal *r.*
general static r. A postural reflex involving various segments of the body.
genital r. Any reflex irritability due to disorder of the genital organs.
Gifford's r. Constriction of the pupil when the orbicularis oculi is contracted, the eyelids being held open.
gluteal r. Contraction of the gluteal muscles induced by stimulation of the overlying skin.
Gonda r. Extension of the great toe when the last two toes are snapped between the examiner's fingers: indicative of a pyramidal tract lesion.
Gordon's r. 1. A paradoxical flexor reflex in diseases of the pyramidal tract, in which there is extension of the great toe or of all the toes on compression of the deep flexor muscles of the leg. Syn., *paradoxic flexor r.* 2. Flexion of the fingers, or thumb and index finger, on squeezing the muscles of the forearm, seen in pyramidal tract disease.
grasp r. A grasping motion of the fingers or of the toes, induced by stimulation of the palm of the hand or the sole of the foot.
great-toe r. A comprehensive term, signifying extension of the great toe, and including the Babinski, Chaddock, Gordon, and Oppenheim reflexes.
Grünfelder's r. Extension of the great toe with a fan-type spreading of the other toes, produced by pressure on the posterior fontanel. Syn., *fontanel r.*
Haab's r. See cerebral cortex *r.*
head retraction r. A test for bilateral pyramidal tract lesions above the cervical cord. The patient relaxes with his head slightly forward. The test is positive if the head is quickly retracted when the middle part of the upper lip is tapped with

the reflex hammer, stretching the flexors and producing an abnormally intense contraction in these latter muscle groups.

Hering-Breuer r. The nervous mechanism which controls respiration by impulses mediated through the pulmonary fibers of the vagus nerves.

Hirschberg's r. Inversion of the foot induced by stimulation of the sole of the foot at the base of the great toe.

Hoffmann's finger r. See Hoffmann's *sign*, digital *r*.

humoral r. See chemical *r*.

hypochondrial r. Sudden inspiration produced by unexpected pressure below the costal border.

hypogastric r. Contraction of the muscles of the lower abdomen induced by stroking of the skin of the inner surface of the thigh.

hypothenar r. Contraction of the palmaris brevis muscle upon stimulation over the pisiform bone.

indirect r. See crossed *r*.

infraspinatus r. Extension of the elbow and lateral rotation of the arm induced by a sudden sharp tap over the infraspinatus muscle.

inguinal r. Contraction of muscle fibers above the inguinal ligament, induced by stimulation of the skin over the upper and inner aspect of the thigh in the female. Syn., *Geigel's r*.

instinctive r. A precise invariable response to a stimulus, inherited and not acquired by association: also called *natural r.*, *unconditioned r.*, *inherited response*. See also conditioned *r*.

intercoronary r. Any reflex arising in vessels of one area of the myocardium and transmitted to those of another.

interscapular r. See scapular *r*.

intersegmental r. Any reflex involving more than one segment of the spinal cord for the completion of its arc.

intestinal r. See myenteric *r*.

intrasegmental r. Any reflex involving only one segment of the spinal cord.

inverted oculocardiac r. Acceleration of the heart rate in response to compression of the eyeballs.

inverted radial r. Flexion of the fingers without flexion of the forearm when the lower end of the radius is tapped; presumed to indicate a lesion involving the fifth cervical segment of the spinal cord.

iris contraction r. Pupillary contraction induced by exposure to light. Syn., *pupillary r.* (a).

Jacobsohn's r. Flexion of the fingers induced by a mild tap on the lower end of the radius or in its neighborhood on the dorsal side of the forearm, formerly considered to indicate pyramidal tract disease, but now considered to be essentially normal, although more distinct in cases of reflex hyperirritability of functional or organic nature.

jaw-jerk r. Clonic contraction of the muscles of mastication and elevation of the mandible, elicited by striking the relaxed and dependent jaw with a percussion hammer, the mouth being open. Observed in disease of the upper motor neurons.

Joffroy's r. Twitching of the gluteal muscles when pressure is made against the nates; observed in spastic paralysis.

Juster's r. Extension of the fingers instead of flexion when the palm of the hand is irritated or stimulated.

Kehrer's r. See auriculopalpebral *r*.

kinetic r. Any reflex which results in movement.

Kisch's r. See auriculopalpebral *r*.

knee-jerk r. See patellar *r*.

Kocher's r. See testicular compression *r*.

labyrinthine r. Reflex initiated by stimulation of the vestibular apparatus of the inner ear.

lacrimal r. Secretion of tears induced by irritation of the corneal conjunctiva.

laryngeal r. A cough resulting from irritation of the larynx.

laughter r. Uncontrollable laughter in response to tickling.

lid r. Conjunctival reflex.

light r. (a) Of the membrana tympani: a cone of light on the anterior and inferior part of the tympanic membrane, with its apex directed toward the umbo. (b) Of the retina: a circular area of light reflected from the retina during retinoscopic examination. (c) Of the pupil: contraction of the pupil in response to light. Also called *Whytt's r*.

lip r. A reflex movement of the lips of sleeping babies, induced by a sudden tap over the angle of the mouth.

long circuit r. A reflex which involves the higher centers in the medulla, midbrain, basal ganglions, or cerebral cortex, as opposed to the segmental reflex.

Lovén's r. Vasodilatation in an organ in response to stimulation of its afferent nerve.

lumbar r. Contraction of the muscles of the back caused by stimulation of the skin over the sacrospinalis muscle. Syn., *dorsal r.*, *erector spinae r.*

lung r. Old term for Hering-Breuer reflex.

Lust's r. Dorsal flexion and eversion of the foot in response to percussion over the common peroneal nerve.

McCarthy's r. See supraorbital *r*.

McCormac's r. Adduction of the opposite leg in response to percussion of one patellar tendon (ligamentum patellae).

Magnus-de Kleyn reflexes. The tonic neck and tonic labyrinthine reflexes.

mandibular r. Jaw-jerk reflex.

Marey r. See Etienne Jules *Marey*.

mark-time r. Rhythmic alternate flexor and extensor reflexes resembling those used in running.

mass r. A complex reflex phenomenon induced by stimulation below the level of a complete transverse lesion of the spinal cord and characterized by simultaneous flexor spasms of the legs, involuntary evacuation of the urinary bladder, defecation, and sweating below the level of the lesion: described by G. Riddoch.

membrana tympani r. See light *r.* (a).

Mendel's dorsal r. of foot. See Bekhterev-Mendel *r*.

middle ear disease r. A reflex phenomenon used to explain the temperature variations which both adults and children occasionally exhibit with mild grades of tympanic inflammation, probably depending on the individual differences in stability of central nervous control.

monosynaptic r. Any reflex involving only one synapse and no internuncial neurons, as the patellar reflex is postulated to be, on the basis of experimental data.

Moro r. A concussion reaction normally observed only in newborn infants, elicited by a sudden sharp noise, such as clapping the hands, or by upsetting the equilibrium, as jarring the surface on which the infant lies: used to test the integrity of the neonate's responses. In the normal response both legs are drawn up and the arms brought up as in an embrace, in contrast to the asymmetric response seen in unilateral brachial palsy.

mucosal r. Contraction of subjacent muscles when mucous membranes are stroked.

myenteric r. Contraction of the intestine above and relaxation below a portion of the intestine that is stimulated through the influence of the myenteric nerve plexus. This action occurs in peristalsis. Syn., *intestinal r.*

myotatic r. See stretch *r.*

nasal r. Sneezing induced by stimulation of the nasal mucosa.

nasomental r. Contraction of the mentalis muscle with consequent elevation of the lower lip and wrinkling of the skin of the chin in response to a light tap on the side of the nose with a percussion hammer.

neck-righting r. Any tonic labyrinthine reflex arising in the neck which tends to keep the body orientated in relation to the head.

negative supporting r. A proprioceptive reflex causing active inhibition of the muscles involved in positive supporting reflex, elicited by flexion of the finger or the hand, or plantar flexion of the toes: observed in the decerebrate animal.

nociceptive r. A reflex initiated by a painful stimulus.

obliquus r. Contraction of the external oblique muscle in response to any stimulus applied to the skin of the thigh below the inguinal ligament. Syn., *hypogastric r.*

oculocardiac r. Slowing of the heart rate in response to pressure upon the eyeballs, a normal reaction when the rate is decreased by 5 to 13 beats per minute.

oculocephalogyric r. The associated movements of the eye, head, and body in the process of focusing visual attention upon an object.

oculopharyngeal r. Rapid movements of deglutition and spontaneous closing of the eyes without apparent contraction of the orbicularis muscle, in response to stimulation of the bulbar conjunctiva.

Onanoff's r. Contraction of the bulbocavernosus muscle in response to compression of the glans penis.

Oppenheim r. Extension of the great toe upon stroking downward along the medial side of the tibia, a sign of corticospinal-tract lesion.

optical righting r. Righting reflex initiated by the visual perception of an improper orientation of the body in reference to the horizon or to familiar objects.

opticofacial r. A defensive reaction characterized by sudden closure of the eyelids when an object is brought suddenly into the field of vision. Syn., *winking r.*

orbicularis oculi r. See supraorbital *r.*

pain r. Nociceptive *r.*

palatal r. (a) Elevation of the soft palate in response to a touch. (b) Swallowing produced by irritation of the palate.

palmar r. Flexion of the fingers when the palm of the hand is irritated.

palm-chin r. Contraction of the muscles of the chin in response to irritation of the thenar eminence of the hand. Also called *palmomental r.*

paradoxic ankle r. An ankle reflex in which percussion over the flexor surface induces an extensor response, and vice versa.

paradoxic flexor r. See Gordon's *r.*

paradoxic patellar r. Contraction of the hamstring muscles in response to tapping of the patellar tendon (ligamentum patellae); sometimes observed in tabes, poliomyelitis, lesions of the femoral nerve, and other lesions affecting the arc of the patellar reflex.

paradoxic pupillary r. Dilatation of the pupil in response to stimulation of the retina by light.

patellar clonus r. Clonic contraction and relaxation of the quadriceps muscle in response to sharp firm pressure against the upper margin of the patella; observed in lesions of the pyramidal tract.

patellar r. Contraction of the quadriceps muscle with extension of the leg at the knee in response to a quick tap against the patellar tendon (ligamentum patellae). Also called *knee-jerk, knee-kick, quadriceps r., patellar tendon r.*

patellar tendon r. Patellar reflex.

patello-adductor r. Crossed adduction of the thigh in response to percussion of the patellar tendon (ligamentum patellae).

pathologic r. Any abnormal reflex indicative of a diseased state.

pectoral r. Adduction and slight internal rotation of the arm in response to a sharp blow against the humeral insertion of the tendon of the pectoralis major muscle.

penile r. Contraction of the bulbocavernosus muscle in response to a moderate tap against the dorsum of the penis. Syn., *bulbocavernosus r.*

periosteal r. Originally considered to be a muscular contraction in response to a blow against the periosteum, but now considered to be a muscle stretch reflex.

peroneal r. Contraction of a peroneal muscle in response to a blow applied to it while it is stretched.

pharyngeal r. Contraction of the constrictor muscles of the pharynx in response to stimulation of the posterior pharyngeal wall or neighboring structures. Syn., *gag r.*

Philipson's r. Extension of the limb opposite to that in which a lengthening reaction is induced.

Pilcz's r. See pupillary *r.* (c).

pilomotor r. Erection of the hairs of the skin (goose flesh) in response to chilling or irritation of the skin or to an emotional stimulus.

placing r. A reaction which organizes postural muscle contractions in anticipation of contact with a solid object.

plantar r. Flexion of the toes in response to irritation of the sole.

plasticity r. The reflex property of maintaining a spastic limb in the position of flexion or extension in which it has been placed; a resistance to change, either lengthening or shortening.

pneocardiac r. A change in the cardiac rhythm or the blood pressure, due to the inhalation of an irritating vapor.

pneopneic r. A change in the respiratory rhythm, due to the inhalation of an irritating vapor.

positive supporting r. Contraction of extensor muscles to support posture, observed in a decerebrate animal.

postural r. Any one of many reflexes which are associated in establishing posture of the individual.

prepotent r. The reflex elicited first when two antagonistic stimuli impinge simultaneously upon an organism.

pressor r. A reflex increase in arterial pressure due to nervous stimulation of the vasomotor center.

proprioceptive r. Any reflex elicited by stimulation of a proprioceptor. The reflex arc is probably a two-neuron arc. Also see proprioceptive *impulses.*

protective r. Any response to defend the body from harm, as winking caused by an object rapidly approaching the eye.

psychocardiac r. Increase in the heart rate induced by recollection of a previous emotional experience.

psychogalvanic r. A variation in the electric conductivity of the skin in response to emotional stimuli. Due to changes in blood circulation, secretion of sweat, and skin temperature changes.

pulmonary r. Old term for Hering-Breuer reflex.

pupillary r. (a) Contraction of the pupil in response to stimulation of the retina by light: also called *Whytt's r.* (b) Contraction of the pupil on accommodation for close vision and dilatation of the pupil on accommodation for distant vision. Syn., *accommodation r.* (c) Reflex contraction of the pupil of one eye in response to stimulation of the other eye by light. Syn., *consensual light r.* (d) Contraction of the pupil on attempted closure of the eye. Syn., *Westphal's pupillary r.* Also called *Westphal-Pilcz r.*

purposive reflexes. Those which provide the mechanism for the preservation of the individual.

quadriceps r. See patellar *r.*

quadrupedal extensor r. An associated movement of extension of the flexed arm in hemiplegia which is sometimes evoked by causing the patient, when standing or kneeling, to lean forward and throw his weight on to the observer's supporting hand placed beneath his chest. See Brain's *r.*

radial r. A muscle stretch reflex characterized by flexion of the forearm and occasionally by flexion of the fingers in response to a light blow against the lower end of the radius.

rectum r. The mechanism by which the accumulated feces are evacuated from the rectum, characterized by peristaltic contraction of the rectal musculature and relaxation of the internal and external sphincters of the anus: also called *defecation r.*

red r. The red glow of light seen to emerge from the pupil when the interior of the eye is illuminated, due to the reflected light having passed through the choroid.

renorenal r. The mechanism by which disease or injury of one kidney may produce pain in, or impair the function of, the opposite kidney.

retinal r. A round light area reflected from the retina when the retinoscope is employed.

Riddoch's mass r. See mass *r.*

righting r. Any of a chain of reflexes which operate to bring, or to maintain, an animal right side up; included are labyrinthine righting reflexes, body righting reflexes acting upon the head, body righting reflexes acting upon the body, neck righting reflexes, and optical righting reflexes.

Roger's r. Salivation on irritation of the esophagus. See esophagosalivary *r.*

Rossolimo's r. A stretch reflex of the plantar muscles of the foot, characterized by flexion of the second to fifth toes in response to tapping of the plantar surfaces of the toes; its intensity varies with the degree of muscle tonus.

scapular r. Contraction of the scapular muscles in response to a stimulus applied between the scapulas. Syn., *interscapular r.*

scapulohumeral r. Contractions of various muscles of the shoulder girdle and arm in response to tapping the vertebral border of the scapula. Syn., *scapuloperiosteal r.*

scapuloperiosteal r. See scapulohumeral *r.*

Schäffer's r. Extension of the great toe in response to pinching of the Achilles tendon.

scratch r. Reflex scratching movements designed to remove an irritating agent from the surface of the skin; the ease with which this reflex may be initiated in experimental animals has made it one of the most commonly studied forms of reflex activity.

scrotal r. Slow vermicular contraction of the dartos muscle in response to stimulation of the perineum by stroking or by cold application. Syn., *dartos muscle r.*

segmental r. See intrasegmental *r.*

segmental static r. A postural reflex involving a whole segment of the body, as both forelimbs or the neck muscles.

sexual r. Erection and ejaculation in response to direct or psychic stimulation of the genitalia.

shivering r. A reflex, occurring in response to cold, causing rhythmic contraction of muscles.

simple r. An uncomplicated reflex, as one acting on a single muscle.

sneezing r. See nasal *r.*

Snellen's r. Congestion of the ear on the same side in response to stimulation of the distal end of the divided auriculotemporal nerve.

spinal r. Any reflex whose arc connects with a center in the spinal cord.

static r. Any one of a series of reflexes which are involved in the establishment of muscular tone for postural purposes.

Stookey's r. Flexion of the leg in response to tapping the tendons of the semimembranosus and semitendinosus muscles while the leg is semiflexed at the knee.

stretch r. Contraction of a muscle in response to sudden brisk longitudinal stretching of the same muscle. Syn., *myotatic r.*

Strümpell's r. See Strümpell's *sign.*

sucking r. Sucking movements of the lips, tongue, and jaw in infants in response to contact of an object with the lips.

superficial r. Any reflex occurring in response to superficial stimulation, as of the skin.

supinator jerk r. Contraction of the supinator muscle when the styloid process of the radius is struck a blow; a stretch reflex.

supinator longus r. Flexion of the forearm in response to a brisk tap on the tendon of the brachioradialis muscle (*O.T.* supinator longus muscle).

supraorbital r. Contraction of the obicularis oculi muscle in response to a tap over the frontal region. Syn., *McCarthy's r., orbicularis oculi r.*

suprapatellar r. A sudden upward movement of the patella produced by contraction of the quadriceps muscle in response to a sharp blow upon a finger which is placed against the upper border of the patella, with the leg extended.

suprapubic r. Deflection of the linea alba toward the stroked side when the abdomen is stroked above the inguinal ligament.

swallowing r. The chain of reflexes involved in the mechanism of deglutition which may be evoked by stimulation of the palate or pharynx. See palatal *r.*

tactile reflexes. Reflex movements from stimulation of the tactile end organs.

tarsophalangeal r. See Bekhterev-Mendel *r.*

tendo Achillis r. See Achilles tendon *r.*

tendon r. Contraction of a muscle in response to sudden stretching of the muscle by a brisk tap against its tendon. Syn., *deep r.*

testicular compression r. Contraction of the abdominal muscles in response to compression or squeezing of a testis. Syn., *Kocher's r.*

tonic labyrinthine reflexes. The acceleratory and righting reflexes.

tonic neck reflexes. Rotation or deviation of the head causes extension of the limbs on the same side as the chin, and flexion of the opposite extremities. Dorsiflexion of the head produces increased extensor tonus of upper extremities and relaxation of the lower limbs, and ventroflexion of the head the reverse. Seen in incomplete forms in the young infant, and thereafter in cases where there is a lesion at midbrain level or above.

tonic r. Any reflex involved in the establishment and maintenance of posture or attitude of the individual.

trace-conditioned reflexes. Reflex responses

occurring at a considerable interval after the time that the conditioned stimulus was given.

triceps r. Extension of the forearm in response to a brisk tap against the triceps tendon, with the forearm at right angles to the arm. Syn., *elbow r.*

unconditioned r. See instinctive *r.*

urinary r. See vesical *r.*

vagopressor r. Reflex rise in blood pressure resulting from the stimulation of afferent fibers of the vagus nerve. The afferents probably include nerve fibers that are normally stimulated by changes in distention of the great veins.

vascular r. See vasomotor *r.*

vasomotor r. Constriction or dilatation of a blood vessel in response to psychic or physical stimulation. Syn., *vascular r.*

vasovagal r. Reflex vagal stimulation from peripheral blood vessels.

vertebra prominens r. Relaxation of all four limbs produced by pressure on the lower cervical spinal column.

vesical r. The reflex or automatic response of the urinary bladder to empty itself, induced by distension of the organ to a certain capacity or degree, normally controlled by voluntary inhibition and release: also called *urinary r.*, *vesicourethral r.*

vesicourethral r. Vesical *r.*

vestibular reflexes. The responses of the autonomic nervous system to strong stimulation of the vestibular nucleus: pallor, nausea, vomiting, and quasi-shock symptoms.

vestibulo-ocular r. A statokinetic reflex, observed as a rotation of the eyes in the opposite direction when the head is quickly rotated.

virile r. (a) See penile *r.* (b) A sudden downward movement of the penis when the prepuce or glans of the relaxed organ is pulled upward. Also called *Hughes r.*

visceral r. Any reflex induced by some irritation of an internal organ.

viscerocardiac r. Alteration in the activity of the heart in response to stimulation of an internal organ.

visceromotor r. Tenseness of skeletal muscles evoked by painful stimuli originating in the viscera.

viscerosensory r. A form of referred pain in which irritating stimuli within the viscera give rise to a painful sensation in some superficial region of the body.

vomiting r. Vomiting induced by tickling the fauces or pharynx.

Wernicke's hemianopic pupillary r. See Wernicke's *sign.*

Westphal's pupillary r. See pupillary *r.* (c).

Whytt's r. See light *r.* (c); pupillary *r.* (a).

winking r. Sudden closure of the eyelids in response to the unexpected appearance of any object within the field of vision.

wrist r. Flexion of the fingers induced by percussion of the wrist tendons.

zygomatic r. Movement of the lower jaw toward the percussed side when the zygoma is tapped with a percussion hammer.

re·flex′i·o. See *reflection.*

r. palpebrarum. See *ectropion.*

re·flex″o·gen′ic [L. *reflexus,* from *reflectere;* G. *genesthai,* from *gignesthai,* to be produced]. Causing or increasing a tendency to reflex action; producing reflexes.

re·flex′o·graph″ [*reflexus;* G. *graphein,* to write]. An instrument for graphically recording a reflex.

re″flex·om′e·ter [*reflexus;* G. *metron,* a measure]. An instrument used to measure the force required to produce myotatic movement.

re·flex″o·ther′a·py [*reflexus;* G. *therapeia,* treatment]. A form of therapeutics based on stimulation by manipulation, anesthetization, or cauterization of areas more or less distant from the affected lesion. Also called *zone therapy, spinal therapeutics.*

re′flux [L. *refluxum,* from *refluere,* to flow back]. A return flow, as in a reflux condenser, which returns the condensate to the original fluid.

pancreatic r. The flow of pancreatic fluid in reverse direction through the common duct so that pancreatic fluid is present in the biliary tract. Also called *biliary-pancreatic r.*

re·fract′ [L. *refractum,* from *refringere,* to break up]. 1. Bend back. 2. Change direction by refraction. 3. Estimate the degree of ametropia, heterophoria, and strabismus present in an eye.

re·frac′ta do′si (ri·frack′tah do′sigh, do′see) [L.]. In broken or divided doses.

re·frac′tion [L. *refractum,* from *refringere,* to break up]. 1. The act of refracting or bending back. 2. The deviation of a ray of light from a straight line in passing obliquely from one transparent medium to another of different density. 3. The state of refractive power, especially of the eye; the ametropia, emmetropia, or muscle imbalance present. 4. The act or process of correcting errors of ocular refraction.

angle of r. The angle formed by a refracted ray of light with the perpendicular at the point of refraction.

coefficient of r. The quotient of the sine of the angle of refraction into the sine of the angle of incidence.

double r. Birefringence. The property of having more than one refractive index, according to the direction of the traversing light. It is possessed by all except isometric crystals; by transparent substances which have undergone internal strains (e.g., glass); and by substances which have different structures in different directions (e.g., fibers).

dynamic r. The static refraction of the eye, plus that secured by the action of the accommodative apparatus.

equivalent r. See specific refractive *power.*

errors of r. Departures from the power of producing a normal or well-defined image upon the retina, because of ametropia.

r. of the eye. The influence of the ocular media upon a cone or beam of light, whereby a normal or emmetropic eye produces a proper image of the object upon the retina.

static r. That of the eye when accommodation is at rest.

re·frac′tion·ist [*refractum*]. One who corrects errors of ocular refraction.

re·frac′tive [*refractum*]. Refracting; capable of refracting or bending back; pertaining to refraction.

re″frac·tiv′i·ty [*refractum*]. Power of refraction; ability to refract.

re″frac·tom′e·ter [*refractum;* G. *metron,* a measure]. 1. An instrument for measuring the refraction of the eye. 2. An instrument for the determination of the refractive index of a liquid.

re·frac′to·ry [*refractum*]. 1. Resisting treatment. 2. Resisting the action of heat; slow to melt. 3. Resisting stimulation, said of a muscle or nerve immediately after responding to a stimulation.

re·frac′ture (ree·frack′chur) [*refractum*]. The breaking again of fractured bones that have united by faulty union.

re·fran″gi·bil′i·ty [L. *refringere,* to break up]. Capability of undergoing refraction. —**refran′gible,** *adj.*

re·fresh′ [OF. *refreschier*]. *In surgery,* give to an old lesion the character of a fresh wound. Also see *débridement.*

re·frig′er·ant (ri·fridj′ur·unt) [L. *refrigerare,* to make cold]. Cooling; lessening fever.

re·frig′er·ant. A medicine or agent having cooling properties or lowering body temperature.

re·frig″er·a′tion [L. *refrigeratio,* from *refrigerare*]. The act of lowering the temperature of a body by conducting away its heat to a surrounding cooler substance.

re·frin′gent. See *refractive.*

ref′use [L. *refusum,* from *refundere,* to pour back]. Waste from manufacturing or other establishments, or any discarded matter.

re·fu′sion [*refundere*]. Injection of blood into the circulation after its removal from the same patient.

Regaud, Claude [*French surgeon,* 1870–1940]. Introduced a fixing fluid called Regaud's fixing fluid. See also *Regaud's theory* under electrosome *theory,* and Regaud's *stain.*

re·gen′er·ate [L. *regenerare,* to bring forth again]. Form anew; reproduce, after loss.

re·gen″er·a′tion [L. *regeneratio,* from *regenerare*]. 1. The new growth or repair of structures or tissues lost by disease or by injury. 2. *In chemistry,* the process of obtaining from the by-products or end products of an operation a substance which was employed in the earlier part of the operation.

Wolffian r. The regeneration of a new lens from the upper margin of the iris after removal of the original lens in amphibians.

reg′i·men (redj′i·men) [L., rule]. A systematic course or plan including food, sanitary arrangements, and medication, to maintain or improve health. For specific regimens, see under *diet.*

stir-up r. Encouragement of the patient to breathe deeply and cough frequently, to prevent postanesthetic pulmonary atelectasis.

re′gion [L. *regio,* region]. One of the divisions of the body possessing either natural or arbitrary boundaries. —**regional,** *adj.*

abdominal r. One of the nine regions of the abdomen artificially formed by two horizontal and two parasagittal lines. The horizontal lines are tangent to the cartilages of the ninth ribs and iliac crests, respectively, while the parasagittal lines are drawn vertically on each side from the middle of the inguinal ligament. The regions are, from above: the right hypochondriac region, the epigastric region, the left hypochondriac region, the right lumbar region, the umbilical region, the left lumbar region, the right inguinal region, the hypogastric region, and the left inguinal region.

anterior cubital r. The triangular area distal to the elbow, bounded above by a line joining the two humeral epicondyles, medially by the pronator teres muscle, and laterally by the brachioradialis muscle; the antecubital fossa.

axillary r. A region upon the lateral aspect of the thorax, extending from the axilla to a line drawn from the lower border of the mammary region to that of the scapular region.

ciliary r. The zone around the cornea of the eye, corresponding to the position of the ciliary body.

deltoid r. The proximal part of the lateral aspect of the upper arm.

epigastric r. See abdominal *r.*

femoral r. That portion of the lower extremity associated with the femur. See Plate 4.

foveal r. of the retina. The fovea.

gluteal r. The region over the gluteal muscles.

gustatory r. The tip, margins, and root of the tongue in the neighborhood of the vallate papillae; also the lateral parts of the soft palate and the anterior surface of the glossopalatine arches.

hypochondriac r. See abdominal *r.*

hypogastric r. See abdominal *r.*

iliac r. The region of the ilium. Also see inguinal *r.*

inferior sternal r. That part of the sternal region lying below the margins of the third costal cartilages.

infraaxillary r. The space between the anterior and posterior axillary lines.

infraclavicular r. The area bounded superiorly by the lower border of the clavicle, inferiorly by the lower border of the third rib, on one side by a line extending from the acromion to the pubic spine, and on the other side by the edge of the sternum.

infrahyoid r. The space below the hyoid bone, between the sternocleidomastoid muscles and the sternum.

inframammary r. The area immediately below each breast and above the costal margin.

infrascapular r. A region on either side of the vertebral column below a horizontal line drawn through the inferior angle of each scapula. Also called *subscapular r.*

infraspinous r. The region corresponding to the infraspinous fossa of the scapula.

infratemporal r. The area below the temporal fossa and deep to the ramus of the mandible.

inguinal r. The right and left inguinal or iliac regions are two of the nine abdominal regions. The right includes the abdominal surface covering the cecum and the vermiform process, the ureter, and the spermatic vessels; the left, that covering the sigmoid flexure of the colon, the ureter, and the spermatic vessels. Also called *iliac r.* See Plate 4.

interscapular r. The space between the scapulas.

ischiorectal r. The region corresponding to the posterior part of the pelvic outlet, between the ischium and the rectum.

lumbar r. See abdominal *r.*

mammary r. The space on the anterior surface of the chest between a line drawn through the lower border of the third rib, and one drawn through the upper border of the xiphoid cartilage.

olfactory r. The area on and above the superior conchae and on the adjoining nasal septum where the mucous membrane has olfactory epithelium and olfactory (Bowman's) glands: also called *pars olfactoria.*

parasternal r. The region between the sternal margin and the parasternal line.

parotid r. The area of the face anterior to the ear lying over the parotid gland.

pelvic r. The region within the true pelvis.

perineal r. The region of the perineum. See *perineum,* 2.

popliteal r. See popliteal *space.*

precordial r. The surface of the chest covering the heart.

preoptic r. Small region of the hypothalamus anterior to the optic lobes, the stimulation of which causes contraction of the urinary bladder and occasionally other evidences of parasympathetic activity: also called *preoptic area.*

pretectal r. A zone of transition between the thalamus and tectum, rostral to the superior colliculi. The optic fibers entering it subserve the pupillary reflex, which is abolished by bilateral lesions of the region.

pulmocardiac r. The region of the left thorax in which the left lung overlaps the heart.

pulmogastric r. The portion of the left thorax in which the lung overlaps the stomach.

pulmohepatic r. The portion of the right thorax in which the lung overlaps the liver.

pulmovascular r. The part of the thorax in which the lung overlaps the origins of the larger vessels.

respiratory r. of the nose. The portion of the

nasal passages having to do with the act of respiration.

retromaxillary r. The space behind the maxilla.

scapular r. The region of the back corresponding to the position of the scapula, the spine of which divides it into a supraspinous and an infraspinous region.

sensitive r. See sensitive *volume.*

sternal r. The region overlying the sternum.

strip r. Area 4S of Brodmann's areas.

sublingual r. That part of the floor of the mouth lying below the tongue.

submaxillary r. The region between the mandible and the anterior and posterior bellies of the digastric muscle. The triangle so bounded contains the submaxillary or submandibular gland. Also called *submandibular triangle.*

submental r. The region just beneath the chin.

subthalamic r. The ventral or motor part of the thalamus concerned largely with extrapyramidal pathways.

superior sternal r. That portion of the sternal region lying above the lower margins of the third costal cartilages.

supraclavicular r. The space between the upper margin of the clavicle and the lower borders of the omohyoid and sternocleidomastoid muscles.

suprahyoid r. The region between the mandible and the hyoid bone.

suprainguinal r. That bounded by the rectus abdominis muscle, the inguinal ligament, and a horizontal line through the iliac crest.

supraspinous r. The region corresponding to the supraspinous fossa of the scapula.

suprasternal r. See suprasternal *notch.*

thyrohyoid r. The region around the thyroid cartilage and the hyoid bone.

umbilical r. See abdominal *r.*

vertebral r. Relating to the region over the vertebral column.

reg'is·ter [ML. *registrum,* from L. *regerere,* to carry back]. The compass of a voice; also a subdivision of its compass, consisting in a series of tones produced in the same way and of a like character.

reg'is·trar [*regerere*]. 1. An official custodian of records. 2. An officer in charge of hospital registry office.

reg"is·tra'tion [*regerere*]. The act of recording, as of deaths, births, etc.

reg'is·try [*regerere*]. Office listing nurses available for general or special services.

regitine. Trade-mark for *phentolamine.*

reg"le·men·ta'tion [F. *réglementation,* from L. *regula,* rule]. The legal restriction or regulation of prostitution.

re·gres'sion [L. *regressio,* from *regredi,* to turn back]. 1. A turning back. 2. The tendency for children to deviate less from the average of the population than their parents. Also called *filial r.* 3. *In psychology,* a mental state and a mode of adjustment to difficult and unpleasant situations, characterized by behavior of a type that had been satisfying and appropriate at an earlier stage of development but which no longer befits the age and social status of the individual. A terminal state in some forms of schizophrenia. 4. *In mathematics,* the tendency for a group equated in one trait to have a mean value closer to the general mean in a related trait. 5. See *retrogression.*

re·gres'sive [*regredi*]. Going back to a former state; subsiding, said of symptoms.

reg'u·lar [L. *regularis,* from *regula,* rule]. 1. According to rule or custom. 2. Colloquial term for menstruating at normal time.

reg"u·la'tion [*regula*]. The ability of a developing organism to continue normal development in spite of experimental interference, such as ablation, implantation, or transplantation.

bathmotropic r. Regulation of the excitability of the atrial and ventricular myocardium by sympathetic and parasympathetic stimulation.

dromotropic r. The regulation of the rate of conduction and duration of the refractory period of the heart, by sympathetic and parasympathetic influences.

reg'u·la"tive [*regula*]. *In embryology,* descriptive of development of eggs in which the cells of the early stages can be affected by inducing agents from the surrounding parts; opposed to mosaic development. See *mosaic,* 2.

regulin. Trade-mark of a preparation of agar and psyllium, used in the treatment of constipation.

reg'u·lus [L., petty king]. A metal reduced from its ore to the metallic state.

re·gur'gi·tant [L. *re-,* back; *gurgitare,* to flood]. Flowing backward.

re·gur"gi·ta'tion [*re-; gurgitare*]. 1. A backflow of blood through a heart valve that is defective. 2. The return of food from the stomach to the mouth soon after eating, without the ordinary efforts at vomiting.

aortic r. That of the blood through the aortic orifice, due to incompetence of the aortic valve.

duodenal r. The return of chyme from the duodenum into the stomach.

functional r. A form of mitral or tricuspid regurgitation, due to dilatation of the muscular rings surrounding the respective valves.

mitral r. Imperfect closure of the mitral valve during the cardiac systole, permitting blood to be forced back into the left atrium.

re"ha·bil"i·ta'tion [L. *re-,* again; *habilitas,* ability]. The restoration to a disabled individual of maximum independence commensurate with his limitations by developing his residual capacities. *In medicine,* it implies prescribed training and employment of many different methods and professional workers.

re"ha·la'tion [*re-;* L. *halare,* to breathe]. Rebreathing; the inhalation of air which has been inspired previously; sometimes used in anesthesia.

Rehberg, Poul Brandt (1895–). Danish physiologist who devised a test for renal function based on the excretion of creatinine, called *Rehberg's test.*

Rehfuss, Martin Emil [*American physician,* 1887–]. Introduced the fractional method of test meal examination. A test meal of two slices of toast (35 gm.) and 8 ounces (250 cc.) of weak tea is called a *Rehfuss test meal.* A narrow flexible tube fitted with a perforated tip at the lower end and a syringe at the upper end is called the *Rehfuss tube.* The tube is passed into the stomach after the meal. At 15-minute intervals, small quantities of gastric content are withdrawn by means of the syringe and examined, called the *Rehfuss method.*

Rehn, Ludwig [*German surgeon,* 1849–1930]. First performed thyroidectomy for exophthalmic goiter (1880). Introduced an operation for rectal prolapse, in which he resected the protruding mucous membrane with infolding of the muscularis by suture; called *Rehn's operation, Rehn-Delorme operation.*

Reichel's duct. See cloacal *duct.*

Reichert, Karl Bogislaus (1811–1883). German anatomist who described the skeletal elements of the embryo which become the styloid processes, the stylohyoid ligaments, and the lesser cornua of the hyoid bone, called *Reichert's cartilages.* He was noted also for his contributions to the knowledge of amphibian craniums. Also see Reichert's *membrane.*

Reichert-Meissl num′ber. See under *number*.

Reichmann, Mikolaj [*Polish physician*, 1851–1918]. Remembered for his description of a chronic disease of the stomach associated with continuous hypersecretion of the gastric juice (1882); called *gastrosuccorrhea, Reichmann's disease.*

Reichstein, Tadeus (1897–). Swiss chemist and physiologist known for his research in the synthesis of vitamin C and the isolation of compounds from the adrenal cortex. In 1950 he shared the Nobel prize in physiology and medicine with Edward C. Kendall and Philip Hench for the synthesis of cortisone and the description of its chemical structure and biological effects.

Reid, Robert William [*Scottish anatomist*, 1851–1939]. Described an imaginary line passing from the infraorbital ridge through the external auditory meatus to the midline of the occiput, useful in marking the level of the base of the skull; called *Reid's base line.*

Reil, Johann Christian [*Dutch physiologist*, 1759–1813]. Distinguished for his many contributions in both physiology and anatomy. Described a number of structures in the brain. The insula of the cerebral hemisphere was formerly called the *island of Reil.*

re″im·plan·ta′tion [L. *re-*, again; *in*, in; *plantare*, to set]. *In dentistry*, the replacing of an extracted tooth into its socket.

Rein's thermostromuhr. See *thermostromuhr of Rein.*

Reinecke's crystals. Rod-shaped crystalloids in the interstitial cells of the testis.

rei′neck·e salt (rye′neck·uh). Ammonium reineckate, $NH_4[Cr(NH_3)_2(SCN)_4].H_2O$. Dark-red crystals or crystalline powder, moderately soluble in cold water. Aqueous solutions are unstable. Used as a precipitant of amines.

re″in·fec′tion [*re-;* L. *infectio*, from *inficere*, to infect]. A second infection with the same kind of organism.

re″in·force′ment [from F. *renforcement*]. 1. The act of reinforcing. 2. Any augmentation of force.
r. of reflexes. Increased myotatic irritability (or reflex response) when muscular or mental actions are synchronously carried out, or other stimuli are coincidentally brought to bear upon parts of the body other than that concerned in the reflex arc.

re″in·fu′sion [L. *re-*, back; *infusio*, from *infundere*, to pour into]. The reinjection of blood serum, or cerebrospinal fluid.

Reinhart method. See Shinowara, Jones, and Reinhart *method.*

Reinhold's method. See Letonoff and Reinhold's *method;* Reinhold and Shiels *method.*

re″in·ner·va′tion [L. *re-*, again; *in-*, in; *nervus*, nerve]. Nerve grafting where the motor nerve supply to a muscle has been lost.

re″in·oc″u·la′tion [*re-;* L. *inoculatio*, from *inoculare*, to inoculate]. Inoculation a second time with the same kind of organism.

Reinsch's test. See under *test.*

re·in″te·gra′tion [*re-;* L. *integrare*, to make whole]. *In psychiatry*, the restoration to harmonious mental functioning after disintegration of the personality by mental illness.

re″in·ver′sion (ree″in·vur′shun, ·zhun) [*re-;* L. *inversio*, from *invertere*, to turn about]. The act of reducing an inverted uterus by the application of pressure to the fundus.

Reisinger's method. See Farley, St. Clair, and Reisinger's *method.*

Reisseisen, Franz Daniel [*German anatomist*, 1773–1828]. Remembered for his description of the muscular fibers of the bronchi (1804); called *Reisseisen's muscles.*

Reissner's membrane. See under *membrane.*

Reiter, Hans [*German physician*, 1881–]. Known for his description of a syndrome, possibly of spirochetal origin, characterized by arthritis, nonspecific urethritis, frequently by an accompanying conjunctivitis, and sometimes by other symptoms; called *Reiter's syndrome.*

re·ju″ve·nes′cence [L. *re-*, again; *juvenescere*, to grow young again]. 1. A renewal of youth; a renewal of strength and vigor; specifically a restoration of sexual vigor. 2. *In biology*, a method of cell formation in which the entire protoplasm of an old cell escapes by rupture of the cell wall and then develops a new cell wall.

re·lapse′ [L. *relapsum*, from *relabi*, to fall back]. Return of symptoms of a disease after convalescence has begun.

re·la′tion [L. *relatio*, a carrying back]. 1. Interdependence; mutual influence or connection between organs or parts. 2. Connection by consanguinity; kinship. 3. *In anatomy*, the position of parts of the body as regards each other.
centric r. The condition in which the mandibular condyles rest unstrained in their most posterior position in the mandibular fossae and from which position all mandibular movements are initiated.
dentofacial r. The relation which the teeth and alveoli bear to the face.

re·lax′ [L. *relaxare*, to loosen]. 1. Loosen or make less tense. 2. Cause a movement of the bowels.

re″lax·a′tion [L. *relaxatio*, from *relaxare*]. A diminution of tension in a part; a diminution in functional activity, as relaxation of the skin.

re·lax′in. Water-soluble hormone found in human serum and the serums of certain other animals during pregnancy; probably acting with progesterone and estrogen, it causes relaxation of pelvic ligaments in the guinea pig.

re·lief′ [OF.]. The partial removal of anything distressing; alleviation of pain or discomfort.

re·lieve′ [OF. *relever*, from L. *relevare*, to raise up]. Free from pain, discomfort, or distress.

REM, rem *R*oentgen *e*quivalent *m*an.

Remak, Ernst Julius [*German neurologist*, 1849–1911]. The son of Robert Remak. He described a flexion of the toes following irritation of the anterior portion of the thigh. *Remak's reflex* is said to be of significance in indicating lesion of the spinal cord.

Remak, Robert [*German physiologist and neurologist*, 1815–65]. Discoverer of the peripheral nonmedullated nerve fibers; called *fibers of Remak* (1838). Discoverer of the group of nerve cells in the coronary sinus where it joins the heart, called *Remak's ganglion.* Pioneer in the use of galvanic current for nerve and muscle therapy. The axis cylinder of a nerve fiber is called *Remak's band.*

re·me′di·al [L. *remedialis*, from *remedium*, remedy]. Having the nature of a remedy; relieving; curative.

rem′e·dy [*remedium*]. Anything used in the treatment of disease.

Re·mij′i·a (ri·midj′ee·uh) [NL., after the surgeon *Remijo*]. A genus of shrubs and trees of the Rubiaceae closely related to cinchona. Some of them yield quinine and related alkaloids but are not commercially collected.

re″min·er·al·i·za′tion [L. *re-*, again; ML. *mineralis*, from *minera*, ore]. Supposed restoration of the body's lost mineral constituents, or those of any tissue.

re·mis′sion [L. *remissio*, a sending back]. 1. Abatement or subsidence of the symptoms of disease. 2. The period of diminution thereof.

re·mit′tence [L. *remittere*, to send back]. Temporary abatement or cessation of symptoms. —**remittent,** *adj.*

ren (pl. *renes*) [L.]. The kidney. —**ren'iform,** *adj.*

r. mobilis. Floating kidney.

r. unguiformis. Horseshoe kidney.

re'nal [L. *renalis*, of the kidneys]. Pertaining to the kidneys.

r. clearance. See kidney function *test.*

Renaut, Joseph Louis [*French physician*, 1844–1917]. Described a thin hyaline membrane, possibly hypothetical, separating the epidermis from the corium, called *Renaut's layer.*

Rendu, Henri Jules Louis (1844–1902). French physician who described hereditary hemorrhagic telangiectasis, also called *Osler-Rendu-Weber's disease* (1896). He also described a hysterical tremor provoked or increased by volitional movements, known as *Rendu's tremor.*

re'nes (ree'neez). Plural of ren.

ren'i·form [L. *ren*, kidney; *forma*, form]. Kidney-shaped.

re'nin, ren'in [L. *ren*, kidney]. A kidney protein which acts as a protease on renin substrate, to liberate angiotonin. In vivo, intravenously injected, it exhibits pressor activity.

r. substrate. A constituent of the α_2 globulin of plasma which is the substrate on which the enzyme renin works. Also called *hypertensinogen, renin-activator.*

ren'i·punc"ture (ren'i·punk"chur, ree'ni·, ren"i-punk'chur, ree"ni·) [*ren;* L. *punctura*, a pricking]. Puncture of the capsule of a kidney.

ren'net [ME. *rennen*, to run]. 1. Rennin. 2. A preparation of the lining of the calf stomach used as a source of rennin.

ren'nin [*rennen*]. The milk-coagulating enzyme found in the gastric juice of the fourth stomach of the calf.

ren·nin'o·gen, ren'no·gen [*rennen;* G. *genesthai*, from *gignesthai*, to be produced]. The zymogen of rennin, found in the wall of the fourth stomach of the calf. Also called *prorennin.*

Rénon, Louis [*French physician*, 1863–1922]. Remembered for his description of thyro-ovarian deficiency and overactive pituitary gland, with acromegaly (1908); called *Rénon-Delille syndrome.*

ren"o·tro'phic (ren"o·tro'fick, ree"no·) [L. *ren*, kidney; G. *trephein*, to nourish]. Pertaining to the ability of certain compounds, such as testosterone, to produce hypertrophy of the kidney.

ren"o·va'tion [L. *renovatio*, from *renovare*, to restore]. The repair or renewal of that which has been impaired.

Renucci, Simon François [*French physician*, nineteenth century]. Described *Sarcoptes scabiei*, the cause of scabies (1835).

re"or·gan·i·za'tion [L. *re-*, again; G. *organon*, instrument]. Healing by the development of tissue elements similar to those lost through some morbid process.

REP, rep *R*oentgen *e*quivalent *p*hysical.

rep. *Repetatur;* let it be repeated.

re·pair' [OF. *reparer*, from L. *repatriare*, to return to one's country]. Restoration to a normal state after injury.

re·pel'lent [L. *repellere*, to drive back]. 1. Driving back. 2. Causing resolution of morbid processes.

re·pel'lents [*repellere*]. Various chemicals employing usually bland oils as vehicles and used to repel or kill external parasites, such as mosquitoes, chiggers, ticks.

re·pel'ler [*repellere*]. An instrument used in large animal obstetrics to push back the fetus so head and limbs can be placed for normal delivery.

re"per·co·la'tion [L. *re-*, again; *percolatio*, from *percolare*, to strain through]. Repeated percolation.

re"per·cus'sion [*re-;* L. *percussio*, from *percutere* to strike through]. 1. Ballottement. 2. A driving in, or dispersion of, a tumor or eruption.

re"per·cus'sive [*re-; percutere*]. 1. Repellent. 2. A repellent drug.

re·pet'i·tive fir'ing. Ability of a tissue to emit, after excitation, a succession of accelerating or decrementing impulses.

re·place'ment [F.]. The act of replacing.

complementary r. See retinal *rivalry.*

reciprocal r. See retinal *rivalry.*

re"plan·ta'tion [L. *re-*, again; *plantare*, to set]. The act of planting again.

r. of the teeth. The replacement of teeth which have been extracted or otherwise removed from their alveolar sockets, usually after appropriate treatment such as filling the root canals and scraping the roots.

re·ple'tion [L. *repletio*, from *replere*, to fill up]. The condition of being, or the act of making, full. —**replete',** *adj.*

re"pli·ca'tion [L. *replicare*, to fold back]. 1. Theoretical multiplication of bacteriophage in bacterium: the phage loses its identity after entering bacterium, and shortly before lysis of the bacterium new phages of adult size and consistency appear. 2. The repetition of an experiment under the same conditions to check for possible error due to personal factors of the observer. 3. A folding back of a part; reduplication. *Rare.* See also *reproduction.*

re·po"lar·i·za'tion (ree·po"lur·i·zay'shun, ·eye-zay'shun) [L. *re-*, again; *polus*, pole]. Restoration of the polarized state in nerve or muscle fiber during recovery from conduction of an excitatory process.

re"po·si'tion (ree"po·zish'un, rep"o·zish'un) [L. *repositio*, from *reponere*, to set back]. The return of an abnormally placed part, organ, or fragment to its proper position.

re·pos'i·tor (ri·poz'i·tur) [*reponere*]. An instrument for replacing parts that have become displaced, especially for replacing a prolapsed umbilical cord. *Obs.*

re·pous"soir' (ruh·pōō"swahr'. *See* NOTES § 35) [F.]. An instrument for extracting the roots of teeth.

re·pres'sion [L. *repressum*, from *reprimere*, to press back]. *In psychopathology*, a psychic mechanism whereby impulses or desires, incompatible or in conflict with the individual's conscious self-image or motives, are forcibly and automatically dismissed from consciousness by superego pressure. The psychic energy with which these impulses are loaded becomes part of the unconscious. Also see *suppression.*

re"pro·duc'tion [L. *re-*, again; *producere*, to produce]. A fundamental property of protoplasm by which organisms give rise to other organisms of the same kind.

re"pro·duc'tive [*re-; producere*]. Pertaining to the capacity of organisms to produce other organisms of the same kind.

re·pul'sion [L. *repulsio*, from *repellere*, to push back]. Act of repelling or driving back or apart.

RES Reticuloendothelial system.

re·saz'u·rin (ri·zazh'ur·in) (C.C.). $C_{12}H_7NO_4$; a tricyclic compound, so-called *diazoresorcinol*, occurring in dark-red crystals with a greenish luster, insoluble in water, soluble in dilute solutions of alkali hydroxides: used in histologic staining as a neutralization indicator, also for detection of hyposulfite (sulfoxylate).

res·cin'na·mine. $C_{35}H_{42}N_2O_9$; a hypotensive and sedative alkaloid, closely related to reserpine, present in *Rauwolfia serpentina.*

re·sect′ [L. *resectum*, from *resecare*, to cut off]. 1. Cut out a portion of a tissue or organ. 2. Cut away the end of one or more of the bones entering into a joint.

re·sec′tion [L. *resectio*, from *resecare*]. The operation of cutting out, as the removal of a section or segment of an organ.

window r. Submucous resection of part of the nasal septum.

re·sec′to·scope [*resecare;* G. *skopein*, to examine]. A tubelike instrument by means of which small structures may be divided within a body cavity without an opening other than that made by the instrument itself.

re·ser′pine. $C_{33}H_{40}N_2O_9$; an alkaloid, from *Rauwolfia serpentina* and other species of *Rauwolfia*, which reduces blood pressure in hypertensive states, slows pulse rate, and possesses sedative and tranquilizing properties. See *serpasil*.

re·serve′ (ri·zurv′) [L. *reservare*, to save up]. A remainder; a capacity or potentiality, retained as an additional store.

alkali r. The components of the blood which are capable of neutralizing acids. These include sodium bicarbonate, dipotassium phosphate, and proteins.

cardiac r. Ability of the heart to do more work in pumping larger amounts of blood per beat.

diminished cardiac r. Condition in which a cardiac patient develops dyspnea on performing ordinary muscular effort but has none at rest.

res′i·dent phy·si′cian. A physician living in the hospital for further training after an internship. Also called *resident*.

re·sid′u·al [L. *residuus*, that is left behind]. Pertaining to that which cannot be evacuated or discharged, as residual air in the lungs, residual urine in the bladder.

re·sid′u·al. A remainder.

res′i·due [*residuus*]. That which remains after a part has been removed; remainder.

res′i·dues [*residuus*]. 1. The amino acids or polypeptides resulting from hydrolysis of a protein. 2. The amino-acid building blocks of a protein. The term is also used for the acid after deaminization.

re·sil′i·ence [L. *resilire*, to spring back]. The quality of being elastic or resilient.

re·sil′i·ent [*resilire*]. Rebounding; elastic.

res′in (rez′in) [L. *resina*, resin]. 1. One of a class of vegetable substances exuding from various plants; generally soluble in alcohol, in ether, and in the volatile oils, and insoluble in water; readily fusible and inflammable. They may represent oxidation products of terpenes, and are composed largely of esters and ethers of organic acids with complex alcohols known as resinols, along with acids and acid anhydrides. 2. A class of pharmaceutical preparations (*resinae*) made by extracting resin-containing drugs with alcohol, concentrating the liquid and adding it to water, whereby the resin and other water-insoluble principles precipitate and may be collected and dried. —**resinous,** *adj.*

acrylic r. A synthetic resin, usually a polymer of methyl methacrylate. Used in dentistry and medicine for the manufacture of artificial dentures, artificial eyes, or splints. See *acrylics*.

anion exchange r. A highly polymerized synthetic organic compound containing amine groups; the basic form has the property of withdrawing acid from a liquid medium in which the resin is placed, and for this reason is utilized as a gastric antacid to control symptoms in simple hyperacidity and in peptic ulcer. See *polyamine-methylene resin*.

cation exchange r. A highly polymerized synthetic organic compound consisting of a large nondiffusible anion and a simple diffusible cation, which latter can be exchanged for a cation in the medium in which the resin is placed. *In medicine* such a resin, often modified to avoid disturbance in the balance of other physiologically important ions, is used to remove sodium ions from the body in treating conditions resulting from abnormal retention of sodium. See *carbacrylamine resins, carbacrylic resin, potassium carbacrylate*.

ion exchange r. A synthetic polymer containing fixed ionizable groups which exchange ions of the opposite charge.

ipomea r. (*resina ipomoeae*). A powerful cathartic with a tendency toward griping. Dose, 0.13–0.32 Gm. (2–5 gr.). Also called *Mexican scammony r.*

jalap r. (*resina jalapae*). A drastic cathartic. Dose, 0.13–0.32 Gm. (2–5 gr.).

podophyllum r. See *podophyllum* resin.

res′in·oid (rez′i·noyd) [*resina;* G. *eidos*, form]. A substance which has some of the properties of a resin. —**res′inoid,** *adj.*

resinol. 1. A proprietary ointment used to allay itching in minor skin disorders. 2. General term for the complex alcohols found in resins.

re·sist′ance [L. *resistere*, to withstand]. 1. Opposition to force or external impression. 2. *In electricity*, the opposition offered by a conductor to the passage of the current. Abbreviated, R. 3. *In psychoanalysis*, the reluctance of the subject to give up habitual patterns of thinking, feeling, and acting to take on less neurotic and newer modes of adaptation.

essential r. The resistance to conduction within the battery itself. Also called *internal r.*

extraordinary r. The resistance to conduction in the circuit outside of the battery. Also called *external r.*

natural r. See native *immunity*.

re″sis·to·my′cin. $C_{23}H_{18}O_6$; a weakly acid antibiotic substance, prepared from *Streptomyces resistomycificus*, active against *Staphylococcus aureus*, *Bacillus subtilis*, and *Mycobacterium tuberculosis*.

res″o·lu′tion [L. *resolutio*, from *resolvere*, to loosen]. 1. The subsidence of inflammation; as in pneumonia, the stage of dissolving the exudate due to proteolytic enzymes. 2. The ability of the eye or a lens to register small detail, the resolution of the human eye being 1 minute of arc. 3. The separation of an optically inactive mixture of isomers into its optically active components. Syn., *mesotomy*.

re·solve′ (ri·zolv′) [*resolvere*]. 1. Return to the normal state after some pathologic process. 2. Separate anything into its component parts.

re·sol′vent (ri·zol′vunt) [*resolvere*]. Causing solution or dissipation of tissue.

re·sol′vent. An agent causing resolution.

re·solv′ing pow′er. The capability of a lens to make clear the finest details of an object.

res′o·nance (rez′o·nuns) [L. *resonare*, to resound]. 1. The attribute of relatively long duration possessed by certain sounds. 2. Normal resonance; in physical diagnosis, the prolonged, nonmusical, composite sound which results from vibration of the normal chest. It consists of a mixture of fundamental tones, most of which are within the range of 90 to 130 vibrations per second, and hence varies but little in pitch. 3. *In chemistry*, the phenomenon of a compound simultaneously having the characteristics of two structural forms of the compound, i.e., resonating between the two structures, thereby conferring greater stability upon it than if it possessed either of the two structures involved. Benzene represents such a resonance hybrid of two forms differing only in the alternation of double bonds in the ring.

amphoric r. A tympanitic percussion note containing overtones which give it the sound of air blown across the mouth of an empty bottle or jar.

bandbox r. See tympanitic *r*.

cracked-pot r. A characteristic clinking sound which can be elicited occasionally by percussion over tuberculous cavities, especially when the percussion is forcible and the patient's mouth is open. Also called *cracked-pot sound.*

skodaic r. Tympanitic resonance in the area above the region of a lung compressed by pleural effusion.

tympanitic r. (a) The prolonged musical sound heard on percussion over the stomach, colon, or other air-containing cavity with flexible walls. In contrast with normal resonance, its sounds vary widely in pitch. (b) A percussion note which exhibits in varying proportion the characteristics of both resonance and tympany. Also called *bandbox r., hyperresonance, Skoda's r.*

vesicular r. That which is contingent upon the existence of air-containing lung vesicles. Also called *normal r.*

vocal r. The vibrations of the spoken voice transmitted through the lungs and the chest wall and detected by auscultation. Abbreviated, V. R.

res'o·nant [*resonare*]. Possessing, or capable of producing, resonance.

res'o·na"tor (rez'o·nay"tur) [*resonare*]. Any physical body capable of being set into vibration in unison with another vibrating body. The thoracic cage, lung, and other human structures possess this capacity in limited degree.

re·sorb'ent [L. *resorbere,* to suck back]. Absorbing.

re·sorb'ent. A drug which aids in the process of resorption.

re·sor'cin (ri·zor'sin). Resorcinol.

re·sor'cin·ol (ri·zor'sin·ole, ·ol, ·awl) [L. *resina,* resin; It. *orcello,* archil]. $C_6H_4(OH)_2$; *meta*-dihydroxybenzene; white needle-shaped crystals or powder, very soluble in water: used in treatment of skin diseases for its antiseptic, keratolytic, exfoliative, and antifungal properties, and also as a reagent.

r. blue. Lacmoid.

r. monoacetate. $C_6H_4.OH.OCOCH_3$; a viscous, pale-yellow or amber liquid, sparingly soluble in water, soluble in alcohol, which slowly liberates resorcinol by hydrolysis: used in treating various diseases of the skin and scalp. See *euresol.*

re·sor"cin·ol·phthal'ein. Fluorescein.

re·sorp'tion [L. *resorbere,* to suck back]. The removal by absorption.

re·spir'a·ble (ri·spy'ruh·bul, res'pi·ruh·bul) [L. *respirare,* to breathe back]. Capable of being inspired and expired; capable of furnishing the gaseous interchange in the lungs necessary for life. —**respirabil'ity,** *n.*

res"pi·ra'tion [L. *respiratio,* from *respirare*]. 1. The interchange of gases of the living and the gases of the medium in which they live, through any channel, as cutaneous respiration. 2. The act of breathing with the lungs; the taking of air into, and its expulsion from, the lungs. It consists of two acts: inspiration, or the taking in of the atmospheric air, and expiration, or the expelling of the modified air. Expired air contains less oxygen and more carbon dioxide than inspired air. The volume of air taken into the lungs and given out during an ordinary respiration (tidal air) is 500 cc.; the volume that can be inspired in addition by a forcible inspiration (complemental air) is 1500 cc.; that which can be exhaled after a normal expiration (reserve or supplemental air) is 1500 cc.; the amount remaining in the chest after the most complete expiration (residual air) is from 1200 to 1600 cc. The volume of air that can be forcibly expelled after the most forcible inspiration is termed vital or respiratory capacity and is equal to the tidal air, complemental air, and reserve air, or about 3500 cc. —**respir'atory,** *adj.*

abdominal r. A type of respiration caused by the contraction of the diaphragm and the elasticity of the abdominal walls and viscera.

absent r. Suppression of respiratory sounds.

amphoric r. A blowing respiration engendered in large cavities with firm walls. Its peculiar character is due to an echo from the walls of the cavity.

apneustic r. Breathing characterized by prolonged deep inspirations.

artificial r. See *artificial respiration.*

Biot's r. Respiration associated with abruptly alternating periods of apnea and hyperpnea, in contrast to the gradually alternating phases of Cheyne-Stokes respirations. Seen in meningitis and medullary disease.

blowing r. See bronchial *r*.

bronchial r. Respiration as heard over the trachea or bronchial tubes in health; it is high in pitch, equal in inspiration and expiration, blowing in character (especially the expiratory element), and marked by a brief pause between inspiration and expiration. It is also heard over other parts of the lungs which are the seat of consolidation.

bronchocavernous r. A form intermediate in character between bronchial and cavernous respiration.

bronchovesicular r. Respiration having the characters of both bronchial and vesicular respiration. It is heard over areas of consolidation surrounded by patches of healthy lung tissue.

cavernous r. A blowing respiration of low pitch, circumscribed, alternating with gurgling, and deriving its chief character from the nature of the cavity in which it is generated.

cerebral r. A shallow blowing respiration seen often in the presence of fever.

Cheyne-Stokes r. Periods of stertorous respiration interrupted by periods of apnea seen in cerebral arteriosclerosis, senility, heart disease, and a few other similar conditions.

cogwheel r. See interrupted *r*.

collateral r. Passage of air between lobules within the same lobe of a lung, allowing ventilation of a lobule whose bronchiole is obstructed.

costal r. Respiration in which the chest movement predominates over the diaphragmatic.

diaphragmatic r. See abdominal *r*.

direct r. Respiration in which the living substance of an organism, as an ameba, takes oxygen directly from the surrounding medium, and returns carbon dioxide directly to it, no respiratory blood being present.

dyspneic r. See *dyspnea.*

electrophrenic r. Respiration induced, increased, or controlled temporarily by electrical stimulation of one phrenic nerve.

exaggerated r. An increase in intensity, without alteration in character or rhythm of the respiratory movements.

external r. The interchange of gases between the atmosphere and air in lungs and between the air in lungs and pulmonary capillaries.

feeble r. Diminution in the intensity without alteration in the character or rhythm of the respiratory movements.

fetal r. The interchange of gases between the fetal and the maternal blood through the medium of the placenta.

forced r. Respiration induced by blowing air into

the lungs by means of a bellows, or in some other way, as in physiologic experiments.

harsh r. See bronchovesicular *r.*

hissing r. An increased vesicular murmur causing a hissing sound.

hollow r. See amphoric *r.*

indirect r. Respiration in which the living substance of the organism, as in all the higher mammals, gets rid of carbon dioxide and obtains oxygen by means of a circulating respiratory blood.

internal r. The exchange of gases between the systemic blood and tissues.

interrupted r. Respiration in which either inspiration or expiration is divided into two or more parts. It is most often heard at the apex of the right lung, anteriorly.

intrauterine r. Respiration by the fetus before delivery.

jerking r. See interrupted *r.*

Kussmaul's r. The deep gasping respiration characteristic of severe acidosis.

labored r. Respiration in which, owing to lack of ability on the part of the ordinary muscles of respiration to aerate the blood sufficiently, the auxiliary muscles of respiration are called into play.

laryngeal r. The widening of the glottis during inspiration and its narrowing during expiration.

nasal r. Nose breathing.

nervous r. See cerebral *r.*

normal r. Respiration as it occurs in a normal individual in a state of rest or moderate action.

paradoxical r. In open pneumothorax, a condition in which the lung on the side of the pleural opening fills on exhalation and empties on inhalation.

pharyngeal r. Rhythmic expansions and contractions of the pharynx in connection with other movements of respiration. The expansion is preinspiratory and the contraction inspiratory.

placental r. See fetal *r.*

pneumotoxic r. Breathing characterized by complete irregularity in rate and amplitude.

prenatal r. See fetal *r.*

puerile r. Exaggerated expiratory breath sounds, prolonged and high pitched, heard in healthy children.

pulmonary r. Respiration in which the interchange of gas between the blood and air occurs in the lungs.

stertorous r. The sound produced by breathing through the nose and mouth at the same time, causing vibration of the soft palate between the two currents of air.

subsibilant r. A dull, whistling sound heard over the bronchi, and due to obstruction by mucus.

tracheal r. The respiratory murmur heard in a normal individual by placing a stethoscope over the suprasternal fossa.

uremic r. See Cheyne-Stokes *r.*

vesicular r. A soft, gradual, low-pitched inspiration immediately followed by a shorter and less distinct expiration sound heard over the normal lung during respiration.

vesiculobronchial r. See bronchovesicular *r.*

vesiculocavernous r. Respiration that is both vesicular and cavernous.

wavy r. See interrupted *r.*

res′pi·ra″tor [*respirare*]. A device for producing artificial respiration. Except for the head, the body is hermetically enclosed in a cabinet and respiratory movements are produced by introducing alternately pressure and suction.

Both r. A cabinet of wood enclosing the body, except for the head, with a rubber collar about the patient's neck. A small motor drives a bellows connected with the chamber by a flexible pipe, By means of a valve the bellows acts as a sucker. extracting and letting in air alternately.

Drinker r. A power-driven breathing apparatus similar in type to the Both respirator, the cabinet being of metal.

re·spire′ [*respirare*]. Breathe.

res″pi·rom′e·ter [*respirare;* G. *metron*, a measure]. A device to determine the character of respiration.

res″pi·rom′e·try. The quantitative study of respiration.

capillary r. A method to determine changes in the volume of gases in a capillary tube which leads from a chamber filled with a respiring sample to a chamber containing only media and reagents. The capillary tube contains an index droplet, the displacement of which serves to determine the changes in gas volume.

re·sponse′ [L. *responsum*, from *respondere*, to reply]. The reaction or movement of a muscle or other part due to the application of a stimulus. See also *reflex.*

antichromatic responses. Nervous mechanisms postulated to deal with fringe colors which are seen as black and white if they subtend small visual angles.

conditioned r. See conditioned *reflex.*

inherited r. See instinctive *reflex.*

triple r. See *triple response.*

re·spon″si·bil′i·ty [*respondere*]. 1. *In legal medicine*, the accountability for professional acts. 2. The capacity to differentiate right from wrong.

rest [AS.]. 1. Cessation of labor or action; repose. 2. An epithelial remnant persisting after its developmental activity has ceased. Also called *epithelial debris.* See fetal *r.*

bed r. (a) A device to support patients in bed. (b) The keeping of a patient in bed continually.

caudal medullary r. A remnant of the medullary coccygeal vesicle that normally disappears about the sixth fetal month, but may give rise to sacrococcygeal cysts or fistulas.

cell r. See fetal *r.*

epithelial r. One of the cords of cells in the periodontal membrane representing remnants of the epithelial sheath of the enamel organ: also called *epithelial cord, epithelial debris* (of Malassez), *epithelial remnant.*

fetal r. A portion of embryonic tissue, or cells, which is misplaced in another tissue during development.

res′ti·form [L. *restis*, cord; *forma*, form]. Corded or cordlike.

rest′ing [AS. *restan*]. Ceasing from motion; at rest.

res″ti·tu′ti·o ad in′te·grum (res″ti·tew′shee·o ad in′ti·grum) [L.]. Complete restoration to a healthy condition.

res″ti·tu′tion [L. *restitutio*, from *restituere*, to restore]. 1. The act of restoring. 2. *In obstetrics*, a rotation of the fetal head immediately after its birth. See Plate 42. 3. *In psychiatry*, the psychic mechanism whereby the individual seeks to relieve himself of unconscious guilt by benevolent acts which undo, make good, or repair some harm.

res″to·ra′tion [L. *restauratio*, from *restaurare*, to restore]. The return to a state of health or a normal condition. —**restor′ative,** *adj.*

re·stor′a·tive [*restaurare*]. A remedy that is efficacious in restoring health and strength.

re·straint′ [OF. *restrainte*, from L. *restringere*, to draw back tightly]. 1. Hindrance of any action, physical, moral, or mental. 2. The state of being controlled; confinement.

mechanical r. Restraining the insane by mechanical means.

medicinal r. The use of narcotics and sedatives in quieting the mentally deranged.

re·stric'tion of e'go. *In psychology,* a defense mechanism for escaping anxiety by avoiding those situations consciously perceived as dangerous or uncomfortable, as in the many phobias of childhood and in those adults whose sphere of movement is severely limited by their need to avoid anxiety.

re·strin'gent [*restringere*]. An astringent or styptic.

restrol. A trade-mark for the synthetic estrogen dienestrol.

re"sub·li·ma'tion [L. *re-*, again; *sublimatio*, from *sublimare*, to raise]. The process of subliming a drug for the second time.

re·sul'tant. That which results; specifically, any product of a chemical reaction.

re·su'pi·nate [*re-;* L. *supinare*, to bend backward]. Turned in a direction opposite to normal.

res"ur·rec'tion·ist [L. *resurrectio*, from *resurgere*, to raise oneself again]. One who steals dead bodies from the grave as subjects for dissection. *Obs.*

re·sus"ci·ta'tion [L. *resuscitatio*, from *resuscitare*, to revive]. The prevention of asphyxial death by artificial respiration. —**resus'citate,** *v.*

Drinker-Collins r. The use of a negative pressure cabinet where respiration is to be maintained over a long period.

Flagg r. The use of controlled suction and insufflation through a laryngoscope; using the Flagg machine.

re·sus"ci·ta'tion cage. An electrically heated metal cage or cradle which covers at least three-quarters of the patient; used in surgical shock.

re·sus'ci·ta"tor [L., from *resuscitare*]. A device for forcing oxygen or oxygen-carbon dioxide mixtures into the lungs for resuscitation.

re·su'ture (ree·sue'chur) [L. *re-*, again; *sutura*, suture]. Secondary suture; suture of a wound some time after a first suture has been made.

resyl. Trade name for a syrup containing guaiacol glyceryl ester.

re·tain'er [L. *retinere*, to hold back]. A dental appliance for holding in position teeth which have been moved.

re·tard'er. A negative catalyst, i.e., one acting to retard a reaction.

retch [AS. *reccan*]. Strain, as in vomiting. —**retch'-ing,** *n.*

re'te (ree'tee) (pl. *retia*) [L., net]. Any network or decussation and interlacing, especially of capillary blood vessels.

dorsal carpal r. An arterial network on the back of the wrist formed by branches of the dorsal interosseous and the volar interosseous arteries and terminal branches of the ulnar and radial arteries.

r. articulare genus. One formed by the anastomosis of the arteries over the anterior and lateral surfaces of the knee. See Plate 7.

r. calcaneum. An arterial anastomosis over the calcaneus.

r. cutaneum. The network of vessels at the boundary between corium and superficial fascia.

r. dorsale pedis. An arterial network on the dorsum of the foot, formed by branches of the tarsal and metatarsal arteries joined by perforating plantar branches.

r. mirabile. A capillary plexus intercalated in the path of an artery.

r. mucosum. Old term for the germinative layer of the epidermis.

r. olecrani. The network of vessels around the olecranon and at the back of the elbow, formed by the divisions of the profunda brachii and other arteries.

r. ovarii. Vestigial tubules or cords of cells near the hilus of the ovary, corresponding with the rete testis, but not connected with the mesonephric duct.

r. patellae. Plexus of vessels surrounding patella.

r. peg. Prolongation of the epidermis between the papillae of the corium; interpapillary epithelium.

r. subpapillare. The network of vessels between the papillary and reticular layers of the corium.

r. testis. The network of anastomosing tubules in the mediastinum testis.

re'tene, ret'ene. $C_{18}H_{18}$. 1-Methyl-7-isopropylphenanthrene. Occurs in the higher boiling fractions of wood tar.

re·ten'tion [L. *retentio*, from *retinere*, to hold back]. 1. The act of retaining or holding back, as the holding of urine in the bladder due to some hindrance to urination. 2. *In dentistry,* holding moved teeth in their new positions until stability of their investing tissues is established.

nitrogen r. Azotemia.

re·tic'u·la. Plural of reticulum.

re·tic'u·lar [L. *reticulum*, little net]. Resembling a net; formed by a network, as reticular tissue.

re·tic'u·la"ted [L. *reticulatus*, made like a net]. Having netlike meshes or formed like a web. —**reticula'tion,** *n.*

re·tic'u·lin [L. *reticulum*, little net]. A protein isolated from the fibers of reticular tissue.

re·tic'u·lo·cyte" [*reticulum;* G. *kytos*, cell]. 1. An immature or young erythrocyte containing ribonucleoprotein demonstrable on supravital staining, usually with brilliant cresyl blue, as a granular or filamentous network. It is larger than a normal erythrocyte and usually constitutes less than 1% (range: 0.5–2.5%) of the total. There is an increase during active erythrocytopoiesis. In Wright-Giemsa stained blood films these cells appear as polychromatophilic erythrocytes. Also called *reticulated erythrocyte, proerythrocyte, pronormocyte, granule cell, granulophil, skein cells.* 2. A cell of reticular tissue. Syn., *reticular cell.*

re·tic"u·lo·cy"to·pe'ni·a [*reticulum; kytos;* G. *penia*, poverty]. Decrease of reticulocytes in the circulating blood.

re·tic"u·lo·cy·to'sis (ri·tick"yoo·lo·sigh·to'sis) [*reticulum; kytos;* G. *-ōsis*, condition]. Condition in which reticulocytes are present in excess in the peripheral blood.

re·tic"u·lo·en"do·the'li·al [*reticulum;* G. *endon*, within; *thēlē*, nipple]. Pertaining to cells which are grouped under the reticuloendothelial system.

re·tic"u·lo·en"do·the"li·o'ma. See reticulum-cell *sarcoma.*

re·tic"u·lo·en"do·the"li·o'sis [*reticulum; endon; thēlē;* G. *-ōsis*, condition]. A disease of the reticuloendothelial system characterized by an extensive, irreversible, and systematized proliferation of histiocytes. Diagnosis rests on biopsy of involved organs (liver, spleen, and bone marrow), but the blood picture does not show the atypical cells until late or fulminating stages, when the condition is called *Schilling type of monocytic leukemia.* Clinically the manifestations are protean, but in general either visceral or cutaneous involvement predominates. A form seen in infancy and early childhood is called *Letterer-Siwe disease.* Syn., *malignant r., histiocytic, histiomonocytic,* or *malignant reticulosis.*

nonlipid r. See Letterer-Siwe *disease.*

reticulogen. Trade-mark for a brand of purified liver extract.

re·tic"u·lo·pe'ni·a. See *reticulocytopenia.*

re·tic"u·lo·sar·co'ma. See reticulum-cell *sarcoma.*

re·tic"u·lo'sis. Reticuloendotheliosis.

lipomelanotic r. A form of lymph-node hyperplasia characterized by preservation of the architectural structure, inflammatory exudate, and hyperplasia of the reticulum cells which show phagocytosis of hemosiderin, melanin, and occasionally fat. It is often secondary to an extensive dermatitis. Syn., *lipomelanotic reticular hyperplasia, dermatopathic lymphadenitis.*

re·tic"u·lo·the"li·o'ma. See *retothelioma.*

re·tic'u·lum (pl. *reticula*) [L.]. 1. A fine network. 2. *In veterinary medicine,* the second division of the ruminant stomach. —**reticulose,** *adj.*

nuclear r. The network of linin and chromatin of a nucleus.

stellate r. That portion of the pulp of the enamel organ in which the cells form a network with large, fluid-filled spaces between them.

re'ti·fism. A sexual perversion in which a shoe or foot possesses the same value as the genital organs.

re'ti·form, ret'i·form [L. *rete,* net; *forma,* form]. Net-shaped; reticular.

ret'i·na [*rete*]. The light-receptive layer and terminal expansion of the optic nerve in the eye. It extends from the point of exit of the nerve forward to the ora serrata. It consists of the following layers, named from behind forward: the pigment layer; the neuroepithelial layer, comprising the layer of rods and cones (bacillary layer), the outer limiting membrane, and the outer nuclear layer; the outer reticular layer (outer granular layer), the inner nuclear layer, the inner reticular layer (inner granular layer), the ganglionic layer, the nerve fiber layer. These layers are united and supported by neuroglial elements, most prominent of which are the radial fibers of Müller. See Plate 19. —**retinal,** *adj.*

coarctate r. The condition caused by an effusion of liquid between the retina and the choroid; it gives the retina a funnel shape.

cortical r. The projection of retinal points upon the striate area, the visual center in the cerebral cortex. Of particular interest is the large cortical area representing the macula compared with the small part representing the periphery. This area is at the calcarine fissure.

detachment of r. Separation of the retina from the choroid.

shot silk r. A retina with the appearance of changeable, glistening reflections; seen sometimes in young persons.

tigroid r. The spotted retina of retinitis pigmentosa.

ret"i·nac'u·lum (pl. *retinacula*) [L., that which holds back]. A special fascial thickening which holds back an organ or part. Also called *r. tendineum.*

extensor r. A thickening of deep fascia on the dorsum of the wrist and forearm attached to the radius laterally and the ulna, carpus, and medial ligament of the wrist medially. It overlies the compartments which transmit the extensor tendons of the wrist and fingers.

flexor r. of the ankle. The fibrous band that stretches between the medial malleolus and medial tubercle of the calcaneus, binding down the tendons of the tibialis posterior, the flexor digitorum longus, and the flexor hallucis longus.

flexor r. of the wrist. A thickened band of deep fascia on the volar surface of the hand and forearm, attached laterally to the navicular and greater multangular bones and medially to the pisiform and hamate bones. It binds down the tendon of the flexor pollicis longus and the flexor tendons of the fingers. Also called *transverse carpal ligament.*

inferior extensor r. A thickened band of deep fascia which binds down the tendons as they enter the dorsum of the foot.

inferior peroneal r. The band of fascia in the ankle which by its attachment to the peroneal tubercle holds the tendons of the peroneus longus and peroneus brevis to the lateral surface of the calcaneus.

patellar r. Either of the tendinous expansions from the vastus muscles and fascia lata which pass from the patella to the condyles of the tibia. Depending upon the side to which they pass, they are called medial or lateral patellar retinacula. See Plate 2.

r. cutis. A fibrous band connecting the corium with the underlying fascial structure.

r. of the hip joint. Any one of three deep longitudinal bands of the articular capsule which reflect upward along the neck of the femur from the femoral attachment toward the articular margin.

superior extensor r. The broad fibrous band which stretches across the front of the leg between the distal parts of the tibia and fibula. It binds the tendons of the tibialis anterior and extensor muscles of the toe.

superior peroneal r. The retinaculum of the ankle which binds down the tendons of the peroneus longus and the peroneus brevis.

ret'i·nal cor"re·spond'ence. The relation in the two eyes of the retinal areas at which associated retinal images are formed.

abnormal r. c. A condition found in concomitant strabismus, in which the retinal image formed at the macula of the fixing eye is associated with the image formed at an extramacular area of the retina of the squinting eye. Also called *binocular false projection, retinal incongruity.*

normal r. c. The normal condition in which the retinal image formed at the macula of one eye is associated with that formed at the macula of the other eye.

ret'i·nal pur'ple. See *rhodopsin.*

ret'i·nene [L. *rete,* net]. A pigment of the rods of the retina; chemically, vitamin A aldehyde. Two forms are known, retinene$_1$ and retinene$_2$, corresponding to vitamin A_1 and vitamin A_2. On illumination with white light, rhodopsin (visual purple) is converted to retinene$_1$ and the protein opsin; the retinene$_1$ is then reduced to vitamin A_1. In the dark vitamin A_1 reacts with opsin to form retinene$_1$ and then rhodopsin. In freshwater vertebrates, retinene$_2$ undergoes similar reaction with porphyropsin.

ret'i·nene re·duc'tase. The enzyme responsible for the reduction of retinene to vitamin A; it may be identical with alcohol dehydrogenase.

ret"i·ni'tis [*rete;* G. *-itis,* inflammation]. Retinal inflammation.

arteriospastic r. A form due to persistent contraction of the retinal arteries, usually associated with nephritis.

central punctate r. That seen most often in the aged. A great number of striae or white spots are visible in the fundus.

choroidoretinitis. A form of retinitis with cellular infiltration, exudation, atrophy, and proliferation of the pigment epithelium in the choroid, between the choroid and retina, and in the retinal layers.

diabetic r. See under *retinopathy.*

diffuse r. See *r.* serosa.

leukemic r. A form characterized by pallor of the retinal vessels and optic disk, the boundary of the latter being indistinct. Hemorrhages appear at various points of the membrane, while numerous white patches and round bodies are visible about the disk in the retina.

purulent r. A form in which there are small circumscribed white spots near the papilla and in the macular region.

renal r. See vascular *retinopathy.*

r. albuminurica. See vascular *retinopathy.*

r. apoplectica. Retinal apoplexy.

r. circinata. Retinitis in which there is a wreath of white spots around the macula, a degeneration due to deep hemorrhages.

r. circumpapillaris. A form in which there is proliferation of the outer layers of the retina around the disk.

r. disciformis. A degeneration of the macula consisting of a slightly raised, irregularly pigmented, circular or oval lesion.

r. exudativa. The response of histiocytes and fixed tissues to any subretinal hemorrhage, resulting in the production of a pigmented fibrous nodule containing fat-laden histiocytes; it is not a specific disease: also called *Coats's disease.*

r. gravidarum. See vascular *retinopathy.*

r. hemorrhagica. A form in which there is swelling of the papilla and opaque infiltration of the surrounding retina; there are distended, dark, and tortuous veins, and the arteries are small; there are hemorrhages, linear or irregular and round.

r. nephritica. See vascular *retinopathy.*

r. nyctalopia. A diffused, streaked opacity of the retina and swelling of the disk, with central scotoma or color scotoma, and more or less marked amblyopia. It indicates retrobulbar neuritis.

r. paralytica. Retinitis caused by paralysis affecting the optic nerve.

r. pigmentosa. An affection involving all the layers of the retina, and consisting of a slowly progressing connective-tissue and pigment-cell proliferation of the entire membrane, with wasting of its nerve elements.

r. proliferans. A development of connective tissue with the formation of dense bluish-white masses within the retina, and extending into the vitreous body.

r. punctata albescens. See central punctate *r.*

r. serosa. A form characterized by an infiltration, most marked in the nerve fiber and ganglionic layer of the retina, creating opacity, edema, and hyperemia.

r. simplex. See *r.* serosa.

r. sympathetica. Retinitis of sympathetic origin, attended with retinal hyperemia, redness of the disk, engorgement of the veins, and great disturbance of vision.

septic r. See purulent *r.*

simple syphilitic r. A form of syphilitic retinitis in which the ophthalmoscope shows a gray opacity surrounding the papilla, which is discolored and cloudy, and the veins darker than normal.

solar r. Retinal change from the effect of sunlight.

syphilitic r. The form occurring in syphilis; it is chronic, diffuse, and a late manifestation of the systemic disease.

ret″i·no·blas·to′ma [*rete;* G. *blastos,* shoot; *-ōma,* tumor]. Neuroepithelioma of the retina.

ret″i·no·cho″roid·i′tis (ret″i·no·kor″oy·dye′tis) [*rete;* G. *chorioeidēs,* choroid; *-itis,* inflammation]. Inflammation of the retina and choroid.

r. juxtapapillaris. See under Edmund *Jensen.*

ret″i·no·cy·to′ma. Neuroepithelioma of the retina.

ret′i·nol [*rete*]. $C_{32}H_{16}$. A liquid hydrocarbon obtained in the destructive distillation of resin. It is used as a solvent and was formerly employed in gonorrhea.

ret″i·no·pap″il·li′tis [*rete;* L. *papilla,* nipple; G. *-itis,* inflammation]. Inflammation of the retina and the optic disk.

ret″i·nop′a·thy [*rete;* G. *pathos,* disease]. Any morbid condition of the retina.

diabetic r. Retinal manifestations of diabetes mellitus characterized by small punctate hemorrhages generally acknowledged to be associated with characteristic microaneurysms (capillary dilatations) and sharply defined punctate exudates, located in the external plexiform layer of the retina: formerly called *diabetic retinitis.*

hypertensive r. A vascular *r.*

vascular r. Retinal manifestations of such diseases as arterial hypertension, chronic nephritis, eclampsia, and advanced arteriosclerosis, characterized by various combinations and degrees of hemorrhages, exudates, vascular sclerosis, and sometimes by papilledema (malignant hypertension): formerly called *renal retinitis, retinitis albuminurica, r. gravidarum, r. nephritica.*

ret″i·nos′co·py [*rete;* G. *skopein,* to examine]. An objective method of determining the refraction of the eye by observation of the movements of the shadow phenomena produced and observed by means of an instrument called the retinoscope (also called the skiascope). The principle is that of conjugate foci, whereby the image-point is conjugate with the object-point. If rotation of the illuminated mirror of the retinoscope causes the shadow in the *illuminated* pupil to move "with" the retinoscope, the patient's retina is conjugate with a point beyond the instrument (the emergent rays are divergent) and the eye is hyperopic, and the dioptric strength of the lens selected to abolish motion of the shadow is the amount of the hyperopia. If the reflex moves "against" (opposite in direction to) the mirror, the conjugate focus is between the retinoscope and the patient's eye (the emergent rays are convergent) and the eye is myopic, and the dioptric strength of the lens selected to abolish motion of the shadow is the amount of the myopia. Also called *skiascopy.*

ret″i·no·ski·as′co·py (ret″i·no·sky·ass′ko·pee). Retinoscopy.

re·tir′ing board. In the Armed Forces of the United States (Army, Navy, and Air Force), a board of not less than five commissioned officers, of whom two are required to be medical officers. It is the function of the board to determine whether or not officers ordered before it for presumed physical or mental unfitness to perform duty shall be retired from the service for disability. The findings of a retiring board are practically binding under appropriate statutes. At the present writing, retiring boards are composed of Army, Navy, or Air Force officers for the particular department concerned.

re·tort′ [L. *retortum,* from *retorquere,* to twist back]. A distilling vessel consisting of an expanded globular portion and a long neck.

ret″o·the″li·o′ma. See reticulum-cell *sarcoma.*

ret″o·the″li·o·sar·co′ma. See reticulum-cell *sarcoma.*

re·tract′ [L. *retractum,* from *retrahere,* to draw back]. Draw back; contract; shorten.

re″trac·til′i·ty [*retrahere*]. The power of retracting or drawing back. —**retrac′tile,** *adj.*

re·trac′tion [L. *retractio,* from *retrahere*]. The act of retracting or drawing back, as a retraction of the muscles after amputation.

re·trac′tor [*retrahere*]. 1. A surgical instrument for holding back the edges of a wound to give access to deeper parts or regions. It consists ordinarily of a handle with a right-angle flange. 2. O.T. for *flexor.*

abdominal r. A large, heavy instrument, often with a curved flange, to give greater retractive power.

block tin r. A flexible instrument which can be bent to a desired shape.

nerve r. A delicate instrument adapted to isolating nerves during operations.

periosteal r. A toothed instrument for holding periosteum.

self-retaining r. A special instrument having two retractor arms clamped to a bar and adjusted by means of setscrews. Some are equipped with a third arm for retraction of the pubic portion of the urinary bladder during bladder and prostatic operations.

toothed r. A retractor having sharp or blunt teeth.

re·tra′hens au′rem (ri·tray′henz aw′rem, ret′-ruh·henz) [L.]. Old term for posterior auricular muscle.

ret′ro-, re′tro- [L., back]. A combining form meaning *back, backward,* or *behind.*

ret″ro·ac′tion [L. *retroactum,* from *retroagere,* to drive back]. Reverse action.

ret″ro·an″ter·o·am·ne′si·a (ret″ro·an″tur·o·am-nee′zhuh, ·zee·uh, ree″tro·). See retroanterograde *amnesia.*

ret″ro·an′ter·o·grade [L. *retro,* back; *anterior,* that is before; *gradi,* to go]. Reversing the usual order of a succession.

ret″ro·bul′bar [L. *retro,* behind; *bulbus,* bulb]. 1. Situated or occurring behind the eyeball. 2. Behind the medulla oblongata.

ret″ro·car′di·ac [*retro;* G. *kardia,* heart]. Posterior to the heart.

ret″ro·ce′cal [*retro;* L. *caecus,* blind]. Pertaining to the back of the cecum.

ret′ro·cele [*retro;* G. *kēlē,* tumor]. Persistence of the postanal part of the embryonic hindgut. Also called *congenital retrocele.*

ret″ro·chei′li·a. A condition in which a lip is farther posterior than is normal. Cf. *procheilia.*

ret″ro·col′ic [*retro;* G. *kolon,* colon]. Behind the colon.

ret″ro·col′lic [*retro;* L. *collum,* neck]. Pertaining to the muscles at the back of the neck.

ret″ro·col′lis. Torticollis.

ret″ro·con′dy·lism [*retro;* G. *kondylos,* knuckle]. Posterior deviation of the mandibular condyles.

ret″ro·cop″u·la′tion [*retro;* L. *copulatio,* from *copulare,* to unite]. The act of copulating from behind or aversely.

ret″ro·de″vi·a′tion [L. *retro,* back; *devius,* out of the way]. Any backward displacement; a retroflexion or retroversion.

ret″ro·dis·place′ment [*retro;* F. *déplacement,* displacement]. Backward displacement of a part or organ, especially uterine displacement. See *retroversion.*

ret″ro·e″so·phag′e·al (ret″ro·ee″so·fadj′ee·ul, ·fay′jee·ul, ree″tro·) [L. *retro,* behind; G. *oisophagos,* gullet]. Located behind the esophagus.

ret′ro·flex [L. *retroflexus,* from *retroflectere,* to bend back]. Turn back abruptly.

ret′ro·flexed″ [*retroflexus*]. Bent backward; in a permanent, backward malposition, as in retroflexion of the uterus.

ret″ro·flex′ion [*retroflexus*]. The state of being bent backward.

r. of the uterus. A condition in which the uterus is bent backward upon itself, producing a sharp angle in its axis.

ret″ro·gas·se′ri·an. Behind the semilunar or gasserian ganglion.

ret″ro·gnath′ism [*retro;* G. *gnathos,* jaw]. Posterior deviation of the mandible.

ret′ro·grade [L. *retrogradi,* to go backward]. Going backward; undoing.

re·trog′ra·phy [L. *retro,* back; G. *graphein,* to write]. Backward writing; mirror writing.

ret″ro·gres′sion [L. *retrogressus,* retrogression]. 1. *In biology,* the passing from a higher to a lower type of structure in the development of an animal. 2. *In medicine,* a going backward; degeneration, involution, or atrophy, as of tissue. 3. The subsidence of a disease or its symptoms.

ret″ro·jec′tion [*retro;* L. *iacere,* to throw]. The washing out of a cavity from within outward.

ret″ro·jec′tor, ret′ro·jec″tor [*retro; iacere*]. An instrument for washing out the uterus.

ret″ro·len′tal [*retro;* L. *lens,* lentil]. Behind the lens of the eye.

ret″ro·lin′gual [*retro;* L. *lingua,* tongue]. Relating to that part of the pharynx behind the tongue.

ret″ro·mor′pho·sis (ret″ro·mor′fo·sis, ·mor·fo′sis, ree″tro·) [*retro;* G. *morphōsis,* a shaping]. Catabolism; retrograde metamorphosis; catabolic change.

ret″ro·na′sal (ret″ro·nay′zul, ree″tro·) [L. *retro,* behind; *nasus,* nose]. Situated behind the nose or nasal cavities; postnasal.

ret″ro·per″i·to·ne′al [*retro;* G. *peritonaion,* membrane which contains the lower viscera]. Situated behind the peritoneum.

ret″ro·per″i·to·ni′tis [*retro; peritonaion;* G. *-itis,* inflammation]. Inflammation of the retroperitoneal structures.

ret″ro·pha·ryn′ge·al (·fa·rin′jul, ·jee·ul, ·far″in-jee′ul) [*retro;* G. *pharygx,* pharynx]. Situated behind the pharynx, as retropharyngeal abscess.

ret″ro·phar″yn·gi′tis [*retro; pharygx;* G. *-itis,* inflammation]. Inflammation of the retropharyngeal tissues.

ret″ro·phar′ynx [*retro; pharygx*]. The posterior portion of the pharynx.

ret″ro·pla·cen′tal [*retro;* L. *placenta,* cake]. Behind the placenta.

ret″ro·pla′si·a (ret″ro·play′zhuh, ·zee·uh, ree″tro·) [L. *retro,* back; G. *plassein,* to form]. Retrograde change in a tissue; degeneration.

ret′ro·posed (ret′ro·pozed, ree′tro·) [*retro;* OF. *poser,* to place]. Displaced backward.

ret″ro·po·si′tion [*retro;* L. *positio,* from *ponere,* to place]. Backward displacement of the uterus without flexion or version.

ret″ro·pul′sion [*retro;* L. *pulsio,* from *pellere,* to drive]. 1. A driving or turning back, as of the fetal head. 2. A running backward; a form of walking sometimes seen in parkinsonism.

ret″ro·stal′sis [*retro;* G. *stalsis,* checking]. Reversed peristalsis; peristaltic action that tends to drive the intestinal contents cephalad instead of caudad.

ret″ro·tar′sal [L. *retro,* behind; G. *tarsos,* edge of the eyelid]. Situated behind the tarsus, as the retrotarsal fold of the conjunctiva.

ret″ro·tra′che·al (ret″ro·tray′kee·ul, ·tra·kee′ul, ree″tro·) [*retro;* G. *trachys,* rough]. Situated or occurring behind the trachea.

ret″ro·vac″ci·na′tion [L. *retro,* back; *vaccinus,* of cows]. Vaccination with virus from a cow that has been inoculated with the virus of smallpox from a human subject.

ret″ro·ver″si·o·flex′ion (·vur″sho·fleck′shun, ·vur″see·o·fleck′shun) [*retro;* L. *versum,* from *vertere,* to turn; *flexio,* from *flectere,* to bend]. Combined retroversion and retroflexion.

ret″ro·ver′sion [*retro; vertere*]. A turning back.

r. of uterus. A condition in which the uterus is tilted backward without curvature of its axis.

ret″ro·vert′ed [*retro; vertere*]. Tilted or turned backward, as a retroverted uterus.

re·trude′ [L. *retrudere,* to thrust back]. Force inward or backward, as to correct protruding teeth.

re·tru′sion [L. *retrusum,* from *retrudere*]. 1. *In dentistry,* the act or process of pressing teeth backward. 2. That condition which is characterized by backward or retroposed teeth, particularly the anterior teeth.

Retterer's stain. See under *stain.*

Retzius, Anders Adolf [*Swedish anatomist,* 1796–1860]. Universally known for his description of the prevesical space, also called *space of Retzius.* Described the veins forming anastomoses with the mesenteric veins and the inferior vena cava, called *Retzius' veins, retroperitoneal veins.* See also *gyri Andreae Retzii* under *gyrus.*

Retzius, Magnus Gustaf [*Swedish histologist,* 1842–1919]. Described brownish concentric lines in tooth enamel (1837); the *lines of Retzius* are thought to indicate the contour of the enamel at different stages of its development. With E. A. H. Key, described sensory nerve endings, resembling Herbst's corpuscles, seen in the skin of the beaks of certain birds; called *corpuscles of Key and Retzius.* With Key, described the lateral apertures of the fourth ventricle; called *foramens of Key and Retzius, foramens of Luschka.* See under *aperture.*

re·un′ion [L. *re-,* again; *unire,* to unite]. In fractures, the securing of union following its interruption by violence or disease.

Reuss, August Ritter von [*Austrian ophthalmologist,* 1841–1924]. Introduced charts for testing color vision; *Reuss's color tables* consist of colored letters on colored backgrounds.

Reuss test. A test for atropine in which the substance to be tested is heated with sulfuric acid and an oxidizing agent. In the presence of atropine an odor of roses and orange flowers is given off.

re″vac·ci·na′tion [L. *re-,* again; *vaccinus,* of cows]. Renewed or repeated vaccination.

re·vel′lent. See *revulsive.*

re·ver″ber·a′tion [L. *reverberare,* to strike back]. A repetitive discharge of impulses due to the development of transient automaticity of ventral horn cells. The impulses pass in circuits from cell to cell.

Reverdin, Albert [*Swiss surgeon,* 1881–1929]. Son of J. L. Reverdin. Originator of the carrier or aneurysm needle with an eye near the point; *Reverdin's needle* is mounted on a handle and opened and closed by means of a lever.

Reverdin, Jacques Louis [*Swiss surgeon,* 1842–1908]. Widely known for his extensive work in skin grafting. Originated the method of free grafting by means of small points of skin transferred to a clean, granulating surface. These become the starting points of new skin areas; known as *Reverdin's method.* Made studies of myxedema, producing the disease by removal of the thyroid gland (1882).

rev′er·ie [F.]. A state of dreamy abstraction; visionary mental or ideational movement, the mind itself, at least so far as volition is concerned, being passive.

re·ver′sal [L. *reversum,* from *reverti,* to turn back]. 1. *In psychoanalysis,* the change from a love instinct to one of hate; a change of the content of an instinct. 2. The change of the aim of an instinct into its opposite, as from sadism into masochism.

re·verse′ [*reversum*]. In bandaging, a half-turn employed to change the direction of a bandage.

re·ver′sion (ri·vur′shun, ·zhun) [L. *reversio,* from *reverti,* to turn back]. The reappearance of long-lost ancestral traits; a throwback.

Revilliod, Léon [*Swiss physician,* 1835–1919]. Described a sign indicative of facial nerve paralysis, consisting of inability of the person affected to close the eye on the paralyzed side alone; called *Revilliod's sign.*

re″vi·tal·i·za′tion (ree″vye·tul·i·zay′shun, ·eye-zay′shun, ree·vye″tul·) [L. *re-,* again; *vitalis,* from *vita,* life]. The act or process of refreshing.

re·vive′ [L. *revivere,* to live again]. Return to life after seeming death; return to consciousness or strength.

re·viv″i·fi·ca′tion [*revivere;* L. *facere,* to make]. Restoration of life after apparent death.

rev′o·lute [L. *revolutum,* from *revolvere,* to roll back]. Turned backward or downward.

re·vul′sant [L. *revulsum,* from *revellere,* to tear away]. Revulsive.

re·vul′sant. A medicine or agent that, by irritation, draws the blood from a distant part of the body.

re·vul′sive [*revellere*]. Causing revulsion.

re·vul′sive. An agent that causes revulsion.

Reynals. See *Duran-Reynals.*

R. F. A. Right frontoanterior position of the fetus.

R. F. P. Right frontoposterior position of the fetus.

Rh Chemical symbol for rhodium.

Rh Pertaining to or denoting an agglutinogen first found in the red blood cells of the *rh*esus monkey by K. Landsteiner and A. Wiener (1937). See *blood groups, Rh factors, Rh genes, Rh sensitization, Rh testing, Rh typing.*

Rhab·di′tis [G. *rhabdos,* rod; *-itis,* inflammation]. A genus of nematode worms a few species of which are parasitic in man but of doubtful pathogenicity.

Rhab″di·toi′de·a [*rhabdos; -itis;* G. *eidos,* form]. The name given a superfamily of the Nematoda, of which *Strongyloides stercoralis* is the most important species which infests man.

rhab′do·cyte. See band *cell.*

rhab′doid [*rhabdos;* G. *eidos,* form]. Rodlike.

rhab″do·my·o·blas·to′ma. Rhabdomyosarcoma.

embryonal r. 1. A granular-cell myoblastoma. 2. A malignant mesenchymoma.

rhab″do·my·o′ma (rab″do·migh·o′muh) [*rhabdos;* G. *mys,* muscle; *-ōma,* tumor]. A rare tumor of striated muscle, considered by some authorities to be benign, but usually classified as malignant: also called *myoma striocellulare.* See *rhabdomyosarcoma.*

congenital r. of the heart. A developmental anomaly, and not a tumor. Myocardial lesions show characteristic large vacuolated cells containing glycogen and often showing radial or transverse striation of their peripheral cytoplasm. It is often accompanied by other congenital abnormalities.

embryonal r. A mesenchymoma.

r. uteri. A malignant polypoid tumor of the vagina in children, and of the cervix in adults. A mesodermal mixed tumor in which the striated muscle may represent metaplasia of connective-tissue cells. Also called *sarcoma botryoides.*

rhab″do·my″o·sar·co′ma [*rhabdos; mys;* G. *sarkōma,* fleshy excrescence]. A rare malignant tumor of skeletal muscle, usually involving the muscles of the extremities or torso, microscopically composed of myoblasts which may vary greatly in appearance and differentiation. Occasionally transverse striations may be seen in their cytoplasm. Also called *malignant rhabdomyoma, rhabdomyoblastoma.*

embryonal r. A malignant mesenchymoma.

Rhab″do·ne′ma [*rhabdos;* G. *nēma,* thread]. A genus of parasitic roundworms.

rhab″do·pho′bi·a [*rhabdos;* G. *phobos,* fear]. A morbid dread of being beaten; unreasoning fear aroused by the sight of a stick.

rha′chi·o- (ray′kee·o-), **rha′chi-.** See *rachio-.*

rha′cous [G. *rhakos,* tattered]. Wrinkled; lacerated; fissured.

rhag′a·des (rag′uh·deez) [G. *rhagas,* fissure]. Linear cracks or fissures occurring in skin that has lost its elasticity through infiltration and thickening:

observed in syphilis, intertrigo, keratoderma, and other affections.

rha·ga′di·a. See *rhagades.*

rha·gad′i·form [*rhagas;* L. *forma,* shape]. Fissured.

-rha′gi·a. See *-rrhagia.*

rhag′i·o·crin, rhag′i·o·crine (radj′ee·o·krin) [G. *rhagion,* dim. of *rhax,* grape; *krinein,* to separate]. A term applied to colloid-filled vacuoles in the cytoplasm of secretory cells representing a stage in the development of secretory granules.

r. cell. See *histiocyte.*

rhag′oid [*rhax;* G. *eidos,* form]. Resembling a grape.

rham′ne·gin. A glycoside, $C_{34}H_{42}O_{20}$, found in buckthorn berries. Also called *rhamnoxanthin, xanthorhamnin.*

rham′ne·tin. $C_{16}H_{12}O_7$; 3,3′,4′,5-tetrahydroxy-7-methoxyflavone or 7-methylquercetin, the aglycone of xanthorhamnin; a yellow, crystalline powder, slightly soluble in hot water: has been used as a dye.

rham′ni·nose. A reducing trisaccharide obtained by hydrolysis of xanthorhamnin; hydrolysis of rhamninose yields one molecule of galactose and two molecules of rhamnose.

rham′ni·tol. $CH_3(CHOH)_4CH_2OH$. An alcohol resulting from the reduction of the sugar rhamnose. See *inositol.*

rham″no·ca·thar′tin. A glycoside, $C_{27}H_{30}O_{14}$.-$\frac{1}{2}H_2O$, found in buckthorn berries.

rham″no·ga·lac′to·side. A glycoside, such as xanthorhamnin, which yields the sugars rhamnose and galactose on hydrolysis.

rham″no·glu′co·side. A glycoside, such as rutin, which yields the sugars rhamnose and D-glucose on hydrolysis.

rham′nose (ram′nose). CHO.HCOH.HCOH.HO-CH.HOCH.CH_3; L-rhamnose, or 6-desoxy-L-mannose; a desoxysugar occurring free in poison sumac and in glycoside combination in many plants. It occurs in α- and β-forms. Syn., *iso-dulcitol.*

rham′no·side. A glycoside, such as quercetin, which yields the sugar rhamnose on hydrolysis.

rham″no·xan′thin. See *frangulin.*

Rham′nus [L., from G. *rhamnos,* a prickly shrub]. A genus of trees and shrubs which yield cascara (**R. purshiana**), buckthorn bark (**R. frangula**), and buckthorn berries (**R. cathartica**).

rhan′ter. The inner canthus.

rha·pha′ni·a. See *raphania.*

rha·phid′i·o·spore. Sporozoite.

rha·pon′tic [NL. *rhaponticum,* rhubarb]. Pertaining to rhubarb.

rhat′a·ny. See *krameria.*

Rhazes (Abū Bakr Muhammad ibn Zakariyā al-Rāzi) [*Arabian medical writer,* 850–923]. Said to be the first to distinguish measles from smallpox. One of the earliest writers on nervous diseases. Introduced the use of mercurial ointment. His *Opuscula* is one of the earliest printed medical books.

rhe The unit of fluidity, being the reciprocal of the centipoise or one-hundredth of a poise.

rhe′a·dine (ree′uh·deen, ·din). $C_{21}H_{21}NO_6$. An alkaloid from opium.

rhe″bo·cra′ni·a. Torticollis. *Obs.*

rhe″bo·sce′li·a (ree″bo·see′lee·uh) [G. *rhaibos,* crooked; *skelos,* leg]. The condition of being bow-legged. —**rhe″bo·sce′lic,** *adj.*

rheg′ma [G., breakage]. A rupture of the walls of a vessel or of the containing membrane of an organ or region, as the coats of the eye, the walls of the peritoneum. Also, the bursting of an abscess. *Rare.*

rhe′in. A dihydroxyanthraquinone-carboxylic acid, $C_{15}H_8O_6$, present in senna leaves and rhubarb. It has been stated to lack purgative action.

rhem·bas′mus (rem·baz′mus) [G. *rhembasmos,* a roaming about]. Mental distraction; indecision.

rhe′ni·um [L. *Rhenus,* the Rhine]. Re = 186.31. An element of the manganese group; occurs as a minor constituent in many ores.

rhe′o- [G. *rheos,* anything flowing]. A combining form denoting *pertaining to a current.*

rhe′o·base [*rheos;* G. *basis,* base]. The minimum electric potential necessary for stimulation.

rhe″o·car″di·og′ra·phy. The recording of differences in electrical conductivity of the body synchronous with the cardiac cycle. The patient is connected so that he forms one arm of a Wheatstone bridge. Variations in voltage due to alterations in conductivity are amplified after rectification and recorded by an electrocardiograph.

rhe′o·cord [*rheos;* G. *chordē,* cord]. A rheostat.

rhe·ol′o·gy [G. *rheos,* flow; *logos,* study of]. The science of deformation and flow of matter in such a state that it exhibits a tendency to be deformed by the application of stress, e.g., the flow of blood through the heart and vessels or the deformation of the aorta during systole.

rhe·om′e·ter [*rheos;* G. *metron,* a measure]. 1. A galvanometer. 2. An apparatus for measuring the velocity of the blood current.

rhe′o·nome [*rheos;* G. *nomos,* law]. An instrument for the application to excitable tissues of electric currents of different intensity.

rhe′o·pex″y [*rheos;* G. *pēxis,* a fixing]. A special kind of thixotropy consisting of internal-phase particles of a laminar or fibrillar shape, the gelation being greatly hastened by slow but pronounced elliptical stirring.

rhe′o·phore [*rheos;* G. *phoros,* bearing]. An electrode.

rhe′o·scope [*rheos;* G. *skopein,* to examine]. An instrument for demonstrating the existence of an electric current.

rhe′o·stat [*rheos;* G. *statos,* standing]. An instrument introduced into an electric circuit and offering a known resistance, for the purpose of altering the intensity of the current.

rhe″os·to′sis. See *osteopetrosis.*

rhe″o·ta·chyg′ra·phy (ree″o·ta·kig′ruh·fee) [*rheos;* G. *tachys,* swift; *graphein,* to write]. The registration of the curve of variation in electromotive action of muscles.

rhe″o·tax′is [*rheos;* G. *taxis,* arrangement]. The reaction of a body to mechanical stimulation by a current of fluid, whereby that body is induced to move either with or against the current of the fluid.

rhe′o·tome [*rheos;* G. *tomos,* cutting]. An instrument used for breaking and making a galvanic circuit.

differential r. One for indicating the negative variation in muscle currents.

rhe′o·trope [*rheos;* G. *trepein,* to turn]. An apparatus for reversing the direction of an electric current. Also called *commutator.*

rhe·ot′ro·pism. Rheotaxis.

rhe′um. See *rhubarb.*

rheu·mat′ic [G. *rheumatikos,* subject to a flux]. Pertaining to, of the nature of, or affected with, rheumatism.

rheu·mat′ic fe′ver. An acute or chronic inflammatory process initiated by a preceding Group A hemolytic streptococcic infection. The inflammation is disseminated in the connective tissues of many organs and, when pronounced, is manifested by myocarditis, valvulitis, arthritis, serositis, subcutaneous nodules, or rashes, and by generalized and nonspecific manifestations such as fever and elevated erythrocyte sedimentation rate (ESR). It occurs most commonly in childhood and tends to multiple recurrences. Formerly called *Bouillaud's syndrome.*

rheu′ma·tism [G. *rheumatismos*, that which flows]. 1. A general term indicating diseases of muscle, tendon, joint, bone, or nerve, resulting in discomfort and disability. It is often used to include rheumatoid arthritis, degenerative joint disease, spondylitis, bursitis, fibrositis, myositis, neuritis, lumbago, sciatica, and gout. 2. Acute rheumatic fever.

acute articular r. Acute rheumatic fever.

acute r. Acute rheumatic fever.

Bougainville r. See epidemic tropical acute *polyarthritis.*

chronic r. Chronic form of any of the above-mentioned types, but usually one of those leading to joint deformity such as rheumatoid arthritis, degenerative joint disease, or chronic gout.

gonorrheal r. Arthritis due to the gonococcus.

nonarticular r. See *fibrositis* (b).

palindromic r. An acute arthritis and periarthritis occurring in multiple, afebrile, irregularly spaced attacks lasting only a few hours or days and disappearing completely. There are pain, swelling, redness, and disability of usually only one joint. It attacks adults of either sex. The cause is not known.

psychogenic r. Aches and pains, stiffness and soreness in different parts of the body without demonstrable organic change, arising as a result of psychic stimuli.

tuberculous r. Tuberculous arthritis.

rheu′ma·toid [G. *rheuma*, that which flows; *eidos*, form]. Resembling rheumatism.

rheu″ma·tol′o·gy. The study of rheumatism. —**rheumatolog′ic,** *adj.;* **rheumatol′ogist,** *n.*

rheu″mo·crin·ol′o·gy. A study of the endocrine aspects of rheumatic disease, particularly rheumatoid arthritis.

rhex′is [G., a breaking]. Rupture of a blood vessel or of an organ.

Rh fac′tors. Structures on the surface of the erythrocyte responsible for the reactions with animal or human anti-Rh serums. Of the three factors, Rh_0, rh′, and rh″, the Rh_0 factor, which corresponds to the original one discovered in the rhesus monkey, is the most potent antigen and its presence or absence in blood is referred to as *Rh positive* and *Rh negative.* Syn., *Rh agglutinogens* or *antigens.* Also see *blood groups.*

Rh genes. The series of allelic genes which determine the various sorts of Rh agglutinogens and Rh blood types. Eight standard genes have been identified (Wiener): Rh_0, Rh_1, Rh_2, Rh_1Rh_2 (Rh positive) and rh, rh′, rh″, rh′rh″ (Rh negative). See *blood groups.*

rhic·no′sis [G. *rhiknōsis*, a shriveling]. A wrinkling of the skin, the result of muscular or subdermal elastic tissue atrophy.

rhin-. See *rhino-.*

rhi′nal [G. *rhis*, nose]. Pertaining to the nose.

rhi·nal′gi·a (rye·nal′juh, ·jee·uh) [*rhis;* G. *algos*, pain]. Pain in the nose.

rhi″nan·tral′gi·a [*rhis;* G. *antron*, cave; *algos*]. Pain in, or referred to, the walls of the cavities of the nose.

rhi·nel′cos (rye·nel′koss) [*rhis;* G. *helkos*, ulcer]. A nasal ulcer.

rhi″nen·ceph′a·lon [*rhis;* G. *egkephalos*, brain]. That portion of the cerebrum concerned with reception and integration of olfactory impulses, and with regulation of appropriate motor activities in response to such impulses. It comprises the archipallium (hippocampal formation) and paleopallium (olfactory lobe and pyriform lobe). —**rhinencephal′ic,** *adj.*

rhi″nen·chy′sis (rye″neng·kigh′sis, rye·neng′ki-sis) [*rhis;* G. *egchysis*, a pouring in]. Douching of the nasal passages. *Obs.*

rhi″neu·ryn′ter [*rhis;* G. *eurynein*, to make broad]. A distensible bag or sac which is inflated after insertion into a nostril.

rhin·he″ma·to′ma (rin·hee″muh·to′muh, ·hem″-uh·to′muh) [*rhis;* G. *haima*, blood; *-ōma*, tumor]. An effusion of blood around the nasal cartilages.

rhi·ni′a·try (rye·nigh′uh·tree). See *rhinology.*

rhin′i·on [*rhis*]. The point at the distal end of the internasal suture.

rhi′nism, rhi·nis′mus (rye·niz′mus) [*rhis*]. A nasal quality of the voice.

rhi·ni′tis (rye·nigh′tis) [*rhis;* G. *-itis*, inflammation]. Inflammation of the nasal mucous membrane.

acute r. Coryza; cold in the head; the common cold.

allergic r. Rhinitis which may be caused by any allergen, but which is frequently called hay fever.

atrophic r. That followed by atrophy of the mucous membrane; it may also occur in swine: clinically, also called *ozena.*

chronic r. A form usually due to repeated attacks of acute rhinitis, and producing in the early stages hypertrophy of the mucous membrane (hypertrophic rhinitis) and in the later stages atrophy (atrophic rhinitis), and the presence of dark, offensive-smelling crusts (ozena).

fibrinous r. A rare form characterized by the development of a false membrane in the nose.

hypertrophic r. That marked by hypertrophy of the nasal mucous membrane.

perennial r. See allergic *r., hay fever.*

periodic r. Allergic rhinitis.

polypoid r. See nasal *polyp.*

pseudomembranous r. See fibrinous *r.*

r. sicca. See *ozena.*

syphilitic r. A chronic form due to syphilis, and usually attended by ulceration and caries of the bones and an offensive discharge (ozena).

tuberculous r. That due to the tubercle bacillus; it is usually associated with ulceration and caries of the bones.

vasomotor r. (a) Allergic rhinitis. (b) Hay fever. Also called *vasomotor catarrh, perennial r.*

rhi′no-, rhin- [*rhis*]. A combining form meaning *the nose.*

rhi″no·an·tri′tis [*rhis;* G. *antron*, cave; *-itis*, inflammation]. Inflammation of the nasal mucous membrane and of the maxillary sinus.

rhi″no·by′on (rye″no·buy′on, rye·no′bee·on) [*rhis;* G. *byein*, to plug with]. A nasal plug or tampon.

rhi″no·ce·pha′li·a. See *rhinocephaly.*

rhi″no·ceph′a·lus [*rhis;* G. *kephalē*, head]. A monster exhibiting rhinocephaly.

rhi″no·ceph′a·ly, rhi″no·ce·pha′li·a [*rhis; kephalē*]. A form of cyclopia in which the nose is a tubular proboscis situated above the fused orbits.

rhi″no·chei′lo·plas″ty (rye″no·kigh′lo·plas″tee) [*rhis;* G. *cheilos*, lip; *plassein*, to form]. Plastic surgery of the nose and upper lip.

rhi″no·clei′sis (rye″no·klye′sis) [*rhis;* G. *kleisis*, a closing]. Nasal obstruction.

rhi″noc·nes′mus (rye″nock·nez′mus) [*rhis;* G. *knēsmos*, itching]. Itching of the nose.

rhi″no·dac′ry·o·lith [*rhis;* G. *dakryon*, tear; *lithos*, stone]. A calculus in the nasolacrimal duct.

rhi″no·der′ma. See *keratosis* pilaris.

rhi″no·dym′i·a [*rhis;* G. *didymos*, twin]. A mild form of diprosopia in which, although there is doubling of the skeletal parts of both nose and upper jaw, the face appears only unusually wide with a broad space between the eyes and a thick, wide nose.

rhi·nod'y·mus (rye·nod'i·mus) [*rhis; didymos*]. An individual exhibiting rhinodymia.

rhi"no·dyn'i·a (rye"no·din'ee·uh, ·dye'nee·uh) [*rhis;* G. *odynē*, pain]. Any pain in the nose.

Rhi·noes'trus (rye·nes'trus) [*rhis;* G. *oistros*, gadfly]. A genus of flies of the Oestridae; species of this genus deposit hatched larvae in the nares, on the conjunctiva, and occasionally in the mouths of mammals. The species **R. purpureus,** the Russian gadfly, frequently invades the nasopharyngeal region of horses and cattle and occasionally causes human ophthalmomyiasis.

rhi·nog'e·nous (rye·nodj'i·nus) [*rhis;* G. *genesthai*, from *gignesthai*, to be produced]. Having its origin in the nose.

rhi"no·ky·pho'sis (rye"no·kigh·fo'sis) [*rhis;* G. *kyphōsis*, being humpbacked]. The condition of having a nose with a prominent bridge.

rhi"no·la'li·a [*rhis;* G. *lalia*, talk]. A nasal tone in the voice due to undue closure (**rhinolalia clausa**) or to undue patulousness (**rhinolalia aperta**) of the choanae.

rhi"no·lar"yn·gi'tis [*rhis;* G. *larygx*, larynx; *-itis*, inflammation]. Simultaneous inflammation of the mucosa of the nose and larynx.

rhi"no·lar"yn·gol'o·gy [*rhis; larygx;* G. *logos*, word]. The science of the anatomy, physiology, and pathology of the nose and larynx.

rhi'no·lite. See *rhinolith*.

rhi'no·lith [*rhis;* G. *lithos*, stone]. A nasal calculus.

rhi"no·li·thi'a·sis [*rhis;* G. *lithiasis*, disease of the stone]. The formation of nasal calculi.

rhi·nol'o·gist (rye·nol'o·jist) [*rhis;* G. *logos*, word]. A specialist in the treatment of diseases of the nose.

rhi·nol'o·gy (rye·nol'o·jee) [*rhis; logos*]. The science of the anatomy, functions, and diseases of the nose. —**rhinolog'ic,** *adj.*

rhi"no·ma·nom'e·ter [*rhis;* G. *manos*, rare; *metron*, a measure]. A manometer used for measuring the amount of nasal obstruction.

rhi·nom'e·ter (rye·nom'i·tur) [*rhis; metron*]. An instrument for measuring the nose.

rhi"no·mi·o'sis (rye"no·migh·o'sis) [*rhis;* G. *meiōsis*, diminution]. Operative shortening of the nose.

rhi"nom·mec'to·my [*rhis;* G. *omma*, eye; *ektomē*, excision]. Excision of the inner canthus of the eye.

rhi"no·my·co'sis (rye"no·migh·ko'sis) [*rhis;* G. *mykēs*, fungus; *-ōsis*, condition]. The presence of fungi in the mucous membrane and secretion of the nose.

rhi"no·ne·cro'sis [*rhis;* G. *nekrōsis*, mortification]. Necrosis of the nasal bones.

rhi·nop'a·thy (rye·nop'uth·ee) [*rhis;* G. *pathos*, disease]. Any disease of the nose.

rhi"no·pha·ryn'ge·al (rye"no·fa·rin'jul, ·jee·ul, ·far"in·jee'ul) [*rhis;* G. *pharygx*, pharynx]. Pertaining to the nose and pharynx, or to the nasopharynx.

rhi"no·phar"yn·gi'tis [*rhis; pharygx;* G. *-itis*, inflammation]. Inflammation of the nose and pharynx, or of the nasopharynx.

r. mutilans. See *gangosa*.

rhi"no·pha·ryn'go·lith [*rhis; pharygx;* G. *lithos*, stone]. A nasopharyngeal calculus.

rhi"no·phar'ynx [*rhis; pharygx*]. See *nasopharynx*.

rhi"no·pho'ni·a [*rhis;* G. *phōnē*, sound]. A nasal tone in the speaking voice.

rhi"no·phy'ma [*rhis;* G. *phyma*, tumor]. A form of acne rosacea of the nose characterized by a marked hypertrophy of the blood vessels, sebaceous glands, and connective tissue, producing a lobulated appearance of the end of the nose. May be markedly disfiguring. Also called *toper's nose, whisky nose.*

rhi'no·plas"ty [*rhis;* G. *plassein*, to form]. A plastic operation upon the nose. This may be accomplished in a variety of ways, such as the so-called Italian method of rotating bone and skin-lined pedicle flap from the forehead, by flaps from the cheeks, by the transplantation of costal cartilage, etc. —**rhinoplas'tic,** *adj.*

rhi"no·pol'yp, rhi"no·pol'y·pus [*rhis;* G. *polypous*, many-footed]. Polyp of the nose.

rhi·nop'si·a (rye·nop'see·uh) [*rhis;* G. *opsis*, vision]. Convergent strabismus.

rhi"nor·rha'gi·a [*rhis;* G. *rhēgnynai*, to burst forth]. Hemorrhage from the nose. Syn., *epistaxis*.

rhi·nor'rha·phy (rye·nor'uh·fee) [*rhis;* G. *rhaphē*, suture]. A plastic reduction in the size of the nose, in which redundant nasal tissue is removed by section, followed by approximation and suture of the wound edges.

rhi"nor·rhe'a [*rhis;* G. *rhoia*, flow]. 1. A mucous discharge from the nose. 2. Escape of cerebrospinal fluid through the nose.

rhi·nos'chi·sis (rye·nos'ki·sis) [*rhis;* G. *schisis*, a cleavage]. Congenital cleft nose.

rhi"no·scle·ro'ma [*rhis;* G. *sklērōma*, induration]. A new growth of almost stony hardness, affecting the anterior nares and adjacent parts. The disease commences in the skin of the nasal vestibule and about the nares, the lesions consisting of flat, isolated, or coalescent nodules.

rhi'no·scope [*rhis;* G. *skopein*, to examine]. An instrument for examining nasal cavities.

rhi·nos'co·py (rye·nos'ko·pee) [*rhis; skopein*]. Examination of the nasal cavities by means of the rhinoscope; that of the nares is termed **anterior rhinoscopy;** that of the choanae, **posterior rhinoscopy.** —**rhinoscop'ic,** *adj.*

rhi"no·si"nus·o·path'i·a [*rhis;* L. *sinus*, hollow; G. *pathos*, disease]. The diseases of the nose and paranasal sinuses.

rhi"no·spo·rid"i·o'sis [*rhis;* dim. from G. *spora*, seed; *-ōsis*, condition]. An infection caused by *Rhinosporidium seeberi*. The causative agent has not been cultured but, because of similar morphology in tissue, is thought to be a fungus.

Rhi"no·spo·rid'i·um [*rhis; spora*]. A pathogen to man not yet precisely classified but thought to be a fungus.

R. kinealyi. Synonym for *R. seeberi*.

R. seeberi. That species which is the causative agent of rhinosporidiosis.

rhi"no·ste·no'sis [*rhis;* G. *stenos*, narrow]. Permanent constriction of the nose or nasal cavity.

rhi'no·thrix [*rhis;* G. *thrix*, hair]. A hair growing in the nostril.

rhi·not'o·my (rye·not'o·mee) [*rhis;* G. *tomē*, a cutting]. Incision of the nose.

Rhi"pi·ceph'a·lus (rye"pi·sef'uh·lus, rip"i·) [G. *rhipis*, fan; *kephalē*, head]. A genus of ticks of the superfamily Ixodoidea. Many species act as vectors of such diseases as spotted fever, Q fever, and tularemia to man and lower animals.

R. sanguineus. The most common species incriminated in the transmission of disease.

rhip·tas'mus (rip·taz'mus). See *ballism*.

rhit"i·do'sis [G. *rhytidōsis*, a wrinkling]. See *rhytidosis*.

rhi·zag'ra (ri·zag'ruh, ·zay'gruh, rye·) [G. *rhiza*, root; *agra*, a seizing]. An obsolete instrument for extracting the roots of teeth.

rhi'zo-, rhiz- [*rhiza*]. A combining form meaning *root*.

rhi"zo·don'tro·py [*rhiza;* G. *odous*, tooth; *trepein*, to turn]. The pivoting of an artificial crown upon the root of a tooth.

rhi"zo·don'try·py [*rhiza; odous;* G. *trypē*, hole]. Surgical puncture of the root of a tooth.

Rhi″zo·gly′phus. A genus of mites causing coolie itch.

rhi′zoid [*rhica;* G. *eidos*, form]. 1. Slender, rootlike filaments, the organs of attachment in many cryptogams. 2. A bacterial plate culture of an irregular branched or rootlike character. —**rhi′-zoid,** *adj.*

rhi′zome (rye′zohm, rye·zohm′) [G. *rhizōma*, mass of roots of a tree]. An underground stem, or rootstock.

rhi″zo·mel′ic [G. *rhiza*, root; *melos*, limb]. Affecting or relating to the roots of the extremities; pertaining to the hip or shoulder joints.

rhi″zo·mor′phoid [*rhiza;* G. *morphoeidēs*, in form and proportion]. Having the form of a root.

rhi′zo·neure [*rhiza;* G. *neuron*, nerve]. One of the cells that form nerve roots.

rhi″zo·nych′i·a (rye″zo·nick′ee·uh), **rhi″zo-nych′i·um** (rye″zo·nick′ee·um) [*rhiza;* G. *onyx*, nail]. The root of a nail. *Obs.*

rhi′zo·pod [*rhiza;* G. *pous*, foot]. A member of the Rhizopoda, a division of Protozoa.

Rhi·zop′o·da (rye·zop′o·duh) [*rhiza; pous*]. A class of the Protozoa which includes those amebas, characterized by the possession of pseudopodia, which parasitize man.

rhi·zop′ter·in. $C_{15}H_{12}N_6O_4$; the formyl derivative (at the nitrogen atom of the *p*-aminobenzoic acid component) of pteroic acid. It appears to be a precursor in the biogenesis of folic acid or of compounds having folic acid activity, possibly by conversion to formylfolic acid through conjugation with glutamic acid. Syn., *formylpteroic acid.*

Rhi′zo·pus (rye′zo·pus, rye·zo′pus) [*rhiza; pous*]. A genus of the Phycomycetes whose species may act as common allergens and as laboratory contaminants.

R. nigricans. A species of fungus which causes rots of various fruits and is commonly found as a saprophyte on dung.

rhi·zot′o·my (rye·zot′o·mee) [*rhiza;* G. *tomē*, a cutting]. Surgical division of any root, as of a nerve or tooth: also called *radicotomy.*

anterior r. Surgical division of the anterior motor nerve roots within the dura.

posterior r. Surgical division of the posterior sensory roots of the spinal nerves within the dura.

Rh negative. See *Rh factors, blood groups.*

rho′dal·line (ro′duh·leen, ·lin, ro·dal′een, ·in). See *thiosinamine.*

rho′da·mine. Any of a group of red dyes of the xanthene type, closely related to fluorescein.

r. B $C_{28}H_{31}ClN_2O_3$; tetraethylrhodamine; a dye producing a bluish-red solution: used as a dye, also as a reagent for many metals.

rho′da·nate. A thiocyanate.

rho·dan′ic ac′id. See *rhodanine.*

rho′da·nine. $C_3H_3ONS_2$, an organic compound; rhodanic acid.

Rhode reaction. See Voisenet-Rhode *reaction.*

rho″de·o·re′tin. See *convolvulin.*

rho′de·ose. D-Fucose, 6-desoxy-D-galactose, a naturally occurring monosaccharide obtained from the glycosides convolvulin and jalapin.

rho′di·um [G. *rhodon*, rose]. Rh = 102.91. A rare metal of the platinum group.

Rhod′ni·us. A genus of bugs whose species are capable of transmitting *Trypanosoma cruzi.*

rho″do·ci′din. A violet antibiotic pigment produced by *Streptomyces phoenix;* it inhibits Gram-positive and Gram-negative bacteria.

rho″do·gen′e·sis [*rhodon;* G. *genesis*, production]. The regeneration of visual purple which has been bleached by light.

rho″do·my·ce′tin. An antibiotic substance elaborated by a red-pigmented mutant of *Streptomyces griseus;* a dark-red powder, red in acid solution, blue in alkaline solution. It appears to have no activity in vivo.

rho″do·my′cin. A red antibiotic substance obtained from cultures of *Streptomyces purpurascens.*

rho′do·phane [*rhodon;* G. *phainein*, to appear]. Red pigment in the retinal cones.

rho″do·phy·lax′is (ro″do·fi·lack′sis, ·figh·lack′sis) [*rhodon;* G. *phylaxis*, a watching]. The property possessed by the retinal epithelium of producing rhodogenesis. —**rhodophylac′tic,** *adj.*

rho′do·pin. $C_{40}H_{58}O$ or $C_{40}H_{56}O$; a red pigment from *Rhodovibrio* and *Thiocystis* bacteria.

rho·dop′sin [*rhodon;* G. *opsis*, vision]. Visual purple; a retinal substance the color of which is preserved by darkness, but bleached by daylight; it is contained in the retinal rods.

rho″do·vi″o·las′cin. $C_{42}H_{60}O_2$; a dark red carotenoid pigment from *Rhodovibrio* and *Thiocystis* bacteria.

rho″do·xan′thin. $C_{40}H_{50}O_2$; a deep-purple, carotenoid pigment widely distributed in nature, conveniently isolated from arils of the English yew *Taxus baccata.*

rhoe′a·dine (ree′uh·deen, ·din). $C_{21}H_{21}NO_6$. A crystallizable alkaloid obtained from *Papaver rhoeas* (corn poppy).

rhoeb·de′sis (reb·dee′sis) [G. *rhoibdēsis*, a whistling, piping, from *rhoibdein*, to move with a rustling sound, to suck down]. Absorption, resorption. *Obs.*

rhom″ben·ceph′a·lon [G. *rhombos*, magic wheel; *egkephalos*, brain]. The caudalmost of the three primary brain vesicles of the embryo; it divides into myelencephalon and metencephalon. Syn., *hindbrain.*

rhom′bo·coele. Cavity of the rhombencephalon.

rhom′boid [*rhombos;* G. *eidos*, form]. Having a shape similar to that of a rhomb, a quadrilateral figure with opposite sides equal and parallel and oblique angles; said of the rhomboid ligament and rhomboid muscle.

rhom·boi′de·us [*rhombos; eidos*]. Either of the rhomboid muscles, arising from the spines of the lower cervical and upper thoracic vertebrae, and inserted on the vertebral margin of the scapula. See Table of Muscles in the Appendix.

r. occipitalis. A variant of the rhomboideus minor muscle extending from the occipital bone to the scapula.

rhom′bo·mere″ [*rhombos;* G. *meros*, part]. A neuromere of the rhombencephalon. *Obs.*

rhon′chus (rong′kus) (pl. *rhonchi*) [G. *rhogchos*, wheezing]. A coarse, snoring type of rale, caused by secretions in the larger bronchi or in the trachea, sometimes palpable, as fremitus. —**rhon-chial, rhonchal,** *adj.*

rho′ta·cism [G. *rhōtakizein*, to make overmuch or wrong use of the letter rho]. Mispronunciation, or overuse, of the letter r.

Rh pos′i·tive. See *Rh factors, blood groups.*

Rh sen″si·ti·za′tion. The act of becoming sensitive to the D (Rh_0) antigen specifically, and generally, also to C (rh′) and E (rh″) antigens.

Rh test′ing. Examination of blood for the main Rh factor, using either anti-Rhesus serum or anti-Rh_0 serum alone.

Rh typ′ing. Classification of individuals within one of the eight Rh types with the aid of anti-Rh_0, anti-Rh′, and anti-Rh″ serums.

rhu′barb [ML. *rhabarbarum*, barbarian rhubarb, from G. *rha*, rhubarb] (*rheum*). The dried rhizome and roots of *Rheum officinale, R. palmatum*, or other species growing in China and Tibet, deprived of periderm tissue. It owes its purgative properties to certain derivatives of anthraquinone. Dose, laxative and stomachic, 0.3–0.6 Gm. (5–10 gr.); purgative, 1.3–2.0 Gm. (20–30 gr.).

aromatic r. syrup (*syrupus rhei aromaticus*). One prepared from rhubarb, cinnamon, clove, and myristic. Dose, 4–12 cc. (1–3 fluidrachms).

aromatic r. tincture (*tinctura rhei aromatica*). Dose, 2–4 cc. (½–1 fluidrachm).

compound r. powder (*pulvis rhei compositus*). A laxative antacid composed of rhubarb, magnesium oxide, and ginger. Dose, child, 0.3–0.6 Gm. (5–10 gr.); adult, 2–4 Gm. (½–1 dr.). Also called *Gregory's powder*.

r. and soda mixture (*mistura rhei et sodae*). Prepared from rhubarb fluidextract, ipecac fluidextract, sodium bicarbonate, peppermint spirit, and water. A mild laxative used especially for infantile colic. Dose, infants, 2–4 cc. (½–1 fluidrachm).

torrefied r. Rhubarb which has had its purgative powers diminished by roasting; its astringency is not so affected.

rhulitol. A proprietary liquid containing chiefly tannic acid for use in the relief of local symptoms of poison ivy dermatitis.

Rhus [G. *rhous*, sumac]. Sumac, a genus of shrubs or small trees of the Anacardiaceae. Poison ivy, poison oak, and poison sumac were formerly classified under this genus. See *Toxicodendron*.

R. toxicodendron. Old name for poison ivy.

rhyn·choph'yl·line, rhyn"cho·phyl'line. $C_{19}H_{22}N_2O(OCH_3)(OCOCH_3)$; an alkaloid obtained from various *Mitragyna* and *Ourouparia* species, including *O. rynchophylla* (*Nauclea rynchophylla*). It lowers blood pressure and paralyzes sympathetic nerve endings.

rhy·poph'a·gy (rye·pof'uh·jee) [G. *rhypos*, filth; *phagein*, to eat]. The eating of filth or excrement.

rhy"po·pho'bi·a [*rhypos;* G. *phobos*, fear]. A morbid dread of filth.

rhy·se'ma (rye·see'muh) [G., wrinkle]. A wrinkle or corrugation.

-rhy'sis [G., a flow]. A combining form meaning *flowing out*.

rhythm [G. *rhythmos*, any regular recurring motion]. 1. Action recurring at regular intervals. 2. A method of contraception, in which continence is practiced during the ovulatory phase of the menstrual cycle.

alpha r. *In electroencephalography*, the dominant rhythm from the adult cortex. The oscillations are smooth, regular, and occur at a rate of 8–12 per second; they are best obtained from the occipital region with the subject at rest. The discharges tend to disappear when the subject concentrates. Syn., *Berger r.*, *Berger wave, alpha wave.*

atrial r. The heart rhythm in which an ectopic focus in the atrial muscle is the pacemaker: also called *auricular r.*

atrioventricular r. See nodal *r.*

Berger r. See alpha *r.*

beta r. *In electroencephalography*, low potential fast waves, 18 to 35 cycles per second, that are more constant in the frontal lobes of the brain, related to the sensory-motor system.

bigeminal r. Bigeminy.

cardiac r. The normal regularity in the recurrence of heart sounds; also, recognized abnormalities of this regularity.

delta r. *In electroencephalography*, a succession of slow waves with a frequency of six or less per second. Observed frequently during normal sleep.

ectopic r. Rhythmic series of beats originating from ectopic impulses. See ectopic *beat*.

gallop r. The cadence produced when three loud sounds recur in successive cardiac cycles. The extra heart sound may occur in systole or diastole (if early, protodiastolic; if late, presystolic). The protodiastolic third sound is usually of greater significance. Syn., *triple heart r.*

gamma r. *In electroencephalography*, very fast waves whose functional significance is unknown; 40 to 50 per second recorded from the anterior head regions.

heterogenetic r. Cardiac rhythm caused by an impulse arising in the heart outside the specialized tissues.

homogenetic r. Cardiac rhythm caused by an impulse arising in the heart in the specialized tissues.

idioventricular r. The heart rhythm in which an ectopic focus below the atrioventricular node is the pacemaker.

nodal r. A succession of systoles arising from the atrioventricular node at a rate normally between 50 and 60 per minute. The P wave of the electrocardiogram is inverted in leads 2 and 3, and may occur before, during, or after the QRS deflections, depending upon whether the excitation reaches the atria before, during, or after it has reached the ventricles.

parasystolic r. A regular sequence of extrasystoles (atrial or ventricular), representing the rhythm of an ectopic center protected by a zone of unidirectional block.

quadruple r. A cardiac cadence in which four sounds recur in successive cycles.

reciprocal r. *In electrocardiography*, retrograde atrial excitation in A-V nodal rhythm, followed by ventricular excitation when the R-P interval is sufficiently long.

sinus r. The heart rhythm in which the sinoatrial node is the pacemaker.

theta r. *In electroencephalography*, a rhythm, best recorded from the temporal region, having a frequency of 4–7 cycles per second.

triple heart r. See gallop *r.*

triple r. A cardiac cadence in which three sounds recur in successive cycles; it may be normal or abnormal.

ventricular r. See idioventricular *r.*

rhyth'mic [G. *rhythmikos*, rhythmical]. Pertaining to or having the quality of rhythm, as rhythmic segmentations, Cannon's term for repetitive localized contractions occurring in the small intestine during digestion.

rhyth·mic'i·ty (rith·miss'i·tee, rith·) [*rhythmikos*]. The property of rhythmic recurrence, as of symptoms in undulant fever or malaria.

rhyt"i·do·plas'ty [G. *rhytidos*, a wrinkling; *plassein*, to form]. A plastic operation for the removal of skin wrinkles, particularly those of the face and neck.

rhyt"i·do'sis [G., a wrinkling]. A wrinkling, particularly of the cornea. Syn., *rhitidosis*.

riasol. A proprietary liquid containing a mercury soap, phenol, and cresol, used in the treatment of psoriasis.

rib [AS.]. One of the 24 long, flat, curved bones forming the wall of the thorax. See Table of Bones in the Appendix. See Plate 1.

abdominal ribs. (a) The floating ribs. (b) Ossifications of the inscriptiones tendineae.

asternal ribs. The false ribs.

cervical ribs. Occasional riblike processes extending ventrally from the cervical vertebrae.

false r. One of the five lower ribs on each side not attached to the sternum directly.

floating r. One of the last two ribs which have the anterior end free.

rocker r. A first rib which is abnormally bent downward at the subclavian sulcus.

slipping r. Excessive mobility of the lower intercostal joints.

sternal ribs. The true ribs.

true r. One of the seven upper ribs on each side that are attached to the sternum.

vertebrochondral ribs. The highest three false ribs on each side; they are united in front by their costal cartilages.

ri′ba·zole. α-Ribazole; 1-α-D-ribofuranosido-5,6-dimethylbenzimidazole, obtained as one of the products of acid hydrolysis of vitamin B_{12} (cyanocobalamin).

Ribera y Sans, José [*Spanish surgeon,* 1853–1912]. Introduced an artificial anemia of the lower limbs by means of elastic bandages; called *Ribera's method.*

Ribes. See *Champetier de Ribes.*

Ribes, François [*French physician,* 1800–67]. Described the alleged upper termination of the sympathetic nerve which surrounds the anterior communicating artery of the brain; called *Ribes's ganglion.*

ribex. A proprietary vitamin-B complex tablet.

ri′bi·tol. D-Ribitol; $CH_2OH.HCOH.HCOH.HCOH.CH_2OH$; a reduction product of D-ribose; a component of the molecule of riboflavin.

ri″bo·des′ose. Desoxyribose; a pentose sugar present in thymonucleic acid.

ri″bo·fla′vin (rye″bo·flay′vin, ·flav′in, rib″o·) (*riboflavinum*). Constituent of the vitamin-B complex; 6,7-dimethyl-9-(D-1′-ribityl)-isoalloxazine ($C_{17}H_{20}N_4O_6$); constituent of flavoproteins, and thus essential for cellulose oxidations; orange yellow, crystalline powder soluble to the extent of 1 mg. in 10 cc. of water; affected by light, especially when in solution and in the presence of alkalies. Riboflavin deficiency in man produces cheilosis, scaly seborrheic desquamation at the alae nasi, in the ears, and around the eyes; glossitis; photophobia; corneal opacities; and proliferation of the corneal vessels. Principal dietary sources: liver, kidney, heart, milk, cheese, eggs, spinach. Dose, prophylactic, 1 mg. ($\frac{1}{60}$ gr.); therapeutic, 5–15 mg. ($\frac{1}{12}$–$\frac{1}{4}$ gr.) daily. 1 mg. is equivalent to 400 Sherman-Bourquin units. Syn., *vitamin* B_2, *lactoflavin, vitamin G.* See Table of Vitamins in the Appendix.

r. adenine dinucleotide. Flavin adenine dinucleotide.

ri″bo·fla′vin-5′-phos′phate. $C_{17}H_{21}N_4O_9P$; the phosphoric acid ester of riboflavin in which linkage is effected through the CH_2OH group of riboflavin; the prosthetic group of a number of flavoproteins, including Warburg's old yellow enzyme. It functions by being reversibly reduced to a dihydro derivative; its sodium and monodiethanolamine salts are relatively soluble in water and are sometimes used to prepare water-soluble injectable forms of riboflavin. Syn., *flavin phosphate, flavin mononucleotide, isoalloxazine mononucleotide, vitamin-*B_2 *phosphate.*

ri″bo·nu′cle·ase. An enzyme present in various body tissues which depolymerizes ribonucleic acid (yeast nucleic acid) to give mononucleotides.

ri″bo·nu·cle′ic ac′id. Nucleic acid occurring in cell cytoplasm and the nucleolus, first isolated from plants but later found also in animal cells, containing phosphoric acid, D-ribose, adenine, guanine, cytosine, and uracil: also called *ribose nucleic acid, yeast nucleic acid, plasmonucleic acid.* Formerly erroneously called *plant nucleic acid.* Abbreviated, RNA.

ri′bose. $CHO.HCOH.HCOH.HCOH.CH_2OH$; D-ribose; a pentose sugar occurring as a structural component of riboflavin, ribonucleic acid, diphosphopyridine nucleotide, and other nucleotides.

r. nucleic acid. Ribonucleic acid.

ri′bo·side. Any glycoside containing ribose as the sugar component.

ribothiron. Trade-mark for a combination of ferrous sulfate, thiamine hydrochloride, and riboflavin, available as elixir or tablets.

ribranex elixir. Trade-mark for an elixir of vitamin-B complex containing rice bran extract.

rice [It. *riso,* from G. *oryza,* rice]. A plant, *Oryza sativa,* of the Gramineae; also its seed. Used as a food and, occasionally, as a demulcent.

r. bran. Rice polishings.

r. polishings (*perpolitiones oryzae*). The fine, flaky pericarp and spermoderm fragments, the embryo, aleurone layer, and outer adhering cells of the starchy endosperm of rice. Used in the manufacture of the extract.

r. polishings extract (*extractum perpolitionum oryzae*). A hydroalcoholic extract prepared from rice polishings; a dark brown liquid containing not less than 0.06 mg. of vitamin B_1 per cubic centimeter: widely used in certain countries for treatment of beriberi and other forms of vitamin-B_1 deficiency.

Richet, Charles Robert [*French physiologist,* 1850–1935]. In his description, with P. J. Portier, of the phenomenon, he originated the term anaphylaxis for the state of increased susceptibility in an animal following parenteral injection of an antigen (1902). Nobel laureate (1913).

Richet, Didier Dominique Alfred [*French surgeon,* 1816–91]. Described an operation for relief of ectropion, in which the cicatrix at the outer side of the lower lid is excised; after the lids have been sutured, the gap is filled by raising two tongue-shaped flaps; called *Richet's operation.*

Richter, August Gottlieb (1742–1812). German surgeon who described a strangulated partial enterocele, called *Richter's hernia.*

ri′cin (rye′sin, ris′in) [L. *ricinus,* castor oil plant]. A highly toxic albumin in the seed of *Ricinus communis.*

ric′i·nine (ris′i·neen, ·nin). A toxic alkaloid, $C_8H_8N_2O_2$, in the seeds and leaves of the castor plant, *Ricinus communis.*

ric′in·ism (ris′in·iz·um) [*ricinus*]. Poisoning from the seeds of *Ricinus communis.* It is marked by hemorrhagic gastroenteritis and icterus.

ric″in·o′le·ic ac′id (ris″i·no′lee·ick, ris″in·o·lee′·ick). $CH_3(CH_2)_5.CHOH.CH{:}CH(CH_2)_7COOH$. The characteristic acid of the glycerides of castor oil.

ric″in·o′le·in (ris″i·no′lee·in). Glyceryl ricinoleate, the chief constituent of castor oil.

Ric′i·nus (ris′i·nus) [L.]. A genus of the Euphorbiaceae. **R. communis** is the source of castor oil.

rick′ets [apparently from G. *rhachis,* spine]. A deficiency disease occurring during skeletal growth, due to concurrent lack of vitamin D and insufficient exposure to ultraviolet radiation (sunshine), resulting in altered calcium and phosphorus metabolism, which is reflected in defective bone growth. Syn., *infantile r., rachitis.*

adult r. See *osteomalacia.*

celiac r. Rickets resulting from lack of absorption of vitamin D and loss of calcium in the stool, associated with the celiac syndrome: sometimes called *pancreatic r.* Also see *osteomalacia.*

fetal r. See *achondroplasia.*

late r. See resistant *r.*

pancreatic r. See celiac *r.*

refractory r. See resistant *r.*

renal r. Rickets resulting from the failure of the kidney to maintain a normal ratio of calcium to phosphate in the blood. It may be of the glomerular (high phosphate) or tubular (low phosphate) type, or the entire nephron may be involved. Also called *renal osteodystrophy, pseudorickets.*

resistant r. Rickets which fails to respond to administration of ordinary therapeutic doses of vitamin D but which responds to very large amounts. A hereditary factor appears to be involved. Syn., *vitamin-D-refractory r.*

scurvy r. See infantile *scurvy.*

Ricketts, Howard Taylor [*American pathologist,* 1871–1910]. Remembered for his researches in the field of immunity and serum therapy. With John F. Anderson, studied Rocky Mountain spotted fever and demonstrated the wood tick to be a vector (1906).

Rick·ett′si·a [*Ricketts*]. A generic name applied to a group of microorganisms smaller than bacteria but larger than the filtrable viruses; usually found in the arthropods, ticks, fleas, and lice. —**rickett′sial,** *adj.*

R. akamushi. Synonym for *R. tsutsugamushi.*

R. akari. That species which is the causative agent of rickettsialpox.

R. burnetii. A species which is the etiologic agent of Q fever. Synonym for *Coxiella burnetii.*

R. conorii. Synonym for *Coxiella conorii.*

R. diaporica. Synonym for *Rickettsia burnetii.*

R. melophagi. A nonpathogenic species found in the sheep tick *Melophagus ovinus.*

R. mooseri. The etiological agent of murine, flea-borne typhus.

R. muricola. Synonym for *R. prowazekii mooseri.*

R. nipponica. Synonym for *R. tsutsugamushi.*

R. orientalis. The etiologic agent of tsutsugamushi disease. Syn., *R. tsutsugamushi.*

R. pediculi. Synonym for *Rickettsia quintana.*

R. prowazeki. The etiological agent of louse-borne typhus and Brill's disease.

R. prowazeki mooseri. Old term for *R. mooseri.*

R. prowazeki prowazeki. Old term for *R. prowazeki.*

R. psittaci. Name proposed by Lillie for the causative organism of psittacosis, but which has not been accepted because no arthropod host has been demonstrated.

R. quintana. That species which is the causative agent of trench fever.

R. rickettsii. That species which is the causative agent of Rocky Mountain spotted fever. See *Dermacentroxenus.*

R. ruminantium. The causative organism of heartwater disease.

R. tsutsugamushi. The etiologic agent of tsutsugamushi disease. Also called *R. orientalis.*

R. wolhynica. Synonym for *Rickettsia quintana.*

rick·ett′si·al·pox″ [*Ricketts;* ME. *pokkes*]. A disease caused by *Rickettsia akari* characterized by regional lymphadenopathy, fever, chills, headache, secondary rash, and leukopenia following an initial papule at the locale of the bite of the mite *Allodermanyssus sanguineus,* which is the vector. The reservoir is *Mus musculus,* the house mouse. No deaths or sequelae have been recorded.

rick·ett″si·o′ses. Diseases caused by Rickettsii.

rick′et·y [G. *rhachis,* spine]. Affected with or distorted by rickets; rachitic.

Ricord, Philippe [*French urologist and dermatologist,* 1800–89]. Celebrated for his contributions in the fields of urology and syphilology. Described chancre and divided syphilis into three stages (1838). Demonstrated that syphilis and gonorrhea are separate diseases. The initial sore of syphilis is sometimes called *Ricord's chancre.* His operation for circumcision is called *Ricord's method.*

Riddoch, George (1889–1947). English neurologist known for his investigation of the reflex functions of the completely transected spinal cord (1917); see mass *reflex.* He described the automatic bladder (1918).

Rideal, Samuel [*English chemist,* 1863–1929]. Devised a method of standardization of disinfectants, with J. T. A. Walker (1903). The *Rideal-Walker method* consists of checking the amount of the unknown disinfectant required to kill an organism against the amount of carbolic acid necessary to accomplish the same thing in the same time. The resulting value is called the *Rideal-Walker coefficient* or *phenol coefficient.*

rid′er's bone. An osseous deposit in the adductor muscles of the leg, from long-continued pressure of the leg against the saddle.

ridge [AS. *hrycg*]. An extended elevation or crest.

alveolar r. The ridge left after resorption of the alveolar process in an edentulous jaw.

basal r. Cingulum, 4.

bicipital r. Either one of the crests of bone delimiting the bicipital groove of the humerus.

carotid r. The sharp ridge between the inferior aperture of the carotid canal and the jugular fossa.

dental r. An elevation which forms a cusp or margin of a tooth.

endocardial r. One of a pair of internal spiral ridges in the embryonic bulbus cordis whose fusion initiates the division of the bulbus into aortic and pulmonary trunks as well as forming part of the septum membranaceum.

epipericardial r. Paired areas of loose subpharyngeal mesenchyme above the embryonic pericardial cavity; said to form the pathway for migration of occipital premuscle masses and the hypoglossal nerve to the tongue.

ganglion r. Neural crest.

genital r. A medial ridge or fold on the ventromedial surface of the mesonephros in the embryo produced by growth of the peritoneum; the primordium of the gonads and their ligaments.

germ r. Genital ridge.

gluteal r. The bony ridge on the linea aspera for the attachment of the gluteus maximus.

interosseous r. The sharp ridge along the shaft of a bone such as the ulna or fibula, for the attachment of the interosseous ligament. Also called *interosseous crest.*

interureteric r. See *bar of bladder.*

mammary r. A longitudinal elevation of thickened ectoderm between the bases of the limb buds in the embryo from which develop the mammary glands. Syn., *milk r.*

marginal ridges. The elevations forming the mesial and distal margins of occlusal surfaces of premolars and molars, and of lingual surfaces of upper incisors and canines.

mastoid r. The bony ridge on the mastoid process for the attachment of the sternocleidomastoid muscle.

mesonephric r. A ridge or fold of the dorsal coelomic wall in the embryo lateral to the mesentery produced by growth of the mesonephros.

milk r. See mammary *r.*

oblique r. (a) A ridge on the grinding surface of an upper molar tooth. (b) See trapezoid *r.*

palatine ridges. The central ridge (raphe) together with the lateral corrugations of the mucosa (rugae) of the hard palate; in man they are especially prominent in the fetus.

primitive ridges. Those bounding the primitive groove. Syn., *primitive folds.*

pronator r. The bony ridge on the lower anterior surface of the ulna for the attachment of the pronator teres muscle.

pulmonary r. A minor ridge in the embryo on the coelomic surface of the bulging fold formed by the growth of the common cardinal veins that develops into the pleuropericardial membrane.

superciliary r. Supraorbital ridge.

supracondylar r. Either of the two ridges, lateral or medial, above the condyles of the humerus, which serve for muscular attachment.

supraorbital r. The curved prominential margin forming the upper boundary of the orbit.

temporal r. That extending from the external angular process of the frontal bone, across the frontal and parietal bones, and terminating in the posterior root of the zygomatic process.

trapezoid r. A bony ridge on the clavicle for the attachment of the trapezoid ligament. Also called *oblique r.* (b).

urogenital r. The longitudinal peritoneal fold in the embryo produced by growth of the mesonephros and gonad. Syn., *Wolffian r.*

Wolffian r. See urogenital *r.*

ridge′ling [*hrycg*]. A common term applied to cryptorchism in domestic animals.

ri′ding of bones. *In surgery,* the displacement of the fractured ends of bones which are forced past each other by muscular contraction, instead of remaining in end-to-end apposition.

Riedel, Bernhard Moritz Carl Ludwig [*German surgeon,* 1846–1916]. Described a tongue-shaped process of the liver extending downward, occurring infrequently; called *congenital abnormal lobulation of the liver, Riedel's process* or *lobe.* Described chronic thyroiditis (1896); also called *ligneous thyroiditis, Riedel's disease* or *struma.*

Rieder, Hermann [*German pathologist,* 1858–1932]. Remembered for his description of an undifferentiated leukocyte having an indented nucleus, found in acute leukemia and considered by some hematologists as a pathologic myeloblast, and by some an abnormal lymphoblast, called *Rieder's cell.*

Riegel's test. See under *test.*

Riehl, Gustav [*Austrian dermatologist,* 1855–1943]. Described a pigmentary disturbance (1917) usually seen upon the face and neck. See Riehl's *melanosis.* Advocated the use of blood transfusions to prevent shock after severe burns (1925).

Ries-Clark operation. A type of radical hysterectomy, similar to that of Ernst Wertheim, for carcinoma of the uterus.

Riesman, David [*American physician,* 1867–1940]. Well-known clinician and medical historian. Author of *History of Medicine in the Middle Ages* (1935). Described degenerative noninflammatory fibrotic disease of the myocardium; also called *Riesman's myocardosis.*

Rieux, Léon [*French surgeon,* nineteenth century]. Described retrocecal hernia (1853), also called *Rieux's hernia.*

Riga, Antonio [*Italian physician,* contemporary]. Described an oral disease of infancy occurring during dentition, in which the frenulum of the tongue becomes indurated; called *Fede-Riga disease.* See cachetic *aphthae.*

Riggs, John M. [*American dentist,* 1810–85]. Introduced (1876) a method of treating alveolar pyorrhea, called *Riggs's disease.*

Riggs and Stadie method. See under *method.*

right [AS. *riht*]. Dextral. Abbreviated, R.

rig′id [L. *rigidus,* stiff]. Stiff, hard.

ri·gid′i·tas [L.]. Stiffness; rigidity.

r. articulorum. Spurious ankylosis.

r. cadaverica. Rigor mortis.

ri·gid′i·ty [*rigiditas*]. Stiffness; inflexibility; immobility; tonic contraction of muscles.

anatomic r. of the cervix uteri. Rigidity in which the cervix, though neither edematous nor tender, is not wholly effaced in labor, but retains its length and dilates only to a certain extent, beyond which the contractions of the uterus are without effect.

cadaveric r. Rigor mortis.

cerebellar r. Rigidity of the spinal muscles, due to lesion of the middle lobe of the cerebellum. The head is drawn backward, the spine curved, and the arms and legs made rigid.

clasp-knife r. Lengthening reaction, especially that observed in the hemiplegic patient.

cogwheel r. The rigidity or rhythmic contractions noted on passive stretching of the muscles in paralysis agitans.

decerebrate r. Exaggerated postural tonics in the antigravity muscles resulting from interruption of extrapyramidal axons from the motor and premotor areas of the cerebral cortex, or from destruction of cortical neurons in those areas.

hemiplegic r. Spastic rigidity of the paralyzed limbs in hemiplegia.

muscular r. See *myotonia* congenita.

pathologic r. of the cervix uteri. Rigidity due to organic disease or cicatricial contraction.

postmortem r. Rigor mortis.

spasmodic r. of the cervix uteri. Rigidity due to spasmodic contraction of the cervix.

rig′or [L., stiffness]. Chill.

r. mortis. Stiffening and rigidity of muscle, particularly skeletal and cardiac, which occurs after death. Cessation of circulation in the muscle determines increase in content of acids, especially sarcolactic, with resultant swelling of muscle colloid and precipitation of insoluble myosin in the substance of the muscle.

ri′ma (ree′muh) (pl. *rimae*) [L., cleft]. A chink or cleft. —**rimal,** *adj.*

r. glottidis. The cleft between the true vocal folds; the glottis.

r. oris. The line formed by the junction of the lips.

r. palpebrarum. The palpebral fissure.

r. pudendi. The fissure between the labia majora.

r. vulvae. See *r.* pudendi.

rimifon. Trade-mark for a brand of isoniazid.

ri″mo·ci′din. An antibiotic substance isolated from cultures of *Streptomyces rimosus;* it possesses fungistatic properties.

ri′mose (rye′moce, rye·moce′) [L. *rimosus,* full of cracks]. *In biology,* marked by many crevices or furrows.

rin′der·pest [Ger., cattle plague]. A contagious, epidemic disease of cattle, sometimes affecting sheep and goats; caused by a filtrable virus and characterized by fever and ulcerative, diphtheritic lesions of the intestinal tract.

ring [AS. *hring*]. A circular opening or the structure surrounding it. Also see *annulus.*

abdominal inguinal r. Annulus inguinalis abdominalis [BNA]; the abdominal opening of the inguinal canal, bounded below by the inguinal ligament, medially by the inferior epigastric vessels, and laterally and above by the lower border of the transversus abdominis muscle. Syn., *deep inguinal r.* [BR]. Formerly called *internal abdominal r.* See Plate 4.

amniotic r. The ring formed by the attached margin of the amnion at the umbilicus.

anal r. A ring-shaped ridge about the embryonic anal orifice produced by growth and fusion of the anal tubercles.

Braune's r. See retraction *r.*, 1.

Cabot's rings. See *ring bodies* under *body.*

cholane r. *In chemistry,* a tetracyclic, saturated ring system.

ciliary r. Boundary between the iris and the choroid of the eye.

conjunctival r. Annulus conjunctivae [BNA]; a ring of denser tissue marking the attachment of the bulbar conjunctiva to the corneoscleral limbus.

constriction r. See retraction *r.*, 1.

contraction r. Retraction ring.

crural r. See femoral *r.*

deep inguinal r. Synonym for abdominal inguinal ring, the upper and lateral opening of the inguinal canal.

external abdominal r. Subcutaneous inguinal *r.*

femoral r. Annulus femoralis [BNA]; the abdominal opening of the femoral canal. Formerly called *annulus cruralis, crural r.*

fibrous r. Annulus fibrosus.

greater r. of the iris. Annulus iridis major [BNA]; the outer of two concentric zones of the iris separated by the circulus arteriosus minor.

hemorrhoidal r. A circular swelling of the wall of the anal canal at the level of the external sphincter muscle; it contains the internal hemorrhoidal plexus. When enlarged, it forms hemorrhoids (piles). Also called *annulus haemorrhoidalis.*

internal abdominal r. See abdominal inguinal *r.*

Kayser-Fleischer r. A ring of golden brown or brownish green pigment behind the limbic border of the cornea, observed in hepatolenticular degeneration (Wilson's disease) and the pseudosclerosis of Westphal.

Landolt r. *In ophthalmology*, an incomplete ring used as a test object for visual acuity.

lesser r. of the iris. Annulus iridis minor [BNA]; the inner of two concentric zones of the iris separated by the circulus arteriosus minor.

lymphatic r. Ring of lymphatic tissue, including the tonsils, surrounding the pharynx. Also called *Waldeyer's tonsillar r.*

pathologic r. See retraction *r.*, 2.

physiologic r. See retraction *r.*, 1.

retraction r. 1. When physiologic, the ridge on the inner uterine surface which constitutes the boundary line between the upper and lower uterine segments. It results from the process of normal labor, which causes thinning of the lower uterine segment and concomitant thickening of the upper uterine segment. Syn., *constriction r.*, *Braune's r.* 2. When pathologic, the abnormally thickened ridge of uterine musculature lying between the upper and lower uterine segments, resulting from mechanically obstructed labor and associated with extreme thinning of the lower uterine segment: also called *contraction r. of Bandl, Lusk, Schroeder*, or *White.*

rings of the heart valves. See *annulus fibrosus* (b), *skeleton of the heart.*

subchorial closing r. The remnant of the cytotrophoblast of the chorionic plate found between Langhans' stria and the chorionic connective tissue. Once incorrectly called the *decidua subchorialis.*

subcutaneous inguinal r. Annulus inguinalis subcutaneus [BNA]; external opening of the inguinal canal; an obliquely placed, triangular opening in the aponeurosis of the external oblique muscle giving passage to the ilioinguinal nerve and to the spermatic cord in the male or the round ligament of the uterus in the female. See Plate 4.

tracheal r. One of the C-shaped cartilages in the framework of the trachea.

tympanic r. Annulus tympanicus [BNA]; at the time of birth, an incomplete osseous ring; it develops into the tympanic part of the temporal bone.

umbilical r. Annulus umbilicalis [BNA]; margin of the opening in the ventral body wall of the fetus; line of attachment of the umbilical cord. It gives passage to the umbilical vessels.

urethral r. Annulus urethralis [BNA]; a mass of smooth muscle around the internal urethral orifice of the urinary bladder; the internal sphincter of the urinary bladder.

ring'bone" [*hring;* AS. *bān*]. A chronic, hypertrophic osteitis of the pastern or first and second phalanges of the foot in the horse. It is caused by inflammatory changes of long duration.

ring com'pound. A compound in which the atoms form a ring or closed chain.

ringed hair. A rare form of canities, due to the alternate formation of medulla and no medulla, in which the hairs appear silvery gray and dark in alternating bands. Usually seen in several members of a family. Also called *pili annulati.*

Ringer's solution. See under *solution.* See also Locke-Ringer's *solution.*

ring'hals" [S. Afr. D.]. A South African cobra of the genus *Hemachatus*, family Elapidae.

ring'worm" [AS. *hring; wyrm*]. An infestation of the skin, hair, or nails, with various fungi. Also called *dermatomycosis, tinea, trichophytosis.*

Burmese r. Tinea imbricata.

Rinne's test. See under *test.*

ri'no·lite. See *rhinolith.*

riodine. Trade-mark for a 66% solution in oil of an iodine addition product of castor oil, representing about 17% of iodine. The solution is used as a substitute for inorganic iodides.

Río Hortega, Pío del (1882–1945). Spanish neuroanatomist who introduced a silver sodium carbonate method for staining nerve cells (1918) and proposed the names *microglia* and *oligodendroglia.* He did fundamental research in the histology of tumors of the nervous system. See *Hortega's silver method* under *stain.*

Riolan, Jean (1580–1637). French anatomist and physiologist who described an arterial arcade, called *Riolan's arc.* The ossicles sometimes found in the suture between the inferior border of the occipital bone and the mastoid portion of the temporal bone are called *Riolan's bones, ossicles.* He is remembered for his description of the ciliary portion of the orbicularis oculi, called *ciliary muscle, Riolan's muscle.*

riona. A proprietary capsule containing propadrine hydrochloride, acetophenetidin, and aspirin.

Ripault, Louis Henri Antonin [*French physician*, 1807–56]. Described a change in the shape of the pupil on pressure upon the eye, transitory during life but permanent after death; called *Ripault's sign.*

ripe [AS. *rīpe*]. Mature, completed.

Risley's rotary prism. See under *prism.*

ri·so'ri·us (ri·sor'ee·us, rye·) [L. *risum*, from *ridere*, to laugh]. A muscle of the cheek inserted into the angle of the mouth. See Table of Muscles in the Appendix.

ri'sus [L., laughter]. A grin or laugh.

r. caninus. See *r.* sardonicus.

r. sardonicus. The sardonic grin, a peculiar grinning distortion of the face produced by spasm of the muscles about the mouth, seen in tetanus.

Ritchie, William Thomas [*Scottish physician*, 1873–1945]. Described heart block and was one of the first to recognize atrial flutter (1905).

Ritchie-Sneath stim'u·la·tor. An apparatus used for testing the electrical conducting power of a muscle or for therapeutic muscle stimulation.

Ritgen, Ferdinand August Marie Franz [*German gynecologist*, 1787–1867]. Advocated symphysiotomy as a surgical procedure in obstetric surgery. Introduced a technic in obstetric delivery in which he pressed upward upon the fetal head through the posterior portion of the perineum; called *Ritgen's maneuver.*

Ritter, Jacob. Nineteenth-century Swiss physician who described psittacosis in man (1879).

Ritter, Johann Wilhelm [*German physicist,* 1776–1810]. With Eusebio Valli, elaborated a law that section of a living nerve is followed first by increased irritability, then by loss of irritability, the response traveling toward the periphery. Called *Ritter-Valli law.* See also Ritter's *tetanus.*

Ritter von Rittershain, Gottfried [*Austrian dermatologist,* 1820–83]. The first to describe dermatitis exfoliativa in the newborn (1870); also called *Ritter's disease.*

Riva-Rocci, Scipione [*Italian physician,* 1863–1943]. Widely known for his invention of a practical type of sphygmomanometer (1896). Called *Riva-Rocci's method.*

ri'val·ry [L. *rivalis,* competitor]. A struggle for supremacy.

binocular r. See retinal *r.*

retinal r. The continuous physiological process of alternation in consciousness between stimuli falling on the two eyes. When this process is studied by artificially presenting different stimuli to each eye, the alternation is found to be unpredictable in timing and areas involved and dependent on the strength of stimulus to each eye. Also called *r. of visual fields, strife r., complementary* or *reciprocal replacement.*

r. of colors. Retinal rivalry, where colors are the stimuli.

r. of contours. Retinal rivalry, where the contours of two objects are the stimuli.

r. of visual fields. See retinal *r.*

strife r. See retinal *r.*

Rivalta, Sebastiano [*Italian veterinary surgeon,* 1852–93]. Introduced a method for differentiating exudate from transudate, in which one allows a drop of the fluid to fall into a solution of distilled water to which one drop of 50% acetic acid has been added. If the drop sinks and leaves a turbidity, the test is positive for exudate. Called *Rivalta's test.*

rivanol. Trade-mark for a brand of ethodin, chemically ethoxydiamino-acridine lactate; yellow, crystalline powder, soluble in about 15 parts of water; a bactericide in strengths of 0.1–0.2%.

Rivinus, Augustus Quirinus (1652–1723). German anatomist and botanist who described the minor sublingual ducts, called *Rivinian ducts.* He is known for his description of the notch at the upper border of the tympanic sulcus, also called *incisura tympanica, Rivinus' notch.* The sublingual gland was once known as *Rivinus' gland.*

riz'i·form [F. *riz,* rice; L. *forma,* form]. Resembling grains of rice.

ri'zine (rye'zeen) [*riz*]. Rice that has been acted upon by superheated steam.

R. M. A. Right mentoanterior position of the fetus.

R. M. P. Right mentoposterior position of the fetus.

R. N. Registered Nurse.

Rn Chemical symbol for radon.

RNA Ribonucleic acid.

R. O. A. Right occipitoanterior position of the fetus.

roar'ing [AS. *rārung*]. A disease of horses characterized by respiratory distress and a roaring noise, due to paralysis of the intrinsic muscles of the larynx.

robalate. A trade-mark for the gastric antacid substance dihydroxyaluminum aminoacetate.

Robbins, Frederick Chapman (1916–). American pediatrician, who with J. F. Enders and T. H. Weller shared the Nobel prize (1954) in physiology and medicine for their discovery of the ability of the poliomyelitis virus to grow in cultures of different tissues. He is also known for his work on Q fever.

Robert pelvis. See under *pelvis.*

Roberts' reagent. See under *reagent.*

Roberts' test. See under *test.*

Robertson. See *Argyll Robertson.*

Robin, Charles Philippe [*French physician,* 1821–85]. Described osteoclasts, also called *Robin's myeloplaxes.* Described the perivascular spaces, called *Robin's spaces, spaces of Virchow-Robin.*

ro'bin [after Jean *Robin,* French botanist, 1550–1629]. A toxic albuminoid from the bark of the locust tree, *Robinia pseudoacacia;* its action is similar to that of abrin and ricin.

ro'bin·in. A glycoside from the flowers of the locust tree, *Robinia pseudoacacia.*

ro'bin·ose. A trisaccharide obtained from the glycoside robinin, yielding upon hydrolysis one mole of galactose and two of rhamnose.

Robinson, Andrew Rose [*American dermatologist,* 1845–1924]. Gave the first description of hidrocystoma (1884); also called *Robinson's disease.*

Robinson, Byron [*American surgeon and anatomist,* 1857–1910]. Described a circle formed by the uterine, ovarian, hypogastric, and common iliac arteries. Called *Robinson's circle.*

Robinson, Robert (1886–). English chemist noted for his research on certain vegetable products of great biological importance, particularly alkaloids. Nobel laureate in chemistry (1947).

Robinson, Victor [*American physician and medical historian,* 1886–1947]. Remembered for his devotion to historical medicine.

Robiquet, Pierre Jean [*French physician,* 1780–1840]. Isolated codeine (1832).

rob'o·rant (rob'o·runt, ro'bo·runt) [L. *roborare,* to strengthen]. Tonic, strengthening. **—rob'-orant,** *n.*

Robson. See *Mayo-Robson.*

Roc·cel'la (rock·sel'uh) [NL., from It. *rocca,* rock]. A genus of lichens of the Parmeliaceae. Several species yield coloring principles used in litmus and cudbear.

roc·cel'lic ac'id. $C_{17}H_{32}O_4$; α-dodecyl-β-methylsuccinic acid; an antibiotic substance occurring in lichens, including *Lecanora sordida.* It occurs in crystals, is insoluble in water, and forms a water-soluble sodium salt.

Ro·chelle' salt (ro·shell'). Potassium sodium tartrate.

Rockey's sign. See under *sign.*

rock'ing meth'od. See *Eve's method* under *artificial respiration.*

Rock'y Moun'tain spot'ted fe'ver. A form of fever with a characteristic rash occurring throughout the Western Hemisphere, formerly thought to be limited to the Rocky Mountain area. The causative organism is *Dermacentroxenus rickettsii,* and it is transmitted to man by several varieties of ticks, principally *Dermacentor andersoni* and *D. variabilis* in the United States.

rod [AS. *rodd*]. One of numerous, slender, bacillary structures, as in the retina.

enamel r. See enamel *prism.*

r. nuclear cell. See band *cell.*

rods of Corti. The columnar cells lining the tunnel of Corti. See *organ* of Corti.

rods of the retina. One of the two types of photosensitive cells in the retina. Also called *rod cells.*

ro·den'ti·cide [L. *rodere,* to gnaw; *caedere,* to kill]. A preparation that is poisonous to, or destroys, rodents: used as an agent against rats or mice.

ro'dent ul'cer. See rodent *ulcer.*

rodilone. Trade name for 4,4'-di(acetylamino)-diphenylsulfone, $C_{16}H_{16}N_2O_4S$, a drug of the sulfonamide group especially active against streptococci. It has cured experimental toxoplasmosis in mice.

Rodman, William Louis [*American surgeon,* 1858–1916]. Celebrated surgeon, best remembered for his description of his incision for radical amputation of the breast in cancer. This was described as a pear-shaped skin cut encircling the breast, extending upward to a point in the axilla; called *Rodman's incision.*

ro″do·nal′gi·a [G. *rhodon,* rose; *algos,* pain]. Erythromelalgia.

Roe-Kahn method. See under *method.*

Roederer, Johann Georg [*German obstetrician,* 1727–63]. Remembered for his description of pleural and pericardial hemorrhage from the capillaries of the newborn who have attempted to breathe in utero; called *Roederer's ecchymoses.* Described flexion of the chin when the head is engaged at the superior pelvic strait during labor; called *Roederer's obliquity.*

Roenne's na′sal step. A visual field defect typical of glaucoma, caused by asymmetrical nerve fiber damage on either side of the horizontal raphe of the eye.

roent′gen (rent′ghin, runt′ghin, runt′yin. *See* Notes §§ 1, 19, 35) [after *Röntgen*]. Roentgen unit. Symbol, r.

gamma r. That amount of radium which will produce in air the same amount of ionization as would one roentgen of gamma rays. Syn., *gamma-ray roentgen.*

r. e·quiv′a·lent man. That quantity of radiation which, when absorbed by man, produces an effect equivalent to the absorption by man of 1 roentgen of x- or gamma-radiation. Abbreviated, REM, rem.

r. e·quiv′a·lent phys′i·cal. The amount of ionizing radiation which is capable of producing 1.615×10^{12} ion pairs per gram of tissue or that will suffer an absorption in tissue of 93 ergs per gram. This unit is employed primarily to measure beta-radiation. Abbreviated, REP, rep.

roent′gen cin″e·ma·tog′ra·phy. Cinematography of shadows as they appear on the fluoroscopic screen.

roent″gen·i·za′tion (rent″ghin·i·zay′shun, ·eye-zay′shun) [*Röntgen*]. Exposure or subjection to the action of roentgen rays. *Obs.* —**roent′genize,** *v.*

roent″gen·o·der′ma. See roentgen *dermatitis.*

roent′gen·o·gram″. A roentgen-ray photograph.

roent′gen·o·graph″ [*Röntgen;* G. *graphein,* to write]. Make a roentgenogram.

roent″gen·og′ra·phy [*Röntgen; graphein*]. Radiography. —**roentgenograph′ic,** *adj.*

roent″gen·o·ky′mo·gram. A radiographic record of the changes in the size of the heart.

roent″gen·o·ky·mog′ra·phy [*Röntgen;* G. *kyma,* wave; *graphein,* to write]. A roentgenographic procedure for recording changes in the size of the heart by interposing an impermeable sheet of metal, with slits, between the patient and the film moving at right angles to the slits during exposure.

roent″gen·ol′o·gist [*Röntgen;* G. *logos,* word]. A physician specializing in the practice of roentgenology.

roent″gen·ol′o·gy [*Röntgen; logos*]. The branch of medical science which deals with the diagnostic and therapeutic application of roentgen rays. Also called *radiology.* —**roentgenolog′ic,** *adj.*

roent″gen·o·lu′cent. Allowing the passage of roentgen rays, as roentgenolucent material.

roent″gen·om′e·try [*Röntgen;* G. *metron,* a measure]. Measurement of the quality and quantity of roentgen rays.

roent″gen·o·paque′. Not permitting the passage of roentgen rays, as roentgenopaque material.

roent″gen·os′co·py [*Röntgen;* G. *skopein,* to examine]. Examination with roentgen rays by means of a fluorescent screen. —**roent′genoscope,** *n.*

roent′gen rays. See under *ray.*

roent″gen·ther′a·py [*Röntgen;* G. *therapeia,* treatment]. The treatment of disease by means of roentgen rays.

Roese-Gottlieb method. See under *method.*

roe′theln, rö′teln (ret′eln. *See* Notes § 35). See *rubella.*

Roger, Henri Louis [*French physician,* 1809–91]. Known for his description of congenital abnormal communication between the ventricles of the heart; called *Roger's disease, maladie de Roger.*

Roger of Palermo [*Italian surgeon,* late twelfth century]. Author of a practice of surgery (1180), in which end-to-end intestinal anastomosis is described. He is known to have used mercury by inunction; also used seaweed in the preoperative treatment of goiter.

Roger's reflex. See under *reflex.*

Rogers, Leonard [*English physician,* 1868–]. Advocated treatment of amebic dysentery by hypodermic injection of salts of emetine. Demonstrated Leishman-Donovan bodies in kala-azar (1904). See also Rogers' *treatment* for cholera and leprosy.

Rohr, Karl [*German anatomist,* 1863–]. Described a fibrinoid formed on the maternal surface of the intervillous spaces and on the villi, called *stria of Rohr.*

Rokitansky, Carl von [*Austrian pathologic anatomist,* 1804–78]. One of the greatest pathologists. Described spondylolisthesis (1839). Described postnecrotic cirrhosis of the liver (1842), sometimes called *Rokitansky's disease.* See *Rokitansky-Aschoff sinuses* under *sinus.*

Rolando, Luigi [*Italian anatomist,* 1773–1831]. Remembered for his investigations of the anatomy of the central nervous system. Described the external arcuate fibers of the medulla oblongata, called *Rolando's fibers.* Described the longitudinal prominence on either side of the lower part of the medulla oblongata, called *Rolando's funiculus. Rolando's area* is the motor area in the cerebral cortex comprising pre- and postcentral gyri. See also central *sulcus;* formerly called *fissure of Rolando, Rolandic sulcus.* See also *substantia* gelatinosa Rolandi, also called *Rolando's gelatinous substance.*

rol′ler (ro′lur). See roller *bandage.*

Roller's nucleus. See *nucleus* of Roller.

Rolleston, Humphrey Davy (1862–1944). English physician, famous in English historical medicine, who made many important studies in the history of development of knowledge in hematology and cavdiovascular diseases.

Rollet, Alexander [*Austrian physiologist,* 1834–1903]. Described large acidophil cells of the fundic glands of the gastric mucous membrane; called *Rollet's cells, acid cells, parietal cells.* These are thought to secrete hydrochloric acid. Described an insoluble spongy network forming the structure of an erythrocyte within whose interstices is embedded the hemoglobin; called *Rollet's stroma, stromatin.*

Rollett, Joseph Pierre [*French physician,* 1824–94]. Well-known expert on venereal diseases and one of the first to recognize mixed lesions of chancre and other lesions. The mixed chancre is called *Rollett's disease.*

Rollier, Auguste [*Swiss physician,* 1874–]. Introduced the method of treatment of extrapulmonary tuberculosis by sunlight (1903); called *Rollier's method.*

Romana's sign. See under *sign.*

ro·man'o·scope (ro·man'o·scope, ro'mun·o·) [L. *Romanus,* Roman; G. *skopein,* to examine]. A speculum for examining the sigmoid flexure. *Obs.*

Romanovsky, Dmitri Leonidovich [*Russian physician,* 1861–1921]. Remembered for his important studies on the malarial parasite (1891). Introduced methylene blue-eosin blood cell stain used for malarial and other organisms. See Romanovsky *stain.* Described a chromatin stain (1891) modified later (1898) by Nocht; see Nocht-Romanovsky *stain.*

Romberg, Moritz Heinrich [*German physician and neurologist,* 1795–1873]. Noted for his extensive study of the physiology and pathology of diseases of the nervous system. Described achondroplasia (1817). He described progressive facial hemiatrophy or trophoneurosis along the distribution of the fifth cranial nerve (1846), also called *Romberg's disease.* See also Romberg's *sign,* Howship-Romberg *syndrome.*

ron"geur' (rawn·zhur'. *See* NOTES §§ 21, 35) [F.]. A bone-cutting forceps.

ron'go·lite. See *formaldehyde.*

roniacol. Trade-mark for 3-pyridinemethanol; $C_5H_4N.CH_2OH$; the alcohol corresponding to nicotinic acid; it has a vasodilating action resembling that of nicotinic acid and is used in treating various peripheral vascular disorders.

ronone. A proprietary product consisting of 2% of rotenone in a mucilage base, intended for external application in the treatment of scabies.

Röntgen, Wilhelm Konrad [*German physicist,* 1845–1923]. Discovered x-rays (1895) and laid the foundation for the sciences of roentgenology and radiology. See also roentgen *rays.* Nobel laureate (1901).

Roonhuyze, Hendrik van [*Dutch surgeon and gynecologist,* 1622–72]. Author of one of the earliest works on operative gynecology and obstetrics. He is known to have performed Cesarean section and to have operated successfully on vesicovaginal fistulas.

root [AS. *rōt*]. 1. The descending axis of a plant. 2. The part of an organ embedded in the tissues, as the root of a tooth. 3. The beginning or proximal portion of a structure, especially one of two bundles of nerve fibers, the posterior and anterior emerging from the central nervous system and joining to form a nerve trunk.

anatomic r. of tooth. The part of a human tooth covered by cementum.

anterior r. A bundle of efferent nerve fibers emerging from the anterior part of the spinal cord to form a spinal nerve. Syn., *motor r., ventral r.*

clinical r. The part of a tooth apically from the gingival sulcus.

descending vestibular r. See descending vestibular *tract.*

dorsal r. See posterior *r.*

motor r. See anterior *r.*

posterior r. A bundle of afferent nerve fibers arising from the nerve cells in a spinal ganglion and passing to the central nervous system. Syn., *dorsal r., sensory r.*

r. of the lung. The axis formed by the bronchus, pulmonary vessels, lymphatics, and nerves in the hilus, connecting the lung with the heart and trachea. Also called *radix pulmonis.*

r. of the mesentery. The parietal attachment of the mesentery extending from the duodenojejunal flexure to the ileocecal junction. Also called *radix mesentericus.*

r. of the nail. The small proximal region of the nail plate covered entirely by the nail wall. Also called *radix unguis.*

r. of the nose. The part at the forehead between the eyes, from which emerges the dorsum of the nose. Also called *radix nasi.*

r. of the tongue. The pharyngeal, fixed part of the tongue, posterior to the sulcus terminalis. Syn., *basis linguae.*

sensory r. See posterior *r.*

spinal vestibular r. See descending vestibular *tract.*

ventral r. See anterior *r.*

root ca·nal'. A small channel running from the pulp chamber to the apex of the tooth, normally filled with pulp tissue.

root feet. Fine digitations of basal cells of the epidermis into the underlying connective tissue of the corium at the dermoepidermal junction. Syn., *basalzellfüsschen.*

R. O. P. Right occipitoposterior position of the fetus.

Roque's sign. See under *sign.*

Rorschach, Hermann [*Swiss psychiatrist,* 1884–1922]. Described a test which measures the more qualitative, nonintellectual traits of personality, based on the subject's interpretation of 10 ink blots of varying designs and colors. See Rorschach *test.*

ro·sa'ce·a (ro·zay'see·uh). See *acne* rosacea.

ro·sa'ce·i·form" [L. *rosaceus,* made of roses; *forma,* form]. Resembling acne rosacea. Having a dusky red, telangiectatic appearance.

ro·sa'li·a (ro·say'lee·uh) [L. *rosa,* rose]. 1. Scarlet fever. 2. Measles. 3. Erythema.

ros·an'i·line (ro·zan'i·leen, ·lin, ·lyne). $C_{20}H_{21}N_3O$. Brownish red crystals, slightly soluble in water; soluble in acids, alcohol. Used as a stain and in the manufacture of dyes.

r. hydrochloride. Red crystals, soluble in water. See *fuchsin.*

Rose, Anton Richard [*American biochemist,* 1877–1948]. With W. G. Exton, developed a glucose tolerance test, called *Exton and Rose's test.*

Rose, Edmund [*German physician,* 1836–1914]. Known for his description of a position taken by the patient on the operating table in which he is dorsally recumbent, the head being over the end of the table in full extension; the object is to prevent body fluids from entering the trachea during operation upon the mouth and fauces, called *Rose's position.*

Rose, William [*English surgeon,* 1847–1910]. Devised various operations for harelip, called *Rose's operations.*

rose [L. *rosa*]. Any plant or flower of the genus *Rosa.*

attar of r. Rose oil.

cabbage r. See pale *r.*

cottage r. *R. alba;* a source of rose oil.

damask r. *R. damascena;* a source of rose oil.

dog r. *R. canina.* See *rose hips.*

French r. *R. gallica* or red rose.

pale r. *R. centifolia,* whose fragrant petals are used in cosmetics and as a flavoring agent.

red r. *R. gallica.* The dried petals are used as a flavoring agent and perfume.

r. oil (*oleum rosae*). The volatile oil distilled with steam from the fresh flowers of *R. gallica, R. damascena, R. alba,* and *R. centifolia,* and varieties of these species. A perfume and flavoring agent. Also called *otto of r., attar of r.*

r. water (*aqua rosae*). A freshly prepared mixture of equal parts of stronger rose water and distilled water used as a vehicle.

r. water ointment (*unguentum aquae rosae*). A popular emollient and vehicle sometimes referred to as cold cream; it contains spermaceti, white wax, expressed almond or persic oil, sodium borate, rose oil, rose water, and water.

stronger r. water (*aqua rosae fortior*). A saturated solution of the odorous principles of *R. centifolia* flowers; prepared by distillation.

rose ben′gal (beng′gawl, ben′gawl) (C.C.). Dichlortetraiodofluorescein, or tetrachlortetraiodofluorescein, used as a bacterial stain. The rate of disappearance of the dye from the blood stream following its intravenous administration is a test of liver function.

rose cold. An allergic manifestation due to sensitivity to rose pollens. It is a form of hay fever.

rose fe′ver. A form of hay fever.

rose hips. The ripe fruit of the dog rose, *Rosa canina;* contains invert sugar combined with citric and malic acids, salts of these acids, a considerable amount of ascorbic acid and a trace of tannin: used for making pill masses. A syrup of rose hips has been used in vitamin-C therapy.

ro′se·in (ro′zee·in, roz′ee·in), **ro′se·ine** (ro′zee·een, ·in, roz′ee·). Fuchsin.

ro·sel′la (ro·sell′uh). See *rubella.*

rose′mar″y [L. *rosmarinus*, rosemary]. *Rosmarinus officinalis*, a plant of the Labiatae.

r. oil. The volatile oil distilled with steam from the fresh flowering tops of rosemary. Contains at least 1.5% of esters calculated as bornyl acetate and 10% of total borneol, free and as esters. Used as a carminative and in rubefacient liniments. Dose, 0.2–0.4 cc. (3–6 min.).

Rosenau, Milton Joseph [*American pathologist and hygienist*, 1869–1946]. Known for his many contributions to the knowledge of epidemiology and public health.

Rosenbach, Anton Julius Friedrich [*German physician and bacteriologist*, 1842–1923]. Noted for his studies in wound infection (1884) in which he isolated causative organisms. Erysipeloid is sometimes known as *Rosenbach's disease.*

Rosenbach, Ottomar [*German physician*, 1851–1907]. Heberden's disease, or nodes, are also called *Rosenbach's disease* or *nodes.* Enunciated a law that, in lesions of the nerve centers or trunks, paralysis starts in the extensor before it starts in the flexor muscles; called *Rosenbach's law.* Described a number of signs found in neurasthenia and goiter. See also Rosenbach's *test.*

Rosenheim bismuth test. See under *test.*

Rosenheim's iodopotassium iodide solution. See under *solution.*

Rosenmueller, Johann Christian [*German anatomist*, 1771–1826]. Described the parovarium, also called *organ of Rosenmueller*, and the palpebral portion of the lacrimal gland, called *Rosenmueller's gland.* A lymph node in the femoral ring is also called *Rosenmueller's gland.* See also lateral pharyngeal *fossa*, called *Rosenmueller's fossa* or *recess.*

Rosenow, Edward Carl [*American bacteriologist*, 1875–]. Introduced a staining technic for demonstrating bacterial capsules, consisting of successive applications of tannic acid solution, gentian violet, Lugol's solution, alcohol and eosin solution. Called *Rosenow's method.*

Rosenthal, Friedrich Christian [*German anatomist*, 1780–1829]. Described the basal cerebral vein, also called *Rosenthal's vein.*

Rosenthal, Isidor [*German physiologist*, 1836–1915]. Described the spiral canal of the cochlea, also called *Rosenthal's canal.*

Rosenthal-Rowntree test. See under *test.*

ro·se′o·la (ro·zee′o·luh) [L. *roseus*, rosy]. 1. A name given to any rose-colored eruption. 2. See *rubella.*

epidemic r. Rubella.

r. cholerica. An eruption sometimes appearing in cholera.

r. infantum. See *exanthema* subitum.

r. scarlatiniforme. See *erythema* scarlatiniforme.

r. syphilitica. An eruption of rose-colored spots appearing early in secondary syphilis.

r. typhosa. The eruption of typhoid or typhus fever.

r. vaccinia. A general rose-colored eruption occurring about ten days after vaccination. It is of short duration.

ro·se′o·lous (ro·zee′o·lus) [*roseus*]. Having the character of roseola.

ro″se·o·thri′cin. An antibiotic substance, similar to streptothricin, obtained from *Streptomyces roseochromogenus.*

Roser, Wilhelm [*German surgeon*, 1817–88]. Described a sign indicative of cerebral lesion or tumor, in which pulsation of the dura mater is absent; called *Roser's* or *Roser-Braun's sign.*

ro·sette′ (ro·zet′) [F.]. 1. Groups of cells from the neuroepithelial layer of the retina described by Wintersteiner as a characteristic of glioma of the retina. They correspond to the external limiting membrane of the retina, with rudimentary rods and cones projecting into the central cavity. 2. A spherical group of fine red vacuoles surrounding the cytocentrum of monocytes, which can be seen after supravital staining.

ros′in (roz′in) [L. *resina*, resin] (*resina*). The residue left after the volatile oil is distilled from turpentine. It consists chiefly of various modifications of anhydrides of abietic acid with varying quantities of hydrocarbons. Also called *colophony.*

compound r. cerate (*ceratum resinae compositum*). Consists of 23% of rosin and 12% of turpentine in a base of yellow wax, prepared suet, and linseed oil. Also called *Deshler's salve.*

r. cerate (*ceratum resinae*). Consists of 35% of rosin in a base of yellow wax and lard. Also called *resin cerate, basilicon ointment.*

ro·sol′ic ac′id (ro·zol′ick, ·sol′ick). A mixture of triphenylmethane derivatives occurring as a reddish brown powder with green luster. Insoluble in water, soluble in alcohol. An acid-base indicator. Also called *aurin, corallin.*

Ross, Edward Halford [*English pathologist*, 1875–1928]. Described *Lymphocytozoon pallidum*, small, round bodies found in the blood and tissue fluids in syphilis. They are copper colored, with dark granules, and sometimes exhibit ameboid movements. Called *Ross's bodies.*

Ross, Hugh Campbell [*English pathologist*, 1875–1926]. Introduced a test for syphilis using an agar solution, Unna's polychrome blue, sodium bicarbonate, and sterile water. When a thin film of this is spread on a slide and allowed to solidify, the material under question is dropped gently on to it. If the test is positive, the spirochetes will stain. Called *Ross test.*

Ross, Philip Hedgeland [*English physician*, 1876–1929]. With A. D. Milne, discovered the cause of African tick (relapsing) fever (1904).

Ross, Ronald [*English pathologist and parasitologist*, 1857–1932]. First demonstrated that the mosquito is responsible for the transmission of malaria. Studied the life cycle of the malarial parasite; see exogenous *cycle.* Nobel laureate (1902).

Ross's in vitro method. A method of microscopical study of phenomena of living cells, on glass slides covered with nutrient jelly.

Ross-Jones test. See under *test.*

Rossbach, Michael Joseph [*German physician*, 1842–94]. Described a neurosis of the stomach attended by hyperchlorhydria; formerly called *Rossbach's disease, gastroxynsis.*

Rossman, Isadore [*American physician*, 1913–]. Developed a fixative consisting of one part neutral formalin in nine parts of saturated picric acid in absolute alcohol, used for the fixation of glycogen in tissues. Called *Rossman's fluid.*

Rossolimo's reflex. See under *reflex.*

Rostan, Léon [*French physician,* 1790–1866]. Remembered for his early description of cardiac asthma (1817), also called *Rostan's asthma.*

ros·tel'lum [L., little beak]. A little beak, especially the hook-bearing portion of the head of certain worms.

ros'tra. Plural of rostrum.

ros'tral [L. *rostrum,* beak]. 1. Pertaining to, or resembling, a rostrum. 2. Cephalic.

ros'trum (pl. *rostra*) [L.]. A beak; a projection or ridge.

r. corporis callosi. The anterior tapering portion of the corpus callosum.

r. sphenoidale. The vertical ridge on the inferior aspect of the body of the sphenoid bone, which is received in the upper grooved border of the vomer.

rot [AS. *rotian*]. 1. Putrefactive fermentation; decay; decomposition. 2. A disease of the feet of sheep in which the hoofs are destroyed. —**rot,** *v.*

grinder's r. Fibrosis of the lungs occurring in grinders, especially knife grinders. Also called *grinder's asthma.*

jungle r. See *jungle rot.*

liver r. See *fascioliasis.*

ro'ta·me"ter [L. *rota,* wheel; *metron,* a measure]. A device for the measurement of mean blood flow in arteries or veins.

ro'tate [L. *rotare,* to swing around]. Wheel-shaped.

ro'ta·ting (ro'tay·ting) [*rotare*]. Revolving, as rotating devices, appliances for correcting torsion of teeth.

ro·ta'tion [L. *rotatio,* from *rotare*]. 1. The act of turning about an axis passing through the center of a body, as rotation of the eye, rotation of the head. 2. *In dentistry,* the operation by which a malturned tooth is turned or twisted into its normal position. 3. The phenomenon whereby every third or fourth impulse is carried over the cochlear nerve when the exciting impulse is above 1800 cycles. See *alternation,* 2. 4. *In obstetrics,* one of the stages of labor, consisting in a rotary movement of the fetal head or other presenting part, whereby it is accommodated to the birth canal. It may be internal, occurring before the birth of the presenting part, or external, occurring afterward. See Plate 42.

optical r. (a) Optical activity. (b) The number of degrees of rotation of the plane of vibration of polarized light produced by the substance under examination.

specific r. The optical rotation, expressed in angular degrees, of a solution representing 1 Gm. of solute in 1 cc. of solution, and referred to a tube 1 decimeter in length.

wheel r. Helmholtz's method, the tilting of the vertical meridians of the eye.

ro·ta'tion ther'a·py. Radiation therapy during which either the patient is rotated before the source of radiation or the source is revolved around the patient, thereby providing a larger dose of radiation at the center of rotation than on any area of the skin.

ro·ta·to'res. Small deep muscles of the back which extend and rotate the vertebrae, sometimes divided into rotatores breves and longi, depending on their length.

r. spinae. The rotatores muscles.

ro·ta·to'ri·a. See cursive *epilepsy.*

Rotch, Thomas Morgan [*American pediatrician,* 1848–1914]. Widely known in his time for his introduction of percentage modification of milk (protein, fat, and carbohydrate) for individual infant feeding; called *Rotch's method.* See also Rotch's *sign.*

ro'te·none (ro'ti·nohn, rot'i·nohn). $C_{23}H_{22}O_6$. An insecticidal principle derived from derris root and other plant roots; insoluble in water, soluble in ether. Harmless to birds and mammals.

Roth, Moritz [*Swiss physician,* 1839–1914]. Described an inconstant diverticulum of the middle portion of the rete testis; called *Roth's vas aberrans.* Also described white spots on the retina seen in septic retinitis; called *Roth's spots.*

Roth's disease. See *meralgia* paresthetica, also called *Roth-Bernhardt disease.*

Roth's method. See under *method.*

Rothberg-Evans sugar tube. A tube similar to the Folin sugar tube, used in sugar determinations.

Rothera's test. See under *test.*

Rotter, H. [*Hungarian physician,* contemporary]. Introduced a rapid clinical test for vitamin-C deficiency in man, using dichlorophenol-indophenol sodium injected intradermally. If decolorization does not occur within ten minutes, a deficiency may be assumed. Called *Rotter's test.*

rot'tler·a (rot'lur·uh). See *kamala.*

rot'tler·in. A bitter principle from kamala; used as an anthelmintic.

Rouelle, Hilaire Marie [*French pharmacologist,* 1718–79]. Discovered urea (1773).

Rouget, Charles Marie Benjamin [*French physiologist,* 1824–1904]. Described contractile cells on the walls of the capillaries of the frog and salamander; called *Rouget cells.*

rough'age [AS. *rūh*]. Food residue in the colon, usually composed for the most part of cellulose.

Rougnon de Magny, Nicolas François [*French physician,* 1727–99]. Described what appears to have been angina pectoris (1768). Heberden reported and described the disease at the same time, giving it the name, but published only in 1772. Angina pectoris was formerly called *Rougnon-Heberden's disease.*

rou·leau' (roo·lo') [F.]. A roll of red blood cells resembling a roll of coins.

round shoul'ders. Faulty posture in which dropping of the shoulders and increased convexity of the thoracic spine are conspicuous, the postural abnormalities not being limited to the shoulder girdle and chest.

round'worm" [L. *rotundus;* AS. *wyrm*]. A worm of the order Nematoda.

roup (ro͞op) [probably imitative in origin]. An infectious disease of fowls characterized by inflammation of the upper air passages and sinusitis.

Rous, Francis Peyton [*American physician,* 1879–]. Known for his experimental work on the virus causation of tumors; a chicken sarcoma is called *Rous tumor* or *sarcoma.*

Roussy, Gustave [*French pathologist,* 1874–1948]. Known for his description, with J. J. Dejerine, of the thalamic syndrome (1906). He also described dermatofibrosarcoma, a tumor of the skin occurring singly or as multiple nodules, with a wide variation in malignancy, called *Darier-Roussy sarcoid.* See also Lévy-Roussy *syndrome.*

Roux, César [*Swiss surgeon,* 1857–1926]. Developed an operation for excision of the esophagus for carcinoma, in which he performed esophagojejunogastroanastomosis in stages; called *Roux's operation.* Introduced an operation for gastroenterostomy "en Y," the jejunum being divided, the distal end anastomosed to the side of the stomach, and the proximal end to the side of the jejunum at a lower level; called *Roux's gastroenterostomy.*

Roux, Jules [*French surgeon,* 1807–77]. Devised an operation for exstrophy of the bladder, in which he made a closure by means of flaps, one dissected from the abdomen above and another from the scrotum below; called *Roux's operation.*

Roux, Pierre Paul Emile [*French bacteriologist,* 1853–1933]. Co-worker with Pasteur in many of his studies of the bacterial cause of disease. With Pasteur and Chamberland, demonstrated the rabies virus in the blood (1884). With Yersin, proved the existence of a soluble diphtheria toxin by passing the culture through a porcelain filter (1888). Developed an antitetanic serum known as *Roux's serum.* With Nocard, published an early study on filtrable viruses (1898). Also see Elie *Metchnikoff.*

Rovsing, Niels Thorkild [*Danish surgeon,* 1862–1927]. Described a sign said to be of value in the diagnosis of acute appendicitis: pressure on the ascending colon on a level with McBurney's point elicits pain at the point; called *Rovsing's sign.*

Rowe, Albert Holmes (1889–). American physician and author of books on allergy, particularly food allergy; he instituted a regimen of elimination diets for the study of food allergy, called *Rowe elimination diets.*

row'ing meth'od. See under *artificial respiration.*

Rowntree, Leonard George [*American internist,* 1883–]. With J. T. Geraghty, introduced the phenolsulfonphthalein test for kidney function (1910); called *Rowntree-Geraghty test.* See also *Rosenthal-Rowntree test* (*for liver function*) under *test.* With Geraghty and N. M. Keith, introduced a method of estimating the blood and plasma volume (1915).

roxenol. A trade-mark for the British Pharmacopoeia solution of chloroxylenol.

R. Q. Respiratory quotient.

-rrha'gi·a [G. *rhēgnynai,* to burst forth]. *In medicine,* a combining form signifying *abnormal* or *excessive discharge.*

-rrha'phy. *In surgery,* a combining form meaning a sewing or suturing, usually of an immediate or recent injury or laceration.

R. S. A. Right sacroanterior position of the fetus.

R. S. P. Right sacroposterior position of the fetus.

R. T. Registered technician; certificate awarded to qualified x-ray technicians by the American Registry of X-Ray Technicians.

Ru Chemical symbol for ruthenium.

rub'ber [ME. *rubben*]. The *elastica* of the U.S.P. The prepared milk juice of several species of *Hevea.* Also called *caoutchouc, India rubber, Pará rubber.*

ru·be'do [L., redness]. Any diffuse redness of the skin.

ru"be·fa'cient (rōō"bi·fay'shunt) [L. *rubefacere,* to make red]. Causing redness of the skin. —**rubefa'cient,** *n.*

ru"be·fac'tion [*rubefacere*]. 1. Redness of the skin due to the action of an irritant. 2. The act of causing redness of the skin.

ru·bel'la [L. *rubellus,* reddish]. German measles. An acute, contagious, eruptive disease, of short duration and mild character. After a period of incubation varying from one to three weeks, the disease sets in abruptly with sore throat and slight fever. The eruption appears at the end of the first day, and consists of red maculopapular lesions, and disappears usually without desquamation in about three days. The disease is associated with enlargement of the superficial cervical and posterior auricular lymph nodes. Also called *epidemic roseola, French measles, German measles, rötheln.*

ru·be'o·la, ru"be·o'la. See *measles.*

ru·be'o·lin. A name given to the so-called specific toxin of measles.

ru"be·o'sis i'rid·is. Increased vascularization of the iris, seen most often in diabetes mellitus. Such an iris appears grossly pink to reddish.

ru'ber [L.]. Red.

ru·be·ryth'ric ac'id. $C_{25}H_{26}O_{13}$; a glycosidal constituent of the root of madder which yields on hydrolysis alizarin and dextrose. Syn., *rubianic acid.*

ru·bes'cence [L. *rubescere,* to grow red]. The state or quality of redness; a flushed or blushing countenance. —**rubescent,** *adj.*

ru'bi·a [L., madder]. The *Rubia tinctorum* or dyers' madder, containing the coloring principles alizarin and purpurin; used as a dye.

ru"bi·an'ic ac'id. Ruberythric acid.

ru·bid'i·um [L. *rubidus,* red]. Rb = 85.48. An alkali metal resembling potassium in appearance. It reacts violently with water and is kept under a liquid hydrocarbon. Used in photoelectric cells.

r. bromide. RbBr. A colorless, crystalline, soluble powder; has been used like potassium bromide.

r. iodide. RbI. White, crystalline, very soluble powder; has been used like potassium iodide.

ru·big'i·nous (rōō·bidj'i·nus) [L. *rubigo,* rust]. Rust-colored.

ru"bi·jer'vine. An alkaloidal constituent, being an alkanolamine, of veratrum viride and veratrum album; it is practically inert physiologically.

Rubin, Isidor Clinton (1883–). American gynecologist, known for his test for the patency of the uterine tubes (1919). See tubal *insufflation.*

ru'bin. Basic fuchsin.

Rubner, Max [*German physiologist,* 1854–1932]. Known for his investigations on the metabolism of foods (1902). With O. J. L. Heubner, determined the caloric requirements of infants. Introduced a test for lactose in the urine, called *Rubner's test.* Enunciated two laws, each called *Rubner's law:* (a) The law of constant energy consumption states that the rapidity of growth is proportional to the intensity of the metabolic process. (b) The law of constant growth quotient states that the same fractional part of the entire energy is used for growth: most young mammals use approximately 34% and an adult man about 4%. Found that metabolism is proportional to body area.

ru'bor [L.]. Redness due to inflammation.

ru·bres'e·rine (rōō·bress'ur·een, ·in, rōō"bri·seer'·een, ·in). A red decomposition product of physostigmine; it accounts for part of the color which develops in physostigmine solutions on aging and indicates a decrease in potency.

ru'bri·blast [L. *ruber,* red; G. *blastos,* germ]. A cell, in the earliest stage of formation of red blood cells, in which the chromatin is fine and stippled. Nucleoli are usually present. See *proerythroblast, erythroblast.*

ru'bri·cyte [*ruber;* G. *kytos,* cell]. A cell, in the formative stages of red blood cells, with a definite chromatin pattern, but no nucleolus. See *erythroblast, normoblast.*

ru"bro·sta'sis. See under *peristasis.*

ru'brum scar"la·ti'num [L.]. Scarlet red.

ruc·ta'tion [L. *ructatio,* belching]. Eructation; belching.

ruc'tus [L., belching]. A belching of gas from the stomach.

r. hystericus. Hysteric belching, the gas escaping with a loud, sobbing, gurgling noise.

Rudbeck, Olof [*Swedish anatomist,* 1630–1702]. Discovered the intestinal lymphatics and their connection with the thoracic duct (1653). Prior discovery was also claimed by Thomas Bartholin who was certainly the first to appreciate the significance of the lymph system as a whole.

ru'di·ment [L. *rudimentum,* first trial]. That which is but partially developed. —**rudimen'tary,** *adj.*

amnioembryonic r. The inner cell mass of the early blastocyst from which the amnion and the blastoderm differentiate. Also called *intrachorionic r.*

ru"di·men'ta·ry [*rudimentum*]. Undeveloped; unfinished; incomplete.

ru"di·men'tum (pl. *rudimenta*) [L.]. A rudiment.

rue [L. *ruta*, rue]. A plant, *Ruta graveolens*, of the family Rutaceae, yielding a volatile oil consisting chiefly of methyl-nonyl-ketone, $CH_3.CO.C_9H_{19}$, and acting as a potent local irritant.

Ruffini, Angelo [*Italian anatomist*, 1864–1929]. Author of important studies on gastrulation. Described nerve endings in the subcutaneous tissue of the fingers, made up of terminal arborization of one or more nerve fibers within a fibrous framework, called *Ruffini's corpuscle, end organ, cell.*

ru'fous [L. *rufus*, red]. Reddish; ruddy.

Rufus' pill. A pill of aloes and myrrh.

ru'ga (pl. *rugae*) [L.]. A wrinkle, fold, elevation, or ridge, as in the mucosa of the stomach, vagina, and palate.

rugar. Trade-mark for a radiopaque medium containing chiefly barium sulfate.

Ruggi, Giuseppe [*Italian surgeon*, 1844–1925]. Described an operation for radical cure of femoral hernia using the inguinal approach (1893). Used sympathectomy for cure of pelvic pain.

ru·gi'tus (rōō·jye'tus, rōō'ji·tus) [L., rumbling]. Rumbling of the intestines.

ru'gose, ru·gose' [L. *rugosus*, wrinkled]. Characterized by many folds.

ru·gos'i·ty [L. *rugositas*, the state of being wrinkled]. A condition exhibiting many folds in a tissue or integument.

ru'gous. See *rugose.*

Ruhmkorff, Heinrich Daniel [*German physicist*, 1823–87]. Invented an induction coil in which the secondary coil is fixed at the point of maximum intensity; called *Ruhmkorff's coil.*

rule [L. *regula*, a model]. An established guide for action or procedure.

Goodsall's r. *In proctology*, fistulas with external openings in the posterior half of the perianal area have their primary opening in the posterior half of the anus, usually at or near the posterior commissure; fistulas with external openings in the anterior perineum usually have their primary opening in the anterior quadrant of the anus.

Haase's r. A clinical rule for the approximation of crown-heel length of the fetus in centimeters by the use of the lunar month of gestation, and vice versa. Calculated by squaring the lunar month through 5 months (e.g., $5 \times 5 = 25$ cm) or taking the square root of length up to 25 cm ($\sqrt{25} = 5$ lunar mo.), and thereafter multiplying the lunar month by 5 (e.g., $7 \times 5 = 35$ cm) or dividing length by 5 (35 cm $\div$ 5 = 7 lunar mo.).

Hardy-Schulze r. The higher the valence, the greater the coagulating effect of added ions of charge opposite to that of the suspended particles of a colloidal system.

r. of nines. A rule for the estimate of the percentage of body surface according to which the head and upper extremities each represent 9%, the trunk, anterior and posterior, and the lower extremities, each 18%, and the perineum 1%. It is of particular usefulness in judging the severity and extent of burns; in second or third degree burns, involvement of 15% of body surface may produce shock in adults, or of 10% in children.

Traube's r. The extent to which members of a homologous series are adsorbed from aqueous solution increases as the number of CH_2 groups in the molecule increases or as the molecular weight increases.

Young's r. Child's dose (for children over 2 years of age) $= \frac{\text{lbs. body weight} \times \text{adult dose}}{\text{age} + 12}$. See also Thomas *Young.*

rum'bling. See *borborygmus.*

ru'men [L., gullet]. First compartment of the stomach of the ruminant, where food is temporarily stored while undergoing fermentation prior to regurgitation and remastication. Also called *paunch.*

ru"men·ot'o·my [*rumen;* G. *tomē*, a cutting]. A laparotomy operation in which the rumen is exposed and incised for the correction of certain diseases of the organ.

Ru'mex [L., sorrel]. A genus of plants of the Polygonaceae. Yellow dock, the root of **R. crispus,** is a mild laxative and astringent.

ru'mi·nant [L. *ruminare*, to chew over again]. One of an order of animals possessing an arrangement of the fore-stomach whereby food is regurgitated and remasticated. An animal which chews the cud.

ru"mi·na'tion [L. *ruminatio*, from *ruminare*]. 1. A characteristic of ruminants in which food is regurgitated and remasticated in preparation for true digestion. Syn., *merycism.* 2 *In psychiatry*, an obsessional preoccupation with a single idea or system of ideas which dominates the mind despite all efforts to dislodge it. Observed in anxiety states and in psychasthenia.

Rummo, Gaetano [*Italian physician*, 1853–1917]. Described cardioptosis or drop heart (1898); also called *Rummo's disease.*

rump [ME. *rumpe*]. The region near the end of the backbone; the buttocks or nates.

Rumpel, Theodor [*German physician*, 1862–1923]. Described a sign observed in scarlet fever and some other exanthemas, consisting of petechiae following the application of constriction applied to the arm. Called *Rumpel-Leede sign, phenomenon.*

run [AS. *rinnan*]. To discharge, as pus or purulent matter from a diseased part.

run'-a·round". A paronychia extending completely around a nail.

Ruotte's operation. Venoperitoneostomy.

ru'pi·a [G. *rhypos*, filth]. A form of eruption characterized by the formation of large, dirty-brown, stratified, conic crusts, that resemble oyster shell; commonly, a type of eruption seen in syphilis. —**rupial,** *adj.*

ru"po·pho'bi·a. See *rhypophobia.*

rup'ti·o (rup'shee·o) [L., a breaking]. Rupture of a vessel or organ.

rup'ture [L. *ruptura*, a break]. 1. A forcible tearing of a part, as rupture of the uterus, rupture of the urinary bladder. 2. Hernia.

rup'tured [*ruptura*]. Burst; broken; forcibly torn; affected with hernia.

Rush, Benjamin [*American physician*, 1745–1813]. Surgeon of the Continental Army. Described dengue (1780), yellow fever, cholera infantum, and rheumatism. Author of the first American book on psychiatry (1812).

Russell, Frederick Fuller [*American bacteriologist*, 1870–]. Widely known for his work, while a member of the United States Army Medical Corps, in the control of typhoid fever and syphilis. With P. H. Hiss, reported a type of *Shigella paradysenteriae* (1903). See Hiss and Russell's Y *bacillus.*

Russell, Patrick [*Irish physician of the East India Company*, 1727–1805]. Author of a comprehensive work on the venomous serpents of India. See *Russell's viper* under *Viperidae;* also see *Vipera russellii.*

Russell, William (1852–1940). Scottish pathologist who described small, spherical, fuchsinophil bodies found in carcinomatous and other conditions, by some considered to be of etiologic significance, and called *Russell's bodies, Unna bodies* or *cells.*

Russell's method. See Frame, Russell, and Wilhelmi's *method.*

Rus'sian in"ter·mit'tent fe'ver. See trench *fever.*

Rust, Johann Nepomuk [*German physician,* 1755–1840]. Described tuberculous spondylitis of the cervical region (1834); also called *Rust's disease.* See also Rust's *phenomenon.*

rust [AS. *rūst*]. 1. A product consisting of the oxide, hydroxide, and carbonate of iron, formed on the surface of iron exposed to moist air. 2. A group of parasitic fungi (Uredinales) causing discoloration on plants. They are common allergens.

rut [L. *rugitus,* roaring]. 1. A period of heightened sexual excitement and its accompanying behavior in males, especially that occurring annually in wild ungulates. 2. In loose usage, heat; estrus.

Ru·ta'ce·ae (roo·tay'see·ee) [L. *ruta,* rue]. A family including herbs, trees, and shrubs. The genus *Citrus* belongs to this group.

ru"te·car'pine. $C_{18}H_{13}N_3O$; an alkaloid from the fruit of *Evodia rutaecarpa,* also synthesized. It causes increased arterial pressure. Also written *rutaecarpine.*

Rut'gers 612. Ethohexadiol.

Ruth, Charles Edward [*American surgeon,* 1861–1930]. Devised a method of reduction of fracture of the femoral neck, a modification of the Leadbetter method using outward traction on the thigh by an assistant. Called *Ruth's method.*

ru·the'ni·um [ML. *Ruthenia,* Russia]. Ru = 101.1. A rare metal of the platinum group.

r. chloride. $RuCl_3$. Brownish red, deliquescent crystals.

r. red. Ammoniated ruthenium oxychloride. Brownish red powder used in microscopy as a stain and as a reagent for pectin and gum.

Rutherford, Daniel [*Scottish physicist,* 1749–1819]. Discoverer of nitrogen (1772).

Rutherford, Ernest [*English physicist,* 1871–1937]. Known for atomic research and investigations into radioactivity. Nobel laureate (1908).

ruth'er·ford (ruth'ur·furd) [after *E. Rutherford*]. A unit of radioactivity representing 10^6 disintegrations per second. Abbreviated, rd.

ru'tin. $C_{27}H_{30}O_{16}.3H_2O$. A rhamno-glycoside of quercetin which occurs in several plants; occurs as a bright yellow powder; it is difficultly soluble in water and insoluble in ether and chloroform; it is soluble in alcohol and alkalies. It has the property, in certain cases, of decreasing capillary fragility in cases of increased fragility. Dose, 20 mg., (⅓ gr.) t.i.d. Also called *eldrin, melin, myrticolorin, osyritin, phytomelin, violaquercitrin.*

ru'tin·ose. $C_{12}H_{22}H_{10}$. A disaccharide produced by enzymatic or controlled acid hydrolysis of rutin or hesperidin. Rutinose yields one molecule each of glucose and rhamnose on hydrolysis.

rutonal. Trade-mark for 5-methyl-5-phenylbarbituric acid; $C_{11}H_{10}N_2O_3$: recommended as a sedative and hypnotic.

Ruttan and Hardisty's test. See under *test.*

Ruysch, Frederik [*Dutch anatomist,* 1638–1731]. Described a minute tubular cavity in the nasal septum in front of the incisive canal, called *Ruysch's tube;* later called *Jacobsen's organ.*

Ry·a'ni·a. A genus of tropical American shrubs and trees, of which the wood of several species is insecticidal.

ry·an'o·dine. An alkaloid, isolated from the stem and root of *Ryania speciosa* Vahl., having a high degree of insecticidal activity.

Rydygier, Ludwig von [*German surgeon,* 1850–1920]. Introduced a method of fixation of the spleen in a peritoneal pouch, called *Rydygier's operation.*

rye [AS. *ryge*]. The plant *Secale cereale* and its grain. The grain is used for making bread and whisky.

r. smut. Ergot.

spurred r. Ergot.

Rynd, Francis [*Irish physician,* 1801–61]. Inventor of an apparatus for administering fluid by injection into a nerve for the treatment of neuralgia (1845). He is sometimes credited with the invention of the hypodermic syringe.

rythmin. Trade name for a solution of active principles obtained from coral snakes and copperheads, intended for use as an anticonvulsant in epilepsy and other disorders.

ryzamin-B. A proprietary rice-polishings concentrate in syrup form used in vitamin-B_1 therapy.

S

S 1. Chemical symbol for sulfur. 2. *In electrocardiography,* abbreviation for spatial vector: also written $\hat{S}$.

S. 1. Abbreviation for *signa,* sign; used in prescriptions to mean "write." 2. Abbreviation for spherical or spherical lens.

$\hat{S}$ See *S,* 2.

s. 1. *Sinister,* left. 2. *Semis,* half.

S.A. Sinoatrial.

Sa Chemical symbol for samarium.

Saathoff method. See Pappenheim-Saathoff methyl green-pyronin *stain.*

sab"a·dil'la [Sp. *cebadilla,* from *cebada,* barley]. The dried ripe seeds of *Schoenocaulon officinale* (*Asagraea officinalis*). Contains the alkaloids cevadine (crystallized veratrine), cevine (sabadinine), veratridine (amorphous veratrine), cevadilline (sabadilline), and sabadine. An acrid, drastic emetocathartic; formerly used as a taeniacide and to destroy vermin in the hair. Syn., *cevadilla.*

sa·bad'i·nine (sa·bad'i·neen, ·nin). See *cevine.*

sab'al, sa'bal. See *serenoa.*

Sabaneev, I. F. [*Russian surgeon,* nineteenth century]. Remembered for his operation of gastrostomy. He made an incision five inches long through the middle of the left rectus muscle, a second incision one or two inches long being placed at the same time through the skin just above the left costal margin in the midclavicular line, the two being connected subcutaneously. The anterior stomach wall was drawn out through the smaller incision after being passed through the larger one. It was attached to the skin by sutures, a purse string suture placed in the cone of the stomach wall, and an opening made to admit a catheter. The latter was transfixed and sutured securely to the stomach. This is similar to the operation devised by Frank and is also called *Sabaneev-Frank operation.*

Sab·ba'ti·a (sa·bay'shee·uh, sa·bat'ee·uh) [NL.,

after Liberatus *Sabbati*, Italian botanist]. A genus of the Gentianaceae.

S. angularis. The American centaury; has been used as a febrifuge.

sab′ba·tin. A glycoside obtained from *Sabbatia elliottii*, quinine flower; has been used as an antiperiodic and antipyretic.

Sa″be·thi′ni. Mosquitoes of a tribe of Diptera known to transmit jungle yellow fever.

Sabin, Albert Bruce [*American bacteriologist*, 1906–]. Introduced a method of typing pneumococcus, called *Sabin's rapid method, agglutination method.*

Sabin, Florence Rena (1871–1953). American anatomist who investigated the embryological origin of blood vessels and lymphatics, and living human blood cells and their development.

Sabouraud, Raymond Jacques Adrien [*French dermatologist*, 1864–1938]. Known for his study of fungi (1894). Cultivated the acne bacillus (1897). Contributed to knowledge of *Trichophyton* and introduced the treatment of ringworm by radiology (1904); called *Sabouraud's method.* He prepared a nutrient agar containing peptone and maltose, called *French proof*, or *Sabouraud's agar.*

sab′u·lous [L. *sabulum*, coarse sand]. Gritty; sandy.

sac [L. *saccus*, from G. *sakkos*, sack]. A pouch; a baglike covering of a natural cavity, hernia, cyst, or tumor.

air s. Old term for pulmonary alveolus.

allantoic s. The distal enlarged part of the allantois, especially in Sauropsida. Also called *allantoic vesicle.*

alveolar s. A terminal group of pulmonary alveoli; one of the branches of an alveolar duct.

amniotic s. The amnion.

aortic s. The saclike dilatation distal to the bulbus arteriosus from which the aortic arches arise, more or less comparable to a ventral aorta.

conjunctival s. That formed by reflection of the palpebral conjunctiva.

dental s. The connective tissue that encloses the developing tooth. Also called *dental follicle.*

endolymphatic s. The bulblike terminal enlargement of the endolymphatic duct.

greater s. The peritoneum forming the main peritoneal cavity.

hernial s. The pouch or protrusion of peritoneum containing a herniated organ or part, formed gradually by pressure against a defect in the containing wall or present at birth.

lacrimal s. The dilated upper portion of the nasolacrimal duct. See Plate 19.

lesser s. The omental bursa; that part of the peritoneal sac located behind the stomach, lesser omentum, and the caudal lobe of the liver and within the greater omentum; it communicates with the greater sac through the epiploic foramen.

olfactory sacs. The deepened olfactory pits extending from the embryonic nares to the bucconasal membranes.

omental s. The sac formed between the ascending and descending portions of the greater omentum.

otic s. The auditory vesicle.

pericardial s. That formed by the pericardium. Also called *heart s.*

peritoneal s. That formed by the peritoneum.

pleural s. That formed by the pleura.

tooth s. See dental *s.*

vaginal s. Vaginal process of the peritoneum.

vitelline s. Yolk sac.

yolk s. An extraembryonic membrane composed of endoderm and splanchnic mesoderm enclosing the yolk mass in reptiles, birds, and monotremes, or a cavity in higher mammals. Also called *umbilical vesicle, saccus omphaloentericus.*

sac′cha·rase (sack′uh·race, ·raze) [G. *sakchar*, sugar, from the Sanskrit]. An enzyme occurring in plants and microorganisms, particularly yeasts, and capable of hydrolyzing disaccharides to monosaccharides; more specifically the enzyme which is responsible for hydrolysis of sucrose to dextrose and levulose. Also called *invertase, invertin, sucrase, β-h-fructosidase.*

sac′cha·rate (sack′uh·rate) [*sakchar*]. A salt of saccharic acid.

sac′cha·ra″ted [*sakchar*]. Containing sugar.

s. ferric oxide (*ferri oxidum saccharatum*). Each 100 Gm. contains the equivalent of 3 Gm. of iron. Used as a mild chalybeate. Dose, 2 Gm. (30 gr.). Also called *soluble ferric oxide, eisenzucker.*

s. ferrous carbonate (*ferri carbonas saccharatus*). A light, olive-gray, odorless powder, containing 15 Gm. of ferrous carbonate in each 100 Gm. The oxidation of the ferrous carbonate is materially reduced by the presence of sugar. Used as a source of iron in the treatment of anemia. Dose, 0.6–2 Gm. (10–30 gr.).

s. pepsin. Contains 10% pepsin and 90% lactose.

sac″char·eph″i·dro′sis [*sakchar*; G. *ephidrōsis*, superficial perspiration]. A form of hyperhidrosis, characterized by the excretion of sugar in the sweat.

sac·char′ic ac′id (sa·kar′ick). 1. A product obtained by oxidizing an aldose with nitric acid so that both the aldehyde and primary alcohol groups are converted to carboxyl groups. 2. COOH.HCOH.HOCH.HCOH.HCOH.COOH; the saccharic acid obtained by oxidation of D-glucose with nitric acid. Syn., *D-glucosaccharic acid.*

sac′cha·ride [*sakchar*]. A compound of a base with sugar. A sucrate.

sac·char″i·fi·ca′tion [*sakchar*; L. *facere*, to make]. The act of converting into sugar.

sac·char′i·fy (sa·kar′i·figh) [*sakchar*; *facere*]. 1. Make sweet. 2. Convert into sugar.

sac″cha·rim′e·ter [*sakchar*; G. *metron*, a measure]. An apparatus for determining the amount of sugar in solutions. It may be in the form of a hydrometer, which indicates the strength in sugar by the specific gravity of the solution; a polarimeter, which indicates the strength in sugar by the number of degrees of rotation of the plane of polarization; or a fermentation tube, which indicates the strength in sugar by the amount of gas formed during fermentation.

sac″cha·rim′e·try [*sakchar*; *metron*]. The determination of the optically active sugar content of a solution, from its optical activity.

sac′cha·rin [*sakchar*] (*saccharinum*). $C_7H_5O_3NS$; anhydro-*o*-sulfaminebenzoic acid; occurs as white crystals or a white, crystalline powder; 1 Gm. dissolves in 290 cc. of water and in 31 cc. of alcohol. It is used in medicine as a sweetening agent in diseases such as diabetes and obesity, where sugar is contraindicated; 0.06 Gm. (1 gr.) of saccharin is approximately equal in sweetening power to 30 Gm. of sucrose. Also called *benzosulfimide, gluside, garantose, saccharinol, saccharinose, saccharol, sykose.* See *saxin.* —**sac′charine,** *adj.*

s. sodium (*saccharinum sodicum*). $C_7H_4O_3NSNa.2H_2O$. The sodium salt of saccharin; occurs as white crystals or a white, crystalline powder; 1 Gm. dissolves in about 1.5 cc. of water and in about 50 cc. of alcohol. It is used, like saccharin, as a sweetening agent, but has the advantage of being more freely soluble in water. Also called *soluble saccharin, soluble gluside, sodium benzosulfimide.*

sac′cha·ro- (sack′uh·ro-), **sacchar-** [*sakchar*]. A combining form denoting *sugar* or *saccharine.*

sac″cha·ro·bi′ose. $C_{12}H_{22}O_{11}$. A disaccharide.

sac″cha·ro·ga·lac″tor·rhe′a [*sakchar;* G. *gala*, milk; *rhoia*, flow]. The secretion of milk which contains an excess of sugar.

sac′cha·roids [*sakchar;* G. *eidos*, form]. Sugarlike substances. The term is generally applied to polysaccharides of high molecular weight which do not ferment, but which yield fermentable sugars on hydrolysis.

sac″cha·ro·me·tab′o·lism [*sakchar;* G. *metabolē*, change]. The metabolism of sugar. —**saccharometabol′ic,** *adj.*

sac″cha·rom′e·ter. See *saccharimeter.*

Sac″cha·ro·my′ces (sack″uh·ro·migh′seez) [*sakchar;* G. *mykēs*, fungus]. A genus of yeasts which includes baker's and brewer's yeasts.

S. hominis. Synonym for *Cryptococcus histolyticus.*

sac″cha·ro·my·ce′tic (·migh·see′tick, ·migh·set′-ick) [*sakchar; mykēs*]. Pertaining to, or caused by, *Saccharomyces.*

sac″cha·ro·my·co′sis (sack″uh·ro·migh·ko′sis) [*sakchar; mykēs;* G. *-ōsis*, condition]. A pathologic condition due to yeasts or *Saccharomyces.*

sac″cha·ror·rhe′a [*sakchar;* G. *rhoia*, flow]. Glycosuria.

sac′cha·rose (sack′uh·roce, ·roze) [*sakchar*]. 1. Sucrose, cane sugar. $C_{12}H_{22}O_{11}$. A crystalline carbohydrate occurring in the juice of many plants, chiefly in sugar cane, sugar beets, and some varieties of maple. It is not fermentable without preliminary hydrolysis and does not reduce alkaline copper solutions. 2. A term used in the classification of carbohydrates as: **monosaccharose,** a simple carbohydrate of formula $C_6H_{12}O_6$; **disaccharose,** a carbohydrate of formula $C_{12}H_{22}O_{11}$ formed from two monosaccharose units with the elimination of a molecule of water.

sac″cha·ro·su′ri·a [*sakchar;* G. *ouron*, urine]. The presence of saccharose in the urine.

sac′cha·rum [*sakchar*]. See *sucrose.*

sac′ci·form (sack′si·form) [L. *saccus*, from G. *sakkos*, sack; L. *forma*, form]. Resembling a sac.

sac′cu·lar [L. *sacculus*, little sac]. Sac-shaped.

sac′cu·la″ted [*sacculus*]. Divided into small sacs.

sac″cu·la′tion [*sacculus*]. 1. The state of being sacculated. 2. The formation of small sacs.

sac′cule [*sacculus*]. 1. A small sac. 2. The smaller of two vestibular sacs of the membranous labyrinth of the ear. Also called *sacculus labyrinthi.*

s. of the larynx. A blindly ending diverticulum of mucous membrane extending from the laryngeal ventricle upward between the ventricular fold and the inner surface of the thyroid cartilage. Syn., *appendix of the laryngeal ventricle.*

sac″cu·lo·coch′le·ar (sack″yoo·lo·cock′lee·ur) [*sacculus;* L. *cochlea*, snail]. Relating to the saccule of the vestibule and the cochlea.

sac′cu·lus [L.]. 1. A saccule. 2. The saccule of the vestibule.

sac′cus (pl. *sacci*) [L.]. Sac.

s. endolymphaticus. See endolymphatic *sac.*

s. omphaloentericus. The yolk sac.

s. vaginalis. Vaginal process of the peritoneum.

Sacher-Masoch. See *masochism.*

Sachs, Bernard Parney [*American neurologist*, 1858–1944]. Known for his description of amaurotic familial idiocy (1887).

Sachs, Hans [*German bacteriologist*, 1877–1945]. With Walter Georgi, introduced a variation on the Wassermann test used in the diagnosis of syphilis, known as *Georgi-Sachs reaction* or *test.*

Sacks, Benjamin [*American physician*, 1896–]. With Libman, described a form of nonrheumatic, nonbacterial endocarditis, called *Osler-Libman-Sacks disease* or *syndrome.* See atypical verrucous *endocarditis.*

sa′cra. Plural of sacrum.

sa·cral′gi·a. Pain in the region of the sacrum.

sa″cral·i·za′tion [L. *sacer*, sacred]. Fusion of the sacrum to the fifth lumbar vertebra, leading to proneness to rupture of the disc between the fourth and fifth lumbar vertebrae: formerly called *Bertolloti's syndrome.*

sa·crec′to·my [*sacer;* G. *ektomē*, excision]. Excision of part of the sacrum.

sa′cro- (say′kro-) [*sacer*]. A combining form meaning *relating to the sacrum.*

sa″cro·an·te′ri·or [*sacer;* L. *anterior*, foremost]. A fetal position, with the sacrum directed forward.

sa″cro·coc·cyg′e·al (say″kro·cock·sidj′ee·ul) [*sacer;* G. *kokkyx*, cuckoo]. Pertaining to the sacrum and the coccyx.

sa″cro·coc·cyg′e·us (·cock·sidj′ee·us) [*sacer; kokkyx*]. One of two inconstant thin muscles extending from the lower sacral vertebrae to the coccyx.

s. anterior. That on the anterior surfaces of the sacrum and coccyx, inserted into the anterior sacrococcygeal ligament.

s. posterior. That on the posterior surfaces of the sacrum and coccyx, lying beneath the superficial layer of the sacrotuberous ligament.

sa″cro·cox·al′gi·a. See sacroiliac *disease.*

sa″cro·cox·i′tis. See sacroiliac *disease.*

sa″cro·dyn′i·a (say″kro·din′ee·uh, ·dye′nee·uh) [*sacer;* G. *odynē*, pain]. Pain in the sacrum.

sa″cro·il′i·ac (say″kro·il′ee·ack) [*sacer;* L. *ilium*, flank]. Pertaining to the sacrum and the ilium, as sacroiliac disease. See Table of Joints and Ligaments in the Appendix.

sa″cro·lum·ba′lis. Old name for iliocostalis lumborum muscle.

sa″cro·lum′bar [*sacer;* L. *lumbus*, loin]. Pertaining to the sacrum and the loins. Syn., *lumbosacral.*

sa″cro·pos·te′ri·or [*sacer;* L. *posterior*, that comes after]. A fetal position with the sacrum directed backward.

sa″cro·sci·at′ic (say″kro·sigh·at′ick) [*sacer;* G. *ischiadikos*, of the hips]. Pertaining to the sacrum and the ischium, as the sacrosciatic notch, sacrosciatic ligaments. *O.T.*

sa″cro·spi·na′lis (say″kro·spy·nah′lis, ·nay′lis) [*sacer;* L. *spinalis*, of the spine] [BNA]. A large muscle arising from the posterior aspect of the sacrum and inserted above on the spine and ribs. See Table of Muscles in the Appendix.

sa″cro·u′ter·ine (say″kro·yoo͞′tur·in, ·yne, sack″-ro·) [*sacer;* L. *uterus*, uterus]. Pertaining to the sacrum and the uterus, as sacrouterine ligament, old term for uterosacral ligament.

sa′crum (pl. *sacra*) [*sacer*]. A curved triangular bone composed of five united vertebrae, situated between the last lumbar vertebra above, the coccyx below, and the innominate bones on each side, and forming the posterior boundary of the pelvis. See Table of Bones in the Appendix. See Plates 1, 2, 14. —**sacral,** *adj.*

sac″to·sal′pinx. Hydrosalpinx.

sad′ism, sa′dism [after Count de *Sade*, 1740–1814]. Sexual perversion in which pleasure is derived from inflicting cruelty upon another. —**sadis′tic,** *adj.*

sad′ist, sa′dist [*Sade*]. One affected with sadism.

sad″o·mas′o·chism. The coexistence of sadism and masochism, i.e., both aggressiveness and passivity in social and sexual relationships; a strong tendency to hurt others and to invite being hurt.

Saemisch, Edwin Theodor [*German ophthalmologist*, 1833–1909]. Known for his description of serpiginous corneal ulcer (1870), called *Saemisch's ulcer.* He described vernal conjunctivitis (1876). Introduced an operation for hypopyon ulcer in which he transfixed the cornea and the base of the ulcer, known as *Saemisch's operation.*

Saenger, Max [*German gynecologist,* 1853–1903]. Known for his introduction of the classic, but now obsolete, operation of Cesarean section in which he delivered the uterus through a long abdominal incision, extracting the fetus before returning the uterus to the cavity (1882). Known as *Saenger's operation.* Described his sign of gonorrheal vulvitis, a red spot marking the orifice of the duct of the major vestibular gland.

Safář, Karl [*German ophthalmologist,* contemporary]. Known for his introduction of a method of treating retinal detachment by diathermy, using multiple electrodes (1932).

saf′fron [Ar. *za'farān,* saffron]. Crocus.

saf′ra·nine (saf′ruh·neen, ·nin), **saf′ra·nin** [*za'farān*]. A basic aniline dye of the azine group, used as a biologic stain. The commonest form is **safranin O,** C.C., which is used as a nuclear stain, and as a counterstain in Gram's stain for bacteria.

saf′ra·no·phile (saf′ruh·no·file), **saf′ra·no·phil** (·fill) [*za'farān;* G. *philein,* to love]. Pertaining to tissue elements which stain readily with safranine.

saf′role, saf′rol. $C_{10}H_{10}O_2$; 4-allyl-1,2-methylenedioxybenzene; the preponderant liquid constituent of sassafras oil, present also in other volatile oils.

sa′fu (sah′foo). A reticulated vitiligo of the legs. seen in the Pacific area. Some cases seem to be hereditary.

sage. See *salvia.*

sage′brush″ [L. *salvia,* sage; OF. *broche*]. Any of several members of the genus *Artemisia;* its pollen is among the more important causes of hay fever in the Mountain and Pacific States.

sage femme (sahzh fahm′· *See* Notes §§ 21, 35) [F.]. A midwife.

sag′it·tal (sadj′i·tul) [L. *sagitta,* arrow]. 1. Arrow-like, as the sagittal suture of the skull. 2. Pertaining to the anteroposterior median plane of the body.

Sagnac rays. See *rays of Sagnac* under *ray.*

sa′go [Malay *sagu*]. A starch derived from the pith of certain East Indian and Malaysian palms; used as a food and as a demulcent.

sag′u·lum [L., cloak]. A cell-poor layer of the superficial gray matter lateral to the inferior colliculus.

Sahli, Hermann [*Swiss physician,* 1856–1933]. Introduced a method of ascertaining the functional activity of the stomach (1891), known as *Sahli's test.* See also Sahli *method.*

Sahyun method. See under *method.*

Sai·gon′ cin′na·mon (sigh·gohn′. *See* Notes §§ 15, 35). Cinnamon.

Saint Agatha's disease. Disease of the female breast.

Saint Agnan's disease. Ringworm, tinea.

Saint Aman's disease. Pellagra.

Saint Anthony's dance. Chorea.

Saint Anthony's fire. Erysipelas or gangrene; ergotism.

Saint Apollonia's disease. Toothache.

Saint Blaize's disease. Quinsy.

St. Clair's method. See Farley, St. Clair, and Reisinger's *method.*

Saint Erasmus' disease. Colic.

Saint Fiacre's disease. Hemorrhoids.

Saint Gervasius' disease. Rheumatism.

Saint Gothard's disease. Ancylostomiasis.

Saint Guy's dance. Chorea.

Saint Guy's disease. Chorea.

Saint Ignatius' bean. See *Ignatia.*

Saint Ignatius' itch. Pellagra.

St. John Long, John [*English painter and charlatan,* 1800–37]. Said to have introduced a liniment of turpentine and acetic acid, called *St. John Long's liniment.*

Saint Main's evil. Itch.

Saint Martin's disease. Dipsomania.

Saint Roche's disease. Bubonic plague.

Saint Sebastian's disease. Plague.

Saint Valentine's disease. Epilepsy.

Saint Vitus' dance. Chorea.

Saint Zachary's disease. Mutism.

Saissy, Jean Antoine [*French otologist,* 1756–1822]. Wrote on diseases of the tympanum and auditory tube. Described a bougie for the auditory tube (1829).

sajodin. Trade-mark for a brand of calcium iodobehenate.

Sakaguchi test. See under *test.*

Sakel, Manfred [*American psychiatrist,* 1900–]. Known for his important contribution in the treatment of schizophrenia and other mental disorders with insulin shock (1929); known as *Sakel's method.*

sal [L.]. 1. Salt. 2. Any substance resembling salt.

s. acetosellae. Potassium binoxalate.

s. aeratus. (a) Sodium bicarbonate. (b) Potassium bicarbonate.

s. amarum. Magnesium sulfate.

s. ammoniac. Ammonium chloride.

s. diureticus. Potassium acetate.

s. fossile. Sodium chloride.

s. Glauberi. Sodium sulfate.

s. kissingense. A salt obtained from the mineral springs of Kissingen, in Bavaria.

s. marinum. Sodium chloride.

s. mirabile. Sodium sulfate.

s. prunella. (a) A fused mixture of potassium nitrate, 128 parts, and sulfur, 1 part. (b) Fused potassium nitrate. Also called *s. prunelle.*

s. rupium. Rock salt.

s. seignette. Potassium sodium tartrate.

s. soda. Sodium carbonate.

s. vegetabile. Potassium tartrate.

s. volatile. Ammonium carbonate.

sa·la′cious [L. *salax,* lustful]. Lustful. **—salac′ity,** *n.*

sal·az′o·lon. Antipyrine salicylate.

sal′ep, sa′lep [Ar. *sahlab,* from *khusa al-tha'lab,* fox's testes]. The dried tubers of various species of the genus *Orchis* and the genus *Eulophia.* Used as a food, like sago and tapioca, or as a demulcent.

sal″e·ra′tus. Potassium bicarbonate or sodium bicarbonate. Syn., *sal aeratus.*

salethyl. Trade-mark for ethyl salicylate.

salethyl carbonate. Trade-mark for the carbonic acid ester of ethyl salicylate. The substance occurs as white, odorless crystals; insoluble in water, slightly soluble in alcohol. Used as an antipyretic and analgesic.

Saliceto, Gulielmus de (Salicetti; William of Salicet) [*Italian surgeon,* ca. 1201–77]. Renowned for his skill and teaching abilities. Known to have sutured divided tendons. Author of a work on surgery in the thirteenth century (published 1476). Described dropsy due to contracted kidneys, also called *dropsy of Salicetus.*

sal′i·cin (*salicinum*). $C_{13}H_{18}O_7$; a glycoside of orthohydroxybenzyl alcohol found in several species of willow and poplar; occurs as shining needles or prisms or as a white, crystalline powder; 1 Gm. dissolves in about 25 cc. of water and in about 90 cc. of alcohol. Salicin is rapidly absorbed and partly decomposed in the system, thus acting as an uncertain form of salicylic acid. Used in rheumatism, but since its conversion is uncertain it is inferior to the salicylates. Dose, 0.6–2.0 Gm. (10–30 gr.).

salicionyl. Trade-mark for a granular effervescent salt containing sodium salicylate, sodium bicarbonate, with salts of calcium, potassium, sodium, and magnesium. The salt is used as an antipyretic and antirheumatic.

salicitrin. See *novaspirin.*

sal′i·cyl. 1. The radical, $C_6H_4.OH.CO$—, of salicylic acid: also called *salicylyl.* 2. The radical C_6H_4OH— (*ortho*). 3. The radical $C_6H_4.OH.CH_2$—.

s. alcohol. $C_6H_4OHCH_2OH$; *o*-hydroxybenzyl alcohol; occurs as a white, crystalline powder; soluble in water and alcohol. It has marked local anesthetic powers and is practically nontoxic. It is also used as an antipyretic. See *saligenin, saligenol.*

sal′i·cyl-. See *salicylo-.*

sal″i·cyl·al′de·hyde. $C_6H_4.(OH).CHO$; *o*-hydroxybenzaldehyde; an oily liquid, slightly soluble in water, having an odor resembling that of bitter almond oil: used in perfumery. Syn., *salicylic aldehyde.*

sal″i·cyl·am′ide. $C_6H_4(OH)CONH_2$; *o*-hydroxybenzamide; a white, crystalline powder, slightly soluble in cold water: used as an analgesic, antipyretic, and antirheumatic.

sal″i·cyl·an′i·lide. $C_6H_5NH.CO.C_6H_4.OH$, occurring in white or slightly pink crystals, slightly soluble in water; an antimildew and antifungal agent, used in treatment of tinea capitis due to *Microsporon audouini.*

sal′i·cyl″ate (sal′i·sil″ate, sa·liss′i·late, sal″i·sil′ate). A salt of salicylic acid.

sal″i·cyl·a′zo·sul″fa·pyr′i·dine. $COOH(OH)$-$C_6H_3.N{:}N.C_6H_4.SO_2NH.C_5H_4N$; 5-[*p*-(2-pyridylsulfamyl)phenylazo]salicylic acid; a brownish-yellow powder, practically insoluble in water. It shares the actions of related sulfonamide compounds; because of special affinity for connective tissue it is used in chronic ulcerative colitis. See *azulfidine.*

sal″i·cyl′ic ac′id (*acidum salicylicum*). $C_6H_4.OH.$-$COOH$. *o*-Hydroxybenzoic acid; occurs as white crystals, usually in fine needles, or as a white, fluffy, crystalline powder; 1 Gm. dissolves in about 460 cc. of water and in 3 cc. of alcohol. Internally, the salts of salicylic acid are used as urinary antiseptics, analgesics, antipyretics, and in the treatment of various forms of rheumatism. Salicylic acid is used only for its local effect. It is widely used in the form of dusting powders, lotions, and ointments in the treatment of various skin diseases, especially chronic eczemas. Its action in these conditions is due in part to its antiseptic and fungicidal effect and in part to its softening action upon the corneous layer of the skin.

benzoic and s. a. ointment. One which formerly contained 12% benzoic acid and 6% salicylic acid in a base of wool fat and petrolatum; now, 6% benzoic acid and 3% salicylic acid in polyethylene glycol ointment base: used in the treatment of ringworm and other parasitic skin diseases. Also called *Whitfield's ointment.*

zinc oxide paste with s. a. (*pasta zinci oxidi cum acido salicylico*). Contains salicylic acid, 2 Gm.; zinc oxide paste, a sufficient quantity to make 100 Gm. The paste adds to the protective action and antiseptic action of the salicylic acid. Also called *Lassar's zinc paste with salicylic acid.*

sal″i·cyl′ic al′de·hyde. Salicylaldehyde.

sal′i·cyl·ism [L. *salix*, willow; G. *hylē*, material]. A toxic condition, produced by full doses of salicylates; characterized chiefly by tinnitus, hebetude, nausea, and vomiting.

sal″i·cyl′o-, salicyl- [*salix; hylē*]. *In chemistry*, a combining form denoting *salicylic.*

sal″i·cyl·sal″i·cyl′ic ac′id. $OH.C_6H_4.COO.C_6H_4.$-$COOH$; a crystalline powder, almost insoluble in water: used for the same purposes as acetylsalicylic acid but yields twice as much salicylate ion. See *diplosal, salysal.*

sal″i·cy·lu′ric ac′id. $C_6H_4.OH.CO.NH.CH_2COOH$. A detoxication product of salicylic acid found in the urine.

sal′i·fi″a·ble. Forming a salt by union with an acid.

saligenin. Trade name for salicyl alcohol.

saligenol. Trade name for salicyl alcohol.

sa·lim′e·ter [L. *sal*, salt; G. *metron*, a measure]. A hydrometer used to determine the density of salt solutions.

sa′line (say′lyne) [*sal*]. 1. Saltlike in character. 2. Containing sodium chloride.

sa′lines [*sal*]. Salts of the alkalies or of magnesium; used as hydragogue cathartics. Magnesium sulfate and citrate, sodium sulfate, and Rochelle salt are examples.

sal″i·py·raz′o·lone (sal″i·pye·raz′o·lone). See *antipyrine* salicylate.

salipyrin. A brand of antipyrine salicylate.

sa·li′va [L.]. The mixed secretions of the parotid, submaxillary, sublingual, and other glands of the mouth. It is opalescent, tasteless, and weakly alkaline. Its most important constituent is ptyalin. The functions of saliva are to moisten the food and lubricate the bolus, to dissolve certain substances, to facilitate tasting, to aid in deglutition and articulation, and to digest starches, which it converts into maltose, dextrin, and glucose. —**sal′ivary, salivous,** *adj.*

chorda s. That produced by stimulation of the chorda tympani nerve.

ganglionic s. That produced by stimulating the submaxillary ganglion.

resting s. The saliva found in the mouth between meals.

s. ejector. See saliva *ejector.*

sympathetic s. That produced by stimulation of a sympathetic nerve.

sal′i·vant [L. *salivare*, to spit out]. Stimulating the secretion of saliva.

sal′i·vant. A drug which increases the flow of saliva.

sal″i·va′tion [L. *salivatio*, from *salivare*]. An excessive secretion of saliva; a condition produced by mercury, pilocarpine, and by nervous disturbances. In severe cases of mercurial salivation, ulceration of the gums and loosening of the teeth may occur. —**sal′ivate,** *v.*

sal′i·va″tor [*salivare*]. An agent causing salivation. —**saliva′tory,** *adj.*

sal″i·vo·li·thi′a·sis [L. *saliva*, saliva; G. *lithiasis*, disease of the stone]. Presence of a salivary calculus.

sa′lix [L., willow]. The bark of several species of *Salix* (willow). The active constituent of all species of *Salix* is salicin.

Salk, Jonas Edward (1914–). American bacteriologist associated with the development of a poliomyelitis vaccine.

Salkowski test. See under *test.*

sal′len·ders. See *malanders.*

sal·mes′ter. See *mesotan.*

sal′mine (sal′meen, ·min) [L. *salmo*, salmon]. A protamine obtained from the spermatozoa of salmon.

Salmon, Daniel Elmer [*American pathologist*, 1850–1914]. With Theobald Smith he studied immunity. Discovered that dead virus induces immunity against living virus. A genus of Enterobacteriaceae is called *Salmonella* after him.

sal′mone. A histone obtained from the spermatozoa of salmon.

Sal″mo·nel′la [NL., after *Salmon*]. A genus of bacteria of the tribe Salmonelleae, family Enterobacteriaceae, and now including the former genus *Eberthella*. The organisms are non-lactose-fermenting, Gram-negative, motile rods which are commonly called paratyphoid bacilli. Infection produces an acute gastroenteritis called the food-poisoning type or a typhoidlike group of symptoms. Many species are causes of diarrhea in domestic animals.

S. abortus equi. A natural pathogen for mares, causing abortion. It is infectious also for guinea pigs, rabbits, goats, and cows, producing abortion. Also called *Salmonella abortivoequina*.

S. abortus ovis. A pathogen causing abortion in sheep, and not known to infect any other animal.

S. aertrycke. Synonym for *S. typhimurium*.

S. choleraesuis. A species occasionally found in epidemics of acute gastroenteritis. Syn., *Bacterium cholerae-suis*. Also called *hog cholera bacillus*.

S. enteritidis. A species causing gastroenteritis in man, isolated also from the horse, hog, mouse, rat, and duck: formerly called *Bacterium enteritidis*.

S. foetida. A small, Gram-negative coccobacillus, variably motile and doubtfully considered the etiologic agent of ozena: formerly called *Coccobacillus foetidus ozaenae*, *Escherichia foetida*, *Perez' bacillus*.

S. gallinarum. A species causing fowl typhoid, a diarrhea of domestic fowl, especially adult birds.

S. hirschfeldii. An aerobic, motile, Gram-negative rod causing enteric fever in man: formerly called *Bacterium paratyphosum C*, *S. paratyphi C*.

S. icteroides. A bacillus isolated from persons dying with yellow fever, formerly called *Bacillus icteroides*, *Bacterium icteroides*, *Sanarelli's bacillus*.

S. oranienburg. A species isolated from feces of normal carriers, feces of food-poisoning cases, and from abscesses: often found in dried-egg products.

S. paratyphi A. Old term for *S. paratyphosa*.

S. paratyphi B. Old term for *S. schottmülleri*.

S. paratyphi C. Old term for *S. hirschfeldii*.

S. paratyphosa. An aerobic, motile, Gram-negative rod with peritrichous flagella; a natural pathogen of man, causing an enteric fever: formerly called *Bacterium paratyphosum A*, *S. paratyphi A*.

S. pullorum. A species causing pullorum disease or bacillary white diarrhea of chicks. Transmission can occur through the egg.

S. schottmülleri. A motile, Gram-negative rod with peritrichous flagella; a natural pathogen of man, causing an enteric fever: found (rarely) in cattle, sheep, swine, chickens, and lower primates. Formerly called *Bacterium paratyphosum B*, *S. paratyphi B*.

S. suipestifer. A species found commonly in hogs and at one time thought to be the cause of hog cholera. It occasionally causes enteritis in man. Syn., *S. choleraesuis*.

S. typhi. *S. typhosa*.

S. typhimurium. A species commonly causing diarrhea in mice, rats, and birds and gastroenteritis in man. The most commonly isolated bacterium in outbreaks of food poisoning in the United States and Great Britain.

S. typhosa. A species causing typhoid fever, the symptoms being produced largely by endotoxins liberated upon destruction of the organisms. In culture, glucose is fermented to acid but not to gas. Also called *Bacterium typhosum*, *Eberthella typhosa*, *S. typhi*.

Sal″mo·nel′le·ae (sal″mo·nel′ee·ee) [*Salmonella*]. A tribe of the family Enterobacteriaceae.

S. sp. Any serotype that has not yet been assigned to a definite species.

sal″mo·nel·lo′sis [*Salmonella;* G. *-osis*, condition]. Infection with an organism of the genus *Salmonella*. It may be food-poisoning, gastroenteritic, typhoidal, or septicemic.

sal′ol. Phenyl salicylate.

salophen. Trade-mark for a brand of phenetsal.

sal″pin·gec′to·my [G. *salpigx*, trumpet; *ektomē*, excision]. Excision of a uterine tube.

sal″pin·gem·phrax′is [*salpigx;* G. *emphraxis*, stoppage]. Closure of the auditory or uterine tube.

sal″pin·gi′tis [*salpigx;* G. *-itis*, inflammation]. 1. Inflammation of the uterine tube. 2. Inflammation of the auditory tube. —**salpingit′ic,** *adj.*

chronic parenchymatous s. Chronic interstitial inflammation and thickening of the muscular coat of the uterine tube.

chronic vegetating s. Excessive hypertrophy of the mucosa of the uterine tube.

eustachian s. Inflammation of the eustachian tube between the middle ear and the nasopharynx.

gonococcic s., gonorrheal s. That of the uterine tube due to infection with gonococci.

hemorrhagic s. Hematosalpinx.

interstitial s. That marked by excessive formation of connective tissue.

isthmic nodular s. Follicular inflammation of the small constricted portion (isthmus) of the oviduct, with formation of small nodules of muscular and connective tissue: also called *productive glandular nodular s.*, *adenomyohyperplasia*, *adenomyosalpingitis*, *adenomyosis of fallopian tube*, *adenosalpingitis*, *diverticulosis of fallopian tube*, *epitheliomyosis*. Syn., *endosalpingiosis*.

mural s. See chronic parenchymatous *s*.

nodular s. A form marked by formation of solid nodules.

pneumococcic s. That due to infection with pneumococci.

productive glandular nodular s. See isthmic nodular *s*.

pseudofollicular s. Adenomyoma originating in the epithelium of the uterine tube.

purulent s. Salpingitis, 1, in which there is collection of pus; pyosalpinx.

pyogenic s. That of the uterine tube caused by pus-producing organisms.

tuberculous s. That marked by the infiltration of the lining membrane and walls of a uterine tube with tuberculous nodules.

sal·pin′go- (sal·ping′go-, sal′ping·go-), **salping-** [*salpigx*]. A combining form meaning *a trumpet;* used to denote *relation to an auditory tube* or *to a uterine tube*.

sal·pin″go·cath′e·ter·ism [*salpigx;* G. *kathetēr*, anything let down into]. Catheterization of an auditory tube.

sal·pin′go·cele [*salpigx;* G. *kēlē*, hernia]. Hernia of an oviduct.

sal·pin″go·cy·e′sis (sal·ping″go·sigh·ee′sis) [*salpigx;* G. *kyēsis*, pregnancy]. Tubal pregnancy.

sal″pin·gol′y·sis [*salpigx;* G. *lysis*, a loosing]. The breaking down of adhesions of a uterine tube.

sal·pin″go-o″o·pho·rec′to·my (-o″o·fo·reck′to·mee, -o″off·o·reck′to·mee). Excision of a uterine tube and an ovary.

sal·pin″go-o″o·pho·ri′tis. Inflammation of the uterine tubes and the ovaries.

sal·pin″go-o·oph′o·ro·cele (-o·off′o·ro·seel, -o″o·for′o·seel). Hernial protrusion of an ovary and oviduct.

sal·pin″go-o″o·the·cec′to·my. See *salpingo-oophorectomy*.

sal·pin″go-o″o·the·ci′tis. See *salpingo-oophoritis*

sal·pin″go-o″o·the′co·cele. See *salpingo-oophorocele.*

sal·pin″go·o·va″ri·ec′to·my. See *salpingo-oophorectomy.*

sal·pin″go·o·va″ri·ot′o·my. See *salpingo-oophorectomy.*

sal·pin″go-o″va·ri′tis. See *salpingo-oophoritis.*

sal·pin″go·pal′a·tine (sal·ping″go·pal′uh·tyne, ·tin) [*salpigx;* L. *palatum,* palate]. Pertaining to the auditory tube and the palate.

sal·pin″go·per″i·to·ni′tis [*salpigx;* G. *peritonaion,* membrane which contains the lower viscera; *-itis,* inflammation]. Inflammation of the peritoneum and uterine tube.

sal·pin′go·pex″y [*salpigx;* G. *pēxis,* a fixing]. Operative fixation of one or both uterine tubes.

sal·pin″go·pha·ryn′ge·al (sal·ping″go·fa·rin′jul, ·jee·ul, ·far″in·jee′ul) [*salpigx;* G. *pharygx,* pharynx]. Pertaining to the auditory tube and the pharynx, as the salpingopharyngeal muscle.

sal·pin″go·phar″yn·ge′us (·far″in·jee′us, ·fa·rin′-jee·us) [*salpigx; pharygx*]. A muscular bundle passing from the auditory tube downward to the constrictors of the pharynx. See Table of Muscles in the Appendix.

sal·pin′go·plas″ty [*salpigx;* G. *plassein,* to form]. Surgery of a uterine tube.

sal″pin·gor′rha·phy. [*salpigx;* G. *rhaphē,* suture]. Suture of a uterine tube.

sal·pin″go·sal″pin·gos′to·my [*salpigx; salpigx;* G. *stoma,* mouth]. The operation reuniting an oviduct after removal of an intervening section.

sal·pin′go·scope [*salpigx;* G. *skopein,* to examine]. Old term for nasopharyngoscope.

sal·pin″go·sten″o·cho′ri·a (sal·ping″go·sten″o-kor′ee·uh) [*salpigx;* G. *stenochōria,* narrowness of space]. Stenosis or stricture of the auditory tube.

sal·pin″go·sto·mat′o·my. Salpingostomy.

sal″pin·gos′to·my [*salpigx;* G. *stoma,* mouth]. 1. The operation of making an artificial fistula between a uterine tube and the body surface. 2. Any plastic operation for opening the uterine tube.

sal″pin·got′o·my [*salpigx;* G. *tomē,* a cutting]. The operation of cutting into a uterine tube.

sal″pin·gys″ter·o·cy·e′sis (sal″pin·jis″tur·o·sigh-ee′sis) [*salpigx;* G. *hystera,* womb; *kyēsis,* pregnancy]. Interstitial pregnancy.

sal′pinx [*salpigx*]. A tube, especially the auditory or the uterine tube.

salt [AS. *sealt*]. 1. Sodium chloride. 2. A group of substances that result from the reaction between acids and bases; a compound of a metal or positive radical and a nonmetal or negative radical. 3. A mixture of several salts, as artificial salt and effervescent salt.

acid s. A salt that contains unreplaced hydrogen atoms of the acid from which the salt was formed, as $NaHCO_3$.

amphoteric s. A salt that has both acid and basic properties.

artificial s. A mixture of the more important chemical salts naturally present in several of the well-known mineral springs of Europe.

basic s. A salt that contains unreplaced hydroxyl groups of the base from which it was formed.

buffer s. The salt of a weak acid and strong base, or of a strong acid and a weak base which, in solution, tends to resist a change in reaction upon addition of acid or alkali, respectively.

complex s. A salt made up of more than one simple acid or metallic radical, but which ionizes in solution into only two types of ions; as $K_4Fe(CN)_6$.

effervescent s. A mixture of one or more active chemical salts with an effervescent base. The base usually consists of sodium bicarbonate, citric and tartaric acids. The salts formed are usually in the form of coarse granules or powder.

Epsom s. Magnesium sulfate.

Mohr's s. Ferrous ammonium sulfate.

Monsel's s. Ferric subsulfate.

neutral s. A salt whose solution has a neutral reaction, as sodium chloride.

normal s. A salt of an acid and base that have completely neutralized each other. The reaction in solution may be neutral, acid, alkaline, or amphoteric.

rock s. Sodium chloride as obtained in the solid form by mining.

sal·ta′tion [L. *saltatio,* from *saltare,* to dance]. Dancing or leaping as in chorea.

sal′ta·to″ry, sal″ta·tor′ic [L. *saltatorius,* of dancing]. Dancing or leaping.

Salter, Samuel James Augustus [*English dentist,* 1825–97]. Described the incremental lines of the dentin, called *Salter's lines, Owen's lines.*

salt′ing out. A method of precipitating proteins and other substances by the use of aqueous solutions of neutral salts.

salt″pe′ter, salt″pe′tre [ML. *sal petrae,* rock salt]. Potassium nitrate.

Chile s. Sodium nitrate.

salts. A saline cathartic, especially magnesium sulfate, sodium sulfate, or Rochelle salt.

salt′-sen″si·tive. Characterized by a tendency to agglutinate in normal saline solution; said of certain bacteria.

sa·lu′bri·ty [L. *salubritas,* healthfulness]. The state or quality of being wholesome, conducive to physical well-being. —**salubrious,** *adj.*

sal′u·tar″y (sal′yoo·terr″ee) [L. *salutaris,* healthful]. Promoting health.

salvarsan. Trade-mark for a brand of arsphenamine.

s. glucose solution. An aqueous solution of arsphenamine diglucoside solution containing 10% of salvarsan base. Used as a spirocheticide.

silver-s. Trade-mark for silver arsphenamine.

salve [AS. *sealf*]. Ointment.

Deshler's s. Compound rosin cerate.

sal′vi·a [L., the herb sage] (*salvia*). The dried leaf of *Salvia officinalis.* Both the leaves and flowering tops contain a volatile oil. It also contains several terpenes, thujone, ordinary camphor, and an unidentified hydrocarbon, salvene. It is claimed to possess secretion-inhibitory and spasmolytic actions. Also called *garden sage.*

salyrgan. Trade-mark for a brand of mersalyl.

salyrgan-theophylline solution. Trade-mark for a brand of mersalyl and theophylline injection.

salysal. Trade-mark for *salicylsalicylic acid.*

Sam″a·de′ra, Sa·mad′er·a [NL.]. A genus of old-world trees of the Simarubaceae.

S. indica. Produces a niepa bark which has been used as a bitter tonic.

sa·ma′ri·um [after Colonel *Samarski,* Russian mine official]. Sm (or Sa) = 150.43. A metallic element belonging to the didymium group.

sam·bu′cus [L., elder-tree] (*sambucus*). The air-dried flower of *Sambucus canadensis,* or of *Sambucus nigra.* The flowers yield, on distillation, a small portion of volatile oil. It also contains eldrin, which is identical with rutin. It has been used as a diaphoretic and diuretic, in febrile conditions, syphilis, and rheumatism. Also called *elder flowers.*

sam′ple [L. *exemplum,* model]. A specimen or part to show the quality of the whole.

random s. A finite number of individuals, cases, or measurements chosen from a larger group in such a manner that each individual, case, or measurement has an equal and independent chance of being selected.

Sampson, John Albertson [*American surgeon*, 1873–1946]. Described ovarian endometriomas, noted by him in his work on chocolate cysts (1921); called *endometrial implants, Sampson's implants, endometriosis.*

Sanarelli, Giuseppe [*Italian bacteriologist*, 1864–1940]. *Salmonella icteroides* is sometimes called *Sanarelli's bacillus.* He made experimental observations (1924) of a phenomenon interpreted by him as "hemorrhagic allergy" of intestinal epithelium (epithalaxia). See Shwartzman *phenomenon*, Sanarelli *virus.*

san″a·to′ri·um [L. *sanare*, to heal]. An establishment for the treatment of the chronic diseases; especially, a private hospital or place having conditions which are natural therapeutic agents.

san′a·to″ry [*sanare*]. Health-giving. *Obs.*

san′dal·wood″ [Skr. *candana*, from *candra*, shining]. 1. White sandalwood (*Santalum album*). The heartwood of *Santalum album.* Its therapeutic use is due solely to the volatile oil which it contains. The wood is not used medicinally. Also called *white saunders, white santal.* 2. Red sandalwood (*Santalum rubrum*). The heartwood of *Pterocarpus santalinus.* It contains a coloring principle called santalin. The wood is employed solely for the purpose of imparting color. It is used in compound tincture of lavender. Also called *red saunders, red santal.*

s. oil. The volatile oil distilled with steam from the dried heartwood of *Santalum album.* It contains two isomeric sesquiterpine alcohols, alpha-santalol and beta-santalol. Other less important constituents are isovaleric aldehyde, santene, santenone, teresantol, santalone, and santalene. It is largely used as a perfume. *In medicine*, its chief use has been in gonorrheal urethritis; it was also sometimes used in chronic bronchitis and cystitis. Also called *santal oil.*

san′da·rac [G. *sandarakē*, realgar]. A white, transparent resin produced by *Callitris quadrivalvis*, a tree of North Africa.

s. varnish. *In dentistry*, a solution of sandarac in alcohol used as a separating medium in making plaster casts.

sand crack. *In veterinary medicine*, a fissure in the hoof of a horse, from the coronet to the sole; due to disease of the horn-secreting membrane.

Sander, Wilhelm [*German psychiatrist*, 1838–1922]. Described a type of paranoia appearing in youth (1868), called *Sander's disease* or *paranoia.*

Sanders, Clarence Elmer [*American physician*, 1885–1949]. Devised a bed for treatment of peripheral vascular disease which automatically shifts the patient from a head-up to a head-down position; called *oscillating bed, vaso-oscillator bed, Sanders' bed.*

Sanders, James [*English physician*, 1777–1843]. Described the undulatory character of the cardiac impulse in the epigastric region, indicative of adherent pericardium; called *Sanders' sign.* (The classic description of adherent pericardium was given by John Broadbent in 1897.) Described epidemic keratoconjunctivitis; also called *Sanders' syndrome, Sanders-Hogan syndrome.*

san′ders. Sandalwood.

Sanderson. See *Burdon-Sanderson.*

sand flea. See *Tunga penetrans.*

sand′fly [AS. *sand; flyge*]. Any member of the genus *Phlebotomus*, especially the *Phlebotomus papatasii.*

sand′fly fe′ver. See pappataci *fever.*

sandoptal. Trade-mark for 5-allyl-5-isobutylbarbituric acid, officially designated allylbarbituric acid; a white, crystalline powder, slightly soluble in water: used as a sedative and hypnotic.

Sandström, Ivar Victor [*Swedish anatomist*, 1852–89]. Described the parathyroids (1880); called *Sandström's bodies, Gley's glands.*

Sandwith, Fleming Mant [*English physician*, 1853–1918]. Described bald tongue sometimes seen in late stages of pellagra; called *Sandwith's bald tongue.*

sane [L. *sanus*, healthy]. Of sound mind.

Sanford, Arthur Hawley (1882–). American clinical pathologist who, with Magath, introduced a graduated tube for the hematocrit reading, called *Sanford and Magath's centrifuge tube.* He introduced an erythrocyte fragility test. See *Sheard-Sanford photelometer* under Charles *Sheard.* See also Sanford, Sheard, and Osterberg *method.*

san·guic′o·lous (sang·gwick′o·lus) [L. *sanguis*, blood; *colere*, to inhabit]. Living in the blood, as a parasite.

san·guif′er·ous [*sanguis;* L. *ferre*, to bear]. Carrying, or conveying, blood.

san″gui·fi·ca′tion [*sanguis*]. The formation of blood; conversion into blood.

san″gui·na′ri·a (sang″gwi·nair′ee·uh) [L. *sanguinarius*, of the blood] (*sanguinaria*). The dried rhizome of *Sanguinaria canadensis.* It contains several alkaloids, of which chelerythrine and sanguinarine are present in greatest quantity. It is an active local irritant, in large doses producing nausea and vomiting. It has been used as an expectorant in the treatment of subacute or chronic bronchitis. It is an ingredient in compound syrup of white pine and in the compound syrup with codeine. Also called *bloodroot.*

san·guin′a·rine. $C_{20}H_{15}NO_5$; an alkaloid from sanguinaria. Syn., *pseudochelerythrine.*

san′guine (sang′gwin) [L. *sanguis*, blood]. 1. Resembling blood; bloody. 2. Hopeful, active, as sanguine temperament.

san·guin′e·ous [L. *sanguineus*, of blood]. 1. Pertaining to the blood; containing blood. 2. Sanguine.

san·guin′o·lent [L. *sanguinolentus*, full of blood]. Tinged with blood.

san′guis [L.]. Blood.

san″gui·suc′tion [*sanguis;* L. *suctum*, from *sugere*, to suck]. Abstraction of blood by suction, as by a leech or other parasite.

san″gui·su′ga. See *leech.*

sa′ni·es (say′nee·eez) [L., bloody matter]. A thin, fetid, greenish, seropurulent fluid discharged from an ulcer, wound, or fistula. —**sanious,** *adj.*

san″i·ta′ri·an [L. *sanitas*, health]. One skilled in sanitary science and matters of public health.

san″i·ta′ri·um. See *sanatorium.*

san′i·tar″y [*sanitas*]. Pertaining to health.

san′i·tar″y a′re·a. *In military medicine*, a section in a theater of operations in charge of a medical officer regulating sanitation in the area.

san′i·tar″y or′der. *In military medicine*, a general order, issued by the headquarters of a command, setting down sanitary measures to be carried out within the whole command.

san′i·tar″y re·port′. *In military medicine*, the report of the medical inspector or surgeon of a unit to the commanding officer regarding the health and sanitation of the command.

san′i·tar″y sur′vey. *In military medicine*, a study of health conditions in an area occupied by troops, made for the purpose of taking measures that will prevent disease or its spread.

san″i·ta′tion [*sanitas*]. The act of securing a healthful condition; the application of sanitary measures.

san′i·tize [*sanitas*]. Make sanitary; a term proposed by Walter to describe the process of boiling instruments, solutions, etc., to destroy organisms; distinguished from sterilize. *Rare.*

san'i·ty [*sanitas*]. Soundness of mind.

sanocrysin. Trade-mark for gold and sodium thiosulfate.

Sansom, Arthur Ernest [*English physician*, 1838–1907]. Described a number of signs, as extension of dullness in the second and third interspaces in pericardial effusion; a rhythmic murmur of possible diagnostic value in aortic aneurysm; a reduplication of the second sound of the heart heard at the base in mitral stenosis. These were once called *Sansom's signs.*

Sanson, Louis Joseph [*French physician*, 1790–1841]. Described, contemporaneously with Johannes Purkinje, a set of three images called *Purkinje-Sanson images.* See under *image.*

san'tal. Sandalwood.

san'ta·lin. See under *sandalwood.*

san'ta·lol. $C_{15}H_{26}O$. See under *sandalwood* oil.

san'ta·lum. See under *sandalwood.*

san·ton'i·ca [G. *santonikon*, wormwood]. The unexpanded flower heads of several species of *Artemisia.* The most important constituent is santonin. It also contains a volatile oil and another crystalline principle, artemisin. Also called *wormseed, Levant wormseed.*

san·ton'ic ac'id. $C_{15}H_{20}O_4$. An acid obtained by heating santonin with alkali; it is isomeric with santoninic acid.

san'to·nin (*santoninum*). $C_{15}H_{18}O_3$. The inner anhydride of santoninic acid; occurs as colorless crystals, or a white, crystalline powder, almost insoluble in water, 1 Gm. dissolves in about 45 cc. of alcohol. Used as a vermifuge, especially against the ascarids. Coarse crystals are preferred as they are less readily dissolved and therefore less likely to be absorbed. Dose, for three-year-old child, 0.015–0.03 Gm. (¼–½ gr.) followed by a cathartic; for adults, 0.06–0.2 Gm. (1–3 gr.).

san"to·nin'ic ac'id. $C_{15}H_{20}O_4$. The acid of which santonin is the inner anhydride.

san'ton·ism. [*santonikon*]. Poisoning from overdosage of santonin. Symptoms: yellow vision, gastrointestinal, renal, and vesical irritation, weakness, hallucinations, convulsions, coma.

Santorini, Giovanni Domenico (**Santorinus**) (1681–1739). Italian anatomist; one of the great anatomists of his time; author of *Anatomic Observations* (1724). He described the cartilaginous nodules on the tips of the arytenoid cartilages, called *Santorini's cartilages, corniculate cartilages.* He is remembered for his description of the accessory pancreatic duct, called *Santorini's duct.* The risorius muscle was once called *Santorini's muscle.* Other structures associated with his name are the muscles of the external ear, called *Santorini's muscles;* the papilla of the duodenum; the vesicoprostatic venous plexus in the male; and the emissary veins between the sinuses of the dura mater and the veins of the scalp.

Santos, Reynaldo dos [*Portuguese surgeon and radiologist*, 1880–]. With Chaldas, introduced thorotrast used in arteriography (1931). Inventor of a pistol-shaped instrument with tiny jaws at one end, manipulated from the handle, used in connection with fluoroscopy for removing small particles of metal from tissues, called *Santos' foreign body remover.*

santyl. Trade-mark for santalyl salicylate. The substance occurs as a yellowish, oily liquid insoluble in water, soluble in alcohol; it has been used as a urinary sedative and analgesic.

sap [AS. *saep*]. Plant juice. The watery solution which circulates through the vascular tissues of a plant.

cell s. Hyaloplasm.

nuclear s. The fluid material within a nucleus, occupying the space not taken by nucleolus, linin or chromatin.

sa·phe'na [ML. *saphena*, from Ar. *sāfin*]. One of two large veins of the leg—the great or long and the small or short saphena.

sa·phe'nous, saph'e·nous [*sāfin*]. Apparent; superficial; manifest; applied to two veins of the lower limb, the great or long saphenous vein and the small or short saphenous vein, situated just beneath the surface; also applied to the nerves accompanying these veins. See Tables of Nerves and of Veins in the Appendix.

sap'id [L. *sapidus*, flavorful]. Capable of being tasted.

sa'po [L.]. Soap.

sa·pog'e·nin (sa·podj'i·nin, sap"o·jen'in). The nonsugar or aglycone component of a saponin.

sap"o·na'ceous [*sapo*]. Having the nature of soap.

Sap"o·na'ri·a [*sapo*]. A genus of plants of the order Caryophylleae. **S. officinalis,** or soapwort, bouncing Bet, is a species growing wild abundantly in the United States and Europe. Formerly employed in treatment of gout, syphilis, and as an expectorant. It contains saponin, sapotoxin, sapogenin, etc.

sa·pon"i·fi·ca'tion [*sapo;* L. *facere*, to make]. The conversion of an ester into an alcohol and a salt; in particular, the conversion of a fat into a soap and glycerin by means of an alkali. —**sapon'ify,** *v.*

sa·pon'i·form [*sapo;* L. *forma*, form]. Soaplike in appearance and consistency.

sap'o·nin, sa·po'nin [*sapo*]. 1. A glycoside usually obtained from *Quillaja* or *Saponaria.* The commercial saponin occurs as a white to brownish, amorphous powder. Used in liquid soaps, cosmetic preparations, and in many industrial processes. 2. One of a group of glycosidal principles which have the property of foaming when shaken with water and dissolving red blood cells. Saponins are widely distributed in nature. Because of their ability to lower surface tension, they form emulsions with oils and resinous substances. They tend to alter the permeability of cell walls and, therefore, exert a general toxicity on all organized tissues. Certain of the saponins possess powerful physiologic properties which are quite different from those due to the general surface tension effects of the group.

Saporta, Antoine [*French physician*, d. 1573]. Said to have given the first description of aneurysm of the aorta (1554).

sap"o·tox'in [L. *sapo*, soap; G. *toxikon*, poison]. A name sometimes given to the more toxic saponins.

Sappey, Marie Philibert Constant [*French anatomist*, 1810–96]. Author of an important work on the lymphatics (1874). Best known for his description of the accessory portal veins; called *venae parumbilicales, Sappey's accessory portal veins.* Described smooth muscular fibers found in the check ligaments of the eyeball, called *Sappey's ligaments.* See *muscle* of Sappey.

sap'phism (saf'iz·um) [G. *Sapphō*, Greek poetess]. Female homosexuality.

Sap·pin'i·a dip·loi'de·a. A free-living ameba found in decaying feces.

sa·pre'mi·a, sa·prae'mi·a [G. *sapros*, putrid; *haima*, blood]. The intoxication produced by absorption of the products of putrefaction.

sa·pre'mic [*sapros; haima*]. Affected with, of the nature of, or pertaining to, sapremia.

sap'rine (sap'reen, ·rin) [*sapros*]. A product or products of growth when saprophytic or simple parasitic bacteria grow upon diseased or injured tissues.

sap'ro-, sapr- [*sapros*]. A combining form meaning

rotten; used to denote *dead* or *decaying organic matter* or *saprophytic*.

sap′ro·gen [*sapros;* G. *genesthai*, from *gignesthai*, to be produced]. A putrefactive microorganism.

sap″ro·gen′ic, sa·prog′e·nous (sa·prodj′i·nus) [*sapros; genesthai*]. 1. Causing putrefaction. 2. Produced by putrefaction.

sa·proph′a·gous [*sapros;* G. *phagein*, to eat]. Subsisting on decaying matter.

sap′ro·phyte [*sapros;* G. *phyton*, plant]. An organism living on dead organic matter. —**sapro-phyt′ic,** *adj.*

sap″ro·zo′ic [*sapros;* G. *zōion*, living being]. Characterizing an organism which lives upon decaying organic matter.

sar′a·pus [G. *sarapous*, splay-footed]. A flat-footed person.

Sar′ci·na [L. *sarcina*, bundle]. A genus of the family Micrococcaceae. Cell division occurs in three planes forming cubical groups.

sar·ci′tis [G. *sarx*, flesh; *-itis*, inflammation]. Inflammation of fleshy tissue; especially inflammation of muscle.

sar′co-, sarc- [*sarx*]. A combining form meaning *flesh*.

sar″co·ad″e·no′ma. See *adenosarcoma*.

sar″co·bi′ont [*sarx;* G. *bioun*, to live]. Living on flesh.

sar′co·blast [*sarx;* G. *blastos*, germ]. A cell developing into a muscle cell or fiber. Syn., *myoblast*.

sar″co·car″ci·no′ma. See *carcinosarcoma*.

sar′co·cele [*sarx;* G. *kēlē*, tumor]. A tumor of the testis resembling muscle.

Sar″co·cys′tis [*sarx;* G. *kystis*, bladder]. A group of the sporozoa.

S. lindemanni. Genus of the order Sarcosporidia. A rare parasite of man, in various muscles. Sarcosporidiosis is common in lower animals.

sar′code [G. *sarkōdēs*, fleshy]. An early term used by Dujardin to designate the living substance of the cell, the protoplasm.

Sar″co·di′na [*sarkōdēs*]. A class of protozoa moving and feeding by means of pseudopodia. Syn., *Rhizopoda*.

sar″co·en″do·the·li·o′ma. A malignant mesothelioma.

synovial s. Malignant synovioma.

sar″co·gen′ic [G. *sarx*, flesh; *genesthai*, from *gignesthai*, to be produced]. Producing muscle.

sar″co·hy′dro·cele [*sarx;* G. *hydōr*, water; *kēlē*, tumor]. A sarcocele complicated with hydrocele of the tunica vaginalis.

sar′coid [G. *sarkoeidēs*, fleshlike]. Resembling flesh.

sar′coid. The characteristic lesion seen in sarcoidosis.

Boeck′s s. See *sarcoidosis*.

Spiegler-Fendt s. See *lymphocytoma* cutis.

sar″coid·o′sis [*sarkoeidēs;* G. *-ōsis*, condition]. A disease of young adults and sometimes of older persons, of unknown etiology; characterized by granulomatous lesions, somewhat resembling true tubercles, but showing little or no necrosis, affecting lymph nodes, skin, lungs, bones in distal parts of the extremities (osteitis cystica of Jüngling) and other structures. Iridocyclitis and uveoparotid fever may occur. Usually shows periods of activity, and recovery may take place. Also called *Boeck's sarcoid, Besnier-Boeck disease, Besnier-Boeck-Schaumann disease, lupus pernio of Besnier, lymphogranulomatosis of Schaumann, benign lymphogranulomatosis*.

sar″co·lac′tic ac′id. $CH_3.CHOH.COOH$. An isomeric form of lactic acid occurring in muscle. Also called *paralactic acid*.

sar″co·lem′ma [G. *sarx*, flesh; *lemma*, husk]. The delicate sheath enveloping a muscle fiber. —**sarcolemmic,** *adj.*

sar″co·leu·ke′mi·a. See *leukosarcoma*.

sar·co′ma [G. *sarkōma*, fleshy excrescence]. A malignant tumor composed of cells derived from nonepithelial tissues, mainly connective tissue. May be divided into those made up of immature cells including undifferentiated spindle cells or round cells and those made up of differentiated cells of such nature that the tumor may be so designated, for instance, fibrosarcoma, chondrosarcoma, osteosarcoma, liposarcoma, etc.

alveolar soft-part s. See malignant granular-cell *myoblastoma*.

ameloblastic s. Ameloblastosarcoma.

botryoid s. See *s.* botryoides.

carotid-body s. See carotid-body *tumor*.

endothelial s. 1. Hemangioendothelioma. 2. Ewing's *s.* 3. A malignant mesothelioma.

Ewing's s. A primary malignant tumor of bone, showing no osteogenic potentialities and usually arising as a central tumor in long bones. It is composed of sheets of cells with little cytoplasm and fairly large, uniform nuclei showing scattered chromatin. It occurs usually in the second decade of life and responds temporarily to radiation therapy, but prognosis is poor. Also called *angioendothelioma of bone, hemendothelioma of bone, endothelial myeloma*. Syn., *Ewing's tumor*.

giant-cell s. (a) Giant-cell tumor of bone, usually benign. (b) Epulis in malignant form. (c) Synovial sarcoma.

histiocytic s. See reticulum-cell *s.*

Hodgkin's s. See Hodgkin's *disease* (c).

intracanalicular s. See *cystosarcoma* phylloides.

Jensen's s. A transmissible spindle-cell type of neoplasm which grows in a high percentage of inoculated rats and recedes in a large proportion after a few weeks' growth.

Kaposi's s. See multiple idiopathic hemorrhagic *s.*

lymphangioendothelial s. Lymphangiosarcoma.

lymphocytic s. See *lymphosarcoma*.

melanotic s. See *melanoma*.

meningeal s. See *meningioma*.

mesothelial s. A malignant mesothelioma.

multiple idiopathic hemorrhagic s. A mesodermal tumor, characterized by the occurrence of multiple bluish-red or brown nodules and plaques, usually on the extremities. In the early granulomatous lesions, which occasionally involute spontaneously, tumor is not evident; in later stages, the histologic picture resembles angiosarcoma or fibrosarcoma. Extravasated erythrocytes and hemosiderin granules are inconspicuous but constant features; infrequently, viscera may be involved. Syn., *Kaposi's s., s. cutaneum telangiectaticum multiplex, multiplex angiosarcoma*.

myelocytic s. See *myeloma*.

myeloid s. See giant-cell *tumor*, 1.

neurogenic s., neurogenous s. See malignant *schwannoma*.

osteoblastic s. See osteogenic *s.*

osteogenic s. A primary malignant tumor of bone, derived from osteoblastic cells, or occasionally via a cartilaginous stage, and usually occurring in younger age groups. Histologically the tumor exhibits a high degree of variability, but is characterized essentially by a sarcomatous stroma, and osteoid and osseous transformation; it is variously subdivided on basis of location as *medullary, subperiosteal, periosteal, capsular*, and *parosteal*. When osteogenesis predominates, it is also called *osteoblastic s., sclerosing osteogenic s.*, and *osteoblastoma;* when osteolysis is the predominating feature, it is called *osteolytic s., tetangiectatic s., malignant bone aneurysm, osteo-*

aneurysm, and *malignant bone cyst*. Syn., *osteosarcoma*.

osteolytic s. See osteogenic *s.*

paraganglion caroticum s. See carotid-body *tumor*.

periductal s. See *cystosarcoma* phylloides.

plasmacytic, plasmocytic s. See *myeloma*.

pleomorphic granular-cell s. See malignant granular-cell *myoblastoma*, 1.

pleural s. Malignant mesothelioma of the pleura.

polymorphous s. See malignant granular-cell *myoblastoma*.

reticulocytic s. Reticulum-cell sarcoma.

reticuloendothelial s. See reticulum-cell *s.*

reticulum-cell s. A type of lymphoma in which the predominant cell type is probably derived from the reticuloendothelium; the cells seen are larger than endothelial cells and have a large nucleus with a single nucleolus and pale-staining, poorly defined cytoplasm. Multinucleated cells occur and mitotic figures may be numerous. Also called *histiocytic s.*, *reticulocytic s.*, *reticuloendothelial s.*, *reticuloendothelioma*, (*diffuse syncytial*, *trabecular syncytial*, or *lymphoblastic*) *reticulosarcoma*, *retotheliosarcoma*, *retothelioma*, *reticulum-cell lymphosarcoma*, *endothelioma of lymph node*, *clasmocytoma*, *clasmatocytic lymphoma*. See also *lymphosarcoma*.

Rous s. A transplantable tumor of fowls caused by a filtrable virus.

s. of bone. Osteogenic *s.*

s. botryoides. Mesenchymoma (mesenchymal or mesodermal mixed tumor) of the fundus uteri of older women or cervix of children, characterized grossly by polypoid nodular appearance: also called *s. colli uteri hydropicum capillare*, *botryoid tumor*, *grapelike tumor*.

s. capitis. See *cylindroma*.

s. colli uteri hydropicum capillare. A *s.* botryoides.

s. cutaneum telangiectaticum multiplex. See multiple idiopathic hemorrhagic *s.*

s. epithelioides. Epithelioma of the lymph nodes.

s. myxomatodes. One in which there are foci of mucoid degeneration.

s. of peripheral nerve. See malignant *schwannoma*.

s. phylloides. See *cystosarcoma* phylloides.

sclerosing osteogenic s. See osteogenic *s.*

serocystic s. See *cystosarcoma* phylloides.

spindle-cell s. A malignant connective-tissue tumor composed of spindle-shaped cells.

synovial s. See under *synovioma*.

telangiectatic s. See osteogenic *s.*

thymic s. A rare form of thymoma made up largely of spindle cells, sometimes myxomatous.

Walker s. A transplantable, solid, mixed-cell sarcoma of rats.

sar·co″ma·to′sis [*sarkōma;* G. *-ōsis*, condition]. The formation of multiple sarcomatous growths in various parts of the body.

meningeal s. See meningeal *gliomatosis*.

sar·co′ma·tous, sar·com′a·tous [*sarkōma*]. Of the nature of, or resembling, sarcoma.

sar′co·mere [G. *sarx*, flesh; *meros*, part]. One of the segments into which a muscle fibril appears to be divided by Z disks.

sar″co·mes″o·the·li·o′ma. A malignant mesothelioma.

synovial s. Malignant synovioma.

sar″co·my′ces (sahr″ko·migh′seez) [*sarx;* G. *mykēs*, fungus]. A fleshy growth of a fungous appearance.

Sar″co·phag′i·dae (sahr″ko·fadj′i·dee) [*sarx;* G. *phagein*, to eat]. A large cosmopolitan family of the Diptera, commonly known as flesh flies, blowflies, and scavenger flies. They normally deposit their eggs or larvae on the decaying flesh of dead animals, but sometimes also in open wounds and sores of man. The important genera are *Sarcophaga* and *Wohlfahrtia*. The maggots of *W. vigil* are known to cause cutaneous myiasis in young children. *W. magnifica* is said to be a great pest to wounded soldiers in Europe and Asia.

sar′co·plasm [*sarx;* G. *plasma*, anything formed]. The hyaline or finely granular interfibrillar material of muscle tissue; the term is opposed to the myofibrils or contractile substance. —**sar-coplas′mic,** *adj.*

sar′co·plast. See *sarcoblast*, *myoblast*.

sar″co·poi·et′ic [*sarx;* G. *poiētikos*, capable of making]. Producing muscle.

Sar·cop′tes (sahr·cop′teez) [*sarx;* G. *koptein*, to cut]. A genus of minute, rounded, short-legged, flattened mites which cause scabies in man and mange in many kinds of animals.

S. scabiei. The arachnid which causes scabies in man; the itch mite.

Sar·cop′ti·dae (sahr·cop′ti·dee) [*sarx; koptein*]. A family of the order Acarina, including the genera *Sarcoptes* and *Notoedres*.

sar·cop′toid [*sarx; koptein;* G. *eidos*, form]. Referring to the Sarcoptoidea.

Sar″cop·toi′de·a [*sarx; koptein; eidos*]. A superfamily of the parasitic mites; the mange and itch mites of the genus *Sarcoptes* are included.

sar′co·sine (sahr′ko·seen, ·sin). $CH_3NH.CH_2.COOH$; N-methylglycine or N-methylaminoacetic acid; deliquescent crystals, very soluble in water. It occurs naturally in certain higher animals and is a product of hydrolysis of peanut proteins.

dimethyl s. Betaine.

Sar″co·spo·rid′i·a [*sarx;* dim. from G. *spora*, seed]. An order of sporozoa which includes the genus *Sarcocystis*.

sar″co·spo·rid″i·o′sis [*sarx; spora;* G. *-ōsis*, condition]. A disease of warm-blooded animals caused by sporozoa of the order Sarcosporidia; it is rare in man. The parasites usually encyst in striated muscle and produce few symptoms.

sar′co·style. O.T. for myofibril.

sar″co·thla′sis [*sarx;* G. *thlasis*, a bruising]. Old term for a bruise or hematoma.

sar′cous [*sarx*]. Pertaining to flesh or muscle.

sar·don′ic grin. See *risus* sardonicus.

sar·men″to·cy·mar′in. A cardioactive, steroidal glycoside from the seeds of *Strophanthus sarmentosus*. See *sarmentogenin*, *sarmentose*.

sar″men·tog′e·nin. $C_{23}H_{34}O_5$; the steroidal aglycone of sarmentocymarin. It is isomeric with digoxigenin and is characterized by having a hydroxyl group at carbon atom number 11.

sar′men·tose. $C_7H_{14}O_4$; the methyl ether of a 2-desoxyhexomethylose; a sugar obtained by hydrolysis of sarmentocymarin; it is isomeric with cymarose.

sar′sa. Sarsaparilla.

sar″sa·pa·ril′la [Sp. *zarzaparilla*] (*sarsaparilla*). The dried root of *Smilax aristolochiaefolia*, *Smilax regelii*, or of undetermined species of *Smilax*. The most important principles in sarsaparilla are at least three saponins: smilasaponin, sarsasaponin, and parillin, which on hydrolysis yield the steroidal sapogenins *smilagenin*, *sarsasapogenin*, and *parigenin*. Sarsaparilla was formerly used in chronic rheumatism, skin diseases, and syphilis.

compound s. syrup (*syrupus sarsaparillae compositus*). Contains fluidextracts of sarsaparilla and glycyrrhiza, oils of sassafras and anise, methyl salicylate, syrup, and alcohol: used as a vehicle especially for the iodides and other saline drugs.

sar″sa·sa·pog′e·nin. $C_{27}H_{44}O_3$; the steroidal aglycone of sarsasaponin, a glycoside of sarsaparilla; a starting compound for synthesis of desoxycorticosterone, progesterone, and certain other steroid hormones. It is identical with parigenin.

sar″sa·sap′o·nin. A glycoside from sarsaparilla. On hydrolysis it yields the aglycone sarsasapogenin.

sar·to′ri·us [L. *sartor*, patcher]. The tailor's muscle, so called from being concerned in crossing one leg over the other. See Table of Muscles in the Appendix.

sas′sa·fras [Sp. *sasafrás*] (*sassafras*). The dried bark of the root of *Sassafras albidum.* Contains a volatile oil, and has been used as a mild aromatic and carminative.

s. oil (*oleum sassafras*). The volatile oil distilled with steam from the root of *Sassafras albidum.* As it is much less irritant to mucous membranes than other volatile oils, it is less useful as a carminative. The oil contains safrol, pinene, phellandrene, and dextrogyrate camphor. Dose, 0.12–0.4 cc. (2–6 min.).

s. pith. Formerly used, because of the delicate quality of its mucilage, in the preparation of collyriums.

sas′sa·frol. Safrol. See *sassafras* oil.

sas′so·lin. Old term for boric acid extracted from the deposits in lagoons of Tuscany.

sas′sy bark. The bark of *Erythrophleum.* Syn., *casca bark.*

sat. Saturated.

sat′el·lite. See satellite *cell.*

perineural s. See *oligodendroglia.*

perivascular s. See *oligodendroglia.*

sat″el·li·to′sis (sat″i·lye·to′sis, ·li·to′sis) [L. *satelles*, attendant; G. *-ōsis*, condition]. *In neuropathology*, a condition in which there is an increase of satellite cells around the nerve cells of the central nervous system in inflammatory and degenerative diseases. These satellite cells usually represent phagocytic neuroglia cells.

sa·ti′e·ty [L. *satietas*, sufficiency]. Fullness beyond desire; a condition of gratification beyond desire or need.

Sato and Shoji's stain. See under *stain.*

sat. sol. Saturated solution.

Satterthwaite's method. See under *artificial respiration.*

Sattler, Hubert [*Austrian ophthalmologist*, 1844–1928]. Described a thin layer of elastic fibers lying between the layer of large vessels and the lamina choriocapillaris of the choroid of the eye; called *Sattler's elastic layer.*

sat′u·ra″ted [L. *saturatus*, saturated]. 1. Having all the atoms of molecules linked so that only single bonds exist. 2. Having sufficient substance, either solid or gaseous, dissolved in a solution so that no more of that substance can be dissolved. Abbreviated, sat.

s. compound. An organic compound with no free valence, and in which there are neither double nor triple bonds.

sat″u·ra′tion. *In optics*, the quality of visual sensation which distinguishes between colors of the same dominant wavelength but different purities.

sat′ur·nine (sat′ur·nyne) [L. *Saturnus*, Saturn]. 1. Pertaining to or produced by lead. 2. Of gloomy nature.

sat′ur·nism [*Saturnus*]. Chronic lead poisoning; plumbism.

sat″y·ri′a·sis [G.]. 1. Excessive venereal desire in man. Also called *satyromania.* See *priapism.* 2. Old term for leprosy.

sat′yr tip. The posteriorly directed pointed portion of the superior part of the helix: also called *satyr tubercle.*

sau′cer·ize [OF. *saussier*]. Shape bone cavity in the operation for chronic osteomyelitis, in order to eliminate sharp angles and overhanging walls, thus permitting soft parts to fill it completely during the process of healing; to gutter.

Saucerotte, Nicolas [*French physician*, 1741–1814]. Credited with having given the first clinical description of acromegaly (1772). The case was included among the five reported by Pierre Marie a century later.

Sauerbruch, Ernst Ferdinand [*German surgeon*, 1875–1951]. With E. Schumacher, devised paravertebral thoracoplasty for chronic pulmonary tuberculosis. Invented a negative pressure chamber for use in chest operations. See S.H.G. *diet.*

Saunders, Edward Watt [*American physician*, 1854–1927]. Described an acute gastric disturbance in infants caused by carbohydrate excess in the diet; called *Saunders' disease.*

saun′ders. See under *sandalwood.*

sau·ri′a·sis [G. *sauros*, lizard; NL. *-iasis*, condition]. Ichthyosis.

Sau·rop′si·da [*sauros;* G. *opsis*, appearance]. A superclass of vertebrates comprising the birds and reptiles.

sau·rox′ine (saw·rock′seen, ·sin). An alkaloid obtained from *Lycopodium saururus.* See *piligan.*

sau·ru′rine (saw·roor′een, ·in). An alkaloid obtained from *Lycopodium saururus.* See *piligan.*

sau′sar·ism [G. *sausarismos*, paralysis of the tongue]. 1. Paralysis of the tongue. 2. Dryness of the tongue.

Sauter, Johann Nepomuk [*German surgeon*, 1766–1840]. Pioneer in performing vaginal hysterectomy, leaving ovaries and uterine tubes *in situ;* called *Sauter's operation.*

Sauvineau, Charles [*French ophthalmologist*, 1862–]. Described an ophthalmoplegia in which there is paralysis of the medial rectus muscle of one side and spasm of the lateral rectus muscle on the opposite side; called *Sauvineau's ophthalmoplegia.*

Savill, Thomas Dixon [*English physician*, 1856–1910]. Said to have been the first to describe epidemic exfoliative dermatitis; called *Savill's disease.*

sav′in. The evergreen shrub *Juniperus sabina*, from the tops of which a volatile oil may be obtained and a fluidextract prepared, both formerly used for emmenagogue, vermifuge, and antirheumatic effects.

sa′vo·ry [L. *sapor*, flavor]. Having a pleasant odor or flavor.

saw [AS. *sagu*]. An instrument having a thin blade with sharp teeth on one edge, and used for dividing bones and other hard substances.

Adams' s. A small straight saw with a long handle.

Albee's s. An electrically operated, double rotary circular saw with adjustable blades, for use in preparing bone grafts.

Butcher's s. One in which the blade can be fixed at any angle.

chain s. One in which the teeth are set in links movable upon each other, the saw being moved by pulling alternately upon one and the other handle.

crown s. See *trephine.*

Gigli's s. A flexible wire saw operated by handles at either end, which pass through loops. Adapted to cranial and other bone operations.

Hey's s. A serrated disk affixed to a handle, and used for enlarging an opening in a bone.

nasal s. A small, narrow instrument used for removing nasal spurs and turbinate bones.

saw pal·met'to. See *serenoa.*

Sawyer, Wilbur Augustus [*American epidemiologist,* 1879–1951]. With Kitchen and Lloyd, prepared a vaccine for prophylactic immunization against yellow fever (1932). Introduced a yellow fever test. See Sawyer and Lloyd serum protection *test.*

sax'i·frage [L. *saxum,* stone; *frangere,* to break]. Any plant of the genus *Saxifraga. S. crassifolia* and other species contain a crystalline bitter principle, bergenin. *Saxifraga ligulata,* containing tannic acid, is used in India for dysentery.

saxin. Trade-mark for a brand of saccharin.

Saxtorph, Mathias [*Danish obstetrician,* 1740–1800]. Described a technic for extracting the fetus, in which he applied strong downward pressure with one hand on the lock of the obstetric forceps, while using the other for horizontal traction; called *Saxtorph's maneuver.*

Sayre, Lewis Albert [*American surgeon,* 1820–1900]. Known especially for his work in orthopedic surgery. Performed resection of the hip joint (1855). Said to have been the first to use a plaster of Paris jacket as a support for the spine (1877). Inventor of a device for suspending a patient during the application of a plaster jacket, called *Sayre's apparatus.*

Sb Chemical symbol for antimony (stibium).

Sc Chemical symbol for scandium.

scab [ME., from L. *scabere,* to scratch]. 1. Dried exudate covering an ulcer or wound. Syn., *crust.* 2. A disease of sheep caused by a mite.

scab'bard [ME. *scaubert*]. A veterinary term for the prepuce of the horse.

scabbed [L. *scabere,* to scratch]. Crusted.

sca'bi·cide [L. *scabies,* the itch; *caedere,* to kill]. Any agent or drug which kills *Sarcoptes scabiei,* the causative organism of scabies.

sca'bi·es (skay'bee·eez, skay'beez) [L., the itch]. A contagious disorder of the skin caused by *Sarcoptes scabiei;* characterized by multiform lesions with intense itching which occurs chiefly at night. The female insect, burrowing beneath the skin to lay eggs, causes the irritation. Also called *itch, seven-year itch.*

camel s. A form acquired from the camel. Runs a limited course as the parasite does not live long on human skin. Various similar organisms live on other animals in conditions which are called *canary s., cat s., horse s.,* etc.

s. crustosa. An extreme form of general scabies of the body resulting in fish-scalelike desquamation. Also called *Boeck's s., Norway itch.*

s. papuliformis. A form marked by papular efflorescence. Also called *rank itch, s. papulosa.*

s. pustulosa. That in which there is formation of large pustules resembling those of smallpox, occurring on the wrists and buttocks of children. Seen more commonly in warm weather.

sca"bi·o·pho'bi·a [*scabies;* G. *phobos,* fear]. Morbid fear of scabies.

sca'bi·ous [L. *scabiosus,* rough]. 1. Scabby or scaly. 2. Pertaining to scabies.

sca'brin. $C_{22}H_{35}NO$; N-isobutyl-2,4,6,10 (or 12),-14-octadecapentaenamide; a constituent of the roots of *Heliopsis scabra* (rough heliopsis) and other *Heliopsis* species; an insecticide.

sca·bri'ti·es (ska·brish'ee·eez) [L., roughness]. Roughness; scabbiness.

s. unguium syphilitica. Abnormal thickening and roughness of the nails, seen in syphilis.

sca'la (pl. *scalae*) [L., ladder]. A subdivision of the cavity of the cochlea; especially, one of the perilymphatic spaces.

s. media. Old term for cochlear duct.

s. tympani. The perilymphatic space below the osseous spiral lamina and the basilar membrane. See Plate 20.

s. vestibuli. The perilymphatic space above the osseous spiral lamina and the vestibular membrane. See Plate 20.

scald [ME. *scalden,* from L. *calidus,* warm]. The burn caused by hot liquids or vapors.

scald'ing [*scalden*]. Burning pain in urination.

scale [ME.]. 1. An instrument bearing marks or graduations at regular intervals and used as a standard in measuring, as barometric scale, thermometric scale. 2. The dry, semiopaque lamina of horny epidermis that is shed from the skin, usually as a result of imperfect cornification, a secondary skin lesion. Also called *squama.*

Bellevue s. See *Wechsler-Bellevue intelligence scale* under *test.*

Binet-Simon intelligence s. See Binet-Simon *test.*

Cattell infant intelligence s. See under *test.*

Cornell-Coxe performance-ability s. See Ethel Letitia *Cornell.*

Haldane s. A standard for establishing hemoglobin levels in which 13.8 Gm. in 100 cc. of blood equals 100 per cent.

Minnesota preschool s. See under *test.*

Vineland social maturity s. See under *test.*

Wechsler-Bellevue intelligence s. See under *test.*

sca·lene' (skay·leen', skay'leen) [G. *skalēnos,* uneven]. Having unequal sides, as scalene muscle.

sca"le·nec'to·my [*skalēnos;* G. *ektomē,* excision]. Excision of the scalene muscles, particularly the scalenus anterior.

sca"le·not'o·my [*skalēnos;* G. *tomē,* a cutting]. Severing of the fibers of a scalene muscle.

sca·le'nus [*skalēnos*]. One of three muscles in the neck, arising from the transverse processes of the cervical vertebrae, and inserted on the first two ribs. See Table of Muscles in the Appendix.

s. minimus. An inconstant muscle of the scalene group arising from the anterior tubercle of the sixth or sixth and seventh ribs, inserted into the first rib, and attached to the dome of the pleura.

s. pleuralis. That part of the scalenus minimus muscle attached to the pleura.

sca'ler [ME. *scale*]. 1. An instrument for removing calcareous deposits from the teeth. 2. An electronic instrument for counting and recording electrical impulses, as those produced by such detectors of radioactivity as the Geiger-Müller tube and the scintillation probe.

sca'ling [*scale*]. Desquamating; producing scales.

sca'ling. A pharmaceutical process consisting of drying concentrated solutions of drugs on glass plates.

s. the teeth. An operation, in dentistry, which consists in the removal of deposits of calculus from the teeth.

sca'ling cir'cuit. One which permits mechanical recording of electrical impulses which are produced at a high frequency, by counting only every 2^n or 10^n impulse; such a circuit is employed in a scaler, 2.

scalp [ME.]. The hairy integument covering the cranium.

scal'pel [L. *scalpellum,* small surgical knife]. A surgical knife with a short blade, a convex or straight cutting edge, rounded or pointed at the end.

sca'ly [ME. *scale*]. 1. Resembling scales; characterized by scales. 2. Covered with, or possessing, scales.

scam'mo·ny. See *ipomea.*

scan'di·um [L. *Scandia,* Scandinavia]. Sc = 44.96. A rare metal belonging to the aluminum group.

scan·sor′i·us [L. *scansor*, climber]. The small anterior gluteal muscle.

Scanzoni, Friedrich Wilhelm [*German obstetrician*, 1821–91]. Introduced a procedure to convert a posterior vertex presentation to an anterior position by the use of double forceps application; called *Scanzoni's maneuver* or *operation*.

sca′pha [BNA] [L., skiff, from G. *skaphē*, boat]. The furrow of the auricle between the helix and antihelix.

scaph″o·ceph′a·ly (skaf″o·sef′uh·lee, skay″fo·) [*skaphē;* G. *kephalē*, head]. A condition of the skull, characterized by a projecting, keel-like sagittal suture, due to its premature closure. —**scaphocephal′ic, scaphocephalous,** *adj.*

scaph′oid [*skaphē;* G. *eidos*, form]. Boat-shaped.

scaph′oid. A boat-shaped bone of the tarsus and of the carpus. Old term for navicular. See Table of Bones in the Appendix.

scap′u·la [L.]. The shoulder blade, the large, flat, triangular bone forming the back of the shoulder. See Table of Bones in the Appendix. See Plates 1, 2, 14. —**scapular,** *adj.*

alar s. See *angel's wing.*

winged s. See *angel's wing.*

scap″u·lal′gi·a [*scapula;* G. *algos*, pain]. Pain in the region of the scapula.

scap″u·lec′to·my [*scapula;* G. *ektomē*, excision]. Surgical removal of a scapula.

scap′u·lo- [*scapula*]. A combining form denoting *relation to the shoulder* or *scapula.*

scap″u·lo·cla·vic″u·la′ris. A variable muscle extending from the coracoid process to the lateral third of the clavicle.

scap′·u·lo·cos″tal. Of or pertaining to the scapula and the ribs. Syn., *costoscapular.*

scap″u·lo·hu′mer·al [*scapula;* L. *humerus*, upper bone of the arm]. Pertaining to the scapula and the humerus, or to the shoulder joint, as scapulohumeral amputation.

scap′u·lo·pex″y (skap′yoo·lo·peck″see, skap″yoo·lo·peck′see) [*scapula;* G. *pēxis*, a fixing]. Fixation of the scapula to the ribs, as in cases of paralysis of scapular muscles.

scar [OF. *escare*, from G. *eschar*, hearth, scab]. A permanent mark resulting from a wound or disease process in tissue, especially the skin.

scar″a·bi′a·sis (skar″uh·buy′uh·sis) [L. *scarabaeus;* N.L. *-iasis*, condition]. A condition occurring usually in children in which the intestine is invaded by the dung beetle. Characterized by anorexia, emaciation, and gastrointestinal disturbances. Also called *beetle disease.*

scarf′skin″ [AS. *scearfe;* ON. *skinn*]. The epidermis or cuticle.

scar″i·fi·ca′tion [L. *scarificare*, to scratch open]. The operation of making numerous small, superficial incisions in skin or other tissue. —**scar′ify,** *v.*

scar′i·fi·ca″tor [*scarificare*]. An instrument used in scarification, consisting of a number of small lancets operated by a spring.

scar″la·ti′na (skahr″luh·tee′nuh). Scarlet fever. —**scarlatinal, scarlatinous,** *adj.*

scar″la·ti·nel′la. See fourth *disease.*

scar″la·ti′ni·form (skahr″luh·tee′ni·form, ·tin′i·form) [ME. *scarlet;* L. *forma*, form]. Resembling scarlet fever.

scar″la·ti′noid (skahr″luh·tee′noyd, skahr·lat′i·noyd) [*scarlat;* G. *eidos*, form]. Scarlatiniform.

scar′let fe′ver. An acute, contagious, febrile disease, having a period of incubation varying from several hours to a week, setting in with vomiting or chill, which is followed by high fever, rapid pulse, sore throat, cervical adenitis, and the appearance of a punctiform, scarlet-red eruption from one to five days thereafter. The tongue, at first heavily coated and red at the tip and edges, soon shows prominence of the papillae, which are red and swollen (strawberry tongue). The eruption, at the appearance of which all the symptoms become intensified, gradually fades after five or six days, and is followed by a scaly desquamation. A peculiarity of scarlet fever is its tendency to involve the kidneys. The causal agent is a hemolytic streptococcus. See Dick *test.* Also called *scarlatina.*

anginal s. f. Scarlet fever with marked inflammation of the throat.

gastric s. f. Scarlet fever complicated with gastroenteritis.

hemorrhagic s. f. Scarlet fever, or, more usually, septic fever with hemorrhagic spots.

latent s. f. Scarlet fever without eruptions.

malignant s. f. A form characterized by an abrupt onset, high fever, convulsions, coma, and death, often before the appearance of the eruption.

papular s. f. Scarlet fever in which there are prominent papules, due to involvement of the hair follicles.

puerperal s. f. Littré's name for a rash resembling that of scarlet fever sometimes followed by vesication and pustulation of the affected parts, but without fever; observed in puerperants. Also called *erythema diffusum, porphyra.*

pustular s. f. Scarlet fever with a pustular eruption.

s. f. sine angina. Scarlet fever without throat symptoms.

s. f. sine eruptione. Scarlet fever without the rash.

s. f. streptococcus antitoxin (*antitoxinum scarlatinae streptococcicum*). A sterile aqueous solution of antitoxic substances obtained from the blood serum or plasma of a healthy animal which has been immunized against the toxin produced by the streptococcus regarded as the causative agent of scarlet fever. It is used in the treatment of scarlet fever, and occasionally for producing a temporary passive immunity in persons exposed to the infection. It is also used to distinguish the rash of scarlet fever from other rashes. Dose, prophylactic: 2000 units; therapeutic: 6000 units. Also called *s. f. antitoxin, refined s. f. antitoxin, concentrated s. f. antitoxin, anti-scarlet-fever globulins.*

s. f. streptococcus toxin (*toxinum scarlatinae streptococcicum*). A sterile solution in a medium containing not more than 1% of peptone but no meat extractive, of certain products including a soluble toxin, resulting from the growth in the broth of suitable strains of hemolytic streptococci (*Streptococcus pyogenes*). Used either as a diagnostic agent or as a therapeutic agent against scarlet fever. As a diagnostic agent, the toxin is greatly diluted with a buffered diluent isotonic with the blood and the pH adjusted to 7.5. Dose, diagnostic, 0.1 cc. of the dilution, intracutaneously; as an immunizing agent, graded hypodermic doses, starting at 500 to 650 S.T.D., given at proper intervals until a negative Dick test is obtained. Also called *s. f. toxin for immunization and for the Dick test.*

septic s. f. A grave form of scarlet fever characterized by symptoms of septic intoxication.

simple s. f. Mild scarlet fever.

traumatic s. f. The eruption of scarlet fever, accompanied by febrile symptoms, which sometimes follow wounds or surgical operations infected with hemolytic streptococcus.

scar′let red (*rubrum scarlatinum*). $C_{24}H_{20}N_4O$. An azo dye, *o*-tolyl azo-*o*-tolyl azo-*β*-naphthol; occurs as a dark, brownish red powder; almost insoluble in water, slightly soluble in alcohol. Scarlet red has the power of stimulating the proliferation of epithelial cells. It is used to promote the growth of epithelium in the treatment of burns, wounds, chronic ulcers, etc. It is generally used in the form of an ointment. Also called *s. r., medicinal; Biebrich s. r.*

s. r. ointment (*unguentum rubri scarlatini*). Contains 5% of scarlet red in a base consisting of olive oil, wool fat, and petrolatum.

s. r. sulfonate. The sodium salt of azobenzenedisulfonic acid azobetanaphthol; the sulfonic acid derivative of scarlet red. It differs from scarlet red in that the two CH_3 groups are replaced by the SO_3Na group; occurs as a dark, brownish red powder; it is soluble in water and only slightly soluble in organic solvents. Used for the same purposes as scarlet red. Also called *soluble s. r.*

Scarpa, Antonio [*Italian anatomist and surgeon*, 1752–1832]. Described the ganglion of the vestibular nerve, called *Scarpa's ganglion.* Described the triangular space having for its base the inguinal ligament, and for its apex the point of intersection of the sartorius and adductor longus muscles, called *Scarpa's triangle*, and the median incisive foramen, called *foramen of Scarpa.*

scat″a·cra′ti·a (skat″uh·kray′shuh, ·shee·uh). See *scoracratia.*

sca·te′mi·a [G. *skōr*, dung; *haima*, blood]. Intestinal toxemia.

scat′ol, sca′tol. See *skatole.*

scat″o·lo′gi·a, sca·tol′o·gy [*skōr;* G. *logos*, word]. The study of excreta. —**scatolog′ic,** *adj.*

sca·to′ma [*skōr;* G. *-ōma*, tumor]. A mass of fecal matter in the colon resembling, on palpation, an abdominal tumor.

sca·toph′a·gous [*skōr;* G. *phagein*, to eat]. Excrement-eating.

sca·toph′a·gy [*skōr; phagein*]. The eating of excrement.

sca·tos′co·py [*skōr;* G. *skopein*, to examine]. Inspection of the excreta.

scat′ter [ME. *scateren*]. 1. The spreading of rays, as x-rays. 2. *In psychology*, the range of levels through which an individual passes on an intelligence test.

back s. Roentgen rays scattered backward within irradiated tissues and reemerging through the area of incidence.

scat′ter·ing. *In nuclear science*, the change in direction of a particle or photon as a result of a collision with another particle or system.

scav′en·ger [ONF. *escauwage*, inspection]. A macrophage: also called *scavenger cell.*

scav′en·ging. *In nuclear chemistry*, the formation of an unspecific precipitate to remove from a solution, by adsorption or coprecipitation, a substantial proportion of one or more undesirable radioactive ions. Hydrous ferric oxide is frequently so used being then called *a scavenger.*

Sc. D. Doctor of Science.

Sc. D. A. Right scapuloanterior position of the fetus.

Sc. D. P. Right scapuloposterior position of the fetus.

scent [OF. *sentir*, to smell]. An effluvium from any body capable of affecting the olfactory sense; odor; fragrance.

Schachowa, Seraphina [*Russian histologist*, nineteenth century]. Described the section of a uriniferous tubule lying between the proximal convolution and the loop of Henle; called *Schachowa's spiral tubule.*

Schachter, Rubin Joseph [*American physiologist*, 1904–]. Has made valuable contributions to the study of shock, adrenals, antibiotics, antihistamines, thyroid, and parasympathetic drugs. 5 mg. of acetylcholine chloride dissolved in 0.025 cc. of bicarbonate Ringer's solution at pH 7.4 and 38° C., in the presence of cholinesterase, liberating 1 mm.^{3} of CO_2 per minute, is *Schachter's unit of cholinesterase.*

Schaeffer, Jacob Parsons [*American anatomist*, 1878–]. Authority on paranasal sinuses. Author of monographs and papers on anatomy and embryology. Editor-in-Chief of Morris' *Textbook of Human Anatomy.*

Schaeffer-Fulton stain. See *Schaeffer-Fulton modification of Wirtz method*, under *stain.*

Schafer, Edward Albert Sharpey. See *Sharpey-Schafer.*

Schaffer, Károly (Karl) (1864–1939). Hungarian neuropathologist known for his work on hereditary diseases of the nervous system and the three criteria he established for these: (1) ectodermal defect, (2) localization determined by the neuraxial defect, (3) system selectivity, which are called *triad of Schaffer.*

Schäffer's reflex. See under *reflex.*

Schales and Schales method. See under *method.*

Schamberg, Jay Frank (1870–1934). American dermatologist who first (1901) described progressive pigmentary dermatosis (Schamberg's disease) and acarodermatitis urticaroides, and wrote on the etiology of psoriasis.

Schanz, Alfred [*German orthopedic surgeon*, 1868–1931]. Described a syndrome of fatigue, pain on pressure over the spinal processes, pain when lying down, spinal curvature, as indicative of spinal weakness; called *Schanz's syndrome.*

Schardinger reaction. See under *reaction.*

Schaudinn, Fritz Richard [*German bacteriologist*, 1871–1906]. Noted for his discovery, with P. E. Hoffmann, of the *Spirochaeta pallida* or *Treponema pallidum*, the cause of syphilis (1905).

Schaudinn's fixing fluid. See under *fixing fluid.*

Schaumann, Jörgen (1879–1953). Swedish dermatologist known for his fundamental work in sarcoidosis, sometimes called *Schaumann's disease.* He described (1941) the inclusion bodies in giant cells in sarcoidosis and berylliosis, called *Schaumann inclusion bodies.*

Schauta, Friedrich [*Austrian gynecologist*, 1849–1919]. Remembered for his operation of radical hysterectomy called *Schauta's operation.* An operation for cystocele is called *Schauta-Wertheim operation.*

Schede, Max [*German surgeon*, 1844–1902]. Devised a method of treating bone caries by curetting the cavity and allowing it to fill with blood clot; called *Schede's method.* Best known for his extrapleural pneumonolysis, now obsolete; called *Schede's operation.*

Scheele, Karl Wilhelm [*Swedish chemist*, 1742–86]. Isolated oxygen (ca. 1772); see also *Lavoisier* and *Priestley.* Discovered barium, chlorine, and manganese. A brilliant green pigment, an acid copper arsenite, is known as *Scheele's green.* Isolated uric acid from urine (1776).

Scheerer. See Goldstein-Scheerer *test.*

Scheiner, Christoph [*German physicist*, 1575–1650]. Famous for his many discoveries and observations in physiologic optics. Demonstrated the changes in the curvature of the crystalline lens during accommodation. Demonstrated the manner in which images strike the retina. Devised a pinhole test illustrating refraction and accommodation of the eye (1619), called *Scheiner's test.*

Schellong-Strisower phenomenon. A fall of systolic blood pressure on assuming the erect position from recumbency.

sche′ma (skee′muh) [G., figure]. 1. A simple design

to illustrate a complex mechanism. 2. An outline of a subject. —**schemat'ic,** *adj.*

sche'mo·graph (skee'mo·graf) [*schēma;* G. *graphein,* to write]. An apparatus for tracing the outline of the field of vision; the measurement of the field is made with the perimeter.

Schenck, Benjamin Robinson [*American surgeon,* 1842–1920]. The first to describe sporotrichosis, called *Schenck's disease.*

Schenk, Samuel Leopold [*Austrian physiologist,* 1840–1902]. Described a method of determination of the sex of infants based on the theory that, by regulation of the mother's diet before and during pregnancy, the sex can be controlled. When no sugar is secreted, he believed that the ovum would be qualified to develop into a male child. Called *Schenk's method* or *theory.*

Scherer's test. See under *test.*

sche·ro'ma (ski·ro'muh). Xerophthalmia.

Scheuermann, Holger Werfel (1877–). Danish surgeon who described osteochondrosis of the vertebral epiphyses in children (1921), called *Scheuermann's disease.*

Schick, Bela (1877–). Austrian pediatrician known for his development of a reliable skin test for the determination of susceptibility to diphtheria (1913). See Schick *test.* Earlier (1905) he made, with C. P. Pirquet von Cesenatico, a study of serum sickness and its importance to medicine. Together they introduced the term *allergy.*

Schiff's reagent. See under *reagent.*

Schilder, Paul Ferdinand [*German physician,* 1886–1940]. Remembered for his description of encephalitis periaxialis diffusa (1912), also known as *Schilder's disease, Huebner-Schilder's disease, progressive subcortical encephalopathy.*

Schiller, Walter (1887–). American pathologist who introduced his test for carcinoma of the uterine cervix in which he painted the suspected area with Lugol's solution. The appearance of whitish spots indicates the possibility of carcinoma, the change being due to loss of glycogen in the epithelium (1933). See Schiller *test.*

Schilling, Victor (1883–). Austrian hematologist who modified Arneth's classification of the neutrophils (1911) by dividing them into four groups, tabulated from left to right: (1) myelocytes or younger-than-juveniles; (2) juveniles with indented nuclei; (3) band forms with unsegmented but T-, V-, or U-shaped nuclei; (4) segmented mature neutrophils: also called *Schilling's blood count, hemogram* or *method.* He set up an index of nuclear shift and further modified immature neutrophils by describing a degenerative shift (failure of neutrophils to mature) and a regenerative shift (temporary increase in immature cells due to increased production in response to acute infection). See under *shift.* See also monocytic *leukemia.*

Schimmelbusch, Curt [*German surgeon,* 1860–95]. Described adenosis of the breast, called *Schimmelbusch's disease.*

schin"dy·le'sis (skin"di·lee'sis) [G., a cleaving into small pieces]. A form of articulation in which a plate of one bone is received into a fissure of another.

Schiötz, Hjalmar [*Norwegian ophthalmologist,* 1850–1927]. Known for his invention (1881) of an ocular tonometer; called *Schiötz's tonometer.* With Louis Emile Javal, modified the Helmholtz ophthalmometer (1881); called *Schiötz's ophthalmometer.*

-schi'sis (ski'sis) [G. *schisis,* a cleaving]. A combining form meaning *cleft, split, fissure.*

schis'to- (skis'to-) [G. *schistos,* cleft]. A combining form meaning *split, fissured.*

schis"to·ce'li·a [*schistos;* G. *koilia,* cavity]. Celosoma.

schis"to·ceph'a·lus [*schistos;* G. *kephalē,* head]. 1. A monster with a fissured skull. 2. Gurlt's general term for cleft in any part of the head. —**schistocephal'ic,** *adj.*

schis"to·cor'mus [*schistos;* G. *kormos,* trunk]. A monstrosity having a cleft thorax (**schistocormus fissisternalis**), neck (**schistocormus fissicollis**), or abdominal wall (**schistocormus fissiventralis**).

schis"to·cys'tis [*schistos;* G. *kystis,* bladder]. Fissure of the urinary bladder: also called *vesical ectopia, exstrophy of the bladder.*

schis'to·cyte [*schistos;* G. *kytos,* cell]. A fragmented part of an erythrocyte containing hemoglobin.

schis"to·cy·to'sis (skis"to·sigh·to'sis) [*schistos; kytos;* G. *-ōsis,* condition]. The presence of large numbers of schistocytes in the blood.

schis"to·glos'si·a [*schistos;* G. *glōssa,* tongue]. Cleft tongue.

schis·tom'e·lus [*schistos;* G. *melos,* limb]. An individual with a cleft extremity.

schis·tom'e·ter [*schistos;* G. *metron,* a measure]. A device for measuring the distance between the vocal cords.

schis"to·pro·so'pi·a, schis"to·pros'o·py [*schistos;* G. *prosōpon,* face]. Congenital fissure of the face. —**schistopros'opous,** *adj.*

schis"to·pros'o·pus (skis"to·pros'o·pus, ·pro·so'pus) [*schistos; prosōpon*]. A monster having a fissure of the face.

schis·tor'rha·chis, schis·tor'ra·chis (skis·tor'uh·kis) [*schistos;* G. *rhachis,* spine]. Spina bifida; rachischisis.

schis·to'sis [*schistos;* G. *-ōsis,* condition]. Fibrosis of the lungs occurring in slate cutters. Also see *silicosis.*

Schis"to·so'ma [*schistos;* G. *sōma,* body]. The genus of blood flukes infesting man.

S. haematobium. The adults are found in the vessels of the urinary bladder; common in Africa.

S. japonicum. The adults are found in the mesenteric veins; widely distributed in Japan and China.

S. mansoni. The adults are found in the mesenteric veins and portal vein; found in parts of Africa, South America, and the West Indies.

schis"to·so·mi'a·sis [*schistos; sōma;* NL. *-iasis,* condition]. 1. Infestation with *Schistosoma.* Syn., *bilharziasis.* 2. A papular and pustular dermatitis occurring on the skin of persons wading or swimming in fresh-water lakes of the northern United States and Canada. A self-limited disease caused by the penetration of one of the cercarial larvae which are parasites of snails. Also called *swimmer's itch, swamp itch.*

Schis"to·so·mo·phor'a hy"dro·bi·op'sis. A fresh-water snail, the intermediate host of *Schistosoma japonicum.*

schis"to·so'mus [*schistos; sōma*]. A monster in which there is a lateral or median eventration extending the whole length of the abdomen, one or both lower extremities being absent or rudimentary.

schis"to·ster'ni·a [*schistos;* G. *sternon,* breast]. Sternal fissure.

schis"to·tho'rax [*schistos;* G. *thōrax,* thorax]. Fissure of the thorax.

schis"to·tra'che·lus (skis"to·tray'ki·lus, ·tra·kee'lus) [*schistos;* G. *trachēlos,* neck]. Cervical fissure. Also called *tracheloschisis.*

schiz·am'ni·on (skiz·am'nee·on) [G. *schizein,* to cleave; *amnion,* membrane around the fetus]. An amnion developing by cavity formation in the inner cell mass.

schiz·ax′on (skiz·acks′on) [*schizein;* G. *axōn,* axis]. An axon which divides in its course into equal, or nearly equal, branches.

schiz′o- (skiz′o-), **schiz-** [*schizein*]. A combining form denoting *split* or *cleft.*

schiz″o·ble·pha′ri·a [*schizein;* G. *blepharon,* eyelid]. Fissure of the eyelid.

schiz′o·cyte. See *schistocyte.*

schiz″o·cy·to′sis (skiz″o·sigh·to′sis). See *schistocytosis.*

schiz″o·gen′e·sis [*schizein;* G. *genesis,* production]. Reproduction by fission.

schiz″o·gnath′ism (skiz″o·nath′iz·um) [*schizein;* G. *gnathos,* jaw]. Cleavage of the jaw.

schi·zog′o·ny (ski·zog′o·nee, sky·) [*schizein;* G. *gonē,* offspring]. 1. Schizogenesis. 2. Multiple division in which the contents of the oocyst eventually split into swarm spores. —**schizogon′ic,** *adj.*

schiz″o·gy′ri·a (skiz″o·jye′ree·uh, ·jirr′ee·uh) [*schizein;* G. *gyros,* circle]. Cerebral deformity marked by partial separation of the gyri.

schiz′oid [*schizein;* G. *eidos,* form]. Resembling schizophrenia. —**schiz′oid,** *n.*

schiz″o·ma′ni·a [*schizein;* G. *mania,* madness]. A mental disorder presenting features of both schizophrenia and mania.

Schiz″o·my·ce′tes (skiz″o·migh·see′teez) [*schizein;* G. *mykēs,* fungus]. A class of fungi; the fission fungi or bacteria.

schiz″o·my·co′sis (skiz″o·migh·ko′sis) [*schizein; mykēs;* G. *-ōsis,* condition]. A disease due to schizomycetes, a disease caused by bacteria.

schiz′ont [*schizein*]. A stage in the asexual life cycle of *Plasmodium,* covering the period from beginning of division of nuclear material until the mature merozoites are formed. See Plates 27, 28, 29.

schi·zon′ti·cide. A substance destructive to schizonts.

schiz″o·nych′i·a (skiz″o·nick′ee·uh) [*schizein;* G. *onyx,* nail]. Disease of the nails characterized by irregular splitting.

schiz″o·pha′si·a (skiz″o·fay′zhuh, ·zee·uh) [*schizein;* G. *phasis,* utterance]. Word-salad; scrambled speech which may occur in schizophrenia.

schiz″o·phre′ni·a [*schizein;* G. *phrēn,* mind]. Bleuler's term for dementia precox, now classified as *schizophrenic reaction.* —**schizophren′ic,** *n., adj.*

schiz″o·phren′ic re·ac′tion. One of a group of psychotic reactions, often beginning after adolescence or in young adulthood, characterized by fundamental disturbances in reality relationships and concept formations, with associated affective, behavioral, and intellectual disturbances in varying degrees and mixtures. These reactions are marked by a tendency to withdraw from reality, inappropriate mood, unpredictable disturbances in stream of thought, regressive tendencies to the point of deterioration, and often hallucinations and delusions.

catatonic type of s.r. A form characterized by disturbances in motor behavior, varying from generalized inhibition (stupor, mutism, negativism, and waxy flexibility) to frenzied activity. The patient may regress completely, so that bodily requirements, as feeding and elimination, must be cared for by others.

childhood type of s.r. A schizophrenic or schizophreniclike reaction, occurring before puberty, which may vary from the more differentiated forms because of the immaturity of the patient. It includes psychotic reactions in young children who are markedly withdrawn and introspective, and may include infantile autism.

hebephrenic type of s.r. A form in which there is marked silliness, posturing and mannerisms, playing with words, and regressive behavior; delusions and hallucinations, though present, are not predominant features.

paranoid type of s.r. A form in which delusions of persecution or of grandeur or both, hallucinations, and ideas of reference predominate and sometimes are systematized. The patient is often more intact and less bizarre in other areas, but generally is hostile, grandiose, excessively religious, and sometimes hypochondriacal.

residual type of s.r. Recognizable residual disturbance of thought, affect, or behavior shown by patients who, after a definite psychotic schizophrenic reaction, have improved sufficiently to be able to get along in the general community.

schizoaffective type of s.r. A psychotic reaction of combined schizophrenic and affective reactions. Mental content may be predominantly schizophrenic, accompanied by marked manic or depressive moods.

simple type of s.r. A form characterized by general loss of interest in people and external affairs, leading to apathy and typically a progressive course resistant to treatment, with apparent mental deterioration, occasional delusions, and hallucinations.

undifferentiated type of s.r. A form with mixed symptomatology, unclassifiable as one of the more distinct forms. It includes all early, as yet undifferentiated forms at the first attack, and may be *acute,* appearing suddenly and disappearing within a brief period though often recurring; or *chronic,* including latent, incipient, or prepsychotic forms not classifiable as of another type.

schiz″o·so′ma si″ren·oid′es (sigh″ren·oy′deez). Lateral abdominal cleft with absence of the leg on that side.

schiz″o·tho′rax. See *schistothorax.*

schiz″o·thy′mic [*schizein;* G. *thymos,* soul]. Having a schizoid personality or temperament. —**schizothymia,** *n.*

schiz″o·trich′i·a (skiz″o·trick′ee·uh) [*schizein;* G. *thrix,* hair]. Splitting of the hair.

schiz″o·tryp″a·no·so·mi′a·sis (skiz″o·trip″uh-no·so·my′uh·sis, skiz″o·try″puh·no·) [*schizein;* G. *trypanon,* auger; *sōma,* body; NL. *-iasis,* condition]. Infection with *Trypanosoma cruzi.*

schiz′o·type. Coined abbreviation for schizophrenic phenotype.

Schlaer test. See Hecht-Schlaer night vision *test.*

Schlange's sign. See under *sign.*

Schlatter, Carl [*Swiss surgeon,* 1864–1934]. Said to have been the first to excise the stomach (1897). He described a painful lesion observed in the tibial tuberosity in the young, which had been noted earlier (1903) by R. B. Osgood. Osteochondrosis of tuberosity of the tibia is known as *Osgood-Schlatter disease.*

Schleich, Carl Ludwig [*German surgeon,* 1859–1922]. Remembered for his development of infiltration anesthesia (1894–95). Made use of a cocaine solution.

Schleiden, Matthias Jakob [*German scientist and botanist,* 1804–81]. Recognized as the discoverer of the universality of the cell in plant structure. He considered plant growth due to increase in the number of cells (1838). It was due to similar research in animal life that Theodor Schwann was able to evolve a like theory in regard to the animal cell.

Schlemm, Friedrich S. [*German anatomist,* 1795–1858]. Known for his description of the canal at the sclerocorneal junction, called *Schlemm's* canal, or *venous sinus of the sclera.* See under *sinus.*

Schlesinger's sign. See Pool-Schlesinger's *sign.*

Schlesinger's test. See under *test.*

Schloffer, Hermann [*German surgeon,* 1868–1937]. Said to have been the first to operate for the relief of acromegaly by removing a pituitary tumor (1906). Developed a method of operating upon pituitary tumors by the nasal route (1907) called *Schloffer's operation.* Described an inflammatory swelling of the abdominal wall following surgical repair of inguinal hernia (1908); called *Schloffer's tumor.*

Schlösser, Carl [*German ophthalmologist,* 1857–1925]. First to employ deep alcohol injections in neuralgia (1903); called *Schlösser's treatment.*

Schmelzer method. See *Tirmann-Schmelzer method for ionic iron* under *stain.*

Schmidel, Casimir Christoph [*German anatomist,* 1718–92]. Abnormal communications between the vena cava and the portal system are sometimes called *Schmidel's anastomoses.*

Schmidt, Eduard Oskar [*German anatomist,* 1823–86]. Described his blood coagulation theory, that paraglobulin, under the influence of fibrin ferment, combines with fibrinogen to produce fibrin; called *Schmidt's coagulation theory.* Serum globulin is sometimes called *Schmidt's fibrinoplastic.*

Schmidt nuclei test. See under *test.*

Schmidt's test for urobilin. See under *test.*

Schmidt-Lantermann incisures. See *inciurse* of Schmidt-Lantermann.

Schmiedeberg, Johann Ernst Oswald [*German pharmacologist,* 1838–1921]. Did important work in pharmacology, especially in the effects of poisons on the circulation. Described digitalinum verum (1913), later studied by Kiliani; sometimes called *Schmiedeberg's digitalis.*

Schmincke's tumor. See *lymphoepithelioma.*

Schmitz's bacillus. See *Shigella ambigua.*

Schmorl, Christian G. [*German pathologist,* 1861–1932]. Described herniation of the nucleus pulposus, called *Schmorl's nodules.* See also *Schmorl's method for bone sections* under *stain.*

Schmorl's alizarin SX method for calcium. See under *stain.*

Schneider, Conrad Victor [*German anatomist,* 1614–80]. Remembered for his description of the origin of nasal mucus in the nasal mucous membrane (1660), which is called *Schneider's membrane, Schneiderian membrane.*

Schneider, Edward Christian [*American physiologist,* 1874–]. Introduced a test of physiologic fitness according to cardiovascular rating; called *Schneider's index.* With Haldane, Douglas, and Henderson, studied the effect of atmospheric pressure at high altitudes.

Schneider's acetocarmine stain. See *acetocarmine* under *stain.*

Schoenbein's test for cyanide. See under *test.*

Schoenheimer, Rudolf [*American biochemist,* 1898–1941]. Introduced the use of isotopic and radioactive tracer compounds in studies of fat and amino acid metabolism. Developed the modern concept of the dynamic state with the continuous, random destruction and resynthesis of the formed elements of the body. With Sperry, devised a method for analysis of blood cholesterol; see Schoenheimer and Sperry's *method.*

Schönberg. See *Albers-Schönberg.*

Schönlein, Johann Lucas (1793–1864). German physician who described a form of nonthrombocytopenic purpura associated with joint or limb pains, called *Schönlein's purpura* (1837). He also discovered a fungus, *Achorion schoenleini* or *Trichophyton schoenleini,* to be the cause of favus (1839).

Schott, Theodor [*German physician,* 1852–1921]. Remembered for his advocacy of a method of treating heart disease by resisted exercise and special forms of baths. *Schott's method* is a system of gymnastic movements combined with Nauheim salt baths used for chronic rheumatic affections as well as for diseases of the heart.

Schottmüller, Hugo [*German physician and bacteriologist,* 1867–1936]. The first to isolate *Streptococcus viridans* as the cause of bacterial endocarditis (1910); also called *Schottmüller's bacillus.* The bacillus of paratyphoid is called *Salmonella schottmuelleri, Schottmüller's bacillus.* Paratyphoid is called *Schottmüller's disease.* Isolated *Streptothrix muris ratti* as a cause of rat bite fever (1914).

Schreger's lines. See *lines of Schreger* under *line.*

Schridde, Hermann [*German pathologist,* 1875–]. Described thick, coarse, dark hairs found occasionally in the beard and on the temples of cancerous or cachectic patients; called *Schridde's cancer hairs.* Congenital generalized dropsy is called *Schridde's disease.*

Schröder, Karl Ernst [*German gynecologist,* 1838–87]. Excised the mucous membrane of the cervix for chronic endometritis; called *Schröder's operation.* See also retraction *ring.*

Schroeder's method. See under *artificial respiration.*

Schüffner, Wilhelm August Paul [*German pathologist,* 1867–1949]. Known for his description of small, round, pink or reddish yellow granules which appear in red blood cells, stained with the Romanovsky stain, concomitantly with the developing malarial parasite. Called *Schüffner's dots, granules, stippling.* See Plate 28.

Schüller, Artur (1874–). Austrian neurologist who described a syndrome (1915) similar to one noted earlier by Alfred Hand (1893) and characterized fully by Henry A. Christian (1919). See Hand-Schüller-Christian *disease.*

Schüller, Karl Heinrich Anton Ludwig Max [*German surgeon,* 1843–1907]. Introduced a method of artificial respiration in which the thorax is raised rhythmically, the fingers being hooked under the ribs. Called *Schüller's method.*

Schultes, Johann (Scultetus; Scultet) [*German surgeon,* 1595–1645]. See scultetus *bandage.*

Schultz, Werner (1878–1945). German physician who described agranulocytosis, called *Schultz's syndrome* or *disease.* See also Schultz-Charlton blanching *test,* Schultz-Dale *test.*

Schultz's sterol reaction method for cholesterol. See under *stain.*

Schultze, Friedrich [*German neurologist,* 1848–1934]. Described a type of acroparesthesia (1893), which is also called *Schultze's paresthesia.*

Schultze, Maximilian Johann Sigismund [*German anatomist and histologist,* 1825–74]. Showed the role of the cell in muscle tissue (1865). Best known for his description of the olfactory cells and of the nerve endings in the retina (1866). Described descending fibers of the dorsal root, which form a plug-shaped bundle lying about the middle of the dorsal funiculus of the cervical and thoracic cords; called the *comma tract of Schultze, fasciculus interfascicularis.*

Schultze's method. See under *artificial respiration.*

Schütz, E. [*German biochemist,* 1900–]. Known for his law stating that the rate of an enzymatic reaction may be in direct proportion to the square root of the enzyme concentration; known as *Schütz rule, Schütz-Borissov rule.*

Schwabach's test. See under *test.*

Schwalbe, Gustav [*German anatomist,* 1844–1916]. Remembered for his description of the medial vestibular nucleus; also called *nucleus of Schwalbe.* Described supercentral and anterior occipital fissures, called *fissures of Schwalbe.* Described lymph spaces along the outer surface of the dural sheath of the optic nerve; called *Schwalbe's spaces*.

Schwalbe, Marcus Walter [*German neurologist*, 1883–]. Described dystonia musculorum deformans (1908), later described by Oppenheim and Ziehen, called *torsion spasm*.

Schwann, Theodor [*German anatomist*, 1810–82]. Widely known for his application of Schleiden's theories to animal life. Regarded as the founder of theories of putrefaction and fermentation. Demonstrated pepsin in gastric juice (1836). Discovered the yeast cell (1837). Made important studies concerning the action of bile on digestion (1844). Described the neurilemma of a nerve fiber, which is also called *sheath of Schwann*. See *myelin*. See also *neurilemma*, 1.

schwan'no·gli·o'ma. Neurilemmoma.

schwan·no'ma (shvon·o'muh). A neurilemmoma. **malignant s.** A malignant tumor of peripheral nerves derived from Schwann cells, possibly associated with neurofibromatosis but not with neurilemmoma: also called *fibrosarcoma of nerve sheath, malignant neurilemmoma, malignant neurinoma, malignant neurofibroma, malignant peripheral glioma, neurilemmosarcoma, neurofibrosarcoma, neurogenic (neurogenous) sarcoma, sarcoma of peripheral nerve, schwannosarcoma*.

schwan"no·sar·co'ma. See malignant *schwannoma*.

Schwartz-McNeil test for gonorrhea. See under *test*.

Schwartze, Hermann Hugo Rudolf [*German otologist*, 1837–1910]. With Eysell, revived mastoidectomy. A procedure using hammer and chisel is known as *Schwartze's operation*.

Schweigger-Seidel, Franz [*German physiologist*, 1834–71]. Remembered for his demonstration of the nucleus and cytoplasm of the spermatozoon (1865). See also *sheath* of Schweigger-Seidel.

Schweinfurth green. Paris green.

Schweinitz, George Edmund de [*American ophthalmologist*, 1858–1938]. Long regarded as the leader in ophthalmology in the United States of America.

Schweitzer reagent. See under *reagent*.

Schweizer-Foley Y-plasty. See *Y-plasty of Schweizer-Foley*.

Schweninger, Ernst [*German physician*, 1850–1924]. Introduced his method for reducing, based on the restriction of fluids in the diet, called *Schweninger's method*.

sci·age' (see·ahzh', see'ahzh) [F.]. A sawing movement in massage, practiced with the ulnar border, or with the dorsum of the hand.

sci·ap'o·dy (sigh·ap'o·dee) [G. *Skiapodes*, shade-footed people]. Gigantism of the foot. Also called *macropodia, pes gigas*.

sci"as·co'pi·a, sci·as'co·py (sigh·ass'ko·pee). See *retinoscopy*.

sci·at'ic (sigh·at'ick) [G. *ischion*, hip-joint]. 1. Pertaining to the ischium, as the sciatic notch. 2. Pertaining to the sciatic nerve, as sciatic neuralgia. See Table of Nerves in the Appendix.

sci·at'i·ca (sigh·at'i·kuh) [*ischion*]. A disease characterized by neuralgic pain along the course of the sciatic nerve. It is dependent upon inflammation or injury to the nerve. In addition to pain, there are numbness, tingling, and tenderness along the course of the nerve, and eventually wasting of the muscles innervated by it.

sci"e·ro'pi·a [G. *skieros*, shady; *ōps*, eye]. Defective vision in which all objects appear dark.

scil'la. See *squill*.

scil"la·bi'ose. $C_{12}H_{22}O_{11}$; glucosidorhamnose; a disaccharide obtained by hydrolysis of the squill glycoside known by the trade-marked name *scillaren-A*.

scillaren. Trade-mark for a mixture of the natural glycosides, **scillaren-A** and **scillaren-B** (the latter a mixture) occurring in fresh squill, *Urginea maritima*, in the proportions in which they exist in the fresh crude drug; namely, about 2 parts of scillaren-A to 1 part of scillaren-B. The substance is used as a cardiac stimulant and as a diuretic.

scil'le·nin. See under *squill*.

scil"li·a·zu'ro·side. A cardioactive glycoside present in the fraction of squill glycosides identified by the trade-marked name *scillaren-B*.

scil"li·co·el'o·side. A cardioactive glycoside present in the fraction of squill glycosides identified by the trade-marked name *scillaren-B*.

scil"li·cryp'to·side. A cardioactive glycoside present in the fraction of squill glycosides identified by the trade-marked name *scillaren-B*.

scil"li·cy·an'o·side. A cardioactive glycoside present in the fraction of squill glycosides identified by the trade-marked name *scillaren-B*.

scil"li·di"u·ret'in. See under *squill*.

scil"li·glau'co·side. A cardioactive glycoside present in the fraction of squill glycosides identified by the trade-marked name *scillaren-B*.

scil"li·mar'in. See under *squill*.

scil'lin. See under *squill*.

scil"li·phe'o·side. A cardioactive glycoside present in the fraction of squill glycosides identified by the trade-marked name *scillaren-B*.

scil"li·pic'rin. See under *squill*.

scil·li'ro·side. $C_{32}H_{44}O_{12}$; a glycoside from red squill, the red variety of *Urginea maritima*. Its sugar component is D-glucose.

scil'lism [L. *scilla*, squill, from G. *skilla*]. Poisoning from preparations of squill; characterized by vomiting, retarded pulse, cardiac arrhythmia, and ventricular fibrillation.

scil'li·tin. See under *squill*.

scil"li·tox'in. See under *squill*.

scil"lo·ceph'a·lus [*scilla*; G. *kephalē*, head]. A person exhibiting scillocephaly.

scil"lo·ceph'a·ly [*scilla; kephalē*]. Congenital deformity of the head, in which it is small and conically pointed.

scin'ti·gram. A printed or penned record, consisting of horizontal rows of short vertical lines, variably spaced, which in the aggregate shows the distribution of a radioactive tracer substance in intact tissue and also the profile of the tissue. It is obtained by automatic scanning of the region of the body in which the tissue is located by means of a directional scintillation counter called a *scintiscanner*.

scin·til'la·scope [L. *scintilla*, spark; G. *skopein*, to examine]. An instrument for observing minute flashes of light upon a fluorescent screen struck by alpha particles, emitted from a small source of radioactive material.

scin"til·la'tion [L. *scintillatio*, from *scintilla*]. 1. An emission of sparks. 2. A subjective visual sensation, as of sparks.

scin"til·la'tion coun'ter. A counter in which radioactive particles cause scintillations on a fluorescent screen that are picked up by the photosensitive electrode of a multiplier tube and amplified into electric signals that can be registered on a meter.

scin'ti·scan"ner. A directional scintillation counter which automatically scans an object or region of the body to determine the distribution of a radioactive tracer substance and obtain a profile of the radioactive area, simultaneously recording the information in the form of a scintigram.

scir'rhoid (skirr'oyd, sirr'oyd) [G. *skiros*, hard; *eidos*, form]. Resembling a scirrhus.

scir'rhous (skirr'us, sirr'us) [*skiros*]. Hard.

scir'rhus (skirr'us, sirr'us) [*skiros*]. A hard carcinoma.

scis'sion. 1. A splitting or dividing, as of a living cell or a molecule. 2. Fission of the nucleus of an atom.

scis'sors [ME. *sisours*, from L. *caedere*, to cut]. An instrument consisting of two blades held together on a pivot, and crossing each other so that in closing they cut the object placed between them. The blades may be straight, angular, or curved, blunt, sharp, or probe-pointed.

canalicular s. Delicate scissors, one blade of which is probe-pointed; used in slitting the lacrimal canaliculus.

craniotomy s. A strong S-shaped instrument used in craniotomy for perforating the skull and cutting away portions of bone.

iris s. One having flat blades bent in such a manner that they may be applied to the eyeball.

Smellie's s. Craniotomy scissors.

scis·su'ra [L., a tearing]. A fissure; a splitting.

scis'sure. Scissura.

scle'ra [G. *sklēros*, hard]. The sclerotic coat of the eye; the firm, fibrous, outer layer of the eyeball, continuous with the sheath of the optic nerve behind and with the cornea in front. See Plate 19. —**scleral,** *adj.*

scler·ac'ne (skli·rack'nee). See *acne* indurata.

scle"ra·ti'tis, scler"a·ti'tis. See *scleritis.*

scle"ra·tog'e·nous (skleer"uh·todj'i·nus, sklerr"-uh·). See *sclerogenous.*

scler"ec·ta'si·a (sklerr"eck·tay'zhuh, ·zee·uh, ·shuh, ·see·uh, skleer"eck·) [*sklēros;* G. *ektasis*, extension]. Localized bulging of the sclera.

scle·rec"to·ir"i·dec'to·my [*sklēros;* G. *ektomē*, excision; *iris*, iris; *ektomē*]. Excision of a portion of the sclera and of the iris, for glaucoma.

scle·rec'to·my [*sklēros; ektomē*]. Excision of a portion of the sclera.

scler"e·de'ma a"dul·to'rum (sklerr"i·dee'muh, skleer"i·dee'muh). An affection characterized by indurated edema, often beginning on the head and later involving larger areas of the body surface. Terminates after weeks or months, leaving no sequela. Often follows some acute general infection. Also called *Buschke's scleredema.*

scle·re'ma [*sklēros*]. Sclerosis, or hardening, especially of the skin.

s. adiposum. See *s.* neonatorum.

s. cutis. Scleroderma.

s. edematosum. A generally fatal form of edema of the skin with induration, impairment of muscular action, and subnormal temperature. Also called *edema neonatorum.*

s. neonatorum. A disease of the newborn characterized by a hardening of the subcutaneous tissue, especially of the legs and feet. Dryness of the skin is marked, so that little fluid exudes on incision.

scle·re'mi·a, scle·re'mus. See *sclerema.*

scle"ren·ce·pha'li·a, scle"ren·ceph'a·ly [*sklēros;* G. *egkephalos*, brain]. Sclerosis of brain tissue.

scle·ren'chy·ma (skli·reng'ki·muh) [*sklēros;* G. *egchyma*, instillation]. The hard, fibrous, woody tissue or covering of plants. —**sclerenchym'-atous,** *adj.*

scle·rer'yth·rin, scler"e·ryth'rin [*sklēros;* G. *erythros*, red]. A red coloring matter in ergot.

scle·ri'a·sis. Scleroderma.

scle·rit'ic [*sklēros*]. Sclerous.

scle·ri'tis [*sklēros;* G. *-itis*, inflammation]. Inflammation of the sclerotic coat of the eye. It may exist alone (simple scleritis or episcleritis), or involve the cornea, iris, or choroid.

annular s. Inflammation of the sclera at the limbus.

scle'ro- (skleer'o-, sklerr'o-) [*sklēros*]. 1. A combining form meaning *hard.* 2. A combining form denoting *connection with the sclera.*

scle"ro·a·troph'ic [*sklēros;* G. *atrophia*, want of food]. Pertaining to fibrosis associated with atrophy.

scle"ro·blas·te'ma [*sklēros;* G. *blastēma*, offspring]. Embryonic tissue from which bones are formed. —**scleroblastem'ic,** *adj.*

scle"ro·cat"a·rac'ta [*sklēros;* G. *kataraktēs*, cataract]. A hard cataract.

scle"ro·cho"roid·i'tis (skleer"o·kor"oy·dye'tis, sklerr"o·) [*sklēros;* G. *chorioeidēs*, choroid; *-itis*, inflammation]. Inflammation of the choroid and sclerotic coats of the eye.

scle"ro·con"junc·ti'val (·kon"junk·ty'vul, ·kon-junk'ti·vul) [*sklēros;* L. *conjunctivus*, connective]. Pertaining conjointly to the sclerotic coat of the eye and the conjunctiva.

scle"ro·con·junc"ti·vi'tis [*sklēros; conjunctivus;* G. *-itis*, inflammation]. Simultaneous conjunctivitis and scleritis.

scle"ro·cor'ne·a [*sklēros;* L. *corneus*, horny]. The sclera and cornea regarded as one. Syn., *corneosclera.* —**sclerocorneal,** *adj.*

scle"ro·dac·tyl'i·a, scle"ro·dac'ty·ly [*sklēros;* G. *daktylos*, finger]. Scleroderma of the fingers. It is often symmetrical, occurs chiefly in women, and leads to marked deformity.

scle"ro·der'ma [*sklēros;* G. *derma*, skin]. A disease characterized by induration of the skin in localized patches or diffuse areas, and associated with atrophy of the epidermis and pigmentation. Vasomotor disturbances, myosclerosis, and calcinosis may occur. Also called *scleriasis, dermatosclerosis, chorionitis.* Also see *acrosclerosis.*

scle"ro·der"ma·ti'tis [*sklēros; derma;* G. *-itis*, inflammation]. Inflammatory thickening and hardening of the skin: also spelled *sclerodermitis.*

scle·rog'e·nous (skli·rodj'i·nus) [*sklēros;* G. *genesthai*, from *gignesthai*, to be produced]. Producing a hard substance.

scle'roid [*sklēros;* G. *eidos*, form]. Hard or bony in texture.

scle"ro·i·ri'tis (skleer"o·eye·rye'tis, sklerr"o·) [*sklēros;* G. *iris*, iris; *-itis*, inflammation]. Inflammation of the sclera and the iris.

scle"ro·ker"a·ti'tis [*sklēros;* G. *keras*, horn; *-itis*]. Inflammation of the sclera and cornea.

scle"ro·ker"a·to·i·ri'tis (·kerr"uh·to·eye·rye'tis) [*sklēros; keras;* G. *iris*, iris; *-itis*]. Combined inflammation of the sclera, cornea, and iris.

scle·ro'ma [G. *sklērōma*, induration]. Abnormal hardness or induration of a part.

respiratory s. Rhinoscleroma.

scle"ro·ma·la'ci·a (skleer"o·ma·lay'shee·uh, ·see·uh, sklerr"o·) [G. *sklēros*, hard; *malakia*, softening]. Softening of the sclera.

s. perforans. Softening of the sclera with perforation.

scle'ro·mere [*sklēros;* G. *meros*, part]. The caudal half of a sclerotome, a primitive vertebra.

scle·rom'e·ter [*sklēros;* G. *metron*, a measure]. 1. A device for determining hardness. 2. Obsolete instrument for determining penetration or quality of x-rays.

scle"ro·nych'i·a (skleer"o·nick'ee·uh, sklerr"o·) [*sklēros;* G. *onyx*, nail]. Induration and thickening of the nails.

scle"ro·nyx'is [*sklēros;* G. *nyxis*, a pricking]. Operative puncture of the sclera.

scle"ro-o"o·pho·ri'tis (-o"o·fo·rye'tis, -o"off·o-rye'tis). Sclerosis of the ovary.

scle'ro·plas"ty [*sklēros;* G. *plassein*, to form]. Plastic surgery on the sclera.

scle"ro·pro'te·in [*sklēros;* G. *prōteios*, of first rank].

The term used in the British classification of proteins corresponding to the term albuminoid in the American classification. See American Classification of Proteins in the Appendix.

scle·ro′sant. A chemical irritant producing an inflammatory reaction and subsequent fibrosis.

scle·rose′ (skli·roze′, skli·roce′, skleer′oze) [*sklēros*]. Affect with sclerosis; become affected with sclerosis. —**sclerosed′,** *adj.*

scle·ro′sis [G. *sklērōsis*, hardening]. Hardening, especially of a part by overgrowth of fibrous tissue; applied particularly to hardening of the nervous system from atrophy or degeneration of the nerve elements and hyperplasia of the interstitial tissue; also to a thickening of the coats of arteries, produced by proliferation of fibrous connective tissue and deposit of lipids and calcium salts.

amyotrophic lateral s. A degenerative disease of the pyramidal tracts and lower motor neurons, characterized by motor weakness and a spastic condition of the limbs associated with muscular atrophy, fibrillary twitching, and final involvement of nuclei in the medulla.

annular s. A chronic myelitis, in which the sclerosis extends about the spinal cord like a ring.

arterial s. See *arteriosclerosis.*

arteriolar s. That involving irregularly distributed hardening of arterioles with uneven reduction of the caliber of the lumens. See generalized arteriolar *s.*

atrophic s. Sclerosis with atrophy.

calcific nodular valvular s. See valvular *s.*

cerebrospinal s. See multiple *s.*

combined s. Simultaneous sclerosis of the posterior and lateral columns of the spinal cord.

diffuse hyperplastic s. See generalized arteriolar *s.*

diffuse s. One extending through a large part of the brain and spinal cord.

disseminated s. See multiple *s.*

dorsal s. Old term for degeneration of the posterior white columns of the spinal cord, or for sclerosis involving the thoracic (dorsal) levels of the spinal cord.

dorsolateral s. See subacute combined *degeneration* of spinal cord.

endocardial s. See endocardial *fibrosis.*

focal s. One confined to a particular region of the brain and cord.

generalized arteriolar s. That affecting the arterioles of the kidney, liver, brain, meninges, gastrointestinal tract, skeletal muscle, adrenal, pancreas, and other organs; more frequent and severe in hypertensive subjects. Also called *diffuse arteriolar s., diffuse hyperplastic s.*

general s. A connective-tissue hyperplasia affecting an entire organ.

hereditary cerebellar s. See hereditary cerebellar *ataxia.*

hereditary spinal s. See Friedreich's *ataxia.*

insular s. See multiple *s.*

lateral s. See amyotrophic lateral *s.*, primary lateral *s.*

lobar s. Gliosis and atrophy of a lobe of the cerebrum, resulting in dementia. Also called *lobar atrophy, convolutional atrophy of the brain, walnut brain.* See also circumscribed cerebral *atrophy.*

miliary s. Small sclerotic patches such as have been observed in the spinal cord in some cases of pernicious anemia.

Mönckeberg's aortic s. See valvular *s.*

multilocular s. See multiple *s.*

multiple cerebral s. Multiple sclerosis affecting only the brain.

multiple cerebrospinal s. Multiple sclerosis affecting both the brain and the spinal cord.

multiple s. Chronic induration occurring in patches in different parts of the nervous system. The principal symptoms are *i*ntention tremor, *n*ystagmus, *s*canning speech, *u*rogenital disturbances, *l*abile emotions, *a*taxia, and *r*etrobulbar *r*etinitis (mnemonic: *insular* sclerosis). Syn., *insular s.*

neural s. Sclerosis attended by chronic neuritis.

posterior spinal s. See *tabes* dorsalis.

posterolateral s. See subacute combined *degeneration* of spinal cord.

presenile s. A degeneration of the cortical cells of the brain, characterized by an abnormal bunching and distortion of the neurofibrils within the cytoplasm; this is associated with the appearance of large, star-shaped plaques, scattered through the cortex, which contain masses of argentophilic material surrounded by a homogeneous nonstaining area; these changes are noted both in presenile and senile dementia. Also called *Alzheimer's disease.*

primary ascending s. of the aortic valve. See valvular *s.*

primary lateral s. A sclerotic disease of the crossed pyramidal tracts of the cord, characterized by paralysis of the limbs, with rigidity, increased tendon reflexes, and absence of sensory and nutritive disorders. A peculiar characteristic jerking gait is produced, and clonus of the lower limbs may be readily excited. It is usually a spinal form of multiple sclerosis.

progressive muscular s. See pseudohypertrophic muscular *paralysis.*

Putnam's type of spinal s. See subacute combined *degeneration* of spinal cord.

renal s. See *nephrosclerosis.*

s. corii. Old term for scleroderma.

s. dermatis. Old term for scleroderma.

s. ossium. See condensing *osteitis.*

subacute combined s. See subacute combined *degeneration* of spinal cord.

tuberous s. A syndrome consisting of mental deficiency, epileptic attacks, adenoma sebaceum, nodular sclerosis of the cerebral cortex, and tumors of the kidney and other organs: generally congenital. Also called *Bourneville's disease.*

ulcerating s. The primary lesion of syphilis; chancre.

valvular s. Primary nonrheumatic degenerative changes of aortic cusps, producing rigidity, calcification, and deformity of the valves. This may result in stenosis, with or without insufficiency. Syn., *calcific nodular valvular sclerosis, calcareous valvular disease, Mönckeberg's aortic sclerosis, primary ascending sclerosis of the aortic valve.*

vascular s. Sclerosis of the walls of the blood vessels; arteriosclerosis.

venous s. See *phlebosclerosis.*

scle″ro·ste·no′sis [G. *sklēros*, hard; *stenōsis*, a being straitened]. Hardening with contracture of a part or closure of an orifice.

s. cutanea. Scleroderma.

scle·ros′to·my [*sklēros;* G. *stoma*, mouth]. Making an artificial opening in the sclera for the relief of glaucoma.

scle″ro·ther′a·py. The deposition or injection of an irritant into a tissue to produce fibrosis, as in the treatment of varicose veins or hemorrhoids.

scle′ro·thrix [*sklēros;* G. *thrix*, hair]. Abnormal brittleness of the hair.

scle·ro′ti·a [*sklēros*]. Firm, small, compact masses of hyphal cells which develop in grain when the ergot fungus grows under unfavorable conditions.

scle·rot′ic [*sklēros*]. 1. Hard; indurated. 2. Pertaining to the outer coat of the eye, as the sclerotic coat, or sclera. 3. Related to or derived from ergot.

scle·rot′ic. The sclera.

blue sclerotics. A congenital, often hereditary, condition of unknown cause in which the sclerae are deep blue indigo sometimes fading with age: often associated with osteogenesis imperfecta, but may occur in the absence of bone fragility.

scle·rot′i·ca. See *sclera*.

scle·rot″i·cec′to·my [*sklēros;* G. *ektomē*, excision]. The removal of a part of the sclera.

scle·rot″i·co·cho″roid·i′tis (·kor″oy·dye′tis). See *sclerochoroiditis*.

scle·rot″i·co·nyx′is. See *scleronyxis*.

scle·rot″i·co·punc′ture. Scleronyxis.

scle·rot″i·cot′o·my. See *sclerotomy*.

scle·rot″i·dec′to·my. See *sclerectomy*.

scle·ro′tis [*sklēros*]. The ergot of rye.

scle″ro·ti′tis. See *scleritis*.

scle·ro′ti·um (skli·ro′shee·um) [*sklēros*]. A thick mass of mycelium constituting a resting stage in the development of some fungi, as the ergot.

scle′ro·tome [*sklēros;* G. *tomos*, cutting]. 1. A knife used in sclerotomy. 2. The fibrous tissue separating successive myotomes in certain of the lower vertebrates. 3. That part of a mesodermal somite which enters into the formation of the vertebrae. —**sclerotom′ic,** *adj.*

scle·rot′o·my [*sklēros;* G. *tomē*, a cutting]. The operation of incising the sclera.

anterior s. The making of an incision through the sclera anterior to the ciliary body, and entering the anterior chamber, as in glaucoma.

posterior s. Sclerotomy by an incision through the sclera behind the ciliary body, and entering the vitreous chamber.

scle″ro·to·nyx′is [*sklēros;* G. *nyxis*, a pricking]. An operation for cataract formerly practiced, in which a broad needle was introduced into the sclera, behind the ciliary region, passed between the iris and the lens, and the latter depressed into the vitreous body.

scle″ro·trich′i·a (skleer″o·trick′ee·uh, sklerr″o·) [*sklēros;* G. *thrix*, hair]. A harsh and dry state of the hair.

scle′rous [*sklēros*]. Hard; indurated.

sco′bi·nate [L. *scobis*, powder produced by scraping]. Having a rough surface.

sco·lec′i·form (sko·less′i·form, sko·lee′si·form) [G. *skōlēx*, earthworm; L. *forma*, form]. Having the form or character of a scolex.

scol′e·coid, sco′le·coid [G. *skōlēkoeidēs*, worm-shaped]. Vermiform.

sco′lex (pl. *scolices*) [G.]. The head of a tapeworm by means of which it attaches to the intestinal wall.

sco″li·o·lor·do′sis [G. *skolios*, crooked; *lordōsis*, curvature of the spine which is convex in front]. Combined scoliosis and lordosis.

sco″li·o·si·om′e·try [G. *skoliōsis*, obliquity; *metron*, a measure]. The estimation of the degree of deformity in scoliosis.

sco″li·o′sis [G.]. Lateral curvature of the spine, named according to location and direction of the convexity, as right thoracic. Usually there are two curves, the original and a compensatory curve, as an original right thoracic with a compensating left lumbar curve. —**scoliot′ic,** *adj.*

congenital s. One due to a congenital defect in the development of the spine, such as a hemivertebra.

functional s. One due to persistent faulty posture, such as standing on one leg or with one shoulder held lower than the other or with the head tilted. Early, this is a mobile scoliosis, that is, one which can be voluntarily straightened, but if the faulty posture is long continued, it may become a structural scoliosis. Also called *habit s.*

organic s. That due to a disease process, as one which affects the spine, such as rickets or infections; one which affects the muscles which support the spine, such as paralysis; due to deformities of the thoracic cage, as following empyema; or due to disease of the hip or leg.

structural s. One in which a series of vertebrae remain constantly deviated from the normal spinal axis and accompanied by some degree of rotation of the vertebrae with corresponding changes in the thoracic cage. Organic and congenital forms are structural, and the functional type may become so.

sco″li·o·som′e·ter [*skoliōsis;* G. *metron*, a measure]. An instrument for measuring the amount of deformity in scoliosis.

sco′li·o·tone″ [G. *skolios*, crooked; *tonos*, a stretching]. An apparatus for elongating the spine and lessening the rotation in lateral curvature.

Scol″o·pen′dra. A genus of centipedes.

scom′brine (skom′breen, ·brin) [G. *skombros*, mackerel]. A protamine obtained from mature spermatozoa of mackerel.

scom′brone [*skombros*]. A histone obtained from spermatozoa of mackerel.

scoop [ME. *scope*]. An instrument resembling a spoon, for the extraction of bodies from cavities, as an ear scoop, lithotomy scoop.

sco·pa′rin. $C_{22}H_{22}O_{11}$; a glycosidal principle from scoparius, occurring in yellow crystals, soluble in hot water.

sco·pa′ri·us [L. *scopa*, broom]. The dried tops of *Cytisus scoparius*, a shrub of the family Leguminosae; they contain the alkaloid sparteine, and a glycoside, scoparin. Scoparius has been used as a diuretic and cathartic. Also called *broom-tops*.

-scope [G. *skopein*, to examine]. A combining form denoting *an instrument for seeing* or *examining*.

sco′po·la, sco·po′la [after G. A. *Scopoli* of Pavia, 1723–88]. The dried rhizome of *Scopolia carniolica*. It yields approximately 0.6% of total alkaloids, of which about 80% is hyoscyamine and the rest scopolamine and nor-hyoscyamine. The physiologic action and therapeutic effects closely resemble those of belladonna. It is little used as an internal medicine but is employed as a commercial source of scopolamine and hyoscyamine.

sco·pol′a·mine (sko·pol′uh·meen, ·min, sko·po′-luh·, sko″po·luh·meen′, sko″po·lam′in). $C_{17}H_{21}NO_4$. An alkaloid obtained from various plants of the Solanaceae. It occurs as a syrupy liquid, if obtained from a chloroform solution; as crystals, if obtained from an ether solution. It is slightly soluble in water; soluble in alcohol, chloroform, and ether.

s. hydrobromide (*scopolaminae hydrobromidum*). $C_{17}H_{21}NO_4.HBr.3H_2O$. The hydrobromide of levorotatory scopolamine obtained from plants of the Solanaceae; occurs as colorless or white crystals or a white, granular powder; 1 Gm. dissolves in 1.5 cc. of water and in 20 cc. of alcohol. Scopolamine paralyzes the peripheral endings of the parasympathetic nerves, acting like atropine but less powerfully and without stimulating the medullary centers. It also appears to act frequently as a cerebral depressant and tends to promote sleep. It has slight analgesic properties, but greatly enhances the effect of other narcotics, such as morphine. When locally applied it will cause dilation of the pupil. It is used mainly as a sedative in psychiatry and surgery. As a mydriatic it is much quicker and less permanent in its effects than atropine. For the relief of pain it is advantageously combined with morphine. In doses of

0.5–1.0 mg. of scopolamine with 10 mg. of morphine it is used for producing anesthesia, especially for obstetric purposes. Great care must be exercised when used in this manner. Dose, 0.3–0.8 mg. ($\frac{1}{200}$–$\frac{1}{80}$ gr.). Also called *hyoscine hydrobromide.*

scopolamine stable. Trade-mark for an aqueous solution of levorotatory scopolamine hydrobromide with 10% of mannite to prevent decomposition. The substance is used in surgery as preanesthesia medication and in obstetrics for the production of twilight sleep; it is also used in psychiatry as a cerebral sedative in acute mania, delirium tremens, drug addiction, alcoholism, and similar disturbances. See *scopomannit.*

sco″po·le′tin, sco·po′le·tin. $C_{10}H_8O_4$; β-methylesculetin or 6-methoxy-7-hydroxycoumarin; the aglycone of scopolin.

sco·po′lin. A glycoside from certain species of *Scopolia;* on hydrolysis it yields scopoletin and D-glucose.

sco·po′line. $C_8H_{13}NO_2$; a decomposition product of scopolamine. Syn., *oscine.*

scopomannit. Trade name for an aqueous solution of scopolamine hydrobromide, protected against decomposition by the addition of 10% of mannite See *scopolamine stable.*

sco·pom′e·ter [G. *skopein*, to examine; *metron*, a measure]. An optical instrument with an optical wedge for visual measurement of turbidity or opalescence, by observation of the disappearance of an illuminated target.

sco·pom′e·try [*skopein; metron*]. A branch of nephelometry; matching colors or turbidities by comparing an illuminated line against a field of constant intensity.

sco″po·pho′bi·a [*skopein;* G. *phobos*, fear]. Morbid dread of being seen.

Scop″u·la″ri·op′sis [L. *scopula*, broom; *opsis*, vision]. A genus of fungi.

S. brevicaule. One of the species of fungi which cause aspergillosis.

-scopy [G. *skopein*, to examine]. A combining form denoting *inspection* or *examination.*

scor″a·cra′ti·a (skor″uh·kray′shee·uh) [G. *skōr*, dung; *akrateia*, want of power]. Involuntary evacuation of feces.

scor·bu″ti·gen′ic [ML. *scorbutus*, scurvy; G. *genesthai*, from *gignesthai*, to be produced]. Causing scurvy.

scor·bu′tus. See *scurvy.*

scor″di·ne′ma [G., stretching]. Yawning.

scor″e·te′mi·a. See *scatemia.*

Scor′pi·o [L., from G. *skorpios*, scorpion]. A genus of the order Scorpionida (scorpions).

S. maurus. A poisonous species of scorpion found in Egypt and Tunis.

scor′pi·on [*skorpios*]. An arachnid of the order Scorpionida which injects poison by a sting located on the end of the tail. The venom is a neurotoxin similar in action to cobra venom. See *Buthus, Centruroides, Euscorpius, Scorpio, Tityus.*

scot″o·din′i·a (skot″o·din′ee·uh, ·dye′nee·uh, sko″-to·) [G. *skotos*, darkness; *dinos*, whirling]. Vertigo associated with the appearance of black spots before the eyes.

scot′o·gram (skot′o·gram, sko′to·) [*skotos;* G. *gramma*, letter]. An impression made on a photographic plate by a radioactive substance without the intervention of an opaque object.

sco·to′ma [G., dizziness]. An area of absent or depressed vision in the visual field, surrounded by an area of normal or less depressed vision.

absolute s. Scotoma with perception of light entirely absent.

annular s. A partial or complete area of blindness in the form of a ring. Also called *ring s.*

Bjerrum's s. See Jannik Peterson *Bjerrum.*

central s. One limited to the region of the visual field corresponding to the macula lutea.

color s. Colorblindness limited to a part of the visual field; may exist without interruption of the field for white light.

negative s. A defect, due to the destruction of the retinal center; not noticeable to the patient.

positive s. A scotoma perceptible to the patient as a dark spot before his eyes.

relative s. A scotoma within which perception of light is only partially impaired.

scintillating s. A scotoma with serrated margins extending peripherally and producing a large defect in the visual field.

sco·to′ma·graph [*skotōma;* G. *graphein*, to write]. An instrument for recording the size and shape of a scotoma.

sco·tom′e·ter [G. *skotos*, darkness; *metron*, a measure]. An instrument for detecting, locating, and measuring scotomas.

scot″o·phil′i·a. See *nyctophilia.*

scot″o·pho′bi·a (skot″o·fo′bee·uh, sko″to·) [*skotos;* G. *phobos*, fear]. A morbid fear of darkness.

sco·to′pi·a [*skotos;* G. *ōps*, eye]. The ability to see in the dark; dark adaptation. —**scotop′ic,** *adj.*

sco·top′sin. A name proposed for the protein moiety of rhodopsin.

sco·tos′co·py. See *retinoscopy.*

sco·to′sis. See *scotoma.*

scour′ing. A nonscientific term for diarrhea in horses and cattle and usually attributed to excesses in eating green fodder and unripe fruit.

scours. An infectious diarrhea of horses and cattle.

scra′per [AS. *scrapian*]. An instrument used to produce an abrasion.

scrap′ie (scrap′ee, skray′pee) [*scrapian*]. A form of dysentery in sheep caused by *Mycobacterium paratuberculosis* (*Johne's bacillus*).

scra′pings [*scrapian*]. Epithelial or nail fragments removed from dermal lesions for microscopical examination for the presence of fungi.

screen [ME. *scren*]. That which cuts off, shelters, or protects.

fluorescent s. A screen covered with substances which become fluorescent on exposure to rays which are normally invisible to the eye.

intensifying s. A sheet of cardboard coated with a fluorescent material, such as calcium tungstate, placed in contact with an x-ray film. When roentgen rays pass through film and screen, the fluorescent light from the screen supplements the effect of the roentgen rays on the film, thus reducing the necessary exposure time.

screen mem′o·ry. *In psychoanalysis*, an unimportant memory recalled in place of an associated important one.

scrive′ner's pal′sy. See writer's *cramp.*

scro·bic′u·lus [L., little ditch]. A small pit. —**scrobiculate,** *adj.*

scrof′u·la [L. *scrofa*, breeding sow]. Tuberculosis of cervical lymph nodes. —**scrofulous,** *adj.*

scrof″u·lo·der′ma [*scrofa;* G. *derma*, skin]. Lesions of the skin produced by the local action of the *Mycobacterium tuberculosis* by direct extension from some focus of infection beneath the skin, usually on the neck from draining lymph nodes, resulting in ulceration, draining sinuses, and scar formation.

scroph″u·la′ri·a [*scrofa*]. The leaves of *Scrophularia marilandica*, figwort; formerly used internally and externally as a cure-all, but probably without definite value.

scro·tec′to·my [L. *scrotum*, scrotum; G. *ektomē*, excision]. Resection of the scrotum or a part of it.

scro′to·plas″ty [*scrotum;* G. *plassein*, to form]. Plastic surgery on the scrotum.

scro′tum [L.]. The pouch containing the testes, consisting of skin and subcutaneous tissue, dartos, external spermatic fascia, cremasteric fascia, internal spermatic fascia, and parietal tunica vaginalis propria. See Plate 44. —**scrotal,** *adj.*

bilobate s. A congenital failure of the lateral halves of the scrotum to fuse at the line of the median raphe, resulting in a separate pouch for each testis.

scrub ty′phus. See tsutsugamushi *disease.*

scru′ple [L. *scrupulus*, small stone]. A unit of apothecaries' weight represented by the symbol ℈, and equal to 20 grains.

scru″pu·los′i·ty [L. *scrupulosus*, careful]. An over-precision, or morbid conscientiousness as to one's thoughts, words, and deeds. A prominent personality trait in those persons predisposed to psychasthenia or obsessive compulsive reaction and to certain schizophrenic reactions.

Scudder, Charles Locke [*American surgeon*, 1860–1949]. Known for his reduction of supracondylar fracture of the femur. Author of an important textbook on fractures in 11 editions (1900–39).

Scultet's bandage. See scultetus *bandage.*

scurf [AS.]. A branlike desquamation of the epidermis, especially from the scalp; dandruff.

scur′vy [*scurf*]. A nutritional disorder caused by deficiency of vitamin C; characterized by extreme weakness, spongy gums, and a tendency to develop hemorrhages under the skin, from the mucous membranes, and under the periosteum.

infantile s. An acute form, characterized by subperiosteal hemorrhage, especially of the long bones, with painful swellings: also called *Moeller-Barlow disease.*

land s. See idiopathic thrombocytopenic *purpura.*

scute [L. *scutum*, shield]. 1. An external plate or scale, as that of reptiles, fish, and certain insects. 2. Old term for tegmen tympani.

scu″tel·la′ri·a [L. *scutella*, tray] (*scutellaria*). The dried overground portion of *Scutellaria lateriflora.* It contains a yellow, crystalline substance, scutellarin. Formerly used in neuralgia, epilepsy, chorea, and other nervous diseases. Dose, 2–6 Gm. (30–90 gr.). Also called *skullcap.*

scu·tel′la·rin, scu″tel·la′rin. See under *scutellaria.*

scu·tel′lum [dim. from L. *scutum*, shield]. Small plate or squamous structure.

scu′tu·late [*scutum*]. Shaped like a lozenge.

scu′tu·lum [*scutum*]. 1. Any one of the thin crusts of the eruption of favus. Syn., *godet.* 2. The scapula. —**scutular,** *adj.*

scu′tum [L.]. A shieldlike plate of bone. —**scutate,** *adj.*

s. tympanicum. The semilunar plate of bone separating the attic of the tympanum from the outer mastoid cells.

scyb′a·lum (sib′uh·lum) (pl. *scybala*) [G. *skybalon*, dung]. A mass of abnormally hard fecal matter. —**scybalous,** *adj.*

scyl′li·tol. $C_6H_6(OH)_6$; an alcohol isomeric with inositol, often described as an inositol, identified as a constituent of dogfish liver and cartilage, and also of several plants.

scy′phi·form (sigh′fi·form) [G. *skyphos*, cup; L. *forma*, form]. Cup-shaped.

scy·ti′tis (sigh·tight′is) [G. *skytos*, skin; *-itis*, inflammation]. Inflammation of the skin; dermatitis.

SD Streptodornase.

Se Chemical symbol for selenium.

Seaborg, Glenn Theodore (1912–). American chemist known for his work on neutron and nuclear reactions; with E. M. McMillan, he shared the Nobel prize (1951) in chemistry for the discovery and creation of transuranium elements.

seam. See *suture, raphe.*

sea on′ion. Squill.

Seashore, Carl Emil [*American psychologist*, 1866–1949]. Widely known for his research in esthetics, acoustics, motor skills, etc. Devised a much used test to measure native musical aptitude; see Seashore *test.*

sea′sick″ness [AS. *sǣ; sēoc*]. A condition produced in some persons by the rolling of a ship; characterized by vertigo, nausea, retching, and prostration. A similar state may be induced by riding in cars, elevators, airplanes.

seat′worm. *Enterobius vermicularis.*

se·ba″ce·o·fol·lic′u·lar [L. *sebaceus*, a tallow candle; *folliculus*, follicle]. Relating to a pilosebaceous apparatus.

se·ba′ceous [*sebaceus*]. Pertaining to sebum; secreting sebum.

se·bac′ic ac′id (si·bas′ick, si·bay′sick). COOH-$(CH_2)_8$COOH; decanedioic acid or 1,8-octanedicarboxylic acid, obtained by decomposition of certain fatty acids; it occurs in white leaflets, slightly soluble in water.

se·bas″to·ma′ni·a [G. *sebastos*, venerable; *mania*, madness]. Religious psychosis. *Obs.*

se·bif′er·ous [L. *sebum*, tallow, grease; *ferre*, to bear]. See *sebiparous.*

se·bip′a·rous [*sebum;* L. *parere*, to bring forth]. Secreting sebum.

seb″o·cys″to·ma·to′sis. See *steatocystoma multiplex.*

seb′o·lith [*sebum;* G. *lithos*, stone]. A concretion in a sebaceous gland.

seb″or·rha′gi·a. See *seborrhea.*

seb″or·rhe′a, seb″or·rhoe′a [*sebum;* G. *rhoia*, flow]. A functional disease of the sebaceous glands, characterized by an excessive secretion or disturbed quality of sebum, which collects upon the skin in the form of an oily coating or of crusts or scales. —**seborrheic, seborrheal,** *adj.*

s. capitis. Seborrhea of the scalp.

s. congestiva. Lupus erythematosus.

s. corporis. Seborrheic dermatitis of the trunk.

s. furfuracea. See *dermatitis* seborrheica.

s. ichthyosis. A variety characterized by the formation of large, platelike crusts.

s. nasi. Seborrhea of the sebaceous glands of the nose.

s. nigricans. Chromhidrosis in which there is a dark, greasy-looking discoloration of the eyelids and adjacent skin.

s. oleosa. A form characterized by an excessive oiliness of the skin, especially about the forehead and nose.

s. sicca. See *dermatitis* seborrheica.

se′bum (pl. *seba*) [L.]. The secretion of the sebaceous glands, composed of fat, keratohyalin granules, keratin, and cellular debris.

s. palpebrale. The dried secretion of the sebaceous glands of the eyelids.

s. praeputiale. Smegma praeputii.

sec′a·line. $(CH_3)_3N$; trimethylamine. Traces are found in ergot. It has no medicinal importance.

se·cern′ment [L. *secernere*, to separate]. Secretion: applied to the function of a gland.

se·clu′sion of pu′pil. Annular or posterior synechia.

se″co·bar′bi·tal so′di·um. Generic name for the barbiturate introduced under the trade-marked name seconal sodium. Syn., *quinalbarbitone sodium.*

sec′o·dont (seck′o·dont, see′ko·) [L. *secare*, to cut; G. *odous*, tooth]. Possessing molar teeth which have cusps with cutting edges.

seconal sodium. Trade-mark for monosodium 5-allyl-5-(1-methylbutyl) barbiturate, a short-acting hypnotic and sedative.

sec′ond·ar″y [L. *secundarius*, secondary]. 1. Second in the order of time or development, as the secondary lesions of syphilis. 2. Second in relation; subordinate; produced by a cause considered primary.

se·cre′ta [L. *secretum*, from *secernere*, to separate]. The substances secreted by a gland, follicle, or other organ; products of secretion.

se·cre′ta·gogue (si·kree′tuh·gog), **se·cre′to·gogue** [*secretum;* G. *agōgos*, leading]. A substance promoting or causing secretion, as certain hormones.

se·crete′ [*secretum*]. Separate; specifically, to separate from blood, or form out of materials furnished by the blood, a certain substance termed secretion. **—secret′ing,** *adj.*

se·cre′tin [*secretum*]. A hormone produced in the epithelial cells of the duodenum by the contact of acid. It is absorbed from the cells by the blood and excites the pancreas to activity; it has been isolated as secretin picrolonate. See Table of Hormones in the Appendix.

se·cre′tin·ase. An enzyme present in blood serum which inactivates the hormone secretin.

se·cre′tion [L. *secretio*, from *secernere*, to separate]. 1. The act of secreting or forming, from materials furnished by the blood, a certain substance which is either eliminated from the body (excretion) or used in carrying on special functions. 2. The substance secreted.

antilytic s. That arising in a control salivary gland as the result of experimental denervation of the gland of the opposite side. Syn., *antiparalytic s.*

external s. A secretion thrown out upon any epithelial surface of the body.

gastric s. The secretion of the glands of the stomach.

internal s. A secretion that is not thrown out upon a surface, but is absorbed into the blood.

paralytic s. That occurring in a gland or organ after denervation, as in the stomach after vagotomy.

salivary s. The secretion of the salivary glands.

se·cre′tor. A person who secretes demonstrable amounts of the A or B antigen or both in his saliva and gastric juice. This characteristic is a Mendelian dominant.

se·cre′to·ry [L. *secretum*, from *secernere*, to separate]. Pertaining to secretion; performing secretion.

sec·ta′ri·an [ML. *sectarius*]. Old term for one who, in the practice of medicine, follows a dogma, tenet, or principle based on the authority of its promulgator to the exclusion of demonstration and experience.

sec′tile (seck′tyle, ·til) [L. *sectilis*, cut]. Capable of being cut.

sec′tion [L. *sectio*, a cutting]. 1. A cutting or dividing. 2. A cut or slice. **—section,** *v.*

abdominal s. Incision into the abdominal cavity.

Cesarean s. See *Cesarean section.*

coronal s. One in a vertical and frontal plane making 90-degree angle with the sagittal plane of the head.

cross s. See *cross section.*

frontal s. One dividing the body or the head into dorsal and ventral parts.

frozen s. In the teaching of anatomy, one of a series of divisions of the body or a part which has been frozen before being sectioned. See *frozen sections.*

parasagittal s. One in a plane which is parallel to the sagittal plane.

perineal s. External urethrotomy.

Pitres sections. A series of sections made through the brain for post-mortem examination.

sagittal s. One made in the sagittal suture and hence in the median plane of the body, dividing it into equal halves. See Plate 12.

sec′tion cut′ter. A microtome, particularly one to be held in the hand.

sec·to′ri·al [L. *sectum*, from *secare*, to cut]. Having cutting edges, as the molar teeth of carnivorous animals.

se·cun″di·grav′i·da [L. *secundus*, second; *gravidus*, pregnant]. A woman pregnant the second time.

sec″un·di′na (seck″un·dye′nuh, ·dee′nuh, see″-kun·). See *secundines.*

sec′un·dines (seck′un·dynz, ·deenz, ·dinz, si·kun′-dynz) [*secundus*]. The placenta and membranes discharged from the uterus after birth.

sec″un·dip′a·ra (seck″un·dip′uh·ruh, see″kun·) [*secundus;* L. *parere*, to bring forth]. A woman who has borne two children, not twins. **—secundiparous,** *adj.;* **secundipar′ity,** *n.*

se·cun′dum ar′tem [L.]. In the approved professional manner. *Obs.*

SED Skin erythema dose.

sed′a·tine (sed′uh·teen, ·tin). See *antipyrine.*

se·da′tion [L. *sedatio*, from *sedare*, to soothe]. 1. A state of lessened functional activity. 2. The production of a state of lessened functional activity.

sed′a·tive [*sedare*]. Quieting function or activity. **—sed′ative,** *n.*

sed′en·tar″y [L. *sedentarius*, sedentary]. Occupied in sitting. Pertaining to the habit of sitting.

Sedillot, Charles Emmanuel [*French surgeon*, 1804–83]. One of the first to perform gastrostomy (1849).

sed′i·ment [L. *sedimentum*, a sinking down]. The material settling to the bottom of a liquid. **—sedimen′tary,** *adj.*

sed″i·men·ta′tion [*sedimentum*]. The process of producing the deposition of a sediment, especially the rapid deposition by means of a centrifugal machine. See sedimentation *rate.*

sed″i·men·tom′e·ter [*sedimentum;* G. *metron*, a measure]. An apparatus for recording the sedimentation rate of blood.

sedobrol. Trade-mark for a preparation in cube form containing 17 grains of sodium bromide with concentrated vegetable extractives and condiments. A cube dissolved in boiling water yields a broth in which the taste of the bromide is masked. Used in conditions where bromides are indicated.

se″do·hep′tu·lose. $CH_2OH.CO.HOCH.HCOH.HCOH.HCOH.CH_2OH$; a ketoheptose found in plants of the genus *Sedum* of the stonecrop family; under certain conditions, a product of photosynthesis.

sedormid. Trade-mark for allyl-isopropyl-acetyl-carbamide. The substance occurs as a white, crystalline powder slightly soluble in water: used as a sedative and hypnotic.

seed [AS. *sǣd*]. A fertilized and ripened ovule produced by flowering plants, along with reserve nutritive material and protective covering. It is primarily a sporophyte in a resting stage.

radon s. A small capillary tube, of glass, containing radon, suitable for implantation in tissues; the tube may be placed inside a small gold tube.

Seeligmueller, Otto Ludwig Gustav Adolf [*German neurologist*, 1837–1912]. Described bilateral neuralgia of the auriculotemporal nerves. See Seeligmueller's *neuralgia.* Mydriasis on the side of the face affected is called *Seeligmueller's sign.*

Seessel, Albert [*American embryologist*, 1850–1910]. Described a small diverticulum which persists as a vestige of the preoral gut that extended cephalic to the point of rupture of the stomodeal plate. It indicates the point at which the stomodeal ectoderm and fore-gut entoderm became continuous upon rupture of the oral plate; called *Seessel's pocket.*

seg'ment [L. *segmentum,* a piece cut off]. 1. A small piece cut along the radii of anything regarded as circular; a part bounded by a natural or imaginary line. 2. A natural division, resulting from segmentation; one of a series of homologous parts, as a myotome; the part of a limb between two consecutive joints. A subdivision, ring, lobe, somite, or metamere of any cleft or articulated body.

body s. A somite or a division of the body derived from an embryonic somite. Syn., *metamere.*

bronchopulmonary s. The portion of lung supplied by any bronchus.

interannular s. The portion of a nerve included between two consecutive nodes of Ranvier. *Obs.*

intermediate s. of a cilium. The isotropous, delicately striated portion of a cilium between the cilium proper and its pedicle. *Obs.*

lower uterine s. The isthmus of the uterus which expands as pregnancy progresses, and whose muscle fibers are stretched passively during labor, together with the cervix, allowing the upper uterine musculature to retract and thus to expel the fetus. See also retraction *ring.*

mesodermal s. A somite.

muscle s. A myotome.

P-R s. The interval between the end of the P wave and the beginning of the QRS complex.

primitive s. A somite.

R(S)-T s. In an electrocardiogram, that portion of the ECG from R(S)-T which is usually isoelectric. It may be slightly elevated or depressed normally. It corresponds to the period when depolarization is complete.

S-T s. In an electrocardiogram, that interval between the end of the S wave and the beginning of the T wave.

T-P s. The interval from the end of the T wave to the beginning of the P wave.

upper uterine s. The upper and major portion of the uterine musculature, which actively contracts and thickens during labor. See also retraction *ring.*

seg·men'tal [*segmentum*]. 1. Pertaining to a segment; made up of segments. 2. Undergoing or resulting from segmentation.

seg"men·ta'tion [*segmentum*]. 1. The process of cleavage or cell division, especially as applied to the fertilized ovum and blastomeres. 2. The division of an organism into somites or metameres.

complete s. Holoblastic cleavage.

unequal s. Segmentation producing blastomeres of unequal size, those of the animal pole being smaller and more numerous than those of the vegetal pole.

Seg"men·ti'na [*segmentum*]. A fresh-water snail; the intermediate host of *Fasciolopsis buski.*

seg'ment·ing bod'y. The sporulating malaria parasite, when the schizont breaks up into the merozoites.

seg"re·ga'tion [L. *segregatio,* from *segregare,* to separate]. The reappearance of contrasted Mendelian characters in the offspring of heterozygotes, or the separation of the paired maternal and paternal genes at meiosis in the formation of gametes.

s. apparatus. See internal reticular *apparatus.*

seg're·ga"tor [*segregare*]. An instrument by means of which urine from each kidney may be secured without admixture.

Séguin, Edouard [*American psychiatrist,* 1812–80]. Described the involuntary muscular contraction occurring just before an attack of Jacksonian epilepsy; called *Séguin's sign.*

Seidel, Erich [*German ophthalmologist,* 1882–1946]. Known for his description of a sign of early glaucoma. He observed an increase in the normal size of the blind spot in the retina, characterized by irregular, wedge-shaped extensions at the periphery; called *Seidel's sign.*

Seidelin, Harold [*English physician,* contemporary]. Described *Paraplasma flavigenum* bodies which he observed in the red blood cells of yellow fever patients. He considered them parasites and of etiologic significance. Called *Seidelin's bodies.*

Seid'litz pow'ders. Two powders, one commonly in a blue paper, containing potassium sodium tartrate and sodium bicarbonate, the other in a white paper, containing tartaric acid. On mixing solutions of the powders effervescence occurs; the solution is taken for cathartic effect. Syn., *compound effervescent powders.*

sei"es·the'si·a (sigh"ess·thee'zhuh, ·zee·uh) [G. *seiein,* to shake; *aisthēsis,* perception]. Perception of concussion.

Seignette, Pierre [*French apothecary,* 1660–1719]. Said to have introduced the use of potassium sodium tartrate as a laxative; known as *Rochelle salt;* once called *Seignette salt.*

seis"mo·ther'a·py (size"mo·therr'uh·pee, sice"-mo·) [G. *seismos,* earthquake; *therapeia,* treatment]. The therapeutic use of mechanical vibration.

Seitz filter. See under *filter.*

sei'zure [OF. *seisir*]. 1. The sudden onset of a disease or an attack. 2. *In surgery,* the grasping of a part to be operated upon. 3. Specifically, an epileptic or epileptoid attack. See *epilepsy.*

akinetic s. An epileptic seizure marked by sudden loss of consciousness and of motor power resulting in head nodding or body slumping; and usually lasting a few seconds to a few minutes.

larval seizures. *In electroencephalography,* subliminal seizures which produce no clinical symptoms but which are recognized by abnormal brain wave discharges.

se·junc'tion [L. *sejunctio,* from *sejungere,* to separate]. *In psychology,* the interruption of the continuity of association complexes, tending to break up personality.

se"la·pho'bi·a [G. *selas,* light; *phobos,* fear]. Morbid fear of flashing light.

se·lec'tion [L. *selectio,* from *seligere,* to choose out]. *In biology,* choosing for survival or elimination.

artificial s. Process in which man, for his own purposes, picks out some individuals in a group of organisms for survival, others for elimination.

natural s. Darwin's theory of evolution, according to which organisms tend to produce progeny far above the means of subsistence; a struggle for existence ensues which results in the survival of those with favorable variations. Since the favorable variations accumulate as the generations pass, the descendants tend to diverge markedly from their ancestors, and to remain adapted to the conditions under which they live.

sexual s. The view that the differences between males and females, other than the presence of ovaries or testes, have originated as the result of preferential mating, regarded usually as a preference of the females for the males showing the differentiated traits.

se·lec'tor [*selectum,* from *seligere*]. A device for selecting or separating.

switch s. A switch arranged so that an electric conductor connection may be connected to any one of several other conductors.

se·le'ne (si·lee'nee) [G. *selēnē,* moon]. The white

spot sometimes occurring on the finger nails. Also see *lunula*, 1.

se·le′ni·ate (si·lee′nee·ate, si·len′ee·ate). A salt of selenic acid.

se·le′nic (si·lee′nick, si·len′ick). A compound of hexavalent (sometimes tetravalent) selenium.

se·le′nic ac′id. H_2SeO_4. A crystalline acid, soluble in water, forming a corrosive liquid.

sel″e·nif′er·ous [*selēnē;* L. *ferre*, to bear]. Containing selenium.

se·le′ni·ous ac′id. H_2SeO_3. The acid formed by tetravalent selenium.

sel′e·nite, se′le·nite. 1. A salt of selenious acid. 2. A translucent form of calcium sulfate.

se·le′ni·um [*selēnē*]. Se = 78.96. A poisonous element resembling sulfur. Plants grown in seleniferous soil may prove fatal to cattle feeding upon them.

se·le′no·dont [*selēnē;* G. *odous*, tooth]. Possessing molar teeth with crescent-shaped ridges.

se·le″no·gam′i·a [*selēnē;* G. *gamos*, marriage]. Somnambulism. *Obs.*

se·le·no′sis. Selenium poisoning.

self″-ab·sorp′tion. Absorption of radiation by the source material itself.

self″-a·buse′. See *masturbation.*

self″-di·ges′tion. See *autodigestion.*

self″-fer·men·ta′tion. See *autolysis.*

self″-fer·ti·li·za′tion. The impregnation of the ovules by pollen of the same flower or of the ova by sperm of the same animal.

self″-hyp·no′sis. Hypnosis by autosuggestion; autohypnosis.

self″-in·duc′tance. The property of a conductor to oppose changes in current by the development of a counter electromotive force.

self″-in·fec′tion. See *autoinfection.*

self″-in·oc″u·la′tion. See *autoinoculation.*

self″-lim′it·ed. Denoting a disease which runs a definite course in a specific time.

self″-pol·lu′tion. See *masturbation.*

self″-sug·ges′tion. See *autosuggestion.*

self″-sus·pen′sion. Suspension of the body by the head for the purpose of stretching or making extension on the vertebral column.

Seliwanoff's test. See under *test.*

sel′la (pl. *sellae*) [L., seat]. A saddle. —**sellar,** *adj.*

s. turcica. The superior portion of the body of the sphenoid bone that surrounds the hypophyseal fossa. It includes the tuberculum sellae, anterior clinoid processes, and the dorsum sellae with its posterior clinoid processes.

Sellards, Andrew Watson [*American physician,* 1884–1942]. Introduced a test for acidosis based on alkaline tolerance, called *Sellards' test.*

sel′len·ders. Sallenders.

Selter, Paul (1866–1941). German pediatrician who described erythredema polyneuropathy.

Selye, Hans (1907–). Canadian endocrinologist who investigated the functions and pathology of the endocrine glands (particularly the adrenals), the pharmacology of steroid hormones and of pregnancy and lactation. He described the general adaptation syndrome as a response to severe or prolonged physiological stress.

se·man′tics [G. *sēmantikos*, significant]. The branch of linguistic science that treats of problems of meaning, both current and historical.

general s. A study or theory of living which stresses a scientific approach to problems and life; emphasizes the way in which language is used as an important factor in adjustment; used in treating certain psychologic maladjustments.

Semb, Carl [*Norwegian surgeon,* 1895–]. Known for his thoracoplasty with extrafascial apicolysis for pulmonary tuberculosis, called *Semb's operation.*

se″mei·og′ra·phy, se″mi·og′ra·phy (see″migh-og′ruh·fee, see″mee·, sem″ee·) [G. *sēmeion*, sign; *graphein*, to write]. Symptomatology. *Obs.*

se″mei·ol′o·gy, se″mi·ol′o·gy (see″migh·ol′o·jee, see″mee·, sem″ee·) [*sēmeion;* G. *logos*, word]. Symptomatology. *Obs.* —**semeiolog′ic,** *adj.*

se″mei·ot′ics, se″mi·ot′ics (see″migh·ot′icks, see″mee·, sem″ee·) [G. *sēmeiōtikos*, observant of signs]. Symptomatology. *Obs.* —**semeiotic,** *adj.*

se′men [L.]. 1. A seed. 2. The fluid produced by the male reproductive organs, carrying the male germ cells or spermatozoa. —**sem′inal,** *adj.*

sem″e·nu′ri·a. See *seminuria.*

sem′i- [L., half-]. A prefix denoting *half.*

sem″i·a·ceph′a·lus. See *anencephalus.*

sem″i·ca·nal′ [*semi-;* L. *canalis*, channel]. A canal open on one side; a sulcus or groove.

s. for the auditory tube. The groove in the temporal bone in which the auditory tube lies.

s. for tensor tympani muscle. The groove in the temporal bone in which the tensor tympani muscle lies.

sem″i·ca·nal′is (sem″i·ka·nal′is, ·nay′lis) (pl. *semicanales*) [*semi-; canalis*]. See *semicanal.*

sem″i·car′ba·zide. $NH_2.NHCO.NH_2$; an organic compound formed by the reaction of cyanic acid with hydrazine or by electrolytic reduction of nitrourea: used for the detection of aldehydes and ketones in tissues. Also called *hydrazinoformamide* or *carbazinamide.*

s. hy″dro·chlo′ride. $NH_2.NHCO.NH_2.HCl$; carbamylhydrazine hydrochloride or aminourea hydrochloride; a crystalline salt freely soluble in water: used as a reagent for ketones and aldehydes.

sem′i·car′ba·zone. A colored compound formed by reaction of aldehydes or ketones with semicarbazide.

sem″i·car″ti·lag′i·nous (·kahr″ti·ladj′i·nus) [*semi-;* L. *cartilagineus*, cartilaginous]. Gristly; partly cartilaginous.

sem″i·co′ma [*semi-;* G. *kōma*, deep sleep]. A condition of mild or partial coma.

sem″i·com′a·tose (·kom′uh·toce, ·toze, ·ko′muh·) [*semi-; kōma*]. Partially comatose.

sem″i·con′scious [*semi-;* L. *conscius*, knowing of something with another]. Half conscious; partially conscious.

semikon hydrochloride. A trade-marked name for *methapyrilene hydrochloride.*

sem″i·lu′nar [*semi-;* L. *luna*, moon]. Resembling a half moon in shape.

sem″i·lu′nar. One of the carpal bones. Old term for *lunate.* See Table of Bones in the Appendix.

sem″i·lux·a′tion [*semi-;* L. *luxatio*, from *luxare*, to dislocate]. Subluxation.

sem″i·mem″bra·no′sus [*semi-;* L. *membrana*, membrane]. One of the hamstring muscles, arising from the ischial tuberosity, and inserted into the tibia. See Table of Muscles in the Appendix.

sem″i·mem′bra·nous [*semi-; membrana*]. Partly membranous, as semimembranous muscle.

sem′i·nal [L. *semen*, seed]. Pertaining to the semen.

sem′i·nal ve·sic′u·lo·gram. A radiograph of the seminal vesicles, made by injecting a radiopaque substance into them via the ejaculatory ducts.

sem″i·na′tion [L. *seminatio*, from *seminare*, to sow]. The intromission of semen into the uterus or vagina. Also called *insemination.*

sem″i·nif′er·ous (sem″i·nif′ur·us, see″mi·) [L. *semen*, seed; *ferre*, to bear]. Producing or carrying semen, as the seminiferous tubules of the testis.

sem″i·no′ma, se″mi·no′ma [*semen;* G. *-ōma*, tumor]. A testicular tumor of low malignancy, made up of characteristic large, uniform cells with clear cytoplasm which resemble spermatogonia:

also called *dysgerminoma, seminal carcinoma, spermatocytoma.*

pineal s. See *pinealoma.*

sem″i·nor′mal [L. *semi-*, half; *norma*, rule]. Half-normal, as seminormal solution, a solution which contains one-half of an equivalent weight of the active reagent, in grams, in one liter of solution. It is written 0.5 N or N/2.

sem″i·nu′ri·a (sem″i·new′ree·uh, see″mi·) [L. *semen*, seed; G. *ouron*, urine]. The discharge of semen in the urine.

se″mi·og′ra·phy. See *semeiography.*

se″mi·ol′o·gy. See *semeiology.*

se″mi·ot′ics. See *semeiotics.*

sem″i·pen′ni·form [L. *semi-*, half; *penna*, wing; *forma*, form]. Penniform on one side only.

sem″i·ple′gi·a. See *hemiplegia.*

sem″i·pro·na′tion [*semi-*; L. *pronare*, to bend forward]. The assumption of a semiprone or partly prone position; an attitude of semisupination. —**semiprone′,** *adj.*

sem″i·pto′sis (sem″i·to′sis, sem″ip·to′sis) [*semi-*; G. *ptōsis*, a falling]. Partial ptosis.

se′mis [L.]. Half; abbreviated in prescriptions to ss, which is placed after the sign indicating the measure. Sometimes abbreviated, s.

sem″i·sid″e·ra′ti·o (sem″i·sid″uh·ray′shee·o). See *hemiplegia.*

sem″i·som′nus [L. *semi-*, half; *somnus*, sleep]. Coma. —**semisomnous,** *adj.*

sem″i·so′por [*semi-*; L. *sopor*, sleep]. Partial coma.

sem″i·spi·na′lis (sem″i·spy·nah′lis, ·nay′lis) [*semi-*; L. *spinalis*, of the spine]. One of the longitudinal muscles of the back, attached to the vertebrae. See Table of Muscles in the Appendix.

se·mis′sis. Semis.

sem″i·su″pi·na′tion [*semi-*; L. *supinatio*, from *supinare*, to bend backward]. A position halfway between supination and pronation.

sem″i·ten″di·no′sus [*semi-*; L. *tendere*, to stretch]. One of the hamstring muscles, arising from the ischium and inserted into the tibia. See Table of Muscles in the Appendix.

sem″i·ten′di·nous [*semi-*; *tendere*]. Partly tendinous, as a semitendinous muscle.

Semmelweis, Ignaz Philipp [*Hungarian obstetrician*, 1818–65]. The first to recognize the septicemic character of puerperal fever, and to attribute its spread to contamination by the hands of attending physicians.

Semon, Felix [*English laryngologist*, 1849–1921]. Known for his observations on myxedema and cretinism and their relationship (1883). Studied carcinoma of the thyroid gland and noted the impaired mobility of the vocal cords in this disease; called *Semon's symptom.* Believed that, in progressive organic lesions of the motor laryngeal nerves, the abductor muscles of the vocal cords are the first, and sometimes the only, muscles affected, called *Semon's, Semon-Rosenbach's law.*

sem″per·vi′rine. An alkaloid from gelsemium.

Semple, David [*English physician*, 1856–1937]. Introduced an inoculation against rabies called *Semple's treatment.* The vaccine used is made from 4% inoculated rabbit brain attenuated with 0.5% phenol; called *Semple's vaccine.*

Sendroy method. See under *method.*

Senear, Francis Eugene [*American dermatologist*, 1889–]. With B. Usher, described a dermatitis combining features of pemphigus and lupus erythematosus. See *pemphigus erythematosus.*

Se·ne′ci·o (si·nee′shee·o, ·see·o) [L.]. Groundsel; a genus of composite-flowered plants, said to contain 960 species, many of which have been used medicinally. **S. aureus** is the common liferoot. **S. canicida,** yerba del Puebla, a Mexican species, is diuretic. **S. cineraria** is a species of South America; the fresh juice of the leaves, stems, and flowers has been recommended in treatment of diseases of the eye. **S. jacoboea,** ragwort, is astringent.

se·ne′ci·o·nine (si·nee′shee·o·neen, ·nin, si·nee′-see·o·). An alkaloid, $C_{18}H_{25}NO_5$, from various species of South African *Senecio.*

se·nec′ti·tude [L. *senectus*, old age]. Old age.

sen′e·ga (*senega*). The dried root of *Polygala senega.* The active principles of senega belong to the group of saponins. The names senegin and polygalic acid have been applied to them. Used in various preparations as an expectorant in bronchitis and in asthma.

sen′e·gin. See under *senega.*

se·nes′cence [L. *senescere*, to grow old]. A growing old; aging. —**senescent,** *adj.*

se′nile (see′nile, ·nil) [L. *senilis*, aged]. Pertaining to, caused by, or characteristic of, old age or the infirmities of old age. —**senil′ity,** *n.*

se′nil·ism (see′nigh·liz·um, see′ni·) [*senilis*]. Senility, especially when premature.

se′ni·um [L., the feebleness of age]. Old age.

s. precox. Premature senility, considered clinically to occur in individuals under the age of 55 who exhibit senile manifestations, and associated with pseudocirrhosis and presenile sclerosis: also called *presenile dementia.*

Senn, Nicholas [*American surgeon*, 1844–1908]. Described a method of detecting intestinal perforation by rectal insufflation (1888); called *Senn's test.* Used decalcified bone plates in intestinal anastomosis and devised a two-stage operation for pancreatic cyst, both called *Senn's operation.*

sen′na [Ar. *sana*] (*senna*). The dried leaflets of *Cassia acutifolia*, or of *C. angustifolia.* It has been reported to contain the anthraquinone derivatives, either free or in glycosidal combination, rhein and aloe-emodin. A substance, sennanigrin, which yielded chrysophanol and emodin has also been found; more recently the glycosides sennoside A and sennoside B have been isolated and claimed to be the laxative principles. Other substances which have been found, but which probably are not connected with its purgative properties, are sennacrol, sennapicrin, sennarhamnetin, kaempferol and its glycoside kaempferin, and a small amount of volatile oil. Senna is a cathartic; its action is chiefly upon the lower bowel. Its tendency to gripe may be obviated by combining it with aromatics or with a saline laxative. Dose, 2–8 Gm. (½–1 dr.). Also called *senna leaves.*

compound s. powder (*pulvis sennae compositus*). Contains senna, 180 Gm.; glycyrrhiza, 236 Gm.; washed sulfur, 80 Gm.; fennel oil, 4 Gm.; sucrose, 500 Gm. Used as a laxative for the relief of habitual constipation. Dose, 2–4 Gm. (30–60 gr.). Also called *compound licorice powder.*

sen′na·crol. See under *senna.*

sen″na·pic′rin. See under *senna.*

Sennert, Daniel [*German physician*, 1572–1637]. Author of an important monograph on fevers (1627). Noted for his early description of scarlet fever, scurvy, and dysentery (1641).

sen′no·side. See under *senna.*

se·no′pi·a [G. *senex*, old; *ōps*, eye]. The change of vision in the aged, in which persons formerly myopic acquire what seems to be normal vision because of presbyopia.

sen·sa′tion [L. *sensatus*, gifted with sense]. A feeling or impression produced by the stimulation of an afferent nerve. Also see *sensibility.*

cincture s. Zonesthesia.

correlative s. Stimulation of the cerebrum by a sensation carried by a single sensory nerve.

cutaneous s. A sensation produced through the medium of the skin.
eccentric s. The conception of locality.
external s. A sensation transmitted from a peripheral sense organ.
general s. One of the body sensations, as pain, touch, heat, cold.
internal s. A sensation from viscera, such as hunger, thirst, fullness.
kinesthetic sensations. Sensations of motion.
psychovisual sensations. Those of sight without the stimulation of the retina; visions.
radiating s. See secondary *s.*
secondary s. (a) Mueller's name for the excitement of one sensation by another, or the extension of morbid sensations in disease to unaffected parts. (b) Synesthesia; a sensation of one type attending a sensation of another type.
special s. Any sensation produced by the special senses. See *sense.*
subjective s. One not caused by external stimuli.
tactile s. One produced through the sense of touch.
transference of s. Clairvoyance.

sen·sa′tion lev′el. A scale of the strength of a stimulus necessary to produce the minimal or threshold subjective sensation, used chiefly as a decibel scale in measuring sound intensity.

sense [L. *sensus*, sense]. Any one of the faculties by which stimuli from the external world or from within the body are received and transformed into sensations. The faculties receiving impulses from the external world are the senses of sight, hearing, touch, smell, and taste, which are the special senses, and the muscular and dermal senses. Those receiving impulses from the internal organs, the visceral senses, are the hunger sense, thirst sense, and others.
body s. Impressions from somatic structures which orient with regard to the body or its parts in space or which concern contacts or degrees of contact.
chemical s. Perception of chemical agents in the neighborhood of or in contact with the body; as smell, taste, and the detection of irritating chemicals on the mucous membranes.
color s. *In ophthalmology*, the faculty of distinguishing light of various wave lengths.
dermal s. The faculty of perceiving heat, cold, pain, or pressure mediated through receptors in the skin.
form s. *In ophthalmology*, acuteness of vision; the faculty of perceiving the shape or form of objects.
genesic s. The sexual instinct.
light s. *In ophthalmology*, the faculty of perceiving light and recognizing gradations of its intensity.
muscular s. Deep sensibility; proprioception.
posture s. The capability of recognizing (without seeing) the position in which a limb has been placed.
pressure s. The sense by which knowledge is obtained of the amount of weight or of pressure which is exerted upon a part of the body.
s. organs. Structures capable of detecting the presence of some specific type of agent in the environment of the body and reacting to this agent by sending impulses up their afferent nerves to the central nervous system.
seventh s. Visceral sense. *Obs.*
sixth s. Muscular sense. *Obs.*
space s. The faculty of orienting environmental objects in space.
temperature s. The sense by which differences in temperature are appreciated, consisting of a sense for cold, cryesthesia, and a heat sense, thermesthesia. These are represented on the surface by different nerve-endings, the so-called cold and hot points.
vibratory s. A modification of the touch sense with possible response from pressure receptors, elicited by a vibrating body (e.g. a tuning fork) in contact with parts of the human body: not a sense modality per se.

sense or′gan. A specialized sensory nerve terminal giving rise to a specific sensation, but responding to any adequate stimulus.

sen·sib′a·mine (sen·sib′uh·meen, ·min, sen″si-bam′een). A name given to an alkaloid of ergot, but later found to be an equimolecular mixture of ergotamine and ergotaminine.

sen″si·bil′i·ty [L. *sensibilis*, that which can be perceived by the senses]. 1. The ability to receive and feel impressions. 2. The ability of a nerve or end organ to receive and transmit impulses.
deep s. Perception of pressure, tension, and pain in the muscles, joints, tendons, and deep layers of the skin, as contrasted with sensations derived from the superficial layers of the skin.
electromuscular s. Responsiveness of muscles to electric stimulus.
epicritic s. The ability to appreciate and localize fine degrees of light touch, pain, and temperature stimuli.
gnostic s. The perception of epicritic sensations as contrasted with sensations from the viscera, which are called paleosensations. Also called *neo-sensibility.*
two-point s. See two-point *discrimination.*

sen″si·bil″i·za′tion. See *sensitization.*

sen′si·bi·li″zer [*sensibilis*]. 1. An agent that renders an enzyme active. 2. An amboceptor.

sen′si·ble [*sensibilis*]. Perceptible by the senses, as sensible perspiration; capable of receiving an impression through the senses; endowed with sensation.

sen·sim′e·ter [L. *sensus*, sense; G. *metron*, a measure]. An instrument for determining the sensitiveness of the skin.

sen″si·tiv′i·ty. 1. Capacity to feel or to transmit sensation. 2. Power to react to a stimulus. —**sen′-sitive,** *adj.*
tuberculin type s. See tuberculin type of *hypersensitivity.*

sen″si·ti·za′tion [*sentire*]. 1. Rendering cells sensitive by the action of an amboceptor. 2. The process of rendering an individual sensitive to a given protein.
Rh s. See *Rh sensitization.*

sen′si·tized [*sentire*]. Rendered sensitive to subthreshold stimuli or ordinarily ineffective agents, as in allergy. —**sen′sitize,** *v.*

sen′si·ti″zer [*sentire*]. The intermediary body of Ehrlich, by some called **hemotoxic sensitizer.**

sen″so·mo′tor. Sensorimotor.

sen″so·pa·ral′y·sis [L. *sensus*, sense; G. *paralysis*, paralysis]. Paralysis of a sensory nerve. *Obs.*

sen″so·ri·mo′tor [*sensus;* L. *motor*, from *movere*, to move]. Both sensory and motor; concerned with the perception of sensory impulses and with motor impulses, as sensorimotor centers.

sen·so′ri·um [*sensus*]. A center for sensations, especially the part of the brain which receives and combines impressions conveyed to the individual sensory centers. Also called *perceptorium.*

sen′so·ry [*sensus*]. Pertaining to, or conveying, sensation.

sen′su·al·ism [*sensus*]. The condition or character of one who is controlled by the more primitive instincts or emotions.

sen′sus [L.]. Sense; feeling.

sen′tient (sen′shunt, ·shee·unt) [L. *sentire*, to feel]. Having sensation; capable of feeling.

sen′ti·ment [*sentire*]. *In psychology,* a mental attitude characterized by feeling; an emotional disposition toward some object or objects.

sep′a·ra″tor [L. *separare*, to separate]. 1. Anything that separates, especially an instrument for separating the teeth. 2. An instrument for detaching periosteum: also called *periosteal elevator*.

sep′sine (sep′seen, ·sin). A poisonous ptomaine obtained from decomposed yeast and blood.

sep′sis [G., putrefaction]. A general reaction, usually febrile, the result of action of bacteria or their products or both; the organisms may be parasites or saprophytes.

gas s. That due to presence of *Clostridium welchii* or other gas-forming anaerobes.

puerperal s. That occurring as a complication or sequel of pregnancy; due to infection, usually streptococcal, in the birth canal, especially in the uterus.

s. agranulocytica. See *agranulocytosis*.

sep·tec′to·my [L. *saeptum*, fence; G. *ektomē*, excision]. Excision of part of the nasal septum.

sep·te′mi·a, sep·tae′mi·a. See *septicemia*.

sep″ten·tri″o·nal′ine. $C_{33}H_{46}N_2O_9$; an alkaloid isolated from *Aconitum septentrionale*.

sep′tic [G. *sēptikos*, putrefactive]. Relating to sepsis; affected by pathogenic organisms or their toxins.

sep″ti·ce′mi·a [*sēptikos;* G. *haima*, blood]. A systemic disease produced by microorganisms and their poisonous products in the blood stream. —**septicemic,** *adj.*

puerperal s. A febrile state caused by infection of the blood stream of the mother through the genital tract before, during, or following delivery. Also called *puerperal sepsis*.

sep″ti·co·phle·bi′tis [*sēptikos;* G. *phleps*, vein; *-itis*, inflammation]. Inflammation of veins secondary to infection of the blood stream.

sep′tic tank. In sewage disposal, a closed chamber through which sewage passes slowly to permit bacterial action.

sep″ti·grav′i·da [L. *septem*, seven; *gravidus*, pregnant]. A woman who is pregnant for the seventh time.

sep″ti·me·tri′tis [G. *sēptikos*, putrefactive; *mētra*, womb; *-itis*, inflammation]. Infection of the uterus.

sep·tip′a·ra [L. *septem*, seven; *parere*, to bring forth]. A woman who has borne seven children.

sep″to·mar′gi·nal [L. *saeptum*, fence; *margo*, edge]. Relating to the margin of a septum, as septomarginal tract.

sep·tom′e·ter [*saeptum;* G. *metron*, a measure]. An instrument for determining the thickness of the nasal septum.

sep·tom′e·ter [G. *sēptikos*, putrefactive; *metron*]. An apparatus for determining organic impurities in the air.

sep′to·tome [L. *saeptum*, fence; G. *tomos*, cutting]. An instrument for cutting the nasal septum.

sep·tot′o·my [*saeptum;* G. *tomē*, a cutting]. The operation of cutting the nasal septum.

sep′tu·lum (pl. *septula*) [dim. from *saeptum*]. A small septum.

septula of the pia mater. Thin septal processes from the pia mater which enter the substance of the white matter of the spinal cord.

septula testis. The interlobular septums of the testis.

sep′tum (pl. *septums, septa*) [*saeptum*]. A partition; a dividing wall between two spaces or cavities. —**septal, septile,** *adj.*

aortico-pulmonary s. See bulbar *s.*

atrial s. The septum between the right and left atria of the heart.

bronchial s. The ridge at the bifurcation of the trachea. See *carina* tracheae.

bulbar s. A septum, formed from the paired bulbar endocardial ridges, that divides spirally the bulbus cordis into aortic and pulmonary trunks. Also called *aortico-pulmonary s., aortic s.*

bulbourethral s. A partial median fibrous septum of the urethral bulb.

cartilaginous s. The angular cartilage plate forming the anterior part of the nasal septum.

cloacal s. See urorectal *s.*

dorsal median s. A glial partition continuous with the dorsal median sulcus and extending into the gray matter of the spinal cord.

femoral s. The layer of areolar tissue closing the femoral ring.

gingival s. The mucous membrane projecting into the interproximal space between two teeth.

hanging s. A broad alar cartilage overlying the anterior nasal septum abnormally.

interalveolar s. A bony septum between the tooth sockets.

interatrial s. See atrial *s.*

interdental s. The alveolar process between adjoining teeth.

intermediate cervical s. The septum formed by the union of the cervical spinal arachnoid and dura mater in the posterior midline.

intermuscular s. A connective-tissue septum between muscles, particularly one from which the muscles take origin, as the septum between the brachialis and the triceps muscles in the arm.

interradicular s. The bony partition between the roots of a tooth.

intersegmental s. The space intervening between two mesodermal somites.

interventricular s. The wall between the ventricles of the heart, largely muscular, partly membranaceous. Syn., *ventricular s.*

intraalveolar s. A bony projection within the tooth socket.

lingual s. The vertical median partition of the tongue which divides the muscular tissue into halves.

mediastinal s. See *mediastinum*.

mobile s. See nasal membranous *s.*

nasal membranous s. The most anterior and inferior part of the nasal septum, consisting of fibrous membrane and the medial crura of the alar cartilages; the movable part of the nasal septum.

nasal s. The septum between the two nasal cavities.

orbital s. A membranous sheet attached to the anterior edge of the orbit where it is continuous with the periosteum.

pectiniform s. The septum between the corpora cavernosa of the penis or clitoris.

pontine s. The median raphe of the pons, formed by the decussation of nerve fibers and by neuroglia fibers.

posterior intermediate s. The septum between the fasciculus gracilis and the fasciculus cuneatus.

posterior median s. The septum between the two posterior funiculi of the spinal cord.

posterior s. See subarachnoid *s.*

rectovaginal s. The tissue forming the partition between the rectum and the vagina.

s. crurale. Old term for femoral septum.

s. lucidum. Old term for septum pellucidum.

s. membranaceum. The superior part of the interventricular septum, composed of fibrous connective tissue.

s. mobile nasi. See nasal membranous *s.*

s. of musculotubarius canal. See cochleariform *process*.

s. pellucidum. A thin, translucent septum forming the internal boundary of the lateral ventricles of the brain and enclosing between its two laminas the so-called fifth ventricle. See Plate 18.

s. primum. The first incomplete interatrial septum of the embryo.

s. secundum. The second incomplete interatrial septum of the embryo containing the foramen ovale; it develops to the right of the septum primum and fuses with it to form the adult atrial septum.

s. spurium. A fold on the anterodorsal wall of the embryonic right atrium, formed by the fusion of the ends of the right and left valves of the sinus venosus.

sigmoidal s. A thin membrane that occupies the mandibular notch and separates the masseter from the external pterygoid muscles.

subarachnoid s. A partition formed by bands of fibroelastic tissue attaching the spinal arachnoid to the pia mater along the dorsal midline.

transverse s. The embryonic partition between the ventral part of the pericardial cavity and the peritoneal cavity that contributes to the formation of the diaphragm, the capsule and connective tissue of the liver, as well as the lesser omentum.

tubal s. See cochleariform *process*.

urorectal s. The embryonic horizontal connective-tissue septum that divides the cloaca into the rectum and primary urogenital sinus. Syn., *cloacal s.* Formerly called *Douglas' s.*

ventricular s. See interventricular *s.*

sep'tu·plet, sep·tu'plet [L. *septem*, seven; after trip*let*]. One of seven offspring born from a single gestation.

sep'ul·ture [L. *sepultura*, burial]. The disposal of the dead by burial.

Séquard. See Charles Edouard *Brown-Séquard.*

se·que'la, se·quel'a (pl. *sequelae*) [L. *sequi*, to follow]. An abnormal condition following a disease upon which it is directly or indirectly dependent.

se'quence [L. *sequi*, to follow]. 1. The order of occurrence, as of symptoms. 2. A sequela. —**sequen'tial,** *adj.*

se·ques'ter [L. *sequester*, depository]. Sequestrum.

se·ques'ter·ing a'gent. Any substance which will inactivate a metallic ion in solution, as by formation of a complex compound, and keep the resulting compound in solution.

se"ques·tra'tion [L. *sequestratio*, from *sequestrare*, to give up for safekeeping]. 1. The formation of a sequestrum. 2. The isolation of persons suffering from disease for purposes of treatment or for the protection of others.

se"ques·trec'to·my [L. *sequester*, depository; G. *ektomē*, excision]. The operative removal of a sequestrum.

sequestrene. A trade-mark for ethylenediaminetetraacetic acid and various of its salts.

se"ques·trot'o·my [*sequester;* G. *tomē*, a cutting]. See *sequestrectomy.*

se·ques'trum (pl. *sequestrums, sequestra*) [L., deposit]. A detached or dead piece of bone within a cavity, abscess, or wound. —**sequestral,** *adj.*

primary s. That entirely detached and requiring removal.

secondary s. One that is partially detached, and that, unless very loose, may be pushed into place.

tertiary s. That which is cracked or partially detached and remaining firmly in place.

se"ral·bu'min [L. *serum*, whey; *albus*, white]. Serum albumin, the albumin fraction of serum.

se·rem'pi·on. A form of epidemic measles occurring in the West Indies, which causes great mortality, especially among children.

serenium. Trade-mark for the hydrochloride of 2,4-diamino-4'-ethoxy-azobenzene, an organic azo dye. The substance is used as an urinary antiseptic, most active in acid medium.

ser"e·no'a (*serenoa*). The partially dried ripe fruit of *Serenoa repens*. The drug yields on pressure a brownish yellow to dark red oil, which is composed of about 63% of free fatty acids and about 37% of ethyl esters of these acids. It exerts a stimulating action upon the mucous membranes of the genitourinary tract and has been used in chronic and subacute cystitis. Also called *saw palmetto berries, sabal.*

ser'i·ceps [L. *sericum*, silk; *caput*, head]. A device made of loops of ribbon for making traction upon the fetal head.

se'ries [L.]. 1. A succession or a group of compounds, objects, or numbers, arranged systematically according to a rule. 2. *In taxonomy,* the sample of a population which forms the basic working unit in modern systematics. 3. *In hematology,* the succession of cell types in the development of a cell of the circulating blood. Classification and terminology vary widely among investigators in the field. There may be considered to be five series: (a) the **myeloid** or **granulocytic series** composed of the myeloblast, myelocyte, unsegmented or nonfilamentous polymorphonuclear leukocyte, and the neutrophil, eosinophil, or basophil granulocyte; (b) the **lymphoid** or **lymphocytic series** composed of the lymphoblast, young lymphocyte, and adult lymphocyte; (c) the **monocytic series** composed of the monoblast, immature monocyte, and adult monocyte; (d) the **erythrocytic series,** the megaloblast, erythroblast, normoblast, reticulocyte, and adult erythrocyte; and (e) the **blood platelet** or **thrombocytic series,** the megakaryoblast, megakaryocyte, and blood platelet or thrombocyte.

acetylene s. Straight-chained hydrocarbons with a triple linkage.

aliphatic s. The series of organic compounds in which the linkages of successive carbon atoms are terminated, as in an open chain.

aromatic s. The series of organic compounds derived from benzene and characterized by the presence of a number of the carbon atoms arranged in the form of a closed chain.

closed chain s. A series of organic compounds characterized by linkages between successive atoms as in a closed chain.

contact s. A series of metals ranged in such an order that each becomes positively electrified by contact with the one that follows it.

homologous s. A group of compounds differing from one another by a definite radical or group.

lyotropic s. An arrangement of the ions in the order of their behavior, such as their effect in salting-out of proteins, or on the viscosity of colloids. Also called *Hofmeister s.*

open chain s. A series of organic compounds characterized by linkages between successive atoms as in an open chain.

ser'i·flux, se'ri·flux [L. *serum*, whey; *fluxus*, flow]. Any serous or watery discharge, or a disease characterized by such a discharge. *Obs.*

ser'ine, se'rine. $CH_2OH.CHNH_2.COOH$. α-Amino-β-hydroxypropionic acid; hydroxyalanine, an amino acid; occurs as a colorless, crystalline powder; soluble in water, insoluble in alcohol or ether. It is a constituent of many proteins.

se'ro-, ser- [*serum*]. A combining form denoting *relating to serum* or *serous.*

serobacterin. Trade-mark for emulsions of killed bacteria which have been sensitized by treatment with a specific immune serum and which more rapidly produce immunity.

se·roche′ (seh·roshe′). See chronic mountain *sickness.*

se′ro·chrome [*serum;* G. *chrōma,* color]. Gilbert's name for the pigments which serve to give color to normal serum.

se″ro·co·li′tis [*serum;* G. *kolon,* colon; *-itis,* inflammation]. Inflammation of the serous covering of the colon. *Obs.*

se′ro·cul″ture [*serum;* L. *cultura,* cultivation]. A bacterial culture on blood serum.

se″ro·der″ma·ti′tis [*serum;* G. *derma,* skin; *-itis,* inflammation]. An inflammatory skin affection attended with serous effusion.

se″ro·der″ma·to′sis [*serum; derma; -ōsis,* condition]. A skin disease characterized by serous effusion into or onto the skin.

se″ro·der·mi′tis. See *serodermatitis.*

se″ro·di″ag·no′sis [*serum;* G. *diagnōsis,* a deciding]. Diagnosis based upon the reaction of blood serum of patients.

se″ro·en″ter·i′tis [*serum;* G. *enteron,* intestine; *-itis,* inflammation]. Inflammation of the serous covering of the small intestine. *Obs.*

se″ro·fi′brin·ous [*serum;* L. *fibra,* fiber]. 1. Composed of serum and fibrin, as a serofibrinous exudate. 2. Characterized by the production of a serofibrinous exudate, as a serofibrinous inflammation.

se″ro·lem′ma [*serum;* G. *lemma,* husk]. Old term for the serosa or false amnion, especially in *Sauropsida.* Syn., *chorion.*

se″ro·li′pase (seer″o·lye′pace, ·lip′ace). Lipase as found in blood serum.

se·rol′o·gist [*serum;* G. *logos,* word]. One versed in serology.

se·rol′o·gy [*serum; logos*]. That branch of science which deals with serum. —**serolog′ic, serolog′ical,** *adj.*

se·rol′y·sin, se″ro·ly′sin [*serum;* G. *lysis,* a loosing]. Bactericidal substance contained in normal blood serum.

se″ro·mem′bra·nous [*serum;* L. *membrana,* membrane]. Pertaining to a serosa.

se″ro·mu′cous [*serum;* L. *mucus,* mucus]. Having the nature of or containing both serum and mucus, as a glandular cell which has the characteristics of both a serous cell and a mucous cell.

seromycin. A name assigned to *cycloserine.*

se″ro·per″i·to·ne′um [*serum;* G. *peritonaion,* membrane which encloses the lower viscera]. Hydroperitoneum, ascites.

se″ro·prog·no′sis [*serum;* G. *prognōsis,* foreknowledge]. Prognosis of disease as determined by seroreactions.

se″ro·pu′ru·lent [*serum;* L. *purulentus,* purulent]. Composed of serum and pus, as a seropurulent exudate.

se″ro·re·ac′tion [*serum;* L. *re-,* again; *agere,* to act]. A reaction performed with serum.

se″ro·re·sis′tance. Persistent positive serologic reaction for syphilis despite prolonged intensive treatment; the patient is said to be *Wassermann-fast.* —**seroresis′tant,** *adj.*

se·ro′sa [*serum*]. 1. A serous membrane composed of mesothelium and subjacent connective tissue, lining the pericardial, pleural, and peritoneal cavities and covering their contents. Also called *tunica s.* 2. The chorion of birds and reptiles.

se·ro″sa·mu′cin. A protein resembling mucin found in ascitic fluid.

se″ro·san·guin′e·ous [L. *serum,* whey; *sanguineus,* bloody]. Having the nature of, or containing, both serum and blood.

se″ro·se′rous [*serum; serum*]. Pertaining jointly to two serous surfaces.

se″ro·si′tis [*serum;* G. *-itis,* inflammation]. Inflammation of a serous membrane.

adhesive s. See fibrous *adhesion.*

multiple s. See *polyserositis.*

se″ro·syn″o·vi′tis (seer″o·sin″o·vy′tis, ·sigh″no·vy′tis) [*serum;* NL. *synovia; -itis*]. A synovitis with increase of synovial fluid.

se″ro·ther′a·py [*serum;* G. *therapeia,* treatment]. The treatment of disease by means of human or animal blood serum containing antibodies.

ser″o·to′nin. A substance present in the blood stream which imparts vasoconstrictor activity to the latter. It has been isolated in crystalline form, but its chemical structure has not been determined.

ser′o·trin. A glycoside from the leaves of the wild black cherry (*Prunus serotina*); on hydrolysis it yields D-glucose and quercetin. Sometimes written *serotin.*

se′rous [*serum*]. 1. Pertaining to, characterized by, or resembling serum. 2. Producing serum, as a serous gland; containing serum, as a serous cyst.

se′ro·zyme. See *prothrombin.*

serpasil. Trade-mark for *reserpine.*

ser′pens (sur′penz) [L., a creeping thing]. Serpentine, sinuous; creeping.

ser″pen·ta′ri·a [*serpens*]. The dried rhizome and roots of *Aristolochia serpentaria* or of *A. reticulata.* It contains a volatile oil and a bitter principle. The volatile oil consists mainly of an ester of borneol and a terpene. The drug is classed among the aromatic bitters and in moderate dose acts as a gastric stimulant.

ser′pen·tine. An alkaloid from *Rauwolfia serpentina.*

ser·pent′i·nine. An alkaloid isolated from *Rauwolfia serpentina:* sometimes called *isorauwolfine.*

ser·pig′i·nous (sur·pidj′i·nus) [L. *serpere,* to creep]. Creeping; having an irregular but arched and serpentine shape; applied to skin lesions.

ser·pyl′lum [L.]. The wild thyme, *Thymus serpyllum,* used by the homeopaths as a bronchial antispasmodic.

ser′ra [L.]. *In biology,* a saw or sawlike structure, as the saw of a sawfish.

Ser·ra′ti·a (seh·ray′shee·uh) [*serra*]. A genus of bacilli commonly found in water.

S. marcescens. A motile, Gram-negative organism which produces a deep-red pigment. It may be found in stool cultures, but has no clinical significance. Formerly called *Bacillus prodigiosus.*

ser·ra′tion [*serra*]. The state or condition of being toothed or having a toothed margin. —**ser′rate,** *adj.*

ser·ra′tus [L., from *serra*]. Serrated; said of muscles arising or inserted by a series of processes like teeth of a saw, as serratus anterior muscle. See Table of Muscles in the Appendix.

s. magnus. Old name for the anterior serratus muscle.

Serres, Antoine Etienne Rênaud Augustin [*French physician,* 1786–1868]. Remembered for his description of pearl-like epithelial masses found on the gums of infants. Called *Serres, glands, gingival glands.* Described the metafacial angle, also called *Serres' angle.*

Sertoli, Enrico [*Italian histologist,* 1842–1910]. Known for his exploration of the origin and histology of the sustentacular cells of the seminiferous tubules; called *cells of Sertoli.*

Sertürner, Friedrich Wilhelm Adam [*German pharmacologist,* 1784–1841]. Isolated morphine (1806).

se′rum (pl. *serums, sera*) [L., whey]. 1. The amber-colored fluid which exudes from coagulated blood as the clot shrinks and then no longer contains fibrinogen. Serum is of a complex nature and is made up of water, albumin, globulins, metabolites, catabolites, lipids, hormones, salts, enzymes, etc. Serum proteins are antigenic and may be toxic for members of a different species. Serum may carry agglutinating, precipitating, neutralizing, opsonic, bactericidal, hemolytic, bacteriolytic, complementary, vasoconstrictive, sensitizing, and other properties. Serum proteins have been designated by Tiselius as albumin, α-globulin, β-globulin, and γ-globulin on the basis of their electrophoretic mobilities. In human serum, the albumin comprises about 55% to 60% of the total serum proteins, the α-globulin about 10% to 15%, the β-globulin varies from 9% to 13%, and the γ-globulin from 9% to 12%. The fact that the serums of immunized animals and of man contain antibodies, etc., has resulted in extensive use of serums for diagnosis, prophylaxis, and therapy. See Table of Normal Values of Blood Constituents in the Appendix. —**serous, serumal,** *adj.*

antianthrax s. A serum prepared by immunizing horses against virulent anthrax bacilli (*Bacillus anthracis*). Used in the treatment of human anthrax. Dose, a minimum of 50 cc., intramuscularly or intravenously.

antibotulinus s. An antitoxin prepared from animals which have been immunized by botulinus toxin-antitoxin or toxoid. Dose, 20–40 cc. intravenously early in the disease, or 10 cc. intramuscularly for prophylaxis.

antidysenteric s. The serum (polyvalent) of horses immunized against the Shiga bacillus (*Shigella dysenteriae*), its products of growth, and other types of the dysentery bacilli. Dose, 20–100 cc., subcutaneously or intramuscularly.

antierysipelas s. A serum containing the antibodies and antibacterial properties for hemolytic streptococci from erysipelas. The serum is obtained from horses immunized with strains of hemolytic streptococci obtained from human cases of erysipelas. Since chemotherapeutic preparations are now available, this serum is rarely used.

antierysipeloid s. A serum containing the antibodies and antibacterial properties for *Erysipelothrix rhusiopathiae* (suis). It is prepared from horses subjected to increasing subcutaneous injections of live cultures of the organism. It is used in cases of erysipeloid. Dose, 10–20 cc., subcutaneously or intramuscularly.

antiglobulin s. An immune serum containing globulin antibodies produced in rabbits by repeated injection of human serum or gamma-globulin of human serum: used in the antiglobulin test. Syn., *Coombs' s.*

antimeningococcic s. (*serum antimeningococcicum*). A serum obtained from the blood of an animal immunized with cultures of the several types of meningococci (*Neisseria meningitidis*) which prevail in the United States. It has been supplemented or supplanted by the newer chemotherapeutic agents. Dose, intravenously, 50 cc. for children and up to 100 cc. for adults; intrathecally, 30 cc. Also called *antimeningococcus s., meningococcus s., meningitis s.*

antiphage s. A serum produced against a given bacteriophage. See *bacteriophage*.

antiplague s. Immune serum obtained by injecting an animal with *Pasteurella pestis* or its products. Its use in cases of plague has been disappointing.

antipneumococcic s.-type specific (*serum antipneumococcicum*). A serum obtained from the blood of an animal which has been immunized with cultures of a pneumococcus (*Diplococcus pneumoniae*) of one of the types for which a serum has been prepared and which has been standardized, or is released, by the National Institute of Health of the United States Public Health Service and complies with the requirements of that agency of the government. It is used primarily in the treatment of pneumococcic pneumonias. Dose, parenteral, therapeutic, from 20,000 to 100,000 units. Also called *antipneumococcus s., pneumonia s.*

antireticular cytotoxic s. See *ACS*.

anti-Rh serums. Immune serums prepared in rabbits, guinea pigs, goats, and other animals by injecting them with the blood of rhesus monkeys.

antitetanic s. See *tetanus* antitoxin.

convalescent s. Blood serum taken from a person who is convalescing from some acute, infectious disease. It is injected as a prophylactic or curative measure.

Coombs' s. See antiglobulin *s.*

despeciated bovine s. A bovine serum altered in such a manner that its species specificity is reduced. Also called *DBS.*

gastrotoxic s. An immune serum which when injected damages the gastric cells, allowing ulceration of the mucosa by the gastric juice: produced by using gastric cells to immunize an animal.

Hiss's s. water. Serum diluted with two or three times its volume of distilled water. It is used in bacteriology to aid the growth of fastidious organisms.

horse s. One obtained from the blood of a horse. It may be normal or immune serum. Many of the therapeutically useful serums are obtained from horses immunized against a specific organism or its toxin. The serum obtained from an immunized animal is known as **immune horse serum** as distinguished from the **normal horse serum** obtained from an unimmunized animal.

human measles immune s. (*serum immune morbillosi humanum*). Sterile serum obtained from the blood of a healthy human who has survived an attack of measles. This serum is administered during the incubation period to prevent or modify the expected attack of measles. Dose, children 6 years or under, 10 cc., intramuscularly, within five days after exposure; for children between 7 and 12 years of age, 15 cc.; and for older children and adults, 20 cc. Also called *measles convalescent s.*

human scarlet fever immune s. (*serum immune scarlatinae humanum*). A sterile serum obtained from the blood of a healthy human who has survived an attack of scarlet fever. It is of value in transferring passive immunity to a patient exposed to scarlet fever. Dose, children under 6 years of age, 10 cc.; for children between 6 and 12 years of age, 15 cc.; and for children over 12 years and for adults, 15 to 20 cc. are given intramuscularly. Also called *scarlet fever convalescent s.*

immune s. The sterile serum of an immunized animal or person, which carries antibodies naturally or artificially produced.

normal human s. (*serum humanum normale*). The sterile serum obtained by pooling approximately equal amounts of serum from eight or more healthy humans. Its chief use is in the treatment of bacterial infections, in the treatment of surgical and traumatic shock, and in the treatment of burns. Dose, 500 cc., intravenously or subcutaneously. Also called *human s.*

North American antisnakebite s. An antitoxic serum prepared by immunizing animals against the venom of snakes of the crotalus family. Dose, 50 cc. administered intramuscularly or subcutaneously; in late cases or in the presence of severe symptoms, it may be given intravenously. Also called *crotalus antivenin, crotalus antitoxin.*

pooled s. Mixed serum from a number of persons.

pregnant mare's s. The source for the manufacture of various sex hormones.

purified antidiphtheritic s. See *diphtheria* antitoxin.

purified antitetanic s. See *tetanus* antitoxin.

Rh blocking s. One able to react with blood containing the Rh factor without producing agglutination, though blocking the action of subsequently added anti-Rh serums; i.e., Rh positive blood treated with Rh blocking serum can no longer be agglutinated by anti-Rh serum. Blocking antibodies of only one specificity, anti-Rh_0, are known.

truth s. See *narcoanalysis.*

se'rum ac·cel'er·a·tor glob'u·lin. See *accelerin.*

se'rum pro'te·ase. See *plasmin.*

se'rum pro·throm'bin con·ver'sion ac·cel'er·a·tor (SPCA). See *convertin.*

se'rum rash. See serum *sickness.*

se'rum tryp'sin, tryp'tase. See *plasmin.*

se'rum tryp'to·gen. See *plasminogen.*

se'rum ur"ti·ca'ri·a. An anaphylactic reaction to the injection of a serum.

Servetus, Michael [*Spanish theologian and physician,* 1511–53]. Celebrated in medical history for his early concept of the pulmonary circulation (1546), sometimes referred to as the *circulation of Servetus.*

ser'vo-mech'an·ism. A control system such that small continuous mechanical displacements involving small expenditures of power by the controller cause proportionate displacements involving large amounts of power at a distance in the device being controlled.

ser'yl. The univalent radical, $HOCH_2CH(NH_2)$-CO—, of the amino acid serine.

ses'a·me (sess'uh·mee) [G.]. An herb, *Sesamum indicum;* yields sesame oil.

ses'a·moid [G. *sēsamē,* sesame; *eidos,* form]. Resembling a sesame seed, as in sesamoid bone, a small bone developed in a tendon subjected to much pressure (see Table of Bones in the Appendix) and sesamoid cartilages, small cartilages in the alae of the nose.

ses"a·moid·i'tis [*sēsamē; eidos;* G. *-itis,* inflammation]. An inflammation of the sesamoid bones which may involve the articular surfaces and cause lameness.

Se·sar'ma. A genus of fresh water crabs found in Asia. **S. dehaani** and **S. sinensis** are intermediate hosts of the lung fluke, *Paragonimus westermani.*

ses'qui- [L., more by a half]. A combining form indicating *one and one-half, the proportion of two* of one radical or element *to three* of another.

ses"qui·chlo'ride. A compound of chlorine and another element containing three parts of chlorine to two of the other element, as Fe_2Cl_3.

ses"qui·ho'ra [*sesqui;* L. *hora,* hour]. An hour and a half.

ses"qui·ox'ide. A compound of three parts of oxygen to two of another element, as Al_2O_3.

ses'qui·salt. A salt containing one and one-half times as much of the acid as of the radical or base, as $Fe_2(SO_4)_3$.

ses"qui·sul'fide. A compound of sulfur and another element containing three parts of sulfur to two of the other element, as Sb_2S_3.

ses"qui·ter'pene. One of a group of terpenes of the general formula $C_{15}H_{24}$.

ses'sile (sess'il) [L. *sessilis,* of sitting]. Attached by a broad base; not pedunculated, as a sessile tumor.

set [AS. *settan*]. 1. To reduce the displacement in a fracture and apply bandages suitably arranged for fixation. 2. To harden, solidify, as a cement, amalgam, or plaster.

set, mental s. The attitude, interest, or intent of an observer which may influence his perception.

se'ta (pl. *setae*) [L. *saeta,* bristle]. A stiff, stout, bristlelike appendage; a chaeta, vibrissa. —**se·ta'ceous,** *adj.*

Se·ta'ri·a [*saeta*]. A genus of grasses including millet, *Setaria italica.*

se'ton [*saeta*]. A thread or skein of threads drawn through a fold of the skin, so as to produce a fistulous tract; used as a counterirritant. *Obs.*

Sever, James Warren [*American orthopedic surgeon,* 1878–]. Known for his numerous contributions to the knowledge of orthopedic surgery. Described epiphysitis of the calcaneus; also called *Sever's disease.* Originated *Sever's operation* for obstetric paralysis.

se·vip'a·rous [L. *sevum,* tallow; *parere,* to bring forth]. Sebiparous; fat-producing.

se'vum [L.]. Suet.

sew'age [OF. *sewiere*]. The heterogeneous substances constituting the excreta and waste matter of domestic economy and the contents of drains.

sew'er [*sewiere*]. A canal for the removal of sewage.

sew'er·age [*sewiere*]. 1. The collection and removal of sewage. 2. The system of pipes, etc., for the removal of sewage.

sex [L. *sexus,* sex]. The state or condition of an organism which comes to expression in the production of ova, as in the female, or of sperm cells, as in the male, or both ova and sperm cells, as in certain hermaphroditic invertebrates.

sex- [L. *sex,* six]. A combining form meaning *six.*

sex chro'mo·some. An odd or accessory chromosome having a special relation to determining whether a fertilized egg develops into a male or a female. The X and Y chromosomes. When other conditions are normal, a fertilized egg with two X's becomes a female; one with the XY combination becomes a male.

sex de·ter"mi·na'tion. The process which determines the sex of an individual. See *sex chromosome.*

sex"i·dig'i·tal (seck"si·didj'i·tul), **sex"i·dig'i·tate** (seck"si·didj'i·tayt) [*sex;* L. *digitus,* finger]. Having six fingers or six toes.

sex'-in'ter·grade". An intersex.

sex'-lim'it·ed. Appearing in, or affecting, one sex only.

sex'-linked". Applied to genes located on the X chromosome, and to the characteristics, which may occur in either sex, conditioned by such genes.

sex'o-es·thet'ic in·ver'sion. The adoption of the habits, manners, and costume of the opposite sex. Also see *eonism, transvestitism.*

sex·ol'o·gy [L. *sexus,* sex; G. *logos,* word]. The science or study of sex and sex relations. —**sex·olog'ic,** *adj.*

sex re·ver'sal. A change of characteristics in an individual of one sex to those of the opposite sex.

sex"ti·grav'i·da [L. *sextus,* sixth; *gravidus,* pregnant]. A woman who is pregnant for the sixth time.

sex·tip'a·ra [*sextus;* L. *parere,* to bring forth]. A woman who has borne six children.

sex'tu·plet, sex·tu'plet [*sextus;* after trip*let*]. One of the six offspring of a single gestation.

sex'u·al [L. *sexualis,* of sex]. Pertaining to or characteristic of sex, as the sexual organs. —**sexual'ity,** *n.*

sex'ual de·vi·a'tion. *In psychiatry,* a sociopathic personality disturbance characterized by deviant or aberrant sexuality which is not part of any more extensive disorder such as the schizophrenic or obsessional reactions. It includes the various forms and practices of homosexuality, transvestitism, pedophilia, fetishism, and sexual sadism (assault and rape, mutilation).

Sgambati, O. [*Italian physician*, contemporary]. Described a test for peritonitis. If nitric acid and chloroform are added to urine and a red tint results, the reaction is said to be positive; called *Sgambati's test* or *reaction.*

S. G. O. Surgeon General's Office.

SH Sulfhydryl.

shad'ow [ME. *shadowe*]. A hemolyzed erythrocyte consisting only of stroma. Also called *phantom cell, ghost cell, blood shadow.*

Shaffer method. See Folin-Shaffer *method.*

Shaffer's theory of oxidation catalysis. See under *theory.*

shaft [AS. *sceaft*]. The trunk of any columnar mass, especially the diaphysis of a long bone.

hair-s. A hair, particularly that portion of it imbedded in the hair follicle.

sha'king [AS. *scacan*]. A type of massage imparting a vibration to the tissues.

sham rage. Paroxysms of reactions in decorticate animals, giving the appearance of rage, which are evoked by very mild stimuli. The reactions, such as erection of hairs, dilatation of the pupil, protrusion of claws, struggling and biting, are in considerable part those which are controlled by the autonomic nervous system.

shank [AS. *sceanca*]. The leg from the knee to the ankle; the tibia.

Sharpey, William [*English physiologist and anatomist*, 1802–80]. Celebrated founder of English physiology. Made many important anatomic studies including research on the ossicles of the ear and the histology of bone.

Sharpey-Schafer, Edward Albert [*English physiologist*, 1850–1935]. With George Oliver, discovered the existence of an adrenal pressor substance (1894), later named epinephrine by Abel. See also *Schafer* (*prone pressure*) *method* under *artificial respiration.*

sha'ven-beard ap·pear'ance. A spotted pigmentation of the intestinal mucosa, especially the colon; the spots are discrete, a millimeter or less in diameter, and closely approximated, suggesting the appearance of a freshly shaved, heavy beard. The pigment is usually hemosiderin but may be other pigments, such as bismuth or a protein combination with hydrogen sulfide.

Sheard, Charles (1883–). American biophysicist who introduced, with Sanford, a photoelectric colorimeter called *Sheard-Sanford photelometer.* He designed and introduced the spectrophotelometer. See also Sanford, Sheard, and Osterberg *method.*

shears [AS. *sceran*]. A large pair of scissors.

bandage s. Strong shears for cutting bandages, the blades usually bent at an angle with the shaft.

sheath [AS. *scǣth*]. 1. An envelope; a covering. 2. *In anatomy,* the connective tissue covering vessels, muscles, nerves, tendons, etc. 3. A condom.

arachnoidean s. A delicate partition lying between the pial sheath and the dural sheath of the optic nerve.

bast s. Phloem sheath.

carotid s. The fibrous sheath about the carotid arteries and associated structures.

cellular s. See *epineurium.*

crural s. The femoral sheath.

dentinal s. The structure lining the dentinal tubules.

dural s. A strong fibrous membrane forming the external investment of the optic nerve. See *dura mater.*

epithelial s. of Hertwig. That portion of the enamel organ which forms no enamel, but serves as a mold for the shape of the root of a tooth.

femoral s. A continuation downward of the fasciae that line the abdomen. It contains the femoral vessels.

fibril s. A sheath formed by connective-tissue fibrils and surrounding individual nerve fibers.

Hertwig s. See epithelial *s.* of Hertwig.

Huxley's s. See *layer* of Huxley.

lamellar s. See *perineurium.*

Mauthner's s. See *axolemma.*

medullary s. The myelin sheath.

mucous s. Tendon sheath.

myelin s. A glistening white sheath of myelinated nerve fibers, immediately around the axis cylinder. Consists of a complex lipoid mixture and is a poor electric conductor.

nerve s. See *perineurium.*

Neumann's s. See dentinal *s.*

neural s. See myelin *s.*

phloem s. *In botany,* a layer of thin-walled cells surrounding the phloem tissue; bast sheath; periphloem; vascular bundle sheath.

pial s. The extension of the pia which closely invests the surface of the optic nerve. See *pia.*

primitive s. See *neurilemma.*

root s. That portion of the hair follicle derived from the epidermis; it surrounds the root of the hair and consists of the **internal root sheath,** three layers of cells immediately surrounding the root, and the **external root sheath,** a stratified layer adjacent to the dermal portion of the hair follicle.

Schwalbe's s. The delicate sheath which covers elastic fibers.

s. of Henle. The endoneurium. See *layer* of Henle.

s. of rectus. That formed by the aponeuroses of the external and internal oblique and transversus abdominis muscles. See Plate 4.

s. of Schwann. See *neurilemma.*

s. of Schweigger-Seidel. The thickening of the arterial wall in the sheathed arteries of the splenic penicilli.

s. of the optic nerve. See dural *s.*

synovial s. A synovial membrane which lines the cavity through which a tendon glides.

tendon s. In particular, the synovial sheath surrounding a tendon crossing the wrist or ankle joints.

shed [AS. *scādan*]. Throw off.

shed'ding [*scādan*]. 1. Casting off. 2. *In dentistry,* the natural process of resorption of the roots and the subsequent loss of deciduous teeth.

sheep pox. *In veterinary medicine,* a contagious disease of sheep characterized by vesicopustular lesions of the skin. Found only in central Asia and Europe.

shell. 1. A hard outer covering, as for an animal, egg, fruit, seed, or the like. 2. *In nuclear physics,* an orbit of electrons at the same energy level around the nucleus of an atom.

equipotential s. A surface at every point of which the potential energy is equal, and having a contour everywhere normal to the force or flow lines of the field.

shel·lac'. See *lac,* 2.

shells [AS. *scell*]. Tinted spectacles, for protection of the eyes; coquilles.

shell'shock. 1. Old term for battle fatigue. 2. Concussion produced by the bursting of a shell.

shel'tered work'shop". A workshop for disabled ambulatory individuals. Type of work, machinery, and tempo are modified so that the handicapped may cope with their jobs successfully.

Shenstone, Norman Strahan [*Canadian surgeon,*

1881–]. Known for his introduction of an operation for the closure of bronchial fistula, in which he implanted intercostal muscle into the fistulous tract. Two ribs are resected to give proper access and to allow a pedicle graft to be made from the muscle. Called *Shenstone's operation.*

Shepherd, Francis J. [*British surgeon,* 1851–1929]. Described a type of fracture of the lateral process of the talus, called *Shepherd's fracture.*

Sherman, Harry Mitchell [*American orthopedic surgeon,* 1854–1921]. Vanadium steel bone plates for internal fixation of fractures are called *Sherman plates.* Vanadium steel tap screws used for attaching them are called *Sherman screws.*

Sherman, Henry Clapp [*American chemist,* 1875–]. With Hazel E. Munsell, introduced the rat growth unit, which is the daily requirement of vitamin A necessary to maintain a weekly gain of 3 Gm. in test rats previously depleted of vitamin A; called *Sherman-Munsell unit.* See also Bourquin-Sherman *unit.*

Sherman and Chase assay t. See under *test.*

Sherrington, Charles Scott (1857–1952). English neurophysiologist who established neurophysiology as a discipline by numerous and epochal contributions to the experimental knowledge, nomenclature, and concepts of this field. He analyzed the distribution of the ventral and dorsal nerve roots, established the sensory innervation of striated muscles, laid the foundation of our knowledge of the proprioceptive system (1894), described decerebrate rigidity (1897), and introduced the term *synapse* (1897). His classic work, *The Integrative Action of the Nervous System* (1906), introduced the classification of the senses into *proprio-, extero-, intero-, tele-,* and *nociceptors* and established the concept of the nervous system implied in the term *integrative action.* He mapped the cerebral cortex, studied special reflexes, and discovered the stretch reflex (1927). Nobel laureate in physiology and medicine, with E. D. Adrian, 1932.

she′ster·in. $C_{26}H_{30}O_{13}$; a glycoside from the berries of *Rhamnus cathartica.*

Shevsky's test. See Addis and Shevsky's *test.*

Shibley, Gerald Spencer [*American internist,* 1890–]. Described a sign useful in the diagnosis of consolidation of the lung or of a collection of fluid in the pleural cavity. When bronchial or tracheal voice is heard through the stethoscope, the vowels spoken are carried to the ear of the examiner as "Ah!" Called *Shibley's sign, "e" to "a" sign.*

shield [AS. *scild*]. 1. A protective structure or apparatus. 2. *In biology,* a protective plate, scute, lorica, or carapace. 3. A structure having the shape of a shield.

antithermic s. A protective covering of the cautery to prevent destruction of the tissues about the field of operation.

cytherean s. A condom.

embryonic s. The shield-shaped bilaminar blastodisk from which develops the embryo proper.

nipple s. A protective covering for sore nipples.

Shiels method. See Reinhold and Shiels *method.*

shift [AS. *sciftan,* to divide]. A change of direction or position.

axis s. Axis deviation.

basal s. A dislocation of the brain beneath the arch of the falx cerebri, due to increased pressure.

chloride s. The movement of chloride ions from plasma into the red blood cells when the blood is giving up oxygen and receiving carbon dioxide. When hemoglobin is reduced it becomes more basic, therefore a shift of negative ions into the cell is required to maintain ionic equilibrium. The chloride shift frees base (Na^+) in the plasma. This unites with part of the CO_2 entering the blood to form bicarbonate which together with carbonic acid constitutes an acid-salt buffer pair. The buffers prevent serious changes in pH with respiratory gas exchanges in the tissues and the lungs.

degenerative s. to left. A term used by Schilling to designate a depression of bone-marrow function characterized by delivery into the circulation of immature neutrophils and degenerative changes in the cells such as pyknotic nuclei, vacuoles, and irregularities in staining. Such cells, it is assumed, can mature no further. See *s. to left.*

index of nuclear s. The ratio of the percentages of immature to mature neutrophils, based on Schilling's classification. Normal values are 1:10 or less.

left axis s. Left axis deviation.

regenerative s. to left. A term used by Schilling to describe the presence of many immature neutrophils in the peripheral blood, as a result of rapid delivery from the bone marrow in reaction to an acute need, as in an infection. See *s. to left.*

right axis s. Right axis deviation.

s. to left. A marked increase in the percentage of immature neutrophils (those having a single or bilobed nucleus) in the peripheral blood, occurring in granulocytic leukemia, in acute infective diseases, and also in pernicious anemia. The term is based on Arneth's classification of neutrophils. See also *degenerative* and *regenerative s. to left.*

s. to right. A marked increase in the percentage of mature neutrophils (those having nuclei with three or more lobes) in the peripheral blood, frequently occurring in diseases of the liver and in pernicious anemia. The term is based on Arneth's classification of neutrophils.

Shiga, Kiyoshi [*Japanese bacteriologist,* 1870–]. Collaborated with Paul Ehrlich. Studied leprosy, beriberi, tuberculosis. Especially known for his work on bacillary dysentery. See *Shigella* dysenteriae, Shiga *bacillus.*

Shi·gel′la (shi·jel′uh, shi·ghel′uh) [after *Shiga*]. The genus of the dysentery bacillus of the family Enterobacteriaceae, tribe Salmonelleae. They are non-lactose-fermenting, nonmotile, Gram-negative rods. **S. ambigua** (Schmitz's bacillus), **S. madampensis, S. sonnei** (Duval's bacillus), and the strains of **S. paradysenteriae** (Flexner, Strong, and Hiss) have been isolated from human cases of dysentery.

S. dysenteriae, Shiga bacillus, is the most virulent, as these organisms elaborate a neurotropic exotoxin in addition to the endotoxin common to all members of the *Shigella* group. Also called *Bacillus dysenteriae.*

Boyd's types of S. A classification of the large Flexner group of *Shigella* which is gaining acceptance. It includes three new pathogenic types which exist in India.

S. alkalescens. A species found associated with enteric disease of sporadic nature; identified by fermentation of dulcitol.

shi″gel·lo′sis (shy″ji·lo′sis, shig″i·lo′sis) [*Shiga;* G. *-ōsis,* condition]. Bacillary dysentery caused by bacteria of the genus *Shigella.*

shi·kim′ic ac′id. $C_6H_9O_3.COOH$; 3,4,5-trihydroxy-Δ-1,6-cyclohexene-1-carboxylic acid, found in plant tissues. It serves as a precursor of phenylalanine, tyrosine, tryptophan, and para-aminobenzoic acid for certain strains of *E. coli* and *Neurospora.*

shi″ma-mu′shi (shee″mah-mōō′shee). Japanese river fever, or tsutsugamushi disease.

shi″mu-mu′shi. See *shima-mushi.*

shin [AS. *scinu*]. The sharp anterior margin of the tibia.

saber s. A condition seen in congenital syphilis, in which the anterior border of the tibia has a sharp convex edge; due to periosteal proliferation.

shin′gles. See *herpes* zoster.

Shinowara, Jones, and Reinhart method. See under *method.*

shiv′er [ME. *chiveren*]. A slight tremor or shaking of the body due to cold, etc.

Shock and Hastings method. See under *method.*

shock [F. *choquer*, to shock]. 1. The clinical manifestations of an inadequate volume of circulating blood accompanied by physiologic adjustments of the organism to a progressive discrepancy between the capacity of the arterial tree and the volume of blood to fill it. Signs include marked decrease in blood pressure, weak thready pulse, pale cold skin with ashen-gray cyanosis, and thirst relieved only by transfusion. Shock may be classified according to mechanism as *cardiogenic, vasogenic, neurogenic,* or *hematogenic.* Also called *peripheral circulatory failure, shock syndrome.* See also *countershock,* general adaptation *syndrome, photoshock, shellshock.* 2. A physical or emotional trauma. 3. *In physiology,* electric *s.* 4. The first phase of the alarm reaction in the general adaptation syndrome. —**shock,** *v.*

anaphylactic s. The syndrome following the reintroduction of an antigen in an animal previously sensitized to it. See *anaphylaxis.*

anaphylactoid s. A shock syndrome resembling anaphylactic shock but independent of antigen-antibody reactions and produced by the injection of a variety of substances, including certain colloids such as peptone, into the body.

cardiogenic s. Shock caused by inadequate pumping of blood into the arterial tree owing to left-ventricular failure, tamponade, or pulmonary embolism.

colloidoclastic s. See anaphylactoid *s. Obs.*

electric s. (a) The sudden violent effect of the passage of an electric current through the body. (b) A therapeutic measure in psychosis. Also see electroshock *therapy.*

gravity s. Circulatory failure resulting from prolonged maintenance of a vertical position of the body, particularly when muscle tension is absent.

hematogenic s. Shock caused by reduced blood volume which may be due to loss of blood or plasma as in burns, the crush syndrome, perforating gastrointestinal wounds, or other wounds. Syn., *wound s.*

insulin s. Hypoglycemia with coma as a result of overdosage of insulin in diabetes or as a therapeutic measure in psychoses. Also see insulin shock *therapy.*

irreversible s. A late stage of shock from which recovery cannot be achieved by any known form of therapy.

nervous s. An acute nervous collapse, typically accompanied by syncope, that is produced by severe physical or psychic trauma.

neurogenic s. That caused by vasodilatation leading to low blood pressure and reduction in venous return and in cardiac output: due to such causes as injury to the central nervous system, spinal anesthesia, or reflex.

osmotic s. A phenomenon observed in certain bacteriophages, in which (when the salt solution medium is rapidly diluted and osmotic pressure suddenly reduced) the bacteriophages swell and burst and only their outer membranes can be demonstrated.

peptone s. See anaphylactoid *s.*

primary s. The type of shock manifested immediately after an injury.

secondary s. The type of shock appearing several hours after an injury.

serum s. An anaphylactic reaction resulting from the injection of a serum into a sensitive individual. It may be in the nature of an accident, with death (serum accident); or a reaction, with cyanosis, feeble pulse, fall in blood pressure, cold clammy skin, chills, and high fever. Sometimes adenitis, urticarial rashes, joint pains, etc., will occur in a protein-sensitive individual after he has been given the homologous protein to which he is sensitive.

spinal s. Temporary condition of flaccid paralysis and areflexia following functional transection of the spinal cord rostral to the motor outflow to the affected muscles.

systolic s. That occurring in association with a diastolic impact when the heart pounds against the thorax.

therapeutic s. See Jarisch-Herxheimer *reaction.*

vasogenic s. Shock caused by paralysis and dilatation of small arteries, arterioles, and capillaries, with no loss of blood volume but increased vascular-tree capacity, as seen in overwhelming toxic infections or due to histamine.

wound s. See hematogenic *s.*

shoe boil [AS. *scōh;* L. *bulla,* bubble]. A hard, fibrous mass formed on the sole of a horse's hoof, caused by poorly fitting shoes.

Shohl and King method. See under *method.*

Shoji's stain. See Sato and Shoji's *stain.*

Shorr trichrome stain. See under *stain.*

short cir′cuit. 1. A circuit in which an electric current encounters an abnormally small resistance. 2. *In surgery,* an intestinal anastomosis whereby a segment of bowel, in which is located a tumor or other obstruction, is isolated and the fecal current diverted beyond the point of obstruction or pathologic process. It is generally a palliative or temporary procedure.

shoul′der [AS. *sculdor*]. The region where the arm joins the trunk, formed by the meeting of the clavicle, scapula, humerus, and the overlying soft parts. See Table of Joints and Ligaments in the Appendix. See Plates 2, 4.

frozen s. A chronic tenosynovitis of unknown cause associated with increased vascularity, degeneration, and fibrosis of collagen fibers in and about the shoulder joint, and characterized by pain and limitation of motion: also called *adhesive capsulitis, periarthritis of the shoulder, scapulohumeral periarthritis.*

noisy s. A grating over the scapula on moving the shoulder up and down, believed to be due to a snapping tendon or bursitis.

painful s. See frozen *s.*

slipped s. A dislocated humerus.

shoul′der slip. Upward displacement of the scapula in the horse caused by excessive impact of the front leg with the ground.

show [AS. *scēawian*]. A bloody discharge from the birth canal prior to labor or to a menstrual flow.

Shrady, George Frederick [*American surgeon,* 1837–1907]. Well known in his time as surgeon, medical writer, and editor. Inventor of a surgical saw to be used through a cannula which enabled the surgeon to cut through bone in a subcutaneous operation; called *Shrady's saw.*

Shrapnell, Henry Jones [*English anatomist,* 1761–1841]. Described the flaccid portion of the tympanic membrane (1851), called *pars flaccida.* See Shrapnell's *membrane.*

shreds [AS. *scrēade*]. Slender strands of mucus visible grossly in urine, denoting inflammation of the urethra, urinary bladder, or prostate.

shriv′el [cf. Swed. dial, *skryvla*]. Shrink in bulk and wrinkle.

shud′der [ME. *shoderen*]. A convulsive momentary tremor, caused by fright, disgust, or nervous shock.

Shunk's stain. See under *stain.*

shunt [ME. *shunten*]. 1. *In medicine*, an alternate pathway, bypass or sidetrack; an anastomosis, either occurring as a natural anatomic feature or established by surgical means. 2. *In electricity*, a branch of a circuit parallel with other parts of it.

Oxford s. See Trueta's *s.*

peritoneosubarachnoid s. Surgical communication between the lumbar subarachnoid space and the peritoneal cavity, for relief of hydrocephalus: also called *peritoneothecal s.*

portacaval s. A surgical connection between the portal vein and inferior vena cava.

portarenal s. A surgical connection between the left renal vein and the portal system, usually the splenic vein.

renal s. See Trueta's *s.*

salpingothecal s. Surgical communication between the lumbar subarachnoid space and an oviduct, for drainage of cerebrospinal fluid into the peritoneal cavity.

Trueta's s. A part of the renal circulation in which blood passes through the juxtamedullary glomeruli into the capillary beds of the medulla, bypassing the cortex. It results in greatly decreased production of urine and may be of special significance under certain abnormal circulatory conditions, as hemorrhage and shock. Also called *Oxford s.*, *renal s.*

ureterothecal s. See *arachnoid-ureterostomy.*

ventriculoperitoneal s. Surgical communication between a lateral ventricle and the peritoneal cavity by means of a plastic or rubber tube, for the relief of hydrocephaly.

Shwartzman phenomenon, reaction. See under *phenomenon.*

Si Chemical symbol for silicon.

Sia's test. See under *test.*

si″a·go·nag′ra (sigh″uh·go·nag′ruh, ·nay′gruh) [G. *siagōn*, jaw-bone; *agra*, a seizure]. Gouty pain in the maxilla.

si·al′a·den (sigh·al′uh·den) [G. *sialon*, saliva; *adēn*, gland]. A salivary gland.

si″al·ad″e·ni′tis [*sialon; adēn;* G. *-itis*, inflammation]. Inflammation of a salivary gland.

si·al′a·gogue (sigh·al′uh·gog), **si·al′a·gog** [*sialon;* G. *agōgos*, leading]. A drug producing a flow of saliva. —**sialagog′ic,** *adj.*, *n.*

si″a·lan″gi·og′ra·phy, si″a·lo·an″gi·og′ra·phy. See *sialography.*

si″al·a·po′ri·a [*sialon;* G. *aporia*, difficulty]. Deficiency in the amount of saliva.

si·al′ic (sigh·al′ick), **si′a·line** (sigh′uh·lyne, ·leen) [*sialon*]. Having the nature of saliva.

si″a·li·thot′o·my [*sialon;* G. *lithos*, stone; *tomē*, a cutting]. Incision of a salivary gland or duct for removal of a calculus.

si′al·o-, si′al-. Combining form meaning *saliva.*

si″a·lo·ad″e·nec′to·my [*sialon;* G. *adēn*, gland; *ektomē*, excision]. Surgical removal of a salivary gland.

si″a·lo·ad″e·ni′tis [*sialon; adēn;* G. *-itis*, inflammation]. Sialadenitis.

si″a·lo·ad″e·not′o·my [*sialon; adēn;* G. *tomē*, a cutting]. Incision of a salivary gland.

si″a·lo·a″er·oph′a·gy [*sialon;* G. *aēr*, air; *phagein*, to eat]. The habit of constantly swallowing and thus taking saliva and air into the stomach.

si″a·lo·an·gi′tis [*sialon;* G. *aggeion*, vessel; *-itis*, inflammation]. Inflammation of a salivary duct.

si″a·lo·do·chi′tis (sigh″uh·lo·do·kigh′tis) [*sialon;* G. *dochos*, receptacle; *-itis*]. Inflammation of a salivary duct.

si″a·lo·do′chi·um (·do′kee·um) [*sialon; dochos*]. A salivary duct.

si″a·lo·do′cho·plas″ty (·do′ko·plas″tee) [*sialon; dochos;* G. *plassein*, to form]. Plastic surgery of a salivary gland duct.

si″a·log′e·nous (sigh″uh·lodj′i·nus) [*sialon;* G. *genesthai*, from *gignesthai*, to be produced]. Generating saliva.

si·al′o·gram (sigh·al′o·gram) [*sialon;* G. *gramma*, letter]. Roentgenogram of a salivary duct.

si″a·log′ra·phy [*sialon;* G. *graphein*, to write]. Radiographic examination of a salivary gland following injection of an opaque substance into its duct.

si′a·loid [*sialon;* G. *eidos*, form] Pertaining to, or like, saliva.

si·al′o·lith″ (sigh·al′o·lith″, sigh′uh·lo·lith″) [*sialon;* G. *lithos*, stone]. A salivary calculus.

si″a·lo·li·thi′a·sis [*sialon; lithos;* NL. *-iasis*, condition]. The presence of salivary calculi.

si″a·lo·li·thot′o·my [*sialon; lithos;* G. *tomē*, a cutting]. Surgical incision into a salivary duct or salivary gland for the removal of a calculus.

si′a·lon [G.]. Saliva.

si″a·lor·rhe′a, si″a·lor·rhoe′a [*sialon;* G. *rhoia*, flow]. Salivation.

pancreatic s. A flow of pancreatic juice.

si″a·los′che·sis [*sialon;* G. *schesis*, retention]. Suppression of the secretion of saliva.

si″a·lo·se″mei·ol′o·gy (sigh″uh·lo·see″migh·ol′o·jee) [*sialon;* G. *sēmeion*, sign; *logos*, word]. Diagnosis based upon examination of the saliva.

si″a·lo′sis. See *salivation.*

si″a·lo·ste·no′sis [*sialon;* G. *stenōsis*, a being straitened]. Stricture of a salivary duct.

si″a·lo·syr′inx (sigh″uh·lo·sirr′inks, ·sigh′rinks) [*sialon;* G. *syrigx*, pipe]. 1. A salivary fistula. 2. A syringe for washing out the salivary ducts. 3. A drainage tube for a salivary duct.

sib, sibling [AS. *sibb*]. One of a group of children of the same parents; a brother or sister.

sib′i·lant [L. *sibilare*, to hiss]. Hissing or whistling, as a sibilant rale.

sib″i·la′tion [L. *sibilatio*, from *sibilare*]. Pronunciation in which the *s* sound predominates.

sib″i·lis′mus (sib″i·liz′mus) [*sibilare*]. 1. A hissing sound. 2. A sibilant rale.

s. aurium. Tinnitus.

sib′i·lus [L., a hissing]. A sibilant rale.

sib′ship [*sibb;* AS. *-scipe*]. All the brothers and sisters in a family regarded as a single group.

Sibson, Francis [*English anatomist*, 1814–76]. Remembered for his description of a furrow formed in some individuals by a prominence of the lower border of the pectoralis major muscle; called *Sibson's furrow.* See also Sibson's *fascia.*

Sicard, Jean Athanase [*French physician and radiologist*, 1872–1929]. Used lipiodol in roentgenology (1921). Described his method of treating varicose veins by injecting sodium salicylate (1922). Described a syndrome of retroparotid-space injury (similar to Villaret's syndrome) in which there is homolateral paralysis of the last four cranial nerves.

sic′cant, sic′ca·tive [L. *siccare*, to make dry]. Drying; tending to make dry. —**sic′cant, sic′ca·tive,** *n.*

sic·cha′si·a (si·kay′zhuh, ·zee·uh) [G., loathing]. Nausea.

sic′cus [L., dry]. Dry.

sick [AS. *sēoc*]. Ill; not well. Also used colloquially for nauseated.

sick call. *In military medicine*, the assembly of the sick at a dispensary, hospital, or other point for examination and disposition by the military surgeon in charge; a term used in the United States Army. Also see *sick parade*.

veterinary s. c. *In military medicine*, a routine inspection and treatment of sick animals assembled daily at a veterinary dispensary or station hospital.

sick″la·ne′mi·a. See sickle-cell *anemia*.

sick′le-form″. Descriptive of certain forms of malarial parasites and of blood cells.

sick′le-hocked″. Excessive flexion of the hock of a horse due to strained ligaments and tendons of the tarsus.

sick·le′mi·a (sick·lee′mee·uh, sick″ul·ee′mee·uh). See sickle-cell *anemia*.

sick list. A list of persons, especially in military or naval service, who are disabled by sickness.

sick′ness [*sēoc*]. Disease; illness.

African horse s. A highly infectious virus disease of horses and mules probably carried by mosquitoes. It is characterized by fever, constitutional symptoms, and edematous swellings.

air s. See *airsickness*.

altitude s. See chronic mountain *s*.

black s. See *kala-azar*.

bleeding s. Hemophilia.

bush s. Enzootic marasmus; a cobalt deficiency disease of herbivorous animals in New Zealand causing severe anemia and emaciation.

car s. See motion *s*.

Ceylon s. Beriberi.

chronic mountain s. A disease occurring in persons living at high altitudes when homeostatic adjustments to the lowered atmospheric oxygen tension fail or develop disproportionately. The *erythremic type*, in which the hematopoietic system is the primary reacting tissue, is characterized by great increase in erythrocytes (polycythemia). Symptoms include cyanosis, vasodilatation, clubbing of fingers, and epistaxis. In the *emphysematous type*, symptoms may include dyspnea on slight effort, reduction in vital capacity, and respiratory acidosis. Reversible disturbances of vision and mental and physical depression also are common. Syn., *high-altitude disease, Monge's disease, high-altitude erythremia, seroche.*

compressed-air s. See caisson *disease*.

creeping s. Chronic ergotism.

decompression s. Aeroembolism.

fainting s. Old term for epilepsy.

falling s. Epilepsy.

green s. Chlorosis.

Indian s. Gangrenous proctitis.

milk s. An acute disease with weakness, anorexia, and vomiting due to ingestion of milk or flesh of animals which have a disease called trembles.

miner's s. See *ancylostomiasis*.

monthly s. Menstruation.

morning s. Nausea of early pregnancy.

motion s. Vertigo, nausea, and vomiting occurring during travel by auto, airplane, or train.

mountain s. See chronic mountain *s*.

painted s. See *pinta*.

radiation s. (a) Illness due to the effects of therapeutic irradiation with roentgen rays or radium and comprising symptoms of nausea, vomiting, headache, cramps, and diarrhea. (b) The effect of radiant energy following the explosion of an atomic bomb, the resultant effects of which include alopecia, loss of teeth, decrease in red and white blood cells, and prolonged hemorrhage.

sea s. See *seasickness*.

serum s. An anaphylactic reaction following serum therapy, characterized by urticaria, arthritis, edema, fever, and prostration.

sleeping s. Lethargic encephalitis or trypanosomiasis.

sweating s. See miliary *fever*.

sick pa·rade′. A term used in the British military service for sick call.

sick re·port′. *In military medicine*, a daily organization record that lists the personnel of a command who require medical treatment; a similar report for sick animals.

Si′da [G. *sidē*]. A genus of plants of the Malvaceae.

S. paniculata. A species of Peru, reputed to be an active vermifuge. Its action is believed to be due to the very minute but resisting bristles which cover its leaves.

S. rhombifolia. Queensland hemp, which contains a great amount of mucilage; is used in Australia for snake bite, pulmonary disease, and in making poultices.

Siddall, Alcines Clair [*American gynecologist and obstetrician*, 1897–]. Introduced (1928) a hormone test for early or late pregnancy, using an immature virgin white mouse. For four or five days, serum from the woman is injected into the mouse. At the end of that time, if the ratio between the mouse's body weight and the weight of its uterus and ovaries is less than 400, the test is positive; known as *Siddall's test for pregnancy.*

side [AS. *sīde*]. The lateral aspect of any body or organ.

side′bone″ [*side;* AS. *bān*]. *In veterinary medicine*, ossification of the lateral cartilages of the pedal bone in the horse, resulting in lameness.

sid″er·a′tion [L. *sideratio*, disease produced by a constellation]. Obsolete term for a sudden stroke, as in apoplexy.

sid′er·ism [G. *sidēritis*, loadstone]. The curative influences long supposed to be exerted over the body by the lodestone. *Obs.*

sid′er·ite. Native ferrous carbonate, $FeCO_3$.

sid′er·o·cyte″ [G. *sidēros*, iron; *kytos*, cell]. An erythrocyte which contains iron in other forms than hematin; probably an aging erythrocyte.

sid″er·o·dro″mo·pho′bi·a (sid″ur·o·dro″mo·fo′bee·uh, ·drom″o·) [*sidēros;* G. *dromos*, course; *phobos*, fear]. Morbid dread of traveling by railway; fear of trains.

sid″er·o·fi·bro′sis (sid″ur·o·figh·bro′sis) [*sidēros;* L. *fibra*, fiber; G. *-ōsis*, condition]. Fibrosis associated with deposits of iron-bearing pigments. Usually seen in the reticuloendothelial system.

sid″er·o·pe′ni·a [*sidēros;* G. *penia*, want]. Deficiency of iron, especially in the blood.

sid′er·o·phil, sid′er·o·phile [*sidēros;* G. *philein*, to love]. A cell or tissue having affinity for iron. —**sid′erophil,** *adj.*

sid″er·o·phil′in. A pseudoglobulin of blood, having a molecular weight of about 90,000, capable of combining with two atoms of ferric iron to form a compound which serves as a transport form of iron in blood. Syn., *transferrin.*

sid″er·oph′i·lous [*sidēros; philein*]. Having an affinity for iron; applied to erythrocytes or other cells. Syn., *siderophil.*

sid′er·o·scope″ [*sidēros;* G. *skopein*, to examine]. An instrument for the detection of particles of iron or steel in the eyes.

sid″er·o·sil″i·co′sis [*sidēros;* L. *silex*, flint; G. *-ōsis*, condition]. Diffuse fibrosis of the lungs due to the prolonged inhalation of dusts containing silicon dioxide and iron salts.

sid″er·o′sis [*sidēros; -ōsis*]. Chronic inflammation of the lungs due to prolonged inhalation of dust containing iron salts; occurs in iron miners and arc welders. It is characterized by inflammatory tissue reaction mainly in the lymphatic tissues of the lungs and by diffuse, nodular shadows in the x-ray film. Also called *arc-welder's disease, arc-welder's nodulation.* —**siderot'ic,** *adj.*

Siebold, Adam Elias von [*German obstetrician,* 1775–1826]. Celebrated clinician. Noted for his classic account of uterine cancer (1824).

Siebold, Eduard Caspar Jacob von [*German obstetrician,* 1801–61]. Popularized pubic symphysiotomy for difficult delivery in Germany. The operation was first proposed by Pieter Camper and introduced in 1777 by Jean Sigault. Called *Siebold's* or *Sigault's operation.*

Siebold, Karl Theodor Ernst von [*German zoologist and parasitologist,* 1804–85]. First to establish definitely the life cycle of a parasite (1854). In his study of sheep gid he found that the causative organism, *Taenia coenurus,* is the larval stage of *Taenia multiceps* which spends its adult life in the intestine of the dog.

Siegemundin, Justine Ditrichin [*German midwife,* 1650–1705]. Widely known as the most celebrated midwife of her time. Advocated puncture of the amniotic sac to arrest hemorrhage in placenta previa.

Siegert, Ferdinand [*German pediatrician,* 1865–1946]. Observed that in mongolism the terminal phalanges of the little fingers are short and curved inward; this is known as *Siegert's sign.*

Siegfried's hypothesis. See Kossel and Siegfried's protamine nucleus *hypothesis.*

Siegle, Emil [*German otologist,* 1833–1900]. Inventor of an otoscope in which compressed air was employed to give mobility to the tympanum while under observation; called *Siegle's otoscope* or *speculum.*

Siemens, Hermann Werner [*German dermatologist,* 1891–]. Known for his description of congenital ectodermal dysplasia; also called *Siemens' syndrome.*

sig. Abbreviation for *signa,* label it; *signetur,* let it be labeled.

Sigault, Jean René [*French surgeon,* b. 1740]. Introduced pubic symphysiotomy (1777); also called *Sigault's operation.* See also under Eduard Caspar Jacob von *Siebold.*

Sigerist, Henry Ernest [*Swiss medical historian,* 1891–]. Well-known writer on medical history.

sigh [AS. *sīcan*]. A prolonged and deep inspiration followed by a shorter expiration. Also called *suspirium.* —**sigh,** *v.*

sight [AS. *gesiht*]. 1. The act of seeing. 2. The special sense concerned in seeing.

aging s. Presbyopia.

day s. Hemeralopia.

far s. Hypermetropia.

short s. Myopia.

weak s. Asthenopia.

sig'ma·tism [G. *sigma,* Σ, eighteenth letter of the Greek alphabet]. 1. Lisping. 2. The too frequent use of the *s* sound in speech.

sigmodal. A trade-mark for secondary amyl-β-bromallylbarbituric acid. The substance is used in the form of a solution of the sodium salt.

sig'moid [G. *sigmoeidēs,* shaped like the letter sigma]. 1. Shaped like the letter S. 2. Pertaining to the sigmoid flexure of the colon, as the sigmoid artery (see Table of Arteries in the Appendix), the sigmoid mesocolon. —**sigmoid,** *n.*

sig"moid·ec'to·my [*sigmoeidēs;* G. *ektomē,* excision]. Excision of a part or all of the sigmoid flexure of the colon.

sig"moid·i'tis [*sigmoeidēs;* G. *-itis,* inflammation]. Inflammation of the sigmoid flexure of the colon.

sig·moi'do-, sigmoid- [*sigmoeidēs*]. A combining form meaning *sigmoid.*

sig·moi'do·pex"y [*sigmoeidēs;* G. *pēxis,* a fixing]. An operation for prolapse of the rectum; colopexy; fixation of the sigmoid colon by obliterating the intersigmoid fossa and shortening the mesosigmoid by suture, through an abdominal incision.

sig·moi"do·proc·tos'to·my [*sigmoeidēs;* G. *prōktos,* anus; *stoma,* mouth]. Anastomosis of the sigmoid flexure of the colon with the rectum.

sig·moi"do·rec·tos'to·my [*sigmoeidēs;* L. *rectus,* straight; *stoma*]. Formation by surgical means of an artificial anus at the sigmoid flexure of the descending colon, at its junction with the rectum; sigmoidostomy; low colostomy.

sig·moi'do·scope [*sigmoeidēs;* G. *skopein,* to examine]. An appliance for the inspection, by artificial light, of the sigmoid flexure; it differs from the proctoscope in its greater length and diameter. —**sigmoidos'copy,** *n.*

sig"moid·os'co·py [*sigmoeidēs; skopein*]. Visual inspection of the sigmoid flexure, with the aid of special instruments.

sig·moi"do·sig"moid·os'to·my [*sigmoeidēs; sigmoeidēs;* G. *stoma,* mouth]. Surgical anastomosis between two portions of the sigmoid colon.

sig"moid·os'to·my [*sigmoeidēs; stoma*]. The formation of an artificial anus in the sigmoid flexure of the colon; sigmoid colostomy.

sig"moid·ot'o·my [*sigmoeidēs;* G. *tomē,* a cutting]. Incision into the sigmoid colon.

sig'mo·scope. See *sigmoidoscope.*

Sigmund, Karl Ludwig [*Austrian physician,* 1810–83]. Described epitrochlear lymph nodes; called *Sigmund's glands.*

sign [L. *signum*]. 1. A mark or objective evidence; in a restricted sense, a physical manifestation of disease. For any sign not listed here see under the individual whose name it bears; see also under *reflex.*

abdominocardiac s. A sign for hypotonia in which the right area of cardiac dullness becomes larger on stimulation of the abdominal aortic plexus, as when the patient changes from the reclining to the erect position: also called *Livierato's s.,* or *orthostatic s.*

accessory s. A nonpathognomonic sign.

Allis' s. When the neck of the femur is fractured, the fascia between the greater trochanter and the crest of the ilium is less tense than normally.

André Thomas' s. In patients with disease of the cerebellum, a rebound phenomenon; if the patient is directed to raise his arm and then suddenly asked to let it fall, the arm will rebound.

antecedent s. A sign which precedes an attack of a disease.

Argyll Robertson s. See Argyll Robertson *pupil.*

Arnoux's s. See Emile *Arnoux.*

assident s. See accessory *s.*

Auenbrugger's s. A sign of pericardial effusion in which there is bulging of the epigastrium.

Babinski's s. See Joseph F. F. *Babinski.*

Baccelli's s. A sign for pleural effusion in which whispered voice sounds are heard over the chest.

Ballance's s. A sign for rupture of the spleen in which the dullness in the right flank will shift with position but not that on the left.

Barré's s. The patient lies prone and his legs are flexed at the knee. If there is disease of the corticospinal tracts, the patient is unable to hold his legs in the vertical position.

Battle's s. A sign for fracture of the posterior cranial fossa in which discoloration appears over the tip of the mastoid process.

Beevor's s. The umbilicus is higher than normal due to paralysis of the inferior portion of the rectus abdominis muscle.

Bezold's s. Swelling below the apex of the mastoid process; considered a sign of mastoiditis.
Bjerrum's s. See Jannik Peterson *Bjerrum.*
Blumberg's s. A sign of peritoneal inflammation in which sudden release of the examiner's hand from the right iliac fossa produces pain.
Boas' s. A sign for cholecystitis in which there is an area of hyperesthesia over the lower right ribs posteriorly.
Boston's s. An eye sign for exophthalmic goiter in which the upper lid does not follow the downward motion of the eye smoothly, but jerks.
Bragard's s. Aggravated pain or muscle spasm elicited by strong dorsiflexion of the foot after the production of a positive Lasègue's sign.
Braxton Hicks's s. See Hicks's *s.*
Broadbent's s. A systolic retraction in the back at the eleventh or twelfth rib on the left side; seen when there are adhesions between the pericardium and the diaphragm.
Brudzinski's signs. A group of signs frequently seen in meningeal irritation, especially meningitis: (1) **neck sign.** Passive flexion of the head is followed by flexion of both thighs and legs. (2) **contralateral leg signs.** (a) Passive flexion of one thigh is accompanied by flexion of the opposite hip and knee. (b) When one leg and thigh are flexed and the other extended, lowering of the flexed limb is followed by flexion of the contralateral one. (3) **cheek sign.** Pressure on both cheeks just below the zygomatic arch causes flexion of both elbows and rapid lifting of the arms. (4) **symphysis sign.** Pressure on the symphysis pubis is followed by flexion of both lower extremities.
Brun's s. See hand *s.* of Brun.
Bryant's s. When the humerus is dislocated, the anterior and posterior boundaries of the axillary fossa are lowered.
Carman's meniscus s. See meniscus *s.*
Chvostek's s. A sign for tetany in which tapping of the face in front of the ear produces spasm of the facial muscles.
Claybrook's s. A sign for rupture of the intestine in which the heart and respiratory sounds are transmitted over the abdominal area.
coin s. See bell *sound.*
commemorative s. A sign of some previous disease.
coughing s. of Huntington. Flexion of the thigh and extension of the paralyzed leg on coughing, when the patient is recumbent with legs hanging over the edge of the table.
Cowen's s. A jerky pupillary reaction on eliciting the consensual light reaction.
Crichton-Browne's s. A sign seen early in paralytic dementia in which there is twitching of the outer corners of the eyes and lips.
Crowe's s. In patients with lateral sinus thrombosis, the retinal vessels are engorged if the internal jugular vein is compressed on the normal side.
Cruveilhier's s. A sign for saphenous varix in which a tremor can be palpated when the patient coughs.
Cullen's s. A sign for ruptured ectopic pregnancy in which a bluish discoloration is seen about the umbilicus.
Dalrymple's s. Widening of the palpebral fissures sometimes seen in hyperthyroidism.
Dance's s. A sign for intussusception consisting of an empty feeling in the right iliac fossa.
D'Espine's s. A sign for tracheobronchial adenitis or mediastinal tumor in which whispered voice sounds are heard over the upper thoracic vertebrae.
diaphragmatic s. The movement of the diaphragm during respiratory excursions causing an altered contour of the chest wall. If the patient is observed by means of oblique illumination, a shadow is seen moving up or down the side of the chest. Also called *Litten's shadow.*
drawer s. A sign diagnostic of rupture of the cruciate ligaments of the knee, in which, with the knee flexed to a right angle, there is increased anterior or posterior glide of the tibia in rupture of the anterior or posterior ligaments, respectively.
Duroziez's s. A to-and-fro hum heard with the stethoscope placed over the femoral artery; occurs in aortic insufficiency.
echo s. The involuntary repetition of the last syllable, word, or clause of a sentence.
Ely's s. A sign of irritation of the psoas muscle or of hip-joint disease, elicited by having the patient lie prone with feet hanging over the edge of the table. The heel is approximated to the buttock and the thigh is hyperextended. Inability to complete the movement is a positive response.
Enroth's s. Puffy, edematous swelling of the eyelid, often found in thyrotropic exophthalmos.
Erb's s. A sign for tetany in which hyperexcitability can be determined by the use of a galvanic current.
"e" to "a" s. See Gerald S. *Shibley.*
Ewart's s. Dullness, increased fremitus, and bronchial breathing at the left lung base in pericardial effusion.
fanning s. of Babinski. See Joseph F. F. *Babinski.*
fontanel s. Constant bulging of the anterior fontanel in infants observed in acute meningeal infections and in the condition where the intracranial pressure is increased.
Friedreich's s. A sign for cavitation of the lungs in which there is a change in the percussion note during inspiration and expiration.
Froment's s. In ulnar paralysis, the thumb of the affected limb is involuntarily flexed by the flexor pollicis longus.
Gerhardt's s. A sign for cavitation of the lungs in which there is a change in percussion note with change in the patient's position from upright to recumbent.
Gifford's s. Inability to evert the upper eyelid in the early stages of exophthalmic goiter.
Goodell's s. Softening of the cervix of the uterus, considered to be evidence of pregnancy.
Gordon's s. See Gordon's *reflex.*
Graefe's s. See von Graefe's *s.*
Griesinger's s. In patients with transverse sinus thrombosis, a swelling behind the mastoid process.
Grocco's s. A sign for pleural effusion in which there is paravertebral dullness on the opposite side.
Haenel's s. Analgesia to pressure on the eyeball in tabes dorsalis.
Hamilton's s. Long hairs growing on the antitragus of the ear, typical of males with normal androgenic function after the age of 25 or 30.
hand s. of Brun. Genital grasping by patients (especially children) with vesical stones or foreign bodies to prevent involuntary escape of urine. The hands may become lacerated and have a strong ammoniacal odor.
Hefke-Turner s. See obturator *s.*
Hertoghe s. A trichomadesis characterized by frontal alopecia with oily scales and loss of the outer third of the eyebrows, seen most frequently in myxedema, and also in syphilis, thallium poisoning, and other types of hair loss.
Hicks's s. A sign of pregnancy after the third month in which rhythmic uterine contractions can be detected.

Hoehne's s. If uterine contractions disappear during delivery, rupture of the uterus may have occurred.
Hoffmann's s. A test for overactive tendon reflexes in which tapping the nail of the index or middle finger causes flexion of the thumb. Syn., *digital reflex.*
Homan's s. Pain in the calf on strong passive dorsiflexion of the foot, indicating deep venous thrombosis of calf.
Horsley's s. A sign for middle meningeal hemorrhage in which the axillary temperature is higher on the paralyzed side.
Hutchinson's s. Interstitial keratitis, eighth-nerve deafness, and notched teeth occurring in a patient with congenital syphilis. Also called *Hutchinson's triad.*
Jackson's s. In patients with pulmonary tuberculosis, a prolonged expiratory sound heard over the affected area.
Jellinek-Tillais' s. In toxic diffuse goiter, pigmentation of the area surrounding the eyes.
Joffroy's s. A sign for exophthalmic goiter in which the forehead does not wrinkle when the patient looks up with the head bent down.
Kanavel's s. A sign for ulnar bursitis in which there is a point of maximal tenderness in the center of the hypothenar eminence.
Kashida's s. The appearance of paresthesias with the application of cold and warm stimuli to the skin of the involved area in tetany.
Kayser-Fleischer s. See Kayser-Fleischer *ring.*
Kehr's s. A sign for rupture of the spleen in which there is an area of hyperesthesia over the left shoulder due to the presence of blood under the left diaphragm.
Kérandel's s. A delayed hyperesthesia in which pain occurs after a few minutes following pressure or a slight knock. Seen in African trypanosomiasis.
Kernig's s. A sign for meningeal irritation in which an attempt to completely extend the leg at the knee with the thigh flexed at a right angle causes pain or meets resistance.
Kerr's s. A peculiar thickening of the skin in levels below a spinal-cord lesion.
Knies' s. Unequal dilatation of the pupils, found in thyrotoxicosis and other conditions.
Kocher's s. When the patient looks up, his upper lid retracts faster than the globe is raised, thus exposing the sclera above the cornea: found in thyrotoxicosis. Syn., *globe lag.*
Koplik's s. Small red spots surrounded by quite white areas seen in the mucous membrane of the mouth in the prodromal stage of measles. Also called *Koplik's spots.*
Kussmaul's s. Air hunger seen in patients with severe diabetes.
Larrey's s. A sign for sacroiliac joint disease in which pain in the joint is felt when the patient sits down abruptly on a hard seat.
Lasègue's s. A sign elicited in certain types of muscle spasm of the lower extremity. The patient is placed supine and the entire extremity is raised, keeping the knee in full extension. The sign becomes positive at whatever angle of elevation pain or muscle spasm is produced.
leg s. of Neri. *In clinical neurology,* the patient is asked to bend forward, whereupon the paralyzed leg flexes at the knee while the other leg remains extended.
Leudet's s. In catarrhal or nervous diseases of the ear, the patient hears a fine, crackling sound in the ear.
Lhermitte's s. Flexion of the neck is accompanied by the sensation of an electric shock shooting into the extremities in certain cases of multiple sclerosis, and rarely in other conditions associated with a thickening of the cervical meninges.
Litten's s. See diaphragmatic *s.*
Livierato's s. See abdominocardiac *s.*
Lockwood's s. A sign for chronic appendicitis in which flatus can be palpated trickling through the ileocecal valve.
McBurney's s. A sign for early acute appendicitis in which the area of maximum tenderness is over McBurney's point.
Macewen's s. Increased resonance on combined percussion and auscultation of the skull in certain gross lesions of the intracranial contents, as in cerebral abscess or overdistended lateral ventricles.
McMurray's s. A sign for posterior tears of the lateral and medial menisci of the knee in which, with the knee fully flexed, a finger flattened along the joint line feels a click when the torn meniscus moves in and out on internal and external rotation of the tibia respectively as the joint is extended.
meniscus s. Roentgenographic concavoconvex filling defect of the stomach, valued as an aid in the diagnosis of carcinoma.
Milian's ear s. A sign to differentiate facial erysipelas from subcutaneous inflammations; involvement of the ear occurs in the former and not in the latter.
Möbius' s. Inability to maintain convergence of the eyes in exophthalmic goiter.
moulage s. *In radiology,* lack of the normal delicate, feathery appearance of the small intestine after a barium meal: often seen in sprue.
Murphy's s. A sign for cholecystitis in which the thumb presses over the area of the gallbladder and on expiration causes pain and catching of the breath.
Myerson's s. A series of reflex blinking movements following a tap on the forehead or a quick thrust towards the eyes, frequently seen in parkinsonism.
Negro's s. See cogwheel *rigidity.*
Neri's s. 1. Faradic stimulation of the sole of the foot causes extension of the great toe in sciatica; in a normal condition, flexion results. 2. See leg *s.* of Neri.
Nikolsky's s. The ready removal of epidermis upon the slightest injury, found between lesions (bullae) on the seemingly unaffected skin. It may be disclosed by (1) pulling the ruptured wall of the blister, or (2) rubbing off the epidermis between bullae by slight friction without breaking the surface of the skin. It occurs in pemphigus and epidermolysis bullosa. Described by Peter S. Nikolsky (1896).
objective s. One apparent to the observer.
obturator s. A widening and a change in the contour of the x-ray shadow of the obturator foramen indicative of a pathologic condition of the hip joint: also called *Hefke-Turner s.*
Oliver's s. See William S. *Oliver.*
Orroya's s. Delay of the contraction of the pupil to light; a symptom of status lymphaticus. See also *lymphatism,* Sergent's *s.*, Schriddle's *s.*
orthocardiac s. See abdominocardiac *s.*
Pardee's s. See Harold E. B. *Pardee.*
Pastia's s. See *Pastia's lines* under *line.*
physical s. One of the phenomena observed on inspection, palpation, percussion, auscultation, mensuration, or combinations of these methods.
Pool-Schlesinger's s. The production of painful extensor spasm at the knee joint and tonic spasm at the ankle by flexion of the affected leg at the hip with the knee extended; seen in tetany.
Queckenstedt's s. See Queckenstedt-Stookey *test.*

Rockey's s. A sign for depression of the zygomatic bone in which there is a difference in the angle on the two sides where two straight edges are placed from the outer edge of the orbit to the prominence of the zygomatic bone.

Romana's s. Unilateral edema of the face seen early in an acute attack of Chagas' disease. Usually seen in children.

Romberg's s. (a) A sign for obturator hernia in which there is pain radiating to the knee. (b) A sign for tabes dorsalis in which the patient cannot maintain equilibrium when standing with feet together and eyes closed.

Roque's s. Unilateral dilation of the pupil of the eye and elevation of the upper eyelid, due to compression of the cervical sympathetic chain by a tuberculous lesion at the apex of the lung.

Rosenbach's s. Fibrillary tremor of the closed eyelids sometimes seen in hyperthyroidism.

Rotch's s. Obliteration of the cardiohepatic angle in pericardial effusion; dullness on percussion over the right fifth intercostal space.

Rovsing's s. A sign for acute appendicitis in which pressure over the right iliac fossa causes pain in the left iliac fossa.

Schlange's s. Fecal blocking; the intestine is dilated above the obstruction and peristaltic movements are absent below that point.

Schriddle's s. Prominence of lymphoid follicles on the pharyngeal wall between the tonsils; a symptom of status lymphaticus. See also *lymphatism,* Orroya's *s.*, Sergent's *s.*

Sergent's s. Delay or failure of the skin of the chest or abdomen to redden when lightly scratched; a symptom of status lymphaticus. See also *lymphatism,* Orroya's *s.*, Schriddle's *s.*

Spalding's s. The roentgenographic finding in a fetus of overlapping of the skull bones at several sutures, associated with distinct signs of shrinkage of the cerebrum: observed in some cases of fetal death.

stairs s. Difficulty in descending stairs; one of the early symptoms of tabes dorsalis.

Stellwag's s. A sign for exophthalmic goiter in which the upper eyelid is retracted.

sternomastoid s. Spasm of the sternomastoid muscle manifested by increased tenseness of its tendinous attachment to the manubrium sterni in cases of pulmonary disease causing either displacement or traction of the mediastinum toward the same side.

Strümpell's s. Dorsal flexion of the foot when the thigh is flexed; seen in paralysis. Also called *tibialis s.*

subjective s. One recognized only by the patient.

Suker's s. Inability to maintain fixation on extreme lateral rotation of the eye: seen in thyrotoxicosis.

Szabo's s. Sensory changes restricted to the skin below the lateral malleolus in sciatica.

Thomas' s. A test for flexion fixation of the hip joint in which the examiner flexes the sound hip until the lumbar lordosis is reduced and then the amount of flexion observed in the affected limb can be estimated.

tibialis s. See Strümpell's *s.*

Tinel's s. A sign to indicate nerve regeneration in which tapping the nerve below the point of injury causes a tingling sensation in the distal parts.

Troisier's s. A sign for late abdominal carcinoma in which the left supraclavicular lymph nodes are enlarged.

Trousseau's s. A sign for tetany in which carpal spasm can be elicited by compressing the upper arm.

Vedder's s. In patients with beriberi, pressure on the calf muscles causes pain.

von Graefe's s. A sign for exophthalmic goiter in which the upper eyelid lags when the patient looks down.

Wartenberg's s. Decreased swinging of the leg or legs affected by parkinsonism after the patient's legs are placed so they can swing freely and caused to do so: also called *pendulousness of the legs test.*

Wernicke's s. A reaction obtained in some cases of hemianopsia in which a pencil of light thrown on the blind side of the retina gives rise to no movement in the iris, but, when thrown upon the normal side, produces contraction of the iris. It indicates that the lesion producing the hemianopsia is situated at or anterior to the geniculate bodies.

Westphal's s. Absence of the knee jerk.

Wintrich's s. A sign for cavitation of the lungs in which there is a change in percussion note when the mouth is closed or open.

sig′na. 1. Plural of signum. 2. Used in prescriptions to mean "write"; abbreviated, S., sig.

sig′na·ture [L. *signare,* to mark]. 1. The part of the prescription that is placed on the label, containing directions to the patient. 2. A distinguishing character.

doctrine of signatures. A theory that the medicinal uses of a plant can be determined from its fancied physical resemblance to normal or diseased organs (liverwort, lungwort, orchis).

sig·nif′i·cant dif′fer·ence. A difference between two statistical constants, calculated from two separate samples, which is of such magnitude that it is unlikely to have occurred by chance alone. Usually this probability must be less than 0.05 (5%) before a difference is accepted as significant. The smaller the probability, the more significant is the difference.

sig′num (pl. *signa*) [L.]. A mark, sign, or indication.

si′lent. *In clinical medicine,* progressing without signs or symptoms: said of pathological processes.

sil′i·ca [L. *silex,* flint]. Silicon dioxide, SiO_2, occurring in nature in the form of quartz, flint, and other minerals.

s. gel. A precipitated and dried silicic acid in the form of granules, used as a dehydrating agent and for absorption of various vapors.

sil′i·cate. A salt or ester of silicic acid.

sil″i·ca·to′sis [*silex;* G. *-ōsis,* condition]. Chronic inflammation of the lungs caused by the prolonged inhalation of dust containing silicates. A form of pneumonoconiosis. The only recognized example is asbestosis.

si·li′ceous, si·li′cious (si·lish′us) [*silex*]. Having the nature of, or containing, silicon.

si·lic′ic ac′id (si·liss′ick). Approximately H_2SiO_3. A white, amorphous powder.

si·lic″i·co′lin. A tumor-damaging substance, shown to be identical with desoxypodophyllotoxin, obtained from the dried needles of *Juniperus silicicola,* the southern red cedar.

si·li′ci·um (si·lish′ee·um, si·liss′ee·um). Silicon.

sil″i·co·flu′o·ride. A compound of silicon and fluorine with some other element.

sil′i·con [*silex*]. Si = 28.09. A nonmetallic element of the carbon group. It occurs in several allotropic modifications. Like carbon, it forms many complex compounds that are an essential part of the earth's surface.

s. carbide. See *carborundum.*

s. dioxide. SiO_2; silica. See purified siliceous *earth.*

silicone. Trade-mark for a class of synthetic polymers having the composition of a polyorganosiloxane.

si″li·co·si″der·o′sis. A type of pneumonoconiosis occurring among hematite miners. The lungs are bright brick red owing to the presence of hematite. Silica is also present in amounts up to 1.6% in fatal cases. Fibrosis of the lungs is diffuse, but occasionally nodular. There is often an associated tuberculosis. This disease has only recently been recognized and is probably caused by modern mining methods which greatly increase the dust in the atmosphere.

sil″i·co′sis [*silex;* G. *-ōsis,* condition]. Diffuse fibrosis of the lungs caused by the inhalation, through a period of years, of dust having a significant content of silicon dioxide particles less than 10μ in diameter. A form of pneumonoconiosis. Also called *chalicosis, lithosis, schistosis, miner's phthisis, miner's asthma, grinder's asthma, grinder's rot, potter's asthma, potter's rot, potter's consumption.*

conglomerate s. That form in which, in addition to discrete nodules, there are single or multiple fibrous masses of larger size. It is also known as silicosis with infection, based on the concept that infection, either obsolete, latent, or active, is an essential etiologic factor in the development of the conglomerate masses. Conglomerate silicosis may be indistinguishable from tuberculosilicosis.

simple s. Fibrosis in the form of discrete nodules, usually not exceeding 5 mm. in diameter and tending toward uniformity in size and in distribution.

sil″i·co·tu·ber″cu·lo′sis [*silex;* L. *tuberculum,* small swelling; *-ōsis*]. Silicosis with tuberculosis; any manifestation of tuberculous infection in a silicotic lung.

sil″i·co·tung′stic ac′id. $SiO_2.12WO_3.26H_2O$. In white or yellowish crystals, used as a reagent for alkaloids.

si·lique′ (si·leek′, sil′ick) [F., from L. *siliqua,* pod]. *In biology,* the slender, two-valved capsule of some plants, as the mustard.

sil′i·quose [*siliqua*]. Resembling a silique.

silloid. Trade-mark for a brand of mild silver protein containing about 20% of silver. The substance is used in various inflammations of the mucous membranes in strengths of from 5–10%.

sil″lo·neur′ (see″yo·nur′. *See* NOTES § 35) [F.]. A three-bladed scalpel used by ophthalmologists.

Silvatico, Giambattista [*Italian physician,* 1550–1621]. Said to have written the earliest work on malingering (1595).

sil′ver [AS. *seolfor*] (*argentum*). Ag = 107.880. A white, soft, ductile, and malleable metal. Metallic silver is insoluble in water, HCl, and most other acids in the cold, but dissolves in dilute nitric acid; dissolves slowly in hot concentrated sulfuric acid and is dissolved by solutions of alkali cyanides. Silver compounds are used in medicine to secure caustic, astringent, and antiseptic effects. The results are brought about by free silver ions. For caustic and astringent effects, silver nitrate is the drug of choice. For antiseptic effects, colloidal silver preparations are used, as the antiseptic action of silver nitrate is accompanied with irritation, pain, astringency, and corrosion. The colloidal silver compounds are used mainly on mucous membranes for antisepsis. The long-continued use of any silver preparation may produce irremediable discoloration of the skin or mucous membrane.

ammoniacal s. nitrate solution. See under *solution.*

colloidal s. chloride. See *lunosol.*

colloidal s. iodide. See *neo-silvol.*

mild s. protein (*argentum proteinicum mite*). Silver rendered colloidal by the presence of, or combination with, protein. It contains between 19% and 23% of silver; occurs as dark brown or almost black, shining scales or granules; freely soluble in water, but almost insoluble in alcohol. Used in medicine, especially in the treatment of infections of mucous membranes. Possibilities of argyria from its continued use must be kept in mind. Also called *mild protein s., mild protargin.*

s. acetate. CH_3COOAg; a white to slightly grayish crystalline powder, sparingly soluble in water: used as a reagent.

s. arsphenamine. The sodium salt of silver-diamino-dihydroxy-arseno-benzene; contains not less than 19% of arsenic and 12–14% of silver; occurs as a brownish black powder, unstable in air; readily soluble in water. Silver arsphenamine has been used for the same purposes as arsphenamine. Also called *sodium s. arsphenamine, s. diarsenol.* See *silver-salvarsan.*

s. bromide. AgBr; a yellowish powder, insoluble in water; the basis of light-sensitive emulsions used in photography.

s. chloride. AgCl; a white powder, practically insoluble in water: used in preparing antiseptic silver preparations.

s. citrate. $C_6H_5Ag_3O_7$; a white, crystalline powder, very slightly soluble in water. It has been used as an antiseptic dusting powder for wounds.

s. iodate. $AgIO_3$; a white, crystalline powder, very slightly soluble in water: used as a reagent.

s. iodide. AgI; a light-yellow powder, practically insoluble in water: used, especially in colloidal form, as a mild local antiseptic.

s. lactate. $AgC_3H_5O_3.H_2O$. The silver salt of lactic acid; occurs as crystalline needles, granular masses, or crystalline powder; it dissolves in about 15 parts of water. It is used as an active antiseptic. See *actol.*

s. nitrate (*argenti nitras*). $AgNO_3$. Occurs as colorless or white crystals; 1 Gm. is soluble in 0.4 cc. of water and in 30 cc. of alcohol. It is used locally as an astringent and germicide, especially in infections of the mucous membranes. The strength varies according to the location and nature of the infection. It is also used as a prophylactic against ophthalmia neonatorum. Silver nitrate has been employed as an astringent in the treatment of various types of gastritis, especially in ulcer of the stomach. Dose, 0.016–0.032 Gm. (¼–½ gr.).

s. nucleate. Trade name for a brand of mild silver protein.

s. nucleinate. Silver nucleate.

s. oxide. Ag_2O; a brownish-black powder, practically insoluble in water, formerly used in human medicine. In veterinary practice it is employed locally as a general germicide and parasiticide.

s. picrate. $(NO_2)_3.C_6H_2.OAg.H_2O$; yellow crystals, sparingly soluble in water: used locally in treatment of urethritis and vaginitis.

s. potassium cyanide. $AgK(CN)_2$; white crystals, soluble in water. It has been used as a bactericide. Syn., *potassium argenticyanide.*

s. sulfate. Ag_2SO_4; colorless crystals or a white, crystalline powder, slightly soluble in water: used as a reagent.

s. trinitrophenolate. Silver picrate.

strong s. protein (*argentum proteinicum forte*). Contains from 7.5% to 8.5% of silver; occurs as a brown, odorless powder; freely soluble in water, but almost insoluble in alcohol. It is used in the same conditions for which the mild compound is used. It differs from the mild compound in that it has irritating properties, which are practically absent in the mild compound, even in concentrated solution; this is because strong silver protein contains more ionizable silver than the mild variety. Possibilities of argyria from its continued use must be kept in mind. Also called *strong protein s., strong protargin.*

toughened s. nitrate (*argenti nitras induratus*). Silver nitrate toughened by the addition of a small proportion of hydrochloric acid, sodium chloride, or potassium nitrate; occurs in the form of white, hard pencils or cones. Used as a means of applying silver nitrate locally in concentrated form where an escharotic and germicidal action is desired. Also called *molded s. nitrate, fused s. nitrate, s. nitrate pencils, lunar caustic.*

silver-salvarsan. Trade-mark for *silver arsphenamine.*

Silvester's method. See under *artificial respiration.*

silvol. Trade-mark for a brand of mild silver protein.

Sim″a·ru′ba [Galabi *simarouba*]. A genus of trees of the family Simarubaceae. The bark of the root of **S. officinalis** has been used as a simple bitter.

sim″a·ru′bi·din. $C_{22}H_{32}O_9$; a principle, probably a glycoside, in the bark and wood of *Simaruba amara.*

sim′i·an [L. *simia*, ape]. Apelike; pertaining to or characteristic of apes or monkeys.

sim′i·le phe·nom′e·non. See *homeopathy*, simile *phenomenon.*

si·mil′i·a si·mil′i·bus cu·ran′tur [L.]. Likes are cured by likes; a sophism formulated by Hippocrates, then by Paracelsus (simile similis cura, non contrarium). See *homeopathy.*

si·mil′i·mum [L. *simillimus*, superl. of *similis*, like]. The homeopathic remedy which will produce the symptom complex most like that of a given disease.

Simmonds, Morris [*German physician*, 1855–1925]. Described hypopituitary cachexia, also called *hypophyseal cachexia, Simmonds' disease.*

Simmons, James Stevens (1890–1954). American physician and bacteriologist who demonstrated that dengue virus as it exists in *Aëdes aegypti* is filtrable, incriminated *Aëdes albopictus* as vector, and proved that *Anopheles punctimacula* and other mosquitoes are malaria vectors (1934).

Simon, Gustav [*German surgeon*, 1824–76]. Repaired vesicovaginal fistula and lacerated perineum by colpocleisis (1854); called *Simon's operation.* Revived extirpation of the spleen (1854), which had been performed previously by C. F. Quittenbaum (1836). Probably the first in Europe to excise the kidney (1870). See also Simon's *position.*

Simon, John [*English physician*, 1816–1904]. Recognized as one of the great sanitarians of the nineteenth century. First medical health officer of the city of London. Originator of the English Public Health Act (1848).

Simon, Théodore [*French psychologist*, 1873–]. Developed, with Alfred Binet, a well-known intelligence test for children in current use today; called *Binet-Simon test.* See Alfred *Binet.*

Simonart, Pierre Joseph Cécilien [*Belgian obstetrician*, 1817–47]. Remembered for his description of the amniotic bands formed by adhesions between the fetus and the amnion; called *Simonart's bands* or *threads.*

sim′ple [L. *simplex*, simple]. 1. Not complex; consisting of but one substance, or containing only one active substance; not compound. 2. Wanting in intellect.

sim′ple. A medicinal plant, thought of as possessing a single medicinal substance; also, any drug consisting of but one vegetable medicinal ingredient.

sim′plex′in. An antibiotic substance derived from *Bacillus simplex*, active against Gram-negative and Gram-positive bacteria and against fungi.

Simpson, James Young [*Scottish obstetrician*, 1811–70]. The first to promote the use of chloroform in England, especially in obstetrics (1847). In this he was closely followed by John Snow, who, however, preferred ether. Inventor of a number of obstetric and gynecologic instruments including a forceps called *Simpson's forceps.*

Simpson, William Kelly [*American laryngologist*, 1855–1914]. Devised a shaped cotton tampon cut to fit the nasal cavity, and used to retain the parts and to control epistaxis following operation; called *Simpson's nasal splint.*

Sims, James Marion [*American surgeon*, 1813–83]. Noted for his distinguished contributions to gynecology and to general surgery. Developed a successful operation for the closure of vesicovaginal fistula, in which he used sutures of silver wire (1858). Introduced his operation for amputation of the uterine cervix (1861). Performed cholecystectomy for hydrops of the gallbladder (1870). Invented the duckbill vaginal speculum, called *Sims's speculum.* See a so Sims's *position.*

si′mul [L.]. At once; at the same time.

sim″u·la′tion [L. *simulatio*, from *simulare*, to pretend]. The feigning or counterfeiting of disease; malingering.

sim′u·la″tor. See *malingerer.*

Si·mu′li·um [*simulare*]. A genus of small, robust, humpbacked Diptera with short legs and broad wings, commonly called black flies or buffalo gnats. They are worldwide in distribution. The females are vicious bloodsuckers.

S. columbaczense. A migratory species of Europe; kills cattle and has been known to kill children.

S. damnosum. An intermediate host of the nematode worm, *Onchocerca volvulus;* other transmitters of this parasite are *S. metallicum, S. ochraceum* and *S. callidum.*

S. griseicollis. Known as the nimetti; a pest in the African Sudan.

S. pecuarum. A small black fly which is an important scourge of man and cattle in the Mississippi Valley.

S. venustum. A small black fly of northern New England, New York, and Canada, most bothersome to man in June and July.

si″mul·tag·no′si·a (of Wol′pert). A form of visual agnosia in which the patient is able to perceive parts but not the whole of a pattern or picture; the result of bilateral lesions of the occipital lobes (area 19, and perhaps also 18, of Brodmann).

sin·al′bin. A glycoside found in white mustard, which on enzymatic hydrolysis yields glucose, parahydroxybenzylisothiocyanate, choline, and sinapinic acid.

sinan. Trade-mark for *mephenesin.*

si·na′pis [G. *sinapi*]. Mustard.

sin″a·pis′co·py [*sinapi;* G. *skopein*, to examine]. The use of mustard as a test of sensory disturbances.

sin′a·pism [*sinapi*]. A mustard plaster.

sin′ca·line (sing′kuh·leen, ·lin). See *choline.*

sin′ci·put (sin′sip·ut) [L., half a head]. 1. The top of the head; the bregma. 2. Old term for the superior and anterior part of the head. —**sincip′ital,** *adj.*

sin′ew (sin′yōō) [AS. *sinu*]. A tendon.

weeping s. See *ganglion*, 2.

Singleton, Albert Olin [*American surgeon*, 1882–1947]. Introduced an incision for upper abdominal operations, called *Singleton's incision.*

sin·gul′tus [L., a sobbing]. A hiccup. —**singultous,** *adj.;* **singulta′tion,** *n.*

sin′i·grin. $KC_{10}H_{16}O_9NS_2.H_2O$; potassium myronate, a glycoside found in black mustard, *Brassica nigra.* Under the influence of myrosin, an albuminous ferment which is also in black mustard, the glycoside is hydrolyzed, yielding allyl isothiocyanate, acid potassium sulfate, and glucose.

sin′is·ter (sin′is·tur, si·nis′tur), **si·nis′tra, si·nis′trum** [L.]. Left. Abbreviated, s.

sin′is·trad, sin·is′trad [*sinister;* L. *ad,* to, toward]. Toward the left.

sin′is·tral, sin·is′tral [*sinister*]. 1. On the left side. 2. Showing preference for the left hand, eye, or foot for certain acts or functions. —**sinistral′ity,** *n.*

sin′is·tral. A left-handed individual.

sin″is·tra′tion [*sinister*]. 1. A turning to the left. 2. Development of dominance of the right side of the cerebral hemisphere in left-handed persons: the opposite of *dextralization.*

sin″is·trau′ral [*sinister;* L. *auris,* ear]. Left-eared; the opposite of *dextraural.*

sin′is·tro- (sin′is·tro-, si·nis′tro-), **sinistr-** [*sinister*]. A combining form denoting *left* or *toward the left side.*

sin″is·tro·car′di·al [*sinister;* G. *kardia,* heart]. Having the heart displaced to the left.

sin″is·tro·cer′e·bral [*sinister;* L. *cerebrum,* brain]. 1. Located in the left cerebral hemisphere. 2. Functioning preferentially with the left side of the brain; the opposite of *dextrocerebral.*

sin″is·troc′u·lar [*sinister;* L. *oculus,* eye]. Left-eyed; the opposite of *dextrocular.*

sin″is·tro·gy·ra′tion (sin″is·tro·jye·ray′shun, si-nis″tro·) [*sinister;* G. *gyros,* circle]. Turning or twisting to the left; as the plane of polarization, or a movement of the eye. —**sinistrogy′ric,** *adj.*

sin″is·tro·man′u·al [*sinister;* L. *manualis,* of the hand]. Left-handed.

sin″is·trop′e·dal (sin″is·trop′i·dul, sin″is·tro·pee′-dul, si·nis″tro·) [*sinister;* L. *pedalis,* of the foot]. Left-footed.

sin″is·tro·phor′i·a. See *levophoria.*

sin′is·trorse [*sinister;* L. *versus,* from *vertere,* to turn]. *In biology,* turning from right to left, as certain twining stems.

sin″is·tro′sis [*sinister;* G. *-ōsis,* condition]. Shell-shock.

sin″is·tro·tor′sion [*sinister;* L. *torsio,* from *torquere,* to twist]. A twisting or turning toward the left; the opposite of *dextrotorsion.*

sin′is·trous, sin·is′trous [*sinister*]. Awkward; unskilled; the reverse is dextrous, skilled, expert.

sink′a·lin, sink′a·line, sink′o·line. See *choline.*

si′no- [L. *sinus,* fold, curve]. A combining form denoting *sinus.*

si″no·a′tri·al [*sinus;* L. *atrium,* atrium]. Pertaining to the region between the atrium and the sinus venosus, as the sinoatrial node.

si″no·au·ric′u·lar. See *sinoatrial.*

si″no·bron·chi′tis. Inflammation of the bronchi and the paranasal sinuses.

si·nom′e·nine. $C_{19}H_{23}NO_4$; an alkaloid from *Sinomenium acutum* or orientvine, having a morphinelike structure but not the sedative or analgesic properties of morphine; a convulsive poison.

sin′u- [*sinus*]. A combining form signifying *sinus.*

sin″u·i′tis. See *sinusitis.*

sin″u·ot′o·my. See *sinusotomy.*

sin′u·ous [L. *sinuosus,* curving]. Wavy; applied especially to tortuous fistulas and sinuses.

si′nus [L.]. 1. A hollow or cavity; a recess or pocket. 2. A large channel containing blood, especially venous blood. 3. A suppurating tract. 4. A cavity within a bone. —**sinal, sinusal,** *adj.*

accessory nasal sinuses. See *paranasal sinuses* under *sinus.*

air s. A cavity containing air within a bone, especially one communicating with the nasal passages; a paranasal sinus.

anal s. The anal pit or proctodeum.

aortic s. One of the pouchlike dilatations of the aorta opposite the cusps of the semilunar valves. Also called *s. of Valsalva.*

basilar s. See basilar *plexus.*

carotid s. 1. A slight dilatation of the common carotid artery at its bifurcation, the walls of which are innervated by the intercarotid or sinus branch of the glossopharyngeal nerve. It is concerned with the regulation of systemic blood pressure. 2. An extension of the cavernous sinus into the carotid canal.

cavernous s. An irregularly shaped sinus of the dura mater, located on the side of the body of the sphenoid bone, and extending from the superior orbital fissure in front to the apex of the petrous bone behind. See Table of Veins in the Appendix. See Plate 10.

cervical s. A triangular depression caudal to the hyoid arch containing the posterior visceral arches and grooves; it is obliterated superficially by the growth of the hyoid arch and forms the cervical vesicle.

circular s. That consisting of the two cavernous sinuses and their communications across the median line by means of the anterior and posterior intercavernous sinuses, all of which surround the hypophysis.

coccygeal s. The coccygeal fovea.

coronary s. A venous sinus which drains most of the cardiac veins, opens into the right atrium, and is located in the lower part of the atrioventricular sulcus of the heart. It is derived from the transverse portion of the embryonic sinus venosus. See Table of Veins in the Appendix. See Plate 5.

cortical s. A lymph sinus in the cortex of a lymph node.

costomediastinal s. Bilateral spaces between the reflection of the costal pleura upon the anterior mediastinum into which the border of the lung advances on inspiration.

definitive urogenital s. The distal part of the primitive urogenital sinus forming a common chamber for the openings of the primary urethra and the mesonephric and paramesonephric ducts.

dural s. See *s.* of the dura.

ethmoidal sinuses. The ethmoidal cells. See Plate 12.

frontal s. The paranasal sinus situated in the frontal bone. See Plates 12, 20.

inferior petrosal s. A sinus of the dura running posteriorly from the cavernous sinus along the line of the petro-occipital suture to the beginning of the internal jugular vein at the jugular foramen. See Table of Veins in the Appendix.

inferior sagittal s. A sinus of the dura which extends along the posterior half of the lower border of the falx cerebri and terminates in the straight sinus. See Table of Veins in the Appendix. See Plates 10, 18.

intercavernous sinuses. Sinuses of the dura running across the median line of the hypophyseal fossa in front of and behind the hypophysis, connecting the cavernous sinuses of each side. See Table of Veins in the Appendix.

lactiferous s. A dilatation of a lactiferous duct where milk may accumulate. See Plate 43.

laryngeal s. See laryngeal *ventricle.*

lateral s. Transverse sinus of the dura. See Plate 17.

longitudinal s. Sagittal sinus. See inferior sagittal *s.*, superior sagittal *s.*

lymph s. One of the tracts of diffuse lymphatic

tissue between the cords and nodules, and the septa and capsule of a lymph node.

marginal s. (a) An enlarged venous sinus incompletely encircling the margin of the placenta. (b) One of the bilateral, small sinuses of the dura which skirt the edge of the foramen magnum, usually uniting posteriorly to form the occipital sinus. (c) Terminal sinus.

mastoid s. See mastoid *cell.*

maxillary s. The paranasal sinus in the maxilla. Also called *antrum of Highmore.* See Plate 12.

medullary s. A lymph sinus in the medulla of a lymph node.

nasal sinuses. See *paranasal sinuses* under *sinus.*

oblique s. of the pericardium. An arched reflection of pericardium forming a pocket that extends upward on the posterior aspect of the atria.

occipital s. A sinus of the dura running in the attached margin of the falx cerebelli from the foramen magnum to the confluence of the sinuses. See Table of Veins in the Appendix. See Plates 10, 17.

oral s. The stomodeum.

paranasal sinuses. Air cavities lined by mucous membrane which communicate with the nasal cavity: the ethmoidal, frontal, sphenoidal, and maxillary sinuses. See Plate 12.

parasinoidal s. Any one of a number of irregular spaces in the dura mater found on either side of the superior sagittal sinus and communicating with the latter. The arachnoid granulations project into the sinuses. Also called *lateral lacuna.*

petrosquamous s. An inconstant sinus of the dura at the junction of the petrous and squamous parts of the temporal bone, opening into the transverse sinus posteriorly.

phrenicocostal s. Bilateral space between the reflection of the costal pleura upon the diaphragm into which the inferior edge of the lung advances on inspiration.

pilonidal s. A congenital anomaly in the sacral region which may be cystic, consisting of a tract leading to the exterior. Also called *pilonidal cyst.*

piriform, pyriform s. See piriform *recess.*

pleural sinuses. See costomediastinal *s.*, phrenicocostal *s.*

precervical s. See cervical *s.*

primitive urogenital s. The larger part of the cloaca ventral to the urorectal septum. Also called *urogenital tube.*

prostatic s. The groove on each side of the urethral crest into which open the ducts of the prostate gland.

pyriform s. See piriform *recess.*

rectal s. One of the depressions between the rectal columns in the anal canal.

renal s. The potential space surrounded by the mass of the kidney and occupied by the renal pelvis, calyxes, vessels, and parts of the renal capsule.

rhomboidal s. The opening in the extreme posterior end of the embryonic spinal cord which forms the terminal ventricle of the adult.

Rokitansky-Aschoff sinuses. Small outpouchings of the mucosa of the gallbladder, lined and continuous with the surface epithelium, and extending through the lamina propria and muscular layer.

sagittal s. See inferior sagittal *s.*, superior sagittal *s.*

sigmoid s. The S-shaped part of the transverse sinus which lies on the mastoid portion of the temporal bone and the jugular portion of the occipital bone. See Table of Veins in the Appendix. See Plate 17.

s. alae parvae. The sphenoparietal sinus.

s. of external jugular vein. The portion of the external jugular vein between two sets of valves in the distal part of the vessel; this area is often dilated.

s. of the dura. Any endothelially lined, venous blood space situated between the periosteal and meningeal layers of the dura mater. One of the channels by which the blood is conveyed from the cerebral veins, and from some of the veins of the meninges and diploë, into the veins of neck.

s. of the epididymis. See digital *fossa.*

s. of Valsalva. See aortic *s.*

s. pocularis. Old term for prostatic utricle.

s. venarum. That portion of the adult right atrium behind the crista terminalis.

s. venosus. (a) The chamber of the lower vertebrate heart to which the veins return blood from the body. (b) The vessel in the transverse septum of the embryonic mammalian heart into which open the vitelline and allantoic veins, and the ducts of Cuvier.

sphenoidal s. The paranasal sinus in the body of the sphenoid bone. See Plates 12, 20.

sphenoparietal s. A sinus of the dura located along the posterior border of the lesser wing of the sphenoid bone.

straight s. A sinus of the dura running from the inferior sagittal sinus along the junction of the falx cerebri and tentorium to the transverse sinus. See Table of Veins in the Appendix. See Plates 10, 17, 18.

subcapsular s. A lymph sinus between the capsule and the cortex of a lymph node.

superior petrosal s. A sinus of the dura running in a groove in the petrous portion of the temporal bone from the cavernous sinus to the transverse sinus. See Table of Veins in the Appendix.

superior sagittal s. A sinus of the dura which runs along the upper edge of the falx cerebri, beginning in front of the crista galli and terminating at the confluence of the sinuses. See Table of Veins in the Appendix. See Plates 10, 17.

terminal s. That bounding the area vasculosa of the blastoderm of a meroblastic ovum. Syn., *marginal s.*

transverse s. (a) A sinus of the dura running from the internal occipital protuberance, following for part of its course the attached margin of the tentorium cerebelli, then over the jugular process of the occipital bone to reach the jugular foramen. Also called *lateral s.* See Table of Veins in the Appendix. See Plate 10. (b) A dorsal communication between the right and left sides of the pericardial cavity between the reflections of the epicardium at the arterial and venous attachments of the heart, passing behind the aorta and pulmonary artery and in front of the superior vena cava and left atrium.

tympanic s. A deep recess in the labyrinthine wall of the tympanic cavity whose inferior border is formed by the subiculum promontorii.

urogenital s. See definitive urogenital *s.*, primitive urogenital *s.*

uterine s. A venous sinus in the wall of the gravid uterus.

venous s. of the sclera. A canal in the sclera close to the sclerocorneal junction running circularly around the periphery of the cornea. It gives rise to the anterior ciliary veins. Also called *Schlemm's canal.*

vertebral s. See vertebral *plexus* (b).

si″nus·i′tis (sigh″nuh·sigh′tis, sin″yoo·, sigh″new·) [*sinus;* G. *-itis,* inflammation]. Inflammation of a sinus. May affect any of the paranasal sinuses, as **ethmoidal, frontal,** or **maxillary.**

adenomatous s. Glandular *s.*

follicular s. A type of pathologic lesion in chronically infected sinuses, characterized by numerous lymph follicles.

glandular s. An extensive hyperplasia of the seromucinous glands of the nose, which in the advanced stage may become cystic: also called *adenomatous s.*

papillary s. Papillary hypertrophy of the mucosa of any of the paranasal sinuses.

si′nus·oid [*sinus;* G. *eidos,* form]. One of the relatively large spaces or tubes constituting part of the venous circulatory system in the suprarenal gland, liver, and other viscera. —**si′nusoid,** *adj.*

si″nus·oi′dal [*sinus; eidos*]. 1. Varying in proportion to the sine of an angle or of a time function. 2. Pertaining to a sinus.

si″nus·oi″dal·i·za′tion (sigh″nuh·soy″dul·i·zay′-shun, ·eye·zay′shun) [*sinus; eidos*]. The medical application of a sinusoidal current.

si″nus·ot′o·my (sigh″nus·ot′o·mee, sigh″new·sot′-o·mee) [*sinus;* G. *tomē,* a cutting]. The production of an artificial opening into a paranasal sinus, to promote drainage.

siomine. Trade-mark for $(CH_2)_6N_4I_4$; hexamethylenetetramine tetraiodide or methenamine tetraiodide. The substance occurs as an amorphous red powder; insoluble in water, slightly soluble in alcohol. It is decomposed in the intestines with formation of methenamine and iodide, and is used for the effects of the iodide. The methenamine serves only to render the substance insoluble.

si′phon [G.]. A tube bent at an angle, one arm of which is longer than the other; used for the purpose of removing liquids from a cavity or vessel, by means of atmospheric pressure.

si′phon·age [*siphōn*]. The action of a siphon, such as washing out the stomach, drainage of wounds, by the use of atmospheric pressure.

Si″pho·nap′ter·a [*siphōn;* G. *pteron,* wing]. An order of insects, commonly called fleas. They have small, hard, laterally compressed bodies without wings, and the mouth parts are adapted for piercing and sucking. They feed exclusively upon the blood of birds and mammals and so become important disease vectors. The important genera are *Ctenocephalides, Echidnophaga, Pulex, Tunga,* and *Xenopsylla.*

Si·phun″cu·la′ta (sigh·funk″yoo·lay′tuh, ·lah′tuh) [L. *siphunculus,* a little pipe]. Suborder of Anoplura; the sucking lice.

Si·phun″cu·li′na (sigh·funk″yoo·lye′nuh) [*siphunculus*]. A genus of flies found in India.

S. funicola. The common eye fly of India which is responsible for transmitting conjunctivitis.

Sippy, Bertram Welton [*American physicina,* 1866–1924]. Widely known for his advocacy of a diet adapted to the treatment of gastric and duodenal ulcer. The *Sippy diet* consisted of alternately taking Sippy's powders (see under *powder,* 2), and a milk-cream mixture.

si′ren [G. *seirēn,* siren]. *In teratology,* sirenomelus.

si′ren-limb. See *sympus.*

si″re·no·me′li·a, si″re·nom′e·ly [*seiren; melos,* limb]. The condition of having fused lower extremities and no feet.

si″ren·om′e·lus [*seirēn; melos*]. A monster whose lower extremities are intimately fused, the feet being absent. Also called *sympus apus.*

si·ri′a·sis [G. *seiriasis,* heatstroke]. Sunstroke. *Obs.*

sir′up. See *syrup.*

sis″mo·ther′a·py. See *seismotherapy.*

Sisto, Genaro [*Argentinian pediatrician,* d. 1923]. Observed that constant crying is a sign of hereditary syphilis in infants; called *Sisto's sign.*

Sis·tru′rus [G. *seistron,* rattle; *oura,* tail]. A genus of small rattlesnakes.

site [L. *situs,* placed]. Situation.

placental s. The area to which the placenta is attached.

sit′fast″ [AS. *sittan; faest*]. *In veterinary medicine,* a form of dry gangrene, resulting from pressure on a circumscribed area of the skin, with firm adherence of the dead tissue to the living tissue below, through its continuity with fibrous elements of the underlying structures; affects horses.

sit″i·eir′gi·a (sit″ee·ire′jee·uh, ·eer′jee·uh) [G. *sitos,* food; *eirgein,* to shut out]. Hysterical anorexia. *Obs.*

sit″i·ol′o·gy (sit″ee·ol′o·jee, sigh″tee·). See *sitology.*

sit″i·o·pho′bi·a. See *sitophobia.*

si·tol′o·gy (sigh·tol′o·jee) [*sitos;* G. *logos,* word]. The science of foods; dietetics.

si″to·ma′ni·a [*sitos;* G. *mania,* madness]. An abnormal craving for food: also spelled *sitiomania.*

si″to·pho′bi·a [*sitos;* G. *phobos,* fear]. Morbid aversion to food; morbid fear of eating.

si′to·stane, si·tos′tane. $C_{29}H_{52}$. A steroid hydrocarbon, probably the parent substance of sitosterols.

si·tos′ter·ol. Any one of the principal sterols of plants, probably derivatives of sitostane.

si″to·ther′a·py [*sitos;* G. *therapeia,* treatment]. Dietotherapy.

sit′ting height. *In anthropometry,* a measurement taken vertically from the table on which the subject is sitting to the vertex, with the anthropometer behind the subject. Enough pressure is applied to compress the hair.

si′tus [L.]. A position.

s. inversus. Altered location or position.

s. inversus viscerum. An anomaly in which the viscera are changed from the normal to the opposite side of the body. Also called *s. mutatus, s. transversus.*

s. perversus. Malposition of one or more of the viscera.

Sjögren, Tage Anton Ultimus [*Swedish surgeon,* 1859–1939]. The first to employ successfully radiation therapy in carcinoma and sarcoma (1899–1904).

SK Streptokinase.

skat′ole, ska′tole. C_9H_9N, methyl indole. A nitrogenous decomposition product of proteins, formed from tryptophan in the intestine. It contributes to the characteristic, disagreeable odor of feces.

skat·ox′yl. C_9H_9ON. A product of the oxidation of skatole. It occurs as the sulfuric acid ester in the urine in cases of disease of the intestine or in excessive intestinal putrefaction.

skein (skane). See *spireme.*

ske·lal′gi·a [G. *skelos,* leg; *algos,* pain]. Pain in the leg.

skel′e·tal trac′tion. Traction exerted directly upon the long bones themselves by means of pins, wire, tongs, and other mechanical devices which are attached to, or passed through, the bones by operative procedures.

skel″e·ti·za′tion [G. *skeletos,* dried up]. The process of converting into a skeleton; gradual wasting of the soft parts, leaving only the skeleton.

skel′e·to- [*skeletos*]. A combining form meaning *skeleton.*

skel′e·ton [*skeletos*]. A supporting structure, especially the bony framework supporting and protecting the soft parts of an organism. See Plates 1, 24. —**skeletal,** *adj.*

appendicular s. The skeleton of the pectoral and pelvic girdles and limbs.

axial s. The skeleton of the head and trunk.

cartilaginous s. The cartilaginous precursor of most of the bony skeleton.

dermal s. The exoskeleton.

s. of the heart. The fibrous rings (*annuli fibrosi*) surrounding the four valvular orifices of the heart. The four rings are conjoined and attached to the upper membranous part of the interventricular septum (*pars membranacea septi*). All heart muscles arise from the cardiac skeleton and eventually return to be inserted therein.

Skene, Alexander Johnston Chalmers [*American gynecologist*, 1838–1900]. Remembered for his description of the tubular mucous glands in the female urethra opening just within the urinary meatus (1880); called *Skene's glands, paraurethral glands*. The duct of each is known as *Skene's duct*.

ske·nei'tis, ske·ni'tis [after A. J. C. *Skene;* G. *-itis*, inflammation]. Inflammation of the paraurethral glands, or Skene's ducts.

skene'o·scope" (skee'no·scope") [*Skene;* G. *skopein*, to examine]. An endoscope for use in examining Skene's glands.

ske·ni'tis. See *skeneitis.*

ske"o·cy·to'sis (skee"o·sigh·to'sis). See *shift* to left.

skep"to·phy·lax'i·a, skep"to·phy·lax'is. See *tachyphylaxia.*

skew de"vi·a'tion. A condition in which one eyeball is deviated upward and outward, the other inward and downward; sometimes observed in cerebellar disease.

skew'foot". Metatarsus adductovarus.

skiabaryt. Trade-mark for barium sulfate and for mixtures of barium sulfate, sugar, and tragacanth suitable for use in roentgen examinations.

ski'a·gram [G. *skia*, shadow; *gramma*, letter]. The finished, printed roentgen-ray picture.

ski·ag'ra·phy [*skia;* G. *graphein*, to write]. Radiography.

ski·am'e·try (sky·am'i·tree) [*skia;* G. *metron*, a measure]. 1. Shadow mensuration applied to a method of determining the density of x-ray shadow. 2. The measurement of x-ray intensity, for the determination of exposure time. 3. The measurement of accommodation by retinoscopy.

dynamic s. Refraction in which retinoscopy is performed with the accommodation active but controlled.

ski"a·po·res'co·py. See *retinoscopy.*

ski'a·scope [*skia;* G. *skopein*, to examine]. An instrument employed in retinoscopy.

ski·as'co·py (sky·ass'ko·pee) [*skia; skopein*]. 1. Examination with a retinoscope. 2. Examination with a fluoroscope.

ski"a·ther'a·py [*skia;* G. *therapeia*, treatment]. Old term for x-ray therapy.

skim"mi·an'ine. $C_{14}H_{13}NO_4$; an alkaloid from *Skimmia japonica* and other *Skimmia* species: identical with β-fagarine.

skin [ON. *skinn*]. The covering of the body, composed of the epidermis **(scarfskin)**, or cuticle, and the corium **(true skin)**, or derma. The epidermis consists of a deep layer, the stratum germinativum, and three superficial layers: the stratum granulosum, the stratum lucidum, and the stratum corneum. The corium, derma, or true skin consists of a papillary and reticular layer (stratum papillare and stratum reticulare), the former projecting upward in the form of papillae. The true skin is made up of fibroelastic connective tissue and, in some regions, smooth muscle (the arrectores pilorum). The subcutaneous tissue consists of fibroelastic and adipose tissue, blood vessels, and sweat glands in its upper portion. The appendages of the skin are the nails, hairs, and sweat, sebaceous and mammary glands, which are derivatives of the epithelial layer of the skin. In the skin are also placed terminal nerve organs subserving the senses of touch, pain, and temperature.

anserine s. Goose flesh; cutis anserina.

atrophic s. A wasting or retrogressive change in the skin. Also called *dermatrophia.*

bronzed s. See *adrenal cortical hypofunction.*

congestive s. Engorgement of the blood vessels of the skin. Also called *dermathemia.*

deciduous s. Keratolysis.

edematous s. Effusion of serum into the areolar tissue of the skin. Also called *dermatoclysis.*

farmer's s. See sailor's *s.*

fish s. See *ichthyosis.*

glossy s. A peculiar shiny skin seen in conditions in which the trophic nerve supply to the skin is cut off, as after injury to a nerve.

goldbeater's s. A thin tenacious sheet from the cecum of cattle, occasionally used as a surgical dressing.

goose s. See goose *flesh.*

indiarubber s. See *cutis* hyperelastica.

parchment s. Atrophy of the skin.

piebald s. See *vitiligo.*

pigmentation of the s. Coloration of the skin due to natural body pigments, or to the deposition of foreign substances in the skin. Natural pigments include melanin, hemosiderin, carotene, and bile salts. Foreign pigments include atabrine and silver salts.

sailor's s. A condition seen in exposed areas in elderly persons. There is pigmentation and senile keratosis, frequently leading to epitheliomas: also called *farmer's s.*

shark s. See *dyssebacia.*

toad s. A dry, roughened skin associated with vitamin-A deficiency.

true s. The corium.

skin graft'ing. The application of portions of the skin, either the outer layers or the full thickness, to a granulating wound to promote healing, to fill a defect, to replace scar tissue for plastic repair. Also see *graft.*

skin'ny [*skinn*]. 1. Cutaneous. 2. Emaciated.

skin trac'tion. Traction exerted by direct attachment to the skin, using adhesive plaster or linen or gauze strips cemented to the skin.

skiodan sodium. Trade-marked name for the radiopaque substance methiodal sodium.

skle·ri'a·sis. See *scleroderma.*

Sklowsky, E. L. [*German physician*, contemporary]. Introduced a method of distinguishing a varicella vesicle from the vesicles of smallpox and herpes. A very light pressure of the index finger near and then over the lesion will easily rupture the former, while greater pressure is necessary to rupture the latter. This is known as *Sklowsky's symptom.*

Skoda, Josef [*Austrian physician*, 1805–81]. First to attempt systematic investigation of pulmonary disease on the basis of sounds observed in examination by percussion. Tympanitic resonance is also called *Skoda's resonance* or *tympany.*

sko"li·o'sis. See *scoliosis.*

sko"li·o·som'e·ter. See *scoliosometer.*

Skop'tsy. Religious sect in Russia whose members practice castration.

skull [ME. *skulle*]. 1. The entire bony framework of the head, consisting of the cranium and the face. The cranium is made up of the occipital, frontal, sphenoid, and ethmoid bones, and the two parietal and two temporal bones. The face is composed of two nasal, two lacrimal, two zygomatic, two palate, and two inferior turbinate bones, two maxillas, the vomer, and the mandible. Sometimes loosely used to include only the fixed bones, excluding the mandible. See Table of Bones in the Appendix. See Plate 1. 2. *In embryology*, neurocranium (fixed bones of head and face listed in 1) and viscerocranium (derivatives of the visceral arches, such as the hyoid bone).

fenestrated s. Osteoporosis of the skull, as from osteomyelitis.

lacuna s. A congenital bony defect of the skull, restricted to the diploë and the inner table. See *craniofenestria.*

open-roofed s. See *cranioschisis.*

steeple s. See *oxycephaly.*

tower s. See *oxycephaly.*

skull'cap" [*skulle;* AS. *caeppe*]. 1. The bones comprising the vault of the skull; calvaria. 2. See *scutellaria.*

skunk cab'bage. *Symplocarpus foetidus,* the rhizome of which has been used as a stimulant, antispasmodic, and narcotic in asthma, rheumatism, hysteria, and dropsy.

Skutsch, Felix [*German gynecologist,* 1861–1951]. Remembered for his operation of salpingostomy in which he excised an oval portion of tissue from the abdominal end of the uterine tube, uniting the mucous and serous surfaces with silk sutures around the opening, the new ampulla being sutured to the ovary; called *Skutsch's operation.*

slake [AS. *slacian*]. 1. Quench or appease. 2. Disintegrate by the action of water.

slap'ping. *In massage,* percussion movements in which the hands with palms open come down alternately in a sharp series of blows. The movement is carried out chiefly from the wrist.

slav'er [cf. Icel. *slafra*]. Drivel; saliva, especially that which is discharged involuntarily.

sleep [AS. *slǣp*]. The periodic state of rest in which there is diminution of consciousness and activity.

hypnotic s. See *hypnotism.*

paroxysmal s. See *narcolepsy.*

sleep'ing sick'ness. Lethargic encephalitis.

sleep'less·ness. See *insomnia.*

sli'cer [ME. *slice*]. Tissue slicers for making fresh tissue slices for studies of respiration include such types as Martin, Stadie-Riggs, template, Terry, Thomas De Eds. See *microtome.*

slide [AS. *slīdan*]. A piece of glass on which objects are examined by use of the microscope.

sling [ME.]. A bandage, usually slung from the neck, to support the arm or wrist.

sling and swathe. A dressing for fractures of the humerus at the upper end. It consists of a three-cornered handkerchief sling holding the arm at the side, the forearm flexed at 90°, with an axillary pad, the swathe passing about the body and arm from shoulder to elbow and secured by pins.

slit [AS. *slītan*]. A narrow opening; a visceral cleft; the separation between any pair of lips.

genitourinary s. The urogenital opening.

Sloan, Guy Arthur [*American surgeon,* 1889–]. Introduced an incision for upper abdominal surgery called *Sloan's incision.*

slough (sluff) [ME. *slughe*]. A mass of necrotic tissue in, or separating from, living tissue, as in a wound or ulcer.

slows. See *trembles.*

Sluder, Greenfield [*American laryngologist,* 1865–1928]. Introduced a snare for use in tonsillectomy, called *Sluder's snare.* His operation, in which he used this snare to excise completely the tonsil in its capsule, is called *Sluder's method* or *operation.* The syndrome of sphenopalatine ganglion neuralgia is called *Sluder's syndrome* or *neuralgia.*

sludge. Sewage deposit.

slum'ber [AS. *slūma*]. Light sleep. —**slum'ber,** *v.*

Slye, Maud [*American pathologist,* 1879–1954]. Noted for her work on cancer and heredity (1928). Her selective breeding of mice, both resistant to and capable of developing cancer, has shown that there is hereditary influence determining susceptibility to cancer type, site of malignancy, and age at which it is likely to occur.

Sm Chemical symbol for samarium.

small'pox" [AS. *smael; pocc*]. A contagious infectious disease, often fatal, ushered in with severe febrile symptoms, which, in the course of two or three days, are followed by a papular eruption appearing over all parts of the body. The eruption passes successively through the states of maculation, vesiculation, pustulation, and later crust formation; after this a pitted appearance of the skin (pock-marks) is produced. The period of incubation is twelve to twenty-one days. The papules appear about the third day, pustules the sixth day, crusting the twelfth day.

black s. See hemorrhagic *s.*

bovine s. Vaccinia.

coherent s. A form in which the pustules coalesce but retain their individuality.

confluent s. A severe form in which the pustules spread and run together.

discrete s. A form in which the pustules preserve their distinct individuality.

equine s. Horsepox.

hemorrhagic s. Smallpox in which hemorrhage occurs into the vesicles, which gives them a blackish appearance.

malignant s. A severe hemorrhagic type with high mortality.

modified s. See *varioloid.*

s. inoculation. A method formerly used for protecting or attempting to protect against a severe attack of smallpox in adult life, by the direct transfer of the virus from a sick patient to a well person.

s. vaccine. See under *vaccine.*

smear [AS. *smeoru*]. Preparation of secretions or blood for microscopical study, made by spreading them on a glass slide.

Smee, Alfred [*English surgeon,* 1818–77]. Described an electric cell composed of one zinc plate and one of platinized silver in dilute sulfuric acid; called *Smee cell.*

smeg'ma [G., soap, unguent]. Sebum. —**smegmatic,** *adj.*

s. clitoridis. The substance secreted by the sebaceous glands of the clitoris and labia minora.

s. embryonum. See *vernix caseosa.*

s. praeputii. The substance secreted by the sebaceous glands of the prepuce.

smell [ME. *smellen*]. 1. The perception of odor. 2. Odor.

Smellie, William [*English obstetrician,* 1697–1763]. Devised several types of obstetric forceps, some with lock and curved blades, called *Smellie's forceps.* Developed craniotomy scissors, called *Smellie's scissors.* His method of delivery of the aftercoming head with the child resting on the physician's forearm is known as the *Smellie method, Smellie-Veit method, Mauriceau's method.*

smell'ing salts. A preparation containing ammonium carbonate and stronger ammonia water, usually scented with aromatic substances.

smi'la·cin. A saponin from sarsaparilla, identical with parillin.

smi·lag'e·nin. $C_{27}H_{44}O_3$; the steroidal aglycone of smilasaponin, a glycoside of sarsaparilla; an isomer of sarsasapogenin. Syn., *isosarsasapogenin.*

smi"la·sap'o·nin. A glycoside from sarsaparilla; on hydrolysis it yields the aglycone smilagenin.

smi'lax. See *sarsaparilla.*

Smith, Edwin [*American Egyptologist,* nineteenth century]. Remembered for his acquisition (1862) of the oldest known medical writing of ancient Egypt, the manuscript dating from the seventeenth century B.C. It has been published in facsimile with translation by James Henry Breasted, as the *Edwin Smith papyrus.*

Smith, Grafton Elliot (1871–1937). English neuroanatomist known for his fundamental work in comparative anatomy and in the study of the evolution of the nervous system, particularly comparative analyses of the fissural pattern of the cerebral cortex. He furthered the understanding of the development of speech and of binocular vision.

Smith, Henry [*English surgeon of the Indian medical service,* 1862–1948]. Famous throughout the world for his original clinical work on the extraction of immature cataract within the capsule (ca. 1900); known as *Smith's operation.*

Smith, John Blackburn [*English surgeon,* 1865–1928]. Devised a method for staining flagella; known as *Smith-Pitfield method.*

Smith, Nathan [*American surgeon,* 1762–1829]. Wrote extensively on typhus (1824). Performed oophorectomy (1822). Described amputation at the knee, using a large anterior and smaller posterior flap; called *Smith's operation.* Described osteomyelitis (1827).

Smith, Richard Root [*American surgeon,* 1869–1940]. Remembered for his ingenuity in devising a type of skin closure after radical amputation of the breast. The operation is done through a long incision from below the center of the clavicle, around the inner border of the breast, vertically downward to the costal margin, and laterad five or six inches. A second incision joins the first, completing the circle around the breast. By mobilizing the flaps thus formed, a plastic skin repair can be made with closure of the defect through the transference of large skin areas to new positions. Called *Smith's incision.*

Smith, Theobald [*American pathologist,* 1859–1934]. With D. E. Salmon, demonstrated that dead virus can give immunity against living virus (1884). Discovered the parasite of Texas cattle fever and that it is transmitted by the tick (1893). Differentiated human and bovine tuberculosis (1898). Sensitization to specific foreign proteins on inoculation is called *Theobald Smith phenomenon.* Richet gave it the name of *anaphylaxis.*

Smith, Thomas [*English pathologist,* 1833–1909]. Reported a case of craniohypophyseal xanthomatosis, later called *Hand-Schüller-Christian disease* (1865).

Smith, Walter George [*Irish physician,* 1844–1932]. Devised a test for bile in the urine. A positive test is the appearance of a green color at the intersurface between the urine and tincture of iodine; called *Smith's test.*

Smith's method. See erythrocyte sedimentation *test.*

Smith-Dietrich stain. See under *stain.*

Smith-Hodge pessary. See retroversion *pessary.*

Smith-Petersen, Marius Nygaard [*American physician,* 1886–1953]. Outstanding authority on fractures. Devised a supraarticular subperiosteal approach to the hip joint (1917), called *Smith-Petersen's incision.* Devised a flanged metal nail used for intracapsular fractures of the neck of the femur, called *Smith-Petersen's nail.*

Smithwick, Reginald Hammerick [*American surgeon,* 1899–]. Known for his introduction of an operation for hypertension, in which he resected the greater splanchnic nerve and the sympathetic chain from the ninth thoracic through the first lumbar ganglion, through a transdiaphragmatic extrapleural incision; called *lumbodorsal splanchnicectomy, Smithwick's operation.*

smudge cells. See *basket cells* under *cell.*

smudg'ing [ME. *smogen*]. A form of defective speech in which the difficult consonants are dropped.

smut [LG. *smutt*]. 1. A fungous disease of plants involving the grains wheat, rye, oats, and corn. 2. A fungus producing such a disease; a common allergen.

Sn Chemical symbol for tin.

SN 7618 See *chloroquine.*

SN 13,274 Isopentaquine.

SN 13,276 See *pentaquine.*

snail [AS. *snaegel*]. An invertebrate of the order Gastropoda, phylum Mollusca. Important as hosts of many of the flukes.

snake [AS. *snaca*]. An elongate reptile covered with scales and without limbs, external ears, or functional eyelids; a serpent.

black s. A poisonous snake of Australia. See *Pseudechis porphyriacus.*

brown s. A venomous snake of New Guinea and Australia. See *Pseudechis scutellatus.*

copperhead s. See *Ancistrodon mokasen.*

coral s. A small, brightly colored snake found in America; the venom is a neurotoxin. See *Leptomicrurus, Micrurus.*

cottonmouth s. A thick-bodied pit viper found in or near water; the water moccasin. See *Ancistrodon piscivorus.*

poisonous snakes. The venom-producing snakes, which are divided into four families: Elapidae, the cobras and coral snakes; Hydrophidae, the sea snakes; Crotalidae, the pit vipers; and Viperidae, the true vipers. All have large, hypodermic-like front fangs by which venom is injected.

sea s. A venomous snake found in the ocean near northern Australia and southern Asia. See *Hydrophidae.*

tiger s. An important poisonous snake of Australia which is named for its marking, dark bands on yellow-buff. See *Notechis scutatus.*

snake'root" [*snaca;* AS. *rōt*]. Any of various plants, such as species of *Asarum, Cimicifuga racemosa,* or *Eupatorium rugosum,* most of which have been used as remedies for snakebite.

snap [MD. *snappen*]. A short, abrupt sound heard in auscultation of the heart in certain cardiac diseases. Also applied to the sound made by the action of a tendon on contraction of its muscle.

snare [AS. *sneare*]. An instrument designed to hold a wire loop which can be constricted by means of a mechanism in the handle, and used to remove tonsils, polyps, and small growths having a narrow base or pedicle.

sneeze [ME. *snesen*]. A sudden, noisy, spasmodic expiration through the nose. It is caused by irritation of nasal nerves or overstimulation of the optic nerve by a very bright light. —**sneeze,** *v.*

Snell, Simeon [*English ophthalmologist,* 1851–1909]. Known for his laws of refraction. (1) With any two adjacent mediums, the sine of the angle of incidence bears a fixed ratio to the sine of the angle of refraction, the ratio varying with different mediums; called *Snell's* or *Descartes' law.* (2) The incident and the refracted ray are in the same plane, which is perpendicular to the surface separating the two mediums; called *Snell's law.*

Snell-Strong method. See under *method.*

Snellen, Hermann [*Dutch ophthalmologist,* 1834–1908]. Introduced a number of ophthalmic procedures, including operations for ectropion and entropion. An operation for ptosis in which he shortened the levator tendon by section or tucking is called *Snellen's operation.* An ophthalmologic test chart which measures the degree of visual acuity is called the *Snellen chart.* See also Snellen's *reflex,* test *type,* Snellen *test.*

snore [ME. *snoren*]. Breathe through the nose in such a manner as to cause a vibration of the soft palate, thereby producing a rough, audible sound.

Snow, John [*English physician*, 1813–58]. Contributed valuable study on the water-borne character of cholera (1849). He was a pioneer anesthetist, using extensively both chloroform and ether (1848–58).

snow′blind″ness. Photophobia and conjunctivitis due to exposure of the eyes to ultraviolet rays: also spelled *snow blindness.*

snuff′box″. See *anatomist's snuffbox.*

soap [AS. *sāpe*]. A salt of one or more of the higher fatty acids with an alkali or metal. Soaps may be divided into two classes, soluble and insoluble. The soluble soaps are the detergent or cleansing soaps, and usually are prepared from the alkali metals, sodium and potassium. The insoluble soaps are salts of the fatty acids and metals of other groups. Soap is used chiefly as a detergent and in solution as a vehicle for liniments. In constipation, a solution of soap forms a useful enema. In skin conditions, soap is useful, not merely because of its detergent action but also because it softens the horny layer of the epidermis and has distinct germicidal power. *In pharmacy,* soap is an excellent emulsifying agent when the mixture is intended for external use. Soap is also used in making pills, liniments, and plasters.

castile s. A hard soap usually prepared from sodium hydroxide and olive oil. Much commercial castile soap contains coconut oil soap to increase its lathering quality.

compound green s. tincture. Compound soft soap liniment.

compound soft s. liniment (*linimentum saponis mollis compositum*). Contains soft soap, 150 Gm.; juniper tar, 20 cc.; alcohol, a sufficient quantity to make 1000 cc. Used as a detergent in parasitic skin diseases. Also called *compound green s. tincture.*

curd s. A soap usually made from sodium hydroxide and animal fats and oils. It is used largely for domestic purposes.

disinfectant s. A soap containing some form of disinfectant, such as phenol, cresol, or some salt of mercury.

floating s. A soap in which air bubbles have been incorporated.

green s. See medicinal soft *s.*

green s. tincture. Soft soap liniment.

hard s. (*sapo durus*). A soap made with sodium hydroxide. Hard soap occurs as a white solid in the form of bars, or a white or yellowish white fine powder. Hard soap is used in the following preparations: camphor and soap liniment, chloroform liniment, aloe pills, and N.F. dentifrice.

hard water s. Marine soap.

hexachlorophene s. One containing the anti-infective agent hexachlorophene.

liquid s. A solution of soap used as an economical and sanitary substitute for soap in public places.

marine s. A soap for use with sea water or with water containing calcium or magnesium salts. Ordinary soap is unsatisfactory with such water, as the soap is precipitated by the salts contained therein. Marine soaps usually contain coconut or palm kernel oil. Also called *salt water soap.*

medicinal soft s. (*sapo mollis medicinalis*). A potassium soap made by the saponification of vegetable oils, excluding coconut oil and palm kernel oil, without the removal of glycerin; occurs as a soft, unctuous, yellowish white to brownish or greenish yellow, transparent to translucent, mass; a 1 in 20 solution is alkaline to indicators. Soft soap possesses the detergent properties of soap in general, but because of its alkaline reaction has active medical virtues as a topical remedy. It is useful in many forms of skin diseases. Also called *green s., soft s.*

potash s. A soft soap. See medicinal soft *s.*

s. liniment. See *camphor* and soap liniment.

soda s. See hard *s.*

soft s. liniment (*linimentum saponis mollis*). Contains medicinal soft soap, 650 Gm.; lavender oil, 20 cc.; alcohol, a sufficient quantity to make 1000 cc. Used as a detergent and largely employed for cleansing the skin preceding surgical operations. It is also used in certain skin diseases. It exerts a mild germicidal action because of its alcohol and alkalinity. Also called *green s. tincture*

solid s. liniment (*linimentum saponis spissum*). A liniment made into solid form by sodium stearate and containing camphor, oils of thyme and rosemary, diluted solution of ammonia and alcohol. Used as a mild stimulating liniment. Also called *solid opodeldoc, camphorated s. liniment.*

transparent s. Soap made transparent by the presence of glycerin, alcohol, or sucrose.

sob [ME. *sobben*]. A convulsive inspiration due to contraction of the diaphragm and spasmodic closure of the glottis. —**sob,** *v.*

sobisminol mass. A complex organic bismuth product obtained by the interaction of sodium bismuthate, triisopropanolamine, and propylene glycol; it contains approximately 20% of bismuth; occurs as a red-brown to chocolate-brown pasty mass; soluble in water and alcohol. It has been used in the treatment of syphilis.

so·cal′o·in. Aloin obtained from Socotrine aloes.

so′cial [L. *socialis*, belonging to companionship]. Gregarious; growing near, or together.

so′cial med′i·cine. See social *medicine.*

so′ci·a pa·rot′i·dis (so′shee·uh, so′see·uh) [L.]. Old term for a small, separate lobe of the parotid gland.

so·ci′e·ty screw. The screw at the lower end of the drawtube or body-tube of a microscope for receiving the objective.

Socin, August [*Swiss surgeon*, 1837–99]. An advocate of radical cure of inguinal hernia by ligature and excision of the sac; sometimes called *Socin's operation.* Incised through healthy thyroid tissue and enucleated neoplasms to avoid cachexia strumipriva; also called *Socin's operation.*

so″ci·ol′o·gy [L. *socius*, companion; G. *logos*, word]. The science of mutual relations of people and of social organization.

so″ci·o·med′i·cal [*socius;* L. *medicus*, medical]. Referring to the relationship between social welfare and medicine.

so″ci·o·path′ic per″son·al′i·ty dis·turb′ance. See under *personality.*

sock′et [AF. *soket*]. The concavity into which a movable part is inserted.

dry s. Alveolitis after tooth extraction; without suppuration, but associated with pain.

tooth s. The alveolus in which the tooth is fixed.

so·cor′di·a [L., folly]. Hallucination.

so′da [Ar. *sudā'*, splitting headache]. Sodium carbonate.

baking s. Sodium bicarbonate.

caustic s. Sodium hydroxide.

chlorinated s. solution. Sodium hypochlorite solution.

sal s. Sodium carbonate.

s. ash. Commercial sodium carbonate; essentially anhydrous but containing more or less impurity.

s. lime (*calx sodica*). A mixture in granular form of calcium hydroxide with sodium hydroxide or potassium hydroxide or both; occurs as white or grayish white granules. Used to absorb carbon dioxide in basal metabolism tests, in rebreathing anesthesia machines, and in oxygen therapy. Also used to absorb carbon dioxide in various chemical manipulations.

s. lye. Sodium hydroxide.
s. mint. Solution of soda and mint.
s. niter. Sodium nitrate.
s. water. Water charged with carbon dioxide gas.
washing s. Sodium carbonate.

so'da·mide, sod·am'ide. $NaNH_2$; sodium amide, prepared by the interaction of sodium and gaseous or liquid ammonia; a white crystalline powder, decomposable by water to sodium hydroxide and ammonia: used in various syntheses.

so'di·o- [*sudā'*]. A combining form denoting *a compound containing sodium.*

so'di·um [*sudā'*] (*natrium*). Na = 22.991. A metallic element of the alkali group of metals. Light, silver-white, and lustrous when freshly cut, but rapidly oxidizes when exposed to air, becoming dull and gray. Sodium violently decomposes water, forming sodium hydroxide and hydrogen. It also decomposes alcohol and other liquids containing hydroxyl groups. It is usually stored under kerosene in tightly stoppered containers. Sodium metal and its salts are widely used in industry and in medicine. The sodium ion is the least toxic of all the metallic ions, and is therefore the base of choice when it is desired to obtain the effects of various acid ions. See Table of Normal Values of Blood Constituents in the Appendix.

anticoagulant s. citrate solution. A solution of 4 Gm. of sodium citrate in sufficient water for injection to make 100 cc.

aromatic s. perborate (*sodii perboras aromaticus N.F.*). Sodium perborate containing 0.4% each of soluble saccharin and peppermint oil. Used as a dentifrice, and in solution as a mouthwash and gargle.

compound s. borate solution (*liquor sodii boratis compositus*). Contains sodium borate 15 Gm., sodium bicarbonate 15 Gm., liquefied phenol 3 cc., glycerin 35 cc., distilled water a sufficient quantity to make 1000 cc. Used as a nonirritant wash for the mucous membranes. Also called *Dobell's solution.*

dextrose and s. chloride injection (*injectio dextrosi et sodii chloridi*). A sterile solution of dextrose and sodium chloride in water for injection. Administered parenterally when dextrose is required, to supply fluid, to sustain blood volume temporarily, or to produce diuresis.

diluted s. hypochlorite solution (*liquor sodii hypochloritis dilutus*). Each 100 cc. contains 0.45–0.50 Gm. of NaOCl, equivalent to 0.43–0.48 Gm. of available Cl; occurs as a colorless or faintly yellow liquid. This solution possesses powerful germicidal action and is applied by a method of continuous irrigation. Also called *modified Dakin's solution.*

effervescent s. phosphate (*sodii phosphas effervescens*). Sodium phosphate made into an effervescent salt by the addition of citric and tartaric acids and sodium bicarbonate. Used as a pleasant means of administering sodium phosphate. Dose, 8–15 Gm. (2–4 dr.).

exsiccated s. arsenate (*sodii arsenas exsiccatus*). Na_2HAsO_4. Occurs as an amorphous, white powder; 1 Gm. dissolves in about 3.5 cc. of water; slightly soluble in alcohol. The arsenic in this compound is reduced in the body to exert an effect similar to that of trivalent arsenic. It is usually administered in solution. Dose, 1.6–4.0 mg. ($\frac{1}{40}$–$\frac{1}{50}$ gr.). Also called *dried s. arsenate.*

exsiccated s. phosphate (*sodii phosphas exsiccatus*). Sodium phosphate rendered free of its water of crystallization. Used in preparing the effervescent salt. Also called *dried s. phosphate.*

exsiccated s. sulfite (*sodii sulfis exsiccatus*). Na_2SO_3. Occurs as a white powder; 1 Gm. dissolves in about 4 cc. of water; sparingly soluble in alcohol. It is used as a preservative in tannic acid glycerite.

isotonic s. chloride solution (*liquor sodii chloridi isotonicus*). Contains 0.9 Gm. of NaCl in each 100 cc. This solution provides a simple, watery fluid, which is approximately isotonic with the body fluids and free from drug action. Used for washing mucous membranes and raw surfaces and as a nonirritating solvent for parenteral injection of drugs. It is also used, by parenteral injection, for the restoration of the body water in dehydration or for the temporary replacement of the circulating blood volume. Also called *normal saline solution, physiological salt solution, physiological s. chloride solution.* The injectable preparation, made with water for injection, is called *sodium chloride injection.*

monohydrated s. carbonate (*sodii carbonas monohydratus*). $Na_2CO_3.H_2O$. Occurs as colorless crystals or a white, granular powder; 1 Gm. dissolves in 3 cc. of water; insoluble in alcohol. It is used primarily for pharmaceutical purposes; in medicine it is used chiefly in the preparation of alkaline baths and occasionally as an antacid. Dose, 0.3–2.0 Gm. (5–30 gr.).

one-sixth molar s. r-lactate. Sodium lactate is oxidized in the body to a carbonate. This solution is used in the treatment of acidosis. It is approximately isotonic with the blood. Also used for the purpose of alkalizing the urine. Dose, subcutaneously or intravenously, a rate not greater than 300 cc. per hour (60 drops per minute). Also called *sodium lactate injection* (*injectio sodii lactatis*).

s. acetate (*sodii acetas*). $NaC_2H_3O_2.3H_2O$. Occurs as colorless, transparent crystals or a granular, crystalline powder; 1 Gm. is soluble in about 9.8 cc. of water and about 19 cc. of alcohol. It is diuretic, acting much like potassium acetate. Dose, 1.3–8.0 Gm. (20–120 gr.).

s. ac''e·tri·zo'ate. Official generic name for sodium 3-acetylamino-2,4,6-triiodobenzoate; $C_9H_5I_3NNaO_3$; a contrast medium. See *urokon sodium.*

s. acid phosphate. See *s.* biphosphate.

s. acid sulfate. Sodium bisulfate.

s. acid tartrate. Sodium bitartrate.

s. alginate. The sodium salt of alginic acid. A gelatinous substance obtained from various seaweeds. In cold water it dissolves to form a mucilage similar to acacia, but more viscous. Used in pharmaceutical compounding as a suspending agent.

s. alizarin sulfonate. Alizarin red S.

s. aluminate. $NaAlO_2$; in white, granular masses, very soluble in water: used as a water softener and in many industrial applications.

s. alurate. See under *alurate.*

s. amide. Sodamide.

s. ammonium phosphate. $NaNH_4HPO_4.4H_2O$; colorless crystals or white granules, freely soluble in water: used as a reagent for determination of magnesium. Syn., *microcosmic salt.*

s. amytal. See under *amytal.*

s. antimony tartrate. Antimony sodium tartrate.

s. arsanilate. Atoxyl.

s. arsenate. $Na_2HAsO_4.7H_2O$; colorless, efflorescent crystals, freely soluble in water, also available as exsiccated sodium arsenate. It has been used therapeutically for the effect of arsenic.

s. arsenate solution (*liquor sodii aresenatis*). An aqueous solution of sodium arsenate containing 1 Gm. of Na_2HAsO_4 in each 100 cc. Dose, 0.2–0.3 cc. (3–5 min.).

s. arsenite. Approximately $NaAsO_2$; a white or grayish-white powder, freely soluble in water; an insecticide.

s. ascorbate. $C_6H_7O_6Na$. The sodium salt of ascorbic acid. This salt possesses the activity of ascorbic acid and is used when parenteral therapy is indicated.

s. aurothiomalate. Gold sodium thiomalate. See *myochrysine*.

s. azide. NaN_3. A compound which has inhibiting action on many Gram-negative bacteria and can be used to allow growth of Gram-positive organisms in a mixture.

s. barbital. See *barbital* sodium.

s. benzoate (*sodii benzoas*). $C_6H_5.COONa$. Occurs as a white, granular salt or a crystalline powder; 1 Gm. dissolves in 2 cc. of water and in 50 cc. of a mixture of 47.5 cc. of alcohol and 3.7 cc. of water. Occasionally used in the treatment of rheumatism, either acute or chronic, but less efficient than the salicylates. Also used as a urinary antiseptic, but the ammonium salt is generally preferred. By intravenous injection, it is used as a liver function test. Also used as a food preservative. Dose, 1–2 Gm. (15–30 gr.); intravenously, for liver function test, 20 cc. of solution containing 1.77 Gm. (27 gr.) of sodium benzoate.

s. benzosulfimide. See *saccharin* sodium.

s. biborate. Sodium borate.

s. bicarbonate (*sodii bicarbonas*). $NaHCO_3$. Occurs as a white, crystalline powder; 1 Gm. dissolves in 10 cc. of water; insoluble in alcohol. Used as a mild alkali for the relief of hyperacidity of the stomach, blood, or urine. As a local remedy its solution is used for washing the nose or mouth. A saturated solution is used as an application for minor burns. *In pharmacy*, it is used in the preparation of effervescent salts. Dose, 0.6–4.0 Gm. (10–60 gr.). Syn., *baking soda*.

s. bichromate. Sodium dichromate.

s. biphosphate (*sodii biphosphas*). $NaH_2PO_4.H_2O$. Occurs as colorless crystals or a white, crystalline powder; freely soluble in water but almost insoluble in alcohol. Used for the purpose of increasing the acidity of the urine. Dose, 0.6–2.0 Gm. (10–30 gr.). Also called *s. dihydrogen phosphate, monosodium orthophosphate, s. acid phosphate*.

s. bismuthate. $NaBiO_3$; a yellow to yellowish-brown powder which slowly decomposes, especially in the presence of moisture; a reagent. It has been used in treating syphilis.

s. bismuth iodide. See *s.* iodobismuthite.

s. bismuth thioglycollate. See *thio-bismol*.

s. bismuthyl tartrate. See *bismuth* and sodium tartrate.

s. bisulfate. $NaHSO_4.H_2O$; colorless crystals, very soluble in water; a reagent having many important industrial uses. Syn., *s. acid sulfate*.

s. bisulfite. The substance known by this name, corresponding to the formula $NaHSO_3$, actually has the composition $Na_2S_2O_5$, corresponding to sodium metabisulfite or (International Pharmacopoeia) sodium pyrosulfite; a white, crystalline powder, freely soluble in water. It has been used internally as an antiseptic in gastric fermentation, externally in treatment of parasitic diseases. It prevents oxidative deterioration of certain injections.

s. bitartrate. $NaHC_4H_4O_6.H_2O$; white crystals, freely soluble in water: used as a reagent and in nutrient media. Syn., *sodium acid tartrate*.

s. borate (*sodii boras*). $Na_2B_4O_7.10H_2O$. Occurs as colorless, transparent crystals or white, crystalline powder; 1 Gm. dissolves in 16 cc. of water and in about 1 cc. of glycerin; insoluble in alcohol. Used as a wash for ulcers and abscesses, and for inflammatory conditions of the mucous membranes. Syn., *borax, s. tetraborate*.

s. bromate. $NaBrO_3$; colorless crystals or white granules or powder, freely soluble in water: used as an oxidizing agent.

s. bromide (*sodii bromidum*). NaBr. Occurs as white crystals or a white, crystalline powder; 1 Gm. dissolves in 1.2 cc. of water and 16 cc. of alcohol. Its action and uses are similar to those of potassium bromide. Dose, 0.6–4.0 Gm. (10–60 gr.).

s. cacodylate (*sodii cacodylas*). $Na(CH_3)_2AsO_2.3H_2O$. Sodium dimethylarsonate; occurs as white crystals or a white, crystalline powder; 1 Gm. dissolves in about 0.5 cc. of water and in about 2.5 cc. of alcohol. Like other pentavalent arsenicals, it is changed in the body into the trivalent state and becomes therapeutically active. Its uses are similar to those of arsenic. Its advantages over arsenic lie in its lower toxicity and in that it can be given hypodermically. Dose, 0.016–0.130 Gm. (¼–2 gr.).

s. carbonate. (a) $Na_2CO_3.10H_2O$. Usually in colorless, transparent, efflorescent crystals; soluble in water, insoluble in alcohol. Occasionally used in pharmacy and medicine like monohydrated sodium carbonate. Syn., *soda, washing soda, sal soda*. (b) $Na_2CO_3.H_2O$. Monohydrated sodium carbonate. (c) Na_2CO_3. Anhydrous or exsiccated sodium carbonate, sometimes used like monohydrated sodium carbonate.

s. carboxymethylcellulose. $ROCH_2COONa$, where R represents cellulose; a white to light buff, hygroscopic powder, forming viscous solutions with water; a synthetic hydrophilic colloid gum, used to increase viscosity of aqueous systems, as a protective colloid, and in medicine as a colloid laxative and antacid.

s. cevitamate. Sodium ascorbate.

s. chlorate. $NaClO_3$; colorless crystals or white granules, freely soluble in water; an oxidizing agent and weed killer.

s. chloride (*sodii chloridum*). NaCl. Occurs as colorless crystals or a white, crystalline powder; 1 Gm. dissolves in 2.8 cc. of water; slightly soluble in alcohol. Sodium chloride constitutes the greater part of the inorganic constituents of blood serum and, therefore, is the salt preferred for making solutions isotonic with the blood. Externally, sodium chloride in saturated solution tends to relieve congestion and exudation and is useful in sprains and bruises.

s. chromate. $Na_2CrO_4.4H_2O$; yellow, somewhat deliquescent crystals, very soluble in water: used as a reagent and to protect iron against corrosion and rusting.

s. citrate (*sodii citras*). $Na_3C_6H_5O_7.2H_2O$. Occurs as colorless crystals or a white, crystalline powder; 1 Gm. dissolves in 1.5 cc. of water; insoluble in alcohol. It is used, like potassium citrate, to restore the carbonate reserve of the blood and to overcome excessive acidity of the urine. Also used as a diuretic, expectorant, and sudorific, and as an anticoagulant in the indirect transfusion of blood. Dose, 1–4 Gm. (15–30 gr.).

s. citrate, acid. $C_7H_7O_7Na.H_2O$; monosodium citrate; a white powder, soluble in water, having the uses of sodium citrate, but its solutions are not alkaline in reaction.

s. citrate solution (*liquor sodii citratis*). Each 100 cc. contains 2.75 Gm. of $Na_3C_6H_5O_7.2H_2O$; it is prepared from citric acid 2.0 Gm., sodium bicarbonate 2.5 Gm., and distilled water a sufficient quantity to make 100 cc. Dose, 15 cc. (4 fluidrachms).

s. cobaltinitrite. $Na_3Co(NO_2)_6$; a yellow to

brownish-yellow crystalline powder, very soluble in water; a reagent for detection of potassium.

s. cyanide. NaCN; white granules or fused pieces, freely soluble in water; the aqueous solution is markedly alkaline and quickly decomposes: used as a fumigant and in industry.

s. deficit. A deficit of water and of some electrolytes results if sodium chloride is withdrawn from the diet.

s. dehydrocholate. The sodium salt of dehydrocholic acid; occurs as a fine, colorless, crystalline powder; soluble in water and alcohol. It is useful for its ability to increase the volume of the bile to encourage drainage of the bile ducts for the removal of mucus, inspissated bile, and debris, and to prevent the ascent of infection in these structures. It is also useful in the determination of the arm to tongue circulation time as a diagnostic aid in certain conditions affecting the velocity of the blood flow.

s. dichromate. $Na_2Cr_2O_7.2H_2O$; red, somewhat deliquescent crystals, very soluble in water: used as an oxidizing agent. Syn., *sodium bichromate.*

s. diethylbarbiturate. Barbital sodium.

s. diethyldithiocarbamate. $(C_2H_5)_2N.CS_2Na$; colorless or white crystals, freely soluble in water: used as a reagent for determining small amounts of copper.

s. dihydrogen phosphate. Sodium biphosphate.

s. diphenylhydantoin, s. diphenylhydantoinate. See *diphenylhydantoin sodium.*

s. estrone sulfate. An oral estrogenic hormone.

s. ethoxide. Sodium ethylate.

s. ethylate. C_2H_5ONa; a white or yellowish powder, decomposable by water into sodium hydroxide and alcohol. An alcoholic solution has been used as an escharotic. Syn., *sodium ethoxide.*

s. ethylmercurithiosalicylate. Thimerosal.

s. fluoride. NaF; colorless crystals or white powder, soluble in water: used as an insecticide and for disinfecting fermentation apparatus, preserving wood, and fluoridating drinking water.

s. fluoroacetate. A rodenticide. Also called *compound 1080.*

s. fluosilicate. Sodium silicofluoride.

s. folate. $C_{19}H_{18}N_7NaO_6$; the form in which folic acid is prepared to obtain water-soluble solutions for injection; a yellow to orange-yellow solution having a pH of 8.5 to 11. It has the actions of folic acid.

s. formaldehyde sulfoxylate. $CH_2OHSO_2Na.2H_2O$. Occurs as a white, crystalline powder; soluble in water but sparingly soluble in alcohol. It has been used as an antidote for poisoning by bichloride of mercury.

s. formate. HCOONa; white, deliquescent granules or crystalline powder, freely soluble in water: used in industry and as a reagent; in medicine it has been used as a caustic and astringent.

s. glutamate. Monosodium glutamate.

s. glycerophosphate (*sodii glycerophosphas*). $Na_2C_3H_5(OH)_2PO_4.5\frac{1}{2}H_2O$. Occurs as white, scalelike crystals or a white powder; 1 Gm. dissolves in about 1.5 cc. of water; it is nearly insoluble in alcohol. It has been used as a nerve tonic but clinical evidence shows its usefulness to be slight.

s. glycocholate. The sodium salt of glycocholic acid, usually containing also some sodium taurocholate; a constituent of the bile of man and of herbivora; a white to yellowish powder, hygroscopic, soluble in water: used as a choleretic and cholagogue.

s. gold thiosulfate. Gold sodium thiosulfate.

s. hexametaphosphate. See under *s.* metaphosphate.

s. hydnocarpate. The sodium salts of the fatty acids of chaulmoogra oil; a yellowish powder, soluble in water: used in the treatment of Hansen's disease (leprosy).

s. hydrosulfite. 1. $Na_2S_2O_4$; a white or grayish-white, crystalline powder, very soluble in water: used as a reducing agent. Syn., *sodium sulfoxylate.* 2. $NaHSO_2$; a white powder, soluble in water.

s. hydroxide (*sodii hydroxidum*). NaOH. Occurs as fused masses, small pellets, flakes, or sticks; 1 Gm. dissolves in 1 cc. of water; it is freely soluble in alcohol. Rarely used as an internal remedy. Its most important medicinal use is as a caustic. Its chief use is in various chemical and pharmaceutical manipulations. Syn., *caustic soda.*

s. hypochlorite solution (*liquor sodii hypochloritis*). Contains 5% of NaOCl; occurs as a pale, clear, greenish yellow liquid. This solution possesses the germicidal value of its available chlorine. Used for the disinfection of various utensils which are not injured by its bleaching action, such as clinical thermometers, glass, or china ware. This solution is not suitable for application to wounds. See also diluted *s.* hypochlorite solution.

s. hypophosphite (*sodii hypophosphis*). $NaH_2PO_2.H_2O$. Occurs as white plates or scales or a white powder; 1 Gm. dissolves in about 1 cc. of water; soluble in alcohol. The hypophosphites have been used as tonics, but reliable evidence indicates they are inert. Dose, 0.6–1.3 Gm. (10–20 gr.).

s. hyposulfite. Sodium thiosulfate.

s. indigotindisulfonate (*sodii indigotindisulfonas*). Indigo carmine.

s. iodate. $NaIO_3$; a white, crystalline powder, freely soluble in water. It is an oxidizing agent and has been used locally in treating inflammatory conditions of mucous membranes.

s. iodide (*sodii iodidum*). NaI. Occurs as colorless crystals or a white, crystalline powder; 1 Gm. dissolves in 0.6 cc. of water and about 2 cc. of alcohol. Its uses are practically identical with those of potassium iodide. Dose, 0.3–2.0 Gm. (5–30 gr.).

s. iodoacetate. $CH_2.I.COONa$. See under *iodoacetic acid.*

s. iodobismuthite. A compound formed by the interaction of bismuth chloride and sodium iodide in ethyl acetate solution, consisting essentially of hydrated sodium iodobismuthite, Na_2BiI_5, with inorganic salts. It is claimed that this compound penetrates readily into the cerebrospinal canal, for which reason it has been used in cases of nerve syphilis. Syn., *s. bismuth iodide.*

s. iodohippurate. See *hippuran.*

s. iodomethamate. $C_8H_3I_2NNa_2O_5$; disodium 1-methyl-3,5-diiodo-4-pyridone-2,6-dicarboxylate; a white powder, freely soluble in water: used as a radiopaque medium for urography and retrograde pyelography. Syn., *iodoxyl.* See *neo-iopax.*

s. lactate. $CH_3.CHOH.COONa$. Occurs as a clear or faintly yellow, viscous liquid, containing about 70% of sodium lactate; soluble in water and alcohol. Has been used as a substitute for glycerin in making cataplasm of kaolin. In the form of an injection (see one-sixth molar *sodium* r-lactate), it is administered parenterally in acidosis.

s. lauryl sulfate (*sodii laurylis sulfas*). Chiefly $CH_3(CH_2)_{10}CH_2OSO_3Na$. Occurs as white crystals; soluble in water. Used as a wetting agent and substitute for soap; not affected by hard water. It has been used in treatment of gastric ulcers. See *duponol C.*

s. malate. $Na_2C_4H_4O_5.\frac{1}{2}H_2O$. Occurs as white, granular powder; soluble in water. Because of its salty taste it is used in place of table salt to render food more palatable in salt-free diets.

s. mandelate. $C_6H_5.CHOH.COONa$; a white, crystalline powder, freely soluble in water: used as a urinary antiseptic.

s. metabisulfite. $Na_2S_2O_5$: commonly, though incorrectly, called *sodium bisulfite.*

s. metaphosphate. Any of several salts of the composition $(NaPO_3)_n$, where n is 2 or more; the most common is *sodium hexametaphosphate*, where n is 6. The salts occur as colorless, hygroscopic sticks, or white flakes or powder, soluble in water to form alkaline solutions. Sodium metaphosphates are used as water softeners.

s. molybdate. $Na_2MoO_4.2H_2O$; a white crystalline powder, freely soluble in water: used as a reagent, especially for alkaloids.

s. molybdophosphate. Sodium phosphomolybdate.

s. morrhuate. A mixture of the sodium salts of the saturated and unsaturated fatty acids occurring in cod liver oil; occurs as a pale, yellowish, granular powder; soluble in water. It is a sclerosing agent. It is used in solution with addition of a local anesthetic for the obliteration of varicose veins. Dose, 0.5–1.0 cc. of a 5% solution, injected into the lumen of the vein.

s. nicotinate. $C_5H_4N.COONa.1\frac{1}{2}H_2O$; a white crystalline powder, freely soluble in water. It has the actions and is used for the effects of nicotinic acid, especially when the latter is to be administered by injection.

s. nitrate. $NaNO_3$. Colorless, transparent crystals, white granules or powder; 1 Gm. is soluble in 1.1 cc. of water. Formerly used in the treatment of dysentery. Syn., *Chile saltpeter, soda niter.*

s. nitrite (*sodii nitris*). $NaNO_2$. Occurs as a white to slightly yellow, granular powder; 1 Gm. dissolves in 1.5 cc. of water; sparingly soluble in alcohol. Used to dilate the general arterial system for the purpose of lowering the general blood pressure in hypertension and in cardiac weakness, and to increase secretions from the sweat glands or kidneys. Also used to relieve local spasm in angina pectoris and in Raynaud's syndrome, and to relieve spasms in asthma. Has been found useful in intestinal spasms not caused by inflammatory conditions, and in seasickness. Dose, 0.06–0.2 Gm. (1–3 gr.).

s. nitroferricyanide. $Na_2Fe(CN)_5NO.2H_2O$; ruby-red, transparent crystals, freely soluble in water: used as a reagent for many organic compounds, alkali sulfides, and zinc. Syn., *sodium nitroprusside.*

s. nitroprusside. Sodium nitroferricyanide.

s. oleate. Approximately $C_{17}H_{33}COONa$; a white powder, freely soluble in water: formerly used as a choleretic agent.

s. oxalate. $Na_2C_2O_4$; a white crystalline powder, soluble in water: used as a reagent and industrially.

s. para-aminobenzoate. $NH_2.C_6H_4.COONa$; colorless crystals, freely soluble in water, having the actions and uses of para-aminobenzoic acid.

s. para-aminosalicylate. $NH_2.C_6H_3.OH.COONa.2H_2O$; white to cream-colored, crystalline powder; 1 Gm. dissolves in about 2 cc. of water; solutions decompose slowly. It has the actions and uses of para-aminosalicylic acid. Also called *s. aminosalicylate.*

s. paratoluenesulfonchloramide. See *chloramine-T.*

s. pentothal. See *pentothal sodium.*

s. perborate (*sodii perboras*). $NaBO_3.4H_2O$. Occurs as white, crystalline granules or as a white powder; 1 Gm. dissolves in about 40 cc. of water. It is used for its antiseptic action. It may be employed in solution or as a dusting powder. It is most frequently used for the preparation of mouth washes and dentifrices.

s. perchlorate. $NaClO_4.H_2O$; white deliquescent crystals, very soluble in water: used as a reagent and in explosives.

s. peroxide. Na_2O_2. The sodium compound analogous to hydrogen peroxide; occurs as a white or yellowish powder; it is soluble in water, with decomposition and evolution of heat, forming an alkaline solution and liberating oxygen. A powerful oxidizing agent. Used in acne, applied in the form of a paste prepared with liquid petrolatum, or as a soap to remove comedones. Also called *s. superoxide.*

s. persulfate. $Na_2S_2O_8$; a white crystalline powder, soluble in water: used as an oxidizing agent.

s. phenolsulfonate. $OH.C_6H_4.SO_3Na.2H_2O$; a white crystalline powder, freely soluble in water. It has been used internally and externally for supposed antiseptic action. Syn., *sodium sulfocarbolate.*

s. phosphate (*sodii phosphas*). $Na_2HPO_4.7H_2O$. Occurs as a colorless or white, granular salt; 1 Gm. dissolves in 4 cc. of water; it is very slightly soluble in alcohol. Used as a mild saline cathartic and has a less disagreeable taste than magnesium or sodium sulfate. Dose, 4–15 Gm. (1–4 dr.). Also called *dibasic s. phosphate, disodium hydrogen phosphate.*

s. phosphate solution (*liquor sodii phosphatis*). Contains exsiccated sodium phosphate 400 Gm., citric acid 130 Gm., glycerin 150 cc., distilled water a sufficient quantity to make 1000 cc. This solution affords a convenient way of administering sodium phosphate. Dose, 4–12 cc. (1–3 fluidrachms).

s. phosphomolybdate. $Na_3PO_4.12MoO_3$; white crystals, freely soluble in water: used as a reagent in various chemical determinations. Syn., *sodium molybdophosphate.*

s. phosphotungstate. $2Na_2O.P_2O_5.12WO_3.18H_2O$; white crystals, freely soluble in water: used as a reagent in various chemical determinations.

s. potassium bismuthyl tartrate. A basic water-soluble sodium potassium bismuth tartrate; occurs as a white, heavy powder. Used as a means of obtaining the systemic effects of bismuth in the treatment of syphilis.

s. propionate (*sodii propionas*). CH_3CH_2COONa. Occurs as colorless crystals or a granular powder; 1 Gm. dissolves in about 1 cc. of water and in about 24 cc. of alcohol. This salt has been shown to possess antibacterial and fungicidal properties; used in the control of athlete's foot, tinea cruris, and other mycoses.

s. psylliate. The sodium salt of the liquid fatty acids of psyllium oil (plantago-seed oil), available as an aqueous solution, commonly of 5% concentration: used as a sclerosing agent for obliteration of varicose veins. See *sylnasol.*

s. pyrophosphate. $Na_4P_2O_7.10H_2O$; white granules or colorless crystals, soluble in water: used for removing rust stains, in industry, and has been used as a laxative.

s. pyrosulfite. The International Pharmacopoeia name for sodium metabisulfite: commonly, though incorrectly, known as *sodium bisulfite.*

s. rhodanate. Sodium thiocyanate.

s. ricinate. A mixture of the sodium salts of the fatty acids from castor oil, chiefly ricinoleic; occurs as a white or yellowish powder; soluble in water and in alcohol. This compound has the property of detoxifying bacterial toxins and is used in various types of intestinal intoxication. Dose, 0.3 Gm. (5 gr.) t.i.d. Also called *s. ricinoleate, s. oleoricinate.*

s. salicylate (*sodii salicylas*). $C_6H_4.OH.COONa$. Occurs as a white, microcrystalline powder; it has not more than a faint pink tinge; 1 Gm. dissolves in 1 cc. of water and in 10 cc. of alcohol. Its actions and uses are those of salicylic acid, except that it is not locally irritating and is more rapidly absorbed. It is used as an antirheumatic, antipyretic, and analgesic. It has also been recommended as a sclerosing agent in the treatment of varicose veins. Dose, 0.6–2.0 Gm. (10–30 gr.).

s. silicate. Any of several compounds representing combinations of Na_2O and SiO_2, as Na_2SiO_3, $Na_6Si_2O_7$, and $Na_2Si_3O_7$, with variable amounts of water. They occur as colorless to white or grayish-white crystal-like pieces or lumps, insoluble or very slightly soluble in cold water, but dissolved by heating with water under pressure. The common sodium silicate solution contains about 40% $Na_2Si_3O_7$. It is used as a dressing in fractures, as a detergent, fireproofing and waterproofing material, and in industry.

s. silicofluoride. Na_2SiF_6; a white, granular powder, slightly soluble in water: used as a source of fluoride in fluoridation of municipal water supplies, and as an insecticide and rodenticide and in industry. Also called *s. fluosilicate.*

s. silver arsphenamine. Silver arsphenamine.

s. stearate (*sodii stearas*). A mixture of varying proportions of sodium stearate ($NaC_{18}H_{35}O_2$) and sodium palmitate ($NaC_{16}H_{31}O_2$). Occurs as a fine, white powder; it is slightly soluble in cold water and alcohol, but readily soluble when these solvents are hot. Used in the preparation of glycerin suppositories.

s. stibogluconate. A pentavalent antimony derivative, of indefinite composition, prepared by interaction of a pentavalent inorganic antimony compound, gluconic acid, and sodium hydroxide; a colorless powder, soluble in water: used in the treatment of leishmaniasis. See *pentostam, solustibosan.*

s. succinate. $COONa.CH_2.CH_2.COONa$; a white, crystalline or granular powder, freely soluble in water. It has been variously used in medicine, e.g., to awaken patients after barbiturate anesthesia.

s. sulfate (*sodii sulfas*). $Na_2SO_4.10H_2O$. Occurs as large, colorless, transparent crystals or a granular powder; 1 Gm. dissolves in 1.5 cc. of water; insoluble in alcohol. In large doses it is an efficient hydragogue cathartic; in smaller doses it is aperient and diuretic. Dose, 8–30 Gm. (2 dr.–1 oz.). Also called *Glauber's salt.*

s. sulfide. $Na_2S.9H_2O$; colorless, deliquescent crystals, very soluble in water to form a strongly alkaline solution: used as a reagent and for many industrial purposes.

s. sulfite. $Na_2SO_3.7H_2O$; colorless, efflorescent crystals, freely soluble in water, prepared also in anhydrous form. It has been used for treatment of parasitic skin diseases and widely in industry, chiefly because of its reducing property.

s. sulfocarbolate. Sodium phenolsulfonate.

s. sulfocyanate. Sodium thiocyanate.

s. sulfoxylate. Sodium hydrosulfite, 1.

s. superoxide. Sodium peroxide.

s. tartrate. $Na_2C_4H_4O_6.2H_2O$; white crystals or granules, freely soluble in water: formerly used as a laxative.

s. taurocholate. The sodium salt of taurocholic acid, usually containing also some sodium glycocholate; a constituent of the bile of carnivora; a yellowish-gray powder, soluble in water: used as a choleretic and cholagogue.

s. tetraborate. Sodium borate.

s. tetradecyl sulfate. $C_{14}H_{29}SO_4Na$; a white, waxy solid, soluble in water: variously used as a wetting agent.

s. thiocyanate (*sodii thiocyanas*). NaSCN. Occurs as white or colorless crystals; it is hygroscopic; 1 Gm. dissolves in about 0.7 cc. of water and in about 4 cc. of alcohol. Used in hypertension. Dose, 0.06–0.3 Gm. (1–5 gr.). Syn., *s. sulfocyanate, s. rhodanate.*

s. thiosulfate (*sodii thiosulfas*). $Na_2S_2O_3.5H_2O$. Occurs as large, colorless crystals or a coarse, crystalline powder; 1 Gm. dissolves in 0.5 cc. of water; insoluble in alcohol. Intravenously it is used against the late toxic action of arsphenamine. Also used as an antidote in other metallic poisons. Has also been used, internally, in the treatment of nonarsenical skin diseases such as eczema and urticaria. Dose, 0.6–2.0 Gm. (10–30 gr.), larger doses are used in mercuric chloride poisoning; intravenously, 0.5–1.0 Gm. (8–15 gr.) in about a 3% solution, injected slowly, once a day. Also called *s. hyposulfite.*

s. tungstate. $Na_2WO_4.2H_2O$; a white, crystalline powder or colorless crystals, freely soluble in water: used as a reagent, especially to precipitate alkaloids, and in industry.

sulfobromophthalein s. (*sulfobromophthaleinum sodicum*). $C_{20}H_8Br_4O_{10}S_2Na_2$. The disodium salt of phenoltetrabromophthalein disulfonic acid; occurs as a white, crystalline powder; soluble in water but insoluble in alcohol. In aqueous solution (sulfobromophthalein sodium injection) it is used as a test of the functional capacity of the liver. Dose, 2 mg. per kilo of body weight. Also called *bromtetragnost.* See also *bromsulphalein.*

tribasic s. phosphate. $Na_3PO_4.12H_2O$. Occurs as colorless or white crystals; soluble in water, insoluble in alcohol. This sodium salt of phosphoric acid is not used medicinally, but has many industrial uses.

so′do·ku (so′do·kōō, so·do′kōō). See rat-bite *fever.*

sod′om·ist. See *sodomite.*

sod′om·ite [*Sodom*]. One who practices sodomy. Syn., *sodomist.*

sod′om·y [*Sodom*]. 1. Sexual intercourse by the anus, usually considered as between males. See also *pederasty.* 2. Bestiality, 2.

so·do′sha. See rat-bite *fever.*

Soemmering, Samuel Thomas [*German anatomist,* 1755–1830]. Classified the cranial nerves (1778). Said to have been the first to describe achondroplasia (1791). The marginal process of the zygomatic bone is called *Soemmering's bone.* The fovea centralis is called *Soemmering's foramen.* The substantia nigra is called *Soemmering's ganglion.* The suspensory ligament of the lacrimal gland is called *Soemmering's ligament.* The pudendal nerve is called *Soemmering's nerve.* The macula lutea is called *Soemmering's spot.*

sof′ten·ing [AS. *sōfte*]. The act of becoming less cohesive, firm, or resistant.

anemic s. Disintegration and liquefaction of the brain substance from lack of blood supply.

colliquative s. Condition in which the affected tissues liquefy.

gray s. An inflammatory softening of the brain or cord with a gray discoloration.

green s. A purulent softening of nervous matter.

hemorrhagic s. The softening of parts involved in a hemorrhage.

mucoid s. Myxomatous degeneration.

red s. That of the brain when hemorrhage accompanies the ischemic softening, and the products of disintegration of the blood mingle with the nerve substance, giving it a red hue.

s. of the bones. Osteomalacia.

s. of the brain. Encephalomalacia.

s. of the heart. Myomalacia cordis.

s. of the spinal cord. Various stages in myelitis.

s. of the stomach. Gastromalacia, consequent upon highly acid contents with a feeble circulation in the walls, but usually a post-mortem phenomenon.

white s. Softening of nerve substance in which the affected area presents a whitish color due to fatty degeneration following anemia.

so′ja bean (so′yah, so′jah). See *soybean.*

so·ko′sho. See rat-bite *fever.*

sol. 1. A colloidal solution. A sol consists of a suitable dispersion medium, which may be gas, liquid, or solid, and the colloidal substance, the disperse phase, which is distributed throughout the dispersion medium. The disperse phase may be gas, liquid, or solid. To indicate the nature of the dispersion medium a prefix is often added, thus, hydrosol, alcosol, aerosol. 2. Abbreviation for solution.

Sol″a·na′ce·ae [L. *solanum,* nightshade]. A family of herbs, shrubs, and trees comprising approximately 75 genera and 1,800 species and including the potato and tomato plants, and also plants from which are derived such drugs as belladonna, hyoscyamus, scopola, and stramonium. —**solana′ceous,** *adj.*

so·lan′i·dine (so·lan′i·deen, ·din). $C_{27}H_{43}NO$; the alkaloidal aglycone, having a steroid structure, obtained by hydrolysis of solanine. Syn., *solatubine.*

so·lan′i·dine-S. Solasodine.

sol′a·nine (sol′uh·neen, ·nin, so′luh·). $C_{45}H_{73}NO_{15}$; a glycosidal alkaloid from *Solanum tuberosum,* the potato, and other *Solanum* species. On hydrolysis it yields glucose, galactose, rhamnose, and the steroidal aglycone solanidine. Syn., *solatunine.*

sol′a·nine-S. Solasonine.

So·la′num [L., nightshade]. A genus of the Solanaceae, including the tomato, potato, bittersweet, and black nightshade.

so·lap′sone. British generic name for the agent, used in the treatment of leprosy, supplied under the trade-mark *sulphetrone.*

solargentum. Trade-mark for a brand of mild silver protein.

so″lar·i·za′tion [L. *solaris,* of the sun]. The application of solar or electric light for therapeutic purposes. —**so′larize,** *v.*

so′lar plex′us. Celiac plexus.

solarson. Trade-mark for ammonium heptenchlorarsonate, $CH_3(CH_2)_4CCl{:}CH.AsO.OH.ONH_4$, a brand of chlorarsenol: used as a substitute for arsenous oxide in the treatment of anemia, skin disease, malaria, and neuroses.

so·las′o·dine. $C_{27}H_{43}NO_2$; the alkaloidal aglycone, having a steroid structure, obtained by hydrolysis of solasonine. Syn., *solanidine-S.*

so·las′o·nine. $C_{45}H_{73}NO_{16}$; a glycosidal alkaloid from certain *Solanum* species. On hydrolysis it yields glucose, galactose, rhamnose, and the steroidal aglycone solasodine. Syn., *solanine-S.*

so·la′tion. Conversion of a gel into a sol.

so″la·tu′bine. Solanidine.

so″la·tu′nine. Solanine.

so″laur·ic′i·dine. $C_{27}H_{43}NO_2$; the alkaloidal aglycone, having a steroid structure, obtained by hydrolysis of solauricine.

so·laur′i·cine. $C_{45}H_{73}NO_{16}.2H_2O$; a glycosidal alkaloid from *Solanum auriculatum,* violet nightshade. On hydrolysis it yields glucose, rhamnose, galactose, and the aglycone solauricidine.

solbrol. Trade-mark for methyl parahydroxybenzoate. See *methylparaben.*

sol′dier's heart. See neurocirculatory *asthenia.*

sole [L. *solea,* sole]. The plantar surface of the foot.

So″le·nog′ly·pha [G. *sōlēn,* channel; *glyphein,* to engrave]. One of the two groups of the important venomous snakes, includes the family Crotalidae (pit vipers) and Viperidae (true vipers).

sole-plate. End-plate.

Solera reaction. See under *reaction.*

so′le·us, so·le′us [L. *solea,* sole]. A flat muscle of the calf. See Table of Muscles in the Appendix.

s. accessorius. A small anomalous muscle running from the head of the fibula to the medial surface of the calcaneus.

solganal. Trade-mark for a suspension in oil of aurothioglucose.

sol′id [L. *solidus*]. 1. Firm; dense; not fluid or gaseous. 2. Not hollow.

so·lid″i·fi·ca′tion [*solidus;* L. *facere,* to make]. The act of becoming solid.

sol′i·ped [L. *solus,* alone; *pes,* foot]. An animal having a solid, undivided hoof, as the horse, donkey, zebra.

sol′ip·sism [*solus;* L. *ipse,* self]. The doctrine that any organism can know only itself and its own conception of its environment.

sol′i·tar″y [L. *solitarius*]. Single; existing separately; not collected together, as solitary fasciculus, a strand of nerve fibers in the medulla, the central processes of the sensory fibers of the seventh, ninth, and tenth cranial nerves; and solitary follicles, minute lymphatic nodules in the mucous membrane of the intestine.

Sollmann, Torald Hermann [*American pharmacologist,* 1874–]. Known for his *Manual of Pharmacology* (1917–48). Described the carotid sinus depressor reflex (1912).

sol′-lu′nar [L. *sol,* sun; *luna,* moon]. Influenced by, or relating to, the sun and the moon.

Sol·pu′gi·da [L. *solpuga,* a venomous spider]. An order of the Arachnida which are hairy and spiderlike in external appearance but in structure show closer relationship to the scorpions. They lack poison glands, but have powerful fangs capable of inflicting severe wounds that are liable to secondary infections. They live in warm countries in sandy regions, as in the southwestern United States.

sol″u·bil′i·ty [L. *solubilis,* that may be loosed]. The extent to which a substance (solute) dissolves in a liquid (solvent) to produce a homogeneous system (solution). The degree of solubility is the concentration of a saturated solution at a given temperature.

s. product. The product of the concentrations of the ions of a solute, each raised to the power of the number of such ions in a molecule of the solute, in a saturated solution of the substance. Also called *precipitation value.*

sol′u·ble [*solubilis*]. Capable of mixing with a liquid (dissolving) to form a homogeneous mixture (solution).

s. gluside. Saccharin sodium.

s. saccharin. Saccharin sodium.

so′lum tym′pa·ni (tim′puh·nigh) [L.]. The floor of the tympanic cavity.

sol″u·sep′ta·sine (sol″yoo·sep′tuh·seen, ·sin). Disodium-*p*-(γ-phenylpropylamino)-benzenesulfonamide-α,γ-disulfonate, a white, crystalline powder, soluble in water. It is used, by intravenous injection, in scarlet fever and streptococcal tonsillitis; locally, in the treatment of varicose ulcers, skin infections, and infected wounds.

solustibosan. Trade-mark for *sodium stibogluconate.*

sol′ute (sol′yōōt, so′lute, so·lute′). The dissolved substance in a solution.

so·lu′tion [L. *solutio*, a loosing]. 1. A homogeneous mixture of a solid, liquid, or gaseous substance (the solute) in a liquid (the solvent) from which the dissolved substance can be recovered by crystallization or other physical processes. The formation of a solution is not accompanied by permanent chemical change, and is thus commonly considered a physical phenomenon. For solutions not defined here, see qualifying word. Abbreviated, sol. 2. *In physical chemistry,* any homogeneous phase consisting of two or more compounds.

alkaline aromatic s. (*liquor aromaticus alkalinus*). Contains potassium bicarbonate 20 Gm., sodium borate 20 Gm., thymol 0.5 Gm., eucalyptol 1 cc., methyl salicylate 0.5 cc., amaranth solution 14 cc., alcohol 50 cc., glycerin 100 cc., purified water a sufficient quantity to make 1000 cc. It occurs as a clear, bright red liquid, is used as a wash for the nasal or pharyngeal cavities, and as a pleasant mouth wash.

Alsever's s. A blood-preservative mixture used in blood banks, containing trisodium citrate, citric acid, sodium chloride, sucrose, and water.

ammoniacal silver nitrate s. (*liquor argenti nitratis ammoniacalis*). An aqueous solution of silver diammino nitrate. Prepared from silver nitrate 70.4 Gm., purified water 24.5 cc., strong ammonia solution about 68 cc., to make about 100 cc. Occurs as a clear, colorless, almost odorless liquid. Used by dentists to deposit silver in exposed dentin or to fill up minute crevices in the teeth. After application of the solution it should be followed by some reducing agent, as eugenol or formaldehyde, to cause the precipitation of the metallic silver. Also called *Howe's ammoniacal silver nitrate.*

Benedict's s. A solution containing an easily reduced copper salt; used for the determination of glucose.

Bielschowsky-Maresch diammine silver s. See under *stain.*

buffer s. A solution prepared from a weak acid and a salt of the weak acid, or a weak base and a salt of the weak base, which resists any appreciable change in pH on the addition of small amounts of acid or alkali or by dilution with water.

Burow's s. Aluminum acetate solution.

Butler's s. A hypotonic solution of the electrolytes of plasma, containing 30 mEq./L sodium, 25 mEq./L chloride, 20 mEq./L potassium, 20 mEq./L lactate, and 5 mEq./L phosphorus.

Cajal's gold-sublimate s. *Stock solution A:* Gold chloride (brown or yellow crystals) 1 Gm., distilled water 100 cc. *Stock solution B:* $HgCl_2$ 5 Gm., distilled water at 60° C. 100 cc. To use, mix 5 cc. of solution A, 5 cc. of solution B, and 30 cc. of distilled water.

chlorinated soda s. (*liquor sodae chlorinatae*). A solution of sodium hypochlorite containing 2.5% of available chlorine; used as a disinfectant and antiseptic. Also called *Labarraque's s.* See *sodium* hypochlorite solution.

colloidal s. A macroscopically homogeneous system consisting of either single, large molecules or aggregations of smaller molecules (the dispersed phase) suspended in a liquid (the continuous phase). Colloidal dispersions are frequently called sols.

Darrow's s. A solution of the electrolytes of plasma, containing added amounts of potassium, used in fluid therapy. It contains 122 mEq./L sodium, 104 mEq./L chloride, 35 mEq./L potassium, and 53 mEq./L lactate.

Dobell's s. See compound *sodium* borate solution.

Fehling's s. A solution containing an easily reduced copper salt; used for the determination of glucose.

Fowler's s. Potassium arsenite solution.

G s. A buffered acid solution (pH 4) used in the dissolution of urinary calculi and incrustations.

Gower's s. A dilution fluid used in the erythrocyte count, made up of 12.5 Gm. sodium sulfate and 33.3 ml. glacial acetic acid dissolved in 200 ml. distilled water. It is superior to Hayem's solution because it prevents rouleaux formation and will not cause protein to precipitate in cases of hyperglobulinemia.

Hayem's s. See Georges *Hayem.*

hypertonic s. A solution which produces a change in the tone of a tissue immersed in it through passage of water from the tissue into the solution. With reference to erythrocytes, a hypertonic solution of sodium chloride is one which contains more than 0.9 Gm. of sodium chloride in each 100 cc.

hypotonic s. A solution which produces a change in the tone of a tissue immersed in it through passage of water from the solution into the tissue. With reference to erythrocytes, a hypotonic solution of sodium chloride is one which contains less than 0.9 Gm. of sodium chloride in each 100 cc.

isohydric s. A solution having the same hydrogen-ion concentration as another so that no change in the concentration of this ion takes place when the solutions are mixed.

isosmotic s. A solution which has the same osmotic pressure as that of a selected reference solution: commonly accepted as synonymous with *isotonic solution* but the two are identical only when there is no diffusion of solute across the membrane of a tissue immersed in the solution. Also spelled *isoosmotic s.*

isotonic s. A solution which causes no change in the tone of a tissue, such as erythrocytes, immersed in the solution. In the absence of solute diffusing through the tissue membrane, a solution which is isotonic is isosmotic with the fluid phase of the tissue.

Labarraque's s. Chlorinated soda solution.

Locke-Ringer's s. Sodium chloride 9 Gm.; potassium chloride 0.42 Gm.; calcium chloride 0.24 Gm.; magnesium chloride 0.2 Gm.; sodium bicarbonate 0.5 Gm.; dextrose 0.5 Gm.; water, recently distilled, to make 1000 cc.

M s. A buffered acid solution (pH 4.4) used in the dissolution of urinary calculi and incrustations.

MIF stain-preservative s. A solution composed of tincture of *m*erthiolate, Lugol's *i*odine, and *f*ormaldehyde: used as a stain and preservative of fecal material for identification of intestinal protozoa.

modified Dakin's s. Diluted sodium hypochlorite solution. See under *sodium.*

molal s. A solution which contains one gram-molecular weight or mole of reagent dissolved in 1000 Gm. of solvent.

molar s. A solution which contains a gram-molecular weight or mole of reagent in 1000 cc. of solution.

Monsel's s. Ferric subsulfate solution.

N.F. antiseptic s. (*liquor antisepticus N.F.*). Contains boric acid 25 Gm.; thymol, chlorothymol, and menthol 0.5 Gm. each; eucalyptol 0.1 cc.; methyl salicylate 0.2 cc.; thyme oil 0.01 cc.; alcohol 300 cc.; purified water a sufficient quantity to make 1000 cc. Occurs as a clear, colorless liquid Used as a mouth wash.

normal oxidizing s. A solution containing sufficient oxidizing agent per liter to increase the positive valence or decrease the negative valence of a gram-formula weight of reducing agent by one.

normal reducing s. The opposite of normal oxidizing solution.

normal saline s. See isotonic *sodium* chloride solution.

normal salt s. See isotonic *sodium* chloride solution.

normal s. One containing one gram-equivalent weight of reagent in 1000 cc. of solution.

physiological salt s. Isotonic sodium chloride solution.

Ringer's s. (*liquor Ringeri*). Contains sodium chloride 8.6 Gm., potassium chloride 0.30 Gm., calcium chloride 0.33 Gm., and purified water a sufficient quantity to make 1000 cc. Used in all forms of dehydration but particularly in cases in which loss of gastrointestinal secretions has resulted from vomiting, diarrhea, or fistulas when sodium, potassium, and calcium have been diminished. Also used in acidosis or alkalosis for improvement of circulation and stimulation of renal activity. Also called *isotonic solution of three chlorides.* When prepared with water for injection for parenteral administration it is called *Ringer's injection.*

Rosenheim's iodopotassium iodide s. Dissolve 272 Gm. of potassium iodide in water and add 80 Gm. of bismuth subnitrate dissolved in 200 Gm. of nitric acid (sp. gr. 1.18). Permit the potassium nitrate to crystallize out, then filter it off and make the filtrate up to 1 liter with water.

saturated s. One that normally contains the maximum amount of substance able to be dissolved. Abbreviated, sat. sol.

seminormal s. A solution which contains one-half of an equivalent weight of the active reagent in grams, in one liter of solution. It is written 0.5N or N/2.

soda and mint s. (*liquor sodae et menthae*). Contains sodium bicarbonate 50 Gm., aromatic ammonia spirit 20 cc., spearmint water or peppermint water a sufficient quantity to make 1000 cc. Used occasionally as a mild gastric antacid. Dose, 8–15 cc. (2–4 fluidrachms).

s. pressure. The tendency of the molecules or ions to leave the surface of a solute and pass into the solvent. It varies in different solute-solvent combinations.

standard s. One that contains a definite amount of substance, as a molar or normal solution.

Suby's s. See G *s.*

sulfurated lime s. (*liquor calcis sulfuratae*). Prepared from lime 165 Gm., sublimed sulfur 250 Gm., water a sufficient quantity to make 1000 cc. Occurs as a clear, brownish red liquid, with a slight odor of hydrogen sulfide. Used as a means of obtaining the action of the sulfides in the treatment of various skin diseases. It should be diluted with from five to ten volumes of water before using. Also called *Vleminckx's solution, Vleminckx's lotion.*

supersaturated s. One that contains a greater quantity of solid than can normally be dissolved at a given temperature. It is an unstable system.

Takayama s. A mixture of 3 ml. of 10% NaOH, 3 ml. of pyridine, 3 ml. of saturated solution of glucose, and 7 ml. of water. The solution works rapidly in the cold if at least 24 hours old. With a fresh solution, warming or more time is necessary.

test s. A reagent solution. Abbreviated, T. S.

Tyrode s. A solution containing sodium chloride 8 Gm., calcium chloride 0.2 Gm., potassium chloride 0.2 Gm., sodium bicarbonate 1 Gm., glucose 1 Gm., magnesium chloride 0.1 Gm., sodium diphosphate 0.05 Gm., and distilled water to make 1000 cc.

volumetric s. A standard solution containing 1, ½, ⅒, etc., gram-equivalent of a substance in 1000 cc. of solution. Used in volumetric analysis. Abbreviated, V. S.

sol'vate. A compound formed between solute and solvent in a solution.

sol·va'tion. The process of forming a solvate.

sol'vent. 1. That component of a homogeneous mixture which is in excess. 2. A liquid which dissolves another substance (solute), without any change in chemical composition, as sugar or salt in water. 3. A liquid which reacts chemically with a solid and brings it into solution, as acids which dissolve metals.

so'ma [G.]. 1. The entire body with the exclusion of the germ cells. 2. A term used loosely for the body without the limbs. —**somal,** *adj.*

som'a·lin. A cardiac glycoside from the root of *Adenium somalense.* It may be hydrolyzed to digitoxigenin and cymarose.

so"mas·the'ni·a [G. *sōma*, body; *astheneia*, weakness]. Old term for bodily deterioration and exhaustion.

so"ma·tes·the'si·a (so"muh·tess·thee'zhuh, ·zee·uh) [*sōma;* G. *aisthēsis*, perception]. Bodily sensation, the consciousness of the body.

so·mat'ic [G. *sōmatikos*, of the body]. 1. Pertaining to the body. 2. Pertaining to the framework of the body and not to the viscera, as the somatic musculature, the muscles of the body wall or somatopleure, as distinguished from those of the splanchnopleure, the splanchnic musculature.

so·mat"i·co·splanch'nic (·splank'nick). See *somaticovisceral.*

so·mat"i·co·vis'cer·al [*sōmatikos;* L. *viscera*, internal organs]. Relating to the body and the viscera.

so'ma·tist [G. *sōma*, body]. A psychiatrist who regards any psychoneurosis or psychosis as of physical origin.

so"ma·ti·za'tion. *In psychiatry*, a psychoneurotic displacement of emotional conflicts onto muscles and sensory apparatus innervated by the voluntary nervous system, in distinction from *psychosomatic reaction*, in which displacement occurs onto organs and viscera innervated by the autonomic nervous system; a conversion reaction. See also *psychophysiologic autonomic and visceral disorders.*

so·mat'o·chrome", so'mat·o·chrome" [*sōma;* G. *chrōma*, color]. Term applied by Nissl to a group of nerve cells possessing a well-defined cell body completely surrounding the nucleus on all sides, the cytoplasm having a distinct contour, and readily taking a stain.

so"ma·to·did'y·mus [*sōma;* G. *didymos*, twin]. Conjoined twins united by their trunks.

so"ma·to·dym'i·a [*sōma; didymos*]. A general term for union of the trunks of conjoined twins.

so"ma·tog'e·ny (so"muh·todj'i·nee) [*sōma;* G. *genesthai*, from *gignesthai*, to be produced]. The acquirement of bodily characters, especially the acquirement of characters due to environment. —**somatogen'ic,** *adj.*

so"ma·tol'o·gy [*sōma;* G. *logos*, word]. The study of the development, structure, and functions of the body. —**somatolog'ic,** *adj.*

so'ma·tome [*sōma;* G. *tomos*, cutting]. 1. A transverse segment of an organized body; a somite. 2. An embryotome. *O.T.* —**somatom'ic,** *adj.*

so"ma·to·meg'a·ly [*sōma;* G. *megas*, large]. Gigantism.

so"ma·tom'e·try [*sōma;* G. *metron*, a measure]. Measurement of the human body with the soft parts intact. —**somatomet'ric,** *adj.*

so"ma·top'a·gus [*sōma;* G. *pagos*, that which is fixed]. Conjoined twins with their trunks more or less in common.

so″ma·to·path′ic [*sōma;* G. *pathos,* disease]. Disordered in body.

so′ma·to·plasm″ (so′muh·to·plaz″um, so·mat′o·) [*sōma;* G. *plasma,* anything formed]. The protoplasm of the body cells; that form of living matter which composes the mass of the body, as distinguished from germ plasm, which composes the reproductive cells.

so′ma·to·pleure″ (so′muh·to·ploor″, so·mat′o·) [*sōma;* G. *pleura,* rib]. The body wall composed of ectoderm and somatic mesoderm, as contrasted with splanchnopleure. —**somatopleur′al,** *adj.*

so″ma·to·psy′chic (so″muh·to·sigh′kick) [*sōma;* G. *psychē,* soul]. Pertaining to both the body and mind.

somatose. Trade-mark for an artificially digested meat albumin containing deutero- and hetero-albuminoses and peptone; the substance occurs as a yellowish powder; soluble in water.

so″ma·to·splanch″no·pleu′ric (·splank″no-ploor′ick) [*sōma;* G. *splagchnon,* inner parts; *pleura,* rib]. Relating to the somatopleure and the splanchnopleure.

so″ma·to·to′ni·a [*sōma;* G. *tonos,* tension]. The behavioral counterpart of component II (mesomorphy) of the somatotype, manifested in desire for expenditure of energy through vigorous bodily assertiveness and the enjoyment of muscular activity. —**somatoton′ic,** *adj.*

so″ma·to·top″ag·no′si·a. Inability to identify or orient the body or its parts. There may be loss of identification of and amnesia for a limb or other body part, or of one half of the body. *Autotopagnosia* is a special form. The condition occurs in lesions of the thalamoparietal pathways or the cortex at the subparietal sulcus.

so″ma·to·top′ic. Pertaining to the correspondence between a body part and a particular area of the cerebral cortex, or other region of the brain, to which sensory pathways from the body part are projected, or from which motor pathways to the part take origin.

so″ma·to·trid′y·mus [*sōma;* G. *tridymos,* three-fold]. A monster with three trunks or bodies.

so″ma·to·tro′phin. See *somatotropin.*

so″ma·to·tro′pin [*soma;* G. *tropos,* turn, turning]. The growth hormone: formerly spelled *somatotrophin.*

so′ma·to·type″ [*sōma;* G. *typos,* impression]. The body type; the quantitative description of the morphological structure of an individual by a series of three numerals representing the primary components: I. *endomorphy;* II. *mesomorphy;* III. *ectomorphy.* On the behavioral level, these are termed *viscerotonia, somatotonia,* and *cerebrotonia.* See also *aplasia,* 2, *dysmorphic, dysplasia, gynandromorphy,* t *component.*

midrange s. Any individual whose somatotype includes only the midrange numerical evaluation of the three primary components: also called *midranger.*

Somers method. See Sumner-Somers *method.*

so″mes·the′si·a (so″mess·thee′zhuh, ·zee·uh) [*sōma;* G. *aisthēsis,* perception]. Sensibility to bodily sensations.

so″mes·thet′ic [*sōma;* G. *aisthētikos,* of perception]. Pertaining to proprioceptive and tactile sensation, as the somesthetic area of the parietal cortex, Brodmann's areas 1,2,3.

so″mes·the″tog·no′sis. Somesthesia.

so″mes·the″to·psy′chic (·sigh′kick) [*sōma; aisthētikos;* G. *psychē,* soul]. Pertaining to the somesthetic association area of the parietal cortex, Brodmann's areas 5, 7.

so′mite [*sōma*]. A segment of the body of an embryo; one of a series of paired segments of the paraxial mesoderm composed of dermatome, myotome, and sclerotome. —**somit′ic,** *adj.*

occipital s. Three or four indistinct somites in the occipital region, part of which form the tongue muscles innervated by the hypoglossal nerve.

preotic s. Condensation of mesenchyme that forms the eye muscles; believed to represent head somites.

som·nam′bu·lance. See *somnambulism.*

som·nam″bu·la′tion. See *somnambulism.*

som·nam′bu·lism [L. *somnus,* sleep; *ambulare,* to walk]. 1. Sleepwalking; a condition in which the individual walks during sleep. 2. The type of hypnotic sleep in which the subject is possessed of all his senses, often having the appearance of one awake, but his consciousness is under the control of the hypnotizer.

som·nam·bu·lis′me pro·vo·qué′ (sohm·nam-bew·leess′muh pro·vo·kay′. *See* Notes § 35) [F.]. Sleepwalking induced by hypnotism.

som·nam′bu·list [*somnus; ambulare*]. One who walks in his sleep: also called *somnambulator.*

som′ni·al [L. *somnialis,* dream-bringing]. Relating to dreams. *Rare.*

som″ni·a′tion [L. *somniare,* to dream]. Dreaming. *Obs.*

som′ni·a″tive [*somniare*]. Somnial. *Rare.*

som·nic′u·lous [L. *somniculosus,* sleepy]. Drowsy; sleepy. *Obs.*

som″ni·fa′cient [L. *somnus,* sleep; *facere,* to make]. A medicine producing sleep; a hypnotic. —**somnifa′cient,** *adj.*

som·nif′er·ous [*somnus;* L. *ferre,* to bring]. Producing sleep.

som·nif′ic [*somnus;* L. *facere,* to make]. Causing sleep.

som·nif′u·gous [*somnus;* L. *fugere,* to flee]. Driving away sleep.

som·nil′o·quence. See *somniloquism.*

som·nil′o·quism [*somnus;* L. *loqui,* to speak]. The act of talking during sleep.

som·nil′o·quist [*somnus; loqui*]. One given to talking during sleep.

som·nil′o·quy [*somnus; loqui*]. Talking in one's sleep.

som·nip′a·thist [*somnus;* G. *pathos,* disease]. One affected by somnipathy.

som·nip′a·thy [*somnus; pathos*]. 1. Any disorder of sleep. 2. Hypnotic somnambulism.

som″no·cin″e·mat′o·graph [*somnus;* G. *kinēma,* movement; *graphein,* to write]. Apparatus for recording, experimentally, movements made during sleep.

som′no·form [*somnus;* L. *forma,* form]. An anesthetic consisting of ethyl chloride 60%, methyl chloride 35%, methyl bromide 5%.

som′no·lence [L. *somnulentia,* sleepiness]. A condition of drowsiness or sleep. —**som′nolent,** *adj.*

som″no·len′ti·a (som″no·len′shee·uh) [L. *somnulentia,* sleepiness]. 1. Sleep-drunkenness, a condition of incomplete sleep in which a part of the faculties are abnormally excited, while the others are in repose. 2. Somnolence.

som″no·les′cent [L. *somnus,* sleep]. 1. Drowsy. 2. Inducing drowsiness.

som′no·lism [*somnus*]. Hypnotism.

som·nop′a·thist. See *somnipathist.*

som·nop′a·thy. See *somnipathy.*

som″no·vig′il (som″no·vidj′il). See *coma* **vigil.**

som′nus [L.]. Sleep.

Somogyi, Michael (1883–). American biochemist who has contributed studies on insulin action, on amylase action, and on a method for determination of true sugar in blood. He furnished the basis for large-scale preparation of insulin (1922). See Somogyi's *method,* Somogyi's *unit.*

sone [L. *sonus*, noise]. The unit of loudness.

son′i·tus. See *tinnitus*.

Sonne, Carl [*Danish bacteriologist*, 1882–1948]. Described a strain of the *Shigella* group which ferments mannitol and lactose; called *Sonne's bacillus*.

so′no·chem″is·try. The study of chemical reactions brought about by sound waves, especially those in the ultrasonic range. —**sonochem′ical,** *adj*.

so·nom′e·ter [L. *sonus*, noise; G. *metron*, a measure]. An instrument for determining the pitch of sounds and their relation to the musical scale.

son′to·chin. $C_{19}H_{28}ClN_3$; 7-chloro-4-(4-diethylamino-1-methylbutylamino)-3-methylquinoline; a suppressive antimalarial drug with action similar to that of chloroquine: also written *santochin, sontoquin, santoquin*.

so′nus. See *sound*.

soor (soor, sor). See *thrush*.

soor′pilz. See *moniliasis*.

so·phis″ti·ca′tion [G. *sophistikos*, of a sophist]. The adulteration or imitation of a substance.

soph″o·ma′ni·a [G. *sophos*, wise; *mania*, madness]. Megalomania in which the patient believes himself to excel in wisdom.

So·pho′ra [Ar. *sufayrā′*]. A genus of the Leguminosae; grows mainly in warm regions. Yields poisonous seeds. **S. sericea** is a poisonous plant of the United States; its seeds contain sophorine. **S. speciosa,** a tree of Texas, and **S. tomentosa,** of the East Indies, also contain sophorine. The seeds of *Sophora* have been used as a remedy for cholera and diarrhea.

so·pho″ra·bi′o·side. $C_{27}H_{30}O_{14}.3H_2O$; a glycoside from *Sophora japonica*. On hydrolysis it yields D-glucose, rhamnose, and genistein (4′,5,7-trihydroxyisoflavone).

so·pho′ri·co·side. $C_{21}H_{20}O_{10}$; a glycoside from *Sophora japonica*. On hydrolysis it yields D-glucose and genistein (4′,5,7-trihydroxyisoflavone).

soph′o·rine (sof′o·reen, ·rin, so′fo·). $C_{11}H_{14}ON_2$. A paralyzant, poisonous alkaloid which exists in the seeds of some species of *Sophora, Cytisus*, and *Baptisia*.

soph″ro·nis′tae den′tes (sof″ro·nis′tee den′teez) [L.]. Wisdom teeth. *Obs*.

so′por [L.]. Sleep, especially the profound sleep symptomatic of a morbid condition.

sop′o·rate, so′po·rate [L. *soporare*, to cast into sleep]. Stupefy; render drowsy. *Obs*.

so″po·rif′er·ous. See *soporific*.

so″po·rif′ic, sop″o·rif′ic [L. *sopor*, sleep; *facere*, to make]. 1. Producing sleep. 2. Narcotic. —**soporif′ic,** *n*.

sop′o·rose, so′po·rose [*sopor*]. Sleepy; characterized by morbid sleep.

sor″be·fa′cient [L. *sorbere*, to suck in; *facere*, to make]. A medicine or agent that induces absorption. *Obs*. —**sorbefa′cient,** *adj*.

sor′bic [L. *sorbus*, service-tree]. Pertaining to, or derived from, the mountain ash.

sor′bic ac′id. $CH_3.CH{:}CH.CH{:}CH.COOH$; 2,4-hexadienoic acid, from the berries of *Sorbus aucuparia*, European mountain ash; white crystals, very slightly soluble in water.

sor′bic al′co·hol. $CH_3.CH{:}CH.CH{:}CH.CH_2OH$; 2,4-hexadien-1-ol, in crystals, practically insoluble in water. It has been proposed for use in treatment of burns.

sor′bi·tan. An anhydride, also called *inner ether*, produced when a molecule of water is eliminated from sorbitol. Several such derivatives are possible.

sor′bite. Sorbitol.

sor′bi·tol. $CH_2OH.HCOH.HOCH.HCOH.HCOH$-$CH_2OH$; D-sorbitol; a hexahydric alcohol isomeric with mannitol; occurs as colorless or white, sweet crystals; soluble in water, sparingly soluble in alcohol. Used as an osmotic dehydrating agent and diuretic, usually administered in a 50% solution. It is also recommended as a sweetening agent for diabetics in place of sugar.

sor′bose. $CH_2OH.CO.HOCH.HCOH.HOCH.CH_2$-$OH$; L-sorbose, a ketohexose obtained by oxidative fermentation of D-sorbitol by certain organisms: used in the synthesis of ascorbic acid.

Sorby's cell. See under *cell*.

sor′des (sor′deez) [L.]. Filth, dirt, especially the crusts that accumulate on the teeth and lips in continued fevers.

sor′did [L. *sordidus*, dirty]. *In biology*, of a dull or dirty color.

sore [AS. *sar*]. Painful; tender.

sore. An ulcer or wound.

bed s. See *bedsore*.

canker s. Small ulceration of the mucous membrane of the mouth. Some may be due to a food allergy.

coldsore. Herpes facialis.

date s. Leishmaniasis.

Delasoa s. See *oriental sore*.

Delhi s. See *oriental sore*.

desert s. See *veldt sore*.

hard s. Chancre.

Kandahar s. See *oriental sore*.

Naga s. See tropical *ulcer*.

Natal s. See *veldt sore*.

oriental s. See *oriental sore*.

pressure s. See *bedsore*.

primary s. The initial lesion, chancre, of syphilis. Also called *hard s*.

soft s. Chancroid.

tropical s. See *oriental sore*.

veldt s. See *veldt sore*.

venereal s. See *chancre*.

Sørensen, Søren Peter Lauritz [*Danish chemist*, 1868–1939]. Introduced the symbol pH, used in expressing hydrogen-ion concentration; called *Sørensen's symbol*. *Sørensen's indicators* are the indicators of hydrogen-ion concentration.

Sørensen's method. See Henriques-Sørensen *method* for amino-acid nitrogen.

Soret, Celestin [*French radiologist*, d. 1931]. Described an absorption band in the extreme violet end of the spectrum of blood, characteristic of hemoglobin; called *Soret's band*.

sor′ghum [It. *sorgo*]. A group of annual fodder grasses of the family Gramineae from which a sugar and syrup are obtained.

soricin. Trade-mark for certain preparations containing purified sodium ricinoleate: used as detoxicants and to prevent absorption of toxins.

so·ro″ri·a′tion [L. *soror*, sister]. The development which takes place in the female breasts at puberty.

sor′rel [OF. *sur*, sour]. A plant of the genus *Rumex*, containing oxalates.

salt of s. Potassium binoxalate.

S. O. S. *Si opus sit*, if necessary.

sotradecol. Trade-mark for solutions of sodium tetradecyl sulfate for use as a sclerosing agent.

Sottas, Jules [*French neurologist*, 1866–1943]. Described, with J. J. Dejerine, progressive hypertrophic interstitial neuropathy (1893); also called *Dejerine-Sottas disease* or *neuropathy*.

souf′fle (sōō′ful) [F.]. A blowing sound; an auscultatory murmur.

cardiac s. See *heart murmur*.

fetal s. An inconstant murmur heard over the uterus during pregnancy.

funic s. A hissing sound, synchronous with the fetal heart sounds, heard over the abdomen of a pregnant woman, and supposed to be produced in the umbilical cord.

placental s. Old term for uterine souffle; the sound erroneously believed to be produced by circulation of blood through the placenta.

splenic s. A sound said to be audible over the spleen in cases of malaria and leukemia.

uterine s. A soft, blowing sound, synchronous with the maternal heart, heard over the abdomen at the sides of the uterus. The sound is due to the circulation of the blood in the large uterine arteries and veins. Its value as a diagnostic sign of pregnancy is doubtful.

sou'ma (sōō'muh). An acute infection in cattle, horses, mules, and sheep, marked by hemorrhages and serous exudates in the body cavities. It may become chronic, with anemia and subcutaneous edema.

sound [L. *sonus*, sound]. The sensation produced by stimulation of the auditory nerve by vibrations transmitted by the endolymph.

anasarcous s. A moist bubbling sometimes heard on auscultation when the skin is edematous.

bandbox s. The resonant percussion note sometimes heard in emphysema.

bellows s. An endocardial murmur which sounds like a bellows.

bell s. That produced in pneumothorax by striking a coin, placed flat upon the chest, with another coin. It can be heard through a stethoscope placed over the affected side. Also called *bell tympany, coin s.*

blowing s. A blowing murmur.

bottle s. See amphoric *respiration.*

breath sounds. The sounds heard during respiration when ausculting the lungs under all possible pathologic and normal conditions.

bronchial s. The large, harsh sound of bronchial respiration.

cardiac sounds. See *heart sounds* under *sound.*

cracked-pot s. A type of tympanitic resonance indicative of a cavity.

fetal heart sounds. The sounds produced by the beating of the fetal heart, best heard near the umbilicus of the mother.

flapping s. The clap made by the closure of the cardiac valves.

friction s. The sound heard in auscultation, as a result of the rubbing together of adjacent parts, as of the pleural folds, the pericardium, or the peritoneum, when the layers are dry or roughened.

funicular bellows s. See *souffle.*

heart sounds. See *heart sounds.*

humming-top s. See venous *hum.*

kettle-singing s. A chest sound sometimes heard in early pulmonary tuberculosis. It resembles the sound of water boiling in a kettle.

Korotkov sounds. See Nikolai S. *Korotkov.*

mediastinal emphysematous sounds. Crackling or popping noises in the mediastinum caused by the heart moving against air caught in the mediastinum. It sometimes occurs with conditions such as interstitial pulmonary emphysema or trauma.

metamorphosing breath s. A sound due to the passage of air through a narrow opening into and out of a pulmonary cavity.

muscle s. The sound heard through the stethoscope when placed over a muscle while it is contracting; susurrus.

osseous s. A high-pitched, intense, auscultatory sound having a slightly metallic timbre.

pulmonary s. The respiratory murmur.

respiratory s. Respiratory murmur.

sawing s. A cardiac murmur resembling the sound produced by sawing.

shadow s. The interference with a sound wave caused by an object being placed between the ear and the source of sound.

subjective s. See *phonism.*

to-and-fro s. The friction sound of pericarditis and pleuritis.

tubular s. The sound of tracheal respiration.

white s. A noise made up of pure tones, harmonics, and discordants throughout the range of human hearing in equal parts and at equal intensities. It is used as a background noise in speech intelligibility tests.

xiphosternal crunch s. See *xiphosternal crunch.*

sound [OF. *sonde*]. An instrument for introduction into a channel or cavity, for determining the presence of constriction, foreign bodies, or other morbid conditions, and for treatment.

esophageal s. A long flexible sound for examination of the esophagus.

lacrimal s. A fine sound for exploring or dilating the lacrimal canaliculus.

urethral s. An elongated steel instrument, usually slightly conical, for examination and dilatation of the urethra.

uterine s. A graduated probe for measurement of the uterine cavity.

Souques' sign. See *kinesis paradoxa.*

Sourdille, Maurice [*French otologist,* 1885–]. Known for his operation for the restoration of hearing in otosclerosis, in which he made a fistula into the horizontal semicircular canal, covering it with a plastic skin flap attached to the tympanum; called *fenestration operation, Sourdille's operation.*

sour'wood" [AS. *sūr; wudu*]. *Oxydendrum arboreum,* a tree of the Ericaceae. The leaves have a sour taste; has been used as a diuretic.

south'ern·wood" [AS. *sūth; wudu*]. *Artemisia abrotanum,* related to absinthium. The leaves have been used as a bitter tonic and anthelmintic.

Soxhlet, Franz von [*German chemist,* 1848–1926]. Known for his invention of an apparatus for sterilizing milk (1886). Best known for his apparatus for extracting fats in foods and for analysis of fat in tissues.

soy'bean", so'ya bean. The seed of *Glycine soja* (*Glycine hispida, Soja hispida*), a legume native to Asia but now cultivated in other regions, particularly the United States, because of the high food and commercial value of its seeds. The bean and flour are used in dietetics for their high protein and relatively low carbohydrate content. The bean contains protein, fixed oil, carbohydrates, crude fiber, and several enzymes. The meal is used as a feed, in the manufacture of a number of industrial products, and in some articles of food.

Soy'mi·da. A genus of the Meliaceae. **S. febrifuga** is an East Indian tree that furnishes rotun bark, which has been used as a tonic and antiperiodic.

so"zo·i·od'o·late (so"zo·eye·od'o·late, ·eye'o·dolate). A salt of sozoiodolic acid.

so"zo·i"o·dol'ic ac'id. $C_6H_2I_2(SO_3H)OH$. A crystalline, odorless powder used as an antiseptic, disinfectant, and parasiticide, chiefly in the form of its salts. Also called *sozoiodole.*

sp. *Spiritus,* spirit.

spa [after a place of this name in Belgium which has mineral springs]. A mineral spring, especially one having medicinal value and visited as a health resort.

space [L. *spatium,* space]. A delimited area or region. —**spa'tial,** *adj.*

air s. The space in tissues filled with air or other gases.

antecubital s. The triangular space in front of the elbow, often used as the site of venepuncture.

anterior perforated s. Anterior perforated substance.
Bogro's s. A potential space between the parietal peritoneum and the transversalis fascia, situated in the lower anterior abdominal wall; the retroinguinal space.
bregmatic s. The anterior fontanel.
chloride s. A theoretical volume of body fluid containing all the body chloride at a concentration equal to that in a plasma ultrafiltrate.
circumlental s. The interspace between the ciliary body and the equator of the lens.
complemental s. The portion of the pleural cavity, just above the attachments of the diaphragm, which is not filled with lung during ordinary inspiration.
corneal spaces. Spaces in the interstitial cement substance between the lamellas of the substantia propria of the cornea.
dead s. (a) A cavity left after the closure of a wound. (b) **Anatomical d. s.** is that space in the trachea, bronchi, and air passages in general which contains air that does not reach the alveoli during respiration, the amount of air being about 140 cc. The **physiological d. s.** is a calculated expression of the anatomical plus whatever degree of overventilation or underperfusion is present. It is alleged to reflect the relationship of ventilation to pulmonary capillary perfusion. The formula is:

$$\text{Physiological dead space} = \text{tidal volume} \times \frac{\text{arterial } {}_{\text{p}}CO_2 - \text{expired } {}_{\text{p}}CO_2}{\text{arterial } {}_{\text{p}}CO_2}$$

distal closed s. The fascial space overlying the palmar surface of a distal phalanx, covered by fascia attached to the tip, lateral margins, and base of the distal phalanx.
endolymphatic s. The space containing the endolymphatic sac, situated behind the petrous portion of the temporal bone and communicating with the vestibular aqueduct.
epidural s. The space between the spinal dura and the periosteum lining the canal.
epitympanic s. See epitympanic *recess.*
fascial spaces. Potential spaces between layers of fascia, as fascial spaces of the foot.
Fontana's spaces. A series of small spaces formed by the interlacing of the connective-tissue fibers of the framework of the peripheral processes of the iris, situated in the angle of the anterior chamber, and serving as a medium for the transudation of the aqueous humor from the posterior to the anterior chamber of the eye. Also called *Fontana's canal.*
freeway s. The distance between the occluding surfaces of the upper and lower teeth when the mandible is at rest.
Gerota's s. See Dumitru *Gerota.*
hypothenar s. A potential space in the fascia surrounding the muscles of the hypothenar eminence in the hand.
image s. The space around an optical system each point of which is an image of a corresponding point in the object space. Properties relating to the image are said to be in the image space, and properties relating to the object are said to be in the object space.
intercellular spaces. Cavities between adjacent cells.
intercostal s. The space between two adjacent ribs.
interfascial s. See *s.* of Tenon.
interglobular s. A region of incompletely calcified dentin bounded by calcified spherules. Preferably called interglobular dentin.
interpeduncular s. The region between the cerebral peduncles.
interpleural s. The mediastinum.
interproximate s. *In dentistry,* the V-shaped space between the proximal surfaces of the teeth and the alveolar septum which is filled by the gum.
intersepto-valvular s. A narrow cleft between the left valve of the sinus venosus and the septum primum after the latter develops.
intervaginal spaces. The subdural and subarachnoid spaces of the optic sheaths.
intervillous spaces. Spaces within the placenta developed from the trophoblastic lacunas and the dilated maternal veins, with which the maternal vessels communicate.
ischiorectal s. See ischiorectal *fossa.*
lateral midpalmar s. A deep fascial space on the radial side of the palm; thenar space.
lymph s. Lymph sinus; a tract of loose lymphatic tissue in a lymph node.
marrow s. A marrow-filled space between the trabeculae of cancellous bone.
medial palmar s. See midpalmar *s.*
mediastinal s. The mediastinum.
meningeal spaces. The subdural and subarachnoid spaces.
midpalmar s. A deep fascial space beneath the flexor tendons on the ulnar side of the palm. Syn., *medial palmar s.*
Nuel's s. A space between the outer pillars and the outer hair cells.
object s. The space around an optical system each point of which is considered as a possible source of radiation of light.
palmar spaces. The lateral and medial potential fascial spaces in the hand between the thenar and hypothenar areas, separated by a fibrous septum and filled with areolar tissue.
perichoroidal s. A potential space between the sclera and the choroid.
perilenticular s. The space surrounding the crystalline lens holding the ciliary zonule.
perilymphatic spaces. Small, irregular cavities filled with perilymph, between the membranous and bony labyrinths of the internal ear.
perineural spaces. Spaces within the sheaths of cranial nerve roots, through which passes cerebrospinal fluid.
perineuronal spaces. The tissue spaces surrounding neurons.
periotic spaces. See perilymphatic *spaces.*
perisinusoidal s. Lymphatic space of the liver, bounded on one side by the endothelium of the sinusoids and on the other by the walls of the liver cells: also called *space of Disse.*
peritoneal spaces. Potential spaces within the peritoneum formed by the various reflections from the parietes and abdominal viscera.
perivascular spaces. Fluid-filled spaces between the adventitia of the blood vessels of the brainsubstance and the pial limiting membrane, lined with endothelial cells, connecting with the subarachnoid space. Also called *spaces of Virchow-Robin.*
perivitelline s. In mammalian ova, the space formed between the ovum and the zona pellucida at the time of maturation, into which the polar bodies are given off.
placental blood spaces. The intervillous lacunas of the placenta.
popliteal s. A diamond-shaped space at the back of the knee joint.
portal s. The area between hepatic lobules, containing connective tissue, arteries, veins, bile ducts, nerves, and lymphatics.
posterior triangular s. The space lying above

the clavicle and between the sternomastoid and the trapezius muscles and the occiput.

preputial s. A potential space between the prepuce and glans penis represented by two shallow fossae on either side of the frenulum.

prevesical s. A space lying immediately above the pubis and between the peritoneum and the posterior surface of the rectus abdominis. Also called *s. of Retzius, retropubic s.*

prezonular s. The space of the eye enclosed by the iris, lens, ciliary body, and vitreous body.

Prussak's s. See *recess* of tympanic cavity (b). See also Alexander *Prussak.*

quadrangular s. The lateral division of the triangular space of the shoulder which contains the axillary nerve and the posterior humeral circumflex artery.

quadrilateral s. (a) The anterior and posterior triangles of the neck taken together. (b) The deep fascial space of the wrist beneath the annular ligament and flexor tendons, above the pronator quadratus muscle.

rectovesical s. The rectovesical pouch; the space between the urinary bladder and the rectum.

retroparotid s. A potential space situated between the medial surface of the parotid gland and the upper lateral wall of the pharynx.

retroperitoneal s. That behind the peritoneum, but in front of the spinal column and lumbar muscles; in it lie the kidneys, the aorta, the inferior vena cava, and the sympathetic trunk.

retropharyngeal s. That behind the pharynx, containing areolar tissue.

retropubic s. See prevesical *s.*

semilunar s. A percussion area on the left anterior portion of the thorax, overlying the stomach. Also called *Traube's s.*

small triangular s. The medial division of the triangular space of the shoulder through which pass the circumflex scapular vessels.

snuffbox s. Anatomist's snuffbox.

s. of Burns. See suprasternal *s.*

s. of Disse. See perisinusoidal *s.*

s. of Retzius. See prevesical *s.*

s. of Tenon. The space between the sclera and the capsule of Tenon.

spaces of Littré. The potential spaces between the liver cell cords and the lining cells of the sinusoids; characteristically enlarged and filled with transudate in edema of the liver.

spaces of Virchow-Robbins. See perivascular *spaces.*

subarachnoid s. The space between the arachnoid and the pia proper, containing subarachnoid trabeculae and filled with cerebrospinal fluid.

subdural s. The space between the dura and the arachnoid which normally contains only a capillary layer of fluid.

subphrenic s. One of the two spaces, right and left, between the diaphragm and the liver, on either side of the falciform ligament.

subumbilical s. A triangular space in the body cavity having its apex at the umbilicus.

suprasternal s. The triangular space above the manubrium, enclosed by the layers of the deep cervical fascia which are attached to the front and back of this bone. Formerly called *s. of Burns.*

supravaginal s. A continuation of the space of Tenon along the external side of the dural sheath of the optic nerve.

temporal s. The temporal fossa.

thenar s. A deep fascial space beneath the flexor tendons of the index and, occasionally, of the middle finger and overlying the second metacarpal bone. Syn., *lateral midpalmar s.*

tissue s. A cavity or space in connective tissue.

Traube's s. See semilunar *s.*

triangular s. A space of triangular form in the posterior wall of the axilla, bounded by the latissimus dorsi, teres minor, and subscapular muscles and the surgical neck of the humerus; it is divided by the long head of the triceps into the quadrangular and small triangular spaces.

tunnel s. See *tunnel* of Corti.

undefended s. of Peacock. The thin membranous portion of the interventricular septum of the heart.

vitelline s. See perivitelline *s.*

zonular spaces. Those between the zonular fibers; a part of the posterior chamber of the eye. Also called *canals of Petit.*

space med'i·cine. A division of aviation medicine concerned with the physiologic and pathologic effects of flying at extremely high altitudes and at supersonic speeds.

spa·gyr'ic [G. *span*, to draw; *ageirein*, to assemble]. Pertaining to the obsolete chemical, alchemistic, or Paracelsian school of medicine. —**spag'yrist,** *n.*

spag'y·rism (spadj'i·riz·um) [*span; ageirein*]. The Paracelsian, or spagyric, school or doctrine of medicine.

Spallanzani, Lazaro [*Italian physiologist*, 1729–99]. Remembered for his investigations on fertilization, circulation, and digestion. He opposed the doctrine of spontaneous generation. Made a number of important observations on the character of gastric juice; his experiments included the obtaining of specimens from the living by the use of a sponge attached to a cord which was swallowed (1780). Observed that the regenerative power of cells is in proportion to the age of the individual; known as *Spallanzani's law.*

spal·la'tion. The process of bombarding various elements with extremely high energy protons, deuterons, or alpha particles, whereby extensive alteration of the bombarded nucleus results.

span"i·o·car'di·a [G. *spanios*, scanty; *kardia*, heart]. Bradycardia.

Span'ish col'lar. Paraphimosis.

Span'ish wind'lass. An improvised tourniquet consisting of a handkerchief knotted about a limb and tightened by means of a stick which is twisted.

spans. Trade-mark for a series of long chain fatty acid partial esters of hexitol anhydrides such as those of sorbitol and mannitol. The substances are used as wetting agents, emulsifiers, and solubilizing agents. See *tweens.*

spar'a·drap [It. *sparadrappo*]. A plaster spread on cotton, linen, silk, leather, paper; adhesive plaster.

spa'ras·sol. $C_{10}H_{12}O_4$; 6-hydroxy-4-methoxy-2-methylbenzoic acid methyl ester; an antibiotic substance produced by the fungus *Sparassis ramosa* and also obtained in extracts of the lichen *Evernia prunasti.*

spar"ga·no'sis [G. *sparganon*, swaddling-clothes; *-ōsis*, condition]. Infestation with *Sparganum*, which is a larval stage of the fish tapeworms.

Spar·ga'num, Spar'ga·num (pl. *Spargana*) [*sparaganon*]. A generic name applied to the plerocercoid larva of *Diphyllobothrium*, especially if the adult form is unknown.

S. mansoni. A species seen in the Far East, which is frequently found in the eye. Infestation probably follows contact with freshly killed frogs.

S. mansonoides. A species which infests mice and has also been reported in the muscles and subcutaneous tissues of man.

S. proliferum. A species which proliferates in the tissues of the host by branching and budding off large numbers of spargana. The adult form is unknown.

spar·go′sis [G., swelling]. Enlargement or distention, as of the breasts due to accumulation of milk.

spark [AS. *spaerca*]. A light flash, usually electric in origin, as that emanating from an electrode through which a current is passing.

Sparkman's test for urobilin. See under *test.*

spar′te·ine (spahr′tee·een, ·in, spahr′teen). $C_{15}H_{26}N_2$. A liquid alkaloid obtained from *Cytisus scoparius;* occurs as a colorless, oily liquid; slightly soluble in water but soluble in alcohol.

s. sulfate (*sparteinae sulfas*). $C_{15}H_{26}N_2.H_2SO_4.5H_2O$; occurs as colorless crystals or a white, crystalline powder; 1 Gm. dissolves in about 1.1 cc. of water, and in about 3 cc. of alcohol. Has been used chiefly in the treatment of irregularities of the heart, such as tachycardia and functional palpitation. Dose, 0.01–0.12 Gm. (1/6–2 gr.).

spasm [G. *spasmos*]. A sudden muscular contraction.

Bell's s. Convulsive facial tic.

bronchial s. Asthma.

cadaveric s. Early, or at times immediate, appearance of rigor mortis; seen after death from certain causes. The muscle spasm actually causes movements of the limbs.

carpopedal s. A spasm of the hands and feet, or of the thumbs and great toes; associated with tetany.

clonic s. (a) A spasm broken by relaxations of the muscles. (b) In the area of the accessory nerve it is called spasmodic torticollis. (c) In the area of the facial nerve it is called painless tic.

cynic s. A contraction of the facial muscles upon one side, so as to expose the teeth.

facial s. A peculiar clonic contraction of the muscles surrounding the eye, or else involving one entire side of the face.

fatigue spasms. A group of affections characterized by spasmodic contractions, either clonic or tonic, brought about by voluntary movement, the exciting cause being limited to some particular action. Also called *business spasms, coordinated business neuroses, functional spasms, handicraft spasms, movement spasms, occupational spasms, professional spasms.*

fixed s. Permanent or continuous tetanic rigidity of one or more muscles.

Friedreich's spasms. See *paramyoclonus multiplex.*

functional spasms. See *fatigue spasms* under *spasm.*

habit s. Half voluntary spasmodic movements, the result of habit, sometimes called *habit chorea.*

histrionic s. A condition in which local involuntary twitchings of the face, acquired in childhood, persist during adult life, and are increased by emotional causes.

idiopathic muscular s. See *tetany.*

inspiratory s. A spasmodic contraction of nearly all the inspiratory muscles.

laryngeal congenital s. A peculiar stridor developing at birth, and disappearing after one or two years.

lingual s. See *aphthongia.*

lock s. A form of writer's cramp in which the fingers become locked on the pen.

masticatory s. of the face. See *trismus.*

mimic s. Facial tic.

mobile s. Slow, irregular movements following hemiplegia.

movement spasms. See *fatigue spasms* under *spasm.*

myopathic s. One attending a disease of muscles.

nodding s. Eclampsia nutans; spasmus nutans.

occupation spasms. See *fatigue spasms* under *spasm.*

pantomimic s. See painless *tic.*

phonic s. A spasm of the laryngeal muscles occurring on attempting to speak.

retrocollic s. Spasm of the muscles at the back of the neck, causing retraction of the head.

salaam s. Clonic spasm causing bowing movements. See also *eclampsia* nutans and *spasmus* nutans.

saltatory s. A clonic spasm that causes the patient to leap or jump when he attempts to stand.

sewing s. An occupational spasm seen in tailors, seamstresses, and shoemakers.

smith's s. An occupational spasm with associated hemiplegia: also called *hephestic hemiplegia.*

s. of accommodation. Spasm of the ciliary muscles, in attempting accommodation for objects nearby.

s. of the glottis. See *laryngismus* stridulus.

stutter s. See *laliophobia.*

synclonic s. Tremulous agitation.

tailor's s. An occupational neurosis occurring in tailors, characterized by spasm of the muscles of the arm and hand. Also called *tailor's cramp.*

telegrapher's s. An occupational spasm. See *fatigue spasms* under *spasm.*

tetanic s. See tonic *s.*

tonic s. A spasm that persists without relaxation for some time.

torsion s. See *dystonia* musculorum deformans.

toxic s. One due to poison.

winking s. A habit tic of spasmodic twitching or blinking of the eyelids. Also called *spasmus nictitans.*

spasmalgin. Trade-mark for a tablet or injection containing papaverine hydrochloride, pantopon, and atrinal. The preparations are used as an analgesic and antispasmodic.

spas′mo- (spaz′mo-) [*spasmos*]. A combining form denoting *pertaining to a spasm.*

spas·mod′ic (spaz·mod′ick) [G. *spasmōdēs*, convulsive]. Pertaining to, or characterized by, spasm.

spas·mol′o·gy (spaz·mol′o·jee) [G. *spasmos*, spasm; *logos*, word]. The sum of scientific knowledge of the nature and causes of spasms and convulsions.

spas″mo·lyg′mus. See *hiccup.*

spas″mo·lyt′ic. Antispasmodic.

spas″mo·phe′mi·a [*spasmos;* G. *phēmis*, speech]. Stuttering. *Obs.*

spas″mo·phil′i·a [*spasmos;* G. *philein*, to love]. A morbid tendency to convulsions, and to tonic spasms, such as those observed in tetany. —**spasmophilic,** *adj.*

spas′mous (spaz′mus) [*spasmos*]. Having the nature of a spasm. *Rare.*

spas′mus (spaz′mus) [*spasmos*]. A spasm.

s. bronchialis. See *asthma.*

s. glottidis. Spasm of the glottis or larynx; laryngismus stridulus.

s. intestinorum. See *enteralgia.*

s. muscularis. See *cramp.*

s. nictitans. Spasmodic action of the orbicularis oculi muscle, causing a winking movement of the lid.

s. nutans. Rhythmic nodding and eye jerking frequently seen in rachitic and debilitated children: also called *gyrospasm, nodding spasm.*

s. oculi. See *nystagmus.*

spas′tic [G. *spastikos*, drawing in]. Pertaining to, or characterized by, spasm; produced by spasm.

spas·tic′i·ty (spas·tiss′i·tee) [*spastikos*]. An increased tonus or tension of a muscle which is associated with an exaggeration of deep reflexes, and frequently with clonus and a partial or complete loss of voluntary control.

cerebral s. That due to organic disease of the brain.

clasp-knife s. The resistance of a muscle to passive extension followed by a sudden relaxation, like the snapping of a clasp-knife blade.

spa′ti·um (spay′shee·um). Space.

spat′u·la [L. dim. from *spatha*, flat wooden instrument]. A flexible blunt blade; used for spreading ointment. —**spatulate,** *adj.*

Spatz, Hugo [*German neurologist,* 1888–]. Described a progressive degenerative disease of childhood, characterized by an extrapyramidal syndrome of athetosis, mental deterioration, and speech defect; called *Hallervorden-Spatz syndrome.*

spav′in [OF. *esparvain*]. Disease of the hock of a horse. Also see *hock.*

s. bog. An enlargement due to distention of the capsular ligament, prominent on the inner aspect of the joint.

s. bone. An enlargement due to an exostosis of the tarsal bones, termed high or low depending on its position.

spay [AF. *espeier*]. Remove the ovaries.

SPCA Serum prothrombin conversion accelerator. See *convertin.*

S.P.C.A. Society for the Prevention of Cruelty to Animals.

spear′mint [ME. *spere;* G. *mintha,* mint] (*mentha viridis*). The dried leaf and flowering top of *Mentha spicata* (*Mentha viridis*) containing a volatile oil which is found in the external glandular hairs.

s. oil (*oleum mentha viridis*). A volatile oil distilled with steam from fresh, overground parts of the flowering plant of *Mentha spicata* (*Mentha viridis*); occurs as a colorless, yellow, or greenish yellow liquid; soluble in an equal volume of 80% alcohol. It contains about 50% of *l*-carvone. Other constituents are phellandrene, *l*-limonene, pinene, dihydrocarvol acetate, dihydrocuminic acetate. The oil as well as the plant is little used except as a flavoring agent.

s. spirit (*spiritus menthae viridis*). An alcoholic solution containing 10% of spearmint oil.

s. water (*aqua menthae viridis*). A clear, saturated solution of spearmint oil in distilled water. Used as a vehicle.

spe′cial·ist [L. *specialis,* individual]. One who limits his practice to certain diseases, or to the diseases of a single organ or class, or to a certain type of therapy; specifically, a diplomate of one of the American specialty boards in medicine, such as the American Board of Surgery.

spe′cial·ty [*specialis*]. The branch of medicine or surgery pursued by a specialist.

spe′cies (spee′sheez) [L., appearance]. 1. A group of individuals, similar in certain morphologic and physiologic characteristics which distinguish them from other groups with which they may be united on the basis of other characters into a higher group, the genus; the species also may fall into groups of minor rank, as subspecies, varieties, races. 2. A name sometimes applied to certain mixtures of herbs used in making decoctions and infusions.

spe·cif′ic [*species;* L. *facere,* to make]. 1. Of or pertaining to a species, or to that which distinguishes a thing or makes it of the species to which it belongs. 2. Produced by a certain microorganism, as a specific disease; in a restricted sense, syphilitic.

spe·cif′ic. A medicine that has a distinct curative influence on a particular disease, as quinine in malaria or mercury in syphilis.

spec″i·fic′i·ty (spess″i·fiss′i·tee) [*species; facere*]. The quality of being specific.

compound s. The qualitative and quantitative differences in physiologic behavior of various compounds of similar structure on the same animal organism.

species s. The difference in physiologic response to one or more compounds by different species of animals.

spec′ta·cles [L. *spectaculum,* sight]. Framed or mounted lenses for aiding vision where there are optical or muscular defects of the eye. See *lens.*

bifocal s. See *bifocal.*

orthoscopic s. See *orthoscopic.*

pantoscopic s. Bifocal spectacles.

prismatic s. Spectacles with prismatic lenses, either alone or combined with spherical or cylindrical lenses.

protective s. Lenses that shield the eyes from light, dust, heat.

telescopic s. Spectacles that magnify the retinal image: useful for persons with cloudy media, partial cataracts, or impaired retinal sensitivity.

trifocal s. See under *glasses.*

spec′tro- [L. *spectrum,* appearance]. A combining form denoting *relating to a spectrum.*

spec″tro·col″or·im′e·ter (·kul″ur·im′i·tur) [*spectrum;* L. *color,* color; G. *metron,* a measure]. Combination of spectroscope and ophthalmoscope for the detection of colorblindness to one spectral color.

spec′tro·gram. A graphical record of a spectrum.

spec′tro·graph [*spectrum;* G. *graphein,* to write]. A spectroscope which records a spectrum on a photographic plate.

mass s. An instrument used for determining the mass of atoms or molecules by producing charged ions and measuring their deflection in a magnetic field.

spec·trom′e·ter [*spectrum;* G. *metron,* a measure]. A spectroscope provided with equipment for measuring the deviations of light and other electromagnetic rays and therewith the wavelengths of spectral lines. —**spectrometry,** *n.*

Beckman s. One in which the spectrum is produced by the use of a quartz prism.

Coleman s. One in which the spectrum is produced by a diffraction grating.

spec″tro·mi′cro·scope. See *microspectroscope.*

spec″tro·pho″te·lom′e·ter. A device combining a spectrometer and photoelectric cell for the accurate identification and quantitation of unknown material.

spec″tro·pho·tom′e·ter [*spectrum;* G. *phōs,* light; *metron*]. Combination of spectrometer and photometer for making quantitative measurements in various parts of the visible, ultraviolet, or infrared spectrum. —**spectrophotometry,** *n.*

flame s. A device used to quantitate emission spectra derived from heating a solid or solution in a flame. See flame *photometry.*

spec″tro·po″lar·im′e·ter [*spectrum;* L. *polus,* pole; *metron*]. Combination of a spectrometer and polariscope; used for measuring optical rotation produced by certain solutions.

spec′tro·scope [*spectrum;* G. *skopein,* to examine]. An instrument for dispersing radiations by various methods, such as a prism, diffraction gratings, and crystals, and for observing the resultant spectrum. —**spectroscop′ic,** *adj.*

spec·tros′co·py. Study of spectra; use of the spectroscope.

microwave s. The study of interactions between matter and radio waves of wavelengths between a few meters and a few tenths of a millimeter; such study provides information concerning the molecular and nuclear structure of matter.

spec′trum (pl. *spectrums, spectra*) [L.]. 1. The series of images resulting when a beam of electromagnetic waves (such as electric waves, infrared, visible light, ultraviolet, or x-rays), is dispersed and the constituent waves are arranged according to their frequencies or wavelengths. 2. Figuratively, any series of entities arranged according to the quantitative variation of a given common property; a range. —**spectral,** *adj.*

absorption s. Spectrum of radiation, which has passed through some selectively absorbing substance, as white light after it has passed through a vapor.

antibiotic s. The range of activity of an antibiotic against different bacteria: also called *bacteriostatic s., antibacterial s., antimicrobial s.*

auditory s. See *phonism, photism.*

bacterial s. The susceptibility of a range of microorganisms to a particular chemotherapeutic or antibiotic agent.

comparison s. The arrangement side by side of the spectrums of two different substances.

continuous s. A spectrum without sudden variations, representing a continuous variation of wavelengths from one end to the other.

electromagnetic s. See electromagnetic *radiation.*

emission s. Spectrum of the radiation which a substance emits. The opposite of absorption spectrum.

fortification s. Scintillating scotoma.

solar s. The spectrum afforded by the refraction of sunlight.

spec′u·lum [L., mirror]. An instrument for dilating the opening of a cavity of the body in order that the interior may be more easily visible.

anal s. An instrument of varying design similar to a nasal speculum, but with longer blades which allows examination of the lower portion of the rectum: also called *rectal s.*

aural s. A small, hollow instrument with an expanded end, which may be introduced into the ear for examination of the external auditory canal and the tympanic membrane.

duckbill s. A bivalve vaginal speculum with flat, broad blades.

eye s. An instrument for retracting the eyelids.

nasal s. A small bivalve instrument with handles, which dilates the nostril and allows examination of the nasal passages.

Spee, Ferdinand von (1855–1937). German embryologist who described a curved line which extends along the summits of the buccal cusps from the first premolar to the third molar, called *Spee's curve.*

speech [AS. *spǣc*]. 1. The faculty of expressing thought by spoken words; the act of speaking. 2. The words spoken.

ataxic s. The intermittent, explosive speech resulting from cerebellar disorders.

bulbar s. The thick speech occurring when the nuclei of the medulla concerned with speech are damaged or when there is injury to both corticobulbar tracts.

echo s. Echolalia.

esophageal s. Speech produced after laryngectomy by swallowing air into the esophagus and expelling it with an eructation past the pharyngeal opening to produce a sound which is then modulated by the lips, tongue, and palate.

interjectional s. The expression of emotions by inarticulate sounds.

laryngeal s. Speech produced by means of an artificial larynx following laryngectomy: now less commonly employed.

mirror s. Defective speech characterized by pronouncing words or syllables backward.

scanning s. A slow and measured form of speech with pauses between syllables. Characteristic of diffuse lesions of the cerebellum and brain stem, particularly common in multiple sclerosis.

slurred s. The tremulous, feeble, careless speech which is characteristic of lesions of the basal ganglions.

staccato s. See scanning *s.*

syllabic s. A form of dysphasia with halting, stumbling articulation.

spe·le·os′to·my. See *cavernostomy.*

Spemann, Hans [*German embryologist,* 1869–1941]. Demonstrated that the structural development of the embryo is the result of the physicochemical interaction between different regions of tissue, thereby introducing the concept of the organizer. Nobel laureate (1935).

Spencer, Roscoe Roy (1888–). American physician who developed, with R. R. Parker, Rocky Mountain spotted-fever vaccine.

Spencer's bright-line counting chamber. A double membrane counting chamber.

Spencer Wells. See Thomas Spencer *Wells.*

Spengler, Carl [*Swiss physician,* 1861–1937]. Described small, spheroidal bodies found in the sputum of tuberculous patients; called *Spengler's fragments.*

Spens, Thomas [*Scottish physician,* 1764–1842]. Reported a case of what was undoubtedly heart block (1792). Morgagni had earlier described a similar case. The classic descriptions are those of Robert Adams (1826) and William Stokes (1846). Stokes-Adams syndrome is sometimes called *Spens syndrome.*

sperm [G. *sperma,* seed]. 1. A spermatozoon; the mature male germ cell. Syn., *sperm cell.* 2. An inexact term for the seminal fluid.

sper″ma·cet′i (spur″muh·set′ee, ·see′tee) [*sperma;* G. *kētos,* sea-monster] (*cetaceum*). A waxy substance obtained from the head of the sperm whale, *Physeter macrocephalus.* The chief constituent is cetyl palmitate or cetin. Cetyl alcohol is also present in appreciable amounts. There are also small amounts of the esters of lauric, myristic, palmitic, and stearic acids, and also of dodecyl, tetradecyl, and octadodecyl alcohols. Used chiefly to add firmness to ointment bases. An ingredient in rose water ointment.

sperm′al·ist [*sperma*]. A preformationist who held the view that the animalcule was in the sperm cell rather than in the egg. Syn., *spermist.*

sperm as′ter. The radiating structure which precedes the sperm nucleus as it advances within the egg.

sper″ma·ta·cra′si·a (spur″muh·tuh·kray′zhuh, ·zee·uh) [*sperma;* G. *akrasia,* absence of mixture]. Deficiency or decrease of spermatozoa in the semen. Also called *spermacrasia.*

sper·mat′ic [L. *spermatikos,* of seed]. 1. Pertaining to the semen or spermatozoa; conveying semen, as the spermatic cord. See Plate 4. 2. Pertaining to the spermatic cord, as the spermatic fascia.

sper′ma·tid [*sperma*]. A male germ cell immediately before assuming its final typical form.

sper′ma·to-, spermat- [*sperma*]. A combining form meaning *seed, germ.*

sper′ma·to·cele″ (spur′muh·to·seel″, spur·mat′o·) [*sperma;* G. *kēlē,* hernia]. Cystic dilatation of a duct in the head of the epididymis or in the rete testis. Rupture into the tunica vaginalis produces spermatic hydrocele.

sper″ma·to·ce·lec′to·my [*sperma; kēlē;* G. *ektomē,* excision]. Excision of a spermatocele, or cyst of the epididymis.

sper″ma·to·ci′dal [*sperma;* L. *caedere,* to kill]. Destructive to spermatozoa: also spelled *spermaticidal.*

sper′ma·to·cide″ [*sperma; caedere*]. An agent that destroys spermatozoa.

sper′ma·to·cyst″ (spur′muh·to·sist″, spur·mat′o·). See seminal *vesicle.* —**spermatocys′tic,** *adj.*

sper″ma·to·cys·tec′to·my. See *vesiculectomy.*

sper″ma·to·cys·ti′tis [*sperma;* G. *kystis,* bladder; *-itis,* inflammation]. Inflammation of the seminal vesicles.

sper″ma·to·cys·tot′o·my [*sperma; kystis;* G. *tomē,* a cutting]. Surgical incision of a seminal vesicle.

sper′ma·to·cyte″ (spur′muh·to·sight″, spur·mat′o·) [*sperma;* G. *kytos,* cell]. A cell of the last or next to the last generation of cells which divide to form mature male germ cells.

primary s. A developing sperm cell in the growth phase preceding the first meiotic division.

secondary s. One of the two cells produced by the first meiotic division.

sper″ma·to·cy·to′ma. Seminoma.

sper″ma·to·gen′e·sis [*sperma;* G. *genesis,* production]. The phenomena involved in the production of mature male germ cells, sometimes restricted to denote the process of meiosis in the male.

sper″ma·to·gen′ic [*sperma;* G. *genesthai,* from *gignesthai,* to be produced]. Producing spermatozoa, as the spermatogenic cells of the testis. Also called *spermatogenous.*

sper″ma·to·go′ni·um (pl. *spermatogonia*) [*sperma;* G. *gonē,* offspring]. One of the primitive male germ cells. The primary spermatocytes arise from the last generation of spermatogonia by an increase in size.

sper′ma·toid [*sperma;* G. *eidos,* form]. Resembling a sperm cell.

sper″ma·tol′y·sin (spur″muh·tol′i·sin, spur″muh-to·lye′sin) [*sperma;* G. *lysis,* a loosing]. A substance causing dissolution of sperm cells.

sper″ma·tol′y·sis [*sperma; lysis*]. The process of dissolution of sperm cells. —**spermatolyt′ic,** *adj.*

sper″ma·top′a·thy [*sperma;* G. *pathos,* disease]. Disease of the sperm cells or of their secreting mechanism.

sper′ma·to·phore″, sper·mat′o·phore″ [*sperma;* G. *phoros,* bearing]. A special capsule or pocket containing male germ cells; found in certain annelids, mollusks, crustacea, and vertebrates, but especially remarkable in the cephalopods.

sper″ma·tor·rhe′a, sper″ma·tor·rhoe′a [*sperma;* G. *rhoia,* flow]. Involuntary discharge of semen without orgasm.

false s. That occurring when spermatozoa are not in the fluid. Also called *prostatorrhea.*

s. dormientum. A nocturnal emission of semen.

sper″ma·tox′in, sper″ma·to·tox′in. See *spermolysin.*

sper″ma·to·zo′i·cide [*sperma;* G. *zōion,* living being; L. *caedere,* to kill]. An agent destructive to spermatozoa. Syn., *spermicide, spermatocide.*

sper″ma·to·zo′id [*sperma; zōion*]. *In botany,* a motile male germ cell found in certain algae, in mosses and ferns, and in certain gymnosperms. Also called *spermatozooid.*

sper″ma·to·zo′on (pl. *spermatozoa*) [*sperma; zōion*]. The mature male germ cell. See Plate 41. —**spermatozoal,** *adj.*

sper″ma·tu′ri·a [*sperma;* G. *ouron,* urine]. The presence of semen in the urine.

sperm cell. A spermatozoon. Syn., *sperm.*

sperm cen′ter. The centrosome which precedes the sperm nucleus as it advances within the egg. In flagellate spermatozoa it arises from the middle piece.

sper·mec′to·my [*sperma;* G. *ektomē,* excision]. Resection of part of the spermatic duct.

sperm head. The head of a spermatozoon.

sper′mi·cide [*sperma;* L. *caedere,* to kill]. An agent that destroys spermatozoa. Syn., *spermatocide.*

sper′mi·dine. $H_2N(CH_2)_3NH(CH_2)_4NH_2$; a polyamino compound found in semen and other animal tissues.

sper′min, sper′mine [*sperma*]. Diaminopropyltetramethylene-diamine, $H_2N(CH_2)_3NH(CH_2)_4NH(CH_2)_3NH_2$, found in the form of a phosphate in semen and other animal fluids and tissues; its exact function is unknown. Has been used in the treatment of nervous disorders.

sperm′ism [*sperma*]. A form of the theory of preformation, which held that the sperm cell contains the animalcule. —**spermist,** *n.*

sper′mo·lith [*sperma;* G. *lithos,* stone]. A calculus in a spermatic duct or seminal vesicle.

sper·mol′y·sin, sper″mo·ly′sin [*sperma;* G. *lysis,* a loosing]. A cytolysin produced by inoculation with spermatozoa. Syn., *spermatoxin.*

sper·mol′y·sis. See *spermatolysis.*

sper″mor·rhe′a. See *spermatorrhea.*

Sperry's method. See Schoenheimer and Sperry's *method.*

sp. g., sp. gr. Specific gravity.

sph. Spherical or spherical lens.

sphac″e·la′tion (sfass″i·lay′shun) [G. *sphakelos,* gangrene]. Necrosis, gangrene, mortification. —**sphac′elate,** *v.*

sphac′e·lism (sfass′i·liz·um) [*sphakelos*]. The condition of being affected by sphacelus.

sphac″e·lo·der′ma (sfass″i·lo·dur′muh) [*sphakelos;* G. *derma,* skin]. Gangrene of the skin from many different causes.

sphac′e·lus (sfass′i·lus) [*sphakelos*]. A slough. —**sphac′eloid, sphac′elous,** *adj.*

spha″gi·as′mus (sfay″jee·az′mus) [G. *sphagiasmos,* a slaying]. Epileptic spasm of the muscles of the neck.

spha·gi′tis [G. *sphagē,* throat; *-itis,* inflammation]. 1. Inflammation of a jugular vein. 2. Sore throat.

sphe′ni·on [G. *sphēn,* wedge]. The point at the anterior extremity of the sphenoparietal suture.

sphe′no-, sphen- [*sphēn*]. A combining form meaning *wedge;* used to denote *pertaining to the sphenoid bone.*

sphe″no·bas′i·lar. Spheno-occipital.

sphe″no·ceph′a·lus [*sphēn;* G. *kephalē,* head]. 1. In Isidore Geoffroy Saint-Hilaire's classification, a variety of monster with separated eyes, the ears united under the head, the jaws and mouth distinct, and the sphenoid bone altered in shape. 2. In Blanc's classification, a monster in which the lower jaw is absent or rudimentary, the fauces are occluded, with severe defects in the upper jaw and sphenoid region, and with various degrees of synotia. The upper face is nearly normal, as in Geoffrey Saint-Hilaire's sphenocephalus. 3. An individual having a wedge-shaped, narrow head, resulting from compensatory enlargement of the anterior fontanel after premature sagittal sutural union.

sphe″no·ceph′a·ly [*sphēn; kephalē*]. The condition of having a wedge-shaped head.

sphe″no·eth′moid [*sphēn;* G. *ēthmoeidēs,* perforated]. Relating to both the sphenoid and the ethmoid bones.

sphe′noid [G. *sphēnoeidēs,* wedge-shaped]. Wedge-shaped, as the sphenoid bone.

sphe′noid. The sphenoid bone. See Table of Bones in the Appendix. —**sphenoid′al,** *adj.*

sphe″noid·i′tis [*sphēnoeidēs;* G. *-itis,* inflammation]. Inflammation of the sphenoid air sinus.

sphe″noid·ot′o·my [*sphēnoeidēs;* G. *tomē,* a cutting]. Incision into the sphenoid air sinus.

sphe″no·man·dib′u·lar [G. *sphēn,* wedge; L.

mandibula, jaw]. Pertaining to the sphenoid and mandibular bones, as sphenomandibular ligament.

sphe″no·max′il·lar″y (sfee″no·mack′si·lerr″ee) [*sphēn;* L. *maxilla*, jawbone]. Pertaining to the sphenoid and maxillary bones, as the sphenomaxillary fossa.

sphe″no-oc·cip′i·tal (-ock·sip′i·tul). Pertaining to the sphenoid and the occipital bones; sphenobasilar.

sphen·op′a·gus par″a·sit′i·cus. See *episphenoid.*

sphe″no·pal′a·tine (sfee″no·pal′uh·tyne, ·tin, ·teen) [*sphēn;* L. *palatum*, palate]. Pertaining to the sphenoid bone and the palate, as the sphenopalatine foramen.

sphe″no·pa·ri′e·tal [*sphēn;* L. *paries*, wall]. Pertaining to the sphenoid and parietal bones.

sphe″no·pe·tro′sal. Pertaining to the sphenoid bone and the petrous portion of the temporal bone.

sphe·no′sis [G., a closing up]. The wedging of the fetus in the pelvis.

sphe″no·tre′si·a (sfee″no·tree′zhuh, ·zee·uh, ·shuh, ·see·uh) [G. *sphēn*, wedge; *trēsis*, perforation]. A variety of craniotomy in which the basal portion of the fetal skull is perforated.

sphe′no·tribe [*sphēn;* G. *tribein*, to rub]. An instrument for crushing the basal portion of the fetal skull.

sphe′no·trip″sy [*sphēn;* G. *tripsis*, a rubbing]. Crushing of the fetal skull.

sphere [G. *sphaira*, ball]. 1. A ball or globe. 2. A space. —**spher′ic, spher′ical,** *adj.*

attraction s. A clear spot in the cytoplasm, outside and close to the nucleus of an ovum undergoing mitosis. It contains the centrosome, and is the center of the formation of the amphiasters in karyokinesis.

vitelline s. The mulberrylike mass of cells that results from the fission of the substance of the ovum after fertilization. Also called *yolk s.*

sphe″res·the′si·a, sphe″raes·the′si·a (sfeer″ess·thee′zhuh, ·zee·uh) [*sphaira;* G. *aisthēsis*, perception]. Globus hystericus.

sphe″ro·ceph′a·lus [*sphaira;* G. *kephalē*, head]. Blanc's term for a monster with absent or rudimentary lower jaw, occlusion of the fauces, approximation of the ears, lack of the bones of the face, marked deficiencies in the frontal and sphenoid bones, and with a vesicular brain.

sphe″ro·cyl′in·der [*sphaira;* G. *kylindros*, cylinder]. Bifocal lens combining a spherical with a cylindrical surface.

sphe′ro·cyte [*sphaira;* G. *kytos*, cell]. An erythrocyte which is spherical in form rather than biconcave and having the microscopic appearance of a hyperchromatic microcyte.

sphe″ro·cy′tic. Pertaining to a blood picture in which the mean corpuscular volume (MCV) or volume index is within ±2 standard deviations of the mean normal, but the mean corpuscular diameter is more than 2 standard deviations below the mean normal as determined by the same method on the bloods of healthy persons of the patient's age or sex group.

sphe″ro·cy·to′sis (sfeer″o·sigh·to′sis) [*sphaira; kytos;* G. *-ōsis*, condition] A preponderance in the blood of spherocytes as observed microscopically.

hereditary s. A chronic, congenital disorder of the erythrocytopoietic system characterized by spherocytosis, increased osmotic fragility, a variable degree of intracorpuscular hemolytic anemia, and splenomegaly. The manifestations vary widely in severity, and hence in time of recognition. Also called *congenital hemolytic anemia, chronic acholuric jaundice, chronic familial jaundice* or *icterus, familial acholuric jaundice, familial hemolytic jaundice* or *icterus, familial jaundice, hemolytic splenomegaly.*

sphe′roid, sphe·roi′dal [*sphaira;* G. *eidos*, form]. Resembling a sphere.

sphe′roid. A solid resembling a sphere.

oblate s. One in which the polar axis is less than the equatorial diameter.

prolate s. One in which the polar axis exceeds the equatorial diameter.

sphe·rom′e·ter [*sphaira;* G. *metron*, a measure]. An instrument for determining the degree of curvature of a sphere or part of a sphere, especially of optical lenses, or of the tools used for grinding them.

spher′ule [dim. from *sphaira*]. A minute sphere.

sphinc′ter [G. *sphigktēr*, that which binds tight]. A muscle surrounding and closing an orifice. See Table of Muscles in the Appendix. —**sphincter′ic,** *adj.*

anal s. Either of the sphincter ani muscles.

cardiac s. The circular muscle fibers around the cardiac end of the esophagus.

pyloric s. The thickened ringlike band of the circular layer of smooth muscle at the lower end of the pyloric canal of the stomach.

s. ampullae. The occasionally present network of smooth muscle of the ampulla of Vater.

s. ani. (a) The **sphincter ani externus,** composed of bundles of striate muscle fibers surrounding the anus. (b) The **sphincter ani internus,** a thickening of the inner circular (smooth) muscle layer of the anal canal.

s. choledochus. The annular smooth muscle of the common bile duct just before its junction with the pancreatic duct.

s. of Boyden. That strong muscular part of the sphincter of Oddi around the preampullary part of the bile duct, which remains contracted during interdigestive phases, allowing the gallbladder to be filled.

s. of Oddi. The intricate arrangement of smooth muscle about the ductus choledochus and pancreatic duct in the wall of the duodenum.

s. pancreaticus. The inconstant band of smooth muscle encircling the pancreatic duct just before it joins the ampulla of Vater.

s. urethrae. (a) The **sphincter urethrae membranaceae,** composed of bundles of voluntary muscle which surround the membranous portion of the urethra in the male; in the female the analogous muscle fibers surround the proximal portion of the urethra. (b) The **sphincter vesicae,** composed of bundles of smooth muscle which are a part of the tunica muscularis of the bladder; the fibers are looped around the neck of the bladder, thus forming an involuntary urethral sphincter.

urethral s. See *s.* urethrae.

vaginal s. The bulbocavernosus muscle in the female.

sphinc″ter·al′gi·a [*sphigktēr;* G. *algos*, pain]. Pain in the sphincter ani muscle, or about the anus.

sphinc″ter·ec′to·my [*sphigktēr;* G. *ektomē*, excision]. Oblique blepharotomy; Stellwag's operation for the dilatation of the palpebral fissure, or for blepharospasm.

sphinc″ter·is′mus (sfink″tur·iz′mus) [*sphigktēr*]. A spasmodic contraction of the sphincter ani muscle, usually attendant upon fissure or ulcer of the anus, but occasionally occurring independently of such lesion.

sphinc″ter·i′tis [*sphigktēr;* G. *-itis*, inflammation]. Inflammation of a sphincter, especially the anal sphincter.

sphinc″ter·ol′y·sis [*sphigktēr;* G. *lysis*, a loosing]. The operation of freeing the iris in anterior synechia.

sphinc′ter·o·plas″ty [*sphigktēr;* G. *plassein,* to form]. A plastic or reparative operation on a sphincter muscle.

sphinc″ter·ot′o·my [*sphigktēr;* G. *tomē,* a cutting]. The operation of incising a sphincter.

sphin′gol. Sphingosine.

sphin″go·my′e·lin. A phospholipid occurring in brain, kidney, liver, and egg yolk. It is composed of choline, sphingosine, phosphoric acid, and a fatty acid. The latter is usually lignoceric acid but probably several sphingomyelins exist which contain other fatty acids, such as stearic and nervonic acids.

sphin′go·sine (sfing′go·seen, ·sin). A basic, unsaturated amino-alcohol occurring in sphingomyelin and the cerebrosides. It has the probable composition, $CH_3(CH_2)_{12}CH{=}CH.CHOH.CH$-$NH_2.CH_2OH$. Syn., *sphingol.*

sphyg′mic, sphyg′mic·al [G. *sphygmos,* pulse]. Pertaining to the pulse.

sphyg′mo- [*sphygmos*]. A combining form meaning *pulse.*

sphyg″mo·bo·lom′e·ter [*sphygmos;* G. *bolē,* stroke; *metron,* a measure]. An instrument for measuring and recording the force of the pulse. —**sphygmobolometry,** *n.*

sphyg″mo·chron′o·graph (sfig″mo·kron′o·graf, ·kro′no·graf) [*sphygmos;* G. *chronos,* time; *graphein,* to write]. A registering sphygmograph.

sphyg″mo·chro·nog′ra·phy [*sphygmos; chronos; graphein*]. The registration of the extent and oscillations of the pulse wave.

sphyg·mod′ic (sfig·mod′ick, ·mo′dick) [G. *sphygmōdēs,* like the pulse]. Like the pulse; throbbing.

sphyg″mo·dy″na·mom′e·ter (·dye″na·mom′i·tur, ·din″uh·) [G. *sphygmos,* pulse; *dynamis,* power; *metron,* a measure]. An instrument for measuring the force of the pulse.

sphyg′mo·gram″ [*sphygmos;* G. *gramma,* letter]. The tracing made by the sphygmograph.

sphyg′mo·graph″ [*sphygmos;* G. *graphein,* to write]. An instrument for recording graphically the features of the pulse and the variations in blood pressure. —**sphygmograph′ic,** *adj.*

sphyg·mog′ra·phy [*sphygmos; graphein*]. A description of the pulse, its pathologic variations and their significance.

sphyg′moid [*sphygmos;* G. *eidos,* form]. Resembling or having the nature of continuous pulsation.

sphyg″mo·ma·nom′e·ter [*sphygmos;* G. *manos,* rare; *metron,* a measure]. An instrument for measuring the tension of the blood current or arterial pressure. —**sphygmomanometry,** *n.*

sphyg·mom′e·ter. See *sphygmograph.*

sphyg″mo-os″cil·lom′e·ter [*sphygmos;* L. *oscillare,* to swing; *metron*]. A form of sphygmomanometer in which the systolic and diastolic blood pressures are indicated by an oscillating device.

sphyg″mo·pal·pa′tion [*sphygmos;* L. *palpatio,* from *palpare,* to touch softly]. The palpation of the pulse.

sphyg′mo·phone [*sphygmos;* G. *phōnē,* sound]. A sphygmograph in which the vibrations of the pulse produce a sound.

sphyg′mo·scope [*sphygmos;* G. *skopein,* to examine]. A pulse pressure recorder in which the force of arterial pressure is made visible. There are numerous mechanical devices for accomplishing this result.

sphyg·mos′co·py [*sphygmos; skopein*]. 1. The art of tracing the pulse curve by the sphygmoscope. 2. Examination of the pulse.

sphyg″mo·sys′to·le (sfig″mo·sis′to·lee) [*sphygmos;* G. *systolē,* contraction]. That part of the sphygmogram produced under the influence of the cardiac systole upon the pulse.

sphyg′mo·tech″ny (sfig′mo·teck″nee, sfig″mo·teck′nee) [*sphygmos;* G. *technē,* art]. The art of diagnosis and prognosis by means of the pulse.

sphyg″mo·to′no·graph [*sphygmos;* G. *tonos,* tension; *graphein,* to write]. An instrument which records pulsations from an inflatable rubber cuff; systolic and diastolic pressures are read by this means.

sphyg″mo·to·nom′e·ter [*sphygmos; tonos;* G. *metron,* a measure]. An instrument for measuring human blood pressure.

sphyg′mus [*sphygmos*]. The pulse; a pulsation. —**sphygmous,** *adj.*

sphynx-neck. The webbed neck seen in Turner's syndrome.

spi′ca [L.]. 1. A spike or spur. 2. A spiral bandage with reversed turns. See Plate 34.

spice [L. *species,* sort]. An aromatic vegetable substance used for flavoring; a condiment.

spic′u·la, spic′ule. 1. A small spike-shaped bone or fragment of bone. 2. A needle-shaped body; a spike. —**spicular,** *adj.*

spi′der [AS. *spinnan,* to spin]. An animal of the order Araneida of the class Arachnida, characterized by having four pairs of legs, usually eight eyes, and an unsegmented abdomen.

black widow s. The species *Latrodectus mactans,* a black spider with globose abdomen. The adult has an hourglass-shaped red or yellow spot on the ventral side. The female is about 0.5 in. long, the male about half as big as the female. Its bite has been fatal in about 5% of the reported cases. Also called *knoppie s.*

Menarody s. A poisonous species of *Latrodectus* found in Madagascar.

spi′der burst. Old term for the telangiectatic areas in the skin of the legs associated with varicose veins.

Spiegler's test for albumin. See under *test.*

Spielmeyer, Walter [*German neurologist,* 1879–1935]. Described juvenile amaurotic familial idiocy; also called *Spielmeyer-Vogt disease.* The retinal atrophy observed in this disease is known as *Spielmeyer-Stock disease.*

Spielmeyer's myelin stain. See under *stain.*

Spies, Tom Douglas [*American physician,* 1902–]. Distinguished for contributions in the field of vitamins and vitamin deficiency diseases. Demonstrated that folic acid is an erythrocyte maturation factor (1945–46). See also Spies *test.*

Spi·ge′li·a (spy·jee′lee·uh) [L., after Adriaan van der *Spieghel,* Belgian botanist and anatomist, 1578–1625]. Pinkroot, a genus of plants of the family Loganiaceae. The rhizome and rootlets of **S. marilandica** formerly were used as a vermifuge.

Spigelian hernia. See under *hernia.*

Spigelian lobe. See caudate *lobe.*

Spigelius' line. Linea semilunaris; see semilunar *line.*

spike [L. *spica,* spike]. *In electroencephalography,* a sporadic, rapid wave appearing suddenly out of a slower wave rhythm. Duration, about 0.02 sec.

spike-and-wave. *In electroencephalography,* a complex consisting of a spike followed by a slow wave.

spike′nard (spike′nurd, ·nard) [*spica;* L. *nardus,* nard]. 1. A name given to the rhizome of various species of *Valeriana* or closely related genera. Used as an aromatic and a perfume among ancient Oriental peoples. 2. American spikenard. See *Aralia racemosa.*

spill [AS. *spillan,* to destroy]. An overflow, especially that of blood. Also applied to certain forms of cellular metastasis in malignant disease.

Spiller, William Gibson [*American neurologist,* 1863–1940]. With C. H. Frazier, introduced intracranial neurotomy of the sensory root of the trigeminal nerve for the relief of trigeminal neuralgia or tic douloureux (1901), called *Spiller's* or *Frazier's operation.* He also described epidural ascending spinal paralysis, called *Spiller's syndrome.*

spi·lo′ma (spy·lo′muh). Nevus.

spi″lo·pla′ni·a [G. *spilos*, spot; *planos*, a wandering]. A condition characterized by transient maculas of the skin.

spi′lus [*spilos*]. A mole or colored mark on the skin; nevus.

spi′na (pl. *spinae*) [L., thorn]. A sharp projection. See *spine.*

s. bifida. A congenital defect in the closure of the spinal canal with hernial protrusion of the meninges of the cord. The hernial sac contains cerebrospinal fluid and sometimes nervous tissue. Most common in the lumbosacral region. Also called *rachischisis.*

s. bifida occulta. A defect in the closure of the spinal canal without hernial protrusion of the meninges, usually diagnosed only by x-ray.

s. ventosa. Tuberculous infection of the long bones of the hand or foot, involving rarefaction of the compacta and subperiosteal formation of new bone to produce a spindle-shaped enlargement of the shaft. Syn., *tubercular dactylitis.*

spin′a·cene. Squalene.

spi′nal ac·ces′so·ry nerve. See accessory *nerve.*

spi′nal cord. See under *cord.* See Plate 16.

spi·na′lis (spy·nah′lis, ·nay′lis) [L. *spinalis*, spinal]. A muscle attached to the spinous processes of the vertebrae. See Table of Muscles in the Appendix.

spi′nal man. A patient in a prolonged state of spinal shock, following a complete transection of the spinal cord.

spin·as′ter·ol. A phytosterol obtained from spinach.

spin′dle [AS. *spinel*]. 1. A tapering rod. A fusiform shape. 2. That part of the achromatic figure in mitosis between the centrosomes or asters, consisting of modified cytoplasm and spindle fibers.

achromatic s. A protoplasmic framework of achromatin. See nuclear *s.*, *karyokinesis.* Syn., *amphiaster.*

central s. A central group of fibers extending between the asters, in contrast to the peripheral ones attached to chromosomes.

cleavage s. A spindle formed during cleavage of the ovum or blastomeres.

enamel s. A space in the dental enamel due to growth of an odontoblastic process into the ameloblastic layer before enamel formation.

Krukenberg's s. A pigmented line seen with the corneal slit lamp on the endothelium of the cornea.

muscle s. See neuromuscular *s.*

neuromuscular s. Small fusiform sensory end-organs found in almost all the muscles of the body.

neurotendinal s. See tendon *s.*

nuclear s. A spindle formed from nuclear substance, especially in some types of anastral mitoses.

sleep s. *In electroencephalography*, the bursts of about 14-per-second waves that occur during sleep.

s. cataract. A form of cataract characterized by a spindle-shaped opacity extending from the posterior surface of the anterior portion of the capsule to the anterior surface of the posterior portion of the capsule, with a central dilatation.

s. cell. See under *cell.*

tendon s. A specialized, encapsulated sensory nerve end-organ in tendon adjacent to muscular tissue. Also called *neurotendinal s.*

spin′dle tree. See *euonymus.*

spine [L. *spina*, thorn]. 1. A sharp process of bone. 2. The backbone or spinal column. Also see *tubercle.* —**spi′nous, spi′nal,** *adj.*

angular s. A downward projection from the posterior extremity of the great wing of the sphenoid, giving attachment to the sphenomandibular ligament and some fibers of the tensor veli palatini muscle.

anterior nasal s. A median, sharp process formed by the forward prolongation of the two maxillas at the lower margin of the anterior aperture of the nose.

bifid s. A complete or incomplete congenital cleft of the vertebral column; a posterior fusion defect of the vertebral arches. Also called *spina bifida.*

cervical s. Loosely, the spinous process of a cervical vertebra.

Civinini's s. A small process on the lateral pterygoid plate.

ethmoid s. The spine of the sphenoid bone articulating with the cribriform plate of the ethmoid bone.

frontal s. A sharp, medial, downward projection from the nasal process of the frontal bone; nasal spine.

helical s. An anterior projection of the cartilage of the auricle of the ear in the region of the helix.

hemal s. The part that closes in the hemal arch of a typical vertebra, e.g. in a fish's tail.

Henle's s. The suprameatal spine.

iliac spines. Four spines of the ilium. The anterior extremity of the iliac crest forms the **anterior superior iliac spine;** the posterior extremity, the **posterior superior iliac spine.** The **anterior inferior iliac spine** is that on the anterior border of the ilium, and the **posterior inferior iliac spine** is that on the posterior border, separated from the respective posterior superior spine by a notch.

mental s. Spina mentalis [BNA]. The single or double tubercle on each side of the body of the mandible near the midline, for origin of the genioglossus and geniohyoid muscles. Syn., *genial tubercle.*

nasal s. (a) A sharp, medial process projecting downward from the nasal process of the frontal bone into the nasal septum and articulating with the crests of the nasal bones and the perpendicular plate of the ethmoid. (b) See anterior nasal *s.* (c) See posterior nasal *s.*

neural s. The part that closes in the neural arch of the typical vertebra.

occult bifid s. A simple variety of spinal nonunion in the lumbar or thoracolumbar region, with few or no symptoms. Often revealed only by the presence of a dimple in the skin. Also called *spina bifida occulta.*

palatine s. See posterior nasal *s.*

pharyngeal s. A small elevation near the middle of the inferior surface of the basilar process of the occipital bone, for the superior attachment of the median raphe of the pharynx.

posterior nasal s. A process formed by the united, projecting, medial ends of the posterior borders of the two palate bones, giving attachment to the muscle of the uvula.

pubic s. The pubic tubercle on the superior border of the pubis.

railway s. Traumatic neurosis following concussion injury with spinal symptoms and without demonstrable pathology. *Obs.*

sphenoid s. (a) See angular *s.* (b) See ethmoid *s.*

s. of ischium. A pointed eminence on the posterior border of the body of the ischium. It forms the lower border of the greater sciatic notch. Also called *ischial s.*

s. of the scapula. The strong, triangular plate of bone attached obliquely to the dorsum of the scapula and dividing it into two unequal parts, the supraspinous and infraspinous fossae.

s. of the tibia. Intercondyloid eminence.

suprameatal s. A small tubercle projecting from the posterosuperior margin of the external auditory meatus of the temporal bone.

trochlear s. A small projection on the upper medial wall of the orbit, for attachment of the fibrocartilaginous pulley for the superior oblique muscle.

typhoid s. A neurosis sometimes following typhoid, characterized by acute pains in the vertebral column on the slightest movement.

vertebral s. See spinous *process* of a vertebra.

spinocain. Trade-mark for a 10% solution of novocain in a solvent of a specific gravity lower than that of the spinal fluid. The solution is used in spinal anesthesia by the method of Dr. George P. Pitkin.

spi″no·cel′lu·lar [*spina;* L. *cellula,* small storeroom]. Pertaining to, or like, prickle cells.

spi″no·gal″va·ni·za′tion [*spina;* Luigi *Galvani*]. Galvanization of the spinal cord.

spi′no·gram″. See *myelogram.*

spi′no·graph″ [*spina;* G. *graphein,* to write]. A radiograph of the spine.

spi″no·tec′tal [*spina;* L. *tectum,* roof]. Pertaining to the spinal cord and the corpora quadrigemina, as the spinotectal tract.

spi″no·trans″ver·sa′ri·us [*spina;* L. *transversarius,* transverse]. Old term for any of the rotator muscles of the spine.

spin·thar′i·scope. Scintillascope.

spin′ther·ism [G. *spinthēr,* spark]. Sensation of sparks before the eyes. See scintillating *scotoma.*

spin″u·lo′sin, spin′u·lo·sin [L. *spinula,* little thorn]. $C_8H_8O_5$; 3,6-dihydroxy-5-methoxy-*p*-toluquinone or hydroxyfumigatin; an antibiotic substance produced by *Penicillium spinulosum* and *Aspergillus fumigatus,* occurring in purple-black crystals, slightly soluble in cold water, and having some activity against Gram-positive organisms.

spi·rad″e·ni′tis sup″pu·ra·ti′va (spy·rad″i·nigh′-tis). See *hidradenitis suppurativa.*

spi′ral [*speira*]. Winding screwlike, as a spiral bandage; helical. **—spi′ral,** *n.*

Curschmann's spirals. See Heinrich *Curschmann.*

spi′reme (spy′reem, spy·reem′) [G. *speirēma,* coil]. The skein or ribbon of chromatin in the prophase of meiosis or mitosis which segments and condenses to form the chromosomes.

spir″il·li·ci′dal (spirr″il·i·sigh′dul, spy·ril″i·) [*speira;* L. *caedere,* to kill]. Capable of destroying spirilla.

spir″il·lo′sis (spirr″i·lo′sis, spy″ri·) [*speira;* G. *-ōsis,* condition]. A disease caused by infection with one of the spiral bacilli. See rat-bite *fever, Spirillum.*

Spi·ril′lum (spy·ril′um) (pl. *spirilla*) [*speira*]. A genus of spiral bacilli of the family Pseudomonadaceae.

S. minus. The causative agent of rat-bite fever.

spir′it [L. *spiritus,* breath]. 1. An alcoholic solution of a volatile principle, formerly prepared by distillation but now generally prepared by dissolving the volatile substance in alcohol. 2. Any distilled liquid. Abbreviated, sp.

cologne s. Ethanol.

colonial s. Methanol.

columbian s. Methanol.

methylated s. Denatured ethanol.

perfumed s. (*spiritus odoratus*). Contains the volatile oils from bergamot, lemon, rosemary, lavender, and orange flower, ethyl acetate, water, and alcohol. Used as a pleasant perfume and sometimes used externally for the relief of neuralgia. Also called *cologne water.*

s. of wine. Alcohol, 2.

sweet s. of niter. Ethyl nitrite spirit.

spi′ro-, spir- [G. *speira,* a coil]. A combining form meaning *a coil;* used to denote *spiral.*

spi′ro- [L. *spirare,* to breathe]. A combining form denoting *respiration.*

Spi″ro·chae′ta (spy″ro·kee′tuh) [G. *speira,* a coil; *chaitē,* hair]. A genus of spiral microorganisms of the family Spirochaetaceae.

S. cuniculi. See *Treponema cuniculi.*

S. icterogenes. See *Leptospira icterohaemorrhagiae.*

S. icterohaemorrhagiae. See *Leptospira icterohaemorrhagiae.*

S. morsus muris. See *Spirillum minus.*

S. nodosa. See *Leptospira icterohaemorrhagiae.*

S. obermeieri. See *Borrelia recurrentis.*

S. pallida. See *Treponema pallidum.*

S. sogdiana. Old name for *Borrelia recurrentis.*

Spi″ro·chae·ta′ce·ae (spy″ro·ki·tay′see·ee) [*speira; chaitē*]. A family of spiral microorganisms which includes the genera *Spirochaeta, Saprospira,* and *Cristispira.* The family is nonpathogenic for man; a few species of *Cristispira* are parasites of crustaceans, all other species are free-living forms.

Spi″ro·chae·ta′les (spy″ro·ki·tay′leez) [*speira; chaitē*]. An order of spiral microorganisms which includes the families Spirochaetaceae and Treponemataceae.

spi″ro·chae·to′sis ic″te·ro·hae″mor·rhag′i·ca. See spirochetal *jaundice.*

spi′ro·chete (spy′ro·keet) [*speira; chaitē*]. Any of the spiral microorganisms belonging to the order Spirochaetales. **—spiroche′tal,** *adj.*

spi″ro·che·te′mi·a (spy″ro·ki·tee′mee·uh) [*speira; chaitē;* G. *haima,* blood]. The presence of spirochetes in the blood.

spi″ro·che′ti·cide (spy″ro·kee′ti·side) [*speira; chaitē;* L. *caedere,* to kill]. An agent which kills spirochetes.

spi″ro·che·tol′y·sis (spy″ro·ki·tol′i·sis) [*speira; chaitē;* G. *lysis,* a loosing]. Destruction of spirochetes by lysis.

spi″ro·che·to′sis [*speira; chaitē;* G. *-ōsis,* condition]. Any of the diseases caused by infection with one of the spirochetes, such as syphilis, relapsing fever, spirochetal jaundice. **—spirochetot′ic,** *adj.*

spirocid. Trade-mark for a brand of acetarsone.

spiroform. Trade-mark for phenyl acetylsalicylate.

spi′ro·gram″ [L. *spirare,* to breathe; G. *gramma,* letter]. A recorded tracing of the movements and excursion of the chest in respiration.

spi′ro·graph″ [*spirare;* G. *graphein,* to write]. An instrument for registering respiration.

spi·rom′e·ter (spy·rom′i·tur) [*spirare;* G. *metron,* a measure]. An instrument for measuring the vital capacity or volumes of inhaled and exhaled air. Syn., *gasometer.* **—spiromet′ric,** *adj.;* **spirometry,** *n.*

Tissot s. See *Tissot spirometer.*

spis′sa·ted (spis′ay·tid) [L. *spissus,* thick]. Inspissated.

spis′si·tude [L. *spissitudo,* thickness]. The state of being inspissated.

spitz′en·stoss″ [Ger. *Spitze,* point; *Stoss,* beat]. The apex beat in contradistinction to *herzstoss.* See *point* of maximal impulse.

Spitzer, Alexander [*Austrian anatomist,* 1868–1946]. Proposed a phylogenetic theory of heart development, accounting for anomalies by faulty degrees of torsion; called *Spitzer's phylogenetic theory.*

Spitzka, Edward Charles [*American neurologist*, 1852–1914]. Said to have discovered the dorsolateral tract one year before Lissauer; called *Spitzka's* or *Lissauer's tract* or *zone*.

Spix, Johann Baptist [*German anatomist*, 1781–1826]. Described the lingula mandibulae, the spine at the medial border of the mandibular foramen, to which the sphenomandibular ligament is attached. Called *Spix's spine*.

splanch'na (splank'nuh) [G. *splagchna*, inward parts]. 1. The intestines. 2. The viscera.

splanch"nec·to'pi·a (splank"neck·to'pee·uh) [*splagchna;* G. *ektopos*, away from a place]. The abnormal position or dislocation of a viscus.

splanch"nem·phrax'is [*splagchna;* G. *emphraxis*, stoppage]. Obstruction of the intestine.

splanch"nes·the'si·a (splank"ness·thee'zhuh, ·zee·uh) [*splagchna;* G. *aisthēsis*, perception]. Visceral sensation. —**splanchnesthet'ic,** *adj.*

splanch"neu·rys'ma (splank"new·riz'muh) [*splagchna;* G. *eurynein*, to make wide]. Distention of the intestine.

splanch'nic [*splagchna*]. Pertaining to, or supplying, the viscera.

splanch"ni·cec'to·my [*splagchna;* G. *ektomē*, excision]. The surgical excision of the splanchnic nerves.

splanch"ni·cot'o·my [*splagchna;* G. *tomē*, a cutting]. Surgical division of a splanchnic nerve.

splanch'no- (splank'no-), **splanchn-** [*splagchna*]. A combining form denoting *pertaining to the viscera.*

splanch'no·cele [*splagchna;* G. *kēlē*, hernia]. A protrusion of any abdominal viscus.

splanch'no·coele (splank'no·seel) [*splagchna;* G. *koilos*, hollow]. That part of the coelom which persists in the adult, and gives rise to the pericardial, pleural, and abdominal cavities; the ventral coelom, or pleuroperitoneal space. It appears as a narrow fissure in the lateral mesoderm.

splanch"no·di·as'ta·sis (·dye·ass'tuh·sis) [*splagchna;* G. *diastasis*, separation]. Displacement or separation of the viscera.

splanch·nog'ra·phy [*splagchna;* G. *graphein*, to write]. The descriptive anatomy of the viscera.

splanch'no·lith [*splagchna;* G. *lithos*, stone]. Calculus of a viscus.

splanch"no·li·thi'a·sis [*splagchna;* G. *lithiasis*, disease of the stone]. The condition of having a calculus of the intestine.

splanch·nol'o·gy [*splagchna;* G. *logos*, word]. The branch of medical science pertaining to the viscera.

splanch"no·meg'a·ly [*splagchna;* G. *megas*, large]. Abnormal enlargement of the viscera.

splanch"no·mi'cri·a (splank"no·migh'kree·uh, ·mick'ree·uh) [*splagchna;* G. *mikros*, small]. Generalized smallness of the visceral organs.

splanch·nop'a·thy [*splagchna;* G. *pathos*, disease]. Disease of the viscera.

splanch'no·pleure [*splagchna;* G. *pleura*, side]. The wall of the gut, composed of endoderm and the splanchnic layer of lateral mesoderm. —**splanchnopleu'ral,** *adj.*

splanch"nop·to'sis (splank"nop·to'sis, splank"-no·), **splanch"nop·to'si·a** (splank"nop·to'shuh, ·see·uh, ·zhuh, ·zee·uh, splank"no·) [*splagchna;* G. *ptōsis*, a falling]. A condition of abnormal relaxation of the abdominal viscera.

splanch"no·scle·ro'sis [*splagchna;* G. *sklērōsis*, a hardening]. Visceral induration.

splanch·nos'co·py [*splagchna;* G. *skopein*, to examine]. Visual examination of the viscera.

splanch"no·skel'e·ton [*splagchna;* G. *skeletos*, dried up]. 1. That portion of the skeleton related to the viscera. *Obs.* 2. The visceral skeleton.

splanch"no·so·mat'ic [*splagchna;* G. *sōmatikos*, of the body]. Pertaining to the viscera and the body.

splanch·not'o·my [*splagchna;* G. *tomē*, a cutting]. Dissection of the viscera.

splanch'no·tribe [*splagchna;* G. *tribein*, to rub]. An instrument for crushing a segment of the intestine and so occluding its lumen, previous to resecting it.

spleen [G. *splēn*]. One of the abdominal viscera, located immediately below the diaphragm on the left side; the largest lymphatic organ of the body. It is covered by a fibromuscular capsule continuous with trabeculae which radiate through the organ from the hilus, the portal of entry and exit of the splenic vessels. Between the trabeculae is white pulp, ensheathing branches of the splenic artery and composed of cords and nodules of lymphatic tissue, and red pulp composed of atypical lymphatic tissue, the splenic cords, filling the spaces between venous sinuses. See Plates 8, 10, 13, 14.

accessory s. Small mass of splenic tissue found either isolated or connected to the spleen by thin bands of splenic tissue. Also called *supernumerary s.*

ague cake s. That which is the seat of chronic, long-standing malarial splenomegaly.

bacon s. One with areas of amyloid degeneration, appearing like fried bacon on cut surface.

flecked s. One containing multiple areas of nonembolic anemic necrosis.

floating s. An abnormally movable and perhaps displaced spleen. Also called *wandering s.*

Gandy-Gamna s. An enlarged siderotic spleen.

iced s. One with a clear, translucent, pearl-gray or pale blue hyalinized capsule occurring most often in chronic syphilitic hyperplasia. Also called *sugar-coated s., zuckerguss s.*

lardaceous s. One affected with diffuse amyloid degeneration. Also called *waxy s.*

porphyry s. One which is affected by multiple nodular infiltrations.

sago s. One in which amyloid is present in the follicles showing on cut section numerous small glassy areas transmitting the red color of the spleen.

wandering s. See floating *s.*

sple·nal'gi·a [*splēn;* G. *algos*, pain]. Pain originating in the spleen.

sple·nec'to·my [*splēn; ektomē*]. Excision of the spleen. —**splenec'tomize,** *v.*

splen"ec·to'pi·a (splen"eck·to'pee·uh, splee"-neck·), **sple·nec'to·py** [*splēn;* G. *ektopos*, away from a place]. Displacement of the spleen.

sple·net'ic [*splēn*]. 1. Pertaining to the spleen. 2. Having a diseased spleen.

splen'ic, sple'nic [*splēn*]. Pertaining to the spleen.

splen"i·co·pan"cre·at'ic [G. *splēnikos*, of the spleen; *pagkreas*, pancreas]. Belonging, or pertaining, to both the spleen and the pancreas.

splen'i·form, sple'ni·form [*splēn;* L. *forma*, form]. Resembling the spleen.

sple·ni'tis [G., disease of the spleen]. Inflammation of the spleen.

sple'ni·um [G. *splēnion*, pad of linen]. 1. Old term for a bandage. 2. The rounded posterior extremity of the corpus callosum. See Plate 18.

sple'ni·us [*splēnion*]. One of two muscles of the back of the neck, splenius capitis and splenius cervicis. See Table of Muscles in the Appendix. —**splenial,** *adj.*

s. cervicis accessorius. A variant of the splenius cervicis muscle.

splen"i·za'tion [G. *splēn*, spleen]. The stage of consolidation in the development of pneumonia during which lung tissue, grossly, takes on an appearance resembling that of the normal spleen or liver, thus also called hepatization.

sple′no- (splee′no-, splen′o-), **splen-** [*splēn*]. A combining form denoting *pertaining to the spleen.*

sple′no·cele [*splēn;* G. *kēlē,* hernia]. 1. Hernia of the spleen. 2. A tumor of the spleen.

sple″no·clei′sis (·kly′sis) [*splēn;* G. *kleisis,* a closing]. Causing the production of new fibrous tissue on the spleen.

sple′no·cyte [*splēn;* G. *kytos,* cell]. A monocyte, regarded as developing from the pulp of the spleen.

sple″no·dyn′i·a (splee″no·din′ee·uh, ·dye′nee·uh, splen″o·) [*splēn;* G. *odynē,* pain]. Pain in the spleen.

sple″no·gran″u·lo″ma·to′sis sid″er·ot′i·ca. A rare, slowly progressive splenomegaly of southern Europe, generally considered a form of chronic congestive splenomegaly. Histologically the spleen is granulomatous with heavy hemosiderin deposition. Syn., *Gamna's disease, mycotic splenomegaly.*

sple″no·hep″a·to·meg′a·ly [*splēn;* G. *hēpar,* liver; *megas,* large]. Enlargement of the liver and spleen.

sple′noid [*splēn;* G. *eidos,* form]. Resembling the spleen.

sple·nol′y·sis, splen″o·ly′sis [*splēn;* G. *lysis,* a loosing]. Destruction of splenic tissue.

sple″no·ma·la′ci·a (·ma·lay′shee·uh, ·see·uh) [*splēn;* G. *malakia,* softness]. Softening of the spleen.

sple″no·meg′a·ly [*splēn;* G. *megas,* large]. Enlargement of the spleen; occurs in brucellosis, histoplasmosis, malaria, and other diseases.

chronic congestive s. A syndrome associated with portal hypertension, in which there is leukopenia and splenomegaly which may precede the anemia present. The degree and type of anemia vary with duration of the syndrome, the presence of cirrhosis of the liver, and the amount of hemorrhage. Lymphadenopathy is absent. Probably synonymous with *Banti's syndrome.* Also called *splenic anemia, hepatolienal fibrosis.* See also *splenogranulomatosis siderotica.*

Egyptian s. Large spleen probably due to *Schistosoma mansoni.*

hemolytic s. See hereditary *spherocytosis.*

mycotic s. See *splenogranulomatosis siderotica.*

Stengel-Wolbach s. See splenic *anemia.*

tropical s. Enlarged spleen due to kala-azar.

sple·nop′a·thy [*splēn;* G. *pathos,* disease]. Any disease of the spleen.

sple′no·pex″y [*splēn;* G. *pēxis,* a fixing]. Fixation of the spleen to the abdominal wall by means of sutures.

sple″no·pneu·mo′ni·a [*splēn;* G. *pneumōn,* lung]. The stage of pneumonia producing splenization or hepatization of lung tissue.

sple″nop·to′sis [*splēn;* G. *ptōsis,* a falling]. Downward displacement of the spleen, due to abnormal mobility.

sple·nor′rha·phy [*splēn;* G. *rhaphē,* suture]. Suture of the spleen.

sple·not′o·my [*splēn;* G. *tomē,* a cutting]. 1. The operation of incising the spleen. 2. Dissection of the spleen.

sple″no·tox′in (splee″no·tock′sin, splen″o·) [*splēn;* G. *toxikon,* poison]. A cytotoxin with specific action on the cells of the spleen.

sple″no·ty′phoid [*splēn;* G. *typhos,* cloud; *eidos,* form]. Typhoid fever with splenic complication. *Obs.*

splen′u·lus [L., dim. from *splēn*]. Accessory spleen or rudimentary spleen.

splice [D. *splissen*]. Join by suture, as to splice a tendon.

splint [MD. *splinte*]. 1. A piece of wood, metal, plastic, wire, or other material for immobilizing the ends of a fractured bone or for restricting the movement of any movable part. 2. *In veterinary medicine,* a form of periostitis in the foreleg of the horse.

acrylic s. (a) *In dental surgery,* an apparatus or stent of plastic material used in fracture of the mandible and maxilla, or to give support in bone grafts of the jaws. (b) *In facial surgery,* one used to give support in fractures of the nasal bones and septum.

airplane s. A special type which holds the arm in abduction with the forearm midway in flexion; generally of wire with an axillary strut and frequently incorporated in a plaster body support.

ambulatory s. See ambulatory *traction.*

anchor s. A special type used in dentistry in fracture of the jaw, equipped with metal loops fitting about the teeth.

Anderson s. One used in fracture of the femur. Also see under Roger *Anderson.*

angular s. One formed by two flat splints united at an angle, or a wire or other metal or plastic splint forming an angle appropriate to the condition to be treated.

Balkan s. See *Balkan frame.*

banjo s. A hand splint usually made of wire in the shape of a banjo or racket, attached to the forearm and sometimes incorporated in plaster. It is used generally for the attachment of rubber band traction devices for overriding and comminuted phalangeal bones; the rubber bands are said to resemble the strings of a banjo.

Böhler's s. A wire extension splint used in the treatment of fractured fingers.

Bolles' s. One used in the treatment of fracture of the coronoid process of the ulna.

caliper s. One designed for the leg, consisting of two metal rods from a posterior thigh band or a padded ischial ring to a metal plate attached to the sole of the shoe at the instep. Also called *walking caliper.*

coaptation s. A series of narrow splints of uniform size placed parallel to one another and held by adhesive plaster or leather, used to envelop a limb, such as the upper arm or thigh, where uniform and complete support is desired in the area covered.

cockup s. A hand splint for immobilizing the hand in hyperextension during wound healing.

divided dental s. One constructed in sections, lingual and buccal, joined together by wire hinges or ligatures and used in jaw fractures to retain bony fragments in apposition.

flange s. *In dentistry,* one of cast silver, with a high flange pointed upward to ride upon the buccal surface of the opposing upper teeth. The splint is cemented to several posterior teeth of the lower jaw in a dentulous fragment of a mandibular fracture.

Fulton s. One used in the treatment of dislocation of the radius.

Hodgen s. A splint used in the treatment of fractures of the shaft of the femur.

interdental s. A dental apparatus for holding the ends of fractured maxillas or mandibles in place by means of wires passing about the teeth.

Jones s. A hinged arm splint of the Thomas type. See traction *s.*

Keller-Blake s. A hinged, half-ring splint of the Thomas type for the lower extremity.

ladder s. One with cross bars resembling a ladder.

Magnuson s. An abduction splint used in the treatment of fractures of the humerus.

pillow s. A pillow support used as an emergency dressing for fractures of the lower leg. The pillow is compressed on either side and posteriorly with board splints held by several straps so as to exert firm pressure upon the leg.

plastic s. One made of plastic material which can be molded into the form desired.

sectional s. See divided dental *s.*

Stader's s. A metal bar with pins affixed at right angles. The pins are driven into the fragments of a fracture, and the bar maintains the alignment.

Thomas s. One used to maintain traction in fractures of the humerus or femur, consisting of a ring which fits around the upper arm or thigh and two long metal rods extending from the ring on either side of the extremity. The rods are joined by a crosspiece below the hand or foot, and traction or fixation is applied to the crosspiece. Also used as an emergency splint for safe transportation in such injuries.

traction s. One so devised that traction can be exerted on the distal fragment of a fracture to overcome muscle pull and maintain proper alignment of the fractured bone, such as the banjo, Thomas, or caliper splint.

T s. One used to hold back the shoulders, and adapted by bandaging to hold the fragments in apposition in clavicular fractures.

splint'age [*splinte*]. The application of splints.

splin'ter [MD.]. *In veterinary medicine*, a vestigial second or fourth metacarpal or metatarsal of the horse; one of the splint bones extending, in the forelimb, from the "knee" and, in the hindlimb, from the hock, toward the fetlock.

splint'ing [MD. *splinte*]. Application of a splint.

split-prod'uct. A decomposition product, as the aglycone produced by hydrolysis of a glycoside.

split'ters of Speng'ler. Fragments of Spengler. See Carl *Spengler.*

split'ting [MD. *splitten*]. A chemical change in which a compound is changed into two or more simpler bodies, as by hydrolysis.

spo"di·o·my"e·li'tis (spo"dee·o·migh"i·lye'tis, spod"ee·o·) [G. *spodios*, gray; *myelos*, marrow; *-itis*, inflammation]. Old term for acute anterior poliomyelitis.

spo'di·um [G. *spodos*, wood-ashes]. Old term for animal charcoal.

spo'do·gram. A photograph or diagram picturing the distribution of mineral ash of a cell or tissue section following microincineration.

spoke'shave" [AS. *spaca; scafan*]. A ring knife, devised by Carmalt Jones, for use in operations on the nasal cavities.

spondyl-. See *spondylo-.*

spon"dy·lal'gi·a [G. *spondylos*, vertebra; *algos*, pain]. Pain referred to a vertebra.

spon"dy·lar·throc'a·ce (spon"di·lahr·throck'uh-see) [*spondylos;* G. *arthron*, joint; *kakē*, badness]. Caries of a vertebra.

spon"dy·li'tis [*spondylos;* G. *-itis*, inflammation]. Inflammation of one or more vertebrae. —**spondylit'ic,** *adj.*

ankylosing s. Arthritis of the spine affecting the apophyseal and the sacroiliac joints leading to bony ankylosis with complete stiffness of the back. The costovertebral joints are included in the process when it involves the thoracic spine. Ossification of the anterior, lateral, and posterior, or yellow, ligaments produces the so-called bamboo spine. The intervertebral disks are not affected. It usually affects young men and is accompanied by severe debility. The peripheral joints, except for the hips, are usually spared. Also called *bamboo spine, rhizomelic spondylosis, spondylitis ankylopoietica, spondyloarthritis ankylopoietica, rheumatoid arthritis of the spine, poker back, poker spine, deforming spondylitis, Strümpell-Marie disease, Bekhterev's disease.*

deforming s. (a) Ankylosing spondylitis. (b) Degenerative joint disease of the spine characterized by spur formation. It results, in part at least, from trauma with injury and deformity of the intervertebral disks. Limitation of motion is due to bony block, not to bony ankylosis.

ochronotic s. See *osteoarthritis.*

rheumatoid s. See ankylosing *s.*

tuberculous s. Tuberculosis of the vertebral bodies leading to bone destruction, vertebral collapse, and kyphosis, healing by fusion of adjacent vertebrae. There may be accompanying psoas abscess and compression of the spinal cord. Also called *Pott's disease.*

spon"dy·li·ze'ma (spon"di·li·zee'muh, ·lye·zee'-muh) [*spondylos;* G. *hizēma*, a sinking]. The settling of a vertebra into the place of a subjacent one that has been destroyed. *Obs.*

spon'dy·lo-, spondyl- [*spondylos*]. A combining form signifying *pertaining to a vertebra.*

spon"dy·lo·ar·thri'tis an"ky·lo·poi·et'i·ca. See ankylosing *spondylitis.*

spon"dy·loc'a·ce (spon"di·lock'uh·see). See *spondylarthrocace.*

spon"dy·lo·di·dym'i·a [*spondylos;* G. *didymos*, twin]. The condition of union of conjoined twins united by their vertebrae. See *rachipagus.*

spon"dyl·od'y·mus [*spondylos; didymos*]. Conjoined twins united by the vertebrae.

spon"dy·lo·dyn'i·a (spon"di·lo·din'ee·uh, ·dye'-nee·uh) [*spondylos;* G. *odynē*, pain]. Pain in a vertebra.

spon"dy·lo·lis·the'sis [*spondylos;* G. *olisthēsis*, a slipping and falling]. Forward displacement of a vertebra upon the one below as a result of bilateral defect in the vertebral arch, or erosion of the articular surface of the posterior facets due to degenerative joint disease. It occurs most commonly between the fifth lumbar vertebra and the sacrum.

spon"dyl·ol'y·sis [*spondylos;* G. *lysis*, a loosing]. Dissolution or destruction of a vertebra.

spon"dyl·op'a·thy [*spondylos;* G. *pathos*, disease]. Any disease of the vertebrae.

spon"dy·lo·py·o'sis (spon"di·lo·pye·o'sis) [*spondylos;* G. *pyōsis*, suppuration]. Suppurative inflammation of one or more vertebrae.

spon"dy·lo'sis [*spondylos;* G. *-ōsis*, condition]. Vertebral ankylosis.

rhizomelic s. Spondylose rhizomélique; Marie's term for ankylosing *spondylitis.*

spon"dy·lo·syn·de'sis. Spinal fusion.

spon"dy·lot'o·my [*spondylos;* G. *tomē*, a cutting]. Section of a vertebra in correcting a deformity.

spon'dy·lus [*spondylos*]. Old term for a vertebra. —**spondylous,** *adj.*

sponge [G. *spoggos*]. A marine animal of the phylum Porifera. Some of the class semospongia have a porous, horny skeleton. Also the skeleton itself, used as an absorbent. —**spon'giform,** *adj.*

gauze s. A flat folded piece of gauze of varying size, used by a surgical assistant to mop blood from the wound during the process of an operation.

gelatin s. Sheet of gelatin, prepared to check bleeding when applied to a raw surface.

sponge hold'er. An instrument consisting of a rod which serves as a handle, furnished at the distal end with a device for clasping a sponge.

spon'gi·o·blast" (spon'jee·o·blast", spun'jee·o·) [G. *spoggia*, sponge; *blastos*, germ]. A nonnervous cell derived from the ectoderm of the embryonic neural tube, and later forming the neuroglia, the ependymal cells, the neurilemma sheath cells, the satellite cells of ganglions, and Müller's fibers of the retina.

spon″gi·o·blas·to′ma. Astroblastoma.

s. multiforme. See *glioblastoma multiforme.*

s. polare. See *astroblastoma.*

s. primitivum. See *ependymoma.*

s. unipolare. See *astroblastoma.*

spon′gi·o·cyte″ [*spoggia;* G. *kytos,* cell]. 1. A neuroglia cell. 2. A cell, in the fasciculate zone of the adrenal cortex, which appears spongy because of the solution of lipoids during preparation of the tissue for microscopical study.

spon″gi·o·cy·to′ma. See *astrocytoma.*

spon′gi·oid (spon′jee·oyd, spun′·) [*spoggia;* G. *eidos,* form]. Spongiform.

spon″gi·o·neu″ro·blas·to′ma. See *neuroastrocytoma.*

spon′gi·o·plasm [*spoggia;* G. *plasma,* anything formed]. The fine protoplasmic threads forming the reticulum of cells after certain fixations. *Obs.*

spon′gi·ose [*spoggia*]. Full of pores, like a sponge.

spon″gi·o′sis. Accumulation of fluid in the intercellular spaces of the epidermis causing an increase in the width of the spaces and stretching out of the intercellular bridges; intercellular edema.

spon″gi·o·si′tis [*spoggia;* G. *-itis,* inflammation]. Inflammation of the corpus spongiosum.

spon′gy (spun′jee) [G. *spoggos,* sponge]. Having the texture of sponge; very porous.

spon·ta′ne·ous gen″er·a′tion. The view that living matter may arise at the present time from nonliving matter. Syn., *abiogenesis. Obs.*

spoon [AS. *spōn,* chip]. An instrument, usually made of metal, with a circular or oval bowl attached to a handle. A spoon is considered full when the contained liquid comes up to, but does not show a curve above, the upper edge or rim of the bowl. Household spoons are popularly used to measure the dose of medicines on the generally incorrect assumption that a teaspoon holds 4 cc. (1 drachm), a tablespoon 15 cc. (half an ounce), and a dessertspoon 8 cc. (2 drachms). Medicine glasses are graduated on this basis. The actual spoons vary quite widely, teaspoons from 2 to 8 cc., averaging doses of 5 rather than of 4 cc.

cataract s. A small spoon-shaped instrument used to remove the lens in cataract operations.

s. nail. A fingernail with a concave outer surface.

surgical s. A surgical instrument consisting of an oval or circular bowl fixed to a handle; it is used to scrape away dead tissue, granulations, etc.

spoon′er·ism [after the Rev. Wm. A. *Spooner,* of England, 1844–1930]. A psychic speech or writing defect characterized by the tendency to transpose letters or syllables of two or more words.

spo·rad′ic [G. *sporadikos,* scattered]. Scattered; occurring in an isolated manner.

spo·ran′gi·o·phore″ [G. *spora,* seed; *aggeion,* vessel; *phoros,* bearing]. A specialized hyphal branch of a fungus which bears a sporangium.

spo·ran′gi·o·spore″ [*spora; aggeion; spora*]. A fungus spore borne within a sporangium.

spo·ran′gi·um (pl. *sporangia*) [*spora; aggeion*]. A specialized structure of a fungus; the enlarged end of a hypha within which spores develop.

resting s. *In biology,* Pringsheim's term for peculiar resting cells formed by the mycelium of a few fungi (such as *Saprolegnia*), in which zoospores are produced.

spore [*spora*]. A reproductive cell of a protozoan, bacterium, or higher plant. There is usually a thick cell wall enabling the cell to survive in adverse environments.

asexual s. A spore formed without previous fusion of nuclear material.

resting s. *In biology,* a spore, invested with a firm cell wall, which remains dormant during adverse environmental conditions before it germinates.

sexual s. A spore formed subsequent to the union of two nuclei.

spo′ri·cide [*spora;* L. *caedere,* to kill]. Any agent which destroys spores. —**sporici′dal,** *adj.*

spo′ro-, spor- [*spora*]. A combining form signifying *relating to a spore* or *seed.*

spo″ro·ag·glu″ti·na′tion [*spora;* L. *agglutinare,* to glue]. Agglutination of spores by antiserum.

spo′ro·cyst [*spora;* G. *kystis,* bladder]. 1. The oocyst of certain protozoa, e.g., plasmodia and coccidia, in which sporozoites develop. 2. The larval stages of flukes in snails, from which cercariae develop.

spo′ro·cyte″. A single binucleated cell formed in the life cycle of protozoa of the orders *Myxosporidia* and *Actinomyxidia.*

spo″ro·gen′e·sis [*spora;* G. *genesis,* production]. Production of spores.

spo·rog′e·ny [*spora;* G. *gignesthai,* to be produced]. Reproduction by spores; especially spore formation in Sporozoa following encystment of a zygote.

spo′ront [*spora;* G. *ōn,* pres. part. of *einai,* to be]. In Sporozoa, a cell which forms spores by encystment and subsequent division.

spo′ro·phyte. The asexual, spore-producing phase in plants having alternation of generations.

spo·rot′ri·chin (spo·rot′ri·kin) [*spora;* G. *thrix,* hair]. An antigenic filtrate of a culture of *Sporotrichum;* used for diagnostic complement fixation test.

spo″ro·tri·cho′sis (spor″o·tri·ko′sis, ·try·ko′sis) [*spora; thrix;* G. *-ōsis,* condition]. A subacute or chronic granulomatous disease caused by the fungus *Sporotrichum.* The lesions are usually cutaneous and spread along lymph channels; occasionally the internal organs and bones may be involved. The disease is reported among farmers, florists, and others working in soil. Also called *de Beurmann-Gougerot disease, Schenck's disease.*

Spo″ro·trich′um (spo″ro·trick′um) [*spora; thrix*]. A genus of fungi, the causative agents of sporotrichosis; short, blunt, cigar-shaped to spherical, partially Gram-positive bodies which occur singly or in groups, either in pus or in tissue. They may be free in the necrotic material or phagocytized by macrophages. **S. beurmanni** and **S. schencki** are the species most frequently isolated from cases of human infestation.

Spo″ro·zo′a [*spora;* G. *zōion,* living being]. A class of parasitic Protozoa; the orders Coccidia, Sarcosporidia, and Haemosporidia are parasites of man.

spo″ro·zo′an [*spora; zōion*]. Pertaining to Sporozoa. —**sporozo′an,** *n.*

spo″ro·zo′ite [*spora; zōion*]. 1. The organism resulting from sexual multiplication of the Sporozoa. 2. An animal spore.

spo″ro·zo′on [*spora; zōion*]. *In biology,* a member of the Sporozoa.

sport [ME. *desport*]. An individual organism which differs from its parents to an unusual degree; a mutation.

spor′u·late [*spora*]. To eject spores from a sporangium.

spot [ME.]. A small circumscribed area, differing in appearance or function from the surrounding area.

acoustic spots. See *maculae acusticae* under *macula.*

Bier spots. See A. K. G. *Bier.*

Bitot's spots. Xerosis conjunctivae; silver-gray, shiny, triangular spots on both sides of the cornea, within the region of the palpebral aperature, consisting of dried epithelium, flaky masses, and microorganisms: seen in some cases of nyctalopia,

blind s. of Mariotte. A scotoma in the visual field representing the entrance of the optic nerve, where the rods and cones are absent. Syn., *optic disk, optic papilla.* See Plate 19.

blue s. A bluish discoloration of the skin seen in such nevi as Mongolian spot, blue nevus.

Brushfield's spots. Speckled white or very light yellow, clearly defined pinpoints seen on the irides of infant mongolian idiots, which disappear if later the color of the iris changes to brown; sometimes also seen in normal infants, but their absence may serve to rule out suspected cases of mongolism: so named for Thomas Brushfield, English physician, 1858–1937.

café au lait spots. Light brown or coffee-colored areas of the skin seen independently of tumor nodules in multiple fibromatosis.

Cayenne-pepper s. See papillary *varix.*

cherry-red s. A bright red area seen in the retina in cases of amaurotic familial idiocy.

cold spots. Areas on the surface of the skin overlying the nerve endings that are stimulated by cold.

corneal s. An opacity of the cornea; leukoma.

cribriform spots. The perforations of the wall of the vestibule for the passage of the filaments of the acoustic nerve: also called *maculae cribrosae.*

embryonic s. The nucleolus of the ovum.

focal s. The area of an x-ray-tube target against which the main electron beam strikes.

genital s. An area on the nasal mucosa which has a tendency to bleed during menstruation. The bleeding is called vicarious menstruation.

germinal s. The nucleolus of the egg nucleus.

hot spots. Areas on the surface of the skin overlying the sense organs that are stimulated by heat.

hypnogenetic spots. Surface areas of the body, stimulation of which produces sleep.

itch spots. Small areas of the skin upon stimulation of which the sensation of itching is perceived. They appear to be identical with pain spots.

Koplik's spots. The characteristic exanthema of measles. See Koplik's *sign.*

light s. A cone of light on the anterior and inferior part of the tympanic membrane, with its apex directed inward.

Mariotte's s. The optic disk.

Michel's spots. Black spots of posterior pigment epithelium, seen in the iris through atrophied areas of anterior lamina, and sometimes seen in protracted iritis.

milk s. A patch of thickening and opacity of the epicardium, found post mortem, usually over the right ventricle; of common occurrence in persons who have passed middle life.

milky spots. Small regions of the omentum containing multitudes of fixed and free macrophages.

Mongolian s. A focal bluish-gray discoloration of the skin of the lower back, also aberrantly on the face, present at birth and fading gradually: often seen in members of the Mongolian race.

mother's s. Nevus.

Mueller's spots. Spots seen (rarely) on the iris after an attack of smallpox. Syn., *vitiligo iridis.*

pain spots. Areas on the skin overlying the nerve endings which respond to painful stimuli.

rose spots. A red, papular eruption forming spots from 1 to 5 mm. in size which fade on pressure, occurring mostly on the abdomen and loins during the first seven days of typhoid fever. They are due to inflammation of the papillary layer of the skin from invasion of typhoid bacilli. Also called *typhoid roseola, typhoid spots, taches rosées lenticulaires.*

Roth's spots. See Moritz *Roth.*

soldier's s. See milk *plaque.*

sun spots. See *lentigo.*

temperature spots. Hot and cold spots on the skin.

typhoid spots. See *rose spots* under *spot.*

vesical blind s. *In urology,* the area or areas of the anterior urinary bladder wall which cannot be visualized in cystoscopic examination.

white spots. Grayish or yellowish white elevated spots, from 2–15 mm in diameter, of varying shape and distinctness of outline, often occurring on the ventricular surface of the anterior leaflet of the mitral valve.

wine s. See port-wine *nevus.*

yellow s. See *macula* lutea.

spot grind'ing. *In dentistry,* correction of occlusion by removal of high areas of teeth or prosthetic devices, as disclosed by use of articulating paper.

spot'ting [*spot*]. Small amounts of bloody vaginal discharge, usually intermenstrual, and of significance in certain obstetric and gynecologic conditions.

sprain [OF. *espreindre,* from L. *exprimere,* to press out]. A wrenching of a joint, producing a stretching or laceration of the ligaments.

rider's s. A sprain of the adductor longus muscle of the thigh, resulting from a sudden effort of the horseman to maintain his seat owing to some unexpected movement of his horse.

s. fracture. An injury in which a tendon, together with a shell of bone, is torn from its attachment.

spray [ME. *sprayen*]. 1. A stream of air and finely divided liquid produced with an atomizer, nebulizer, or other device. 2. A liquid pharmaceutical preparation intended for applying medication to the nose, throat, or other cavities by spraying from an atomizer or nebulizer; may be aqueous or oily in character. Light liquid petrolatum is usually employed as the vehicle for oily sprays.

spread'ing [AS. *sprǣdan*]. Growth of bacteria beyond the line of inoculation.

Sprengel, Otto Gerhard Karl [*German surgeon,* 1852–1915]. Described congenital elevation of the scapula (1891); also called *Sprengel's deformity.* This was first noted by M. M. Eulenburg (1863) as congenital high scapula, but never received his name.

spring'fin"ger. See under *finger.*

spring'halt", spring hock. See *stringhalt.*

Spritz bottle. A wash bottle for laboratory use.

sprue [D. *sprouw*]. 1. An afebrile, chronic disease characterized by the passage of voluminous, mushy, and often frothy stools, weakness, emaciation, changes in the tongue, and anemia. Common in white people in southeastern Asia, East Indies, Ceylon, West Indies. Originally the disease was thought to be caused by the yeast *Monilia psilosis,* but recent work tends to show that the disease is basically a deficiency disease. Vedder stated that sprue may occur in individuals who have excellent diets. The question of defective absorption has been considered. Vedder also suggested that dysfunction of the anterior pituitary gland may be associated with the disturbed absorption from the intestine. Also called *aphthous cachexia, psilosis, Ceylon sore mouth, diarrhea alba, Cochin-China diarrhea, tropical sprue.* 2. *In dentistry,* a wire or other object used to produce a vent in a mold for casting.

indigenous s. See celiac *disease.*

nontropical s. A form of celiac syndrome seen in adults.

para-sprue. A dietary disease characterized by chronic watery diarrhea, weight loss, a sore red tongue, and macrocytic anemia. It differs from true sprue in showing less emaciation, no swollen lower abdomen, dry skin, dysphagia, and pale, frothy stools with the fat content above 40%.

spud [ME.]. A dull flattened blade used in surgery.

spur [AS. *spura*]. 1. A sharp projection. Also called *calcar*. 2. *In biology*, a pointed, spinelike outgrowth, either of the integument or of a projecting appendage.

calcaneal s. A painful exostosis of the heel due to trauma, static conditions of the foot, improper shoes, or systemic infections. Also called *heel s.*

s. of the septum. An outgrowth of the nasal septum.

spur'gall" (spur'gawl") [*spura;* ME. *galle*, sore spot]. A calloused and hairless place on the side of a horse, caused by the use of a spur.

spurge [L. *expurgare*, to purge]. A general name for plants of the genus *Euphorbia*.

spurge flax. See *mezereum.*

spu'tum (pl. *sputums, sputa*) [L., spittle]. Material discharged from the surface of the air passages, throat, or mouth, and removed chiefly by spitting but in lesser degree by swallowing. It may consist of saliva, mucus, or pus, either alone or in any combination. It may also contain microorganisms, fibrin, blood or its decomposition products, or inhaled particulate foreign matter.

hailstone s. That containing particles having the appearance of hailstones.

mucopurulent s. That consisting of a mixture of mucus and pus.

mucous s. Sputum consisting chiefly of mucus, often erroneously designated as mucoid sputum.

nummular s. Sputum containing small, round, flattened masses of heavy material.

purulent s. That consisting chiefly of pus.

rusty s. That colored by various decomposition products of blood; seen chiefly in lobar pneumonia. Also called *prune-juice s., icteric s.*

squa'lene. $C_{30}H_{50}$; 2,6,10,15,19,23-hexamethyl-2,6,-10,14,18,22-tetracosahexaene; an unsaturated hydrocarbon occurring in large proportion in shark-liver oil and in smaller proportion in various vegetable oils; an oil, insoluble in water, sparingly soluble in alcohol, and freely soluble in ether: believed to be an intermediate in the biological synthesis of cholesterol. Syn., *spinacene.*

synthetic s. A product obtained in an attempt to prepare natural squalene, differing from it probably in the position of double bonds.

squa'ma (pl. *squamae*) [L., scale]. A scale or scale-like mass, as the squama of the temporal bone.

s. frontalis. The vertical portion of the frontal bone.

s. occipitalis. Posterior part of the occipital bone.

s. temporalis. The squamosa.

squame (pl. *squames*) [*squama*]. A flat plate, scale, or platelike cell.

squa'mo- [*squama*]. A combining form denoting *relating to the squamous portion of the occipital or temporal bone.*

squa"mo-oc·cip'i·tal (skway"mo-ock·sip'i·tul). Pertaining to the squamous portion of the occipital bone, or to the suture between the squamosa and the occipital bone.

squa·mo'sa [L. *squamosus*, scaly]. The squamous portion of the temporal bone.

squa"mo·sphe'noid [L. *squama*, scale; G. *sphēnoeidēs*, wedge-shaped]. Pertaining to the squamous portion of the temporal bone and to the sphenoid bone.

squa"mo·tym·pan'ic [*squama;* G. *tympanon*, drum]. Pertaining to the squamosal and tympanic parts of the temporal bone.

squa'mous [L. *squamosus*, scaly]. Of the shape of a scale, as the squamous portion of the temporal bone, or squamous epithelium, epithelium consisting of flat, scalelike cells.

squill [G. *skilla*] (*scilla*). The cut and dried fleshy inner scale of the bulb of the white variety of *Urginea maritima*, or of *Urginea indica*. The active principles of squill have been variously reported as scillipicrin, scillitoxin, scillin, scillenin, scillimarin, scillitin, and scillidiuretin. In many cases, these have been obtained from the dry drug. Investigations on the fresh drug first led to separation of the crystalline glycoside known by the trade-marked name *scillaren-A* and an amorphous fraction known as *scillaren-B*. Later studies showed the amorphous fraction to contain glucoscillaren A, scillipheoside, glucoscillipheoside, scillicryptoside, scilliglaucoside, scillicyanoside, scillicoeloside, and scilliazuroside. Its action and uses are similar to those of digitalis. Squill has been used as a nauseant and an expectorant.

compound s. syrup (*syrupus scillae compositus*). Contains fluidextracts of squill and senega, of each 80 cc.; antimony and potassium tartrate, 2 Gm.; sucrose, 720 Gm.; distilled water, a sufficient quantity to make 1000 cc. It was originally introduced as a remedy for croup or hives. It has expectorant and diaphoretic properties. Dose, children, 0.12–1.3 cc. (2–20 min.); adults, 1.3–2 cc. (20–30 min.).

s. fluidextract (*fluidextractum scillae*). Chiefly employed as a nauseating expectorant. It is an ingredient in expectorant mixtures. Dose, 0.06–0.2 cc. (1–3 min.).

s. syrup (*syrupus scillae*). Contains squill vinegar, 450 cc.; sucrose, 800 Gm.; distilled water, a sufficient quantity to make 1000 cc. Used as an expectorant. Dose, 2–4 cc. (½–1 fluidrachm).

squint. See *strabismus.*

squir'rel corn. See *corydalis.*

squirt'ing cu'cum·ber. See *elaterium.*

Sr Chemical symbol for strontium.

s̄s̄, ss. *Semis*, one-half.

SSS. Specific soluble substance.

S.T. Surface tension.

S.T. 37. Trade-mark for 1:1000 solution of hexylresorcinol in glycerin and water, having a surface tension of 37 dynes per cm.; also used for certain related products.

stab. 1. A puncture wound. 2. Path formed by plunging an inoculation needle into nutrient media. 3. See band *cell.* —**stab,** *v.*

sta'bile (stay'bil, stab'il) [L. *stabilis*, stable]. Stationary; immobile; maintaining a fixed position.

sta'bi·li"zer [*stabilis*]. 1. A retarding agent, or a substance that counteracts the effect of a vigorous accelerator and preserves a chemical equilibrium. 2. A substance added to a solution to render it more stable, as acetanilid to hydrogen peroxide solution.

froth s. Certain oils and chemicals which produce stable froths in water; they function best in the presence of finely divided solids.

sta'ble [*stabilis*]. Unlikely to break down or dissolve; in the case of a compound, likely to retain its composition under the application of physical or chemical forces.

sta'ble com·po'nent. See *convertin.*

sta'ble pro·throm'bin con·ver'sion ac·cel"er·a'tor (SPCA). See *convertin.*

stac·ca'to (sta·kah'to) [It., detached]. Denoting an abrupt, jerky manner of speech with a noticeable interval between words.

stach'y·drine. $C_7H_{13}NO_2$. N-Methylproline-methylbetaine, an alkaloid occurring in *Stachys tuberifera* and other plants.

stach'y·ose. A tetrasaccharide obtained from the tubers of *Stachys tuberifera* and some other plants. On complete hydrolysis it yields one molecule each of fructose and glucose and two of galactose. Also called *mannotetrose, lupeose.*

Stacke, Ludwig [*German otologist*, 1859–1918].

Introduced excision of the ossicles of the ear. Made important improvements in the technic of radical mastoidectomy. Devised an operation in which the tympanum and external acoustic meatus were connected, in chronic suppurative disease of the middle ear; called *Stacke's operation.*

Stader's splint. See under *splint.*

Stadie method. See Riggs and Stadie *method.*

sta'di·um (pl. *stadia*) [G. *stadion,* race-course]. Stage.

s. acmes. The height of a disease.

s. amphiboles. See amphibolic *stage.*

s. annihilationis. The convalescent stage.

s. augmenti. The period in which there is increase in the intensity of the disease.

s. caloris. The period during which there is fever.

s. contagii. The prodromal stage of an infectious disease.

s. convalescentiae. The period of recovery from disease.

s. decrementi. Defervescence of a febrile disease; the period in which there is a decrease in the severity of the disease.

s. decrustationis. The stage of an exanthematous disease in which the lesions form crusts.

s. desquamationis. The period of desquamation in an exanthematous fever.

s. eruptionis. That period of an exanthematous fever in which the exanthema appears.

s. exsiccationis. See *s.* decrustationis.

s. floritionis. The stage of an eruptive disease during which the exanthema is at its height.

s. frigoris. The cold or algid stage of a fever.

s. incrementi. The stage of increase of a fever or disease.

s. incubationis. See *stage* of latency.

s. maniacale. The last stage of excitement in mania, after which the nervous manifestations gradually subside.

s. nervosum. The paroxysmal stage of a disease.

s. prodromorum. The stage immediately prior to the appearance of the signs and symptoms of disease.

s. sudoris. The sweating stage.

s. suppurationis. The period in the course of smallpox in which suppuration occurs.

s. ultimum. The final stage of a febrile affection.

staff [AS. *staef*]. 1. An instrument for passing through the urethra to the urinary bladder, used as a guide in operations on the bladder or for stricture. It is usually grooved. 2. The personnel concerned with the care of patients in a hospital.

consulting s. Specifically, a body of physicians, surgeons, or specialists attached to a hospital or medical unit, who serve only in an advisory capacity.

house s. The interns and residents living in the hospital.

visiting s. The nonresident physicians and surgeons who supervise the care of patients in a hospital.

stage [L. *stare,* to stand]. 1. A definite period of a disease characterized by certain symptoms; a condition in the course of a disease. 2. The horizontal plate projecting from the pillar of a microscope for supporting the slide or object.

algid s. A condition characterized by subnormal temperature, feeble, flickering pulse, and various nervous symptoms. It occurs in cholera and other diseases marked by exhausting intestinal discharges.

amphibolic s. The stage of a disease intervening between its height and its decline.

asphyxial s. The preliminary stage of Asiatic cholera, marked by extreme thirst, muscular cramps, etc., due to loss of water from the blood.

cold s. The rigor or chill of an attack of a malarial paroxysm.

defervescent s. Stage of declining temperature.

eruptive s. That in which an exanthema makes its appearance.

expulsive s. The stage of labor which begins when dilatation of the cervix uteri is complete and during which the child is expelled from the uterus.

first s. That stage of labor in which the molding of the fetal head and the dilatation of the cervix are effected.

hot s. The febrile stage of a malarial paroxysm.

mechanical s. A fixture on a microscope stage with two horizontal screw adjustments at right angles to each other which permit the specimen to be moved as desired. Some have vernier scales for reading the amount of displacement to 0.1 mm.

microscope s. The platform under the microscope tube which carries the specimen and is usually mounted permanently on the microscope pillar; it may be mounted on a rack and pinion.

placental s. The period of labor occupied by the expulsion of the placenta and fetal membranes.

pre-eruptive s. The period of an eruptive fever following infection and prior to the appearance of the eruption.

pyrogenic s. The stage of invasion in febrile diseases. Also called *pyrogenetic s.*

resting s. *In biology,* the period of dormancy of a plant or germ.

second s. See expulsive *s.*

s. of invasion. The period in the course of a disease in which the body comes under the influence of the infective agent.

s. of latency. The incubation period of an infectious disease, or that period intervening between the entrance of the agent and the manifestations of the symptoms to which it gives rise.

sweating s. The third or terminal stage of a malarial paroxysm, during which sweating occurs.

third s. See placental *s.*

stag'gers [ON. *stakra,* to push]. A term applied to various diseases which are manifested by lack of coordination in movement and a staggering gait, as gid and sturdy of sheep, encephalomyelitis of horses, botulism, loco poisoning, and some cerebral affections of livestock.

stag'ing a're·a. A military camp near a port of embarkation where troop units are assembled en route to overseas stations to await embarkation. Such areas include station hospitals and dispensary service, where immunizations against infectious disease are accomplished if necessary.

stag·na'tion [L. *stagnare,* to form a pool of standing water]. 1. A cessation of motion. 2. *In pathology,* a cessation of motion in any fluid; stasis. —**stag'nate,** *v.*

Stahl, Friedrich Karl [*German physician,* 1811–73]. Described a congenital deformity of the ear consisting of a broadening of the helix. The fossa antihelicis and upper part of the scaphoid fossa are practically obliterated; called *Stahl's ear.*

Stahl, Georg Ernst [*German physiologist and chemist,* 1660–1734]. Described lacrimal fistula and its causation (1702). Expounded a theory (now obsolete) that the body is presided over by the sensitive soul which regulates its activities by motion; called *animism, Stahl's theory.* With Johann Becher, postulated the phlogiston theory of combustion.

Stahli's pigment line. A horizontal brown line in the lower part of the cornea, found in senile degeneration; also called *Hudson's line.*

stain [L. *dis-,* denoting reversal; *tingere,* to color]. (For a list of Special Stains and Staining Methods,

see below.) 1. A discoloration produced by absorption of, or contact with, foreign matter. 2. *In microscopy,* a pigment or dye used (a) to render minute and transparent structures visible, (b) to differentiate tissue elements, or (c) to produce specific microchemical reactions.
acid s. A dye in which the anion is colored and does the staining. Acid stains are the common stains for cytoplasm and cytoplasmic inclusions.
acid-fast s. See Ziehl-Neelsen *method.*
basic s. A dye in which the cation is colored and does the staining. Basic stains are the common stains for chromatin in nuclei, for nucleoproteins, for mucins, and for calcium-salt deposits in tissues.
celestin blue s. An aqueous solution of iron alum and celestin blue, useful as a nuclear stain.
chrome hematoxylin. A stain for lipofuscins, containing equal parts of 1% aqueous hematoxylin and 2% aqueous chrome alum.
Commission Certified s. A stain which has been certified by the Biological Stain Commission. Abbreviated, C.C.
contrast s. A double stain in which certain cell constituents take one stain and other constituents take the contrasting stain.
counterstain. A second stain, usually a contrasting one, which is used after one which stains nuclei or desired constituents.
double s. A mixture of two dyes of contrasting colors, usually an acid stain and a basic stain, or a method involving the successive use of contrasting stains. See contrast *s.*
fluorescent s. method. A staining method using a fluorescent dye, such as the method for demonstrating *Mycobacterium tuberculosis* in smears using auramine O, and a fluorescence microscope.
Gram-Claudius s. A stain for fungi in tissue sections.
intravital s. A dye, introduced by injection into the body of man or animal, which stains certain tissues or cells selectively; the stain must be nontoxic so as not to kill any of the cells.
inversion s. A process in which, under the influence of a mordant, a basic aniline dye behaves as a plasma or acid dye.
metachromatic s. A stain which changes apparent color when absorbed by certain cell constituents, as mucin staining red instead of blue with toluidine blue.
neutral s. A compound produced by the interaction of an acid and a basic dye, insoluble in pure water, and therefore employed in alcoholic solution when used as a stain.
nuclear s. A stain, usually a basic dye, which stains nuclei selectively.
Papanicolaou's stains. A group of stains (e.g., hematoxylin, light green–Bismarck brown–eosin yellowish) used in a staining technique which is efficacious for the detailed study of exfoliated cells, particularly those from the vagina.
Paschen's s. A stain used to make a presumptive diagnosis of smallpox from a smear of the material from skin lesions.
rhodamine B. A stain used in the fluorescent microscopy of the *Mycobacterium tuberculosis.* It minimizes the chance of error, since artifacts do not take on an orange tinge.
Southgate's mucicarmine s. A stain used in the diagnosis of carcinoma of the stomach, particularly that with unicellular diffuse infiltration and secondary carcinomatous nodules.
substantive s. A histologic stain obtained by direct absorption of the pigment from the solution in which the tissue is immersed. Dyes that combine directly with the substance acted on are called substantive dyes.
supravital s. A stain applied to living cells removed from a living animal or to still living cells within a recently killed animal; the stain may be perfused through the blood vessels of the animal.
triple s. See Mallory's triple *s.*, Masson's trichrome *s.*
vital s. A nontoxic coloration of tissues produced by injection of a nontoxic dye into a living organism. Also called *intravital s.*

SPECIAL STAINS AND STAINING METHODS

Abbott's staining method (*for staining spores*). Cover the preparation with Loeffler's alkaline methylene blue, heat to boiling, and maintain at that temperature for one minute. Wash and decolorize with acid alcohol (2% nitric acid in 80% alcohol) until all traces of blue disappear. Wash and counterstain with 10% eosin for 8–10 seconds. Wash, dry, and mount. The spores appear blue while the bacteria are pink or red.
acetocarmine (Belling's). Acetocarmine to which an iron salt is added; one of the best stains for chromosomes in fresh tissue.
acetocarmine (Schneider). A saturated solution of powdered carmine in 45% acetic acid.
Achucárro's silver tannin method (*for astrocytes*). Place sections in 3% aqueous tannic acid at 50° C. for 5 minutes; wash in a 1% dilution of 28% ammonia water until sections are pliable; impregnate in three changes of diamine silver hydroxide—sections become yellowish brown when sufficiently impregnated; wash in three changes of distilled water, tone 20 minutes at 40° C. in 0.2% gold chloride solution; wash in water; fix in 5–10% sodium thiosulfate for 2–5 minutes. Astrocytes are stained dark gray to violet.
acid alizarin blue modification (*for connective tissue*). *Staining solution A:* Acid alizarin blue 2B (C.I. No. 1063), 0.25 Gm.; $Al_2(SO_4)_3$ (Baker's analyzed, dried), 5 Gm.; distilled water, 50 cc. Boil 5 min., cool, filter, and restore to original volume. Buffer to pH 2.25 with 20 cc. of Sørensen's citrate solution. *Staining solution B:* Aniline blue W.S. (C.C.), 0.5 Gm.; orange G (C.C.), 2 Gm.; distilled water, 100 cc.; glacial acetic acid, 8 cc. Bring to a boil, cool, and filter. After stain A, 5% phosphotungstic acid is used as a mordant.
acid fuchsin (C.C.). An acid dye of the triphenylmethane series, the sulfonated derivative of basic fuchsin, widely used as a cytoplasmic stain; a 0.5%–1.0% aqueous solution of acid fuchsin (70% dye content) is employed. Also called *acid magenta; acid rubin; fuchsin S, SN, SS, ST,* or *SIII.*
acid green. See *light green SF yellowish* under *Special Stains.*
acid polychrome methylene blue (Goodpasture's). Mix 1 Gm. of methylene blue, 1 Gm. of potassium carbonate, and 400 cc. of distilled water. Boil for one-half hour. Cool, add 3 cc. of glacial acetic acid, and shake well. Boil down to 200 cc. and cool.
acid violet. Any one of several triphenylmethane dyes; an inaccurate designation for various violet-colored dyes.
acridine stains. Dyes formed from acridine; they include acriflavine and phosphine.
acriflavine. A yellow dye used as a disinfectant or bacteriostatic agent. Mixed with methyl and crystal violets to make acriviolet. Also called *a. base, neutral a.*
Albert's s. (*for diphtheria bacilli*). Dissolve 0.15 Gm. of toluidine blue (85% dye content) and 0.2 Gm. of methyl green (55% dye content) in 100 cc. of distilled water. Add 1 cc. of glacial acetic acid and 2 cc. of alcohol. Filter after 24 hours. Stain the

heat-fixed film for 5 minutes, drain, and, without washing, apply iodine solution (2 Gm. of iodine and 3 Gm. of potassium iodide in 300 cc. of water) for one minute.

alizarin red S (C.C.). An acid aniline dye, sodium alizarin sulfonate; an ingredient in some mitochondrial staining methods such as Benda's stain. Used as a stain for bone. Also called *alizarin red, water soluble; alizarin carmine.*

alizarin red S and toluidine blue (*for mammalian embryos*). This alizarin red method employs a blue counterstain, made as follows: Toluidine blue (C.C.), 0.25 Gm.; 70% alcohol, 100 cc.; 0.5% HCl, 2 cc. Let stand for 24 hours, filter, and keep tightly corked.

Altmann's aniline-acid fuchsin-picric acid s. (*for mitochondria*). A stain which gives the mitochondria a crimson color against a bright yellow cytoplasm. The sections are stained first in the aniline acid fuchsin, and then differentiated and counterstained in picric acid.

alum hematoxylin. See *Delafield's*, *Ehrlich's*, and *Harris' hematoxylins* and *Mayer's hemalum* under *Special Stains.*

Alzheimer's s. A modification of Mann's eosin-methyl blue stain.

aniline blue, water soluble (C.C.). An acid aniline dye of the triphenylmethane series, a mixture of trisulfonates of diphenylrosaniline and triphenylpararosaniline. Used to stain collagenous fibers, and as a general stain. Usually a 0.2%–1.0% solution of aniline blue in water or in 90% alcohol. Also called *china blue, soluble blue 3M* or *2R, marine blue V, cotton blue, water blue, Berlin blue.*

aniline-fuchsin-methyl green method (*for mitochondria*). A modification of Altmann's stain using methyl green as the counterstain instead of picric acid. The mitochondria are stained red against a green background. Also called *Bensley's stain* (for mitochondria).

Anthony's method (*for bacterial capsules*). Air-dried smears are stained with 1% aqueous crystal violet (C.C.) and washed with 20% aqueous $CuSO_4.5H_2O$.

auramine O (C.C.). A basic aniline dye of the diphenylmethane series, used chiefly as a drug, but of use in fluorescence microscopy. Also called *canary yellow, pyoktanin yellow, pyoktaninum aureum.*

azan s. See *Heidenhain's azocarmine*, under *stain.*

azocarmine G (C.C.). A basic azine dye used in tissue staining; a constituent of Heidenhain's (azan) stain. Also called *azocarmine GX, rosazine, rosindulin GXF.*

azure. A basic thiazine dye; used in blood and connective-tissue stains.

azure A (C.C.). Asymmetrical dimethyl thionine; used in 0.1%–1.5% aqueous solution as a nuclear stain for sections of fixed tissue, or in combination with other dyes.

azure B (C.C.). The trimethyl derivative of thionine.

azure C. A basic dye, monomethyl thionine.

azure I. Trade name for a mixture of azure A and azure B. Syn., *methylene azure.*

azure II. A mixture of equal parts of azure I and methylene blue.

Bailey's method (*for bacterial flagella*). *Mordant solution A:* Mix 18 cc. of 10% aqueous tannic acid with 6 cc. of 6% aqueous $FeCl_3.6H_2O$. *Mordant solution B:* To 3.5 cc. of solution A, add: 0.5% alcoholic basic fuchsin (C.C.), 0.5 cc.; conc. HCl, 0.5 cc.; formalin, 2 cc. After mordanting, Ziehl's carbolfuchsin is used as a stain.

basic fuchsin (C.C.). A basic dye, or group of dyes, of the triphenylmethane group; mixtures of pararosaniline and rosaniline and magenta II of varying proportions, used as a bacterial stain and in general histologic work; a 0.6% aqueous solution of basic fuchsin (90% dye content is employed). Also called *diamond fuchsin, magenta, aniline red, rubin.*

Bauer's method (*for glycogen*). Stain for 15 min. in Schiff reagent: 1 Gm. of basic fuchsin (C.C.) in 100 cc. of hot (80°–100° C.) distilled water. Filter at 60°–80° C. Cool, add 2 Gm. of $NaHSO_3$ and 10 cc. of N/1 HCl. Stopper tightly, let stand 18–24 hours in the dark. Add 300 mg. of finely ground charcoal, shake 1 min., store at 0°–5° C. Wash in M/20 $NaHSO_3$ and water, counterstain with acid hemalum.

Benda's alizarin red S s. 1 cc. of a saturated aqueous solution of alizarin red S diluted with 80–100 cc. of distilled water. Originally used in Benda's stain for mitochondria, but more recently used in the gross staining of skeletons.

Benda's method (*for mitochondria*). Crystal violet and alizarin are employed to stain the mitochondria a deep violet in a rose background. A method more complicated than iron hematoxylin or aniline acid fuchsin, and now not much used.

Bensley's crystal violet-acid fuchsin s. (*for cytoplasmic granules*). A saturated and filtered aqueous solution of acid fuchsin is added to a similar solution of crystal violet. The precipitate is collected, washed with distilled water, dried, and dissolved in absolute alcohol to saturation, for a stock solution. A 1:9 dilution with 20% alcohol (made from absolute) is used for staining.

Bensley's method (*for glycogen*). Fixation of material in 10 parts of neutral formalin diluted either with 90 parts of 100% alcohol or with 90 parts of saturated picric acid solution in 100% alcohol. Stain in Best's carmine.

Bensley's neutral safranin s. A neutral dye, composed of safranin O and acid violet, used to stain mitochondria and antecedents of secretions.

Berlin blue. Aniline blue.

Best's carmine (*for glycogen*). Prepare a stock solution by mixing 2 Gm. of carmine, 1 Gm. of potassium carbonate, 5 Gm. of potassium chloride, and 60 cc. of distilled water. Boil gently until color darkens, cool, and add 20 cc. of concentrated ammonia. A test for the selectivity of the glycogen staining is the pretreatment of the section with saliva, which digests the glycogen; Best's carmine should then stain nothing in the section.

Biebrich scarlet. An acid disazo dye used as a plasma stain.

Bielschowsky silver methods (*for nervous system*). Various modifications, the essentials of which are: fixation, usually in formol, silver impregnation, washing, treating with ammoniacal silver solution, washing, and reducing in formol. Different modifications selectively stain nerve cells or neuroglia. Bielschowsky methods are also used for the demonstration of reticular fibers in other organs.

Bielschowsky-Maresch diamine silver solution. Add 5 drops of 40% NaOH to 10 cc. of 10% $AgNO_3$ solution. Brown precipitate is redissolved by constant shaking while adding 28% ammonia water drop by drop (about 1 cc.). It is best to leave the last few granules undissolved as excess NH_3 inhibits impregnation. Dilute to 25 cc. with distilled water for use. Use once. See *Ogata and Ogata's silver method*, under *Special Stains.*

Biondi's s. A triple histologic stain consisting of orange G, methyl green, and acid fuchsin. Now not much used. Also called *Ehrlich-Biondi-Heidenhain stain.*

Bismarck brown with methyl green. Stain for mucin, cartilage, and goblet cells with 1% aqueous Bismarck brown (C.C.) followed by rinsing in alcohol and subsequent staining with 0.5% aqueous methyl green (C.C.).

Bismarck brown Y (C.C.). An aniline dye of the azo series; used in aqueous or saturated alcoholic solution as a contrast stain, as a mucin stain, for vital staining, and for staining in bulk. Also called *Vesuvin; phenylene brown; Manchester brown; Excelsior brown; leather brown; basic brown G, GX*, or *GXP; aniline brown.*

Bodian method. A method of staining nerve fibers in paraffin sections. The sections are saturated with a copper protargol solution, the colloidal silver proteinate then being reduced with hydroquinone, and the sections finally toned in gold.

Böhmer's hematoxylin. An alum hematoxylin stain. Largely of historical interest.

borax carmine (Grenacher). Make a concentrated solution of carmine in borax (2%–3% carmine in 4% aqueous solution of borax) by boiling for 30 min. Allow to stand 2–3 days with occasional stirring. Dilute with equal volume 70% alcohol. Again allow to stand, and filter; used for staining tissues in bulk or in section.

Bordeaux red. An acid monoazo dye; used as a plasma stain. Also called *acid Bordeaux; archelline 2B; azo-Bordeaux; cerasin R; fast red B, BN*, or *P*.

Bowie's ethyl violet-Biebrich scarlet s. A neutral stain made from ethyl violet and Biebrich scarlet, used for staining pepsinogen granules in sections of stomach.

brazalum s. A good nuclear stain made by the formula for hemalum, but by using brazilin instead of hematoxylin.

brazilin. A dye extracted from Brazilian redwood; similar in properties and uses to hematoxylin.

brilliant cresyl blue (C.C.). A basic dye of the oxazine group, having highly metachromatic properties; used chiefly for staining blood to demonstrate the platelets and reticulated erythrocytes. Also called *brilliant blue C; cresyl blue 2RN* or *BBS*.

brilliant green (C.C.). A basic dye of the triphenylmethane series used to color culture media. Also called *ethyl green, malachite green G.*

Buzaglo's s. (*for connective tissue*). Staining solutions used are glycocyanin, orcein, acid alizarin blue, and alizarin-veridine. Nuclei stain dark blue; elastic fibers, red brown; muscle and epithelium, pale blue violet; collagen, mucus, and cartilage, shades of green; myelin sheaths, rose; axis cylinders, dark blue; and erythrocytes, red-brown.

Cajal's gold-sublimate method (*for astrocytes*). Impregnate sections 3–4 hours in Cajal's gold-sublimate solution at 25° C. If impregnation is satisfactory, sections acquire an over-all purple coloration. Wash in distilled water. Fix in 5–10% sodium thiosulfate solution for 5–10 minutes. Wash thoroughly in several changes of tap water. Dehydrate in alcohol, clear, and mount.

Cajal's silver methods (*for nerve tissue*). These are based upon silver impregnations reduced by a photographic developer such as hydroquinone. There are many variations; some have a high selectivity for certain cells of the nervous system, others for various types of nerve fibers.

carbol-aniline fuchsin s. (*for Negri bodies*). 1 cc. of phenol and 1 cc. of aniline oil are added to 100 cc. of 0.5% basic fuchsin in 20% alcohol. Sections are stained for 10–30 minutes, washed, decolorized in alcohol, and counterstained with methylene blue. Negri bodies are stained crimson. Also called *Goodpasture's s.*

carbol-crystal violet (Nicolle). Dissolve 1.0 Gm. of crystal violet (85% dye content) in 10 cc. of 95% alcohol, and 1 Gm. of phenol in 100 cc. of distilled water; mix the solutions and filter.

carbolfuchsin. Basic fuchsin, saturated alcoholic solution (about 6%–7%) 10 cc.; carbolic acid, 5% aqueous, 90 cc.

carbolfuchsin (Kinyoun). Basic fuchsin 4 Gm., phenol 8 Gm., alcohol 95% 20 cc., distilled water 100 cc.

carbolfuchsin solution (*for Mycobacterium tuberculosis*). A staining fluid composed of basic fuchsin 0.3 Gm., alcohol 10 cc., liquefied phenol 5 cc., distilled water 95 cc. Used primarily for the staining of tubercle bacilli. Formerly called *Ziehl-Neelsen's carbolfuchsin.*

carbol-thionine (King) (*for Nissl bodies*). A saturated alcoholic solution of thionine in 1% aqueous carbolic acid.

carbol-thionine (Nicolle). Thionine (90% dye content) 0.125 Gm., phenol 1 Gm., distilled water 100 cc. Filter before use.

Carey's method (*for motor end-plates*). Muscles are fixed in full-strength, fresh, filtered lemon juice for 10–15 minutes, placed into 1% aqueous solution of gold chloride until golden in color (10 minutes to one hour), and then reduced in 25% formic acid. End-plates are stained black.

carmalum. Carmine; a stain consisting of carminic acid 1, potassium alum 10, water 100 parts. It is well adapted for sections cut on the freezing microtome and for staining of small embryos *in toto*. Also called *Mayer's carmalum.*

carmine (C.C.). A bright red coloring matter prepared from cochineal, the active staining principle being carminic acid; of use in staining *in toto*, for staining tissues in bulk which are later sectioned; used as a specific stain for glycogen and for mucus and as a counterstain for blue vital dyes.

Casares Gil's s. (*for flagella*). Carbolfuchsin is used to stain the smears which have been treated with a special mordant composed of tannic acid (hydrated), aluminum chloride, zinc chloride, basic fuchsin, and alcohol (60%).

Champy-Kull's method (*for mitochondria*). Aniline acid fuchsin is used as in Altmann's method, but toluidine blue and aurantia are used as counterstains.

chlorazol black E (C.C.). An acid poly-azo dye; used as a vital dye and as a nuclear stain. Also called *Erie black GXOO, Pontamine black E.*

chromaffin reaction. A brown coloration of a tissue, as adrenal medulla, when fixing fluids containing dichromate salts are used.

chromotrope aniline blue s. A stain made up of 1 Gm. phosphotungstic acid dissolved in 100 cc. 0.02 *N* hydrochloric acid, to which 0.5 Gm. aniline blue is added and dissolved by means of gentle heat. After cooling, 2 Gm. chromotrope is added and the solution is allowed to stand for several hours and then filtered. It is useful in staining Mallory bodies, pituitary cells, and renal glomeruli.

Congo red (C.C.). An acid aniline dye of the azo group; used as a histologic stain and as an indicator, usually in 0.1% aqueous solution, for estimating free mineral acids, especially in the presence of organic acids. It is also used to test for amyloidosis, in the determination of plasma and blood volumes, and as a cytoplasmic stain. Also called *Congo; cotton red A, B*, or *C; direct red C, R*, or *Y*.

Conn's technic (*for soil bacteria*). Rose bengal (C.C.), 1 Gm.; $CaCl_2$, 0.01 Gm. more or less; 5% aqueous phenol, 100 cc.

cresyl violet (C.C.). A basic dye of the oxazine group, having strongly metachromatic properties;

used for staining nervous tissue and fresh tumor tissue. Also called *cresylecht violet, cresyl fast violet.*

crystal violet (C.C.). A basic dye of the triphenylmethane group, hexamethyl pararosaniline. A constituent of all the bluer shades of methyl violet and gentian violet; may be used in nearly all procedures calling for gentian violet, being of more constant composition than gentian violet. Also called *hexamethyl violet, methyl violet 10B, gentian violet.*

crystal violet s. (*for amyloid*). Pathologic tissue stain of crystal violet (C.C.), 1.0 Gm.; methyl violet 2B (C.C.), 0.5 Gm.; 10% alcohol, 100 cc.

Custer's method (*for bone marrow in sections*). *Solution A:* Eosin Y (C.C.), 0.1% aqueous. *Solution B:* Azure II (C.C.), 0.1% aqueous. *Solution C:* Mix: 20 cc. of solution A, 10 cc. of solution B, and 80 cc. of distilled water. Filter through cotton.

da Fano's cobalt nitrate method (*for Golgi apparatus*). Fix in 1 Gm. of cobalt nitrate ($Co(NO_3)_2.6H_2O$), 100 cc. of distilled water, 6–15 cc. of formalin, for 3–18 hours. Vary the amount of formalin and time according to the type of tissue. Rinse in distilled water. Impregnate 1–2 days in 1–2% $AgNO_3$ (1% for very small, easily permeable fragments, 2% for fatty and central nervous tissues). Rinse in distilled water. Cut blocks thinner than 2 mm. Reduce in fresh Ramón y Cajal's developer for 12–24 hours. Wash in distilled water 30 minutes. Dehydrate, clear, and imbed in paraffin. For greater permanence, bring sections to water, tone 1–2 hours in 0.1 to 0.2% gold chloride, wash, counterstain with alum carmine. Result: Golgi apparatus black.

D'Antoni s. One containing powdered reagent iodine crystals and accurately standardized 1% potassium iodide solution; used to stain intestinal parasites and their ova.

Davenport's alcoholic silver nitrate method (*for nerve tissue*). See *Cajal's silver methods,* under *Special Stains.*

Delafield's hematoxylin. An excellent nuclear stain. Dissolve 4 Gm. of hematoxylin in 25 cc. of absolute alcohol, and add 400 cc. of saturated aqueous solution of ammonium alum; expose to light and air for 3–4 days; filter; add to the filtrate 100 cc. each of glycerin and methyl alcohol; allow to ripen before use and dilute with water as desired.

del Río Hortega's silver method. See *Hortega's silver method* under *Special Stains.*

Dominici s. A blood stain, especially for sectioned material, using eosin-orange G (eosin 0.5 Gm., orange G 0.5 Gm., distilled water 100 cc.) and toluidine blue (0.5% aqueous) solutions. Stain 5–7 minutes in the eosin-orange G; rinse briefly in distilled water; stain about 30 seconds in toluidine blue; rinse in water; differentiate in 95% alcohol.

Donaldson's method (*for protozoan cysts in feces*). A staining procedure for cysts in feces using an eosin, iodine, and potassium iodide solution.

Dorner's spore s. A solution containing nigrosin, formalin, and water; used in staining bacteria. The bacteria are stained with Ziehl-Neelsen carbolfuchsin with the aid of heat, decolorized with 95% alcohol, washed in water, and treated with a saturated aqueous solution of nigrosin. Spores are stained red, other parts of bacilli colorless against a dark gray background.

Dunn-Thompson s. (*for hemoglobin*). Stain 15 minutes in unacidified alum hematoxylin, wash in tap water, mordant 1 minute in 4% iron alum, rinse in tap water, stain 15 minutes in a picrofuchsin solution (13 cc. of 1% acid fuchsin and 87 cc. of saturated aqueous picric acid solution), dehydrate, and mount. Hemoglobin casts, phagocytized particles, and erythrocytes are stained green.

Ehrlich's acid hematoxylin. Used for staining sections and in the mass. Dissolve 1 Gm. of hematoxylin in 30 cc. of alcohol and add 50 cc. each of glycerin and water, alum in excess, and 4 cc. of glacial acetic acid. Allow the mixture to stand in the light until it acquires a deep red color. Stains nuclei, mucin, and calcium deposits deep blue. One of the most frequently used hematoxylin stains.

Ehrlich's aniline gentian violet solution. Shake 2 cc. of aniline with 98 cc. of distilled water, allow the mixture to stand several minutes, and filter until clear. Dissolve 1.2 Gm. of crystal violet (85% dye content) in 12 cc. of alcohol. Mix the two solutions.

Ehrlich-Biondi-Heidenhain s. A triple stain, the constituent dyes of which are acid fuchsin, methyl green, and orange G.

Einarson's gallocyanin chrome alum method (*for Nissl bodies*). *Stain:* Dissolve 10 Gm. of chrome alum—$KCr(SO_4)_2.12H_2O$—in 200 cc. of distilled water. Add 300 mg. of gallocyanin. Heat slowly to boiling and boil 15–25 minutes, with frequent shaking. Cool slowly and filter. *Technic:* Deparaffinize and bring down to water the usual way. Stain 24–48 hours, depending upon fixative used. Dehydrate in alcohol, clear in xylol, and mount. See also *gallocyanin,* under *Special Stains.*

eosin. Tetrabromofluorescein, an acid dye which occurs in red or yellowish crystals. Commercially several rose-colored fluorescein dyes of the xanthine series are called eosins: eosin Y, ethyl eosin, eosin B, phloxine, and rose bengal.

eosin, bluish (C.C.). Dinitro-dibromofluorescein, a useful counterstain for hematoxylin. Also called *eosin BN, B, BW,* or *DKV; saffrosin; eosin scarlet B* or *BB; scarlet J, JJ,* or *V; napolinG; imperial red.*

eosin J. Erythrosin, bluish.

eosin-methylene blue s. (Mallory's). See phloxine-methylene blue *s.*

eosin S (C.C.). The ethyl ester of eosin Y. Dissolve 1 Gm. of erythrosin B (78% dye content) in 100 cc. of 95% alcohol. Also called *ethyl eosin.*

eosin Y. Tetrabromofluorescein, a valuable stain; used most frequently as a counterstain for hematoxylin and the green or blue basic dyes. Dissolve 0.1–1.0 Gm. of eosin Y (85% dye content) in 100 cc. of distilled water. Also called *water-soluble yellowish eosin; eosin W* or *WS.*

Erie garnet B s. Acid dye used with basic azure A to form a polychromatic stain for freshly incised frozen tissue. Add 4 parts of filtered 1% aqueous solution azure A to 1 part filtered 0.5% aqueous solution Erie garnet B; filter; then stain the tissue for 10–15 seconds.

erythrosin. A red dye, an iodine derivative of fluorescein.

erythrosin BB (C.C.). Phloxine.

erythrosin, bluish (C.C.). Tetraiodofluorescein; used as a counterstain. Also called *bluish erythrosin, dianthin B, eosin J, iodoeosin B, pyrosin B.*

erythrosin, yellowish. Di-iodofluorescein; a valuable counterstain after Delafield's hematoxylin or methylene blue. Also called *dianthinG; erythrosin R* or *G; iodoeosin G; pyrosin J.*

ethyl violet. Hexaethyl pararosaniline, a basic dye used in staining glands.

fast green FCF (C.C.). An acid dye of the diaminotriphenylmethane series; used as a counterstain.

fat stains in supersaturated isopropanol alcohol. Sudan IV (C.C.), Sudan brown, oil red 4B in 99% isopropanol. After various stainings these are mounted in Apathy's gum syrup.

Feulgen reaction. See under *reaction.*

Foley's combined method (*for nerve fibers, sheaths, cells*). A modification of the Bodian method, dependent on special reducing and counterstaining techniques.

Fontana's s. (*for Treponema pallidum*). (a) *Fixing solution:* 1 cc. of glacial acetic acid, 2 cc. of formalin, 100 cc. of distilled water. (b) *Mordant:* 1 cc. of phenol (liquid crystals), 5 Gm. of tannic acid, 100 cc. of distilled water. (c) A 0.25% silver nitrate solution. *T. pallidum* appears dark brown or black on a light brown background.

Foot's ammoniated silver carbonate method (*for brain tissue*). See *Bielschowsky silver methods,* under *Special Stains.*

Foot's methods. The method for the staining of reticular fibers is a modification of a Bielschowsky method. That for the staining of nerve fibers is a modification of a Cajal method.

fuchsin. $C_{20}H_{19}N_3C_2H_4O_2$. Rosaniline hydrochloride or acetate; a lustrous, green, crystalline salt, imparting an intense red color to solutions; used as a stain in microscopy. There are two main types: acid fuchsin and basic fuchsin.

fuchsin NB. New fuchsin.

Gabbett's s. (*for Mycobacterium tuberculosis*). Stain the dried and fixed preparation with a carbolfuchsin solution with heat; wash in distilled water; and counterstain with Gabbett's methylene blue solution (2 Gm. of methylene blue, 100 cc. of 25% sulfuric acid); then wash and mount.

gallocyanin. A basic oxazine dye; used in an aqueous solution with chromalum as a stain for Nissl bodies; sometimes used as a nuclear stain.

gentian violet. A violet aniline dye, a mixture of methylated pararosanilines composed of pentamethyl or hexamethyl pararosaniline or either of these compounds alone. It is a biologic stain having many histologic and cytologic applications, including its use in Gram's stain. Also used as an antiseptic, anthelmintic, and bactericide, having a selective action on Gram-positive organisms. Crystal violet is now used where old formulas call for gentian violet, since it is of more definite composition.

Giemsa s. (C.C.). A neutral stain used in staining blood, and as a general cytologic stain. It is the compound formed from eosin with one of the derivatives of methylene blue, known as azure II. A stock solution may be prepared by dissolving 0.5 Gm. of Giemsa powder in 33 cc. of glycerin, C.P., and after several hours adding 33 cc. of absolute alcohol. Also called *azure II-eosin.*

gold chloride. Recommended for tracing nerve endings in fresh tissues and for staining connective tissue and cartilage cells.

Golgi's silver method. Fresh pieces of nervous tissue are immersed in a solution containing potassium bichromate and osmic acid, and then in silver nitrate, producing a black deposit of reduced silver salt in and around the processes and cell bodies of many of the neurons. The original of all the silver staining methods for nerve cells, and still very useful.

Gomori's acid phosphatase method. Remove sections from water and incubate in lead nitrate sodium glycerophosphate solution (5 cc. of molar acetate buffer pH 4.7, 2 cc. of 5% lead nitrate, 6 cc. of 2% sodium glycerophosphate, 87 cc. of distilled water) at 37° C. for 1½–24 hours. Rinse in distilled water, then in 2–3% acetic acid and again thoroughly in distilled water. Immerse 1 minute in 1:40 or 1:50 dilution of yellow ammonium sulfide. Wash thoroughly in tap water. Counterstain as desired. Results: sites of phosphatase activity are shown by dark brown deposits of lead sulfide.

Gomori's alkaline phosphatase method. The method depends on the action of alkaline phosphatase on organic phosphates in the presence of Ca ions to form calcium phosphate *in situ,* followed by the replacement of the Ca by Ag. *Technic:* deparaffinize in two changes of xylol, pass through two changes of absolute alcohol, soak in 0.5–1% ether alcohol solution of collodion or nitrocellulose for 5–10 minutes. Drain 1 minute, harden in 80% alcohol 5 minutes, and transfer to water. Incubate 8–14 hours at 37° C. in 6 cc. of 3.2% aqueous solution of Na glycerophosphate, 9 cc. of 2% aqueous $Ca(NO_3)_2$, 6 cc. of 10% Na barbital, 6 cc. of 2.465% $MgSO_4$, 33 cc. of distilled water. Calcium control sections should be run concurrently, incubating these in 0.1% $Ca(NO_3)_2$ solution at the same temperature for the same length of time. Rinse in distilled water treated with 5% $AgNO_2$ in a strong light for 15–60 minutes. Counterstain. Dehydrate with acetone and clear. Mount. Results: alkaline phosphatase appears as black deposits in nuclei and cytoplasm.

Gomori's lipase method. The method involves the hydrolysis of water-soluble palmitic or stearic acid esters of certain polymer glycols or hexitans in the presence of 2% anhydrous calcium chloride and the calcium soaps formed *in situ* are converted into lead soaps by treatment with 2% lead nitrate solution. Lead soaps are converted to black lead sulfide with 1:100 dilution of yellow ammonium sulfide in distilled water. Counterstain in alum hematoxylin. Dehydrate clear in dichloroethylene or ligroin. Mount. Result: sites of lipase activity in dark brown deposits of lead sulfide.

Goodpasture's s. (*for bacteria in sections*). A combined tissue and bacterial stain, the staining constituents of which are basic fuchsin, picric acid, and Stirling's gentian violet. Gram-negative bacteria stain red; Gram-positive, blue; tissue, red and blue; fibrin, deep blue.

Goodpasture's s. (*for peroxidase granules*). Cover a dried blood smear with a solution containing 0.05 Gm. of sodium nitroprusside dissolved in 2 cc. of distilled water, 0.05 cc. of benzidine, 0.05 Gm. of basic fuchsin, and 0.5 cc. of hydrogen peroxide in 100 cc. of 95% alcohol. After one minute add an equal volume of distilled water plus hydrogen peroxide, 3–4 minutes. Rinse. Peroxidase granules are colored blue.

Graham alphanaphthol pyronin method (*for oxidase granules*). 1–2 minute fixation of fresh air-dried smears in fresh 10% formalin alcohol. Wash in water. Stain 4–5 minutes in 1 Gm. of alphanaphthol dissolved in 100 cc. of 40% alcohol to which 0.2 cc. of 3% H_2O_2 is added shortly before using. Wash 15 minutes in running water. Stain 2 minutes in 0.1 Gm. of pyronin (C.I. No. 739-Y or 741-B), 4 cc. of anilin, and 96 cc. of 40% alcohol. Wash in water. Stain 30–60 seconds in 0.5% aqueous methylene blue. Wash in water, blot, dry, and mount. Results: neutrophil granules, giving oxidase reaction, are purplish red, eosinophil granules lighter red, basophil granules deep purple. All nuclei blue, cytoplasm pale blue, erythrocytes greenish yellow to pink.

Gram's iodine. See *Lugol's solution,* under *Special Stains.*

Gram's s. (*for staining bacteria*). Smear material to be examined on a glass slide, dry, and fix with heat. Stain with carbol-gentian violet for one-half minute. Wash with water. Stain with Gram's iodine for 1½ minutes. Wash with water. Destain with 95% ethyl alcohol for 2–3 minutes. Wash with water. Stain with 1% safranin for one-half to one minute. Wash with water, dry, and mount. Gram-positive organisms are dark violet or purple. Gram-negative organisms are faint pink. Numerous modifications are used.

Gram-Weigert staining method (*for bacteria in sections*). Stain paraffin sections which have been fixed in Zenker's solution in alum hematoxylin, 1% aqueous eosin, and aniline methyl violet, washing with water after each. Mordant with Lugol's solution, wash, blot, dehydrate, clear, and mount.

Gray's s. (*for flagella*). Carbolfuchsin is used to stain the smears which have been treated with a special mordant composed of: (a) *Solution A:* potassium alum, saturated aqueous solution; tannic acid and mercuric chloride; (b) *Solution B:* saturated alcoholic solution of basic fuchsin.

Gutstein's s. An aqueous solution of 1% methyl violet and 2% sodium bicarbonate, used to stain smears of the material from skin lesions of smallpox.

Harris' hematoxylin. Dissolve 1 Gm. of hematoxylin in 10 cc. of alcohol and add to 200 cc. of a saturated aqueous solution of alum; heat to boiling and add 0.5 Gm. of mercuric oxide. When the solution turns a dark purple, remove from the flame and cool quickly. For use dilute to the color of port wine with aqueous solution of alum.

Heidenhain's (azan) azocarmine. A 2% aqueous solution of azocarmine G in distilled water. When used as a tissue stain it is acidified strongly with glacial acetic acid. Aniline blue and orange G are used as counterstains in Heidenhain's modification of the Mallory connective-tissue stain.

Heidenhain's iron hematoxylin s. See *iron hematoxylin (Heidenhain's)*, under *Special Stains.*

hemalum. A solution of hematoxylin containing an alum salt for a mordant. Hematoxylin ordinarily will not stain tissues readily unless they are previously mordanted or unless a mordant is added to the hematoxylin solution.

hematoxylin (C.C.). $C_{16}H_{14}O_6$. A crystalline glycoside derived by extracting logwood with water in the presence of ether. It is oxidized to hematein which yields a deep blue coloration. An excellent nuclear stain. Various types are chrome hematoxylin, Harris' hematoxylin, iron hematoxylin, Mallory's ferric chloride hematoxylin, Mallory's phosphomolybdic acid hematoxylin, Mallory's phosphotungstic acid hematoxylin.

hematoxylin-eosin method. Stain sections with hematoxylin (Harris'). Rinse with tap water, decolorize in 0.5% acid alcohol, washing thoroughly afterward with tap water, then with 0.5% ammonia water and again with tap water. Rinse in 70% alcohol, stain with alcoholic eosin, and rinse with 95% alcohol. Dehydrate in absolute alcohol, clear in carbolxylol and xylol, and mount. Many modifications are employed, such as the use of other hematoxylin solutions, or of water-soluble eosin.

Herxheimer's technic (*for staining fat*). See the various Sudan stains.

Hetherington's pinacyanol supravital mitochondria s. Make a stock 0.1% solution in 100% alcohol of pinacyanol (C.I. No. 808). Dilute this 1:40 in 100% alcohol (1 drop per cc.) for use. *Technic:* flame clean slide, flood with dilute alcohol pinacyanol, and drain. Let slide dry, then place on it a small drop of blood, cover with clean cover glass, let spread, and ring cover with petrolatum. Mitochondria soon color a deep blue to violet in living and motile cells. Addition of a similar quantity of neutral red will stain nuclei and other cell granules. See *pinacyanol*, under *Special Stains.*

Hiss method (*for capsules of bacteria*). Films are prepared from fresh material or by mixing cultures of organisms with animal serum. Dry in air. Apply staining solution (Ziehl-Neelsen carbolfuchsin or a gentian violet solution). Heat until steam appears and allow to stain for 1–2 minutes. Wash off the stain with a 20% copper sulfate solution. Blot dry or examine wet under a cover slip. The capsule should show a lighter color than the rest of the organism.

Hortega's silver method (*for oligodendrocytes*). Wash in 1:100 dilution of 28% ammonia water and then distilled water, impregnate 1–5 minutes in an ammoniacal silver carbonate solution, wash 15 seconds in distilled water, reduce 30 seconds in a 1:100 dilution of strong formalin, wash in tap water, tone in 0.2% gold chloride until gray, fix in 5–10% sodium thiosulfate 2–5 minutes, wash in tap water, dehydrate and mount. Cytoplasm and processes of oligodendrocytes stain black.

Huber's toluidine blue s. (*for Nissl bodies*). Paraffin sections of tissues which have been fixed in a mixture of 95% alcohol, trichloroacetic acid, and mercuric chloride are stained with a 0.1% aqueous solution of toluidine blue, and washed in distilled water and a weak aqueous solution of lithium carbonate. Differentiate in 70% alcohol and 95% alcohol, dehydrate, clear, and mount.

Hucker's ammonium oxalate crystal violet s. (*used in Hucker's modification of the Gram stain*). 2 or 4 Gm. of crystal violet (85% dye content) in 20 cc. of 95% ethyl alcohol; 0.8 Gm. of ammonium oxalate in 80 cc. of distilled water. Mix the two solutions and filter. The concentration of the crystal violet may be varied as desired.

Huntoon's s. (*for capsules*). *Solution I:* 100 cc. of a 3% sodium caseinate solution (nutrose) and 5 cc. of 2% phenol solution. *Solution II:* 100 cc. of 2% phenol solution; 0.25–0.5 cc. of concentrated lactic acid; 1 cc. of 1% acetic acid; 1 cc. of saturated alcoholic basic fuchsin solution; 1 cc. of carbolfuchsin. Mix the organisms to be stained with a drop of solution I; spread a thin film; and dry in air without fixing. Stain with solution II for 30 seconds, wash, and dry.

Huntoon's s. (*for spores*). *Staining solution:* The filtrate obtained upon filtering a mixture of acid fuchsin in 50 cc. of 2% acetic acid and 2 Gm. of methylene blue in 50 cc. of 2% acetic acid. A rather thick smear, after drying and fixing, is stained with the aid of heat, and washed in water, the film appearing bright red. It is then dipped a few times into a weak sodium carbonate solution, and, as soon as it turns blue, washed again with water, dried, and mounted.

India ink method. A method of making spirochetes and other organisms visible under the microscope by means of India ink. Negative staining. The background is black with India ink, and the spirochetes, being unstained, show up clearly.

indigo blue. Indigo carmine.

indigo carmine (C.C.). A blue dye, sodium or potassium indigo-disulfonate, very sensitive to oxidizing agents; used in urologic work and as a test for kidney function; as a coloring for foods, drugs, and cosmetics. Sometimes used as a cytoplasmic stain. Also called *indigotine Ia.*

iron hematoxylin (Heidenhain's). Tissues are mordanted in a 5% aqueous solution of ferric ammonium sulfate (iron alum), rinsed in distilled water, stained with 1% aqueous hematoxylin, and differentiated in 1% aqueous iron alum.

iron hematoxylin (Weigert's). *Solution A:* 1% alcoholic hematoxylin solution. *Solution B:* Ferric chloride 30% solution 4 cc., hydrochloric acid 1 cc., and distilled water to make 100 cc. For use, mix equal parts of solutions A and B.

Janus green B (C.C.). A basic aniline dye, diethyl safranin-azodimethylaniline chloride; used as a supravital stain for mitochondria and as an oxidation-reduction indicator. Useful in the flocculation reaction for syphilis. Also called *diazin green S.*

jelly method of in vitro staining. The use of an agar solution containing a dye and other ingredients, spread on a glass slide, in studying living cells under the microscope.

Jenner's s. (C.C.) (*for blood*). The eosinate of methylene blue, precipitated from aqueous solution and redissolved in methanol. For use, dissolve 0.5 Gm. of powder (Jenner's stain) in 100 cc. of acetone-free methanol.

Kornhauser's quadruple s. (*for connective tissue*). (A) Orcein, synthetic (C.C.), 0.4 Gm.; conc. HNO_3, C.P., 0.4 cc.; 90% ethyl alcohol, 100 cc. (B) Acid alizarin blue 2B, 0.35 Gm.; ammonia alum, 5 Gm.; N/10 acetic acid, 82 cc.; N/10 sodium acetate, 18 cc. Boil gently for 10 min. in a flask covered with a watch crystal. Cool, filter. (C) Orange G (C.C.), 2 Gm.; fast green FCF (C.C.), 0.2 Gm.; glacial acetic acid, 2 cc.; distilled water, 100 cc. (D) Phosphotungstic acid C.P. crystals, 4 Gm.; phosphomolybdic acid C.P. crystals, 1 Gm.; distilled water, 100 cc.

Krajian's Congo s. (*for elastic fibers*). Congo red staining followed by aniline blue gives red elastic fibers, other fibers blue.

Krajian's rapid staining. The principle of the modification of staining with hematoxylin and eosin consists in the dehydration of the section before counterstaining and the application of eosin as a solution in carbolxylol. Then, since the tissue passes afterward through xylol only, there is no opportunity for decolorization. Alcohol is saved because dehydration can be commenced in the stronger alcohol, discarding the lower gradations. The solution of eosin in carbolxylol which constitutes the principal element of modification may be called, for convenience, "eosinol."

Kultschitzky's hematoxylin. The stock solution of 10% hematoxylin in absolute alcohol is ripened at least 6 months, and diluted for use as follows: stock solution 10 cc., 2% acetic acid 90 cc. A valuable myelin-sheath stain. Used in the Smith-Dietrich stain for lipoids.

Kultschitzky's myelin s. *Technic:* stain celloidin sections 12–24 hours at 15°–20° C. in Kultschitzky's hematoxylin. Differentiate in Kultschitzky's decolorizer (10 cc. of 1% potassium ferricyanide, 100 cc. of saturated aqueous Li_2CO_3) three to four changes during a period of 4–12 hours. Wash thoroughly. Dehydrate, clear, and mount.

lactophenol blue s. An aqueous solution of 1 part phenol crystals, 1 part lactic acid, and 2 parts glycerol, for the mounting of fungi in routine or permanent wet preparations.

Laidlaw's s. Silver stain for normal ectodermal cells except basal epidermal cells and Schwann cells. It also stains ectodermal tumors.

Leishman's s. (*for blood*). A Romanovsky type of stain, the eosinate of polychrome methylene blue, available as a dry powder which is dissolved for use in pure methyl alcohol in the proportion of 0.15 Gm. to 100 cc.

leuko-basic fuchsin s. When to an aqueous solution of basic fuchsin, hydrochloric acid and sodium bisulfite are added, in that order, sulfurous acid is liberated and the magenta dye becomes colorless.

Levaditi's method (*for Treponema pallidum in sections*). A modification of Cajal's method of staining nerve fibers; a silver nitrate solution is used, which stains the treponema a dense black.

Liebermann-Burchardt cholesterol test. See *Schultz's sterol reaction method* (for cholesterol) under *Special Stains.*

Liefson's method (*for bacterial flagella*). A modification of Gray's stain.

light green SF yellowish (C.C.). An acid dye of the triphenylmethane series, a sulfonated derivative of brilliant green and a valuable counterstain for safranin; used in 0.5% aqueous solution. Also called *light green 2G, 3G, 4G,* or *2GN; acid green; fast acid green N.*

Lillie's acid hemalum. See *Mayer's acid hemalum modified by Lillie* under *Special Stains.*

Lillie's azure eosinates in buffered solutions (*for staining bacteria in tissues*). These are mixtures of azure A (C.C.), or C (C.C.), eosin Y or B in distilled water, from which the precipitated filtrate is dissolved in methanol and glycerol. Buffer solutions of M/10 citric acid and M/5 $NaHPO_4$ are prepared and the stains are used in a solution of stain, 1 cc.; buffer mixture, 2 cc.; acetone (C.P.), 5 cc.; distilled water, 32 cc.

Lillie's azure-eosin method. Stain 3–5 minutes in alum hematoxylin, wash in water, stain 1 hour in azure eosinate solution, rinse in distilled water, dehydrate with acetone, and mount. Nitrocellulose sections or collodion-coated sections require 2–2½ hours' staining in the azure eosinate solution. See *Lillie's azure eosinates in buffered solutions* under *Special Stains.*

Lillie's combined myelin and fat s. An iron hematoxylin method, followed by a Sudan II (C.I. No. 73)-isopropanol stain, differentiated with borax-$K_3Fe(CN)_6$.

Lillie's oil blue N or NA. Saturated oil blue N or NA in 60% isopropanol. Dilute to 40% or 50% isopropanol with distilled water for use. Counterstain with Janus green B, Bismarck brown Y, Bismarck brown R, or pyronin Y. For fat in animal tissue.

lithium carmine (Orth's). Contains 2.5–5.0 Gm. of carmine in 100 cc. of saturated aqueous lithium carbonate. It is used to stain histologic sections, the nuclei being stained bright red, and as a vital stain.

Ljubinsky's s. (*for bacterial granules*). Methyl violet 2B or crystal violet in 5% acetic acid; counterstain, Bismarck brown, 0.1% aqueous solution.

Loeffler's alkaline methylene blue. Add 30 cc. of a concentrated alcoholic methylene blue solution to 100 cc. of a caustic potash solution (0.01:100). Filter before using.

Loeffler's s. (*for flagella*). Treat air-dried film with freshly filtered mordant (100 cc. of 20% aqueous solution of tannic acid, 50 cc. of saturated aqueous solution of ferrous sulfate, 10 cc. of saturated basic fuchsin in 95% alcohol), heating gently for one-half to one minute; stain with carbolfuchsin.

Lorrain Smith's s. (*for fatty acids*). See *Nile blue A* under *Special Stains.*

Lugol's solution (*liquor iodi compositus*). Iodine 5 Gm., potassium iodide 10 Gm., water 100 cc. Gram's iodine solution may be made from this by adding 14 times its volume of water. For staining smears for protozoan cysts, dilute solutions may be used, such as iodine 1 part, potassium iodide 2 parts, and distilled water 100 parts.

MacCallum's s. (*for influenza bacilli and Gram-positive organisms in tissues*). A combination of Goodpasture's stain with gentian violet.

Macchiavello's s. (*for Rickettsiae*). See *basic fuchsin* under *Special Stains.*

MacNeal's tetrachrome s. A blood stain containing eosin, methylene azure A, methylene blue, and methylene violet in methyl alcohol; it is used like Wright's stain.

malachite green (C.C.). A weakly basic dye of the triphenylmethane series, commonly used as a counterstain for safranin or carmine. A 1% aqueous solution may be used. Has also been used in the treatment of trypanosomiasis. Also called *emerald green, new Victoria green, diamond green, solid green, light green N.*

Mallory's acid fuchsin s. (*for connective tissue*). Zenker fixation, paraffin sections. Stain in a 1% aqueous solution of acid fuchsin overnight at room temperature or for one hour at 54° C. Differentiate in a 0.1% potassium permanganate solution for 40–60 seconds, dehydrate, clear, and mount. Nuclei and fibroglia fibrils stain red; elastic fibrils, bright lemon yellow; collagen, pale reddish yellow; red blood corpuscles, purplish red.

Mallory's connective-tissue s. (*for collagen*). Zenker fixation, paraffin or celloidin sections. Remove mercury from sections with iodine or 0.5% sodium hyposulfite. Stain in 0.5% aqueous acid fuchsin, 1–5 minutes. Drain off and put in: aniline blue, water soluble, 0.5 Gm.; orange G, 2 Gm.; 1% aqueous phosphotungstic acid, 100 cc., for 20 minutes or longer. Rinse in 95% alcohol, dehydrate, clear, and mount. For celloidin sections, reduce staining time and pass from 95% alcohol to terpineol and mount. Collagenous fibers, blue; myoglia fibrils, neuroglia, and fibroglia, red; elastic fibers, pink or yellow. Numerous modifications of this stain are in use. Heidenhain's azan stain using azocarmine instead of acid fuchsin is the most popular modification.

Mallory's eosin-methylene blue s. See phloxine-methylene blue *s.*

Mallory's ferric chloride hematoxylin. Mordant in 10% ferric chloride for 5 minutes; rinse quickly and stain in 1% hematoxylin for 5 minutes; differentiate in 0.25% ferric chloride.

Mallory's phosphomolybdic acid hematoxylin. Mix 10% phosphomolybdic acid solution 1 part, hematoxylin 1 part, water 100 parts, chloral from 6 to 10 parts. Expose to sunlight for a week. Filter before using, and save the used portions. Stain sections for from 10 minutes to one hour; wash in 40%–50% alcohol, changing it two or three times. Dehydrate and mount. If the solution does not stain readily, add a little hematoxylin. The stain is blue, and in its general effect similar to nigrosin. It is recommended for preparations of the central nervous system.

Mallory's phosphotungstic acid hematoxylin. Dissolve 0.1 Gm. of hematoxylin and 2 Gm. of phosphotungstic acid crystals in 100 cc. of water. Ripen with 10 cc. of 0.25% aqueous potassium permanganate or 0.2 cc. of hydrogen peroxide. An excellent stain for muscle tissue.

Mallory's triple s. (*for connective tissue*). See Mallory's connective-tissue *s.* (for collagen).

Mann's eosin-methyl blue s. Composed of 35 cc. of 1% aqueous methyl blue and 45 cc. of 1% aqueous eosin in 100 cc. of distilled water. Used for inclusions caused by viruses and for protozoa.

Marchi's method. Used to demonstrate early degeneration of nerves. After hardening in Mueller's fluid, place the tissue in a large quantity of a mixture of Mueller's fluid 2 parts, 1% osmic acid 1 part. The myelin sheaths of degenerated fibers are stained black; the normal are yellow or uncolored.

Martius yellow (C.C.). An acid nitro dye used as a stain and in preparing certain light filters for photomicrography. Also called *Manchester yellow, naphthol yellow.*

Masson's trichrome s. (*for connective tissue*). Paraffin sections are stained in (a) Regaud's hematoxylin, (b) a mixture of 0.3% acid fuchsin and 0.7% ponceau de xylidine in 1% acetic acid, and (c) saturated aniline blue in 2% acetic acid.

Maximow's hematoxylin-azure II-eosin method (*for blood-forming organs*). Stain sections with alum hematoxylin, wash in water, stain 18–24 hours in azure II-eosin (dilute 5 cc. of 1:1000 eosin Y with 40 cc. of distilled water and add 5 cc. of 1:1000 azure II), differentiate in 95% alcohol, dehydrate, and mount.

May-Grünwald s. (*for blood*). A saturated solution of methylene blue eosinate in methyl alcohol. Syn., *Jenner's s.*

Mayer's acid carmine. Add 4 Gm. of carmine to 20 cc. of distilled water and 30 drops of hydrochloric acid and boil to dissolve. Add 100 cc. of 80% alcohol, filter, and neutralize with ammonia (until carmine reprecipitates); add 4 drops of ammonia, and filter again.

Mayer's acid hemalum modified by Lillie. A modified formula for nuclei. Dissolve 5.0 Gm. of hematoxylin (C.C.) in 700 cc. of distilled water overnight. Add 50.0 Gm. of ammonia alum and 1 Gm. of $NaIO_3$; after these are dissolved add 300 cc. of glycerin (C.P.) and 20 cc. of glacial acetic acid.

Mayer's carmalum. Take 1 Gm. of carminic acid, 10 Gm. of alum, and 200 cc. of distilled water; heat the mixture and filter, adding an antiseptic to keep it clear. The fluid is light red in color, shading toward violet, and is said to have good penetrating powers, even in osmium preparations, and to be better than alum carmine for staining *in toto.*

Mayer's hemalum. An excellent stain for large objects. It consists of two solutions: (a) hematein, or ammonium hematein, 1 Gm., dissolved by the aid of heat in 50 cc. of 90% alcohol; (b) alum 50 Gm. and distilled water 1 liter. The solutions are mixed, left to cool, and then filtered. A crystal of thymol may be added to prevent the formation of mold. For most purposes it is advisable to dilute this stain with water or alum solution. Hemalum plus 2% glacial acetic acid gives a more precise nuclear stain. *Later modified formula:* Dissolve 1 Gm. of hematoxylin in 1 liter of water. To the solution add 0.2 Gm. of sodium iodate and 50 Gm. of alum. When the latter is dissolved, add 1 Gm. of citric acid and 50 Gm. of chloral hydrate.

Mayer's hemalum and indigo carmine. Add 1 volume of a 0.05% aqueous solution of indigo carmine to 4 volumes of hemalum.

Mayer's paracarmine. Dissolve carminic acid 1 Gm., aluminium chloride 0.5 Gm., calcium chloride 4 Gm., in 100 cc. of 70% alcohol, with or without heat. Filter, after precipitation, and the solution will have a clear red color.

medicinal methylene blue. Methylthionine chloride. It is free of zinc, hence less toxic than commercial methylene blue. It is used as a urinary antiseptic, and for a kidney-function test. Also an antidote for carbon monoxide and cyanide poisoning.

methyl blue. An acid dye of the triphenylmethane series, used as a counterstain and in Mann's stain. Also called *cotton blue, Helvetia blue.*

methylene azure. Azure I.

methylene blue. An aniline dye of the thiazine series, tetramethylthionine chloride, widely used as a histologic and bacteriologic stain, a 1% aqueous solution being commonly used. Also called *Swiss blue*.

methylene blue, Med. U.S.P. Methylene blue which is zinc-free, less toxic, and superior as a stain.

methylene blue N. A basic dye of the thiazine series, of a greener shade than the true methylene blue. Also called *methylene blue NN*.

methylene blue O. Toluidine blue O.

methylene violet (C.C.). A weakly basic thiazine dye, one of the oxidation products of methylene blue, and a constituent of polychrome methylene blue; used in MacNeal's tetrachrome blood stain.

methyl green (C.C.). A basic triphenylmethane dye, readily decomposed to crystal violet, used as a biologic stain in aqueous solution. Also called *double green, light green*.

methyl green pyronin s. (*for bacteria in sections*). Methyl green (C.C.), 1 Gm.; pyronin Y or B (C.C.), 0.25 Gm.; 95% alcohol, 5 cc.; glycerol, 20 cc.; 2% aqueous phenol, 100 cc.

methyl orange (C.C.). A weakly acid dye of the azo series used as an acid-base indicator; used occasionally as a histologic counterstain. Also called *orange III, helianthin, gold orange, tropaeolin D*.

methyl violet. A basic aniline dye of the triphenylmethane series, which is a mixture of tetramethyl, pentamethyl, and hexamethyl rosanilines or pararosanilines. The shade of blue varies with the degree of methylation; the greater the degree, the more blue is the shade; used as a general biologic stain and as a stain for amyloid tissue. Also called *dahlia B, gentian violet, Paris violet, pyoktaninum coeruleum, methylrosaniline chloride*.

methyl violet 2B (C.C.). A bluish shade of methyl violet; used as a substitute for methyl or gentian violet.

modified Gallego elastic tissue s. A fuchsin procedure dependent on a special mordant prepared as follows: conc. HNO_3, 1.5 cc.; conc. formalin, 1 cc.; 50% aqueous $FeCl_3$ (U.S.P.), 1.5 cc.; distilled water, 200 cc.

modified Warthin-Starry method (*for leptospiroses*). This stain depends on an acidulated water, buffered; Walpole's buffer solution; $AgNO_3$ in the acidulated water; $AgNO_3$ in the buffer solution; and developers using $AgNO_3$ in acidulated water, gelatin in hot acidulated water, and hydroquinone in buffer.

Moeller's method (*for staining spores*). Make thin smears, dry, and fix. Wash in chloroform and then in water. Apply a 5% chromic acid solution and wash again in water. Apply carbolfuchsin and heat to boiling. Decolorize in a 5% sulfuric acid solution. Wash in water, and stain with a 1% aqueous solution of methylene blue or malachite green. Wash, dry, and mount.

Mollier's quadruple s. (*for connective tissue*). (A) Dissolve 1 Gm. of orcein (C.C.) in 100 cc. of 70% alcohol, then add 1 cc. of conc. HCl. (B) Dissolve 0.1 Gm. of azocarmine G (C.C.) in 100 cc. of distilled water by bringing to a boil; cool to room temp., filter at once through medium paper. Add 1.0 cc. of glacial acetic acid. (C) Dissolve 1 Gm. of naphthol green B in 100 cc. of distilled water and 1 cc. of glacial acetic acid.

muchematein (Mayer's) (*for mucin*). (a) *Alcoholic:* Dissolve 0.2 Gm. of hematein and 0.1 Gm. of aluminum chloride in 100 cc. of 70% alcohol. Two drops of nitric acid may be added. (b) *Aqueous:* Pulverize 0.2 Gm. of hematein with a few drops of glycerin; add 0.1 Gm. of aluminum chloride, 40 cc. of glycerol, and 60 cc. of water.

mucicarmine (Mayer's) (*for mucin*). A stain made up of carmine and aluminum hydroxide in 50% alcohol, diluted for use 1:10 with water or 50% alcohol; used after alum hematoxylin.

mucicarmine with hematoxylin and metanil yellow (*for connective tissue*). (A) Mucicarmine: Dissolve 1 Gm. of carmine (C.C.) with 0.5 Gm. of anhydrous $AlCl_3$ in 2 cc. of distilled water by gentle heat for 2 min., stirring until mixture becomes dark. Add 100 cc. of 50% alcohol, stirring continuously. After standing 24 hours, filter. Dilute 1 volume of this stock with 10 vols. of distilled water or preferably 50%–70% alcohol for use. (B) Place 0.25 Gm. of metanil yellow on filter paper in a funnel and pour over it 100 cc. of 0.25% acetic acid.

myelin stains. Staining technics for myelin sheaths include the following methods: Kultschitzky, Pal, Spielmeyer, Weigert, Wolters, Wright. See under *stain* for these methods.

negative staining of bacteria. Nigrosin (C.C.) 10 Gm., 100 cc. of distilled water; heat for 30 min. over a water bath, replace water lost by evaporation, add 0.5 cc. of formalin. Filter. Useful when India ink is not available.

Neisser's s. (*for demonstration of granules in diphtheria bacilli*). *Solution 1:* 0.1 Gm. of methylene blue (90% dye content), 2 cc. of alcohol, 5 cc. of glacial acetic acid, and distilled water to make 100 cc. *Solution 2:* 1.0 Gm. of crystal violet (85% dye content), 10 cc. of alcohol, and 300 cc. of distilled water. *Solution 3:* 1.0–2.0 Gm. of chrysoidin Y in 300 cc. of distilled water. For use mix two parts of Solution 1 with one part of Solution 2 and counterstain with Solution 3.

neutral red (C.C.). A weakly basic, nontoxic amino-azine dye, usually a chloride; used as an indicator and in staining as a vital stain and a general histologic stain, a 1% aqueous solution of neutral red (55% dye content) being employed. Also called *toluylene red*.

new fuchsin. A basic dye, similar in staining properties to basic fuchsin; triamino-tritolylmethane chloride.

Nile blue A (C.C.). A basic oxazine dye, of value as a biologic stain because of its property of staining fatty acids blue; used as a 0.5% alcoholic solution or a 2% aqueous solution. Also called *Nile blue sulfate*.

Nissl's methylene blue. Methylene blue 3.75 parts, Venice soap 1.75 parts, distilled water 1000 parts. Used for the staining of Nissl substance in nerve cells.

Nocht-Romanovsky s. This requires two solutions: (a) Methylene blue 1.0 Gm., sodium carbonate 0.5 Gm., distilled water 100 Gm. Heat at 60° C. for two days until solution shows a slight purplish color. (b) Eosin soluble, yellowish, 1.0 Gm., distilled water 100 cc. Mix a few drops of each of these solutions with about 10 cc. of distilled water in an Esmarch dish; the smear, which has previously been fixed in absolute methyl alcohol, is then floated on this mixture for about 10 minutes.

Nonidez chloral hydrate method (*for nerve tissue*). Method dependent on fixation 1–3 days in: chloral hydrate, 25 Gm.; 50% alcohol, 100 cc. Reducer: pyrogallol, 2.5–3.0 Gm.; formalin, 8 cc.; distilled water, 100 cc.

Ogata and Ogata's silver method (*for chromaffin cells*). *Technic:* Treat fresh tissue for 1–2 hours in the dark in 1% dilution of 28% ammonia water (1 cc. and 99 cc.). Place blocks in Bielschowsky-Maresch diammine silver solution, diluted with an equal volume of distilled water, for 3–5 hours in the dark. Transfer to several changes of 1:100 dilution of ammonia water, during 30 minutes, in the dark. Fix 1 hour in 3% sodium thiosulfate in the dark. Wash 1 hour in running water. Fix 1–2 days in 10% formalin. Cut frozen sections, float onto slides, dehydrate, clear, and mount. See *Bielschowsky-Maresch diamine silver solution* under *Special Stains.*

orange G (C.C.). An acid monoazo dye, widely used as a counterstain with various nuclear stains. Also called *wool orange 2G.*

orange II (C.C.). An acid monoazo dye used as a histologic stain. Also called *gold orange; orange A, P,* or *R; acid orange; orange extra; mandarin G; tropaeolin OOO No. 2.*

orcein (C.C.). A weakly acid dye obtained from certain lichens. It is violet in color and has metachromatic effects, which make it useful as a biologic stain, staining nuclei blue, cytoplasm pink. Dissolve 2 Gm. of orcein in 2% acetic acid. Especially used for staining elastic fibers. See *Unna's orcein method* (for elastic tissue) under *Special Stains.*

osmic acid. Osmium tetroxide used in fixing fluids blackens many fatty inclusions in cells, and is used to stain the Golgi apparatus. It also stains degenerating myelin, as used in Marchi's method.

Pal's myelin s. Celloidin sections stained in combined Weigert's lithium hematoxylin 6–48 hours at 15°–20° C. Wash in water and 2–3 drops of saturated aqueous Li_2CO_3. Differentiate in 0.25% $KMnO_4$ for 15–20 seconds followed by a few seconds in Pal's bleach (0.5 Gm. of oxalic acid, 0.5 Gm. of potassium sulfite, 100 cc. of distilled water). Wash thoroughly. Counterstain in carmine optional. Dehydrate, clear, and mount.

Pal-Weigert method (*for nerve tissue*). See *Weigert's method* under *Special Stains.*

panchrome s. (*for blood*). A modification by Pappenheim of the Giemsa stain, available as a powder (Grübler).

Pappenheim's method (*for Mycobacterium tuberculosis*). Stain the fixed smear by steaming with carbolfuchsin (Ziehl-Neelsen). Pour off the dye, and, without washing, apply Pappenheim's solution 4–5 times. Wash, dry, and mount.

Pappenheim's solution. Dissolve 1.0 Gm. of rosolic acid in 100 cc. of alcohol; add 1.3 Gm. of methylene blue and shake until dissolved. Add 20 cc. of glycerin, mix well, and filter.

Pappenheim-Saathoff methyl green-pyronin s. Dissolve 1.0 Gm. of methyl green (55% dye content) in 5 cc. of 95% ethyl alcohol. Mix 20 cc. of glycerin with 100 cc. of distilled water, and dissolve 0.25 Gm. of pyronin and 2.0 Gm. of phenol in the mixture. Mix the two solutions and filter. This solution is used as a stain for chromatin, for granules in mast cells, for gonococci in smears of exudates, and for lymphocytes and plasma cells in tissue sections.

Penfield's method (*for glia*). Increase the volume of the silver solution in Hortega's silver method from 45–75 cc. with distilled water and take out sections after 20, 45, and 120 seconds in the silver. The rest of the technic is the same. Glia cells dark gray to black and background pale. See also *Hortega's silver method* under *Special Stains.*

Perdrau's method (*for reticulum*). A modification of Bielschowsky's method.

peroxidase s. A stain used for distinguishing between leukocytes of myeloid origin and those of lymphatic origin. See Goodpasture's *s.*, Sato and Shoji's *s.* under *Special Stains.*

phloxine (C.C.). An acid dye of the xanthine series, used as a counterstain with certain blue dyes of the thiazine series; usually a 1%–5% solution in water or in 90% alcohol is employed. Also called *erythrosin BB, new pink.*

phloxine-methylene blue s. (**Mallory's**). Deparaffinize sections of Zenker fixed material. Remove mercury, and wash in water. Stain sections in 2.5% aqueous solution of phloxine or a 5% aqueous solution of eosin overnight in the cold or for one hour at 55° C. Cool and then wash off in water. Take 5 cc. of 1% methylene blue in 1% borax, 5 cc. of 1% aqueous azure II, add 90 cc. of distilled water, filter onto the sections, and pour the solution on and off several times. Differentiate in absolute alcohol, clear, and mount. Nuclei and bacteria, blue; collagen, etc., bright rose. This method has modifications for celloidin sections or formol-fixed tissues.

phosphine. A mixture of nitrates of chrysaniline, used following methylene blue to stain bacterial nucleoproteins yellow. Also used as a microchemical test for nucleoproteins.

phosphomolybdic acid hematoxylin. See *Mallory's phosphomolybdic acid hematoxylin* under *Special Stains.*

phosphotungstic acid hematoxylin. See *Mallory's phosphotungstic acid hematoxylin* under *Special Stains.*

picrocarmine. A large number of solutions of carmine, picric acid, and an alkali are called picrocarmine. One formula is prepared as follows: Dissolve 1 Gm. of carmine in a mixture of 5 cc. of ammonia and 50 cc. of distilled water; then add 50 cc. of a saturated aqueous solution of picric acid. Expose the mixture to light and air for 2 days and filter.

picro-indigo carmine. Three parts saturated indigo carmine in 70% alcohol and one part saturated picric acid, also in 70% alcohol.

picronigrosin (*for muscle*). After Bouin or alcohol fixation, stain sections in a saturated solution of nigrosin in saturated aqueous picric acid. Muscle is stained yellow, connective tissue black.

pinacyanol. A basic xanthine dye of the cyanine group, used as a supravital stain for mitochondria, and for the staining of frozen sections.

polychrome methylene blue. Methylene blue partially oxidized into its lower homologs, methylene violet and the azures, with an increase in metachromatic properties; prepared by allowing methylene blue to age or by boiling a methylene blue solution with alkali.

ponceau de xylidine. Probably the same as the dye sold in the United States as ponceau 2R or brilliant ponceau G. Used in Masson's trichrome stain.

Ponder-Kinyoun s. (*for diphtheria bacilli*). Dissolve 100 mg. of toluidine blue (85% dye content), 10 mg. of azure A (80% dye content), and 10 mg. of methylene blue (90% dye content) in 5 cc. of alcohol; add 120 cc. of distilled water and 1 cc. of glacial acetic acid. Use after 24 hours. Stain the heat-fixed film for 2–7 minutes.

Proescher's oil red-pyridine (*for lipids*). Oil red O, 3–5 Gm.; 70% pyridine, 100 cc. Let stand for 1 hr. at room temperature, stirring occasionally. Keep in a glass-stoppered bottle in the dark. Delafield's hematoxylin is used as counterstain.

protargol. A proprietary protein silver compound, used for staining nervous tissue. See *Bodian method* under *Special Stains.*

Prussian blue. $Fe_4[Fe(CN_6)]_3$. Ferric ferrocyanide. Used in injection media for demonstrating blood vessels.

purpurin (*for calcium deposits*). Schmorl stains material fixed in 80%–90% alcohol in saturated alcoholic purpurin, 5–10 minutes, washes 3–5 minutes in 0.75% aqueous NaCl, then in 70% alcohol until color clouds no longer appear.

pyridine-silver method (*for neurons, axis cylin-*

ders, and neurofibrils). See *Cajal's silver methods* under *Special Stains.*

pyronin (C.C.). A basic triphenylmethane dyestuff.

pyronin B. Tetraethyldiamino-xanthine; used as a histologic stain.

pyronin G or Y. Tetramethyldiamino-xanthine; used as a stain in certain special procedures, as in the Pappenheim-Saathoff stain in combination with methyl green, and as a supravital stain for the duct system of the pancreas.

Ramón y Cajal's gold-sublimate method. See *Cajal's gold-sublimate method* under *Special Stains.*

Ranson's pyridine silver s. A modification of a Cajal method for staining nerve fibers, in which the tissue is treated with pyridine before being immersed in the silver nitrate solution.

Ranvier's gold chloride method. For a modern modification of this staining method, see *Carey's method* under *Special Stains.*

Regaud's s. (*for mitochondria*). An iron hematoxylin method similar to Heidenhain's, after fixation of the tissue in Regaud's fluid, a formalin-potassium dichromate mixture.

resazurin (C.C.). A dye occurring in the form of dark red crystals with a greenish luster; soluble in dilute alkali hydroxides. Also called *diazoresorcinol, resazoin.*

resorcin-fuchsin. See Weigert's resorcin-fuchsin *s.* under *Special Stains.*

Retterer's s. (*for muscle*). Stain sections of tissue which has been fixed in 80% alcohol 10 parts, formic acid 1 part, with alum carmine. Muscle bright red, all connective tissue unstained.

Romanovsky s. Polychrome methylene blue eosinates used for staining blood. The modifications include the Leishman, Giemsa, Wright, MacNeal, and Jenner stains.

rose bengal (C.C.). An acid dye, dichlor-tetraiodo, or tetrachlor-tetraiodo, fluorescein; used as a bacterial stain.

safranin. A basic aniline dye of the azine group used as a biologic stain.

safranin O (C.C.). A mixture of di-methyl and tri-methyl phenosafranins; used as a nuclear stain, in making neutral stains, and as a counterstain in the Gram technic. Dissolve 0.25 Gm. of safranin O (90% dye content) in 10 cc. of alcohol and add 100 cc. of distilled water and mix. Also called *cotton red; gossypimine; safranin Y* or *A.*

Sato and Shoji's s. (*for peroxidase granules*). Flood dry blood smears with solution A (0.5% copper sulfate). After one minute, without washing, apply solution B (a saturated aqueous solution of benzidine to which hydrogen peroxide has been added) for 2 minutes. Wash, and stain with solution C (1% aqueous safranin solution), one minute. Wash and dry. Peroxidase granules are colored blue in granular leukocytes and the nuclei orange-red.

Schaeffer-Fulton modification of Wirtz method (*for spores*). Stain the flame-fixed smear with a 5% aqueous solution of malachite green for 30–60 seconds, heating to steam 3–4 times. Wash and stain with a 0.5% aqueous solution of safranin for 30 seconds. Spores, green; remainder of the cells, red.

Scharlach R stain. A stain utilizing scarlet red solution with subsequent staining with hematoxylin. Used to demonstrate fat in tissue sections. Fat globules stain brilliant red, nuclei dark blue.

Schmorl's alizarin SX method (*for calcium*). Sections are deparaffinized and brought through 100% alcohol into saturated alcohol stain for 5–10 minutes. Alizarin SX solution should contain also 1% NaCl and a trace of ammonia water. Wash in 0.75% aqueous NaCl solution for 3–5 minutes. Wash thoroughly in 70% alcohol until no more color comes out of sections. Dehydrate, clear, and mount as usual.

Schmorl's method (*for bone sections*). A method employing carbol-thionine (Nicolle) and a thionine in alcohol-water.

Schultz's sterol reaction method (*for cholesterol*). An application of the Liebermann-Burchardt cholesterol test. Mordant thin frozen sections of formalin-fixed tissue in a closely stoppered bottle 3 days at 37° C. in 2.5% iron alum solution. Rinse in distilled water, float onto slides, and blot dry. Treat with a few drops of acetic sulfuric mixture (2–5 cc. of glacial acetic acid with an equal volume of concentrated H_2SO_4, mixture made while tube is in ice water). Place cover glass and examine at once. Preparation may be kept a few days if sealed with petrolatum. At least 2 or 3 sections should be tested before considering test negative. Results: a blue-green color appears in a few seconds, becoming stronger in the first few minutes and often turning to brown in ½ hr. Positive controls, such as sections from tissue, other sections of which had been treated previously, should always be used.

Shorr trichrome s. (*for vaginal epithelium*). An alcoholic solution of Biebrich scarlet (water soluble), orange G, fast green FCF, aniline blue (water soluble), phosphomolybdic acid, phosphotungstic acid, and glacial acetic acid. It differentiates between cornified (brilliant orange-red) and noncornified (blue-green) cells.

Shunk's s. (*for flagella*). Smears are mordanted with a special reagent composed of two solutions—(*Solution A*, tannic acid, saturated aqueous solution, 3 parts; ferric chloride, 5% aqueous solution, 1 part; *Solution B*, aniline, 1 part; 95% alcohol, 4 parts)—and stained with Loeffler's methylene blue solution (30 cc. mixed with 3 cc. of solution B or mordant), carbolfuchsin, 1% safranin in 50% alcohol, or aniline gentian violet may be used.

silver method (*for Treponema pallidum*). A method for staining spirochetes, based upon the principle of the precipitation of metallic silver from silver nitrate solution onto the body of the organisms, causing them to appear black.

silver nitrate method (*for calcium deposits*). Lillie treats formalin-fixed tissue 4–5 days in 2.0–2.5% $AgNO_3$ solution, decalcifies in Ebner's fluid. Sections are variously counterstained. See also *Von Kóssa's $AgNO_3$ method* under *Special Stains.*

Smith-Dietrich s. (*for lipoids*). Staining in Kultschitzky's hematoxylin after mordanting in potassium dichromate. Lipoid droplets are stained dark blue.

Spielmeyer's myelin s. Used on formol-fixed tissues. Frozen sections taken into 2–5% iron alum 6 minutes followed by Spielmeyer's hematoxylin (4 cc. of 5% alcohol hematoxylin *aged* in 36 cc. of distilled water), staining 10–24 hours at 20° C. Rinse. Differentiate in 2.5% iron alum under microscopic observation. Wash in two changes of distilled water, and 1–2 hours in tap water. Dehydrate, clear, and mount.

Stirling's aniline-gentian violet solution. Mix 2 cc. of aniline with 10 cc. of alcohol, and dissolve 5 Gm. of crystal violet (85% dye content) in the mixture; add 88 cc. of distilled water, mix well, let stand for at least 24 hours, and filter.

Stovall and Black s. (*for Negri bodies in sections*). (A) 1% ethyl eosin (C.C.) in 95% ethyl alcohol adjusted to pH 3.0 with N/10 HCl. If this eosin fails to stain Negri bodies, add about 1% acetic acid. (B) Dissolve 0.3 Gm. of methylene blue (C.C.) in 30 cc. of 95% ethyl alcohol, mix with 100 cc. of distilled water. Adjust to pH 5.5 by adding 2 cc. of acetate-acetic acid buffer to 60 cc. of fluid. Differentiation must be in water acidulated by adding 13 drops of acetic acid to 60 cc. of distilled water.

Sudan. $C_{20}H_{14}N_{12}O$. A disazo compound from alpha-naphthalamine with naphthol; a brown powder used as a stain; soluble in alcohol, ether, fats, and oils. Also called *pigment brown.*

Sudan black. A valuable stain for fat.

Sudan R. A stain suggested for use in the Kahn reaction for syphilis. Also called *oil vermilion.*

Sudan II. An acid monoazo dye; used to stain fat in sections.

Sudan III (C.C.). A weakly acid, disazo, fat-soluble dye which colors fat orange. Use a saturated solution in 70% alcohol for staining. (Herxheimer's Sudan III, equal parts of 70% alcohol and acetone saturated with Sudan III.) Also called *Sudan G; Tony red; scarlet G* or *B; fat ponceau G; oil red; cerasin red.*

Sudan IV (C.C.). A weakly acid disazo dye, a dimethyl derivative of Sudan III; may be used as a stain by dissolving an excess in equal parts of 70% alcohol and acetone or as a saturated solution in 70% alcohol alone. Also called *Scharlach red, oil red IV, scarlet red, ponceau 2B, fat ponceau.*

tetrachrome s. (MacNeal's) (C.C.) (*for blood*). A solution containing eosin, methylene blue, methylene violet, and methylene azure A in methyl alcohol; employed like Wright's stain.

thiazine red R. An acid monoazo dye used especially as a counterstain after iron hematoxylin.

thionine (C.C.). A basic thiazine dye, highly metachromatic, the uses and technic of which are the same as for methylene blue; use a 0.5% solution in 20% alcohol. Also called *Lauth's violet.*

thionine "end point" staining (*for chromophilic substance of nerve cells*). (A) *Stock dye solution:* thionine (C.C.), 1 Gm.; distilled water, 100 cc. (B) *Buffer, acid component:* glacial acetic acid (98%–100%), 6 cc.; distilled water to make 1000 cc. (C) *Buffer, basic component:* $NaC_2H_3O_2.3H_2O$ crystals, 13.6 Gm.; distilled water to make 1000 cc. (D) *Staining solution:* Mix 90 cc. of solution B with 10 cc. of solution C and add 2.5 cc. of solution A, getting pH *ca.* 3.7. (E) *Staining solution:* Mix 60 cc. of solution B with 40 cc. of solution C, and add 2.5 cc. of solution A, getting pH *ca.* 4.5.

Tirmann-Schmelzer method (*for ionic iron*). This method is based on the formation of ferrous ferricyanide from the ferrous sulfide by treatment with ferricyanide and acid. Impregnate sections for 1–2 hours (may be as long as 1–2 days) in strong, slightly yellow ammonium sulfide solution. Wash thoroughly in distilled water. Soak 15 minutes in equal volumes of 1% hydrochloric acid and 20% potassium ferricyanide, freshly mixed. Wash thoroughly in distilled water. Counterstain in 0.5% basic fuchsin in 50% alcohol for 5–20 minutes. Wash in water. Differentiate in alcohol. Dehydrate with alcohol, clear, and mount.

toluidine blue O (C.C.). A basic dye of the thiazine series used in Albert's stain for the diphtheria organism, in the panchrome stain of Pappenheim, and for many other purposes. Also called *methylene blue O.* Also see under *toluidine.*

trypan blue. An acid disazo dye of the benzopurpurin series used in vital staining, and also as a trypanocide.

tubercle bacilli, staining of. The smear is stained with hot carbolfuchsin for 1–2 minutes, then rinsed with water, then decolorized with a 10% aqueous solution of sodium sulfite for 30–60 seconds, then rinsed with water, then counterstained with malachite green (50 cc. of saturated aqueous solution of malachite green in 100 cc. of distilled water) for 15–30 seconds; the tubercle bacilli appear as dark red rods on a green background. Also see *carbolfuchsin solution* (for tubercle bacilli) under *Special Stains.*

Turnbull's blue. $Fe_3[Fe_2(C3N_3)]_4$. Ferrous ferricyanide.

universal s. (Strumia's). A mixture of the Giemsa and May-Grünwald stains in 1% aqueous solution of sodium carbonate.

Unna's alkaline polychrome methylene blue. A 0.5% methylene blue solution in distilled water plus 0.5 Gm. of potassium carbonate per 100 cc.

Unna's orcein method (*for elastic tissue*). Stain sections in orcein 1 Gm., absolute alcohol 100 cc., and hydrochloric acid 1 cc. for several hours. Wash in 70% alcohol and destain in 95% alcohol plus a trace of hydrochloric acid to sharpen the brown coloration. Wash in 95% alcohol, dehydrate, clear, and mount. Methylene blue may be used as a counterstain.

Unna's orcein method (*for muscle*). A modification of the stain for elastic tissue may be used: After sublimate fixation, stain sections for 24 hours in aniline blue 0.25 Gm., absolute alcohol 60 cc., orcein 1 Gm., glycerin 10 cc., water 30 cc.; wash in 70% alcohol, dehydrate, clear, and mount. Muscle purple, elastic connective tissues red, collagenous tissue blue.

Van Gieson's s. (*for connective tissue*). Saturated aqueous solution of picric acid 100 cc., with 5 cc. of a 1% solution of acid fuchsin. Used after hematoxylin.

Verhoeff's s. (*for elastic tissue*). 1 Gm. of hematoxylin crystals, 20 cc. of absolute alcohol, 8 cc. of 10% aqueous solution of ferric chloride, and 8 cc. of Lugol's solution. Eosin may be used as a counterstain. Elastic fibers are stained black, while collagenous fibers, myelin, fibrin, myoglia fibrils, and neuroglia fibrils take the eosin stain.

Victoria blue. A basic triphenylmethane dye used for staining viruses.

vital red. An acid disazo dye frequently used in the determination of plasma and blood volumes. Also called *acid Congo R, azidine scarlet R, brilliant Congo R, brilliant dianil red D, brilliant vital red.*

Von Kóssa's $AgNO_3$ method (*for demonstration of calcification*). Remove sections from water and immerse in 5% $AgNO_3$ for 5 minutes exposed to bright daylight. Wash well in distilled water. Treat for 2–3 minutes in 5% aqueous sodium thiosulfate solution. Wash in water. Counterstain 20–60 seconds in 0.5%–1.0% aqueous safranin O (C.I. No. 841). Differentiate and dehydrate in 95% and 100% alcohol. Clear with 100% alcohol and xylene and two changes of xylene. Mount.

Weigert's iron hematoxylin with safranin. The standard Weigert iron hematoxylin method with basophil granules counterstained by 0.5% aqueous safranin O (C.C.).

Weigert's method (*for myelin sheaths*). Used on formol-fixed tissues of the central nervous system to show the arrangement of the gray and white matter and to demonstrate the fiber tracts. Four special solutions are required: a primary mordant (Weigert's rapid mordant), a secondary mordant (copper mordant, Weigert's neuroglia mordant), hematoxylin stain, and a differentiating fluid. There are several variants.

Weigert's resorcin-fuchsin s. (*for elastic fibers*). Boil 200 cc. of distilled water with 2 Gm. of basic fuchsin and 4 Gm. of resorcin in an enamel dish, and while boiling add 25 cc. of 29% aqueous ferric chloride. Collect the precipitate, and, after drying, dissolve in 95% alcohol (200 cc.) and add 4 cc. of hydrochloric acid.

Weil and Davenport's modified Stern method (*for brain*). See *Bielschowsky silver methods*, under *Special Stains*.

Weil-Davenport method (*for gliomas*). (A) *Stain:* Dissolve 8 Gm. of $AgNO_3$ (Merck's reagent) in 10 cc. of distilled water, add 90 cc. of 95% alcohol. (B) *Reducer:* Dissolve 5 Gm. of pyrogallic acid in 95 cc. of 95% alcohol, add 5 cc. of commercial formalin. Dilute with alcohol to control intensity of staining. Control settling of precipitate with a solution of 3 vols. of distilled water to 1 vol. of commercial corn syrup, applied at the rate of 1 cc. of corn solution to 100 cc. of reducer.

Weil's rapid method (*for myelin sheaths*). An iron hematoxylin method with original methods of destaining.

Wolters' myelin s. Used on formol-fixed tissue. Stain celloidin sections 24 hours in warm Wolters' hematoxylin (2 Gm. of hematoxylin dissolved in 10–20 cc. of alcohol, 2 cc. of glacial acetic acid, diluted to 100 cc. with distilled water). Wash for a few seconds in Müller's fluid. Differentiate and mount according to Pal's variation of myelin stain. See Müller's *fixing fluid*.

Wright's myelin s. Used on formol-fixed tissues. Take frozen sections into 10% $FeCl_3$ for 5 minutes followed by Wright's hematoxylin (a few crystals in 15 cc. of distilled water), staining 30 minutes at 20° C. Rinse and differentiate in 10% $FeCl_3$ briefly. Wash thoroughly. Dehydrate, clear, and mount.

Wright's s. (C.C.) (*for blood*). Wright's stain powder (methylene blue, polychromated with sodium bicarbonate and heat, to which eosin is added) 0.3 Gm., 100 cc. of absolute methyl alcohol (acetone free). Filter; let filtrate stand. Cover the dried film of blood for one minute. Add distilled water or buffered water (pH 6.4–7.0) for 4–10 minutes, the time for staining varying with different batches of stain. Wash with distilled water and dry. The nuclei of the leukocytes should stain a dark purple, the eosinophilic granules a bright red, and the erythrocytes an orange or buff.

Ziehl-Neelsen s. (*for Mycobacterium tuberculosis*). See *carbolfuchsin solution* under *Special Stains*.

stair'case phe·nom'e·non. See under *phenomenon*.

stal"ag·mom'e·ter [G. *stalagmos*, a dropping; *metron*, a measure]. An instrument for measuring the size of drops, or the number of drops in a given volume of liquid. It is used to measure the surface tension of liquids.

sta'ling [ME. *stalen*]. Urination in farm animals.

stalk [ME. *stalke*]. Any lengthened support to an organ.

allantoic s. The narrow proximal part of the allantoic vesicle. Syn., *allantoic duct*.

auditory s. The temporary epithelial connection between auditory vesicle and superficial ectoderm. Syn., *placodal s.*

body s. The extraembryonic mesoderm connecting the chorion and the caudal region of the amnio-embryonic vesicle. It forms a path for the allantoic blood vessels and the connective tissue of the future umbilical cord.

cerebellar s. One of the peduncles of the cerebellum.

Meckel's s. The yolk stalk or vitelline duct.

optic s. The narrow median part of the optic vesicle and cup which forms a pathway for the developing optic nerve.

placodal s. See auditory *s.*

s. of the neurohypophysis. That part of the neurohypophysis between the pars nervosa and the median eminence of the tuber cinereum, transmitting fibers of the hypothalamo-hypophyseal tract and supplied with clusters of capillaries: also called *infundibulum, infundibular stem.*

yolk s. The narrow, ductlike part of the yolk sac uniting it to the midgut. Syn., *Meckel's s., vitelline duct.*

sta'men [L., thread]. The male organ of the flower, consisting of stalk or filament and an anther containing pollen.

stam'i·na [L., plural of *stamen*]. Natural strength of constitution; vigor; inherent force.

Stamm, Martin [*American surgeon*, 1847–1918]. Devised an operation for gastrostomy in which he withdrew a cone of gastric wall through a left rectus muscle incision, perforating the apex of the cone, and introducing a rubber catheter by inverting the stomach wall. Several concentric purse string sutures were applied for retention purposes.

stam'mer·ing [AS. *stamerian*]. Interrupted or hesitating speech. Syn., *anarthria, battarism, psellism.* —**stammer,** *v.;* **stammerer,** *n.*

urinary s. See stammering *bladder*.

stamp'er [ME. *stampen*]. Colloquial term for one affected with tabes dorsalis, from the stamping gait incident to it.

stamyl. Trade-mark for a pancreatic extract containing trypsin, amylopsin, and steapsin with hemicellulase and ox gall. The preparation is used in intestinal indigestion due to insufficiency of pancreas secretion, in chronic gastroenteritis, and in fermentative and putrefactive dyspepsia.

stand'ard [OF. *estandart*]. 1. An established form of quality or quantity. 2. A substance of known strength used for determining the strength of an unknown by comparison.

albumin standards. See under F. *Kingsbury*.

Harris and Benedict standards. Multiple prediction equations and tables based on a statistical study of the available data for the basal metabolism of normal men and women.

reference standards. Substances of defined purity used for comparison in conducting certain assays of the United States Pharmacopeia or National Formulary.

stand'ard con·di'tions. In gas analysis, an atmospheric pressure of 760 mm., and a temperature of 0° C., at latitude 45°. It is sometimes abbreviated S.T.P. (= standard temperature and pressure).

stand'ard de"vi·a'tion. Sigma (σ). The square root of the arithmetic average of the squares of the differences of each observation in a series from the mean of the series. The most commonly used measure of variation. Also called *the root-mean squared deviation from the mean.*

stand'ard er'ror. A measure of the variability which any statistical constant would be expected to show in taking repeated random samples of a given size from the same universe of observations.

stand"ard·i·za'tion [*estandart*]. The procedure necessary to bring a preparation to an established or known quality, as the adjustment of a standard solution in volumetric analysis.

biological s. The standardization of drugs or biological products, which cannot be chemically analyzed, by their pharmacologic action on animals. Also called *physiologic standardization, biological assaying.*

stand'ard·ized death rate. *In biometry*, the number of deaths per 1000 which would have occurred in some standard population with a known age-specific death rate. The rate may be standardized for race, sex, or other variables with known death rates.

stand'ard mil'lion. A population of one million divided into age groups in the same proportion as found in a designated population, as the age distribution of England and Wales in 1901 or the age distribution of the United States as shown in the census of 1940. Used in calculating standardized death rates.

stand′still [AS. *standan; stille*]. A state of quiescence dependent upon suspended action.

atrial s. Complete sinoatrial block; atrial paralysis. Also called *auricular s.*

cardiac s. Cessation or suspension of heartbeats.

expiratory s. Suspension of action at the end of expiration.

inspiratory s. A halt in the respiratory cycle at the end of inspiration when the lungs are filled with air. The condition can be produced by stimulating the central end of the cut vagus.

respiratory s. Suspended respiration.

Stanford achievement test. See under *test.*

Stanford revision of Binet-Simon test. See under *test.*

Stanford scientific aptitude test. See under *test.*

Stanford-Binet test. See under *test.*

Stanley, Wendell Meredith [*American biochemist,* 1904–]. Isolated tobacco mosaic virus in crystalline form (1935), and found it to be a nucleoprotein. Subsequently he isolated other viruses in purified form, demonstrated that virus strains can exist in the form of similar, yet different, nucleoproteins, prepared centrifuge-type influenza vaccine, and laid the foundation for studies of the chemistry of viruses. Nobel laureate in chemistry with J. H. Northrop (1946).

stan′nate. A salt of stannic acid.

stan′nic [L. *stannum,* tin]. Pertaining to stannum, or tin; containing tin in the tetravalent state.

stan′nic ac′ids. A series of acids which vary in composition from H_2SnO_3 to H_4SnO_4.

stan·nic oxide. SnO_2. Its inhalation for long periods may produce benign, symptomless pneumonoconiosis.

Stannius, Hermann Friedrich [*German physiologist,* 1808–83]. A constriction placed between the sinus venosus and the atrium in the frog is called *Stannius' first ligature.* A constriction tied around the atrioventricular groove is called *Stannius' second ligature.* Using these ligatures, he demonstrated that the muscle tissues of the atria and ventricles have independent, spontaneous rhythm; called *Stannius' experiment.* His work suggests the role of the sinus venosus as pacemaker of the heart.

stan′nous [L. *stannum,* tin]. Containing tin as a bivalent element.

stannoxyl. Trade-mark for a preparation containing metallic tin and oxide of tin.

stan′num. See *tin.*

sta″pe·dec′to·my [LL. *stapes,* stirrup; G. *ektomē,* excision]. Resection of a stapes.

sta′pe·des (stay′pi·deez). Plural of stapes.

sta·pe′di·al [*stapes*]. 1. Shaped like a stirrup. 2. Relating to the stapes.

sta·pe″di·o·te·not′o·my [*stapes;* G. *tenōn,* tendon; *tomē,* a cutting]. Cutting of the tendon of the stapedius muscle.

sta·pe″di·o·ves·tib′u·lar [*stapes;* L. *vestibulum,* entrance-court]. Relating to the stapes and the vestibule.

sta·pe′di·us [*stapes*]. A muscle in the middle ear, inserted into the stapes. See Table of Muscles in the Appendix.

sta′pes (stay′peez) (pl. *stapedes*) [LL.]. The stirrup-shaped bone of the middle ear, articulating with the incus and the fenestra ovalis. It is composed of the head, the crura or legs, and the foot plate. See Table of Bones in the Appendix. See Plate 20.

staph″is·a′gri·a (staf″iss·ay′gree·uh, ·ag′ree·uh) [G. *staphis agria,* stavesacre]. The ripe seed of *Delphinium staphisagria.* It contains the alkaloids delphinine and its isomer, delphisine, delphinoidine, and staphisagroine. It is used for the destruction of lice in the hair. Also called *stavesacre.*

staph″y·la′grum, staph″y·la′gra (staf″i·lay′·gruh, ·lag′ruh, sta·fil′uh·gruh) [G. *staphylagra,* forceps for taking hold of the uvula]. An instrument formerly used to hold the uvula during amputation of that body.

staph′y·le (staf′i·lee) [G. *staphylē,* bunch of grapes, uvula]. Old term for the uvula.

staph″y·lec′to·my [*staphylē;* G. *ektomē,* excision]. Operation for removal of the uvula.

staph″yl·e·de′ma [*staphylē;* G. *oidēma,* swelling]. Edema of the uvula; any enlargement of the uvula.

staph″y·le′us [*staphylē*]. Pertaining to the uvula.

staph″yl·he″ma·to′ma, staph″yl·hae″ma·to′ma (staf″il·hee″muh·to′muh, ·hem″uh·to′·muh) [*staphylē;* G. *haima,* blood; *-ōma,* tumor]. An extravasation of blood into the uvula.

staph′y·line (staf′i·lyne, ·leen) [*staphylē*]. Pertaining to the uvula or to the entire palate.

staph″y·li″no·pha·ryn′ge·us (staf″i·lye″no·fa·rin′jee·us [*staphylē;* G. *pharygx,* pharynx]. Old term for the pharynopalatinus muscle.

staph″y·li′nus [*staphylē*]. Old term for palatal.

s. externus. *O.T.* The tensor veli palatini muscle.

s. internus. *O.T.* The levator veli palatini muscle.

s. medius. *O.T.* The uvular muscle.

sta·phyl′i·on [G., dim. from *staphylē*]. The point where the straight line, that is drawn tangent to the two curved posterior borders of the horizontal plates of the palatine bones, intersects the interpalatine suture.

staph″y·li′tis [*staphylē;* G. *-itis,* inflammation]. Inflammation of the uvula.

staph′y·lo-, staphyl- [*staphylē*]. A combining form denoting *relating to the uvula.*

staph″y·lo·coc′cal [*staphylē;* G. *kokkos,* berry]. Pertaining to, or caused by, staphylococci.

staph″y·lo·coc·ce′mi·a, staph″y·lo·coc·cae′·mi·a (staf″i·lo·cock·see′mee·uh) [*staphylē; kokkos;* G. *haima,* blood]. A morbid condition due to the presence of staphylococci (*Micrococci pyogenes*) in the blood.

staph″y·lo·coc′cic (staf″i·lo·cock′sick) [*staphylē; kokkos*]. Pertaining to, or caused by, staphylococci.

Staph″y·lo·coc′cus [*staphylē; kokkos*]. A genus of cocci officially classified with *Micrococcus* by American bacteriologists.

S. albus. *Micrococcus pyogenes* var. *albus.*

S. aureus. *Micrococcus pyogenes* var. *aureus.*

S. citreus. *Micrococcus citreus.*

staph″y·lo·coc′cus (pl. *staphylococci*) [*staphylē; kokkos*]. Any coccus of the genus *Micrococcus* (*Staphylococcus*).

s. antitoxin. An antitoxin prepared by immunizing horses with staphylococcus toxoid and/or staphylococcus toxin. Its use is suggested in the treatment of acute and severe staphylococcic infections with or without septicemia. The antitoxin should be supplemented with normal or immune donors in the more severe infections. Dose, localized infections, 10,000 units; more severe infections, 30,000 to 100,000 units in divided doses during first day, followed by 20,000 to 100,000 units daily.

s. toxin. See *staphylotoxin.*

s. toxoid. Univalent or polyvalent, potently hemolytic and dermonecrotic toxins of *Staphylococcus aureus* and *albus* altered by the formaldehyde-detoxifying process of Burnet (modified from Ramon). Antigenicity is maintained but toxicity is greatly diminished. Used in the prophylaxis and therapy of various staphylococcic pyodermas and localized pyogenic processes due to *S. aureus* and *albus*. Dose, 0.1 cc. injected subcutaneously at the insertion of the deltoid. Subsequent doses, at weekly intervals, of 0.1 to 0.2 cc.

staph″y·lo·co′sis [*staphylē;* G. *ōsis*, condition]. Infection by staphylococci. *Obs.*

staph″y·lo·der″ma·ti′tis [*staphylē;* G. *derma*, skin; *-itis*, inflammation]. Dermatitis due to staphylococci (*Micrococcus pyogenes*).

staph″y·lo·di·al′y·sis (staf″i·lo·dye·al′i·sis) [*staphylē;* G. *dialysis*, separation]. Relaxation of the uvula. *Obs.*

staph″y·lo·e·de′ma [*staphylē;* G. *oidēma*, swelling]. Edema of the uvula. *Obs.*

staph″y·lo·ki′nase. A factor isolated from strains of *Micrococcus pyogenes* (staphylococci) which can convert plasminogen to plasmin.

staph″y·lol′y·sin (staf″i·lol′i·sin, staf″i·lo·lye′sin) [*staphylē;* G. *lysis*, a loosing]. A hemolysin produced by staphylococci (*Micrococcus pyogenes*).

staph″y·lo′ma [G.]. A bulging of the cornea or sclera of the eye. —**staphylomat′ic, staphylom′atous,** *adj.*

anterior s. See *keratoglobus.*

ciliary s. One in the region of the ciliary body.

equatorial s. Staphyloma of the sclera in the equatorial region.

intercalary s. One developing in that region of the sclera which is united with the periphery of the iris. See *buphthalmia.*

posterior s. A backward bulging of the sclerotic coat at the posterior pole of the eye.

s. corneae. A bulging of the cornea due to a thinning of the membrane with or without previous ulceration.

s. uveale. Thickening of the iris. Syn., *iridoncosis.*

staph″y·lon′cus [G. *staphylē*, bunch of grapes, uvula; *ogkos*, mass]. Swelling of the uvula. *Obs.*

staph″y·lo·pha·ryn′ge·us (staf″i·lo·fa·rin′jee·us, ·far″in·jee′us) [*staphylē;* G. *pharygx*, pharynx]. Old term for the palatopharyngeus muscle.

staph″y·lo·phar″yn·gor′rha·phy [*staphylē; pharygx;* G. *rhaphē*, suture]. A plastic operation on the palate and pharynx, as for repair of a cleft palate.

staph′y·lo·plas″ty [*staphylē;* G. *plassein*, to form]. A plastic operation on the soft palate or uvula.

staph″y·lop·to′sis [*staphylē;* G. *ptōsis*, a falling]. Abnormal elongation of the uvula.

staph″y·lor′rha·phy [*staphylē;* G. *rhaphē*, suture]. Repair of a cleft palate by plastic operation and suture.

staph″y·los′chi·sis (staf″i·los′ki·sis) [*staphylē;* G. *schisis*, cleavage]. Cleft uvula, or cleft soft palate.

staph′y·lo·tome″ [*staphylē;* G. *tomos*, cutting]. A cutting instrument used in staphylotomy.

staph″y·lot′o·my [*staphylē;* G. *tomē*, a cutting]. 1. The operation of incising the uvula. 2. *In ophthalmology*, the operation of incising a staphyloma.

staph″y·lo·tox′in [*staphylē;* G. *toxikon*, poison]. One of the toxins elaborated by the Staphylococci. Hemolysin, leukocidin, coagulase, fibrinolysin, necrotizing enterotoxin, and a lethal exotoxin are some of the toxins which have been identified.

staph·yl″y·gro′ma. See *staphyledema.*

star. *In biology*, any of various radiate structures, granules, cells, groups of cells, or organisms.

fibrin s. See fibrin *aster.*

lens s. The starlike arrangement of the lens sutures, having three to nine rays, produced by the growth of the lens fibers.

Winslow's stars. Capillary whorls which form the beginning of the vorticose veins of the choroid.

star an′ise. See *illicium.*

star′blind″ [*steorra;* AS. *blind*]. Half blind; blinking.

starch [AS. *stercan*, to stiffen]. 1. Any one of a group of carbohydrates or polysaccharides occurring as organized or structural granules of varying size and markings in many plant cells. Starch is especially abundant in the cereals (as barley, corn, oats, rice, rye, and wheat), in the legumes (as peas and beans), in seeds (as acorns, chestnuts, and other nuts), in many rhizomes or roots (as arrowroot, potatoes, and yams), and in some stems. The ordinary starch occurs as a white, soft, amorphous powder or as irregular, angular masses. It is insoluble in cold water and alcohol. It hydrolyzes to several forms of dextrin and glucose. Its chemical structure is not completely known, but the granules consist of at least two fractions: an inner portion called amylose or granulose, relatively soluble in water, and an outer portion called amylopectin, which is practically insoluble in water. Iodine produces a characteristic blue coloration with starch. The mechanism of this reaction is not clearly understood. 2. (*amylum*). Consists of the granules separated from the grain of *Zea mays;* occurs as irregular, angular, white masses or as a fine powder; insoluble in cold water and alcohol. Powdered and dusted upon the skin, it is of value to absorb irritant or excessive secretions. Also used as a diluent in pastes and ointments, and in the preparation of powdered extracts. Has many technical applications in industry. Also called *cornstarch.*

animal s. Glycogen.

soluble s. Starch transformed into water-soluble dextrins by heating to about 200° C.

s. glycerite (*glyceritum amyli*). Contains starch 10 Gm., benzoic acid 0.2 Gm., distilled water 20 cc., glycerin 70 cc. to make about 100 Gm.; occurs as a translucent, jellylike mass. Used directly as an emollient, or as a vehicle for other substances to be employed locally.

s. syrup. A commercial product obtained by the acid hydrolysis of starch, and containing dextrins, maltose, and dextrose, and variously designated as commercial glucose, glucose syrup, and corn syrup.

starch su′gar. See *dextrose.*

star grass. Aletris, the dried rhizomes of *Aletris farinosa;* has been used as a tonic. Also called *starwort, bitter grass, blazing star.*

Starling, Ernest Henry [*English physiologist*, 1866–1927]. Expressed the fundamental principle of cardiac behavior: that the energy set free at each contraction is a simple function of cardiac filling; called *Starling's law of the heart.* With W. M. Bayliss, demonstrated that secretin stimulates pancreatic secretion (1902). With E. B. Vernay, demonstrated the reabsorption of water by the tubules of the kidney (1924).

start′er [ME. *sterten*]. A pure culture of bacteria employed to start a particular fermentation, as in ripening of cream.

star·va′tion [ME. *sterven*, to die]. 1. Deprivation of food. 2. The state produced by deprivation of food. —**starve,** *v.*

Stas, Jean Servais [*Belgian chemist*, 1813–91]. Introduced a method of extracting alkaloids using successively alcohol, water, and ether compounds. Called *Stas-Otto method.*

stas″i·bas″i·pho′bi·a (stas″i·bas″i·fo′bee·uh) [G. *stasis*, standing; *basis*, stepping; *phobos*, fear]. A morbid fear of walking or of standing.

stas″i·pho′bi·a (stas″i·fo′bee·uh, stay″si·) [*stasis; phobos*]. A morbid fear of standing upright.

sta′sis [G.]. In blood vessels, complete cessation of the blood flow. The vessels are dilated and completely filled with a mass of red blood corpuscles. There is no transudation of fluid through the capillary walls and no diapedesis of erythrocytes.

biliary s. Stasis of the bile in the bile ducts and capillaries.

diffusion s. Stasis in which there occurs diffusion of serum or lymph.

duodenal s. Stasis of the duodenal contents.

intestinal s. An undue delay in the passage of fecal matter along the intestines.

pressure s. The discoloration of the head and neck when the upper torso undergoes sudden and severe compression.

venous s. Stasis due to venous congestion.

state [L. *status*, a standing]. A condition.

anxiety s. See anxiety *reaction*.

cataleptoid s. A condition due to neuromuscular excitability and differing from true catalepsy in that the limbs must be held in fixed attitudes for a few seconds before they maintain themselves and then function causes them to become limp.

central excitatory s. The state of supernormal excitability of a motoneuron, corresponding to the negative afterpotential, produced by stimuli each of which alone is incapable of exciting the motoneuron. Abbreviated c.e.s.

central inhibitory s. The state of subnormal excitability of a neuron, corresponding to the positive afterpotential, produced by one or more stimuli. Abbreviated c.i.s.

convulsive s. See *status* convulsivus.

depressive states. Certain mental disorders characterized by extreme depression. See also depressive *reaction*.

dream s. A state of disturbed consciousness of psychogenic origin in which the patient perceives his environment inadequately or may be wholly disoriented. Auditory and visual hallucinations are common. Dream states usually last a few minutes to a few days, and on regaining full consciousness the patient may feel he has dreamed and remember little. It is associated often with hysterical dissociative reactions and epilepsy. Syn., *twilight s.*

fatigue s. See *neurasthenia*.

hypnoidal s. The state between sleeping and waking.

metastable s. An excited state of an atomic system such that its energy of excitation cannot be radiated as electromagnetic energy.

nascent s. The active state.

resting s. *In biology*, a state of suspended activity, the condition of perennial plants (bulbs, seeds) and spores during their period of dormancy.

steady s. in muscular exercise. The condition in which the rate of oxygen consumption and the rate of energy release are metabolically equal.

twilight s. See dream *s.*

typhoid s. A condition of stupor and hebetude, with dry, brown tongue, sordes on the teeth, rapid, feeble pulse, incontinence of feces and urine, and rapid wasting; seen in typhoid fever and other continued fevers.

state′ment [*status*]. A declaration.

ante-mortem s. A declaration made immediately before death, which, if made with the consciousness of impending death, is legally held as binding as a statement sworn to.

stat′ic [G. *statikos*, causing to stand]. At rest. In equilibrium. Pertaining to the laws of statics.

s. breeze. A method of administration of static electricity, consisting in the withdrawal of a static charge from a patient by means of a pointed electrode.

staticin. A trade-mark applied to *carinamide*.

stat′ics [*statikos*]. That science which deals with bodies at rest or at equilibrium relative to some given state of reference.

stat″i·den·sig′ra·phy. Measurement of the quantity of roentgen rays passing through a subject onto a radioscopic screen provided with a photoelectric cell: used to determine the local density of the lung.

stat′im, sta′tim [L.]. Immediately; at once.

sta′tion [L. *statio*, from *stare*, to stand]. 1. Standing position or attitude. 2. A place where first aid or treatment is given, as a dressing station, rest station.

aid s. *In U. S. Army medicine*, a medical treatment facility where emergency treatment, sorting, classification, and evacuation of sick and wounded to the next higher channel in the chain of evacuation are accomplished.

clearing s. *In U. S. Army medicine*, a medical installation which receives casualties from collecting stations and gives additional treatment to, classifies, and makes further disposition of those patients.

collecting s. *In U. S. Army medicine*, a medical station in the forward combat zone where casualties are treated, sorted, returned to duty if fit, or prepared for evacuation to a clearing station in the rear.

NP treatment s. *In U. S. Army medicine*, a field army medical treatment facility normally located in the forward part of the field army service area, serving as a principal focal point for the reception of NP (neuropsychiatric) casualties from the division, from corps, and from field army units and installations. Usually all NP casualties pass through one of these stations prior to evacuation from the field army area.

personnel decontamination s. *In military medicine*, an installation intended for decontamination of personnel, located as far forward as the tactical situation permits, near a medical aid station and where water for bathing is available.

sta′tion hos′pi·tal. See under *hospital*.

sta·tis′ti·cal con′stant. A value such as the arithmetic mean, the standard error, or any other measure which characterizes a particular series of quantitative observations. Used as an estimate of the corresponding value for the universe from which the observations were chosen.

sta·tis′tics [ML. *statisticus*]. A numerical collection of facts relating to any subject.

medical s. That part of statistics relating to facts and data concerning human diseases.

vital s. A term usually limited to data concerning births, marriages, and deaths; a branch of biostatistics.

stat″o·ki·net′ic (stat″o·ki·net′ick, ·kigh·net′ick) [G. *statos*, standing; *kinētikos*, of motion]. Pertaining to the position of the body or its parts during movement, as in locomotion.

stat′o·lith. Otolith.

sta·tom′e·ter [*statos;* G. *metron*, a measure]. An instrument for measuring the degree of exophthalmos.

stat′ure [L. *statura*, stature]. The height of any animal when standing. In quadrupeds, it is measured at a point over the shoulders. In man, it is the measured distance from the sole to the top of the head.

sta′tus [L.]. A state or condition; often, a severe or intractable condition.

s. anginosus. A severe or prolonged attack of angina pectoris, due to extreme coronary insufficiency with or without thrombosis of a coronary artery.

s. arthriticus. The nervous manifestations preceding an attack of gout.

s. asthmaticus. Intractable asthma characterized by extreme dyspnea, cyanosis, and exhaustion, lasting from a few days to a week or longer; sometimes fatal.

s. catarrhalis. A condition characterized by a succession of inflammatory processes of a mucosa.

s. convulsivus. A transient state of uncontrollable motor activity, focal or generalized, alternating with rigidity or atonia; it may be associated with diminution or loss of consciousness.

s. cribrosus. A scarcely macroscopic sievelike condition of the brain or nerve substance, due to dilatation of perivascular spaces: probably a postmortem effect.

s. dysmyelinicus. See Hallervorden-Spatz *syndrome.*

s. dysmyelinisatus of Vogt. A syndrome of cerebral degeneration, similar to the Hallervorden-Spatz syndrome but differing from it by not being a heredofamilial condition, and pathologically by showing less increase of pigmentation of the globus pallidus and other structures.

s. dysraphicus. A developmental defect in closure of the neural tube, associated with anomalies of the spinal cord, spine, and sternum.

s. epilepticus. A condition in which epileptic attacks occur in rapid succession, the patient not regaining consciousness during the interval.

s. lymphaticus. See *s.* thymicolymphaticus.

s. marmoratus. The gross pathological appearance of the striatum suggesting a marbled surface, as described by C. and O. Vogt, in a form of athetosis characterized by hyperkinesis and rigidity. The ganglion cells show spotty atrophy, being replaced by a network of myelinated fibers. Syn., *état marbré.*

s. parathyreoprivus. A pathologic state caused by complete loss of parathyroid tissue.

s. praesens. The state of a patient at the time of examination.

s. raptus. Ecstasy.

s. thymicolymphaticus. A condition formerly held to be the cause of sudden and otherwise unexplained death in children, in which the only pathologic finding was relative enlargement of the thymus and lymphoid tissues. The diagnosis is held by many to be untenable. Syn., *lymphatism, s. lymphaticus. s. thymicus.*

s. vertiginosus. Persistent vertigo.

sta″tu·vo′lence, sta·tu′vo·lence [*status;* L. *volens,* from *velle,* to be willing]. Autohypnotism; voluntary somnambulism or clairvoyance; a trance into which one voluntarily enters without aid from another. *Obs.*

Staub, Hans [*Swiss internist,* 1890–]. Demonstrated that a second administration of dextrose one hour after the first will not raise the blood sugar level; called *Staub-Traugott phenomenon* or *effect.*

stau′ri·on [G. *stauros,* cross]. The craniometric point located at the intersection of the median palatine and transverse palatine sutures.

staves′a″cre (stayvz′ay″kur). See *staphisagria.*

stax′is [G., a dropping]. Obsolete term for hemorrhage, or dribbling of urine.

S.T.D. Abbreviation for standard test dose of scarlet fever toxin. A skin test dose is the least amount of standard scarlet fever streptococcus toxin which, when injected intracutaneously into a person known to be susceptible to the toxin, will induce a red area in the skin measuring 1 cm. in diameter when observed 18 to 24 hours after the injection. The reaction is compared with that made by a control injection of the same amount of the material which has been heated to 100° C. for two hours. See Dick *test.*

stead′y state. See *homeostasis,* steady *state* in muscular exercise.

steam [AS. *stēam*]. The vapor of water; water in a gaseous state.

steap′sin (steep′sin). A lipase present in pancreatic juice and capable of hydrolyzing fats to glycerin and fatty acids: also called *pancreatic lipase.*

stear′ate (steer′ate). An ester or salt of stearic acid, as stearin (glyceryl stearate) or sodium stearate.

ste·ar′ic ac′id (stee·ar′ick, steer′ick) (*acidum stearicum*). A mixture of solid acids obtained from fats; consists chiefly of stearic acid, $CH_3(CH_2)_{16}COOH$, and palmitic acid, $CH_3(CH_2)_{14}COOH$; occurs as a hard, white, or faintly yellowish, somewhat glossy and crystalline solid, or a white or yellowish powder; 1 Gm. dissolves in about 20 cc. of alcohol; it is almost insoluble in water. It was formerly used in making glycerin suppositories but is now replaced by sodium stearate. It is used as an ingredient of the so-called vanishing cream used as an ointment base.

ste·ar′i·form [G. *stear,* fat; L. *forma,* form]. Having the appearance of, or resembling, fat.

stear′in (steer′in). $C_3H_5O_3(C_{17}H_{35}CO)_3$. Tristearin, glyceryl tristearate. The glyceryl ester of stearic acid, occurring in many of the solid animal fats.

stear″o·der′mi·a [*stear;* G. *derma,* skin]. An affection of the sebaceous glands of the skin.

stearodine. A trade-mark for *calcium iodostearate.*

stear·op′ten. That portion of a volatile oil, usually consisting of oxygenated substances, which is solid at ordinary temperatures.

ste″ar·rhe′a. See *seborrhea.*

s. flavescens. A seborrhea in which the sebaceous matter turns yellow after being deposited upon the skin.

s. nigricans. See *chromhidrosis.*

s. simplex. Seborrhea oleosa.

stear′yl. The monovalent radical, $C_{17}H_{35}CO—$, of stearic acid.

stear′yl al′co·hol. $CH_3(CH_2)_{16}CH_2OH$; a white unctuous solid, occurring as flakes or granules, insoluble in water, soluble in alcohol. The official substance of this name is a mixture of alcohols, composed chiefly of the preceding. It is an ingredient of ointment bases and creams.

ste′a·tin. 1. Stearin. 2. Any cerate containing a considerable proportion of tallow.

ste″a·ti′num. Certain pharmaceutical preparations similar to cerates. Their use is now obsolete.

ste″a·ti′tis [*stear;* G. *-itis,* inflammation]. Inflammation of adipose tissue.

ste′a·to-, steat- [*stear*]. A combining form meaning *fat.*

ste″a·to·cryp·to′sis [*stear;* G. *kryptein,* to hide; *-ōsis,* condition]. Abnormal function of the sebaceous glands.

ste″a·to·cys·to′ma mul′ti·plex. An uncommon skin disorder characterized by various-sized cystic lesions over the trunk, back, arms, or thighs. Usually occurs in young men who, as a rule, do not have acne or seborrhea. Also called *sebocystomatosis.*

ste″a·tog′e·nous (stee″uh·todj′i·nus) [*stear;* G. *genesthai,* from *gignesthai,* to be produced]. Producing steatosis.

ste″a·tol′y·sis [*stear;* G. *lysis,* a loosing]. The emulsifying process by which fats are prepared for absorption and assimilation. **—steatolyt′ic,** *adj.*

ste″a·to′ma [G., sebaceous tumor]. 1. A sebaceous cyst. *Obs.* 2. A lipoma. *Obs.*

ste″a·to·py′gi·a (stee″uh·to·pye′jee·uh, ·pidj′ee·uh) [G. *stear,* fat; *pygē,* buttocks]. Excessive accumulation of fat on the buttocks. **—steatop′ygous,** *adj.*

ste″a·tor·rhe′a [*stear;* G. *rhoia,* flow]. 1. An

increased flow of the secretion of the sebaceous follicles; see *seborrhea*. 2. Fatty stools.

chronic idiopathic s. See celiac *disease*.

congenital pancreatic s. See pancreatic *fibrosis*.

s. simplex. Excess of sebaceous excretion of the face.

ste″a·to′sis [*stear;* G. *-ōsis*, condition]. An old term formerly used loosely for fatty degeneration, or disease of sebaceous glands.

corneal s. Deposits of fat in the cornea.

steclin. Trade-mark for the antibiotic substance tetracycline, commonly supplied as the hydrochloride.

steel [AS. *stēl*]. Iron chemically combined with a certain proportion of carbon. It holds an intermediate position between white cast iron and wrought iron, partaking of the most valuable qualities of both. Steel of good quality is fine-grained, elastic, and tough.

stainless s. A steel which contains elements such as nickel and/or chromium; it does not tarnish on exposure and is extensively used in the manufacture of high-grade cutlery.

Steell, Graham [*English physician*, 1851–1942]. Described the murmur of pulmonary valve incompetence: it may occur in mitral stenosis and cardiac insufficiency; called *Graham Steell murmur*.

Steenbock, Harry (1886–). American physiologist and biochemist known for his researches in nutrition, e.g., the correlation of vitamin-A activity with the occurrence of yellow plant pigments, the role of copper in the prevention of anemia, and the effect of ultraviolet irradiation on calcium and phosphorus metabolism. He invented vitamin-D milk and the synthesis of vitamin D by the irradiation of certain sterols.

stee′ple skull. Oxycephaly.

steg·no′sis [G., a making watertight]. The closing of a passage. **—stegnot′ic,** *adj.*

Steg″o·my′ia, Ste″go·my′ia [G. *stegos*, roof; *myia*, fly]. A genus of mosquitoes or *Culicidae*, represented in most tropical and subtropical countries. See *Aëdes aegypti. Obs.*

Stehle gasometric method (for urea). See under *method*.

Stein, Stanislav Aleksandr Fyodorovich von [*Russian otologist*, b. 1855]. Remembered for his test for labyrinthine disease. If the patient closes his eyes, he will be unable to stand or hop on one foot. Called *Stein's test*.

Stein-McCarthy prostatic electrotome. See Joseph Francis *McCarthy*.

Steinach, Eugen [*Austrian physiologist*, 1861–1944]. Widely known for his rejuvenation operation in which he occluded the ductus deferens, called *Steinach's method* or *operation*.

Steindler, Arthur (1878–). American orthopedic surgeon who made many contributions to kinesiology and orthopedic surgery. His methods for fusion of the shoulder joint, the stripping of the calcaneus, and plastic repair of the elbow paralyzed by poliomyelitis are called *Steindler operations*.

Steinmann, Fritz [*Swiss surgeon*, 1872–1932]. Remembered for his invention of a surgical nail inserted in distal portions of such bones as the femur or tibia for skeletal traction; called *Steinmann's pin* or *nail*.

stel′la len′tis hy″a·loi′de·a. Posterior pole of the lens of the eye.

stel′la len′tis i·rid′i·ca. The anterior pole of the lens of the eye.

stel′late [L. *stellatus*, starry]. Star-shaped, or with parts radiating from a center.

stellite. Trade-mark for an acid-resistant alloy, containing cobalt, chromium, tungsten, and molybdenum: used in certain surgical instruments.

Stellwag von Carion, Carl [*Austrian ophthalmologist*, 1823–1904]. Known for his description of a sign of exophthalmic goiter: absence or diminution in frequency of the winking movements of the eyelids with abnormal width of the palpebral aperture indicates the disease. Called *Stellwag's sign*.

stem [AS. *stemm*]. 1. The pedicle or stalk of a tumor. 2. A supporting stalk, as of a leaf or plant.

brain s. The portion of the brain remaining after the cerebral hemispheres and cerebellum have been removed. See Plates 17, 18.

infundibular s. See *stalk* of the neurohypophysis.

ste·nag′ma [G.]. Sigh. *Rare.*

ste·nag′mus [G. *stenagmos*, a sighing]. Sighing. *Rare.*

Stender dish. A covered cylindrical glass vessel used in histologic technic.

Stenger test. See Wells-Stenger *test*.

ste′ni·on, sten′i·on (pl. *stenia*) [G. *stenos*, narrow]. That point on the sphenosquamosal suture which is located most medially.

Steno, Nicolaus (Nils). See Nicolaus *Stensen*.

sten′o- [*stenos*]. A combining form meaning *narrow* or *constricted*.

sten″o·car′di·a [*stenos;* G. *kardia*, heart]. Angina pectoris. *Obs.*

sten″o·ceph′a·ly, sten″o·ce·pha′li·a [*stenos;* G. *kephalē*, head]. Unusual narrowness of the head. **—stenocephalous,** *adj.*

sten″o·chas′mus (sten″o·kaz′mus) [*stenos;* G. *chasma*, chasm]. Lissauer's term for a skull with a small angle, 94° to 74°, of the nasopharynx. The angle is included between two lines drawn, respectively, from the posterior nasal spine and basion to the point on the rostrum of the sphenoid where it is included between the alae vomeris.

sten″o·cho′ri·a (sten″o·kor′ee·uh) [G., narrowness of space]. Narrowing; partial obstruction, particularly of a lacrimal duct.

sten″o·co·ri′a·sis [G., unnatural contraction of the pupil]. Narrowing of the pupil.

sten″o·crot′a·phy (sten″o·krot′uh·fee, ·kro′tuh·fee) [G. *stenos*, narrow; *krotaphos*, temple]. Abnormal narrowness of the skull in the pterionic region, probably due to hypoplasia of the sphenoidal angles of the parietal bones, and of the great wings of the sphenoid bone.

sten′o·dont [*stenos;* G. *odous*, tooth]. Provided with narrow teeth.

sten″o·mer′ic [*stenos;* G. *mēros*, thigh]. *In osteometry*, designating a femur with no anteroposterior compression of the proximal portion of the diaphysis. There may be considerable mediolateral compression of the same portion as is indicated by the platymeric index of 100.0 or more. Stenomeric femurs are abnormal, normal femurs being either platymeric or eurymeric.

sten″o·myc·te′ri·a [*stenos;* G. *myktēr*, nostril]. Nasal stenosis. *Obs.*

sten″o·pe′ic [*stenos;* G. *opē*, hole]. A device of metal or other opaque substance with a very fine slit or minute hole or holes. Held before defective eyes, it facilitates vision. Duke-Elder's device enables a presbyope who has lost his glasses to read in an emergency. The slitted stenopeic (long used by Eskimos) protects from ultraviolet radiation from sunlight on snow or ice.

sten″o·pe′ic. Pertaining to a narrow slit or minute hole.

ste·nosed′ (sti·noced′, ·nozed′, sten′ozed) [*stenos*]. Constricted, narrowed.

ste·no′sis [G.]. Constriction or narrowing, especially

of a channel or aperture. —**steno′sal, stenot′ic,** *adj.*

aortic s. A narrowing of the aortic orifice at the base of the heart or a narrowing of the aorta itself.

aqueduct s. Stenosis of the cerebral aqueduct, usually at the junction of the upper and middle third: also called *atresia of iter.*

bronchial s. See *bronchostenosis.*

cicatricial s. Stenosis due to a contracted cicatrix.

Dittrich's s. Stenosis of the conus arteriosus.

granulation s. Narrowing caused by encroachment or contraction of granulations.

mitral s. Disease of the mitral valve causing obstruction to the flow of blood through the left atrioventricular opening. It is a late (remote) effect of acute rheumatic fever.

post-tracheotomy s. Stenosis after tracheotomy.

pulmonary s. A disease of the pulmonary valve in which congenital obstruction and other anomalies are usually present.

pyloric s. Congenital obstruction of the pyloric orifice of the stomach caused by hypertrophy of the pyloric muscle.

tricuspid s. Narrowing of the tricuspid valve, with resultant resistance to flow of blood into the right ventricle. There is an elevation of right-atrial and venous pressure, with hypertrophy of the right atrium and distention of the veins.

valvular s. Narrowing of the orifice of a valve.

sten″o·sto′mi·a [G. *stenostomos,* narrow-mouthed]. A reduction in the orifice of the mouth as a result of cicatrization. —**stenostom′atous,** *adj.*

ste·nos′to·my [*stenostomos*]. Contracture of any mouth or aperture.

sten″o·ther′mal [G. *stenos,* narrow; *thermē,* heat]. Capable of resisting a small range of temperature.

sten″o·tho′rax [G., narrow-chested]. An unusually narrow chest.

Stensen, Nicolaus (1638–1686). Danish anatomist who discovered the parotid duct and the lateral incisive foramen: variously called *Nils* or *Niels Stensen* or *Steno.*

stent. 1. A compound used for immobilizing some forms of skin graft. 2. A mold made of stent, used for immobilizing some forms of skin graft.

sten″to·roph′o·nous [G. *Stentōr,* a Greek at Troy famous for his loud voice; *phōnē,* voice]. Having a loud voice.

ste·pha′ni·on (sti·fay′nee·on, sti·fan′ee·on) [G. *stephanos,* wreath]. The point where the coronal suture crosses the linea temporalis inferior. —**stephanial, stephan′ic,** *adj.*

Stephanus. See Charles *Estienne.*

step′page gait. The peculiar high-stepping gait seen in tabes dorsalis and certain forms of multiple neuritis, or neuropathy. It also occurs in toe drop.

ster″co·bi′lin. The chief constituent of the brown pigment found in feces. Derived from bilirubin by reduction due to bacteria in the intestine. Also called *hydrobilirubin, urobilin.*

ster″co·bi·lin′o·gen (stur″ko·buy·lin′o·jin, ·bi·lin′-o·jin). A reduction product of stercobilin which occurs in the feces. Stercobilinogen is a colorless compound which becomes brown on oxidation. It is probably identical with urobilinogen.

ster′co·lith [L. *stercus,* dung; G. *lithos,* stone]. A calcified, fecal concretion.

ster″co·ra′ceous [*stercus*]. Fecal; having the nature of or containing feces, as stercoraceous vomiting.

ster′co·ral, ster′co·rous. See *stercoraceous.*

ster′co·rar″y (stur′ko·rerr″ee) [L. *stercorarius,* of dung]. Fecal.

ster″co·ro′ma [*stercus;* G. *-ōma,* tumor]. Fecalith; a hard fecal mass usually in the rectum.

Ster·cu′li·a [L. *Sterculius,* deity who presided over manuring]. A large genus of tropical trees. **S. urens** of India and **S. tragacantha** of Africa afford karaya gum, which has been substituted for tragacanth. **S. acuminata** (*Cola nitida*) produces the kola nut.

ster′cus [L.]. Feces.

stere (steer, stair) [G. *stereos,* solid]. A measure of 1000 liters; a kiloliter.

ster″e·a·tron′ics. The science of the controllable electronic performance of solids.

ster′e·o- (sterr′ee·o-, steer′ee·o-), **ster′e-** [*stereos*]. A combining form meaning *solid.*

ster″e·o·ag·no′sis. See *astereognosis.*

ster″e·o·an″es·the′si·a [*stereos;* G. *anaisthēsia,* lack of sensation]. Inability to ascertain the form or size of objects by feeling them.

ster″e·o·ar·throl′y·sis [*stereos;* G. *arthron,* joint; *lysis,* a loosing]. Loosening stiff joints by operation or manipulation in cases of ankylosis.

ster″e·o·blas′tu·la [*stereos;* NL. dim. from G. *blastos,* sprout]. A solid blastula, not having a blastocoele, but having all its cells bounding the external surface.

equal s. One having cells of the same size derived from equal cleavage.

unequal s. One with small cells in one pole or hemisphere and large cells in the other.

ster″e·o·cam·pim′e·ter. An instrument for measuring the extent of the visual field of both eyes simultaneously. Syn., *stereoscopic campimeter.*

ster″e·o·chem′is·try [*stereos;* G. *chymos,* juice]. A branch of science that investigates the spatial arrangement of the atoms in a molecule.

ster″e·o·cil′i·a [*stereos;* L. *cilium,* eyelid]. Non-motile cilia.

ster″e·o·en·ceph′a·lo·tome. A device for localizing exactly any point within the brain, for the operation of stereoencephalotomy.

ster″e·o·en·ceph″a·lot′o·my. Selective destruction, by cautery or electrolysis, of cerebral tracts or nuclei, using the pineal body or posterior commissure as the point of reference or zero point on the stereotaxic coordinates.

ster″e·og·no′sis [*stereos;* G. *gnōsis,* knowledge]. The faculty of recognizing the size and shape of objects by the sense of touch. —**stereognos′tic,** *adj.*

ster′e·o·gram″ [*stereos;* G. *gramma,* letter]. 1. A two-dimensional picture which represents an object with the impression of three dimensions, by means of contour lines or shading. 2. A stereoscopic picture.

ster′e·o·graph″ [*stereos;* G. *graphein,* to write]. An instrument devised by Broca for drawing geometric contours of skulls in the various normae.

ster″e·og′ra·phy [*stereos; graphein*]. That phase of craniometry which consists of making geometric projections of a skull held rigidly in a predetermined plane, thus producing drawings so accurate that lines and angles may be measured on them.

ster″e·o·i′so·mer [*stereos;* G. *isomerēs,* equally divided]. A compound containing the same number and kind of atoms as another compound, but with the atoms grouped differently in the molecule. A stereoisomer is optically active and contains one or more asymmetric atoms.

ster″e·o·i·som′er·ism (sterr″ee·o·eye·som′ur·iz·um, steer″ee·o·) [*stereos; isomerēs*]. The condition in which two or more substances having the same molecular formulas have different properties; these differences are due to the different relative positions of the atoms in the molecule.

ster″e·o·mon′o·scope [*stereos;* G. *monos,* alone; *skopein,* to examine]. An instrument which projects two stereoscopic images upon the same spot on a ground glass screen by means of two lenses, the combined image giving the impression of solidity.

ster″e·o-oph·thal′mo·scope. See under *ophthalmoscope.*

ster″e·o·phan′to·scope [*stereos;* G. *phantos,* visible; *skopein*]. A panoramic stereoscope using rotating disks in place of pictures. *Obs.*

ster″e·o·phor′o·scope [*stereos;* G. *phoros,* bearing; *skopein*]. A stereoscopic stroboscope, an instrument for producing a series of images apparently in motion; used in tests of visual perception.

ster′e·o·plasm [*stereos;* G. *plasma,* anything formed]. The solid part of the protoplasm of cells. *Obs.*

ster″e·op′sis [*stereos;* G. *opsis,* vision]. Stereoscopic vision.

ster′e·op″ter [*stereos;* G. *optēr,* one who looks]. An instrument to provide a rapid quantitative test for depth perception.

ster″e·o·ra″di·og′ra·phy [*stereos;* L. *radius,* ray; G. *graphein,* to write]. Taking of two radiographs with the roentgen-ray tube in two positions, about six inches apart, and viewing of these two films in such a manner that the stereoscopic picture appears three-dimensional.

ster″e·o·roent″gen·og′ra·phy (sterr″ee·o·rent″-ghin·og′ruh·fee, steer″ee·o·) [*stereos; Röntgen; graphein*]. A roentgenographic procedure for making stereoscopic roentgenograms.

ster″e·o·roent″gen·om′e·ter. Apparatus for determining the solid dimensions of a radiopaque object from its stereoscopic roentgenograms.

ster″e·o·roent″gen·om′e·try (·rent″ghin·om′i-tree) [*stereos; Röntgen;* G. *metron,* a measure]. The use of the stereoscope in the study of stereoroentgenograms.

ster′e·o·scope [*stereos;* G. *skopein,* to examine]. An instrument by which two similar pictures of the same object are so mounted that the images are seen as one, thereby giving a three-dimensional impression. —**stereoscop′ic,** *adj.;* **stereos′copy,** *n.*

ster″e·o·stro′bo·scope [*stereos;* G. *strobos,* a whirling round; *skopein*]. An apparatus for the study of points moving in three dimensions.

ster″e·o·tax′i·a [*stereos;* G. *taxis,* arrangement]. The production of electrolysis in a definite circumscribed area within the brain, with minimal damage to the remainder of the organ. —**stereotax′ic,** *adj.*

ster″e·o·tax′is. Taxis in response to touch or contact, especially with respect to a solid body. Syn., *thigmotaxis.*

ster″e·ot′ro·pism [*stereos;* G. *trepein,* to turn]. Growth or movement toward a solid body (**positive stereotropism**) or away from a solid body (**negative stereotropism**). Syn., *thigmotropism.* —**stereotrop′ic,** *adj.*

ster′e·o·ty″py (sterr′ee·o·tye″pee, steer′ee·o·) [*stereos;* G. *typos,* impression]. Morbid persistence of a volitional impulse when once started.

ster″e·o·vec″tor·car′di·o·graph″. Dual-beam oscillograph for instantaneous registration of third-dimensional vectocardiogram.

ster′ic. Relating to the arrangement of atoms in space.

ster′ic hin′drance. *In chemistry,* the power ascribed to bulky atoms or bulky groups of atoms of interfering with the normal mobility of molecules or parts thereof. According to the theory, if the bulky group is close to the site of the reaction, it may interfere with the attack by a reagent and may retard or prevent the reaction or permit a competing process to occur. The presence of bulky groups in a molecule may also interfere with the free rotation around single bonds. This can increase the number of stable stereoisomeric forms and can decrease the stabilization of the molecule by resonance.

ster′id. A substance that is either a sterol or a steroid.

Ster″ig·mat″o·cys′tis [G. *stērigma,* support; *kystis,* bladder]. A genus of molds belonging to the family Mucoraceae. It is occasionally a parasite of man.

S. cinnamomina. A species found in mycetoma and occasionally producing a generalized infection similar to aspergillosis.

ster′ile [L. *sterilis*]. 1. Not fertile; not capable of reproducing. 2. Free from germs.

ste·ril′i·ty. Involuntary total inability to reproduce.

facultative s. Sterility caused by the prevention of conception.

idiopathic s. See *azoospermia.*

one-child s. Sterility occurring in a woman after she has given birth to one child.

relative s. Inability to produce a viable child.

sterility clinic. See *fertility clinic.*

ster″i·li·za′tion [L. *sterilis,* sterile]. 1. The destruction of all forms of life. Substances may be sterilized by the use of physical or chemical agents, heat being the most important. Moist heat, at temperatures above the boiling point of water, will kill the most resistant spores formed by microorganisms within a relatively short period of time. Fractional or intermittent sterilization consists of the successive application of moist heat to destroy vegetative cells with intervening periods of sufficient duration to permit spores to germinate. 2. Any procedure which renders an individual incapable of reproduction.

ster′i·lize [*sterilis*]. 1. Render sterile or free from bacteria. 2. Render incapable of procreation.

ster′i·li″zer [*sterilis*]. An instrument for the destruction of all forms of life. The Arnold sterilizer utilizes steam at atmospheric pressure. The autoclave or pressure cooker uses steam under pressure at temperatures above the boiling point of water.

Stern potential. See under *potential.*

ster·nal′gi·a [G. *sternon,* breast; *algos,* pain]. Pain in the sternum.

ster·na′lis (stur·nah′lis, ·nay′lis) [*sternon*]. A rare muscle over the sternum. See Table of Muscles in the Appendix.

Sternberg, Carl (1872–1935). German pathologist who described the large polynuclear cells characteristic of Hodgkin's disease, in America called *Reed-Sternberg cells.* Leukosarcoma is sometimes called *Sternberg's disease,* and Hodgkin's disease is sometimes called *Paltauf-Sternberg disease.*

Sternberg, George Miller (1838–1915). American Army medical officer; pioneer bacteriologist who discovered the pneumococcus independently of its discovery by Louis Pasteur. He was the first to photograph the *Mycobacterium tuberculosis.*

ster′ne·bra. Embryological segment of the body of the sternum; there are usually four, of which the lower two or three arise from paired ossification centers.

ster′no- [G. *sternon,* breast]. A combining form denoting *breast* or *connection with the sternum.*

ster″no·chon″dro·scap″u·lar′is (stur″no·kon″-dro·skap″yoo·lair′is) [*sternon;* G. *chondros,* cartilage; L. *scapula,* shoulder]. A rare muscle arising from the sternum and the first costal cartilage, and extending to the upper border of the scapula.

ster″no·cla·vic′u·lar [*sternon;* L. *clavicula,* small key]. Pertaining to the sternum and the clavicle, as the sternoclavicular joint. See Table of Joints and Ligaments in the Appendix.

ster″no·cla·vic″u·lar′is. A rare variant slip of the subclavius muscle.

ster″no·clei″do·mas′toid (stur″no·kly″do·mas′-toyd) [*sternon;* G. *kleis,* hook; *mastoeidēs,* like a breast]. Pertaining to the sternum, the clavicle, and the mastoid process, as the sternocleidomastoid muscle. See Table of Muscles in the Appendix.

ster″no·cos·ta′lis. BR name for the transversus thoracis muscle.

ster″no·dym′i·a [*sternon;* G. *didymos,* twin]. A form of conjoined twins in which the union is in the sternum. Also called *sternopagia.*

ster·nod′y·mus [*sternon; didymos*]. Twin monsters united at the anterior wall of the thorax; sternopagus.

ster″no·dyn′i·a (stur″no·din′ee·uh, ·dye′nee·uh) [*sternon;* G. *odynē,* pain]. Sternalgia; pain in the sternum.

ster″no·hy′oid [*sternon;* G. *hyoeidēs,* shaped like the letter upsilon]. Pertaining to the sternum and the hyoid bone, as the sternohyoid muscle. See Table of Muscles in the Appendix.

ster″no·hy·oid′e·us a′zy·gos. A rare muscle of the neck extending from the posterior surface of the manubrium of the sternum to the hyoid.

ster″no·mas′toid [*sternon;* G. *mastoeidēs,* like a breast]. Unofficial term for sternocleidomastoid muscle.

ster″no-om·phal″o·dym′i·a. A form of conjoined twins in which the union is in both the sternal and the umbilical regions.

ster″no·pa′gi·a, ster·nop′a·gy [*sternon;* G. *pagos,* that which is fixed]. The condition of being a sternopagus.

ster·nop′a·gus [*sternon; pagos*]. Conjoined twins united at the sternum. Also called *ectopagus, thoracopagus.*

ster″no·per″i·car′di·al [*sternon;* G. *perikardios,* around the heart]. Pertaining to the sternum and the underlying pericardium.

ster·nos′chi·sis (stur·nos′ki·sis) [*sternon;* G. *schisis,* cleavage]. Congenital cleft or fissure of the sternum: also called *fissura sterni.*

ster″no·thy′roid [*sternon;* G. *thyreoeidēs,* shield-shaped]. Pertaining to the sternum and thyroid cartilage, as the sternothyroid muscle. See Table of Muscles in the Appendix.

ster·not′o·my [*sternon;* G. *tomē,* a cutting]. Cutting through the sternum.

ster′num [*sternon*]. The flat, narrow bone in the median line in the front of the chest, composed of three portions—the manubrium, the body, and the xiphoid process. See Table of Bones in the Appendix. See Plates 1, 13. —**sternal,** *adj.*

cleft s. Congenital fissure of the sternum.

ster″nu·ta′tion [L. *sternutatio*]. The act of sneezing.

ster′nu·ta″tor [L. *sternutare,* to sneeze]. A substance capable of inducing sneezing, as certain war gases. See also vomiting *gas.*

ster″o·chem′is·try. See *stereochemistry.*

ster′oid, ste′roid [G. *stereos,* solid; *eidos,* form]. The generic name for the compounds comprising the sterols, bile acids, heart poisons, saponins, and sex hormones. See Table of Hormones in the Appendix.

ster′ol, ste′rol. Any saturated or unsaturated alcohol derived from cyclopentanoperhydrophenanthrene; the alcohols occur both free and combined as esters or glycosides, and usually are obtained as principal constituents of the nonsaponifiable fraction of fixed oils and fats. *Zoosterols* are sterols of animal origin; *phytosterols* are sterols from higher plants; *mycosterols* are the sterols of fungi.

ster′one, ste′rone. A steroid possessing one or more ketone groups.

ster′tor [L. *stertere,* to snore]. Sonorous breathing or snoring; the rasping, rattling sound produced when the larynx and the air passages are partially obstructed by mucus. —**stertorous,** *adj.*

steth·ar″te·ri′tis [G. *stēthos,* breast; *artēria,* artery; *-itis,* inflammation]. Inflammation of the arteries of the thorax. *Rare.*

steth′o-, steth- [*stēthos*]. A combining form meaning *breast* or *chest.*

ste·thog′ra·phy [*stēthos;* G. *graphein,* to write]. See *phonocardiography.*

steth′o·phone [*stēthos;* G. *phōnē,* sound]. 1. Stethoscope. A more accurate term than stethoscope, but now obsolete. 2. An electric stethoscope capable of transmitting heart murmurs and lung sounds to a large group of listeners.

steth″o·pol′y·scope [*stēthos;* G. *polys,* many; *skopein,* to examine]. A stethoscope having several tubes for the simultaneous use of several listeners.

steth′o·scope [*stēthos; skopein*]. An instrument for the detection and study of sounds arising within the body. Invented by Laennec. The early type was a slender wooden tube with a flange on each end. The modern stethoscope has a bell or cup-shaped end piece of metal or hard rubber connected with rubber tubing, which conducts the sound to both ears of the examiner.

binaural s. One which connects to both ears of the user.

steth″o·scop′ic [*stēthos; skopein*]. Pertaining to, or detected by means of, a stethoscope.

ste·thos′co·py [*stēthos; skopein*]. Examination with the aid of the stethoscope.

Stevens, William [*Scottish surgeon,* 1786–1868]. Remembered for his successful ligation of the internal iliac artery for gluteal aneurysm (1812). This is said to have been the first case of the kind on record. Called *Stevens' operation.*

Stewart, Francis Torrens [*American surgeon,* 1877–1920]. Remembered for his incision for radical mastectomy by means of two transverse incisions meeting laterally and at the sternum to form a pointed oval around the breast; called *Stewart's incision.*

Stewart-Holmes phenomenon. Rebound phenomenon.

Stewart-Morel syndrome. See metabolic *craniopathy.*

STH Abbreviation for somatotropic hormone.

sthe′ni·a [G. *sthenos,* strength]. Normal or excessive force or vigor; opposed to *asthenia.*

sthen′ic [*sthenos*]. Strong; active.

stib′a·mine glu′co·side. A nitrogen glucoside of sodium *p*-aminophenylstibonate, a pentavalent antimony compound used in the treatment of kala-azar.

stib″i·ac′ne (stib″ee·ack′nee) [G. *stibi,* antimony; perhaps G. *achnē,* chaff]. Acne caused by the use of antimony. *Rare.*

stib′i·al·ism [*stibi*]. Antimonial poisoning.

stib′ine (stib′een, ·in). Antimonous hydride, SbH_3.

stib′i·um [L., from *stibi*]. Antimony.

sti·bo′ni·um. The monovalent radical, SbH_4^+, analogous to ammonium.

stib′o·phen. $(NaO_3S)_2C_6H_2O_2{:}SbOC_6H_2(ONa)(SO_3Na)_2.7H_2O$. Sodium antimony-bispyrocatechol-3,5-sodium disulfonate; employed as a remedy in venereal lymphogranuloma and schistosomiasis. Dose, intramuscularly, a total of 40 cc., in divided portions, of a 6.3% solution. See *fuadin.*

stich′o·chrome (stick′o·krohm) [G. *stichos,* row; *chrōma,* color]. Applied by Nissl to a nerve cell in which the chromophilic substance is arranged in striae running in the same direction as, and usually parallel with, the contour of the cell body. *Obs.*

Sticker, Georg (1860–). German physician and epidemiologist, known for his many writings on the history of medicine. He described erythema infectiosum (1899), also called *Sticker's disease.*

stic'ta [G. *stiktos,* spotted, pricked]. A lichen, *Sticta pulmonaria;* used in rheumatism and chronic coughs by homeopaths and eclectics.

stic·tac'ne (stick·tack'nee) [*stiktos;* perhaps G. *achnē,* chaff]. Acne punctata; acne in which the pustules are tiny and surround a comedone.

Stieda, Alfred [*German surgeon,* 1869–1945]. Known for his description of medial condylar fracture of the femur, called *Stieda's fracture.* Posttraumatic calcification of the medial collateral ligament of the knee is called *Pellegrini-Stieda disease.*

Stieda, Ludwig [*German anatomist,* 1837–1918]. Described the posterior process of the talus, also called *Stieda's process.*

stiff [AS. *stīf*]. Inflexible, unyielding, immovable in continuity; applied especially to normally movable parts.

sti'fle [ME. *stuflen*]. Choke; kill by impeding respiration.

sti'fle bone. The patella of the horse.

sti'fle joint. The true knee joint of the hind leg of the horse, corresponding to the knee joint of man.

stig'ma (pl. *stigmas, stigmata*) [G., tattoo-mark]. 1. A small spot or mark, especially a spot of hemorrhage in the palm or sole, occurring in hysterical persons. 2. Any one of the marks or signs characteristic of a condition, as hysterical stigmas. 3. That part of a pistil which receives the pollen. 4. An opening between cells, especially one between the endothelial cells of a capillary, now considered an artifact. A stoma. —**stig'mal, stigmat'ic,** *adj.*

baker's stigmas. Corns on the fingers from kneading dough.

follicular s. The thin, nonvascular area of the ovary overlying the mature follicle marking the spot at which rupture of the follicle will occur; also the point of rupture.

hereditary stigmas. Psychic stigmas resembling those of an ancestor and supposed to be inherited.

hysterical stigmas. The specific, peculiar phenomena or symptoms of hysteria, as anesthesia, hyperesthesia, hysterogenic zones, reversal of the color field, contraction of the visual field, the phenomena of transport amblyopia, impairment of the senses of hearing and of taste and of muscular sense, etc.

neurasthenic stigmas. See *hysterical stigmas* under *stigma.*

psychic stigmas. Certain mental states characterized by susceptibility to particular suggestions.

somatic stigmas. The objective signs of certain nervous affections.

s. of the Graafian follicle. The point of rupture through which the ovum escapes.

stigmata of Beneke. Acute ulcers along the greater curvature of the stomach.

stigmata nigra. The black spots caused by the presence of grains of gunpowder in the skin.

stig·mas'ter·ol. $C_{29}H_{46}O$. A sterol derived from the soybean.

stig'ma·tism [*stigma*]. 1. A condition of the refractive media of the eye in which rays of light from a point are accurately brought to a focus on the retina. Also see *astigmatism.* 2. The condition of having stigmas.

stig"ma·ti·za'tion [*stigma*]. The formation of stigmas.

stig'ma·tose [*stigma*]. Marked with stigmas.

stigmonene bromide. Trade-marked name for the benzpyrinium bromide, a cholinergic agent.

stil·bam'i·dine (stil·bam'i·deen, ·din). NH:C-(NH$_2$).C$_6$H$_4$.CH:CH.C$_6$H$_4$.(NH$_2$)C:NH; 4:4'-diamidinostilbene. One of a group of diamidines possessing trypanocidal activity. It has been used in the treatment of kala-azar and of multiple myeloma.

stil'bene. $C_6H_5.CH{=}CH.C_6H_5$. The parent hydrocarbon from which the synthetic estrogen diethylstilbestrol may be considered to be derived.

stil·bes'trol, stil·boes'trol (stil·bes'trole, ·trol, ·trawl). Diethylstilbestrol.

Stiles, Charles Wardell [*American bacteriologist and parasitologist,* 1867–1941]. Known for his extensive work in ancylostomiasis in America. Discovered its cause, the American hookworm, *Necator americanus* or *Uncinaria americana* (1902).

sti·let', sti·lette' (sti·let', sty·let', sty'let). See *stylet.*

Still, Andrew Taylor [*American osteopathic physician,* 1828–1917]. Widely known as the founder of osteopathy.

Still, George Frederic [*English pediatrician,* 1868–1941]. Described a form of polyarthritis affecting children; called Still's disease. Author of a *History of Pediatrics.*

still'birth" [AS. *stille;* ME. *burth*]. The birth of a dead child.

still'born" [*stille;* AS. *beran*]. Born dead.

Stiller, Berthold (1837–1922). German physician who described an asthenic body-build (1907) associated with enteroptosis, called *Stiller's disease.* The attribution of enteroptosis and gastroptosis to universal asthenia is called *Stiller's theory.* He noted the marked mobility or fluctuation of the tenth rib in neurasthenia and enteroptosis; this is known as *Stiller's sign.*

stil"li·cid'i·um [L., a liquid which falls drop by drop]. Old term for the flow of a liquid drop by drop.

s. lacrimarum. Overflow of tears from obstruction of the lacrimal ducts; epiphora. *Obs.*

s. urinae. Dribbling of urine. *Obs.*

Stilling, Benedict [*German anatomist,* 1810–79]. Described the central canal of the spinal cord, called *Clarke's* or *Stilling's canal.* The scattered cells lying along its anterior aspect are called *Stilling's nucleus.* The gelatinous substance, surrounding the central canal, is also called *Stilling's nucleus.* The hyaloid canal of the vitreous body is called *Cloquet's* or *Stilling's canal.* See also Stilling's *raphe.*

Stilling's test. See under *test.*

stil·lin'gi·a [after Benjamin *Stillingfleet,* English botanist, 1702–71]. The dried root of *Stillingia sylvatica.* It contains a volatile oil, an acrid resin termed sylvacrol, and an acrid fixed oil. Formerly used in syphilitic and scrofulous conditions. Syn., *queensroot.*

stilpalmitate. Trade-mark for the di-palmitic acid ester of diethylstilbestrol, used in oil solution like diethylstilbestrol; the ester has prolonged therapeutic effect because of slower absorption.

stilrone. Trade-mark for a brand of diethylstilbestrol.

Stimson, Lewis Atterbury [*American surgeon,* 1844–1917]. Described a method of reducing dislocated hip; called *Stimson's method.* See Plate 38.

stim'u·lant [L. *stimulare,* to goad]. An agent that causes stimulation. —**stim'ulant,** *adj.*

diffusible s. One that has a prompt but transient effect.

local s. One acting directly on the end organs of the sensory nerves of the skin.

stim'u·late [*stimulare*]. Quicken; stir up; excite; increase functional activity.

stim"u·la'tion [L. *stimulatio,* from *stimulare*]. 1. The act of stimulating. 2. The effect of a stimulant.

stim'u·lin [L. *stimulus*, a goad]. Metchnikoff's name for substances supposed to stimulate the phagocytes to destroy germs. *Obs.*

stim'u·lus (pl. *stimuli*) [L.]. An excitant or irritant; an alteration in the environment of any living thing (cell, tissue, organism) producing a response.

adequate s. A physical or chemical change in the environment to which there is a preferential response, e.g., rods and cones of the eye respond preferentially to the electromagnetic vibrations between 400 and 800 mμ and with a much higher threshold to mechanical stimuli (inadequate stimulus).

chemical s. One due to, or produced by, chemical means.

conditioned s. One to which a conditioned reflex response has been developed.

heterologous s. One acting upon the nervous elements of the sensory apparatus along their entire course.

homologous s. One acting only upon the end organ.

inadequate s. 1. One unable to produce a response; a subthreshold s. 2. One to which a response occurs at a much higher threshold than to an adequate stimulus.

liminal s. See threshold *s.*

maximal s. A stimulus, increase above which produces no additional action.

mechanical s. One acting by mechanical means, as pinching or striking.

minimal s. See threshold *s.*

nocuous stimuli. Stimuli of injurious nature.

subliminal s. See subthreshold *s.*

subminimal s. See subthreshold *s.*

subthreshold s. One too weak to produce any obvious effect. Syn., *subliminal s.*, *subminimal s.*

summation of stimuli. See under *summation.*

thermal s. One acting through change in temperature.

threshold s. The smallest stimulus which produces an effect. Syn., *subliminal s.*, *subminimal s.*

sting [AS. *stingan*]. 1. The acute burning sensation caused by pricking, striking, or chemically stimulating the skin or a mucous membrane. 2. The wound caused. 3. The organ or part causing the wound, e.g., the sting of a bee. —**sting,** *v.*

stip"i·tat'ic ac'id. $C_7H_3O(OH)_2COOH$; a 7-membered cyclic compound produced by the mold *Penicillium stipitatum.*

stip'pling [D. *stippelen*]. 1. A change of a surface whereby the presence of tiny nodules produces an appearance like that of a pebbled paper, as slight deposits of fibrin on a serous surface. 2. A change in erythrocytes whereby minute droplets with affinity for basic dyes occur in erythrocytes, as in lead poisoning.

Stirling's aniline-gentian violet solution. See under *stain.*

stir'pi·cul"ture [L. *stirps*, stock, family; *cultura*, culture]. The improvement of animal stocks by scientific breeding. —**stirpicul'tural,** *adj.*

stir'rup bone. Old term for the stapes.

stitch [AS. *stice*]. 1. A sudden, sharp, lancinating pain. 2. See *suture*, 2.

glover's s. The continuous suture used especially in wounds of the intestines. See Plate 40.

s.-abscess. A pustular infection in the skin, about a suture.

Stitt, Edward Rhodes [*American naval medical officer*, 1867–1948]. Known for his lifelong devotion to problems of bacteriology, tropical medicine, and hematology. Author, with R. P. Strong, of a standard work on tropical diseases and parasitology.

Stock, Wolfgang [*German ophthalmologist*, 1874–]. Described retinal atrophy in juvenile amaurotic familial idiocy; called *Spielmeyer-Stock disease.*

stock [AS. *stocc*]. 1. A quantity of solution, or other material, kept on hand ready for use. 2. A line of descent, ethnic or linguistic; lineage.

Stockert phenomenon. See von Stockert *phenomenon.*

Stockholm and Koch method. See under *method.*

stock"i·net' [*stocc*]. Cotton material or shirting, woven like a stocking, but of uniform caliber and used according to size to cover extremities or the body preparatory to the application of a fixed dressing, as plaster, splints.

stock'ing [*stocc*]. A close-fitting covering for the leg and foot, sometimes designed and fitted for a special hygienic or therapeutic purpose; usually made of knitted or woven goods that sometimes contains an elastic thread.

elastic s. One containing rubber so that it exerts a continuous pressure on the part.

Stoddard and Drury method. See under *method.*

Stoerk, Carl [*Austrian laryngologist*, 1832–99]. Described chronic catarrh of the upper air passages which is first purulent, then dry, and leads to hypertrophy of the mucous membrane; called *Stoerk's blennorrhea.*

Stoerk, Oscar [*German physician*, 1870–1926]. With Hans Eppinger, described electrocardiographic changes in bundle-branch block. Described a primitive loop of the developing nephron, a part of which forms Henle's loop; called *Stoerk's loop.*

Stoffel, Adolf [*German orthopedic surgeon*, 1880–1937]. Devised an operation for the relief of spastic paralysis, in which he resected a portion of the bundles of the nerve trunk supplying the affected area; called *Stoffel's operation.*

stoi"chi·om'e·try (stoy"kee·om'i·tree) [G. *stoicheion*, element; *metron*, a measure]. The branch of chemistry that deals with the numerical relationship between elements or compounds (atomic weights), the determination of the proportions in which the elements combine (formulas), and the weight relations in reactions (equations). —**stoichiomet'ric,** *adj.*

Stokes, Charles Francis [*American naval medical officer*, 1863–1931]. Invented an open basket type of litter used in the United States Navy; called *Stokes litter.*

Stokes, Whitley [*Irish physician*, 1763–1845]. First to describe ecthyma gangrenosum or dermatitis gangrenosa infantum (1807).

Stokes, William [*Irish physician*, 1804–78]. Author of classic works on diseases of the chest and heart, and on the use of the stethoscope. Described the characteristic syndrome of heart block which had been noted earlier by Morgagni and Spens, and classically described by Adams (1846), called *Spens syndrome*, or *Stokes-Adams syndrome.* See Cheyne-Stokes *respiration*, Stokes's *liniment.*

Stokes, William Royal [*American bacteriologist*, 1870–1930]. Introduced a reagent for reducing oxyhemoglobin to hemoglobin. See Stokes's *reagent.*

Stokes's law. See under *law.*

Stokes operation. See Gritti-Stokes *amputation.*

Stokvis, Barend Joseph E. [*Dutch physician*, 1834–1902]. Introduced the term enterogenous cyanosis for cyanosis due to intestinal disturbance of long standing. It is associated with methemoglobin and sulfhemoglobin in the blood. Called *Stokvis' disease.*

Stoll's method. See under *method.*

sto'lon [L. *stolo*, a shoot]. 1. *In biology*, a creeping stem or runner capable of taking root or bearing a bud, where it forms one or more new plants. 2. An analogous budding stock in certain lower animals.

Stoltz, Joseph [*French gynecologist*, 1803–96]. Known for his purse-string operation for cystocele, called *Stoltz's operation.*

sto'ma [G., mouth]. A minute opening or pore in a surface; particularly, one of the stigmas, or minute openings, of a peritoneal surface, presumably for the drainage of fluid into lymphatics.

sto·mac'a·ce (sto·mack'uh·see) [*stoma;* G. *kakē*, badness]. Ulcerative stomatitis.

sto"ma·ceph'a·lus [*stoma;* G. *kephalē*, head]. A combination of the ethmocephalic type of cyclopia with agnathia or micrognathia. Microstomia (or astomia) and a variable degree of synotia are associated. Also called *stomatocephalus.*

stom'ach [G. *stomachos*, gullet]. The most dilated part of the alimentary canal, situated below the diaphragm in the left hypochondriac, the epigastric, and part of the right hypochondriac regions. It is continuous at the cardiac end with the esophagus, at the pyloric end with the duodenum. Its wall consists of four coats: mucous, submucous, muscular, and serous. The mucous coat contains the gastric glands—cardiac, fundic, and pyloric—which secrete the gastric juice and mucus. See Plates 8, 10, 13. —**stomachic,** *adj.*

accessory s. See gastroenteric *cyst.*

cascade s. That due to hypertrophy of the circular muscle fibers between the pyloric antrum and the body of the stomach; characterized by filling of the cardiac portion followed by spilling into the pyloric segment. Also called *cup and spill s.*

dumping s. See dumping *syndrome.*

fishhook s. See J *s.*

hourglass s. One divided more or less completely into two compartments by an equatorial constriction.

J s. A long, vertically located stomach.

leather-bottle s. The small stomach with markedly thickened wall seen in chronic interstitial gastritis or scirrhous carcinoma.

powdered s. (*stomachus pulveratus*). Powdered stomach is the dried and powdered, defatted wall of the stomach of the hog, *Sus scrofa* var. *domesticus;* occurs as a granular substance with a slight, not unpleasant, meaty odor, and is practically insoluble in water. It contains factors which cause an increase in the number of red blood cells in the blood of persons suffering from pernicious anemia. The activity is readily destroyed when the preparation is suspended in a hot liquid. It is used solely in the treatment of anemia, especially pernicious anemia. Also called *dried stomach.* See *ventriculin.*

primitive s. The endoderm-lined cavity of the gastrula; archenteron.

steerhorn s. A high, transversely located stomach. Also called *cow horn s.*

thoracic s. Congenital herniation of the stomach above the diaphragm due to imperfect development of the diaphragm.

sto·mach'ic (sto·mack'ick) [*stomachos*]. One of a class of substances which may stimulate the secretory activity of the stomach.

sto"ma·tal'gi·a [G. *stoma*, mouth; *algos*, pain]. Pain in the mouth.

sto·mat'ic [G. *stomatikos*, good for the mouth]. Relating or belonging to the mouth.

sto"ma·ti'tis (sto"muh·tye'tis, stom"uh·) [G. *stoma*, mouth; *-itis*, inflammation]. Inflammation of the soft tissues of the mouth.

aphthous s. A form characterized by the presence of small white vesicles in the mouth, occurring chiefly in children under three years.

arsenical s. Necrotic stomatitis due to arsenical poisoning.

catarrhal s. A simple or nonulcerative form characterized by swelling.

epidemic s. An acute, infectious stomatitis common in epidemics.

epizootic s. See foot-and-mouth *disease.*

erythematous s. Simple inflammation of the oral mucous membrane.

exudative s. Inflammation of the oral mucosa characterized by swelling and redness. Also called *fetid s.*

gangrenous s. Stomatitis characterized by necrosis. See *noma.*

herpetic s. That characterized by fever blisters or cold sores.

membranous s. Stomatitis with the formation of an adventitious membrane.

mercurial s. Stomatitis due to the excessive absorption of mercury.

mycotic s. See *thrush*, 1.

parasitic s. See *thrush*, 1.

scorbutic s. That associated with scurvy.

s. venenata. One caused by drugs.

syphilitic s. Inflammation associated with the oral lesions of syphilis.

traumatic s. That due to mechanical injury.

ulcerative s. Stomatitis characterized by the formation of ulcers and necrosis of oral tissues.

vesicular s. Bednar's aphthae, two symmetrically placed ulcers, one on each side of the median line, seen at times on the hard palate of cachectic infants.

Vincent's s. An extension of necrotizing ulcerative gingivitis to other oral tissues. See also Vincent's *angina.*

sto'ma·to- (sto'muh·to-, stom'uh·to-), **stomat-** [*stoma*]. A combining form meaning *mouth.*

sto"ma·toc'a·ce (sto"muh·tock'uh·see, stom"uh·) [*stoma;* G. *kakē*, badness]. Ulcerative stomatitis.

sto"ma·to·ca·thar'sis. Salivation. *Obs.*

sto"ma·to·ceph'a·lus. See *stomacephalus.*

sto"ma·to·dyn'i·a [*stoma;* G. *odynē*, pain]. Pain in the mouth.

sto"ma·to·dy·so'di·a (sto"muh·to·di·so'dee·uh, stom"uh·to·) [*stoma;* G. *dysōdia*, foul smell]. Ill-smelling breath.

sto"ma·to·gas'tric [*stoma;* G. *gastēr*, belly]. 1. Pertaining to the mouth and the stomach. 2. Pertaining to the nerves which supply the anterior end of the digestive tract in various invertebrates.

sto"ma·tol'o·gy (sto"muh·tol'o·jee, stom"uh·) [*stoma;* G. *logos*, word]. That branch of medical science which treats of the anatomy, physiology, pathology, therapeutics, and hygiene of the oral cavity, of the tongue, teeth, and adjacent structures and tissues, and of the relationship of that field to the entire body. —**stomatolog'ic,** *adj.*

sto"ma·to·ma·la'ci·a (·ma·lay'shee·uh, ·see·uh) [*stoma;* G. *malakia*, softness]. Sloughing or degeneration of the structures of the mouth.

sto"ma·to·me'ni·a [*stoma;* G. *mēn*, month]. Vicarious bleeding in the mouth, associated with menstrual disorders.

sto"ma·to'mi·a (sto"muh·to'mee·uh, stom"uh·) [*stoma;* G. *temnein*, to cut]. A general term for the incision of a mouth, as of the uterus.

sto·mat'o·my [*stoma;* G. *tomē*, a cutting]. Incision of the os uteri.

sto"ma·to·my·co'sis (sto"muh·to·migh·ko'sis, stom"uh·to·) [*stoma;* G. *mykēs*, fungus; *-ōsis*, condition]. A disease of the mouth due to fungi, especially *Candida albicans.* See *thrush*, 1.

sto″ma·to·ne·cro′sis. See gangrenous *stomatitis*.

sto″ma·to·no′ma [*stoma;* G. *nomē*, a feeding]. Gangrene of the mouth: also called *stomatonecrosis*.

sto″ma·top′a·thy (sto″muh·top′uth·ee, stom″uh·) [*stoma;* G. *pathos*, disease]. Any disease of the mouth.

sto′ma·to·plas″ty (sto′muh·to·plas″tee, stom′uh·to·, sto·mat′o·) [*stoma;* G. *plassein*, to form]. A plastic operation upon the mouth. —**stomatoplas′tic,** *adj*.

sto″ma·tor·rha′gi·a (·ray′juh, ·jee·uh, ·radj′uh, ·radj′ee·uh) [*stoma;* G. *rhēgnynai*, to burst forth]. Copious hemorrhage from the mouth.

sto′ma·to·scope″ (sto′muh·to·scope″, stom′uh·to·, sto·mat′o·) [*stoma;* G. *skopein*, to examine]. An instrument used for inspecting the cavity of the mouth.

sto″ma·to′sis [*stoma;* G. *-ōsis*, condition]. Disease of the mouth.

sto″ma·tot′o·my [*stoma;* G. *tomē*, a cutting]. Incision of the os uteri.

sto·men″or·rha′gi·a (sto·men″o·ray′juh, ·jee·uh, ·radj′uh, ·radj′ee·uh, sto″men·o·) [*stoma;* G. *mēn*, month; *rhēgnynai*, to burst forth]. Vicarious bleeding in the mouth, associated with abnormal menstruation.

sto″mo·de′um (sto″mo·dee′um, stom″o·) [*stoma;* G. *hodaios*, on the way]. The primitive oral cavity of the embryo; an ectodermal fossa formed by the growth of the facial processes about the buccopharyngeal membrane. —**stomodeal,** *adj*.

sto·mos′chi·sis (sto·mos′ki·sis) [*stoma;* G. *schisis*, a cleavage]. Fissure of the mouth. There are the following special types: cheiloschisis, cleft lip; gnathoschisis, cleft jaw; uranoschisis or palatoschisis, cleft palate; staphyloschisis, cleft soft palate; uvula fissa, cleft uvula.

Sto·mox′ys [*stoma;* G. *oxys*, sharp]. A genus of bloodsucking flies of the family Muscidae. It is similar to the common house fly.

S. calcitrans. The common stable fly which aids in the transmission of trypanosomiasis and anthrax, and serves as an intermediate host of the nematode *Habronema*, parasitic in the stomach of the horse.

Stone, Harvey Brinton [*American surgeon*, 1882–]. Known for his operation for the relief of anal incontinence, in which he used strips of fascia lata, passing them through the gluteal muscles and encircling the anus by two loops running in opposite directions. The patient uses the action of the gluteal muscles for control.

stone [AS. *stān*]. 1. A hardened mass of mineral matter. See *calculus*. 2. An English unit of weight, 14 lb.

blue s. Copper sulfate crystals.

kidney s. See under *kidney*.

pulp s. See *denticle*, 2.

stone′cut″ter′s dis·ease′. See *silicosis*.

stone search′er. An instrument equipped with a porcelain tip, used to explore the urinary bladder, bile duct, etc., for concretions; now little used.

Stookey, Byron Polk (1887–). American neurosurgeon who described a test for spinal subarachnoid block, called Queckenstedt-Stookey *test*. See also Stookey's *reflex*.

stool [AS. *stōl*]. 1. Evacuation of the bowels. Also see *allochezia*. 2. In the plural, feces.

acholic stools. (a) Light gray or clay-colored stools having the consistency of putty, which follow obstruction of the flow of bile into the duodenum. The color is due to the presence of the normal urobilin. The stools show, under the microscope, an abnormal amount of fat. This form of acholic stool is accompanied by icterus and choluria. (b) Stools of the same color may occur in noninterference with the flow of bile, but then the stools do not contain an excessively large amount of fat and fatty acids.

bilious stools. The discharge is green-colored, as after large doses of calomel.

caddy stools. Yellow fever stools which resemble fine, dark, sandy mud.

fatty stools. Stools in which fat is present; due to pancreatic disease.

lead-pencil stools. Fecal discharges of very small caliber. Usually due to general nervousness causing local intestinal spasm, or to stricture or stenosis of the descending colon, sigmoid, or rectum. Also called *ribbon stools*.

mucous stools. Stools containing mucus. They indicate the existence of intestinal inflammation.

pea-soup stools. The peculiar liquid evacuation of typhoid fever.

rice-water stools. The stools of cholera, in which there is a copious serous exudation containing detached epithelium.

sheep-dung stools. The small, round, fecal masses, similar to the dung of sheep, due to atony of the intestine; this form of passage may occur in the so-called starvation or hunger evacuation which is found in cases of inanition.

tarry stools. Stools having the color and consistency of tar, usually due to hemorrhage into the intestinal tract but also produced by iron, bismuth, barium, or other medication.

stop′cock″ [AS. *stoppian; cocc*]. A turning cock, connected with a pipe, for regulating the flow of gases or liquids.

stop′page [*stoppian*]. Cessation of flow or action; closure or stenosis.

sto′rax [L., from G. *styrax*] (*styrax*). A balsam obtained from the trunk of *Liquidambar orientalis*, or of *L. styraciflua;* occurs as a semiliquid, grayish to grayish brown, sticky, opaque mass, or a semisolid, sometimes a solid mass, softened by gentle warming; insoluble in water, but is soluble, usually incompletely, in an equal weight of warm alcohol. It consists largely of storesin, which is present in two forms—alpha and beta storesin—both free and in the form of a cinnamic ester. Cinnamic acid and its esters are also present. Of the esters, cinnamyl cinnamate, or styracin, is present in greater proportion. Other esters present are phenylpropyl cinnamate, ethyl cinnamate, and benzyl cinnamate. It also contains a hydrocarbon called styrol or styrene, a small amount of a levorotatory oil, and traces of vanillin. Storax is a stimulating expectorant and was at one time used in various catarrhs, but is now seldom used except as an ingredient of compound benzoin tincture. Externally, as an ointment, it has been used as a parasiticide in scabies and other parasitic infections. Also called *liquid s.*

sto·res′in (sto·rez′in). A hard resin from storax.

storm [AS.]. Term sometimes used for sudden exacerbation of symptoms or crisis in a disease.

renal s. A peculiar form of neurosal attack referred to the kidney, frequently seen in patients suffering from aortic regurgitation. There is a sudden excruciating pain over the region of the kidney like renal colic, but without nausea or retraction of the testis and with the passage of normal urine.

thyroid s. Severe, acute thyrotoxicosis.

stovaine. Trade-mark for *amylocaine hydrochloride*.

Stovall and Black stain. See under *stain*.

stovarsol. Trade-mark for acetarsone.

STP *S*tandard *t*emperature and *p*ressure.

STPD *S*tandard *t*emperature, *p*ressure, *d*ry (0° C., 760 mm Hg).

stra″bi·lis′mus (stray″bi·liz′mus, strab″i·). See *strabismus.*

stra′bism (stray′biz·um, strab′iz·um). See *strabismus.*

stra″bis·mom′e·ter. Strabometer.

stra″bis·mom′e·try. Strabometry.

stra·bis′mus (stra·biz′mus) [*strabismos*]. Squint; that abnormality of the eyes in which the visual axes do not meet at the desired objective point, in consequence of incoordinate action of the extrinsic ocular muscles. Syn., *heterotropia.* —**strabismal, strabismic,** *adj.*

alternating s. One in which either eye fixes alternately.

anoopsia s. See sursumvergent *s.*

apparent s. A subjective strabismus in which the patient sees angle alpha as too large or too small according to his degree of myopia or hyperopia.

bilateral s. See alternating *s.*

concomitant s. One in which the squinting eye has full range of movement.

convergent s. Esotropia; the squinting eye is turned to the nasal side.

divergent s. Exotropia; the squinting eye is turned to the temporal side.

external s. See divergent *s.*

Hirschberg's test for s. A rough estimate of the amount of strabismus. See under Julius *Hirschberg.*

internal s. See convergent *s.*

paralytic s. Due to paralysis of one or more muscles.

penile s. See Peyronie's *disease.*

spastic s. Due to a spastic contraction of an ocular muscle.

sursumvergent s. One in which the visual axis is directed upward.

vertical concomitant s. A squint in which one eye turns up, the deviation remaining constant in all fields of vision.

stra·bom′e·ter [G. *strabos*, squinting; *metron*, a measure]. An instrument for the measurement of the deviation of the eyes in strabismus. Syn., *strabismometer.*

stra·bom′e·try [*strabos; metron*]. The determination of the degree of ocular deviation in strabismus. Syn., *strabismometry.*

strab′o·tome [*strabos;* G. *tomos*, cutting]. A knife used for strabotomy. *Obs.*

stra·bot′o·my [*strabos;* G. *tomē*, a cutting]. An operation for the correction of strabismus. *Obs.*

strag′u·lum. A layer of gray matter lying lateral to the brachium conjunctivum and containing several small fiber tracts.

strain [OF. *estraindre*, from L. *stringere*, to draw tight]. 1. Excessive stretching; overuse of a part. 2. The condition produced in a part by overuse or wrong use, as eyestrain. 3. A group of organisms closely related to each other, characterized by a common peculiarity.

Flury s. A rabies strain 3, used in prophylactic vaccination of dogs. It has been modified by prolonged cultivation in chick embryos.

Lansing s. A mouse-adapted strain of the type II (Lansing) poliomyelitis virus.

ventricular s. A term used in electrocardiography as either (a) **left-ventricular strain,** designating the effect of increased left-ventricular work as caused by hypertension or aortic valve disease, possibly reversible if the hypertension is removed (see left axis *deviation*); or (b) **right-ventricular strain,** designating the effect of increased right-ventricular work as caused by pulmonary embolism (acute) or pulmonary disease or pulmonic stenosis (chronic). See right axis *deviation.*

strain. *In pharmacy,* to separate insoluble substances from liquid; to filter.

strait [OF. *estrait*, from L. *stringere*]. A narrow or constricted passage, as the inferior or superior strait of the pelvis.

strait′jack″et. A strong jacket placed on the insane or delirious to prevent injury to themselves or others.

stramid. Trade name for a brand of sulfanilamide.

stra·mo′ni·um [NL.] (*stramonium*). The dried leaf and flowering top of *Datura stramonium* (including *Datura tatula*). It contains the alkaloid daturine, which is identical with hyoscyamine, and traces of scopolamine. The general physiologic and therapeutic action of stramonium is similar to that of belladonna. Stramonium has also been used in the treatment of asthma by smoking in cigarettes or by mixing with potassium nitrate and burning and inhaling the vapors. Dose, 0.06–0.2 Gm. (1–3 gr.). Syn., *Jamestown weed, Jimson weed.*

stran′gle [G. *straggalē*, halter]. Choke or throttle by compression of the glottis or trachea.

stran′gles [*straggalē*]. An infectious disease of solipeds involving the nasal passages and related structures; characterized by a purulent inflammation with involvement of the lymphatic system of the head and, in some instances, accompanied by difficult breathing. Caused by the organism *Streptococcus equi.*

stran″gu·la′tion [L. *strangulatio*, from *straggalē*]. 1. Asphyxiation due to obstruction of the air passages, as by external pressure on the neck. 2. Constriction of a part producing arrest of the circulation, as strangulation of a hernia. —**stran′gulated,** *adj.*

stran′gu·ry [G. *stragx*, drop; *ouron*, urine]. Painful urination, the urine being voided drop by drop.

strap [AS. *stropp*, from G. *strophos*, band]. A long band, as of adhesive plaster.

strap. To compress or support a part by means of bands, especially bands of adhesive plaster.

Strassmann, Paul Ferdinand [*German gynecologist*, 1866–1938]. Described a reaction which indicates that the placenta has not become detached in the third stage of labor. Pressure on the fundus uteri is transmitted to the umbilical vein, which becomes engorged; called *Strassmann's phenomenon.*

strat″i·fi·ca′tion [L. *stratum*, a covering; *facere*, to make]. Arrangement in layers.

strat′i·fied [*stratum; facere*]. Arranged in layers.

stra·tig′ra·phy. Sectional radiography.

strat′o·sphere (strat′o·sfeer, stray′to·) [*stratum;* G. *sphaira*, sphere]. The atmosphere above the tropopause, where temperature changes are small and winds essentially horizontal.

strat′um (strat′um, stray′tum) (pl. *strata*) [L.]. A layer.

central gray s. The layer of gray matter surrounding the cerebral aqueduct in the midbrain, and continuous with the gray matter surrounding the fourth ventricle and that covering the rhomboid fossa.

optic s. The third layer of superior colliculus, composed of optic fibers from the retina and lateral geniculate body which enter through the brachium of the superior colliculus and end mainly in the stratum cinereum.

s. basale. The basal layer of the endometrium not subject to loss during menstruation or at the termination of pregnancy.

s. cinereum. The second layer of the superior colliculus, composed of radially arranged cells which receive the corticotectal fibers and most of the optic fibers.

s. compactum. The surface layer (about one-fourth) of the decidua parietalis.

s. corneum. The layer of keratinized cells of the epidermis.

s. cylindricum. The basal-cell layer of a stratified epithelium, especially of a stratified squamous epithelium, as the epidermis.

s. disjunctum. The outermost layer of desquamating cells of the stratum corneum of the epidermis.

s. germinativum. The deeper layer of the epidermis in which cell proliferation and growth take place. Syn., *Malpighian layer.* Formerly called *s. mucosum, rete mucosum.*

s. granulosum. A layer of minute cells or one of cells containing many granules, especially the layer containing keratohyalin granules in volar epidermis.

s. intermedium. The thin zone of the enamel pulp which lies next to the ameloblasts and consists of cells which do not become part of the stellate reticulum.

s. lemnisci. The deepest layer of the superior colliculus, composed of cell bodies and nerve fibers, which receives the spinocollicular tract and sends out fibers mainly to the reticular formation, oculomotor nucleus, medulla oblongata, and spinal cord.

s. lucidum. A translucent layer of the epidermis consisting of irregular transparent cells with traces of nuclei.

s. Malpighii. See *s.* germinativum.

s. papillare. The zone of fine-fibered connective tissue within and immediately subjacent to the papillae of the corium.

s. reticulare. The coarse-fibered connective tissue of the corium.

s. spinosum. Prickle-cell layer.

s. spongiosum. The deeper layer (about three-fourths) of the decidua parietalis.

s. submucosum. The thin layer of smooth muscle of the myometrium adjacent to the endometrium.

s. subserosum. The thin layer of smooth muscle of the myometrium adjacent to the serous coat.

s. supravasculare. The layer of muscle of the myometrium between the stratum vasculare and the stratum subserosum.

s. vasculare. The thickest layer of muscle in the myometrium next to the stratum submucosum.

s. zonale of midbrain. The most superficial layer of the superior colliculus, composed of fibers which arise from the occipital cortex and enter the colliculus through the brachium of the superior colliculus.

s. zonale of thalamus. A thin plate of nerve fibers covering the thalamus and giving it a whitish color.

Straus reaction. See under *reaction.*

Strauss's phenomenon. The administration of fatty foods by mouth results in an increase of fatty constituents in the effusion of chylous ascites.

Strauss's test for lactic acid. See under *test.*

Straus test for glanders. See under *test.*

straw′ber″ry mark. A congenital hemangioma clinically characterized by its raised, bright-red, soft, often lobulated appearance. Syn., *nevus vasculosus.*

streak [AS. *strica*]. 1. A furrow, line, or stripe. 2. *In bacteriology,* the process of distributing the inoculum over the surface of a solid culture medium. Cultures thus obtained are called streak cultures.

angioid s. A dark, linear streak seen in the retina with the ophthalmoscope, in individuals having pseudoxanthoma elasticum. Occasionally followed by complete degeneration of the macula.

medullary s. See medullary *plate.*

meningitic s. See *tache* cérébrale.

primitive s. A dense, opaque band of ectoderm in the bilaminar blastoderm associated with the morphogenetic movements and proliferation of the mesoderm and notochord. It indicates the first trace of the embryo.

reflex s. A shining, white streak running along the vessels in the retina. It is due to the reflection of light from the anterior surface of the column of blood.

stream [AS. *strēam*]. Flow, especially in a definite direction; applied to movement in protoplasm.

Streatfield, John Fremlyn [*English ophthalmologist,* 1828–86]. Described his operation for entropion in which he removed a wedge-shaped strip from the tarsal plate; called *Streatfield's operation.*

Streeter, George Linius [*American anatomist and embryologist,* 1873–1948]. Described his theory stating that the cause of intrauterine amputation is intrinsic and due to focal deterioration, not the result of constriction by the umbilical cord or by amniotic bands; called *Streeter's theory.* Made other notable contributions to embryology and the study of placentation.

strem′ma [G., a twist]. A sprain. *Obs.*

streph″o·sym·bo′li·a (stref″o·sim·bo′lee·uh, ·sim·bol′ee·uh) [G. *strephein,* to twist; *symbolon,* symbol]. Difficulty of children in learning to read; inability to distinguish between similar letters, as *p* and *q* or *n* and *u.* It is the result of mixed motor dominance of right and left cerebral hemispheres.

strep′i·tus [L.]. A sound, a noise.

coriaceous s. An auscultatory sound resembling the creaking of leather.

s. aurium. See *tinnitus.*

s. uteri. See uterine *souffle.*

s. uterinus. Uterine bruit.

strep″o·gen′in. A factor, possibly a peptide derivative of glutamic acid, reported to exist in certain proteins, acting as a growth stimulant to bacteria and mice in the presence of completely hydrolyzed protein: also called *streptogenin.*

streptamide. Trade name for a brand of sulfanilamide.

strep″ti·ce′mi·a [G. *streptos,* curved; *sēptikos,* putrefactive; *haima,* blood]. Streptococcal septicemia.

strep′ti·dine. $C_8H_{18}N_6O_4$. 1,3-Diguanidino-2,4,5,6-tetrahydroxycyclohexane, obtained when streptomycin undergoes acid hydrolysis; in the streptomycin molecule it is glycosidally linked to streptobiosamine.

strep′tin. An antibiotic substance derived from a species of *Streptomyces.* Its action is similar to that of streptothricin, but it is more active against staphylococci and micrococci.

strep′to-, strept- [*streptos*]. A combining form meaning *twisted* or *curved* or *streptococcal.*

strep″to·an·gi′na (strep″to·an·jye′nuh, ·an′ji·nuh) [*streptos;* L. *angina,* quinsy]. Streptococcal sore throat; septic sore throat; a pseudomembranous deposit in the throat due to streptococci.

strep″to·ba·cil′lus [*streptos;* L. *bacillum,* little stick]. A bacillus which remains attached end to end, resulting in the formation of chains. It is a constant characteristic of some strains and appears atypically in others.

strep″to·bi·o′sa·mine. $C_{13}H_{23}NO_9$. A nitrogen-containing disaccharide obtained when streptomycin undergoes acid hydrolysis; in the streptomycin molecule it is glycosidally linked to streptidine.

streptocide. Trade-mark for a brand of sulfanilamide.

strep″to·coc′cal, strep″to·coc′cic (strep″to·

cock′sick) [*streptos;* G. *kokkos,* berry]. Relating to, or due to, streptococci.

strep″to·coc·ce′mi·a (·cock·see′mee·uh) [*streptos; kokkos;* G. *haima,* blood]. The presence of streptococci in the blood.

strep″to·coc′ci. Members of the genus *Streptococcus.* The streptococci have been classified into (1) *alpha, beta,* and *gamma s.* by type of reaction of colonies on blood agar (Brown); (2) groups A through O (Lancefield method) by the specific antigenic complex carbohydrates (**C-substance**) elaborated; (3) *hemolytic s., viridans s., enterococci,* and *Streptococcus lactis* by their immunologic, biochemical, and physiologic characters.

alpha s. A group which produces a greenish or brownish discoloration of blood agar. Syn., *green s.* See also *viridans s.*

beta s. A group which produces clear hemolysis on blood agar. See also hemolytic *s.*

gamma s. A group which produces no change on blood agar, including organisms of low pathogenicity and many anaerobic strains, often isolated as secondary invaders. Syn., *Streptococcus anhemolyticus, indifferent s.*

green s. Alpha *s.*

hemolytic s. A group which produces complete hemolysis on blood agar. It includes Lancefield groups A, B, C, E, F, G, H, K, L, M, O. Occasionally strains not producing complete hemolysis elaborate C-substance identical with the above Lancefield groups, and are therefore classified in this group. Group A and less commonly groups C and G are pathogenic for man. Group A is subdivided into 40 or more types on the basis of a type-specific protein (**M-substance**) produced by matt colonies; specifically, types 12 and 4 are thought to be associated with acute glomerulonephritis. Members of this group also cause scarlet fever, erysipelas, rheumatic fever, sore throat, and other infections. Syn., *Streptococcus pyogenes, Streptococcus epidemicus.*

indifferent s. Gamma *s.*

viridans s. A group including strains not causing beta hemolysis, although many members cause alpha hemolysis; they do not elaborate a C-substance and therefore cannot be classified by the Lancefield method. Both pathogenic and saprophytic organisms are involved, the former often being isolated from subacute bacterial endocarditis, bronchopneumonia, urinary-tract infections, and focal inflammations. See also alpha *s.*

Strep″to·coc′cus [*streptos; kokkos*]. A genus of Gram-positive, chain-forming bacteria of the tribe Streptococcacea, family Lactobacteriaceae. See *streptococci.*

S. anhemolyticus. See gamma *streptococci.*

S. epidemicus. See hemolytic *streptococci.*

S. lactis. A group all the members of which produce group N C-substance and are nonpathogenic for man. They readily coagulate milk and are very important in the dairy industry.

S. pyogenes. Old term for hemolytic streptococci.

strep″to·co·ly′sin [*streptos; kokkos;* G. *lysis,* a loosing]. See *streptolysin.*

strep″to·der″ma·ti′tis [*streptos;* G. *derma,* skin; *-itis,* inflammation]. Inflammation of the skin due to streptococci.

strep″to·dor′nase. An enzyme, occurring in filtrates of cultures of certain hemolytic streptococci, capable of hydrolyzing desoxyribonucleoproteins and desoxyribonucleic acid: used, along with streptokinase, for enzymatic debridement of infected tissues. Syn., *Streptococcal desoxyribonuclease.* Abbreviated, SD. See *varidase.*

strep″to·gen′in. See *strepogenin.*

strep″to·he·mo·ly′sin. See *streptolysin.*

strep″to·hy′dra·zid. A product obtained by condensation of streptomycin and isoniazid; in tuberculosis protection studies in animals, it has been found to be at least as effective as combined therapy with streptomycin and isoniazid.

strep″to·ki′nase. A catalytic enzyme, a component of the fibrinolysin occurring in cultures of certain hemolytic streptococci. The enzyme activates the fibrinolyzing system present in the euglobulin fraction of human blood. With streptodornase, it is used for enzymatic debridement of infected tissues. Abbreviated, SK. See *varidase.*

strep′to·lin. An antibiotic agent isolated from cultures of an actinomycetes designated as *Streptomyces* No. 11. It has been separated into two components, designated *streptolin A* and *streptolin B.* The antibiotic is active against a wide range of Gram-positive and Gram-negative bacteria, but appears to be too toxic to be therapeutically useful.

strep″to·ly′sin (strep″to·lye′sin, strep·tol′i·sin) [*streptos;* G. *lysis,* a loosing]. A group of hemolysins produced by *Streptococcus pyogenes.* **Streptolysin O** is one of a group of oxygen-labile and antigenically related toxins, including the theta toxin of *Clostridium perfringens,* the tetanolysin of *Clostridium perfringens,* and the pneumolysin of *Diplococcus pneumoniae.* **Streptolysin S** is an oxygen-stable hemolysin, probably not antigenic, and separable from the streptococcal cells by serum extraction.

Strep″to·my′ces [*streptos;* G. *mykēs,* fungus]. An aerobic genus of fungus whose species are saprophytic soil forms. Several species are sources of antibiotics. **S. aureofaciens** elaborates chlortetracycline (aureomycin); **S. erythreus,** erythromycin; **S. fradiae,** neomycin; **S. griseocarneus,** hydroxystreptomycin; **S. griseus,** streptomycin; **S. lavendulae,** streptothricin; **S. rimosus,** oxytetracycline (terramycin); **S. venezuelae,** chloramphenicol (chloromycetin).

strep″to·my′cin [*streptos;* G. *mykēs,* fungus]. $C_{21}H_{39}N_7O_{12}$. A water-soluble antibiotic obtained from *Streptomyces griseus.* It consists of a hydroxylated base, streptidine, glycosidally linked to the disaccharidelike molecule streptobiosamine. It is active against a variety of organisms including *Mycobacterium tuberculosis,* and has been successfully employed in the treatment of tularemia, *Hemophilus influenza* infections, certain types of meningitis, bacteremia due to Gram-negative organisms, certain urinary-tract infections, and tuberculosis. Resistant strains of organisms have appeared. The antibiotic may produce toxic effects, of which those involving the eighth nerve are the most serious. It is administered subcutaneously, intramuscularly, intrathecally, and, sometimes, by intravenous drip; various salts, such as the hydrochloride, sulfate, or calcium chloride complex, are used therapeutically.

strep″to·sep″ti·ce′mi·a [*streptos;* G. *sēptikos,* putrefactive; *haima,* blood]. Septicemia due to streptococci.

strep″to·so′mus [*streptos;* G. *sōma,* body]. A nonhuman form of celosoma in which the spine is twisted so that the legs are displaced laterally.

strep″to·thri′cin (strep″to·thry′sin, ·thriss′in) [*streptos;* G. *thrix,* hair]. An antibiotic substance from *Streptomyces lavendulae.* It is an organic base and is soluble in water, dilute mineral acids, and acid alcohol. It is insoluble in ether and chloroform. Streptothricin is active against various Gram-negative and some Gram-positive bacteria. Its toxicity is limited and it is active in vivo.

strep″to·thri·co′sis [*streptos; thrix;* G. *-ōsis,* condition]. A disease resulting from infection with a streptothrix.

Strep′to·thrix [*streptos; thrix*]. A genus which is not clearly differentiated from *Actinomyces.*

S. muris ratti. Causative agent of epidemic arthritic erythema. Also called *Actinomyces muris ratti, Streptobacillus moniliformis,* and *Actinomyces muris.*

strep″to·thry′cin. Streptothricin.

streptozone. Trade-mark for a brand of sulfanilamide.

stress [L. *stringere,* to bind tight]. 1. Force exerted by load, pull, pressure, or other mechanical means; also the exertion of such force. 2. *In medicine,* any stimulus or succession of stimuli of such magnitude as to tend to disrupt the homeostasis of the organism; when mechanisms of adjustment fail or become disproportionate or incoordinate, the stress may be considered an injury, resulting in disease, disability, or death. See also general adaptation *syndrome, injury.* 3. *In dentistry,* the force exerted by the lower teeth against the upper during mastication.

stress in·con′ti·nence. See under *incontinence.*

stress phe·nom′e·non. See general adaptation *syndrome.*

stretch [AS. *streccan*]. Draw out to full length.

stretch′er [*streccan*]. See *litter.*

Neil Robertson s. A canvas litter strengthened with slats of split bamboo. It is used to transport an injured man aboard a vessel.

stri′a (pl. *striae*) [L., *furrow*]. 1. Streak, stripe, narrow band. 2. Fibrinoid.

lateral longitudinal s. The lateral one of the two long bundles of fibers on the upper surface of the corpus callosum.

medial longitudinal s. The medial one of the two long bundles of fibers on the upper surface of the corpus callosum. Syn., *stria Lancisii.*

s. albicans gravidarum. Stria atrophica due to pregnancy.

s. atrophica. See *lineae albicantes* under *linea.*

s. cerebellaris. See *s.* medullaris.

striae acusticae. Inaccurate term for several fiber strands (striae medullares) transversely crossing the intermediate portion of the floor of the fourth ventricle. The true acoustic fibers lie ventral to the visible fibers. Also called *striae of Piccolomini.*

striae gravidarum. See *lineae albicantes* under *linea.*

s. Lancisii. Medial longitudinal stria.

s. medullaris. Any of the white fibers originating in the acoustic tubercle and the surrounding region which traverse the intermediate portion of the rhomboid fossa to pass over the dorsal surface of the restiform body and area acoustica and disappear in the median sulcus of the fossa: formerly called *s. of Held, s. of Monakov;* also called *s. acustica, s. cerebellaris, s. medullaris acustica.*

s. medullaris thalami. A band of white matter on the dorsal surface of the thalamus.

s. of Baillarger. One of two well-defined, white bands in the cerebral cortex, containing large numbers of myelinated nerve fibers running parallel to the surface of the cortex; in the region of the calcarine fissure, the outer band is known as the stripe of Gennari, the inner band being absent. Formerly called *lines of Baillarger.*

s. of Gennari. See under *Gennari.*

s. of Held. Old term for *stria medullaris.*

s. of Lancisi. Medial longitudinal stria.

s. of Langhans. The discontinuous zone of fibrinoid on the chorionic plate present during the first half of pregnancy.

s. of Monakov. Old term for *stria medullaris.*

s. of Nitabuch. The first fibrinoid to appear in the placenta, located in the decidua basalis and capsularis below the exposed surface at the boundary of the fetal and maternal tissues.

s. of Rohr. The fibrinoid found on the maternal surface of the intervillous spaces and on the villi.

s. olfactoria. One of the two divisions, lateral and medial, of the olfactory tract, containing fibers continued from the tract and covered by a thin layer of gray matter: also called *medial* and *lateral olfactory gyri.*

s. semicircularis. See *s.* terminalis.

s. terminalis. A longitudinal bundle of nerve fibers lying in the terminal sulcus. It arises in the amygdaloid nucleus and terminates mainly in the preoptic region and hypothalamus, although some fibers cross in the anterior commissure to the amygdaloid nucleus of the opposite side. Syn., *s. semicircularis.*

s. vascularis. The vascular upper part of the spiral ligament of the ductus cochlearis: also called *s. vascularis of Huschke.*

stri′a·ted (stry′ay·tid) [L. *striare,* to furnish with channels]. Striped, as striated muscle.

stri·a′tum (stry·ay′tum) [*striare*]. The corpus striatum. —**striatal,** *adj.*

Stricker, Salomon [*German pathologist,* 1834–98]. Contributed to the knowledge of tissue anatomy, cell proliferation, and the histology of the cornea. The first to describe vasodilatation following stimulation of the posterior nerve roots (1876).

stric′ture [L. *strictura,* compression]. A narrowing of the lumen of a canal or hollow organ, as the esophagus, pylorus, ureter, or urethra, the result of inflammatory or other changes in its walls, and, occasionally, of external pressure. It may be temporary or permanent, depending upon the cause and the course of the disease producing it.

annular s. A ringlike obstruction produced by a contracture which involves the entire circumference of a canal, intestine, etc.

bridle s. A stricture caused by a delicate band stretched across the urethral lumen.

spasmodic s. That involving the membranous urethra and caused by muscular spasm of the sphincter muscle, and usually associated with urethritis.

stri′dor [L., harsh sound]. A peculiar, harsh, vibrating sound produced during respiration.

congenital laryngeal s. Respiratory croaking, heard in babies.

inspiratory s. The sound heard in inspiration through a spasmodically closed glottis.

laryngeal s. Stridor due to laryngeal stenosis.

s. dentium. Grinding of the teeth.

s. serraticus. A sound like sharpening a saw, sometimes produced by expiration through a tracheotomy tube.

strid′u·lous [L. *stridulus,* creaking]. Characterized by stridor; as stridulous laryngismus.

strin′gent [L. *stringere,* to bind]. Binding.

string-gal″va·nom′e·ter. Instrument for measuring intensity and direction of minute currents. See *electrocardiograph.*

string′halt″ (string′hawlt″) [AS. *streng; healt*]. An involuntary, convulsive movement of muscles in the hind leg of the horse; the leg is suddenly raised from the ground and lowered again with unnatural force. Also called *springhalt.*

strip [AS. *strȳpan*]. Press with a milking movement so as to force out the contents of a canal or duct.

stripe [MD.]. A streak; a discolored mark.

strip′ping [AS. *strȳpan*]. 1. Uncovering; unsheathing. 2. In the plural, the last and richest milk given at any one milking; so called because it is slowly removed by the milker, who strips the teats between the fingers.

s. of the pleura. Removal of the lining membrane of the thorax of an animal used for food, to remove the traces of pleurisy and of tuberculosis.

strob′ic [G. *strobos*, a whirling round]. Resembling, or pertaining to, a top.

stro·bi′la [G. *strobilos*, anything twisted]. 1. The segmented body of the adult tapeworm. 2. The whole adult tapeworm including the scolex.

strob″i·la′tion [*strobilos*]. The formation of zooids, disks, or joints by metameric division, gemmation, or fission.

strob′ile (strob′il, ·ile, stro′bil, ·bile) [*strobilos*]. 1. A multiple fruit whose seeds are enclosed by prominent scales, as a pine cone. 2. A strobila.

strob′il·oid, stro′bil·oid [*strobilos;* G. *eidos*, form]. Like a strobile.

stro·bi′lus [*strobilos*]. The adult tapeworm.

stro′bo·scope, strob′o·scope [*strobos;* G. *skopein*, to examine]. A device by which a moving object may appear to be at rest; a rapid motion may appear to be slowed, or motion can be depicted by a series of still pictures. The effect depends upon an accurately controlled, intermittent source of light or periodically interrupted vision. —**stroboscop′ic,** *adj.*

strob″o·ster′e·o·scope. See *stereostroboscope.*

Stroganoff, Vasilii Vasilievich [*Russian obstetrician,* 1857–1938]. Known for his important contributions to the knowledge of the pathology and treatment of puerperal eclampsia (1900). Advocated conservative measures and the use of narcotics to arrest convulsions; called *Stroganoff's method.*

stroke [ME. *strok*]. 1. A sudden and severe seizure or fit of disease. 2. A popular term for apoplexy.

apoplectic s. See *apoplexy.*

back s. The recoil of the ventricles of the heart at the moment the blood is discharged into the aorta.

heat s. See heat *prostration.*

light s. Narcosis or death due to exposure to light.

paralytic s. Sudden loss of muscular power from lesion of the brain or spinal cord.

s. volume. The volume of blood ejected by the left ventricle during a single systole.

stro′ma [G., bed]. The supporting framework of an organ, including its connective tissue, vessels, and nerves, as contrasted with the epithelial or other tissues performing the special function of the organ, the parenchyma. —**stromal,** *adj.*

stro′mal my·o′sis. See stromal *endometriosis.*

stro′ma·tin, stro·ma′tin. The protein of the stroma of erythrocytes.

stro″ma·to′sis. See stromal *endometriosis.*

Stromeyer, Georg Friedrich Ludwig [*German military surgeon,* 1804–76]. Advocated tenotomy of the Achilles tendon for clubfoot (1833). Described a hinged leg splint, called *Stromeyer's splint.* An operation for liver abscess in which the pus is located by a cannula is called *Stromeyer's operation.*

stro′muhr (stro′moor) [Ger.]. An instrument for measuring the velocity of blood flow.

Strong, Richard Pearson [*American physician and pathologist,* 1872–1948]. Author, with E. R. Stitt, of a standard work on tropical diseases and parasitology. A bacillus belonging to *Shigella paradysenteriae* is called *Strong's bacillus.*

Strong method. See Snell-Strong *method.*

Stron″gy·loi′de·a [G. *stroggylos*, curved; *eidos*, form]. A superfamily of roundworms, of the suborder Strongylinae, order Rhabditida. The genera *Ancylostoma* and *Necator* are included.

Stron″gy·loi′des (stron″ji·loy′deez) [*stroggylos; eidos*]. A genus of nematode worms.

S. stercoralis. An intestinal parasite of man with the same distribution as hookworm. Other species are parasites of lower animals. Also called *S. intestinalis.*

stron″gy·loi·di′a·sis [*stroggylos; eidos;* NL. *-iasis*, condition]. Infestation with one of the roundworms of the genus *Strongyloides.* Formerly called *anguilluliasis.*

stron″gy·loi·do′sis. See *strongyloidiasis.*

stron″gy·lo′sis. See *strongyloidiasis.*

stron′ti·a (stron′shee·uh). Strontium oxide.

stron′ti·um (stron′shee·um, stron′tee·um) [from *Strontian*, Scotland]. Sr = 87.63. A silver-white to pale yellow, malleable, ductile metal; decomposes in water and alcohol. Its salts color a nonluminous flame brilliant crimson. It is stored under petroleum or other liquids not containing oxygen. Strontium is used only as a carrier of therapeutically active acids.

s. bromide (*strontii bromidum*). $SrBr_2.6H_2O$; occurs as colorless crystals; 1 Gm. dissolves in about 0.35 cc. of water; soluble in alcohol. Used in the treatment of epilepsy and allied conditions. It depends for its action upon the bromide ion. Dose, 1–2 Gm. (15–30 gr.).

s. iodide. $SrI_2.6H_2O$; occurs as colorless crystals or white granular powder; soluble in water. Sometimes used as a substitute for other iodides. See also under *amniography.*

s. peroxide. SrO_2; occurs as a white, odorless powder; almost insoluble in water but decomposed by it gradually with the evolution of oxygen. Used externally as an antiseptic in the form of a dusting powder or an ointment.

s. salicylate (*strontii salicylas*). $(C_6H_4.OH.COO)_2$-$Sr.2H_2O$; occurs as a white, crystalline powder; 1 Gm. dissolves in about 19 cc. of water and in about 61 cc. of alcohol. Its use is identical with that of sodium salicylate, over which it has no advantage. Dose, 0.3–2.0 Gm. (5–30 gr.).

stro·phan′thi·din. $C_{23}H_{32}O_6$; a cardioactive, steroidal aglycone obtained by hydrolysis of glycosides, found in varieties of *Strophanthus* and related plants. Strophanthin and cymarin are two such glycosides that yield strophanthidin.

stro·phan′thin (*strophanthinum*). A glycoside or a mixture of glycosides obtained from *Strophanthus kombé;* occurs as a yellowish white powder; soluble in water and dilute alcohol. Strophanthin is extremely poisonous. It can be separated into two portions, a crystalline and an amorphous fraction. The crystalline fraction can be separated into the glycosides *K-strophanthin-α*, and *K-strophanthin-β.* The amorphous fraction consists of glycosides, and the mixture is referred to as *amorphous K-strophanthin.* It is a cardiac stimulant, used like digitalis, but principally in emergencies by intravenous injection. Dose, intravenously, 0.25–0.5 mg. ($\frac{1}{240}$–$\frac{1}{120}$ gr.).

G-s. See *ouabain.*

s. injection (*injectio strophanthini*). A sterile solution of strophanthin in water for injection. The commercially available injections of strophanthin vary in potency from 0.25 mg. to 1 mg. per cc.

stro·phan″tho·bi′ose. Disaccharide present in strophanthus.

strophanthone. Trade-mark for a preparation containing the active principles of strophanthus.

stro·phan′thus [G. *strophos*, a twisted band; *anthos*, flower]. The dried ripe seed of *Strophanthus kombé*, or of *Strophanthus hispidus*, deprived of the awns. The activity of strophanthus is due to several glycosides. See *strophanthin.* Strophanthus belongs to that group of cardiac drugs of which digitalis is the type. Its effects upon the circulation are similar to that drug. It is more rapid in its action and less permanent than digitalis. It is used solely for its influence on the circulation, especially in cases of chronic heart disease. In urgent cases, the effects of strophanthus can be obtained almost immediately by intravenous injection of its active principles. It is absorbed from the intestinal tract with much less regularity than digitalis and is, therefore, less certain in its effects. Dose, 0.016–0.065 Gm. (1/4–1 gr.). Also called *s. seed.*

stroph″o·ceph′a·lus [*strophos;* G. *kephalē*, head]. A monster exhibiting strophocephaly.

stroph″o·ceph′a·ly [*strophos; kephalē*]. A form of cyclopia in which there is marked deformity of the lower face, with partial or complete agnathia and synotia, astomia, and severe disturbance in the maxillary, sphenoid, and temporal regions.

stroph′u·lus [dim. from *strophos*]. A form of miliaria occurring in infants, and often unilateral. Also called *red gum.*

s. pruriginosus. An eruption characterized by disseminated, intensely itching papules. Also called *prurigo.*

struck. An acute disease of sheep occurring in England, caused by *Clostridium perfringens,* type C.

struc′ture [L. *structura*, from *struere*, to erect]. 1. The manner or method of the building up, arrangement, and formation of the different tissues and organs of the body or of a complete organism. 2. An organ, a part, or a complete organic body. —**structural,** *adj.*

stru′ma [L., scrofulous tumor]. Goiter.

cast iron s. A rare form of chronic thyroiditis characterized by extreme fibrosis and fixation of the surrounding tissues.

Hashimoto's s. See *s.* lymphomatosa.

metastasizing s. See follicular *carcinoma* of thyroid.

Riedel's s. Chronic thyroiditis. Also called *ligneous thyroiditis, woody thyroiditis, Riedel's disease.*

s. aberrata. A goiter of an accessory thyroid gland.

s. androblastoma of ovary. See adrenocorticoid *adenoma* of the ovary.

s. cibaria. Goiter due to the ingestion of goitrogens, such as cabbage and rape seed.

s. congenita. Congenital goiter.

s. lingualis. The presence of thyroid glandular tissue in the region of the foramen caecum (linguae).

s. lymphomatosa. A very rare type of diffuse thyroid enlargement of unknown origin characterized by atrophy of the thyroid parenchyma, fibrosis, and lymphoid hyperplasia. Also called *Hashimoto's s., lymphadenoid goiter.*

s. maligna. See follicular *carcinoma* of thyroid.

s. medicamentosa. Goiter due to medicine, as potassium thiocyanate.

s. ovarii. A rare teratoma of the ovary containing thyroid tissue.

s. ovarii luteinocellularis. See *luteoma.*

Strumia, Max Maurice [*American pathologist,* 1896–]. Introduced a modification of Giemsa's stain. See universal *stain.*

stru′mi·form [*struma;* L. *forma*, form]. Having the appearance of struma.

stru″mi·priv′al (strōō″mi·priv′ul, stroo·mip′-riv·ul), **stru″mi·pri′vous** (strōō″mi·pry′vus, stroo·mip′ri·vus) [*struma;* L. *privare*, to deprive]. Deprived of the thyroid; due to removal of the thyroid; thyroprival.

stru·mi′tis [*struma;* G. *-itis*, inflammation]. Inflammation of a goitrous thyroid gland.

stru′mous [*struma*]. 1. Goitrous. 2. Scrofulous. *Rare.*

Strümpell, Ernst Adolf Gustav Gottfried [*German physician,* 1853–1925]. Described ankylosing spondylitis, also called *Strümpell-Marie disease.* Described acute encephalitis of infancy, called *Strümpell's* or *Strümpell-Leichtenstern's disease.* Described pseudosclerosis, called *Strümpell-Westphal pseudosclerosis.* See also Strümpell's *sign.*

strych′ni·a (strick′nee·uh). See *strychnine.*

strych′nine (strick′nin, ·neen, ·nyne) (*strychnina*). $C_{21}H_{22}O_2N_2$; an alkaloid obtained chiefly from nux vomica; occurs as a white, crystalline powder or as colorless, transparent crystals; 1 Gm. dissolves in about 6420 cc. of water and in about 136 cc. of alcohol. Strychnine is a powerful stimulant to the central nervous system, especially to the spinal cord and medullary centers. The effects on the cerebrum are relatively slight. Used as a stimulant in cases of poisoning by the respiratory depressants. As a circulatory stimulant, it is used in a wide variety of conditions, such as surgical shock, poisoning by depressants as ether or alcohol, etc. Like other bitters, strychnine improves the appetite and digestion, but its use in this respect has been abused. Dose, 1–3 mg. (1/60–1/20 gr.).

s. nitrate (*strychninae nitras*). $C_{21}H_{22}O_2N_2.HNO_3$; occurs as colorless needles or a white, crystalline powder; 1 Gm. dissolves in about 45 cc. of water and in about 150 cc. of alcohol.

s. phosphate (*strychninae phosphas*). $C_{21}H_{22}N_2O_2.H_3PO_4.2H_2O$; occurs as white crystals or a white powder; 1 Gm. is slowly soluble in about 30 cc. of water; it is slightly soluble in alcohol.

s. sulfate (*strychninae sulfas*). $(C_{21}H_{22}N_2O_2)_2.H_2SO_4.5H_2O$; occurs as colorless or white crystals or a white, crystalline powder; 1 Gm. dissolves in 35 cc. of water and in 85 cc. of alcohol. Dose, 1–4 mg. (1/60–1/15 gr.).

strych″nin·i·za′tion (strick″nin·i·zay′shun, ·eye-zay′shun) [G. *strychnon*, sleepy nightshade]. 1. The condition produced by large doses of strychnine or nux vomica. 2. Topical application of strychnine to areas of the central nervous system to increase nervous excitability and thus facilitate the study of neuron connections. See also physiological *neuronography.*

Strych′nos (strick′nos) [*strychnon*]. A genus of the Loganiaceae of which the most important is *S. nux-vomica.* See *nux* vomica.

stul·ti′ti·a (stul·tish′ee·uh) [L.]. Foolishness; dullness of intellect. *Obs.*

stump [ME. *stumpe*]. The extremity, pedicle, or basis of the part left after surgical amputation, excision, or ablation.

s. of eyeball. The remainder of the globe after excision of an anterior staphyloma or after other capital operation on the globe that deprives it of vision.

s. of tooth. That part remaining after removal or destruction of the crown.

stun [OF. *estoner*]. Render temporarily insensible, as by a blow.

stunt′ing. The arrest of the normal growth and development of an organism. See also *dwarf.*

stupe [G. *styppē*, the coarse fiber of hemp]. A cloth used for applying heat or counterirritation; especially a cloth wrung out of hot water and sprinkled with a counterirritant, as turpentine-stupe.

stu″pe·fa′cient [L. *stupefacere*, to make senseless]. Narcotic.

stu″pe·fac′tion [*stupefacere*]. 1. Stupor. 2. The process of succumbing to stupor.

stu″pe·ma′ni·a [L. *stupere*, to be struck senseless; G. *mania*, madness]. Mental stupor. *Obs.*

stu·pid′i·ty. See *asynesia.*

stu′por [L.]. 1. The condition of being but partly conscious or sensible; or a condition of insensibility. 2. Mutism without lack of sensorial clarity. —**stuporous,** *adj.*

anergic s. Stupor with immobility. Syn., *stuporous insanity.*

delusional s. Melancholic dullness of mind, with delusions.

epileptic s. The stupor following an epileptic convulsion.

lethargic s. See *trance.*

s. formicans. Formication.

s. melancholicus. The stupor found in association with melancholia.

s. miliaris. Paresthesia of the fingers and toes in connection with miliary fever.

s. vigilans. Catalepsy.

stur′dy. See *staggers.*

Sturge-Weber-Dimitri disease. See nevoid *amentia.*

Sturgis, Cyrus Cressey [*American physician,* 1891–]. Demonstrated, with Raphael Isaacs, that the stomach contains a factor which is of benefit in the treatment of pernicious anemia (1929).

stu′rine (stew′reen, ·rin). A protamine obtained from the spermatozoa of the sturgeon.

Sturmdorf, Arnold [*American gynecologist,* 1861–1934]. Introduced an operation for diseased endocervix, by conical excision of the diseased area. Called *Sturmdorf's operation.*

stut′ter·er [ME. *stutten*]. One who stutters. The **interiorized stutterer** wants to avoid stuttering; the **exteriorized stutterer** wants to express himself. —**stut′ter,** *v.*

stut′ter·ing [*stutten*]. A hesitation in speech due to an inability to enunciate the syllables without repeated efforts. See *stammering.*

urinary s. Hesitancy and involuntary interruptions in urination.

Stuttgart disease. See under *disease.*

sty, stye. See *hordeolum.*

sty′let (sty′lit, sty·let′) [G. *stylos,* pillar]. 1. A wire inserted into a soft catheter or cannula to secure rigidity. 2. A fine wire inserted into a hollow hypodermic needle or other hollow needle to maintain patency.

sty′lo-, styl- [*stylos*]. A combining form meaning *pillar;* used to denote *connection with the styloid process of the temporal bone.*

sty″lo·glos′sus [*stylos;* G. *glōssa,* tongue]. A muscle arising from the styloid process of the temporal bone, and inserted into the tongue. See Table of Muscles in the Appendix. —**styloglossal,** *adj.*

sty″lo·hy′oid [*stylos;* G. *hyoeidēs,* shaped like the letter upsilon]. Pertaining to the styloid process of the temporal bone and the hyoid bone, as the stylohyoid muscle. See Table of Muscles in the Appendix.

sty″lo·man·dib′u·lar [*stylos;* L. *mandibula,* jaw]. Pertaining to the styloid process and the mandible, as stylomandibular ligament.

sty″lo·mas′toid [*stylos;* G. *mastoeidēs,* like a breast]. Relating to the styloid and mastoid processes.

sty″lo·pha·ryn′ge·us (sty″lo·fa·rin′jee·us, ·far″in-jee′us) [*stylos;* G. *pharygx,* pharynx]. A muscle arising from the styloid process of the temporal bone, and inserted into the pharynx. See Table of Muscles in the Appendix.

sty′lus [*stylos*]. A pointed device in the form of a holder for applying medicines, as caustic potash. —**styloid,** *adj.*

sty′ma. See *priapism. Obs.*

sty″ma·to′sis [G. *styma,* priapism; *-ōsis,* condition]. A violent erection of the penis attended with hemorrhage. *Obs.*

styph′nic ac′id. $(NO_2)_3C_6H(OH)_2$; 2,4,6-trinitroresorcinol; yellow crystals, soluble in water: used for identification of various organic compounds through formation of styphnates.

styp′tic [G. *styptikos,* astringent]. An agent that checks hemorrhage by causing contraction of the blood vessels, as alum, tannic acid.

stypticin. Trade-mark for cotarnine chloride.

styptol. Trade-mark for cotarnine phthalate.

styr′a·cin (stirr′uh·sin, sty′ruh·sin). Cinnamyl cinnamate, a constituent of storax and Peruvian balsam.

sty′rax. See *storax.*

sty′rol. $C_6H_5CH{=}CH_2$. Phenylethylene. A liquid hydrocarbon found in storax: also called *styrene,* or *cinnamene.*

sty′ro·lene. Styrol.

sub- [L., under]. 1. A prefix denoting *under, beneath, deficient.* 2. *In chemistry,* a prefix denoting the *lower of two compounds of the same element* or *basic.*

sub″ab·dom′i·nal [*sub;* L. *abdomen,* belly]. Beneath the abdomen.

sub·ac′e·tate (sub·ass′i·tayt). A basic acetate, as lead subacetate.

sub″a·cro′mi·al [*sub;* G. *akrōmia,* point of the shoulder]. Beneath the acromion, as the subacromial bursa.

sub″a·cute′ [*sub;* L. *acutus,* pointed]. The stage of a disease when it is intermediate between an acute and a chronic form.

sub·al″i·men·ta′tion [*sub;* L. *alimentum,* food]. Inadequate or deficient nourishment.

sub·an″co·ne′us. A variable muscle arising from the posterior distal surface of the humerus and inserted into the posterior aspect of the capsule of the elbow joint.

sub·ap′i·cal (sub·ap′i·kul, ·ay′pi·kul) [*sub;* L. *apex,* summit]. Beneath an apex.

sub″ap·o·neu·rot′ic [*sub;* G. *aponeurōsis,* end of the muscle]. Beneath an aponeurosis.

sub·a′que·ous [*sub;* L. *aqua,* water]. Occurring beneath the water.

sub″a·rach′noid (sub″a·rack′noyd) [*sub;* G. *arachnoeidēs,* like a cobweb]. Beneath the arachnoid membrane, as the subarachnoid space.

sub″a·re′o·lar [*sub;* L. *areola,* small, open space]. Situated, or occurring, beneath the mammary areola.

sub″as·trin′gent [*sub;* L. *astringere,* to draw together]. Only slightly astringent.

sub″a·tom′ic [*sub;* G. *atomos,* uncut]. Pertaining to the structure or components of atoms.

sub″au·di′tion (sub″aw·dish′un) [*sub;* L. *auditio,* from *audire,* to hear]. The act or ability of comprehending what is not expressed.

sub·au′ral. Subauricular.

sub″au·ric′u·lar [*sub;* L. *auricula,* external ear]. Below the auricle or external ear.

sub·brach″y·ce·phal′ic (sub·brack″i·si·fal′ick, sub·bray″ki·) [*sub;* G. *brachys,* broad; *kephalē,* head]. *In craniometry,* once used to characterize the mild degree of brachycephaly embracing cephalic indexes between 80.00 and 83.32; *in cephalometry,* indexes between 82.01 and 85.33.

sub″cal·ca′re·ous [*sub;* L. *calcarius,* pertaining to lime]. Somewhat calcareous.

sub·cal′ca·rine (sub·kal′kuh·rin, ·ryne, ·reen) [*sub;* L. *calcar,* spur]. Situated beneath the calcarine fissure, as the subcalcarine gyrus.

sub″cal·lo′sal [*sub;* L. *callosus,* hard-skinned]. Below the corpus callosum.

sub·cap′su·lar [*sub;* L. *capsula,* small box]. Beneath a capsule.

sub·car′bon·ate. A basic carbonate.

sub·chlo′ride. That chloride of a series which contains relatively the least chlorine.

sub·chon′dral. Situated beneath cartilage.

sub·chron′ic [*sub;* G. *chronikos,* of time]. More nearly chronic than is indicated by the term subacute.

sub·cla′vi·an [*sub;* L. *clavis,* key]. Lying under the clavicle, as the subclavian artery. See Table of Arteries in the Appendix.

sub·cla′vi·us [*sub; clavis*]. A small muscle attached to the clavicle and the first rib. See Table of Muscles in the Appendix.

s. posterior. A variant of the subclavius.

sub·clin′i·cal [*sub;* G. *klinikos,* of a bed]. Pertaining to a disease, in which manifestations are so slight as to be unnoticeable and even not demonstrable.

sub″col·lat′er·al [*sub;* L. *cum,* with; *lateralis,* of the side]. Ventrad of the collateral fissure of the brain.

sub″con·junc·ti′val (sub″kon·junk·ty′vul, ·kon-junk′ti·vul) [*sub;* L. *conjunctivus,* serving to connect]. Situated beneath the conjunctiva.

sub·con′scious [*sub;* L. *conscius,* knowing something with another]. *In psychiatry,* pertaining to material outside the range of clear consciousness, but which is capable of producing or determining conscious mental or physical reactions.

sub·con′scious. *In psychoanalysis,* that portion of the unconscious containing mental experiences which are not in the focus of immediate attention, but which may be recalled to consciousness.

sub·con′scious·ness [*sub; conscius*]. Imperfect consciousness; that state in which mental processes take place without the mind being distinctly conscious of its own activity.

sub″con·tin′u·ous [*sub;* L. *continuus,* continuous]. Almost continuous.

sub·cor′a·coid [*sub;* G. *korakoeidēs,* like a raven]. Situated below the coracoid process, as subcoracoid dislocation of the humerus.

sub·cor′ti·cal [*sub;* L. *cortex,* bark]. Beneath the cortex of the cerebrum.

sub·cos′tal [*sub;* L. *costa,* rib]. Lying beneath a rib or the ribs.

sub·cos′tal. Any of certain variable small muscles associated with the lower ribs.

sub″cos·tal′gi·a [*sub; costa;* G. *algos,* pain]. Pain beneath the ribs, or over a subcostal nerve.

sub·crep′i·tant [*sub;* L. *crepitare,* to creak]. Almost crepitant, as subcrepitant rale.

sub″crep·i·ta′tion [*sub; crepitare*]. An indistinctly crepitant sound.

sub·cru′re·us. Old name for the articularis genus muscle.

sub·cul′ture [*sub;* L. *cultura,* cultivation]. *In microbiology,* the procedure of transferring organisms from one culture to fresh culture medium; also, the resulting culture.

sub″cu·ta′ne·ous [*sub;* L. *cutis,* skin]. Beneath the skin; hypodermic.

sub″cu·tic′u·lar [*sub;* L. *cuticula,* skin]. Beneath the epidermis, as a subcuticular suture.

sub·cu′tis [*sub;* L. *cutis,* skin]. The superficial fascia below the skin or cutis. Also called *hypodermis, tela subcutanea.*

sub″de·lir′i·um [*sub;* L. *delirium,* madness]. A slight or muttering delirium, with lucid intervals.

sub·del′toid [*sub;* G. *deltoeidēs,* delta-shaped]. Beneath the deltoid muscle, as subdeltoid bursa.

sub·den′tal [*sub;* L. *dens,* tooth]. Situated beneath the teeth.

sub·der′mal. See *subcutaneous.*

sub·der′mic [*sub;* G. *derma,* skin]. Hypodermic.

sub″di·a·phrag·mat′ic (sub″dye·uh·frag·mat′ick) [*sub;* G. *diaphragma,* diaphragm]. Under the diaphragm, as subdiaphragmatic abscess.

sub″di·vi′ded [*sub;* L. *dividere,* to divide]. Redivided; making secondary or smaller divisions.

sub·dol″i·cho·ce·phal′ic (sub·dol″i·ko·si·fal′ick) [*sub;* G. *dolichos,* long; *kephalē,* head]. *In craniometry,* once used to characterize the lower range of the mesocephalic group, with cephalic indexes between 75.00 and 77.76; *in cephalometry,* indexes between 77.01 and 79.77.

sub·duct′ [L. *subducere,* to withdraw]. Draw downward.

sub·duc′tion [*subducere*]. Maddox's term for deorsumduction.

sub·du′ral [L. *sub,* under; *durus,* hard]. Beneath the dura mater.

sub″e·pen″dy·mo′ma. A tumor found in the fourth ventricle of the brain, and believed to be derived from the subependymal cell plate. Macroscopically, this tumor is similar to an ependymoma, but microscopically it is composed of nests of small polygonal cells surrounded by fibroglial bands.

su·ber′ic ac′id. $COOH(CH_2)_6COOH$; octanedioic acid; a metabolic product of capric acid, also obtained by heating castor oil or cork with nitric acid.

su′ber·in [L. *suber,* cork-tree]. A waxy substance found in the cork cells of plants.

sub·fam′i·ly [L. *sub,* under; *familia,* family]. In the classification of plants or animals, a lower division of a family.

sub·fas′cial (sub·fash′ul, ·fash′ee·ul) [*sub;* L. *fascia,* band]. Beneath fascia.

sub·ga′le·al [*sub;* L. *galea,* helmet]. Beneath the galea aponeurotica.

sub·gal′late. A basic salt of gallic acid. See *bismuth* subgallate.

sub·ger′mi·nal [*sub;* L. *germen,* sprout]. Situated beneath a germinal structure or blastoderm.

sub·gle′noid [*sub;* G. *glēnoeidēs,* like a socket]. Beneath the glenoid fossa, as subglenoid dislocation of the humerus.

sub″glos·si′tis [*sub;* G. *glōssa,* tongue; *-itis,* inflammation]. Inflammation of the tissues under the tongue. See *ranula.*

sub″grun·da′tion [F. *subgrondation*]. The intrusion of one fragment of a cranial bone beneath another part in a fracture.

su·bic″u·lum [L.]. The dorsal part of the hippocampal gyrus near the hippocampal fissure. —**subicular,** *adj.*

s. promontorii. (a) Support of the promontory. (b) Posterior boundary of the fenestra cochleae.

sub″in·ci′sion (sub″in·sizh′un) [L. *sub,* under; *incisio,* from *incidere,* to cut into]. Making a permanent opening into the urethra through the under surface of the penis, a practice common in some primitive tribes, especially those of central Australia. It does not impair coitus or cause sterility.

sub″in·fec′tion [*sub;* L. *infectio,* from *inficere,* to infect]. A slight degree of infection.

sub″in·vo·lu′tion [*sub;* L. *involutio,* from *involvere,* to roll up]. Imperfect return to normal size after functional enlargement.

s. of the uterus. The imperfect involution of the uterus after delivery.

sub·i′o·dide. That iodide of a series containing the least iodine.

sub·ja′cent [L. *subjacere,* to lie under]. Lying beneath.

sub·jec′tive [L. *subjectivus,* subjective]. 1. Pertaining to the individual himself. 2. Referring to symptoms, experienced by the patient himself, and not amenable to physical exploration.

sub·jec′to·scope [*subjectivus;* G. *skopein,* to examine]. An instrument for examining subjective visual sensations.

sub·la′tion [L. *sublatio,* removal]. Removal, ablation.

sub·le′thal [L. *sub*, under; *letalis*, deadly]. Less than fatal, as a sublethal dose of poison.

sub′li·mate [L. *sublimare*, to elevate]. A solid or condensed substance obtained by heating a material, which passes directly from the solid to the vapor phase and then back to the solid state.
corrosive s. Mercury bichloride.

sub′li·mate. *In psychiatry*, to express or externalize instinctual impulses in a socially acceptable or conventional manner; to purify instinctual modes of expression.

sub″li·ma′tion [*sublimare*]. 1. The transformation of a solid to the gaseous state, followed by condensation to the solid state. It is used to purify substances such as iodine, mercuric chloride. 2. *In psychiatry*, a psychic device whereby undesirable primitive cravings and impulses gain outward expression by converting their energies into socially acceptable activities.

sub·lime′ [*sublimare*]. To successively volatilize and condense a solid.

sub·lim′i·nal [L. *sub*, under; *limen*, threshold]. Below the threshold of consciousness or of sensation. See *threshold*.

sub·lim′i·nal fringe. Neurons that are in close functional association with active neurons so that their excitability is momentarily increased even though they are not directly stimulated.

sub·li′mis [L.]. Elevated; superficial, a qualification applied to certain muscles, as the flexor digitorum sublimis.

sub·lin′gual [L. *sub*, under; *lingua*, tongue]. 1. Lying beneath the tongue. 2. Pertaining to the parts lying beneath the tongue.

sub″lin·gui′tis [*sub; lingua;* G. *-itis*, inflammation]. Inflammation of a sublingual gland.

sub″lux·a′tion [*sub;* L. *luxatio*, dislocation]. Incomplete dislocation; sprain.

sub″mal·le′o·lar [*sub;* L. *malleolus*, small hammer]. Under the malleoli, as submalleolar amputation, removal of the foot at the ankle joint.

sub″man·dib′u·lar [*sub;* L. *mandibula*, jaw]. Below or beneath the mandible, as the submandibular gland.

sub′ma·rine, sub″ma·rine′ [*sub;* L. *marinus*, of the sea]. A dental term applied to conditions or materials which may be employed effectively while in contact with oral fluids.

sub·max″il·lar·i′tis [*sub;* L. *maxilla*, jaw; G. *-itis*, inflammation]. Inflammation of a submaxillary gland.

sub·max′il·lar″y (sub·mack′si·lerr″ee) [*sub; maxilla*]. 1. Lying beneath the lower maxilla (*O.T.*), or mandible, as the submaxillary gland. 2. Pertaining to the submaxillary gland. Syn., *submandibular* (*B.R.*).

sub·men′tal [*sub;* L. *mentum*, chin]. Situated under the chin.

sub·mes″a·ti·ce·phal′ic [*sub;* G. *mesatos*, midmost; *kephalē*, head]. The lower division in the category, mesaticephalic, of Paul Topinard's (1885) classification of human head form, embracing cephalic indices of 75 to 76.

sub″me·tal′lic [*sub;* G. *metallon*, mine]. Metallic to a certain extent.

sub·mi′cron [*sub;* G. *mikros*, small]. A colloid particle visible by aid of the ultramicroscope.

sub″mi·cro·scop′ic (sub″migh·kro·skop′ick) [*sub; mikros;* G. *skopein*, to examine]. Pertaining to a particle which is below the limit of resolution of the optical microscope.

sub·mor′phous [*sub;* G. *morphē*, form]. Having a structure intermediate between amorphous and true crystalline. Often applied to the indefinite, partially crystalline structure of calculi.

sub″mu·co′sa [*sub;* L. *mucosus*, mucous]. The layer of fibrous connective tissue that attaches a mucous membrane to its subjacent parts. —**submu′cous,** *adj.*

sub″nar·cot′ic [*sub;* G. *narkōtikos*, benumbing]. Moderately narcotic.

sub·ni′trate. A basic nitrate.

sub·nor′mal [*sub;* L. *norma*, rule]. Below normal.

sub″nor·mal′i·ty [*sub; norma*]. The condition of being subnormal.

sub·no″to·chor′dal (sub·no″to·kor′dul) [*sub;* G. *nōton*, back; *chordē*, chord]. Below the notochord.

sub·nu′cle·us [*sub;* L. *nucleus*, kernel]. Any one of the smaller groups of cells into which a large nerve nucleus is divided by the passage through it of nerve bundles. *O.T.*

sub″nu·tri′tion (sub″new·trish′un) [*sub;* L. *nutrire*, to nourish]. Defective nutrition.

sub″oc·cip′i·tal (sub″ock·sip′i·tul) [*sub;* L. *occiput*, back part of the head]. Situated beneath the occiput, as a suboccipital triangle.

sub″o·per′cu·lum [*sub;* L. *operculum*, lid]. A gyrus of the brain between the presylvian and subsylvian fissures; the orbital operculum.

sub·or″di·na′tion [*sub;* L. *ordinatio*, an arranging]. The condition of being under subjection or control; the condition of organs that depend upon or are controlled by other organs.

sub·ox′ide. That oxide of an element which contains the lowest proportion of oxygen.

sub·pap′u·lar [*sub;* L. *papula*, pustule]. Indistinctly papular.

sub·par″a·lyt′ic [*sub;* G. *paralytikos*, paralytic]. Slightly paralytic.

sub″per·i·os′te·al [*sub;* G. *periosteos*, round the bones]. Beneath the periosteum.

sub″per·i·to·ne′al [*sub;* G. *peritonaion*, membrane which contains the lower viscera]. Beneath the peritoneum.

sub·phren′ic. See *subdiaphragmatic.*

sub″pla·cen′ta [*sub;* L. *placenta*, cake]. The decidua parietalis.

sub″pla·cen′tal [*sub; placenta*]. 1. Situated beneath the placenta. 2. Pertaining to the decidua parietalis.

sub·plan′ti·grade [*sub;* L. *planta*, sole; *gradi*, to walk]. Incompletely plantigrade; walking with the heel slightly elevated.

sub·pu′bic [*sub;* L. *pubes*, private parts]. Situated beneath the pubic arch or symphysis.

sub″sar·to′ri·al [*sub;* L. *sartor*, patcher]. Situated beneath the sartorius muscle, as the subsartorial plexus.

sub·scap′u·lar [*sub;* L. *scapula*, shoulder]. 1. Beneath the scapula, as the subscapular muscle, or subscapularis. 2. Pertaining to the subscapular muscle.

sub″scap·u·la′ris [*sub; scapula*]. A muscle arising from the anterior surface of the scapula and inserted on the lesser tubercle of the humerus. See Table of Muscles in the Appendix.

sub·scrip′tion [L. *subscriptio*, anything written underneath]. That part of a prescription containing the directions to the pharmacist, indicating how the ingredients are to be mixed and prepared.

sub″sen·sa′tion [L. *sub*, under; *sensus*, sense]. A subordinate sensation.

sub·se′rous [*sub;* L. *serum*, whey]. Beneath a serous membrane.

sub·sib′i·lant [*sub;* L. *sibilare*, to hiss]. Having a sound like a muffled whistling.

sub·si′dence, sub′si·dence [L. *subsidere*, to settle down]. The gradual cessation and disappearance of the manifestations of disease.

sub·sig′moid [L. *sub*, under; G. *sigmoeidēs*, of the shape of a sigma]. Under the sigmoid flexure.

sub·sist′ence [L. *subsistentia*, from *subsistere*, to

subsist]. That which nourishes or gives support; food.

sub·spi′nous [L. *sub*, under; *spina*, thorn]. 1. Beneath a spine, as subspinous dislocation, luxation of the head of the humerus below the spine of the scapula. 2. Beneath the spinal column.

sub′stage″ [*sub;* L. *stare*, to stand]. The parts beneath the stage of a microscope, including the diaphragm, condenser, mirror, and other accessories.

sub′stance [L. *substantia*, material]. 1. The material of which anything is composed. 2. A tissue. 3. A factor.

anterior perforated s. A depressed area of gray matter at the base of the brain, rostral to the optic tract, containing numerous small foramens transmitting arteries to the basal ganglions: also called *olfactory area.*

anterior pituitarylike s. Chorionic gonadotropin; a hormone derived from the chorionic villi of the placenta, similar to the gonadotropic hormone of the pituitary gland; but active only in the presence of the pituitary gland and having a chiefly luteinizing effect on the ovaries. Also called *pregnancy urine hormone* (*P.U.*). See also *A.P.L.*

antiketogenic s. A substance which, when ingested, is antagonistic to the production of ketone bodies.

central gelatinous s. See *substantia* grisea centralis.

chromophil s. A nucleoprotein in the cytoplasm of many cells staining deeply with basic dyes: also called *chromidial substance, tigroid bodies.*

depressor s. One whose pharmacodynamic action results in a lowering of arterial pressure.

desiccated ovarian s. See *ovary*, 2.

gonadotropic s. See *gonadotropin.*

gray s. That part of the central nervous system composed of nerve cell bodies, their dendrites, and the proximal and terminal unmyelinated portions of axons; gray matter.

ground s. Homogeneous matrix or intercellular substance of a tissue in which the cellular elements and fibers are imbedded.

group-specific s. 1. A substance, isolated from a tryptic digest of hog gastric mucin, which reduces the anti-A antibody in group O and B bloods. 2. A substance, obtained from the glandular portion of the horse gastric mucosa, which can reduce the anti-B agglutinin in group O and A bloods. Syn., *Witebsky's substances.*

G s. Giant molecular complexes of cholesterol with proteins and lipids which may be productive of or associated with development of atherosclerosis.

intercellular s. That part of a tissue which lies between the cells.

interprismatic s. The cementing substance between enamel prisms.

interstitial s. The intercellular and interfibrillar substance of the connective tissue.

intertubular s. The matrix of dentin, containing the dentinal tubules.

isotelic s. One which owes its physiologic action to the occurrence in the molecule of a certain strategic grouping of atoms.

ketogenic s. A foodstuff from which ketone bodies are produced.

Nissl s. The chromophil substance of nerve cells.

perforated s. A part of the base of the brain pierced with many small holes for the passage of blood vessels.

posterior perforated s. A depressed area at the base of the brain, posterior to the mammillary bodies, containing numerous foramens for the passage of blood vessels.

posterior pituitary s. Extracts of the neurohypophysis contain three principles: an oxytocic, a pressor, and an antidiuretic. The oxytocic principle stimulates the uterus, the pressor principle produces peripheral vasoconstriction, and the antidiuretic principle inhibits the renal tubules.

pressor s. One whose pharmacodynamic action results in an elevation of arterial pressure.

proteic s. See *protein.*

reticular s. Mixed white and gray matter in the central nervous system; in the cervical region of the spinal cord, located in the angle between the anterior and posterior columns; reticular formation.

slow-reacting s. A substance having muscle-contracting properties released during anaphylactic shock.

specific soluble s. (SSS). A soluble, type-specific, polysaccharide hapten obtained from the capsule of the pneumococcus.

standard s. A substance used to standardize volumetric solutions.

s. Fa (**Reichstein's**). Cortisone.

vasodilator s. A chemical compound capable of dilating blood vessels.

white s. That part of the central nervous system composed of myelinated nerve fibers; white matter.

Witebsky's substances. See *group-specific s.*

sub·stan′ti·a (sub·stan′shee·uh) (pl. *substantiae*) [L.]. Substance.

s. adamantina. Dental enamel.

s. alba. See white *substance.*

s. compacta. Compact bone.

s. eburnea. Dentin.

s. gelatinosa Rolandi. Translucent, gelatinous gray matter forming the apex of the posterior column of the spinal cord, crescentic or inverted V-shaped in section. A synaptic region for peripheral nerves conveying thermal and pain sensibilities.

s. gliosa. See *s.* grisea centralis.

s. grisea. See gray *substance.*

s. grisea centralis. A condensation of neuroglia around the central canal of the spinal cord. Syn., *central gray matter, central gelatinous substance, substantia gliosa.*

s. nigra. A broad, thick plate of large, pigmented nerve cells separating the basis pedunculi from the tegmentum and extending from the border of the pons through the mesencephalon into the hypothalamus.

s. ossea. Cementum.

s. propria of the cornea. The central, transparent, lamellated layer of dense connective tissue in the cornea.

s. reticularis. Reticular *substance.*

s. spongiosa. Cancellous bone.

sub·ster′nal [L. *sub*, under; G. *sternon*, breast]. Beneath the sternum, as substernal pain.

sub″sti·tu′tion [L. *substitutio*, from *substituere*, to put in place of]. 1. The replacement of one thing by another. 2. *In chemistry*, the replacing of one or more elements or radicals in a compound by other elements or radicals. 3. *In psychiatry*, a defense mechanism whereby alternative or substitutive gratifications are secured to reduce tension resulting from frustration. The substitutes are generally comparable to the pleasures and satisfactions which the individual was frustrated in obtaining.

sub′sti·tu″tive [L. *substitutivus*, from *substituere*]. Effecting a change in symptoms. *Rare.*

sub′strate [L. *substratus*, a spreading under]. 1. An under layer. 2. A substance upon which an enzyme acts.

sub·sul′fate. A basic sulfate.

sub·sul′to·ry [L. *subsultare*, to leap]. Leaping; twitching.

sub·sul′tus [*subsultare*]. A morbid jerking or twitching.

s. tendinum. Involuntary twitching of the muscles, especially of the hands and feet, seen in low fevers: also called *s. clonus*.

sub·ten′o·lin. An antibiotic substance derived from *Bacillus subtilis*, active in vitro against several bacterial species.

sub″ten·to′ri·al [L. *sub*, under; *tentorium*, tent]. Below or beneath the tentorium cerebelli.

sub″te·tan′ic [*sub;* G. *tetanos*, convulsive tension]. Pertaining to convulsions which are not distinctly clonic or tonic.

sub·thal′a·mus [*sub;* G. *thalamos*, chamber]. The ventral, motor portion of the thalamus. —**subthalam′ic,** *adj.*

sub·thy′roid·ism [*sub;* G. *thyreoeidēs*, shield-shaped]. Obsolete term for hypothyroidism.

sub′ti·lin. An antibiotic substance obtained from *Bacillus subtilis*, active against Gram-positive bacteria.

sub·til′y·sin. An antibiotic substance obtained from *Bacillus subtilis*, active against Gram-negative and Gram-positive bacteria.

subtosan. Trade-mark for *polyvinylpyrrolidone*.

sub·to′tal [*sub;* L. *totus*, all]. Less than complete.

sub·tro·chan·ter′ic. Below a trochanter.

sub·trop′i·cal [*sub;* G. *tropikos*, of the solstice]. Pertaining to regions almost tropical in climate.

sub·u′ber·es (sub·yōō′bur·eez) [*sub;* L. *uber*, breast]. Children at the breast; suckling children.

sub·un′gual [*sub;* L. *unguis*, nail]. Beneath the nail.

sub·vir′ile (sub·virr′il, ·vy′ril) [*sub;* L. *virilis*, manly]. Deficient in virility.

sub·vi″ta·min·o′sis B_1. See *beriberi*.

sub″vo·lu′tion [*sub;* L. *volvere*, to roll]. A method of operating for pterygium, in which a flap is turned over so that an outer or cutaneous surface comes in contact with a raw, dissected surface. Adhesions are thus prevented.

sub·wa′king [*sub;* AS. *wacan*]. Pertaining to the condition between sleeping and complete wakefulness.

sucaryl calcium. Trade-marked name for *cyclamate calcium*.

sucaryl sodium. Trade-marked name for *cyclamate sodium*.

suc″ce·da′ne·ous (suck″si·day′nee·us) [L. *succedaneus*, that follows after]. 1. Relating to, or acting as, a substitute. 2. Pertaining to that which follows after, as a permanent tooth that replaces a deciduous tooth.

suc″cen·tu′ri·ate [L. *succenturiare*, to substitute]. Old term for accessory.

suc·cif′er·ous [L. *succus*, sap; *ferre*, to bear]. Producing sap.

suc′ci·nate. A salt of succinic acid.

suc″cin·chlo′ri·mide. $C_4H_4O_2NCl$. Occurs as white crystals or a crystalline powder, soluble in water, with decomposition forming hypochlorous acid. Possesses powerful germicidal activity. Used as a water decontaminant.

suc·cin′ic ac′id. $COOH.CH_2.CH_2.COOH$. A dibasic, crystalline acid occurring in amber and certain other resins; the sodium salt has been used as an analeptic in counteracting barbiturate poisoning. Succinates may possess protective action against depression of tissue metabolism by various noxious agents.

suc″cin·im′ide. $CH_2.CO.NH.CO.CH_2$ (the two CH_2 groups joined by a bond); an interaction product of succinic acid and ammonia, occurring in colorless crystals, soluble in water.

suc·cin″o·de·hy′dro·gen·ase. The enzyme which catalyzes the oxidation of succinic acid to fumaric acid.

suc″cin·yl·cho′line chlo′ride.

$$\begin{array}{l}CH_2COOCH_2CH_2N(CH_3)_3Cl\\ |\\ CH_2COOCH_2CH_2N(CH_3)_3Cl\end{array}$$

A powerful inhibitor of neuromuscular transmission which on intravenous injection produces complete muscular relaxation in about 1 minute, the effect lasting only 2 to 4 minutes because of rapid destruction of the agent in the body by esterases. It is useful clinically in conditions requiring profound but brief muscular relaxation.

suc″cin·yl·sul″fa·thi′a·zole (*succinylsulfathiazolum*). $HOOC.(CH_2)_2CO.NH.C_6H_4.SO_2.NHC_3H_2NS.H_2O$; 2-(*p*-succinylaminobenzenesulfonamide) thiazole monohydrate; occurs as a white or yellowish white, crystalline powder; 1 Gm. dissolves in about 4800 cc. of water; soluble in solutions of sodium bicarbonate and alkali hydroxides; sparingly soluble in alcohol. Exerts a sulfonamide bacteriostatic action, chiefly on the intestinal contents, as it is poorly absorbed. Used for preoperative and postoperative treatment of intestinal operations, prophylaxis and treatment of bacillary dysentery and carriers. Dose, 0.06 Gm. per kg. of body weight, four times daily for one or two weeks.

suc″cor·rhe′a, suc″cor·rhoe′a [*succus;* G. *rhoia*, flow]. An excessive flow of a secretion.

pancreatic s. A pathologic increase of the pancreatic juice when the secretory activity of the gland is exaggerated.

suc′cu·bus [L. *succuba*, one who lies under]. 1. Nightmare. *Obs.* 2. A heavy mental burden. 3. A female demon said to have sexual intercourse with sleeping men. *Obs.* See *incubus*.

suc′cu·lent [L. *succulentus*, full of juice]. Juicy.

suc·cur′sal [L. *succurrere*, to assist]. Subsidiary.

suc′cus (pl. *succi*) [L.]. 1. A vegetable juice. 2. An animal secretion.

s. entericus. The intestinal juice, secreted by the glands of the intestinal mucous membrane. It is thin, opalescent, alkaline, and has a specific gravity of 1.011. It contains an amylolytic and a proteolytic ferment.

s. gastricus. The gastric juice.

s. intestinalis. See *s.* entericus.

s. pancreaticus. The pancreatic juice.

s. prostaticus. The prostatic fluid, a constituent of the semen.

s. spissatus. Any extract prepared by evaporation of the natural juice of a plant.

suc·cuss′ [L. *succutire*, to fling up from below]. To make succussion.

suc·cus′sion (suh·kush′un) [L. *succussio*, from *succutire*]. A shaking, especially of the individual, from side to side, for the purpose of determining the presence of fluid in a cavity or hollow organ of the body.

s. sound. The splashing sound heard when the patient is shaken; occurs in hydropneumothorax, pyopneumothorax, or in cases of dilated stomach containing fluid.

suck [AS. *sūcan*]. To take nourishment at the breast.

suck′er ap″pa·ra′tus. A contrivance for evacuating fluid from body cavities, operating by means of negative pressure. Syn., *suction apparatus*.

suck′ing [*sūcan*]. Nursing; drawing with the mouth.

suck′le [freq. from *sūcan*]. To nurse at the breast.

suck′ling [*sūcan*]. A nursling.

cross s. Reciprocal foster nursing.

su′crase. See *saccharase*.

su′crate. A salt of saccharic acid.

su'crol. Trade name for *dulcin.*

su'crose (*sucrosum*). $C_{12}H_{22}O_{11}$. A sugar obtained from *Saccharum officinarum, Beta vulgaris,* and other sources; occurs as colorless or white crystals, crystalline masses or blocks, or a white, crystalline powder; 1 Gm. dissolves in 0.5 cc. of water and in 170 cc. of alcohol. Used as a sweetening agent and preservative in syrups and other preparations. Also called *saccharum, sugar.*

s. octaacetate. $C_{28}H_{38}O_{19}$; a white, hygroscopic powder, sparingly soluble in water, soluble in alcohol: used as a denaturant for alcohol.

su"cro·su'ri·a [*sucrosum;* G. *ouron,* urine]. A rare condition in which sucrose is not metabolized in the intestine and is excreted in the urine.

suc'tion [L. *suctum,* from *sugere,* to suck]. The act of sucking.

Bier's s. A first-aid treatment for snakebites which employs suction tubes over the wound to draw out the toxic material.

posttussive s. A sucking sound heard on auscultation over certain pulmonary cavities during the brief interval between a cough and the succeeding inspiration.

suc'tion ap"pa·ra'tus. See *sucker apparatus.*

Suc·to'ri·a [*sugere*]. 1. A synonym for *Siphonaptera,* the fleas. 2. A class of Protozoa, closely related to the Ciliata, without cilia in the mature stage, but possessing processes called tentacles, some of which are suctorial in function. A few species are parasitic on fish and other aquatic animals.

suc·to'ri·al [*sugere*]. Pertaining to, or suitable for, sucking.

su·da'men (pl. *sudamina*) [L. *sudare,* to sweat]. An eruption of translucent, whitish vesicles, due to a noninflammatory disturbance of the sweat glands, consisting in a collection of sweat in the ducts of the sweat glands. Is very transitory and occurs after excessive sweating. Syn., *miliaria crystallina.* —**sudam'inal,** *adj.*

Su·dan'. Any of a number of chemically related biological stains.

S. II. $(CH_3)_2C_6H_3.N{:}N.C_{10}H_6OH$. A fat stain. Also called *oil scarlet, fat ponceau.*

S. III (C.C.). $C_6H_5N{:}N.C_6H_4N{:}N.C_{10}H_6OH$. A fat-soluble, diazo dye; used as a fat stain. Also called *fat ponceau G., oil red, Sudan G.*

S. IV (C.C.). $CH_3.C_6H_4.N{:}N.C_6H_3(CH_3).N{:}N.C_{10}H_6OH$. A dimethyl derivative of Sudan III; a fat stain, more intense than Sudan III. Also called *fat ponceau, oil red IV.*

S. R $CH_3O.C_6H_4.N{:}N.C_{10}H_6OH$; a stain suggested for use in the Kahn reaction for syphilis: also called *oil vermilion.*

su·dan'o·phil. A leukocyte which, owing to fatty degeneration, is stained readily by Sudan III.

su·da'tion [L. *sudatio,* from *sudare,* to sweat]. The act of sweating.

su"da·to'ri·a. Hyperhidrosis.

su"da·to'ri·um [L., a sweating-room]. 1. A hot-air bath. 2. A room for the administration of a hot-air bath.

Sudeck, Paul Herman Martin [*German surgeon,* 1866–1938]. Known for his description of acute bone atrophy or aseptic necrosis following injury; called *Sudeck's atrophy, traumatic osteoporosis.*

su·do"lor·rhe'a. See *dermatitis* seborrheica.

su"do·mo'tor [L. *sudor,* sweat; *motor,* from *movere,* to move]. Sudoriferous.

su'dor [L.]. Sweat. —**sudoral,** *adj.*

s. nocturnus. Night sweat.

s. sanguinosus. See *hemathidrosis.*

su"do·re'sis [*sudor*]. Excessive sweating.

su"dor·if'er·ous [*sudor;* L. *ferre,* to bear]. Producing sweat.

su"dor·if'ic. Inducing sweating.

su"dor·if'ic. An agent inducing sweating.

su"dor·i·ker"a·to'sis [*sudor;* G. *keras,* horn; *-ōsis,* condition]. Keratosis of the sweat glands.

su"dor·ip'a·rous [*sudor;* L. *parere,* to bring forth]. Secreting sweat.

su'et [L. *sebum,* tallow, suet]. 1. The internal fat of the abdomen of sheep or cattle. 2. Prepared suet.

mutton s. See prepared *s.*

prepared s. (*sebum praeparatum*). The internal fat of the abdomen of the sheep, *Ovis aries,* purified by melting and straining; occurs as a white, solid fat, having when fresh a slight characteristic odor and a bland taste. It becomes rancid on exposure to air; insoluble in water and cold alcohol. It consists approximately of 70% of stearin and palmitin and 30% of olein. Used as an ointment base. Syn., *mutton s.*

suf'fo·cate [L. *suffocare,* to choke]. Asphyxiate.

suf"fo·ca'tion [L. *suffocatio,* from *suffocare*]. Interference with the entrance of air into the lungs.

suf·frag'i·nis (suh·fradj'i·nis) [L. *suffrago,* ham]. The large pastern or proximal phalangeal bone of the horse. Contraction of *os suffraginis.*

suf·fu'sion [L. *suffusio,* from *suffundere,* to suffuse]. 1. A spreading or flow of any fluid of the body into surrounding tissue; an extensive superficial extravasation of blood. 2. The pouring of water upon a patient as a remedial measure.

sug'ar [OF. *sucre,* from Skr. *ṣarkarā*]. 1. Any carbohydrate having a sweet taste and the general formula $C_nH_{2n}O_n$ or $C_nH_{2n-2}O_{n-1}$. 2. Sucrose.

acid of s. Oxalic acid.

acorn s. Quercite.

beet s. Sucrose.

blood s. The carbohydrate of the blood, chiefly glucose.

brain s. Cerebrose; galactose.

brown s. Partially refined cane sugar.

cane s. Sucrose.

corn s. Glucose.

date s. The sugar from the fruit of the date, *Phoenix dactylifera.*

fruit s. Levulose or fructose.

grape s. Glucose.

gum s. Arabinose.

honey s. Glucose.

invert s. A mixture of approximately equal parts of glucose and levulose obtained by hydrolysis of sucrose.

lead s. See *lead* acetate.

liver s. Glycogen.

malt s. Maltose.

maple s. The mixture of carbohydrates, chiefly sucrose, obtained from the sap of the sugar maple.

meat s. Inositol.

milk s. Lactose.

mucin s. Levulose.

muscle s. Inositol.

pectin s. Arabinose.

refined s. Purified cane sugar.

wood s. Xylose.

sug'ar·ine (shŏŏg'ur·een, ·in). Methylbenzol-sulfinide, a compound said to have 500 times greater sweetening power than sugar.

sug·gest"i·bil'i·ty [L. *suggerere,* to suggest]. The condition of being readily influenced by another; an abnormal state when the individual conforms with unusual readiness, as patients who too readily accept ideas of health or illness.

negative s. Active negativism.

sug·gest'i·ble [*suggerere*]. Amenable to suggestion.

sug·ges'tion [L. *suggestio,* from *suggerere*]. 1. The artificial production of a certain psychic state in which the individual experiences such sensations as are suggested to him or ceases to experience those which he is instructed not to feel. 2. The thing suggested.

hypnotic s. A suggestion made to an individual in the hypnotic state.

posthypnotic s. The command to do certain acts given the subject while in the hypnotic stage, and causing him to execute these acts after his return to his normal condition.

self-s. See *autosuggestion.*

sug·ges′tion·ist [*suggerere*]. One who treats disease by means of suggestion. **—suggestionize,** *v.t.*

sug″gil·la′tion (sug″ji·lay′shun, sudj″i·) [L. *sugillatio*, a black-and-blue mark]. An ecchymosis or bruise.

su′i·cide [L. *sui*, of oneself; *caedere*, to kill]. 1. Self murder; intentionally taking one's own life. 2. One who takes his own life. —**suicid′al,** *adj.*

su′int (sue′int, swint) [L. *sudare*, to sweat]. A soapy substance rich in potassium salts of higher fatty acids and in cholesterol, derived from sheep's wool. Also called *wool-soap.*

sulamyd. Trade-mark for *sulfacetimide.*

sul′cus (pl. *sulci*) [L., furrow]. A furrow or linear groove, as in bone. When applied to linear depressions on the cerebral hemisphere, the term indicates a less deep depression than a fissure. Sulci in the brain separate the convolutions or gyri. See also *fissure.* See Plate 18. —**sulcal, sulcate,** *adj.*

ampullary s. The external transverse groove on each membranous ampulla for the entrance of the ampullary nerve.

angular s. See angular *incisure.*

anterior longitudinal cardiac s. A groove situated on the sternocostal surface of the heart, separating the ventricles.

anterolateral spinal s. A broad, shallow groove on the anterolateral surface of the spinal cord, corresponding to the line of the origin of the ventral nerve roots.

anterolateral s. of the medulla oblongata. The continuation cephalad of the anterolateral spinal sulcus, from which emerge the roots of the hypoglossal nerves.

aortic s. A vertical groove on the medial aspect of the left lung lodging the thoracic aorta.

atrioventricular s. See coronary *s.*

basilar s. A groove along the median line of the ventral surface of the pons lodging the basilar artery.

bulboventricular s. The groove formed by the loop of the embryonic cardiac tube in the pericardial cavity.

calcaneal s. The groove along the medial aspect of the calcaneus adjacent to the posterior articular surface lodging the interosseous talocalcaneal ligament.

calcarine s. See calcarine *fissure.*

callosal s. The groove separating the corpus callosum from the overlying cingulate gyrus.

callosomarginal s. See cingulate *s.*

central s. A groove situated about the middle of the lateral surface of the cerebral hemisphere, separating the frontal from the parietal lobe: also called *Rolandic sulcus, fissure of Rolando.* See Plate 18.

chiasmatic s. The optic groove of the sphenoid bone.

cingulate s. One on the medial aspect of the cerebral hemisphere separating the superior frontal gyrus and paracentral lobule from the cingulate gyrus below; it terminates by dividing into subparietal and marginal portions. Also called *callosomarginal s.* or *fissure, cingulate fissure, s. cinguli.*

circular s. A limiting furrow surrounding the base of the insula, separating it from the operculum. Formerly called *limiting s. of Reil.*

collateral s. See collateral *fissure.*

coronary s. A groove separating the atria from the ventricles, containing the trunks of the nutrient vessels of the heart: also called *atrioventricular s.*

costal s. The groove along the inferior aspect of the rib for the intercostal vessels and nerves.

cruciate s. One of the grooves on the dorsal surface of the mesencephalon between the corpora quadrigemina.

cuticular s. One of many little furrows on the skin which intersect so that they bound polygonal areas. Also called *s. cutis.*

diagonal s. A short, oblique furrow traversing the opercular portion of the inferior frontal gyrus.

dorsolateral s. See posterolateral spinal *s.*

fimbriodentate s. A groove on the superior medial aspect of the temporal lobe, separating the hippocampal fimbria from the dentate gyrus.

frontal s. One of three longitudinal grooves separating the superior, middle, and inferior frontal gyri. See Plate 18.

gingival s. The space between the free gingiva and the surface of a tooth: formerly called *gingival crevice.*

gluteal s. See gluteal *fold.*

hemispheric s. A shallow, circular groove separating the embryonal telencephalon from the diencephalon.

hippocampal s. See hippocampal *fissure.*

horizontal cerebellar s. A deep groove encircling the cerebellum and separating the superior and inferior surfaces.

hypothalamic s. A groove on the lower medial surface of each thalamus at the level of the third ventricle. Formerly called *s. of Monro.*

interatrial s. The superficial groove separating the two embryonic atria.

intermediate s. A slight groove on the greater curvature of the stomach, opposite the angular incisure, separating the pyloric antrum and vestibule.

interparietal s. See intraparietal *s.*

intertubercular s. See bicipital *groove.*

intraparietal s. A well-marked furrow separating the superior and inferior parietal lobules. This furrow has a complex and variable form having the following subdivisions: superior postcentral sulcus, inferior postcentral sulcus, and transverse occipital sulcus. Formerly called *interparietal s.* See Plate 18.

lacrimal s. See nasolacrimal *groove.*

lateral cerebral peduncular s. A longitudinal furrow on the lateral surface of each peduncle separating it from the tegmentum dorsally: also called *lateral mesencephalic s.*

lateral occipital s. The longitudinal groove dividing the lateral surface of the occipital lobe into a superior and an inferior gyrus. Syn., *s. lunatus.* See Plate 18.

malleolar s. A shallow groove on the posterior border of the medial malleolus for the passage of the tendons of the tibialis posterior and flexor digitorum longus muscles.

marginal s. A branch of the cingulate sulcus which comes off at the level of the splenium and goes to the dorsal margin of the hemisphere behind the central sulcus.

medial lingual s. A narrow median groove on the dorsum of the tongue.

median posterior s. A longitudinal groove incompletely dividing the spinal cord posteriorly into two symmetrical parts.

median s. The longitudinal groove in the floor of the fourth ventricle of the brain.
nasofrontal s. The groove between the frontal process and nasal process in the developing face.
nymphocaruncular s. A groove between the labium minus and the hymen.
oculomotor s. A longitudinal furrow on the medial surface of the cerebral peduncle from which emerge the roots of the oculomotor nerve.
olfactory s. A well-defined anteroposterior groove on the medial orbital gyrus for the passage of the olfactory tract.
orbital s. An H-shaped groove on the inferior surface of the frontal lobe dividing it into four orbital gyri.
paracentral s. A branch of the cingulate sulcus, sometimes reaching the dorsal margin of the cerebral hemisphere.
paraglenoidal s. One of many slight grooves inferior to and in front of the auricular surface of the iliac bone for the attachment of the sacroiliac and interosseous ligaments.
parallel s. Synonym for superior temporal sulcus.
paramedial s. A series of irregular furrows on the lateral surface of the superior frontal gyrus, dividing it into a superior and an inferior part.
parieto-occipital s. The upper limb of the calcarine fissure between the precuneus of the parietal lobe and the cuneus of the occipital lobe. Also called *parieto-occipital fissure.* See Plate 18.
parolfactory s. The **anterior parolfactory sulcus** separates the superior frontal gyrus from the parolfactory area and the **posterior parolfactory sulcus** separates the subcallosal gyrus from the parolfactory area.
polar s. One of several small grooves at the distal end of the calcarine fissure.
postcentral s. The first sulcus of the parietal lobe lying behind and roughly parallel to the central sulcus.
posterior longitudinal cardiac s. A groove situated on the diaphragmatic surface of the heart, between the ventricles.
posterior median s. of spinal cord. A narrow groove extending the entire length of the spinal cord posteriorly in the midline.
posterolateral spinal s. A narrow, deep groove on the posterolateral surface of the spinal cord, corresponding to the line of origin of the dorsal nerve roots.
posterolateral s. of the medulla oblongata. The extension cephalad of the posterolateral spinal sulcus.
postolivary s. A deep groove on the dorsolateral border of the inferior olive; it may be considered as the laterally shifted continuation of the posterolateral sulcus.
precentral s. A groove separating the horizontal frontal gyri from the anterior central gyrus. See Plate 18.
prenodular s. A groove on the posterolateral surface of the embryonal cerebellum separating the vermis from the flocculus.
prepyramidal s. of the cerebellum. A groove lying between the middle lobe of the cerebellum and the pyramids.
pterygopalatine s. A groove on the perpendicular part of the palatine bone, which, with the corresponding groove in the maxilla, forms the pterygopalatine canal.
radial s. A groove on the lateral surface of the shaft of the humerus for the transmission of the radial nerve and profunda brachii artery.
Rolandic s. See central *s.*
sagittal s. A shallow groove in the midline on the cerebral surface of the frontal squama, lodging the superior sagittal sinus.
scleral s. A shallow groove at the junction of the sclera and the cornea.
semicircular s. See terminal *s.*
sigmoid s. A deep, S-shaped groove on the inner surface of the mastoid portion of the temporal bone, lodging part of the transverse sinus: also called *sigmoid groove.*
spiral s. A concave groove below the membrana tectoria of the floor of the cochlear duct. Sometimes called *inner spiral s.* A groove where the basilar membrane is attached to the bony cochlear canal is called *outer spiral s.*
subclavian s. A shallow groove on the upper surface of the first rib, lodging the subclavian artery.
subparietal s. A groove separating the precuneus of the parietal lobe from the cingulate gyrus. Syn., *suprasplenial s.*
s. brevis. One of several short furrows seen on the insula of the cerebrum.
s. carpi. The broad groove seen in the articulated carpal bones on the anterior aspect of the wrist between the pisiform and hamulus of the hamate.
s. cinguli. See cingulate *s.*
s. limitans. A longitudinal groove on the middle of the inner surface of the lateral wall of the neural tube, dividing it into a dorsal alar plate and a ventral basal plate.
s. lunatus. See lateral occipital *s.*
s. of auditory tube. A groove between the petrous part of the temporal bone and the great wing of the sphenoid, lodging the cartilaginous part of the auditory tube.
s. primarius. See primary *fissure.*
suprasplenial s. See subparietal *s.*
talar s. A deep groove on the inferior surface of the body of the talus, separating the posterior and middle calcaneal articular surfaces.
temporal s. One of the three grooves (superior, middle, and inferior), dividing the temporal lobe into superior, middle, inferior, and fusiform gyri. See Plate 18.
terminal cardiac s. A groove on the external surface of the right atrium, extending from the right side of the superior vena cava to the right side of the inferior vena cava, the embryonic right boundary of the sinus venosus.
terminal lingual s. The shallow, V-shaped groove, with its apex directed backward, on the dorsum of the tongue; it separates the oral and pharyngeal parts of the organ.
terminal s. A furrow between the dorsal surface of the thalamus and caudate nucleus, lodging the terminal vein and stria terminalis. Syn., *semicircular s.*
transverse occipital s. The groove continuous with the posterior end of the occipital ramus of the intraparietal sulcus, extending over the superior portion of the occipital lobe. See Plate 18.
transverse sulci (*of nail*). Transverse grooves in the nails resulting from disease.
tympanic s. The groove in the osseous portion of the external auditory meatus in which the circumference of the tympanic membrane is attached; it is deficient superiorly at the tympanic notch.
uvulonodular s. One separating the uvula from the nodulus of the cerebellum.
ventrolateral s. See anterolateral spinal *s.*
ventrolateral s. of the medulla. See anterolateral *s.* of the medulla oblongata.
vermicular s. The groove between the vermis and a cerebellar hemisphere.

sul″fa·cet′a·mide. $NH_2.C_6H_4.SO_2.NH.CH_3CO$. Para-aminobenzenesulfonacetamide; a crystalline powder, soluble in about 100 parts of water. Used in a variety of infections, particularly those of the urinary tract; its sodium derivative is used for treatment of ophthalmic infections because of rarity of sensitization reactions. Dose, 3–4 Gm. (45–60 gr.) daily. Also called *sulfacetimide.* See *albucid, sulamyd.*

sulf·ac′id. 1. A thioacid. 2. A sulfonic acid.

sul·fac′tin. An antibiotic substance derived from a species of *Actinomyces,* active in vitro against a number of bacterial species.

sulfactol. Trade-mark for a brand of sodium thiosulfate used in the prevention and treatment of toxic reactions during arsenic, bismuth, and mercury administration, and in poisoning by these metals, as well as in eczema.

sul″fa·di′a·zine (sul″fuh·dye′uh·zeen, ·zin, ·dye-az′een, ·in, ·dye·ay′zeen, ·zin) (*sulfadiazinum*). $NH_2.C_6H_4.SO_2.NH.C_4H_3N_2$; *p*-amino-N-2-pyrimidylbenzene sulfonamide or 2-sulfanilylamidopyrimidine; occurs as a white or slightly yellow powder; 1 Gm. dissolves in about 13,000 cc. of water; it is sparingly soluble in alcohol. An anti-infective agent of the sulfonamide group, effective against a variety of organisms; it is used in the treatment of pneumococcic pneumonia, hemolytic streptococcus infections, staphylococcic infections, and meningococcic meningitis. It causes fewer toxic reactions than sulfanilamide, sulfapyridine, or sulfathiazole. Dose, oral, 0.1 Gm. per kg. of body weight initially, then 1.0 to 1.5 Gm. every 4 hours until temperature becomes normal.

sterile s. sodium (*sulfadiazinum sodicum sterile*). Sterile sulfadiazine sodium contained in tight containers so closed that the sterility of the product is maintained until the container is opened for use. This is intended for preparing solutions for intravenous injection. Average dose, intravenous, 2 Gm. (30 gr.). Also called *sterile sodium sulfadiazine.*

s. sodium (*sulfadiazinum sodicum*). $C_{10}H_9N_4O_2SNa$. Occurs as a white powder; 1 Gm. dissolves in about 2 cc. of water; it is slightly soluble in alcohol.

sul″fa·di′me·tine. Generic name for N′-(2,6-dimethyl-4-pyrimidyl)-sulfonamide, a sulfonamide characterized by a very low degree of acetylation in the body and by maintenance of high blood and urine levels with moderate dosage. See *elkosin.*

sul′fa drugs. A family of drugs of the sulfonamide type which have marked bacteriostatic properties. The more important sulfa drugs are sulfanilamide, sulfathiazole, sulfaguanidine, and sulfadiazine. All are soluble in dilute acid or acetone, insoluble in ether.

sul″fa·guan′i·dine (sul″fuh·gwan′i·deen, ·din, ·gwah′ni·deen, ·din) (*sulfaguanidinum*). $NH_2.C_6H_4.SO_2.NH.C(NH)NH_2.H_2O$; *p*-aminobenzenesulfonylguanidine monohydrate; occurs as a white, needlelike, crystalline powder; 1 Gm. dissolves in about 1000 cc. of water; it is sparingly soluble in alcohol. Used primarily in the treatment of certain intestinal bacillary infections. Dose, 0.05 Gm. per kg. of body weight initially, then 0.05 Gm. per kg. every 4 to 8 hours. Also called *sulfanilylguanidine monohydrate.*

sul″fa·mer′a·zine (sul″fuh·merr′uh·zeen, ·zin) (*sulfamerazinum*). 2-Sulfanilamido-4-methylpyrimidine; the 4-(mono)methyl derivative of sulfadiazine; it is more soluble in water than sulfadiazine. Its therapeutic uses are similar to those of sulfadiazine. Adult dose, oral, 3 to 4 Gm. initially followed by 1 Gm. every 8 hours.

sul″fa·meth′a·zine (sul″fuh·meth′uh·zeen, ·zin). 2-Sulfanilamido-4,6-dimethylpyrimidine; the dimethyl derivative of sulfadiazine. Used like sulfadiazine, but its acetyl derivative is more soluble than that of sulfadiazine.

sul″fa·mez′a·thine (sul″fuh·mez′uh·theen, ·thin). Sulfamethazine.

sul·fam′ic ac′id. $HO.SO_2.NH_2$. A colorless, crystalline acid; has been used in the treatment of cholera.

sulfamidyl. Trade-mark for a brand of sulfanilamide.

sul″fa·min′ic ac′id. Sulfamic acid.

sulfamylon. Trade-mark for the hydrochloride of marfanil.

sul″fa·nil′a·mide (*sulfanilamidum*). $NH_2.C_6H_4.SO_2.NH_2$; *p*-aminobenzenesulfonamide; occurs as white crystals, granules, or powder; 1 Gm. dissolves in about 125 cc. of water and in about 37 cc. of alcohol. It exerts a potent antibacterial effect against many organisms, being of chemotherapeutic value in treating infections caused by beta hemolytic streptococci, meningococci, and gonococci. Other, less toxic, sulfonamides are now preferred. Sulfanilamide has been supplied under various names, including sulfamidyl, sulfonamide-P, prontylin, prontosil album, streptamide, streptozone, streptocide, stramid, colsulanyde, lysococcine. It may act as an allergen. Dose, oral, 0.1 Gm. per kg. of body weight initially, followed by one-sixth this amount every 4 hours until temperature becomes normal.

sul·fan′i·late. A salt of sulfanilic acid.

sul″fa·nil′ic ac′id. $NH_2C_6H_4SO_3H$. Para-aminobenzene sulfonic acid, occurring in colorless, water-soluble crystals. Used as a reagent for bile pigments and other substances, also in organic synthesis.

sul″fa·pyr′a·zine (sul″fuh·pirr′uh·zeen, ·zin). $NH_2.C_6H_4.SO_2.NH.C_4H_3N_2$. *p*-Amino-N-2-pyrazinylbenzenesulfonamide, isomeric with sulfapyridine; 1 Gm. dissolves in about 20,000 cc. of water. Appears to be as effective as sulfadiazine in pneumococcal, hemolytic streptococcal, and *Escherichia coli* infections; it also appears to be effective against *Shigella paradysenteriae.* Dose, for adults, 2–4 Gm. (30–60 gr.) initially, then 1 Gm. every 4–6 hours.

sul″fa·pyr′i·dine (sul″fuh·pirr′i·deen, ·din) (*sulfapyridinum*). $NH_2.C_6H_4.SO_2.NH.C_5H_4N$; 2-(*p*-aminobenzenesulfonamido) pyridine. Occurs as white or faintly yellowish white crystals, granules, or powder; 1 Gm. dissolves in about 3500 cc. of water and in about 440 cc. of alcohol. Originally it was used especially in lobar pneumonia and in gonorrheal infections; it is now little used except in treating dermatitis herpetiformis. The range of dose is 0.5–1 Gm.

sul″fa·quin·ox′a·line. $C_{14}H_{12}N_4O_2S$; 2-sulfanilamidoquinoxaline, practically insoluble in water but soluble in alkaline solutions: used in veterinary medicine to control outbreaks of cecal and intestinal coccidiosis of chickens and turkeys.

sulfarsenol. A trade-mark for a brand of sulfarsphenamine.

sulf·ars″phen·a·mine′ (sulf·ars″fen·uh·meen′, ·ars″fen·am′een, ·in, ·ars·fen′uh·meen, ·min) (*sulfarsphenamina*). Consists chiefly of disodium 3,3′-diamino-4,4′-dihydroxyarsenobenzene-N-di-methylenesulfonate; it contains not less than 19% of arsenic; occurs as a yellow powder; it is very soluble in water but slightly soluble in alcohol. Used in the treatment of syphilis. Dose, 0.25–0.45 Gm. (4–7 gr.) intravenously or intramuscularly at about one-week intervals.

s. bismuth. See *bismarsen.*

sulfasuxidine. Trade-mark for a brand of succinylsulfathiazole.

sul′fa·tase. Any enzyme which hydrolyzes an ethereal sulfate (ester sulfate).

sul′fate. A salt of sulfuric acid of the type M_2SO_4.

sulfathalidine. Trade-mark for phthalylsulfathiazole, a poorly absorbed sulfonamide useful for suppressing growth of bacteria in the large intestine.

sul″fa·thi′a·zole (*sulfathiazolum*). $NH_2.C_6H_4.SO_2.$-$NH.C_3H_2NS$; 2-(*p*-aminobenzenesulfonamido) thiazole; occurs as white or faintly yellowish white crystals, granules, or powder; 1 Gm. dissolves in about 1700 cc. of water and in about 200 cc. of alcohol. It was formerly widely used in the treatment of pneumococcal, staphylococcal, and urinary-tract infections; it has been largely replaced by less toxic sulfonamides.

sulf″he·mo·glo′bin (sulf″hee·mo·glo′bin, ·hem·o-glo′bin). A greenish substance derived from hemoglobin by the action of hydrogen sulfide. It may appear in the blood following the ingestion of sulfanilamide. Syn., *sulfmethemoglobin.*

sulf·he″mo·glo″bi·ne′mi·a (sulf·hee″mo·glo″bi-nee′mee·uh, ·hem″o·). A condition in which sulfhemoglobin is present in the blood; the symptoms are similar to those present in methemoglobinemia. Diagnosis is made by spectroscopic examination. Also see *methemoglobinemia.*

sulf·hy′drate. A compound of a base with the univalent radical sulfhydryl, SH.

sulf″hy′dryl. The univalent radical SH, usually attached to a carbon chain. The presence of active sulfhydryl groups is important for the activity of many enzymes. Often written *SH group.*

sul′fide. A compound of sulfur with an element or basic radical.

sul′fine. Sulfonium.

sul″fi·sox′a·zole. Generic title for the sulfonamide supplied under the trade-marked name gantrisin. Syn., *sulphafurazole.*

sul′fite. A salt of sulfurous acid of the type M_2SO_3.

sulf″met·he″mo·glo′bin (sulf″met·hee″mo·glo′-bin, ·hem″o·glo′bin). Sulfhemoglobin.

sul′fo- [L. *sulfur*, brimstone]. A combining form generally indicating *the presence of divalent sulfur* or *the sulfo- group, —SO₃H.*

sul″fo·ac′id (sul″fo·ass′id, sul′fo·ass″id). 1. A thioacid. 2. A sulfonic acid.

sul″fo·bro″mo·phthal′e·in so′di·um. $C_{20}H_8Br_4$-$O_{10}S_2Na_2$; disodium phenoltetrabromophthalein sulfonate; a white, crystalline powder, hygroscopic, soluble in water: used as a reagent for liver function tests. See *bromsulphalein.*

sul″fo·car′bo·late. A salt of phenolsulfonic acid.

sul″fo·car·bol′ic ac′id. Phenolsulfonic acid.

sul″fo·cy′a·nate. Thiocyanate.

sul″fo·cy·an′ic ac′id. Thiocyanic acid.

sul′fo·nal. Sulfonmethane.

sul′fo·nal·ism (sul′fo·nul·iz·um, sul·fon′ul·iz·um). A group of symptoms said to be occasioned by the prolonged administration of sulfonal. *Obs.*

sul·fon′a·mide (sul·fon′uh·mide, ·mid, sul·fo′nuh·, sul″fo·nam′ide, ·id). Any of a group of compounds derived from sulfanilamide, $H_2N.C_6H_4.SO_2.NH_2$, and used in the treatment of various bacterial infections. The various members of the group vary with respect to activity, degree and rate of absorption, metabolic alteration and excretion, and the toxic manifestations produced. Prominent among the toxic effects encountered is renal damage, particularly of the type caused by the crystallization of the drugs and their N^4-acetyl derivatives in the urinary tract; many other toxic effects have been noted, of which some can be attributed to sensitization. Prior to the advent of the antibiotics, such as penicillin, the sulfonamides revolutionized the treatment of pneumonia, hemolytic streptococcal infections, gonorrhea, and many other infectious diseases. The action of sulfonamides is blocked by *p*-aminobenzoic acid.

sulfonamide-P. Trade-mark for a brand of sulfanilamide.

sul′fon·ate. Treat an aromatic hydrocarbon with fuming sulfuric acid.

sul′fon·ate. 1. A sulfuric acid derivative. 2. The ester of a sulfonic acid.

sul″fo·na′tion. A chemical process resulting in the introduction in a compound of one or more sulfo groups.

sul′fone. An oxidation product of thio-compounds containing the group SO_2 attached to a hydrocarbon group.

sul″fone·phthal′e·in. Any one of a group of organic compounds made by the interaction of phenols with acid chlorides or anhydrides of orthosulfobenzoic acid and its derivatives, such as thymolsulfonephthalein and phenolsulfonephthalein.

sul″fon·eth″yl·meth′ane (*sulfonethylmethanum*). $CH_3.C_2H_5.C.(SO_2C_2H_5)_2$. Diethylsulfonemethylethylmethane; occurs as colorless, lustrous, crystalline scales; 1 Gm. dissolves in about 200 cc. of water; it is soluble in alcohol. The sulfone group of hypnotics, which includes this drug and sulfonmethane, have little action on the system except to depress the cerebral centers. A therapeutic dose has almost no effect except to produce sleep; it has been used as a hypnotic. Syn., *methylsulfonal.*

sul·fon′ic ac′id. An organic acid containing the $—SO_3H$ or $—SO_2OH$ group.

sul·fo′ni·um. The univalent, electropositive radical $R_3S—$, in which R is an organic radical. Syn., *sulfine.*

sul″fon·meth′ane (*sulfonmethanum*). $(CH_3)_2C.$-$(SO_2C_2H_5)_2$; diethylsulfonedimethylmethane; occurs as white crystals, or a white powder; 1 Gm. dissolves in about 365 cc. of water and in about 60 cc. of alcohol. The physiologic action of sulfonmethane is similar to that of sulfonethylmethane, but it is more slowly absorbed and less readily eliminated. It has been used as a hypnotic. Also called *sulfonal.*

sul′fo·nyl. The bivalent radical $—SO_2—$.

sul″fo·phe′nate, sul″fo·phen′yl·ate. 1. Phenolsulfonate, a salt or ester of phenolsulfonic acid, $C_6H_4(OH)SO_3H$. 2. Phenylsulfate, a salt of phenylsulfuric acid, $C_6H_5OSO_3H$.

sul″fo·phen′yl·ate. Sulfophenate.

sul″fo·sal″i·cyl′ic ac′id. $SO_3H.C_6H_3.OH.COOH.$-$2H_2O$. A white or nearly white, crystalline powder, used as a reagent for albumin.

sul′fo·salt″ (sul′fo·sawlt″). A salt of sulfonic acid.

sul″fo·vi′nic ac′id (sul″fo·vy′nick, ·vin′ick). C_2H_5-HSO_4, ethylsulfuric acid formed by the interaction of sulfuric acid and ethyl alcohol.

sulf·ox′ide. 1. The divalent radical=SO. 2. An organic compound of the type of R_2SO or $R.SO.R'$, where R and R′ are organic radicals.

sulf·ox′one so′di·um. Generic name for disodium [sulfonylbis(*p*-phenyleneimino)] dimethanesulfinate tetrahydrate; $SO_2(C_6H_4.NHCH_2SO_2Na)_2.$-$4H_2O$, supplied under the trade-marked name diasone sodium. The substance was introduced for treatment of tuberculosis but was not found clinically satisfactory; later it was found to be useful in the treatment of leprosy.

sul′fur [L.]. S = 32.066. A solid, nonmetallic element. Occurs as a yellow, brittle mass or in transparent monoclinic or rhombic crystals and exists in a number of modifications. It is insoluble in water, slightly soluble in alcohol and ether, and soluble in carbon disulfide. The solubility varies with the modification. Sulfur, in contact with living tissue, forms hydrogen sulfide. Due to its local irritant action upon the mucous membrane, hydrogen sulfide provokes intestinal peristalsis, and, therefore, sulfur exerts a laxative influence. The hydrogen sulfide formed may exert a toxic action on intestinal parasites, and sulfur has been recommended in the treatment of enterobiasis. The most important uses of sulfur are external. In contact with the skin, especially in the presence of alkalies, there forms either hydrogen sulfide or a polythionic acid. The compound formed is an active poison to various pathogenic parasites; and, therefore, sulfur is used in diseases such as scabies, ringworm, and favus. Sulfur is also used in a number of nonparasitic diseases of the skin, such as acne, psoriasis, and seborrhea. Sulfur also has many uses in industry. Precipitated sulfur, sublimed sulfur, and washed sulfur are official.

colloidal s. This form of sulfur may have some therapeutic action analogous, when injected intravenously, to that of foreign protein injections. Colloidal sulfur is available on the market under a number of trade names.

compound s. ointment (*unguentum sulfuris compositum*). Contains calcium carbonate, 10 Gm.; sublimed sulfur, 15 Gm.; juniper tar, 15 Gm.; soft soap, 30 Gm.; solid petroxolin, 30 Gm.; to make 100 Gm. Also called *Wilkinson's ointment, Hebra's itch ointment.*

flowers of s. Sublimed sulfur.

milk of s. Precipitated sulfur.

precipitated s. (*sulfur praecipitatum*). The form of sulfur obtained by adding hydrochloric acid to a solution prepared by boiling sublimed sulfur and lime with water. Because it is finely subdivided it is more readily suspended in liquids than are other forms of sulfur.

sublimed s. (*sulfur sublimatum*). The form of sulfur obtained by subliming native sulfur. Syn., *flowers of s.*

s. dioxide. SO_2. A colorless, noninflammable gas with a strong suffocating odor; with water it forms sulfurous acid. It is a powerful bleaching agent, due to its reducing properties. If inhaled in the concentrated state, it proves fatal. Its use as a disinfectant, by burning in a closed room, has been practically abandoned. It is used for the preservation of dried fruits to prevent darkening during the drying. It is also used for its bleaching properties in many industrial processes.

s. ointment (*unguentum sulfuris*). Contains 10% of precipitated sulfur in a base of liquid petrolatum and white ointment.

s. trioxide. SO_3, sulfuric anhydride, existing in three forms, two being solid, and one liquid, at room temperature. It is an intermediate in the manufacture of sulfuric acid and is used in chemical syntheses.

washed s. (*sulfur lotum*). Sublimed sulfur which has been washed with a dilute solution of ammonia to remove traces of acid. It is the preferred form for internal administration. Dose, 4–12 Gm. (1–3 drachms).

sul'fu·ra"ted. Combined with sulfur.

sul'fu·ra"tor. An apparatus for applying sulfur fumes for purposes of disinfection.

sul·fu'ric ac'id (*acidum sulfuricum*). An aqueous solution containing about 96% of H_2SO_4; occurs as a colorless, odorless liquid of oily consistency; it is miscible with water and alcohol with the evolution of much heat, and is very caustic and corrosive. It is widely employed in the arts and sciences. Also called *oil of vitriol.*

diluted s. acid (*acidum sulfuricum dilutum*). An aqueous solution containing 10 Gm. of H_2SO_4 in each 100 cc.; occurs as a colorless, odorless liquid. It is used like other acids in gastric hypoacidity except that it is also astringent. Dose, 0.6–2 cc. (10–30 min.) taken through a glass tube.

sul'fu·rous. 1. Of the nature of sulfur. 2. Combined with sulfur; derived from sulfur dioxide.

sul'fu·rous ac'id. H_2SO_3. A solution of SO_2 in water. It has been used internally as a gastric antiseptic, and externally in the treatment of various skin diseases.

Sulkowitch reagent. See under *reagent.*

Sulkowitch's test. See under *test.*

sul'lage [OF. *soillage*]. Sewage.

Sullivan's test. See under *test.*

sul"pha·dim'i·dine, sul"pha·di'mi·dine. British Pharmacopoeia name for sulfamethazine.

sul"pha·fu'ra·zole. British generic name for the sulfonamide supplied under the trade-marked name gantrisin. Syn., *sulfisoxazole.*

sul'phate. Sulfate.

sul·phe"mo·glo"bi·ne'mi·a. Sulfhemoglobinemia.

sulphetrone. A trade-mark for 4,4′-bis(γ-phenyl-*n*-propylamino)-diphenylsulfone-tetrasodium sulfonate, a crystalline, water-soluble compound: used in the treatment of leprosy. See *solaprone.*

sul'phur. This spelling has been changed to *sulfur*, which is now official in the U. S. Pharmacopeia and in the publications of the American Chemical Society.

sum. *Sume*, take; *sumendus*, to be taken; used as direction in prescriptions.

su'mac, su'mach (sue'mack, shoo'mack) [Ar. *summāq*]. A name applied to various species of *Rhus* and *Toxicodendron.* Among the substances to which the irritant properties of the poison sumacs are ascribed are toxicodendrol, toxicodendrin, lobinol, urushiol. There is also present much tannin and fixed oil, resin, wax. Also see *poison sumac, poison sumac extract.*

s. wax. Japan wax.

sum'bul [Ar. *sunbul*] (*sumbul*). Consists of the dried rhizome and roots of *Ferula sumbul*, or of other closely related species of *Ferula* possessing a characteristic musklike odor. It contains resinous matter and a small portion of volatile oil. Formerly used in treatment of various hysterical conditions.

sum·ma'tion [L. *summa*, sum]. The accumulation of effects, especially of those of muscular, sensory, or mental stimuli. **—summational,** *adj.*

spatial s. Additive effect of subthreshold stimuli infringing on one neuron, resulting in a discharge from the neuron.

s. of stimuli. See spatial *s.*, temporal *s.*

temporal s. Cumulative effect of successive subthreshold stimuli on excitable tissue, resulting in a response. Most phenomena formerly believed to be due to temporal summation can be explained by spatial summation.

sum'mer e·rup'tion. Miliaria.

recurrent s. e. Hydroa vacciniforme.

Summerson-Barker method. See under *method.*

Sumner, F. W. [*English surgeon*, contemporary]. Discovered a sign indicative of cystic calculi, appendicitis, or a twisted pedicle of an ovarian cyst. A slight increase in abdominal muscle tonus is detected by very gentle palpation of the iliac fossa; this is known as *Sumner's sign.*

Sumner, James Batcheller (1887–1955). American biochemist known for being the first to crystallize enzymes. Nobel laureate (1946).

Sumner method. See under *method.*

Sumner-Somers method. See under *method.*

sun'burn" [AS. *sunne; baernan*]. 1. Discoloration of the skin due to exposure to the sun. 2. Inflammation of the skin, due to the action of the sun's rays, which may be of the first or second degree. **—sun'burn,** *v.*

sun lamp. A lamp designed to give off radiations similar to those received from the sun. A mercury arc produces radiations ranging in wavelength from infrared to visible and ultraviolet. A quartz bulb absorbs all ultraviolet radiations shorter than 2800 angstroms which are not present in sunlight.

sun spots. See *lentigo.*

sun'stroke" [*sunne;* ME. *strok*]. A form of heat stroke occurring on exposure to the sun. The body temperature rises because of faulty heat dissipation due to high environmental temperature and humidity as well as absorption of solar radiant energy. Rectal temperatures may go from 106° F. to 110° F. Syn., *insolation.*

su'per- [L., above]. A prefix denoting *above, upon,* or *excessive.*

su"per·ab·duc'tion [*super;* L. *abductio,* a forcible carrying off]. Excessive abduction; hyperabduction.

su"per·ac'id [*super;* L. *acidus,* sour]. 1. Excessively acid. 2. More acid than normal, as gastric contents.

su"per·a·cid'i·ty. Hyperacidity.

su"per·ac·tiv'i·ty [*super;* L. *activus,* active]. Hyperactivity.

su"per·a·cute' [*super;* L. *acutus,* pointed]. Extremely acute.

su"per·al·bu"mi·no'sis [*super;* L. *albus,* white; *-ōsis,* condition]. The overproduction of albumin.

su"per·al"i·men·ta'tion [*super;* L. *alimentum,* food]. Overfeeding; feeding beyond ordinary metabolic requirements.

su"per·al"ka·lin'i·ty [*super;* Ar. *al-kili,* ashes of saltwort]. Excessive alkalinity.

su·per'bus. Old name for the mentalis muscle.

su"per·cer"e·bel'lar [*super;* L. *cerebellum,* small brain]. Situated in the upper part of the cerebellum.

su"per·cil'i·um [L., eyebrow]. The eyebrow. —**superciliary,** *adj.*

su"per·di·crot'ic (·dye·krot'ick) [L. *super,* above; G. *dikrotos,* double-beating]. Hyperdicrotic.

su"per·dis·ten'tion [*super;* L. *distentio,* from *distendere,* to stretch out]. Excessive distention; hyperdistention.

su"per·duct' [L. *superducere,* to lead over]. Elevate; lead upward.

su"per·duc'tion [L. *superductio,* from *superducere*]. Maddox's term for sursumduction.

su"per·e'go [L. *super,* above; *ego,* I]. *In psychoanalysis,* that subdivision of the psyche which acts as the conscience of the unconscious. Its components are derived from both the id and the ego.

su"per·e·vac"u·a'tion [*super;* L. *evacuare,* to evacuate]. Excessive evacuation.

su"per·ex"ci·ta'tion [*super;* L. *excitatio,* from *excitare,* to rouse up]. Excessive excitement.

su"per·ex·ten'sion [*super;* L. *extensio,* from *extendere,* to stretch out]. Excessive extension; hyperextension.

su"per·fam'i·ly [*super;* L. *familia,* household]. *In biology,* a classification group which ranks next above a family.

su"per·fe"cun·da'tion [*super;* L. *fecundus,* fertile]. The fertilization of two or more ova, ovulated more or less simultaneously, by two or more successive coital acts not necessarily involving the same male.

su"per·fe·cun'di·ty [*super;* L. *fecunditas,* fertility]. Superabundant fertility.

su"per·fe·ta'tion, su"per·foe·ta'tion [*super;* L. *fetus,* fetus]. The production or development of a second fetus after one is already present in the uterus.

su"per·fi'cial (sue"pur·fish'ul) [L. *superficies,* outer surface]. Confined to or pertaining to the surface, as superficial fascia, a sheet of fatty areolar tissue under the skin.

su"per·fi'ci·es (sue"pur·fish'ee·eez, ·fish'eez) [L.]. The outer surface.

su"per·im"preg·na'tion [L. *super,* over; *in-,* in; *praegnans,* pregnant]. 1. Superfetation. 2. Superfecundation.

su"per·in·duce' [*super;* L. *inducere,* to bring into]. Add a new factor or a complication of a condition already existing.

su"per·in·fec'tion [*super;* L. *infectio,* from *inficere,* to infect]. A second or subsequent infection by the same microorganism, as seen in tuberculosis.

su"per·in"vo·lu'tion [*super;* L. *involutio,* from *involvere,* to roll up]. Hyperinvolution; excessive rolling up; return of the uterus after labor to less than normal size.

su·pe'ri·or [L., higher]. *In anatomy,* higher; denoting the upper of two parts; toward the vertex.

su·pe"ri·or'i·ty com'plex. A general attitude or character trait, often pathologic and usually arising out of an underlying feeling of inferiority, which is characterized by the occurrence of some form of real or assumed ascendancy and by feelings of conceit, vanity, envy, jealousy, or revenge.

su"per·lac·ta'tion [L. *super,* over; *lactare,* to give suck]. 1. Excess of the secretion of milk. 2. Excessive continuance of lactation.

su"per·le'thal [*super;* L. *letalis,* deadly]. Highly lethal or death dealing.

su"per·mo'ron [*super;* G. *mōros,* dull]. A person whose mentality is slightly below normal, but who is of higher grade than a moron.

su'per·nate [L. *supernans,* swimming above]. The fluid which remains after the removal of suspended matter by centrifugation or other physical or chemical means. —**superna'tant,** *adj.*

su"per·nor'mal [L. *super,* over; *norma,* rule]. 1. Pertaining to a faculty or phenomenon which is beyond the level of ordinary experience. 2. Superior to the average.

su"per·nu'mer·ar"y (sue"pur·new'mur·err"ee) [L. *supernumerarius,* supernumerary]. Existing in more than the usual number, as supernumerary mammary gland.

su"per·nu·tri'tion [L. *super,* over; *nutrire,* to nourish]. Excessive nourishment; hypernutrition. Nourishment in excess of ordinary metabolic requirements.

su'per·ol. See *oxyquinoline* sulfate.

su"per·ox'i·dized. Having an excess of oxygen above the usual amount which satisfies the combining capacities of the other elements of a body.

superoxol. Trade-mark for a 30% solution of hydrogen peroxide.

su"per·ox"y·gen·a'tion. Excessive oxygenation.

su"per·par'a·site [*super;* G. *parasitos,* parasite]. *In biology,* a parasite of parasites.

su"per·par"a·sit'ic [*super; parasitos*]. Pertaining to superparasitism.

su"per·par'a·si·tism (sue"pur·par'uh·sigh·tiz·um) [*super; parasitos*]. The infestation of parasites by other parasites.

su"per·phos'phate. An acid phosphate.

su"per·pig"men·ta'tion [*super;* L. *pigmentum,* color]. Excessive pigmentation.

su'per·salt" (sue'pur·sawlt"). An acid salt.

su"per·sat'u·rate. Saturate to excess; add more of a substance than a liquid can normally and permanently dissolve.

su"per·scrip'tion [L. *superscriptio,* superscription]. The sign ℞ (abbreviation of Latin *recipe,* take), at the beginning of a prescription.

su"per·se·cre'tion [L. *super,* over; *secretio,* from *secernere,* to separate]. Excessive secretion.

su"per·sen'si·tive [*super;* L. *sentire,* to feel]. Abnormally sensitive.

su"per·sen"si·ti·za'tion [*super; sentire*] Excessive

susceptibility to the action of a protein following its injection.

su″per·son′ic, su″pra·son′ic [*super;* L. *sonus,* sound]. Referring to waves of too high a frequency to produce sound that is audible to the human ear.

su″per·spi·na′tus (·spy·nay′tus) [*super;* L. *spina,* thorn]. *In veterinary medicine,* an extensor of the humerus which has no exact homolog in man.

su″per·ten′sion [*super;* L. *tendere,* to stretch]. Extreme tension. See *hypertension.*

su″per·ve·nos′i·ty [*super;* L. *venosus,* venous]. The condition in which the blood has become venous to a high degree.

su″per·ven′tion [L. *superventio,* from *supervenire,* to come upon, to be added to]. That which is added; a new, extraneous, or unexpected condition added to another, as the supervention of septicemia, or other complication in disease.

su″per·ver′sion. See *sursumversion.*

su′per·vi″sor. A supervising or head nurse.

su″pi·na′tion 1. The turning of the palm of the hand upward. 2. See *inversion* of the foot. 3. The condition of being supine; lying on the back. —**su′pinate,** *v.*

su′pi·na″tor, su″pi·na′tor [*supinare*]. A muscle of the forearm, which turns the radius outward. See Table of Muscles in the Appendix.

s. brevis. Old name for the supinator muscle.

su·pine′ [L. *supinus,* thrown backward]. Lying on the back face upward; or of the hand, palm upward: the opposite of *prone.*

sup″pe·da′ne·ous [L. *sub,* under; *pedaneus,* of the size of a foot]. Pertaining to the sole of the foot.

sup″pe·da′ne·um [L., footstool]. An application to the sole of the foot.

sup″ple·men′tal [L. *supplementum,* a filling up]. Additional.

sup·port′ [L. *supportare,* to carry]. 1. The act of holding anything in its position. 2. Any appliance acting as a support, as an arch support.

sup·port′er [*supportare*]. An apparatus intended to hold in place a low-hanging or prolapsed organ, as the uterus, the scrotum and its contents, the abdomen, etc., or to limit the use of certain joints, as the knee, ankle. See *pessary, jockey strap, binder, suspensory.*

sup·pos′i·to″ry (suh·poz′i·tor″ee) [L. *suppositorius,* that is placed underneath]. A medicated solid body of varying weight and shape, intended for introduction into different orifices of the body. Usually suppositories melt or are softened at body temperature; in some instances release of medication is effected through use of a hydrophilic vehicle. Typical vehicles or bases are theobroma oil, glycerinated gelatin, sodium stearate, and propylene glycol monostearate. Rectal suppositories weigh about 2 Gm. and are tapered. Urethral suppositories are pencil-shaped, pointed at one end, and are either 7 cm. in length, weighing about 2 Gm., or 14 cm. in length, weighing about 4 Gm. Vaginal suppositories are globular or oviform in shape and weigh about 5 Gm.

glycerin s. (*suppositoria glycerini*). Contains glycerin, 93 Gm.; sodium stearate, 9 Gm. to make about 30 adult rectal suppositories or 50 infant rectal suppositories. Used to produce fecal discharges in constipation. They act by locally irritating the mucous membranes of the rectum.

sup·pres′sion [L. *suppressio,* from *supprimere,* to press down]. 1. A sudden cessation of secretion, as of the urine, or of a normal process, as the menses. 2. *In psychiatry,* a mode of adjustment to urges and desires that are considered to be unacceptable, untenable, or unworthy, through attempting, consciously and thoughtfully, to control or prevent their occurrence or expression in consciousness. Also see *repression.*

sup′pu·rant [L. *suppurare,* to suppurate]. Promoting suppuration. —**sup′pu·rant,** *n.*

sup″pu·ra′tion [L. *suppuratio,* from *suppurare*]. The formation of pus. —**sup′purate,** *v.*

sup′pu·ra″tive [*suppurare*]. Producing pus. —**sup′purative,** *n.*

su′pra- [L., above]. A prefix signifying *upon* or *above.*

su″pra·cho′roid (sue″pruh·kor′oyd) [*supra;* G. *chorioeidēs,* choroid]. Situated above or upon the choroid coat of the eye.

su″pra·cla·vic′u·lar [*supra;* L. *clavicula,* little key]. Above the clavicle, as supraclavicular nerves. See Table of Nerves in the Appendix.

su″pra·cla·vic″u·lar′is pro′pri·us. A rare muscle extending from the acromial end of the clavicle and lying superficial to the trapezius and sternocleidomastoid muscles.

su″pra·cla·vic′u·lar mus′cle. A rare muscle, better called cleido-occipital muscle.

su″pra·con′dy·lar [*supra;* G. *kondylos,* knuckle]. Above a condyle, as the supracondylar ridge of the femur.

su″pra·con′dy·lism [*supra; kondylos*]. Upward deviation of the mandibular condyles.

su″pra·cos·ta′lis. One of a number of rare variant muscles associated with the serratus muscles; they may be anterior or posterior.

su″pra·gle′noid [*supra;* G. *glēnoeidēs,* like a socket]. Above the glenoid cavity, as the supraglenoid tubercle of the scapula.

su″pra·glot′tic [*supra;* G. *glōssa,* tongue]. Above the glottis.

su″pra·hy′oid [*supra;* G. *hyoeidēs,* shaped like the letter upsilon]. Above the hyoid bone, as a suprahyoid muscle.

su″pra·lim′i·nal [*supra;* L. *limen,* threshold]. Lying above a threshold.

su″pra·mar′gin·al [*supra;* L. *margo,* edge]. Above an edge or margin, as the supramarginal gyrus of the brain.

su″pra·mas′toid [*supra;* G. *mastoeidēs,* like a breast]. Above the mastoid process of the temporal bone.

su″pra·oc·clu′sion [*supra;* L. *occludere,* to close up]. That condition created by the abnormal elongation of teeth in their sockets.

su″pra·om″pha·lo·dym′i·a [*supra;* G. *omphalos,* navel; *didymos,* twin]. A form of conjoined twins in which the union is in the superior umbilical region. Syn., *gastropagus.*

su″pra·or′bit·al [*supra;* L. *orbita,* track]. 1. Above the orbit, as the supraorbital nerve. See Table of Nerves in the Appendix. 2. Pertaining to the supraorbital nerve.

su″pra·pa·tel′lar [*supra;* L. *patella,* small pan]. Above the patella.

su″pra·pu′bic [*supra;* L. *pubes,* private parts]. Above the pubes, as suprapubic prostatectomy.

su″pra·ren′-. For words beginning with *supraren-* not found here, see words beginning *adren-.*

su″pra·re′nal [*supra;* L. *renalis,* of the kidneys]. 1. The suprarenal gland. See adrenal *gland.* 2. (*suprarenalum.*) The dried, partially defatted and powdered suprarenal gland of cattle, sheep, or swine; occurs as a light yellow to brown amorphous powder; it is only partially soluble in water. Various investigations have led to the isolation of over twenty crystalline derivatives from adrenal cortical extracts. These compounds have been demonstrated to be steroid derivatives which are closely related to the hormones derived from the reproductive system. Among the more potent are aldosterone, desoxycorticosterone, and corticosterone. Also called *desiccated suprarenal, dried adrenal substance.*

su″pra·re″nal·ec′to·my [*supra; renalis;* G. *ektomē,* excision]. Adrenalectomy; removal of an adrenal or suprarenal gland.

su″pra·ren′al·in (sue″pruh·ren′ul·in, ·ree′nul·in). Epinephrine.

su″pra·re·na′lis ab″er·ra′ta of the o′va·ry. See adrenocorticoid *adenoma* of the ovary.

su″pra·re′nal·ism. See *adrenalism.*

su″pra·re″nal·op′a·thy [*supra; renalis;* G. *pathos,* disease]. A disordered condition resulting from disturbed function of the adrenal glands.

suprarenin. Trade-mark for a brand of epinephrine.

su″pra·scap′u·la [*supra;* L. *scapula,* shoulder blade]. An anomalous bone occasionally found between the superior border of the scapula and the spines of the lower cervical or first thoracic vertebrae, present in some cases of congenital elevation of the scapula: also called *omovertebral bone.*

su″pra·scap′u·lar [*supra;* L. *scapula,* shoulder]. Above or in the upper part of the scapula, as the suprascapular nerve. See Table of Nerves in the Appendix.

su″pra·scle′ral [*supra;* G. *sklēros,* hard]. Situated at or upon the outer surface of the sclera.

su″pra·sel′lar [*supra;* L. *sella,* seat]. Situated upon or above the sella turcica of the sphenoid bone.

su″pra·son′ic. See *supersonic.*

su″pra·spi·na′tus (sue″pruh·spy·nay′tus) [*supra;* L. *spina,* thorn]. A muscle originating above the spine of the scapula and inserted on the greater tubercle of the humerus. See Table of Muscles in the Appendix.

su″pra·spi′nous [*supra; spina*]. Above the spinous process of the scapula or of a vertebra.

su″pra·ster′nal [*supra;* G. *sternon,* breast]. Above the sternum, as suprasternal notch.

su″pra·ster′ol, su″pra·ste′rol. A type of sterol produced by the irradiation of ergosterol. Suprasterols are toxic.

su″pra·ton′sil·lar [*supra;* L. *tonsillae,* tonsils]. Above a tonsil, as supratonsillar abscess.

su″pra·troch′le·ar (sue″pruh·trock′lee·ur) [*supra;* L. *trochlea,* case containing pulleys]. Above the trochlea or pulley of the superior oblique muscle.

su″pra·ver′gence [*supra; vergere*]. Divergence of the two eyes in a vertical plane, measured by a prism of 2°–3°: also called *sursumvergence.* —**supraverge′,** *v.*

right s. The ability to overcome prisms, base down before the right eye, or base up before the left eye.

su″pra·vi′tal stain′ing. A method whereby cells may be stained and studied in the living state, of especial value in studying the immature leukocytes found in leukemia. Janus green, brilliant cresyl blue, and neutral red are stains commonly employed.

su′ra [L.]. The calf of the leg. —**sural,** *adj.*

sur″al·i·men·ta′tion [F. *sur,* from L. *super,* above; *alimentum,* food]. The method of forced feeding or overalimentation sometimes employed in pulmonary tuberculosis and other diseases.

sur·am′in, su′ram·in. $C_{51}H_{34}N_6O_{23}S_6Na_6$. British Pharmacopoeia title for the substance originally introduced as Bayer 205. It is the symmetrical urea of the sodium salt of *m*-benzoyl-*m*-amino-*p*-methylbenzoyl-1-aminonaphthalene-4,6,8-trisulfonic acid. A white or faintly cream-colored powder used in various trypanosome infections, especially African sleeping sickness, and in pemphigus. Toxic degeneration of the liver, spleen, kidneys, and adrenals has been reported from its use, as has agranulocytosis. Dose, 0.5 Gm. (7½ gr.) intravenously every other day, increased cautiously to 1 Gm. (15 gr.). Trade names are germanin, Fourneau 309, naganol, moranyl, and Bayer 205.

s. sodium. Name used in the United States for suramin. See *naphuride sodium.*

sur′di·tas. See *deafness.*

s. verbalis. See *aphasia.*

surd′i·ty [L. *surditas,* deafness]. Deafness.

sur″ex·ci·ta′tion (sur″eck·sigh·tay′shun) [*sur;* L. *excitatio,* from *excitare,* to rouse up]. Excessive excitement.

sur′face [F., from L. *superficies,* surface]. 1. The exterior of a body. 2. The face or faces of a body; a term frequently used in anatomy in the description of various structures.

buccal s. That of the crown of a tooth next the cheek.

contact s. That of a tooth facing an adjoining tooth mesially or distally; proximal surface.

distal s. That of the crown of a tooth away from the midline.

fixation s. A curved surface the points of which occupy, in the two monocular fields, positions which are identical horizontally, regardless of vertical disparity.

labial s. That of the crown of a tooth toward the lips.

lingual s. That of the crown of a tooth next the tongue.

mesial s. That of the crown of a tooth toward the midline.

occlusal s. That of the crown of a tooth toward its antagonists.

respiratory s. The entire surface of pulmonary tissue coming in contact with the respired air.

sur′face ten′sion. The contractile surface of a liquid by which it tends to assume a spherical form and to present the least possible surface (e.g., the formation of a meniscus). Abbreviated, S.T.

sur′geon [G. *cheirourgos,* working by hand]. 1. One who practices surgery. The term implies the possession of a medical degree and license and is used irrespective of the field or limitation of practice. 2. In the United States Army, the ranking officer of the Medical Corps in a military command.

attending s. One associated with the staff of a hospital, visiting the patients at specific times, performing major surgical operations, and supervising the postoperative care through directions to the house surgeon.

aural s. An otologist.

chief s. 1. The senior surgeon of a hospital or of a surgical team. 2. *In U. S. Army medicine,* the senior medical officer assigned to a general headquarters or to an expeditionary force as a staff officer.

contract s. *In military medicine,* a civilian who performs the professional and administrative functions of a medical officer, but without military rank or commission.

dental s. (a) One who limits his field to the surgery of the mouth and jaws. (b) *In U. S. Army medicine,* the military staff officer of the Dental Corps in charge of the dental service of an area command, unit, or installation. He performs his staff, professional, command, and administrative duties under the commanding officer or general of such area, unit, or installation to which he is assigned, and advises in matters of dental supply, operation, and training.

house s. A resident surgeon in a hospital.

plastic s. One who specializes in plastic surgery.

s. general. In the United States Armed Forces and Public Health Service, the ranking officer and head of the Medical Service or Department. In foreign armies, in some cases, the title denotes the chief medical officer of a department or command.

veterinary s. One whose practice is limited to the treatment of domestic, large and small animals, or to meat and food inspections on behalf of the national or state governments.

visiting s. A surgeon whose duties require regular attendance at a hospital or dispensary as well as emergency visits to operate upon or care for patients himself or to supervise the care given by house surgeons.

sur′ger·y [G. *cheirourgia*, a working by hand]. The branch of medicine dealing with diseases requiring operative procedure, including manipulation. See also *chemosurgery.* —**surgical,** *adj.*

antiseptic s. The application of antiseptic methods in the treatment of wounds.

aseptic s. Operative procedure in the absence of germs, everything coming in contact with the wound being sterile.

aural s. That pertaining to the ear.

battle s. Urgent surgery during active military operations in a forward area.

brain s. That pertaining to any part within the cranium.

cautery s. Use of cautery in surgical procedures, usually applied to benign and malignant growths of the skin.

clinical s. The practice of surgery in teaching.

conservative s. Measures directed to the preservation rather than the removal of a part.

dental s. That pertaining to the teeth and jaws.

general s. Surgery as a whole and not confined to a particular specialty.

major s. That in which the operations are important and involve risk to life.

military s. That pertaining to gunshot wounds and other injuries peculiar to military life.

minor s. That part of surgery including procedures not involving serious hazard to life and usually not requiring general anesthesia; examples are bandaging, application of splints and casts, suturing of superficial lacerations, excision, incision, and drainage of superficial structures.

operative s. That which refers to the performance of operations.

ophthalmic s. That pertaining to the eye and its appendages.

oral s. That branch of dental science which is concerned with surgical procedures involving structures concerned with the oral cavity, particularly the teeth and jaws.

orthopedic s. The remedy of skeletal deformities by manual and instrumental measures.

pelvic s. Surgery limited to the pelvic area.

plastic s. Repair of absent or defective tissue by transference of tissue from another part or person.

reparative s. Plastic surgery.

veterinary s. The surgery of animals.

sur′gi·cal team. 1. The group of individuals that carries out a surgical operation: it usually consists of a chief surgeon, assistants, surgical nurses, and anesthesiologist. 2. A team of doctors working as a unit who are proficient in certain surgical procedures.

Su″ri·nam′ bark (soor″i·nahm′, ·nam′). Cabbage tree bark; the bark of *Andira retusa*, which has been used as an anthelmintic in the West Indies.

surital sodium. Trade-mark for *thiamylal sodium.*

sur′ra (soor′uh, surr′uh) [Marathi *sūrra*, wheezing sound]. A term applied to those trypanosomiases of domestic animals in southeastern Asia which are caused by *Trypanosoma evansi.*

sur′ro·gate [L. *surrogare*, to substitute]. Any medicine used as a substitute for a more expensive one, or for one to which there is a special objection in any particular case.

sur″sum·duc′tion [L. *sursum*, upward; *ducere*, to lead]. 1. The power of the two eyes of fusing two images when one eye has a prism placed vertically before it. 2. See *supravergence.* 3. A movement of either eye alone upward.

right s. The absolute power that the right eye has to rotate upward.

sur″sum·ver′gence [*sursum;* L. *vergere*, to turn]. The turning of the eyes upward; supravergence. Anoopsia.

sur″sum·ver′sion [*sursum;* L. *vertere*, to turn]. The upward movement of both eyes.

sur·vi′vor·ship [L. *supervivere*, to survive]. *In legal medicine*, the living of one of two or more persons after the death of the other or others.

SUSA fixing fluid. See under *fixing fluid.*

sus·cep″ti·bil′i·ty [L. *suscipere*, to take up]. The opposite of immunity. A characteristic rendering an individual liable to acquire a disease if exposed to the causative agent. Susceptibility may be increased by certain traits, as racial, familial.

sus·cep′ti·ble [*suscipere*]. Sensitive to impression or influence. *In immunology*, said especially of one who has neither natural nor acquired immunity to a disease.

sus″cep·tiv′i·ty. Susceptibility.

sus′ci·tate [L. *suscitare*, to arouse]. Increase activity, stimulate.

sus·pend′ed [L. *suspendere*, to hang]. 1. Hanging; applied to any structure attached to or hanging from another structure, and attached by a pedicle or cord. 2. Interrupted.

sus·pen′sion [L. *suspensio*, from *suspendere*]. 1. Hanging or fixation in a higher position; a method of treatment, as suspension of the uterus. 2. *In chemistry and pharmacy*, a dispersion of solid particles throughout the body of a liquid.

tendon s. Tenodesis.

sus·pen′soid. An apparent solution which is seen, by the microscope, to consist of small particles of the solute in active Brownian movement.

sus″pen·so′ri·um [*suspendere*]. Old term for that upon which anything hangs for support.

s. hepatis. The coronary ligament of the liver.

s. testis. The cremaster muscle.

s. vesicae. The superior false ligament of the urinary bladder.

sus·pen′so·ry [*suspendere*]. Serving for suspension or support, as suspensory ligament, or suspensory bandage.

sus·pen′so·ry. 1. A device for suspending a part, as the scrotum. 2. A jockey strap.

sus″pi·ra′tion [L. *suspiratio*, from *suspirare*, to sigh]. 1. A sigh. 2. The act of sighing.

sus″ten·tac′u·lum [L., support]. A support. —**sustentacular,** *adj.*

s. tali. A process of the calcaneus supporting the talus.

su″sur·ra′tion [L. *susurratio*, from *susurrare*, to murmur]. A murmur, or susurrus.

su·sur′rus [L., a murmuring]. A soft murmur in aneurysm, cardiac diseases, contracting muscle, etc.

s. aurium. See *tinnitus.*

Sutton, Henry Gawen [*English physician*, 1837–1891]. Described arteriocapillary fibrosis. Generalized arteriosclerosis is called *Gull and Sutton's disease.*

Sutton, Richard Lightburn [*American dermatologist*, 1878–]. With his son, R. L. Sutton, Jr., author of standard works in dermatology. Described a type of leukoderma called *Sutton's disease, leukoderma acquisitum centrifugum.*

su·tu′ra (pl. *suturae*) [L., a sewing together]. A suture.

s. dentata. One with toothlike interlocking processes, as the suture between the parietal bones.
s. harmonia. One in which there is simple apposition of contiguous rough surfaces.
s. limbosa. An interlocking suture, with beveling and overlapping of the articular surfaces, as in the coronal suture.
s. notha. A false suture; includes sutura squamosa and sutura harmonia.
s. serrata. One in which the edges of the bones are saw-toothed.
s. squamosa. One formed by the overlapping of contiguous bones by broad, beveled margins.
s. vera. A true suture, one in which the margins of the bones are connected by a series of processes and indentations interlocked together.

u'tur·al (sue'chur·ul) [*sutura*]. Pertaining to, or having the nature of, a suture.

u'ture. To close a wound by sewing.

u'ture [*sutura*]. 1. *In osteology*, a line of junction or closure between bones, as a cranial suture. 2. *In surgery*, fine, cordlike structures used to close a wound. The term may mean either the material used, as gut, silk, etc., or the method of using the suture, as interrupted, mattress, etc. There are two main types of materials: absorbable, such as catgut, which are placed in deep tissue, and nonabsorbable, which usually are removed, as silk, linen, wire, etc., though some are used and left in deep tissue. See Plate 40.
approximating s. One placed in deep tissue to pull together the edges of the wound.
basilar s. That formed by the junction of the basilar process of the occipital bone with the posterior surface of the body of the sphenoid.
bulb s. Technic employed where, after resection, the nerve cannot be sutured without undue tension. The neighboring joint is flexed and the untrimmed nerve ends are laid side by side with as much overlap as possible, and united by strong sutures; the wound is closed, and gradual extension is then effected with elongation of the nerve.
buried s. One completely covered by, and not involving, the skin.
button s. A mattress suture which includes a button on either side of the wound to prevent cutting of the skin by the suture.
catgut s. One in which the material employed is catgut.
chainstitch s. One made with the sewing machine stitch.
circular s. One that is applied to the entire circumference of a divided part, as the intestine.
coapting s. One which brings the divided skin edges accurately together.
continuous s. One in which the suture material is continued from one end of the wound to the other; may be of several types, the plain over-and-over sewing stitch being most common. See Plate 40.
coronal s. The union of the frontal with the parietal bones transversely across the vertex of the skull.
Czerny's s. See Vincenz *Czerny*.
dentate s. An irregular notched suture, as that between the parietal bones.
dermal s. A fine linen suture impregnated with various chemicals used when a fine scar is desired.
ethmofrontal s. The union between the frontal and ethmoid bones.
ethmolacrimal s. The union between the lacrimal and ethmoid bones.
ethmosphenoidal s. See sphenoethmoidal *s.*
false s. Any suture in which there is interlocking of the bones without serration.
frontal s. A suture which at birth joins the two frontal bones from the vertex to the root of the nose, but which afterward becomes obliterated. Syn., *metopic s.*
frontoethmoidal s. One between the frontal and ethmoid bones.
frontomalar s. The union between the frontal and zygomatic bones.
frontomaxillary s. The union between the maxillary and the frontal bones.
frontonasal s. The union between the nasal and frontal bones.
frontoparietal s. See coronal *s.*
frontosphenoid s. See sphenofrontal *s.*
frontotemporal s. The union between the temporal and frontal bones.
frontozygomatic s. The union between the frontal and zygomatic bones.
harelip s. One in which the edges of the wound are transfixed with pins and approximation secured by twisting or wrapping the ends of the pins with thread.
incisive s. That between the premaxilla and maxilla in the embryo and fetus; union usually occurs before birth. It is rarely visible in the adult.
intermaxillary s. The union between the maxillary bones.
internasal s. The union between the nasal bones.
interparietal s. The sagittal suture, or that formed by the approximation of the parietal bones.
interrupted s. A type in which each stitch is tied and cut individually. See Plate 40.
lambdoid s. The union between the two superior borders of the occipital and the parietal bones.
longitudinal s. See sagittal *s.*
mattress s. One in which the needle, after being drawn through both skin edges, is reinserted on the same side and drawn through the original side again. This may be continuous or interrupted. See Plate 40.
maxillolacrimal s. The union between the lacrimal and maxillary bones.
metopic s. The frontal suture, between the two vertical halves of the frontal bone. Syn., *frontal s.*
nasofrontal s. The frontonasal suture.
nasomaxillary s. The union between the maxillary and nasal bones.
occipital s. See lambdoid *s.*
occipitomastoid s. The union between the mastoid portion of the temporal bone and the occipital bone.
occipitoparietal s. See lambdoid *s.*
palatine s. The union between the palate bones.
palatomaxillary s. A suture between the horizontal part of the os palatinum and the palatine process of the maxilla.
parietomastoid s. The union between the mastoid portion of the temporal bone and the parietal bone.
petro-occipital s. The union between the occipital bone and the petrous portion of the temporal.
petrosphenoid s. The union between the great wing of the sphenoid bone and the petrous portion of the temporal: also called *sphenopetrosal s.*
plicating s. A running stitch which is pulled together as a gathering string to shorten the distance between two points.
primary s. One done at the time of injury or operation.
purse-string s. A running stitch placed in a circle and pulled together to close an opening.
quill s. Similar to a button suture except that the sutures are tied over a quill, or a roll of cotton.
relaxing s. One placed deep to and at a distance from the wound to relieve tension.
rhabdoid s. The sagittal suture.

sagittal s. The union between the superior borders of the parietal bones.

secondary s. One done some time after the time of injury or operation. Also called *delayed s.*

shotted s. One in which each end of the suture is passed through a perforated shot and then drawn tight.

sphenoethmoidal s. The union between the sphenoid and ethmoid bones.

sphenofrontal s. The union between a great wing of the sphenoid bone and the frontal bone.

sphenomalar s. The union between the zygomatic bone and the great wing of the sphenoid.

sphenopalatine s. A cranial suture between the sphenoid and palatine bones.

sphenoparietal s. The union between the great wing of the sphenoid bone and the parietal bone.

sphenosquamosal s. That between the great wing of the sphenoid and the squamous portion of the temporal bone.

sphenotemporal s. The union between the temporal and the sphenoid bones.

sphenozygomatic s. The union between the zygomatic bone and the great wing of the sphenoid.

squamoparietal s. The union between the squamous portion of the temporal bone and the parietal bone. Also called *squamosal s.*

squamosphenoid s. The union between the great wing of the sphenoid and the squamous portion of the temporal bone: also called *sphenosquamosal s.*

subcuticular s. A buried, continuous suture in which the needle is passed horizontally into the true skin back and forth until the wound is closed.

tension s. One made at a distance from the wound edge and through the deeper tissues, to lessen the strain on the skin suture.

transfixion s. A method of closing a wound by the use of a pin or needle which is placed through both wound edges and held by winding suture material over both ends in a figure-of-eight fashion. Also called *figure-of-eight s., harelip s. Rare.*

Svedberg, Theodor (1884–). Swedish chemist who developed an ultracentrifuge and a procedure for determining large molecular weights of organic substances, e.g., proteins and resins, by measuring the sedimentation equilibrium in the ultracentrifuge. Nobel laureate in chemistry, 1926. See Svedberg flotation *unit*, Folin and Svedberg's *method.*

swab [D. *zwabber*]. A piece of cloth, sponge, or cotton upon the end of a stick, used in feeding the sick, making applications to the throat, cleansing the mouth and teeth, etc.

NIH s. A small square of cellophane folded around the end of a glass rod and held in place by a rubber band, developed by the National Institutes of Health and used in collecting the ova of *Enterobius* or other ova from the perianal region.

swab stick. A rod or shaft, one extremity of which is to be wound with cotton; a cotton stick.

swage [OF. *souage*]. A counter-die used in shaping thin metal. See *swaging.* —**swage,** *v.*

swag′ing [*souage*]. Conforming a thin metal plate to the shape of a model, cast, or die by the aid of a counter-die, the swage.

swal′low·ing [AS. *swelgan*]. Deglutition; the act of taking into the stomach through the esophagus.

air s. See *aerophagia.*

tongue s. A condition in which there is an abnormal flaccidity of the tongue, so that it falls backward, giving rise to danger of suffocation.

Swammerdam, Jan [*Dutch physician and naturalist,* 1637–80]. Pioneer microscopist, said to have been the first to observe the red blood cells. Discovered the valves of the lymphatics (1664). Made important entomologic studies.

sway′-back″. See *lordosis.*

sweat [AS. *swǣtan*]. The secretion of the sudoriferous glands, consisting of a transparent, colorless, aqueous fluid, holding in solution neutral fats, volatile fatty acids, traces of albumin and urea, free lactic acid, sodium lactate, sodium chloride, potassium chloride, and traces of alkaline phosphates, sugar, ascorbic acid, etc. Its excretion, largely by the cooling effect of evaporation, helps regulate the temperature of the body.

bloody s. See *hemathidrosis.*

blue s. Perspiration which has a blue color.

colliquative s. A profuse clammy sweat.

colored s. Chromhidrosis.

excessive s. Hyperhidrosis.

fetid s. See *bromhidrosis.*

green s. Sweat having a bluish or greenish color, seen mainly in copper workers; may be due to copper taken into the system.

night s. Drenching perspiration occurring at night or whenever the patient sleeps, in the course of pulmonary tuberculosis or other diseases.

phosphorescent s. A very rare peculiarity of the sweat, in which it becomes phosphorescent; it has been observed in some cases of malaria and after eating fish containing phosphorescent microorganisms.

red s. A peculiar, red perspiration noted in the axillas and genital region, and due to microorganisms which have developed on the hairs of these warm, moist parts. See *trichomycosis* rubra.

Swediaur, François Xavier [*Austrian physician,* 1748–1824]. Described inflammation of the Achilles bursa, called *achillodynia, Albert's disease, Swediaur's disease.*

Swe′dish move′ments. Gymnastics according to a system originating in Sweden and adapted to the health needs of individuals, especially for those having postural deformities.

swee′ny [perhaps from Ger. dial. *schweine*]. A wasting or atrophy of the scapular muscles of the horse, usually due to an injury of the nerve supply. Also called *swinney.*

swel′ling [AS. *swellan*]. 1. Any morbid enlargement, inflation, or abnormal protuberance. 2. *In embryology,* a small eminence or ridge.

arytenoid s. An eminence on either side of the primitive embryonic glottis that fuses with the hypobranchial eminence.

bulbar s. One of the endocardial ridges of the embryonic bulbus cordis.

Calabar swellings. Edematous, egg-shaped, distended areas occurring in different parts of the body of natives of Calabar and other parts of West Africa. It is thought to be produced by the action of *Filaria loa* in the subcutaneous tissues.

cloudy s. Parenchymatous degeneration; a retrogressive change in cytoplasm of parenchymatous cells, as glandular epithelium, endothelial cells, and leukocytes, whereby the cell enlarges, the outline becomes irregular. In fresh tissue the nucleus is obscured, and the cytoplasm becomes coarsely granular. The basic change is imbibition of water, with agglomeration of protein particles and dispersal of lipid protein combinations.

genital s. See labioscrotal *s.*

glassy s. Amyloid degeneration.

labioscrotal s. The eminence or ridge on either side of the base of the embryonic phallus that is the primordium of half the scrotum in the male or of a labium majus in the female: also called *labial s., torus genitalis.*

lateral lingual s. One of the paired swellings of

the floor of the first visceral arch that form the primordia of the oral part of the tongue.

sexual s. See labioscrotal *s.*

white s. *In orthopedics*, enlargement of a joint or part without increased local heat or redness; usually due to tuberculosis.

Swift, W. Contemporary Australian physician who described acrodynia, also called *Swift's disease, pink disease.* See *erythredema polyneuropathy.*

Swift-Ellis treatment. See under *treatment.*

swine plague. 1. The term applied to hemorrhagic septicemia of swine caused by *Pasteurella suiseptica.* The disease is characterized by a pleuropneumonia with focal necrosis and occasionally by septicemia. 2. Hog cholera.

swiv'el stir'rup. An apparatus fashioned like a stirrup and used by attaching it to a Steinmann pin for traction in leg fractures.

sy·co'ma (sigh·ko'muh) [G., ulcer resembling a fig]. A condyloma, or wart.

sy'cose. Saccharin.

sy·co'si·form (sigh·ko'si·form) [G. *sykōsis*, ulcer resembling a fig; L. *forma*, form]. Resembling sycosis.

sy·co'sis (sigh·ko'sis) [G.]. An inflammatory disease affecting the hair follicles, particularly of the beard, and characterized by papules, pustules, and tubercles, perforated by hairs, together with infiltration of the skin and crusting. Also called *s. coccogenica, s. staphylogenes, folliculitis barbae, s. mentagra.* See Plate 31.

hypertrophic s. See keloid *s.*

hyphogenic s. Tinea barbae, the inflammation excited by the trichophyta, usually of the ectothrix type.

keloid s. Sycosis in which keloid degeneration occurs in the cicatrices resulting from the follicular inflammation. Also called *ulerythema sycosiforme.*

lupoid s. See keloid *s.*

nonparasitic s. Sycosis due to the presence of coccogenic organisms.

parasitic s. See *s.* parasitica.

s. barbae. Sycosis of the beard.

s. capillitii. Dermatitis papillaris capillitii, of Kaposi; sycosis framboesiformis, of Hebra; acne keloid, of Bazin.

s. contagiosa. See *s.* parasitica.

s. framboesiformis. See *dermatitis* papillaris capillitii.

s. palpebrae marginalis. Sycosis affecting the edge of the eyelids.

s. parasitica. Achor barbaratus, barbers' itch; a disease of the hair follicles, usually affecting the region covered by the beard and due to the presence of various trichophyta. Also see hyphogenic *s.*

s. vulgaris. A pustular, follicular lesion caused by a staphylococcus.

Sydenham, Thomas [*English physician*, 1624–89]. Described measles and differentiated it from scarlet fever. Wrote a classic description of gout. See also *chorea.*

syl·lab'ic ut'ter·ance. Scanning speech, as in multiple sclerosis; words are enunciated slowly and separately and there may be a staccato accentuation of some syllables.

syl'la·ble-stum'bling. A form of dysphasia wherein each sound and syllable can be distinctly uttered, but the word as a whole is spoken with difficulty. Occurs in dementia paralytica.

syl'la·bus [erron. reading from G. *sittyba*, strip of parchment]. 1. A compendium containing the heads of a discourse. 2. The main propositions of a course of lectures. 3. An abstract.

syl·lep"si·ol'o·gy [G. *syllēpsis*, pregnancy; *logos*, word]. The physiology of conception and pregnancy. *Obs.*

syl·lep'sis [G.]. Conception, or impregnation. *Obs.*

sylnasol. Trade-mark for an aqueous solution containing 5% of sodium psylliate: used as a sclerosing agent for obliteration of varicose veins.

syl·vat'ic plague. A name used in the U.S.A. for a bubonic plague transmitted by fleas from squirrels, chipmunks, and other rodents in California, Montana, and other western states. The disease is gradually spreading eastward among wild rodents, according to reports of the United States Public Health Service.

Sylvius, Franciscus (de le Boë) [*Dutch physician*, 1614–72]. Wrote classic description of pulmonary tuberculosis. Described the cerebral aqueduct, called *aqueduct of Sylvius.* See also Sylvian *angle;* lateral cerebral *fissure.*

Sylvius, Jacobus (Jacques Du Bois) [*French anatomist*, 1478–1555]. Described the lenticular process, called *Sylvian ossicle* or *bone.* Probably the first to describe the auditory tube, which was called the *Sylvian valve.* Said to have been a teacher of Vesalius. He is often confused with Franciscus Sylvius.

sym-. See *syn-.*

sym·bal'lo·phone [G. *symballein*, to throw together; *phōnē*, sound]. A stethoscope equipped with two chest pieces for simultaneous use as a special aid in localizing or in comparing sounds.

sym'bi·on, sym'bi·ont [G. *symbios*, living together]. An organism living in symbiosis.

sym"bi·o'sis [G., a living together with]. A more or less intimate association or union between organisms of different species. In the restricted sense of the term, the organisms are mutually benefited and sometimes so dependent on each other that life apart is impossible. Symbiosis includes commensalism in which neither organism is injured and one may receive benefit, and parasitism in which the relation is detrimental to one organism, the host, and beneficial to the other, the parasite. Various gradations occur so that rigid classification cannot be maintained. —**symbiot'ic,** *adj.*

sym·bleph'a·ron [G. *syn*, with; *blepharon*, eyelid]. Adhesions of the eyelids to the eyeball.

anterior s. Occurs when the edge of the lid is adherent.

posterior s. Occurs when the adhesion is near the conjunctival fornix.

total s. Occurs when the entire lid is adherent.

sym·bleph"a·ro'sis [*syn; blepharon;* G. *-ōsis*, condition]. Adhesion of the eyelids to the globe of the eye or to each other.

sym'bol [G. *symbolon*, pledge]. 1. A sign or character denoting an idea. See Table of Medical Signs and Symbols in the Appendix. 2. *In chemistry*, a conventional abbreviation of the name of an element, generally consisting of the initial letter or letters of the name in Latin or English. It denotes one atom of the element.

sym·bo'li·a [*symbolon*]. The ability to recognize an object by the sense of touch.

sym'bol·ism [*symbolon*]. The delusional or hallucinational interpretation of all events or objects as having a mystic significance, a habit not uncommon in certain forms of insanity.

sym"bol·i·za'tion [*symbolon*]. *In psychiatry*, the process by which mental disorder is expressed by substitute devices, as in dreams, the meaning of which is not clear to the conscious mind.

Syme, James [*Scottish surgeon*, 1799–1870]. Early advocate of ether anesthesia (1847–48). Operated for stricture of the urethra and perineal fistula (1849) and for iliac aneurysm (1862). See also Syme's *amputation.*

sy·me'li·a [G. *syn*, with; *melos*, limb]. A coalescence of the lower extremities. See *sympodia, sympus.*

sym′e·lus, sym′me·lus. Sympus.

sym′me·try [G. *symmetria*, symmetry]. *In anatomy*, a harmonious correspondence of parts; also the relation of homologous parts at opposite sides or ends of the body. —**symmet′ric,** *adj.*

bilateral s. Correspondence of both halves of an organism.

sym″pa·ral′y·sis [*syn;* G. *paralysis*, paralysis]. Conjugate paralysis, a term given to the abolition of certain synkineses of the eye.

sym″pa·thec′to·my, sym·path″i·cec′to·my [G. *sympathein*, to feel for; *ektomē*, excision]. Excision of a portion of the autonomic or sympathetic nervous system.

lumbodorsal s. Surgical removal of a portion or all of the lumbar and thoracic ganglia of the sympathetic trunk.

sym·path″e·o·neu·ri′tis [*sympathein;* G. *neuron*, nerve; *-itis*, inflammation]. See *sympathiconeuritis.*

sym″pa·thet′ic [*sympathein*]. 1. Pertaining to or produced by sympathy. 2. Pertaining to the sympathetic nervous system.

sym″pa·thet′ic. The sympathetic nervous system.

sym″pa·thet″i·co·mi·met′ic (·mi·met′ick, ·mighmet′ick) [*sympathein;* G. *mimētikos*, imitative]. See *sympathomimetic.*

sym″pa·thet″i·co·to′ni·a. See *sympathicotonia.*

sym″pa·thet″i·co·ton′ic [*sympathein;* G. *tonos*, tension]. Pertaining to the state of sympathicotonia.

sym″pa·thet″i·co·to′nus. See *sympathicotonia.*

sym″pa·thet′o·blast [*sympathein;* G. *blastos*, germ]. Sympathoblast.

sym·path′ic. See *sympathetic.*

sym·path″i·cec′to·my. See *sympathectomy.*

sym·path″i·co·blas·to′ma. A malignant tumor, composed of embryonal sympathetic nerve cells, which characteristically grows rapidly and metastasizes freely. Some tumors concentrate metastases in lymph nodes and liver (**Pepper type**); others metastasize to bone, particularly in the cranium, sometimes resulting in orbital tumors which displace the globe (**Hutchinson type**). Histologically the cells are collected into groups which have a supportive fibrous framework between them. Sympathicoblastomas show a wide range of differentiation, variously called *typical s.* (those with pseudorosettes) or *atypical s.*, *sympathogonioma* (undifferentiated type), *gangliosympathicoblastoma,* (*sympathetic*) *neuroblastoma, neurocytoma, sympathicogonioma, sympathoblastoma, sympathoma* (*embryonale*).

sym·path″i·co·cy·to′ma. See *ganglioneuroma.*

sym·path″i·co·go″ni·o′ma. See *sympathicoblastoma.*

sym·path″i·co·neu·ri′tis [*sympathein;* G. *neuron*, nerve; *-itis*, inflammation]. Inflammation of the sympathetic system, particularly the sympathetic ganglionated chain.

sym·path″i·cop′a·thy [*sympathein;* G. *pathos*, disease]. A disordered condition resulting from disturbance of the sympathetic nervous system.

sym·path″i·co·to′ni·a [*sympathein;* G. *tonos*, tension]. Domination of body functions by the sympathetic nervous system, manifested by goose flesh, increased blood pressure, vascular spasm.

sym·path′i·co·trip″sy (sim·path′i·ko·trip″see, sim·path″i·ko·trip′see) [*sympathein;* G. *tripsis*, a rubbing]. Surgically crushing the superior cervical ganglion. *Obs.*

sym·path″i·co·trop′ic [*sympathein;* G. *trepein*, to turn]. Possessing affinity for the sympathetic nervous system.

sym·path′i·cus [*sympathein*]. The sympathetic nervous system.

sym′pa·thin [*sympathein*]. A hormone similar to epinephrine, believed to be formed in the muscle cells by nerve impulses. Causes augmentation of blood pressure and heart rate.

s. E A postulated form of sympathin causing excitation and formed by combination of a chemical mediator released at sympathetic nerve endings with a hypothetical substance in excited effector cells. It is probably norepinephrine.

s. I A postulated form of sympathin causing inhibition; formed by combination of a chemical mediator released at sympathetic nerve endings with a hypothetical substance in inhibited effector cells.

sym′pa·thism [*sympathein*]. Susceptibility to hypnotic suggestion. —**sympathist,** *n.*

sym′pa·thi″zer [*sympathein*]. An eye with sympathetic ophthalmia.

sym·path′o·blast [*sympathein;* G. *blastos*, germ]. Embryonic sympathetic nerve cell which differentiates into the characteristic sympathetic ganglion cell. It is larger than the sympathogonia, with a less dense nucleus, more cytoplasm, and often a short cytoplasmic process.

sym·path″o·blas·to′ma. See *sympathicoblastoma.*

sym·path″o·chro′maf·fin (sim·path″o·kro′muhfin, ·kro·maf′in, sim″puth·o·) [*sympathein;* G. *chrōma*, color; L. *affinis*, taking part in]. Pertaining to sympathetic nerve cells which exhibit a chromaffin reaction.

sym·path″o·go′ni·a [*sympathein;* G. *gonē*, offspring]. Primitive cells of the sympathetic nervous system derived from neuroblasts of the ganglionic crest of the neural tube. They have dense nuclei, rich in chromatin, and only a thin rim of cytoplasm, and differentiate to form along one line ganglion cells and along another line chromaffin cells. Also called *sympathogone.*

sym·path″o·go″ni·o′ma. See *sympathicoblastoma.*

sym·path″o·lyt′ic [*sympathein;* G. *lysis*, a loosing]. Pertaining to an effect antagonistic to the activity produced by stimulation of the sympathetic system; the opposite of sympathomimetic.

sym·pa·tho′ma. See *sympathicoblastoma.*

sym·path″o·mi·met′ic (sim·path″o·mi·met′ick, ·migh·met′ick, sim″puth·o·) [*sympathein;* G. *mimētikos*, imitative]. Having the power to cause physiologic changes similar to those produced by action of the sympathetic nervous system.

sym′pa·thy [G. *sympatheia*, sympathy]. The mutual relation between parts more or less distant, whereby a change in the one has an effect upon the other.

sym·pet′al·ous [G. *syn*, with; *petalon*, leaf]. *In botany*, having the petals united.

sym·pex′i·on [G. *sympēxis*, a putting together, coagulation]. A concretion found in the seminal vesicles. Also called *sympexis.*

sym·phal′an·gism [G. *syn*, with; *phalagx*, finger]. Inherited condition of stiff fingers, or ankylosed finger joints.

sym″phy·o·ceph′a·lus [G. *symphyein*, to grow together; *kephalē*, head]. Conjoined twins united by their heads. Also called *cephalopagus, craniopagus, syncephalus.*

sym″phy·si·ec′to·my (sim″fiz·ee·eck′to·mee) [G. *symphysis*, a growing together; *ektomē*, excision]. Excision of the symphysis pubis for the purpose of facilitating delivery. *Obs.*

sym·phys′i·on (sim·fiz′ee·on) [*symphysis*]. The most anterior point of the alveolar process of the lower jaw, used as a craniometric point.

sym″phy·si·or′rha·phy (sim″fiz·ee·or′uh·fee) [*symphysis;* G. *rhaphē*, suture]. Suture of a divided symphysis.

sym·phys′i·o·tome″ (sim·fiz′ee·o·tome″) [*symphysis;* G. *tomos*, cutting]. An instrument used in performing symphysiotomy.

sym″phy·si·ot′o·my (sim″fiz·ee·ot′o·mee) [*symphysis;* G. *tomē,* a cutting]. The dividing of the symphysis pubis for the purpose of increasing the diameters of the pelvic canal and facilitating labor. *Obs.*

sym′phy·sis (sim′fi·sis) (pl. *symphyses*) [G., a growing together]. A synarthrosis, especially one in the sagittal plane. —**symphys′eal,** *adj.*

s. cartilaginosa. Synchondrosis.

s. ligamentosa. Syndesmosis.

s. mandibulae. The midline osteochondral union of the halves of the mandible.

s. pubis. The fibrocartilaginous union (synchondrosis) of the pubic bones. See Plates 2, 13.

sym″phy·so·dac·tyl′i·a (sim″fi·so·dack·til′ee·uh, sim″fi·zo·). See *syndactyly.*

sym″phy·sop′si·a (sim″fi·zop′see·uh). See *cyclopia.*

sym″phy·so·ske′li·a [*symphysis;* G. *skelos,* leg]. The condition in which the lower extremities are united. See *sympus.*

sym′plasm. A multinucleate protoplasmic mass resulting from the coalescence of originally separate cells, as in certain giant cells.

sym·po′di·a [G. *sympous,* with the feet together]. The condition of united lower extremities. See *sympus.*

symp′tom [G. *symptōma,* anything that happens]. A phenomenon of disease which leads to complaints on the part of the patient; a subjective sign in contrast to one which is objective.

accessory s. A minor symptom. Also called *assident s.*

accidental s. One intervening in the course of a disease without having any connection with it.

concomitant symptoms. Accessory phenomena occurring in connection with the essential phenomena of a disease.

constitutional s. One produced by the effect of the disease on the whole body. Also called *general s.*

delayed s. See *shock,* 1.

direct s. One depending directly upon disease.

dissociation s. Anesthesia to pain and to heat and cold, with preservation of tactile sensibility and of the muscular sense; observed in syringomyelia.

equivocal s. One of doubtful significance.

focal s. One occurring at a given site.

halo s. The colored circles seen around lights in glaucoma.

indirect s. One only indirectly due to disease.

labyrinthine symptoms. A group of symptoms due to lesion or disease of the internal ear.

local s. One indicating the concentration of a disease in a certain part of the body.

negatively pathognomonic s. One which never occurs in a certain disease and therefore by its presence shows the absence of that disease.

passive s. See static *s.*

pathognomonic s. A symptom which exhibits itself only in a certain disease and therefore undeniably proves its presence.

signal s. The first disturbance of sensation preceding a more extensive convulsion, as the aura heralding an attack of epilepsy.

static s. A symptom which indicates the condition in a single organ without reference to the rest of the body.

sympathetic symptoms. Symptoms for which no adequate cause can be given other than so-called sympathy.

withdrawal symptoms. See withdrawal *syndrome.*

symp″to·mat′ic [G. *symptōmatikos,* accidental]. 1. Pertaining to, or of the nature of, a symptom. 2. Affecting symptoms, as symptomatic treatment.

symp″tom·a·tog′ra·phy [G. *symptōma,* anything that happens; *graphein,* to write]. A written or printed description of symptoms.

symp″tom·a·tol′o·gy [*symptōma;* G. *logos,* word], 1. The science of symptoms. 2. In common usage. the symptoms of disease taken together as a whole. —**symptomatolog′ic,** *adj.*

symp′tom com′plex. The ensemble of symptoms of a disease. Also see *syndrome.*

Avellis' s. c. Paralysis of one half of the soft palate, associated with a recurrent laryngeal nerve paralysis on the same side.

Bernhardt-Roth's s. c. See *meralgia* paresthetica.

Erb-Goldflam's s. c. Myasthenia gravis.

Escherich's s. c. See *pseudotetanus.*

Friedmann's vasomotor s. c. A train of symptoms following injury to the head, consisting of headache, vertigo, nausea, and intolerance of mental and physical exertions and of galvanic excitation; it is occasionally associated with ophthalmoplegia and mydriasis. These phenomena may subside and recur with greater intensity, with fever, unconsciousness, and paralysis of the cranial nerves, ending in fatal coma. They are probably due to an encephalitis of slow development with acute exacerbations.

Hoppe-Goldflam s. c. Old term for myasthenia gravis.

Putnam-Dana's s. c. Subacute combined degeneration of the spinal cord.

Roth's s. c. See *meralgia* paresthetica.

Wilks's s. c. Old term for myasthenia gravis.

symp′tom group′ing, symp′tom group. See *symptom complex.*

symp·to′sis [G., a falling together]. Wasting; emaciation; collapse.

sym′pus [G. *sympous,* with the feet together]. A monster characterized by greater or less fusion of the legs, rotation of the legs, and marked deficiencies of the pelvic region and genitalia. Also called *cuspidate fetus, symelus, symmelus, sirenoform fetus, mermaid fetus.*

s. apus. One lacking feet. Syn., *sirenomelus.*

s. dipus. A sympus with two more or less complete feet.

s. monopus. One with but one more or less complete foot. Syn., *uromelus.*

sym·sep′a·lous [G. *syn,* with; NL. *sepalum*]. *In biology,* having the sepals united.

syn- [G.]. A prefix signifying *with* or *together.*

syn″ac·to′sis [G. *synaktos,* collected; *-ōsis,* condition]. Malformations caused by the abnormal growing together of parts.

syn″a·del′phus [G. *synadelphos,* from *syn, adelphos,* brother]. Equal conjoined twins having eight limbs with but one head and trunk. Not observed in man. Also called *cephalothoracoiliopagus.*

syn·al′gi·a [G. *synalgein,* to share in suffering]. Pain felt in a distant part from an injury or stimulation of another part. —**synalgic,** *adj.*

syn″an·as″to·mo′sis [G., supposed communications between arteries and veins]. The joining of several blood vessels. *Rare.*

sy·nan′che (si·nang′kee, sigh·nang′kee) [G. *synagchē,* sore throat]. Severe sore throat with choking, often caused by diphtheria organisms. Syn., *diphtheria.*

syn·an′the·ma (si·nan′thi·muh, sin″an·theem′uh) [G. *synanthein,* to blossom together]. A group of elementary skin lesions of the same type.

syn·an′throse. See *levulose.*

syn′apse (sin′aps, si·naps′) [G. *synapsis,* contact]. 1. The region of communication between neurons; the point at which an impulse passes from an axon of one neuron to a dendrite or to the cell body of another. The relation between the neurons is probably one of contiguity of plasma membranes, rather than one of continuity of protoplasm. A synapse is polarized, that is, nerve impulses are transmitted only in one direction, and is characterized by fatigability. Also spelled *synapsis*. 2. The fusion of the male and female chromosome pairs. This occurs either side-to-side or end-to-end without either univalent chromosome losing its identity. A bivalent chromosome results and is responsible for transmitting mixed characteristics from the parents to the offspring. Also spelled *synapsis*.

axodendritic s. A type in which the end-feet of the axon of one nerve are in contact with the dendrites of another neuron.

axomatic s. A type in which the end-feet of the axon of one nerve are in contact with the cell body of another neuron.

syn′apse. To make a connection with a neuron.

syn·ap′tase (si·nap′tace, ·taze). See *emulsin.*

syn·ap′tene. See *amphitene.*

syn·ap″to·lem′ma [G. *synaptos*, fastened together; *lemma*, that which is peeled off]. The membrane at the synapse, separating the axonic ending from the body of the nerve cell.

syn″ar·thro′di·a. See *synarthrosis.* —**synarthrodial,** *adj.*

syn″ar·thro·phy′sis [G. *syn*, with; *arthron*, joint; *physis*, growth]. Progressive ankylosis of the joints.

syn″ar·thro′sis [*syn;* G. *arthrōsis*, jointing]. A form of articulation in which the bones are immovably bound together without any intervening synovial cavity. The forms are sutura, in which processes are interlocked; schindylesis, in which a thin plate of one bone is inserted into a cleft of another; and gomphosis, in which a conical process is held by a socket.

syncaine. Trade name for *procaine hydrochloride.*

syn·can′thus [*syn;* G. *kanthos*, corner of the eye]. Adhesions between the orbital tissues and the eyeball.

syn·car′y·on [*syn;* G. *karyon*, nut]. See *synkaryon.*

syn·ceph′a·lus [*syn;* G. *kephalē*, head]. Conjoined twins united by their heads. This group includes the various types of craniopagus (cephalopagus) and cephalothoracopagus.

s. asymmetros. See *iniops.*

syn·chi′li·a, syn·chei′li·a (sin·kigh′lee·uh) [*syn;* G. *cheilos*, lip]. Fusion of the lips.

syn″chon·dro′sis (sing″kon·dro′sis) [G., junction of two bones by cartilage]. A joint in which the surfaces are connected by a plate of cartilage. —**synchondrosial,** *adj.*

sacroiliac s. The union between the sacrum and the ilium.

syn″chon·drot′o·my (sing″kon·drot′o·mee) [G. *syn*, with; *chondros*, cartilage; *tomē*, a cutting]. A division of the cartilage uniting bones, especially of that of the symphysis pubis.

syn″cho·pex′i·a (sing″ko·peck′see·uh). See *tachycardia.*

syn″chro·cy′clo·tron. Modification of the cyclotron to produce particles of higher kinetic energy in discontinuous streams. The frequency of the electric field is varied as the orbit of the particle increases in diameter.

syn′chro·nism, syn·chro′ni·a [G. *sygchronos*, contemporaneous]. Concurrence in time of two or more events. —**syn′chronous,** *adj.*

syn′chro·tron. Instrument in which electrons or protons are accelerated first by the betatron principle and then by the cyclotron principle, to gain more kinetic energy.

syn′chy·sis scin′til·lans (sing′ki·sis sin′ti·lanz, sin·til′anz). The presence of bright, shining particles in the vitreous body of the eye.

syn″ci·ne′sis. See *synkinesis.*

syn′ci·put. Sinciput.

syn·clei′sis (sin·kly′sis) [G. *syn*, with; *kleisis*, a closing]. Obsolete term for occlusion.

syn′cli·tism [G. *sygklinein*, to lean]. A condition marked by parallelism or similarity of inclination; parallelism between the pelvic planes and those of the fetal head. —**synclit′ic,** *adj.*

syn′clo·nus [G. *syn*, with; *klonos*, agitation]. 1. Tremor, or clonic spasm, of several muscles at the same time. 2. A disease thus characterized, as chorea.

s. ballismus. Paralysis agitans.

s. tremens. General tremor.

syn′co·pe (sing′ko·pee) [G. *sygkopē*, sudden loss of strength]. Swooning or fainting; temporary suspension of consciousness from cerebral anemia. —**syncopal, syncop′ic,** *adj.*

cardiac s. One due to extreme bradycardia and asystole, or to tachycardia.

carotid sinus s. Spontaneous attacks of unconsciousness and convulsions caused by a hyperactive carotid sinus. See also carotid sinus *syndrome.*

laryngeal s. Spasm of the larynx associated with vertigo and loss of consciousness.

local s. Sudden pallor and insensibility of a part.

s. anginosa. Synonym of angina pectoris.

tussive s. Fainting following a severe coughing episode.

vasovagal s. That developing in persons with unstable vasomotor systems; emotional strain or pressure on the vagus causes a lowering of blood pressure and slowing of the pulse. Also see carotid sinus *s.*

syn″co·pex′i·a, syn′co·pex″y. See *tachycardia.*

syncurine. A trade-marked name for decamethonium bromide.

syn·cyt″i·o·ly′sin (sin·sit″ee·o·lye′sin, sin·sish″-ee·o·, sin·sit″ee·ol′i·sin, sin·sish″ee·) [G. *syn*, with; *kytos*, cell; *lysis*, a loosing]. A cytolysin produced by injections of an emulsion made from placental tissue.

syn·cyt″i·o′ma. See *choriocarcinoma.*

syn·cyt″i·o·tox′in (sin·sit″ee·o·tock′sin, sin·sish″-ee·o·) [*syn; kytos;* G. *toxikon*, poison]. A cytotoxin with specific action on syncytial cells.

syn·cyt″i·o·troph′o·blast (·tro′fo·blast, trof′o-blast) [*syn; kytos;* G. *trophē*, nourishment; *blastos*, germ]. Syncytial trophoblast. An irregular sheet or net of deeply staining cytoplasm in which nuclei are irregularly scattered; it lies outside of the cytotrophoblast. Also called *syncytium, plasmoditrophoblast.*

syn·cyt′i·um (sin·sish′ee·um, sin·sit′ee·um) [*syn; kytos*]. A mass of cytoplasm with numerous nuclei. —**syncyt′ial,** *adj.*

syn·dac′tyl [*syn;* G. *daktylos*, finger]. Having the fingers or toes joined together.

syn·dac′ty·lus [*syn; daktylos*]. A person with webbed fingers or toes.

syn·dac′ty·ly, syn·dac′tyl·ism, syn″dac·tyl′i·a [*syn; daktylos*]. Adhesion of fingers or toes; webbed fingers or webbed toes. —**syndactylous,** *adj.*

syn′de·sis, syn·de′sis [G., a binding together]. The state of being bound together.

syn·des″mec·to′pi·a (sin·dess″meck·to′pee·uh, sin·dez″·) [G. *syndesmos*, bond; *ektopos*, away from a place]. Ligamentous displacement.

syn″des·mi′tis (sin″dess·my′tis, sin″dez·) [*syndesmos;* G. *-itis*, inflammation]. 1. Inflammation of a ligament. 2. Conjunctivitis.

syn·des″mo·cho′ri·al (sin·dess″mo·kor′ee·ul, sin-dez″mo·) [*syndesmos;* G. *chorion*, membrane that encloses the fetus]. Pertaining to maternal connective tissue and chorionic ectoderm. See *placenta.*

syn·des″mo·di·as′ta·sis (·dye·ass′tuh·sis) [*syndesmos;* G. *diastasis,* separation]. Separation of ligaments.

syn″des·mol′o·gy [*syndesmos;* G. *logos,* word]. The study of ligaments.

syn·des′mo·pex″y [*syndesmos;* G. *pēxis,* a fixing]. The attachment of a ligament in a new position.

syn″des·mor′rha·phy [*syndesmos;* G. *rhaphē,* suture]. Suture or repair of ligaments.

syn″des·mo′sis [*syndesmos;* G. *-ōsis,* condition]. A form of articulation in which the bones are connected by fibrous connective tissue.

tympanostapedial s. The joint between the foot plate of the stapes and fenestra vestibuli (oval window).

syn″des·mot′o·my [*syndesmos;* G. *tomē,* a cutting]. The division of a ligament.

syn′det. Generic name for synthetic detergents.

syn′drome (sin′drohm, sin′dro·mee″) [G. *syndromos,* a running together]. A group of symptoms and signs, which, when considered together, characterize a disease or lesion. —**syndrom′ic,** *adj.*

For any syndrome not listed here, see the individual name and under *disease.*

abstinence s. See withdrawal *s.*

Achard-Thiers s. Diabetes of bearded women; a rare condition in which features of the adrenogenital and Cushing's syndromes are combined.

Adair-Dighton s. A familial symptom complex characterized by fragility of the bones, blue scleras, and deafness.

Adams-Stokes s. See Stokes-Adams *s.*

Adie's s. Impairment of pupillary reaction to light and of accommodation associated with decrease or loss of the deep reflexes of the extremities: also called *pupillotonic pseudotabes.* See Adie's *pupil.*

adiposogenital s. See adiposogenital *dystrophy.*

adrenal s. See Waterhouse-Friderichsen *s.*

adrenogenital s. A clinical condition associated with hypersecretion of androgenic hormones by adrenal cortical tissue. Effects vary with time of development. *In the female,* in fetal life, pseudohermaphroditism results; in childhood, precocious puberty; in sexual maturity, virilism. *In the male,* the condition is usually recognizable only if it occurs before puberty and is characterized by sexual and somatic precocity. Also called *corticosexual s.*

adrenosympathetic s. Episodes of paroxysmal hypertension, glycosuria, tachycardia, pallor or flushing or both, headache, nausea, vomiting; occurs at irregular intervals and resembles the effects of toxic doses of epinephrine; associated with pheochromocytoma. Hypertension is rarely persistent.

adversive s. A type of motion sickness in which there are compulsive pivoting and circling motions. Dramamine (dimenhydrinate) acts in an atropinelike fashion to control it.

Albright-McCune-Sternberg s. See Fuller *Albright,* fibrous *dysplasia.*

amnestic s. A syndrome observed in organic brain disorders, characterized by retro- and anterograde amnesia, defects in retention and recall of ideas or facts, disorientation, and confabulation, seen in varying degrees of severity. Common causes are senile sclerosis, alcoholic (Korsakoff's) psychosis, electroshock therapy, and bilateral prefrontal lobotomy. Syn. *amnestic-confabulatory s.*

amyostatic s. See hepatolenticular *degeneration.*

anginal s. Retrosternal pain during exercise, emotion, digestion, or exposure to cold due to decreased coronary artery circulation.

angiospastic s. One characterized by segmental spasm of peripheral blood vessels, as Raynaud's phenomenon or acroparesthesia: frequently associated with psychogenic factors. Syn., *vasospastic s.* See also *angioneurosis.*

anterior cornual s. Muscular atrophy due to motor paralysis caused by lesions of the anterior horn of the spinal cord.

anterior tibial s. Traumatic necrosis of and hemorrhage into pretibial muscles following vigorous exercise, clinically characterized by acute swelling of the muscles involved, pain, and even paralysis.

Anton's s. A form of anosognosia in which the patient denies his blindness: usually accompanied by confabulation, with the patient claiming to see objects in the blind field.

Apert's s. See *acrocephalosyndactylia.*

auriculotemporal s. A local redness and sweating of the cheek with pain anterior to the tragus, produced during mastication of food or tasting; following a suppuration and fistulation of the parotid gland. Also called *Frey's s.*

Avelli's s. See ambiguospinothalamic *paralysis.*

Ayerza's s. See Ayerza's *disease.*

Banti's s. See chronic congestive *splenomegaly.* See also Guido *Banti.*

Bardet-Biedl s. See Lawrence-Moon-Biedl *s.*

Behcet's s. Recurrent retinitis or iridocyclitis, aphthous ulcers of the mouth and ulcerations of the genitalia, and in some cases erythema nodosum: also called *triple symptom complex of Behcet.*

Benedikt s. Hemianesthesia and involuntary movements of a choreiform nature in the extremities on the side opposite to the lesion which is caused by occlusion of the vessels and subsequent softening in the medial lemniscus and region of the red nucleus. Also called *tegmental mesencephalic paralysis.*

Bernheim's s. Partial occlusion of the right ventricle of the heart, caused by a deviated interventricular septum.

Bertolloti's s. Sacralization. *Obs.*

Bland-White-Garland s. Anomalous origin of the left coronary artery from the pulmonary artery, accompanied by hypertrophy and dilatation of the left ventricle and severe myocardial necrosis and fibrosis. Attacks simulate angina pectoris; the ECG is abnormal; death occurs in the first year of life.

Blount-Barber s. See *osteochondrosis deformans tibiae.*

blue-sclera s. Blue sclerotics occurring in osteogenesis imperfecta. See also Van der Hoeve's *s.*

Bouillaud's s. See *rheumatic fever.*

Brown-Séquard s. See Charles Edward *Brown-Séquard.*

Budd-Chiari s. Thrombosis of the hepatic veins associated with right upper quadrant abdominal pain, hepatomegaly, splenomegaly, ascites, edema of the lower extremities, and formation of collateral venous channels.

Burnett's s. See pathologic *calcification* (c).

Caffey's s. See infantile cortical *hyperostosis.*

capsular thrombosis s. Hemiplegia with rigidity resulting from a lesion of the internal capsule due to occlusion of striatal branches of the middle cerebral artery.

capsulothalamic s. Hemianesthesia and partial hemiplegia with emotional instability following lesions in the thalamus and internal capsule.

carotid sinus s. Overirritability of the carotid sinus causing attacks of dizziness, fainting, and sometimes convulsions. During the attack there is a fall in arterial blood pressure and a marked slowing or standstill of the heart. Attacks may come on spontaneously, may follow an emotional upset, or may be caused by pressure over the carotid sunis.

carpal tunnel s. A symptom complex due to compression of the median nerve within the carpal tunnel, characterized by disturbances of sensation in the area of skin supplied by the median nerve, edema of the fingers, tense and shiny skin, and atrophy of the thenar muscles.

cavernous sinus s. A group of symptoms produced by thrombosis of the cavernous sinus and marked by palsy of the muscles supplied by the third, fourth, and sixth cranial nerves, with edema of the face and eyelids.

celiac s. A syndrome in which intestinal malabsorption of fat results in bulky, loose, foul-smelling stools, high in fatty acid content. Failure to gain weight, weakness, anorexia, and consequent vitamin deficiencies with their accompanying symptoms result. Causes may be (in addition to primary defects in intestinal absorption of fat) obstruction of digestive and absorptive pathways, as in Whipple's disease, giardiasis, and tuberculous and lymphomatous infiltration of mesenteric nodes.

cerebellopontine-angle tumor s. The progressive manifestations of neoplastic growth at the cerebellopontine angle. Varying with the site of the lesion and direction of growth, the signs include tinnitus, impairment and loss of hearing, ipsilateral paralysis of the sixth and seventh cranial nerves, involvement of the trigeminal (fifth cranial) nerve, vertigo and nystagmus, and signs of cerebellar disturbances, such as vomiting and ataxia. Also see acoustic nerve *tumor*.

cervical radicular s. A syndrome similar to the shoulder-hand syndrome, due to radiculitis of the lower cervical nerves and the first thoracic, and characterized by neuralgia, alterations in sensation, and muscle weakness and atrophy in the corresponding dermatomes. Syn., *shoulder-neck s.* See also shoulder-girdle *s.*

Charlin's s. of the nasal nerve. A triad of inflammation of the anterior segment of the eye, neuralgic pain at the inner angle of the eye, and profuse rhinorrhea.

Chauffard-Minkowski s. Congenital form of hemolytic jaundice.

chiasma s. A group of symptoms due to a lesion in the optic chiasm and marked by impaired vision, headache, vertigo, and limitation of the visual field.

compression s. Crush *s.*

corpus striatum s. See *status* marmoratus.

corticometabolic s. Cushing's *s.*

corticosexual s. Adrenogenital *s.*

Costen's s. See temporomandibular *s.*

cough s. Giddiness (not true vertigo) or occasionally unconsciousness following strenuous coughing. This usually occurs in middle-aged obese men with a tendency towards chronic laryngitis or bronchitis, and in men who smoke and/or use liquor to excess. Syn., *laryngeal vertigo s.*

crocodile-tears s. See crocodile *tears.*

crus s. Hemiparetic symptoms homolateral with a cerebral lesion, usually found when a chronic subdural hematoma, brain tumor, or brain abscess has caused dislocation of the brain stem in such a manner as to force the contralateral crus cerebri against the tentorium: also called *Kernohan-Woltman s.*

crush s. Lower nephron nephrosis consequent to crush injuries of the extremities.

Cruveilhier-Baumgarten s. Distention of the periumbilical veins of the abdominal wall, accompanied by a hum: associated with portal hypertension and usually with a patent umbilical vein.

Cushing's s. A clinical condition characterized by obesity confined chiefly to the trunk and face, thin plethoric skin with purplish striae in areas of tension, easy bruisability, osteoporosis, hypertension, and impairment of glucose tolerance: frequently associated with glycosuria, polycythemia, hirsutism, and amenorrhea in females or impotence in males. It appears to result from a prolonged excess of adrenocortical hormones, particularly the 17-hydroxycorticosteroids. It may be associated with diffuse hyperplasia of the adrenal cortex, benign or malignant tumors of the adrenal cortex, basophilic adenoma of the pituitary, or prolonged administration of large doses of adrenocorticotropic hormone (ACTH), cortisone, or hydrocortisone.

Da Costa's s. See neurocirculatory *asthenia.*

Danlos s. See Ehlers-Danlos *s.*

Debré-de Toni-Fanconi s. See amino *diabetes.*

Debré-Semelaigne s. A symptom complex observed in cretinous children, characterized by enlarged muscles, reduced strength, easy fatigability, and slowness of movements.

Dejerine-Rousy s. See thalamic *s.*

de Lange's s. A form of congenital muscular hypertrophy accompanied by signs of extrapyramidal motor disturbances and mental deficiency. Death usually ensues early. At autopsy, polygyria, microgyria, and failure of basal ganglia to develop have been noted.

de Toni-Fanconi s. See amino *diabetes.*

diencephalic s. A syndrome characterized by disturbances of consciousness and of the autonomic nervous system, emotional upheavals, and frequently by epilepsylike seizures. This condition is difficult to distinguish from other psychic disturbances, such as the schizophrenic reaction, manic-depressive reactions, or epilepsy.

Dresbach's s. 1. Ovalocytosis. 2. Erroneously, sickle-cell anemia.

Duane's retraction s. See Alexander *Duane.*

dumping s. A symptom complex of a feeling of warmth, weakness, sweating, vertigo, tightness or pain in the epigastrium, nausea, palpitation, and in some cases collapse, seen in patients who have had partial or complete removal of the stomach.

duodenal loop triad s. A symptom complex seen in cases of duodenitis with associated disease of the gallbladder and pancreas, characterized by indigestion, a feeling of fullness in the epigastrium, gaseous eructations and heartburn, often biliary colic or a tender gallbladder, and sometimes umbilical pain radiating to the left shoulder, nausea, vomiting, and weakness.

dyskinetic s. Symptoms associated with congestive heart failure.

effort s. A group of reactions evoked by moderate physical exercise and consisting principally of an abnormal degree of dyspnea, rapid heart action, palpitation, substernal oppression, and sometimes pain. It is usually described in connection with neurocirculatory asthenia, but is manifest also in other cardiac disorders.

egg-white s. See *egg-white injury.*

Ehlers-Danlos s. See Meekrin-Ehlers-Danlos *s.*

Eisenmenger's s. See Eisenmenger's *complex.*

Ellis-van Creveld s. See chondroectodermal *dysplasia.*

epiphyseal s. See Pellizzi's *s.*

exhaustion s. A somewhat ill-defined syndrome with the characteristics of muscular, nervous, and circulatory asthenia and poor appetite. It has been ascribed to hypoadrenia. Also called *hypoadrenalemia.*

exophthalmic s. A condition of unknown cause, not necessarily associated with hyperthyroidism or thyroid hyperplasia, in which there is unilateral or bilateral exophthalmos. When progressive to a severe degree the condition is termed *malignant exophthalmos.* Also called *hyperophthalmopathic Graves's disease.*

facet s. A form of traumatic arthritis involving the articular facets of the spinal column, usually in the lumbar region. The symptoms are sudden in onset, with low back pain relieved in certain postures and exaggerated in others, the pain being described as of the locking type.

Felty's s. Splenomegaly, leukopenia, and chronic atrophic arthritis of the rheumatoid type; a form of hypersplenism.

flocculonodular s. Cerebellar deficiency characterized by disturbances in gait and the tendency to lose balance.

Frey's s. Auriculotemporal *s.*

Froehlich's s. See adiposogenital *dystrophy.*

Froin's s. See loculation *s.*

Ganser s. A mental syndrome in which questions are given nonsensical answers, from which a hidden relevancy may be inferred. Observed in prisoners who wish to gain leniency by simulating mental clouding; may be deliberate, neurotic, or both.

Garcin's s. The collection of signs and symptoms when all the cranial nerves of one side are affected by tumor.

general adaptation s. The sum of all nonspecific systemic reactions of the body which ensue upon long-continued exposure to systemic stress. It is divided into three stages: (1) *Alarm reaction,* the sum of all nonspecific phenomena elicited by sudden exposure to stimuli which affect large portions of the body and to which the organism is quantitatively or qualitatively not adapted. This stage is divided into phases of *shock* and *countershock* and is of short duration, usually no more than 24 hours. (2) *Stage of resistance,* the sum of all nonspecific systemic reactions elicited by prolonged exposure to stimuli to which the organism has acquired adaptation; it may last weeks to months. (3) *Stage of exhaustion,* the sum of all nonspecific systemic reactions which ultimately develop as a result of prolonged overexposure to stimuli to which adaptation has been developed but can no longer be maintained. It is of indefinite duration. Term introduced by Hans Selye.

Godtfredsen's s. A symptom complex consisting of total ophthalmoplegia, amaurosis, trigeminal neuralgia, and symptoms referable to paralysis of the twelfth cranial nerve. See Jacod's *triad.*

Gougerot-Houwers-Sjögren s. See Sjögren's *s.*

Groenblad-Strandberg s. See *pseudoxanthoma elasticum.*

Guillain-Barré s. A spreading paralysis, sometimes reversible, due to involvement of nerves, nerve roots, cord, brain, and meninges, separately or combined. The unique symptom is bilateral peripheral facial palsy. Other symptoms besides paralysis include painful, tactile, and thermal hyperesthesia, usually aural in distribution, or hypoesthesia and tenderness of muscles. Cerebrospinal fluid shows elevated protein without corresponding increase in cells. Syn., *infective meningomyeloneuritis.* Also called *polyradiculoneuritis, infective neuritis* or *neuronitis.*

gynecomastia-and-small-testes s. See Klinefelter's *s.*

Hallervorden-Spatz s. A symmetrical glial proliferation and demyelinization of the globus pallidus and zona incerta which may extend into the central nucleus of the thalamus, dentate nucleus, and ventral nucleus of the thalamus, with increased pigmentation in these structures; a heredofamilial condition producing symptoms of progressive bilateral rigidity, speech difficulties, dementia, and sometimes optic atrophy and hyperkinesis. Syn., *status dysmyelinicus.*

hand-shoulder s. See shoulder-hand *s.*

Harada's s. Vogt-Koyanagi syndrome, complicated by retinal detachment.

Hedblom's s. Acute primary diaphragmitis. Rare.

Heller-Nelson s. A rare form of hypogonadism due to anorchism or a destructive lesion of the interstitial cells and spermatic tubules, exhibiting some of the changes seen in prepuberal eunuchoidism and Klinefelter's syndrome, but characterized by the absence of eunuchoidal skeletal changes and the presence of a high titer of urinary gonadotropins.

hepatorenal s. Renal failure allegedly due to hepatic injury: a term widely used without adequate pathologic basis.

Hoffman's s. A symptom complex similar to the Debré-Semelaigne syndrome, seen in myxedematous adults.

Horner's s. Unilateral ptosis, miosis, enophthalmos, diminished sweating, and flushing of the face, due to destruction of the cervical sympathetics of the same side.

Horton's s. Histaminic cephalalgia: unilateral, intense headache believed to be due to the release of histamine and its action on cerebral arteries.

Howship-Romberg s. Pain on the medial aspect of the thigh down to and usually most marked at the knee, as a result of pressure on the obturator nerve by an obturator hernia.

Hurler's s. See *gargoylism.*

Hutchinson's s. See Hutchinson's *triad.* See also Jonathan *Hutchinson.*

hyperabduction s. See Wright's *s.*

hyperkinetic s. Effort syndrome.

hyperventilation s. Respiratory alkalosis occurring as a result of overbreathing. It may be due to intense psychological stimuli (as in anxiety reactions), anesthetics or other drugs, organic brain disease, or excessive artificial respiration. The condition is clinically characterized by cerebral symptoms, including dizziness or even loss of consciousness, by peripheral signs such as tingling and numbness, and by tetanic or clonic motor responses.

hypokinetic s. One in which various forms of acute circulatory failure occur, regardless of cause.

inferior mediastinal s. See inferior vena cava *s.*

inferior vena cava s. Edema of the lower extremities and distention of the superficial veins of the legs and abdomen, or hepatic congestion, as a result of obstruction of the vena cava inferior, as by thrombosis, neoplasm, aneurysm, or adhesions.

internal derangement s. See internal *derangement* of the knee.

Jackson's s. See John H. *Jackson.*

Jeghers-Peutz s. See hereditary multiple *polyposis.*

Kartagener's s. A hereditary symptom complex consisting of complete transposition of the viscera, sinusitis, and bronchiectasis: also called *K.'s triad.*

Kast's s. Multiple cavernous hemangiomas associated with chondromas or dyschondroplasia. Some patients show pigmentary skin changes. It is thought to be a variant of Maffucci's syndrome.

Kimmelstiel-Wilson s. See *intercapillary glomerulosclerosis.*

Klinefelter's s. A form of testicular dysfunction

of unknown cause associated with hyalinization of the seminiferous tubules and characterized by the presence of gynecomastia, aspermia, and elevated urinary excretion of gonadotropin.

Klippel-Feil s. Congenital fusion of the bodies of two or more cervical vertebrae; the spines are small, deficient, or bifid; atlanto-occipital fusion is common. As a result the neck is short and head movements are markedly limited.

Korsakoff's s. Polyneuritis with loss of memory, a retrograde amnesia associated with tendency to confabulation, caused by alcohol and severe deficiency of food intake.

labyrinthine s. See Ménière's *s.*

laryngeal-vertigo s. See cough *s.*

Laurence-Moon-Biedl s. An inherited endocrine disturbance of the pituitary or other hypothalamic structures characterized by girdle-type obesity, hypogenitalism, mental retardation, polydactyly, and pigmentary retinal degeneration.

Leriche s. Intermittent claudication of the lower extremities with pain extending to the hips and buttocks, easy fatiguability of the lower extremities, and in males, impotence, due to arteriosclerotic thrombotic obliteration of the abdominal aorta at its bifurcation or of the iliac arteries.

Lermoyez s. Attacks or episodes of diminished hearing followed by attacks of vertigo, after which hearing improves or returns to normal. Cause and mechanism are unclear.

Leschke's s. A group of symptoms, which may be found in hemochromatosis or xanthoma diabeticorum, characterized by hyperglycemia, many brown macules on the skin, and general weakness: also called *dystrophia pigmentosa.*

Lévy-Roussy s. One exhibiting the classical signs and symptoms of peroneal muscular atrophy plus scoliosis and a mild degree of cerebellar ataxia. These cases are considered to be transitional forms between peroneal muscular atrophy and Friedreich's ataxia.

Libman-Sacks s. See atypical verrucous *endocarditis.*

loculation s. A change in the consistency and circulatory activity of the lumbar spinal fluid in which a yellow color appears attended by rapid coagulation, large amounts of globulin, and increased number of lymphocytes. Characteristic of isolation of the lumbar spinal fluid from communication with the ventricles of the brain. Also called *Froin's s.*

Loeffler's s. A disease of unknown cause characterized by extensive pulmonary infiltration of eosinophils and eosinophilia of peripheral blood. Syn., *eosinophilic pneumonitis.*

Looser-Milkman s. See Milkman's *s.*

Lorain-Levi s. Panhypopituitarism occurring before puberty; dwarfism or infantilism in association with destructive lesions of the pituitary gland. Rare.

lower-leg s. See post-thrombotic *s.*

lower nephron s. See lower nephron *nephrosis.*

low-salt s. A clinical syndrome characterized by a low serum sodium concentration, occurring acutely in heat exhaustion or water intoxication, also in chronic cardiac or renal disease, especially with prolonged restriction in sodium chloride intake. There may be oliguria, azotemia, muscle cramps, and prostration.

Lubarsch-Pick s. Atypical amyloidosis frequently associated with a diffuse enlargement of the tongue (amyloid macroglossia), involvement of the skeletal muscles, and scleroderma.

Luetscher s. A form of hyperosmolarity of body fluids occurring in occasional patients during recovery from the anuric stage of lower nephron nephrosis resulting from sulfathiazole administration. See *hyperosmolarity, hypernatremia.*

Maffucci's s. Cutaneous hemangiomas associated with dyschondroplasia. Involvement is unilateral or extremely asymmetric. See Kast's *s.*

Mallory-Weiss s. Gastrointestinal hemorrhage caused by lacerations at the cardiac orifice of the stomach induced by protracted retching and vomiting, or even violent hiccuping. Common associated factors are alcoholism, atrophic gastritis, and nutritional cirrhosis.

Marchiafava-Micheli s. Nocturnal hemoglobinuria.

Mauriac s. Hepatomegaly, retarded growth, and obesity, in association with diabetes mellitus. Its cause is not understood.

Mediterranean hemolytic syndromes. Thalassemia major and minor.

Meekrin-Ehlers-Danlos s. One including hyperelastic skin, hyperflexible joints, fragile skin and blood vessels, subcutaneous nodules, and pseudotumors following trauma.

Meigs's s. Ovarian fibroma with ascites and hydrothorax.

Melkersson's s. A disease, usually of young people, characterized by recurrent peripheral facial paralysis, swelling of the face and lips, and deep furrows in the tongue. Prognosis is good.

Ménière's s. A disease of the internal ear characterized by deafness, vertigo, and tinnitus, frequently accompanied by nausea, vomiting, and nystagmus. The process may be an allergy because the mechanism is similar to angioneurotic edema. Also called *labyrinthine s.*

metameric s. See segmentary *s.*

middle-lobe s. Inflammatory disease, bronchiectasis, or atelectasis, secondary to extrinsic obstruction of middle-lobe bronchus. The obstruction is usually secondary to severe lymphadenitis

milk-drinker's s. See pathologic *calcification* (c).

Milkman's s. A condition occurring frequently when skeletal bones have been sufficiently decalcified, particularly in osteomalacia. There are bone pain and tenderness, and x-ray examination reveals multiple incomplete pseudofractures, often characterized by Looser's zone, with a tendency to be bilateral and symmetrically placed. Also called *Looser-Milkman's s.*

Millard-Gubler s. See Auguste L. J. *Millard.*

Morgagni-Stewart-Morel s. See metabolic *craniopathy.*

Morgagni-Stokes-Adams s. Stokes-Adams *s.*

Morton's s. A condition characterized by tenderness at the base of the second metatarsal bone, callosities beneath the second and third metatarsals, and hypertrophy of the second metatarsal, due to a short first metatarsal bone: described by Dudley J. Morton.

Moschkowitz's s. See thrombotic thrombocytopenic *purpura.*

motor s. One due to a lesion of Brodmann's area four of the cerebral cortex, with resulting flaccidity of the affected muscles, sometimes exaggerated tendon reflexes, and loss of motor power.

Müller's s. A symptom complex characterized by hypercholesterolemia, xanthelasma, xanthomas, and angina pectoris.

Naffziger s. See scalenus anterior *s.*

neocerebellar s. Cerebellar deficiency characterized by hypotonia, intention tremor, and disorders of range, direction, and timing of movements.

neuroanemic s. The various nervous symptoms associated with pernicious anemia.

neurocutaneous s. The formation of skin lesions

associated with skeletal deformities and symptoms indicative of degenerative lesions of the nervous system.

neuropituitary s. See adiposogenital *dystrophy.*

nitritoid s. A severe reaction with dyspnea, flushed face, cough, and precordial pain following the administration of arsphenamine, named from its resemblance to the symptoms following the administration of a toxic dose of amyl nitrite. Also called *nitritoid crisis.*

Nonne-Marie s. See hereditary cerebellar *ataxia.*

orbital apex s. The irregular paresis and neuralgia resulting from invasion of the apex of the orbit and associated branches of the cranial nerves by a malignant tumor of the nasopharynx.

organic brain s. A generalized disturbance of cerebral function, residual to widespread brain damage, usually of traumatic, toxic, or degenerative origin. Commonest manifestations are emotional instability, deterioration of intellect, gross defects in memory, judgment, and orientation, undue mental and physical fatigability, paroxysmal headache, and dizziness on exertion. Preexisting neurotic reactions contribute to greatly increased severity of these symptoms.

Osler-Libman-Sacks s. Disseminated lupus erythematosus.

Osler-Rendu-Weber s. See hereditary hemorrhagic *telangiectasis.*

ovarian short-stature s. See Turner's *s.*

paleostriatal s. Parkinsonism in juveniles.

Pancoast s. The combination of a malignant or nonmalignant (e.g., tuberculous) invasion of the thoracic inlet and Horner's syndrome, osteolytic involvement of the first two ribs and sometimes of vertebral bodies, pain, sensory and motor disturbances of the upper extremities, and sometimes vocal-fold paralysis. Syn., *superior pulmonary sulcus s.*

paratrigeminal s. A rare syndrome due to lesion of the semilunar ganglion and related sympathetic fibers from the carotid plexus, characterized by trigeminal neuralgia, often followed by sensory loss on the affected side of the face, weakness and atrophy of the muscles of mastication, miosis, and ptosis of the upper eyelid.

Parinaud's s. Conjunctivitis associated with palpable preauricular lymph nodes.

Parkes Weber s. Hypertrophy of a limb due to congenital hemangiectasis.

Parkinson's s. Parkinsonism.

Pautrier-Woringer s. (1937). A form of chronic hyperplastic lymphadenitis (called *lipomelanotic reticulosis*) accompanying certain generalized dermatoses. See dermatopathic *lymphadenopathy.*

Pellizzi's s. A tumor of the pineal gland occurring usually in male children, occasionally accompanied by precocious genital development and adiposity or general overgrowth, which, with symptoms of internal hydrocephalus, make up the syndrome designated by Pellizzi as *macrogenitosomia precox.* Syn., *epiphyseal syndrome.*

Peutz-Jeghers s. See hereditary multiple *polyposis.*

peritubal s. The collection of symptoms caused by the infiltration of certain cranial nerves or their branches by a malignant tumor of the nasopharynx, characterized by ipsilateral deafness without objective signs in the ear, temporofacial neuralgia, and palatal paresis. Syn., *Potter's triad.*

pineal s. A rare syndrome due to a pinealoma or other pathological condition in or about the pineal body, resulting in increased intracranial pressure and associated neurologic disturbances, and at times in precocious sexual development.

Plummer-Vinson s. The syndrome of dysphagia, glossitis, and hypochromic anemia which probably is due to an iron deficiency: also called *sideropenic dysphagia.*

pontocerebellar-angle tumor s. See cerebellopontine-angle tumor *s.*

postconcussion s. Symptoms chiefly of a subjective nature which follow brain concussion, namely headache, head noises, dizziness, insomnia, irritability, and an aversion to commotion or emotional excitement. Also called *posttraumatic constitution, Marie's head-wound s.*

postphlebitic s. A syndrome following thrombophlebitis of deep veins. See post-thrombotic *s.*

post-thrombotic s. A condition resulting from deep venous thrombosis of the lower extremity, characterized by edema, pain, stasis dermatitis, stasis cellulitis, varicose veins, pigmentation of the skin, and eventually chronic ulceration of the lower leg.

premotor s. One due to a destruction of the cerebral cortex in Brodmann's area six, with disturbance of skilled movements, spasticity such as forced grasping, and vasomotor disturbances of the involved extremity.

Putnam-Dana s. See subacute combined *degeneration* of spinal cord.

pyloric s. Gastritis in which the symptoms are like those of chronic peptic ulcer. Ulceration does not occur.

radiation s. See radiation *sickness.*

Raynaud's s. A syndrome of unknown cause, characterized clinically by pallor, cyanosis, and engorgement and pain of the extremities, especially the digits: usually bilateral and symmetrical. It occurs commonly in females who exhibit emotional and autonomic instability. Attacks may be brought on by cold or emotional upsets. In advanced cases pain and necrosis may become prominent.

Reiter's s. See under Hans *Reiter.*

release s. See crush *s.*

retrolenticular capsule s. Hemiplegia, hemianesthesia and hemihypalgesia, and hemianopsia due to occlusion of the branch of the posterior cerebral artery which supplies the posterior part of the internal capsule.

retroparotid s. See Maurice *Villaret.*

Riley-Day s. See *dysautonomia.*

Rothmund's s. A genodermatosis appearing in infancy with disturbances limited to ectodermal structures. There is erythema, telangiectases, and pigmentation and atrophy of the skin. Marmorization of the skin and cataracts occur. There is linkage to congenital ectodermal dysplasia with bony deformities.

scalenus anterior s. A symptom complex due to compression of the brachial plexus by the scalenus anterior muscle, characterized by pain, numbness, or weakness of the arm: described by H. C. Naffziger. Also called *scalenus anticus s.*

scapulocostal s. One characterized by the insidious onset of pain in the superior or posterior aspect of the shoulder girdle with radiation into the neck, occiput, upper or lower arm, or chest, and often accompanied by tingling and numbness in the fingers. It is due to long-standing alterations in the relationships between the scapula and the posterior thoracic wall. Also called *fatigue-postural paradox.*

Schmidt's s. See vagoaccessory *s.*

Schüller-Christian s. See Hand-Schüller-Christian *disease.*

Seabright-Bantam s. A phenomenon, first observed in the Seabright-Bantam rooster, in which there is unresponsiveness of the target organ to a hormone: sometimes applied to human physiology, as in the case of pseudohypoparathyroidism.

segmentary s. Signs and symptoms which indicate a lesion of the spinal cord at a certain level.

Selye's s. See general adaptation *s.*

Senear-Usher s. See *pemphigus* erythematosus.

Sheehan's s. Postpartum pituitary deficiency, generally associated with severe hemorrhage and shock during or following childbirth, which produces, apparently by thrombosis, an extensive necrosis of the adenohypophysis: also called *postpartum pituitary necrosis.*

shock s. See *shock.*

short-stature s. See Turner's *s.*

shoulder-girdle s. Atrophy of the shoulder girdle accompanied by sudden onset of acute pain in the shoulder which may radiate to the arm or neck: also called *acute brachial radiculitis.*

shoulder-hand s. A syndrome characterized by severe constant intractable pain in the shoulder and arm, limited joint motion, diffuse swelling of the distal part of the upper extremity, fibrosis and atrophy of muscles, and decalcification of underlying bones. The cause is not well understood. It is similar to and may be identical with, or may be a form of, causalgia (reflex sympathetic dystrophy). Syn., *hand-shoulder s.*

shoulder-neck s. See cervical radicular *s.*

Sicard's s. See Jean A. *Sicard.*

Sjögren's s. A symptom complex described by Sjögren (1933) as consisting of keratoconjunctivitis sicca, laryngopharyngitis sicca, rhinitis sicca, xerostomia, enlargement of the parotid gland, and polyarthritis: also called *xerodermosteosis.*

Spiller's s. See epidural ascending spinal *paralysis.*

splenic-flexure s. Left-upper-quadrant abdominal pain, referred heart pain, dyspnea, palpitations, and feelings of apprehension: probably psychogenic in origin.

Stein-Leventhal s. A group of symptoms and findings characterized by amenorrhea and/or abnormal uterine bleeding, enlarged polycystic ovaries, hirsutism frequently, and occasionally retarded breast development and obesity: first described by I. F. Stern and M. L. Leventhal (1935).

Stevens-Johnson s. A severe form of erythema multiforme, characterized by constitutional symptoms and marked involvement of the conjunctiva and oral mucosa.

Stewart-Morel s. See metabolic *craniopathy.*

Stewart-Treves s. See postmastectomy *lymphangiosarcoma.*

Stokes-Adams s. A slowed pulse with syncopal attacks or convulsive seizures, usually epileptiform in character. The slowed cardiac action is a result of heart block; the cerebral symptoms are a direct result of the bradycardia.

Sturge-Weber s. Nevoid amentia.

superior pulmonary sulcus s. See Pancoast's *s.*

superior vena cava s. Blockage of the superior vena cava, as by thrombosis, neoplasm, aneurysm, or mediastinitis, resulting in elevation of venous pressure of the upper extremities, head, and neck.

sweat-retention s. Inability to sweat because of plugging of sweat pores, followed by the classic clinical and histological signs of prickly heat, which may persist after heat rash has subsided: also called *thermogenic anhidrosis, tropical anhidrotic asthenia.*

s. of rudimentary ovaries. See Turner's *s.*

Taussig s. A congenital heart condition with transposed aorta, large pulmonary artery arising primarily from the right ventricle and partially overriding the ventricular septum, a high ventricular septal defect, and right-ventricular hypertrophy: also called *Taussig-Bing s.*

Teacher Collins s. Mandibulofacial dysostosis.

tegmental s. An old term for hemiplegia associated with disturbance of eye movements, indicative of a lesion in the tegmentum of the midbrain.

temporomandibular s. A rare degenerative disease of the temporomandibular joint, manifested as tinnitus, deafness, pain in the ear, and headache: also called *Costen's s.*

thalamic s. A symptom complex produced by a lesion of the posterior portion of the lateral nuclear mass of the thalamus. It includes contralateral partial hemianesthesia and hemiplegia, contralateral severe paroxysmal pain over the entire half of the body, contralateral increased response to stimuli, slight hemiataxia, and occasional hemichorea. Also called *Dejerine-Roussy s., thalamic hyperesthetic anesthesia.*

Tietze's s. A benign, self-limiting disease of unknown etiology characterized by painful nonsuppurative swelling of the costal cartilages, frequently preceded or accompanied by upper respiratory tract infection. The tenderness disappears in a few days or weeks, but the swelling may persist for months or even years.

traumatic vasospastic s. A form of Raynaud's phenomenon resulting from the use of vibrating tools, unilateral at first and sometimes precipitated by exposure to cold. Syn. *pneumatic-hammer disease.*

Turner's s. A syndrome associated with ovarian agenesis, short stature, webbing of the neck, and cubitus valgus. Other congenital defects, e.g., coarctation of the aorta, may be present. Also called *ovarian short-stature s., s. of rudimentary ovaries, short-stature s.*

vagoaccessory s. Homolateral paralysis of the soft palate, pharynx, and larynx, with flaccidity and atrophy of the sternocleidomastoid and part of the trapezius muscle of the same side, due to a lesion of the nucleus ambiguus and nucleus of the spinal accessory nerve or their root fibers: also called *Schmidt's s.*

Van der Hoeve's s. Osseous fragility, blue sclerotics, and deafness. See also *osteogenesis imperfecta.*

vasospastic s. Angiospastic *s.*

Villaret's s. See Maurice *Villaret.*

Vogt-Koyanagi s. Bilateral uveitis, poliosis, vitiligo, alopecia, and dysacousia.

Vogt s. See double *athetosis.*

Waldenström s. See *macroglobulinanemia.*

Waterhouse-Friderichsen s. A syndrome of acute collapse associated with hemorrhages into the adrenal glands, occurring in fulminating infections, particularly in acute meningococcemia. It is also associated with acute trauma, asphyxia, or heparin therapy.

Weber's s. See Hermann D. *Weber.*

Werner's s. Progeria of adults.

Wernicke's s. Presbyophrenia.

withdrawal s. The physical and psychological disturbances observed in addicts upon complete withdrawal of the addicting agent. Severity of the autonomic and psychomotor disturbances varies in part with length of addiction and size of dosage.

Wittmaack-Ekbom s. See *restless legs* under *leg.*

Wolff-Parkinson-White s. A usually benign condition in which there exists one or several accessory muscular bridges, in addition to the normal bundle of His, for transmission of excitation from atria to ventricles. In the electrocardiogram it is diagnosed by a short P-R interval and a prolonged QRS complex. Patients with this syndrome may be subject to paroxysmal atrial tachycardia, probably due to a reentry phenomenon.

Wright's s. A neuromuscular syndrome produced by prolonged hyperabduction of the arms causing pinching of the subclavian artery and the trunks of the brachial plexus, which produces paresthesias, numbness, and tingling, followed by gangrene in protracted cases.

syn·ech'i·a (si·neck'ee·uh, si·nee'kee·uh, sin"i-kigh'uh) [G. *synecheia*, continuity]. A morbid union of parts; especially, adhesion of the iris to a neighboring part of the eye.

annular s. Exclusion of the pupil.

anterior s. Adhesion between the iris and transparent cornea.

posterior s. Adhesion between the iris and crystalline lens.

total s. Adhesion of the entire surface of the iris to the lens. See *iris* bombé.

syn·ech'o·tome (si·neck'o·tome) [G. *synechein*, to hold together; *tomos*, cutting]. An instrument for the division of adhesions, particularly of the tympanic membrane.

syn"ech·ot'o·my (sin"i·kot'o·mee) [*synechein;* G. *tomē*, a cutting]. The division of a synechia.

syn"en·ceph'a·lo·cele [G. *syn*, with; *egkephalos*, brain; *kēlē*, hernia]. An encephalocele with adhesions.

syn·er'e·sis [G. *synairesis*, a drawing together]. 1. Contraction of a clot (as blood, milk). 2. *In colloid chemistry*, the exudation of the liquid constituent of gels irrespective of the vapor pressure imposed upon the system. Lowered vapor pressure aids the process.

syn"er·get'ic [G. *synergētikos*, cooperative]. Exhibiting synergy; working together; synergic.

syn'er·gism (sin'ur·jiz·um, si·nur'jiz·um) [G. *synergos*, working together]. 1. The harmonious and cooperative action of two or more agents or organs, as two muscles cooperating to produce a movement which neither alone could effect. 2. The joint action of two types of microorganisms on a carbohydrate medium, leading to the production of gas that is not formed by either organism when grown separately. 3. The production of a therapeutic effect, with a combination of two or more drugs, which is more intense or more prolonged than that obtained when any component is used alone. Sometimes the term is used to designate an effect greater than the sum of the effects when the components are used separately, which is more generally referred to as *potentiation.* —**synergis'tic,** *adj.*

syn'er·gist [*synergos*]. An agent cooperating with another.

syn'er·gy [*synergos*]. The cooperative action of two or more agents or organs. —**syner'gic,** *adj.*

syn"es·the'si·a, syn"aes·the'si·a (sin"ess·thee'-zhuh, ·zee·uh) [G. *synaisthēsis*, joint sensation]. A secondary sensation or subjective impression accompanying an actual perception, as a sensation of color or sound aroused by a sensation of taste.

syn"es·the"si·al'gi·a, syn"aes·the"si·al'gi·a (sin"ess·thee"zee·al'juh, ·jee·uh) [*synaisthēsis;* G. *algos*, pain]. A painful sensation secondary to, and of a different quality from, that of a primary irritation.

Syn'ga·mus [G. *syggamos*, married]. A genus of nematode worms of the family Syngamidae which inhabits the upper respiratory tract of fowl and mammals.

S. laryngeus. A species which is usually a parasite of ruminants; incidental infestation of man has occurred.

S. trachealis. A species which causes gapeworm in chickens.

syn'ga·my [*syggamos*]. Conjugation or union of gametes in fertilization. —**syngamous, syngam'ic,** *adj.*

syn"gen·e'si·o·plas"ty. Plastic surgery employing homografts taken from parents, siblings, or offspring. —**syngenesioplas'tic,** *adj.*

syn"ge·ne'sious [G. *syn-*, together; *genesis*, generation]. Of, or derived from, an individual of the same family or species, as a tissue transplant. See also *homograft, homotransplantation, syngenesioplasty.*

syn·gig'no·scism (sin·jig'no·siz·um, sin·ghig'·) [G. *syggignōskein*, to know together with]. Hypnotism.

syn·hex'yl. 1-Hydroxy-3-*n*-hexyl-6,6,9-trimethyl-7,8,9,10-tetrahydro-6-dibenzopyran, a synthetic analog of a tetrahydrocannabinol; a pale yellow, translucent, viscous and odorless resin, insoluble in water but soluble in organic solvents. Employed as a euphoriant in the thalamic syndrome in doses of 15 to 90 mg. Syn., *parahexyl, pyrahexyl.*

syn"hi·dro'sis [G. *synidrōsis*, excessive perspiration]. Concurrent sweating; the association of perspiration with another condition.

syn"i·ze'sis [G., collapse]. Closure.

s. pupillae. Closure of the pupil.

synkamin. Trade-mark for 2-methyl-4-amino-1-naphthol hydrochloride; referred to as vitamin K_5, a water-soluble, active vitamin-K compound. See *menadione.*

syn·kar'y·on [G. *syn*, with; *karyon*, nut]. The diploid zygotic nucleus formed by the fusion of two haploid nuclei, especially in the lower fungi. Also spelled *syncaryon.*

synkavite. Trade-mark for *menadiol sodium diphosphate.*

syn"ki·ne'si·a, syn"ki·ne'sis [G., commotion]. Coincidental movement of muscles or limb along with the leading or essential movements, such as the swinging of the arms while walking. Syn., *associated automatic movement, accessory movement, synkinetic movement.* —**synkinet'ic,** *adj.*

syn·oph'rys [G., with meeting eyebrows]. Meeting of the eyebrows.

syn"oph·thal'mi·a [G. *syn*, with; *ophthalmos*, eye]. A condition characterized by fused orbits and various degrees of fusion of the eyes. Also called *cyclopia.*

syn"oph·thal'mus [*syn; ophthalmos*]. A monster exhibiting synophthalmia.

synophylate. Trade-mark for *theophylline sodium glycinate.*

syn·op'si·a [G. *synopsis*, a seeing all together]. Congenital fusion of the eyes. See *cyclopia.*

syn·or'chid·ism (sin·or'kid·iz·um), **syn·or'chism** (sin·or'kiz·um) [G. *syn*, with; *orchis*, testis]. Partial or complete fusion of the two testes within the abdomen or scrotum.

syn·os'che·os (sin·os'kee·os) [*syn;* G. *oscheos*, scrotum]. A condition of adherence between the skin of the penis and that of the scrotum. *Rare.*

syn·os'te·o·phyte" [*syn;* G. *osteon*, bone; *phyton*, plant]. Congenital bony ankylosis. Syn., *synostosis congenita.*

syn·os"te·o'sis. See *synostosis.*

syn'os·tosed (sin'os·toced, ·tozed, sin·os·toced', ·tozed') [*syn; osteon*]. Joined in bony union.

syn"os·to'sis [*syn; osteon;* G. *-ōsis*, condition]. A union of originally separate bones by osseous material. —**synostot'ic,** *adj.*

s. congenita. See *synosteophyte.*

tribasilar s. Shortening of the base of the skull

and consequent curvature of the basal parts of the brain caused by fusion in infancy of the three bones at the base of the skull.

syn·o′ti·a (si·no′shee·uh) [*syn;* G. *ous*, ear]. Approximation or union of the ears in the anterior cervical region in the absence, or marked reduction, of the lower jaw.

syn·o′tus [*syn; ous*]. A monster characterized by fused ears.

syn″o·vec′to·my (sin″o·veck′to·mee, sigh″no·) [NL. *synovia;* G. *ektomē*, excision]. Excision of synovial membrane.

syn·o′vi·a (si·no′vee·uh, sigh·no′vee·uh) [NL.]. The clear fluid which is normally present in joint cavities. See synovial *fluid.* —**synovial,** *adj.*

syn·o″vi·al·o′ma (si·no″vee·uh·lo′muh, sigh·no″·). See *synovioma.*

syn·o″vi·o·en″do·the″li·o′ma. See *synovioma.*

syn·o″vi·o′ma (si·no″vee·o′muh, sigh·no″·) [*synovia;* G. *-ōma*, tumor]. A tumor of the synovial membranes of joints, tendon sheaths, and bursas. Affects younger age groups, especially in the knee, ankle, metatarsal joints, and elbow. It grows slowly and may metastasize. Accordingly it is often named *synovial sarcoma.* Microscopically it is composed of spindle, cuboidal, and round cells of fairly large size, arranged in sheets, papillary structures, and pseudoacini, sometimes accompanied by production of hyaluronic acid. When benign it is also called *fibroendothelioma of joint, synovialoma, synovioendothelioma,* and *tenosynovioma;* when malignant, *synovial sarcoendothelioma* or *sarcomesothelioma.*

syn″o·vi′tis (sin″o·vy′tis, sigh″no·) [*synovia;* G. *-itis*, inflammation]. Inflammation of a synovial membrane.

acute suppurative s. A very acute, purulent form of infectious or traumatic origin. Syn., *pyarthrosis.*

chronic purulent s. Fungous arthritis.

chronic serous s. Hydrarthrosis.

dry s. Synovitis with little if any exudate.

exanthematous s. Synovitis secondary to the exanthemas.

fibrinous s. See dry *s.*

fungous s. Fungous arthritis.

gonorrheal s. Gonorrheal arthritis.

lipomatous s. Synovitis in which there is fatty degeneration.

metritic s. A synovitis secondary to uterine infection.

puerperal s. Synovitis occurring after childbirth, and due to septic infection.

purulent s. Synovitis with suppuration.

scarlatinal s. Synovitis occurring in an attack of scarlet fever.

s. hyperplastica. Fungous arthritis.

syphilitic s. Synovitis due to syphilitic inflammation.

tendinous s. Inflammation of the synovial sheath surrounding a tendon.

tuberculous s. Synovitis due to tuberculosis.

urethral s. Synonym of gonorrheal arthritis.

villous s. A type of synovitis in which villous growths develop within the articular cavity.

syn′ta·sis [G., tension]. A stretching, or tension.

syn·tax′is [G., a putting together]. 1. Articulation. *Obs.* 2. Reduction; taxis. *Obs.*

syn′tha·lin. $NH_2.C{:}NH.NH(CH_2)_{12}NH.C{:}NH.NH_2.2HCl$. The dihydrochloride of decamethylene bisguanidine, having hypoglycemic action through stimulation of insulin secretion by pancreas. Its use has been abandoned because of harmful effects.

syn′the·sis [G., a putting together]. 1. *In chemistry,* the processes and operations necessary to build up a compound. In general, a reaction, or series of reactions, in which a complex compound is obtained from elements or simple compounds. 2. The formation of a complex concept by the combination of separate ideas. 3. *In psychiatry,* the process in which the ego accepts unconscious ideas and feelings and amalgamates them within itself more or less consciously.

syn·thet′ic [G. *synthetikos*, skilled in putting together]. Produced by artificial means.

synthobilin. Trade-mark for a choleretic consisting of the diethanolamine salt of the camphoric ester of *p*-tolylmethylcarbinol.

syn·tho′rax. See *thoracopagus.*

syn·ton′ic [G. *syntonos*, strained tight]. Pertaining to a type of personality in which there is an appropriate harmony of thinking, feeling, and behavior.

syn′to·nin. 1. A metaprotein obtained by the action of dilute acid on more complex proteins. 2. The specific metaprotein thus obtained from the myosin of muscle.

syntopherol acetate. Trade-mark for the acetate ester of alpha-tocopherol.

syntrogel. Trade-mark for a tablet containing aluminum hydroxide, syntropan, bismuth subcarbonate, calcium carbonate, and flavored with peppermint oil. The drug is used to neutralize excess gastric acidity, to relieve flatulence, and to overcome spasm and hypersecretion.

syntropan. Trade-mark for the phosphate of the *dl*-tropic acid ester of 3-diethylamino-2,2-dimethyl-1-propanol. The substance occurs as a white, crystalline powder; freely soluble in water, slightly soluble in alcohol. It is used for its antispasmodic action on smooth muscle.

syn·troph′o·blast. See *syncytiotrophoblast.*

syn′tro·phus [G. *syntrophos*, brought up together]. A congenital disease.

syn″u·lo′sis [G. *synoulōsis*, complete cicatrization]. Cicatrization; cicatrix. *Obs.*

syn″u·lot′ic [G. *synoulōtikos*, promoting cicatrization]. Promoting cicatrization.

Sy·pha′ci·a (sigh·fay′see·uh). A genus of nematode worms belonging to the family Oxyuridae.

S. obvelata. A species commonly found in rats and mice; man is very rarely infested.

syph″il·el′cos [NL. *syphilis*, from the title of a poem by Fracastoro, 1530, the hero of which was the shepherd Syphilus; G. *helkos*, wound]. Syphilitic ulcer; chancre: also spelled *syphilelcus.*

syph″il·e′mi·a [*syphilis;* G. *haima*, blood]. The presence of *Treponema pallidum* in the blood stream.

syph′i·lid, syph′i·lide [*syphilis*]. A skin eruption due to syphilis. Nearly any type of skin lesion can be produced by *Treponema pallidum.*

secondary s. Any syphilid occurring during the early stage of syphilis.

tertiary s. Any syphilid occurring during the late stage of syphilis.

syph″i·lid·oph·thal′mi·a [*syphilis;* G. *ophthalmos*, eye]. Syphilitic ophthalmia. *Obs.*

syph″il·i·on′thus [*syphilis;* G. *ionthos*, eruption on the face]. Any copper-colored scaly eruption in syphilis.

syph′i·lis [NL.]. A prenatal or acquired chronic, systemic infection with *Treponema pallidum*, most often contracted in sexual intercourse. Lesions may occur in any tissue or vascular organ of the body, and the disease may give rise to symptoms characteristic of other diseases. Hence syphilis is called "the great imitator." When untreated the clinical course of the infection progresses through early (primary and secondary) stages, exhibiting the primary lesion or chancre and skin eruption, a latency period of variable duration, and the late (tertiary) phase. Also called *lues.* See Plates 31, 32.

acquired s. The reaction of man to *Treponema pallidum*, most commonly acquired by sexual intercourse, in which there is a tissue reaction at the inoculation site known as *primary syphilis* or the chancre. This is followed in about six weeks by a generalized skin eruption, *syphiloderm*. The mucous membranes, the eyes, and the central nervous system are often diseased in these early stages (under four years from the onset of the infection). Late acquired syphilis (over four years after infection) is characterized by greater localization of the lesions and destruction of the tissues. Benign late syphilis includes disease of the skin, bones, and mucous membranes. Late disabling syphilis of more vital organs includes disease of the central nervous system, eye, heart, and large blood vessels.

cardiovascular s. One of the late disabling lesions of acquired syphilis. Definite clinical signs appear usually from 20 to 30 years after infection. The first lesion is aortitis. Destruction of the elastic tissue leads to dilation of the aorta, which produces aortic insufficiency or aneurysm. The root of the aorta is involved and may effect occlusion of the coronary arteries. This in turn produces symptoms of angina pectoris and coronary insufficiency.

congenital s. See prenatal *s.*

early s. Primary, secondary, or latent infection of less than four years' duration. See acquired *s.*

extragenital s. Syphilis in which the first lesion is situated elsewhere than on the genital organs.

late s. Infection, latent or active, of greater than four years' duration: formerly called *tertiary s.* See acquired *s.*

latent s. Absence of clinical disease in syphilis, which occurs after spontaneous healing of early syphilis. The period of latency varies from a few months to a lifetime, during which there is no overt evidence of infection and the existence of the disease is recognized only by serologic or spinal-fluid tests.

marital s. Syphilis acquired in lawful wedlock.

meningovascular s. Syphilis of the central nervous system involving the leptomeninges and the cerebral arteries causing the formation of large or small gummas and an endarteritis; parenchymatous changes in brain or spinal-cord tissue occur only secondary to vascular disease.

nonvenereal s. Syphilis not acquired during sexual intercourse.

prenatal s. Infection of a fetus with *Treponema pallidum* by placental transfer from the mother. If the fetus dies, it is usually a macerated one. If born alive, it may, when untreated, progress through the various lesions seen in acquired syphilis, both early and late, except for the absence of the chancre and cardiovascular syphilis. Syn., *congenital s.*, *s. hereditaria.*

primary s. The first tissue reaction of early syphilis, usually characterized by the hard ulcer or chancre and regional adenopathy.

secondary s. Early syphilis; formerly, any of the manifestations of the disease after the primary complex and up to the end of the fourth year of infection, most often the syphiloderm.

s. alopecia. A patchy loss of hair in syphilis.

s. d'emblée. The invasion of syphilis without a local lesion.

s. hereditaria. See prenatal *s.*

s. insontium. Syphilis acquired in an innocent manner; nonvenereal syphilis.

s. technica. Syphilis acquired in following one's occupation, as by physicians, midwives, nurses.

tertiary s. Late syphilis, including all the symptoms of disease occurring after the fourth year of infection. See acquired *s.*

tests for s. See under *test.*

venereal s. Syphilis acquired in sexual intercourse.

syph″i·lit′ic [*syphilis*]. Pertaining to, or affected with, syphilis. Syn., *luetic.*

syph″i·li·za′tion [*syphilis*]. 1. Inoculation with *Treponema pallidum.* 2. The state produced by inoculation with the *Treponema pallidum.*

syph′i·lo-, syphil- [*syphilis*]. A combining form for *syphilis.*

syph′i·lo·derm, syph″i·lo·der′ma [*syphilis;* G. *derma*, skin]. Skin manifestations of syphilis. They are common, of many forms, and often diagnostic problems. While occurring in any stage of the disease, they are more frequent during the first two years of the infection. Early lesions are usually a dull- to ham-red color and appear symmetrically over the body, palms, and soles. **—syphiloder′matous,** *adj.*

syph″i·lo·gen′e·sis [*syphilis;* G. *genesis*, production]. The origin or development of syphilis.

syph″i·log′ra·pher [*syphilis;* G. *graphein*, to write]. One who writes about syphilis.

syph″i·log′ra·phy [*syphilis; graphein*]. A treatise on syphilis; any writing about the disease.

syph′i·loid [*syphilis;* G. *eidos*, form]. Resembling syphilis.

syph′i·loid. A disease resembling syphilis.

syph″i·lol′o·gist [*syphilis;* G. *logos*, word]. One who has made a study of syphilis; an expert in the diagnosis and treatment of the disease.

syph″i·lol′o·gy [*syphilis; logos*]. The sum of knowledge regarding the origin, nature, and treatment of syphilis.

syph″i·lo′ma [*syphilis;* G. *-ōma*, tumor]. 1. A syphilitic gumma. 2. Tumor due to syphilis. **—syphilom′atous,** *adj.*

cylindrical s. A rare growth in a segment of the urethra due to syphilis, occurring as a regular, cylindrical mass composed mainly of sclerotic tissue.

syph″i·lo·ma′ni·a [*syphilis;* G. *mania*, madness]. A mental disorder resulting from syphilophobia.

syph″i·lo·nych′i·a (sif″i·lo·nick′ee·uh) [*syphilis;* G. *onyx*, nail]. An onychia of syphilitic origin.

s. exulcerans. Syphilitic onychia with ulceration.

s. sicca. Syphilis of the nail bed.

syph″i·lop′a·thy [*syphilis;* G. *pathos*, disease]. Any syphilitic disease.

syph′i·lo·phobe″ [*syphilis;* G. *phobos*, fear]. One affected with syphilophobia.

syph″i·lo·pho′bi·a [*syphilis; phobos*]. Morbid fear of syphilis.

syph″i·lo·phy′ma [*syphilis;* G. *phyma*, growth]. 1. Syphiloma of the skin. 2. Any growth due to syphilis.

syph″i·lo·ther′a·py. Treatment for syphilis.

syr. *Syrupus*, syrup.

syrette. Trade-mark for a small hypodermic syringe containing a dose of the drug to be administered.

sy·rig″mo·pho′ni·a [G. *syrigma*, sound of a pipe; *phōnē*, sound]. 1. A piping or whistling state of the voice. 2. A sibilant rale.

sy·rig′mus [*syrigma*]. Any subjective hissing, murmuring, or tinkling sound heard in the ear.

syr″ing·ad″e·no′ma [G. *syrigx*, pipe; *adēn*, gland; *-ōma*, tumor]. A sweat-gland tumor.

syr″ing·ad″e·no′sus [*syrigx; adēn*]. Pertaining to the sweat glands.

syr′inge [*syrigx*]. An apparatus of metal, glass, or plastic material, consisting of a nozzle, a barrel, and a plunger or a rubber bulb; used to inject a liquid into a cavity or under the skin.

aural s. One used to wash out the external auditory canal.

hypodermic s. One used to administer drugs, as opiates, under the skin.

penis s. See urethral *s.*

rectal s. A large syringe used to administer an enema.

urethral s. One adapted to force liquid into the male urethra.

sy·rin″go·bul′bi·a [*syrigx;* L. *bulbus*, bulb]. The presence of cavities in the medulla oblongata similar to syringomyelia.

sy·rin″go·car″ci·no′ma. Sweat-gland tumor.

sy·rin′go·cele, sy·rin″go·coe′li·a (si·ring″go·see′-lee·uh) [*syrigx;* G. *koilia*, hollow]. Old term for the cavity or central canal of the spinal cord.

sy·rin″go·cyst′ad·e·no′ma. Syringoma.

sy·rin″go·cys·to′ma. Syringoma.

sy·rin′goid [*syrigx;* G. *eidos*, form]. Like a tube.

syr″in·go′ma. A multiple nevoid tumor of sweat glands, occurring most often in females and developing after puberty. Histologically the derma contains numerous small cystic ducts with commalike tails of epithelium. Also called *syringocystadenoma, syringocystoma.*

sy·rin″go·me·nin′go·cele. See *syringomyelocele.*

sy·rin″go·my·e′li·a (si·ring″go·migh·ee′lee·uh) [*syrigx;* G. *myelos*, marrow]. A chronic disease characterized pathologically by the presence of long cavities surrounded by gliosis, which are situated in relation to the central canal of the spinal cord and frequently extend up into the medulla (syringobulbia).

sy·rin″go·my′e·lo·cele″ [*syrigx; myelos;* G. *kēlē*, hernia]. Spina bifida with protrusion of a meningeal sac containing a portion of the spinal cord whose central canal is greatly distended with cerebrospinal fluid.

syr′inx [*syrigx*]. 1. Old term for a fistula or tube. 2. The posterior larynx of birds, found within the thorax at the tracheal bifurcation; the organ of voice in birds.

syr′up [Ar. *sharāb*, a drink] (*syrupus*). 1. A concentrated solution of sugar in aqueous fluids, with the addition of medicating or flavoring ingredients. 2. The U.S.P. preparation containing sucrose, 850 Gm.; purified water, a sufficient quantity to make 1000 cc. Used in the preparation of other medicated or flavored syrups and preparations and in pharmaceutical operations where sucrose in solution is required. Abbreviated, syr. Syn., *sirup.* Also called *simple s.* —**syrupy,** *adj.*

sys″sar·co′sis [G. *syn*, with; *sarkōsis*, growth of flesh]. The failure of union of bones after fracture by the interposition of muscular tissue. —**syssarcot′ic,** *adj.*

sys·so′ma [*syn;* G. *sōma*, body]. A double monstrosity with two separate heads, but with the bodies fused in more or less intimate union. —**sysso′mic,** *adj.*

sys·so′mus [*syn; sōma*]. A double monster joined by the trunks.

sys·tal′tic [G. *systaltikos*, depressing]. Pulsatory; contracting; having a systole.

sys′ta·sis [G., a bringing together]. Consistency, density. *Obs.*

sys′tem [G. *systēma*, system]. 1. A methodical arrangement. 2. A combination of parts into a whole, as the digestive system, the nervous system. 3. The body as a whole. —**system′ic, systemat′ic,** *adj.*

alimentary s. The alimentary canal with its accessory glands.

arch-loop-whorl s. of fingerprints. See fingerprint *s.*

autonomic nervous s. An aggregation of ganglia, nerves, and plexuses through which the viscera, heart, blood vessels, smooth muscles, and glands receive their motor innervation. It is divided into the *craniosacral* or *parasympathetic system*, and the *thoracicolumbar* or *sympathetic system.* Also called *vegetative nervous s.*

Bertillon s. of identification. See under *identification.*

brain stem activating s. See reticular activating *s.*

cardiovascular s. The heart and blood vessels.

centimeter-gram-second s. The system based upon the use of the centimeter, gram, and second as units of length, mass, and time, respectively.

central nervous s. The brain and spinal cord, including the dorsal root ganglions. Abbreviated, C.N.S.

cerebrospinal s. The central nervous *s.*

corticopontocerebellar s. See extrapyramidal *s.*

corticostrionigral s. See extrapyramidal *s.*

craniosacral s. That part of the autonomic nervous system composed of nerve fibers in cranial nerves III, VII, IX, X, and sacral nerves II, III, and IV, which go to the outlying parasympathetic ganglions, and which in turn send motor fibers to the effector organs. Syn., *parasympathetic s.*

digestive s. The digestive tract from mouth to anus and usually considered as the alimentary canal.

endocrine s. The ductless glands or glands of internal secretion considered as a whole.

exterofective s. That part of the nervous system that is concerned with adapting the body to changes in its external environment.

extrapyramidal s. A widespread and complicated system of descending fiber tracts arising in the cortex and subcortical motor centers; in the widest sense it includes all nonpyramidal motor tracts, such as corticopontine tracts and tracts from globus pallidus to the midbrain nuclei. It acts as a servomechanism for the control and adjustment of the final common pathway.

fingerprint s. A scientific system for the identification of persons in the military service, for the apprehension of criminals, and for the identification of the dead. A modern development of the Bertillon system.

Galton s. of identification. See under *identification.*

genital s. See reproductive *s.*

Haversian s. The concentric layers of bone about the blood vessels in the Haversian canals of compact bone.

hematopoietic, hemopoietic s. The system concerned with the formation of blood cells. It includes the marrow and lymphatic organs.

hepatic duct s. The biliary tract including the hepatic ducts, gallbladder, cystic duct, and common bile duct.

hexaxial reference s. *In electrocardiography*, a six-line star coordinate graft formed by the triaxial reference system on which is superimposed a similar star in relative rotation of 30° μ: used for plotting the bipolar and unipolar limb-lead voltages of the electrocardiogram.

His-Tawara s. The conduction system of the heart, composed of the atrioventricular node (of Tawara) and the atrioventricular bundle (of His).

hydrophilic colloidal s. A colloidal solution whose external phase is water and which has affinity for water.

hydrophobic colloidal s. A colloidal suspension whose external phase is water but which shows no affinity for water.

integumentary s. That pertaining to the body covering, as the skin, hair, nails, etc.

locomotor s. The extremities and their parts, as the bones, muscles, and joints concerned with locomotion, or the motor activities of the body.

lymphatic s. A system of vessels and nodes accessory to the blood vascular system, conveying lymph. It begins as innumerable capillaries in interspaces of tissues. These form plexuses studded with lymph nodes that act as filters and finally all those below the diaphragm unite in the cisterna chyli on the second lumbar vertebra. From this the thoracic duct leads upward to empty into the junction of the left subclavian and internal jugular veins. The lymph from the upper left half of the body also empties here. The lymph from the upper right half of the body and head enters the right lymphatic duct, which empties into the junction of the right internal jugular and subclavian veins. See Plate 11.

lymphoreticular s. See reticuloendothelial *s.*

orthosympathetic s. The thoracicolumbar system, in contrast to the craniosacral or parasympathetic system.

osseous s. The bony skeleton of the body.

parasympathetic nervous s., parasympathetic s. See craniosacral *s.*

portal s. The portal circulation, 1; specifically, the portal vein and its tributaries. See portal *circulation*, 2. See also hypophysioportal *circulation.*

projection systems. The name given to the pathways connecting the cerebral cortex with the periphery.

Purkinje s. See *Purkinje fibers* under *fiber.*

pyramidal s. The corticospinal and corticobulbar tracts.

redox s. (*red*uctant-*ox*idant). A simple oxidation-reduction system in which two substances react reversibly with each other. The oxidized material is a reductant; the reduced material, an oxidant.

renal pressor s. The interaction of renin and renin substrate with formation and coincident destruction of angiotonin.

reproductive s. The generative apparatus, as a whole, consisting in man of the penis, testes, deferential ducts, seminal vesicles, and prostate, and in woman of the vagina, uterus, uterine tubes (oviducts), and ovaries.

respiratory s. All the passages by which air is conducted to, and including, the parts of the lungs where an exchange of oxygen and carbon dioxide takes place, such as the nasal cavities, pharynx, larynx, trachea, bronchi, bronchioles, and the pulmonary lobules with their alveoli. Other accessory structures, for example the diaphragm and muscles concerned with respiration, are included.

reticular activating s. The reticular formation of the superior levels of the brain stem and the adjacent subthalamus, hypothalamus, and medial thalamus, which has been shown in animal experiments to play a basic role in regulating the background activity of the rest of the central nervous system. It is connected by collaterals in parallel with long afferent and efferent nervous pathways, and is thus stimulated by and acts upon them: caudal influences upon spinal cord levels contribute to optimum motor performance; cephalic influences upon the cerebral hemispheres form the basis of the initiation, maintenance, and degree of the state called wakefulness on which higher nervous functions depend. Many hypnotics block transmission of impulses from this area, and lesions of it result in states similar to coma in man. See also arousal *reaction.*

reticular s. See reticuloendothelial *s.*

reticuloendothelial s. The macrophage system, which includes all the phagocytic cells of the body, except the leukocytes. These cells, diverse morphologically, all have the capacity for the elective storage of certain colloidal dyes. They include: the histiocytes and macrophages of loose connective tissue, the reticular cells of lymphatic and myeloid tissues, the endotheliumlike littoral cells lining lymphatic sinuses and sinusoids of bone marrow, the Kupffer cells of hepatic sinusoids, the cells lining the sinusoids of the adrenal and hypophysis, and the dust cells of the lungs. Abbreviated, RES.

supraopticohypophysial s. Supraoptic nucleus with the supraopticohypophyseal tract to the neurohypophysis. A dual neuroglandular mechanism whose normal function is control of water balance in the tissues and secretion of urine.

sympathetic nervous s., sympathetic s. 1. The thoracicolumbar system. 2. Formerly, the autonomic nervous system as a whole.

s. of Batson. The vertebral venous *s.*

thoracicolumbar s., thoracolumbar s. The part of the autonomic nervous system composed of nerve fibers in the thoracic and the superior two lumbar nerves which go to the ganglions of the sympathetic trunk and which in turn send motor fibers to the effector organs. Syn., *sympathetic s.* Also called *orthosympathetic s.*

triaxial reference s. A means for the determination of the mean electric axis of any wave of depolarization or repolarization from the electrocardiogram.

urinary s. The system made up of the kidneys, ureters, urinary bladder, and urethra, whose function is the elaboration and excretion of urine.

urogenital s. The combined urinary and genital systems which are intimately related embryologically and anatomically.

vascular s. See cardiovascular *s.*

vasomotor s. The nerve supply of the blood vessels.

vegetative nervous s. The autonomic nervous system.

vertebral venous s. A group of venous anastomoses which pass through the intervertebral foramens to connect the veins of the pelvic cavity, of the pelvic girdle, of the shoulder girdle, and of the body wall with the vertebral veins and thus with the sinuses of the dura: also called *s. of Batson.*

sys'tem·oid [*systēma;* G. *eidos*, form]. A term applied to tumors composed of a number of tissues resembling a system of organs.

sys'to·le (sis'to·lee) [G., a drawing together]. The contraction phase of the cardiac cycle.

aborted s. A premature cardiac systole. Systolic ejection is small because of the short preceding diastolic filling.

arterial s. The expansion and elongation of the arteries following cardiac systole.

auricular s. Atrial contraction.

electric s. QT interval.

premature s. A systole resulting from a premature impulse discharged by the sinus node.

ventricular s. The contraction of the ventricles.

sys·tol'ic [*systolē*]. Pertaining to the systole; occurring during systole.

sys·trem'ma (pl. *systremmata*) [G., anything twisted up together]. Cramp in the muscles of the leg.

syz'y·gy (siz'i·jee) [G. *syzygos*, yoked]. End-to-end union of the sporonts of certain gregarines. **—syzyg'ial,** *adj.*

Szabo's sign. See under *sign.*

Szent-Györgyi, Albert (1893–). Hungarian

biochemist, known for his isolation of ascorbic acid (vitamin C) and postulation of vitamin P. He performed miscellaneous studies on cellular oxidation, including the discovery of the catalytic role of C_4-dicarboxylic acids in tissue respiration, which eventually gave rise to present knowledge of the tricarboxylic acid cycle, and won the Nobel prize in physiology and medicine (1937). His later studies of cellular-structure proteins culminated in the discovery of the contractility of actomyosin. See also Szent-Györgyi *test*.

Szymanowski, Julius von [*Russian surgeon*, 1829–68]. Developed a form of blepharoplasty called *Szymanowski's operation*. Developed operations for the restoration of the auricle, for ectropion, for restoration of the upper lip by lateral flaps brought together in the midline; also called *Szymanowski's operations*.

T

T Tension, temperature.

T Symbol for transmittance.

T 1824 See *Evans blue.*

T. A. Toxin-antitoxin.

Ta Chemical symbol for tantalum.

tab″a·co′sis [Taino *tabaco*, roll of tobacco leaves; G. *-ōsis*, condition]. A toxic state produced by the excessive use of tobacco, or by the inhalation of tobacco dust.

ta·ba′cum. See *tobacco.*

tab′a·gism (tab′uh·jiz·um). Tabacosis.

tab′a·nid [L. *tabanus*, gadfly]. Any representative of the family Tabanidae.

Ta·ban′i·dae (ta·ban′i·dee) [*tabanus*]. A family of the Diptera, which includes the horseflies, deer flies, and gadflies. They are medium to large size, robust flies, world-wide in distribution. The females of the well-known species are blood suckers which attack man and warm-blooded animals generally. Certain species distribute diseases such as anthrax among cattle and sheep; others transmit the trypanosomes of animals, especially the *Trypanosoma evansi*, the cause of surra in horses and cattle. The important genera are *Chrysops*, *Haematopota*, *Tabanus*, and *Pangonia*.

ta″bar·dil′lo (tah″bahr·deel′yo). Term used in Mexico for both epidemic and murine typhus.

ta″ba″tière′ an″a·to·mique′. See *anatomist's snuffbox.*

ta·bel′la [L., little table]. A medicated troche or tablet.

ta′bes (tay′beez) [L.]. A wasting or consumption: used as a synonym for tabes dorsalis.

diabetic t. A peripheral neuritis affecting diabetics.

optic t. Old term for optic atrophy resulting from syphilis.

spastic t. Combined cord disease or posterolateral cord disease producing ataxia and spasticity of the lower extremities.

t. coxaria. Wasting from hip disease.

t. diuretica. See *diabetes* mellitus.

t. dolorosa. A form in which pain is the dominating feature.

t. dorsalis. Locomotor ataxia, a disease dependent upon sclerosis of the posterior columns of the spinal cord. The symptoms are lightning pains; unsteadiness and incoordination of voluntary movements, extending to the upper extremities; disorders of vision, as the Argyll Robertson pupil; cutaneous anesthesia; pain crises in the gastric, laryngeal, and rectal zones; trophic disorders of the joints; abolition of the patellar reflex; diminution of sexual desire; and disturbance of the sphincters.

t. ergotica. A toxemia resulting from the use of ergot; its symptomatology closely simulates that of tabes dorsalis.

t. mesenterica. Tuberculous mesenteric lymphadenitis.

ta·bes′cence [L. *tabescere*, to waste away]. Wasting; marasmus; emaciation. *Obs.* —**tabescent,** *adj.*

ta·bet′ic [L. *tabes*, a wasting]. 1. Affected with tabes; of, or pertaining to, tabes. 2. Pertaining to, or affected with, tabes dorsalis.

ta·bet′i·form [*tabes;* L. *forma*, form]. Resembling tabes.

tab′ic, tab′id. *Obs.* See *tabetic.*

ta′ble [L. *tabula*, board]. 1. A flat-topped piece of furniture, as an operating table, examining table. 2. A flat plate, especially one of bone, as the inner or outer table (of compact bone) of a flat bone of the cranium. 3. A presentation of numerical data in the form of rows and columns.

ta′ble·spoon″ [*tabula;* AS. *spōn*, a chip]. A large spoon, holding about 15 cc. or 4 fluidrachms. Abbreviated, tbsp.

tab′let [dim. from *tabula*]. A friable solid dosage form. Hypodermic tablets must be readily soluble in water.

tabloid. Trade-mark for a compressed or other medicinal tablet.

ta″bo·pa·ral′y·sis [L. *tabes*, a wasting; G. *paralysis*, paralysis]. A condition in which tabes is associated with general paralysis and with primary optic atrophy.

ta″bo·pa·re′sis (tay″bo·pa·ree′sis, ·par′i·sis). See *taboparalysis.*

tab′u·lar [L. *tabula*, board]. Having the form of a table, as a tabular bone.

tac′a·ma·hac, tac″a·ma·hac′a [Sp. *tacamaca*, from the Nahuatl]. Common name for poplar bud.

TACE Trade-mark for tri-*p*-anisylchloroethylene or chlorotrianisene, a synthetic estrogen employed in the treatment of prostatic carcinoma.

tache (tahsh) (pl. *taches*) [OF.]. A spot.

t. bleuâtre. A spot of a delicate blue tint, sometimes observed in the skin of typhoid fever patients.

t. cérébrale. The red line made when the fingernail is drawn over the skin, due to vasomotor reaction and occurring especially in connection with meningeal irritation. Also called *t. meningeale.*

t. motrice. An eminence of sarcoplasm within the sarcolemma where the nerve fibers pierce the latter; a motor end-plate.

t. noire. The primary painless lesion of the tick-bite fevers of Africa, manifested by a raised red area with typical black necrotic center which appears at the site of the tick bite.

taches blanches. Certain white spots described by Hanot as occurring on the liver, especially on its convex surfaces, in infectious diseases. Microscopically, they present a leukocytic infiltration and bacteria.

taches du café au lait. See *café au lait spots* under *spot.*

t. spinale. A bullalike spot seen in certain diseases of the spinal cord.

tach″e·om′e·ter (tack″ee·om′i·tur). See *hemotachometer.*

ta·chet′ic (ta·ket′ick) [*tache*]. Relating to the formation of reddish blue or purple patches (taches).

ta·chis′to·scope (ta·kis′to·scope) [G. *tachistos*, swiftest; *skopein*, to examine]. An instrument used in psychophysiology to observe the time rate and time conditions for apperception; also an instrument used in orthoptics for visual training, especially to overcome the suppression area in amblyopia ex anopsia. —**tachistoscop′ic,** *adj.*

tach′o·gram (tack′o·gram) [G. *tachos*, swiftness; *gramma*, letter]. The record made in tachography.

ta·chog′ra·phy (ta·kog′ruh·fee) [*tachos;* G. *graphein*, to write]. The estimation of the rate of flow of arterial blood by means of a flowmeter, or tachygraph.

ta·chom′e·ter (ta·kom′i·tur). See *hemotachometer.*

tach′y- (tack′i-) [G. *tachys*, swift]. A combining form meaning *swift.*

tach″y·aux·e′sis [*tachys;* G. *auxēsis*, increase]. Heterauxesis in which the part grows more rapidly than the whole organism.

tach″y·car′di·a [*tachys;* G. *kardia*, heart]. Excessive rapidity of the heart's action.

atrial t. Rapid and regular succession of P waves which are normal or are abnormal in form. The QRS group may be normal, or slightly or markedly aberrant. The rate is usually 160–200 per minute.

atrioventricular t. Rapid and regular succession of systoles arising from the atrioventricular node at a rate over 100 per minute; may be as fast as 270 per minute. In some records the P waves cannot be recognized. In others there is retrograde block and the basic atrial rhythm is undisturbed (His's bundle tachycardia or idioventricular tachycardia).

auricular t. See atrial *t.*

essential t. That occurring in paroxysms, and due to functional disturbance of the cardiac nerves.

His's bundle t. Atrioventricular paroxysmal tachycardia with retrograde block.

idioventricular t. Atrioventricular paroxysmal tachycardia with retrograde block.

junctional t. Paroxysmal tachycardia originating in the A-V node.

paroxysmal sinus t. Paroxysm of rapid heart action due to ectopic focus in or near the sinoatrial node.

paroxysmal supraventricular t. Paroxysm of rapid heart action due to ectopic focus in the atria or atrioventricular node.

paroxysmal t. Tachycardia occurring periodically in paroxysms.

reflex t. Tachycardia due to causes other than those producing essential tachycardia.

supraventricular t. One in which the origin of the P waves cannot be classified definitely, and the pacemaker is above the point where the bundle of His branches. The main characteristics are the same as those in atrial tachycardia.

t. strumosa exophthalmica. The tachycardia occurring in exophthalmic goiter.

ventricular t. A rapid succession of beats, each with the characteristics of a ventricular systole, occurring at rates from 150–250 per minute, regular or slightly irregular. The atrial rhythm, if recognized, is not disturbed.

tach″y·car′di·ac [*tachys; kardia*]. Pertaining to, or suffering from, tachycardia.

tach′y·graph [*tachys;* G. *graphein*, to write]. An instrument for measuring the rate of blood flow.

ta·chyg′ra·phy (ta·kig′ruh·fee) [*tachys; graphein*]. The estimation of the rate of flow of arterial blood by means of the tachygraph.

tach″y·i·a′tri·a (tack″ee·eye·ay′tree·uh, ·at′-ree·uh) [*tachys;* G. *iatreia*, healing]. The art of curing quickly. *Obs.*

tach″y·lo′gi·a [*tachys;* G. *logos*, word]. Morbid rapidity or volubility of speech; occurs in the manic phase of manic-depressive psychosis. Syn., *logorrhea, tachyphrasia, tachyphemia.*

ta·chym′e·ter (ta·kim′i·tur) [*tachys;* G. *metron*, a measure]. An instrument for measuring the rate of speed of a moving object.

tach″y·pha′gi·a [*tachys;* G. *phagein*, to eat]. Rapid eating.

tach″y·pha′si·a. See *tachylogia.*

tach″y·phe′mi·a. See *tachylogia.*

tach″y·phra′si·a. See *tachylogia.*

tach″y·phre′ni·a [*tachys;* G. *phrēn*, mind]. Morbidly accelerated mental activity.

tach″y·phy·lax′ia, tach″y·phy·lax′is [*tachys;* G. *phylaxis*, a watching]. Injection of small quantities of toxic organ extracts which will protect animals; also, doses of the same extract administered shortly afterward. The protection is transitory and lasts for a few hours only. Also called *skeptophylaxia, skeptophylaxis.*

tach″yp·ne′a, tach″yp·noe′a [*tachys;* G. *pnoē*, a breathing hard]. Abnormal frequency of respiration.

nervous t. Respiration of 40 or more to the minute accompanying neurotic disorders, particularly hysteria and neurasthenia.

tach″y·rhyth′mi·a [*tachys;* G. *rhythmos*, rhythm]. 1. Tachycardia. 2. *In electroencephalography*, an increase in the normal brain wave frequency up to 12–50 per second.

ta·chys′ter·ol (ta·kis′tur·ole, ·ol, ·awl, tack″i-steer′·). The precursor of calciferol in the irradiation of ergosterol. It is an isomer of ergosterol.

tach″y·sys′to·le (tack″i·sis′to·lee) [*tachys;* G. *systolē*, contraction]. Tachycardia.

tac′tile (tack′til) [L. *tactilis*, that may be touched]. Pertaining to the sense of touch.

tac′toid. A type of colloidal structure showing intense birefringence in which elongated particles are oriented in a group and parallel to a central axis; a cigar-shaped colloidal particle.

tae′di·um vi′tae (tee′dee·um vy′tee) [L.]. Weariness of life, a symptom occurring in many cases of depressive reactions; it is sometimes a precursor of suicide.

Tae′ni·a (tee′nee·uh) [G. *tainia*, band, tapeworm]. A genus of parasitic worms of the class Cestoda; they are ribbonlike segmental flatworms. The adult is an intestinal parasite of vertebrates; the larvae parasitize both vertebrate and invertebrate tissues. The adult consists of a scolex, an undifferentiated germinal neck, and two or more hermaphroditic segments or proglottids which contain fertile ova when mature.

T. coenurus. A tapeworm occurring in the small intestine of the dog. The intermediate stage, *Multiceps multiceps*, develops in the brain and spinal cord of sheep, goats, cattle, horses, and has also been found in man.

T. echinococcus. See *Echinococcus granulosus.*

T. nana. See *Hymenolepis nana.*

T. saginata. A tapeworm which passes its larval stages in cattle, its adult stage in the intestine of man. The human infestation is acquired by eating insufficiently cooked infested beef. Syn., *beef tapeworm.*

T. solium. The larval stages occur in hogs; the adult is found in the intestine of man. Ingestion of ova may result in larval infestation in man; the larvae are then called *Cysticercus cellulosae.* Infestation is usually acquired by ingestion of viable larvae in pork. Syn., *pork tapeworm.*

tae′ni·a (pl. *taeniae*) [*tainia*]. 1. A band or bandlike structure. 2. See *tapeworm.*

mesocolic t. The longitudinal muscle band corresponding to the insertion of the mesocolon.

t. choroidea. The bands appearing at the lateral boundaries of the fourth or third ventricle when their telae choroideae are removed, respectively called *t. of fourth ventricle* and *t. of third ventricle* or *t. thalami.*

t. coli. One of the three tapelike bands of the longitudinal layer of the tunica muscularis of the colon. See Plate 13.

t. of fourth ventricle (*t. ventriculi quarti*). See *t. choroidea.*

t. of third ventricle (*t. ventriculi tertii*). See *t. choroidea.*

t. pontis. See *filum lateralis pontis.*

t. thalami. See *t. choroidea.*

tae′ni·a·cide″ [*tainia;* L. *caedere,* to kill]. Destructive of tapeworms. —**tae′niacide,** *n.*

tae′ni·a·fuge″ [*tainia;* L. *fugere,* to flee]. Expelling tapeworms. —**tae′niafuge,** *n.*

tae·ni′a·sis (tee·nigh′uh·sis, ti·nigh′·) [*tainia;* NL. *-iasis,* condition]. The symptoms caused by infestation with any of the species of *Taenia.*

tae′ni·form [*tainia;* L. *forma,* form]. Having a segmented, ribbonlike form; resembling a tapeworm.

tae′ni·oid [*tainia;* G. *eidos,* form]. Taeniform.

tae″ni·o·pho′bi·a [*tainia;* G. *phobos,* fear]. Morbid dread of becoming the host of a tapeworm.

Taenzer, Paul [*German dermatologist,* 1858–1919]. Described ulerythema ophryogenes (1889); also called *Taenzer's disease, keratosis pilaris.*

tag [prob. Scand. in origin]. A flap or appendage.

epithelial t. A mass of epithelial cells projecting from the urethral groove on the glans of the embryonic phallus. Syn., *epithelial tubercle.*

tagathen •citrate. Trade-marked name for the antihistaminic substance chlorothen citrate.

Tagliacozzi, Gasparo [*Italian surgeon,* 1546–99]. He developed a form of rhinoplasty in which he formed a new nose from a pedicle flap taken from the arm. Called *Italian* or *Tagliacozzi's operation.*

tag′ma [G., arrangement]. An aggregate of molecules.

tail [AS. *taegel*]. 1. The caudal extremity of an animal. 2. Anything resembling a tail.

tai′lor's spasm. See under *spasm.*

taint [L. *tingere,* to dye]. 1. Hereditary predisposition to disease; affection by disease without outspoken manifestations. 2. Putrefaction or infestation, as tainted meat. 3. Local discoloration, as a blemish.

tai′pan. *Pseudechis scutellatus;* giant brown snake, largest venomous snake of Australia and New Guinea, belonging to the Elapidae.

Tait, Robert Lawson [*English surgeon and gynecologist,* 1845–99]. One of the first to operate for ruptured ectopic pregnancy (1883). Believed that all cases of dangerous or crippling pelvic or abdominal lesions should be surgically explored; called *Tait's law.* Introduced a flap-splitting procedure for plastic repair, especially of the perineum (1891); called *Tait's operation* or *Tait's method.*

taka-diastase. Trade-mark for a powdered vegetable diastase, obtained by the action of *Aspergillus oryzae* on wheat bran; the substance is capable of liquefying 450 times its weight of starch in 10 minutes. Used in cases of faulty starch digestion.

Takaki, Kanehiro [*Japanese physician,* 1849–1915]. One of the first to demonstrate the dietary origin of Japanese beriberi or kakke (1885).

Takamine, Jôkichi [*Japanese chemist in the United States,* 1854–1922]. Isolated epinephrine in crystalline form (1901). Takadiastase is named for him.

Takata reaction. See under *reaction.*

Takata-Ara test. See under *test.*

Takayama solution. See under *solution.*

takazyme. Trade-mark for an antacid and starch digestant consisting of calcium carbonate, magnesium carbonate, bismuth subcarbonate, and taka-diastase.

take [AS. *tacan*]. In *medicine,* a successful inoculation, as by a vaccine.

ta·lal′gi·a [L. *talus,* ankle; G. *algos,* pain]. Pain in the ankle.

Talbot's solution, diluted. See iodine and *zinc* iodide glycerite.

talc, tal′cum. A native, hydrous magnesium silicate sometimes containing a little aluminum silicate. It occurs in various grades and degrees of purity, as potstone, soapstone, steatite, French chalk.

purified t. (*talcum purificatum*). Talc, purified by acid washing. A fine, white, crystalline powder, unctuous to the touch. Used as filtering medium and as dusting powder.

tal′i·pes (tal′i·peez) [L. *talus,* ankle; *pes,* foot]. Any one of a variety of deformities of the human foot, especially those of congenital origin, such as clubfoot or equinovarus. Also embraces paralytic deformities and the numerous simple varieties of foot distortion, according to whether the forefoot is inverted or everted and whether the Achilles tendon is shortened or lengthened. Combinations of the various types occur, called talipes equinovalgus, talipes equinovarus, talipes calcaneovalgus, talipes calcaneovarus, etc.

equinocavus t. A deformity of the foot characterized by fixed plantar flexion and a high longitudinal arch.

equinovarus t. A deformity of the foot characterized by fixed plantar flexion and a turning inward of the foot.

flaccid t. A foot in which there is a complete flaccid type paralysis.

t. arcuatus. See *t.* cavus.

t. calcaneocavus. A calcaneus deformity of the foot in which there is also a cavus; a dorsal rotation of the calcaneus with a relative plantar tilting of the forefoot.

t. calcaneovalgus. A calcaneus deformity of the foot with associated valgus deviation.

t. calcaneus. Talipes in which the patient walks upon the heel alone.

t. cavus. An increased curvature of the arch of the foot.

t. equinus. Talipes in which the heel is elevated and the weight thrown upon the anterior portion of the foot.

t. percavus. Excessive plantar curvature.

t. planus. Flatfoot; splay foot.

t. spasmodica. Noncongenital talipes due to muscular spasm.

t. valgus. Talipes in which the outer border of the foot is everted, with inward rotation of the tarsus and flattening of the plantar arch. Also called *flatfoot, splay foot, pes planus, weak foot.*

t. varus. A variety in which the foot is inverted, the weight falling on the outer border. If the inversion is extreme, with rotation of the forefoot, the condition is known as clubfoot.

tal″i·pom′a·nus (tal″i·pom′uh·nus, tal″i·po·may′·nus) [*talus; pes;* L. *manus,* hand]. Clubhand.

Tallerman, Lewis A. [*English inventor,* contemporary]. Devised an apparatus for the local application of superheated dry air in the treatment of joint diseases, the affected part being enclosed in a cylinder. Called *Tallerman's apparatus.* Treatment using the apparatus is called *Tallerman's treatment.*

tal'low [ME. *talgh*]. The fat extracted from suet, the solid fat of cattle, sheep, and other ruminants. It consists largely of stearin and palmitin.

Tallqvist, Theodor Waldemar [*Finnish physician,* 1871–1927]. Remembered for his description of a method for hemoglobin determination. *Tallqvist's method,* or *scale,* is only approximate.

Tallqvist hemoglobin measurement. The measurement of hemoglobin concentration in whole blood. The test solution is compared with a series of color-saturation standards. The measurement is not very precise, and is most useful as a screening test.

Talma, Sape [*Dutch surgeon,* 1847–1918]. Independently of Morison, described omentopexy to relieve ascites associated with cirrhosis of the liver, called *Talma's operation* or *Talma-Morison operation.*

ta'lo- [L. *talus,* ankle]. A combining form denoting *pertaining to the talus* or *astragalus.*

tal'ose. $C_6H_{12}O_6$. A monosaccharide isomeric with dextrose.

ta'lus [L.]. The bone of the ankle which articulates with the bones of the leg. The old term is *astragalus.* See Table of Bones in the Appendix.

ta'ma, tam'a [L.]. Swelling of the feet and legs.

tam'a·rind [Ar. *tamr hindi,* Indian date]. The fruit of the *Tamarindus indica,* a tree of the Leguminosae. The preserved pulp of the fruit (tamarindus) is laxative and refrigerant.

tam'bour (tam'boor, tam·boor') [F.]. A drum; a drumlike instrument used in physiologic experiments for recording. It consists of a metal cylinder over which is stretched an elastic membrane, and to which passes a tube for transmitting changes in air pressure. Recording is done optically by means of a small mirror on the membrane, or mechanically by a stylus attached to the membrane.

tam'pan. *Ornithodorus moubata;* a parasitic tick infesting birds, small mammals, domestic animals, and occasionally man; an important vector of relapsing fever. Also called *bibo, mabata.*

tampax. Trade-mark for an intravaginal, absorbent menstruation plug.

tam'pi·cin. A purgative resin, $C_{34}H_{54}O_{14}$, from the root of the Mexican plant, *Ipomoea simulans,* or Tampico jalap.

tam'pon [F.]. A plug of cotton, sponge, or other material inserted into the vagina, nose, or other cavity.

tam'pon. To plug with a tampon.

tam"pon·ade' [*tampon*]. The act of plugging with a tampon.

cardiac t. Symptoms due to large accumulation of pericardial fluid, pyo- or hemopericardium, or to extensive compression scar of the pericardium. Pressure on lungs, mediastinal contents, superior and inferior venae cavae, and the mouths of the hepatic veins results in a quiet heart, small-volume paradoxical pulse, enlarged liver, and high venous pressure.

tam'pon·ing, tam'pon·ment (tam'pun·mint, tam·pon'mint) [*tampon*]. The act of inserting a pack or plug within a cavity for checking hemorrhage, etc.

tan [OF. *tanner*]. To color the skin by exposure to sun or wind (or artificially, by use of a sun lamp).

tan"a·ce'tin (tan"uh·see'tin, tan·ass'i·tin). A bitter principle, $C_{11}H_{16}O_4$, in the seeds, leaves, and flowers of *Tanacetum vulgare,* or tansy.

tan"a·ce'tone (tan"uh·see'tone, tan·ass'i·tone). The chief constituent in the volatile oil of tansy. It is identical with thujone.

tanexin. A proprietary antiseptic tannic acid ointment.

tan'ghi·nin (tang'ghi·nin, tan·ghin'in) [Malagasy *voa tanging*]. The toxic neutral principle of the ordeal bean *Tanghinia madagascariensis,* Apocynaceae. Its action resembles that of strophanthin.

tannalbin. Trade-mark for an albumin tannate, an astringent in diarrhea.

tan'nase (tan'ace, ·aze). An enzyme found in cultures of *Penicillium* and *Aspergillus* which converts tannic acid to gallic acid.

tan'nic ac'id (*acidum tannicum*). A tannin usually obtained from nutgalls, the excrescences formed on the young twigs of *Quercus infectoria* and allied species. Yellow to light brown powder of astringent taste; very soluble in water, alcohol, or glycerin. A styptic and astringent; a local dressing for burns; a chemical antidote for poisoning by alkaloids and heavy metals; in diarrhea it lessens secretion. Syn., *gallotannic acid, tannin, digallic acid.*

t. a. glycerite (*glyceritum acidi tannici*). A stable 20% solution in glycerin with sodium citrate and exsiccated sodium sulfite. Also called *tannin glycerite.*

t. a. ointment (*unguentum acidi tannici*). A 20% ointment used as an astringent.

tannigen. Trade-mark for *acetyltannic acid.*

tan'nin. 1. Tannic acid. 2. Any one of a group of astringent plant principles characterized by their ability to precipitate collagen and to produce dark-colored compounds with ferric salts. The source is frequently identified by a prefix, as gallotannin, quercitannin, etc.

tannismut. Trade-mark for *bismuth bitannate.*

tannoform. Trade-mark for a condensation product of tannin and formaldehyde: formerly used internally in diarrhea and enteritis and as an astringent local application in powder or ointment form.

Tanret reagent. See under *reagent.*

Tanret-Mayer test. See under *test.*

tan'sy (tan'zee) [G. *athanasia,* immortality]. 1. A perennial herb, *Tanacetum vulgare,* of the family Compositae. 2. An aromatic bitter and irritant narcotic; has been used in malaria, in hysteria and as an emmenagogue and anthelmintic. In overdoses it produces abdominal pain, vomiting, epileptiform convulsions, and death from failure of respiration. Dose, 2–4 Gm. (30–60 gr.). See *tanacetin, tanacetone.*

tan'ta·lum [named for the Phrygian king *Tantalus* because of the difficulties in isolating it]. Ta = 180.95. A rare metal element; silver-white, very hard, malleable, and ductile. Unaffected by water, acids, or alkalies, and useful wherever resistance to corrosion is important. It is used in surgery, implants of the metal being used to cover skull defects and the foil being employed as a wound covering. **Tantalum oxide** has been used as a dusting powder for wounds.

tan'trum. An expression of uncontrollable anger, sometimes accompanied by acts of violence.

tap [M.E. *tappen*]. 1. A sudden slight blow. 2. Withdrawal of fluid by the use of a trochar or hollow needle.

dry t. A *tap,* 2, in which no fluid can be obtained.

tapazole. Trade-marked name for *methimazole.*

ta·pe'tum (pl. *tapeta*) [L. *tapete,* carpet]. 1. The layer forming the roof of the posterior horn of the lateral ventricle of the brain. It is composed of fibers from the corpus callosum. 2. The brilliant layer that makes the eyes of nocturnal animals visible by reflected light at night. —**tapet'al,** *adj.*

t. alveoli. The alveolar periosteum.

tape'worm" [AS. *taeppe; wyrm*]. Any of the species of the class Cestoidea; segmented, ribbonlike flatworms which are parasites of man and other animals. See *Bertiella, Diphyllobothrium, Dipylidium, Echinococcus, Hymenolepis, Multiceps, Raillietina, Sparganum, Taenia.*

beef t. See *Taenia saginata.*

broad t. See *Diphyllobothrium latum.*

dog t. See *Dipylidium caninum.*

dwarf t. See *Hymenolepis nana.*

fish t. See *Diphyllobothrium latum.*

mouse t. See *Hymenolepis diminuta.*

pork t. See *Taenia solium.*

taph″e·pho′bi·a [G. *taphos*, tomb; *phobos*, fear]. Morbid fear of being buried alive.

Tapia, Antonio Garcia [*Spanish physician*, b. 1875]. Described palatopharyngolaryngeal hemiplegia (1905); also called *Tapia's syndrome*. The tongue, larynx, and sternocleidomastoid muscle on the same side are involved.

tap″i·no·ceph′a·ly [G. *tapeinos*, low-lying; *kephalē*, head]. Flatness of the top of the cranium; flat top. —**tapinocephal′ic,** *adj.*

tap″i·o′ca [Tupi and Guarani, *typyóca*]. A variety of starch obtained from the cassava or manioc plant, *Jatropha manihot*. Used as a food.

ta′pir mouth, lip. The peculiarly loose, thickened, protruding lips of facies myopathica. The patient is unable to smile or whistle.

ta′pir·oid (tay′pur·oyd, tap′ur·) [Tupi *tapyra*, any large mammal; G. *eidos*, form]. Referring to an elongated cervix uteri, so called from its resemblance to a tapir's snout.

ta″pote″ment′ (tah″poht″mahng′. *See* NOTES § 35) [F.]. In massage, the operation of percussing. See *percussion movements* under *movement.*

tap′ping [AS. *taeppa*]. 1. Paracentesis of the abdomen, pleural cavity, hydrocele sac, etc. 2. *In massage*, percussion movements in which the tips of the fingers are used.

tap′root [*taeppa;* AS. *rōt*]. The main root or downward continuation of a plant axis.

tar [AS. *teru*]. A thick brown to black liquid consisting of a mixture of hydrocarbons and their derivatives obtained by the destructive distillation of many kinds of carbonaceous matter.

coal t. (*pix carbonis*). A thick, nearly black, complex liquid of characteristic odor and taste; slightly soluble in water and incompletely soluble in organic solvents. An antipruritic. Prolonged application may lead to dermatitis, and, eventually, to a precancerous or cancerous lesion.

juniper t. (*pix juniperi*). The empyreumatic volatile oil from the wood of the prickly juniper, *Juniperus oxycedrus*. A thick, dark brown liquid, slightly soluble in water, soluble in 9 volumes of alcohol. It is used in skin diseases. Syn., *cade oil.*

pine t. (*pix pini*). Obtained by the destructive distillation of the wood of species of *Pinus*. A viscid brownish black liquid of terebinthinate odor and sharp taste. A stimulating expectorant in bronchitis; externally it is used in skin diseases. Also called *Stockholm t.*

rectified t. oil (*oleum picis rectificatum*). The volatile oil of pine tar rectified by steam distillation. It contains chiefly phenolic constituents. Used internally in chronic bronchitis and externally in skin diseases.

t. weed. Grindelia.

wood t. A product obtained by destructive distillation of wood. See pine *t.*

tar″a·ba′gan. The marmot *Arctomys bobac*, a disease carrier among fur-bearing animals. Also called *tarbagan.*

Tar″ak·tog′e·nos (tar″ack·todj′i·nos) [G. *taraktos*, disturbed; *genos*, race]. A genus of trees of India.

T. Kurzii. A species from the seeds of which chaulmoogra oil is obtained.

tar′ant·ism, tar″an·tis′mus (tar″un·tiz′mus) [It. *tarantismo*, from *Taranto*, city in southern Italy]. A choreic affection, ascribed to the bite of a tarantula, and supposed to be cured by dancing.

ta·ran′tu·la [*Taranto*]. A large, hairy spider of the family Aviculariidae. The bite may be very painful, but is seldom dangerous to man, although small animals may be killed.

ta·ran′tu·lism. See *tarantism.*

ta·ras′sis [G. *tarassein*, to disturb]. Hysteria occurring in the male. *Obs.*

ta·rax′a·cum. Dandelion root. The dried rhizomes and roots of *Taraxacum officinale* or *T. laevigatum*, family Compositae. Formerly used as a cholagogue and diuretic.

ta·rax′is [G., irritation of the eye]. A slight conjunctivitis, or eye trouble.

tar′bag·an plague (tahr′bag·un). A local name for bubonic plague in Siberia and Mongolia; derived from local name of a rodent. See *tarabagan.*

tarbonis cream. A proprietary ointment of solution of coal tar and menthol in a vanishing-cream base, used in dermatitis.

Tarchanoff, Ivan Romanovich (Tarkhanoff) [*Russian physiologist*, 1848–1909]. Described the psychogalvanic reflex (1890).

Tardieu, Auguste Ambroise [*French physician*, 1818–79]. Known as a medicolegal writer, especially upon the legal aspects of poisoning (1867). Best remembered for his description of ecchymotic spots found beneath the pleura after death from strangulation or suffocation (1859); called *Tardieu's ecchymoses.*

tard′ive. Tending to be late; tardy.

tare [Ar. *tarḥah*, that which is thrown away]. 1. A counterweight. 2. A deduction made for the weight of a container. 3. Counterbalance.

tared [*tarḥah*]. 1. Allowed for, as a tare or deduction; having the weight previously ascertained, as a tared filter. 2. Counterbalanced. Used in pharmacy and chemistry.

targesin. Trade-mark for an antiseptic and astringent product prepared from silver and diacetyltannin-albumin.

tar′get [OF. *targette*, of Teutonic origin]. 1. The point of metal in a roentgen-ray tube upon which the electrons are directed and from which the roentgen rays arise. 2. Mire.

targot. Trade-mark for a tyrothricin emulsion for veterinary use, especially in mastitis.

Tarin, Pierre [*French anatomist*, ca. 1725–61]. Described a number of anatomic structures, the best known being the fascia dentata or gyrus dentatus, also called *Tarin's fascia*, and the interpeduncular fossa, also called *fossa of Tarin.*

ta·rir′ic ac′id. $CH_3(CH_2)_{10}C\vdots C(CH_2)_4COOH$. An unsaturated acid occurring as a glyceride in the fat of tariri seeds.

Tarnier, Étienne Stéphane [*French obstetrician*, 1828–97]. Remembered for his early adoption of antiseptic measures in the practice of obstetrics. The inventor of axis-traction forceps (1877), called *Tarnier's forceps*. Described a sign of inevitable abortion—effacement of the angle between the upper and lower segments of the uterus; called *Tarnier's sign.*

ta′ro (tah′ro) [Tahitian and Maori]. The starchy root of *Colocasia antiquorum* or Indian kale. Used as a food in certain Pacific islands.

tars·ad″e·ni′tis [G. *tarsos*, edge of the eyelid; *adēn*, gland; *-itis*, inflammation]. Inflammation of the tarsal glands and tarsal plate.

tars·al′gi·a [G. *tarsos*, flat of the foot; *algos*, pain]. Pain, especially of neuralgic character, in the tarsus of the foot.

tars·ec′to·my [*tarsos;* G. *ektomē*, excision]. Excision of a tarsal bone or bones.

tar·si′tis [G. *tarsos*, edge of the eyelid; *-itis*, inflammation]. 1. Inflammation of the tarsus of the eyelid. 2. See *blepharitis.* 3. Inflammation of the tarsus of the foot.

syphilitic t. Syphilitic infection of a tarsal bone.

tuberculous t. Tuberculous infection of a tarsal bone.

tar′so-, tars- [G. *tarsos*, flat of the foot, edge of the eyelid]. A combining form denoting *pertaining to a tarsus.*

tar″so·chei′lo·plas″ty (tahr″so·kigh′lo·plas″tee) [G. *tarsos*, edge of the eyelid; *cheilos*, lip; *plassein*, to form]. Plastic surgery of the edge of the eyelid.

tar″so·ma·la′ci·a (tahr″so·ma·lay′shee·uh, ·see·uh) [*tarsos;* G. *malakia*, softness]. Softening of the tarsus of the eyelid.

tar″so·met″a·tar′sal [G. *tarsos*, flat of the foot; *meta*, between; *tarsos*]. Relating to the tarsus and the metatarsus.

Tar″so·nem′i·dae (tahr″so·nem′i·dee) [*tarsos;* G. *nēma*, thread]. A family of soft-bodied mites which are parasites of plants.

tar″so·phy′ma [G. *tarsos*, edge of the eyelid; *phyma*, tumor]. Any morbid growth or tumor of the tarsus of the eye.

tar″so·pla′si·a (tahr″so·play′zhuh, ·zee·uh, ·shuh, ·see·uh) [*tarsos;* G. *plassein*, to form]. Tarsoplasty.

tar′so·plas″ty [*tarsos; plassein*]. Plastic surgery of the eyelid; blepharoplasty.

tar″sop·to′si·a (tahr″sop·to′shuh, ·see·uh, ·zhuh, ·zee·uh) [G. *tarsos*, flat of the foot; *ptōsis*, a falling]. Flatfoot.

tar·sor′rha·phy [G. *tarsos*, edge of the eyelid; *rhaphē*, a suture]. 1. The operation of sewing the eyelids together for a part or the whole of their extent. Also called *blepharorrhaphy.* 2. Suture of tarsal plate.

tar·sot′o·my [*tarsos;* G. *tomē*, a cutting]. Operation upon the tarsal plate.

tar·sot′o·my [G. *tarsos*, flat of the foot; *tomē*]. Operation upon the tarsus of the foot.

tar′sus (pl. *tarsi*) [*tarsos*]. 1. The instep, or ankle, consisting of the calcaneus, talus or astragalus, cuboid, navicular or scaphoid, first, second, and third cuneiform bones. See Table of Bones in the Appendix. 2. The dense connective tissue forming the support of an eyelid; the tarsal plate. See Plate 19. —**tarsal,** *adj.*

tar′tar [ML. *tartarum*]. 1. A hard deposit on the inside of wine casks, consisting mainly of acid potassium tartrate (cream of tartar). 2. That accretion, properly termed *dental calculus*, which is deposited on the surface of the teeth. Its composition varies, but it consists of organic secretion and food particles into which are deposited various salts, as calcium carbonate, calcium phosphate, and ferric phosphate.

cream of t. Potassium bitartrate.

soluble t. Potassium tartrate.

t. emetic. Antimony potassium tartrate.

tar·tar′ic ac′id (tahr·tar′ick, tahr·tahr′ick) (*acidum tartaricum*). Any of four substances of the composition COOH(CHOH)$_2$COOH, differentiated as follows: (1) Dextrotartaric acid or *d*-tartaric acid (in accordance with new rules of nomenclature known as L(+)-tartaric acid, COOH.HCOH.-HOCH.COOH) is ordinary tartaric acid, dextrorotatory in aqueous solution. (2) Levotartaric acid or *l*-tartaric acid (known also as D(−)-tartaric acid, COOH.HOCH.HCOH.COOH) has the same properties as the preceding, but is levorotatory in solution. (3) Racemic tartaric acid or *dl*-tartaric acid, a mixture of (1) and (2), differs in several physical properties, and is optically inactive in solution. Syn., *racemic acid.* (4) Mesotartaric acid, an optically inactive form, in which the dextrorotatory tendency of one of the asymmetric carbon atoms is compensated by the levorotatory tendency of the other; it is not resolvable into optically active components, as is (3). Ordinary tartaric acid, (1), is a white crystalline powder, soluble in 0.8 part of water. It is prepared from the argol and lees formed in the manufacture of wine. It is not oxidized in the body, but appears in the urine unchanged. The acid is used in preparing effervescent medicinal preparations and various salts, and has wide industrial usage.

tar′trate. Any salt or ester of tartaric acid.

tar′tra·zine (tahr′truh·zeen, ·zin). $C_{16}H_9N_4O_9S_2Na_3$. Water-soluble yellow color suitable for use in foods, drugs, and cosmetics.

tar·tron′ic ac′id. COOH.CHOH.COOH. Hydroxymalonic acid, a product of oxidation, under certain conditions, of dextrose and several other substances.

Tashkend ulcer. See *oriental sore.*

taste [OF. *taster*, to feel]. A sensation produced by stimulation of special sense organs in the tongue and pharynx by sweet, sour, bitter, or salty substances.

aftertaste. A secondary taste perceived after the immediate taste has ceased.

contrast t. Greater sensitivity to one form of taste stimulus when presented immediately after, or simultaneously with, another form, as a sour substance following a sweet substance.

metallic t. A sensation recognized by some in addition to the usual categories of sweet, sour, bitter, and salty tastes.

taste blind′ness. Inability to recognize the acid, bitter, salty, or sweet flavor of substances, readily detected by others; especially the inability to detect the bitter flavor of phenylthiocarbamide. Syn., *ageusia.*

tat·too′ing [Polynesian in origin]. The production of permanent colors in the skin by the introduction of foreign substances, vegetable or mineral, directly into the corium.

electrolytic t. The treatment of skin diseases by introducing the negative pole of a galvanic current into the lesions. Drugs may be driven into the skin to treat certain diseases.

t. of the cornea. A method of hiding leukomatous spots.

Tauber test. See under *test.*

Tauber and Kleiner modification of Barfoed's test. See under *test.*

tau′rine (taw′reen, ·rin). Aminoethanesulfonic acid, NH$_2$.CH$_2$.CH$_2$.SO$_2$.OH. Occurs in bile combined with the cholic acids. Found also in small quantities in lung and muscle tissue. White or yellowish crystals.

tau′ro-, taur- [L. *taurus*, bull]. A combining form meaning *bull.*

tau″ro·chol·an″o·poi·e′sis (taw″ro·ko·lan″o·poy·ee′sis). The synthesis of taurocholic acid, which is dependent on a supply of amino acids containing sulfur.

tau″ro·cho′lic ac′id (taw″ro·ko′lick, ·kol′ick). $C_{26}H_{45}NSO_7$. An acid resulting from the conjugation of cholic acid with taurine and found in bile.

taur′yl. The univalent radical, H$_2$NCH$_2$CH$_2$SO$_2$—, of taurine.

Taussig, Helen Brooke (1898–). American pediatrician, known for her work in congenital malformations of the heart, and for her association with Alfred Blalock in the development of his operation for congenital malformations of the heart with pulmonary stenosis or atresia, called

Blalock operation, Blalock-Taussig operation. See Alfred *Blalock.* She also described a congenital heart condition, called *Taussig syndrome.*

tau″to·me′ni·al [G. *to auto,* the same; *mēn,* month]. Relating to the same menstrual period.

tau·tom′er·al [*to auto;* G. *meros,* part]. Applied to neurons of the spinal cord, the axons of which pass into the white matter of the cord on the same side in which they are located.

tau″to·mer′ic [*to auto; meros*]. 1. Relating to tautomerism. 2. Tautomeral.

tau·tom′er·ism [*to auto; meros*]. The property of existing in a state of equilibrium between two isomeric forms and capable of reacting as either one.

Tawara, Sunao (1873–). Japanese pathologist who first described the atrioventricular node, also called *Tawara node.*

tax′ine (tack′seen, ·sin). A poisonous alkaloid from the leaves and seeds of the *Taxus baccata,* or yew tree. Formerly used in epilepsy.

tax′is [G., arrangement]. 1. A manipulation of an organ whereby it is brought into normal position; specifically, the reduction of a hernia by manual methods. 2. The involuntary response of an organism involving change of place toward (**positive taxis**) or away from (**negative taxis**) stimulus. Also see *tropism.*

tax·o′di·um [G. *taxos,* yew; *eidos,* form]. The common bald or black cypress of the southern United States and Mexico; said to be useful in hepatic diseases, in rheumatism, and as a diuretic.

tax′on (pl. *taxa*). Taxonomic group.

tax·on′o·my [G. *taxis,* arrangement; *nomos,* law]. The science of the classification of organisms. —**taxonom′ic,** *adj.*

Tax′us [G. *taxos,* yew]. A genus of cone-bearing trees, the yews.

T. baccata. The common European yew tree. Its leaves and seeds are poisonous and said to have sedative qualities.

Tay, Warren [*English physician,* 1843–1927]. Remembered for his description of the ocular changes (choroiditis guttata) in amaurotic familial idiocy, called *Tay's choroiditis.* The disease is called *Tay-Sachs disease;* see *amaurotic* familial idiocy. The cherry-red spot edged with white which is seen at the macula lutea in this condition is called *Tay's spot.*

Taylor, Charles Fayette [*American orthopedist,* 1827–99]. Introduced a steel back brace for support in cases of tuberculosis of the spine, called *Taylor brace* or *apparatus.*

Taylor, Robert William [*American dermatologist,* 1842–1908]. Remembered for his description of idiopathic localized atrophy of the skin (1875); called *Taylor's disease.* The same condition was described (1902) by Herxheimer and Hartmann as acrodermatitis atrophicans chronica.

TB Tuberculosis.

Tb Chemical symbol for terbium.

t. b. Tubercle bacillus, *Mycobacterium tuberculosis.*

tbsp. Tablespoon.

Tc Chemical symbol for technetium.

Te 1. Chemical symbol for tellurium. 2. Abbreviation for tetanic contraction.

tea [from the Chinese]. 1. The leaves of *Camellia sinensis* (*Thea sinensis*), family Theaceae. Tea contains 1–5% of caffeine, 5–15% of tannin, and a fragrant volatile oil. An infusion is used as a stimulating beverage. 2. An infusion or decoction prepared from the leaves of *C. sinensis.* 3. Any vegetable infusion or decoction used as a beverage.

black t. Prepared by exposing the dried leaves to air at a temperature of 35–40° C. for about 12 hours, to permit a partial fermentation to occur whereby the characteristic color is developed. Some of the aromatic principle is volatilized and some tannin is destroyed.

green t. Prepared by heating the leaves in open pans with agitation.

teamster's t. A decoction prepared from *Ephedra nebrodensis.* Formerly used in urogenital diseases.

t. oil. The expressed oil from the seeds of several species of *Camellia.* Also called *t. seed oil.*

TEAB Tetraethylammonium bromide.

tea′ber″ry. See *gaultheria.*

teach′ers′ nodes. Singer's nodes.

Teal test. See under *test.*

Teale, Thomas Pridgin [*English surgeon,* 1801–67]. Best remembered for his amputations in which he used a long anterior and a short posterior rectangular flap (1858); called *Teale's method* or *amputation.*

tears [AS. *tēar*]. 1. The secretion of the lacrimal gland. 2. Hardened lumps, or drops, of any resinous or gummy drug.

crocodile t. A profuse, paroxysmal flow of tears observed in certain patients with facial paralysis, when they taste food. Also called *gustolacrimal reflex.*

tease [AS. *tǣsan*]. Tear or gently separate into its component parts, by the use of needles, a tissue which it is desired to examine microscopically.

tea′spoon″ [*tea;* AS. *spōn*]. A spoon commonly assumed to hold about 4 cc or 1 fluidrachm, but usually holding about 5 cc. Abbreviated, tsp.

teat [OF. *tete*]. A nipple.

tech·ne′ti·um (teck·nee′shee·um) [G. *technetos,* artificial]. Tc. Element number 43, prepared in 1937 by neutron or deuteron bombardment of molybdenum and later found among the fission products of uranium. Formerly called masurium.

tech·nic′. Technique.

tech·ni′cian [G. *technikos,* skillful]. A person trained and expert in the technical details of certain medical fields, as bacteriology, pathology, roentgenology.

tech·nique′, tech·nic′ (tek·neek′). The method of procedure in operations or manipulations of any kind.

Engström t. Roentgen absorption histospectroscopy. See under *histospectroscopy.*

tec′no·cyte [G. *teknon,* child; *kytos,* cell]. A young metamyelocyte: also called *juvenile metagranulocyte.*

tec′ti·form [L. *tectum,* roof; *forma,* form]. Roof-shaped.

tec″to·ceph′a·ly [*tectum;* G. *kephalē,* head]. The condition of having a roof-shaped skull.

tec·to′ri·al [L. *tectorium,* covering]. Serving as a roof or covering, as a tectorial membrane, a membrane in the cochlear duct.

tec″to·spi′nal [NL. *tectospinalis*]. Pertaining to the spinal cord and the corpora quadrigemina, as tectospinal tract.

tec′tum [L.]. A roof or covering.

te′di·ous [L. *taediosus,* tedious]. Unduly protracted, as tedious labor.

tedral. A proprietary tablet containing ephedrine hydrochloride, phenobarbital, and theophylline.

teel oil. See sesame *oil.*

teeth′ing [AS. *tōth*]. The eruption of the deciduous teeth; the process of dentition.

Teevan, William Frederick [*English surgeon,* 1834–87]. Enunciated a law that skull fracture occurs in the line of expansion and not of compression; called *Teevan's law.*

tegin. Trade-mark for a brand of glyceryl monostearate used as an emulsifying agent in ointments, lotions, or similar substances.

teg′men [L., a covering]. A cover.

t. mastoideum. The roof of the mastoid cells.

t. tympani. The roof of the tympanic cavity.

t. ventriculi quarti. The roof of the fourth ventricle.

teg·men′tum (pl. *tegmenta*) [L., a covering]. A covering; specifically, the dorsal portion of the midbrain, exclusive of the corpora quadrigemina and the central gray substance. —**tegmental,** *adj.*

tegosept. Trade-mark for a brand of preservatives, consisting of esters of parahydroxybenzoic acid.

Teichmann, Ludwig T. Stawiarski [*German histologist,* 1825–95]. Described hemin crystals, also called *Teichmann's crystals.* See Teichmann's *test.*

tei·chop′si·a (tye·kop′see·uh) [G. *teichos,* wall; *opsis,* vision]. Temporary amblyopia, with subjective visual images.

tek′no·cyte. See *tecnocyte.*

te′la (pl. *telae*) [L., web]. A web or tissue.

t. adiposa. Adipose tissue.

t. choroidea. The membranous roof of the third and fourth ventricles of the brain including the choroid plexuses.

t. subcutanea. The subcutaneous connective tissue; the superficial fascia.

t. submucosa. The layer of connective tissue which lies between a mucous membrane and subjacent tissues. Also called *tunica submucosa.*

tel·al′gi·a [G. *tēle,* far off; *algos,* pain]. Referred pain.

tel·an″gi·ec′ta·sis, tel·an″gi·ec·ta′si·a (tel·an″-jee·eck·tay′zhuh, ·zee·uh, ·shuh, ·see·uh) [G. *telos,* end; *aggeion,* vessel; *ektasis,* extension]. Dilatation of groups of capillaries. They form elevated, dark red, wartlike spots, varying in size from 1 to 7 mm. —**telangiectat′ic,** *adj.*

hereditary hemorrhagic t. A hereditary disease characterized by multiple telangiectases and a tendency to habitual hemorrhages, most commonly epistaxis, described by Rendu (1896), Osler (1901), and Frederick Parkes Weber (1907).

t. faciei. Acne rosacea.

t. lymphatica. Lymphangiectasis.

tel·an″gi·ec·to′des (tel·an″jee·eck·to′deez) [*telos; aggeion; ektasis;* G. *eidos,* form]. Characterized by telangiectasis.

tel·an″gi·i′tis [*telos; aggeion;* G. *-itis,* inflammation]. Inflammation of capillaries.

tel·an″gi·o′ma [*telos; aggeion;* G. *-ōma,* tumor]. A tumor composed of dilated capillaries.

tel·an′gi·on [*telos; aggeion*]. A terminal arteriole.

tel·an″gi·o′sis [*telos; aggeion;* G. *-ōsis,* condition]. Disease of minute blood vessels.

tel″e·an″gi·ec′ta·sis. See *telangiectasis.*

tel″e·car′di·o·gram″ [G. *tēle,* far off; *kardia,* heart; *gramma,* letter]. Telelectrocardiogram.

tel″e·car′di·o·phone″ [*tēle; kardia;* G. *phōnē,* sound]. An apparatus amplifying heart sounds.

tel″e·cep′tor. A sense organ which receives stimuli from distant objects, e.g., nose, eye, and cochlea. Syn., *teloreceptor.*

tel″e·ci·ne′sis. See *telekinesis.*

tel″e·den′drite. See *telodendron.*

tel″e·di″as·tol′ic [G. *telos,* end; *diastolē,* dilatation]. Relating to the last phase of a diastole.

tel″e·flu″or·os′co·py. The procedure by which the usual distortion of a fluoroscopic picture by divergence of the roentgen rays is eliminated by placing the source of the rays two meters or more from the area to be fluoroscoped.

te·leg′o·ny [G. *tēle,* far off; *gonē,* offspring]. The erroneous belief that a male once mated with a female will affect the subsequent progeny of the same female mated with a different male.

tel″e·ki·ne′sis (tel″eh·ki·nee′sis, ·kigh·nee′sis) [*tēle;* G. *kinēsis,* movement]. The power claimed by some people of causing objects to move without touching them.

tel″e·lec″tro·car′di·o·gram″ [*tēle;* G. *ēlektron,* amber; *kardia,* heart; *gramma,* letter]. An electrocardiogram taken in a laboratory, the galvanometer being connected by a wire with the patient who is elsewhere.

tel″e·lec″tro·ther″a·peu′tics (tel″eh·leck″tro-therr″uh·pew′ticks) [*tēle; ēlektron;* G. *therapeutikos,* inclined to serve]. The treatment of hysterical paralysis by a series of electric discharges near the patient without actual contact.

tel″en·ceph′a·lon [G. *telos,* end; *egkephalos,* brain]. The anterior subdivision of the primary forebrain that develops into olfactory lobes, cerebral cortex, and corpora striata. Syn., *endbrain.* —**telencephal′ic,** *adj.*

tel″e·neu′rite [*telos;* G. *neuron,* nerve]. Old term for one of the terminal filaments of the main stem of an axis cylinder process.

tel″e·neu′ron [*telos; neuron*]. Old term for a neuron forming the terminus of an impulse in a physiologic act involving the nervous system.

tel″e·o·den′dron. See *telodendron.*

tel″e·ol′o·gy (tel″ee·ol′o·jee, tee″lee·) [*telos; logos*]. The doctrine that explanations of phenomena are to be sought in terms of final causes, purpose, or design in nature. —**teleolog′ic,** *adj.*

tel″e·op′si·a [G. *tēle,* far off; *opsis,* vision]. A disorder in visual perception of space characterized by an excess of depth, or the illusion that close objects are far away.

tel″e·o·roent′gen·o·gram″ (tel″ee·o·rent′ghin·o-gram″, tee″lee·o·) [*tēle; Röntgen;* G. *gramma,* letter]. A radiograph, usually of the heart, made at a distance of about 6 feet, to avoid distortion.

teleostol. Trade-mark for a biologically standardized mixture of fish liver oils used as a source of vitamins A and D.

tel″e·o·ther″a·peu′tics (tel″ee·o·therr″uh·pew′-ticks, tee″lee·o·) [*tēle;* G. *therapeutikos,* inclined to serve]. Suggestive therapeutics.

telepaque. Trade-mark for *iodopanoic acid.*

te·lep′a·thist [*tēle;* G. *pathos,* disease]. One who is versed in telepathy.

te·lep′a·thy [*tēle; pathos*]. The direct awareness of what is taking place in another person's mind.

tel″e·ra″di·og′ra·phy [*tēle;* L. *radius,* ray; G. *graphein,* to write]. Radiography with the tube about 6 feet from the body to avoid distortion.

tel″e·ra′di·um [*tēle; radius*]. Radium which is used in a radium cannon for accurate directing of the emanations on a region. See teleradium *therapy.*

tel″e·re·cep′tor. See *teleceptor.*

tel′er·gy [*tēle;* G. *ergon,* work]. Automatism.

tel″e·roent″gen·og′ra·phy (tel″i·rent″ghin·og′-ruh·fee) [*tēle; Röntgen;* G. *graphein,* to write]. Teleradiography.

tel″e·ster″e·o·roent″gen·og′ra·phy (tel″i·sterr″-ee·o·rent″ghin·og′ruh·fee, tel″i·steer″ee·o·) [*tēle;* G. *stereos,* solid; *Röntgen; graphein*]. A stereogram made with the tube about 6 feet from the object.

tel″es·the′si·a, tel″aes·the′si·a (tel″ess·thee′-zhuh, ·zee·uh) [*tēle;* G. *aisthēsis,* perception]. 1. Distant perception. 2. A perception of objects or conditions independently of the recognized channels of sense. See *telepathy.*

tel″e·sys·tol′ic [G. *telos,* end; *systolē,* contraction]. Pertaining to the last phase of systole.

tel″e·ther′a·py [G. *tēle,* far off; *therapeia,* treatment]. Absent treatment.

tel·lu′ri·um [L. *tellus,* earth]. Te = 127.61. A non-metallic element of bluish white color, obtained chiefly as a by-product in the refining of copper and lead. Salts of the element have been used for their antisyphilitic effect; certain of its compounds are bactericidal. Absorbable salts are poisonous. Prolonged use leads to a garlicky breath.

Tellyesniczky, Kálmán [*Hungarian histologist*, 1868–1932]. Introduced a tissue-hardening fluid containing 3% potassium dichromate solution in water, to which 5% glacial acetic acid is added just before use; called *Tellyesniczky's fluid*.

tel′o·coele. Cavity of the telencephalon.

tel″o·den′dron [G. *telos*, end; *dendron*, tree]. The terminal arborization of an axon.

tel′o·gen. See under *telomerization*.

tel″og·no′sis. Diagnosis by telephone-transmitted roentgenograms.

tel″o·lec′i·thal (tel″o·less′i·thul) [*telos;* G. *lekithos*, yolk]. An ovum having a large mass of yolk placed eccentrically.

tel″o·lem′ma [*telos;* G. *lemma*, sheath]. The membrane over a motor end-plate of a skeletal muscle fiber.

tel′o·mer. See under *telomerization*.

tel·om″er·i·za′tion. A type of polymerization reaction in which a compound XY dissociates and unites with another compound R, containing unsaturated groups, to form a large molecule $X(R)_nY$. The compound XY is called a *telogen;* the large polymerized compound is a *telomer*.

tel′o·phase (tel′o·faze) [*telos;* G. *phasis*, appearance]. 1. The final stage of mitosis in which the chromosomes reorganize to form an interstage nucleus. 2. The final phase of any process.

tel″o·re·cep′tor. See *teleceptor*.

Tel″o·spo·rid′i·a [*telos;* G. *sporē*, seed]. A subclass of Sporozoa, characterized by spore formation after the sporozoon has completed its growth. The orders included are Gregarinida, Coccidia, and Haemosporidia.

tel″o·syn·ap′sis [*telos;* G. *synapsis*, contact]. The end-to-end union of homologous chromosomes at the time of the maturation of the germ cells, in contrast to the side-by-side union as in parasynapsis.

TEM Abbreviation for triethylene melamine.

tem′per [AS. *temprian*]. Make metals hard and elastic by heating them and then suddenly cooling them.

tem′per. The hardness or brittleness of a metal, as induced by heating and suddenly cooling.

spring t. A quality induced in steel by hardening and tempering in the ordinary way and then reheating until the steel assumes a bright blue color (about 570° F.), which increases the upper limit of elasticity of the steel.

tem′per·a·ment [L. *temperamentum*, a mixing in due proportion]. *In constitutional medicine*, the mixture of motivational drives in a personality. The level of personality just above physiologic function and just below acquired attitudes and beliefs. The quantitative patterning of viscerotonia, somatotonia, and cerebrotonia in a personality.

tem′per·ance [L. *temperantia*, moderation]. Moderation in satisfying desire, especially in the use of alcoholic beverages.

tem′per·ate [L. *temperare*, to be moderate]. Moderate; without excess.

tem′per·a·ture [L. *temperatura*]. The degree of intensity of heat of a body, especially as measured by the scale of a thermometer. Abbreviated, T.

absolute t. That reckoned from the absolute zero, estimated at −273° C.

basal t. That of the healthy body after a sufficient period of rest, usually obtained in the fasting state before arising after at least eight hours of relaxed sleep: used particularly in the detection of ovulation.

body t. The temperature of the body. Elevation above normal constitutes fever.

critical t. The temperature at which a gas can, by pressure, be reduced to a liquid.

dry-bulb t. The actual air temperature, with the exclusion of variations due to radiation or conduction.

inverse t. Variations of body temperature through the day, opposite to normal, so that the morning temperature is higher than the evening temperature.

maximum t. The temperature above which bacterial growth does not occur.

mean t. The average temperature for a given period of time.

minimum t. That below which bacterial growth ceases.

normal t. The temperature of the body in health (37° C. or 98.6° F.).

optimum t. That most favorable for cultivating microorganisms.

wet-bulb t. That obtained when a current of air is passed over a thermometer bulb which is enclosed by a damp jacket. Increasing moisture impedes evaporation, and the cooling effect decreases.

tem′ple [L. *tempora*, temples, plural of *tempus*]. The portion of the head anterior to the ear and above the zygomatic arch.

tem′plin oil. A volatile oil obtained from the cones of *Pinus mugo*.

tem′po·ral [*tempora*]. 1. Pertaining to the temple, as the temporal bone, the temporal artery. See Tables of Arteries, of Bones, and of Muscles in the Appendix. 2. Pertaining to time. 3. Pertaining to the temporal lobe.

tem′po·ral″is su″per·fi·ci·al′is. A portion of the auricularis anterior muscle.

tem′po·rar″y [L. *temporarius*, lasting but for a time]. Not permanent.

tem″po·ri·za′tion [L. *tempus*, time]. The expectant treatment of disease.

tem′po·ro- [L. *tempora*, plural of *tempus*]. A combining form denoting *pertaining to the temple* or *to the temporal lobe of the cerebral hemisphere*.

tem″po·ro·man·dib′u·lar [*tempora;* L. *mandibula*, jaw]. Pertaining to the temporal bone and the mandible, used specifically for a ligament of the mandibular joint.

tem″po·ro-oc·cip′i·tal (tem″po·ro-ock·sip′i·tul). Pertaining to the temporal and occipital bones, regions, or lobes of the cerebrum.

tem″po·ro·pa·ri′e·tal [*tempora;* L. *paries*, wall]. 1. Pertaining to the temporal and parietal bones. 2. Pertaining to the temporal and parietal lobes of the brain.

tem″po·ro·pon′tile (·pon′tile, ·til) [*tempora;* L. *pons*, bridge]. Pertaining to the temporal lobe and the pons.

tem′u·lence, tem″u·len′ti·a [L. *temulentia*, intoxication]. Inebriety; drunkenness. *Obs.*

te·na′cious [L. *tenax*, holding fast]. 1. Tough. 2. Cohesive.

te·nac′i·ty (ti·nass′i·tee) [L. *tenacitas*, a holding fast]. Toughness.

te·nac′u·lum [L., an instrument for holding]. A slender, hook-shaped instrument with a long handle for seizing and holding parts, approximating incised edges, etc., during surgical operations.

ten·al′gi·a. See *tenodynia*.

t. crepitans. See *tenosynovitis* crepitans.

ten′der·ness [L. *tener*, soft]. The condition of abnormal sensitiveness to touch; soreness.

ten′din·o·plas″ty [L. *tendere*, to stretch; G. *plassein*, to form]. Plastic surgery of tendons. Also see *tenoplasty*. —**tendinoplas′tic,** *adj.*

ten′di·nous [*tendere*]. Pertaining to, or having the nature of, tendon.

ten′do (pl. *tendines*) [ML., from *tendere*]. A tendon.

t. achillis. The Achilles tendon or common tendon of the gastrocnemius and soleus muscles inserted into the heel. Also called *tendo calcaneus.*

ten·dol′y·sis, ten″do·ly′sis. [*tendere;* G. *lysis,* a loosing]. The freeing of adhesions about a tendon.

ten″do·mu′cin, ten″do·mu′coid [*tendere;* L. *mucus,* mucus]. A mucoid found in tendons.

ten′don [*tendere*]. A band of dense fibrous tissue forming the termination of a muscle and attaching the latter to a bone. See Plate 2.

central t. The aponeurosis in the center of the diaphragm.

conjoined t. The fused tendon of insertion of the internal oblique abdominal and transverse abdominal muscles into the pubis. In many bodies muscle fibers are present and a tendon as such is not demonstrable.

cricoesophageal t. The tendon of origin of the longitudinal and part of the circular striated musculature of the esophagus, attached to the posterior medial surface of the cricoid cartilage.

patellar t. See patellar *ligament.*

slipped t. A deficiency disease of growing poultry characterized by a deformity of the tibia-metatarsal joint causing the tendon of the gastrocnemius muscle to slip from its normal position. The principal factor is manganese deficiency, although lack of biotin, niacin, or choline may also be involved. Also called *perosis.*

t. of conus arteriosus. A band of fibrous tissue extending from the fibrous trigone of the heart and fibrous ring about the right atrioventricular opening to the posterior surface of the conus arteriosus.

trefoil t. Old term for the central tendon of the diaphragm.

ten″do·syn″o·vi′tis (ten″do·sin″o·vy′tis, ·sigh″no·). See *tenosynovitis.*

ten″do·vag″i·ni′tis (·vadj″i·nigh′tis) [*tendere;* L. *vagina,* sheath; *-itis,* inflammation]. Inflammation of a tendon and its sheath; tenosynovitis.

t. crepitans. See *tenosynovitis* crepitans.

t. granulosa. Tuberculosis of tendon sheaths, the sheaths being filled with granulation or fungous tissue.

t. stenosans. See Fritz de *Quervain.*

Te·neb′ri·o [L., one who shuns the light]. A genus of beetles.

T. molitor. The meal worm. The larva of this species acts as an intermediate host for the tapeworm, *Hymenolepis diminuta.*

te·nec′to·my [G. *tenōn,* tendon; *ektomē,* excision]. 1. Excision of a lesion, as a ganglion or xanthoma, of a tendon or tendon sheath. 2. Tenoplasty.

te·nes′mus (tuh·nez′mus, tuh·ness′mus) [*teinesmos*]. A straining, especially the painful straining to empty the bowels or bladder without the evacuation of feces or urine. —**tenes′mic,** *adj.*

teni-. For words beginning with *teni-* not found here, see words beginning *taeni-.*

ten·i′o·la (ti·nigh′o·luh, ti·nee′o·luh) [dim. from G. *tainia,* ribbon]. A small ribbon.

t. cinerea. A thin, grayish ridge separating the striae of the fourth ventricle from the cochlear division of the acoustic nerve. *O.T.*

ten′nis arm, ten′nis el′bow. An acute or chronic synovitis of the radiohumeral articulation common in tennis players. Radiohumeral bursitis.

ten′o-, ten- [G. *tenōn,* tendon]. A combining form meaning *pertaining to a tendon.*

ten″o·de′sis [*tenōn;* G. *desis,* a binding together]. Fixation of a tendon, as to a bone.

ten″o·dyn′i·a (ten″o·din′ee·uh, ·dye′nee·uh) [*tenōn;* G. *odynē,* pain]. Pain in a tendon.

ten″o·fi′bril [*tenōn;* L. *fibra,* fiber]. A small, delicate fibril connecting one epithelial cell with another; a tonofibril.

ten″o·my′o·plas″ty [*tenōn;* G. *mys,* muscle; *plassein,* to form]. Tenontomyoplasty.

ten″o·my·ot′o·my (ten″o·migh·ot′o·mee) [*tenōn; mys;* G. *tomē,* a cutting]. *In ophthalmology,* a procedure for the treatment of squint, devised to enfeeble the action of one of the rectus muscles by incising portions of its tendon near the sclerotic insertion.

Tenon, Jacobus René [*French anatomist and surgeon,* 1724–1816]. Instrumental in bringing about hospital reform in eighteenth century Paris. See also Tenon's *capsule, space* of Tenon.

ten″o·nec′to·my [G. *tenōn,* tendon; *ektomē,* excision]. Excision of a portion of a tendon.

ten″on·i′tis [after J. R. *Tenon;* G. *-itis,* inflammation]. Inflammation of Tenon's capsule.

ten″on·i′tis [G. *tenōn,* tendon; *-itis*]. Inflammation of a tendon sheath.

ten″o·nom′e·ter [G. *teinein,* to stretch; *metron,* a measure]. An instrument for measuring the tension of the eyeball.

ten″o·nos·to′sis. See *tenostosis.*

te·non″to·my′o·plas″ty [G. *tenōn,* tendon; *mys,* muscle; *plassein,* to form]. Reparative surgery involving both tendon and muscle; used particularly for hernia.

te·non″to·my·ot′o·my (ti·non″to·migh·ot′o·mee) [*tenōn; mys;* G. *tomē,* a cutting]. Surgical division of tendons and muscles.

te·non″to·the·ci′tis. See *tenosynovitis.*

t. prolifera calcarea. Necrobiosis of the tendons in their sheaths with calcareous deposit.

ten′o·phyte [*tenōn;* G. *phyton,* plant]. A bony or cartilaginous growth on a tendon.

ten′o·plas″ty [*tenōn;* G. *plassein,* to form]. Reparative or plastic surgery of a tendon. —**teno·plas′tic,** *adj.*

ten·or′rha·phy [*tenōn;* G. *rhaphē,* suture]. The uniting of a divided tendon by sutures.

ten″os·to′sis [*tenōn;* G. *osteon,* bone; *-ōsis,* condition]. Ossification of a tendon.

ten″o·su′ture. Tenorrhaphy.

ten″o·syn″o·vec′to·my (ten″o·sin″o·veck′to·mee, ·sigh″no·) [*tenōn;* NL. *synovia,* synovia; G. *ektomē,* excision]. Excision of a tendon sheath.

ten″o·syn·o·vi·o′ma. See *synovioma.*

ten″o·syn″o·vi′tis (·sin″o·vy′tis, ·sigh″no·) [*tenōn; synovia;* G. *-itis,* inflammation]. Inflammation of a tendon and its sheath.

adhesive t. An inflammatory reaction of a tendon sheath which produces adhesions between tendon and tendon sheath.

t. crepitans. That form associated with cracking sounds during muscular activity.

tuberculous t. A slow and progressively destructive tuberculosis of the sheaths of the tendons. The tendons of the wrist are the ones most commonly involved. Treatment is synovectomy and excision of the surrounding tuberculous tissue.

villous t. A chronic inflammatory reaction of a tendon sheath producing hypertrophy of the lining with the formation of redundant folds and villi.

ten′o·tome [*tenōn;* G. *tomos,* cutting]. A small, narrow-bladed knife mounted on a slender handle; a tenotomy knife.

te·not′o·mize [*tenōn; tomos*]. Perform tenotomy.

te·not′o·my [*tenōn;* G. *tomē,* a cutting]. The operation of cutting a tendon.

graduated t. Specifically, cutting a part of the fibers of the tendon of an ocular muscle for heterophoria or slight degrees of strabismus.

tarsal t. Division of the peroneal tendon in the horse for the relief of spavin.

ten″o·vag″i·ni′tis (ten″o·vadj″i·nigh′tis) [*tenōn;* L. *vagina,* sheath; G. *-itis,* inflammation]. Inflammation of the sheath of a tendon.

tensilon chloride. Trade-marked name for (3-hydroxylphenyl) dimethylethylammoniumchloride, a specific anticurare agent.

ten″si·om′e·ter [L. *tensio*, from *tendere*, to stretch; G. *metron*, a measure]. An apparatus for measuring tension, as in the eyeball or blood vessels.

ten′sion [*tensio*]. 1. The act of stretching; the state of being stretched or strained. 2. *In electricity*, the power of overcoming resistance. Abbreviated, T. 3. The partial pressure exerted by a gas.

arterial t. The strain in the arterial walls at the height of the pulse wave.

elastic t. Stretching by means of an elastic material.

gaseous t. The tendency of a gas to expand, due to the mutual repulsion of its molecules.

interfacial t. A measure of the work which must be done in increasing the interface between two phases by a given unit of surface. When one of the phases is gas, then the interfacial tension is commonly called the surface tension.

intraocular t. The tension of the coats of the eyeball, produced by the pressure of the intraocular fluid. It may be estimated by means of an instrument called a tonometer, or by palpation with the fingers.

intravenous t. The strain to which the wall of a vein is subjected by the pressure of the blood.

muscular t. The state of muscular contraction which occurs when muscles are passively stretched.

premenstrual t. The increased emotional tension and nervous or circulatory symptoms associated with the period in the human menstrual cycle which precedes menstruation.

surface t. The force operating at surfaces (commonly at the interface of a liquid and a gas) which is due to the unequal molecular attraction on either side of the molecules at the surface. The contractile force in the surface of a liquid by virtue of which the surface tends to shrink and assume the smallest area possible. The surface tension of water against air at 20° C. is 72.5 dynes per centimeter. Abbreviated, S.T.

ten′si·ty [L. *tensus*, from *tendere*]. Tenseness, the condition of being stretched.

ten′sive [*tensus*]. Giving the sensation of stretching or contraction.

ten′sor [*tensus*]. A muscle that serves to make a part tense, as the tensor tympani. See Table of Muscles in the Appendix.

t. capsularis articulationis metacarpophalangei digiti quinti. A variant of the opponens digiti quinti muscle.

t. laminae posterioris vaginae musculae recti abdominis. Rare variant insertion of certain fibers of the transversus abdominis muscle.

t. ligamenti annularis. Variant parts of the supinator muscle. There may be anterior or posterior bands.

ten′sure [L. *tensura*, a stretching]. Tension, a stretching or straining.

tent [OF. *tente*, from L. *tendere*, to stretch]. 1. A plug or stuffing of soft material, such as gauze, sponge, or felt, that increases in volume by wetting; it is used for dilating an orifice or canal and for keeping a wound or sinus open. Except in gynecologic practice, the term in its strictest sense has almost disappeared from medical literature. 2. A portable shelter or covering.

laminaria t. A cone-shaped plug made from *Laminaria digitata*, a seaweed. When wet, the plug dilates: sometimes used in gynecologic and surgical procedures.

oxygen t. An airtight chamber, enclosing the patient's head and shoulders, in which the oxygen content of the atmosphere can be maintained at a higher than normal level.

sponge t. One made of compressed sponge, for dilating the os uteri.

ten′ta·tive [L. *tentare*, to try]. Empirical; experimental.

tenth′me″ter. One ten-millionth of a millimeter, or one angstrom.

ten·tig′i·nous (ten·tidj′i·nus) [L. *tentigo*, lust]. Characterized by insane lust.

ten·ti′go [L.]. Lust, satyriasis.

t. prava. See *lupus*.

t. venerea. See *nymphomania*.

ten·to′ri·al pres′sure cone. See *pressure cone*.

ten·to′ri·um (pl. *tentoria*) [L., tent]. A partition of dura mater, roofing over the posterior cranial fossa, separating the cerebellum from the cerebral hemispheres. Also called *t. cerebelli*. See Plate 17. —**tentorial,** *adj.*

t. of the hypophysis. Old term for the diaphragm of the sella, the circular fold of dura mater attached to the margins of the hypophyseal fossa; it covers the hypophysis and has an opening in the center through which passes the stalk of the hypophysis.

ten′u·ate [L. *tenuare*, to make thin]. Make thin.

ten·u′i·ty [L. *tenuitas*, thinness]. Thinness; the condition of being thin.

ten′u·ous [L. *tenuis*, thin]. Thin; minute.

teph″ro·my″e·li′tis [G. *tephros*, ash-colored; *myelos*, marrow; *-itis*, inflammation]. Inflammation of the gray matter of the cord; poliomyelitis.

tep′id [L. *tepidus*, lukewarm]. About blood heat.

TEPP Tetraethylpyrophosphate.

ter- (tur-) [L., thrice]. A combining form meaning *three* or *threefold*.

ter″ab·del′la (terr″ab·dell′uh) [G. *terein*, to bore; *bdella*, leech]. An artificial leech.

ter″a·mor′phous (terr″uh·mor′fus) [G. *teras*, monster; *morphē*, form]. Of the nature of a monstrosity.

te′ras (teer′ass, terr′us) (pl. *terata*) [G.]. A monster. For terata listed by name, see Table of Representative Monstrosities and Anomalies in the Appendix. See Plate 25. —**terat′ic,** *adj.*

ter′a·tism [*teras*]. A congenital anomaly or monstrosity.

acquired t. Deformity which is the result of disease, violence, or operation.

atresic t. Deformity in which the natural openings are occluded.

casemic t. Deformity in which parts which should be united remain in their primitive, fissured state.

ectogenic t. One in which certain parts of the body are absent or defective.

ectopic t. One in which there is displacement of one or more parts.

hypergenetic t. One in which certain organs are disproportionately large.

symphysic t. One in which certain organs or parts are abnormally fused.

ter″a·to·blas·to′ma [*teras;* G. *blastos*, germ; *-ōma*, tumor]. See *teratoma*.

ter″a·to·car″ci·no′ma. A malignant teratoma.

t. of testis. See embryonal *carcinoma* of testis.

ter″a·tog′e·ny (terr″uh·todj′i·nee), **ter″a·to·gen′e·sis** [*teras;* G. *genesis*, production]. The formation, or bringing forth, of monsters.

ter′a·toid [*teras;* G. *eidos*, form]. Resembling a monster.

ter″a·tol′o·gy [*teras;* G. *logos*, word]. The science of malformations and monstrosities. —**teratolog′ic,** *adj.;* **teratologist,** *n.*

ter″a·to′ma (pl. *teratomata, teratomas*) [*teras;* G. *-ōma*, tumor]. A true tumor or neoplasm composed of multiple tissues, as teeth, hair, or other material not found in the part wherein it grows, and resulting from an embryonic misplacement of tissue or from the enclosure of parts of a rudimentary fetus: also called *bidermoma, cholesteatoma of ovary, dermoid cyst, hairy cyst, mixed cyst, teratoid cyst, teratomatous cyst, dermoid, dysembryoma, embryoma, monodermoma, teratoblastoma, tridermoma, compound ovarian tumor, ectopic ovarian tumor, Nelaton's tumor, teratoid tumor.* —**teratom'atous,** *adj.*

malignant t. The malignant variation, usually involving all components, but occasionally only one: also called *embryonic carcinoma, teratocarcinoma, teratoid carcinoma.*

ter"a·to·pho'bi·a [*teras;* G. *phobos,* fear]. 1. Morbid fear of monsters or of deformed people. 2. Morbid dread, on the part of a pregnant woman, of giving birth to a monstrosity.

ter"a·to'sis [*teras;* G. *-ōsis,* condition]. 1. A congenital deformity. 2. Teratism.

ter"a·to·zo·o·sper'mi·a. Abnormal sperm morphology.

ter'bi·um [*Ytterby,* in Sweden]. Tb = 158.93. A rare metallic element.

terchlorethylene. Tetrachloroethylene.

tercinin. A brand of clavacin.

te're [L., imperative of *terere,* to rub]. Rub. Used in writing prescriptions.

ter'e·bene. A mixture of hydrocarbons, chiefly dipentene and terpinene, prepared by the action of sulfuric acid on turpentine oil followed by steam distillation. A pale yellow liquid of terebinthinate taste; soluble in 3 volumes of alcohol. A stimulant expectorant. Useful in flatulence and dyspepsia.

ter"e·bin'thi·nate [G. *terebinthos,* turpentine]. Containing or resembling turpentine.

ter"e·bin'thism (terr"i·binth'iz·um) [*terebinthos*]. Poisoning with turpentine oil.

ter"e·bra·che'sis (terr"i·bra·kee'sis) [L. *teres,* round; G. *brachys,* short]. The operation of shortening the round ligament of the uterus.

ter"e·phthal'ic ac'id. $COOH.C_6H_4.COOH$; *p*-phthalic acid, occurring in crystals, insoluble in water: used as an analytical reagent.

te'res (teer'eez) (pl. *teretes*) [L.]. Cylindrical.

te'res. A muscle having a cylindrical shape, as teres major, teres minor. See Table of Muscles in the Appendix.

ter in die [L.]. Three times a day; abbreviated, t.i.d.

term [L. *terminus,* boundary]. 1. A limit; the time during which anything lasts. 2. The time of expected delivery.

Terman, Lewis Madison [*American psychologist,* 1877–]. Known for his modification of the Binet-Simon tests for measuring intelligence, called *Terman's collective test, Stanford revision of the Binet-Simon test.* He has also contributed genetic studies on genius.

ter'mi·nal [L. *terminalis,* of a boundary]. 1. Pertaining to the end; placed at or forming the end.

ter'mi·nal. The pole of a battery or other electric source, or the end of the conductors or wires connected thereto.

Wilson central t. *In electrocardiography,* an indifferent electrode of near zero potential obtained by connecting the three limbs of the subject to a central terminal through resistances of 5000 ohms each.

ter'mi·nal crest. See *crista terminalis.*

ter"mi·na'tion [L. *terminatio,* a fixing of limits]. Cessation; the end or ending.

ter"mi·nol'o·gy [L. *terminus,* boundary; G. *logos,* word]. Nomenclature; a system of technical names or terms.

terms [*terminus*]. The menses.

ter'na·ry. Of chemical compounds, made up of three elements or radicals.

Ter'ni·dens (tur'ni·denz) [L. *terni,* three; *dens,* tooth]. A genus of strongyloid nematode worms, a species of which, **T. diminutus,** sometimes infests man.

teropterin. A trade-mark for sodium pteroyltriglutamate, a derivative of folic (pteroylglutamic) acid, investigated for possible usefulness in the treatment of leukemia.

terpane. Eucalyptol.

ter'pene. Any hydrocarbon of the general formula $C_{10}H_{16}$, sometimes represented as a condensation of two isoprene (C_5H_8) units. By extension the term may include compounds representing any multiple of C_5H_8 units. Terpenes occur naturally in volatile oils and other plant sources; they are generally insoluble in water but soluble in alcohol and other organic liquids. **Sesquiterpenes** are hydrocarbons of the formula $C_{15}H_{24}$ or $(C_5H_8)_3$; **diterpenes** are hydrocarbons of the formula $C_{20}H_{32}$ or $(C_5H_8)_4$; **triterpenes** are hydrocarbons of the formula $C_{30}H_{48}$ or $(C_5H_8)_6$; **polyterpenes** are hydrocarbons of the formula $(C_5H_8)_n$. The term **hemiterpene** is sometimes applied to the hydrocarbon of the formula C_5H_8 (isoprene).

ter'pen·ism. Poisoning by terpene from internal use or inhalation.

ter'pi·lene di"hy·dro·chlo'ride (dye"high·dro-klor'ide). Eucalypteol.

ter·pin'e·ol. $C_{10}H_{17}OH$. A colorless, viscous liquid of lilac odor, occurring in many volatile oils and prepared from terpin hydrate; used in perfumes.

ter'pin hy'drate (*terpini hydras*). $C_{10}H_{20}O_2.H_2O$. Colorless crystals prepared by the action of nitric acid on turpentine oil in the presence of alcohol. Soluble in 200 parts of water or in 13 of alcohol. An expectorant. Dose, 0.13–0.32 Gm. (2–5 gr.).

t. h. elixir (*elixir terpini hydratis*). Contains 1.7% of terpin hydrate. Dose, 4–8 cc. (1–2 fluidrachms).

ter'pin·ol. An oily liquid, chiefly $C_{10}H_{16}$ and $C_{10}H_{18}O$, obtained by the action of dilute mineral acids on terpin hydrate with heat; soluble in alcohol. Formerly used in bronchial affections.

ter'ra (pl. *terrae*) [L., land]. Earth.

t. alba. Kaolin.

t. sigillata. Sealed earth; kaolin. In medieval Europe, earth guaranteed to be genuine through the use of a seal.

terramycin. Trade-mark for the antibiotic substance oxytetracycline, marketed in the form of the hydrochloride salt.

Terry's method. See under *method.*

ter'tian [L. *tertianus,* tertian]. Recurring every other day, as tertian fever.

double t. Quotidian.

ter'ti·ar·ism (tur'shee·ur·iz"um) [L. *tertiarius,* containing a third part]. Tertiary syphilis.

ter'ti·ar"y [*tertiarius*]. Third in order.

ter'ti·ar"y al'co·hol. An alcohol which contains the trivalent group COH.

ter·tip'a·ra [L. *tertius,* third; *parere,* to bring forth]. A woman who has borne three children.

ter·va'lence. See *trivalence.*

Tesla current. See under *current.*

test [L. *testum,* earthen vessel]. 1. A trial or examination. 2. A procedure to identify a constituent, to detect changes of a function, or to establish the true nature of a condition. 3. The reagent for producing a special reaction. For methods of performing quantitative tests, see *method.* For any test not listed here, see under *method* or *reaction,* or under the proper name.

Abderhalden's t. (*for pregnancy*). A test depending upon certain changes occurring in the blood serum in pregnancy. *Obs.*

abortin t. See brucellergin *t.*

Abridged A. O. color vision t. (Abridged version of American Optical Company's Charts.) A group of pseudo-isochromatic plates designed to detect color-vision deficiency.

absorption t. (*for differentiating bacteria*). The test consists of adding separately to agglutinative serums the various bacteria in the group in order to remove separately the partial agglutinins. Often used to differentiate between typhoid and paratyphoid fevers.

acetic acid and boiling t. See heat and acid *t.*

acetoacetic acid t. See Gerhardt's *t.*, Rothera's *t.*

acetone t. See Behre's *t.*, Legal's *t.*, Lieben's *t.*

acetylmethylcarbinol t. A test for the differentiation of the aerogenes group and colon group of bacteria. An equal volume of the reagent (copper sulfate, ammonium hydroxide, sodium hydroxide, and distilled water) is added to the culture. The development of a red color in 10 to 20 minutes is a positive test, indicating the presence of the aerogenes group.

acid serum phosphatase t. A measurement of the activity of phosphatase in an acid substrate either by its ability to liberate phenol from disodium phenylphosphate or phosphorus from glycerophosphate. Highly elevated values are diagnostic for prostatic carcinoma with metastases.

acrolein t. (*for glycerol and fats*). The suspected substance is heated with an equal quantity of potassium bisulfate. If glycerin or fats are present, acrolein is given off and is recognized by its characteristic irritating odor.

Addis and Shevky's t. (*for kidney function*). A concentration test based upon the specific gravity of urine passed during the last 12 hours of a 24-hour period of fluid deprivation.

adhesion t. (*for infectious jaundice*). The serum of the patient is added to a mixture of *Leptospira icterohaemorrhagiae* and either bacilli or blood platelets; it is examined after a short time with the dark-field microscope. The test is considered positive when the bacilli or platelets are found adherent to the spirochetes.

afterimage t. *In ophthalmology*, a measurement of abnormal retinal correspondence in strabismus. The patient looks at a horizontal luminous filament with the left eye and at a vertical one with the right. If the afterimages cross, correspondence is normal and binocular vision probably can be restored following correction of the strabismus.

agglutination t. (a) A test in which an agglomeration or clumping of particles produces masses which may be seen either with the unaided eye (**macroscopic agglutination test**) or with the aid of a microscope (**microscopic agglutination test**). The test also may be used for the identification of bacteria. (b) A test for the presence of specific antibodies (agglutinins) in the blood serum of infected individuals which will produce clumping of the specific bacteria causing the infection.

albumin t. See Heller's *t.*, Nonne-Apelt's *t.*, Osgood-Haskins *t.*, Parnum's *t.*, Purdy's *t.*, Roberts' *t.*, Spiegler's *t.*, sulfosalicylic acid *t.*

alcohol-turbidity t. A flocculation test for liver function.

Alexander's t. See *Hemophilus influenzae* antibody *t.*

alkaline serum phosphatase t. A measurement of the activity of phosphatase in an alkaline substrate either by its ability to liberate phenol from disodium phenylphosphate or phosphorous from glycerophosphate. Elevated values are found in obstructive liver disease, malignant bone tumors, rickets, pregnancy, and Paget's disease.

Allen's t. (*for phenol.*) To 2 parts of the unknown add 5 parts of hydrochloric acid and 1 part nitric acid. A cherry red color indicates the presence of phenol. (*for tinea versicolor.*) Paint the skin lesion with compound solution of iodine. The diseased portion will stain deep brown or mahogany color if the eruption is tinea.

allergy t. Any test used to demonstrate the presence of allergy, such as the conjunctival test, nasal test, patch test, or skin test.

alpha t. A series of eight types of intelligence tests designed for group application and for rapid scoring; first used by the U. S. Army in World War I.

Althausen t. See galactose tolerance *t.*

Althausen-Mancke's t. See insulin-glucose-water tolerance *t.*

amino-acid tolerance t. (*for liver function*). A test based upon the theory that in liver disease there is a significant delay in the removal from the blood of injected amino acids.

ammonium sulfide t. (*for lead*). A drop or two of residue from evaporated urine is allowed to fall into a tall glass full of ammonium sulfide. If lead is present, a white trail will develop in the fluid as the drop descends.

amylase t. See Fabricus-Moller urine *t.*, Somogyi's *t.*

amyloid t. See Congo red *t.*

Anderson-Nightingale dilution t. (*for vitamin A*). The material to be tested is diluted with chloroform until the blue color, formed after addition of antimony trichloride, is just visible.

aniline t. (*for vitamin D*). Liver oils and irradiated provitamin D give a red color with a mixture of aniline and hydrochloric acid.

animal protection t. A test of aid in the diagnosis of certain diseases, performed by injecting tissue extract or wound secretion and various antiserums into a series of animals. The animals protected by the specific antiserums indicate the nature of the organism to be identified. Also see serum protection *t.*

anoxemia t. See hypoxemia *t.*

antiglobulin t. A test originally developed for the detection of univalent Rh antibodies. It depends on the fact that the univalent antibodies coating the erythrocytes consist of human serum globulins. A potent precipitating rabbit antihuman serum is used. It will detect human globulin coating a particle (examples: erythrocytes, brucella organisms). Syn., *direct Coombs t.*, *direct developing t.*, *Race-Coombs t.*

antimony t. See Marsh's *t.*

antimony t. for kala-azar. A test in which a solution of a pentavalent antimony compound is stratified beneath a mixture of blood and potassium acetate. A flocculent precipitate forms immediately in advanced cases of kala-azar, but may take as long as 15 minutes in new cases.

antimony trichloride t. (*for provitamin D*). Provitamin D dissolved in chloroform and mixed with a solution of antimony trichloride in chloroform yields a red color.

antitrypsin t. A test based on the ability of blood serum to inhibit the action of trypsin. It is said to be of value in the diagnosis of carcinoma, nephritis, and other conditions.

aptitude t. A psychologic test given to determine a student's aptitude or ability for medicine or other pursuits. Also see Oseretsky *t.*, Stanford scientific aptitude *t.*

arm deviation t. Test for disease of the nervous system. The patient stands with his arms outstretched in front of him, and the examiner stands the same way with his fingertips supporting those of the patient. The patient then closes his eyes, with his arms still outstretched and the examiner moves away. The following deviations may occur: if pyramidal lesion is present, the arms move downward; if extrapyramidal lesion, the arms move downward and inward; if cerebellar lesion, the arms move strongly outward and upward; if parietal lobe lesion, the arms move slightly downward, and the fingers exhibit involuntary athetoid movements.

arm-lung time t. One in which the time is measured from the injection of ether into a vein until the odor of ether appears in the breath.

arm-tongue time t. One in which the time is measured from the injection of a substance into a vein until the taste of it is noticed in the mouth.

arsenic t. See Bettendorff's *t.*, Fleitmann's *t.*, Gutzeit's *t.*, Marsh's *t.*, Reinsch's *t.*

Aschheim-Zondek t. (*for pregnancy*). Urine from a woman is injected subcutaneously into immature white mice. If the woman is pregnant the ovaries of the mice will be enlarged, hyperemic, and hemorrhagic, and will show maturation of the ovarian follicles.

Ascoli t. A precipitin test for the detection of anthrax bacilli in meat, performed by overlaying antianthrax serum with the meat extract. A white ring of precipitation is a positive test.

associated movement of thumb t. A test for spastic paralysis of the hand. If the thumb is adducted when the patient tightly grasps with his four fingers those of the examiner, the test is positive. Also called *associated movements t.*

association t. *In psychoanalysis,* the procedure used in the diagnosis of certain abnormal mental states; sometimes used in crime detection. The test is oral and consists of presenting the patient with a predetermined series of words and noting his word associations and his reaction time.

auditory acuity t. The determination of the threshold of a person's hearing by the use of tuning forks or, preferably, an audiometer.

Ayala t. (*for cerebrospinal fluid*). A test, expressed as a quotient, used to determine whether the spinal fluid is in a large reservoir, as in hydrocephalus, or in a small reservoir, as in subarachnoid block. Also called *Ayala quotient.*

azorubin S t. (*for liver function*). A delay in the appearance of injected azorubin S in the bile or prolonged urinary excretion indicates impaired liver function.

Babcock-Levy t. An examination designed to measure intellectual deterioration by testing vocabulary, general information, symbol substitution, and the copying of designs with respect to correctness, speed, and accuracy; useful in organic cerebral deteriorative conditions.

Bachman t. (*for trichinosis*). A solution of powdered trichina larvae is injected intradermally. If the patient has trichinosis an area of edema at the site of injection develops in 1 to 2 weeks.

Bacillus proteus pregnancy t. A test based upon the fact that the serum from a pregnant woman will agglutinate *B. proteus* strain OX19.

Bárány's pointing t. The patient points with finger or toe at a fixed object alternately with eyes open and closed. A constant error in pointing with the eyes closed in the presence of vertigo indicates peripheral labyrinthine disease or an intracranial lesion.

Bárány's t. See caloric *t.*

Barberio's t. (*for semen*). A drop of spermatic fluid or an aqueous extract of spermatic stain, when treated with a saturated aqueous solution of picric acid, shows a precipitate of yellow refractile crystals.

Barfoed's t. (*for monosaccharides*). A copper reduction test formerly used for glucose in urine.

basophilic aggregation t. (*for lead poisoning*). Stippled erythrocytes normally do not constitute more than 1% of the total number of erythrocytes, but in lead poisoning they may constitute 2% or more of the total.

Bauer's t. See galactose tolerance *t.*

Baumann and Goldmann's t. (*for cystine*). If a solution of cystine is shaken in caustic soda with benzoyl chloride, a voluminous precipitate of benzoyl cystine will be produced.

Beer dye t. A test for renal function in which methylene blue, given orally or intravenously, is normally cleared after many hours. In chronic pyelonephritis, coincident with rupture of the dye-stained abscesses, the urine becomes blue periodically after original clearance is reached.

beer t. One in which the patient drinks a quantity of beer or other alcoholic drink in order to encourage reactivation of a chronic gonorrhea.

Behre's t. (*for acetone*). Vapor from hot urine containing acetone reacts with salicylic aldehyde and sodium hydroxide to produce a pink to rose color.

Bence Jones protein t. A test in which a precipitate, appearing when urine is heated to 50° to 60° C., disappearing at the boiling point, and reappearing on cooling, indicates Bence Jones protein.

Benda's t. Injection of epinephrine causes, in normal persons, an outpouring of young cells from the marrow, but in aplastic anemia it has no such effect; monocytes, however, may arise.

Bender gestalt t. A diagnostic and experimental psychological test in which the subject reproduces a series of designs. Deviations from the originals are interpreted in terms of Gestalt laws of perception and organization. Syn., *Bender visual motor gestalt t.*

Benedict's quantitative t. See Benedict's *method* for glucose.

Benedict's t. (*for glucose*). Eight drops of urine are added to 5 cc. of Benedict's qualitative sugar reagent (sodium citrate, copper sulfate, sodium carbonate, distilled water). Boil vigorously for 3 minutes. A green, yellow, or red precipitate indicates glucose.

Bennhold's t. See Congo red *t.*

benzidine t. (*for blood*). To 3 cc. of a saturated solution of benzidine in glacial acetic acid add 1 cc. of 3% hydrogen peroxide and 1 cc. of the unknown. A blue or green color indicates blood.

benzodioxane t. (*for pheochromocytoma*). Benzodioxane, an adrenergic blocking agent, is injected intravenously over a two-minute period in dosages of 10 mg per square meter of body surface. A hypotensive effect for ten minutes or longer is characteristic of pheochromocytoma.

Bernreuter personality inventory. A test designed to measure neurotic tendency, self-sufficiency, introversion, dominance, sociability, and confidence.

betahydroxybutyric acid t. See Black's *t.*

beta t. An intelligence test used, instead of the alpha test, for illiterates; carried out with signs and pictures.

Bettendorff's t. (*for arsenic*). The suspected liquid is mixed with hydrochloric acid and stannous chloride solution and a piece of tinfoil are added. A brown color or precipitate indicates arsenic.

Bial's t. (*for pentose*). Glucose must be removed from the urine by fermentation. Add a strongly acidified solution of orcinol to urine, and, if pentose is present, a green flocculent precipitate of furfural is formed.

bile acid t. See Pettenkofer's *t.*, Hay's *t.*, Bischoff's *t.*

bile pigment t. See Gmelin's *t.*, Huppert's *t.*, iodine *t.* (for bile pigments), Rosenbach's *t.*

bile solubility t. (*for Diplococcus pneumoniae*). A test for identifying pneumococci based on the fact that they dissolve in bile or bile salts.

bilirubin clearance t. (*for liver function*). A test based upon the ability of the liver to remove injected bilirubin from the blood.

bilirubin t. See Gmelin's *t.*, Huppert's *t.*, iodine *t.* (for bile pigments), Rosenbach's *t.*, van den Bergh's *t.*

Binet-Simon t. A method of estimating the intellectual capacity or measuring intelligence and expressing it as an intelligence quotient (IQ): also called *Binet's test.*

biologic t. See serum *t.*

biological t. of Wiener. The comparison of the icterus index of blood plasma or serum of the patient before and one hour after the injection of 50 cc of blood to test for blood compatibility.

Bischoff's t. (*for bile acids*). Bile acids heated with dilute sulfuric acid and cane sugar produce a red color.

bitterling t. (*for pregnancy*). A test made by placing a bitterling (a small carplike fish of Japan) in water to which some of the woman's urine has been added. If pregnancy is present, there is an outgrowth of the oviduct from the body of the fish.

biuret t. (*for proteins*). Add concentrated potassium hydroxide solution and a few drops of dilute copper sulfate solution to the unknown. A violet color indicates the presence of proteins.

Black's t. (*for betahydroxybutyric acid*). Black's reagent (ferric chloride, ferrous chloride, water) and hydrogen peroxide are added to an extract of urine which has been treated with plaster of Paris, ether, hydrochloric acid, and barium carbonate. The development of a rose color is a positive test.

bleeding time t. See Duke's *t.*, Ivy *t.*

blind t. A comparison of two methods of treatment in which both the patient and the observer are ignorant of the identity until the results have been recorded.

blood t. See benzidine *t.*, Gregersen's *t.*, guaiac *t.*, phenolphthalein *t.*, Ruttan and Hardisty's *t.*, serum *t.*, Teichmann's *t.*

blood urea clearance t. See urea clearance *t.*

Blyth's t. (*for lead in water*). The addition of a 1% alcoholic tincture of cochineal to water containing lead results in the formation of a precipitate.

Boas' t. (*For intestinal atony.*) In cases of intestinal atony a splashing sound can be obtained on pressure upon the abdominal wall after the injection of a small quantity (200–300 cc.) of water into the bowel. (*For hydrochloric acid in the gastric contents.*) A glass rod dipped in the solution (alcohol, resorcinol, and sucrose) is applied to a drop of the filtrate from the stomach and a deep scarlet streak is produced if hydrochloric acid is present.

Boerner, Jones, and Lukens t. A flocculation test for syphilis.

Boerner-Lukens t. (*for syphilis*). A modification of the Wassermann test.

bone conduction t. The testing of hearing threshold by placing a tuning fork or audiometer oscillator directly against the mastoid process. The **absolute bone conduction test** is a similar test done when the external auditory meatus is blocked by any of several means.

Bordet's t. See serum *t.*

bromsulphalein t. (*for liver function*). A test based upon the ability of the liver to remove injected bromsulphalein from the blood. Delayed removal indicates hepatic dysfunction.

Brown personality inventory. A psychologic test designed for the detection of psychoneurotic problem children.

Brown's t. See cold pressor *t.*

Brown's t. (*for arteriovenous fistula*). Blood withdrawn from a surface vein containing a considerable admixture of oxygenated arterial blood indicates arteriovenous fistula.

brucellergin t. An allergic skin test of aid in the diagnosis of brucellosis, made by the intradermal injection of brucellergin.

brucellosis t. See brucellergin *t.*, Huddleson's *t.*, opsonocytophagic *t.*

Bufo arenarum Hensel t. See male-toad *t.*

cadmium sulfate t. A flocculation test for the determination of liver damage.

calcium t. See Sulkowitch's *t.*

Calmette t. A tuberculin test in which dilute tuberculin is applied to the conjunctiva: rarely used.

caloric t. In the normal individual, nystagmus is produced by irrigating the external ear canal with hot (110°–120° F.) or cold (68° F.) water. When the vestibular nerve or labyrinth is destroyed, no nystagmus is produced upon testing the diseased side.

cancer t. See Schiller *t.*

candle t. (*for diplopia*). One performed by placing a red glass over one eye of the patient and a green one over the other eye, then noting what the patient sees as he looks at a candle in all the cardinal positions of gaze. Also see red lens *t.*

capillary resistance t. A test of the tendency for blood capillaries to break down and produce petechial hemorrhages. Two general procedures are used, a tourniquet *t.*, and a suction *t.*

carbon monoxide t. See tannic acid *t.*

Casoni's t. (*for echinococcus disease*). Sterile hydatid fluid from echinococcic cysts of lung or liver of sheep is injected intracutaneously. An urticarial wheal surrounded by a zone of erythema appearing rapidly and an area of erythema and edema lasting 2–3 days is indicative of echinococcic disease.

catatorulin t. (*for vitamin B_1*). A test which measures in vitro the uptake of oxygen by brain tissues from avitaminotic pigeons. Addition of vitamin B_1 proportionally increases the amount of oxygen consumed.

catoptric t. The diagnosis of cataract by means of the reflection of the Purkinje images from the cornea and lens capsules.

Cattell infant intelligence scale. A modification of the revised Stanford-Binet test adapted for infants from 3–30 months of age.

cat t. (*for staphylococcus enterotoxin*). A test to determine the production of enterotoxin produced by micrococci recovered in cultures of foods. The production of characteristic signs in a cat injected intravenously with the culture indicates the presence of enterotoxin.

cephalin-cholesterol flocculation t. (*for liver function*). A test which measures the capacity of serum of persons with hepatic disease to flocculate a colloidal suspension of cephalin cholesterol complex. The result, if positive, is expressed in graded form.

Cherry and Crandall's t. (*for lipase*). A test in which pancreatic lipase in serum is allowed to act on a substrate of olive oil, lipase then being determined by the amount of fatty acid liberated.

Chi-square t. A test used to determine the probability that the difference between an actual and a theoretical distribution or between two or more distributions is the result of chance alone.

chloral hydrate t. (*for provitamin D*). Crystals of

provitamin D, when heated slowly with crystals of chloral hydrate, melt above 50° C. and the mixture becomes first red, then green, and finally deep blue.

cholesterol t. See Liebermann-Burchard *t.*

Chopra's t. See antimony *t.* for kala-azar.

cinchophen oxidation t. (*for liver function*). A test based on the 24-hour excretion of oxycinchophen in the urine after the ingestion of a standard oral dose of 0.45 Gm. of cinchophen. Patients with hepatic dysfunction show a higher excretion than normal.

circulation time t. See arm-lung time *t.*, arm-tongue time *t.*

clearance t. (*For kidney function.*) A test of the excretory efficiency of the kidneys based upon the amount of blood cleared of a substance in 1 minute as determined by the ratio of the substance in the blood to the amount excreted in the urine during a fixed time. (*For liver function.*) A test based on the ability of the liver to remove a substance from the blood.

coagulase t. One used to determine the virulence of staphylococci, performed by incubating the bacteria in citrated or oxalated blood plasma. The development of coagulation is a positive test.

coccidioidin t. An allergic skin test of aid in the diagnosis of coccidioidomycosis made by the intradermal injection of coccidioidin which is prepared from cultures of *Coccidioides immitis.*

coin t. The use of silver coins as plexor and pleximeter in percussion while the examiner auscults the opposite side of the hemithorax. A clear, silver-bell note indicates the presence of pneumothorax. A dull, muffled note is the normal sound.

cold agglutination t. (*for primary atypical pneumonia*). A test for the detection of the autohemagglutinins or so-called cold agglutinins which may occur in high titer in the serums of individuals with primary atypical pneumonia.

cold pressor t. The rise in blood pressure is observed after the immersion of one hand in ice water for 1 minute. Individuals showing an excessive rise or unusual delay in return to normal are called hyperreactors and are thought likely to develop hypertension.

colloidal benzoin t. A colloidal suspension of Sumatra benzoin resin is added to varying saline dilutions of cerebrospinal fluid. The degree of precipitation in the various tubes is read in 24 hours. The principle and interpretation of the test are the same as for Lange's colloidal gold test.

colloidal gold t. See Lange's *t.*

colloidal red t. A liver function test which gives results almost identical with the colloidal gold test. The reagent is prepared from alcoholic Scharlach red.

color threshold t. A lantern type test of the ability of color-vision-deficient individuals to identify colored light signals at intensities ranging from the normal chromatic thresholds to 100 times as great.

color vision t. See Abridged A. O. color vision *t.*, color threshold *t.*, Ishihara's *t.*

colostrum t. (*for pregnancy*). One in which 0.02 cc. of equal parts of human colostrum and saline solution are injected intradermally. No areola or a slight areola under 1 inch in diameter indicates pregnancy.

complement-fixation t. A test based on the complement-fixation reaction in which antigen uniting with its antibody combines with the complement and thus inactivates or fixes it.

completed t. (*for Escherichia coli in water*). Organisms from atypical colonies of a confirmed test are transferred to lactose broth and agar slants. The formation of gas in the lactose broth and the demonstration of Gram-negative non-spore-forming bacilli in the agar culture is a positive test.

concentration t. (*for kidney function*). A test of kidney function based upon their normal ability to concentrate or dilute urine. See Addis and Shevky's *t.*, Fishberg's *t.*, Lashmet and Newburgh's *t.*, Mosenthal *t.*, Volhard's and Fahr's *tests.*

confirmed t. (*for Escherichia coli in water*). Eosin-methylene blue plates are incubated with water from a positive presumptive test. The development of typical colonies in 24 hours is a positive test, but in the case of atypical colonies a *completed test* is performed.

confusion t. A test to detect malingering used in eye injuries and based upon the fact that vision in the injured eye is recorded while the patient thinks the healthy eye is being examined.

conglutination t. An antigen-antibody reaction in which a conglutinin is added.

Congo red t. (*for amyloidosis*). Congo red is injected intravenously. In normal persons, 30% of the dye disappears from the blood within an hour, but in amyloid disease from 40 to 100% disappears.

conjunctival t. A test for allergy in which the antigen is instilled into the conjunctival sac. A positive test consists of injection of the conjunctival vessels with itching and lacrimation. Syn., *ophthalmic t.*

contact t. See patch *t.*

contrast t. A test performed or reaction elicited in one area and contrasted with the response of another area to simultaneous and identical application of excitant.

Coombs t. See antiglobulin *t.*, Rh blocking *t.*

Cowie's t. See guaiac *t.*

cross-match t. See *cross-matching.*

cutaneous t. See skin *t.*

Cutler-Power-Wilder t. A test of aid in the diagnosis of adrenal insufficiency (Addison's disease). The patient is given additional potassium in the diet with restriction of sodium and water. In the presence of the disease, the urinary excretion of chlorides is much higher than normal.

Cutting's colloidal mastic t. See mastic *t.*

cyanide t. See Liebig's *t.*, Prussian blue *t.*, Schoenbein's *t.*

cyanine dye t. (*for vitamin B_6*). A color reaction obtained by converting vitamin B_6 into a pyridinium compound. On heating this product with potassium hydroxide and chloroform, a violet cyanine dye is obtained.

cystine t. See Baumann and Goldmann's *t.*, Liebig's *t.*, Müller's *t.*

cytoplasm-modifying t. See dye *t.*

Davidsohn differential t. (*for infectious mononucleosis*). A test to determine if the heterophil antibodies (antisheep agglutinins) in the serum are absorbed by a suspension of guinea pig kidney. The heterophil antibodies produced in infectious mononucleosis are not absorbed, whereas those produced in serum disease are readily absorbed.

Davidsohn presumptive t. (*for infectious mononucleosis*). An agglutination test for the presence of heterophil agglutinin which is characteristically produced in the serum of patients with infectious mononucleosis.

dermal t. See scratch *t.*

dextrose t. See Barfoed's *t.*, Benedict's *t.*, Fehling's *t.*, fermentation *t.*, Folin-McEllroy *t.*, Haines's *t.*, Moore's *t.*, Nylander's *t.*, phenylhydrazine *t.*

dextrose tolerance t. See glucose tolerance *t.*

diacetic acid t. See Gerhardt's *t.*, Rothera's *t.*

diagnostic t. An examination or trial in which, if

certain responses or reactions are present, a diagnosis of a specific disease may be presumed.

Dick t. (*for susceptibility or immunity to scarlet fever*). An immunologic skin test in which development of a local area of redness of the skin 18 to 24 hours after the intracutaneous injection of the filtrate of a culture of specific hemolytic streptococcus indicates susceptibility, and the absence of redness indicates immunity, to scarlet fever.

dilution t. (*for kidney function*). See concentration *t.*

dilution turbidity t. A flocculation test for liver function.

diodrast clearance t. (*for kidney function*). The rate of renal excretion of diodrast in relation to the blood level is used as a test of renal function and as an approximate measure of renal blood flow.

direct Coombs t. See antiglobulin *t.*, Rh blocking *t.*

direct developing t. See antiglobulin *t.*, Rh blocking *t.*

Doerfler-Stewart t. A test for psychogenic deafness performed by measuring the amount of background noise required to reduce the speech intelligibility threshold of a deafened person by 50%.

Donath-Landsteiner t. (*for paroxysmal hemoglobinuria*). A test based upon a thermolabile isohemolysin occurring in the blood of patients with paroxysmal hemoglobinuria which unites with the red cells at low temperatures and causes hemolysis after the cells are warmed to 37° C.: also called *Donath-Landsteiner phenomenon.*

Donné's t. (*for pus in urine*). Decant, filter, or centrifuge urine and put a small piece of sodium hydroxide on the sediment. If pus is present, the sediment will become slimy and tough.

Duke t. (*for bleeding time*). A test performed by puncturing the lobe of the ear and determining the time which elapses until bleeding stops.

dye t. (*for toxoplasmosis*). A test based on the observation that the cytoplasm of *Toxoplasma*, when acted on by a specific antibody and complement-like accessory factor, loses its affinity for methylene blue at pH 11. Serial dilutions of serum are made, and to a given amount an equal aliquot of a heparinized *Toxoplasma*-accessory-factor dye mixture is added. After incubation, one drop from each tube is examined microscopically, and the number of extracellular *Toxoplasma* with stained or unstained cytoplasm determined. The highest dilution of serum leaving 50% or more of the organisms unstained is the titer. Syn., *dye-inhibition t.*

Eagle t. (a) A complement-fixation test for syphilis. (b) A flocculation test for syphilis.

echinococcus t. See Casoni's *t.*

Ehrlich's t. (*for urobilinogen*). Bilirubin-free, undiluted urine is added to a solution of paradimethylaminobenzaldehyde in hydrochloric acid. A deep cherry-red color indicates urobilinogen.

electrophoresis t. See electrophoresis *method.*

Ellsworth-Howard t. A test to distinguish pseudohypoparathyroidism from hypoparathyroidism. Failure of injected parathyroid extract to produce a phosphate diuresis is a positive reaction, indicating pseudohypoparathyroidism.

epinephrine hypersensitiveness t. See Emil *Goetsch.*

epinephrine t. See Benda's *t.*

erythrocyte fragility t. A measure of the resistance of red blood cells to osmotic hemolysis in hypotonic salt solutions of graded dilutions.

erythrocyte sedimentation t. When citrated or oxalated blood is allowed to stand in a column, the erythrocytes settle to the bottom. The rate of this sedimentation varies in different pathologic conditions and may be determined by any of the different methods, such as Cutler's, Westergren's, Smith's, Wintrobe's, etc.

estrogen t. See Fluhmann's *t.*

exercise tolerance t. (*for angina pectoris*). A test performed in a constant temperature room in which the patient climbs and descends a standard two-step staircase until an attack of angina pectoris is precipitated.

Exton's t. (*for albumin*). Equal volumes of clear urine and Exton's reagent (sodium sulfate, sulfosalicylic acid, bromphenol blue, water) are mixed in a test tube. Cloudiness appearing upon heating indicates albumin.

Exton and Rose's t. A modification of the glucose tolerance test.

Fabricus-Moller urine t. (*for amylase*). Urine is incubated with graded dilutions of starch solution. The amount of digestion is then determined by using iodine as an indicator.

Falls's t. See colostrum *t.*

fat t. See acrolein *t.*

Fehling's t. (*for glucose*). Equal volumes of copper sulfate solution and alkaline tartrate solution are mixed. Equal volumes of this mixture (Fehling's solution) and urine are boiled. In the presence of glucose the solution turns green, yellow, or red depending on the amount present.

fermentation t. (*for glucose*). A test based on the production of carbon dioxide and alcohol when yeast is added to a glucose solution. Commonly applied to urine.

ferric chloride t. (*for diacetic acid*). See Gerhardt's *t.*

ferric chloride t. for vitamin A. Ferric chloride reacts with vitamin A to give a characteristic color which can be compared colorimetrically.

finger-finger t. A cerebellar function test in which the patient is asked to bring his index fingers together from a position in which the arms are outstretched, or to place his index finger on the examiner's index finger with eyes open. Normally this is carried out smoothly.

finger-nose t. A cerebellar function test in which the patient is asked to put the index finger of each hand on the nose alternately in rapid succession with eyes open. Normally this is carried out smoothly.

Fishberg's t. (*for kidney function*). A concentration test in which urinary specific gravity is determined 12 hours after fluid deprivation.

five-glass t. See glass *t.*

Fleck's leukergy t. See leukergy *t.*

Fleitmann's t. (*for arsenic*). Hydrogen generated from zinc and potassium hydroxide is passed through the suspected solution and then over filter paper moistened with a solution of silver nitrate. Upon heating, the filter paper will turn black if an inorganic arsenic compound is present.

flicker fusion t. A test of the minimal frequency of standard flashes of light which will be seen as a steady illumination; used as a test for fatigue and for tolerance to anoxia; also used for diagnosing high blood pressure and some forms of heart disease, as angina pectoris.

flocculation t. A test in which the antibody reacts directly with the antigen to produce flocculi rather than to form a combination for the inactivation of complement as in a complement-fixation test.

Florence's t. (*for semen*). Semen treated with a strong solution of iodine and potassium iodide yields brown crystals in the shape of needles or plates.

Fluhmann's t. A test for the blood estrogen

level performed by injecting blood serum into spayed mice, and using the degree of histologic change in the vaginal epithelium as a guide.

foam t. (*for bile pigments*). To 5 ml. of diluted bile add 3–4 drops of a very dilute aqueous solution of furfural. Shake the tube until a thick foam is formed, then add 2–3 drops of concentrated sulfuric acid to the foam and a dark pink coloration is produced.

Foerster's cutaneous numeral t. A method of drawing numerals on various areas of body skin for the patient to identify; a test of topognostic sensibility.

Folin-McEllroy t. (*for glucose*). A copper reduction test used for glucose in the urine.

Folin-Wu t. A method for the quantitative estimation of urea in the blood, utilizing urease.

formol-gel t. See Napier's aldehyde *t.*

Foshay's t. (*for tularemia*). A skin test of aid in diagnosis of tularemia made by the intradermal injection of a dilute suspension of *Pasteurella tularensis*. A local erythema is considered a positive reaction.

fragility t. See erythrocyte fragility *t.*

Francis t. An immunologic skin test for the presence or absence of antibody in pneumococcal pneumonia performed by the intradermal injection of the type specific capsular polysaccharide.

Frei t. An allergic skin test of aid in the diagnosis of venereal lymphogranuloma made by the intradermal injection of an antigen obtained from a bubo, the brain of an infected mouse, or infected chick embryo.

Friedman t. (*for pregnancy*). The intravenous injection of urine from a pregnant woman into a female rabbit will bring about the formation of corpora hemorrhagica and corpora lutea in the ovaries of the rabbit.

frog t. (*for pregnancy*). If urine from a pregnant woman is injected into the female African frog (*Xenopus laevis*), five or more eggs will be deposited within 12 hours.

fructose t. See Seliwanoff's *t.*

fundus reflex t. See *retinoscopy.*

galactose t. See Tollens' *t.*, mucic acid *t.*

galactose tolerance t. (*for liver function*). A test of the glycogenic function of the liver, performed by administering 40 Gm. of galactose to a fasting individual. The elimination of more than 3 Gm. of galactose over a 5-hour period indicates hepatic dysfunction.

gallbladder function t. See sodium tetraiodophenolphthalein *t.*

Garrod's t. for porphyrins in urine. To 100 cc. of urine add 20 cc. of 10 per cent sodium hydroxide. Separate the precipitate by centrifugation or filtration, wash thoroughly with water, and dissolve in 5 cc. of alcohol containing 5 to 10 drops of hydrochloric acid. A pink to red solution indicates the presence of acid hematoporphyrin which may be confirmed by spectroscopic examination for the characteristic absorption bands.

Georgi-Sachs t. A method for testing anticomplementary serums as part of a serodiagnostic test for syphilis.

Gerhardt's t. (*for diacetic acid*). Urine containing diacetic acid produces a Bordeaux red color when ferric chloride is added.

Gesell developmental schedule. A test of the mental growth of the preschool child which includes motor development, adaptive behavior, language development, and personal-social behavior.

Gibbon-Landis t. See Landis-Gibbon *t.*

Gibbs's t. (*for vitamin B_6*). A vitamin-B_6 solution mixed with a barbiturate buffer and a butanol solution of 2,6-dichloroquinone chlorimide yields a blue color which may be compared colorimetrically.

glass t. A gross test for infection of the urinary tract in which the urine is voided in fractions into two or more glass containers for the purpose of localizing the site of inflammatory disease.

globulin t. See Nonne-Apelt's *t.*

glucose t. See Barfoed's *t.*, Benedict's *t.*, Fehling's *t.*, fermentation *t.*, Folin-McEllroy *t.*, Haines's *t.*, Moore's *t.*, Nylander's *t.*, phenylhydrazine *t.*

glucose tolerance t. (*for liver function*). A test based on the ability of the liver to convert glucose to glycogen. It is useful in measuring the approximate severity of diabetes mellitus.

glycerol t. See acrolein *t.*

glyoxylic acid t. Given by most proteins. The solution is treated with a small amount of a solution containing a salt of glyoxylic acid. For Benedict's modification of this reagent a suspension of powdered magnesium in distilled water is treated under cooling with an excess of saturated oxalic acid solution and the mixture is filtered to remove magnesium oxidate. The filtrate is acidified with acetic acid and diluted. The mixture of protein solution and glyoxylate is stratified above concentrated H_2SO_4. A positive reaction is the formation of a violet ring at the zone of contact. The reaction is due to the presence of the indole group in the tryptophan residues of the protein. Proteins lacking tryptophan give no color in this reaction. Also called *Hopkins-Cole reaction.*

Gmelin's t. (*for bile pigment*). Urine is stratified over concentrated nitric acid. In the presence of bile pigment various colored rings are seen at the junction of the two fluids.

Gofman t. An ultracentrifuge analysis of the low-density beta-lipoproteins of serum, based on the relationship of specific classes of serum cholesterol-bearing lipoproteins and atherosclerosis: used as an index of atherosclerogenic potentialities.

Goldstein-Scheerer t. A test which measures the impairment of brain function with respect to abstract and concrete thinking; useful for studying patients with brain injuries.

gonorrhea t. See Schwartz-McNeil *t.*, two glass *t.*

Gordon's t. (*for Hodgkin's disease*). The intracerebral inoculation of rabbits with suspensions of the lymph nodes from a patient with Hodgkin's disease produces encephalitis. The reaction may be due to the presence of eosinophils. The test is seldom used.

Graham-Cole t. See *cholecystography.* See also sodium tetraiodophenolphthalein *t.*

Gregersen's t. (*for occult blood*). A modification of the benzidine test used for testing feces.

guaiac t. (*for blood*). An acetic acid or alcoholic solution of guaiac resin and hydrogen peroxide is mixed with the unknown. The development of a blue color is a positive test.

Gudernatsch's t. (*for thyroid activity*). If active thyroid is fed to young frogs, metamorphosis is accelerated, resulting in dwarf frogs.

gum mastic t. See mastic *t.*

Günzberg t. (*for free hydrochloric acid*). A stirring rod moistened in the unknown solution is drawn through dried Günzberg reagent which turns a purplish red color in the presence of free hydrochloric acid.

Gutzeit's t. (*for arsenic*). Zinc, stannous chloride, and sulfuric acid are added to the sample in a container. If present, arsenic is reduced to arsine and evolved as a gas which imparts a characteristic stain to paper previously impregnated with silver nitrate or mercuric chloride.

Haines's t. A copper reduction test used for glucose in the urine.
Hamburger's t. A tuberculin skin test which consists of rubbing tuberculin ointment over the skin of the sternum. A positive result is indicated by a crop of papules in from two to seven days.
Hanger's t. See cephalin-cholesterol flocculation *t.*
Harrison spot t. (*for bilirubin*). Bilirubin is concentrated on filter paper by precipitating it with barium chloride and filtering. A drop of Fouchet's reagent (ferric chloride in a dilute solution of trichloracetic acid) is added. A green color indicates the presence of bilirubin, which is oxidized to biliverdin.
Harrower-Erickson t. A modification of the Rorschach test.
Hay's t. (*for bile acids*). Finely pulverized sulfur is sprinkled upon the surface of urine. If the sulfur sinks to the bottom, bile acids are present.
head-bending t. Test for infection of the meninges or the nerve roots. While the patient is sitting, his head is bent forward by the examiner. The test is positive if the patient feels pain. The location of the pain indicates the area affected.
head-dropping t. A test for early parkinsonism. The patient lies on a table, and the examiner lifts his head suddenly and allows it to drop. In the normal person, the head falls quickly; but in a patient with parkinsonism the tightened neck muscles cause the head to drop slowly.
hearing t. See bone conduction *t.*, Rinne's *t.*, Schwabach's *t.*, Teal *t.*, Weber's *t.*
heat and acid t. (*for protein*). Urine is boiled in a test tube for 1 or 2 minutes and then 3 to 5 drops of 5% acetic acid are added. A white precipitate indicates protein.
Hecht-Schlaer night vision t. A low brightness adaptometer for measuring both light and form discrimination below the cone threshold.
heel-to-knee-to-toe t. A test for nonequilibratory coordination in which the patient is asked to place the heel of one foot on the opposite knee, then push the heel along the shin to the big toe. Normally, this is done smoothly and accurately.
Heller's t. (*for albumin*). Stratify clear urine over concentrated nitric acid in a test tube. A white zone at the junction of the fluids indicates albumin.
hemagglutination t. Any test in which hemagglutination is used as an indicator.
hemin t. See Teichmann's *t.*
hemolysin t. One used for identification of streptococci performed by incubating the bacteria with blood agar and then noting the type of hemolysis produced.
Hemophilus influenzae antibody t. An immunologic skin test for the presence or absence of antibody in influenzal infections such as meningitis or pneumonia.
Hench and Aldrich's t. (*for urea*). A test for retention of urea in the blood by measuring the amount of urea in the saliva.
Henry's melano-flocculation t. (*for malaria*). A test which depends upon changes in the serum proteins, especially an increase in euglobulin. The test gives a high percentage of positive reactions in malaria, but sometimes is positive in syphilis and other diseases.
hepatic function t. See liver function *t.*
heterophil antibody t. See Paul-Bunnell *t.*
Hines and Brown t. See cold pressor *t.*
Hinton t. A macroscopic flocculation test for syphilis.
hippuric acid t. (*for liver function*). A test based upon the ability of the liver to synthesize glycine and to conjugate it with benzoic acid to form hippuric acid. Given 6 Gm. of sodium benzoate, in 4 hours a normal person will eliminate 3 or more Gm. of hippuric acid in the urine, whereas a person with liver dysfunction will eliminate less than 3 Gm.
histamine cutaneous t. Intradermal injections of histamine are made at various points along a limb. Normally a wheal with an erythematous areola appears within 5 minutes. Absence of these phenomena indicates insufficient pressure in skin vessels or arterial spasm or nonfunctioning sensory nerves of the skin.
histamine t. (a) The subcutaneous injection of histamine stimulates the gastric secretion of hydrochloric acid. (b) The precipitation of an attack of histaminic cephalalgia (vasomotor headache) by the injection of histamine done for purposes of diagnosis.
histidine t. (*for pregnancy*). A test for the diagnosis of pregnancy based on the amount of histidine in the urine: not specific and rarely used.
histoplasmin t. Cutaneous injection of histoplasmin will effect a positive skin reaction if the subject has been or is infected with *Histoplasma capsulatum* and has been sensitized to the organism. Cross reaction may also occur in cases of blastomycosis and coccidioidomycosis.
Hoffman's t. (*for tyrosine*). The brilliant red color given by tyrosine when treated with Millon's reagent.
Hogben t. See frog *t.*
Holmgren t. A test for color vision in which the subject is required to separate a number of pieces of wool yarn according to their color.
hormone t. See Abderhalden's *t.*, Aschheim-Zondek *t.*, bitterling *t.*, Fluhmann's *t.*, Friedman *t.*, frog *t.*
Howard-Dolman depth perception t. A test of the average error in setting a moving rod equidistant to a fixed rod at a distance of 20 feet. All clues to depth perception other than those furnished by binocular vision are eliminated.
Huddleson's t. (*for brucellosis*). An agglutination test for brucellosis in humans or cattle, using *Brucella abortus* as an antigen.
Huggins t. See iodoacetate *index.*
Huggins-Miller-Jensen t. See iodoacetate *index.*
Hunt's t. See opsonocytophagic *t.*
Huppert's t. A test for bile pigments based upon their oxidation by concentrated hydrochloric acid to produce a green-colored derivative.
Hurtley's t. (*for diacetic acid*). Concentrated hydrochloric acid, sodium nitrite, ammonium hydroxide, and ferrous sulfate are added to urine. The development of a violet or purple color indicates diacetic acid.
hydrochloric acid t. See Boas' *t.*, Töpfer's *t.*
hydrostatic t. A live birth is indicated if the lungs of a dead infant float in water.
hypoxemia t. An electrocardiographic (ECG) test to determine the functional capacity of the coronary circulation by having the subject breathe a mixture of 10% oxygen and 90% nitrogen.
icterus index t. A colorimetric test in which blood serum is compared with a standard solution of sodium dichromate.
indican t. See Obermayer's *t.*
indigo carmine t. A test of kidney function. Indigo carmine should appear in the urine 7 minutes after intravenous injection if the kidney is functioning normally.
indirect Coombs t. See Rh blocking *t.*
indirect developing t. See Rh blocking *t.*

indole t. See oxalic acid paper *t.*

infectious mononucleosis t. See Davidsohn differential *t.*, Davidsohn presumptive *t.*, Paul-Bunnell *t.*

inkblot t. See Rorschach *t.*

inositol t. See Scherer's *t.*

insulin-glucose-water tolerance t. (*for liver function*). A test in which 20 units of insulin, 50 Gm. of glucose, and 1500 cc. of water are administered. Terminal hypoglycemia within 3 hours is said to be indicative of liver damage.

insulin tolerance t. (*for liver function*). A test based upon the comparison of depression of blood sugar levels and rapidity of recovery from relative hypoglycemia following a standard intravenous dose of insulin as compared to the response of normal individuals.

intelligence t. See alpha *t.*, Babcock-Levy *t.*, beta *t.*, Binet-Simon *t.*, Cattell infant intelligence scale (under *test*), Gesell developmental schedule (under *test*), Goldstein-Scheerer *t.*, Kent mental *t.*, Minnesota preschool scale (under *test*), Stanford-Binet *t.*, Wechsler-Bellevue intelligence scale (under *test*).

intradermal vitamin-C t. One based upon the length of time that an intradermal injection of dichlorophenolindophenol takes to decolorize.

iodine t. (*for bile pigments*). Tincture of iodine is slowly poured into urine. The development of a greenish blue color indicates bile pigments.

iodine t. (*for starch*). A potassium iodide solution of iodine reacts with starch to produce a blue color.

iodine tolerance t. (*for hyperthyroidism*). A test based on the observation that in patients with hyperthyroidism the total blood iodine is only slightly increased as compared to normal by the oral administration of iodine.

iodoform t. (*for acetone*). See Lieben's *t.*

Ishihara's t. A color vision test made by using a series of plates upon which are printed round dots of various sizes, colors, and combinations.

Ito-Reenstierna t. An allergic skin test of aid in the diagnosis or exclusion of chancroid performed by the intradermal injection of a vaccine of killed *Hemophilus ducreyi.*

Ivy t. (*for bleeding time*). A test performed by making a small puncture wound in a relatively avascular forearm and determining the time which elapses until bleeding stops.

Jaffé's t. Creatinine forms a red compound with picric acid in alkaline solution.

Jezler-Takata t. See Takata-Ara *t.*

Kahn t. A macroscopic flocculation test for syphilis.

Kajdi t. A test for scurvy used for infants; the vitamin-C storage capacity is determined by noting the difference between the fasting plasma ascorbic acid level and the plasma level four hours after the intramuscular injection of 200 mg. of ascorbic acid. A rise to 0.2 mg. per cent is considered positive.

kala-azar t. See antimony *t.* for kala-azar, Napier's aldehyde *t.*, Sia's *t.*

Kasanin-Vigotsky t. A psychologic test used to demonstrate difficulty in conceptual thinking which may indicate organic cerebral disease or a schizophrenic disorder.

Kay-Graham pasteurization t. The destructive effect of heat on the natural phosphatase in raw milk is used as a basis for testing the efficiency of pasteurization. Phosphatase activity is measured by the hydrolysis of disodium phenyl phosphate and colorimetric estimation of the released phenol by means of Folin-Ciocalteu's reagent.

Kelling's t. (*for lactic acid*). Ferric chloride added to gastric juice produces a deep yellow color if lactic acid is present.

Kent mental t. An oral test for intelligence consisting of 25 questions for emergency use in clinics.

kidney function t. See Addis and Shevky's *t.*, clearance *t.*, concentration *t.*, diodrast clearance *t.*, Fishberg's *t.*, indigo carmine *t.*, Mosenthal *t.*, Lashmet and Newburgh's *t.*, phenolsulfonphthalein *t.*, urea clearance *t.*, Volhard's and Fahr's *tests.*

Kingsbury's t. A test for albumin concentration performed by adding 3% sulfosalicylic acid to urine and comparing turbidity with a set of standards.

Kline t. A microscopic flocculation test for syphilis.

knee-dropping t. A simple test for the early detection of hemiplegia. The relaxed patient lies supine on a hard surface with legs drawn into a flexed position (slightly more than 45° at the knees); on the side of the pyramidal lesion, the knee drops continuously and evenly, with speed proportionate to severity of lesion, until the leg lies flat. The knee-drop should occur on successive examinations before the test may be considered positive.

Kolmer's t. (a) A complement-fixation test for syphilis. (b) A complement-fixation test for bacterial, spirochetal, viral, protozoal, or metazoal diseases.

Kossel's t. (*for hypoxanthine*). The unknown solution is treated with hydrochloric acid, zinc, and sodium hydroxide. A ruby red color indicates the presence of hypoxanthine.

Kunkel t. A test for the estimation of gamma-globulin in serum, in which the turbidity resulting on addition of zinc sulfate solution is compared with suitable standards.

Kveim t. See Nickerson-Kveim *t.*

lability t. A test for glaucoma in eyes of normal pressure; it consists of placing one of the patient's hands in ice-cold water and simultaneously raising the venous pressure in the head and maintaining it at 40 mm. Hg for one minute. The results are positive when ocular pressure increases, or increases and levels off, negative when it decreases, and indeterminate when it is already normal and neither ncreases nor decreases.

labyrinthine t. See Bárány's pointing *t.*, caloric *t.*

lactic acid t. See Kelling's *t.*, MacLean's *t.*, Strauss's *t.*, Uffelmann's *t.*

lactic acid tolerance t. See sodium *d*-lactate clearance *t.*

lactose t. See Rubner's *t.*

Landis-Gibbon t. A test for the evaluation of vasospasm in peripheral vascular disease, based on reflex vasodilatation. After the patient has reached temperature stability in a cool room, one of his uninvolved extremities, his trunk, or abdomen is exposed to heating, and the skin temperature of the digits of the involved extremity is recorded. In the presence of obliterative vascular disease, little or no rise in temperature occurs.

Landolt's broken C t. A test for visual acuity described by Landolt (1888) wherein the subject is to determine in which segment the gap in the ring (or letter C) lies, a factor which is determined by the size of the image of the gap on the retina.

Lange's t. A test based on the fact that normal cerebrospinal fluid does not visibly precipitate a colloidal gold suspension but that in syphilis of the central nervous system and other affections of the central nervous system precipitation may occur.

laryngeal mirror t. A tuberculin test used to

replace the usual sputum test where the patient swallows the sputum. A laryngeal mirror is placed in the back of the throat so that the vocal folds may be seen. The patient coughs, and the sputum on the mirror is examined for acid-fast bacilli.

Lashmet and Newburgh's t. (*for kidney function*). A concentration test based upon the specific gravity of urine voided during the day with the patient on a special diet with no fluids.

Lassaigne t. (*for organic nitrogen*). The organic compound containing nitrogen is fused with sodium to form sodium cyanide. This, when heated with ferrous sulfate in alkaline solution, forms sodium ferrocyanide. The sodium ferrocyanide reacts with ferric ion, to form the blue ferric ferrocyanide.

Laughlen t. A flocculation test for syphilis.

Leach t. (*for formaldehyde*). 10 ml. of the solution to be tested is mixed with 10 ml. of concentrated hydrochloric acid containing about 1 ml. of 10% ferric chloride solution to each 500 ml. of acid. The temperature of the mixture is raised, on a water bath, nearly to boiling and if formaldehyde is present a violet color is produced. A brown color develops in the absence of formaldehyde.

lead t. See Blyth's *t.*, ammonium sulfide *t.*

Lee's t. (*for rennin*). A test for rennin in gastric juice based upon its ability to coagulate the protein of milk.

Legal's t. (*for acetone*). An alkaline urine distillate containing acetone produces a red color in the presence of sodium nitroprusside.

leishmanin t. An intradermal test of great practical value to indicate past or present infection with *Leishmania brasiliensis* or *L. tropica*.

leprolin t. An intradermal test with a vaccine used as a diagnostic procedure in leprosy.

lepromin t. The intradermal injection of lepromin as a skin test, useful in the classification and prognosis of leprosy, generally positive in the tuberculoid and negative in the lepromatous form. First described by Mitsuda (1916).

L.E. t. See under *lupus erythematosus*.

leukergy t. Increased agglomeration of leukocytes in citrated blood, as a test for rheumatic disease. Syn., *Fleck's leukergy t.*

Levinson t. (*for tuberculous meningitis*). A test based on the observation that a characteristic ratio may be obtained between the alkaloidal precipitate formed by sulfosalicylic acid and the metallic precipitate formed by mercuric chloride in tuberculous meningitis.

levulose t. See Seliwanoff's *t.*

levulose tolerance t. (*for liver function*). A test based on the observation that the blood sugar level is normally unaffected by the oral administration of levulose, whereas it is increased in the presence of hepatic disease.

lid vibration t. (*for facial paralysis*). Diminished vibration of the upper lid of the closed eye against resistance, as an index of facial paralysis.

Lieben's t. (*for acetone in urine*). To a urine distillate, sodium hydroxide and Lugol's iodine solution are added. Turbidity changing to a yellow precipitate of iodoform is a positive test.

Liebermann-Burchard t. (*for cholesterol*). Dissolve the unknown in acetic anhydride and add concentrated sulfuric acid. A violet color turning to green indicates the presence of cholesterol.

Liebig's t. (*for cyanide*). To a distillate prepared from the suspected material, add yellow ammonium sulfide and evaporate to dryness. Add hydrochloric acid and ferric chloride solution to the residue. A deep red color indicates the presence of cyanide.

Liebig's t. (*for cystine*). Boil the substance with caustic alkali containing lead oxide. In the presence of cystine a precipitate of black lead sulfide is formed.

line t. Developed to study the progress of rickets. The bone is split lengthwise, immersed briefly in 3% $AgNO_3$, washed in water, and exposed to bright light. A black deposit of metallic silver appears in the epiphyseal region and is proportional to the degree of calcification. In extreme rickets no silver will appear in the epiphysis but when healing has begun the calcium deposits are so located that the corresponding silver stain appears along a distinct line.

lipase t. See Cherry and Crandall's *t.*

liver function t. See amino-acid tolerance *t.*, azorubin S *t.*, bilirubin clearance *t.*, bromsulfalein *t.*, cephalin-cholesterol flocculation *t.*, cinchophen oxidation *t.*, galactose tolerance *t.*, glucose tolerance *t.*, hippuric acid *t.*, insulin tolerance *t.*, insulin-glucose-water tolerance *t.*, levulose tolerance *t.*, phenoltetrachlorophthalein *t.*, rose bengal *t.*, Rosenthal-Rowntree *t.*, sodium *d*-lactate clearance *t.*, sodium tetraiodophenolphthalein *t.*, Takata-Ara *t.*

MacLean's t. (*for lactic acid*). To gastric juice, add a reagent containing ferric chloride, mercuric chloride, and hydrochloric acid. A yellow color indicates lactic acid.

malaria t. See Henry's melano-flocculation *t.*, Proske and Watson's *t.*

male-toad t. A biologic pregnancy test. When urine containing chorionic gonadotropin is injected into the toad (*Bufo arenarum Hensel*), spermatozoa migrate into the urinary bladder, and are demonstrable in the toad's urine within three hours after injection.

mallein t. An intradermal test used in the detection of chronic and latent glanders.

Mancke-Sommer t. (*for liver function*). A modification of the Takata-Ara *t.*

manometric t. See Queckenstedt-Stookey *t.*

Mantoux t. A tuberculin test in which the substance is injected intradermally. Also called intracutaneous tuberculin *t.*, Mendel's *t.*

Marsh's t. (*for arsenic or antimony*). Introduce the substance into a flask with dilute sulfuric acid and zinc. Light a jet, and permit it to impinge on cold porcelain, or heat the delivery tube, when a steel-white mirror of metallic arsenic is deposited. This may be distinguished from a similar deposit of antimony by the solubility of the arsenical mirror in potassium hypochlorite.

mastic t. A test similar in principle to Lange's colloidal gold test but using a colloidal suspension of gum mastic as the reagent with varying dilutions of cerebrospinal fluid.

Mazzini t. A microscopic flocculation test for syphilis.

mechanical fragility t. A test of the susceptibility of erythrocytes to hemolysis by mechanical trauma. Trauma is induced arbitrarily by rotating a small volume of blood in a flask with glass beads for an arbitrary period of time. Mechanical fragility is always increased when osmotic fragility is increased, and is increased in some clinical conditions (sickle-cell anemia) when the osmotic fragility is normal or decreased.

median nerve t. A test for loss of function of the median nerve. A pyramid is formed by placing the fingertips in contact, with the thumbs abducted and at right angles to the palms. If there is loss of function of the median nerve the patient is unable to abduct the thumb on the affected side as far downward as that on the normal side.

medicolegal tests for blood. (a) Microscopical identification of the erythrocytes, (b) spectroscopic identification of blood solutions, (c) the guaiac or benzidine reaction, (d) preparation of hemin crystals, and (e) precipitin and other immunologic tests.

Meinicke's t. A flocculation test for syphilis.

melanin t. See von Jaksch-Pollak's *t.*, Zeller's *t.*

Mendel's t. See Mantoux *t.*

mercury t. See Reinsch's *t.* (for mercury).

methylene blue reduction t. A simple method of assessing the general hygienic quality of raw mixed milk by measuring the reducing substances produced by the organisms present in the milk.

methylene blue t. (*for renal permeability*). An injected solution of methylene blue normally appears in the urine in about 30 minutes. A longer interval indicates impaired renal permeability. Also called *Achard-Castaigne method.* (*For vitamin C*) Vitamin C in the unknown is extracted with trichloroacetic acid or sulfosalicylic acid and then determined by its capacity to reduce methylene blue to the leuko-compound. (*For urinary bilirubin*) To 5 ml. of urine are added 5 drops of 0.2% aqueous methylene blue solution. Green color with transmitted light is positive indication of bilirubin; normal urine is blue: not an absolutely specific test, but valuable as a screening test.

methyl red t. A test for the differentiation of the aerogenes group and the colon group of bacteria performed by incubating the bacteria in a special medium and testing with methyl red indicator.

Michailow's t. (*for protein*). Add ferrous sulfate to the suspected solution and underlay with concentrated sulfuric acid; then add a drop or two of nitric acid. A brown ring and red coloration indicate the presence of protein.

Middlebrook-Dubois t. A test for antibodies in human serum against the products of the tubercle bacillus. Washed sheep erythrocytes are sensitized with aqueous extracts of *Mycobacterium tuberculosis.* The treated cells are thereby made agglutinable by the antibodies in the serum of tuberculous patients.

Minnesota multiphasic personality inventory. A psychologic test designed to provide, in a single interview, scores on all the more important traits of personality, consisting of over 500 questions which the subject places into three categories as they apply to him. Abbreviated, MPI.

Minnesota preschool scale. A test for measuring the learning ability of children from 18 months to 6 years of age. Being both verbal and nonverbal, it is particularly valuable in differentiating between the specific kinds of intellectual abilities.

Mitsuda's t. See lepromin *t.*

Molisch's t. (*for glucose*). (a) An alcoholic solution of naphthol and concentrated sulfuric acid is added to the unknown. The development of a deep violet color and, upon the addition of water, the formation of a violet precipitate indicate the presence of glucose. (b) If a solution of thymol is used instead of naphthol, the color produced is ruby red which changes to carmine on dilution with water.

Möller, McIntosh, and Van Slyke's t. See urea clearance *t.*

Moloney t. A test to determine hypersensitivity to diphtheria toxoid performed by the intradermal injection of a small amount of the toxoid. A positive reaction consists in the development of a characteristic patch about 2 cm. in diameter.

Montenegro's t. (*for leishmaniasis*). An intradermal test of aid in the diagnosis of leishmaniasis.

Moore's t. (*for reducing sugars*). Equal volumes of a sugar solution and concentrated sodium hydroxide are boiled. If a reducing sugar is present, the solution darkens and finally becomes brown.

Mörner's t. A test for tyrosine, which consists in the development of a green color on boiling with H_2SO_4 containing formaldehyde. See Mörner's *reagent.*

Moro t. A skin test performed by inunction of 50% O. T., Koch, in an ointment base. A local erythematous reaction appearing in from 24 to 48 hours indicates present or past infection with tubercle bacilli.

Mosenthal t. (*for kidney function*). A test in which the variability of specific gravity of the urine is measured through a 24-hour period of controlled dietary intake.

mucic acid t. (*for galactose*). To the unknown add concentrated nitric acid and heat. Let stand overnight. If galactose is present a crystalline precipitate of mucic acid is formed.

Mulder's t. (*for proteins*). See xanthoproteic *t.*

Müller's t. (*for cystine*). Boil the substance with potassium hydroxide; when cold, dilute with water and add a solution of sodium nitroprusside. A violet color changing rapidly to yellow is produced if cystine is present.

murexide t. Guanine or uric acid treated with HNO_3 gives a yellow compound which turns purple upon the addition of KOH or NH_4OH. Adenine does not respond to this test. See *murexide.*

Mylius modification of Pettenkofer's t. (*for bile acids*). To 5 ml. of diluted bile in a test tube add 3 drops of a very dilute aqueous solution of furfural. Carefully pour 2–3 ml. of concentrated sulfuric acid down the side of the tube and note the red ring at the point of contact.

Naegeli t. Described by Naegeli of Berne, by Jaeger and by Tucker and Thomas in the United States. Consists essentially of the application of patch tests to lightly scarified or abraded skin areas, instead of to normal skin. Often produces reactions when the patch test is negative.

Naffziger's t. Pressure on the jugular veins increases the intraspinal tension which increases the pain in cases of herniated nucleus pulposus.

Nagel's t. A test for color vision performed by using an instrument in which the patient attempts to match spectral yellow by a mixture of red and green.

Naiman's t. (*for vitamin* B_1). A test depending upon the production of an orange-red precipitate with vitamin B_1 when bismuth potassium iodide is added.

Napier's aldehyde t. (*for kala-azar*). A test based upon the increase of euglobulin which occurs in kala-azar. Solidification and opacity of serum to which formalin has been added is a positive test.

nasal t. An allergy test in which the allergen is applied to the nasal mucosa.

Neill-Mooser t. A test demonstrating the occurrence of forms, often within cells, closely resembling *Rickettsia prowazekii,* in the exudate on the surface of the testes in guinea pigs and rats, when the virus inoculated is from the typhus of Mexico, southeastern United States, or Europe.

Nelson's t. *Treponema pallidum* immobilization *t.*

Neufeld quellung t. Capsular swelling of pneumococci appearing as a sharply outlined halo, observed microscopically when pneumococci in dilute suspension are mixed with specific antiserum in the presence of Loeffler's alkaline methylene blue: generally employed for rapid pneumococcus typing directly from sputum.

Nickerson-Kveim t. (*for sarcoidosis*). 0.1 cc of Kveim antigen is injected intradermally, and skin biopsies are made from 3 to 6 weeks later. A positive finding of typical tubercles with giant cells indicates sarcoidosis. Emulsion of normal human spleen has been used for injection, and frequently gives the same reaction.

nitric acid t. (*for protein*). See Heller's *t.*

nitrobrucine t. (*for vitamin C*). Nitrobrucine (cacotheline) produces in hydrochloric acid solution a lilac color with vitamin C and other reducing agents. Not a specific test.

nitroprusside t. (*For acetone.*) See Legal's *t.* (*For diacetic acid.*) See Rothera's *t.*

Noguchi's t. (*for syphilis*). Luetin injected intradermally into a syphilitic patient results in the development in 6 to 24 hours of a papule surrounded by a bluish red area. Unreliable.

Nonne-Apelt's t. A test for excess albumin or globulin in spinal fluid in which saturated ammonium sulfate is used as the reagent.

nucleus t. (*for pancreatic function*). A test based on the fact that cell nuclei are digested by pancreatic juice and not gastric juice. See Schmidt nuclei *t.*

Nylander's t. A bismuth reduction test used for glucose in the urine.

Obermayer's t. (*for indican*). Urine is treated with ferric chloride and concentrated hydrochloric acid and then extracted with chloroform. A pale blue to deep blue or violet color indicates indican.

occult blood t. See benzidine *t.*, Gregersen's *t.*, phenolphthalein *t.*, Ruttan and Hardisty's *t.*

Ochsner-Mahorner t. Test for demonstration of incompetent valves in perforating veins lying between the deep and superficial venous systems of the leg.

oidiomycin t. An intradermal test with oidiomycin vaccine said to be of aid in the diagnosis of infections due to *Monilia albicans*, but often positive in other fungous infections.

ophthalmic t. Conjunctival *t.*

opsonocytophagic t. (*for brucellosis and tularemia*). A test in which the capacity of the leukocytes to phagocytize the causative organisms of tularemia and brucellosis is determined. If the phagocytosis is marked, the patient is supposedly immune to the disease.

orcinol t. See Bial's *t.*

orthotoluidine t. (*for blood*). See Ruttan and Hardisty's *t.*

osazone t. (*for sugars*). See phenylhydrazine *t.*

Oseretsky t. A psychologic test designed to measure the motor proficiency of an individual.

Osgood-Haskins t. (*for albumin*). Add one volume of 50% acetic acid and 3 volumes of saturated sodium chloride solution to 5 volumes of urine. A precipitate appearing after addition of the acid indicates bile salts, urates, or resin acids. A precipitate appearing after adding the salt solution suggests Bence-Jones protein. Heat, and Bence-Jones protein, if present, will dissolve; if albumin or globulin is present a precipitate will form.

osmotic fragility t. See erythrocyte fragility *t.*

Ott precipitation t. (*for nucleoprotein*). A solution of 25 ml. is mixed with an equal volume of a saturated solution of sodium chloride; Almen's reagent is slowly added. In the presence of nucleoprotein, a precipitate forms.

oxalic acid paper t. (*for indole in cultures*). Filter paper impregnated with oxalic acid is suspended over the medium in a culture tube. A pink color on the paper indicates the production of indole.

oxygen debt t. A determination of the amount of excess oxygen absorbed after cessation of exercise. A B.M.R. is taken both before and after exercise. The exercise is standardized, i.e., the patient climbs a stairway one meter high at the rate of 100 steps per minute. The percentage increase in oxygen is the oxygen debt. From 2% to 45% is normal.

oxyphenylsulfonic acid t. (*for protein*). Urine is added to an aqueous solution of oxyphenylsulfonic acid and salicylsulfonic acid. A white, transparent precipitate indicates the presence of protein.

pancreatic function t. One of several pancreatic function tests. The two most common are a study of the pancreatic and gastric juices aspirated from the duodenum and stomach by means of a double-lumened tube to keep them separate, and an analysis of the stool.

Pandy's t. (*for protein*). One cc. of the reagent (phenol and distilled water) is placed in a test tube and one drop of spinal fluid is added. If increased protein is present, a bluish white ring or cloud is formed.

Pangborn t. A flocculation test for syphilis.

para-aminohippuric acid t. (*for renal clearance*). Given in its sodium salt form, para-aminohippuric acid is well adapted to measurement of effective renal plasma flow, the clearance being identical with diodrast. It does not penetrate the red cells in man even after prolonged infusion and is nontoxic. Chemical determination is extremely simple.

parallax t. One used to locate opacities in the cornea, lens, and vitreous. It is used with the plane mirror at 10 to 12 inches. A body situated anterior to the plane of the pupil will move in the direction taken by the eye, while one posterior to the plane of the lens will move against the direction taken by the eye. Bodies lying about the same plane as the pupil will show little if any movement.

parentage t. See paternity *t.*

Parnum's t. (*for albumin*). To filtered urine add one-sixth of its volume of a concentrated solution of magnesium or sodium sulfate. On acidifying with acetic acid and boiling, albumin is precipitated.

passive transfer t. A method of demonstrating allergic antibodies in the blood of a patient, performed by sensitizing a local area of the skin of a nonallergic individual by the intracutaneous injection of the serum of an allergic individual. Also called *Prausnitz-Küstner reaction.*

patch t. An allergy test in which material is applied to an intact skin surface in order to demonstrate tissue sensitivity.

paternity t. The determination of the blood groups of an identified mother, an identified child, and a putative father in order to determine hereditary blood characters and to establish nonpaternity.

patting t. A cerebellar function test in which the patient pats with each hand his knee or the examiner's hand. Normally this is carried out with even amplitude and a smooth rhythm.

Paul's t. (*for smallpox*). The scarified cornea of a rabbit is inoculated with material from a suspected lesion. If the lesion is smallpox, a typical keratitis develops in about 50% of the cases.

Paul-Bunnell t. A test for the presence of heterophil antibodies in the serum produced in infectious mononucleosis.

Pels-Macht t. The phytopharmacological method of testing the toxicity of human serum for plant protoplasm: of historical interest.

pendulousness of the legs t. See Wartenberg's *sign.*

penicillin sensitivity t. A test to determine what bacteria are inhibited by penicillin. The usual method is to place a disk of penicillin in an agar plate. The growth of penicillin-sensitive bacteria will be inhibited in the area around the disk where the penicillin has diffused into the agar.

pentose t. See Bial's *t.*
percussion t. (*for varicose veins*). See Schwartz *t.*
personality t. See Bernreuter personality inventory, Brown personality inventory, Minnesota multiphasic personality inventory (all under *test*), Rorschach *t.*, thematic apperception *t.*
Perthes t. One testing the patency of the deep veins of the leg.
Pettenkofer's t. (*for bile acids*). Urine containing bile acids, mixed with sucrose and sulfuric acid, produces a red color.
phenolphthalein t. (*for occult blood*). Add a boiled suspension of feces to phenolphthalein reagent (phenolphthalein, potassium hydroxide, powdered zinc, and distilled water). Add hydrogen peroxide; a resulting pink to red color is a positive test.
phenolsulfonphthalein t. (*for kidney function*). A test based upon the ability of the kidneys to excrete phenolsulfonphthalein which has been injected intravenously or intramuscularly. Abbreviated, P.S.P.
phenol t. See Allen's *t.* (for phenol).
phenoltetrachlorophthalein t. (*for liver function*). After the intravenous injection of phenoltetrachlorophthalein, the feces have a bright color. Delay in the appearance of brightness of the color is said to indicate deficiency of liver function.
phenylhydrazine t. (*for sugars*). A test in which a sugar combines with phenylhydrazine to produce an osazone of definite crystalline form which is typical for that sugar. Commonly used to identify glucose in urine.
phlorhizin t. If no sugar appears in the urine within half an hour after the injection of phlorhizin, it is probable that renal insufficiency is present.
phloroglucinol-hydrochloric acid t. See Tollens' *t.*
phytopharmocologic t. A test of the toxicity of blood serum on plant seedlings.
Pirquet t. See von Pirquet *t.*
plasma L.E. t. A test for disseminated lupus erythematosus. From the cellular layer of a preparation containing 0.5 cc of the patient's plasma and 1 cc heparinized dog bone-marrow, smears are made and stained with Wright's stain; rosettes of clumped leukocytes and/or L.E. cells indicate a positive test. The patient's own peripheral blood may also be used by remixing the cells with the plasma. See *L.E. cell* under *lupus*.
platelet antibody t. An in-vitro test for antibodies which agglutinate or dissolve platelets: used to distinguish idiopathic thrombocytopenic purpura from other purpuric disorders.
pneumococcus antibody t. See Francis *t.*
pneumococcus type t. A precipitation test performed by layering centrifuged or filtered pneumococcus exudate over immune serum. A turbid ring will form at the junction of the fluids in the tube containing serum homologous with the pneumococcus type causing the infection. Also see Neufeld quellung *t.*
Pohl's t. (*for globulins*). The suspected solution is treated with ammonium sulfate which precipitates the globulins.
pointing t. See Bárány's pointing *t.*
potassium tolerance t. (*for Addison's disease*). A test based on the observation that a person with hypoadrenalism shows an increased rise and duration of the serum potassium as compared to normal after the oral ingestion of a potassium salt.
Prausnitz-Küstner t. Local passive sensitization of human skin by intracutaneous injection of human serum containing a particular antibody. The site so sensitized shows an immediate type of reaction (wheal and flare) when tested with the respective allergen.
precipitation t. A test in which a positive reaction depends upon the formation of a precipitate.
precipitin t. See precipitation *t.*, serum *t.*
pregnancy t. Any procedure, usually biologic or chemical, used to determine the presence of pregnancy state. Biologic tests usually depend upon the level of chorionic gonadotropin in the pregnant woman. See Abderhalden's *t.*, Aschheim-Zondek *t.*, *Bacillus proteus* pregnancy *t.*, bitterling *t.*, Friedman *t.*, frog *t.*, male toad *t.*, Porges-Pollatschek *reaction*, Q *t.*(a), prostigmine *t.*
presumptive t. (*for Escherichia coli in water*). Fermentation tubes containing lactose broth are inoculated with the water to be tested. If more than 10% of the fermentation tube contains gas at the end of 24 hours, the test is positive and a *confirmed test* should be performed.
Preyer's t. A spectroscopic test for the presence of carbon monoxide in the blood.
pronation-supination t. A cerebellar function test in which the arms, extended in front, are rapidly pronated and supinated. Normally the movements are of equal amplitude, smooth and even.
Proske and Watson's t. (*for malaria*). A tyrosine colorimetric test used to measure the increase of euglobulin which occurs in malaria.
prostigmine t. (*for pregnancy*). The failure of injected prostigmine to bring about menstrual bleeding in the presence of amenorrhea is indicative of pregnancy.
protein t. See Bence-Jones protein *t.*, biuret *t.*, heat and acid *t.*, Pandy's *t.*, Ross-Jones *t.*
prothrombin time t. See Quick's *t.*
provitamin D t. See antimony trichloride *t.*, chloral hydrate *t.*
Prussian blue t. (*for cyanide*). Sodium hydroxide, ferrous sulfate, ferric chloride, and hydrochloric acid are added to a distillate of the suspected material. If cyanide is present, a precipitate of Prussian blue develops. (*For vitamin C*) Vitamin C converts an acid ferricyanide solution to Prussian blue which may be compared colorimetrically. (*For ferric iron*) Ferric iron converts ferrocyanide to Prussian blue.
psychologic t. A planned situation in which an individual's behavior can be characterized by a numerical value or score. Also see aptitude *t.*, intelligence *t.*, personality *t.*
psychomotor t. An apparatus test, in contrast to a paper and pencil test, usually necessitating some form of muscular coordination and speed of reaction and often requiring certain perceptual abilities.
Pugh's t. A visual test for fusion which uses a stereoscope by means of which pictures seen separately by each eye are superimposed.
Purdy's t. (*for albumin*). To a test tube two-thirds full of urine, add one-sixth of its volume of a saturated solution of sodium chloride and 5 to 10 drops of 50% acetic acid. Mix, boil the upper portion, and watch for white cloud.
pus t. See Donné's *t.*, guaiac *t.*
push t. (*for parkinsonism*). The patient stands, feet apart, and the examiner gives him a gentle backward push. The normal person lifts his toes to maintain balance, but the person with parkinsonism keeps his feet entirely on the floor.
pyridoxine t. See cyanine dye *t.*, Gibbs's *t.*
Q t. (a) A pregnancy test in which a small amount of sterile colostrum is injected intracutaneously; inflammation after 1 hour indicates nonpregnancy. (b) Abbreviation also used for Quick's prothrombin test. See Quick's *t.*
Queckenstedt-Stookey t. Pressure on the jugular veins normally causes a prompt rise in cerebro-

spinal fluid pressure: not seen in partial or total subarachnoid block or lateral sinus thrombosis.
quellung t. See Neufeld quellung *t.*
Quick's hippuric acid synthesis t. See hippuric acid *t.*
Quick's t. (*for prothrombin*). Oxalated plasma is added to an excess of thromboplastin and then recalcified with a definite quantity of calcium chloride. The coagulation time is then an inverse measure of prothrombin concentration.
Race-Coombs t. See antiglobulin *t.*, Rh blocking *t.*
Ramon's flocculation t. See Gaston *Ramon.*
Raygat's t. See hydrostatic *t.*
Rayleigh t. A test for red-green colorblindness.
reactive hyperemia t. (*for arterial occlusion*). After temporary circulatory arrest there is an increase in the normal flow of blood which is complete within 3 seconds. A lengthened interval indicates arterial occlusion of the involved extremity.
recruitment t. *In otology,* the measurement of the span between the threshold of a deafened person's hearing and the level of discomfort. This span is much shorter in perception cases than in conduction cases, and explains the greater problem in fitting a perception case with a hearing aid.
red lens t. A test for diplopia and suppression utilizing a red lens and a light source of 75 cm. in all cardinal positions of gaze.
red t. See phenolsulfonphthalein *t.*
reduction t. A test indicating the presence of a substance (glucose) by its property of reducing the oxides of heavy metals in alkaline solution. Examples are Benedict's test and Fehling's test.
Reinsch's t. (*For arsenic.*) A piece of bright copper foil is placed into acidified urine which is then heated to the boiling point. If arsenic is present it is deposited on the copper. The copper is then dried, placed in a test tube, and heated, whereupon the arsenic volatilizes and is condensed upon the upper portion of the tube in the form of arsenic trioxide crystals which may be recognized. (*For mercury*) Similar to the test for arsenic except that the mixture is not heated to boiling and the end product is metallic mercury.
renal function t. See kidney function *t.*
rennin t. See Lee's *t.*, Riegel's *t.*
reversed Prausnitz-Küstner t. An urticarial reaction appearing at an injection site when reagin-containing serum is injected into the skin of a person in whom the allergen is already present; the reaction which appears when Prausnitz-Küstner antibody is administered, not before, but after, the administration of the antigen.
Rh blocking t. A test for the detection of Rh antibody in plasma wherein erythrocytes having the Rh antigen are incubated in the patient's serum so that the antibodies may be adsorbed on these cells, which are then employed in the antiglobulin test. Syn., *indirect developing t., indirect Coombs t.*
Rh testing. Examination of blood for the Rh factor, using either anti-Rhesus serum or anti-Rh_0 serum alone.
Riegel's t. (*for rennin*). Neutralized gastric juice is incubated with fresh milk. Coagulation will occur in 10–15 minutes if rennin is present in normal amount.
Rinne's t. A hearing test which compares the duration of bone conduction with that of air conduction. Normally air conduction is longer than bone conduction (Rinne positive; symbol, +R). Alteration in this relationship (Rinne negative; symbol, −R) indicates a lesion of the sound-conducting apparatus.
Roberts' t. (*for albumin*). Overlay urine upon Roberts' reagent (saturated solution of magnesium sulfate and concentrated nitric acid). A white ring at the zone of contact indicates albumin.
Robinson-Kepler-Power t. A test for adrenal cortical insufficiency or Addison's disease by measuring the urea clearance, chloride clearance, and water diuresis.
Rorschach t. A psychologic test in which the subject describes what he sees on a series of 10 standard ink blots. The subject's responses indicate personality patterns, special interests, general intelligence, deviations of affect, and neurotic or psychotic tendencies. Also called *Rorschach diagnosis.*
rose bengal t. (*for liver function*). A test based on the ability of the liver to remove injected rose bengal (tetraiodotetrachlorfluorescein) from the blood. Delayed removal indicates hepatic dysfunction.
Rosenbach's t. (*for bile pigment*). Filter urine and put a drop of concentrated nitric acid on the filter paper. If bile pigment is present a succession of colors will be seen as in Gmelin's test.
Rosenheim bismuth t. (*for choline*). Prepare an alcoholic extract of the fluid under examination and after evaporation apply Rosenheim's iodopotassium iodide solution to a little of the residue. In a short time dark brown plates and prisms of choline periodide begin to form and may be detected by means of the microscope.
Rosenthal-Rowntree t. (*for liver function*). A modification of the phenoltetrachlorophthalein test in which the amount of dye remaining in the blood is measured.
Ross-Jones t. (*for protein*). Spinal fluid is stratified over saturated ammonium sulfate reagent. A turbid ring at the junction of the fluids indicates increased protein.
rotation t. The study of the reaction of the semicircular canals by rotating the patient with the head fixed in certain planes.
Rothera's t. (*for diacetic acid*). To urine saturated with ammonium sulfate, add concentrated ammonium hydroxide and sodium nitroprusside. The appearance of a purple tinge is a positive test.
Roth-Kvale t. (*for pheochromocytoma*). A test employing the intravenous injection of histamine phosphate, which, in cases of pheochromocytoma, is followed by a very marked elevation in blood pressure and the acute paroxysm typical of the condition: infrequently used.
Rubin t. (*for tubal patency*). See tubal *insufflation.*
Rubner's t. (*for lactose*). To urine saturated with lead acetate add concentrated ammonium hydroxide and boil. If lactose is present, the solution turns brick-red with a precipitate.
Ruttan and Hardisty's t. (*for blood*). Blood in the presence of an acetic acid solution of orthotoluidine and hydrogen peroxide yields a blue color. Used for testing urinary sediment.
Sakaguchi t. A color reaction of arginine, using α-naphthol and NaOBr.
salicylic aldehyde t. (*for acetone*). See Behre's *t.*
Salkowski t. (*for cholesterol*). Dissolve a few crystals of cholesterol in a little chloroform and add an equal volume of concentrated sulfuric acid. A play of colors from bluish-red to cherry red and purple is noted in the chloroform, while the acid assumes a marked green fluorescence.
salt t. An intradermal test to determine the deficiency in the peripheral circulation of the extremities. Injections of 0.2 cc. of physiological saline are made and the wheals observed by inspection and palpation. Under normal conditions they disappear in one hour. The disappearance in 5 to 10

minutes suggests an area of gangrene, while a 10- to 20-minute interval indicates deficient circulation.

Sanford's t. See erythrocyte fragility *t.*

Savino t. (*for renal fixity*). A pyelographic examination made after complete expiration and then after complete inspiration, to determine renal fixation. Perirenal inflammatory diseases fix the kidney, and the roentgenogram is not blurred.

Sawyer and Lloyd serum protection t. A test used in epidemiologic investigations to determine whether individuals have ever had yellow fever or whether vaccinated persons have been successfully immunized.

scarification t. See scratch *t.*

scarlet fever t. See Dick *t.*, Schultz-Charlton blanching *t.*

Scherer's t. (*for inositol*). Ammonium hydroxide and calcium chloride are added to partially evaporated acidified urine and the whole is evaporated. In the presence of inositol a bright red color is obtained.

Schick t. (*for immunity to diphtheria*). An immunologic skin test performed by the intracutaneous injection of an amount of diluted diphtheria toxin equal to one-fiftieth of the minimal lethal dose. A positive reaction is interpreted on the fifth to seventh day. It consists of local erythema with edema, and indicates the lack of immunity.

Schiller's t. A test using aqueous iodine and potassium iodine solution to delineate areas of epithelium which do not contain glycogen and therefore do not take the stain. It aids in localizing areas of the uterine cervix where biopsy studies should be taken to exclude malignancy.

Schirmer t. Test for deficiency of tear formation: a strip of filter paper 5 mm × 30 mm is hooked over the lower lid; tears in normal individuals moisten at least 15 mm in 5 minutes.

Schlesinger's t. (*for urobilin*). Lugol's solution and a saturated alcoholic solution of zinc acetate are added to urine which is then filtered. A greenish fluorescence in the filtrate under strong light indicates urobilin.

Schmidt nuclei t. (*for pancreatic sufficiency*). A test in which beef or thymus, hardened in alcohol, is passed through the intestinal tract. If the nuclei are undigested on microscopic examination, pancreatic insufficiency may be assumed.

Schmidt's t. (*for urobilin*). A test based upon the formation of hydro-bilirubin-mercury with the production of a red color.

Schoenbein's t. (*for cyanide*). A strip of filter paper impregnated with guaiac and copper sulfate is suspended over a distillate of the suspected material. No change in color of the paper indicates the absence of cyanide; a blue color indicates that cyanide may be present and a specific test is then performed.

Schultz-Charlton blanching t. An immunologic skin test of aid in the diagnosis of scarlet fever performed by the intracutaneous injection of convalescent scarlet fever serum. A positive reaction which occurs in scarlet fever consists of blanching of the rash in a zone surrounding the point of injection.

Schultz-Dale t. The specific production of contraction of an excised intestinal loop (Schultz) or of the excised (virginal) uterine strip (Dale) of the anaphylactic guinea pig, when the excised tissue is exposed to the anaphylactogen. The intestinal or uterine preparation must also be shown to be susceptible to specific desensitization.

Schultz t. (*for cholesterol*). A histochemical adaptation of the Liebermann-Burchard *t.*

Schwabach's t. A hearing test which compares the duration of bone conduction appreciation of the pathologic ear to the normal.

Schwartz-McNeil t. (*for gonorrhea*). A complement-fixation test for gonorrhea using an antigen which is an autolysate of a number of strains of gonococci.

Schwartz t. (*for varicose veins*). With the patient standing, the examiner puts one hand along the inner surface of the groin, and percusses the vein in the calf with the other hand. A wave of fluid is palpated at the groin if the vein is varicose. Syn., *percussion t.*

scratch t. An allergic skin test performed by scratching the epidermis and then applying the allergen to the scratch. Syn., *dermal t.*

Seashore t. One designed to measure musical talent with respect to pitch, loudness, time, timbre, rhythm, and tonal memory.

sedimentation t. See agglutination *t.*, erythrocyte sedimentation *t.*

Seliwanoff's t. (*for fructose*). To a resorcinol-hydrochloric acid mixture add urine. The production of a red color and the separation of a red precipitate indicate fructose.

semen t. See Barberio's *t.*, Florence's *t.*

serologic t. One for testing blood serum.

serology t. (*for syphilis*). Any test on serum for the diagnosis of syphilis.

serum cholinesterase t. A test to determine the amount of cholinesterase in serum. Since hepatic cells elaborate cholinesterase, its level in the serum is indicative of liver function.

serum colloidal gold t. The addition of an electrolyte (NaCl) to a colloidal suspension of gold chloride will precipitate the gold chloride with characteristic color changes. The colloids in normal cerebrospinal fluid exert a protective action on the gold which prevents precipitation. In many pathological states, however, the fluid loses this protective power so that precipitation of the gold follows.

serum protection t. A test in which each animal of a group is given a known immune serum. This is followed by inoculation of these and an equal number of control animals with an organism, the identity of which it is desired to establish. If the animals receiving the immune serum survive, this identifies the organism. The test may also be used to determine the virulence of organisms and to demonstrate specific antibodies in serum. Also see animal protection *t.*

serum t. (*for blood, meat, etc.*). An antigen is injected at intervals into a rabbit. The serum of the rabbit is then added to a saline solution of the suspected material. The solution becomes cloudy if the suspected material is of the same species as the antigen used. Also called biologic *t.*, Bordet's *t.*, precipitin *t.*, Uhlenhuth's *t.*

seven-glass t. See glass *t.*

shadow t. See *retinoscopy.*

Sherman and Chase assay t. (*for thiamine hydrochloride*). Rats, depleted of their thiamine hydrochloride reserves by means of a vitamin B_1-free basal diet, are fed graded supplements of thiamine hydrochloride in the form of the standard or test materials. The relative growth responses to the doses of assay material and of pure thiamine hydrochloride constitute the basis for evaluation.

shoulder-shaking t. A test for extrapyramidal rigidity and cerebellar lesions. When the examiner swings the patient's arms from the shoulders, the swinging is lessened by extra-pyramidal rigidity, and increased by cerebellar affections.

Shumm t. (*for methemalbumin*). To 9 volumes of plasma covered with ether, 1 volume of concentrated ammonium sulfide is added and mixed;

presence of methemalbumin is indicated by the appearance of the sharp band of hemochromogen at 558μ on spectrometric examination.

Sia's t. (*for kala-azar*). A test in which the patient's blood is mixed with distilled water. The formation of a precipitate constitutes a positive reaction.

Simms-Huhner t. An examination of sperm obtained from the vaginal fornix and cervical canal during a certain interval following coitus: used in fertility studies.

skin t. Any test depending upon the production of an inflammatory or irritative reaction in the skin, usually performed for immunologic or allergic purposes.

Snellen t. One testing central vision in which the subject stands a certain distance from a standard chart and reads the letters on the chart. It is based upon the fact that objects may be seen by the normal eye when they subtend an angle of one minute.

sodium benzoate t. See hippuric acid *t.*

sodium d-lactate clearance t. (*for liver function*). A test based on the ability of the liver to convert injected sodium *d*-lactate into glycogen. Delayed conversion indicates hepatic dysfunction.

sodium tetraiodophenolphthalein t. (*for liver and gallbladder function*). Normal persons have less than 15% of 2.5 Gm. of injected sodium tetraiodophenolphthalein in the blood at the end of 30 minutes and less than 5% at the end of 60 minutes. Retention of more than this may indicate liver damage. Also, the concentration of the dye in the gallbladder with its subsequent evacuation may be determined by x-ray examination. Also called *Graham-Cole t.*

Somogyi's t. (*for amylase*). See Somogyi's *method.*

space perception t. Psychological test used to measure the ability to estimate space differences.

Sparkman's t. (*for urobilinogen in feces and urine*). A modification of Ehrlich's test based on the development of a red color on the addition of an acid solution of paradimethylaminobenzaldehyde to solutions containing urobilinogen.

spectroscopic t. A procedure for the detection of compounds by observing the characteristic absorption spectrums that they produce.

Spiegler's t. (*for albumin*). Overlay clear acidulated urine upon Spiegler's reagent (mercuric chloride, tartaric acid, glycerin, distilled water). Opalescence at the junction of the fluids indicates albumin.

Spies t. (*for pellagra*). A chemical test performed on the urine that is positive in pellagra and certain other intestinal-tract dysfunctions.

spot t. Any test using small quantities of a reagent and substance tested, as on a plate or sheet of paper, for the determination of the presence of a substance.

Stanford achievement t. A group test covering achievement at a variety of school grades: named for Stanford University.

Stanford-Binet t. A modification of the original Binet intelligence test; considered the standard individual test for pre-adult levels.

Stanford revisions of Binet-Simon t. Revisions of the Binet-Simon test (1916, 1937). The last revision provides for more adequate sampling of intelligence at upper and lower levels by employing two new scales, by procedures for the administration and scoring of the test which have been defined more meticulously, and by standardization based upon larger and more representative samples of the population.

Stanford scientific aptitude t. A test to detect the traits which comprise an aptitude for a science.

starch t. See iodine *t.* (for starch).

star t. A test for determining whether under- or overcorrection exists in the microscope system, and for determining the proper tube length for a microscope.

Stein t. (*for bile pigments*). A histochemical method, staining with iodine reagent, decolorizing with sodium hyposulfite, and counterstaining with alum carmine. Bile pigments appear emerald green.

Stilling's t. A color vision test now used as Ishihara's modification.

straight-leg-raising t. See Lasègue's *sign.*

Straus t. The development of an acute orchitis in male guinea pigs after the intraperitoneal inoculation of diseased tissues from a case of glanders.

Strauss's t. (*for lactic acid*). To an ether extract of gastric juice, add a solution of ferric chloride. A light green or yellow color indicates lactic acid.

suction t. A test for capillary resistance in which suction is applied to the skin for a measured interval of time, and the number of petechiae which result are counted. Syn., *Dalldorf method.*

sugar t. See Barfoed's *t.*, Benedict's *t.*, Bial's *t.*, Fehling's *t.*, fermentation *t.*, Folin-McEllroy *t.*, Haines's *t.*, Moore's *t.*, mucic acid *t.*, Nylander's *t.*, phenylhydrazine *t.*, Seliwanoff's *t.*, Tollens' *t.*

sulfosalicylic acid t. (*for albumin*). 1 cc. of urine is put into a test tube with 1 cc. of sulfosalicylic acid reagent. Cloudiness developing after 10 minutes indicates albumin.

Sulkowitch's t. (*for calcium*). Equal parts of clear urine and Sulkowitch's reagent (oxalic acid, ammonium oxalate, glacial acetic acid, distilled water) are mixed. A fine white precipitate indicates normal serum calcium; no precipitate indicates reduced calcium; and a milky precipitate indicates increased serum calcium.

Sullivan's t. (*for cystine*). With sodium-β-naphthoquinone-4-sulfonate, cystine develops a red color in the presence of alkali.

surface fixation t. A test for brucellosis, utilizing the diffusion of the patient's serum in blotting paper.

sweating t. An objective, easily elicited test of sympathetic innervation. The skin of the entire body, or the area to be tested, is covered with a mixture of iodine and starch which, on becoming moist, turns blue-black (see iodine *test* for starch). Other nontoxic powders, or cobalt blue paper changing color when moist, are used less frequently. Sweating may be produced by heat, emotional disturbances, by highly spiced foods, drugs, and by other methods. In areas where there is impairment of innervation or absence of sweat glands, no color change is marked.

syphilis t. See Boerner, Jones, and Lukens *t.*, Boerner-Lukens *t.*, colloidal benzoin *t.*, Eagle *t.*, Hinton *t.*, Kahn *t.*, Kline *t.*, Kolmer's *t.* (a), Lange's *t.*, Laughlen *t.*, mastic *t.*, Mazzini *t.*, Meinicke's *t.*, Noguchi's *t.*, Pangborn *t.*, Wassermann's *t.*

Szent-Györgyi t. (*for vitamin C*). A test based on the violet coloration upon the addition of ferrous sulfate to an alkaline solution of ascorbic acid (vitamin C).

Takata-Ara t. (*for liver function*). A test based on the assumption that in hepatic dysfunction there is a diminution of the colloid protective action in the blood serum due to an increase in the globulin content.

tannic acid t. (*for carbon monoxide in blood*). Blood is mixed with distilled water and a tannic acid solution is added. The development of a cherry red color indicates the presence of carbon monoxide.

Tanret-Mayer t. One for determining the presence of quinine in the urine.

Tauber t. (*for pentose*). To 0.1 ml. of urine add 0.5 ml. of a 4% solution of benzidine in glacial acetic acid. Heat to vigorous boiling, cool under the cold water tap, and add 1 ml. of water. The presence of pentose is indicated by the immediate appearance of a pink to red color. If pentoses are absent, the mixture has a yellowish brown color.

Tauber and Kleiner modification of Barfoed's t. A monosaccharide, heated with copper reagent in a boiling water bath, will yield a blue color when Benedict's or Folin's phosphomolybdic reagent is added.

Teal t. A hearing test to determine actual or simulated air conduction loss when normal bone conduction is admitted. It is done with two similar tuning forks, one inactive on the mastoid and the other active close to the tested ear. The patient admitting hearing tone actually hears by air and this is evidence of simulated deafness.

Teichmann's t. (*for blood*). A crystal of sodium chloride and glacial acetic acid are added to the suspected liquid under a cover glass and the whole is heated without boiling and then cooled. The appearance of rhombic crystals of hemin indicates blood.

tendon palpation t. Decreased resistance to palpation of a tendon as an index of cerebellar or peripheral nervous system disease.

t. for atabrine. One which determines the presence of atabrine in the urine; devised by Tropp and Weise.

t. meal. See *test meal.*

tetraiodophenolphthalein t. See sodium tetraiodophenolphthalein *t.*

thematic apperception t. (TAT). A test using a set of pictures from which the subject constructs a story, designed to reveal to the trained interpreter some of the dominant drives, emotions, sentiments, complexes, and conflicts of personality; one of the projective-type tests.

therapeutic t. A test in which the response to specific therapy is used to aid in the establishment of a diagnosis, such as liver extract in pernicious anemia and Lugol's solution in hyperthyroidism.

Thorn t. (*for adrenal cortex activity*). A test of adrenocortical reserve, as manifested by changes in circulating eosinophils, following administration of adrenocorticotropic hormone (ACTH).

three glass t. See glass *t.*

thymol flocculation t. A modification of the thymol turbidity test in which the mixture is allowed to stand overnight and the amount of flocculation is measured. Normal limits are 0-+.

thymol turbidity t. A test for liver function, particularly useful in determining biliary obstruction; 0.1 cc serum are added to 6.0 cc thymol reagent. The result is read in units on a colorimeter, 0 to 2 units being normal.

tinea versicolor t. See under Allen's *t.*

toad t. See frog *t.*, male toad *t.*

Tobey-Ayer t. See George Loring *Tobey*, Jr.

tolerance t. See clearance *t.*

Tollens' t. (*for galactose*). To equal volumes of the unknown and hydrochloric acid, add phloroglucinol, and heat the mixture. Galactose, pentose, or glycuronic acid will be indicated by the appearance of a red color. Differentiate by means of spectroscopic examination.

toluidine t. (*for blood*). See Ruttan and Hardisty's *t.*

Töpfer's t. (*for free hydrochloric acid in gastric contents*). A few drops of a 1% alcoholic solution of *p*-dimethylaminoazobenzene give a cherry-red color to a fluid containing free hydrochloric acid.

tourniquet t. (*for capillary resistance*). A blood pressure cuff about the upper arm is used to occlude the veins effectively for a measured number of minutes, after which the skin of the forearm and hand is examined for petechiae. In various techniques the pressure applied, the duration of its application, and the number of petechiae which result in the normal individual vary.

toxoplasmin t. A cutaneous test for toxoplasmosis by the intradermal injection of toxoplasmin. Observation of a hypersensitivity reaction with a negative reaction in a control injection indicates past or persistent infection.

TPI t. See *Treponema pallidum* immobilization *t.*

Trendelenburg's t. (a) One designed to demonstrate the incompetence of the saphenous vein valves and the efficiency of the communicating veins at different levels. (b) A dipping of the pelvis to the opposite side when the patient stands on the affected limb; seen in congenital dislocation of the hip and certain other conditions.

Treponema pallidum immobilization t. (*for syphilis*). An immunologically specific in vitro reaction employing *Treponema pallidum* in a special maintenance medium, antibody and complement resulting in immobilization and death of the spirochetes. The reaction may be employed for the specific serological diagnosis of syphilis. The antibody involved apparently is distinct from that detected in the Wasserman type of reaction.

Trommer's t. A test for reducing sugars involving $CuSO_4$ in a solution of KOH. Fehling's test is similar but can detect smaller concentrations of sugar.

tryptophan t. (*for tuberculous meningitis*). Sodium nitrate solution is overlaid a mixture of spinal fluid, hydrochloric acid, and formalin. A violet ring at the junction of the fluids is a positive reaction.

t test. A test of significance of differences between statistical constants calculated from small samples.

tuberculin t. The introduction of measured quantities of tuberculin into superficial tissues of the body to establish the presence or absence of infection by the tubercle bacillus. A positive tuberculin reaction which may consist of erythema, edema, or necrosis indicates infection. Also see Calmette *t.*, Mantoux *t.*, Moro *t.*, Vollmer patch *t.*, von Pirquet *t.*

tuning fork t. See bone conduction *t.*, Rinne's *t.*, Schwabach's *t.*, Teal *t.*, Weber's *t.*

two glass t. See glass *t.*

two-step t. Repeated ascents over two nine-inch steps as a simple exercise test of cardiovascular function: also called *Master's two-step t.*

Tzanck t. The demonstration of degenerative changes in epidermal cells in bullae of pemphigus by microscopic examination of a smear made from the base of an early intact bulla and stained with Giemsa stain.

Uffelmann's t. (*for lactic acid*). To gastric juice, add a reagent consisting of ferric chloride solution and phenol. Lactic acid produces a canary yellow color whereas hydrochloric acid decolorizes the reagent.

Uhlenhuth's t. See serum *t.*

urea clearance t. (*for kidney function*). The excretory efficiency of the kidneys is tested by the amount of blood cleared of urea in 1 minute as determined by the ratio of the blood urea to the amount of urea excreted in urine during a fixed time.

urobilinogen t. See Ehrlich's *t.*, Sparkman's *t.*

urobilin t. See Schlesinger's *t.*, Schmidt's *t.*

vaccine t. A skin test made with a suspension of killed bacteria in measured concentration.

van den Bergh's t. (*The direct test.*) Diluted serum is added to diazo reagent. A bluish violet color becoming maximal in 10 to 30 seconds is an *immediate direct reaction* supposedly indicating uncombined bilirubin and therefore the presence of obstructive jaundice. A red color beginning after 1 to 15 minutes and gradually turning to violet is a *delayed direct reaction*, indicating impaired liver function. A red color appearing at once and changing to violet is a biphasic direct reaction. (*The indirect test.*) Alcohol is added to serum which is then centrifuged. The diazo reagent is added to the supernatant fluid. An immediate violet-red color supposedly indicates bilirubin combined with protein and signifies a hemolytic jaundice. The tests are now used as a modification in which diazotized serum or plasma is compared with a standard solution of diazotized bilirubin.

Verhoeff depth perception t. A small portable test of stereopsis in which the separation of the test objects is constant. Given at different distances, the difficulty varies as the square of the testing distance. False monocular size clues are introduced.

vestibular t. A series of tests and observations on the vestibular system, including observations on postural nystagmus, vertigo, and a tendency to fall, plus such other tests as the caloric and rotation tests. Although not absolutely diagnostic of brain tumors, this test is often used to aid or supplement such a diagnosis.

Vineland social maturity scale. A psychologic test designed to measure social maturity.

vision t. See Abridged A. O. color vision *t.*, afterimage *t.*, candle *t.*, color threshold *t.*, confusion *t.*, Hecht-Schlaer night vision *t.*, Holmgren *t.*, Ishihara's *t.*, Nagel's *t.*, Pugh's *t.*, red lens *t.*, Snellen *t.*, Stilling's *t.*, Verhoeff depth perception *t.*

Visscher-Bowman t. (*for pregnancy*). See Frank Evert *Visscher*.

vital capacity t. A test of pulmonary function. See vital *capacity*.

vitamin-A t. See Anderson-Nightingale dilution *t.*, ferric chloride *t.* for vitamin A.

vitamin-B_1 t. See catatorulin *t.*

vitamin-B_6 t. See cyanine dye *t.*, Gibbs's *t.*

vitamin-C t. See intradermal vitamin-C *t.*, methylene blue *t.* (for vitamin C), nitrobrucine *t.*, Prussian blue *t.* (for vitamin C).

vitamin-D t. See aniline *t.*

vitamin-K t. A liver-function test in which 2 mg. of menadione are administered intramuscularly. If the prothrombin level rises more than 20% in 24 hours, liver function is normal.

Volhard's and Fahr's tests. (a) Test of the kidney's ability to concentrate urine. After withholding all fluids for 33 hours and giving a dry food for 24 hours, urine samples are collected at three-hour intervals for 12 hours and one 12-hour sample is collected. Normally, at least one sample will have a specific gravity of at least 1.025. With progressive renal impairment, concentrating power is reduced until the specific gravity usually becomes fixed at about 1.010. (b) Test of the kidney's ability to secrete dilute urine. In a fasting state, the patient drinks 1500 cc. of water, and urine specimens are collected at 30-minute intervals. Normally, at least one specimen will have a specific gravity as low as 1.003. In severe kidney disease, the specific gravity becomes fixed at about 1.010.

Vollmer patch t. A tuberculin test in which gauze saturated with tuberculin is applied to an intact skin surface under adhesive plaster.

von Aldor's t. (*for proteoses*). Phosphotungstic acid is added to urine and the precipitate is washed with absolute alcohol, dissolved in potassium hydroxide, and the biuret test is applied.

von Jaksch-Pollak's t. (*for melanin*). Ferric chloride is added to urine. If melanin is present, there develops a gray color and a dark precipitate of phosphates and adhering melanin.

von Pirquet t. A tuberculin test in which the substance is applied to a superficial abrasion of the skin.

von Udránszky t. See foam *t.*

Vulpian t. Epinephrine gives a green color with $FeCl_3$ in slightly acid solution.

Wang's t. (*for indican*). Indican, if present, is converted into indigosulfuric acid and titrated with potassium permanganate solution.

Wassermann's t. A complement-fixation test for syphilis now used only as a modification of the original test.

water-drinking t. A test for glaucoma in which the patient drinks water. Increase in ocular pressure of more than 6 mm. Hg when the initial tension is 30 mm., or of more than 9 mm. Hg when initial tension is less than 30 mm., is indicative of a positive reaction. Osmotic changes in blood serum are responsible for the amount of ocular tension.

water-gurgle t. The swallowing of water causes a gurgling sound heard on auscultation in cases of stricture of the esophagus.

water-pitressin t. A combination of water intoxication induced by forced liquid intake, with administration of pitressin to detect the existence of epilepsy in a patient. A seizure will be produced in about 50% of all persons predisposed to convulsions. The test is valuable in differentiating hysteria from idiopathic epilepsy.

water t. (*for Addison's disease*). A test based on the fact that patients with Addison's disease do not have a normal diuresis following the rapid intake of a large quantity of water.

Waugh-Ruddick t. A procedure reputed to test a tendency toward thromboembolic disease in which the clotting time of a mixture of whole blood and serial dilutions of heparin is measured.

Weber's t. A hearing test in which the vibrations from a tuning fork placed on the forehead of a normal person are referred to the midline and heard equally in both ears. In unilateral middle-ear deafness, the sound is heard in the diseased ear. In deafness due to disease of the auditory nerve on one side, it is heard better in the normal ear.

Wechsler-Bellevue intelligence scale. A verbal and performance test of information, comprehension, arithmetical reasoning, digit memory, similarities, configurational grasp, visual completion, object assembly, and vocabulary.

Weil-Felix t. An agglutination test used in the diagnosis of certain rickettsial diseases, based upon the fact that the serum of a patient with a rickettsial disease will agglutinate certain strains of *Proteus vulgaris*.

Weisz t. (*for urochromogen*). A 1% solution of potassium permanganate is added to diluted urine. In the presence of urochromogen a yellow tint will appear due to the oxidation of the urochromogen.

Wells-Stenger t. A test for determining actual or simulated unilateral deafness. A tuning fork stem is inserted into a 30-in. length of rubber tubing having an earpiece at the other end. The fork is set in vibration. The earpiece is inserted into the deaf ear and the fork is approximated to the good, or normal, ear. If it is not heard until much closer than was the case in previous tests indicating normal hearing distance, the deafness is simulated.

Weltmann's t. A serum coagulation test used to indicate whether a lesion is of an exudative inflammatory nature or a fibrotic nature: of diagnostic aid in subacute bacterial endocarditis and acute rheumatic endocarditis.

Weyl's t. (*for creatinine*). Ruby-red color, then yellow, when solution containing creatinine is treated with sodium nitroprusside and sodium hydroxide.

Widal t. (*for typhoid fever*). An agglutination test for typhoid fever, using a living agglutinable culture of the typhoid bacillus as an antigen. The test is now performed by using H (formalized) and O (alcoholic) antigens.

Wilder t. See Cutler-Power-Wilder *t.*

Windaus digitonin t. A histochemical method for 3-cis-OH sterols, such as cholesterol, vitamin-D compounds, and isoandrosterone, using digitonin solution to produce needle-shaped birefringent crystals observed under the polarizing microscope.

Wolff-Eisner t. See Calmette *t.*

worsted t. See Holmgren *t.*

Wurster's t. (*For hydrogen dioxide.*) Paper saturated with a solution of tetramethylparaphenylenediamine turns bluish violet if hydrogen dioxide is present. (*For tyrosine.*) Dissolve the suspected substance in boiling water and add quinone. A ruby red color changing slowly to brown indicates tyrosine.

xanthoproteic t. (*for proteins*). Nitric acid which turns proteins yellow is added to the suspected substance. Upon alkalinizing the color turns to an orange yellow.

Xenopus pregnancy t. See frog *t.*

Yensen allness t. A psychologic test to determine to what extent an individual tends to react in an all-or-none fashion.

Yvon's t. (*for acetanilid*). Urine is extracted with chloroform and the residue heated with mercurous nitrate. A green color indicates acetanilid.

Zeller's t. (*for melanin*). Equal volumes of urine and bromine water are mixed. In the presence of melanin a yellow precipitate will form and gradually become black.

zinc sulfate turbidity t. A flocculation test for liver function, resembling the thymol turbidity test but using zinc sulfate as the precipitating agent and a buffer of lower ionic strength. It reliably differentiates obstructive and hepatocellular jaundice in the early stages. Normal limits are 0-4 units.

Zondek-Aschheim t. See Aschheim-Zondek *t.*

Zwemer's t. See potassium tolerance *t.*

tes·ta′ceous [L. *testaceus*, consisting of bricks or tiles]. Pertaining to a shell.

tes′ti·cle [L. *testiculus*, testis]. See *testis.*

tes·tic′u·lar [*testiculus*]. Pertaining to the testis.

tes′tis (pl. *testes*) [L.]. One of the pair of male reproductive glands, after sexual maturity the source of the spermatozoa; a male gonad. See Plates 44, 45.

abdominal t. One which is undescended and remains in the abdominal cavity.

displaced t. A testis in an abnormal situation, as in the pelvic cavity.

femoral t. One which has nearly descended into the scrotum, but remains in the inguinal canal near or over the femoral ring.

inguinal t. An undescended testis remaining in the inguinal canal.

inverted t. A testis which is so placed in the scrotum that the epididymis is attached to the anterior part of the gland.

migrating t. A freely movable inguinal testis which may be moved even into the abdominal cavity and predisposes to torsion of the spermatic cord.

perineal t. One that is situated outside the scrotum in the perineal region.

puboscrotal t. One that is situated over the pubic tubercle.

undescended t. The condition in which a testis remains either in the pelvis or in the inguinal canal.

tes·ti′tis. See *orchitis.*

test meal. A specified quantity and type of food which, at a certain interval after ingestion, is removed from the stomach by means of a tube; the contents are studied chemically to ascertain the function of the stomach.

motor t. m. A test for pyloric obstruction. When the stomach is empty, the patient eats a meal consisting of 100 Gm. each of boiled potato, spinach, carrots, raw apple, an egg, a slice of bread, a pat of butter, 15 Gm. of dried tea leaves, and a beverage. Upon aspiration several hours later, the stomach should normally yield only 60 cc. of liquid and some tea leaves.

Rehfuss t. m. See Martin Emil *Rehfuss.*

tes′toid. Pertaining to any substance, natural or synthetic, which is androgenic, i.e., capable of producing secondary male-sex characters.

tes·tos′te·rone. $C_{19}H_{28}O_2$. Δ^4-Androstene-17(α)-ol-3-one. An androgenic hormone isolated first from the testis of the bull; also obtained by synthesis; a white crystalline powder, insoluble in water: used therapeutically principally in the treatment of deficiency or absence of the testicular hormone, also in palliation of metastatic carcinoma of the female breast. Administration is by intramuscular injection, subcutaneous implantation, or by buccal absorption. See Table of Hormones in the Appendix.

tes·tos′te·rone pro′pi·o·nate (*testosteroni propionas*). The propionic acid ester of testosterone; white or slightly yellow crystals, insoluble in water but soluble in organic solvents and in vegetable oils; the form of testosterone commonly used in preparing solutions in oil for injection.

test type. See under *type.*

te′ta·ine. An antibiotic substance produced by a strain of *Bacillus pumilus.*

tet′a·nal, te·tan′ic [G. *tetanos*, convulsive tension, tetanus]. 1. Pertaining to, or resembling, tetanus. 2. Producing tetanus.

te·ta′ni·a. See *tetany.*

te·tan′i·form [*tetanos;* L. *forma*, form]. Resembling tetanus.

tet″a·nig′e·nous (tet″uh·nidj′i·nus) [*tetanos;* G. *genesthai*, from *gignesthai*, to be produced]. Causing tetanus or tetanic spasms.

tet″a·nil′la [dim. from *tetanos*]. A mild form of tetanus.

tet′a·nin. $C_{14}H_{30}N_2O_4$. A ptomaine obtained from cultures of the bacillus of tetanus in beef broth and from the tissues of patients suffering from tetanus.

tet′a·nism [*tetanos*]. A more or less continuous hypertonicity of muscle.

tet″a·ni·za′tion [*tetanos*]. Production of tetanus or of tetanic spasms. —**tet′anize,** *v.*

tet′a·no- [*tetanos*]. A combining form denoting *relating to tetanus.*

tet″a·no·can′na·bin [*tetanos;* G. *kannabis*, hemp]. A substance found in some samples of cannabis, or hemp, producing strychninelike symptoms.

tet′a·node [G. *tetanōdēs*, of the nature of tetanus].

The quiescent interval in tetanus, between the tonic spasms.

tet′a·noid [G. *tetanos*, convulsive tension, tetanus; *eidos*, form]. A spastic condition producing symptoms like tetanus.

tet″a·no·ly′sin (tet″uh·no·lye′sin, tet″uh·nol′i·sin) [*tetanos;* G. *lysis*, a loosing]. The lytic toxin of *Clostridium tetani.*

tet″a·no·ly′sis. Lysis of erythrocytes in vitro by one of two exotoxins produced by tetanus bacilli.

tet″a·nom′e·ter [*tetanos;* G. *metron*, a measure]. An instrument for measuring tetanic spasms.

tet″a·no·mo′tor [*tetanos;* L. *motor*, from *movere*, to move]. An instrument for stimulating a nerve mechanically and producing tetanus of the supplied muscle.

tet″a·no·pho′bi·a [*tetanos;* G. *phobos*, fear]. A morbid fear of tetanus.

tet″a·no·spas′min (tet″uh·no·spaz′min) [*tetanos;* G. *spasmos*, spasm]. A toxin produced by the tetanus bacillus which causes tetanic convulsions.

tet′a·nus [*tetanos*]. 1. An infectious disease, usually fatal, characterized by tonic spasm of the voluntary muscles, an intense exaggeration of reflex activity, and convulsions. It is due to the toxin produced by the tetanus bacillus, *Clostridium tetani*, which enters through a wound. Since the tetanus bacillus can grow only in the absence of oxygen, the character of the wound is important, the most dangerous being puncture, penetrating, and crushing injuries. Commonly called lockjaw. 2. A tense, contracted state of a muscle, especially when caused experimentally.

acoustic t. Tetanus produced in a muscle-nerve preparation by rapidly repeated induction shocks, the period of which is determined by a tuning fork.

artificial t. That produced by a drug.

ascending t. A type in which the muscular spasms are first noted at the site of injury, then spread to the rest of the body.

cephalic t. A special form of tetanus occasionally observed following head injuries, especially those in the neighborhood of the eyebrow; trismus and facial paralysis occur at the site of the injury; there are dysphagia and epileptiform seizures, an early appearance of the disease, and usually a rapid fatal termination. Also called *cerebral t.*, *kopf t.*

chronic t. That occurring when a latent infection in a healed wound is reactivated by reopening the wound. Also called *delayed t.*

descending t. A type in which the muscle spasms are first noted about the jaw and throat, later spreading to the rest of the body.

hydrophobic t. Tetanus characterized by violent spasm of the muscles of the throat.

idiopathic t. Tetanus in which there is no history of injury.

imitative t. Hysteria which simulates tetanus.

localized t. Tetanic spasm of a part.

puerperal t. That following labor.

remittent t. See *tetany.*

Ritter's t. The series of contractions, or apparent tetanus, observed on the opening or interrupting of an electric current which has been passing through the nerve for some time; opening tetanus.

surgical t. That following operation, from contamination by infected catgut or feces.

t. antitoxin. Antitoxin produced in man or animals by the injection of tetanus toxin or tetanus toxoid. For therapeutic use a refined concentrated antitoxin obtained from the serum of immunized horses is given at the time of injury to prevent the development of tetanus. Dose, 1500 units, or in larger and repeated doses for treatment of the disease.

t. neonatorum. That due to infection of the umbilical stump: also called *t. infantum.*

t. toxoid. Inactivated tetanus toxin used to produce active immunity against the disease. Dose, 1 cc. repeated after four to six weeks and as a booster shot at the time of a subsequent injury.

toxic t. Tetanus produced by an overdose of nux vomica or its alkaloids.

traumatic t. Tetanus following an injury.

Wundt's t. A prolonged tetanic contraction induced in a frog's muscle by injury or the passage of a strong current.

tet′a·ny [*tetanos*]. A disease characterized by intermittent, bilateral, painful, tonic spasms of the muscles, in children and young adults. It is due to an abnormal calcium metabolism. Occurs in deficiency of parathyroid secretion, alkalosis, vitamin-D deficiency, and after extirpation of the parathyroid glands.

duration t. A continuous tetanic spasm occurring in degenerated muscles when a strong continuous current is applied. Abbreviated, D.t.

epidemic t. A form seen in large portions of Europe, especially in the winter season. It is acute, lasting only two or three weeks, and rarely proves fatal.

grass t. Tetany in lactating cows first turned out to pasture. Probably due to magnesium deficiency. Also called *lactation t.*

gutturotetany. A stammering due to tetanoid spasm of the laryngeal muscles.

hyperventilation t. Tetany due to alkalosis from washing out of carbon dioxide from the blood following hyperventilation. See respiratory *alkalosis.*

parathyreoprival, parathyroprival t. See parathyroid *t.*

parathyroid t. Tetany following removal of the parathyroid glands.

rheumatic t. See epidemic *t.*

thyreoprival, thyroprival t. A form following removal of the thyroid gland when the parathyroids have also been removed.

tet′ar·cone. Tetartocone.

te·tar″ta·no′pi·a, te·tar″ta·nop′si·a [G. *tetartos*, fourth; *opsis*, vision]. Loss of vision in a homonymous quadrant in each field of vision.

te·tar′to·cone [*tetartos;* G. *kōnos*, cone]. Distolingual cone; the fourth or distolingual cusp of an upper molar tooth.

te·tar″to·co′nid (te·tahr″to·ko′nid, ·kon′id) [*tetartos; kōnos*]. Distolingual or fourth cusp of a lower molar tooth.

tet·i″o·thal′ein so′di·um. Iodophthalein sodium.

tet′mil. Ten millimeters.

tet′ra-, tetr- [G. *tetra-*, four]. A combining form meaning *four.*

tet″ra·ba′sic [*tetra-;* G. *basis*, base]. Having four atoms of replaceable hydrogen.

tet″ra·bo′ric ac′id. $H_2B_4O_7$. An acid obtained from boric acid by heating. Syn., *pyroboric acid.*

tet″ra·bra′chi·us (tet″ruh·bray′kee·us) [*tetra-;* G. *brachiōn*, arm]. Having four arms.

tet″ra·bro″mo·phthal′ein so′di·um (tet″ruh·bro″mo·thal′in, ·thal′ee·in, ·fthal′in, ·ee·in). Sulfobromophthalein sodium.

tet′ra·caine hy″dro·chlo′ride. $C_4H_9.NH.C_6H_4.CO.O.CH_2.CH_2.N(CH_3)_2.HCl$. The hydrochloride of the *p-n*-butylaminobenzoic ester of β-dimethylaminoethanol; very soluble in water. A powerful local anesthetic similar in its action to, but more potent than, procaine hydrochloride, employed in the eye, nose and throat, and also intraspinally. Recognized by the B.P. as *amethocaine hydrochloride.* See also *pantocaine, pontocaine hydrochloride.*

tet″ra·chei′rus (tet″ruh·kigh′rus) [G. *tetracheir*, four-handed]. Having four hands.

tet″ra·chlo″ro·eth′ane. $CHCl_2.CHCl_2$. A highly toxic solvent for fats, oils, waxes, resins, etc.

***sym*.-tet″ra·chlo″ro·eth′ane.** Acetylene tetrachloride.

tet″ra·chlo″ro·eth′yl·ene (*tetrachloroaethylenum*). $Cl_2C{:}CCl_2$. Clear, colorless liquid of characteristic ethereal odor used as an anthelmintic, especially for the hookworm. Dose, 1–3 cc. (15–45 min.) in capsule, followed by saline cathartic. Also called *ethylene tetrachloride, perchloroethylene.*

tet″ra·chlo″ro·meth′ane. Carbon tetrachloride.

tet″ra·coc′cus [*tetra-;* G. *kokkos*, berry]. A coccus which divides in two planes and forms a group of four cells.

tet″ra·cy′cline. Generic name for the four-ring skeleton common to the antibiotic substances chlortetracycline and oxytetracycline, better known under their trade-marked names *aureomycin* and *terramycin*, respectively. Tetracycline, prepared by reductive dehalogenation of chlortetracycline, is itself a potent antibiotic. In the form of the hydrochloride it is supplied under the trade-marked names *achromycin, panmycin, polycycline, steclin, tetracyn.*

tetracyn. Trademark for *tetracycline.*

tet′rad [*tetra-*]. 1. An element having a valence of four. 2. A group of four chromatids which arises during meiosis from the pairing and splitting of maternal and paternal homologous chromosomes.

tet″ra·dac′tyl [G. *tetradaktylos*, four-toed]. Having four digits on each limb.

tet″ra·eth″yl·am·mo′ni·um. The univalent cation $(C_2H_5)_4N^+$, used in the form of the bromide or chloride salt, which on intramuscular or intravenous injection produces reversible blockade of impulses of both sympathetic and parasympathetic divisions of the autonomic nervous system. Used diagnostically or therapeutically in treating peripheral vascular diseases, hypertension, and other disorders in which peripheral circulation is disturbed. See *etamon chloride, TEAB.*

tet″ra·eth′yl·lead. A poisonous liquid, $Pb(C_2H_5)_4$, used in gasoline as an antiknock agent.

tet″ra·eth″yl·py″ro·phos′phate. $(C_2H_5)_4P_2O_7$; a synthetic substance having the power to inhibit cholinesterase, for which reason it is used as an insecticide and also clinically, especially in treatment of myasthenia gravis. A colorless, hygroscopic liquid, both water-soluble and lipid-soluble, it is probably the predominant active component of hexaethyltetraphosphate. Abbreviated, TEPP.

tet″ra·eth″yl·thi′u·ram di·sul′fide. $(C_2H_5)_2N.CS.S.S.CS.N(C_2H_5)_2$. A white or slightly yellow powder, insoluble in water; useful in treating alcoholism. Ingestion of alcohol following oral use of drug produces a series of disagreeable symptoms, including nausea, through increased conversion of alcohol to aldehyde. Available under trade-marked name *antabuse.*

tet″ra·gen′ic [G. *tetra-*, four; *genesthai*, from *gignesthai*, to be produced]. Referring to genotypes of polysomic or polyploid organisms which contain four different alleles for any given locus.

te·trag′e·nous (teh·tradj′i·nus) [*tetra-; genesthai*]. *In bacteriology,* pertaining to organisms which divide in two planes and form groups of four cells.

tet″ra·hy′dric. Containing four replaceable atoms of hydrogen.

tet″ra·hy″dro·can·nab′in·ol. Any one of a group of substances obtained from cannabis possessing to a great degree the activity of that drug.

β-tet″ra·hy″dro·naph·thyl′a·mine (·naf·thil′uh-meen, ·min, ·naf″thil·am′een, ·in, ·naf″thil·uh-meen′). $C_{10}H_{11}NH_2$. A substance causing a rise in body temperature when injected subcutaneously.

tet″ra·i·o″do·eth′yl·ene. See *diiodoform.*

tet″ra·i·o″do·phe″nol·phthal′ein. Iodophthalein.

tet″ra·i·o″do·phthal′ein so′di·um. Iodophthalein sodium.

tet″ra·i·o″do·thy′ro·nine. Thyroxin.

tetralin. Trade-mark for tetrahydronaphthalene, $C_{10}H_{12}$, a colorless liquid of penetrating odor used as a solvent for fats, oils, waxes, etc., and in cleaning and degreasing fabrics.

tetralogy of Fallot. A quadruple malformation of the heart, consisting of a high ventricular septal defect, dextroposition of the aorta so that it overrides and receives blood from both ventricles, stenosis of the pulmonary artery or atresia of the pulmonary valve, and hypertrophy of the right ventricle.

tet″ra·mas′ti·a [*tetra-;* G. *mastos*, breast]. The condition of having four breasts.

tet″ra·mas′ti·gote [*tetra-;* G. *mastix*, whip]. Having four flagella.

tet″ra·ma′zi·a [*tetra-;* G. *mazos*, breast]. The presence of four breasts.

te·tram′e·lus. Tetrascelus.

te·tram′er·ism [*tetra-;* G. *meros*, part]. *In biology,* division into four parts. —**tetramerous,** *adj.*

tet″ra·meth″yl·ene·di·am′ine (tet″ruh·meth″il-een·dye·am′een, ·in, ·dye′uh·meen, ·min, ·dye″-uh·meen′). $NH_2(CH_2)_4NH_2$. Putrescine.

tet″ra·meth″yl·pu·tres′cine (·pew·tress′een, ·in). $C_8H_{20}N_2$. A poisonous base from putrescine.

tet″ra·ni′trol. Erythrityl tetranitrate.

tet″ra·nop′si·a [*tetra-;* G. *a-*, not; *opsis*, vision]. A contraction of the field of vision limited to one quadrant.

tet″ra·nu′cle·o·tide. The name sometimes given to nucleic acid from yeast from the fact that it contains four constituent nucleotides.

tet″ra·oph·thal′mus, tet″roph·thal′mus [*tetra-;* G. *ophthalmos*, eye]. Having four eyes. See *diprosopus.*

tet″ra·o′tus. See *tetrotus.*

tet″ra·pep′tide. A polypeptide composed of four amino-acid groups.

tet″ra·ple′gi·a. See *quadriplegia.*

tet′ra·ploid [G. *tetraploos*, fourfold; *eidos*, form]. Having four haploid sets of chromosomes.

tet′ra·pus [G. *tetrapous*, four-footed]. Having four feet.

tet″ra·sac′cha·ride (tet″ruh·sack′uh·ride, ·rid). A polysaccharide hydrolyzable into four molecules of monosaccharide.

te·tras′ce·lus (teh·trass′i·lus) [G. *tetra-*, four; *skelos*, leg]. Having four legs.

tet″ra·so′mic [*tetra-;* G. *sōma*, body]. Having four chromosomes of a given kind, but only two of each of the other chromosomes of a haploid set; hence an individual with 2n + 2 chromosomes.

te·tras′ter [*tetra-;* G. *astēr*, star]. The achromatic figure in an abnormal mitosis when four centrosomes are present, as in dispermic eggs.

tet″ra·sti·chi′a·sis (tet″ruh·sti·kigh′uh·sis) [G. *tetrastichos*, in four rows; NL. *-iasis*, condition]. Arrangement of the eyelashes in four rows.

tet″ra·thi′o·nate. The bivalent ion $S_4O_6^{--}$. See *tetrathione.*

tet″ra·thi′o·nate re·duc′tion. The reduction of a tetrathionate compound; used in bacteriologic isolations. The chemistry may be represented thus:

$$S_4O_6^{--} + 2H = 2S_2O_3^{--} + 2H^+$$

It is valuable for isolating typhoid-paratyphoid organisms from feces.

tetrathione. Trade-mark for a brand of sodium tetrathionate, $Na_2S_4O_6.H_2O$, used in the treatment of certain peripheral circulatory diseases.

tet″ra·tom′ic. 1. Containing four atoms. 2. Having four hydroxyl radicals.

tet″ra·vac′cine (tet″ruh·vack′seen, ·sin, tet′ruh·vack″seen, ·sin) [G. *tetra-*, four; L. *vaccinus*, of cows]. A polyvalent vaccine containing four different cultures, as one containing typhoid, paratyphoid A and B, and cholera.

tet″ra·va′lent. See *quadrivalent.*

tet′ra·zole. 1. Either of two isomeric heterocyclic compounds in which three nitrogen atoms and one CH and one NH are joined in a ring. 2. Any derivative of the preceding.

tet″ra·zo′li·um salts. Generic term for certain salt-type derivatives of a tetrazole; some are water-soluble, colorless compounds which are reduced to highly pigmented, water-insoluble compounds in the presence of metabolic activity of living cells.

tet·relle′ [F., dim. of *tetin*, nipple]. An appliance for enabling a weakly infant to obtain milk from its mother. It consists of a nipple shield and two tubes; the mother sucks one of the latter, and the milk flows to the infant's mouth through the other. *Obs.*

tet·rod′o·nine (tet·rod′o·neen, ·nin, tet″ro·don′een, ·in). Poisonous principle of the fish roe of *Tetrodon.*

tet′ro·nal. $(C_2H_5)_2.C.(C_2H_5SO_2)_2$; diethylsulfonediethylmethane; a white crystalline powder, insoluble in water: used as a hypnotic.

tet′rose. A monosaccharide whose molecule contains only four atoms of carbon, as erythrose, $C_4H_8O_4$.

te·tro′tus [G. *tetra-*, four; *ous*, ear]. Having four ears. See *diprosopus.*

te·trox′ide, te·trox′id. A binary compound containing four atoms of oxygen.

tet′ryl. 1. See *butyl.* 2. Tetranitromethylaniline, picrylmethyl-nitramine, $C_7H_5N_5O_8$. Yellow powder used as explosive and as pH indicator. Also called *nitramine.*

tet′ter [AS. *teter*]. Any of various skin eruptions, particularly herpes, eczema, and psoriasis.

tex′is [G.]. Childbearing.

text blind′ness. See *alexia.*

tex′ti·form [L. *textum*, web; *forma*, form]. Reticular, forming a mesh.

tex″to·blas′tic [*textum;* G. *blastos*, germ]. Forming regenerative tissue.

tex′ture [L. *textura*, web, texture]. 1. Any organized substance or tissue of which the body is composed. 2. The arrangement of the elementary parts of tissue. *O.T.* —**textural,** *adj.*

tex′tus. A tissue. *O.T.*

Th Chemical symbol for thorium.

Thackrah, Charles Turner [*English physician*, 1795–1833]. First to investigate brass founder's ague, dust diseases. Author of first systematic English book on industrial disease (1831).

Thaddeus of Florence. See *Alderotti.*

thal″a·men·ceph′a·lon. See *thalamus.*

thal′a·mo- [G. *thalamos*, chamber]. A combining form denoting *relating to the thalamus.*

thal″a·mo·cor′ti·cal [*thalamos;* L. *cortex*, bark]. Pertaining to the thalamus and the cortex of the brain, as thalamocortical fibers, sensory projection fibers to the cerebral cortex.

thal″a·mo·len·tic′u·lar [*thalamos;* L. *lenticula*, lentil]. Pertaining to the thalamus and the lenticular nucleus.

thal″a·mo·mam′mil·lar″y (thal″uh·mo·mam′i·lerr″ee) [*thalamos;* L. *mammilla*, breast]. Pertaining to the thalamus and the mammillary bodies.

thal″a·mo·teg·men′tal [*thalamos;* L. *tegumentum*, covering]. Relating to the thalamus and tegmentum.

thal″a·mot′o·my [*thalamos;* G. *tomē*, a cutting]. Bilateral destruction of the medial thalamic nuclei for treatment of depressive states, such as manic depression.

thal′a·mus (pl. *thalami*) [*thalamos*]. A mass of gray matter at the base of the brain, developed from the wall of the vesicle of the third ventricle, and forming part of the wall of the latter cavity. The posterior part is called the pulvinar. The thalamus sends projection fibers to the primary sensory areas of the cortex. The thalamus receives fibers from all parts of the cortex, and is also connected with the tegmentum and with fibers of the optic tract. —**thalam′ic,** *adj.*

tha·las″sa·ne′mi·a [G. *thalassa*, sea; *anaimia*, want of blood]. Thalassemia.

tha·las·se′mi·a. A chronic hemolytic anemia, with erythroblastosis, occurring in Mediterranean families and due to a specific gene influencing hemoglobin production. The classic condition **thalassemia major,** due to homozygous genes and first described by Thomas B. Cooley, is characterized by insidious onset commencing in early life, underdevelopment, mongoloid facies, and splenomegaly. The blood picture shows a hypochromic microcytic anemia, bizarre cells, many target cells, reticulocytosis, erythroblastosis, leukocytosis, stippling, decreased osmotic fragility of the erythrocytes, and slight bilirubinemia. **Thalassemia minor,** a carrier state due to a heterozygous condition, is characterized by hypochromic and microcytic erythrocytes exhibiting marked morphologic abnormalities (stippling, target cells) but no erythroblastosis and rarely anemia. Also called *thassanemia, Mediterranean disease, hemolytic syndrome.* Syn., *thalassanemia, Cooley's anemia* or *disease* (*major* and *minor*), *familial erythroblastic* or *microcytic anemia, target-cell anemia, hereditary leptocytosis.*

tha·las″so·pho′bi·a [*thalassa;* G. *phobos*, fear]. A morbid fear of the sea.

tha·las″so·ther′a·py [*thalassa;* G. *therapeia*, treatment]. Treatment of disease by sea voyages, sea bathing, sea air.

thal′grain [G. *thallos*, young shoot; L. *granum*, grain]. Grain mixed with thallium sulfate and used as a poison for the destruction of rodents.

tha·lic′trine (tha·lick′treen, ·trin, thal′ick·). A poisonous alkaloid obtained from *Thalictrum macrocarpum.*

Tha·lic′trum [G. *thaliktron*, meadow-rue]. A genus of plants of the Ranunculaceae. Some species are cardiac poisons.

thal·lei′o·quin. The green substance produced when quinine or its salts is treated with a solution of chlorine or bromine followed by ammonia (called the *thalleioquin reaction*). Sometimes spelled *thalleoquin, thalleoquine.*

thal′line (thal′een, ·in). A synthetic alkaloid, tetrahydro-para-methoxyquinoline, $C_{10}H_{13}NO$, having antiseptic and antipyretic action but not used because of its toxicity.

thal′li·um [G. *thallos*, young shoot]. Tl = 204.39. A bluish white metallic element; used in the manufacture of alloys, special glasses, and artificial gems. Salts of the metal have been used for epilation and for destruction of rodents; both uses are dangerous to humans since thallium is highly toxic.

Thal·loph′y·ta [*thallos;* G. *phyton*, plant]. The phylum of plants having a thallus and no true roots, stems, and leaves; it includes the algae and the fungi.

thal′lo·spore [*thallos;* G. *spora*, seed]. An asexual reproductive spore formed by the thallus or mycelium of lower plants. Types of thallospores include arthrospores, blastospores, and chlamydospores.

thal″lo·tox″i·co′sis [*thallos;* G. *toxikon*, poison;

-*ōsis*, condition]. Poisoning by thallium or its derivatives.

thal'lus [*thallos*]. The simple type of plant structure without root, stem, and leaf, characteristic of members of the phylum Thallophyta.

tha·mu'ri·a [G. *thama*, often; *ouron*, urine]. Frequent urination.

than'a·to- [G. *thanatos*, death]. A combining form meaning *death*.

than"a·to·bi"o·log'ic (than"uh·to·buy"o·lodj'ick) [*thanatos;* G. *bios*, life; *logos*, word]. Pertaining to life and death.

than"a·to·gno·mon'ic (than"uh·to·no·mon'ick, than"uh·tog"no·) [*thanatos;* G. *gnōmōn*, interpreter]. Indicative of death.

than"a·tog'ra·phy [*thanatos;* G. *graphein*, to write]. 1. A dissertation on death. 2. A description of symptoms and feelings while dying.

than'a·toid [*thanatos;* G. *eidos*, form]. Resembling death.

than"a·tol'o·gy [*thanatos;* G. *logos*, word]. The study of the phenomena of somatic death.

than"a·to·ma'ni·a [*thanatos;* G. *mania*, madness]. Death by autosuggestion, as in individuals who believe they are under the spell of a sorcerer.

than"a·to·pho'bi·a [*thanatos;* G. *phobos*, fear]. A morbid fear of death.

than'a·top·sy [*thanatos;* G. *opsis*, vision]. Autopsy, necropsy. *Obs.*

than'a·tos [G.]. *In psychoanalysis*, all the instinctive tendencies which lead the organism toward death or senescence. Also called *death instinct*.

Thane, George Dancer [*English anatomist*, 1850–1930]. Remembered for his contributions to human anatomy. Described his method of locating the central sulcus preparatory to a cerebral operation, in which he used the middle point of an imaginary line passing from the root of the nose to the occipital protuberance. The upper extremity of the fissure lies one-half inch beyond this point.

thantis lozenge. A proprietary lozenge containing mercurochrome and salicyl alcohol.

Thap'si·a [G., deadly carrot]. A genus of plants of the Umbelliferae. The resin of various species has been used as a counterirritant and vesicant.

thas·sa·ne'mi·a. See *thalassemia*.

thau'ma·trope [G. *thauma*, wonder; *trepein*, to turn]. A device containing figures, on opposite sides of a rotating board, which blend when in motion. It shows the duration of visual impressions.

thau·mat'ro·py. See *metaplasia*.

Thayer, Sidney Allen [*American physician*, 1902–]. Known for his isolation, with Edward Adelbert Doisy and C. D. Veler, of a crystalline ovarian hormone from the urine of pregnant women. See also mouse *unit*.

Thayer, William Sydney [*American biochemist*, 1864–1932]. Discovered, with G. A. Blumer, that the gonococcus may cause ulcerative endocarditis and septicemia (1896). Best remembered for his clinical study of trichinosis, typhoid fever, and cardiology, to all of which he contributed material knowledge.

Thaysen, Thorvald Einar Hess [*Danish physician*, 1883–1936]. Studied nontropical sprue, or celiac disease, which he called idiopathic steatorrhea.

The'a [G. *thea*, goddess]. A genus of plants, now more properly named *Camellia*, from species of which tea is obtained. See *tea*.

theamin. Trade-mark for theophylline monoethanolamine, a vasodilator and diuretic. See *theophylline*.

the·ba'ic [G. *Thēbaikos*, of Thebes]. Pertaining to, or derived from, opium. *Obs.*

the'ba·ine (theeb'uh·een, thi·bay'een, ·in). $C_{19}H_{21}NO_3$. An alkaloid found in opium; it causes spasms like strychnine. Also called *paramorphine*.

Thebesius, Adam Christian [*German physician*, 1686–1732]. Gave the first description of the coronary valves, also called *Thebesian valves*. See also *Thebesian veins* under *vein*.

the'ca (pl. *thecae*) [G. *thēkē*, chest, a case]. A sheath, especially one of a tendon.

t. folliculi. The capsule of a growing or mature ovarian (Graafian) follicle consisting of an inner vascular, cellular layer, the **theca interna,** and an outer fibrous layer, the **theca externa.** —**thecal,** *adj.*

the·ci'tis [*thēkē;* G. *-itis*, inflammation]. Inflammation of the sheath of a tendon.

the'co·dont [*thēkē;* G. *odous*, tooth]. Characterizing a tooth which is fixed in a separate socket, or a dentition composed of such teeth.

the·co'ma [*thēkē;* G. *-ōma*, tumor]. A tumor of the ovary composed of cells derived from the ovarian stroma, in some instances resembling the thecal elements of the follicle: also called *thelioma*.

the"co·so'ma, the"co·so'mum. See *Schistosoma*.

the"co·steg·no'sis [*thēkē;* G. *stegnōsis*, a making watertight]. The shrinking or contraction of the sheath of a tendon.

the'e·lin (thee'uh·lin, thee'lin). See *estrone*.

the'e·lol (thee'uh·lohl, ·lol, ·lawl). See *estriol*.

Theiler, Max (1899–). South African physician and bacteriologist known for his extensive research on yellow fever, proving it is a virus disease, on dengue fever, spirochetal jaundice, and Japanese encephalitis. In 1951 he received the Nobel prize in medicine and physiology for the development of two vaccines against yellow fever.

Theiler's virus. See under *virus*.

Thei·le'ri·a (thigh·leer'ee·uh) [after Arnold *Theiler*, Swiss bacteriologist, 1867–1936]. A genus of Protozoa, parasites of cattle, transmitted by a tick.

thei"le·ri'a·sis (thigh"li·rye'uh·sis) [*Theiler;* NL. *-iasis*, condition]. Infection with *Theileria*. A disease of cattle in South Africa. Also called *East Coast fever*, *Rhodesian tick fever*.

the'ine (thee'een, ·in, tee'·) [G. *thea*, goddess]. Caffeine.

Theis method. See Benedict and Theis's *method*.

Theis and Benedict's method for blood phenols. See under *method*.

the'ism [*thea*]. Old term for the toxic condition produced by the excessive use of tea.

the·lal'gi·a [G. *thēlē*, nipple; *algos*, pain]. Pain in a nipple.

the·las'is, the·las'mus (thi·laz'mus) [*thēlē*]. The act of sucking.

The·la'zi·a. A genus of threadlike nematodes with a predilection for the eye of their hosts. A few cases have been reported in man.

T. californiensis. A parasite of dogs and cats which is found on the west coast of the U. S. A.

T. callipaeda. A parasite of dogs which is found in India and China.

the"la·zi'a·sis [*Thelazia;* NL. *-iasis*, condition]. An affection of the eye produced by infestation by worms of the genus *Thelazia*.

the'le·plas"ty, thel'y·plas"ty [G. *thēlē*, nipple; *plassein*, to form]. Plastic surgery of a nipple.

the·ler'e·thism [*thēlē;* G. *erethisma*, provocation]. Erection of a nipple.

thelestrin. Trade-mark for a preparation of estrogenic substances in sesame oil.

the"li·o'ma. See *thecoma*.

the·li'tis [*thēlē;* G. *-itis*, inflammation]. Inflammation of a nipple: also called *mammillitis*.

puerperal t. Postpartum inflammation of the nipple of the breast.

the'li·um [*thēlē*]. 1. A papilla. 2. The nipple.

the·lon′cus [*thēlē;* G. *ogkos,* tumor]. Tumor of a nipple.

the″lo·phleb″o·stem′ma [*thēlē;* G. *phleps,* vein; *stemma,* wreath]. Venous circle around a nipple.

the″lor·rha′gi·a (theel″o·ray′juh, ·jee·uh, ·radj′uh, ·radj′ee·uh) [*thēlē;* G. *rhēgnynai,* to burst forth]. Hemorrhage from a nipple.

the′lo·thism [*thēlē;* G. *ōthismos,* a pushing]. Projection of a nipple, caused by contraction of its smooth muscle.

thel″y·ot′o·ky [G. *thēlys,* female; *tokos,* childbirth]. Parthenogenetic reproduction of females only. Also called *thelytocia.*

the′nar [G., palm]. 1. The palm of the hand. 2. The fleshy prominence of the palm corresponding to the base of the thumb.

the′nar. Pertaining to the palm, as thenar muscles.

Thénard, Baron Louis Jacques [*French chemist,* 1777–1857]. Known for his discovery of hydrogen peroxide (1818).

thenardol. Trade-mark for a glycerin solution of urea peroxide which slowly liberates urea and hydrogen peroxide when applied to wounds and infected areas. The hydrogen peroxide is germicidal, the urea stimulates wound healing, and the glycerin draws plasma from deeper parts of the wound.

thenfadil hydrochloride. Trade-marked name for *thenyldiamine hydrochloride.*

then″yl·di′a·mine hy″dro·chlo′ride. 2-[(2-Dimethylaminoethyl)-3-thenylamino]pyridine hydrochloride; $C_{14}H_{19}N_3S.HCl$; an antihistaminic substance. See *thenfadil hydrochloride.*

thenylene hydrochloride. A trade-marked name for *methapyrilene hydrochloride.*

then″yl·pyr′a·mine (then″il·pirr′uh·meen, ·min). N,N-dimethyl-N′(2-thenyl)-N′(2-pyridyl)-ethylenediamine; $(CH_3)_2NCH_2CH_2N(C_5H_4N)$-$(C_4H_3SCH_2)$, or methapyrilene: used in the form of its hydrochloride salt as an antihistaminic agent.

then″yl·pyr′a·mine hy″dro·chlo′ride. Methapyrilene hydrochloride.

The″o·bro′ma [G. *theos,* god; *brōma,* food]. A genus of trees of the Sterculiaceae. The seeds of **T. cacao** yield a fixed oil (theobroma oil) and contain the alkaloid theobromine. The seeds are used in the preparation of chocolate and cocoa.

the″o·bro′ma oil (*oleum theobromatis*). A yellowish white solid consisting chiefly of the glycerides of stearic, palmitic, oleic, and lauric acids, obtained from the roasted seeds of *T. cacao.* It melts between 30° and 35° C. and is used in the preparation of suppositories, in ointments, and as an emollient. Also called *cocoa butter, cacao butter.*

the″o·bro′mine (thee″o·bro′meen, ·min). An alkaloid, 3,7-dimethylxanthine, $C_7H_8N_4O_2$, differing from theophylline only in the position of the methyl groups, found in cacao beans and kola nuts and usually obtained as a by-product in the manufacture of cocoa and chocolate. A diuretic and myocardial stimulant. Dose, 0.3–0.5 Gm. (5–8 gr.).

t. calcium salicylate. A mixture of theobromine and calcium salicylate, representing 44% of theobromine, more soluble than theobromine.

t. sodium acetate. An approximately equimolecular mixture of theobromine sodium and sodium acetate representing from 55–65% of theobromine. It is a white, crystalline, hygroscopic powder which absorbs carbon dioxide from the air with the liberation of theobromine. One Gm. dissolves in about 1.5 cc. of water. See *thesodate.*

t. sodium salicylate. An approximately equimolecular mixture of theobromine sodium and sodium salicylate, representing about 46.5% of theobromine. See *diuretin.*

theocalcin. Trade-mark for a brand of theobromine calcium salicylate.

theocin. Trade-mark for *theophylline.*

theocin soluble. Trade-mark for *theophylline sodium acetate.*

theoglycinate. Trade-mark for *theophylline sodium glycinate.*

the″o·ma′ni·a [*theos;* G. *mania,* madness]. 1. Religious mania. 2. Mental disorder in which the individual believes himself to be a divine being. —**theomaniac,** *n.*

theominal. Trade-mark of a tablet containing luminal and theobromine.

the″o·pho′bi·a [*theos;* G. *phobos,* fear]. Morbid fear of God.

the″o·phyl′line (thee″o·fil′een, ·in, thee·off′il·een, ·in, thee″o·fi·leen′). An alkaloid, 1,3-dimethylxanthine, $C_7H_8N_4O_2.H_2O$, obtained from tea leaves and also prepared synthetically. It differs chemically from theobromine only in the position of the methyl groups. It is a white, crystalline, odorless, bitter-tasting powder, soluble in about 120 parts of water; freely soluble in alkali hydroxides and ammonia. It is a diuretic and vasodilator; it also relaxes bronchial spasms. Dose, 0.2–0.3 Gm. (3–5 gr.).

t. calcium salicylate. An approximately equimolecular mixture of theophylline calcium and calcium salicylate, representing about 48% of theophylline.

t. diethanolamine. A compound of 1 mol of theophylline with 1 or 2 mols of diethanolamine.

t. ethylenediamine. Aminophylline.

t. isopropanolamine. Represents approximately 70% of theophylline. Dose, 0.06 Gm. (1 gr.) t.i.d. See *theopropanol.*

t. methylglucamine. A mixture of theophylline and methylglucamine.

t. monoethanolamine. A white, crystalline powder representing about 75% of anhydrous theophylline. Dose, 0.2–0.5 Gm. (3–8 gr.).

t. sodium acetate. An approximately equimolecular mixture of theophylline sodium and sodium acetate, representing about 60% of theophylline.

t. sodium glycinate. An equilibrium mixture containing theophylline sodium ($C_7H_7N_4NaO_2$) and glycine in approximately molecular proportions buffered with an additional mole of glycine; it has the actions of theophylline but is less irritating than other soluble derivatives. See *cinaphyl, dorsaphyllin, glynazan, glytheonate, synophylate, theoglycinate.*

the″o·ple′gi·a [*theos;* G. *plēgē,* stroke]. Apoplexy.

theopropanol. Trade-mark for theophylline isopropanolamine. See under *theophylline.*

the″o·ret′i·cal [G. *theorētikos,* speculative]. Based on theory; speculative.

the′o·ry [G. *theōria,* a beholding, speculation]. The abstract principles of a science. Also, a reasonable supposition or assumption, generally better developed and more probable than a mere hypothesis.

alternation t. A theory on the nature of antigen-antibody reactions which assumes that the antigen is multivalent and the antibody is bivalent. According to the theory, the secondary phase of antigen-antibody reactions, such as agglutination and precipitation, is due to the action of specific chemical forces operating between the antigen and antibody molecules. The theory assumes that the primary and secondary stages of antigen-antibody reactions are produced by the same phenomena, for example, chemical. Therefore, aggregates of antigen and antibody molecules would be bound together by specific chemical linkages. One antigen molecule would be united with two or more antibody molecules within the mass, or one molecule of antibody would be united with one or at the most two molecules of antigen. Also called *lattice t., framework t., multivalent t.*

antichromatic t. A theory, proposed by Hartridge, postulating a suppressor mechanism in the retina or brain which depresses the sensitivity to both blue and yellow, to explain the correction of chromatic aberrations, i.e., the blue and yellow fringes surrounding images on the retina.

backward failure t. An attempt to explain the origin of the symptoms and signs of congestive heart failure by increased peripheral and pulmonary venous pressures.

cell t. The theory that the cell is the unit of organic structure, and that cell formation is the essential process of life and its phenomena. Also called *cell doctrine.*

closed circulation t. The theory that in the spleen blood moves directly from the arteries of the ellipsoids, through capillaries, into the venous sinusoids. Blood escapes into the pulp through openings in the walls of the sinusoids.

Cohnheim t. A classical theory of the origin of tumors. Rests of embryonic cells are misplaced, remain dormant, and later may go on to produce neoplasms. Also called *fetal rest-cell t., embryonal t.*

cytocrine t. The postulated transfer of pigment granules from melanocytes directly into epidermal cells: opposed to *exocrine* or *endocrine* transfer.

dichromatic t. According to Hering, when two of the four basic-color sensations are missing, most frequently the red-green, wavelength is discriminated along the visible spectrum in terms of two-color processes.

dualist t. of hematopoiesis. A polyphyletic theory of hemopoiesis involving two stem cells, myeloblast and lymphoblast, each having different potencies.

duplicity t. See *duplicity theory.*

electrosome t. Regaud's theory that the mitochondria are the centers of specific chemical action in cells, capable of synthesizing certain substances from materials selected from the cytoplasm.

embryonal t. See Cohnheim *t.*

extravascular t. of erythrocyte formation. A theory that erythrocytes are formed in the reticular mesh of bone marrow outside of the circulatory system and enter it through sinusoids.

fetal rest-cell t. See Cohnheim *t.*

Folin t. The bulk of excreted nitrogen is of exogenous origin and does not arise by the metabolism of tissue protein.

germ-layer t. A young embryo establishes three superimposed cellular plates, the primary germ layers, which are called ectoderm, mesoderm, and entoderm. According to the germ-layer theory, the skin, nervous system and sense organs are derived from ectoderm, the inner lining of the primitive digestive canal from entoderm, and muscles, blood vessels, connective tissues and organs of excretion and reproduction from mesoderm.

germ t. The theory that all contagious and infectious diseases are caused by microorganisms.

intravascular t. of erythrocyte formation. A theory that erythrocytes are formed inside delicate blood vessels in bone marrow from the lining of these vessels.

Knoop's t. The theory that fats are metabolized by β-oxidation.

lock and key t. An enzyme to be effective must fit the molecule of the substrate somewhat as a key fits into a lock. Some enzymes appear to be "master keys" in that they fit into a considerable number of substrates. This analogy of enzyme specificity was suggested by Emil Fischer.

Meyer-Overton t. An explanation of the action of anesthetics. The intensity of a narcotic action of an anesthetic may depend on the physical affinity between the anesthetic, the lipids, and other cell constituents, particularly water. It is the partition coefficient which indicates how a substance disseminates in an emulsion of fat and water.

monochromatic t. A theory postulating colorblindness, absence of color perception, because of arrested development of receptors at an early age. The red-green and yellow-blue mechanisms are blocked in otherwise intact cones with normal luminosity mechanism.

monophyletic t. of hematopoiesis. Unitarian theory.

neounitarian t. of hematopoiesis. A concept that the lymphocyte of normal blood does not develop into all other cell types but that, under proper environmental conditions as in tissue cultures or in pathologic states, the lymphocyte or cells that morphologically resemble lymphocytes can become multipotent.

neuron t. See *neuron doctrine.*

omega oxidation t. A theory predicting that oxidation of certain fatty acids of medium chain length occurs at the end methyl group, originally postulated to explain the formation of dicarboxylic acids from monocarboxylic acids in vivo.

open circulation t. The theory that in the spleen blood moves from the arteries of the ellipsoids into the tissue of the pulp cords, and is transfused back into the vascular system through openings in the walls of the venous sinusoids.

open-closed circulation t. The theory that in the spleen the circulation of blood can be either open or closed, depending on circumstances.

Petzval t. A theory which states that the sum of the product of the refractive indexes and focal lengths of two thin lenses must equal zero in order to attain a fairly flat field free from astigmatic conditions.

place t. of hearing. The theory that each frequency of sound is detected by a structure having a specific location on the basilar membrane of the inner ear. Also see resonance *t.* of hearing.

polychromatic t. A theory of color vision, advanced by Hartridge (1941), postulating seven types of receptors possessing eight response curves: (1) crimson, (2) orange, (3) yellow, (4) green, (5) blue-green, (6) blue, (7) blue-violet.

polyphyletic t. of hematopoiesis. A hypothesis concerning the mode of origin of blood cells which assumes the development of a specific parental cell for each cell type.

quantum t. According to Max Planck, radiant energy is given off from atoms or molecules in small discrete lots called quanta, and is absorbed in a like manner. The discharge of energy from an atom accompanies the passing of an electron from a high energy level to a lower level (from a larger to a smaller orbit), and the passage of an electron from a smaller to a greater orbit is accompanied by an absorption of energy. The energy discharged is equal to $h\nu$, where h is the Planck constant and ν is the frequency of the radiated energy. See quantum *constant.*

quantum t. of color vision. The theory that a retinal cone, when stimulated by light, possesses the power of transmitting along its nerve fibers impulses of different kinds, depending upon the quantum number or wavelength of the light; that is, light from the violet end of the spectrum would evoke nerve impulses different from those generated by rays from the red end of the spectrum.

recapitulation t. The theory that the individual organism in its development from the ovum passes through a series of stages which resemble a series of ancestral types through which the species passed in its evolutionary history. This is also called the *biogenetic law.* Haeckel recognized a difference between those structures which are adaptive to the embryonic, larval, or fetal mode of life and those which may be regarded as inherited from the ancestral types. The former he included under cenogenesis and the latter under palingenesis.

Reed-Frost t. (*of epidemics*). *In epidemiology,* a theory, intended to cover acute communicable diseases, based on an expression of the probable number of cases at time $T + 1$ in terms of known facts at time T. The theory is one that proceeds stepwise in time and does not give a continuous time curve; it is not expected to describe the course of a particular epidemic, but allows the exploration of a variety of epidemiologic principles.

resonance t. of hearing. The theory that the inner ear contains tuned resonators that stimulate specific nerve endings when a tone of their resonant frequency enters the ear. Usually associated with place theory of hearing.

Shaffer's t. of oxidation catalysis. A theory advanced by P. A. Shaffer to explain why catalytic amounts of certain ions are needed to establish a steady potential in electromotively sluggish systems. In its broader aspects it has important implications for the mechanism of biological oxidation-reduction systems.

side-chain t. A chemical theory explaining the phenomena of immunity by the action of antibodies which, when circulating in an organism, unite with and render harmless the antigen and thereby prevent the antigen from attaching itself to the chemical system of the protoplasm.

sound pattern t. The basilar membrane is supposed to vibrate as a whole, but with "nodes," or lines of rest, in different places according to the pitch of the note.

static t. Goltz's theory that every position of the head causes the endolymph of the semicircular canals to exert greatest pressure upon some part of the canals, thus in varying degree exciting the nerve endings of the ampullae.

telephone t. of hearing. The theory that the auditory nerve transmits nerve impulses to the brain having the same frequency as the sound waves striking the ear.

theories of hematopoiesis. The dualist, neounitarian, polyphyletic, trialist, and unitarian theories of hematopoiesis. See extravascular and intravascular *t.* of erythrocyte formation.

trialist t. A polyphyletic theory of hemopoiesis involving three stem-cells, each having different potencies; usually, lymphoblast, myeloblast, monoblast.

tritubercular t. The theory of Cope, later modified by Osborn, that mammalian molar teeth are derived phylogenetically from primitive three-cusped teeth.

unitarian t. A theory of blood-cell formation which supposes that all blood cells come from a single parental blood cell, the hemocytoblast. Syn., *monophyletic t. of hematopoiesis.*

unitarian t. of antibodies. One opposed to the belief that each different serologic reaction is based on a separate antibody, maintaining to the contrary that the same antibody can perform all or most of these functions. Of necessity it holds that the number of hypothetical entities is limited.

Wieland t. of hydrogen activation. Certain hydrogen atoms of the metabolite (substance oxidized) are "activated" by an enzyme (dehydrogenase) so that they may be removed by a "hydrogen-acceptor," which can be molecular oxygen or other oxidizing agent.

the″o·ther′a·py [G. *theos*, god; *therapeia*, treatment]. The treatment of disease by prayer and religious exercises.

thephorin. A trade-mark for a brand of the antihistaminic substance phenindamine.

thephyldine. A trade-mark for *aminophylline.*

theranates. A trade-mark for a tonic preparation containing mixed glycerophosphates and thiamine hydrochloride.

ther″a·peu′sis (therr″uh·pew′sis) [G., treatment]. Therapeutics.

ther″a·peu′tic [G. *therapeutikos*, inclined to serve]. Pertaining to therapeutics; curative.

ther″a·peu′tics [*therapeutikos*]. The branch of medical science dealing with the treatment of disease. Also see *therapy, treatment.*

ther″a·peu′tist [*therapeutikos*]. One skilled in therapeutics.

the″ra·pi′a ste·ril′i·sans mag′na (therr″uh-pye′uh sti·ril′i·zanz mag′nuh, thi·ray′pee·uh) [L.]. Ehrlich's aim of treatment by destruction of the parasites in the body of a patient without doing serious harm to the patient; it is accomplished by the administration, in one large dose, of a sufficient quantity of a drug having a special affinity for the parasite causing the disease.

ther′a·pist. Therapeutist.

physical t. An individual professionally trained in the utilization of physical agents for therapeutic purposes.

ther′a·pist-vec′tor. *In psychoanalysis,* the mature affect expressed by a person in response to the immature needs of another person.

ther′a·py [G. *therapeia*, treatment]. Treatment. Also see *treatment.*

anticoagulant t. The use of drugs that prevent the clotting of blood, such as heparin and dicoumarin, in the treatment of thrombosis.

biologic t. The use of biologic products such as serums, vaccines, antitoxins, and antibiotics.

Chaoul t. See contact *t.*

chemical t. See *chemotherapy.*

cold t. The use of cold in any form as a therapeutic agent.

collapse t. The treatment of pulmonary tuberculosis by any surgical procedure designed to decrease lung volume, such as artificial pneumothorax, extrapleural thoracoplasty, or interruption of the phrenic nerve.

contact t. Superficial x-ray therapy which is delivered by a special low-voltage x-ray tube. The beam is emitted generally from one end of the tube. The tube is shockproof and small, and may be placed in direct contact with the skin or introduced into body cavities.

corrective t. *In physical medicine,* a medically supervised program of physical exercise and activities for the purpose of improving or maintaining the health of the patient through individual or group participation. Specifically, techniques have been designed to conserve and increase neuromuscular strength and skill, to reestablish or improve ambulation, to improve habits of personal health, and to promote relaxation by adjustment to physical and mental stresses.

Curie t. Treatment of diseases with rays emanating from radioactive substances.

diathermic t. Use of electromagnetic radiation. See *diathermy.*

electroshock t. Treatment of mental patients, particularly those suffering with melancholia, mania, or catatonia, by passing a current through the brain (temple to temple), 85 to 110 volts and

500 milliamperes for 1/10 to 1/5 of a second. The patient does not recall the treatment. Better and safer than the metrazol shock therapy.

endocrine t. The treatment of disease by the administration of extracts of the endocrine glands.

fangotherapy. Treatment of the extremities by immersing them in hot mud.

fever t. Treatment of disease by artificially induced fever.

fluid t. Administration of fluids to dehydrated patients; determinations must be made as to the degree of dehydration and amount of electrolyte imbalance. Fluids may be given orally or intravenously depending upon circumstances; subcutaneous administration is rarely used.

fluorine t. The use of fluorine, as a fluoride, for the control of dental caries. The term covers topical application of fluorine to the teeth, the addition of fluorine to water supplies, or the internal administration of fluorine.

glandular t. The treatment of disease by glandular extracts, especially those obtained from organs which furnish internal secretions necessary to the bodily economy.

gold t. The injection of various preparations of gold such as inorganic or organic salts or as a colloid for the treatment of lupus erythematosus, various dermatologic tuberculids, and rheumatoid arthritis.

group t. *In psychoanalysis,* the therapy given to a group of patients by a professional therapist, and based on the effect of the group upon the individual and his interaction with the group.

heat t. The treatment of disease with heat by means of hot baths, short-wave electric fields, heat lamps, hot-air cabinets.

hormone t. The treatment of disease with hormones.

immunization t. Use of vaccines or antiserums to produce immunity against a specific disease.

insulin shock t. Treatment of nervous disease by large doses of insulin.

interstitial irradiation t. Radium therapy with various types of implants or seeds filled with radium salts or radon.

intracavitary irradiation t. Radium therapy by means of tubes, single or in strings of two or more, inserted into a cavity of the body.

intravenous t. Introduction of therapeutic agents into the blood stream through a vein.

isotope t. Therapy with substances made artificially radioactive by bombardment with positive ions or neutrons.

maggot t. The treatment of osteomyelitis by the introduction of live larvae of the bluebottle fly into the open wound. The larvae clean the wound by eating the necrotic material. Also called *Baer's treatment.*

malarial t. The artificial induction of malaria for its therapeutic effect in central nervous system syphilis.

metrazol shock t. Treatment of persons suffering with melancholia and with catatonic forms of schizophrenia with an intravenous injection of metrazol, which causes convulsions and produces temporary brain changes resulting in elevation of the mood to normal levels and promotion of normal mental animation. Also see electroshock *t.*

metric occupational t. A form of occupational therapy in which the amount of work a patient does in a given time is measured to help form a basis for an estimate of the amount of work he can or should do (*work tolerance*): most useful with chronically ill patients with limited physical capacities. Syn., *measured work t.*

mucin t. The administration of mucin to protect the gastric mucosa against the action of pepsin and hydrochloric acid by protective coating and the neutralization of the hydrochloric acid.

multiple t. *In psychoanalysis,* the therapy given to one patient by a group of therapists.

musical t. The use of music for therapeutic effect, especially in treating mental disorders.

neutron t. Irradiation with neutrons for therapeutic purposes.

nonspecific protein t. The therapeutic use of any protein which causes a response in the body other than one to which the patient is allergic.

nonspecific t. That used for its general constitutional effect instead of removing or neutralizing the etiologic agent.

occupational t. Any prescribed mental or physical activity, such as hobbies, crafts, light household tasks, gardening, or simple trades, designed to aid the patient in his recovery from, or during the chronic course of, any disease or disabling condition.

oxygen t. The administration of oxygen by means of nasal catheter, face mask, or oxygen tent. It has also been given subcutaneously and intravenously.

physical t. The treatment of disease and injury by physical means, such as light, heat, cold, water, electricity, massage, and exercise, performed by trained personnel under the prescription of a physician.

protein shock t. The injection of a foreign protein subcutaneously or intravenously for the therapeutic effect of the resulting reaction.

radiant light t. The use in physical therapy of curative rays derived from the sun or artificial sources as ultraviolet and infrared radiation.

radiation t. The treatment of disease with any type of radiation, but most commonly with ionizing radiation, including use of roentgen rays, radium, or other radioactive substances; such use of ionizing radiation is usually called *radiotherapy.*

radium t. Exposure of a part to high-voltage radium emanations, usually for their destructive effect on malignant tissues.

replacement t. The use of endocrine therapy to replace a function which has been destroyed surgically or has ceased naturally.

roentgen t. Treatment with roentgen rays. Syn., *x-ray t.*

rotation t. A type of radiation therapy in which either the patient or the source of radiation is in continuous rotation during exposure.

shock t. The treatment of psychiatric patients by inducing coma, with or without convulsions, by means of drugs as insulin or metrazol or by passing an electric current through the brain. Also see electroshock *t.*, insulin shock *t.*, metrazol shock *t.*

solar t. Treatment of disease by exposing the body to the direct rays of the sun or by the use of a sun lamp; heliotherapy.

specific t. One having a proved destructive effect against a specific etiologic factor or having a definite curative effect upon a particular disease.

substitutional t. The use in treatment of substances the secretion of which has failed in whole or in part, or which, being formed, are unavailable to the body.

suggestion t. Treating disordered states by means of suggestion.

supplementary x-ray t. The irradiation of affected areas with x-ray in addition to the use of radium in the treatment of carcinoma.

telecurie t. Therapy in which the radioactive substance is located at some distance from the lesion to be treated.

teleradium t. External radium therapy with the radium source at some distance from the skin.

tissue t. of Filatov. Implantation of small pieces of refrigerated placentas from mothers with negative Wassermann reactions in the subconjunctiva of patients with various eye diseases: useful for keratitis and iridocyclitis.

vaccine t. The attempt to produce active immunity against disease by the use of specific antigens. See *vaccination.*

work t. See occupational *t.*

x-ray t. Therapy with roentgen rays.

ther″en·ceph′a·lous [G. *thēr*, beast of prey; *egkephalos*, brain]. A term applied to a skull in which the lines from the inion and nasion to the hormion make an angle of from 116° to 129°.

the·ri′a·ca [G. *thēriakos*, concerning venomous beasts]. Treacle.

t. Andromachi. Venice treacle, a compound containing nearly 70 ingredients, and used as an antidote against poisons. *Obs.*

The″ri·di′i·dae (theer″i·dye′i·dee) [G. *thēridion*, small animal]. A family of spiders which includes the genus *Latrodectus* or black widow spider.

the″ri·od′ic [G. *thēriōdēs*, full of wild beasts, malignant]. Malignant.

the″ri·o′ma [G. *thērion*, wild animal; *-ōma*, tumor]. A malignant ulcer or tumor.

the″ri·o·mim′ic·ry [*thērion;* G. *mimos*, mime]. Imitation of animals.

therm [G. *thermē*, heat]. Small calorie.

ther′mal [*thermē*]. Pertaining to heat.

ther″mal·ge′si·a [*thermē;* G. *algēsis*, sense of pain]. Pain caused by heat.

ther·mal′gi·a. See *causalgia.*

therm·an″al·ge′si·a. See *thermoanalgesia.*

therm·an″es·the′si·a. See *thermoanesthesia.*

ther″ma·tol′o·gy [*thermē;* G. *logos*, word]. The scientific use or understanding of heat or of the waters of thermal springs in the cure of disease. **—thermatolog′ic,** *adj.*

therm″es·the′si·a (thurm″ess·thee′zhuh, ·zee·uh) [*thermē;* G. *aisthēsis*, sensation]. 1. Temperature sense for heat. 2. Sensitiveness to heat.

therm″es·the″si·om′e·ter (thurm″ess·thee″zee·om′i·tur, ·see·om′i·tur) [*thermē; aisthēsis;* G. *metron*, a measure]. An instrument for measuring the sensibility to heat of different regions of the skin.

ther′mic [*thermē*]. Pertaining to heat.

ther′min. Tetrahydro-β-naphthylamine hydrochloride, $C_{10}H_{11}NH_2.HCl$. A white, crystalline compound once used as a mydriatic. It is pyrogenic.

ther′mite. Finely powdered aluminum mixed with iron oxide and capable of being ignited with a magnesium ribbon; the resulting reaction produces a temperature of about 3000° C.; used in welding.

ther′mo- [*thermē*]. A combining form meaning *heat.*

ther″mo·al·ge′si·a. See *thermalgesia.*

ther″mo·an″al·ge′si·a (thur″mo·an″al·jee′zee·uh, ·see·uh) [*thermē;* G. *analgēsia*, want of feeling]. Insensibility to heat or to contact with heated objects.

ther″mo·an″es·the′si·a (thur″mo·an″ess·thee′zhuh, ·zee·uh) [*thermē;* G. *anaisthēsia*, lack of sensation]. Loss of the perception of thermal impressions, a condition sometimes present in syringomyelia, severed nerve diseases and leprosy.

ther″mo·cau′ter·y [*thermē;* G. *kautērion*, branding-iron]. A cautery which depends for its action upon heat delivered to the metal end of the instrument, either by a direct action of flame, aided by the passage of a current of hot air as in the Paquelin cautery, or by the passage of electric current.

ther″mo·chem′is·try [*thermē;* G. *chymos*, juice]. That branch of chemical science which treats of the mutual relations of heat and chemical changes.

ther″mo·chro′ism [*thermē;* G. *chroia*, color]. The property of transmitting some thermal radiations while absorbing or changing others.

ther″mo·co·ag″u·la′tion [*thermē;* L. *coagulare*, to cause a fluid to curdle]. 1. A method of destroying tissue by means of electrocautery or high-frequency current. 2. A method by which one or several layers of the cerebral cortex in a desired area can be destroyed without alteration of the surrounding tissue.

ther′mo·cou″ple (thur′mo·cup″ul) [*thermē;* L. *copula*, bond]. A pair of metallic plates or wires forming a junction, in which a thermoelectromotive force is formed under the influence of heat. Thermocouple principle is also applied in the measurement of skin temperature.

ther″mo·du′ric [*thermē;* L. *durus*, hard]. Capable of resisting high temperatures.

ther″mo·dy·nam′ics (thur″mo·dye·nam′icks, ·di·nam′icks) [*thermē;* G. *dynamis*, power]. The science which treats of the relations of heat and other forms of energy.

ther″mo·es·the′si·a. See *thermesthesia.*

ther″mo·es·the″si·om′e·ter. See *thermesthesiometer.*

ther″mo·ex·ci′to·ry [*thermē;* L. *excitare*, to rouse up]. Exciting the production of heat.

ther″mo·gen′ic, ther″mo·ge·net′ic [*thermē;* G. *genesthai*, from *gignesthai*, to be produced]. Pertaining to thermogenics; producing heat.

ther″mo·gen′ics [*thermē; genesthai*]. The science of the production of heat.

ther·mog′e·nous (thur·modj′i·nus) [*thermē; genesthai*]. Thermogenic.

ther″mo·hy″per·al·ge′si·a (·al·jee′zee·uh, ·see·uh) [*thermē;* G. *hyper*, over; *algēsis*, sense of pain]. The condition in which the application of heat causes excessive pain.

ther″mo·hy″per·es·the′si·a (·ess·thee′zhuh, ·zee·uh) [*thermē; hyper;* G. *aisthēsis*, sensation]. Abnormal sensitiveness to the application of heat.

ther″mo·hy″pes·the′si·a [*thermē;* G. *hypo*, under; *aisthēsis*]. Abnormal indifference or insensibility to heat or to contact with heated objects.

ther″mo·hy″po·es·the′si·a. See *thermohypesthesia.*

ther″mo·in·hib′i·to″ry [*thermē;* L. *inhibere*, to restrain]. Inhibiting the production of heat.

ther″mo·la′bile (thur″mo·lay′bil) [*thermē;* L. *labilis*, slipping]. Destroyed or changed by heat.

ther·mol′y·sis [*thermē;* G. *lysis*, a loosing]. 1. Dissipation of animal heat. 2. Chemical decomposition by means of heat. **—thermolyt′ic,** *adj.*

ther″mo·mas·sage′ (thur″mo·ma·sahzh′) [*thermē;* F. *massage*]. Massage with application of heat.

ther·mom′e·ter [*thermē;* G. *metron*, a measure]. An instrument for measuring temperatures or thermal states, generally consisting of a substance capable of expanding and contracting with different temperatures, and a graduated scale by means of which variations in the expansion of the substance can be determined.

air t. One in which the expansive substance is air.

alcohol t. One in which the expansive substance is alcohol.

centigrade t. One in which the freezing point for water is at 0° and the boiling point at 100°. The interval is divided into 100 parts of 1° each. Also called *Celsius t.*

clinical t. One used to ascertain the body temperature, so constructed that the maximum reading remains stationary after removal of thermometer from the patient.

electric t. A clinical thermometer consisting of a resistance thermometer or a thermocouple with calibrated indicating or recording meters.

Fahrenheit t. One in which the interval between the freezing point and the boiling point for water is divided into 180 equal parts, each called a degree. 32° F. represents the freezing point and 212° F. the boiling point of water.

fever t. A clinical thermometer.

homigrade t. A thermometer which is not now in use, which is so calibrated that zero represents freezing, 100° represents normal body temperature (98.6° F. or 37° C.), and 270° the boiling point.

kata t. See *katathermometer.*

maximum and minimum t. One which registers the maximum and minimum temperatures to which it has been exposed.

mercurial t. One in which the expansive substance is mercury.

Réaumur t. One in which the freezing point of water is 0° and the boiling point 80° with an interval of 80 points or degrees.

self-registering t. See maximum and minimum *t.*

spirit t. One in which alcohol or ether is used.

surface t. One for registering the surface temperature of any portion of the body.

wet and dry bulb t. A device for determining the relative humidity. It consists of two thermometers, the bulb of one of which is kept saturated with water vapor. The evaporation of water vapor has a cooling effect which depresses the temperature. The temperature difference between the two thermometers depends upon the relative humidity.

ther″mo·met′ric [*thermē; metron*]. Pertaining to a thermometer or to thermometry.

ther·mom′e·try [*thermē; metron*]. Measuring temperature with the thermometer.

ther″mo·neu·ro′sis [*thermē;* G. *neuron,* nerve; *-ōsis,* condition]. Pyrexia of vasomotor origin.

ther·moph′a·gy [*thermē;* G. *phagein,* to eat]. The habit of swallowing very hot food.

ther′mo·phile (thur′mo·file, ·fil) [*thermē;* G. *philein,* to love]. A microorganism for which the optimum temperature for growth is between 50°–55° C.; found in soil and water, especially hot springs.

ther″mo·phil′ic [*thermē; philein*]. Pertaining to a microorganism which grows best at high temperatures.

ther″mo·pho′bi·a [*thermē;* G. *phobos,* fear]. Morbid dread of heat.

ther′mo·phore [*thermē;* G. *phoros,* bearing]. Any appliance adapted to hold heat; as used in local treatment, a receptacle for hot water.

ther″mo·phyl′ic, ther″mo·phy′lic [*thermē;* G. *phyl*assein, to guard]. Resistance to the effect of heat.

ther′mo·pile [*thermē;* L. *pila,* pillar]. An instrument for measuring temperatures; it consists of a series of thermocouples which permit measurement of minute temperature effects.

ther″mo·ple′gi·a [*thermē;* G. *plēgē,* stroke]. Sunstroke.

ther″mo·pol″yp·ne′a [*thermē;* G. *polys,* many; *pnoē,* breathing hard]. Rapid respiration due to high temperature. —**thermopolypneic,** *adj.*

ther″mo·reg″u·la′tion [*thermē;* L. *regulare,* to regulate]. The regulation of heat production and heat loss to maintain normal temperature, as of the human body.

ther″mo·reg′u·la″tor. See *thermostat.*

ther′mo·scope [*thermē;* G. *skopein,* to examine]. An instrument for detecting changes or differences in temperature.

ther″mo·sta′ble [*thermē;* L. *stabilis,* stable]. Resistant to temperatures above a certain critical temperature, 56° C. —**thermostabil′ity,** *n.*

ther′mo·stat [*thermē;* G. *statos,* standing]. A device for automatically regulating and maintaining a constant temperature.

ther″mo·ste·re′sis [*thermē;* G. *sterēsis,* deprivation]. Deprivation of heat.

thermostromuhr of Rein. A flowmeter which measures the changes in the temperature of the blood resulting from its passage over a small heated coil surrounding a vessel.

ther″mo·sys·tal′tic [*thermē;* G. *systaltikos,* depressing]. Contracting under the influence of heat; pertaining to muscular contraction due to heat. —**thermosys′taltism,** *n.*

ther″mo·tac′tic op′ti·mum. That part of a room, cage, or floor which is most preferable in temperature, and to which an animal will go for comfort; the assumption is that the temperature stimuli on the skin of the feet control the response.

ther″mo·tax′is [*thermē;* G. *taxis,* arrangement]. 1. The regulation and correlation of heat production and heat dissipation. 2. Thermotropism. —**thermotactic, thermotaxic,** *adj.*

ther″mo·ther′a·py [*thermē;* G. *therapeia,* treatment]. Treatment of disease by heat of any kind.

ther″mo·to·nom′e·ter [*thermē;* G. *tonos,* a stretching; *metron,* a measure]. An apparatus for determining the amount of muscular contraction induced by thermic stimuli.

ther″mo·tox′in [*thermē;* G. *toxikon,* poison]. A poison produced by heat in the body.

ther″mo·tra″che·ot′o·my (thur″mo·tray″kee·ot′-o·mee) [*thermē;* G. *trachys,* rough; *tomē,* a cutting]. Tracheotomy by means of the actual cautery.

ther·mot′ro·pism [*thermē;* G. *trepein,* to turn]. That property possessed by some cells and organisms of moving or growing toward, or away from, heat.

the′ro·morph [G. *thēr,* beast of prey; *morphē,* form]. 1. One of an extinct order of reptiles, the Theromorpha, possible ancestors of the mammals. 2. A monster resembling an animal.

the″ro·mor′phi·a, the″ro·mor′phism [*thēr; morphē*]. Apparent reversion, in a human subject, to an animal form of lower type.

the·sau″ris·mo′sis [G. *thēsauros,* treasury; *-ōsis,* condition]. A storage disease, characterized by excess deposition of exogenous or endogenous substances within the body.

the′sis [G., a placing]. A dissertation. Usually, the essay presented by the candidate for a degree.

thesodate. Trade-mark for a brand of theobromine sodium acetate.

the′tin, the′tine. Any of a group of sulfur compounds, structurally resembling the betaines, having the general formula R_2:S.CH_2.COO, where R is commonly an alkyl group, as dimethyltetin.

thev′e·tin [after André *Thevet,* French author and traveler, 1502–90]. A poisonous glucoside with digitalislike action, from the seed of *Thevetia neriifolia.*

thi″a·ce′ta·zone, thi″a·cet′a·zone. British generic name for *amithiozone.*

thialixir. A proprietary thiamine hydrochloride elixir.

thi′a·min, thi′a·mine. See *thiamine hydrochloride.*

thi′a·min·ase. An enzyme, present in raw fish and in certain bacteria, which catalyzes cleavage of thiamine into pyramin (a pyrimidine derivative) and a thiazole derivative.

thi′a·min chlo′ride. Thiamine hydrochloride.

thi′a·mine hy″dro·chlo′ride (thigh′uh·meen, ·min) (*thiaminae hydrochloridum*). $C_{12}H_{17}ClN_4OS$.-HCl. White crystals or powder, soluble in water. An essential vitamin occurring in many natural sources, especially the seed coats of cereal grains; frequently it occurs in the form of the pyrophosphoric acid ester known as cocarboxylase. Commercial thiamine hydrochloride is largely synthetic. A deficiency of this vitamin is evidenced chiefly in the nervous system, the circulation, and the alimentary tract. Among the symptoms are irritability, emotional disturbances, multiple neuritis, increased pulse rate, dyspnea, edema, loss of appetite, reduced intestinal motility. A normal adult requires about 3 mg. (1/20 gr.) daily. Syn., *thiamin chloride, vitamin B_1, aneurin, aneurine hydrochloride.* Also called *thiamin* and *thiamine*, although these names are sometimes given to the basic form of the vitamin. See Table of Vitamins in the Appendix.

t. h. unit. Three micrograms of thiamine hydrochloride represent one International Unit.

thia·mine mon″o·ni′trate. $C_{12}H_{17}N_5O_4S$; a salt of thiamine, soluble in water, having in certain formulations greater stability than the hydrochloride; aqueous solutions are neutral; those of the hydrochloride are acid.

thi′a·mine py″ro·phos′phate. Cocarboxylase.

thi·am′y·lal so′di·um. Generic name for sodium 5-allyl-5-(1-methylbutyl)-2-thiobarbiturate, $C_{12}H_{17}N_2NaO_2S$, an intravenously administered, ultra-short-acting barbiturate, supplied under the trade-marked name *surital sodium.*

thiantoin. Trade-marked name for *phethenylate.*

thi′a·zine. Any of a group of heterocyclic compounds containing one nitrogen atom and one sulfur atom in the ring.

thi′a·zole. 1. Either of two isomeric heterocyclic compounds in which a sulfur atom, a nitrogen atom, and three CH groups are joined in the ring. 2. Any derivative of the preceding.

Thibierge, Georges [*French dermatologist,* 1856–1926]. Described calcinosis, called *Thibierge-Weissenbach syndrome.*

thick′wind″. See *heaves.*

Thiers, Joseph [*French physician,* 1885–]. Described, with E. C. Achard, the syndrome of hirsutism associated with diabetes (1921); called *Achard-Thiers syndrome.*

Thiersch, Carl [*German surgeon,* 1822–95]. Studied cancer, and advanced a theory of its epithelial origin (1865). Introduced a method of skin grafting in which strips of epithelium are sliced away by a razor and transferred directly to a granulating area; called *Thiersch* or *Ollier-Thiersch graft.* Contributed numerous procedures to plastic surgery, including repair of epispadias and closure of defect of the hard palate, each called *Thiersch's operation.*

thigenol. Trade-mark for a solution of the sodium salts of sulfo-oleic acids; the solution is used as a mild antiseptic and antipruritic, usually as 20% ointment.

thigh [AS. *thīoh*]. That part of the lower extremity from the pelvis to the knee.

thig″mes·the′si·a. Superficial touch sensibility.

thig″mo·tax′is. See *stereotaxis.*

thig·mot′ro·pism. Stereotropism.

thi·mer′o·sal. $C_6H_4.(COONa).SHgC_2H_5$; sodium ethylmercurithiosalicylate; a light cream-colored crystalline powder, freely soluble in water, bacteriostatic and fungistatic: used for disinfecting tissue surfaces and as a preservative of biological preparations. See *merthiolate.*

thi′o-, thi- [G. *theion,* brimstone]. A combining form denoting *the presence of sulfur.*

thi′o ac′id. An organic acid in which sulfur replaces oxygen.

thi′o al′co·hol. An alcohol in which sulfur replaces oxygen; a mercaptan.

thi″o·aur′in. A crystalline antibiotic substance isolated from cultures of an unclassified *Streptomyces.* It inhibits Gram-positive and Gram-negative bacteria, but shows little promise as a chemotherapeutic agent.

thi″o·bac·te′ri·a [*theion;* G. *baktērion,* little staff]. Bacteria which grow where decaying organic material releases hydrogen sulfide. Found in stagnant water and at the bottom of the sea. They are not pathogenic to man or animals.

thi″o·bar′bi·tal. 5,5-Diethylthiobarbituric acid; $C_8H_{12}N_2O_2S$; has been suggested for the control of hyperthyroidism.

thi″o·bar·bit′u·rate. A derivative of thiobarbituric acid, differing from the barbiturates only in the replacement of one oxygen atom by sulfur; they are analogous in their effects.

thi″o·bar″bi·tu′ric ac′id. $C_4H_4N_2O_2S$; malonyl thiourea, the parent compound of the thiobarbiturates. It represents barbituric acid in which the oxygen atom of the urea component has been replaced by sulfur.

thio-bismol. Trade-mark for sodium bismuth thioglycollate, of the approximate formula $Bi(SCH_2COONa)_3$, containing about 38% of bismuth: used as an antisyphilitic by intramuscular injection.

thi″o·car·bam′ide (thigh″o·kahr·bam′id, ·ide, thigh″o·kahr′buh·mid, ·mide). See *thiourea.*

thi″o·car·ban′i·lide. Any of a class of compounds of the general formula $R.C_6H_4.NH.CS.NH.C_6H_4.R'$, where R and R′ are various substituent groups. Several such compounds have antituberculous activity.

thi′o·chrome. $C_{12}H_{14}N_4OS$. A fluorescent oxidation product of thiamine hydrochloride or other derivatives of the basic form of the vitamin.

t. assay. A procedure for the analysis of thiamine hydrochloride or other derivatives of the basic form of the vitamin based on the intensity of the fluorescence produced by the thiochrome obtained by oxidation of the sample.

thiocol. Trade-mark for a brand of potassium guaiacolsulfonate.

thiocresol. *p*-Thiocresol. $C_6H_4SH.CH_3$. Crystalline leaflets of unpleasant odor, practically insoluble in water, soluble in alcohol; has been used as cell proliferant in wounds, ulcers.

thi·oc′tic ac′id. Any of several dithio-*n*-octanoic acids, particularly 6-thioctic acid which is 6,8-dithio-*n*-octanoic acid (also called *lipoic acid*) all of which are more or less able to promote oxidative decarboxylation of pyruvic acid by certain bacteria.

thi″o·cy′a·nate. Any compound containing the monovalent radical, —SCN. The sodium and potassium salts are used in the control of hypertension, but not without danger.

thi″o·cy·an′ic ac′id. HCNS; an unstable liquid acid, the potassium salt of which is employed therapeutically; several of its salts are useful analytical reagents. Syn., *sulfocyanic acid.*

thiodine. Trade-mark for certain antiseptic preparations containing ammonium ichthosulfonate, iodine tincture, boric acid, hydrastine, phenol, and glycerin.

thi′o e′ther. An ether containing sulfur instead of oxygen.

thi″o·glyc′er·ol (thigh″o·gliss′ur·ole, ·ol, ·awl). $CH_2OH.CHOH.CH_2SH$. Yellowish, viscous liquid, slightly soluble in water, miscible with alcohol; has been applied to wounds or ulcers as a 1:5000 suspension in tragacanth mucilage or in glycerin to promote healing.

thi′ol. 1. The univalent radical —SH, when occurring in organic compounds. 2. Any organic compound containing the —SH radical.

thi″ol·his′ti·dine. $C_3H_3SN_2.CH_2.CH(NH_2)-COOH$. Histidine in which a hydrogen atom in the imidazole group is replaced by a —SH (thiol) group. See *thioneine.*

thi′ol·prive. A substance reacting or interfering with the thiol activity of biologically functional molecules.

thi″o·lu′tin. An antibiotic substance isolated from several strains of *Streptomyces albus;* it inhibits, in vitro, Gram-negative and Gram-positive bacteria and many fungi.

thiomerin sodium. Trade-marked name for the mercurical diuretic *mercaptomerin sodium.*

thi″o·ne′ine. $C_9H_{15}N_3O_2S$. An amino-acid derivative, the betaine of thiolhistidine, which was first isolated from ergot and later shown to be a normal constituent of blood and especially of blood cells. Also known as *ergothioneine.*

thi·on′ic (thigh·on′ick) [*theion*]. Pertaining to sulfur.

thi′o·nine (thigh′o·neen, ·nin), **thi′o·nin.** $C_{12}H_{10}N_3S.HCl$. A dark green powder, solutions of which are purple; used as a stain in microscopy. Has been suggested for use in methemoglobinemia.

thi″o·pan′ic ac′id. Pantoyltaurine.

thi″o·pen′tal so′di·um. The U. S. Pharmacopeia title for the barbiturate available under the trade-marked name pentothal sodium.

thi″o·pen′tone so′di·um. The British Pharmacopoeia title for the barbiturate available under the trade-marked name pentothal sodium.

thi′o·phene. C_4H_4S; heterocyclic substance in coal tar and technical benzene; a liquid of slightly aromatic odor, insoluble in water.

t. diiodide. $C_4H_2I_2S$; has been used as an antiseptic dusting powder or ointment.

thi′o·phile (thigh′o·file, ·fil) [*theion;* G. *philein,* to love]. Loving sulfur; applied to microorganisms which require sulfur compounds for metabolism.

thi″o·phil′ic [*theion; philein*]. 1. Pertaining to, or characteristic of, a thiophile. 2. Thriving in sulfur.

thi″o·sem″i·car′ba·zone. A condensation product of an aldehyde or ketone with thiosemicarbazide, $NH_2.NH.CS.NH_2$. Certain thiosemicarbazones, such as amithiozone, possess a chemotherapeutic effect against tuberculosis.

thi″o·sin·am′ine (thigh″o·sin·am′een, ·in, ·sin′uh-meen, ·min, ·sin″uh·meen′). Allyl thiourea, $CH_2:CH.CH_2.NH.CS.NH_2$. White crystals of bitter taste and garlic odor, soluble in about 30 parts of water. It has been used to promote absorption of cicatrices. Syn., *rhodalline.* See *fibrolysin.*

thi″o·sul′fate. Any salt containing the divalent radical, S_2O_3.

thi″o·sul·fur′ic ac′id. $H_2S_2O_3$. An unstable acid, readily decomposing to sulfurous acid and sulfur.

thi″o·u′ra·cil. NH.CS.NH.CO.CH:CH (ring closed between the first NH and the terminal CH). White, crystalline powder, odorless, soluble in 2000 parts of water; readily soluble in alkalies. Used in the treatment of thyrotoxicosis. It interferes with the formation of thyroxin. See also *propylthiouracil.*

thi″o·u·re′a. $H_2N.CS.NH_2$. White crystals soluble in 11 parts of water. Has been used in the treatment of thyrotoxicosis. A photographic fixative. Syn., *thiocarbamide.* Also called *sulfocarbamide.*

thirst [AS. *thurst*]. A sensation associated with the need of the body for water. The sensory nerve endings for thirst are principally in the mucous membrane of the pharynx, and less than normal water content in this region supposedly produces thirst. Prolonged deprivation with dehydration of tissues produces severe unpleasant sensations probably of wide origin. These are more than thirst.

Thiry, Ludwig [*Austrian physiologist,* 1817–97]. Remembered for his production of a fistula, usually in a dog, for obtaining intestinal juices by means of a separated segment of gut, closed at one end and communicating with the exterior at the other (1865). A somewhat similar, but not identical, method was described by Luigi Vella (1881); called *Thiry fistula, Thiry-Vella fistula.*

thix·ot′ro·py [G. *thixis,* a touching; *trepein,* to turn]. The property of some gels, when mechanically agitated, to undergo a reversible isothermal solution and reconversion to a gel when allowed to stand. The tobacco mosaic virus has this property of thixotropy. —**thixotrop′ic,** *adj.*

thizodrin. Trade-mark for a nasal bacteriostat and vasoconstrictor containing sodium sulfathiazole and desoxyephedrine.

thlip″sen·ceph′a·lus [G. *thlipsis,* a crushing; *egkephalos,* brain]. A type of anencephalus in which the cranial vault is lacking; there is some degree of cervical spina bifida, and the brain is merely a spongy, vascular mass.

Thoma, Richard [*German histologist,* 1847–1923]. Invented an instrument for counting red and white cells, consisting of a chamber ruled into squares on a glass slide; called *Thoma-Zeiss counting chamber* or *cell, hemocytometer, Abbe-Zeiss counting cell.* Developed a pipet with an ampulla for collecting and diluting blood, called *Thoma's pipet.* Described the supposed dilatations at the terminations of the penicillar arteries of the spleen, called the *ampullae of Thoma.*

Thomas, André. See André Thomas' *sign.*

Thomas, Hugh Owen [*English orthopedist,* 1834–91]. Founder of orthopedic surgery in Great Britain and renowned internationally for his inventiveness in constructing orthopedic apparatus. Invented a number of iron splints, adapted to immobilizing tuberculous hip and knee joints; see Thomas *splint.* See also Thomas' *sign.*

Thomas, James William Tudor [*English ophthalmologist,* contemporary]. Known for his research, including experimental work, on transplantation of the cornea (1930). *Thomas' operation* for corneal transplantation consists of outlining a disk on the cornea with a trephine, and removing it with trephine and scissors in such a way that the endothelial surface is smaller than the epithelial. A clear disk is removed from the donor eye in the same way and is then sutured into place.

Thomas, Theodore Gaillard [*American physician,* 1832–1902]. Author of an outstanding textbook on diseases of women (1868). He is said to have performed the first vaginal oophorectomy (1870).

Thomas skin reaction test. See Naegeli *test.*

Thompson, Henry [*English surgeon,* 1820–1904]. Eminent urologist and teacher. Described an operation for urinary bladder tumors (1884), called *Thompson's operation.*

Thompson stain. See Dunn-Thompson *stain.*

Thomsen, Asmus Julius Thomas [*Danish physician,* 1815–96]. Described myotonia congenita (1876); also called *Thomsen's disease.*

Thomson, Allen [*Scottish anatomist,* 1809–84]. Described a fascia of yellow fibers which covers the inner half of the subcutaneous inguinal ring, called *Thomson's fascia.*

Thomson, Elihu [*American physicist and inventor,* 1853–1937]. Made the first practical application of the stereoscope to roentgenology (1896).

Thomson, Frederick Holland [*English physician,* 1867–1938]. Described a sign in scarlet fever in which two or three pink or red lines are present in the fold of the elbow; the lines first appear in the preeruptive stage, continuing through the course of the disease: called *Thomson's* or *Pastia's sign.*

Thomson, William. See *kelvin.*

Thom·so′ni·an·ism [after Samuel *Thomson,* American physician, 1769–1843]. A system of medicine which insisted on the use of vegetable remedies only.

thon·zyl'a·mine hy"dro·chlo'ride. 2-[(2-Dimethylaminoethyl)(*p*-methoxybenzyl)amino]pyrimidine hydrochloride; $C_{16}H_{22}N_4O.HCl$; an antihistaminic substance. See *neohetramine hydrochloride.*

tho"ra·cec'to·my [G. *thōrax*, thorax; *ektomē*, excision]. Resection of a rib.

tho"ra·cen·te'sis [*thōrax;* G. *kentēsis*, a pricking]. Aspiration of the chest cavity for removal of fluid, usually for hydrothorax or empyema.

tho·rac'ic. Pertaining to the thorax.

tho"ra·ci·co·lum'bar. Same as *thoracolumbar.*

tho·ra"ci·co·lum'bar sys'tem. See under *system.*

tho'ra·co-, thorac-, tho·rac'ic·o- [*thōrax*]. A combining form denoting *the thorax.*

tho"ra·co·a·ceph'a·lus [*thōrax;* G. *a-*, not; *kephalē*, head]. Thoracopagus parasiticus in which the parasite has no head. See *heteradelphus.*

tho"ra·co·a·cro'mi·al [*thōrax;* G. *akrōmia*, point of the shoulder]. Pertaining to the acromion and the chest, as thoracoacromial artery.

tho"ra·co·ce·los'chi·sis (·si·los'ki·sis) [*thōrax;* G. *koilia*, cavity; *schisis*, cleavage]. Congenital fissure of the chest and abdomen. Syn., *thoracogastroschisis.*

tho"ra·co·cen·te'sis. See *thoracentesis.*

tho"ra·co·cyl·lo'sis [*thōrax;* G. *kyllōsis*, from *kylloun*, to crook]. Deformity of the thorax.

tho"ra·co·cyr·to'sis (·sur·to'sis) [*thōrax;* G. *kyrtōsis*, convexity]. Excessive curvature of the thorax.

tho"ra·co·del'phus. See *thoradelphus.*

tho"ra·co·did'y·mus [*thōrax;* G. *didymos*, twin]. Thoracopagus.

tho"ra·co·dyn'i·a [*thōrax;* G. *odynē*, pain]. Pain in the chest.

tho"ra·co·gas"tro·did'y·mus [*thōrax;* G. *gastēr*, belly; *didymos*, twin]. A twin monstrosity united by the thorax and abdomen.

tho"ra·co·gas·tros'chi·sis (thor"uh·ko·gas·tros'ki·sis, tho·ray"ko·) [*thōrax; gastēr;* G. *schisis*, cleavage]. Congenital fissure of the thorax and abdomen. Syn., *thoracoceloschisis.*

tho"ra·co·lap"a·rot'o·my [*thōrax;* G. *lapara*, soft part of the body between the ribs and the hip; *tomē*, a cutting]. An operation in which both the thorax and the abdomen are opened. *Obs.*

tho"ra·co·lum'bar [*thōrax;* L. *lumbus*, loin]. Pertaining to the thoracic and lumbar portions of the spine, or to thoracic and lumbar ganglions and fibers of the autonomic nervous system.

tho"ra·col'y·sis. See *pneumonolysis.*

tho"ra·com'e·lus [*thōrax;* G. *melos*, limb]. A parasitic limb attached to the thorax of the host.

tho"ra·com'e·try [*thōrax;* G. *metron*, a measure]. Measurement of the chest.

tho"ra·cop'a·gus [*thōrax;* G. *pagos*, that which is fixed]. Conjoined twins united by their thoraxes or epigastric regions. See Plate 25. —**thoracopagous,** *adj.*

t. parasiticus. A more or less complete parasitic twin united with the thorax or epigastrium of the host.

t. tribrachius. Conjoined thoracopagous twins with two of the upper limbs coalescent.

t. tripus. Conjoined thoracopagous twins with two of the lower limbs coalescent.

tho"ra·co·par"a·ceph'a·lus [*thōrax;* G. *para*, beside; *kephalē*, head]. A thoracopagus parasiticus in which the parasite has a rudimentary head.

t. pseudoacormus. A thoracopagus parasiticus in which the parasite is little more than a head. See *heterodymus.*

tho"ra·co·par"a·si'tus [*thōrax;* G. *parasitos*, parasite]. Taruffi's term for thoracopagus parasiticus.

tho'ra·co·plas"ty [*thōrax;* G. *plassein*, to form]. The mobilization of the chest wall by the resection of any number of ribs, wholly or in part, in order to produce collapse of the chest wall and obliteration of the pleural cavity. The operation is commonly extrapleural and may be partial or complete, the latter involving segments of the first to eleventh ribs. It is also referred to by location, as anterior, lateral, posterior, apical, etc.

tho"ra·co·pneu'mo·plas"ty. See *thoracoplasty.*

tho"ra·cos'chi·sis (thor"uh·kos'ki·sis) [*thōrax;* G. *schisis*, cleavage]. Congenital fissure of the thorax.

tho·ra'co·scope, tho·rac'o·scope [*thōrax;* G. *skopein*, to examine]. An electrically lighted, tubular instrument designed for insertion between ribs into a pneumothorax space. Used for visual examination of the pleural surfaces and for the severance of pleural adhesion bands by electrocautery.

tho"ra·cos'co·py [*thōrax; skopein*]. Examination of the pleural cavity in the presence of a pneumothorax by means of a thoracoscope. Syn., *pleuroscopy.*

tho"ra·cos'to·my [*thōrax;* G. *stoma*, mouth]. Opening the chest; particularly, the removal of some ribs for drainage, or for access to the pleural cavity.

tho"ra·cot'o·my [*thōrax;* G. *tomē*, a cutting]. Incision of the thoracic wall.

tho"ra·del'phus [*thōrax;* G. *adelphos*, brother]. A double monster united above the umbilicus, with one head, four lower and two upper extremities. Also called *cephalothoracopagus dibrachius.*

Thoraeus filter. See under *filter.*

tho'rax (pl. *thoraxes, thoraces*) [G.]. The chest; that portion of the trunk above the diaphragm and below the neck; the framework of bones and soft tissues bounded by the diaphragm below, the ribs and sternum in front, the ribs and thoracic portion of the vertebral column behind, and above by the structures in the lower part of the neck, and containing the heart enclosed in the pericardium, the lungs invested by the pleura, and the mediastinal structures. —**thorac'ic,** *adj.*

thorazine hydrochloride. A trade-marked name for *chlorpromazine hydrochloride.*

Thorek, Max (1880–). American surgeon known for his technique of mammaplasty with free transplantation of the nipple, called *Thorek's mammaplasty*, and his operation for electrosurgical obliteration of the gallbladder.

tho'ri·um [*Thor*, Norse god of thunder]. Th = 232.05. A radioactive, grayish white, lustrous metal, the parent of a series of radioactive elements.

t. formate. Has been used in diarrhea and dysentery. See *thoroxyl.*

t. nitrate. $Th(NO_3)_4.4H_2O$. Has been used as a local astringent and antiparasitic.

t. oxide. ThO_2; white powder used as contrast medium for roentgenography; it may cause tissue damage. See *thorotrast, umbrathor.*

t. sodium citrate. Employed as a radiopaque medium for the preparation of cystograms.

t. sodium tartrate. Has been suggested as a diagnostic agent for the gastrointestinal tract.

t. X. An isotope of radium formed in the disintegration of thorium: used in dermatology in treatment of superficial conditions where irradiation is indicated.

Thorn, Wilhelm [*German gynecologist*, 1857–1913]. Described his method of converting a face presentation into a vertex by combined external and internal version; called *Thorn's method.*

thorn'-ap"ple. See *stramonium.*

Thornwaldt. See *Tornwaldt.*

tho'ron [*Thor*, Norse god of thunder]. Tn = 220. A gaseous, radioactive element evolved from thorium X, one of the disintegration products of thorium. Also called *thorium emanation.*

thorotrast. A proprietary stabilized suspension of thorium dioxide injected for radiologic visualization of the blood vessels, brain ventricles, liver, and spleen.

thor′ough·joint″. Diarthrosis or arthrodia. *Obs.*

thor′ough·pin″ [ME. *thoru;* AS. *pinn*]. A bursitis occurring over the tuber calcis of the hock joint of a horse.

thor′ough·wort. See *Eupatorium.*

thoroxyl. Trade-mark for a brand of thorium formate.

thor′ter ill. See *louping ill.*

thought read′ing. See *telepathy.*

thought trans·fer′ence. See *telepathy.*

thread [AS. *thrǣd*]. The spun and twisted fibers of cotton, linen, silk, etc.

mycelial threads. The hyphae of a mycelium.

nuclear threads. Chromatin fibrils of the cell nucleus.

Simonart's threads. See amniotic *band.*

thread′ed wire. Wire with screw threads: also called *Kirschner wire.*

thread′worm″. See *Nematoda, Trichuris, Enterobius.*

threm″ma·tol′o·gy [G. *thremma,* nursling; *logos,* word]. The breeding of plants and animals under domestication. *Obs.*

thre′o·nine (three′o·neen, ·nin). α-Amino-β-hydroxybutyric acid, $CH_3CHOH.CHNH_2.COOH$. An amino acid essential to human nutrition.

thre′o·nyl. The univalent radical, $CH_3CH(OH)$-$CH(NH_2)CO$—, of the amino acid threonine.

thre′ose. $CHO.HOCH.HCOH.CH_2OH$. A monosaccharide having a spatial configuration similar to that of threonine, the latter having for this reason been named after the former substance.

threp·sol′o·gy [G. *threpsis,* a nourishing; *logos*]. The science of nutrition.

thresh′old [AS. *therscwold*]. 1. The lower limit of stimulus capable of producing an impression upon consciousness or of evoking a response in an irritable tissue. 2. The entrance of a canal.

absolute t. The lowest limit of perception of a sensation.

auditory t. The minimum perceptible sound.

differential t. The lowest limit at which two stimuli can be discriminated.

double point t. The smallest distance apart at which two points can be felt as two.

excretion t. The critical concentration of a substance in the blood, above which the substance is excreted by the kidneys.

flicker-fusion t. The minimal frequency of standard flashes of light which will be seen as steady illumination. See *flicker-fusion test.*

ketosis t. The critical ratio at which ketone substances can be oxidized by the tissues as they are put forth by the liver. Ketosis occurs when the ketosis threshold has been passed and the liver is spilling out ketone substances faster than they can be oxidized by the tissues.

neuron t. See *neuron.*

pain t. The lowest limit of perceiving the sensation of pain.

relational t. The ratio of two stimuli when their difference is just perceptible.

stimulus t. See absolute *t.*

thrill [ME. *thrillen,* to pierce]. A fine vibration felt by the hand. A thrill may be felt on palpation over an aneurysm, over a heart which is the seat of valvular disease, and over certain cysts.

diastolic t. The vibration felt in the region of the heart during the diastole of the ventricle.

presystolic t. A thrill which can sometimes be felt before the systole when the hand is placed over the apex beat (mitral stenosis).

purring t. A thrill resembling that felt when the hand is placed on the back of a purring cat.

thrix an″nu·la′ta. Hairs with alternating light and dark segments.

throat [AS. *throte*]. The pharynx and the fauces.

sore t. Pharyngitis and/or tonsillitis.

throb [ME. *throbben,* imitative in origin]. A pulsation or beating.

throe [AS. *thrauu*]. A violent pang, as in parturition.

throm′base [G. *thrombos,* lump]. Thrombin.

throm″bas·the′ni·a [*thrombos;* G. *astheneia,* weakness]. Hemorrhagic disease dependent on an abnormality of the blood platelets.

hereditary hemorrhagic t. See hereditary hemorrhagic *diathesis.*

throm·bec′to·my [*thrombos;* G. *ektomē,* excision]. Excision of a thrombus.

throm′bin [*thrombos*]. An enzyme elaborated in shed blood from an inactive precursor, prothrombin. It induces clotting by converting fibrinogen to fibrin, possibly by proteolysis, and is used therapeutically as a topical hemostatic agent. Also called *thrombase;* formerly called *fibrin ferment.*

throm·bin′o·gen. See *prothrombin.*

throm′bo-, thromb- [*thrombos*]. A combining form denoting *pertaining to a thrombus.*

throm″bo·an″gi·i′tis [*thrombos;* G. *aggeion,* vessel; *-itis,* inflammation]. Thrombosis with inflammation of the intima of a vessel.

t. obliterans. A disease characterized by minute, widespread, fugitive phlebitis with perivascular fibrosis involving the accompanying arteries and nerves. Seen chiefly in young or middle-aged males. Also called *Buerger's disease.*

throm″bo·ar″te·ri′tis [*thrombos;* G. *artēria,* artery; *-itis*]. Inflammation of an artery associated with thrombosis.

t. obliterans. See *thromboangiitis* obliterans.

throm′bo·blast [*thrombos;* G. *blastos,* germ]. The precursor of the thrombocyte; megakaryocyte.

throm·boc′la·sis [*thrombos;* G. *klasis,* a breaking]. Breaking up or destruction of a thrombus; thrombolysis. —**thromboclas′tic,** *adj.*

throm′bo·cyte [*thrombos;* G. *kytos,* cell]. Blood platelet; a small, colorless disk in the circulating blood of all mammals; it contains thromboplastin and is important in the clotting of blood. Normally, 1 cu. mm. of blood contains 250,000 to 500,000 platelets. Syn., *platelet, blood platelet.* —**thrombocyt′ic,** *adj.*

throm″bo·cy·the′mi·a. See *thrombocytopenia.*

throm″bo·cyt′ic se′ries. The series of cells concerned in the origin of blood platelets (thrombocytes), including the megakaryoblasts and megakaryocytes which occur normally in bone marrow.

throm″bo·cy′to·crit [*thrombos; kytos;* G. *krinein* to distinguish]. A glass tube introduced by Van Allen for counting blood platelets. Blood diluted with sodium oxalate is centrifuged in a special spherical sedimentation chamber so that the platelets are seen layered above the red cells. This volume can be measured. Normal is 0.35 to 0.67 per cent.

throm″bo·cy″to·ly′sin. A substance which disrupts platelets.

throm″bo·cy″to·path′i·a. A hemorrhagic state in which the blood platelets are functionally abnormal.

throm″bo·cy″to·pe′ni·a [*thrombos; kytos;* G. *penia,* want]. A condition in which there is a decrease in the number of blood platelets below normal. —**thrombocytopenic,** *adj.*

tropical t. See *onyalai.*

throm″bo·cy·to′sis (throm″bo·sigh·to′sis) [*thrombos; kytos;* G. *-ōsis,* condition]. A condition marked by the presence of a large number of thrombocytes in the blood.

throm″bo·em″bo·li·za′tion [*thrombos;* G. *embolē,* a putting in]. The occlusion of a blood vessel by the lodgment of a portion of a thrombus.

throm″bo·en″dar·ter·ec′to·my. See *endarterectomy.*

throm″bo·en″do·car·di′tis [*thrombos;* G. *endon,* within; *kardia,* heart]. Bacterial or nonbacterial thrombotic vegetations on heart valves.

throm′bo·gen. See *prothrombin.*

throm″bo·gen′ic [*thrombos; genesthai*]. 1. Producing thrombi. 2. Relating to thrombogen.

throm″bo·kin′ase (throm″bo·kin′ace, ·kigh′nace). A substance, probably an enzyme, obtainable from plasma globulins and also found in some crude tissue extracts, having the capacity of activating prothrombin to thrombin. It is considered by some to be identical with thromboplastin, but the latter may instead be an important accessory factor, along with calcium ions, in converting prothrombin to thrombin. Thrombokinase appears to exist in an inactive form called *prothrombokinase.* See *thrombozym.*

thrombol. Trade-mark for a hemostatic containing blood-clotting principles extracted from fresh tissue. The substance is used locally in hemorrhage.

throm″bo·lym″phan·gi′tis [*thrombos;* L. *lympha,* water; G. *aggeion,* vessel; *-itis,* inflammation]. Lymphangitis with thrombosis.

throm·bol′y·sis [*thrombos;* G. *lysis,* a loosing]. Destruction or dissolution of a thrombus; thromboclasis. —**thrombolyt′ic,** *adj.*

throm·bop′a·thy [*thrombos;* G. *pathos,* disease]. Disease characterized by disturbance of platelet formation and consequent interference with the formation of blood clots.

constitutional t. See hereditary hemorrhagic *diathesis.*

throm″bo·pe′ni·a [*thrombos;* G. *penia,* want]. A decrease in platelets. —**thrombopenic,** *adj.*

throm″bo·phil′i·a [*thrombos;* G. *philein,* to love]. A tendency to form thrombi.

essential t. Diffuse thrombosis of the arteries and veins not accounted for by infection, stasis, or local inflammatory lesions. An increase of the coagulability of the plasma seems to be the primary factor.

throm″bo·phle·bi′tis [*thrombos;* G. *phleps,* vein; *-itis,* inflammation]. Inflammation of a vein associated with thrombosis.

throm″bo·plas′tic [*thrombos;* G. *plassein,* to form]. Causing or hastening the coagulation of the blood.

throm″bo·plas′tin [*thrombos; plassein*]. Commonly, any of a group of diverse preparations, obtained from blood platelets or fixed tissue (including brain phosphatide) extracts, which accelerate appearance of thrombin in prothrombin-containing systems, regardless of mode of action. Some consider thromboplastin to be the factor which activates prothrombin, thereby making it identical with thrombokinase. Also called *thromboplastic substance.*

throm″bo·plas·tin′o·gen. A protein precursor in plasma which is necessary for the elaboration of plasma thromboplastic activity, distinct from plasma thromboplastin antecedent (PTA) and plasma thromboplastin component (PTC). Syn., *antihemophilic globulin, globulin substance, antihemophilic factor.*

throm″bo·plas″tin·o·pe′ni·a [*thrombos; plassein;* G. *penia,* want]. A deficiency of thromboplastin in the blood.

throm″bo·poi·e′sis [*thrombos;* G. *poiēsis,* production]. The production of blood platelets and other elements necessary for thrombus formation.

throm′bose. To form or become a thrombus.

throm′bosed [*thrombos*]. 1. Affected with thrombosis. 2. Clotted.

throm′bo·sin [*thrombos*]. Old term for thrombin.

throm·bo′sis [G., a becoming curdled]. The formation of a thrombus. —**thrombot′ic,** *adj.*

atrophic t. That due to general malnutrition.

cardiac t. Thrombosis in the heart.

cavernous sinus t. Inflammation of a cavernous sinus with thrombus formation, usually secondary to staphylococcus infection of the nares and upper lip.

coagulation t. That caused by fibrin coagulation.

compression t. That due to compression of a vessel, as by a tumor.

coronary t. Thrombosis of the coronary arteries of the heart.

dilatation t. That which results from the slowing of the blood current next to the vessel walls as the result of dilatation of a vessel (as in aneurysms, varices) or of the heart.

intervillous t. Coagulation of blood in the intervillous spaces of the placenta, usually seen near the end of pregnancy: also called *placentosis.*

lateral sinus t. Thrombosis of a lateral sinus due to extension of infection from mastoid air cells. The thrombus may be attached to the wall (mural thrombus) or it may completely obliterate the sinus.

marantic t. See atrophic *t.*

marasmic t. See atrophic *t.*

placental t. That of the uterine veins at the site of a placenta.

plate t. See blood plate *thrombus.*

puerperal venous t. Puerperal thrombosis of pelvic veins.

throm″bo·sta′sis [G. *thrombos,* lump; *stasis,* a standing]. Stasis of blood leading to formation of a thrombus.

throm′bo·zym. A substance, occurring in plasma and in tissue extracts, which is active in bringing about the clotting of blood. It may be identical with, or contain, thrombokinase.

throm′bus (pl. *thrombi*) [*thrombos*]. A clot of blood formed within the heart or blood vessels, due usually to a slowing of the circulation or to alteration of the blood or vessel walls. —**thromboid,** *adj.*

annular t. One involving the whole circumference of a vessel but not entirely occluding it.

ante-mortem t. An intravascular blood clot which occurs before death.

autochthonous t. See blood plate *t.*

ball t. A small or large, rounded, ante-mortem clot found in the heart, especially in an atrium.

ball-valve t. See ball *t.*

blood plate t. That ascribed by Eberth to agglutination of blood plates.

coronary t. One that affects a branch of a coronary artery.

currant-jelly t. A soft, reddish, postmortem clot.

fibrolaminar t. See stratified *t.*

globoid t. See ball *t.*

hyaline t. One found in the smaller blood vessels, as a glossy fibrinous mass. Probably due to toxic injuries to the intima.

Laennec's t. A globular thrombus formed in the heart, especially in cases where the latter is the seat of fatty degeneration.

lateral t. A clot attached to a vessel wall, and not completely obstructing the lumen.

marantic t. One occurring in an area of retarded flow, as the atria.

mixed t. See stratified *t.*

mural t. One attached to the wall of a blood vessel or mural endocardium: also called *lateral t., parietal t.*

obstructing t. One completely obstructing the lumen of a vessel.

parietal t. One adherent to the wall of a vessel or the heart and not entirely occluding the lumen.

progressive t. One that grows into the lumen of a vessel.

red t. One composed principally of red cells and fibrin intimately mixed, commonly formed by clotting of blood in an occluded vessel.

saddle t. A Y-shaped clot straddling the bifurcation of a vessel: also called *riding t.*

stratified t. One in which there are successive layers of fibrin and red cells to produce a mixture of colors. Syn., *fibrolaminar t., mixed t.*

t. neonatorum. See *cephalhematoma.*

t. vulvae. Hematoma of a labium majus.

white t. One composed principally of a deposit of fibrin, such as those seen on the chordae tendinae in the heart.

throt′tle [dim. from AS. *throte*]. The throat.

throt′tle. To choke; to suffocate.

through drain′age. A method of drainage in which a perforated tube is carried through the cavity to be drained, so that the latter can be flushed through and through by the injection of fluid into one end of the tube.

throw′back″ [ME. *throwen;* AS. *baec*]. A reversion to an ancestral type. See *atavism.*

thrush [D. *tröske*]. 1. A form of moniliasis due to infection by *Candida albicans.* It occurs most often in children and is characterized by small, whitish spots on the tip and sides of the tongue and the buccal mucous membrane. Syn., *mycotic stomatitis, parasitic stomatitis.* 2. A diseased condition of the frog of the horse's foot, with a fetid discharge.

sheep t. See *orf.*

thrush fun′gus. *Candida albicans.* A fungus of low pathogenicity which inhabits the mucous membranes.

Thu′ja (thew′jah, thew′yah) [G. *thyia,* odorous cedar]. A genus of trees of the Pinaceae. The leafy young twigs of **T. occidentalis** were once used as an antipyretic, expectorant, and anthelmintic.

thu″ja·pli′cin. $C_7H_4.CH(CH_3)_2.O.(OH)$; any of three isomeric substance, designated α-, β-, and γ-thujaplicin, being isopropyl derivatives of tropolone. They occur naturally in various woods, and have antibiotic properties against organisms harmful to trees.

thu′jic ac′id. $C_7H_5(CH_3)_2COOH$; a substance, characterized by a 7-membered cyclic structure, isolated from *Thuja plicata,* the so-called western red cedar, which is antibiotic to wood-destroying fungi and is presumably responsible for the great durability of the wood.

thu′jone. A cyclic ketone, $C_{10}H_{16}O$, found in thuja, tansy, wormwood, and sage oils. It is convulsant in large doses.

thu′li·um [L. *Thule,* northernmost limit of the habitable world]. Tm = 168.94. A rare earth metal.

thumb [AS. *thūma*]. The digit on the radial side of the hand, differing from the other digits in having but two phalanges, and in that its metacarpal bone is freely movable.

thumps [imitative in origin]. 1. A disease of swine caused by the larvae of *Ascaris lumbricoides* in the lungs. 2. An affection in the horse, similar to hiccup in man, due to spasmodic contraction of the diaphragm.

Thunberg and Ahlgren method. See under *method.*

thus [L.]. 1. True frankincense or olibanum. 2. Turpentine of pine trees.

thydron. A proprietary syrup and tablet containing ferrous sulfate and thiamine hydrochloride.

thy″la·ken′trin (thigh″luh·ken′trin). Follicle-stimulating hormone: old term.

thyloquinone. Trade-mark for a brand of menadione.

thyme (time) [G. *thymon,* thyme]. The dried leaves and flowering tops of *Thymus vulgaris* (family Lamiaceae) yielding not less than 1.5% of volatile oil. A diaphoretic and carminative; used in coughs and as a condiment.

t. camphor. Thymol.

t. oil (*oleum thymi*). The volatile oil from the flowering plant. It yields not less than 20% of phenols, chiefly thymol. A germicide.

thy·mec′to·my (thigh·meck′to·mee) [G. *thymos,* mind, soul; *ektomē,* excision]. Excision of the thymus. —**thymectomize,** *v.*

thy′mene (thigh′meen, tigh′meen). $C_{10}H_{16}$. A terpene in thyme oil, identical with *l*-pinene found in turpentine oil from certain species of *Pinus.*

thy″mer·ga′si·a (thigh″mur·gay′zhuh, ·zee·uh) [*thymos;* G. *ergasia,* a working]. *In psychiatry,* Meyer's term for the affective-reaction psychoses such as manic-depressive psychosis and involutional melancholia. —**thymergasic,** *adj.*

-thy′mi·a [*thymos*]. A combining form denoting *a condition of mind.*

thy′mic (tigh′mick) [G. *thymon,* thyme]. Pertaining to, or contained in, thyme.

thy′mic (thigh′mick) [G. *thymos,* mind, soul]. Pertaining to the thymus.

thy′mic nu·cle′ic ac′id. See *desoxyribonucleic acid.*

thy″mi·co·lym·phat′ic [*thymos;* L. *lympha,* water]. Affecting the thymus and lymphatic structures such as spleen, lymph nodes, and lymphoid aggregates, as thymicolymphatic state.

thy′mi·dine. $C_{10}H_{14}N_2O_5$; thymine-2-desoxyriboside; a nucleoside obtained from thymonucleic acid, essential for growth of certain organisms in media devoid of vitamin B_{12} and folic acid.

thy′mine (thigh′meen, ·min). 2,4-Dihydroxy-5-methylpyrimidine; a substance, first isolated from the thymus, which may be of value in nutritional macrocytic anemia.

thy′mi·on [G., large wart]. A wart; a condyloma.

thy·mi′tis [G. *thymos,* mind, soul; *-itis,* inflammation]. Inflammation of the thymus.

thy′mo-, thym- [G. *thymon,* thyme]. A combining form denoting *thymol;* also referring to *thymus.*

thy″mo·cres′cin [G. *thymos,* mind, soul; L. *crescere,* to grow]. A principle, claimed to be present in extracts of the thymus, that has growth-promoting properties.

thy′mo·cyte [*thymos;* G. *kytos,* cell]. A lymphocyte formed in the thymus.

thy″mo·hy″dro·qui·none′ (thigh″mo·high″dro-kwi·nohn′, ·kwin′ohn). A substance occurring in the urine after the ingestion of thymol, producing a greenish color of the urine.

thy″mo·ke′sis [*thymos*]. Abnormal persistence or enlargement of the thymus.

thy′mol (thigh′mole, ·mol, ·mawl, tigh′·). Methyl-propyl-phenol. A crystalline phenol, $C_{10}H_{14}O$, obtained from the volatile oils of many plants including *Thymus vulgaris, Monarda punctata, Trachyspermum ammi,* and others. It is also synthesized. It is a bactericide and fungicide, and has been used as an intestinal antiseptic. As an anthelmintic its therapeutic dose too closely approximates the toxic dose.

t. blue. Thymolsulfonphthalein. $C_{27}H_{30}O_5S$. Brownish green, crystalline powder soluble in alcohol. An indicator covering the pH ranges 1.2 to 2.8 and 8.0 to 9.6.

t. carbonate. $(C_{10}H_{13}O_2)CO$: formerly used as an anthelmintic.

t. iodide (*thymolis iodidum*). A mixture of iodine derivatives of thymol, chiefly dithymoldiiodide, $(C_6H_2.CH_3.C_3H_7.OI)_2$. A reddish yellow powder, affected by light; insoluble in water, slightly soluble in alcohol. Soluble in fixed and volatile oils. Used as an antiseptic dusting powder. See *aristol.*

thy″mol·phthal′ein (·thal′in, ·thal′ee·in, ·fthal′·). A compound, analogous to phenolphthalein, used as an indicator; it is colorless below pH 9.3 and blue at pH 10.5.

thy″mol·sul″fon·phthal′e·in, thy″mol·sul″fone·phthal′e·in. Thymol blue.

thy·mo′ma (thigh·mo′muh) [*thymos;* G. *-ōma,* tumor]. A primary tumor of the thymus. Frequently associated with myasthenia gravis, but no clear interrelationship is established. Also see thymic *carcinoma,* thymic *sarcoma.*

thy″mo·no′ic [*thymos;* G. *nous,* mind]. Pertaining to thoughts and ideas which are strongly influenced by deviations in mood.

thy″mo·nu·cle′ic ac′id. Desoxyribonucleic acid.

thy·mop′a·thy (thigh·mop′uth·ee) [*thymos;* G. *pathos,* disease]. Any disease of the thymus.

thy′mo·pex″y [*thymos;* G. *pēxis,* a fixing]. The fixation into a new position of thymus. *Obs.*

thy″mo·priv′ic [*thymos;* L. *privus,* deprived of]. Related to, or caused by, removal of or premature involution of the thymus.

thy·mop′riv·ous. See *thymoprivic.*

thy′mus [*thymos*]. An organ situated in the anterior superior mediastinum. It continues to develop until the second year of life, afterward remains stationary until about the fourteenth, and then undergoes fatty metamorphosis and atrophy. It consists of lobules largely composed of lymphatic tissue in which are found minute concentric bodies, the remnants of epithelial structures, or thymic corpuscles. See Plate 45.

thy′mus nu·cle′ic ac′id. See *desoxyribonucleic acid.*

thyractin. Trade-mark for a preparation from the thyroid gland containing about 0.6% iodine and used in conditions where thyroid medication is indicated.

thy′re·o-. For words beginning with *thyreo-* not found here, see words beginning *thyro-*.

thy″re·o·a·pla′si·a con·gen′i·ta (thigh″ree·o·a·play′zhuh, ·zee·uh, ·shuh, ·see·uh). Anomalies found in congenital defects of the thyroid gland and in deficient thyroid secretion.

thy″re·o·gen′ic. Of thyroid origin, as thyreogenic obesity (obesity due to thyroid deficiency).

thy′ro- [G. *thyreoeidēs,* shield-shaped]. A combining form signifying *thyroid.*

thy″ro·ad″e·ni′tis [*thyreoeidēs;* G. *adēn,* gland; *-itis,* inflammation]. Inflammation of the thyroid gland.

thy″ro·ar″y·te′noid [*thyreoeidēs;* G. *arytainoeidēs,* shaped like a ladle]. Pertaining to the thyroid and arytenoid cartilages, as the thyroarytenoid ligaments, thyroarytenoid muscle.

thy″ro·car′di·ac [*thyreoeidēs;* G. *kardia,* heart]. Pertaining to thyroid disease with cardiac symptoms predominating.

thy′ro·cele [*thyreoeidēs;* G. *kēlē,* tumor]. A tumor affecting the thyroid gland; goiter.

thy″ro·chon·drot′o·my (thigh″ro·k on·drot′o·mee) [*thyreoeidēs;* G. *chondros,* cartilage; *tomē,* a cutting]. Incision of the thyroid cartilage; laryngotomy.

thy″ro·cri·cot′o·my (thigh″ro·cry·cot′o·mee, ·kri·cot′o·mee) [*thyreoeidēs;* G. *krikos,* ring; *tomē*]. Tracheotomy performed through the cricothyroid membrane.

thy″ro·ep″i·glot′tic [*thyreoeidēs;* G. *epiglōttis,* epiglottis]. Pertaining to the thyroid cartilage and the epiglottis, as the thyroepiglottic muscle.

thy·rog′en·ous, thy″ro·gen′ic. Thyreogenic.

thy″ro·glob′u·lin [*thyreoeidēs;* L. *globulus,* little ball]. The iodine-protein of the thyroid, secreted by it and lodged in the colloid substance. See Table of Hormones in the Appendix.

thy″ro·glos′sal [*thyreoeidēs;* G. *glōssa,* tongue]. Pertaining to the thyroid and the tongue.

thy″ro·hy′al [*thyreoeidēs;* G. *hyoeidēs,* shaped like the letter upsilon]. The greater cornu of the hyoid bone.

thy″ro·hy′oid [*thyreoeidēs; hyoeidēs*]. Pertaining to the thyroid cartilage and hyoid bone, as the thyrohyoid membrane.

thy′roid [*thyreoeidēs*]. 1. Shield-shaped. 2. Pertaining to the thyroid gland. 3. Pertaining to the thyroid cartilage. See Plates 13, 45.

thy′roid. 1. The thyroid gland. See Plates 13, 45. 2. The cleaned, dried, and powdered thyroid gland previously deprived of connective tissue and fat; it is obtained from domesticated animals that are used for food by man. Contains 0.17 to 0.23 per cent iodine in thyroid combination, especially as thyroxin. Administered orally in the treatment of thyroid deficiency states. Dose, 60 mg. (1 gr.).

thy″roid·ec′to·my [*thyreoeidēs;* G. *ektomē,* excision]. Partial or complete excision of the thyroid gland.

thy′roid·ism [*thyreoeidēs*]. 1. Disturbances produced by hypertrophy of the thyroid gland. 2. A series of phenomena due to continued use of thyroid preparations.

thy″roid·i′tis [*thyreoeidēs;* G. *-itis,* inflammation]. Inflammation of the thyroid gland. See Riedel's *struma.*

thy″roid·i·za′tion [*thyreoeidēs*]. Treatment with thyroid gland preparations.

thy″roid·ot′o·my [*thyreoeidēs;* G. *tomē,* a cutting]. Incision of the thyroid gland.

thy·roid″o·tox′in (thigh·roy″do·tock′sin) [*thyreoeidēs;* G. *toxikon,* poison]. A substance specifically toxic for the cells of the thyroid gland.

thy″ro·i′o·dine (thigh″ro·eye′o·dyne, ·deen, ·din). A substance, now known not to be a chemical entity, formerly thought to be the active principle of thyroid. Syn., *iodothyrine.*

thy′ro·nyl. The univalent radical, p-$(p$-$HOC_6H_4O)$-$C_6H_4CH_2CH(NH_2)CO$—, of thyronine, the amino acid resulting when the iodine atoms in thyroxine are replaced by hydrogen atoms.

thy″ro·par″a·thy″roid·ec′to·my. Excision of the thyroid and parathyroid glands.

thy″ro·phar·yn·ge′us. A portion of the inferior constrictor muscle of the pharynx.

thy″ro·pri′val (thigh″ro·pry′vul, thigh·rop′ri·vul) [*thyreoeidēs;* L. *privus,* deprived of]. Pertaining to loss of function, or removal, of the thyroid gland.

thy″ro·pri′vus [*thyreoeidēs privus*]. Deprived of the thyroid gland.

thy″ro·pri′vus. A disease due to loss of thyroid activity.

thy″ro·pro′te·in (thigh″ro·pro′tee·in, ·pro′teen) [*thyreoeidēs;* G. *prōteios,* of first rank]. A protein from the thyroid gland.

thy″rop·to′sis [*thyreoeidēs;* G. *ptōsis,* a falling]. Displacement of a goitrous thyroid so that it is partially or completely concealed in the thorax.

thy·ro′sis (thigh·ro′sis) [*thyreoeidēs;* G. *-ōsis,* condition]. Any disorder caused by abnormal function of the thyroid gland.

thy″ro·ther′a·py [*thyreoeidēs;* G. *therapeia,* treatment]. Treatment of disease by thyroid gland preparations.

thy·rot'o·my (thigh·rot'o·mee) [*thyreoeidēs;* G. *tomē*, a cutting]. Incision or splitting of the thyroid cartilage.

thy"ro·tox'ic [*thyreoeidēs;* G. *toxikon*, poison]. Pertaining to disease caused by excessive activity of the thyroid gland or excessive thyroid hormone action.

thy"ro·tox"i·co'sis [*thyreoeidēs; toxikon;* G. *-ōsis*, condition]. Hyperthyroidism of any type.

thy"ro·tox'in [*thyreoeidēs; toxikon*]. Any substance which is toxic to the thyroid cells.

thy·rot'ro·phin (thigh·rot'ro·fin). See *thyrotropin.*

thy·rot'ro·pin. A thyroid-stimulating hormone (TSH) produced by the adenohypophysis: formerly spelled *thyrotrophin.*

thy·rox'in (thigh·rock'sin), **thy·rox'ine** (thigh·rock'seen, ·sin). $HOC_6H_2I_2OC_6H_2I_2CH_2CH(NH_2)COOH$. An active physiologic principle obtained from the thyroid gland or prepared synthetically; contains about 64 per cent iodine. Occurs as white crystals, insoluble in water. It is used for the same purposes as thyroid, but the latter is preferred. Dose, 0.5 mg. ($\frac{1}{120}$ gr.). Until recently the synthetic form was the racemic product; now the L-form, identical with natural thyroxin, is prepared by synthesis and advocated for therapeutic use. See Table of Hormones in the Appendix.

thy·rox"in·so'di·um. Thyroxin treated with sodium. Also spelled *thyroxine-sodium.*

Ti Chemical symbol for titanium.

ti·ba'tin, tib'a·tin. 4,4'-Diaminodiphenylsulfone bis-*d*-galactoside: said to be effective against *β*-hemolytic streptococci. It has been used experimentally to combat tuberculosis.

tib'i·a [L.]. The larger of the two bones of the leg, commonly called the shinbone, articulating with the femur, fibula, and talus. See Table of Bones in the Appendix. See Plates 1, 2. —**tibial,** *adj.*

saber t. Anterior bowing and thickening of the tibia due to periostitis caused by congenital syphilis or yaws. Also called *saber shin, boomerang leg.*

tib"i·al'gi·a [*tibia;* G. *algos*, pain]. Pain in the tibia.

tib"i·a'lis (tib"ee·ah'lis, ·ay'lis) [L., of the shinbone]. One of two muscles of the leg, **tibialis anterior** and **tibialis posterior.** See Table of Muscles in the Appendix.

t. secundus. An occasional small muscle arising from the lower third of the body of the fibula and inserted into the capsule of the ankle joint.

tib'i·o- [L. *tibia*, shinbone]. A combining form signifying *tibia.*

tib"i·o·fib'u·lar [*tibia;* L. *fibula*, clasp]. Pertaining to the tibia and the fibula.

tibione. Trade-mark for *amithiozone.*

tic [F.]. A twitching, especially of the facial muscles; a habit spasm.

convulsive t. Spasm of the facial muscles.

diaphragmatic t. Rapid regular contraction of the diaphragm, often mimicking angina pectoris. Syn., *diaphragmatic flutter.*

painless t. The occurrence, at intervals, of sudden rapid involuntary contraction in a muscle or group of muscles.

t. douloureux. Paroxysmal neuralgia of the trigeminal nerve.

t. rotatoire. Spasmodic torticollis, spinal accessory spasm; a spasm of certain muscles by which the head and neck are forcibly rotated to one side or from one side to the other.

Tichy, Vladimir Leslie [*American surgeon,* 1899–]. With Claude Schaeffer Beck, performed cardiomyopexy and cardiopericardipexy as an experimental study in providing collateral circulation to the heart (1935).

tick [ME. *tike*]. An arthropod of the order Acarina infesting vertebrate animals. They are important vectors and reservoirs of rickettsial diseases. They also transmit many viral, bacterial, and protozoal diseases. Toxins produced by the female before oviposition produce tick paralysis. The important genera are *Amblyomma, Argas, Boöphilus, Dermacentor, Haemaphysalis, Hyalomma, Ixodes, Ornithodorus,* and *Rhipicephalus.*

tick'ling. A rapid series of light, tactile stimulations of skin or mucous membrane arousing a tingling sensation.

tic"po·lon'ga. See *Vipera russellii.*

tic·tol'o·gy [G. *tiktein*, to bring forth; *logos*, word]. Obstetrics.

t. i. d. *Ter in die,* three times a day.

ti'dal drain'age. Drainage of a paralyzed urinary bladder with an automatic irrigation apparatus.

tide [AS. *tīd*]. A definite period of time.

acid t. A period of increased excretion of acid radicals by the kidney after meals, while excessive alkali is secreted into the duodenum.

alkaline t. The transient increase in the alkalinity of the urine during gastric digestion, presumably related to the secretion of hydrochloric acid into the stomach and the resulting relative excess of base in the blood. It is diminished or absent in achlorhydria.

Tiedemann, Friedrich [*German anatomist,* 1781–1861]. Remembered for his description of the greater vestibular glands; also called *Tiedemann's glands,* but more often *Bartholin's glands.* Described a plexus of nerve fibers derived from the ciliary nerves and surrounding the central artery of the retina; called *Tiedemann's nerve.*

Tietze, Alexander [*German surgeon,* 1864–1927]. Described painful, nonsuppurative swelling of the rib cartilages, called *Tietze's disease.*

ti'ger lil'y ap·pear'ance. The speckled appearance of the myocardium observed in pernicious anemia.

ti·gog'e·nin (ti·godj'i·nin). The aglycone of tigonin.

tig'o·nin. A saponin from *Digitalis purpurea.* On acid hydrolysis it yields the steroid aglycone tigogenin, glucose, galactose, and rhamnose.

ti'groid [G. *tigroeidēs*, like a tiger]. A term applied to masses of chromophil substance in nerve cells.

ti·grol'y·sis (tye·grol'i·sis) [*tigroeidēs;* G. *lysis*, a loosing]. Disintegration of the chromophil substance in a nerve cell.

ti'ki·ti'ki (tee'kee·tee'kee). See *rice* polishings.

Tilbury Fox. See William Tilbury *Fox.*

Til'i·a [L., linden]. A genus of trees—the linden or basswood.

til·i'a·cin [*tilia*]. A glucoside found in the leaves of the linden tree.

Tillaux, Paul Jules [*French surgeon,* 1834–1904]. With B. G. Phocas, described a form of chronic mastitis associated with small, fibrous nodules; called *Tillaux-Phocas disease, Phocas' disease.*

tim'bre. The peculiar quality of a tone, other than pitch and intensity, that makes it distinctive. It depends upon the overtones of the vibrating body.

time [AS. *tīma*]. The duration of an event or phenomenon. For specific time measurements, see under the qualifying noun or adjective.

inertia t. In the stimulation of a muscle or sense organ the latent time required to overcome the inertia of the muscle or organ after the reception of the stimulus through the nerve.

L D 50 t. Median lethal time.

median lethal t. The amount of time required for 50 per cent of the organisms in a large group to die following a specific dose of a drug, infective agent, or radiation.

persistence t. Time that responses to a stimulus may persist, as persistence of a retinal image.

recognition t. The time required for the recognition of the kind of stimulus after its application.

thermal death t. The time required to kill microorganisms when kept at a given temperature.

utilization t. (*temps utile*). The period of time during which a given stimulus is effective in causing excitation of a tissue.

tim'o·thy [after *Timothy* Hanson, who brought the seed to Carolina from New York about 1720]. A common name for the most important meadow grass in America. It flowers during June and July, shedding quantities of pollen which is one of the more common causes of hay fever.

tin [AS.] (*stannum*). Sn = 118.70. An element and silver-white metal; used in alloys and the manufacture of tin salts.

t. chloride. Stannous chloride, $SnCl_2.2H_2O$; used in chemical procedures as a reducing agent.

t. oxide. Stannic oxide, SnO_2; used in combination with metallic tin for the treatment of furunculosis.

tin'cal. Crude or native borax.

tinc·to'ri·al [L. *tinctorius*, of dyeing]. Pertaining to staining or dyeing.

tinc·tu'ra [L., a dyeing]. Tincture. Abbreviated, tr.

tinc'ture [L. *tinctura*, a dyeing]. Alcoholic or hydroalcoholic solutions of medicinal substances, generally representing 10% or 20% (w/v) of drug and usually prepared by maceration or percolation of the drug with suitable menstruum. Abbreviated, tr.

ammoniated t. One prepared with aromatic ammonia spirit as the menstruum.

ethereal t. One prepared with ether spirit as the menstruum.

mother t. *In homeopathy*, a tincture, usually representing 10% of the drug, from which the standard dilutions are made.

tine [AS. *tind*]. A fine pointed instrument, used in dentistry to explore fine crevices and cavities: commonly called an *explorer*.

tin'e·a [L., a gnawing worm]. The lesions of dermatophytosis; ringworm.

t. amiantacea. A chronic scalp condition characterized by areas of dry heavy scales binding together the bases of the hairs. It is not a fungus infection.

t. barbae. Ringworm of the bearded areas of the face and neck, caused by various species of *Trichophyton* and *Microsporum*: also called *barber's itch, t. sycosis*.

t. capitis. Fungus infection of the scalp and hair. Caused by several species of *Trichophyton* and *Microsporum*. Also called *t. tonsurans*.

t. corporis. A fungus infection involving the glabrous skin. Caused by various species of *Trichophyton* and *Microsporum*. Also called *t. circinata, t. glabrosa*.

t. cruris. A fungus infection involving the skin of the groin, perineum, and perianal regions. Caused by *Epidermophyton floccosum* and several species of *Trichophyton*. Also called *gym itch, jockey itch, laundryman's itch*.

t. favosa. A chronic fungus infection which usually is limited to the scalp. Caused by *Trichophyton schoenleini* and *T. violaceum*. Also called *favus, honeycomb ringworm*.

t. imbricata. A superficial fungus disease of the tropics characterized by the presence of concentric rings of papulosquamous patches scattered over the body. Caused by *Trichophyton concentricum*. Also called *gogo, scaly ringworm, Tokelau ringworm, tropical tinea circinata*.

t. kerion. See *kerion celsi*.

t. manus. Fungus infection of the hand, usually chronic, due to *Trichophyton purpureum*.

t. nigra. A contagious cutaneous fungus infection caused by *Cladosporium mansoni* in the East and *Cladosporium wernecki* in the Americas, clinically characterized by its black or dark-brown coloration and its predominant occurrence on the trunk, neck, or palmar regions, though other sites may be involved: also called *keratomycosis, keratomycosis nigrans palmaris, cladosporiosis epidermica, pityriasis nigra, microsporosis nigra*.

t. nodosa. See *piedra*.

t. pedis. A fungus infection of the feet, especially the webs of the toes and the soles. Caused by *Epidermophyton floccosum*, various species of *Trichophyton*, and rarely by *Microsporum*. Also called *athlete's foot*.

t. unguium. A chronic fungus infection involving the nails of the hands and feet. Caused by *Epidermophyton floccosum*, various species of *Trichophyton*, and *Candida albicans*.

t. versicolor. A chronic superficial fungus infection of the skin, usually of the trunk. It is caused by *Malassezia furfur*.

Tinel, Jules [*French neurosurgeon*, 1879–1952]. Author of a treatise on gunshot wounds of the nerves (1916). Described a sign of nerve regeneration, in which percussion over the course of a regenerating nerve trunk causes sensations up to, but not beyond, the actual site of regeneration, called *Tinel's sign*.

tin'gle. A pricking or stinging sensation; the feeling of a slight, sharp, and sudden thrill, as of pain; acanthesthesia.

tin·ni'tus, tin'ni·tus [L.]. A ringing in one or both ears. It may also be like a roaring or hissing sound. Syn., *tinnitus aurium*.

objective t. Tinnitus audible to the examiner as well as to the subject, usually caused by organic vascular disease in the head or neck, such as an arteriovenous aneurysm or a venous hum. Syn., *pseudotinnitus*.

subjective t. Tinnitus audible only to the subject.

telephone t. That believed to be caused by continual use of the telephone.

t. cranii. A subjective sound in the head, poorly localized and lacking the specific character of true ear noises.

tin·tom'e·ter. An apparatus used in hemoglobinometry. A film of whole blood is arranged between two glass plates, and compared with a series of tinted glasses mounted on a disk.

tin·tom'e·try [L. *tinctum*, from *tingere*, to dye; G. *metron*, a measure]. Estimation of the amount of coloring matter in a liquid.

tip [ME.]. The point or summit of anything.

Woolner's t. The apex of the helix of the ear.

Ti·pu'li·dae (ti·pew'li·dee) [L. *tipula*, water spider]. A family of the order Diptera, the crane flies. Their importance as disease vectors is not established.

ti"queur' (tee"kur') [F.]. One exhibiting tics.

tire [AS. *tȳrian*]. Weary; become exhausted; fag. The term is used extensively by the medical profession and laymen alike in reference to muscular and brain fatigue, general bodily and mental exhaustion, etc.

tires. See *trembles*.

Tirmann-Schmelzer method for ionic iron. See under *stain*.

ti·sane' (ti·zan', tee"zahn'. *See* NOTES § 35) [F.]. Any decoction or beverage having slight curative or restorative qualities. *Obs.*

Tisdall method. See Kramer-Tisdall *method*.

Tiselius, Arne [*Swedish biochemist*, 1902–]. Described a method for the separation of proteins from body fluids by means of electrophoresis. The apparatus used is called *Tiselius apparatus.* Nobel laureate (1948).

Tissot spirometer. A large bell-type spirometer (capacity 100 liters or more) used for basal metabolism determination. The subject inspires atmospheric air and expires into the spirometer. At the end of the test period the total volume of expired air is measured and samples analyzed for CO_2 and O_2. The apparatus can be used to measure maximum breathing capacity (MBC). Syn., *Tissot gasometer.*

tis′sue [OF. *tissu*, from L. *texere*, to weave]. An aggregation of similar cells and their intercellular substance.

adenoid t. Old term for lymphatic tissue.

adipose t. A form of connective tissue consisting of fat cells lodged in areolar tissue and arranged in lobules along the course of small blood vessels.

areolar t. A form of loose connective tissue composed of cells and delicate collagenous and elastic fibers interlacing in all directions.

blubbery tissues. The distended tissues of the extremities found in filariasis and formed by blockage of lymphatic drainage.

cartilaginous t. See *cartilage.*

cavernous t. Erectile tissue.

celluloadipose t. Tissue infiltrated by fat but retaining some of its original cellular structure.

chondroid t. Embryonic cartilage.

cicatricial t. Scar tissue.

connective t. A general term for all those tissues of the body that support the specialized elements or parenchyma. The most important varieties are adipose tissue, areolar tissue, osseous tissue, cartilaginous tissue, elastic tissue, fibrous connective tissue, and lymphatic tissue.

elastic t. Connective tissue which is composed predominantly of yellow elastic fibers.

embryonic connective t. Mucoid tissue.

epithelial t. See *epithelium.*

erectile t. A spongelike system of vascular spaces in the penis and clitoris which becomes filled with blood causing enlargement and rigidity of the organ.

fibrous connective t. The densest connective tissue of the body. Collagenous fibers form the main constituent and are arranged in parallel bundles between which are rows of connective-tissue cells. It includes tendons, ligaments, and fibrous membranes, as the dura mater.

gelatinous t. See mucoid *t.*

glandular t. A group of epithelial cells which elaborate secretions.

granulation t. The mixture of newly formed capillaries and fibroblasts in inflammation, especially of exudative character, representing the early stages of healing. Followed by a growth into exudate or destroyed tissue, the process becomes one of organization. As it progresses to cicatrization by atrophy of blood vessels and maturation of connective tissue, inflammatory foci are cicatrized, or such foci or foreign bodies are encapsulated; on surfaces, especially serous, fibrous adhesions are formed; wounds are healed.

hematopoietic t. Blood-cell-forming tissue consisting of reticular fibers and primitive reticular cells which can be converted into all types of blood and connective-tissue cells.

hemopoietic t. See hematopoietic *t.*

homologous tissues. Those identical in type of structure.

indifferent t. Undifferentiated tissue.

inflammatory t. Tissue in which there is exudation or proliferation as a result of injury.

interstitial t. The intercellular connective tissue.

keratinized t. Tissue found in the nails, hair, or epidermis.

lymphatic t. Tissue consisting of networks of reticular and collagenous fibers and lymphocytes.

lymphoid t. Lymphatic tissue, especially that occurring where it is not normally present.

mesenchymal t. Undifferentiated embryonic tissue composed of branching cells between which is a ground substance of coagulable fluid. See also *mesenchyme.*

metanephrogenic t. The caudal part of the nephrogenic tissue giving rise to the metanephros or definitive kidney.

mucoid t. A form of loose connective tissue found in many parts of the embryo, as in the umbilical cord of the human fetus. The tissue is characterized by the presence of large, stellate fibroblasts surrounded by a soft, homogeneous intercellular substance which takes a basic stain.

mucous t. Old term for mucoid tissue.

muscular t. The tissue of which muscles are composed. See *muscle,* 1.

myeloid t. Red bone marrow consisting of reticular cells attached to argyrophile fibers which form wide meshes containing scattered fat cells, erythroblasts, myelocytes, and mature myeloid elements.

nephrogenic t. The tissue of the nephrogenic cord derived from the nephrotome plate that forms the blastema or primordium from which the embryonic and definitive kidneys develop.

nervous t. The nerve cells, their processes and accessory cells, such as the neuroglia.

nodal t. The sinoatrial node, the atrioventricular node and bundle and its branches, which serve for the origin and transmission of impulses in the heart. This system is made up of a dense network of Purkinje fibers.

osseous t. See *bone.*

parenchymal t. The epithelial components of an organ or, in the case of lymphatic organs, the lymphatic tissue, as contrasted with the supporting and nutritive framework of the organ, the stroma.

pseudoerectile t. The submucosa of the nasal conchae, with its rich venous plexus.

reticular t. Connective tissue in which reticular fibers are the conspicuous element, forming a branching nonelastic network.

scar t. Contracted dense connective tissue, the end result of healing.

shock t. See shock *organ.*

subcutaneous t. The layer of loose connective tissue under the dermis. Also called *hypodermis.*

white fibrous t. See fibrous connective *t.*

yellow elastic t. See elastic *t.*

tis′sue throm″bo·plas′tic fac′tor. See *thromboplastin.*

ti·ta′ni·um (tye·tay′nee·um, ti·tay′nee·um) [G. *Titanes*, Titans, sons of the earth]. Ti = 47.90. A very hard, dark gray, lustrous, metallic element used in certain alloys to impart toughness.

t. dioxide. TiO_2; extensively used as a white pigment in paints, plasters, etc.

ti′ter, ti′tre (ty′tur, tee′tur). 1. *In chemistry,* a titration figure. 2. An expression of the strength of a volumetric solution, usually grams of active constituent per cubic centimeter of solution. 3. The amount of one substance which corresponds to, reacts with, or is otherwise equivalent to a stated quantity of another substance.

tit″il·la′tion [L. *titillatio*, from *titillare*, to tickle]. The act of tickling; the sensation produced by tickling.

ti·tra′tion. An operation involving the measurement of the concentration or volume of a standard solution required to react chemically or immunologically with a substance being analyzed or standardized. —**ti′trate,** *v.*

electrometric t. A method of titration in which the end point is detected by measuring the change in potential of a suitable electrode or the change of electric conductance during titration.

ti'tre. See *titer*.

tit"u·ba'tion [L. *titubatio*, from *titubare*, to stagger]. A staggering gait seen especially in diseases of the cerebellum.

lingual t. Stammering; stuttering.

Tit'y·us. A genus of Scorpionida.

T. servulatus. A poisonous species of Brazil.

T. trinitalis. A poisonous black scorpion of Trinidad.

tivrim. A proprietary multivitamin and mineral product comprising minerals in wafer form and encapsulated vitamins.

TKD Abbreviation for tokodynamometer.

TKG Abbreviation for tokograph.

Tl Chemical symbol for thallium.

Tm Chemical symbol for thulium.

Tn Chemical symbol for thoron.

TNT Abbreviation for trinitrotoluene.

T.O. Original, or old, tuberculin. Also abbreviated O.T.

toad'head" [AS. *tādie; hēafod*]. The head of an anencephalus.

toad poi'sons. Toxic constituents of the skin glands of various toads, chiefly bufotoxins, bufagins, and bufotalins, all closely related to the digitalis principles in structure and action. Some contain the alkaloids bufotenin, bufotenidine, and bufothionine. Several tropical species yield epinephrine.

toad'skin" [*tādie;* ON. *skinn*]. Abnormal dryness, scaling, and fissuring of the skin resulting from vasomotor disturbances. Seen in vitamin deficiencies and syringomyelia.

to·bac'co [Taino *tabaco*, roll of tobacco leaves]. A plant, *Nicotiana tabacum*, of the family Solanaceae, the dried leaves of which contain an alkaloid, nicotine. It was formerly employed as an enema to overcome intestinal obstruction.

Indian t. Lobelia.

Tobey, George Loring, Jr. [*American otolaryngologist*, 1881–1947]. With J. B. Ayer, devised a test for lateral sinus thrombosis, based on changes in the pressure of the spinal fluid during compression of one or both jugular veins; called *Tobey-Ayer test.*

Tobruk plaster. A combination of the long Thomas splint with plaster fixation of the thigh, leg, and foot for the emergency transportation of patients with wounds and fractures of the lower extremity.

toco-. See *toko-*.

tocopherex. Trade-mark for a distillate of vegetable oils containing mixed tocopherols.

to·coph'er·ol [G. *tokos*, birth; *pherein*, to bear]. Any one of four substances, α-, β-, γ-, and δ-tocopherol, possessing vitamin-E activity, the α-variety being the most potent. Wheat-germ oil is a rich source; contained also in cottonseed oil and lettuce.

alpha-tocopherol. 5,7,8-Trimethyltocol; $C_{29}H_{50}O_2$, sometimes referred to as vitamin E although the latter substance probably has a multiple nature. Obtained from natural sources or prepared synthetically. Light yellow, viscous, odorless, oily liquid, miscible with alcohol. It is destroyed by light and air. See Table of Vitamins in the Appendix.

alpha-tocopherol acetate. The acetate ester of alpha-tocopherol, more stable than the free alcohol: also spelled *alpha-tocopheryl acetate.*

toc'o·sine (tock'o·seen, ·sin). Tyramine hydrochloride.

to'cus [*tokos*]. Childbirth.

Todd, John Lancelot [*English physician*, 1876–1949]. With J. E. Dutton, demonstrated that the cause of relapsing fever in monkeys is a spirillum, *Spirillum duttoni* (1905).

Todd's paralysis. See under *paralysis.*

toe [ME. *too*]. A digit of the foot.

hammer t. See *hammertoe.*

Morton's t. See *metatarsalgia.*

overlapping t. A congenital variation characterized by dorsal displacement of the fifth toe over the fourth.

tofaxin. Trade-mark for a distillate of vegetable oils containing mixed tocopherols.

Toison, J. [*French histologist*, 1858–1950]. Introduced a stain for red blood cells made with 0.025 Gm. of methyl violet (6B), 1.0 Gm. of sodium chloride, 8.0 Gm. of sodium sulfate, 30 cc. of glycerine in 300 cc. of water.

To"ke·la'u ring'worm (to"keh·lah'ōō). See *tinea* imbricata.

to'ko-, to'co- [G. *tokos*, birth]. Combining form meaning *birth.*

tok"o·dy"na·mom'e·ter [G. *tokos*, birth; *dynamis*, power; *metron*, a measure]. An instrument for measuring the amplitude, duration, and frequency of uterine muscular contraction, as during labor. Abbreviated, TKD.

tok'o·graph [*tokos; graphein*, to write]. A record taken by a tokodynamometer. Abbreviated, TKG.

to·kog'ra·phy. The making and interpreting of graphic recordings of the amplitude, duration, and frequency of uterine muscular contractions during labor.

to·kol'o·gy [*tokos;* G. *logos*, word]. The science of obstetrics.

tok"o·ma'ni·a (tock"o·may'nee·uh, to"ko·) [*tokos;* G. *mania*, madness]. Puerperal insanity; psychosis in a woman at the time of childbirth.

to·kom'e·try. A study of the amplitude, duration, and frequency of the uterine muscular contractions, as during labor, with a tokodynamometer. —**tokom'eter,** *n.*

tokophin. Trade-mark for a brand of synthetic alpha-tocopherol.

tok"o·pho'bi·a (tock"o·fo'bee·uh, to"ko·) [*tokos;* G. *phobos*, fear]. Undue dread of childbirth.

to'kos. Childbirth.

tol·az'o·line. Official generic name for 2-benzylimidazoline or benzazoline, an adrenergic-blocking agent, the hydrochloride of which is supplied under the trade-marked name *priscoline* (formerly priscol) *hydrochloride.*

tol'er·ance, tol"er·a'tion [L. *tolerantia*, from *tolerare*, to endure]. The ability of enduring the influence of a drug or poison, particularly when acquired by a continued use of the substance.

sugar t. The tolerance of a diabetic patient for ingested sugar. It is measured by the maximum amount of sugar intake which does not produce glycosuria.

work t. *In medicine*, the amount of work a certain category of chronically ill patient can or should do, e.g., most patients are discharged from tuberculosis sanatoriums with a daily work tolerance of four hours.

tol'er·ant [*tolerare*]. Withstanding the action of a drug without harm.

tol"er·a'tion. Tolerance.

Tollens' test. See under *test.*

to·lo'ni·um chlo'ride. Generic name for the antiheparin-active dye toluidine blue O. See *blutene chloride.*

tolserol. A trade-marked name for *mephenesin.*

to·lu' bal'sam (to·lōō' bawl'sum) (*balsamum tolutanum*). Obtained from *Myroxylon Balsamum*, a South American tree of the Leguminosae. It contains cinnamic and benzoic acids, esters of these acids and resins. A mild stimulant expectorant used in the form of a tincture or syrup.

tol′u·ene. Methylbenzene. $C_6H_5.CH_3$. A colorless liquid obtained chiefly from coal tar. Used as a solvent and reagent.

tol″u·ene·sul″fon·di″chlor·am′ide (para). Dichloramine-T. Also spelled *p-toluenesulfondichloroamide, p-toluenesulfonedichloramide, p-toluenesulfonedichloroamide.*

to·lu′ic ac′id. Any of four isomeric, crystalline acids: *o*-toluic, *m*-toluic, *p*-toluic, all represented by the formula $CH_3.C_6H_4.COOH$, and α-toluic, of the formula $C_6H_5CH_2COOH$, better known as phenylacetic acid.

to·lu′i·dine (to·lew′i·deen, ·din). Aminotoluene. $H_2N.C_6H_4.CH_3$. The *o*- and *m*- varieties are liquids; the *p*- is a solid.

t. blue O (C.C.). $C_{15}H_{16}ClN_3S$; 3-amino-7-dimethylamino-2-methylphenazathionium chloride; a basic thiazine dye, used as a nuclear stain, for Nissl substance in the staining of nerve cells, and for bacteriologic staining. Systemic administration reduces bleeding tendency in certain hemorrhagic conditions associated with excessive amounts of heparinoid substances in the blood; it has been used also for detection of corneal defects. Syn., *tolonium chloride.* See *blutene chloride.*

tol′u·ol. Toluene.

tol′u·yl·ene, tol·u′yl·ene. Stilbene.

t. red. Aminodimethylamino-toluphenazine hydrochloride. $C_{15}H_{16}N_4.HCl$. An indicator covering the pH range 6.8–8.0. Suggested for use in a test of gastric function. Syn., *neutral red.*

tol′yl. The univalent radical $C_6H_4.CH_3$.

tolysin. Trade-mark for a brand of *neocinchophen.*

to·mat′i·dine. The aglycone portion, chemically a steroid secondary amine, resulting from hydrolysis of tomatine.

to·ma·tine. A glycosidal alkaloid, isolated from the tomato plant, having antifungal activity.

-tome [G. *tomē*, a cutting; *tomos*, cutting]. 1. A combining form denoting *a part* or *a section.* 2. A combining form denoting *an instrument for cutting.*

to·men′tum [L.]. A lock of wool.

t. cerebri. The network of small blood vessels of the pia penetrating the cortex of the brain.

Tomes's fibers. See under *fiber.*

Tomes's granular layer. See under *layer.*

Tomes's process. See ameloblastic *process.*

Tommaselli, Salvatore [*Italian physician,* 1830–1902]. Described a syndrome of hematuria and pyrexia due to overdose of quinine; called *Tommaselli's syndrome.*

to′mo·gram [*tomos;* G. *gramma*, letter]. A roentgenogram obtained by sectional radiography.

to·mog′ra·phy. See sectional *radiography.*

to″mo·to′ci·a (to″mo·to′shee·uh, ·see·uh, tom″o·) [*tomos;* G. *tokos*, birth]. Cesarean section.

-tomy [G. *tomē*, a cutting]. A combining form denoting *a cutting operation.*

to′nal is′lands. Isolated areas in the range of human hearing in which some persons with practically no hearing have an appreciation of pure tones at maximum intensity.

to″na·pha′si·a (to″nuh·fay′zhuh, ·zee·uh, ton″uh·) [G. *tonos*, tone; *aphasia*, speechlessness]. Loss of the ability to sing (due to a cerebral lesion).

tone [*tonos*]. 1. A distinct sound. 2. The normal state of tension of a part or of the body.

summational tones. Supposed production of new tones by the summation or addition of the number of vibrations of existing tones.

to·neph′in. See *pitressin.*

ton′ga. A mixture of barks, formerly used in the treatment of neuralgia.

tongue [AS. *tunge*]. The movable muscular organ attached to the floor of the mouth, and concerned in tasting, masticating, swallowing, and speaking. It consists of a number of muscles, and is covered by mucous membrane from which project numerous papillae, and in which are placed the terminal organs of taste. See Plate 12.

bifid t. A tongue the anterior portion of which is cleft in the median line.

black, hairy t. A tongue with a brown, furlike patch on the dorsum, due to hypertrophied filiform papillae and the presence of pigment. Also called *hyperkeratosis linguae, lingua nigra.*

black t. 1. In dogs, a deficiency disease. See *blacktongue.* 2. Black, hairy tongue.

cleft t. See bifid *t.*

fern-leaf pattern t. One presenting a well-marked median sulcus with lateral branches.

filmy t. One with whitish, symmetrical patches on both sides.

fissured t. A condition of the tongue in which there are deep furrows in the mucous membrane. Also called *furrowed t., lingua plicata.*

frog t. Ranula.

furred t. A tongue the papillae of which are coated, giving the mucous membrane the appearance of a whitish fur.

geographic t. One with localized thickening of the epithelium, giving to the surface the appearance of a map.

hairy t. One with a hyperplasia of the papillae, giving rise to hairlike projections.

magenta t. The rosy-colored glossitis of ariboflavinosis in which lesions of the mucosa of the lip develop, redness and swelling of the mucosa follow, and the papillae of the tongue become lower and assume a mushroom appearance.

parrot t. A shriveled, dry tongue that cannot be protruded, found in typhus.

scrotal t. Fissured tongue, lingua plicata.

strawberry t. A hyperemic tongue, the fungiform papillae of which are very prominent; it is seen especially in scarlet fever.

wooden t. One which is the seat of actinomycosis.

tongue′-tie″. A congenital abnormality of the frenulum of the tongue, interfering with its mobility. Syn., *ankyloglossia.*

ton′ic [G. *tonikos*, of stretching]. 1. Pertaining to tone; producing normal tone or tension. 2. Characterized by continuous tension or contraction, as a tonic spasm, tonic convulsion.

ton′ic. An agent or drug given to improve the normal tone of an organ or of the patient generally.

cardiac t. One which strengthens the heart muscle.

to·nic′i·ty (to·niss′i·tee) [*tonikos*]. The condition of normal tone or tension of organs.

ton″i·co·clon′ic (ton″i·ko·klon′ick, to″nick·o·) [*tonikos;* G. *klonos*, confused motion]. Both tonic and clonic, pertaining to muscular spasms.

ton″i·tro·pho′bi·a (ton″i·tro·fo′bee·uh, to″ni·tro·) [L. *tonitrus*, thunder; G. *phobos*, fear]. Morbid fear of thunder. Also called *astrapophobia.*

ton′ka bean. The seed of *Dipteryx odorata*, a tree of South America; it contains coumarin, and is used as a flavoring agent.

ton″o·clon′ic. See *tonicoclonic.*

to″no·fi′brils (to″no·figh′brilz, ton′o·) [G. *tonos*, tension; dim. from L. *fibra*, fiber]. Delicate fibrils found particularly in epithelial cells, between which they run across intercellular bridges.

to′no·gram (to′no·gram, ton′o·) [*tonos;* G. *gramma*, letter]. A record made by a tonograph.

to′no·graph (to′no·graf, ton′o·) [*tonos;* G. *graphein*, to write]. A term formerly applied to a device for determining or recording blood pressure.

to·nom'e·ter [*tonos;* G. *metron,* a measure]. An instrument to measure tension, as that of the eyeball, or an instrument used to equilibrate samples of fluid, as blood, with gases at known tensions.

Gaertner's t. One used for estimating blood pressure.

Musken's t. One used for measuring the tonicity of the Achilles tendon.

to'no·plasts (to'no·plasts, ton'o·) [*tonos;* G. *plassein,* to form]. Small intracellular bodies which build up strongly osmotic substances within themselves and in this way swell to small vacuoles.

to·nos"cil·log'ra·phy [*tonos;* L. *oscillare,* to swing; G. *graphein,* to write]. Method of automatic blood-pressure recording of extremities.

to'no·scope (to'no·scope, ton'o·) [*tonos;* G. *skopein,* to examine]. An instrument for examination of the interior of the cranium by means of sound.

ton'quin bean (tong'kin). Tonka bean.

ton'sil [L. *tonsillae,* tonsils]. 1. Aggregated lymph nodules and associated lymph vessels surrounding crypts or depressions of the pharyngeal mucosa. 2. A small lobe of the cerebellar hemisphere, on its inferior medial aspect. —**tonsillar,** *adj.*

Gerlach's tubal t. See tubal *t.*

lingual t. Accumulations of lymphatic tissue more or less closely associated with crypts which serve also as ducts of the mucous glands of the base of the tongue.

Luschka's t. See pharyngeal *t.*

nasal t. Old term for pharyngeal tonsil, which is located in the nasopharynx.

palatine t. One found on each side of the isthmus of the fauces and between the glossopalatine and pharyngopalatine arches, in the tonsillar sinus; almond-shaped and separated from the pharyngeal musculature by a well-defined thin capsule.

pharyngeal t. An unpaired tonsil found on the posterior wall of the nasopharynx, in folds of the mucosa, with grooves between, which simulate crypts; more prominent during childhood; when hypertrophied forms the "adenoids." See Plate 12.

tubal t. Minor and variable aggregations of lymphatic tissue about the pharyngeal orifice of each pharyngo-tympanic (auditory) tube: also called *Gerlach's tubal tube.*

ton·sil'la (pl. *tonsillae*) [*tonsillae*]. Tonsil.

t. cerebelli. Tonsil of the cerebellum.

ton"sil·lec'tome [*tonsillae;* G. *ektomē,* excision]. An instrument for the performance of tonsillectomy.

ton"sil·lec'to·my [*tonsillae; ektomē*]. Removal of the palatine tonsils.

ton"sil·li'tis [*tonsillae;* G. *-itis,* inflammation]. Inflammation of the tonsils. —**tonsillit'ic,** *adj.*

acute t. Inflammation of the tonsils with sudden onset, pyrexia, constitutional symptoms, and intense sore throat.

follicular t. A form in which the crypts are involved and their contents project as whitish spots from the surface of the tonsil.

herpetic t. A form characterized by an eruption of herpetic vesicles, which soon rupture, leaving small, circular ulcers that coalesce and become covered with a fibrinous exudation. The disease has an acute onset, a continuous fever, and a critical decline, affects those subject to herpes elsewhere, and tends to recur.

lacunar t. See follicular *t.*

mycotic t. Tonsillitis due to fungi.

pustular t. A form characterized by the formation of pustules, as in smallpox.

ton·sil'lo·lith, ton'sil·lo·lith [*tonsillae;* G. *lithos,* stone]. A concretion within the tonsil.

ton·sil'lo·tome, ton'sil·lo·tome [*tonsillae;* G. *tomos,* cutting]. An instrument for removing a tonsil.

ton"sil·lot'o·my [*tonsillae;* G. *tomē,* a cutting]. The operation of cutting away the whole or a part of a tonsil.

ton·sil"lo·ty'phoid (ton·sil"o·ty'foyd, ton"sil·o·) [*tonsillae;* G. *typhōdēs,* delirious]. Typhoid fever complicated with a membranous or pseudomembranous deposit on the tonsils.

ton"sil·sec'tor [*tonsillae;* L. *sector,* cutter]. A tonsillotome consisting of a pair of circular or oval scissor blades moving inside a guarding ring.

ton'sure [L. *tonsura,* a shearing]. The shaving or removal of the hair from the crown of the head.

to'nus [G. *tonos,* a stretching]. The slight degree of contraction usually present in muscles when not undergoing active movement. In skeletal muscles, tonus is a reflex response to motor nerve impulses of low frequency. In smooth muscle, it is an inherent property of the muscle cells.

Tooth, Howard Henry [*English physician,* 1856–1925]. Described a peroneal type of progressive neuropathic muscular atrophy (1886), sometimes called *Tooth's muscular atrophy.* See also Charcot-Marie-Tooth *disease.*

tooth (pl. *teeth*) [AS. *tōth*]. One of the calcified organs supported by the alveolar processes and gums of both jaws, serving to masticate food, aid speech, and influence facial contour. Each tooth consists of: (1) a main mass of dentin surrounding a pulp cavity which contains the dental pulp with its nerves and vessels, (2) a coronal portion (crown) covered by enamel, (3) a radicular portion (root), which may be single, bifid, or trifid, covered by bone called cementum, (4) a cervical portion (neck), the junction of crown and root.

antagonistic t. One which meets a tooth or teeth of the opposite dental arch during mastication or in occlusion.

artificial teeth. A denture or bridgework; dental prosthesis; the porcelain, acrylic, or metallic imitations of the crowns of teeth used in dental prosthesis.

auditory teeth. The toothlike projections on the edge of the limbus laminae spiralis of the ear. They extend between the epithelial cells and give the limbus an uneven, highly refracting surface.

bicuspid t. See premolar *t.*

buck t. A protruding tooth.

canine t. A tooth with a conical crown, situated between the lateral incisor and the first premolar in each quadrant of the jaws. Also called *cuspid t.*

cheek teeth. The molar teeth.

cheoplastic teeth. Artificial teeth without pins, but with undercuts adapted to the reception and retention of molten metal as a means of attachment to a cheoplastic base.

Corti's teeth. See *auditory teeth,* under *tooth.*

cuspid t. See canine *t.*

deciduous teeth. The 20 temporary or milk teeth; those replaced by succedaneous permanent teeth. There are eight incisors, four canines, and eight molars. See Plate 21.

Huschke's teeth. See *auditory teeth* under *tooth.*

Hutchinson's teeth. See Jonathan *Hutchinson.*

impacted t. See *impacted,* 2.

incisor t. One of the two cutting teeth nearest the midline in each quadrant of the dentition.

milk teeth. The deciduous teeth.

molar t. A multicuspidate tooth used for crushing, grinding, or triturating food. In the human deciduous dentition there are two in each quadrant immediately behind the canine; in the permanent dentition, three, behind the premolars.

multicuspid teeth. The molar teeth.

notched teeth. Those with irregular incisal edges due to imperfect fusion or hypoplasia of the developmental lobes.

permanent t. One of the 32 teeth of the second dentition. There are eight incisors, four canines, eight premolars, and 12 molars. See Plate 22.

pivot t. An artificial crown doweled to the root of a natural tooth.

premolar t. One of the two teeth with two cusps situated between the canine and the first molar in each quadrant of the permanent dentition. Also called *bicuspid t.*

sectorial t. One of the cutting teeth of the Carnivora.

stomach t. The lower canine tooth.

succedaneous t. One of the permanent teeth which takes the place of a deciduous tooth.

supernumerary t. One which is additional to the normal complement.

temporary teeth. (a) The teeth of the first dentition; milk teeth; deciduous teeth. (b) A provisional set of artificial teeth.

wisdom t. The third molar tooth in man: formerly called *dens serotinus, dens sapientia.*

tooth′ache″ [*tōth;* AS. *acan*]. Any pain in or about a tooth; odontalgia.

tooth′ache″ tree. A tree whose bark, xanthoxylum, has been used as a masticatory in toothache.

toothed [*tōth*]. Having teeth or indentations; dentate.

tooth′paste″. See *dentifrice.*

top″ag·no′sis [G. *topos*, place; *agnōstos*, unknown]. Loss of localization sensibility.

to·pal′gi·a [*topos;* G. *algos*, pain]. Localized pain, common in neurasthenia and hysteria; often appears suddenly after emotional disturbances.

to·pec′to·my [*topos;* G. *ektomē*, excision]. Excision of a portion of the cerebral cortex, usually in the frontal area, as applied in the treatment of certain mental disorders or intractable pain.

top″es·the′si·a, top″aes·the′si·a (top″ess·thee′zhuh, ·zee·uh, to″pess·) [*topos;* G. *aisthēsis*, sensation]. Local tactile sensibility.

Töpfer's reagent. See under *reagent.*

Töpfer's test. See under *test.*

to·pha′ceous [L. *tophus*, tufa]. Of the nature of tophi; sandy, or gritty.

to′phus (pl. *tophi*) [L.]. A mineral concretion in the body, especially about the joints. A sodium urate deposit in the skin about a joint, in the ear, or in bone, in gout.

top′ic, top′i·cal [G. *topos*, place]. Local.

topicillin. Trade-mark for a brand of penicillin preparations for topical use.

Topinard, Paul [*French anthropologist*, 1830–1911]. Described the angle formed at the anterior nasal spine by lines from the glabella and the auricular point; called *Topinard's angle.*

top′o- (top′o-, to′po-), **top-** [G. *topos*, place]. A combining form meaning *place;* used to signify *localized.*

top″o·al′gi·a. See *topalgia.*

top″o·an″es·the′si·a (·an″ess·thee′zhuh, ·zee·uh) [*topos;* G. *anaisthēsia*, lack of sensation]. Inability to locate exactly a cutaneous sensation.

top″o·gen′e·sis, to″po·gen′e·sis. See *morphogenesis.*

top″og·no′sis. See *topesthesia.*

top″og·nos′tic [*topos; gnōsis*, a recognizing]. Pertaining to the recognition of changes, positions, or symptoms of parts of the body, as topognostic sensibility.

to·pog′ra·phy [*topos;* G. *graphein*, to write]. A study of the regions of the body or its parts, as cerebral topography. —**topograph′ic,** *adj.*

top·ol′o·gy [*topos;* G. *logos*, word]. 1. Topographic anatomy. 2. The relation of the presenting part of the fetus to the pelvic canal.

top″o·nar·co′sis [*topos;* G. *narkōsis*, a benumbing]. Local insensibility or anesthesia.

top″o·neu·ro′sis [*topos;* G. *neuron*, nerve; *-ōsis*, condition]. A localized neurosis.

top″o·pho′bi·a [*topos;* G. *phobos*, fear]. Morbid dread of certain places.

top′o·phone [*topos;* G. *phōnē*, sound]. An instrument to determine the direction of a source of sound.

torantil. A proprietary histaminase-containing tablet prepared from desiccated kidney and extract of intestinal mucosa of hogs. Used in prophylaxis and treatment of allergies.

tor′cu·lar He·roph′i·li (hi·rof′i·lye). Old term for confluens sinuum, or confluence of the sinuses.

Torek, Franz [*American surgeon*, 1861–1938]. Remembered for his ingenuity in devising a technic of orchiopexy (1909), called *Torek's operation.* Performed the first successful resection for cancer of the esophagus, also called *Torek's operation.*

Torkildsen procedure. See *ventriculocisternostomy.*

tor·men′tum [L., an engine for hurling missiles]. An old name for various obstructive disorders of the intestine.

t. intestinorum. See *dysentery.*

tor′mi·na (sing., *tormen*) [L., griping of the bowels]. Griping pains in the bowel.

post-partum t. The afterpains of parturition.

t. alvi. Colic.

t. Celsi. Dysentery.

t. intestinorum. Dysentery.

t. ventriculi nervosa. See *hyperperistalsis.*

tor′mi·nal, tor′mi·nous [*tormina*]. Affected with tormina.

Tornwaldt, Gustav Ludwig (Thornwaldt) [*German physician*, 1843–1910]. Described nasopharyngeal bursitis, accompanied by the formation of a cystic cavity in the pharyngeal mucosa containing pus or mucopus (1885); called *Tornwaldt's bursitis.* This had been described by Hermann Wendt as an inflammation of the pharyngeal tonsil (1874).

torocol. A proprietary tablet containing bile salts, cascara sagrada extract, phenolphthalein, and capsicum oleoresin. Used as a cholagogue cathartic.

Toronto unit. The anticoagulant activity of 0.01 mg. of a standard barium heparin employed at the University of Toronto.

tor·pes′cence [L. *torpescere*, to grow stiff]. Numbness; torpidity. *Rare.*

tor′pid [L. *torpidus*, benumbed]. Affected with torpor.

tor·pid′i·ty. See *torpor.*

tor′por [L., numbness]. Sluggishness; inactivity.

t. intestinorum. Constipation.

t. retinae. Dulled perceptive power of the retina.

torque [L. *torquere*, to twist]. The measure of the effectiveness of a force in producing the rotation of a body about an axis; the *moment* of force, i.e., the magnitude of the force times the perpendicular distance from the axis to the line of action of the force.

Torricellian vacuum. See under *vacuum.*

tor″si·om′e·ter [L. *torquere*, to twist; G. *metron*, a measure]. An instrument for measuring ocular torsion.

tor′sion [*torquere*]. 1. A twisting; also, the rotation of the eye about the visual axis. 2. The tilting of the vertical meridian of the eye.

t. of an artery. Twisting of the free end of an artery to check hemorrhage.

t. of teeth. The forcible turning of teeth in their alveoli for the purpose of correcting irregularity in position.

t. of the umbilical cord. The spontaneous twisting of the umbilical cord. From eight to ten twists are normal; great torsion may occur after the death of the fetus.

tor′sive (tor′siv) [*torquere*]. Twisted; twisting.

tor″si·ver′sion. Rotated position of a tooth in its alveolus.

tor′so [It.]. The trunk; the body without head or limbs.

tor″soc·clu′sion [L. *torquere*, to twist; *occludere*, to shut]. Occlusion, 4, occurring when a tooth is rotated on its long axis.

tort [*torquere*]. To tilt the vertical meridian of the eye; **extort,** to tilt the vertical meridian outward; **intort,** inward.

Torti, Francesco [*Italian physician*, 1658–1741]. Said to have introduced the term malaria. Probably the first in Italy to use cinchona bark for its treatment.

tor″ti·col′lar [L. *torquere*, to twist; *collum*, neck]. Affected with wryneck, or torticollis.

tor″ti·col′lis [*torquere; collum*]. Wryneck, a contraction of the sternocleidomastoid muscle, usually of one side, resulting in an abnormal position of the head.

hysterical t. See psychogenic *t.*

intermittent t. See spasmodic *t.*

psychogenic t. Spasmodic torticollis associated with an anxiety reaction, with spread often beyond the sternocleidomastoid muscle, resulting in blepharospasm and spasm of other facial or shoulder muscles.

rheumatic t. Old term for stiff neck, a form due to myositis of the sternocleidomastoid or other muscle of the neck.

spasmodic t. Spasmodic contraction of the muscles of the neck of one side, especially the sternocleidomastoid, causing a drawing of the head toward the opposite side. The spasm may be tonic or clonic. Also called *torticollis spastica.*

tor′tu·ous [L. *tortuosus*, twisting]. Twisted, sinuous.

Tor′u·la [L. *torulus*, small elevation]. A genus of fungi which reproduce by budding.

T. histolytica. See *Cryptococcus histolyticus.*

torulexin. Trade-mark for a proprietary vitamin-B complex capsule.

Tor″u·lop′sis ne″o·for′mans (nee″o·for′manz). See *Cryptococcus histolyticus.*

tor″u·lo′sis. See *cryptococcosis.*

tor′u·lus [*torulus*]. An elevation.

to′rus (pl. *tori*) [L., a bulging]. 1. A surface having a regular curvature with two principal meridians of dissimilar curvature at right angles to each other. 2. An elevation or prominence.

buccal t. An inconstant slight ridge along the buccal raphe.

mandibular t. Ridge of the mandible situated in the anterior portion of the inner aspect of the bone approximately at the junction between the body and the alveolar process in the region of the incisors, canines, and premolars, rarely in the molar region, due to an overgrowth of the bone.

occipital t. See transverse occipital *t.*

supraorbital t. Extreme development of the supraorbital region.

t. levatorius. An elevation of the lateral part of the upper surface of the soft palate caused by the underlying levator veli palatini muscle.

t. palatinus. A nodular elevation along the median suture of the hard palate; due to an exostosis.

t. pubicus. A low vertical elevation overlying the pelvic margin of the fibrocartilagenous disk of the pubic symphysis.

t. tubarius. The arcuate elevation of the mucous membrane of the pharynx over the medial end of the cartilage of the auditory tube, above and behind the pharyngeal orifice of the tube. Also called *Eustachian cushion, tubal elevation.*

t. uretericus. A ridge in the urinary bladder wall connecting the ureteral orifices.

t. uterinus. A transverse fold on the posterior aspect of the cervix of the uterus formed as an extension of the uterosacral ligaments.

transverse occipital t. An occasional elevation found on the occipital bone which includes the external occipital protuberance and the adjacent area.

tos″yl·chlor·am′ide so′di·um. International Pharmacopoeia name for chloramine-T.

to′ta·quine (to′tuh·kween, ·kwin) (*totaquina*). A mixture of alkaloids from the bark of species of *Cinchona.* It contains not less than 10% of anhydrous quinine and a total of 70–80% of the anhydrous alkaloids cinchonidine, cinchonine, quinidine, and quinine. Yellowish white to gray powder affected by light. An antimalarial. Dose, 0.12–0.6 Gm. (2–10 gr.).

Toti, Addeo [*Italian otolaryngologist*, b. 1861]. Described his operation of dacryocystorhinostomy; also called *Toti's operation.*

to·tip′o·tence [L. *totus*, whole; *potentia*, power]. The capacity of a cleavage cell to give rise to a complete embryo. —**totipo′tent,** *adj.*

touch [F. *toucher*]. 1. Tactile sense. 2. Judging by the tactile sense; palpation. 3. *In obstetrics*, digital examination of the internal genitalia through the vagina.

abdominal t. Application of the hands to the abdomen for the diagnosis of intraabdominal conditions.

after t. The sensation which persists for a short time after contact with an object has ceased.

double t. Combined vaginal and abdominal or vaginal and rectal palpation.

rectal t. Examination made by the finger in the rectum.

royal t. The laying on of the hands by a king, formerly believed to be efficacious in scrofula or king's evil.

vaginal t. Digital examination of the genital organs through the vagina.

vesical t. Examination through the urinary bladder.

tour de mai′tre (toor de may′truh. *See* Notes §35) [F.]. A method of passing a catheter into the male urinary bladder in which it is introduced into the urethra with the convexity upward. The shaft lies obliquely across the left thigh of the patient, and as the point enters the bulb, the handle is swept around toward the abdomen, when the beak passes into the membranous urethra. It is carried into the urinary bladder by depressing the shaft between the patient's thighs.

Tourette. See Georges *Gilles de la Tourette.*

Tournay's sign. Unilateral dilatation of the pupil of the abducted eye in extreme lateral fixation.

tour′ne·sol′ (toorn′sawl′. *See* Notes § 35). Litmus.

tour′ni·quet [F.]. Any apparatus for controlling hemorrhage from, or circulation in, a limb or part of the body, where direct pressure can be brought upon the blood vessels by means of straps, cords, rubber tubes, or pads. Tourniquets are made in a multiplicity of forms, from the simplest emergency adaptation of a handkerchief or piece of clothing wound about the limb and tightened with a stick, to elaborate instruments where pressure is made by means of screws acting upon metal pads or where a rubber hose encircling the limb is distended with air by means of a pump.

tous-les-mois′ (too-lay-mwah′). A variety of arrowroot starch prepared from *Canna edulis;* canna starch.

Touton cells. Multinucleated giant cells resembling those of epulis, sometimes containing fatty crystals or masses, observed in xanthoma.

tow [AS.]. The coarse part of flax or hemp; used as an absorbent.

Townsend, David [*American orthopedic surgeon,* 1875–1950]. Introduced his operation for flatfoot, in which he performed arthrodesis of the talonavicular joint with transference of the anterior tibial tendon and lengthening of the Achilles tendon; called *Townsend's operation.*

tox-. See *toxico-.*

tox·ae′mi·a. See *toxemia.*

tox″al·bu′min [G. *toxikon*, poison; L. *albus*, white]. A poisonous protein, obtained from cultures of bacteria and from certain plants.

tox·al′bu·mose. A toxic albumose.

tox′a·phene. A product obtained by chlorination of camphene to an average composition of $C_{10}H_{10}Cl_8$; an amber-colored, waxy solid, insoluble in water but soluble in organic liquids: used as a toxicant against many agricultural insect pests. Syn., *chlorinated camphene.*

tox·e′mi·a [*toxikon;* G. *haima*, blood]. A condition in which the blood contains poisonous products, either those produced by the body cells or those due to the growth of microorganisms. It is a general involvement in which the blood contains toxins but not bacteria.

acute toxemias of pregnancy. See *eclampsia*, 2.

eclamptogenic t. See *eclampsia*, 2.

t. of pregnancy. See *eclampsia*, 2.

tox·e′mic [*toxikon; haima*]. Pertaining to, affected with, or caused by toxemia.

tox·en′zyme, tox′en·zyme [*toxikon;* G. *en*, in; *zymē*, leaven]. A toxic enzyme.

tox′ic [*toxikon*]. Poisonous.

toxic-. See *toxico-.*

tox′i·cant [*toxikon*]. Poisonous or toxic.

tox′i·cant. A poisonous agent.

tox″i·ce′mi·a. See *toxemia.*

tox′i·cide [*toxikon;* L. *caedere*, to kill]. A remedy or principle that destroys toxic agents.

tox·ic′i·ty (tock·sis′i·tee) [*toxikon*]. 1. The quality of being toxic. 2. The kind and amount of poison or toxin produced by a microorganism.

tox′i·co′, toxic-, tox′o-, tox- [*toxikon*]. A combining form meaning *poison.*

tox″i·co·den′drol [*toxikon;* G. *dendron*, tree]. A toxic nonvolatile oil from poison ivy and poison oak.

Tox″i·co·den′dron. A genus of plants and shrubs, formerly classified as *Rhus*, including poison ivy, *T. radicans*, poison oak, *T. quercifolium*, poison sumac, *T. vernix*, and other species.

tox″i·co·der′ma [*toxikon;* G. *derma*, skin]. Disease of the skin due to poison.

tox″i·co·der″ma·ti′tis [*toxikon; derma;* G. *-itis*, inflammation]. Skin inflammation due to poison.

tox″i·co·der″ma·to′sis [*toxikon; derma;* G. *-ōsis*, condition]. Toxicoderma.

tox″i·co·gen′ic [*toxikon;* G. *genesthai*, from *gignesthai*, to be produced]. Producing poisons.

tox′i·coid [*toxikon;* G. *eidos*, form]. Resembling a poison or a toxin.

tox″i·col′o·gist [*toxikon;* G. *logos*, word]. One versed in toxicology.

tox″i·col′o·gy [*toxikon; logos*]. The science of the nature and effects of poisons, their detection, and treatment of their effects. —**toxicolog′ic, toxicolog′ical,** *adj.*

tox″i·co·ma′ni·a [*toxikon;* G. *mania*, madness]. Morbid desire to consume poison. —**toxicomaniac,** *n.*

tox″i·co·mu′cin [*toxikon;* L. *mucus*, mucus]. A toxic substance from cultures of tubercle bacilli.

tox″i·co·path′ic [*toxikon;* G. *pathos*, disease]. Pertaining to any morbid condition due to the action of a poison.

tox″i·co·phid′i·a [*toxikon;* G. *ophidion*, small serpent]. Poisonous serpents. *Rare.*

Tox″i·co·phloe′a (tock″si·ko·flee′uh) [*toxikon;* G. *phloios*, bark]. *Acokanthera.*

tox″i·co·pho′bi·a [*toxikon;* G. *phobos*, fear]. Morbid dread of being poisoned.

tox″i·co′sis [*toxikon;* G. *-ōsis*, condition]. A state of poisoning.

endogenic t. That due to toxic substances produced within the body; autointoxication.

exogenic t. One with clinical symptoms induced by the action of toxic bases taken into the system from without, as in botulism.

retention t. One with clinical symptoms due to the retention of waste products, as in uremia.

tox″i·co·ta·bel′la. See *toxitabella.*

tox″i·der·ma·to′sis. Toxicoderma.

tox″i·der·mi′tis. See *toxicodermatitis.*

tox·if′er·ous [*toxikon;* L. *ferre*, to bear]. Producing or conveying poison.

tox″i·ge·nic′i·ty [*toxikon;* G. *genesthai*, from *gignesthai*, to be produced]. The degree of ability of an organism to produce toxicity or disease.

tox·ig′e·nous (tock·sidj′i·nus) [*toxikon; genesthai*]. Producing toxins.

tox″i·mu′cin. See *toxicomucin.*

tox′in [*toxikon*]. A poisonous product of animal or vegetable cells which, on injection into animals or man, causes the formation of antibodies, called antitoxins. The most important toxins are those produced by bacteria. Phytotoxins, produced by plants, include ricin, from the castor bean, and abrin, from the seed of the Indian licorice, *Abrus praecatorius;* the zootoxins, produced by animals include snake venoms and spider poisons. —**toxin′ic,** *adj.*

Amanita t. A toxin produced by *Amanita phalloides.*

dermonecrotic t. An exotoxin of *Micrococcus pyogenes* which produces necrosis of the skin on intradermal injection: perhaps identical with alpha hemolysin.

diphtheria t. That produced by the *Corynebacterium diphtheriae.* See *diphtheria.*

erythrogenic t. That produced by certain hemolytic streptococci, which is responsible for the rash of scarlet fever. Five antigenetically distinct substances, producing the same clinical reaction, are known. Also called *Dick t.*

fatigue t. A supposed toxic material arising from tissue disintegration in excessive fatigue.

kappa t. See *collagenase.*

tox′in-an″ti·tox′in. Abbreviated, T. A. See *diphtheria* toxin-antitoxin.

tox″in·fec′tion [*toxikon;* L. *infectum*, from *inficere*, to infect]. Infection by means of a toxin, the causative microorganism not being recognized.

tox·in′i·cide [*toxikon;* L. *caedere*, to kill]. Any substance that destroys a toxin.

tox″i·no′sis. See *toxicosis.*

tox″i·pho′bi·a. Toxicophobia. *Obs.*

tox″i·res′in (tock″si·rez′in) [*toxikon;* L. *resina*, resin]. A poisonous decomposition product of digitalis, resulting when the latter is treated with dilute acids or heated to 240° C.

tox·is′ter·ol. A product of the excessive irradiation of ergosterol. Although isomeric with calciferol, it has little antirachitic action and is highly toxic.

tox″i·ta·bel′la [*toxikon;* L. *tabella*, small tablet]. A poison tablet, of an angular shape, and having the word poison and the skull and crossbones design distinctly stamped upon it.

tox″i·ther′a·py [*toxikon;* G. *therapeia*, treatment]. The therapeutic use of antitoxins.

tox″i·tu·ber′cu·lide [*toxikon;* L. *tuberculum*, small

swelling]. A skin lesion due to the action of tuberculous toxin.

tox′o-, tox-. See *toxico-*.

Tox″o·ca′ra (tock″so·kah′ruh) [G. *toxon*, bow; *kara*, head]. A genus of ascarid worms; a few species have been reported in cases of human infestation.

T. canis. The common ascarid of dogs.

T. cati. The common ascarid of cats.

tox′oid [G. *toxikon*, poison; *eidos*, form]. A toxin detoxified by moderate heat and chemical treatment (formaldehyde) but with antigenic properties intact. The toxoids of diphtheria and tetanus are used frequently for immunization.

aluminum hydroxide adsorbed t. One similar to alum precipitated toxoid except that aluminum hydroxide is used to adsorb the toxoid.

alum precipitated t. A detoxified toxin, precipitated with alum, effective in producing active immunity with even a single inoculation, due to its prolonged antigenic stimulus.

tox″o·in·fec′tion. Toxinfection.

tox″o·lec′i·thin (tock″so·less′i·thin) [*toxikon;* G. *lekithos*, yolk]. A mixture of a venom with a lecithin, the latter behaving as a complement for the former.

tox″on·o′sis [*toxicon;* G. *-ōsis*, condition]. An affection resulting from a poison.

tox′o·phil, tox′o·phile (tock′so·file, ·fil) [*toxikon;* G. *philein*, to love]. Having an affinity for toxins or poisons.

tox′o·phore [*toxikon;* G. *phoros*, bearing]. That complex of atoms of a toxin unit which is the poisonous element of a toxin.

t. group. That part of the toxin molecule which exerts the poisonous effects. —**toxoph′orous,** *adj.*

Tox″o·plas′ma (tock″so·plaz′muh) [*toxikon;* G. *plasma*, anything formed]. A genus of parasitic protozoans.

T. gondii. The causative agent of toxoplasmosis.

tox″o·plas·mat′ic (tock″so·plaz·mat′ick) [*toxikon; plasma*]. Relating to infection with *Toxoplasma.*

tox″o·plas′min. The *Toxoplasma* antigen, usually derived from the sediment of the peritoneal fluid of mice highly infected with *Toxoplasma:* used in a cutaneous test for toxoplasmosis.

tox″o·plas·mo′sis (tock″so·plaz·mo′sis) [*toxikon; plasma;* G. *-ōsis*, condition]. The disease caused by infection with the protozoan, *Toxoplasma.* In infants and children the disease usually is characterized by an encephalomyelitis. In adults a form clinically resembling a spotted fever has been reported. Diagnosis is aided by biopsy studies and identification of *Toxoplasma*, skin tests, (toxoplasmin and dye tests).

congenital t. Toxoplasmosis in children, manifested as disseminated encephalomyelitis accompanied by ventricular enlargement, cerebral calcification, and bilateral focal retinochoroiditis.

tox·o′sis. See *toxonosis.*

Toynbee, Joseph [*English otologist*, 1815–66]. One of the outstanding English otologists and author of a classic text on diseases of the ear (1860). Described the corneal corpuscles, also called *Toynbee's corpuscles.* Described the tensor tympani muscle and its sheath, also called *Toynbee's ligament.* Devised a special otoscope, called *Toynbee's otoscope.* See *Gull-Toynbee law* under William Withey *Gull.*

TPI *Treponema pallidum* immobilization. See under *test.*

TPN Triphosphopyridine nucleotide.

TPN.2H Abbreviation for the reduced form of triphosphopyridine nucleotide or dihydrocoenzyme II.

tr. *Tinctura;* tincture.

tra·bec′u·la (pl. *trabeculae*) [L., little beam]. 1. Any one of the fibrous bands extending from the capsule into the interior of an organ. 2. One of the variously shaped spicules of bone in cancellous bone. —**trabecular,** *adj.*

trabeculae carneae. The interlacing muscular columns projecting from the inner surface of the ventricles of the heart. Also called *trabeculae cordis.*

trace el′e·ments. Substances or elements essential to plant or animal life, but present in extremely small amounts. Also called *trace substances.*

tra′cer [OF. *trace*, from L. *tractus*, a drawing]. An isotope which, because of its unique physical properties, can be detected in extremely minute quantity, and hence is used to trace the chemical behavior of the natural element. As isotopes of the same element differ in physical properties only, but have identical chemical properties (with a few exceptions), an isotope detectable by physical properties may be used to trace the pattern of biochemical reactions. Such use of isotopes is referred to as a tracer study. The isotope itself is a tracer. Stable (by measurement of isotopic ratios) or unstable (by detection of their ionizing radiation) isotopes may be used. Also called *t. element.*

tra′che·a (tray′kee·uh, tra·kee′uh) [G. *trachys*, rough]. The windpipe; the cartilaginous and membranous tube extending from the lower end of the larynx to its division into the two bronchi. See Plates 12, 13, 45. —**tracheal,** *adj.*

tra″che·a·ec′ta·sy (tray″kee·uh·eck′tuh·see) [*trachys;* G. *ektasis*, extension]. Dilatation of the trachea.

tra″che·al′gi·a [*trachys;* G. *algos*, pain]. 1. Pain in the trachea. 2. Croup.

tra″che·i′tis [*trachys;* G. *-itis*, inflammation]. Inflammation of the trachea.

trachel-. See *trachelo-.*

trach″e·lag′ra (track″i·lag′ruh) [G. *trachēlos*, neck; *agra*, a seizing]. Rheumatic or gouty pain in the neck.

trach″e·lec′to·my (track″i·leck′to·mee) [*trachēlos;* G. *ektomē*, excision]. Excision of the neck of the uterus.

trach″e·le″ma·to′ma [*trachēlos;* G. *haima*, blood; *-ōma*, tumor]. A hematoma of the neck, or in the sternocleidomastoid muscle.

trach″e·lis′mus (track″i·liz′mus, ·liss′mus) [G. *trachēlismos*, a seizing by the neck]. Spasmodic contraction of the muscles of the neck.

trach″e·li′tis (track″i·lye′tis). [G. *trachēlos*, neck; *-itis*, inflammation]. Inflammation of the neck of the uterus. Also see *cervicitis.*

trach′e·lo- (track′i·lo-), **trachel-** [*trachēlos*]. A combining form meaning *neck.*

trach″e·lo·cyl·lo′sis [*trachēlos;* G. *kyllōsis*, from *kyllos*, crooked]. Torticollis.

trach″e·lo·dyn′i·a [*trachēlos;* G. *odynē*, pain]. Pain in the neck.

trach″e·lo·ky·pho′sis (·kigh·fo′sis) [*trachēlos;* G. *kyphōsis*, a being humpbacked]. An abnormal anterior curvature of the cervical portion of the spinal column.

tra″che·lo·mas′toid. Longissimus capitis muscle: old term.

trach″e·lo·par″a·si′tus [*trachēlos;* G. *parasitos*, parasite]. Taruffi's term for any parasitic growth upon the neck or jaws. See *deromelus, epignathus, pleonotus.*

trach″e·lo·pex′i·a [*trachēlos;* G. *pēxis*, a fixing]. Surgical fixation of the neck of the uterus.

trach″e·lo·plas″ty [*trachēlos;* G. *plassein*, to form]. Plastic operation on the neck of the uterus.

trach″e·lor′rha·phy (track″i·lor′uh·fee) [*trachēlos;* G. *rhaphē*, suture]. Repair of a laceration of the cervix uteri.

trach″e·lor·rhec′tes (·reck′teez) [*trachēlos;* G. *rhēktēs*, a breaker]. An instrument for crushing the cervical vertebrae; used in embryotomy.

trach″e·los′chi·sis (track″i·los′ki·sis) [*trachēlos;* G. *schisis*, cleavage]. A congenital fissure of the neck.

trach″e·lo·syr″in·gor′rha·phy [*trachēlos;* G. *syrigx*, pipe; *rhaphē*, suture]. An operation for vaginal fistula with stitching of the cervix uteri.

trach″e·lot′o·my (track″i·lot′o·mee) [*trachēlos;* G. *tomē*, a cutting]. Incision into the cervix uteri.

tra′che·o- (tray′kee·o-, tra·kee′o-), **tra′che-** [G. *trachys*, rough]. A combining form denoting *connection with*, or *relation to, the trachea.*

tra″che·o·blen″nor·rhe′a [*trachys;* G. *blenna*, mucous discharge; *rhoia*, flow]. A profuse discharge of mucus from the trachea.

tra″che·o·bron′chi·al (·brong′kee·ul) [*trachys;* G. *brogchos*, windpipe]. Pertaining to the trachea and a bronchus or the bronchi.

tra″che·o·bron·chi′tis (·brong·kigh′tis) [*trachys; brogchos;* G. *-itis*, inflammation]. Inflammation of the trachea and bronchi.

tra″che·o·bron·chos′co·py (tray″kee·o·brong-kos′ko·pee, tra·kee″o·) [*trachys; brogchos;* G. *skopein*, to examine]. Inspection of the interior of the trachea and bronchi.

tra′che·o·cele [*trachys;* G. *kēlē*, hernia]. A hernia of the mucous membrane of the trachea.

tra″che·o·fis′sure [*trachys;* L. *fissura*, fissure]. Congenital longitudinal cleft of the trachea.

tra″che·o·la·ryn′ge·al (·la·rin′jul, ·jee·ul, ·lar″in-jee′ul) [*trachys;* G. *larygx*, larynx]. Pertaining to the trachea and the larynx.

tra″che·o·lar″yn·got′o·my [*trachys; larygx;* G. *tomē*, a cutting]. Incision into the larynx and trachea; combined tracheotomy and laryngotomy.

tra″che·o·path′i·a os″te·o·plas′ti·ca [L.]. A deposit of cartilage and bone in the mucosa of the trachea.

tra″che·oph′o·ny (tray″kee·off′o·nee) [*trachys;* G. *phōnē*, sound]. The sound heard over the trachea on auscultation.

tra′che·o·plas″ty [*trachys;* G. *plassein*, to form]. Plastic surgery of the trachea.

tra″che·o·py·o′sis (tray″kee·o·pye·o′sis, tra-kee″o·) [*trachys;* G. *pyōsis*, suppuration]. Purulent tracheitis.

tra″che·or·rha′gi·a [*trachys;* G. *rhēgnynai*, to burst forth]. Hemorrhage from the trachea.

tra″che·or′rha·phy [*trachys;* G. *rhaphē*, suture]. Suturing of the trachea.

tra″che·os′chi·sis (tray″kee·os′ki·sis) [*trachys;* G. *schisis*, cleavage]. Congenital fissure of the trachea.

tra″che·os′co·py [*trachys;* G. *skopein*, to examine]. Inspection of the interior of the trachea by means of a laryngoscopic mirror and reflected light, or through a bronchoscope. —**tracheoscop′ic,** *adj.*

tra″che·o·ste·no′sis [*trachys;* G. *stenōsis*, a being straitened]. Abnormal constriction or narrowing of the trachea.

tra″che·os′to·my [*trachys;* G. *stoma*, mouth]. The formation of an opening into the trachea, and suturing the edges of the opening to an opening in the skin of the neck, as in laryngectomy.

tra′che·o·tome [*trachys;* G. *tomos*, cutting]. A cutting instrument used in tracheotomy; a tracheotomy knife.

tra″che·ot′o·mist [*trachys; tomos*]. One skilled in tracheotomy.

tra″che·ot′o·mize [*trachys; tomos*]. Perform tracheotomy upon a living subject.

tra″che·ot′o·my (tray″kee·ot′o·mee) [*trachys;* G. *tomē*, a cutting]. The operation of cutting into the trachea.

inferior t. One performed below the isthmus of the thyroid gland.

superior t. One performed above the isthmus of the thyroid gland. The cut may be extended to include the cricoid cartilage. See *laryngotomy.*

tra″chi·el·co′sis (tray″kee·el·ko′sis) [*trachys;* G. *helkōsis*, ulceration]. Ulceration of the trachea.

tra″chi·el′cus [*trachys;* G. *helkos*, ulcer]. A tracheal ulcer.

tra·chi′tis (tra·kigh′tis). See *tracheitis.*

tra·cho′ma (tra·ko′muh) [G.]. An infectious disease of the conjunctiva and cornea, producing photophobia, pain, and excessive lacrimation, caused by *Chlamydozoon trachomatis.* The lesion is characterized initially by inflammation and later by pannus and follicular and papillary hypertrophy of the conjunctiva. Syn., *Egyptian conjunctivitis, Egyptian ophthalmia, conjunctivitis granulosa, granular lids.* —**trachom′atous,** *adj.*

Arlt's t. Granular trachoma.

brawny t. A late stage in which the conjunctiva is thickened due to lymphoid infiltration.

diffuse t. A form in which large growths cover the tarsal conjunctiva.

granular t. The usual form of trachoma. Also called *follicular t.*

papillary t. That in which the granulations are red and papillary.

t. deformans. A form of kraurosis vulvae at the stage when it results in diffuse scar tissue.

t. of the vocal cords. Nodular swellings on the vocal folds; singers' nodes.

Türck's t. See dry *laryngitis.*

tra″chy·chro·mat′ic [G. *trachys*, rough; *chrōma*, color]. Deeply staining, as certain nuclei.

tra″chy·o·nych′i·a. An inflammation of the proximal portion of the nail matrix causing the nail to become covered with an opaque, corrugated, lamellated, grayish superficial layer.

tra″chy·pho′ni·a (tray″ki·fo′nee·uh, track″i·) [*trachys;* G. *phōnē*, voice]. Rough or hoarse voice.

trac′ing [OF. *trace*, from L. *tractus*, a drawing]. A recording or marking out of a movement, design, or action.

gothic arch t. A registration of mandibular movement.

tract [*tractus*]. 1. A pathway or course. 2. A bundle or collection of nerve fibers. 3. Any one of the nervous pathways of the spinal cord or brain as an anatomic and functional entity. 4. A group of parts or organs serving some special purpose.

afferent t. A nerve tract of the spinal cord conveying impulses toward the brain: also called *ascending t.*

alimentary t. The alimentary canal.

biliary t. The entire hepatic duct system, including hepatic ducts, gallbladder, cystic duct, and common bile duct.

central tegmental t. Nerve fibers which arise in the red nucleus and reticular formation and end in the inferior olives.

cerebellobulbar t. See fastigiobulbar *t.*

cerebellovestibular t. Efferent fibers arising in the fastigial nuclei and ending in the ipsilateral vestibular nuclei; part of the fastigiobulbar tract.

colliculorubral t. See tectorubral *t.*

comma t. A tract, comma-shaped in cross section, in the dorsal funiculus of the spinal cord. Also called *fasciculus interfascicularis.*

commissurospinal t. Descending nerve fibers arising from the nucleus of the posterior commissure and entering the medial longitudinal fasciculus.

corticobulbar t. Fibers of the pyramidal system that originate in the motor cortex, pass through the internal capsule, and terminate in the motor nuclei of the cranial nerves: also called *corticonuclear tract.*

corticocollicular t. Part of the posterior commissure; nerve fibers which arise in the cerebral cortex and go to the stratum zonale of the superior colliculus.

corticogeniculate t. Nerve fibers arising in the calcarine area of the cerebral cortex and ending in the lateral geniculate body.

corticohabenular t. See *fornix,* 2.

corticohypothalamic t. Nerve fibers which arise in the premotor and posterior orbital areas and end directly in the hypothalamus.

corticomammillary t. See *fornix,* 2.

corticonigral t. A component of the extrapyramidal system; fibers arise principally from areas four and six of the cortex, with some contribution from temporal and parietal lobes, and pass through the stratum intermedium of the cerebral peduncle to synapse with the cells of the substantia nigra.

corticonuclear t. See corticobulbar *t.*

corticopallidal t. Nerve fibers which arise in the premotor area of the cerebral cortex and end in the globus pallidus.

corticopontile t. Fibers of the frontopontile, temporopontile, parietopontile, and occipitopontile tracts which descend from the cortex, pass through the internal capsule, and terminate in the pontine nuclei. The fibers receive various designations depending on whether they arise in the frontal, temporal, parietal, or occipital lobes of the cerebrum. Also called *corticopontine tract.*

corticorubral t. A component of the extrapyramidal system; fibers arise principally from areas four and six, with some contribution from areas three and five of the parietal lobe of the cortex, pass through the posterior limb of the internal capsule, and enter the superior radiation of the red nucleus.

corticospinal tracts. Efferent tracts which descend from the frontal cortex through the internal capsule, cerebral peduncles, pons and medulla, where they undergo incomplete decussation to form the lateral and ventral corticospinal tracts. They are concerned in finely coordinated voluntary movements. The ventral corticospinal tract is also called *fasciculus of Türck.* Syn., *pyramidal tracts.*

corticothalamic t. See *thalamic radiations* under *radiation.*

dentatoreticular t. Nerve fibers which arise from the dentate nucleus, separate from the superior cerebellar peduncle just before and beyond its decussation, and descend as crossed and uncrossed fibers in the reticular formation.

dentatorubral t. Part of the superior cerebellar peduncle; nerve fibers which arise in the dentate nucleus and terminate in the contralateral red nucleus.

dentatothalamic t. The largest component of the superior cerebellar peduncle; nerve fibers which arise in the ventrolateral part of the dentate nucleus and end in the lateral ventral thalamic nucleus.

descending t. A collection of nerve fibers conducting impulses down the spinal cord. Syn., *efferent t.*

descending vestibular t. The descending branches of the vestibular root which end in the spinal and lateral vestibular nuclei: also called *spinal vestibular tract, descending* or *spinal vestibular root.*

digestive t. The alimentary canal.

direct cerebellar t. Old term for dorsal spinocerebellar tract.

dorsal longitudinal t. of Schütz. See periventricular *t.*

dorsal spinocerebellar t. A nerve tract which arises from the cells of the dorsal nucleus of Clark, ascends the spinal cord in the lateral funiculus, and reaches the cerebellum by way of the restiform body; it conveys subconscious proprioceptive impulses.

dorsal t. of Schütz. See periventricular *t.*

dorsolateral t. The narrow bridge of white substance between the apex of the dorsal horn and the periphery of the spinal cord; it is traversed by some of the root fibers. Syn., *Lissauer's t.*

efferent t. See descending *t.*

fastigiobulbar t. A tract arising in the fastigial nuclei, containing crossed and uncrossed fibers, which descends medial to the restiform body into the medulla oblongata: also called *cerebellobulbar tract.*

Flechsig's t. See Paul Emil *Flechsig.*

frontopontile t. See corticopontile *t.*

gastrointestinal t. The alimentary canal.

generative t. Old term for the female genital system which consists of ovaries, tubes, uterus, vagina, and the external genitalia. See Plate 41.

geniculocalcarine t. A nerve tract arising from the lateral geniculate body and terminating in the striate area or visual cortex; it conveys visual impulses. Also called *optic radiation.*

geniculotemporal t. See auditory *radiation.*

genitourinary t. The urogenital system.

Goll's t. Fasciculus gracilis.

Gowers' t. See William Richard *Gowers.*

habenulopeduncular t. See *fasciculus* retroflexus.

Helweg's t. See olivospinal *t.*

hypothalamicohypophyseal t. A tract of nerve fibers, with cells of origin in the supraoptic and paraventricular nuclei of the hypothalamus and also in the tuber cinereum, which runs through the median eminence and infundibular stem to the neurohypophysis and which distributes fibers to these parts. Injury to this tract or its nuclei of origin is associated with diabetes insipidus. Its component parts are also referred to as *supraopticohypophyseal t., paraventriculohypophyseal t.,* and *tuberohypophyseal t.,* respectively.

iliotibial t. A thickened portion of fascia lata extending from the lateral condyle of the tibia to the iliac crest. Formerly called *Maissiat's band.*

interstitiospinal t. Descending nerve fibers which arise in the interstitial nucleus of Cajal and enter the medial longitudinal fasciculus.

lateral corticospinal t. Fibers of the corticospinal tract which have formed the pyramidal decussation and descend in the lateral funiculus of the spinal cord, terminating in the gray matter of the same side.

lateral spinothalamic t. A tract of nerve fibers which arise from cells of the posterior column, cross in the anterior white commissure, ascend in the lateral funiculus, and terminate in the thalamus; it conducts pain and temperature impulses.

lenticulothalamic t. Fibers from the lenticular nucleus to the thalamus.

Lissauer's t. See dorsolateral *t.*

Loewenthal's t. See tectospinal *t.*

mammillotegmental t. Nerve fibers which arise in the mammillary bodies and end in the tegmental nuclei of the midbrain.

mammillothalamic t. A tract of nerve fibers passing from the mammillary body to the anterior nucleus of the thalamus. Also called *Vicq d'Azyr's bundle* or *fasciculus.*

mesencephalic t. of trigeminal nerve. Nerve

fibers which arise in cells located in the lateral portion of the central gray matter of the upper fourth ventricle and the cerebral aqueduct and join the motor root of the trigeminal nerve.
motor t. Any descending tract of the central nervous system, terminating in primary motor nuclei.
nigroreticular t. Nerve fibers which arise in the substantia nigra and end in the reticular formation by way of the basis pedunculi and the tegmentum.
nigrorubral t. Nerve fibers which arise in the substantia nigra and end in the red nucleus by way of the tegmentum.
nigrostriatal t. Nerve fibers which arise in the substantia nigra and end in the corpus striatum.
occipitopontile t. See corticopontile *t.*
olfactohabenular t. Nerve fibers which arise in the basal olfactory nuclei, curve dorsally, and, entering the stria medullaris thalami, go to the habenular nucleus of the same and opposite side.
olfactohypothalamic t. See basal olfactory *fasciculus.*
olfactory t. A narrow band of white substance originating in the olfactory bulb and extending posteriorly in the olfactory sulcus, to the anterior perforated substance where it enlarges to form the olfactory trigone and divides into two roots, the lateral and medial olfactory striae. See Plates 17, 18.
olfactotegmental t. See basal olfactory *fasciculus.*
olivocerebellar t. A tract of nerve fibers from the inferior and accessory olivary nuclei of the same and opposite sides, which reaches the cerebellum by way of the restiform body.
olivospinal t. A tract composed of fibers arising in the medulla oblongata, perhaps in the inferior olivary nucleus, and ending in the gray matter of the spinal cord; formerly called *Helweg's tract* or *bundle.*
optic t. A band of nerve fibers running around the lateral side of a cerebral peduncle from the optic chiasma to the lateral geniculate body and midbrain.
pallidohypothalamic t. Nerve fibers which arise in the globus pallidus and end in the hypothalamus.
pallidoreticular t. Nerve fibers which arise in the globus pallidus and end in the reticular formation of the midbrain, pons, and medulla.
pallidosubthalamic t. Nerve fibers which arise in the globus pallidus, traverse the basis pedunculi, and end in the subthalamic nucleus.
pallidothalamic t. Nerve fibers which arise in the globus pallidus and go to the anterior ventral nucleus and perhaps also to some of the medial thalamic nuclei.
paraventriculohypophyseal t. See hypothalamicohypophyseal *t.*
parietopontile t. See corticopontile *t.*
periependymal t. See periventricular *t.*
periventricular t. Nerve fibers which arise in the posterior hypothalamic nucleus and tuberal and supraoptic nuclei. Some end in the dorsomedial thalamic nucleus and in some of the midline nuclei. Some descend dorsally to the cerebral aqueduct and end in the tectum of the midbrain. Others descend ventrally to the aqueduct in the subependymal portion of the central gray matter and end in the vestibular nuclei and the dorsal nucleus of the vagus; these fibers form the periependymal tract. Also called *dorsal t. of Schütz* or *dorsal longitudinal t. of Schütz.*
pontocerebellar t. See middle cerebellar *peduncle.*
pyramidal tracts. See *corticospinal* and *corticobulbar tracts* under *tract.*
respiratory t. The respiratory organs in continuity. See Plate 12.
reticulobulbar t. Nerve fibers which arise in cells of the reticular formation and go to the motor nuclei of the cranial nerves in the medulla.
reticulo-olivary t. Part of the central tegmental tract; nerve fibers which arise in the reticular formation and end in the inferior olive.
reticuloreticular t. Nerve fibers which arise in the reticular formation and end in it at lower levels.
reticulospinal t. Nerve fibers descending from large cells of the reticular formation of pons and medulla into the spinal cord. It is a component of the extrapyramidal system mediating brain stem and spinal reflexes.
rubrobulbar t. Nerve fibers which arise in the red nucleus, cross in the ventral tegmental decussation, descend in the reticular formation, and go to the nuclei of the cranial nerves in the medulla.
rubro-olivary t. Nerve fibers which arise in the red nucleus and end in the homolateral inferior olive.
rubroreticular t. Nerve fibers descending from the red nucleus and terminating in the nuclei of the reticular formation.
rubrospinal t. A nerve tract descending from the red nucleus into the spinal cord which, in man, has been largely replaced in function by the phylogenetically newer, reticulospinal tract. It is a component of the extrapyramidal system concerned with tonic and automatic associative control. Also called *Monakow's bundle, fibers, tract.*
rubrothalamic t. Nerve fibers which arise in the red nucleus and go mainly to the lateral ventral nucleus of the thalamus.
sensory t. Any tract of fibers conducting sensory impulses to the brain.
septomarginal t. A nerve tract composed of descending fibers of intraspinal and dorsal root origin, located in the posterior funiculus of the thoracic region.
solitary t. See *tractus* solitarius.
spinal t. of the trigeminal nerve. A nerve tract located in the medulla, composed of sensory fibers of the trigeminal nerve which terminate in the nucleus of the spinal tract of the trigeminal nerve.
spinal vestibular t. See descending vestibular *t.*
spinocerebellar t. See dorsal spinocerebellar *t.*, ventral spinocerebellar *t.*
spino-olivary t. A tract composed of fibers running from the spinal cord to the inferior olivary nucleus of the medulla oblongata: also called *spino-olivary fasciculus.*
spinospinal t. See *fasciculus* proprius.
spinothalamic t. See lateral spinothalamic *t.*, ventral spinothalamic *t.*
strionigral t. Nerve fibers which arise in the putamen and caudate nucleus and go to the substantia nigra.
striothalamic t. See lenticulothalamic *t.*
supraopticohypophyseal t. See hypothalamicohypophyseal *t.*
tectobulbar t. See tectospinal *t.*
tectocerebellar t. A bundle of fibers arising in the tectum or roof of the midbrain and descending to the cerebellum.
tectorubral t. Nerve fibers which arise in the superior colliculus and go to the red nucleus by way of the dorsal tegmental decussation. Syn., *colliculorubral t.*
tectospinal t. A nerve tract which descends from large cells in the tectum of the mesencephalon,

decussates, gives off fibers to the motor nuclei of the brain stem, and synapses with motor cells of the spinal cord, chiefly in the cervical region. It includes the tectobulbar tract. Also called *Loewenthal's t.*

tegmento-olivary t. A tract arising in the midbrain and terminating in the inferior olivary nucleus.

temporopontile t. See corticopontile *t.*

thalamocortical t. See *thalamic radiations* under *radiation.*

t. of Allen. The tractus solitarius.

t. of Schütz. See periventricular *t.*

trigeminothalamic t. Trigeminal lemniscus.

tuberohypophyseal t. See hypothalamicohypophyseal *t.*

urinary t. The passage for the urine, including the kidneys, renal pelves, ureters, urinary bladder, and urethra.

urogenital t. Old term for urogenital system. See Plates 43, 44.

uveal t. The iris, ciliary body, and choroid.

ventral corticospinal t. Fibers of the corticospinal tract which, without decussating, descend directly in the ventral funiculus, normally to the upper thoracic region.

ventral spinocerebellar t. A nerve tract which arises from cells of the dorsal column of the same and opposite sides, and ascends in the lateral funiculus of the spinal cord to reach the cerebellum by way of the brachium conjunctivum.

ventral spinothalamic t. A tract of nerve fibers which arise from cells in the posterior column, cross in the anterior white commissure, ascend in the ventral funiculus, and terminate in the thalamus; it conducts impulses from touch and pressure stimuli.

vestibulocerebellar t. A nerve tract of vestibular root fibers and secondary vestibular fibers which reach the fastigial nuclei in the cerebellum by way of the restiform body.

vestibulo-ocular t. A tract of homolateral and contralateral nerve fibers arising from the superior and medial vestibular nuclei, which ascends in the median longitudinal fasciculus to the nuclei of the oculomotor, trochlear, and abducens nerves; it mediates reflex movements of head and eyes.

vestibulospinal t. A nerve tract which originates principally from the lateral vestibular nucleus and descends in the anterior funiculus of the spinal cord; it mediates impulses concerned with static equilibrium.

trac'tion [*tractus*]. The act of drawing or pulling.

ambulatory t. That exerted by a walking splint or brace so that the pull is maintained upon the fractured limb or inflamed joint while the patient is up and about.

axis t. Traction in the axis or direction of a channel, as of the pelvis, through which a body is to be drawn.

bed t. Any form of traction in which the patient is of necessity confined to bed.

elastic t. Traction exerted by means of rubber bands, usually employed in phalangeal fractures treated with some form of wire frame or plaster splint, and in connection with certain dental splints.

head t. That exerted upon the head, usually employed in the treatment of injuries of the cervical spine.

weight t. That exerted by means of a weight, connected to the injured limb.

trac'to·graph [*tractus;* G. *graphein,* to write]. An apparatus used to make traction tests.

trac'tor [*tractus*]. An instrument for making traction.

trac·tot'o·my [*tractus;* G. *tomē,* a cutting]. The surgical resection of a nerve-fiber tract of the central nervous system, usually for relief of pain.

medullary t. Surgical incision of the spinothalamic tract in the medulla or of the descending of spinal root of the trigeminal nerve: also called *bulbar t.*

mesencephalic t. See *mesencephalotomy.*

spinal t. See *chordotomy.*

trac'tus [L.]. Tract.

t. genitalis. See genital *cord.*

t. solitarius. The sensory fibers in the medulla of the seventh, ninth, and tenth nerves which bend caudally to form a descending bundle and terminate in the dorsal sensory nucleus of the vagus and the nucleus of the solitary tract. Also called *t. of Allen.*

Tracy method. See Welker and Tracy *method.*

trade-mark. A name or mark applied to a substance or product whereby its origin as of a particular producer is indicated; such a name or mark, which may or may not be officially registered, is the property of the producer. A name in this category is frequently called a *trade-marked name.*

trade name. A name, commonly not descriptive or invested with ownership rights, by which a substance or product is known in commerce and industry. If it is intended to indicate the origin of the substance or product as of a particular producer, it is preferably called a *trade-mark* or *trade-marked name.*

trag'a·canth [G. *tragakantha,* tragacanth]. A gummy exudation from various Asiatic species of *Astragalus,* of the family Leguminosae. Almost white ribbons or powder; swells with 50 parts of water to make a stiff opalescent mucilage. A soluble portion is said to consist chiefly of uronic acid and arabinose; the insoluble portion which swells in water is largely bassorin, $(C_{11}H_{20}O_{10})_n$. Used as a suspending agent for insoluble powders and in the manufacture of troches.

tra'gi (tray'jye) [G. *tragos,* goat]. Hairs of the external auditory meatus.

Tra'gi·a [NL.]. A genus of poisonous plants; some species have been used in folk medicine as a purgative, diuretic, and caustic.

tra'gi·cus [G. *tragos,* goat]. Vestigial muscle associated with the tragus of the external ear.

trag"o·mas·chal'i·a (trag"o·mas·kal'ee·uh) [*tragos;* G. *maschalē,* armpit]. Bromhidrosis of one or both axillas.

trag"o·pho'ni·a, tra·goph'o·ny. See *egophony.*

tra'gus [*tragos*]. 1. The small prominence of skin-covered cartilage projecting over the meatus of the external ear. 2. One of the hairs at the external auditory meatus.

trail'er. See trailing *hand.*

train'ing [OF. *trainer,* to draw]. Systematic exercise for physical development or for some special attainment.

auricular t. The training of a person with handicapped hearing in the full use of the hearing that he has available.

train'ing school. A school of nursing.

trait [F., from L. *tractus,* a drawing]. Any characteristic, quality, or property of an individual.

Cooley's t. Thalassemia minor.

sickle-cell t. See sickle-cell *anemia.*

trance [L. *transire,* to pass over]. 1. The hypnotic state; resembles sleep. See *hypnosis.* 2. A form of catalepsy, characterized by a prolonged condition of abnormal sleep, in which the vital functions are depressed and from which the patients ordinarily cannot be aroused. The breathing is almost imperceptible, and sensation abolished. The onset and awakening are both very sudden.

ecstatic t. Catalepsy.

hysterical t. The trancelike condition sometimes met with in hysteria.

trans- (trans-, tranz-) [L., through, across]. A combining form denoting *through* or *across*.

trans"am·i·da'tion. See *transdeamination*.

trans·am'i·nase. The enzyme that catalyzes the transfer of the amino group of a dicarboxylic amino acid to a keto acid, to form another amino acid.

trans"am·i·na'tion. 1. The transfer of one or more amino groups from one compound to another. 2. The transposition of an amino group within a single compound.

trans·an"i·ma'tion [*trans;* L. *animare*, to fill with breath]. The performing of artificial respiration on a newborn infant.

trans·au'di·ent [*trans-;* L. *audire*, to hear]. Allowing the transmission of sound.

trans·ca'lent [*trans-;* L. *calere*, to be warm]. Permeable to radiant heat rays.

trans·cav'i·tar"y. Through or across a cavity: usually referring to metastasis of tumor cells, most often in the peritoneal cavity.

trans·con'dy·lar [*trans-;* G. *kondylos*, knuckle]. Across or through condyles.

trans"de·am"i·na'tion. The transference of amino groups from amino acids to other molecules.

trans"de·hy"dro·an·dros'ter·one. See *dehydroisoandrosterone*.

trans·duc'tion. The process of transferring energy from one system to another; the transferred energy may be of the same or of a different form, e.g., a steam engine converting thermal energy to mechanical energy. —**transduc'er,** *n.*

tran·sec'tion [*trans-;* L. *sectio*, a cutting]. A section made across the long axis of a part, as transection of the spinal cord.

trans·fer'ence [L. *transferre*, to convey over]. *In psychoanalysis*, that aspect of the patient's feelings and reactions toward the analyst, based upon seeing in him the reimbodiment of some important figure of his childhood, usually father or mother. Transference may be *positive*, when the feelings and reactions are affectionate, friendly, or loving; it may be *negative*, when these feelings and reactions are hostile. Understanding of transference forms a basic part of psychoanalytic technique.

trans·fer'rin. Siderophilin.

trans·fix'ion [L. *transfixum*, from *transfigere*, to pierce through]. 1. The act of piercing through and through. 2. A method of amputation in which the knife is passed directly through the soft parts, the cutting being done from within outward. —**transfix,** *v.*

trans"fo·ra'tion [L. *transforatio*, a boring through]. The act of perforating the fetal skull. —**trans'-forate,** *v.*

trans'for·a"tor [*transforatio*]. An instrument for perforating the fetal head.

trans"for·ma'tion [L. *transformatio*, from *transformare*, to transform]. A marked change in form, structure, or function.

trans·form'er. An electrical apparatus for the transformation of lower potentials to higher potentials or vice versa. It consists of a laminated iron core on which are wound two coils, a primary and a secondary core, properly insulated from each other. The primary coil is energized by an alternating current at a given voltage, which induces in the secondary coil a voltage related to that in the primary by the ratio of the number of windings in the two coils.

closed core t. Doughnut-shaped core of a high-voltage transformer, with primary coil windings on one side and secondary coil windings on the opposite side.

filament t. A step-down transformer to provide current for the cathode filament in x-ray tubes.

step-down t. A transformer to decrease voltage.

step-up t. A transformer to increase voltage.

trans·fuse' [L. *transfusum*, from *transfundere*, to transfuse]. Perform transfusion.

trans·fu'sion [L. *transfusio*, from *transfundere*]. 1. A transfer of blood into the veins. 2. The introduction into a vessel of the body of blood, saline solution, or other liquid. 3. The pouring of liquid from one vessel to another.

arterial t. Transfusion of blood into an artery.

blood t. Transfer of blood from one individual to another. The blood of donor and recipient must be of the same type.

bone-marrow t. That into a bone-marrow cavity, usually of the sternum, femur, or tibia.

citrate method of t. An indirect method of blood transfusion; the donor's blood is collected in a bottle and mixed with sodium citrate to prevent clotting.

direct t. The transfusion of blood from one person to another without exposure of the blood to the air. Also called *immediate t.*

indirect t. The introduction of blood that was first drawn into a vessel. Also called *mediate t.*

peritoneal t. Transfusion into the peritoneal cavity.

reciprocal t. The exchange of equal volumes of blood between a patient suffering from a febrile disease and one who is convalescent from that disease.

replacement t. A transfusion technic used in the newborn with erythroblastosis foetalis in which the greater part of the total blood volume is replaced in small amounts at a time with Rh negative donor blood, the theory being that the Rh positive antibodies remaining will be minimal.

sternal t. Bone-marrow transfusion into the sternum.

venous t. Transfusion into a vein.

trans·fu'sion·ist [*transfusio*]. One skilled in the transfusion of blood.

trans·fu'so-vac ap"pa·ra'tus. A blood transfusion apparatus originating in Canada, and adapted especially to field use. It consists of a flask containing the appropriate amount of sodium citrate solution, in a partial vacuum, and a special perforation connected with a length of rubber tubing, to the distal end of which an intravenous needle is attached.

tran'sient der"ma·to·zo·o·no'sis. Any skin disease in which the parasite attacks, but does not attach itself to, the skin; if its larvae are left upon the skin to embed themselves within it, the resulting disease is classified as *endodermatozoonosis*. Syn., *transito-zoonosis*.

tran'sient or'ange. An unstable carotenoid pigment formed by the breakdown of visual purple exposed to light, which is rapidly transformed to indicator yellow and then to retinene.

tran'sient sit"u·a'tion·al per"son·al'i·ty dis·or'der. *In psychiatry*, a form of personality disorder, more or less transient, and generally an acute symptom response to a specific situation, without persistent personality disturbance. The acute symptoms, representing attempts to deal with overwhelming situations, generally recede as stress diminishes; repeated failure to do so indicates more severe disturbance. See gross stress, adult situational, adjustment *reaction*.

trans·il'i·ac [L. *trans-*, across; *ilium*, flank]. Passing across from one ilium to the other, as the transiliac diameter or axis.

trans″il·lu″mi·na′tion [*trans-;* L. *illuminare,* to illumine]. 1. Illumination of an object by transmitted light. 2. Illumination of the paranasal sinuses by means of a light placed in the patient's mouth. Also spelled *translumination.*

tran·sis′tor. A device, considerably smaller than a vacuum tube used similarly, for amplifying electric currents through utilization of the semiconductor property of germanium containing minute amounts of other elements.

tran·si′tion·al (tran·zish′un·ul, tran·sish′·) [L. *transitio,* a going across]. Denoting change.

tran·si′tion·al. Ehrlich's name for a monocyte having a U-shaped nucleus, which he regarded as a transitional form in the development of a polymorphic granulocyte; now considered to be an older form of monocyte.

tran′si·to-zo·o·no′sis. Transient-dermatozoonosis.

trans·lu′cent [L. *trans-,* through; *lucere,* to shine]. Permitting a partial transmission of light; somewhat transparent.

trans·lu′cid [*trans-;* L. *lucidus,* shining]. Semitransparent.

trans·meth″yl·a′tion. A type of metabolic chemical reaction in which a methyl group is transferred from a donor to a receptor compound. Methionine and choline are important sources of methyl groups.

trans″mi·gra′tion (trans″migh·gray′shun, ·migray′shun, tranz″·) [L. *transmigratio,* from *transmigrare,* to transmigrate]. A wandering across or through, as transmigration of an ovum, transmigration of white blood cells. See *diapedesis.*

external t. The passage of an ovum from one ovary to the opposite oviduct without transversing the uterus.

internal t. The passage of an ovum through its proper oviduct into the uterus and across to the opposite oviduct.

trans·mis″si·bil′i·ty [L. *transmissum,* from *transmittere,* to send across]. The capability of being transmitted or communicated from one person to another. —**transmis′sible,** *adj.*

trans·mis′sion [L. *transmissio,* from *transmittere*]. The communication or transfer of anything, especially disease, from one person or place to another.

duplex t. The movement of impulses along a nerve in two directions.

humoral t. Transmission of impulse over a synapse by means of chemical substances secreted at the synapse.

placental t. The conveyance of drug and disease products through the placental circulation from mother to offspring.

saltatory t. See saltatory *conduction.*

trans·mit′tance. *In applied spectroscopy,* the ratio of the radiant power transmitted by a sample to the radiant power incident on the sample, both measurements being made at the same spectral position and with the same slit width. Symbol, *T.*

relative t. *In applied spectroscopy,* the ratio of the transmittance of the photographic image of a spectrum line to the transmittance of an adjacent clear (unexposed but developed) portion of the photographic emulsion.

trans″mu·ta′tion [L. *transmutatio,* from *transmutare,* to change]. 1. The evolution of one species into another. *Obs.* 2. *In physics,* any process by which an atomic nucleus is converted into another of different atomic number.

trans·oc′u·lar [L. *trans-,* across; *oculus,* eye]. Extending across the eye.

trans′o·nance [*trans-;* L. *sonare,* to sound]. Transmitted resonance; the transmission of sounds through an organ, as of the cardiac sounds through the lungs and chest wall.

trans·par′ent [*trans-;* L. *parere,* to appear]. Permitting the passage of light rays without material obstruction, so that objects beyond the transparent body can be seen.

trans″phos·phor′yl·ase. One of a group of enzymes, widely distributed in living organisms, which catalyze transfer of phosphate from one compound to another.

tran·spi′ra·ble [*trans-;* L. *spirare,* to breathe]. Capable of passing in a gaseous state through the respiratory epithelium or the skin.

tran″spi·ra′tion (tran″spi·ray′shun, tran″spy-ray′shun) [*trans-; spirare*]. 1. Exhalation of fluid through the skin. 2. The material exhaled.

pulmonary t. The exhalation of water vapor from the lungs.

trans′plant [L. *transplantare,* to transplant]. Tissue removed from any portion of the body and placed in a different site. —**transplant′,** *v.*

trans″plan·ta′tion [*transplantare*]. The operation of transplanting or of applying to a part of the body tissues taken from another body or from another part of the same body. Also see *graft.*

autoplastic t. The exchange of different parts within the same individual.

heteroplastic t. See *heterotransplantation.*

heterotopic t. That in which the graft is transplanted to a different location in the host than it had in the donor.

homoioplastic t. See *homotransplantation.*

homoiotopic t. See homotopic *t.*

homoplastic t. See *homotransplantation.*

homotopic t. That in which the graft is transplanted to the same location in the host that it had in the donor.

isoplastic t. See *homotransplantation.*

tendon t. The removal of a tendon from its normal location and its reinsertion in another place, used to substitute a functioning muscle for a paralyzed one by transplanting its tendon.

tenoplastic t. The exchange of parts from individuals belonging to widely different genera.

t. of cornea. See *keratoplasty.*

trans·pose′ [L. *transpositum,* from *transponere,* to set across]. Displace; change about, as tissue from one location to another by operation.

trans″po·si′tion (trans″po·zish′un) [*transponere*]. A change of position.

t. of the great vessels of the heart. A congenital abnormality which may vary from complete transposition, in which the aorta and pulmonary artery arise from reversed ventricles, to partial transposition, in which both large vessels arise from a common ventricle but in a reversed relation.

t. of the viscera. A change in the position of the viscera to the side opposite to that normally occupied.

trans″sub·stan″ti·a′tion (trans″sub·stan″shee-ay′shun) [L. *trans-,* over; *substantia,* substance]. The replacement of one tissue by another.

tran′su·date [*trans-;* L. *sudare,* to sweat]. A liquid or other substance produced by transudation.

tran″su·da′tion [*trans-; sudare*]. The passing of fluid through a membrane, especially of blood serum through the vessel walls. —**transu′datory,** *adj.;* **transude′,** *v.*

trans″u·ra′nic el′e·ment. An element with an atomic number greater than that of uranium (92).

trans″u·re′thral [*trans-;* G. *ourēthra,* urethra]. Via the urethra, as transurethral operation.

trans·vag′i·nal (trans·vadj′i·nul, ·va·jy′nul, tranz·) [*trans-;* L. *vagina,* vagina]. Across, or through, the vagina.

trans″ver·sa′lis (·vur·sah′lis, ·say′lis) [L. *transversus,* turned across]. Transverse, as transversalis fascia, the fascia on the inner surface of the transversus abdominis muscle between the latter and the peritoneum.

t. sterni. The transverse thoracic muscle.

trans·verse′ [*transversus*]. Crosswise; at right angles to the longitudinal axis of the body.

trans″ver·sec′to·my [*transversus;* G. *ektomē*, excision]. Excision of a transverse process of a vertebra; specifically, in orthopedic practice, the removal of the transverse process of the fifth lumbar vertebra for pain due to irritation of the lower spinal nerve roots.

trans·ver′sus [L.]. Transverse, as transversus abdominis muscle, a muscle of the anterior abdominal wall. See Table of Muscles in the Appendix.

t. nuchae. The occipitalis minor muscle.

trans·ves′ti·tism [L. *trans-*, over; *vestire*, to clothe]. The morbid desire to dress in the clothing of the opposite sex. See *eonism*, *sexo-esthetic inversion.*

trap [AS. *treppe*]. A device for preventing the foul vapors from sewers and waste pipes from entering a house. It generally consists of ∽-shaped pipes, filled with water; some are provided also with valves.

trapadin. A proprietary high-potency, multivitamin capsule.

tra·pe′zi·um [G. *trapezion*, small table]. The multangulum majus, the first bone of the second row of the carpal bones. See Table of Bones in the Appendix.

tra·pe′zi·us [*trapezion*]. A muscle arising from the occipital bone, the nuchal ligament, and the spines of the thoracic vertebrae, and inserted into the clavicle, acromion, and spine of the scapula. See Table of Muscles in the Appendix.

trap′e·zoid [G. *trapezoeidēs*, table-shaped]. 1. A geometrical, four-sided figure having two parallel and two diverging sides. 2. The multangulum minus, the second bone of the second row of the carpus. See Table of Bones in the Appendix.

Trapp, Julius [*Russian pharmacist*, 1815–1908]. Introduced a formula for the determination of solids in the urine, called *Trapp's formula, Trapp-Haeser formula.* Also see *Haeser.*

trasentine. Trade-mark for a brand of adiphenine; chemically diphenylacetyl-diethylaminoethanol hydrochloride, $(C_6H_5)_2CH.CO.O.CH_2.CH_2.N(C_2H_5)_2.HCl$. The substance is used as an antispasmodic in spasms of an involuntary muscle.

tras′si. A preparation of fermented fish used as food in eastern Asia.

t ratio. The ratio of a statistical constant to its standard error. Also called *t function.*

Traube, Ludwig (1818–1876). German physician who described phantom blood corpuscles, sometimes called *Traube's corpuscles.* A double sound heard over the peripheral arteries, especially the femoral, in aortic insufficiency or mitral stenosis is called *Traube's sign.* See also *Traube-Hering waves* under *wave;* semilunar *space.*

Traube's rule. See under *rule.*

Traugott, Carl [*German internist*, 1885–]. See Hans *Staub* for the *Staub-Traugott phenomenon.*

trau′ma (trou′muh) (pl. *traumas, traumata*) [G.]. A form of injury; commonly, injury by mechanical agents; broadly, injury produced by any physical agent; also, severe psychic injury.

auditory t. Impairment of hearing due to degeneration in the middle or inner ear produced by unusual or prolonged sounds. Also called *acoustic t.*

occlusal t. Injury to the periodontium associated with abnormal or damaging forces of occlusion.

trau·mat′ic (trou·mat′ick) [G. *traumatikos*, of wounds]. Pertaining to, or caused by, a wound or injury.

trau·mat′ic ac′id. $COOH.CH{:}CH(CH_2)_8COOH$. A dibasic acid found in certain plants after they have been cut or bruised; stimulates resumption of division of mature cells.

trau·mat′i·cin (traw·mat′i·sin). A solution of gutta-percha in chloroform used for closing superficial wounds.

trau′ma·tism (trou′muh·tiz·um) [G. *trauma*, a wound]. The general or local condition produced by a wound or injury. —**traumatize,** *v.*

periodontal t. Injury of periodontium due to excessive occlusal, operative, accidental, or orthodontic stress.

trau″ma·tol′o·gy [*trauma;* G. *logos*, word]. The science or description of wounds and injuries, especially as they occur in industry and transportation.

trau″ma·top′a·thy [*trauma;* G. *pathos*, disease]. Pathologic condition due to wounds or other violence.

trau″ma·top·ne′a [*trauma;* G. *pnoē*, breathing]. The passage of respiratory air through a wound in the chest wall.

trau″ma·to′sis [*trauma;* G. *-ōsis*, condition]. Traumatism.

Trautmann's triangle. See under *triangle.*

trav′ail (trav′ail, trav′ul) [F.]. Labor of childbirth.

travamin. Trade-mark for an enzymatic hydrolysate of bovine plasma used for the nutritive effect of the constituent amino acids. See *plasma hydrolysate.*

trav′el ra′tion. See under *ration.*

Travers, Benjamin [*English surgeon*, 1783–1858]. Tied the common carotid artery for aneurysm of the orbit (1811). Made an early study of intestinal sutures. Author of an early treatise on diseases of the eye.

tray [AS. *trēg*]. A flat, shallow vessel of glass, hard rubber, or metal, for holding instruments during a surgical operation.

impression t. *In dentistry*, a metal receptacle used to hold wax or other plastic material used for making impressions of the teeth and gums.

tread (tred) [AS. *tredan*]. *In veterinary medicine*, injury to the coronet of a horse's hoof, due to striking with the shoe of the opposite side.

treat [L. *tractare*, to treat]. Combat disease by the application of remedies.

treat′ment [*tractare*]. The means employed in effecting the cure of disease; the management of disease or of diseased patients. Also see *therapy.*

active t. That which is vigorously applied to the disease.

Ascoli t. One form of treatment for malaria which consists of daily injections of adrenalin. The treatment should be used in conjunction with cinchona alkaloids.

Baer's t. In an ankylosed joint, the adhesions are broken and sterile oil is then injected to prevent the re-forming of the adhesions.

Carrel-Dakin t. The frequent and regularly repeated irrigation of open wounds with a solution of chlorinated soda and sodium bicarbonate.

causal t. That which is directed to the removal of the cause of a disease.

closed plaster t. A general descriptive term for a procedure in which plaster is used over a recent operative wound, the cast complementing the operation in the treatment. The encasement of the wound is carried out without suture. Except over the prominent bony points, plaster is applied directly to the skin over a petroleum jelly gauze. Joints proximal and distal to the wound are immobilized. Ordinarily, the dressing is not changed before a week or ten days.

conservative t. Treatment which is entirely

expectant and abstains from any interference until absolutely necessary; in surgical cases, it aims at preservation rather than mutilation.

crossfire t. A method of arranging treatment beams in roentgen-ray deep therapy in such a manner that they overcross in the depth of the body at the site of the tumor without overloading the skin.

definitive t. Treatment which includes generally accepted procedures necessary to produce ultimately recovery of the patient, as the repair of a perforated intestine.

dietetic t. That depending entirely on the control of the type and amount of food.

drip t. The continuous injection of fluid into the blood or a body cavity so slowly that the rate is measured in drops.

drug t. That depending on the use of drugs.

electric light t. The therapeutic application of electric light by means of cabinets in which the patient sits with the light directed upon the affected part. Its therapeutic effect depends on heat. Used in rheumatism, neuralgia, etc.

electric shock t. See electroshock *therapy.*

Elliott t. Treatment cf pelvic infections by use of a special apparatus which delivers circulating hot water of the desired temperature to the vagina or rectum.

emergency medical t. Medical treatment administered by trained U. S. Army Medical Service personnel prior to definitive treatment.

empiric t. One based on practical observation rather than on scientific reasoning.

expectant t. Watching the progress of a disease, and not interfering unless special symptoms arise.

fever t. See fever *therapy.*

holistic t. Treatment of the patient as a whole.

hot air t. The local application of superheated dry air, the affected part being introduced into a cylinder or chamber.

hypoglycemic shock t. Treatment used in certain types of mental diseases, in which shock and unconsciousness are produced by large doses of insulin.

light t. Treatment by sunlight or artificial light.

palliative t. That which is directed toward relief of symptoms rather than the cure of disease.

perennial t. Treatment carried on throughout the year, as for seasonal hay fever, in contradistinction to preseasonal or coseasonal treatment.

preseasonal t. Prophylactic treatment by injection of pollen extract before the onset of hay fever.

Proetz's t. See Arthur Walter *Proetz.*

rational t. One based on scientific reasoning rather than practical observation or empiricism.

Rogers' t. for cholera. This treatment employs two solutions—hypertonic and alkaline saline—which are given intravenously in amounts proportional to the rise in specific gravity of the blood.

root canal t. The opening, cleansing, and sterilization of a root canal preparatory to root canal filling.

specific t. A treatment having a proved destructive effect against a specific etiologic factor or having a definite curative effect upon a particular disease.

starvation t. In diabetes, certain days of fasting followed by a limited diet with very little carbohydrate.

surgical t. One requiring manipulation or operative procedure.

Swift-Ellis t. Treatment of central nervous system syphilis by injecting the patient's own serum into the subarachnoid space. For this purpose, the blood is drawn one-half hour after an intravenous injection of arsphenamine.

tonic t. Treatment of disease by tonics.

vibration t. Massage by rapid shaking of the body or a part, maintained by a mechanical machine or oscillator.

Wagner-Jauregg t. Treatment of central nervous system syphilis by fever of artificially induced malaria.

Winkelstein's t. A method for controlling gastric acidity in ulcer patients. A fluid pabulum which contains an antacid is introduced into the stomach by means of the Penrose, latex nasogastric tube. This intragastric drip is continuous, and is prescribed for one, two, or three weeks.

treburon. Trade-mark for the sodium salt of sulfated polygalacturonic acid methyl ester methyl glycoside, an anticoagulant having heparinlike activity, with the advantage of less toxicity: administered intravenously or intramuscularly.

tree [ME. from AS. *trēo*]. 1. A perennial woody plant with one main stem and numerous branches. 2. *In medicine*, a structure resembling a tree; a system or organ with many branches.

bronchial t. The arborization of the bronchi of the lung, considered as a structural and functional unit: also called *respiratory t.*

spindle t. See *euonymus.*

tre·ha'la (tri·hah'luh, tri·hay'luh) [*Turk.*]. Turkish manna; a variety of manna derived from the cocoons of *Larinus maculatus*, an insect that feeds upon an Asiatic thistle, *Echinops persicus.*

tre'ha·lose (tree'huh·loce, tri·hal'oce). $C_{12}H_{22}O_{11}.2H_2O$; a sugar found in trehala manna and widely distributed in fungi; 1-α-D-glucopyranosyl-α-D-glucopyranoside, yielding on hydrolysis two molecules of D-glucose.

Treitz, Wenzel [*Austrian physician and anatomist*, 1819–72]. Best known for his description of retroperitoneal hernia through the duodenojejunal fossa (1857), called *Treitz's hernia.* Described the inferior duodenal fossa, which is known as *Treitz's fossa.* Described a fold of peritoneum extending from the duodenojejunal junction to the left crus of the diaphragm, called *ligament of Treitz.* See also *muscle* of Treitz.

tre'ma [G. *trēma*, hole]. 1. A foramen. 2. The vulva.

Trem"a·to'da (trem"uh·to'duh) [G. *trēmatōdēs*, from *trēma*, hole; *eidos*, form]. A class of flatworms; the digenetic species are endoparasites of man. The life cycle is complex, involving sexual and asexual reproduction; two intermediate hosts are required. Some of the genera seen most often are *Clonorchis, Fasciola, Fasciolopsis, Opisthorchis, Paragonimus, Schistosoma,* and *Troglotrema.* Also called *fluke.* —**trem'atode, trem'atoid,** *adj., n.*

trem"a·to·di'a·sis [*trēmatōdēs;* NL. *-iasis*, condition]. Infestation with a trematode.

trem'bles [L. *tremulus*, trembling]. A disease occurring in humans who have ingested milk, butter, or possibly beef of animals with the disease. Animals are affected from eating white snakeroot, *Eupatorium urticaefolium*, or the rayless goldenrod, *Aplopappus heterophyllus.* The disease is afebrile, but there are weakness, anorexia, vomiting, and sometimes death. Also called *milk sickness.*

trem'bling [*tremulus*]. A tremor; quivering.

trem'bling. Affected with involuntary muscular agitation. —**tremble,** *v.*

trem'bling-ill". Louping-ill.

trem'el·loid, trem'el·lose [L. *tremere*, to tremble; G. *eidos*, form]. Gelatinous; resembling the spore-producing organ of the fungus, *Tremella.*

trem'e·tol [*tremere*]. A toxic unsaturated alcohol from white snakeroot; produces trembles in cattle and sheep that eat the plant.

trem′o·gram (trem′o·gram, tree′mo·) [*tremere;* G. *gramma*, letter]. The tracing of tremor made by means of the tremograph.

trem′o·graph (trem′o·graf, tree′mo·) [*tremere;* G. *graphein*, to write]. A device for recording tremor.

tre″mo·la′bile (tree″mo·lay′bil, ·lab′il, trem″o·) [*tremere;* L. *labilis*, slipping]. Easily inactivated or destroyed by agitation.

trem′o·lo. An irregular, exaggerated vibrato; a voice tremor, symptomatic of psychogenic disturbance, old age, or diseases affecting the organs of respiration and phonation or their nervous control.

tre″mo·pho′bi·a (tree″mo·fo′bee·uh, trem″o·) [*tremere;* G. *phobos*, fear]. A morbid fear of trembling.

trem′or (trem′ur, tree′mur) [L., from *tremere*]. A trembling of the voluntary muscles; involuntary rhythmic movements, involving the entire muscle, or only a circumscribed group of muscle bundles.

arsenical t. The result of arsenical intoxication.

asynergic family t. See essential *t.*

coarse t. One with not more than six or seven vibrations per second.

continuous t. A form of tremor which resembles that of paralysis agitans; it is, however, likely to be remittent, and may be diminished or arrested by voluntary effort.

convulsive t. See *paramyoclonus multiplex.*

effort t. Intention tremor.

epileptoid t. Intermittent clonus with tremor.

essential t. A familial tremor, associated with no other stigmas, which is exaggerated by action and emotional tension; it begins in childhood or adolescence and becomes progressive in old age. Syn., *heredofamilial tremor.*

fascicular t. See fibrillary *t.*

fibrillary t. Tremor caused by consecutive contractions of separate muscle fibers.

fine t. One with ten or twelve vibrations per second.

forced t. The convulsive movements persisting during repose after voluntary motion, due to an intermittent and rhythmic irritation of the nervous centers.

heredofamilial t. See essential *t.*

Hunt's t. See striocerebellar *t.*

hysterical t. The tremor observed in hysteria, due to the irregularity of nervous impulses.

intention t. A slow, coarse tremor of the limbs which is intensified upon voluntary movement and may cease on rest. It is present in certain diseases of the nervous system, notably multiple sclerosis.

intermittent t. The tremor commonly observed in hemiplegics on any attempt at voluntary motion.

lenticulostriate t. That which is caused by degenerative disease of the basal ganglions.

mercurial t. A peculiar form of tremor observed among smelters and others exposed to the fumes of mercury. It is sudden or gradual in onset, and usually is unaccompanied by excessive salivation. The arms are first involved, and then the entire muscular system. If allowed to go on, paralysis and dementia may result.

Minor's t. See essential *t.*

muscular t. Slight, oscillating, rhythmic muscular contractions.

passive t. A static tremor.

physiologic t. A tremor in normal individuals, due to fatigue, apprehension, or overexposure to cold.

pill-rolling t. The behavior of the hand in parkinsonism or shaking palsy; the action is due to static tremor and the exaggerated flexion of the metacarpophalangeal joints.

purring t. See purring *thrill.*

Rendu's t. A hysterical tremor provoked or increased by volitional movements.

resting t. A static tremor.

senile t. Involuntary, rhythmic, oscillatory movements developing with age; moderate movements are apparently physiologic changes.

static t. That which is present while the muscles involved are at rest, usually with three or four vibrations per second and disappearing when the muscles are moved voluntarily or with sleep or anesthesia. Syn., *passive t.*, *resting t.*

striocerebellar t. That which is present while muscles are either at rest or in voluntary movement and which is associated with ataxia and hypotonia.

t. artuum. Paralysis agitans.

t. capitis. Tremor affecting the muscles of the neck and head.

t. coactus. See forced *t.*

t. cordis. A sudden rapid fluttering of the heart, the ordinary full pulse of health suddenly dropping to a mere tremulous thread. A symptom often met in neurotic persons.

t. metallicus. See mercurial *t.*

t. potatorum. Delirium tremens.

t. saturninus. The tremor of lead poisoning.

t. tendinum. See *subsultus* tendinum.

vibratile t. See *fremitus.*

volitional t. A trembling of the entire body during voluntary effort, as observed in multiple sclerosis. See intention *t.*

zinc poisoning tremors. Brass founder's ague.

trem″o·sta′ble [*tremere;* L. *stabilis*, stable]. Not easily inactivated or destroyed by agitation.

trem″u·la′tion [L. *tremulus*, shaking]. A tremulous condition.

trem′u·lous [*tremulus*]. Trembling, quivering, as tremulous iris.

trench foot. A condition of the feet somewhat like frostbite; it occurs in those exposed in the trenches.

trench mouth. See necrotizing ulcerative *gingivitis.*

Trendelenburg, Friedrich [*German surgeon*, 1844–1924]. Ligated the saphenous vein for treatment of varicose veins of the leg (1890). Proposed operation for relief of hydronephrosis. Attempted pulmonary embolectomy (1908) and led the way to its successful performance by Kirschner (1924). See also Trendelenburg's *position*, Trendelenburg's *test.*

Trenner's automatic pipet. An automatic pipet of the glass bulb type used for collecting and diluting blood.

tre·pan′. See *trephine.*

trep″a·na′tion [G. *trypan*, to bore]. The operation of trephining. *Obs.*

trep′a·nize [*trypan*]. Trephine.

tre·pan′ning [*trypan*]. Boring; using the trephine.

tre·phine′ (tre·fine′, tre·feen′) [*trypan*]. A circular instrument with sawlike edges for cutting out a disk of bone, usually from the skull. —**trephine′**, *v.*

conical t. A trephine with a truncated, cone-shaped crown, and provided with oblique ridges on its outer surface to stop its progress as soon as the bone is penetrated.

corneal t. A small cutting trephine used to remove a circular section from the summit of a conical cornea.

nasal t. An instrument made of a steel shaft ending in a small, fenestrated tube, having a knife or saw edge.

tympanic t. An instrument made of a small steel shaft ending in a small, polished tube, 2 mm. ni diameter, with a cutting edge.

tre·phin′ing (tre·figh′ning, tre·fee′ning) [*trypan*]. The operation of cutting bone with a trephine; usually applied to removing a disk of cortical bone by means of a special sawlike instrument.

sclerocorneal t. The removal of a portion of the sclera by means of a specially devised instrument, for the relief of excessive intraocular pressure in chronic simple glaucoma.

treph'one [G. *trephein*, to nourish]. A growth-promoting hormone produced by leukocytes, said to stimulate fibroblastic activity.

trep'i·dant [L. *trepidare*, to tremble at]. Trembling.

trep"i·da'ti·o (trep"i·day'shee·o) [L., from *trepidare*]. State of agitation.

t. cordis. Palpitation of the heart.

trep"i·da'tion [*trepidatio*]. 1. Trembling. 2. Fear; trembling anxiety.

Trep"o·ne'ma [G. *trepein*, to turn; *nēma*, thread]. A genus of spiral organisms of the family Treponemaceae. See Table of the Most Common Microorganisms Pathogenic to Man in the Appendix.

oral T. Organisms, such as *T. macrodentium*, *T. microdentium*, and *T. mucosum*, of no proved pathogenicity, which are found in the mouth.

T. carateum. The organism which causes pinta. Also called *T. americanum*, *T. herrijoni*, *T. pictor*, *T. pintae*.

T. cuniculi. The organism which causes a venereal disease of rabbits called pallidoidosis.

T. pallidum. The organism which causes syphilis.

T. pertenue. The organism which causes yaws.

Trep"o·ne·ma'ce·ae (trep"o·ni·may'see·ee) [*trepein; nēma*]. The family of spiral microorganisms which includes the genera *Borrelia*, *Leptospira*, and *Treponema*.

trep"o·ne"ma·to'sis [*trepein; nēma;* G. *-ōsis*, condition]. Infection caused by *Treponema*.

trep"o·ne·mi'a·sis [*trepein; nēma;* NL. *-iasis*, condition]. Infection caused by *Treponema*.

trep"o·ne"mi·cid'al (trep"o·nee"mi·sigh'dul, ·nem"i·sigh'dul) [*trepein; nēma;* L. *caedere*, to kill]. 1. Destructive to any treponema. 2. Antisyphilitic.

trep'o·ne'min. An antigen prepared from formalin-killed *Treponema pallidum:* used in a skin test for syphilis.

trep·op'ne·a [*trepein;* G. *pnein*, to breathe]. A respiratory distress present in one recumbent posture and absent in another.

trep'pe (tre'eh) [Ger.). See staircase *phenomenon*.

Tresilian, Frederick James [*English physician*, 1862–1926]. Described a sign of mumps, in which the opening of the parotid duct on the inner surface of the cheek, opposite the second upper molar, appears as a bright red papilla; called *Tresilian's sign*.

Treves's bloodless fold. See ileocecal *fold*.

tri- (trye-) [G. and L. *tri-*, three]. A combining form denoting *three*.

tri·ac'e·tin (trye·ass'i·tin). Glyceryl triacetate.

tri'ad [G. *trias*, the number three]. 1. A set of three related elements, objects, or symptoms. 2. *In chemistry*, a trivalent atom or radical.

Charcot t. Nystagmus, intention tremor, and staccato speech, occurring in multiple sclerosis.

chronic anal ulcer t. Hypertrophied papillae, ulcer, and sentinel pile.

Hutchinson's t. The combination of notched teeth, interstitial keratitis, and eighth nerve deafness, found in subjects with prenatal syphilis.

Jacod's t. A triad consisting of total ophthalmoplegia, amaurosis, and trigeminal neuralgia, caused by tumor involvement of cranial nerves II, III, IV, V, and VI.

Kartagener's t. See Kartagener's *syndrome*.

Luciani's t. Asthenia, atonia, and ataxia as manifestations of cerebellar disease.

portal t. The three main structures found in each portal canal, a branch of the hepatic artery and of the portal vein, and a tributary to the common bile duct.

Potter's t. See peritubal *syndrome*.

t. of Schaffer. See Károly *Schaffer*.

t. of Whipple. The three conditions which together are diagnostic of hyperinsulinism: (1) attacks invariably occur after a meal, (2) fasting blood sugar is below 50 mg. per cent, (3) immediate recovery from an acute attack upon administration of glucose.

tri·age' (tree·ahj') [F.]. *In military medicine*, the process of sorting sick and wounded on the basis of urgency and type of condition presented, so that they can be properly routed to medical installations appropriately situated and equipped.

tri"a·kai"de·ka·pho'bi·a (try"uh·ky"di·kuh·fo'-bee·uh) [G. *tria kai deka*, thirteen; *phobos*, fear]. Superstitious fear of thirteen. Also called *triskaidekaphobia*.

tri'al [AF.]. The act of trying or testing.

tri·al"kyl·a·mine' (trye·al"kil·uh·meen', trye·al"-kil·am'in). See *alkylamine*.

tri'an"gle [L. *triangulus*, having three corners]. 1. A geometrical figure having three sides and three angles. 2. A three-sided area or region having natural or arbitrary boundaries. —**trian'gular,** *adj.*

anal t. One with the base between the two ischial tuberosities and the apex at the coccyx. Syn., *rectal t.*

anterior neck t. One bounded in front by the median line of the neck, behind by the anterior margin of the sternocleidomastoid, and above by the lower border of the body of the mandible and a line extending from the angle of the mandible to the mastoid process; it is divided into the inferior carotid, superior carotid, submaxillary, and suprahyoid triangles.

aortic t. One formed below by the upper border of the aortic arch, posteriorly by the upper thoracic spine, and anteriorly by the left subclavian artery, seen on the left antero-oblique view of the heart.

Assézat's t. See facial *t.*

bladder t. The triangle formed by the openings of the ureters and the urethra. Syn., *trigone*.

Bryant's t. See iliofemoral *t.*

cardiohepatic t. One in the right fifth intercostal space separating the heart and the upper surface of the liver.

carotid t. See superior carotid *t.*

Codman's t. The little trumpet-shaped cuff of reactive periosteal bone which surrounds the upper limit of a bone tumor and which appears in an x-ray as a triangular space beneath the uplifted periosteal edge. This signifies subperiosteal, extracortical involvement. Syn., *reactive t.*

digastric t. See submaxillary *t.*

Einthoven's t. Triangle used to show that the algebraic sum of the potential differences of electrocardiographic leads I and III equals that of lead II.

facial t. One bounded by lines between the alveolar point, the basion, and the nasion.

femoral t. One formed laterally by the medial margin of the sartorius, medially by the lateral margin of the adductor longus, and superiorly by the inguinal ligament. Also called *Scarpa's t.*

Garland's t. Area of relative resonance in the low back near the spine, found on the same side as pleurisy with effusion.

Grocco's t. See paravertebral *t.*

Hesselbach's t. One bounded laterally by the inferior epigastric artery, medially by the rectus abdominis, and inferiorly by the medial half of the inguinal ligament.

iliofemoral t. One formed by a line from the anterior superior iliac spine to the top of the greater trochanter, a horizontal line from the anterior superior iliac spine, and a vertical line from the top of the greater trochanter. Also called *Bryant's t.*

inferior carotid t. One bounded by the median line of the neck, the sternocleidomastoid muscle, and the superior belly of the omohyoid muscle. Also called *t. of necessity, muscular t., tracheal t.*

Kiesselbach's t. See Wilhelm *Kiesselbach.*

Lesser's t. One bounded above by the hypoglossal nerve and below by the anterior and posterior bellies of the digastric muscle.

lumbar t. Lateral abdominal wall triangle bounded by the iliac crest below, the external oblique in front, the latissimus dorsi behind, and floored by the internal oblique. Also called *Petit's t., trigonum lumbale.*

lumbocostal t. (*of Bochdalek*) An area of potential weakness in the left half of the diaphragm, bounded medially by the lateral margin of the lumbar part of the diaphragm, laterally by the posterior margin of the costal part, and posteriorly by the lateral arcuate ligament. In the embryo it is occupied by the left pleuroperitoneal canal. Also called *vertebrocostal t.*

Macewen's t. See suprameatal *t.*

muscular t. See inferior carotid *t.*

occipital t. One bounded in front by the sternocleidomastoid, behind by the trapezius, and below by the omohyoid.

paravertebral t. A triangular area of dullness on the back on the side opposite to that containing a pleural effusion. Also called *Grocco's t.*

pectineal t. One bounded anteriorly by the anterior abdominal wall, laterally by the external iliac vessels, and medially by the pelvic brim.

Petit's t. See lumbar *t.*

posterior neck t. One bounded in front by the sternocleidomastoid, behind by the anterior margin of the trapezius, its base being formed by the middle third of the clavicle, its apex by the occipital bone; divided by the omohyoid into the occipital and subclavian triangles.

reactive t. See Codman's *t.*

rectal t. See anal *t.*

Reinke's t. The space beneath the epithelial border of the vocal folds, allowing some freedom of motion of the margins of the true folds.

Scarpa's t. See femoral *t.*

subclavian t. One bounded above by the inferior belly of the omohyoid, below by the clavicle, and in front by the posterior border of the sternocleidomastoid.

submaxillary t. One bounded above by the lower border of the body of the mandible and a line drawn from its angle to the mastoid process, below by the posterior belly of the digastric and the stylohyoid, and in front by the anterior belly of the digastric. Syn., *digastric t.*

submental t. See suprahyoid *t.*

suboccipital t. One bounded by the posterior major rectus capitis, the superior oblique, and the inferior oblique muscles.

superior carotid t. Triangle bounded above by the posterior belly of the digastric and the stylohyoid, behind by the sternocleidomastoid, and below by the omohyoid. Also called *t. of election, carotid t.*

suprahyoid t. A triangle limited behind by the anterior belly of the digastric, in front by the middle line of the neck, and below by the body of the hyoid bone. Syn., *submental t.*

suprameatal t. Area between the posterior wall of the external acoustic meatus and the posterior root of the zygomatic process. Also called *Macewen's t.*

surgical t. Any triangular area in which surgically important nerves and arteries are found.

tracheal t. The inferior carotid triangle.

Trautmann's t. One with its anterior angle at the labyrinthine prominence, limited behind by the lateral sinus and above by the temporal line.

t. of auscultation. Area limited above by the trapezius, below by the latissimus dorsi, and laterally by the vertebral border of the scapula.

t. of Calot. One bounded above by the cystic artery and on either side by the cystic and hepatic ducts, and found in about 60 per cent of cases in which the cystic artery arises from the right hepatic artery: also called *cystic t.*

t. of election. See superior carotid *t.*

t. of necessity. See inferior carotid *t.*

t. of Phillippe-Gombault. A small triangle, in the dorsomedian border of the spinal cord at the sacral level, occupied by the septomarginal fasciculus.

urogenital t. One with the base between the two ischial tuberosities and the apex below the symphysis pubis.

vertebrocostal t. See lumbocostal *t.*

vesical t. The trigone.

tri·an″gu·la′ris. 1. Old name for triquetrum. See Table of Bones in the Appendix. 2. A muscle of facial expression. See Table of Muscles in the Appendix.

Tri·at′o·ma (trye·at′o·muh) [G. *tri-*, three; *atomos*, uncut]. A genus of bloodsucking Hemiptera, commonly called conenosed bugs. The most important species is **T. megista,** the chief carrier of *Trypanosoma cruzi.* Other species are **T. sordida, T. dimidiata,** and **T. infestans.**

tri″a·tom′ic. 1. Consisting of three atoms. 2. Having three atoms of replaceable hydrogen.

tri·ax′i·al ref′er·ence sys′tem (trye·ack′see·ul). A simple means for determining the mean electric axis of any wave of depolarization or repolarization from the electrocardiogram.

tri′a·zol 156. Cyclohexyl-ethyl-triazole. A substance related chemically to metrazol; used as a convulsant in the treatment of schizophrenia.

trib′ade (trib′ade, trib′ud) [G. *tribas*, from *tribein*, to rub]. A woman who plays the role of the male in homosexual practices. —**tribadism,** *n.*

tri·ba′sic (trye·bay′sick). Having three hydrogen atoms replaceable by bases.

tri·bas′i·lar (trye·bas′i·lur) [G. *tri-*, three; *basis*, base]. Having three bases, as tribasilar synostosis.

tribe [L. *tribus*, tribe]. *In biology*, a division between a genus and a family.

tri″bo·lu″mi·nes′cence (try″bo·lew″mi·ness′uns, trib″o·) [G. *tribein*, to rub; L. *lumen*, light]. Luminosity induced by friction.

tri·bra′chi·us (trye·bray′kee·us) [G. *tri-*, three; *brachiōn*, arm]. Having three arms.

tri·bro″mo·an′i·line hy″dro·bro′mide (trye-bro″mo·an′i·leen, ·lin). $C_6H_2Br_3.NH_2.HBr$. Formerly used as antipyretic and analgesic.

tri·bro″mo·eth′a·nol (trye·bro″mo·eth′a·nole, ·nol, ·nawl) (*tribromoaethanol*). Tribromoethyl alcohol, Br_3CCH_2OH. White, crystalline powder of slight aromatic odor and taste; unstable in air and light. One gram dissolves in 35 cc. of water; very soluble in amylene hydrate.

t. solution (*liquor tribromoaethanolis*). Each cc. contains 1 Gm. of tribromoethanol in amylene hydrate. A clear, colorless liquid of camphoraceous odor. Used as a basal anesthetic, it decreases the amount of inhalation anesthetic necessary for complete anesthesia. Dose, rectal, 0.06 cc. per kilogram of body weight. The solution should be diluted with 40 times its volume of water at approximately body temperature before injection. Maximum total dose is 6–8 cc. for women and 9–10 cc. for men. See *avertin* with amylene hydrate.

tri·bro″mo·eth′yl al′co·hol. Tribromoethanol.

tri·bro″mo·meth′ane. Bromoform.

tri·bu′ty·rin (trye·bew′ti·rin). A constituent of butterfat. See *butyrin.*

tri·cal′cic (trye·kal′sick). Containing three atoms of calcium. *Obs.*

tri·cal′ci·um phos′phate. See tribasic *calcium* phosphate.

tri·car″bal·lyl′ic ac′id. $COOH.CH_2.CH(COOH).-CH_2.COOH$; 1,2,3-propanetricarboxylic acid; colorless crystals, soluble in water; a constituent of beet-sugar molasses.

tri·cel′lu·lar [L. *tri-*, three; *cellula*, small storeroom]. Having three cells.

tri·ceph′a·lus (trye·sef′uh·lus) [G. *tri-*, three; *kephalē*, head]. A monster with three heads.

tri′ceps [L., having three heads]. Three-headed.

tri′ceps. A muscle having three heads, as triceps brachii. See Table of Muscles in the Appendix.

t. extensor cubiti. Triceps muscle: old term.

Tri″cer·com′o·nas. See *Enteromonas.*

trich- (trick-). See *tricho-.*

trich″an·gi·ec·ta′si·a (trick″an·jee·eck·tay′zhuh, ·zee·uh, ·shuh, ·see·uh) [G. *thrix*, hair; *aggeion*, vessel; *ektasis*, extension]. Dilatation of the capillaries.

trich″a·tro′phi·a [*thrix;* G. *atrophia*, want of food]. A brittle state of the hair from atrophy of the hair bulbs.

trich″es·the′si·a, trich″aes·the′si·a (trick″ess-thee′zhuh, ·zee·uh) [*thrix;* G. *aisthēsis*, perception]. 1. A peculiar form of tactile sensibility in regions covered with hairs. 2. See *trichoesthesia.*

trich·i′a·sis (trick·eye′uh·sis) [G., disease of the eyelids]. An abnormal position of the eyelashes which produces irritation by friction upon the globe. The acquired type usually follows an inflammatory condition that produces distortion.

t. of the anus. An incurvation of the hairs about the anus, consequently irritating the mucous membrane.

Tri·chi′na (tri·kigh′nuh). See *Trichinella.*

Trich″i·nel′la (trick″i·nel′uh) [G. *trichinos*, of hair]. A genus of nematode worms which are parasites of man, hogs, rats, dogs, cats, and many other mammals.

T. spiralis. The species found in man.

trich″i·nel·li′a·sis [*trichinos;* NL. *-iasis*, condition]. Trichinosis.

trich″i·nel·lo′sis [*trichinos;* G. *-ōsis*, condition]. Trichinosis.

trich″i·ni′a·sis. See *trichinosis.*

trich″i·no·pho′bi·a [*trichinos;* G. *phobos*, fear]. Morbid fear of trichinosis.

trich″i·no′sis [*trichinos;* G. *-ōsis*, condition]. A disease produced by the ingestion of pork containing *Trichinella spiralis.* It is characterized by nausea, vertigo, fever, diarrhea, prostration, stiffness and painful swelling of muscles, and edema of the face. The intestinal symptoms are due to the development of the adult stage. The muscular and mental symptoms are due to the larval migration through the tissues.

trich·i′tis [G. *thrix*, hair; *-itis*, inflammation]. Inflammation of the hair bulbs.

tri·chlo″ro·ac″et·al′de·hyde. Chloral, 1.

tri·chlo″ro·a·ce′tic ac′id (trye·klor″o·a·see′tick) (*acidum trichloroaceticum*). $CCl_3.COOH$. Colorless, deliquescent crystals. One gram dissolves in about 0.1 cc. of water. A caustic in the pure state or in concentrated solution. Astringent in strengths of 0.1–1%.

tri·chlo″ro·bu′tyl al′co·hol. Chlorobutanol.

tri·chlo″ro·bu″tyl·al′de·hyde. Butyl-chloral hydrate.

tri″chlo·ro·bu·tyl′i·dene gly′col. Butyl-chloral hydrate.

tri·chlo″ro·eth′yl·ene (*trichloroaethylenum*). $CHCl{:}CCl_2$. A clear, colorless liquid of characteristic odor. An anesthetic administered by inhalation in trigeminal neuralgia, migraine, and angina pectoris. It is available in frangible ampuls containing 1 cc. (15 min.); dose, one ampul crushed in a handkerchief and the fumes inhaled.

tri·chlo″ro·meth′ane. Chloroform.

tri·chlo″ro·phe′nol. $C_6H_2Cl_3(OH)$. White crystals of pronounced germicidal power.

trich′o- (trick′o-), **trich-** [*thrix*]. A combining form meaning *hair.*

trich″o·be′zoar [*thrix;* Per. *pād-zahr*, protecting against poison]. A hair ball or concretion in the stomach or intestine. See *egagropilus.*

Tri·cho·bil·har′zi·a oc·el·la′ta. A parasite of wild and domesticated ducks in Europe and North America whose cercaria (*Cercaria elvae*) may cause schistosome dermatitis.

trich″o·car′di·a [*thrix;* G. *kardia*, heart]. Inflammation of the pericardium with pseudomembranous elevations.

trich″o·ceph″a·li′a·sis. See *trichuriasis.*

Trich″o·ceph′a·lus. See *Trichuris.*

trich·oc′la·sis, trich″o·cla′si·a. See *trichorrhexis* nodosa.

trich″o·clas·ma′ni·a [*thrix;* G. *klasis*, a breaking; *mania*, madness]. An affection characterized by an abnormal desire to break off the hair, usually that of the scalp.

trich″o·cryp·to′sis [*thrix;* G. *kryptein*, to hide; *-ōsis*, condition]. Any disease of the hair follicles.

trich′o·cyst [*thrix;* G. *kystis*, bladder]. *In biology*, a small vesicle containing a thread, which can be shot out rapidly; found in the ectoplasm of the Infusoria and in some of the Flagellata.

Trich″o·dec′tes (trick″o·deck′teez) [*thrix;* G. *dektēs*, beggar]. A genus of the suborder Mallophaga or biting lice. They do not infest man.

T. canis. The dog louse; an intermediate host of the dog tapeworm, *Dipylidium caninum.*

Trich″o·der′ma [*thrix;* G. *derma*, skin]. A genus of fungi which is a common laboratory contaminant.

trich″o·ep″i·the″li·o′ma [*thrix;* G. *epi*, on; *thēlē*, nipple; *ōma*, tumor]. A tumor characterized by many pin-headed to pea-sized, round, yellow or skin-colored papules chiefly on the central face. It may be associated with syringoma or cylindroma. Also called *epithelioma adenoides cysticum, Brooke tumor, multiple benign cystic epithelioma, acanthoma adenoides cysticum.*

t. papulosum multiplex. Multiple benign cystic epithelioma.

trich″o·es·the′si·a (trick″o·ess·thee′zhuh, ·zee·uh) [*thrix;* G. *aisthēsis*, perception]. The sensation received when a hair is touched.

trich″o·es·the″si·om′e·ter (·ess·thee″zee·om′i-tur, ·ess·thee″see·om′i·tur) [*thrix; aisthēsis;* G. *metron*, a measure]. An electric appliance for determining the amount of sensation when a hair is touched.

trich′o·gen (trick′o·jen) [*thrix;* G. *genesthai*, from *gignesthai*, to be produced]. A substance that stimulates growth of hair.

trich″o·glos′si·a [*thrix;* G. *glōssa*, tongue]. Hairy tongue, a lengthening of the filiform papillae, producing an appearance as if the tongue were covered with hair.

trich″o·hy′a·lin [*thrix;* G. *hyalos*, glass]. The hyalin of the hair which is like keratohyalin.

trich′oid (trick′oyd) [G. *trichoeidēs*, like a hair]. Resembling hair.

trich″o·kryp″to·ma′ni·a [*thrix;* G. *kryptos*, hidden; *mania*, madness]. Trichorrhexomania.

trich′o·lith [G. *thrix*, hair; *lithos*, stone]. A calcified hair ball within the stomach or intestines.

trich″o·lo′gi·a [*thrix;* G. *legein*, to pick up]. 1. Carphology; floccillation. 2. The plucking out of one's hair.

tri·chol′o·gy [*thrix; legein*]. Trichologia.

trich·ol′o·gy [*thrix;* G. *logos*, word]. The science of the hair and its diseases.

trich·o′ma [G., growth of hair]. 1. Trichomatosis. 2. Trichiasis.

tri·cho″ma·de′sis. The falling out of hair which may lead to alopecia.

trich″o·ma′ni·a. See *trichotillomania*.

trich·o′ma·tose [*trichōma*]. Matted together.

trich″o·ma·to′sis [*trichōma;* G. *-ōsis*, condition]. An affection of the hair characterized by a matted condition, a result of neglect, filth, and the invasion of parasites. See *plica* polonica.

trich′ome (trick′ohm) [*trichōma*]. A hair or other appendage of the epidermis.

t. dermatitis. Dermatitis due to irritation by spicules, hairs, and scales of the epidermis of plants.

trich″o·mo′na·cide. An agent effective in killing *Trichomonas*.

trich″o·mo′nad (trick″o·mo′nad, ·mon′ad) [G. *thrix*, hair; *monas*, unit]. Resembling the flagellates belonging to the genus *Trichomonas*. —**trichomo′nad,** *n.*

Trich″o·mo′nas (trick″o·mo′nas) [*thrix; monas*]. A genus of flagellate protozoa, belonging to the class Mastigophora. Three to five flagella, a thick rodlike axostyle extending throughout the pear-shaped body, and an undulating membrane characterize members of the genus.

T. hominis. The intestinal form found in man; it is not pathogenic.

T. vaginalis. The vaginal form which has been implicated in vaginitis.

trich″o·mo·ni′a·sis [*thrix; monas;* NL. *-iasis*, condition]. The presence of *Trichomonas*.

Trich″o·my·ce′tes (trick″o·migh·see′teez) [*thrix;* G. *mykēs*, fungus]. Fungi of the family Actinomycetaceae, having very narrow filaments, usually much longer than bacteria and often branched; regarded as an intermediate group linking bacteria and higher fungi.

trich″o·my·co′sis (trick″o·migh·ko′sis) [*thrix; mykēs;* G. *-ōsis*, condition]. A disease of the hair produced by fungi.

t. axillaris. Nodules formed on the axillary hairs by the saprophytic growth of species of *Nocardia* and bacteria: also called *trichonocardiosis axillaris*. Syn., *chromotrichomycosis*.

t. barbae. See *sycosis* parasitica.

t. capillitii. See *t.* circinata.

t. circinata. Ringworm of the scalp.

t. favosa. See *favus*.

t. flava nigra. A yellow-red variety of trichomycosis nodosa.

t. nodosa. A peculiar but common condition, generally nodose in character, affecting the hairs of the axilla and scrotum and due to the growth of masses of fungous and bacterial material along the hair. Also called *lepothrix*.

t. palmellina. A disease affecting the hairy parts of the trunk; trichomycosis nodosa.

t. pustulosa. A pustular, parasitic disease affecting hairy regions.

t. rubra. A red variety of trichomycosis nodosa. Red cocci are found in the gelatinous nodules.

trich″o·no·car″di·o′sis (trick″o·no·kahr″dee·o′sis) [*thrix;* after Edmond *Nocard; -ōsis*]. Nodular appearance of the hair due to a species of *Nocardia;* axillary hair is most often affected.

t. axillaris. Trichomycosis axillaris.

trich″o·no·do′sis [*thrix;* L. *nodus*, knot; *-ōsis*]. A pseudoknotting and fraying of the hair associated with thinning and breaking of the hair shaft. At times true knots occur and one case is described in which all were in half-hitch knots. Also called *knotting hair*.

trich″o·no′sis (trick″o·no′sis) [*thrix;* G. *nosos*, disease]. Any disease of the hair.

t. cana. See *canities*.

t. discolor. See *canities*.

trich″o·path″o·pho′bi·a [*thrix;* G. *pathos*, disease; *phobos*, fear]. Undue anxiety and fear regarding the hair, its growth, color, or diseases.

trich·op′a·thy (trick·op′uth·ee) [*thrix; pathos*]. Any disease of the hair. —**trichopath′ic,** *adj.*

trich·oph′a·gy (trick·of′uh·jee), **trich″o·pha′gi·a** [*thrix;* G. *phagein*, to eat]. The eating of hair.

trich″o·pho′bi·a [*thrix;* G. *phobos*, fear]. 1. A morbid fear of hair. 2. Trichopathophobia.

trich″o·phy′ta [*thrix;* G. *phyton*, plant]. A fungus of the genus *Trichophyton*.

trich″o·phy′tid, trich·oph′y·tid [*thrix; phyton*]. A dermophytid caused by *Trichophyton* fungi. There are many varieties. It is due to the absorption of dead fungi or their end products.

trich″o·phy′tin, trich·oph′y·tin [*thrix; phyton*]. A fungous extract made from *Trichophyton* organisms. Used as antigen for a skin test to show the presence of existing or previous infection with these fungi. It is thought by some to be specific, and has been used to treat trychophytid eruptions.

trich″o·phy″to·be′zoar [*thrix; phyton;* Per. *pādzahr*, protecting against poison]. A ball or concretion in the stomach or intestine, made of hair and fibers of vegetable matter and food detritus.

Trich″o·phy′ton, Trich·oph′y·ton [*thrix; phyton*]. A genus of parasitic fungi which attach to the hair, skin, and nails, and are common allergens. Species are identified by the size and position of the spores and by the appearance of the colonies on artificial mediums. The lesions of these fungi are included in the dermatomycoses or ringworm infections. *In dermatology*, the genus is grouped into three main divisions: **Trichophyton ectothrix,** species which invade the hair shaft but which also form a persistent sheath of spores outside the shaft; **T. endothrix,** species which invade the hair shaft without forming a persistent sheath of spores outside the shaft; **T. neo-endothrix,** species intermediate in character between ectothrix and endothrix species. *In medicine*, the species of particular importance include: **T. acuminatum** (**T. sabouraudi**), **T. concentricum, T. crateriforme, T. epilans** (**T. cerebriforme**), **T. megnini** (**T. rosaceum;** syn., *Achorion gallinar*), **T. mentagrophytes** (**T. gypseum;** syn., *Achorion quinckeanum*), **T. rubrum** (**T. purpureum**), **T. schoenleini** (syn., *Achorion schoenleini*), **T. sulfureum, T. tonsurans,** and **T. violaceum.** Also see *tinea*.

trich″o·phy·to′sis (trick″o·figh·to′sis) [*thrix; phyton;* G. *-ōsis*, condition]. A contagious disease of skin and hair, occurring mostly in children, and due to skin invasion by the *Trichophyton* fungus. It is characterized by circular scaly patches and partial loss of hair.

t. barbae. Tinea barbae.

t. cruris. Tinea cruris.

trich″o·po″li·o′sis. See *canities*.

trich″o·pti·lo′sis (trick″o·tye·lo′sis). See *trichorrhexis* nodosa.

trich″or·rhe′a (trick″o·ree′uh) [*thrix;* G. *rhoia*, flow]. Rapid loss of the hair.

trich″or·rhex′is [*thrix;* G. *rhēxis*, a breaking]. Brittleness of the hair.

t. nodosa. An atrophic condition of the hair, affecting more often the male beard, and characterized by irregular thickenings resembling nodes on the hair shaft that are really partial fractures of the hair. The hairs often break, leaving a brush-like end; a certain amount of alopecia is thus produced.

trich″or·rhex″o·ma′ni·a [*thrix; rhēxis;* G. *mania,* madness]. A compulsion to break off hairs of the scalp or beard with the fingernails.

trich·o′sis [*thrix;* G. *-ōsis,* condition]. Any morbid affection of the hair.

Trich″o·spo′ron, Trich·os′po·ron (trick″o·spor′-on, trick·os′po·ron) [*thrix; spora*]. A genus of fungi which grow on hair shafts. The causative agent of piedra. **T. beigelii, T. giganteum, T. glyophile, T. ovale,** and **T. ovoides** have been recovered from nodules on the hair of persons with piedra.

trich″o·spo·ro′sis [*thrix;* G. *spora,* seed; *-ōsis,* condition]. A fungous infection of the hair shaft. See *piedra.*

trich″o·sta′sis spin″u·lo′sa (trick″o·stay′sis). A condition characterized by dark comedone-like plugs in the hair follicles over the trunk. The plugs are composed of bundles of many tiny hairs.

trich″o·stron″gy·li′a·sis (trick″o·stron″ji·lye′uh-sis) [*thrix;* G. *stroggylos,* round; NL. *-iasis,* condition]. Infestation with *Trichostrongylus.*

Trich″o·stron′gy·lus [*thrix; stroggylos*]. A genus of nematode worms which usually are parasites of ruminants. Man is infested by consuming raw plants grown in contaminated soil. The species identified from human cases are **T. colubriformis, T. orientalis, T. probolurus, T. vitrinus.**

trich″o·the′cin. An antifungal substance produced in cultures of *Trichothecium roseum.*

trich″o·til″lo·ma′ni·a [*thrix;* G. *tillein,* to pluck; *mania,* madness]. An uncontrollable impulse to pull out one's hair.

tri·chot′o·my (try·cot′o·mee) [G. *tricha,* in three parts; *tomē,* a cutting]. Division into three parts.

trich″o·zo′a. Animals with hair. Syn., *pilifera.*

tri′chro·ism [G. *tri-,* three; *chroia,* color]. The property of exhibiting three different colors when viewed in three different aspects. —**trichro′ic,** *adj.*

tri′chro·mat [*tri-;* G. *chrōma,* color]. A person with normal color vision.

tri″chro·mat′ic [*tri-;* G. *chrōmatikos,* of color]. Having three standard colors.

tri″chro·ma·top′si·a [*tri-;* G. *chrōma,* color; *opsis,* vision]. Normal color vision; ability to see the three primary colors.

tri·chro′mic (try·kro′mick) [*tri-; chrōma*]. Able to distinguish the three colors red, blue, and green.

trich″u·ri′a·sis (trick″yoo·rye′uh·sis) [G. *thrix,* hair; *oura,* tail; NL. *-iasis,* condition]. Infestation by *Trichuris trichiura.*

Trich·u′ris [*thrix; oura*]. A genus of nematodes of the superfamily Trichinelloidea.

T. trichiura. The species infesting man. Transmission is from man to man by ingestion of mature ova. Also called *Trichocephalus dispar, Trichocephalus trichiurus, whipworm.*

tri·cre′sol (try·kree′sole, ·sol, ·sawl). Cresol.

t. phosphate. Pale yellow liquid, chiefly tri-orthocresyl phosphate, $(CH_3C_6H_4)_3PO_4$; used as plasticizer in lacquers and varnishes. Its ingestion causes a degeneration of the nerve cells of the anterior horns of the spinal cord, leading to more or less permanent paralysis of the extremities.

tri′cro·tism [G. *trikrotos,* from *tri-,* three; *krotos,* beat]. The condition of having three waves corresponding to one pulse beat. —**tricrot′ic, tricrotous,** *adj.*

tri·cus′pid (try·kus′pid) [L. *tri-,* three; *cuspis,* point]. 1. Having three cusps, as a tricuspid tooth, or the tricuspid valve. 2. Affecting, or producing at, the tricuspid valve.

tri·dac′tyl [G. *tri-,* three; *daktylos,* finger]. Having three digits.

tri′dent [L. *tridens,* having three teeth]. Tridentate.

tri·den′tate (try·den′tayt) [*tridens*]. Three-pronged.

tri·der′mic [G. *tri-,* three; *derma,* skin]. Derived from, or relating to, all germ layers of the embryo.

tri″der·mo′ma. See *teratoma.*

tridione. Trade-mark for trimethadione or 3,5,5-trimethyloxazolidine-2,4-dione,

$$(CH_3)_2C.O.CO.N(CH_3).CO$$

The substance is a white, crystalline powder, soluble in about 20 parts of water. An anticonvulsant useful in petit mal and in myoclonic or akinetic seizures in epilepsy. Usually given orally, but may be administered parenterally. Must be used with caution; it may produce aplastic anemia. Dose, 1–2 Gm. (15–30 gr.) daily.

trid′y·mite. A very hard native silica occurring in volcanic rocks.

trid′y·mus [G. *tridymos,* triplet]. Triplet.

tri″en·ceph′a·lus. See *triocephalus.*

tri·eth″a·nol′am·ine (try·eth″uh·nol′uh·meen, ·min). $N(CH_2.CH_2.OH)_3$; colorless, viscid, hygroscopic liquid miscible with water and alcohol. The commercial article contains up to 15% of diethanolamine and up to 2.5% of monoethanolamine. A solvent and emulsifying agent used in the preparation of emulsions, ointments, lotions, and detergents.

tri·eth″yl·a·mine′ (try·eth″il·uh·meen′, ·am′een, ·am′in). $(C_2H_5)_3N$. A colorless liquid of strong ammoniacal odor. A ptomaine obtained from putrid haddock; also prepared synthetically.

tri·eth′yl·ene gly′col. $HO.CH_2.CH_2.O.CH_2.CH_2.$-$O.CH_2.CH_2.OH$. Colorless, hygroscopic, practically odorless liquid; miscible with water or alcohol. Used extensively in organic syntheses; incorporated in plastics to increase pliability. As an aerosol it is bactericidal in concentration of 0.005 mg. per liter of air.

tri·eth′yl·ene mel′a·mine.

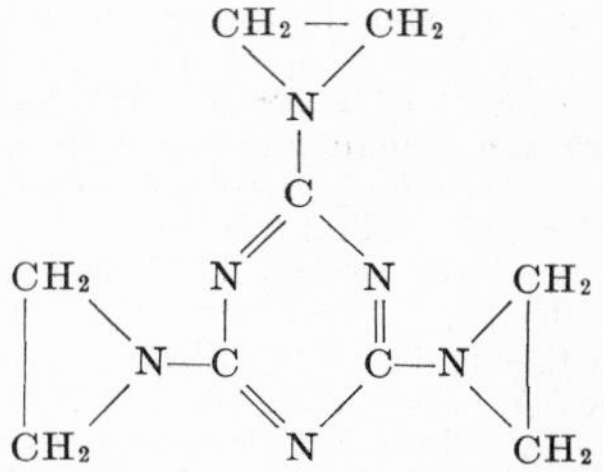

```
              CH2 — CH2
                \   /
                  N
                  |
                  C
                //  \
 CH2            N      N            CH2
 |  \           |      ||          /  |
 |    N — C              C — N        |
 |  /           \\     /           \  |
 CH2               N                CH2
```

2,4,6-Tri(ethylenimino)-*s*-triazine, a white crystalline powder readily soluble in water. It is chemically related to the nitrogen mustard methyl-*bis*-(β-chloroethyl)amine by virtue of the ethyleniminium transformation the latter undergoes in the body. Triethylene melamine appears to be useful for palliative treatment of certain types of neoplastic disease. Abbreviated, TEM.

tri·fa′cial nerve (try·fay′shul). Old term for the fifth cranial nerve, so called because it divides into three main branches that supply the face. See *trigeminal nerve.*

tri′fid [L. *trifidus,* cleft into three parts]. Three-cleft, tripartite.

tri·fo′cal spec′ta·cles. See trifocal *glasses.*

tri·fo″li·o′sis (try·fo″lee·o′sis) [L. *trifolium,* trefoil; G. *-ōsis,* condition]. *In veterinary medicine,* a superficial necrosis of the white markings, caused by exposure to the sun after the animals have been sensitized to light by eating certain substances, chiefly the legumes.

Tri·fo′li·um [L.]. A genus of herbs including the clovers.

T. pratense. Common red clover; used empirically in the treatment of whooping cough.

tri·for′mol. Paraformaldehyde.

tri″fur·ca′tion. Division into three prongs. —**tri′-furcate,** *adj.*, *v.*

tri·gas′tric [G. *tri-*, three; *gastēr*, belly]. Having three fleshy bellies, as certain muscles.

tri·gas′tri·cus. The digastric muscle: variant term.

tri·gem′i·nal [L. *trigeminus*, threefold]. Triple; dividing into three parts, as the trigeminal nerve.

tri·gem′i·nal nerve. The fifth cranial nerve with central attachment at the lateral aspect of the pons. At the semilunar (Gasserian) ganglion it divides into three divisions: (1) *ophthalmic*, which gives sensory innervation to the conjunctiva, forehead, meninges, frontal, ethmoid and sphenoid sinuses, and upper nose; (2) *maxillary*, which gives sensory innervation to the cheeks, upper lip, upper teeth and gums, soft and hard palates, nose, maxillary sinus, and meninges; (3) *mandibular*, which provides sensory innervation to the chin, lower teeth and gums, anterior two-thirds of the tongue, and meninges, and provides motor fibers for the muscles of mastication, the anterior belly of the digastric, mylohyoid, tensor veli palatini, and tensor tympani.

tri·gem′i·nus [L.]. The fifth cranial nerve.

tri·gem′i·ny [*trigeminus*]. Grouping of arterial pulse beats in groups of three.

tri·gen′ic [G. *tri-*, three; *genesthai*, from *gignesthai*, to be produced]. Referring to genotypes of polysomic or polyploid organisms which contain three different alleles for any given locus.

trig′ger-ma·te′ri·al. See *apheter.*

tri·glyc′er·ide. An ester of glycerin in which al three hydroxyl groups of the latter are esterified with an acid; animal and vegetable fixed oils are composed chiefly of triglycerides of fatty acids.

tri′gone [G. *trigōnos*, three-cornered]. 1. Triangle. 2. The smooth triangular area on the inner surface of the urinary bladder between the orifices of the two ureters and the internal urethral orifice: also called *vesical t.*, *t. of the urinary bladder;* formerly called *t. of Lieutaud.* —**trig′onal,** *adj.*

collateral t. A triangular area at the junction of the posterior and inferior horns of the lateral ventricles.

femoral t. See femoral *triangle.*

fibrous t. of the heart. The triangular fibrous base of the heart. The *right trigone* is situated between the right and left atrioventricular openings; the *left*, between the left side of the opening of the aorta and the left atrioventricular opening.

habenular t. A small, medial, triangular area on the dorsal aspect of the thalamus between the stalk of the epiphysis and the superior colliculi, and overlying the habenular nucleus; part of the epithalamus.

hypoglossal t. See *t.* of the hypoglossal nerve.

olfactory t. The lateral root of the olfactory tract.

t. of the hypoglossal nerve. The triangular area of the floor of the fourth ventricle overlying the nucleus of the hypoglossal nerve.

t. of the lemniscus. A slightly elevated area of the tegmentum overlying the lateral lemniscus.

t. of the urinary bladder. See *trigone*, 2.

vesical t. The trigone of the urinary bladder.

Trig″o·nel′la (trig″o·nel′uh, try″go·) [*trigōnos*]. A genus of the Leguminosae.

T. foenum-graecum. Used in plasters and salves and in veterinary medicine.

T. monspeliaca. A decoction of the seeds has been used in Italy in various forms of diarrhea.

tri′go·nid (try′go·nid, trig′o·, try·gon′id) [*trigōnos*]. The first three cusps (viewed as one) of a lower molar tooth.

tri″go·ni′tis [*trigōnos;* G. *-itis*, inflammation]. Inflammation of the trigone of the urinary bladder.

trig″o·no·ceph′a·lus (trig″o·no·sef′uh·lus, tri·go″-no·) [*trigōnos;* G. *kephalē*, head]. An individual exhibiting trigonocephaly.

trig″o·no·ceph′a·ly [*trigōnos; kephalē*]. Triangular or egg-shaped head, due to early synostosis of the metopic suture.

tri·go′num (try·go′num) [L., from *trigōnos*]. Trigone. See *triangle.*

t. acusticum. See *area* acustica.

t. fibrosum cordis (**dextrum** and **sinistrum**). See fibrous *trigone* of the heart.

t. interpedunculare. See interpeduncular *fossa.*

t. lumbale. See lumbar *triangle.*

t. vagi. See *ala* cinerea.

t. vesicae. See *trigone*, 2.

tri″hex·y·phen′i·dyl. The generic name for 3-(1-piperidyl)-1-phenyl-1-cyclohexyl-1-propanol hydrochloride, a synthetic antispasmodic. Sometimes spelled *trihexyphenydyl.* See *artane.*

tri·hy′brid (try·hy′brid) [G. *tri-*, three; *hybris*, violence]. The offspring of parents differing in three pairs of Mendelian characteristics.

tri·hy′dric. Containing three atoms of hydrogen replaceable by metals.

tri·hy′drol. An associated form of water having the composition $(H_2O)_3$.

tri″hy·drox″y·an″thra·qui·none′ (try″high-drock″see·an″thruh·kwi·none′). See *anthragallol.*

tri″hy·drox″y·ben·zo′ic ac′id. Gallic acid.

tri″hy·drox″y·oes′trin (·es′trin). See *estriol.*

tri″hy·drox″y·pro′pane. Glycerin.

tri·in″i·od′y·mus (try·in″ee·od′i·mus) [*tri-;* G. *inion*, occipital bone; *didymos*, twin]. A monster having three heads united posteriorly and attached to a single body.

tri·i″o·do·meth′ane. Iodoform.

tri·i″o·do·thy′ro·nine. An amino acid isolated from human blood and prepared synthetically, similar to, but containing one less iodine atom than, thyroxin and with similar but more rapid biological action.

tri·ke″to·cho·lan′ic ac′id (try·kee″to·ko·lan′ick). 3,7,12-Triketocholanic acid. The compound resulting from the oxidation of the three secondary alcohol groups of cholic acid to ketone linkages.

tri·ke″to·pu′rine. Uric acid.

tri′labe [*tri-;* G. *labē*, handle]. A three-pronged instrument for withdrawing small calculi or other foreign bodies from the urinary bladder, through the urethral passage. *Obs.*

tri·lam′i·nar (try·lam′i·nur) [*tri-;* L. *lamina*, plate]. Three-layered.

trilene. Trade-mark for a brand of trichloroethylene.

tri″li·no′le·in. Glyceryl linoleate, $(C_{18}H_{31}O_2)_3C_3H_5$, occurring in many vegetable oils.

tri·lo′bate (try·lo′bayt) [*tri-;* G. *lobos*, lobe]. Three-lobed.

tri·loc′u·lar [L. *tri-*, three; *loculus*, little place]. *In biology*, having three chambers or cells, as trilocular heart, a congenitally defective heart with three chambers instead of four.

tri·man′u·al [*tri-;* L. *manus*, hand]. Accomplished by the aid of three hands.

tri·mas′ti·gate [G. *tri-*, three; *mastix*, whip]. Having three flagella; triflagellate.

trimax. Trade-mark for a brand of magnesium trisilicate.

tri·men′su·al [*tri-;* G. *mēn*, month]. Occurring at periods of three months.

Trim″er·e·su′rus [G. *trimerēs*, having three parts; *oura*, tail]. A genus of venomous snakes of the family Crotalidae, the pit vipers. **T. flavoviridis** or habu is found in the Ryukyu Islands; **T. gramineus** and **T. mucrosquamatus** are found in Formosa.

tri·mes′ter (try·mes′tur) [L. *trimestris*, of three months]. A stage or period of three months.

tri″meth·a·di′one. Generic name for the substance 3,5,5-trimethyloxazolidine-2,4-dione, available under the trade-marked name *tridione*.

tri·meth″yl·a·ce′tic ac′id. See under *valeric acid*.

tri·meth″yl·a·mine′ (try·meth″il·uh·meen′, ·am′-een, ·am′in). $(CH_3)_3N$. Colorless gas of fishy ammoniacal odor, very soluble in water. Produced by bacterial action on decayed animal matter or synthesized. Used in organic syntheses. Also called *secaline*.

tri·meth′yl·ene. Cyclopropane.

tri·meth″yl·gly′cine (try·meth″il·gly′seen, ·sin, ·gly·seen′). See *betaine*.

tri·meth″yl·xan′thine (try·meth″il·zan′theen, ·thin). Caffeine.

trimeton. Trade-mark for a brand of the antihistaminic substance prophenpyridamine.

tri·mor′phism (try·mor′fiz·um) [G. *tri-*, three; *morphē*, form]. 1. *In biology*, a term used to indicate the fact that hermaphrodite flowers of three different kinds (short-styled, mid-styled, and long-styled) are produced on the same species of plant. 2. Occurrence in three distinct forms, as certain insects. —**trimorphic,** *adj.*

trinesium. Trade-mark for a brand of magnesium trisilicate.

tri·ni″tro·phe′nol (*trinitrophenol*). $C_6H_2(NO_2)_3OH$. 2,4,6-Trinitrophenol, pale yellow crystals of intensely bitter taste; 1 Gm. dissolves in 80 cc. of water and in 12 cc. of alcohol. It is germicidal and astringent and is used locally for these effects; it has been used internally as a vermifuge, antipyretic, and antimalarial. Syn., *carbazotic acid, picric acid.*

t. poisoning. Poisoning by picric acid. Symptoms: dermatitis (''picric itch''); hemolytic anemia; gastric, intestinal, and renal irritation; hepatitis; icterus; darkened urine.

tri·ni″tro·tol′u·ene. $(NO_2)_3C_6H_2.CH_3$; any of six isomers of this formula, but especially 1-methyl-2,4,6-trinitrobenzene, occurring as pale-yellow crystals: used in explosives. Abbreviated, TNT.

tri″o·ceph′a·lus [*tri-;* G. *kephalē*, head]. A monster characterized by an absence of the ocular, nasal, and oral apparatus, the head being merely a small spheroidal mass with no brain.

tri·o′le·in. See *olein*.

trional. Trade-mark for a brand of sulfonethylmethane.

tri′o·nym [*tri-;* G. *onyma*, name]. A name consisting of three terms.

tri″oph·thal′mos [*tri-;* G. *ophthalmos*, eye]. Characterizing that variety of diprosopus in which three eyes are present.

tri″o·pod′y·mus [*tri-;* G. *ōps*, face; *didymos*, twin]. A monster with three faces and but a single head.

tri·or′chid (try·or′kid) [*tri-;* G. *orchis*, testis]. Having three testes.

tri·or′chid. An individual having three testes. —**trior′chidy,** *n.*

tri·or′chis [*tri-; orchis*]. A person with three testes.

tri·or″tho·cres′yl phos′phate. See *tricresol* phosphate.

tri′ose. A monosaccharide containing three carbon atoms in the molecule.

tri″ose·phos·phor′ic ac′id. Triose phosphate. A phosphorylated three-carbon sugar. Several of these compounds are intermediaries in the breakdown of glycogen to pyruvic acid in carbohydrate metabolism.

tri·o·tus [*tri-;* G. *ous*, ear]. Having three ears.

tri·ox″y·meth′yl·ene. Paraformaldehyde.

tri·ox″y·pu′rine (try·ock″si·pew′reen, ·rin). Uric acid.

tri·pal′mi·tin. See *palmitin*.

trip′a·ra [L. *tri-*, three; *parere*, to bear]. A woman who has borne three children.

tri″pel·en′na·mine hy″dro·chlo′ride. Generic name for the antihistaminic substance N,N-dimethyl-N′-benzyl-N′-(α-pyridyl)ethylene-diamine. See *pyribenzamine*.

tri·pep′tide, tri·pep′tid. A protein hydrolysis product representing condensation of three molecules of amino acids.

triphal. Trade-mark for an ampuled product, principally sodium aurothiobenzimidazole carboxylate, C_6H_3N:NHCSAu.COONa, used in lupus erythematosus.

tri″pha·lan′gi·a, tri″pha·lan′gy [G. *tri-*, three; *phalagx*, bone between two joints of the fingers and toes]. The presence of three phalanges in the thumb or great toe. Also called *hyperphalangy*.

tri·phar′ma·con, tri·phar′ma·cum [*tri-;* G. *pharmakon*, drug]. A medicine made up of three ingredients.

tri·pha′sic (try·fay′zick) [*tri-;* G. *phasis*, appearance]. Having three phases or variations.

tri·phen″yl·eth′yl·ene. $(C_6H_5)_2C$:CH(C_6H_5). A proestrogen potentiated as estrogen by passage through the liver.

tri·phen″yl·meth′ane. Rosaniline dye.

2,3,5-tri·phen′yl·tet″ra·zo′li·um chlor′ide. $[C_6H_5.\overline{C:N.N(C_6H_5).N^+(C_6H_5):N}]Cl^-$; colorless crystals, soluble in water; when reduced, as by certain enzymes, it forms the red pigment 2,3,5-triphenyl formazan. See *formazan*. Abbreviated, TTC.

tri·phos″pho·pyr′i·dine nu′cle·o·tide. Coenzyme II. Abbreviated, TPN.

tri·ple′gi·a [*tri-;* G. *plēgē*, stroke]. Hemiplegia with the additional paralysis of one limb on the opposite side.

trip′le point. The single temperature and pressure at which the solid, liquid, and vapor forms of a substance may coexist.

trip′le re·sponse′. Thomas Lewis' term for three stages of normal vasomotor reaction resulting when a pointed instrument is drawn heavily across the skin. They are: reddening of the area stimulated, wide spreading of flush to adjacent skin, and development of wheals. The response is due to a histaminelike substance liberated from tissue by a noxious stimulus.

trip′let [G. *triplous*, triple]. 1. One of three children born at one birth. 2. *In optics*, a system consisting of three lenses.

tri′plex (trip′lecks, try′plecks) [L.]. Triple.

trip″lo·blas′tic [G. *triplous*, triple; *blastos*, germ]. Possessing three germ layers, ectoderm, entoderm, and mesoderm.

trip″lo·ko′ri·a [*triplous;* G. *korē*, pupil]. Having three pupillary openings in one eye.

trip·lo′pi·a [*triplous;* G. *ōps*, eye]. A disturbance of vision in which three images of a single object are seen.

tri·pro′so·pus [G. *tri-*, three; *prosōpon*, face]. A reputed monster in which there is a fusion of three faces in one.

trip′sis [G., a rubbing]. 1. Trituration. 2. Massage.

trip·ter′y·gine. An insecticidal alkaloid fraction from *Tripterygium wilfordi*.

Trip″te·ryg′i·um. A genus of twining vines the root bark of certain species of which, notably *T. wilfordi* Hook, or thunder-god vine, has long been used in China as an insecticide. The individual alkaloids are wilfordine, wilforgine, wilforine, wilfortrine, and wilforzine, all insecticidal.

tri·que′trum (try·kwee′trum, try·kwet′rum) [L. *triquetrus*, three-cornered]. 1. The third carpal bone from the radial side in the proximal row; formerly called *cuneiform bone of the carpus*. See Table of Bones in the Apendix. 2. Any one of the Wormian bones.

tri·sac′cha·ride (try·sack′uh·ride, ·rid). A carbohydrate which, on hydrolysis, yields three molecules of monosaccharides.

tris·kai″dek·a·pho′bi·a (tris·kigh″deck·uh·fo′-bee·uh). Triakaidekaphobia.

tris′mus (triz′mus) [G., a grinding]. 1. Tonic spasm of the muscles of mastication. 2. Old term for lockjaw. See *tetanus*, 1.

trisodarsen. Trade-mark for a trivalent arsenic compound used as an antisyphilitic.

trisogel. Trade-mark for an aqueous suspension of magnesium trisilicate and aluminum hydroxide used as an antacid.

tri·so′mic (try·so′mick) [G. *tri-*, three; *sōma*, body]. Having three chromosomes of a given kind, but otherwise only two of each of the other chromosomes of a haploid set, hence an individual with 2n + 1 chromosomes.

trisomin. Trade-mark for a brand of magnesium trisilicate.

tri·so′mus. More or less conjoined triplets from a single ovum, as a tricephalus.

t. omphaloangiopagus. Monochorionic triplets of which two are more or less normal autosites, the third an omphalosite.

tri·ste′a·rin. See *stearin*.

tris″ti·chi′a·sis (tris″ti·kigh′uh·sis) [*tri-*; G. *stichos*, row; NL. *-iasis*, condition]. The arrangement of the cilia (eyelashes) in three rows.

tris″ti·ma′ni·a [L. *tristis*, sad; G. *mania*, madness]. Melancholia. *Obs.*

tris′tis [L.]. 1. Sad; gloomy. 2. Dull in color.

trit″an·o′pi·a (trit″an·o′pee·uh, try″tan·) [G. *tritos*, third; *a-*, not; *ōps*, eye]. A defect in a third constituent essential for color vision, as in violet blindness. See *dichromatism*.

trit″i·a′tion. The process of introducing into a chemical compound one or more atoms of the hydrogen isotope tritium in place of a like number of atoms of ordinary hydrogen (protium) commonly existing in the compound.

tri·ti′ceous (tri·tish′us) [L. *triticeus*, of wheat]. Having the shape of a grain of wheat, as the triticeous cartilage.

trit′i·cin [L. *triticum*, wheat]. 1. A gumlike substance found in *Triticum repens*. 2. A proprietary food preparation.

tri″ti·co·nu·cle′ic ac′id. A nucleic acid from wheat and having ribose as the sugar component.

Trit′i·cum [L.]. A genus of the Gramineae. **T. sativum** is wheat.

trit′i·cum [L.]. The dried rhizome and roots of *Agropyron repens*, family Gramineae. A diuretic formerly used in genitourinary ailments.

trit′i·um (trit′ee·um, trish′ee·um). The hydrogen isotope with mass three. It is radioactive, displaying a beta-activity with a half-life of 31 years.

trit′o·cone (trit′o·cone) [G. *tritos*, third; *kōnos*, cone]. The distobuccal cusp on a premolar tooth of the upper jaw; not found in humans.

trit″o·co′nid (trit″o·ko′nid) [*tritos*; *kōnos*]. The distolingual cusp on a premolar tooth of the lower jaw; not found in man.

tri′ton (try′ton). The nucleus of the tritium atom. It contains two neutrons and one proton, and thus bears unit positive charge.

trit′o·pine (trit′o·peen, ·pin, ·pyne, try·to′pin). An alkaloid, $C_{20}H_{25}NO_4$, of opium. Syn., *laudanine*.

tri″to·tox′in [*tritos*; G. *toxikon*, poison]. One of the third group into which Ehrlich classifies toxins, according to the avidity with which they combine with antitoxins, tritotoxin combining least readily. See *prototoxin*.

tri″tu·ber′cu·lar [L. *tri-*, three; *tuberculum*, small swelling]. Having three tubercles or cusps; tricuspid.

trit′u·ra·ble [L. *triturare*, to thresh]. Capable of being powdered.

trit′u·rate [*triturare*]. 1. Reduce to a fine powder. 2. Mix powdered substances in a mortar with the aid of a pestle.

trit′u·rate. A finely divided powder.

tablet t. A molded tablet as distinguished from a compressed tablet. Generally prepared in a base of sucrose and lactose; easily friable.

trit″u·ra′tion [L. *trituratio*, from *triturare*]. 1. The process of reducing a solid substance to a powder by rubbing. 2. The product obtained by triturating together 10 Gm. of a powdered medicinal substance and 90 Gm. of powdered lactose.

tri·va′lence (try·vay′luns, triv′uh·luns) [L. *tri-*, three; *valere*, to be strong]. The quality of having a valence of three. —**trivalent,** *adj.*

tri′valve″ [*tri-*; L. *valva*, leaf of a door]. Having three valves or blades, as a speculum.

tri·valv′u·lar (try·valv′yoo·lur) [*tri-*; *valva*]. Having three valves.

tro′car [F. *trocart*, from *trois*, three, *carre*, side of a sword blade]. A surgical instrument for puncturing cavities for the removal of fluid contained therein. It consists of a hollow tube or cannula within which is a snugly fitting bayonet-pointed mandrel or perforating core whose point protrudes beyond the beveled cannula end. The entire instrument is used to puncture a cavity, the perforator being removed when it is desired to begin evacuation of the fluid.

troch. Trochiscus, troche.

tro·chan′ter (tro·can′tur) [G., runner]. One of two processes on the upper extremity of the femur below the neck. The **greater trochanter** is situated on the outer, and the **lesser trochanter** on the inner, side of the bone. See Plates 1, 2. —**trochanter′ic,** *adj.*

t. major. The greater trochanter.

t. minor. The lesser trochanter.

third t. An enlargement of the upper end of the gluteal tuberosity.

tro·chan′tin (tro·can′tin) [*trochantēr*]. 1. Obsolete term for lesser trochanter. 2. The proximal segment of the trochanter of an insect's leg.

tro″chan·tin′i·an (tro″can·tin′ee·un) [*trochantēr*]. Pertaining to the trochantin.

tro′che (tro′kee) [G. *trochos*, wheel]. A lozenge. Abbreviated, troch.

tro″chis·ca′tion (tro″kis·kay′shun) [G. *trochiskos*, small wheel]. The process of making troches from fine powder obtained by elutriation.

tro·chis′cus (tro·kis′kus) (pl. *trochisci*) [*trochiskos*]. Troche. Abbreviated, troch.

troch′le·a (trock′lee·uh) (pl. *trochleae*) [L., mechanical contrivance for raising weights]. A part or process having the nature of a pulley.

t. of the astragalus. Old term for trochlea tali.

t. of the femur. The intercondyloid fossa of the femur.

t. of the humerus. The medial portion of the distal articulation of the humerus; the surface which articulates with the semilunar notch of the ulna.

t. of the obliquus oculi superior. The ligamentous ring or pulley, attached to the upper margin of the orbit, which transmits the tendon of the superior oblique muscle of the eye. See Plate 19.

t. tali. The surface of the talus articulating with the tibia.

troch′le·ar [*trochlea*]. Of the nature of, or pertaining to, a pulley.

troch′le·ar. The trochlear nerve, the fourth cranial nerve whose fibers emerge from the brain on the dorsal surface and go to supply the superior oblique muscle of the eye.

troch″le·a′ris. The superior oblique muscle of the eyeball: old term.

troch″o·car′di·a (trock″o·kahr′dee·uh, tro″ko·) [G. *trochos*, wheel; *kardia*, heart]. Displacement of the heart by rotation on its long axis.

troch″o·ceph′a·lus [*trochos;* G. *kephalē*, head]. A rounded appearance of the head, due to early partial synostosis of the frontal and parietal bones.

troch″o·gin′gly·mus (trock″o·jing′gli·mus, ·ging′-gli·mus, tro″ko·) [*trochos;* G. *gigglymos*, hinge]. A combination of a hinge joint and a pivot joint, as in the humeroradial articulation.

tro′choid (tro′koyd) [G. *trochoeidēs*, circular]. Serving as a pulley or pivot; involving a pivotal action.

troch′o·phore [G. *trochos*, wheel; *phoros*, bearing]. The typical, primitive larval form of annelids.

troch″or·i″zo·car′di·a (trock″or·eye″zo·kahr′-dee·uh) [*trochos;* G. *horizōn*, horizon; *kardia*, heart]. Form of displacement of the heart characterized by rotation and change to horizontal position.

Trog″lo·tre′ma [G. *trōglē*, hole; *trēma*, perforation]. A genus of flukes which are common parasites of fish-eating mammals.

T. salmincola. The species which has been found in cases of human infestation.

Trog″lo·tre·mat′i·dae (trog″lo·tri·mat′i·dee) [*trōglē; trēma*]. A family of flukes which includes the genera *Paragonimus* and *Troglotrema.*

Troisier, Émile [*French physician*, 1844–1919]. Drew attention to the enlargement of the left supraclavicular lymph node, called *Virchow's node* or *gland, gland* or *node of Virchow-Troisier.* See also Troisier's *sign.* Described a syndrome of diabetic cachexia with bronzed skin which is called *Troisier's syndrome.*

Tröltsch, Anton Friedrich von [*German otologist*, 1829–90]. Remembered for his description of corpuscle-like spaces among the radial fibers of the tympanic membrane, called *Tröltsch's corpuscles.* Described two small pockets formed by the mucus membrane which envelops the chorda tympani. One lies in front of and one behind the manubrium of the malleus; called *Tröltsch's recesses* or *spaces.* He is credited with the invention of the modern otoscope.

Trom·bic′u·la. A genus of mites; the larvae are blood suckers and cause a severe dermatitis.

T. akamushi. A vector of *Rickettsia tsutsugamushi*, the cause of tsutsugamushi disease.

T. alfreddugèsi. The species which causes an annoying dermatitis; widely distributed in North America. Also called *chigger, red bug, T. irritans.*

T. holosericeum. A species of acarine mites.

T. irritans. The chigger mite of eastern North America; attacks man and other mammals.

trom·bic″u·lo′sis [*Trombicula;* G. *-ōsis*, condition]. Infestation with *Trombicula.*

trom·bid″i·o′sis [*Trombicula; -ōsis*]. Infestation by a member of Trombidium.

Trom·bid′i·um. A genus of mites of the family Trombidiidae (the chiggers).

tromexan. A trade-marked name for *bis*-3,3′-(4-oxycoumarinyl)ethyl acetate, also known as ethyl biscoumacetate, an anticoagulant.

Trommer's test. See under *test.*

trom″o·ma′ni·a [G. *tromos*, a trembling; *mania*, madness]. Delirium tremens.

tro′na. A native compound of sodium carbonate and sodium bicarbonate. $Na_2.CO_3.NaHCO_3.2H_2O$.

Tronchin, Théodore [*Swiss physician*, 1709–81]. Wrote one of the earliest accounts of lead colic (1757). A pupil of Boerhaave, he is said to have introduced his methods in France.

tro″pa·co·caine′ (tro″puh·ko·kayn′, ·ko′kayn, ·ko′kuh·een, ·in, ·ko·kay′in). Benzoyl-pseudotropine. $C_{15}H_{19}NO_2$. An alkaloid in Java coca leaves; also prepared synthetically.

t. hydrochloride. White crystals soluble in water. A local anesthetic somewhat like cocaine.

tro·pae′o·lin, tro·pe′o·lin. An indefinite name for several dyes used as pH indicators; so called because their colors resemble the flowers of *Tropaeolum*, the garden nasturtium.

t. D. Methyl orange.

t. G. Metanil yellow.

t. O. Sodium azoresorcinol-sulfanilate. $NaSO_3.$-$C_6H_4.N{:}N.C_6H_3(OH)_2$. Brown powder used as indicator. Yellow at pH 11; orange-brown at pH 12.7. Also called *resorcinol yellow.*

t. OO. Sodium *p*-diphenylamine-azobenzenesulfonate. $NaSO_3.C_6H_4.N{:}N.C_6H_4.NH.C_6H_5$. Yellow powder used as indicator. Red at pH 1.4; yellow at pH 2.6.

t. OOO. Sodium azo-α-naphtholsulfanilate. Na-$SO_3.C_6H_4.N{:}N.C_{10}H_6.OH$. Reddish brown powder used as color for foods, drugs, and cosmetics, and as indicator. Brownish yellow at pH 7.6; purple at pH 8.9. Also called *orange I.*

t. R. See *t.* O.

tro′pane. $C_8H_{15}N$; 2,3-dihydro-8-methylnortropidine; a two-ring heterocyclic liquid hydrocarbon from which tropine is derived. Many ester alkaloids, including atropine and cocaine, are referred to as belonging to the tropane group.

tro′pe·ine (tro′pee·een, ·in). An ester of tropine and an organic acid, as atropine and homatropine.

tro·pe′sis [G. *tropē*, a turning]. Inclination.

tro″phe·de′ma, tro″phoe·de′ma (tro″fi·dee′muh, trof″i·) [G. *trephein*, to nourish; *oidema*, swelling]. Localized chronic edema due to damaged nourishment or nerve supply.

hereditary t. See hereditary *edema.*

t. of Basedow. See circumscribed *myxedema.*

troph′e·sy [G. *trophē*, nourishment, from *trephein*]. Defective nutrition of a part from disorder of the nerves regulating nutrition; trophoneurosis. —**trophe′sial, trophe′sic,** *adj.*

troph′ic [*trephein*]. Pertaining to the functions concerned in nutrition, digestion, and assimilation.

tro·phic′i·ty (tro·fiss′i·tee) [*trephein*]. Trophic influence or state.

troph′ism [*trephein*]. 1. Nutrition. 2. Trophicity.

tro′pho-, troph′o-, troph- [*trephein*]. A combining form denoting *relation to nutrition* or *to nourishment.*

tro′pho·blast (tro′fo·blast, trof′o·) [*trephein;* G. *blastos*, germ]. The outer, ectodermal epithelium of the mammalian blastocyst or chorion and chorionic villi. See *cytotrophoblast, syncytiotrophoblast.* —**trophoblas′tic,** *adj.*

tro″pho·blas·to′ma. See *choriocarcinoma.*

tro″pho·chro·mid′i·a [*trephein;* G. *chrōma*, color]. The nutritional chromatin of the cell.

tro′pho·cyte [*trephein;* G. *kytos*, cell]. A Sertoli or sustentacular cell of the testis.

tro′pho·derm [*trephein;* G. *derma*, skin]. 1. The trophoblast or chorionic ectoderm. 2. The growing, active part of the trophoblast in the placental region. Also called *placental trophoblast, ectoplacenta.* —**trophoder'mal,** *adj.*

tro"pho·der"ma·to·neu·ro'sis [*trephein; derma;* G. *neuron,* nerve; *-ōsis,* condition]. Selter's term for acrodynia. See *erythredema polyneuropathy.*

tro"pho·dy·nam'ics (tro"fo·dye·nam'icks, ·di-nam'icks, trof"o·) [*trephein;* G. *dynamis,* power]. That branch of medical science dealing with the forces governing nutrition.

tro·phol'o·gy [*trephein;* G. *logos,* word]. The science of nutrition.

tro"pho·neu·ro'sis [*trephein;* G. *neuron,* nerve; *-ōsis,* condition]. Any disease of a part due to disturbance of the nerves or nerve centers with which it is connected.

disseminated t. See *scleroderma.*

facial t. Progressive facial atrophy.

muscular t. Trophic changes in the muscles in connection with disease of the nervous system.

t. of Romberg. Unilateral atrophy of the face; hemiatrophy.

trophonine X. A proprietary liquid containing B-complex vitamins with amino acids and carbohydrate used as a food supplement.

tro"pho·no'sis. See *trophopathy.*

tro"pho·nu'cle·us [*trephein;* L. *nucleus,* kernel]. The nucleus which is concerned with the nutrition of a unicellular organism and not with its reproduction.

tro·phop'a·thy [*trephein;* G. *pathos,* disease]. A disorder of nutrition.

tro'pho·plasm [*trephein;* G. *plasma,* anything formed]. The alveolar nutritive protoplasm in contrast to the filar, active kinoplasm of a cell. *Obs.*

tro"pho·spon'gi·a (tro"pho·spun'jee·uh, ·spon'-jee·uh, troph"o·) [*trephein;* G. *spoggia,* sponge]. The vascular endometrium forming the outer or maternal layer of the placenta. *Obs.*

tro"pho·spon'gi·um [*trephein; spoggia*]. Intracellular canals of unknown significance; the canalicular apparatus of Holmgren.

tro"pho·tax'is [*trephein;* G. *taxis,* arrangement]. Trophotropism.

tro"pho·ther'a·py [*trephein;* G. *therapeia,* treatment]. Dietotherapy.

tro"pho·trop'ic [*trephein;* G. *trepein,* to turn]. Exhibiting trophotropism.

tro·phot'ro·pism [*trephein; trepein*]. The attraction or repulsion exhibited by certain organic cells to various nutritive solutions.

tro"pho·zo'ite [*trephein;* G. *zōion,* living being]. The final product of sexual multiplication of sporozoa of the genera *Coccidia* and *Plasmodium.* Found within the tissues of a host. See Plates 27, 28, 29.

-trop'ic [G. *tropikos,* from *trepein,* to turn]. A combining form denoting *a turning.*

trop'ic ac'id. $CH_2OH.CH(C_6H_5).COOH$; α-phenyl-β-hydroxypropionic acid.

trop'i·cal [*tropikos*]. Pertaining to the tropical zone of the earth, as the belt lying between the Tropic of Cancer and that of Capricorn.

trop'i·cal sore. See *oriental sore.*

trop'in [G. *trepein,* to turn]. Any one of the substances in the blood serum which make bacteria susceptible to phagocytosis. See *bacteriotropin.*

tro'pine (tro'peen, ·pin). $C_8H_{15}NO$; 3-tropanol; a crystalline alcohol derivative of tropane. It is a product of hydrolysis of atropine and certain other alkaloids.

tro'pi·none. $C_8H_{13}NO$. A substance formed by oxidation of tropine and used in the synthesis of atropine substitutes.

tro'pism [*trepein*]. The involuntary bending, turning, or orientation of an organism toward (**positive tropism**), or away from (**negative tropism**), a stimulus. Various types, depending upon the directing influence, include *chemotropism, galvanotropism, geotropism, phototropism, rheotropism, stereotropism, thermotropism.*

-tro·pism [*trepein*]. A combining form meaning *a tendency to turn, an affinity for.*

tro'po·chrome [*trepein;* G. *chrōma,* color]. A term applied to those special serous cells of the salivary glands not staining with mucin stains after fixation in a formalin-bichromate mixture. Also see *homeochrome.*

trop'o·lone. 1. $C_7H_5O(OH)$; hydroxycycloheptatrienone; a 7-membered cyclic compound, certain derivatives of which occur naturally, notably in plants. 2. Any derivative of $C_7H_5O(OH)$.

tro·pom'e·ter [*trepein;* G. *metron,* a measure]. 1. An instrument for measuring the various rotations of the eyeball. 2. One for estimating the amount of torsion in long bones.

trop'o·pause (trop'o·pawz) [*trepein;* G. *pausis,* a stopping]. The top of the troposphere, just below the stratosphere.

tro'po·sphere. The atmosphere which lies between the stratosphere and the earth's surface, a zone of marked changes in temperature, with ascending and descending air currents and cloud formations.

Trousseau, Armand [*French physician,* 1801–67]. Performed tracheotomy and intubation (1859). Hemochromatosis is also called *Trousseau's disease.* Drew attention to the congested streaks (taches cérébrales) produced by drawing a nail over the skin, in certain nervous and cerebral diseases; called *Trousseau's spots* or *marks.* See also Trousseau's *sign.*

trox'i·done. British generic name for *trimethadione.*

troy weight. See Tables of Weights and Measures in the Appendix.

true [AS. *trēowe*]. Real; not false.

Trueta Raspall, José (contemporary). Spanish surgeon who developed a treatment of war wounds now combined with a method used by H. Winnett Orr. See Orr-Trueta *method.*

trun'cat·ed (trung'kay·tid) [L. *truncare,* to mutilate]. 1. With the top cut off; shortened in height. 2. Deprived of limbs or accessory parts.

trun'cus (pl. *trunci*) [L.]. Trunk.

t. arteriosus. The embryonic arterial trunk arising from the heart. It divides into the aorta and main pulmonary artery. It may persist as an anomalous cardiac defect in which the ventricular centrifugal vessel is placed over a ventricular septal defect, guarded by three to five semilunar valves.

t. costocervicalis. A branch of the subclavian artery: also called *costocervical trunk.* See Plate 8.

t. transversus. Duct of Cuvier.

trunk [*truncus*]. 1. The torso; the body without head or limbs. See Plate 4. 2. The main stem of a blood vessel, lymphatic, or nerve.

bronchomediastinal trunks. Two collecting lymph vessels, right and left, receiving lymph from the heart, lungs, thorax, and upper surface of the liver. The right bronchomediastinal trunk empties into the right lymphatic duct or into the angle of junction of the right subclavian and internal jugular veins; the left bronchomediastinal trunk empties into the thoracic duct or independently into the angle of junction of the left subclavian and internal jugular veins.

costocervical t. A main branch of the subclavian artery. It gives off the deep cervical artery and continues as the highest intercostal artery.

intestinal t. The collecting lymph trunk receiving lymph from the stomach, intestine, pancreas, spleen, and the lower and anterior part of the liver. It empties into the cisterna chyli.

jugular trunks. Two collecting lymph trunks, right and left, draining the head and neck. The right jugular trunk empties into the right lymphatic duct or into the right subclavian vein at its angle of junction with the right internal jugular vein; the left lymphatic trunk empties into the thoracic duct.

lumbar trunks. Two collecting lymph trunks, right and left, receiving lymph from the lower limbs, walls of the pelvis and abdomen, pelvic viscera, kidneys, and adrenal glands, and emptying into the cisterna chyli.

lumbosacral t. That formed by the anterior ramus of the fifth lumbar nerve and the smaller part of the anterior ramus of the fourth, contributing to the sacral plexus.

pulmonary t. The stem of the pulmonary artery.

subclavian trunks. Two collecting lymph vessels draining the upper extremities. The right subclavian trunk empties into the right lymphatic duct, or directly into the right subclavian vein; the left subclavian trunk, into the thoracic duct.

sympathetic t. The chain of interconnected sympathetic ganglions extending along each side of the vertebral column.

thyrocervical t. A main branch of the subclavian artery, dividing into the inferior thyroid, transverse scapular, and transverse cervical arteries.

truss [OF. *trusser*]. Any mechanical apparatus for preventing the recurrence of a hernial protrusion which has been reduced. The term includes simple devices such as a yarn truss for the control of infantile inguinal hernia, as well as complicated pieces of apparatus with pressure pads designed to hold large inguinal or abdominal hernias.

trych″o·phy·to′sis. See *trichophytosis.*

trypaflavin. Trade-mark for *acriflavine.*

acid t. Trade-mark for acriflavine hydrochloride.

tryp′an blue (trip′an, try′pan). $C_{34}H_{24}N_6Na_4O_{14}S_4$; sodium ditolyldisazobis-8-amino-1-naphthol-3,6-disulfonate; a bluish-gray powder forming deep-blue solutions. It has been used in various protozoan infections, being especially effective in piroplasmosis, and is also used as a vital stain.

tryp′a·nide [G. *trypanon*, auger]. Any eruption of the skin observed in trypanosomiasis.

try·pan′o·cide″ (tri·pan′o·side″, trip′uh·no·side″, try′puh·) [*trypanon;* L. *caedere*, to kill]. An agent that destroys trypanosomes. —**trypanoci′dal,** *adj.*

try·pan′o·san (tri·pan′o·san, try·pan′·). A dyestuff of trypanocidal properties when combined with arsenophenylglycine.

Tryp″a·no·so′ma (trip″uh·no·so′muh, try″puh·no·) [*trypanon;* G. *sōma*, body]. A genus of protozoa belonging to the class Mastigophora. They are slender, elongate organisms with a central nucleus, posterior blepharoplast, and an undulatory membrane, from which a free flagellum projects forward. Transmitted by insect vectors.

T. brucei. An organism which causes nagana in equine and other ungulate domestic animals in tropical Africa.

T. cruzi. The cause of Chagas' disease in South America and of American trypanosomiasis.

T. evansi. The cause of surra in horses and cattle.

T. gambiense. The cause of mid-African sleeping sickness.

T. hippicum. An organism which causes murrina.

T. lewisi. A nonpathogenic trypanosome of rats which is transmitted by the rat flea.

T. rhodesiense. An organism which causes East African sleeping sickness.

try·pan′o·some (tri·pan′o·sohm, try·pan′o·) [*trypanon; sōma*]. One of any species of *Trypanosoma.* —**trypanosom′ic,** *adj.*

tryp″a·no·so·mi′a·sis (trip″uh·no·so·my′uh·sis, try″puh·no·) [*trypanon; sōma;* NL. *-iasis*, condition]. Any of several diseases due to infection with various species of *Trypanosoma*, characterized by irregular fever and palpable lymph nodes.

American t. That in which the causative agent is *Trypanosoma cruzi.* Also called *barbiero fever, Brazilian t., Chagas' disease, South American t.*

Gambian t. That in which the causative agent is *Trypanosoma gambiense.* Also called *mid-African sleeping sickness.*

Rhodesian t. That in which the causative agent is *Trypanosoma rhodesiense.* Also called *East African sleeping sickness.*

try·pan′o·so·mide″ (tri·pan′o·so·mide″, ·mid″, ·meed″, try·pan′o·) [*trypanon; sōma*]. A skin lesion in any disease caused by a trypanosome.

tryp″a·no·tox′yl (trip″uh·no·tock′sil, try″puh·no·) A substance (thought to be a reduced glutathione) in the liver or blood, which transforms atoxyl into a trypanocidal agent.

tryp′an red (trip′an, try′pan). A complex azo dye, occurring as a reddish brown powder, recommended in the treatment of trypanosomiasis. Also used in vital staining.

tryp′an·roth. See *trypan red.*

tryp·ars′a·mide (trip·ahr′suh′mid). (HO)OAs-(ONa)C_6H_4.NH.CH_2.CO.NH_2. Sodium N-phenylglycineamide-*p*-arsonate, a white, crystalline powder, soluble in water. Used in treatment of trypanosomiasis and syphilis. Dose, intravenously or intramuscularly, 1–3 Gm. (15–45 gr.) at weekly intervals for 8–16 weeks, followed by a rest period of six or more weeks.

tryp′sin [G. *tryein*, to rub down; *pepsis*, a cooking]. The proteolytic enzyme resulting from the action of the enterokinase of intestinal juice upon the trypsinogen secreted in the pancreatic juice. It catalyzes the hydrolysis of peptide linkages in proteins and partially hydrolyzed proteins, more readily on the latter. Syn., *tryptase.* —**tryptic,** *adj.*

serum t. See *plasmin.*

tryp·sin′o·gen [*tryein; pepsis;* G. *genesthai*, from *gignesthai*, to be produced]. The zymogen of trypsin, occurring in the pancreatic juice and converted to trypsin by enterokinase in the small intestine. Syn., *protrypsin.*

tryp′ta·mine. $C_{10}H_{12}N_2$; the decarboxylation product of tryptophan; an intermediate substance in certain metabolic processes in plants and animals.

tryp′tase. Trypsin.

t. se′rum. See *plasmin.*

tryp″to·lyt′ic [*tryein; pepsin;* G. *lysis*, a loosing]. Of, or pertaining to, the hydrolysis of proteins caused by trypsin.

tryp′to·phan, tryp′to·phane. α-Amino-β-indole propionic acid.

```
        C6H4
       /    \
   HN         C.CH2.CH(NH2).COOH.
       \    //
        CH
```

An essential amino acid widely distributed in animal and some plant proteins.

tryp″to·phan′ase. A bacterial enzyme which catalyzes degradation of tryptophan to indole, pyruvic acid, and ammonia.

tryp′to·phyl. The univalent radical, $C_8H_6NCH_2$-$CH(NH_2)CO$—, of the amino acid tryptophan.

T. S. Test solution.

Tschamer, Anton [*German physician*, nineteenth century]. Said to have given the first description of acute infectious erythema, the so-called fifth disease (1889), also called *Sticker's disease* (1899).

Tscherning's theory of accommodation. See under *accommodation.*

tset′se fly (tset′see, tet′see). Any dipterous insect of the genus *Glossina,* almost wholly restricted to Africa. Glossina flies carry the flagellate trypanosomes, the causative agents of nagana in cattle, and of the African sleeping sickness in man.

TSH Thyroid-stimulating hormone.

tsp. Teaspoon.

Tsuchiya's reagent. See under *reagent.*

Tsu′ga [Jap., larch]. The generic name of the hemlock tree which belongs to the pine family (Pinaceae). Not to be confused with the poison hemlock (*Conium*) which is an herb (Umbelliferae).

tsut″su·ga·mush′i dis·ease′. See under *disease.*

TTC 2,3,5-Triphenyltetrazolium chloride.

tuamine. Trade-mark for the sympathomimetic amine known by the generic name *tuaminoheptane.*

tu′a·mine sul′fate (tew′uh·meen, ·min). Trademark for 2-aminoheptane sulfate, $(C_7H_{15}NH_2)_2.H_2SO_4$, a local vasoconstrictor used in 0.5–2.0% solution in the relief of nasal congestion. The base is employed in an inhaler for treatment of acute rhinologic conditions.

tu″a·mi·no·hep′tane. Generic name for 1-methylhexylamine, also known as 2-aminoheptane; $CH_3(CH_2)_4CH(CH_3)NH_2$; a colorless to pale-yellow liquid, sparingly soluble in water. It is a sympathomimetic amine, and is used for its local vasoconstrictive action by inhalation of vapors of the base and by application of a solution of the sulfate. See *tuamine.*

tu′a-tu′a. See *Jatropha gossypifolia.*

tu′ba (pl. *tubae*) [L., trumpet]. A tube.

t. auditiva. The auditory or eustachian tube.

t. uterina. The uterine or fallopian tube.

tu′bage [F.]. The introduction of a tube or catheter.

t. of the glottis. See *intubation. Obs.*

tu′bal [L. *tubus,* tube]. Pertaining to a tube, especially the uterine or the auditory.

tube [*tubus*]. A hollow, cylindrical structure, especially a uterine tube or an auditory tube.

air t. A bronchial tube.

alimentary t. The alimentary canal.

auditory t. The canal, lined by mucous membrane, with partly bony, partly cartilaginous support, connecting the pharynx with the tympanic cavity on each side. Also called *tuba auditiva* [BNA], *pharyngotympanic tube, eustachian tube.* See Plates 12, 20.

auricular t. The external auditory meatus.

auscultation t. One used to test the acuteness of hearing.

bronchial t. A bronchus, or one of its subdivisions.

capillary t. A tube with minute lumen.

cardiac t. The embryonic heart.

cathode t. An evacuated tube, frequently with a thin window opposite the cathode, to permit cathode rays to emerge from the tube.

Chaoul t. A special roentgen-ray tube used in contact therapy.

Crookes t. A highly exhausted vacuum tube used in producing x-rays.

digestive t. 1. That portion of the digestive system which includes the esophagus, stomach, intestines, and rectum [BNA]. 2. The entire alimentary tract from mouth to anus.

drainage t. A hollow tube of glass, rubber, or other material inserted into a wound or cavity to allow the escape of fluids.

embryonic digestive t. The digestive tube of the embryo. Sometimes used to include the portion of the alimentary canal between the stomodeum and the proctodeum; includes the fore-, mid-, and hindguts.

eustachian, Eustachian t. See auditory *t.* See Plates 12, 20.

fallopian, Fallopian t. A uterine tube. See *oviduct.* See Plate 41.

feeding t. One for introducing food into the stomach.

fermentation t. A glass tube used in the fermentation test for glucose.

Folin sugar t. A special tube for use in blood sugar determinations. It holds more than 25 cc. and in its lower half has a narrow portion (4 cm. long and 8 mm. in diameter) which ends in an expanded bulb holding about 3.0 cc.

fusion t. Priestly Smith's name for a miniature stereoscope by which the two images formed by a straight and a squinting eye may be fused together and seen simultaneously. Also see *heteroscope.*

gas t. Early roentgen-ray tube with a relatively low vacuum.

Geiger-Müller t. A tube which, when attached to a potential source, will produce an electric pulse each time an ionizing particle penetrates its walls.

grenz ray t. A roentgen-ray tube for production of soft roentgen rays operated at low potentials, around 10 kilovolts.

hot cathode t. A modern highly evacuated roentgen-ray tube with a hot filament cathode for the production of an abundant and controllable stream of cathode rays.

intubation t. A tube for insertion into the larynx through the mouth in laryngeal diphtheria, etc.

Levin t. See under Abraham Louis *Levin.*

Linzenmeier's blood sedimentation t. One 70 mm. long with a 5-mm. lumen; calibrated 1 ml. and 6, 12, 18, and 24 mm. below the 1-ml. mark.

Little's t. A curved glass tube 20 to 25 cm. long, introduced by Döderlein and improved by H. M. Little, used to aspirate a specimen of the lochia for laboratory study.

Lyon's t. A glass tube sealed at one end and drawn out at the other end into a capillary pipet with a small hole in the side of the tube to allow the escape of air. Used for collecting small quantities of blood from a skin puncture wound.

Miescher's t. The elongated tubelike sporocysts of the *Sarcosporidia,* in the connective tissue between the muscle fibers of the host.

Miller-Abbott t. An intestinal catheter, approximately 2.5 meters in length, having a double lumen; the smaller lumen is for inflation of a small balloon near the end of the tube which acts as a bolus stimulating peristalsis to carry the tube to the desired location; the larger lumen is for aspiration of intestinal contents. The tube is used for relief of distention due to obstruction in the small intestine.

nasotracheal t. A rubber tube or catheter inserted into the trachea by way of the nasal cavity and pharynx.

neural t. The embryonic tube formed from the ectodermal neural plate that differentiates into brain and spinal cord.

Patton-Johnston t. A four-lumen plastic tube for the treatment of bleeding from esophageal varices. There is one lumen to each of two balloons which inflate separately, one lumen to aspirate the stomach, and one to administer thrombin solution.

Penrose latex nasogastric t. See cigarette *drain.*

Pflüger's t. One of the cellular cortical sex cords or invaginations of the germinal epithelium of the embryonic ovary.

pharyngotympanic t. See auditory *t.*

Pitot t. A device for measuring fluid flow by difference in pressure caused by a simple constriction in the tube; used in the construction of certain flowmeters.

polyethylene t. See *polyethylene.*

pus t. See *pyosalpinx.*

Rehfuss t. See Martin Emil *Rehfuss.*

roentgen t. An evacuated vessel containing a source of electrons and two electrodes, the positive anode and the negative cathode at a considerable potential difference; the cathode contains the source of electrons, as a hot filament, and the anode is of sturdy construction to withstand bombardment by the cathode rays. At the anode the energy of the cathode rays is converted into 98% of heat energy and 2% of roentgen rays.

Sanford and Magath's centrifuge t. A graduated tube used in hematocrit readings.

sediment t. A glass cylinder constricted to a fine point at one end and having both ends open; used in precipitating urine.

Sengstaken-Blakemore t. A large three-lumen rubber tube for the treatment of bleeding from esophageal varices. There is one lumen to each of two balloons and a large central lumen for aspiration of the stomach and for feeding.

Southey's t., Southey-Leech t. A small cannula inserted subcutaneously into edematous tissues, usually of the lower extremities, for the purpose of draining fluid.

stomach t. A flexible tube used for irrigation or evacuation of the stomach.

test t. A cylindrical glass tube with one end open; used for growing cultures of bacteria, or for chemical analysis.

tracheotomy t. A metal tube placed in the opening made in a tracheotomy, and through which breathing is carried on.

t-tube. A rubber or glass tube in the form of the letter T.

urogenital t. The ventral part of the cloaca after division by the urorectal septum. It comprises the vesicourethral primordium and the urogenital sinus. Also called *urogenital canal.*

uterine t. The tuba uterina [BNA]; oviduct.

vacuum t. A sealed glass tube out of which the air has been pumped and which has at each end a piece of platinum wire passed through the glass and entering the tube.

tu·bec'to·my [*tubus;* G. *ektomē,* excision]. Salpingectomy; excision of a tube, specifically a uterine tube.

tube length. In a microscope, the distance between the upper focal point of the objective and the lower focal point of the eyepiece. The tube length of a monocular microscope is measured from the top of the eyepiece tube to the bottom of the nosepiece. In the binocular microscope, a correction is introduced to compensate for the distance added by the system of prisms.

tu'ber (pl. *tubera*) [L., swelling]. 1. A thickened portion of an underground stem. 2. Any rounded swelling. Also see *tuberosity, eminence.*

t. calcanei. The calcaneal tuberosity.

t. cinereum. An area of gray matter extending from the optic chiasma to the mammillary bodies and forming part of the floor of the third ventricle. The stalk of the neurohypophysis is attached to it. See median *eminence* of the tuber cinereum.

t. frontale. The frontal eminence.

t. ischiadicum. The ischial tuberosity.

t. maxillare. The maxillary tuberosity.

t. omentale hepatis. A prominence on the left lobe of the liver, corresponding to the lesser curvature of the stomach.

t. omentale pancreatis. A prominence of the middle part of the pancreas, corresponding to the lesser omentum.

t. parietale. The parietal eminence.

t. vermis. The posterior end of the inferior portion of the vermis of the cerebellum.

tu'ber·cle [L. *tuberculum,* small swelling]. 1. A small nodule. 2. A rounded prominence on a bone. 3. The specific lesion produced by the tubercle bacillus, consisting of a collection of lymphocytes and epithelioid cells, at times with giant cells.

acoustic t. A prominence on the ventrolateral surface of the restiform body produced by the cochlear nuclei: also called *acoustic eminence.*

adductor t. A slight protuberance at the lower end of the medial supracondylar line of the femur, giving attachment to the tendon of the adductor magnus muscle.

amygdaloid t. A projection of gray matter from the roof of the descending cornu of the lateral ventricle, marking the site of the amygdaloid nucleus.

anal t. One of a pair of eminences lateral to the anal opening in the embryo.

anterior obturator t. An occasional projection on the obturator crest of the superior ramus of the pubis; the anterior margin of the obturator groove.

anterior t. A tubercle at the anterior part of the extremity of the transverse process of certain cervical vertebrae.

articular t. The projection upon the zygomatic process of the temporal bone which marks the anterior boundary of the mandibular fossa. Also called *articular eminence* [BR].

auricular t. One of six tubercles on the hyoid and mandibular arches which form the auricle of the ear. See also Darwin's *t.*

Carabelli's t. See Georg *Carabelli.*

carotid t. A prominence of the sixth cervical vertebra on the anterior part of its transverse process, against which the common carotid artery can be compressed. Also called *Chassaignac's t.*

cervical t. A prominence at the junction of the upper part of the neck of the femur and the greater trochanter. It marks the beginning of the intertrochanteric line.

cloacal t. See genital *t.*

condyloid t. A protuberance on the condyle of the mandible to which the temporomandibular ligament attaches.

conglomerate t. A large lesion of tuberculosis formed by the growth and fusion of miliary tubercles.

conoid t. The medial and posterior portion of the coracoid tuberosity to which the conoid portion of the coracoclavicular ligament is attached.

corniculate t. A rounded eminence on each side of the entrance to the laryngeal cavity lying over the corniculate cartilage.

costal t. A roughened elevation found on the dorsal margin of a rib at the junction of the neck and body. It articulates with the tip of the transverse process of the corresponding vertebra.

cuneate t. One of the two ovoid eminences in the caudal end of the fourth ventricle, representing continuations of the fasciculus cuneatus; subjacent to them is the cuneate nucleus.

cuneiform t. A rounded eminence on each side of the entrance to the laryngeal cavity lying over the cuneiform cartilage. Also called *tuberculum of Santorini.*

Darwin's t. A blunt tubercle projecting from the upper free margin of the helix toward the center of the auricle.

deltoid t. See deltoid *tuberosity.*

dental t. A cusp of a tooth.

distomolar t. See under *distomolar.*

ear t. See Darwin's *t.*
epiglottic t. A slight convexity on the dorsal surface of the epiglottis.
epithelial t. The epithelial tag on the urethral groove of the embryonic phallus.
genial t. Mental spine.
genital t. A conical elevation in the midventral line between tail and umbilicus that develops into the embryonic phallus. Also spelled *genitoanal t.*
Ghon t. The primary tubercle of aerogenous tuberculosis formed in the periphery of the lung just beneath the pleura.
greater t. of humerus. A prominence on the upper lateral end of the shaft of the humerus into which are inserted the supraspinatus, infraspinatus, and teres minor muscles.
hyoid t. One of three auricular tubercles on the anterior surface of the hyoid arch of the embryo.
infraglenoid t. See infraglenoid *tuberosity.*
intercondyloid t. One of two sharp elongations on the summit of the intercondyloid eminence of the tibia.
intervenous t. A tubercle formed by the superior limbic band of cardiac muscle developing in the posterior wall of the sinus venosus between the superior and inferior caval openings. Also called *Lower's t.*
jugular tubercles. Paired eminences on the basilar portion of the occipital bone between the foramen magnum and the jugular foramen.
labial t. A small, inconstant median tubercle of the philtrum of the upper lip.
lacrimal t. One of the small papillary prominences at the margin of the eyelids in the center of which is the lacrimal punctum.
laminated t. The cerebellar nodulus.
lateral intercondylar t. The spine on the lateral side of the intercondylar eminence of the tibia.
lesser t. of humerus. A prominence on the upper anterior end of the shaft of the humerus into which is inserted the subscapularis muscle.
Luschka's t. An osteochondroma located at the superior angle of the scapula.
malar t. The blunt, thickened, inferior angle of the zygomatic bone.
mandibular t. One of three auricular tubercles on the posterior surface of the mandibular arch.
medial intercondylar t. The spine on the medial side of the intercondylar eminence of the tibia.
mental t. A raised area on each side of the mental protuberance of the mandible in the midline. See mental *spine.*
miliary tubercles. Tubercles of uniform size, approximating the millet seed, 1.0–2.0 mm. in diameter, distributed rather uniformly throughout an organ or series of organs.
Montgomery's tubercles. The apocrine sweat glands in the areola of the nipple which appear more prominent during pregnancy and lactation. Also called *areolar glands of Montgomery.*
Müller's t. An eminence of the dorsal wall of the urogenital tube at the orifice of the mesonephric and later the Müllerian ducts.
nuchal t. An elevation projecting beneath the skin, produced by the long spinous process of the seventh cervical vertebra.
obturator tubercles. See anterior obturator *t.*, posterior obturator *t.*
olfactory t. A small, oval elevation of the anterior perforated substance lateral to the olfactory trigone.
palatine t. See *tuberosity* of the palatine bone
papillary t. An extension of the caudate lobe of the liver into the portal fossa.
paramolar t. See under *paramolar.*
peroneal t. The trochlear process of the calcaneus.
pharyngeal t. The ridge on the under surface of the basilar process of the occipital bone.
plantar t. A prominence at the base of the first metatarsal bone where the tendon of the peroneus longus muscle is inserted.
posterior obturator t. An occasional projection on the medial border of the ischium, immediately anterior to the acetabular notch; the posterior boundary of the obturator groove.
posterior t. A tubercle at the posterior part of the extremity of the transverse process of certain cervical vertebrae.
postglenoid t. A process of the temporal bone that descends behind the articular fossa and prevents backward displacement of the mandible during mastication.
preglenoid t. A small elevation at the base of the anterior root of the zygomatic process of the temporal bone.
prostatic t. The middle lobe of the prostate.
pterygoid t. A tubercle on the inner surface of the mandible; it gives attachment to the internal pterygoid muscle.
pubic t. A prominent bony point on the superior ramus of the pubis for the attachment of the inguinal ligament.
satyr t. A rare pointed projection from the posterior superior aspect of the helix giving the appearance of pointed ear.
scalene t. A tubercle on the upper surface of the first rib for the insertion of the scalenus anterior muscle. Also called *Lisfranc's t.*
supraglenoid t. See supraglenoid *tuberosity.*
vertebral tubercles. Three elevations, the superior, inferior, and lateral, subdividing the transverse process of the twelfth thoracic vertebra; similar rudimentary prominences are found on the transverse processes of the tenth and eleventh thoracic vertebrae.

tu·ber′cu·lar [*tuberculum*]. Characterized by the presence of small nodules or tubercles: often used erroneously for *tuberculous.*

tu·ber′cu·la″ted [*tuberculum*]. Having tubercles; tuberculose; tubercular.

tu·ber″cu·la′tion [*tuberculum*]. 1. The formation, development, or arrangement of tubercles. 2. The process of affecting a part with tubercles.

tu·ber′cu·lid, tu·ber′cu·lide [*tuberculum*]. A group of varied skin manifestations from tuberculosis of viscera. The skin changes often begin with necrosis in the dermis; later there is involvement of the epidermis followed by ulceration. They are considered to be caused either by bacillary embolisms or by toxins from tubercle bacilli.
micropapular t. An id reaction characterized by many pinhead-sized indurated papules limited to the face, usually brownish-red, although some appear semitranslucent and almost colorless.
papulonecrotic t. An id reaction with the lesion tending to undergo central necrosis and scarring later. The lesions are located on the face and extremities; the trunk may be involved.

tu·ber′cu·lin [*tuberculum*]. A material containing the proteins of the tubercle bacillus, or products derived from such proteins and capable of eliciting an inflammatory reaction in the tissues of a human or animal body which has been sensitized either by tuberculosis or by inoculation with living or dead tubercle bacilli.
old t. A broth culture of tubercle bacilli, sterilized by heat, filtered, and concentrated by evaporation. Abbreviated, O.T., T.O.

tu·ber″cu·lo·der′ma [*tuberculum;* G. *derma*, skin]. A cutaneous manifestation of the action of tubercle bacilli; a tuberculid.

tu·ber″cu·lo·fi′broid [*tuberculum;* L. *fibra,* fiber; G. *eidos,* form]. Relating to a tubercle, 3, that has undergone fibroid degeneration.

tu·ber′cu·loid [*tuberculum; eidos*]. Resembling tuberculosis or a tubercle.

tu·ber″cu·lo′ma [*tuberculum;* G. *-ōma,* tumor]. A conglomerate caseous tubercle, usually solitary, which has attained such a size as to suggest the appearance of a tumor.

t. en plaque. A rare type of chronic tuberculous meningo-encephalitis, characterized by a flat plaque of a granulomatous reaction.

tu·ber″cu·lo·ma′ni·a [*tuberculum;* G. *mania,* madness]. An unalterable and unfounded conviction that one is suffering from tuberculosis.

tu·ber″cu·lo·mu′cin. See *toxicomucin.*

tu·ber″cu·lo·pho′bi·a [*tuberculum;* G. *phobos,* fear]. Morbid fear of tuberculosis.

tu·ber″cu·lo·pro′te·in (·pro′tee·in, ·pro′teen) [*tuberculum;* G. *prōteios,* of first rank]. A variety of proteins not exerting appreciable toxic effect upon the normal body but highly toxic for the tuberculous, hypersensitive individual, leading to necrosis, fever, and severe constitutional symptoms.

tu·ber′cu·lose. Tuberculated.

tu·ber″cu·lo·sil″i·co′sis [*tuberculum;* L. *silex,* flint; *-ōsis,* condition]. Chronic inflammation of the lungs, caused by the combined action of tubercle bacilli and silicon dioxide. This term is preferred in South Africa to silicotuberculosis, which is in common usage. See *silicotuberculosis.*

tu·ber″cu·lo′sis [*tuberculum; -ōsis*]. An infectious disease caused by the *Mycobacterium tuberculosis,* commonly known as the tubercle bacillus. It may affect any organ or tissue of the body, but by far the most deaths are due to tuberculosis of the lungs. It is a leading cause of death. Since the time of Hippocrates it has been known as *phthisis.* The name *tuberculosis* was introduced in 1834 by Schönlein. The two characteristic types of tissue reaction are the exudative, consisting of acute inflammation, and the productive or proliferative, consisting of tubercle formation. Abbreviated, TB.

active t. That which is undergoing change, either progressive or retrogressive, causing, or threatening to cause, clinical symptoms or disability.

acute disseminated t. That in which miliary tubercles are widely distributed through the body as a result of transmission of tubercle bacilli in large numbers through the blood stream: also called *acute generalized miliary t.*

avian t. A form found in birds.

bovine t. A form found in cattle, transmitted to man usually by raw milk from infected cows. Also see glandular *t., t.* of bones and joints.

bronchogenic t. That resulting from extension of infection within the lung by way of the air passages. Also called *bronchogenous t.*

bronchopneumonic t. An exudative reaction in the lung caused by the tubercle bacillus, having the distribution of bronchopneumonia. Also see *pneumonia.*

caseous pneumonic t. Exudative tuberculosis of the lung which has undergone a characteristic type of necrosis, simulating cheese in its gross appearance.

chronic fibroid t. Slowly progressive pulmonary tuberculosis with extensive fibrosis and mild symptoms.

chronic miliary t. A condition in which healing or healed miliary tubercles are distributed through one or more organs as a result of transmission of tubercle bacilli in small numbers through the blood stream.

chronic ulcerative t. The most prevalent type of pulmonary tuberculosis in which necrosis has been followed by the formation of cavities surrounded by varying degrees of fibrosis. It represents a later stage in the evolution of either exudative or proliferative tuberculosis, and may coexist with lesions of either or both of these types.

closed t. Pulmonary tuberculosis not discharging tubercle bacilli; it is therefore not capable of transmission to other persons.

cutaneous t. See *t.* cutis.

endogenous t. That arising from a source within the body; especially disease caused by bacilli transmitted through lymphatic or blood vessels, or both, to another organ, usually to the lungs.

exogenous t. That arising from a source outside the body.

extrapulmonary t. Tuberculosis occurring in any part of the body outside the lungs; most commonly affected are bones, joints, the genitourinary tract, meninges, skin, and the intestines.

far advanced t. (According to the National Tuberculosis Association classification.) That in which there are lesions more extensive than moderately advanced.

fibroid t. Chronic tuberculosis, usually in the upper lobe of the lung, associated with extensive fibrosis.

glandular t. That affecting the lymph nodes, especially the cervical, bronchial, and mesenteric. Usually due to bovine tuberculosis.

hematogenous t. Any manifestation resulting from the transmission of tubercle bacilli through the blood stream.

inactive t. That which is in a state of partial or complete healing, causing no clinical symptoms or disability; it shows no change over a prolonged period of time.

incipient t. The earliest stage of pulmonary tuberculosis in point of time. Often confused with minimal tuberculosis which refers only to the extent of disease.

latent t. That which shows no change over a prolonged period of time, but is incompletely healed and potentially active.

lobar pneumonic t. An exudative reaction in the lung caused by the tubercle bacillus, having the characteristic distribution of lobar pneumonia. Also see *pneumonia.*

lymphogenic t. Metastasis from any focus to another by way of the lymph channels. Also called *lymphogenous t.*

minimal t. (According to the National Tuberculosis Association classification.) Tuberculosis in which there are slight lesions without demonstrable excavation confined to a small part of one or both lungs. The total extent of the lesions, regardless of distribution, shall not exceed the equivalent of the volume of lung tissue which lies above the second chondrosternal junction and the spine of the fourth or the body of the fifth thoracic vertebra on one side.

moderately advanced t. That in which both lungs may be involved, but the total extent of the lesions shall not exceed the following limits: slight disseminated lesions which may extend through not more than the volume of one lung, or the equivalent of this in both lungs; dense and confluent lesions which may extend through not more than the equivalent of one-third the volume of one lung. Any gradation within the above limits. Total diameter of cavities, if present, is estimated not to exceed 4 cm.

open t. Pulmonary tuberculosis in an infectious state; it is capable of transmission to other persons.

pelvic t. Tuberculosis of the uterine tubes which has spread to other pelvic structures or organs.

primary t. The reaction which follows the first implantation of tubercle bacilli in the body. It consists of a caseous focal reaction in the parenchyma of the organ and a similar reaction in the regional lymph node or nodes. Both foci usually run a benign course and undergo healing with calcification. The most frequent site is the lung. Also called *primary phase, primary infection, primary focus* or *complex, childhood type t.*

pulmonary t. Tuberculosis of the lungs.

reinfection t. That which includes all manifestations of tuberculosis other than the primary phase. It exhibits in varying degree the influence of two factors not operative in primary tuberculosis; acquired resistance, and hypersensitivity of the tissues to tuberculin. It is characterized especially by an increased capacity for destruction of tissue, and by acceleration of both the early, exudative reaction and the subsequent, productive reaction. Also called *adult type t.*

t. cutis. That affecting the skin. It occurs in many forms and is more frequent in Europe than in America. Also see *lupus* vegetans, *t.* lichenoides, *tuberculid.*

t. cutis orificialis. Ulcerative tuberculosis of the skin at the body orifices.

t. lichenoides. A skin eruption consisting of groups of papules, usually on the trunk, seen in subjects suffering from tuberculosis, especially the glandular and bone types of the disease. Also called *lichen scrofulosus, chronic miliary t. of the skin.*

t. luposa. See *lupus* vulgaris.

t. of bones and joints. That affecting bones and joints, characterized by bone destruction and the formation of cold abscesses. Usually due to bovine tuberculosis.

t. verrucosa. A type of warty skin eruption, usually on the hands and arms, due to inoculation with the tubercle bacillus from handling meat of infected cattle or infected human material.

tu·ber″cu·lo·ste·ar′ic ac′id. 10-Methylstearic acid, obtained from tubercle bacilli.

tu·ber′cu·lous [*tuberculum*]. Affected with, or caused by, tuberculosis.

tu·ber′cu·lum (pl. *tubercula*) [L.]. Tubercle.

t. acusticum. See acoustic *tubercle.*

t. anterius. (a) The conical prominence on the anterior arch of the atlas. (b) The frontal extremity of the thalamus.

t. articulare. Articular tubercle.

t. auriculae. Darwin's tubercle of the auricle.

t. caudatum. The caudate lobe of the liver.

t. cinereum. A longitudinal elevation between the cuneate fasciculus and tubercle on the one hand and the roots of the ninth, tenth, and eleventh cranial nerves on the other. It is formed by the expansion of the substantia gelatinosa extending into the medulla oblongata and descending fibers derived from the sensory root of the trigeminal nerve.

t. corniculatum. See corniculate *tubercle.*

t. costae. Tubercle of a rib. See costal *tubercle.*

t. cuneiforme. See cuneiform *tubercle.*

t. epiglotticum. Epiglottic tubercle or cushion of the epiglottis.

t. genitale. See genital *tubercle.*

t. impar. The unpaired mass of tissue between the anterior lingual swellings and the copula in the developing tongue.

t. intercondyloideum laterale. A lateral intercondyloid tubercle.

t. intercondyloideum mediale. Medial intercondyloid tubercle.

t. jugulare. See *jugular tubercles* under *tubercle.*

t. linguale laterale. The lateral lingual swelling in the embryo.

t. linguale mediale. See *t.* impar.

t. mentale. Mental tubercle. See mental *spine.*

t. obturatorium anterius. See anterior obturator *tubercle.*

t. obturatorium posterius. See posterior obturator *tubercle.*

t. pharyngeum. Pharyngeal tubercle.

t. posterius. The rudimentary spinous process of the atlas.

t. pubicum. See pubic *tubercle.*

t. scaleni. Scalene tubercle of Lisfranc.

t. sellae. Anterior boundary of the sella turcica.

tu′ber·in [L. *tuber*, swelling]. A simple protein of the globulin type which occurs in potatoes.

tu″ber·os′i·tas. Tuberosity.

tu″ber·os′i·ty [*tuber*]. A protuberance on a bone.

calcaneal t. The posterior extremity of the calcaneus. Syn., *tuber calcanei.*

coracoid t. A rough elevation on the inferior surface of the acromial end of the clavicle, which overhangs the coracoid process of the scapula, and to which the coracoclavicular ligament is attached.

costal t. A rough area on the under surface of the medial end of the clavicle, which gives attachment to the costoclavicular ligament.

deltoid t. A rough elevation about the middle of the anterolateral surface of the humerus for the insertion of the deltoid muscle.

gluteal t. The lateral and upward extension of the linea aspera, which gives attachment to part of the gluteus maximus muscle.

greater t. of femur. The greater trochanter of the femur.

iliac t. A rough, elevated area above the articular surface on the inner aspect of the ala of the ilium, which gives attachment to the posterior sacroiliac ligament, and from which the sacrospinalis and multifidus muscles take origin.

infraglenoid t. A rough impression below the glenoid cavity, from which the long head of the triceps muscle arises.

ischial t. A protuberance on the posterior portion of the superior ramus of the ischium, upon which the body rests in sitting.

lesser t. of femur. The lesser trochanter of the femur.

malar t. See malar *tubercle.*

maxillary t. A protuberance on the lower part of the infratemporal surface of the maxillary bone; the medial side articulates with the pyramidal process of the palatine bone.

parietal t. The parietal eminence.

pyramidal t. See *t.* of the palatine bone.

radial t. The large eminence on the medial side of the upper extremity of the radius, into which the tendon of the biceps brachii muscle is inserted.

sacral t. A rough area on the posterior surface of the sacrum, bearing three deep, uneven impressions for attachment of the posterior sacroiliac ligament.

sciatic t. See ischial *t.*

supraglenoid t. A slight elevation on the upper margin of the glenoid cavity, which gives attachment to the long head of the biceps brachii muscle.

t. of the cuboid bone. An eminence on the lateral side of the cuboid bone; it bears an oval facet on which glides the sesamoid bone or cartilage often found in the tendon of the peroneus longus muscle.

t. of the fifth metatarsal. A rough projection from the lateral surface of the base of the bone, giving attachment to the peroneus brevis muscle on its dorsal surface, and to the flexor digiti quinti brevis muscle on its plantar surface.

t. of the first metatarsal. An oval prominence

on the lateral side of the base of the bone, into which part of the tendon of the peroneus longus muscle is inserted.

t. of the navicular bone. A rounded eminence on the medial surface of the navicular bone of the foot, into which part of the tendon of the tibialis posterior muscle is inserted.

t. of the palatine bone. A backward and laterad projection from the junction of the horizontal and vertical parts of the palatine bone. Syn., *pyramidal process, pyramidal t.*

t. of the second rib. A rough eminence on the lateral surface of the second rib for attachment of part of the first and all of the second digitation of the serratus anterior muscle.

t. of the tibia. An oblong elevation on the anterior surface of the upper extremity of the tibia, to which the patellar ligament is attached.

t. of the ulna. A rough eminence below coronoid process on anterior surface of ulna, which gives insertion to part of the brachialis muscle.

ungual t. The expanded distal end of a terminal phalanx.

tu′bo- [L. *tubus*, tube]. A combining form denoting *pertaining to a tube.*

tu″bo·ab·dom′i·nal [*tubus;* L. *abdomen*, belly]. Pertaining to a uterine tube and to the abdomen.

tu″bo·ad·nex′o·pex″y [*tubus;* L. *annexum*, from *annectere*, to tie to; G. *pēxis*, a fixing]. Surgical fixation of the uterine adnexa.

tu″bo·cu·ra′re (tew″bo·cue·rah′ree). Curare so named because of its tube shape, the result of being packed in hollow bamboo canes.

tu″bo·cu·ra′rine (·cue·rah′reen, ·rin). An alkaloid, $C_{19}H_{21}NO_4$, in tubocurare prepared from *Chondodendron tomentosum.* It is responsible for the typical action of curare. Also called *d-tubocurarine.* See *intocostrin.*

tu″bo·lig″a·men′tous [*tubus;* L. *ligamentum*, tie]. Relating to the oviduct and the broad ligament.

tu″bo-o·va′ri·an. Pertaining to the uterine tube and the ovary.

tu″bo-o·va″ri·ot′o·my. Excision of a uterine tube and ovary.

tu″bo·per″i·to·ne′al [*tubus;* G. *peritonaion*, membrane which contains the lower viscera]. Relating to the oviducts and the peritoneum.

tu″bo·u′ter·ine [*tubus;* L. *uterus*, womb]. Pertaining to the uterine tube and the uterus.

tu″bo·vag′i·nal [*tubus;* L. *vagina*, vagina]. Pertaining to a uterine tube and the vagina.

tu′bu·lar [L. *tubulus*, small tube]. 1. Shaped like a tube. 2. Pertaining to or affecting tubules, as tubular nephritis. 3. Produced in a tube, as tubular breathing.

tu′bule [*tubulus*]. 1. A small tube. 2. *In anatomy*, any minute, tube-shaped structure.

collecting tubules. The ducts conveying the urine from the renal tubules (nephrons) to the minor calyxes of the renal pelvis.

convoluted tubules. (a) The contorted tubules of the testis. (b) The parts of the renal tubule which lie in the cortex, as the proximal and distal convoluted portions of the nephron.

dentinal tubules. Canals in the matrix of dentin occupied by odontoblastic processes.

epigenital t. A mesonephric tubule which becomes one of the ductuli aberrantes.

hepatic t. See *hepatic cords* under *cord.*

mesonephric t. A tubule of the mesonephros.

nephric t. See uriniferous *t.*

paragenital mesonephric tubules. Mesonephric tubules which become the efferent ductules of the testis, the appendix of the epididymis, and the paradidymis.

seminiferous t. Any of the tubules of the testes.

uriniferous t. One of the numerous winding tubules of the kidney; a nephron.

tu″bu·li·za′tion [*tubulus*]. Protection of the ends of nerves, after neurorrhaphy, by an absorbable cylinder.

tu″bu·lo·al·ve′o·lar, tu″bu·lo·ac′i·nous [*tubulus;* L. *alveolus*, dim. of *alveus*, trough]. Consisting of a system of branching tubules which terminate in alveoli, as in the salivary glands.

tu′bu·lo·cyst″ [*tubulus;* G. *kystis*, bladder]. A cystic dilatation in an occluded canal or duct.

tu″bu·lo·rac′e·mose (·rass′i·moce) [*tubulus;* L. *racemosus*, full of clusters]. Denoting a gland that is both tubular and racemose.

tu′bu·lus (pl. *tubuli*) [L.]. A small, tubelike organ; a tubule.

tubuli lactiferi. The excretory ducts of the mammae.

tubuli renales. Renal tubules.

tubuli renales contorti. Convoluted renal tubules.

tubuli renales recti. Straight renal tubules.

tubuli seminiferi contorti. Convoluted seminiferous tubules.

tubuli seminiferi recti. Straight seminiferous tubules.

tu′bus (pl. *tubi*) [L.]. A tube, canal.

t. digestorius. The digestive canal

t. medullaris. The vertebral canal.

t. vertebralis. The spinal or vertebral canal.

Tucker's test. See Naegeli *test.*

Tuffier, Theodore [*French surgeon*, 1857–1929]. Remembered for his description of a surgical operation which he introduced for chronic valvular heart disease (1914). He described a mesenterio-parietal fold, a portion of the mesentery extending into the right iliac fossa, called *Tuffier's inferior ligament.* Spinal anesthesia was once referred to as *Tuffier's method*, because of his use of it before it received general acceptance. Described a syndrome of general debility with relaxation and displacement of organs; once called *Tuffier's syndrome.*

tug, tug′ging [ME. *tuggen*]. A jerking, pulling, or drawing.

tracheal tugging. The downward tugging movement of the larynx, sometimes observed in aneurysm of the aortic arch.

tuinal. Trade-mark for a mixture of equal parts of the substances known by the trade-marked names *seconal sodium* and *sodium amytal*, supplied in capsules.

tu″la·re′mi·a [*Tulare* County, California; G. *haima*, blood]. An infectious disease due to the bacterium, *Pasteurella tularensis*, and transmitted to man by the handling of infected rabbits or other rodents or by the bite of a blood-sucking insect.

oculoglandular t. Infection by *Pasteurella tularensis* which, in addition to the usual symptoms of tularemia, causes swollen eyelids, conjunctivitis, swollen lymph nodes, and ulcers on the conjunctivae.

tu′lip·ine (tew′lip·een, ·in). A poisonous alkaloid from the tulip.

Tulp, Nicholas [*Dutch physician and anatomist*, 1593–1674]. Author of an early description of beriberi (1652). Among the first to describe the ileocecal valve. A noted demonstrator of anatomy, he is the central figure, the Demonstrator, in Rembrandt's *Lesson in Anatomy.*

tum′bu fly (tōōm′bōō, tum′bōō). An African species of the Diptera, *Cordylobia anthropophaga*, whose larvae develop in the skin of man and various mammals, e.g., rats, dogs, cats, monkeys.

tu″me·fa′cient (tew″mi·fay′shunt) [L. *tumefacere*, to swell]. Swelling; swollen, or tending to cause swelling.

tu″me·fac′tion [*tumefacere*]. 1. A swelling. 2. The act of swelling.

tu′me·fy. To swell or cause to swell.

tu·men′ti·a (tew·men′shee·uh) [L., a swelling]. Vasomotor disturbance characterized by irregular swellings in the legs and arms.

tu·mes′cence [L. *tumescere*, to begin to swell]. 1. The condition of growing tumid. 2. A swelling.

tu·mes′cent [*tumescere*]. Swollen or enlarged.

tu′mid [L. *tumidus*, swollen]. Swollen.

tu·mid′i·ty [L. *tumiditas*, a swelling]. The state of being swollen.

tu′mor [L.]. 1. A swelling. 2. Specifically, a new growth of cells or tissues characterized by autonomy, that is, independent of the laws of growth of the host. It is progressive, of unknown cause, and in malignant form limited only by the nutrition provided by the host. —**tumorous, tumoral,** *adj.*

Abrikosov's t. See granular-cell *myoblastoma.*

acoustic-nerve t. A neurilemmoma in which acoustic, and sometimes vestibular, disturbances of the eighth cranial nerve are dominant and early clinical features. Syn., *acoustic neurinoma.*

adenomatoid t. Characteristic, small, benign neoplasms peculiar to the genital tracts of both male and female, composed of fibrous stroma in which are found numerous irregular spaces lined by cells which may resemble endothelium, epithelium, or mesothelium.

adipose t. Lipoma.

adrenal clear-cell t. of ovary. See adrenocorticoid *adenoma* of ovary.

adrenocortical t. of ovary. See adrenocorticoid *adenoma* of ovary.

alveolar (cell) t. See bronchiolar *carcinoma.*

amyloid t. A nonmalignant nodule situated usually on a vocal fold, a few millimeters in diameter, spherical and often pedunculated. Made up principally of a hyaline acidophilic substance which has staining reactions like primary amyloid. Less often found in the wall of the urinary bladder and rarely in other sites.

androgenic hilar-cell t. See adrenocorticoid *adenoma* of ovary.

aortic-body t. A rare benign tumor, resembling the carotid body tumor but occurring at the aortic arch.

argentaffin t. See *carcinoid.*

basal-cell t. of ovary. See granulosa-cell *t.*

basophilic t. of pituitary. See basophilic *adenoma.*

benign t. One that grows by expansion, is usually encapsulated, and does not exhibit the features of malignant tumors.

blood t. See *hematoma.*

botryoid t. See *sarcoma* botryoides.

Brenner t. A solid or cystic tumor of the ovaries, composed of cords or nests of polyhedral, epithelial cells separated by an abundant connective-tissue stroma, generally benign and having no known endocrine activity: also called *oophoroma folliculare* (Brenner), *brenneroma.*

Brooke t. See *trichoepithelioma.*

"brown" t. of hyperparathyroidism. A tumorlike lesion of bone, seen in patients with hyperparathyroidism, histologically resembling the giant-cell tumor of bone.

calcified t. of skin. (a) Any cutaneous neoplasm containing calcium. (b) Calcifying epithelioma.

calcifying giant-cell t. See *chondroblastoma.*

carotid-body t. A benign tumor at the bifurcation of the common carotid artery, composed of nests of ovoid or polygonal cells having a rich cytoplasm and small vesicular or dense nuclei, in a vascular fibrous stroma reduplicating the histologic structure of the carotid body. Clinically it is manifested only by a lump in the neck. Syn., *chemodectoma, inactive* or *nonchromaffin paraganglioma, paraganglion caroticum, potato tumor of neck.*

central giant-cell t. Same as giant-cell *t.* (a).

cerebellopontine angle t. Any tumor located at the cerebellopontine angle; usually, a neurilemmoma of the acoustic nerve or a meningioma.

chordoid t. See *chordoma.*

chromaffin t. Pheochromocytoma; chromophil tumor.

chromophobe t. of pituitary. See chromophobic *adenoma.*

Codman's t. See *chondroblastoma.*

collision t. One in which a sarcoma invades a carcinoma, or vice versa.

colloid ovarian t. See pseudomucinous *cystadenoma.*

compound ovarian t. See *teratoma.*

cystic t. of tendon sheath. See *ganglion*, 2.

dermoid t. See dermoid *cyst.*

desmoid t. A slightly destructive, tumorlike lesion of subcutaneous tissues or of muscle, as of the rectus abdominis, probably a form of fibroma, following injury.

desmoid t. of mediastinum. One composed of sparsely cellular connective tissue; it may attain great size and be locally invasive, but does not metastasize.

ductal t. See ductal *carcinoma.*

dumbbell t. A ganglioneuroma or neurofibroma composed of a mass in both the spinal canal and thorax connected by a narrow band of tumor tissue in the intervertebral foramen. Syn., *hourglass t.*

dysontogenic t. Any tumor exhibiting defective gonadal development and function.

ectopic ovarian t. See *teratoma.*

embryonal mixed t. (*of kidney*). See Wilms's *t.*

eosinophilic t. of pituitary. See eosinophilic *adenoma.*

eosinophilic t. of sweat gland. A sweat-gland tumor characterized by the prominence of eosinophilic apocrinelike cells.

epiphyseal chondromatous giant-cell t. See *chondroblastoma.*

estrogenic t. See feminizing *t.* of ovary.

Ewing's t. See Ewing's *sarcoma.*

feminizing t. of ovary. Any functional tumor of the ovary resulting in an exaggeration of female sex characters. In children, it may produce precocious puberty; in sexually mature females, clinical signs are less apparent; in the postmenopausal patient, uterine bleeding may occur. Morphologically it appears in two predominant forms, *granulosa-cell tumor* and *thecoma*, but foci of one may be found in the other. Also called *estrogenic t., feminizing adenoma, ovarian folliculoma, feminizing mesenchymoma of ovary.*

fibroid t. A fibroma; also often used to mean a fibromyoma of the uterus.

Flexner-Jobling t. See Simon *Flexner.*

follicular t. A sebaceous cyst.

functional cortical t. See cortical *adenoma.*

ganglion nodosum t. A rare tumor of the ganglion nodosum of the vagus, histologically indistinguishable from the carotid-body tumor.

giant-cell t. (a) A distinctive tumor of bone, thought to arise from nonosteogenic connective tissue of marrow, composed of a richly vascularized reticulum of stromal cells interspersed with multinuclear giant cells. It generally appears after the second decade of life near the end of long limb bones and it causes thinning of the compact bone. Also called *central giant-cell t., giant-cell sarcoma of bone, osteoclastoma, myeloid sarcoma,* *myeloplaxic t., chronic hemorrhagic osteomyelitis.* (b) Less specifically: (1) epulis; (2) chondroblastoma; (3) nonosteogenic fibroma; (4) chondromyxoid fibroma of bone; (5) xanthomatous giant-cell tumor of tendon sheath.

glomus jugulare t. A rare tumor, histologically resembling the carotid-body tumor, arising in the vicinity of the middle ear from either the glomus jugulare (of Guild) or the paraganglion tympanicum (of Krause). Clinically there is usually slowly progressing hearing loss, discharge from one ear, and sometimes dizziness. Malignant behavior is fairly common. Syn., *granular-cell myoblastoma of ear canal, nonchromaffin paraganglioma of middle ear.*

glomus t. A tumor derived from an arteriovenous glomus of the skin, especially of the digits. It is usually small, blue, painful, and benign. Also called *angioneuromyoma, glomangioma.*

granular-cell t. of adrenal cortex. See cortical *adenoma.*

granulosa-cell t. An ovarian neoplasm composed of cells resembling those lining the primordial follicle, associated with clinical signs of feminization: also called *diffuse, microcystic* or *microfolliculoid, macrocystic* or *macrofolliculoid, parenchymatous* or *pseudoadenomatous granulosa-cell t.* Syn., *basal-cell t. of ovary, Kahlden's t.*

grapelike t. See *sarcoma* botryoides.

Grawitz t. See clear-cell *carcinoma;* also see *hypernephroma.*

Grawitz t. of ovary. See adrenocorticoid *adenoma* of ovary.

heterologous t. One composed of tissues different from that in which it grows.

hilus-cell t. See adrenocorticoid *adenoma* of ovary.

histioid t. One in which the tumor is made up almost entirely of a single type of cell.

homologous t. A tumor consisting of tissue identical with that of the organ from which it springs.

hourglass t. (*of the spine*). See dumbbell *t.*

Hürthle-cell t. A thyroid tumor composed predominantly or entirely of large, acidophilic, glandular epithelial cells (Hürthle cells) and showing little or no follicular development or colloid; it is usually benign, but malignant forms have been described.

hypernephroid t. A tumor whose cells resemble those of the adrenal gland.

hypernephroid t. of ovary. See adrenocorticoid *adenoma* of ovary.

hypophyseal-duct t. An inclusive term applied to tumors derived from epithelial remnants of the involuted pouch of Rathke. Usually suprasellar, they include the adamantinoma and the so-called craniopharyngioma, which originate in the residual stalk, and cystic neoplasms, which originate from the residual cleft. More frequent in children than in adults.

interstitial-cell t. A tumor of the testis, usually benign, composed of interstitial cells (Leydig cells), which may be associated with hypersecretion of male sex hormones: also called *interstitioma, Leydig-cell t.*

islet-cell t. A tumor arising from cells of the islets of the pancreas, clinically classified as *functioning,* producing hyperinsulinism, or as *nonfunctioning.* Histological distinction between the benign and malignant forms may be difficult. Syn., *islet adenoma, Langerhansian adenoma, islet-cell carcinoma, insulinoma, insuloma.*

Kahlden's t. See granulosa-cell *t.*

Krukenberg t. A malignant tumor of the ovary, secondary to a tumor of the gastrointestinal tract or breast, usually bilateral, characterized histologically by mucus-containing so-called "signet-ring cells": also called *fibrosarcoma ovarii mucocellulare carcinomatodes* (Krukenberg), *carcinoma mucocellulare ovarii.*

Leydig-cell t. See interstitial-cell *t.*

lipid-cell t. of ovary. See *luteoma.*

malignant t. One which grows peripherally, invades and destroys surrounding tissues, may extend directly, and may produce distant secondary tumors by metastasis.

masculinizing t. of ovary. One of a rare group of ovarian tumors, considered together on a clinical and biological basis, and characterized by their production of defemination or virilism. It is chiefly represented by the arrhenoblastoma and by closely related neoplastic growths grouped together as *adrenocorticoid adenomas of ovary.* Syn., *virilizing t. of ovary.*

medullary t. of adrenal. See *pheochromocytoma.*

melanotic t. Malignant melanoma.

mesenchymal (mixed) t. Mesenchymoma.

mesodermal mixed t. See *mesenchymoma.*

metastatic t. A secondary tumor produced by metastasis.

milk t. A swelling of the breast due to the obstruction of milk ducts; not a neoplasm.

mixed t. One composed of two or more tissue types or cell types. More specifically, a tumor originating from one or two of the primary germinal embryonal layers as contrasted with teratomas or teratoid tumors which contain elements of all three germinal layers.

mixed t. of breast. See *cystosarcoma* phylloides.

mixed t. of salivary-gland type. A mixed tumor, similar to the type seen in salivary glands, occasionally found in the skin of almost any part of the body, and containing, in addition to epithelial elements, myxoid tissue and cartilage: variously called *adenochondroma, adenomyxochondrosarcoma, pleomorphic (salivary) adenoma, chondrocarcinoma* (salivary-gland type), *fibromyxoendothelioma, myxopleomorphic epithelioma.*

mucous t. A myxoma.

myeloid t. See *myeloma.*

myeloplaxic t. See giant-cell *t.* (a).

myoepithelial (sweat-gland) t. See *myoepithelioma.*

Nelaton's t. See *teratoma.*

nerve-sheath t. See *neurilemmoma.*

neuromyoarterial glomus t. See glomus *t.*

nonencapsulated sclerosing t. of thyroid. A small nonencapsulated epithelial tumor of the thyroid showing marked sclerosis of stroma which are histologically malignant: thought to be a small papillary carcinoma of very low-grade malignancy.

occupational t. A tumor resulting from prolonged exposure to some physical or chemical agent in the course of one's occupation.

organoid t. One in which the components are so arranged as to resemble the general structure of an organ, as an adenoma.

osteogenic t. Any tumor of bone-forming tissue. See *osteoma,* osteogenic *sarcoma.*

paraganglion caroticus t. See carotid-body *t.*

parvilocular pseudomucinous t. See pseudomucinous *cystadenoma.*

phantom t. A swelling s mulating a tumor produced by the contraction of a muscle or by gaseous distention of the intestine.

pineal t. See *pinealoma.*

potato t. of neck. See carotid-body *t.*

Pott's puffy t. A doughy swelling which appears on the scalp as a result of a subaponeurotic, extradural collection of pus due to osteomyelitis of the skull.

primitive fat-cell t. See *liposarcoma.*

Pringle's t. See *adenoma* sebaceum.

pseudocolloid ovarian t. See pseudomucinous *cystadenoma.*

recurrent t. One recurring after surgical removal.

rhabdomyoblastic mixed t. A malignant mesenchymoma.

sand t. See *psammoma.*

Schmincke's t. Lymphoepithelioma.

Spiegler's t. See *cylindroma.*

splenic t. A term sometimes applied to an enlarged spleen, not necessarily neoplastic, and usually only hyperplastic.

sweat-gland t. A neoplasm derived from sebaceous glands, variously described, as sebaceous adenoma, sebaceous epithelioma, and cystic basal-cell epithelioma.

sympathotropic-cell t. See adrenocorticoid *adenoma* of ovary.

teratoid t. Teratoma.

theca-cell t. of ovary. See *thecoma.*

thoracic-inlet tumors. Infiltrating tumors at the thoracic inlet which produce a symptom complex, commonly known as *Pancoast's syndrome*, most frequently caused by bronchogenic carcinoma but also by the rarer branchiogenic carcinoma, sympathicoblastoma of cervical ganglia, osteogenic sarcomas, metastatic tumors, and such noncancerous conditions as tuberculosis.

tuberous cystic t. of breast. See *cystosarcoma* phylloides.

tuberous t. Any tumor, such as an angioma, which grossly resembles a tuber.

turban t. See *cylindroma.*

virilizing lipoid-cell t. See adrenocorticoid *adenoma* of ovary.

Warthin's t. A benign mixed salivary-gland tumor, usually of the parotid gland, composed of lymphoid interstitial tissue arranged in papillary processes and covered by a layer of epithelium: also called *papillary cystadenoma lymphomatosum.*

Werth's t. See *pseudomyxoma peritonaei.*

Wilms's t. A teratoma of the renal cortex, almost always unilateral, manifesting itself usually in infancy or childhood. Malignant transformation with metastasis to lungs and brain is common. Also called *embryonal mixed tumor of kidney, adenosarcoma (of kidney), nephrogenic dysembryoma, embryoma of kidney, hamartoblastoma of kidney, mesoblastic nephroma.*

xanthomatous giant-cell t. of the tendon sheath. A benign, usually well-defined tumor composed of vacuolated macrophages and multinucleated giant cells set in a collagenic stroma, which varies greatly in amounts.

yellow t. A tumor of the ovary, usually a luteoma: nonspecific term.

tu′mor·af″fin, tu″mor·af′fin [*tumor;* L. *affinis*, related to]. Substances (drugs, radiant energy, etc.) which are supposed to have some special affinity for tumor cells.

tu″mor·i·gen′ic. Tumor-forming.

tu′mor·ous [*tumor*]. Of the nature of a neoplasm or tumor.

tu·mul′tus [L.]. Tumult.

t. cordis. Irregular heart action.

t. sermonis. A stuttering manner of reading, from pathologic cause.

Tun′ga. A genus of fleas which burrow beneath the skin to lay their eggs; serious local inflammation results.

T. penetrans. A species prevalent in the tropical regions of Africa and America: also called *chigoe, jigger.*

tun·gi′a·sis. The cutaneous pustular inflammation caused by the gravid female sandflea, *Tunga penetrans.*

tung′sten [Swed., from *tung*, heavy; *sten*, stone] (*wolframium*). W = 183.92. A heavy metallic element. Used in steel to increase hardness and tensile strength, in the manufacture of filaments for electric lamps, in contact points, and other products where hardness and toughness are demanded. *Wolfram* is an alternative name.

tu′nic [L. *tunica*, tunic]. A coat or membrane.

tu′ni·ca (pl. *tunicae*) [L.]. A tunic.

t. adventitia. The outer connective-tissue coat of an organ where it is not covered by a serous membrane.

t. albuginea oculi. The sclera.

t. albuginea ovarii. The compact connective tissue immediately under the germinal epithelium of the cortex of the ovary.

t. albuginea penis. The fibrous investment of the corpora cavernosa.

t. albuginea testis. The dense fibrous capsule of the testis, deep to the tunica vaginalis propria.

t. dartos. The layers of connective tissue containing smooth muscle in the corium and outer portion of the superficial fascia of the scrotum and penis.

t. externa. The tunica adventitia of a blood or lymph vessel.

t. fibrosa oculi. The sclera and cornea.

t. intima. The inner coat of a blood or lymph vessel: also called *t. interna.*

t. media. The middle coat of a blood or lymph vessel.

t. mucosa. A mucous membrane.

t. muscularis. The muscular coat of certain hollow organs; e.g., the digestive tube.

t. propria mucosae. The connective-tissue coat of a mucous membrane. Syn., *lamina propria.*

t. serosa. The mesothelium and underlying connective tissue forming the visceral and parietal pericardium, pleura, peritoneum, and tunica vaginalis propria testis.

t. uvea. See *t.* vasculosa oculi.

t. vaginalis communis. The internal, middle, and external spermatic fascias of the spermatic cord and scrotum. See Plate 44.

t. vaginalis propria testis. The serous membrane covering the testis and epididymis and lining the serous cavity of the scrotum. See Plate 44.

t. vasculosa lentis. A mesodermal lens capsule in the embryo, vascularized by the hyaloid and annular arteries; the anterior part is the pupillary membrane.

t. vasculosa oculi. The choroid, ciliary body, and iris of the eye.

t. vasculosa testis. A layer of loose connective tissue containing many blood vessels, on the inner surface of the tunica albuginea testis.

tu′ning fork. A two-tined metallic fork capable of vibrating at a rate which will produce a definite tone.

tu′ni·ver oil. Oil from the liver of the tuna fish.

tun′nel [OF. *tonnel*]. A narrow, enclosed passageway.

carpal t. The space between the flexor retinaculum of the wrist and the carpal bones, through which pass the tendons of the long flexors of the fingers and long flexor of the thumb and the median nerve.

t. of Corti. The triangular canal formed by the pillars of Corti, the base of which corresponds to the membrana basilaris. It extends over the entire length of the lamina spiralis. Also called *canal of Corti, tunnel space.*

Tunnicliff, Ruth [*American physician*, 1876–1946]. Introduced a measles prophylactic known as *Tunnicliff's serum.*

tu·ran′ose (tew·ran′oce, too·rahn′oce, tew′ran·oce). A disaccharide yielding on hydrolysis glucose and fructose.

tur′bid [L. *turbidus*, confused]. Cloudy.

tur″bi·dim′e·ter [*turbidus;* G. *metron*, a measure]. An instrument for measuring the degree of turbidity of a liquid. —**turbidimet′ric,** *adj.;* **turbidimetry,** *n.*

Parr t. A turbidimeter designed for the determination of sulfur. The source of light is a filament lamp built into the base of the tube containing a suspension of barium sulfate into which the sulfur is first converted.

tur′bi·nate [L. *turbinatus*, cone-shaped]. A turbinate bone. See *concha*, 2. See Table of Bones in the Appendix.

tur′bi·na″ted [*turbinatus*]. Top-shaped; scroll-shaped, as turbinated bone.

tur″bi·nec′to·my [L. *turbo*, that which whirls around; G. *ektomē*, excision]. Excision of a nasal concha.

tur′bi·no·tome″ [*turbo;* G. *tomos*, cutting]. An instrument used in turbinotomy.

tur″bi·not′o·my [*turbo;* G. *tomē*, a cutting]. Incision into a turbinated bone.

Türck, Ludwig [*Austrian neurologist and laryngologist*, 1810–68]. Established laryngoscopy by means of Garcia's laryngoscope. Described the temporopontile tract, called *Türck's bundle*. The direct pyramidal tracts are sometimes called *Türck's column*. Dry laryngitis is called *Türck's trachoma*.

tur·ges′cence [L. *turgescere*, to swell up]. Swelling.

tur·ges′cent [*turgescere*]. Swollen, tumid.

tur′gid [L. *turgidus*, swollen]. 1. Swollen. 2. Congested; hyperemic.

tur′gor [L., a swelling]. Active hyperemia; turgescence.

t. vitalis. The normal fullness of the blood vessels.

Türk, Wilhelm [*Austrian physician*, 1871–1916]. Remembered for his description of agranulocytosis (1907); also called *Türk's disease*. See Türk's irritation *cell*.

tur′key corn. Popular name for corydalis.

Turlington's balsam. See compound *benzoin* tincture.

tur′mer·ic. See *curcuma*.

turn [L. *tornare*, to turn in a lathe]. 1. Cause to revolve about an axis. 2. Change the position of the fetus so as to facilitate delivery.

Turnbull's blue. See under *stain*.

Turner, Daniel [*English dermatologist*, 1667–1740]. Author of an early textbook in English on dermatology (1714). Introduced a cerate containing calamine; called *Turner's cerate*.

Turner, George Grey (1877–1951). English surgeon and pioneer in the surgery of the esophagus who described local discoloration of the abdominal wall in the flanks as a sign of acute pancreatitis.

turn′ing. See *version*.

turn′key″ [AS. *turnian; cǣg*]. An instrument formerly used for extracting teeth.

tur′pen·tine [G. *terebinthos*, turpentine-tree]. 1. A concrete or liquid oleoresin obtained from coniferous trees. 2. (*terebinthina*). The concrete oleoresin from *Pinus palustris* and other species of *Pinus*. Yellow-orange, opaque masses of characteristic odor and taste. Freely soluble in alcohol. Contains up to 32% of volatile oil. Occasionally used for local irritant effect. Also called *gum thus, gum turpentine*.

acetic t. liniment (*linimentum terebinthinae aceticum*). A rubefacient. Also called *Stokes's liniment*.

Canada t. The liquid oleoresin from the American silver fir, *Abies balsamea*. Commonly used under the name Canada balsam as a mounting medium in microscopy.

Chian t. The oleoresin collected in the island of Chios from the *Pistacia terebinthus*. See *mastic*.

larch t. Venice turpentine.

t. liniment (*linimentum terebinthinae*). Contains 35% of turpentine in rosin cerate. Once used for burns. Also called *Kentish ointment*.

t. oil (*oleum terebinthinae*). The volatile oil distilled from turpentine. Colorless liquid soluble in 5 volumes of alcohol. Consists essentially of terpenes, principally varieties of pinene. A local irritant and feeble antiseptic. The rectified oil (*oleum terebinthinae rectificatum*) has been used as a stimulant expectorant in chronic bronchitis and a carminative in flatulent colic. Externally rubefacient. Also called *t. spirits*.

Venice t. From *Larix decidua*, yielding about 15% of volatile oil. Also called *larch t.*

wood t. Prepared from stumps, roots, sawdust, etc. Not equivalent to the official substance.

tur′peth [Per. *tirbid*]. *Ipomoea turpethum*, a purgative plant resembling jalap, found in Asia.

t. mineral. The yellow subsulfate of mercury, once used as an emetic but discontinued because of its toxicity.

tur′peth·in [*tirbid*]. 1. A resin obtained from turpeth, similar to that of jalap. 2. A glycoside from the resin of turpeth.

turps. Turpentine oil.

tur″ri·ceph′a·ly. See *acrocephaly, oxycephaly*.

tur′tle [corrup. of F. *tortue*]. An aquatic or marine shelled reptile of the order Chelonia.

tusk [AS. *tux*]. A large, projecting tooth.

tus′sal [L. *tussis*, cough]. Pertaining to, or of the nature of, a cough.

tus·se′do [L., cough]. Tussis.

Tus″si·la′go [L., coltsfoot]. A genus of plants of the Compositae. The leaves of **T. farfara,** coltsfoot, and also other parts of the plant have been used as a demulcent in pulmonary affections associated with cough.

tus′sis [L.]. A cough.

t. convulsiva. Whooping cough.

tus′sive [*tussis*]. Pertaining to, or caused by, a cough.

tussol. A trade-mark for *antipyrine mandelate*.

Tuthill's method. See Butler and Tuthill's *method*.

tutocaine hydrochloride. Trade-mark for the local anesthetic *p*-aminobenzoyldimethyl-amino-methyl-butanol hydrochloride. The substance is a light ivory-colored, crystalline powder soluble in 4 parts of water. Used for surface anesthesia in 2% solution in the eye, nose, and throat; in 0.5–1.0% solution for urethral use; for infiltration anesthesia, 0.2% solutions are generally used.

Tuttle, James P. [*American surgeon*, 1857–1913]. Described a rectal speculum with electric light and a device for inflation of the rectum; called *Tuttle's proctoscope*. Known for his one-stage operation for rectal cancer; called *Tuttle's operation*.

twang. A nasal quality of the voice.

tweens. Trade-mark for a series of surface-active agents consisting of partial esters of long-chain fatty acids with polyoxyalkylene derivatives of hexitol anhydride. See *spans*.

tweez′ers [F. *étui*]. Delicate surgical forceps which are capable of seizing without crushing easily damaged structures, as nerves; they are also used for removing eyelashes or hairs.

twig [AS.]. A small branch, especially a nerve filament, or an arteriole.

twi′light sleep. *In obstetrics*, an injection of scopolamine and morphine to produce amnesia and analgesia.

twin [AS. *twinn*]. One of two born at the same birth.

allantoido-angiopagous twins. Uniovular, separate, unequal twins of which one, the omphalosite, is an acardiacus (acardius), hence parasitic on the extraembryonic vessels supplied by the comparatively normal twin, the autosite. Also called *omphaloangiopagous twins.*

conjoined twins. Equal or unequal uniovular twins, united: also called *diplopagi.* See Plate 25 for several types of equal conjoined twins.

fraternal twins. Twins resulting from the simultaneous fertilization of two ova. They may be of the same or opposite sex, have a different genetic constitution, and each has a separate chorion. Also called *biovular twins, dichorial twins, dissimilar twins, dizygotic twins.*

identical twins. Twins which have developed from a single ovum, always of the same sex, have the same genetic constitution, and have the same chorion. Also called *monochorionic twins, uniovular twins, similar twins, enzygotic twins.*

interlocking twins. Those in which the neck of the first child becomes engaged with the head of the second above the superior strait. Such locking is possible when the first is a breech and the second a vertex presentation. The interlocking makes vaginal delivery virtually impossible.

omphaloangiopagous twins. See *allantoido-angiopagous twins* under *twin.*

unequal twins. Those in which only one of the pair is fully developed.

twinge [AS. *twengan*]. A sudden short, sharp pain.

twin′ning [AS. *twinn*]. Production of like structures by division.

twitch [ME. *twicchen*]. Give a short, sudden pull or jerk.

twitch′ing [*twicchen*]. An irregular spasm of a minor extent.

Twort, Frederick William [*English bacteriologist,* 1877–1950]. Known for his investigations in ultramicroscopical viruses (1915). Discovered in the same year an ultramicrobic agent causing transmissible lysis of bacteria. This was observed by d'Herelle (1917) and is called *Twort-d'Herelle phenomenon, bacteriophage, phage.* The agent may be separated from the organisms by filtration and is believed to be particulate and capable of multiplication.

tyl′i·on (til′ee·on, ty′lee·on) [G. *tylē*, a swelling]. A craniometric point in the midline on the anterior border of the optic or chiasmatic groove.

ty·lo′ma (tye·lo′muh) [G. *tylos*, callus; *-ōma*, tumor]. A callus.

ty·lo′sis (tye·lo′sis) [G., a making callous]. 1. A localized patch of hyperkeratotic skin due to chronic pressure and friction. 2. A form of blepharitis with thickening and hardening of the edge of the lid. —**tylot′ic,** *adj.*

t. palmaris et plantaris. An ectodermal anomaly of the palms and soles producing marked hyperkeratosis. Syn., *keratosis palmaris et plantaris.*

ty″lo·ste·re′sis [G. *tylos*, callus; *sterēsis*, deprivation]. Removal of a callosity.

tym″pa·nec′to·my [G. *tympanon*, drum; *ektomē*, excision]. Excision of the tympanic membrane.

tym·pan′i·a. See *tympanites.*

tym·pan′ic nerve. A visceral sensory and parasympathetic nerve attached to the glossopharyngeal. It innervates the mucosa of the middle ear, mastoid air cells, and auditory tube, and sends filaments to the otic ganglion and parotid gland.

tym′pa·nism [*tympanon*]. Distention with gas; tympanites.

tym″pa·ni′tes (tim″puh·nigh′teez) [*tympanon*]. A distention of the abdominal wall from accumulation of gas in the intestine or peritoneal cavity.

tym″pa·nit′ic [*tympanon*]. Caused by, or of the nature of, tympanites.

tym″pa·ni′tis [*tympanon;* G. *-itis*, inflammation]. Inflammation of the tympanum; otitis media.

tym″pa·no·mas′toid [*tympanon;* G. *mastoeidēs*, like a breast]. Relating to the tympanum and the mastoid process or the mastoid cells.

tym″pa·no·mas″toid·i′tis [*tympanon; mastoeidēs*]. Inflammation of the tympanum and mastoid cells.

tym″pa·no′sis [*tympanon;* G. *-ōsis*, condition]. Tympanites.

tym″pa·no·sta·pe′di·al. Relating to the tympanum and stapes, e.g., the tympanostapedial syndesmosis between the base of the stapes and the oval window.

tym″pa·no·sym″pa·thec′to·my [*tympanon;* G. *sympathēs*, sympathetic; *ektomē*, excision]. The removal of the plexus on the medial wall of the middle ear for the relief of tinnitus.

tym″pa·not′o·my [*tympanon;* G. *tomē*, a cutting]. Incision of a tympanic membrane. Syn., *myringotomy.*

tym′pa·nous [*tympanon*]. Distended with gas; relating to tympanism.

tym′pa·num [*tympanon*]. The middle ear. —**tympan′ic,** *adj.*

tym′pa·ny [*tympanon*]. 1. Tympanites. 2. A tympanitic percussion note. See tympanitic *resonance.*

Tyndall blue. See *Tyndall effect.*

Tyndall effect. The scattering of light by small particles suspended in a liquid or gas. The diffused light often appears blue.

Tyn″dal·li·za′tion [after John *Tyndall*, English physicist, 1820–93]. Fractional sterilization by the use of steam at atmospheric pressure. A sufficient period is permitted to elapse between treatments to allow spores of microorganisms to germinate.

type [G. *typos*, impression]. 1. Imprint; emblem; symbol; character. 2. A normal average example. 3. *In pathology,* the grouping of the distinguishing features of a fever, disease, etc., whereby it is referred to its proper class.

body t. See *somatotype.*

test t. A chart of letters, most commonly the Snellen chart or its modifications, used to test the acuity of central vision.

typh·lat′o·ny, typh″la·to′ni·a [G. *typhlos*, blind; *atonia*, slackness]. An atonic condition of the wall of the cecum.

typh″lec·ta′si·a (tif″leck·tay′zhuh, ·zee·uh) [*typhlos;* G. *ektasis*, extension]. Dilatation of the cecum.

typh·lec′to·my [*typhlos;* G. *ektomē*, excision]. Excision of the cecum.

typh·len″ter·i′tis [*typhlos;* G. *enteron*, intestine; *-itis*, inflammation]. Typhlitis.

typh·li′tis [*typhlos; -itis*]. Inflammation of the cecum. *Obs.*

typh′lo-, typhl- [*typhlos*]. A combining form meaning *cecum.*

typh′lo·cele. See *cecocele.*

typh″lo·di″cli·di′tis (tif″lo·dye″kli·dye′tis, ·dick″-li·dye′tis) [*typhlos;* G. *diklis*, double-folding; *-itis*, inflammation]. Inflammation of the ileocecal valve.

typh″lo·em″py·e′ma (tif″lo·em″pye·ee′muh, ·em″pee·ee′muh) [*typhlos;* G. *empyēma*, abscess]. Abscess attending typhlitis or appendicitis.

typh″lo·en″ter·i′tis. See *typhlitis.*

typh′loid [*typhlos;* G. *eidos*, form]. Having defective vision.

typh″lo·lex′i·a [*typhlos;* G. *lexis*, word]. Word blindness. See *aphasia.*

typh″lo·li·thi′a·sis [*typhlos;* G. *lithiasis*, disease of the stone]. The formation of calculi in the cecum.

typh″lo·meg′a·ly [*typhlos;* G. *megas,* large]. Enlarged cecum.

typh″lo·pto′sis (tif″lo·to′sis, tif″lop·to′sis) [*typhlos;* G. *ptōsis,* a falling]. Downward displacement or prolapse of the cecum.

typh·lo′sis [G., a making blind]. Blindness.

typh′lo·sole [*typhlos;* G. *sōlēn,* channel]. A longitudinal internal ridge or fold of the dorsal intestinal wall of certain worms parasitic and nonparasitic, such as the common earthworm; also a fold in the intestinal wall of certain cyclostomes.

typh′lo·spasm [*typhlos;* G. *spasmos,* spasm]. Spasm of the cecum.

typh″lo·ste·no′sis [*typhlos;* G. *stenōsis,* a being straitened]. Stenosis of the cecum.

typh·los′to·my [*typhlos;* G. *stoma,* mouth]. A cecal colostomy.

ty′pho-, typh- [G. *typhos,* delusion]. A combining form denoting *typhus* or *typhoid.*

ty″pho·ba·cil·lo′sis of Lan·dou″zy′. Fulminating septicemia caused by *Mycobacterium tuberculosis,* without the formation of miliary tubercles.

ty″pho·bac′te·rin [*typhos;* G. *baktērion,* little staff]. A vaccine prepared from the typhoid bacillus.

ty′phoid [G. *typhōdēs,* delirious]. 1. An old term for any condition resembling typhus. 2. Typhoid fever, an acute infectious disease caused by *Salmonella typhosa,* which enters the body with food and drinking water, and is found in the intestine, the spleen, and the fecal discharges, but may also occur in the various complicating lesions. The principal lesions of typhoid fever are an enlargement of the spleen and the mesenteric lymph nodes. The mucous membrane of the intestine is also the seat of a catarrhal inflammation. After a period of incubation of from two to three weeks, the disease sets in with weakness, headache, vague pains, the tendency to diarrhea, and nosebleed. The temperature gradually rises, being higher each evening than the previous evening, and reaches its maximum (104°–105° F.) in from one to two weeks. It then remains at this level for from one to two weeks, and finally sinks by lysis. The pulse is soft and dicrotic, but often not so rapid as would be expected from the high temperature. The tongue is at first coated on the dorsum and red at the tip and edges, but soon becomes dry, brown, and tremulous, and, like the teeth and lips, covered with sordes. There is usually complete anorexia, the bowels are loose, and the stools have a peculiar pea-soup color. At times constipation exists. Slight congestion of the lungs with cough is usually present. On the seventh, eighth, or ninth day the peculiar eruption appears; it consists of small, slightly elevated, rose-colored spots, disappearing on pressure, and coming out in successive crops. Nervous symptoms are prominent in typhoid, and consist of headache, slight deafness, stupor, muttering delirium, carphology, subsultus tendinum, and coma vigil. Complications are frequent, the most important being intestinal hemorrhage, perforation of the bowel, peritonitis, pneumonia, and nephritis. Relapses are fairly common, although second attacks are rare. —**typhoid′al,** *adj.*

abortive t. A form characterized by abrupt onset of symptoms, which subside quickly, convalescence following in a few days.

afebrile t. Typhoid fever with the usual symptoms, positive diazo and Widal reaction, presence of rose spots, but no increased temperature.

ambulatory t. Typhoid in which the patient does not take to his bed.

sudoral t. Typhoid fever accompanied by profuse sweating and great prostration.

t. nodules. Characteristic lesions found in the liver after fatal typhoid.

t. vaccine (*vaccinum typhosum*). A sterile suspension of killed typhoid bacilli (*Salmonella typhosa*) of a strain selected for high antigenic efficiency. The vaccine contains not less than 1,000,000,000 typhoid organisms in each cubic centimeter.

walking t. See ambulatory *t.*

ty″pho·ma′ni·a [G. *typhos,* delusion; *mania,* madness]. The lethargic state, with delirium, sometimes observed in typhus, typhoid, and other fevers.

ty″pho·pneu·mo′ni·a [*typhos;* G. *pneumonia,* disease of the lungs]. Pneumonia concurrent with typhoid fever.

ty′phus [*typhos*]. A group of infectious diseases caused by *Rickettsia prowazekii.* The term is commonly applied to classic epidemic typhus or murine typhus.

Brill's t. See recrudescent *t.*

canine t. See Stuttgart *disease.*

classic epidemic t. An epidemic type caused by *Rickettsia prowazekii,* var. *prowazekii,* and characterized by violent headache, a macular or papulomacular rash, neurological symptoms, and a high fever, ending by crisis in 10–14 days. The disease has occurred in the Orient, Russia, southern and central Europe, Africa, Mexico, and Central and South America. Also called *camp fever, classic t., European t. fever, famine fever, hospital fever, jail fever, ship fever, t. fever, war fever, morbus hungaricus, epidemic t., European t., Fleck t., louse-borne t.*

endemic t. See murine *t.*

epidemic t. See classic epidemic *t.*

epidemic t. vaccine. See Cox *vaccine.* See also Castañeda *vaccine.*

European t. See classic epidemic *t.*

flea t. See murine *t.*

Fleck t. See classic epidemic *t.*

Kenya t. See *tick-bite fevers of Africa* under *fever.*

louse-borne t. See classic epidemic *t.*

Malayan t., Malayan scrub t. See tsutsugamushi *disease.*

Mexican t. Murine typhus occurring in Mexico.

mite-borne t. See tsutsugamushi *disease.*

murine t. A relatively mild, acute, febrile illness of 9–15 days' duration caused by *Rickettsia prowazekii,* var. *moosari,* characterized by headache and macular rash, found throughout the world; a natural infection of rats, and sporadically transmitted to man by the flea. Case-fatality rate is about 2 per cent. Also called *endemic t., urban t., shop t., flea t., rat t.*

Nigerian t. See *tick-bite fevers of Africa* under *fever.*

North Queensland tick t. A rickettsial disease probably transmitted by a tick. The principal symptoms are malaise and headache. The fever may be either continuous or intermittent, and is often accompanied by a rash.

rat t. See murine *t.*

recrudescent t. A relatively mild form of classic epidemic typhus, first described by Nathan E. Brill among east-European immigrants (1910), occurring years after initial infection by *Rickettsia prowazekii.* It is postulated that the infection is latent during the interval. Patients with Brill's disease may thus become foci for the epidemic form. Also called *sporadic t.*

rural t. See tsutsugamushi *disease.*

São Paulo t. A disease endemic in São Paulo, Brazil, associated with tick bites and now known to be identical with Rocky Mountain spotted fever due to *Rickettsia rickettsii.*

scrub t. See tsutsugamushi *disease.*

sporadic t. Recrudescent *t.*

Sumatran (mite) t. See tsutsugamushi *disease.*
tropical t. See tsutsugamushi *disease.*
urban t. See murine *t.*

typ′i·cal [G. *typikos*, impressionable]. 1. Constituting a type or form for comparison. 2. Illustrative. 3. Complete.

ty′ping [G. *typos*, impression]. 1. The determination of a specific blood group. 2. The determination of the specific type into which certain bacteria (*e.g.*, *Diplococcus pneumoniae*) have been subdivided.
blood t. The method used to determine to which blood group an individual belongs. This consists of matching the unknown blood cells with known serum, one serum containing α agglutinin for type A cells, and the other serum containing β agglutinin for type B cells. If a corresponding agglutinogen is present on the unknown cells, the red cells will clump together and can be observed under a microscope.

ty′po·scope [*typos;* G. *skopein*, to examine]. A small device to exclude extraneous light, for the use of cataract patients and amblyopes in reading.

ty″ra·mine′ (ty″ruh·meen′, tirr″uh·, tye·ram′een, ·in, ti·). *p*-Hydroxyphenyl-ethylamine. $HO.C_6H_4.CH_2.CH_2NH_2$. An amine present in ergot and formed in putrefied animal tissue; also prepared synthetically. Syn., *tyrosamine.*
t. hydrochloride. White, crystalline powder, soluble in water; used as a vasoconstrictor and heart stimulant in shock, post-partum hemorrhage; occasionally used to stimulate the uterus in labor; stimulates the respiratory center. Dose, 0.02–0.06 Gm. (⅓–1 gr.).

tyr′an·nism [G. *tyrannos*, tyrant]. Cruelty of morbid inception, of which sadism is an erotic variety.

ty·rem′e·sis (tye·rem′i·sis) [G. *tyros*, cheese; *emesis*, vomiting]. The vomiting of caseous or curdy matter, often seen in infants.

ty′ro-, tyr- [*tyros*]. A combining form meaning *cheese* or *cheeselike.*

ty″ro·ci′din, ty″ro·ci′dine. A component of tyrothricin.

Tyrode solution. See under *solution.*

ty·rog′e·nous (tye·rodj′i·nus) [*tyros;* G. *genesthai*, from *gignesthai*, to be produced]. Produced by or in cheese.

Ty·rog′ly·phus (tye·rog′li·fus) [*tyros;* G. *glyphein*, to carve]. A genus of sarcoptoid mites which usually infest dried vegetable products, cheese, and dead or living plants. Occasionally, they produce a temporary pruritus which is named by the occupation of the host. **T. farinor** causes grocer's itch; **T. siro** causes vanillism among handlers of vanilla pods, and **T. longior** causes copra itch and grocer's itch.

ty′roid [G. *tyrōdēs*, like cheese]. Cheeselike.

tyrosamine. Tyramine.

ty′ro·sin·ase (ty′ro·sin·ace, ·aze, tirr′o·, tye·ro′-sin·, tye·ros′in·). A copper-containing enzyme found in plants, molds, crustacea, mollusks, and some bacteria. In the presence of oxygen, it causes the oxidation of mono- and poly-phenols with the introduction of —OH groups and/or formation of quinones. May be identical with monophenol oxidase and perhaps with polyphenol oxidase.

ty′ro·sine (ty′ro·seen, ·sin, tirr′o·, tye·ro′sin). *p*-Hydroxyphenyl alanine. $p\text{-}HO.C_6H_4.CH_2.CH(NH_2)\text{-}COOH$. An amino acid widely distributed in proteins, particularly in casein. It is closely related to, and a probable precursor of, epinephrine, thyroxin, and melanin.

ty″ro·sin·o′sis [G. *tyros*, cheese; *-ōsis*, condition]. Excretion in the urine of unusual amounts of tyrosine and of its first oxidation products.

ty″ro·si·nu′ri·a [*tyros;* G. *ouron*, urine]. The presence of tyrosine in the urine.

ty′ro·syl. The univalent radical, $p\text{-}HOC_6H_4CH_2\text{-}CH(NH_2)CO\text{—}$, of the amino acid tyrosine.

ty″ro·thri′cin. An alcohol-soluble, water-insoluble polypeptide mixture isolated by Dubos from *Bacillus brevis* and consisting of the antibiotic substances gramicidin and tyrocidin; used as a bactericide in infections due to Gram-positive organisms. Applied topically in a concentration of 50 mg. per 100 cc. of sterile distilled water.

ty″ro·tox′in [*tyros;* G. *toxikon*, poison]. A curarelike poison claimed to be present in some specimens of cheese.

Tyrrell, Frederick [*English physician and ophthalmologist*, 1797–1843]. Devised a slender hook used in eye surgery, especially for removing a piece of iris in iridectomy; called *Tyrrell's hook.*

Tyson's glands. See under *gland.*

U

U Chemical symbol for uranium.

U. Abbreviation for unit.

u′ber·ty [L. *ubertas*, fertility]. Fertility; productiveness. —**uberous,** *adj.*

u·cam′bin, u·kam′bin (yōō·kam′bin, ōō·kam′-bin). An African arrow-poison with the effects of strophanthin.

ud′der [AS. *ūder*]. The mammary gland of the cow and other animals.

Udránszky, Lázlô von [*Hungarian physiologist*, 1862–1914]. Remembered for his tests for bile acids and tyrosine, called *Udránszky's tests.* See foam *test.*

Uffelmann's test. See under *test.*

Uhlenhuth, Paul Theodore (1870–). German bacteriologist, discoverer of a method for identification of human and animal blood (see serum *test*). He devised a treatment for spirochetal jaundice, for syphilis with organic arsenic, and for tropical diseases with organic antimony preparations, and also prepared serums against foot-and-mouth disease and hog cholera.

u·kam′bin. See *ucambin.*

u′la [G. *oulon*, gum]. See *oula.*

u·lag″a·nac′te·sis (yōō·lag″uh·nack′ti·sis, ·nack-tee′sis) [*oulon;* G. *aganaktēsis*, physical pain and irritation]. Irritation or uneasy sensations in the gums. *Obs.*

u″la·tro′phi·a, u·lat′ro·phy [*oulon;* G. *atrophia*, want of food]. A shrinkage and recession of the gingivae. *Obs.*

ul′cer [L. *ulcus*, sore]. An interruption of continuity of a surface, with an inflamed base. See Plate 40.
Aden u. See tropical *u.*
amputating u. A penetrating ulcer encircling a part, such as a toe, leading ultimately to loss of the distal portion, as in yaws.
anastomotic u. A jejunal ulcer which most commonly follows a gastroenterostomy.
Annam u. See tropical *u.*

aphthous u. Canker sore of the mouth. The etiology is diverse.
arterial u. An ulcer of a part or surface due to arterial occlusion.
atheromatous u. Ulcer of the intima of the aorta or other artery, due to breakdown of an atheromatous plaque.
atonic u. One which shows little or no disposition to heal.
autochthonous u. Chancre.
Bahia u. See *leishmaniasis* americana.
Bauru u. See *leishmaniasis* americana.
calloused u. See hyperkeratotic *u.*
carious u. One with superimposed gangrene.
chiclero u. See *leishmaniasis* americana.
chrome u. One due to the action of chrome salts; seen in those who work with such material.
cinchophen u. A peptic ulcer produced experimentally in dogs by large oral doses of cinchophen (200 mg. per kg. given daily will cause a chronic ulcer in three weeks, usually in the pyloric region). Cases of gastric ulcer have been discovered in man with cinchophen poisoning.
contact u. A rare superficial ulcer on one or both sides of the larynx, usually on the arytenoid, caused by abuse of the voice or excessive smoking.
coral u. That produced by silica-headed darts from coral, injected into wounds in coral lacerations. The wound becomes secondarily infected, and a painful ulcer appears, accompanied by enlargement of neighboring lymph nodes, cellulitis, and lymphangitis.
crateriform u. A rodent ulcer of conical form, resembling a furuncle with fibrotic border.
creeping u. One which slowly extends peripherally, sometimes with central healing. Syn., *serpiginous u.*
Curling's u. A peptic ulcer of duodenum or stomach which is associated with extensive burns of the body surface.
decubitus u. A bedsore; that is, ulceration of skin and underlying tissue from prolonged pressure; seen especially in the aged or in paralysis.
diabetic u. Ulcer associated with diabetes mellitus.
diphtheritic u. Specifically, an ulcer due to action of *Corynebacterium diphtheriae* or to detachment of a diphtheritic membrane. Also applied loosely to an ulcer, on or about which is a fibrinous exudate. One of the forms of tropical ulcer appears to be due to *C. diphtheriae.*
duodenal u. A chronic ulcer, usually in the anterior wall of the duodenum, near the pylorus. Syn., *peptic u.*
endemic u. One which is frequent in certain regions, as tropical ulcer.
erethistic u. One which is exceedingly tender such, as may occur in the anus or around the fingernails.
esophageal u. A rare type of peptic ulcer, found in the lower third of the esophagus.
exuberant u. One which has an excess of granulation tissue growing from the base.
fistulous u. An ulcer about the orifice of a fistula.
follicular u. An ulcer due to breakdown of a lymphatic aggregate, such as a solitary nodule of the ileum.
fungous u. See exuberant *u.*
funnel u. An ulcer of either of two types: in one the axis of the funnel is perpendicular to the surface of the mucosa and a bleeding or thrombosed blood vessel may be found at the apex of the funnel; in the other, the axis of the funnel tends to parallel the lesser curvature, and the ulcer is characterized by an elevated, undermined margin on the cardiac side and a flat margin on the pyloric side.
Gaboon u. A tropical ulcer, resembling a syphilitic ulcer.
gastric u. One affecting the mucosa of the stomach. May be a peptic ulcer or due to hemorrhagic erosion.
Hunner's u. A chronic ulcer of the urinary bladder, of unknown etiology, found frequently near the vertex and in association with interstitial cystitis: also called *elusive u.* See also interstitial *cystitis.*
hyperkeratotic u. A chronic, nonmalignant, cutaneous ulcer with hyperkeratosis of the margin. The cornified epithelium must be removed before healing can take place. Also called *calloused u.*
hypertrophic u. A chronic nonmalignant skin ulcer with an excess of granulation tissue: also called *proud flesh.*
indolent u. One with little tendency to heal, often accompanied by fibrosis of the base and margins with scanty granulation tissue.
inflamed u. One accompanied by acute inflammation.
irritable u. See erethistic *u.*
Jacob's u. A rodent ulcer of the eyelid.
Jeddah u. See *oriental sore.*
jejunal u. See marginal *u.*
kissing u. One which appears to be due to transmission from one apposing part to another, or due to pressure of apposing parts.
leprous u. One which occurs in leprosy, as in the nares or more often in the skin, due to the breakdown of a cutaneous lesion.
lupoid u. An ulcer of the skin with a resemblance to lupus vulgaris.
Mann-Williamson u. Experimental peptic ulcer occurring in dogs after gastrojejunostomy or adrenalectomy.
marginal u. An ulcer of the jejunum along the stoma of a gastrojejunostomy; due to erosive action of acid gastric juice upon the jejunum.
Marjolin's u. One due to malignant change in an indolent ulcer or in a scar, especially a scar from an old burn or roentgen-ray treatment.
Mozambique u. Tropical ulcer.
neurogenic u. One due to trophic disturbances following interruption of efferent nerve fibers plus the factor of external trauma.
neurotrophic u. Neurogenic ulcer.
papillomatous u. A type found in the stomach of rats afflicted with nutritional gastritis, occurring in small groups as small circular areas with a prominent rough circumference.
penetrating u. One which extends more deeply than the surface originally affected, as a peptic ulcer penetrating into muscular coats.
peptic u. One due in part at least to digestive action of gastric juice, affecting the gastric or duodenal mucosa, or the mucosa of stomach and jejunum associated with gastrojejunal anastomosis.
perforating u. One which extends through all coats of a viscus.
phagedenic u. One accompanied by extensive necrosis or gangrene of neighboring tissues.
phlegmonous u. One accompanied by acute exudative inflammation.
rodent u. See basal-cell *epithelioma.*
round u. A peptic ulcer of the stomach.
saddle u. A peptic ulcer which has elongated so that it partially encircles the lesser curvature of the stomach.
Saemisch's u. An infected ulcer of the cornea.
serpiginous u. See creeping *u.*
stercoraceous u. An ulcer of the skin which is contaminated by feces. *Obs.*
stomal u. See marginal *u.*

UVW

tanner's u. A chronic ulcer occurring on the hands of tanners.

Tashkend u. See *oriental sore.*

trophic u. One due to disturbances of nutrition of a part, such as varicose ulcer.

tropical u. A cutaneous ulcer prevalent in tropical regions, not due to syphilis, yaws, leishmaniasis, or hookworm. May be acute, chronic, or phagedenic. Various microorganisms are associated with different ulcers in different regions, *Corynebacterium diphtheriae* being found most frequently. Syn., *Naga sore, Aden u., Annam u., Mozambique u., Yemen u.*

vagotomy u. An ulcer in the mucosa of the stomach along the lesser curvature in the pyloric antrum following vagotomy. Such ulcers have been produced routinely in rabbits.

varicose u. A chronic ulcer of skin due largely to malnutrition of the skin as a result of varicose veins, especially of the leg. Also called *leg u.*

venereal u. Chancre or chancroid.

Yemen u. Tropical ulcer.

ul'cer·ate [L. *ulcerare,* to make sore]. Become converted into, or affected with, an ulcer.

ul"cer·a'tion [L. *ulceratio,* from *ulcerare*]. The process of formation of an ulcer.

cutis u. A chronic or subacute ulceration of the cutis and underlying subcutaneous tissue of the upper or lower extremity, caused by *Mycobacterium ulcerans.*

ul'cer·a"tive [*ulcerare*]. Pertaining to, or characterized by, ulceration.

ul"cer·o·mem'bra·nous [L. *ulcus,* sore; *membrana,* membrane]. Pertaining to, or characterized by, ulceration, and accompanied by fibrinous inflammation with accompanying formation of a pseudomembrane.

ul'cus (pl. *ulcera*) [L.]. An ulcer.

u. cancrosum. (a) Cancer. (b) Rodent ulcer.

u. cruris. Indolent ulcer of the leg.

u. exedens. Old term for rodent ulcer.

u. induratum. Chancre.

u. molle. Chancroid.

u. phagedaenicum. Phagedenic ulcer.

u. rodens. Rodent ulcer.

u. serpens. An irritating, purulent ulcer of the cornea, often caused by pneumococci; it may lead to perforation or scarring with concomitant loss of vision.

u. tuberculosum. Lupus vulgaris.

u. venereum. (a) Chancre. (b) Chancroid.

u. ventriculi. A gastric ulcer.

vulvae acutum u. A condition of ovoid erosions and ulcers on the female external genitalia, whose cause is not definitely known, although *Bacillus crassus* has been isolated from some cases: This condition probably belongs in the group of atypical erythema multiforme.

u"le·gy'ri·a [G. *oulē,* scar; *gyros,* circle]. Convolutions in the cortex of the brain, made irregular by scar formation.

uleron, uliron. Trade-mark for dimethyldisulfanilamide, $NH_2.C_6H_4.SO_2.NH.C_6H_4.SO_2N(CH_3)_2$, used like sulfanilamide, particularly in the treatment of gonorrhea.

u·ler"y·the'ma [G. *oulē,* scar; *erythēma,* redness]. An erythematous disease marked by the formation of cicatrices.

u. centrifugum. Lupus erythematosus.

u. ophryogenes. Ulerythema of the eyebrows with loss of hair.

u. sycosiforme. Keloid sycosis.

u·let'ic [G. *oulon,* gum]. Pertaining to the gums.

uliron. See *uleron.*

u·li'tis [*oulon;* G. *-itis,* inflammation]. A general inflammation of the gums, as distinguished from simple gingivitis, which is confined to the free margins of the gums.

ul'mus [L., elm]. The inner bark of *Ulmus fulva* (slippery elm); mucilaginous and demulcent; has been used mainly in folk medicine.

ul'na [L., elbow]. The bone on the inner side of the forearm, articulating with the humerus and the head of the radius above and with the radius below. See Table of Bones in the Appendix. See Plate 1. —**ulnar,** *adj.*

ul·no·car'pe·us. The flexor carpi ulnaris brevis muscle.

u·loc'a·ce (yoo·lock'uh·see) [G. *oulon,* gum; *kakē,* badness]. Ulcerative inflammation of the gums.

u"lo·der"ma·ti'tis [G. *oulē,* scar; *derma,* skin; *-itis,* inflammation]. Inflammation of the skin with formation of cicatrices. *Rare.*

u"lo·glos·si'tis [G. *oulon,* gum; *glōssa,* tongue; *-itis*]. Inflammation of gums and tongue.

u'loid [G. *oulē,* scar; *eidos,* form]. Scarlike.

u"lor·rha'gi·a [G. *oulon,* gum; *rhēgnynai,* to burst forth]. Bleeding from the gums.

u·lo'sis [G. *oulē,* scar; *-ōsis,* condition]. Cicatrization.

U"lo·so'ni·a par"vi·cor'nis. A beetle which may act as an intermediate host of *Hymenolepis diminuta,* the rat tapeworm.

u·lot'ic [*oulē*]. Pertaining to, or tending toward, cicatrization.

u·lot'o·my [G. *oulon,* gum; *tomē,* a cutting]. Incision into the gum.

ultex. Trade name of a bifocal lens ground from one piece of glass.

ul"ti·mo·bran'chi·al (ul"ti·mo·brang'kee·ul) [L. *ultimus,* last; G. *bragchia,* gills]. Pertaining to the caudal pharyngeal or branchial pouch derivatives. See *ultimobranchial bodies* under *body.*

ul"ti·mo·gen'i·ture [*ultimus;* L. *genitura,* birth]. The state of being the last born. —**ultimogenitary,** *adj.*

ul'ti·mum mor'i·ens. The right atrium, said to be the last part of the body to cease moving in death; literally, the last dying.

ul'tra- [L., beyond]. A prefix denoting *beyond, excess.*

ul"tra·brach"y·ce·phal'ic (ul"truh·brack"i·si·fal'ick) [*ultra;* G. *brachys,* short; *kephalē,* head]. Having an extremely high cephalic index.

ul"tra·cen'tri·fuge [*ultra;* G. *kentron,* center; L. *fugere,* to flee]. A high-speed centrifuge, developed by Theodor Svedberg, which will produce centrifugal fields up to several hundred thousand time the force of gravity. This centrifuge permits optical observation of the sedimentation of substances in solution, contained in a small cell: used for the determination of particle sizes in proteins. viruses, etc., and for the analysis of such materials in complex fluids as blood plasma. —**ultracentrif'ugal,** *adj.*

ul"tra·fil'ter [*ultra;* ML. *feltrum,* felt]. A filter which will separate colloidal particles from their dispersion mediums and from crystalloids: sometimes called *jelly filter.*

ul"tra·fil·tra'tion [*ultra; feltrum*]. 1. The removal of all but the smallest particles, such as viruses, by filtration. Either positive or negative pressure may be employed. 2. A method for the separation of colloids from their dispersion mediums and dissolved crystalloids by the use of ultrafilters.

fractional u. Separation of colloidal particles into certain magnitude ranges by means of ultrafilters of varied pore size.

ul"tra·mi'cro·scope [*ultra;* G. *mikros,* small; *skopein,* to examine]. A microscope for examination, by powerful side illumination, of objects not apparent with ordinary microscopes. Also called *slit microscope.* —**ultramicroscop'ic,** *adj.;* **ultramicros'copy,** *n.*

ul"tra·phag"o·cy·to'sis. Phagocytosis of colloidal particles.

ul"tra·red' [*ultra;* AS. *rēad*]. Radiations of shorter wavelength than the red of the visible spectrum.

ul"tra·son'ic [*ultra;* L. *sonus,* sound]. Pertaining to sounds with a frequency above that of audible sounds, that is, above 20 kilocycles. Ultrasonic waves of moderate intensity are being applied in such fields as dermatology, neurology, and genetics. Waves of high intensity have been used for the destruction of cells. —**ultrasound',** *n.*

ul"tra·son'o·gram. A record of ultrasonic waves or their echoes. See *ultrasonoscope.*

ul"tra·son'o·scope. An instrument used to detect and locate the position of regions of varying density in a medium by recording the echoes of ultrasonic waves reflected from these regions. The ultrasonic waves, modulated by pulsations, are introduced into the medium usually by means of a piezoelectric transducer. In neurology, the use of this instrument has been suggested for the detection of subcortical brain tumors.

ul"tra·struc'ture [*ultra;* L. *structura,* structure]. The arrangement of ultramicroscopic particles.

ul"tra·vi'rus [*ultra;* L. *virus,* slimy liquid]. A virus which is filtrable in an ultrafilter.

um'ber. A native ferric hydroxide containing manganese dioxide and silicate; occurs as a dark brown to brownish red powder. Used as a pigment.

burnt u. A reddish brown pigment obtained by heating umber.

um"bi·lec'to·my [L. *umbilicus,* middle; G. *ektomē,* excision]. 1. Excision of the umbilicus. 2. An operation for the relief of umbilical hernia.

um·bil'i·cate, um·bil'i·ca"ted [*umbilicus*]. Having a depression like that of the navel.

um·bil"i·ca'tion [*umbilicus*]. 1. A depression like the navel. 2. The state of being umbilicated.

um·bil'i·cus, um"bi·li'cus [L.]. The navel; the round, depressed cicatrix in the median line of the abdomen, marking the site of the aperture which in fetal life gave passage to the umbilical vessels. See Plates 4, 41. —**umbil'ical,** *adj.*

um'bo (pl. *umbos, umbones*) [L., boss]. A boss or bosselation; any central convex eminence, as the umbo of the tympanic membrane.

um·bras'co·py. See *retinoscopy.*

umbrathor. Trade-mark for a 25% suspension of thorium oxide used as a radiopaque medium for the gastrointestinal tract.

un·bal'ance. See *imbalance.*

un'ci·a [L., ounce]. Ounce.

un'ci·form [L. *uncus,* hook; *forma,* form]. Hook-shaped.

un'ci·form. Old name for the hamate. See Table of Bones in the Appendix.

Un"ci·na'ri·a [L. *uncinus,* hook]. A generic name formerly applied to hookworms.

un"ci·na·ri'a·sis. See *ancylostomiasis.*

un'ci·nate [*uncinus*]. Hooked.

un'ci·nate fit. Episodic olfactory hallucinations associated with a peculiar dreamy state and smacking movements of the lips, due to irritative lesions of the uncus. It is generally idiopathic, and may be associated with gross lesions of the uncus and hippocampus.

un"ci·pi"si·for'mis. An occasional band of muscle running from the pisiform to the hamulus of the hamate.

un·con'scious [AS. *un-,* not; L. *conscius,* knowing something with another]. 1. *In psychiatry,* pertaining to behavior or experiences not controlled by the conscious ego. 2. Insensible; in a state lacking conscious awareness and with reflexes abolished. —**uncon'sciousness,** *n.*

un·con'scious. That part of the personality not in the immediate field of awareness.

unc'tion [L. *unctio,* an anointing]. 1. The act of anointing. 2. An ointment.

unc'tu·ous [L. *unctum,* from *unguere,* to anoint]. Greasy; oily.

un'cus [L.]. 1. A hook. 2. The hooklike anterior extremity of the hippocampal gyrus.

un·dec'yl. The univalent organic radical $CH_3(CH_2)_{10}$—. Syn., *hendecyl.*

un·dec"y·len'ic ac'id (un·dess"i·len'ick, ·lee'nick). $CH_3CH{:}CH(CH_2)_7COOH$. An unsaturated acid, melting at 24° C.; used therapeutically, generally in combination with one or more of its salts (copper, sodium, or zinc), as a fungicide.

un"der·weight' [AS.; *wiht*]. A condition of the whole body which is characterized by a deficiency of body tissue, lack of fat being the most obvious. Usually the term is applied to persons whose body weight is at least 10% less than that of the average for persons of the same age, sex, and height.

Underwood, Michael [*English physician and pediatrician,* 1737–1820]. Wrote an early description of infantile poliomyelitis (1789). Scleroma of the newborn is sometimes called *Underwood's disease.*

un·dine' (un·deen', un'dyne) [L. *unda,* a wave]. A glass container for irrigating the eye.

un'din·ism [*unda*]. Old term for a condition in which water, urine, or micturition arouses sexual thoughts or desire.

un·do'ing. *In psychopathology,* a defense mechanism, particularly characteristic of the obsessive-compulsive reaction, in which the patient performs a symbolic act, often repeatedly, to undo or annul in some magic way the possible effects of his unrecognized impulses or of some act for which he has unconscious guilt.

un'du·lant fe'ver. Brucellosis.

un"du·la'tion [L. *undulatus,* undulated]. A wave-like motion; fluctuation.

jugular u. The venous pulse.

respiratory u. The variations in the blood pressure due to respiration.

un'du·la·to"ry [*undulatus*]. Moving like waves; vibratory.

ung. *Unguentum;* ointment.

unguentine. Trade-mark for an ointment containing anhydro-*p*-hydroxy-mercuri-*m*-cresol, zinc oxide, alum compound, phenol, and oils of eucalyptus and red thyme in a petrolatum and oleostearin base: used as an antiseptic dressing for minor burns, cuts, bruises, and skin irritations.

un·guen'tum [L.]. Ointment. Abbreviated, ung.

un'guis (pl. *ungues*) [L., nail]. A fingernail or toenail. —**ungual,** *adj.*

u. incarnatus. Ingrowing nail.

un'gu·la [L., claw]. 1. An instrument for extracting a dead fetus. 2. A hoof; a claw. —**ungulate,** *adj.*

Un"gu·la'ta [*ungula*]. An order of mammals characterized by being herbivorous and having hoofs.

un·health'y [AS. *un-,* not; *hǣlth*]. 1. Lacking health; sickly. 2. Injurious to health.

u'ni- [L. *unus,* one]. A combining form meaning *one.*

u"ni·ar·tic'u·lar [*unus;* L. *articulus,* joint]. Pertaining to a single joint.

u"ni·cam'er·al, u"ni·cam'er·ate. Having only one cavity or chamber.

UNICEF United Nations International Children's Emergency Fund.

u"ni·cel'lu·lar [*unus;* L. *cellula,* small storeroom]. Composed of but one cell.

u"ni·cen'tral [*unus;* L. *centrum,* center]. Having a single center of growth.

u"ni·cor'nous [*unus;* L. *cornu,* horn]. Having one horn or cornu.

u"ni·cus'pid, u"ni·cus'pi·date [*unus;* L. *cuspis,* point]. A tooth with but a single cusp or point. —**unicus'pid, unicus'pidate,** *adj.*

unidigin. A trade-mark for *digitoxin.*

u"ni·fa·mil'i·al [*unus;* L. *familia,* family]. Pertaining to a single family.

u"ni·fi'lar [*unus;* L. *filum,* thread]. Connected by one thread; furnished with one filament.

u"ni·grav'i·da [*unus;* L. *gravidus,* pregnant]. A woman who is pregnant for the first time. Also called *primigravida.*

u"ni·lat'er·al [*unus;* L. *lateralis,* of a side]. Pertaining to, or affecting, but one side.

u"ni·lo'bar [*unus;* G. *lobos,* lobe]. Having one lobe.

u"ni·loc'u·lar [*unus;* L. *loculus,* small place]. Having but one loculus or cavity.

u"ni·nu'cle·ar [*unus;* L. *nucleus,* kernel]. Having but a single nucleus.

u"ni·oc'u·lar [*unus;* L. *oculus,* eye]. 1. Pertaining to, or performed with, one eye. 2. Having only one eye.

un'ion [L. *unio,* union]. A joining; specifically, the consolidation of bone fractures.

immediate u. That by first intention.

vicious u. The healing of a fracture in improper position, with resulting deformity.

u"ni·o'val [*unus;* L. *ovum,* egg]. Formed from one ovum; uniovular.

u"ni·ov'u·lar [*unus; ovum*]. Concerning, or derived from, one egg, as uniovular twins.

u·nip'a·ra [*unus;* L. *parere,* to bring forth]. A woman who has borne but one child.

u"ni·par'i·ens. Uniparous.

u·nip'a·rous [*unus; parere*]. Bearing one offspring, or producing one ovum, at a time.

u"ni·po'lar [*unus;* L. *polus,* pole]. 1. Having but one pole or process. 2. Pertaining to one pole.

u'nip'o·tent. Giving rise to only one cell or tissue type: said of embryonic or multiplying cells. —**unipo'tency,** *n.*, **unipoten'tial,** *adj.*

u"ni·sex'u·al [*unus;* L. *sexus,* sex]. Provided with the sexual organs of one sex only.

u'nit [L. *unitum,* from *unire,* to unite]. 1. A single thing or person or a group considered as a whole, as a hospital unit. 2. A standard of weight or measurement. Abbreviated, U.

angstrom u. See *angstrom.*

antitoxic u. The amount of antitoxin which neutralizes a definite number of minimum lethal doses, generally 100, of a given toxin.

Board of Trade u. (*B.T.U.*). A unit of energy used in Britain equivalent to one kilowatt hour, 3,600,000 joules, or 3,415 American B.T.U.

Bodansky u. The amount of phosphatase required to liberate 1 mg. of phosphorus as the phosphate ion from a sodium beta-glycerophosphate substrate during the first hour of incubation at 37° C. and pH 8.6.

Bourquin-Sherman u. The amount of riboflavin which, when fed daily to rats, will give an average gain of 3 Gm. a week during a test period of 4 to 8 weeks in excess of gains in control rats without riboflavin.

British thermal u. (B.Th.U. in British usage. American usage is B.T.U. In Britain, B.T.U. means Board of Trade unit.) The heat required to raise one pound of water 1° F. One B.T.U. is equivalent to 1,054 joules, 0.002928 kilowatt hours, 777.7 foot-pounds, 0.2520 large calories.

BTU, B.T.U., Btu, B.Th.U. British thermal *u.*

cat u. The amount of digitalis which will kill a cat when injected intravenously, calculated per kilogram of the animal.

centigrade heat u. The quantity of heat required to increase the temperature of 1 lb. of water 1° C. at atmospheric pressure: approximately 454 small calories. Abbreviated CHU.

C.G.S. u. A unit in the centimeter-gram-second system.

clearing u. *In U. S. Army medicine,* a medical organization establishing one or more clearing stations. It receives and classifies casualties, gives them emergency medical treatment, if they are fit, returns them to duty or prepares them for further evacuation.

clinical u. That amount of a substance, e.g. liver extract, which will produce a desired response in a patient. Abbreviated, C.U.

cobalt-60 cancer teletherapy u. A machine for high-energy radiation at a distance, using cobalt-60 in the treatment of cancer in the way that x-rays are now used.

Collip u. One denoting a dose of parathyroid extract; calculated as 1/100 of the amount of calcium necessary to cause a 5-mg. rise in the calcium content of 100 cc. of blood after 15 hours in a dog weighing 20 kg.

Cooke pollen u. See protein nitrogen *u.*

Cornell u. of riboflavin. One Cornell unit of riboflavin = 1γ of riboflavin, defined by the growth effect on chicks.

Dam u. of vitamin K. 10 Dam units of vitamin K = 1 Thayer-Doisy unit.

electric u. One for measuring the strength of an electric current. Three different systems of electric units are used: the electromagnetic, the electrostatic, and the ordinary or practical units. The commonly used practical units are the ampere or unit of current, the volt or unit of electromotive force, the ohm or unit of resistance, the coulomb or unit of quantity, the farad or unit of capacitance, and the watt or unit of power.

electromagnetic units. Fundamental electric units expressed in the electromagnetic system: they are usually characterized by adding *ab-* to the unit, such as abampere, abvolt. Units measured in the electromagnetic system are 3×10^{10} times as large as electrostatic units.

electrostatic units. Fundamental electric units expressed in the electrostatic system; they are usually characterized by adding *stat-* to the unit, such as statampere, statvolt.

e u. See roentgen *u.*

Florey u. See Oxford *u.*

flotation u. See Svedberg flotation *u.*

gravitational u. One gravitational unit equals one pound of force divided by one pound of mass. Abbreviated, G.

heat u. The amount of heat required to raise the temperature of one kilogram of water from 0° to 1° C.; it is technically called a calorie.

hypothetical units. The ultimate vital units of protoplasm, speculatively regarded as molecular aggregates, ultramicroscopic in size, usually endowed with the properties of growth and reproduction, and any other properties depending upon the demands required of them. Also called *organic molecules, physiologic units, gemmules, pangenes, plastidules, micelles, tagmas, inotagmas, microzymas, plasomes, biophores, gemmae, idioblasts, idiosomes, somacules, chondria, bioblasts, protomeres.*

immunizing u. Antitoxic *u.* Abbreviated, I.U.

international u. An arbitrarily defined weight of an international standard of reference adopted by the Permanent Commission on Biological Standardization of the League of Nations. Abbreviated, I.U.

International Units of vitamins. See *vitamin* A, *vitamin* B_1, *vitamin* C, *vitamin* D.

Jukes u. See Bourquin-Sherman *u.*

Kienböck's photometric u. See Robert *Kienböck.*
Lovibond u. One Lovibond unit of vitamin A = 208 international (or U.S.P.) units.
M.K.S. units. Meter-kilogram-second system of fundamental units; mostly used by engineers.
motor u. The axon of an anterior horn cell, or the motor fiber of a cranial nerve, together with the striated muscle fibers innervated by its terminal branches. The proportion of muscle fibers innervated (innervation ratio) varies greatly, muscles carrying out skilled movements having the lowest ratio.
mouse u. That amount of estrus-producing substance which, when injected into a spayed mouse, will produce a characteristic change in the vaginal epithelium: also called *Thayer-Doisy u.*
Noon pollen u. The quantity of pollen extract which contains 0.00001 mg. of total nitrogen.
Oslo u. A unit of vitamin D; 1.66 Oslo units are equal to one international unit.
Oxford u. The minimum quantity of penicillin which, when dissolved in 50 cc. of a meat broth, is sufficient to inhibit completely the growth of a test strain of *Micrococcus aureus.* Syn., *Florey u.*
physiologic u. The ultimate vital unit, as named by Herbert Spencer. See *hypothetical units* under *unit.*
previral u. One related to early stages of intracellular virus multiplication; a number of such units surrounded by a matrix comprise a fully formed virus particle.
protein nitrogen u. The quantity of pollen extract which contains 0.00001 mg. of protein nitrogen. Syn. *Cooke pollen u.*
rat growth u. The amount of vitamin A necessary to maintain a weekly gain of 3 Gm. in test rats previously depleted of vitamin A. Also called *Sherman-Munsell u.*
roentgen u. Unit of x-ray dose in which the quantity of x- or gamma-radiation is such that the associated corpuscular emission per 0.001293 Gm. of air produces, in air, ions carrying one electrostatic unit of quantity of electricity of either sign: also called *roentgen.* Abbreviated r, r.u.
r u. See roentgen *u.*
sensation u. The degree of increase in the intensity of a stimulus just discernible by an individual, chiefly used in audiometry, where the unit measuring an increase in intensity of a tone is not a constant, but the expression of a ratio between two tones whose intensity varies sufficiently to make recognition of difference possible. Also see Fechner's *law,* Weber's *law.*
S_f u. See Svedberg flotation *u.*
Somogyi u. A measure of diastase or amylase activity; the amount of diastase in 100 cc. of plasma, serum, or urine necessary to produce 1 mg. of copper-reducing substance from a starch substrate after 30 minutes of incubation at 40° C.
Steenbock u. The amount of vitamin D which will produce a line of calcification at the distal ulnar and radial epiphysis of rachitic rats within ten days.
Svedberg flotation u. Flotation rate of any molecule in a centrifugal field. Example: $S_f u$ or $S_f 10$ lipoprotein.
Thayer-Doisy u. See mouse *u.*
thermal u. The amount of heat required to raise the temperature of a pound of water one degree F. or C.
Toronto u. The anticoagulant activity of 0.01 mg. of a standard barium heparin employed at the University of Toronto.
toxic u. The smallest dose of a toxin which is capable of proving fatal to an experimental animal, usually a guinea pig, of definite weight, in a specified period of time.
u. character. One of a pair of sharply contrasted traits which are inherited according to the Mendelian law of segregation.
u. of force. The dyne; the force which, when acting for one second, will give to one gram a velocity of one centimeter per second.
u. of heat. The calorie or B.T.U.
u. of length. See Tables of Weights and Measures in the Appendix.
u. of light. Foot-candle. The foot-candle is the illumination equal to one lumen per square foot or the illumination of a surface at a uniform distance of one foot from a point source of one candle.
u. of volume. See Tables of Weights and Measures in the Appendix.
u. of weight. See Tables of Weights and Measures in the Appendix.
u. of work. The erg. Also called *u. of energy.*
U.S.P. u. A certain amount of a substance as standardized by the United States Pharmacopeia.

u′ni·tar″y (yōō′ni·terr″ee) [*unire*]. 1. Pertaining to, or having the qualities of, a unit. 2. Pertaining to monsters having the organs of a single individual.

United Nations International Children's Emergency Fund (UNICEF). An organization, created by and dependent on the General Assembly of the United Nations, which deals with rehabilitation of children in war-ravaged countries, with maternal and child welfare, and, where necessary, with development of a technical and health program particularly as applied to children.

United States Public Health Service. The division of the Federal Security Agency of the United States concerned with the development of a public-health program and the handling of health problems within the jurisdiction of the federal government. It is charged with interstate and foreign quarantine matters, the representation of the United States in international health activities, and the compilation of national vital statistics. Its four statutory bureaus are: the Office of the Surgeon General, responsible for the general administration of Public Health Service activities; the National Institutes of Health, which carry on research; Bureau of Medical Services, which administers a program of medical and hospital care; the Bureau of State Services, which gives assistance to state and local health services upon request. Abbreviated, U.S.P.H.S.

u″ni·va′lent (yōō″ni·vay′lunt) [L. *unus,* one; *valere,* to be strong]. Having a valence of one.

u″ni·ver′sal do′nor. The blood donor of the group O type.

u″ni·ver′sal re·cip′i·ent. An individual of AB blood group. *Obs.*

univis. Trade name for a brand of bifocal lens.

Unna, Paul Gerson [*German dermatologist,* 1850–1929]. One of the foremost figures in dermatology. Originated the idea of using coated pills to provide for local absorption in the intestine (1884). Introduced ichthyol and resorcin into medicine (1886). Described seborrheic eczema (1887); also called *Unna's disease.* For *Unna's hard* and *soft zinc pastes,* see under *paste.* For *Unna's stains,* see under *stain.*

Un′na's paste boot. A sheath or casing for the leg used in treating varicose ulcers and veins by relieving venous hydrostatic pressure. A paste of zinc oxide (Unna's), gelatin, and glycerin is applied to the leg, and a bandage is placed over the paste; commonly three layers of paste and three layers of bandages are applied alternately.

un″of·fi′cial [AS. *un-,* not; L. *officialis,* of office].

Describing a drug or remedy that is not included in the Pharmacopeia or National Formulary.

un·or′gan·ized [*un-;* G. *organon*, organ]. 1. Without organs. 2. Not arranged in the form of an organ or organs.

un·rest′ [*un-;* AS. *rest*]. A condition characterized by general body and mental tension, and especially by vigorous and irregular movements of the gastrointestinal tract.

un·sat′u·ra″ted [*un-;* L. *saturare*, to fill up]. 1. Not saturated. 2. Describing an organic compound having double or triple bonds.

un·sex′ [*un-;* L. *sexus*, sex]. Remove the testes in male, or the ovaries in female, animals.

un·sound′ness [*un-;* L. *sonus*, sound]. The state of being not healthy, diseased, or not properly functioning. —**unsound,** *adj.*

u. of mind. Incapacity to govern one's affairs.

un·stri′a·ted (un·stry′ay·tid) [*un-;* L. *striare*, to furnish with channels]. Not striped, as unstriated muscle.

un″u·ni′ted [*un-;* L. *unire*, to unite]. Not joined, as an ununited fracture.

Unverricht's disease. See Unverricht's familial *myoclonus.*

un·well′ [*un-;* AS. *wel*]. 1. Ill; sick. 2. Menstruating: lay term.

u·ra′chus (yōō·ray′kus) [G. *ourachos*, urachus]. An epithelial tube or cord connecting the apex of the urinary bladder with the allantois, regarded as the stalk of the allantois or as the degenerate apex of the primitive bladder. Its connective tissue forms the median umbilical ligament. See Plate 44. —**urachal,** *adj.*

patent u. A condition in which the urachus of the embryo does not become obliterated, but persists as a tube from the apex of the urinary bladder to the umbilicus.

u′ra·cil. $C_4H_4N_2O_2$; 2,4(1,3)-pyrimidinedione; a pyrimidine base constituent of nucleic acids.

u″ra·cra′si·a, u″ra·cra′ti·a [G. *ouron*, urine; *akrasia*, incontinence]. Incontinence of urine; enuresis.

uradal. Trade-mark for *carbromal.*

u′ra·gogue (yoor′uh·gog) [*ouron;* G. *agōgos*, leading]. A diuretic. —**uragogue,** *adj.*

u′ra·mil. $C_4H_5N_3O_3$; 5-aminobarbituric acid; a derivative of barbituric acid and certain related compounds, occurring as crystals, insoluble in cold water.

u′ra·mine. See *guanidine.*

u′rane. 1. Uranium oxide. 2. A unit of radioactivity. See *kilurane.*

u′ra·nin. See *fluorescein* sodium.

u·ran′i·nite. Pitchblende. Native uranium oxide, a source of radium.

u″ra·nis′co·plas″ty. Uranoplasty. *Obs.*

u″ra·nis·cor′rha·phy [*ouraniskos;* G. *rhaphē*, suture]. Suture of a palatal cleft; staphylorrhaphy. *Obs.*

u″ra·nis′cus [*ouraniskos*]. The palate. *Obs.*

u·ra′ni·um. U = 238.07. A heavy metal of the radium group; occurs as silver-white, lustrous, radioactive crystals or powder. As concentrated from its ores uranium contains 99.3% of the isotope weighing 238, 0.7 per cent of the 235 isotope, and a negligible amount of the 234 isotope. Uranium 235 may be made to undergo fission with the release of a large amount of energy. Uranium 238 can absorb a neutron to produce uranium 239; this spontaneously loses a beta particle to form neptunium, which, in turn, loses another beta particle to form plutonium, the last also being fissionable. In large doses the soluble salts of uranium are violent poisons.

u″ra·no·col″o·bo′ma [G. *ouranos*, vault; *kolobōma*, the part taken away in mutilation]. Cleft hard palate, not involving the alveolar process.

u′ra·no·plas″ty [*ouranos;* G. *plassein*, to form]. A plastic operation for the repair of cleft palate: formerly called *uraniscoplasty.* —**uranoplas′tic,** *adj.*

u″ra·no·ple′gi·a [*ouranos;* G. *plēgē*, stroke]. Paralysis of the muscles of the soft palate.

u″ra·nor′rha·phy [*ouranos;* G. *rhaphē*, suture]. Suture of a cleft palate; staphylorrhaphy.

u″ra·nos′chi·sis (yoor″uh·nos′ki·sis), **u·ran′o·schism** (yoo·ran′o·skiz·um, ·siz·um), **u″ra·no·schis′ma** [*ouranos;* G. *schisis*, cleavage]. 1. Cleft hard palate. 2. Cleft hard palate and alveolar process. Also called *gnathopalatoschisis.*

u″ra·no·staph′y·lo·plas″ty. Uranoplasty.

u″ra·no·staph″y·lor′rha·phy [*ouranos;* G. *staphylē*, bunch of grapes, uvula; *rhaphē*, suture]. Repair of a cleft in both the hard and soft palates.

u′ra·nyl. The bivalent uranium radical UO_2, which forms salts with many acids, as, for example, uranyl acetate, $UO_2(C_2H_3O_2)_2.2H_2O$.

u″ra·ro′ma [G. *ouron*, urine; *arōma*, aromatic herb]. Aromatic odor of urine.

u′rase (yoor′ace, ·aze). Urease.

u′ra·sin [*ouron*]. A ferment derived from urea.

u′rate. A salt of uric acid. —**urat′ic,** *adj.*

u″ra·te′mi·a, u″ra·tae′mi·a [*ouron;* G. *haima*, blood]. The presence of urates in the blood.

u″ra·tu′ri·a [*ouron; ouron*]. The presence of urates in the urine.

Urbach, Erich [*American dermatologist*, 1893–1946]. Described, with Wiethe, a syndrome with cutaneous mucous lesions consisting of yellow-white infiltrations, dystrophies of different types, and disturbances of lipid metabolism often of familial occurrence; called *lipoidosis cutis et mucosae, lipid proteinosis, Urbach-Wiethe disease.* Introduced the term necrobiosis lipoidica diabeticorum, also known as *Oppenheim-Urbach disease.*

ur″ban·i·za′tion [L. *urbanus*, of a city]. A term to express the tendency of modern society to develop cities at the expense of the country population, with a consequent influence upon disease, the death rate, etc.

u·re′a [G. *ouron*, urine] (*urea*). $CO(NH_2)_2$. Carbonyldiamide, found in urine, occurring as colorless to white, prismatic crystals, or as a white, crystalline powder; 1 Gm. dissolves in 1.5 cc. of water and in about 10 cc. of alcohol: used as a diuretic, similar in its mode of action to the saline diuretics, and also used externally in treating infected wounds in 10% solution or by implantation of pure crystals. Dose, 8–20 Gm., several times daily. See Table of Normal Values of Blood Constituents in the Appendix. Syn., *carbamide.* —**ureal,** *adj.*

quinine and u. hydrochloride. A salt employed as a local anesthetic and sclerosing agent.

u. nitrogen. The nitrogen of urea. A term used to distinguish that nitrogen from the nitrogen in the form of protein.

u. peroxide. A solid compound of urea and hydrogen peroxide; in contact with water it liberates urea and hydrogen peroxide. Also called *carbamide peroxide.* See *thenardol.*

u″re·am′e·ter [*ouron;* G. *metron*, a measure]. An apparatus for determining the amount of urea in a liquid by measuring the volume of nitrogen evolved.

u″re·am′e·try [*ouron; metron*]. The determination of the amount of urea in a liquid.

u′re·ase (yoor′ee·ace, ·aze). A urealytic enzyme obtained from the jack bean, the seed of *Canavalia;* occurs as a fine, white, or cream-colored powder; readily soluble in slightly alkaline water. Used in the estimation of urea.

u·rec′chy·sis (yoo·reck′i·sis) [*ouron;* G. *ekchysis*, outflow]. Extravasation of urine into the tissues.

u·rech′i·tin (yoo·reck′i·tin, yoor″i·kigh′tin). $C_{28}H_{42}O_8$. A poisonous glucoside from *Urechites suberecta*, with action similar to strophanthin.

u·rech″i·tox′in (yoo·reck″i·tock′sin, yoor″i·ki·). A highly poisonous principle from the leaves of *Urechites suberecta*, with action similar to urechitin.

urecholine chloride. Trade-marked name for *bethanechol chloride.*

u″re·de′ma [*ouron;* G. *oidēma*, swelling]. Swelling of tissues from extravasation of urine.

u′re·ide. A compound of urea and an acid radical.

u·re′mi·a [*ouron;* G. *haima*, blood]. The retention in the blood of urinary constituents, due to failure of the kidneys to excrete them, and the constitutional symptoms resulting. There may be headache, nausea, vomiting, and coma. —**uremic,** *adj.*

prerenal u. Failure of urinary excretion because of physiologic disturbances outside the urinary tract, such as shock, dehydration, hemorrhage, or electrolyte loss.

u″re·om′e·ter. See *ureameter.*

u″re·om′et·ry. See *ureametry.*

u″re·o·tel′ic [*ouron;* G. *telos*, the end]. Characterizing an animal in which urea is the principal compound of nitrogenous waste, as in mammals. —**ureotelism,** *n.*

ur·er′yth·rin. See *uroerythrin.*

u·re″si·es·the′si·a (yoo·ree″see·ess·thee′zhuh, ·zee·uh) [G. *ourēsis*, a making water; *aisthēsis*, sensation]. The impulse to urinate.

u·re′sis [*ourēsis*]. Urination.

u·re′ter, u′re·ter [G. *ourētēr*, ureter]. Either of the long, narrow tubes conveying the urine from the pelvis of each kidney to the urinary bladder. See Plates 8, 14, 43, 44, 45. —**ure′teral, ureter′ic,** *adj.*

aberrant ureters. Ureters emptying at some point other than into the urinary bladder.

u·re″ter·ec′ta·sis [*ourētēr;* G. *ektasis*, extension]. Dilatation of a ureter.

u·re″ter·ec′to·my [*ourētēr;* G. *ektomē*, excision]. Excision of a ureter.

u·re″ter·i′tis [*ourētēr;* G. *-itis*, inflammation]. Inflammation of a ureter.

cystic u. That characterized by multiple cystic protrusions from the mucosal surface.

u. cystica. Cystic *u.*

u·re′ter·o-, ureter- [*ourētēr*]. A combining form denoting *the ureter.*

u·re′ter·o·cele [*ourētēr;* G. *kēlē*, hernia]. A cystlike dilatation at the termination of a ureter; of congenital origin or due to a narrowing of the terminal orifice. It is identified by cystoscopic examination.

u·re″ter·o·ce·lec′to·my. Surgical removal of a ureterocele.

u·re″ter·o·co·los′to·my [*ourētēr;* G. *kolon*, colon; *stoma*, mouth]. Implantation of a ureter, severed from the urinary bladder, into the colon.

u·re″ter·o·cys′tic [*ourētēr;* G. *kystis*, bladder]. Pertaining to the ureter and urinary bladder.

u·re″ter·o·cys·tos′to·my [*ourētēr; kystis;* G. *stoma*, mouth]. The surgical formation of a communication between a ureter and the urinary bladder.

u·re″ter·o·en·ter′ic [*ourētēr;* G. *enteron*, intestine]. Relating to, or connected with, a ureter and adjacent bowel.

u·re″ter·o·en″ter·os′to·my [*ourētēr; enteron;* G. *stoma*, mouth]. Surgical formation of a passage from a ureter to some portion of the intestine.

u·re″ter·og′ra·phy [*ourētēr;* G. *graphein*, to write]. Radiography of the ureters after the injection of some radiopaque substance.

u·re″ter·o·hem″i·ne·phrec′to·my. Surgical removal of a portion of a kidney and its ureter in cases of reduplication of ureter, pelvis, or the entire upper urinary tract.

u·re″ter·o·hy″dro·ne·phro′sis [*ourētēr;* G. *hydōr*, water; *nephrōsis*, from *nephros*, kidney, *-ōsis*, condition]. Distention of a ureter and the pelvis of its kidney, due to distal obstruction of outflow of urine.

u·re″ter·o-in·tes′ti·nal a·nas″to·mo′sis. Surgical implantation of a ureter into the colon.

u·re′ter·o·lith [*ourētēr;* G. *lithos*, stone]. Calculus in a ureter.

u·re″ter·o·li·thi′a·sis [*ourētēr;* G. *lithiasis*, disease of the stone]. The presence or formation of a calculus in a ureter.

u·re″ter·o·li·thot′o·my [*ourētēr;* G. *lithos*, stone; *tomē*, a cutting]. Incision of a ureter for removal of a calculus.

u·re″ter·ol′y·sis [*ourētēr;* G. *lysis*, a loosing]. Surgical repair of a tortuous or kinked ureter.

u·re″ter·o·ne″o·cys·tos′to·my. Surgical reimplantation of the upper end of a divided ureter into the urinary bladder.

u·re″ter·o·ne″o·py″e·los′to·my [*ourētēr;* G. *neos*, new; *pyelos*, trough; *stoma*, mouth]. Suturing the distal end of a severed ureter into a new opening in the pelvis of its kidney.

u·re″ter·o·ne·phrec′to·my [*ourētēr;* G. *nephros*, kidney; *ektomē*, excision]. Removal of a kidney and its ureter.

u·re″ter·o·pel′vic. Pertaining to a ureter and renal pelvis.

u·re″ter·o·pel′vi·o·plas″ty. A surgical procedure aimed at the correction of abnormalities of the ureter and renal pelvis.

u·re′ter·o·plas″ty [*ourētēr;* G. *plassein*, to form]. A plastic operation on a ureter.

u·re″ter·o·py″e·li′tis [*ourētēr;* G. *pyelos*, trough; *-itis*, inflammation]. Inflammation of a ureter and the pelvis of a kidney.

u·re″ter·o·py″e·log′ra·phy [*ourētēr; pyelos;* G. *graphein*, to write]. Roentgenographic visualization of the upper urinary tract by the injection of contrast mediums.

u·re″ter·o·py″e·lo·ne·os′to·my [*ourētēr; pyelos;* G. *neos*, new; *stoma*, mouth]. Formation of a new passageway from the pelvis of a kidney to its ureter.

u·re″ter·o·py″e·lo·ne·phri′tis [*ourētēr; pyelos;* G. *nephros*, kidney; *-itis*, inflammation]. Inflammation of a ureter and its kidney and pelvis.

u·re″ter·o·py″e·lo·ne·phros′to·my [*ourētēr; pyelos; nephros;* G. *stoma*, mouth]. Surgical anastomosis of the ureter with the pelvis of its kidney.

u·re″ter·o·py′e·lo·plas″ty [*ourētēr; pyelos;* G. *plassein*, to form]. Any plastic operation involving the upper portion of a ureter and the adjacent pelvis of the kidney.

u·re″ter·o·py″e·los′to·my [*ourētēr; pyelos;* G. *stoma*, mouth]. Excision of part of a ureter and implantation of the remaining part into a new aperture made into the pelvis of the kidney.

u·re″ter·or·rha′gi·a [*ourētēr;* G. *rhēgnynai*, to burst forth]. Hemorrhage from a ureter.

u·re″ter·or′rha·phy [*ourētēr;* G. *rhaphē*, suture]. Suture of a ureter.

u·re″ter·o·sig″moid·os′to·my [*ourētēr;* G. *sigmoeidēs*, shaped like the letter sigma; *stoma*, mouth]. Implantation of a ureter, severed from the urinary bladder, into the sigmoid colon.

u·re″ter·os′to·my [*ourētēr; stoma*]. Transplantation of a ureter to the skin; the formation of an external ureteral fistula.

u·re″ter·ot′o·my [*ourētēr;* G. *tomē*, a cutting]. Incision of a ureter.

u·re″ter·o·u·re′ter·al [*ourētēr; ourētēr*]. Pertaining

to both ureters, or to two parts of one ureter, as ureteroureteral anastomosis.

u·re″ter·o·u·re″ter·os′to·my [*ourētēr; ourētēr;* G. *stoma,* mouth]. Surgical formation of a passage between the ureters or between different parts of the same ureter.

u·re″ter·o·u′ter·ine [*ourētēr;* L. *uterus,* womb]. Pertaining to the ureters and the uterus.

u·re″ter·o·vag′i·nal (·vadj′i·nul, ·va·jy′nul) [*ourētēr;* L. *vagina,* vagina]. Pertaining to the ureters and the vagina.

u′re·than, u′re·thane. 1. $C_2H_5O.CO.NH_2$. Ethyl carbamate, occurring as crystals or a white powder; 1 Gm. is soluble in 0.5 cc. of water and in 1 cc. of alcohol. Used as a somnifacient and, recently, in the treatment of myeloid and lymphatic leukemia. Dose, 1–3 Gm. (15–45 gr.). Also called *ethyl urethan.* 2. Any ester of carbamic acid.

u·re′thra [G. *ourēthra,* urethra]. The canal through which the urine is discharged, extending from the neck of the urinary bladder to the external urethral orifice, divided in the male into the prostatic portion, the membranous portion, and the spongy or penile portion, and from 8 to 9 inches long. (See Plate 44.) In the female it is about 1½ inches in length. (See Plates 41, 43.) —**urethral,** *adj.*

membranous u. The part of the urethra between the two layers of the urogenital diaphragm.

phallic u. See urogenital *canal.*

primary u. That part of the urogenital tube between the embryonic bladder and the urogenital sinus; in the female, it forms the definitive urethra; in the male, the proximal part of the prostatic urethra from urinary bladder to ejaculatory ducts.

prostatic u. That portion of the male urethra within the prostate gland.

secondary u. The definitive urethra, especially in the male where it includes the primary urethra as well as the urogenital sinus.

spongy portion of u. That contained in the corpus spongiosum of the penis; the penile urethra: also called *cavernous u.*

u. muliebris. Female urethra.

u. virilis. Male urethra.

u·re′thra·scope. See *urethroscope.*

u″re·threc′to·my [*ourēthra;* G. *ektomē,* excision]. Excision of the urethra or a portion of it.

u″re·thri′tis [*ourēthra;* G. *-itis,* inflammation]. Inflammation of the urethra.

allergic u. A nonspecific type of inflammation, acute or chronic, of the urethral mucosa, which represents a local sensitivity response to a specific antigen or group of antigens.

anterior u. Inflammation of the part situated anterior to the inferior layer of the urogenital diaphragm.

granular u. A type of nonspecific chronic inflammation of the urethral mucosa, characterized by discrete or confluent circumscribed areas of hyperemia and edema located principally about the openings of the paraurethral ducts.

polypoid u. A type of nonspecific chronic inflammation of the urethral mucosa, characterized by edematous bullae and blebs which project into the urethral lumen as inflammatory polyps.

posterior u. Inflammation of the prostatic and membranous portions of the male urethra.

simple u. A nonspecific inflammation of the urethra.

specific u. That due to the gonococcus; gonorrhea.

u. cystica. A condition similar to cystitis cystica, but confined to the urethra.

u. orificii externi. Inflammation of the urethra at the meatus, usually characterized by superficial ulceration about the glans penis: most often seen in male infants.

u. venerea. Gonorrhea.

u·re′thro-, urethr- [*ourēthra*]. A combining form denoting *the urethra.*

u·re″thro·bulb′ar [*ourēthra;* L. *bulbus,* bulb]. Relating to the urethra and the bulb of the corpus spongiosum.

u·re′thro·cele [*ourēthra;* G. *kēlē,* hernia]. A urethral protrusion or diverticulum involving, usually, the female urethra.

u·re″thro·cys·ti′tis [*ourēthra;* G. *kystis,* bladder; *-itis,* inflammation]. Inflammation of the urethra and urinary bladder.

u·re′thro·gram [*ourēthra;* G. *gramma,* letter]. A roentgenographic visualization of the urethra, obtained through the injection of a contrast medium.

u·re′thro·graph [*ourēthra;* G. *graphein,* to write]. A recording urethrometer.

u″re·throg′ra·phy [*ourēthra; graphein*]. Radiography of the urethra performed after the injection of the urethra with an opaque contrast substance.

u″re·throm′e·ter [*ourēthra;* G. *metron,* a measure]. An instrument for determining the caliber of the urethra or for measuring the lumen of a stricture.

u·re″thro·phy′ma [*ourēthra;* G. *phyma,* growth]. Old term for urethral tumor.

u·re′thro·plas″ty [*ourēthra;* G. *plassein,* to form]. Plastic operation upon the urethra; surgical repair of the urethra.

u·re″thro·pro·stat′ic [*ourēthra;* G. *prostatēs,* one who stands before]. Relating to the urethra and the prostate.

u″re·thror′rha·phy [*ourēthra;* G. *rhaphē,* suture]. Surgical restoration of the continuity of the urethra.

u·re″thror·rhe′a [*ourēthra;* G. *rhoia,* flow]. A morbid discharge from the urethra.

u. ex libidine. Old term indicating the normal glandular mucous secretion occurring during sexual excitement preparatory to coitus.

u·re′thro·scope [*ourēthra;* G. *skopein,* to examine]. An instrument for inspecting the interior of the urethra. —**urethroscop′ic,** *adj.*

u″re·thros′co·py [*ourēthra; skopein*]. Inspection of the urethra with the aid of the urethroscope.

u·re′thro·spasm [*ourēthra;* G. *spasmos,* spasm]. Spasmodic contraction of the urethral sphincters.

u·re″thro·ste·no′sis [*ourēthra;* G. *stenōsis,* a being straitened]. Stricture of the urethra.

u″re·thros′to·my [*ourēthra;* G. *stoma,* mouth]. Perineal section with permanent opening of the membranous urethra in the perineum.

u·re′thro·tome [*ourēthra;* G. *tomos,* cutting]. An instrument used for performing urethrotomy.

dilating u. A combined urethrotome and dilator.

u″re·throt′o·my [*ourēthra;* G. *tomē,* a cutting]. The operation of cutting a stricture of the urethra.

external u. Division of a urethral stricture by an incision from without.

internal u. Division of a urethral stricture from within the urethra.

u·re″thro·tri″go·ni′tis. Inflammation of the trigone of the urinary bladder, usually the anterior segment, and the adjacent urethra.

u·re″thro·vag′i·nal (·vadj′i·nul, ·va·jy′nul) [*ourēthra;* L. *vagina,* vagina]. Pertaining to the urethra and the vagina.

Urey, Harold Clayton (1893–). American physical chemist known for isolating deuterium (heavy hydrogen) and scientific work in developing atomic power. Nobel laureate in chemistry (1934).

ur′gen·cy [L. *urgere,* to impel]. Urgent desire to empty the urinary bladder.

Ur·gin′e·a [NL., from the name of an Arab tribe in Algeria]. A genus of the Liliaceae.

U. maritima. The plant that produces the official squill. See *squill.*

urginin. Trade-mark for a mixture of two water insoluble glycosides *urginin-A* and *urginin-B*, derived from squill, in the proportions in which they exist in the drug; the substance occurs as a pale yellow, granular powder; insoluble in water, but soluble in alcohol. The cardiac action of urginin is essentially similar to that of digitalis.

ur″hi·dro′sis (yoor″hi·dro′sis, ·high·dro′sis) [G. *ouron*, urine; *hidrōsis*, a sweating]. A condition in which some of the constituents of the urine, chiefly urea, are excreted in excess of normal with the sweat.

u′ri·an. Urochrome.

u′ric [*ouron*]. Pertaining to the urine, as uric acid.

u′ric ac′id. $C_5H_4N_4O_3$. The end product of purine metabolism in man. It is a normal constituent of the blood and urine. Abnormal metabolism of uric acid with a high blood level and decreased excretion are characteristic of gout. Also called *triketopurine*, 2,6,8-*trioxypurine.* See Table of Normal Values of Blood Constituents in the Appendix.

u″ric·ac″i·de′mi·a (yoor″ick·ass″i·dee′mee·uh) [*ouron;* L. *acidus*, sour; G. *haima*, blood]. The presence of an abnormal amount of uric acid in the blood. Syn., *uricemia.*

u″ric·ac″i·du′ri·a (·ass″i·dew′ree·uh) [*ouron; acidus; ouron*]. The presence of excessive amounts of uric acid in the urine.

u″ri·can′i·case. An enzyme in the liver which catalyzes conversion of urocanic acid to *l*-glutamic acid.

u′ri·case (yoor′i·kace, ·kaze). An enzyme present in the liver, spleen, and kidney of most mammals except man. In the presence of gaseous oxygen, it converts uric acid to allantoin.

u″ri·ce′mi·a. See *uricacidemia.*

u″ri·col′y·sis [*ouron;* G. *lysis*, a loosing]. The disintegration of uric acid.

ur″i·cos·u′ri·a. Urinary excretion of uric acid.

u″ri·cos·u′ric. Promoting uricosuria, as benemid.

u″ri·co·tel′ic [*ouron;* G. *telos*, the end]. Characterizing an animal in which uric acid is the principal compound of nitrogenous waste, as in birds, snakes, and lizards. —**uricotelism,** *n.*

u′ri·dine. Uracil riboside; the nucleoside obtained when phosphoric acid is removed by uridylic acid.

u″ri·dro′sis. See *urhidrosis.*

u″ri·dyl′ic ac′id. A mononucleotide of yeast nucleic acid which yields uracil, ribose, and phosphoric acid upon complete hydrolysis.

u′ri·nal [L. *urina*, urine]. A vessel for receiving urine.

u″ri·nal′y·sis [*urina;* G. *lysis*, a loosing]. Analysis of the urine; in routine examination, this involves description of appearance (color, turbidity), determination of pH, specific gravity, presence or absence of proteins (albumin), sugar, ketone bodies, pus, or crystals, as well as a microscopical examination of the sediment for abnormal constituents such as casts, erythrocytes, leukocytes, and epithelial cells. Abnormal findings are followed by special quantitative and semiquantitative tests. Also spelled *uranalysis.*

u′ri·nate [*urina*]. Discharge urine from the bladder. —**urina′tion,** *n.*

u′ri·na″tive [*urina*]. A drug which stimulates the flow of urine; a diuretic.

u′rine [*urina*]. The fluid excreted by the kidneys. In health, urine has an amber color, a slightly acid reaction, a faint odor, a saline taste, and a specific gravity of 1.005 to 1.030. The quantity excreted in 24 hours varies with the amount of fluids consumed but averages between 1000 and 1500 cc. The amount of solids in the urine varies with the diet, more being excreted on a high protein, high salt diet. Normally between 40–75 Gm. of solids are present in the 24-hour urine, of which approximately 25% is urea, 25% chlorides, 25% sulfate and phosphates, and the remainder organic substances including organic acids, pigments, neutral sulfur, hormones, etc. The most important abnormal constituents present in disease are albumin, sugar, blood, pus, acetone, diacetic acid, fat, chyle, tube-casts, various cells, and bacteria. —**urinary,** *adj.*

incontinence of u. Inability to retain the urine. See *enuresis; incontinence.*

residual u. Any considerable amount of urine remaining in the bladder after urination. The commonest causes are: in the male, prostatic hypertrophy and vesical disease; in the female, cystocele and pressure from uterine tumors.

retention of u. Anuria.

suppression of u. Anuria.

u″ri·nif′er·ous [*urina;* L. *ferre*, to bear]. Carrying or conveying urine, as uriniferous tubule.

u″ri·nif′ic [*urina;* L. *facere*, to make]. Excreting or producing urine.

u″ri·nip′a·rous [*urina;* L. *parere*, to bring forth]. Producing urine.

u′ri·no-, urin- [*urina*]. A combining form denoting *urine.*

u″ri·no·cry·os′co·py (·krye·os′ko·pee) [*urina;* G. *kryos*, icy cold; *skopein*, to examine]. Cryoscopy of the urine.

u′ri·nod [*urina*]. A substance whose formula is said to be C_6H_8O, and upon whose presence the odor of stale urine is said to depend.

u″ri·no·gen′i·tal [*urina;* L. *genitalis*, genital]. Urogenital.

u″ri·nog′e·nous (yoor″i·nodj′i·nus) [*urina;* G. *genesthai*, from *gignesthai*, to be produced]. Urogenous.

u″ri·nol′o·gy [*urina;* G. *logos*, word]. The science of diagnosis of disease by means of urinary analysis. *Obs.*

u″ri·no′ma [*urina;* G. *-ōma*, tumor]. A cyst containing urine.

u″ri·nom′e·ter [*urina;* G. *metron*, a measure]. A hydrometer for ascertaining the specific gravity of urine.

u″ri·nom′e·try [*urina; metron*]. The determination of the specific gravity of urine.

u″ri·no·scop′ic. Pertaining to uronoscopy.

u″ri·nos′co·py. See *uronoscopy.*

u′ri·nose, u′ri·nous [*urina*]. Having the characters of urine, as a urinose or urinous odor.

u″ri·sol′vent [G. *ouron*, urine; L. *solvere*, to loose]. Dissolving uric acid.

u·ri′tis [L. *urere*, to burn; G. *-itis*, inflammation]. Inflammation following a burn. *Rare.*

uritone. Trade-mark for a brand of methenamine.

ur′ning (oor′ning) [Ger.]. A homosexual male. *Obs.*

u′ro-, ur- [G. *ouron*, urine]. A combining form denoting *urine.*

u″ro·ac″i·dim′e·ter (yoor″o·ass″i·dim′i·tur) [*ouron;* L. *acidus*, sour; G. *metron*, a measure]. An instrument for measuring the acidity of urine.

u″ro·am·mo′ni·ac. Relating to, or containing, uric acid and ammonia.

u″ro·an′thel·one. Anthelone derived from urine.

u″ro·az″o·tom′e·ter [G. *ouron*, urine; *a-*, not; *zōē*, life; *metron*, a measure]. An apparatus for quantitative estimation of the nitrogenous substances in urine.

u″ro·ben·zo′ic ac′id. Old term for hippuric acid.

u″ro·bi′lin (yoor″o·buy′lin, ·bil′in) [*ouron;* L. *bilis*, bile]. A bile pigment produced by the putrefaction of bilirubin in the gut and excreted by the kidneys or removed by the liver. A brown, resinous mass, soluble in alcohol, ether, or chloroform; used as a reagent.

u″ro·bi″li·ne′mi·a (·buy″li·nee′mee·uh, ·bil″i·nee′-mee·uh) [*ouron; bilis;* G. *haima,* blood]. The presence of urobilin in the blood.

u″ro·bi″lin·ic′ter·us (·buy″li·nick′tur·us, ·bil″i·) [*ouron; bilis;* G. *ikteros,* jaundice]. Jaundice associated with urobilinemia. *Rare.*

u″ro·bi·lin′o·gen (·buy·lin′o·jen, ·bi·lin′o·jen) [*ouron; bilis;* G. *genesthai,* from *gignesthai,* to be produced]. A chromogen from which urobilin is formed by oxidation when urine is allowed to stand.

u″ro·bi″li·noi′din (·buy″li·noy′din, ·bil″i·) [*ouron; bilis;* G. *eidos,* form]. A form of urinary pigment derived from hematin and resembling urobilin though not identical with it. It occurs in certain pathologic conditions.

u″ro·bi″li·nu′ri·a (·buy″li·new′ree·uh, ·bil″i·) [*ouron; bilis; ouron*]. The presence of an excess of urobilin in urine.

u″ro·can′ic ac′id. $C_3H_3N_2CH{:}CHCOOH$. An acid, found in dog's urine, resulting from deamination of histidine.

u·roch′e·ras (yoo·rock′ur·us) [*ouron;* G. *cherades,* gravel]. Gravel in urine.

u″ro·che′si·a (yoor″o·kee′zhuh, ·zee·uh) [*ouron;* G. *chezein,* to ease oneself]. Discharge of urine through the anus.

u″ro·chlo·ral′ic ac′id. Trichlorethylglycuronic acid; a metabolic product of chloral hydrate which is excreted in the urine after the ingestion of chloral hydrate. It gives a false positive test for sugar.

u′ro·chrome [*ouron;* G. *chrōma,* color]. A yellow pigment in urine.

u″ro·chro′mo·gen [*ouron; chrōma;* G. *genesthai,* from *gignesthai,* to be produced]. A substance occurring in tissues, which is oxidized to urochrome.

u″ro·clep′si·a [*ouron;* G. *kleptein,* to steal]. Involuntary or unconscious urination.

u″ro·cris′i·a (yoor″o·kriz′ee·uh, ·kriss′ee·uh) [*ouron;* G. *krisis,* a distinguishing]. Diagnosis by means of urinary examination and analysis.

u″ro·cri′sis [*ouron; krisis*]. 1. The critical stage of a disease distinguished by the excretion of a large volume of urine. 2. Severe pain in any part of the urinary tract occurring in tabes dorsalis.

u″ro·cy′a·nin. See *uroglaucin.*

u″ro·cy·an′o·gen (yoor″o·sigh·an′o·jen) [*ouron;* G. *kyanos,* blue; *genesthai,* from *gignesthai,* to be produced]. A blue pigment found in urine.

u″ro·cy′a·nose. See *urocyanogen.*

u″ro·cy″a·no′sis [*ouron; kyanos;* G. *-ōsis,* condition]. Blue discoloration of the urine, usually from the presence of excess amounts of indican oxidized to indigo blue; also from drugs such as methylene blue.

u·ro′de·um. The portion of the cloaca into which the urogenital ducts open.

u″roe·de′ma (yoor″i·dee′muh). See *uredema.*

u″ro·er′yth·rin (yoor″o·err′ith·rin, ·i·rith′rin) [*ouron;* G. *erythros,* red]. A red pigment found in urine.

u″ro·fla′vin. A fluorescent compound of unknown structure, with properties similar to riboflavin, excreted in the urine along with the vitamin, following ingestion of riboflavin.

u″ro·fus′cin [*ouron;* L. *fuscus,* dark]. A pigment found occasionally in urine in cases of porphyrinuria.

u″ro·fus″co·hem′a·tin (yoor″o·fus″ko·hem′uh-tin, ·hee′muh·tin) [*ouron; fuscus;* G. *haima,* blood]. A red pigment derived from hematin, occurring in the urine.

u″ro·gas′trone [*ouron;* G. *gastēr,* belly]. A substance extracted from urine which inhibits gastric secretion and motility; probably related to enterogastrone.

u″ro·gen′i·tal [*ouron;* L. *genitalis,* genital]. Pertaining to the urinary and genital organs.

u·rog′e·nous (yoo·rodj′i·nus) [*ouron;* G. *genesthai,* from *gignesthai,* to be produced]. Producing urine.

u″ro·glau′cin (yoor″o·glaw′sin) [*ouron;* G. *glaukos,* bluish green]. A blue pigment sometimes occurring in urine.

u′ro·gram [*ouron;* G. *gramma,* letter]. A radiograph or roentgenographic visualization of the urinary tract made after intravenous or retrograde injection of an opaque contrast substance.

u·rog′ra·phy [*ouron;* G. *graphein,* to write]. Roentgenographic visualization of the urinary tract by the use of contrast mediums.

excretory u. That following intravenous injection of a contrast medium and depending on the ability of the kidney to excrete the medium in concentration sufficient to make the urine radiopaque while passing through the urinary tract.

intravenous u. Excretory *u.*

retrograde u. See retrograde *pyelography.*

u″ro·gra·vim′e·ter. See *urinometer.*

u″ro·hem′a·tin (yoor″o·hem′uh·tin, ·hee′muh·tin) [*ouron;* G. *haima,* blood]. Altered hematin in the urine.

u″ro·hem″a·to·ne·phro′sis (·hem″uh·to·ni·fro′sis, ·hee″muh·to·) [*ouron; haima;* G. *nephros,* kidney; *-ōsis,* condition]. Distention of the pelvis of a kidney with blood and urine.

u″ro·hem″a·to·por′phy·rin [*ouron; haima;* G. *porphyra,* purple]. Urohematin; a urinary pigment occasionally occurring in urine in certain pathologic states.

u″ro·hy″per·ten′sin [*ouron;* G. *hyper,* over; L. *tensio,* a stretching]. A substance derived from urine which increases blood pressure when it is injected intravenously.

u″ro·ki·net′ic (·ki·net′ick, ·kigh·net′ick) [*ouron;* G. *kinētikos,* of putting in motion]. Due to a reflex from the urinary system; a term generally used to denote a form of indigestion secondary to irritation or disease of the urinary tract.

urokon sodium. Trade-marked name for sodium 3-acetylamino-2,4,6-triiodobenzoate, or sodium acetrizoate; $C_9H_5I_3NNaO_3$, prepared in aqueous solution by the interaction of acetrizoic acid and sodium hydroxide: used in 30% or 70% w/v solution as a contrast medium for excretory urography, retrograde pyelography, nephrography, translumbar arteriography, and angiocardiography.

u″ro·leu·kin′ic ac′id. An acid found in the urine in alkaptonuria.

u′ro·lite. See *urolith.*

u′ro·lith [*ouron;* G. *lithos,* stone]. A calculus occurring in urine. —**urolith′ic,** *adj.*

u″ro·li·thi′a·sis [*ouron;* G. *lithiasis,* disease of the stone]. 1. The presence of, or a condition associated with, urinary calculi. 2. The formation of urinary calculi.

u″ro·li·thol′o·gy [*ouron;* G. *lithos,* stone; *logos,* word]. That branch of medicine pertaining to the diagnosis and treatment of disease caused by the presence of urinary calculi. *Obs.*

u″ro·lith·ot′o·my. Removal of a calculus from anywhere in the urinary tract.

u·rol′o·gist [*ouron; logos*]. One skilled in urology; a specialist in the diagnosis and treatment of diseases of the urogenital tract in the male and the urinary tract in the female.

u·rol′o·gy [*ouron; logos*]. The scientific study of the urine. That branch of medical science embracing the study and treatment of the diseases and the abnormalities of the urogenital tract in the male and the urinary tract in the female. —**urolog'ic,** *adj.*

u"ro·lu'te·in [*ouron;* L. *luteus,* yellow]. A yellow pigment sometimes found in urine.

u'ro·man"cy, u"ro·man'ti·a [*ouron;* G. *manteia,* divination]. Diagnosis or prognosis by observation of the urine. *Obs.*

u"ro·mel'a·nin [*ouron;* G. *melas,* black]. A black pigment which sometimes appears in urine as a decomposition product of urochrome.

u·rom'e·lus [G. *oura,* tail; *melos,* limb]. A monster in which there is more or less complete fusion of the legs, with but a single foot. Also called *sympus monopus.*

u·rom'e·ter. See *urinometer.*

u"ro·ne·phro'sis. See *hydronephrosis.*

u·ron'ic ac'id. Any of a group of monobasic sugar acids obtained when the primary alcohol group of an aldose is oxidized to carboxyl, without oxidizing the aldehyde group.

u"ro·nol'o·gy. See *urology.*

u"ron·on·com'e·try [*ouron;* G. *ogkos,* mass; *metron,* a measure]. Measurement of the quantity of urine passed or excreted in a definite period, as 24 hours.

u"ro·nos'co·py [*ouron;* G. *skopein,* to examine]. Examination of urine by inspection and use of the microscope. Syn., *urinoscopy, uroscopy.*

u·rop'a·thy [*ouron;* G. *pathos,* disease]. Old term for any disease involving the urinary tract, as indicated by urinary pathology.

u"ro·pep'sin. The urinary end product of the secretion of pepsinogen into the blood stream by peptic cells, followed by transport to the kidneys and excretion in urine.

u'ro·phan [*ouron;* G. *phainein,* to appear]. A generic name for substances which, taken into the body, appear again unchanged chemically in the urine. —**urophan'ic,** *adj.*

u"ro·phe'in [*ouron;* G. *phaios,* gray]. A gray pigment found in urine.

u"ro·pit'tin [*ouron;* G. *pitta,* pitch]. A resinous decomposition product of urochrome.

u"ro·pla'ni·a [*ouron;* G. *planos,* a wandering]. Urine elsewhere than in the urinary organs; discharge of urine from an orifice other than the urethra.

u"ro·poi·e'sis [*ouron;* G. *poiēsis,* production]. Old term for the production of urine.

u"ro·por'phy·rin [*ouron;* G. *porphyra,* purple]. Any of several isomeric, metal-free porphyrins, occurring in small amounts in normal urine and feces, characterized by having as substituents 4 acetic acid (—CH_2COOH) and 4 propionic acid (—CH_2-CH_2COOH) groups. Increased excretion of uroporphyrin I results in porphyrinuria.

u"ro·psam'mus (yoor"o·sam'us, yoor"op·sam'us) [*ouron;* G. *psammos,* sand]. Urinary gravel or sediment. *Obs.*

u"ro·ro'sein, u"ro·ro'se·in. A urinary pigment which does not occur preformed in the urine, but is present in the form of a chromogen, indoleacetic acid, which is transformed into the pigment upon treatment with a mineral acid. It is said to be identical with urorrhodin.

u"ror·rha'gi·a [*ouron;* G. *rhēgnynai,* to burst forth]. Excessive discharge of urine.

u"ror·rho'din, u"ro·rho'din [*ouron;* G. *rhodon,* rose]. A red pigment found in urine and derived from uroxanthin.

u"ror·rho·din'o·gen [*ouron; rhodon;* G. *genesthai,* from *gignesthai,* to be produced]. The chromogen which by decomposition produces urorrhodin.

u"ro·ru'bin [*ouron;* L. *rubeus,* red]. A red pigment found in urine, seen only in disease.

u·ro'sa·cin. See *urorrhodin.*

u·ros'che·sis (yoo·ros'ki·sis) [*ouron;* G. *schesis,* retention]. Anuria. *Obs.*

u·ros'co·pist [*ouron;* G. *skopein,* to examine]. One who makes a specialty of urinary examinations; a technician who examines urine for evidence of disease.

u·ros'co·py [*ouron; skopein*]. Examination of urine; uronoscopy. —**uroscop'ic,** *adj.*

u·ro'se·in. See *urorrhodin.*

u"ro·se"mi·ol'o·gy (yoor"o·seem"eye·ol'o·jee) [*ouron;* G. *sēmeion,* sign; *logos,* word]. Examination of the urine as an aid to diagnosis. *Obs.*

u"ro·sep'sis [*ouron;* G. *sēpsis,* decay]. A systemic infection originating in the urinary tract. *Rare.* —**uroseptic,** *adj.*

u"ro·spec'trin [*ouron;* L. *spectrum,* image]. A pigment of normal urine.

u"ro·ste'a·lith [*ouron;* G. *stear,* fat; *lithos,* stone]. A fatlike substance occurring in some urinary calculi.

u"ro·the"o·bro'mine. See *paraxanthine.*

u"ro·tox'ic [*ouron;* G. *toxikon,* poison]. 1. Pertaining to poisonous substances eliminated in urine. 2. Pertaining to poisoning by urine or some of its constituents. *Obs.*

u"ro·tox·ic'i·ty (yoor"o·tock·sis'i·tee) [*ouron; toxikon*]. The toxic properties of urine. *Obs.*

u"ro·tox'in [*ouron; toxikon*]. Poison of urine. *Obs.*

u'ro·tox"y, u"ro·tox'i·a [*ouron; toxikon*]. The unit of toxicity of urine; the amount necessary to kill a kilogram of living substance. *Obs.*

urotropin. Trade-mark for a brand of methenamine.

u"ro·xan'thin (yoor"o·zan'thin) [*ouron;* G. *xanthos,* yellow]. A yellow pigment in human urine which yields indigo blue on oxidation.

u·rox'in. See *alloxantin.*

ur'rho·din (yoor'o·din, yoo·ro'din). See *urorrhodin.*

ur·sol'ic ac'id (ur·sol'ick). $C_{30}H_{48}O_3$. A triterpene acid occurring in the waxlike coating of the skin or cuticle of fruits and in the leaves of certain plants. Used as an emulsifying agent in the manufacture of pharmaceuticals and food products.

ur'ti·ca, ur·ti'ca [L.]. 1. A plant of the genus *Urtica;* a nettle. 2. A wheal.

ur"ti·ca'ri·a [*urtica*]. Hives or nettle rash. A skin condition characterized by the appearance of intensely itching wheals or welts with elevated, usually white, centers and a surrounding area of erythema. They appear in crops, widely distributed over the body surface, tend to disappear in a day or two, and usually are unattended by constitutional symptoms. —**urtica'rial,** *adj.*

allergic u. That due usually to the ingestion, more rarely inhalation of or contact with, a substance to which the individual is sensitive. Common food allergens are strawberries, citrus fruits, fish and shellfish, eggs, tomatoes, and chocolate.

caterpillar u. Caterpillar dermatitis.

cholinogenic u. Wheals due to an abnormal response to choline esters.

cold u. A form due to a physical allergy to exposure to cold.

factitious u. Dermographia.

giant u. See angioneurotic *edema.*

u. bullosa. A type with the formation of fluid-filled vesicles or bullae on the surface of the wheals.

u. hemorrhagica. A type of urticaria bullosa in which the vesicles contain bloody fluid.

u. medicamentosa. That due to the ingestion of a drug to which the individual is allergic.

u. papulosa. An intensely pruritic skin eruption seen in children, characterized by recurrent crops of erythematous patches and papules on the extensor surfaces of the extremities. Also called *lichen urticatus, prurigo simplex.*

u. pigmentosa. A rare form of urticarial eruption, marked by more or less persistent, yellowish, brownish, or slate-colored lesions, which may be macules, papules, or nodules.

u. solaris. A type occurring in certain individuals due to exposure to sunlight.

ur'ti·cate [*urtica*]. Characterized by the presence of wheals.

ur"ti·ca'tion [*urtica*]. 1. A sensation as if one had been stung by nettles. 2. Production of wheals. —**ur'ticate,** *v.*

u·ru'shi·ol (yoo·roo'shee·ol). [(Jap. *urushi*]. The irritant principle of poison ivy and poison oak, consisting of one or more derivatives of catechol with an unsaturated 15-carbon side chain.

Usher, Barney David (1899–). Canadian dermatologist who, with F. Senear, described a dermatitis combining features of pemphigus and lupus erythematosus.

Us'ne·a [Ar. *ushnah*, moss]. A genus of lichen.

U. barbata. Yields usnic acid.

us'nic ac'id. $C_{18}H_{16}O_7$; an antibacterial phenolic substance found in lichens, as in *Usnea barbata:* also called *usninic acid, usnein.*

U. S. P. United States Pharmacopeia.

U. S. P. H. S. United States Public Health Service.

us"ti·lag'i·nism (us"ti·ladj'i·niz·um) [L. *ustilago*, a thistlelike plant, from *ustulatus*, burned]. Condition resembling ergot poisoning; caused by eating smutty corn.

Us"ti·la'go [L.]. A genus of parasitic fungi—the smuts.

U. maydis. Corn smut, a fungus parasitic upon maize or Indian corn. In properties it resembles ergot of rye.

us'tin. An antibiotic substance produced by *Aspergillus ustus.*

us'tion [L. *ustio*, a burning]. *In surgery*, cauterization.

u'ta. See *leishmaniasis* americana.

u"ter·al'gi·a [L. *uterus*, womb; G. *algos*, pain]. Pain in the uterus.

u'ter·ine (yoo'tur·in, yoo'tuh·ryne) [*uterus*]. Pertaining to the uterus.

u"ter·is'mus (yoo"tur·iz'mus) [*uterus*]. Uterine contraction of a spasmodic and painful character.

u"ter·i'tis [*uterus;* G. *-itis*, inflammation]. Inflammation of the uterus; metritis.

u'ter·o-, uter- [*uterus*]. A combining form denoting *pertaining to the uterus.*

u"ter·o·ab·dom'i·nal [*uterus;* L. *abdomen*, abdomen]. Pertaining to the uterus and the abdomen.

u"ter·o·cer'vi·cal [*uterus;* L. *cervix*, neck]. Relating to the uterus and the cervix of the uterus.

u"ter·o·col'ic [*uterus;* G. *kolon*, colon]. Relating to the uterus and the colon.

u"ter·o·fix·a'tion. See *hysteropexy.*

u"ter·o·ges·ta'tion [*uterus;* L. *gestatio*, a bearing]. Gestation within the cavity of the uterus; normal pregnancy.

u"ter·og'ra·phy [*uterus;* G. *graphein*, to write]. Roentgenographic visualization of the uterine cavity by means of an iodized oil or other contrast medium injected therein through the cervical canal; metrography.

u"ter·o·in·tes'ti·nal [*uterus;* L. *intestinus*, intestine]. Relating to the uterus and the intestine.

u"ter·o·ma'ni·a [*uterus;* G. *mania*, madness]. Mental disorder associated with uterine disorder. *Obs.*

u"ter·om'e·ter [*uterus;* G. *metron*, a measure]. An instrument used to measure the uterus.

u"ter·o-o·va'ri·an. Pertaining to the uterus and the ovaries.

u"ter·o·pa·ri'e·tal [*uterus;* L. *paries*, wall]. Pertaining to the uterus and the abdominal wall.

u"ter·o·pel'vic [*uterus;* L. *pelvis*, basin]. Pertaining to the uterus and the pelvic ligaments.

u"ter·o·pex'i·a, u'ter·o·pex"y. See *hysteropexy.*

u"ter·o·pla·cen'tal [*uterus;* L. *placenta*, cake]. Pertaining to the uterus and the placenta.

u'ter·o·plas"ty [*uterus;* G. *plassein*, to form]. A plastic operation on the uterus.

u"ter·o·rec'tal [*uterus;* L. *rectus*, straight]. Relating to the uterus and the rectum.

u"ter·o·sa'cral [*uterus;* L. *sacer*, sacred]. Pertaining to the uterus and the sacrum.

u"ter·o·sal"pin·gog'ra·phy [*uterus;* G. *salpigx*, trumpet; *graphein*, to write]. Radiographic visualization of the cavities of the uterus and uterine tubes by means of an iodized oil contrast substance injected into the cervical canal under pressure. Also called *hysterosalpingography, metrosalpingography.*

u'ter·o·scope" [*uterus;* G. *skopein*, to examine]. A uterine speculum.

u"ter·ot'o·my. See *hysterotomy.*

u"ter·o·ton'ic [*uterus;* G. *tonos*, tone]. Increasing muscular tone of the uterus.

u"ter·o·trac'tor [*uterus;* L. *tractum*, from *trahere*, to draw]. 1. Old term for uterine tenaculum or volsella forceps. 2. A wide, heavy, sharp-toothed retractor used to make continuous traction on the anterior portion of the cervix of the uterus during surgery.

u"ter·o·tu'bal [*uterus;* L. *tubus*, tube]. Relating to the uterus and the oviducts.

u"ter·o·vag'i·nal (yoo"tur·o·vadj'i·nul, ·va·jy'nul) [*uterus;* L. *vagina*, vagina]. Relating to the uterus and vagina.

u"ter·o·ven'tral [*uterus;* L. *venter*, belly]. Relating to the uterus and the abdomen.

u"ter·o·ves'i·cal [*uterus;* L. *vesica*, bladder]. Relating to the uterus and the urinary bladder.

u'ter·us (pl. *uteri*) [L.]. The womb; the organ of gestation which receives and holds the fertilized ovum, during the development of the fetus, and becomes the principal agent in its expulsion during parturition. It is a pear-shaped, muscular organ, three inches long, two inches wide, and one inch thick, and is divided into three portions: the fundus, the body, and the cervix. The fundus is the upper and broad portion; the body gradually narrows to the neck, which is the contracted portion. The orifice, os uteri, communicates with the vagina. The inner surface is covered with mucous membrane continuous with that of the vagina. The outer surface of the fundus and body is covered with peritoneum. The whole organ is suspended in the pelvis by means of the broad and round ligaments and the uterosacral ligaments. The uterine tubes enter, one on each side of the fundus, at the cornua of the organ. See Plates 41, 43.

anteflexion of u. See *anteflexion* of the uterus.

bipartite u. See *u.* septus.

Couvelaire u. A uterus with a bluish, purplish, coppery coloration, resembling an ovarian cyst with twisted pedicle; this appearance is due to premature separation of the placenta. Also called *uterine apoplexy, uteroplacental apoplexy.*

fetal u. One of defective development, in which the length of the cervical canal exceeds the length of the cavity of the body.

gravid u. A pregnant uterus.

infantile u. A uterus normally formed, but arrested in development.

pubescent u. An abnormality of the uterus in which the characters of that organ peculiar to the epoch preceding puberty persist in the adult.

retroflexion of u. See *retroflexion* of the uterus.

retroversion of u. See *retroversion* of the uterus.

sacculated u. A sacculation of the retroverted pregnant uterus at term.

u. acollis. A uterus in which the vaginal part is abnormally small or absent.

u. arcuatus. A subvariety of uterus bicornis in which there is merely a vertical depression in the middle of the fundus uteri.

u. bicornis. A uterus divided into two horns or compartments due to an arrest of development.

u. bilocularis. See *u.* septus.

u. didelphys. Double uterus from failure of the paramesonephric ducts to fuse. Syn., *u. duplex.*

u. duplex. A uterus that is double from failure of the paramesonephric ducts to unite.

u. masculinus. See *utricle,* 2.

u. parvicollis. A malformation described by Herman in which the vaginal portion is small but the body is normal. Also called *u. acollis.*

u. septus. A uterus in which a median septum more or less completely divides the lumen into halves.

u. unicornis. A uterus having but a single lateral half with usually only one uterine tube; it is the result of faulty development.

Uthoff, Wilhelm [*German ophthalmologist,* 1853–1927]. Described the nystagmus of multiple sclerosis; called *Uthoff's sign.*

u′tri·cle [L. *utriculus,* small skin]. 1. A delicate membranous sac communicating with the semicircular canals of the ear. 2. The uterus masculinus, or prostatic utricle; a vestigial blind pouch in the colliculus seminalis opening into the prostatic urethra. The homolog of a part of the female vagina; derived from the fused distal ends of the paramesonephric ducts. Syn., *utriculus masculinus, sinus pocularis.* See Plate 44. —**utric′-ular,** *adj.*

u·tric″u·li′tis [*utriculus;* G. *-itis,* inflammation]. Inflammation of the prostatic utricle.

u·tric″u·lo·sac′cu·lar [*utriculus;* L. *sacculus,* little sack]. Pertaining to the utricle and saccule of the ear.

u·tric′u·lus [L.]. Utricle.

u. masculinus. The uterus masculinus. See *utricle,* 2.

u′va ur′si (yōō′vuh ur′sigh) (*uva ursi*). The dried leaf of *Arctostaphylos Uva-ursi* or its varieties *coactylis* and *adenotricha.* Contains, besides tannic and gallic acids, quercetin, bitter extractive resin, gum, the glycosides arbutin (ursin) and methylarbutin. Also reported present are ursolic acid (urson), isoquercitrin, and hydroquinone, a decomposition product of arbutin. It has been used in the treatment of inflammations of the urinary tract.

u′ve·a [ML. from L. *uva,* grape]. The pigmented, vascular layer of the eye, the iris, ciliary body, and choroid. —**uveal,** *adj.*

u″ve·i′tis [*uva;* G. *-itis,* inflammation]. Inflammation of the uvea. —**uveit′ic,** *adj.*

u″ve·o·par″o·ti′tis. See uveoparotid *fever.*

uviol. Trade-mark for a glass which is transparent to a large part of the ultraviolet spectrum, as in uviol lamp, a lamp with uviol glass, for supplying ultraviolet rays.

u′vi·o·lize″ [L. *ultra,* beyond; *viola,* violet]. Submit to the action of ultraviolet rays. *Rare.*

u″vi·o·re·sist′ant (yōō″vee·o·ri·zist′unt) [*ultra; viola;* L. *resistere,* to oppose]. Not responding to ultraviolet rays.

u′vu·la [dim. from L. *uva,* grape]. The conical appendix hanging from the free edge of the soft palate, containing the uvular muscle covered by mucous membrane. —**uvular,** *adj.*

bifid u. Cleft uvula.

u. cerebelli. A small lobule of the inferior vermis of the cerebellum, forming the posterior boundary of the fourth ventricle.

u. fissa. Cleft uvula.

u. palatina. The uvula.

u. vermis. The uvula of the vermis; the uvula cerebelli.

u′vu·lae. The muscle of the uvula.

u″vu·lap·to′si·a, u″vu·lap·to′sis. See *uvuloptosis.*

u″vu·lec′to·my [*uva;* G. *ektomē,* excision]. Resection of the uvula.

u″vu·li′tis [*uva;* G. *-itis,* inflammation]. Inflammation of the uvula.

u″vu·lop·to′sis [*uva;* G. *ptōsis,* a falling]. A relaxed and pendulous condition of the uvula.

u′vu·lo·tome, u′vu·la·tome [*uva;* G. *tomos,* cutting]. An instrument used in uvulotomy.

u″vu·lot′o·my, u″vu·lat′o·my [*uva;* G. *tomē,* a cutting]. The operation of cutting off the uvula.

V

V Chemical symbol for vanadium.

V. Abbreviation for vision.

v, v. Volt.

vac′cin. See *vaccine.*

vac·ci′na (vack·sigh′nuh). See *vaccinia.*

vac′ci·na·ble [L. *vaccinus,* of cows]. Susceptible of successful vaccination.

vac′ci·nal (vack′si·nul) [*vaccinus*]. Pertaining to vaccination or to vaccine.

vac′ci·nate [*vaccinus*]. Perform a vaccination.

vac″ci·na′tion [*vaccinus*]. 1. Inoculation with the virus of vaccinia in order to protect against smallpox. 2. Inoculation with any organism to produce immunity against a given disease.

compulsory v. That legally required, as for admission to school or to a foreign country.

Jennerian v. See *vaccination,* 1.

vac′cine (vack′seen, ·sin) [*vaccinus*]. 1. Smallpox vaccine. 2. Any organism used for preventive inoculation against a specific disease.

acne v. One made from organisms cultured from the patient's lesions, or from a mixture of several strains of staphylococci or from the acne bacillus, *Corynebacterium acnes.*

anthrax v. Attenuated cultures of anthrax bacilli used to immunize animals against the disease.

autogenous v. A vaccine made from a culture obtained from the patient himself.

bacterial v. An emulsion of bacteria, killed, living, or attenuated, in normal salt solution used hypodermically for the purpose of raising the immune response of a patient suffering from infection by the same organism.

BCG v. (*B*acillus *C*almette-*G*uérin). One made from cultures of attenuated human tubercle bacilli, used orally to obtain immunity against tuberculosis. It has been suggested that the vaccine might also give some protection against leprosy. Also called *Calmette's v.*

bovine v. That derived from the cow.

brain-tissue v. One prepared from brain tissue.

brucella v. One obtained from *Brucella melitensis, abortus* or *suis:* used in the treatment of brucellosis.

Castañeda v. A vaccine against typhus fever prepared from lungs of mice infected with *Rickettsia prowazekii.*

cholera v. (*vaccinum cholerae*). A sterile suspension of killed cholera vibrios (*Vibrio comma*), of strains selected for high antigenic efficiency, in isotonic sodium chloride solution or other suitable diluent; it shall contain, in each cubic centimeter, at least 8,000,000,000 cholera organisms.

Cox v. A vaccine against classic epidemic typhus, prepared from *Rickettsia prowazekii* cultivated on the allantoic membrane of the developing chick embryo.

epidemic typhus v. Cox *v.;* Castañeda *v.*

Haffkine v. See Waldemar M. W. *Haffkine.*

heterogenous v. One prepared from organisms derived from some source other than the patient in whose treatment they are to be used; the source is usually a stock culture.

homologous v. See autogenous *v.*

humanized v. That obtained from vaccinal vesicles of man.

mixed v. A vaccine prepared from more than one species of bacteria.

multivalent v. See polyvalent *v.*

paratyphoid v. A vaccine made from cultures of *Salmonella schottmülleri* for immunization against paratyphoid.

pertussis v. One made from cultures of *Hemophilus pertussis,* used in the prevention and treatment of whooping cough.

poliomyelitis v. One prepared by cultivation of representative strains of 3 types of poliomyelitis virus, commonly in a monkey kidney tissue culture medium, followed by an inactivation treatment with formaldehyde: used to stimulate immunity against paralytic poliomyelitis in man.

polyvalent v. A bacterial vaccine made from cultures of two or more strains of the same species of bacteria.

rabies v. (*vaccinum rabies*). An uncontaminated suspension of the attenuated, diluted, dried or dead, fixed virus of rabies. The virus is obtained from the tissue of the central nervous system of an animal suffering from fixed virus rabies infection. Rabies vaccine is used exclusively as a prophylactic agent. By treatment with rabies vaccine after the bite of a rabid animal, immunity is often established before the incubation period of the disease is completed.

Rocky Mountain spotted-fever v. A prophylactic vaccine against Rocky Mountain spotted fever prepared from the supernatant fluid secured after grinding and centrifuging infected ticks: also called *Spencer-Parker vaccine.*

Salk v. Poliomyelitis *v.*

sensitized v. One prepared from killed microorganisms, to which has been added material containing homologous antibody material.

smallpox v. (*vaccinum variolae*). A glycerinated suspension of the vesicles of vaccinia or cowpox which have been obtained from healthy vaccinated bovine animals. Smallpox vaccine is used exclusively for the prevention of this disease. Also called *virus vaccinum, glycerinated v. virus, Jennerian v., antismallpox v.* Also see *vaccinia.*

Spencer-Parker v. See Rocky Mountain spotted-fever *v.*

staphylococcus v. One made from *Micrococcus pyogenes* var. *aureus* (*Staphylococcus aureus*), used in the treatment of furunculosis and other infections due to the organism.

stock v. A standard mixture of various bacteria.

streptococcus v. One made from the cultures of streptococci, used in treatment of infections due to the organism.

T.A.B. v. Typhoid-paratyphoid A and B vaccine.

triple v. for typhoid. Typhoid-paratyphoid A and B vaccine.

typhoid-paratyphoid A and B v. One containing organisms of typhoid, and paratyphoid A and B strains, for simultaneous immunization against all three diseases.

typhoid v. A sterile suspension of killed typhoid bacilli used to produce immunity against typhoid.

typhus v. See Cox *v.*, Castañeda *v.*

vac·cin'i·a (vack·sin'ee·uh) [*vaccinus*]. Cowpox, a contagious disease of cows characterized by vesicopustular lesions of the skin which are prone to appear on the teats and udder, and transmissible to man by handling infected cows and by vaccination; it confers immunity against smallpox. In the human subject inoculated with cowpox, a small papule appears at the site of inoculation in from one to three days, which becomes a vesicle about the fifth day, and at the end of the first week is pustular, umbilicated, and surrounded by a red areola. Desiccation begins in the second week and a scab forms, which soon falls off, leaving a white, pitted cicatrix.

vac·cin'i·fer (vack·sin'i·fur) [*vaccinus;* L. *ferre,* to bear]. 1. A person or animal from whom vaccine virus is taken. 2. A vaccine point.

vac·cin'i·form (vack·sin'i·form, vack'sin·i·form) [*vaccinus;* L. *forma,* form]. Resembling vaccinia.

vac·cin"i·o'la (vack·sin"ee·o'luh, vack"sin·eye'o-luh) [*vaccinus*]. A secondary eruption, sometimes following vaccinia, and resembling the eruption of smallpox.

vac'ci·noid [*vaccinus;* G. *eidos,* form]. Resembling vaccinia.

vac"ci·no·pho'bi·a [*vaccinus;* G. *phobos,* fear]. Morbid dread of vaccination.

vac'ci·no·style" (vack'sin·o·style", vack·sin'o·) [*vaccinus;* G. *stylos,* writing instrument]. A small, metallic lance formerly used in smallpox vaccination.

vac"ci·no·ther'a·py [*vaccinus;* G. *therapeia,* treatment]. The therapeutic use of vaccines.

vac'u·o·lar [dim. from L. *vacuum,* empty space]. Pertaining to, or of the nature of, a vacuole.

vac'u·o·late [*vacuum*]. Having, or pertaining to, vacuoles.

vac'u·o·la"ted [*vacuum*]. Containing one or more vacuoles; said of a cell or cytoplasm.

vac"u·o·la'tion [*vacuum*]. The formation of vacuoles; the state of being vacuolated.

vac'u·ole [*vacuum*]. A clear space in a cell.

contractile v. A vacuole in the cytoplasm of certain protozoa, which rhythmically and gradually increases in size and then collapses.

diffusion v. In the in vitro method of examining living cells, a minute droplet of the surrounding colored liquid which has been absorbed by the cell.

plasmocrin v. A crystalloid-filled vacuole in the cytoplasm of a secretory cell.

rhagiocrin v. A colloid-filled vacuole in the cytoplasm of a secretory cell.

vac"u·ol"i·za'tion. See *vacuolation.*

vac'u·ome [*vacuum;* G. *-ōma,* tumor]. The internal reticular apparatus, consisting of vacuoles found singly or forming a canalicular network near the centrosome and stainable with neutral red in living cells.

vac'u·um [L.]. A space from which most of the air has been exhausted.

high v. A vacuum in which the exhaustion of air has been extreme.

Torricellian v. The vacuum above the mercury in the tube of a barometer.

va′gal [L. *vagus*, wandering]. Pertaining to the vagus nerve.

va′gal at·tack′. A condition characterized by a feeling of impending death, dyspnea, cardiac discomfort, and a sinking sensation; supposed to be due to vasomotor spasm.

va′gal es·cape′. One or more spontaneous beats of the heart, occurring in spite of the fact that the function of the sinus node that normally initiates heart beats has been arrested by stimulation of the vagus nerve.

va·gi′na (pl. *vaginas, vaginae*) [L., sheath, vagina]. 1. A sheath. 2. The musculomembranous canal from the vulvar opening to the cervix uteri, ensheathing the latter and the penis during copulation. See Plates 41, 43. —**vag′inal,** *adj.*

mucosa of v. The mucous membrane lining the vagina.

septate v. One more or less completely divided by a longitudinal septum; a congenital abnormality.

v. dentis. Fleshy sheath surrounding the fang in venomous snakes.

v. masculina. See *utricle*, 2.

vag″i·na·lec′to·my. See *vaginectomy*, 2.

va·gi′na·pex″y. See *colpopexy.*

vag″i·nec′to·my (vadj″i·neck′to·mee) [*vagina;* G. *ektomē*, excision]. 1. Excision of the vagina or a portion of it. 2. Excision of the tunica vaginalis.

vag″i·nic′o·line. [*vagina;* G. *colere*, to inhabit]. Living in the vagina, as an animalcule.

vag″i·nif′er·ous (vadj″i·nif′ur·us) [*vagina;* L. *ferre*, to bear]. Producing, or bearing, a vagina.

vag″i·nis′mus (vadj″i·niz′mus, ·nis′mus) [*vagina*]. Painful spasm of the vagina.

mental v. That due to extreme aversion to the sexual act.

perineal v. That due to spasm of the perineal muscles.

posterior v. That due to spasm of the pubococcygeal portion of the levator ani muscle.

vag″i·ni′tis (vadj″i·nigh′tis) [*vagina;* G. *-itis*, inflammation]. 1. Inflammation of the vagina. 2. Inflammation of a sheath.

atrophic v. Inflammation of the vagina occurring after the menopause, surgical or other.

circumscribed v. Inflammation of the mucosa of the vagina which is enclosed in or confined to a certain area of the vagina.

emphysematous v. That characterized by vesicles which contain a gaseous material. Syn., *emphysematous colpitis, colpohyperplasia cystica.*

exfoliative v. That characterized by a peeling away or shedding of large fragments of the surface tissue.

gonococcic v. That caused by infection with gonococci: usually seen only before puberty.

senile v. Inflammation of the vagina occurring after the menopause: properly called *atrophic v.*

Trichomonas vaginalis v. Vaginitis associated with, and thought to be caused by, *Trichomonas vaginalis.*

vag′i·no- (vadj′i·no-), **vagin-** [*vagina*]. A combining form denoting *the vagina.*

vag′i·no·cele. Colpocele.

vag″i·no·dyn′i·a [*vagina;* G. *odynē*, pain]. Neuralgic pain of the vagina.

vag″i·no·fix·a′tion [*vagina;* L. *fixum*, from *figere*, to fix]. Fixation of the uterus to the vagina.

vag″i·no·my·co′sis (vadj″i·no·migh·ko′sis, va·jy″-no·) [*vagina;* G. *mykēs*, fungus; *-ōsis*, condition]. A fungus infection of the vagina, usually by *Candida albicans.*

vag′i·no·plas″ty (vadj′i·no·plas″tee, va·jy′no·, vadj″i·no·plas′tee) [*vagina;* G. *plassein*, to form]. A plastic operation on the vagina.

vag′i·no·scope (vadj′i·no·scope, va·jy′no·) [*vagina;* G. *skopein*, to examine]. A vaginal speculum.

vag″i·nos′co·py [*vagina; skopein*]. Inspection of the vagina.

vag″i·not′o·my [*vagina;* G. *tomē*, a cutting]. Incision of the vagina; colpotomy.

va·gi′tus [L., a crying]. The cry of an infant.

v. uterinus. The cry of a child while still in the uterus.

v. vaginalis. The cry of a child while the head is still in the vagina.

va·got′o·mized [L. *vagus*, wandering; G. *tomē*, a cutting]. Having had the vagus nerves severed.

va·got′o·my [*vagus; tomē*]. Division of the vagus nerve.

va″go·to′ni·a [*vagus;* G. *tonos*, tension]. A condition due to overaction of the vagus nerves and modification of functions in organs innervated by them. —**vagoton′ic,** *adj.*

va·got′o·nin, vag″o·to′nin [*vagus; tonos*]. A hormonal substance from the pancreas which stimulates the parasympathetic system.

va″go·trop′ic (vay″go·trop′ick, vag″o·) [*vagus;* G. *trepein*, to turn]. Having an effect upon, or influencing, the vagus nerve.

va′grant [OF. *waucrant*]. Wandering, as a vagrant cell.

va′gus (pl. *vagi*) [L., wandering]. The tenth cranial nerve; a mixed nerve whose motor fibers arise in the nucleus ambiguus and are distributed to the muscles of larynx and pharynx; parasympathetic fibers from the dorsal motor nucleus of the vagus are widely distributed to autonomic ganglia to function in the regulation of motor and secretory activities of the abdominal and thoracic viscera. Somatic sensory fibers go to the skin of the external auditory meatus and the meninges, and visceral sensory fibers reach the pharynx, larynx, and thoracic and abdominal viscera. Formerly called the *pneumogastric nerve.* See Table of Nerves in the Appendix.

va′gus·stoff. Substance liberated at the terminations of the fibers of the vagus nerve that depresses heart action; now believed to be similar to, or identical with, acetylcholine.

va′lence, va′len·cy [L. *valere*, to be strong]. 1. The capacity of an atom to combine with other atoms in definite proportions. 2. By analogy, also applied to radicals and atomic groups. Valence is measured with the combining capacity of a hydrogen atom taken as unity. —**valent,** *adj.*

coordinate v. Covalence in which one atom or ion contributes both electrons of the pair, and the other atom or ion supplies no electrons.

covalence. The sharing of valence electrons between atoms.

residual v. forces. The unsatisfied forces of ions or molecules which lead to formation of more complex substances from apparently saturated ions or molecules.

Valentin, Gabriel Gustav [*German physician,* 1810–83]. Described, with Purkinje, motion of the cilia of epithelial cells (1835). Named the nucleolus of the cell nucleus (1836).

Valentin's bodies. Small amyloid bodies in nerve tissue. Also called *Valentin's corpuscles.*

Valentin's ganglion. A small ganglionlike enlargement at the junction of the posterior and middle superior alveolar nerves.

Valentine, Ferdinand C. [*American surgeon,* 1851–1909]. Known for his description of a position used in ureteral irrigation. With the patient supine, the hips are flexed by means of a double inclined plane.

val′er·ate. A salt of valeric acid. Also called *valerianate.*

acid ammonium v. (*ammonii valeras acidus*). $NH_4C_5H_9O_2.2HC_5H_9O_2$; occurs as colorless, quadrangular plates; 1 Gm. dissolves in about 0.3 cc. of water and in about 0.6 cc. of alcohol. It has been used as a nerve sedative and euphoric. Also called *ammonium valerianate.*

va·le′ri·an [*valere*] (*valeriana*). The dried rhizome and roots of *Valeriana officinalis.* Contains a volatile oil which consists chiefly of formic, acetic, butyric, and valeric acid esters of borneol, with small amounts of pinene and camphene. The alkaloids valerine and chatinine have also been reported present. It has been used in treatment of hysteria, hypochondriasis, nervous unrest, and similar emotional states. Its action is believed to be psychic due to its strong, persistent odor.

va·le′ri·a·nate. Valerate.

ammonium v. Acid ammonium valerate.

va·ler′ic ac′id (va·lerr′ick, va·leer′ick), **va·le″ri·an′ic ac′id.** $C_5H_{10}O_2$. Four isomeric modifications of this acid are known: 1. Normal valeric or propylacetic acid, $CH_3(CH_2)_3COOH$. 2. Isovaleric or isopropylacetic acid, $(CH_3)_2CH.$-$CH_2.COOH$, the valeric acid of commerce. 3. Methylethylacetic acid, $CH_3(C_2H_5).CH.COOH$. 4. Trimethylacetic acid, $(CH_3)_3C.COOH$.

val′er·o-, valer- [*valere*]. A combining form denoting *valeric.*

val″e·tu″di·na′ri·an [L. *valetudinarius*, sickly]. An invalid.

val″e·tu″di·na′ri·an·ism [*valetudinarius*]. Feeble or infirm state due to invalidism.

val′goid [L. *valgus*, bowlegged; G. *eidos*, form]. Resembling valgus. *Rare.*

val′gus [L.]. A term denoting position; if of the foot it means eversion (talipes valgus); if of the knee it can mean either bowlegged, old term, or knock-kneed, modern usage (genu valgum); if of the hip it refers to an increase in the angle between the neck and the shaft of the femur (coxa valga); if of the great toe it denotes a turning of that toe toward the other toes (hallux valgus). If the term is used alone it generally refers to the foot.

val′ine (val′een, ·in, vay′leen, ·lin). $(CH_3)_2CHCH$-$(NH_2)COOH$; α-aminoisovaleric acid, an amino-acid constituent of many proteins. It is essential to man, as well as to certain animals.

val′late [L. *vallare*, to surround with a rampart]. Surrounded by a walled depression; cupped.

val·lec′u·la (pl. *valleculae*) [dim. from L. *valles*, valley]. A shallow groove or depression.

v. cerebelli. The depression between the cerebellar hemispheres.

v. epiglottica. A depression between the lateral and median glossoepiglottic folds on each side.

v. linguae. See *v.* epiglottica.

v. unguis. The depression in the skin for the root of the nail.

Valleix, François Louis Isidore [*French physician*, 1807–55]. Described tender points found in the course of certain nerves in peripheral neuralgias where they pass through openings in fascia or issue from bony canals; called *Valleix's points douloureux.* See *cachectic aphthae* under *aphtha.*

Vallet's mass. See ferrous carbonate *mass.*

Valsalva, Antonio Maria [*Italian anatomist*, 1666–1723]. Described the tympanic antrum, called *Valsalva's antrum.* The ligaments of the pinna or ligamenta auricularia are also called *Valsalva's ligaments.* He tested the patency of the auditory tubes by the maneuver of inflating the tympanic cavity by holding the mouth and nose while forcible expiratory efforts are made; called *Valsalva's test.* See also aortic *sinus.*

Valsuani, Emilio [*Italian physician*, nineteenth century]. Described progressive pernicious anemia in pregnant and lactating women (1870), called *Valsuani's disease.*

valve [L. *valva*, leaf of a door]. A device in a vessel or passage which prevents reflux of its contents.

anal valves. Valvelike folds in anal mucous membrane which join together the lower ends of the rectal columns.

aortic v. One consisting of three semilunar cusps situated at the junction of the aorta and the left ventricle of the heart.

atrioventricular valves. The mitral and tricuspid valves of the heart.

auriculoventricular valves. See *atrioventricular valves* under *valve.*

bicuspid v. See mitral *v.* See Plate 5.

caval v. The semilunar valve in the right atrium of the heart between the orifice of the inferior vena cava and the right atrioventricular orifice. Syn., *eustachian v., inferior vena caval v.*

colic v. See ileocecal *v.*

congenital urethral v. Modified folds of the mucous membrane of the prostatic urethra which frequently give rise to urinary obstruction.

coronary v. A semicircular fold of the endocardium of the right atrium at the orifice of the coronary sinus. Syn., *Thebesian v.*

eustachian, Eustachian v. See caval *v.*

Gerlach's v. A mucosal fold sometimes surrounding the orifice of the appendix.

Hasner's v. The slitlike opening of the nasolacrimal duct into the inferior meatus of the nose. Also called *plica lacrimalis.*

Houston's valves. Three transverse semilunar folds in the mucous membrane of the rectum.

ileocecal v. The valve at the junction of the terminal ileum and the cecum which consists of a superior and inferior lip and partially prevents reflux from the cecum into the ileum. Syn., *colic v.* Also called *ileocolic v.* Formerly called *Bauhin's v.*

ileocolic v. See ileocecal *v.*

inferior vena caval v. See caval *v.*

mitral v. One containing two cusps, situated between the left atrium and left ventricle. Syn., *bicuspid v.* See Plate 5.

pulmonary v. One consisting of three semilunar cusps situated between the right ventricle and the pulmonary artery.

pyloric v. The fold of mucous membrane at the pyloric end of the stomach together with the underlying pyloric sphincter, a thickened ring of smooth muscle.

rectal valves. See *Houston's valves* under *valve.*

semilunar valves. The valves situated between the ventricles and the aorta or the pulmonary artery. See Plate 5.

spiral v. Coiled mucomembranous folds in the neck of the urinary bladder and cystic duct. Also called *Heister's v.*

Thebesian v. See coronary *v.*

tricuspid v. The three-cusped valve situated between the right atrium and right ventricle. See Plate 5.

utriculoendolymphatic v. That part of the wall of the utriculus which overlies the expansion of the utriculosaccular duct and guards its opening into the utriculus.

v. of the navicular fossa. A mucous membrane fold sometimes occurring in the roof of the navicular fossa of the urethra. Also called *Guérin's v.*

v. of the sinus venosus. One of the right and left folds of the opening of the sinus venosus into the right atrium found in the embryonic heart. The right disappears. The left forms the crista terminalis and portions of the valve of the inferior vena cava and of the valve of the coronary sinus.

v. of Vieussens. See anterior medullary *velum.*

val·vot′o·my [*valva;* G. *tomē*, a cutting]. Surgical incision into a valve, especially one of the rectal folds. Syn., *diclidotomy*.

val′vu·la (pl. *valvulae*) [dim. from *valva*]. A valve. —**valvular,** *adj*.

v. coli. Ileocecal valve.

valvulae conniventes. See *circular folds* under *fold*. Also called *valves of Kerckring*.

v. processus vermiformis. A fold of mucous membrane at the opening of the appendiceal canal.

val″vu·li′tis [*valva;* G. *-itis*, inflammation]. Inflammation of a valve, especially of a cardiac valve.

val′vu·lo·tome [*valva;* G. *tomos*, cutting]. An instrument designed especially for incising the valves of the heart.

val″vu·lot′o·my [*valva;* G. *tomē*, a cutting]. The surgical incision of a valve of the heart, as in mitral stenosis.

val′yl. The univalent radical, $(CH_3)_2CHCH(HN_2)$-CO—, of the amino acid valine.

val′zin. See *dulcin*.

vam′pire [F., from the Slavic]. 1. In worldwide folk belief, a living corpse that rises from its grave at night and sucks the blood of the living. 2. A blood-sucking bat, belonging to the family Phyllostomidae, found in South and Central America and along the southern border of the United States.

vam′pir·ism. 1. Belief in vampires, 1. 2. The acts or practice of vampires; blood sucking. 3. Necrophilism. *Obs*.

van′a·date. A salt of vanadic acid.

va·nad′ic ac′id (va·nad′ick, va·nay′dick). H_3VO_4. An acid derived from vanadium; forms salts called vanadates.

va·na′di·um [ON. *Vanadīs*, a goddess]. V = 50.95. A rare metallic element.

va·na′di·um·ism [*vanadīs*]. A chronic form of intoxication due to the absorption of vanadium; it occurs in workers using the metal or its compounds.

Van Allen, Chester Montague [*American physician*, 1896–   ]. Introduced a glass tube used in measuring blood platelet volume; called *thrombocytocrit, Van Allen's thrombocytocrit*.

Van de Graaff, Robert Jemison (1901–   ). American physicist who invented a high-voltage electrostatic generator using a high-speed belt as a charge conveyer. Such generators, often called *Van de Graaff generators*, are used for research in nuclear physics and as a source of high-voltage x-rays and cathode rays for radiation therapy, food sterilization, and industrial radiography.

van den Bergh's test. See under *test*.

Vanghetti, Giuliano [*Italian orthopedic surgeon*, 1861–1940]. Remembered for his experimental work which introduced cineplastic amputations.

Van Gieson's stain. See under *stain*.

Van Hook, Weller [*American surgeon*, 1862–1933]. Pioneer in end-to-side ureteral anastomosis; called *Van Hook's operation*.

va·nil′la [Sp. *vainilla*, from L. *vagina*, sheath] (*vanilla*). The cured, full-grown, unripe fruit of *Vanilla planifolia*, or *V. tahitensis*. The fresh fruit possesses none of the pleasant odor commonly associated with the fruit. Two enzymes, under the influence of gentle heat and moisture, produce vanillin from two of three glycosides, and perhaps another aromatic substance from a third glycoside. The two glycosides are reported to be glucovanillic alcohol and glycovanillin. The third glycoside, which on hydrolysis yields an ether of strong and pleasant odor, is yet unnamed. Of the enzymes present, one is an oxidase, the other a hydrolyzing enzyme. The flavor of vanilla is probably enhanced by the presence of other aromatic substances. Vanilla is used solely as a flavoring agent. Also called *vanilla bean*.

va·nil′lic ac′id. $CH_3O.C_6H_3(OH)COOH$. 3-Methoxy-4-hydroxybenzoic acid; the crystalline solid resulting from the oxidation of vanillin.

van′il·lin, va·nil′lin (*vanillinum*). $CH_3.C_6H_3$-(OH)CHO. 3-Methoxy-4-hydroxybenzaldehyde; occurs as fine, white to slightly yellow crystals; 1 Gm. dissolves in about 100 cc. of water; it is freely soluble in alcohol. Used as a flavoring agent in place of vanilla.

va·nil′lism [*vainilla*]. A form of contact dermatitis characterized by marked itching; occurring among vanilla workers.

Van Millingen, Edwin [*English ophthalmologist*, 1851–1900]. Devised an operation for trichiasis, in which he covered the wound by mucosa from the patient's lips instead of with skin; called *Van Millingen's operation*.

Van Slyke, Donald Dexter [*American chemist*, 1883–   ]. Devised a test of renal function based upon the rate of urea excretion in the urine as compared with the blood urea concentration; called *blood urea clearance test, Van Slyke's test*. Various modifications of this have been introduced by Austin and McLean. Inventor of a graduated glass buret connected with a mercury leveling bulb, used in volumetric determination of blood gases; called *Van Slyke's apparatus*. Devised, with Cullen, a method of determining alkali reserve; see Van Slyke and Cullen's *method*. Also see Van Slyke's *method* for chlorides, Van Slyke's *method* for acetone bodies, Austin and Van Slyke's *method*, McLean and Van Slyke's *method*, Van Slyke titration *method*, Van Slyke and Kirk *method*, Van Slyke and Neill *method*, Van Slyke and Palmer *method*, Van Slyke, MacFayden, and Hamilton ninhydrin *method*.

van't Hoff's factor i. See under *factor*.

vapex. Trade-mark for a proprietary inhalant, used in coryza, laryngitis, etc.

va″po·cau″ter·i·za′tion [L. *vapor*, steam; *kautērion*, branding iron]. Cauterization by live steam.

va′por [L.]. A gas, especially the gaseous form of a substance which at ordinary temperatures is liquid or solid.

va·po′res u″te·ri′ni. [L.]. Hysteria. *Obs*.

va′por·ish [*vapor*]. 1. Of the nature of vapor. 2. Given to periods of depression or hysteria. *Obs*.

va″por·i·za′tion [*vapor*]. The conversion of a solid or liquid into a vapor. —**va′porize,** *v*.

va′por·i″zer [*vapor*]. An atomizer.

va′pors [*vapor*]. Lowness of spirits; hysteria. *Obs*.

va″po·ther′a·py [*vapor;* G. *therapeia*, treatment]. The therapeutic employment of medicated or nonmedicated vapors, steam, or sprays.

Vaquez, Louis Henri [*French physician*, 1860–1936]. Described small painful nodules in the fingertips found in bacterial endocarditis, called *Osler-Vaquez' nodes*. See primary *polycythemia*.

va″ri·a·bil′i·ty [L. *variabilis*, changeable]. The property of organisms which results in differences among members of the same species, so that no two are alike in all their characteristics.

va′ri·a·ble [*variabilis*]. *In biometry*, a quantity or magnitude which may vary in value under differing conditions. Also see *curve*, 2.

va′ri·ance [L. *variantia*, diversity]. The square of the standard deviation. The second moment when deviations are taken from the mean.

va′ri·ant [L. *variare*, to diversify]. *In bacteriology*, a colony which differs in appearance from the parent colony grown on the same mediums.

va″ri·a′tion [*variare*]. Deviation from a given type as the result of environment, natural selection, or cultivation and domestication; diversity in characteristics among related organisms.

bacterial phase v. The alternation of the flagella

of many Gram-negative bacteria between two antigenic constituents. Phase I was formerly considered to be species specific, and phase II to be group specific.

bacterial v. A hereditary deviation from the modal form of a particular bacterium with regard to morphology, biochemical reactions, pigment production, colonial characteristics, virulence, or toxigenicity. See also *colony*.

biological v. Inherent differences between individuals who, for most purposes, are considered to be within a homogeneous group.

continuous variations. A series of minute variations.

double v. The double current produced in a muscle by the passage of a single induction shock.

meristic variations. Variations in the number of parts.

negative v. The diminution of the muscle current during tetanic contraction.

sampling v. *In biostatistics*, variation in the estimates of some biostatistical value, e.g. mean, between different samples of, or from, the same universe.

var″i·ca′tion [L. *varix*, dilated vein]. 1. The formation of a varix. 2. A system of varices.

var″i·cec′to·my [*varix;* G. *ektomē*, excision]. Excision of a varix or varicose vein, as distinguished from avulsion of a vein.

var″i·cel′la [L. *varius*, various]. Chickenpox.

pustular v. A form of varicella marked by lesions which become pustular.

v. gangraenosa. Varicella in which the eruption leads to a gangrenous ulceration.

v. inoculata. Vaccination of susceptibles with the clear vesicular fluid from varicella lesions.

var″i·cel·la′tion [*varius*]. Preventive inoculation with the virus of varicella.

var″i·cel′li·form [*varius;* G. *forma*, form]. Characterized by vesicles resembling those of varicella.

var″i·cel′loid [*varius;* G. *eidos*, form]. Resembling varicella.

var′i·ces (vair′i·seez, var′i·seez). Plural of varix.

va·ric′i·form (va·riss′i·form, var′i·si·) [L. *varix*, dilated vein; *forma*, form]. Having the form of a varix.

var″i·co·bleph′a·ron [L. *varicosus*, full of dilated veins, from *varix;* G. *blepharon*, eyelid]. A varicosity of an eyelid.

var′i·co·cele″ [*varicosus;* G. *kēlē*, tumor]. Dilatation of the veins of the pampiniform plexus of the spermatic cord, forming a soft, elastic swelling.

ovarian v. Varicosity of the veins of an ovary.

utero-ovarian v. A varicose condition of the veins of the pampiniform plexus in the broad ligament.

var″i·co·ce·lec′to·my [*varicosus; kēlē;* G. *ektomē*, excision]. Excision of dilated spermatic veins, with or without removal of a portion of the scrotum, for the radical cure of varicocele.

var″i·cog′ra·phy [*varicosus;* G. *graphein*, to write]. Roentgenographic visualization of the course and extent of a collection of varicose veins.

var′i·coid [L. *varix*, dilated vein; G. *eidos*, form]. Resembling a varix.

var″ic·om′pha·lus [*varix;* G. *omphalos*, navel]. A varicosity at the navel.

var″i·co·phle·bi′tis [L. *varicosus*, full of dilated veins; G. *phleps*, vein; *-itis*, inflammation]. Inflammation of a varicose vein or veins.

var′i·cose [*varicosus*]. 1. Descriptive of blood vessels that are dilated, knotted, and tortuous. 2. Due to varicose veins, as varicose ulcer.

var″i·co′sis [*varicosus;* G. *-ōsis*, condition]. A constant abnormal dilatation of the veins.

var″i·cos′i·ty [*varicosus*]. A varicose portion of a vein, usually of definite and limited extent.

var″i·cot′o·my [*varicosus;* G. *tomē*, a cutting]. Excision of a varicose vein.

va·ric′u·la [dim. from L. *varix*, dilated vein]. A varix of the conjunctiva.

varidase. Trade-marked name for a purified mixture of streptokinase and streptodornase, enzymes elaborated by hemolytic streptococci. The mixed enzymes cause liquefaction and removal of necrotic tissue and thickened or clotted exudates resulting from wounds or inflammatory processes, thereby promoting normal repair of tissue.

va·ri′e·ty [L. *varietas*, difference]. A subdivision of a species; a stock, strain, breed.

va′ri·form [L. *varius*, various; *forma*, form]. Having diversity of form.

va·ri′o·la (va·rye′o·luh, va·ree′) [L.]. Smallpox.

v. minor. A form of smallpox due probably to a less virulent strain. It has a long incubation period, and the eruptions do not become pustular.

v. notha. Varicella.

v. vera. True smallpox as distinguished from varioloid.

va·ri′o·lar, va·ri′o·lous [L. *varius*, various]. Pertaining to smallpox.

var′i·o·late (vair′ee·o·late, var′ee·o·) [*varius*]. Having small pustules like those of variola.

var″i·o·la′tion (vair″ee·o·lay′shun, var″ee·o·) [*varius*]. Inoculation of unmodified smallpox, usually from human to human; practice forbidden in most countries. —**variolate,** *v.*

var″i·ol′ic (vair″ee·ol′ick, var″ee·) [*varius*]. Pocky, variolous. Referring to lesions similar to those in smallpox.

var″i·o′li·form (vair″ee·o′li·form, ·ol′i·form, var″-ee·, va·ree′o·li·form) [*varius;* L. *forma*, form]. Resembling variola.

var″i·o·li·za′tion (vair″ee·o·li·zay′shun, ·lye·zay′-shun, var″ee·o·, va·ree″o·). See *variolation*.

var′i·o·loid (vair′ee·o·loyd, var′ee·o·) [*varius;* G. *eidos*, form]. A mild form of smallpox following the injection of smallpox virus in persons who previously had been successfully vaccinated or who previously had the disease.

va·ri″o·lo·vac′cine (va·rye″o·lo·vack′seen, ·sin, va·ree″o·lo·) [*varius;* L. *vaccinus*, of cows]. A vaccine obtained from the lymph in lesions produced in a heifer inoculated with smallpox virus. The virus may also be cultivated in a chick embryo by chorioallantoic inoculation.

va·ri″o·lo·vac·cin′i·a [*varius; vaccinus*]. A form of vaccinia or cowpox induced in a heifer by inoculating it with smallpox virus.

var′ix (vair′icks, var′icks) (pl. *varices*) [L.]. A dilated and tortuous vein. See *cirsoid, cirsotomy*.

aneurysmal v. See arteriovenous *aneurysm* (a).

chyle v. A varix of a vessel which transports chyle. A complicated procedure may produce chylocele, chyluria, chylous ascites, or chylous diarrhea.

papillary v. A benign cutaneous tumor consisting of a single dilated blood vessel: occurs after middle age. Syn. *angioma senile, Cayenne-pepper spot*.

v. lymphaticus. Dilatation of the lymphatic vessels, especially that due to the *Filaria sanguinis hominis*.

Varolio, Constanzo [*Italian anatomist*, 1543–75]. Author of an early study of the optic nerve (1573). Described the pons of the brain, also called *pons Varoli*.

va′rus [L., knock-kneed]. A term denoting position; if of the foot it means inversion (talipes varus) or adduction (metatarsus varus); if of the knee it means bowlegged (genu varum); if of the hip it refers to a decrease in the angle between the neck and the shaft of the femur (coxa vara);

if of the great toe it denotes a turning of that toe away from the other toes (hallux varus). Used alone the term generally refers to the foot.

vas (pl. *vasa*) [L.]. A vessel.

vasa aberrantia hepatis. Remnants of the bile ducts in atrophied liver substance sometimes persisting from fetal life, in the left lobe of the liver.

vasa brevia. The gastric branches of the splenic artery. See Table of Arteries in the Appendix.

v. afferens. An afferent lymphatic vessel of a lymph node.

v. afferens glomeruli. The arteriole supplying the capillary loops in a renal corpuscle.

vasa praevia. Presentation of the velamentous vessels across the internal os, seen with a low implantation of the placenta.

vasa vasorum. The blood vessels supplying the walls of arteries and veins having a caliber greater than 1 mm. See Plate 6.

v. deferens. The excretory duct of the testis; the ductus deferens (BNA).

v. efferens. An efferent lymphatic vessel of a lymph node.

v. efferens glomeruli. The precapillary draining the capillary loops in a renal corpuscle.

v. prominens. One of the capillary loops in the ridge of connective tissue which lies above the line of attachment of the basilar membrane to the spiral ligament and extends throughout the cochlea.

v. spirale. The largest of the blood vessels which lie in the connective tissue on the under surface of the basilar membrane.

vas′cu·lar [L. *vasculum*, small vessel]. Consisting of, pertaining to, or provided with, vessels.

vas′cu·lar bed. The total blood supply—arteries, capillaries, and veins—of an organ or region.

cognate v. b. A region normally supplied by a specified artery; contrasted to collateral vascular bed.

vas″cu·lar′i·ty [*vasculum*]. The quality of being vascular.

vas″cu·lar·i·za′tion [*vasculum*]. 1. The process of becoming vascular. 2. The formation and extension of vascular capillaries.

vas″cu·li′tis. See *angiitis*.

vas″cu·lo·gen′e·sis [*vasculum;* G. *genesis*, production]. The formation of the vascular system.

vas·ec′to·my [L. *vas*, vessel; G. *ektomē*, excision]. Resection of the ductus deferens.

vaseline. Trade-mark for a petroleum jelly and certain other products.

vas′i·cine (vass′i·seen, ·sin). *l*-Peganine.

vas″i·fac′tion [*vas;* L. *facere*, to make]. The process of giving rise to new blood vessels.

vas″i·for·ma′tion [*vas;* L. *formare*, to form]. The process by which a structure assumes the appearance of a vessel or duct.

vas·i′tis [*vas;* G. *-itis*, inflammation]. Inflammation of the vas or ductus deferens.

vas′o- (vass′o-, vay′zo-, vay′so-, vaz′o-, vah′zo-), **vas-** [*vas*]. A combining form signifying *the blood vessels, ductus deferens*, or *vasomotor*.

vas″o·con·stric′tion [*vas;* L. *constringere*, to bind]. The constriction of blood vessels.

vas″o·con·stric′tive [*vas; constringere*]. Promoting or stimulating constriction of blood vessels.

vas″o·con·stric′tor [*vas; constringere*]. A nerve or a drug that causes constriction of blood vessels. —**vasoconstric′tor,** *adj.*

vas″o·de·pres′sor [*vas;* L. *deprimere*, to press down]. Lowering blood pressure by relaxing the blood vessels.

vas″o·dil″a·ta′tion (vay″zo·dil″uh·tay′shun, ·dye″luh·tay′shun, vay″so·) [*vas;* L. *dilatare*, to dilate]. Dilatation of the blood vessels.

vas″o·di·la′tin (·dye·lay′tin, ·di·lay′tin) [*vas; dilatare*]. A widely distributed substance which lowers the blood pressure and stimulates gastric secretion. The substance is believed to be identical with histamine.

vas″o·di·la′tor [*vas; dilatare*]. 1. Pertaining to the relaxation of the smooth muscle of the vascular system. 2. Producing dilatation of blood vessels. —**vasodilator,** *n.*

vas″o·ep″i·did″y·mos′to·my (vaz″o·ep″i·did″i·mos′to·mee, vah″zo·) [*vas;* G. *epididymis*, epididymis; *stoma*, mouth]. Anastomosis of a ductus deferens with its epididymal duct.

vas″o·for·ma′tion [*vas;* L. *formare*, to form]. The process in which blood vessels are produced or formed.

vas″o·form′a·tive [*vas; formare*]. Forming or producing vessels.

va·sog′ra·phy [*vas;* G. *graphein*, to write]. Roentgenography of blood vessels.

vas″o·hy″per·ton′ic. Vasoconstrictor, *adj.*

vas″o·hy″po·ton′ic. See *vasodilator*, 1.

vas″o·in·hib′i·tor [*vas;* L. *inhibere*, to check]. A drug or agent tending to inhibit the action of the vasomotor nerves. —**vasoinhibitory,** *adj.*

vas″o·li·ga′tion (vaz″o·lye·gay′shun, vah″zo·) [*vas;* L. *ligare*, to bind]. Surgical ligation of a ductus deferens.

vas″o·mo′tion (vay″zo·mo′shun, vay″so·) [*vas;* L. *motum*, from *movere*, to move]. Increase or decrease of the caliber of a blood vessel.

vas″o·mo′tor [*vas; movere*]. Regulating the contraction (vasoconstriction) and expansion (vasodilatation) of blood vessels.

vas″o·mo·to′ri·al, vas″o·mo′tor·y [*vas; movere*]. Relating to, or capable of effecting, vasomotion.

vas″o·mo″to·tro″pho·neu·ro′sis. Old term for *angioneurosis*.

vas″o·mo·tric′i·ty [*vas; movere*]. The qualities of vasomotor action.

vas″o·neu·ro′sis [*vas;* G. *neuron*, nerve; *-ōsis*, condition]. Angioneurosis.

vas″o-or″chid·os′to·my (vaz″o-or″kid·os′to·mee, vah″zo-) [*vas;* G. *orchis*, testis; *stoma*, mouth]. Surgical anastomosis of a ductus deferens with any portion of its testis.

vas″o·pa·ral′y·sis [*vas;* G. *paralysis*, paralysis]. Paralysis of vasomotor mechanism.

vas″o·pa·re′sis [*vas;* G. *paresis*, slackening]. Paresis affecting the vasomotor nerves.

vas″o·pres′sin. The pressor principle of the posterior pituitary. Also called *beta-hypophamine.* See *pitressin.*

vas″o·punc′ture (vaz″o·punk′chur, vah″zo·) [*vas;* L. *punctura*, a pricking]. Surgical puncture of a ductus deferens.

vas″o·re″lax·a′tion [*vas;* L. *relaxare*, to loosen]. Diminution of vascular tension.

vas·or′rha·phy (vaz·or′uh·fee, vahz·) [*vas;* G. *rhaphē*, suture]. End-to-end or end-to-side suture of a ductus deferens or of a blood vessel.

vas″o·sec′tion [*vas;* L. *sectio*, a cutting]. Severing of a ductus deferens.

vas′o·spasm [*vas;* G. *spasmos*, spasm]. Vasoconstriction, angiospasm.

vas″o·spas′tic [*vas;* G. *span*, to draw]. Angiospastic.

vas″o·stim′u·lant [*vas;* L. *stimulare*, to rouse up]. Inducing or exciting vasomotor action.

vas·os′to·my (va·zos′to·mee, va·sos′to·mee) [*vas;* G. *stoma*, mouth]. The making of an artificial opening into a ductus deferens.

vas·ot′o·my (va·zot′o·mee, va·sot′o·mee) [*vas;* G. *tomē*, a cutting]. Incision of a ductus deferens.

vas″o·ton′ic [*vas;* G. *tonikos*, stretching]. Pertaining to the normal tone or tension of the blood vessels.

vas″o·ton′ic. A vasostimulant.

vas″o·to′nin [*vas;* G. *tenein,* to stretch]. A vasoconstrictor substance present in the blood.

vas′o·tribe. See *angiotribe.*

vas″o·troph′ic (vay″zo·trof′ick, ·tro′fick, vay″so·) [*vas;* G. *trophē,* nourishment]. Concerned in the nutrition of blood vessels.

vas″o·va′gal [*vas;* L. *vagus,* wandering]. Pertaining to the blood vessels and vagus nerve, as paroxysmal vasovagal attacks, or vasovagal syncope.

vas″o·va′gal at·tack′. Loss of consciousness, marked pallor, usually a drop in heart rate and rapid fall in blood pressure, occasionally profuse sweating; due to exaggerated vagal action through abnormal sensitivity of the carotid sinus. If it occurs in epileptiform diseases, it is called **paroxysmal vasovagal attack.** Also see carotid sinus *syncope.*

vas″o·vas·os′to·my [*vas; vas;* G. *stoma,* mouth]. Surgical anastomosis of one portion of a ductus deferens to another.

vas″o·ve·sic″u·lec′to·my [*vas;* L. *vesicula,* vesicle; G. *ektomē,* excision]. Excision of a ductus deferens and seminal vesicle.

vasoxyl hydrochloride. Trade-marked name for the pressor substance methoxamine hydrochloride.

Vassale, Giulio [*Italian physiologist,* 1862–1912]. With E. Sacchi, studied hypophysectomy. With F. Generale, demonstrated that tetany and death follow complete removal of the parathyroids (1896).

vas′tus [L., immense]. A portion of the quadriceps femoris muscle which extends the knee joint. Its origin is from three heads on the femur, its insertion is on the patella and ultimately into the tubercle of the tibia, and it is innervated by the femoral nerve. See Table of Muscles in the Appendix. **—vas′tus,** *adj.*

v. verticalis linguae. The vertical muscle fibers of the intrinsic musculature of the tongue.

Vater, Abraham [*German anatomist,* 1684–1751]. Described the ampulla of the common bile duct (1720), called *ampulla of Vater.* See also Pacinian *corpuscle.*

Vaughan, Victor Clarence [*American bacteriologist,* 1851–1929]. Remembered for his investigations of the poisons produced by bacteria and protein split products.

vault [OF. *vaute,* from L. *volvere,* to roll]. 1. An arched structure, as a dome. 2. Specifically, the vault of the skull; calvaria.

vau″que·line′ (vo″ki·leen′). See *strychnine.*

VD, V.D., vd, v.d. Venereal disease.

V. D. H. Valvular disease of the heart.

Veale, Henry Richard Lobb [*Scottish physician,* 1832–1908]. Described an epidemic of German measles (1866), in which he originated the term rubella.

Veau's operation. A modification of Dieffenbach's operation for the repair of cleft palate.

ve·cor′di·a [L., senselessness]. Any mental disorder. *Obs.*

vec′tion [L., from *vehere,* to carry]. The conveyance of disease germs from the sick to the well.

vec′tis [L., bar]. An instrument similar to the single blade of a forceps, used in hastening the delivery of the fetal head in labor.

vec′tor [L., from *vehere,* to carry]. 1. An arthropod which carries microorganisms from a sick person to some other person. 2. A quantity involving both magnitude and direction, as velocity, force, momentum, which may be represented by a straight line of suitable length and direction. **—vector′ial,** *adj.*

patient vectors. *In psychoanalysis,* immature transference needs expressed between persons when there is some possibility of their satisfaction and resolution.

v. quantity. *In electrocardiography,* magnitude, direction, and sense of the cardiac potential derived from the electrocardiogram.

vec″tor·car′di·o·gram″ [*vector;* G. *kardia,* heart; *gramma,* letter]. A single record or figure which represents the electric forces that are present in the standard leads of the electrocardiogram in such a way that the instantaneous values of the magnitude and direction of the electric phenomena within the heart are clearly shown. Vectorcardiograms may be obtained by the use of the cathode-ray oscillograph or other special apparatus. Also called *monocardiogram.*

vec″tor·car′di·o·graph. Apparatus for making a vectorcardiogram.

Vedder, Edward Bright [*American physician and Army medical officer,* 1878–1952]. Demonstrated the action of emetine against the ameba in the intestinal tract (1911). See also Vedder's *sign.*

veg′e·tal (vedj′i·tul) [L. *vegetus,* lively]. Trophic, rather than mitotically active. See vegetal *pole.*

veg″e·ta′tion [L. *vegetare,* to quicken]. An outgrowth resembling a plant in outline, as the projections on the cardiac valves in endocarditis, papillomas, polypoid growths, etc.

adenoid vegetations. Growths of lymphatic tissue in the nasopharyngeal cavity.

ve′hi·cle [L. *vehiculum,* conveyance]. A liquid or solid substance, generally inactive therapeutically, employed as a medium or carrier for the active component of a medicine.

veil [L. *velum,* veil]. A caul or piece of the amniotic sac covering the face of a newborn infant.

acquired v. An obscuration or imperfection of voice from exposure to cold, catarrhal conditions, overuse, or bad training.

uterine v. A cap fitted over the cervix uteri to prevent the entrance of semen.

Veillon's tube. A glass tube for use in making bacterial cultures. One end is fitted with a rubber stopper, one with a cotton plug.

Veil″lo·nel′la (vay″yo·nel′uh, vah″yo·nel′uh) [after Adrien *Veillon,* French bacteriologist, 1864–1931]. A genus of microorganisms belonging to the family Neisseriaceae; they are small, Gram-negative, anaerobic cocci.

V. gazogenes. A species found in the saliva of man and other animals.

V. parvula. A species found in the mouth and digestive tract of man and other animals.

vein [L. *vena,* vein]. A blood vessel carrying blood from the tissues toward the heart. Veins, like arteries, have three coats, but the media is less well developed; many also possess valves. For veins not listed here, see Table of Veins in the Appendix. See Plates 9, 10.

advehent v. *In embryology,* the portion of the omphalomesenteric vein caudal to the liver and cranial to the transverse anastomoses; it becomes a branch of the portal vein.

afferent veins. Those conveying blood directly to an organ, as the portal vein.

allantoic veins. See *umbilical veins* under *vein.*

anterior cardinal veins. The paired primary veins of the anterior part of the early embryo.

arcuate v. A venous arch at the base of a renal pyramid, accompanying an arcuate artery.

azygos line veins. See *medial sympathetic veins* under *vein.*

central v. (a) The vein in the center of a liver lobule into which the sinusoids empty. (b) That which receives blood from all vessels of the cortex and medulla of the adrenal gland.

cephalic v. See *cephalic vein.*
collecting v. A vein formed by the confluence of several intercalated veins of the liver.
common cardinal veins. Paired primary veins located in the septum transversum, connecting the anterior and posterior cardinals with the sinus venosus. Syn., *ducts of Cuvier.*
diploic v. One of the large, thin-walled veins occupying bony channels in the diploë of cranial bones, and communicating with each other, with meningeal veins and sinuses of the dura, and, through emissary veins, with the veins of the pericranium.
intercalated v. See sublobular *v.*
interlobar v. In the kidney, one of the veins running in the renal columns and draining into the renal vein.
interlobular v. In the kidney, a tributary of an arcuate vein, lying in the cortical substance between the medullary rays.
intralobular v. See central *v.* (a).
lateral sympathetic veins. Longitudinal venous trunks of the embryo lateral to the sympathetic ganglions and dorsomedial to the posterior cardinal veins. The right vein forms the postrenal part of the inferior vena cava. Syn., *paraureteric veins, supracardinal veins.*
medial sympathetic veins. Longitudinal venous channels of the embryo medial to the sympathetic ganglions, forming the azygos and hemiazygos veins. Syn., *azygos line veins, supracardinal veins.*
meningorachidian veins. See *vertebral veins* under *vein.*
oblique v. of Marshall. The small vein passing downward across the posterior surface of the left atrium and draining into the coronary sinus; it represents the remnant of the left common cardinal vein. *O.T.*
omphalomesenteric veins. Embryonic veins uniting yolk sac and sinus venosus; their proximal fused ends form the portal vein. Syn., *vitelline veins.*
paraureteric veins. See *lateral sympathetic veins* under *vein.*
posterior cardinal veins. The paired primary veins of the embryo draining body and mesonephros, located in the dorsolateral part of the urogenital fold; they unite with the anterior cardinal veins to form the common cardinal veins.
primary head veins. The chief veins developing in the head of an early embryo; they are continuous with the anterior cardinal veins and lie medial to the trigeminal, but ventrolateral to the more posterior cranial ganglions.
pulp v. One of the veins draining the venous sinuses of the splenic pulp.
revehent v. *In embryology,* the portion of the omphalomesenteric vein between the liver and the sinus venosus. The veins of the two sides join and form the inferior vena cava.
stellate veins. Radially arranged subcapsular veins of the renal cortex which drain into the interlobular veins.
subcardinal veins. Paired longitudinal veins of the embryo partly replacing the postcardinals; the prerenal part of the inferior vena cava develops largely from the right subcardinal.
sublobular v. A vein formed by the joining of the central veins of several liver lobules. Syn., *intercalated v.*
supracardinal veins. Paired longitudinal venous channels of the embryo that replace the postcardinal and subcardinal veins and form the azygos-hemiazygos system of veins, and, on the right side, most of the postrenal part of the inferior vena cava.
systemic v. One of those conveying venous blood from the systemic circuit to the right atrium of the heart.
Thebesian veins. Small veins from the myocardium which open directly into the atria and ventricles.
trabecular v. In the spleen, a tributary of the splenic vein, formed by the confluence of pulp veins.
umbilical veins. Originally paired veins conveying blood from the placenta to the sinus venosus; the proximal right umbilical vein disappears early in development and the extraembryonic parts fuse to form a single vein in the cord.
varicose veins. Those which have become abnormally dilated and tortuous, due to interference with venous drainage or weakness of their walls.
vertebral veins. The plexus of thin-walled valveless veins situated about the spinal cord within the vertebral canal: also called *meningorachidian veins.*
vitelline veins. See *omphalomesenteric veins* under *vein.*

vein seek′er. A small pipet equipped with a teat-bulb, a glass sight filled with sodium citrate solution, and armed with an infusion needle. The teat is emptied by pressure of the fingers. The point of the needle is inserted under the skin where the vein is suspected, and the pressure released. The teat remains collapsed until a vein is entered, when blood appears in the tube. *Obs.*

ve·la′men [L., covering]. A veil or covering membrane.
v. vulvae. The Hottentot apron.

vel″a·men′tum [L., covering]. A veil, or covering membrane. —**velamentous,** *adj.*

Velden, Reinhard von den [*German physician,* 1880–1941]. Said to have been the first to restore heart action after complete cessation, by intracardiac injection (1919); called *von den Velden's method.*

veldt sore (velt, felt). A disease common in the African desert, but seen also in Australia and Burma; characterized by multiple, shallow, chronic, painful ulcers on exposed parts of the bodies of light-skinned individuals. It usually follows slight trauma, such as an insect bite. Exposure to sunlight is necessary, and there are usually secondary bacterial invaders. Also called *Barcoo disease, desert sore, Natal sore, septic sore.*

ve′li·ger (vee′li·jur, vel′i·jur) [L., sail-bearing]. A larval mollusk with a velum.

vel′li·cate [L. *vellicare,* to twitch]. Twitch spasmodically.

vel″li·ca′tion [*vellicatio,* from *vellicare*]. Spasmodic twitching of muscular fibers.

vel·lo′sine (veh·lo′seen, ·sin, vel′o·). $C_{23}H_{28}N_2O_4$. An alkaloid in Pao-Pereira bark, *Geissospermum vellosii laeve;* it resembles brucine in physiologic action.

Velpeau, Alfred Armand Louis Marie [*French surgeon,* 1795–1867]. Described silver-fork deformity, called *Velpeau's deformity,* which occurs in fractures of the lower end of the radius (Colles' fracture). See also Velpeau's *bandage.*

ve′lum (pl. *vela*) [L.]. A veil or veil-like structure. —**velar,** *adj.*
anterior medullary v. A thin leaf of medullary substance forming the roof of the anterior portion of the fourth ventricle of the brain. Formerly called *valve of Vieussens.*
posterior medullary v. The commissure of the flocculus of the cerebellum.
v. interpositum. The choroid plexus in the roof of the third ventricle of the brain.
v. palati. The posterior portion of the soft palate. Syn., *v. palatinum.*

v. pendulum palati. The soft palate, especially the uvula.

v. terminale. Lamina terminalis.

VEM *V*aso*e*xcitor *m*aterial produced by the kidney: formed anaerobically in normal kidney; formed aerobically and anaerobically in the kidney in hypertensive states.

ve′na (pl. *venae*) [L.]. A vein.

v. cava inferior. A vein formed by the junction of the two common iliac veins and emptying into the right atrium of the heart. It receives the lumbar, right spermatic, renal, suprarenal, phrenic, and hepatic veins. See Plates 5, 8, 9, 10, 14.

v. cava superior. A vein formed by the union of the innominate veins, and conveying the blood from the head, chest wall, and upper extremities to the right atrium. See Plates 5, 9.

venae comitantes. The veins accompanying an artery.

venae cordis minimae. The smallest of the cardiac vessels, entering into the cavities of the heart.

venae Galeni. Two venous trunks in the brain.

venae Thebesii. See *Thebesian veins* under *vein.*

venae vorticosae. The stellate veins of the choroid coat of the eyeball.

venapis. A proprietary preparation of bee venom; has been used in the treatment of arthritis.

ve·na′tion [*vena*]. Distribution of venous circulation of a part or organ.

ven·ec′to·my [*vena;* G. *ektomē*, excision]. Excision of a vein or a portion of one.

ve·nene′. Venin.

ven″e·nif′er·ous (ven″i·nif′ur·us, vee″ni·) [L. *venenum*, poison; *ferre*, to bear]. Conveying poison.

ven″e·no′sa [L. *venenosus*, full of poison]. The venomous snakes.

ven″e·punc′ture. See *venipuncture.*

ve·ne′re·al [L. *Venereus*, from Venus, goddess of love]. Pertaining to, or produced by, sexual intercourse.

ve·ne″re·ol′o·gist [*Venereus;* G. *logos*, word]. An expert in venereal diseases.

ve·ne″re·ol′o·gy [*Venereus; logos*]. The study of venereal diseases.

ve·ne″re·o·pho′bi·a [*Venereus;* G. *phobos*, fear]. Morbid fear of getting venereal disease.

ven′er·y [L. *Venus*, goddess of love]. Copulation.

ven″e·sec′tion (ven″i·seck′shun, vee″ni·) [L. *vena*, vein; *sectio*, a cutting]. The abstraction of blood from the body by incising a vein, popularly known as *bleeding.* In practice, blood is usually removed in measured quantity by the use of a needle or trochar passed into the lumen of a vessel. Locally, a small amount of blood may be removed by scarifying or leeching.

ven″e·su′ture, ven″i·su′ture [*vena;* L. *sutura*, a sewing]. The suturing of a vein.

Ve·ne′tian red. A form of ferric oxide; used as a red pigment.

ven′in. A mixture of the venoms of various poisonous snakes, used in neurasthenia, hysteria, chorea: also spelled *venene.*

ven″i·punc′ture (ven″i·punk′chur, vee″ni·, ven′i·punk″chur, vee′ni·) [*vena;* L. *punctura*, a puncture]. The surgical puncture of a vein.

ve·noc′ly·sis [*vena;* G. *klysis*, a drenching]. Injection of food or drugs into a vein.

ve′no·gram [*vena;* G. *gramma*, a letter]. Roentgenogram of a vein.

ven·og′ra·phy [*vena;* G. *graphein*, to write]. Radiographic examination of veins following injection of an opaque contrast medium.

ven′om [L. *venenum*, poison]. Poison, especially a poison secreted by certain reptiles and arthropods.

snake v. A secretion of the posterior superior labial glands of a poisonous snake, normally yellowish, sometimes colorless, possessing varying degrees of toxicity. Toxic constituents include neurotoxins, cytolysins, proteolysins, hemolysins, and hemocoagulins.

ven″o·mo·sal′i·var″y (ven″o·mo·sal′i·verr″ee) [*venenum;* L. *saliva*, saliva]. *In zoology*, designating the salivary glands of certain animals, that secrete venom instead of saliva.

ve″no·mo′tor [L. *vena*, vein; *motum*, from *movere*, to move]. Causing veins to contract or dilate.

ven′om·ous [L. *venenum*, poison]. Poisonous.

ve″no·per″i·to·ne·os′to·my [L. *vena*, vein; G. *peritonaion*, membrane which contains the lower viscera; *stoma*, mouth]. Surgical implantation of a divided greater saphenous vein into the peritoneal cavity for drainage of ascites. Also called *Ruotte's operation.*

ve″no·pres′sor [*vena;* L. *premere*, to press]. Pertaining to blood pressure in the veins and right side of the heart.

ve″no·scle·ro′sis [*vena;* G. *sklērōsis*, a hardening]. Induration of veins; phlebosclerosis.

ve·nos′i·ty [L. *venosus*, full of veins]. A condition in which the arterial blood shows venous qualities.

ve″no·sta′sis, ve·nos′ta·sis [L. *vena*, vein; G. *statis*, a standing]. Retardation or prevention of the return flow of the blood by compression of veins, obstruction, varicosities, weakness of vessel walls, or lowering of venous pressure.

ve″no·throm·bot′ic [*vena;* G. *thrombos*, clot]. Having the property of producing venous thrombosis.

ve·not′o·my [*vena;* G. *tomē*, a cutting]. Phlebotomy; incision of a vein.

ve′nous [*vena*]. Pertaining to the veins.

ve″no·ve·nos′to·my [*vena; vena;* G. *stoma*, mouth]. The anastomosing of two veins.

vent [L. *findere*, to split]. Any aperture or outlet.

alveolar vents. Communicating pores between neighboring alveoli in the lung.

common v. The cloaca.

vent′er [L.]. 1. The belly or abdomen. 2. The belly of a muscle. 3. The cavity of the abdomen.

ven′ti·late [L. *ventilare*, to brandish in the air]. 1. Renew the air in a place. 2. Oxygenate the blood in the capillaries of the lungs.

ven″ti·la′tion [L. *ventilatio*, from *ventilare*]. 1. The act or process of supplying fresh air, i.e., air whose partial pressure of oxygen is higher and of carbon dioxide lower than in the air being replaced. 2. The act or process of purifying the air of a place.

alveolar v. A calculated expression of the effective ventilation of the diffusing region of the lung. In principle, alveolar ventilation = (tidal volume − physiologic dead space) × respiration rate.

minute v. The volume of air respired in a minute. This depends on degree of activity, strength of the impulses from the respiratory center, and the ability of the respiratory apparatus to respond.

walking v. A test of breathing response to mild exercise. The patient walks at the rate of 2 miles per hour on level ground, and after 4 minutes the expired air is collected and measured. Abbreviated, WV.

ven″ti·lom′e·ter. An apparatus used in a fixed-time hyperventilation test in electroencephalography; it makes possible greater precision of interpretation because the total ventilation volume is kept constant from patient to patient.

ven″ti·lom′e·try. Pneumometry.

ven′tral [L. *venter*, belly]. 1. Pertaining to the belly. 2. Referring to the anterior aspect of the body or to the flexor aspect of the limbs. —**ventrad,** *adv.*

ven′tri·cle [L. *ventriculum*, ventricle]. A small cavity or pouch. —**ventric′ular,** *adj.*

Arantius' v. The terminal depression of the median sulcus of the fourth ventricle immediately ventral to the obex.
fifth v. The cavity of the septum pellucidum: a misnomer.
fourth v. The cavity of the metencephalon and upper half of the myelencephalon, bounded by the brain stem anteriorly and posteriorly by the anterior medullary velum, fastigium of the cerebellum, and tela chorioidea.
laryngeal v. The lateral recess on either side between the true and false vocal folds.
lateral v. The cavity of either cerebral hemisphere communicating with the third ventricle through the interventricular foramen, and consisting of a triangular central cavity or body and three smaller cavities or cornua. See Plates 10, 17.
left v. of the heart. That forcing the blood through the aorta and throughout the body. See Plate 5.
pineal v. One found occasionally within the pineal body; the persisting remnant of the fetal cavity.
right v. of the heart. That forcing the blood through the pulmonary artery into the lungs. See Plate 5.
single v. of the heart. See *cor* triloculare biatrium.
sixth v. The cavum Vergae: a misnomer.
terminal v. The dilated portion of the central canal of the spinal cord in the conus medullaris.
third v. The cavity of the diencephalon, a narrow cleft between the two thalami. See Plate 18.
ventricles of the brain. Cavities in the interior of the brain, comprising the two lateral ventricles and the third and fourth ventricles.

ven·tric′u·lar es·cape′. Single or repeated ventricular beats, arising from the A-V node, usually following a long diastole.

ven·tric′u·lar sep′tal de′fect. Congenital defect of the muscular septum between the ventricles of the heart anterior to the membranous portion of the septum. Syn., *maladie de Roger.*

ventriculin. Trade-mark for a preparation of dried and powdered, defatted, hog gastric tissue. A brand of powdered stomach. The substance is used orally as a hematopoietic drug.

ven·tric″u·li′tis [*ventriculum;* G. *-itis,* inflammation]. Inflammation of the ependymal lining of the ventricles of the brain. Syn., *ependymitis.*

ven·tric″u·lo·cis″ter·nos′to·my. Surgical establishment of communication between the ventricles of the brain and the subarachnoid cisterns; it may be performed by a third ventriculostomy or by the Torkildsen procedure in which communication is established between a lateral ventricle and the cisterna magna.

ven·tric″u·lo·cor·dec′to·my [*ventriculum;* G. *chordē,* cord; *ektomē,* excision]. Excision of the wall of the laryngeal ventricle and part of the vocal folds, for the relief of bilateral abductor paralysis of the vocal folds.

ven·tric′u·lo·gram″ [*ventriculum;* G. *gramma,* letter]. A roentgenogram of the brain after the introduction of air or an opaque medium into the cerebral ventricles through trephine openings in the skull.

ven·tric″u·log′ra·phy [*ventriculum;* G. *graphein,* to write]. A method of demonstrating the ventricles of the brain by roentgenography after the ventricular fluid has been replaced by air or by an opaque medium injected through trephine openings in the skull.

ven·tric″u·lo·mas″toid·os′to·my. A surgical treatment of hydrocephaly in which the temporal horn of a lateral ventricle is connected to the ipsilateral mastoid antrum, usually by a piece of polyethylene tubing.

ven·tric″u·lom′e·try [*ventriculum;* G. *metron,* a measure]. Measurement of the intraventricular pressure.

ven·tric′u·lo·punc′ture [*ventriculum;* L. *punctura,* puncture]. Puncture with a spinal puncture needle of a ventricle of the brain, particularly the lateral ventricle.

ven·tric′u·lo·scope″ [*ventriculum;* G. *skopein,* to examine]. An instrument for inspecting the interior of the cerebral ventricles and for electrocoagulation of the choroid plexus.

ven·tric″u·los′co·py [*ventriculum; skopein*]. Examination of the ventricles of the brain by means of an endoscope.

ven·tric″u·los′to·my [*ventriculum;* G. *stoma,* mouth]. The surgical establishment of drainage of cerebrospinal fluid from the ventricles of the brain.
external v. That accomplished by a communication between a lateral ventricle and an external closed drainage system: the more common procedure.
internal v. See third *v.*
third v. That accomplished by a communication between the third ventricle and basal cistern. Syn., *internal v.*

ven·tric″u·lo·sub″a·rach′noid (·sub″a·rack′-noyd) [*ventriculum;* L. *sub,* under; G. *arachnoeidēs,* like a cobweb]. Of or pertaining to the subarachnoid space and the cerebral ventricles.

ven·tric′u·lus (pl. *ventriculi*) [L.]. 1. Ventricle. 2. Old term for stomach.
v. cerebri. Ventricle of the brain.
v. cordis. Ventricle of the heart.
v. dexter. Right ventricle.
v. lateralis. Lateral ventricle.
v. medius. Middle (third) ventricle.
v. opticus. The lumen of the embryonic optic vesicle, continuous with that of the diencephalon.
v. quartus. Fourth ventricle.
v. sinister. Left ventricle.
v. tertius. Third ventricle.

ven″tri·cum′bent [L. *venter,* belly; *recumbere,* to recline]. Prone.

ven″tri·duc′tion [*venter;* L. *ducere,* to lead]. Drawing a part toward the abdomen.

ven·tril′o·quism [*venter;* L. *loqui,* to speak]. The art of speaking or singing without seeming to use the organs of speech. When the hearer's attention is properly directed, the voice seems to come from elsewhere, as from a dummy.

ven″tri·me′sal (ven″tri·mee′sul) [*venter;* G. *mesos,* in the middle]. In the middle in front.

ven′tro- [*venter*]. A combining form denoting *the abdomen* or *anterior aspect of the body.*

ven″tro·cys·tor′rha·phy. See *marsupialization.*

ven″tro·fix·a′tion [*venter;* L. *fixum,* from *figere,* to fix]. The stitching of a displaced viscus to the abdominal wall; specifically, the operative attachment of the uterus to the anterior abdominal wall for prolapse or displacement.

ven″tro·hys′ter·o·pex″y [*venter;* G. *hystera,* womb; *pēxis,* a fixing]. Ventrofixation of the uterus.

ven″tro·lat′er·al [*venter;* L. *latus,* side]. Relating to the ventral and lateral aspects of a part.

ven″tro·me′di·an [*venter;* L. *medius,* middle]. At the middle of the ventral surface.

ven″trop·to′sis. See *gastroptosis.*

ven·tros′co·py [*venter;* G. *skopein,* to examine]. Direct examination of the abdominal and pelvic cavities by means of an apparatus resembling the cystoscope. Also called *peritoneoscopy.*

ven′trose [*venter*]. Having a belly, or a swelling like a belly (potbelly).

ven·tros′i·ty [*venter*]. Corpulence.

ven″tro·sus·pen′sion [*venter;* L. *suspensio,* from

suspendere, to hang]. The operation of correcting a displacement of the uterus by shortening the round ligaments or attaching them to the anterior abdominal wall.

ven″tro·ves″i·co·fix·a′tion [*venter;* L. *vesica*, bladder; *fixum*, from *figere*, to fix]. Suturing of the uterus to the urinary bladder and abdominal wall.

ven·tu′ri·me·ter. A differential pressure flowmeter used for measuring pulsatile flow.

ven′ule [L. *venula*, small vein]. A small vein.

ve′nus [L., goddess of love]. 1. Old term for sexual intercourse. 2. Alchemic name for copper.

collar of v. A rarely seen, mottled, marblelike skin of the neck; a syphilitic condition. Also called *melanoleucodermia colli, venereal collar*.

crown of v. A syphilitic eruption about the hairline with associated patchy alopecia of the area.

mound of v. See *mons* pubis, *mons* veneris.

ver″a·ce′vine. A nonketonic base, obtainable from veratrum viride, believed to be one of the original alkanolamine bases of veratrum viride alkaloids; it is isomeric with cevine and cevagenine and is probably the precursor of these compounds.

ver·al′bi·dine. $C_{37}H_{61}NO_{12}$; an alkaloid isolated from *Veratrum album*.

ve·rat′ra·mine. $C_{27}H_{39}NO_2$; the aglucone of veratrosine, isolated from veratrum viride.

ve·rat′ric ac′id. $(CH_3O)_2C_6H_3COOH$. Dimethoxybenzoic acid, found in sabadilla seeds.

ver·at′ri·dine (vuh·rat′ri·deen, ·din). $C_{36}H_{51}NO_{11}$; an alkaloid isolated from both sabadilla seed and veratrum viride, formerly considered to be a veratric acid ester of cevine, but now believed to be the same ester of veracevine.

ver′a·trine. 1. Cevadine: original name. 2. A mixture of alkaloids from veratrum viride.

ve·rat″ro·ba′sine. $C_{24}H_{37}NO_3$; an alkaloid isolated from *Veratrum album*.

ve·rat′ro·sine. A glucoside isolated from veratrum viride. On hydrolysis it yields D-glucose and veratramine.

ve·rat″ro·yl·zy″ga·de′nine. An ester alkaloid isolated from *Veratrum fimbriatum* Gray and also from *Zygadenus venenosus* Watson.

ve·ra′trum vi′ri·de. The dried rhizome and roots of green hellebore (*Veratrum viride*). It contains a number of alkaloids, including germidine, germitrine, cevadine, veratridine, jervine, rubijervine, pseudojervine. It is irritant, causes sneezing if inhaled, and vomiting if swallowed in sufficient dose. The outstanding physiologic actions of the drug after a moderately large dose are slowing of the respiration, slowing of the pulse, and fall of blood pressure. Used for the reduction of blood pressure in various conditions of hypertension. Also used to lower the pulse rate in various forms of tachycardia. It has also been widely used by obstetricians in the treatment of puerperal eclampsia. Dose, 0.06–0.13 Gm. (1–2 gr.). Also called *green hellebore, American hellebore*.

Ver·bas′cum [L., mullein]. Mullein; a genus of plants of the family Scrophulariaceae. The leaves and flowers of **V. thapsus** have been used as a demulcent in catarrhal inflammation of mucous membranes and as an application to hemorrhoids.

ver·big″er·a′tion (vur·bidj″ur·ay′shun) [L. *verbigerare*, to chat]. The frequent and uncontrollable repetition of the same word, sentence, or sound without reference to its meaning.

ver′di·gris (vur′di·gree, ·griss) [OF. *vert de Grice*, green of Greece]. 1. A mixture of basic copper acetates. 2. A deposit upon copper, from the formation of cupric salts.

ver′do·fla·vin. A naturally occurring flavin of grass which is said to be chemically identical with riboflavin.

ver″do·glo′bin. Choleglobin.

ver″do·he′min. A green-colored bile pigment; a derivative of hemin in which the porphyrin ring has opened, rendering the iron labile.

ver″do·per·ox′i·dase. A green-colored peroxidase in leukocytes.

ver du Cayor. See *Cordylobia anthropophaga*.

ver′gen·ces (vur′jin·seez) [L. *vergere*, to bend]. A term applied to associated disjunctive movements of the eyes, as convergence, divergence.

ver′gens (vur′jenz) [*vergere*]. Inclining.

v. deorsum. Inclining downward, as of the axis of vision in one eye in strabismus.

v. sursum. Upward inclination.

Verger, Henri (1873–1930). French neurologist who introduced intraneural injection of alcohol for the treatment of neuralgia.

ver′ger prism. An instrument used in the measurement and enlargement of the fusion power of the eyes.

ver′ge·ture. Stria atrophica.

Verheyen, Philippe [*Flemish anatomist*, 1648–1710]. Described the venous plexus of stellate form situated on the surface of the kidney just beneath the capsule; called *Verheyen's stars, stellate veins*.

Verhoeff, Frederick Herman [*American ophthalmologist*, 1874–   ]. Known for his operation for retinal detachment, in which he performed posterior sclerotomy followed by multiple electrolytic punctures. Devised a technic for cataract extraction whereby the lens is grasped above and slid through the corneal incision. In *Verhoeff's operation*, the cataract is removed within the capsule. See Verhoeff depth perception *test*, Verhoeff's *stain*.

veriloid. Trade-mark for the fraction of veratrum viride alkaloids known by the generic name *alkavervir*.

ver′i·tol. $OH.C_6H_4.CH_2.CH(CH_3)NH.CH_3$. Parahydroxyphenyl-isopropylmethylamine; a base isomeric with ephedrine. Its action is more nearly related to that of ephedrine than to that of epinephrine. Used largely in Europe as a stimulant in circulatory failure. It is marketed in the form of the hydrochloride.

ver ma·caque′ (vair mah·kahk′). A club-shaped larval form of the tropical warble fly, *Dermatobia hominis*.

ver″mi·ci′dal [L. *vermis*, worm; *caedere*, to kill]. Destructive of worms.

ver′mi·cide [*vermis; caedere*]. An agent that destroys worms.

ver·mic′u·lar [L. *vermiculus*, little worm]. Wormlike.

ver·mic′u·late [*vermiculus*]. Resembling or shaped like a worm.

ver·mic″u·la′tion [*vermiculus*]. A wormlike motion; peristaltic motion.

ver′mi·cule [*vermiculus*]. A small worm.

ver·mic′u·lose, ver·mic′u·lous [*vermiculus*]. 1. Vermiform, vermicular. 2. Infested with worms or larvae.

ver·mic′u·lus [L.]. A little worm or grub.

ver′mi·form [L. *vermis*, worm; *forma*, form]. Wormshaped, as vermiform process.

ver′mi·fuge [*vermis; fugere*]. Any agent that kills or expels intestinal worms. —**vermif′ugal,** *adj.*

ver″mi·lin′gual [*vermis;* L. *lingua*, tongue]. Having a worm-shaped tongue.

ver′min [*vermis*]. A term applied to animals which are obnoxious or harmful to man, especially those infesting his person, domesticated animals, or buildings, as flies, lice, rats, or mice.

ver″mi·na′tion [L. *verminatio*, from *vermis*]. Infestation with vermin or worms. The multiplication of parasitic vermin by breeding.

ver′min·ous [*vermis*]. Infested with, or pertaining to, vermin.

ver″mi·pho′bi·a [*vermis;* G. *phobos*, fear]. Morbid fear of worms or of worm infestation.

ver′mis [L.]. 1. A worm. 2. The median lobe of the cerebellum, between the hemispheres, or lateral lobes.

inferior v. The inferior portion of the vermis, which includes the lobules called *nodulus, uvula, pyramid,* and *tuber.*

superior v. The superior part of the cerebellar vermis, which includes the lobules called *central lobule,* the *monticulus* consisting of *culmen* and *declive,* and the *folium.*

Vernet, Maurice [*French neurologist,* 1887–]. Described associated laryngeal paralysis due to lesions of the glossopharyngeal, vagus, and spinal accessory nerves; called *Vernet's syndrome.*

Verneuil, Aristide Auguste Stanislaus [*French surgeon and anatomist,* 1823–95]. One of the first to use hemostatic forceps in surgery (1875). Described syphilitic bursitis, also called *Verneuil's disease* or *bursitis.* A plexiform neuroma, or cirsoid neuroma, is also known as *Verneuil's neuroma.*

ver′ni·er [after Pierre *Vernier*, French physicist, 1580–1637]. A device attached to the graduated scale of various instruments which permits subdividing and measuring the smallest unit of this scale into tenths or other fractions.

ver′nine. Guanosine.

ver′nix ca″se·o′sa. A cheesy deposit on the surface of the fetus derived from the stratum corneum, sebaceous secretion, and remnants of the epitrichium.

Ver·no′ni·a [after William *Vernon*, English botanist, seventeenth century]. A genus of plants of the Carduaceae.

V. anthelmintica. That found in East India; the seeds are anthelmintic.

V. nigritiana. That found in West Africa; contains vernonin.

ver′no·nin, ver·no′nin. A glycoside from *Vernonia nigritiana* (Nigerian ironweed); has digitalislike actions.

Verocay, José (1876–1927). Uruguayan pathologist in Czechoslovakia who showed that neurofibromas are derived from the sheath of Schwann cells. See also *Verocay bodies* under *body.*

ver·o′di·gen. Gitalin.

veronal. Trade-mark for a brand of barbital.

v. sodium. Trade-mark for a brand of barbital sodium.

ver·ru′ca (pl. *verrucae*) [L.]. Wart.

venereal v. Condyloma acuminatum.

v. acuminata. A venereal wart occurring on the genitals. May occur in the absence of venereal disease, but usually some discharge is present. Syn., *condyloma acuminatum.*

v. digitata. One usually seen on the scalp or in the beard with fingerlike projections and a horny cap. The lesion is soft.

v. filiformis. A soft, slender, soft-pointed, threadlike lesion usually seen on the face and neck.

v. necrogenica. A warty excrescence found on the fingers of those who frequently handle the tissues of tuberculous subjects. Also called *anatomic tubercle, dissection tubercle.*

v. peruviana, v. peruana. The benign form of bartonellosis (Carrión's disease), endemic in the mountainous areas of northwestern South America, characterized by a skin eruption of purpuric vascular papules interspersed with nodular elements, the proliferation of epithelial cells, and the presence in the lesions of the causative agent, *Bartonella bacilliformis*, usually in the cytoplasm of endothelial cells. It is related etiologically and immunologically to Oroya fever, but the two diseases differ greatly in their clinical picture. Both are associated with the name of Daniel A. Carrión, who first demonstrated their etiologic relationship.

v. plana juvenilis. A smooth, flat, and small type of wart seen most often in children on the back of the hands and face, often arranged in lines.

v. plantaris. A wart on the sole of the foot. It is often quite painful due to ingrowth and pressure. Usually multiple but often grouped. Covered with a callus.

v. senilis. A brownish, pigmented, hypertrophic lesion, usually seen on the skin of the face, chest, and back of older people; it is usually scaly and greasy. While listed with precancerous lesions, it occasionally may become malignant. There is no inflammation, and the crust or scale is soft. Syn., *keratosis seborrheica.*

v. vulgaris. The common wart, a disease caused by a filtrable virus. It is usually seen on the hands, about the nails, or on the arms or legs, and is more common in children. Lesions are horny projections of normal skin color but soon become dark with papillary projections. They are of various sizes but usually are circular and from ⅓ to 2 cm. in diameter.

ver·ru′ci·form [*verruca;* L. *forma*, form]. Wartlike.

ver′ru·coid, ver·ru′coid [*verruca;* G. *eidos*, form]. Resembling a wart.

ver′ru·cose, ver′ru·cous [L. *verrucosus*, full of warts]. Warty; covered with, or having, warts.

ver·ru′ga. See *verruca.*

versene. A trade-mark for various synthetic amino acids and their salts, as ethylenediaminetetraacetic acid and its salts; the substances are used as chelating and sequestering agents.

ver′si·col″or, ver·sic′o·lor [L. *vertere*, to turn; *color*, color]. Denoting change of color.

ver′sion [*vertere*]. Turning; manipulation during delivery to alter the presentation of the fetus.

abdominal v. Manipulations made exclusively through the external abdominal wall. Also called *external v.*

anopelvic v. Manipulation of the pelvis of the fetus with a finger in the mother's rectum.

bimanual v. Manipulation through the abdominal wall with one hand with the aid of one or more fingers of the other within the vagina. Also called *combined v.*

bipolar v. Manipulation of both the pelvis and the vertex of the fetus.

Braxton Hicks v. Manipulation by the bimanual method to bring the fetal head into the pelvis. This has been advocated in treatment of placenta previa and prolapsed cord.

cephalic v. Turning of the fetus to establish a vertex presentation.

combined v. See bimanual *v.*

external v. See abdominal *v.*

forced v. Accouchement forcé.

internal v. Turning of the fetus by introducing the entire hand within the uterus.

pelvic v. Turning the fetus to bring about a breech presentation.

podalic v. One in which one or both feet are brought down to the outlet.

prophylactic v. Converting a vertex into a breech presentation to avoid prolonged pressure on the head. Formerly employed in moderate dystocia.

spontaneous v. Turning of the fetus without artificial assistance.

ver′te·bra (pl. *vertebrae*) [L., joint, vertebra]. One of the 33 bones forming the spinal or vertebral column. A typical vertebra consists of a body and an arch, the latter being formed by two pedicles and two laminas. The arch supports seven processes—four articular, two transverse, and one spinous. See Table of Bones in the Appendix. See Plates 1, 14. —**vertebral,** *adj.*

basilar v. The last lumbar vertebra.

cervical vertebrae. Those of the neck.

false v. One of the sacral or coccygeal vertebrae.

flexion vertebrae. All except the first two cervical vertebrae.

primitive v. The condensed caudal half of an embryonic sclerotome from which develops the greater part of a vertebra. Also called *scleromere.*

rotation vertebrae. The first and second cervical vertebrae.

true v. One of the cervical, thoracic, or lumbar vertebrae.

v. dentata. The axis.

v. magna. The sacrum.

v. prominens. The seventh cervical vertebra, so called because its spinous process projects beyond the others.

ver″te·bra·dym′i·a. See *spondylodidymia.*

ver″te·brar·te′ri·al [*vertebra;* G. *artērion,* artery]. Giving passage to the vertebral artery, as the vertebrarterial foramens in the transverse processes of the cervical vertebrae.

Ver″te·bra′ta [*vertebra*]. One of the most important groups in the animal kingdom, comprising the fishes, amphibians, reptiles, birds, and mammals. They are characterized by a spinal column composed of bony, or, in the case of certain groups of fishes, cartilaginous, vertebrae. The spinal column also contains the spinal cord, which connects with a brain enclosed in a skull. The spinal column develops in embryonic life about a notochord; and the Vertebrata are commonly classified as a subphylum of the Chordata.

ver′te·brate, ver′te·bra″ted [*vertebra*]. 1. Having a vertebral column. 2. Resembling a vertebral column in flexibility, as a vertebrate catheter.

ver″te·brec′to·my [*vertebra;* G. *ektomē,* excision]. Excision of a portion of a vertebra.

ver′te·bro-, vertebr- [*vertebra*]. A combining form denoting *vertebrae* or *vertebral.*

ver″te·bro·di·dym′i·a [*vertebra;* G. *didymos,* twin]. Conjoined twins united by vertebrae.

ver′tex [L., top]. 1. The highest point, in the sagittal plane, on the outer surface of a skull oriented on the Frankfort horizontal plane. 2. The crown. 3. The center of a lens surface; the point on either lens surface which lies on the principal axis.

v. corneae. The central portion of the cornea.

ver′ti·cal [*vertex*]. 1. Pertaining to the vertex. 2. Perpendicular; referring to the position of the long axis of the human body in the erect posture.

ver′ti·cal di·men′sion. See under *dimension.*

ver′ti·cil [L. *verticillus,* the whirl of a spindle]. A whorl; a circle of leaves, tentacles, hairs, organs, or processes radiating from an axis on the same horizontal plane. —**vertic′illate,** *adj.*

Ver″ti·cil′li·um gra′phi·i (vur″ti·sil′ee·um gray′-fee·eye). A mold sometimes found in the external acoustic meatus in otitis externa.

ver·tig′i·nous (vur·tidj′i·nus) [L. *vertigo,* a whirling around]. Resembling or affected with vertigo.

ver′ti·go [L.]. The sensation that the outer world is revolving about the patient (*objective vertigo*) or that he himself is moving in space (*subjective vertigo*). The word frequently is used erroneously as a synonym for dizziness or giddiness to indicate an unpleasant sensation of disturbed relations to surrounding objects in space.

auditory v. See Ménière's *syndrome.*

cerebral v. That due to cerebral disorder.

epileptic v. Vertigo associated with or preceding an attack of epilepsy.

essential v. One not due to any discoverable cause.

gastric v. That arising from dyspepsia.

intestinal v. (a) That caused by intestinal disorder. (b) That caused by pressure on the terminal portions of the intestine by gas or feces, or even when a finger, introduced into the rectum, irritates the intestinal wall.

labyrinthine v. Vertigo, pallor, and aural, ocular, or gastric disturbances due to congestion or inflammation of the semicircular canals. See Ménière's *syndrome.*

lithemic v. A form associated with gout and lithemia.

neurasthenic v. Psychologic vertigo found in neurasthenia.

objective v. One in which objects seem to the patient to move.

ocular v. That due to eye diseases.

organic v. That due to brain lesion.

peripheral v. That due to irritation that is not central.

psychogenic v. See neurasthenic *v.*

stomachal v. Gastric vertigo caused by disorder of the stomach.

subjective v. One in which the patient has a sensation as if he himself were moving.

toxemic v. That due to some poison in the blood.

vertical v. That caused by looking downward from or upward to a height.

v. tenebricosa. That accompanied by dimness of vision and headache.

vestibular v. That due to irritation of or injury to the labyrinth or vestibular nerve.

ver·tig′ra·phy. See sectional *radiography.*

ver″u·mon″ta·ni′tis [L. *veru,* spit; *montanus,* of a mountain; G. *-itis,* inflammation]. Inflammation of the verumontanum.

ver″u·mon·ta′num (verr″oo·mon·tay′num, veer″-oo·) [*veru; montanus*]. The colliculus seminalis.

Vesalius, Andreas [*Flemish anatomist,* 1514–64]. His *De humani corporis fabrica* is one of the great classics of anatomy. Described an inconstant foramen at the base of the skull anterointernal to the foramen ovale; called *Vesalius' foramen.* The emissary vein passing through this foramen from the cavernous sinus is called *Vesalius' vein.* The inguinal ligament was sometimes called *Vesalius' ligament.*

ve·sa′ni·a [L., madness]. Unsoundness of mind. *Obs.* —**vesan′ic,** *adj.*

ves′i·ca [L.]. A bladder.

v. biparta. A urinary bladder which is incompletely reduplicated by partial frontal or sagittal septa.

v. duplex. Reduplication of the urinary bladder.

v. fellea. The gallbladder.

v. umbilicalis. The umbilical vesicle, or yolk sac of mammals.

v. urinaria. The urinary bladder.

ves′i·cal [*vesica*]. Pertaining to a bladder.

ves′i·cant [*vesica*]. 1. A blistering agent. 2. *In military medicine,* blister gas.

ves″i·ca′tion [*vesica*]. The formation of a blister; a blister. —**ves′i·cate,** *v.*

ves′i·ca·to″ry [*vesica*]. Blistering.

ves′i·ca·to″ry. A blistering agent.

ves′i·cle [L. *vesicula,* vesicle]. 1. A small bladder; especially a small sac containing fluid. 2. A small bulla, as seen in herpes simplex or varicella.

air v. An alveolus of the lungs, the ultimate divisions of the air passages.

allantoic v. The allantois. See allantoic *sac.*

amniocardiac v. In lower vertebrates (e.g.,

birds), that part of the coelom which lies below and lateral to the developing heart in its early stages.

amnioembryonic v. The early amnion.

amnionic v. The amnion.

anterior brain v. See *prosencephalon.*

auditory v. The vesicular anlage of the inner ear. Also called *otocyst, otic v.*

blastodermic v. A blastocyst.

brain vesicles. The primary embryonic subdivisions of the brain.

cerebral vesicles. The paired lateral outpouchings of the telencephalon which become the cerebral hemispheres; also called *telencephalic vesicles.*

cervical v. See cervical *sinus.*

chorionic v. The gestation sac covered by chorionic villi and containing the embryo.

germinal v. The special name given (Purkinje, 1825) to the egg nucleus before a nucleus was recognized as a constant feature of all cells (Brown, 1831) and before the egg itself was recognized as a single cell (Gegenbaur, 1861).

Greeff's v. *In histopathology,* a small vesicle of the ciliary process associated with hyaline degeneration of that structure.

lens v. The ectodermal vesicle that differentiates into the lens of the eye.

medullary coccygeal v. The enlarged caudal termination of the spinal cord present in embryos of 10–17 mm.

optic v. The embryonic evagination of the diencephalon from which are derived the pigment and sensory layers of the retina.

otic v. See auditory *v.*

primary brain v. One of the first subdivisions of the embryonic brain; the prosencephalon, mesencephalon, or rhombencephalon.

prosencephalic v. See *prosencephalon.*

seminal v. The contorted, branched, saccular, glandular diverticulum of each ductus deferens with which its duct unites to form an ejaculatory duct. See Plate 44.

umbilical v. The yolk sac.

ves'i·co- [L. *vesica,* bladder]. A combining form denoting *bladder.*

ves"i·co·pro·stat'ic [*vesica;* G. *prostatēs,* one who stands before]. Pertaining to the prostate gland and the urinary bladder.

ves"i·cot'o·my [*vesica;* G. *tomē,* a cutting]. Incision of the urinary bladder; cystotomy.

ves"i·co·u'ter·ine (ves"i·ko·yōō'tur·in, ·yōō'tuh-ryne) [*vesica;* L. *uterus,* womb]. Pertaining to the urinary bladder and the uterus.

ve·sic'u·la (pl. *vesiculae*) [L.]. A vesicle.

v. fellea. The gallbladder.

v. optica inversa. The optic vesicle after it has invaginated to form the optic cup. Also called *cupula optica.*

v. prostatica. The prostatic utricle.

v. seminalis. See seminal *vesicle.*

ve·sic'u·lar [*vesicula*]. 1. Pertaining to, or composed of, vesicles. 2. Produced in air vesicles, as vesicular breathing, vesicular murmur.

ve·sic'u·lase. An enzyme of the prostate gland which coagulates seminal fluid in certain lower animals, not detected as yet in man.

ve·sic"u·la'tion [*vesicula*]. The formation of vesicles; the state of becoming vesiculated.

ve·sic"u·lec'to·my [*vesicula;* G. *ektomē,* excision]. Resection, complete or partial, of the seminal vesicles.

ve·sic"u·li'tis [*vesicula;* G. *-itis,* inflammation]. Inflammation of the seminal vesicles.

ve·sic"u·lo·bul'lous, ves"i·co·bul'lous. Characterized by both vesicles and bullae at the same time.

ve·sic'u·lo·gram" [*vesicula;* G. *gramma,* letter]. A radiograph of the seminal vesicles, made by injecting a radiopaque substance by way of the ejaculatory ducts.

ve·sic"u·log'ra·phy [*vesicula;* G. *graphein,* to write]. Radiography of the seminal vesicles: also called *seminal v.*

ve·sic"u·lo·pap'u·lar [*vesicula;* L. *papula,* pimple]. Consisting of vesicles and papules.

ve·sic"u·lo·pus'tu·lar [*vesicula;* L. *pustula,* blister]. Consisting of vesicles and pustules.

ve·sic"u·lot'o·my [*vesicula;* G. *tomē,* a cutting]. Division of a seminal vesicle.

ves'sel [L. *vascellum,* small vase]. A receptacle for fluids, especially a tube or canal for conveying blood or lymph.

ves'sig·non (vess'ig·non, vess'in·yon, vess·een-yohn'. *See* NOTES §§ 1, 35) [L. *vesica,* bladder]. *In veterinary medicine,* a tumor within the synovial membrane of the hock of a horse.

ves'ti·bule [L. *vestibulum,* vestibule]. An approach; an antechamber. —**vestib'ular,** *adj.*

aortic v. The space formed by the left ventricle adjoining the root of the aorta.

pyloric v. Antrum between the body of the stomach and the duodenal cap.

v. of the ear. The oval cavity of the internal ear, which forms the entrance to the cochlea. See Plate 20.

v. of the mouth. The vestibular space; it is bounded internally by the teeth and gums, externally by the lips and cheeks.

v. of the nose. The skin-lined portion of each nasal cavity, between the naris and the limen nasi.

v. of the vagina. That portion of the vulva bounded by the minor lips.

ves·tib"u·lot'o·my [*vestibulum;* G. *tomē,* a cutting]. A surgical opening into the vestibule of the labyrinth.

ves'tige [L. *vestigium,* footprint]. A trace or remnant of something formerly present or more fully developed; a vestigium. —**vestig'ial,** *adj.*

caudal medullary v. See coccygeal *v.*

coccygeal v. A remnant of the saccular termination of the embryonic neural tube located in the integument near the tip of the coccyx; derived from the medullary coccygeal vesicle.

ves·tig'i·um (ves·tidj'ee·um, ves·tig'ee·um) [L.]. An anatomic relic of fetal or embryonic life; e.g., the thymus becomes in adults a vestigium.

ves"ti·men'tum mor'tis [L. the clothing of death]. The seeming of improvement shortly before death.

ve'ta (vay'tah, vee'tah) [Sp.]. Mountain sickness.

vet"er·i·na'ri·an, vet'er·i·nar"y [L. *veterinarius,* of beasts of burden]. One who practices veterinary medicine.

vet'er·i·nar"y (vet'ur·i·nerr"ee) [*veterinarius*]. Pertaining to the practice of medicine with animals, especially domesticated animals.

Vi Chemical symbol for virginium.

vi'a·ble [F. *vie,* life; cf. L. *vita*]. Capable of living; likely to live; applied to a fetus capable of living outside of the uterus. —**viabil'ity,** *n.*

vi'al [ME. *viole,* G. *phialē*]. A small glass bottle.

Vi-an'ti·gen. An antigen discovered by Felix and Pitt which they thought was related to the virulence of the organism (typhoid). It is similar to the somatic and flagellar antigens and heat labile in water but heat stable in absolute alcohol, acetone, and glycerol. It is present in bacteria isolated from disease but disappears upon repeated culture transfers.

vi'bo·ra de la cruz' (vee'bo·rah day lah krōōss'). A venomous snake. Syn., *Bothrops alternata.*

vi·bra'tion (vye·bray'shun) [L. *vibratio,* from *vibrare*]. Oscillation; also, a rapid fluctuation; a period movement in alternately opposite directions from a position of equilibrium. —**vi′brate,** *v.*

vi′bra·tor [*vibrare*]. A device for conveying mechanical vibration to a part.

vi′bra·to″ry [*vibrare*]. Characterized by vibrations.

Vib′ri·o (vib′ree·o, vib′rye·o) [*vibrare*]. A genus of the Spirillaceae. Short, bent, motile rods, single or united end-to-end in spirals. Many species liquefy gelatin.

V. comma. The causative organism of cholera.

vi·bri·on′ sep·tique′ (vee·bree·ohn′ sep·teek′. *See* Notes § 35). See *Clostridium septicum.*

vi·bris′sa (vye·briss′uh, vi·briss′uh) [L. *vibrissae,* hairs in the nose, from *vibrare*]. 1. One of the hairs in the vestibule of the nose. 2. One of the long, coarse hairs on the face of certain animals.

vi″bro·mas·sage′ [*vibrare;* F. *massage*]. See vibratory *massage.*

vi·brom′e·ter. An instrument which registers at which point on the body surface a sensation is felt.

vi·bur′num o′pu·lus (vye·bur′num o′pew·lus, op′yoo·lus). The dried bark of *Viburnum opulus.* It contains valeric acid, an enzyme, viburnin, and a volatile oil. Preparations containing it have been used empirically in various menstrual disorders, especially those of a painful nature. Also called *high-bush cranberry bark, true cramp bark.*

vi·bur′num pru″ni·fo′li·um [L., the wayfaring tree]. The dried bark of the root or stem of *Viburnum prunifolium* or *V. rufidulum.* It contains a crystalline glycoside, salicin, which has a relaxing action on uterine muscle; other active constituents appear to be present also. It has been used to treat various uterine colics and as a general antispasmodic. Also called *blackhaw.*

vi·car′i·ous (vye·kair′ee·us, vi·) [L. *vicarius,* substituted]. Taking the place of something else; said of a habitual discharge occurring in an abnormal situation, as vicarious menstruation.

vice [L. *vitium*]. 1. A physical defect. 2. Depravity. 3. Immorality. —**vicious,** *adj.*

Vi′chy wa″ter (vish′ee, vee′shee, vee·shee′). A mildly laxative and antacid mineral water obtained from Vichy, France; has been used in rheumatic and gouty conditions and in disorders of the liver.

vi′ci·an·ose. A disaccharide which, on hydrolysis, yields *l*-arabinose and dextrose.

Vicq d'Azyr, Félix [*French anatomist,* 1748–94]. Described a foramen at the upper end of the median groove of the anterior surface of the medulla oblongata; called *cecal foramen of the medulla oblongata, Vicq d'Azyr's foramen.* Inferior laryngotomy is called *Vicq d'Azyr's operation.* See also mammillothalamic *tract.*

Vidal, Jean Baptiste Emil [*French dermatologist,* 1825–93]. Described lichen chronicus simplex, also called *Vidal's disease.* The treatment of lupus vulgaris by scarification is called *Vidal's treatment.*

vid″e·og·no′sis. Television transmission of x-ray pictures; makes possible long distance consultation and diagnosis.

Vidian artery, canal, nerve. See Guido *Guidi.*

Vierordt, Karl [*German physiologist,* 1818–84]. Used a spectroscope in the analysis of blood, bile, and urine (1876). Devised a method of counting blood cells based on essentially modern principles (1852). Developed a sphygmograph (1854) which was probably the first practical instrument for graphic recording of the pulse. Invented a hemotachometer for measuring the rate of blood flow (1858).

Vieussens, Raymond [*French anatomist,* 1641–1715]. Noted for his study of the brain and spinal cord. One of the first to describe the pathology of mitral stenosis and pulse changes in aortic disease. Described aortic regurgitation. Best remembered for his description of the centrum ovale, also called *centrum ovale of Vieussens.* The annulus ovalis is also called *Vieussens' annulus* and the ansa subclavia is also called *ansa of Vieussens.*

vig′il [L., on the watch]. Watchful wakefulness.

coma v. See *coma* vigil.

vig″il·am′bu·lism″ (vidj″il·amb′yoo·liz″um) [*vigil;* L. *ambulare,* to walk]. Ambulatory automatism in the waking state.

vig′i·lance [L. *vigilantia,* wakefulness]. Insomnia, vigil.

Vigotsky. See Kasanin-Vigotsky *test.*

Villaret, Maurice [*French neurologist,* 1877–1946]. Known for his description of a syndrome of the retroparotid space in which there is a paralysis of the faucial muscles and loss of taste in the posterior portion of the tongue with vocal-fold paralysis, called *retroparotid syndrome, Villaret's syndrome.*

Villemin, Jean Antoine [*French physician,* 1827–92]. Proved, by inoculation with tuberculous material (1868), that tuberculosis is transmissible.

vil·lik′i·nine (vi·lick′i·neen, ·nin). The active principle of crude secretin extracts, which produces strong movements of the intestinal villi.

vil·li′tis [L. *villus,* shaggy hair; G. *-itis,* inflammation]. *In veterinary medicine,* inflammation of the laminas of the corium of a horse's hoof.

vil″lo·si′tis [L. *villosus,* hairy; *-itis*]. Inflammation of the villous surface of the placenta.

vil′lous [*villosus*]. Pertaining to a villus; covered with villi; characterized by villuslike projections.

vil′lus (pl. *villi*) [L., shaggy hair]. A minute, elongated projection from the surface of a mucous membrane or other membrane.

anchoring v. One of the placental villi with ends attached to the exposed surface of the decidua basalis by basal ectoderm.

arachnoid v. See *arachnoidal granulations* under *granulation.*

chorionic v. A villus of the chorion or the placenta.

cotyledonary villi. Villi grouped in rosettes and separated by smooth chorion, as in cotyledonary placentas of ruminants.

diffuse villi. Villi evenly spaced over the entire surface of the chorion or placenta.

intestinal villi. The villi of the mucous membrane of the small intestine. Each consists of an epithelially covered, vascular core of connective tissue containing smooth muscle cells and an efferent lacteal end-capillary.

labial villi. Minute, conical projections from the inner aspect (pars villosa) of the fetal lips, sometimes retained until birth.

primary villi. The earliest villi of the embryo, consisting of cordlike masses of trophoblast separated by blood lacunas.

secondary v. A definitive, placental villus having a core of connective tissue and blood vessels. Also called *true v.*

synovial v. One of the processes extending from a synovial membrane into an articular cavity.

zonary villi. Villi restricted to an annular zone about the chorion, as in carnivores.

vil″lus·ec′to·my [*villus;* G. *ektomē,* excision]. Synovectomy; excision of a hypertrophied fold of the synovial membrane of a joint.

vin·bar′bi·tal. 5-Ethyl 5-(1-methyl-1-butenyl) barbituric acid. Delvinal sodium is a trade-mark for a brand of the sodium derivative.

Vincent, Jean Hyacinthe (1862–1950). French bacteriologist who described an angina due to fusiform bacilli (1898). See necrotizing ulcerative *gingivitis,* Vincent's *angina,* Vincent's *stomatitis.*

vin″ce·tox′i·cum [L. *vincere*, to conquer; G. *toxikon*, poison]. The root of *Cynanchum vincetoxicum* (white swallowwort), indigenous to Europe; has been used as an emetic and in menstrual disorders.

vin′cu·lum (pl. *vincula*) [L., bond, chain]. A ligament, frenum.

v. tendinum. One of the slender, tendinous filaments which connect the phalanges with the flexor tendons.

vin′e·gar. 1. A weak (approximately 6%) solution of acetic acid containing coloring matter and other substances (esters, mineral matter, etc.) formed by the fermentation of alcoholic liquids. It is commonly obtained from fruit juices or other sugar-containing liquids that have first undergone alcoholic fermentation. The process involves the oxidation of ethyl alcohol, forming acetic acid as the final product. 2. A pharmaceutical preparation obtained by macerating a drug with diluted acetic acid and filtering.

Vineland social maturity scale. See under *test.*

vinethene. A trade-mark for divinyl ether, CH_2:CH.O.CH:CH_2. The substance occurs as a clear, colorless liquid, with a slight purple fluorescence. Contains 3.5% of absolute alcohol and 0.01% of phenyl-α-naphthylamine. An inhalation anesthetic to be used for short anesthesias; differs from ether in the rapidity of its action. Intended for use in minor surgical operations of short duration, and in dentistry where gas anesthesia is not available. Also useful as an induction anesthetic. It is inflammable and deteriorates on exposure to air and light.

Vinson, Porter Paisley [*American physician*, 1890–]. Described hysterical dysphagia (1922); called *Plummer-Vinson syndrome.*

vi′nyl, vin′yl. The univalent organic radical H_2C:CH—.

v. cyanide. See *acrylonitrile.*

v. ether. See *divinyl ether; vinethene.*

vi′nyl·ene. The bivalent organic radical —CH:CH—.

vi·nyl′i·dene. The bivalent organic radical H_2C:C=.

vioform. A trade-mark for *iodochlorhydroxyquin.*

vi″o·la′ce·in. A dark purple antibiotic substance produced by *Chromobacterium violaceum* (*Bacillus violaceus*).

vi″o·la·quer′cit·rin. Rutin.

vi″o·la′tion [L. *violatio*, from *violare*, to outrage]. Rape; the act of violating or ravishing. In a medicolegal sense, it is sometimes used to indicate the act of coitus without violence or force but by means of deception, by the influence of alcohol, or by intimidation.

vi′o·let [L. *viola*, violet]. 1. A reddish blue color resembling the extreme blue end of the visible spectrum or the purple of violets; possesses the greatest refrangibility of the spectral colors. 2. A dyestuff imparting the above color.

gentian v. Methylrosaniline chloride.

vi′o·let blind′ness. Amianthinopsy.

vi″o·lu′ric ac′id. 5-Isonitroso-barbituric acid.

vi″o·my′cin. An antibiotic substance, isolated from culture filtrates of a violet-colored soil microorganism, *Streptomyces floridae* or *S. puniceus.* It is active against mycobacteria, including tubercle bacilli, and some Gram-negative organisms. It does not inhibit fungi, yeasts, protozoa, or viruses.

vi·os′ter·ol (vye·os′tur·ole, ·ol, ·awl). Activated ergosterol. Ergosterol is the principal sterol of yeast and molds and occurs as a colorless or white solid. On activation (irradiation) with ultraviolet light it undergoes a series of progressive molecular rearrangements forming several sterols of which calciferol possesses the greatest antirachitic activity. Viosterol is also known as vitamin D_2. It is used to fortify fish liver oils, and, as a solution in an edible vegetable oil, is used in the treatment of rickets. Activation of the ergosterol may also be brought about by bombarding the ergosterol with low-velocity electrons.

v. in oil. See synthetic *oleovitamin* D.

vi-penta drops. Trade-mark for a concentrated solution of vitamins A, B_1, B_2 (G), C, and D.

vi-penta perles. Trade-mark for capsules containing vitamins A, B_1, B_2(G), C, and D.

vi′per [L. *vipera*]. A poisonous snake of the genus *Vipera.* —**vi′perine,** *adj.*

Vi′per·a [L.]. A genus of the family Viperidae or true vipers.

V. russellii. One of the most important species of venomous snakes of Asia. Also called *ticpolonga.*

Vi·per′i·dae (vye·perr′i·dee) [*vipera*]. A family of venomous snakes possessing long, curved, movable front fangs which can be erected when striking. Some Viperidae are: *Bitis gabonica,* Gaboon viper; *B. lachesis,* puff adder; *B. nasicornis,* rhinoceros viper; *Echis carinatus,* saw-scaled viper; night adders of the genus *Causus; Aspis cornutus,* horned viper; and the pit viper (see *Crotalidae*). Outstanding representative in southern Asia is *Vipera russellii* (Russell's viper).

vi′per·ine (vy′puh·rin, ·ryne, ·reen) [*vipera*]. A toxalbumin extracted from the venom of vipers.

Virchow, Rudolf Ludwig Karl [*German pathologist,* 1821–1902]. Described leukemia, neuroglia, and thrombosis. The angle formed by the union of a line joining the nasofrontal suture and the most prominent point of the lower edge of the superior alveolar process with a line joining the superior border of the external auditory meatus is called *Virchow's angle.* Established the principle that all cells are derived from preexisting cellular elements, and stated it as a law, called *Virchow's law.* A line from the root of the nose to the lambda is called *Virchow's line.* See also signal *node· perivascular spaces,* under *space.*

vi·re′mi·a. The presence of a virus in the blood stream.

vir′gin [L. *virgo*, maiden]. A female who has never experienced sexual intercourse as normally understood; medicolegally, perforation of the hymen need not have occurred for loss of virginity. —**virginal,** *adj.;* **virgin′ity,** *n.*

vir·gin′i·um [NL. from the state *Virginia*]. Element number 87, symbol Vi, reported in 1930 by Allison and Murphy but not isolated until 1939, by Perey, who named it *francium.*

vir′i·din. $C_{20}H_{16}O_6$; an antibiotic substance produced by the fungus *Trichoderma viride.*

vir′ile (virr′il, vy′ril) [L. *virilis*, manly]. Pertaining to, or characteristic of, the male.

vir″i·les′cence [*virilis*]. The acquiring of characters more or less like those of the male.

vir′i·lism [*virilis*]. 1. Masculinity; the development of male traits or characteristics in the female. 2. A rare form of pseudohermaphroditism in which the subject is female, but has external genitals which appear in some degree like those of a male. Syn., *gynandry.*

vir″i·lis′mus (virr″i·liz′mus) [*virilis*]. Virilism.

vi·ril′i·ty (vi·ril′i·tee, vye·ril′i·tee) [*virilis*]. 1. The condition of being virile. 2. Procreative power.

vi·rip′o·tent (vi·rip′o·tunt, vye·rip′o·tunt) [L. *vir*, man; *potens*, powerful]. Sexually mature.

vi·rol′o·gist (vi·rol′o·jist, vye·) [L. *virus*, slimy liquid; G. *logos*, word]. One who studies viruses and virus diseases.

vi·rol′o·gy (vi·rol′o·jee, vye·) [*virus; logos*]. The study of viruses and virus diseases.

vir″u·ci′din [*virus;* L. *caedere,* to kill]. An agent capable of destroying a virus.

vir′u·lence [L. *virulentus,* poisonous]. Malignancy; noxiousness; infectiousness. The disease-producing power of a microorganism. —**virulent,** *adj.*

vir″u·lif′er·ous [*virulentus;* L. *ferre,* to bear]. Containing, or conveying, a virus.

vi′rus [L.]. 1. A general term for the poison of an infectious disease. 2. One of a group of pathogenic agents smaller than the accepted bacterial forms, some being visible by ordinary microscopical examination; others, also known as ultraviruses, are beyond this range. They are of particulate nature, and in each virus disease they are represented by particles of fairly constant size. They range from 0.2μ (200 mμ) to 0.01μ (10 mμ). Their animate nature was strongly suggested before they were actually seen, because of the results of serial transmission of virus diseases. They multiply in the animal body much like pathogenic bacteria. Unlike bacteria, they have never been cultivated on inanimate media. Virus cultures can be set up with surviving cells or proliferating embryonic cells. Cultivation is carried out in a number of cases on the chorioallantois of the developing chick. The virus of the tobacco mosaic disease has been isolated as a crystalline or paracrystalline protein which retains its infectivity (Stanley, 1935). As small an amount as 1 ml. of a one in ten billion dilution of the protein may produce infection. The virus of the tobacco mosaic disease has a molecular weight of 17×10^6 to 50×10^6. Among the well-known virus diseases of man are: rabies, poliomyelitis, encephalitis lethargica, St. Louis encephalitis, smallpox, chickenpox, herpes facialis, herpes zoster, molluscum contagiosum, common cold, influenza, measles, yellow fever, and mumps. The virus diseases of animals and plants are numerous. —**viral,** *adj.*

alastrim v. See smallpox *v.*

attenuated v. One whose disease-producing ability has been lessened by heat, chemicals, transfer through animals, or other means.

Brunhilde v. Type I poliomyelitis *v.*

Bunyamvera v. An encephalitis virus isolated from *Aëdes* mosquitoes in Uganda and pathogenic for various animals, including man.

Coxsackie viruses. A group of antigenically distinct viruses characterized by the capacity to induce destruction of striated muscle, paralysis, and death in infant mice; some strains cause pancreatitis in adult mice: related to Coxsackie disease of man.

C v. Coxsackie virus.

filtrable v. One capable of passing through a fine filter, such as the porcelain or diatomaceous earth filters. Actually, all specific disease-producing viruses are filtrable. See *virus,* 2.

fixed rabies v. Street rabies virus which is injected into rabbits and passed from one animal to another until it acquires a shorter and more constant incubation period than the naturally occurring virus. It is this fixed virus which is used for immunization. Also see rabies *vaccine.*

hepatitis v. A The virus of infectious hepatitis.

hepatitis v. B The virus of homologous serum hepatitis.

herpes simplex v. The virus responsible for a variety of diseases, as herpes simplex, eczema herpeticum, keratoconjunctivitis, and an encephalitis. Complement-fixing and neutralizing antibodies are developed four to five days after initial infection. In general, the characteristic pathologic finding is that of the large intranuclear inclusion body, called *Lipschütz body* (1921) or *Type A inclusion body* (Cowdry, 1934).

IH v. Infectious hepatitis virus.

Lansing poliomyelitis v. A strain of virus which can infect human beings; it was adapted to the cotton rat and white mouse in 1937, and is useful in serological studies of poliomyelitis.

Lansing v. Type II poliomyelitis *v.*

Leon v. Type III poliomyelitis *v.*

neurotropic v. One that attacks and has its most serious effects upon nerve tissue.

poliomyelitis v. A small (20–25 mμ), relatively stable virus which is the causative agent of poliomyelitis. On an immunological basis, three distinct types have been identified, of which the classical prototypes are: Type I, Brunhilde; Type II, Lansing; Type III, Leon. Type I is most frequently responsible for the epidemic form of the disease.

Sanarelli v. The virus of infectious myxomatosis.

SH v. The virus of homologous serum hepatitis.

smallpox v. That which causes smallpox, one of three major types, all closely related, yet distinguishable by their effects in both man and animals. The viruses are smallpox or variola, alastrim, and vaccinia or cowpox. Smallpox and alastrim viruses, by animal passage, become transformed into vaccinia virus. Various strains of vaccinia virus are in use, the dermal strains, used for vaccine, being maintained by passage through calves, sheep, or rabbits. Recently the virus has been grown in tissue cultures and in the egg.

street rabies v. The virus of rabies as found in dogs in nature or in the street as contrasted with the so-called fixed virus of rabbits.

Theiler's v. A neurotropic virus recovered from the intestines of normal laboratory mice by Theiler in 1936. It is known as mouse poliomyelitis.

tobacco mosaic v. A specific virus causing the mosaic disease of tobacco, frequently used in virus studies.

vaccine v. The virus of vaccinia.

vaccinia v. See smallpox *v.*

Venezuelan v. An immunologically distinct type of virus recovered from the brains of Venezuelan horses affected with equine encephalomyelitis. Infection of man has occurred with this strain.

West Nile v. A virus occurring in central Africa and producing a very mild encephalitis similar to the St. Louis and Japanese B encephalitides.

vi′rus·cytes″. Atypical lymphocytes resembling those seen in infectious mononucleosis, frequently present in a small percentage of cases of various viral diseases, such as influenza, infectious hepatitis, and acute respiratory disease.

vis (pl. *vires*) [L.]. Force; energy; power.

v. a fronte. A force that attracts.

v. a tergo. A force that pushes something before it.

v. conservatrix. The healing power of nature.

v. formativa. Energy manifesting itself in the formation of new tissue to replace that which has been destroyed.

v. inertiae. That force by virtue of which a body at rest tends to remain at rest.

v. in situ. Intrinsic force due to position.

v. medicatrix naturae. The healing power of nature apart from medicinal treatment.

v. vitae. Vital force.

vis·am′min. Khellin: a more recent term.

vis′ce·ra. Plural of viscus. See Plates 13, 14, 44.

cervical v. The cervical portions of the digestive and respiratory tracts, and the thyroid and parathyroid glands: a descriptive term.

vis″cer·al′gi·a [L. *viscera,* inner organs; G. *algos,* pain]. Pain in a viscus.

vis′cer·o- [*viscera*]. A combining form denoting *the viscera.*

vis″cer·o·in·hib′i·to″ry [*viscera;* L. *inhibere,* to check]. Inhibiting the movements of viscera.

vis″cer·o·meg′a·ly. Abnormally large viscera; enlargement of viscera. Syn., *splanchnomegaly.*

vis″cer·op·to′sis [*viscera;* G. *ptōsis,* a falling]. Enteroptosis.

vis″cer·o·sen′so·ry [*viscera;* L. *sensorium,* seat of sensation]. Relating to sensation in the viscera.

vis′cer·o·tome [*viscera;* G. *tomos,* cutting]. 1. An instrument used only in postmortem examinations to secure specimens of the liver. 2. The areas of the viscera supplied with sensory fibers from a single spinal nerve.

vis″cer·ot′o·my [*viscera;* G. *tomē,* a cutting]. The process of cutting out a piece of liver or other organ with the viscerotome.

vis″cer·o·to′ni·a [*viscera;* G. *tonos,* tension]. The behavioral counterpart of component I (endomorphy) of the somatotype, manifested predominantly by a desire for assimilation and the conservation of energy through sociability, relaxation, and love of food. —**visceroton′ic,** *adj.*

vis″cer·o·troph′ic [*viscera;* G. *trophē,* nourishment]. Pertaining to trophic changes induced by visceral conditions.

vis′cid [L. *viscidus,* sticky]. Adhesive; glutinous.

vis·cid′i·ty. See *viscosity.*

vis′co·li″zer [L. *viscosus,* sticky]. A machine used in reduction of size of fat particles, or in homogenization of a mixture or tissue. Also called *homogenizer.*

vis·com′e·ter (vis·kom′i·tur). See *viscosimeter.*

vis″co·sim′e·ter [*viscosus;* G. *metron,* a measure]. An apparatus for determining the degree of viscosity of a fluid.

monolayer v. An instrument used for determining the viscosity of monomolecular films.

Ostwald v. An instrument used for study of the viscosity of lyophilic colloidal systems.

vis·cos′i·ty [*viscosus*]. The resistance which a liquid exhibits to the flow of one layer over another. The property of being glutinous or sticky, and of offering resistance to a change of form, caused by the molecular attraction between the molecules of a liquid.

formula for v. $v = \frac{\pi p r^4 t}{8 l \eta}$ in which the volume of flow of a liquid v is proportional to the pressure p, the fourth power of the radius of the capillary r, the time t, and a constant $\frac{\pi}{8}$, and inversely proportional to the length of the tube l and the viscosity η of the fluid.

vis′cous [*viscosus*]. Glutinous; semifluid; sticky.

vis′cus (pl. *viscera*) [L.]. Any one of the organs enclosed within one of the four great cavities, the cranium, thorax, abdomen, or pelvis; especially an organ within the abdominal cavity. See Plates 13, 14, 44. —**visceral,** *adj.*

vis″i·bil′i·ty lim′it. 1. The maximum distance to which prominent objects, e.g., trees or houses, located in a definite direction and viewed against the horizon sky, are visible to an observer of normal eyesight under existing conditions of atmosphere, light, etc. For an object to be regarded as visible, it must be recognized by the observer, who has previous knowledge of its character from having seen it on occasions when the atmosphere was clear. 2. In *physiologic optics,* (a) *minimum visibile,* (b) *minimum separabile.* Also see under *acuity.*

vis′i·ble [L. *visibilis,* visible]. Capable of being seen. —**visibil′ity,** *n.*

vi′sion [L. *visio*]. The act of seeing; sight. Abbreviated, V. —**vis′ual,** *adj.*

binocular v. The faculty of using both eyes synchronously, without diplopia.

central v. Vision with macula lutea.

chromatic v. That pertaining to the color sense.

double v. See *diplopia.*

gun-barrel v. See tubular *v.*

indirect v. Vision with parts of the retina other than the macula.

multiple v. A condition of the eye wherein more than one image of an object is formed upon the retina.

photopic v. Vision with accurate recognition of color, as occurs when the eyes have become properly adapted to good illumination.

qualitative v. Vision in which there is ability to distinguish objects.

quantitative v. Mere perception of light.

scotopic v. Perception of shape and form without recognition of color, as occurs with very dim illumination.

solid v. The perception of relief or depth of objects obtained by binocular vision. Also called *stereoscopic v.*

tubular v. A hysterical phenomenon in which the constricted visual field defies the laws of physical projection and maintains a uniform small size, despite a change in distance of the patient from the tangent screen or the size of the test object: popularly called *gun-barrel v., tunnel v.*

vis·na′gin, vis·nag′in. $C_{13}H_{10}O_4$; 2-methyl-5-methoxyfuranochromone; a minor constituent of *Ammi visnaga,* from which khellin and khellinin are also obtained. It has been claimed that visnagin has a smooth-muscle-relaxing action, but this is not certain.

Visscher, Frank Evert (1912–). American biologist who, with Donald E. Bowman, described a chemical test for pregnancy in which anterior pituitary hormones are present in the urine: called *Visscher-Bowman test.*

vis′u·al an′gle. The angle at the eye subtended by the limits of the object. The angle is one minute of arc at the threshold of resolution.

vis″u·al·i·za′tion [L. *visualis,* attained by sight]. 1. Perceiving images in the mind with such distinctness that they seem to be seen by the eyes. 2. The act of making visible or of becoming visible, as by means of a microscope, x-ray photograph, otoscope, or other indirect means.

vis′u·al pur′ple. Erythropsin or rhodopsin. An organic pigment of the retina which is bleached to yellow by light. It is a conjugated protein closely related to vitamin A.

vis′u·al yel′low. A substance formed in the retina by visual purple in a photochemical reaction; it breaks up to yield colorless products and vitamin A.

vis″u·o·au′di·to″ry [L. *visus,* vision; *audire,* to hear]. Pertaining to hearing and seeing, as visuoauditory nerve fibers, which connect the visual and auditory centers.

vis″u·o·au′di·to″ry re·vi′val. Treatment in which soldiers suffering from combat neuroses are made to view moving pictures of actual battle scenes with appropriate sound effects; each individual, as he relives his emotional experiences, becomes conscious of the similar behavior of others and realizes that his reactions are universal and natural.

vis″u·og·no′sis (vizh″ōō·og·no′sis, ·o·no′sis) [*visus;* G. *gnōsis,* a knowing]. Appreciation and recognition of visual impressions.

vis″u·om′e·ter [*visus;* G. *metron,* a measure]. An apparatus for determining range of vision.

vis″u·o·psy′chic (vizh″ōō·o·sigh′kick) [*visus;* G. *psychē,* soul]. Pertaining to the visual association areas of the occipital cortex, Brodmann's areas 18, 19.

vis″u·o·sen′so·ry [*visus;* L. *sensorium*, seat of sensation]. Pertaining to the visual projection area of the occipital cortex, Brodmann's area 17.

vi′sus [L.]. Vision.

v. acrior. Night blindness.

v. acris. Acuteness of vision.

v. brevior. Myopia.

v. coloratus. Chromatopsia.

v. debilitas. Asthenopia.

v. decoloratus. Achromatopsia.

v. dimidiatus. Hemianopsia.

v. diurnus. Hemeralopia.

v. duplicatus. Diplopia.

v. hebetudo. Amblyopia.

v. juvenum. Myopia.

v. lucidus. Photopsia.

v. muscarum. Specks before the eyes.

v. senilis. Presbyopia.

vi′ta- [L., life]. A combining form meaning *life.*

vi′ta·gen [L. *vita*, life; G. *genesthai*, from *gignesthai*, to be produced]. A name suggested for one of the nutrients which meet a specific need for vital building material and a general need for fuel substance. These compounds are like vitamins in that a relatively small quantity is required, but are unlike vitamins in that they are utilized in animal metabolism as sources of energy.

vitaglass. Trade-mark for a glass that transmits the ultraviolet rays of sunlight.

vi′tal [L. *vitalis*, vital]. Pertaining to life.

Vitali, Dioscoride [*Italian physician and pharmacologist*, 1832–1917]. Remembered for his tests for alkaloids, for atropine, for bile pigments in the urine, and for the presence of pus in the urine.

vi′tal·ism [*vitalis*]. The theory that the activities of a living organism are under the guidance of an agency which has none of the attributes of matter or energy. —**vitalist,** *n.*

vi·tal′i·ty [L. *vitalitas*, from *vitalis*]. The power to grow, develop, perform living functions; vigor.

vi′tal·ize [*vitalis*]. Endow with the capacity to grow or develop as a living thing.

vitallium. Trade-mark for an alloy of cobalt, chromium, and molybdenum used in certain surgical appliances and procedures.

vi′tal red. A disazo dye, better known commercially as brilliant Congo R; used as a vital stain. Also called *brilliant vital red, acid Congo R, azidine scarlet R,* and *brilliant dianil red R.*

vi′tals [*vitalis*]. The organs essential to life.

vi′tal sen″si·bil′i·ties. The sensations which are of prime importance in self-preservation. Also called *paleo-s., affective s., autonomic s.*

vi′ta·mer [L. *vita*, life]. Any dietary factor or other substance which in a given species can produce a vitamin effect, as carotene in human subjects produces an effect of vitamin A.

vi′ta·min [*vita; am*monia]. One of a group of organic compounds present in variable, minute quantities in natural foodstuffs, required for the normal growth and maintenance of the life of animals, including man, who, as a rule, are unable to synthesize these compounds. They are effective in small amounts and do not furnish energy, but are essential for transformation of energy and for the regulation of the metabolism in the organism. See Table of Vitamins in the Appendix.

antiberiberi v. See *v.* B_1.

antidermatitis v. See *v.* B_6.

antihemorrhagic v. See *v.* K.

antiinfection v. See *v.* A.

antineuritic v. See *v.* B_1.

antipellagra v. Nicotinic acid.

antirachitic v. See *v.* D.

antiscorbutic v. See *v.* C.

antisterility v. See *v.* E.

antixerophthalmic v. See *v.* A.

coagulation v. See *v.* K.

fertility v. See *alphatocopherol* under *tocopherol.*

neo-vitamin A. See *v.* A.

sunshine v. See *v.* D.

synthetic v. K. See *menadione.*

v. A One necessary for maintenance of normal mucosal epithelium and visual acuity. Deficiency leads to atrophy of epithelial cells, and is conducive to susceptibility to local bacterial infections of mucous membranes (eyes, nasopharynx, genitourinary tract), xerophthalmia, and night blindness. It is a highly complex alcohol, plentiful in fish-liver oil, milk fat, and many pigmented vegetables, and is now produced synthetically. The standard unit of vitamin A is the International unit which equals in activity 0.6 microgram of pure β-carotene. One United States Pharmacopeia unit has the same value. Older units are the cod-liver oil unit which equals 208 International units, and the blue unit of Moore which equals 60 International units. Also called *antixerophthalmic v., antiinfection v.* See *oleovitamin* A.

v.-B complex. An association of an unknown number of different vitamins of which the following have been identified: thiamine (vitamin B_1), riboflavin (vitamin B_2), nicotinic acid (niacin), pyridoxine (vitamin B_6), pantothenic acid, inositol, *p*-aminobenzoic acid, biotin, adenylic acid, folic acid, and vitamin B_{12}. The complex occurs in high concentration in yeast and liver.

v. B_c See *folic acid.*

v. B_T A factor required for growth and survival of the mealworm, *Tenebrio molitor*, probably identical with carnitine.

v. B_x Para-aminobenzoic acid.

v. B_1 Thiamine hydrochloride or thiamine, necessary for normal carbohydrate metabolism, especially in nerves, and for maintenance of normal appetite, muscular tissues, reproduction, and lactation. Deficiency leads to peripheral neuropathy and heart failure. It is distributed in whole-grain cereals, meats (especially liver and pork), legumes, and yeast. One United States Pharmacopeia or International unit equals the activity of 3.0 micrograms of thiamine hydrochloride. Also called *aneurin, torulin, antineuritic v., antiberiberi factor.* See *thiamine hydrochloride.*

v. B_2 Riboflavin: found in milk, lean meat, glandular organs, eggs, yeast, and certain leafy vegetables. Also called *lactoflavin, ovoflavin, hepatoflavin, vitamin G.* Also see *riboflavin.*

v. B_3 As yet undetermined heat-labile factor essential for growth and weight maintenance of pigeons. Said to occur in yeast, liver, grain, and malt.

v. B_4 As yet undetermined factor postulated to prevent paralysis in rats and chicks. May be identical with a mixture of arginine, glycine, and cystine, or may be essential for proper utilization of these three amino acids. Said to occur in dried grass, wheat germ, liver, and yeast.

v. B_5 As yet undetermined heat-stable factor essential for maintaining growth in the pigeon. Possibly identical with niacin: also called *Peters' factor.*

v. B_6 Pyridoxine; a vitamin essential to prevent edema and swelling of the skin in the rat, found in rice bran, liver, yeast, and other sources rich in vitamin-B complex. Its deficiency may cause convulsive disorders in infants. Also called *antidermatitis v., antiacrodynia factor, adermin.*

v. B_{12} An essential vitamin needed for the normal

maturation of cells of the erythrocytic series, and also for normal neurological function. When given parenterally it corrects both the hematologic and neurologic symptoms of pernicious anemia. Syn., *antianemia factor, erythrocyte-maturing factor, extrinsic factor, anti-pernicious-anemia factor, maturation factor of liver, animal-protein factor, cyanocobalamin, hydroxocobalamin.*

v. B$_{14}$ An unidentified crystalline compound, isolated from human urine, having high cell-proliferating activity in bone marrow cultures but an inhibitory effect on certain suspensions of cells of neoplastic tissue.

v. C Ascorbic acid, cevitamic acid, cevitaminic acid; necessary for maintenance of intercellular substance of teeth, bones, and vascular walls. Deficiency leads to scurvy. Distributed in fruits, especially of the citrus variety, tomatoes, potatoes, leafy vegetables, and to a lesser degree in everything raw. It is destroyed by heat. One International unit equals the activity of 50 micrograms of ascorbic acid. Also called *antiscorbutin, scorbutanin, antiscorbutic factor.*

v. D One of several vitamins having antirachitic activity, as calciferol (D_2), irradiated 7-dehydrocholesterol (D_3), irradiated 22-dihydroergosterol (D_4), and irradiated 7-dehydrositosterol (D_5). Of these, vitamin D_3 is probably the most abundant in natural sources like fish-liver oils. Vitamin D is necessary for normal deposition of calcium and phosphorus in bones and teeth. Deficiency leads to rickets in children, osteomalacia in adults. Found in fish-liver oils (principally D_3), eggs, salmon, and produced after irradiation of ergosterol (to D_2) and other sterols or foods containing them. The action of sunshine on skin promotes the synthesis of vitamin D in the body, so that exposure to sunshine is also antirachitic. One United States Pharmacopeia or International unit is equal in activity, in standard rachitic rats, to 0.025 microgram of vitamin D_3. One Association of Official Agricultural Chemists unit equals the activity for chicks of one United States Pharmacopeia unit in the United States Pharmacopeia Reference cod-liver oil. One standard unit equals 1,000,000 International units and one clinical unit equals 12.5–17 International units. Also called *antirachitic v., antiricketic v.* See synthetic *oleovitamin* D.

v. E Tocopherol; three tocopherols have vitamin-E activity; α-tocopherol ($C_{29}H_{50}O_2$), β-tocopherol ($C_{28}H_{48}O_2$), and γ-tocopherol ($C_{28}H_{48}O_2$; isomer of β-tocopherol). Vitamin-E deficiency in rats produces muscular dystrophy, degeneration, death and resorption of the fetus in the gravid female, and testicular degeneration in the male. This vitamin appears to be essential for the maturation and differentiation of certain cells. Occurs in wheat-germ oil, cottonseed oil, corn oil, rice-germ oil, lettuce, and alfalfa. One rat unit, or the fertility dose, is equal to 2–3 mg. of α-tocopherol. Also called *antisterility v., tocopherol.*

v. F A term formerly used for essential fatty acids, such as linoleic acid ($C_{18}H_{32}O_2$), linolenic acid ($C_{18}H_{30}O_2$), and arachidonic acid ($C_{20}H_{32}O_2$).

v. G See *v.* B_2.

v. H A water-soluble component of the vitamin-B complex identical with biotin and coenzyme R.

v. H′ Para-aminobenzoic acid.

v. K Group of at least three naphthoquinone derivatives, vitamin K_1, vitamin K_2, and vitamin K_3. Vitamin K is essential for formation of prothrombin. In vitamin-K deficiency, the blood clotting time is markedly prolonged and hemorrhages result. The principal dietary sources are spinach, cabbage, kale, cauliflower, tomatoes, and soybean oil. There is no International unit standard. Also called *antihemorrhagic v., prothrombin factor.* See *menadione.*

v. K$_1$ Phytonadione.

v. K$_2$ 2-Methyl-3-difarnesyl-1,4-naphthoquinone, isolated from putrefied fish meal; it occurs in microorganisms.

v. K$_3$ See *menadione.*

v. L One of a group of lactation vitamins. Evidence indicates that these vitamins are distinct entities, but they have not been characterized chemically or extensively studied.

v. M A factor, probably a member of the vitamin-B complex, believed to be necessary for the prevention of anemia and loss of weight in monkeys. Present in yeast and liver.

v. P-P Nicotinic acid.

v. T A substance extracted from the yeast *Torula utilis* which has a stimulating and regulating effect on growing and regenerating tissues.

v. U A supposed vitamin necessary for growth in the chick.

vi′ta·zyme″. A substance having the properties of both a vitamin and an enzyme. *Obs.*

vit′el·lar″y (vit′i·lerr″ee, vye′ti·) [L. *vitellus,* yolk]. Pertaining to the vitellus. Vitelline.

vi·tel′li·cle (vi·tel′i·kul, vye·tel′·) [*vitellus*]. Old term for the yolk sac or umbilical vesicle.

vi·tel′lin (vi·tel′in, vye·tel′in) [*vitellus*]. A phosphoprotein found in egg yolk.

vi·tel′line (vi·tel′in, ·een, ·yne, vye·tel′·) [*vitellus*]. Pertaining to the vitellus or yolk.

vi·tel″lo·lu′te·in [*vitellus;* L. *luteus,* yellow]. A yellow pigment of yolk.

vi·tel″lo·mes″en·ter′ic (vi·tel″o·mess″en·terr′ick, vye·tel″o·) [*vitellus;* G. *mesos,* middle; *enteron,* intestine]. Omphalomesenteric.

vi·tel″lo·ru′bin [*vitellus;* L. *rubeus,* red]. A reddish pigment obtained from the yolk of egg.

vi·tel′lus (vi·tel′us, vye·tel′us) [L.]. A yolk; specifically, the yolk of the egg of the common fowl, *Gallus domesticus.*

v. ovi. The yolk of an egg.

vi″ti·a′tion (vish″ee·ay′shun) [L. *vitiatio,* from *vitiare,* to spoil]. A change which lessens utility or efficiency or neutralizes an action.

vit″i·lig′i·nes (vit″i·lidj′i·neez) [L. *vitiligo,* cutaneous eruption]. The lineae albicantes.

vit″i·li′go [L.]. A skin disease characterized by an acquired achromia in areas of various sizes and shapes. There is an almost complete lack of pigment with hyperpigmented borders. Lesions are more marked in areas exposed to sun. Also called *leukoderma, piebald skin, lichromia.* **—vitilig′inous, vitil′igoid,** *adj.*

circumnevic v. See *leukoderma* acquisitum centrifugum.

perinevoid v. See *leukoderma* acquisitum centrifugum.

v. acquisita syphilitica. See *vitiligoid.*

v. capitis. Alopecia areata.

vi·til′i·goid [*vitiligo;* G. *eidos,* form]. A rare form of pigmentary syphiloderm in early syphilis, usually occurring on the sides of the neck and more frequent in women. It appears as rounded, discrete or confluent macules of hyperpigmentation (coffee brown), or in a form, simulating vitiligo, in which hypopigmented macules are bordered by slight hyperpigmentation. Also called *leukomelanoderma, leukoderma syphiliticum, vitiligo acquisita syphilitica.*

vit″il·i·goi′de·a [*vitiligo; eidos*]. Old term for xanthoma.

vit′re·in. A complex protein found in the vitreous body of the eye.

vit″re·o·cap″su·li′tis. See *hyalitis.*

vit″re·o·den′tin, vit″re·o·den′tine (vit″ree·o·den′tin) [L. *vitreus*, of glass; *dens*, tooth]. A variety of dentin with but few dentinal tubules.

vit′re·ous [*vitreus*]. Glassy; hyaline.

vit′re·ous. The transparent, gelatinlike substance filling the greater part of the globe of the eye: also called *vitreous body, vitreous humor.* See Plate 19.

vi·tres′cence [*vitreus*]. The condition of becoming hard and transparent like glass.

vit′re·um [*vitreus*]. The vitreous.

vit′ric [L. *vitrum*, glass]. Relating to glass or any vitreous substance.

vi·tri′na (pl. *vitrinae*) [*vitrum*]. The vitreous.

v. auditoria. The endolymph: also called *v. auris.*

v. ocularis. The vitreous.

vit′ri·ol [L. *vitreus*, glassy]. 1. Old term for any substance having a glassy fracture or appearance. 2. Sulfuric acid. Syn., *oil of v.* 3. Any crystalline salt of sulfuric acid. —**vit′riolated, vitriol′ic,** *adj.*

blue v. Copper sulfate.

green v. Ferrous sulfate or copperas.

oil of v. Sulfuric acid.

v. elixir. Aromatic sulfuric acid.

white v. Zinc sulfate.

vit″ri·ol′ic ac′id. Sulfuric acid.

vit·ri′tis [L. *vitrum*, glass; G. *-itis*, inflammation]. Glaucoma.

vit″ro·den′tin, vit″ro·den′tine. 1. Calcified tissue allegedly occurring on or in the scales or teeth of certain lower fishes. 2. Vitreodentin: erroneous.

vit″ro·pres′sion [*vitrum;* L. *pressio*, pressure]. Pressure with a glass slide on the skin to aid in study and diagnosis of skin lesions.

vit′rum [L.]. Glass.

viv″i·dif·fu′sion [L. *vivus*, living; *diffusio*, from *diffundere*, to pour forth]. The passage of diffusible substances from blood of a living animal flowing through collodion tubes into surrounding isotonic saline solution.

viv″i·fi·ca′tion [*vivus;* L. *facere*, to make]. The act of making alive or of converting into living tissue.

vi·vip′a·rous (vye·vip′uh·rus, vi·vip′·) [*vivus;* L. *parere*, to bring forth]. Bringing forth the young alive—distinguished from *oviparous.* —**vivipar′ity,** *n.*

viv″i·sec′tion [*vivus;* L. *sectio*, from *secare*, to cut]. The surgical preparation of anesthetized animals for study of functions or their derangements. —**viv′isect,** *v.*

viv″i·sec′tion·ist [*vivus; secare*]. One who practices or defends experimental work on animals.

viv′i·sec″tor [*vivus; secare*]. One who uses surgical procedures on anesthetized animals to study functions or their derangements.

Vleminckx's solution. See under sulfurated lime *solution.*

vo′cal [L. *vocalis*, vocal]. Pertaining to the voice; pertaining to the organs producing the voice.

vo·ca′lis. The muscle lying beneath the true vocal folds.

Voegtlin, Carl (1879–). American pharmacologist who demonstrated that calcium metabolism is controlled by the parathyroid glands (1909) and contributed to the elucidation of the chemotherapeutic action of arsenicals.

Voges-Proskauer reaction. See under *reaction.*

Vogt, Oskar (1870–). German neurologist, who, with his brother Cecil (b. 1875) described status marmoratus, also called *Vogt's disease* or *syndrome.* A juvenile form of amaurotic familial idiocy is called *Spielmeyer-Vogt disease.*

Vogt, Paul Friedrich Emmanuel [*German surgeon*, 1847–85]. Remembered for his description of a point selected for trephining in traumatic meningeal hemorrhage; *Vogt's point* is found by taking a horizontal line two fingers' breadth above the zygomatic arch, and a vertical line a thumb's breadth behind the sphenofrontal process of the zygoma, the intersection of the two marking the point.

voice [L. *vox*, voice]. The sounds, especially articulate sounds, that are produced by the vibration of the vocal folds and modified by the resonance organs.

esophageal v. See esophageal *speech.*

nasal v. A peculiar, muffled timbre of the voice, especially marked in cases of perforated palate.

void [L. *vacuus*, empty]. Evacuate.

clocked voids. Voidings at stated intervals, usually initiated with assistance of manual pressure over the bladder: part of a regimen for patients with a neurogenic urinary bladder.

Voillemier's point. See under *point.*

Voisenet-Rhode reaction. See under *reaction.*

vo′la [L., palm]. The palm of the hand or the sole of the foot. —**volar,** *adj.*

vol′a·tile [L. *volatilis*, flying]. Readily vaporizing; evaporating. —**volatiliza′tion,** *n.;* **volatilize,** *v.*

v. oils. Essential oils.

vole [Scand. in origin]. Any ratlike rodent belonging to the genus *Microtus.*

vo·le′mic [volume; G. *haima*, blood]. Referring to volume of blood or plasma.

Volhard, Franz [*German physician*, 1872–1950]. Introduced pericardectomy for adhesive pericarditis (1923); also called *cardiolysis.* Devised technics for determining chloride in blood or urine, using silver nitrate; called *Volhard-Arnold method.* See also *Volhard's and Fahr's tests* under *test.* Malignant nephrosclerosis is called *Fahr-Volhard's disease.*

Volhard-Harvey method. See under *method.*

Volhard and Löhlein method. See under *method.*

vo·li′tion [L. *velle*, to will]. The will or determination to act. —**volitional,** *adj.*

Volkmann, Alfred Wilhelm (1800–1877). German physiologist who described the small canals found in compact bone, called *Volkmann's canals*, which transmit blood vessels. Contributed important work on the histology of the central nervous system (1842).

Volkmann, Richard von [*German surgeon*, 1830–89]. Distinguished for having been the first to describe cancer resulting from irritation of the skin by coal tar and paraffin (1873). Excised the rectum for cancer (1878). Described ischemic contracture of the muscles due to pressure or injury accompanied often by muscle degeneration; called *Volkmann's contracture.* The resulting paralysis is called *ischemic paralysis, Volkmann's paralysis.* Originator of a splint with foot piece and two lateral supports, used in fractures of the lower extremity, called *Volkmann's splint.*

vol′ley [L. *volare*, to fly]. Approximately simultaneous discharges, as nerve impulses which travel simultaneously in different axons of a nerve or which are discharged simultaneously from groups of central neurons.

Vollmer patch test. See under *test.*

vol. %. Volume per cent.

vol·sel′la [L., a kind of pincers]. A forceps having one or more hooks at the end of each blade. Also called *vulsella, vulsellum forceps.*

volt [after Alessandro *Volta*, Italian physicist, 1745–1827]. The unit of electromotive force and of electric potential; the electromotive force that, steadily applied to a conductor whose resistance is 1 ohm, will produce a current of 1 ampere. Abbreviated, v, v.

electronvolt. Unit of energy equivalent to the

kinetic energy which an electron acquires in falling through a potential of one volt.

million electronvolts. One million electronvolts; 1.59×10^{-6} erg. Abbreviated, *mev.*

volt′age [*Volta*]. Electromotive force measured in volts.

effective v. For alternating currents, 0.707 of the peak voltage.

inverse v. The voltage between the filament and the plate in a roentgen-ray tube during that part of the cycle that the anode is negatively charged.

volt′a·gram″ [*Volta;* G. *gramma*, letter]. A faradic battery so arranged as to produce an almost continuous current. *Obs.*

vol·ta′ic. Of or pertaining to Alessandra Volta or to voltaism; galvanic.

vol′ta·ism. See *galvanism.*

vol·tam′e·ter [*Volta;* G. *metron*, a measure]. An instrument for ascertaining the electromotive force of a current in volts.

volt′am″me·ter [*Volta;* A. M. *Am*père, French physicist; *metron*]. An instrument for measuring both voltage, or potential, and amperage, or amount of current.

volt′-am′pere. A watt; the rate of working in an electric circuit when the current is one ampere and the potential one volt.

Volterra method. See under *method.*

volt′me″ter [*Volta; metron*]. An instrument for measuring voltage, or electromotive force.

electrostatic v. One for measurement of high voltages; built on the principle that like electric charges repel and unlike charges attract each other.

Voltolini, Friedrich Eduard Rudolph [*German laryngologist and otologist*, 1819–89]. Known for his description of an acute inflammation of the internal ear, of labyrinthine origin, associated with fever and severe constitutional and cerebral symptoms (1867); called *Voltolini's disease.* The first to use the galvanic cautery in laryngeal surgery (1867) and a pioneer in the use of external illumination in laryngeal surgery (1889).

vol′ume [L. *volumen*, roll, volume]. *In physics*, the space which a substance fills. Cubic dimension.

atomic v. The atomic weight of an element divided by the density; it represents the volume in cubic centimeters which would be occupied by the atomic weight of an element taken in grams.

expiratory reserve v. The volume of air that can be expelled after involuntary exhalation at any level of activity. Syn., *reserve air, supplemental air.* See also *respiration.*

inspiratory reserve v. Complemental air. See also inspiratory *capacity, respiration.*

mean cell v. See MCV.

mean corpuscular v. See MCV.

molecular v. The volume of one gram-molecule of substance; in the gaseous state under the same conditions of temperature and pressure, the molecular volumes of all substances are equal.

residual v. Air remaining in the lungs after the most complete expiration possible. It is elevated in diffuse obstructive emphysema and during an attack of asthma. Syn. *residual air* or *capacity.*

sensitive v. *In radiobiology*, a region within a cell which is especially sensitive to radiation. Syn., *sensitive region.*

specific v. The volume occupied by a definite weight of a substance, as the volume in cubic centimeters of 1 Gm. of substance.

tidal v. The amount of air moved by a single breath at any level of activity: normally, at rest, approximates 500 cc. (resting tidal volume). Syn. *tidal air.*

v. per cent. The number of cubic centimeters of a substance contained in 100 cc. of medium. Usually refers to gas (O_2 or CO_2) contained in blood. Symbol, vol. %.

vol″u·met′ric [*volumen;* G. *metron*, a measure]. Pretaining to measurement by volume.

vol′un·tar″y [L. *voluntarius*, voluntary]. Under control of the will; performed by an exercise of the will.

vol′u·tin [L. *volutum*, from *volvere*, to roll]. Inclusion bodies in bacterial and yeast cells.

vol·vu·lo′sis. Onchocerciasis.

vol′vu·lus [*volvere*]. A twisting of the bowel upon itself so as to occlude the lumen, occurring most frequently in the sigmoid flexure.

vo′mer [L., ploughshare]. The thin plate of bone which is situated vertically between the nasal cavities, and which forms the posterior portion of the septum of the nose. See Table of Bones in the Appendix.

vom″er·o·na′sal (vom″ur·o·nay′zul, vo″mur·o·) [*vomer;* L. *nasus*, nose]. Pertaining to the vomer and the nasal cavity.

vom′it [L. *vomitum*, from *vomere*, to vomit]. Matter expelled from the stomach by vomiting.

bilious v. Vomit stained with bile.

black v. A dark fluid consisting of blood and the contents of the stomach.

coffee-ground v. Vomit consisting of altered blood and the contents of the stomach.

vom′it. To expel from the stomach by vomiting.

vom′it·ing [*vomere*]. The forcible ejection of the contents of the stomach through the mouth.

cyclic v. Vomiting recurring at regular periods.

dry v. Persistent nausea with attempts at vomiting, but with ejection of nothing but gas.

epidemic v. of childhood. Epidemic acute non-bacterial gastroenteritis in children.

fecal v. See stercoraceous *v.*

pernicious v. A variety of vomiting occasionally occurring in pregnancy and becoming at times so excessive as to threaten life.

projectile v. A form observed in some diseases of the brain stem; the vomitus is suddenly projected out of the mouth to some distance, usually without nausea.

stercoraceous v. Ejection of fecal matter in vomit, usually due to intestinal obstruction.

vom′i·tive [*vomere*]. Emetic.

vom′i·to ne′gro. Black vomit; a Spanish term for hematemesis in yellow fever.

vom′i·to″ry [L. *vomitorius*, vomiting]. 1. Any agent that induces emesis. 2. A vessel used to receive ejecta.

vom″i·tu·ri′tion (vom″i·tew·rish′un) [L. *vomere*, to vomit]. Ineffectual attempt at vomiting; retching.

vom′i·tus [L.]. 1. Vomited matter. 2. The act of vomiting.

v. cruentus. Bloody vomit.

v. marinus. Seasickness.

v. matutinus. Morning sickness.

v. niger. Black vomit.

von Aldor's test. See under *test.*

vonedrine. Trade-mark for phenylpropylmethyl amine, a nasal vasoconstrictor used by inhalation See *phenylpropylmethylamine.*

von Graefe's knife. A small knife with a long, narrow blade, used in ophthalmic surgery.

Von Kóssa's $AgNO_3$ method. See under *stain.*

Voorhees, James Ditmars [*American obstetrician* 1869–1929]. Introduced a hydrostatic rubber bag useful in dilating the uterine cervix where it is desired to induce labor; called *Voorhees bag.*

vo·ra′cious [L. *vorax*, voracious]. Having an insatiable appetite or desire for food.

Voronoff, Serge [*Russian physiologist*, 1866–1951]. Widely known for his advocacy of rejuvenation by testicular implantations (1919); called *Voronoff's operation.*

vor'tex (pl. *vortices*) [L., a whirl]. A structure having the appearance of being produced by a rotary motion about an axis.

v. coccygeus. The point of convergence of the lanugo hairs over the coccyx.

v. lentis. Lens star.

v. of the heart. The region at the apex of the heart where the superficial layer of muscle of both ventricles (vortex fibers) passes into the deep layer of the ventricles.

vortices pilorum. Hair whorls.

vor'ti·cose [*vortex*]. Whirling; having a whorled appearance.

Vossius ring. See pigmented *cataract.*

vox [L.]. The voice.

v. abscissa. Loss of voice.

v. capitis. The upper register of the voice; falsetto voice.

v. cholerica. A peculiar, faint voice noted in the last stage of cholera.

v. rauca. Hoarse voice.

vo"yeur' (vwah"yur'. *See* NOTES § 35) [F.]. Peeping Tom. One who obtains sexual gratification from witnessing the sexual acts of others or from viewing persons in the nude. —**voyeurism,** *n.*

V. R. Vocal resonance.

V. S. Volumetric solution.

vu"e·rom'e·ter (view"i·rom'i·tur, view·rom'i·tur) [F. *vue*, sight; G. *metron*, a measure]. An apparatus for determining the interpupillary distance.

vul'can·ize [L. *Vulcanus*, the fire god]. Subject rubber to a process wherein it is treated with sulfur at a high temperature, and thereby rendered either flexible or very hard.

vul'ner·a·ble [L. *vulnerabilis*, from *vulnus*, injury]. Susceptible to injury.

vul'ner·ar"y (vul'nur·err"ee) [L. *vulnerarius*, of wounds]. An agent useful in healing wounds. *Rare.* —**vul'nerary,** *adj.*

vul'nus [L.]. A wound. *Obs.*

Vulpian, Edme Félix Alfred [*French physician*, 1826–87]. Described progressive muscular atrophy affecting the muscles of the scapulohumeral region; called *Vulpian's atrophy.* He described a slow, prolonged contraction obtained in denervated lingual muscle by stimulation of the chorda tympani nerve. This was believed to have been caused by a diffusion of acetylcholine from neighboring end organs to the sensitized end plate; called *Vulpian effect.* See also Vulpian-Heidenhain-Sherrington *phenomenon.*

Vulpian test. See under *test.*

vul·pin'ic ac'id. $C_{19}H_{14}O_5$; a yellow pigment found in some rare lichens, used to kill foxes and wolves; it causes pronounced dyspnea, convulsions, and death from respiratory failure.

vul·sel'lum (pl. *vulsella*). See *volsella.*

vul'va [L., covering, womb]. The external genital organs in woman. Syn., *pudendum muliebre.* —**vulvar,** *adj.*

garrulity of v. Flatus vaginalis.

v. connivens. A form of vulva in which the labia majora are in close apposition.

v. hians. The form of vulva in which the labia majora are gaping.

vul·vec'to·my [*vulva;* G. *ektomē*, excision]. Excision of the vulva.

vul·vis'mus (vul·viz'mus). See *vaginismus.*

vul·vi'tis [*vulva;* G. *-itis*, inflammation]. Inflammation of the vulva.

adhesive v. One associated with the sticking together of vulvar structures.

intertriginous v. One secondary to the irritation which follows the rubbing together of adjacent parts.

vul'vo-, vulv- [*vulva*]. A combining form denoting *the vulva.*

vul"vo·vag"i·ni'tis (vul"vo·vadj"i·nigh'tis) [*vulva;* L. *vagina*, vagina; G. *-itis*, inflammation]. Inflammation of the vulva and of the vagina existing at the same time.

W

W Chemical symbol for wolfram.

w, w. Watt.

Waage, Peter [*Norwegian chemist*, 1833–1900]. Described, with C. M. Guldberg, the law of mass action, called *Guldberg-Waage law.*

Wachendorf, Eberhard Jacob von [*Dutch anatomist*, 1703–58]. Remembered for his description of the fetal pupillary membrane; called *Wachendorf's membrane.*

wad'ding [F. *ouate*]. 1. Carded cotton or wool, used for surgical dressings, generally not of the first quality. 2. Cotton batting, sometimes glazed to render it nonabsorbent.

wad'dle [AS. *wadan*, to go]. A clumsy, swaying walk or gait.

Wade's urethral suppositories. Suppositories containing iodoform, bismuth subnitrate, chloral, and morphine.

wa'fer [Teut. in origin]. A thin sheet made by heating moistened flour and used to enclose powders that are taken internally. Also called *cachet.*

Wagner, Ernst Leberecht [*German pathologist*, 1829–88]. Described dermatomyositis (1863). First to describe colloid milium, also called *Wagner's disease.* Made contributions to the knowledge of pathology of uterine cancer (1858).

Wagner, Johann Philip [*German physicist*, 1799–1879]. Devised an instrument for opening and closing a galvanic circuit, called *Wagner's hammer* or *Neef's hammer.*

Wagner, Rudolf [*German physician*, 1805–64]. Remembered for his many contributions to the knowledge of sympathetic nerves, nerve ganglions, and nerve endings (1842–53). With Meissner, described the tactile corpuscles, also called *Wagner's corpuscles;* see Meissner's *corpuscle.*

Wagner, Wilhelm [*German surgeon*, 1848–1900]. Introduced an osteoplastic resection of the skull; called *Wagner's operation.*

Wagner von Jauregg, Julius (1857–1940). Austrian physician who practiced fever therapy as treatment for neurosyphilis and dementia paralytica, using inoculation with malaria, called *Wagner-Jauregg treatment.* Nobel laureate (1927).

Wagstaffe, William Warwick [*English surgeon*, 1843–1910]. Remembered for his description of fracture with separation of the medial malleolus: called *Wagstaffe's fracture.*

Wahl, Eduard von [*German surgeon*, 1833–90]. Described a sign indicative of intestinal obstruction, in which local meteorism appears above the point of obstruction; called *Wahl's sign*.

wa·hoo' bark (wah·hōō', wah'hōō). Euonymus.

waist [ME. *wast*]. The narrowest portion of the trunk above the hips.

waistline. The circumference of the waist.

wa·kam'ba. A vegetable arrow poison, used in Zanzibar.

wake'ful·ness [AS. *wacan*]. Insomnia; continued inability to sleep.

Waksman, Selman A. (1888–). American soil microbiologist known for his extensive research on soil microorganisms, such as actinomycetes and other fungi, the bacteria concerned with the oxidation of sulfur, and the organisms concerned in the formation of antibiotic substances, as well as marine bacteria. He received the Nobel prize in 1952 for the discovery of streptomycin.

Walcher's position. See under *position*.

Waldenström, Johan Anton [*Swedish physician*, 1839–79]. Reported, with A. F. Linstedt, what was probably the first description of a case of volvulus (1878).

Waldenström, Johan Henning [*Swedish surgeon*, 1877–]. Described osteochondritis deformans juvenilis; also described the formation and disappearance of amyloid in man.

Waldeyer-Hartz, Heinrich Wilhelm Gottfried von [*German anatomist*, 1836–1921]. The germinal epithelium is called *Waldeyer's epithelium*. The duodenal fossae are sometimes known as *Waldeyer's fossae*. Described the lymphatic ring formed by the two faucial tonsils, the pharyngeal tonsil, and smaller groups of lymphatic follicles at the base of the tongue and behind the posterior pillars of the fauces; called *Waldeyer's tonsillar ring*. Modified sweat glands at the border of the tarsal plates of the eyelid are known as *Waldeyer's glands*.

Waldschmitz-Leitz method. See Willstätter, Waldschmitz-Leitz, and Hesse *method*.

Walker, J. T. Ainslie (1868–1930). English chemist who introduced, with Samuel Rideal, a method for testing disinfectants (1903) called *Rideal-Walker method*. See under Samuel *Rideal*.

Walker sarcoma. See under *sarcoma*.

walk'ing i'ron. A metal support attached to a splint, shoe, or plaster cast designed to permit walking without the sole of the foot coming in contact with the ground.

walk'ing wound'ed. *In military medicine*, a sick or wounded person who can walk from the place where he became a casualty to the place where he can receive medical treatment; an ambulant case.

wall [L. *vallum*, rampart]. The bounding side or inside surface of a natural or artificial cavity or vessel.

axial walls. Walls of a tooth, or of a cavity in a tooth, which are parallel with the long axis of the tooth.

cell w. (a) The cellulose cell membrane of plant cells. (b) The outer boundary or membrane of some animal cells.

Wallace, Alfred Russel [*English naturalist*, 1823–1913]. Independently developed a theory of natural selection which was in every respect comparable to that of Darwin. The accounts of both were published in a joint paper by the Linnean Society of London (1858).

Wallace and Diamond's method. See under *method*.

Wallenberg, Adolf [*German physician*, 1862–1949]. Described a syndrome involving the lateral portion of the medulla, due to thrombosis in the posterior inferior cerebellar artery. The symptoms include ipsilateral lateropulsion, hemisynergia, hemiataxia, and hemifacial anesthesia; contralateral loss of pain and temperature sensibility in arm, trunk, leg; ipsilateral laryngoplegia and palatoplegia. Called *Wallenberg's syndrome*.

Waller, Augustus Désiré [*English physiologist*, 1856–1922]. First to employ electrodes in research upon action currents and electromotive changes accompanying the heart beat (1887). His experiments had an important bearing upon the development of electrocardiography.

Waller, Augustus Volney [*English physiologist*, 1816–70]. Known for his classic experiments upon the effects of section of the glossopharyngeal and hypoglossal nerves of the frog, which demonstrated nerve degeneration (1850). Demonstrated that a nerve fiber can maintain its anatomic and physiologic integrity only when it is in uninterrupted continuity with its cell of origin, called *Wallerian law, law of Wallerian degeneration*.

wall'eye" [ON. *vagleygr*]. 1. Leukoma of the cornea. 2. Divergent strabismus. —**walleyed,** *adj*.

wall teeth. Molar teeth.

Walter, William Grey (1910–). English physiologist who introduced location of brain tumor by electroencephalography (1936).

Walther, Augustin Friedrich [*German anatomist*, 1688–1746]. Described the coccygeal ganglion, called *Walther's ganglion, ganglion impar*. Described the lateral talomalleolar ligament which was once called *Walther's ligament*.

Walton, Albert James [*English surgeon*, 1881–]. Described an operation for relief of hourglass stomach due to ulcer of the lesser curvature, called *Walton's operation*. He also described an operation for reconstructing the common bile duct.

Walton, Ernest T. S. (1903–). Irish physicist who shared the Nobel prize in 1951 with John D Cockcroft for their work in atom-smashing.

wan'der·ing [AS. *wandrian*]. 1. Moving about, as wandering cells. 2. Abnormally movable, as wandering spleen or kidney.

Wang's test. See under *test*.

Wangensteen, Owen Harding [*American surgeon*, 1898–]. Devised an instrument for relief of gastric and intestinal distention, which consists of a suction apparatus connected with a duodenal tube, called *Wangensteen's apparatus* or *Wangensteen's tube*.

war'bles (wawr'bulz). The disease produced by infestation of domestic animals and man with the larva of the warble fly or botfly, *Dermatobia hominis*.

Warburg, Carl [*Austrian physician*, b. 1804]. Introduced an antiperiodic preparation of various drugs; called *Warburg's tincture*.

Warburg, Otto Heinrich (1883–). German biochemist who conducted penetrating studies on the mechanisms of cellular respiration and photosynthesis, and on the metabolism of tumors, which were of the greatest influence on the development of modern biochemistry. He developed a manometric method for the study of tissue metabolism (see Warburg *manometer*), characterized the oxygen-activating respiratory enzyme, cytochrome oxidase (Warburg's yellow ferment or old yellow enzyme) as a heme-containing compound, and showed that carbon monoxide inhibits intracellular respiration (1926). This inhibition technique and his tissue-slice technique have been used widely in biochemical studies. He isolated several other respiratory and fermentative enzymes and coenzymes. Nobel laureate in physiology and medicine (1931).

ward [AS. *weard*]. A division or room of a hospital.

Wardell method. See Myers and Wardell *method.*

Wardrop, James [*English surgeon,* 1782–1869]. Distal ligation of an artery for aneurysm is sometimes called *Wardrop's operation.* Onychia maligna is called *Wardrop's disease.*

war'far·in [*W*isconsin *A*lumni *R*esearch *F*oundation]. $C_{19}H_{16}O_4$; 3-(α-acetonylbenzyl)-4-hydroxycoumarin; a colorless powder, practically insoluble in water: used as a rodenticide and therapeutically as an anticoagulant.

warm'-blood'ed. Having a relatively high and constant body temperature, as in birds and mammals. Syn., *homothermic, homothermal.*

Warren, John Collins [*American surgeon,* 1842–1927]. Remembered for his incision for breast amputation, in which he made a pear-shaped cut encircling the breast, the stem following the greater pectoral muscle at the axillary border and ending high in the axilla. A bracketlike, two-pronged extension joins the original incision at the external border of the breast. Called *Warren's incision.*

Warren, Jonathan Mason [*American surgeon,* 1811–67]. Introduced a form of uraniscoplasty, in which he dissected the mucous membrane upward, freeing the soft palate by dividing the posterior pillars and placing sutures in the midline; called *Warren's operation.*

wart [AS. *wearte*]. A hyperplasia of the papillae of the skin, forming a small projection. See *verruca.* —**wart'y,** *adj.*

fig w. A papillary growth of filiform or vegetating projections, often covered with an offensive-smelling secretion; usually found on the genitalia. Syn., *verruca acuminata, condyloma acuminatum, venereal w.*

moist w. Condyloma acuminatum.

Peruvian w. See *verruca* peruviana.

plantar w. Verruca plantaris.

venereal w. Condyloma acuminatum.

Wartenberg, Robert (1887–). American neurologist who described chiralgia paresthetica (isolated neuritis of the superficial branch of the radial nerve), brachialgia statica paresthetica (nocturnal arm paresthesias), partial thenar atrophy (abiotrophy of the lateral thenar muscles), sign of facial palsy (diminution of palpebral vibration of the upper lid), sign of ulnar paralysis (abduction position of the little finger), pyramidal sign (flexion of the thumb on flexion of the other fingers against resistance), sign of median-nerve palsy (defective abduction of the thumb), head-retraction reflex (retraction of the head on tapping the upper lip). He introduced the pinwheel for examination of sensibility and of superficial reflexes.

Warthin, Aldred Scott [*American physician,* 1867–1931]. Described pulmonary fat embolism (1913). Warthin's sign consists of exaggerated pulmonary sounds in acute pericarditis. See also *Warthin-Finkeldey giant cells,* under *cell.*

wash [AS. *wascan*]. A lotion; any of a class of pharmaceutical preparations (solutions or mixtures) for local application without friction or rubbing. Mouth and nasal washes also belong to this class.

yellow w. Yellow lotion.

wash'ing so'da. Sodium carbonate, $Na_2CO_3.10H_2O$.

wasp's waist. Atrophy of trunk muscles in muscular dystrophy.

Wassermann, August von [*German bacteriologist,* 1866–1925]. Known internationally for his introduction, with Albert Neisser and Carl Bruck, of a specific blood test for the diagnosis of syphilis (1906). Called *Wassermann reaction* or *test, complement-fixation test.* See Wassermann's *test.*

Was'ser·man-fast. See *seroresistance.*

waste [ONF. *wast*]. 1. Useless matter eliminated from the body. 2. Food no longer suitable for consumption.

waste. To become thin; to pine away.

wast'er (way'stur) [*wast*]. 1. A child suffering from marasmus. 2. An animal affected with tuberculosis, usually bovine types.

watch'ma"ker's cramp. 1. An occupational neuritis characterized by painful cramps of the muscles of the hands. 2. Spasm of the orbicularis oculi muscle, due to holding a jeweler's lens.

wa'ter [AS. *waeter*]. 1. The liquid consisting of molecules of the composition H_2O, or aggregates thereof. 2. Pharmaceutically, any saturated aqueous solution of a volatile oil or other aromatic or volatile substance. Also called *aromatic w.*

activated w. Water containing ions, free atoms, radicals, and molecules in a highly reactive state: the temporary result of passing ionizing radiation through it.

camphor w. A saturated solution of camphor in distilled water.

deep w. Water obtained from a porous layer beneath the first impervious stratum of the ground.

deionized w. Water purified by passage through substances which remove contaminating cations and anions and leave finally a water equivalent to distilled water in purity.

distilled w. (*aqua destillata*). Water purified by distillation.

ground w. See subsoil *w.*

hard w. Water containing soluble calcium or magnesium salts and not readily forming a lather with soap.

heavy w. That which contains double-weight atoms of hydrogen (deuterium) instead of ordinary (light-weight) hydrogen atoms. Syn., *deuterium oxide.*

mineral w. A natural water containing mineral substances in solution.

purified w. The U.S.P. title for water obtained by distillation or deionization.

redistilled w. Distilled water redistilled one or more times. For parenteral use, it is sterilized by a suitable method of sterilization, within two hours after its redistillation, and preserved against contamination. Also called *double-distilled w.*

sterile distilled w. (*aqua destillata sterilis*). Sterile distilled water stored in suitable containers, properly sealed or closed.

subsoil w. Water which has penetrated the soil, and is found immediately above the first impervious stratum.

w. for injection (*aqua pro injectione*). Water for parenteral use, which has been distilled, sterilized, and stored in sealed or other suitable sterile containers, so that it is free and remains free from pyrogens.

w. of crystallization. Water entering into the crystalline structure of a compound in definite molecular proportions. It may often be removed by heating at 100° C. with resultant disruption of the crystal and formation of the anhydrous compound.

w. of hydration. See *w.* of crystallization.

w. on the brain. Hydrocephaly.

wa'ter brash. Watery acid fluid regurgitated from the stomach, accompanied by nausea.

wa'ter-brax"y. A highly fatal disease of the digestive tract of sheep, causing a diffuse, intense inflammation of the abomasum. It is believed to be caused by *Clostridium septicum.*

wa'ter-far"cy. Old term for glanders.

Waterhouse, Rupert (1873–). English physician known for his description of acute collapse associated with hemorrhages into the adrenal glands in acute meningiococcemia. See Waterhouse-Friderichsen *syndrome.*

wa′ter moc′ca·sin. The cottonmouth, a venomous pit viper. See *Ancistrodon piscivorus.*

wa′ters [*waeter*]. Lay term for the liquor amnii; amniotic fluid.

bag of w. The amnion and amniotic fluid.

wa′ter·y eye. Epiphora.

Watson, Benjamin Philip (1880–). American obstetrician and gynecologist who introduced a method for induction of labor by the use of castor oil supplemented by quinine and pituitary extract, called *Watson's method.*

Watson, Cecil James [*American physician*, 1901–]. Devised methods for the estimation of urobilinogen in urine and feces, especially in relation to jaundice and anemia. Called *Watson methods.*

Watson, Edwin M. [*American surgeon*, contemporary]. Known for his method of urethral reconstruction, in which he bridged the gap between the severed ends of the posterior urethra by urethral flaps pedunculated at the proximal limit of the patent urethral canal to form the roof and sides of the urethra, called *Watson's operation.*

Watson, Francis Sedgwick [*American urologist*, 1853–1942]. Performed median perineal prostatectomy (1889), published in 1905.

Watson, William Spencer [*English ophthalmologist*, 1836–1906]. Known for his operation for entropion, in which he transplanted a bridge of skin from the eyelid through to the conjunctival surface.

Watson's test. See Proske and Watson's *test.*

watt [after James *Watt*, Scottish engineer, 1736–1819]. The unit of power, equal to 10 million units of power in the centimeter-gram-second system; the power required to cause an unvarying current of 1 ampere to flow between points differing in potential by 1 volt: also called *volt-ampere.* Abbreviated, w, w.

watt′age [*Watt*]. Consumption or output of an electric device in watts.

watt′me″ter [*Watt;* G. *metron*, a measure]. An instrument for measuring electric power or activity in watts.

wave [AS. *wafian*]. 1. A uniform movement in a body which is propagated with a continuous motion, each part of the body vibrating through a fixed path. 2. The course traced by a lever or a beam of light on a surface moving at right angles to the direction of lever or beam.

activation w. The spread of the electrical impulse over the heart in electrocardiography.

alpha w. See alpha *rhythm.*

A w. Alpha wave. See alpha *rhythm.*

a w. The atrial wave of the venous pulse.

Berger w. See *rhythm.*

brain w. Alpha wave. See *electroencephalography*, alpha *rhythm.*

coronary T w. An inverted T wave with an upward convexity of the first limb, its apex peaked and its second limb rather straight. In some leads it may be upright. Frequently seen in electrocardiograms during various stages of myocardial infarction, but not confined to this exclusively. Also called *cove-plane T w.*

cove-plane T w. See coronary T *w.*

c w. Ventricular contraction or systolic wave of the venous pulse.

deep Q w. A Q wave of large amplitude, as considered in relation to other deflections of the QRS complex.

electrocardiographic waves. P, Q, R, S, T, U are signs arbitrarily chosen to signify various phases of the spread of depolarization and repolarization of cardiac muscle as seen in the electrocardiogram.

excitation w. The wavelike involvement of successive muscle fibers by the excitatory process.

ff waves. The waves of atrial fibrillation seen in the electrocardiogram.

F waves. The waves of atrial flutter seen in the electrocardiogram, consisting of an atrial depolarization wave and an atrial repolarization wave. They are precisely regular in spacing, size, and contour.

Hertzian waves. Original term for radio waves; electromagnetic waves resembling light waves, but having greater wavelength.

P mitrale w. A broad, notched P wave, usually indicating left atrial hypertrophy or dilatation, as a consequence of mitral stenosis or left ventricular failure.

P pulmonale w. A peaked, narrow P wave, usually indicating right atrial hypertrophy or dilatation.

presinus w. One of low amplitude recorded at the sinoatrial node, immediately preceding the action potential of the latter.

pulse w. The progressive expansion followed by contraction due to the flow of blood. It begins with each cardiac systole and is propagated along the aorta and other arteries, ending normally at the capillaries.

P w. of the electrocardiogram. The first wave, due to depolarization of the atria. The average maximum height is 1.25 mm., and the average duration is 0.08 second.

QS w. of the electrocardiogram. First and downward wave of the initial ventricular complex, not followed by an R wave.

Q w. of the electrocardiogram. First and downward wave of the ventricular complex. It represents early ventricular depolarization. It is often absent normally.

R w. of the electrocardiogram. The first upward deflection of the ventricular complex, usually of relatively large amplitude: it represents a major portion of ventricular depolarization.

R′ w. of the electrocardiogram. The second upward deflection of the normal electrocardiogram, if present.

sharp w. *In electroencephalography*, a wave form of relatively short duration, usually showing an abrupt rise but slower fall.

S w. of the electrocardiogram. The first downward deflection of the ventricular complex, following upon an R wave: it is often absent normally.

Ta w. of the electrocardiogram. The deflection representing atrial repolarization. Normally it is opposite in direction to the P wave, which it follows. Usually it cannot be identified in a normal electrocardiogram.

Traube-Hering waves. Rhythmic oscillations in mean blood pressure not correlated with the heart beat nor with respiration.

T w. of the electrocardiogram. The deflection which represents repolarization of the ventricles. In most leads it is normally upright, varying rather widely in amplitude and duration.

U w. of the electrocardiogram. A deflection, usually of low amplitude, following the T wave. It is often absent normally: its causation and significance are not certain.

V w. The stasis or diastolic wave of the venous pulse.

w.-and-spike. *In electroencephalography*, a complex consisting of a slow wave followed by a spike.

w. a of the phlebogram. The first and atrial

wave of the venous pulse observed in the jugular bulb.

w. b or h of the phlebogram. Diastolic wave.

w. c of the phlebogram. Systolic wave.

w. front. A surface at which all vibratory motion is of like phase concurrently.

w. number. The number of waves or cycles of light flux or radiant energy, measured through a distance of 1 cm.

wave'length". The distance in the line of advancement between two points of a (sine, light, radio) wave such that the two points are in the identical phase of the wave cycle. Differences in wavelength distinguish visible light, roentgen rays, and gamma rays from one another. Frequency and wavelength are related by the equation, $C = f\lambda$, where C is the velocity of light and f is the frequency of the radiation. Symbol, λ. Abbreviated, wl, wl.

dominant w. The wavelength of a beam of light which determines its hue.

wax [AS. *weax*]. Any substance, of plant, animal, or mineral origin, consisting of a mixture of one or more of the following constituents: high molecular weight fatty acids, high molecular weight monohydric alcohols, esters of the fatty acids and alcohols, solid hydrocarbons.

earth w. Ceresin.

mineral w. Ceresin.

vegetable w. Japan wax.

white w. (*cera alba*). Bleached yellow wax. For chemical composition and uses, see yellow *w.* Also called *bleached beeswax.*

yellow w. (*cera flava*). The purified wax from the honeycomb of the bee, *Apis mellifera*. It consists chiefly of myricin (myricyl palmitate). It also contains cerotic acid (cerin), melissic acid, and about 6% of hydrocarbons of the paraffin series. It is used in the formation of ointments, cerates, plasters, suppositories, and surgical dressings in which it acts mechanically, either giving stiffness or serving to protect from water. Also called *beeswax.*

WBC, Wbc White blood cell. See *leukocyte.*

wean [AS. *wenian*]. Cease to suckle or nurse offspring at a period when the latter is capable of taking substantial food from sources other than the breast.

weav'ers' bot'tom. Chronic ischial bursitis due to long-continued pressure in a sedentary occupation.

web [AS. *webb*]. A membranelike structure; especially, the skin and underlying tissue between the bases of fingers or toes. See also *patagium.*

Weber, Adolph [*German ophthalmologist,* 1829–1915]. Described operations for cataract extraction, using a curved bistoury, and for lacrimal stricture, a modification of Bowman's operation in which he slit the upper canaliculus, divided the medial palpebral ligament, and dilated the duct with a sound. Introduced a form of rhinoplasty in which he raised an oval flap from the center of the upper lip, attaching it to the freshened edges of the defective ala, called *Weber's operation.*

Weber, Eduard Friedrich Wilhelm [*German physiologist,* 1806–71]. Distinguished for his many accomplishments in the field of the physiology of the nervous system. With E. H. Weber, he determined the velocity of the pulse wave (1825) and discovered the inhibitory action of the vagus (1845). With Wilhelm Eduard Weber, wrote an important work on motion and locomotion (1836).

Weber, Ernst Heinrich [*German anatomist and physiologist,* 1795–1878]. Proponent of the law in physiology that the increase of stimulus necessary to produce the smallest perceptible change in a sensation is proportionate to the strength of a stimulus already acting (1834); called *Weber's law,* or *Fechner-Weber law.* See also Weber's *test.*

Weber, Frederick Parkes (1863–). English physician who described hereditary hemorrhagic telangiectasis (1907), also called *Osler-Rendu-Weber's disease,* and nodular nonsuppurative panniculitis, called *Christian-Weber disease,* and nevoid amentia, called *Sturge-Weber disease.*

Weber, Hermann David [*English physician,* 1823–1918]. Described oculomotor nerve paralysis on the side of a lesion of the cerebral peduncle with contralateral spastic hemiplegia, called *Weber's paralysis.* Alternate hemiplegia of various types is known as *Weber-Gubler syndrome, Millard-Gubler syndrome.* See also *Millard.*

Weber, Wilhelm Eduard [*German physiologist,* 1804–91]. With E. F. W. Weber, wrote an important work on motion and locomotion.

Weber's circles. Circles of points of tactile sense discrimination.

Weber's glands. Racemose glands situated in the posterior portion of the tongue.

Weber's organ or **vesicle.** The prostatic utricle of the male urethra. See *utricle,* 2.

Weber's test. See under *test.*

Webster, John [*English chemist,* 1878–1927]. Described a test for trinitrotoluene in urine; called *Webster's test.*

Webster, John Clarence [*Canadian gynecologist,* 1863–1950]. Developed an operation for the relief of retrodisplaced uterus, in which he drew the round ligaments through perforations in the broad ligaments, suturing them to the posterior surface of the uterus; called *Webster's operation.*

Webster dinner pills. Aloe and mastic pills; also called *Lady Webster dinner pills.*

Webster, Hill, and Eidinow method. See under *method.*

Wechsler-Bellevue intelligence scale. See under *test.*

Wecker, Louis de [*French ophthalmologist,* 1832–1906]. Described a large number of operations on the eye. A procedure for surgical treatment of paralytic strabismus is called *de Wecker's operation.*

Wedensky, Nicolai Igorevich [*Russian neurologist,* b. 1844]. Contributed studies in nerve physiology. Described the following phenomenon: when two stimuli are applied in succession to the motor nerve of a curarized muscle, the end-plate potentials evoked by the volleys, sum, and, if the summated potential reaches a critical intensity, a conducted spike potential will appear and contraction follows. This effect resembles facilitation across a nerve block and is called *Wedensky's facilitation.* See also Wedensky's *inhibition.*

wedge [AS. *wecg*]. An instrument or material used by dentists to separate adjoining teeth.

Weed, Lewis Hill [*American anatomist,* 1886–1952]. Known for his many contributions to the knowledge of the anatomy of the central nervous system. Indicated the pathways of the circulation of cerebrospinal fluid (1916).

Weeks, John Elmer [*American ophthalmologist,* 1853–1949]. Demonstrated that one of the two bacilli discovered by Koch as causative of Egyptian ophthalmia was also the cause of pinkeye. The bacillus, called *Koch-Weeks bacillus,* is a pleomorphic form of *Hemophilus influenzae.* Pinkeye, or acute contagious conjunctivitis, is also called *Koch-Weeks conjunctivitis.*

weep'ing [AS. *wēpan*]. 1. Lacrimation. 2. Exudation or leakage of a fluid.

weep'ing. Exuding: said of raw or excoriated surfaces bathed with a moist discharge.

Wegner, Friedrich Rudolph Georg [*German pathologist,* b. 1843]. Described osteochondritic epiphyseal separation in prenatal syphilis (1870), also called *Wegner's disease.*

Weichselbaum, Anton [*Austrian pathologist,* 1845–1920]. Known for his discovery of the *Micrococcus meningitidis* (1887), the cause of cerebrospinal meningitis; also called *Weichselbaum's coccus, Neisseria meningitidis.*

Weidel reaction. See under *reaction.*

Weigert, Carl [*German pathologist and histologist,* 1845–1904]. Especially known for his development of staining methods and for his discoveries in microchemistry. See *iron hematoxylin* (*Weigert's*) under *stain; Weigert's method for myelin sheaths* under *stain;* Weigert's resorcin-fuchsin *stain; Gram-Weigert staining method* under *stain; Weigert's law* under *overproduction theory.*

weight [AS. *wiht*]. The force with which a body is attracted by the earth. For weights listed by name, see Tables of Weights and Measures in the Appendix.

atomic w. A number representing the relative weight of an atom of an element compared with oxygen (= 16.000). It is the mean value of the isotopic weights of an element. Abbreviated at. wt.

equivalent w. The weight of an element which can replace or combine with a unit weight of hydrogen or is otherwise equivalent to the latter.

molecular w. The weight of a molecule of any substance, representing the sum of the weights of its constituent atoms. Abbreviated, M.

specific w. Specific gravity.

Weigl's method. See under *method.*

Weil, Adolph [*German physician,* 1848–1916]. Remembered for his description of leptospirosis icterohemorrhagica (1886) and his differentiation of it from other forms of acute jaundice; also called *Weil's disease, spirochetal jaundice.*

Weil, Richard [*American physician,* 1876–1917]. Devised a test for syphilis, based on the fact that hemolysis does not occur if an emulsion of the blood of a syphilitic person is mixed with a solution of dried cobra venom; known as *Weil's test.*

Weil's methods. See under *stain.*

Weil-Felix test. See under *test.*

Weinbach method. See under *method.*

Weinbach's modification. See Butler and Tuthill's *method.*

Weinberg, Michel [*French bacteriologist,* 1868–1940]. With P. Séguin, isolated bacteria found in gas gangrene. Devised a complement-fixation test in echinococcus disease; called *Weinberg's method.*

Weir, Robert Fulton [*American surgeon,* 1838–1927]. He developed a lumbar incision for nephrectomy, called *Weir's incision.* A procedure for correction of hallux valgus is called *Weir's operation.* Introduced appendicostomy, also called *Weir's operation.*

Weisbach, Albin W. [*Austrian anthropologist,* 1837–1914]. Described an angle formed by lines starting from the basion and from the middle of the frontal suture and meeting at the alveolar point; called *Weisbach's angle.*

Weisman, Abner Irving [*American obstetrician,* 1907–]. Known for his modification of the Aschheim-Zondek test, in which he used female mice, his gynograph used in radiography and insufflation of the uterine tubes, and his work on the use of the frog in pregnancy diagnosis.

Weismann, August Friedrich Leopold [*German biologist,* 1834–1914]. Proponent of a theory that the hereditary material or germ plasm is distinct from the somatoplasm; that there is a continuity of germ plasm from generation to generation; that a change in the somatoplasm or body cannot affect the germ plasm, which renders it impossible for acquired characteristics to be inherited; that during development the heredity determiners are sorted out to the parts of the body where they give rise to hereidtary characteristics. Called *Weismann's theory.*

Weiss, Leonhard [*German physician,* contemporary]. Devised a combined stain for determining the presence of tubercle bacilli; called *Weiss's stain.*

Weiss, Leopold [*German ophthalmologist,* 1849–1901]. Remembered for his description of a reflex on the nasal side of the optic disk; *Weiss's reflex* is regarded as a prodromal sign of myopia.

Weiss, Nathan [*Austrian physician,* 1851–83]. Known for the sign which bears his name and which is manifested by contraction of the facial muscles when lightly struck; appears in cases of tetany and neurasthenia; called *Weiss's sign.*

Weisz test. See under *test.*

Welch, William Henry [*American pathologist,* 1850–1934]. A founder of the Johns Hopkins Medical School. Discovered, with S. Flexner, pathologic processes arising from action of diphtheria toxins (1891). Discovered *Staphylococcus epidermidis albus,* or *Micrococcus albus.* Advanced knowledge of thrombosis and embolism (1899). With G. H. F. Nuttall, discovered *Bacillus aerogenes capsulatus,* the cause of gas gangrene (1892); also called *Bacillus perfringens, B. achalme, Clostridium welchii, Welch bacillus.*

Welcker, Hermann [*German physiologist,* 1822–97]. Known for his research in the determination of blood volume in experimental animals (1854). Is credited with being the first to determine the total blood volume (1858), called *Welcker's method.*

Welker method. See Marshall and Welker *method,* Welker and Tracy *method.*

Weller, Thomas Huckle (1915–). American authority in tropical medicine and public health, who with J. F. Enders and F. C. Robbins shared the Nobel prize (1954) in physiology and medicine for their discovery that the poliomyelitis virus will grow in cultures of different tissues.

Wells, Horace [*American dentist,* 1815–48]. Celebrated in the history of anesthesia. He first used nitrous oxide as a dental anesthetic (1844). One of the trio which has received credit for the introduction of anesthesia in America, the others being William T. G. Morton and Crawford W. Long.

Wells, Thomas Spencer [*English gynecologist,* 1818–97]. Pioneer ovariotomist. Described the anxious expression of face found in ovarian disease; called *Wells's facies.* A type of surgical forceps is called *Spencer Wells's forceps.*

Wells-Stenger test. See under *test.*

Welsbach, Carl Auer von [*Austrian chemist,* 1858–1929]. Inventor of the *Welsbach burner* which employs a mixture of gas and vapor to incandesce the *Welsbach mantle.*

Weltmann's reaction. See Weltmann's *test.*

Weltmer, Sidney A. [*American,* contemporary]. Founder of a system of treatment by suggestion, based on a theory of harmony between mind and body; called *Weltmerism.*

wen [AS. *wenn*]. A sebaceous cyst. The term is commonly used when the lesion occurs in the scalp.

Wenckebach, Karel Frederik [*Dutch physician,* 1864–1940]. Remembered for his investigations of the value of quinine in cardiac arrhythmia and atrial fibrillation (1914). Conducted important study of beriberi (1934). Described a period, or phenomenon, of cardiac arrhythmias in which he noted that conduction disturbances may be produced by gradually increasing prolongation of the conduction time up to a final omission of the ventricular beat; called *Wenckebach's period, type I.* If produced by periodic lapse of a ventricular beat without delay of conduction, it is known as *type II.*

Wenzel, Michael Jean Baptiste de [*French ophthalmologist*, d. 1790]. Early cataract extractor, renowned for his skill. Introduced a special operation adapted to cases of posterior synechia, called *Wenzel's operation.*

Werdnig, Guido [*Austrian neurologist*, contemporary]. Known for his description of an infantile variety of hereditary familial spinal muscular atrophy (1890), called *Hoffmann-Werdnig syndrome.* This appears to be a rare form of spinal progressive muscular atrophy appearing at an early age in the muscles about the pelvis and terminating fatally within five or six years.

Werlhof's disease. See idiopathic thrombocytopenic *purpura.*

Wernekinck, Friedrich Christian Gregor [*German anatomist*, 1798–1835]. Described the decussating fibers of the middle cerebellar peduncle; called *Wernekinck's commissure.*

Werner, Heinrich (1874–1946). German physician who described trench fever, also called *Werner's syndrome, Werner-His disease, Volhynia fever.*

Wernicke, Carl [*German psychiatrist*, 1848–1905]. Described acute, superior hemorrhagic polioencephalitis, previously noted by C. J. Gayet; called *Wernicke's disease.* Described a form of spastic hemiplegia called *Wernicke-Mann's palsy,* and pseudophthalmoplegia. See also Wernicke's *aphasia*, Wernicke's *sign* (hemianopsic pupillary reaction), Wernicke's *syndrome.*

Wertheim, Ernst [*Austrian gynecologist*, 1864–1920]. Known for his modification of Watkins' operation for procidentia uteri, and for an operation for cystocele; called *Wertheim-Schauta operation.* Also called *Schauta-Wertheim operation.* Introduced a radical operation for complete hysterectomy in uterine carcinoma; called *Wertheim's operation.*

Westberg, Friedrich [*German physician*, nineteenth century]. Described a condition marked by the appearance of white or atrophied spots on the skin; called *Westberg's disease.*

Westergren method. A method of obtaining sedimentation rate of erythrocytes by determining the sinking velocity of the red cells, using a glass tube graduated at 1-mm. intervals. The reading is usually made after one hour. See also under *method.*

Westphal, Carl Friedrich Otto [*German neurologist*, 1833–90]. Described agoraphobia (1871). Drew attention to the value of the knee jerk in diagnosis of disease, especially of tabes (1875). Its absence is called *Westphal's sign.* Described a pseudosclerosis, a cerebral degenerative hepatolenticular condition, in which symptoms resemble those of multiple sclerosis; called *Westphal's disease* or *neurosis, Strümpell-Westphal pseudosclerosis.* See also Edinger-Westphal *nucleus.*

Westphal-Pilcz reflex. See pupillary *reflex.*

wet'ting a'gent. See under *agent.*

Wetzel, Norman Carl [*American pediatrician*, 1897–]. Known for his description of a precision control chart for measuring and guiding growth and development of children from 5 to 18 years. Body build, maturation, nutritional grade, metabolic rate, and caloric intake are all determined by this graphic method. Called *Wetzel's grid.*

Wever-Bray effect. The microphonic response of the cochlea, so called because of resemblance to the electrical phenomena produced by sound waves in microphones. It consists of electrical potentials caused by the stimulation of the cochlea by sound. The exact nature of the cochlear microphonics is not known. Also called *Wever-Bray phenomenon.*

Weyer, Johann (Wierus) [*Swiss physician*, 1515–88]. Celebrated as the founder of medical psychiatry. Author of an important work on diseases of the mind (1563).

Weyl, Theodor [*German chemist*, 1851–1913]. Introduced a test for creatinine, in which he added to the solution to be tested a few drops of a dilute solution of sodium nitroprusside and, drop by drop, a few drops of sodium hydroxide. The development of a ruby-red coloration, changing to a yellow and then to blue on warming with acetic acid, indicates the presence of creatinine. Called *Weyl's test.*

W fac'tor. Biotin.

Wharton, Thomas (1610–1673). English anatomist who wrote a treatise on glands and discovered the submaxillary duct, named for him. See also under *jelly.*

wheal [ME. *whele*]. A primary lesion of the skin that is a circumscribed, edematous, usually transitory elevation that varies in size from a pin-head to that of the palm or larger. Lesions come and go quickly and are accompanied by tingling, burning, or intense itching. They occur classically in urticaria but also occur after insect bites, animal bites, trauma, or even physical agents as heat, cold, or sunlight. Syn., *pomphus, urtica.*

Wheat'stone bridge. See under *bridge.*

Wheelhouse, Claudius Galen [*English surgeon*, 1826–1909]. Remembered for his external urethrotomy in which he divided the stricture on a grooved probe; called *Wheelhouse operation.* The staff used in the operation is known as *Wheelhouse's staff.*

wheeze [ME. *whesen*]. A whistling or sighing noise produced in the act of breathing. Often heard only by stethoscopic examination. It signifies partial obstruction of one or more of the air passages due to spasm, edema, inflammation, foreign body, tumor, or external pressure.

whey [AS. *hwaeg*]. The liquid part of milk separating from the curd.

whiff [ME. *weffe*]. A puff of air.

oral w. A peculiar sound heard during expiration from the open mouth, principally in cases of thoracic aneurysm.

Whipple, Allen Oldfather (1881–). American surgeon who developed an operation for excision of islet-cell tumors of the pancreas by using a wide transverse abdominal incision dividing the great omentum and freeing the duodenum, so that all parts of the pancreas can be palpated to discover the hidden tumor; first to propose with Parsons and Mullins the two-stage procedure for radical pancreaticoduodenectomy for carcinoma of the ampullary area and pancreatic head, and the first to perform radical pancreaticoduodenectomy in one stage.

Whipple, George Hoyt (1878–). American pathologist known for his studies of normal and pathological liver function, his work on the bile and other endogenous pigments, plasma proteins, and iron metabolism. He made important contributions to knowledge of the anemias, and, with G. R. Minot and W. P. Murphy, received the Nobel prize (1934) in physiology and medicine for discovering the beneficial effects of liver therapy against pernicious anemia. He described (1907) intestinal lipodystrophy, also called *Whipple's disease.*

whip'worm [ME. *whippen;* AS. *wyrm*]. *Trichuris trichiura.*

whis'per [AS. *hwisprian*]. A low, soft, sibilant sound produced by the passage of the breath through the glottis without vibrating the vocal folds.

White, Charles [*English surgeon*, 1728–1813]. Said to be first to excise the head of the humerus (1770).

Described phlegmasia alba dolens (1773). To reduce a dislocation of the humerus he advocated a method in which the heel is placed in the axilla and traction is exerted on the arm (1785), called *White's method, Cooper's method.*

White, James Clarke [*American dermatologist,* 1833–1916]. First to hold a chair of dermatology in the United States. Described keratosis follicularis (1889); also called *White's disease, Darier's disease.*

White, James William [*American surgeon,* 1850–1916]. Widely known for his skill in operative surgery. Devised an operation in which he removed the testes for hypertrophy of the prostate; called *White's operation.*

White method. See Lee-White *method.*

white [AS. *hwit*]. Having a color produced by reflection of all the rays of the spectrum: opposed to black.

white. Any white substance, as white of egg.

Whitehead, Walter [*English surgeon,* 1840–1913]. Known in his time for his operation of removal of the hemorrhoidal area from the anal canal; called *Whitehead's operation for hemorrhoids.* His excision of the tongue through the mouth, using only scissors, was also known as *Whitehead's operation.*

Whitehorn's method. See under *method.*

white lo'tion (*lotio alba*). A lotion prepared from zinc sulfate, 40 Gm.; sulfurated potash, 40 Gm.; distilled water, a sufficient quantity to make 1000 cc. Used in the treatment of various types of skin diseases for which sulfur is employed. It may be used full strength or diluted with an equal part of water. Also called *lotio sulfurata.*

white pine (*pinus alba*). The dried inner bark of *Pinus strobus.* It contains a glycoside coniferin, tannin, mucilage, and oleoresin. Used as an ingredient in cough syrups. It is always employed in conjunction with other remedial agents. Also called *white pine bark.*

compound w. p. syrup (*syrupus pini albae compositus*). A syrup prepared by percolation from white pine, wild cherry, aralia, poplar bud, sanguinaria, sassafras, chloroform, sucrose, glycerin, alcohol, and distilled water and colored with either cudbear or amaranth. Used as a mild expectorant in subacute bronchitis. Dose, 4–8 cc. (1–2 fluidrachms).

white'pox" [AS. *hwīt;* ME. *pokkes*]. A varicellalike disease occurring in Brazil.

whites [*hwīt*]. A lay term for leukorrhea.

Whitfield, Arthur [*English dermatologist,* 1867–1947]. Devised an ointment used in treatment of some dermatoses. It consists of benzoic acid 4 Gm., salicylic acid 2 Gm., petrolatum 24 Gm.; often used half strength. Called *Whitfield's ointment.*

whi'ting [*hwīt*]. Prepared chalk or white clay; purified calcium carbonate.

whit'low [perhaps from E. *quickflaw,* sore at the quick]. An old general term for any suppurative inflammation of the end of a finger or toe. See *felon, paronychia.*

melanotic w. A rare melanoma of the nail bed.

Whitman, Royal [*American orthopedic surgeon,* 1857–1946]. Treated fracture of the femoral neck in children by forced abduction. Devised a type of astragalectomy for relief of talipes calcaneus in which he partially removed the malleoli and performed tenoplasty of the peroneal tendons; called *Whitman's operation.*

Whitmore, Alfred [*English surgeon in the Indian Medical Service,* 1876–1946]. First to describe melioidosis, with C. S. Krishnaswami; also called *Whitmore's disease.* The bacillus isolated from the disease is known as *Pfeifferella whitmori, Malleomyces pseudomallei.*

WHO World Health Organization.

whoop (hōōp, whōōp) [OF. *houper*]. The inspiratory crowing sound which precedes or occurs during a coughing paroxysm.

whoop'ing cough (hōōp'ing, hōōp'ing). Pertussis, an infectious catarrhal inflammation of the air passages with peculiar paroxysms of coughing ending in a loud whooping inspiration. Most frequent in children. Caused by *Hemophilus pertussis.*

Whytt, Robert [*Scottish physician,* 1714–66]. Noted that destruction of the corpora quadrigemina abolishes pupillary contraction to light; called *Whytt's reflex.* Described tuberculous meningitis in children, and acute hydrocephaly; both sometimes called *Whytt's disease.*

Wichmann, Johann Ernst [*German physician,* 1740–1802]. First to describe laryngismus stridulus, also called *Wichmann's asthma, Millar's asthma, Kopp's thymic asthma.* Demonstrated the parasitic origin of scabies (1786).

wick'ing [AS. *wēoce*]. Loosely twisted unspun cotton or gauze, employed in packing cavities; a gauze wick.

Widal, Georges Fernand Isidor [*French physician,* 1862-1929]. Investigated, with André Chantemesse, the possibilities of antityphoid inoculation (1888). Best known today for his description of acquired hemolytic jaundice with anemia (1907); called *Widal-Abrami's disease, Hayem-Widal disease.* See also Widal *test.*

Wiegand. See *Wigand.*

Wigand, Justus Heinrich [*German gynecologist,* 1766–1817]. Described a method of extraction of the aftercoming head by pressure above the symphysis with the second hand, the first being under the child's body; called *Wigand's maneuver.*

Wiggers and Dean method. See under *method.*

Wijs method. See under *method.*

Wilbur and Addis method. See under *method.*

Wildbolz, Hans [*Swiss urologist,* 1873–1940]. Described a reaction indicative of tuberculosis. The intradermal injection of a few drops of the patient's urine causes a local reaction known as *Wildbolz's reaction.*

Wilde, William Robert Wills [*Irish surgeon,* 1815–76]. An incision for relief of mastoid periostitis made about half an inch behind the pinna and parallel to it is called *Wilde's incision.*

Wilder, Russell Morse [*American internist,* 1885–]. Described, with Cutler and Power, a test for adrenal insufficiency; see Cutler-Power-Wilder *test.* Author of many contributions on diabetes and hyperinsulinism.

Wilder, William Hamlin [*American ophthalmologist,* 1860–1935]. Described a twitch of the eyeball when the position of the eye is changed from abduction to adduction, or vice versa, as indicative of exophthalmic goiter; called *Wilder's sign.*

Wildermuth, Hermann A. [*German psychiatrist,* 1852–1907]. Described a congenital deformity of the ear in which the antihelix is prominent, the helix being turned downward or badly developed; called *Wildermuth's ear.*

wil·for'dine. An insecticidal alkaloidal constituent of *Tripterygium wilfordi.*

wil·for'gine. An insecticidal alkaloidal constituent of *Tripterygium wilfordi.*

wil·for'ine. An insecticidal alkaloidal constituent of *Tripterygium wilfordi.*

wil·for'trine. An insecticidal alkaloidal constituent of *Tripterygium wilfordi.*

wil·for'zine. An insecticidal alkaloidal constituent of *Tripterygium wilfordi.*

Wilhelmi's method. See Frame, Russell, and Wilhelmi's *method.*

Wilhelmy balance. An apparatus for determining surface tension by means of a glass slide which is weighed as it dips into a liquid.

Wilkinson, J. H. [*English physician*, nineteenth century]. Introduced a compound sulfur ointment known as *Wilkinson's ointment*.

Wilkinson and Peters benzidine peroxidase reaction. See under *reaction*.

Wilks, Samuel [*English physician*, 1824–1911]. Brought Hodgkin's disease to the attention of the profession and named it (1856, 1865). Wrote a classic description of bacterial endocarditis (1870). Myasthenia gravis is sometimes called *Wilks's symptom complex*. Chronic parenchymatous nephritis, one form of large white kidney, is called *Wilks's disease*. Verruca necrogenica is also called *Wilks's disease*.

will [AS. *willa*]. *In psychology*, the faculty by which the mind chooses its ends and directs action in carrying out its purpose.

w. to power. *In psychiatric theory*, the neurotic and excessive aggressiveness of an individual compensating for feelings of inferiority and insecurity (Alfred Adler).

Willan, Robert [*English dermatologist*, 1757–1812]. Distinguished psoriasis as a separate disease entity (1808); called *Willan's lepra*. Described (1796) nonthrombopenic purpura, also called *Henoch's purpura*.

Willebrand, E. A. von [*Finnish physician*, contemporary]. Described hereditary pseudohemophilia or constitutional thrombopathy, a rare disease of unknown etiology. It is characterized by prolonged bleeding time with normal number of platelets and normal coagulation time, and is found in both males and females. Called *von Willebrand's disease*.

Willems, Charles [*Belgian surgeon*, contemporary]. Known for his introduction of a method of treating acute suppurative arthritis by arthrotomy and immediate mobilization; called *Willems' method* or *treatment*.

Williams, Robert Runnels (1886–). American biochemist who determined the structure and developed the synthesis of vitamin B_1 (thiamine).

Williams, Roger John (1893–). American biochemist who separated pantothenic acid from other members of the vitamin-B complex, and identified it chemically.

Williamson, Oliver K. (1866–1941). English physician who described a sign of pleural effusion or pneumothorax in which there is a marked fall in blood pressure in the leg, as compared with that of the arm on the same side; called *Williamson's test* or *sign*.

Williamson, Richard Thomas [*English physician*, 1862–1937]. Introduced a blood test for diabetes using methylene blue and potassium hydroxide. When the tube is placed in boiling water the blue soon disappears from the blood of a diabetic. Called *Williamson's test*.

Willis, David Arthur [*American surgeon*, 1900–1952]. Inventor of a forceps attached to an electric battery and lamp, the forceps blades being insulated from each other. Upon contact with a metallic object, the circuit is completed and the lamp glows. Called *Willis' forceps for foreign body removal*.

Willis, Thomas [*English anatomist and physician*, 1621–1675]. Described epidemic typhus and typhoid (1659). Described diabetes mellitus which is sometimes called *Willis' disease*. The corpora albicantia are called *Willis' glands*. The ophthalmic branch of the fifth cranial (trigeminal) nerve is called *Willis' nerve*. See also *circle* of Willis.

Willis salt flotation method. See under *method*.

Willstätter, Waldschmidt-Leitz, and Hesse method. See under *method*.

Wilmer, Bradford [*English physician*, eighteenth century]. Originator of the Coventry or burnt-sponge treatment for goiter (1779).

Wilms, Max [*German surgeon*, 1867–1918]. Known for his description of embryonal carcinosarcoma of the kidney, observed in early childhood and often bilateral; called *Wilms's tumor*.

Wilson, Frank Norman (1890–1952). American physician who introduced the term *ventricular gradient* in electrocardiography. He introduced unipolar leads using a terminal connected to the three limb electrodes as a point of indifferent or zero potential.

Wilson, Karl Miller [*American obstetrician*, 1885–]. Introduced a test for pregnancy in which urine is injected into the female rabbit. *Wilson's test for pregnancy* is regarded as positive if the rabbit develops corpora hemorrhagica.

Wilson, Samuel Alexander Kinnier (1877–1937). American neurologist in England, known for his description, with Frerichs, of hepatolenticular degeneration (1912), also called *Wilson's disease, Kinnier Wilson's disease*.

Wilson, William James Erasmus [*English dermatologist*, 1809–84]. Remembered for his description of dermatitis exfoliativa, also called *Wilson's disease*.

Winckel's disease. See epidemic *hemoglobinuria*.

wind'age (win'didj) [AS. *wind*]. Compression of air by the passage of a missile, shell, etc., near the body, causing blast injury.

Windaus, Adolf (1876–). German chemist who provided the foundation for the chemistry of the sex hormones and conducted basic studies on digitalis and the biosynthesis of vitamin D; Nobel laureate in chemistry (1928).

wind'-bro"ken. Affected with expiratory dyspnea: said especially of horses.

wind'gall" (wind'gawl") [AS. *wind*; ME. *galle*, sore spot]. A soft tumor or synovial swelling in the region of the fetlock joint of the horse.

wind' kes'sel. Compression-chamber-like action of the aorta and its immediate branches in buffering pressure and flow changes during the cardiac cycle, a function of the large capacity and elastic walls of the vessels.

wind'lass (wind'lus) [Icel. *vindilāss*]. Apparatus for exerting traction upon a limb by means of a winding device attached to the lower end of a splint, turned with a metal key.

Spanish w. A temporary emergency expedient for accomplishing traction upon a limb supported by a splint; consists of cords which are tightened by twisting with a wooden skewer or similar object.

wind'lass trac'tion. A method for exerting traction on an extremity of the body. Extension straps are attached to the skin by means of adhesive tape or to a bone by means of a pin passed through it. The distal ends of the straps are attached to a fixed point, and traction is exerted by winding up the straps with a metal key or other device.

win'dow [ME. *windowe*]. 1. An opening in a wall usually enclosed by a movable frame of glass panes for the admission of light and air. 2. A small aperture in a bone or other unyielding tissue. See *fenestra*. See Plate 20.

wind'pipe". See *trachea*.

wind'-puff". See *windgall*.

wind'stroke" [AS. *wind*; ME. *strok*]. Acute spinal paralysis of a horse.

wind suck'ing. See *cribbing*, 2.

wine'glass" [AS. *win*; *glaes*]. A measure of nearly two fluidounces, or 60 cc.

wine spot. See port-wine *nevus*.

wing. See *ala*.

Winiwarter, Alexander von [*Austrian surgeon*, 1848–1917]. Introduced an operation of cholecystenterostomy in which he first united the gallbladder to the upper portion of the jejunum, fixing the area to the parietal peritoneum. After several days, the second stage was undertaken in which the intestine was incised and a communication established between it and the gallbladder. Called *Winiwarter's operation*.

wink [AS. *wincian*]. Close and open the eyelids quickly.

Winkler, Cornelius (1855–1941). Dutch neuroanatomist known for his experimentation on the neuroanatomy of animals and his laboratory manuals on the brain of the cat and the rabbit.

Winkler reagent. See under *reagent*.

Winslow, Jacques Benigne (Jacobus Benignus) [*French anatomist*, 1669–1760]. Described the uncinate process of the pancreas, called *Winslow's pancreas*. The epiploic foramen is also called *foramen of Winslow*. See also *Winslow's stars* under *star*.

Winterbottom, Thomas Masterman [*English explorer*, 1765–1859]. Wrote an account of his travels in Africa, in which he gave one of the first accounts of sleeping sickness (1803). He noted that the enlarged cervical lymph nodes indicated the probability of infection with the disease, called *Winterbottom's sign*.

win′ter·green″. See *gaultheria*.

win′ter itch. See *pruritus* hiemalis.

Winternitz, Wilhelm [*Austrian physician and hydrotherapist*, 1835–1917]. Invented an apparatus resembling a pulpit which he used for hot and cold needle douches; known as *Winternitz's pulpit*.

Wintersteiner, Hugo [*Austrian physician*, 1865–1918]. Described congeries of cells from the neuroepithelial layer of the retina as a characteristic of glioma of the retina. See *rosette*.

Wintrich's sign. See under *sign*.

Wintrobe, Maxwell Myer (1901–   ). American internist and hematologist known for research in hematology and his classification of anemias, known as *Wintrobe's classification*. He devised a hematocrit, used to determine sedimentation rate, volume of packed red cells, and icterus index, called *Wintrobe tube*. With J. W. Landsberg, developed a standardized technique for blood sedimentation tests called *Wintrobe-Landsberg method*. The standard amount of venous blood mixed with anticoagulant is placed in the tube, which is placed vertically. For average cases the reading is taken after one hour.

Wintrobe method. See under *method*.

wir′ing [AS. *wir*]. Securing in position, by means of wire, the fragments of a broken bone.

continuous loop w. *In dentistry*, a procedure for reduction and immobilization of jaw fractures by the use of a long strand of wire wound around several selected teeth in each fragment.

eyelet w. See single loop *w*.

single loop w. *In dentistry*, a type of intermaxillary wiring used in fractures of the jaw.

Wirsung's canal. See pancreatic *duct*.

Wirsung's duct. See pancreatic *duct*.

wir′y [*wīr*]. Resembling wire; tough and flexible.

wis′dom teeth. The third permanent molars. Also called *dentes sapientes*.

Wiseman, Richard [*English military surgeon*, 1622–76]. Gave an early account of "king's evil," or scrofula. Classified aneurysms. Described tuberculosis of the knee, which he called *tumor albus*.

wish ful·fil′ment. A central theme in psychoanalytic theory, serving to explain the manifestation of repressed wishes in the form of neurotic symptoms, common errors, and (normally) dreams; a partial substitute for the forbidden or unattainable satisfaction.

asymptotic w. f. A psychological state wherein the patient has found the neurotic expression which would resolve his conflicts or compensate for them, but wherein his ego is strong enough to compel him to postpone indefinitely putting the neurotic solution into effect (Freud).

witch ha′zel. See *Hamamelis virginiana*.

witch's milk. Lay term for milk secreted in the breasts of a newborn infant.

Wi·teb′sky's sub′stan·ces. See group-specific *substance*.

with·draw′al. Coitus interruptus.

Withering, William [*English physician*, 1741–99]. Renowned for his introduction of digitalis into medicine (1783–85). Acknowledged as one of the greatest medical botanists of his time. He discovered the virtues of foxglove from noting its use in dropsy when steeped and administered by women experienced in its action. Published a notable treatise on scarlet fever (1779).

with′ers (wiŧħ′urz) [ME. *wither*, resistance]. The ridge above the shoulders of the horse, formed by the spinous processes of the first eight or ten thoracic vertebrae.

wit′kop [S. Afr. D., White head]. A noncontagious favoid condition of the scalp characterized by white, hard, dry, friable, confluent, firmly adherent crusts which give the appearance of a tightly fitting, white skull cap, seen only in prenatal syphilis in natives of South Africa, and described by McArthur and Thornton (1911): also called *diwakwadi, white head*.

Witzel, Friedrich Oskar [*German surgeon*, 1856–1925]. Known for his gastrostomy, in which a catheter is passed through a small opening in the stomach and fixed in place. A tube approximately 5 cm. long is buried in the stomach wall by interrupted sutures, and the stomach is then anchored to the peritoneum. The abdominal wall is well closed about the tube. Called *Witzel's operation*.

wit′zel·sucht″ (vit′sul·zŏŏkt″. *See* NOTES § 35) [Ger.]. A mental condition characterized by silly behavior, shallow facetiousness, and unstable mood; regarded as a symptom of frontal lobe disease such as brain tumor.

wl, wl. Wavelength.

Wöhler, Friedrich [*German chemist*, 1800–82]. Remembered for his discovery that ingested benzoic acid is excreted in the urine as hippuric acid, a fact which became the starting point of modern chemistry of metabolism (1842). He was concerned with a number of important investigations in organic chemistry, including the synthesis of urea (1828).

Wohl·fahr′ti·a (voal·fahr′tee·uh). A genus of flesh flies. See *Sarcophagidae*.

W. magnifica. The Old World flesh fly; the larvae are deposited in cutaneous lesions or in one of the body openings.

W. meigeni. A North American flesh fly.

W. vigil. A North American flesh fly.

Wohlgemuth, Julius [*German physician*, 1874–   ]. Known for his methods of quantitative determination of diastatic ferments in the blood, and of the amylolytic contents of feces; both called *Wohlgemuth method*. They are especially used in determination of pancreatic function.

Wolcott, Erastus Bradley [*American surgeon*, 1804–80]. Performed the first operation for excision of the kidney (1861).

Wolfe, John Reissberg [*Scottish ophthalmologist*, 1824–1904]. Remembered for his operation for ectropion in which he transplanted a full-thickness skin graft (1875), marking the earliest successful technic with this type of graft, which was made without a pedicle. The area to be grafted is prepared by excising all scar, ulcer, and granulation tissue to make a bed to receive the graft which is excised by using an exact pattern, so that it may be sutured accurately into place. Called *Wolfe's method, Wolfe-Krause graft, full-thickness graft.*

Wolfenden, Richard Norris (1854–1925). English laryngologist who introduced a position to induce deglutition when this is impeded by ulceration of the epiglottis. The patient lies prone, head lower than feet, with head and arms hanging over the edge of the bed; called *Wolfenden's position.*

Wolff, Caspar Friedrich [*German anatomist,* 1733–94]. Noted for his advancement of the germ-layer theory (1759). The functional tubules of the mesonephros are called *Wolffian tubules.* Cyst of broad ligament is called *Wolffian cyst.* The mesonephric duct is called *Wolffian duct.* The urogenital ridge is known as *Wolffian ridge.*

Wolff, Julius [*German surgeon and anatomist,* 1836–1902]. Proponent of a law in which he stated that every change in the use or static relations of a bone leads not only to a change in its internal structure and architecture but also to a change in its external form and function (1884). Called *Wolff's law.*

Wolff method. See under *method.*

Wolff-Eisner test. See Calmette *test.*

Wolff-Parkinson-White syndrome. See under *syndrome.*

Wölfler, Anton [*Bohemian surgeon,* 1850–1917]. Remembered for his operation for obstructed pylorus in which he anastomosed the jejunum to the lower part of the stomach; called *Wölfler's operation.*

wolf'ram. Tungsten.

Wolfring, Emilij Franzevic von [*Polish ophthalmologist,* 1832–1906]. Described the posterior tarsal glands of the eyelid; also called *accessory lacrimal glands, Wolfring's glands, Krause's glands.*

wolfs'bane". 1. Aconite. 2. Any plant of the genus *Aconitum,* especially *A. lycoctonum.*

Wollaston, William Hyde [*English physician and physicist,* 1766–1828]. Remembered for his description of gouty and urinary concretions (1797). He invented two planoconvex lenses to be placed in the eyepiece of a microscope, for correction of chromatic aberration; called *Wollaston's doublet.*

Wolters' myelin stain. See under *stain.*

Woltman, Henry William (1889–). American neurologist who, with J. W. Kernohan, described the crus syndrome.

womb (wōōm) [AS. *wamb*]. The uterus.

Women's Medical Specialist Corps. A corps of the U. S. Army Medical Service comprised of female commissioned officers, e.g., dietitians, physical therapists, and occupational therapists.

Women's Medical Specialist Corps Reserve. A section of the U. S. Army Reserve comprised of female commissioned officers, e.g., dietitians, physical and occupational therapists.

Wong's method. See under *method.*

Wood, Robert Williams (1868–). American physicist who developed a light filter, made of glass containing nickel oxide, which transmits only ultraviolet rays. It has been used in the diagnosis of infections by fungi, e.g., tinea capitis, which fluoresce when radiated with ultraviolet light. Also called *Wood's light, Wood's filter.*

Wood, William [*Scottish physician,* 1774–1857]. Usually credited with the first description of neuroma, although it was previously described by D. J. Larrey (1824).

wood [AS. *wudu*]. The hard fibrous part of trees; the part within the bark.

wood al'co·hol. See *methyl alcohol.*

wood sor'rel. *Oxalis acetosella,* a low, tender pubescent herb of North America, Europe, Asia, and Northern Africa. Contains potassium binoxalate, which is sometimes obtained from it and sold as sorrel salt.

wood spir'it. See *methyl alcohol.*

wood sug'ar. Xylose.

wood vin'e·gar. Vinegar obtained by the dry distillation of wood.

wood wool. Prepared fibers of wood. Formerly used as a surgical dressing.

wool fat (*adeps lanae*). The purified, anhydrous, fatlike substance from the wool of sheep, *Ovis aries.* Wool fat is chiefly composed of esters of high molecular weight alcohols, as cholesterol and lanosterol, with fatty acids. It is used as an ointment base, and may cause sensitization. Also called *anhydrous lanolin, refined w. f.*

hydrous w. f. (*adeps lanae hydrosus*). Wool fat containing about 30% of water. Used as an ointment base. Syn., *lanolin.*

Woolner, Thomas [*English sculptor and poet,* 1825–92]. He is remembered medically for his description of the apex of the helix of the auricle. This is known as *Woolner's tip.*

word blind'ness. See *alexia.*

word deaf'ness. See under *deafness.*

word sal'ad. Meaningless words or neologisms emitted by psychotic patients, particularly those with schizophrenia. Syn., *schizophasia.*

work'ing dis'tance. *In microscopy,* the distance between the object and the objective.

World Health Organization (WHO). A specialized agency of the United Nations Organization whose broad purposes in the international health field are primarily to assist governments upon request in the field of health; to promote standards, provide information, and foster research in the field of health; to promote cooperation among scientific and professional groups; to promote and foster activities in the fields of maternal and child health and of mental health; and to study and report on administrative and social techniques as relating to preventive medicine. It has authority to make sanitary and quarantine regulations, to regulate morbidity and mortality nomenclature, and to set standards for purity and potency of biological and pharmaceutical products.

Worm, Ole (Olaus Wormius) [*Danish anatomist,* 1588–1654]. Remembered for his description of the small, supernumerary bones in the sutures of the skull; called *Wormian bones.* See also anterior Wormian *suture.*

worm [AS. *wyrm*]. A member of the phyla Annelida, Nemathelminthes, or Platyhelminthes. The medically important forms belong to the last two phyla.

dragon w. See *Dracunculus medinensis.*

eye w. See *Loa loa.*

Guinea w. See *Dracunculus medinensis.*

hookworm. See *Ancylostoma, Necator.*

kidney w. See *Dioctophyma renale.*

pinworm. See *Enterobius vermicularis.*

roundworm. See *Ascaris.*

screwworm. The larva of *Cochliomyia.*

seatworm. See *Enterobius vermicularis.*

tapeworm. See *tapeworm.*

threadworm. *Enterobius vermicularis.*

tongue w. See *Linguatula.*

whipworm. See *Trichuris trichiura.*

worm'seed. *Santonica.*

w. oil. See chenopodium *oil.*

wound [AS. *wund*]. The disruption of normal anatomical relationships as a result of injury, or more specifically of trauma, as a gunshot wound.

bullet splash w. One caused by a fragmentation of steel armor from the impact of a bullet; this type of wound is small and frequently involves the neck; common in combat airmen.

contused w. One produced by a blunt instrument or weapon.

gunshot w. One made by a projectile from a gun or any small firearm.

incised w. One caused by a cutting instrument.

lacerated w. One in which the tissues are torn.

open w. One having a free external opening.

penetrating w. One that pierces the walls of a cavity or enters into an organ.

punctured w. One made by a pointed instrument.

shell w. Usually a large lacerated one with accompanying devitalization of tissue and resulting from artillery fire or bombing.

spatter w. One which is peppered superficially with a multitude of small splinters from an explosive.

tunnel w. One having a small entrance and a small exit, the wound tract being the same diameter throughout.

Wreden, Robert Robertovich [*Russian otologist,* 1837–93]. Described otomycosis (1867). Introduced a test for live birth, consisting of examination for the presence of gelatinous matter in the middle ear; its absence is regarded as proof that the child was born alive and has breathed; called *Wreden's test.*

Wright, Almroth Edward [*English pathologist and bacteriologist,* 1861–1947]. Widely known for his experimental work in inoculation against typhoid fever (1896). Developed an agglutination test against undulant fever (1897). Best known for demonstration of opsonins in normal and immune serums (1903). His *opsonic index* is a term to indicate the relation between the phagocytic action of a particular serum and that of a normal serum.

Wright, James Homer [*American pathologist,* 1869–1928]. Said to have been the first to observe the origin of the blood platelets. Observed *Leishmania tropica* in Delhi, or oriental, sore (1903). See also Wright's *stain,* Wright's myelin *stain.*

wrin'kles [AS. *wrincle*]. Minute crevices or furrows in the skin caused by habitual frowning, etc., but particularly by old age, due to atrophy of the corium.

Wrisberg, Heinrich August [*German anatomist,* 1739–1808]. Described the medial cutaneous nerve of the arm; also called *nerve of Wrisberg.* Described the pars intermedia of the seventh cranial nerve; called *Wrisberg's nerve* or *Wrisberg's pars intermedia,* now known as nervus intermedius. The cuneiform cartilages were formerly called *Wrisberg's cartilages.*

wrist [AS.]. The part joining forearm and hand. See *carpus* in Table of Bones in the Appendix.

w. joint. The articulation between the forearm and the hand; the radiocarpal articulation.

wri'ting hand. A peculiar position assumed by the hand in paralysis agitans, with an exaggerated flexion of the metacarpophalangeal joints and an extension of the fingers.

wry-head. See *plagiocephaly.*

wry'neck". Old term for torticollis.

w. s. Water soluble.

Wu, H. [*Chinese biochemist,* contemporary]. Devised a test, with Otto Folin, for urea in the blood. See Folin-Wu *test.* Also see Folin and Wu's *method.*

Wuch"er·er'i·a (wŏŏtch"ur·err'ee·uh) [Otto *Wucherer,* German physician, 1820–73]. A genus of filarial worms found in all the warm regions of the world. The larva or microfilaria must be ingested by a mosquito for metamorphosis to take place.

W. bancrofti. A species of filaria of worldwide distribution. Man is the only known definitive host.

W. malayi. A species of filaria infecting man by mosquito bite, endemic in the Far East, and frequently associated with elephantiasis of the upper extremities.

wuch"er·e·ri'a·sis (wŏŏtch"ur·eh·rye'uh·sis) [*Wucherer;* NL. *-iasis,* condition]. The disease caused by worms of the genus *Wuchereria.* The symptoms depend upon the location of the parasite within the body, but are due to obstruction of the lymph vessels by the adult worms. Also called *filariasis, Bancroft's filariasis, elephantiasis.*

Wunderlich, Carl Reinhold August [*German physician,* 1815–77]. Remembered for his observations on body heat in disease (1868). Said to have established clinical thermometry. Proponent of a law or curve in typhoid fever corresponding to the present knowledge of the fever oscillations in the course of that disease; called *Wunderlich's law* or *curve.*

Wundt, Wilhelm Max [*German physiologist,* 1832–1920]. Known for his contributions to experimental physiology and psychology. Described a prolonged tetanic contraction induced in a frog's muscle by injury or the closure of a strong, direct electric current; called *Wundt's tetanus.*

wur'rus [Ar. *wars*]. A powder obtained in Arabia from the fruits of a leguminous plant, *Flemingia congesta;* used as an anthelmintic. Also called *waras, warras.*

Wurster's test. See under *test.*

WV Walking ventilation.

w/v. Weight in volume; indicating that a weighed quantity of a solid substance is contained in solution in a measured volume of liquid.

wyamine. Trade-mark for *amine mephentermine.*

w. sulfate. Trade-mark for *mephentermine sulfate.*

wyanoid. Trade-mark for a hemorrhoidal suppository.

wycillin. Trade-mark for an aqueous suspension of crystalline procaine penicillin G.

wydase. Trade-mark for *hyaluronidase.*

Wyeth, John Allan [*American surgeon,* 1845–1922]. Remembered especially for his important invention of 12-in. steel pins to hold a tourniquet in place in amputation at the hip or shoulder: also called *Wyeth's pins.*

Wylie, Walter Gill [*American gynecologist,* 1848–1923]. Remembered for his operation of shortening the round ligaments of the uterus for relief of retroflexion; called *Wylie's operation.*

Wyllys Andrews. See Edward Wyllys *Andrews.*

X

X. Symbol for the decimal scale of potency or dilution; used by the homeopaths.

xan′tha·line (zan′thuh·leen, ·lin). $C_{20}H_{19}NO_5$. An alkaloid from opium.

xan′thate. A salt of xanthic acid.

xan″the·las′ma (zan″thi·laz′muh, ·lass′muh) [G. *xanthos*, yellow; *elasma*, metal plate]. A type of xanthoma seen on the eyelids.

xan″the·las·moi′de·a (zan″thi·laz·moy′dee·uh, ·lass·moy′dee·uh). See *urticaria* pigmentosa.

xan′thene. 1. $C_{13}H_{10}O$; dibenzopyran; a 3-ring heterocyclic compound resulting from the joining of two benzene rings by a methylene (CH_2) and also an oxygen bridge. Certain derivatives are medicinally important. 2. Any of several derivatives of xanthene, 1.

xan′thic [*xanthos*]. 1. Yellow. 2. Pertaining to xanthine.

xan′thic ac′id. An ester of thiosulfocarbonic acid; an unstable, colorless oil which decomposes at 25° C. into carbon disulfide and alcohol.

xan′thine. $C_5H_4N_4O_2$; 2,6(1,3)-purinedione, or 2,6-dioxopurine; crystals, practically insoluble in water, found in plant and animal tissues; an intermediate product in the transformation of adenine and guanine into uric acid. See also *hypoxanthine.*

xan′thine ox′i·dase. A flavoprotein enzyme catalyzing the oxidation of certain purines.

xan′thin·in. $C_{17}H_{22}O_5$; a crystalline unsaturated keto lactone isolated from the leaves of *Xanthium pennsylvanicum*, or cocklebur; the principle responsible for auxin antagonism of extracts of leaves of the plant.

xan″thi·nu′ri·a, xan″thi·u′ri·a [*xanthos*; G. *ouron*, urine]. The presence of xanthine in urine.

xan′tho-, xanth- [*xanthos*]. A combining form meaning *yellow.*

xan″tho·chroi′a [*xanthos*; G. *chroia*, skin]. Yellow discoloration of the skin.

xan″tho·chro·mat′ic [*xanthos*; G. *chrōma*, color]. Yellow-colored.

xan″tho·chro′mi·a [*xanthos*; *chrōma*]. 1. A yellowish discoloration of the skin. 2. The yellow discoloration of the cerebrospinal fluid, diagnostic of hemorrhage in the spinal cord or brain. —**xanthochromic,** *adj.*

xan·thoch′ro·ous (zan·thock′ro·us) [*xanthos*; G. *chroia*, skin]. Yellow-skinned.

xan″tho·cy″a·no′pi·a, xan″tho·cy″a·nop′si·a [*xanthos*; G. *kyanos*, blue; *ōps*, eye]. A defect of color vision in which yellow and blue are perceived, while red is not perceptible.

xan′tho·cyte [*xanthos*; G. *kytos*, cell]. A cell containing a yellow pigment.

xan″tho·der′ma [*xanthos*; G. *derma*, skin]. A yellow discoloration of the skin.

xan′tho·dont, xan″tho·don′tous [*xanthos*; G. *odous*, tooth]. Having yellow teeth.

xan″tho·gran·u·lo′ma. Xanthoma.

juvenile x. See *nevoxanthoendothelioma.*

xan″tho·gran″u·lo″ma·to′sis [*xanthos*; L. *granulum*, small grain; G. *-ōma*, tumor; *-ōsis*, condition]. A condition characterized by granulomalike deposits of cholesterol, chiefly in the flat bones, sometimes associated with hypercholesteremia. Exophthalmos and diabetes insipidus may occur, depending on the localization of the lipid deposits in the skull. See also Hand-Schüller-Christian *disease.*

xan″tho·ky·an′o·py (zanth″o·kigh·an′o·pee) [*xanthos*; G. *kyanos*, blue; *ōps*, eye]. Red-green blindness, with undiminished spectrum. See *xanthocyanopia.*

xan·tho′ma [*xanthos*; G. *-ōma*, tumor]. A new growth of the skin occurring as flat or slightly raised patches or nodules from 2 to 12 mm. in size, and of a yellowish orange color. Several types are seen and often more than one type is seen in the same patient. They are all due to some disturbance of lipoid metabolism. Histologically, foam or xanthoma cells are seen with giant cells and some infiltrate. Various types of sterol crystals are seen with polariscopic examination. See *xanthelasma.*

giant-cell x. See xanthomatous giant-cell *tumor* of the tendon sheath.

juvenile x. One occurring in children usually as xanthoma tuberosum, but often disseminated. May occur as an evidence of Hand-Schüller-Christian disease.

x. diabeticorum. A rare disease of the skin associated with diabetes mellitus, the lesions of which are denser and firmer than those of true xanthoma, and are dull red, discrete, and solid, being more often seen on the palms and soles.

x. disseminatum. A rare form occurring as papules or plaques diffusely distributed over the face, flexor surfaces, and often the mucous membranes. Other parts of the body may be involved. Diabetes insipidus may be associated.

x. tuberosum. One of the common types. Papules, nodules, plaques, or linear lesions are seen on the extensor surfaces. The yellow color is typical. Lesions are usually grouped together and are often found about the joints. Total blood lipids are usually elevated, as is cholesterol. Tendon sheaths or other internal structures may be involved, giving various and bizarre symptoms.

xan·tho″ma·to′sis [*xanthos*; *-ōma*; G. *-ōsis*, condition]. A condition marked by the deposit of a yellowish or orange lipoid material in the reticuloendothelial cells, the skin, and the internal organs. See *lipoidosis*, Hand-Schüller-Christian *disease.*

xan·thom′a·tous [*xanthos*; *-ōma*]. Of the nature of, or affected with, xanthoma.

xan″tho·my′cin. Either of two antibiotic substances, designated xanthomycin A and xanthomycin B, isolated from cultures of a *Streptomyces* species.

xan′thone. 1. $C_{13}H_8O_2$; dibenzopyrone, or benzophenone oxide, obtained when the CH_2 bridge of xanthene is oxidized to CO. Certain dyes and some yellow flower pigments are derivatives of xanthone. 2. Any of several derivatives of xanthone, 1.

xan′tho·phane [*xanthos*; G. *phainein*, to appear]. A yellow pigment found in the retinal cones.

xan′tho·phore [*xanthos*; G. *phoros*, bearing]. A yellow chromatophore.

xan′tho·phose (zanth′o·foze) [*xanthos*; G. *phōs*, light]. A yellow phose.

xan′tho·phyll. $C_{40}H_{56}O_2$. A yellow vegetable pigment similar to chlorophyll, found in plants.

xan·tho′pi·a. See *xanthopsia.*

xan″tho·pro·te′ic ac′id. The yellow compound

resulting from the treatment of protein with nitric acid.

xan″tho·pro′te·in (zanth″o·pro′tee·in, ·pro′teen) [*xanthos;* G. *prōteios,* of first rank]. A yellowish derivative formed by the action of concentrated nitric acid on proteins.

xan·thop′si·a [*xanthos;* G. *opsis,* vision]. Yellow vision; the condition in which objects look yellow. It sometimes accompanies jaundice.

xan·thop′sin [*xanthos; opsis*]. Visual yellow, produced by the action of light on rhodopsin (visual purple).

xan·thop″sy·dra′ci·a (zan·thop″si·dray′shee·uh, ·see·uh) [*xanthos;* G. *psydrax,* pimple]. The occurrence on the skin of yellow pimples or pustules.

xan·thop′ter·in. $C_6H_5N_5O_2$. A yellow pigment, widely distributed in animal organisms and representing an element of the structure of folic acid; it appears to have some role in hematopoiesis.

xan″tho·rham′nin. $C_{34}H_{42}O_{20}$; the 3-rhamninoside of rhamnetin, obtained from the berries of *Rhamnus infectoria* (*tinctoria*) and other *Rhamnus* species. On hydrolysis it yields rhamninose and the aglycone rhamnetin.

xan″thor·rhe′a, xan″thor·rhoe′a [*xanthos;* G. *rhoia,* flow]. An acrid, purulent, yellow discharge from the vagina.

xan′tho·sine (zanth′o·seen, ·sin). A nucleoside made up of xanthine and ribose.

xan·tho′sis [G., from *xanthos, -ōsis,* condition]. A yellow discoloration of the skin due to a deposit of carotenoid pigment; occurs from eating quantities of carrots, squash, sweet potatoes, etc. The reaction is readily reversible. A similar reaction is seen from another pigmentary deposit in the skin after taking atabrine over a period of time. Also called *aurantiasis cutis.* **—xan′thous,** *adj.*

x. fundi diabetica. A condition, seen in diabetic retinopathy, in which the retinal vessels are extremely well defined and the retina in the posterior part of the eye has a peculiar orange-yellow color.

xan″tho·tox′in. $C_{12}H_8O_4$; the methyl ether of 8-hydroxy-4′,5′,6,7-furocoumarin, obtained from the fruits of *Fagara xanthoxyloides* and identical with ammoidin from *Ammi majus.*

xan·thox′y·lum (zan·thock′si·lum) [*xanthos;* G. *xylon,* wood] (*xanthoxylum*). The dried bark of *Zanthoxylum americanum,* or of *Z. clavaherculis.* Contains xanthoxylin-N, xanthyletin, volatile oil, and resins. It has been used as an internal remedy in rheumatism, as a gastrointestinal stimulant in flatulence and diarrhea, and as a masticatory in toothache. Also called *prickly ash bark.*

x. fruit. The dried, full-grown fruit of *Z. americanum,* or of *Z. clavaherculis.* Contains a volatile oil and hesperidin. It has no therapeutic effect other than that of a mild aromatic. Also called *prickly ash berries.*

xan″thu·re′nic ac′id. A green pigment derived from quinoline found in the urine of rats suffering from pyridoxine deficiency; appears to be a tryptophan metabolic product.

xan·thu′ri·a. See *xanthinuria.*

xan·thy′drol. $C_{13}H_{10}O_2$, an organic compound used for the detection of urea.

xan·thyl′ic [*xanthos;* G. *hylē,* material]. Pertaining to xanthine.

X chro′mo·some. See under *chromosome.*

Xe Chemical symbol for xenon.

xen′o- (zen′o-), **xen-** [G. *xenos,* stranger]. A combining form meaning *strange* or *foreign.*

xen″o·di″ag·no′sis [*xenos;* G. *diagnōsis,* a distinguishing]. The procedure of using a suitable arthropod to transfer a disease from a patient to a susceptible laboratory animal.

xen″o·gen′e·sis [*xenos;* G. *genesis,* production]. 1. Heterogenesis. 2. The hypothetical production of offspring completely unlike the parent. **—xenogenic,** *adj.*

xe·nol′o·gy [*xenos;* G. *logos,* word]. The study of the host relationship of parasites, as of intermediary and definitive hosts.

xen″o·me′ni·a [*xenos;* G. *mēn,* month]. Vicarious menstruation.

xe′non (zee′non, zen′on) [*xenos*]. Xe = 131.3. A chemically inert gaseous element found in the atmosphere.

xen″o·pho′bi·a [*xenos;* G. *phobos,* fear]. A morbid fear of strangers.

xen″oph·thal′mi·a [*xenos;* G. *ophthalmos,* eye]. Conjunctivitis due to injury.

xe″no·plas′ty [*xenos;* G. *plassein,* to form]. Heteroplasty. **—xenoplas′tic,** *adj.*

Xen″op·syl′la [*xenos;* G. *psylla,* flea]. A genus of fleas of the family Pulicidae.

X. cheopis. The Indian rat flea; found in tropical and subtropical regions. A vector for bubonic plague and *Hymenolepis diminuta,* a tapeworm. This flea attacks man and other mammals, in addition to the rat, its natural host. It transmits the organism of murine typhus, *Rickettsia mooseri,* from rat to rat and from rat to man.

Xen′o·pus, Xen·o′pus [*xenos;* G. *pous,* foot]. A genus of African toad belonging to the Pipidae, used in laboratory tests for pregnancy.

xe·ran′tic [G. *xērainein,* to dry up]. Having desiccative properties; drying. **—xeransis,** *n.*

xe·ra′si·a (zi·ray′see·uh) [G., desiccation]. Old term for a disease of the hair marked by cessation of growth and excessive dryness.

xe′ro- (zeer′o-), **xer-** [G. *xēros,* dry]. A combining form meaning *dry.*

xe″ro·der′ma, xe″ro·der′mi·a [*xēros;* G. *derma,* skin]. 1. An abnormal dryness of the skin. 2. Ichthyosis.

follicular x. See *keratosis pilaris.*

x. pigmentosum. A rare disease of the skin usually beginning in childhood, and characterized by disseminated pigment spots, telangiectasis, atrophy, and contraction of the skin. Occurs particularly in areas exposed to sunlight and is made worse by it. Patients have photophobia, and there is a definite familial tendency. Warty and keratolytic lesions occur that soon develop into malignant growths. The skin develops many characteristics of the senile skin in early life. Also called *angioma pigmentosum atrophicum, atrophoderma pigmentosum, Kaposi's disease, melanosis lenticularis progressiva.*

xe″ro·der″mos·te·o′sis. See Sjögren's *syndrome.*

xeroform. Trade-mark for a brand of bismuth tribromphenate.

xe·ro′ma. See *xerophthalmia.*

xe″ro·me′ni·a [*xēros;* G. *mēn,* month]. The presence of the usual constitutional disturbances at the menstrual period but without the menstrual flow of blood.

xe″ro·myc·te′ri·a [*xēros;* G. *myktēr,* nostril]. Lack of moisture in the nasal passages.

xer·on′o·sus [*xēros;* G. *nosos,* disease]. A condition of dryness of the skin.

xe″ro·pha′gi·a, xe·roph′a·gy [*xēros;* G. *phagein,* to eat]. The eating of dry or desiccated food.

xe″roph·thal′mi·a [*xēros;* G. *ophthalmos,* eye]. A dry and thickened condition of the conjunctiva, sometimes following chronic conjunctivitis, disease of the lacrimal apparatus, or vitamin-A deficiency. Also see *xerosis.*

xe″ro·ra″di·og′ra·phy. A rapid method of recording a roentgen image by a totally dry process without the necessity of a darkroom. The pow-

XYZ

dered surface of an electrically charged selenium plate records the roentgen image, and from this a paper print is made.

xe·ro'sis [*xēros;* G. *-ōsis,* condition]. A state of dryness, especially of the skin (see *xeroderma*) or of the conjunctiva (see *xerophthalmia*). Syn., *asteatosis.*

x. conjunctivae. A condition marked by silver-gray, shiny, triangular spots on both sides of the cornea, within the region of the palpebral aperture, consisting of dried epithelium, flaky masses, and microorganisms. The spots are observed in some cases of hemeralopia. See *xerophthalmia.*

x. infantilis. Xerophthalmia marked by a lusterless, grayish white, foamy, greasy, very persistent deposit on the conjunctiva. Also called *keratitis sicca.*

xe"ro·sto'mi·a [*xēros;* G. *stoma,* mouth]. Dry mouth, caused by insufficient secretion of saliva.

xe'ro·tes (zeer'o·teez, zerr'o·teez, zi·ro'teez) [G., dryness]. Dryness of the body.

xe·rot'ic [*xēros*]. Characterized by xerosis; dry.

xe"ro·to'ci·a (zeer"o·to'shee·uh, ·see·uh) [*xēros;* G. *tokos,* childbirth]. Old term for dry labor.

xe"ro·trip'sis [*xēros;* G. *tripsis,* a rubbing]. Dry friction.

xiph-, xiph'i-. See *xipho-.*

xiph"i·ster'num [G. *xiphos,* sword; *sternon,* breast]. The xiphoid cartilage of the sternum. —**xiphister'nal,** *adj.*

xiph'o- (zif'o-, zy'fo-), **xiph-** [*xiphos*]. A combining form signifying *relation to the xiphoid cartilage.*

xiph"o·cos'tal [*xiphos;* L. *costa,* rib]. Pertaining to the xiphoid cartilage and to the ribs.

xiph·od'y·mus (zi·fod'i·mus, zye·fod'i·mus) [*xiphos;* G. *didymos,* twin]. A double monster with two heads, two thoraces, four arms, abdominal and pelvic regions in common, with two legs or occasionally a rudimentary third leg. Also called *dicephalus tetrabrachius.*

xiph"o·dyn'i·a [*xiphos;* G. *odynē,* pain]. Pain in the xiphoid cartilage.

xiph'oid (zif'oyd, zy'foyd) [G. *xiphoeidēs,* sword-shaped]. Sword-shaped; ensiform.

xiph'oid. The xiphoid process.

xiph"oid·i'tis [*xiphoeidēs;* G. *-itis,* inflammation]. Inflammation of the xiphoid process.

xi·phop'a·gus (zi·fop'uh·gus, zye·fop'uh·gus) [*xiphos;* G. *pagos,* that which is fixed]. Conjoined twins united at the inferior end of the sternum; a type of thoracopagus. See Plate 25.

xiph"o·ster'nal crunch. Normal functional systolic sound of a crunching or splitting nature, heard best, when present, to the left and above the xiphoid process: also called *xiphosternal crunch sound.*

x'-ray pho·tog'ra·phy. See *radiography.*

x'-rays. See *roentgen rays* under *ray.*

x-ray serv'ice. The professional service of a medical institution equipped to perform x-ray examinations and in some cases to give radiation therapy.

x'ray u'nit. Any assemblage of equipment primarily for diagnostic or therapeutic use of x-rays.

xy'lan. A hemicellulose of the pentosan type, occurring in woody tissue, corncobs, peanut shells, straw, etc. On hydrolysis it yields xylose.

xy'lem (zy'lem) [G. *xylon,* wood]. The inner or woody portion of a vascular bundle of a plant, as opposed to the phloem.

xy'lene. $C_6H_4(CH_3)_2$; dimethylbenzene, occurring as a colorless, mobile, inflammable liquid. The xylene of commerce is a mixture of the three isomerides—*o-*, *m-*, and *p-*xylenes. It has many industrial uses, and is used as a solvent and clearing agent in microscopy. Syn., *xylol.*

xy'len·ol. $(CH_3)_2.C_6H_3.OH$; dimethylphenol, existing in six isomeric forms, all crystalline and slightly soluble in water: used in the preparation of coal-tar disinfectants.

xy'li·dene. $(CH_3)_2.C_6H_3.NH_2$; aminodimethylbenzene, existing in six isomeric forms, all liquids except one, sparingly soluble in water: used chiefly in the manufacture of dyes.

xy'lo-, xyl- [*xylon*]. A combining form denoting *pertaining to* or *derived from wood.*

xylocaine hydrochloride. Trade-marked name for diethylamino-2,6-acetoxylidide hydrochloride. See *lidocaine hydrochloride, lignocaine.*

xy'lol. See *xylene.*

Xy·lo'pi·a (zye·lo'pee·uh) [*xylon;* G. *pikros,* bitter]. A genus of shrubs. **X. polycarpa** yields a yellow dye; also used as a bitter.

xy'lose. $C_5H_{10}O_5$; wood sugar, obtained from vegetable fibers: used medicinally as a diabetic food.

xy"lo·ther'a·py [*xylon;* G. *therapeia,* treatment]. Suggestion treatment by the application of certain woods to the body.

xy'lyl. 1. The univalent radical $CH_3.C_6H_4.CH_2$—. 2. The univalent radical $(CH_3)_2.C_6H_3$—.

x. bromide. $CH_3.C_6H_4.CH_2Br$; methylbenzylbromide, existing as *o-*, *m-*, and *p-* forms. The mixed isomers are a lacrimatory poison "gas."

xy'ro·spasm [G. *xyron,* razor; *spasmos,* spasm]. Shaving cramp.

xys'ma (ziz'muh) [G., filings]. The flocculent pseudomembrane sometimes seen in the stools in diarrhea.

xys'ter (zis'tur) [G., scraper]. A surgeon's raspatory or scraping instrument. *Obs.*

Y Chemical symbol for yttrium.

ya'kri·ton. A hypothetical substance claimed to be a detoxifying hormone, found in the liver.

Yamagiwa, Katsusaburo [*Japanese physician,* 1863–1930]. Produced the so-called tar cancer (1916), confirming prior observations as to the etiologic relationship of chemicals to the incidence of tumors.

Yasuda method. See under *method.*

yatren. Trade name for *chiniofon.*

yawn [AS. *gānian*]. To gape, to open the mouth widely. Also called *chasma.*

yawn'ing [*gānian*]. A reflex stretching of the muscles accompanied by a deep inspiration, occurring during the drowsy state preceding the onset of sleep. Also called *hiant.*

yaws [Cariban in origin]. An infectious, nonvenereal disease occurring in the hot, moist tropics; caused by *Treponema pertenue;* characterized by an initial cutaneous lesion, the mother yaw, followed by one or more crops of multiple, papillomatous raspberrylike lesions of the skin. Occasionally late destructive lesions occur involving especially skin and bones. This aspect of yaws, if the tissues about the nose and mouth are involved, is called *gangosa.* The spirochetes gain entrance through the skin. Flies, especially species of *Hippelates*, may be vectors. Serologic tests of the blood for syphilis are positive. Syn., *frambesia, pian.*

bosch y. Leishmaniasis americana.

crab y. Hyperkeratosis with fissuring of the soles of the feet, accompanying the secondary lesions of yaws. The resulting peculiarity of gait gives rise to the name.

forest y. See *leishmaniasis americana.*

mother yaw. The primary lesion of yaws. Also called *maman pian.*

Yb Chemical symbol for ytterbium.

Y chro′mo·some. See under *chromosome.*

yeast [AS. *gist*]. The name applied to various species of *Saccharomyces.* Yeast is chiefly employed medicinally because of its richness in the water-soluble vitamins including thiamine, riboflavin, pyridoxine, nicotinic acid, and pantothenic acid.

autolyzed y. Yeast digested by its own proteolytic enzymes: used to correct dietary deficiencies or to replace meat and meat products in special diets.

brewer's y. See dried *yeast.*

compressed y. The moist, living cells of *Saccharomyces cerevisiae* or of other species of *Saccharomyces* combined with a starchy or absorbent base. It contains at least two enzymes: invertase which changes sucrose to monosaccharides, and zymase which converts monosaccharides to alcohol.

dried y. Consists of the dry cells of any suitable strain of *Saccharomyces cerevisiae.* It may be obtained as a by-product from the brewing of beer which has been made from an extract from cereal grains and hops. The yeast cells are washed free of beer and dried. This yeast is commonly known as brewer's dried yeast. Dried yeast may also be obtained by growing suitable strains of yeast, using mediums other than those required for the production of beer. This yeast is commonly known as primary dried yeast. Dried yeast is frequently fortified with vitamins of the B-complex group.

y. extract. Yeast preparations usually prepared by extracting specially cultured dried brewer's yeast with aqueous medium. The extracts are either concentrated to form a liquid and preserved as such, or dehydrated to powder form.

yeast nu′cle·ic ac′id. *Ribonucleic acid.*

yel′low [ME. *yelow*]. Of a color like that of gold; producing such a color.

butter y. See *butter yellow.*

indicator y. A hypothetical intermediary product in the breakdown of visual purple to retinene.

yel′low jack. See yellow *fever.*

yel′low lo′tion (*lotio flava*). A lotion prepared from mercury bichloride 3 Gm., boiling distilled water 35 cc., calcium hydroxide solution a sufficient quantity to make 1000 cc. Yellow lotion is actively germicidal and stimulant and has been used for sluggish skin infections and syphilitic ulcers. Also called *yellow wash.*

yel′low·root″. See *hydrastis.*

Yem′en ul′cer. See tropical *ulcer.*

Yensen allness test. See under *test.*

yer′ba bue′na (yair′bah bway′nah). A labiate herb of the Pacific Coast; has been used as an emmenagogue. *Obs.*

Yersin, Alexandre Emil Jean [*French bacteriologist,* 1863–1943]. With P. P. E. Roux, demonstrated the existence of diphtheria exotoxin (1888). Discovered the plague bacillus independently of Kitasato in the same year (1894).

Y lig′a·ment. The iliofemoral ligament.

yodoxin. Trade-mark for *diiodohydroxyquin.*

yo·him′bé, yo·him′bi. The rubiaceous tree *Corynanthe Yohimbi* (*Pausinystalia Yohimbe*) growing in the southern Cameroons district in Africa. The bark contains several alkaloids of which the most important is yohimbine; both bark and yohimbine have been employed for reputed aphrodisiac effect.

yo·him′bine. $C_{21}H_{26}N_2O_3$; the principal alkaloid of yohimbé, identical with quebrachine. Has been used as an aphrodisiac, also in treating angina pectoris and arteriosclerosis.

yolk [AS. *geolca*]. The nutritive part of an ovum. Also called *deutoplasm.*

yolk of wool. Suint.

yolk sac. An extraembryonic membrane composed of endoderm and splanchnic mesoderm. It encloses the yolk when the latter is present and is also the site of the formation of the primitive blood cells.

Young, Hugh Hampton [*American urologist,* 1870–1945]. Demonstrated vesiculography (1923). Devised operation for amputation of the penis with removal of lymph nodes in both inguinal regions. Devised operation for epispadias in which skin incisions are made on each side of the central groove, dissection is carried through one of them between the corpora to the skin beneath, and a new tube is formed from the groove which is sutured to the lower skin; called *Young's operation.* Devised a cautery punch for removal of prostatic obstruction transurethrally, called *Young's punch.* Perfected a method of reconstructing the posterior urethra, called *Young's method.* Best known for his introduction of perineal prostatectomy, called *Young's operation.*

Young, John Richardson [*American physician,* 1782–1804]. Demonstrated that gastric digestion is due to the solvent action of the gastric juice (1803).

Young, Thomas [*English physician,* 1773–1829]. The first to describe astigmatism and the mechanism of accommodation (1793). His color-vision theory (1803) was modified later by von Helmholtz and is called the *Young-Helmholtz theory.* It states that there are three elements in the retina which are sensitive to the three primary colors, red, green, and blue, which, mixed in equal proportions, make white light. Vision of other colors is due to different intensity of stimulation of these three elements. Developed a formula for determining drug dosage for children over two years, called *Young's rule.*

Youngburg and Folin method. See under *method.*

youth [AS. *geoguth*]. The period between childhood and maturity.

y′per·ite (ee′pur·ite, eye′pur·ite). Di(chloroethyl) sulfide; mustard gas, $(C_2H_4Cl)_2S$. A vesicant liquid or vapor that is intended for use in chemical warfare.

Y-plas′ty of Schweizer-Foley. A surgical urological procedure designed to correct ureteropelvic junction obstruction, utilizing a **Y**-shaped linear incision in the renal pelvis and area of stricture.

yp·sil′i·form (ip·sil′i·form, ip′sil·i·form) [G. *upsilon,* twentieth letter of the Greek alphabet; L. *forma,* form]. Resembling the Greek letter Υ; Y-shaped.

Yt Alternate chemical symbol for yttrium.

yt·ter′bi·um (i·tur′bee·um) [NL., from *Ytterby,* Sweden]. Yb = 173.04. A rare metal.

yt′tri·um (it′ree·um) [*Ytterby*]. Y = 88.92. A rare metallic element.

Yukawa, Hideki (1907–). Japanese physicist, known for his extensive research in theoretical and nuclear physics. In 1949 he received the Nobel prize in physics for his prediction of the existence of the meson.

Yvon, Paul [*French physician and chemist,* 1848–1913]. Described the ratio between the amount of urea and the phosphates in the urine represented by one-eighth; called *Yvon's coefficient* Described a test for acetanilid. See Yvon's *test.*

Z

z *Zwischenscheibe,* intermediate disk. See Z *disk.*

Z. *Zuckung,* contraction; a term used in electrotherapeutics.

Zander, Jonas Gustaf Willem [*Swedish physician,* 1835–1920]. Introduced exercise by passive movements using special apparatus; called *Zander's system.* The apparatus is called *Zander's apparatus.*

Zappert, Julius (1867–1942). Austrian physician, inventor of a blood corpuscle counting chamber, called *Zappert's chamber* or *cell.*

zar·an′than [Heb.]. Scirrhous condition of the breast.

Zaufal, Emanuel [*Austrian rhinologist and otologist,* 1833–1910]. Described saddle nose due to syphilis and believed it to be pathognomonic of the disease if associated with alopecia; called *Zaufal's sign.* Improved and modified the operation of mastoidectomy; also called *Zaufal's operation.*

Z disk. See *z* and also under *disk.*

ze′a [G., one-seeded wheat] (*zea*). Consists of the fresh styles and stigmas of *Zea mays.* Contains maizenic acid, fixed oil, resin, and mucilage. Has been used in acute and chronic cystitis and urethritis. Also called *corn silk.*

ze″a·xan′thine (zee″uh·zan′theen, ·thin). A carotenoid from maize, egg yolk, and many plants.

zed′o·ar″y [Per. *zadwār*]. The dried rhizome of species of *Curcuma;* has actions similar to ginger.

Zeidler, Othmar [*German chemist,* nineteenth century]. Remembered for his experimental work in compounding chloral and brombenzal (1874), now known as DDT, an important insecticide.

ze′in (zee′in, tsee′in) [G. *zea,* one-seeded wheat]. A yellowish, soft, insipid prolamine of maize.

Zeller, Simon [*Austrian obstetrician,* 1746–1816]. Remembered for his operation for webbed fingers in which he dissected a triangular flap on the dorsal aspect of the root of the web, the latter being divided, after which the apex of the flap was drawn down between the fingers and attached to a prepared surface on the palm.

Zeller's test. See under *test.*

zematol. Proprietary ointment used for eczema.

Zenker, Friedrich Albert [*German pathologist,* 1825–98]. Described the muscular and enteric forms of trichinosis (1860). Gave one of the first adequate descriptions of pulmonary embolism (1862). Described a liquefying, degenerative disease of the striated muscles occurring in acute infectious disease; called *Zenker's degeneration.* Described a form of paralysis of parts supplied by the common peroneal nerve; called *Zenker's paralysis.* Best known for his fixing fluid; see Zenker's *fixing fluid.*

Zenker's pouch. See under *pouch.*

ze′o·lite. Any one of a group of hydrated aluminum and calcium or sodium silicates, of the type $Na_2O.2Al_2O_3.5SiO_2$ or $CaO.2Al_2O_3.5SiO_2$, certain of which may be used for water softening by an ion exchange process.

zephiran chloride. Trade-mark for benzalkonium chloride, a quarternary antiseptic.

Zernicke, Fritz (1888–). Dutch physicist who won the Nobel prize in physics (1953) for his invention of the phase-contrast microscope, which proved a major advance in visualization of the living cell.

ze′ro [Ar. *sifr,* cipher]. 1. Any character denoting absence of quantity. 2. The point on thermometers from which temperatures are counted.

absolute z. Approximately −273.2° C. or −459.8° F.

Ziehen, Georg Theodor [*German psychiatrist,* 1862–]. Known for his description of dystonia musculorum deformans (1911); also called *torsion spasm, Ziehen-Oppenheim's disease.*

Ziehl-Neelsen stain. See *carbolfuchsin solution* under *stain.*

Ziemssen, Hugo Wilhelm von [*German physician,* 1829–1902]. Remembered for his use of electricity in medicine and author of a volume on the subject (1857). Described points of election in electrization of muscles corresponding to the points of entrance of motor nerves into the muscles; called *Ziemssen's points.*

Zimmerlin, Franz [*Swiss physician,* 1858–1932]. Described a type of progressive muscular atrophy starting in the upper part of the body; called *Zimmerlin's type of progressive muscular atrophy.*

Zimmermann, Johann Georg [*German physician,* 1728–95]. Remembered for having published an early monograph on what is now known as bacillary dysentery (1767).

zinc [Ger. *zink*] (*zincum*). Zn = 65.38. Occurs as a bluish white, lustrous metal with a crystalline fracture; it is dissolved by dilute hydrochloric, nitric, and sulfuric acids with the evolution of hydrogen. Most of the salts of zinc are astringent and antiseptic and employed as such in medicine.

compound z. sulfate powder (*pulvis zinci sulfatis compositus*). Contains salicylic acid, 5 Gm.; phenol, eucalyptol, menthol, thymol, 1 Gm. of each; zinc sulfate, 125 Gm.; boric acid, 866 Gm.; to make 1000 Gm. Used for making solution for washing out body cavities, especially as a vaginal douche.

iodine and z. iodide glycerite (*glyceritum iodi et zinci iodidi*). Contains zinc iodide, 8 Gm.; iodine, 10 Gm.; glycerin, 55 cc.; distilled water, a sufficient quantity to make 100 cc. An active germicide and astringent used chiefly for local application in gingivitis. Also called *diluted Talbot's solution.*

medicinal z. peroxide. A mixture consisting essentially of zinc peroxide, ZnO_2, with varying amounts of zinc oxide, ZnO, and zinc hydroxide, $Zn(OH)_2$; occurs as a fine, white, crystalline powder; it is insoluble in water but forms a smooth paste which does not cake or harden. Used as an antiseptic deodorant and astringent application to various ulcerated conditions in skin diseases. It is used as a dusting powder, usually with talc, in ointment form, or as a thick suspension or cream in distilled water.

z. acetate (*zinci acetas*). $Zn(C_2H_3O_2)_2.2H_2O$. Occurs as white crystals or granules; 1 Gm. dissolves in 2.5 cc. of water and in 30 cc. of alcohol. Used as a local remedy, principally as an astringent in collyrium in ophthalmia. It has also been used as an injection in gonorrhea, after the acute stage has passed.

z. carbonate. A basic carbonate of variable composition; occurs as a white, amorphous powder; practically insoluble in water or alcohol. Used as a mild astringent and protective. Applied in the form of an ointment or a dusting powder.

z. chloride (*zinci chloridum*). $ZnCl_2$. Occurs as a white, or nearly white, crystalline powder; 1 Gm. dissolves in 0.5 cc. of water and in about 1.5 cc. of alcohol; it is very deliquescent. It is occasionally used for its caustic effect in aphthous stomatitis and venereal ulcers. In dilute solution, it is sometimes used for its astringent action in leukorrhea and is the principal constituent in certain proprietary forms of astringent mouth wash.

z. iodide (*zinci iodidum*). ZnI_2. Occurs as a white, or nearly white, granular powder; it is freely soluble in water and alcohol; it is very deliquescent. Zinc iodide possesses astringent and caustic powers like those of the chloride but is rarely employed. It is used only as an ingredient in iodine and zinc iodide glycerite.

z. ointment. Zinc oxide ointment.

z. oxide (*zinci oxidum*). ZnO. Occurs as a fine, amorphous, white or yellowish white powder; insoluble in water and alcohol; dissolves in dilute acids. Used as a mildly astringent and protective application to excoriated surfaces and in various skin diseases. It may be applied as a dusting powder, usually with talc, in aqueous mixtures, or in the form of an ointment.

z. oxide hard paste (*pasta zinci oxidi dura*). Contains zinc oxide, 25 Gm.; purified siliceous earth, 5 Gm.; benzoinated lard, 70 Gm. Also called *Unna's hard z. paste.*

z. oxide ointment (*unguentum zinci oxidi*). Contains zinc oxide, 20 Gm., liquid petrolatum, 15 Gm., white ointment, 65 Gm.: also called *z. ointment.*

z. oxide paste (*pasta zinci oxidi*). Contains zinc oxide, 25 Gm.; starch, 25 Gm.; white petrolatum, 50 Gm. Also called *Lassar's plain zinc paste.*

z. oxide paste with salicylic acid. See under *salicylic acid.*

z. oxide soft paste (*pasta zinci oxidi mollis*). Contains zinc oxide, 25 Gm.; precipitated calcium carbonate, 25 Gm.; oleic acid, 2.5 Gm.; linseed oil, 25 Gm.; calcium hydroxide solution, 22.5 Gm. Also called *Unna's soft z. paste.*

z. phenolsulfonate (*zinci phenolsulfonas*). $Zn(HOC_6H_4SO_3)_2.8H_2O$. Occurs as colorless, transparent crystals, or as white granules or powder; 1 Gm. dissolves in about 1.6 cc. of water and in 1.8 cc. of alcohol. Used as an antiseptic and astringent application to indolent or foul ulcers, and in subacute inflammations of the mucous membranes. It has also been used as an intestinal antiseptic. Dose, 0.06–0.2 Gm. (1–3 gr.). Also called *z. sulfocarbolate.*

z. stearate (*zinci stearas*). A compound of zinc with variable proportions of stearic and palmitic acids; occurs as a fine, white, bulky powder; insoluble in water and alcohol. Used in eczema and other cutaneous diseases, in the form of powder or made into an ointment.

z. sulfanilate. $Zn[C_6H_4(NH_2)SO_3]_2.4H_2O$. A salt used in 0.25–0.5% aqueous solution or in ointment as an astringent application. See *nizin.*

z. sulfate (*zinci sulfas*). $ZnSO_4.7H_2O$. Occurs as colorless crystals, white granules, or a white powder; 1 Gm. dissolves in 0.6 cc. of water and in about 2.5 cc. of glycerin. It is efflorescent in dry air. Internally, it is used for its emetic action in various poisonings because of its promptness and its comparative freedom from danger. Externally, it is actively astringent and is used as such on the mucous membranes of the eye, nose, throat, or genital tract. Dose, as an emetic, 0.65–2.0 Gm. (10–30 gr.).

z. sulfocarbolate. Zinc phenolsulfonate.

z. undecylenate. $[CH_2{:}CH(CH_2)_8COO]_2Zn$; a fine, white powder, practically insoluble in water: used as a fungicide. See *desenex.*

zinc′ite. 1. A native zinc oxide, orange-yellow to deep red. 2. Any ore of zinc.

zinc′um. See *zinc.*

zin′ger·one (zin′jur·ohn). Gingerol. A pungent ketone, $C_{11}H_{14}O_3$, present in ginger.

zin′gi·ber. See *ginger.*

Zinn, Johann Gottfried [*German anatomist*, 1727–59]. Author of an important atlas of the human eye (1755). Described the suspensory ligament of the lens; also called the *ciliary zonule, zonule of Zinn.* Described the annulus from which arise the superior, inferior, medial, and lateral rectus muscles of the eye, called *Zinn's ligament* or *tendon* or *ring.* Described the central artery of the retina, called *Zinn's central artery.* Described the plexus of small branches of the ciliary artery in the sclera around the entrance of the optic nerve, formerly called *circulus arteriosus halleri, Zinn's circlet* or *corona.*

Zinsser's agar slant tissue culture method. See under *method.*

zir·co′ni·um [NL.]. Zr = 91.22. A metallic element resembling titanium and silicon.

z. dioxide. ZrO_2. Occurs as a heavy white powder. Used in x-ray photography as a substitute for bismuth salts.

Zn Chemical symbol for zinc.

zoalite. Trade name for a device for producing infrared rays.

zo·an′thro·py [G. *zōion*, living being, animal; *anthrōpos*, man]. A form of mental disorder in which the person imagines himself transformed into or inhabited by an animal.

Zoeller, Christian [*French pathologist*, 1888–1939]. One of the first, with G. Ramon, to use tetanus toxoid in immunization of humans (1933). The reaction produced by the use of the toxoid is called *Ramon-Zoeller's reaction.*

Zoellner, Johann Carl Friedrich [*German physicist*, 1834–82]. Remembered for his production of a chart with figures composed of variously arranged lines, designed to illustrate optical illusion; called *Zoellner's lines.*

zo′e·scope. See *stroboscope.*

zo′e·trope. See *stroboscope.*

zo′na [G. *zōnē*, belt]. 1. A belt or girdle. 2. See *herpes* zoster.

z. arcuata. The inner zone of the basilar membrane, extending from the lower edge of the spiral groove of the cochlea to the external edge of the base of the outer rods of Corti.

z. cartilaginea. The limbus of the spiral lamina.

z. ciliaris. The ciliary processes collectively.

z. columnaris recti. The portion of the anal canal in which lie the rectal columns.

z. cutanea recti. The portion of the anal canal lined by skin.

z. denticulata. The inner zone of the basilar membrane, together with the limbus of the spiral lamina.

z. fasciculata. The central portion of the cortex of the suprarenal gland in which the cellular cords are radially disposed.

z. glomerulosa. The outer zone of the adrenal cortex in which the cells are grouped in rounded masses.

z. incerta. The anterior portion of the reticular formation under the thalamus.

z. intermedia recti. The portion of the anal canal which lies between the cutaneous and columnar zones.

z. ophthalmica. Herpes zoster along the course of the ophthalmic division of the fifth nerve.

z. orbicularis. A thickening of the capsular ligament around the acetabulum.

z. pectinata. The outer portion of the basilar membrane, extending from the rods of Corti to the spiral ligament.

z. pellucida. The thick, solid, elastic envelope of the ovum: also called *oolemma.*

z. perforata. The lower edge of the spiral groove of the cochlea.

z. reticularis. 1. The inner zone of the adrenal cortex in which the cellular cords form a network. 2. See reticular *layer.*

z. spongiosa. A thin zone of nerve cells and myelinated fibers, external to the substantia gelatinosa in the posterior column of the spinal cord.

z. tecta. The inner portion of the basilar membrane, bearing the organ of Corti.

Zondek, Bernhard [*German gynecologist in Israel,* 1891–]. Isolated, with S. Aschheim, prolan-A and -B (1928). Author of work on hormones (1931–46). Devised a test, with S. Aschheim, for pregnancy (1928). See Aschheim-Zondek *test, reaction.*

Zondek, Hermann (1887–). German physician in Israel who described the condition of the heart in myxedema (1918), called *myxedema heart,* and introduced small iodine doses into the treatment of Graves' disease (1921).

zone [G.]. A delimited area or region. —**zo'nal,** *adj.*

androgenic z. The hypertrophic, inner zone of the fetal adrenal cortex. It involutes rapidly after birth, has certain hormonal functions similar to the testes, and theoretically serves to protect the fetus against the excessive effect of maternal estrogens. Also called *x-zone, fetal cortex.*

chondrogenic z. The layer of cartilage formation under the deep face of the perichondrium.

ciliary z. The ciliary processes collectively.

cochlear z. Old term for the membranous part of the spiral lamina or basilar membrane: also called *cochlear z. of Zinn.*

Cozzolino's z. See *fissula* ante fenestram.

dentofacial z. That facial area which includes the teeth and their supporting alveolar process. It is subdivided into four sections: upper apical, upper coronal, lower apical, lower coronal.

ectopic z. An area in the prosencephalon surrounding the optic vesicle on its dorsal, cephalic, and ventral aspects. From this zone several parts of the telencephalon and diencephalon take origin. Also called *ectopic z. of Schulte.*

entry z. The parts along the posterior horns of gray matter of the spinal cord where the posterior roots enter the cord.

ependymal z. The internal zone of the embryonic neural tube containing ependymal cells and undifferentiated, proliferative cells.

erotogenic z. Any part of the body which, on being touched, causes sexual feelings.

hepatic zones. The central, midzonal, and peripheral parts of the liver lobule.

hysterogenic z. Painful spots occurring in hysteria, not due to organic disease.

interpalpebral z. That part of the cornea which ordinarily is not covered by the lids when the eye is open.

isoelectric z. The range of pH over which the isoelectric condition prevails. See isoelectric *point.*

latent z. That part of the cerebral cortex in which a lesion produces no recognized symptoms.

limitrophic z. Any area of the cerebral cortex transitional between two neighboring well-defined areas: also called *limitrophic area* or *cortex.*

Looser's zones. Ribbonlike zones of decalcification, or united but uncalcified pseudofractures, characteristically seen on roentgenograms in osteomalacia, including Milkman's syndrome and rickets.

radiary z. A layer in the cortical gray matter of the brain, characterized by radiating nerve fibers.

root entrance z. See Obersteiner-Redlich *area.*

sclerotic z. A condition occurring in iritis, marked by a ring of anastomoses of deep, conjunctival vessels around the periphery of the cornea, which perforate the sclera and anastomose with those of the iris and choroid.

supraradiary z. The layer of cortex immediately above the radiary zone.

trigger z. Any area of hyperexcitability, stimulation of which will precipitate a specific response such as an epileptic seizure or an attack of neuralgia.

x z. See androgenic *z.*

z. of antibody excess. See under *z.* of equivalence.

z. of antigen excess. See under *z.* of equivalence.

z. of equivalence. This term applies to the precipitation reaction in serology. A series of test tubes is prepared containing a constant amount of antiserum in each tube but increasing amounts of the soluble antigen. Precipitation occurs in those tubes in which there is excess antibody and the supernatant fluid contains excess, uncombined antibody (*z. of antibody excess*). Precipitation also occurs when the proper or optimal ratio of antigen and antiserum are mixed so that there is no uncombined antigen or antibody in the supernatant fluid (*z. of equivalence*). When the ratio of antigen to antibody is increased slightly, precipitation still occurs; however, with further increase in the ratio of antigen to antibody, precipitation is inhibited (*z. of inhibition*). Both situations are said to occur in the *z. of antigen excess* where excess antigen is present in the supernatant fluid.

z. of inhibition. See under *z.* of equivalence.

zon"es·the'si·a, zon"aes·the'si·a (zo"ness·thee'-zhuh, ·zee·uh) [*zōnē;* G. *aisthēsis,* sensation]. A sensation like that produced by a tight girdle encircling the waist. Syn., *girdle pain.*

zo·nif'u·gal [*zōnē;* L. *fugere,* to flee]. Pertaining to the tendency to pass out of, or away from, a zone.

zo·nip'e·tal [*zōnē;* L. *petere,* to seek]. Pertaining to the tendency to pass into a zone from without.

zon'ule (zone'yōōl, zon'yōōl) [L. *zonula,* dim. from *zōnē*]. A small band. —**zon'ular,** *adj.*

ciliary z. The suspensory structure supporting the lens of the eye. Also called *z. of Zinn.*

zon"u·li'tis (zone"yoo·lye'tis, zon"yoo·) [*zonula;* G. *-itis,* inflammation]. Inflammation of the ciliary zonule.

zon"u·lot'o·my [*zonula;* G. *tomē,* a cutting]. The severing of the ciliary zonular fibers.

zo'o-, zo- [G. *zōion,* living being, animal]. A combining form denoting *animal* or *pertaining to an animal.*

zo"o·der'mic [*zōion;* G. *derma,* skin]. Pertaining to, or taken from, the skin of some animal other than man; applied to a form of skin grafting.

zo"o·er·as'ti·a [*zōion;* G. *erastēs,* lover]. Sexual intercourse with an animal.

zo"o·ge·og'ra·phy [*zōion;* G. *geographia,* geography]. The study of animals and animal life in various parts of the earth.

zo″o·gle′a (zo″o·glee′uh, zo·og′lee·uh) [*zōion;* G. *gloia*, glue]. Microorganisms which are embedded in a jellylike matrix formed as the result of their metabolic activities. —**zoogleic,** *adj.*

zo·og′o·ny [*zōion;* G. *gonē*, offspring]. The breeding of animals.

zo′o·graft [*zōion;* G. *graphein*, to write]. A graft of tissue taken from an animal.

zo′oid [*zōion*]. An individual member of a metazoan colony.

zo″o·lag′ni·a [*zōion;* G. *lagneia*, coition]. Sexual attraction toward animals.

zo·ol′o·gist [*zōion;* G. *logos*, word]. A scientist who studies animal life.

zo·ol′o·gy [*zōion; logos*]. The study of animals.

zo″o·no′sis (pl. *zoonoses*). A disease which can be transmitted to man by vertebrate animals. —**zoonot′ic,** *adj.*

zo″o·par′a·site [*zōion;* G. *parasitos*, parasite]. An animal parasite.

zo·oph′a·gous [*zōion;* G. *phagein*, to eat]. Subsisting on animal food.

zo·oph′i·lism [*zōion;* G. *philein*, to love]. The love of animals; it is usually immoderate, and toward certain animals, illustrated in the fanaticism of antivivisection.

erotic z. The desire or impulse to stroke or pet animals for sexual excitement.

zo″o·pho′bi·a [*zōion;* G. *phobos*, fear]. Morbid fear of animals.

zo′o·phyte [*zōion;* G. *phyton*, plant]. An invertebrate animal that superficially resembles a plant in appearance, as the sponges, hydroids, bryozoa.

zo′o·plas″ty [*zōion;* G. *plassein*, to form]. The surgical transfer of zoografts; the transplantation of tissue from any of the lower animals to man.

zo·op′si·a [*zōion;* G. *opsis*, vision]. The seeing of animals, as an illusion or as a hallucination or in a dream; occurs commonly in delirium tremens.

zo′o·spore [*zōion;* G. *spora*, seed]. A motile spore.

zo·os′ter·ol. Sterol of animal origin.

zo·o′to·my. Anatomy of animals other than man.

zo″o·tox′in [*zōion;* G. *toxikon*, poison]. A toxin or poison of animal origin.

zos′ter [G., girdle]. An acute inflammatory disease, consisting of grouped vesicles corresponding in distribution to the course of a cutaneous nerve; accompanied by pain or burning, and usually unilateral. Syn., *herpes zoster.*

z. auricularis. A form affecting the ear.

z. brachialis. A form affecting the arm or forearm.

z. facialis. That involving the sensory fibers of the trigeminal nerve distributed over the face. Any or all of the three branches may be involved.

z. femoralis. That occurring over the sacrum and extending down the thighs. The perineal region may be involved.

z. ophthalmicus. An eruption in the course of the ophthalmic division of the fifth nerve.

zos·ter′i·form [*zōstēr;* L. *forma*, form]. Resembling zoster.

zos′ter·oid [*zōstēr;* G. *eidos*, form]. Zosteriform.

Z-plas′ty. See Z-plastic relaxing *operation.*

Zr Chemical symbol for zirconium.

Zsigmondy's movement. See Brownian *movement.*

Zuckerkandl, Emil [*Austrian anatomist*, 1849–1910]. Described retroperitoneal chromaffin bodies close to the main vessels and associated with the sympathetic ganglions; called *Zuckerkandl's bodies.* The gyrus subcallosus is called *Zuckerkandl's convolution.* The pharyngeal (formerly called nasal) tonsil is called *Zuckerkandl's tubercle.*

zuck′ung [Ger.]. Contraction; a term used in electrotherapeutics. Abbreviated, Z.

Zwemer's test. See potassium tolerance *test.*

zwit′ter·i″on. An ion which contains both a positive and a negative charge, but neutral as a whole; a dipolar ion. Amino acids may form such ions by migration of a hydrogen ion from the carboxyl group to the basic nitrogen atom as, for example, when RNH_2COOH is thus converted to $RNH_3^+COO^-$. Also written *zwitter ion.*

Zy″ga·de′nus [G. *zygadēn*, jointly]. A genus of herbs producing a crystalline alkaloid $C_{39}H_{63}NO_{10}$.

Z. venenosus. Death camas, a liliaceous plant; an important forage poison in the western United States. It contains an alkaloid zygatuine, similar to veratrine, producing violent convulsions.

zy″ga·poph′y·sis (zy″guh·pof′i·sis) [G. *zygon*, yoke; *apophysis*, sideshoot]. An articular process of a vertebra. —**zygapophys′eal,** *adj.*

zyg′i·on (zig′ee·on) [*zygon*]. A craniometric point at either end of the greatest bizygomatic diameter.

zy″go·dac′ty·ly. See *syndactyly.*

zy·go′ma (zye·go′muh, zi·go′muh) [G., arcus zygomaticus]. 1. The arch formed by the union of the zygomatic processes of the temporal bone, maxilla, and the zygomatic bone. 2. The cheekbone. See Table of Bones in the Appendix. —**zygomat′ic,** *adj.*

zy″go·mat′ic (zy″go·mat′ik) [*zygōma*]. 1. One of several small subcutaneous muscles arising from, or in relation with, the zygoma. See Table of Muscles in the Appendix. 2. A somatic sensory nerve attached at the maxillary, which innervates the skin in the region of the zygoma and temple.

zy″go·mat′i·co- (zy″go·mat′i·ko-) [*zygōma*]. A combining form denoting *relating to the zygoma.*

zy″go·mat″i·co·fa′cial [*zygōma;* L. *facies*, face]. Pertaining to the zygoma and the face, as zygomaticofacial foramen.

zy″go·mat″i·co·tem′po·ral [*zygōma;* L. *tempus*, temple]. Pertaining to zygoma and temporal bone or fossa, as zygomaticotemporal foramen.

zy″go·mat′i·cus. Muscle of facial expression associated with the zygoma.

zy″go·max″il·la′re (zy″go·mack″si·lair′ee, ·mack′-si·lair·ee) [G. *zygon*, yoke; L. *maxilla*, jawbone]. The point on the zygomaticomaxillary suture that lies most inferior to the horizontal plane.

zy″go·my·ce′tes [*zygon;* G. *mykēs*, fungus]. A group of fungi characterized by sexual reproduction through the union of two similar gametes.

zygon. Trade-mark for a brand of wheat-germ oil.

zy″go·ne′ma [*zygon;* G. *nēma*, thread]. The chromonema when in the zygotene stage of meiosis.

zy′go·spore [*zygon;* G. *spora*, seed]. The spore resulting from the fusion of two similar gametes, as in certain algae and fungi.

zy′gote (zy′goat) [*zygon*]. 1. An organism produced by the union of two gametes. 2. The fertilized ovum before cleavage.

zy′go·tene [*zygon;* G. *tainia*, ribbon]. Characterizing the stage in the prophase of the first maturation division when the chromosomes are undergoing synapsis. Syn., *amphitene, synaptene.*

zylcaine. Trade-mark for a local anesthetic product containing procaine, butesin, and benzyl alcohol in sweet almond oil; used by injection for the relief of painful anal conditions.

zy′mase (zy′mace). 1. An enzyme. 2. An enzyme mixture of yeast causing alcoholic fermentation.

Buchner's z. That expressed from dried yeast; yeast-cell plasma.

zyme [G., leaven]. An organized ferment. *Obs.* —**zymic,** *adj.*

zy′mo-, zym- [*zymē*]. A combining form denoting *pertaining to* or *produced by fermentation.*

zy″mo-ex·ci′tor. An agent which activates a zymogen: a kinase.

zy′mo·gen [*zymē;* G. *genesthai*, from *gignesthai*, to be produced]. The inactive precursor of an enzyme which, on reaction with an appropriate kinase or other chemical agent, liberates the enzyme in active form.

zy″mo·gen′ic, zy·mog′e·nous (zye·modj′i·nus) [*zymē; genesthai*]. 1. Causing fermentation. 2. Pertaining to, or producing, a zymogen.

zy″mo·hex′ase. See *aldolase.*

zy″mo·hy·drol′y·sis (zy″mo·high·drol′i·sis) [*zymē;* G. *hydōr*, water; *lysis*, a loosing]. Hydrolysis produced by the action of an enzyme. Also called *enzymatic hydrolysis.*

zy′moid [G. *zymoeidēs*, like leaven]. Resembling an organized ferment.

zy·mol′o·gy (zye·mol′o·jee) [G. *zymē*, leaven; *logos*, word]. The science of fermentation. —**zymolog′ic,** *adj.*

zy·mol′y·sis. See *zymosis*, 1. —**zymolyt′ic,** *adj.*

zy′mo·lyte. Material upon which an enzyme acts. *Obs.*

zy·mom′e·ter [*zymē;* G. *metron*, a measure]. An instrument for measuring fermentation.

Zy″mo·ne′ma. See *Blastomyces.*

zy″mo·nem″a·to′sis [*zymē;* G. *nēma*, thread; *-ōsis*, condition]. Blastomycosis.

zy′mo·phore [*zymē;* G. *phoros*, bearing]. The active part of an enzyme, that which bears the ferment. That portion of the enzyme which possesses the characteristic activity. —**zymophor′ic,** *adj.*

zy″mo·plas′tic [*zymē;* G. *plassein*, to form]. Enzyme-producing.

zy″mo·pro′te·in (zy″mo·pro′tee·in, ·pro′teen) [*zymē;* G. *prōteios*, of first rank]. Any one of a class of proteins possessing catalytic powers.

zy·mo′sis (zye·mo′sis) [G., fermentation]. 1. Fermentation. 2. An infectious disease due to a fungus. —**zymot′ic,** *adj.*

zy·mos′ter·ol (zye·mos′tur·ole, ·ol, ·awl). $C_{27}H_{44}O$. A sterol from yeast; found in ergosterol residues.

zy′mur·gy [G. *zymourgos*, maker of leaven]. The branch of chemical technology dealing with the application of fermentation or enzymatic action to any industrial process, as the curing of cheese, processing of leather, production of organic solvents, etc.

Z.Z.′Z.″ Increasing strengths of contraction. Also see *Z.*

Appendix

Tables

TABLE OF ARTERIES

(See Plates 7, 8)

NAME	ORIGIN	BRANCHES	DISTRIBUTION
Aberrant	Brachial or axillary		Radial, radial recurrent, or, rarely, ulnar art.
Aberrant	Descending aorta		Anastomoses with an aberrant art. from the right subclavian, costocervical trunk, or superior intercostal art.
Acetabular or **articular**	Obturator		Round ligament of femur, synovial membrane, acetabular fat, head of femur
Acromial	Thoracoacromial		Deltoid m., acromial rete
Acromial	Transverse scapular		Trapezius m., acromial rete
Acromiothoracic	See *Thoracoacromial*		
Afferent	Interlobular of kidney		Glomeruli
Alveolar or **gingival**	Posterior superior alveolar		Gums of posterior portion of upper jaw
Alveolar, anterior superior (anterior superior dental OT)	Infraorbital	Dental, antral	Upper incisor and canine teeth, mucous membrane of maxillary sinus
Alveolar, inferior (inferior dental OT) (see Plate 8)	Internal maxillary	Mylohyoid, lingual, dental, mental, incisive	Mylohyoid m., buccal mucous membrane, lower teeth, mandible, gums
Alveolar, middle superior (inconstant)	Infraorbital		Upper premolar teeth
Alveolar, posterior superior (posterior superior dental OT)	Internal maxillary	Dental, antral, alveolar, muscular	Buccinator m., upper molar and premolar teeth, gums, mucous membrane of maxillary sinus
Anastomotic of inferior gluteal	Inferior gluteal		Anastomoses with first perforating and medial and lateral femoral circumflex art. in what is known as "crucial anastomosis"
Anastomotic of middle meningeal (also called **perforating temporal**)	Middle meningeal		Anastomoses with deep temporal
Anastomotica magna of brachial	See *Collateral, inferior ulnar*		
Angular	External maxillary	Muscular, lacrimal, terminal	Orbicularis oculi, nasalis, angular head of quadratus labii superioris and procerus mm.; lacrimal sac; anastomoses with dorsal nasal branch of ophthalmic
Antral	Anterior and posterior superior alveolar		Mucous membrane of maxillary sinus (antrum of Highmore OT)

TABLE OF ARTERIES—(Continued)

Name	Origin	Branches	Distribution
Aorta, abdominal	Continuation of descending (thoracic) aorta from level of inferior border of twelfth thoracic vertebra	(1) Visceral celiac superior mesenteric inferior mesenteric middle suprarenal renal internal spermatic (ovarian) (2) Parietal inferior phrenic lumbar (4 pairs) middle sacral (3) Terminal common iliac	Diaphragm, body wall, abdominal and pelvic viscera, lower extremities
Aorta, arch of	Continuation of ascending aorta outside pericardium	Innominate, left common carotid, left subclavian (occasionally thyreoidea ima and bronchial art.)	
Aorta, ascending	Base of left ventricle	Right and left coronary	
Aorta, descending (thoracic)	Continuation of arch of aorta at inferior border of left side of fourth thoracic vertebra	(1) Visceral pericardial bronchial esophageal mediastinal (2) Parietal intercostal superior phrenic subcostal (aberrant, vas aberrans)	Body wall, thoracic viscera, diaphragm
Appendicular	Ileocolic	Cecal, appendicular	Apex of cecum, vermiform process
Arciform or **arcuate of kidney**	Interlobar	Interlobular	
Arcuate	Dorsalis pedis	Second, third, and fourth dorsal metatarsal	Dorsal metatarsal portion of foot
Auditory, internal (see Plate 17)	Basilar or anterior inferior cerebellar		Internal ear
Auricular, deep	Internal maxillary	Meatal, tympanic, auricular	Skin of external acoustic meatus, external surface of tympanic membrane, temporomandibular articulation
Auricular, posterior	External carotid	Muscular, auricular, stylomastoid, occipital, parotid	Digastric, stylohyoid, sternocleidomastoid, auricularis posterior, occipitalis, and stapedius mm.; tympanic membrane and cavity, tympanic antrum, mastoid air cells, semicircular canals, auricle, scalp, parotid gland
Axillary (see Plate 7)	Continuation of subclavian	Highest thoracic, thoracoacromial, lateral thoracic, subscapular, posterior humeral circumflex, anterior humeral circumflex	Pectoralis major, pectoralis minor, biceps brachii, coracobrachialis, triceps (long head), subclavius, deltoid, serratus anterior, teres major, teres minor, latissimus dorsi, subscapularis, and infraspinatus mm.; mammary gland, shoulder joint, head of humerus, skin of pectoral region and shoulder, acromial rete

TABLE OF ARTERIES—(Continued)

Name	Origin	Branches	Distribution
Azygos of vagina	Uterine and vaginal		Vagina
Basilar (see Plates 17, 18)	Formed by junction of the two vertebral	Anterior inferior cerebellar, internal auditory, pontine, superior cerebellar, posterior cerebral	Pons, internal ear, cerebellum, pineal body, anterior medullary velum, tela chorioidea of third ventricle, temporal and occipital lobes of cerebrum
Brachial (see Plate 7)	Axillary	Profunda brachii, nutrient, muscular, superior ulnar collateral, inferior ulnar collateral, radial, ulnar	Deltoid, triceps, brachioradialis, biceps brachii, brachialis, coracobrachialis, and anconeus mm.; shaft of humerus, elbow joint, forearm, and hand
Bronchial	(1) Descending (thoracic) aorta (upper and lower left) (2) First aortic intercostal (right) (3) Arch of aorta (occasionally)		Bronchial tubes, areolar tissue of lungs, bronchial lymph nodes, esophagus
Buccal	See *Buccinator*		
Buccinator (see Plate 8)	Internal maxillary		Buccinator m.; skin and mucous membrane of cheek, upper gums
Bulb of urethra, art. of	Internal pudendal	Muscular, glandular, spongiosal	Sphincter urethrae membranaceae m.; bulbourethral gland (Cowper's), bulb of urethra, corpus spongiosum urethrae
Bulb of vestibule, art. of	Internal pudendal	Bulbar, glandular	Major vestibular glands (Bartholin's), bulb of vestibule
Caroticotympanic	Internal carotid		Lining of tympanic cavity
Carotid, common (see Plates 5, 7, 8, 13)	Right from innominate, left from arch of aorta	External and internal carotid, occasionally superior thyroid, ascending pharyngeal, and even vertebral	Region of neck and head
Carotid, external (see Plates 7, 8)	Common carotid	Superior thyroid, ascending pharyngeal, lingual, external maxillary (facial), sternocleidomastoid (occasionally), occipital, posterior auricular, superficial temporal, internal maxillary	Anterior portion of neck, face, scalp, side of head, ear, dura mater
Carotid, internal (see Plates 7, 8, 17, 18)	Common carotid	(1) Petrous portion: caroticotympanic, art. of pterygoid canal (Vidian) (inconstant) (2) Cavernous portion: cavernous, hypophyseal, semilunar, anterior meningeal, ophthalmic (3) Cerebral portion: anterior cerebral, middle cerebral, posterior communicating, choroid	Anterior portion of cerebrum, eye and its appendages, forehead, nose, internal ear, trigeminal nerve, dura mater, hypophysis

TABLE OF ARTERIES—(Continued)

NAME	ORIGIN	BRANCHES	DISTRIBUTION
Celiac	Abdominal aorta	Left gastric, hepatic, splenic	Esophagus, cardia and lesser curvature of stomach, liver, gallbladder, pylorus, duodenum, pancreas, great omentum, spleen
Central art. of retina	Ophthalmic	Superior; nasal, temporal Inferior; nasal, temporal	Retina
Cerebellar, anterior inferior (see Plate 17)	Basilar		Anterior portion of inferior surface of cerebellum
Cerebellar, posterior inferior (see Plate 17)	Vertebral	Bulbar, choroid, nuclear, medial terminal, lateral terminal	Medulla oblongata, choroid plexus of third ventricle, dentate nucleus, nuclei of cranial nerves IX, X, XI
Cerebellar, superior (see Plate 17)	Basilar	Medial, lateral	Vermis cerebelli, superior surface of cerebellum, pineal body, anterior medullary velum, tela chorioidea of third ventricle
Cerebral, anterior (see Plates 17, 18)	Internal carotid	Anterior communicating, orbital, anterior medial frontal, recurrent, intermediate medial frontal, posterior medial frontal	Anterior perforated substance, lamina terminalis, rostrum of corpus callosum, septum pellucidum, head of caudate nucleus, frontal lobe of putamen, frontal lobe of globus pallidus, orbital surface of frontal lobe of cerebrum, gyrus rectus, medial orbital gyrus, olfactory lobe, superior frontal gyrus, middle frontal gyrus, corpus callosum, cinguli, anterior commissure, internal capsule, column of fornix, precuneus, upper part of ascending frontal gyrus, upper part of ascending parietal gyrus, superior parietal lobule
Cerebral, middle (art. fossae Sylvii OT) (see Plate 17)	Internal carotid	Medial striate, lateral striate, inferior lateral frontal, ascending frontal, ascending parietal, parietotemporal, temporal	Putamen, caudate nucleus, globus pallidus, internal capsule, inferior frontal gyrus (Broca's convolution), lateral part of orbital surface of frontal lobe, ascending frontal gyrus, ascending parietal gyrus, lower part of superior parietal lobule, supramarginal gyrus, angular gyrus, posterior parts of superior and middle temporal gyri, lateral surface of temporal lobe
Cerebral, posterior (see Plate 17)	Basilar	Anterior temporal, posterior temporal, posteromedial central, posterolateral central, posterior choroid, calcarine, parieto-occipital	Posterior perforated substance, cerebral peduncle, posterior part of thalamus, mammillary bodies, walls of third ventricle, corpora quadrigemina, medial and lateral geniculate bodies, uncus, hippocampal gyrus, fusiform gyrus, cuneus, precuneus, lingual gyrus, tela chorioidea of third ventricle, choroid plexus, fornix, posterior half of visual path, half of visual center of occipital lobe
Cervical, ascending	Inferior thyroid	Muscular, spinal, phrenic	Longus capitis, scalenus anterior and mm. of nape of neck, spinal medulla and its membranes. vertebrae, phrenic nerve

TABLE OF ARTERIES—(Continued)

Name	Origin	Branches	Distribution
Cervical, deep	Costocervical trunk	Muscular, spinal	Semispinalis cervicis, semispinalis capitis, and adjoining neck mm.; spinal medulla and membranes via intervertebral foramen for eighth cervical nerve
Cervical, superficial	Transverse cervical	Muscular, glandular	Trapezius, levator scapulae, splenius cervicis, splenius capitis mm.; posterior chain of lymph nodes
Cervical, transverse	Thyrocervical trunk	Ascending or superficial cervical, descending	Trapezius, levator scapulae, splenii, rhomboids, latissimus dorsi mm.; posterior chain of lymph nodes
Choroid, anterior (see Plate 17)	Internal carotid	Optic, peduncular, ganglionic, choroid	Optic tract, cerebral peduncle, base of cerebrum, lateral geniculate body, tail of caudate nucleus, globus pallidus, internal capsule, choroid plexus of inferior horn of lateral ventricle
Choroid, posterior	Posterior cerebral		Tela chorioidea of third ventricle, choroid plexus
Ciliary, anterior	Muscular branches of ophthalmic and lacrimal	Episcleral, anterior conjunctival	Iris and conjunctiva
Ciliary, long posterior	Ophthalmic		Ciliary muscle and iris
Ciliary, short posterior	Ophthalmic		Choroid and ciliary processes
Circumflex, anterior humeral	Axillary	Muscular, bicipital, pectoral	Coracobrachialis, biceps brachii, deltoid mm.; head of humerus, shoulder joint, tendons of pectoralis major and long head of biceps brachii mm.
Circumflex, deep iliac	External iliac	Muscular, cutaneous	Psoas, iliacus, sartorius, tensor fasciae latae, obliquus abdominis externus, obliquus abdominis internus, transversus abdominis mm.; skin over course of vessel
Circumflex, lateral femoral	Profunda femoris	Ascending, transverse, descending	Muscles of thigh
Circumflex, medial femoral	Profunda femoris	Muscular, superficial, deep, acetabular	Adductor, gracilis, obturator externus, quadratus femoris mm.; acetabular fat, round ligament of femur, head of femur
Circumflex, posterior humeral	Axillary	Muscular, articular, nutrient, acromial	Deltoid, teres minor, triceps brachii (long and lateral heads) mm.; greater tubercle of humerus, posterior portion of shoulder joint, acromial rete
Circumflex, scapular	Subscapular	Muscular, articular, nutrient	Subscapularis, infraspinatus, teres major, teres minor, deltoid, triceps brachii (long head) mm.; scapula, shoulder joint
Circumflex, superficial iliac (see Plate 7)	Femoral	Muscular, glandular, cutaneous	Sartorius, iliacus, tensor fasciae latae mm.; inguinal lymph nodes, skin over course of vessel

TABLE OF ARTERIES—(Continued)

Name	Origin	Branches	Distribution
Clitoris, deep art. of	Internal pudendal		Corpus cavernosum clitoridis
Clitoris, dorsal art. of	Internal pudendal		Dorsum, glans, corona and prepuce of clitoris
Colic, left (see Plate 8)	Inferior mesenteric	Ascending, descending	Left portion of transverse colon, upper portion of descending colon, splenic flexure
Colic, middle (see Plate 8)	Superior mesenteric	Right, left	Upper portion of ascending colon, hepatic flexure, right portion of transverse colon
Colic, right (see Plate 8)	Superior mesenteric	Ascending, descending	Ascending colon
Collateral, inferior ulnar (anastomotica magna OT)	Brachial	Posterior, anterior	Triceps brachii, brachialis, pronator teres mm.; articular rete of elbow joint
Collateral, middle	Profunda brachii	Muscular, anastomotic	Medial head of triceps brachii m.; articular rete of elbow joint
Collateral, radial	Profunda brachii	Muscular, anastomotic	Triceps brachii, brachioradialis mm.; articular rete of elbow joint
Collateral, superior ulnar (profunda inferior OT) (see Plate 7)	Brachial	Muscular, articular, anastomotic	Triceps brachii m.; skin, elbow joint, articular rete of elbow joint
Comes nervi mediani, art.	See *Median*		
Comes nervi phrenici, art.	See *Pericardiacophrenic*		
Comitans nervi ischiadici, art.	Inferior gluteal		Sciatic nerve
Communicating, anterior (see Plates 17, 18)	Anterior cerebral	Anteromedial	Anterior perforated substance
Communicating, posterior (see Plate 17)	Internal carotid	Hippocampal, middle thalamic	Optic chiasm, optic tract, tuber cinereum, mammillary body, hippocampal gyrus, internal capsule, cerebral peduncle, interpeduncular region, thalamus
Conjunctival, anterior	Episcleral of anterior ciliary		Conjunctiva
Conjunctival, posterior	Medial and lateral palpebral arteries		Conjunctiva
Coronary, left (see Plate 5)	Left posterior aortic sinus	Anterior descending, circumflex, left marginal, left atrial, terminal	Left atrium, root of aorta and pulmonary art., myocardium of both ventricles, interventricular septum
Coronary, right (see Plate 5)	Anterior aortic sinus	Right atrial, posterior descending, right marginal, preventricular, transverse	Right atrium, root of pulmonary art. and aorta, anterior wall of right ventricle, septal myocardium, left ventricle adjoining posterior longitudinal cardiac sulcus

TABLE OF ARTERIES—(Continued)

NAME	ORIGIN	BRANCHES	DISTRIBUTION
Costocervical trunk	Subclavian	Superior intercostal, deep cervical, arteria aberrans on right	First and second intercostal spaces, mm. of neck, spinal cord and its membranes
Cremasteric	See *Spermatic, external*		
Cystic (see Plate 8)	Right hepatic	Superficial, deep	Free surface of gallbladder, attached surface of gallbladder, and liver substance
Deferential	Superior vesical, inferior vesical, or internal iliac	Ascending, descending	Seminal vesicle, ampulla of ductus deferens, ductus deferens, epididymis
Dental, anterior superior	See *Alveolar, anterior superior*		
Dental, inferior	See *Alveolar, inferior*		
Dental, posterior superior	See *Alveolar, posterior superior*		
Digital, common volar	Superficial volar arch	Proper volar digital	Contiguous sides of second to fifth fingers, flexor tendons and tendon sheaths, matrix of nails
Digital, dorsal, of thumb	Radial		Dorsum and sides of thumb
Digital, plantar	Plantar metatarsal arteries		Contiguous sides of toes, flexor tendons and sheaths, joints, skin
Digital, plantar, of lateral side of fifth toe	Lateral plantar		Lateral plantar part of fifth toe
Digital, proper volar, of medial side of little finger	Ulnar		Medial side of little finger, flexor tendon and sheath, matrix of nail
Digital, radial dorsal, of index finger	Radial		Radial dorsal surface of index finger
Dorsalis pedis (see Plate 7)	Anterior tibial	Cutaneous, lateral tarsal, medial tarsal, arcuate, first dorsal, metatarsal, deep plantar	Anastomoses with lateral plantar to form plantar arterial arch; plantar surface of first and second toes; tarsal, metatarsal, digital portions of dorsum of foot
Epigastric, deep	See *Epigastric, inferior*		
Epigastric, inferior (deep epigastric OT)	External iliac	Cutaneous, muscular, external spermatic (cremasteric in male, art. of round ligament of uterus in female), pubic	Skin and muscles of anterior abdominal wall, cremaster m., spermatic cord (round ligament of uterus in female), peritoneum
Epigastric, superficial	Femoral		Skin of abdominal wall below umbilicus, superficial fascia (Camper's), inguinal lymph nodes
Epigastric, superior	Internal mammary	Cutaneous, muscular, hepatic, peritoneal, phrenic, xiphoid	Skin, fascia, muscles and peritoneum of upper abdominal wall, diaphragm, falciform ligament of liver

TABLE OF ARTERIES—(Continued)

Name	Origin	Branches	Distribution
Episcleral	Anterior ciliary	Anterior conjunctival	Iris, ciliary processes, conjunctiva
Esophageal (4 or 5)	Thoracic aorta		Esophagus
Ethmoidal, anterior	Ophthalmic	Ethmoidal, anterior meningeal, nasal, frontal, cutaneous	Anterior and middle ethmoidal air cells, dura mater of anterior cranial fossa, mucoperiosteum of middle meatus, lateral wall and septum of nose, frontal air sinus, skin of dorsum of nose
Ethmoidal, posterior	Ophthalmic	Ethmoidal, meningeal, nasal	Posterior ethmoidal air cells, dura mater around cribriform plate, superior meatus and superior nasal concha
Facial	See *Maxillary, external*		
Facial, transverse	Superficial temporal	Glandular, muscular, cutaneous	Masseter m.; parotid gland, skin of face
Femoral (see Plates 7, 11, 13)	Continuation of external iliac	Superficial epigastric, superficial iliac circumflex, superficial external pudendal, deep external pudendal, muscular, profunda femoris, highest genicular (art. genus suprema)	Skin of lower part of abdomen and groin, external genitalia, inguinal lymph nodes; mm. of medial, lateral, and anterior aspects of thigh; femur, knee joint
Femoral, deep (see Plate 7)	See *Profunda femoris*		
Fossae Sylvii, art. of	See *Cerebral, middle*		
Frenulum linguae, art. of	Sublingual		Frenulum of tongue
Frontal (see Plate 8)	Ophthalmic		Skin, mm. and pericranium of forehead
Gastric, left (see Plate 8)	Celiac	Esophageal, hepatic (occasionally)	Lesser curvature and cardia of stomach, lower end of esophagus, left lobe of liver (occasionally)
Gastric, right (see Plate 8)	Hepatic		Pyloric portion of stomach
Gastric, short (vasa brevia)	Splenic		Greater curvature of stomach
Gastroduodenal (see Plate 8)	Hepatic	Pylorus, right gastroepiploic, superior pancreaticoduodenal, omental	Pylorus, duodenum, pancreas, great omentum, common bile duct
Gastroepiploic, left (see Plate 8)	Splenic	Gastric, omental	Greater curvature of stomach, great omentum
Gastroepiploic, right (see Plate 8)	Hepatic	Gastric, omental	Greater curvature of stomach, great omentum
Genicular, highest (genus suprema OT)	Femoral	Saphenous, muscular, patellar, articular	Sartorius, gracilis, distal ends of vasti, adductor magnus mm., knee joint, skin of the medial-distal portion of thigh, arterial retia on medial and lateral sides of knee

TABLE OF ARTERIES—(Continued)

Name	Origin	Branches	Distribution
Genicular, lateral inferior	Popliteal		Knee joint, deep articular rete
Genicular, lateral superior	Popliteal	Superficial, deep	Vastus lateralis, vastus intermedius mm., knee joint, femur, patella, deep articular rete
Genicular, medial inferior	Popliteal		Popliteus m., proximal end of tibia, knee joint
Genicular, medial superior	Popliteal		Vastus medialis m., femur, patella, knee joint, deep articular rete
Genicular, middle (azygos articular OT)	Popliteal		Knee joint, cruciate ligaments, patellar synovial and alar folds
Genus suprema	See *Genicular, highest*		
Gluteal, inferior (sciatic OT)	Internal iliac, anterior trunk	Inside pelvis, muscular, vesical; outside pelvis, muscular, coccygeal, anastomotic, articular, comitans nervi ischiadici	Gluteus maximus, piriformis, coccygeus, levator ani, upper portion of hamstrings and mm. of buttocks; perirectal fat, fundus of bladder, seminal vesicle, prostate gland, hip joint, sciatic nerve, crucial anastomosis, skin over buttock, thigh, sacrum, and coccyx
Gluteal, superior	Internal iliac, posterior trunk	Muscular, iliac, superficial, deep	Iliacus, piriformis, obturator internus, gluteus medius, gluteus minimus, tensor fasciae latae mm., hip joint, ilium, skin over sacrum
Hallucis, art. dorsalis	See *Metatarsal, first dorsal*		
Hallucis, art. princeps	See *Metatarsal, first plantar*		
Helicine	Name applied by Müller to tortuous blood vessels in cavernous tissue such as corpora cavernosa penis (clitoridis), uterus, etc.		
Hemorrhoidal, inferior	Internal pudendal		Ischiorectal fat, anal canal, levator ani, sphincter ani externus mm., skin around anus and lower region of buttock
Hemorrhoidal, middle	Internal iliac		Rectum, ductus deferens, seminal vesicle, prostate gland
Hemorrhoidal, superior (see Plate 8)	Inferior mesenteric		Muscular and mucous coats of the pelvic colon and proximal portion of the rectum, mucous coat of distal portion of rectum
Hepatic (see Plates 8, 13)	Celiac	Right gastric, gastroduodenal, cystic, right, left	Lesser and greater curvatures of stomach, pylorus, pancreas, great omentum, gallbladder, liver
Hepatic, accessory	Left gastric		Left lobe of liver

TABLE OF ARTERIES—(Continued)

NAME	ORIGIN	BRANCHES	DISTRIBUTION
Hypogastric (see Plates 7, 8)	See *Iliac, internal*		
Ileocolic (see Plate 8)	Superior mesenteric	Ascending, descending, anterior cecal, posterior cecal, appendicular, ileal	Ascending colon, cecum, vermiform process, lower part of ileum
Iliac, common (see Plates 7, 8)	Abdominal aorta	Internal iliac, external iliac (occasionally accessory renal, internal spermatic, middle sacral, lateral sacral, iliolumbar), small twigs to peritoneum, psoas major m., ureter	Psoas major m., peritoneum, fascia, pelvic viscera, external genitalia, gluteal region, lower extremity
Iliac, external (see Plates 7, 8)	Common iliac	Inferior epigastric, deep iliac circumflex, muscular, glandular, continuing as femoral art.	Psoas major, iliacus, sartorius, tensor fasciae latae, cremaster, and mm. of abdominal wall; external iliac lymph nodes, peritoneum, skin of lower abdominal wall, spermatic cord (round ligament of uterus), lower extremity
Iliac, internal (hypogastric OT)	Common iliac	Anterior trunk, superior vesical, middle vesical, middle hemorrhoidal, obturator, internal pudendal, inferior gluteal; uterine and vaginal in female; posterior trunk, iliolumbar, lateral sacral, superior gluteal	Pelvic wall and contents, gluteal region, medial portion of thigh, external genitalia, anal region
Iliolumbar	Internal iliac, posterior trunk	Iliac, lumbar	Psoas major, quadratus lumborum, iliacus mm.; ilium, cauda equina
Infraorbital (see Plate 8)	Internal maxillary	Orbital, middle superior Alveolar, anterior superior Alveolar, terminal	Inferior rectus, inferior oblique of the eye, levator labii superioris, orbicularis oculi mm.; fat of the orbit, lacrimal gland and sac, upper premolar, canine, and incisor teeth, mucosa of maxillary sinus
Innominate (see Plates 5, 7)	Arch of aorta	Thyreoidea ima (occasionally), thymic, or bronchial (occasionally), right subclavian, right common carotid	Right side of neck and head, right shoulder girdle and arm, occasionally thymus gland, bronchus, inferior portion of thyroid gland
Intercostal, aortic	Descending (thoracic) aorta	Anterior, collateral intercostal Muscular, lateral cutaneous, mammary Posterior, muscular, spinal	Intercostal, pectoral, serratus anterior, iliocostalis, longissimus dorsi, multifidus spinae, semispinalis dorsi mm.; abdominal wall, vertebrae, ribs, mammary gland, skin of body wall and back, contents of vertebral canal
Intercostal, highest	Costocervical trunk	Muscular, spinal	Posterior vertebral mm.; contents of first and second intercostal spaces, contents of vertebral canal
Interlobar of kidney	Renal, primary branches	Arciform	
Interlobular of kidney	Arciform	Afferent glomerular (mostly)	Glomeruli of kidney

TABLE OF ARTERIES—(Continued)

Name	Origin	Branches	Distribution
Interosseous, common	Ulnar	Volar interosseous, dorsal interosseous	Deep mm. of forearm, radius, ulna, median nerve, volar carpal and dorsal carpal retia, rete olecrani
Interosseous, dorsal	Common interosseous	Muscular, interosseous recurrent	Mm. and skin on dorsal surface of forearm, dorsal carpal rete, rete olecrani
Interosseous, recurrent	Dorsal interosseous		Supinator, anconeus mm., rete olecrani
Interosseous, volar	Common interosseous	Muscular, nutrient, median, communicating, volar terminal, dorsal terminal	Flexor digitorum profundus, flexor pollicis longus, pronator quadratus mm.; radius, ulna, median nerve, volar carpal and dorsal carpal retia
Intestinal (vasa intestini tenuis OT) (10–16)	Superior mesenteric	Ileal, jejunal	Jejunum, ileum, mesentery, mesenteric lymph nodes
Labial, inferior (see Plate 8)	External maxillary		Mucous membrane, skin, mm. and glands of lower lip
Labial, posterior	Perineal		Labium majus
Labial, superior (see Plate 8)	External maxillary	Septal, alar	Mucous membrane, skin, mm. and glands of upper lip, nasal septum, ala of nose
Lacrimal	Dorsal nasal		Lacrimal sac
Lacrimal	Ophthalmic	Recurrent, muscular, zygomatic, lateral palpebral, anterior ciliary	Lacrimal gland, superior and lateral rectus mm.; eyelids, conjunctiva, region of cheek, dura mater, temporal fossa, sclera, iris, ciliary processes
Laryngeal, inferior	Inferior thyroid		Constrictor pharyngis inferior m. and mucous membrane of lower part of larynx
Laryngeal, superior	Superior thyroid		Muscles, mucous membrane, and glands of larynx
Lienal	See *Splenic*		
Ligamenti teretis uteri (equivalent to external spermatic in male)	Inferior epigastric		Round ligament of the uterus
Lingual (see Plate 8)	External carotid	Hyoid, dorsal lingual, sublingual, profunda linguae	Intrinsic and extrinsic mm. of tongue, mucous membrane of tongue and mouth, gums, sublingual gland, glossopalatine arch, tonsil, soft palate, epiglottis, frenulum linguae
Lumbalis ima (fifth lumbar)	Middle sacral	Dorsal	Iliacus, gluteus maximus mm., vertebral canal
Lumbar (4 pairs)	Abdominal aorta	Vertebral, muscular, dorsal, renal, spinal	Psoas, quadratus lumborum, obliqui abdominis, sacrospinalis mm.; contents of vertebral canal, capsule of kidney, vertebrae, subperitoneal plexus of Turner
Malleolar, anterior lateral	Anterior tibial		Lateral side of ankle

NAME	ORIGIN	BRANCHES	DISTRIBUTION
Malleolar, anterior medial	Anterior tibial		Medial side of ankle
Malleolar, posterior lateral	Peroneal		Lateral aspect of calcaneus, lateral malleolus
Malleolar, posterior medial	Posterior tibial		Medial side of ankle, medial malleolar rete
Mammary, external	See *Thoracic, lateral*		
Mammary, internal	Subclavian	Pericardiacophrenic, anterior mediastinal, thymic, pericardial, sternal, anterior intercostal, perforating, musculophrenic, superior epigastric	Phrenic nerve, pleura, pericardium, diaphragm, connective tissue of mediastinum, lymph nodes in mediastinum, thymus gland, sternum; transversus thoracis, intercostal, pectoral, rectus abdominis, obliqui abdominis mm.; skin over chest and upper abdomen, mammary gland, falciform ligament, subpleural mediastinal plexus
Masseteric	Internal maxillary		Masseter m.
Maxillary	See *Maxillary, internal*		
Maxillary, external (facial OT) (see Plate 8)	External carotid	Ascending palatine, tonsillar, glandular, submental, muscular, inferior labial, superior labial, lateral nasal, angular	Constrictor mm. of pharynx, styloglossus, stylopharyngeus, pterygoid internus, levator veli palatini, stylohyoid, masseter, buccinator, and mm. of facial expression; tonsil, auditory tube, root of tongue, submaxillary gland, lymph nodes of neck and face, skin of face, ala and dorsum of nose, lacrimal sac, nasal septum
Maxillary, internal (maxillary OT)	External carotid	(1) Mandibular portion anterior tympanic deep auricular middle meningeal accessory meningeal inferior alveolar (2) Pterygoid portion deep temporal pterygoid masseteric buccinator (3) Pterygopalatine portion posterior superior alveolar infraorbital descending palatine artery of pterygoid canal pharyngeal sphenopalatine	Tensor tympani, mylohyoid mm., lining of external acoustic meatus, temporomandibular joint, lining of tympanic cavity, dura mater, skull, facial nerve, semilunar ganglion, lower teeth, mandible, mucous membrane of mouth Temporalis, pterygoid internus pterygoid externus, masseter, buccinator mm.; pericranium, mucous membrane of mouth Rectus inferior, obliquus inferior, quadratus labii superioris, caninus mm.; upper teeth, gums, mucous membrane of roof of mouth, soft palate, palatine tonsil, upper part of pharynx, auditory tube, conchae and meati of nose, nasal septum; mucous membrane of frontal, maxillary, sphenoidal, and ethmoidal air sinuses
Median (comes nervi mediani OT)	Volar interosseous		Median nerve
Median, anterior, of spinal cord	Anterior spinal		Pia mater of spinal cord, substance of spinal cord, cauda equina

TABLE OF ARTERIES—(**Continued**)

NAME	ORIGIN	BRANCHES	DISTRIBUTION
Mediastinal, anterior	Internal mammary		Connective tissue, fat, and lymph nodes of mediastinum, thymus gland
Meningeal, accessory	Internal maxillary		Semilunar ganglion, walls of cavernous sinus, dura mater of middle cranial fossa
Meningeal, anterior	(1) Internal carotid (2) Anterior ethmoidal		Dura mater of anterior cranial fossa
Meningeal, middle	Internal maxillary	Ganglionic, superficial petrosal, superior tympanic, perforating temporal, orbital, anterior terminal, posterior terminal, nutrient	Tensor tympani m.; semilunar ganglion, trigeminal nerve, dura mater of anterior and middle cranial fossae, skull, tympanic cavity, orbit, infratemporal fossa
Meningeal, posterior	Ascending pharyngeal		Dura mater of posterior and middle cranial fossae
Mental (see Plate 8)	Inferior alveolar		Lower lip and chin
Mesenteric, inferior (see Plate 8)	Abdominal aorta	Left colic, sigmoid, superior hemorrhoidal (occasionally hepatic, renal, middle colic)	Transverse colon, splenic flexure, descending colon, sigmoid flexure, proximal portion of rectum
Mesenteric, superior (see Plate 8)	Abdominal aorta	Inferior pancreaticoduodenal, intestinal, ileocolic, right colic, middle colic (occasionally hepatic, splenic, pancreatic, gastric, gastroepiploic, or gastroduodenal)	Pancreas, duodenum, jejunum, ileum, mesentery, mesenteric lymph nodes, cecum, vermiform process, ascending colon, hepatic flexure
Metacarpal, first dorsal	Radial		Adjacent sides of thumb and index finger
Metacarpal, second, third, and fourth dorsal	Dorsal radial carpal	Two dorsal digital, perforating	Adjacent sides of fingers
Metacarpal, volar (3)	Deep volar arch	Perforating	Interosseous and second, third, and fourth lumbrical mm.; common digital of superficial volar arch, metacarpal bones
Metatarsal, first dorsal (dorsalis hallucis OT)	Dorsalis pedis	Two dorsal digital	Adjacent sides of first and second toes
Metatarsal, first plantar (princeps hallucis OT)	Union of deep plantar with lateral plantar	Two plantar digital, medial digital to medial side of great toe	Great toe and medial side of second toe
Metatarsal, second, third, and fourth dorsal	Arcuate	Two dorsal digital, perforating	Adjacent sides of second, third, fourth, and fifth toes
Metatarsal, second, third, and fourth plantar	Plantar arch	Two plantar digital, perforating	Adjacent sides of second, third, fourth, and fifth toes
Musculophrenic	Internal mammary	Phrenic, anterior intercostal, muscular	Mm. of abdominal wall, diaphragm, lower six intercostal spaces
Nasal, dorsal	Ophthalmic	Lacrimal	Dorsum of nose, lacrimal sac

TABLE OF ARTERIES—(Continued)

NAME	ORIGIN	BRANCHES	DISTRIBUTION
Nasal, posterior lateral	Sphenopalatine		Nasal conchae and meati, mucosa of frontal, maxillary, sphenoidal, and ethmoidal air sinuses
Nasopalatine	See *Sphenopalatine*		
Neubauer's	See *Thyreoidea ima*		
Nutrient	Brachial		Shaft of humerus
Nutrient	Volar interosseous		Shaft of radius
Nutrient	Volar interosseous		Shaft of ulna
Nutrient	Second perforating art. of profunda femoris		Shaft of femur
Nutrient	Posterior tibial		Shaft of tibia
Nutrient	Peroneal		Shaft of fibula
Nutrient	Transverse scapular		Shaft of clavicle
Nutrient	Transverse scapular		Scapula
Nutrient	A general term used to designate a branch of any artery that supplies the substance of bone. Usage has lifted a certain number of this type of arterial branch to the status of "artery." This should not make us unmindful of the fact that an artery which lies near bone supplies a number of "nutrient" branches to it.		
Obturator	Internal iliac, anterior trunk	Iliac, vesical, pubic, anterior terminal, posterior terminal, muscular, acetabular	Iliacus, iliopsoas, obturator internus, obturator externus, adductors, pectineus, gracilis, semimembranosus, semitendinosus, biceps femoris (long head) mm.; pubis, hip joint, head of femur, bladder, ilium
Occipital (see Plate 8)	External carotid	Muscular, sternocleidomastoid, auricular, meningeal, descending, mastoid, medial terminal, lateral terminal	Digastric, occipitalis, stylohyoid, splenius capitis, longissimus capitis, sternocleidomastoid, trapezius, semispinalis capitis and cervicis mm.; posterior surface of auricle, mastoid cells, pericranium and scalp of posterolateral surface of the head
Ophthalmic	Internal carotid	Orbital: lacrimal, supraorbital, posterior ethmoidal, anterior ethmoidal, medial palpebral, frontal, dorsal nasal; Ocular: central artery of the retina, short posterior ciliary, long posterior ciliary, anterior ciliary, muscular	Contents of orbit, diploë of frontal bone, mucous membrane of frontal sinus and ethmoidal air cells, dura mater of anterior fossa of skull, superior nasal concha and meatus, lacrimal sac, skin of dorsum of nose
Ovarian (homolog of internal spermatic in male) (see Plates 7, 8)	Abdominal aorta	Ureteric, ligamentous, uterine, tubal	Ovary, ureter, suspensory ligament of ovary, broad ligament of uterus, uterine tube, round ligament of uterus, skin of labium majus and groin

TABLE OF ARTERIES—(Continued)

NAME	ORIGIN	BRANCHES	DISTRIBUTION
Palatine, ascending	External maxillary	Palatine, tonsillar	Styloglossus, stylopharyngeus, superior constrictor of pharynx, levator veli palatini mm., auditory tube, lateral wall of upper part of pharynx, soft palate, palatine tonsil
Palatine, descending	Internal maxillary	Greater palatine, lesser palatine	Soft palate, palatine tonsil, mucous membrane of roof of mouth, gums, palatine glands, palatine bone, maxilla
Palatine, greater	Descending maxillary		Mucous membrane of hard palate, gums, palatine glands, palatine bone, maxilla
Palatine, lesser	Descending palatine		Soft palate, palatine tonsil
Palpebral, inferior medial	Ophthalmic		Conjunctiva, lacrimal caruncle, lacrimal sac, lower eyelid
Palpebral, lateral	Lacrimal		Upper and lower eyelids, conjunctiva
Palpebral, superior medial	Ophthalmic		Upper eyelid
Pancreatica magna	Splenic		Posterior surface of pancreas, following course of pancreatic duct
Pancreaticoduodenal, inferior	Superior mesenteric		Head of pancreas, descending and inferior parts of duodenum
Pancreaticoduodenal, superior	Gastroduodenal		Second part of duodenum, common bile duct, pancreas
Penis (clitoris), deep art. of	Internal pudendal		Corpus cavernosum penis (clitoridis)
Penis (clitoris), dorsal art. of	Internal pudendal		Dorsum of penis (clitoris), prepuce, glans, corpus cavernosum and its fibrous sheath
Perforating (3)	Profunda femoris	(1) Muscular	Pectineus, adductor brevis, adductor magnus, biceps femoris, gluteus maximus mm.; crucial anastomosis
		(2) Nutrient, ascending, descending	Posterior femoral mm., shaft of femur
		(3) Muscular, terminal	Adductor magnus m., posterior femoral mm.
Pericardiacophrenic (comes nervi phrenici OT)	Internal mammary		Phrenic nerve, pleura, pericardium, diaphragm
Perineal	Internal pudendal	Posterior scrotal (labial), transverse perineal	Transversus perinei superficialis, bulbocavernosus, ischiocavernosus mm.; posterior portion of scrotum (labium majus), subcutaneous structures in urogenital triangle
Perineal, transverse	Perineal		Transversus perinei superficialis m., structures between the anus and the bulb of the urethra, skin of perineum

TABLE OF ARTERIES—(Continued)

Name	Origin	Branches	Distribution
Peroneal (see Plate 7)	Posterior tibial	Muscular, nutrient to fibula, perforating communicating, lateral calcaneal, lateral posterior malleolar	Soleus, tibialis posterior, flexor hallucis longus, peroneus longus, peroneus brevis, peroneus tertius, extensor digitorum longus mm.; shaft of fibula, tibiofibular syndesmosis, dorsum of foot, ankle joint, lateral malleolar rete, rete calcaneum
Pharyngeal, ascending	External carotid	Pharyngeal, palatine, prevertebral, inferior tympanic, posterior meningeal	Longus colli, longus capitis, rectus capitis anterior, constrictors of pharynx (superior, medial, inferior), stylopharyngeus mm.; mucous membrane of pharynx, soft palate, palatine tonsil, auditory tube, cervical lymph nodes, tympanic cavity, dura mater of middle and posterior cranial fossae
Phrenic, inferior (see Plate 8)	Abdominal aorta	Right medial, lateral, superior suprarenal, caval, hepatic, pericardial Left medial, lateral superior suprarenal, hepatic, pericardial, esophageal, splenic	Inferior surface of diaphragm, suprarenal gland, vena cava inferior, liver, pericardium (from the right artery), esophagus, spleen (from the left)
Phrenic, superior	Descending (thoracic) aorta		Posterior surface of diaphragm
Plantar arch	Lateral plantar	Perforating (3), plantar metatarsals (4)	Interosseous mm., toes
Plantar, deep	Dorsalis pedis	First plantar metatarsal	Plantar surface of first and second toes, unites with lateral plantar to form plantar arch
Plantar, lateral	Posterior tibial	Calcaneal, muscular, cutaneous, plantar metatarsal (4), perforating (3)	Flexor digitorum brevis, quadratus plantae, abductor digiti quinti, adductor hallucis, interossei mm.; toes, heel, skin on lateral side of foot
Plantar, medial	Posterior tibial	Deep, superficial	Abductor hallucis, flexor digitorum brevis mm., skin on medial surface of sole of foot
Pontine	Basilar		Pons
Popliteal (see Plate 7)	Continuation of femoral	Muscular, superior, sural, cutaneous, medial, superior genicular, lateral superior genicular, middle genicular (azygos articular), medial inferior genicular, lateral inferior genicular	Adductor magnus, semimembranosus, semitendinosus, biceps femoris, gastrocnemius, soleus, vastus lateralis, vastus medialis, vastus intermedius, popliteus, plantaris mm.; femur, patella, tibia, knee joint, rete patellae, rete articulare genus
Preventricular	Right coronary		Anterior wall of right ventricle
Princeps cervicis (OT for descending branch)	Occipital	Superficial, deep	Splenius capitis, semispinalis capitis and cervicis, trapezius mm.
Princeps hallucis	See *Metatarsal, first plantar*		

TABLE OF ARTERIES—(Continued)

NAME	ORIGIN	BRANCHES	DISTRIBUTION
Princeps pollicis	Radial	Volar digital (2)	Dorsal interosseus, adductor pollicis obliquus, opponens pollicis, flexor pollicis brevis, lumbrical mm., sides of volar aspect of the thumb
Profunda brachii	Brachial	Deltoid, middle collateral, radial collateral, nutrient	Triceps (lateral and medial heads), brachioradialis, brachialis, deltoid, coracobrachialis, biceps brachii mm.; radial nerve, articular rete of elbow, shaft of humerus
Profunda femoris (deep femoral OT)	Femoral	Medial femoral circumflex, lateral femoral circumflex, perforating (3), muscular	Quadriceps femoris, iliopsoas, obturator externus, pectineus, tensor fasciae latae, quadratus femoris, adductors, semimembranosus, semitendinosus, biceps femoris, gracilis mm.; hip joint, head of femur, shaft of femur, crucial anastomosis
Profunda linguae (ranine OT)	Lingual		Genioglossus m., intrinsic mm. of the tongue, mucous membrane of inferior surface of tongue
Pterygoid canal, art. of (Vidian OT)	Internal maxillary	Pharyngeal, auditory, tympanic, muscular	Upper portion of pharynx; levator and tensor veli palatini mm.; auditory tube, tympanic cavity
Pudendal, deep external	Femoral	Anterior scrotal	Pectineus, adductor longus mm., scrotum (labium majus), skin of perineum
Pudendal, internal	Internal iliac	Muscular, inferior hemorrhoidal, perineal, art. of urethral bulb, urethral, deep art. of penis (clitoris), dorsal art. of penis (clitoris)	Levator ani, coccygeus, sphincter ani externus, bulbocavernosus, ischiocavernosus, transversus perinei superficialis, transversus perinei profundus, obturator externus, obturator internus, gemelli, quadratus femoris, gluteus maximus mm.; skin of anus and perineum, bulb of urethra, bulbourethral (vestibular gland), urethra, corpus cavernosum penis (clitoridis), dorsum of penis (clitoris), posterior surface of scrotum (labium majus)
Pudendal, superficial external	Femoral		Skin of lower part of abdomen, skin of penis (clitoris), scrotum (labium majus)
Pulmonary (see Plates 5, 9)	Right ventricle of heart	Right, left	Lungs
Radial (see Plate 7)	Brachial	(1) In forearm radial recurrent muscular volar radial carpal superficial volar (2) At wrist dorsal radial carpal first dorsal metacarpal (3) In hand princeps pollicis volaris indicis radialis volar metacarpal (3) perforating (3) recurrent	Pronator teres, flexor pollicis longus, pronator quadratus, supinator, brachialis, brachioradialis, extensor carpi radialis longus, extensor carpi radialis brevis, flexor carpi radialis, flexor digitorum sublimis, interossei, lumbricals, and mm. of thenar eminence; metacarpals, elbow, wrist, and carpal joints; flexor tendon sheaths, volar carpal rete, dorsal carpal rete, superficial volar arch, deep volar arch, radius, skin of dorsum of hand and fingers, skin of volar surface of thumb and lateral side of index finger

TABLE OF ARTERIES—(Continued)

NAME	ORIGIN	BRANCHES	DISTRIBUTION
Radial recurrent	Radial		Supinator, brachialis, brachioradialis, extensor carpi radialis longus, extensor carpi radialis brevis mm.; elbow joint, rete of elbow joint
Radialis, volaris indicis	Radial		Lateral volar aspect of index finger
Ranine	See *Profunda linguae*		
Renal (see Plates 7, 14, 45)	Abdominal aorta	Inferior suprarenal, capsular or perirenal, ureteric, terminal	Suprarenal gland, capsule of kidney, perirenal fat, upper end of ureter, aortic lymph nodes, kidney
Renales, arteriae propriae (4 or 5)	Renal		Kidney proper
Sacral, lateral inferior	Internal iliac	Spinal, rectal	Contents of sacral canal, sacral plexus, rectum; skin; piriformis and mm. on dorsal surface of sacrum; filum terminale
Sacral, lateral superior	Internal iliac		Piriformis and mm. on dorsal surface of sacrum, sacral dura mater, arachnoid, filum terminale, skin on dorsal surface of sacrum
Sacral, middle	Abdominal aorta	Lowest lumbar, lateral sacral, rectal	Iliacus, gluteus maximus mm.; contents of sacral canal, rectum, coccygeal body
Saphenous	Femoral or art. genus suprema	Cutaneous, muscular	Gracilis and sartorius mm.; skin on medial side of leg around knee, saphenous nerve, medial genicular rete
Scapular circumflex	See *Circumflex, scapular*		
Scapular, transverse (suprascapular OT)	Thyrocervical trunk	Nutrient, acromial, articular, subscapular, suprasternal, supraspinous, infraspinous	Sternocleidomastoid, subclavius, trapezius, subscapularis, supraspinatus, infraspinatus, omohyoid (inferior belly) mm.; clavicle, scapula, acromioclavicular and shoulder joints, acromial rete, periosteum, skin over upper part of chest and acromial area
Sciatic	See *Gluteal, inferior*		
Scrotal, anterior	Deep external pudendal		Anterior part of scrotum (labium majus), perineum
Scrotal, posterior	Perineal		Posterior part of scrotum (labium majus)
Septal, posterior	Sphenopalatine		Mucous membrane of posterior superior portion of nasal septum
Sigmoid (2 or 3) (see Plate 8)	Inferior mesenteric		Lower part of descending colon, iliac colon, and sigmoid or pelvic colon
Spermatic, external (cremasteric OT)	Inferior epigastric		Spermatic cord, cremaster m. (round ligament of uterus in female)

TABLE OF ARTERIES—(Continued)

Name	Origin	Branches	Distribution
Spermatic, internal (ovarian in female) (see Plates 7, 8)	Abdominal aorta	Ureteric, cremasteric, epididymal, testicular	Ureter, cremaster m., epididymis, body of testis
Sphenopalatine (nasopalatine OT)	Internal maxillary	Posterolateral nasal, posterior septal	Nasal conchae and meati, mucous membrane of frontal, maxillary, sphenoidal, and ethmoidal air sinuses, posterior portion of nasal septum
Spinal, anterior (see Plate 17)	Vertebral		Spinal cord and its coverings
Spinal, posterior (see Plate 17)	Vertebral		Fasciculi cuneatus and gracilis, spinal cord and its coverings
Splenic (lienal OT) (see Plate 8)	Celiac	Pancreatica magna, left gastroepiploic, short gastric, terminal splenic (or trabecular)	Pancreas, pancreatic duct, fundus of stomach, greater curvature of stomach, both surfaces of great omentum, body of spleen
Stapedial	Stylomastoid		Stapedius m. and tendon
Sternocleidomastoid	Occipital		Sternocleidomastoid m.
Stylomastoid	Posterior auricular	Mastoid, stapedial, posterior tympanic	Mastoid cells, stapes, stapedius m. and tendon, posterior portion of tympanic membrane
Subclavian (see Plates 5, 7, 8)	Right innominate, left arch of aorta	Vertebral, thyrocervical trunk, internal mammary, costocervical trunk	Mm. of neck and upper extremity, cervical vertebrae and canal, skull, brain and meninges, pericardium, pleura, mediastinum, bronchi, sternum, skin over shoulder and anterior body wall, mammary gland, peritoneum
Subcostal (twelfth thoracic OT)	Thoracic aorta	Posterior	Quadratus lumborum, transversus abdominis, obliquus abdominis internus mm.; lumbar vertebrae and contents of canal, skin of back
Sublingual	Lingual	Art. of the frenulum linguae	Mylohyoid, geniohyoid, genioglossus mm.; sublingual gland, frenulum linguae
Submental (see Plate 8)	External maxillary	Superficial, deep	Mylohyoid, digastric (anterior belly), platysma, triangularis, quadratus labii inferioris mm.; submaxillary and sublingual glands, skin over these parts
Subscapular	Axillary	Scapular circumflex, thoracodorsal	Subscapularis, teres minor, teres major, infraspinatus, triceps brachii (long head), latissimus dorsi, serratus anterior, deltoid mm.; scapula, shoulder joint, axillary lymph nodes
Supraduodenal art. of Wilkie	Gastroduodenal	Anterior, posterior	Anterior and posterior surfaces of first part of the duodenum
Supraorbital (see Plate 8)	Ophthalmic	Periosteal, muscular, diploic, trochlear, palpebral	Rectus superior, levator palpebrae superioris mm.; periosteum of roof of orbit, diploë of frontal bone, mucous membrane of frontal sinus, trochlea of obliquus superior m., upper eyelid

TABLE OF ARTERIES—(Continued)

Name	Origin	Branches	Distribution
Suprarenal, inferior	Renal		Suprarenal gland
Suprarenal, middle	Abdominal aorta		Suprarenal gland
Suprarenal, superior	Inferior phrenic		Suprarenal gland
Suprascapular	See *Scapular, transverse*		
Sural (2)	Popliteal		Gastrocnemius, soleus, plantaris mm., skin and fascia of calf of leg
Tarsal, lateral	Dorsalis pedis		Extensor digitorum brevis m., navicular and cuboid bones and joint between them
Tarsal, medial	Dorsalis pedis		Skin of medial surface of foot, tarsal joints
Temporal, deep (see Plate 8) Anterior Posterior	Internal maxillary		Temporal m., orbit, pericranium, skull
Temporal, middle	Superficial temporal		Temporal m., temporal fascia
Temporal, superficial (see Plates 7, 8)	External carotid	Parotid, transverse facial, anterior auricular, middle temporal, zygomatico-orbital, frontal, parietal, articular	Temporal, masseter, frontalis, orbicularis oculi mm.; parotid gland and duct, skin of face, external ear, external acoustic meatus, scalp
Testicular	Internal spermatic		Body of testis
Thalamic, middle	Posterior communicating		Thalamus
Thoracic, highest	Axillary		Pectoralis major, pectoralis minor, intercostal, serratus anterior mm., wall of thorax
Thoracic, lateral (external mammary OT)	Axillary	External mammary	Pectoralis major, pectoralis minor, serratus anterior, subscapularis mm.; axillary lymph nodes, mammary gland
Thoracic, twelfth	See *Subcostal*		
Thoracoacromial (acromiothoracic OT)	Axillary	Pectoral, acromial, clavicular, deltoid	Pectoralis major, pectoralis minor, deltoid, subclavius mm.; mammary gland, sternoclavicular joint, acromial rete
Thoracodorsal	Subscapular		Latissimus dorsi, teres major, serratus anterior mm.
Thymic	Internal mammary		Thymus gland
Thyreoidea ima (Neubauer's art. OT)	Innominate, arch of aorta, right common carotid, right subclavian, or internal mammary		Lower part of thyroid gland
Thyrocervical trunk	Subclavian	Inferior thyroid, transverse scapular (suprascapular), transverse cervical	Mm. of neck, scapular region and upper back; cervical spinal cord, cervical vertebrae, larynx and trachea, esophagus, thyroid gland, pharynx

TABLE OF ARTERIES—(**Continued**)

Name	Origin	Branches	Distribution
Thyroid, inferior (see Plate 8)	Thyrocervical trunk	Muscular, inferior laryngeal, tracheal, esophageal, pharyngeal, ascending cervical, terminal, glandular	Scalenus anterior, longus colli, sternohyoid, sternothyroid, omohyoid, inferior constrictor of pharynx, longus capitis mm.; esophagus, pharynx, larynx, trachea, posterior surface of thyroid gland, vertebrae, contents of vertebral canal
Thyroid, superior (see Plate 8)	External carotid	Hyoid, sternocleidomastoid, superior laryngeal, cricothyroid, muscular, glandular	Thyrohyoid, sternocleidomastoid, sternohyoid, cricothyroid, omohyoid, platysma, inferior constrictor of pharynx, and intrinsic mm. of larynx, mucous membrane of larynx, esophagus, thyroid gland
Tibial, anterior (see Plate 7)	Popliteal	Anterior tibial recurrent, fibular, posterior tibial recurrent, muscular, anterior lateral malleolar, anterior medial malleolar	Popliteus, tibialis anterior, extensor digitorum longus, peroneus tertius, soleus, peroneus longus, extensor hallucis longus mm.; knee joint, proximal tibiofibular joint, ankle joint, medial malleolar rete, lateral malleolar rete, fascia and skin over course of vessel on front of leg
Tibial, anterior recurrent	Anterior tibial		Tibialis anterior, extensor digitorum longus mm.; knee joint, overlying fascia and skin, rete patellae
Tibial, posterior (see Plate 7)	Popliteal	Peroneal, nutrient to tibia, muscular, posterior medial malleolar, communicating, medial calcaneal, medial plantar, lateral plantar	Soleus, tibialis posterior, flexor hallucis longus, flexor digitorum longus, peroneus longus, peroneus brevis mm.; ankle joint, skin of medial and posterior part of leg and tarsus, lateral and medial malleolar retia, rete calcaneum, sole of foot, shaft of tibia, shaft of fibula
Tibial, posterior recurrent	Anterior tibial		Popliteus m., proximal tibiofibular joint
Trabecular	Splenic	Lobular	Substance of spleen
Transverse facial	See *Facial, transverse*		
Transverse perineal	See *Perineal, transverse*		
Tympanic	Art. of pterygoid canal (Vidian OT)		Lining of wall of tympanic cavity
Tympanic, anterior	Internal maxillary		Mucous membrane of tympanic cavity
Tympanic, inferior	Ascending pharyngeal		Lining of medial wall of tympanic cavity
Tympanic, posterior	Stylomastoid		Tympanic membrane
Tympanic, superior	Middle meningeal		Tensor tympani m., lining of wall of tympanic cavity

TABLE OF ARTERIES—(Continued)

Name	Origin	Branches	Distribution
Ulnar (see Plate 7)	Brachial	(1) In forearm anterior ulnar recurrent posterior ulnar recurrent common interosseous muscular (2) At wrist dorsal carpal volar carpal (3) In hand deep volar superficial volar arch	Flexor digitorum sublimis, flexor digitorum profundus, flexor carpi radialis, flexor carpi ulnaris, pronator teres, flexor pollicis longus, brachialis, pronator quadratus, anconeus, supinator, abductor pollicis longus, and superficial and deep extensor mm. of forearm; shafts of radius and ulna, median nerve, ulnar half of hand, dorsal carpal rete, volar carpal rete, carpal joints, skin over course of vessels
Ulnar, recurrent, anterior	Ulnar		Brachialis, pronator teres mm., skin over medial cubital region
Ulnar, recurrent, posterior	Ulnar		Flexor digitorum profundus, flexor digitorum sublimis, flexor carpi ulnaris mm.; cubital rete, elbow joint, ulnar nerve
Uterine (homolog of deferential art. in male)	Internal iliac, anterior trunk	Cervical, tubal, ovarian, vaginal, ligamentous	Uterus, broad ligament of uterus, round ligament of uterus, uterine tube, portion of vagina
Vaginal (corresponds to inferior vesical art. in male)	Internal iliac, anterior trunk	Rectal, vesical, vestibular	Vagina, fundus of bladder, rectum, vestibular bulb
Vasa brevia	See *Gastric, short*		
Vertebral (see Plates 7, 8, 17, 18)	Subclavian	(1) Cervical spinal muscular (2) Cranial meningeal posterior spinal anterior spinal medullary posterior inferior cerebellar	Semispinalis capitis, rectus capitis posterior major and minor, obliquus capitis superior, obliquus capitis inferior mm.; cervical vertebrae, cervical spinal cord and its membranes, intervertebral disks, bone and dura mater of posterior fossa of skull, falx cerebelli, cerebellum, medulla oblongata
Vesical, inferior (corresponds to vaginal art. in female)	Internal iliac	Vesical, prostatic, ureteric, deferential	Fundus of bladder, prostate gland, ductus deferens, seminal vesicle, lower part of ureter
Vesical, middle	Internal iliac, or superior vesical		Fundus of bladder, seminal vesicle
Vesical, superior	Internal iliac	Urachal, ureteric, vesical, deferential	Medial umbilical ligament (vestige of urachus), lower part of ureter, upper part of bladder, ductus deferens
Vidian	See *Pterygoid canal, art. of*		
Volar arch, deep	Radial and deep volar branch of ulnar	Volar metacarpal (3), recurrent, perforating	Interossei and second, third, and fourth lumbrical mm.; metacarpals, joints of fingers
Volar arch, superficial	Ulnar and superficial volar branch of radial	Common volar digital (3)	Flexor tendons and tendon sheaths, joints of fingers, bones of fingers, skin of palm and fingers
Volaris indicis radialis	Radial	Dorsal, communicating	First lumbrical, first dorsal interosseous, adductor pollicis mm., radial side of index finger
Zygomatico-orbital	Superficial temporal or middle temporal	Orbital	Orbicularis oculi m., fat between the two layers of temporal fascia, lateral portion of orbit

TABLE OF BONES

(See Plate 1)

Name	Principal Features	Bones with Which Articulation Occurs and Type of Joint
Anvil	See *Incus*	
Astragalus [OT]	See *Talus*	
Atlas	First cervical vertebra; ringlike; lateral masses; anterior and posterior arches and tubercles; vertebral foramen; articular surfaces; transverse foramens; ossifies in cartilage	Occipital bone, *bilateral gliding* Epistropheus, 3 joints, *bilateral gliding* and *pivot* with dens
Axis [OT; BR]	See *Epistropheus*	
Calcaneus (calcaneum BR) (os calcis OT)	Heel bone; largest tarsal bone, irregularly cuboid; medial process (sustentaculum tali,) lateral process (trochlear process), medial, lateral and anterior tubercles on inferior surface; articular surfaces; ossifies in cartilage	Talus (3 facets), Cuboid, } *gliding*
Calvaria or **calvarium**	Skull cap or upper part of skull	
Capitate (os magnum OT)	Usually largest carpal bone; in distal row of carpal bones; occupies center of wrist; head, neck, body; ossifies in cartilage	Navicular, Lunate, Lesser multangular, Hamate, Second, Third, Fourth } metacarpal, } *gliding*
Carpus (wrist) (see Plate 1)	Consists of 8 short bones: navicular, lunate, triquetrum, pisiform, greater multangular, lesser multangular, capitate, and hamate. See individual bones	
Clavicle	Collarbone; resembles the italic "*f*"; body, medial and lateral extremities; conoid tubercle, trapezoid ridge, coracoid tuberosity, costal tuberosity, subclavian groove; ossifies partly in cartilage and partly in membrane	Sternum, Scapula, Cartilage of first rib, } *gliding*
Coccyx	Last bone of vertebral column; usually composed of 4 small incomplete vertebrae fused together; base, apex, cornua, transverse processes; ossifies in cartilage	Sacrum, *amphiarthrosis*
Concha, inferior nasal (inferior turbinate OT)	Irregular scroll-shaped bone situated on lateral wall of nasal cavity; lacrimal, ethmoidal, and maxillary processes; ossifies in cartilage	Ethmoid, Maxilla, Lacrimal, Palatine, } *synarthroses*
Costae	See *Ribs*	
Coxae (innominate OT)	Hipbone; large broad bone consisting of 3 parts; with its fellow, sacrum, and coccyx forms the bony pelvis or pelvic girdle; acetabulum; obturator foramen; pubic arch; greater and lesser sciatic notches; ossifies in cartilage *Ilium*—broad, expanded upper portion; crest, spines, gluteal lines, fossa, iliopectineal eminence, tuberosity, auricular surface; ⅖ (about) of acetabulum	With its fellow of opposite side (symphysis pubis), *amphiarthrosis* Sacrum, *gliding* (very little movement) Femur, *ball-and-socket*

TABLE OF BONES—(Continued)

Name	Principal Features	Bones with Which Articulation Occurs and Type of Joint
Coxae—(*Continued*)	*Ischium*—heavy, posterior lower portion; body, tuberosity, ramus, spine, notches, lower boundary of obturator foramen; 2/5 (about) of acetabulum *Pubis*—anterior lower portion, body, superior and inferior rami, tubercle, crest, pectineal line, upper boundary of obturator foramen; 1/5 (about) of acetabulum	
Cranium	Brain case; composed of occipital, parietal (2), frontal, temporal (2), sphenoid, and ethmoid. See individual bones Sometimes cranium is used to designate entire skull without mandible	
Cuboid	Roughly cubical bone in lateral part of tarsus; tuberosity; ossifies in cartilage	Calcaneus, Third cuneiform, Fourth and fifth metatarsals, Navicular, } *gliding*
Cuneiform of carpus [OT]	See *Triquetrum*	
Cuneiform, first (inner cuneiform OT) (medial cuneiform BR)	Irregularly wedge-shaped; largest of the three; ossifies in cartilage	Navicular (of foot), Second cuneiform, First and second metatarsals, } *gliding*
Cuneiform, second (middle cuneiform OT) (intermediate cuneiform BR)	Wedge-shaped; smallest of the three; ossifies in cartilage	Navicular (of foot), First cuneiform, Third cuneiform, Second metatarsal, } *gliding*
Cuneiform, third (outer cuneiform OT) (lateral cuneiform BR)	Wedge-shaped; ossifies in cartilage	Navicular (of foot), Second cuneiform, Cuboid, Second, Third, Fourth } metatarsal, } *gliding*
Epistropheus (axis OT; BR)	Second cervical vertebra; body, dens, thick spine, laminas, pedicles, transverse processes, articular surfaces, transverse foramens; vertebral foramen; ossifies in cartilage	Atlas, 3 joints, *bilateral gliding* and *pivot* with dens Third cervical vertebra, *amphiarthrosis*
Ethmoid (see Plate 1)	Irregular shape; situated in anterior part of base of skull and forming medial wall of each orbit and a portion of roof and lateral walls of nasal cavities; horizontal or cribriform plates, nasal slit; perpendicular plate, crista galli, alar processes; labyrinth with air cells; superior and middle nasal conchae; ossifies in cartilage	Sphenoid, Frontal, Nasal (2), Maxilla (2), Lacrimal (2), Palatine (2), Inferior nasal concha (2), Vomer, } *synarthroses*
Face	Consists of nose and jaws; formed by maxilla, zygoma, nasal, lacrimal, palatine, inferior nasal concha, vomer, mandible, and parts of ethmoid and sphenoid	
Femur	Thigh bone; largest, longest, and heaviest bone in the body; shaft, head, neck, greater and lesser trochanters, quadrate tubercle, medial and lateral condyles, linea aspera, epicondylic lines, adductor tubercle; ossifies in cartilage	Coxae, *ball-and-socket* Patella, *gliding* Tibia, combined *hinge* and *gliding*

TABLE OF BONES—(Continued)

Name	Principal Features	Bones with Which Articulation Occurs and Type of Joint
Fibula	Splint bone; lateral bone of leg; head, body, interosseous crest, lateral malleolus; ossifies in cartilage	Tibia, *gliding* Talus with tibia and fibula, *hinge*
Foot	Composed of tarsus, metatarsus, and phalanges	
Frontal (see Plate 1)	Forehead bone; flat bone; frontal part with tuberosities, zygomatic processes, temporal line, sagittal sulcus; orbital part forming upper portion of each orbit, anterior and posterior ethmoidal canals; nasal part, frontal spine; ossifies in membrane	Parietal (2), Sphenoid, Ethmoid, Nasal (2), Maxilla (2), Lacrimal (2), Zygoma (2), } *synarthroses*
Greater multangular or **multangulum majus** (trapezium OT; BR)	In distal row of carpal bones; irregular bone with 6 surfaces, ridge; distal articular facet is saddle-shaped; ossifies in cartilage	Navicular, Lesser multangular, Second metacarpal, } *gliding* First metacarpal, *saddle*
Hamate (unciform OT)	Wedge-shaped; in distal row of carpal bones; hooklike process (hamulus); ossifies in cartilage	Lunate, Fourth and fifth metacarpals, Triquetrum, Capitate, } *gliding*
Hammer	See *Malleus*	
Hand	Composed of carpus, metacarpus, and phalanges	
Humerus	Largest bone of the arm; head, greater and lesser tubercles, intertubercular sulcus, surgical neck, deltoid tuberosity, capitulum, trochlea, coronoid and olecranon fossae; medial and lateral lines, condyles and epicondyles; ossifies in cartilage	Scapula (glenoid cavity), *ball-and-socket* Ulna, *hinge* Radius, *gliding*
Hyoid (see Plate 45)	U-shaped bone in front of neck; body, greater and lesser cornua; ossifies in cartilage	None
Ilium	See *Coxae*	
Incus (anvil)	Resembles a premolar tooth with two roots, body, long and short processes or crura, lenticular process; middle bone of chain of auditory ossicles; ossifies in cartilage	Malleus, *gliding* Stapes, *gliding*
Inferior maxilla [OT]	See *Mandible*	
Inferior turbinate [OT]	See *Concha, inferior nasal*	
Innominate [OT]	See *Coxae*	
Ischium	See *Coxae*	
Lacrimal (see Plate 1)	Small scale of bone resembling a finger nail; situated in anterior medial wall of orbit; crest, descending process, hamulus, groove; ossifies in membrane	Frontal, Ethmoid, Maxilla, Inferior nasal concha, } *synarthroses*
Lesser multangular or **multangulum minus** (trapezoid OT; BR)	Smallest bone of distal row of carpal bones; irregular bone with 6 surfaces; ossifies in cartilage	Navicular, Second metacarpal, Greater multangular, Capitate, } *gliding*

TABLE OF BONES—(Continued)

Name	Principal Features	Bones with Which Articulation Occurs and Type of Joint
Lunate (semilunar OT)	One of proximal row of carpal bones; named from lateral crescent-shaped articular facet; ossifies in cartilage	Radius, *biaxial* Capitate, Hamate, Triquetrum, Navicular, } *gliding*
Magnum [OT]	See *Capitate*	
Malar [OT]	See *Zygoma*	
Malleus (hammer)	Resembles a hammer; head, neck, spur, crista, handle, anterior and lateral processes; ossifies in cartilage	Incus, *gliding*
Mandible (inferior maxilla OT)	Lower jaw; body, 2 rami, coronoid and condyloid processes, symphysis, alveolus, mental protuberance and spine, mylohyoid line and groove, mandibular and mental foramens, notch; ossifies partly in membrane and partly in cartilage	Two temporal bones, combined *gliding* and *hinge*
Maxilla (superior maxilla OT)	Upper jaw; body with infraorbital foramen and canal, maxillary sinus, lacrimal groove, greater palatine foramen and canal; zygomatic process; frontal process, ethmoidal crest; alveolar process, maxillary tuberosity; palatine process, incisive crest, spine and canal, nasal crest; ossifies in membrane	Frontal, Ethmoid, Nasal, Zygoma, Lacrimal, Inferior nasal concha, Palatine, Vomer, Fellow of opposite side, } *synarthroses*
Metacarpus (see Plate 1)	Five bones of hand proper; each with head, shaft, and base; numbered from 1 to 5 beginning on thumb side; styloid process on base of third; each ossifies in cartilage	First metacarpal with greater multangular, *saddle* Four medial metacarpal bases with each other and with distal row of carpal bones, *gliding* Metacarpal heads with corresponding phalanges, *ball-and-socket*
Metatarsus (see Plate 1)	Five bones of foot proper; each with head, shaft, and base; numbered from 1 to 5 beginning on great toe side; tuberosity on lateral side of base of fifth; each ossifies in cartilage	Distal tarsal bones, Metatarsal bases with each other, } *gliding* Metatarsal heads with corresponding phalanges, *ball-and-socket*
Nasal (see Plates 1, 12)	Rectangular plate; two form bridge of nose; ethmoidal sulcus, crest; ossifies in membrane	Frontal, Ethmoid, Maxilla, Nasal (opposite), } *synarthroses*
Navicular (of foot) (scaphoid of foot OT)	Boat-shaped; proximal articular surface markedly concave; plantar process, tuberosity; ossifies in cartilage	Talus, Three cuneiforms, Cuboid, } *gliding*
Navicular (of hand) (scaphoid of hand OT; BR)	Largest bone of proximal row of carpal bones; comma-shaped; tubercle; ossifies in cartilage	Greater multangular, Lesser multangular, Capitate, Lunate, } *gliding* Radius, *biaxial*

TABLE OF BONES—(Continued)

Name	Principal Features	Bones with Which Articulation Occurs and Type of Joint
Occipital (see Plate 1)	Posterior part and base of cranium; saucer-shaped; squamous part with internal and external protuberances, highest, superior and inferior nuchal lines, sagittal and transverse sulci; lateral part with condyles, canal for hypoglossal nerve, condyloid canal, jugular notch, process and tubercle; basal part with pharyngeal tubercle and foramen magnum; squamous part ossifies in membrane, the rest in cartilage	Parietal (2), Temporal (2), Sphenoid, } *synarthroses* Atlas, *bilateral gliding*
Palatine	Forms portions of hard palate, orbits and nasal cavities; irregularly L-shaped; horizontal part, posterior nasal spine, greater palatine foramen, palatine crest, nasal crest; perpendicular part, conchal crest, ethmoidal crest, greater palatine canal, maxillary, pyramidal, orbital and sphenoidal processes, sphenopalatine foramen, lesser palatine canals and foramens; ossifies in membrane	Sphenoid, Ethmoid, Maxilla, Inferior nasal concha, Vomer, Palatine (opposite). } *synarthroses*
Parietal (see Plate 1)	Forms side and roof of cranium; quadrilateral plate of bone; eminence, superior and inferior temporal lines, parietal foramen; sagittal and transverse sulci; ossifies in membrane	Parietal (opposite), Occipital, Frontal, Temporal, Sphenoid, } *synarthroses*
Patella	Knee cap; triangular; largest sesamoid; ossifies in cartilage	Condyles of femur, *gliding*
Pelvis	Pelvic girdle composed of 2 coxae, sacrum, and coccyx	
Phalanges (of foot)	Two of great toe, three of each of others, 14 in all; usually fifth toe has only two; each phalanx is a miniature long bone with head, shaft, and base; each ossifies in cartilage	Proximal row with corresponding metatarsal bones, *ball-and-socket* Interphalangeal joints, *hinge*
Phalanges (of hand)	Two of great toe, three of each of fingers, 14 in all; each phalanx is a miniature long bone with head, shaft, and base; each ossifies in cartilage	Proximal row with corresponding metacarpal bones, *ball-and-socket* Interphalangeal joints, *hinge*
Pisiform	Most medial of proximal row of carpus; smallest carpal; resembles half a pea; ossifies in cartilage	Triquetrum, *gliding*
Pubis	See *Coxae*	
Pyramidal [OT]	See *Triquetrum*	
Radius	Lateral bone of forearm; head, shaft, tuberosity, styloid process, interosseous crest, ulnar notch; ossifies in cartilage	Humerus, *gliding* Ulna, proximal, *pivot* Ulna, distal, *gliding* Lunate, Navicular, Triquetrum, } *biaxial*
Ribs	Twelve on each side; head, neck, body, tubercle, angle, costal groove; first is relatively broad and flattened; second, tubercle; 11 and 12 floating; each ossifies in cartilage	Head with vertebral bodies, Tubercle with transverse process, } *gliding* Sternum with first ribs, *synchondroses* Sternum with others, *amphiarthroses*

Name	Principal Features	Bones with Which Articulation Occurs and Type of Joint
Sacrum	Large triangular bone composed of 5 fused vertebrae; base, apex, foramens, superior articular processes, promontory, auricular surface, sacral canal; ossifies in cartilage	Last lumbar vertebra, Coccyx, *amphiarthroses* Coxae (2), *gliding* (very little movement)
Scaphoid of foot [OT]	See *Navicular* (*of foot*)	
Scaphoid of hand [OT; BR]	See *Navicular* (*of hand*)	
Scapula	Shoulder blade; flat, triangular bone of posterior portion of shoulder; head, neck, body, spine, acromion, coracoid, glenoid cavity, subscapular fossa, supraspinous fossa, infraspinous fossa, crest, greater and lesser scapular notches; ossifies in cartilage	Humerus, *ball-and-socket* Clavicle, *gliding*
Semilunar [OT]	See *Lunate*	
Sesamoid	Small seedlike nodules of bone which develop in muscular tendons where they play against a bone; patella one in each tendon of insertion of flexor hallucis brevis muscle and one in tendon of insertion of flexor pollicis brevis and of adductor pollicis are constant, others are variable; each develops in cartilage	
Skull	See *Cranium*. Sometimes used to include mandible as well	
Sphenoid (see Plate 1)	Forms anterior part of base of skull and portions of cranial, orbital, and nasal cavities; in shape resembles a butterfly with extended wings; body, air sinuses, sella turcica, hypophyseal fossa, dorsum sellae, posterior clinoid processes, optic groove, spine, carotid groove, crest, petrosal process, rostrum; small wings, optic foramen, anterior clinoid processes, superior orbital fissure; great wings, foramen rotundum, foramen ovale, foramen spinosum, pterygoid processes, medial and lateral pterygoid plates, hamulus, scaphoid fossa, pterygoid canal; ossifies partly in cartilage and partly in membrane	Frontal, Parietal (2), Occipital, Temporal (2), Ethmoid, Palatine (2), Zygoma (2), Vomer, *synarthroses*
Stapes (stirrup OT)	Resembles a stirrup; head, neck, base, anterior and posterior crura; smallest of auditory ossicles; ossifies in cartilage	Incus, *gliding* Fenestra ovalis, *gliding*
Sternum	Breastbone; dagger-shaped, manubrium, body, xiphoid process; ossifies in cartilage	Clavicle (2), *gliding* First rib (2), *synchondrosis* Costal cartilages of ribs 2 to 7, *amphiarthroses*
Stirrup [OT]	See *Stapes*	
Superior maxilla [OT]	See *Maxilla*	

TABLE OF BONES—(Continued)

NAME	PRINCIPAL FEATURES	BONES WITH WHICH ARTICULATION OCCURS AND TYPE OF JOINT
Sutural (Wormian OT)	Irregular variable bones occasionally found along cranial sutures; most frequent in lambdoid suture	
Talus (astragalus OT)	Second largest bone of tarsus; head, body, medial and posterior tubercles; ossifies in cartilage	Tibia, Fibula, } *hinge* Calcaneus (3 facets), Navicular (of foot), } *gliding*
Tarsus (see Plate 1)	Posterior portion of foot; consists of 7 bones: calcaneus, talus, cuboid, navicular, and 3 cuneiforms	
Temporal (see Plate 1)	Forms a portion of lateral aspect of skull and part of base of cranium; squamous part, zygomatic process, mandibular fossa, petrotympanic fissure; tympanic part, auditory process, external acoustic meatus, styloid process and sheath, stylomastoid foramen; mastoid part, air cells, notch, foramen, sigmoid sulcus; petrous part, auditory tube, jugular fossa, carotid canal, internal acoustic meatus; ossifies partly in cartilage and partly in membrane	Occipital, Parietal, Sphenoid, Zygoma, } *synarthroses* Mandible, combined *gliding* and *hinge*
Tibia	Shinbone; large medial bone of leg; medial and lateral condyles, tuberosity, popliteal notch, intercondylar eminence, popliteal line, medial malleolus; ossifies in cartilage	Femur, combined *hinge* and *gliding* Fibula, superior, Fibula, inferior, } *gliding* Talus with fibula, *hinge*
Trapezium [OT; BR]	See *Greater multangular*	
Trapezoid [OT; BR]	See *Lesser multangular*	
Triquetrum (cuneiform of carpus OT) (pyramidal OT)	One of proximal row of carpal bones; wedge-shaped; ossifies in cartilage	Lunate, Pisiform, Hamate, } *gliding* Radius, *biaxial*
Turbinate, inferior [OT]	See *Concha, inferior nasal*	
Turbinate, middle [OT]	See *Ethmoid, middle nasal concha.* (Not a separate bone)	
Turbinate, superior [OT]	See *Ethmoid, superior nasal concha.* (Not a separate bone)	
Tympanic	Includes 3 auditory ossicles: incus, malleus, and stapes	
Ulna	Medial bone of forearm; olecranon, coronoid process, radial notch, semilunar notch, tuberosity, shaft, head, styloid process, interosseous crest; ossifies in cartilage	Humerus, *hinge* Radius, proximal, *pivot* Radius, distal, *gliding*
Unciform [OT]	See *Hamate*	
Vertebra	Backbone; composed of 33 in all, cervical 7, thoracic 12, lumbar 5, sacrum 5 (fused), coccyx 4 (fused); each has a body, arch, articular processes, transverse processes, spinous process, foramen; see *Atlas, Epistropheus, Coccyx, Sacrum;* each vertebra ossifies in cartilage	Between vertebral bodies, *amphiarthroses* Between articular processes, *gliding*

TABLE OF BONES—(Continued)

Name	Principal Features	Bones with Which Articulation Occurs and Type of Joint
Vomer	Forms posterior part of nasal septum; alae; ossifies in membrane	Sphenoid, Ethmoid, Maxilla (2), Palatine (2), } *synarthroses*
Wormian [OT]	See *Sutural*	
Wrist	See *Carpus*	
Zygoma (malar OT) (see Plate 1)	Cheekbone; forms cheek and lateral aspect of orbit; tuberosity, zygomatico-facial foramen temporal process, fronto-sphenoidal process, marginal process, orbital process, zygomatic foramen, zygomaticotemporal foramen; ossifies in membrane	Frontal, Sphenoid, Temporal, Maxilla, } *synarthroses*

TABLE OF JOINTS[1] AND LIGAMENTS

(See Plate 2)

Name	Type	Named[2] Ligaments
Acromioclavicular	Gliding	Articular disk (intraarticular fibrocartilage OT) Coracoclavicular (1) Conoid (2) Trapezoid Inferior acromioclavicular Superior acromioclavicular
Ankle	Hinge	Anterior Deltoid (internal lateral OT; medial BR) (1) Anterior talotibial (2) Calcaneotibial (3) Deep talotibial (4) Posterior talotibial (5) Tibionavicular Interosseous membrane of leg Lateral (external lateral OT) (1) Anterior talofibular (2) Calcaneofibular (3) Posterior talofibular Posterior
Atlantoepistrophic	See *Central* and *Lateral atlantoepistrophic*	
Atlanto-occipital	Gliding	Anterior atlanto-occipital membrane (anterior occipitoatlantal ligament OT) Membrana tectoria (occipitoaxial ligament OT) Posterior atlanto-occipital membrane (posterior occipitoatlantal ligament OT)
Calcaneocuboid	Gliding	Dorsal calcaneocuboid Inferior calcaneocuboid (1) Long plantar (2) Plantar calcaneocuboid (short plantar OT; BR) Lateral calcaneocuboid Calcaneocuboid part of bifurcate (internal calcaneocuboid OT; medial calcaneocuboid BR)
Carpal	See *Intercarpal* and *Pisotriquetral*	
Carpometacarpal articulation of the thumb	Saddle	
Carpometacarpal articulations of fingers	Gliding	Dorsal carpometacarpal Interosseous carpometacarpal Volar carpometacarpal (palmar carpometacarpal BR)
Central atlantoepistrophic	Pivot	Alar (check or lateral odontoid OT; alar of odontoid process BR) Apical of dens (middle odontoid OT; apical of odontoid process BR) Cruciate atlantis (cruciform OT) (1) Inferior crus (2) Superior crus (3) Transverse crus (transverse of atlas BR)

[1] This table does not include sutures, synostoses, syndesmoses, synchondroses.
[2] It is understood that every diarthrodial joint has a capsular ligament composed of two layers.

TABLE OF JOINTS[1] AND LIGAMENTS—(Continued)

Name	Type	Named[2] Ligaments
Costotransverse (upper 10 ribs only)	Gliding	Anterior costotransverse (superior costotransverse OT; BR) Ligament of neck of rib (middle costotransverse OT; inferior costotransverse BR) Ligament of tubercle of rib (lateral costotransverse BR) Posterior costotransverse
Cuboideonavicular (cuboideoscaphoid OT) (inconstant)	Gliding	Dorsal cuboideonavicular (dorsal cuboideoscaphoid OT) Interosseous cuboideonavicular (interosseous cuboideoscaphoid OT) Plantar cuboideonavicular (plantar cuboideoscaphoid OT)
Cuneocuboid	Gliding	Dorsal cuneocuboid Interosseous cuneocuboid Plantar cuneocuboid
Cuneometatarsal	See *Intermediate* and *Medial tarsometatarsal*	
Cuneonavicular (cuneoscaphoid OT)	Gliding	Dorsal cuneonavicular (dorsal cuneoscaphoid OT) Plantar cuneonavicular (plantar cuneoscaphoid OT)
Distal radioulnar	Gliding	Anterior radioulnar Interosseous membrane of forearm Posterior radioulnar Triangular articular disk (triangular fibrocartilage OT)
Distal tibiofibular (variable)	When present, is an extension of ankle joint	
Elbow (1) Humeroradial (2) Humeroulnar (3) Proximal radioulnar (sometimes described as a separate joint)	 Gliding Hinge Pivot	Annular (orbicular OT) Anterior Interosseous membrane of forearm Posterior Quadrate [BR] Radial collateral (external lateral OT; lateral BR) Ulnar collateral (internal lateral OT; medial BR)
Heads of ribs	Combined hinge and gliding	Interarticular of head of rib (intervertebral OT; intraarticular BR) Radiate of head of rib (anterior costovertebral or stellate OT)
Hip (see Plate 2)	Ball-and-socket	Iliofemoral (Y-ligament of Bigelow OT) Ischiocapsular (ischiofemoral OT; BR) Labrum glenoidale (cotyloid OT; labrum acetabulare BR) Pubocapsular (pubofemoral OT; BR) Teres (round OT; ligament of head of femur BR) Transverse

[1] This table does not include sutures, synostoses, syndesmoses, synchondroses.
[2] It is understood that every diarthrodial joint has a capsular ligament composed of two layers.

TABLE OF JOINTS[1] AND LIGAMENTS—(Continued)

NAME	TYPE	NAMED[2] LIGAMENTS
Humeroradial	See *Elbow*	
Humeroulnar	See *Elbow*	
Intercarpal (1) Distal (between 4 bones of distal row) (2) Proximal (between 3 bones of proximal row) (3) Transverse (between proximal and distal rows)	Gliding	Dorsal carpal (extensor retinaculum BR) Dorsal intercarpal Interosseous intercarpal Radiate or volar carpal Radial collateral carpal (external lateral OT; lateral BR) Transverse carpal (flexor retinaculum BR) Ulnar collateral carpal (internal lateral OT; medial BR) Volar intercarpal (palmar intercarpal BR)
Intercuneiform	Gliding	Dorsal intercuneiform Interosseous intercuneiform Plantar intercuneiform
Intermediate tarsometatarsal	Gliding	Dorsal tarsometatarsal Interosseous cuneometatarsal Interosseous intercuneiform Plantar tarsometatarsal
Intermetacarpal (4 medial metacarpal bases)	Gliding	Basal dorsal metacarpal (dorsal metacarpal BR) Basal interosseous metacarpal (interosseous metacarpal BR) Basal volar metacarpal (palmar metacarpal BR)
Intermetatarsal (4 lateral metatarsal bases)	Gliding	Basal dorsal metatarsal (dorsal metatarsal BR) Basal interosseous metatarsal (interosseous metatarsal BR) Basal plantar metatarsal (plantar metatarsal BR) Transverse metatarsal
Interphalangeal of fingers	Hinge	Collateral (lateral phalangeal OT)
Interphalangeal of toes	Hinge	Accessory plantar (plantar BR) Collateral (lateral phalangeal OT)
Intertarsal	See *Cuboideonavicular*, *Cuneocuboid*, *Cuneonavicular*, *Intercuneiform*, *Talocalcaneal*, *Talocalcaneonavicular*, *Talonavicular*, and *Transverse tarsal*	
Knee (see Plate 2)	Combined hinge and gliding	Alar folds (alar ligaments OT) Anterior cruciate Arcuate popliteal (arcuate BR) Coronary Fibular collateral (external lateral OT; lateral BR) Lateral meniscus (external semilunar cartilage OT; lateral semilunar cartilage BR)

[1] This table does not include sutures, synostoses, syndesmoses, synchondroses.
[2] It is understood that every diarthrodial joint has a capsular ligament composed of two layers.

TABLE OF JOINTS[1] AND LIGAMENTS—(Continued)

Name	Type	Named[2] Ligaments
Knee—(*Continued*)		Lateral patellar retinaculum [BR] Medial meniscus (internal semilunar cartilage OT; medial semilunar cartilage BR) Medial patellar retinaculum [BR] Oblique popliteal (ligament of Winslow OT; oblique posterior BR) Patellar Patellar synovial fold (ligamentum mucosum OT) Posterior Posterior cruciate Superior patellar retinaculum [BR] Tibial collateral (internal lateral OT; medial BR) Transverse
Lateral atlantoepistrophic	Gliding	Accessory atlantoepistrophic (accessory atlantoaxial BR) Anterior atlantoepistrophic obturator (anterior atloaxoid OT; anterior atlantoaxial BR) Posterior atlantoepistrophic obturator (posterior atloaxoid OT; posterior atlantoaxial BR)
Lateral tarsometatarsal	Gliding	Dorsal tarsometatarsal Interosseous cuneocuboid Plantar tarsometatarsal
Mandibular (temporomandibular OT)	Combined gliding and hinge	Articular disk (intraarticular fibrocartilage OT) Sphenomandibular Stylomandibular Temporomandibular (external lateral OT)
Medial tarsometatarsal	Gliding	Dorsal tarsometatarsal Interosseous cuneometatarsal Plantar tarsometatarsal
Metacarpophalangeal	Ball-and-socket	Accessory volar (glenoid cartilage OT; palmar BR) Collateral (lateral phalangeal OT) Transverse of heads of metacarpals (deep transverse of palm BR)
Metatarsophalangeal	Ball-and-socket	Accessory plantar (glenoid OT; plantar of digits BR) Collateral (lateral phalangeal OT) Transverse of heads of metatarsals (transverse metatarsal OT; deep transverse of sole BR)
Midtarsal [OT]	See *Transverse tarsal*	
Pisotriquetral	Gliding	Pisohamate Pisometacarpal
Proximal radioulnar	See *Elbow*	

[1] This table does not include sutures, synostoses, syndesmoses, synchondroses.
[2] It is understood that every diarthrodial joint has a capsular ligament composed of two layers.

TABLE OF JOINTS[1] AND LIGAMENTS—(Continued)

Name	Type	Named[2] Ligaments
Proximal tibiofibular	Gliding	Anterior of head of fibula (anterior superior tibiofibular OT) Interosseous membrane of leg Posterior of head of fibula (posterior superior tibiofibular OT)
Radioulnar	See *Elbow* and *Distal radioulnar*	
Sacroiliac (see Plate 2)	Gliding	Anterior sacroiliac Iliolumbar Interosseous sacroiliac Long posterior sacroiliac (oblique sacroiliac OT) Sacrotuberous (great or posterior sacrosciatic OT) Sacrospinous (lesser or anterior sacrosciatic OT) Short posterior sacroiliac
Shoulder (see Plate 2)	Ball-and-socket	Coracoacromial Coracohumeral Inferior glenohumeral Labrum glenoidale (glenoid ligament OT) Middle glenohumeral Superior glenohumeral Transverse humeral
Sternoclavicular	Gliding	Anterior sternoclavicular Articular disk (intraarticular fibrocartilage OT) Costoclavicular (rhomboid OT) Interclavicular Posterior sternoclavicular
Talocalcaneal (astragalocalcaneal OT)	Gliding	Anterior talocalcaneal (anterior calcaneoastragaloid OT) Interosseous talocalcaneal (interosseous calcaneoastragaloid OT) Lateral talocalcaneal (external calcaneoastragaloid OT) Medial talocalcaneal (internal calcaneoastragaloid OT) Posterior talocalcaneal (posterior calcaneoastragaloid OT)
Talocalcaneonavicular (anterior calcaneoscaphoastragaloid OT)	Gliding	Calcaneonavicular part of bifurcate (superior calcaneoscaphoid OT; lateral calcaneonavicular BR) Dorsal talonavicular (dorsal astragaloscaphoid OT) Interosseous talonavicular (interosseous astragaloscaphoid OT) Plantar calcaneonavicular or spring (inferior calcaneoscaphoid OT)
Talonavicular (taloscaphoid OT)	A portion of talocalcaneonavicular	

[1] This table does not include sutures, synostoses, syndesmoses, synchondroses.
[2] It is understood that every diarthrodial joint has a capsular ligament composed of two layers.

TABLE OF JOINTS[1] AND LIGAMENTS—(**Continued**)

NAME	TYPE	NAMED[2] LIGAMENTS
Tarsal	See *Cuboideonavicular, Cuneocuboid, Cuneonavicular, Intercuneiform, Talocalcaneal, Talocalcaneonavicular, Talonavicular,* and *Transverse tarsal*	
Tarsometatarsal	See *Intermediate, Lateral,* and *Medial tarsometatarsal*	
Temporomandibular [OT]	See *Mandibular*	
Tibiofibular	See *Distal* and *Proximal tibiofibular*	
Transverse tarsal (**Chopart's**) (midtarsal OT)	Combined calcaneocuboid and talocalcaneonavicular	
Wrist	Biaxial	Dorsal radiocarpal (posterior radiocarpal OT; BR) Radial collateral carpal (external lateral OT; lateral BR) Triangular articular disk (triangular fibrocartilage OT) Ulnar collateral carpal (internal lateral OT; medial BR) Volar radiocarpal (anterior radiocarpal BR)

[1] This table does not include sutures, synostoses, syndesmoses, synchondroses.
[2] It is understood that every diarthrodial joint has a capsular ligament composed of two layers.

TABLE OF MUSCLES

(See Plates 3, 4)

Name	Origin	Insertion	Innervation	Function
Abductor digiti quinti (of foot) (abductor digiti minimi BR)	Medial and lateral tubercles of calcaneus and plantar fascia	Lateral surface of base of proximal phalanx of little toe	Lateral plantar	Abducts little toe
Abductor digiti quinti (of hand) (abductor digiti minimi BR)	Pisiform and tendon of flexor carpi ulnaris	Medial surface of base of proximal phalanx of little finger	Ulnar	Abducts little finger
Abductor hallucis	Medial tubercle of calcaneus and plantar fascia	Medial surface of base of proximal phalanx of great toe	Medial plantar	Abducts and flexes great toe at metatarsophalangeal joint
Abductor ossis metatarsi quinti [BR]	Small variable portion of abductor digiti quinti of foot, inserting into fifth metatarsal			
Abductor pollicis brevis (abductor pollicis OT)	Navicular, ridge of greater multangular, and transverse carpal ligament	Lateral surface of base of proximal phalanx of thumb	Median	Abducts and flexes thumb
Abductor pollicis longus (extensor ossis metacarpi pollicis OT) (see Plate 3)	Posterior aspect of ulna, radius, and interosseous membrane	Lateral aspect of base of first metacarpal and greater multangular	Dorsal interosseous branch of radial	Abducts and extends thumb
Accelerator urinae [OT]	See *Bulbocavernosus*			
Accessorius [OT]	See *Quadratus plantae*			
Accessorius [OT]	See *Iliocostalis dorsi*			
Adductor brevis	Pubis	Proximal part of linea aspera of femur and femur proximal to that line	Obturator	Adducts thigh
Adductor hallucis (1) Oblique head (2) Transverse head (adductor hallucis transversus OT) (transversus pedis OT)	Plantar fascia and bases of second, third, and fourth metatarsals Transverse metatarsal ligament and capsules of 4 lateral metatarsophalangeal joints	Lateral aspect of base of proximal phalanx of great toe	Lateral plantar	Adducts great toe
Adductor hallucis transversus [OT]	See *Adductor hallucis, transverse head*			
Adductor longus (see Plates 3, 4)	Pubis	Linea aspera of femur	Obturator	Adducts thigh
Adductor magnus (see Plate 3)	(1) Inferior ramus of pubis and ramus of ischium (2) Ischial tuberosity	Linea aspera of femur Adductor tubercle of femur	Obturator Tibial	Adducts thigh Extends hip joint
Adductor minimus (variable)	When present is a separate proximal portion of adductor magnus			

TABLE OF MUSCLES—(Continued)

NAME	ORIGIN	INSERTION	INNERVATION	FUNCTION
Adductor pollicis (1) Oblique head	Greater and lesser multangular, capitate, and bases of second, third, and fourth metacarpals	Medial aspect of base of proximal phalanx of thumb	Ulnar	Adducts and opposes thumb
(2) Transverse head (adductor pollicis transversus OT)	Third metacarpal			
Agitator caudae (variable)	Portion of gluteus maximus. Sometimes arises separately from coccyx			
Anconeus (see Plate 3)	Dorsal surface of lateral epicondyle of humerus	Olecranon of ulna	Radial	Extends elbow joint
Antitragicus (vestigial)	Lateral surface of antitragus	Antihelix and cauda helicis	Facial	
Arrectores pilorum (erector pili OT) (smooth muscle)	Found in corium	Hair follicles	Sympathetic	Elevate hairs of skin
Articularis genus (subcrureus OT)	Distal fourth of anterior surface of femur	Synovial membrane of knee joint	Femoral	Draws synovial membrane proximally during extension of knee
Aryepiglottic	Apex of arytenoid cartilage	Lateral margin of epiglottis	Recurrent laryngeal	Closes inlet of larynx
Arytenoepiglotticus [OT]	Continuation of oblique arytenoid			
Arytenoid (1) Oblique portion	Dorsal aspect of muscular process of arytenoid cartilage	Apex of opposite arytenoid cartilage	Recurrent laryngeal	Closes inlet of larynx
(2) Transverse portion		Becomes continuous with thyroarytenoid		Approximates arytenoid cartilages
Attolens aurem [OT] (vestigial)	See *Auricularis superior*			
Attrahens aurem [OT] (vestigial)	See *Auricularis anterior*			
Auricularis (vestigial) (1) Anterior (attrahens aurem OT)	Galea aponeurotica	Helix	Facial	Move external ear
(2) Oblique	Scattered fibers across transverse sulcus of antihelix			
(3) Posterior (retrahens aurem OT)	Mastoid	Auricle		
(4) Superior (attolens aurem OT) (see Plate 3)	Galea aponeurotica	Antihelix		
(5) Transverse	Scattered fibers from concha to scapha			
Axillary arches	Occasional slips of muscle in axillary fascia			

TABLE OF MUSCLES—(Continued)

NAME	ORIGIN	INSERTION	INNERVATION	FUNCTION
Azygos uvulae [OT]	See *Uvulae*			
Biceps brachii (1) Short head (2) Long head (see Plate 3)	Tip of coracoid process of scapula Supraglenoid tuberosity of humerus	Tubercle of radius and deep fascia of forearm	Musculocutaneous	Flexes and supinates forearm
Biceps femoris (1) Short head	Linea aspera of femur	Head of fibula, lateral condyle of femur, and deep fascia on lateral aspect of knee	Peroneal	Flexes knee joint
(2) Long head (see Plates 3, 4)	Ischial tuberosity		Tibial	Flexes knee joint and extends hip joint
Biventer cervicis [OT]	See *Semispinalis capitis*			
Brachialis (brachialis anticus OT) (see Plate 3)	Anterior aspect of humerus	Coronoid process of ulna	Musculocutaneous	Flexes elbow joint
Brachioradialis (supinator longus OT) (see Plate 3)	Lateral supracondylar ridge of humerus	Lower end of radius	Radial	Flexes elbow joint
Buccinator	Alveolar process of maxilla and of mandible and pterygomandibular raphe	Blends about mouth with orbicularis oris	Facial	Compresses cheek and retracts angle of mouth
Buccopharyngeus	Portion of superior constrictor of pharynx			
Bulbocavernosus (accelerator urinae OT) (compressor vaginae OT) (ejaculator urinae OT) (sphincter vaginae OT) (bulbospongiosus BR)	Central point of perineum and median raphe of bulb	Fascia of perineum and of penis (clitoris)	Perineal	In male, compresses urethra. In female, contracts vaginal orifice and compresses vestibular bulbs
Caninus (levator anguli oris BR; OT)	Maxilla	Skin of angle of mouth	Facial	Muscle of facial expression
Cephalopharyngeus [OT]	Portion of superior constrictor of pharynx			
Ceratopharyngeus	Portion of middle constrictor of pharynx			
Cervicalis ascendens [OT]	See *Iliocostalis cervicis*			
Chondroepitrochlearis (variable)	Occasional slip of muscle in axillary fascia			
Chondroglossus (variable portion of hyoglossus)	Lesser cornu of hyoid	Side of tongue	Hypoglossal	Depresses tongue
Chondropharyngeus	Portion of middle constrictor of pharynx			

TABLE OF MUSCLES—(Continued)

Name	Origin	Insertion	Innervation	Function
Ciliary (smooth muscle) Meridional portion Radiated (reticular) portion Circular portion	Scleral spur Sphincter of ciliary body	Ciliary processes	Oculomotor, parasympathetic	Visual accommodation
Coccygeofemoralis (variable)	Occasional slip of gluteus maximus arising separately from coccyx			
Coccygeus (ischiococcygeus)	Ischial spine and sacrospinous ligament	Lateral border of lower sacrum and upper coccyx	Sacral	Helps to form pelvic diaphragm
Complexus [OT]	See *Semispinalis capitis*			
Compressor naris [BR] (compressor nasi OT)	See *Nasalis*			
Compressor urethrae [OT]	See *Sphincter urethrae membranaceae*			
Compressor vaginae [OT]	See *Bulbocavernosus*			
Constrictor of pharynx, inferior	Oblique line of thyroid cartilage, side of cricoid cartilage	Median raphe of posterior wall of pharynx	Accessory via pharyngeal plexus, laryngeal branches of vagus	Constricts pharynx
Constrictor of pharynx, middle	Stylohyoid ligament and both cornua of hyoid	Median raphe of pharynx	Accessory via pharyngeal plexus	Constricts pharynx
Constrictor of pharynx, superior	Medial pterygoid lamina, pterygomandibular raphe, and mylohyoid line of mandible	Pharyngeal tubercle of occiput and median raphe of pharynx	Accessory via pharyngeal plexus	Constricts pharynx
Coracobrachialis (see Plate 4)	Coracoid process of scapula	Medial aspect of shaft of humerus	Musculocutaneous	Flexes and adducts humerus
Coracobrachialis superior or **brevis**	Occasional proximal slip of coracobrachialis			
Corrugator cutis ani (smooth muscle)	Found in skin about anus		Sympathetic	
Corrugator supercilii	Superciliary arch of frontal bone	Skin of forehead	Facial	Muscle of facial expression
Costalis [BR]	See *Iliocostalis dorsi*			
Costocervicalis [BR]	See *Iliocostalis cervicis*			
Costocoracoideus (variable)	Occasional slip of muscle in axillary fascia			
Cremaster	Inferior margin of internal oblique muscle of abdomen	Pubic tubercle	Genitofemoral	Elevates testis

TABLE OF MUSCLES—(Continued)

Name	Origin	Insertion	Innervation	Function
Cricoarytenoid, lateral	Lateral surface of cricoid cartilage	Muscular process of arytenoid cartilage	Recurrent laryngeal	Approximates vocal folds
Cricoarytenoid, posterior	Dorsal surface of cricoid cartilage	Muscular process of arytenoid cartilage	Recurrent laryngeal	Separates vocal folds
Cricopharyngeus	Portion of inferior constrictor of pharynx			
Cricothyroid (see Plate 45)	Arch of cricoid cartilage	Lamina of thyroid cartilage	External branch of superior laryngeal	Tenses vocal cords
Crureus [OT]	See *Vastus intermedius*			
Dartos (smooth muscle)	Found in and beneath the skin of scrotum		Sympathetic	Corrugates skin of scrotum
Deltoid (see Plates 3, 4)	Clavicle, acromion, and spine of scapula	Deltoid tuberosity of humerus	Axillary	Abducts humerus, anterior fibers flex and medially rotate humerus, posterior fibers extend and laterally rotate humerus
Depressor alae nasi	Incisor fossa of maxilla	Ala and septum of nose	Facial	Pulls ala and septum of nose downward. Muscle of facial expression
Depressor anguli oris [BR]	See *Triangularis*			
Depressor epiglottidis [OT]	Fibers of thyroepiglottic			
Depressor labii inferioris [BR; OT]	See *Quadratus labii inferioris*			
Depressor septi [BR]	Portion of depressor alae nasi			
Diaphragm	Xiphoid process of sternum, lower 6 costal cartilages, and lumbar vertebrae	Central tendon	Phrenic	Acts as main muscle of inhalation; aids in expulsive actions such as parturition
Digastric				
(1) Anterior belly	Inner surface of mandible near symphysis	Lesser cornu of hyoid via fascial sling	Nerve to mylohyoid	Elevates and fixes hyoid bone
(2) Posterior belly	Mastoid notch		Facial	
Dilator naris				
(1) Anterior portion	Alar cartilage	Ala	Facial	Muscle of facial expression
(2) Posterior portion	Nasal notch of maxilla			
Dilator naris [BR]	See *Nasalis*			
Dilator pupillae (smooth muscle)	Circumference of iris	Margin of pupil	Sympathetic	Dilates pupil
Dilator tubae [OT]	See *Tensor veli palatini*			

TABLE OF MUSCLES—(Continued)

Name	Origin	Insertion	Innervation	Function
Dorsoepitrochlearis (variable)	Occasional muscle slip in axillary fascia			
Ejaculator urinae [OT]	See *Bulbocavernosus*			
Epicranius (occipito-frontalis OT; BR)				
(1) Anterior belly (frontalis)	Galea aponeurotica	Skin of forehead	Facial	Elevates eyebrows and draws scalp forward
(2) Posterior belly (occipitalis)	Superior nuchal line of occiput	Galea aponeurotica	Facial	Draws scalp backward
Erector clitoridis [OT]	See *Ischiocavernosus*			
Erector penis [OT]	See *Ischiocavernosus*			
Erector pili [OT]	See *Arrectores pilorum*			
Extensor carpi radialis brevis (extensor carpi radialis brevior OT) (see Plate 3)	Lateral epicondyle of humerus	Base of second and third metacarpals	Radial	Extends wrist
Extensor carpi radialis longus (extensor carpi radialis longior OT) (see Plate 3)	Lateral epicondyle of humerus	Base of second metacarpal	Radial	Extends wrist
Extensor carpi ulnaris (see Plate 3)	Lateral epicondyle of humerus and dorsal margin of ulna	Base of fifth metacarpal	Radial	Extends wrist
Extensor digiti quinti proprius (extensor digiti minimi BR)	Lateral epicondyle of humerus	Dorsum of proximal phalanx of little finger	Radial	Extends metacarpophalangeal joint of little finger
Extensor digitorum brevis (of foot)	Dorsal surface of calcaneus	Extensor tendons of first, second, third, and fourth toes	Deep peroneal	Extends toes at metatarsophalangeal joints
Extensor digitorum communis (of hand) (extensor digitorum BR) (see Plate 3)	Lateral epicondyle of humerus	Common extensor tendon of each finger	Dorsal interosseous of forearm	Extends wrist and fingers at metacarpophalangeal joints
Extensor digitorum longus (of foot)	Anterior aspect of fibula, lateral aspect of lateral condyle of tibia, and interosseous membrane	Common extensor tendons of 4 lateral toes	Deep peroneal	Extends toes at metatarsophalangeal joints
Extensor hallucis brevis (most medial portion of extensor digitorum brevis)	Dorsal surface of calcaneus	Base of proximal phalanx of great toe	Deep peroneal	Extends metatarsophalangeal joint of great toe
Extensor hallucis longus (see Plate 3)	Medial surface of fibula and interosseous membrane	Base of terminal phalanx of great toe	Deep peroneal	Dorsiflexes ankle joint and extends great toe
Extensor indicis proprius (extensor indicis BR; OT)	Dorsal surface of ulna	Common extensor tendon of index finger	Dorsal interosseous of forearm	Extends metacarpophalangeal joint of index finger

TABLE OF MUSCLES—(Continued)

NAME	ORIGIN	INSERTION	INNERVATION	FUNCTION
Extensor ossis metacarpi pollicis [OT]	See *Abductor pollicis longus*			
Extensor ossis metatarsi hallucis [OT]	Occasional separate slip of insertion of extensor hallucis longus into first metatarsal			
Extensor pollicis brevis (extensor primi internodii pollicis OT) (see Plate 3)	Dorsal surface of radius and interosseous membrane	Dorsal surface of proximal phalanx of thumb	Dorsal interosseous of forearm	Extends metacarpophalangeal joint of thumb
Extensor pollicis longus (extensor secundi internodii pollicis OT)	Dorsal surface of ulna and interosseous membrane	Dorsal surface of distal phalanx of thumb	Dorsal interosseous of forearm	Extends and abducts thumb
Extensor primi internodii longus hallucis [OT]	Occasional separate slip of insertion of extensor hallucis longus into proximal phalanx of great toe			
Extensor primi internodii pollicis [OT]	See *Extensor pollicis brevis*			
Extensor secundi internodii pollicis [OT]	See *Extensor pollicis longus*			
Flexor carpi radialis (see Plate 3)	Medial epicondyle of humerus	Base of second metacarpal	Median	Flexes wrist joint
Flexor carpi ulnaris (see Plate 3)	Medial epicondyle of humerus and medial border of ulna	Pisiform, hamulus of hamate, and proximal end of fifth metacarpal	Ulnar	Flexes wrist joint
Flexor digiti quinti brevis (of foot) (flexor digiti minimi brevis BR)	Base of fifth metatarsal and plantar fascia	Lateral aspect of base of proximal phalanx of little toe	Lateral plantar	Flexes little toe at metatarsophalangeal joint
Flexor digiti quinti brevis (of hand) (flexor digiti minimi brevis BR) (variable)	Hamulus of hamate and transverse carpal ligament	Medial side of proximal phalanx of little finger	Ulnar	Flexes metacarpophalangeal joint of little finger
Flexor digitorum accessorius [BR]	See *Quadratus plantae*			
Flexor digitorum brevis	Medial tuberosity of calcaneus and plantar aponeurosis	Four tendons, one to middle phalanx of each of 4 lateral toes	Medial plantar	Flexes toes at metatarsophalangeal and proximal interphalangeal joints
Flexor digitorum longus	Posterior aspect of tibia	Four tendons, one to base of distal phalanx of each of 4 lateral toes	Tibial	Flexes toes at metatarsophalangeal and interphalangeal joints
Flexor digitorum profundus	Medial and anterior aspects of ulna and interosseous membrane	Four tendons, one to base of distal phalanx of each finger	Ulnar to medial portion, median to lateral portion	Flexes fingers primarily at distal interphalangeal joints, aids in flexing at wrist and other joints of the fingers

TABLE OF MUSCLES—(Continued)

Name	Origin	Insertion	Innervation	Function
Flexor digitorum sublimis (see Plate 3)	Medial epicondyle of humerus, coronoid process of ulna, and anterior margin of radius	Four tendons, one to base of middle phalanx of each finger	Median	Flexes fingers primarily at proximal interphalangeal joints. Aids in flexing wrist and metacarpophalangeal joints
Flexor hallucis brevis	Plantar aspect of cuboid and plantar fascia	Base of proximal phalanx of great toe	Medial plantar	Flexes metatarsophalangeal joint of great toe
Flexor hallucis longus	Posterior aspect of fibula	Base of distal phalanx of great toe	Tibial	Flexes great toe, plantar flexes foot, supports arches of foot
Flexor ossis metacarpi pollicis [OT]	See *Opponens pollicis*			
Flexor pollicis brevis	Transverse carpal ligament and ridge of greater multangular	Base of proximal phalanx of thumb	Median	Flexes metacarpophalangeal joint of thumb
Flexor pollicis longus	Anterior aspect of radius and interosseous membrane	Base of distal phalanx of thumb	Median	Flexes thumb
Frontalis (see Plate 3)	See *Epicranius*			
Gastrocnemius				
(1) Lateral head	Lateral condyle of femur	Posterior surface of calcaneus via tendo calcaneus (achillis)	Tibial	Plantar flexes ankle joint. Flexes knee joint
(2) Medial head (see Plate 3)	Medial condyle of femur			
Gemellus, inferior	Tuberosity of ischium	Greater trochanter of femur	Nerve to quadratus femoris	Rotates femur laterally
Gemellus, superior	Spine of ischium	Greater trochanter of femur	Nerve to obturator internus	Rotates femur laterally
Genioglossus (geniohyoglossus OT)	Superior genial tubercle of mandible	Hyoid and lateral portion of tongue	Hypoglossal	Protrudes and depresses tongue
Geniohyoid	Inferior genial tubercle of mandible	Body of hyoid	Descendens hypoglossi (first and second cervical)	Elevates and draws hyoid forward
Glossopalatine (palatoglossus OT; BR)	Inferior surface of soft palate	Side of tongue	Accessory	Elevates tongue and constricts anterior fauces
Glossopharyngeus	A portion of superior constrictor of pharynx			
Gluteus maximus (see Plates 3, 4)	Lateral surface of ilium, posterior surface of sacrum and coccyx, and sacrotuberous ligament	Gluteal tuberosity and iliotibial tract	Inferior gluteal	Extends hip joint, extends trunk on legs when raising body from sitting position

TABLE OF MUSCLES—(Continued)

Name	Origin	Insertion	Innervation	Function
Gluteus medius (see Plates 3, 4)	Lateral surface of ilium	Greater trochanter	Superior gluteal	Abducts femur
Gluteus minimus	Lateral surface of ilium	Greater trochanter	Superior gluteal	Abducts and medially rotates femur
Gracilis (see Plates 3, 4)	Pubis	Medial surface of tibia	Obturator	Adducts femur, flexes knee joint
Hamstrings	Include semimembranosus, semitendinosus, and biceps femoris			
Helicis major (vestigial)	Spina helicis	Ascending part of helix	Facial	
Helicis minor (vestigial)	Spina helicis	Crux of helix	Facial	
Hyoglossus	Body and greater cornu of hyoid	Side of tongue	Hypoglossal	Depresses tongue
Iliacus	Iliac fossa and sacrum	Lesser trochanter	Femoral	Flexes hip joint and trunk on lower extremity
Iliacus minor (iliocapsularis) (variable)	Iliac fossa and sacrum	Capsule of hip joint	Femoral	
Iliococcygeus	Portion of levator ani			
Iliocostalis cervicis (costocervicalis BR) (cervicalis ascendens OT)	Upper 6 ribs	Posterior tubercles of transverse processes of fourth, fifth, and sixth cervical vertebrae	Posterior rami of cervical	The iliocostalis muscles form the lateral portion of the sacrospinalis. Extends vertebral column and assists in lateral movements of trunk
Iliocostalis dorsi (accessorius OT) (costalis BR)	Lower 6 ribs	Upper 6 ribs	Posterior rami of thoracic	Extends vertebral column and assists in lateral movements of trunk
Iliocostalis lumborum (sacrolumbalis OT) (iliocostalis BR)	Iliac crest, lumbar vertebrae, sacrum, and lumbodorsal fascia	Lower 6 ribs	Posterior rami of lumbar	Extends vertebral column and assists in lateral movements of trunk
Iliocostocervicalis [BR]	Composed of iliocostalis cervicis and iliocostalis dorsi			
Iliopsoas (see Plates 3, 4)	Combination of iliacus and psoas muscles			
Infracostals [OT]	See *Subcostals*			
Infraspinatus	Infraspinous fossa of scapula	Greater tubercle of humerus	Suprascapular nerve	Rotates humerus laterally

TABLE OF MUSCLES—(Continued)

Name	Origin	Insertion	Innervation	Function
Intercostal, external (11 pairs)	Lower border of rib above	Superior border of rib below	Anterior rami of thoracic	Accessory muscles of respiration (inhalation)
Intercostal, internal (11 pairs)	Lower border of costal cartilage and rib above	Superior border of costal cartilage and rib below	Anterior rami of thoracic	Accessory muscles of respiration (exhalation)
Interossei, dorsal (**of foot**) (4)	Each by two heads from sides of adjacent metatarsals	Extensor tendon of each of 4 lateral toes	Lateral plantar	Abduct toes. Plantar flex at metatarsophalangeal joints and extend at interphalangeal joints
Interossei, dorsal (**of hand**) (4)	Each by two heads from sides of adjacent metacarpals	Extensor tendons of second, third, and fourth fingers	Ulnar	Abduct fingers. Flex at metacarpophalangeal joints, and extend at interphalangeal joints
Interossei, plantar (3)	Medial side of third, fourth, and fifth metatarsals, respectively	Extensor tendons of third, fourth, and fifth toes	Lateral plantar	Adduct toes and assist the dorsal interossei
Interossei, volar (interossei, palmar OT; BR) (3)	Sides of metacarpals	Extensor tendons of second, fourth, and fifth fingers	Ulnar	Adduct fingers and assist dorsal interossei
Interspinales (variable, may be absent in thoracic region)	Spinous process of vertebra above	Spinous process of vertebra below	Posterior rami of spinal	Extend vertebral column
Intertransversarii (intertransversales OT) (may be absent in thoracic region)	Transverse process of vertebra	Transverse process of vertebra	Anterior rami of spinal	Aid in lateral movements of vertebral column
Ischiobulbosus (variable)	Ischium	Perineal raphe	Perineal	Assists bulbocavernosus
Ischiocavernosus (erector penis OT) (erector clitoridis OT)	Ischium	Crus of penis (clitoris)	Perineal	Assists in erection of penis (clitoris)
Ischiofemoralis (variable)	Occasional slip of gluteus maximus arising from ischial tuberosity			
Ischiopubicus (variable)	Portion of sphincter urethrae membranaceae			
Latissimus dorsi (latissimus thoracis BR) (see Plates 3, 4)	Spines of lower 6 thoracic vertebrae, spines of lumbar vertebrae, lumbodorsal fascia, crest of ilium, lower ribs, and inferior angle of scapula	Intertubercular sulcus of humerus	Thoracodorsal	Adducts and extends humerus; used to pull body up in climbing; accessory muscle of respiration
Levator anguli oris [BR; OT]	See *Caninus*			
Levator anguli scapulae [OT]	See *Levator scapulae*			

TABLE OF MUSCLES—(Continued)

Name	Origin	Insertion	Innervation	Function
Levator ani (1) Iliococcygeal portion (2) Pubococcygeal portion	Pelvic surface of ischial spine and pelvic fascia Pubic and pelvic fascia	Central point of perineum, anococcygeal raphe, and coccyx Some fibers form a sling around the upper portion of anal canal	Anterior rami of third and fourth sacral and perineal	Supports pelvic viscera
Levator glandulae thyroideae (variable)	Hyoid	Isthmus of thyroid		
Levator labii superioris [OT; BR]	Portion of quadratus labii superioris			
Levator labii superioris alaeque nasi [OT; BR]	See *Quadratus labii superioris*			
Levator menti [OT]	See *Mentalis*			
Levator palati [OT; BR]	See *Levator veli palatini*			
Levator palpebrae superioris (see Plate 19)	Roof of orbit	Skin of upper eyelid and superior tarsus	Oculomotor	Elevates upper lid
Levator prostatae	Medial fibers of pubococcygeal portion of levator ani			
Levator scapulae (levator anguli scapulae OT) (see Plates 3, 4)	Transverse processes of upper cervical vertebrae	Vertebral margin and medial angle of scapula	Dorsal scapular and anterior rami of third and fourth cervical	Elevates shoulder, rotates inferior angle of scapula medially
Levator veli palatini (levator palati OT; BR) (see Plate 20)	Apex of petrous part of temporal bone and cartilaginous part of auditory tube	Aponeurosis of soft palate	Accessory via pharyngeal plexus	Raises soft palate
Levatores costarum (12 pairs)	Transverse processes of seventh cervical and upper 11 thoracic vertebrae	Medial to angle of corresponding rib below	Anterior rami of thoracic	Aid in raising ribs in inspiration
Lingual, inferior [OT]	See *Longitudinalis, inferior, of tongue*			
Lingual, superior [OT]	See *Longitudinalis, superior, of tongue*			
Longissimus (portion of sacrospinalis) (1) **Capitis** (trachelomastoideus OT) (2) **Cervicis** (transversalis colli OT) (transversus colli OT) (3) **Dorsi** (thoracis BR)	Transverse processes of upper sixth thoracic vertebrae and articular processes of lower 4 cervical vertebrae Transverse processes of upper 6 thoracic vertebrae Iliac crest, sacroiliac ligament, spines of lumbar and sacral vertebrae	Mastoid process of temporal bone Transverse processes of second to sixth cervical vertebrae Ribs and transverse processes of thoracic and upper lumbar vertebrae	Posterior rami of spinal	Longissimus muscles form middle portion of sacrospinalis. Extends vertebral column and assists in rotation and lateral movements of trunk

TABLE OF MUSCLES—(Continued)

Name	Origin	Insertion	Innervation	Function
Longitudinalis, of tongue (1) Inferior (inferior lingual OT) (2) Superior (superior lingual OT)	Base of tongue	Tip of tongue	Hypoglossal	Alters shape of tongue
Longus capitis (rectus capitis anticus major OT)	Transverse processes of third to sixth cervical vertebrae	Basal portion of occipital bone	Anterior rami of upper 4 cervical	Flexes head
Longus colli (longus cervicis BR)				
(1) Inferior oblique portion	Bodies of first 3 thoracic vertebrae	Anterior tubercles of fifth and sixth cervical vertebrae	Anterior rami of cervical	Flexes vertebral column
(2) Superior oblique portion	Transverse processes of third to fifth cervical vertebrae	Anterior tubercle of atlas		
(3) Vertical portion	Bodies of last 3 cervical and first 3 thoracic vertebrae	Bodies of second to fourth cervical vertebrae		
Lumbricals (of fingers) (4)	Tendons of flexor digitorum profundus	One to extensor tendon of each finger	Two lateral by median and two medial by ulnar	Flex at metacarpophalangeal joints and extend at interphalangeal joints
Lumbricals (of toes) (4)	Tendons of flexor digitorum longus	One to extensor tendon of each of 4 lateral toes	Medial one by medial plantar, others by lateral plantar	Flex at metatarsophalangeal joints and extend at interphalangeal joints
Masseter (see Plate 3)	Arch of zygoma	Ramus and angle of mandible	Mandibular	Muscle of mastication. Closes mouth and clenches teeth
Mentalis (levator menti OT)	Incisor fossa of mandible	Skin of chin	Facial	Muscle of facial expression
Multifidus (multifidus spinae OT)	Sacrum, sacroiliac ligament, mammillary processes of lumbar vertebrae, transverse processes of thoracic vertebrae, articular processes of lower 4 cervical vertebrae	Spines of vertebrae	Posterior rami of spinal	Extends and rotates vertebral column
Mylohyoid	Mylohyoid line of mandible	Hyoid	Nerve to mylohyoid	Elevates hyoid and supports floor of mouth
Mylopharyngeal	Portion of superior constrictor of pharynx			
Nasalis (compressor nasi OT) (compressor naris BR) (dilator naris BR) (see Plate 3)	Maxilla	Skin over bridge of nose	Facial	Muscle of facial expression

TABLE OF MUSCLES—(Continued)

Name	Origin	Insertion	Innervation	Function
Obliquus abdominis externus (see Plates 3, 4)	Lower 8 ribs	Xiphoid, linea alba, pubis, crest of ilium	Lower 6 thoracic	Supports abdominal viscera. Flexes vertebral column
Obliquus abdominis internus (see Plate 4)	Lumbodorsal fascia, iliac crest, inguinal ligament	Lower 3 ribs, linea alba, xiphoid, pubis	Lower 6 thoracic and iliohypogastric	Supports abdominal viscera. Flexes vertebral column
Obliquus auriculae (obliquus auris OT) (vestigial)	Helix	Antihelix	Facial	
Obliquus capitis inferior	Spine of epistropheus	Transverse process of atlas	Posterior ramus of first cervical	Aids in extension and lateral movements of head
Obliquus capitis superior	Transverse process of atlas	Occipital bone	Posterior ramus of first cervical	Aids in extension and lateral movements of head
Obliquus oculi inferior (see Plate 19)	Medial aspect of floor of orbit	Sclera	Oculomotor	Rotates eyeball upward and outward
Obliquus oculi superior (trochlearis OT)	Margin of optic foramen	Sclera	Trochlear	Rotates eyeball outward and downward
Obturator externus	Pubis, ischium, and superficial surface of obturator membrane	Trochanteric fossa of femur	Obturator	Rotates femur laterally
Obturator internus	Pubis, ilium, ischium, and deep surface of obturator membrane	Greater trochanter of femur	Nerve to obturator internus	Rotates femur laterally
Occipitalis (see Plate 3)	See *Epicranius*			
Occipitofrontalis [OT; BR]	See *Epicranius*			
Omohyoid (1) Anterior belly (2) Posterior belly (see Plates 3, 4)	 Intermediate tendon Superior margin of scapula	 Hyoid Intermediate tendon	 Descendens cervicis and hypoglossi	 Depresses hyoid
Opponens digiti quinti (of foot) (opponens digiti minimi BR) (variable)	Occasional insertion of flexor digiti quinti brevis into fifth metatarsal			
Opponens digiti quinti (of hand) (opponens digiti minimi BR)	Transverse carpal ligament and hamulus of hamate	Medial aspect of fifth metacarpal	Ulnar	Deepens palm
Opponens hallucis (variable)	Occasional insertion of some fibers of flexor hallucis brevis into shaft of first metatarsal			
Opponens pollicis (flexor ossis metacarpi pollicis OT)	Ridge of greater multangular and transverse carpal ligament	First metacarpal	Median	Opposes thumb

TABLE OF MUSCLES—(Continued)

NAME	ORIGIN	INSERTION	INNERVATION	FUNCTION
Orbicularis oculi (orbicularis palpebrarum OT)	Medial aspect of orbit	Skin about eyelids	Facial	Closes lids
Orbicularis oris (see Plate 3)	Lies in skin about mouth		Facial	Muscle of facial expression; puckers mouth
Orbicularis palpebrarum [OT]	See *Orbicularis oculi*			
Orbitalis (smooth muscle)	Bridges inferior orbital fissure		Sympathetic	
Palatoglossus [OT; BR]	See *Glossopalatine*			
Palatopharyngeus [OT; BR]	See *Pharyngopalatinus*			
Palmaris brevis	Palmar aponeurosis	Skin of medial border of hand	Ulnar	Deepens hollow of hand
Palmaris longus (variable) (see Plate 3)	Medial epicondyle of humerus	Transverse carpal ligament and palmar aponeurosis	Median	Flexes wrist joint
Pectineus (see Plates 3, 4)	Pubis	Femur distal to lesser trochanter	Femoral (occasionally obturator)	Adducts femur and flexes hip joint
Pectoralis major (see Plates 3, 4)	Clavicle, sternum, first 6 ribs, aponeurosis of external oblique muscle of abdomen	Intertubercular sulcus of humerus	Medial and lateral anterior thoracic	Adducts and medially rotates humerus, flexes shoulder joint, depresses shoulder girdle
Pectoralis minor (see Plate 4)	Third to fifth ribs	Coracoid process of scapula	Medial and lateral anterior thoracic	Draws shoulder forward
Peroneocalcaneus (variable)	Occasional separate portion of tibialis posterior			
Peroneocalcaneus externus (variable)	Occasional slip of insertion of peroneus longus or brevis into calcaneus			
Peroneocuboideus (variable)	Occasional slip of insertion of peroneus longus or brevis into cuboid			
Peroneus accessorius (variable)	Occasional extra portion of peroneus longus or brevis			
Peroneus brevis	Lateral surface of fibula	Base of fifth metatarsal	Superficial peroneal	Everts and plantar flexes foot
Peroneus digiti quinti (variable)	Occasional extra slip of insertion of peroneus brevis into fifth toe			

TABLE OF MUSCLES—(Continued)

NAME	ORIGIN	INSERTION	INNERVATION	FUNCTION
Peroneus longus (see Plate 3)	Lateral condyle of tibia and lateral surface of fibula	First cuneiform and first metatarsal	Superficial peroneal	Everts and plantar flexes foot. Supports arches
Peroneus tertius	Medial surface of fibula	Fifth metatarsal	Deep peroneal	Everts and dorsiflexes foot
Pharyngopalatinus (palatopharyngeus OT; BR)	Soft palate and auditory tube	Aponeurosis of pharynx	Accessory via pharyngeal plexus	Aids in swallowing
Piriformis	Second to fourth sacral vertebrae, ilium, and sacrotuberous ligament	Greater trochanter of femur	Anterior rami of first and second sacral	Rotates femur laterally
Plantaris (variable) (see Plate 3)	Lateral condyle of femur	Calcaneus by tendo calcaneus (achillis)	Tibial	Flexes knee joint and plantar flexes ankle joint
Platysma (platysma myoides OT) (see Plate 3)	Deep fascia of cervical region	Mandible and skin around mouth	Facial	Muscle of facial expression
Popliteus	Lateral condyle of femur	Back of tibia	Tibial	Rotates tibia medially, flexes knee joint
Procerus (pyramidalis nasi OT)	Skin over nose	Skin of forehead	Facial	Muscle of facial expression
Pronator quadratus	Volar surface of ulna	Volar surface of radius	Volar interosseous	Pronates forearm
Pronator teres (pronator radii teres OT) (see Plate 3)	(1) Medial epicondyle of humerus (2) Coronoid of ulna	Lateral surface of radius	Median	Pronates forearm
Psoas major (psoas magnus OT)	Lumbar vertebrae and fascia	Lesser trochanter of femur	Anterior rami of second and third lumbar	Flexes hip joint and trunk on lower extremities
Psoas minor (psoas parvus OT) (variable)	Last thoracic and first lumbar vertebrae	Iliopectineal eminence	Anterior ramus of first lumbar	Flexes trunk on pelvis
Pterygoideus externus (pterygoideus lateralis BR)	(1) Sphenoid (2) Lateral pterygoid plate	Neck of mandible and capsule of temporomandibular joint	Mandibular	Muscle of mastication, protrudes mandible
Pterygoideus internus (pterygoideus medialis BR)	(1) Lateral pterygoid plate (2) Tuberosity of maxilla	Medial surface of angle of mandible	Mandibular	Muscle of mastication, clenches teeth
Pterygopharyngeus	Portion of superior constrictor of pharynx			
Pubocavernosus	Occasional slip of ischiocavernosus arising from pubis			
Pubococcygeus	Portion of levator ani			
Puborectalis	Middle fibers of pubococcygeal portion of levator ani			

NAME	ORIGIN	INSERTION	INNERVATION	FUNCTION
Pyramidalis abdominis (variable)	Pubis	Linea alba	Anterior ramus of lowest thoracic	Supports abdominal viscera
Pyramidalis auriculae (vestigial)	Portion of tragicus			
Pyramidalis nasi [OT]	See *Procerus*			
Quadratus femoris	Ischial tuberosity	Quadrate tubercle of femur	Nerve to quadratus femoris	Adducts and laterally rotates femur
Quadratus labii inferioris (depressor labii inferioris BR; OT) (see Plate 3)	Mandible	Skin about mouth	Facial	Muscle of facial expression
Quadratus labii superioris (levator labii superioris alaeque nasi OT; BR) (see Plate 3)	Maxilla	Skin about mouth	Facial	Muscle of facial expression
Quadratus lumborum	Iliac crest, lumbodorsal fascia, and lumbar vertebrae	Last rib	Anterior rami of first 3 lumbar	Assists in lateral movements of vertebral column
Quadratus plantae (flexor digitorum accessorius BR) (accessorius OT)	Calcaneus and plantar fascia	Tendons of flexor digitorum longus	Lateral plantar	Assists in flexion of toes
Quadriceps femoris (quadriceps extensor OT)	Includes rectus femoris and 3 vastus muscles			
Rectus abdominis (see Plate 4)	Pubis	Xiphoid, fifth to seventh costal cartilages	Anterior rami of lower 6 thoracic	Supports abdominal viscera; flexes vertebral column
Rectus capitis anterior (rectus capitis anticus minor OT)	Lateral portion of atlas	Occipital bone	Anterior rami of first and second cervical	Flexes head
Rectus capitis anticus major [OT]	See *Longus capitis*			
Rectus capitis anticus minor [OT]	See *Rectus capitis anterior*			
Rectus capitis lateralis	Transverse process of atlas	Occipital bone	Anterior ramus of first cervical	Assists in lateral movements of head
Rectus capitis posterior major (rectus capitis posticus major OT)	Spine of epistropheus	Occipital bone	Posterior ramus of first cervical	Extends head
Rectus capitis posterior minor (rectus capitis posticus minor OT)	Posterior tubercle of atlas	Occipital bone	Posterior ramus of first cervical	Extends head

TABLE OF MUSCLES—(Continued)

NAME	ORIGIN	INSERTION	INNERVATION	FUNCTION
Rectus femoris (1) Straight head (2) Reflected head (see Plates 3, 4)	Anterior inferior spine of ilium Dorsum ilii	Patella and ultimately into tubercle of tibia	Femoral	Extends knee joint Flexes hip joint
Rectus oculi inferior (see Plate 19)	Lower border of optic foramen	Sclera	Oculomotor	Rotates eyeball downward and somewhat inward
Rectus oculi lateralis (rectus oculi externus OT) (see Plate 19)	Lateral border of optic foramen	Sclera	Abducens	Rotates eyeball laterally
Rectus oculi medialis (rectus oculi internus OT) (see Plate 19)	Medial border of optic foramen	Sclera	Oculomotor	Rotates eyeball medially
Rectus oculi superior (see Plate 19)	Upper border of optic foramen	Sclera	Oculomotor	Rotates eyeball upward and somewhat inward
Retrahens aurem [OT] (vestigial)	See *Auricularis posterior*			
Rhomboideus major (see Plate 3)	Spines of second to fifth thoracic vertebrae	Vertebral margin of scapula	Dorsal scapular	Draws scapula backward and aids in rotating inferior angle of scapula medially
Rhomboideus minor	Spines of seventh cervical and first thoracic vertebrae	Vertebral margin of scapula	Dorsal scapular	Same as rhomboideus major
Risorius (see Plate 3)	Fascia over masseter	Skin at angle of mouth	Facial	Muscle of facial expression
Rotatores (11 pairs)	Transverse process of thoracic vertebra below	Lamina of thoracic vertebra above	Posterior rami of thoracic	Extend and rotate vertebral column
Sacrolumbalis [OT]	See *Iliocostalis lumborum*			
Sacrospinalis	Composed of longissimus, iliocostalis, and spinalis dorsi			
Salpingopharyngeus	Portion of pharyngopalatinus arising from auditory tube			
Sartorius (see Plates 3, 4)	Anterior superior spine of ilium	Tibia	Femoral	Flexes hip and knee joints, rotates femur laterally
Scalenus anterior (scalenus anticus OT) (see Plate 4)	Transverse processes of third to sixth cervical vertebrae	Tubercle of first rib	Anterior rami of third and fourth cervical	Flexes vertebral column laterally, accessory muscle of respiration (inhalation)
Scalenus medius (see Plate 4)	Transverse processes of second to sixth cervical vertebrae	First rib	Anterior rami of third and fourth cervical	Flexes vertebral column laterally, accessory muscle of respiration (inhalation)

TABLE OF MUSCLES—(Continued)

Name	Origin	Insertion	Innervation	Function
Scalenus posterior (scalenus posticus OT) (see Plate 4)	Tubercles of fourth to sixth cervical vertebrae	Second rib	Anterior rami of third and fourth cervical	Flexes vertebral column laterally, accessory muscle of respiration (inhalation)
Semimembranosus (see Plate 3)	Ischial tuberosity	Medial condyle of tibia	Tibial	Flexes knee joint and extends hip joint
Semispinalis capitis (complexus OT) (biventer cervicis OT)	Transverse processes of upper 6 thoracic and articular processes of lower 4 cervical vertebrae	Occipital bone	Posterior rami of spinal	Extends head
Semispinalis cervicis (semispinalis colli OT)	Transverse processes of upper 6 thoracic and lower 4 cervical vertebrae	Spines of second to fifth cervical vertebrae	Posterior rami of spinal	Extends and rotates vertebral column
Semispinalis dorsi (semispinalis thoracis BR)	Transverse processes of lower 6 thoracic vertebrae	Spines of last 2 cervical and first 4 thoracic vertebrae	Posterior rami of thoracic	Extends and rotates vertebral column
Semitendinosus (see Plate 3)	Ischial tuberosity	Medial aspect of proximal portion of tibia	Tibial	Flexes knee joint and extends hip joint
Serratus anterior (serratus anticus OT) (serratus magnus OT) (see Plates 3, 4)	Upper 8 or 9 ribs	Vertebral border of scapula	Long thoracic	Draws scapula forward, draws inferior angle laterally
Serratus posterior inferior (serratus posticus inferior OT)	Lumbodorsal fascia, spines of lowest thoracic and upper lumbar vertebrae	Last 4 ribs	Lower thoracic	Accessory muscle of respiration
Serratus posterior superior (serratus posticus superior OT)	Ligamentum nuchae, spines of seventh cervical and upper thoracic vertebrae	Second to fifth ribs	Second and third thoracic	Accessory muscle of respiration, elevates ribs
Soleus (see Plate 3)	Fibula, popliteal fascia, and tibia	Calcaneus by tendo calcaneus (achillis)	Tibial	Plantar flexes ankle joint
Sphincter ani externus (subdivided into subcutaneous, superficial, and deep portions)	Tip of coccyx	Surrounds anus	Pudendal	Closes anus
Sphincter pupillae	Circular fibers of iris		Oculomotor, parasympathetic portion	Constricts pupil
Sphincter urethrae membranaceae (sphincter urethrae BR) (compressor urethrae OT)	Ramus of pubis	Median raphe	Perineal	Compresses urethra
Sphincter vaginae [OT]	See *Bulbocavernosus*			

TABLE OF MUSCLES—(Continued)

Name	Origin	Insertion	Innervation	Function
Spinalis capitis (variable)	Spines of upper thoracic and lowest cervical vertebrae	Occipital	Posterior rami of spinal	Extends head
Spinalis cervicis (spinalis colli OT) (variable)	Spines of lower cervical and upper thoracic vertebrae	Spines of second to fourth cervical vertebrae	Posterior rami of spinal	Extends vertebral column
Spinalis dorsi (spinalis thoracis BR)	Spines of lower 2 thoracic and upper 2 lumbar vertebrae	Spines of upper thoracic vertebrae	Posterior rami of spinal	Forms medial portion of sacrospinalis, extends vertebral column, and assists in rotation and lateral movements of vertebral column
Splenius capitis (see Plate 3)	Ligamentum nuchae, spines of last cervical and upper thoracic vertebrae	Mastoid process	Posterior rami of spinal	Extends head
Splenius cervicis (splenius colli OT)	Ligamentum nuchae, spines of last cervical and upper thoracic vertebrae	Transverse processes of upper cervical vertebrae	Posterior rami of spinal	Extends vertebral column
Stapedius	Pyramidal eminence	Neck of stapes	Nerve to stapedius	Draws base of stapes toward tympanic cavity
Sternalis (variable)	Fascia of chest wall	Fascia of chest wall	Anterior thoracic	
Sternoclavicularis (variable)	Small separate slip of subclavius occasionally arising from sternum			
Sternocleidomastoid (see Plates 3, 4)	Manubrium of sternum and clavicle	Mastoid process	Accessory and branch from second and third cervical	Flexes head
Sternocostalis [BR]	See *Transversus thoracis*			
Sternohyoid (see Plates 3, 4)	Manubrium of sternum	Hyoid	Descendens cervicis and hypoglossi	Depresses hyoid
Sternothyroid (see Plate 4)	Manubrium of sternum	Thyroid cartilage	Descendens cervicis and hypoglossi	Depresses larynx
Styloglossus	Styloid process	Side of tongue	Hypoglossal	Elevates tongue
Stylohyoid	Styloid process	Hyoid	Facial	Elevates hyoid
Stylopharyngeus	Styloid process	Lateral wall of pharynx	Glossopharyngeal	Pulls pharynx up
Subanconeus (variable)	Posterior distal surface of humerus	Posterior aspect of elbow joint	Radial	Pulls capsule back in extension of elbow joint

TABLE OF MUSCLES—(Continued)

NAME	ORIGIN	INSERTION	INNERVATION	FUNCTION
Subclavius	First costal cartilage and first rib	Clavicle	Nerve to subclavius	Depresses lateral end of clavicle
Subcostals (infracostals OT) (variable)	Lower ribs	Lower ribs	Thoracic	Muscles of respiration
Subcrureus [OT]	See *Articularis genus*			
Subscapularis	Subscapular fossa of scapula	Lesser tubercle of humerus	Subscapular	Rotates humerus medially
Supinator (supinator radii brevis OT)	Lateral epicondyle of humerus, fascia about elbow joint, and shaft of ulna	Radius	Dorsal interosseous of forearm	Supinates forearm
Supinator longus [OT]	See *Brachioradialis*			
Supinator radii brevis [OT]	See *Supinator*			
Supraspinatus	Supraspinous fossa of scapula	Greater tubercle of humerus	Suprascapular	Abducts humerus
Temporal	Temporal fossa	Coronoid process of mandible	Mandibular	Closes mouth, clenches teeth, retracts lower jaw
Tensor fasciae latae (tensor vaginae femoris OT) (see Plates 3, 4)	Iliac crest	Iliotibial tract and ultimately into tibia	Superior gluteal	Abducts leg, flexes hip joint, extends knee joint
Tensor fasciae suralis (variable)	Occasional insertion of long head of biceps femoris into tendo calcaneus (achillis)			
Tensor palati [OT; BR]	See *Tensor veli palatini*			
Tensor tarsi [OT]	Portion of orbicularis oculi			
Tensor tympani	Cartilaginous portion of auditory tube	Manubrium of malleus	Mandibular	Tenses membrana tympani (ear drum)
Tensor vaginae femoris [OT]	See *Tensor fasciae latae*			
Tensor veli palatini (tensor palati OT; BR) (dilator tubae OT)	Scaphoid fossa of sphenoid and wall of auditory tube	Aponeurosis of soft palate	Mandibular	Tenses soft palate and opens auditory tube
Teres major (see Plate 3)	Axillary margin of scapula	Intertubercular sulcus of humerus	Subscapular	Adducts and medially rotates humerus
Teres minor	Axillary margin of scapula	Greater tubercle of humerus	Axillary	Laterally rotates humerus
Thyroarytenoid	Lamina of thyroid cartilage	Muscular process of arytenoid cartilage	Recurrent laryngeal	Relaxes vocal cords; closes vestibule of larynx

TABLE OF MUSCLES—(Continued)

Name	Origin	Insertion	Innervation	Function
Thyroepiglottic (depressor epiglottidis OT)	Lamina of thyroid cartilage	Epiglottis	Recurrent laryngeal	Closes inlet of larynx
Thyrohyoid (see Plate 4)	Thyroid cartilage	Hyoid	Descendens hypoglossi (first and second cervical)	Draws thyroid and hyoid toward each other
Thyropharyngeus	Portion of inferior constrictor of pharynx			
Tibialis anterior (tibialis anticus OT) (see Plate 3)	Tibia and interosseous membrane	First cuneiform and first metatarsal	Deep peroneal	Dorsiflexes and inverts foot
Tibialis posterior (tibialis posticus OT)	Fibula, tibia, and interosseous membrane	Bases of metatarsals and all tarsal bones except talus	Tibial	Plantar flexes and inverts foot, supports arches of foot
Tibiofascialis anterior (variable)	Occasional slip of insertion of tibialis anterior into fascia of dorsum of foot			
Trachelomastoideus [OT]	See *Longissimus capitis*			
Tragicus (vestigial)	Crosses tragus		Facial	
Transversalis colli [OT]	See *Longissimus cervicis*			
Transversus abdominis (transversalis abdominis OT) (see Plate 4)	Costal cartilages of lower 6 ribs, lumbodorsal fascia, iliac crest, and inguinal ligament	Xiphoid, linea alba, inguinal ligament, and pubis	Anterior rami of lower 6 thoracic and iliohypogastric	Supports abdominal viscera and flexes vertebral column
Transversus auriculae (vestigial)	Crosses back of concha		Facial	
Transversus colli [OT]	See *Longissimus cervicis*			
Transversus linguae	Median raphe of tongue	Dorsum and sides of tongue	Hypoglossal	Alters shape of tongue
Transversus pedis [OT]	See *Adductor hallucis, transverse head*			
Transversus perinei profundus	Inferior ramus of ischium	Central point of perineum	Perineal	Supports perineum
Transversus perinei superficialis (variable)	Tuberosity of ischium	Central point of perineum	Perineal	Supports perineum
Transversus thoracis (sternocostalis BR) (triangularis sterni OT)	Mediastinal surface of xiphoid and body of sternum	Second to sixth costal cartilages	Thoracic	
Transversus urethrae (inconstant)	Occasional slip of sphincter urethrae membranaceae			

TABLE OF MUSCLES—(Continued)

Name	Origin	Insertion	Innervation	Function
Transversus vaginae	Muscle in female which corresponds to sphincter urethrae membranaceae			
Trapezius (see Plates 3, 4)	Occipital bone, ligamentum nuchae, spines of seventh cervical and all thoracic vertebrae	Clavicle, acromion, and spine of scapula	Accessory and anterior rami of third and fourth cervical	Rotates inferior angle of scapula laterally, raises shoulder, draws scapula backward
Triangularis (depressor anguli oris BR) (see Plate 3)	Mandible	Skin at angle of mouth	Facial	Muscle of facial expression
Triangularis sterni [OT]	See *Transversus thoracis*			
Triceps brachii				
(1) Long head	Infraglenoid tuberosity	Olecranon of ulna	Radial	Extends elbow joint; long head also aids in adducting humerus
(2) Lateral head	Shaft of humerus			
(3) Medial head (see Plate 3)	Shaft of humerus			
Triceps surae [OT]	Combined gastrocnemius, soleus, and plantaris			
Trochlearis [OT]	See *Obliquus oculi superior*			
Uvulae (azygos uvulae OT)	Posterior nasal spine	Aponeurosis of soft palate	Accessory (pharyngeal plexus)	
Vastus crureus [OT]	See *Vastus intermedius*			
Vastus externus [OT]	See *Vastus lateralis*			
Vastus intermedius (crureus OT) (vastus crureus OT)	Anterior and lateral aspects of femur	Patella and ultimately into tubercle of tibia	Femoral	Extends knee joint
Vastus internus [OT]	See *Vastus medialis*			
Vastus lateralis (vastus externus OT) (see Plates 3, 4)	Capsule of hip joint and lateral aspect of femur	Patella and ultimately into tubercle of tibia	Femoral	Extends knee joint
Vastus medialis (vastus internus OT) (see Plates 3, 4)	Medial aspect of femur	Patella and ultimately into tubercle of tibia	Femoral	Extends knee joint
Verticalis linguae	Dorsal aspect of tongue	Sides and base of tongue	Hypoglossal	Alters shape of tongue
Vocalis (medial fibers of thyroarytenoid)	Thyroid cartilage	Vocal process of arytenoid cartilage	Recurrent laryngeal	Adjusts vocal cords
Zygomatic (zygomaticus major OT; BR) (see Plate 3)	Zygoma	Skin about mouth	Facial	Muscle of facial expression
Zygomaticus major [OT; BR]	See *Zygomatic*			
Zygomaticus minor [OT; BR]	Portion of quadratus labii superioris			

TABLE OF NERVES

(See Plate 16)

NAME	CENTRAL ATTACHMENT	COMPONENTS	BRANCHES	DISTRIBUTION
Abducens (sixth cranial) (see Plate 18)	Brain stem at inferior border of pons	Motor	Muscular filaments	Lateral rectus muscle of eye
Accessory (eleventh cranial) (spinal accessory OT) (see Plates 16, 17)				
(1) Bulbar part	Lateral aspect of medulla oblongata	Motor*	Internal ramus to vagus	Striate muscles of larynx and pharynx
		Parasympathetic		Thoracic and abdominal viscera
(2) Spinal part	Upper 5 or 6 cervical segments of cord	Motor	External ramus to second, third, and fourth cervical (cervical plexus)	Trapezius and sternocleidomastoid muscles
Acoustic (eighth cranial) (auditory OT; BR) (see Plate 17)	See *Cochlear* and *Vestibular*			
Alveolar, anterior superior (anterior superior dental OT; BR)	Infraorbital	Somatic sensory	Filaments	Upper incisor and canine teeth, mucosa of nasal floor
Alveolar, inferior (inferior dental OT; BR)	Mandibular	Motor	N. to mylohyoid muscle	Mylohyoid and anterior belly of digastric muscles
		Somatic sensory	Mental and filaments	Lower teeth, skin of lower lip, and chin
Alveolar, middle superior (middle superior dental OT; BR)	Infraorbital	Somatic sensory	Filaments	Upper premolar teeth
Alveolar, posterior superior (posterior superior dental OT; BR)	Maxillary	Somatic sensory	Filaments	Upper molar teeth and mucosa of maxillary sinus
Ampullary, inferior	Vestibular	Sensory (movement of head in space—dynamic)	Filaments	Ampulla of posterior semicircular duct
Ampullary, lateral	Vestibular	Sensory (movement of head in space—dynamic)	Filaments	Ampulla of lateral semicircular duct
Ampullary, superior	Vestibular	Sensory (movement of head in space—dynamic)	Filaments	Ampulla of superior semicircular duct
Anastomotic, peroneal	See *Peroneal, anastomotic*			
Anococcygeal	Fourth and fifth sacral and coccygeal segments of cord	Somatic sensory	Filaments	Skin in vicinity of coccyx
Arnold, N. of [OT]	See *Auricular*			
Auditory [OT; BR]	See *Acoustic*			
Auricular (N. of Arnold OT)	Vagus	Somatic sensory	Filaments	Skin of auricle and external acoustic meatus

* Nerves to muscles contain proprioceptive sensory fibers in addition to motor fibers; muscular branches of third, fourth, sixth, seventh, and twelfth cranial nerves may be exceptions.

TABLE OF NERVES—(Continued)

Name	Central Attachment	Components	Branches	Distribution
Auricular, great (see Plate 16)	Second and third cervical segments (cervical plexus)	Somatic sensory	Auricular, facial, and mastoid branches	Skin about ear
Auricular, posterior	Facial	Motor	Filaments	Occipitalis and intrinsic muscles of auricle
Auriculotemporal	Mandibular	Somatic sensory	Filaments	Skin of scalp and temple
Axillary (circumflex OT; BR) (see Plate 16)	Fifth and sixth cervical segments of cord (brachial plexus)	Motor Somatic sensory	Muscular, articular, and cutaneous filaments Lateral cutaneous of arm	Deltoid and teres minor muscles Shoulder joint, skin of lateral aspect of shoulder and arm
Bell, N. of [OT]	See *Thoracic, long*			
Bigeminus [OT]	Old term for third sacral nerve			
Buccinator (buccal BR)	Mandibular	Somatic sensory	Filaments	Skin and mucosa of cheek
Calcanean	Medial sural	Somatic sensory	Filaments	Skin of heel
Cardiac, inferior	Inferior cervical ganglion	Sympathetic. Visceral sensory	To cardiac plexuses	Heart
Cardiac, inferior or thoracic	Vagus and recurrent laryngeal	Parasympathetic. Visceral sensory	To cardiac plexuses	Heart
Cardiac, middle	Middle cervical ganglion	Sympathetic. Visceral sensory	To cardiac plexuses	Heart
Cardiac, superior	Superior cervical ganglion	Sympathetic. Visceral sensory	To cardiac plexuses	Heart
Cardiac, superior or cervical	Vagus	Parasympathetic. Visceral sensory	To cardiac plexuses	Heart
Caroticotympanic (small deep petrosal OT) (1) Inferior (2) Superior	Sympathetic plexus on internal carotid artery	Sympathetic	Tympanic plexus	Filaments
Carotid, external	Superior cervical ganglion	Sympathetic	Plexuses on external carotid artery and its branches	Filaments to smooth muscle and glands of head
Carotid, internal	Superior cervical ganglion	Sympathetic	Plexuses on internal carotid artery and its branches. See *Petrosal, deep; Caroticotympanic*	Filaments to smooth muscle and glands of head
Cervical, first (anterior division) (suboccipital OT)	First cervical segment of cord	Motor	Fibers to descendens hypoglossi	Neck muscles

TABLE OF NERVES—(Continued)

Name	Central Attachment	Components	Branches	Distribution
Cervical, first (posterior division) (suboccipital OT)	First cervical segment of cord	Motor	Muscular	Deep muscles of back of neck
Cervical, second (anterior division)	Second cervical segment of cord	Motor. Somatic sensory	Fibers to descendens cervicis and to third cervical	Neck muscles
Cervical, second (posterior division)	Second cervical segment of cord	Motor. Somatic sensory	Greater occipital and communicating to third cervical	Deep muscles of back of neck and skin of back of neck
Cervical, third (anterior division)	Third cervical segment of cord	Motor. Somatic sensory	Lesser occipital, great auricular, supraclavicular, phrenic, and cutaneus colli	Levator scapulae, sternocleidomastoid, trapezius, scalenus medius, and scalenus posterior muscles; skin of neck
Cervical, third (posterior division)	Third cervical segment of cord	Motor. Somatic sensory	Third occipital, muscular	Deep muscles of neck; skin of back of neck
Cervical, fourth (anterior division)	Fourth cervical segment of cord	Motor. Somatic sensory	Phrenic, supraclavicular	Same as anterior division of third cervical
Cervical, fourth to eighth (posterior divisions)	Fourth to eighth cervical segments of cord	Motor. Somatic sensory	Muscular and cutaneous	Deep muscles of neck and upper portion of back; skin of upper back
Cervical, fifth to eighth (anterior divisions)	Fifth to eighth cervical segments of cord	Motor. Somatic sensory	Nerves of brachial plexus	Muscles and skin of upper extremity
Cervical, superficial [OT]	See *Cutaneus colli*			
Chorda tympani	Intermedius	Parasympathetic Sensory (taste)	Filaments	Sublingual and submaxillary salivary glands Taste buds of anterior two-thirds of tongue
Ciliary, long	Nasociliary	Somatic sensory	Filaments	Eyeball
Ciliary, short	Ciliary ganglion Nasociliary	Parasympathetic Somatic sensory	Filaments	Ciliary muscle and constrictor fibers of iris Eyeball
Circumflex [OT; BR]	See *Axillary*			
Cluneal, inferior (gluteal BR)	Posterior cutaneous n. of thigh	Somatic sensory	Filaments	Skin of lower gluteal region
Cluneal, medial (gluteal BR)	First, second, and third sacral (posterior divisions)	Somatic sensory	Filaments	Skin of medial portion of gluteal region
Cluneal, superior (gluteal BR)	First, second, and third lumbar (posterior divisions)	Somatic sensory	Filaments	Skin of upper portion of gluteal region

TABLE OF NERVES—(Continued)

Name	Central Attachment	Components	Branches	Distribution
Coccygeal	Coccygeal segment of cord	Somatic sensory	Anococcygeal	Skin over coccyx
Cochlear (see Plate 20)	Brain stem at lower border of pons	Sensory (hearing)	Filaments	Spiral organ (of Corti) of cochlea
Crural, anterior [OT]	See *Femoral*			
Cutaneous, anterior, of abdomen	Iliohypogastric	Somatic sensory	Filaments	Skin of lower anterior abdomen
Cutaneous, dorsal, of forearm	Radial	Somatic sensory	Filaments	Skin of lower portion of posterior aspect of arm and dorsal aspect of forearm
Cutaneous, dorsal, of hand	Ulnar	Somatic sensory	Filaments	Skin of medial portion of dorsal aspect of hand
Cutaneous, dorsal intermediate, of foot	Superficial peroneal	Somatic sensory	Filaments	Skin of dorsum of foot
Cutaneous, dorsal medial, of foot	Superficial peroneal	Somatic sensory	Filaments	Skin of dorsum of foot
Cutaneous, intermediate, of thigh	Femoral	Somatic sensory	Filaments	Skin of anterior aspect of thigh
Cutaneous, lateral, of arm (upper lateral cutaneous of upper arm BR) (see Plate 16)	Axillary	Somatic sensory	Filaments	Skin of lateral aspect of arm
Cutaneous, lateral, of forearm	Musculocutaneous	Somatic sensory	Filaments	Skin of lateral aspect of forearm
Cutaneous, lateral, of leg (lateral cutaneous of calf or lateral sural)	Common peroneal	Somatic sensory	Filaments	Skin of lateral aspect of leg
Cutaneous, lateral, of thigh (see Plate 16)	Second and third lumbar segments of cord (lumbar plexus)	Somatic sensory	Filaments	Skin of lateral aspect of thigh
Cutaneous, lateral palmar	Median	Somatic sensory	Digital branches	Skin of lateral portion of palm and fingers
Cutaneous, medial, of arm (lesser internal cutaneous OT)	First thoracic segment of cord (brachial plexus)	Somatic sensory	Filaments	Skin of medial aspect of arm
Cutaneous, medial, of forearm (internal cutaneous OT)	Eighth cervical and first thoracic segments of cord (brachial plexus)	Somatic sensory	Filaments	Skin of medial aspect of arm and forearm
Cutaneous, medial, of leg (medial sural) (tibial communicating OT) (sural BR)	Tibial	Somatic sensory	Filaments	Skin of medial aspect of leg
Cutaneous, medial, of thigh	Femoral	Somatic sensory	Filaments	Skin of posterior aspect of buttocks and medial aspect of thigh

TABLE OF NERVES—(Continued)

Name	Central Attachment	Components	Branches	Distribution
Cutaneous, medial palmar	Ulnar	Somatic sensory	Filaments. Digital	Skin of medial aspect of palm and fingers
Cutaneous, perforating (variable)	Second and third sacral segments of cord (pudendal plexus)	Somatic sensory	Filaments	Skin of posterior aspect of buttocks
Cutaneous, posterior, of arm	Radial	Somatic sensory	Filaments	Skin of posterior aspect of arm
Cutaneous, posterior, of thigh (small sciatic OT)	Second, third, and fourth sacral segments of cord (pudendal plexus)	Somatic sensory	Filaments	Skin of posterior aspect of buttocks, thigh, and perineum
Cutaneus colli (anterior cutaneous of neck BR) (superficial cervical OT)	Second and third cervical segments of cord (cervical plexus)	Somatic sensory	Filaments	Skin of anterior triangle of neck
Dental [OT; BR]	See *Alveolar*			
Descendens cervicis	Second and third cervical segments of cord (cervical plexus)	Motor	To ansa hypoglossi	Geniohyoid, thyrohyoid, sternothyroid, sternohyoid, and omohyoid muscles
Descendens hypoglossi	First and second cervical segments of cord (cervical plexus)	Motor	To ansa hypoglossi	Same as above
Digital (of fingers) (see Plate 16)	Median, ulnar, and superficial rami of radial	Somatic sensory	Filaments	Skin of digits
Digital (of toes) (see Plate 16)	Superficial peroneal, deep peroneal, medial plantar, and lateral plantar	Somatic sensory	Filaments	Skin of digits
Dorsal, of penis (clitoris)	Pudendal	Somatic sensory	Filaments	Skin of penis (clitoris)
Ethmoidal, anterior (internal nasal BR)	Nasociliary	Somatic sensory	External nasal, filaments	Mucosa of nasal cavity, mucosa of anterior ethmoidal air sinus
Ethmoidal, posterior	Nasociliary	Somatic sensory	Filaments	Mucosa of sphenoidal and posterior ethmoidal air sinuses
Facial (seventh cranial) (see Plates 16, 17, 20)	Brain stem at inferior border of pons	Motor	Stapedius, posterior auricular, temporal, zygomatic, buccal, mandibular, and cervical rami	Stapedius, stylohyoid, posterior belly of digastric, and muscles of facial expression
		Parasympathetic. Sensory (taste)	See *Intermedius*	

TABLE OF NERVES—(Continued)

Name	Central Attachment	Components	Branches	Distribution
Femoral (anterior crural OT) (see Plate 16)	Second, third, and fourth lumbar segments of cord (lumbar plexus)	Motor. Somatic sensory	Muscular, articular, saphenous, medial, and intermediate cutaneous of thigh	Pectineus, quadriceps femoris, articularis genus muscles; skin of anterior aspect of thigh and medial aspect of leg; hip and knee joints
Frontal (see Plate 16)	Ophthalmic	Somatic sensory	Supraorbital, supratrochlear, and nasociliary	Skin of upper eyelid, forehead, and scalp
Furcalis [OT]	Old term for fourth lumbar nerve			
Genitofemoral (genitocrural OT)	First and second lumbar segments of cord (lumbar plexus)	Somatic sensory	External spermatic and lumboinguinal	Skin of thigh and scrotum (labium majus)
Glossopalatine	See *Intermedius*			
Glossopharyngeal (ninth cranial) (see Plate 17)	Lateral aspect of medulla oblongata	Motor	Muscular, pharyngeal, tonsillar, lingual, tympanic	Stylopharyngeus and muscles of soft palate and pharynx via pharyngeal plexus;
		Visceral sensory		mucosa of posterior one-third of tongue, pharynx, middle ear and mastoid air cells;
		Sensory (taste)		taste buds of posterior one-third of tongue;
		Parasympathetic		parotid gland via otic ganglion
Gluteal [BR] **(cutaneous)**	See *Cluneal*			
Gluteal, inferior	Fifth lumbar, first and second sacral segments of cord (sacral plexus)	Motor	Filaments	Gluteus maximus muscle
Gluteal, superior	Fourth and fifth lumbar and first sacral segments of cord (sacral plexus)	Motor	Filaments	Gluteus medius and minimus and tensor fasciae latae muscles
Hamstrings, N. to	Fourth and fifth lumbar, upper 3 sacral segments of cord (sacral plexus)	Motor	Filaments	Biceps femoris, semimembranosus, semitendinosus, and adductor magnus muscles
Hemorrhoidal, inferior	Pudendal	Motor. Somatic sensory	Filaments	External anal sphincter; skin about anus
Hypogastric	Aortic plexus	Sympathetic	To pelvic plexus	Pelvic viscera
Hypoglossal (twelfth cranial) (see Plate 17)	Medulla oblongata	Motor	Filaments	Intrinsic and extrinsic muscles of tongue

TABLE OF NERVES—(Continued)

Name	Central Attachment	Components	Branches	Distribution
Iliohypogastric	First lumbar segment of cord (lumbar plexus)	Motor. Somatic sensory	Filaments	Muscles of anterior abdominal wall; skin of buttocks and anterior abdominal wall
Ilioinguinal	First lumbar segment of cord (lumbar plexus)	Motor. Somatic sensory	Anterior scrotal (labial). Filaments	Muscles of anterior abdominal wall; skin of anterior abdominal wall and scrotum (labium majus)
Infraorbital (see Plate 16)	Maxillary	Somatic sensory	Anterior and middle superior alveolar, inferior palpebral, external nasal, and superior labial	Upper teeth, mucosa of nasal floor, and skin of face
Infratrochlear	Nasociliary	Somatic sensory	Filaments	Skin of eyelids and root of nose
Intercostobrachial (intercostohumeral OT)	Second thoracic segment of cord (brachial plexus)	Somatic sensory	Filaments	Skin of axilla and medial aspect of arm
Intermedius (glossopalatine) (Wrisberg's OT) (see Plate 17)	Brain stem at inferior border of pons	Parasympathetic. Sensory (taste)	Greater superficial petrosal, chorda tympani, anastomotic ramus with tympanic plexus, external superficial petrosal (inconstant)	Glands of palate and nose, taste buds of anterior two-thirds of tongue, submaxillary and sublingual salivary glands
Interosseous, dorsal, of forearm (posterior interosseous OT; BR)	Radial	Motor. Somatic sensory	Muscular and articular filaments	Extensor carpi radialis brevis, supinator, extensor digitorum communis, extensor digiti quinti proprius, extensor carpi ulnaris; wrist joint
Interosseous, volar, of forearm (anterior interosseous OT; BR)	Median	Motor. Somatic sensory	Muscular and articular filaments	Flexor pollicis longus, flexor digitorum profundus, pronator quadratus; wrist joint
Jugular	Communicating branch of superior cervical ganglion to vagus			
Labial, inferior	Inferior alveolar	Somatic sensory	Filaments	Skin of lower lip
Labial, superior	Infraorbital	Somatic sensory	Filaments	Skin of upper lip and cheek
Lacrimal	Ophthalmic	Somatic sensory	Filaments	Skin of region of lateral commissure of eye

TABLE OF NERVES—(Continued)

Name	Central Attachment	Components	Branches	Distribution
Laryngeal, external [BR]	External branch of superior laryngeal nerve			
Laryngeal, inferior	Recurrent laryngeal	Motor	Filaments	Intrinsic muscles of larynx
Laryngeal, internal [BR]	Internal branch of superior laryngeal nerve			
Laryngeal, recurrent	Vagus	Motor. Parasympathetic	Inferior laryngeal, cardiac, and muscular	Intrinsic muscles of larynx, inferior constrictor of pharynx, trachea, and esophagus
Laryngeal, superior	Vagus	Motor. Visceral sensory	External and internal laryngeal branches	Cricothyroid and inferior constrictor of pharynx, mucosa of larynx, and base of tongue
Lingual	Mandibular	Somatic sensory	Filaments	Mucosa of floor of mouth and anterior two-thirds of tongue
Lumbar (5 pairs)	Lumbar segments of cord	Motor. Somatic sensory. Visceral sensory. Sympathetic (upper segments only)	Anterior and posterior divisions	Posterior divisions to muscles and skin of lower back; anterior divisions, lumbar plexus, to muscles and skin of lower abdomen and lower extremity, pelvic viscera, and genitalia
Lumboinguinal	Genitofemoral	Somatic sensory	Filaments	Skin of anterior aspect of thigh
Malar [OT]	See *Zygomaticofacial*			
Mandibular	Trigeminal	Motor (masticator n.). Somatic sensory	Spinosus, internal pterygoid, auriculotemporal, lingual, inferior alveolar, and branches to external pterygoid, temporal, and masseter muscles	Tensor tympani, tensor veli palatini, mylohyoid, anterior belly of digastric, and muscles of mastication; lower teeth, mucosa of anterior two-thirds of the tongue, floor of mouth, cheek and skin of lower portion of face, meninges
Masticator	Motor portion of trigeminal nerve			
Maxillary	Trigeminal	Somatic sensory	Middle meningeal, posterior superior alveolar, zygomatic, and infraorbital	Meninges, skin of upper portion of face, upper teeth, and mucosa of nose, palate, and cheeks

TABLE OF NERVES—(Continued)

NAME	CENTRAL ATTACHMENT	COMPONENTS	BRANCHES	DISTRIBUTION
Median (see Plate 16)	Fifth to eighth cervical and first thoracic segments of cord (brachial plexus)	Motor. Somatic sensory	Articular, muscular, and volar interosseous	Pronator teres, flexor carpi radialis, palmaris longus, flexor digitorum sublimis, flexor digitorum profundus, small muscles of thumb, two lateral lumbricals; skin of palm, hand, and fingers; elbow, wrist, and hand joints
Meningeal	Vagus	Somatic sensory	Filaments	Meninges
Meningeal, middle (recurrent OT)	Maxillary	Somatic sensory	Filaments	Meninges
Mental	Inferior alveolar	Somatic sensory	Filaments	Skin of lower lip and chin
Musculocutaneous (of lower extremity) [OT; BR]	See *Peroneal, superficial*			
Musculocutaneous (of upper extremity) (see Plate 16)	Fourth, fifth, and sixth cervical segments of cord (brachial plexus)	Motor. Somatic sensory	Lateral cutaneous of forearm, muscular	Coracobrachial, biceps brachii, and brachialis muscles; skin of lateral aspect of forearm
Musculospiral [OT]	See *Radial*			
Mylohyoid, N. to	Inferior alveolar	Motor	Filaments	Mylohyoid and anterior belly of digastric muscles
Nasal, external	Infraorbital	Somatic sensory	Filaments	Skin of side of nose
Nasal, external (anterior nasal OT)	Nasociliary	Somatic sensory	Filaments	Skin of lower half and tip of nose
Nasal, lateral	Nasociliary	Somatic sensory	Filaments	Mucosa of lateral wall of nasal cavity
Nasal, medial	Nasociliary	Somatic sensory	Filaments	Mucosa of nasal septum
Nasal, posterior inferior lateral	Great palatine	Somatic sensory	Filaments	Mucosa of inferior nasal concha
Nasal, posterior superior lateral (short sphenopalatine BR)	Maxillary via sphenopalatine ganglion	Somatic sensory	Filaments	Mucosa of superior and middle nasal conchae
Nasociliary (nasal OT)	Ophthalmic	Somatic sensory	Anterior and posterior ethmoidal, infratrochlear, medial nasal, lateral nasal, external nasal, long and short ciliary	Eyeball, skin and mucosa of eyelids and nose, mucosa of ethmoidal and sphenoidal air cells

TABLE OF NERVES—(Continued)

Name	Central Attachment	Components	Branches	Distribution
Nasopalatine (long sphenopalatine BR)	Maxillary via sphenopalatine ganglion	Somatic sensory	Posterior superior medial nasal rami	Mucosa of nose and hard palate
Obturator (see Plate 16)	Second, third, and fourth lumbar segments of cord (lumbar plexus)	Motor. Somatic sensory	Muscular, cutaneous, and articular filaments	Obturator externus, gracilis, adductor brevis, adductor longus, adductor magnus muscles; skin of medial aspect of thigh; knee and hip joints
Obturator, accessory (variable)	Second, third, and fourth lumbar segments of cord (lumbar plexus)	Motor. Somatic sensory	Muscular and cutaneous filaments	Pectineus muscle, reinforces obturator n.
Obturator internus, N. to	Fifth lumbar, first and second sacral segments of cord (sacral plexus)	Motor. Somatic sensory	Filaments	Obturator internus and superior gemellus muscles; sacroiliac joint
Occipital, greater (see Plate 16)	Second cervical segment of cord	Somatic sensory	Filaments	Skin of posterior portion of scalp
Occipital, lesser (see Plate 16)	Second and third cervical segments of cord (cervical plexus)	Somatic sensory	Filaments	Skin of posterior portion of scalp and posterior aspect of auricle
Occipital, third (occipital minimus OT)	Third cervical segment of cord	Somatic sensory	Filaments	Skin of posterior aspect of neck and scalp
Oculomotor (third cranial) (see Plates 17, 18)	Brain stem in region of posterior perforated substance	Motor. Parasympathetic	Muscular, root to ciliary ganglion	Levator palpebrae superioris, medial rectus, inferior rectus, superior rectus, inferior oblique muscles; ciliary and sphincter pupillae muscles
Olfactory (first cranial)	Olfactory bulb	Sensory (smell)	Filaments	Olfactory mucosa
Ophthalmic	Trigeminal	Somatic sensory	Tentorii, lacrimal, frontal, supratrochlear, nasociliary, communicating to oculomotor, trochlear, and abducens	Skin of forehead, upper eyelids, and anterior portion of scalp; orbit and eyeball; meninges; mucosa of nose, frontal, ethmoidal, and sphenoidal air sinuses
Optic (second cranial) (see Plates 18, 19)	Optic tracts	Sensory (sight)	Filaments	Retina
Orbital	Maxillary via sphenopalatine ganglion	Somatic sensory	Filaments	Orbit
Orbital [OT]	See *Zygomatic*			
Palatine, anterior (great palatine BR) (large posterior palatine OT)	Maxillary via sphenopalatine ganglion	Somatic sensory	Filaments	Mucosa of hard and soft palates

TABLE OF NERVES—(Continued)

NAME	CENTRAL ATTACHMENT	COMPONENTS	BRANCHES	DISTRIBUTION
Palatine, middle (external) (lesser palatine BR) (accessory posterior palatine OT)	Maxillary via sphenopalatine ganglion	Somatic sensory	Filaments	Mucosa of soft palate, uvula, and palatine tonsil
Palatine, posterior (lesser palatine BR) (small posterior palatine OT)	Maxillary via sphenopalatine ganglion	Somatic sensory	Filaments	Mucosa of soft palate, uvula, and palatine tonsil
Palpebral, inferior	Infraorbital	Somatic sensory	Filaments	Lower eyelid
Palpebral, superior	Lacrimal, frontal, and nasociliary	Somatic sensory	Filaments	Upper eyelid
Pathetic [OT]	See *Trochlear*			
Perineal	Pudendal	Motor. Somatic sensory	Filaments	Skin of root of penis and scrotum (labium majus)
Peroneal, anastomotic (communicating fibular OT)	Common peroneal	Somatic sensory	Filaments; fibers may unite with fibers of medial cutaneous of leg	Skin of lateral aspect of leg, heel, and ankle
Peroneal, common (lateral popliteal BR) (external popliteal OT) (see Plate 16)	Fourth and fifth lumbar, first and second sacral segments of cord (sacral plexus)	Motor. Somatic sensory	Articular, muscular, lateral cutaneous of leg, peroneal anastomotic, recurrent peroneal, deep peroneal, and superficial peroneal	Short head of biceps femoris, knee joint
Peroneal, deep (anterior tibial OT; BR)	Common peroneal	Motor. Somatic sensory	Muscular, articular, and cutaneous filaments	Tibialis anterior, extensor hallucis longus, extensor digitorum longus and brevis, and peroneus tertius muscles; skin of region between first and second toes; ankle joint and joints of feet
Peroneal, superficial (musculocutaneous OT; BR)	Common peroneal	Motor. Somatic sensory	Muscular and cutaneous filaments	Peroneus longus and peroneus brevis; skin of lower lateral aspect of leg and dorsum of foot
Petrosal, deep	Plexus on internal carotid artery	Sympathetic	N. of pterygoid canal	Along palatine branches of sphenopalatine ganglion
Petrosal, external superficial (inconstant)	Geniculate ganglion	Not known	Filaments	To plexus on middle meningeal artery
Petrosal, greater superficial	Geniculate ganglion	Visceral sensory. Parasympathetic	N. of pterygoid canal and on to sphenopalatine ganglion	Mucosa and glands of palate

TABLE OF NERVES—(Continued)

Name	Central Attachment	Components	Branches	Distribution
Petrosal, lesser superficial	Formed by union of anastomotic ramus from geniculate ganglion and tympanic branch of glossopharyngeal	Parasympathetic	To otic ganglion	Parotid gland
Petrosal, small deep [OT]	See *Caroticotympanic*			
Pharyngeal	Glossopharyngeal	Visceral sensory	Filaments	Mucosa of pharynx
Pharyngeal	Maxillary via sphenapolatine ganglion	Somatic sensory	Filaments	Mucosa of pharynx
Phrenic (see Plate 16)	Third, fourth, and fifth cervical (cervical plexus)	Motor	Filaments	Diaphragm
Piriformis, N. to	Fourth and fifth lumbar and first sacral segments of cord (sacral plexus)	Motor	Filaments	Piriformis
Plantar, lateral	Tibial	Motor. Somatic sensory	Muscular, cutaneous, and articular filaments	Quadratus plantae, adductor hallucis, small muscles of little toe, interossei, and lateral three lumbrical muscles of foot; skin of lateral aspect of sole; tarsal and metatarsal joints
Plantar, medial	Tibial	Motor. Somatic sensory	Muscular, cutaneous, and articular filaments	Abductor hallucis, flexor digitorum brevis, flexor hallucis brevis, and first lumbrical of foot; skin of medial aspect of sole; tarsal and metatarsal joints
Pneumogastric [OT]	See *Vagus*			
Popliteal, lateral [BR]	See *Peroneal, common*			
Popliteal, medial [BR]	See *Tibial*			
Pterygoid, external	Mandibular	Motor. Somatic sensory	Filaments	External pterygoid muscle; temporomandibular joint
Pterygoid, internal	Mandibular	Motor	Filaments	Internal pterygoid, tensor tympani, and tensor veli palatini muscles
Pterygoid canal, N. of (N. of Vidius OT)	Formed by union of greater superficial and deep petrosal nerves	Parasympathetic. Sympathetic	Filaments along branches of sphenopalatine ganglion	Glands of palate and nose

TABLE OF NERVES—(Continued)

NAME	CENTRAL ATTACHMENT	COMPONENTS	BRANCHES	DISTRIBUTION
Pudendal (pudic OT)	Second, third, and fourth sacral segments of cord (sacral plexus)	Motor. Somatic sensory	Inferior hemorrhoidal, perineal, and dorsal nn. of penis (clitoris)	Muscles and skin of perineal region
Quadratus femoris, N. to	Fourth and fifth lumbar and first sacral segments of cord (sacral plexus)	Motor. Somatic sensory	Filaments	Quadratus femoris and inferior gemellus; hip joint
Radial (musculospiral OT) (see Plate 16)	Fifth, sixth, seventh, and eighth cervical segments of cord (brachial plexus)	Motor. Somatic sensory	Muscular, superficial branch (radial OT), deep branch (posterior interosseous OT), dorsal interosseous, digital and articular	Triceps brachii, anconeus, extensor muscles of forearm, brachioradialis; skin of posterior aspect of arm and dorsal aspect of forearm and hand; elbow, carpal and hand joints
Recurrent	See *Laryngeal, recurrent*			
Recurrent [OT]	See *Spinosus*			
Recurrent [OT]	See *Tentorii*			
Rhomboids, N. to [OT; BR]	See *Scapular, dorsal*			
Saccular	Vestibular root of acoustic	Sensory (position of head in space—static)	Filaments	Macula acustica of saccule
Sacral (5 pairs)	Sacral segments of cord	Motor. Somatic sensory. Parasympathetic. Visceral sensory	Anterior and posterior divisions	Posterior divisions to muscles and skin of lower back and sacral region; anterior divisions to sacral plexus supplying muscles and skin of lower extremity and perineum; branches to hypogastric and pelvic plexuses supplying pelvic viscera and genitalia
Saphenous (see Plate 16)	Femoral	Somatic sensory	Filaments	Skin of medial aspect of leg and foot
Scapular, dorsal (N. to rhomboids OT; BR) (posterior scapular OT)	Fifth cervical segment of cord (brachial plexus)	Motor	Filaments	Levator scapulae, rhomboideus major, and rhomboideus minor
Sciatic (see Plate 16)	Fourth and fifth lumbar; first, second, and third sacral segments of cord (sacral plexus)	Composed of tibial, common peroneal, and n. to hamstrings		
Sciatic, small [OT]	See *Cutaneous, posterior, of thigh*			

TABLE OF NERVES—(Continued)

NAME	CENTRAL ATTACHMENT	COMPONENTS	BRANCHES	DISTRIBUTION
Scrotal, anterior (labial)	Ilioinguinal	Somatic sensory	Filaments	Skin of pubic area and scrotum (labium majus)
Scrotal, posterior (labial)	Perineal	Somatic sensory	Filaments	Skin of posterior portion of scrotum (labium majus)
Spermatic, external	Genitofemoral	Somatic sensory	Filaments	Skin of scrotum (labium majus) and thigh near superficial inguinal ring
Sphenopalatine	Maxillary	Somatic sensory	Nasal and palatine branches of sphenopalatine ganglion	Via sphenopalatine ganglion and palatine nerves to nose and palate
Sphenopalatine, long [BR]	See *Nasopalatine*			
Sphenopalatine, short [BR]	See *Nasal, posterior superior lateral*			
Spinal (31 pairs) (see Plate 17)	See *Cervical, Thoracic, Lumbar, Sacral*, and *Coccygeal*			
Spinal accessory [OT] (see Plate 17)	See *Accessory*			
Spinosus (recurrent OT)	Mandibular	Somatic sensory	Filaments	Meninges and mucosa of mastoid air cells
Splanchnic, greater	Fifth to ninth or tenth sympathetic ganglions	Sympathetic. Visceral sensory	Filaments	Cardiac, pulmonary, esophageal, and celiac plexuses
Splanchnic, lesser	Ninth and tenth sympathetic ganglions	Sympathetic. Visceral sensory	Filaments	Celiac plexus
Splanchnic, lowest	Last thoracic sympathetic ganglion	Sympathetic. Visceral sensory	Filaments	Renal plexus
Stapedius, N. to	Facial	Motor	Filaments	Stapedius muscle
Subclavius, N. to	Fourth, fifth, and sixth cervical (brachial plexus)	Motor	Filaments	Subclavius muscle
Subcostal [BR]	Anterior ramus of twelfth thoracic nerve			
Suboccipital [OT]	See *Cervical, first*			
Subscapular	Fifth and sixth cervical segments of cord (brachial plexus)	Motor	Filaments	Subscapularis and teres major muscles
Supraacromial [OT]	See *Supraclavicular, posterior*			

TABLE OF NERVES—(**Continued**)

Name	Central Attachment	Components	Branches	Distribution
Supraclavicular, anterior (medial supraclavicular BR) (suprasternal OT)	Third and fourth cervical segments of cord (cervical plexus)	Somatic sensory	Filaments	Skin of lower anterior aspect of neck and anterior chest wall; sternoclavicular joint
Supraclavicular, middle (intermediate supraclavicular BR) (supraclavicular OT)	Third and fourth cervical segments of cord (cervical plexus)	Somatic sensory	Filaments	Skin of lower anterior aspect of neck and anterior chest wall
Supraclavicular, posterior (lateral supraclavicular BR) (supraacromial OT)	Third and fourth cervical segments of cord (cervical plexus)	Somatic sensory	Filaments	Skin of lateral aspect of neck and shoulder
Supraorbital (see Plate 16)	Frontal	Somatic sensory	Filaments	Skin of upper eyelid and forehead, mucosa of frontal sinus
Suprascapular	Fourth, fifth, and sixth cervical segments of cord (brachial plexus)	Motor. Somatic sensory	Muscular and articular filaments	Supraspinatus and infraspinatus muscles; shoulder and acromioclavicular joints
Suprasternal [OT]	See *Supraclavicular, anterior*			
Supratrochlear	Frontal	Somatic sensory	Filaments	Skin of medial aspect of forehead, root of nose, and upper eyelid
Sural [BR]	Formed by union of medial sural and anastomotic ramus of common peroneal			
Sural, lateral (**lateral cutaneous n. of calf or leg**)	Common peroneal	Somatic sensory	Filaments	Skin of lateral aspect of leg
Sural, medial (tibial communicating OT)	Tibial	Somatic sensory	Cutaneous and articular filaments	Skin of back of leg; ankle and tarsal joints
Temporomalar [OT]	See *Zygomatic*			
Tentorii (recurrent OT)	Ophthalmic	Somatic sensory	Filaments	Meninges
Terminalis	Medial olfactory tract	Not known	Filaments associated with olfactory n.	Not known
Thoracic (12 pairs)	Thoracic segments of cord	Motor. Somatic sensory. Visceral sensory. Sympathetic	Anterior and posterior divisions	Posterior divisions to muscles and skin of back; anterior divisions to brachial plexus (muscles and skin of upper extremity) and muscles and skin of abdominal wall; sympathetic fibers and visceral sensory fibers for various viscera and blood vessels

TABLE OF NERVES—(Continued)

Name	Central Attachment	Components	Branches	Distribution
Thoracic, lateral anterior (lateral pectoral BR) (external anterior thoracic OT)	Fifth, sixth, and seventh cervical segments of cord (brachial plexus)	Motor	Filaments	Pectoralis major and minor muscles
Thoracic, long (N. to serratus anterior BR) (posterior thoracic OT) (N. of Bell OT)	Fifth, sixth, and seventh cervical segments of cord (brachial plexus)	Motor	Filaments	Serratus anterior muscle
Thoracic, medial anterior (medial pectoral BR) (internal anterior thoracic OT)	Eighth cervical and first thoracic segments of cord (brachial plexus)	Motor	Filaments	Pectoralis major and minor muscles
Thoracodorsal (long subscapular OT)	Sixth, seventh, and eighth cervical segments of cord (brachial plexus)	Motor	Filaments	Latissimus dorsi muscle
Tibial (internal popliteal OT) (medial popliteal BR) (see Plate 16)	Fourth and fifth lumbar and first, second, and third sacral segments of cord (sacral plexus)	Motor. Somatic sensory	Muscular, articular, medial sural, medial, and lateral plantar	Muscles of back of leg and sole of foot; skin of back of leg and foot; knee and ankle joints
Tibial, posterior [BR]	Posterior branch of tibial			
Tibial, recurrent	Common peroneal	Motor. Somatic sensory	Muscular and articular filaments	Tibialis anterior muscle; knee and proximal tibiofibular joints
Trigeminal (fifth cranial) (see Plate 17)	Brain stem at inferior surface of pons. See *Ophthalmic, Maxillary*, and *Mandibular*			
Trochlear (fourth cranial) (pathetic OT) (see Plate 17)	Dorsal surface of midbrain	Motor	Filaments	Superior oblique muscle of eyeball
Tympanic (N. of Jacobson OT)	Glossopharyngeal	Visceral sensory. Parasympathetic	Tympanic plexus	Mucosa of middle ear, mastoid air cells and auditory tube; filaments to otic ganglion and on to parotid gland
Ulnar (see Plate 16)	Eighth cervical and first thoracic segments of cord (brachial plexus)	Motor. Somatic sensory	Muscular, articular, and cutaneous filaments	Flexor carpi ulnaris, flexor digitorum profundus, adductor pollicis, muscles of hypothenar eminence, interossei and medial two lumbricals of hand; skin of medial portion of hand; elbow, wrist, carpal, and metacarpal joints
Ulnar, collateral (inconstant)	Radial	Proprioceptive	Filaments	Brachialis muscle

TABLE OF NERVES—(**Continued**)

NAME	CENTRAL ATTACHMENT	COMPONENTS	BRANCHES	DISTRIBUTION
Utricular	Vestibular	Sensory (position of head in space—static)	Filaments	Macula acustica of utricle
Vagus (**tenth cranial**) (pneumogastric OT) (see Plate 17)	Lateral aspect of medulla oblongata	Motor	Pharyngeal and laryngeal	Striate muscles of pharynx and larynx
		Parasympathetic	Cardiac, esophageal, and abdominal	Cardiac musculature, smooth muscle of thoracic and abdominal viscera
		Somatic sensory	Auricular (N. of Arnold OT), meningeal	Skin of external auditory meatus, meninges
		Visceral sensory	Pharyngeal, laryngeal, thoracic, and abdominal branches	Mucosa of pharynx, larynx, thoracic and abdominal viscera
Vestibular (**part of eighth cranial**) (see Plate 20)	Brain stem near restiform body	Sensory (movement and position of head in space—dynamic and static)	Utricular, ampullary, and saccular	Ampullae of semicircular canals and maculae acusticae of utricle and saccule
Vidius, N. of [OT]	See *Pterygoid canal, N. of*			
Wrisberg's [OT]	See *Intermedius*			
Zygomatic (temporomalar or orbital OT)	Maxillary	Somatic sensory	Zygomaticofacial and zygomaticotemporal	Skin in region of zygoma and temple
Zygomaticofacial (malar OT)	Zygomatic	Somatic sensory	Filaments	Skin over zygoma
Zygomaticotemporal (temporal OT)	Zygomatic	Somatic sensory	Filaments	Skin over anterior portion of temple

TABLE OF VEINS

(See Plates 9, 10)

The following list includes only those veins and venous sinuses and plexuses which have no accompanying artery of the same name, or which differ considerably from an accompanying artery. For all other veins—as, for example, the deep veins of the upper or lower extremity, or of the body wall—see the Table of Arteries for the accompanying artery of the same name; these veins have tributaries with the same distribution as the branches of the accompanying arteries.

Name of Vein	Region or Tributary Drained	Location	Drains into:
Accessory hemiazygos (v. hemiazygos accessoria BNA)	Three or four upper left intercostal spaces	Left side of vertebral column	Either azygos or hemiazygos
Anterior facial (v. facialis anterior BNA)	Continuation of angular vein	Anterior side of face	Joins with posterior facial to form common facial
Anterior jugular (v. jugularis anterior BNA)	Anterior part of neck	Near midline of neck	External jugular or subclavian
Azygos (v. azygos BNA)	Right chest wall; begins from ascending lumbar vein	Right side of vertebral column	Superior vena cava
Basilar plexus (plexus basilaris BNA)	Both inferior petrosal sinuses	Basilar part of occipital bone	Anterior part of vertebral plexus
Basilic (v. basilica BNA)	Ulnar side of hand and forearm	Medial side of biceps muscle	Joins the brachial to form the axillary
Basivertebral (vv. basivertebrales BNA)	Bodies of vertebrae	Bodies of vertebrae	External and internal vertebral plexuses
Cavernous sinus (sinus cavernosus BNA)	Superior ophthalmic	Lateral to sella turcica	Superior and inferior petrosal sinuses
Cephalic (v. cephalica BNA)	Radial side of hand and forearm	Lateral side of arm	Axillary
Common facial (v. facialis communis BNA)	Formed by junction of anterior and posterior facial veins	Below angle of mandible	Internal jugular
Coronary sinus (sinus coronarius BNA)	Most of the veins of the heart	Posterior part of coronary sulcus	Right atrium
Coronary v. of stomach (v. coronaria ventriculi BNA)	Both surfaces of stomach	Lesser curvature of stomach	Portal
Diploic veins (vv. diploicae BNA)	Diploë of cranium	Inside cranial bones	Either internally into the sinuses or externally into veins like the occipital or supraorbital
Emissary veins	Venous sinuses inside cranial cavity, such as the transverse sinus	Apertures in skull, named as follows according to location: condyloid, mastoid, occipital, parietal, and postcondyloid	Veins external to the skull, as the posterior auricular or occipital
External jugular (v. jugularis externa BNA)	Posterior auricular and posterior division of posterior facial	Side of neck	Subclavian
External vertebral plexus (plexus venosi vertebrales externi BNA)	Vertebrae and surrounding muscles	Anterior and posterior to vertebral column	Basivertebral and intervertebral veins
Great cardiac (v. cordis magna BNA)	Anterior side of ventricles	Anterior longitudinal sulcus of heart	Coronary sinus

TABLE OF VEINS—(Continued)

Name of Vein	Region or Tributary Drained	Location	Drains into:
Great cerebral (great v. of Galen) (v. cerebri magna [Galeni] BNA)	Internal cerebral veins	Below and behind splenium of corpus callosum	Straight sinus
Great saphenous (v. saphena magna BNA)	Medial side of leg and thigh	Medial side of leg and thigh	Femoral
Hemiazygos (v. hemiazygos BNA)	Left ascending lumbar	Left side of vertebral column	Azygos
Hemorrhoidal plexus (plexus haemorrhoidalis BNA)	Rectum	Rectum, submucosa, and external to muscular coat	Superior, middle, and inferior hemorrhoidal veins
Hepatic	Substance of the liver	Converge at posterior surface of liver	Inferior vena cava
Inferior ophthalmic (v. ophthalmica inferior BNA)	Lower part of orbit	Floor of orbit	Pterygoid plexus and cavernous sinus
Inferior petrosal sinus (sinus petrosus inferior BNA)	Cavernous sinus	Inferior petrosal sulcus	Internal jugular
Inferior sagittal sinus (sinus sagittalis inferior BNA)	Falx cerebri	Lower edge of falx cerebri	Straight sinus
Inferior vena cava (vena cava inferior BNA)	Common iliac veins, blood from lower extremities and abdomen	Front of vertebral column, right of aorta	Right atrium
Innominate (vv. anonymae dextra et sinistra BNA)	Internal jugular and subclavian	Root of neck	Superior vena cava
Intercavernous sinuses (anterior and posterior) (sinus intercavernosus anterior et posterior BNA)	Connect the two cavernous sinuses		
Internal cerebral (vv. cerebri internae BNA)	Terminal and choroid veins	Beneath splenium of corpus callosum	Great cerebral
Internal jugular (v. jugularis interna BNA)	Brain, face, and neck; transverse sinus	Side of neck	Innominate
Internal vertebral plexus (plexus venosi vertebrales interni BNA)	Vertebrae and meninges	Within the vertebral canal anterior and posterior to the spinal cord	Intervertebral veins
Middle cardiac (v. cordis media BNA)	Posterior side of heart	Posterior longitudinal sulcus of heart	Coronary sinus
Oblique v. of left atrium (oblique v. of Marshall OT) (v. obliqua atrii sinistri BNA)	Left atrium	Back of left atrium	Coronary sinus
Occipital sinus (sinus occipitalis BNA)	Region around foramen magnum	Attached margin of falx cerebelli	Confluence of the sinuses
Parumbilical (vv. parumbilicales [Sappeyi] BNA)	Commences at umbilicus	Round ligament of liver	Portal
Portal (v. portae BNA)	Superior mesenteric and lienal veins	Lesser omentum	Sinusoids of liver
Posterior facial (v. facialis posterior BNA)	Superficial temporal and internal maxillary veins	In parotid gland	Common facial and external jugular veins

TABLE OF VEINS—(Continued)

Name of Vein	Region or Tributary Drained	Location	Drains into:
Posterior v. of left ventricle (v. posterior ventriculi sinistri BNA)	Left ventricle	Diaphragmatic surface of left ventricle of heart	Coronary sinus
Prostatic plexus (plexus prostaticus BNA)	Prostatic veins	Fascial sheath of prostate gland	Pudendal and vesical plexuses
Pterygoid plexus (plexus pterygoideus BNA)	Veins corresponding to branches of internal maxillary artery	Between pterygoid muscles	Internal maxillary
Pudendal plexus (plexus pudendalis BNA)	Deep dorsal vein of penis	Behind symphysis pubis, in front of bladder	Vesical and hypogastric veins
Pyloric (v. coronaria ventriculi BNA)	Stomach	Lesser curvature of stomach	Portal
Sigmoid sinus (sinus transversus BNA)	Transverse sinus	Groove on posterior surface of temporal bone	Internal jugular
Small cardiac (v. cordis parva BNA)	Back of right atrium and ventricle	Coronary sulcus	Coronary sinus
Small saphenous (v. saphena parva BNA)	Leg and foot	Back of leg	Popliteal
Straight sinus (sinus rectus BNA)	Inferior sagittal sinus and great cerebral vein	Junction of falx cerebri with tentorium cerebelli	Transverse sinus
Superior ophthalmic (v. ophthalmica superior BNA)	Tributaries corresponding to branches of ophthalmic artery	Orbit	Cavernous sinus
Superior petrosal sinus (sinus petrosus superior BNA)	Cavernous sinus	Superior petrosal sulcus of temporal	Transverse sinus
Superior sagittal sinus (sinus sagittalis superior BNA)	Superior cerebral veins, diploic veins, and dura mater	Attached margin of falx cerebri	Confluence of the sinuses or transverse sinus
Superior vena cava (vena cava superior BNA)	Head, chest wall, and upper extremities; is formed by junction of two innominate veins	Behind first and second intercostal spaces and right margin of sternum	Right atrium
Transverse sinus (sinus transversus BNA)	The right one is usually continuation of the superior sagittal sinus, the left of the straight sinus	Attached margin of tentorium cerebelli	Internal jugular; the terminal portion is often called the sigmoid sinus
Vesical plexus (plexus vesicalis BNA)	Pudendal and prostatic plexuses	Lower part of bladder and base of prostate gland	Hypogastric
Vorticose (venae vorticosae BNA)	Veins of eyeball	Eyeball	Ciliary and superior ophthalmic veins

TABLE OF NORMAL VALUES OF BLOOD CONSTITUENTS

All values are expressed in mg. per 100 cc. of whole blood unless otherwise stated. Figures represent weighted averages of the observations of several investigators.

Acetone bodies, total (as acetone)	0.5–1.0
Albumin (serum)	3–6 Gm. %
Amino acids (as amino acid N)	5.0–8.0
Amylase (serum or plasma)	40–200 Somogyi units
Ascorbic acid (reduced)	0.6–2.5
Base, total (serum)	150–160 mEq./l.
Bilirubin (serum)	
Direct	0.0–0.4
Total	0.0–1.0
Calcium, total (serum)	9–11 4.5–5.5 mEq./l.
Carbon dioxide combining power (plasma)	55–75 vol. %
Carbon dioxide content (arterial)	45–55 vol. %
Carbon dioxide content (venous)	50–60 vol. % 22–27 mEq./l.
Carotene (plasma or serum)	0.1
Chlorides (as chloride ion) (plasma or serum)	350–380 97–106 mEq./l.
Chlorides as sodium chloride) (plasma or serum)	570–620
Cholesterol, total (plasma or serum)	150–250
Cholesterol esters	60–75% of total cholesterol
Creatine	3–7
Creatinine	1–2
Fat, neutral (serum)	0–370
Fatty acids	190–450
Fibrinogen (plasma)	0.2–0.4 Gm. %
Globulin (serum)	1.5–3 Gm. %
Glucose (Folin Wu method)	70–120
Guanidine	0.1–0.4
Hemoglobin	
For children	13 ± 1 Gm. %
For men	16 ± 2 Gm. %
For women	14 ± 2 Gm. %
Hydrogen-ion concentration	pH 7.3–7.5
Icterus index (serum)	4–6 units
Iodine (total)	3–13 micrograms %
Iron, inorganic (serum)	0.05–0.18
Ketone bodies (same as acetone bodies)	0.5–1.0
Lactic acid	5–20
Lipase (serum) in terms of N/20 NaOH used per cc. of serum	0.2–1 cc.
Lipids, total (serum)	400–800
Magnesium (serum)	1–3
Nitrogen, nonprotein	25–35
Nitrogen, undetermined	4–18
Oxygen capacity	16–24 vol. %
Oxygen content (arterial)	15–23 vol. %
Oxygen content (venous)	10–18 vol. %
Phenols (free)	1–2
Phosphatase (acid)	0.0–1.2 Bodansky units
Phosphatase (alkaline)	
For adults	1–5.4 Bodansky units
For children	5–12 Bodansky units
Phospholipid (serum) (as lecithin)	150–300
Phosphorus (serum), inorganic	
For adults	2.5–4.0
For children	3.5–6.0
Potassium (serum)	16–22 4–6 mEq./l.
Proteins (serum)	6–8 Gm. %
(Also see *Albumin, Globulin*)	
Sodium (serum)	310–335 133–145 mEq./l.
Solids, total	19–23%
Specific gravity	1.055
Specific gravity (plasma)	1.052–1.063
Sugar (see *Glucose*)	
Sulfates, inorganic as S (serum)	0.9–1.5
Urea	11–39
Urea nitrogen	5–18
Uric acid	2–4
Water content	77–81%

TABLE OF ELEMENTS

Name	Symbol	Atomic Weight*,†	Atomic Number
Actinium	Ac	227	89
Alabamine (now *astatine*)	Ab	[210]	85
Aluminum	Al	26.98	13
Americium	Am	[243]	95
Antimony (*stibium*)	Sb	121.76	51
Argentum. See *Silver*.			
Argon	A	39.944	18
Arsenic	As	74.91	33
Astatine (formerly *alabamine*)	At	[210]	85
Aurum. See *Gold*.			
Barium	Ba	137.36	56
Berkelium	Bk	[249]	97
Beryllium (formerly *glucinum*)	Be	9.013	4
Bismuth	Bi	209.00	83
Boron	B	10.82	5
Bromine	Br	79.916	35
Cadmium	Cd	112.41	48
Calcium	Ca	40.08	20
Californium	Cf	[249]	98
Carbon	C	12.011	6
Cerium	Ce	140.13	58
Cesium	Cs	132.91	55
Chlorine	Cl	35.457	17
Chromium	Cr	52.01	24
Cobalt	Co	58.94	27
Columbium (now *niobium*)	Cb	92.91	41
Copper (*cuprum*)	Cu	63.54	29
Cuprum. See *Copper*.			
Curium	Cm	[245]	96
Cyclonium (now *promethium*)	Cy	[145]	61
Dysprosium	Dy	162.51	66
Erbium	Er	167.27	68
Europium	Eu	152.0	63
Ferrum. See *Iron*.			
Florentium (now *promethium*)	Fl	[145]	61
Fluorine	F	19.00	9
Francium (formerly *virginium*)	Fr	[223]	87
Gadolinium	Gd	157.26	64
Gallium	Ga	69.72	31
Germanium	Ge	72.60	32
Glucinum. See *Beryllium*.			
Gold (*aurum*)	Au	197.0	79
Hafnium	Hf	178.50	72
Helium	He	4.003	2
Holmium	Ho	164.94	67
Hydrargyrum. See *Mercury*.			
Hydrogen	H	1.0080	1
Illinium (now *promethium*)	Il	[145]	61
Indium	In	114.82	49
Iodine	I	126.91	53
Iridium	Ir	192.2	77
Iron (*ferrum*)	Fe	55.85	26
Kalium. See *Potassium*.			
Krypton	Kr	83.80	36
Lanthanum	La	138.92	57
Lead (*plumbum*)	Pb	207.21	82
Lithium	Li	6.940	3
Lutetium	Lu	174.99	71
Magnesium	Mg	24.32	12
Manganese	Mn	54.94	25
Masurium (now *technetium*)	Ma	[99]	43
Mendelevium	Mv	[256]	101

* Weights as adopted by International Union of Pure and Applied Chemistry, 1955.

† A value in brackets denotes the mass number of the isotope of longest known half-life.

NOTE: At this time, elements 99 and 100 are reported as having been isolated. The mass number of each of their most stable isotopes known is 253 and 254, respectively.

TABLE OF ELEMENTS—(Continued)

NAME	SYMBOL	ATOMIC WEIGHT*,†	ATOMIC NUMBER
Mercury (*hydrargyrum*)	Hg	200.61	80
Molybdenum	Mo	95.95	42
Natrium. See *Sodium.*			
Neodymium	Nd	144.27	60
Neon	Ne	20.183	10
Neptunium	Np	[237]	93
Nickel	Ni	58.71	28
Niobium (formerly *columbium*)	Nb	92.91	41
Niton. See *Radon.*			
Nitrogen	N	14.008	7
Osmium	Os	190.2	76
Oxygen	O	16	8
Palladium	Pd	106.4	46
Phosphorus	P	30.975	15
Platinum	Pt	195.09	78
Plumbum. See *Lead.*			
Plutonium	Pu	[242]	94
Polonium	Po	210	84
Potassium (*kalium*)	K	39.100	19
Praseodymium	Pr	140.92	59
Promethium (formerly also *cyclonium, florentium, illinium*)	Pm	[145]	61
Protactinium	Pa	231	91
Radium	Ra	226.05	88
Radon	Rn	222	86
Rhenium	Re	186.22	75
Rhodium	Rh	102.91	45
Rubidium	Rb	85.48	37
Ruthenium	Ru	101.1	44
Samarium	Sm	150.35	62
Scandium	Sc	44.96	21
Selenium	Se	78.96	34
Silicon	Si	28.09	14
Silver (*argentum*)	Ag	107.880	47
Sodium (*natrium*)	Na	22.991	11
Stannum. See *Tin.*			
Stibium. See *Antimony.*			
Strontium	Sr	87.63	38
Sulfur, sulphur	S	32.066‡	16
Tantalum	Ta	180.95	73
Technetium (formerly *masurium*)	Tc	[99]	43
Tellurium	Te	127.61	52
Terbium	Tb	158.93	65
Thallium	Tl	204.39	81
Thorium	Th	232.05	90
Thulium	Tm	168.94	69
Tin (*stannum*)	Sn	118.70	50
Titanium	Ti	47.90	22
Tungsten (*wolfram*)	W	183.86	74
Uranium	U	238.07	92
Vanadium	V	50.95	23
Virginium (now *francium*)	Vi	[223]	87
Wolfram. See *Tungsten*			
Xenon	Xe	131.30	54
Ytterbium	Yb	173.04	70
Yttrium	Y	88.92	39
Zinc (*zincum*)	Zn	65.38	30
Zincum. See *Zinc.*			
Zirconium	Zr	91.22	40

* Weights as adopted by International Union of Pure and Applied Chemistry, 1955.

† A value in brackets denotes the mass number of the isotope of longest known half-life.

‡ Because of natural variations in the relative abundances of the isotopes of sulfur, the atomic weight of sulfur has a range of ±0.003.

NOTE: At this time, elements 99 and 100 are reported as having been isolated. The mass number of each of their most stable isotopes known is 253 and 254, respectively

TABLE OF ENZYMES*

Name and Class	Distribution	Substrate	End Products
Hydrolases			
Carbohydrases		Carbohydrates	
1. Amylases	Pancreas, saliva, malt, etc.	Starch, dextrin, etc.	Maltose and dextrins
2. Lactase	Intestinal juice and mucosa	Lactose	Dextrose and galactose
3. Maltase	Intestinal juice, yeast, etc.	Maltose	Dextrose
4. Saccharase (sucrase, invertase)	Intestinal juice, yeast, etc.	Sucrose	Dextrose and levulose
5. Emulsin (glucosidase)	Plants	β-Glucosides	Dextrose, etc.
6. Cellulase	Molds, bacteria, and snails	Cellulose	Various carbohydrate fragments
Nucleases		Nucleic acid and derivatives	
1. Polynucleotidase	Pancreatic juice, intestinal juice, etc.	Nucleic acid	Nucleotides
2. Nucleotidase	Intestinal juice, and other tissues	Nucleotides	Nucleosides and phosphoric acid
3. Nucleosidase	Animal tissues	Nucleosides	Carbohydrate and bases
Amidases		Amino compounds and amides	
1. Arginase	Liver	Arginine	Ornithine and urea
2. Urease	Bacteria, soybean, jack bean, etc.	Urea	Carbon dioxide and ammonia
3. Glutaminase	Liver, etc.	Glutamine	Glutamic acid and ammonia
4. Transaminase	Animal tissues	Glutamic acid and oxalacetic acid, etc.	α-Ketoglutaric acid, aspartic acid, etc.
Purine Deaminases		Purine bases and derivatives	
1. Adenase	Animal tissues	Adenine	Hypoxanthine and ammonia
2. Guanase	Animal tissues	Guanine	Xanthine and ammonia
Peptidases		Peptides	
1. Aminopolypeptidase	Yeast, intestines, etc.	Polypeptides	Simpler peptides and amino acids
2. Carboxypeptidase	Pancreas	Polypeptides	Simpler peptides and amino acids
3. Dipeptidase	Plant and animal tissues and bacteria	Dipeptides	Amino acids
4. Prolinase	Animal tissues and yeast	Proline peptides	Proline and simpler peptides
Proteinases		Proteins	
1. Pepsin	Gastric juice	Proteins	Proteoses, peptones, etc.
2. Trypsin	Pancreatic juice	Proteins, proteoses, and peptones	Polypeptides and amino acids
3. Cathepsin	Animal tissues	Proteins	Proteoses and peptones
4. Rennin	Calf stomach	Casein	Paracasein
5. Chymotrypsin	Pancreatic juice	Proteins, proteoses, and peptones	Polypeptides and amino acids
6. Papain	Papaya, other plants	Proteins, proteoses, and peptones	Polypeptides and amino acids
7. Ficin	Fig sap	Proteins	Proteoses, etc.
8. Enterokinase	Intestinal juice	Trypsinogen	Trypsin
Esterases		Esters	Alcohols and acids
1. Lipase	Pancreas, castor bean, etc.	Fats	Glycerol and fatty acids
2. Esterases	Liver, etc.	Ethyl butyrate, etc.	Alcohols and acids
3. Phosphatases	Plant and animal tissues	Esters of phosphoric acid	Phosphate and alcohol

* Modified from Hawk, Oser, and Summerson's *Practical Physiological Chemistry*, 13th ed., New York, Blakiston Division, McGraw-Hill Book Company, Inc.

TABLE OF ENZYMES—(Continued)

Name and Class	Distribution	Substrate	End Products
Esterases (Continued)			
4. Sulfatases.............	Animal and plant tissues	Esters of sulfuric acid	Sulfuric acid and alcohol
5. Cholinesterase.........	Blood	Acetylcholine	Choline and acetic acid
6. Cholineacetylase.......	Brain and other animal tissues	Choline	Acetylcholine
7. Lecithinases...........	Kidney, brain, intestinal mucosa, and snake venom	Lecithin	Diglycerides, choline, and phosphate
Iron Enzymes			
1. Catalase..............	All living organisms except a few species of microorganisms	Hydrogen peroxide	Water and oxygen
2. Cytochrome oxidase....	All living organisms except a few species of microorganisms	Reduced cytochrome C in the presence of oxygen	Oxidized cytochrome C and water
3. Peroxidase............	Nearly all plant cells	A large number of phenols, aromatic amines, etc., in the presence of H_2O_2	Oxidation product of substrate and water
Copper Enzymes			
1. Tyrosinase (polyphenol oxidase, monophenol oxidase)	Plant and lower animal tissues	Various phenolic compounds	Oxidation product of substrate
2. Ascorbic acid oxidase...	Plant tissues	Ascorbic acid in the presence of oxygen	Dehydroascorbic acid
Enzymes Containing Coenzymes I and/or II			
1. Alcohol dehydrogenase	Animal and plant tissues	Ethyl alcohol and other alcohols	Acetaldehyde and other aldehydes
2. Malic dehydrogenase...	Animal and plant tissues	*l*(−)Malic acid	Oxalacetic acid
3. Isocitric dehydrogenase	Animal and plant tissues	*l*-Isocitric acid	Oxalosuccinic acid
4. Lactic dehydrogenase...	Animal tissues and yeast	Lactic acid	Pyruvic acid
5. β-Hydroxybutyric dehydrogenase	Liver, kidneys, and heart	*l*-β-Hydroxybutyric acid	Acetoacetic acid
6. Glucose dehydrogenase	Animal tissues	*d*-Glucose	*d*-Gluconic acid
7. Robison ester dehydrogenase	Erythrocytes and yeast	Robison ester (hexose-6-phosphate)	Phosphohexonic acid
8. Glycerophosphate dehydrogenase	Animal tissues	Glycerophosphate	3-Phosphoglyceric aldehyde
Enzymes Which Reduce Cytochrome			
1. Succinic dehydrogenase (as ordinarily prepared)	Plants, animals, and microorganisms	Succinic acid	Fumaric acid
Yellow Enzymes			
1. Warburg's old yellow enzyme	Yeast	Reduced coenzyme II	Oxidized coenzyme II and reduced yellow enzyme
2. Diaphorase............	Bacteria, yeasts, higher plants, and animals	Reduced coenzyme I	Oxidized coenzyme I and reduced diaphorase
3. Haas enzyme..........	Yeast	Reduced coenzyme II	Oxidized coenzyme II and reduced yellow enzyme
4. Xanthine oxidase.......	Animal tissues	Hypoxanthine, xanthine, aldehydes, reduced coenzyme I, etc.	Xanthine, uric acid, acids, oxidized coenzyme I, etc. In presence of air, H_2O_2
5. D-Amino acid oxidase...	Animal tissues	D-Amino acids + O_2	α-Keto-acids + NH_3 + H_2O_2

TABLE OF ENZYMES—(Continued)

Name and Class	Distribution	Substrate	End Products
Yellow Enzymes (Continued)			
6. L-Amino acid oxidases..	Animals and snake venom	L-Amino acids	Keto acids and ammonia
7. TPN-Cytochrome C reductase	Yeast and liver	Reduced coenzyme II and cytochrome C	Oxidized coenzyme II and reduced cytochrome C
8. DPN-Cytochrome C reductase	Liver and yeast	Reduced coenzyme I and cytochrome C	Oxidized coenzyme I and reduced cytochrome C
Hydrases			
1. Fumarase............	Living organisms in general	Fumaric acid + H_2O	L-Malic acid
2. Aconitase............	Animals and plants	Citric acid	*cis*-Aconitic acid and L-isocitric acid
3. Enolase............	Animal tissues and yeast	2-Phosphoglyceric acid	Phosphopyruvic acid + H_2O
4. Aspartase............	Bacteria	Aspartic acid	Fumaric acid and ammonia
5. Serine deaminase.......	Animal tissues	Serine	Pyruvic acid and ammonia
Mutases			
1. Aldehyde mutase.......	Liver and yeast	2 Acetaldehyde + H_2O	Acetic acid and ethyl alcohol
2. Glyoxalase...........	Living organisms in general	Methylglyoxal and other substituted glyoxals	D(−)Lactic acid
Desmolases			
1. Zymohexase (aldolase)..	All cells	Fructose-1,6-diphosphate	Dihydroxyacetone phosphoric acid and phosphoglyceric acid
2. Carboxylase..........	Plant tissues	Pyruvic acid	Acetaldehyde and CO_2
3. β-Keto carboxylases....	Animals, bacteria, and plants	β-Keto acids	α-Keto acids
4. Amino acid decarboxylases	Plants, animals, and bacteria	L-Amino acids	Amines and CO_2
5. Carbonic anhydrase....	Erythrocytes	Carbonic acid	CO_2 + H_2O
Other Enzymes			
1. Phosphorylase.........	Animal and plant tissues	Starch or glycogen and phosphate	Glucose-1-phosphate
2. Phosphohexoisomerase .	Animal and plant tissues	Glucose-6-phosphate	Fructose-6-phosphate
3. Hexokinase...........	Yeast and animal tissues	Adenosinetriphosphate + glucose	Adenosinediphosphate + glucose-6-phosphate
4. Phosphoglucomutase ...	Plants and animals	Glucose-1-phosphate	Glucose-6-phosphate

TABLE OF HORMONES

A. Steroid Hormones

Hormone	Source	Physiologic Action	Structure
Testosterone	Testis	Androgenic	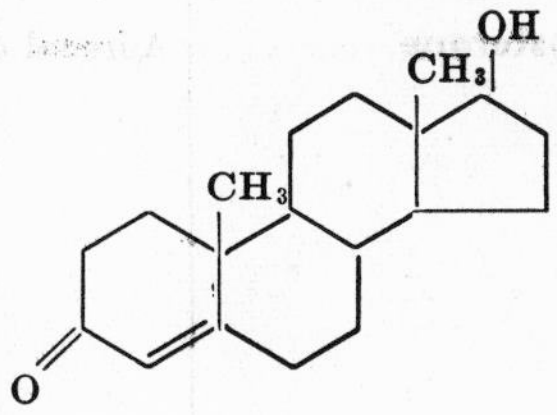
Adrenosterone	Adrenal cortex	Androgenic	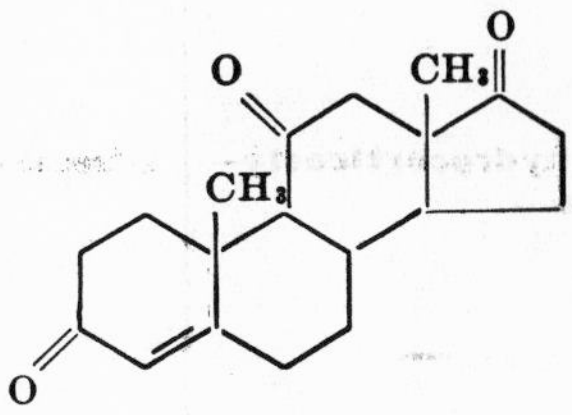
Estrone	Ovary Placenta Adrenal cortex	Estrogenic	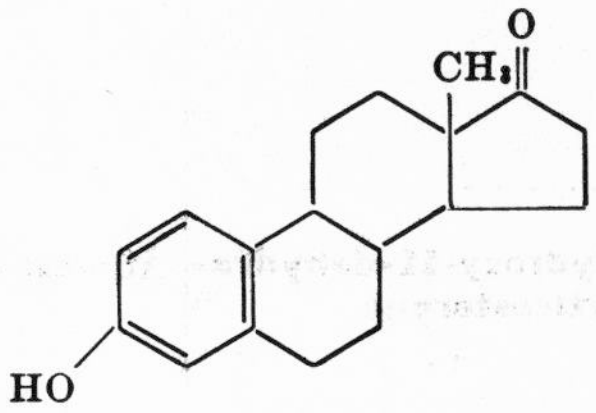
Estriol	Placenta	Estrogenic	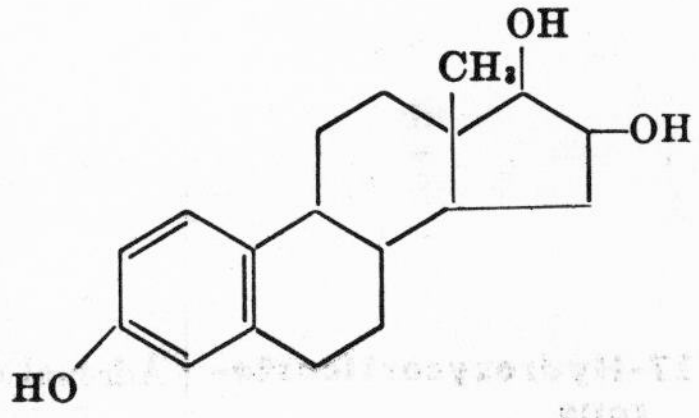
Estradiol	Ovary Placenta	Estrogenic	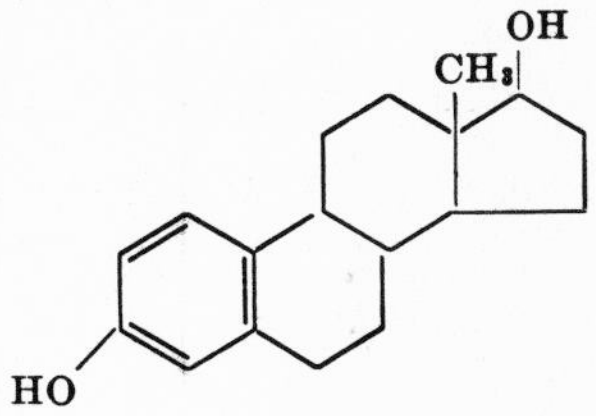
Progesterone	Placenta Corpus luteum Adrenal cortex	Progestational activity	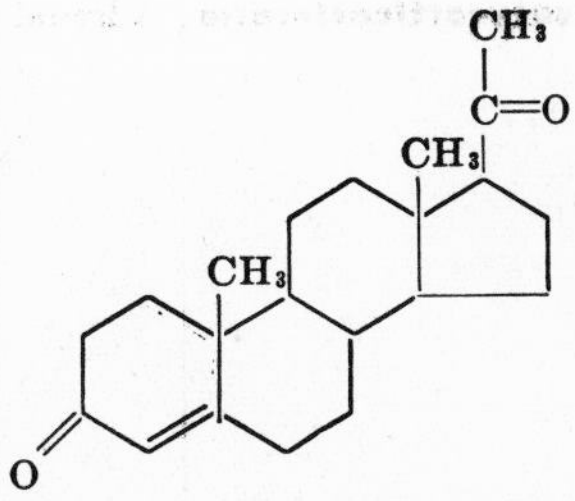

TABLE OF HORMONES—(Continued)

A. Steroid Hormones—(Continued)

Hormone	Source	Physiologic Action	Structure
Corticosterone	Adrenal cortex	Effects in adrenalectomized animals: 1. Maintains life 2. Influences carbohydrate metabolism 3. Protects against stress, such as poisons, cold, heat, etc. 4. Influence on electrolyte metabolism 5. Influence on muscular efficiency	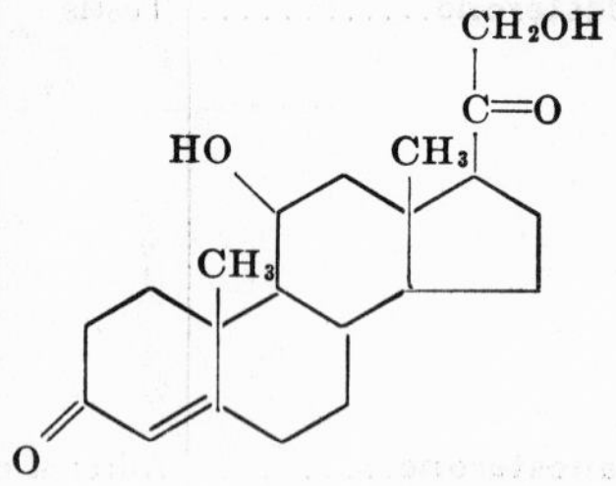
11-Dehydrocorticosterone	Adrenal cortex	See *Corticosterone*	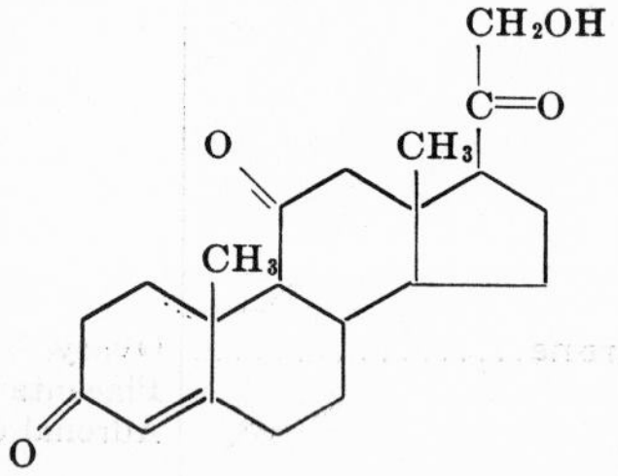
17-Hydroxy-11-dehydrocorticosterone	Adrenal cortex	See *Corticosterone* Antiarthritic (?)	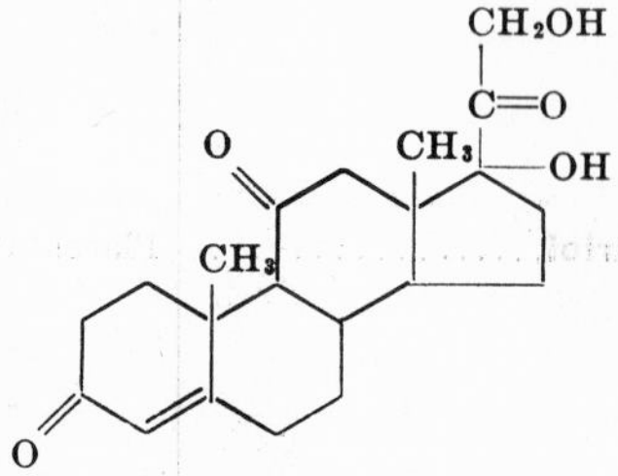
17-Hydroxycorticosterone	Adrenal cortex	See *Corticosterone*	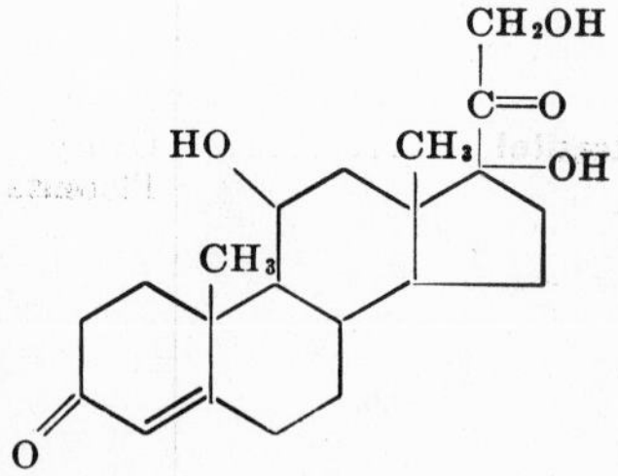
11-Desoxycorticosterone	Adrenal cortex	Effects in adrenalectomized animals: 1. Maintains life 2. Influence on electrolyte metabolism	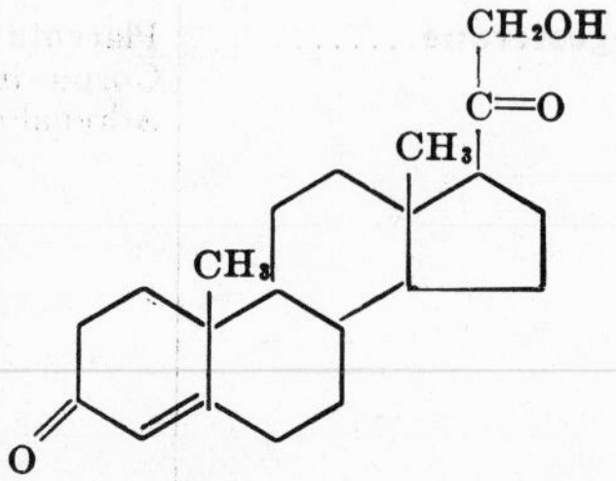

TABLE OF HORMONES—(Continued)

A. Steroid Hormones—(Continued)

Hormone	Source	Physiologic Action	Structure
17-Hydroxy-11-desoxy-corticosterone	Adrenal cortex	See *11-Desoxycorticosterone*	(structural formula: CH_2OH, C=O, CH_3, OH, CH_3, O)
Aldosterone .... **(Electrocortin)**	Adrenal cortex	1. In very small amounts, maintains life of adrenalectomized animals 2. Potent regulator of metabolism of sodium and potassium 3. Less effective regulator of carbohydrate metabolism	(structural formula: CH_2OH, C=O, HO, OCH, CH_3, O)

B. Protein and Protein-derivative Hormones

Hormone	Source	Physiologic Action	Molecular Weight	Presence of Carbohydrate
Luteinizing hormone (LH)	Anterior pituitary	Stimulates interstitial cells. Produces corpora lutea	100,000 (Hog) 40,000 (Sheep)	Present
Follicle-stimulating hormone (FSH)	Anterior pituitary	*Male:* Increase in size of testes and stimulates spermatogenesis *Female:* Increase in size of ovary and follicular growth	..	Present
Pregnant mare's serum hormone (PMS)	Placenta	Produces effects of both LH and FSH	30,000?	Present
Prolactin	Anterior pituitary	Produces lactation after previous alveolar development	32,000	Absent
Growth hormone	Anterior pituitary	A factor in somatic growth	44,000	Absent
Thyrotropic hormone	Anterior pituitary	Regulation of thyroid	10,000 (Beef) 35,000 (Sheep)	..
Adrenotropic hormone	Anterior pituitary	Regulation of adrenal cortex	20,000 (Hog and Sheep)	Absent
Oxytocin	Posterior pituitary	Oxytocic activity Milk-ejecting activity	1,007	Absent
Vasopressin	Posterior pituitary	Antidiuretic activity Pressor activity	1,084? (Beef)	Absent
Parathyroid hormone (parathyrin)	Parathyroid	Control of calcium and phosphorus metabolism	..	Absent
Insulin	Pancreas	Regulates oxidation of carbohydrates in tissues and storage of glycogen in liver	12,000?	Absent

TABLE OF HORMONES—(Continued)

B. Protein and Protein-derivative Hormones—(Continued)

Hormone	Source	Physiologic Action	Molecular Weight	Presence of Carbohydrate
Epinephrine	Adrenal medulla	Sympathomimetic activity	183.2	Absent
Thyroxin	Thyroid	Controls metabolic rate, etc.	776.9	Absent
Diiodotyrosine	Thyroid	See *Thyroxin*	433.0	Absent
Thyroglobulin	Thyroid	See *Thyroxin*	675,000	Absent
Secretin	Intestinal mucosa	Stimulates flow of pancreatic juice	..	..
Cholecystokinin	Intestinal mucosa	Stimulates contraction of gallbladder	..	..
Enterogastrone	Intestinal mucosa	Inhibits contractions and secretion of stomach	..	..
Enterocrinin	Intestinal mucosa	Stimulates secretion of glands of small intestine	..	..

TABLE OF RADIOACTIVE AND OTHER ISOTOPES COMMONLY USED IN MEDICINE*

Name and Symbol†	Radiation: Type and Energy‡	Radioactive Half-life	Medical Uses
Deuterium (hydrogen, heavy) $_1H^2$	None; naturally occurring		*Investigative:* tracer studies
Tritium $_1H^3$	Beta (0.02)	12.5 years	*Investigative:* tracer studies
Carbon 13 $_6C^{13}$	None; naturally occurring		*Investigative:* tracer studies
Carbon 14 $_6C^{14}$	Beta (0.154)	5,700 years	*Investigative:* tracer studies
Nitrogen 15 $_7N^{15}$	None; naturally occurring		*Investigative:* tracer studies
Oxygen 18 $_8O^{18}$	None; naturally occurring		*Investigative:* tracer studies
Sodium 24 $_{11}Na^{24}$	Beta (1.39) Gamma (1.38, 2.76)	14.9 hours	*Diagnostic:* study of peripheral vascular disease, extracellular fluid volume, formation of cerebrospinal fluid, and sodium metabolism
Phosphorus 32 $_{15}P^{32}$	Beta (1.71)	14.3 days	*Therapeutic:* chronic myeloid leukemia, polycythemia vera, lymphomas, and widespread carcinomatosis *Diagnostic:* determination of blood volume; study of peripheral vascular disease; localization of brain tumors
Sulfur 35 $_{16}S^{35}$	Beta (0.167)	87.1 days	*Investigative:* tracer studies
Potassium 42 $_{19}K^{42}$	Beta (3.56, 2.04) Gamma (1.51)	12.5 hours	*Diagnostic:* localization of brain tumors; determination of intracellular fluid volume; study of potassium metabolism
Chromium 51 $_{24}Cr^{51}$	Gamma (0.32)	26 days	*Diagnostic:* study of blood volume with radioactively labeled erythrocytes
Iron 59 $_{26}Fe^{59}$	Beta (0.26, 0.46) Gamma (1.1, 1.3)	46 days	*Diagnostic:* study of blood volume, iron metabolism, and blood transfusion
Cobalt 60 $_{27}Co^{60}$	Beta (0.31) Gamma (1.17, 1.33)	5.2 years	*Therapeutic:* source of teleoroentgen therapy and interstitial radiation for malignancies sensitive to gamma radiation
Strontium 90 $_{38}Sr^{90}$	Beta (0.65)	25 years	*Therapeutic:* benign conditions of the eye such as pterygia, traumatic corneal ulceration, corneal scars, vernal conjunctivitis, and hemangioma of the eyelid and in preparation for corneal transplant
Ruthenium 106 $_{44}Ru^{106}$	Beta (0.04)	330 days	*Therapeutic:* same as *strontium 90*

TABLE OF RADIOACTIVE AND OTHER ISOTOPES COMMONLY USED IN MEDICINE*—(Continued)

Name and Symbol†	Radiation: Type and Energy‡	Radioactive Half-life	Medical Uses
Iodine 131 $_{53}I^{131}$	Beta (0.60, 0.3) Gamma (0.364, 0.636, 0.284, 0.080)	8 days	*Therapeutic:* cancer of the thyroid, hyperthyroidism, and severe heart disease *Diagnostic:* study of thyroid and antithyroid drugs; determination of thyroid activity When incorporated in diiodofluorescein, used to localize brain tumors With iodinated serum globulin, studies of blood volume, cardiac output
Gold 198 $_{79}Au^{198}$	Beta (0.965) Gamma (0.411)	2.69 days	*Therapeutic:* widespread abdominal carcinomatosis with ascites; carcinomatosis of the pleural cavity; lymphomas; and lymphatic metastases from other malignant tumors
Lead 210 (radium D) $_{82}Pb^{210}$	Beta (0.028) Gamma (0.046, 0.0078, 0.0258) Naturally occurring	22 years	*Therapeutic:* same as *strontium 90*
Radon $_{86}Rn^{222}$	Alpha (5.486) Naturally occurring	3.8 days	*Therapeutic:* treatment of malignancies by interstitial radiation; used in cancer of uterine cervix and fundus, oral pharynx, urinary bladder, skin, and in metastatic cancer of the lymph nodes
Radium $_{88}Ra^{226}$	Alpha (4.79, 4.61) Gamma (0.19) Naturally occurring	1,620 years	*Therapeutic:* same as *radon*

* This table is organized on the basis of atomic number. See Table of Elements (pages 1426–1427) for the atomic number of any element in question.

† The subscript preceding the nomial abbreviation is the atomic number of the isotope. The superscript following the nomial abbreviation is the atomic weight; in common practice, it is this number which characterizes the isotope, thus $_6C^{14}$ is often called carbon 14.

‡ Alpha (α) radiation refers to emission of helium nuclei consisting of two protons and two neutrons; beta (β) radiation refers to emission of electrons; gamma (γ) radiation refers to emission of gamma rays. The energy of the characteristic radiation is given in million electron volts (mev); two or more values indicate two or more components of the radiation.

TABLE OF MEDICAL SIGNS AND SYMBOLS

āā, āa	of each
A, Å	angstrom unit
C′	complement
E_0	electroaffinity
F_1	first filial generation
F_2	second filial generation
L_+	limes death
L_0	limes zero
Q_{O_2}	oxygen consumption
m-	meta-
o-	ortho-
p-	para-
℞	[*L. recipe*]. Take
S.	[*L. signa*]. Write
c̄, c	[*L. cum*]. With
s̄s̄, ss	[*L. semis*]. One-half
m̄, M̶	[*L. misce*]. Mix
O.	[*L. octarius*]. Pint
C.	[*L. congius*]. Gallon
C.	Centigrade
F.	Fahrenheit
°	degree
♏	minim
℈	scruple
ʒ	drachm (apothecaries')
fʒ	fluidrachm
oz.	ounce (avoirdupois)
℥	ounce (troy)
f℥	fluidounce
μ	micron
$\mu\mu$	micromicron

σ	1/1000 of a second
π	3.1416—ratio of circumference of a circle to its diameter
lb.	pound (usually avoirdupois)
℔.	pound (usually apothecaries')
Gm.	gram
mEq.	milliequivalent
®	registered trade-mark status
mg. %	milligrams per cent
vol. %	volume per cent
mμ	millimicron, micromillimeter
μg.	microgram
cm.	centimeter
cc.	cubic centimeter
l.	liter
ml.	milliliter
gr.	grain
□, ♂	male
○, ♀	female
*	birth
†	death
−	negative
+	positive
±	either positive or negative, not definite
⇋	denotes a reversible reaction
#	number
^	value considered as a vector in electrocardiography
w/v	weight in volume

TABLE OF THE MOST COMMON MICROORGANISMS PATHOGENIC TO MAN

A. Bacteria (See Plate 30)

Name	Resulting Disease
Bacillus anthracis	Anthrax
Bartonella bacilliformis	Oroya fever
Borrelia duttonii	Tick-borne relapsing fever
Borrelia recurrentis	Louse-borne relapsing fever
Borrelia vincentii	Vincent's angina
Brucella abortus **Brucella melitensis** **Brucella suis**	Undulant fever
Clostridium botulinum	Botulism Food poisoning
Clostridium septicum	Gas gangrene
Clostridium tetani	Lockjaw Tetanus
Clostridium welchii	Gas gangrene
Corynebacterium diphtheriae	Diphtheria
Coxiella burnetii	Q fever
Diplococcus pneumoniae	Lobar pneumonia
Eberthella typhosa	Typhoid fever
Escherichia coli	Peritonitis Urinary-tract infection
Fusobacterium plauti-vincenti	Vincent's angina
Gaffkya tetragena	Pus producer
Hemophilus ducreyi	Chancroid
Hemophilus influenzae	Acute respiratory infections Conjunctivitis Influenzal meningitis
Hemophilus pertussis	Whooping cough
Klebsiella pneumoniae	Lobar pneumonia
Leptospira icterohaemorrhagiae	Spirochetal jaundice
Malleomyces mallei	Glanders
Micrococcus albus **Micrococcus aureus**	Local suppurative inflammation, occasionally generalized
Moraxella lacunata	Conjunctivitis
Mycobacterium leprae	Leprosy
Mycobacterium tuberculosis	Tuberculosis
Neisseria gonorrhoeae	Arthritis Cervicitis Conjunctivitis Urethritis
Neisseria meningitidis	Epidemic cerebrospinal meningitis
Pasteurella pestis	Plague
Pasteurella tularensis	Tularemia
Proteus vulgaris	Internal infection (secondary invader)
Pseudomonas aeruginosa	Wound infections (usually as secondary invader)

TABLE OF THE MOST COMMON MICROORGANISMS PATHOGENIC TO MAN—(Continued)

A. Bacteria—(Continued)

Name	Resulting Disease
Rickettsia prowazekii	Typhus fever
Rickettsia quintana	Trench fever
Rickettsia rickettsii	Rocky Mountain spotted fever
Rickettsia tsutsugamushi	Tsutsugamushi disease
Salmonella choleraesuis **Salmonella enteritidis** **Salmonella typhimurium**	Food poisoning Gastroenteritis Paratyphoid fever
Salmonella schottmuelleri	Paratyphoid fever
Shigella dysenteriae **Shigella paradysenteriae** **Shigella sonnei**	Bacillary dysentery
Spirillum minus	Rat-bite fever
Streptococcus mitis	Subacute bacterial endocarditis Local suppurative inflammation
Streptococcus pyogenes	Septic sore throat Scarlet fever Local and generalized suppurative inflammation
Treponema carateum	Pinta
Treponema pallidum	Syphilis
Treponema pertenue	Yaws
Vibrio comma	Cholera

B. Fungi

Name	Resulting Disease
Actinomyces bovis Also called *ray fungus*	Actinomycosis Streptothricosis
Aspergillus fumigatus	Aspergillosis
Blastomyces dermatitidis	North American blastomycosis Gilchrist's disease
Candida albicans Also called *thrush fungus*	Thrush
Coccidioides immitis	Coccidioidomycosis San Joaquin Valley fever
Cryptococcus histolyticus Also called *Torula histolytica*	Cryptococcosis (torulosis)
Epidermophyton	Dermatophytosis Tinea
Histoplasma capsulatum	Histoplasmosis
Microsporum	Dermatophytosis
Sporotrichum schencki	Sporotrichosis
Trichophyton	Dermatophytosis

TABLE OF THE MOST COMMON MICROORGANISMS PATHOGENIC TO MAN—(Continued)

C. Protozoa

Name	Resulting Disease
Endamoeba histolytica	Amebic dysentery
Leishmania braziliensis	Mucocutaneous leishmaniasis Leishmaniasis americana
Leishmania donovani	Visceral leishmaniasis Kala-azar
Leishmania tropica	Cutaneous leishmaniasis Oriental sore Delhi boil
Plasmodium falciparum	Malignant tertian malaria Estivo-autumnal malaria
Plasmodium malariae	Quartan malaria
Plasmodium vivax	Benign tertian malaria
Toxoplasma gondii	Encephalomyelitis Toxoplasmosis
Trichomonas vaginalis	Vaginitis
Trypanosoma cruzi	American trypanosomiasis Chagas' disease
Trypanosoma gambiense	Gambian trypanosomiasis Mid-African sleeping sickness
Trypanosoma rhodesiense	East African sleeping sickness

TABLE OF REPRESENTATIVE MONSTROSITIES AND ANOMALIES (TERATA)*

(See Plate 25)

Type, or Parts Involved	Name, or Examples (Synonymous Terms in Parentheses)
Single Individual Involved:	
1. Affecting the whole, or nearly the whole, body	Pantasomatous terata
Excessive size	Gigantism (Macrosomia)
Markedly less than normal size	Dwarfism (Microsomia; Nanism; Nanosomia)
Marked discrepancy of size of lateral halves of body	Hemihypertrophy. Hemiatrophy
Altered form of whole body	Fetus cylindricus. Fetus papyraceus. Lithopedion. Achondroplasia (Chondrodystrophy)
Anomalies of color (pigmentation):	
Complete or partial deficiency	Albinism
Generalized or local excess	Melanism
2. Affecting regions, parts, or organs	Merosomatous terata
Cranium and contents:	
Cleft or fissure	Cranioschisis
Complete or partial absence	Acrania
Cleft with protrusion of meninges	Meningocele
Cleft with protrusion of brain	Encephalocele
Cleft with protrusion of brain and meninges	Encephalomeningocele (Meningoencephalocele)
Herniation of brain with fluid in the ventricles	Hydrencephalocele (Hydroencephalocele)
Herniation of brain with fluid in the meninges	Hydromeningocele
Abnormal amount of fluid in ventricles or meninges	Hydrocephaly (Hydrencephaly; Macrocephaly)
Complete or partial lack of brain	Anencephaly
Deficiency or absence of olfactory lobes	Arrhinencephaly. *Cf.* Ethmocephaly
Abnormal smallness of brain and cranium	Microcephaly (Micrencephaly)
Altered shape due to premature sutural union	Acrocephaly. Pachycephaly. Scaphocephaly. Sphenocephaly (see *sphenocephalus*, 1). Trigonocephaly. Plagiocephaly
Occipital and cervical spinal cleft with herniation of brain and spinal cord	Iniencephaly
Spine and spinal cord:	
Cleft or fissure of spine	Rachischisis (Spina bifida)
Cleft with herniation of meninges	Rachicele (Spinal meningocele)
Cleft with herniation of spinal cord	Myelocele
Cleft with herniation of meninges and spinal cord	Myelomeningocele (Meningomyelocele)
Herniation of spinal cord with fluid in central canal	Myelocystocele (Syringomyelocele)
Excessive fluid in central canal	Hydromyelia
Absence of spinal cord	Amyelia
Occipital and cervical spinal cleft with herniation of brain and spinal cord	Iniencephaly
Cleft of entire cranium and spine with marked deficiency of brain and spinal cord	Holorachischisis
Face and sense organs:	
Complete or partial absence of olfactory lobes with major defect of ethmoidal region	Ethmocephaly. *Cf.* Arrhinencephaly
Complete or partial fusion of orbits and eyes with ethmoidal defect	Cyclopia (Synopsia)
Ethmoidal and nasal defects with approximation of orbits	Cebocephaly

* In compiling this table, no one classification was followed exclusively—rather, those terms were adopted which most generally have been accepted in American usage. The strongest influence was the terminology used by Schwalbe (*Die Morphologie der Missbildungen des Menschen und der Tiere*), who, in turn, was influenced by Förster (*Die Missbildungen des Menschen systematisch dargestellt*) and by Ahlfeld (*Die Missbildungen des Menschen, usw., mit Atlas*). Isidore Geoffroy St.-Hilaire also exerted a strong influence, but his classification into orders, genera, and species was abandoned as being antedated and unsatisfactory. Ballantyne (*Manual of Antenatal Pathology and Hygiene—I. The Embryo*), and his exposition of Taruffi's cumbersome terminology, probably played the next most important role. Wilder ("Duplicate Twins and Double Monsters") made some contribution, chiefly in regard to orderly arrangement of conjoined twins.

The form of this table was planned in particular for the use of those whose acquaintance with teratology is limited. The key will make it possible to identify an unknown specimen, or at least to localize it in the proper teratologic class.

TABLE OF REPRESENTATIVE MONSTROSITIES AND ANOMALIES (TERATA)—(Continued)

Type, or Parts Involved	Name, or Examples (Synonymous Terms in Parentheses)
Absence of eyes	Anophthalmia
Absence of eyelids	Ablepharia (Ablepharon)
Absence of palpebral fissure	Cryptophthalmia
Absence of iris	Aniridia (Irideremia)
Absence of lens	Aphakia
Absence of nose	Arrhinia
Absence of mouth	Astomia
Absence of eyes, nose, and mouth	Triocephaly (Aprosopia)
Absence of teeth	Anodontia
Absence of tongue	Aglossia
Absence of lower jaw	Agnathia
Approximation or fusion of ears (associated with agnathia)	Synotia. Otocephaly
Cyclopia, with agnathia and synotia	Cyclotia
Marked sphenoidal defect with partial synotia	Sphenocephaly (see *sphenocephalus*, 2)
Abnormally small face	Microprosopia
Abnormally large face	Macroprosopia
Abnormally small eye(s)	Microphthalmia
Abnormally large eye(s)	Megalophthalmia (Buphthalmus; Hydrophthalmus congenitus)
Abnormally small eyelids	Microblepharia (Microblephary)
Abnormally small palpebral fissure	Blepharophimosis
Abnormally small mouth	Microstomia
Abnormally large mouth	Macrostomia
Abnormally small ears	Microtia
Abnormally small lower jaw	Micrognathia
Abnormally large lower jaw	Macrognathia
Abnormally small teeth	Microdontia
Abnormally large teeth	Macrodontia
Abnormally small tongue	Microglossia
Abnormally large tongue	Macroglossia
Clefts of the face and jaws:	
From palpebral fissure to nasal cavity	Oblique facial cleft (Type I)
From palpebral fissure to philtrum of lip	Oblique facial cleft (Type II)
From level of mandibular joint to angle of mouth	Transverse facial cleft (Cleft cheek; Genal cleft; Macrostomia)
Vertical cleft of one or both eyelids	Coloboma palpebrae or palpebrarum (Blepharocoloboma)
Cleft of iris, lens, choroid, etc	Coloboma of iris, lens, choroid, etc.
Cleft nose	Rhinoschisis
Cleft lip	Cheiloschisis
Cleft jaw	Gnathoschisis
Cleft palate	Palatoschisis (Uranoschisis)
Cleft uvula	Staphyloschisis (Uvula fissa)
Cleft lip, jaw, and palate	Cheilognathopalatoschisis
Absence of nasal septum, philtrum of lip, and premaxilla	False median cleft of upper jaw
Cleft tongue	Bifid tongue. Trifid tongue
Neck:	
Median cleft or fissure	Tracheloschisis
Retention of pharyngeal pouches and grooves, or branchial ducts	Cervical cysts, diverticula, or fistulas
Congenital goiter	Struma congenita
Thorax and contents:	
Median cleft or fissure	Thoracoschisis (Sternoschisis)
Lateral cleft or fissure	Pleurosoma
Median cleft with herniation of heart	Ectopia cordis
Absence of breasts	Amastia
Supernumerary breast(s)	Polymastia (Hypermastia)
Absence of nipple(s)	Athelia
Supernumerary nipple(s)	Polythelia
Hypoplasia of breasts	Micromastia
Hyperplasia of breasts	Macromastia
Transposition of thoracic viscera	Situs inversus viscerum

TABLE OF REPRESENTATIVE MONSTROSITIES AND ANOMALIES (TERATA)—(Continued)

TYPE, OR PARTS INVOLVED	NAME, OR EXAMPLES (SYNONYMOUS TERMS IN PARENTHESES)
Herniation of abdominal viscera into thorax	Diaphragmatic hernia
Various anomalies of skeleton, muscles, vessels, nerves, and viscera of the thorax.	*E.g.*, Dextrocardia; Patent foramen ovale; Patent ductus arteriosus; Right aortic arch; Cardiac lobe of lung; etc.
Abdomen and contents:	
Cleft or fissure of abdomen	Gastroschisis (Celosoma)
Herniation of viscera into umbilical cord	Umbilical hernia
Herniation through lumbar triangle	Lumbar hernia
Herniation through inguinal canal	Inguinal hernia
Herniation through diaphragm	Diaphragmatic hernia
Various anomalies of skeleton, muscles, vessels, nerves, and viscera of abdomen.	*E.g.*, Congenital cystic kidney; Horseshoe kidney; Pelvic kidney; Double renal pelvis or ureter; Diverticula of gut; Stenosis and atresia of gut; Volvulus, etc.
Pelvis and contents:	
Cleft or fissure of pelvis	Pelvis fissa
Pelvic cleft with extroversion of bladder	Ectopia vesicae (Exstrophy of the bladder)
Rectum opens into bladder	Rectovesical fistula (Anus vesicalis)
Urogenital system:	
Double penis or clitoris	Diphallus (see *duplicity*)
Adhesion of prepuce	Phimosis
Urethra opens on dorsum of penis	Epispadias
Urethra opens on ventral side of penis	Hypospadias
Absence of testes	Anorchism (Anorchidism)
Absence of one testis	Monorchism (Monorchidism)
Failure of testes to descend	Cryptorchism (Cryptorchidism)
Accessory testis or testes	Polyorchidism
Fusion of testes	Synorchidism
Absence of ovaries	Anovarism
Uterus divided by septum	Uterus septus
Uterus possessing two horns	Uterus bicornis
Halves of uterus completely separate	Uterus duplex (Uterus didelphys)
Only one lateral half of uterus formed	Uterus unicornis
Ovarian and testicular tissue present in the same individual	Hermaphroditism
Male genitalia simulate female type	Pseudohermaphroditismus masculinus (Androgyny)
Female genitalia simulate male type	Pseudohermaphroditismus femininus (Gynandry)
Rectum opens into vagina or vulva	Atresia ani vaginalis (Vulvar anus)
Extremities:	
Congenital absence of all extremities	Amelia (Amelus)
Congenital absence of one, two, or three extremities, or their imperfect development	Ectromely (Ectromelus)
Distal portion of one or more limbs absent or markedly deficient	Hemimely (Peromely)
Proximal portion of one or more limbs lacking or rudimentary	Phocomely (Phocomelus)
Limbs normal in form, but abnormally small	Micromely (Micromelus)
Arms only thus	Microbrachius
Legs only thus	Micropus
Inversion (rotation) and fusion of legs	Sympodia (Symelia)
With feet lacking	Sympus apus (Sirenomelus)
One foot present	Sympus monopus (Uromelus)
Two feet present	Sympus dipus (Symelus)
Skin only between limbs	Patagium
Complete or partial absence of one or more digits	Ectrodactyly
Absence of digits II–IV	Bidactyly ("Lobster-claw"; Cleft hand or foot)
Abnormally short digits	Brachydactyly
Abnormally long digits	Arachnodactyly
More than normal number of digits	Polydactyly
Accessory thumb (or great toe)	Prepollex (or Prehallux)
Fusion of digits	Syndactyly
Web of skin between digits	Patagium

TABLE OF REPRESENTATIVE MONSTROSITIES AND ANOMALIES (TERATA)—(Continued)

Type, or Parts Involved	Name, or Examples (Synonymous Terms in Parentheses)
More than normal number of phalanges	Hyperphalangism
Less than normal number of phalanges	Hypophalangism
Congenital hypertrophy of hand	Chiromegaly
Congenital hypertrophy of foot	Pes gigas (Macropody)
Duplication (partial) of hand	Dichirus
Congenital distortion of foot	Talipes (Clubfoot)
Congenital distortion of hand	Talipomanus (Clubhand)
Free, Completely Separated Individuals	Twins (Gemini); Triplets; Quadruplets; Quintuplets; etc.
1. Individuals of equal or nearly equal size	Equal twins, etc. (Gemini aequales)
Derived from separate fertilized ova	False, or fraternal, twins (Not terata)
Derived from one ovum; common chorion	True, identical, monochorionic, or uniovular twins (Gemini monochorii)
2. Individuals markedly discrepant in size	Unequal twins (Gemini inaequales)
Derived from separate fertilized ova	Retarded development of one of fraternal twins
Derived from one ovum; one twin (the autosite) normal, or nearly so, the other (the omphalosite) small, markedly defective, with defective heart or no heart; dependent on the circulation furnished by the autosite by way of the placenta	Acardius (Acardiacus; Placental parasite)
Two or More More or Less Complete Individuals More or Less Intimately United	Conjoined twins (Diplopagi; Double monsters)
1. Component individuals, or parts of individuals, of nearly equal size	Symmetrical conjoined twins (Gemini monochorii aequales)
Union chiefly by heads or chiefly by heads and thoraces; duplicity involves at least infraumbilical parts	Inferior duplicity (Terata anadidyma)
Union by heads only	Craniopagus (Cephalopagus)
Dorsal union in occipital region	Craniopagus occipitalis (Iniopagus)
End-to-end union by vertices	Craniopagus parietalis (Acrocephalopagus)
Ventral union in frontal region	Craniopagus frontalis (Metopagus)
Ventral union by heads and thoraces	Cephalothoracopagus (Syncephalus)
With but one laterally directed face, or a major lateral face with parts of another opposite	Cephalothoracopagus monosymmetros
With two equal, laterally directed faces	Cephalothoracopagus disymmetros (Janus monster; Janiceps)
Lateral union at least by heads and thoraces, grading into an individual single except in pelvic region	Dipygus
Double penis or clitoris	Diphallus
With more or less complete third (median) lower extremity	Dipygus tripus
With four lower extremities	Dipygus tetrapus
Parts of body below umbilicus mostly single; duplicity involves mostly supraumbilical parts	Superior duplicity (Terata katadidyma)
Partial or complete doubling of hypophysis	Double hypophysis
Partial or complete doubling of face	Diprosopus
Partial or complete doubling of nose	Rhinodymus (Diprosopus diophthalmus)
Double nose; more or less complete third (median) eye	Diprosopus triophthalmus
Two noses; four eyes; facial skeleton more or less duplicated	Diprosopus tetrophthalmus (Iniodymus)
Two faces; third, more or less complete, median ear	Diprosopus triotus
Two faces; four ears; heads nearly separate	Diprosopus tetrotus
Two complete heads	Dicephalus
Two heads; necks fused, or a single neck	Dicephalus monauchenos
Two heads on separate necks	Dicephalus diauchenos
Two heads; partly double thorax; two arms	Dicephalus dibrachius
Two heads; partly double thorax; more or less complete third, median arm	Dicephalus tribrachius
Two heads; two thoraces; four arms	Dicephalus tetrabrachius

TABLE OF REPRESENTATIVE MONSTROSITIES AND ANOMALIES (TERATA)—(Continued)

Type, or Parts Involved	Name, or Examples (Synonymous Terms in Parentheses)
Parts of body both above and below the umbilicus show duplicity	Superior and inferior duplicity (Terata anakatadidyma)
Ventral union by heads and thoraces, but head somewhat doubled	Some forms of Cephalothoracopagus (see above under Inferior duplicity)
Ventral union by faces and thoraces	Prosopothoracopagus
Extensive ventral union chiefly by thoraces	Thoracopagus
Ventral union chiefly by sterna	Sternopagus
Ventral union in xiphoid region only	Xiphopagus
Lateral union by thoraces and hips	Iliothoracopagus
Lateral union in iliac region	Iliopagus
Dorsal union in sacral region	Pygopagus
End-to-end union by buttocks	Ischiopagus
2. One member of conjoined twins (the autosite) complete and normal, or nearly so; the other (the parasite) markedly smaller and more or less imperfect, often represented by only a part or parts of an individual, or by an amorphous mass of tissues (teratoma)	Asymmetrical conjoined twins (Gemini monochorii inaequales)
Parasite attached to head of autosite	Craniopagus parasiticus (Epicomus)
Parasite attached to upper jaw or base of cranium of autosite	Epignathus
Attached to the maxilla	Epignathus (sensu strictu)
Attached to the palate	Epipalatum
Attached to the sphenoid region	Episphenoid
Parasite attached to neck of autosite	Tracheloparasitus
Accessory limb attached to the neck	Deromelus
Parasite attached to thorax of autosite	Thoracopagus parasiticus
Parasite attached to epigastrium of autosite	Epigastrius (Epigastrius parasiticus)
Parasite attached below umbilicus	Dipygus parasiticus
Parasite attached in sacral region	Pygopagus parasiticus
Parasite attached in ischial region	Ischiopagus parasiticus
Parasite attached in iliac region	Iliopagus parasiticus
Parasite within body of autosite	Fetus in fetu
Within skin of autosite	Dermocyma
Within body wall of autosite	Endocyma

TABLE OF PHOBIAS

Substitute the combining form *-philia* for *-phobia* to obtain the antonym of fear

Fear	Phobia
afraid, being	phobophobia
air currents	aerophobia
alarmed, being	phobophobia
alone, being	monophobia
angina pectoris	anginophobia
animals	zoophobia
animals' skin or fur, touching	doraphobia
animals' teeth	odontophobia
bacilli	bacillophobia
bacteria	bacteriophobia
beaten, being	rhabdophobia
bees	apiphobia
	melissophobia
blood, sight of	hematophobia
	hemophobia
blushing	ereuthophobia
	erythrophobia
bodies, dead	necrophobia
body, left side of, objects on	levophobia
naked	gymnophobia
right side of, objects on	dextrophobia
body odors	bromhidrosiphobia
books	bibliophobia
bound, being	merinthophobia
bridges, crossing	gephyrophobia
buried alive, being	taphephobia
cadavers	necrophobia
cancer	cancerophobia
	cancerphobia
cats	ailurophobia
	galeophobia
	gatophobia
celestial space	astrophobia
childbirth	maieusiophobia
	tocophobia
children	pedophobia
choking	pnigophobia
cholera	cholerophobia
clawed, being	amychophobia
cliffs	cremnophobia
coitus	coitophobia
cold	cheimaphobia
	psychrophobia
colors, certain	chromatophobia
	chromophobia
red	ereuthophobia
	erythrophobia
confined space, being in	claustrophobia
contact, physical	aphephobia
	haphephobia
	haptephobia
contamination	molysmophobia
	mysophobia
crossing bridges	gephyrophobia
crossing the street	agyiophobia
crowds	ochlophobia
darkness	achluophobia
	nyctophobia
	scotophobia
daylight	phengophobia
dead bodies	necrophobia
death	necrophobia
	thanatophobia
defecation	coprophobia
deformity	dysmorphophobia
	teratophobia
deity	theophobia
demons	demonophobia

Fear	Phobia
depths	bathophobia
devils	demonophobia
diabetic, becoming	diabetophobia
dirt	mysophobia
disease	nosophobia
heart	cardiophobia
skin	dermatopathophobia
venereal	cypridophobia
	venereophobia
disorder	ataxiophobia
dogs	cynophobia
drafts	aerophobia
	anemophobia
drink	dipsophobia
dust	amathophobia
eating	sitophobia
electricity	electrophobia
empty spaces, large	kenophobia
error	hamartophobia
everything	pantophobia
exhaustion	kopophobia
exposure to sun's rays	heliophobia
failure	kakorrhaphiophobia
falling asleep	hypnophobia
fatigue	kopophobia
fears, one's own	phobophobia
feces	coprophobia
fever	febriphobia
	pyrexeophobia
filth	rhypophobia
finger, being touched by	aichmophobia
fire	pyrophobia
fish	ichthyophobia
floods	antlophobia
flowers	anthophobia
flutes	aulophobia
fog	homichlophobia
food	cibophobia
	sitophobia
forests	hylophobia
fur, animals', touching	doraphobia
gaiety	cherophobia
glare of light	photaugiophobia
glass	crystallophobia
	hyalophobia
God	theophobia
gravity	barophobia
hair	trichopathophobia
	trichophobia
happiness	cherophobia
hearing a certain name	onomatophobia
heart disease	cardiophobia
heat	thermophobia
heights	acrophobia
	hypsophobia
hell	hadephobia
high objects	batophobia
home	oikophobia
house, being in a	domatophobia
human society	anthropophobia
hydrophobia	hydrophobophobia
	lyssophobia
ideas	ideophobia
infants	pedophobia
infection	molysmophobia
venereal	cypridophobia
	venereophobia
infestation, with lice	pediculophobia
with worms	helminthophobia
	vermiphobia

TABLE OF PHOBIAS—(Continued)

Fear	Phobia
infinity	apeirophobia
insane, becoming	lyssophobia
insects	entomophobia
stinging	melissophobia
intercourse, sexual	coitophobia
kleptomaniac, becoming a	kleptophobia
laceration	amychophobia
left side of body, objects on	levophobia
leprosy	leprophobia
lice	pediculophobia
	phthiriophobia
lies, telling	mythophobia
light	photophobia
flashing	selaphobia
glare of	photaugiophobia
lightning	astraphobia
	astrapophobia
	keraunophobia
lights, northern	auroraphobia
liquids	hygrophobia
liquors, alcoholic	dipsophobia
locked in, being	cleithrophobia
lockjaw	tetanophobia
lonely, being	eremophobia
love, sexual	erotophobia
many things	polyphobia
marriage	gamophobia
matter, fecal	coprophobia
medicine, mercurial	hydrargyrophobia
taking	pharmacophobia
men	androphobia
meningitis	meningitophobia
mercurial medicines	hydrargyrophobia
metals	metallophobia
microbes	bacillophobia
	microbiophobia
	microphobia
microorganisms	bacteriophobia
missiles	ballistophobia
mites	acarophobia
moisture	hygrophobia
money	chrematophobia
monster, giving birth to a	teratophobia
motion	kinesophobia
movement	kinesophobia
nakedness	gymnophobia
name, hearing a certain	onomatophobia
needles	belonephobia
newness	cainophobia
	kainophobia
	neophobia
night	noctiphobia
	nyctophobia
noise	phonophobia
northern lights	auroraphobia
novelty	cainophobia
	kainophobia
	neophobia
number 13	triskaidekaphobia
objects, metal	metallophobia
small	microphobia
ocean	thalassophobia
odors	osmophobia
body	bromhidrosiphobia
oneself	autophobia
pain	algophobia
	odynoph bia
parasites	parasitophobia
people	anthropophobia
deformed	teratophobia

Fear	Phobia
people—(*Continued*)	
naked	gymnophobia
strange	xenophobia
pins	belonephobia
places, certain	topophobia
desolate	eremophobia
open	agoraphobia
steep	cremnophobia
pleasure	hedonophobia
pointed objects	aichmophobia
poisoned, being	toxicophobia
poisons	iophobia
precipices	cremnophobia
projectiles	ballistophobia
rabies	lyssophobia
railroad traveling	siderodromophobia
rain	ombrophobia
rays of sun, exposure to	heliophobia
red colors	ereuthophobia
	erythrophobia
reptiles	ophidiophobia
responsibility	hypengyophobia
ridicule	catagelophobia
right side of body, objects on	dextrophobia
roaming about	dromophobia
robbers	harpaxophobia
	kleptophobia
room, closed, being in	claustrophobia
ruin	atephobia
sacred things	hierophobia
scabies	scabiophobia
scratched, being	amychophobia
sea	thalassophobia
seen, being	scopophobia
sex	genophobia
female	gynephobia
male	androphobia
sexual love	erotophobia
sexual union	coitophobia
sharp-pointed objects	aichmophobia
	belonephobia
shock	hormephobia
sin	hamartophobia
sitting down	kathisophobia
skin, animals', touching	doraphobia
skin diseases	dermatopathophobia
sleep	hypnophobia
small objects	microphobia
smells	osmophobia
personal	bromhidrosiphobia
snakes	ophidiophobia
snow	chionophobia
society, human	anthropophobia
solitude	autophobia
sounds	acousticophobia
	phonophobia
sourness	acerbophobia
	acerophobia
space, celestial	astrophobia
confined, being in	claustrophobia
spaces, large empty	kenophobia
open	agoraphobia
speech	laliophobia
	lalophobia
	phonophobia
spiders	arachnephobia
staircases	climacophobia
standing upright	basophobia
	stasibasiphobia
	stasiphobia

TABLE OF PHOBIAS—(Continued)

Fear	Phobia
stared at, being	ophthalmophobia
stars	astrophobia
steep places	cremnophobia
sticks	rhabdophobia
stillness	eremiophobia
stinging insects	melissophobia
stings, bee	apiphobia
strangers	xenophobia
streets	agyiophobia
string	linonophobia
stuttering	laliophobia lalophobia
sunlight	heliophobia
syphilis	syphilophobia
talking	laliophobia lalophobia
tapeworms, harboring	taeniophobia
taste	geumaphobia
teeth, animals', seeing	odontophobia
telling untruths	mythophobia
tetanus	tetanophobia
thieves	harpaxophobia kleptophobia
thinking	phronemophobia
thirteen	triskaidekaphobia
thunder	brontophobia tonitrophobia
thunderstorms	astraphobia astrapophobia
tied up, being	merinthophobia
time	chronophobia
touched, being	aphephobia haphephobia haptephobia
touching animals' skin or fur	doraphobia
touching metals	metallophobia
trains	siderodromophobia
travel	hodophobia
traveling, railroad	siderodromophobia
trembling	tremophobia
trichinosis	trichinophobia
tuberculosis	phthisiophobia tuberculophobia
uncleanliness, personal	automysophobia
union, sexual	coitophobia
untruths, telling	mythophobia
vaccination	vaccinophobia
vehicles, being in	amaxophobia
venereal infection	cypridophobia venereophobia
voice, one's own	phonophobia
vomiting	emetophobia
walking	basiphobia stasibasiphobia
wandering	dromophobia
water	hydrophobia
sheets of	potamophobia
weakness	asthenophobia
weariness	kopophobia
winds	anemophobia
women	gynephobia
woods	hylophobia
words, hearing certain	onomatophobia
work	ergasiophobia ergophobia
worms	helminthophobia vermiphobia
writing	graphophobia

ELY'S TABLE OF THE DURATION OF PREGNANCY

(See Plate 41)

Explanation.—In the upper horizontal row of numbers, find the date of last menstruation; the number beneath, set in *italics*, will show the expiration of 280 days or ten months of 28 days each.

January	1	2	3	4	5	6	7	8	9	10	11	12	13	14	15	16	17	18	19	20	21	22	23	24	25	26	27	28	29	30	31	
October	*8*	*9*	*10*	*11*	*12*	*13*	*14*	*15*	*16*	*17*	*18*	*19*	*20*	*21*	*22*	*23*	*24*	*25*	*26*	*27*	*28*	*29*	*30*	*31*	*1*	*2*	*3*	*4*	*5*	*6*	*7*	*November*
February	1	2	3	4	5	6	7	8	9	10	11	12	13	14	15	16	17	18	19	20	21	22	23	24	25	26	27	28				
November	*8*	*9*	*10*	*11*	*12*	*13*	*14*	*15*	*16*	*17*	*18*	*19*	*20*	*21*	*22*	*23*	*24*	*25*	*26*	*27*	*28*	*29*	*30*	*1*	*2*	*3*	*4*	*5*				*December*
March	1	2	3	4	5	6	7	8	9	10	11	12	13	14	15	16	17	18	19	20	21	22	23	24	25	26	27	28	29	30	31	
December	*6*	*7*	*8*	*9*	*10*	*11*	*12*	*13*	*14*	*15*	*16*	*17*	*18*	*19*	*20*	*21*	*22*	*23*	*24*	*25*	*26*	*27*	*28*	*29*	*30*	*31*	*1*	*2*	*3*	*4*	*5*	*January*
April	1	2	3	4	5	6	7	8	9	10	11	12	13	14	15	16	17	18	19	20	21	22	23	24	25	26	27	28	29	30		
January	*6*	*7*	*8*	*9*	*10*	*11*	*12*	*13*	*14*	*15*	*16*	*17*	*18*	*19*	*20*	*21*	*22*	*23*	*24*	*25*	*26*	*27*	*28*	*29*	*30*	*31*	*1*	*2*	*3*	*4*		*February*
May	1	2	3	4	5	6	7	8	9	10	11	12	13	14	15	16	17	18	19	20	21	22	23	24	25	26	27	28	29	30	31	
February	*5*	*6*	*7*	*8*	*9*	*10*	*11*	*12*	*13*	*14*	*15*	*16*	*17*	*18*	*19*	*20*	*21*	*22*	*23*	*24*	*25*	*26*	*27*	*28*	*1*	*2*	*3*	*4*	*5*	*6*	*7*	*March*
June	1	2	3	4	5	6	7	8	9	10	11	12	13	14	15	16	17	18	19	20	21	22	23	24	25	26	27	28	29	30		
March	*8*	*9*	*10*	*11*	*12*	*13*	*14*	*15*	*16*	*17*	*18*	*19*	*20*	*21*	*22*	*23*	*24*	*25*	*26*	*27*	*28*	*29*	*30*	*31*	*1*	*2*	*3*	*4*	*5*	*6*		*April*
July	1	2	3	4	5	6	7	8	9	10	11	12	13	14	15	16	17	18	19	20	21	22	23	24	25	26	27	28	29	30	31	
April	*7*	*8*	*9*	*10*	*11*	*12*	*13*	*14*	*15*	*16*	*17*	*18*	*19*	*20*	*21*	*22*	*23*	*24*	*25*	*26*	*27*	*28*	*29*	*30*	*1*	*2*	*3*	*4*	*5*	*6*	*7*	*May*
August	1	2	3	4	5	6	7	8	9	10	11	12	13	14	15	16	17	18	19	20	21	22	23	24	25	26	27	28	29	30	31	
May	*8*	*9*	*10*	*11*	*12*	*13*	*14*	*15*	*16*	*17*	*18*	*19*	*20*	*21*	*22*	*23*	*24*	*25*	*26*	*27*	*28*	*29*	*30*	*31*	*1*	*2*	*3*	*4*	*5*	*6*	*7*	*June*
September	1	2	3	4	5	6	7	8	9	10	11	12	13	14	15	16	17	18	19	20	21	22	23	24	25	26	27	28	29	30		
June	*8*	*9*	*10*	*11*	*12*	*13*	*14*	*15*	*16*	*17*	*18*	*19*	*20*	*21*	*22*	*23*	*24*	*25*	*26*	*27*	*28*	*29*	*30*	*1*	*2*	*3*	*4*	*5*	*6*	*7*		*July*
October	1	2	3	4	5	6	7	8	9	10	11	12	13	14	15	16	17	18	19	20	21	22	23	24	25	26	27	28	29	30	31	
July	*8*	*9*	*10*	*11*	*12*	*13*	*14*	*15*	*16*	*17*	*18*	*19*	*20*	*21*	*22*	*23*	*24*	*25*	*26*	*27*	*28*	*29*	*30*	*31*	*1*	*2*	*3*	*4*	*5*	*6*	*7*	*August*
November	1	2	3	4	5	6	7	8	9	10	11	12	13	14	15	16	17	18	19	20	21	22	23	24	25	26	27	28	29	30		
August	*8*	*9*	*10*	*11*	*12*	*13*	*14*	*15*	*16*	*17*	*18*	*19*	*20*	*21*	*22*	*23*	*24*	*25*	*26*	*27*	*28*	*29*	*30*	*31*	*1*	*2*	*3*	*4*	*5*	*6*		*September*
December	1	2	3	4	5	6	7	8	9	10	11	12	13	14	15	16	17	18	19	20	21	22	23	24	25	26	27	28	29	30	31	
September	*7*	*8*	*9*	*10*	*11*	*12*	*13*	*14*	*15*	*16*	*17*	*18*	*19*	*20*	*21*	*22*	*23*	*24*	*25*	*26*	*27*	*28*	*29*	*30*	*1*	*2*	*3*	*4*	*5*	*6*	*7*	*October*

TABLE OF THE MORE COMMON LATIN OR GREEK TERMS AND ABBREVIATIONS USED IN PRESCRIPTION WRITING

Term or Abbreviation	Latin or Greek	Translation
āā, āa	ana	of each
a.c.	ante cibum	before meals
ad	ad	to, up to
add.	adde; addantur; addendum; addendo	add (thou); let them be added; to be added; by adding
ad lib.	ad libitum	at pleasure
admov.	admove; admoveatur; admoveantur	apply (thou); let it be applied; let them be applied
ad part. dolent.	ad partes dolentes	to the painful parts
agit.	agita	shake (thou), stir (thou)
alb.	albus	white
alter	alter	the other
alternis horis	alternis horis	every other hour
ante	ante	before
aq.	aqua	water
aq. bull.	aqua bulliens	boiling water
aq. comm.	aqua communis	common water
aq. dest.	aqua destillata	distilled water
aq. ferv.	aqua fervens	hot water
aut	aut	or
baccillum	baccillum	a bougie
bene	bene	well
bib.	bibe	drink (thou)
b.i.d.	bis in die, bis in dies	twice daily
bis	bis	twice
bol.	bolus	a large pill
c̄, c	cum	with
calefactus	calefactus	warmed
cap.	capiat	let him (her) take
caps.	capsula	a capsule
caute	caute	cautiously
cera	cera	wax
cerat.	ceratum	cerate
chart.	charta	a paper
chart. cerat.	charta cerata	waxed paper
chartula	chartula	a small paper
cibus	cibus	food
cito disp.	cito dispensetur	let it be dispensed quickly
co.	compositus	a compound, compounded
coch., cochleat.	cochlear, cochleare; cochleatim	a spoonful; by spoonfuls
coch. amp.	cochleare amplum	a tablespoonful
coch. mag.	cochleare magnum	a large spoonful (about ½ oz.)
coch. med.	cochleare medium, cochleare modicum	a dessertspoonful (about 2 fluidrachms)
coch. parv.	cochleare parvum	a teaspoonful (about 1 fluidrachm)
col.	cola	strain (thou)
colat.	colatus	strained
colent.	colentur	let them be strained
colet.	coletur	let it be strained
coll.	collyrium	an eyewash
collunarium	collunarium	a nose wash
collut.	collutorium	a mouth wash
collyr.	collyrium	an eyewash
coloretur	coloretur	let it be colored
commisce	commisce	mix (thou) together
comp.	compositus	compounded
conf.	confectio	a confection
confricamentum	confricamentum	a liniment
cong.	congius	a gallon
cons.	conserva	a conserve; keep (thou)
consperg.	consperge	dust (thou), sprinkle (thou)
contra	contra	against
cont. rem.	continuantur remedia	let the medicines be continued
contusus	contusus	bruised
cor	cor	the heart
cordis	cordis	the heart
cort.	cortex	the bark

TABLE OF THE MORE COMMON LATIN OR GREEK TERMS AND ABBREVIATIONS USED IN PRESCRIPTION WRITING—(Continued)

Term or Abbreviation	Latin or Greek	Translation
cotula	cotula	a measure
cuj.	cujus; cujuslibet	of which; of any
d.	da	give (thou)
de	de	of, from
dec.	decanta	pour (thou) off
decem	decem	ten
decimus	decimus	the tenth
de d. in d.	de die in diem	from day to day
deglut.	deglutiatur	may be swallowed, let be swallowed
dein	dein	thereupon
det.	detur	let be given
detur in duplo	detur in duplo	let twice as much be given
dexter	dexter	the right
dextra	dextra	the right
dieb. alt.	diebus alternis	every other day
dieb. tert.	diebus tertiis	every third day
digere	digere	digest (thou)
dil.	dilue; dilutus	dilute (thou); diluted
dim.	dimidius	one-half
d. in p. aeq.	dividatur in partes aequales	let it be divided into equal parts
direc. prop.	directione propria	with a proper direction
divid.	divide	divide (thou)
dividendus, -a, -um	dividendus, -a, -um	to be divided
donec	donec	until
D.P.	directione propria	with a proper direction
d.t.d. No. iv	dentur tales doses No. iv	let 4 such doses be given
e.	ex, e	from, one of
eadem (*fem.*)	eadem	the same
ejusd.	ejusdem	of the same
elect.	electuarium	an electuary
elix.	elixir	an elixir
e.m.p.	ex modo prescripto	after the manner prescribed; as directed
emp.	emplastrum	a plaster
emulgens	emulgens	an emulsifying agent
en.	enema	an enema, a clyster
enem.	enema	an enema
enemata	enemata	clysters
epistom.	epistomium	a stopper
et	et	and
etiam	etiam	also, besides
ext.	extende	spread (thou)
f.	fac; fiat; fiant	make (thou); let it be made; let them be made
farina	farina	flour
febris	febris	fever
ferv.	fervens	boiling
fiat pulvis in chartulas xii dividenda	fiat pulvis in chartulas xii dividenda	let 12 powders be made
filt.	filtra	filter (thou)
flav.	flavus	yellow
fldxt.	fluidextractum	fluidextract
fol.	folium	a leaf
f. pil. xi	fac pilulas xi	make (thou) 11 pills
ft.	fac; fiat; fiant	make (thou); let it be made; let them be made
ft. cataplasm.	fiat cataplasma	let a poultice be made
ft. cerat.	fiat ceratum	let a cerate be made
ft. chart. vi	fiant chartulae vi	let 6 powders be made
ft. collyr.	fiat collyrium	let an eyewash be made
ft. emuls.	fiat emulsio	let an emulsion be made
ft. enema	fiat enema	let an injection be made [for rectum]
ft. garg.	fiat gargarisma	let a gargle be made
ft. infus.	fiat infusum	let an infusion be made
ft. injec.	fiat injectio	let an injection be made [for urethra]
ft. linim.	fiat linimentum	let a liniment be made
ft. mas.	fiat massa	let a mass be made

TABLE OF THE MORE COMMON LATIN OR GREEK TERMS AND ABBREVIATIONS USED IN PRESCRIPTION WRITING—(Continued)

Term or Abbreviation	Latin or Greek	Translation
ft. mas. div. in pil. xiv	fiat massa et divide in pilulas xiv; or, fiat massa in pilulas xiv dividenda	let 14 pills be made
ft. mist.	fiat mistura	let a mixture be made
ft. pil. xxiv	fiant pilulae xxiv	let 24 pills be made
ft. pulv.	fiat pulvis	let a powder be made
ft. pulv. et div. in char. xii	fiat pulvis et divide in chartulas xii; or, fiat pulvis in chartulas xii dividenda	let 12 powders be made
ft. solut.	fiat solutio	let a solution be made
ft. suppos.	fiat suppositorium	let a suppository be made
ft. suppos. iv	fiant suppositoria iv	let 4 suppositories be made
ft. ung.	fiat unguentum	let an ointment be made
garg.	gargarisma	a gargle
gland.	glandula	a gland
glyc.	glyceritum	glycerite
gradatim	gradatim	by degrees, gradually
grana	grana	grains
granum	granum	a grain
gtt.	gutta(e)	drop(s)
H.	hora	an hour
haec	haec	this
haust.	haustus	a draught
H.D.	hora decubitus	at the hour of going to bed
herba	herba	an herb
hic	hic	this
hoc	hoc	this
hor. som.	hora somni	at bedtime
H.S.	hora somni	at bedtime
idem	idem	the same
identidem	identidem	repeatedly
in d.	in dies	from day to day, daily
inde	inde	therefrom
inf.	infusum	an infusion
inger in capsulas	inger in capsulas	put (thou) in capsules
inject.	injectio	an injection
inter	inter	between
involve gelatina	involve gelatina	coat (thou) with gelatin
ita	ita	in such manner
lac	lac	milk
lamella	lamella	leaf, scale
leniter terendo	leniter terendo	by rubbing gently
leviter	leviter	lightly
lin.	linimentum	a liniment
liq.	liquor	a solution
lot.	lotio	a lotion
M.	misce	mix (thou)
m.	minimum	a minim
mag.	magnus	large
massa	massa	a mass
massa pilularis	massa pilularis	a pill mass
min.	minimum	a minim
minutum	minutum	a minute
mist.	mistura	a mixture
mitt.	mitte	send (thou)
mittatur	mittatur	let it be sent
mitt. tal.	mitte talis	send (thou) of such (or this)
mod. praesc.	modo praescripto	in the manner prescribed
more dict.	more dictu	in the manner directed
more sol.	more solito	in the usual manner
nisi	nisi	unless
no.	numero, numerus	number
noctis	noctis	of the night
non	non	not
non rep.	non repetatur	do not repeat
nox	nox	night
nunc	nunc	now
O.	octarius	a pint

TABLE OF THE MORE COMMON LATIN OR GREEK TERMS AND ABBREVIATIONS USED IN PRESCRIPTION WRITING—(Continued)

Term or Abbreviation	Latin or Greek	Translation
obduce	obduce	cover (thou), conceal (thou), coat (thou)
octavus	octavus	eighth
octo	octo	eight
oculus	oculus	the eye
O.D.	oculus dexter	the right eye
O.L.	oculus laevus	the left eye
ol.	oleum	oil
omn. bih.	omni bihorio	every 2 hours
omn. hor.	omni hora	every hour
omn. 2 hor.	omni secunda hora	every 2 hours
omni mane	omni mane	every morning
omni nocte	omni nocte	every night
omn. quadr. hor.	omni quadrante horae	every quarter of an hour
O.S.	oculus sinister	the left eye
p.	pondere	by weight
p. ae.	partes aequales	equal parts
pars	pars	a part
partis	partis	of part
part. vic.	partitis vicibus	in divided doses
parvulus	parvulus	an infant
parvus	parvus	little
p.c.	post cibos; post cibum	after eating; after food
per	per	through, by
perinde	perinde	in the same manner as before
pes	pes	the foot
pil.	pilula(e)	pill(s)
placebo	placebo	a substance which pleases
pocill.	pocillum	a little cup
pocul.	poculum	a cup
pondus medicinale	pondus medicinale	medicinal (apothecaries') weight
potus	potus	a drink
prand.	prandium	dinner
primus	primus	the first
prius	prius	before, former
p.r.n.	pro re nata	as occasion arises, occasionally
pro	pro	for
proratione aetatis	proratione aetatis	according to the age of the patient
proximo	proximo	nearest
pulv.	pulvis; pulveres; pulveratus	powder; powders; powdered
pyxis	pyxis	a pill box
q.h.	quaque hora	each hour, every hour
q. 2 h.	quaque secunda hora	every 2 hours
q. 3 h.	quaque tertia hora	every 3 hours
q. 4 h.	quaque quarta hora	every 4 hours
q.i.d.	quater in die	4 times a day
q.l.	quantum libet	as much as is desired
q.p.	quantum placet	as much as you please
Q.Q.	quaque; quoque	each, every; also
q.s.	quantum sufficit; quantum sufficiat; quantum satis	a sufficient quantity; as much as is sufficient
quam libet	quam libet	as much as you wish
quartus	quartus	fourth
quater	quater	4 times
quatuor	quatuor	four
quibus	quibus	from which
qui libet	qui libet	whatever you please
quinque	quinque	five
quintus	quintus	the fifth
quor.	quorum	of which
quotidie	quotidie	daily
quoties	quoties	as often as
q.v.	quantum vis, quantum volueris	as much as you wish
℞	recipe	take (thou)
ratio	ratio	proportion
rec.	recens	fresh
recipe	recipe	take (thou)

TABLE OF THE MORE COMMON LATIN OR GREEK TERMS AND ABBREVIATIONS USED IN PRESCRIPTION WRITING—(Continued)

Term or Abbreviation	Latin or Greek	Translation
rep.	repetatur; repetantur	let it be repeated; let them be repeated
rub.	ruber	red, ruddy
S.	signa; signetur	write (thou); let it be written; label (thou)
S.A.	secundum artem	according to art
secundus	secundus	second
semel	semel	once
semidr.	semidrachma	half a drachm
semih.	semihora	half an hour
septem	septem	seven
septimana	septimana	a week
sescuncia	sescuncia	an ounce and a half
sesquihora	sesquihora	an hour and a half
sex	sex	six
sextus	sextus	sixth
si	si	if
siccus	siccus	dry, dried
sig.	signa; signetur	write (thou); let it be written; label
simul	simul	together
sine	sine	without
si op. sit	si opus sit	if necessary
sit	sit	let it be
S.N.	secundum naturam	according to nature
sol.	solutio	a solution
solutus	solutus	dissolved
solve	solve	dissolve (thou)
solvere	solvere	to dissolve
solvo	solvo	to dissolve
somnus	somnus	sleep
S.O.S.	si opus sit	if necessary
sp.	spiritus	spirit
spiritus vini tenuis	spiritus vini tenuis	proof spirit
spiritus vinosus	spiritus vinosus	ardent spirit of any strength
spissus	spissus	dense, hard
spt.	spiritus	spirit
ss, $\overline{\text{ss}}$	semis	a half
st.	stet; stent	let it stand; let them stand
stat.	statim	immediately
stillatim	stillatim	by drops; in small quantities
subinde	subinde	frequently
subtilis	subtilis	fine, smooth, nice
succus	succus	juice, sap
sum.	sume; sumat; sumatur; sumantur; sumendus	take (thou); let him take; let it be taken; let them be taken; to be taken
suppos.	suppositorium	a suppository
supra	supra	above
S.V.R.	spiritus vini rectificatus	rectified spirit of wine (alcohol)
syr.	syrupus	syrup
tabel.	tabella (dim. of *tabula*, a table)	a lozenge
talis	talis	such; like this
t.d.	ter die	3 times a day
tenuis	tenuis	fine, thin
ter	ter	3 times
ter.	tere	rub (thou)
tertius	tertius	third
t.i.d.	ter in die	3 times a day
tinct.	tinctura	a tincture
tr.	tinctura	a tincture
tres	tres	three
triduum	triduum	3 days
trit.	tritura	triturate
troch.	trochiscus	a troche
ubi	ubi	where, wherever, whenever
uncia	uncia	an ounce
ung.	unguentum	an ointment

TABLE OF THE MORE COMMON LATIN OR GREEK TERMS AND ABBREVIATIONS USED IN PRESCRIPTION WRITING—(Continued)

Term or Abbreviation	Latin or Greek	Translation
ut dict.	ut dictum	as directed
utend.	utendum	to be used
uti	uti	to make use of
uto	uto	to make use of
vehiculum	vehiculum	a vehicle
vel	vel	or
venenosus	venenosus	poisonous, a poison
verus	verus	true, genuine
vesp.	vesper	the evening
vin.	vinum	wine
vitreum	vitreum	glass
vitrum	vitrum	glass

AMERICAN CLASSIFICATION OF PROTEINS

I. SIMPLE PROTEINS—*Substances that yield only α-amino acids or their derivatives on hydrolysis.*

a. **Albumins**—Soluble in pure water or dilute salt solution and coagulable by heat.
- ovalbumin.................................from egg white
- serum albumin.............................from blood serum
- lactalbumin...............................from milk
- vegetable albumin.........................from plant tissues

b. **Globulins**—Insoluble in pure water, soluble in salt solutions, and coagulable by heat.
- ovoglobulin...............................from egg white
- serum globulin............................from blood serum
- edestin...................................from hemp seed
- amandin...................................from fruit kernels

c. **Glutelins**—Insoluble in neutral solvents, soluble in dilute acids and bases, and coagulable by heat.
- glutenin..................................from wheat

d. **Prolamines** (or **gliadins**)—Soluble in 80 per cent alcohol; insoluble in water, absolute alcohol, or neutral solvents.
- zein......................................from corn
- gliadin...................................from wheat
- hordein...................................from barley
- bynin.....................................from malt

e. **Albuminoids** (sometimes called **scleroproteins**)—Insoluble in all neutral solvents.
- elastin...................................from ligament
- collagen..................................from tendon
- keratin...................................from horn and hoofs

f. **Globins**—Soluble in water, acids, and alkalis and coagulable by heat.
- globin....................................from hemoglobin

g. **Histones**—Soluble in water or dilute acids, precipitated or insoluble in ammonia.
- scombrone.................................from mackerel spermatozoa
- thymus histone............................from thymus gland

h. **Protamines**—Soluble in water, uncoagulable by heat. Simplest proteins or polypeptides.
- salmine...................................from salmon spermatozoa
- sturine...................................from sturgeon spermatozoa
- clupeine..................................from herring spermatozoa

II. CONJUGATED PROTEINS—*Substances that consist of protein combined with some other substance (the prosthetic molecule).*

a. **Nucleoproteins**—Compounds of one or more proteins with nucleic acid.
- cytoglobulin..............................from white blood cells
- nucleohistone.............................from cell nuclei

b. **Glycoproteins**—Compounds of protein with carbohydrates and certain derivatives such as hexoseamine.
- mucin.....................................from mucus
- osseomucoid...............................from bone
- tendomucin................................from tendon
- ichthulin.................................from fish eggs
- helicoprotein.............................from snails

c. **Phosphoproteins**—Compounds of proteins with a phosphorus compound other than lecithin or nucleic acid.
- casein....................................from milk
- ovovitellin...............................from egg yolk

d. **Chromoproteins** (**hemoglobins**)—Compounds of proteins with a chromophoric group (or pigments).
- hemoglobin................................from mammalian blood
- hemocyanin................................from blood of invertebrates
- chlorophyll...............................from green plants

e. **Lecithoproteins**—Compounds of proteins with lecithins.

f. **Lipoproteins**—Compounds of proteins with fatty acids.

g. **Metalloproteins**—Protein enzymes containing metals as an inherent portion of their molecule.

III. DERIVED PROTEINS—*Primary and secondary split products of proteins.*

a. **Proteans**—Insoluble products due to the action of water, dilute acids, or enzymes.
- myosan....................................from myosin
- edestan...................................from edestin

b. **Metaproteins**—Products resulting from the action of acids or bases.

c. **Coagulated proteins**—Resulting from the action of heat or alcohol on proteins.

d. **Proteoses**—Products resulting from further hydrolysis. They are soluble in water and not coagulable by heat, and are precipitated by saturating their solutions with ammonium or zinc sulfate.

e. **Peptones**—Soluble in water, noncoagulable by heat, not precipitated by saturating their solutions with ammonium or zinc sulfate.

f. **Peptides**—Compounds of two or more amino acids possessing one or more —CO.NH— or peptide groups.

TABLE OF THERMOMETRIC EQUIVALENTS*

Centigrade to Fahrenheit Scales

$\frac{9}{5}$ C. ° + 32 = F. °

C. °	F. °	C. °	F. °	C. °	F. °	C. °	F. °	C. °	F. °
−20	−4.0	21	69.8	61	141.8	101	213.8	141	285.8
−19	−2.2	22	71.6	62	143.6	102	215.6	142	287.6
−18	−0.4	23	73.4	63	145.4	103	217.4	143	289.4
−17	1.4	24	75.2	64	147.2	104	219.2	144	291.2
−16	3.2	25	77.	65	149.	105	221.	145	293.
−15	5.	26	78.8	66	150.8	106	222.8	146	294.8
−14	6.8	27	80.6	67	152.6	107	224.6	147	296.6
−13	8.6	28	82.4	68	154.4	108	226.4	148	298.4
−12	10.4	29	84.2	69	156.2	109	228.2	149	300.2
−11	12.2	30	86.	70	158.	110	230.	150	302.
−10	14.	31	87.8	71	159.8	111	231.8	151	303.8
−9	15.8	32	89.6	72	161.6	112	233.6	152	305.6
−8	17.6	33	91.4	73	163.4	113	235.4	153	307.4
−7	19.4	34	93.2	74	165.2	114	237.2	154	309.2
−6	21.2	35	95.	75	167.	115	239.	155	311.
−5	23.	36	96.8	76	168.8	116	240.8	156	312.8
−4	24.8	37	98.6	77	170.6	117	242.6	157	314.6
−3	26.6	38	100.4	78	172.4	118	244.4	158	316.4
−2	28.4	39	102.2	79	174.2	119	246.2	159	318.2
−1	30.2	40	104.	80	176.	120	248.	160	320.
0	32.	41	105.8	81	177.8	121	249.8	161	321.8
1	33.8	42	107.6	82	179.6	122	251.6	162	323.6
2	35.6	43	109.4	83	181.4	123	253.4	163	325.4
3	37.4	44	111.2	84	183.2	124	255.2	164	327.2
4	39.2	45	113.	85	185.	125	257.	165	329.
5	41.	46	114.8	86	186.8	126	258.8	166	330.8
6	42.8	47	116.6	87	188.6	127	260.6	167	332.6
7	44.6	48	118.4	88	190.4	128	262.4	168	334.4
8	46.4	49	120.2	89	192.2	129	264.2	169	336.2
9	48.2	50	122.	90	194.	130	266.	170	338.
10	50.	51	123.8	91	195.8	131	267.8	171	339.8
11	51.8	52	125.6	92	197.6	132	269.6	172	341.6
12	53.6	53	127.4	93	199.4	133	271.4	173	343.4
13	55.4	54	129.2	94	201.2	134	273.2	174	345.2
14	57.2	55	131.	95	203.	135	275.	175	347.
15	59.	56	132.8	96	204.8	136	276.8	176	348.8
16	60.8	57	134.6	97	206.6	137	278.6	177	350.6
17	62.6	58	136.4	98	208.4	138	280.4	178	352.4
18	64.4	59	138.2	99	210.2	139	282.2	179	354.2
19	66.2	60	140.	100	212.	140	284.	180	356.
20	68.								

* Courtesy, *The Pharmacopeia of the United States of America.*

TABLE OF THERMOMETRIC EQUIVALENTS—(Continued)

Fahrenheit to Centigrade Scales

(F. ° − 32) × 5/9 = C. °

F. °	C. °	F. °	C. °	F. °	C. °	F. °	C. °	F. °	C. °
0	−17.78	51	10.56	101	38.33	151	66.11	201	93.89
1	−17.22	52	11.11	102	38.89	152	66.67	202	94.44
2	−16.67	53	11.67	103	39.44	153	67.22	203	95.
3	−16.11	54	12.22	104	40.	154	67.78	204	95.56
4	−15.56	55	12.78	105	40.56	155	68.33	205	96.11
5	−15.	56	13.33	106	41.11	156	68.89	206	96.67
6	−14.44	57	13.89	107	41.67	157	69.44	207	97.22
7	−13.89	58	14.44	108	42.22	158	70.	208	97.78
8	−13.33	59	15.	109	42.78	159	70.56	209	98.33
9	−12.78	60	15.56	110	43.33	160	71.11	210	98.89
10	−12.22	61	16.11	111	43.89	161	71.67	211	99.44
11	−11.67	62	16.67	112	44.44	162	72.22	212	100
12	−11.11	63	17.22	113	45.	163	72.78	213	100.56
13	−10.56	64	17.78	114	45.56	164	73.33	214	101.11
14	−10.	65	18.33	115	46.11	165	73.89	215	101.67
15	−9.44	66	18.89	116	46.67	166	74.44	216	102.22
16	−8.89	67	19.44	117	47.22	167	75.	217	102.78
17	−8.33	68	20.	118	47.78	168	75.56	218	103.33
18	−7.78	69	20.56	119	48.33	169	76.11	219	103.89
19	−7.22	70	21.11	120	48.89	170	76.67	220	104.44
20	−6.67	71	21.67	121	49.44	171	77.22	221	105.
21	−6.11	72	22.22	122	50.	172	77.78	222	105.56
22	−5.56	73	22.78	123	50.56	173	78.33	223	106.11
23	−5.	74	23.33	124	51.11	174	78.89	224	106.67
24	−4.44	75	23.89	125	51.67	175	79.44	225	107.22
25	−3.89	76	24.44	126	52.22	176	80.	226	107.78
26	−3.33	77	25.	127	52.78	177	80.56	227	108.33
27	−2.78	78	25.56	128	53.33	178	81.11	228	108.89
28	−2.22	79	26.11	129	53.89	179	81.67	229	109.44
29	−1.67	80	26.67	130	54.44	180	82.22	230	110.
30	−1.11	81	27.22	131	55.	181	82.78	231	110.56
31	−0.56	82	27.78	132	55.56	182	83.33	232	111.11
32	0.	83	28.33	133	56.11	183	83.89	233	111.67
33	0.56	84	28.89	134	56.67	184	84.44	234	112.22
34	1.11	85	29.44	135	57.22	185	85.	235	112.78
35	1.67	86	30.	136	57.78	186	85.56	236	113.33
36	2.22	87	30.56	137	58.33	187	86.11	237	113.89
37	2.78	88	31.11	138	58.89	188	86.67	238	114.44
38	3.33	89	31.67	139	59.44	189	87.22	239	115.
39	3.89	90	32.22	140	60.	190	87.78	240	115.56
40	4.44	91	32.78	141	60.56	191	88.33	241	116.11
41	5.	92	33.33	142	61.11	192	88.89	242	116.67
42	5.56	93	33.89	143	61.67	193	89.44	243	117.22
43	6.11	94	34.44	144	62.22	194	90.	244	117.78
44	6.67	95	35.	145	62.78	195	90.56	245	118.33
45	7.22	96	35.56	146	63.33	196	91.11	246	118.89
46	7.78	97	36.11	147	63.89	197	91.67	247	119.44
47	8.33	98	36.67	148	64.44	198	92.22	248	120.
48	8.89	99	37.22	149	65.	199	92.78	249	120.56
49	9.44	100	37.78	150	65.56	200	93.33	250	121.11
50	10.								

TABLE OF CHARACTERIZED VITAMINS*

Vitamins		Principal Vitamers	
Common Name	*Principal Synonyms*	*Natural*	*Synthetic*
***p*-Aminobenzoic acid**	Chromotrichia factor Vitamin B_x Anti-gray-hair factor		
Ascorbic acid	Vitamin C Antiscorbutic vitamin Cevitamic acid	Dehydroascorbic acid	6-Desoxyascorbic acid Isoascorbic acid L-Fucoascorbic acid
Bioflavonoids	Vitamin P Permeability vitamin	Eriodictin Hesperidin	Eriodictyol Hesperetin
Biotin	Vitamin H Skin factor Anti-egg-white injury factor Bios IIb Coenzyme R	Desthiobiotin	Sulfoxide of biotin Esters Desthiobiotin
Cholecalciferol	See *Vitamin D*		
Choline	Sinkalin Bilineurine Fagin Amanitin	Methionine + ethanolamine Betaine + ethanolamine	Analog containing phosphorus instead of nitrogen Arsenocholine Methyl-diethyl homolog Triethyl homologs
Cobalamin	See *Vitamin B_{12}*		
Cyanocobalamin	See *Vitamin B_{12}*		
Ergocalciferol	See *Vitamin D*		
Hydroxocobalamin	See *Vitamin B_{12}*		
Inositol	Bios I Mouse antialopecia factor Rat anti-spectacled-eye factor	Phytin Soybean cephalin	Methyl inositol Inositol hexa-acetate
Nicotinic acid	Niacin P-P factor Antipellagra factor Anti-black-tongue factor	Nicotinamide (Niacinamide) Coenzyme I Coenzyme II N^1-methylnicotinamide	Nikethamide Esters of nicotinic acid
Nitrosocobalamin	See *Vitamin B_{12}*		
Pantothenic acid	Chick antidermatitis factor Filtrate factor		Esters
Pteroylglutamic acid	Folic acid Antianemia factor Vitamin B_c	*Lactobacillus casei* factor Fermentation *L. casei* factor Liver *L. casei* factor	Pteroic acid derivatives
Pyridoxine	Antidermatitis factor Antiacrodynia factor Adermin (Eur.)	Pyridoxal Pyridoxamine Pyridoxal phosphate	
Riboflavin	Vitamin B_2 Vitamin G Lacto-, ovo-, verdo-, or hepatoflavin	Riboflavin mononucleotide Riboflavin dinucleotide	7-Methyl-9-(D,1′-ribityl)-isoalloxazine 6-Methyl-9-(D,1′-ribityl)-isoalloxazine 6-Ethyl-7-methyl-9-(D,1′-ribityl)-isoalloxazine

* Modified from Hawk, Oser, and Summerson's *Practical Physiological Chemistry*, 13th ed., New York. Blakiston Division, McGraw-Hill Book Company, Inc.

TABLE OF CHARACTERIZED VITAMINS—(Continued)

Vitamin		Principal Vitamers	
Common Name	*Principal Synonyms*	*Natural*	*Synthetic*
Thiamine	Vitamin B_1 Aneurin (Brit.) Antineuritic factor Antiberiberi factor	Thiamine pyrophosphate (cocarboxylase) Thiamine orthophosphate	Vitamin B_1 disulfide Analog with methyl group in position 6 instead of 2 in pyrimidine ring
α-Tocopherol	Vitamin E Antisterility vitamin Fertility vitamin	β-, γ-, and δ- Tocopherols Esters	Esters Analogs with ethyl substituents in place of methyl Analog with NH_2 in place of OH
Vitamin A	Axerophthol (Eur.) Antixerophthalmic factor Antixerotic factor Vitamin A_1	α-, β-, and γ-Carotene Cryptoxanthin Vitamin A esters Vitamin A_2 Neovitamin A	Vitamin A acid Vitamin A ketone Vitamin A esters
Vitamin B_c	See *Pteroylglutamic acid*		
Vitamin B_x	See *p-Aminobenzoic acid*		
Vitamin B_1	See *Thiamine*		
Vitamin B_2	See *Riboflavin*		
Vitamin B_6	See *Pyridoxine*		
Vitamin B_{12}	Cyanocobalamin Anti-pernicious-anemia vitamin Extrinsic factor	Vitamin B_{12a} (= B_{12b}) = Hydroxocobalamin	B_{12c} (Nitroso)
Vitamin C	See *Ascorbic acid*		
Vitamin D	Antirachitic vitamin	Vitamin D_2 (Calciferol [ergocalciferol]) Vitamin D_3 (Cholecalciferol)	Ergocalciferol (D_2, irradiated ergosterol) Cholecalciferol (D_3, irradiated 7-dehydrocholesterol) Irradiated 22-dihydroergosterol (D_4) Irradiated 7-dehydrositosterol (D_5)
Vitamin E	See *α-Tocopherol*		
Vitamin G	See *Riboflavin*		
Vitamin H	See *Biotin*		
Vitamin K	Vitamin K_1 Phylloquinone Phytonadione Antihemorrhagic vitamin Coagulation vitamin	Vitamin K_2	Menadione (K_3) Menadione sodium bisulfite Esters of the hydroquinone forms
Vitamin P	See definitions of *citrin, bioflavonoids*		

TABLES OF WEIGHTS AND MEASURES

Troy Weight

1 pound = 22.816 cubic inches of distilled water at 62° F.

Grains gr.		*Pennyweights* dwt.		*Ounces* oz.		*Pound* lb.
24	=	1				
480	=	20	=	1		
5760	=	240	=	12	=	1

Avoirdupois Weight

1 pound = 1.2153 pounds troy

Grains gr.		*Drachms* dr.		*Ounces* oz.		*Pound* lb.
27.34375	=	1				
437.5	=	16	=	1		
7000	=	256	=	16	=	1

Apothecaries' Weight

Grains gr.		*Scruples* ℈		*Drachms* ʒ		*Ounces* ℥		*Pound* lb.
20	=	1						
60	=	3	=	1				
480	=	24	=	8	=	1		
5760	=	288	=	96	=	12	=	1

Apothecaries' Measure

Minims ♏		*Fluidrachms* fʒ		*Fluidounces* f℥		*Pints* O.		*Gallon* C.
60	=	1						
480	=	8	=	1				
7,680	=	128	=	16	=	1		
61,440	=	1024	=	128	=	8	=	1

Metric Weights

1 gram = 1 cubic centimeter of distilled water at 4° C.

		Grams		*Grains*		*Av. Ounces*
Milligram	=	0.001	=	0.01543		
Centigram	=	0.01	=	0.15432		
Decigram	=	0.1	=	1.54324		
Gram	=	1.	=	15.43248	=	.03528
Decagram	=	10.	=		=	.3528
Hectogram	=	100.	=		=	3.52758
Kilogram	=	1,000.	=		=	35.2758

Comparative Values of Standard and Metric Measures of Length

Inches	*Centimeters*	*Inches*	*Millimeters*
1	2.54	1/25	1.00
2	5.08	1/12	2.12
3	7.62	1/8	3.18
4	10.16	1/4	6.35
5	12.70	1/3	8.47
6	15.24	1/2	12.70
7	17.78	5/8	15.88
8	20.32	2/3	16.93
9	22.86	3/4	19.05
10	25.40	5/6	21.16
11	27.94	7/8	22.22
12	30.48	11/12	23.28

Comparative Values of Avoirdupois and Metric Weights

Av. Ounces	*Grams*	*Av. Pounds*	*Grams*
1/16	1.772	1	453.59
1/8	3.544	2	907.18
1/4	7.088	2.2	1000.00
1/2	14.175	3	1360.78
1	28.350	4	1814.37
2	56.699	5	2267.96
3	85.049	6	2721.55
4	113.398	7	3175.15
5	141.748	8	3628.74
6	170.097	9	4082.33
7	198.447	10	4535.92
8	226.796		
9	255.146		
10	283.495		
11	311.845		
12	340.194		
13	368.544		
14	396.893		
15	425.243		

Comparative Values of Apothecaries' and Metric Liquid Measures

Minims	*Cubic Centimeters*	*Fluidrachms*	*Cubic Centimeters*	*Fluidounces*	*Cubic Centimeters*
1	0.06	1	3.70	1	29.57
2	0.12	2	7.39	2	59.15
3	0.19	3	11.09	3	88.72
4	0.25	4	14.79	4	118.29
5	0.31	5	18.48	5	147.87
6	0.37	6	22.18	6	177.44
7	0.43	7	25.88	7	207.01
8	0.49			8	236.58
9	0.55			9	266.16
10	0.62			10	295.73
11	0.68			11	325.30
12	0.74			12	354.88
13	0.80			13	384.45
14	0.86			14	414.02
15	0.92			15	443.59
16	0.99			16	473.17
17	1.05			17	502.74
18	1.11			18	532.31
19	1.17			19	561.89
20	1.23			20	591.46
25	1.54			21	621.03
30	1.85			22	650.60
35	2.16			23	680.18
40	2.46			24	709.75
45	2.77			25	739.32
50	3.08			26	768.90
55	3.39			27	798.47
				28	828.04
				29	857.61
				30	887.19
				31	916.76
				32	946.33
				48	1419.49
				56	1656.08
				64	1892.66
				72	2129.25
				80	2365.83
				96	2839.00
				112	3312.16
				128	3785.32

TABLES OF WEIGHTS AND MEASURES—(Continued)

Metric Linear Measure

		Meter		*U. S. Inches*		*Feet*		*Yards*		*Miles*
Millimeter	=	.001	=	.03937	=	.00328				
Centimeter	=	.01	=	.3937	=	.03280				
Decimeter	=	.1	=	3.937	=	.32808	=	.10936		
Meter	=	1.	=	39.37	=	3.2808	=	1.0936		
Decameter	=	10.	=		=	32.808	=	10.936		
Hectometer	=	100.	=		=	328.08	=	109.36	=	.062137
Kilometer	=	1,000.	=		=	3,280.8	=	1,093.6	=	.62137

Comparative Values of Metric Liquid and Apothecaries' Measures

Cubic Centimeters	*Fluidounces*	*Cubic Centimeters*	*Fluidrachms*	*Cubic Centimeters*	*Minims*
30	1.01	5	1.35	0.05	0.81
50	1.69	6	1.62	0.07	1.14
75	2.54	7	1.89	0.09	1.46
100	3.38	8	2.17	1	16.23
200	6.76	9	2.43	2	32.5
300	10.15	10	2.71	3	48.7
400	13.53	25	6.76	4	64.9
473	16.00				
500	16.91				
600	20.29				
700	23.67				
800	27.05				
900	30.43				
1000	33.82				

Table for Converting Metric Weights into Apothecaries' Weights

Grams	*Exact Equivalents in Grains*	*Grams*	*Exact Equivalents in Grains*
0.01	0.1543	12.0	185.189
0.02	0.3086	13.0	200.621
0.03	0.4630	14.0	216.054
0.04	0.6173	15.0	231.486
0.05	0.7716	16.0	246.918
0.06	0.9259	17.0	262.351
0.07	1.0803	18.0	277.783
0.08	1.2346	19.0	293.216
0.09	1.3889	20.0	308.648
0.1	1.543	21.0	324.080
0.2	3.086	22.0	339.513
0.3	4.630	23.0	354.945
0.4	6.173	24.0	370.378
0.5	7.716	25.0	385.810
0.6	9.259	26.0	401.242
0.7	10.803	27.0	416.674
0.8	12.346	28.0	432.107
0.9	13.889	29.0	447.538
1.0	15.432	30.0	462.971
2.0	30.865	31.0	478.403
3.0	46.297	32.0	493.835
4.0	61.730	40.0	617.294
5.0	77.162	45.0	694.456
6.0	92.594	50.0	771.618
7.0	108.027	60.0	925.942
8.0	123.459	70.0	1080.265
9.0	138.892	80.0	1234.589
10.0	154.324	90.0	1388.912
11.0	169.756	100.0	1543.236

Table for Converting Apothecaries' Weights into Metric Weights

Grains	*Grams*	*Grains*	*Grams*
1/50	0.00130	50	3.240
1/32	0.00202	51	3.305
1/20	0.00324	52	3.370
1/18	0.00360	53	3.434
1/16	0.00405	54	3.499
1/15	0.00432	55	3.564
1/12	0.00540	56	3.629
1/10	0.00648	57	3.694
1/8	0.00810	58	3.758
1/6	0.01080	59	3.823
1/5	0.01296	60	3.888
1/4	0.01620	61	3.953
1/3	0.02160	62	4.018
1/2	0.03240	63	4.082
3/4	0.04860	64	4.147
1	0.0648	65	4.212
2	0.1296	66	4.277
3	0.1944	67	4.342
4	0.2592	68	4.406
5	0.3240	69	4.471
6	0.3888	70	4.536
7	0.4536	71	4.601
8	0.5184	72	4.666
9	0.5832	73	4.730
10	0.6480	74	4.795
11	0.7128	75	4.860
12	0.7776	76	4.925
13	0.8424	77	4.990
14	0.9072	78	5.054
15	0.9720	79	5.119
16	1.037	80	5.184
17	1.102	81	5.249
18	1.166	82	5.314
19	1.231	83	5.378
20	1.296	84	5.443
21	1.361	85	5.508
22	1.426	86	5.573
23	1.490	87	5.638
24	1.555	88	5.702
25	1.620	89	5.767
26	1.685	90	5.832
27	1.749	91	5.897
28	1.814	92	5.962
29	1.879	93	6.026
30	1.944	94	6.091
31	2.009	95	6.156
32	2.074	96	6.221
33	2.138	97	6.286
34	2.203	98	6.350
35	2.268	99	6.415
36	2.333	100	6.480
37	2.398	120	7.776
38	2.462	150	9.720
39	2.527	180	11.664
40	2.592	200	12.958
41	2.657	480	31.103
42	2.722	500	32.396
43	2.786	600	38.875
44	2.851	700	45.354
45	2.916	800	51.833
46	2.981	900	58.313
47	3.046	960	62.207
48	3.110	1000	64.799
49	3.175		

Metric Doses with Approximate Apothecary Equivalents

The approximate dose equivalents in the following table represent the quantities that would be prescribed, under identical conditions, by physicians trained, respectively, in the metric or in the apothecary system of weights and measures.

When prepared dosage forms such as tablets, capsules, pills, etc., are prescribed in the metric system, the pharmacist may dispense the corresponding approximate equivalent in the apothecary system, and vice versa. However, this does not authorize the alternative use of the approximate dose equivalents given below for specific quantities on a prescription that requires compounding, nor in converting a pharmaceutical formula from one system of weights or measures to the other system; for such purposes exact equivalents must be used.

Liquid Measures

Metric	*Approximate Apothecary Equivalents*
1000 cc.	1 quart
750 cc.	1½ pints
500 cc.	1 pint
250 cc.	8 fluidounces
200 cc.	7 fluidounces
100 cc.	3½ fluidounces
50 cc.	1¾ fluidounces
30 cc.	1 fluidounce
15 cc.	½ fluidounce (4 fluidrachms)
10 cc.	2½ fluidrachms
8 cc.	2 fluidrachms
5 cc.	75 minims (1¼ fluidrachms)
4 cc.	1 fluidrachm
3 cc.	45 minims
2 cc.	30 minims
1 cc.	15 minims
0.75 cc.	12 minims
0.6 cc.	10 minims
0.5 cc.	8 minims
0.3 cc.	5 minims
0.25 cc.	4 minims
0.2 cc.	3 minims
0.1 cc.	1½ minims
0.06 cc.	1 minim

Weights

Metric	*Approximate Apothecary Equivalents*
30 Gm.	1 ounce
15 Gm.	4 drachms
10 Gm.	2½ drachms
7.5 Gm.	2 drachms
6 Gm.	90 grains
5 Gm.	75 grains
4 Gm.	60 grains (1 drachm)
3 Gm.	45 grains
2 Gm.	30 grains (½ drachm)
1.5 Gm.	22 grains
1 Gm.	15 grains
0.75 Gm.	12 grains
0.6 Gm.	10 grains
0.5 Gm.	7½ grains
0.45 Gm.	7 grains
0.4 Gm.	6 grains
0.3 Gm.	5 grains
0.25 Gm.	4 grains
0.2 Gm.	3 grains
0.15 Gm.	2½ grains
0.12 Gm.	2 grains
0.1 Gm.	1½ grains
75 mg.	1¼ grains
60 mg.	1 grain
50 mg.	¾ grain
40 mg.	⅔ grain
30 mg.	½ grain
25 mg.	⅜ grain
20 mg.	⅓ grain
15 mg.	¼ grain
12 mg.	⅕ grain
10 mg.	⅙ grain
8 mg.	⅛ grain
6 mg.	1/10 grain
5 mg.	1/12 grain
4 mg.	1/15 grain
3 mg.	1/20 grain
2 mg.	1/30 grain
1.5 mg.	1/40 grain
1.2 mg.	1/50 grain
1 mg.	1/60 grain
0.8 mg.	1/80 grain
0.6 mg.	1/100 grain
0.5 mg.	1/120 grain
0.4 mg.	1/150 grain
0.3 mg.	1/200 grain
0.25 mg.	1/250 grain
0.2 mg.	1/300 grain
0.15 mg.	1/400 grain
0.1 mg.	1/600 grain

NOTE: A cubic centimeter (cc.) is the approximate equivalent of a milliliter (ml.).